BNF *for Children*

2020 2021

September 2020 – 21

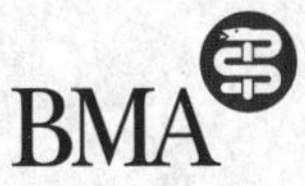

ROYAL PHARMACEUTICAL SOCIETY

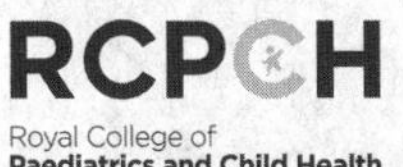

Royal College of
Paediatrics and Child Health
Leading the way in Children's Health

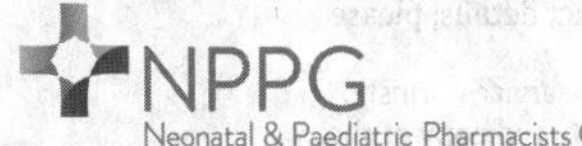

Neonatal & Paediatric Pharmacists Group

Published jointly by
BMJ Group
Tavistock Square, London, WC1H 9JP, UK

and

Pharmaceutical Press
Pharmaceutical Press is the publishing division of the Royal Pharmaceutical Society.
66-68 East Smithfield, London E1W 1AW, UK

ISBN: 978 0 85711 372 6

ISBN: 978 0 85711 373 3 (NHS edition)

ISBN: 978 0 85711 374 0 (ePDF)

Printed by GGP Media GmbH, Pößneck, Germany

Typeset by Data Standards Ltd, UK

Text design by Peter Burgess

A catalogue record for this book is available from the British Library.

Requesting copies of BNF publications

Paper copies may be obtained through any bookseller or direct from:

Pharmaceutical Press
c/o Macmillan Distribution (MDL)
Hampshire International Business Park
Lime Tree Way
Basingstoke
Hampshire
RG24 8YJ
Tel: +44 (0) 1256 302 699
Fax: +44 (0) 1256 812 521
direct@macmillan.co.uk

or via our website www.pharmpress.com

For all bulk orders of more than 20 copies:
Tel: +44 (0) 207 572 2266
pharmpress-support@rpharms.com

BNFC is available as a mobile app, online (bnfc.nice.org.uk/) and also through MedicinesComplete; a PDA version is also available. In addition, *BNFC* content can be integrated into a local formulary by using *BNFC* on FormularyComplete; see www.bnf.orgfor details.

Distribution of printed BNFCs
In **England**, NICE purchases print editions of *BNFC* for distribution within the NHS. For details of who is eligible to receive a copy and further contact details, please refer to the NICE website: www.nice.org.uk/about/what-we-do/evidence-services/british-national-formulary. If you are entitled to a shared copy of the BNFC, please call (0)1268 495 609 or email: BNF@wilmingtonhealthcare.com.

In **Scotland**, email:
nss.psd-bnf@nhs.net

In **Wales**, email:
nwssp-primarycareservices@wales.nhs.uk

In **Northern Ireland**, email:
ni.bnf@hscni.net

About BNFC content
The *BNF for Children* is for rapid reference by UK health professionals engaged in prescribing, dispensing, and administering medicines to children. *BNF for Children* has been constructed using robust procedures for gathering, assessing and assimilating information on paediatric drug treatment, but may not always include all the information necessary for prescribing and dispensing. It is expected that the reader will be relying on appropriate professional knowledge and expertise to interpret the contents in the context of the circumstances of the individual child. *BNF for Children* should be used in conjunction with other appropriate and up-to-date literature and, where necessary, supplemented by expert advice. Information is also available from Medicines Information Services.

Special care is required in managing childhood conditions with unlicensed medicines or with licensed medicines for unlicensed uses. Responsibility for the appropriate use of medicines lies solely with the individual health professional.

Please refer to digital versions of *BNF for Children* for the most up-to-date content. *BNF for Children* is published in print but interim updates are issued and published in the digital versions of *BNF for Children*. The publishers work to ensure that the information is as accurate and up-to-date as possible at the date of publication, but knowledge and best practice in this field change regularly. *BNF for Children's* accuracy and currency cannot be guaranteed and neither the publishers nor the authors accept any responsibility for errors or omissions. While considerable efforts have been made to check the material in this publication, it should be treated as a guide only. Prescribers, pharmacists and other healthcare professionals are advised to check www.bnf.orgfor information about key updates and corrections.

Pharmaid
Numerous requests have been received from developing countries for *BNFCs*. The Pharmaid scheme of the Commonwealth Pharmacists Association will dispatch old *BNFCs* to certain Commonwealth countries. For more information on this scheme see commonwealthpharmacy.org/what-we-do/pharmaid/.
If you would like to donate your copy, email:
admin@commonwealthpharmacy.org

Preface

BNF for Children aims to provide prescribers, pharmacists, and other healthcare professionals with sound up-to-date information on the use of medicines for treating children.

A joint publication of the British Medical Association, the Royal Pharmaceutical Society, the Royal College of Paediatrics and Child Health, and the Neonatal and Paediatric Pharmacists Group, BNF for Children ('BNFC') is published under the authority of a Paediatric Formulary Committee which comprises representatives of these bodies, the Department of Health for England, and the Medicines and Healthcare products Regulatory Agency.

Many areas of paediatric practice have suffered from inadequate information on effective medicines. BNFC addresses this significant knowledge gap by providing practical information on the use of medicines in children of all ages from birth to adolescence. Information in BNFC has been validated against emerging evidence, best-practice guidelines, and crucially, advice from a network of clinical experts.

Drawing information from manufacturers' literature where appropriate, BNFC also includes a great deal of advice that goes beyond marketing authorisations (product licences). This is necessary because licensed indications frequently do not cover the clinical needs of children; in some cases, products for use in children need to be specially manufactured or imported. Careful consideration has been given to establishing the clinical need for unlicensed interventions with respect to the evidence and experience of their safety and efficacy; local paediatric formularies, clinical literature and national information resources have been invaluable in this process.

BNFC has been designed for rapid reference and the information presented has been carefully selected to aid decisions on prescribing, dispensing and administration of medicines. Less detail is given on areas such as malignant disease and the very specialist use of medicines generally undertaken in tertiary centres. BNFC should be interpreted in the light of professional knowledge and it should be supplemented as necessary by specialised publications. Information is also available from Medicines Information Services (see inside front cover).

It is **important** to use the most recent BNFC information for making clinical decisions. The print edition of *BNF for Children* is updated in September each year. Monthly updates are provided online via the BNF Publications website www.bnf.org, MedicinesComplete and the NHS Evidence portal. The more important changes listed under Changes p. xvii are cumulative (from one print edition to the next), and can be printed off each month to show the main changes since the last print edition as an aide memoire for those using print copies.

The website (www.bnf.org) includes additional information of relevance to healthcare professionals. Other digital formats of BNFC—including versions for mobile devices and integration into local formularies—are also available.

BNF Publications welcomes comments from healthcare professionals. Comments and constructive criticism should be sent to:

British National Formulary,
Royal Pharmaceutical Society,
66–68 East Smithfield
London
E1W 1AW
editor@bnf.org

The contact email for manufacturers or pharmaceutical companies wishing to contact BNF Publications is manufacturerinfo@bnf.org

Contents

Acknowledgements

The Paediatric Formulary Committee is grateful to individuals and organisations that have provided advice and information to the *BNF for Children* (BNFC).

Contributors for this update were:

M.N. Badminton, S. Bailey, G.D.L. Bates, H. Bedford, M.W. Beresford, R.M. Bingham, L. Brook, K.G. Brownlee, I.F. Burgess, A. Cant, R. Carr, T.D. Cheetham, A.G. Cleary, A.J. Cotgrove, J.B.S. Coulter, B.G. Craig, J.H. Cross, A. Dhawan, P.N. Durrington, A.B. Edgar, J.A. Edge, D.A.C. Elliman, N.D. Embleton, A. Freyer, P.J. Goadsby, J. Gray, J.W. Gregory, P. Gringras, J.P. Harcourt, C. Hendriksz, R.F. Howard, R.G. Hull, H.R. Jenkins, S. Jones, B.A. Judd, E. Junaid, P.T. Khaw, J.M.W. Kirk, E.G.H. Lyall, P.S. Malone, S.D. Marks, D.F. Marsh, P. McHenry, P.J. McKiernan, L.M. Melvin, E. Miller, S. Moledina, R.E. Morton, P. Mulholland, C. Nelson-Piercy, J.M. Neuberger, K.K. Nischal, C.Y. Ng, J.Y. Paton, G.A. Pearson, J. Puntis, J. Rogers, K.E. Rogstad, J.W. Sander, N.J. Scolding, M.R. Sharland, N.J. Shaw, O.F.W Stumper, A.G. Sutcliffe, E.A. Taylor, S. Thomas, M.A. Thomson, J.A. Vale, S. Vijay, J.O. Warner, N.J.A. Webb, A.D. Weeks, R. Welbury, W.P. Whitehouse, A. Wright, Z. Zaiwalla, and S.M. Zuberi.

Valuable advice has been provided by the following expert groups: Advisory Committee on Malaria Prevention, Association of British Neurologists, British Association of Dermatologists' Therapy & Guidelines Sub-committee, British Geriatrics Society, British Paediatric Neurology Association, British Society of Gastroenterology, British Society for Paediatric Endocrinology and Diabetes, British Society of Paediatric Gastroenterology, Hepatology and Nutrition, College of Mental Health Pharmacy, Faculty of Sexual and Reproductive Healthcare, Neonatal and Paediatric Pharmacists Group, Royal College of Anaesthetists, Royal College of Obstetricians and Gynaecologists, Royal College of Paediatrics and Child Health, Royal College of Physicians, Royal College of Psychiatrists, Society for Endocrinology, Vascular Society.

The MHRA have provided valuable assistance.

Correspondents in the pharmaceutical industry have provided information on new products and commented on products in the BNFC.

Numerous doctors, pharmacists, nurses, and others have sent comments and suggestions.

The BNF team are grateful for the support and access to in-house expertise at Pharmaceutical Press and acknowledge the assistance of K. Baxter, A. Naylor, J. Macdonald, N. Potter and their teams.

T. Ali, J. Chen, R. Gupta, E. Kim, O. Komolafe, E. Olaoke, A. Paul, D. Usop provided considerable assistance during the production of this update of the BNF.

This edition of the BNF carries a rainbow in recognition of the work and dedication of all frontline healthcare workers throughout the COVID-19 pandemic.

BNF Staff

ASSOCIATE CONTENT DIRECTOR (BNF PUBLICATIONS)
Kate Towers *BPharm (AU), GCClinPharm (AU)*

SENIOR EDITORIAL STAFF
Kiri Aikman *BPharm (NZ), PGDipClinPharm (NZ), ARPharmS*

Alison Brayfield *BPharm, MRPharmS*

Robert Buckingham *BSc, SRPharmS*

Catherine Cadart *BPharm (AU), BA(Hons), GradDipHospPharm (AU), MRPharmS*

Mahinaz Harrison *BPharm, DipPharmPract, IP, MRPharmS*

Holly Hayne *BSc (Pharmacology) (NZ), BPharm (NZ)*

Rebecca Luckhurst *BSc, MSc*

Alexander McPhail *MPharm, PGDipClinPharm*

Claire McSherry *BPharm (NZ), PGCertClinPharm (NZ)*

Claire Preston *BPharm, PGDipMedMan, MRPharmS*

EDITORIAL STAFF
Mohammed Abou Daya *MPharm, PGDipGPP, MRPharmS*

Hannah Arnold *BPharm (NZ)*

Natasha Bell-Asher *BPharm (NZ), PGDipClinPharm (NZ)*

Lucía Camañas Sáez *MPharm (ESP), PGDipClinPharm, PGCertPsychTherap, MRPharmS*

Rochelle Chin *BPharm (AU)*

Kathleen Eager *BPharm*

Emily Henderson *BPharm (NZ), PGCertClinPharm (NZ)*

Sue Ho *BPharm (AU), MRPharmS*

Elizabeth King *MAPharmT*

Sonal Ladani *MPharm, PGDipGPP, MRPharmS*

David Lipanovic *BPharm (NZ), PGCertClinPharm (NZ)*

Jean MacKershan *BSc, PgDip*

John Martin *BPharm, PhD, MRPharmS*

Angela McFarlane *BSc, DipClinPharm*

Deirdre McGuirk *BComm, MPharm*

Anna McLachlan *BPharm (NZ), PGCertClinPharm (NZ)*

Liliana Moreira Vilas Boas *MPharm(PT), PGDipHPS(PT), PGCertHSDM(PT), PGCertGPP, MRPharmS*

Nalwenga Mutambo *MPharm*

Merusha Naidoo *BPharm (NZ), PGCertClinPharm (NZ)*

Hana Numan *BPharm (NZ), PGDipClinPharm (NZ)*

Barbara Okpala *MPharm, PGDipHospPharm*

Heenaben Patel *MPharm, PGDipClinPharm, MRPharmS*

Laura Pham *BPharm(Hons) (AU)*

Catherine Pitt *MPharm, PGDipClinPharm, MRPharmS*

Stephanie Powell *MBioSci*

Rebekah Raymond *BSc, DipPharmPrac, MRPharmS*

Caraliese Rebello *BPharm (NZ), PGDipClinPharm (NZ)*

Sharyl Rodrigues *BPharm (NZ), PGDipClinPharm (NZ)*

Jannah Ryan *BSc(Hons)*

Harpreet Sandhu *MPharm, MRPharmS*

Beejal Shah *MPharm, PGDipClinPharm, IP*

Lucy Sheed *BPharm (NZ)*

Tadeh Tahmasi *MPharm, MRPharmS*

Hannah Tan *BPharm (AU)*

Julia Webb *MPharm, PGCertPharmPrac*

SUPPORT STAFF
Matt Bradbury *BSc(Hons)*

Darren Chan *BSc, MSc*

Lauren Cheetham *BA(Hons)*

Filsane Haji *BSc, MSc*

Rebecca Harwood *BSc(Hons)*

Nick Judd *BA(Hons), MA*

Philip Lee *BSc, PhD*

Olivia Maskill *BSc(Hons)*

Tom Mathew *BSc, MSc*

Vicky Pollington *BSc(Hons)*

Carina Redig de Campos

Elisabetta Stramiglio *BSc, MSc*

Louise Symmons *BSc(Hons), MSc*

Nikolaos Tsimplis *BSc, MRes*

Paediatric Formulary Committee

CHAIR
David Tuthill
MB, BCh, FRCPCH

DEPUTY CHAIR
Neil A. Caldwell
BSc, MSc, MRPharmS, FFRPS

COMMITTEE MEMBERS
Indraneel Banerjee
MB BS, MD, FRCPCH
Martin G. Duerden
BMedSci, MB BS, DRCOG, MRCGP, DipTher, DPH
Emily Lam (lay member)
James H. Larcombe
MB, ChB, PhD, FRCGP, DipAdvGP
Alison Lockley (lay member)
Cert Ed, MA, MA (Econ)
Poonam Lumb
MPharm(Hons), PGDipGPP, IP, MRPharmS
John Marriott
BSc, PhD, MRPharmS, FHEA
E. David G. McIntosh
MB BS, MPH, LLM, PhD, FAFPHM, FRACP, FRCPCH, FFPM, DRCOG, DCH, DipPharmMed
Gary Meager
Dip HE (Child), BSc, PGCert, FHEA
Angeliki Siapkara
MSc, MD, CCST (Ortho)
Andrew Wignell
MPharm, PGDipClinPharm, IP, MRPharmS

Dental Advisory Group

CHAIR
Sarah Manton
BDS, FDSRCS Ed, FHEA, PhD, FDFTEd

COMMITTEE MEMBERS
Rebecca Bloor
BPharm (NZ)
Andrew K. Brewer
BSc, BchD, MFDS (Glas)
Alexander Crighton
BDS, MB, ChB, FDS, OM
Hannah Giles
BPharm (NZ)
Michelle Moffat
BDS MFDS RCS Ed, M Paed Dent RCPS, FDS (Paed Dent) RCS Ed
Barbara Okpala
MPharm, PGDipHospPharm
Wendy Thompson
BSC(Hons), BDS(Hons), MJDF
Kate Towers
BPharm (AU), GCClinPharm (AU)

SECRETARY
Arianne J. Matlin
MA, MSci, PhD

ADVICE ON DENTAL PRACTICE
The **British Dental Association** has contributed to the advice on medicines for dental practice through its representatives on the Dental Advisory Group.

Nurse Prescribers' Advisory Group

CHAIR
Molly Courtenay
PhD, MSc, Cert Ed, BSc, RGN

COMMITTEE MEMBERS
Penny M. Franklin
RN, RCN, RSCPHN(HV), MA, PGCE
Matt Griffiths
BA(Hons), FAETC, RGN, Cert A&E, NISP, PHECC
Tracy Hall
BSc, MSc, Cert N, Dip N, RGN, DN, NIP, QN
Penny Harrison
BSc(Hons)
Julie MacAngus
BSc(Hons), RGN, RM, PGCE
Joan Myers
MSc, BSc, RGN, RSCN, Dip DN
Fiona Peniston-Bird
BSc(Hons), NIP, RHV, RGN
Kathy Radley
BSc, RGN
Kate Towers
BPharm (AU), GCClinPharm (AU)

How BNF Publications are constructed

Overview

The BNF *for Children* (BNFC) is an independent professional publication that addresses the day-to-day prescribing information needs of healthcare professionals involved in the care of children. Use of this resource throughout the health service helps to ensure that medicines are used safely, effectively, and appropriately.

Hundreds of changes are made between print editions, and are published monthly in some digital formats. The most clinically significant updates are listed under Changes p. xvii.

BNFC is unique in bringing together authoritative, independent guidance on best practice with clinically validated drug information.

Information in BNFC has been validated against emerging evidence, best-practice guidelines, and advice from a network of clinical experts. BNFC includes a great deal of advice that goes beyond marketing authorisations (product licences or summaries of product characteristics). This is necessary because licensed indications frequently do not cover the clinical needs of children; in some cases, products for use in children need to be specially manufactured or imported. Careful consideration has been given to establishing the clinical need for unlicensed interventions with respect to the evidence and experience of their safety and efficacy.

Validation of information follows a standardised process. Where the evidence base is weak, further validation is undertaken through a process of peer review. The process and its governance are outlined in greater detail in the sections that follow.

Paediatric Formulary Committee

The Paediatric Formulary Committee (PFC) is responsible for the content of BNFC. The PFC comprises pharmacy, medical and nursing representatives with a paediatric background, and lay representatives who have worked with children or acted as a carer of a paediatric patient; there are also representatives from the Medicines and Healthcare products Regulatory Agency (MHRA) and the Department of Health for England. The PFC decides on matters of policy and reviews amendments to BNFC in the light of new evidence and expert advice.

Dental Advisory Group

The Dental Advisory Group oversees the preparation of advice on the drug management of dental and oral conditions; the group includes representatives from the British Dental Association and a representative from the UK Health Departments.

Nurse Prescribers' Advisory Group

The Nurse Prescribers' Advisory Group oversees the list of drugs approved for inclusion in the Nurse Prescribers' Formulary; the group includes representatives from a range of nursing disciplines and stakeholder organisations.

Expert advisers

BNFC uses about 80 expert clinical advisers (including doctors, pharmacists, nurses, and dentists) throughout the UK to help with the clinical content. The role of these expert advisers is to review existing text and to comment on amendments drafted by the clinical writers. These clinical experts help to ensure that BNFC remains reliable by:

- commenting on the relevance of the text in the context of best clinical practice in the UK;
- checking draft amendments for appropriate interpretation of any new evidence;
- providing expert opinion in areas of controversy or when reliable evidence is lacking;
- advising on the use of unlicensed medicines or of licensed medicines for unlicensed uses ('off-label' use);
- providing independent advice on drug interactions, prescribing in hepatic impairment, renal impairment, pregnancy, breast-feeding, neonatal care, palliative care, and the emergency treatment of poisoning.

In addition to consulting with regular advisers, BNFC calls on other clinical specialists for specific developments when particular expertise is required.

BNFC also works closely with a number of expert bodies that produce clinical guidelines. Drafts or pre-publication copies of guidelines are often received for comment and for assimilation into BNFC.

Editorial team

BNFC clinical writers have all worked as pharmacists or possess a pharmacy degree and further, relevant post-graduate qualification, and have a sound understanding of how drugs are used in clinical practice. A number of the clinical writers have specific experience of paediatric practice. As a team, the clinical writers are responsible for editing, maintaining, and updating BNFC content. They follow a systematic prioritisation process in response to updates to the evidence base in order to ensure the most clinically important topics are reviewed as quickly as possible. In parallel the team of clinical writers undertakes a process of rolling revalidation, aiming to review all of the content in the BNF over a 3- to 4-year period.

Amendments to the text are drafted when the clinical writers are satisfied that any new information is reliable and relevant. A set of standard criteria define when content is referred to expert advisers, the Joint Formulary Committee or other advisory groups, or submitted for peer review.

Clinical writers prepare the text for publication and undertake a number of validation checks on the knowledge at various stages of the production.

Sources of BNFC information

BNFC uses a variety of sources for its information; the main ones are shown below.

Summaries of product characteristics

BNFC reviews the summaries of product characteristics (SPCs) of all new products as well as revised SPCs for existing products. The SPCs are a key source of product information and are carefully processed. Such processing involves:

- verifying the approved names of all relevant ingredients including 'non-active' ingredients (BNFC is committed to using approved names and descriptions as laid down by the Human Medicines Regulations 2012);
- comparing the indications, cautions, contra-indications, and side-effects with similar existing drugs. Where these are different from the expected pattern, justification is sought for their inclusion or exclusion;
- seeking independent data on the use of drugs in pregnancy and breast-feeding;
- incorporating the information into BNFC using established criteria for the presentation and inclusion of the data;
- checking interpretation of the information by a second clinical writer before submitting to a content manager; changes relating to doses receive a further check;
- identifying potential clinical problems or omissions and seeking further information from manufacturers or from expert advisers;
- constructing, with the help of expert advisers, a comment on the role of the drug in the context of similar drugs.

Much of this processing is applicable to the following sources as well.

Literature

Clinical writers monitor core medical, paediatric, and pharmaceutical journals. Research papers and reviews relating to drug therapy are carefully processed. When a difference between the advice in BNFC and the paper is noted, the new information is assessed for reliability (using tools based on SIGN methodology) and relevance to UK clinical practice. If necessary, new text is drafted and discussed with expert advisers and the Paediatric Formulary Committee. BNFC enjoys a close working relationship with a number of national information providers.

In addition to the routine process, which is used to identify 'triggers' for changing the content, systematic literature searches are used to identify the best quality evidence available to inform an update. Clinical writers receive training in critical appraisal, literature evaluation, and search strategies.

Consensus guidelines

The advice in BNFC is checked against consensus guidelines produced by expert bodies. The quality of the guidelines is assessed using adapted versions of the AGREE II tool. A number of bodies make drafts or pre-publication copies of the guidelines available to BNFC; it is therefore possible to ensure that a consistent message is disseminated. BNFC routinely processes guidelines from the National Institute for Health and Care Excellence (NICE), the All Wales Medicines Strategy Group (AWMSG), the Scottish Medicines Consortium (SMC), and the Scottish Intercollegiate Guidelines Network (SIGN).

Reference sources

Paediatric formularies and reference sources are used to provide background information for the review of existing text or for the construction of new text. The BNFC team works closely with the editorial team that produces *Martindale: The Complete Drug Reference*. BNFC has access to *Martindale* information resources and each team keeps the other informed of significant developments and shifts in the trends of drug usage.

Peer review

Although every effort is made to identify the most robust data available, inevitably there are areas where the evidence base is weak or contradictory. While the BNF has the valuable support of expert advisers and the Paediatric Formulary Committee, the recommendations made may be subject to a further level of scrutiny through peer review to ensure they reflect best practice.

Content for peer review is posted on bnf.org and interested parties are notified via a number of channels, including the BNF e-newsletter.

Statutory information

BNFC routinely processes relevant information from various Government bodies including Statutory Instruments and regulations affecting the Prescription only Medicines Order. Official compendia such as the British Pharmacopoeia and its addenda are processed routinely to ensure that BNFC complies with the relevant sections of the Human Medicines Regulations 2012.

BNFC maintains close links with the Home Office (in relation to controlled drug regulations) and the Medicines and Healthcare products Regulatory Agency (including the British Pharmacopoeia Commission). Safety warnings issued by the Commission on Human Medicines (CHM) and guidelines on drug use issued by the UK health departments are processed as a matter of routine.

Relevant professional statements issued by the Royal Pharmaceutical Society are included in BNFC as are guidelines from bodies such as the Royal College of Paediatrics and Child Health.

Medicines and devices

NHS Prescription Services (from the NHS Business Services Authority) provides non-clinical, categorical information (including prices) on the medicines and devices included in BNFC.

Comments from readers

Readers of BNFC are invited to send in comments. Numerous letters and emails are received by the BNF team. Such feedback helps to ensure that BNFC provides practical and clinically relevant information. Many changes in the presentation and scope of BNFC have resulted from comments sent in by users.

Comments from industry

Close scrutiny of BNFC by the manufacturers provides an additional check and allows them an opportunity to raise issues about BNFC's presentation of the role of various drugs; this is yet another check on the balance of BNFC advice. All comments are looked at with care and, where necessary, additional information and expert advice are sought.

Market research

Market research is conducted at regular intervals to gather feedback on specific areas of development.

Assessing the evidence

From January 2016, recommendations made in BNFC have been evidence graded to reflect the strength of the recommendation. The addition of evidence grading is to support clinical decision making based on the best available evidence.

The BNFC aims to revalidate all content over a rolling 3- to 4-year period and evidence grading will be applied to recommendations as content goes through the revalidation process. Therefore, initially, only a small number of recommendations will have been graded.

Grading system

The BNFC has adopted a five level grading system from A to E, based on the former SIGN grading system. This grade is displayed next to the recommendation within the text.

Evidence used to make a recommendation is assessed for validity using standardised methodology tools based on AGREE II and assigned a level of evidence. The recommendation is then given a grade that is extrapolated from the level of evidence, and an assessment of the body of evidence and its applicability.

Evidence assigned a level 1- or 2- score has an unacceptable level of bias or confounding and is not used to form recommendations.

Levels of evidence

- **Level 1++**
  High quality meta-analyses, systematic reviews of randomised controlled trials (RCTs), or RCTs with a very low risk of bias.
- **Level 1+**
  Well-conducted meta-analyses, systematic reviews, or RCTs with a low risk of bias.
- **Level 1–**
  Meta-analyses, systematic reviews, or RCTs with a high risk of bias.
- **Level 2++**
  High quality systematic reviews of case control or cohort studies; or high quality case control or cohort studies with a very low risk of confounding or bias and a high probability that the relationship is causal.
- **Level 2+**
  Well-conducted case control or cohort studies with a low risk of confounding or bias and a moderate probability that the relationship is causal.
- **Level 2–**
  Case control or cohort studies with a high risk of confounding or bias and a significant risk that the relationship is not causal.
- **Level 3**
  Non-analytic studies, e.g. case reports, case series.
- **Level 4**
  Expert advice or clinical experience from respected authorities.

Grades of recommendation

- **Grade A: High strength**
  NICE-accredited guidelines; or guidelines that pass AGREE II assessment; or at least one meta-analysis, systematic review, or RCT rated as 1++, and directly applicable to the target population; or a body of evidence consisting principally of studies rated as 1+, directly applicable to the target population, and demonstrating overall consistency of results.
- **Grade B: Moderate strength**
  A body of evidence including studies rated as 2++, directly applicable to the target population, and demonstrating overall consistency of results; or extrapolated evidence from studies rated as 1++ or 1+.
- **Grade C: Low strength**
  A body of evidence including studies rated as 2+, directly applicable to the target population and demonstrating overall consistency of results; or extrapolated evidence from studies rated as 2++.
- **Grade D: Very low strength**
  Evidence level 3; or extrapolated evidence from studies rated as 2+; or tertiary reference source created by a transparent, defined methodology, where the basis for recommendation is clear.
- **Grade E: Practice point**
  Evidence level 4.

How to use BNF Publications in print

How to use the BNF *for Children* in print

This edition of the BNF *for Children* (BNFC) continues to display the fundamental change to the structure of the content that was first shown in BNFC 2015-2016. The changes were made to bring consistency and clarity to BNFC content, and to the way that the content is arranged within print and digital products, increasing the ease with which information can be found.

For reference, the most notable changes to the structure of the content include:

- Drug monographs – where possible, all information that relates to a single drug is contained within its drug monograph, moving information previously contained in the prescribing notes. Drug monographs have also changed structurally: additional sections have been added, ensuring greater regularity around where information is located within the publication.
- Drug class monographs – where substantial amounts of information are common to all drugs within a drug class (e.g. macrolides p. 352), a drug class monograph has been created to contain the common information.
- Medicinal forms – categorical information about marketed medicines, such as price and pack size, continues to be sourced directly from the Dictionary of Medicines and Devices provided by the NHS Business Services Authority. However, clinical information curated by the BNF team has been clearly separated from the categorical pricing and pack size information and is included in the relevant section of the drug monograph.
- Section numbering – the BNF and BNFC section numbering has been removed. This section numbering tied the content to a rigid structure and enforced the retention of defunct classifications, such as mercurial diuretics, and hindered the relocation of drugs where therapeutic use had altered. It also caused constraints between the BNF and BNFC, where drugs had different therapeutic uses in children.
- Appendix 4 – the content has been moved to individual drug monographs. The introductory notes have been replaced with a new guidance section, Guidance on intravenous infusions p. 16.

Introduction

In order to achieve the safe, effective, and appropriate use of medicines, healthcare professionals must be able to use the BNFC effectively, and keep up to date with significant changes in the BNFC that are relevant to their clinical practice. This *How to Use the BNF for Children* is key in reinforcing the details of the new structure of the BNFC to all healthcare professionals involved with prescribing, monitoring, supplying, and administering medicines, as well as supporting the learning of students training to join these professions.

As with previous editions, the BNFC provides information on the use of medicines in children ranging from neonates (including preterm neonates) to adolescents. The terms infant, child, and adolescent are not used consistently in the literature; to avoid ambiguity actual ages are used in the dose statements in BNFC. The term neonate is used to describe a newborn infant aged 0–28 days. The terms child or children are used generically to describe the entire range from infant to adolescent in BNFC.

Structure of the BNFC

This BNFC edition continues to broadly follow the high level structure of earlier editions of the BNFC (i.e. those published before BNFC 2015-2016):

Front matter, comprising information on how to use the BNFC, the significant content changes in each edition, and guidance on various prescribing matters (e.g. prescription writing, the use of intravenous drugs, particular considerations for special patient populations).

Chapters, containing drug monographs describing the uses, doses, safety issues and other considerations involved in the use of drugs; drug class monographs; and treatment summaries, covering guidance on the selection of drugs. Monographs and treatment summaries are divided into chapters based on specific aspects of medical care, such as Chapter 5, Infections, or Chapter 16, Emergency treatment of poisoning; or drug use related to a particular system of the body, such as Chapter 2, Cardiovascular.

Within each chapter, content is organised alphabetically by therapeutic use (e.g. Airways disease, obstructive), with the treatment summaries first, (e.g. Asthma, acute p. 158), followed by the monographs of the drugs used to manage the conditions discussed in the treatment summary. Within each therapeutic use, the drugs are organised alphabetically by classification (e.g. Antimuscarinics, Beta $_2$-agonist bronchodilators) and then alphabetically within each classification (e.g. Formoterol fumarate, Salbutamol, Salmeterol, Terbutaline sulfate).

Appendices, covering interactions, borderline substances, and cautionary and advisory labels.

Back matter, covering the lists of medicines approved by the NHS for Dental and Nurse Practitioner prescribing, proprietary and specials manufacturers' contact details, and the index. Yellow cards are also included, to facilitate the reporting of adverse events, as well as quick reference guides for life support and key drug doses in medical emergencies, for ease of access.

Navigating the *BNF for Children*

The contents page provides the high-level layout of information within the BNFC; and in addition, each chapter begins with a small contents section, describing the therapeutic uses covered within that chapter. Once in a chapter, location is guided by the side of the page showing the chapter number (the *thumbnail*), alongside the chapter title. The top of the page includes the therapeutic use (the *running head*) alongside the page number.

Once on a page, visual cues aid navigation: treatment summary information is in black type, with therapeutic use titles similarly styled in black, whereas the use of colour indicates drug-related information, including drug classification titles, drug class monographs, and drug monographs.

Although navigation is possible by browsing, primarily access to the information is via the index, which covers the titles of drug class monographs, drug monographs and treatment summaries. The index also includes the names of branded medicines and other topics of relevance, such as abbreviations, guidance sections, tables, and images.

Content types

Treatment summaries

Treatment summaries are of three main types;

- an overview of delivering a drug to a particular body system (e.g. Skin conditions, management p. 764),
- a comparison between a group or groups of drugs (e.g. beta-adrenoceptor blockers (systemic) p. 109),
- an overview of the drug management or prophylaxis of common conditions intended to facilitate rapid appraisal of options (e.g. Hypertension p. 104, or Malaria, prophylaxis p. 420).

In order to select safe and effective medicines for individual children, information in the treatment summaries must be used in conjunction with other prescribing details about the drugs and knowledge of the child's medical and drug history.

Monographs

Overview

In earlier editions (i.e. before BNFC 2015-2016), a systemically administered drug with indications for use in different body systems was split across the chapters relating to those body systems. So, for example, codeine phosphate p. 293 was found in chapter 1, for its antimotility effects and chapter 4 for its analgesic effects. However, the monograph in chapter 1 contained only the dose and some selected safety precautions.

Now, all of the information for the systemic use of a drug is contained within one monograph, so codeine phosphate p. 293 is now included in chapter 4. This carries the advantage of providing all of the information in one place, so the user does not need to flick back and forth across several pages to find all of the relevant information for that drug. Cross references are included in chapter 1, where the management of diarrhoea is discussed, to the drug monograph to assist navigation.

Where drugs have systemic and local uses, for example, chloramphenicol p. 385, and the considerations around drug use are markedly different according to the route of administration, the monograph is split, as with earlier editions, into the relevant chapters.

This means that the majority of drugs are still placed in the same chapters and sections as earlier editions, and although there may be some variation in order, all of the relevant information will be easier to locate.

One of the most significant changes to the monograph structure is the increased granularity, with a move from around 9 sections to over 20 sections; sections are only included when relevant information has been identified. The following information describes these sections and their uses in more detail.

Nomenclature

Monograph titles follow the convention of recommended international non-proprietary names (rINNs), or, in the absence of a rINN, British Approved Names. Relevant synonyms are included below the title and, in some instances a brief description of the drug action is included. Over future editions these drug action statements will be rolled out for all drugs.

In some monographs, immediately below the nomenclature or drug action, there are a number of cross references used to signpost the user to any additional information they need to consider about a drug. This is most common for drugs formulated in combinations, where users will be signposted to the monographs for the individual ingredients (e.g. senna with ispaghula husk p. 52) or for drugs that are related to a drug class monograph (see Drug class monographs, below).

Indication and dose

User feedback has highlighted that one of the main uses of the BNFC is identifying indications and doses of drugs. Therefore, indication and dose information has been promoted to the top of the monograph and highlighted by a coloured panel to aid quick reference.

The indication and dose section is more highly structured than in earlier editions, giving greater clarity around which doses should be used for which indications and by which route. In addition, if the dose varies with a specific preparation or formulation that dosing information has been moved out of the preparations section and in to the indication and dose panel, under a heading of the preparation name.

Doses are either expressed in terms of a definite frequency (e.g. 1 g 4 times daily) or in the total daily dose format (e.g. 6 g daily in 3 divided doses); the total daily dose should be divided into individual doses (in the second example, the child should receive 2 g 3 times daily).

Doses for specific patient groups (e.g. neonates) may be included if they are different to the standard dose. Doses for children can be identified by the relevant age range and may vary according to their age or body-weight.

Selecting the dose

The dose of a drug may vary according to different indications, routes of administration, age, body-weight, and body surface area. The right dose should be selected for the right age and body-weight (or body surface area) of the child, as well as for the right indication, route of administration, and preparation.

In earlier editions of the BNFC, age ranges and weight ranges overlapped. For clarity and to aid selection of the correct dose, wherever possible these age and weight ranges now do not overlap. When interpreting age ranges it is important to understand that a child is considered to be 11 up until the point of their 12 thbirthday, meaning that an age range of child 12 to 17 years is applicable to a child from the day of their 12 thbirthday until the day before their 18 thbirthday. All age ranges should be interpreted in this way. Similarly, when interpreting weight ranges, it should be understood that a weight of up to 30 kg is applicable to a child up to, but not including, the point that they tip the scales at 30 kg and a weight range of 35 to 59 kg is applicable to a child as soon as they tip the scales at 35 kg right up until, but not including, the point that they tip the scales at 60 kg. All weight ranges should be interpreted in this way.

A pragmatic approach should be applied to these cut-off points depending on the child's physiological development, condition, and if weight is appropriate for the child's age.

For some drugs (e.g. vancomycin p. 349) the neonatal dose varies according to the *corrected gestational* age of the neonate. Corrected gestational age is the neonate's total age expressed in weeks from the start of the mother's last menstrual period. For example, a 3 week old baby born at 27 weeks gestation is treated as having a corrected gestational age of 30 weeks. A term baby has a corrected gestational age of 37–42 weeks when born. For most other drugs, the dose can be based on the child's actual date of birth irrespective of corrected gestational age. However, the degree of prematurity, the maturity of renal and hepatic function, and the clinical properties of the drug need to be considered on an individual basis.

Many children's doses in BNFC are standardised by *body-weight*. To calculate the dose for a given child the weight-standardised dose is multiplied by the child's weight (or occasionally by the child's ideal weight for height). The calculated dose should not normally exceed the maximum recommended dose for an adult. For example, if the dose is 8 mg/kg (max. 300 mg), a child of 10 kg body-weight should receive 80 mg, but a child of 40 kg body-weight should receive 300 mg (rather than 320 mg). Calculation by body-weight in the overweight child may result in much higher doses being administered than necessary; in such cases, the dose should be calculated from an ideal weight for height.

Occasionally, some doses in BNFC are standardised by *body surface area* because many physiological phenomena correlate better with body surface area. In these cases, to calculate the dose for a given child, the body surface area-standardised dose is multiplied by the child's body surface area. The child's body surface area can be estimated from his or her weight using the tables for Body surface area in children (image) p. 1192.

Wherever possible, doses are expressed in terms of a definite frequency (e.g. if the dose is 1 mg/kg twice daily, a child of body-weight 9 kg would receive 9 mg twice daily).

Typical layout of a monograph and associated medicinal forms

❶ Class Monographs and drug monographs
In most cases, all information that relates to an individual drug is contained in its drug monograph and there is no symbol. Class monographs have been created where substantial amounts of information are common to all drugs within a drug class, these are indicated by a flag symbol in a circle:

Drug monographs with a corresponding class monograph are indicated by a tab with a flag symbol: 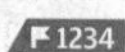

The page number of the corresponding class monograph is indicated within the tab. For further information, see How to use BNF Publications

❷ Drug classifications
Used to inform users of the class of a drug and to assist in finding other drugs of the same class. May be based on pharmacological class (e.g. opioids) but can also be associated with the use of the drug (e.g. cough suppressants)

❸ Review date
The date of last review of the content

❹ Specific preparation name
If the dose varies with a specific preparation or formulation it appears under a heading of the preparation name

Class monograph ❶

CLASSIFICATION ❷

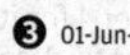

Drug monograph ❶

❸ 01-Jun-2017

(Synonym) another name by which a drug may be known

- DRUG ACTION how a drug exerts its effect in the body

- **INDICATIONS AND DOSE**
Indications are the clinical reasons a drug is used. The dose of a drug will often depend on the indications
Indication
▸ ROUTE
▸ Age groups: [Neonate/Child]
Dose and frequency of administration (max. dose)
SPECIFIC PREPARATION NAME ❹
Indication
▸ ROUTE
▸ Age groups: [Neonate/Child]
Dose and frequency of administration (max. dose)
DOSE ADJUSTMENTS DUE TO INTERACTIONS dosing information when used concurrently with other drugs
DOSES AT EXTREMES OF BODY-WEIGHT dosing information for patients who are overweight or underweight
DOSE EQUIVALENCE AND CONVERSION information around the bioequivalence between formulations of the same drug, or equivalent doses of drugs that are members of the same class
PHARMACOKINETICS how the body affects a drug (absorption, distribution, metabolism, and excretion)
POTENCY a measure of drug activity expressed in terms of the concentration required to produce an effect of given intensity

- UNLICENSED USE describes the use of medicines outside the terms of their UK licence (off-label use), or use of medicines that have no licence for use in the UK

IMPORTANT SAFETY INFORMATION
Information produced and disseminated by drug regulators often highlights serious risks associated with the use of a drug, and may include advice that is mandatory

- CONTRA-INDICATIONS circumstances when a drug should be avoided
- CAUTIONS details of precautions required
- INTERACTIONS when one drug changes the effects of another drug; the mechanisms underlying drug interactions are explained in Appendix 1
- SIDE-EFFECTS listed in order of frequency, where known, and arranged alphabetically
- ALLERGY AND CROSS-SENSITIVITY for drugs that carry an increased risk of hypersensitivity reactions
- CONCEPTION AND CONTRACEPTION potential for a drug to have harmful effects on an unborn child when prescribing for a woman of childbearing age or for a man trying to father a child; information on the effect of drugs on the efficacy of latex condoms or diaphragms

- **PREGNANCY** advice on the use of a drug during pregnancy
- **BREAST FEEDING** [EvGr] advice on the use of a drug during breast feeding ⟨A⟩ ❺
- **HEPATIC IMPAIRMENT** advice on the use of a drug in hepatic impairment
- **RENAL IMPAIRMENT** advice on the use of a drug in renal impairment
- **PRE-TREATMENT SCREENING** covers one off tests required to assess the suitability of a patient for a particular drug
- **MONITORING REQUIREMENTS** specifies any special monitoring requirements, including information on monitoring the plasma concentration of drugs with a narrow therapeutic index
- **EFFECTS ON LABORATORY TESTS** for drugs that can interfere with the accuracy of seemingly unrelated laboratory tests
- **TREATMENT CESSATION** specifies whether further monitoring or precautions are advised when the drug is withdrawn
- **DIRECTIONS FOR ADMINISTRATION** practical information on the preparation of intravenous drug infusions; general advice relevant to other routes of administration
- **PRESCRIBING AND DISPENSING INFORMATION** practical information around how a drug can be prescribed and dispensed including details of when brand prescribing is necessary
- **HANDLING AND STORAGE** includes information on drugs that can cause adverse effects to those who handle them before they are taken by, or administered to, a patient; advice on storage conditions
- **PATIENT AND CARER ADVICE** for drugs with a special need for counselling
- **PROFESSION SPECIFIC INFORMATION** provides details of the restrictions certain professions such as dental practitioners or nurse prescribers need to be aware of when prescribing on the NHS
- **NATIONAL FUNDING/ACCESS DECISIONS** details of NICE Technology Appraisals, SMC advice and AWMSG advice
- **LESS SUITABLE FOR PRESCRIBING** preparations that are considered by the Paediatric Formulary Committee to be less suitable for prescribing
- **EXCEPTION TO LEGAL CATEGORY** advice and information on drugs which may be sold without a prescription under specific conditions

---

- **MEDICINAL FORMS**

  Form

  CAUTIONARY AND ADVISORY LABELS if applicable

  EXCIPIENTS clinically important but not comprehensive [consult manufacturer information for full details]

  ELECTROLYTES if clinically significant quantities occur

  ▸ Preparation name (Manufacturer/Non-proprietary)

  Drug name and strength pack sizes [PoM] ❻ Prices

Combinations available this indicates a combination preparation is available and a cross reference page number is provided to locate this preparation

❺ Evidence grading

Evidence grading to reflect the strengths of recommendations will be applied as content goes through the revalidation process. A five level evidence grading system based on the former SIGN grading system has been adopted. The grades ⟨A⟩ ⟨B⟩ ⟨C⟩ ⟨D⟩ ⟨E⟩ are displayed next to the recommendations within the text, and are preceded by the symbol: [EvGr]

For further information, see How BNF Publications are constructed

❻ Legal categories

[PoM] This symbol has been placed against those preparations that are available only on a prescription issued by an appropriate practitioner. For more detailed information see *Medicines, Ethics and Practice*, London, Pharmaceutical Press (always consult latest edition)

[CD1] [CD2] [CD3] [CD4-1] [CD4-2] [CD5] These symbols indicate that the preparations are subject to the prescription requirements of the Misuse of Drugs Act

For regulations governing prescriptions for such preparations, see Controlled Drugs and Drug Dependence

Not all monographs include all possible sections; sections are only included when relevant information has been identified

Occasionally, it is necessary to include doses in the total daily dose format (e.g. 10 mg/kg daily in 3 divided doses); in these cases the total daily dose should be divided into individual doses (in this example a child of body-weight 9 kg would receive 30 mg 3 times daily).

Most drugs can be administered at slightly irregular intervals during the day. Some drugs, e.g. antimicrobials, are best given at regular intervals. Some flexibility should be allowed in children to avoid waking them during the night. For example, the night-time dose may be given at the child's bedtime.

Special care should be taken when converting doses from one metric unit to another, and when calculating infusion rates or the volume of a preparation to administer. Where possible, doses should be rounded to facilitate administration of suitable volumes of liquid preparations, or an appropriate strength of tablet or capsule.

Other information relevant to Indication and dose

The dose panel also contains, where known, an indication of **pharmacokinetic considerations** that may affect the choice of dose, and **dose equivalence** information, which may aid the selection of dose when switching between drugs or preparations.

The BNFC includes **unlicensed use** of medicines when the clinical need cannot be met by licensed medicines; such use should be supported by appropriate evidence and experience. When the BNFC recommends an unlicensed medicine or the 'off-label' use of a licensed medicine, this is shown below the indication and dose panel in the unlicensed use section.

Minimising harm and drug safety

The drug chosen to treat a particular condition should minimise the patient's susceptibility to adverse effects and, where co-morbidities exist, have minimal detrimental effects on the patient's other diseases. To achieve this, the *Contra-indications*, *Cautions* and *Side-effects* of the relevant drug should be reviewed.

The information under Cautions can be used to assess the risks of using a drug in a patient who has co-morbidities that are also included in the Cautions for that drug—if a safer alternative cannot be found, the drug may be prescribed while monitoring the patient for adverse-effects or deterioration in the co-morbidity. Contra-indications are far more restrictive than Cautions and mean that the drug should be avoided in a patient with a condition that is contra-indicated.

The impact that potential side-effects may have on a patient's quality of life should also be assessed. For instance, in a child who has constipation, it may be preferable to avoid a drug that frequently causes constipation.

The *Important safety advice* section in the BNFC, delineated by a coloured outline box, highlights important safety concerns, often those raised by regulatory authorities or guideline producers. Safety warnings issued by the Commission on Human Medicines (CHM) or Medicines and Healthcare products Regulatory Agency (MHRA) are found here.

Drug selection should aim to minimise drug interactions. If it is necessary to prescribe a potentially serious combination of drugs, patients should be monitored appropriately. The mechanisms underlying drug interactions are explained in Appendix 1, followed by details of drug interactions.

Use of drugs in specific patient populations

Drug selection should aim to minimise the potential for drug accumulation, adverse drug reactions, and exacerbation of pre-existing hepatic or renal disease. If it is necessary to prescribe drugs whose effect is altered by hepatic or renal disease, appropriate drug dose adjustments should be made, and patients should be monitored adequately. The general principles for prescribing are outlined under *Prescribing in hepatic impairment* p. 17, and *Prescribing in renal impairment* p. 17. Information about drugs that should be avoided or used with caution in hepatic disease or renal impairment can be found in drug monographs under *Hepatic impairment* and *Renal impairment* (e.g. fluconazole p. 407).

Similarly, drug selection should aim to minimise harm to the fetus, nursing infant, and mother. The infant should be monitored for potential side-effects of drugs used by the *mother during pregnancy or breast-feeding*. The general principles for prescribing are outlined under Prescribing in pregnancy p. 19 and Prescribing in breast-feeding p. 19. The Treatment Summaries provide guidance on the drug treatment of common conditions that can occur during pregnancy and breast-feeding (e.g. Asthma, acute p. 158). Information about the use of specific drugs during pregnancy and breast-feeding can be found in their drug monographs under *Pregnancy*, and *Breast-feeding* (e.g. fluconazole p. 407).

A new section, *Conception and contraception*, containing information around considerations for females of childbearing potential or men who might father a child (e.g. isotretinoin p. 809) has been included.

Administration and monitoring

When selecting the most appropriate drug, it may be necessary to screen the patient for certain genetic markers or metabolic states. This information is included within a section called *Pre-treatment screening* (e.g. abacavir p. 451). This section covers one-off tests required to assess the suitability of a patient for a particular drug.

Once the drug has been selected, it needs to be given in the most appropriate manner. A *Directions for administration* section contains the information about intravenous administration previously located in Appendix 4. This provides practical information on the preparation of intravenous drug infusions, including compatibility of drugs with standard intravenous infusion fluids, method of dilution or reconstitution, and administration rates. In addition, general advice relevant to other routes of administration is provided within this section (e.g. fentanyl p. 296) and further details, such as masking the bitter taste of some medicines.

Whenever possible, intramuscular injections should be **avoided** in children because they are painful.

After selecting and administering the most appropriate drug by the most appropriate route, patients should be monitored to ensure they are achieving the expected benefits from drug treatment without any unwanted side-effects. The *Monitoring* section specifies any special monitoring requirements, including information on monitoring the plasma concentration of drugs with a narrow therapeutic index (e.g. theophylline p. 178). Monitoring may, in certain cases, be affected by the impact of a drug on laboratory tests (e.g. hydroxocobalamin p. 621), and this information is included in *Effects on laboratory tests*.

In some cases, when a drug is withdrawn, further monitoring or precautions may be advised (e.g. clonidine hydrochloride p. 108); these are covered under *Treatment cessation*.

Choice and supply

The prescriber, the child's carer, and the child (if appropriate) should agree on the health outcomes desired and on the strategy for achieving them (see *Taking Medicines to Best Effect*). Taking the time to explain to the child (and the child's carer if appropriate) the rationale and the potential adverse effects of treatment may improve adherence. For some medicines there is a special need for counselling (e.g. appropriate posture during administration of doxycycline p. 381, or recognising signs of blood, liver, or skin disorders with carbamazepine p. 209); this is shown in *Patient and carer advice*.

Other information contained in the latter half of the monograph also helps prescribers and those dispensing medicines choose medicinal forms (by indicating information such as flavour or when branded products are not interchangeable e.g. modified-release theophylline p. 178), assess the suitability of a drug for prescribing, understand the NHS funding status for a drug (e.g. sildenafil p. 125), or assess when a patient may be able to purchase a drug without prescription (e.g. loperamide hydrochloride p. 54).

Medicinal forms

In the BNFC, preparations follow immediately after the monograph for the drug that is their main ingredient.

In earlier editions, when a particular preparation had safety information, dose advice or other clinical information specific to the product, it was contained within the preparations section. This information has been moved to the relevant section in the main body of the monograph under a heading of the name of the specific medicinal form (e.g. peppermint oil p. 40).

The medicinal forms (formerly preparations) section provides information on the type of formulation (e.g. tablet), the amount of active drug in a solid dosage form, and the concentration of active drug in a liquid dosage form. The legal status is shown for prescription-only medicines and controlled drugs, as well as pharmacy medicines and medicines on the general sales list. Practitioners are reminded, by a statement under the heading of "Medicinal Form" that not all products containing a specific drug ingredient may be similarly licensed. To be clear on the precise licensing status of specific medicinal forms, practitioners should check the product literature for the particular product being prescribed or dispensed.

Details of all medicinal forms available on the dm+d for each drug in BNF Publications appears online on MedicinesComplete. In print editions, due to space constraints, only certain branded products are included in detail. Where medicinal forms are listed they should not be inferred as equivalent to the other brands listed under the same form heading. For example, all the products listed under a heading of "Modified release capsule" will be available as modified release capsules, however, the brands listed under that form heading may have different release profiles, the available strengths may vary and/or the products may have different licensing information. As with earlier editions of the BNFC, practitioners must ensure that the particular product being prescribed or dispensed is appropriate.

As medicinal forms are derived from dm+d data, some drugs may appear under names derived from that data; this may vary slightly from those in earlier BNFC versions, e.g. sodium acid phosphate, is now sodium dihydrogen phosphate anhydrous.

Children should be prescribed a preparation that complements their daily routine, and that provides the right dose of drug for the right indication and route of administration. When dispensing liquid preparations, a sugar-free preparation should always be used in preference to one containing sugar. Patients receiving medicines containing cariogenic sugars should be advised of appropriate dental hygiene measures to prevent caries.

Earlier editions of the BNFC only included excipients and electrolyte information for proprietary medicines. This information is now covered at the level of the dose form (e.g. tablet). It is not possible to keep abreast of all of the generic products available on the UK market, and so this information serves as a reminder to the healthcare professional that, if the presence of a particular excipient is of concern, they should check the product literature for the particular product being prescribed or dispensed.

Cautionary and advisory labels that pharmacists are recommended to add when dispensing are included in the medicinal forms section. Details of these labels can be found in Appendix 3, Guidance for cautionary and advisory labels p. 1138. These labels have now been applied at the level of the dose form.

In the case of compound preparations, the prescribing information for all constituents should be taken into account.

Prices in the BNFC

Basic NHS **net prices** are given in the BNFC to provide an indication of relative cost. Where there is a choice of suitable preparations for a particular disease or condition the relative cost may be used in making a selection. Cost-effective prescribing must, however, take into account other factors (such as dose frequency and duration of treatment) that affect the total cost. The use of more expensive drugs is justified if it will result in better treatment of the patient, or a reduction of the length of an illness, or the time spent in hospital.

Prices are regularly updated using the Drug Tariff and proprietary price information published by the NHS dictionary of medicines and devices (dm+d, www.nhsbsa.nhs.uk/pharmacies-gp-practices-and-appliance-contractors/dictionary-medicines-and-devices-dmd). The weekly updated dm+d data (including prices) can be accessed using the dm+d browser of the NHS Business Services Authority (apps.nhsbsa.nhs.uk/DMDBrowser/DMDBrowser.do). Prices have been calculated from the net cost used in pricing NHS prescriptions and generally reflect whole dispensing packs. Prices for extemporaneously prepared preparations are not provided in the BNFC as prices vary between different manufacturers.

BNFC prices are not suitable for quoting to patients seeking private prescriptions or contemplating over-the-counter purchases because they do not take into account VAT, professional fees, and other overheads.

A fuller explanation of costs to the NHS may be obtained from the Drug Tariff. Separate drug tariffs are applicable to England and Wales (www.ppa.org.uk/ppa/edt_intro.htm), Scotland (www.isdscotland.org/Health-Topics/Prescribing-and-Medicines/Scottish-Drug-Tariff/), and Northern Ireland (www.hscbusiness.hscni.net/services/2034.htm); prices in the different tariffs may vary.

Drug class monographs

In earlier editions of the BNFC, information relating to a class of drug sharing the same properties (e.g. tetracyclines p. 380), was contained within the prescribing notes. In the updated structure, drug class monographs have been created to contain the common information; this ensures such information is easier to find, and has a more regularised structure.

For consistency and ease of use, the class monograph follows the same structure as a drug monograph. Class monographs are indicated by the presence of a flag (e.g. beta-adrenoceptor blockers (systemic) p. 109). If a drug monograph has a corresponding class monograph, that needs to be considered in tandem, in order to understand the full information about a drug, the monograph is also indicated by a flag 1234 (e.g. metoprolol tartrate p. 113). Within this flag, the page number of the drug class monograph is provided (e.g. 1234), to help navigate the user to this information. This is particularly useful where occasionally, due to differences in therapeutic use, the drug monograph may not directly follow the drug class monograph (e.g. sotalol hydrochloride p. 85).

Evidence grading

The BNF has adopted a five level evidence grading system (see How BNF Publications are constructed p. viii). Recommendations that are evidence graded can be identified by a symbol appearing immediately before the recommendation. The evidence grade is displayed at the end of the recommendation.

Other content

Nutrition

Appendix 2 includes tables of ACBS-approved enteral feeds and nutritional supplements based on their energy and protein content. There are separate tables for specialised formulae for specific clinical conditions. Classified sections on foods for special diets and nutritional supplements for metabolic diseases are also included.

Other useful information

Finding significant changes in the BNFC

- ***Changes***, provides a list of significant changes, dose changes, classification changes, new names, and new preparations that have been incorporated into the BNFC, as well as a list of preparations that have been discontinued and removed from the BNFC. Changes listed online are cumulative (from one print edition to the next), and can be printed off each month to show the main changes since the last print edition as an aide memoire for those using print copies. So many changes are made for each update of the BNFC, that not all of them can be accommodated in the *Changes* section. We encourage healthcare professionals to review regularly the prescribing information on drugs that they encounter frequently;
- ***Changes to the Dental Practitioners' Formulary***, are located at the end of the Dental List;
- ***E-newsletter***, the BNF & BNFC e-newsletter service is available free of charge. It alerts healthcare professionals to details of significant changes in the clinical content of these publications and to the way that this information is delivered. Newsletters also review clinical case studies, provide tips on using these publications effectively, and highlight forthcoming changes to the publications. To sign up for e-newsletters go to www.bnf.org.

Using other sources for medicines information

The BNFC is designed as a digest for rapid reference. Less detail is given on areas such as malignant disease and anaesthesia since it is expected that those undertaking treatment will have specialist knowledge and access to specialist literature. The BNFC should be interpreted in the light of professional knowledge and supplemented as necessary by specialised publications and by reference to the product literature. Information is also available from medicines information services.

Changes

Monthly updates are provided online via Medicines Complete and the NHS Evidence portal. The changes listed below are cumulative (from one print edition to the next).

Significant changes

Significant changes that appear in the print edition of *BNF for Children* 2020—2021:

- Adrenaline/epinephrine auto-injectors p. 143 (*Emerade*®): all strengths of auto-injector pens have been recalled from patients due to failure to activate. Healthcare professionals are advised to ensure that patients who have previously been prescribed an *Emerade*®150, 300 or 500 microgram pen are supplied with a prescription for an alternative brand—see the MHRA website for full details [MHRA/CHM advice] (updated June 2020).
- Adrenaline/epinephrine auto-injectors p. 143: recent action taken to support safety [MHRA/CHM advice] (updated December 2019).
- Adrenaline/epinephrine p. 143 (*Emerade*®) pre-filled auto-injector: update on failure to activate [MHRA/CHM advice] (updated April 2020).
- Antimicrobial stewardship p. 27: new guidance.
- Asthma, acute p. 158: updated guidance on management.
- Asthma, chronic p. 154: updated guidance on management.
- Bacillus Calmette-Guérin vaccine p. 831: updated guidance in-line with Public Health England recommendations.
- Benzodiazepines: reminder of risk of potentially fatal respiratory depression [MHRA/CHM advice] (advice in clobazam, clonazepam, diazepam, lorazepam, midazolam, temazepam; see example in diazepam p. 236).
- Cannabidiol p. 208 with clobazam for treating seizures associated with Dravet syndrome [NICE guidance].
- Cannabidiol p. 208 with clobazam for treating seizures associated with Lennox–Gastaut syndrome [NICE guidance].
- Contraceptives, hormonal p. 532: updated guidance on combined hormonal contraceptives.
- COVID-19 p. 433: new guidance incorporating a collection of resources.
- Crohn's disease p. 30: updated guidance on management.
- Depression p. 251: updated guidance on management.
- Diabetic foot infections, antibacterial therapy p. 324: new guidance on management.
- Domperidone p. 278 for nausea and vomiting: lack of efficacy in children; reminder of contra-indications in adults and adolescents [MHRA/CHM advice].
- Etonogestrel p. 552 (*Nexplanon*®) contraceptive implants: new insertion site to reduce rare risk of neurovascular injury and implant migration [MHRA/CHM advice].
- Fingolimod p. 568 (*Gilenya*®): increased risk of congenital malformations; new contra-indication during pregnancy and in women of childbearing potential not using effective contraception [MHRA/CHM advice].
- *Flutiform*®50 microgram/ 5 microgram inhaler (fluticasone with formoterol p. 171): age range extension to include children aged 5 to 12 years for the prophylaxis of asthma.
- Gastro-oesophageal reflux disease p. 64: updated guidance.
- Human papillomavirus vaccine p. 834 updated guidance in-line with Public Health England recommendations.
- Hypoglycaemia p. 501: updated guidance on management.
- Immunisation schedule p. 831: changes to infant schedule for pneumococcal polysaccharide conjugate vaccine in-line with Public Health England recommendations.
- Immunisation schedule p. 831: updated national human papillomavirus immunisation programme in-line with Public Health England recommendations.
- Lanadelumab p. 193 for preventing recurrent attacks of hereditary angioedema [NICE guidance].
- Magnesium sulfate p. 646: risk of skeletal adverse effects in the neonate following prolonged or repeated use in pregnancy [MHRA/CHM advice].
- Malaria, prophylaxis p. 420: updated country recommendations in the recommended regimens for prophylaxis against malaria in-line with Public Health England.
- Malaria, prophylaxis p. 420: updated guidance in-line with Public Health England recommendations.
- Mecasermin p. 515 (*Increlex*®▼): risk of benign and malignant neoplasia [MHRA/CHM advice].
- Medicines optimisation p. 25: new guidance.
- Montelukast p. 174 (*Singulair*®): reminder of the risk of neuropsychiatric reactions [MHRA/CHM advice].
- Newborn life support image (see Life support algorithm (image) p. 1189) updated.
- Nusinersen p. 700 for treating spinal muscular atrophy [NICE guidance].
- Ondansetron p. 281: small increased risk of oral clefts following use in the first 12 weeks of pregnancy [MHRA/CHM advice].
- Opioids: reminder of risk of potentially fatal respiratory depression [MHRA/CHM advice] (advice in alfentanil, buprenorphine, codeine phosphate, diamorphine hydrochloride, dihydrocodeine tartrate, fentanyl, hydromorphone hydrochloride, methadone hydrochloride, morphine, oxycodone hydrochloride, pethidine hydrochloride, remifentanil, tapentadol, tramadol hydrochloride; see example in morphine p. 299).
- Oral retinoid medicines (acitretin p. 800, isotretinoin p. 809, and tretinoin p. 599): revised and simplified pregnancy prevention educational materials for healthcare professionals and women [MHRA/CHM advice].
- Parenteral nutrition supplements p. 669: light protection required to reduce the risk of serious adverse effects in premature neonates [MHRA/CHM advice].
- Pneumococcal vaccine p. 838: updated guidance in-line with Public Health England recommendations.
- Poisoning, emergency treatment p. 891: updated guidance on the management of beta-blockers poisoning in-line with TOXBASE recommendations.
- Poisoning, emergency treatment p. 891: updated guidance on the management of paracetamol poisoning in-line with TOXBASE recommendations.
- Respiratory system infections, antibacterial therapy p. 327: updated guidance for community-acquired pneumonia.
- Respiratory system infections, antibacterial therapy p. 327: updated guidance for hospital-acquired pneumonia.
- Rotavirus vaccine p. 841: updated guidance in-line with Public Health England recommendations.
- Skin infections, antibacterial therapy p. 329: updated guidance for management of cellulitis and erysipelas.
- Skin infections, antibacterial therapy p. 329: updated guidance on management of impetigo.
- Sodium valproate p. 223: updated Pregnancy Prevention Programme [MHRA/CHM advice].
- Tocilizumab p. 691 (*RoActemra*®): rare risk of serious liver injury including cases requiring transplantation [MHRA/CHM advice].
- Tuberculosis p. 392: updated guidance on management.
- Typhoid vaccine p. 843: updated guidance in-line with Public Health England recommendations.
- Ulcerative colitis p. 32: updated guidance on management.
- Urinary-tract infections p. 400: updated guidance on management.

- Valproic acid p. 228: updated Pregnancy Prevention Programme [MHRA/CHM advice].
- Yellow fever vaccine, live p. 860: stronger precautions in people with weakened immunity and in those aged 60 years or older [MHRA/CHM advice].
- Yellow fever vaccine p. 843: updated guidance in-line with Public Health England recommendations.

Dose changes

Changes in dose statements that appear in the print edition of *BNF for Children* 2020—2021:

- Benzoin tincture, compound p. 200 [updated child age range].
- Betamethasone with clioquinol p. 791 [updated child age range].
- Co-fluampicil p. 369 [update to dosing information].
- Digoxin p. 86 [clarification of maximum doses for children 5-9 years].
- Emicizumab p. 88 [alternative dosing for existing indications added].
- *Epipen*® preparations (adrenaline/epinephrine p. 143) [body-weight ranges for children's dosing updated].
- Eucalyptus with menthol p. 200 [frequency of dosing].
- Eucalyptus with menthol p. 200 [updated child age range].
- Fluocinolone acetonide with clioquinol p. 793 [updated dosing frequency].
- Glucagon p. 502 [update to age ranges for hypoglycaemia].
- Human papillomavirus vaccines p. 855: Dosing now includes male patients.
- Idursulfase p. 660 [updated age range].
- Iloprost p. 127 [expression of rate of intravenous infusion updated; dosing recommendation unchanged].
- Paracetamol with buclizine hydrochloride and codeine phosphate p. 308 [child age ranges].
- *Qvar*® (beclometasone dipropionate p. 167) [age-range extension].
- *Seretide* 50 *Evohaler*® (fluticasone with salmeterol p. 171) [age-range extension].
- *Seretide* 100 *Accuhaler*® (fluticasone with salmeterol p. 171) [age-range extension].
- Sodium fluoride p. 757 [updating dosing for prophylaxis of dental caries].
- Typhoid vaccine p. 851 [booster dose added].

New preparations

New preparations included that appear in the print edition of *BNF for Children* 2020—2021:

- Benzathine benzylpenicillin p. 363.
- Cannabidiol p. 208.
- *Combisal*®25/50 [fluticasone with salmeterol p. 171].
- *Combisal*®25/125 [fluticasone with salmeterol p. 171].
- *Combisal*®25/250 [fluticasone with salmeterol p. 171].
- *Cuprior*® [trientine dihydrochloride p. 667].
- *Cytotect*® [cytomegalovirus immunoglobulin p. 824].
- *Dupixent*® [dupilumab p. 799].
- *Fusacomb* 50/250 *Easyhaler*® [fluticasone with salmeterol p. 171].
- *Fusacomb* 50/500 *Easyhaler*® [fluticasone with salmeterol p. 171].
- *Gardasil* 9® [human papillomavirus vaccines p. 855].
- *Gilenya*® [fingolimod p. 568].
- *Mimpara*® granules [cinacalcet p. 640].
- *Mozobil*® [plerixafor p. 627].
- *Nyxoid*® [naloxone hydrochloride p. 901].
- *Orkambi*® granules [lumacaftor with ivacaftor p. 197].
- *Renapime*® [cefepime p. 346].
- *Renoxitin*® [cefoxitin p. 340].
- *Takhzyro*® [lanadelumab p. 193].
- *Vitrakvi*® [larotrectinib p. 607].
- *Zalkya*® [dienogest p. 517].
- *Zinforo*® [ceftaroline fosamil p. 347].

Guidance on prescribing

General guidance

Medicines should be given to children only when they are necessary, and in all cases the potential benefit of administering the medicine should be considered in relation to the risk involved. This is particularly important during pregnancy, when the risk to both mother and fetus must be considered.

It is important to discuss treatment options carefully with the child and the child's carer. In particular, the child and the child's carer should be helped to distinguish the adverse effects of prescribed drugs from the effects of the medical disorder. When the beneficial effects of the medicine are likely to be delayed, this should be highlighted.

For guidance on medicines optimisation, see Medicines optimisation p. 25.

Never Events Never events are serious and avoidable medical errors for which there should be preventative measures in place to stop their occurrence.

The NHS Never Events policy and framework can be viewed at: improvement.nhs.uk/documents/2265/Revised_Never_Events_policy_and_framework_FINAL.pdf.

For never events related to single drugs or drug classes, BNF Publications contain information within the monographs, in the important safety information section.

Prescribing competency framework The Royal Pharmaceutical Society has published a Prescribing Competency Framework that includes a common set of competencies that form the basis for prescribing, regardless of professional background. The competencies have been developed to help healthcare professionals be safe and effective prescribers with the aim of supporting patients to get the best outcomes from their medicines. It is available at www.rpharms.com/resources/frameworks/prescribers-competency-framework.

Transitional services for chronic conditions

The process of moving from paediatric to adult services can lead to a loss of continuity in care and provoke anxiety in children and their carers. EvGr Practitioners should start planning for adult care when the child reaches the age of 13 or 14 at the latest and a child-centred approach should be taken. Consider designating a named practitioner among those providing care to the child to take a coordinating role and to act as an advocate for the child, maintaining a link between the various practitioners involved in care (including a named GP). ⟨A⟩

Drug treatment in children

Children, and particularly neonates, differ from adults in their response to drugs. Special care is needed in the neonatal period (first 28 days of life) and doses should always be calculated with care; the risk of toxicity is increased by a reduced rate of drug clearance and differing target organ sensitivity. The terms infant, child and adolescent are used inconsistently in the literature. However, **for reference purposes only**, the terms generally used to describe the paediatric stages of development are:

Preterm neonate	Born at < 37 weeks gestation
Term neonate	Born at 37 to 42 weeks gestation
Post-term neonate	Born at ≥42 weeks gestation
Neonate	From 0 up to 28 days of age (or first 4 weeks of life)
Infant	From 28 days up to 24 months of age
Child	From 2 years up to 12 years of age
Adolescent	From 12 years up to 18 years of age

In *BNF for Children*, the term neonate is used to describe a newborn infant aged 0–28 days. The terms child or children are used generically to describe the entire range from infant to adolescent (1 month–17 years). An age range is specified when the dose information applies to a narrower age range than a child from 1 month–17 years.

Administration of medicines to children

Children should be involved in decisions about taking medicines and encouraged to take responsibility for using them correctly. The degree of such involvement will depend on the child's age, understanding, and personal circumstances.

Occasionally a medicine or its taste has to be disguised or masked with small quantities of food. However, unless specifically permitted (e.g. some formulations of pancreatin p. 77), a medicine should **not** be mixed with large quantities of food because the full dose might not be taken and the child might develop an aversion to food if the medicine imparts an unpleasant taste. Medicines should not be mixed or administered in a baby's feeding bottle.

Children under 5 years (and some older children) find a liquid formulation more acceptable than tablets or capsules. However, for long-term treatment it may be possible for a child to be taught to take tablets or capsules.

An oral syringe should be used for accurate measurement and controlled administration of an oral liquid medicine. The unpleasant taste of an oral liquid can be disguised by flavouring it or by giving a favourite food or drink immediately afterwards, but the potential for food-drug interactions should be considered.

Advice should be given on dental hygiene to those receiving medicines containing cariogenic sugars for long-term treatment; sugar-free medicines should be provided whenever possible.

Children with nasal feeding tubes in place for prolonged periods should be encouraged to take medicines by mouth if possible; enteric feeding should generally be interrupted before the medicine is given (particularly if enteral feeds reduce the absorption of a particular drug). Oral liquids can be given through the tube provided that precautions are taken to guard against blockage; the dose should be washed down with warm water. When a medicine is given through a nasogastric tube to a neonate, **sterile water** must be used to accompany the medicine or to wash it down.

The intravenous route is generally chosen when a medicine cannot be given by mouth; reliable access, often a central vein, should be used for children whose treatment involves irritant or inotropic drugs or who need to receive the medicine over a long period or for home therapy. The subcutaneous route is used most commonly for insulin administration. Intramuscular injections should preferably be **avoided** in children, particularly neonates, infants, and young children. However, the intramuscular route may be advantageous for administration of single doses of medicines when intravenous cannulation would be more problematic or painful to the child. Certain drugs, e.g. some vaccines, are only administered intramuscularly.

The intrathecal, epidural and intraosseous routes should be used **only** by staff specially trained to administer medicines by these routes. Local protocols for the management of intrathecal injections must be in place.

Managing medicines in school

Administration of a medicine during schooltime should be avoided if possible; medicines should be prescribed for once or twice-daily administration whenever practicable. If the medicine needs to be taken in school, this should be discussed with parents or carers and the necessary arrangements made in advance; where appropriate, involvement of a school nurse should be sought. *Managing Medicines in Schools and Early Years Settings* produced by the Department of Health and Social Care provides guidance on using medicines in schools (www.gov.uk/government/organisations/department-of-health-and-social-care).

Patient information leaflets

Manufacturers' patient information leaflets that accompany a medicine, cover only the licensed use of the medicine. Therefore, when a medicine is used outside its licence, it may be appropriate to advise the child and the child's parent or carer that some of the information in the leaflet might not apply to the child's treatment. Where necessary, inappropriate advice in the patient information leaflet should be identified and reassurance provided about the correct use in the context of the child's condition.

Biological medicines

Biological medicines are medicines that are made by or derived from a biological source using biotechnology processes, such as recombinant DNA technology. The size and complexity of biological medicines, as well as the way they are produced, may result in a degree of natural variability in molecules of the same active substance, particularly in different batches of the medicine. This variation is maintained within strict acceptable limits. Examples of biological medicines include insulins and monoclonal antibodies. EvGr Biological medicines must be prescribed by brand name and the brand name specified on the prescription should be dispensed in order to avoid inadvertent switching. Automatic substitution of brands at the point of dispensing is not appropriate for biological medicines. Ⓐ

Biosimilar medicines

A **biosimilar medicine** is a biological medicine that is highly similar and clinically equivalent (in terms of quality, safety, and efficacy) to an existing biological medicine that has already been authorised in the European Union (known as the reference biological medicine or originator medicine). The active substance of a biosimilar medicine is similar, but not identical, to the originator biological medicine. Once the patent for a biological medicine has expired, a biosimilar medicine may be authorised by the European Medicines Agency (EMA). A biosimilar medicine is not the same as a generic medicine, which contains a simpler molecular structure that is identical to the originator medicine.

Therapeutic equivalence EvGr Biosimilar medicines should be considered to be therapeutically equivalent to the originator biological medicine within their authorised indications. Ⓐ Biosimilar medicines are usually licensed for all the indications of the originator biological medicine, but this depends on the evidence submitted to the EMA for authorisation and must be scientifically justified on the basis of demonstrated or extrapolated equivalence.

Prescribing and dispensing The choice of whether to prescribe a biosimilar medicine or the originator biological medicine rests with the clinician in consultation with the patient. EvGr Biological medicines (including biosimilar medicines) must be prescribed by brand name and the brand name specified on the prescription should be dispensed in order to avoid inadvertent switching. Automatic substitution of brands at the point of dispensing is not appropriate for biological medicines. Ⓐ

Safety monitoring Biosimilar medicines are subject to a black triangle status (▼) at the time of initial authorisation. EvGr It is important to report suspected adverse reactions using the Yellow Card Scheme (see Adverse reactions to drugs p. 13). For all biological medicines, adverse reaction reports should clearly state the brand name and the batch number of the suspected medicine. Ⓐ
UK Medicines Information centres have developed a validated tool to determine potential safety issues associated with all new medicines. These 'in-use product safety assessment reports' will be published for new biosimilar medicines as they become available, see www.sps.nhs.uk/home/medicines/.

National funding/access decisions The Department of Health has confirmed that, in England, NICE can decide to apply the same remit, and the resulting technology appraisal guidance, to relevant biosimilar medicines which appear on the market subsequent to their originator biological medicine. In other circumstances, where a review of the evidence for a particular biosimilar medicine is necessary, NICE will consider producing an evidence summary (see *Evidence summary: new medicines*, www.nice.org.uk/about/what-we-do/our-programmes/nice-advice/evidence-summaries-new-medicines).

National information In England, see www.nice.org.uk/Media/Default/About/what-we-do/NICE-guidance/NICE-technology-appraisals/biosimilars-statement.pdf.
In Northern Ireland, see niformulary.hscni.net/ManagedEntry/bios/Pages/default.aspx.
In Scotland, see www.scottishmedicines.org.uk/About_SMC/Policy_statements/Biosimilar_Medicines.
In Wales, see www.wales.nhs.uk/sites3/Documents/814/BIOSIMILARS-ABUHBpositionStatement%5BNov2015%5D.pdf.

Availability The following drugs are available as a biosimilar medicine:

- Adalimumab p. 693
- Enoxaparin sodium p. 101
- Epoetin alfa p. 612
- Epoetin zeta p. 614
- Etanercept p. 696
- Filgrastim p. 625
- Infliximab p. 38
- Insulin glargine p. 496
- Insulin lispro p. 493
- Rituximab p. 574
- Somatropin p. 513

Complementary and alternative medicine

An increasing amount of information on complementary and alternative medicine is becoming available. Where appropriate, the child and the child's carers should be asked about the use of their medicines, including dietary supplements and topical products. The scope of *BNF for Children* is restricted to the discussion of conventional medicines but reference is made to complementary treatments if they affect conventional therapy (e.g. interactions with St John's wort). Further information on herbal medicines is available at www.gov.uk/government/organisations/medicines-and-healthcare-products-regulatory-agency.

BNF for Children and marketing authorisation

Where appropriate the *doses, indications, cautions, contra-indications,* and *side-effects* in *BNF for Children* reflect those in the manufacturers' Summaries of Product Characteristics (SPCs) which, in turn, reflect those in the corresponding marketing authorisations (formerly known as Product Licences). *BNF for Children* does not generally include proprietary medicines that are not supported by a valid Summary of Product Characteristics or when the marketing authorisation holder has not been able to supply essential information. When a preparation is available from more than one manufacturer, *BNF for Children* reflects advice that is the most clinically relevant regardless of any variation in the marketing authorisation. Unlicensed products can be obtained from 'special-order' manufacturers or specialist importing companies.

As far as possible, medicines should be prescribed within the terms of the marketing authorisation. However, many children require medicines not specifically licensed for paediatric use. Although medicines cannot be promoted outside the limits of the licence, the Human Medicines Regulations 2012 do not prohibit the use of unlicensed medicines.

BNF for Children includes advice involving the use of unlicensed medicines or of licensed medicines for unlicensed uses ('off-label' use). Such advice reflects careful consideration of the options available to manage a given condition and the weight of evidence and experience of the unlicensed intervention, and limitations of the marketing authorisation should not preclude unlicensed use where clinically appropriate. Where an unlicensed drug or 'off-label' use is included, this is indicated in the unlicensed use section of the drug monograph.

Prescribing unlicensed medicines Prescribing unlicensed medicines or medicines outside the recommendations of their marketing authorisation alters (and probably increases) the prescriber's professional responsibility and potential liability. The prescriber should be able to justify and feel competent in using such medicines, and also inform the patient or the patient's carer that the prescribed medicine is unlicensed.

Drugs and skilled tasks

Prescribers and other healthcare professionals should advise children and their carers if treatment is likely to affect their ability to perform skilled tasks (e.g. driving). This applies especially to drugs with sedative effects; patients should be warned that these effects are increased by alcohol. General information about a patient's fitness to drive is available from the Driver and Vehicle Licensing Agency at www.gov.uk/government/organisations/driver-and-vehicle-licensing-agency.

A new offence of driving, attempting to drive, or being in charge of a vehicle, with certain specified controlled drugs in excess of specified limits, came into force on 2nd March 2015. This offence is an addition to the existing rules on drug impaired driving and fitness to drive, and applies to two groups of drugs—commonly abused drugs, including amfetamines, cannabis, cocaine, and ketamine p. 879, and drugs used mainly for medical reasons, such as opioids and benzodiazepines. Anyone found to have any of the drugs (including related drugs, for example, apomorphine hydrochloride) above specified limits in their blood will be guilty of an offence, whether their driving was impaired or not. This also includes prescribed drugs which metabolise to those included in the offence, for example, selegiline hydrochloride. However, the legislation provides a statutory "medical defence" for patients taking drugs for medical reasons in accordance with instructions, *if their driving was not impaired*—it continues to be an offence to drive if actually impaired. Patients should therefore be advised to continue taking their medicines as prescribed, and when driving, to carry suitable evidence that the drug was prescribed, or sold, to treat a medical or dental problem, and that it was taken according to the instructions given by the prescriber, or information provided with the medicine (e.g. a repeat prescription form or the medicine's patient information leaflet). Further information is available from the Department for Transport at www.gov.uk/government/collections/drug-driving.

Oral syringes

An **oral syringe** is supplied when oral liquid medicines are prescribed in doses other than multiples of 5 mL. The oral syringe is marked in 0.5-mL divisions from 1 to 5 mL to measure doses of less than 5 mL (other sizes of oral syringe may also be available). It is provided with an adaptor and an instruction leaflet. The 5-*mL spoon* is used for doses of 5 mL (or multiples thereof).

Excipients

Branded oral liquid preparations that do not contain *fructose, glucose,* or *sucrose* are described as 'sugar-free' in *BNF for Children*. Preparations containing hydrogenated glucose syrup, mannitol, maltitol, sorbitol, or xylitol are also marked 'sugar-free' since they do not cause dental caries. Children receiving medicines containing cariogenic sugars, or their carers, should be advised of dental hygiene measures to prevent caries. Sugar-free preparations should be used whenever possible, particularly if treatment is required for a long period.

Where information on the presence of *alcohol, aspartame, gluten, sulfites, tartrazine, arachis (peanut) oil* or *sesame oil* is available, this is indicated in *BNF for Children* against the relevant preparation.

Information is provided on *selected excipients* in skin preparations, in vaccines, and on *selected preservatives* and *excipients* in eye drops and injections.

The presence of *benzyl alcohol* and *polyoxyl castor oil* (polyethoxylated castor oil) in injections is indicated in *BNF for Children*. Benzyl alcohol has been associated with a fatal toxic syndrome in preterm neonates, and therefore, parenteral preparations containing the preservative should not be used in neonates. Polyoxyl castor oils, used as vehicles in intravenous injections, have been associated with severe anaphylactoid reactions.

The presence of *propylene glycol* in oral or parenteral medicines is indicated in *BNF for Children*; it can cause adverse effects if its elimination is impaired, e.g. in renal failure, in neonates and young children, and in slow metabolisers of the substance. It may interact with metronidazole p. 358.

The *lactose* content in most medicines is too small to cause problems in most lactose-intolerant children. However in severe lactose intolerance, the lactose content should be determined before prescribing. The amount of lactose varies according to manufacturer, product, formulation, and strength.

Important In the absence of information on excipients in *BNF for Children* and in the product literature (available at www.medicines.org.uk/emc/), contact the manufacturer if it is essential to check details.

Health and safety

When handling chemical or biological materials particular attention should be given to the possibility of allergy, fire, explosion, radiation, or poisoning. Care is required to avoid sources of heat (including hair dryers) when flammable substances are used on the skin or hair. Substances, such as corticosteroids, some antimicrobials, phenothiazines, and many cytotoxics, are irritant or very potent and should be handled with caution; contact with the skin and inhalation of dust should be avoided. Healthcare professionals and carers should guard against exposure to sensitising, toxic or irritant substances if it is necessary to crush tablets or open capsules.

EEA and Swiss prescriptions

Pharmacists can dispense prescriptions issued by doctors and dentists from the European Economic Area (EEA) or Switzerland (except prescriptions for controlled drugs in Schedules 1, 2, or 3, or for drugs without a UK marketing authorisation). Prescriptions should be written in ink or otherwise so as to be indelible, should be dated, should state the name of the patient, should state the address of the prescriber, should contain particulars indicating whether the prescriber is a doctor or dentist, and should be signed by the prescriber.

Security and validity of prescriptions

The Councils of the British Medical Association and the Royal Pharmaceutical Society have issued a joint statement on the security and validity of prescriptions.

In particular, prescription forms should:

- not be left unattended at reception desks;
- not be left in a car where they may be visible;
- when not in use, be kept in a locked drawer within the surgery and at home.

Where there is any doubt about the authenticity of a prescription, the pharmacist should contact the prescriber. If this is done by telephone, the number should be obtained from the directory rather than relying on the information on the prescription form, which may be false.

Patient group direction (PGD)

In most cases, the most appropriate clinical care will be provided on an individual basis by a prescriber to a specific child. However, a Patient Group Direction for supply and administration of medicines by other healthcare professionals can be used where it would benefit the child's care without compromising safety.

A Patient Group Direction is a written direction relating to the supply and administration (or administration only) of a licensed prescription-only medicine (including some Controlled Drugs in specific circumstances) by certain classes of healthcare professionals; the Direction is signed by a doctor (or dentist) and by a pharmacist. Further information on Patient Group Directions is available in Health Service Circular HSC 2000/026 (England), HDL (2001) 7 (Scotland), and WHC (2000) 116 (Wales); see also the Human Medicines Regulations 2012.

NICE, Scottish Medicines Consortium and All Wales Medicines Strategy Group

Advice issued by the National Institute for Health and Care Excellence (NICE), the Scottish Medicines Consortium (SMC) and the All Wales Medicines Strategy Group (AWMSG) is included in *BNF for Children* when relevant. Details of the advice together with updates can be obtained from: www.nice.org.uk, www.scottishmedicines.org.uk and www.awmsg.org.

Specialised commissioning decisions

NHS England develops specialised commissioning policies that define access to specialised services for particular groups of patients to ensure consistency in access to treatments nationwide. For further information, see www.england.nhs.uk/specialised-commissioning-document-library/routinely-commissioned-policies/.

NHS England also commissions treatments for patients aged less than 18 years where specific commissioning conditions within a NICE Technology Appraisal or NHS England policy are met, see www.england.nhs.uk/publication/commissioning-medicines-for-children-specialised-services/.

Prescription writing

Shared care

In its guidelines on responsibility for prescribing (circular EL (91) 127) between hospitals and general practitioners, the Department of Health has advised that legal responsibility for prescribing lies with the doctor who signs the prescription.

Requirements

Prescriptions should be written legibly in ink or otherwise so as to be indelible (it is permissible to issue carbon copies of NHS prescriptions as long as they are signed in ink), should be dated, should state the name and address of the patient, the address of the prescriber, an indication of the type of prescriber, and should be signed in ink by the prescriber (computer-generated facsimile signatures do not meet the legal requirement). The age and the date of birth of the patient should preferably be stated, and it is a legal requirement in the case of prescription-only medicines to state the age for children under 12 years. These recommendations are acceptable for **prescription-only medicines**. Prescriptions for controlled drugs have additional legal requirements.
Wherever appropriate the prescriber should state the current weight of the child to enable the dose prescribed to be checked. Consideration should also be given to including the dose per unit mass e.g. mg/kg or the dose per m^2 body-surface area e.g. mg/m^2 where this would reduce error.
The following should be noted:

- The strength or quantity to be contained in capsules, lozenges, tablets etc. should be stated by the prescriber. In particular, strength of liquid preparations should be clearly stated (e.g. 125 mg/5 mL).
- The unnecessary use of decimal points should be avoided, e.g. 3 mg, not 3.0 mg. Quantities of 1 gram or more should be written as 1 g etc. Quantities less than 1 gram should be written in milligrams, e.g. 500 mg, not 0.5 g. Quantities less than 1 mg should be written in micrograms, e.g. 100 micrograms, not 0.1 mg. When decimals are unavoidable a zero should be written in front of the decimal point where there is no other figure, e.g. 0.5 mL, not.5 mL. Use of the decimal point is acceptable to express a range, e.g. 0.5 to 1 g.
- 'Micrograms' and 'nanograms' should **not** be abbreviated. Similarly 'units' should **not** be abbreviated.
- The term 'millilitre' (ml or mL) is used in medicine and pharmacy, and cubic centimetre, c.c., or cm^3 should not be used. (The use of capital 'L' in mL is a printing convention throughout the BNF; both 'mL' and 'ml' are recognised SI abbreviations).
- Dose and dose frequency should be stated; in the case of preparations to be taken 'as required' a **minimum dose interval** should be specified. Care should be taken to ensure children receive the correct dose of the active drug. Therefore, the dose should normally be stated in terms of the mass of the active drug (e.g. '125 mg 3 times daily'); terms such as '5 mL' or '1 tablet' should be avoided except for compound preparations. When doses other than multiples of 5 mL are prescribed for *oral liquid preparations* the dose-volume will be provided by means of an **oral syringe**, (except for preparations intended to be measured with a pipette). Suitable quantities:
  - Elixirs, Linctuses, and Paediatric Mixtures (5-mL dose), 50, 100, or 150 mL
  - Adult Mixtures (10 mL dose), 200 or 300 mL
  - Ear Drops, Eye drops, and Nasal Drops, 10 mL (or the manufacturer's pack)
  - Eye Lotions, Gargles, and Mouthwashes, 200 mL
- The names of drugs and preparations should be written clearly and **not** abbreviated, using approved titles **only**; **avoid** creating generic titles for modified-release preparations.
- The quantity to be supplied may be stated by indicating the number of days of treatment required in the box provided on NHS forms. In most cases the exact amount will be supplied. This does not apply to items directed to be used as required—if the dose and frequency are not given then the quantity to be supplied needs to be stated. When several items are ordered on one form the box can be marked with the number of days of treatment provided the quantity is added for any item for which the amount cannot be calculated.
- Although directions should preferably be in **English without abbreviation**, it is recognised that some Latin abbreviations are used.

Sample prescription

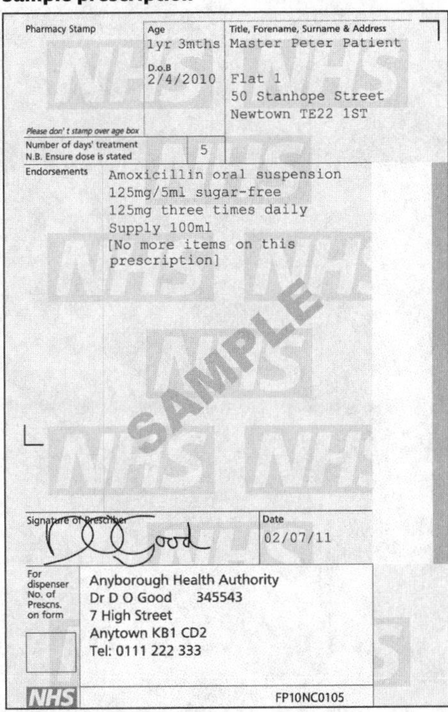

Pharmacy Stamp
Age: 1yr 3mths
D.o.B: 2/4/2010
Title, Forename, Surname & Address: Master Peter Patient, Flat 1, 50 Stanhope Street, Newtown TE22 1ST
Please don't stamp over age box
Number of days' treatment N.B. Ensure dose is stated: 5
Endorsements
Amoxicillin oral suspension
125mg/5ml sugar-free
125mg three times daily
Supply 100ml
[No more items on this prescription]
SAMPLE
Signature of Prescriber
Date: 02/07/11
For dispenser No. of Prescns. on form
Anyborough Health Authority
Dr D O Good 345543
7 High Street
Anytown KB1 CD2
Tel: 0111 222 333
NHS FP10NC0105

Abbreviation of titles In general, titles of drugs and preparations should be written *in full*. Unofficial abbreviations should **not** be used as they may be misinterpreted.

Non-proprietary titles Where non-proprietary ('generic') titles are given, they should be used for prescribing. This will enable any suitable product to be dispensed, thereby saving delay to the patient and sometimes expense to the health service. The only exception is where there is a demonstrable difference in clinical effect between each manufacturer's version of the formulation, making it important that the child should always receive the same brand; in such cases, the brand name or the manufacturer should be stated.

Non-proprietary names of compound preparations Non-proprietary names of **compound preparations** which appear in *BNF for Children* are those that have been compiled

by the British Pharmacopoeia Commission or another recognised body; whenever possible they reflect the names of the active ingredients. Prescribers should avoid creating their own compound names for the purposes of generic prescribing; such names do not have an approved definition and can be misinterpreted.
Special care should be taken to avoid errors when prescribing compound preparations; in particular the hyphen in the prefix 'co-' should be retained. Special care should also be taken to avoid creating generic names for **modified-release** preparations where the use of these names could lead to confusion between formulations with different duration of action.

Supply of medicines

Overview

When supplying a medicine for a child, the pharmacist should ensure that the child and the child's carer understand the nature and identity of the medicine and how it should be used. The child and the carer should be provided with appropriate information (e.g. how long the medicine should be taken for and what to do if a dose is missed or the child vomits soon after the dose is given).

Safety in the home

Carers and relatives of children must be warned to keep all medicines out of the reach and sight of children. Tablets, capsules and oral and external liquid preparations must be dispensed in a reclosable *child-resistant container* unless:

- the medicine is in an original pack or patient pack such as to make this inadvisable;
- the child's carer will have difficulty in opening a child-resistant container;
- a specific request is made that the product shall not be dispensed in a child-resistant container;
- no suitable child-resistant container exists for a particular liquid preparation.

All patients should be advised to dispose of *unwanted medicines* by returning them to a pharmacy for destruction.

Labelling of prescribed medicines

There is a legal requirement for the following to appear on the label of any prescribed medicine:

- name of the patient;
- name and address of the supplying pharmacy;
- date of dispensing;
- name of the medicine;
- directions for use of the medicine;
- precautions relating to the use of the medicine.

The Royal Pharmaceutical Society recommends that the following also appears on the label:

- the words 'Keep out of the sight and reach of children';
- where applicable, the words 'Use this medicine only on your skin'.

A pharmacist can exercise professional skill and judgement to amend or include more appropriate wording for the name of the medicine, the directions for use, or the precautions relating to the use of the medicine.

Unlicensed medicines

A drug or formulation that is not covered by a marketing authorisation may be obtained from a pharmaceutical company, imported by a specialist importer, manufactured by a commercial or hospital licensed manufacturing unit, or prepared extemporaneously against a prescription.
The safeguards that apply to products with marketing authorisation should be extended, as far as possible, to the use of unlicensed medicines. The safety, efficacy, and quality (including labelling) of unlicensed medicines should be assured by means of clear policies on their prescribing, purchase, supply, and administration. Extra care is required with unlicensed medicines because less information may be available on the drug and any formulation of the drug.
The following should be agreed with the supplier when ordering an unlicensed or extemporaneously prepared medicine:

- the specification of the formulation;
- documentation confirming the specification and quality of the product supplied (e.g. a certificate of conformity or of analysis);
- for imported preparations product and licensing information should be supplied in English.

Extemporaneous preparations

A product should be dispensed extemporaneously only when no product with a marketing authorisation is available. Every effort should be made to ensure that an extemporaneously prepared product is stable and that it delivers the requisite dose reliably; the child should be provided with a consistent formulation regardless of where the medicine is supplied to minimise variations in quality. Where there is doubt about the formulation, advice should be sought from a medicines information centre, the pharmacy at a children's hospital, a hospital production unit, a hospital quality control department, or the manufacturer.
In many cases it is preferable to give a licensed product by an unlicensed route (e.g. an injection solution given by mouth) than to prepare a special formulation. When tablets or capsules are cut, dispersed, or used for preparing liquids immediately before administration, it is important to confirm uniform dispersal of the active ingredient, especially if only a portion of the solid content (e.g. a tablet segment) is used or if only an aliquot of the liquid is to be administered.
In some cases the child's clinical condition may require a dose to be administered in the absence of full information on the method of administration. It is important to ensure that the appropriate supporting information is available at the earliest opportunity.
Preparation of products that produce harmful dust (e.g. cytotoxic drugs, hormones, or potentially sensitising drugs such as neomycin sulfate p. 743) should be **avoided** or undertaken with appropriate precautions to protect staff and carers.
The BP direction that a preparation must be *freshly prepared* indicates that it must be made not more than 24 hours before it is issued for use. The direction that a preparation should be *recently prepared* indicates that deterioration is likely if the preparation is stored for longer than about 4 weeks at 15–25°C.
The term **water** used without qualification means either potable water freshly drawn direct from the public supply and suitable for drinking or freshly boiled and cooled purified water. The latter should be used if the public supply is from a local storage tank or if the potable water is unsuitable for a particular preparation.

Emergency supply of medicines

Emergency supply requested by member of the public

Pharmacists are sometimes called upon by members of the public to make an emergency supply of medicines. The Human Medicines Regulations 2012 allows exemptions from the Prescription Only requirements for emergency supply to be made by a person lawfully conducting a retail pharmacy business provided:

a) that the pharmacist has interviewed the person requesting the prescription-only medicine and is satisfied:
   i) that there is immediate need for the prescription-only medicine and that it is impracticable in the circumstances to obtain a prescription without undue delay;
   ii) that treatment with the prescription-only medicine has on a previous occasion been prescribed for the person requesting it;
   iii) as to the dose that it would be appropriate for the person to take;
b) that no greater quantity shall be supplied than will provide 5 days' treatment of phenobarbital p. 232, *phenobarbital sodium*, or Controlled Drugs in Schedules 4 or 5 (doctors or dentists from the European Economic Area and Switzerland, or their patients, cannot request an emergency supply of Controlled Drugs in Schedules 1, 2, or 3, or drugs that do not have a UK marketing authorisation) or 30 days' treatment for other prescription-only medicines, except when the prescription-only medicine is:
   i) insulin, an ointment or cream, or a preparation for the relief of asthma in an aerosol dispenser when the smallest pack can be supplied;
   ii) an oral contraceptive when a full cycle may be supplied;
   iii) an antibiotic in liquid form for oral administration when the smallest quantity that will provide a full course of treatment can be supplied;
c) that an entry shall be made by the pharmacist in the prescription book stating:
   i) the date of supply;
   ii) the name, quantity and, where appropriate, the pharmaceutical form and strength;
   iii) the name and address of the patient;
   iv) the nature of the emergency;
d) that the container or package must be labelled to show:
   i) the date of supply;
   ii) the name, quantity and, where appropriate, the pharmaceutical form and strength;
   iii) the name of the patient;
   iv) the name and address of the pharmacy;
   v) the words 'Emergency supply';
   vi) the words 'Keep out of the reach of children' (or similar warning);
e) that the prescription-only medicine is not a substance specifically excluded from the emergency supply provision, and does not contain a Controlled Drug specified in Schedules 1, 2, or 3 to the Misuse of Drugs Regulations 2001 except for phenobarbital p. 232 or *phenobarbital sodium* for the treatment of epilepsy: for details see *Medicines, Ethics and Practice,* London, Pharmaceutical Press (always consult latest edition). Doctors or dentists from the European Economic Area and Switzerland, or their patients, cannot request an emergency supply of Controlled Drugs in Schedules 1, 2, or 3, or drugs that do not have a UK marketing authorisation.

Emergency supply requested by prescriber

Emergency supply of a prescription-only medicine may also be made at the request of a doctor, a dentist, a supplementary prescriber, a community practitioner nurse prescriber, a nurse, pharmacist, or optometrist independent prescriber, or a doctor or dentist from the European Economic Area or Switzerland, provided:

a) that the pharmacist is satisfied that the prescriber by reason of some emergency is unable to furnish a prescription immediately;
b) that the prescriber has undertaken to furnish a prescription within 72 hours;
c) that the medicine is supplied in accordance with the directions of the prescriber requesting it;
d) that the medicine is not a Controlled Drug specified in Schedules 1, 2, or 3 to the Misuse of Drugs Regulations 2001 except for phenobarbital p. 232 or *phenobarbital sodium* for the treatment of epilepsy: for details see *Medicines, Ethics and Practice,* London, Pharmaceutical Press (always consult latest edition); (Doctors or dentists from the European Economic Area and Switzerland, or their patients, cannot request an emergency supply of Controlled Drugs in Schedules 1, 2, or 3, or drugs that do not have a UK marketing authorisation).
e) that an entry shall be made in the prescription book stating:
   i) the date of supply;
   ii) the name, quantity and, where appropriate, the pharmaceutical form and strength;
   iii) the name and address of the practitioner requesting the emergency supply;
   iv) the name and address of the patient;
   v) the date on the prescription;
   vi) when the prescription is received the entry should be amended to include the date on which it is received.

Royal Pharmaceutical Society's guidelines

1. The pharmacist should consider the medical consequences of not supplying a medicine in an emergency.
2. If the pharmacist is unable to make an emergency supply of a medicine the pharmacist should advise the patient how to obtain essential medical care.

For conditions that apply to supplies made at the request of a patient see Medicines, Ethics and Practice, London Pharmaceutical Press, (always consult latest edition).

Controlled drugs and drug dependence

Regulations and classification

The Misuse of Drugs Act, 1971 as amended prohibits certain activities in relation to 'Controlled Drugs', in particular their manufacture, supply, and possession (except where permitted by the 2001 Regulations or under licence from the Secretary of State). The penalties applicable to offences involving the different drugs are graded broadly according to the *harmfulness attributable to a drug when it is misused* and for this purpose the drugs are defined in the following three classes:

- **Class A** includes: alfentanil p. 877, cocaine, diamorphine hydrochloride p. 294 (heroin), dipipanone hydrochloride, fentanyl p. 296, lysergide (LSD), methadone hydrochloride p. 317, 3, 4-methylenedioxymethamfetamine (MDMA, 'ecstasy'), morphine p. 299, opium, oxycodone hydrochloride p. 302, pethidine hydrochloride p. 304, phencyclidine, remifentanil p. 878, and class B substances when prepared for injection.
- **Class B** includes: oral amfetamines, barbiturates, cannabis, *Sativex*®, codeine phosphate p. 293, dihydrocodeine tartrate p. 295, ethylmorphine, glutethimide, ketamine p. 879, nabilone p. 277, pentazocine, phenmetrazine, and pholcodine p. 199.
- **Class C** includes: certain drugs related to the amfetamines such as benzfetamine and chlorphentermine, buprenorphine p. 291, mazindol, meprobamate, pemoline, pipradrol, most benzodiazepines, tramadol hydrochloride p. 305, zaleplon, zolpidem tartrate, zopiclone, androgenic and anabolic steroids, clenbuterol, chorionic gonadotrophin (HCG), non-human chorionic gonadotrophin, somatotropin, somatrem, somatropin p. 513, gabapentin p. 213, and pregabalin.

The Misuse of Drugs (Safe Custody) Regulations 1973 as amended details the storage and safe custody requirements for Controlled Drugs.

The Misuse of Drugs Regulations 2001 (and subsequent amendments) defines the classes of person who are authorised to supply and possess Controlled Drugs while acting in their professional capacities and lays down the conditions under which these activities may be carried out. In the 2001 regulations, drugs are divided into five Schedules, each specifying the requirements governing such activities as import, export, production, supply, possession, prescribing, and record keeping which apply to them.

- **Schedule 1** includes drugs not used medicinally such as hallucinogenic drugs (e.g. LSD), ecstasy-type substances, raw opium, and cannabis. A Home Office licence is generally required for their production, possession, or supply. A Controlled Drug register must be used to record details of any Schedule 1 Controlled Drugs received or supplied by a pharmacy.
- **Schedule 2** includes opiates (e.g. diamorphine hydrochloride p. 294 (heroin), morphine p. 299, methadone hydrochloride p. 317, oxycodone hydrochloride p. 302, pethidine hydrochloride p. 304), major stimulants (e.g. amfetamines), quinalbarbitone (secobarbital), cocaine, ketamine p. 879, and cannabis-based products for medicinal use in humans. Schedule 2 Controlled Drugs are subject to the full Controlled Drug requirements relating to prescriptions, safe custody (except for quinalbarbitone (secobarbital) and some liquid preparations), and the need to keep a Controlled Drug register, (unless exempted in Schedule 5). Possession, supply and procurement is authorised for pharmacists and other classes of persons named in the 2001 Regulations.
- **Schedule 3** includes the barbiturates (except secobarbital, now Schedule 2), buprenorphine p. 291, gabapentin p. 213, mazindol, meprobamate, midazolam p. 239, pentazocine, phentermine, pregabalin, temazepam p. 879, and tramadol hydrochloride p. 305. They are subject to the special prescription requirements. Safe custody requirements do apply, except for any 5,5 disubstituted barbituric acid (e.g. phenobarbital), gabapentin p. 213, mazindol, meprobamate, midazolam p. 239, pentazocine, phentermine, pregabalin, tramadol hydrochloride p. 305, or any stereoisomeric form or salts of the above. Records in registers do not need to be kept (although there are requirements for the retention of invoices for 2 years).
- **Schedule 4** includes in Part I drugs that are subject to minimal control, such as benzodiazepines (except temazepam p. 879 and midazolam p. 239, which are in Schedule 3), non-benzodiazepine hypnotics (zaleplon, zolpidem tartrate, and zopiclone) and *Sativex*®. Part II includes androgenic and anabolic steroids, clenbuterol, chorionic gonadotrophin (HCG), non-human chorionic gonadotrophin, somatotropin, somatrem, and somatropin p. 513. Controlled drug prescription requirements do not apply and Schedule 4 Controlled Drugs are not subject to safe custody requirements. Records in registers do not need to be kept (except in the case of *Sativex*®).
- **Schedule 5** includes preparations of certain Controlled Drugs (such as codeine, pholcodine p. 199 or morphine p. 299) which due to their low strength, are exempt from virtually all Controlled Drug requirements other than retention of invoices for two years.

Since the Responsible Pharmacist Regulations were published in 2008, standing operation procedures for the management of Controlled Drugs, are required in registered pharmacies.

The Health Act 2006 introduced the concept of the 'accountable officer' with responsibility for the management of Controlled Drugs and related governance issues in their organisation. Most recently, in 2013 The Controlled Drugs (Supervision of Management and Use) Regulations were published to ensure good governance concerning the safe management and use of Controlled Drugs in England and Scotland.

Prescriptions

Preparations in Schedules 1, 2, 3, 4 and 5 of the Misuse of Drugs Regulations 2001 (and subsequent amendments) are identified throughout the BNF and BNF *for children* using the following symbols:

CD1	for preparations in Schedule 1
CD2	for preparations in Schedule 2
CD3	for preparations in Schedule 3
CD4-1	for preparations in Schedule 4 (Part I)
CD4-2	for preparations in Schedule 4 (Part II)
CD5	for preparations in Schedule 5

The principal legal requirements relating to medical prescriptions are listed below (see also Department of Health Guidance at www.gov.uk/dh).

Prescription requirements Prescriptions for Controlled Drugs that are subject to prescription requirements (all preparations in Schedules 2 and 3) must be indelible, must be *signed* by the prescriber, include the *date* on which they were signed, and specify the prescriber's *address* (must be within the UK). A machine-written prescription is acceptable, but the prescriber's signature must be handwritten. Advanced electronic signatures can be accepted for Schedule 2 and 3 Controlled Drugs where the Electronic Prescribing Service (EPS) is used. All prescriptions for Controlled Drugs that are subject to the prescription requirements must always state:

- the name and address of the patient (use of a PO Box is not acceptable);
- in the case of a preparation, the form (the dosage form e.g. tablets must be included on a Controlled Drugs prescription irrespective of whether it is implicit in the proprietary name e.g. *MST Continus*, or whether only one form is available), and, where appropriate, the strength of the preparation (when more than one strength of a preparation exists the strength required must be specified); to avoid ambiguity, where a prescription requests multiple strengths of a medicine, each strength should be prescribed separately (i.e. separate dose, total quantity, etc);
- for liquids, the total volume in millilitres (in both words and figures) of the preparation to be supplied; for dosage units (tablets, capsules, ampoules), state the total number (in both words and figures) of dosage units to be supplied (e.g. 10 tablets [of 10 mg] rather than 100 mg total quantity);
- the dose, which must be clearly defined (i.e. the instruction 'one as directed' constitutes a dose but 'as directed' does not); it is not necessary that the dose is stated in both words and figures;
- the words 'for dental treatment only' if issued by a dentist.

A pharmacist is **not** allowed to dispense a Controlled Drug unless all the information required by law is given on the prescription. In the case of a prescription for a Controlled Drug in Schedule 2 or 3, a pharmacist can amend the prescription *if* it specifies the total quantity only in words or in figures or if it contains minor typographical errors, provided that such amendments are indelible and clearly attributable to the pharmacist (e.g. name, date, signature and GPhC registration number). The prescription should be marked with the date of supply at the time the Controlled Drug supply is made.

The Department of Health and the Scottish Government have issued a strong recommendation that the maximum quantity of Schedule 2, 3 or 4 Controlled Drugs prescribed should not exceed 30 days; exceptionally, to cover a justifiable clinical need and after consideration of any risk, a prescription can be issued for a longer period, but the reasons for the decision should be recorded on the patient's notes.

A prescription for a Controlled Drug in Schedules 2, 3, or 4 is valid for 28 days from the date stated thereon (the prescriber may forward-date the prescription; the start date may also be specified in the body of the prescription). Schedule 5 prescriptions are valid for 6 months from the appropriate date.

Medicines that are not Controlled Drugs should not be prescribed on the same form as a Schedule 2 or 3 Controlled Drug.

See sample prescription:

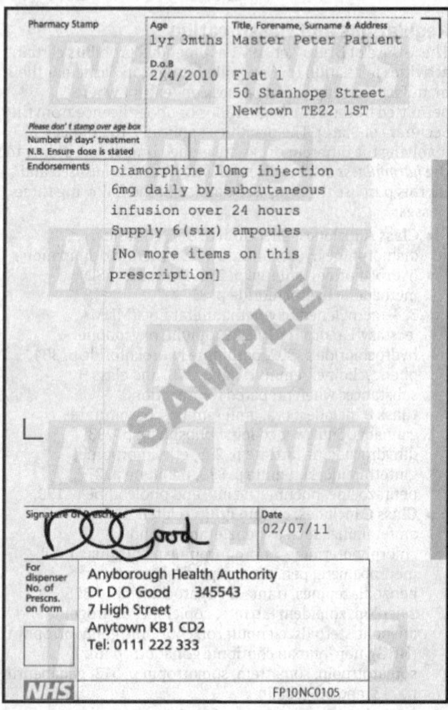
Pharmacy Stamp
Age: 1yr 3mths
D.o.B: 2/4/2010
Title, Forename, Surname & Address: Master Peter Patient, Flat 1, 50 Stanhope Street, Newtown TE22 1ST
Please don't stamp over age box
Number of days' treatment N.B. Ensure dose is stated
Endorsements
Diamorphine 10mg injection
6mg daily by subcutaneous
infusion over 24 hours
Supply 6(six) ampoules
[No more items on this
prescription]
SAMPLE
Signature of Prescriber
Date: 02/07/11
For dispenser No. of Prescns. on form
Anyborough Health Authority
Dr D O Good 345543
7 High Street
Anytown KB1 CD2
Tel: 0111 222 333
NHS
FP10NC0105

Instalments and repeatable prescriptions Prescriptions for Schedule 2 or 3 Controlled Drugs can be dispensed by instalments. An instalment prescription must have an instalment direction including both the dose and the instalment amount specified separately on the prescription, and it must also state the interval between each time the medicine can be supplied.

The first instalment must be dispensed within 28 days of the appropriate day (i.e. date of signing unless the prescriber indicates a date before which the Controlled Drug should not be dispensed) and the remainder should be dispensed in accordance with the instructions on the prescription. The prescription must be marked with the date of each supply.

The instalment direction is a legal requirement and needs to be complied with, however, for certain situations (e.g. if a pharmacy is closed on the day an instalment is due) the Home Office has approved specific wording which provides pharmacists some flexibility for supply. For details, see Medicines, Ethics and Practice, London, Pharmaceutical Press (always consult latest edition) or see Home Office approved wording for instalment prescribing (Circular 027/2015), available at www.gov.uk/.

Repeatable prescriptions are prescriptions which contain a direction that they can be dispensed more than once (e.g. repeat × 3). Only Schedule 4 and 5 Controlled Drugs are permitted on repeatable prescriptions.

Private prescriptions Private prescriptions for Controlled Drugs in Schedules 2 and 3 must be written on specially designated forms which are provided by local NHS England area teams in England (form FP10PCD), local NHS Health Boards in Scotland (form PPCD) and Wales (form W10PCD); in addition, prescriptions must specify the *prescriber's identification number* (or a NHS prescriber code in Scotland).

Prescriptions to be supplied by a pharmacist in hospital are exempt from the requirements for private prescriptions.

Dependence and misuse

The most common drugs of addiction are **crack cocaine** and **opioids**, particularly **diamorphine hydrochloride p. 294 (heroin)** . For arrangements for prescribing of diamorphine hydrochloride, dipipanone, or cocaine for addicts, see *Prescribing of diamorphine (heroin), dipipanone, and cocaine for addicts* below.

Along with traditional stimulants, such as amfetamine and cocaine, there has been an emerging use of methamphetamine and a range of psychoactive substances with stimulant, depressant or hallucinogenic properties such as lysergide (lysergic acid diethylamide, LSD), ketamine or gamma-hydroxybutyrate (sodium oxybate, GHB).

Benzodiazepines and z-drugs (i.e. zopiclone, zolpidem tartrate) have their own potential for misuse and dependence and are often taken in combination with opiates or stimulants.

Cannabis-based products for medicinal use are Schedule 2 Controlled Drugs and can be prescribed only by clinicians listed on the Specialist Register of the General Medical Council. Cannabis with no approved medicinal use is a Schedule 1 Controlled Drug and cannot be prescribed. It remains the most frequently used illicit drug by young people and dependence can develop in around 10% of users. Cannabis use can exacerbate depression and it may cause an acute short-lived toxic psychosis which resolves with cessation, however paranoid symptoms may persist in chronic users; withdrawal symptoms can occur in some users and these can contribute to sleep problems, agitation and risk of self-harm.

Supervised consumption

Supervised consumption is not a legal requirement under the 2001 Regulations. Nevertheless, when supervised consumption is directed on the prescription, the Department of Health recommends that any deviation from the prescriber's intended method of supply should be documented and the justification for this recorded.

Individuals prescribed opioid substitution therapy can take their daily dose under the supervision of a doctor, nurse, or pharmacist during the dose stabilisation phase (usually the first 3 months of treatment), after a relapse or period of instability, or if there is a significant increase in the dose of methadone. Supervised consumption should continue (in accordance with local protocols) until the prescriber is confident that the patient is compliant with their treatment. It is good practice for pharmacists to alert the prescriber when a patient has missed consecutive daily doses.

Prescribing drugs likely to cause dependence or misuse

The prescriber has three main responsibilities:

- To avoid creating dependence by introducing drugs to patients without sufficient reason. In this context, the proper use of the morphine-like drugs is well understood. The dangers of other Controlled Drugs are less clear because recognition of dependence is not easy and its effects, and those of withdrawal, are less obvious.
- To see that the patient does not gradually increase the dose of a drug, given for good medical reasons, to the point where dependence becomes more likely. This tendency is seen especially with hypnotics and anxiolytics. The prescriber should keep a close eye on the amount prescribed to prevent patients from accumulating stocks. A minimal amount should be prescribed in the first instance, or when seeing a patient for the first time.
- To avoid being used as an unwitting source of supply for addicts and being vigilant to methods for obtaining medicines. Methods include visiting more than one doctor, fabricating stories, and forging prescriptions.

Patients under temporary care should be given only small supplies of drugs unless they present an unequivocal letter from their own doctor. Doctors should also remember that their own patients may be attempting to collect prescriptions from other prescribers, especially in hospitals. It is sensible to reduce dosages steadily or to issue weekly or even daily prescriptions for small amounts if it is apparent that dependence is occurring.

Prescribers are responsible for the security of prescription forms once issued to them. The stealing and misuse of prescription forms could be minimised by the following precautions:

- records of serial numbers received and issued should be retained for at least three years;
- blank prescriptions should never be pre-signed;
- prescription forms should not be left unattended and should be locked in a secure drawer, cupboard, or carrying case when not in use;
- doctors', dentists' and surgery stamps should be kept in a secure location separate from the prescription forms;
- alterations are best avoided but if any are made and the prescription is to be used, best practice is for the prescriber to cross out the error, initial and date the error, then write the correct information;
- if an error made in a prescription cannot be corrected, best practice for the prescriber is to put a line through the script and write 'spoiled' on the form, or destroy the form and start writing a new prescription;
- prescribers and pharmacists dispensing drugs prone to abuse should ensure compliance with all relevant legal requirements specially when dealing with prescriptions for Controlled Drugs (see *Prescription requirements* and *Instalments* above);
- at the time of dispensing, prescriptions should be stamped with the pharmacy stamp and endorsed by the pharmacist or pharmacy technician with what has been supplied; where loss or theft is suspected, the police should be informed immediately.

Travelling abroad

Prescribed drugs listed in Schedule 4 Part II (CD Anab) for self-administration and Schedule 5 of the Misuse of Drugs Regulations 2001 (and subsequent amendments) are not subject to export or import licensing. A personal import/export licence is required for patients travelling abroad with Schedules 2, 3, or 4 Part I (CD Benz) and Part II (CD Anab) Controlled Drugs if, they are carrying more than 3 months' supply or are travelling for 3 calendar months or more. A Home Office licence is required for any amount of a Schedule 1 Controlled Drug imported into the UK for personal use regardless of the duration of travel. Further details can be obtained at www.gov.uk/guidance/controlled-drugs-licences-fees-and-returns or from the Home Office by contacting DFLU.ie@homeoffice.gsi.gov.uk. In cases of emergency, telephone (020) 7035 6330.

Applications for obtaining a licence must be supported by a cover letter signed by the prescribing doctor or drug worker, which must confirm:

- the patient's name and address;
- the travel itinerary;
- the names of the prescribed Controlled Drug(s), doses and total amounts to be carried.

Applications for licences should be sent to the Home Office, Drugs & Firearms Licensing Unit, Fry Building, 2 Marsham Street, London, SW1P 4DF.

Alternatively, completed application forms can be emailed to DFLU.ie@homeoffice.gsi.gov.uk. A minimum of 10 days should be allowed for processing the application.

Patients travelling for less than 3 months or carrying less than 3 months supply of Controlled Drugs do not require a personal export/import licence, but are advised to carry a cover letter signed by the prescribing doctor or drug worker. Those travelling for more than 3 months are advised to make arrangements to have their medication prescribed by a practitioner in the country they are visiting.

Doctors who want to take Controlled Drugs abroad while accompanying patients may similarly be issued with licences. Licences are not normally issued to doctors who want to take Controlled Drugs abroad solely in case a family emergency should arise.

Personal export/import licences do not have any legal status outside the UK and are issued only to comply with the Misuse of Drugs Act 2001 and to facilitate passage through UK Customs and Excise control. For clearance in the country to be visited it is necessary to approach that country's consulate in the UK.

Notification of patients receiving structured drug treatment for substance dependence

In **England**, doctors should report cases where they are providing structured drug treatment for substance dependence to their local National Drug Treatment Monitoring System (NDTMS) Team. General information about NDTMS can be found at www.gov.uk/government/collections/alcohol-and-drug-misuse-prevention-and-treatment-guidance.

Enquiries about NDTMS, and how to submit data, should initially be directed to:
EvidenceApplicationteam@phe.gov.uk

In **Scotland**, doctors should report cases to the Substance Drug Misuse Database. General information about the Scottish Drug Misuse Database can be found in www.isdscotland.org/Health-Topics/Drugs-and-Alcohol-Misuse/Drugs-Misuse/Scottish-Drug-Misuse-Database/. Enquiries about reporting can be directed to:
nss.isdsubstancemisuse@nhs.net

In **Northern Ireland**, the Misuse of Drugs (Notification of and Supply to Addicts) (Northern Ireland) Regulations 1973 require doctors to send particulars of persons whom they consider to be addicted to certain Controlled Drugs to the Chief Medical Officer of the Ministry of Health and Social Services. The Northern Ireland contact is:

Public Health Information & Research Branch
Department of Health
Annexe 2, Castle Buildings, Stormont, Belfast BT4 3SQ
028 9052 2340
phirb@health-ni.gov.uk

Public Health Information & Research Branch also maintains the Northern Ireland Drug Misuse Database (NIDMD) which collects detailed information on those presenting for treatment, on drugs misused and injecting behaviour; participation is not a statutory requirement.

In **Wales**, doctors should report cases where they are providing structured drug treatment for substance dependence on the Welsh National Database for Substance Misuse; enquiries should be directed to: substancemisuse-queries@wales.nhs.uk.

Prescribing of diamorphine (heroin), dipipanone, and cocaine for addicts

The Misuse of Drugs (Supply to Addicts) Regulations 1997 require that **only** medical practitioners who hold a special licence issued by the Home Secretary (or Scottish Government's Chief Medical Officer) may prescribe, administer, or supply diamorphine hydrochloride p. 294, dipipanone, or cocaine for *the treatment of drug addiction*. Medical prescribers, pharmacists independent prescribers, nurses independent prescribers and supplementary prescribers do not require a special licence for prescribing diamorphine hydrochloride p. 294, dipipanone, or cocaine for patients (including addicts) for relieving pain from organic disease or injury.

Adverse reactions to drugs

Yellow card scheme

Any drug may produce unwanted or unexpected adverse reactions. Rapid detection and recording of adverse drug reactions is of vital importance so that unrecognised hazards are identified promptly and appropriate regulatory action is taken to ensure that medicines are used safely. Healthcare professionals and coroners are urged to report suspected adverse drug reactions directly to the Medicines and Healthcare products Regulatory Agency (MHRA) through the Yellow Card Scheme using the electronic form at www.mhra.gov.uk/yellowcard. Alternatively, prepaid Yellow Cards for reporting are available from the address below and are also bound in the inside back cover of *BNF for Children*.

Send Yellow Cards to:

FREEPOST YELLOW CARD
(No other address details required).
Tel: 0800 731 6789

Suspected adverse drug reactions to any therapeutic agent should be reported, including drugs (*self-medication* as well as those *prescribed*), blood products, vaccines, radiographic contrast media, complementary and herbal products. For biosimilar medicines and vaccines, adverse reaction reports should clearly state the brand name and the batch number of the suspected medicine or vaccine.

Suspected adverse drug reactions should be reported through the Yellow Card Scheme at www.mhra.gov.uk/yellowcard. Yellow Cards can be used for reporting suspected adverse drug reactions to medicines, vaccines, herbal or complementary products, whether self-medicated or prescribed. This includes suspected adverse drug reactions associated with misuse, overdose, medication errors or from use of unlicensed and off-label medicines. Yellow Cards can also be used to report medical device incidents, defective medicines, and suspected fake medicines.

Report all suspected adverse drug reactions that are:

- **serious, medically significant or result in harm**. Serious events are fatal, life-threatening, a congenital abnormality, disabling or incapacitating, or resulting in hospitalisation;
- associated with **newer drugs and vaccines**; the most up to date list of black triangle medicines is available at:www.mhra.gov.uk/blacktriangle

If in doubt whether to report a suspected adverse drug reaction, please complete a Yellow Card.

The identification and reporting of adverse reactions to drugs in children and neonates is particularly important because:

- the action of the drug and its pharmacokinetics in children (especially in the very young) may be different from that in adults;
- drugs may not have been extensively tested in children;
- many drugs are not specifically licensed for use in children and are used either 'off-label' or as unlicensed products;
- drugs may affect the way a child grows and develops or may cause delayed adverse reactions which do not occur in adults;
- suitable formulations may not be available to allow precise dosing in children or they may contain excipients that should be used with caution in children;
- the nature and course of illnesses and adverse drug reactions may differ between adults and children.

Even if reported through the British Paediatric Surveillance Unit's Orange Card Scheme, any identified suspected adverse drug reactions should also be submitted to the Yellow Card Scheme.

Spontaneous reporting is particularly valuable for recognising possible new hazards rapidly. An adverse reaction should be reported even if it is not certain that the drug has caused it, or if the reaction is well recognised, or if other drugs have been given at the same time. Reports of overdoses (deliberate or accidental) can complicate the assessment of adverse drug reactions, but provide important information on the potential toxicity of drugs.

A freephone service is available to all parts of the UK for advice and information on suspected adverse drug reactions; contact the National Yellow Card Information Service at the MHRA on 0800 731 6789. Outside office hours a telephone-answering machine will take messages.

The following Yellow Card Centres can be contacted for further information:

Yellow Card Centre Northwest
2nd Floor, 70 Pembroke Place, Liverpool, L69 3GF
Tel: (0151) 794 8122

Yellow Card Centre Wales
All Wales Therapeutics and Toxicology Centre, Academic Building, University Hospital Llandough, Penlan Road, Penarth, Vale of Glamorgan, CF64 2XX
Tel: (029) 2074 5831

Yellow Card Centre Northern & Yorkshire
Regional Drug and Therapeutics Centre, 16/17 Framlington Place, Newcastle upon Tyne, NE2 4AB
Tel: (0191) 213 7855

Yellow Card Centre West Midlands
City Hospital, Dudley Road, Birmingham, B18 7QH
Tel: (0121) 507 5672

Yellow Card Centre Scotland
CARDS, Royal Infirmary of Edinburgh, 51 Little France Crescent, Old Dalkeith Road, Edinburgh, EH16 4SA
Tel: (0131) 242 2919
YCCScotland@luht.scot.nhs.uk

The MHRA's database facilitates the monitoring of adverse drug reactions. More detailed information on reporting and a list of products currently under additional monitoring can be found on the MHRA website: www.mhra.gov.uk.

MHRA Drug Safety Update *Drug Safety Update* is a monthly newsletter from the MHRA and the Commission on Human Medicines (CHM); it is available at www.gov.uk/drug-safety-update.

Self-reporting

Patients and their carers can also report suspected adverse drug reactions to the MHRA. Reports can be submitted directly to the MHRA through the Yellow Card Scheme using the electronic form at www.mhra.gov.uk/yellowcard, by telephone on 0808 100 3352, or by downloading the Yellow Card form from www.mhra.gov.uk. Alternatively, patient Yellow Cards are available from pharmacies and GP surgeries. Information for patients about the Yellow Card Scheme is available in other languages at www.mhra.gov.uk/yellowcard.

Prescription-event monitoring

In addition to the MHRA's Yellow Card Scheme, an independent scheme monitors the safety of new medicines using a different approach. The Drug Safety Research Unit identifies patients who have been prescribed selected new medicines and collects data on clinical events in these patients. The data are submitted on a voluntary basis by general practitioners on green forms. More information about the scheme and the Unit's educational material is available from www.dsru.org.

Newer drugs and vaccines

Only limited information is available from clinical trials on the safety of new medicines. Further understanding about the safety of medicines depends on the availability of information from routine clinical practice.
The black triangle symbol identifies newly licensed medicines that require additional monitoring by the European Medicines Agency. Such medicines include new active substances, biosimilar medicines, and medicines that the European Medicines Agency consider require additional monitoring. The black triangle symbol also appears in the Patient Information Leaflets for relevant medicines, with a brief explanation of what it means. Products usually retain a black triangle for 5 years, but this can be extended if required.

Medication errors

Adverse drug reactions where harm occurs as a result of a medication error are reportable as a Yellow Card or through the local risk management systems into the National Reporting and Learning System (NRLS). If reported to the NRLS, these will be shared with the MHRA. If the NRLS is not available and harm occurs, report using a Yellow Card.

Adverse reactions to medical devices

Suspected adverse reactions to medical devices including dental or surgical materials, intra-uterine devices, and contact lens fluids should be reported. Information on reporting these can be found at: www.mhra.gov.uk.

Side-effects in the *BNF for Children*

The *BNF for Children* includes clinically relevant side-effects for most drugs; an exhaustive list is not included for drugs that are used by specialists (e.g. cytotoxic drugs and drugs used in anaesthesia). Where causality has not been established, side-effects in the manufacturers' literature may be omitted from the *BNF for Children*.
Recognising that hypersensitivity reactions (including anaphylactic and anaphylactoid reactions) can occur with virtually all drugs, this effect is not generally listed, unless the drug carries an increased risk of such reactions or specific management advice is provided by the manufacturer.
Administration site reactions have been omitted from the *BNF for Children* (e.g. pain at injection site). The *BNF for Children* also omits effects that are likely to have little clinical consequence (e.g. transient increase in liver enzymes). Drugs that are applied locally or topically carry a theoretical or low risk of systemic absorption and therefore systemic side-effects for these drugs are not listed in the *BNF for Children* unless they are associated with a high risk to patient safety. Infections are a known complication of treatment with drugs that affect the immune system (e.g. corticosteroids or immunosuppressants); this side-effect is listed in the *BNF for Children* as 'increased risk of infection'. Symptoms of drug withdrawal reactions are not individually listed, but are collectively termed 'withdrawal syndrome'.

Description of the frequency of side-effects	
Very common	greater than 1 in 10
Common	1 in 100 to 1 in 10
Uncommon [formerly 'less commonly' in BNF publications]	1 in 1000 to 1 in 100
Rare	1 in 10 000 to 1 in 1000
Very rare	less than 1 in 10 000
Frequency not known	frequency is not defined by product literature or the side-effect has been reported from post-marketing surveillance data

For consistency, the terms used to describe side-effects are standardised using a defined vocabulary across all of the drug monographs in the *BNF for Children* (e.g. postural hypotension is used for the term orthostatic hypotension).

Special problems

Symptoms Children may be poor at expressing the symptoms of an adverse drug reaction and parental opinion may be required.

Delayed drug effects Some reactions (e.g. cancers and effects on development) may manifest months or years after exposure. Any suspicion of such an association should be reported directly to the MHRA through the Yellow Card Scheme.

Congenital abnormalities When an infant is born with a congenital abnormality or there is a malformed aborted fetus, doctors are asked to consider whether this might be an adverse reaction to a drug and to report all drugs (including self-medication) taken during pregnancy.

Prevention of adverse reactions

Adverse reactions may be prevented as follows:

- never use any drug unless there is a good indication. If the patient is pregnant do not use a drug unless the need for it is imperative;
- allergy and idiosyncrasy are important causes of adverse drug reactions. Ask if the child has had previous reactions to the drug or formulation;
- prescribe as few drugs as possible and give very clear instructions to the child, parent, or carer;
- whenever possible use a familiar drug; with a new drug be particularly alert for adverse reactions or unexpected events;
- consider if excipients (e.g. colouring agents) may be contributing to the adverse reaction. If the reaction is minor, a trial of an alternative formulation of the same drug may be considered before abandoning the drug;
- obtain a full drug history including asking if the child is already taking other drugs *including over-the-counter medicines*; interactions may occur;
- age and hepatic or renal disease may alter the metabolism or excretion of drugs, particularly in neonates, which can affect the potential for adverse effects. Genetic factors may also be responsible for variations in metabolism, and therefore for the adverse effects of the drug;
- warn the child, parent, or carer if serious adverse reactions are liable to occur.

Drug allergy (suspected or confirmed)

Suspected drug allergy is any reaction caused by a drug with clinical features compatible with an immunological mechanism. All drugs have the potential to cause adverse drug reactions, but not all of these are allergic in nature. A reaction is more likely to be caused by drug allergy if:

- The reaction occurred while the child was being treated with the drug, or
- The drug is known to cause this pattern of reaction, or
- The child has had a similar reaction to the same drug or drug-class previously.

A suspected reaction is less likely to be caused by a drug allergy if there is a possible non-drug cause or if there are only gastro-intestinal symptoms present.
The following signs, allergic patterns and timing of onset can be used to help decide whether to suspect drug allergy:
Immediate, rapidly-evolving reactions (onset usually less than 1 hour after drug exposure)

- Anaphylaxis, with erythema, urticaria or angioedema, and hypotension and/or bronchospasm. See also

Antihistamines, allergen immunotherapy and allergic emergencies p. 180
- Urticaria or angioedema without systemic features
- Exacerbation of asthma e.g. with non-steroidal anti-inflammatory drugs (NSAIDs)

*Non-immediate reactions, **without** systemic involvement* (onset usually 6–10 days after first drug exposure or 3 days after second exposure)
- Cutaneous reactions, e.g. widespread red macules and/or papules, or, fixed drug eruption (localised inflamed skin)

*Non-immediate reactions, **with** systemic involvement* (onset may be variable, usually 3 days to 6 weeks after first drug exposure, depending on features, or 3 days after second exposure)
- Cutaneous reactions with systemic features, e.g. drug reaction with eosinophilia and systemic signs (DRESS) or drug hypersensitivity syndrome (DHS), characterised by widespread red macules, papules or erythroderma, fever, lymphadenopathy, liver dysfunction or eosinophilia
- Toxic epidermal necrolysis or Stevens–Johnson syndrome
- Acute generalised exanthematous pustulosis (AGEP)

EvGr Suspected drug allergy information should be clearly and accurately documented in clinical notes and prescriptions, and shared among all healthcare professionals. Children and parents or carers should be given information about which drugs and drug-classes to avoid and encouraged to share the drug allergy status.
If a drug allergy is suspected, consider stopping the suspected drug and advising the child and parent or carer to avoid this drug in future. Symptoms of the acute reaction should be treated, in hospital if severe. Children presenting with a suspected anaphylactic reaction, or a severe or non-immediate cutaneous reaction, should be referred to a specialist drug allergy service. Children presenting with a suspected drug allergic reaction or anaphylaxis to NSAIDs, and local and general anaesthetics may also need to be referred to a specialist drug allergy service, e.g. in cases of anaphylactoid reactions or to determine future treatment options. Children presenting with a suspected drug allergic reaction or anaphylaxis associated with beta-lactam antibiotics should be referred to a specialist drug allergy service if their disease or condition can only be treated by a beta-lactam antibiotic or they are likely to need beta-lactam antibiotics frequently in the future (e.g. immunodeficient children). ⟨A⟩ For further information see Drug allergy: diagnosis and management. NICE Clinical Guideline 183 (September 2014) www.nice.org.uk/guidance/cg183.

Defective medicines

During the manufacture or distribution of a medicine an error or accident may occur whereby the finished product does not conform to its specification. While such a defect may impair the therapeutic effect of the product and could adversely affect the health of a patient, it should **not** be confused with an Adverse Drug Reaction where the product conforms to its specification.
The Defective Medicines Report Centre assists with the investigation of problems arising from licensed medicinal products thought to be defective and co-ordinates any necessary protective action. Reports on suspect defective medicinal products should include the brand or the non-proprietary name, the name of the manufacturer or supplier, the strength and dosage form of the product, the product licence number, the batch number or numbers of the product, the nature of the defect, and an account of any action already taken in consequence. The Centre can be contacted at:

The Defective Medicines Report Centre
Medicines and Healthcare products Regulatory Agency,
151 Buckingham Palace Road, London, SW1W 9SZ
Tel: (020) 3080 6574
dmrc@mhra.gsi.gov.uk

Guidance on intravenous infusions

Intravenous infusions for neonatal intensive care

Intravenous policy A local policy on the dilution of drugs with intravenous fluids should be drawn up by a multi-disciplinary team and issued as a document to the members of staff concerned.

Centralised additive services are provided in a number of hospital pharmacy departments and should be used in preference to making additions on wards.

The information that follows should be read in conjunction with local policy documents.

Guidelines

- Drugs should only be diluted with infusion fluid when constant plasma concentrations are needed or when the administration of a more concentrated solution would be harmful.
- In general, only one drug should be mixed with an infusion fluid in a syringe and the components should be compatible. Ready-prepared solutions should be used whenever possible. Drugs should not normally be added to blood products, mannitol, or sodium bicarbonate. Only specially formulated additives should be used with fat emulsions or amino-acid solutions.
- Solutions should be thoroughly mixed by shaking and checked for absence of particulate matter before use.
- Strict asepsis should be maintained throughout and in general the giving set should not be used for more than 24 hours (for drug admixtures).
- The infusion syringe should be labelled with the neonate's name and hospital number, the name and quantity of drug, the infusion fluid, and the expiry date and time. If a problem occurs during administration, containers should be retained for a period after use in case they are needed for investigation.
- Administration using a suitable motorised syringe driver is advocated for preparations where strict control over administration is required.
- It is good practice to examine intravenous infusions from time to time while they are running. If cloudiness, crystallisation, change of colour, or any other sign of interaction or contamination is observed the infusion should be discontinued.

Problems

Microbial contamination The accidental entry and subsequent growth of micro-organisms converts the infusion fluid pathway into a potential vehicle for infection with micro-organisms, particularly species of Candida, Enterobacter, and Klebsiella. Ready-prepared infusions containing the additional drugs, or infusions prepared by an additive service (when available) should therefore be used in preference to making extemporaneous additions to infusion containers on wards etc. However, when this is necessary strict aseptic procedure should be followed.

Incompatibility Physical and chemical incompatibilities may occur with loss of potency, increase in toxicity, or other adverse effect. The solutions may become opalescent or precipitation may occur, but in many instances there is no visual indication of incompatibility. Interaction may take place at any point in the infusion fluid pathway, and the potential for incompatibility is increased when more than one substance is added to the infusion fluid.

Common incompatibilities Precipitation reactions are numerous and varied and may occur as a result of pH, concentration changes, 'salting-out' effects, complexation or other chemical changes. Precipitation or other particle formation must be avoided since, apart from lack of control of dosage on administration, it may initiate or exacerbate adverse effects. This is particularly important in the case of drugs which have been implicated in either thrombophlebitis (e.g. diazepam) or in skin sloughing or necrosis caused by extravasation (e.g. sodium bicarbonate and parenteral nutrition). It is also especially important to effect solution of colloidal drugs and to prevent their subsequent precipitation in order to avoid a pyrogenic reaction (e.g. amphotericin).

It is considered undesirable to mix beta-lactam antibiotics, such as semi-synthetic penicillins and cephalosporins, with proteinaceous materials on the grounds that immunogenic and allergenic conjugates could be formed.

A number of preparations undergo significant loss of potency when added singly or in combination to large volume infusions. Examples include ampicillin in infusions that contain glucose or lactates.

Blood Because of the large number of incompatibilities, drugs should not be added to blood and blood products for infusion purposes. Examples of incompatibility with blood include hypertonic mannitol solutions (irreversible crenation of red cells), dextrans (rouleaux formation and interference with cross-matching), glucose (clumping of red cells), and oxytocin (inactivated).

If the giving set is not changed after the administration of blood, but used for other infusion fluids, a fibrin clot may form which, apart from blocking the set, increases the likelihood of microbial growth.

Intravenous fat emulsion These may break down with coalescence of fat globules and separation of phases when additions such as antibacterials or electrolytes are made, thus increasing the possibility of embolism. Only specially formulated products such as *Vitlipid N*® may be added to appropriate intravenous fat emulsions.

Other infusions Infusions that frequently give rise to incompatibility include amino acids, mannitol, and sodium bicarbonate.

Method

Ready-prepared infusions should be used whenever available. When dilution of drugs is required to be made extemporaneously, any product reconstitution instructions such as those relating to concentration, vehicle, mixing, and handling precautions should be strictly followed using an aseptic technique throughout. Once the product has been reconstituted, further dilution with the infusion fluid should be made immediately in order to minimise microbial contamination and, with certain products, to prevent degradation or other formulation change which may occur; e.g. reconstituted ampicillin injection degrades rapidly on standing, and also may form polymers which could cause sensitivity reactions.

It is also important in certain instances that an infusion fluid of specific pH be used (e.g. **furosemide** injection requires dilution in infusions of pH greater than 5.5).

When drug dilutions are made it is important to mix thoroughly; additions should not be made to an infusion container that has been connected to a giving set, as mixing is hampered. If the solutions are not thoroughly mixed, a concentrated layer of the drug may form owing to differences in density. **Potassium chloride** is particularly prone to this 'layering' effect when added without adequate mixing to infusions; if such a mixture is administered it may have a serious effect on the heart.

A time limit between dilution and completion of administration must be imposed for certain admixtures to

Prescribing in pregnancy

Overview

Drugs can have harmful effects on the embryo or fetus at any time during pregnancy. It is important to bear this in mind when prescribing for a woman of *childbearing age* or for men *trying* to *father* a child.

During the *first trimester* drugs can produce congenital malformations (teratogenesis), and the period of greatest risk is from the third to the eleventh week of pregnancy.

During the *second* and *third trimesters* drugs can affect the growth or functional development of the fetus, or they can have toxic effects on fetal tissues.

Drugs given shortly before term or during labour can have adverse effects on labour or on the neonate after delivery.

Not all the damaging effects of intra-uterine exposure to drugs are obvious at birth, some may only manifest later in life. Such late-onset effects include malignancy, e.g. adenocarcinoma of the vagina after puberty in females exposed to diethylstilbestrol in the womb, and adverse effects on intellectual, social, and functional development.

The BNF and *BNF for Children* identify drugs which:

- may have harmful effects in pregnancy and indicate the trimester of risk
- are not known to be harmful in pregnancy

The information is based on human data, but information from *animal* studies has been included for some drugs when its omission might be misleading. Maternal drug doses may require adjustment during pregnancy due to changes in maternal physiology but this is beyond the scope of the *BNF* and *BNF for Children.*

Where care is needed when prescribing in pregnancy, this is indicated under the relevant drug in the BNF and *BNF for Children.*

Important

Drugs should be prescribed in pregnancy only if the expected benefit to the mother is thought to be greater than the risk to the fetus, and all drugs should be avoided if possible during the first trimester. Drugs which have been extensively used in pregnancy and appear to be usually safe should be prescribed in preference to new or untried drugs; and the smallest effective dose should be used. Few drugs have been shown conclusively to be teratogenic in humans, but no drug is safe beyond all doubt in early pregnancy. Screening procedures are available when there is a known risk of certain defects.

Absence of information does not imply safety. It should be noted that the BNF and *BNF for Children* provide independent advice and may not always agree with the product literature.

Information on drugs and pregnancy is also available from the UK Teratology Information Service. www.uktis.org
Tel: 0344 892 0909 (09.00–17:00 Monday to Friday; urgent enquiries only outside these hours).

MHRA/CHM advice: Medicines with teratogenic potential: what is effective contraception and how often is pregnancy testing needed? (March 2019)

Guidance is available on contraceptive methods and frequency of pregnancy testing to reduce inadvertent exposures during pregnancy in a woman taking a medicine of teratogenic potential. When using these medicines, a woman should be advised of the risks and encouraged to use the most effective contraceptive method taking into account her personal circumstances. The likelihood of pregnancy should be assessed before each prescription of a medicine with known teratogenic potential, by performing a pregnancy test if required. If pregnancy cannot be excluded, the decision to start or continue treatment will depend on individual circumstances, such as the urgency for treatment and alternative treatment options. If feasible, treatment with a medicine with teratogenic potential should be delayed until pregnancy has been excluded by a repeat test.

Information on pregnancy testing and contraception for pregnancy prevention during treatment with medicines of teratogenic potential is available at: www.gov.uk/drug-safety-update/medicines-with-teratogenic-potential-what-is-effective-contraception-and-how-often-is-pregnancy-testing-needed#download-print-and-use-new-table

Prescribing in breast-feeding

Overview

Breast-feeding is beneficial; the immunological and nutritional value of breast milk to the infant is greater than that of formula feeds.

Although there is concern that drugs taken by the mother might affect the infant, there is very little information on this. In the absence of evidence of an effect, the potential for harm to the infant can be inferred from:

- the amount of drug or active metabolite of the drug delivered to the infant (dependent on the pharmacokinetic characteristics of the drug in the mother);
- the efficiency of absorption, distribution, and elimination of the drug by the infant (infant pharmacokinetics);
- the nature of the effect of the drug on the infant (pharmacodynamic properties of the drug in the infant).

Most medicines given to a mother cause no harm to breast-fed infants and there are few contra-indications to breast-feeding when maternal medicines are necessary. However, administration of some drugs to nursing mothers can harm the infant. In the first week of life, some such as preterm or jaundiced infants are at a slightly higher risk of toxicity.

Toxicity to the infant can occur if the drug enters the milk in pharmacologically significant quantities. The concentration in milk of some drugs (e.g. fluvastatin p. 139) may exceed the concentration in maternal plasma so that therapeutic doses in the mother can cause toxicity to the infant. Some drugs inhibit the infant's sucking reflex (e.g. phenobarbital p. 232) while others can affect lactation (e.g. bromocriptine). Drugs in breast milk may, at least theoretically, cause hypersensitivity in the infant even when concentration is too low for a pharmacological effect. *BNF for Children* identifies drugs:

- which should be used with caution or which are contra-indicated in breast-feeding for the reasons given above;
- which, on present evidence, may be given to the mother during breast-feeding, because they appear in milk in amounts which are too small to be harmful to the infant;

- which are not known to be harmful to the infant although they are present in milk in significant amounts.

Where care is needed when prescribing in breast-feeding, this is indicated under the relevant drug in the *BNF for Children*.

Important

For many drugs insufficient evidence is available to provide guidance and it is advisable to administer only essential drugs to a mother during breast-feeding. Because of the inadequacy of information on drugs in breast-feeding, absence of information does not imply safety.

Prescribing in palliative care

Overview

Palliative care is the active and total approach to the care of children and young adults with life-limiting and life-threatening conditions, embracing physical, emotional, social, and spiritual elements of their care. It focuses on enhancing the quality of life for the child and support for their family, and includes the management of distressing symptoms, provision of respite, and care following death and bereavement.

Effective palliative care requires a broad multidisciplinary approach that includes the whole family, and ideally should start as soon as possible after diagnosis or recognition of a life-threatening condition.

Drug treatment The number of drugs should be as few as possible. Oral medication is usually appropriate unless there is severe nausea and vomiting, dysphagia, weakness, or coma, when parenteral medication may be necessary.

For further information on the use of medicines in paediatric palliative care, see the Association for Paediatric Palliative Medicine (APPM) Master Formulary available at www.appm.org.uk/10.html.

Pain

Pain management in palliative care is focused on achieving control of pain by administering the right drug in the right dose at the right time. Analgesics can be divided into three broad classes: non-opioid (paracetamol p. 288, NSAID), opioid (e.g. codeine phosphate p. 293 'weak', morphine p. 299 'strong') and adjuvant (e.g. antidepressants, antiepileptics). Drugs from the different classes are used alone or in combination according to the type of pain and response to treatment. Analgesics are more effective in preventing pain than in the relief of established pain; it is important that they are given regularly.

Paracetamol p. 288 or a NSAID given regularly will often be sufficient to manage mild pain. If non-opioid analgesics alone are not sufficient, then an opioid analgesic alone or in combination with a non-opioid analgesic at an adequate dosage, may be helpful in the control of moderate pain. Codeine phosphate p. 293 or tramadol hydrochloride p. 305 can be considered for moderate pain. If these preparations do not control the pain then morphine is the most useful opioid analgesic. Alternatives to morphine, including transdermal buprenorphine p. 291, transdermal fentanyl p. 296, hydromorphone hydrochloride p. 299, methadone hydrochloride p. 317, or oxycodone hydrochloride p. 302, should be initiated by those with experience in palliative care. Initiation of an opioid analgesic should not be delayed by concern over a theoretical likelihood of psychological dependence (addiction).

Bone metastases In addition to the above approach, radiotherapy and bisphosphonates may be useful for pain due to bone metastases.

Neuropathic pain Patients with neuropathic pain may benefit from a trial of a tricyclic antidepressant, most commonly amitriptyline hydrochloride p. 255, for several weeks. An antiepileptic such as carbamazepine p. 209, may be added or substituted if pain persists. Ketamine p. 879 is sometimes used under specialist supervision for neuropathic pain that responds poorly to opioid analgesics. Pain due to nerve compression may be reduced by a corticosteroid such as dexamethasone p. 475, which reduces oedema around the tumour, thus reducing compression. Nerve blocks can be considered when pain is localised to a specific area. Transcutaneous electrical nerve stimulation (TENS) may also help.

Pain management with opioids

Oral route Treatment with morphine p. 299 is given by mouth as immediate-release or modified-release preparations. During the titration phase the initial dose is based on the previous medication used, the severity of the pain, and other factors such as presence of renal impairment or frailty. The dose is given either as an immediate-release preparation 4-hourly (for starting doses, see Morphine), or as a 12-hourly modified-release preparation, in addition to rescue doses. If replacing a weaker opioid analgesic (such as codeine phosphate p. 293), starting doses are usually higher.

If pain occurs between regular doses of morphine ('breakthrough pain'), an additional dose ('rescue dose') of immediate-release morphine should be given. An additional dose should also be given 30 minutes before an activity that causes pain, such as wound dressing. The standard dose of a strong opioid for breakthrough pain is usually one-tenth to one-sixth of the regular 24-hour dose, repeated every 2–4 hours as required (up to hourly may be needed if pain is severe or in the last days of life). Review pain management if rescue analgesic is required frequently (twice daily or more). Each child should be assessed on an individual basis.

Formulations of fentanyl p. 296 that are administered nasally, buccally or sublingually are not licensed for use in children; their usefulness in children is also limited by dose availability.

Children often require a higher dose of morphine in proportion to their body-weight compared to adults.

Children are more susceptible to certain adverse effects of opioids such as urinary retention (which can be eased by bethanechol chloride), and opioid-induced pruritus.

When adjusting the dose of morphine, the number of rescue doses required and the response to them should be taken into account; increments of morphine should not exceed one-third to one-half of the total daily dose every 24 hours. Thereafter, the dose should be adjusted with careful assessment of the pain, and the use of adjuvant analgesics should also be considered. Upward titration of the dose of morphine stops when either the pain is relieved or unacceptable adverse effects occur, after which it is necessary to consider alternative measures.

Once their pain is controlled, children started on 4-hourly immediate-release morphine can be transferred to the same total 24-hour dose of morphine given as the modified-release preparation for 12-hourly or 24-hourly administration. The first dose of the modified-release preparation is given with, or within 4 hours of the last dose of the immediate-release preparation. For preparations suitable for 12-hourly or 24-hourly administration see modified-release preparations under morphine. Increments should be made to the dose, not to the frequency of administration. The patient must be monitored closely for efficacy and side-effects, particularly constipation, and nausea and vomiting. A suitable laxative should be prescribed routinely.

Oxycodone hydrochloride p. 302 can be used in children who require an opioid but cannot tolerate morphine. If the child is already receiving an opioid, oxycodone hydrochloride should be started at a dose equivalent to the current analgesic. Oxycodone hydrochloride immediate-release preparations can be given for breakthrough pain.

Equivalent doses of opioid analgesics

This table is only an **approximate** guide (doses may not correspond with those given in clinical practice); children should be carefully monitored after any change in medication and dose titration may be required.

Analgesic/Route	Dose
Codeine: PO	100 mg
Diamorphine: IM, IV, SC	3 mg
Dihydrocodeine: PO	100 mg
Hydromorphone: PO	2 mg
Morphine: PO	10 mg
Morphine: IM, IV, SC	5 mg
Oxycodone: PO	6.6 mg
Tramadol: PO	100 mg

PO = by mouth; IM = intramuscular; IV = intravenous; SC = subcutaneous

Parenteral route Diamorphine hydrochloride p. 294 is preferred for injection because, being more soluble, it can be given in a smaller volume. The equivalent subcutaneous dose is approximately a third of the oral dose of morphine p. 299. Subcutaneous infusion of diamorphine hydrochloride via a continuous infusion device can be useful (for details, see Continuous Subcutaneous Infusions).
If the child can resume taking medicines by mouth, then oral morphine may be substituted for subcutaneous infusion of diamorphine hydrochloride. See the table *Approximate Equivalent doses of Morphine and Diamorphine*.

Rectal route Morphine p. 299 is also available for rectal administration as suppositories.

Transdermal route Transdermal preparations of fentanyl p. 296 and buprenorphine p. 291 [not licensed for use in children] are available; they are not suitable for acute pain or in those children whose analgesic requirements are changing rapidly because the long time to steady state prevents rapid titration of the dose. Prescribers should ensure that they are familiar with the correct use of transdermal preparations (see under fentanyl p. 296) because inappropriate use has caused fatalities.
The following 24-hour oral doses of morphine p. 299 are considered to be *approximately* equivalent to the buprenorphine and fentanyl p. 296 patches shown, however when switching due to possible opioid-induced hyperalgesia, reduce the calculated equivalent dose of the new opioid by one-quarter to one-half.

Buprenorphine patches are *approximately* equivalent to the following 24-hour doses of oral morphine

morphine salt 12 mg daily	≡ buprenorphine '5' patch
morphine salt 24 mg daily	≡ buprenorphine '10' patch
morphine salt 36 mg daily	≡ buprenorphine '15' patch
morphine salt 48 mg daily	≡ buprenorphine '20' patch
morphine salt 84 mg daily	≡ buprenorphine '35' patch
morphine salt 126 mg daily	≡ buprenorphine '52.5' patch
morphine salt 168 mg daily	≡ buprenorphine '70' patch

Formulations of transdermal patches are available as 72-hourly, 96-hourly and 7-day patches, for further information see buprenorphine in BNF. Conversion ratios vary and these figures are a guide only. Morphine equivalences for transdermal opioid preparations have been approximated to allow comparison with available preparations of oral morphine.

72-hour Fentanyl patches are *approximately* equivalent to the following 24-hour doses of oral morphine

morphine salt 30 mg daily	≡ fentanyl '12' patch
morphine salt 60 mg daily	≡ fentanyl '25' patch
morphine salt 120 mg daily	≡ fentanyl '50' patch
morphine salt 180 mg daily	≡ fentanyl '75' patch
morphine salt 240 mg daily	≡ fentanyl '100' patch

Fentanyl equivalences in this table are for children on well-tolerated opioid therapy for long periods; fentanyl patches should not be used in opioid naive children. Conversion ratios vary and these figures are a guide only. Morphine equivalences for transdermal opioid preparations have been approximated to allow comparison with available preparations of oral morphine.

Symptom control

Unlicensed indications or routes Several recommendations in this section involve unlicensed indications or routes.

Anorexia Anorexia may be helped by prednisolone p. 478 or dexamethasone p. 475.

Anxiety Anxiety can be treated with a long-acting benzodiazepine such as diazepam p. 236, or by continuous infusion of the short-acting benzodiazepine midazolam p. 239. Interventions for more acute episodes of anxiety (such as panic attacks) include short-acting benzodiazepines such as lorazepam p. 238 given sublingually or midazolam given subcutaneously. Temazepam p. 879 provides useful night-time sedation in some children.

Capillary bleeding Capillary bleeding can be treated with tranexamic acid p. 87 by mouth; treatment is usually continued for one week after the bleeding has stopped but it can be continued at a reduced dose if bleeding persists. Alternatively, gauze soaked in tranexamic acid 100 mg/mL p. 87 or adrenaline/epinephrine solution 1 mg/mL (1 in 1000) p. 143 can be applied to the affected area.
Vitamin K may be useful for the treatment and prevention of bleeding associated with prolonged clotting in liver disease. In severe chronic cholestasis, absorption of vitamin K may be impaired; either parenteral or water-soluble oral vitamin K should be considered.

Constipation Constipation is a common cause of distress and is almost invariable after administration of an opioid analgesic. It should be prevented if possible by the regular administration of laxatives. Suitable laxatives include osmotic laxatives (such as lactulose p. 46 or macrogols), stimulant laxatives (such as co-danthramer p. 50 and senna p. 52) or the combination of lactulose and a senna preparation. Naloxone hydrochloride p. 901 given by mouth may help relieve opioid-induced constipation; it is poorly absorbed but opioid withdrawal reactions have been reported.

Convulsions Intractable seizures are relatively common in children dying from non-malignant conditions. Phenobarbital p. 232 by mouth or as a continuous subcutaneous infusion may be beneficial; continuous infusion of midazolam p. 239 is an alternative. Both cause drowsiness, but this is rarely a concern in the context of intractable seizures. For breakthrough convulsions diazepam p. 236 given rectally (as a solution), buccal midazolam p. 239, or paraldehyde p. 237 as an enema may be appropriate.
See *Continuous subcutaneous infusions*, below, for the use of midazolam by subcutaneous infusion using a continuous infusion device.

Dry mouth Dry mouth may be caused by certain medications including opioid analgesics, antimuscarinic drugs (e.g. hyoscine), antidepressants and some antiemetics;

if possible, an alternative preparation should be considered. Dry mouth may be relieved by good mouth care and measures such as chewing sugar-free gum, sucking ice or pineapple chunks, or the use of artificial saliva. Dry mouth associated with candidiasis can be treated by oral preparations of nystatin p. 763 or miconazole p. 762, alternatively, fluconazole p. 407 can be given by mouth.

Dysphagia A corticosteroid such as dexamethasone p. 475 may help, temporarily, if there is an obstruction due to tumour. See also *Dry mouth*, above.

Dyspnoea Breathlessness at rest may be relieved by regular oral morphine p. 299 in carefully titrated doses. Diazepam p. 236 may be helpful for dyspnoea associated with anxiety. Sublingual lorazepam p. 238 or subcutaneous or buccal midazolam p. 239 are alternatives. A nebulised short-acting beta$_2$ agonist or a corticosteroid, such as dexamethasone p. 475 or prednisolone p. 478, may also be helpful for bronchospasm or partial obstruction.

Excessive respiratory secretion Excessive respiratory secretion (death rattle) may be reduced by hyoscine hydrobromide patches p. 283 or by subcutaneous or intravenous injection of hyoscine hydrobromide p. 283, however, care must be taken to avoid the discomfort of dry mouth. Alternatively, glycopyrronium bromide p. 803 may be given.
Hyoscine hydrobromide p. 283 can be administered by subcutaneous or intravenous infusion using a continuous infusion device.

Fungating tumours Fungating tumours can be treated by regular dressing and antibacterial drugs; systemic treatment with metronidazole p. 358 is often required to reduce malodour, but topical metronidazole is also used.

Gastro-intestinal pain The pain of bowel colic may be reduced by loperamide hydrochloride p. 54. Hyoscine hydrobromide p. 283 may also be helpful in reducing the frequency of spasms; it is given sublingually as *Kwells*® tablets and also by subcutanous infusion.
Gastric distension pain due to pressure on the stomach may be helped by a preparation incorporating an antacid with an antiflatulent and a prokinetic such as domperidone before meals.

Hiccup Hiccup due to gastric distension may be helped by a preparation incorporating an antacid with an antiflatulent.

Insomnia Children with advanced cancer may not sleep because of discomfort, cramps, night sweats, joint stiffness, or fear. There should be appropriate treatment of these problems before hypnotics are used. Benzodiazepines, such as temazepam p. 879, may be useful.

Intractable cough Intractable cough may be relieved by moist inhalations or by regular administration of oral morphine p. 299 every 4 hours. Methadone hydrochloride linctus p. 317 should be avoided because it has a long duration of action and tends to accumulate.

Mucosal bleeding Mucosal bleeding from the mouth and nose occurs commonly in the terminal phase, particularly in a child suffering from haemopoeitic malignancy. Bleeding from the nose caused by a single bleeding point can be arrested by cauterisation or by dressing it. Tranexamic acid p. 87 may be effective applied topically or given systemically.

Muscle spasm The pain of muscle spasm can be helped by a muscle relaxant such as diazepam p. 236 or baclofen p. 701.

Nausea and vomiting Nausea and vomiting are common in children with advanced cancer. Ideally, the cause should be determined before treatment with an antiemetic is started. Nausea and vomiting with opioid therapy are less common in children than in adults but may occur particularly in the initial stages and can be prevented by giving an antiemetic. An antiemetic is usually necessary only for the first 4 or 5 days and therefore combined preparations containing an opioid with an antiemetic are not recommended because they lead to unnecessary antiemetic therapy (and associated side-effects when used long-term).
Metoclopramide hydrochloride p. 278 has a prokinetic action and is used by mouth for nausea and vomiting associated with gastritis, gastric stasis, and functional bowel obstruction. Drugs with antimuscarinic effects antagonise prokinetic drugs and, if possible, should not therefore be used concurrently.
Haloperidol p. 261 is used by mouth or by continuous intravenous or subcutaneous infusion for most metabolic causes of vomiting (e.g. hypercalcaemia, renal failure).
Cyclizine p. 276 is used for nausea and vomiting due to mechanical bowel obstruction, raised intracranial pressure, and motion sickness.
Ondansetron p. 281 is most effective when the vomiting is due to damaged or irritated gut mucosa (e.g. after chemotherapy or radiotherapy).
Antiemetic therapy should be reviewed every 24 hours; it may be necessary to substitute the antiemetic or to add another one.
Levomepromazine p. 285 can be used if first-line antiemetics are inadequate. Dexamethasone by mouth p. 475 can be used as an adjunct.
See *Continuous subcutaneous infusions*, below, for the administration of antiemetics by subcutaneous infusion using a continuous infusion device.

Pruritus Pruritus, even when associated with obstructive jaundice, often responds to simple measures such as application of emollients. Ondansetron p. 281 may be effective in some children. Where opioid analgesics cause pruritus it may be appropriate to review the dose or to switch to an alternative opioid analgesic. In the case of obstructive jaundice, further measures include administration of colestyramine p. 136.

Raised intracranial pressure Headache due to raised intracranial pressure often responds to a high dose of a corticosteroid, such as dexamethasone p. 475, for 4 to 5 days, subsequently reduced if possible; dexamethasone should be given before 6 p.m. to reduce the risk of insomnia.
Treatment of headache and of associated nausea and vomiting should also be considered.

Restlessness and confusion Restlessness and confusion may require treatment with haloperidol p. 261.
Levomepromazine p. 285 is also used occasionally for restlessness.

Continuous subcutaneous infusions

Although drugs can usually be administered *by mouth* to control symptoms in palliative care, the parenteral route may sometimes be necessary. Repeated administration of *intramuscular injections* should be avoided in children, particularly if cachectic. This has led to the use of portable continuous infusion devices such as syringe drivers to give a *continuous subcutaneous infusion*, which can provide good control of symptoms with little discomfort or inconvenience to the patient.
Indications for the **parenteral route** are:

- inability to take medicines by mouth owing to *nausea and vomiting*, *dysphagia*, *severe weakness*, or *coma*;
- *malignant bowel obstruction* for which surgery is inappropriate (avoiding the need for an intravenous infusion or for insertion of a nasogastric tube);
- refusal by the child to take regular medication by mouth.

Syringe driver rate settings Staff using syringe drivers should be **adequately trained** and different rate settings should be **clearly identified** and **differentiated**; incorrect use of syringe drivers is a common cause of medication errors.

Bowel colic and excessive respiratory secretions Hyoscine hydrobromide p. 283 effectively reduces respiratory secretions and is sedative (but occasionally causes paradoxical agitation); it is given in a *subcutaneous* or *intravenous infusion*. Glycopyrronium bromide p. 803 may also be used.
Hyoscine butylbromide p. 67 is effective in bowel colic, is less sedative than hyoscine hydrobromide p. 283, but is not always adequate for the control of respiratory secretions; it is given by *subcutaneous infusion* (**important**: *hyoscine butylbromide p.* 67 must not be confused with *hyoscine hydrobromide p.* 283, above).

Confusion and restlessness Haloperidol p. 261 has little sedative effect. Levomepromazine p. 285 has a sedative effect. Midazolam p. 239 is a sedative and an antiepileptic that may be suitable for a very restless patient.

Convulsions If a child has previously been receiving an antiepileptic drug *or* has a primary or secondary cerebral tumour *or* is at risk of convulsion (e.g. owing to uraemia) antiepileptic medication should not be stopped. Midazolam p. 239 is the benzodiazepine antiepileptic of choice for *continuous subcutaneous infusion*.

Nausea and vomiting Levomepromazine p. 285 causes sedation in about 50% of patients. Haloperidol p. 261 has little sedative effect.
Cyclizine p. 276 is particularly likely to precipitate if mixed with diamorphine hydrochloride p. 294 or other drugs (see under *Mixing and compatibility*); it is given by *subcutaneous infusion*.

Pain control Diamorphine hydrochloride p. 294 is the preferred opioid since its high solubility permits a large dose to be given in a small volume (see under *Mixing and compatibility*). The table shows approximate equivalent doses of morphine p. 299 and diamorphine hydrochloride.

Mixing and compatibility The general principle that injections should be given into separate sites (and should not be mixed) does not apply to the use of syringe drivers in palliative care. Provided that there is evidence of compatibility, selected injections can be mixed in syringe drivers. Not all types of medication can be used in a subcutaneous infusion. In particular, chlorpromazine hydrochloride p. 261, prochlorperazine p. 285, and diazepam p. 236 are **contra-indicated** as they cause skin reactions at the injection site; to a lesser extent cyclizine p. 276 and levomepromazine p. 285 also sometimes cause local irritation.
In theory injections dissolved in water for injections are more likely to be associated with pain (possibly owing to their hypotonicity). The use of physiological saline (sodium chloride 0.9% p. 636) however increases the likelihood of precipitation when more than one drug is used; moreover subcutaneous infusion rates are so slow (0.1–0.3 mL/hour) that pain is not usually a problem when water is used as a diluent.

Compatibility with diamorphine Diamorphine can be given by *subcutaneous infusion* in a strength of up to 250 mg/mL; up to a strength of 40 mg/mL either *water for injections* or *physiological saline* (sodium chloride 0.9%) is a suitable diluent—above that strength only *water for injections* is used (to avoid precipitation).
The following can be mixed with *diamorphine*:

- **Cyclizine**, may precipitate at concentrations above 10 mg/mL *or* in the presence of sodium chloride 0.9% *or* as the concentration of diamorphine relative to cyclizine increases; mixtures of diamorphine and cyclizine are also likely to precipitate after 24 hours.
- **Dexamethasone**, special care is needed to avoid precipitation of dexamethasone when preparing it.
- **Haloperidol**, mixtures of haloperidol and diamorphine are likely to precipitate after 24 hours if haloperidol concentration is above 2 mg/mL.
- **Hyoscine butylbromide**
- **Hyoscine hydrobromide**
- **Levomepromazine**
- **Metoclopramide**, under some conditions infusions containing metoclopramide become discoloured; such solutions should be discarded.
- **Midazolam**

Subcutaneous infusion solution should be monitored regularly both to check for precipitation (and discolouration) and to ensure that the infusion is running at the correct rate.

Problems encountered with syringe drivers The following are problems that may be encountered with syringe drivers and the action that should be taken:

- if the subcutaneous infusion runs *too quickly* check the rate setting and the calculation;
- if the subcutaneous infusion runs *too slowly* check the start button, the battery, the syringe driver, the cannula, and make sure that the injection site is not inflamed;
- if there is an *injection site reaction* make sure that the site does not need to be changed—firmness or swelling at the site of injection is not in itself an indication for change, but pain or obvious inflammation is.

Equivalent doses of morphine sulfate and diamorphine hydrochloride given over 24 hours

These equivalences are *approximate only* and should be adjusted according to response

ORAL MORPHINE	PARENTERAL MORPHINE	PARENTERAL DIAMORPHINE
Oral morphine sulfate over 24 hours	Subcutaneous infusion of morphine sulfate over 24 hours	Subcutaneous infusion of diamorphine hydrochloride over 24 hours
30 mg	15 mg	10 mg
60 mg	30 mg	20 mg
90 mg	45 mg	30 mg
120 mg	60 mg	40 mg
180 mg	90 mg	60 mg
240 mg	120 mg	80 mg
360 mg	180 mg	120 mg
480 mg	240 mg	160 mg
600 mg	300 mg	200 mg
780 mg	390 mg	260 mg
960 mg	480 mg	320 mg
1200 mg	600 mg	400 mg

If breakthrough pain occurs give a subcutaneous injection equivalent to one-tenth to one-sixth of the total 24-hour subcutaneous infusion dose. With an intermittent subcutaneous injection absorption is smoother so that the risk of adverse effects at peak absorption is avoided (an even better method is to use a subcutaneous butterfly needle). To minimise the risk of infection no individual subcutaneous infusion solution should be used for longer than 24 hours.

Drugs and sport

Anti-doping

UK Anti-Doping, the national body responsible for the UK's anti-doping policy, advises that athletes are personally responsible should a prohibited substance be detected in their body. Information regarding the use of medicines in sport is available from:

UK Anti-doping
Fleetbank House
2-6 Salisbury Square
London
EC4Y 8AE
(020) 7842 3450
ukad@ukad.org.uk
www.ukad.org.uk

Information about the prohibited status of specific medications based on the current World Anti-Doping Agency Prohibited List is available from Global Drug Reference Online: www.globaldro.com/UK/search

General Medical Council's advice

Doctors who prescribe or collude in the provision of drugs or treatment with the intention of improperly enhancing an individual's performance in sport contravene the GMC's guidance, and such actions would usually raise a question of a doctor's continued registration. This does not preclude the provision of any care or treatment where the doctor's intention is to protect or improve the patient's health.

Medicines optimisation

Overview

Medicines are the most common intervention in healthcare for the prevention, treatment and/or management of many illnesses. As life expectancy increases and as the population ages, more people are living with several long-term conditions that are being managed with an increasing number of medicines. Medicines use can be complex and how patients can take their medicines safely and effectively is a challenge for the health service.

Multimorbidity (the presence of 2 or more long-term conditions) is associated with a greater use of health services, higher mortality, higher treatment burden (due to polypharmacy or multiple appointments), and reduced quality of life. The risk of patients suffering harm from their medicines increases with polypharmacy, and treatment regimens (including non-pharmacological treatments) can very easily become burdensome for patients with multimorbidity and can lead to care becoming fragmented and uncoordinated. Prescribers should consider the risks and benefits of treatments recommended from guidance for single health conditions, as the evidence for these recommendations is regularly drawn from patients without multimorbidity and who are taking fewer prescribed regular medicines. The management of risk factors for future disease can also be a major treatment burden for patients with multimorbidity and should be taken into consideration.

Medicines optimisation encompasses many aspects of medicines use and helps to ensure that they are taken as intended, thus supporting the management of long-term conditions, multimorbidities, and appropriate polypharmacy. Through the adoption of a patient-focused approach to safe and effective medicines use, medicines optimisation changes the way patients are supported to get the best possible outcomes from their medicines. The use of shared decision-making informed by the best available evidence to guide decisions, ensures all patients have the opportunity to be involved in decisions about their medicines, taking into account their needs, preferences and values.

To reduce the risk of harm, ensure patients taking multiple medicines are receiving the most appropriate treatments for their needs, and to manage the spend on medicines, the Department of Health and Social Care are reviewing over-prescribing in the NHS.

Optimisation tools

Medicines optimisation includes aspects of care such as clinical assessment, clinical audits, disease prevention, health education, individual reviews and monitoring, and risk management. Having effective processes and systems in place can minimise the risk of preventable medicines-related problems (such as interactions with other medicines or comorbidities, and side-effects). Health and social care organisations should consider the use of multiple methods for identifying medicines-related patient safety incidents; learning from these incidents is important for guiding practice and minimising patient harm.

When optimising patient care, areas of intervention to consider include: deprescribing; medicines reconciliation, reviews and repeat prescribing; problematic polypharmacy; reducing medication waste and errors; and self-management plans. Self-management plans can be led by the child and their parents/carers or health professional, and vary in their content depending on the individual needs of the child, with the aim of supporting both them and their parents/carers involvement and empowerment in managing their condition.

Medication reviews involve a structured critical examination of a child's medicines to optimise treatment, minimise the number of medication-related problems, and reduce waste. These should be led by an appropriate health professional with effective communication skills, technical knowledge in the processes for managing medicines, and therapeutic knowledge on medicines use. Reviews can be carried out in different care settings, such as Primary Care Networks utilising pharmacists within the GP practice. For further information on review services available from community pharmacists, such as the 'New Medicines Service' and 'Medicines Use Review', see *Advanced pharmacy services*.

To support the medicines optimisation agenda, The Royal Pharmaceutical Society have produced good practice guidance for health professionals, which details four guiding principles for medicines optimisation. These are:

- Aim to understand the patient's experience;
- Evidence-based choice of medicines;
- Ensure medicines use is as safe as possible;
- Make medicines optimisation part of routine practice.

For further guidance around medicines optimisation and tools to use, NHS England have compiled useful links as part of **RightCare**; NICE have produced guidelines on **Medicines optimisation** and **Multimorbidity**; and the Scottish Government have produced a guideline on **Polypharmacy**, see *Useful resources*.

Advanced Pharmacy Services Advanced Services are provided as part of the NHS Community Pharmacy Contractual Framework, and include services such as the New Medicines Service and Medicines Use Review service. These services are provided by accredited community pharmacists, with the aim of targeting specific children to help manage their medicines more effectively, improve adherence, and reduce medicines wastage.

New Medicines Service The New Medicines Service (NMS) provides education and support to children who are newly prescribed a medicine to manage a long-term condition. The service is split into three stages; patient engagement, intervention and follow-up. As of 2018, this service is available for children living in England who have either been prescribed a new medicine for one of the following conditions – asthma, type 2 diabetes or hypertension, or have been prescribed a new antiplatelet or anticoagulant. Children can be offered the service by prescriber referral, or opportunistically by the community pharmacy. For further information, see: psnc.org.uk/services-commissioning/advanced-services/nms/.

Medicines Use Review The Medicines Use Review (MUR) service consists of structured adherence-centred reviews with children on multiple medicines, particularly those receiving medicines for long-term conditions. The service is undertaken periodically, not usually more than once a year, and can also be prompted when an adherence issue is identified during the dispensing service.

The pharmacist providing the MUR service must ensure that at least 70% of all MURs undertaken in a year are for children who fall within the two national target groups. The national target groups for MURs in England are:

- children taking high-risk medicines (NSAIDs, anticoagulants (including low molecular weight heparin), antiplatelets, or diuretics);
- children recently discharged from hospital who have had changes made to their medicines while they were in hospital.

For further information, see: psnc.org.uk/services-commissioning/advanced-services/murs/.

Wales, Northern Ireland, and Scotland have variations on this service, including different national target groups.

In Wales, see: www.cpwales.org.uk/Contract-support-and-IT/Advanced-Services.aspx.

In Northern Ireland, see: www.hscbusiness.hscni.net/services/2427.htm.

In Scotland, see: www.cps.scot/nhs-services/core/medicines-care-review/.

Communication

As health professionals from various disciplines and specialties may be caring for the same child at the same time, good communication is required between health professionals in order to avoid fragmentation of care. Medication reviews may be carried out by health professionals other than the prescriber; therefore the prescriber should be informed of the review and its outcome—particularly if difficulties with adherence were discussed and further review is required.

There is a greater risk of poor communication and unintended medication changes when children transfer between different care providers (such as when a child is admitted to or discharged from hospital). To support high-quality care when moving from one care setting to another, relevant information about medicines should be shared with children, their parents/carers, and between health and social care practitioners using robust and transparent processes. Information should be securely shared between health and social care practitioners ideally within 24 hours of patient transfer.

Good communication between health professionals, children and their parents/carers is needed for shared decision-making and supporting adherence. Information about their condition and possible treatments should be provided in a format that meets the child's and their parent's/carer's individual needs and preferences. The use of patient decision aids during consultations can help support a shared decision-making approach, and ensure children and their parents/carers are able to make well-informed choices that are consistent with their values and preferences.

For further guidance around communication between health professionals, children and their parents/carers, NICE have produced a guideline on **Medicines optimisation** (see *Useful resources*). For guidance on the transition from paediatric to adult services, see *Transitional services for chronic conditions* in Guidance on prescribing p. 1.

Organisations such as the 'NHS Specialist Pharmacy Service' help support medicines optimisation across the NHS by joining health professionals together through online networks (e.g. Regional Medicines Optimisation Committees and the English Deprescribing Network). This is available at: www.sps.nhs.uk/home/networks/.

Useful resources

Medicines optimisation: the safe and effective use of medicines to enable the best possible outcomes. National Institute for Health and Care Excellence. NICE guideline 5. March 2015.
www.nice.org.uk/guidance/ng5

Multimorbidity: clinical assessment and management. National Institute for Health and Care Excellence. NICE guideline 56. September 2016.
www.nice.org.uk/guidance/ng56

Medicines Optimisation. NHS RightCare. NHS England.
www.england.nhs.uk/rightcare/useful-links/medicines-optimisation/

Polypharmacy Guidance, Realistic Prescribing. Scottish Government Polypharmacy Model of Care Group. 3rd Edition. 2018.
www.therapeutics.scot.nhs.uk/wp-content/uploads/2018/09/Polypharmacy-Guidance-2018.pdf

Medicines Optimisation: Helping patients to make the most of medicines. Royal Pharmaceutical Society. May 2013.
www.rpharms.com/resources/pharmacy-guides/medicines-optimisation-hub

Antimicrobial stewardship

Overview

Effective antimicrobials are required for preventive and curative measures, protecting patients from potentially fatal diseases, and ensuring that complex procedures can be provided at low risk of infection. Antimicrobial resistance (AMR) is the loss of antimicrobial effectiveness, and although it evolves naturally, this process is accelerated by the inappropriate or incorrect use of antimicrobials. Direct consequences of infection with resistant microorganisms can be severe and affect all areas of health, such as prolonged illnesses and hospital stays, increased costs and mortality, and reduced protection for patients undergoing operations or procedures. AMR is an international problem with an increasing prevalence that has consequences for the whole of society. The UK Government has recognised AMR as a significant area of concern and have committed global action to address this as a priority. For information and resources on the UK's plans for AMR, see the Public Health England (PHE) collection: **Antimicrobial resistance** (www.gov.uk/government/collections/antimicrobial-resistance-amr-information-and-resources).

Antimicrobial stewardship (AMS) refers to an organisational or healthcare system-wide approach to promoting and monitoring judicious use of antimicrobials to preserve their future effectiveness. Addressing AMR through improving stewardship is a national medicines optimisation priority, led by NHS England and supported by PHE.

AMR can be managed by a combination of interventions that address:

- A political commitment to prioritise AMR;
- Monitoring antimicrobial use and resistance in microbes;
- Development of new drugs, treatments, and diagnostics;
- Individuals' behaviour relating to infection prevention and control, antimicrobial use, and AMR;
- Healthcare professionals' prescribing decisions.

Guidance for organisations (commissioners and providers)

Commissioners (clinical commissioning groups and local authorities) and providers (e.g. hospitals, GPs, out-of-hours services, dentists, and social enterprises) of health or social care services should establish an AMS programme, taking into account the resources needed to support AMS across all care settings. An AMS programme should take into consideration monitoring and evaluating antimicrobial prescribing, regular feedback to individual prescribers, education and training for health and social care staff, and integrating audits into existing quality improvement programmes.

Commissioners should work collaboratively to provide consistent information and advice to the public and health professionals that reduces inappropriate antimicrobial demand and use, and limits the spread of infection. Local authority public health teams should ensure that information and resources (such as posters, leaflets and digital resources) are made available through multiple routes to provide a coordinated system of information. Information should include simple and practical steps such as scrupulous personal and safe food hygiene practices.

Organisations should involve lead health and social care staff in establishing processes for developing, reviewing, updating, and implementing local antimicrobial guidelines in line with national guidance and informed by local prescribing data and resistance patterns.

Organisations should also consider establishing processes for reviewing national horizon scanning to plan for the availability of new antimicrobials and to use an existing local decision-making group to consider the introduction of new antimicrobials locally.

Guidance for health and social care staff

Health and social care staff should assist with the implementation of local or national guidelines and recognise the significance of them for AMS.

Health professionals should be familiar with current AMS campaigns and programmes. For further information, see PHE and Health Education England's e-learning session **All Our Health: Antimicrobial Resistance** (portal.e-lfh.org.uk/Component/Details/571263), PHE guidance **Health matters: antimicrobial resistance** (www.gov.uk/government/publications/health-matters-antimicrobial-resistance), and the PHE campaigns **Antibiotic Guardian** (antibioticguardian.com/) and **Keep Antibiotics Working** (campaignresources.phe.gov.uk/resources/campaigns/58-keep-antibiotics-working).

Health professionals should be aware of resources and services that can help individuals minimise infections such as travel vaccination clinics, screening programmes, sexual health services, immunisation programmes, and other local referral pathways or schemes. The benefits of good hygiene, vaccination, and other preventative measures to reduce the risk of acquiring infections should be discussed with individuals, and individuals referred to further information or services if necessary.

Those involved in providing care should be educated about the standard principles of infection prevention and control. They should be trained in hand decontamination, the use of personal protective equipment, and the safe use and disposal of sharps. For further information, see NICE guideline: **Healthcare-associated infections** (see *Useful resources*).

Guidance on antimicrobial prescribing

National antimicrobial prescribing and stewardship competencies have been developed to improve the quality of antimicrobial treatment and stewardship. For further information, see Antimicrobial Resistance and Healthcare Associated Infections and PHE guidance: **Antimicrobial prescribing and stewardship competencies** (see *Useful resources*).

National toolkits to support the implementation of AMS best practice include the Royal College of General Practitioners' **TARGET antibiotics toolkit** (www.rcgp.org.uk/TARGETantibiotics) for primary care, and PHE's **Start smart - then focus** (www.gov.uk/government/publications/antimicrobial-stewardship-start-smart-then-focus) for secondary care, and **Dental antimicrobial stewardship: toolkit** (www.gov.uk/guidance/dental-antimicrobial-stewardship-toolkit) for dentists.

Clinical syndrome-specific guidance and advice to help slow the development of AMR have been developed by NICE, in collaboration with PHE, and are available at www.nice.org.uk/.

Considerations for antimicrobial prescribing When deciding whether or not to prescribe an antimicrobial, undertake a clinical assessment and consider the risk of AMR for individual patients and the population as a whole. An immediate antimicrobial prescription for a patient who is likely to have a self-limiting condition is not recommended. Document in the patient's records (electronically wherever possible) the decisions related to antimicrobial use, including the plan as discussed with the patient, and their family and/or carers (if appropriate), and reason for prescribing/not prescribing an antimicrobial.

In hospital, microbiological samples should be taken before initiating an antimicrobial for patients with suspected infection. In primary care, consider taking microbiological samples when prescribing an antimicrobial for patients with recurrent or persistent infections. The choice of antimicrobial should be reviewed when microbiological results are available. For non-severe infections, consider taking microbiological samples before making a decision about prescribing an antimicrobial, providing it is safe to withhold treatment until the results are available.

Follow local or national guidelines on prescribing the shortest effective course and most appropriate dose and route of administration. Review intravenous antimicrobials within 48 hours (taking into account response to treatment and microbiological results) and consider stepping down to oral antimicrobials where possible. If prescribing outside of local or national guidelines, document in the patient's records the reasons for the decision.

Patients on antimicrobial treatment should be appropriately monitored to reduce side-effects and be assessed on the continued need for treatment. Repeat antimicrobial prescriptions are not recommended, unless needed for a particular clinical condition or indication. Avoid issuing a repeat prescription for longer than 6 months without review.

Advice for patients and their family and/or carers

Prescribers, primary care and community pharmacy teams should provide patients with resources educating them about not asking for antimicrobials as a preventive measure against becoming ill or as a stand-by measure, unless the patient has a specific condition or a specific risk that requires antimicrobial prophylaxis.

Prescribers should discuss with patients, and their family and/or carers (if appropriate) the likely nature of the condition, their views on antimicrobials, benefits and harms of antimicrobial prescribing, and why prescribing an antimicrobial may not always be the best option.

Information should be provided about what to do if their symptoms worsen or if problems arise as a result of treatment. Written information should be provided if needed.

If antimicrobial treatment is not the most appropriate option, prescribers should advise patients, and their family and/or carers (if appropriate) about other options (as appropriate), such as self-care with over-the-counter preparations, back-up (delayed) prescribing, or other non-pharmacological interventions. Prescribers, primary care and community pharmacy teams should verbally emphasise and provide written advice about managing self-limiting infections.

If antimicrobials are prescribed or supplied, prescribers, primary care and community pharmacy teams should provide patients with verbal and written information on the correct use of antimicrobials. Advice should encourage people to:

- Take, or use antimicrobials only when recommended by a suitably qualified health professional;
- Obtain antimicrobials only from a health professional;
- Take, or use antimicrobials as instructed (right dose for the duration specified and via the right route);
- Return any unused antimicrobials to a pharmacy for safe disposal.

Useful resources

Antimicrobial prescribing and stewardship competencies. Antimicrobial Resistance and Healthcare Associated Infections (ARHAI) and Public Health England guideline. October 2013.
www.gov.uk/government/publications/antimicrobial-prescribing-and-stewardship-competencies

Antimicrobial resistance (AMR): applying All Our Health. Public Health England guideline. April 2015 (updated June 2019).
www.gov.uk/government/publications/antimicrobial-resistance-amr-applying-all-our-health

Antimicrobial stewardship: systems and processes for effective antimicrobial medicine use. National Institute for Health and Care Excellence. NICE guideline 15. August 2015.
www.nice.org.uk/guidance/NG15

Antimicrobial stewardship: changing risk-related behaviours in the general population. National Institute for Health and Care Excellence. NICE guideline 63. January 2017.
www.nice.org.uk/guidance/NG63

Healthcare-associated infections: prevention and control in primary and community care. National Institute for Health and Care Excellence. Clinical guideline 139. March 2012 (updated February 2017).
www.nice.org.uk/guidance/cg139

Prescribing in dental practice

General guidance

Advice on the drug management of dental and oral conditions has been integrated into the main text. For ease of access, guidance on such conditions is usually identified by means of a relevant heading (e.g. Dental and Orofacial Pain) in the appropriate sections.
The following is a list of topics of particular relevance to dentists.

Chapter 1
Gastro-intestinal system

CONTENTS

1 Chronic bowel disorders

1.1 Coeliac disease

Coeliac disease

25-Jul-2016

Description of condition

Coeliac disease is an autoimmune condition which is associated with chronic inflammation of the small intestine. Dietary proteins known as gluten, which are present in wheat, barley and rye, activate an abnormal immune response in the intestinal mucosa, which can lead to malabsorption of nutrients.

Aims of treatment

The management of coeliac disease is aimed at eliminating symptoms (such as diarrhoea, bloating and abdominal pain) and reducing the risk of complications, including those resulting from malabsorption.

Non-drug treatment

EvGr The only effective treatment for coeliac disease is a strict, life-long, gluten-free diet. A range of gluten-free products is available for prescription (see *Borderline substances*). ⟨A⟩

Drug treatment

EvGr Children who have coeliac disease are at an increased risk of malabsorption of key nutrients (such as calcium and vitamin D). Supplementation of key nutrients may be required if dietary intake is insufficient.

Carers of children who have coeliac disease should be advised **not** to medicate with over-the-counter vitamin or mineral supplements. Initiation of supplementation should involve a discussion with a member of the child's healthcare team in order to identify the individual needs of the patient and to allow for appropriate ongoing monitoring. ⟨A⟩

Useful Resources

Coeliac disease: recognition, assessment and management. National Institute for Health and Care Excellence. Clinical guideline 20. September 2015.
www.nice.org.uk/guidance/ng20

1.2 Inflammatory bowel disease

Inflammatory bowel disease

Chronic inflammatory bowel diseases include Ulcerative colitis p. 32 and Crohn's disease below.

Drugs used in inflammatory bowel disease

Aminosalicylates

Sulfasalazine p. 36 is a combination of 5-aminosalicylic acid ('5-ASA') and sulfapyridine; sulfapyridine acts only as a carrier to the colonic site of action but still causes side-effects. In the newer aminosalicylates, mesalazine p. 34 (5-aminosalicylic acid), balsalazide sodium p. 34 (a prodrug of 5-aminosalicylic acid) and olsalazine sodium p. 36 (a dimer of 5-aminosalicylic acid which cleaves in the lower bowel), the sulfonamide-related side-effects of sulfasalazine are avoided, but 5-aminosalicylic acid alone can still cause side-effects including blood disorders and lupus-like syndrome also seen with sulfasalazine.

Drugs affecting the immune response

Folic acid p. 620 should be given to reduce the possibility of methotrexate toxicity. Folic acid is usually given once weekly on a different day to the methotrexate p. 588; alternative regimens may be used in some settings.

Cytokine modulators

Infliximab p. 38 and adalimumab p. 693 are monoclonal antibodies which inhibit the pro-inflammatory cytokine, tumour necrosis factor alpha. Cytokine modulators should be used under specialist supervision.

Crohn's disease

20-Dec-2016

Description of condition

Crohn's disease is a chronic, inflammatory bowel disease that mainly affects the gastro-intestinal tract. It is characterised by thickened areas of the gastro-intestinal wall with inflammation extending through all layers, deep ulceration and fissuring of the mucosa, and the presence of granulomas; affected areas may occur in any part of the gastro-intestinal tract, interspersed with areas of relatively normal tissue. Crohn's disease may present as recurrent attacks, with acute exacerbations combined with periods of remission or less active disease. Symptoms depend on the site of disease but may include abdominal pain, diarrhoea, fever, weight loss, and rectal bleeding.

Complications of Crohn's disease include intestinal strictures, abscesses in the wall of the intestine or adjacent structures, fistulae, anaemia, malnutrition, colorectal and small bowel cancers, and growth failure and delayed puberty in children. Crohn's disease may also be associated with extra-intestinal manifestation: the most common are arthritis and abnormalities of the joints, eyes, liver and skin. Crohn's disease is also a cause of secondary osteoporosis and those at greatest risk should be monitored for osteopenia and assessed for the risk of fractures.

Up to a third of patients with Crohn's disease are diagnosed before the age of 21 years but there is a lack of evidence regarding treatment for children. Paediatric practice is often based on extrapolation from adult studies.

Fistulating Crohn's disease

Fistulating Crohn's disease is a complication that involves the formation of a fistula between the intestine and adjacent structures, such as perianal skin, bladder, and vagina. It occurs in about one quarter of patients, mostly when the disease involves the ileocolonic area.

Aims of treatment

Treatment is largely directed at the induction and maintenance of remission and the relief of symptoms. Active treatment of acute Crohn's disease should be distinguished from preventing relapse. The aims of drug treatment are to reduce symptoms and maintain or improve quality of life, while minimising toxicity related to drugs over both the short and long term. Drug treatment should always be initiated by a paediatric gastroenterologist.

In fistulating Crohn's disease, surgery and medical treatment aim to close and maintain closure of the fistula.

Non-drug treatment

EvGr In addition to drug treatment, management options for Crohn's disease include Smoking cessation p. 313 and attention to nutrition, which plays an important role in supportive care. Surgery may be considered in certain children with early disease limited to the distal ileum and in severe or chronic active disease. Ⓐ

Drug treatment

Treatment of acute disease

Monotherapy

EvGr A corticosteroid (either prednisolone p. 478 or methylprednisolone p. 478 or intravenous hydrocortisone p. 476), is used to induce remission in children with a first presentation or a single inflammatory exacerbation of Crohn's disease in a 12-month period.

Enteral nutrition is an alternative to a corticosteroid when there is concern about growth or side effects.

In children with distal ileal, ileocaecal or right-sided colonic disease, in whom a conventional corticosteroid is unsuitable or contra-indicated, budesonide p. 37 [unlicensed] may be considered. Budesonide is less effective but may cause fewer side-effects than other corticosteroids, as systemic exposure is limited. Aminosalicylates (such as sulfasalazine p. 36 and mesalazine p. 34) are an alternative option in these children. They are less effective than a corticosteroid or budesonide [unlicensed], but may be preferred because they have fewer side-effects. Aminosalicylates and budesonide are not appropriate for severe presentations or exacerbations. Ⓐ

Add-on treatment

EvGr Add on treatment is prescribed if there are two or more inflammatory exacerbations in a 12-month period, or the corticosteroid dose cannot be reduced.

Azathioprine p. 558 or mercaptopurine p. 587 [unlicensed indications] can be added to a corticosteroid or budesonide to induce remission. In children who cannot tolerate azathioprine or mercaptopurine or in whom thiopurine methyltransferase (TPMT) activity is deficient, methotrexate p. 588 can be added to a corticosteroid.

Under specialist supervision, the tumour necrosis factor-alpha inhibitors adalimumab p. 693 and infliximab p. 38 are options for the treatment of severe, active Crohn's disease, following inadequate response to conventional therapies or in those who are intolerant of or have contra-indications to conventional therapy. Ⓐ See also *National funding/access decisions* for adalimumab and infliximab.

EvGr Adalimumab and infliximab can be used as monotherapy or combined with an immunosuppressant, although there is uncertainty about the comparative effectiveness. Ⓐ There are concerns about the long-term safety of adalimumab and infliximab in children; malignancies, including hepatosplenic T- cell lymphoma, have been reported.

Maintenance of remission

EvGr Children, and their parents or carers, should be made aware of the risk of relapse with and without drug treatment, and symptoms that may suggest a relapse (most frequently unintended weight loss, abdominal pain, diarrhoea and general ill-health). For those who choose not to receive maintenance treatment during remission, a suitable follow up plan should be agreed upon and information provided on how to access healthcare if a relapse should occur.

Azathioprine or mercaptopurine [unlicensed indications] as monotherapy can be used to maintain remission when previously used with a corticosteroid to induce remission. They may also be used in children who have not previously received these drugs (particularly those with adverse prognostic factors such as early age of onset, perianal disease, corticosteroid use at presentation, and severe presentations). Methotrexate [unlicensed] can be used to maintain remission only in children who required methotrexate to induce remission, or who are intolerant of or are not suitable for azathioprine or mercaptopurine for maintenance. Corticosteroids or budesonide should not be used. Ⓐ

Maintaining remission following surgery

EvGr Azathioprine in combination with up to 3 months' postoperative metronidazole p. 358 [unlicensed indication] should be considered to maintain remission in children with ileocolonic Crohn's disease who have had complete macroscopic resection within the previous 3 months. Azathioprine alone should be considered for patients who cannot tolerate metronidazole p. 358. Ⓐ Aminosalicylates are no longer recommended due to the lack of clinical efficacy. NICE do not consider mercaptopurine to be a cost-effective treatment and do not recommend its use.

EvGr Biologic therapies should no longer be used to maintain remission after complete macroscopic resection of ileocolonic Crohn's disease because of limited evidence. Budesonide should also not be used in these patients. Ⓐ

Other treatments

EvGr Loperamide hydrochloride p. 54 can be used to manage diarrhoea associated with Crohn's disease in children who do not have colitis. Ⓐ Colestyramine p. 136 is licensed for the relief of diarrhoea associated with Crohn's disease. See also Diarrhoea (acute) p. 53.

Fistulating Crohn's disease

Perianal fistulae are the most common occurrence in children with fistulating Crohn's disease. EvGr Treatment may not be necessary for simple, asymptomatic perianal fistulae. When fistulae are symptomatic, local drainage and surgery may be required in conjunction with medical therapy.

Metronidazole p. 358 or ciprofloxacin p. 377 [unlicensed indications], alone or in combination, can improve symptoms of fistulating Crohn's disease but complete healing occurs rarely. Metronidazole should be given for at least 6 weeks but no longer than 3 months because of concerns about peripheral neuropathy. Other antibacterials should be given if specifically indicated (e.g. in sepsis associated with fistulae and perianal disease) and for managing bacterial overgrowth in the small bowel.

Either azathioprine p. 558 or mercaptopurine p. 587 [unlicensed indications] is used to control the inflammation in perianal and enterocutaneous fistulating Crohn's disease and they are continued for maintenance.

Infliximab p. 38 is recommended for children with perianal and enterocutaneous active fistulating Crohn's disease who have not responded to conventional therapy (including antibacterials, drainage and immunosuppressive treatments), or who are intolerant of or have contra-indications to conventional therapy. Infliximab should be used after ensuring that all sepsis is actively draining.

Abscess drainage, fistulotomy, and seton insertion may be appropriate, particularly before infliximab treatment.

Azathioprine, mercaptopurine or infliximab should be continued as maintenance treatment for at least one year.

For the management of non-perianal fistulating Crohn's disease (including entero-gynaecological and enterovesical fistulae) surgery is the only recommended approach. (A)

Useful Resources

Crohn's disease: management. National Institute for Health and Care Excellence. Clinical guideline 129. May 2019. www.nice.org.uk/guidance/ng129

Ulcerative colitis

20-Feb-2017

Description of condition

Ulcerative colitis is a chronic inflammatory condition, characterised by diffuse mucosal inflammation—it has a relapsing-remitting pattern. It is a life-long disease that is associated with significant morbidity. Ulcerative colitis is more common in adults; however in children it predominately presents between the ages of 5 and 16 years.

The pattern of inflammation is continuous, extending from the rectum upwards to a varying degree. Inflammation of the rectum is referred to as **proctitis**, and inflammation of the rectum and sigmoid colon as **proctosigmoiditis**. **Left-sided colitis** refers to disease involving the colon distal to the splenic flexure. **Extensive colitis** affects the colon proximal to the splenic flexure, and includes pan-colitis, where the whole colon is involved. Child-onset ulcerative colitis is classified as extensive in 60–80% of all cases. Common symptoms of active disease or relapse include bloody diarrhoea, an urgent need to defaecate, and abdominal pain.

Complications associated with ulcerative colitis include an increased risk of colorectal cancer, secondary osteoporosis, venous thromboembolism, and toxic megacolon. Growth and pubertal development can be affected in children.

Aims of treatment

Treatment is focussed on treating active disease to manage symptoms and to induce and maintain remission.

Drug treatment

Overview

Management of ulcerative colitis is dependent on factors such as clinical severity, extent of disease, and the child's preference. As limited distal disease is uncommon in children, paediatric treatment strategy depends mainly on disease severity rather than the extent of disease. Clinical and laboratory investigations are used to determine the extent and severity of disease and to guide treatment. Severity is classified as mild, moderate or severe (or in remission) by using the Paediatric Ulcerative Colitis Activity Index to assess bowel movement, limitations on daily activity and the presence of abdominal pain or melaena—see the NICE guideline for Ulcerative Colitis for further information (see *Useful resources*).

EvGr The extent of disease should be considered when choosing the route of administration for aminosalicylates and corticosteroids; whether oral treatment, topical treatment or both are to be used. (A)

If the inflammation is distal, a rectal preparation is adequate, but if the inflammation is extended, systemic medication is required. Either suppositories or enemas can be offered, taking into account the child's preferences.

EvGr Rectal foam preparations and suppositories can be used when children have difficulty retaining liquid enemas.

Diarrhoea that is associated with active ulcerative colitis is sometimes treated with anti-diarrhoeal drugs (such as loperamide hydrochloride p. 54 [unlicensed under 4 years]) on the advice of a specialist; however their use is contra-indicated in acute ulcerative colitis as they can increase the risk of toxic megacolon.

A macrogol-containing osmotic laxative (such as macrogol 3350 with potassium chloride, sodium bicarbonate and sodium chloride p. 47) may be useful for proximal faecal loading in proctitis. (E)

Oral aminosalicylates for the treatment of ulcerative colitis are available in different preparations and release forms. EvGr The preparation and dosing schedule should be chosen taking into account the delivery characteristics and suitability for the patient. When used to maintain remission, single daily doses of oral aminosalicylates can be more effective than multiple daily dosing, but may result in more side-effects.

The duration of corticosteroid course (usually 4 to 8 weeks) depends on the corticosteroid chosen. (A)

Treatment of acute mild-to-moderate ulcerative colitis

Proctitis

EvGr A topical aminosalicylate is recommended as first-line treatment for children with a mild-to-moderate initial presentation or inflammatory exacerbation of proctitis. If remission is not achieved within 4 weeks, adding an oral aminosalicylate should be considered. If the response remains inadequate, consider adding a topical or an oral corticosteroid for 4 to 8 weeks.

Monotherapy with an oral aminosalicylate can be considered in children who prefer not to use enemas or suppositories, although this may not be as effective. If remission is not achieved within 4 weeks, adding a topical or an oral corticosteroid for 4 to 8 weeks should be considered.

A topical or an oral corticosteroid for 4 to 8 weeks should be considered for children in whom aminosalicylates are unsuitable. (A)

Proctosigmoiditis and left-sided ulcerative colitis

EvGr A topical aminosalicylate is recommended as first-line treatment for children with a mild-to-moderate initial presentation or inflammatory exacerbation of proctosigmoiditis or left-sided ulcerative colitis. If remission is not achieved within 4 weeks, consider adding a high-dose oral aminosalicylate, or switching to a high-dose oral aminosalicylate and 4 to 8 weeks of a topical corticosteroid. If response remains inadequate, stop topical treatment and offer an oral aminosalicylate and 4 to 8 weeks of an oral corticosteroid.

Monotherapy with a high-dose oral aminosalicylate can be considered for children who prefer not to use enemas or suppositories, although this may not be as effective. If remission is not achieved within 4 weeks, an oral corticosteroid for 4 to 8 weeks in addition to the high-dose aminosalicylate should be offered.

A topical or an oral corticosteroid for 4 to 8 weeks should be considered for children in whom aminosalicylates are unsuitable. ⟨A⟩

Extensive ulcerative colitis

EvGr A topical aminosalicylate and a high-dose oral aminosalicylate is recommended as first-line treatment for children with a mild-to-moderate initial presentation or inflammatory exacerbation of extensive ulcerative colitis. If remission is not achieved within 4 weeks, stop topical aminosalicylate treatment and offer a high-dose oral aminosalicylate and 4 to 8 weeks of an oral corticosteroid. An oral corticosteroid for 4 to 8 weeks should be considered for children in whom aminosalicylates are unsuitable. ⟨A⟩

Treatment of acute severe ulcerative colitis

Acute severe ulcerative colitis of any extent can be life-threatening and is regarded as a medical emergency. EvGr Immediate hospital admission is required for treatment.

Intravenous corticosteroids (such as hydrocortisone p. 476 or methylprednisolone p. 478) should be given to induce remission in children with acute severe ulcerative colitis (whether it is a first presentation or an inflammatory exacerbation) while assessing the need for surgery. If intravenous corticosteroids are contra-indicated, declined or cannot be tolerated, then intravenous ciclosporin p. 559 [unlicensed indication], or surgery should be considered. A combination of intravenous ciclosporin with intravenous corticosteroids, or surgery is second line therapy for children who have little or no improvement within 72 hours of starting intravenous corticosteroids or in children whose symptoms worsen despite treatment with a corticosteroid. ⟨A⟩

EvGr Alternatively, infliximab p. 38 can be used on specialist advice in children over 6 years, if there is little or no improvement within 72 hours of starting intravenous corticosteroids or in children whose symptoms worsen despite treatment with a corticosteroid.

In patients who experience an initial response to steroids followed by deterioration, stool cultures should be taken to exclude pathogens; cytomegalovirus activation should be considered. ⟨E⟩

Infliximab for ulcerative colitis

EvGr Infliximab can be used to treat acute severe active ulcerative colitis in children over 6 years who have had an inadequate response to conventional treatment (including corticosteroids and azathioprine p. 558 or mercaptopurine p. 587) or if conventional treatment is not tolerated or contra-indicated. Treatment with these agents is continued into the maintenance phase if effective and tolerated. See also *National funding/access decisions* for infliximab.

Infliximab can also be used to treat acute exacerbations of severely active ulcerative colitis in children over 6 years, if ciclosporin p. 559 is contra-indicated or clinically inappropriate. ⟨A⟩

Maintaining remission in mild, moderate or severe ulcerative colitis

EvGr To reduce the chances of relapse occurring, maintenance therapy with an aminosalicylate is recommended in most children. Corticosteroids are **not** suitable for maintenance treatment because of their side-effects.

After a mild-to-moderate inflammatory exacerbation of *proctitis* or *proctosigmoiditis*, a rectal aminosalicylate can be started alone or in combination with an oral aminosalicylate, administered daily or as part of an intermittent regimen (such as twice to three times weekly or the first seven days of each month). An oral aminosalicylate can be used alone in children who prefer not to use enemas or suppositories, although this may not be as effective.

A low dose of oral aminosalicylate is given to maintain remission in children after a mild-to-moderate inflammatory exacerbation of *left-sided or extensive* ulcerative colitis.

When used to maintain remission, single daily dosing of oral aminosalicylates can be more effective than multiple daily dosing, but may result in more side-effects.

Oral azathioprine or mercaptopurine [unlicensed indications] can be considered to maintain remission, if there has been two or more inflammatory exacerbations in a 12-month period that require treatment with systemic corticosteroids or if remission is not maintained by aminosalicylates, or following a single acute severe episode. ⟨A⟩ EvGr Oral azathioprine or mercaptopurine is usually required in these cases as an aminosalicylate alone may be ineffective in more severe disease. ⟨E⟩

There is no evidence to support the use of methotrexate p. 588 to induce or maintain remission in ulcerative colitis though its use is common in clinical practice.

Non-drug treatment

EvGr Surgery may be necessary as emergency treatment for severe ulcerative colitis that does not respond to drug treatment. Patients can also choose to have elective surgery for unresponsive or frequently relapsing disease that is affecting their quality of life. ⟨A⟩

Useful Resources

Ulcerative colitis: management. National Institute for Health and Care Excellence. Clinical guideline 130. May 2019. www.nice.org.uk/guidance/NG130

AMINOSALICYLATES

Aminosalicylates 

● **SIDE-EFFECTS**

▶ **Common or very common** Arthralgia · cough · diarrhoea · dizziness · fever · gastrointestinal discomfort · headache · leucopenia · nausea · skin reactions · vomiting

▶ **Uncommon** Alopecia · depression · dyspnoea · myalgia · photosensitivity reaction · thrombocytopenia

▶ **Rare or very rare** Agranulocytosis · bone marrow disorders · cardiac inflammation · hepatitis · neutropenia · pancreatitis · peripheral neuropathy · renal impairment · respiratory disorders

▶ **Frequency not known** Angioedema · eosinophilia · haemolytic anaemia · nephritis tubulointerstitial · oligozoospermia (reversible) · ulcerative colitis aggravated

SIDE-EFFECTS, FURTHER INFORMATION A blood count should be performed and the drug stopped immediately if there is suspicion of a blood dyscrasia.

● **ALLERGY AND CROSS-SENSITIVITY** Contra-indicated in salicylate hypersensitivity.

● **RENAL IMPAIRMENT**

Monitoring Renal function should be monitored more frequently in renal impairment.

● **MONITORING REQUIREMENTS** Renal function should be monitored before starting an oral aminosalicylate, at 3 months of treatment, and then annually during treatment.

● **PATIENT AND CARER ADVICE**

Blood disorders Patients receiving aminosalicylates, and their carers, should be advised to report any unexplained bleeding, bruising, purpura, sore throat, fever or malaise that occurs during treatment.

Balsalazide sodium

F 33

29-Apr-2020

● **INDICATIONS AND DOSE**

Treatment of mild to moderate ulcerative colitis, acute attack

▶ BY MOUTH

▸ Child 12–17 years: 2.25 g 3 times a day until remission occurs or for up to maximum of 12 weeks

Maintenance of remission of ulcerative colitis

▶ BY MOUTH

▸ Child 12–17 years: 1.5 g twice daily (max. per dose 3 g), adjusted according to response; maximum 6 g per day

● **UNLICENSED USE** Not licensed for use in children under 18 years.

● **CAUTIONS** History of asthma

● **INTERACTIONS** → Appendix 1: balsalazide

● **SIDE-EFFECTS** Blood disorder · cholelithiasis · lupus-like syndrome

● **PREGNANCY** Manufacturer advises avoid.

● **BREAST FEEDING** Diarrhoea may develop in the infant. **Monitoring** Monitor breast-fed infants for diarrhoea.

● **HEPATIC IMPAIRMENT** Manufacturer advises caution; avoid in severe impairment (no information available).

● **RENAL IMPAIRMENT** Manufacturer advises avoid in moderate to severe impairment.

● **MEDICINAL FORMS** There can be variation in the licensing of different medicines containing the same drug.

Capsule

CAUTIONARY AND ADVISORY LABELS 21, 25

▸ Colazide (Almirall Ltd)
Balsalazide disodium 750 mg Colazide 750mg capsules | 130 capsule PoM £30.42 DT = £30.42

Mesalazine

F 33

29-Apr-2020

● **INDICATIONS AND DOSE**

DOSE EQUIVALENCE AND CONVERSION

There is no evidence to show that any one oral preparation of mesalazine is more effective than another; however, the delivery characteristics of oral mesalazine preparations may vary.

ASACOL ® MR 400MG TABLETS

Treatment of mild to moderate ulcerative colitis, acute attack

▶ BY MOUTH

▸ Child 12–17 years: 800 mg 3 times a day

Maintenance of remission of ulcerative colitis and Crohn's ileo-colitis

▶ BY MOUTH

▸ Child 12–17 years: 400–800 mg 2–3 times a day

ASACOL ® FOAM ENEMA

Treatment of acute attack of mild to moderate ulcerative colitis affecting the rectosigmoid region

▶ BY RECTUM

▸ Child 12–17 years: 1 g daily for 4–6 weeks, to be administered into the rectum

Treatment of acute attack of mild to moderate ulcerative colitis, affecting the descending colon

▶ BY RECTUM

▸ Child 12–17 years: 2 g once daily for 4–6 weeks, to be administered into the rectum

ASACOL ® SUPPOSITORIES

Treatment and maintenance of remission of ulcerative colitis affecting the rectosigmoid region

▶ BY RECTUM

▸ Child 12–17 years: 250–500 mg 3 times a day, last dose to be administered at bedtime

OCTASA ®

Treatment of mild to moderate ulcerative colitis, acute attack

▶ BY MOUTH

▸ Child 6–17 years (body-weight 40 kg and above): 2.4–4 g daily in divided doses

Maintenance of remission of ulcerative colitis and Crohn's ileo-colitis

▶ BY MOUTH

▸ Child 6–17 years (body-weight 40 kg and above): 1.2–2 g once daily, alternatively daily in divided doses

PENTASA ® GRANULES

Treatment of mild to moderate ulcerative colitis, acute attack

▶ BY MOUTH

▸ Child 5–17 years (body-weight up to 40 kg): 10–20 mg/kg 3 times a day

▸ Child 5–17 years (body-weight 40 kg and above): 1–2 g twice daily, total daily dose may alternatively be given in 3–4 divided doses

Maintenance of remission of ulcerative colitis

▶ BY MOUTH

▸ Child 5–17 years (body-weight up to 40 kg): 7.5–15 mg/kg twice daily, total daily dose may alternatively be given in 3 divided doses

▸ Child 5–17 years (body-weight 40 kg and above): 2 g once daily

PENTASA ® RETENTION ENEMA

Treatment of acute attack of mild to moderate ulcerative colitis affecting the rectosigmoid region

▶ BY RECTUM

▸ Child 12–17 years: 1 g once daily, dose to be administered at bedtime

PENTASA ® SUPPOSITORIES

Treatment of acute attack, ulcerative proctitis

▶ BY RECTUM

▸ Child 12–17 years: 1 g daily for 2–4 weeks

Maintenance, ulcerative proctitis

▶ BY RECTUM

▸ Child 12–17 years: 1 g daily

PENTASA ® TABLETS

Treatment of mild to moderate ulcerative colitis, acute attack

▶ BY MOUTH

▸ Child 5–17 years (body-weight up to 40 kg): 10–20 mg/kg 3 times a day

▸ Child 5–17 years (body-weight 40 kg and above): 1–2 g twice daily, total daily dose may alternatively be given in 3 divided doses

Maintenance of remission of ulcerative colitis

▶ BY MOUTH

▸ Child 5–17 years (body-weight up to 40 kg): 7.5–15 mg/kg twice daily, total daily dose may alternatively be given in 3 divided doses

▸ Child 5–17 years (body-weight 40 kg and above): 2 g once daily

SALOFALK® ENEMA

Treatment of acute attack of mild to moderate ulcerative colitis or maintenance of remission

▶ BY RECTUM

- Child 12–17 years: 2 g once daily, dose to be administered at bedtime

SALOFALK® GRANULES

Treatment of mild to moderate ulcerative colitis, acute attack

▶ BY MOUTH

- Child 5–17 years (body-weight up to 40 kg): 30–50 mg/kg once daily, dose preferably given in the morning, alternatively 10–20 mg/kg 3 times a day
- Child 5–17 years (body-weight 40 kg and above): 1.5–3 g once daily, dose preferably given in the morning, alternatively 0.5–1 g 3 times a day

Maintenance of remission of ulcerative colitis

▶ BY MOUTH

- Child 5–17 years (body-weight up to 40 kg): 7.5–15 mg/kg twice daily, total daily dose may alternatively be given in 3 divided doses
- Child 5–17 years (body-weight 40 kg and above): 500 mg 3 times a day

SALOFALK® RECTAL FOAM

Treatment of mild ulcerative colitis affecting sigmoid colon and rectum

▶ BY RECTUM

- Child 12–17 years: 2 g once daily, dose to be administered into the rectum at bedtime, alternatively 2 g daily in 2 divided doses

SALOFALK® SUPPOSITORIES

Treatment of acute attack of mild to moderate ulcerative colitis affecting the rectum, sigmoid colon and descending colon

▶ BY RECTUM

- Child 12–17 years: 0.5–1 g 2–3 times a day, adjusted according to response, dose to be given using 500 mg suppositories

SALOFALK® TABLETS

Treatment of mild to moderate ulcerative colitis, acute attack

▶ BY MOUTH

- Child 5–17 years (body-weight up to 40 kg): 10–20 mg/kg 3 times a day
- Child 5–17 years (body-weight 40 kg and above): 0.5–1 g 3 times a day

Maintenance of remission of ulcerative colitis

▶ BY MOUTH

- Child 5–17 years (body-weight up to 40 kg): 7.5–15 mg/kg twice daily, total daily dose may alternatively be given in 3 divided doses
- Child 5–17 years (body-weight 40 kg and above): 500 mg 3 times a day

● **UNLICENSED USE**
- With oral use *Asacol®* (all preparations) not licensed for use in children under 18 years. *Pentasa®* tablets not licensed for use in children under 15 years. *Pentasa®* granules and *Salofalk®* tablets and granules not licensed for use in children under 6 years.
- With rectal use *Asacol®* (all preparations) and *Salofalk®* enema not licensed for use in children under 18 years. *Salofalk®* suppositories and *Pentasa®* suppositories not licensed for use in children under 15 years. *Salofalk®* rectal foam no dose recommendations for children (age range not specified by manufacturer).

● **CONTRA-INDICATIONS**
- With oral use Blood clotting abnormalities

● **CAUTIONS** Maintain adequate fluid intake · pulmonary disease

● **INTERACTIONS** → Appendix 1: mesalazine

● **SIDE-EFFECTS**

GENERAL SIDE-EFFECTS

- **Rare or very rare** Cholestasis exacerbated · drug fever · flatulence · nephritis

SPECIFIC SIDE-EFFECTS

- **Rare or very rare**
- With rectal use Constipation

● **PREGNANCY** Negligible quantities cross placenta.

● **BREAST FEEDING** Diarrhoea reported in breast-fed infants, but negligible amounts of mesalazine detected in breast milk.

Monitoring Monitor breast-fed infant for diarrhoea.

● **HEPATIC IMPAIRMENT** Manufacturer advises caution in mild to moderate impairment; avoid in severe impairment.

● **RENAL IMPAIRMENT** Use with caution. Avoid if estimated glomerular filtration rate less than 20 mL/minute/1.73 m^2.

● **DIRECTIONS FOR ADMINISTRATION**

PENTASA® TABLETS Tablets may be halved, quartered, or dispersed in water, but should not be chewed.

PENTASA® GRANULES Granules should be placed on tongue and washed down with water or orange juice without chewing.

Contents of one sachet should be weighed and divided immediately before use; discard any remaining granules.

SALOFALK® GRANULES Granules should be placed on tongue and washed down with water without chewing.

● **PRESCRIBING AND DISPENSING INFORMATION** There is no evidence to show that any one oral preparation of mesalazine is more effective than another; however, the delivery characteristics of oral mesalazine preparations may vary.

Flavours of granule formulations of *Salofalk®* may include vanilla.

● **PATIENT AND CARER ADVICE** If it is necessary to switch a patient to a different brand of mesalazine, the patient should be advised to report any changes in symptoms. Some products may require special administration advice; patients and carers should be informed.

Medicines for Children leaflet: Mesalazine (oral) for inflammatory bowel disease www.medicinesforchildren.org.uk/mesalazine-oral-inflammatory-bowel-disease

Medicines for Children leaflet: Mesalazine foam enema for inflammatory bowel disease www.medicinesforchildren.org.uk/mesalazine-foam-enema-inflammatory-bowel-disease

Medicines for Children leaflet: Mesalazine liquid enema for inflammatory bowel disease www.medicinesforchildren.org.uk/mesalazine-liquid-enema-inflammatory-bowel-disease

Medicines for Children leaflet: Mesalazine suppositories for inflammatory bowel disease www.medicinesforchildren.org.uk/mesalazine-suppositories-inflammatory-bowel-disease

● **MEDICINAL FORMS** There can be variation in the licensing of different medicines containing the same drug.

Modified-release tablet

CAUTIONARY AND ADVISORY LABELS 21 (does not apply to Pentasa® tablets), 25 (does not apply to Pentasa® tablets)

- Pentasa (Ferring Pharmaceuticals Ltd)

  Mesalazine 500 mg Pentasa 500mg modified-release tablets | 100 tablet [PoM] £30.74 DT = £30.74

  Mesalazine 1 gram Pentasa 1g modified-release tablets | 60 tablet [PoM] £36.89 DT = £36.89

Foam

EXCIPIENTS: May contain Cetostearyl alcohol (including cetyl and stearyl alcohol), disodium edetate, hydroxybenzoates (parabens), polysorbates, propylene glycol, sodium metabisulfite

- Salofalk (Dr. Falk Pharma UK Ltd)
  Mesalazine 1 gram per 1 application Salofalk 1g/application foam enema | 14 dose PoM £30.17 DT = £30.17

Gastro-resistant tablet

CAUTIONARY AND ADVISORY LABELS 5 (does not apply to Octasa®), 25

- Asacol MR (Allergan Ltd)
  Mesalazine 400 mg Asacol 400mg MR gastro-resistant tablets | 84 tablet PoM £27.45 DT = £27.45 | 168 tablet PoM £54.90
- Octasa MR (Tillotts Pharma Ltd)
  Mesalazine 400 mg Octasa 400mg MR gastro-resistant tablets | 90 tablet PoM £16.58 DT = £16.58 | 120 tablet PoM £22.10
  Mesalazine 800 mg Octasa 800mg MR gastro-resistant tablets | 90 tablet PoM £40.38 | 180 tablet PoM £80.75 DT = £80.75
- Salofalk (Dr. Falk Pharma UK Ltd)
  Mesalazine 250 mg Salofalk 250mg gastro-resistant tablets | 100 tablet PoM £16.19 DT = £16.19
  Mesalazine 500 mg Salofalk 500mg gastro-resistant tablets | 100 tablet PoM £32.38 DT = £32.38

Suppository

- Pentasa (Ferring Pharmaceuticals Ltd)
  Mesalazine 1 gram Pentasa 1g suppositories | 28 suppository PoM £40.01 DT = £40.01
- Salofalk (Dr. Falk Pharma UK Ltd)
  Mesalazine 500 mg Salofalk 500mg suppositories | 30 suppository PoM £14.81 DT = £14.81
  Mesalazine 1 gram Salofalk 1g suppositories | 30 suppository PoM £29.62

Modified-release granules

CAUTIONARY AND ADVISORY LABELS 25 (does not apply to Pentasa® granules)

EXCIPIENTS: May contain Aspartame

- Pentasa (Ferring Pharmaceuticals Ltd)
  Mesalazine 1 gram Pentasa 1g modified-release granules sachets sugar-free | 50 sachet PoM £30.74 DT = £30.74
  Mesalazine 2 gram Pentasa 2g modified-release granules sachets sugar-free | 60 sachet PoM £73.78 DT = £73.78
- Salofalk (Dr. Falk Pharma UK Ltd)
  Mesalazine 1 gram Salofalk 1g gastro-resistant modified-release granules sachets sugar-free | 50 sachet PoM £28.74 DT = £28.74
  Mesalazine 1.5 gram Salofalk 1.5g gastro-resistant modified-release granules sachets sugar-free | 60 sachet PoM £48.85 DT = £48.85
  Mesalazine 3 gram Salofalk 3g gastro-resistant modified-release granules sachets sugar-free | 60 sachet PoM £97.70 DT = £97.70

Enema

- Pentasa (Ferring Pharmaceuticals Ltd)
  Mesalazine 10 mg per 1 ml Pentasa Mesalazine 1g/100ml enema | 7 enema PoM £17.73 DT = £17.73
- Salofalk (Dr. Falk Pharma UK Ltd)
  Mesalazine 33.9 mg per 1 ml Salofalk 2g/59ml enema | 7 enema PoM £29.92 DT = £29.92

F 33

Olsalazine sodium

- **INDICATIONS AND DOSE**

Treatment of acute attack of mild ulcerative colitis

▶ BY MOUTH

- Child 2–17 years: 500 mg twice daily, dose to be taken after food, then increased if necessary up to 1 g 3 times a day, dose to be increased over 1 week

Maintenance of remission of mild ulcerative colitis

▶ BY MOUTH

- Child 2–17 years: Maintenance 250–500 mg twice daily, dose to be taken after food

- **UNLICENSED USE** Not licensed for use in children under 12 years.
- **INTERACTIONS** → Appendix 1: olsalazine
- **SIDE-EFFECTS**

▶ **Uncommon** Paraesthesia · tachycardia

▶ **Frequency not known** Palpitations · vision blurred

- **PREGNANCY** Manufacturer advises avoid unless potential benefit outweighs risk.
- **BREAST FEEDING**

Monitoring Monitor breast-fed infants for diarrhoea.

- **RENAL IMPAIRMENT** Use with caution; manufacturer advises avoid in significant impairment.
- **DIRECTIONS FOR ADMINISTRATION** Capsules can be opened and contents sprinkled on food.

- **MEDICINAL FORMS** There can be variation in the licensing of different medicines containing the same drug. Forms available from special-order manufacturers include: oral suspension, oral solution

Tablet

CAUTIONARY AND ADVISORY LABELS 21

- Olsalazine sodium (Non-proprietary)
  Olsalazine sodium 500 mg Olsalazine 500mg tablets | 60 tablet PoM £161.00 DT = £161.00

Capsule

CAUTIONARY AND ADVISORY LABELS 21

- Olsalazine sodium (Non-proprietary)
  Olsalazine sodium 250 mg Olsalazine 250mg capsules | 112 capsule PoM £144.00 DT = £144.00

F 33

Sulfasalazine

29-Apr-2020

(Sulphasalazine)

- **INDICATIONS AND DOSE**

Treatment of acute attack of mild to moderate and severe ulcerative colitis | Active Crohn's disease

▶ BY MOUTH

- Child 2–11 years: 10–15 mg/kg 4–6 times a day (max. per dose 1 g) until remission occurs; increased if necessary up to 60 mg/kg daily in divided doses
- Child 12–17 years: 1–2 g 4 times a day until remission occurs

▶ BY RECTUM

- Child 5–7 years: 500 mg twice daily
- Child 8–11 years: 500 mg, dose to be administered in the morning and 1 g, dose to be administered at night
- Child 12–17 years: 0.5–1 g twice daily

Maintenance of remission of mild to moderate and severe ulcerative colitis

▶ BY MOUTH

- Child 2–11 years: 5–7.5 mg/kg 4 times a day (max. per dose 500 mg)
- Child 12–17 years: 500 mg 4 times a day

▶ BY RECTUM

- Child 5–7 years: 500 mg twice daily
- Child 8–11 years: 500 mg, dose to be administered in the morning and 1 g, dose to be administered at night
- Child 12–17 years: 0.5–1 g twice daily

Juvenile idiopathic arthritis

▶ BY MOUTH

- Child 2–11 years: Initially 5 mg/kg twice daily for 1 week, then 10 mg/kg twice daily for 1 week, then 20 mg/kg twice daily for 1 week; maintenance 20–25 mg/kg twice daily; maximum 2 g per day
- Child 12–17 years: Initially 5 mg/kg twice daily for 1 week, then 10 mg/kg twice daily for 1 week, then 20 mg/kg twice daily for 1 week; maintenance 20–25 mg/kg twice daily; maximum 3 g per day

- **UNLICENSED USE** Not licensed for use in children for juvenile idiopathic arthritis.

IMPORTANT SAFETY INFORMATION

SAFE PRACTICE

Sulfasalazine has been confused with sulfadiazine; care must be taken to ensure the correct drug is prescribed and dispensed.

- **CONTRA-INDICATIONS** Child under 2 years of age

- **CAUTIONS** Acute porphyrias p. 652 · G6PD deficiency · history of allergy · history of asthma · maintain adequate fluid intake · risk of haematological toxicity · risk of hepatic toxicity · slow acetylator status
- **INTERACTIONS** → Appendix 1: sulfasalazine
- **SIDE-EFFECTS**
  - **Common or very common** Insomnia · stomatitis · taste altered · tinnitus · urine abnormalities
  - **Uncommon** Face oedema · seizure · vasculitis · vertigo
  - **Frequency not known** Anaemia · appetite decreased · ataxia · cyanosis · encephalopathy · haematuria · hallucination · hepatic failure · hypoprothrombinaemia · lymphadenopathy · macrocytosis · meningitis aseptic · methaemoglobinaemia · nephrotic syndrome · parotitis · periorbital oedema · pseudomembranous enterocolitis · serum sickness · severe cutaneous adverse reactions (SCARs) · smell disorders · systemic lupus erythematosus (SLE) · yellow discolouration of body fluids

  SIDE-EFFECTS, FURTHER INFORMATION Incidence of side-effects increases with higher doses.

  Blood disorders Haematological abnormalities occur usually in the first 3 to 6 months of treatment—discontinue if these occur.
- **PREGNANCY** Theoretical risk of neonatal haemolysis in third trimester; adequate folate supplements should be given to mother.
- **BREAST FEEDING** Small amounts in milk (1 report of bloody diarrhoea); theoretical risk of neonatal haemolysis especially in G6PD-deficient infants.
- **HEPATIC IMPAIRMENT** Manufacturer advises caution.
- **RENAL IMPAIRMENT** Risk of toxicity, including crystalluria, in moderate impairment—ensure high fluid intake. Avoid in severe impairment.
- **MONITORING REQUIREMENTS**
  - Blood disorders Close monitoring of full blood counts (including differential white cell count and platelet count) is necessary initially, and at monthly intervals during the first 3 months.
  - Renal function Although the manufacturer recommends renal function tests in rheumatic diseases, evidence of practical value is unsatisfactory.
  - Liver function Liver function tests should be performed at monthly intervals for first 3 months.
- **PATIENT AND CARER ADVICE**

  Contact lenses Some soft contact lenses may be stained.

- **MEDICINAL FORMS** There can be variation in the licensing of different medicines containing the same drug. Forms available from special-order manufacturers include: oral suspension

Oral suspension

CAUTIONARY AND ADVISORY LABELS 14

EXCIPIENTS: May contain Alcohol

- **Sulfasalazine (Non-proprietary)**
  Sulfasalazine 50 mg per 1 ml Sulfasalazine 250mg/5ml oral suspension sugar free sugar-free | 500 ml PoM £50.67 DT = £47.13

Gastro-resistant tablet

CAUTIONARY AND ADVISORY LABELS 5, 14, 25

- **Sulfasalazine (Non-proprietary)**
  Sulfasalazine 500 mg Sulfasalazine 500mg gastro-resistant tablets | 112 tablet PoM £10.11 DT = £8.01
- **Salazopyrin EN** (Pfizer Ltd)
  Sulfasalazine 500 mg Salazopyrin EN-Tabs 500mg | 112 tablet PoM £8.43 DT = £8.01
- **Sulazine EC** (Genesis Pharmaceuticals Ltd)
  Sulfasalazine 500 mg Sulazine EC 500mg tablets | 112 tablet PoM £6.74 DT = £8.01

Tablet

CAUTIONARY AND ADVISORY LABELS 14

- **Sulfasalazine (Non-proprietary)**
  Sulfasalazine 500 mg Sulfasalazine 500mg tablets | 112 tablet PoM £8.94 DT = £6.21
- **Salazopyrin** (Pfizer Ltd)
  Sulfasalazine 500 mg Salazopyrin 500mg tablets | 112 tablet PoM £6.97 DT = £6.21

Suppository

CAUTIONARY AND ADVISORY LABELS 14

- **Salazopyrin** (Pfizer Ltd)
  Sulfasalazine 500 mg Salazopyrin 500mg suppositories | 10 suppository PoM £3.30 DT = £3.30

CORTICOSTEROIDS

472

Budesonide

12-Jun-2019

- **DRUG ACTION** Budesonide is a glucocorticoid, which exerts significant local anti-inflammatory effects.

- **INDICATIONS AND DOSE**

BUDENOFALK® CAPSULES

Mild to moderate Crohn's disease affecting the ileum or ascending colon

- BY MOUTH
  - Child 12–17 years: 3 mg 3 times a day for up to 8 weeks, reduce dose gradually over 2 weeks following treatment

ENTOCORT® CAPSULES

Mild to moderate Crohn's disease affecting the ileum or ascending colon

- BY MOUTH
  - Child 12–17 years: 9 mg once daily for up to 8 weeks; reduce dose for the last 2–4 weeks of treatment, to be taken in the morning

ENTOCORT® ENEMA

Ulcerative colitis involving rectal and recto-sigmoid disease

- BY RECTUM
  - Child 12–17 years: 1 enema daily for 4 weeks, to be administered at bedtime

- **UNLICENSED USE** Not licensed for use in children for Crohn's disease or ulcerative colitis.
- **INTERACTIONS** → Appendix 1: corticosteroids
- **SIDE-EFFECTS**
  - **Common or very common**
  - With oral use Muscle twitching · oedema · oral disorders
  - With rectal use Diarrhoea · gastrointestinal disorders
- **HEPATIC IMPAIRMENT** For *Budenofalk®* manufacturer advises avoid in cirrhosis (risk of increased exposure, limited information available).
- **MONITORING REQUIREMENTS** Manufacturer advises when used in autoimmune hepatitis, liver function tests should be monitored every 2 weeks for 1 month, then at least every 3 months.
- **DIRECTIONS FOR ADMINISTRATION** Capsules can be opened and the contents mixed with apple or orange juice.
- **PRESCRIBING AND DISPENSING INFORMATION**
  ENTOCORT® CAPSULES Dispense modified-release capsules in original container (contains desiccant).

- **MEDICINAL FORMS** There can be variation in the licensing of different medicines containing the same drug.

Gastro-resistant capsule

CAUTIONARY AND ADVISORY LABELS 5, 10, 22, 25

- **Budenofalk** (Dr. Falk Pharma UK Ltd)
  Budesonide 3 mg Budenofalk 3mg gastro-resistant capsules | 100 capsule PoM £75.05 DT = £75.05

Modified-release capsule

CAUTIONARY AND ADVISORY LABELS 5, 10, 25

- **Entocort CR** (Tillotts Pharma Ltd)
  Budesonide 3 mg Entocort CR 3mg capsules | 50 capsule PoM £37.53 | 100 capsule PoM £75.05 DT = £75.05

Enema

- Entocort (Tillotts Pharma Ltd)
  Budesonide 20 microgram per 1 ml Entocort 2mg/100ml enema | 7 enema PoM £33.66 DT = £33.66

IMMUNOSUPPRESSANTS > TUMOR NECROSIS FACTOR ALPHA (TNF-α) INHIBITORS

Infliximab

20-Nov-2019

- **INDICATIONS AND DOSE**

Severe active Crohn's disease

- BY INTRAVENOUS INFUSION
- Child 6–17 years: Initially 5 mg/kg, then 5 mg/kg after 2 weeks, then 5 mg/kg after 4 weeks, then maintenance 5 mg/kg every 8 weeks, interval between maintenance doses adjusted according to response; discontinue if no response within 10 weeks of initial dose

Fistulating Crohn's disease

- BY INTRAVENOUS INFUSION
- Child 6–17 years: Initially 5 mg/kg, then 5 mg/kg after 2 weeks, followed by 5 mg/kg after 4 weeks, if condition has responded consult product literature for guidance on further doses

Severe active ulcerative colitis

- BY INTRAVENOUS INFUSION
- Child 6–17 years: Initially 5 mg/kg, then 5 mg/kg after 2 weeks, followed by 5 mg/kg after 4 weeks, then 5 mg/kg every 8 weeks, discontinue if no response within 8 weeks of initial dose

- **UNLICENSED USE** Not licensed for fistulating Crohn's disease in children.

IMPORTANT SAFETY INFORMATION
Adequate resuscitation facilities must be available when infliximab is used.

- **CONTRA-INDICATIONS** Moderate or severe heart failure · severe infections
- **CAUTIONS** Demyelinating disorders (risk of exacerbation) · dermatomyositis · development of malignancy · hepatitis B virus—monitor for active infection · history of malignancy · history of prolonged immunosuppressant or PUVA treatment in patients with psoriasis · mild heart failure (discontinue if symptoms develop or worsen) · predisposition to infection (discontinue if new serious infection develops) · risk of delayed hypersensitivity reactions if drug-free interval exceeds 16 weeks (re-administration after interval exceeding 16 weeks not recommended)

CAUTIONS, FURTHER INFORMATION

- Infection Manufacturer advises patients should be up-to-date with current immunisation schedule before initiating treatment.
- Tuberculosis Manufacturer advises to evaluate patients for active and latent tuberculosis before treatment. Active tuberculosis should be treated with standard treatment for at least 2 months before starting infliximab. If latent tuberculosis is diagnosed, treatment should be started before commencing treatment with infliximab. Patients who have previously received adequate treatment for tuberculosis can start infliximab but should be monitored every 3 months for possible recurrence. In patients without active tuberculosis but who were previously not treated adequately, chemoprophylaxis should ideally be completed before starting infliximab. In patients at high risk of tuberculosis who cannot be assessed by tuberculin skin test, chemoprophylaxis can be given concurrently with infliximab. Patients should be advised to seek medical attention if symptoms suggestive of tuberculosis develop (e.g. persistent cough, weight loss and fever).
- Hypersensitivity reactions Hypersensitivity reactions (including fever, chest pain, hypotension, hypertension, dyspnoea, transient visual loss, pruritus, urticaria, serum sickness-like reactions, angioedema, anaphylaxis) reported during or within 1–2 hours after infusion (risk greatest during first or second infusion or in patients who discontinue other immunosuppressants). Manufacturer advises prophylactic antipyretics, antihistamines, or hydrocortisone may be administered.

- **INTERACTIONS** → Appendix 1: monoclonal antibodies
- **SIDE-EFFECTS**
- **Common or very common** Abscess · alopecia · anaemia · arrhythmias · arthralgia · chest pain · chills · constipation · decreased leucocytes · depression · diarrhoea · dizziness · dyspnoea · eye inflammation · fatigue · fever · gastrointestinal discomfort · gastrointestinal disorders · haemorrhage · headache · hepatic disorders · hyperhidrosis · hypertension · hypotension · increased risk of infection · infusion related reaction · insomnia · lymphadenopathy · myalgia · nausea · neutropenia · oedema · pain · palpitations · respiratory disorders · sensation abnormal · sepsis · skin reactions · vasodilation · vertigo
- **Uncommon** Anxiety · cheilitis · cholecystitis · confusion · drowsiness · healing impaired · heart failure · hypersensitivity · lupus-like syndrome · lymphocytosis · memory loss · neoplasms · nerve disorders · pancreatitis · peripheral ischaemia · pulmonary oedema · seborrhoea · seizure · syncope · thrombocytopenia · thrombophlebitis
- **Rare or very rare** Agranulocytosis · circulatory collapse · cyanosis · demyelinating disorders · granuloma · haemolytic anaemia · hepatitis B reactivation · meningitis · pancytopenia · pericardial effusion · sarcoidosis · severe cutaneous adverse reactions (SCARs) · transverse myelitis · vasculitis · vasospasm
- **Frequency not known** Bone fracture · dermatomyositis exacerbated · hepatosplenic T-cell lymphoma (increased risk in inflammatory bowel disease) · myocardial infarction · myocardial ischaemia · ulcerative colitis aggravated · vision loss

- **CONCEPTION AND CONTRACEPTION** Manufacturer advises adequate contraception during and for at least 6 months after last dose.
- **PREGNANCY** Use only if essential.
- **BREAST FEEDING** Amount probably too small to be harmful.
- **PRE-TREATMENT SCREENING**
  Tuberculosis Manufacturer advises patients should be evaluated for tuberculosis before treatment.
- **MONITORING REQUIREMENTS**
  - Monitor for infection before, during, and for 6 months after treatment.
  - All patients should be observed carefully for 1–2 hours after infusion and resuscitation equipment should be available for immediate use (risk of hypersensitivity reactions).
  - Monitor for symptoms of delayed hypersensitivity if re-administered after a prolonged period.
  - Manufacturer advises periodic skin examination for non-melanoma skin cancer, particularly in patients with risk factors.
- **DIRECTIONS FOR ADMINISTRATION** For *intravenous infusion* reconstitute each 100-mg vial of powder with 10 mL Water for Injections; to dissolve, gently swirl vial without shaking; allow to stand for 5 minutes; dilute required dose with Sodium Chloride 0.9% to a final volume of 250 mL and give through a low protein-binding filter (1.2 micron or less) over at least 2 hours; start infusion within 3 hours of reconstitution.
- **PRESCRIBING AND DISPENSING INFORMATION** Infliximab is a biological medicine. Biological medicines must be prescribed and dispensed by brand name, see *Biological*

medicines and *Biosimilar medicines*, under Guidance on prescribing p. 1.

- **PATIENT AND CARER ADVICE**

Tuberculosis Patients and carers should be advised to seek medical attention if symptoms suggestive of tuberculosis (e.g. persistent cough, weight loss, and fever) develop.

Blood disorders Patients and carers should be advised to seek medical attention if symptoms suggestive of blood disorders (such as fever, sore throat, bruising, or bleeding) develop.

Hypersensitivity reactions Patients and carers should be advised to keep Alert card with them at all times and seek medical advice if symptoms of delayed hypersensitivity develop.

Alert card An alert card should be provided.

- **NATIONAL FUNDING/ACCESS DECISIONS**

NICE decisions

▸ **Infliximab for Crohn's disease (May 2010)** NICE TA187

In children over 6 years of age, infliximab is recommended for the treatment of severe active Crohn's disease that has not responded to conventional therapy (including corticosteroids and other drugs affecting the immune response, and primary nutrition therapy) or when conventional therapy cannot be used because of intolerance or contra-indications.

Infliximab should be given as a planned course of treatment for 12 months or until treatment failure, whichever is shorter. Treatment should be continued beyond 12 months only if there is evidence of active disease—in these cases the need for treatment should be reviewed at least annually. If the disease relapses after stopping treatment, infliximab can be restarted.

www.nice.org.uk/guidance/ta187

▸ **Infliximab, adalimumab and golimumab for treating moderately to severely active ulcerative colitis after the failure of conventional therapy (February 2015)** NICE TA329

Infliximab is an option for treating severely active ulcerative colitis in children aged 6–17 years whose disease has responded inadequately to conventional therapy including corticosteroids and mercaptopurine or azathioprine, or who are intolerant to or have contra-indications for conventional therapies.

Infliximab should be given as a planned course of treatment until treatment fails (including the need for surgery) or until 12 months after starting treatment, whichever is shorter. Treatment should be continued only if there is clear evidence of a response. Patients who continue treatment should be reassessed every 12 months to determine whether ongoing treatment is still clinically appropriate.

www.nice.org.uk/guidance/ta329

- **MEDICINAL FORMS** There can be variation in the licensing of different medicines containing the same drug.

Powder for solution for infusion

CAUTIONARY AND ADVISORY LABELS 10

- Flixabi (Biogen Idec Ltd) ▼
  Infliximab 100 mg Flixabi 100mg powder for concentrate for solution for infusion vials | 1 vial PoM £377.00 (Hospital only)
- Inflectra (Pfizer Ltd)
  Infliximab 100 mg Inflectra 100mg powder for concentrate for solution for infusion vials | 1 vial PoM £377.66 (Hospital only)
- Remicade (Merck Sharp & Dohme Ltd)
  Infliximab 100 mg Remicade 100mg powder for concentrate for solution for infusion vials | 1 vial PoM £419.62 (Hospital only)
- Remsima (Napp Pharmaceuticals Ltd)
  Infliximab 100 mg Remsima 100mg powder for concentrate for solution for infusion vials | 1 vial PoM £377.66 (Hospital only)
- Zessly (Sandoz Ltd) ▼
  Infliximab 100 mg Zessly 100mg powder for concentrate for solution for infusion vials | 1 vial PoM £377.66 (Hospital only)

1.3 Irritable bowel syndrome

Irritable bowel syndrome 24-Feb-2016

Description of condition

Irritable bowel syndrome (IBS) is a gastrointestinal disorder characterised by abdominal pain or discomfort that may be relieved by defaecation. It can also be associated with the passage of mucus, bloating, and disordered defaecation; either diarrhoea, constipation, or alternating diarrhoea and constipation. Constipation presents with straining, urgency, and a sensation of incomplete evacuation. Before a diagnosis of IBS is made, the symptoms should be present at least once per week for at least 2 months and other potential pathological causes of the symptoms should be excluded. IBS symptoms are often aggravated by psychological factors, such as anxieties, emotional stress, and fear.

Aims of treatment

Treatment of IBS is focused on symptom control in order to improve quality of life, including minimising abdominal pain and normalising the frequency and consistency of stools.

Non-drug treatment

EvGr There is no evidence of the effectiveness of any form of dietary advice or increased fibre intake in children and it is not known whether dietary advice recommended to adult patients is of benefit to children. (A)

EvGr Eating regularly, limiting fresh fruit intake, and, reducing intake of 'resistant starch' and insoluble fibre (e.g. bran) can be recommended. If an increase in dietary fibre is required, soluble fibre such as oats, ispaghula husk p. 45, or sterculia p. 46 can be recommended. Ensuring a sufficient intake of fluids can also be recommended. (E)

Drug treatment

EvGr Clinicians should only prescribe drugs for children with IBS in cases of severe symptoms that have not responded to non-drug approaches. Treatment options include laxatives, antimotility drugs or antispasmodic drugs. (A)

EvGr A laxative can be used to treat abdominal pain if the underlying cause is suspected to be constipation. An osmotic laxative, such as a macrogol or lactulose p. 46, is preferred; lactulose may cause flatulence during the first few days of treatment. Loperamide hydrochloride p. 54 may relieve diarrhoea and antispasmodic drugs may relieve pain. (E)

ANTISPASMODICS

Mebeverine with ispaghula husk

19-May-2020

The properties listed below are those particular to the combination only. For the properties of the components please consider, mebeverine hydrochloride p. 69, ispaghula husk p. 45.

- **INDICATIONS AND DOSE**

Irritable bowel syndrome

▸ BY MOUTH

▸ Child 12–17 years: 1 sachet twice daily, in water, morning and evening, 30 minutes before food and 1 sachet daily if required, taken 30 minutes before midday meal

- **DIRECTIONS FOR ADMINISTRATION** Contents of one sachet should be stirred into a glass (approx. 150 mL) of cold water and drunk immediately.

- **PATIENT AND CARER ADVICE** Patients or carers should be given advice on how to administer ispaghula husk with mebeverine granules.

- **MEDICINAL FORMS** There can be variation in the licensing of different medicines containing the same drug.

Effervescent granules

CAUTIONARY AND ADVISORY LABELS 13, 22
EXCIPIENTS: May contain Aspartame
ELECTROLYTES: May contain Potassium

- Fybogel Mebeverine (Reckitt Benckiser Healthcare (UK) Ltd)
  Mebeverine hydrochloride 135 mg, Ispaghula husk
  3.5 gram Fybogel Mebeverine effervescent granules sachets orange sugar-free | 10 sachet [P] £5.44 DT = £5.44

Peppermint oil

19-May-2020

- **INDICATIONS AND DOSE**

COLPERMIN®

Relief of abdominal colic and distension, particularly in irritable bowel syndrome

- BY MOUTH
- Child 15–17 years: 1–2 capsules 3 times a day for up to 3 months if necessary, capsule to be swallowed whole with water

- **CAUTIONS** Sensitivity to menthol
- **INTERACTIONS** → Appendix 1: peppermint
- **SIDE-EFFECTS** Ataxia · bradycardia · gastrointestinal discomfort · gastrooesophageal reflux disease · headache · nausea · paraesthesia · rash erythematous · tremor · vomiting
- **PREGNANCY** Not known to be harmful.
- **BREAST FEEDING** Significant levels of menthol in breast milk unlikely.
- **DIRECTIONS FOR ADMINISTRATION** Capsules should not be broken or chewed because peppermint oil may irritate mouth or oesophagus.

- **MEDICINAL FORMS** There can be variation in the licensing of different medicines containing the same drug.

Modified-release capsule

CAUTIONARY AND ADVISORY LABELS 5, 22, 25
EXCIPIENTS: May contain Arachis (peanut) oil

- Colpermin (Johnson & Johnson Ltd)
  Peppermint oil 200 microlitre Colpermin gastro-resistant modified-release capsules | 20 capsule [GSL] £3.77 | 100 capsule [GSL] £14.33 DT = £14.33

1.4 Short bowel syndrome

Short bowel syndrome

31-Aug-2016

Description of condition

Children with a shortened bowel due to large surgical resection (with or without stoma formation) may require medical management to ensure adequate absorption of nutrients and fluid. Absorption of oral medication is also often impaired.

Aims of treatment

The management of short bowel syndrome focuses on ensuring adequate nutrition and drug absorption, thereby reducing the risk of complications resulting from these effects.

Drug treatment

Nutritional deficiencies

[EvGr] Children with a short bowel may require replacement of vitamins and minerals depending on the extent and position of the bowel resection. Deficiencies in vitamins A, B_{12}, D, E, and K, essential fatty acids, zinc and selenium can occur.

Hypomagnesaemia is common and is treated with oral or intravenous magnesium supplementation (see Magnesium imbalance p. 644), though administration of oral magnesium may cause diarrhoea. Occasionally the use of oral alfacalcidol p. 680 and correction of sodium depletion may be useful. Nutritional support can range from oral supplements to parenteral nutrition, depending on the severity of intestinal failure. ⟨A⟩

Diarrhoea and high output stomas

Diarrhoea is a common symptom of short bowel syndrome and can be due to multiple factors. [EvGr] The use of oral rehydration salts can be considered in order to promote adequate hydration. Oral intake influences the volume of stool passed, so reducing food intake will lessen diarrhoea, but will also exacerbate the problems of undernutrition. A child may require parenteral nutrition to allow them to eat less if the extent of diarrhoea is unacceptable.

Pharmacological treatment may be necessary, with the choice of drug depending on the potential for side-effects and the degree of resection. ⟨A⟩

Antimotility drugs

[EvGr] Loperamide hydrochloride p. 54 reduces intestinal motility and thus exerts antidiarrhoeal actions. Loperamide hydrochloride is preferred over other antimotility drugs as it is not sedative and does not cause dependence or fat malabsorption. High doses of loperamide hydrochloride [unlicensed] may be required in children with a short bowel due to disrupted enterohepatic circulation and a rapid gastro-intestinal transit time.

Co-phenotrope p. 53 has traditionally been used alone or in combination with other medications to help decrease faecal output. Co-phenotrope crosses the blood–brain barrier and can produce central nervous system side-effects, which may limit its use; the potential for dependence and anticholinergic effects may also restrict its use. ⟨A⟩

Colestyramine

[EvGr] In children with an intact colon and less than 100 cm of ileum resected, colestyramine p. 136 can be used to bind the unabsorbed bile salts, which reduces diarrhoea. When colestyramine is given to these children, it is important to monitor for evidence of fat malabsorption (steatorrhoea) or fat-soluble vitamin deficiencies. ⟨A⟩

Antisecretory drugs

[EvGr] Drugs that reduce gastric acid secretion reduce jejunostomy output. Omeprazole p. 63 is readily absorbed in the duodenum and upper small bowel, but if less than 50 cm of jejunum remains, it may need to be given intravenously. Use of a proton pump inhibitor alone does not eliminate the need for further intervention for fluid control (such as antimotility agents, intravenous fluids, or oral rehydration salts). ⟨A⟩

Growth factors

Growth factors can be used to facilitate intestinal adaptation after surgery in children with short bowel syndrome, thus enhancing fluid, electrolyte, and micronutrient absorption.

Teduglutide p. 41 is an analogue of endogenous human glucagon-like peptide 2 (GLP-2) which is licensed for use in the management of short bowel syndrome in children aged one year and over. It may be considered after a period of stabilisation following surgery, during which intravenous fluids and nutritional support should have been optimised.

Drug absorption

For *Prescribing in children with stoma* see Stoma care p. 78.

EvGr Many drugs are incompletely absorbed by children with a short bowel and may need to be prescribed in much higher doses than usual (such as levothyroxine, warfarin, oral contraceptives, and digoxin) or may need to be given intravenously. (A)

Several factors can alter the absorption of drugs taken by mouth in children with a compromised gastrointestinal system. The most important factors are the length of intestine available for drug absorption, and which section has been removed. The small intestine, with its large surface area and high blood flow, is the most important site of drug absorption. The larger the amount of the small intestine that has been removed, the higher the possibility that drug absorption will be affected. Other factors such as gastric emptying and gastric transit time also affect drug handling.

EvGr Enteric-coated and modified-release preparations are unsuitable for use in patients with short bowel syndrome, particularly in children with an ileostomy, as there may not be sufficient release of the active ingredient.

Dosage forms with quick dissolution (such as soluble tablets) should be used. Uncoated tablets and liquid formulations may also be suitable. (A) EvGr Before prescribing liquid formulations, prescribers should consider the osmolarity, excipient content, and volume required. Hyperosmolar liquids and some excipients (such as sorbitol) can result in fluid loss. The calorie density of oral supplements should also be considered, as it will influence the volume to be taken. (E)

AMINO ACIDS AND DERIVATIVES

Teduglutide

29-Apr-2020

- **DRUG ACTION** Teduglutide is an analogue of human glucagon-like peptide-2 (GLP-2), which preserves mucosal integrity by promoting growth and repair of the intestine.

- **INDICATIONS AND DOSE**

Short bowel syndrome (initiated under specialist supervision)

▸ BY SUBCUTANEOUS INJECTION

▸ Child 1–17 years: 0.05 mg/kg once daily, dose to be administered to alternating quadrants of the abdomen; alternatively the thigh can be used, for optimal injection volume per body weight and when to review treatment, consult product literature

- **CONTRA-INDICATIONS** Active or suspected malignancy · history of gastro-intestinal malignancy (in previous 5 years)
- **CAUTIONS** Abrupt withdrawal of parenteral support (reduce gradually with concomitant monitoring of fluid status) · cardiac insufficiency · cardiovascular disease · colo-rectal polyps · hypertension

CAUTIONS, FURTHER INFORMATION

▸ Colo-rectal polyps Manufacturer advises faecal occult blood testing before initiation of treatment and yearly thereafter; colonoscopy or sigmoidoscopy should be performed if unexplained blood in stool. Manufacturer also advises colonoscopy or sigmoidoscopy after 1 year of treatment and then every 5 years thereafter.

- **SIDE-EFFECTS**

▸ **Common or very common** Anxiety · appetite decreased · congestive heart failure · cough · dyspnoea · fluid imbalance · gallbladder disorders · gastrointestinal discomfort · gastrointestinal disorders · gastrointestinal stoma complication · headache · influenza like illness · insomnia · nausea · pancreatitis · peripheral oedema · respiratory tract infection · vomiting

▸ **Uncommon** Syncope

- **ALLERGY AND CROSS-SENSITIVITY** Manufacturer advises caution in patients with tetracycline hypersensitivity.
- **PREGNANCY** EvGr Specialist sources indicate use if necessary—no human data available. (D)
- **BREAST FEEDING** Manufacturer advises avoid—toxicity in *animal* studies.
- **RENAL IMPAIRMENT**

Dose adjustments Manufacturer advises use half the daily dose in moderate or severe impairment and end-stage renal disease.

- **MONITORING REQUIREMENTS** Manufacturer advises monitoring of small bowel function, gall bladder, bile ducts and pancreas during treatment.
- **TREATMENT CESSATION** Caution when discontinuing treatment—risk of dehydration.
- **PATIENT AND CARER ADVICE** Patients with cardiovascular disease should seek medical attention if they notice sudden weight gain, swollen ankles or dyspnoea—may indicate increased fluid absorption.
- **NATIONAL FUNDING/ACCESS DECISIONS**

Scottish Medicines Consortium (SMC) decisions

SMC No. 1139/16

The *Scottish Medicines Consortium* has advised (April 2018) that teduglutide (*Revestive*®) is accepted for restricted use within NHS Scotland for the treatment of short bowel syndrome, initiated in paediatric patients aged 1 to 17 years. Patients should be stable following a period of intestinal adaptation after surgery. This advice is contingent upon the continuing availability of the patient access scheme in NHS Scotland or a list price that is equivalent or lower.

- **MEDICINAL FORMS** There can be variation in the licensing of different medicines containing the same drug.

Powder and solvent for solution for injection

▸ Revestive (Shire Pharmaceuticals Ltd) ▼

Teduglutide 1.25 mg Revestive 1.25mg powder and solvent for solution for injection vials | 28 vial PoM £7,307.70

Teduglutide 5 mg Revestive 5mg powder and solvent for solution for injection vials | 28 vial PoM £14,615.39

2 Constipation and bowel cleansing

2.1 Bowel cleansing

Other drugs used for Bowel cleansing Bisacodyl, p. 50 · Docusate sodium, p. 49 · Magnesium sulfate, p. 646

DIAGNOSTIC AGENTS > RADIOGRAPHIC CONTRAST MEDIA

Meglumine amidotrizoate with sodium amidotrizoate

(Diatrizoates)

- **DRUG ACTION** Meglumine amidotrizoate with sodium amidotrizoate is a radiological contrast medium with high osmolality.

- **INDICATIONS AND DOSE**

Uncomplicated meconium ileus

▸ BY RECTUM

▸ Neonate: 15–30 mL for 1 dose.

continued →

Distal intestinal obstruction syndrome in children with cystic fibrosis

- BY MOUTH, OR BY RECTUM
- Child 1–23 months: 15–30 mL for 1 dose
- Child (body-weight 15–25 kg): 50 mL for 1 dose
- Child (body-weight 26 kg and above): 100 mL for 1 dose

Radiological investigations

- Child: Dose to be recommended by radiologist

- UNLICENSED USE Not licensed for use in distal intestinal obstruction syndrome.
- CONTRA-INDICATIONS Hyperthyroidism
- CAUTIONS Asthma · benign nodular goitre · dehydration · electrolyte disturbance (correct first) · enteritis · history of allergy · in children with oesophageal fistulae (aspiration may lead to pulmonary oedema) · latent hyperthyroidism · risk of anaphylactoid reactions increased by concomitant administration of beta-blockers
- SIDE-EFFECTS

GENERAL SIDE-EFFECTS Abdominal pain · cardiac arrest · consciousness impaired · diarrhoea · dizziness · dyspnoea · electrolyte imbalance · face oedema · fever · fluid imbalance · gastrointestinal disorders · headache · hyperhidrosis · hypersensitivity · hyperthyroidism · hypotension · nausea · pneumonia aspiration · pulmonary oedema · respiratory disorders · shock · skin reactions · tachycardia · toxic epidermal necrolysis · vomiting

SPECIFIC SIDE-EFFECTS

- With oral use Oral blistering

- ALLERGY AND CROSS-SENSITIVITY Hypersensitivity to iodine.
- PREGNANCY Manufacturer advises caution.
- BREAST FEEDING Amount probably too small to be harmful.
- DIRECTIONS FOR ADMINISTRATION Intravenous prehydration is essential in neonates and infants. Fluid intake should be encouraged for 3 hours after administration. *By mouth*, for child bodyweight under 25 kg, dilute *Gastrografin*® with 3 times its volume of water or fruit juice; for child bodyweight over 25 kg, dilute *Gastrografin*® with twice its volume of water or fruit juice. *By rectum*, administration must be carried out slowly under radiological supervision to ensure required site is reached. For child under 5 years, dilute *Gastrografin*® with 5 times its volume of water; for child over 5 years dilute *Gastrografin*® with 4 times its volume of water.

- MEDICINAL FORMS There can be variation in the licensing of different medicines containing the same drug.

Oral solution

EXCIPIENTS: May contain Disodium edetate

- Gastrografin (Bayer Plc)
Sodium amidotrizoate 100 mg per 1 ml, Meglumine amidotrizoate 660 mg per 1 ml Gastrografin oral solution sugar-free | 1000 ml [P] £175.00 DT = £175.00

LAXATIVES > OSMOTIC LAXATIVES

Citric acid with magnesium carbonate

16-Mar-2020

(Formulated as a bowel cleansing preparation)

- INDICATIONS AND DOSE

Bowel evacuation for surgery, colonoscopy or radiological examination

- BY MOUTH
- Child 5–9 years: One-third of a sachet to be given at 8 a.m. the day before the procedure and, one-third of a sachet to be given between 2 and 4 p.m. the day before the procedure
- Child 10–17 years: 0.5–1 sachet, given at 8 a.m. the day before the procedure and 0.5–1 sachet, given between 2 and 4 p.m. the day before the procedure

- CONTRA-INDICATIONS Acute intestinal or gastric ulceration · acute severe colitis · gastric retention · gastro-intestinal obstruction · gastro-intestinal perforation · toxic megacolon
- CAUTIONS Debilitated · hypovolaemia (should be corrected before administration of bowel cleansing preparations) · patients with fluid and electrolyte disturbances

CAUTIONS, FURTHER INFORMATION Adequate hydration should be maintained during treatment.

- INTERACTIONS → Appendix 1: bowel cleansing preparations
- SIDE-EFFECTS
  - **Common or very common** Gastrointestinal discomfort · nausea · vomiting
  - **Uncommon** Dehydration · dizziness · electrolyte imbalance · headache

SIDE-EFFECTS, FURTHER INFORMATION Abdominal pain is usually transient and can be reduced by taking preparation more slowly.

- PREGNANCY Use with caution.
- BREAST FEEDING Use with caution.
- RENAL IMPAIRMENT Avoid if estimated glomerular filtration rate less than 30 mL/minute/1.73 m^2—risk of hypermagnesaemia.
- MONITORING REQUIREMENTS Renal function should be measured before starting treatment in patients at risk of fluid and electrolyte disturbances.
- DIRECTIONS FOR ADMINISTRATION One sachet should be reconstituted with 200 mL of hot water; the solution should be allowed to cool for approx. 30 minutes before drinking.
- PRESCRIBING AND DISPENSING INFORMATION Reconstitution of one sachet containing 11.57 g magnesium carbonate and 17.79 g anhydrous citric acid produces a solution containing magnesium citrate with 118 mmol Mg^{2+}.

Flavours of oral powders may include lemon and lime.

- PATIENT AND CARER ADVICE Low residue or fluid only diet (e.g. water, fruit squash, clear soup, black tea or coffee) recommended before procedure (according to prescriber's advice) and copious intake of clear fluids recommended until procedure. Patient or carers should be given advice on how to administer oral powder.

- MEDICINAL FORMS There can be variation in the licensing of different medicines containing the same drug.

Effervescent powder

CAUTIONARY AND ADVISORY LABELS 13, 10

ELECTROLYTES: May contain Magnesium

- Citramag (Sanochemia Diagnostics UK Ltd)
Magnesium carbonate heavy 11.57 gram, Citric acid anhydrous 17.79 gram Citramag effervescent powder sachets sugar-free | 10 sachet [P] £20.50 DT = £20.50

Macrogol 3350 with anhydrous sodium sulfate, potassium chloride, sodium bicarbonate and sodium chloride

10-Mar-2020

(Formulated as a bowel cleansing preparation)

● **INDICATIONS AND DOSE**

Bowel cleansing before radiological examination, colonoscopy, or surgery

▶ INITIALLY BY MOUTH

▸ Child 12–17 years: Initially 2 litres daily for 2 doses: first dose of reconstituted solution taken on the evening before procedure and the second dose on the morning of procedure, alternatively (by mouth) initially 250 mL every 10–15 minutes, reconstituted solution to be administered, alternatively (by nasogastric tube) initially 20–30 mL/minute, starting on the day before procedure until 4 litres have been consumed

Distal intestinal obstruction syndrome

▶ BY MOUTH, OR BY NASOGASTRIC TUBE, OR BY GASTROSTOMY TUBE

▸ Child 1–17 years: 10 mL/kilogram/hour for 30 minutes, then increased to 20 mL/kilogram/hour for 30 minutes, then increased if tolerated to 25 mL/kilogram/hour, max. 100 mL/kg (or 4 litres) over 4 hours, repeat 4 hour treatment if necessary

● **UNLICENSED USE** *Klean-Prep®* not licensed for use in children.

● **CONTRA-INDICATIONS** Acute severe colitis · gastric retention · gastro-intestinal obstruction · gastro-intestinal perforation · toxic megacolon

● **CAUTIONS** Colitis · debilitated patients · fluid and electrolyte disturbances · heart failure (avoid if moderate to severe) · hypovolaemia (should be corrected before administration of bowel cleansing preparations) · impaired gag reflex or possibility of regurgitation or aspiration

● **INTERACTIONS** → Appendix 1: bowel cleansing preparations

● **SIDE-EFFECTS** Angioedema · arrhythmia · chills · confusion · dehydration · dizziness · dyspnoea · electrolyte imbalance · fever · flatulence · gastrointestinal discomfort · headache · malaise · nausea · palpitations · seizure · skin reactions · thirst · vomiting

SIDE-EFFECTS, FURTHER INFORMATION Abdominal pain is usually transient and can be reduced by taking preparation more slowly.

● **PREGNANCY** Manufacturers advise use only if essential—no information available.

● **BREAST FEEDING** Manufacturers advise use only if essential—no information available.

● **MONITORING REQUIREMENTS** Renal function should be measured before starting treatment in patients at risk of fluid and electrolyte disturbances.

● **DIRECTIONS FOR ADMINISTRATION** 1 sachet should be reconstituted with 1 litre of water. Flavouring such as clear fruit cordials may be added if required. After reconstitution the solution should be kept in a refrigerator and discarded if unused after 24 hours.

● **PRESCRIBING AND DISPENSING INFORMATION** Each *Klean-Prep®* sachet provides Na^+ 125 mmol, K^+ 10 mmol, Cl^- 35 mmol and HCO^{3-} 20mmol when reconstituted with 1 litre of water.

● **PATIENT AND CARER ADVICE** Solid food should not be taken for 2 hours before starting treatment. Adequate hydration should be maintained during treatment. Treatment can be stopped if bowel motions become watery and clear.

● **MEDICINAL FORMS** There can be variation in the licensing of different medicines containing the same drug.

Powder

CAUTIONARY AND ADVISORY LABELS 10, 13

EXCIPIENTS: May contain Aspartame

ELECTROLYTES: May contain Bicarbonate, chloride, potassium, sodium

▸ Klean-Prep (Forum Health Products Ltd)
Potassium chloride 742.5 mg, Sodium chloride 1.465 gram, Sodium bicarbonate 1.685 gram, Sodium sulfate anhydrous 5.685 gram, Polyethylene glycol 3350 59 gram Klean-Prep oral powder 69g sachets sugar-free | 4 sachet [P] £10.48

LAXATIVES › STIMULANT LAXATIVES

Magnesium citrate with sodium picosulfate

13-Mar-2020

(Formulated as a bowel cleansing preparation)

● **INDICATIONS AND DOSE**

PICOLAX® SACHETS

Bowel evacuation on day before radiological procedure, endoscopy, or surgery

▶ BY MOUTH

▸ Child 1 year: 0.25 sachet taken before 8 a.m, then 0.25 sachet after 6–8 hours

▸ Child 2–3 years: 0.5 sachet taken before 8 a.m, then 0.5 sachet after 6–8 hours

▸ Child 4–8 years: 1 sachet taken before 8 a.m, then 0.5 sachet after 6–8 hours

▸ Child 9–17 years: 1 sachet taken before 8 a.m, then 1 sachet after 6–8 hours

PHARMACOKINETICS

▸ For *Picolax®*: Acts within 3 hours of first dose.

● **CONTRA-INDICATIONS** Acute severe colitis · ascites · congestive cardiac failure · gastric retention · gastro-intestinal obstruction · gastro-intestinal perforation · gastro-intestinal ulceration · toxic megacolon

● **CAUTIONS** Cardiac disease · children · colitis · debilitated patients · fluid and electrolyte disturbances (avoid in severe dehydration or hypermagnesaemia) · hypovolaemia (should be corrected before administration) · recent gastro-intestinal surgery

● **SIDE-EFFECTS**

▶ **Common or very common** Gastrointestinal discomfort · headache · nausea

▶ **Uncommon** Confusion · electrolyte imbalance · gastrointestinal disorders · seizures · skin reactions · vomiting

● **PREGNANCY** Caution.

● **BREAST FEEDING** Caution.

● **HEPATIC IMPAIRMENT** Avoid in hepatic coma if risk of renal failure.

● **RENAL IMPAIRMENT** Avoid if estimated glomerular filtration rate less than 30 mL/minute/1.73 m^2—risk of hypermagnesaemia.

● **DIRECTIONS FOR ADMINISTRATION** One sachet of sodium picosulfate with magnesium citrate powder should be reconstituted with 150 mL (approx. half a glass) of cold water; patients should be warned that heat is generated during reconstitution and that the solution should be allowed to cool before drinking.

PICOLAX® SACHETS One sachet should be reconstituted with 150 mL (approx. half a glass) of cold water.

● **PRESCRIBING AND DISPENSING INFORMATION** Flavours of oral powder formulations may include lemon.

PICOLAX® SACHETS One reconstituted sachet contains K^+ 5 mmol and Mg^{2+} 87 mmol.

- PATIENT AND CARER ADVICE Low residue diet recommended on the day before procedure and copious intake of water or other clear fluids recommended during treatment. Patients and carers should be given advice on how to administer oral powder; they should be warned that heat is generated during reconstitution and that the solution should be allowed to cool before drinking.

- MEDICINAL FORMS There can be variation in the licensing of different medicines containing the same drug.

Powder

CAUTIONARY AND ADVISORY LABELS 10, 13

ELECTROLYTES: May contain Magnesium, potassium

▸ Picolax (Ferring Pharmaceuticals Ltd)

Sodium picosulfate 10 mg, Magnesium oxide 3.5 gram, Citric acid anhydrous 12 gram Picolax oral powder 16.1g sachets sugar-free | 2 sachet [P] £3.39

2.2 Constipation

Constipation

06-Jun-2017

Description of condition

Constipation is defaecation that is unsatisfactory because of infrequent stools, difficult stool passage, or seemingly incomplete defaecation. It can occur at any age and is common in childhood.

Overview

Before prescribing laxatives it is important to be sure that the child *is* constipated and that the constipation is not secondary to an underlying undiagnosed complaint. Early identification of constipation and effective treatment can improve outcomes for children. Without early diagnosis and treatment, an acute episode of constipation can lead to anal fissure and become chronic. In children with secondary constipation caused by a drug, the drug should be reviewed.

Laxatives

Bulk-forming laxatives

Bulk-forming laxatives include bran, ispaghula husk p. 45, methylcellulose p. 45 and sterculia p. 46. They are of particular value in children with small hard stools if fibre cannot be increased in the diet. [EvGr] They relieve constipation by increasing faecal mass, which stimulates peristalsis; children and their carers should be advised that the full effect may take some days to develop. Adequate fluid intake must be maintained to avoid intestinal obstruction, though this may be difficult for children. (A)

Methylcellulose, ispaghula husk and sterculia may be used in patients who cannot tolerate bran. Methylcellulose also acts as a faecal softener.

Stimulant laxative

Stimulant laxatives include bisacodyl p. 50, sodium picosulfate p. 52, and members of the anthraquinone group, senna p. 52, co-danthramer p. 50 and co-danthrusate p. 51. Stimulant laxatives increase intestinal motility and often cause abdominal cramp; they should be avoided in intestinal obstruction.

The use of co-danthramer and co-danthrusate is limited to constipation in terminally ill patients because of potential carcinogenicity (based on animal studies) and evidence of genotoxicity.

Docusate sodium p. 49 is believed to act as both a stimulant laxative and as a faecal softener (below). Glycerol suppositories act as a lubricant and as a rectal stimulant by virtue of the mildly irritant action of glycerol.

Faecal softeners

Faecal softeners are claimed to act by decreasing surface tension and increasing penetration of intestinal fluid into the faecal mass. Docusate sodium, and glycerol suppositories p. 51 have softening properties. Enemas containing arachis oil p. 49 (ground-nut oil, peanut oil) lubricate and soften impacted faeces and promote a bowel movement. Liquid paraffin has also been used as a lubricant for the passage of stool but manufacturer advises that it should be used with caution because of its adverse effects, which include anal seepage and the risks of granulomatous disease of the gastro-intestinal tract or of lipoid pneumonia on aspiration.

Osmotic laxatives

Osmotic laxatives increase the amount of water in the large bowel, either by drawing fluid from the body into the bowel or by retaining the fluid they were administered with.

Lactulose p. 46 is a semi-synthetic disaccharide which is not absorbed from the gastro-intestinal tract. It produces an osmotic diarrhoea of low faecal pH, and discourages the proliferation of ammonia-producing organisms. It is therefore useful in the treatment of hepatic encephalopathy.

Macrogols (such as macrogol 3350 with potassium chloride, sodium bicarbonate and sodium chloride p. 47) are inert polymers of ethylene glycol which sequester fluid in the bowel; giving fluid with macrogols may reduce the dehydrating effect sometimes seen with osmotic laxatives.

Macrogols are an effective non-traumatic means of evacuation in children with faecal impaction and can be used in the long-term management of chronic constipation.

Bowel cleansing preparations

Bowel cleansing preparations are used before colonic surgery, colonoscopy, or radiological examination to ensure the bowel is free of solid contents; examples include macrogol 3350 with anhydrous sodium sulfate, potassium chloride, sodium bicarbonate and sodium chloride p. 43, citric acid with magnesium carbonate p. 42, magnesium citrate with sodium picosulfate p. 43 and sodium acid phosphate with sodium phosphate p. 48. Bowel cleansing preparations are not treatments for constipation.

Management

[EvGr] The first-line treatment for children with constipation requires the use of a laxative in combination with dietary modification or with behavioural interventions. Diet modification alone is not recommended as first-line treatment.

In children, an increase in dietary fibre, adequate fluid intake and exercise is advised. Diet should be balanced and contain fruits, vegetables, high-fibre bread, baked beans and wholegrain breakfast cereals. Unprocessed bran (which may cause bloating and flatulence and reduces the absorption of micronutrients) is **not** recommended.

If faecal impaction is not present (or has been treated), the child should be treated promptly with a laxative. A macrogol (such as macrogol 3350 with potassium chloride, sodium bicarbonate and sodium chloride) is preferred as first-line management. If the response is inadequate, add a stimulant laxative or change to a stimulant laxative if the first-line therapy is not tolerated. If stools remain hard, lactulose or another laxative with softening effects, such as docusate sodium can be added.

In children with chronic constipation, laxatives should be continued for several weeks after a regular pattern of bowel movements or toilet training is established. The dose of laxatives should then be tapered gradually, over a period of months, according to response. Some children may require laxative therapy for several years.

A shorter duration of laxative treatment may be possible in some children with a short history of constipation.

Laxatives should be administered at a time that produces an effect that is likely to fit in with the child's toilet routine. (A)

Faecal impaction

EvGr Treatment of faecal impaction may initially increase symptoms of soiling and abdominal pain. In children over 1 year of age with faecal impaction, an oral preparation containing a macrogol (such as macrogol 3350 with potassium chloride, sodium bicarbonate and sodium chloride) is used to clear faecal mass and to establish and maintain soft well-formed stools, using an escalating dose regimen depending on symptoms and response. If disimpaction does not occur after 2 weeks, a stimulant laxative can be added or if stools are hard, used in combination with an osmotic laxative such as lactulose. Long-term regular use of laxatives is essential to maintain well-formed stools and prevent recurrence of faecal impaction; intermittent use may provoke relapses.

Suppositories and enemas should not be used in primary care unless all oral medications have failed and preferably only then following specialist advice. If the impacted mass is not expelled following treatment with macrogols and a stimulant laxative, a sodium citrate enema p. 49 can be administered. Although rectal administration of laxatives may be effective, this route is frequently distressing for the child and may lead to persistence of withholding. A sodium acid phosphate with sodium phosphate enema may be administered under specialist supervision if disimpaction does not occur after a sodium citrate enema. Manual evacuation under anaesthetic may be necessary if disimpaction does not occur after oral and rectal treatment, or if the child is afraid. Children undergoing disimpaction should be reviewed within one week. Maintenance treatment should be started as soon as the bowel is disimpacted. (A)

Useful Resources

Constipation in children and young People: Diagnosis and management of idiopathic childhood constipation in primary and secondary care. National Institute for Health and Care Excellence. Clinical guideline 99. May 2010.
www.nice.org.uk/guidance/cg99

LAXATIVES > BULK-FORMING LAXATIVES

Ispaghula husk

09-Mar-2020

- **DRUG ACTION** Bulk-forming laxatives relieve constipation by increasing faecal mass which stimulates peristalsis.

- **INDICATIONS AND DOSE**

Constipation

▶ BY MOUTH

▶ Child 1 month–5 years: 2.5–5 mL twice daily, dose to be taken only when prescribed by a doctor, as half or whole level spoonful in water, preferably after meals, morning and evening

▶ Child 6–11 years: 2.5–5 mL twice daily, dose to be given as a half or whole level spoonful in water, preferably after meals, morning and evening

▶ Child 12–17 years: 1 sachet twice daily, dose to be given in water preferably after meals, morning and evening

Constipation (dose approved for use by community practitioner nurse prescribers)

▶ BY MOUTH

▶ Child 6–11 years: 2.5–5 mL twice daily, dose to be given as a half or whole level spoonful in water, preferably after meals, morning and evening

▶ Child 12–17 years: 1 sachet twice daily, dose to be given in water preferably after meals, morning and evening

DOSE EQUIVALENCE AND CONVERSION

▶ 1 sachet equivalent to 2 level 5 ml spoonsful.

- **CONTRA-INDICATIONS** Colonic atony · faecal impaction · intestinal obstruction · reduced gut motility · sudden change in bowel habit that has persisted more than two weeks · undiagnosed rectal bleeding
- **CAUTIONS** Adequate fluid intake should be maintained to avoid oesophageal or intestinal obstruction
- **SIDE-EFFECTS** Abdominal distension · bronchospasm · conjunctivitis · gastrointestinal disorders · hypersensitivity · rhinitis · skin reactions
- **DIRECTIONS FOR ADMINISTRATION** Dose to be taken with at least 150 mL liquid.
- **PRESCRIBING AND DISPENSING INFORMATION** Flavours of soluble granules formulations may include plain, lemon, or orange.
- **HANDLING AND STORAGE** Ispaghula husk contains potent allergens. Individuals exposed to the product (including those handling the product) can develop hypersensitivity reactions such as rhinitis, conjunctivitis, bronchospasm and in some cases, anaphylaxis.
- **PATIENT AND CARER ADVICE** Manufacturer advises that preparations that swell in contact with liquid should always be carefully swallowed with water and should not be taken immediately before going to bed. Patients and their carers should be advised that the full effect may take some days to develop and should be given advice on how to administer ispaghula husk.

- **MEDICINAL FORMS** There can be variation in the licensing of different medicines containing the same drug.

Effervescent granules

CAUTIONARY AND ADVISORY LABELS 13

EXCIPIENTS: May contain Aspartame

▶ **Fybogel** (Reckitt Benckiser Healthcare (UK) Ltd)

Ispaghula husk 3.5 gram Fybogel 3.5g effervescent granules sachets plain SF sugar-free | 30 sachet GSL £2.83 DT = £2.83
Fybogel Orange 3.5g effervescent granules sachets SF sugar-free | 30 sachet GSL £2.83 DT = £2.83
Fybogel Lemon 3.5g effervescent granules sachets SF sugar-free | 30 sachet GSL £2.83 DT = £2.83

▶ **Fybogel Hi-Fibre** (Reckitt Benckiser Healthcare (UK) Ltd)

Ispaghula husk 3.5 gram Fybogel Hi-Fibre Orange 3.5g effervescent granules sachets sugar-free | 10 sachet GSL £2.26 sugar-free | 30 sachet GSL £4.85 DT = £2.83
Fybogel Hi-Fibre Lemon 3.5g effervescent granules sachets sugar-free | 10 sachet GSL £2.26

▶ **Ispagel** (Bristol Laboratories Ltd)

Ispaghula husk 3.5 gram Ispagel Orange 3.5g effervescent granules sachets sugar-free | 10 sachet GSL £1.92 sugar-free | 30 sachet GSL £2.45 DT = £2.83

Granules

CAUTIONARY AND ADVISORY LABELS 13

EXCIPIENTS: May contain Aspartame

▶ **Ispaghula husk (Non-proprietary)**

Ispaghula husk 3.5 gram Ispaghula husk 3.5g granules sachets gluten free | 30 sachet GSL £2.83

Combinations available: *Senna with ispaghula husk*, p. 52

Methylcellulose

10-Mar-2020

- **DRUG ACTION** Bulk-forming laxatives relieve constipation by increasing faecal mass which stimulates peristalsis.

- **INDICATIONS AND DOSE**

Constipation | Diarrhoea

▶ BY MOUTH USING TABLETS

▶ Child 7–11 years: 2 tablets twice daily

▶ Child 12–17 years: 3–6 tablets twice daily

- **UNLICENSED USE** No age limit specified by manufacturer.
- **CONTRA-INDICATIONS** Colonic atony · difficulty in swallowing · faecal impaction · infective bowel disease · intestinal obstruction · severe dehydration
- **CAUTIONS** Adequate fluid intake should be maintained to avoid oesophageal or intestinal obstruction

CAUTIONS, FURTHER INFORMATION It may be necessary to supervise debilitated patients or those with intestinal narrowing or decreased motility to ensure adequate fluid intake.

- SIDE-EFFECTS Abdominal distension · gastrointestinal disorders
- DIRECTIONS FOR ADMINISTRATION In constipation the dose should be taken with at least 300 mL liquid. In diarrhoea, ileostomy, and colostomy control, avoid liquid intake for 30 minutes before and after dose.
- PATIENT AND CARER ADVICE Patients and their carers should be advised that the full effect may take some days to develop. Preparations that swell in contact with liquid should always be carefully swallowed with water and should not be taken immediately before going to bed.

- MEDICINAL FORMS There can be variation in the licensing of different medicines containing the same drug.

Tablet

- Celevac (Advanz Pharma)
  Methylcellulose "450" 500 mg Celevac 500mg tablets | 112 tablet GSL £3.22 DT = £3.22

Sterculia

10-Mar-2020

- DRUG ACTION Sterculia is a bulk-forming laxative. It relieves constipation by increasing faecal mass which stimulates peristalsis.

- INDICATIONS AND DOSE

Constipation

- BY MOUTH
- Child 6–11 years: 0.5–1 sachet 1–2 times a day, alternatively, half to one heaped 5-mL spoonful once or twice a day; washed down without chewing with plenty of liquid after meals
- Child 12–17 years: 1–2 sachets 1–2 times a day, alternatively, one to two heaped 5-mL spoonfuls once or twice a day; washed down without chewing with plenty of liquid after meals

- CONTRA-INDICATIONS Colonic atony · difficulty swallowing · faecal impaction · intestinal obstruction
- CAUTIONS Adequate fluid intake should be maintained to avoid oesophageal or intestinal obstruction

CAUTIONS, FURTHER INFORMATION It may be necessary to supervise debilitated patients or those with intestinal narrowing or decreased motility to ensure adequate fluid intake.

- SIDE-EFFECTS Diarrhoea · gastrointestinal discomfort · gastrointestinal disorders · nausea
- DIRECTIONS FOR ADMINISTRATION May be mixed with soft food (e.g. yoghurt) before swallowing, followed by plenty of liquid.
- PATIENT AND CARER ADVICE Patients and their carers should be advised that the full effect may take some days to develop. Preparations that swell in contact with liquid should always be carefully swallowed with water and should not be taken immediately before going to bed.

- MEDICINAL FORMS There can be variation in the licensing of different medicines containing the same drug.

Granules

CAUTIONARY AND ADVISORY LABELS 25, 27

- Normacol (Forum Health Products Ltd)
  Sterculia 620 mg per 1 gram Normacol granules 7g sachets | 60 sachet GSL £6.67 DT = £6.67
  Normacol granules | 500 gram GSL £7.92 DT = £7.92

Sterculia with frangula

The properties listed below are those particular to the combination only. For the properties of the components please consider, sterculia above.

- INDICATIONS AND DOSE

Constipation

- BY MOUTH
- Child 6–11 years: 0.5–1 sachet 1–2 times a day, alternatively, 0.5–1 heaped 5-mL spoonful once or twice a day; washed down without chewing with plenty of liquid after meals
- Child 12–17 years: 1–2 sachets 1–2 times a day, alternatively, 1–2 heaped 5 mL spoonfuls once or twice a day; washed down without chewing with plenty of liquid after meals

- PREGNANCY Manufacturer advises avoid.
- BREAST FEEDING Manufacturer advises avoid.
- PATIENT AND CARER ADVICE Patients and their carers should be advised that the full effect may take some days to develop. Preparations that swell in contact with liquid should always be carefully swallowed with water and should not be taken immediately before going to bed.

- MEDICINAL FORMS There can be variation in the licensing of different medicines containing the same drug.

Granules

- Normacol Plus (Forum Health Products Ltd)
  Frangula 80 mg per 1 gram, Sterculia 620 mg per 1 gram Normacol Plus granules 7g sachets | 60 sachet GSL £7.12 DT = £7.12
  Normacol Plus granules | 500 gram GSL £8.45 DT = £8.45

LAXATIVES > OSMOTIC LAXATIVES

Lactulose

10-Mar-2020

- INDICATIONS AND DOSE

Constipation

- BY MOUTH
- Child 1–11 months: 2.5 mL twice daily, adjusted according to response
- Child 1–4 years: 2.5–10 mL twice daily, adjusted according to response
- Child 5–17 years: 5–20 mL twice daily, adjusted according to response

Hepatic encephalopathy (portal systemic encephalopathy)

- BY MOUTH
- Child 12–17 years: Adjusted according to response to 30–50 mL 3 times a day, subsequently adjusted to produce 2–3 soft stools per day

Constipation (dose approved for use by community practitioner nurse prescribers)

- BY MOUTH
- Child 1–11 months: 2.5 mL twice daily, adjusted according to response
- Child 1–4 years: 5 mL twice daily, adjusted according to response
- Child 5–10 years: 10 mL twice daily, adjusted according to response
- Child 11–17 years: Initially 15 mL twice daily, adjusted according to response

PHARMACOKINETICS

- Lactulose may take up to 48 hours to act.

- UNLICENSED USE Not licensed for use in children for hepatic encephalopathy.
- CONTRA-INDICATIONS Galactosaemia · gastro-intestinal obstruction · gastro-intestinal perforation · risk of gastro-intestinal perforation

- **CAUTIONS** Lactose intolerance
- **SIDE-EFFECTS**
  - **Common or very common** Abdominal pain · diarrhoea · flatulence · nausea · vomiting
  - **Uncommon** Electrolyte imbalance
- **PREGNANCY** Not known to be harmful.
- **PATIENT AND CARER ADVICE**
  Medicines for Children leaflet: Lactulose for constipation www.medicinesforchildren.org.uk/lactulose-constipation

---

- **MEDICINAL FORMS** There can be variation in the licensing of different medicines containing the same drug.

Oral solution

- Lactulose (Non-proprietary)
  Lactulose 666.667 mg per 1 ml Lactulose 10g/15ml oral solution 15ml sachets sugar-free | 10 sachet [P] £2.51 DT = £2.51
  Lactulose 10g/15ml oral solution 15ml sachets unflavoured sugar-free | 10 sachet [P] £2.50 DT = £2.51
  Lactulose 10g/15ml oral solution 15ml sachets plum sugar-free | 10 sachet [P] £2.60 DT = £2.51
  Lactulose 680 mg per 1 ml Lactulose 3.1-3.7g/5ml oral solution | 300 ml [P] £1.37–£5.50 | 500 ml [P] £6.50 DT = £2.90
- Duphalac (Mylan)
  Lactulose 680 mg per 1 ml Duphalac 3.35g/5ml oral solution | 200 ml [P] £1.92 | 300 ml [P] £2.88 | 500 ml [P] £4.80 DT = £2.90

Macrogol 3350 with potassium chloride, sodium bicarbonate and sodium chloride

18-Apr-2018

- **INDICATIONS AND DOSE**

Chronic constipation (dose for 'paediatric' sachets) | Prevention of faecal impaction (dose for 'paediatric' sachets)

- BY MOUTH
  - Child 1–11 months: 0.5–1 sachet daily
  - Child 12–23 months: 1 sachet daily, adjust dose to produce regular soft stools; maximum 4 sachets per day
  - Child 2–5 years: 1 sachet daily, adjust dose to produce regular soft stools; maximum 4 sachets per day
  - Child 6–11 years: 2 sachets daily, adjust dose to produce regular soft stools; maximum 4 sachets per day

Faecal impaction (dose for 'paediatric' sachets)

- BY MOUTH
  - Child 1–11 months: 0.5–1 sachet daily
  - Child 12–23 months: 2 sachets on first day, then 4 sachets daily for 2 days, then 6 sachets daily for 2 days, then 8 sachets daily, total daily dose to be taken over a 12-hour period, after disimpaction, switch to maintenance laxative therapy
  - Child 2–4 years: 2 sachets on first day, then 4 sachets daily for 2 days, then 6 sachets daily for 2 days, then 8 sachets daily, total daily dose to be taken over a 12-hour period, after disimpaction, switch to maintenance laxative therapy
  - Child 5–11 years: 4 sachets on first day, then increased in steps of 2 sachets daily, total daily dose to be taken over a 12-hour period, after disimpaction, switch to maintenance laxative therapy; maximum 12 sachets per day

Chronic constipation (dose for 'half-strength' sachets)

- BY MOUTH
  - Child 12–17 years: 2–6 sachets daily in divided doses usually for up to 2 weeks; maintenance 2–4 sachets daily

Faecal impaction (dose for 'half-strength' sachets)

- BY MOUTH
  - Child 12–17 years: 8 sachets on first day, then increased in steps of 4 sachets daily, total daily dose to be drunk within a 6 hour period, after disimpaction, switch to maintenance laxative therapy if required; maximum 16 sachets per day

Chronic constipation (dose for 'full-strength' sachets)

- BY MOUTH
  - Child 12–17 years: 1–3 sachets daily in divided doses usually for up to 2 weeks; maintenance 1–2 sachets daily

Faecal impaction (dose for 'full-strength' sachets)

- BY MOUTH
  - Child 12–17 years: 4 sachets on first day, then increased in steps of 2 sachets daily, total daily dose to be drunk within a 6 hour period, after disimpaction, switch to maintenance laxative therapy if required; maximum 8 sachets per day

DOSE EQUIVALENCE AND CONVERSION

- Each 'paediatric' sachet contains 6.563 g of macrogol 3350; each 'half-strength' sachet contains 6.563 g of macrogol 3350; each 'full-strength' sachet contains 13.125 g of macrogol 3350.

MOVICOL® READY TO TAKE SACHETS

Chronic constipation

- BY MOUTH
  - Child 12–17 years: 1–3 sachets daily in divided doses usually for up to 2 weeks; maintenance 1–2 sachets daily

Faecal impaction

- BY MOUTH
  - Child 12–17 years: 4 sachets on first day, then increased in steps of 2 sachets daily, total daily dose to be drunk within a 6 hour period; patients should also take an additional 1 litre of fluid daily, after disimpaction, switch to maintenance laxative therapy if required; maximum 8 sachets per day

MOVICOL® LIQUID

Chronic constipation

- BY MOUTH
  - Child 12–17 years: 25 mL 1–3 times a day usually for up to 2 weeks; maintenance 25 mL 1–2 times a day

- **UNLICENSED USE** Macrogol 3350 with potassium chloride, sodium bicarbonate and sodium chloride may be used as detailed below, although these situations are considered outside the scope of its licence:
  - [EvGr] chronic constipation/prevention of faecal impaction in children aged under 2 years;
  - dose for chronic constipation/prevention of faecal impaction in children aged 6 years;
  - faecal impaction in children aged under 5 years;
  - dose titration schedule for faecal impaction in children aged 12–17 years ⟨A⟩.
- **CONTRA-INDICATIONS** Intestinal obstruction · intestinal perforation · paralytic ileus · severe inflammatory conditions of the intestinal tract (including Crohn's disease, ulcerative colitis and toxic megacolon) · use of 'paediatric' sachets for faecal impaction in impaired cardiovascular function (no information available)
- **CAUTIONS** Cardiovascular impairment (should not take more than 2 'full-strength' sachets or 4 'half-strength' sachets in any one hour) · impaired consciousness (with high doses) · impaired gag reflex (with high doses) · reflux oesophagitis (with high doses)
- **SIDE-EFFECTS** Electrolyte imbalance (discontinue if symptoms occur) · flatulence · gastrointestinal discomfort · nausea · vomiting
- **PREGNANCY** Manufacturers advise may be used—limited data available.
- **RENAL IMPAIRMENT** Manufacturers advise avoid use of 'paediatric' sachets for faecal impaction—no information available.

- **DIRECTIONS FOR ADMINISTRATION** Manufacturers advise dissolve contents of each 'half-strength' sachet of oral powder in 62.5 mL of water, and each 'full-strength' sachet of oral powder in 125 mL of water; after reconstitution the solution should be kept in a refrigerator—for further information consult product literature.
  Manufacturers advise dissolve contents of each 'paediatric' sachet of oral powder in 62.5 mL of water; after reconstitution the solution should be kept in a refrigerator—for further information consult product literature.
  MOVICOL® LIQUID Manufacturer advises dilute 25 mL of oral concentrate with 100 mL of water; after dilution the solution should be discarded if unused after 24 hours.
- **PATIENT AND CARER ADVICE** Patients or carers should be counselled on how to take the oral powder and oral solution.
  Medicines for Children leaflet: Movicol for constipation www.medicinesforchildren.org.uk/movicol-constipation

- **MEDICINAL FORMS** There can be variation in the licensing of different medicines containing the same drug.

Oral solution

CAUTIONARY AND ADVISORY LABELS 13
ELECTROLYTES: May contain Bicarbonate, chloride, potassium, sodium

- Movicol (Forum Health Products Ltd)
  Macrogol '3350' 105 gram per 1 litre, Potassium 5.4 mmol per 1 litre, Bicarbonate 17 mmol per 1 litre, Chloride 53 mmol per 1 litre, Sodium 65 mmol per 1 litre Movicol Liquid sugar-free | 500 ml [P] £5.41 DT = £5.41
  Macrogol '3350' 13.125 gram, Potassium 27 mmol per 1 litre, Bicarbonate 85 mmol per 1 litre, Chloride 267 mmol per 1 litre, Sodium 325 mmol per 1 litre Movicol Ready to Take oral solution 25ml sachets sugar-free | 30 sachet [P] £7.72 DT = £7.72

Powder

CAUTIONARY AND ADVISORY LABELS 10, 13
ELECTROLYTES: May contain Bicarbonate, chloride, potassium, sodium

- Macrogol 3350 with potassium chloride, sodium bicarbonate and sodium chloride (Non-proprietary)
  Macrogol '3350' 105 gram per 1 litre, Potassium 5.4 mmol per 1 litre, Bicarbonate 17 mmol per 1 litre, Chloride 53 mmol per 1 litre, Sodium 65 mmol per 1 litre Macrogol compound oral powder sachets sugar-free | 20 sachet [P] £2.47–£4.45 sugar-free | 30 sachet [P] £6.68 DT = £3.71
  Macrogol compound oral powder sachets plain sugar-free | 20 sachet [P] £3.11 sugar-free | 30 sachet [P] £3.76 DT = £3.71
  Macrogol compound oral powder sachets citrus sugar-free | 30 sachet [P] £4.38 DT = £3.71
- CosmoCol (Stirling Anglian Pharmaceuticals Ltd)
  Macrogol '3350' 105 gram per 1 litre, Potassium 5.4 mmol per 1 litre, Bicarbonate 17 mmol per 1 litre, Chloride 53 mmol per 1 litre, Sodium 65 mmol per 1 litre CosmoCol Paediatric oral powder 6.9g sachets sugar-free | 30 sachet [PoM] £2.99 DT = £4.38
  CosmoCol Orange Flavour oral powder sachets sugar-free | 20 sachet [P] £2.75 sugar-free | 30 sachet [P] £3.95 DT = £3.71
  CosmoCol Lemon and Lime Flavour oral powder sachets sugar-free | 20 sachet [P] £2.75 sugar-free | 30 sachet [P] £3.95 DT = £3.71
  CosmoCol Orange Lemon and Lime oral powder sachets sugar-free | 30 sachet [P] £3.95 DT = £3.71
  CosmoCol Plain oral powder sachets sugar-free | 30 sachet [P] £3.95 DT = £3.71
- Laxido (Galen Ltd)
  Macrogol '3350' 105 gram per 1 litre, Potassium 5.4 mmol per 1 litre, Bicarbonate 17 mmol per 1 litre, Chloride 53 mmol per 1 litre, Sodium 65 mmol per 1 litre Laxido Orange oral powder sachets sugar-free | 20 sachet [P] £2.75 sugar-free | 30 sachet [P] £3.95 DT = £3.71
  Laxido Paediatric Plain oral powder 6.9g sachets sugar-free | 30 sachet [PoM] £2.99 DT = £4.38
- Molaxole (Mylan)
  Macrogol '3350' 105 gram per 1 litre, Potassium 5.4 mmol per 1 litre, Bicarbonate 17 mmol per 1 litre, Chloride 53 mmol per 1 litre, Sodium 65 mmol per 1 litre Molaxole oral powder sachets sugar-free | 20 sachet [P] £3.78 sugar-free | 30 sachet [P] £5.68 DT = £3.71
- Movicol (Forum Health Products Ltd, Norgine Pharmaceuticals Ltd)
  Macrogol '3350' 105 gram per 1 litre, Potassium 5.4 mmol per 1 litre, Bicarbonate 17 mmol per 1 litre, Chloride 53 mmol per 1 litre, Sodium 65 mmol per 1 litre Movicol Chocolate oral powder 13.9g sachets sugar-free | 30 sachet [P] £8.11 DT = £3.71
  Movicol Paediatric Plain oral powder 6.9g sachets sugar-free | 30 sachet [PoM] £4.38 DT = £4.38
  Movicol oral powder 13.8g sachets lemon & lime sugar-free | 20 sachet [P] £5.41 sugar-free | 30 sachet [P] £8.11 DT = £3.71 sugar-free | 50 sachet [P] £13.49
  Movicol Paediatric Chocolate oral powder 6.9g sachets sugar-free | 30 sachet [PoM] £4.38 DT = £4.38
  Movicol Plain oral powder 13.7g sachets sugar-free | 30 sachet [P] £8.11 DT = £3.71 sugar-free | 50 sachet [P] £13.49

Magnesium hydroxide

09-Mar-2020

- **INDICATIONS AND DOSE**

Constipation

▶ BY MOUTH

- Child 3–11 years: 5–10 mL as required, dose to be given mixed with water at bedtime
- Child 12–17 years: 30–45 mL as required, dose to be given mixed with water at bedtime

- **CONTRA-INDICATIONS** Acute gastro-intestinal conditions
- **CAUTIONS** Debilitated patients
- **INTERACTIONS** → Appendix 1: magnesium
- **HEPATIC IMPAIRMENT** Avoid in hepatic coma if risk of renal failure.
- **RENAL IMPAIRMENT** Increased risk of toxicity in renal impairment.
  Dose adjustments Avoid or reduce dose.
- **PRESCRIBING AND DISPENSING INFORMATION** When prepared extemporaneously, the BP states Magnesium Hydroxide Mixture, BP consists of an aqueous suspension containing about 8% hydrated magnesium oxide.

- **MEDICINAL FORMS** There can be variation in the licensing of different medicines containing the same drug.

Oral suspension

- Magnesium hydroxide (Non-proprietary)
  Magnesium hydroxide 79 mg per 1 ml Magnesium hydroxide 7.45-8.35% oral suspension BP | 500 ml [GSL] £5.31
  Magnesium hydroxide 80 mg per 1 ml Magnesium hydroxide 8% oral suspension | 500 ml [GSL] £8.05 DT = £8.05
- Brands may include Phillips' Milk of Magnesia

Sodium acid phosphate with sodium phosphate

17-Mar-2020

- **INDICATIONS AND DOSE**

Constipation (using Phosphates Enema BP Formula B) | Bowel evacuation before abdominal radiological procedures, endoscopy, and surgery (using Phosphates Enema BP Formula B)

▶ BY RECTUM

- Child 3–6 years: 45–65 mL once daily
- Child 7–11 years: 65–100 mL once daily
- Child 12–17 years: 100–128 mL once daily

Constipation, using Phosphates Enema BP Formula B (dose approved for use by community practitioner nurse prescribers)

▶ BY RECTUM

- Child 3–17 years: Reduced according to body-weight

Constipation, using Phosphates Enema (Cleen Ready-to-Use) (dose approved for use by community practitioner nurse prescribers)

▶ BY RECTUM

- Child 3–11 years: On doctor's advice only

- Child 12-17 years: 118 mL

FLEET ® READY-TO-USE ENEMA

Constipation | Bowel evacuation before abdominal radiological procedures | Bowel evacuation before endoscopy | Bowel evacuation before surgery

- BY RECTUM
- Child 3-6 years: 40–60 mL once daily
- Child 7-11 years: 60–90 mL once daily
- Child 12-17 years: 90–118 mL once daily

- CONTRA-INDICATIONS Conditions associated with increased colonic absorption · gastro-intestinal obstruction · inflammatory bowel disease
- CAUTIONS Ascites · congestive heart failure · debilitated patients · fluid and electrolyte disturbances · uncontrolled hypertension
- INTERACTIONS → Appendix 1: bowel cleansing preparations
- SIDE-EFFECTS
- **Rare or very rare** Chills · dehydration · electrolyte imbalance · gastrointestinal discomfort · metabolic acidosis · nausea · pain · vomiting
- RENAL IMPAIRMENT Use with caution.
- PRESCRIBING AND DISPENSING INFORMATION When prepared extemporaneously, the BP states Phosphates Enema BP Formula B consists of sodium dihydrogen phosphate dihydrate 12.8 g, disodium phosphate dodecahydrate 10.24 g, purified water, freshly boiled and cooled, to 128 mL.

- MEDICINAL FORMS There can be variation in the licensing of different medicines containing the same drug.

Enema

- Sodium acid phosphate with sodium phosphate (Non-proprietary)
  Disodium hydrogen phosphate dodecahydrate 80 mg per 1 ml, Sodium dihydrogen phosphate dihydrate 100 mg per 1 ml Phosphates enema (Formula B) 128ml long tube | 1 enema [P] £27.93 DT = £27.93
  Phosphates enema (Formula B) 128ml standard tube | 1 enema [P] £27.93 DT = £27.93
- Fleet Ready-to-use (Casen Recordati S.L.)
  Disodium hydrogen phosphate dodecahydrate 80 mg per 1 ml, Sodium dihydrogen phosphate dihydrate 181 mg per 1 ml Cleen Ready-to-use 133ml enema | 1 enema [P] £1.95 DT = £1.95

Sodium citrate

18-May-2020

- INDICATIONS AND DOSE

Constipation (dose approved for use by community practitioner nurse prescribers)

- BY RECTUM
- Child 3-17 years: 5 mL for 1 dose

MICOLETTE ®

Constipation

- BY RECTUM
- Child 3-17 years: 5–10 mL for 1 dose

MICRALAX ®

Constipation

- BY RECTUM
- Child 3-17 years: 5 mL for 1 dose

RELAXIT ®

Constipation

- BY RECTUM
- Child 1 month-2 years: 5 mL for 1 dose, insert only half the nozzle length
- Child 3-17 years: 5 mL for 1 dose

- CONTRA-INDICATIONS Acute gastro-intestinal conditions
- CAUTIONS Sodium and water retention in susceptible individuals
- INTERACTIONS → Appendix 1: sodium citrate
- SIDE-EFFECTS Polyuria

- MEDICINAL FORMS There can be variation in the licensing of different medicines containing the same drug.

Enema

- Micolette Micro-enema (Pinewood Healthcare)
  Sodium citrate 90 mg per 1 ml Micolette Micro-enema 5ml | 12 enema [P] £4.50
- Micralax Micro-enema (RPH Pharmaceuticals AB)
  Sodium citrate 90 mg per 1 ml Micralax Micro-enema 5ml | 12 enema [P] £4.87
- Relaxit (Supra Enterprises Ltd)
  Sodium citrate 90 mg per 1 ml Relaxit Micro-enema 5ml | 12 enema £5.21

LAXATIVES > SOFTENING LAXATIVES

Arachis oil

09-Mar-2020

- INDICATIONS AND DOSE

To soften impacted faeces

- BY RECTUM
- Child 3-6 years (under close medical supervision): 45–65 mL as required
- Child 7-11 years (under close medical supervision): 65–100 mL as required
- Child 12-17 years (under close medical supervision): 100–130 mL as required

- UNLICENSED USE Licensed for use in children (age range not specified by manufacturer).
- CONTRA-INDICATIONS Inflammatory bowel disease (except under medical supervision)
- CAUTIONS Hypersensitivity to soya · intestinal obstruction
- ALLERGY AND CROSS-SENSITIVITY Contra-indicated if history of hypersensitivity to arachis oil or peanuts.
- DIRECTIONS FOR ADMINISTRATION Warm enema in warm water before use.

- MEDICINAL FORMS There can be variation in the licensing of different medicines containing the same drug.

Enema

- Arachis oil (Non-proprietary)
  Arachis oil 1 ml per 1 ml Arachis oil 130ml enema | 1 enema [P] £47.50 DT = £47.50

Docusate sodium

16-Mar-2020

(Dioctyl sodium sulphosuccinate)

- INDICATIONS AND DOSE

Chronic constipation

- BY MOUTH
- Child 6-23 months: 12.5 mg 3 times a day, adjusted according to response, use paediatric oral solution
- Child 2-11 years: 12.5–25 mg 3 times a day, adjusted according to response, use paediatric oral solution
- Child 12-17 years: Up to 500 mg daily in divided doses, adjusted according to response
- BY RECTUM
- Child 12-17 years: 120 mg for 1 dose

Adjunct in abdominal radiological procedures

- BY MOUTH
- Child 12-17 years: 400 mg, to be administered with barium meal
- BY RECTUM
- Child 12-17 years: 120 mg for 1 dose

continued →

PHARMACOKINETICS
- Oral preparations act within 1–2 days; response to rectal administration usually occurs within 20 minutes.

- **UNLICENSED USE** *Adult oral solution and capsules* not licensed for use in children under 12 years.
- **CONTRA-INDICATIONS** Avoid in intestinal obstruction
- **CAUTIONS** Do not give with liquid paraffin · excessive use of stimulant laxatives can cause diarrhoea and related effects such as hypokalaemia · rectal preparations not indicated if haemorrhoids or anal fissure
- **INTERACTIONS** → Appendix 1: docusate sodium
- **SIDE-EFFECTS**
- **Rare or very rare**
- With oral use Abdominal cramps · nausea · rash
- **PREGNANCY** Not known to be harmful—manufacturer advises caution.
- **BREAST FEEDING**
- With oral use Manufacturer advises caution—present in milk following oral administration.
- With rectal use Rectal administration not known to be harmful.
- **DIRECTIONS FOR ADMINISTRATION** For administration *by mouth*, solution may be mixed with milk or squash.

- **MEDICINAL FORMS** There can be variation in the licensing of different medicines containing the same drug.

Oral solution
- Docusate sodium (Non-proprietary)
  Docusate sodium 2.5 mg per 1 ml Docusate 12.5mg/5ml oral solution sugar-free | 300 ml [P] £8.96 DT = £8.96
  Docusate sodium 10 mg per 1 ml Docusate 50mg/5ml oral solution sugar-free | 300 ml [P] £9.19 DT = £9.19
- Docusol (Typharm Ltd)
  Docusate sodium 2.5 mg per 1 ml Docusol Paediatric 12.5mg/5ml oral solution sugar-free | 125 ml [P] £4.46

Enema
- Norgalax (Essential Pharma Ltd)
  Docusate sodium 12 mg per 1 gram Norgalax 120mg/10g enema | 6 enema [P] £28.00 DT = £28.00

Capsule
- Dioctyl (UCB Pharma Ltd)
  Docusate sodium 100 mg Dioctyl 100mg capsules | 30 capsule [P] £2.09 DT = £2.09 | 100 capsule [P] £6.98

Combinations available: ***Co-danthrusate***, p. 51

LAXATIVES > STIMULANT LAXATIVES

Bisacodyl

16-Mar-2020

- **INDICATIONS AND DOSE**

Constipation
- BY MOUTH
- Child 4–17 years: 5–20 mg once daily, adjusted according to response, dose to be taken at night
- BY RECTUM
- Child 2–17 years: 5–10 mg once daily, adjusted according to response

Bowel clearance before radiological procedures and surgery
- INITIALLY BY MOUTH
- Child 4–9 years: 5 mg once daily for 2 days before procedure, dose to be taken at bedtime and (by rectum) 5 mg if required, dose to be administered 1 hour before procedure
- Child 10–17 years: 10 mg once daily for 2 days before procedure, dose to be taken at bedtime and (by rectum) 10 mg if required, dose to be administered 1 hour before procedure

Constipation (dose approved for use by community practitioner nurse prescribers)
- BY MOUTH
- Child 4–17 years: 5–20 mg once daily, adjusted according to response, dose to be taken at night (on doctor's advice only)
- BY RECTUM
- Child 4–9 years: 5 mg once daily, adjusted according to response
- Child 10–17 years: 10 mg once daily, dose to be taken in the morning

PHARMACOKINETICS
- Tablets act in 10–12 hours; suppositories act in 20–60 minutes.

- **UNLICENSED USE**
- With rectal use [EvGr] Bisacodyl may be used in children aged under 10 years for the management of constipation, ⟨A⟩ but the higher dose option is not licensed in this age group.
- With oral use [EvGr] Bisacodyl may be used in children for the management of constipation, ⟨A⟩ but the higher dose option is not licensed.
- **CONTRA-INDICATIONS** Acute abdominal conditions · acute inflammatory bowel disease · intestinal obstruction · severe dehydration
- **CAUTIONS** Excessive use of stimulant laxatives can cause diarrhoea and related effects such as hypokalaemia · prolonged use may harm intestinal function · risk of electrolyte imbalance with prolonged use
- **SIDE-EFFECTS**
- **Common or very common** Gastrointestinal discomfort · nausea
- **Uncommon** Haematochezia · vomiting
- **Rare or very rare** Angioedema · colitis · dehydration
- **PREGNANCY** May be suitable for constipation in pregnancy, if a stimulant effect is necessary.

- **MEDICINAL FORMS** There can be variation in the licensing of different medicines containing the same drug. Forms available from special-order manufacturers include: oral suspension, suppository

Gastro-resistant tablet
CAUTIONARY AND ADVISORY LABELS 5, 25
- Bisacodyl (Non-proprietary)
  Bisacodyl 5 mg Bisacodyl 5mg gastro-resistant tablets | 60 tablet [P] £5.66 DT = £2.86 | 100 tablet [P] £3.45–£5.60 | 500 tablet [P] £25.73–£50.00 | 1000 tablet [P] £51.45–£100.00
- Dulco-Lax (bisacodyl) (Sanofi)
  Bisacodyl 5 mg Dulcolax 5mg gastro-resistant tablets | 40 tablet [P] £2.44 | 100 tablet [P] £3.60

Suppository
- Bisacodyl (Non-proprietary)
  Bisacodyl 10 mg Bisacodyl 10mg suppositories | 12 suppository [P] £3.53 DT = £3.53
- Dulco-Lax (bisacodyl) (Sanofi)
  Bisacodyl 5 mg Dulcolax 5mg suppositories for children | 5 suppository [P] £1.04 DT = £1.04
  Bisacodyl 10 mg Dulcolax 10mg suppositories | 12 suppository [P] £2.35 DT = £3.53

Co-danthramer

16-Mar-2020

- **INDICATIONS AND DOSE**

Constipation in palliative care (standard strength capsules)
- BY MOUTH USING CAPSULES
- Child 6–11 years: 1 capsule once daily, dose should be taken at night
- Child 12–17 years: 1–2 capsules once daily, dose should be taken at night

Constipation in palliative care (strong capsules)
- ▶ BY MOUTH USING CAPSULES
- ▸ Child 12–17 years: 1–2 capsules once daily, dose should be given at night

Constipation in palliative care (standard strength suspension)
- ▶ BY MOUTH USING ORAL SUSPENSION
- ▸ Child 2–11 years: 2.5–5 mL once daily, dose should be taken at night
- ▸ Child 12–17 years: 5–10 mL once daily, dose should be taken at night

Constipation in palliative care (strong suspension)
- ▶ BY MOUTH USING ORAL SUSPENSION
- ▸ Child 12–17 years: 5 mL once daily, dose should be taken at night

DOSE EQUIVALENCE AND CONVERSION
- ▸ Co-danthramer (standard strength) capsules contain dantron 25 mg with poloxamer '188' 200 mg per capsule.
- ▸ Co-danthramer (standard strength) oral suspension contains dantron 25 mg with poloxamer '188' 200 mg per 5 mL.
- ▸ Co-danthramer **strong** capsules contain dantron 37.5 mg with poloxamer '188' 500 mg.
- ▸ Co-danthramer **strong** oral suspension contains dantron 75 mg with poloxamer '188' 1 g per 5 mL.
- ▸ Co-danthramer suspension 5 mL = one co-danthramer capsule, **but** strong co-danthramer suspension 5 mL = two strong co-danthramer capsules.

- **CONTRA-INDICATIONS** Acute abdominal conditions · acute inflammatory bowel disease · intestinal obstruction · severe dehydration
- **CAUTIONS** Excessive use of stimulant laxatives can cause diarrhoea and related effects such as hypokalaemia · may cause local irritation · *rodent* studies indicate potential carcinogenic risk

CAUTIONS, FURTHER INFORMATION
- ▸ Local irritation Avoid prolonged contact with skin (incontinent patients or infants wearing nappies—risk of irritation and excoriation).

- **SIDE-EFFECTS** Abdominal cramps · asthenia · gastrointestinal disorders · hypermagnesaemia · skin reactions · urine red
- **PREGNANCY** Manufacturers advise avoid—limited information available.
- **BREAST FEEDING** Manufacturers advise avoid—no information available.
- **PRESCRIBING AND DISPENSING INFORMATION**
  Palliative care For further information on the use of co-danthramer in palliative care, see www.medicinescomplete.com/#/content/palliative/stimulant-laxatives.

- **MEDICINAL FORMS** There can be variation in the licensing of different medicines containing the same drug.

Oral suspension

CAUTIONARY AND ADVISORY LABELS 14 (urine red)
- ▸ Co-danthramer (Non-proprietary)
  Dantron 5 mg per 1 ml, Poloxamer 188 40 mg per 1 ml Co-danthramer 25mg/200mg/5ml oral suspension sugar-free | 300 ml [PoM] £180.00 DT = £180.00
  Dantron 15 mg per 1 ml, Poloxamer 188 200 mg per 1 ml Co-danthramer 75mg/1000mg/5ml oral suspension sugar-free | 300 ml [PoM] £367.50 DT = £367.50

Co-danthrusate

16-Mar-2020

- **INDICATIONS AND DOSE**

Constipation in palliative care
- ▶ BY MOUTH USING ORAL SUSPENSION
- ▸ Child 6–11 years: 5 mL once daily, to be taken at night
- ▸ Child 12–17 years: 5–15 mL once daily, to be taken at night

DOSE EQUIVALENCE AND CONVERSION
- ▸ Co-danthrusate suspension contains dantron 50 mg and docusate sodium 60 mg per 5 mL.

- **CONTRA-INDICATIONS** Acute abdominal conditions · acute inflammatory bowel disease · intestinal obstruction · severe dehydration
- **CAUTIONS** Excessive use of stimulant laxatives can cause diarrhoea and related effects such as hypokalaemia · may cause local irritation · *rodent* studies indicate potential carcinogenic risk

CAUTIONS, FURTHER INFORMATION
- ▸ Local irritation Avoid prolonged contact with skin (incontinent patients—risk of irritation and excoriation).

- **INTERACTIONS** → Appendix 1: docusate sodium
- **SIDE-EFFECTS** Gastrointestinal disorders · skin reactions · urine orange
- **PREGNANCY** Manufacturers advise avoid—limited information available.
- **BREAST FEEDING** Manufacturers advise avoid—no information available.

- **MEDICINAL FORMS** There can be variation in the licensing of different medicines containing the same drug.

Oral suspension

CAUTIONARY AND ADVISORY LABELS 14 (urine orange)
- ▸ Co-danthrusate (Non-proprietary)
  Dantron 10 mg per 1 ml, Docusate sodium 12 mg per 1 ml Co-danthrusate 50mg/60mg/5ml oral suspension sugar-free | 200 ml [PoM] £202.50 DT = £202.50

Glycerol

10-Mar-2020

(Glycerin)

- **INDICATIONS AND DOSE**

Constipation
- ▶ BY RECTUM
- ▸ Child 1–11 months: 1 g as required
- ▸ Child 1–11 years: 2 g as required
- ▸ Child 12–17 years: 4 g as required

- **DIRECTIONS FOR ADMINISTRATION** Moisten suppositories with water before insertion.
- **PRESCRIBING AND DISPENSING INFORMATION** When prepared extemporaneously, the BP states Glycerol Suppositories, BP consists of gelatin 140 mg, glycerol 700 mg, purified water to 1 g.
- **PATIENT AND CARER ADVICE**
  Medicines for Children leaflet: Glycerin (glycerol) suppositories for constipation www.medicinesforchildren.org.uk/glycerin-glycerol-suppositories-constipation

- **MEDICINAL FORMS** There can be variation in the licensing of different medicines containing the same drug. Forms available from special-order manufacturers include: suppository

Suppository
- ▸ Glycerol (Non-proprietary)
  Glycerol 700 mg Glycerol 1g suppositories | 12 suppository [GSL] £1.75 DT = £1.67
  Glycerol 1400 mg Glycerol 2g suppositories | 12 suppository [GSL] £1.78 DT = £1.70
  Glycerol 2800 mg Glycerol 4g suppositories | 12 suppository [GSL] £1.31 DT = £1.29

1 Gastro-intestinal system

Senna

10-Mar-2020

- **DRUG ACTION** Senna is a stimulant laxative. After metabolism of sennosides in the gut the anthrone component stimulates peristalsis thereby increasing the motility of the large intestine.

- **INDICATIONS AND DOSE**

Constipation

▶ BY MOUTH USING TABLETS
- Child 2–3 years: 3.75–15 mg once daily, adjusted according to response
- Child 4–5 years: 3.75–30 mg once daily, adjusted according to response
- Child 6–17 years: 7.5–30 mg once daily, adjusted according to response

▶ BY MOUTH USING SYRUP
- Child 1 month–3 years: 3.75–15 mg once daily, adjusted according to response
- Child 4–17 years: 3.75–30 mg once daily, adjusted according to response

Constipation (dose approved for use by community practitioner nurse prescribers)

▶ BY MOUTH USING TABLETS
- Child 6–17 years: 7.5–30 mg once daily, adjusted according to response

▶ BY MOUTH USING SYRUP
- Child 2–3 years: 3.75–15 mg once daily, adjusted according to response
- Child 4–17 years: 3.75–30 mg once daily, adjusted according to response

PHARMACOKINETICS
- Onset of action 8–12 hours.

- **UNLICENSED USE** *Tablets* not licensed for use in children under 6 years. *Syrup* not licensed for use in children under 2 years.
  Doses in *BNFC* adhere to national guidelines and may differ from those in product literature.
- **CONTRA-INDICATIONS** Atony · intestinal obstruction · undiagnosed abdominal pain
- **SIDE-EFFECTS** Albuminuria · diarrhoea · electrolyte imbalance · fluid imbalance · gastrointestinal discomfort · haematuria · pseudomelanosis coli · skin reactions · urine discolouration

  SIDE-EFFECTS, FURTHER INFORMATION Prolonged or excessive use can cause hypokalaemia.
- **PREGNANCY** EvGr Specialist sources indicate suitable for use in pregnancy. ◇D◇
- **BREAST FEEDING** EvGr Specialist sources indicate suitable for use in breast-feeding in infants over 1 month. ◇D◇
- **PATIENT AND CARER ADVICE**
  Medicines for Children leaflet: Senna for constipation www.medicinesforchildren.org.uk/senna-constipation
- **NATIONAL FUNDING/ACCESS DECISIONS**
  NHS restrictions *Senokot*® tablets are not prescribable in NHS primary care.
- **EXCEPTIONS TO LEGAL CATEGORY** Senna is on sale to the public for use in children over 12 years; doses on packs may vary from those in BNF Publications.

- **MEDICINAL FORMS** There can be variation in the licensing of different medicines containing the same drug.

Oral solution
- Senokot (Forum Health Products Ltd, Reckitt Benckiser Healthcare (UK) Ltd)
  Sennoside B (as Sennosides) 1.5 mg per 1 ml Senokot 7.5mg/5ml Syrup Pharmacy sugar-free | 500 ml P £5.98 DT = £5.98
  Senokot 7.5mg/5ml syrup sugar-free

Tablet
- Senna (Non-proprietary)
  Sennoside B (as Sennosides) 7.5 mg Senna 7.5mg tablets | 20 tablet P £1.00 | 60 tablet P £2.11 DT = £2.09 | 100 tablet P £2.15
- Senokot (Reckitt Benckiser Healthcare (UK) Ltd, Forum Health Products Ltd)
  Sennoside B (as Sennosides) 15 mg Senokot Max Strength 15mg tablets | 24 tablet GSL £3.23 | 48 tablet GSL £5.69 DT = £5.69

Senna with ispaghula husk

23-Apr-2020

The properties listed below are those particular to the combination only. For the properties of the components please consider, senna above, ispaghula husk p. 45.

- **INDICATIONS AND DOSE**

Constipation

▶ BY MOUTH
- Child 12–17 years: 5–10 g once daily, to be taken at night, up to 2–3 times a week

DOSE EQUIVALENCE AND CONVERSION
- 5 g equivalent to one level spoonful of granules.

- **PREGNANCY** Manufacturer advises avoid during first trimester. To be used only intermittently and only if dietary and lifestyle changes fail.
- **DIRECTIONS FOR ADMINISTRATION** Take at night with at least 150 mL liquid.

- **MEDICINAL FORMS** There can be variation in the licensing of different medicines containing the same drug.

Granules

CAUTIONARY AND ADVISORY LABELS 25
EXCIPIENTS: May contain Sucrose
- Manevac (Mylan)
  Senna fruit 124 mg per 1 gram, Ispaghula 542 mg per 1 gram Manevac granules | 400 gram P £9.50 DT = £9.50

Sodium picosulfate

10-Mar-2020

(Sodium picosulphate)

- **DRUG ACTION** Sodium picosulfate is a stimulant laxative. After metabolism in the colon it stimulates the mucosa thereby increasing the motility of the large intestine.

- **INDICATIONS AND DOSE**

Constipation

▶ BY MOUTH
- Child 1 month–3 years: 2.5–10 mg once daily, adjusted according to response
- Child 4–17 years: 2.5–20 mg once daily, adjusted according to response

Constipation (dose approved for use by community practitioner nurse prescribers)

▶ BY MOUTH
- Child 1 month–3 years: 250 micrograms/kg once daily (max. per dose 5 mg), adjusted according to response, (on doctor's advice only); dose to be taken at night
- Child 4–10 years: 2.5–5 mg once daily, adjusted according to response, (on doctor's advice only); dose to be taken at night
- Child 11–17 years: 5–10 mg once daily, adjusted according to response, dose to be taken at night

PHARMACOKINETICS
- Onset of action 6–12 hours.

- **UNLICENSED USE** Sodium picosulfate doses in BNF Publications adhere to national guidelines and may differ from those in product literature.
- **CONTRA-INDICATIONS** Intestinal obstruction · undiagnosed abdominal pain

- **INTERACTIONS** → Appendix 1: sodium picosulfate
- **SIDE-EFFECTS**
  - **Common or very common** Diarrhoea · gastrointestinal discomfort
  - **Uncommon** Dizziness · nausea · vomiting
  - **Frequency not known** Angioedema · skin reactions · syncope

  SIDE-EFFECTS, FURTHER INFORMATION Prolonged or excessive use can cause diarrhoea and related effects such as hypokalaemia.
- **PREGNANCY** Manufacturer states evidence limited but not known to be harmful.
- **BREAST FEEDING** EvGr Specialist sources indicate suitable for use in breast-feeding in infants over 1 month—not known to be present in milk. ⟨D⟩
- **PATIENT AND CARER ADVICE**

  Medicines for Children leaflet: Sodium picosulfate for constipation www.medicinesforchildren.org.uk/sodium-picosulfate-constipation
- **MEDICINAL FORMS** There can be variation in the licensing of different medicines containing the same drug.

Oral solution

EXCIPIENTS: May contain Alcohol

- Sodium picosulfate (Non-proprietary)

  Sodium picosulfate 1 mg per 1 ml Sodium picosulfate 5mg/5ml oral solution sugar-free | 100 ml P £2.69 sugar-free | 300 ml P £8.08 DT = £8.08
- Laxoberal (Sanofi)

  Sodium picosulfate 1 mg per 1 ml Dulcolax Pico 5mg/5ml liquid sugar-free | 100 ml P £1.94 sugar-free | 300 ml P £4.62 DT = £8.08

3 Diarrhoea

Diarrhoea (acute)

01-Aug-2017

Description of condition

Diarrhoea is the abnormal passing of loose or liquid stools, with increased frequency, increased volume, or both. Acute diarrhoea is that which lasts less than 14 days, but symptoms usually spontaneously resolve within 2–4 days. It can result from infection, as a side-effect of a drug, or as an acute symptom of a chronic gastro-intestinal disorder (such as Inflammatory bowel disease p. 30 or Irritable bowel syndrome p. 39). It may also occur when intestinal motility or morphology is altered.

Prompt investigation is required to identify or exclude any serious underlying cause if the child has any red flag symptoms as such unexplained weight loss, rectal bleeding, persistent diarrhoea, a systemic illness, has received recent hospital treatment or antibiotic treatment, or following foreign travel (other than to Western Europe, North America, Australia or New Zealand).

Aims of treatment

The priority in acute diarrhoea treatment, as in gastro-enteritis, is the prevention or reversal of fluid and electrolyte depletion and the management of dehydration when it is present. This is particularly important in infants, when excessive water and electrolyte loss and dehydration can be life-threatening.

Treatment

Most episodes of acute diarrhoea will settle spontaneously without the need for any medical treatment. EvGr Oral rehydration therapy (ORT,) such as disodium hydrogen citrate with glucose, potassium chloride and sodium chloride p. 639; potassium chloride with sodium chloride p. 636; potassium chloride with rice powder, sodium chloride and sodium citrate p. 639) is the mainstay of treatment to prevent or correct diarrhoeal dehydration and to maintain the appropriate fluid intake once rehydration is achieved—see Fluids and electrolytes p. 631.

However, in children with severe dehydration and in those unable to drink, immediate admission to hospital and urgent replacement treatment with an intravenous rehydration fluid is recommended—see Fluids and electrolytes p. 631.

ORT is recommended for children at *increased risk of dehydration* and for those *with clinical dehydration* (including hypernatraemic dehydration). If the child is unable to drink the ORT, or vomits persistently, consider giving the solution via a nasogastric tube.

In infants, after rehydration, encourage breast-feeding, other milk feeds and fluid intake. In older children, after rehydration, give full-strength milk straight away, reintroduce the child's usual solid food, and avoid giving fruit juices and carbonated drinks until the diarrhoea has stopped.

In children with gastroenteritis, but *without clinical dehydration*, encourage fluid intake, continue breast-feeding and other milk feeds, and discourage the drinking of fruit juices and carbonated drinks.

In general, antidiarrhoeal drugs have no practical benefit for children with acute or persistent diarrhoea and their use is generally not recommended (side-effects include drowsiness, abdominal distension and ileus). ⟨A⟩

Racecadotril is licensed, as an adjunct to rehydration, for the symptomatic treatment of uncomplicated acute diarrhoea in children over 3 months; it should only be used when supportive measures, including oral rehydration, are insufficient to control the condition.

Antibacterial drugs for acute diarrhoea

EvGr Antibacterial treatment is **not** recommended *routinely* for children with acute diarrhoea. Antibacterial treatment is recommended in cases of extra-intestinal spread of bacterial infection; *Clostridioides difficile*-associated pseudomembranous colitis; giardiasis, dysenteric shigellosis, dysenteric amoebiasis, or cholera; in children under 6 months with salmonella gastroenteritis; in children who are malnourished or immunocompromised; and in children with suspected or confirmed septicaemia. For children who have recently been abroad, seek specialist advice about antibacterial therapy. ⟨A⟩

Related drugs

Other drugs used for diarrhoea: codeine phosphate p. 293, co-phenotrope below, methylcellulose p. 45.

Other drugs used for Diarrhoea Colestyramine, p. 136

ANTIDIARRHOEALS ›
ANTIPROPULSIVES

F 290

Co-phenotrope

02-Jul-2018

- **INDICATIONS AND DOSE**

Adjunct to rehydration in acute diarrhoea

- BY MOUTH
  - Child 2-3 years: 0.5 tablet 3 times a day
  - Child 4-8 years: 1 tablet 3 times a day
  - Child 9-11 years: 1 tablet 4 times a day
  - Child 12-15 years: 2 tablets 3 times a day
  - Child 16-17 years: Initially 4 tablets, followed by 2 tablets every 6 hours until diarrhoea controlled

Control of faecal consistency after colostomy or ileostomy

- BY MOUTH
  - Child 2-3 years: 0.5 tablet 3 times a day
  - Child 4-8 years: 1 tablet 3 times a day
  - Child 9-11 years: 1 tablet 4 times a day

continued →

- Child 12–15 years: 2 tablets 3 times a day
- Child 16–17 years: Initially 4 tablets, then 2 tablets 4 times a day

- **UNLICENSED USE** Not licensed for use in children under 4 years.
- **CONTRA-INDICATIONS** Gastro-intestinal obstruction · intestinal atony · myasthenia gravis (but some antimuscarinics may be used to decrease muscarinic side-effects of anticholinesterases) · paralytic ileus · pyloric stenosis · severe ulcerative colitis · significant bladder outflow obstruction · toxic megacolon · urinary retention
- **CAUTIONS** Presence of subclinical doses of atropine may give rise to atropine side-effects in susceptible individuals or in overdosage · young children are particularly susceptible to **overdosage**; symptoms may be delayed and observation is needed for at least 48 hours after ingestion
- **INTERACTIONS** → Appendix 1: atropine · opioids
- **SIDE-EFFECTS** Abdominal discomfort · angioedema · angle closure glaucoma · appetite decreased · cardiac disorder · depression · dysuria · fever · gastrointestinal disorders · malaise · mucosal dryness · mydriasis · restlessness · vision disorders
- **PREGNANCY** Manufacturer advises caution.
- **BREAST FEEDING** May be present in milk.
- **HEPATIC IMPAIRMENT** Manufacturer advises caution; avoid in jaundice.
- **DIRECTIONS FOR ADMINISTRATION** For administration *by mouth* tablets may be crushed.
- **PRESCRIBING AND DISPENSING INFORMATION** A mixture of diphenoxylate hydrochloride and atropine sulfate in the mass proportions 100 parts to 1 part respectively.
- **EXCEPTIONS TO LEGAL CATEGORY** Co-phenotrope 2.5/0.025 can be sold to the public for adults and children over 16 years (provided packs do not contain more than 20 tablets) as an adjunct to rehydration in acute diarrhoea (max. daily dose 10 tablets).

- **MEDICINAL FORMS** There can be variation in the licensing of different medicines containing the same drug. Forms available from special-order manufacturers include: tablet

Tablet

- Co-phenotrope (Imported)
  Atropine sulfate 25 microgram, Diphenoxylate hydrochloride 2.5 mg Lomotil 2.5mg/25microgram tablets | 100 tablet PoM CD5
  Lofenoxal 2.5mg/25microgram tablets | 20 tablet PoM CD5

Loperamide hydrochloride

10-Mar-2020

- **INDICATIONS AND DOSE**

Symptomatic treatment of acute diarrhoea

- BY MOUTH
- Child 4–7 years: 1 mg 3–4 times a day for up to 3 days only
- Child 8–11 years: 2 mg 4 times a day for up to 5 days
- Child 12–17 years: Initially 4 mg, followed by 2 mg for up to 5 days, dose to be taken after each loose stool; usual dose 6–8 mg daily; maximum 16 mg per day

Chronic diarrhoea

- BY MOUTH
- Child 1–11 months: 100–200 micrograms/kg twice daily, to be given 30 minutes before feeds; increased if necessary up to 2 mg/kg daily in divided doses
- Child 1–11 years: 100–200 micrograms/kg 3–4 times a day (max. per dose 2 mg), increased if necessary up to 1.25 mg/kg daily in divided doses; maximum 16 mg per day
- Child 12–17 years: 2–4 mg 2–4 times a day; maximum 16 mg per day

- **UNLICENSED USE** Not licensed for use in children for chronic diarrhoea. *Capsules* not licensed for use in children under 8 years. *Syrup* not licensed for use in children under 4 years.

> **IMPORTANT SAFETY INFORMATION**
>
> MHRA/CHM ADVICE: REPORTS OF SERIOUS CARDIAC ADVERSE REACTIONS WITH HIGH DOSES OF LOPERAMIDE ASSOCIATED WITH ABUSE OR MISUSE (SEPTEMBER 2017)
>
> Serious cardiovascular events (such as QT prolongation, torsades de pointes, and cardiac arrest), including fatalities, have been reported in association with large overdoses of loperamide.
>
> Healthcare professionals are reminded that if symptoms of overdose occur, naloxone can be given as an antidote. The duration of action of loperamide is longer than that of naloxone (1–3 hours), so repeated treatment with naloxone might be indicated; patients should be monitored closely for at least 48 hours to detect possible CNS depression.
>
> Pharmacists should remind patients not to take more than the recommended dose on the label.

- **CONTRA-INDICATIONS** Active ulcerative colitis · antibiotic-associated colitis · bacterial enterocolitis · conditions where abdominal distension develops · conditions where inhibition of peristalsis should be avoided
- **CAUTIONS** Not recommended for children under 12 years
- **INTERACTIONS** → Appendix 1: loperamide
- **SIDE-EFFECTS**
  - **Common or very common** Gastrointestinal disorders · headache · nausea
  - **Uncommon** Dizziness · drowsiness · dry mouth · gastrointestinal discomfort · skin reactions · vomiting
  - **Rare or very rare** Angioedema · consciousness impaired · coordination abnormal · fatigue · miosis · muscle tone increased · severe cutaneous adverse reactions (SCARs) · urinary retention
- **PREGNANCY** Manufacturers advise avoid—no information available.
- **BREAST FEEDING** Amount probably too small to be harmful.
- **HEPATIC IMPAIRMENT** Manufacturer advises caution—risk of reduced first pass metabolism leading to central nervous system toxicity.
- **PATIENT AND CARER ADVICE**
  Medicines for Children leaflet: Loperamide for diarrhoea www.medicinesforchildren.org.uk/loperamide-diarrhoea
- **EXCEPTIONS TO LEGAL CATEGORY** Loperamide can be sold to the public, for use in adults and children over 12 years, provided it is licensed and labelled for the treatment of acute diarrhoea.

- **MEDICINAL FORMS** There can be variation in the licensing of different medicines containing the same drug. Forms available from special-order manufacturers include: oral suspension, oral solution

Tablet

- Loperamide hydrochloride (Non-proprietary)
  Loperamide hydrochloride 2 mg Loperamide 2mg tablets | 30 tablet PoM £1.76 DT = £1.54
- Norimode (Tillomed Laboratories Ltd)
  Loperamide hydrochloride 2 mg Norimode 2mg tablets | 30 tablet PoM £2.15 DT = £1.54

Oral solution

- Imodium (Janssen-Cilag Ltd)
  Loperamide hydrochloride 200 microgram per 1 ml Imodium 1mg/5ml oral solution sugar-free | 100 ml PoM £1.17 DT = £1.17

Capsule

- Loperamide hydrochloride (Non-proprietary)
  Loperamide hydrochloride 2 mg Loperamide 2mg capsules | 30 capsule P £1.34–£3.66 DT = £0.98

▸ Imodium (McNeil Products Ltd)
Loperamide hydrochloride 2 mg Imodium Original 2mg capsules | 6 capsule GSL £2.15 | 12 capsule GSL £3.55
Imodium Classic 2mg capsules | 12 capsule P £3.75 | 18 capsule P £4.73

Orodispersible tablet

▸ Imodium (McNeil Products Ltd)
Loperamide hydrochloride 2 mg Imodium Instant Melts 2mg orodispersible tablets sugar-free | 12 tablet P £4.38 sugar-free | 18 tablet P £5.85 DT = £5.85

Loperamide with simeticone

24-Apr-2020

The properties listed below are those particular to the combination only. For the properties of the components please consider, loperamide hydrochloride p. 54, simeticone p. 57.

● **INDICATIONS AND DOSE**

Acute diarrhoea with abdominal colic

▸ BY MOUTH

▸ Child 12–17 years: Initially 1 tablet, then 1 tablet, after each loose stool, for up to 2 days; maximum 4 tablets per day

● **INTERACTIONS** → Appendix 1: loperamide

● **MEDICINAL FORMS** There can be variation in the licensing of different medicines containing the same drug.

Tablet

▸ Imodium Plus (McNeil Products Ltd)
Loperamide hydrochloride 2 mg, Dimeticone (as Simeticone) 125 mg Imodium Plus caplets | 12 tablet P £4.21 DT = £4.21

4 Disorders of gastric acid and ulceration

4.1 Dyspepsia

Dyspepsia

03-Jan-2019

Description of condition

Dyspepsia covers upper abdominal pain, fullness, early satiety, bloating, and nausea. It can occur with gastric and duodenal ulceration, gastro-oesophageal reflux disease, gastritis, and upper gastro-intestinal motility disorders, but most commonly it is of uncertain origin.

Non-drug treatment

Patients with dyspepsia should be advised about lifestyle changes (avoidance of excess alcohol and of aggravating foods such as fats); other measures include weight reduction, Smoking cessation p. 313, and raising the head of the bed.

Drug treatment

Some medications may cause dyspepsia—these should be stopped, if possible.

A compound alginate preparation may provide relief from dyspepsia; persistent dyspepsia requires investigation. Treatment with a H_2-receptor antagonist or a proton pump inhibitor should be initiated only on the advice of a hospital specialist.

Helicobacter pylori may be present in children with dyspepsia. *H. pylori* eradication therapy should be considered for persistent dyspepsia if it is ulcer-like. However, most children with functional (investigated, non-ulcer) dyspepsia do not benefit symptomatically from *H. pylori* eradication.

ANTACIDS

Antacids

Overview

Antacids (usually containing aluminium or magnesium compounds) can often relieve symptoms in *ulcer dyspepsia* and in *non-erosive gastro-oesophageal reflux* ; they are also sometimes used in functional (non-ulcer) dyspepsia but the evidence of benefit is uncertain.

Aluminium- and **magnesium**-containing antacids, being relatively insoluble in water, are long-acting if retained in the stomach. They are suitable for most antacid purposes. Magnesium-containing antacids tend to be laxative whereas aluminium-containing antacids may be constipating; antacids containing both magnesium and aluminium may reduce these colonic side-effects.

Complexes such as **hydrotalcite** confer no special advantage.

Calcium-containing antacids can induce rebound acid secretion; with modest doses the clinical significance of this is doubtful, but prolonged high doses also cause hypercalcaemia and alkalosis.

Simeticone

Simeticone p. 57 (activated dimeticone) is used to treat infantile colic, but the evidence of benefit is uncertain.

Simeticone is added to an antacid as an antifoaming agent to relieve flatulence. These preparations may be useful for the relief of hiccup in palliative care.

Alginates

Alginates taken in combination with an antacid increases the viscosity of stomach contents and can protect the oesophageal mucosa from acid reflux. Some alginate-containing preparations form a viscous gel ('raft') that floats on the surface of the stomach contents, thereby reducing symptoms of reflux. Alginate-containing preparations are used in the management of mild symptoms of dyspepsia and gastro-oesophageal reflux disease.

The amount of additional ingredient or antacid in individual preparations varies widely, as does their sodium content, so that preparations may not be freely interchangeable.

ANTACIDS › ALGINATE

Alginic acid

23-Apr-2020

● **INDICATIONS AND DOSE**

GAVISCON INFANT® POWDER SACHETS

Management of gastro-oesophageal reflux disease

▸ BY MOUTH

▸ Neonate (body-weight up to 4.5 kg): 1 dose as required, to be mixed with feeds (or water, for breast-fed infants); maximum 6 doses per day.

▸ Neonate (body-weight 4.5 kg and above): 2 doses as required, to be mixed with feeds (or water, for breast-fed infants); maximum 12 doses per day.

▸ Child 1–23 months (body-weight up to 4.5 kg): 1 dose as required, to be mixed with feeds (or water, for breast-fed infants); maximum 6 doses per day

▸ Child 1–23 months (body-weight 4.5 kg and above): 2 doses as required, to be mixed with feeds (or water, for breast-fed infants); maximum 12 doses per day

● **CONTRA-INDICATIONS** Intestinal obstruction · preterm neonates · where excessive water loss likely (e.g. fever, diarrhoea, vomiting, high room temperature)

GAVISCON INFANT® POWDER SACHETS Concurrent use of preparations containing thickening agents

- **RENAL IMPAIRMENT** In patients with fluid retention, avoid antacids containing large amounts of sodium.
- **PRESCRIBING AND DISPENSING INFORMATION** Each half of the dual-sachet is identified as 'one dose'.
  To avoid errors prescribe with directions in terms of 'dose'.
- **MEDICINAL FORMS** There can be variation in the licensing of different medicines containing the same drug.

Powder

ELECTROLYTES: May contain Sodium

- Gaviscon Infant (Forum Health Products Ltd)
  Magnesium alginate 87.5 mg, Sodium alginate 225 mg Gaviscon Infant oral powder sachets sugar-free | 30 sachet [P] £5.32 DT = £5.32

Sodium alginate with potassium bicarbonate

The properties listed below are those particular to the combination only. For the properties of the components please consider, alginic acid p. 55.

- **INDICATIONS AND DOSE**

Management of mild symptoms of dyspepsia and gastro-oesophageal reflux disease

- BY MOUTH USING CHEWABLE TABLETS
  - Child 6–11 years (under medical advice only): 1 tablet, to be chewed after meals and at bedtime
  - Child 12–17 years: 1–2 tablets, to be chewed after meals and at bedtime
- BY MOUTH USING ORAL SUSPENSION
  - Child 2–11 years (under medical advice only): 2.5–5 mL, to be taken after meals and at bedtime
  - Child 12–17 years: 5–10 mL, to be taken after meals and at bedtime

- **PRESCRIBING AND DISPENSING INFORMATION** Flavours of oral liquid formulations may include aniseed or peppermint.
- **MEDICINAL FORMS** There can be variation in the licensing of different medicines containing the same drug.

Oral suspension

ELECTROLYTES: May contain Potassium, sodium

- Acidex Advance (Wockhardt UK Ltd)
  Potassium bicarbonate 20 mg per 1 ml, Sodium alginate 100 mg per 1 ml Acidex Advance oral suspension peppermint sugar-free | 250 ml [P] £1.92 sugar-free | 500 ml [P] £3.84 DT = £5.12
  Acidex Advance oral suspension aniseed sugar-free | 250 ml [P] £1.92 sugar-free | 500 ml [P] £3.84 DT = £5.12
- Gaviscon Advance (Reckitt Benckiser Healthcare (UK) Ltd)
  Potassium bicarbonate 20 mg per 1 ml, Sodium alginate 100 mg per 1 ml Gaviscon Advance oral suspension aniseed sugar-free | 150 ml [P] £3.88 sugar-free | 250 ml [P] £2.56 sugar-free | 300 ml [P] £6.46 sugar-free | 500 ml [P] £5.12 DT = £5.12
  Gaviscon Advance oral suspension peppermint sugar-free | 250 ml [P] £2.56 sugar-free | 300 ml [P] £6.46 sugar-free | 500 ml [P] £5.12 DT = £5.12

Chewable tablet

EXCIPIENTS: May contain Aspartame

ELECTROLYTES: May contain Potassium, sodium

- Gaviscon Advance (Reckitt Benckiser Healthcare (UK) Ltd)
  Potassium bicarbonate 100 mg, Sodium alginate 500 mg Gaviscon Advance Mint chewable tablets sugar-free | 24 tablet [GSL] £4.46 sugar-free | 60 tablet [GSL] £3.07 DT = £3.07

ANTACIDS > ALUMINIUM AND MAGNESIUM

Co-magaldrox

17-Apr-2020

The properties listed below are those particular to the combination only. For the properties of the components please consider, magnesium hydroxide p. 48.

- **INDICATIONS AND DOSE**

MAALOX®

Dyspepsia

- BY MOUTH
  - Child 14–17 years: 10–20 mL, to be taken 20–60 minutes after meals, and at bedtime or when required

MUCOGEL®

Dyspepsia

- BY MOUTH
  - Child 12–17 years: 10–20 mL 3 times a day, to be taken 20–60 minutes after meals, and at bedtime, or when required

- **INTERACTIONS** → Appendix 1: antacids · magnesium
- **SIDE-EFFECTS**
  - **Uncommon** Constipation · diarrhoea
  - **Rare or very rare** Electrolyte imbalance
  - **Frequency not known** Abdominal pain · hyperaluminaemia
- **RENAL IMPAIRMENT** There is a risk of accumulation and aluminium toxicity with antacids containing aluminium salts. Absorption of aluminium from aluminium salts is increased by citrates, which are contained in many effervescent preparations (such as effervescent analgesics).
- **PRESCRIBING AND DISPENSING INFORMATION** Co-magaldrox is a mixture of aluminium hydroxide and magnesium hydroxide; the proportions are expressed in the form x/y where x and y are the strengths in milligrams per unit dose of magnesium hydroxide and aluminium hydroxide respectively.
  MAALOX® Maalox® suspension is low in sodium.
  MUCOGEL® Mucogel® suspension is low in sodium.
- **MEDICINAL FORMS** There can be variation in the licensing of different medicines containing the same drug.

Oral suspension

- Maalox (Sanofi)
  Aluminium hydroxide 35 mg per 1 ml, Magnesium hydroxide 40 mg per 1 ml Maalox 175mg/200mg/5ml oral suspension sugar-free | 250 ml [GSL] £2.33 DT = £2.33
- Mucogel (Chemidex Pharma Ltd)
  Magnesium hydroxide 39 mg per 1 ml, Aluminium hydroxide gel dried 44 mg per 1 ml Mucogel oral suspension sugar-free | 500 ml [GSL] £2.99 DT = £2.99

Co-simalcite

17-Apr-2020

- **INDICATIONS AND DOSE**

Dyspepsia

- BY MOUTH
  - Child 8–11 years: 5 mL, to be taken between meals and at bedtime
  - Child 12–17 years: 10 mL, to be taken between meals and at bedtime

- **CONTRA-INDICATIONS** Infants · neonates
  CONTRA-INDICATIONS, FURTHER INFORMATION Aluminium-containing antacids should not be used in neonates and infants because accumulation may lead to increased plasma-aluminium concentrations.
- **RENAL IMPAIRMENT** Aluminium-containing antacids should not be used in children with renal impairment,

because accumulation may lead to increased plasma-aluminium concentrations.

Dose adjustments Antacids containing magnesium salts should be avoided or used at a reduced dose because there is an increased risk of toxicity.

- **PRESCRIBING AND DISPENSING INFORMATION** *Altacite Plus®* is low in Na^+.

- **MEDICINAL FORMS** There can be variation in the licensing of different medicines containing the same drug.

Oral suspension

- Altacite Plus (Peckforton Pharmaceuticals Ltd)
  Simeticone 25 mg per 1 ml, Hydrotalcite 100 mg per 1 ml Altacite Plus oral suspension sugar-free | 100 ml [P] £4.00 sugar-free | 500 ml [P] £5.20 DT = £5.20

Simeticone with aluminium hydroxide and magnesium hydroxide

04-May-2020

The properties listed below are those particular to the combination only. For the properties of the components please consider, simeticone below.

- **INDICATIONS AND DOSE**

Dyspepsia

- BY MOUTH
- Child 2–4 years: 5 mL 3 times a day, to be taken after meals and at bedtime, or when required
- Child 5–11 years: 5 mL 3–4 times a day, to be taken after meals and at bedtime, or when required
- Child 12–17 years: 5–10 mL 4 times a day, to be taken after meals and at bedtime, or when required

- **INTERACTIONS** → Appendix 1: antacids
- **SIDE-EFFECTS**
- **Uncommon** Constipation · diarrhoea
- **Rare or very rare** Electrolyte imbalance
- **Frequency not known** Abdominal pain · hyperaluminaemia
- **RENAL IMPAIRMENT** There is a risk of accumulation and aluminium toxicity with antacids containing aluminium salts. Absorption of aluminium from aluminium salts is increased by citrates, which are contained in many effervescent preparations (such as effervescent analgesics).

- **MEDICINAL FORMS** There can be variation in the licensing of different medicines containing the same drug.

Oral suspension

- Maalox Plus (Sanofi)
  Simeticone 5 mg per 1 ml, Magnesium hydroxide 39 mg per 1 ml, Aluminium hydroxide gel dried 44 mg per 1 ml Maalox Plus oral suspension sugar-free | 250 ml [GSL] £2.91

ANTACIDS > MAGNESIUM

Magnesium trisilicate with magnesium carbonate and sodium bicarbonate

22-Apr-2020

The properties listed below are those particular to the combination only. For the properties of the components please consider, magnesium trisilicate, magnesium carbonate, sodium bicarbonate p. 634.

- **INDICATIONS AND DOSE**

Dyspepsia

- BY MOUTH
- Child 5–11 years: 5–10 mL 3 times a day, alternatively as required, dose to be made up with water
- Child 12–17 years: 10–20 mL 3 times a day, alternatively as required, dose to be made up with water

- **CONTRA-INDICATIONS** Hypophosphataemia · severe renal failure
- **CAUTIONS** Heart failure · hypermagnesaemia · hypertension · metabolic alkalosis · respiratory alkalosis
- **INTERACTIONS** → Appendix 1: antacids · sodium bicarbonate
- **HEPATIC IMPAIRMENT** In patients with fluid retention avoid antacids containing large amounts of sodium. Avoid antacids containing magnesium salts in hepatic coma if there is a risk of renal failure.
- **RENAL IMPAIRMENT** Magnesium trisilicate and magnesium carbonate mixtures have high sodium content; avoid in patients with fluid retention.
- **PRESCRIBING AND DISPENSING INFORMATION** When prepared extemporaneously, the BP states Magnesium Trisilicate Mixture, BP consists of 5% each of magnesium trisilicate, light magnesium carbonate, and sodium bicarbonate in a suitable vehicle with a peppermint flavour.

- **MEDICINAL FORMS** There can be variation in the licensing of different medicines containing the same drug.

Oral suspension

- Magnesium trisilicate with magnesium carbonate and sodium bicarbonate (Non-proprietary)
  Magnesium carbonate light 50 mg per 1 ml, Magnesium trisilicate 50 mg per 1 ml, Sodium bicarbonate 50 mg per 1 ml Magnesium trisilicate oral suspension | 200 ml [GSL] £1.65 DT = £1.65

ANTIFOAMING DRUGS

Simeticone

(Activated dimeticone)

- **DRUG ACTION** Simeticone (activated dimeticone) is an antifoaming agent.

- **INDICATIONS AND DOSE**

DENTINOX®

Colic | Wind pains

- BY MOUTH
- Neonate: 2.5 mL, to be taken with or after each feed; may be added to bottle feed; maximum 6 doses per day.
- Child 1 month–1 year: 2.5 mL, to be taken with or after each feed; may be added to bottle feed; maximum 6 doses per day

INFACOL®

Colic | Wind pains

- BY MOUTH
- Neonate: 0.5–1 mL, to be taken before feeds.
- Child 1 month–1 year: 0.5–1 mL, to be taken before feeds

- **PRESCRIBING AND DISPENSING INFORMATION**
  DENTINOX® The brand name *Dentinox®* is also used for other preparations including teething gel.
- **PATIENT AND CARER ADVICE**
  INFACOL® Patients or carers should be given advice on use of the *Infacol®* dropper.
- **LESS SUITABLE FOR PRESCRIBING**
  INFACOL® *Infacol®* is less suitable for prescribing (evidence of benefit in infantile colic uncertain).
  DENTINOX® *Dentinox®* colic drops are less suitable for prescribing (evidence of benefit in infantile colic uncertain).

- **MEDICINAL FORMS** There can be variation in the licensing of different medicines containing the same drug.

Oral suspension

- Infacol (Teva UK Ltd)
  Simeticone 40 mg per 1 ml Infacol 40mg/ml oral suspension sugar-free | 55 ml [GSL] £3.20 DT = £3.20 sugar-free | 85 ml [GSL] £4.66 DT = £4.66

Oral drops

- Dentinox Infant (Dendron Ltd)
  Simeticone 8.4 mg per 1 ml Dentinox Infant colic drops | 100 ml [GSL] £2.01 DT = £2.01

Combinations available: *Co-simalcite*, p. 56 · *Simeticone with aluminium hydroxide and magnesium hydroxide*, p. 57

4.2 Gastric and duodenal ulceration

Peptic ulceration

Overview

Peptic ulceration commonly involves the stomach, duodenum, and lower oesophagus; after gastric surgery it involves the gastro-enterostomy stoma. Healing can be promoted by general measures, Smoking cessation p. 313 and taking antacids and by antisecretory drug treatment, but relapse is common when treatment ceases. Nearly all duodenal ulcers and most gastric ulcers not associated with NSAIDs are caused by *Helicobacter pylori*.

Helicobacter pylori infection

Eradication of *Helicobacter pylori* reduces the recurrence of gastric and duodenal ulcers and the risk of rebleeding. The presence of *H. pylori* should be confirmed before starting eradication treatment. If possible, the antibacterial sensitivity of the organism should be established at the time of endoscopy and biopsy. Acid inhibition combined with antibacterial treatment is highly effective in the eradication of *H. pylori*; reinfection is rare. Antibiotic-associated colitis is an uncommon risk.

Treatment to eradicate *H. pylori* infection in children should be initiated under specialist supervision. One week triple-therapy regimens that comprise omeprazole p. 63, amoxicillin p. 366, and either clarithromycin p. 353 or metronidazole p. 358 are recommended. Resistance to clarithromycin or to metronidazole is much more common than to amoxicillin and can develop during treatment. A regimen containing amoxicillin and clarithromycin is therefore recommended for initial therapy and one containing amoxicillin and metronidazole is recommended for eradication failure or for a child who has been treated with a macrolide for other infections. There is usually no need to continue antisecretory treatment (with a proton pump inhibitor or H_2-receptor antagonist); however, if the ulcer is large, or complicated by haemorrhage or perforation then antisecretory treatment is continued for a further 3 weeks. Lansoprazole p. 62 may be considered if omeprazole is unsuitable. Treatment failure usually indicates antibacterial resistance or poor compliance.

Two-week triple-therapy regimens offer the possibility of higher eradication rates compared to one-week regimens, but adverse effects are common and poor compliance is likely to offset any possible gain.

Two-week dual-therapy regimens using a proton pump inhibitor and a single antibacterial produce low rates of *H. pylori* eradication and are **not** recommended.

See under *NSAID-associated ulcers* for the role of *H. pylori* eradication therapy in children starting or taking NSAIDs.

Test for *Helicobacter pylori*

^{13}C-Urea breath test kits are available for confirming the presence of gastro-duodenal infection with *Helicobacter pylori*. The test involves collection of breath samples before and after ingestion of an oral solution of ^{13}C-urea; the samples are sent for analysis by an appropriate laboratory. The test should not be performed within 4 weeks of treatment with an antibacterial or within 2 weeks of treatment with an antisecretory drug. A specific ^{13}C-Urea breath test kit for children is available (*Helicobacter Test INFAI for children of the age* 3–11®). However the appropriateness of testing for *H. pylori* infection in children has not been established. Breath, saliva, faecal, and urine tests for *H. pylori* are frequently unreliable in children; the most accurate method of diagnosis is endoscopy with biopsy.

NSAID-associated ulcers

Gastro-intestinal bleeding and ulceration can occur with NSAID use. Whenever possible, NSAIDs should be **withdrawn** if an ulcer occurs.

Children at high risk of developing gastro-intestinal complications with a NSAID include those with a history of peptic ulcer disease or serious upper gastro-intestinal complication, those taking other medicines that increase the risk of upper gastro-intestinal side-effects, or those with serious co-morbidity. In children at risk of ulceration, a proton pump inhibitor can be considered for protection against gastric and duodenal ulcers associated with non-selective NSAIDs; high dose ranitidine p. 59 is an alternative.

NSAID use and *H. pylori* infection are independent risk factors for gastro-intestinal bleeding and ulceration. In children already taking a NSAID, eradication of *H. pylori* is unlikely to reduce the risk of NSAID-induced bleeding or ulceration. However, in children about to start long-term NSAID treatment who are *H. pylori* positive and have dyspepsia or a history of gastric or duodenal ulcer, eradication of *H. pylori* may reduce the overall risk of ulceration.

If the NSAID can be *discontinued* in a child who has developed an ulcer, a proton pump inhibitor usually produces the most rapid healing; alternatively the ulcer can be treated with an H_2-receptor antagonist.

If *NSAID treatment needs to continue*, the ulcer is treated with a proton pump inhibitor.

GASTROPROTECTIVE COMPLEXES AND CHELATORS

Chelates and complexes

Sucralfate

Sucralfate below is a complex of aluminium hydroxide and sulfated sucrose that appears to act by protecting the mucosa from acid-pepsin attack; it has minimal antacid properties.

Sucralfate

- **INDICATIONS AND DOSE**

Benign gastric ulceration | Benign duodenal ulceration

- BY MOUTH
  - Child 1 month–1 year: 250 mg 4–6 times a day
  - Child 2–11 years: 500 mg 4–6 times a day
  - Child 12–14 years: 1 g 4–6 times a day
  - Child 15–17 years: 2 g twice daily, dose to be taken on rising and at bedtime, alternatively 1 g 4 times a day for 4–6 weeks, or in resistant cases up to 12 weeks, dose to be taken 1 hour before meals and at bedtime; maximum 8 g per day

Prophylaxis of stress ulceration in child under intensive care
- BY MOUTH
- Child 1 month–1 year: 250 mg 4–6 times a day
- Child 2–11 years: 500 mg 4–6 times a day
- Child 12–14 years: 1 g 4–6 times a day
- Child 15–17 years: 1 g 6 times a day; maximum 8 g per day

- **UNLICENSED USE** Not licensed for use in children under 15 years. Tablets not licensed for prophylaxis of stress ulceration.
- **CAUTIONS** Patients under intensive care (**Important**: reports of bezoar formation)

CAUTIONS, FURTHER INFORMATION
- Bezoar formation Following reports of bezoar formation associated with sucralfate, caution is advised in seriously ill patients, especially those receiving concomitant enteral feeds or those with predisposing conditions such as delayed gastric emptying.

- **INTERACTIONS** → Appendix 1: sucralfate
- **SIDE-EFFECTS**
  - **Common or very common** Constipation
  - **Uncommon** Dry mouth · nausea
  - **Rare or very rare** Bezoar · rash
  - **Frequency not known** Back pain · bone disorders · diarrhoea · dizziness · drowsiness · encephalopathy · flatulence · headache · vertigo
- **PREGNANCY** No evidence of harm; absorption from gastro-intestinal tract negligible.
- **BREAST FEEDING** Amount probably too small to be harmful.
- **RENAL IMPAIRMENT** Use with caution; aluminium is absorbed and may accumulate.
- **DIRECTIONS FOR ADMINISTRATION** Administration of sucralfate and enteral feeds should be separated by 1 hour and for administration by *mouth*, sucralfate should be given 1 hour before meals. *Oral suspension* blocks fine-bore feeding tubes. Crushed *tablets* may be dispersed in water.
- **PRESCRIBING AND DISPENSING INFORMATION** Flavours of oral liquid formulations may include aniseed and caramel.

- **MEDICINAL FORMS** There can be variation in the licensing of different medicines containing the same drug. Forms available from special-order manufacturers include: tablet, oral suspension

Tablet

CAUTIONARY AND ADVISORY LABELS 5
- **Sucralfate (Imported)**
  Sucralfate 1 gram Sulcrate 1g tablets | 100 tablet [CD]
  Carafate 1g tablets | 100 tablet [CD]

Oral suspension

CAUTIONARY AND ADVISORY LABELS 5
- **Carafate (Imported (United States))**
  Sucralfate 100 mg per 1 ml Carafate 1g/10ml oral suspension sugar-free | 420 ml PoM [CD]
- **Sucralfate (Non-proprietary)**
  Sucralfate 200 mg per 1 ml Sucralfate 1g/5ml oral suspension sugar-free | 200 ml PoM £73.75

H_2-RECEPTOR ANTAGONISTS

H_2-receptor antagonists

Overview

Histamine H_2-receptor antagonists heal *gastric and duodenal ulcers* by reducing gastric acid output as a result of histamine H_2-receptor blockade; they are also used to relieve symptoms of *dyspepsia* and *gastro-oesophageal reflux disease*. H_2-receptor antagonists should not normally be used for *Zollinger–Ellison syndrome* because proton pump inhibitors are more effective.

Maintenance treatment with low doses has largely been replaced in *Helicobacter pylori* positive children by eradication regimens.

H_2-receptor antagonist therapy can promote healing of *NSAID-associated ulcers*.

Treatment with a H_2-receptor antagonist has not been shown to be beneficial in haematemesis and melaena, but prophylactic use reduces the frequency of bleeding from *gastroduodenal erosions in hepatic coma*, and possibly in other conditions requiring intensive care. Treatment also reduces the risk of *acid aspiration* in obstetric patients at delivery (Mendelson's syndrome).

H_2-receptor antagonists are also used to reduce the degradation of pancreatic enzyme supplements in children with cystic fibrosis.

H_2-receptor antagonists 

- **SIDE-EFFECTS**
  - **Common or very common** Constipation · diarrhoea · dizziness · fatigue · headache · myalgia · skin reactions
  - **Uncommon** Confusion · depression · erectile dysfunction · gynaecomastia · hallucination · hepatic disorders · leucopenia · nausea · tachycardia
  - **Rare or very rare** Agranulocytosis · alopecia · arthralgia · atrioventricular block · fever · galactorrhoea · pancytopenia · thrombocytopenia · vasculitis

above

Ranitidine

- **INDICATIONS AND DOSE**

Benign gastric ulceration | Duodenal ulceration
- BY MOUTH
- Neonate: 2 mg/kg 3 times a day (max. per dose 3 mg/kg 3 times a day), oral absorption is unreliable.
- Child 1–5 months: 1 mg/kg 3 times a day (max. per dose 3 mg/kg 3 times a day)
- Child 6 months–2 years: 2–4 mg/kg twice daily
- Child 3–11 years: 2–4 mg/kg twice daily (max. per dose 150 mg)
- Child 12–17 years: 150 mg twice daily, alternatively 300 mg once daily, dose to be taken at night

Prophylaxis of stress ulceration
- INITIALLY BY SLOW INTRAVENOUS INJECTION
- Neonate: 0.5–1 mg/kg every 6–8 hours.
- Child 1 month–11 years: 1 mg/kg every 6–8 hours (max. per dose 50 mg), may be given as an intermittent infusion at a rate of 25 mg/hour
- Child 12–17 years: 50 mg every 8 hours, dose to be diluted to 20 mL and given over at least 2 minutes, then (by mouth) 150 mg twice daily, may be given when oral feeding commences

Reflux oesophagitis and other conditions where gastric acid reduction is beneficial
- BY MOUTH
- Neonate: 2 mg/kg 3 times a day (max. per dose 3 mg/kg 3 times a day), oral absorption is unreliable.
- Child 1–5 months: 1 mg/kg 3 times a day (max. per dose 3 mg/kg 3 times a day)
- Child 6 months–2 years: 2–4 mg/kg twice daily
- Child 3–11 years: 2–4 mg/kg twice daily (max. per dose 150 mg); increased to up to 5 mg/kg twice daily (max. per dose 300 mg), dose increase for severe gastro-oesophageal disease

continued →

- Child 12–17 years: 150 mg twice daily, alternatively 300 mg once daily, dose to be taken at night, then increased if necessary to 300 mg twice daily for up to 12 weeks in moderate to severe gastro-oesophageal reflux disease, alternatively increased if necessary to 150 mg 4 times a day for up to 12 weeks in moderate to severe gastro-oesophageal reflux disease

- BY SLOW INTRAVENOUS INJECTION
- Neonate: 0.5–1 mg/kg every 6–8 hours.
- Child: 1 mg/kg every 6–8 hours (max. per dose 50 mg), may be given as an intermittent infusion at a rate of 25 mg/hour

- **UNLICENSED USE** *Oral* preparations not licensed for use in children under 3 years. *Injection* not licensed for use in children under 6 months.
- **INTERACTIONS** → Appendix 1: H2 receptor antagonists
- **SIDE-EFFECTS**

GENERAL SIDE-EFFECTS
- **Rare or very rare** Bone marrow depression · bradycardia · breast conditions · dyskinesia · nephritis acute interstitial · pancreatitis acute · vision blurred
- **Frequency not known** Dyspnoea

SPECIFIC SIDE-EFFECTS
- **Rare or very rare**
- With parenteral use Anaphylactic shock · cardiac arrest

- **PREGNANCY** Manufacturer advises avoid unless essential, but not known to be harmful.
- **BREAST FEEDING** Significant amount present in milk, but not known to be harmful.
- **RENAL IMPAIRMENT**

Dose adjustments Use half normal dose if estimated glomerular filtration rate less than 50 mL/minute/1.73 m^2.
- **DIRECTIONS FOR ADMINISTRATION** For *slow intravenous injection* dilute to a concentration of 2.5 mg/mL with Glucose 5% or Sodium Chloride 0.9%; give over at least 3 minutes.
- **PATIENT AND CARER ADVICE** In fat malabsorption syndrome, give oral doses 1–2 hours before food to enhance effects of pancreatic enzyme replacement.
Medicines for Children leaflet: Ranitidine for acid reflux www.medicinesforchildren.org.uk/ranitidine-acid-reflux
- **EXCEPTIONS TO LEGAL CATEGORY** Ranitidine can be sold to the public for adults and children over 16 years (provided packs do not contain more than 2 weeks' supply) for the short-term symptomatic relief of heartburn, dyspepsia, and hyperacidity, and for the prevention of these symptoms when associated with consumption of food or drink (max. single dose 75 mg, max. daily dose 300 mg).

- **MEDICINAL FORMS** There can be variation in the licensing of different medicines containing the same drug. Forms available from special-order manufacturers include: oral suspension, oral solution, infusion

Tablet
- Ranitidine (Non-proprietary)

Ranitidine (as Ranitidine hydrochloride) 150 mg Ranitidine 150mg tablets | 60 tablet PoM £8.99 DT = £1.54
Ranitidine (as Ranitidine hydrochloride) 300 mg Ranitidine 300mg tablets | 30 tablet PoM £6.80 DT = £1.55

Solution for injection
- Ranitidine (Non-proprietary)

Ranitidine (as Ranitidine hydrochloride) 25 mg per 1 ml Ranitidine 50mg/2ml solution for injection ampoules | 5 ampoule PoM £2.69–£49.00 DT = £3.30
- Zantac (GlaxoSmithKline UK Ltd)

Ranitidine (as Ranitidine hydrochloride) 25 mg per 1 ml Zantac 50mg/2ml solution for injection ampoules | 5 ampoule PoM £2.82 DT = £3.30

Effervescent tablet
CAUTIONARY AND ADVISORY LABELS 13
ELECTROLYTES: May contain Sodium
- Ranitidine (Non-proprietary)

Ranitidine (as Ranitidine hydrochloride) 150 mg Ranitidine 150mg effervescent tablets | 60 tablet PoM £145.82 DT = £34.99
Ranitidine (as Ranitidine hydrochloride) 300 mg Ranitidine 300mg effervescent tablets | 30 tablet PoM £145.82 DT = £35.02

Oral solution
EXCIPIENTS: May contain Alcohol
- Ranitidine (Non-proprietary)

Ranitidine (as Ranitidine hydrochloride) 15 mg per 1 ml Ranitidine 75mg/5ml oral solution sugar-free | 100 ml PoM £2.20–£2.30 sugar-free | 300 ml PoM £21.55 DT = £5.15
Ranitidine (as Ranitidine hydrochloride) 30 mg per 1 ml Ranitidine 150mg/5ml oral solution sugar-free | 150 ml PoM £5.50–£7.65 DT = £7.65
- Zantac (GlaxoSmithKline UK Ltd)

Ranitidine (as Ranitidine hydrochloride) 15 mg per 1 ml Zantac 150mg/10ml syrup sugar-free | 300 ml PoM £20.76 DT = £5.15

PROTON PUMP INHIBITORS

Proton pump inhibitors

Overview

Omeprazole p. 63 is an effective short-term treatment for *gastric* and *duodenal ulcers*; it is also used in combination with antibacterials for the eradication of *Hellicobacter pylori*. An initial short course of omeprazole is the treatment of choice in *gastro-oesophageal reflux disease* with severe symptoms; children with endoscopically confirmed *erosive, ulcerative, or stricturing oesophagitis* usually need to be maintained on omeprazole.

Omeprazole is also used for the prevention and treatment of NSAID-associated ulcers. In children who need to continue NSAID treatment after an ulcer has healed, the dose of omeprazole should not normally be reduced because asymptomatic ulcer deterioration may occur.

Omeprazole is effective in the treatment of the *Zollinger-Ellison syndrome* (including cases resistant to other treatment). It is also used to reduce the degradation of pancreatic enzyme supplements in children with cystic fibrosis.

Lansoprazole p. 62 is not licensed for use in children, but may be considered when the available formulations of omeprazole are unsuitable.

Esomeprazole p. 61 can be used for the management of gastro-oesophageal reflux disease when the available formulations of omeprazole and lansoprazole are unsuitable.

Proton pump inhibitors 

- **DRUG ACTION** Proton pump inhibitors inhibit gastric acid secretion by blocking the hydrogen-potassium adenosine triphosphatase enzyme system (the 'proton pump') of the gastric parietal cell.

IMPORTANT SAFETY INFORMATION

MHRA ADVICE: PROTON PUMP INHIBITORS (PPIS): VERY LOW RISK OF SUBACUTE CUTANEOUS LUPUS ERYTHEMATOSUS (SEPTEMBER 2015)

Very infrequent cases of subacute cutaneous lupus erythematosus (SCLE) have been reported in patients taking PPIs. Drug-induced SCLE can occur weeks, months or even years after exposure to the drug.

If a patient treated with a PPI develops lesions—especially in sun-exposed areas of the skin—and it is accompanied by arthralgia:
- advise them to avoid exposing the skin to sunlight;
- consider SCLE as a possible diagnosis;
- consider discontinuing PPI treatment unless it is imperative for a serious acid-related condition; a

patient who develops SCLE with a particular PPI may be at risk of the same reaction with another;
- in most cases, symptoms resolve on PPI withdrawal; topical or systemic steroids might be necessary for treatment of SCLE only if there are no signs of remission after a few weeks or months.

- **CAUTIONS** May increase the risk of gastro-intestinal infections (including *Clostridioides difficile* infection) · patients at risk of osteoporosis

CAUTIONS, FURTHER INFORMATION

▸ Risk of osteoporosis Patients at risk of osteoporosis should maintain an adequate intake of calcium and vitamin D, and if necessary, receive other preventative therapy.

- **SIDE-EFFECTS**

▸ **Common or very common** Abdominal pain · constipation · diarrhoea · dizziness · dry mouth · gastrointestinal disorders · headache · insomnia · nausea · skin reactions · vomiting

▸ **Uncommon** Arthralgia · bone fractures · confusion · depression · drowsiness · leucopenia · malaise · myalgia · paraesthesia · peripheral oedema · thrombocytopenia · vertigo · vision disorders

▸ **Rare or very rare** Agranulocytosis · alopecia · gynaecomastia · hallucination · hepatic disorders · hyperhidrosis · hyponatraemia · nephritis tubulointerstitial · pancytopenia · photosensitivity reaction · severe cutaneous adverse reactions (SCARs) · stomatitis · taste altered

▸ **Frequency not known** Hypomagnesaemia (more common after 1 year of treatment, but sometimes after 3 months of treatment) · subacute cutaneous lupus erythematosus

- **MONITORING REQUIREMENTS** Measurement of serum-magnesium concentrations should be considered before and during prolonged treatment with a proton pump inhibitor, especially when used with other drugs that cause hypomagnesaemia or with digoxin.
- **PRESCRIBING AND DISPENSING INFORMATION** A proton pump inhibitor should be prescribed for appropriate indications at the lowest effective dose for the shortest period; the need for long-term treatment should be reviewed periodically.

F 60

Esomeprazole

26-Nov-2019

- **INDICATIONS AND DOSE**

Gastro-oesophageal reflux disease (in the presence of erosive reflux oesophagitis)

▸ BY MOUTH

▸ Child 1–11 years (body-weight 10–19 kg): 10 mg once daily for 8 weeks

▸ Child 1–11 years (body-weight 20 kg and above): 10–20 mg once daily for 8 weeks

▸ Child 12–17 years: Initially 40 mg once daily for 4 weeks, continued for further 4 weeks if not fully healed or symptoms persist; maintenance 20 mg daily

▸ BY INTRAVENOUS INJECTION, OR BY INTRAVENOUS INFUSION

▸ Child 1–11 years (body-weight up to 20 kg): 10 mg once daily, injection to be given over at least 3 minutes

▸ Child 1–11 years (body-weight 20 kg and above): 10–20 mg once daily, injection to be given over at least 3 minutes

▸ Child 12–17 years: 40 mg daily, injection to be given over at least 3 minutes

Gastro-oesophageal reflux disease (in the absence of oesophagitis)

▸ BY MOUTH

▸ Child 1–11 years (body-weight 10 kg and above): 10 mg once daily for up to 8 weeks

▸ Child 12–17 years: 20 mg once daily for up to 4 weeks

▸ BY INTRAVENOUS INJECTION, OR BY INTRAVENOUS INFUSION

▸ Child 1–11 years: 10 mg once daily, injection to be given over at least 3 minutes

▸ Child 12–17 years: 20 mg once daily, injection to be given over at least 3 minutes

- **UNLICENSED USE** Tablets and capsules not licensed for use in children 1–11 years.
- **INTERACTIONS** → Appendix 1: proton pump inhibitors
- **SIDE-EFFECTS**

GENERAL SIDE-EFFECTS

▸ **Uncommon** Encephalopathy

▸ **Rare or very rare** Aggression · agitation · bronchospasm · increased risk of infection · muscle weakness

SPECIFIC SIDE-EFFECTS

▸ **Rare or very rare**

▸ With parenteral use Renal failure

▸ **Frequency not known**

▸ With parenteral use Electrolyte imbalance · vitamin B12 deficiency

- **PREGNANCY** Manufacturer advises caution—no information available.
- **BREAST FEEDING** Manufacturer advises avoid—no information available.
- **HEPATIC IMPAIRMENT** Manufacturer advises caution in severe impairment.

Dose adjustments Manufacturer advises in children 1–11 years, max. 10 mg daily in severe impairment.

Manufacturer advises in children 12–17 years, max. 20 mg daily in severe impairment.

- **RENAL IMPAIRMENT** Manufacturer advises caution in severe renal insufficiency.
- **DIRECTIONS FOR ADMINISTRATION**

▸ With intravenous use For *intravenous infusion*, dilute reconstituted solution to a concentration not exceeding 800 micrograms/mL with Sodium Chloride 0.9%; give over 10–30 minutes.

▸ With oral use Do not chew or crush capsules; swallow whole *or* mix capsule contents in water and drink within 30 minutes. Do not crush or chew tablets; swallow whole *or* disperse in water and drink within 30 minutes. Disperse the contents of each sachet of gastro-resistant granules in approx. 15 mL water. Stir and leave to thicken for a few minutes; stir again before administration and use within 30 minutes; rinse container with 15 mL water to obtain full dose. For administration through a gastric tube, consult product literature.

- **PATIENT AND CARER ADVICE** Counselling on administration of gastro-resistant capsules, tablets, and granules advised.

- **MEDICINAL FORMS** There can be variation in the licensing of different medicines containing the same drug. Forms available from special-order manufacturers include: oral suspension

Gastro-resistant capsule

▸ Esomeprazole (Non-proprietary)

Esomeprazole (as Esomeprazole magnesium dihydrate) 20 mg Esomeprazole 20mg gastro-resistant capsules | 28 capsule PoM £12.95 DT = £2.19

Esomeprazole (as Esomeprazole magnesium dihydrate) 40 mg Esomeprazole 40mg gastro-resistant capsules | 28 capsule PoM £17.63 DT = £2.30

▸ Emozul (Consilient Health Ltd)

Esomeprazole (as Esomeprazole magnesium dihydrate) 20 mg Emozul 20mg gastro-resistant capsules | 28 capsule PoM £5.30 DT = £2.19

Esomeprazole (as Esomeprazole magnesium dihydrate) 40 mg Emozul 40mg gastro-resistant capsules | 28 capsule PoM £6.37 DT = £2.30

▸ Ventra (Ethypharm UK Ltd)
Esomeprazole (as Esomeprazole magnesium dihydrate) 20 mg Ventra 20mg gastro-resistant capsules | 28 capsule PoM £2.55 DT = £2.19
Esomeprazole (as Esomeprazole magnesium dihydrate) 40 mg Ventra 40mg gastro-resistant capsules | 28 capsule PoM £2.97 DT = £2.30

Gastro-resistant tablet
▸ Esomeprazole (Non-proprietary)
Esomeprazole 20 mg Esomeprazole 20mg gastro-resistant tablets | 28 tablet PoM £18.50 DT = £2.46
Esomeprazole 40 mg Esomeprazole 40mg gastro-resistant tablets | 28 tablet PoM £25.19 DT = £3.48
▸ Nexium (AstraZeneca UK Ltd, Pfizer Consumer Healthcare Ltd)
Esomeprazole 20 mg Nexium 20mg gastro-resistant tablets | 28 tablet PoM £18.50 DT = £2.46
Esomeprazole 40 mg Nexium 40mg gastro-resistant tablets | 28 tablet PoM £25.19 DT = £3.48

Powder for solution for injection
▸ Esomeprazole (Non-proprietary)
Esomeprazole (as Esomeprazole sodium) 40 mg Esomeprazole 40mg powder for solution for injection vials | 1 vial PoM £3.07–£3.13 (Hospital only)
▸ Nexium (AstraZeneca UK Ltd)
Esomeprazole (as Esomeprazole sodium) 40 mg Nexium I.V 40mg powder for solution for injection vials | 1 vial PoM £4.25 (Hospital only) | 10 vial PoM £42.50 (Hospital only)

Gastro-resistant granules
CAUTIONARY AND ADVISORY LABELS 25
▸ Nexium (AstraZeneca UK Ltd)
Esomeprazole (as Esomeprazole magnesium trihydrate) 10 mg Nexium 10mg gastro-resistant granules sachets | 28 sachet PoM £25.19 DT = £25.19

60

Lansoprazole

26-Nov-2019

● **INDICATIONS AND DOSE**

Benign gastric ulcer
▶ BY MOUTH
▸ Child (body-weight up to 30 kg): 0.5–1 mg/kg once daily (max. per dose 15 mg once daily), doses to be taken in the morning
▸ Child (body-weight 30 kg and above): 15–30 mg once daily, doses to be taken in the morning

Duodenal ulcer
▶ BY MOUTH
▸ Child (body-weight up to 30 kg): 0.5–1 mg/kg once daily (max. per dose 15 mg once daily), doses to be taken in the morning
▸ Child (body-weight 30 kg and above): 15–30 mg once daily, doses to be taken in the morning

NSAID-associated duodenal ulcer | NSAID-associated gastric ulcer
▶ BY MOUTH
▸ Child (body-weight up to 30 kg): 0.5–1 mg/kg once daily (max. per dose 15 mg once daily), doses to be taken in the morning
▸ Child (body-weight 30 kg and above): 15–30 mg once daily, doses to be taken in the morning

Gastro-oesophageal reflux disease
▶ BY MOUTH
▸ Child (body-weight up to 30 kg): 0.5–1 mg/kg once daily (max. per dose 15 mg once daily), doses to be taken in the morning
▸ Child (body-weight 30 kg and above): 15–30 mg once daily, doses to be taken in the morning

Acid-related dyspepsia
▶ BY MOUTH
▸ Child (body-weight up to 30 kg): 0.5–1 mg/kg once daily (max. per dose 15 mg once daily), doses to be taken in the morning
▸ Child (body-weight 30 kg and above): 15–30 mg once daily, doses to be taken in the morning

Fat malabsorption despite pancreatic enzyme replacement therapy in cystic fibrosis
▶ BY MOUTH
▸ Child (body-weight up to 30 kg): 0.5–1 mg/kg once daily (max. per dose 15 mg once daily), doses to be taken in the morning
▸ Child (body-weight 30 kg and above): 15–30 mg once daily, doses to be taken in the morning

● **UNLICENSED USE** Not licensed for use in children.

● **INTERACTIONS** → Appendix 1: proton pump inhibitors

● **SIDE-EFFECTS**
▶ **Common or very common** Dry throat · fatigue
▶ **Uncommon** Eosinophilia · oedema
▶ **Rare or very rare** Anaemia · angioedema · appetite decreased · erectile dysfunction · fever · glossitis · oesophageal candidiasis · pancreatitis · restlessness · tremor

● **PREGNANCY** Manufacturer advises avoid.

● **BREAST FEEDING** Avoid—present in milk in *animal* studies.

● **HEPATIC IMPAIRMENT** Manufacturer advises caution in moderate to severe impairment (risk of increased exposure).
Dose adjustments Manufacturer advises dose reduction of 50% in moderate to severe impairment.

● **DIRECTIONS FOR ADMINISTRATION** Orodispersible tablets should be placed on the tongue, allowed to disperse and swallowed, or may be swallowed whole with a glass of water. Alternatively, tablets can be dispersed in a small amount of water and administered by an oral syringe or nasogastric tube.

● **PATIENT AND CARER ADVICE** Counselling on administration of orodispersible tablet advised.
Medicines for Children leaflet: Lansoprazole for gastro-oesophageal reflux disease (GORD) and ulcers www.medicinesforchildren.org.uk/lansoprazole-gastro-oesophageal-reflux-disease-gord-and-ulcers

● **MEDICINAL FORMS** There can be variation in the licensing of different medicines containing the same drug. Forms available from special-order manufacturers include: oral suspension, oral solution, powder

Gastro-resistant capsule
CAUTIONARY AND ADVISORY LABELS 5, 22, 25
▸ Lansoprazole (Non-proprietary)
Lansoprazole 15 mg Lansoprazole 15mg gastro-resistant capsules | 28 capsule PoM £12.93 DT = £0.97
Lansoprazole 30 mg Lansoprazole 30mg gastro-resistant capsules | 28 capsule PoM £23.63 DT = £1.27

Orodispersible tablet
CAUTIONARY AND ADVISORY LABELS 5, 22
EXCIPIENTS: May contain Aspartame
▸ Lansoprazole (Non-proprietary)
Lansoprazole 15 mg Lansoprazole 15mg orodispersible tablets | 28 tablet PoM £3.05 DT = £2.98
Lansoprazole 30 mg Lansoprazole 30mg orodispersible tablets | 28 tablet PoM £4.95 DT = £4.62
▸ Zoton FasTab (Pfizer Ltd)
Lansoprazole 15 mg Zoton FasTab 15mg | 28 tablet PoM £2.99 DT = £2.98
Lansoprazole 30 mg Zoton FasTab 30mg | 28 tablet PoM £5.50 DT = £4.62

60

Omeprazole

26-Nov-2019

- **INDICATIONS AND DOSE**

Helicobacter pylori **eradication in combination with amoxicillin and clarithromycin; or in combination with amoxicillin and metronidazole; or in combination with clarithromycin and metronidazole**

▶ BY MOUTH
- Child 1-5 years: 1–2 mg/kg once daily (max. per dose 40 mg)
- Child 6-11 years: 1–2 mg/kg once daily (max. per dose 40 mg)
- Child 12-17 years: 40 mg once daily

Treatment of duodenal ulcers including those complicating NSAID therapy | Treatment of benign gastric ulcers including those complicating NSAID therapy

▶ BY MOUTH
- Neonate: 700 micrograms/kg once daily for 7–14 days, then increased if necessary to 1.4–2.8 mg/kg once daily.
- Child 1 month-1 year: 700 micrograms/kg once daily, increased if necessary to 3 mg/kg once daily (max. per dose 20 mg)
- Child 2-17 years (body-weight 10-19 kg): 10 mg once daily, increased if necessary to 20 mg once daily
- Child 2-17 years (body-weight 20 kg and above): 20 mg once daily, increased if necessary to 40 mg once daily

▶ BY INTRAVENOUS INJECTION, OR BY INTRAVENOUS INFUSION
- Child 1 month-11 years: Initially 500 micrograms/kg once daily (max. per dose 20 mg), increased if necessary to 2 mg/kg once daily (max. per dose 40 mg), injection to be given over 5 minutes
- Child 12-17 years: 40 mg once daily, injection to be given over 5 minutes

Zollinger–Ellison syndrome

▶ BY MOUTH
- Neonate: 700 micrograms/kg once daily for 7–14 days, then increased if necessary to 1.4–2.8 mg/kg once daily.
- Child 1 month-1 year: 700 micrograms/kg once daily, increased if necessary to 3 mg/kg once daily (max. per dose 20 mg)
- Child 2-17 years (body-weight 10-19 kg): 10 mg once daily, increased if necessary to 20 mg once daily
- Child 2-17 years (body-weight 20 kg and above): 20 mg once daily, increased if necessary to 40 mg once daily

▶ BY INTRAVENOUS INJECTION, OR BY INTRAVENOUS INFUSION
- Child 1 month-11 years: Initially 500 micrograms/kg once daily (max. per dose 20 mg), increased if necessary to 2 mg/kg once daily (max. per dose 40 mg), injection to be given over 5 minutes
- Child 12-17 years: 40 mg once daily, injection to be given over 5 minutes

Gastro-oesophageal reflux disease

▶ BY MOUTH
- Neonate: 700 micrograms/kg once daily for 7–14 days, then increased if necessary to 1.4–2.8 mg/kg once daily.
- Child 1 month-1 year: 700 micrograms/kg once daily, increased if necessary to 3 mg/kg once daily (max. per dose 20 mg)
- Child 2-17 years (body-weight 10-19 kg): 10 mg once daily, increased if necessary to 20 mg once daily, in severe ulcerating reflux oesophagitis, maximum 12 weeks at higher dose
- Child 2-17 years (body-weight 20 kg and above): 20 mg once daily, increased if necessary to 40 mg once daily, in severe ulcerating reflux oesophagitis, maximum 12 weeks at higher dose

▶ BY INTRAVENOUS INJECTION, OR BY INTRAVENOUS INFUSION
- Child 1 month-11 years: Initially 500 micrograms/kg once daily (max. per dose 20 mg), increased if necessary to 2 mg/kg once daily (max. per dose 40 mg), injection to be given over 5 minutes
- Child 12-17 years: 40 mg once daily, injection to be given over 5 minutes

Acid-related dyspepsia

▶ BY MOUTH
- Neonate: 700 micrograms/kg once daily for 7–14 days, then increased if necessary to 1.4–2.8 mg/kg once daily.
- Child 1 month-1 year: 700 micrograms/kg once daily, increased if necessary to 3 mg/kg once daily (max. per dose 20 mg)
- Child 2-17 years (initiated by a specialist) (body-weight 10-19 kg): 10 mg once daily, increased if necessary to 20 mg once daily
- Child 2-17 years (initiated by a specialist) (body-weight 20 kg and above): 20 mg once daily, increased if necessary to 40 mg once daily

▶ BY INTRAVENOUS INJECTION, OR BY INTRAVENOUS INFUSION
- Child 1 month-11 years: Initially 500 micrograms/kg once daily (max. per dose 20 mg), increased if necessary to 2 mg/kg once daily (max. per dose 40 mg), injection to be given over 5 minutes
- Child 12-17 years: 40 mg once daily, injection to be given over 5 minutes

Fat malabsorption despite pancreatic enzyme replacement therapy in cystic fibrosis

▶ BY MOUTH
- Neonate: 700 micrograms/kg once daily for 7–14 days, then increased if necessary to 1.4–2.8 mg/kg once daily.
- Child 1 month-1 year: 700 micrograms/kg once daily, increased if necessary to 3 mg/kg once daily (max. per dose 20 mg)
- Child 2-17 years (body-weight 10-19 kg): 10 mg once daily, increased if necessary to 20 mg once daily
- Child 2-17 years (body-weight 20 kg and above): 20 mg once daily, increased if necessary to 40 mg once daily

▶ BY INTRAVENOUS INJECTION, OR BY INTRAVENOUS INFUSION
- Child 1 month-11 years: Initially 500 micrograms/kg once daily (max. per dose 20 mg), increased if necessary to 2 mg/kg once daily (max. per dose 40 mg), injection to be given over 5 minutes
- Child 12-17 years: 40 mg once daily, injection to be given over 5 minutes

- **UNLICENSED USE** *Capsules and tablets* not licensed for use in children except for severe ulcerating reflux oesophagitis in children over 1 year. *Injection* not licensed for use in children under 12 years.
- **INTERACTIONS** → Appendix 1: proton pump inhibitors
- **SIDE-EFFECTS**

▶ **Rare or very rare** Aggression · agitation · bronchospasm · encephalopathy · gastrointestinal candidiasis · muscle weakness

- **PREGNANCY** Not known to be harmful.
- **BREAST FEEDING** Present in milk but not known to be harmful.
- **HEPATIC IMPAIRMENT**

Dose adjustments No more than 700 micrograms/kg (max. 20 mg) once daily.

- **DIRECTIONS FOR ADMINISTRATION** For administration by *mouth*, swallow whole, or disperse *Losec MUPS®* tablets in water, *or* mix capsule contents or *Losec MUPS®* tablets with fruit juice or yoghurt. Preparations consisting of an e/c tablet within a capsule should **not** be opened.

For administration through an *enteral feeding tube*, use *Losec MUPS®* or the contents of a capsule containing omeprazole dispersed in a large volume of water, or in 10 mL Sodium Bicarbonate 8.4% (1 mmol Na^+/mL). Allow to stand for 10 minutes before administration.

For *intermittent intravenous infusion*, dilute reconstituted solution to a concentration of 400 micrograms/mL with Glucose 5% or Sodium Chloride 0.9%; give over 20–30 minutes.

● **PRESCRIBING AND DISPENSING INFORMATION** The RCPCH and NPPG recommend that, when a liquid special of omeprazole is required, the following strength is used: 20 mg/5 mL.

● **PATIENT AND CARER ADVICE**

▸ With oral use Counselling on administration advised. Medicines for Children leaflet: Omeprazole for gastro-oesophageal reflux disease (GORD) www.medicinesforchildren.org.uk/omeprazole-gastro-oesophageal-reflux-disease-gord

● **PROFESSION SPECIFIC INFORMATION**

Dental practitioners' formulary

Gastro-resistant omeprazole capsules may be prescribed.

● **MEDICINAL FORMS** There can be variation in the licensing of different medicines containing the same drug. Forms available from special-order manufacturers include: oral suspension, oral solution

Gastro-resistant capsule

▸ Omeprazole (Non-proprietary)

Omeprazole 10 mg Omeprazole 10mg gastro-resistant capsules | 28 capsule [PoM] £9.30 DT = £1.05

Omeprazole 20 mg Omeprazole 20mg gastro-resistant capsules | 28 capsule [PoM] £9.86 DT = £1.06 | 250 capsule [PoM] £8.50

Omeprazole 40 mg Omeprazole 40mg gastro-resistant capsules | 7 capsule [PoM] £6.96 DT = £0.79 | 28 capsule [PoM] £2.48–£19.72

▸ Losec (AstraZeneca UK Ltd)

Omeprazole 10 mg Losec 10mg gastro-resistant capsules | 28 capsule [PoM] £11.16 DT = £1.05

Omeprazole 20 mg Losec 20mg gastro-resistant capsules | 28 capsule [PoM] £16.70 DT = £1.06

Omeprazole 40 mg Losec 40mg gastro-resistant capsules | 7 capsule [PoM] £8.35 DT = £0.79

▸ Mepradec (Dexcel-Pharma Ltd)

Omeprazole 10 mg Mepradec 10mg gastro-resistant capsules | 28 capsule [PoM] £0.84 DT = £1.05

Gastro-resistant tablet

CAUTIONARY AND ADVISORY LABELS 25

▸ Omeprazole (Non-proprietary)

Omeprazole 10 mg Omeprazole 10mg gastro-resistant tablets | 28 tablet [PoM] £18.91 DT = £7.90

Omeprazole 20 mg Omeprazole 20mg gastro-resistant tablets | 28 tablet [PoM] £28.56 DT = £6.57

Omeprazole 40 mg Omeprazole 40mg gastro-resistant tablets | 7 tablet [PoM] £14.28 DT = £6.77

▸ Losec MUPS (AstraZeneca UK Ltd)

Omeprazole (as Omeprazole magnesium) 10 mg Losec MUPS 10mg gastro-resistant tablets | 28 tablet [PoM] £9.30 DT = £9.30

Omeprazole (as Omeprazole magnesium) 20 mg Losec MUPS 20mg gastro-resistant tablets | 28 tablet [PoM] £13.92 DT = £13.92

Omeprazole (as Omeprazole magnesium) 40 mg Losec MUPS 40mg gastro-resistant tablets | 7 tablet [PoM] £6.96 DT = £6.96

▸ Mezzopram (Sandoz Ltd)

Omeprazole (as Omeprazole magnesium) 10 mg Mezzopram 10mg dispersible gastro-resistant tablets | 28 tablet [PoM] £6.58 DT = £9.30

Omeprazole (as Omeprazole magnesium) 20 mg Mezzopram 20mg dispersible gastro-resistant tablets | 28 tablet [PoM] £9.86 DT = £13.92

Omeprazole (as Omeprazole magnesium) 40 mg Mezzopram 40mg dispersible gastro-resistant tablets | 7 tablet [PoM] £4.93 DT = £6.96

Oral suspension

▸ Omeprazole (Non-proprietary)

Omeprazole 2 mg per 1 ml Omeprazole 10mg/5ml oral suspension sugar-free | 75 ml [PoM] £92.17 DT = £92.17

Omeprazole 4 mg per 1 ml Omeprazole 20mg/5ml oral suspension sugar-free | 75 ml [PoM] £178.35 DT = £178.35

Powder for solution for infusion

▸ Omeprazole (Non-proprietary)

Omeprazole (as Omeprazole sodium) 40 mg Omeprazole 40mg powder for solution for infusion vials | 5 vial [PoM] £6.50–£29.23 DT = £26.00 (Hospital only)

4.3 Gastro-oesophageal reflux disease

Gastro-oesophageal reflux disease

31-Oct-2019

Description of condition

Gastro-oesophageal reflux is the passage of gastric contents into the oesophagus and occurs as a result of transient lower oesophageal sphincter relaxation. It is considered physiological in infants when symptoms are absent or not troublesome. Regurgitation is the voluntary or involuntary movement of part or all of the stomach contents up the oesophagus at least as far as the mouth and often emerging from the mouth. It is common in infants under the age of 1 year and considered normal, and usually resolves without treatment before 1 year of age. Gastro-oesophageal reflux disease (GORD) occurs when reflux results in complications, or symptoms are severe enough to require medical treatment.

In infants up to 1 year of age symptoms suggestive of GORD include excessive crying, crying when feeding, unusual neck posture, hoarseness, chronic cough, faltering growth and feeding difficulties such as gagging, choking or refusal. In older children symptoms include heartburn, retrosternal and epigastric pain.

Risk factors for developing GORD include premature birth, hiatus hernia and neurodisability. Complications that might occur include reflux oesophagitis, aspiration pneumonia, dental erosions and recurrent otitis media.

In children with vomiting and regurgitation problems, look for 'red flag symptoms' such as frequent and forceful vomiting, bile-stained vomit, or blood in vomit or stools, that may suggest disorders other than GORD.

Aims of treatment

The aim of treatment is to manage symptoms of GORD in children and raise awareness of symptoms that need investigating.

Non-drug treatment

[EvGr] Parents and carers of well infants should be reassured that most symptoms of uncomplicated gastro-oesophageal reflux are common and resolve without treatment before 1 year of age.

In breast-fed infants with frequent regurgitation and marked distress, ensure that a person with appropriate expertise and training carries out a breastfeeding assessment.

In formula-fed infants with frequent regurgitation and marked distress use a stepped care approach with review of feeding history, reduction of feed volumes if excessive for the infant's weight, and then a 1–2 week trial of smaller and more frequent feeds. If symptoms are still not improving give a trial of thickened formula for another 1–2 weeks.

Children and adolescents who are obese should be advised that weight reduction may help with their symptoms.

Surgery may be considered under specialist advice for children with severe, intractable GORD where medical treatment has been unsuccessful, or feeding regimens to manage symptoms have proved impractical. ⟨A⟩

Drug treatment

Initial management

EvGr If non-pharmacological methods fail for breast-fed infants, consider alginic acid p. 55 for 1–2 weeks. If successful, this should be continued but consider withholding it at intervals to see if the infant has recovered.

If non-pharmacological methods fail for formula-fed infants, the thickened formula should be stopped and a trial of alginic acid for 1–2 weeks should be used. If successful, it should be continued, but consider withholding it at intervals to see if the infant has recovered.

Acid-suppressing drugs, such as Proton pump inhibitors p. 60 or H2-receptor antagonists p. 59 should not be used to treat regurgitation in children occurring as an isolated symptom. Ⓐ

Follow up management

EvGr For children who are unable to communicate about their symptoms (e.g. infants, young children and those with communication difficulties), a 4-week trial of a proton pump inhibitor (PPI) or histamine$_2$-receptor antagonist (H_2-receptor antagonist) should be considered in those who have regurgitation with one or more of the following symptoms: unexplained feeding difficulties, distressed behaviour or faltering growth.

For children and young people with persistent heartburn, retrosternal or epigastric pain, a 4-week trial of a PPI or H_2-receptor antagonist should be considered.

When choosing between a PPI or H_2-receptor antagonist availability of age-appropriate preparations, patient/carer preference should be taken into account.

Response to treatment should be reviewed after 4 weeks and referral for endoscopy considered if the symptoms did not resolve, or recur after stopping treatment.

Treatment of gastro-oesophageal reflux or GORD with metoclopramide hydrochloride p. 278 (unlicensed), domperidone p. 278 (unlicensed), or erythromycin p. 355 (unlicensed) should only be offered when the benefits outweigh the risk of side-effects, other interventions have been tried, and there is specialist paediatric agreement for its use.

Infants, children and young people with endoscopy-proven reflux oesophagitis should be offered treatment with a PPI or H_2-receptor antagonist, and repeat endoscopic examination performed as necessary to guide subsequent treatment. Ⓐ

Enteral tube feeding

EvGr Enteral tube feeding should only be considered as an option to promote weight gain in infants and children with regurgitation and faltering growth if other pathologies have been ruled out, and/or the recommended feeding and medical management is unsuccessful.

A specific and individualised nutrition plan must be in place for these children with a strategy to reduce it as soon as possible. Oral stimulation is encouraged by continuing oral feeding as tolerated, ensuring that the intended target weight is achieved and sustained. Enteral tube feeding should be reduced and stopped as soon as possible.

Jejunal feeding can be considered in patients who need enteral tube feeding but cannot tolerate intragastric feeds because of regurgitation or if reflux-related pulmonary aspiration is a concern. Ⓐ

For advice on specialised formula feeds, see Enteral nutrition p. 671.

GORD in pregnancy

EvGr Heartburn and acid reflux are symptoms of Dyspepsia p. 55 in pregnancy commonly caused by GORD. Dietary and lifestyle advice should be given as first-line management. If this approach fails to control symptoms, an antacid or an alginate can be used. If this is ineffective or symptoms are severe omeprazole p. 63 or ranitidine p. 59 (unlicensed) may help to control symptoms. Ⓐ

Useful Resources

Gastro-oesophageal reflux disease in children and young people: diagnosis and management. National Institute for Health and Care Excellence. NICE guideline 1. January 2015, updated October 2019.
www.nice.org.uk/guidance/ng1

Other drugs used for Gastro-oesophageal reflux disease
Esomeprazole, p. 61 · Lansoprazole, p. 62

ANTACIDS > ALGINATE

Sodium alginate with calcium carbonate and sodium bicarbonate

24-Apr-2020

The properties listed below are those particular to the combination only. For the properties of the components please consider, alginic acid p. 55, sodium bicarbonate p. 634, calcium carbonate p. 641.

● **INDICATIONS AND DOSE**

Gastro-oesophageal reflux disease

▸ BY MOUTH
▸ Child 6-11 years: 5–10 mL, to be taken after meals and at bedtime
▸ Child 12-17 years: 10–20 mL, to be taken after meals and at bedtime

● **INTERACTIONS** → Appendix 1: calcium salts · sodium bicarbonate

● **PRESCRIBING AND DISPENSING INFORMATION** Flavours of oral liquid formulations may include aniseed or peppermint.

● **PATIENT AND CARER ADVICE**
Medicines for Children leaflet: Gaviscon for gastro-oesophageal reflux disease www.medicinesforchildren.org.uk/gaviscon-gastro-oesophageal-reflux-disease

● **MEDICINAL FORMS** There can be variation in the licensing of different medicines containing the same drug.

Oral suspension

ELECTROLYTES: May contain Sodium

▸ Acidex (Pinewood Healthcare)
Calcium carbonate 16 mg per 1 ml, Sodium bicarbonate 26.7 mg per 1 ml, Sodium alginate 50 mg per 1 ml Acidex oral suspension aniseed sugar-free | 500 ml GSL £2.56 DT = £1.95
Acidex oral suspension peppermint sugar-free | 150 ml GSL £1.21 DT = £2.58 sugar-free | 500 ml GSL £2.56 DT = £1.95

▸ Entrocalm Heartburn and Indigestion Relief (Galpharm International Ltd)
Calcium carbonate 16 mg per 1 ml, Sodium bicarbonate 26.7 mg per 1 ml, Sodium alginate 50 mg per 1 ml Entrocalm Heartburn and Indigestion Relief oral suspension sugar-free | 150 ml GSL ✕ DT = £2.58

▸ Gaviscon (Reckitt Benckiser Healthcare (UK) Ltd)
Calcium carbonate 16 mg per 1 ml, Sodium bicarbonate 26.7 mg per 1 ml, Sodium alginate 50 mg per 1 ml Gaviscon Original Aniseed Relief sugar-free | 150 ml GSL £2.58 DT = £2.58 sugar-free | 300 ml GSL £4.33 DT = £4.33 sugar-free | 600 ml GSL £7.11 DT = £7.11

▸ Gaviscon Liquid Relief (Reckitt Benckiser Healthcare (UK) Ltd)
Calcium carbonate 16 mg per 1 ml, Sodium bicarbonate 26.7 mg per 1 ml, Sodium alginate 50 mg per 1 ml Gaviscon Peppermint Liquid Relief sugar-free | 150 ml GSL £2.58 DT = £2.58 sugar-free | 300 ml GSL £4.33 DT = £4.33 sugar-free | 600 ml GSL £7.11 DT = £7.11

▸ Peptac (Teva UK Ltd)
Calcium carbonate 16 mg per 1 ml, Sodium bicarbonate 26.7 mg per 1 ml, Sodium alginate 50 mg per 1 ml Peptac liquid peppermint sugar-free | 500 ml GSL £1.95 DT = £1.95
Peptac liquid aniseed sugar-free | 500 ml GSL £1.95 DT = £1.95

- Rennie (Bayer Plc)
  Calcium carbonate 16 mg per 1 ml, Sodium bicarbonate 26.7 mg per 1 ml, Sodium alginate 50 mg per 1 ml Rennie Liquid Heartburn Relief oral suspension sugar-free | 150 ml GSL £2.52 DT = £2.58 sugar-free | 250 ml GSL £3.47

4.4 Helicobacter pylori diagnosis

DIAGNOSTIC AGENTS

Urea (13C)

● **INDICATIONS AND DOSE**

Diagnosis of gastro-duodenal *Helicobacter pylori* infection
- BY MOUTH
- Child: (consult product literature)

● **MEDICINAL FORMS** There can be variation in the licensing of different medicines containing the same drug.

Soluble tablet
- Pylobactell (Torbet Laboratories Ltd)
  Urea [13-C] 100 mg Pylobactell breath test kit | 1 kit PoM £20.75 DT = £20.75

Powder
- Helicobacter Test INFAI (INFAI UK Ltd)
  Urea [13-C] 45 mg Helicobacter Test INFAI for children breath test kit sugar-free | 1 kit PoM £19.10 DT = £19.10
  Urea [13-C] 75 mg Helicobacter Test INFAI breath test kit sugar-free | 1 kit PoM £21.70 DT = £21.70 sugar-free | 50 kit PoM £955.00

Tablet
- Diabact UBT (HFA Healthcare Products Ltd)
  Urea [13-C] 50 mg diabact UBT 50mg tablets | 1 tablet PoM £21.25 DT = £21.25 | 10 tablet PoM £78.75 (Hospital only)

5 Food allergy

Food allergy

15-Dec-2016

Description of condition

Food allergy is an adverse immune response to a food, commonly associated with cutaneous and gastro-intestinal reactions, and less frequently associated with respiratory reactions and anaphylaxis. It is distinct from food intolerance which is non-immunological. Cow's milk, hen's eggs, soy, wheat, peanuts, tree nuts, fish, and shellfish are the most common allergens. Cross-reactivity between similar foods can occur (e.g. allergy to other mammalian milk in patients with cow's milk allergy).

Management of food allergy

EvGr Allergy caused by specific foods should be managed by strict avoidance of the causal food. Sodium cromoglicate p. 176 is licensed as an adjunct to dietary avoidance in children with food allergy. Educating the child or their carer about appropriate nutrition, food preparation, and the risks of accidental exposure is recommended, such as food and drinks to avoid, ensuring adequate nutritional intake, and interpreting food labels. For children in whom elimination diets might affect growth, a consultation with a nutritionist is recommended to identify alternative dietary sources. Ⓐ

Drug treatment

EvGr There is low quality evidence to support the use of antihistamines to treat acute, **non-life-threatening** symptoms (such as flushing and urticaria) if accidental ingestion of allergenic food has occurred (see *Antihistamines*, under Antihistamines, allergen immunotherapy and allergic emergencies p. 180). Chlorphenamine maleate p. 186 is licensed for the symptomatic control of food allergy. In case of food-induced anaphylaxis, adrenaline/epinephrine p. 143 is the first-line immediate treatment (see also *Allergic emergencies*, under Antihistamines, allergen immunotherapy and allergic emergencies p. 180). Carers and children (of an appropriate age) who are at risk of anaphylaxis should be trained to use self-injectable adrenaline/epinephrine. Ⓐ

Cow's milk allergy

EvGr Parents of infants with suspected allergy to cow's milk should be informed about the most appropriate hypoallergenic formula or milk substitute. Cow's milk avoidance is recommended for the mothers of breast-fed infants who have cow's milk allergy. Children who are allergic to milk should receive alternative dietary sources of calcium and vitamin D. Ⓐ

Useful Resources

Food allergy in under 19s: assessment and diagnosis. National Institute for Health and Care Excellence. Clinical guideline 116. February 2011
www.nice.org.uk/guidance/cg116

6 Gastro-intestinal smooth muscle spasm

Antispasmodics

19-Feb-2020

Antimuscarinics

The intestinal smooth muscle relaxant properties of antimuscarinic and other antispasmodic drugs may be useful in *irritable bowel syndrome*.

Antimuscarinics (formerly termed 'anticholinergics') reduce intestinal motility. They are occasionally used for the management of *irritable bowel syndrome*.

Antimuscarinics that are used for gastro-intestinal smooth muscle spasm includes the tertiary amine dicycloverine hydrochloride p. 67 and the quaternary ammonium compounds propantheline bromide p. 68 and hyoscine butylbromide p. 67. The quaternary ammonium compounds are less lipid soluble than atropine and are less likely to cross the blood-brain barrier; they are also less well absorbed from the gastro-intestinal tract.

Dicycloverine hydrochloride, may also have some direct action on smooth muscle. Hyoscine butylbromide is advocated as a gastro-intestinal antispasmodic, but it is poorly absorbed; the injection may be useful in endoscopy and radiology.

Other indications for antimuscarinic drugs include asthma and airways disease, motion sickness, urinary frequency and enuresis, mydriasis and cycloplegia, premedication, palliative care and as an antidote to organophosphorus poisoning.

Other antispasmodics

Alverine citrate p. 68, mebeverine hydrochloride p. 69, and peppermint oil p. 40 are believed to be direct relaxants of intestinal smooth muscle and may relieve pain in *irritable bowel syndrome*, and *primary dysmenorrhoea*. They have no serious adverse effects but, like all antispasmodics, should be avoided in paralytic ileus.

Motility stimulants

Domperidone is a dopamine receptor antagonist which stimulates gastric emptying and small intestinal transit, and enhances the strength of oesophageal sphincter contraction. The MHRA and CHM have released important safety information and restrictions regarding the use of domperidone, and a reminder of contra-indications. For further information, see *Important safety information* for domperidone p. 278.

A low dose of erythromycin p. 355 stimulates gastro-intestinal motility and may be used on the advice of a paediatric gastroenterologist to promote tolerance of enteral feeds; erythromycin may be less effective as a prokinetic drug in preterm neonates than in older children.

ANTIMUSCARINICS

F 527

Dicycloverine hydrochloride

23-Apr-2020

(Dicyclomine hydrochloride)

● **INDICATIONS AND DOSE**

Symptomatic relief of gastro-intestinal disorders characterised by smooth muscle spasm

▶ BY MOUTH

- Child 6–23 months: 5–10 mg 3–4 times a day, dose to be taken 15 minutes before feeds
- Child 2–11 years: 10 mg 3 times a day
- Child 12–17 years: 10–20 mg 3 times a day

● **CONTRA-INDICATIONS** Child under 6 months

● **INTERACTIONS** → Appendix 1: dicycloverine

● **SIDE-EFFECTS** Appetite decreased · fatigue · thirst

● **PREGNANCY** Not known to be harmful; manufacturer advises use only if essential.

● **BREAST FEEDING** Avoid—present in milk; apnoea reported in infant.

● **EXCEPTIONS TO LEGAL CATEGORY** Dicycloverine hydrochloride can be sold to the public provided that max. single dose is 10 mg and max. daily dose is 60 mg.

● **MEDICINAL FORMS** There can be variation in the licensing of different medicines containing the same drug.

Oral solution

- Dicycloverine hydrochloride (Non-proprietary)
  Dicycloverine hydrochloride 2 mg per 1 ml Dicycloverine 10mg/5ml oral solution | 120 ml PoM £196.36 DT = £174.40

Tablet

- Dicycloverine hydrochloride (Non-proprietary)
  Dicycloverine hydrochloride 10 mg Dicycloverine 10mg tablets | 100 tablet PoM £221.82 DT = £220.26
  Dicycloverine hydrochloride 20 mg Dicycloverine 20mg tablets | 84 tablet PoM £234.11 DT = £232.91

Dicycloverine hydrochloride with aluminium hydroxide, magnesium oxide and simeticone

28-Apr-2020

The properties listed below are those particular to the combination only. For the properties of the components please consider, dicycloverine hydrochloride above, simeticone p. 57.

● **INDICATIONS AND DOSE**

Symptomatic relief of gastro-intestinal disorders characterised by smooth muscle spasm

▶ BY MOUTH

- Child 12–17 years: 10–20 mL every 4 hours as required

● **INTERACTIONS** → Appendix 1: antacids · dicycloverine

● **SIDE-EFFECTS** Anticholinergic syndrome

● **RENAL IMPAIRMENT** There is a risk of accumulation and aluminium toxicity with antacids containing aluminium salts. Absorption of aluminium from aluminium salts is increased by citrates, which are contained in many effervescent preparations (such as effervescent analgesics).

● **MEDICINAL FORMS** There can be variation in the licensing of different medicines containing the same drug.

Oral suspension

- Kolanticon (Peckforton Pharmaceuticals Ltd)
  Dicycloverine hydrochloride 500 microgram per 1 ml, Simeticone 4 mg per 1 ml, Magnesium oxide light 20 mg per 1 ml, Aluminium hydroxide dried 40 mg per 1 ml Kolanticon gel sugar-free | 200 ml P £4.00 sugar-free | 500 ml P £6.00

F 527

Hyoscine butylbromide

12-Sep-2019

● **INDICATIONS AND DOSE**

Symptomatic relief of gastro-intestinal or genito-urinary disorders characterised by smooth muscle spasm

▶ BY MOUTH

- Child 6–11 years: 10 mg 3 times a day
- Child 12–17 years: 20 mg 4 times a day

Acute spasm | Spasm in diagnostic procedures

▶ INITIALLY BY INTRAMUSCULAR INJECTION, OR BY SLOW INTRAVENOUS INJECTION

- Child 2–5 years: 5 mg, then (by intramuscular injection or by slow intravenous injection) 5 mg after 30 minutes if required, dose may be repeated more frequently in endoscopy; maximum 15 mg per day
- Child 6–11 years: 5–10 mg, then (by intramuscular injection or by intravenous injection) 5–10 mg after 30 minutes if required, dose may be repeated more frequently in endoscopy; maximum 30 mg per day
- Child 12–17 years: 20 mg, then (by intramuscular injection or by slow intravenous injection) 20 mg after 30 minutes if required, dose may be repeated more frequently in endoscopy; maximum 80 mg per day

Excessive respiratory secretions in palliative care

▶ BY MOUTH

- Child 1 month–1 year: 300–500 micrograms/kg 3–4 times a day (max. per dose 5 mg)
- Child 2–4 years: 5 mg 3–4 times a day
- Child 5–11 years: 10 mg 3–4 times a day
- Child 12–17 years: 10–20 mg 3–4 times a day

▶ BY INTRAMUSCULAR INJECTION, OR BY INTRAVENOUS INJECTION

- Child 1 month–4 years: 300–500 micrograms/kg 3–4 times a day (max. per dose 5 mg)
- Child 5–11 years: 5–10 mg 3–4 times a day
- Child 12–17 years: 10–20 mg 3–4 times a day

Bowel colic in palliative care

▶ BY MOUTH

- Child 1 month–1 year: 300–500 micrograms/kg 3–4 times a day (max. per dose 5 mg)
- Child 2–4 years: 5 mg 3–4 times a day
- Child 5–11 years: 10 mg 3–4 times a day
- Child 12–17 years: 10–20 mg 3–4 times a day

▶ BY INTRAMUSCULAR INJECTION, OR BY INTRAVENOUS INJECTION

- Child 1 month–4 years: 300–500 micrograms/kg 3–4 times a day (max. per dose 5 mg)
- Child 5–11 years: 5–10 mg 3–4 times a day
- Child 12–17 years: 10–20 mg 3–4 times a day

PHARMACOKINETICS

- Administration by mouth is associated with poor absorption.

- **UNLICENSED USE** *Tablets* not licensed for use in children under 6 years. *Injection* not licensed for use in children (age range not specified by manufacturer).

> **IMPORTANT SAFETY INFORMATION**
>
> MHRA/CHM ADVICE: HYOSCINE BUTYLBROMIDE (*BUSCOPAN*®) INJECTION: RISK OF SERIOUS ADVERSE EFFECTS IN PATIENTS WITH UNDERLYING CARDIAC DISEASE (FEBRUARY 2017)
>
> The MHRA advises that hyoscine butylbromide injection can cause serious adverse effects including tachycardia, hypotension, and anaphylaxis; several reports have noted that anaphylaxis is more likely to be fatal in patients with underlying coronary heart disease. Hyoscine butylbromide injection is contra-indicated in patients with tachycardia and should be used with caution in patients with cardiac disease; the MHRA recommends that these patients are monitored and that resuscitation equipment and trained personnel are readily available.

- **CONTRA-INDICATIONS**
  - With intramuscular use or intravenous use Tachycardia
- **INTERACTIONS** → Appendix 1: hyoscine
- **SIDE-EFFECTS**
  GENERAL SIDE-EFFECTS Dyspnoea
  SPECIFIC SIDE-EFFECTS
  - With parenteral use Feeling hot · hypotension · mydriasis · sweat changes
- **PREGNANCY** Manufacturer advises avoid.
- **BREAST FEEDING** Amount too small to be harmful.
- **DIRECTIONS FOR ADMINISTRATION**
  - With oral use For administration by *mouth*, injection solution may be used; content of ampoule may be stored in a refrigerator for up to 24 hours after opening.
  - With intravenous use For *intravenous injection*, may be diluted with Glucose 5% or Sodium Chloride 0.9%; give over at least 1 minute.
- **PRESCRIBING AND DISPENSING INFORMATION**
  Palliative care For further information on the use of hyoscine butylbromide in palliative care, see www.medicinescomplete.com/#/content/palliative/hyoscine-butylbromide.
- **EXCEPTIONS TO LEGAL CATEGORY** Hyoscine butylbromide tablets can be sold to the public for medically confirmed irritable bowel syndrome, provided single dose does not exceed 20 mg, daily dose does not exceed 80 mg, and pack does not contain a total of more than 240 mg.

- **MEDICINAL FORMS** There can be variation in the licensing of different medicines containing the same drug. Forms available from special-order manufacturers include: oral suspension, oral solution

Solution for injection

- Buscopan (Sanofi)
  Hyoscine butylbromide 20 mg per 1 ml Buscopan 20mg/1ml solution for injection ampoules | 10 ampoule PoM £2.92 DT = £2.92

Tablet

- Buscopan (Sanofi)
  Hyoscine butylbromide 10 mg Buscopan 10mg tablets | 56 tablet PoM £3.00 DT = £3.00 | 100 tablet PoM £5.35

F 527

Propantheline bromide

- **INDICATIONS AND DOSE**

Symptomatic relief of gastro-intestinal disorders characterised by smooth muscle spasm

- BY MOUTH
  - Child 1 month–11 years: 300 micrograms/kg 3–4 times a day (max. per dose 15 mg), dose to be taken at least one hour before food
  - Child 12–17 years: 15 mg 3 times a day, dose to be taken at least one hour before food and 30 mg, dose to be taken at night; maximum 120 mg per day

- **UNLICENSED USE** Not licensed for use in children.
- **INTERACTIONS** → Appendix 1: propantheline
- **SIDE-EFFECTS** Arrhythmias · bronchial secretion decreased · mydriasis
- **PREGNANCY** Manufacturer advises avoid unless essential—no information available.
- **BREAST FEEDING** May suppress lactation.
- **HEPATIC IMPAIRMENT** Manufacturer advises caution.
- **RENAL IMPAIRMENT** Manufacturer advises caution.

- **MEDICINAL FORMS** There can be variation in the licensing of different medicines containing the same drug. Forms available from special-order manufacturers include: oral suspension, oral solution

Tablet

CAUTIONARY AND ADVISORY LABELS 23

- Pro-Banthine (Kyowa Kirin Ltd)
  Propantheline bromide 15 mg Pro-Banthine 15mg tablets | 112 tablet PoM £20.74 DT = £20.74

ANTISPASMODICS

Alverine citrate

19-May-2020

- **INDICATIONS AND DOSE**

Symptomatic relief of gastro-intestinal disorders characterised by smooth muscle spasm | Dysmenorrhoea

- BY MOUTH
  - Child 12–17 years: 60–120 mg 1–3 times a day

- **CONTRA-INDICATIONS** Intestinal obstruction · paralytic ileus
- **SIDE-EFFECTS** Dizziness · dyspnoea · headache · jaundice (reversible on discontinuation) · nausea · skin reactions · wheezing
- **PREGNANCY** Manufacturer advises avoid—limited information available
- **BREAST FEEDING** Manufacturer advises avoid—limited information available.
- **PATIENT AND CARER ADVICE**
  Driving and skilled tasks Dizziness may affect performance of skilled tasks (e.g. driving).

- **MEDICINAL FORMS** There can be variation in the licensing of different medicines containing the same drug.

Capsule

- Alverine citrate (Non-proprietary)
  Alverine citrate 60 mg Alverine 60mg capsules | 100 capsule PoM £10.50–£19.49 DT = £11.26
  Alverine citrate 120 mg Alverine 120mg capsules | 60 capsule PoM £23.29 DT = £23.29
- Audmonal (Teva UK Ltd)
  Alverine citrate 60 mg Audmonal 60mg capsules | 100 capsule P £14.80 DT = £11.26
  Alverine citrate 120 mg Audmonal Forte 120mg capsules | 60 capsule P £17.75 DT = £23.29
- Spasmonal (Mylan)
  Alverine citrate 60 mg Spasmonal 60mg capsules | 20 capsule P £3.29 | 100 capsule P £16.45 DT = £11.26
  Alverine citrate 120 mg Spasmonal Forte 120mg capsules | 60 capsule P £19.42 DT = £23.29

Mebeverine hydrochloride

12-Feb-2019

● **INDICATIONS AND DOSE**

Adjunct in gastro-intestinal disorders characterised by smooth muscle spasm

▶ BY MOUTH USING IMMEDIATE-RELEASE MEDICINES

- ▶ Child 3 years: 25 mg 3 times a day, dose preferably taken 20 minutes before meals
- ▶ Child 4–7 years: 50 mg 3 times a day, dose preferably taken 20 minutes before meals
- ▶ Child 8–9 years: 100 mg 3 times a day, dose preferably taken 20 minutes before meals
- ▶ Child 10–17 years: 135–150 mg 3 times a day, dose preferably taken 20 minutes before meals

Irritable bowel syndrome

▶ BY MOUTH USING MODIFIED-RELEASE MEDICINES

- ▶ Child 12–17 years: 200 mg twice daily

● **UNLICENSED USE** *Suspension* not licensed for use in children under 10 years. *Tablets* and *modified-release capsules* not licensed for use in children.

● **CONTRA-INDICATIONS** Paralytic ileus

● **SIDE-EFFECTS** Angioedema · face oedema · skin reactions

● **PREGNANCY** Not known to be harmful—manufacturers advise avoid.

● **BREAST FEEDING** Manufacturers advise avoid—no information available.

● **PATIENT AND CARER ADVICE** Patients or carers should be given advice on the timing of administration of mebeverine hydrochloride tablets and oral suspension.
Medicines for Children leaflet: Mebeverine for intestinal spasms www.medicinesforchildren.org.uk/mebeverine-intestinal-spasms

● **MEDICINAL FORMS** There can be variation in the licensing of different medicines containing the same drug. Forms available from special-order manufacturers include: oral suspension

Oral suspension

▶ Mebeverine hydrochloride (Non-proprietary)
Mebeverine hydrochloride (as Mebeverine pamoate) 10 mg per 1 ml Mebeverine 50mg/5ml oral suspension sugar-free | 300 ml [PoM] £187.00 DT = £187.00

Modified-release capsule

CAUTIONARY AND ADVISORY LABELS 25

▶ Mebeverine hydrochloride (Non-proprietary)
Mebeverine hydrochloride 200 mg Mebeverine 200mg modified-release capsules | 60 capsule [PoM] £10.14 DT = £9.22

▶ Aurobeverine MR (Milpharm Ltd)
Mebeverine hydrochloride 200 mg Aurobeverine MR 200mg capsules | 60 capsule [PoM] £6.92 DT = £9.22

▶ Colofac MR (Mylan)
Mebeverine hydrochloride 200 mg Colofac MR 200mg capsules | 60 capsule [PoM] £6.92 DT = £9.22

Tablet

▶ Mebeverine hydrochloride (Non-proprietary)
Mebeverine hydrochloride 135 mg Mebeverine 135mg tablets | 100 tablet [PoM] £20.00 DT = £5.11

▶ Colofac (Mylan)
Mebeverine hydrochloride 135 mg Colofac 135mg tablets | 100 tablet [PoM] £9.02 DT = £5.11

7 Liver disorders and related conditions

7.1 Biliary disorders

Cholestasis

01-May-2017

Description of condition

Cholestasis is an impairment of bile formation and/or bile flow, which may clinically present with fatigue, pruritus, dark urine, pale stools and, in its most overt form, jaundice and signs of fat soluble vitamin deficiencies.

Treatment

[EvGr] Ursodeoxycholic acid p. 71 [unlicensed] and colestyramine p. 136 [unlicensed under 6 years] are used to relieve cholestatic pruritus in children, even if evidence to support their use is limited.

Colestyramine is an anion-exchange resin that is not absorbed from the gastro-intestinal tract. It relieves pruritus by forming an insoluble complex in the intestine with bile acids and other compounds—the reduction of serum bile acid levels reduces excess deposition in the dermal tissue with a resultant decrease in pruritus.

Under specialist supervision, other drugs which may be used as an alternative treatment for **intractable** cholestatic pruritus include rifampicin p. 396 [unlicensed indication], phenobarbital p. 232 [unlicensed indication] and opioid antagonists [unlicensed indication]. However, they should be used with caution and under expert guidance as these children usually have severe liver disease—careful monitoring is required. ⟨E⟩

Inborn errors of primary bile acid synthesis

27-Apr-2018

Description of condition

Inborn errors of primary bile acid synthesis are a group of diseases in which the liver does not produce enough primary bile acids due to enzyme deficiencies. These acids are the main components of the bile, and include cholic acid and chenodeoxycholic acid.

Treatment

Cholic acid p. 70 is licensed for the treatment of inborn errors of primary bile acid synthesis due to an inborn deficiency of two specific liver enzymes. It acts by replacing some of the missing bile acids, therefore relieving the symptoms of the disease.

Chenodeoxycholic acid p. 70 is licensed for the treatment of inborn errors of primary bile acid synthesis due to a deficiency of one specific enzyme in the bile acid synthesis pathway when presenting as cerebrotendinous xanthomatosis.

Ursodeoxycholic acid p. 71 [unlicensed indication] has been used to treat inborn errors in primary bile acid synthesis, but there is an absence of evidence to recommend its use.

Primary biliary cholangitis

30-May-2017

Description of condition

Primary biliary cholangitis (or primary biliary cirrhosis) is a chronic cholestatic disease which develops due to progressive destruction of small and intermediate bile ducts within the liver, subsequently evolving to fibrosis and cirrhosis.

Treatment

EvGr Ursodeoxycholic acid p. 71 is recommended for the management of primary biliary cholangitis, including those with asymptomatic disease. It slows disease progression, but the effect on overall survival is uncertain. (A)

Smith-Lemli-Opitz syndrome

30-May-2017

Description of condition

Smith-Lemli-Opitz syndrome is an inborn error of cholesterol synthesis. It is characterised by multiple congenital anomalies, intellectual deficit, growth delay, microcephaly, and behavioural problems. The disease is present at birth, but may be detected in later childhood or adulthood in mild forms. Hypoglycaemia due to adrenal insufficiency can present as an acute manifestation.

Aims of treatment

There is currently no cure for Smith-Lemli-Opitz syndrome. Management is aimed at symptom relief and alleviation of functional disabilities.

Treatment

EvGr Children with Smith-Lemli-Opitz syndrome are treated with dietary cholesterol supplementation, including high cholesterol foods (such as egg yolks) or a suspension of pharmaceutical grade cholesterol p. 71 (available from Special-order manufacturers p. 1152 or specialist importing companies) to help improve growth failure and photosensitivity. (E) However, it is not clear who will benefit most from cholesterol treatment or how long it should continue.

EvGr In some cases bile acid supplements, such as chenodeoxycholic acid below [unlicensed] and ursodeoxycholic acid p. 71 [unlicensed indication] have been also used for this condition, but their use is not generally recommended. (E)

BILE ACIDS

Chenodeoxycholic acid

05-Apr-2018

- **INDICATIONS AND DOSE**

Cerebrotendinous xanthomatosis (specialist use only)

▶ BY MOUTH

- Child: Initially 5 mg/kg daily in 3 divided doses, adjusted according to response; maximum 15 mg/kg per day; maximum 1000 mg per day

Defective synthesis of bile acid (specialist use only)

▶ BY MOUTH

- Neonate: Initially 5 mg/kg 3 times a day, reduced to 2.5 mg/kg 3 times a day.
- Child: Initially 5 mg/kg 3 times a day, reduced to 2.5 mg/kg 3 times a day

Smith-Lemli-Opitz syndrome (specialist use only)

▶ BY MOUTH

- Neonate: 7 mg/kg once daily, alternatively 7 mg/kg daily in divided doses.
- Child: 7 mg/kg once daily, alternatively 7 mg/kg daily in divided doses

- **UNLICENSED USE** Not licensed for defective synthesis of bile acid. Not licensed for Smith-Lemli-Opitz syndrome.
- **CONTRA-INDICATIONS** Non-functioning gall bladder · radio-opaque stones
- **INTERACTIONS** → Appendix 1: chenodeoxycholic acid
- **SIDE-EFFECTS** Constipation
- **PREGNANCY** Manufacturer advises avoid—fetotoxicity reported in *animal* studies.
- **HEPATIC IMPAIRMENT** Manufacturer advises monitor—no information available.
- **RENAL IMPAIRMENT** Manufacturer advises monitor—no information available.
- **MONITORING REQUIREMENTS** Manufacturer advises to monitor serum cholestanol levels and/or urine bile alcohols every 3 months during the initiation of therapy and dose adjustment, and then at least annually; liver function should also be monitored during initiation of therapy and then at least annually; additional or more frequent investigations may need to be undertaken to monitor therapy during periods of fast growth or concomitant disease.
- **DIRECTIONS FOR ADMINISTRATION** For administration *by mouth* in patients who are unable to swallow capsules and/or need to take a dose below 250 mg, manufacturer advises to add capsule contents to sodium bicarbonate solution 8.4%—for further information, consult product literature.

- **MEDICINAL FORMS** There can be variation in the licensing of different medicines containing the same drug.

Capsule

▶ Chenodeoxycholic acid (non-proprietary) ▼
Chenodeoxycholic acid 250 mg Chenodeoxycholic acid 250mg capsules | 100 capsule PoM £14,000.00 DT = £9,999.99

Cholic acid

12-Jul-2018

- **DRUG ACTION** Cholic acid is the predominant primary bile acid in humans, which can be used to provide a source of bile acid in patients with inborn deficiencies in bile acid synthesis.

- **INDICATIONS AND DOSE**

Inborn errors of primary bile acid synthesis (initiated by a specialist)

▶ BY MOUTH

- Child (body-weight up to 10 kg): 50 mg daily, then increased in steps of 50 mg daily in divided doses; usual dose 5–15 mg/kg daily in divided doses, dose to be given with food at the same time each day
- Child (body-weight 10 kg and above): Usual dose 5–15 mg/kg daily; increased in steps of 50 mg daily in divided doses if required, dose to be given with food at the same time each day; Usual maximum 500 mg/24 hours

- **INTERACTIONS** → Appendix 1: cholic acid
- **SIDE-EFFECTS** Cholelithiasis (long term use) · diarrhoea · pruritus

  SIDE-EFFECTS, FURTHER INFORMATION Patients presenting with pruritus and/or persistent diarrhoea should be investigated for potential overdose by a serum and/or urine bile acid assay.
- **PREGNANCY** Limited data available—not known to be harmful, manufacturer advises continue treatment.
  Monitoring Manufacturer advises monitor patient parameters more frequently in pregnancy.
- **BREAST FEEDING** Present in milk but not known to be harmful.
- **HEPATIC IMPAIRMENT** Manufacturer advises caution and stop treatment if there are signs of severe hepatic failure—limited information available (no experience with impairment from causes not related to inborn errors of primary bile acid synthesis).

Dose adjustments Manufacturer advises adjust dose as the degree of impairment improves during treatment.

- **MONITORING REQUIREMENTS** Manufacturer advises monitor serum and/or urine bile-acid concentrations every 3 months for the first year, then every 6 months for three years, then annually; monitor liver function tests at the same or greater frequency.
- **DIRECTIONS FOR ADMINISTRATION** Manufacturer advises capsules may be opened and the content added to infant formula, juice, fruit compote, or yoghurt for administration.
- **PATIENT AND CARER ADVICE** Counselling advised on administration.

- **MEDICINAL FORMS** There can be variation in the licensing of different medicines containing the same drug.

Capsule

CAUTIONARY AND ADVISORY LABELS 25

▸ Orphacol (Laboratoires CTRS) ▼

Cholic acid 50 mg Orphacol 50mg capsules | 30 capsule PoM £1,860.00

Cholic acid 250 mg Orphacol 250mg capsules | 30 capsule PoM £6,630.00

Ursodeoxycholic acid

05-May-2020

- **INDICATIONS AND DOSE**

Cholestasis

▸ BY MOUTH

▸ Neonate: 5 mg/kg 3 times a day (max. per dose 10 mg/kg 3 times a day), adjusted according to response.

▸ Child 1–23 months: 5 mg/kg 3 times a day (max. per dose 10 mg/kg 3 times a day), adjusted according to response

Improvement of hepatic metabolism of essential fatty acids and bile flow, in children with cystic fibrosis

▸ BY MOUTH

▸ Child: 10–15 mg/kg twice daily, total daily dose may alternatively be given in 3 divided doses

Cholestasis associated with total parenteral nutrition

▸ BY MOUTH

▸ Neonate: 10 mg/kg 3 times a day.

▸ Child: 10 mg/kg 3 times a day

Sclerosing cholangitis

▸ BY MOUTH

▸ Child: 5–10 mg/kg 2–3 times a day (max. per dose 15 mg/kg 3 times a day), adjusted according to response

- **UNLICENSED USE** Not licensed for use in children for the treatment of cholestasis, sclerosing cholangitis, cholestasis associated with total parenteral nutrition or the improvement of hepatic metabolism of essential fatty acids and bile flow in cystic fibrosis.
- **CONTRA-INDICATIONS** Acute inflammation of the gall bladder · frequent episodes of biliary colic · inflammatory diseases and other conditions of the colon, liver or small intestine which interfere with enterohepatic circulation of bile salts · non-functioning gall bladder · radio-opaque stones
- **INTERACTIONS** → Appendix 1: ursodeoxycholic acid
- **SIDE-EFFECTS**

▸ **Common or very common** Diarrhoea · pale faeces

▸ **Rare or very rare** Abdominal pain upper · cholelithiasis calcification · hepatic cirrhosis exacerbated · skin reactions

▸ **Frequency not known** Nausea · vomiting

- **PREGNANCY** No evidence of harm but manufacturer advises avoid.
- **BREAST FEEDING** Not known to be harmful but manufacturer advises avoid.
- **HEPATIC IMPAIRMENT** Avoid in chronic liver disease (but used in primary biliary cirrhosis).
- **PATIENT AND CARER ADVICE** Patients should be given dietary advice (including avoidance of excessive cholesterol and calories).

Medicines for Children leaflet: Ursodeoxycholic acid for cholestasis and sclerosing cholangitis www.medicinesforchildren.org.uk/ursodeoxycholic-acid-cholestasis-and-sclerosing-cholangitis

---

- **MEDICINAL FORMS** There can be variation in the licensing of different medicines containing the same drug. Forms available from special-order manufacturers include: oral suspension, oral solution

Oral suspension

CAUTIONARY AND ADVISORY LABELS 21

▸ Ursofalk (Dr. Falk Pharma UK Ltd)

Ursodeoxycholic acid 50 mg per 1 ml Ursofalk 250mg/5ml oral suspension sugar-free | 250 ml PoM £26.98 DT = £26.98

Tablet

CAUTIONARY AND ADVISORY LABELS 21

▸ Ursodeoxycholic acid (Non-proprietary)

Ursodeoxycholic acid 150 mg Ursodeoxycholic acid 150mg tablets | 60 tablet PoM £19.02 DT = £19.02

Ursodeoxycholic acid 300 mg Ursodeoxycholic acid 300mg tablets | 60 tablet PoM £63.97 DT = £56.06

▸ Cholurso (HFA Healthcare Products Ltd)

Ursodeoxycholic acid 250 mg Cholurso 250mg tablets | 60 tablet PoM £18.00 DT = £18.00

Ursodeoxycholic acid 500 mg Cholurso 500mg tablets | 60 tablet PoM £45.00

▸ Destolit (Norgine Pharmaceuticals Ltd)

Ursodeoxycholic acid 150 mg Destolit 150mg tablets | 60 tablet PoM £18.39 DT = £19.02

▸ Ursofalk (Dr. Falk Pharma UK Ltd)

Ursodeoxycholic acid 500 mg Ursofalk 500mg tablets | 100 tablet PoM £80.00 DT = £80.00

▸ Ursonorm (PRO.MED.CS Praha a.s.)

Ursodeoxycholic acid 500 mg Ursonorm 500mg tablets | 60 tablet PoM £45.00 | 100 tablet PoM £49.00 DT = £80.00

Capsule

CAUTIONARY AND ADVISORY LABELS 21

▸ Ursodeoxycholic acid (Non-proprietary)

Ursodeoxycholic acid 250 mg Ursodeoxycholic acid 250mg capsules | 60 capsule PoM £29.00 DT = £12.23 | 100 capsule PoM £26.61

▸ Ursofalk (Dr. Falk Pharma UK Ltd)

Ursodeoxycholic acid 250 mg Ursofalk 250mg capsules | 60 capsule PoM £30.17 DT = £12.23 | 100 capsule PoM £31.88

▸ Ursonorm (PRO.MED.CS Praha a.s.)

Ursodeoxycholic acid 250 mg Ursonorm 250mg capsules | 60 capsule PoM £29.00 DT = £12.23

LIPIDS > STEROLS

Cholesterol

- **INDICATIONS AND DOSE**

Smith-Lemli-Opitz syndrome

▸ BY MOUTH

▸ Neonate: 5–10 mg/kg 3–4 times a day.

▸ Child: 5–10 mg/kg 3–4 times a day, doses up to 15 mg/kg 4 times daily have been used

- **UNLICENSED USE** Not licensed.
- **CONTRA-INDICATIONS**

CONTRA-INDICATIONS, FURTHER INFORMATION For contra-indications, consult product literature.

- **CAUTIONS**

CAUTIONS, FURTHER INFORMATION For advice on cautions, consult product literature.

- **DIRECTIONS FOR ADMINISTRATION** Cholesterol powder can be mixed with a vegetable oil before administration.

- **MEDICINAL FORMS** Forms available from special-order manufacturers include: oral suspension, powder

7.2 Oesophageal varices

Other drugs used for Oesophageal varices Vasopressin, below

PITUITARY AND HYPOTHALAMIC HORMONES AND ANALOGUES > VASOPRESSIN AND ANALOGUES

Terlipressin acetate

- **INDICATIONS AND DOSE**

GLYPRESSIN ® INJECTION

Adjunct in acute massive haemorrhage of gastro-intestinal tract or oesophageal varices (specialist use only)

▶ BY INTRAVENOUS INJECTION

- Child 12–17 years (body-weight up to 50 kg): Initially 2 mg every 4 hours until bleeding controlled, then reduced to 1 mg every 4 hours if required, maximum duration 48 hours
- Child 12–17 years (body-weight 50 kg and above): Initially 2 mg every 4 hours until bleeding controlled, reduced if not tolerated to 1 mg every 4 hours, maximum duration 48 hours

VARIQUEL ® INJECTION

Adjunct in acute massive haemorrhage of gastro-intestinal tract or oesophageal varices (specialist use only)

▶ BY INTRAVENOUS INJECTION

- Child 12–17 years (body-weight up to 50 kg): Initially 1 mg, then 1 mg every 4–6 hours for up to 72 hours, to be administered over 1 minute
- Child 12–17 years (body-weight 50–69 kg): Initially 1.5 mg, then 1 mg every 4–6 hours for up to 72 hours, to be administered over 1 minute
- Child 12–17 years (body-weight 70 kg and above): Initially 2 mg, then 1 mg every 4–6 hours for up to 72 hours, to be administered over 1 minute

- **UNLICENSED USE** Unlicensed for use in children.
- **CAUTIONS** Arrhythmia · electrolyte and fluid disturbances · heart disease · history of QT-interval prolongation · respiratory disease · septic shock · uncontrolled hypertension · vascular disease
- **SIDE-EFFECTS**

▶ **Common or very common** Abdominal cramps · arrhythmias · diarrhoea · headache · hypertension · hypotension · pallor · peripheral ischaemia · vasoconstriction

▶ **Uncommon** Chest pain · cyanosis · fluid overload · heart failure · hot flush · hyponatraemia · intestinal ischaemia · ischaemic heart disease · lymphangitis · myocardial infarction · nausea · pulmonary oedema · respiratory disorders · seizure · skin necrosis · uterine disorders · vomiting

▶ **Rare or very rare** Dyspnoea · hyperglycaemia · stroke

- **PREGNANCY** Avoid unless benefits outweigh risk—uterine contractions and increased intra-uterine pressure in early pregnancy, and decreased uterine blood flow reported.
- **BREAST FEEDING** Avoid unless benefits outweigh risk—no information available.
- **RENAL IMPAIRMENT** Use with caution in chronic renal failure.
- **MEDICINAL FORMS** There can be variation in the licensing of different medicines containing the same drug.

Solution for injection

▶ Glypressin (Ferring Pharmaceuticals Ltd)

Terlipressin acetate 120 microgram per 1 ml Glypressin 1mg/8.5ml solution for injection ampoules | 5 ampoule PoM ⊠

▶ Variquel (Alliance Pharmaceuticals Ltd)

Terlipressin acetate 200 microgram per 1 ml Variquel 1mg/5ml solution for injection vials | 5 vial PoM £89.98 (Hospital only)

Vasopressin

- **INDICATIONS AND DOSE**

Adjunct in acute massive haemorrhage of gastrointestinal tract or oesophageal varices (specialist use only)

▶ BY CONTINUOUS INTRAVENOUS INFUSION

- Child: Initially 0.3 unit/kg (max. per dose 20 units), dose to be administered over 20–30 minutes, then 0.3 unit/kg/hour, adjusted according to response (max. per dose 1 unit/kg/hour), if bleeding stops, continue at same dose for 12 hours, then withdraw gradually over 24–48 hours; max. duration of treatment 72 hours, dose may alternatively be infused directly into the superior mesenteric artery

- **UNLICENSED USE** Not licensed for use in children.
- **CONTRA-INDICATIONS** Chronic nephritis (until reasonable blood nitrogen concentrations attained) · vascular disease (especially disease of coronary arteries) unless extreme caution
- **CAUTIONS** Asthma · avoid fluid overload · conditions which might be aggravated by water retention · epilepsy · heart failure · hypertension · migraine
- **SIDE-EFFECTS** Abdominal pain · angina pectoris · bronchospasm · cardiac arrest · chest pain · diarrhoea · flatulence · fluid imbalance · gangrene · headache · hyperhidrosis · hypertension · musculoskeletal chest pain · nausea · pallor · peripheral ischaemia · tremor · urticaria · vertigo · vomiting
- **PREGNANCY** Oxytocic effect in third trimester.
- **BREAST FEEDING** Not known to be harmful.
- **DIRECTIONS FOR ADMINISTRATION** For *intravenous infusion* (argipressin); dilute with Glucose 5% or Sodium Chloride 0.9% to a concentration of 0.2–1 unit/mL.
- **MEDICINAL FORMS** There can be variation in the licensing of different medicines containing the same drug. Forms available from special-order manufacturers include: solution for injection

Solution for injection

▶ Argipressin (Advanz Pharma)

Argipressin 20 unit per 1 ml Argipressin 20units/1ml solution for injection ampoules | 10 ampoule PoM £754.86-£950.00 (Hospital only)

8 Obesity

Obesity

01-Jun-2016

Description of condition

Obesity is directly linked to many health problems including cardiovascular disease, type 2 diabetes, and obstructive sleep apnoea syndrome. It can also contribute to psychological and psychiatric morbidities.

In children and adolescents, body mass index (BMI) should be used as a practical estimation of body fat. However, it should be interpreted with caution as it is not a direct measure of adiposity. Assessing the BMI of children is more complicated than for adults because it changes as they grow and mature, with different growth patterns seen between boys and girls.

Public Health England advises that the British 1990 (UK90) growth reference charts should be used to determine the weight status of children. A child ≥ the 91st centile is classified as overweight, and as obese if ≥ the 98th centile. Waist circumference is not recommended as a routine measure, but should be used as an additional predictor for risk of developing other long-term health problems. Children who are overweight or obese and have significant comorbidities or complex needs should be considered for specialist referral.

Aims of treatment

Children who are overweight or obese and are no longer growing taller will ultimately need to lose weight and maintain weight loss to improve their BMI. However, preventing further weight gain while making lifestyle changes, may be an appropriate short-term aim.

Overview

[EvGr] The goals of management of obesity should be agreed together with the child and their parents or carers; parents or carers should be encouraged to take responsibility for lifestyle changes of their children. Referral to a specialist can be considered for children who are overweight or obese and have significant comorbidities or complex needs (e.g. learning disabilities). Children should be assessed for comorbidities such as hypertension, hyperinsulinaemia, dyslipidaemia, type 2 diabetes, psychosocial dysfunction, and exacerbation of conditions such as asthma.

An initial assessment should consider potential underlying causes (e.g. hypothyroidism) and a review of the appropriateness of current medications, which are known to cause weight gain, e.g. atypical antipsychotics, beta-adrenoceptor blocking drugs, insulin (when used in the treatment of type 2 diabetes), sodium valproate, and tricyclic antidepressants. ⟨A⟩

Lifestyle changes

[EvGr] Obese children should be encouraged to engage in a sustainable weight management programme which includes strategies to change behaviour, increase physical activity and improve diet and eating behaviour. These changes should be encouraged within the whole family. Any dietary changes should be age appropriate and consistent with healthy eating recommendations. Surgical intervention is not generally recommended in children or adolescents. ⟨A⟩

Drug treatment

[EvGr] Drug treatment is not generally recommended for children younger than 12 years, unless there are exceptional circumstances, such as if severe comorbidities are present. In children over 12 years, drug treatment is only recommended if physical comorbidities, such as orthopaedic problems or sleep apnoea, or severe psychological comorbidities are present. Drug treatment should **never** be used as the sole element of treatment and should be used as part of an overall weight management plan. Orlistat below [unlicensed use] is the only drug currently available in the UK that is recommended specifically for the treatment of obesity; it acts by reducing the absorption of dietary fat. Treatment should be started and monitored in a specialist paediatric setting by experienced multidisciplinary teams. An initial 6–12 month trial is recommended, with regular review to assess effectiveness, adverse effects and adherence.

Treatment may also be used to maintain weight loss rather than to continue to lose weight. A vitamin and mineral supplement may also be considered if there is concern about inadequate micronutrient intake, particularly for younger children who need vitamins and minerals for growth and development. ⟨A⟩

Useful Resources

Obesity: identification, assessment and management. Clinical Guideline 189. National Institute for Health and Care Excellence. November 2014.
www.nice.org.uk/guidance/cg189

Measuring and interpreting BMI in Children. Public Health England.
webarchive.nationalarchives.gov.uk/20170210161227/www.noo.org.uk/NOO_about_obesity/measurement/children

PERIPHERALLY ACTING ANTIOBESITY PRODUCTS › LIPASE INHIBITORS

Orlistat

- **DRUG ACTION** Orlistat, a lipase inhibitor, reduces the absorption of dietary fat.

- **INDICATIONS AND DOSE**

Adjunct in obesity

▸ BY MOUTH

▸ Child 12–17 years (initiated by a specialist): 120 mg up to 3 times a day, dose to be taken immediately before, during, or up to 1 hour after each main meal, continue treatment beyond 12 weeks only under specialist supervision, if a meal is missed or contains no fat, the dose of orlistat should be omitted

- **UNLICENSED USE** Not licensed for use in children.
- **CONTRA-INDICATIONS** Cholestasis · chronic malabsorption syndrome
- **CAUTIONS** Chronic kidney disease · may impair absorption of fat-soluble vitamins · volume depletion

  CAUTIONS, FURTHER INFORMATION Vitamin supplementation (especially of vitamin D) may be considered if there is concern about deficiency of fat-soluble vitamins.
- **INTERACTIONS** → Appendix 1: orlistat
- **SIDE-EFFECTS**

▸ **Common or very common** Abdominal pain (may be minimised by reduced fat intake) · anxiety · diarrhoea · gastrointestinal disorders

▸ **Frequency not known** Anorectal haemorrhage · bullous dermatitis · cholelithiasis · diverticulitis · hepatitis · oxalate nephropathy · pancreatitis · renal failure

- **PREGNANCY** Use with caution.
- **BREAST FEEDING** Avoid—no information available.

- **MEDICINAL FORMS** There can be variation in the licensing of different medicines containing the same drug.

Capsule

▸ Orlistat (Non-proprietary)
Orlistat 120 mg Orlistat 120mg capsules | 84 capsule [PoM] £35.43 DT = £27.30

▸ Alli (GlaxoSmithKline Consumer Healthcare)
Orlistat 60 mg Alli 60mg capsules | 84 capsule [P] £30.70 DT = £30.70

▸ Beacita (Actavis UK Ltd)
Orlistat 120 mg Beacita 120mg capsules | 84 capsule [PoM] £21.95 DT = £27.30

▸ Orlos (Crescent Pharma Ltd)
Orlistat 60 mg Orlos 60mg capsules | 84 capsule [P] £16.95 DT = £30.70

▸ Xenical (Cheplapharm Arzneimittel GmbH)
Orlistat 120 mg Xenical 120mg capsules | 84 capsule [PoM] £31.63 DT = £27.30

9 Rectal and anal disorders

Other drugs used for Rectal and anal disorders Diltiazem hydrochloride, p. 152

9.1 Anal fissures

Anal fissure

31-Aug-2016

Description of condition

An anal fissure is a tear or ulcer in the lining of the anal canal, immediately within the anal margin. Clinical features of anal fissure include bleeding and persistent pain on defecation, and a linear split in the anal mucosa. Constipation (passage of hard stools) is the most common cause in children. The majority of anal fissures are posterior, and an underlying cause should be considered (secondary anal fissure) if fissures are multiple, occur laterally, and are refractory to treatment.

EvGr Suspect sexual abuse if a child has an anal fissure, and if constipation, Crohn's disease or passing hard stools have been excluded as the cause (see also *Useful resources* below). Ⓐ

Aims of treatment

The aim of treatment is to relieve pain and promote healing of the fissure.

Drug treatment

EvGr Initial management of acute anal fissures should focus on ensuring that stools are soft and easily passed. Osmotic laxatives, such as lactulose p. 46 or macrogols (macrogol 3350 with potassium chloride, sodium bicarbonate and sodium chloride p. 47), are recommended. A simple analgesic (such as paracetamol p. 288 or ibuprofen p. 707, may be offered for prolonged burning pain following defecation.

Children should be referred to a paediatric specialist if the anal fissure has not healed following two weeks of initial management, or earlier if there is significant pain. Ⓐ

Useful Resources

Child maltreatment: when to suspect maltreatment in under 18s. National Institute for Health and Care Excellence. Clinical guideline 89. July 2009.
www.nice.org.uk/guidance/cg89

9.2 Haemorrhoids

Haemorrhoids

01-Dec-2016

Description of condition

Haemorrhoids, or piles, are abnormal swellings of the vascular mucosal anal cushions around the anus. Internal haemorrhoids arise above the dentate line and are usually painless unless they become strangulated. External haemorrhoids originate below the dentate line and can be itchy or painful. Haemorrhoids in children are rare but may occur in infants with portal hypertension.

Aims of treatment

The aims of treatment are to reduce the symptoms (pain, bleeding and swelling), promote healing, and prevent recurrence.

Non-drug treatment

EvGr Stools should be kept soft and easy to pass (to minimise straining) by increasing dietary fibre and fluid intake. Advice about perianal hygiene is helpful to aid healing and reduce irritation and itching. Ⓐ

Drug treatment

EvGr If constipation is present, it should be treated, see Constipation p. 44.

A simple analgesic, such as paracetamol p. 288, can be used for pain relief. NSAIDs should be avoided if rectal bleeding is present.

Symptomatic treatment with a locally applied preparation is appropriate for short periods. Ⓔ Manufacturer advises preparations containing local anaesthetics (lidocaine, cinchocaine, and pramocaine [unlicensed]) should only be used for a few days as they may cause sensitisation of the anal skin— local anaethestic ointments can be absorbed through the rectal mucosa (with a theorectical risk of systemic effects) and very rarely may cause increased irritation; excessive application should be **avoided** in infants and children.

Topical preparations combining corticosteroids with local anaesthetics and soothing agents are available for the management of haemorrhoids. Manufacturer advises long-term use of corticosteroid creams can cause ulceration and permanent damage due to thinning of the perianal skin and should be avoided. Continuous or excessive use carries a risk of adrenal suppression and systemic corticosteroid effects (particularly in infants).

EvGr Topical preparations containing corticosteroids must not be used if infection is present (such as perianal streptococcal infection, *herpes simplex* or perianal thrush).

Recurrent symptoms, should be referred to secondary care for further investigation and management. Ⓔ

Related drugs

Topical preparations used for haemorrhoids: lidocaine hydrochloride p. 884, benzyl benzoate with bismuth oxide, bismuth subgallate, hydrocortisone acetate, peru balsam and zinc oxide below, cinchocaine hydrochloride with fluocortolone caproate and fluocortolone pivalate p. 75, cinchocaine with hydrocortisone p. 75, cinchocaine with prednisolone p. 76.

CORTICOSTEROIDS

Benzyl benzoate with bismuth oxide, bismuth subgallate, hydrocortisone acetate, peru balsam and zinc oxide

21-Dec-2017

● **INDICATIONS AND DOSE**

Haemorrhoids | Pruritus ani

▶ BY RECTUM USING OINTMENT
- Child 12–17 years: Apply twice daily for no longer than 7 days, to be applied morning and night, an additional dose should be applied after a bowel movement

▶ BY RECTUM USING SUPPOSITORIES
- Child 12–17 years: 1 suppository twice daily for no longer than 7 days, to be inserted night and morning, additional dose after a bowel movement

IMPORTANT SAFETY INFORMATION

MHRA/CHM ADVICE: CORTICOSTEROIDS: RARE RISK OF CENTRAL SEROUS CHORIORETINOPATHY WITH LOCAL AS WELL AS SYSTEMIC ADMINISTRATION (AUGUST 2017)

See Corticosteroids, general use p. 470.

- **CAUTIONS** Local anaesthetic component can be absorbed through the rectal mucosa (avoid excessive application, particularly in children and infants) · local anaesthetic component may cause sensitisation (use for short periods only—no longer than a few days)
- **PRESCRIBING AND DISPENSING INFORMATION** A proprietary brand *Anusol Plus HC*® (ointment and suppositories) is on sale to the public.

- **MEDICINAL FORMS** There can be variation in the licensing of different medicines containing the same drug.

Ointment

- Anusol-HC (Church & Dwight UK Ltd)
  Hydrocortisone acetate 2.5 mg per 1 gram, Bismuth oxide 8.75 mg per 1 gram, Benzyl benzoate 12.5 mg per 1 gram, Peru Balsam 18.75 mg per 1 gram, Bismuth subgallate 22.5 mg per 1 gram, Zinc oxide 107.5 mg per 1 gram Anusol HC ointment | 30 gram PoM £2.49

Suppository

- Anusol-HC (Church & Dwight UK Ltd)
  Hydrocortisone acetate 10 mg, Bismuth oxide 24 mg, Benzyl benzoate 33 mg, Peru Balsam 49 mg, Bismuth subgallate 59 mg, Zinc oxide 296 mg Anusol HC suppositories | 12 suppository PoM £1.74

Cinchocaine hydrochloride with fluocortolone caproate and fluocortolone pivalate

21-Dec-2017

- **INDICATIONS AND DOSE**

Haemorrhoids | Pruritus ani

- BY RECTUM USING OINTMENT
  - Child: Apply twice daily for 5–7 days, apply 3–4 times a day if required, on the first day of treatment, then apply once daily for a few days after symptoms have cleared
- BY RECTUM USING SUPPOSITORIES
  - Child 12–17 years: Initially 1 suppository daily for 5–7 days, to be inserted after a bowel movement, then 1 suppository once daily on alternate days for 1 week

Haemorrhoids (severe cases) | Pruritus ani (severe cases)

- BY RECTUM USING SUPPOSITORIES
  - Child 12–17 years: Initially 1 suppository 2–3 times a day for 5–7 days, then 1 suppository once daily on alternate days for 1 week

IMPORTANT SAFETY INFORMATION

MHRA/CHM ADVICE: CORTICOSTEROIDS: RARE RISK OF CENTRAL SEROUS CHORIORETINOPATHY WITH LOCAL AS WELL AS SYSTEMIC ADMINISTRATION (AUGUST 2017)

See Corticosteroids, general use p. 470.

- **CAUTIONS** Local anaesthetic component can be absorbed through the rectal mucosa (avoid excessive application) · local anaesthetic component may cause sensitisation (use for short periods only—no longer than a few days)

- **MEDICINAL FORMS** There can be variation in the licensing of different medicines containing the same drug.

Ointment

- Ultraproct (Meadow Laboratories Ltd)
  Fluocortolone pivalate 920 microgram per 1 gram, Fluocortolone caproate 950 microgram per 1 gram, Cinchocaine hydrochloride 5 mg per 1 gram Ultraproct ointment | 30 gram PoM £8.27

Suppository

- Ultraproct (Meadow Laboratories Ltd)
  Fluocortolone pivalate 610 microgram, Fluocortolone caproate 630 microgram, Cinchocaine hydrochloride 1 mg Ultraproct suppositories | 12 suppository PoM £4.06

Cinchocaine with hydrocortisone

21-Dec-2017

- **INDICATIONS AND DOSE**

PROCTOSEDYL® OINTMENT

Haemorrhoids | Pruritus ani

- TO THE SKIN, OR BY RECTUM
  - Child: Apply twice daily, to be administered morning and night and after a bowel movement. Apply externally or by rectum. Do not use for longer than 7 days

PROCTOSEDYL® SUPPOSITORIES

Haemorrhoids | Pruritus ani

- BY RECTUM
  - Child 12–17 years: 1 suppository, insert suppository night and morning and after a bowel movement. Do not use for longer than 7 days

UNIROID-HC® OINTMENT

Haemorrhoids | Pruritus ani

- TO THE SKIN, OR BY RECTUM
  - Child 1 month–11 years (under medical advice only): Apply twice daily, and apply after a bowel movement, apply externally or by rectum, do not use for longer than 7 days
  - Child 12–17 years: Apply twice daily, and apply after a bowel movement, apply externally or by rectum, do not use for longer than 7 days

UNIROID-HC® SUPPOSITORIES

Haemorrhoids | Pruritus ani

- BY RECTUM
  - Child 12–17 years: 1 suppository, insert twice daily and after a bowel movement. Do not use for longer than 7 days

IMPORTANT SAFETY INFORMATION

MHRA/CHM ADVICE: CORTICOSTEROIDS: RARE RISK OF CENTRAL SEROUS CHORIORETINOPATHY WITH LOCAL AS WELL AS SYSTEMIC ADMINISTRATION (AUGUST 2017)

See Corticosteroids, general use p. 470.

- **CAUTIONS** Local anaesthetic component can be absorbed through the rectal mucosa (avoid excessive application, particularly in children and infants) · local anaesthetic component may cause sensitisation (use for short periods only—no longer than a few days)

- **MEDICINAL FORMS** There can be variation in the licensing of different medicines containing the same drug.

Ointment

- Proctosedyl (Sanofi)
  Cinchocaine hydrochloride 5 mg per 1 gram, Hydrocortisone 5 mg per 1 gram Proctosedyl ointment | 30 gram PoM £10.34 DT = £10.34
- Uniroid HC (Chemidex Pharma Ltd)
  Cinchocaine hydrochloride 5 mg per 1 gram, Hydrocortisone 5 mg per 1 gram Uniroid HC ointment | 30 gram PoM £4.23 DT = £10.34

Suppository

- Proctosedyl (Sanofi)
  Cinchocaine hydrochloride 5 mg, Hydrocortisone 5 mg Proctosedyl suppositories | 12 suppository PoM £5.08 DT = £5.08
- Uniroid HC (Chemidex Pharma Ltd)
  Cinchocaine hydrochloride 5 mg, Hydrocortisone 5 mg Uniroid HC suppositories | 12 suppository PoM £1.91 DT = £5.08

Cinchocaine with prednisolone

21-Dec-2017

● **INDICATIONS AND DOSE**

Haemorrhoids | Pruritus ani

▶ BY RECTUM USING OINTMENT

▸ Child: Apply twice daily for 5–7 days, apply 3–4 times a day on the first day if necessary, then apply once daily for a few days after symptoms have cleared

▶ BY RECTUM USING SUPPOSITORIES

▸ Child 12–17 years: 1 suppository daily for 5–7 days, to be inserted after a bowel movement

Haemorrhoids (severe cases) | Pruritus ani (severe cases)

▶ BY RECTUM USING SUPPOSITORIES

▸ Child 12–17 years: Initially 1 suppository 2–3 times a day, then 1 suppository daily for a total of 5–7 days, to be inserted after a bowel movement

IMPORTANT SAFETY INFORMATION

MHRA/CHM ADVICE: CORTICOSTEROIDS: RARE RISK OF CENTRAL SEROUS CHORIORETINOPATHY WITH LOCAL AS WELL AS SYSTEMIC ADMINISTRATION (AUGUST 2017)

See Corticosteroids, general use p. 470.

● CAUTIONS Local anaesthetic component can be absorbed through the rectal mucosa (avoid excessive application) · local anaesthetic component may cause sensitisation (use for short periods only—no longer than a few days)

● MEDICINAL FORMS There can be variation in the licensing of different medicines containing the same drug.

Ointment

▸ Scheriproct (LEO Pharma)
Prednisolone hexanoate 1.9 mg per 1 gram, Cinchocaine hydrochloride 5 mg per 1 gram Scheriproct ointment | 30 gram PoM £3.23 DT = £3.23

Suppository

▸ Scheriproct (LEO Pharma)
Cinchocaine hydrochloride 1 mg, Prednisolone hexanoate 1.3 mg Scheriproct suppositories | 12 suppository PoM £1.52 DT = £1.52

Hydrocortisone with lidocaine

21-Dec-2017

● **INDICATIONS AND DOSE**

Haemorrhoids | Pruritus ani

▶ BY RECTUM USING AEROSOL SPRAY

▸ Child 2–13 years (under medical advice only): 1 spray up to 3 times a day, spray once over the affected area

▸ Child 14–17 years: 1 spray up to 3 times a day for no longer than 7 days without medical advice, spray once over the affected area

▶ BY RECTUM USING OINTMENT

▸ Child: Apply several times daily, for short term use only

IMPORTANT SAFETY INFORMATION

MHRA/CHM ADVICE: CORTICOSTEROIDS: RARE RISK OF CENTRAL SEROUS CHORIORETINOPATHY WITH LOCAL AS WELL AS SYSTEMIC ADMINISTRATION (AUGUST 2017)

See Corticosteroids, general use p. 470.

● CAUTIONS Local anaesthetic component can be absorbed through the rectal mucosa (avoid excessive application) · local anaesthetic component may cause sensitisation (use for short periods only—no longer than a few days)

● MEDICINAL FORMS There can be variation in the licensing of different medicines containing the same drug.

Ointment

▸ Xyloproct (Aspen Pharma Trading Ltd)
Hydrocortisone acetate 2.75 mg per 1 gram, Lidocaine 50 mg per 1 gram Xyloproct 5%/0.275% ointment | 20 gram PoM £4.19 DT = £4.19

Spray

▸ Perinal (Dermal Laboratories Ltd)
Hydrocortisone 2 mg per 1 gram, Lidocaine hydrochloride 10 mg per 1 gram Perinal spray | 30 ml P £6.11 DT = £6.11

Hydrocortisone with pramocaine

21-Dec-2017

● **INDICATIONS AND DOSE**

Pain and irritation associated with local, non-infected anal or perianal conditions

▶ BY RECTUM

▸ Child 12–17 years: 1 applicatorful 2–3 times a day and 1 applicatorful, after a bowel movement, do not use for longer than 7 days; maximum 4 applicatorfuls per day

IMPORTANT SAFETY INFORMATION

MHRA/CHM ADVICE: CORTICOSTEROIDS: RARE RISK OF CENTRAL SEROUS CHORIORETINOPATHY WITH LOCAL AS WELL AS SYSTEMIC ADMINISTRATION (AUGUST 2017)

See Corticosteroids, general use p. 470.

● CAUTIONS Local anaesthetic component can be absorbed through the rectal mucosa (avoid excessive application) · local anaesthetic component may cause sensitisation (use for short periods only—no longer than a few days)

● MEDICINAL FORMS No licensed medicines listed.

10 Reduced exocrine secretions

Exocrine pancreatic insufficiency

14-Dec-2016

Description of condition

Exocrine pancreatic insufficiency is characterised by reduced secretion of pancreatic enzymes into the duodenum.

The main clinical manifestations are maldigestion and malnutrition, associated with low circulating levels of micronutrients, fat-soluble vitamins and lipoproteins. Children also present with gastro-intestinal symptoms, such as diarrhoea, abdominal cramps and steatorrhoea.

Exocrine pancreatic insufficiency can result from cystic fibrosis, coeliac disease, Zollinger-Ellison syndrome, and gastro-intestinal or pancreatic surgical resection.

Aims of treatment

The aim of treatment is to relieve gastro-intestinal symptoms and to achieve a normal nutritional status.

Drug treatment

EvGr Pancreatic enzyme replacement therapy with pancreatin p. 77 is the mainstay of treatment for children with exocrine pancreatic insufficiency. (A)

Pancreatin contains the three main groups of digestive enzymes: lipase, amylase and protease. These enzymes respectively digest fats, carbohydrates and proteins into their basic components so that they can be absorbed and utilised by the body. EvGr Pancreatin should be administered with meals and snacks. The dose should be adjusted, as necessary, to the lowest effective dose according to the symptoms of maldigestion and malabsorption. (A)

Fibrosing colonopathy has been reported in children with cystic fibrosis taking high dose pancreatic enzyme replacement therapy (in excess of 10 000 units/kg/day of lipase). Possible risk factors are gender (boys are at greater risk than girls), more severe cystic fibrosis, and concomitant use of laxatives. The peak age for developing fibrosing colonopathy is between 2 and 8 years. Manufacturers of *Pancrease HL*® and *Nutrizym 22*® recommend that the total dose of pancreatin used in patients with cystic fibrosis should not usually exceed 10 000 units/kg/day of lipase. Manufacturers recommend that if a patient taking pancreatin develops new abdominal symptoms (or any change in existing abdominal symptoms) the patient should be reviewed to exclude the possibility of colonic damage.

There is limited evidence that acid suppression may improve the effectiveness of pancreatin. EvGr Acid-suppressing drugs (proton pump inhibitors or H_2-receptor antagonists) may be trialled in children who continue to experience symptoms despite high doses of pancreatin.

Levels of fat-soluble vitamins and micronutrients (such as zinc and selenium) should be routinely assessed and supplementation recommended whenever necessary. (A)

Pancreatin preparations

Preparation	Protease units	Amylase units	Lipase units
Creon® 10 000 capsule, e/c granules	600	8000	10 000
Creon® Micro e/c granules (per 100 mg)	200	3600	5000
Pancrex® granules (per gram)	300	4000	5000
Pancrex V® capsule, powder	430	9000	8000
Pancrex V '125'® capsule, powder	160	3300	2950
Pancrex V® e/c tablet	110	1700	1900
Pancrex V® Forte e/c tablet	330	5000	5600
Pancrex V® powder (per gram)	1400	30 000	25 000

Higher-strength pancreatin preparations

Preparation	Protease units	Amylase units	Lipase units
Creon® 25 000 capsule, e/c pellets	1000	18 000	25 000
Creon® 40 000 capsule, e/c granules	1600	25 000	40 000
Nutrizym 22® capsule, e/c minitablets	1100	19 800	22 000
Pancrease HL® capsule, e/c minitablets	1250	22 500	25 000

Non-drug treatment

EvGr Dietary advice should be provided. Food intake should be distributed between three main meals per day, and two or three snacks. Food that is difficult to digest should be avoided, such as legumes (peas, beans, lentils) and high-fibre foods. Alcohol should be avoided completely. Reduced fat diets are not recommended. (A)

Medium-chain triglycerides (see MCT oil, in *Borderline substances*), which are directly absorbed by the intestinal mucosa, were thought to be useful in some children. However evidence has shown that MCT-enriched preparations offer no advantage over a normal balanced diet.

PANCREATIC ENZYMES

Pancreatin

16-Mar-2020

- **DRUG ACTION** Supplements of pancreatin are given to compensate for reduced or absent exocrine secretion. They assist the digestion of starch, fat, and protein.

- **INDICATIONS AND DOSE**

CREON ® 10000

Pancreatic insufficiency

▶ BY MOUTH

▸ Child: Initially 1–2 capsules, dose to be taken with each meal either taken whole or contents mixed with acidic fluid or soft food (then swallowed immediately without chewing)

CREON ® 25000

Pancreatic insufficiency

▶ BY MOUTH

▸ Child 2–17 years: Initially 1–2 capsules, dose to be taken with each meal either taken whole or contents mixed with acidic fluid or soft food (then swallowed immediately without chewing)

CREON ® 40000

Pancreatic insufficiency

▶ BY MOUTH

▸ Child 2–17 years: Initially 1–2 capsules, dose to be taken with each meal either taken whole or contents mixed with acidic fluid or soft food (then swallowed immediately without chewing)

CREON ® MICRO

Pancreatic insufficiency

▶ BY MOUTH

▸ Neonate: Initially 100 mg, for administration advice, see *Directions for administration*.

▸ Child: Initially 100 mg, for administration advice, see *Directions for administration*

DOSE EQUIVALENCE AND CONVERSION

▸ For *Creon ® Micro* : 100 mg granules = one measured scoopful (scoop supplied with product).

NUTRIZYM 22 ® GASTRO-RESISTANT CAPSULES

Pancreatic insufficiency

▶ BY MOUTH

▸ Child 15–17 years: Initially 1–2 capsules, dose to be taken with meals and 1 capsule as required, dose to be taken with snacks, doses should be swallowed whole or contents taken with water, or mixed with acidic fluid or soft food (then swallowed immediately without chewing)

PANCREASE HL ®

Pancreatic insufficiency

▶ BY MOUTH

▸ Child 15–17 years: Initially 1–2 capsules, dose to be taken during each meal and 1 capsule, to be taken with snacks, all doses either taken whole or contents mixed with slightly acidic liquid or soft food (then swallowed immediately without chewing)

PANCREX ® V

Pancreatic insufficiency

▶ BY MOUTH

▸ Child 1–11 months: 1–2 capsules, contents of capsule to be mixed with feeds

▸ Child 1–17 years: 2–6 capsules, dose to be taken with each meal either swallowed whole or sprinkled on food

PANCREX ® V CAPSULES '125'

Pancreatic insufficiency

▶ BY MOUTH

▸ Neonate: 1–2 capsules, contents of capsule to be given in each feed (or mixed with feed and given by spoon).

continued →

PANCREX ® V POWDER

Pancreatic insufficiency

▶ BY MOUTH

▸ Neonate: 250–500 mg, dose to be taken with each feed.

▸ Child: 0.5–2 g, to be taken before or with meals, washed down or mixed with milk or water

- CONTRA-INDICATIONS

PANCREASE HL ® Should not be used in children aged 15 years or less with cystic fibrosis

NUTRIZYM 22 ® GASTRO-RESISTANT CAPSULES Should not be used in children aged 15 years or less with cystic fibrosis

- CAUTIONS Can irritate the perioral skin and buccal mucosa if retained in the mouth · excessive doses can cause perianal irritation
- INTERACTIONS → Appendix 1: pancreatin
- SIDE-EFFECTS

▶ **Common or very common** Abdominal distension · constipation · nausea · vomiting

▶ **Uncommon** Skin reactions

▶ **Frequency not known** Fibrosing colonopathy

- PREGNANCY Not known to be harmful.
- DIRECTIONS FOR ADMINISTRATION Pancreatin is inactivated by gastric acid therefore manufacturer advises pancreatin preparations are best taken with food (or immediately before or after food). Since pancreatin is inactivated by heat, excessive heat should be avoided if preparations are mixed with liquids or food; manufacturer advises the resulting mixtures should not be kept for more than one hour and any left-over food or liquid containing pancreatin should be discarded. Enteric-coated preparations deliver a higher enzyme concentration in the duodenum (provided the capsule contents are swallowed whole without chewing). Manufacturer advises gastro-resistant granules should be mixed with slightly acidic soft food or liquid such as apple juice, and then swallowed immediately without chewing. Capsules containing enteric-coated granules can be opened and the granules administered in the same way. For infants, *Creon® Micro* granules can be mixed with a small amount of milk on a spoon and administered immediately—granules should not be added to the baby's bottle. Manufacturer advises *Pancrex® V* powder may be administered via nasogastric tube or gastrostomy tube—consult local and national official guidelines.
- PRESCRIBING AND DISPENSING INFORMATION Preparations may contain pork pancreatin—consult product literature.
- HANDLING AND STORAGE Hypersensitivity reactions have occasionally occurred in those handling the powder.
- PATIENT AND CARER ADVICE Patients or carers should be given advice on administration. It is important to ensure adequate hydration at all times in patients receiving higher-strength pancreatin preparations.

Medicines for Children leaflet: Pancreatin for pancreatic insufficiency www.medicinesforchildren.org.uk/pancreatin-pancreatic-insufficiency

- MEDICINAL FORMS There can be variation in the licensing of different medicines containing the same drug.

Gastro-resistant capsule

▸ Creon (Mylan)

Protease 600 unit, Amylase 8000 unit, Lipase 10000 unit Creon 10000 gastro-resistant capsules | 100 capsule [P] £12.93

Protease 1000 unit, Amylase 18000 unit, Lipase 25000 unit Creon 25000 gastro-resistant capsules | 100 capsule [PoM] £28.25

▸ Nutrizym (Merck Serono Ltd)

Protease 1100 unit, Amylase 19800 unit, Lipase 22000 unit Nutrizym 22 gastro-resistant capsules | 100 capsule [PoM] £33.33

▸ Pancrease (Janssen-Cilag Ltd)

Protease 1250 unit, Amylase 22500 unit, Lipase 25000 unit Pancrease HL gastro-resistant capsules | 100 capsule [PoM] £40.38

Gastro-resistant granules

CAUTIONARY AND ADVISORY LABELS 25

▸ Creon (Mylan)

Protease 200 unit, Amylase 3600 unit, Lipase 5000 unit Creon Micro Pancreatin 60.12mg gastro-resistant granules | 20 gram [P] £31.50

Powder

▸ Pancrex (Essential Pharmaceuticals Ltd)

Protease 1400 unit, Lipase 25000 unit, Amylase 30000 unit Pancrex V oral powder sugar-free | 300 gram [P] £224.00

Capsule

▸ Pancrex (Essential Pharmaceuticals Ltd)

Protease 160 unit, Lipase 2950 unit, Amylase 3300 unit Pancrex V 125mg capsules | 300 capsule [P] £42.07

Protease 430 unit, Lipase 8000 unit, Amylase 9000 unit Pancrex V capsules | 300 capsule [P] £53.20

11 Stoma care

Stoma care

24-Feb-2016

Description of condition

A stoma is an artificial opening on the abdomen to divert flow of faeces or urine into an external pouch located outside of the body. This procedure may be temporary or permanent. Colostomy and ileostomy are the most common forms of stoma but a gastrostomy, jejunostomy, duodenostomy or caecostomy may also be performed. Understanding the type and extent of surgical intervention in each patient is crucial in managing the patient's pharmaceutical needs correctly.

Overview

Prescribing for patients with stoma calls for special care due to modifications in drug delivery, resulting in a higher risk of sub-optimal absorption. The following is a brief account of some of the main points to be borne in mind.

Enteric-coated and modified-release medicines are **unsuitable**, particularly in patients with an ileostomy, as there may not be sufficient release of active ingredient. Soluble tablets, liquids, capsules or uncoated tablets are more suitable due to their quicker dissolution. When a solid-dose form such as a capsule or a tablet is given, the contents of the ostomy bag should be checked for any remnants.

Preparations containing sorbitol as an excipient should be avoided, due to its laxative side effects.

Analgesics

Opioid analgesics may cause troublesome constipation in colostomy patients. When a non-opioid analgesic is required, paracetamol is usually suitable. Anti-inflammatory analgesics may cause gastric irritation and bleeding; faecal output should be monitored for traces of blood.

Antacids

The tendency to diarrhoea from magnesium salts or constipation from aluminium or calcium salts may be increased in patients with stoma.

Antisecretory drugs

The gastric acid secretion often increases stoma output. Proton pump inhibitors and somatostatin analogues (octreotide p. 504) are often used to reduce this risk.

Antidiarrhoeal drugs

Loperamide hydrochloride p. 54 and codeine phosphate p. 293 reduce intestinal motility and decrease water and sodium output from an ileostomy. Loperamide hydrochloride circulates through the enterohepatic circulation, which is disrupted in patients with a short bowel; high doses of loperamide hydrochloride may be required. Codeine phosphate can be added if response with loperamide hydrochloride alone is inadequate.

Digoxin

Children with a stoma are particularly susceptible to hypokalaemia. This predisposes children on digoxin p. 86 to digoxin toxicity; potassium supplements or a potassium-sparing diuretic may be advisable.

Diuretics

Diuretics should be used with caution in patients with an ileostomy or with urostomy as they may become excessively dehydrated and potassium depletion may easily occur. It is usually advisable to use a potassium-sparing diuretic.

Iron preparations

Iron preparations may cause loose stools and sore skin in these patients. If this is troublesome and if iron is definitely indicated, an intramuscular iron preparation should be used. Modified-release preparations should be avoided for the reasons given above.

Laxatives

Laxatives should be used in children with stoma only under specialist supervision; they should be prescribed with caution for those with an ileostomy as they may cause rapid and severe loss of water and electrolytes.

Colostomy patients may suffer from constipation and whenever possible it should be treated by increasing fluid intake or dietary fibre. If a laxative is required, it should generally be used for short periods only.

Care of stoma

Patients and their carers are usually given advice about the use of cleansing agents, protective creams, lotions, deodorants, or sealants whilst in hospital, either by the surgeon or by stoma care nurses. Voluntary organisations offer help and support to patients with stoma.

Chapter 2
Cardiovascular system

CONTENTS

1 Arrhythmias

Arrhythmias

Overview

Management of an arrhythmia requires precise diagnosis of the type of arrhythmia; electrocardiography and referral to a paediatric cardiologist is essential; underlying causes such as heart failure require appropriate treatment.

Bradycardia

Adrenaline/epinephrine p. 143 is useful in the treatment of symptomatic bradycardia in an infant or child.

Supraventricular tachycardia

In supraventricular tachycardia adenosine p. 84 is given by rapid intravenous injection. If adenosine is ineffective, intravenous amiodarone hydrochloride p. 83, flecainide acetate p. 82, or a beta-blocker (such as esmolol hydrochloride p. 113) can be tried; verapamil hydrochloride p. 116 can also be considered in children over 1 year. Atenolol p. 112, sotalol hydrochloride p. 85 and flecainide acetate are used for the prophylaxis of paroxysmal supraventricular tachycardias.

The use of d.c. shock and vagal stimulation also have a role in the treatment of supraventricular tachycardia.

Syndromes associated with accessory conducting pathways

Amiodarone hydrochloride, flecainide acetate, or a beta-blocker is used to prevent recurrence of supraventricular tachycardia in infants and young children with these syndromes (e.g. Wolff-Parkinson-White syndrome).

Atrial flutter

In atrial flutter without structural heart defects, sinus rhythm is restored with d.c. shock or cardiac pacing; drug treatment is usually not necessary. Amiodarone hydrochloride is used in atrial flutter when structural heart defects are present or after heart surgery. Sotalol hydrochloride may also be considered.

Atrial fibrillation

Atrial fibrillation is very rare in children. To restore sinus rhythm d.c. shock is used; beta-blockers, alone or together with digoxin p. 86 may be useful for ventricular rate control.

Ectopic tachycardia

Intravenous amiodarone hydrochloride is used in conjunction with body cooling and synchronised pacing in postoperative junctional ectopic tachycardia. Oral amiodarone hydrochloride or flecainide acetate are used in congenital junctional ectopic tachycardia.

Amiodarone hydrochloride, flecainide acetate, or a beta-blocker are used in atrial ectopic tachycardia; amiodarone hydrochloride is preferred in those with poor ventricular function.

Ventricular tachycardia and ventricular fibrillation

Pulseless ventricular tachycardia or ventricular fibrillation require resuscitation, see Paediatric Advanced Life Support algorithm. Amiodarone hydrochloride is used in resuscitation for pulseless ventricular tachycardia or ventricular fibrillation unresponsive to d.c. shock; lidocaine hydrochloride p. 81 can be used as an alternative only if amiodarone hydrochloride is not available.

Amiodarone hydrochloride is also used in a haemodynamically stable child when drug treatment is required; lidocaine hydrochloride can be used as an alternative only if amiodarone hydrochloride is not available.

Torsade de pointes

Torsade de pointes is a form of ventricular tachycardia associated with long QT syndrome, which may be congenital or drug induced. Episodes may be self-limiting, but are frequently recurrent and can cause impairment or loss of consciousness. If not controlled, the arrhythmia can progress to ventricular fibrillation and sometimes death. Intravenous magnesium sulfate can be used to treat torsade de pointes (dose recommendations vary—consult local guidelines). Anti-arrhythmics can further prolong the QT interval, thus worsening the condition.

Anti-arrhythmic drugs

Anti-arrhythmic drugs can be classified clinically into those that act on supraventricular arrhythmias (e.g. verapamil hydrochloride), those that act on both supraventricular and ventricular arrhythmias (e.g. amiodarone hydrochloride), and those that act on ventricular arrhythmias (e.g. lidocaine hydrochloride).

Anti-arrhythmic drugs can also be classified according to their effects on the electrical behaviour of myocardial cells during activity (the Vaughan Williams classification) although this classification is of less clinical significance:

- Class I: membrane stabilising drugs (e.g. lidocaine, flecainide)
- Class II: beta-blockers
- Class III: amiodarone; sotalol (also Class II)
- Class IV: calcium-channel blockers (includes verapamil but not dihydropyridines)

The negative inotropic effects of anti-arrhythmic drugs tend to be additive. Therefore special care should be taken if two or more are used, especially if myocardial function is impaired. Most drugs that are effective in countering arrhythmias can also provoke them in some circumstances; moreover, hypokalaemia enhances the arrhythmogenic (pro-arrhythmic) effect of many drugs.

Adenosine is the treatment of choice for terminating supraventricular tachycardias, including those associated with accessory conducting pathways (e.g. Wolff-Parkinson-White syndrome). It is also used in the diagnosis of supraventricular arrhythmias. It is not negatively inotropic and does not cause significant hypotension. The injection should be administered by rapid intravenous injection into a central or large peripheral vein.

Amiodarone hydrochloride is useful in the management of both supraventricular and ventricular tachyarrhythmias. It can be given by intravenous infusion and by mouth, and causes little or no myocardial depression. Unlike oral amiodarone hydrochloride, intravenous amiodarone hydrochloride acts relatively rapidly. Intravenous amiodarone hydrochloride is also used in cardiopulmonary resuscitation for ventricular fibrillation or pulseless ventricular tachycardia unresponsive to d.c. shock.

Amiodarone hydrochloride has a very long half-life (extending to several weeks) and only needs to be given once daily (but high doses may cause nausea unless divided). Many weeks or months may be required to achieve steady state plasma-amiodarone concentration; this is particularly important when drug interactions are likely.

Beta-blockers act as anti-arrhythmic drugs principally by attenuating the effects of the sympathetic system on automaticity and conductivity within the heart. Sotalol hydrochloride has a role in the management of ventricular arrhythmias.

Oral administration of digoxin slows the ventricular rate in atrial fibrillation and in atrial flutter. However, intravenous infusion of digoxin is rarely effective for rapid control of ventricular rate.

Flecainide acetate is useful for the treatment of resistant re-entry supraventricular tachycardia, ventricular tachycardia, ventricular ectopic beats, arrhythmias associated with accessory conducting pathways (e.g. Wolff-Parkinson- White syndrome), and paroxysmal atrial fibrillation. Flecainide acetate crosses the placenta and can be used to control fetal supraventricular arrhythmias.

Lidocaine hydrochloride can be used in cardiopulmonary resuscitation in children with ventricular fibrillation or pulseless ventricular tachycardia unresponsive to d.c. shock, but only if amiodarone hydrochloride is not available. Doses may need to be reduced in children with persistently poor cardiac output and hepatic or renal failure.

Verapamil hydrochloride can cause severe haemodynamic compromise (refractory hypotension and cardiac arrest) when used for the acute treatment of arrhythmias in neonates and infants; it is contra-indicated in children under 1 year. It is also contra-indicated in those with congestive heart failure, syndromes associated with accessory conducting pathways (e.g. Wolff-Parkinson-White syndrome) and in most receiving concomitant beta-blockers. It can be useful in older children with supraventricular tachycardia.

Advanced Pharmacy Services

Children with an arrhythmia may be eligible for the New Medicines Service / Medicine Use Review service provided by a community pharmacist. For further information, see *Advanced Pharmacy Services* in Medicines optimisation p. 25.

Other drugs used for Arrhythmias Metoprolol tartrate, p. 113

ANTIARRHYTHMICS › CLASS IB

Lidocaine hydrochloride

11-Dec-2019

(Lignocaine hydrochloride)

- **INDICATIONS AND DOSE**

Ventricular arrhythmias | Pulseless ventricular tachycardia | Ventricular fibrillation

▶ INITIALLY BY INTRAVENOUS INJECTION, OR BY INTRAOSSEOUS INJECTION

- ▶ Neonate: Initially 0.5–1 mg/kg, followed immediately by (by intravenous infusion) 0.6–3 mg/kg/hour, alternatively (by intravenous injection or by intraosseous injection) 0.5–1 mg/kg repeated at intervals of not less than 5 minutes if infusion is not immediately available following initial injection, until infusion can be initiated; maximum 3 mg/kg per course.
- ▶ Child 1 month–11 years: Initially 0.5–1 mg/kg, followed immediately by (by intravenous infusion) 0.6–3 mg/kg/hour, alternatively (by intravenous injection or by intraosseous injection) 0.5–1 mg/kg repeated at intervals of not less than 5 minutes if infusion is not immediately available following initial injection, until infusion can be initiated; maximum 3 mg/kg per course
- ▶ Child 12–17 years: Initially 50–100 mg, followed by (by intravenous infusion) 120 mg, dose to be given over 30 minutes, then (by intravenous infusion) 240 mg, dose to be given over 2 hours, then (by intravenous infusion) 60 mg/hour, reduce dose further if infusion is continued beyond 24 hours, if infusion not immediately available following initial injection, the initial injection dose may be repeated at intervals of not less than 5 minutes (to a maximum 300 mg dose in 1 hour) until infusion can be initiated

Neonatal seizures

▶ BY INTRAVENOUS INFUSION

- ▶ Neonate: Initially 2 mg/kg, dose to be given over 10 minutes, followed by 6 mg/kg/hour for 6 hours; reduced to 4 mg/kg/hour for 12 hours, then reduced to 2 mg/kg/hour for a further 12 hours, preterm neonates may require lower doses.

- **UNLICENSED USE** Not licensed for use in children under 1 year.
- **CONTRA-INDICATIONS** All grades of atrioventricular block · severe myocardial depression · sino-atrial disorders
- **CAUTIONS** Acute porphyrias p. 652 (consider infusion with glucose for its anti-porphyrinogenic effects) · congestive cardiac failure (consider lower dose) · post cardiac surgery (consider lower dose)
- **INTERACTIONS** → Appendix 1: antiarrhythmics
- **SIDE-EFFECTS** Anxiety · arrhythmias · atrioventricular block · cardiac arrest · circulatory collapse · confusion · dizziness · drowsiness · euphoric mood · headache · hypotension (may lead to cardiac arrest) · loss of consciousness · methaemoglobinaemia · muscle twitching · myocardial contractility decreased · nausea · neurological effects · nystagmus · pain · psychosis · respiratory disorders · seizure · sensation abnormal · temperature sensation altered · tinnitus · tremor · vision blurred · vomiting

SIDE-EFFECTS, FURTHER INFORMATION
Methaemoglobinaemia Methylthioninium chloride can be used for the acute symptomatic treatment of drug-induced methaemoglobinaemia.

- **PREGNANCY** Crosses the placenta but not known to be harmful in *animal* studies—use if benefit outweighs risk.
- **BREAST FEEDING** Present in milk but amount too small to be harmful.
- **HEPATIC IMPAIRMENT** Manufacturer advises caution (risk of increased exposure).
  Dose adjustments ▸ With intravenous use Manufacturer advises slower infusion rate.
- **RENAL IMPAIRMENT** Possible accumulation of lidocaine and active metabolite; caution in severe impairment.
- **MONITORING REQUIREMENTS** Monitor ECG and have resuscitation facilities available.
- **DIRECTIONS FOR ADMINISTRATION** For *intravenous infusion*, dilute with Glucose 5% or Sodium Chloride 0.9%.

- **MEDICINAL FORMS** There can be variation in the licensing of different medicines containing the same drug. Forms available from special-order manufacturers include: solution for injection

Solution for injection

▸ Lidocaine hydrochloride (Non-proprietary)
Lidocaine hydrochloride 5 mg per 1 ml Lidocaine 50mg/10ml (0.5%) solution for injection ampoules | 10 ampoule PoM £7.00
Lidocaine hydrochloride 10 mg per 1 ml Lidocaine 100mg/10ml (1%) solution for injection Mini-Plasco ampoules | 20 ampoule PoM £1.15–£11.21
Lidocaine 100mg/10ml (1%) solution for injection ampoules | 10 ampoule PoM £5.00 DT = £5.00
Lidocaine 200mg/20ml (1%) solution for injection vials | 10 vial PoM £22.00 DT = £22.00
Lidocaine 200mg/20ml (1%) solution for injection ampoules | 10 ampoule PoM £10.00–£11.00 DT = £11.00
Lidocaine 50mg/5ml (1%) solution for injection ampoules | 10 ampoule PoM £3.00–£12.00 DT = £3.00
Lidocaine 200mg/20ml (1%) solution for injection Mini-Plasco ampoules | 20 ampoule PoM ⊠
Lidocaine 20mg/2ml (1%) solution for injection ampoules | 10 ampoule PoM £12.00 DT = £2.50
Lidocaine 50mg/5ml (1%) solution for injection Mini-Plasco ampoules | 20 ampoule PoM £6.50
Lidocaine 50mg/5ml (1%) solution for injection Sure-Amp ampoules | 20 ampoule PoM £6.00
Lidocaine hydrochloride 20 mg per 1 ml Lidocaine 100mg/5ml (2%) solution for injection ampoules | 10 ampoule PoM £3.20–£12.00 DT = £3.20
Lidocaine 400mg/20ml (2%) solution for injection vials | 10 vial PoM £23.00 DT = £23.00
Lidocaine 200mg/10ml (2%) solution for injection Mini-Plasco ampoules | 20 ampoule PoM £14.95 DT = £14.95
Lidocaine 400mg/20ml (2%) solution for injection Mini-Plasco ampoules | 20 ampoule PoM ⊠
Lidocaine 40mg/2ml (2%) solution for injection ampoules | 10 ampoule PoM £12.00 DT = £2.70
Lidocaine 100mg/5ml (2%) solution for injection Mini-Plasco ampoules | 20 ampoule PoM £7.50
Lidocaine 400mg/20ml (2%) solution for injection ampoules | 10 ampoule PoM £11.00–£11.40 DT = £11.40

ANTIARRHYTHMICS › CLASS IC

Flecainide acetate

14-May-2020

- **INDICATIONS AND DOSE**

Resistant re-entry supraventricular tachycardia | Ventricular ectopic beats or ventricular tachycardia | Arrhythmias associated with accessory conduction pathways (e.g. Wolff-Parkinson-White syndrome) | Paroxysmal atrial fibrillation (initiated under direction of hospital consultant)

▸ BY MOUTH

▸ Neonate: 2 mg/kg 2–3 times a day, adjusted according to response, also adjust dose according to plasma-flecainide concentration.

▸ Child 1 month–11 years: 2 mg/kg 2–3 times a day, adjusted according to response, also adjust dose according to plasma-flecainide concentration; maximum 8 mg/kg per day; maximum 300 mg per day
▸ Child 12–17 years: Initially 50–100 mg twice daily; increased if necessary up to 300 mg daily, maximum 400 mg daily for ventricular arrhythmias in heavily built children

DOSE ADJUSTMENTS DUE TO INTERACTIONS
▸ Manufacturer advises reduce dose by half with concurrent use of amiodarone.

- **UNLICENSED USE** Not licensed for use in children under 12 years.
- **CONTRA-INDICATIONS** Abnormal left ventricular function · atrial conduction defects (unless pacing rescue available) · bundle branch block (unless pacing rescue available) · distal block (unless pacing rescue available) · haemodynamically significant valvular heart disease · heart failure · history of myocardial infarction and either asymptomatic ventricular ectopics or asymptomatic non-sustained ventricular tachycardia · long-standing atrial fibrillation where conversion to sinus rhythm not attempted · second-degree or greater AV block (unless pacing rescue available) · sinus node dysfunction (unless pacing rescue available)
- **CAUTIONS** Atrial fibrillation following heart surgery · patients with pacemakers (especially those who may be pacemaker dependent because stimulation threshold may rise appreciably)
- **INTERACTIONS** → Appendix 1: antiarrhythmics
- **SIDE-EFFECTS**

▸ **Common or very common** Arrhythmias · asthenia · dizziness · dyspnoea · fever · oedema · vision disorders
▸ **Uncommon** Alopecia · appetite decreased · constipation · diarrhoea · flatulence · gastrointestinal discomfort · nausea · skin reactions · vomiting
▸ **Rare or very rare** Anxiety · confusion · corneal deposits · depression · drowsiness · flushing · hallucination · headache · hepatic disorders · hyperhidrosis · inflammation · insomnia · memory loss · movement disorders · peripheral neuropathy · photosensitivity reaction · respiratory disorders · seizure · sensation abnormal · syncope · tinnitus · tremor · vertigo
▸ **Frequency not known** Altered pacing threshold · atrioventricular block · cardiac arrest · chest pain · heart failure · hypotension · palpitations · QT interval prolongation

- **PREGNANCY** Used in pregnancy to treat maternal and fetal arrhythmias in specialist centres; toxicity reported in *animal* studies; infant hyperbilirubinaemia also reported.
- **BREAST FEEDING** Significant amount present in milk but not known to be harmful.

- **HEPATIC IMPAIRMENT**
Dose adjustments Avoid or reduce dose in severe impairment.
Monitoring Monitor plasma-flecainide concentration.
- **RENAL IMPAIRMENT**
Dose adjustments Reduce dose by 25–50% if estimated glomerular filtration rate less than 35 mL/minute/1.73 m^2.
Monitoring Monitor plasma-flecainide concentration.
- **MONITORING REQUIREMENTS**
   - Plasma-flecainide concentration for optimal response 200–800 micrograms/litre; blood sample should be taken immediately before next dose.
- **DIRECTIONS FOR ADMINISTRATION** For administration *by mouth*, milk, infant formula, and dairy products may reduce absorption of flecainide—separate doses from feeds. Liquid has a local anaesthetic effect and should be given at least 30 minutes before or after food. Do not store liquid in refrigerator as precipitation occurs.
- **PATIENT AND CARER ADVICE**
Medicines for Children leaflet: Flecainide for arrhythmias www.medicinesforchildren.org.uk/flecainide-arrhythmias

---

- **MEDICINAL FORMS** There can be variation in the licensing of different medicines containing the same drug. Forms available from special-order manufacturers include: oral suspension, oral solution

Tablet

- Flecainide acetate (Non-proprietary)
Flecainide acetate 50 mg Flecainide 50mg tablets | 60 tablet [PoM] £7.68 DT = £4.20
Flecainide acetate 100 mg Flecainide 100mg tablets | 60 tablet [PoM] £8.06 DT = £4.07
- Tambocor (Teva UK Ltd)
Flecainide acetate 50 mg Tambocor 50mg tablets | 60 tablet [PoM] £11.57 DT = £4.20

ANTIARRHYTHMICS > CLASS III

Amiodarone hydrochloride

30-Mar-2020

- **INDICATIONS AND DOSE**

Supraventricular and ventricular arrhythmias (initiated in hospital or under specialist supervision)

- BY MOUTH
   - Neonate: Initially 5–10 mg/kg twice daily for 7–10 days, then reduced to 5–10 mg/kg daily.
   - Child 1 month–11 years: Initially 5–10 mg/kg twice daily (max. per dose 200 mg) for 7–10 days, then reduced to 5–10 mg/kg once daily; maximum 200 mg per day
   - Child 12–17 years: 200 mg 3 times a day for 1 week, then 200 mg twice daily for 1 week, then usually 200mg daily adjusted according to repsonse
- INITIALLY BY INTRAVENOUS INFUSION
   - Neonate: Initially 5 mg/kg, then (by intravenous infusion) 5 mg/kg every 12–24 hours, dose to be given over 30 minutes.
   - Child: Initially 5–10 mg/kg, dose to be given over 20 minutes to 2 hours, then (by continuous intravenous infusion) 300 micrograms/kg/hour, adjusted according to response; (by continuous intravenous infusion) increased if necessary up to 1.5 mg/kg/hour; maximum 1.2 g per day

Ventricular fibrillation or pulseless ventricular tachycardia refractory to defibrillation (for cardiopulmonary resuscitation)

- INITIALLY BY INTRAVENOUS INJECTION
   - Neonate: 5 mg/kg, dose to be given over at least 3 minutes.
   - Child: 5 mg/kg (max. per dose 300 mg), dose to be given over at least 3 minutes

- **UNLICENSED USE** Not licensed for use in children under 3 years.

> **IMPORTANT SAFETY INFORMATION**
> MHRA/CHM ADVICE: SOFOSBUVIR WITH DACLATASVIR; SOFOSBUVIR AND LEDIPASVIR (MAY 2015); SIMEPREVIR WITH SOFOSBUVIR (AUGUST 2015): RISK OF SEVERE BRADYCARDIA AND HEART BLOCK WHEN TAKEN WITH AMIODARONE
> Avoid concomitant use unless other antiarrhythmics cannot be given.

- **CONTRA-INDICATIONS**
GENERAL CONTRA-INDICATIONS
Avoid in severe conduction disturbances (unless pacemaker fitted) · avoid in sinus node disease (unless pacemaker fitted) · avoid rapid loading after cardiac surgery · iodine sensitivity · sino-atrial heart block (except in cardiac arrest) · sinus bradycardia (except in cardiac arrest) · thyroid dysfunction
SPECIFIC CONTRA-INDICATIONS
   - With intravenous use Avoid bolus injection in cardiomyopathy · avoid bolus injection in congestive heart failure · avoid in circulatory collapse · avoid in severe arterial hypotension · avoid in severe respiratory failure
- **CAUTIONS**
GENERAL CAUTIONS Acute porphyrias p. 652 · conduction disturbances (in excessive dosage) · heart failure · hypokalaemia · severe bradycardia (in excessive dosage)
SPECIFIC CAUTIONS
   - With intravenous use Avoid benzyl alcohol containing injections in neonates · moderate and transient fall in blood pressure (circulatory collapse precipitated by rapid administration or overdosage) · severe hepatocellular toxicity
- **INTERACTIONS** → Appendix 1: antiarrhythmics
- **SIDE-EFFECTS**
GENERAL SIDE-EFFECTS
   - **Common or very common** Arrhythmias · hepatic disorders · hyperthyroidism · nausea · respiratory disorders · skin reactions
   - **Rare or very rare** Bronchospasm (in patients with severe respiratory failure) · headache · idiopathic intracranial hypertension · nerve disorders · SIADH
   - **Frequency not known** Angioedema · confusion · delirium · pancreatitis · severe cutaneous adverse reactions (SCARs)

SPECIFIC SIDE-EFFECTS
   - **Common or very common**
      - With oral use Constipation · corneal deposits · hypothyroidism · movement disorders · photosensitivity reaction · sleep disorders · taste altered · vomiting
      - With parenteral use Hypotension (following rapid injection)
   - **Uncommon**
      - With oral use Cardiac conduction disorders · dry mouth · myopathy (usually reversible on discontinuation) · peripheral neuropathy (usually reversible on discontinuation)
   - **Rare or very rare**
      - With oral use Alopecia · aplastic anaemia · epididymo-orchitis · erectile dysfunction · haemolytic anaemia · pulmonary haemorrhage · thrombocytopenia · vertigo
      - With parenteral use Hot flush · hyperhidrosis
   - **Frequency not known**
      - With oral use Altered smell sensation · appetite decreased · parkinsonism · vasculitis
      - With parenteral use Agranulocytosis · libido decreased · neutropenia

SIDE-EFFECTS, FURTHER INFORMATION **Corneal microdeposits** Patients taking amiodarone may develop corneal microdeposits (reversible on withdrawal of treatment). However, if vision is impaired or if optic neuritis or optic neuropathy occur, amiodarone must be stopped to prevent blindness and expert advice sought.

Thyroid function Amiodarone contains iodine and can cause disorders of thyroid function; both hypothyroidism and hyperthyroidism can occur. Hypothyroidism can be treated with replacement therapy without withdrawing amiodarone if it is essential; careful supervision is required.

Hepatotoxicity Amiodarone is also associated with hepatotoxicity and treatment should be discontinued if severe liver function abnormalities or clinical signs of liver disease develop.

Pulmonary toxicity Pneumonitis should always be suspected if new or progressive shortness of breath or cough develops in a patient taking amiodarone.

- PREGNANCY Possible risk of neonatal goitre; use only if no alternative.
- BREAST FEEDING Avoid; present in milk in significant amounts; theoretical risk of neonatal hypothyroidism from release of iodine.
- MONITORING REQUIREMENTS
  - Thyroid function tests should be performed before treatment and then every 6 months. Clinical assessment of thyroid function alone is unreliable. Thyroxine (T4) may be raised in the absence of hyperthyroidism; therefore tri-iodothyronine (T3), T4, and thyroid-stimulating hormone (thyrotrophin, TSH) should all be measured. A raised T3 and T4 with a very low or undetectable TSH concentration suggests the development of thyrotoxicosis.
  - Liver function tests required before treatment and then every 6 months.
  - Serum potassium concentration should be measured before treatment.
  - Chest x-ray required before treatment.
  - Pulmonary function tests required before treatment.
  - With intravenous use ECG monitoring and resuscitation facilities must be available. Monitor liver transaminases closely.
- DIRECTIONS FOR ADMINISTRATION
  - With intravenous use Intravenous administration via central venous catheter recommended if repeated or continuous infusion required, as infusion via peripheral veins may cause pain and inflammation. For *intravenous infusion*, dilute to a concentration of not less than 600 micrograms/mL with Glucose 5%. Incompatible with Sodium Chloride infusion fluids; avoid equipment containing the plasticizer di-2-ethylhexphthalate (DEHP).
  - With oral use For administration *by mouth*, tablets may be crushed and dispersed in water; injection solution should **not** be given orally (irritant).
- PATIENT AND CARER ADVICE Because of the possibility of phototoxic reactions, patients should be advised to shield the skin from light during treatment and for several months after discontinuing amiodarone; a wide-spectrum sunscreen to protect against both long-wave ultraviolet and visible light should be used.
  Medicines for Children leaflet: Amiodarone for abnormal heart rhythms www.medicinesforchildren.org.uk/amiodarone-abnormal-heart-rhythms-0

- MEDICINAL FORMS There can be variation in the licensing of different medicines containing the same drug. Forms available from special-order manufacturers include: oral suspension, oral solution

Tablet

CAUTIONARY AND ADVISORY LABELS 11

- Amiodarone hydrochloride (Non-proprietary)
  Amiodarone hydrochloride 100 mg Amiodarone 100mg tablets | 28 tablet PoM £4.25 DT = £1.63
  Amiodarone hydrochloride 200 mg Amiodarone 200mg tablets | 28 tablet PoM £7.80 DT = £1.91
- Cordarone X (Sanofi)
  Amiodarone hydrochloride 100 mg Cordarone X 100 tablets | 28 tablet PoM £4.28 DT = £1.63
  Amiodarone hydrochloride 200 mg Cordarone X 200 tablets | 28 tablet PoM £6.99 DT = £1.91

Solution for injection

EXCIPIENTS: May contain Benzyl alcohol

- Amiodarone hydrochloride (Non-proprietary)
  Amiodarone hydrochloride 30 mg per 1 ml Amiodarone 300mg/10ml solution for injection pre-filled syringes | 1 pre-filled disposable injection PoM £14.68 DT = £14.68
  Amiodarone hydrochloride 50 mg per 1 ml Amiodarone 150mg/3ml concentrate for solution for injection ampoules | 5 ampoule PoM £7.75 (Hospital only) | 10 ampoule PoM £17.00
- Cordarone X (Sanofi)
  Amiodarone hydrochloride 50 mg per 1 ml Cordarone X 150mg/3ml solution for injection ampoules | 6 ampoule PoM £9.60

ANTIARRHYTHMICS > OTHER

Adenosine

20-Jan-2020

- INDICATIONS AND DOSE

Used in conjunction with radionuclide myocardial perfusion imaging in patients who cannot exercise adequately or for whom exercise is inappropriate

- BY INTRAVENOUS INFUSION
- Child: (consult product literature)

Termination of supraventricular tachycardias, including those associated with accessory conducting pathways (e.g. Wolff-Parkinson-White syndrome) | Diagnosis of supraventricular arrhythmias

- BY RAPID INTRAVENOUS INJECTION
- Neonate: Initially 150 micrograms/kg, then increased in steps of 50–100 micrograms/kg every 1–2 minutes if required, dose to be repeated until tachycardia terminated or maximum single dose of 300 micrograms/kg given.
- Child 1–11 months: Initially 150 micrograms/kg, then increased in steps of 50–100 micrograms/kg every 1–2 minutes if required, dose to be repeated until tachycardia terminated or maximum single dose of 500 micrograms/kg given
- Child 1–11 years: Initially 100 micrograms/kg, then increased in steps of 50–100 micrograms/kg every 1–2 minutes if required, dose to be repeated until tachycardia terminated or maximum single dose of 500 micrograms/kg (max.12 mg) given
- Child 12–17 years: Initially 3 mg, followed by 6 mg after 1–2 minutes if required, followed by 12 mg after 1–2 minutes if required, in some children over 12 years 3 mg dose ineffective (e.g. if a small peripheral vein is used for administration) and higher initial dose sometimes used; however, those with *heart transplant* are **very sensitive** to the effects of adenosine, and should **not** receive higher initial doses

- UNLICENSED USE *Adenocor*® licensed for treatment of paroxysmal supraventricular tachycardia in children; not licensed for diagnosis in children; *Adenoscan*® not licensed in children.
- CONTRA-INDICATIONS Asthma · decompensated heart failure · long QT syndrome · second- or third-degree AV block and sick sinus syndrome (unless pacemaker fitted) · severe hypotension
- CAUTIONS Atrial fibrillation · atrial fibrillation with accessory pathway (conduction down anomalous pathway may increase) · atrial flutter · atrial flutter with accessory pathway (conduction down anomalous pathway may increase) · autonomic dysfunction · bundle branch block ·

first-degree AV block · heart transplant · left main coronary artery stenosis · left to right shunt · pericardial effusion · pericarditis · QT-interval prolongation · recent myocardial infarction · severe heart failure · stenotic carotid artery disease with cerebrovascular insufficiency · stenotic valvular heart disease · uncorrected hypovolaemia

- **INTERACTIONS** → Appendix 1: antiarrhythmics
- **SIDE-EFFECTS**
- ▸ **Common or very common** Abdominal discomfort · arrhythmias · atrioventricular block · chest discomfort · chest pain (discontinue) · dizziness · dry mouth · dyspnoea · flushing · headache · hypotension (discontinue if severe) · pain · paraesthesia · throat discomfort
- ▸ **Uncommon** Asthenia · back discomfort · bradycardia (discontinue if asystole or severe bradycardia occur) · hyperhidrosis · limb discomfort · nervousness · taste metallic
- ▸ **Rare or very rare** Drowsiness · nasal congestion · nipple tenderness · respiratory disorders · respiratory failure (discontinue) · tinnitus · tremor · urinary urgency · vision blurred
- ▸ **Frequency not known** Apnoea · cardiac arrest · loss of consciousness · nausea · seizure · syncope · vomiting
- **PREGNANCY** Large doses may produce fetal toxicity; manufacturer advises use only if potential benefit outweighs risk.
- **BREAST FEEDING** No information available—unlikely to be present in milk owing to short half-life.
- **MONITORING REQUIREMENTS** Monitor ECG and have resuscitation facilities available.
- **DIRECTIONS FOR ADMINISTRATION** For *rapid intravenous injection* give over 2 seconds into central or large peripheral vein followed by rapid Sodium Chloride 0.9% flush; injection solution may be diluted with Sodium Chloride 0.9% if required.

- **MEDICINAL FORMS** There can be variation in the licensing of different medicines containing the same drug. Forms available from special-order manufacturers include: solution for injection, infusion, solution for infusion

Solution for injection

ELECTROLYTES: May contain Sodium

- ▸ Adenosine (Non-proprietary)

  Adenosine 3 mg per 1 ml Adenosine 6mg/2ml solution for injection pre-filled syringes | 10 pre-filled disposable injection PoM ⊠ (Hospital only)

  Adenosine 6mg/2ml solution for injection vials | 5 vial PoM £20.00 (Hospital only) | 6 vial PoM £26.70–£29.24 (Hospital only)

  Adenosine 12mg/4ml solution for injection pre-filled syringes | 10 pre-filled disposable injection PoM ⊠ (Hospital only)
- ▸ Adenocor (Sanofi)

  Adenosine 3 mg per 1 ml Adenocor 6mg/2ml solution for injection vials | 6 vial PoM £6.45 (Hospital only)

Solution for infusion

ELECTROLYTES: May contain Sodium

- ▸ Adenosine (Non-proprietary)

  Adenosine 3 mg per 1 ml Adenosine 30mg/10ml solution for infusion vials | 5 vial PoM £30.00 (Hospital only) | 6 vial PoM £70.00–£85.57 (Hospital only)
- ▸ Adenoscan (Sanofi)

  Adenosine 3 mg per 1 ml Adenoscan 30mg/10ml solution for infusion vials | 6 vial PoM £16.05

BETA-ADRENOCEPTOR BLOCKERS › NON-SELECTIVE

F 109

Sotalol hydrochloride

12-Dec-2019

- **INDICATIONS AND DOSE**

Life-threatening arrhythmias including ventricular tachyarrhythmias

▸ BY MOUTH

- ▸ Child 12–17 years: Initially 80 mg once daily, alternatively initially 40 mg twice daily, then increased to 80–160 mg twice daily, dose to be increased gradually at intervals of 2–3 days; higher doses of 480–640 mg daily may be required for life-threatening ventricular arrhythmias (under specialist supervision)

Ventricular arrhythmias, life-threatening ventricular tachyarrhythmia and supraventricular arrhythmias (initiated under specialist supervision)

▸ BY MOUTH

- ▸ Neonate: Initially 1 mg/kg twice daily, increased if necessary up to 4 mg/kg twice daily, dose to be increased at intervals of 3–4 days.

Atrial flutter, ventricular arrhythmias, life-threatening ventricular tachyarrhythmia and supraventricular arrhythmias (initiated under specialist supervision)

▸ BY MOUTH

- ▸ Child 1 month–11 years: Initially 1 mg/kg twice daily, then increased if necessary up to 4 mg/kg twice daily (max. per dose 80 mg twice daily), dose to be increased at intervals of 2–3 days
- ▸ Child 12–17 years: Initially 80 mg once daily, alternatively initially 40 mg twice daily, increased to 80–160 mg twice daily, dose to be increased gradually at intervals of 2–3 days

- **UNLICENSED USE** Not licensed for use in children under 12 years.

> **IMPORTANT SAFETY INFORMATION**
>
> Sotalol may prolong the QT interval, and it occasionally causes life threatening ventricular arrhythmias (**important**: manufacturer advises particular care is required to avoid hypokalaemia in patients taking sotalol—electrolyte disturbances, particularly hypokalaemia and hypomagnesaemia should be corrected before sotalol started and during use).
>
> Manufacturer advises reduce dose or discontinue if corrected QT interval exceeds 550 msec.

- **CONTRA-INDICATIONS** Long QT syndrome (congenital or acquired) · torsade de pointes
- **CAUTIONS** Diarrhoea (severe or prolonged)
- **INTERACTIONS** → Appendix 1: beta blockers, non-selective
- **SIDE-EFFECTS**
- ▸ **Common or very common** Anxiety · arrhythmia · chest pain · dyspepsia · fever · flatulence · hearing impairment · mood altered · muscle spasms · oedema · palpitations · sexual dysfunction · taste altered · torsade de pointes (increased risk in females)
- **BREAST FEEDING** Water soluble beta-blockers such as sotalol are present in breast milk in greater amounts than other beta blockers.
- **RENAL IMPAIRMENT** Avoid if estimated glomerular filtration rate less than 10 mL/minute/1.73 m^2.

  Dose adjustments Halve normal dose if estimated glomerular filtration rate 30–60 mL/minute/1.73 m^2; use one-quarter normal dose if estimated glomerular filtration rate 10–30 mL/minute/1.73 m^2.

2 Cardiovascular system

- **MONITORING REQUIREMENTS** Measurement of corrected QT interval, and monitoring of ECG and electrolytes required; correct hypokalaemia, hypomagnesaemia, or other electrolyte disturbances.
- **DIRECTIONS FOR ADMINISTRATION** For administration *by mouth*, tablets may be crushed and dispersed in water.

- **MEDICINAL FORMS** There can be variation in the licensing of different medicines containing the same drug. Forms available from special-order manufacturers include: oral suspension, oral solution

Tablet

CAUTIONARY AND ADVISORY LABELS 8

- Sotalol hydrochloride (Non-proprietary)
  Sotalol hydrochloride 40 mg Sotalol 40mg tablets | 28 tablet PoM £1.26 DT = £1.24
  Sotalol hydrochloride 80 mg Sotalol 80mg tablets | 28 tablet PoM £3.75 DT = £1.32 | 56 tablet PoM £2.83
  Sotalol hydrochloride 160 mg Sotalol 160mg tablets | 28 tablet PoM £5.95 DT = £4.87
- Beta-Cardone (Advanz Pharma)
  Sotalol hydrochloride 200 mg Beta-Cardone 200mg tablets | 28 tablet PoM £2.40 DT = £2.40
- Sotacor (Cheplapharm Arzneimittel GmbH)
  Sotalol hydrochloride 80 mg Sotacor 80mg tablets | 30 tablet PoM £3.28

CARDIAC GLYCOSIDES

Cardiac glycosides

Digoxin-specific antibody

Serious cases of digoxin toxicity should be discussed with the National Poisons Information Service (see further information, under Poisoning, emergency treatment p. 891). Digoxin-specific antibody fragments p. 900 are indicated for the treatment of known or strongly suspected life-threatening digoxin toxicity associated with ventricular arrhythmias or bradyarrhythmias unresponsive to atropine sulfate p. 869 and when measures beyond the withdrawal of digoxin below and correction of any electrolyte abnormalities are considered necessary.

Digoxin

Digoxin is most useful in the treatment of supraventricular tachycardias, especially for controlling ventricular response in persistent atrial fibrillation. Digoxin has a limited role in children with chronic heart failure.

For the management of atrial fibrillation, the maintenance dose of digoxin is determined on the basis of the ventricular rate at rest, which should not be allowed to fall below an acceptable level for the child.

Digoxin is now rarely used for rapid control of heart rate, even with intravenous administration, response may take many hours; persistence of tachycardia is therefore not an indication for exceeding the recommended dose. The intramuscular route is **not** recommended.

In children with heart failure who are in sinus rhythm, a loading dose may not be required.

Unwanted effects depend both on the concentration of digoxin in the plasma and on the sensitivity of the conducting system or of the myocardium, which is often increased in heart disease. It can sometimes be difficult to distinguish between toxic effects and clinical deterioration because the symptoms of both are similar. The plasma-digoxin concentration alone cannot indicate toxicity reliably, but the likelihood of toxicity increases progressively through the range 1.5 to 3 micrograms/litre for digoxin. Renal function is very important in determining digoxin dosage.

Hypokalaemia predisposes the child to digitalis toxicity and should be avoided; it is managed by giving a potassium-sparing diuretic or, if necessary, potassium supplements.

If toxicity occurs, digoxin should be withdrawn; serious manifestations require urgent specialist management. Digoxin-specific antibody fragments are available for reversal of life-threatening overdosage.

Digoxin

28-Apr-2020

- **DRUG ACTION** Digoxin is a cardiac glycoside that increases the force of myocardial contraction and reduces conductivity within the atrioventricular (AV) node.

- **INDICATIONS AND DOSE**

Supraventricular arrhythmias | Chronic heart failure

▶ BY MOUTH

- Neonate (body-weight up to 1.5 kg): Initially 25 micrograms/kg in 3 divided doses for 24 hours, then 4–6 micrograms/kg daily in 1–2 divided doses.
- Neonate (body-weight 1.5–2.5 kg): Initially 30 micrograms/kg in 3 divided doses for 24 hours, then 4–6 micrograms/kg daily in 1–2 divided doses.
- Neonate (body-weight 2.6 kg and above): Initially 45 micrograms/kg in 3 divided doses for 24 hours, then 10 micrograms/kg daily in 1–2 divided doses.
- Child 1 month–1 year: Initially 45 micrograms/kg in 3 divided doses for 24 hours, then 10 micrograms/kg daily in 1–2 divided doses
- Child 2–4 years: Initially 35 micrograms/kg in 3 divided doses for 24 hours, then 10 micrograms/kg daily in 1–2 divided doses
- Child 5–9 years: Initially 25 micrograms/kg in 3 divided doses for 24 hours, maximum 750 micrograms per day, then 6 micrograms/kg daily in 1–2 divided doses, maximum 250 micrograms per day
- Child 10–17 years: Initially 0.75–1.5 mg in 3 divided doses for 24 hours, then 62.5–250 micrograms daily in 1–2 divided doses, higher doses may be necessary

▶ BY INTRAVENOUS INFUSION

- Neonate (body-weight up to 1.5 kg): Initially 20 micrograms/kg in 3 divided doses for 24 hours, then 4–6 micrograms/kg daily in 1–2 divided doses.
- Neonate (body-weight 1.5–2.5 kg): Initially 30 micrograms/kg in 3 divided doses for 24 hours, then 4–6 micrograms/kg daily in 1–2 divided doses.
- Neonate (body-weight 2.6 kg and above): Initially 35 micrograms/kg in 3 divided doses for 24 hours, then 10 micrograms/kg daily in 1–2 divided doses.
- Child 1 month–1 year: Initially 35 micrograms/kg in 3 divided doses for 24 hours, then 10 micrograms/kg daily in 1–2 divided doses
- Child 2–4 years: Initially 35 micrograms/kg in 3 divided doses for 24 hours, then 10 micrograms/kg daily in 1–2 divided doses
- Child 5–9 years: Initially 25 micrograms/kg in 3 divided doses for 24 hours, maximum 500 micrograms per day, then 6 micrograms/kg daily in 1–2 divided doses, maximum 250 micrograms per day
- Child 10–17 years: Initially 0.5–1 mg in 3 divided doses for 24 hours, then 62.5–250 micrograms daily in 1–2 divided doses, higher doses may be necessary

DOSE ADJUSTMENTS DUE TO INTERACTIONS

- Manufacturer advises reduce dose by half with concurrent use of amiodarone, dronedarone and quinine.

DOSE EQUIVALENCE AND CONVERSION
- Dose may need to be reduced if digoxin (or another cardiac glycoside) has been given in the preceding 2 weeks.
- When switching from intravenous to oral route may need to increase dose by 20–33% to maintain the same plasma-digoxin concentration.

- **UNLICENSED USE** Digoxin is licensed for use in heart failure and supraventricular arrhythmias.
- **CONTRA-INDICATIONS** Constrictive pericarditis (unless to control atrial fibrillation or improve systolic dysfunction—but use with caution) · hypertrophic cardiomyopathy (unless concomitant atrial fibrillation and heart failure—but use with caution) · intermittent complete heart block · myocarditis · second degree AV block · supraventricular arrhythmias associated with accessory conducting pathways e.g. Wolff-Parkinson-White syndrome (although can be used in infancy) · ventricular tachycardia or fibrillation
- **CAUTIONS** Hypercalcaemia (risk of digitalis toxicity) · hypokalaemia (risk of digitalis toxicity) · hypomagnesaemia (risk of digitalis toxicity) · hypoxia (risk of digitalis toxicity) · recent myocardial infarction · severe respiratory disease · sick sinus syndrome · thyroid disease
- **INTERACTIONS** → Appendix 1: digoxin
- **SIDE-EFFECTS**
- **Common or very common** Arrhythmias · cardiac conduction disorder · cerebral impairment · diarrhoea · dizziness · eosinophilia · nausea · skin reactions · vision disorders · vomiting
- **Uncommon** Depression
- **Rare or very rare** Appetite decreased · asthenia · confusion · gastrointestinal disorders · gynaecomastia · headache · malaise · psychosis · thrombocytopenia

  Overdose If toxicity occurs, digoxin should be withdrawn; serious manifestations require urgent specialist management.
- **PREGNANCY**
  Dose adjustments May need dosage adjustment.
- **BREAST FEEDING** Amount too small to be harmful.
- **RENAL IMPAIRMENT**
  Dose adjustments Use half normal dose if estimated glomerular filtration rate is 10–50 mL/minute/1.73 m^2 and use a quarter normal dose if estimated glomerular filtration rate is less than 10 mL/minute/1.73 m^2.
  Monitoring Monitor plasma-digoxin concentration in renal impairment.
- **MONITORING REQUIREMENTS**
- For plasma-digoxin concentration assay, blood should be taken at least 6 hours after a dose.
- Plasma-digoxin concentration should be maintained in the range 0.8–2 micrograms/litre.
- Monitor serum electrolytes and renal function. Toxicity increased by electrolyte disturbances.
- **DIRECTIONS FOR ADMINISTRATION**
- With intravenous use Avoid rapid intravenous administration (risk of hypertension and reduced coronary flow). For *intravenous infusion*, dilute with Sodium Chloride 0.9% or Glucose 5% to a max. concentration of 62.5 micrograms/mL; loading doses should be given over 30–60 minutes and maintenance dose over 10–20 minutes.
- With oral use For *oral* administration, oral solution must **not** be diluted.
- **PATIENT AND CARER ADVICE** Patient counselling is advised for digoxin elixir (use pipette).
- **MEDICINAL FORMS** There can be variation in the licensing of different medicines containing the same drug. Forms available from special-order manufacturers include: oral suspension, oral solution, solution for injection

Tablet
- Digoxin (Non-proprietary)
  Digoxin 62.5 microgram Digoxin 62.5microgram tablets | 28 tablet PoM £9.99 DT = £1.52
  Digoxin 125 microgram Digoxin 125microgram tablets | 28 tablet PoM £4.99 DT = £1.52
  Digoxin 250 microgram Digoxin 250microgram tablets | 28 tablet PoM £4.99 DT = £1.55
- Lanoxin (Aspen Pharma Trading Ltd)
  Digoxin 62.5 microgram Lanoxin PG 62.5microgram tablets | 500 tablet PoM £8.09
  Digoxin 125 microgram Lanoxin 125 tablets | 500 tablet PoM £8.09
  Digoxin 250 microgram Lanoxin 250microgram tablets | 500 tablet PoM £8.09

Solution for injection
EXCIPIENTS: May contain Alcohol, propylene glycol
- Digoxin (Non-proprietary)
  Digoxin 100 microgram per 1 ml Lanoxin Injection Pediatric 100micrograms/1ml solution for injection ampoules | 10 ampoule PoM [X]

Solution for infusion
- Digoxin (Non-proprietary)
  Digoxin 250 microgram per 1 ml Digoxin 500micrograms/2ml solution for infusion ampoules | 10 ampoule PoM £7.00
- Lanoxin (Aspen Pharma Trading Ltd)
  Digoxin 250 microgram per 1 ml Lanoxin 500micrograms/2ml solution for infusion ampoules | 5 ampoule PoM £3.30

Oral solution
- Lanoxin (Aspen Pharma Trading Ltd)
  Digoxin 50 microgram per 1 ml Lanoxin PG 50micrograms/ml elixir | 60 ml PoM £5.35 DT = £5.35

2 Bleeding disorders

Antifibrinolytic drugs and haemostatics

Overview

Fibrin dissolution can be impaired by the administration of tranexamic acid below, which inhibits fibrinolysis. It can be used to prevent bleeding or treat bleeding associated with excessive fibrinolysis (e.g. in surgery, dental extraction, obstetric disorders, and traumatic hyphaema) and in the management of menorrhagia; it may also be used in hereditary angioedema, epistaxis, and thrombolytic overdose. Tranexamic acid can also be used in cardiac surgery to reduce blood loss and to reduce the need for use of blood products.

Desmopressin p. 468 is used in the management of mild to moderate haemophilia and von Willebrand's disease. It is also used for fibrinolytic response testing.

ANTIHAEMORRHAGICS > ANTIFIBRINOLYTICS

Tranexamic acid

10-Mar-2020

- **INDICATIONS AND DOSE**

Inhibition of fibrinolysis
- BY MOUTH
- Child: 15–25 mg/kg 2–3 times a day (max. per dose 1.5 g)
- BY SLOW INTRAVENOUS INJECTION
- Child: 10 mg/kg 2–3 times a day (max. per dose 1 g), dose to be given over at least 10 minutes
- BY CONTINUOUS INTRAVENOUS INFUSION
- Child: 45 mg/kg, dose to be given over 24 hours

continued →

Menorrhagia
- ▶ BY MOUTH
- ▶ Child 12–17 years: 1 g 3 times a day for up to 4 days, to be initiated when menstruation has started; maximum 4 g per day

Hereditary angioedema
- ▶ BY MOUTH
- ▶ Child: 15–25 mg/kg 2–3 times a day (max. per dose 1.5 g), for short-term prophylaxis of hereditary angioedema, tranexamic acid is started several days before planned procedures which may trigger an acute attack of hereditary angioedema (e.g. dental work) and continued for 2–5 days afterwards
- ▶ BY SLOW INTRAVENOUS INJECTION
- ▶ Child: 10 mg/kg 2–3 times a day (max. per dose 1 g), dose to be given over at least 10 minutes
- ▶ BY CONTINUOUS INTRAVENOUS INFUSION
- ▶ Child: 45 mg/kg, dose to be given over 24 hours

Prevention of excessive bleeding after dental procedures (e.g. in haemophilia)
- ▶ BY INTRAVENOUS INJECTION
- ▶ Child 6–17 years: 10 mg/kg (max. per dose 1.5 g), dose to be given pre-operatively
- ▶ BY MOUTH
- ▶ Child 6–17 years: 15–25 mg/kg (max. per dose 1.5 g), dose to be given pre-operatively, then 15–25 mg/kg 2–3 times a day (max. per dose 1.5 g) for up to 8 days, dose to be given postoperatively

Prevention of excessive bleeding after dental procedures (e.g. in haemophilia) with mouthwash 5% solution (specialist use only)
- ▶ BY MOUTH
- ▶ Child 6–17 years: 5–10 mL 4 times a day for 2 days, rinse mouth with solution; the solution should not be swallowed

Reduction of blood loss during cardiac surgery
- ▶ BY SLOW INTRAVENOUS INJECTION, OR BY INTRAVENOUS INFUSION
- ▶ Child: (consult local protocol)

- **UNLICENSED USE** Not licensed for reduction of blood loss during cardiac surgery; injection not licensed for use in children under 1 year or for administration by intravenous infusion.
- **CONTRA-INDICATIONS** Fibrinolytic conditions following disseminated intravascular coagulation (unless predominant activation of fibrinolytic system with severe bleeding) · history of convulsions · thromboembolic disease
- **CAUTIONS** Irregular menstrual bleeding (establish cause before initiating therapy) · massive haematuria (avoid if risk of ureteric obstruction) · patients receiving oral contraceptives (increased risk of thrombosis)

CAUTIONS, FURTHER INFORMATION
- ▶ Menorrhagia Before initiating treatment for menorrhagia, exclude structural or histological causes or fibroids causing distortion of uterine cavity.

- **INTERACTIONS** → Appendix 1: tranexamic acid
- **SIDE-EFFECTS**

GENERAL SIDE-EFFECTS
- ▶ **Common or very common** Diarrhoea (reduce dose) · nausea · vomiting
- ▶ **Uncommon** Allergic dermatitis
- ▶ **Rare or very rare** Colour vision change (discontinue) · embolism and thrombosis
- ▶ **Frequency not known** Seizure (more common at high doses) · visual impairment (discontinue)

SPECIFIC SIDE-EFFECTS
- ▶ With intravenous use Hypotension · malaise (on rapid intravenous injection)

- **PREGNANCY** No evidence of teratogenicity in *animal* studies; manufacturer advises use only if potential benefit outweighs risk—crosses the placenta.
- **BREAST FEEDING** Small amount present in milk—antifibrinolytic effect in infant unlikely.
- **RENAL IMPAIRMENT** Avoid in severe impairment.
  Dose adjustments Reduce dose in mild to moderate impairment.
- **MONITORING REQUIREMENTS** Regular liver function tests in long-term treatment of hereditary angioedema.
- **DIRECTIONS FOR ADMINISTRATION** For *intravenous administration*, dilute with Glucose 5% *or* Sodium chloride 0.9%.
- **PATIENT AND CARER ADVICE**
  Medicines for Children leaflet: Tranexamic acid for heavy bleeding during periods www.medicinesforchildren.org.uk/tranexamic-acid-heavy-bleeding-during-periods
  Medicines for Children leaflet: Tranexamic acid for the treatment or prevention of bleeding www.medicinesforchildren.org.uk/tranexamic-acid-treatment-or-prevention-bleeding

---

- **MEDICINAL FORMS** There can be variation in the licensing of different medicines containing the same drug. Forms available from special-order manufacturers include: oral suspension, oral solution

Tablet
- ▶ Tranexamic acid (Non-proprietary)
  Tranexamic acid 500 mg Tranexamic acid 500mg tablets | 60 tablet [PoM] £32.10 DT = £6.20
- ▶ Cyklokapron (Mylan)
  Tranexamic acid 500 mg Cyklokapron 500mg tablets | 60 tablet [PoM] £14.30 DT = £6.20

Solution for injection
- ▶ Tranexamic acid (Non-proprietary)
  Tranexamic acid 100 mg per 1 ml Tranexamic acid 500mg/5ml solution for injection ampoules | 5 ampoule [PoM] £7.50 DT = £7.50 (Hospital only) | 10 ampoule [PoM] £15.47 DT = £15.47 (Hospital only)
- ▶ Cyklokapron (Pfizer Ltd)
  Tranexamic acid 100 mg per 1 ml Cyklokapron 500mg/5ml solution for injection ampoules | 10 ampoule [PoM] £15.47 DT = £15.47

ANTIHAEMORRHAGICS > HAEMOSTATICS

Emicizumab

09-May-2018

- **DRUG ACTION** Emicizumab is a monoclonal antibody that bridges activated factor IX and factor X to restore function of missing activated factor VIII, which is needed for haemostasis.

- **INDICATIONS AND DOSE**

Prophylaxis of haemorrhage in haemophilia A (initiated by a specialist)
- ▶ BY SUBCUTANEOUS INJECTION
- ▶ Child: Initially 3 mg/kg once weekly for 4 weeks, then maintenance 1.5 mg/kg once weekly, alternatively maintenance 3 mg/kg every 2 weeks, alternatively maintenance 6 mg/kg every 4 weeks

- **CAUTIONS** Children under 1 year · concomitant bypassing agent · risk factors for thrombotic microangiopathy

CAUTIONS, FURTHER INFORMATION
- ▶ Concomitant bypassing agent Manufacturer advises discontinue bypassing agents the day before starting emicizumab; if a bypassing agent is required—consult product literature.

- **SIDE-EFFECTS**
- ▶ **Common or very common** Arthralgia · diarrhoea · fever · headache · myalgia

- ▶ **Uncommon** Cavernous sinus thrombosis · embolism and thrombosis · skin necrosis · thrombotic microangiopathy
- ● **CONCEPTION AND CONTRACEPTION** Manufacturer advises effective contraception during and for 6 months after treatment in women of childbearing potential.
- ● **PREGNANCY** Manufacturer advises use only if potential benefit outweighs risk—no information available.
- ● **BREAST FEEDING** Manufacturer advises avoid—no information available.
- ● **EFFECT ON LABORATORY TESTS** Manufacturer advises to avoid intrinsic pathway clotting-based laboratory tests or use with caution as results may be misinterpreted—consult product literature.
- ● **DIRECTIONS FOR ADMINISTRATION** Manufacturer advises max. 2 mL per injection site; rotate injection site and avoid skin that is tender, damaged or scarred. Patients or their caregivers may self-administer *Hemlibra*® after appropriate training.
- ● **PRESCRIBING AND DISPENSING INFORMATION** Emicizumab is a biological medicine. Biological medicines must be prescribed and dispensed by brand name, see *Biological medicines* and *Biosimilar medicines*, under Guidance on prescribing p. 1; manufacturer advises to record the brand name and batch number after each administration.
- ● **PATIENT AND CARER ADVICE**

Missed doses Manufacturer advises if a dose is missed, the missed dose may be taken up to a day before the next scheduled dose. The next dose should then be taken on the usual scheduled dosing day.

- ● **MEDICINAL FORMS** There can be variation in the licensing of different medicines containing the same drug.

Solution for injection

- ▸ Hemlibra (Roche Products Ltd) ▼

Emicizumab 30 mg per 1 ml Hemlibra 30mg/1ml solution for injection vials | 1 vial PoM £2,415.30

Emicizumab 150 mg per 1 ml Hemlibra 150mg/1ml solution for injection vials | 1 vial PoM £12,076.50

Hemlibra 105mg/0.7ml solution for injection vials | 1 vial PoM £8,453.55

Hemlibra 60mg/0.4ml solution for injection vials | 1 vial PoM £4,830.60

2.1 Coagulation factor deficiencies

BLOOD AND RELATED PRODUCTS › COAGULATION PROTEINS

Dried prothrombin complex 30-Jan-2020

(Human prothrombin complex)

- ● **INDICATIONS AND DOSE**

Treatment and peri-operative prophylaxis of haemorrhage in patients with congenital deficiency of factors II, VII, IX, or X if purified specific coagulation factors not available | Treatment and peri-operative prophylaxis of haemorrhage in patients with acquired deficiency of factors II, VII, IX, or X (e.g. during warfarin treatment)

- ▸ BY INTRAVENOUS INFUSION
- ▸ Child: (consult haematologist)

- ● **CONTRA-INDICATIONS** History of heparin induced thrombocytopenia · myocardial infarction within the last 3 months (no information available) · unstable angina within the last 3 months (no information available)
- ● **CAUTIONS** Disseminated intravascular coagulation · history of myocardial infarction or coronary heart disease · postoperative use · risk of thrombosis · vaccination against hepatitis A and hepatitis B may be required
- ● **SIDE-EFFECTS**
- ▶ **Common or very common** Embolism and thrombosis
- ▶ **Uncommon** Anxiety · device thrombosis · haemorrhage · hepatic function abnormal · hypertension · respiratory disorders
- ▶ **Frequency not known** Cardiac arrest · chills · circulatory collapse · disseminated intravascular coagulation · dyspnoea · heparin-induced thrombocytopenia · hypotension · nausea · skin reactions · tachycardia · tremor
- ● **HEPATIC IMPAIRMENT** Manufacturer advises caution (risk of thromboembolic complications).

Monitoring Monitor closely in hepatic impairment (risk of thromboembolic complications).

- ● **PRESCRIBING AND DISPENSING INFORMATION** Dried prothrombin complex is prepared from human plasma by a suitable fractionation technique, and contains factor IX, together with variable amounts of factors II, VII, and X.

Available from CSL Behring (*Beriplex*® *P/N*), Octapharma (*Octaplex*®).

- ● **MEDICINAL FORMS** No licensed medicines listed.

Factor VIIa (recombinant) 30-Jan-2020

(Eptacog alfa (activated))

- ● **INDICATIONS AND DOSE**

Treatment and prophylaxis of haemorrhage in patients with haemophilia A or B with inhibitors to factors VIII or IX, acquired haemophilia, factor VII deficiency, or Glanzmann's thrombasthenia

- ▸ BY INTRAVENOUS INJECTION
- ▸ Child: (consult haematologist)

- ● **CAUTIONS** Disseminated intravascular coagulation · risk of thrombosis
- ● **SIDE-EFFECTS**
- ▶ **Uncommon** Embolism and thrombosis · fever · hepatic disorders · intestinal ischaemia · skin reactions
- ▶ **Rare or very rare** Angina pectoris · cerebrovascular insufficiency · coagulation disorders · headache · myocardial infarction · nausea · peripheral ischaemia
- ▶ **Frequency not known** Angioedema · flushing
- ● **MEDICINAL FORMS** There can be variation in the licensing of different medicines containing the same drug.

Powder and solvent for solution for injection

- ▸ NovoSeven (Novo Nordisk Ltd)

Eptacog alfa activated 50000 unit NovoSeven 1mg (50,000units) powder and solvent for solution for injection pre-filled syringes | 1 pre-filled disposable injection PoM £525.20 (Hospital only)

NovoSeven 1mg (50,000units) powder and solvent for solution for injection vials | 1 vial PoM £525.20 (Hospital only)

Eptacog alfa activated 100000 unit NovoSeven 2mg (100,000units) powder and solvent for solution for injection vials | 1 vial PoM £1,050.40 (Hospital only)

NovoSeven 2mg (100,000units) powder and solvent for solution for injection pre-filled syringes | 1 pre-filled disposable injection PoM £1,050.40 (Hospital only)

Eptacog alfa activated 250000 unit NovoSeven 5mg (250,000units) powder and solvent for solution for injection pre-filled syringes | 1 pre-filled disposable injection PoM £2,626.00 (Hospital only)

NovoSeven 5mg (250,000units) powder and solvent for solution for injection vials | 1 vial PoM £2,626.00 (Hospital only)

Eptacog alfa activated 400000 unit NovoSeven 8mg (400,000units) powder and solvent for solution for injection vials | 1 vial PoM £4,201.60 (Hospital only)

NovoSeven 8mg (400,000units) powder and solvent for solution for injection pre-filled syringes | 1 pre-filled disposable injection PoM £4,201.60 (Hospital only)

Factor VIII fraction, dried 05-Feb-2020

(Human coagulation factor VIII, dried)

● **INDICATIONS AND DOSE**

Treatment and prophylaxis of haemorrhage in congenital factor VIII deficiency (haemophilia A), acquired factor VIII deficiency | Von Willebrand's disease

▶ BY INTRAVENOUS INJECTION, OR BY INTRAVENOUS INFUSION, OR BY CONTINUOUS INTRAVENOUS INFUSION

▶ Child: (consult haematologist)

● **CAUTIONS** Risk of intravascular haemolysis after large or frequently repeated doses in patients with blood groups A, B, or AB (in products containing isoagglutinins) · vaccination against hepatitis A and hepatitis B may be required (consult product literature)

● **SIDE-EFFECTS**

▶ **Uncommon** Angioedema · cardiac discomfort · chills · flushing · headache · hypersensitivity · hypotension · lethargy · nausea · paraesthesia · restlessness · skin reactions · tachycardia · vomiting · wheezing

▶ **Rare or very rare** Fever

● **MONITORING REQUIREMENTS** Monitor for development of factor VIII inhibitors.

● **PRESCRIBING AND DISPENSING INFORMATION** Dried factor VIII fraction is prepared from human plasma by a suitable fractionation technique; it may also contain varying amounts of von Willebrand factor. *Optivate*®, *Fanhdi*®, and *Octanate*® are not indicated for use in von Willebrand's disease.

Recombinant human coagulation factor VIII including octocog alfa, moroctocog alfa, and simoctocog alfa are not indicated for use in von Willebrand's disease.

● **MEDICINAL FORMS** There can be variation in the licensing of different medicines containing the same drug.

Powder and solvent for solution for injection

▶ Factor viii fraction, dried (non-proprietary) ▼

Factor VIII 500 unit Dried Factor VIII Fraction type 8Y 500unit powder and solvent for solution for injection vials | 1 vial [PoM] £210.00

▶ Advate (Baxalta UK Ltd)

Octocog alfa 250 unit Advate 250unit powder and solvent for solution for injection vials | 1 vial [PoM] £177.50

Octocog alfa 500 unit Advate 500unit powder and solvent for solution for injection vials | 1 vial [PoM] £355.00

Octocog alfa 1000 unit Advate 1,000unit powder and solvent for solution for injection vials | 1 vial [PoM] £710.00

Octocog alfa 2000 unit Advate 2,000unit powder and solvent for solution for injection vials | 1 vial [PoM] £1,420.00

▶ Alphanate (Grifols UK Ltd)

Factor VIII high purity 1000 unit, von Willebrand factor 1200 unit Alphanate 1,000unit powder and solvent for solution for injection vials | 1 vial [PoM] £330.00

Factor VIII high purity 1500 unit, von Willebrand factor 1800 unit Alphanate 1,500unit powder and solvent for solution for injection vials | 1 vial [PoM] £495.00

Factor VIII high purity 2000 unit, von Willebrand factor 2400 unit Alphanate 2,000unit powder and solvent for solution for injection vials | 1 vial [PoM] £780.00

▶ Elocta (Swedish Orphan Biovitrum Ltd) ▼

Efmoroctocog alfa 250 unit Elocta 250unit powder and solvent for solution for injection vials | 1 vial [PoM] [H] (Hospital only)

Efmoroctocog alfa 500 unit Elocta 500unit powder and solvent for solution for injection vials | 1 vial [PoM] [H] (Hospital only)

Efmoroctocog alfa 750 unit Elocta 750unit powder and solvent for solution for injection vials | 1 vial [PoM] [H] (Hospital only)

Efmoroctocog alfa 1000 unit Elocta 1,000unit powder and solvent for solution for injection vials | 1 vial [PoM] [H] (Hospital only)

Efmoroctocog alfa 1500 unit Elocta 1,500unit powder and solvent for solution for injection vials | 1 vial [PoM] [H] (Hospital only)

Efmoroctocog alfa 2000 unit Elocta 2,000unit powder and solvent for solution for injection vials | 1 vial [PoM] [H] (Hospital only)

Efmoroctocog alfa 3000 unit Elocta 3,000unit powder and solvent for solution for injection vials | 1 vial [PoM] [H] (Hospital only)

Efmoroctocog alfa 4000 unit Elocta 4,000unit powder and solvent for solution for injection vials | 1 vial [PoM] [H] (Hospital only)

▶ Fanhdi (Grifols UK Ltd)

Factor VIII high purity 500 unit Fanhdi 500unit powder and solvent for solution for injection vials | 1 vial [PoM] £165.00 (Hospital only)

Factor VIII high purity 1000 unit Fanhdi 1,000unit powder and solvent for solution for injection vials | 1 vial [PoM] £330.00 (Hospital only)

Factor VIII high purity 1500 unit Fanhdi 1,500unit powder and solvent for solution for injection vials | 1 vial [PoM] £495.00

▶ Haemoctin (Biotest (UK) Ltd)

Factor VIII high purity 250 unit Haemoctin 250unit powder and solvent for solution for injection vials | 1 vial [PoM] £150.00 (Hospital only)

Factor VIII high purity 500 unit Haemoctin 500unit powder and solvent for solution for injection vials | 1 vial [PoM] £300.00 (Hospital only)

Factor VIII high purity 1000 unit Haemoctin 1,000unit powder and solvent for solution for injection vials | 1 vial [PoM] £600.00 (Hospital only)

▶ Kogenate Bayer (Bayer Plc)

Octocog alfa 1000 unit Kogenate Bayer 1,000unit powder and solvent for solution for injection vials | 1 vial [PoM] £630.00

▶ Nuwiq (Octapharma Ltd)

Simoctocog alfa 250 unit Nuwiq 250unit powder and solvent for solution for injection vials | 1 vial [PoM] £190.00

Simoctocog alfa 500 unit Nuwiq 500unit powder and solvent for solution for injection vials | 1 vial [PoM] £380.00

Simoctocog alfa 1000 unit Nuwiq 1,000unit powder and solvent for solution for injection vials | 1 vial [PoM] £760.00

Simoctocog alfa 2000 unit Nuwiq 2,000unit powder and solvent for solution for injection vials | 1 vial [PoM] £1,520.00

▶ Octanate LV (Octapharma Ltd)

Factor VIII high purity 500 unit Octanate LV 500unit powder and solvent for solution for injection vials | 1 vial [PoM] £300.00 (Hospital only)

Factor VIII high purity 1000 unit Octanate LV 1,000unit powder and solvent for solution for injection vials | 1 vial [PoM] £600.00 (Hospital only)

▶ ReFacto (Pfizer Ltd)

Moroctocog alfa 250 unit ReFacto AF 250unit powder and solvent for solution for injection vials | 1 vial [PoM] £125.55 (Hospital only)

ReFacto AF 500unit powder and solvent for solution for injection pre-filled syringes | 1 pre-filled disposable injection [PoM] £251.10 (Hospital only)

ReFacto AF 250unit powder and solvent for solution for injection pre-filled syringes | 1 pre-filled disposable injection [PoM] £125.55 (Hospital only)

Moroctocog alfa 500 unit ReFacto AF 500unit powder and solvent for solution for injection vials | 1 vial [PoM] £251.10 (Hospital only)

Moroctocog alfa 1000 unit ReFacto AF 1,000unit powder and solvent for solution for injection vials | 1 vial [PoM] £502.20 (Hospital only)

ReFacto AF 1,000unit powder and solvent for solution for injection pre-filled syringes | 1 pre-filled disposable injection [PoM] £502.20 (Hospital only)

Moroctocog alfa 2000 unit ReFacto AF 2,000unit powder and solvent for solution for injection pre-filled syringes | 1 pre-filled disposable injection [PoM] £1,004.40 (Hospital only)

ReFacto AF 2,000unit powder and solvent for solution for injection vials | 1 vial [PoM] £1,004.40 (Hospital only)

Moroctocog alfa 3000 unit ReFacto AF 3,000unit powder and solvent for solution for injection pre-filled syringes | 1 pre-filled disposable injection [PoM] £1,506.60 (Hospital only)

▶ Voncento (CSL Behring UK Ltd)

Factor VIII 500 unit, von Willebrand factor 1200 unit Voncento 500unit/1,200unit powder and solvent for solution for injection vials | 1 vial [PoM] £385.00

Factor VIII 1000 unit, von Willebrand factor 2400 unit Voncento 1,000unit/2,400unit powder and solvent for solution for injection vials | 1 vial [PoM] £770.00

Powder and solvent for solution for infusion

▶ Advate (Baxalta UK Ltd)

Octocog alfa 1500 unit Advate 1,500unit powder and solvent for solution for infusion vials | 1 vial [PoM] £1,065.00

Octocog alfa 3000 unit Advate 3,000unit powder and solvent for solution for infusion vials | 1 vial [PoM] £2,130.00

▶ Optivate (Bio Products Laboratory Ltd)

Factor VIII 250 unit, von Willebrand factor 430 unit Optivate 250unit powder and solvent for solution for infusion vials | 1 vial [PoM] £90.00

- Wilate 1000 (Octapharma Ltd)
  Factor VIII 1000 iu, von Willebrand factor 1000 iu Wilate 1000 powder and solvent for solution for infusion vials | 1 vial PoM £500.00
- Wilate 500 (Octapharma Ltd)
  Factor VIII 500 iu, von Willebrand factor 500 iu Wilate 500 powder and solvent for solution for infusion vials | 1 vial PoM £250.00

Factor IX fraction, dried

30-Jan-2020

● **INDICATIONS AND DOSE**

Treatment and prophylaxis of haemorrhage in congenital factor IX deficiency (haemophilia B)

- BY INTRAVENOUS INJECTION, OR BY CONTINUOUS INTRAVENOUS INFUSION
- Child: (consult haematologist)

● **CONTRA-INDICATIONS** Disseminated intravascular coagulation

● **CAUTIONS** Risk of thrombosis—principally with low purity products · vaccination against hepatitis A and hepatitis B may be required (consult product literature)

● **SIDE-EFFECTS**

- **Common or very common** Anxiety · back pain · dyspnoea · hypersensitivity · nausea · sensation abnormal · skin reactions · vasodilation
- **Rare or very rare** Angioedema · cardiac discomfort · chills · disseminated intravascular coagulation · embolism and thrombosis · headache · hypotension · lethargy · myocardial infarction · tachycardia · vomiting · wheezing
- **Frequency not known** Nephrotic syndrome

● **PRESCRIBING AND DISPENSING INFORMATION** Dried factor IX fraction is prepared from human plasma by a suitable fractionation technique; it may also contain clotting factors II, VII, and X.

● **MEDICINAL FORMS** There can be variation in the licensing of different medicines containing the same drug.

Powder and solvent for solution for injection

- AlphaNine (Grifols UK Ltd)
  Factor IX high purity 1000 unit AlphaNine 1,000unit powder and solvent for solution for injection vials | 1 vial PoM £390.00
  Factor IX high purity 1500 unit AlphaNine 1,500unit powder and solvent for solution for injection vials | 1 vial PoM ☒
- Haemonine (Biotest (UK) Ltd)
  Factor IX high purity 500 unit Haemonine 500unit powder and solvent for solution for injection vials | 1 vial PoM £300.00 (Hospital only)
  Factor IX high purity 1000 unit Haemonine 1,000unit powder and solvent for solution for injection vials | 1 vial PoM £600.00 (Hospital only)
- Replenine-VF (Bio Products Laboratory Ltd)
  Factor IX high purity 500 unit Replenine-VF 500unit powder and solvent for solution for injection vials | 1 vial PoM £180.00
  Factor IX high purity 1000 unit Replenine-VF 1,000unit powder and solvent for solution for injection vials | 1 vial PoM £360.00

Powder and solvent for solution for infusion

- BeneFIX (Pfizer Ltd)
  Nonacog alfa 250 unit BeneFIX 250unit powder and solvent for solution for infusion vials | 1 vial PoM £151.80 (Hospital only)
  Nonacog alfa 500 unit BeneFIX 500unit powder and solvent for solution for infusion vials | 1 vial PoM £303.60 (Hospital only)
  Nonacog alfa 1000 unit BeneFIX 1,000unit powder and solvent for solution for infusion vials | 1 vial PoM £607.20 (Hospital only)
  Nonacog alfa 2000 unit BeneFIX 2,000unit powder and solvent for solution for infusion vials | 1 vial PoM £1,214.40 (Hospital only)
  Nonacog alfa 3000 unit BeneFIX 3,000unit powder and solvent for solution for infusion vials | 1 vial PoM £1,821.60 (Hospital only)

Factor XIII fraction, dried

30-Jan-2020

(Human fibrin-stabilising factor, dried)

● **INDICATIONS AND DOSE**

Congenital factor XIII deficiency

- BY INTRAVENOUS INJECTION, OR BY INTRAVENOUS INFUSION
- Child: (consult haematologist)

● **CAUTIONS** Vaccination against hepatitis A and hepatitis B may be required

● **SIDE-EFFECTS**

- **Rare or very rare** Anaphylactoid reaction · dyspnoea · skin reactions

● **MEDICINAL FORMS** There can be variation in the licensing of different medicines containing the same drug.

Powder and solvent for solution for injection

- Fibrogammin P (CSL Behring UK Ltd)
  Factor XIII 250 unit Fibrogammin 250unit powder and solvent for solution for injection vials | 1 vial PoM £106.58
  Factor XIII 1250 unit Fibrogammin 1,250unit powder and solvent for solution for injection vials | 1 vial PoM £532.90

Fibrinogen, dried

30-Jan-2020

(Human fibrinogen)

● **INDICATIONS AND DOSE**

Treatment of haemorrhage in congenital hypofibrinogenaemia or afibrinogenaemia

- BY INTRAVENOUS INJECTION, OR BY INTRAVENOUS INFUSION
- Child: (consult haematologist)

● **CAUTIONS** Risk of thrombosis · vaccination against hepatitis A and hepatitis B may be required

● **SIDE-EFFECTS**

- **Common or very common** Fever · thromboembolism
- **Frequency not known** Chest pain · chills · cough · dyspnoea · nausea · skin reactions · tachycardia · vomiting

● **PREGNANCY** Manufacturer advises not known to be harmful—no information available.

● **BREAST FEEDING** Manufacturer advises avoid—no information available.

● **PRESCRIBING AND DISPENSING INFORMATION** Fibrinogen is prepared from human plasma.

● **MEDICINAL FORMS** There can be variation in the licensing of different medicines containing the same drug.

Powder for solution for infusion

- Riastap (CSL Behring UK Ltd)
  Fibrinogen 1 gram Riastap 1g powder for solution for infusion vials | 1 vial PoM £400.00

Protein C concentrate

30-Jan-2020

● **INDICATIONS AND DOSE**

Congenital protein C deficiency

- BY INTRAVENOUS INJECTION
- Child: (consult haematologist)

● **CAUTIONS** Hypersensitivity to heparins · vaccination against hepatitis A and hepatitis B may be required

● **SIDE-EFFECTS**

- **Rare or very rare** Dizziness · fever · skin reactions
- **Frequency not known** Haemothorax · hyperhidrosis · restlessness

● **PRESCRIBING AND DISPENSING INFORMATION** Protein C is prepared from human plasma.

- **MEDICINAL FORMS** There can be variation in the licensing of different medicines containing the same drug.

Powder and solvent for solution for injection

- Ceprotin (Baxalta UK Ltd)
  Protein C 500 unit Ceprotin 500unit powder and solvent for solution for injection vials | 1 vial PoM £2,000.00
  Protein C 1000 unit Ceprotin 1000unit powder and solvent for solution for injection vials | 1 vial PoM £1,000.00

BLOOD AND RELATED PRODUCTS › HAEMOSTATIC PRODUCTS

Factor VIII inhibitor bypassing fraction

30-Jan-2020

- **INDICATIONS AND DOSE**

Treatment and prophylaxis of haemorrhage in patients with congenital factor VIII deficiency (haemophilia A) and factor VIII inhibitors | Treatment of haemorrhage in non-haemophiliac patients with acquired factor VIII inhibitors

- BY INTRAVENOUS INFUSION, OR BY INTRAVENOUS INJECTION
- Child: (consult haematologist)

- **CONTRA-INDICATIONS** Disseminated intravascular coagulation
- **CAUTIONS** Risk of thrombosis · vaccination against hepatitis A and hepatitis B may be required
- **SIDE-EFFECTS**
- **Common or very common** Dizziness · headache · hypersensitivity · hypotension · skin reactions
- **Frequency not known** Abdominal discomfort · anamnestic reaction · angioedema · chest discomfort · chills · cough · diarrhoea · disseminated intravascular coagulation · drowsiness · dyspnoea · embolism and thrombosis · fever · flushing · hypertension · ischaemic stroke · malaise · myocardial infarction · nausea · paraesthesia · respiratory disorders · restlessness · tachycardia · taste altered · vomiting
- **PRESCRIBING AND DISPENSING INFORMATION** Preparations with factor VIII inhibitor bypassing activity are prepared from human plasma.

- **MEDICINAL FORMS** There can be variation in the licensing of different medicines containing the same drug.

Powder and solvent for solution for injection

- FEIBA Imuno (Baxalta UK Ltd)
  Factor VIII inhibitor bypassing fraction 500 unit FEIBA 500unit powder and solvent for solution for injection vials | 1 vial PoM £390.00

Powder and solvent for solution for infusion

- FEIBA Imuno (Baxalta UK Ltd)
  Factor VIII inhibitor bypassing fraction 1000 unit FEIBA 1,000unit powder and solvent for solution for infusion vials | 1 vial PoM £780.00

BLOOD AND RELATED PRODUCTS › PLASMA PRODUCTS

Fresh frozen plasma

30-Jan-2020

- **INDICATIONS AND DOSE**

Replacement of coagulation factors or other plasma proteins where their concentration or functional activity is critically reduced

- BY INTRAVENOUS INFUSION
- Child: (consult haematologist)

- **CONTRA-INDICATIONS** Avoid use as a volume expander · IgA deficiency with confirmed antibodies to IgA
- **CAUTIONS** Cardiac decompensation · pulmonary oedema · risk of thrombosis · severe protein S deficiency (avoid products with low protein S activity e.g. *OctaplasLG®*) · vaccination against hepatitis A and hepatitis B may be required
- **SIDE-EFFECTS**
- **Common or very common** Skin reactions
- **Uncommon** Fever · hypersensitivity · hypoxia · nausea · sensation abnormal · vomiting
- **Rare or very rare** Abdominal pain · anxiety · arrhythmias · back pain · cardiac arrest · chest discomfort · chills · circulatory collapse · citrate toxicity · dizziness · dyspnoea · flushing · haemolytic anaemia · haemorrhage · hyperhidrosis · hypertension · hypotension · localised oedema · malaise · procedural complications · pulmonary oedema · respiratory disorders · thromboembolism
- **PRESCRIBING AND DISPENSING INFORMATION** Fresh frozen plasma is prepared from the supernatant liquid obtained by centrifugation of one donation of whole blood.

A preparation of solvent/detergent treated human plasma (frozen) from pooled donors is available from Octapharma (*OctaplasLG®*).

Children under 16 years should only receive virucidally inactivated preparations of fresh frozen plasma, sourced from 'low prevalence BSE regions' such as the USA.

- **MEDICINAL FORMS** There can be variation in the licensing of different medicines containing the same drug.

Infusion

- OctaplasLG (Octapharma Ltd)
  Human plasma proteins 57.5 mg per 1 ml OctaplasLG Blood Group A infusion 200ml bags | 1 bag PoM £75.00
  OctaplasLG Blood Group B infusion 200ml bags | 1 bag PoM £75.00
  OctaplasLG Blood Group AB infusion 200ml bags | 1 bag PoM £75.00
  OctaplasLG Blood Group O infusion 200ml bags | 1 bag PoM £75.00

2.2 Subarachnoid haemorrhage

CALCIUM-CHANNEL BLOCKERS

Nimodipine

F 114

14-Feb-2020

- **DRUG ACTION** Nimodipine is a dihydropyridine calcium-channel blocker.

- **INDICATIONS AND DOSE**

Treatment of vasospasm following subarachnoid haemorrhage (specialist use only)

- BY INTRAVENOUS INFUSION
- Child 1 month–11 years: Initially 15 micrograms/kg/hour (max. per dose 500 micrograms/hour), increased after 2 hours if no severe decrease in blood pressure; increased to 30 micrograms/kg/hour (max. per dose 2 mg/hour), continue for at least 5 days (max. 14 days), use initial dose of 7.5 micrograms/kg/hour if blood pressure unstable
- Child 12–17 years (body-weight up to 70 kg): Initially 0.5 mg/hour, increased after 2 hours if no severe decrease in blood pressure; increased to 1–2 mg/hour, continue for at least 5 days (max. 14 days)
- Child 12–17 years (body-weight 70 kg and above): Initially up to 1 mg/hour, use dose if blood pressure stable; increased after 2 hours if no severe decrease in blood pressure; increased to 1–2 mg/hour, continue for at least 5 days (max. 14 days)

Prevention of vasospasm following subarachnoid haemorrhage

- BY MOUTH
- Child: 0.9–1.2 mg/kg 6 times a day (max. per dose 60 mg), started within 4 days of haemorrhage and continued for 21 days

● **UNLICENSED USE** Not licensed for use in children.

> **IMPORTANT SAFETY INFORMATION**
> SAFE PRACTICE
> Nimodipine has been confused with amlodipine; care must be taken to ensure the correct drug is prescribed and dispensed.

● **CAUTIONS** Cerebral oedema · hypotension · severely raised intracranial pressure

● **INTERACTIONS** → Appendix 1: calcium channel blockers

● **SIDE-EFFECTS**
▸ **Uncommon** Thrombocytopenia · vasodilation
▸ **Rare or very rare** Bradycardia · ileus

● **PREGNANCY** Manufacturer advises use only if potential benefit outweighs risk.

● **BREAST FEEDING** Manufacturer advises avoid—present in milk.

● **HEPATIC IMPAIRMENT**
▸ With oral use Manufacturer advises consider avoiding in severe impairment.
Dose adjustments ▸ With oral use In adults, manufacturer advises dose reduction—consult product literature.

● **RENAL IMPAIRMENT**
Monitoring ▸ With intravenous use Manufacturer advises monitor renal function closely in renal impairment.

● **DIRECTIONS FOR ADMINISTRATION** Avoid concomitant administration of nimodipine infusion and tablets.
▸ With oral use For administration *by mouth*, tablets may be crushed or halved but are light sensitive—administer immediately.
▸ With intravenous use For *continuous intravenous infusion*, administer undiluted via a Y-piece on a central venous catheter connected to a running infusion of Glucose 5%, or Sodium Chloride 0.9%; not to be added to an infusion container; incompatible with polyvinyl chloride giving sets or containers; protect infusion from light. Polyethylene, polypropylene, or glass apparatus should be used.

● **MEDICINAL FORMS** There can be variation in the licensing of different medicines containing the same drug. Forms available from special-order manufacturers include: oral suspension

Solution for infusion
▸ Nimotop (Bayer Plc)
Nimodipine 200 microgram per 1 ml Nimotop 0.02% solution for infusion 50ml vials | 1 vial PoM £13.60 (Hospital only)

Tablet
▸ Nimotop (Bayer Plc)
Nimodipine 30 mg Nimotop 30mg tablets | 100 tablet PoM £40.00 DT = £40.00

3 Blood clots

3.1 Blocked catheters and lines

ANTITHROMBOTIC DRUGS > TISSUE PLASMINOGEN ACTIVATORS

Fibrinolytic drugs

Overview

Alteplase below, streptokinase p. 94 and urokinase p. 94 are used in children to dissolve intravascular thrombi and unblock occluded arteriovenous shunts, catheters, and indwelling central lines blocked with fibrin clots. Treatment should be started as soon as possible after a clot has formed and discontinued once a pulse in the affected limb is detected, or the shunt or catheter unblocked.

The safety and efficacy of treatment remains uncertain, especially in neonates. A fibrinolytic drug is probably only appropriate where arterial occlusion threatens ischaemic damage; an anticoagulant may stop the clot getting bigger. Alteplase is the preferred fibrinolytic in children and neonates; there is less risk of adverse effects including allergic reactions.

Fibrinolytics 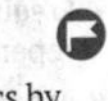

● **DRUG ACTION** Fibrinolytic drugs act as thrombolytics by activating plasminogen to form plasmin, which degrades fibrin and so breaks up thrombi.

● **CONTRA-INDICATIONS** Acute pancreatitis · aneurysm · aortic dissection · arteriovenous malformation · bacterial endocarditis · bleeding diatheses · coagulation defects · coma · history of cerebrovascular disease (especially recent events or with any residual disability) · neoplasm with risk of haemorrhage · oesophageal varices · pericarditis · recent gastro-intestinal ulceration · recent haemorrhage · recent surgery (including dental extraction) · recent trauma · severe hypertension

● **CAUTIONS** Conditions with an increased risk of haemorrhage · hypertension · risk of bleeding (including that from venepuncture or invasive procedures)

● **SIDE-EFFECTS**
▸ **Common or very common** Anaphylactic reaction · angina pectoris · cardiac arrest · cardiogenic shock · chills · CNS haemorrhage · ecchymosis · fever · haemorrhage · haemorrhagic stroke · heart failure · hypotension · ischaemia recurrent (when used in myocardial infarction) · nausea · pericarditis · pulmonary oedema · vomiting
▸ **Uncommon** Aphasia · mitral valve incompetence · myocardial rupture · pericardial disorders · reperfusion arrhythmia (when used in myocardial infarction) · seizure
SIDE-EFFECTS, FURTHER INFORMATION Serious bleeding calls for discontinuation of the thrombolytic and may require administration of coagulation factors and antifibrinolytic drugs.

● **PREGNANCY** Thrombolytic drugs can possibly lead to premature separation of the placenta in the first 18 weeks of pregnancy. There is also a risk of maternal haemorrhage throughout pregnancy and post-partum, and also a theoretical risk of fetal haemorrhage throughout pregnancy.

● **HEPATIC IMPAIRMENT** Manufacturers advise avoid in severe impairment.

above

Alteplase
15-Nov-2019

(rt-PA; Tissue-type plasminogen activator)

● **INDICATIONS AND DOSE**

Intravascular thrombosis
▸ BY INTRAVENOUS INFUSION
▸ Neonate: 100–500 micrograms/kg/hour for 3–6 hours, use ultrasound assessment to monitor effect before considering a second course of treatment (consult local protocol).
▸ Child: 100–500 micrograms/kg/hour for 3–6 hours, use ultrasound assessment to monitor effect before considering a second course of treatment; maximum 100 mg per day

ACTILYSE CATHFLO ®

Thrombolytic treatment of occluded central venous access devices (including those used for haemodialysis)
▸ BY INTRAVENOUS INJECTION
▸ Child: (consult product literature)

- **UNLICENSED USE** *Actilyse®* not licensed for use in children.
- **CONTRA-INDICATIONS** Recent delivery
- **INTERACTIONS** → Appendix 1: alteplase
- **SIDE-EFFECTS**
- ▶ **Uncommon** Haemothorax
- ▶ **Rare or very rare** Agitation · confusion · delirium · depression · epilepsy · psychosis · speech disorder
- ▶ **Frequency not known** Brain oedema (caused by reperfusion)
- **ALLERGY AND CROSS-SENSITIVITY** Contra-indicated if history of hypersensitivity to gentamicin (residue from manufacturing process).
- **DIRECTIONS FOR ADMINISTRATION** For *intravenous infusion* (*Actilyse®*), dissolve in Water for Injections to a concentration of 1 mg/mL or 2 mg/mL and infuse intravenously; alternatively dilute further in Sodium Chloride 0.9% to a concentration of not less than 200 micrograms/mL; not to be diluted in Glucose.

- **MEDICINAL FORMS** There can be variation in the licensing of different medicines containing the same drug. Forms available from special-order manufacturers include: solution for injection

Powder and solvent for solution for injection

▸ Actilyse (Boehringer Ingelheim Ltd)

Alteplase 10 mg Actilyse 10mg powder and solvent for solution for injection vials | 1 vial PoM £172.80

Alteplase 20 mg Actilyse 20mg powder and solvent for solution for injection vials | 1 vial PoM £259.20

Powder and solvent for solution for infusion

▸ Actilyse (Boehringer Ingelheim Ltd)

Alteplase 50 mg Actilyse 50mg powder and solvent for solution for infusion vials | 1 vial PoM £432.00

F 93

Streptokinase

23-Jan-2020

- **INDICATIONS AND DOSE**

Intravascular thrombosis

▶ INITIALLY BY INTRAVENOUS INFUSION

- ▸ Child 1 month–11 years: Initially 2500–4000 units/kg, dose to be given over 30 minutes, followed by (by continuous intravenous infusion) 500–1000 units/kg/hour for up to 3 days until reperfusion occurs
- ▸ Child 12-17 years: Initially 250 000 units, dose to be given over 30 minutes, followed by (by continuous intravenous infusion) 100 000 units/hour for up to 3 days until reperfusion occurs

- **UNLICENSED USE** Not licensed for use in children.
- **CAUTIONS** Atrial fibrillation · cavernous pulmonary disease · cerebrovascular disease · mitral valve defect · recent delivery or abortion · recent streptococcal infections · septic thrombotic disease
- **INTERACTIONS** → Appendix 1: streptokinase
- **SIDE-EFFECTS**
- ▶ **Common or very common** Arrhythmias · asthenia · diarrhoea · epigastric pain · headache · malaise · pain
- ▶ **Uncommon** Respiratory arrest · splenic rupture
- ▶ **Rare or very rare** Arthritis · eye inflammation · hypersensitivity · nephritis · nerve disorders · neurological effects · pulmonary oedema non-cardiogenic (caused by reperfusion) · shock · vasculitis
- **ALLERGY AND CROSS-SENSITIVITY** Contra-indicated if previous allergic reaction to either streptokinase or anistreplase (no longer available). Prolonged persistence of antibodies to streptokinase and anistreplase (no longer available) can reduce the effectiveness of subsequent treatment; therefore, streptokinase should not be used again beyond 4 days of first administration of either streptokinase or anistreplase.
- **DIRECTIONS FOR ADMINISTRATION** For *intravenous infusion*, reconstitute with Sodium Chloride 0.9%, then dilute further with Glucose 5% or Sodium Chloride 0.9% after reconstitution. Monitor fibrinogen concentration closely; if fibrinogen concentration less than 1 g/litre, stop streptokinase infusion and start unfractionated heparin; restart streptokinase once fibrinogen concentration reaches 1 g/litre.

- **MEDICINAL FORMS** There can be variation in the licensing of different medicines containing the same drug.

Powder for solution for infusion

▸ Streptokinase (Non-proprietary)

Streptokinase 1.5 mega unit Streptokinase 1.5million unit powder for solution for infusion vials | 1 vial PoM £195.00

Streptokinase 250000 unit Streptokinase 250,000unit powder for solution for infusion vials | 1 vial PoM £97.50

Streptokinase 750000 unit Streptokinase 750,000unit powder for solution for infusion vials | 1 vial PoM £49.35

F 93

Urokinase

15-Nov-2019

- **INDICATIONS AND DOSE**

Occluded arteriovenous shunts, catheters, and indwelling central lines

▶ TO THE DEVICE AS A FLUSH

- ▸ Neonate: 5000–25 000 units, inject directly into occluded catheter or central line, dilute dose in sodium chloride 0.9% to fill catheter dead space **only**. Leave for 20–60 minutes then aspirate the lysate and flush with sodium chloride 0.9%.
- ▸ Child: 5000–25 000 units, inject directly into occluded catheter or central line, dilute dose in sodium chloride 0.9% to fill catheter dead space **only**. Leave for 20–60 minutes then aspirate the lysate and flush with sodium chloride 0.9%

- **CAUTIONS** Atrial fibrillation · cavernous pulmonary disease · mitral valve defect · recent delivery · septic thrombotic disease · severe cerebrovascular disease
- **INTERACTIONS** → Appendix 1: urokinase
- **SIDE-EFFECTS**
- ▶ **Common or very common** Artery dissection · embolism and thrombosis · stroke
- ▶ **Uncommon** Renal failure
- ▶ **Rare or very rare** Vascular pseudoaneurysm
- **BREAST FEEDING** Manufacturer advises avoid—no information available.
- **DIRECTIONS FOR ADMINISTRATION** May be diluted, after reconstitution, with Sodium Chloride 0.9%.

- **MEDICINAL FORMS** There can be variation in the licensing of different medicines containing the same drug.

Powder for solution for injection

▸ Syner-KINASE (Syner-Med (Pharmaceutical Products) Ltd)

Urokinase 10000 unit Syner-KINASE 10,000unit powder for solution for injection vials | 1 vial PoM £35.95 (Hospital only)

Urokinase 25000 unit Syner-KINASE 25,000unit powder for solution for injection vials | 1 vial PoM £45.95 (Hospital only)

Urokinase 100000 unit Syner-KINASE 100,000unit powder for solution for injection vials | 1 vial PoM £112.95 (Hospital only)

Urokinase 250000 unit Syner-KINASE 250,000unit powder for solution for injection vials | 1 vial PoM ⊠ (Hospital only)

Urokinase 500000 unit Syner-KINASE 500,000unit powder for solution for injection vials | 1 vial PoM ⊠ (Hospital only)

3.2 Thromboembolism

Venous thromboembolism 26-Jul-2018

Venous thromboembolism prophylaxis

Low-dose heparin (unfractionated) p. 101 by subcutaneous injection is used to prevent thrombotic episodes in 'high-risk' patients; laboratory monitoring of APTT or anti-Factor Xa concentration is also required in prophylactic regimens in children. Low molecular weight heparins, aspirin (antiplatelet dose) p. 98, and warfarin sodium p. 103 can also be used for prophylaxis.

The following guidance on reducing the risk of venous thromboembolism applies to children over 16 years and is based on NICE guideline 89 (www.nice.org.uk/guidance/ng89).

EvGr All children over 16 years old should undergo a risk assessment to identify their risk of venous thromboembolism and bleeding on admission to hospital. (A) Commonly used risk assessment tools can be found at www.nice.org.uk/guidance/ng89/resources. Children over 16 years old considered to be at high risk of venous thromboembolism include those who are anticipated to have a substantial reduction in mobility, those with obesity, malignant disease, history of venous thromboembolism and thrombophilic disorder. Pregnancy and the postpartum period are also risk factors for venous thromboembolism.

There are two methods of thromboprophylaxis: mechanical and pharmacological. Options for mechanical prophylaxis are anti-embolism stockings that provide graduated compression and produce a calf pressure of 14–15 mmHg, and intermittent pneumatic compression. EvGr Anti-embolism stockings should be worn day and night until the child is sufficiently mobile; they should not be offered to children over 16 years old admitted with conditions such as severe leg oedema, or local conditions (e.g. gangrene, dermatitis).

When using pharmacological prophylaxis, in most cases, it should start as soon as possible or within 14 hours of admission. Children over 16 years of age with risk factors for bleeding (e.g. thrombocytopenia, acquired or untreated inherited bleeding disorders) should *only* receive pharmacological prophylaxis when their risk of venous thromboembolism outweighs their risk of bleeding. Children over 16 years of age receiving anticoagulant therapy who are at high risk of venous thromboembolism should be considered for prophylaxis if their anticoagulant therapy is interrupted, for example during the peri-operative period. (A)

Surgical patients

EvGr To reduce the risk of venous thromboembolism in surgical patients over 16 years old, regional anaesthesia over general anaesthesia should be used if possible.

Mechanical prophylaxis (e.g. anti-embolism stockings or intermittent pneumatic compression) should be offered to children over 16 years old with major trauma, or undergoing cranial, abdominal, bariatric, thoracic, maxillofacial, ear, nose, and throat, cardiac or elective spinal surgery. Prophylaxis should continue until the child is sufficiently mobile or discharged from hospital (or for 30 days in spinal injury, elective spinal surgery or cranial surgery). (A) Choice of mechanical prophylaxis depends on factors such as the type of surgery, suitability for the child, and their condition.

EvGr Pharmacological prophylaxis should be considered in children over 16 years old undergoing general or orthopaedic surgery when the risk of venous thromboembolism outweighs the risk of bleeding. (A) The choice of prophylaxis will depend on the type of surgery, suitability for the patient, and local policy. EvGr A low molecular weight heparin is suitable in all types of general and orthopaedic surgery; heparin (unfractionated) is preferred in patients with renal impairment. Fondaparinux sodium [unlicensed] is an option for children over 16 years old undergoing abdominal, bariatric, thoracic or cardiac surgery, or for patients with lower limb immobilisation or fragility fractures of the pelvis, hip or proximal femur.

Pharmacological prophylaxis in general surgery should usually continue for at least 7 days post-surgery, or until sufficient mobility has been re-established. Pharmacological prophylaxis should be extended to 28 days after major cancer surgery in the abdomen, and to 30 days in spinal surgery.

Mechanical prophylaxis with intermittent pneumatic compression should be considered when pharmacological prophylaxis is contra-indicated in children over 16 years old undergoing lower limb amputation, or those with major trauma or fragility fractures of the pelvis, hip or proximal femur. (A)

Medical patients

The choice of prophylaxis will depend on the medical condition, suitability for the patient, and local policy. EvGr Acutely ill medical patients over 16 years old who are at high risk of venous thromboembolism should be offered pharmacological prophylaxis. Children over 16 years old should be given either a low molecular weight heparin as a first-line option, or fondaparinux sodium [unlicensed] as an alternative, for a minimum of 7 days. Children over 16 years old with renal impairment should be given either a low molecular weight heparin or heparin (unfractionated) and the dose should be adjusted as necessary.

Mechanical prophylaxis can be considered when pharmacological prophylaxis is contra-indicated; their use should be continued until the child is sufficiently mobile. (A)

Thromboprophylaxis in pregnancy

EvGr All pregnant young women over 16 years old (who are not in active labour), or young women over 16 years old who have given birth, had a miscarriage or termination of pregnancy during the past 6 weeks, with a risk of venous thromboembolism that outweighs the risk of bleeding should be considered for pharmacological prophylaxis with a low molecular weight heparin during hospital admission. In pregnant young women over 16 years old, prophylaxis should be continued until there is no longer a risk of venous thromboembolism, or until discharge from hospital. Young women over 16 years old who have given birth, had a miscarriage or termination of pregnancy during the past 6 weeks, should start thromboprophylaxis with a low molecular weight heparin 4–8 hours after the event, unless contra-indicated, and continue for a minimum of 7 days.

Additional mechanical prophylaxis should be considered for young women over 16 years old who are likely to be immobilised or have significantly reduced mobility and continued until the young woman is sufficiently mobile or discharged from hospital. Intermittent pneumatic compression should be used as the first-line option and anti-embolism stockings as an alternative. (A)

Treatment of venous thromboembolism

For the initial treatment of thrombotic episodes heparin (unfractionated) is given as an intravenous loading dose, followed by continuous intravenous infusion (using an infusion pump) or by intermittent subcutaneous injection; the use of intermittent intravenous injection is no longer recommended. Alternatively, a low molecular weight heparin may be given for initial treatment. If an oral anticoagulant (usually warfarin sodium) is also required, it may be started at the same time as the heparin (the heparin needs to be continued for at least 5 days and until the INR has been in the therapeutic range for 2 consecutive days). Laboratory monitoring of coagulation activity, preferably on a daily basis, involves determination of the activated partial thromboplastin time (APTT) (for heparin (unfractionated) p. 101 only) or of the anti-Factor Xa concentration (for low molecular weight heparins). Local guidelines on recommended APTT for neonates and children should be followed; monitoring of APTT should be discussed with a specialist prior to treatment for thrombotic episodes in neonates.

Treatment of venous thromboembolism in pregnancy
Heparins are used for the management of venous thromboembolism in pregnancy because they do not cross the placenta. Low molecular weight heparins are preferred because they have a lower risk of osteoporosis and of heparin-induced thrombocytopenia. Low molecular weight heparins are eliminated more rapidly in pregnancy, requiring alteration of the dosage regimen for drugs such as dalteparin sodium p. 100, enoxaparin sodium p. 101 and tinzaparin sodium p. 102; see also under individual drugs. Treatment should be stopped at the onset of labour and advice sought from a specialist on continuing therapy after birth.

Extracorporeal circuits

Heparin (unfractionated) is also used in the maintenance of extracorporeal circuits in cardiopulmonary bypass and haemodialysis.

Haemorrhage

If haemorrhage occurs it is usually sufficient to withdraw unfractionated or low molecular weight heparin (unfractionated), but if rapid reversal of the effects of the heparin (unfractionated) is required, protamine sulfate p. 900 is a specific antidote (but only partially reverses the effects of low molecular weight heparin (unfractionated)).

Advanced Pharmacy Services

Children with, or at risk of venous thromboembolism may be eligible for the New Medicines Service / Medicines Use Review service provided by a community pharmacist. For further information, see *Advanced Pharmacy Services* in Medicines optimisation p. 25.

Oral anticoagulants

Overview

The main use of anticoagulants is to prevent thrombus formation or extension of an existing thrombus in the slower-moving venous side of the circulation, where the thrombus consists of a fibrin web enmeshed with platelets and red cells.

Anticoagulants are of less use in preventing thrombus formation in arteries, for in faster-flowing vessels thrombi are composed mainly of platelets with little fibrin.

Oral anticoagulants antagonise the effects of vitamin K and take at least 48 to 72 hours for the anticoagulant effect to develop fully; if an immediate effect is required, unfractionated or low molecular weight heparin must be given concomitantly.

Uses
Warfarin sodium p. 103 is the drug of choice for the treatment of systemic thromboembolism in children (not neonates) after initial heparinisation. It may also be used occasionally for the treatment of intravascular or intracardiac thrombi. Warfarin sodium is used prophylactically in those with chronic atrial fibrillation, dilated cardiomyopathy, certain forms of reconstructive heart surgery, mechanical prosthetic heart valves, and some forms of hereditary thrombophilia (e.g. homozygous protein C deficiency).

Unfractionated or a low molecular weight heparin (see under Parenteral anticoagulants p. 97) is usually preferred for the prophylaxis of venous thromboembolism in children undergoing surgery; alternatively warfarin sodium can be continued in selected children currently taking warfarin sodium and who are at a high risk of thromboembolism (seek expert advice).

Dose

The base-line prothrombin time should be determined but the initial dose should not be delayed whilst awaiting the result.

An induction dose is usually given over 4 days. The subsequent maintenance dose depends on the prothrombin time, reported as INR (international normalised ratio) and should be taken at the same time each day.

Target INR

The following indications and target INRs for adults for warfarin take into account recommendations of the British Society for Haematology Guidelines on Oral Anticoagulation with warfarin—fourth edition. *Br J Haematol* 2011; **154**: 311–324:

An INR which is within 0.5 units of the target value is generally satisfactory; larger deviations require dosage adjustment. Target values (rather than ranges) are now recommended.

INR 2.5 for:

- treatment of deep-vein thrombosis or pulmonary embolism (including those associated with antiphospholipid syndrome or for recurrence in patients no longer receiving warfarin sodium)
- atrial fibrillation
- cardioversion—target INR should be achieved at least 3 weeks before cardioversion and anticoagulation should continue for at least 4 weeks after the procedure (higher target values, such as an INR of 3, can be used for up to 4 weeks before the procedure to avoid cancellations due to low INR)
- dilated cardiomyopathy
- mitral stenosis or regurgitation in patients with either atrial fibrillation, a history of systemic embolism, a left atrial thrombus, or an enlarged left atrium
- bioprosthetic heart valves in the mitral position (treat for 3 months), or in patients with a history of systemic embolism (treat for at least 3 months), or with a left atrial thrombus at surgery (treat until clot resolves), or with other risk factors (e.g. atrial fibrillation or a low ventricular ejection fraction)
- acute arterial embolism requiring embolectomy (consider long-term treatment)
- myocardial infarction

INR 3.5 for:

- recurrent deep-vein thrombosis or pulmonary embolism in patients currently receiving anticoagulation and with an INR above 2;

Mechanical prosthetic heart valves:

- the recommended target INR depends on the type and location of the valve, and patient-related risk factors
- consider increasing the INR target or adding an antiplatelet drug, if an embolic event occurs whilst anticoagulated at the target INR.

Haemorrhage

The main adverse effect of all oral anticoagulants is haemorrhage. Checking the INR and omitting doses when appropriate is essential; if the anticoagulant is stopped but not reversed, the INR should be measured 2–3 days later to ensure that it is falling. The cause of an elevated INR should be investigated. The following recommendations (which take into account the recommendations of the British Society for Haematology Guidelines on Oral Anticoagulation with Warfarin—fourth edition. *Br J Haematol* 2011; **154**: 311–324) are based on the result of the INR and whether there is major or minor bleeding; the recommendations apply to adults taking warfarin:

- Major bleeding—stop warfarin sodium; give phytomenadione (vitamin K_1) p. 687 by slow intravenous injection; give dried prothrombin complex (factors II, VII, IX, and X) p. 89; if dried prothrombin complex unavailable, fresh frozen plasma can be given but is less effective; recombinant factor VIIa is not recommended for emergency anticoagulation reversal
- INR >8.0, minor bleeding—stop warfarin sodium; give phytomenadione (vitamin K_1) by slow intravenous injection; repeat dose of phytomenadione if INR still too high after 24 hours; restart warfarin sodium when INR <5.0
- INR >8.0, no bleeding—stop warfarin sodium; give phytomenadione (vitamin K_1) by mouth using the intravenous preparation orally [unlicensed use]; repeat dose of phytomenadione if INR still too high after 24 hours; restart warfarin sodium when INR <5.0
- INR 5.0–8.0, minor bleeding—stop warfarin sodium; give phytomenadione (vitamin K_1) by slow intravenous injection; restart warfarin sodium when INR <5.0
- INR 5.0–8.0, no bleeding—withhold 1 or 2 doses of warfarin sodium and reduce subsequent maintenance dose
- Unexpected bleeding at therapeutic levels—always investigate possibility of underlying cause e.g. unsuspected renal or gastro-intestinal tract pathology

Advanced Pharmacy Services

Children taking oral anticoagulants may be eligible for the New Medicines Service / Medicines Use Review service provided by a community pharmacist. For further information, see *Advanced Pharmacy Services* in Medicines optimisation p. 25.

Parenteral anticoagulants

Anticoagulants

Although thrombotic episodes are uncommon in childhood, anticoagulants may be required in children with congenital heart disease; in children undergoing haemodialysis; for preventing thrombosis in children requiring chemotherapy and following surgery; and for systemic venous thromboembolism secondary to inherited thrombophilias, systemic lupus erythematosus, or indwelling central venous catheters.

Heparin

Heparin initiates anticoagulation rapidly but has a short duration of action. It is now often referred to as being **standard** or heparin (unfractionated) p. 101 to distinguish it from the **low molecular weight heparins**, which have a longer duration of action. For children at high risk of bleeding, heparin (unfractionated) is more suitable than low molecular weight heparin because its effect can be terminated rapidly by stopping the infusion.

Heparins are used in both the treatment and prophylaxis of thromboembolic disease, mainly to prevent further clotting rather than to lyse existing clots—surgery or a thrombolytic drug may be necessary if a thrombus obstructs major vessels.

Low molecular weight heparins

Dalteparin sodium p. 100, enoxaparin sodium p. 101, and tinzaparin sodium p. 102 are low molecular weight heparins used for treatment and prophylaxis of thrombotic episodes in children. Their duration of action is longer than that of heparin (unfractionated) and in adults and older children *once-daily subcutaneous* dosage is sometimes possible; however, younger children require relatively higher doses (possibly due to larger volume of distribution, altered heparin pharmacokinetics, or lower plasma concentrations of antithrombin) and twice daily dosage is sometimes necessary. Low molecular weight heparins are convenient to use, especially in children with poor venous access.

Heparinoids

Danaparoid sodium p. 99 is a heparinoid that has a role in children who develop heparin-induced thrombocytopenia, providing they have no evidence of cross-reactivity.

Heparin flushes

The use of heparin flushes should be kept to a minimum. For maintaining patency of peripheral venous catheters, sodium chloride injection 0.9% is as effective as heparin flushes. The role of heparin flushes in maintaining patency of arterial and central venous catheters is unclear.

Epoprostenol

Epoprostenol (prostacyclin) p. 126 can be given to inhibit platelet aggregation during renal dialysis when heparins are unsuitable or contra-indicated. It is a potent vasodilator and therefore its side-effects include flushing, headache and hypotension.

Other drugs used for Thromboembolism Alteplase, p. 93 · Streptokinase, p. 94

ANTITHROMBOTIC DRUGS > ANTIPLATELET DRUGS

Antiplatelet drugs

Overview

Antiplatelet drugs decrease platelet aggregation and inhibit thrombus formation in the arterial circulation, because in faster-flowing vessels, thrombi are composed mainly of platelets with little fibrin.

Aspirin p. 98 has limited use in children because it has been associated with Reye's syndrome. Aspirin-containing preparations should not be given to children and adolescents under 16 years, unless specifically indicated, such as for Kawasaki disease, for prophylaxis of clot formation after cardiac surgery, or for prophylaxis of stroke in children at high risk.

If aspirin causes dyspepsia, or if the child is at a high risk of gastro-intestinal bleeding, a proton pump inhibitor or a H_2-receptor antagonist can be added.

Dipyridamole p. 98 is also used as an antiplatelet drug to prevent clot formation after cardiac surgery and may be used with specialist advice for treatment of persistent coronary artery aneurysms in Kawasaki disease.

Kawasaki disease

Initial treatment is with high dose aspirin and a single dose of intravenous normal immunoglobulin; this combination has an additive anti-inflammatory effect resulting in faster resolution of fever and a decreased incidence of coronary artery complications. After the acute phase, when the patient is afebrile, aspirin is continued at a lower dose to prevent coronary artery abnormalities.

Advanced Pharmacy Services

Children taking antiplatelet drugs may be eligible for the New Medicines Service / Medicines Use Review service provided by a community pharmacist. For further information, see *Advanced Pharmacy Services* in Medicines optimisation p. 25.

2

Cardiovascular system

Aspirin

03-Mar-2020

(Acetylsalicylic Acid)

● **INDICATIONS AND DOSE**

Antiplatelet | Prevention of thrombus formation after cardiac surgery

▶ BY MOUTH

- Neonate: 1–5 mg/kg once daily.
- Child 1 month–11 years: 1–5 mg/kg once daily (max. per dose 75 mg)
- Child 12–17 years: 75 mg once daily

Kawasaki disease

▶ BY MOUTH

- Neonate: Initially 8 mg/kg 4 times a day for 2 weeks *or* until afebrile, followed by 5 mg/kg once daily for 6–8 weeks, if no evidence of coronary lesions after 8 weeks, discontinue treatment or seek expert advice.
- Child 1 month–11 years: Initially 7.5–12.5 mg/kg 4 times a day for 2 weeks *or* until afebrile, then 2–5 mg/kg once daily for 6–8 weeks, if no evidence of coronary lesions after 8 weeks, discontinue treatment or seek expert advice

Mild to moderate pain (dose approved for use by community practitioner nurse prescribers) | Pyrexia (dose approved for use by community practitioner nurse prescribers)

▶ BY MOUTH

- Child 16–17 years: 300–600 mg every 4–6 hours as required, maximum 2.4 g per day without doctor's advice

● **UNLICENSED USE** Not licensed for use in children under 16 years.

● **CONTRA-INDICATIONS** Active peptic ulceration · bleeding disorders · children under 16 years (risk of Reye's syndrome) · haemophilia · previous peptic ulceration (analgesic dose) · severe cardiac failure (analgesic dose)

CONTRA-INDICATIONS, FURTHER INFORMATION

▶ **Reye's syndrome** Owing to an association with Reye's syndrome, manufacturer advises aspirin-containing preparations should not be given to children under 16 years, unless specifically indicated, e.g. for Kawasaki disease.

● **CAUTIONS** Allergic disease · anaemia · asthma · dehydration · G6PD deficiency · preferably avoid during fever or viral infection in children (risk of Reye's syndrome) · previous peptic ulceration (but manufacturers may advise avoidance of low-dose aspirin in history of peptic ulceration) · thyrotoxicosis · uncontrolled hypertension

● **INTERACTIONS** → Appendix 1: aspirin

● **SIDE-EFFECTS**

GENERAL SIDE-EFFECTS

▶ **Rare or very rare** Asthmatic attack · bronchospasm

SPECIFIC SIDE-EFFECTS

▶ **Common or very common** Dyspepsia · haemorrhage
▶ **Uncommon** Dyspnoea · rhinitis · severe cutaneous adverse reactions (SCARs) · skin reactions
▶ **Rare or very rare** Aplastic anaemia · erythema nodosum · gastrointestinal haemorrhage (severe) · granulocytosis · haemorrhagic vasculitis · intracranial haemorrhage · menorrhagia · nausea · thrombocytopenia · vomiting
▶ **Frequency not known** Fluid retention · gastrointestinal disorders · headache · hearing loss · hepatic failure · hyperuricaemia · iron deficiency anaemia · renal impairment · sodium retention · tinnitus · vertigo

Overdose The main features of salicylate poisoning are hyperventilation, tinnitus, deafness, vasodilatation, and sweating. Coma is uncommon but indicates very severe poisoning.

For specific details on the management of poisoning, see Aspirin, under Emergency treatment of poisoning p. 891.

● **ALLERGY AND CROSS-SENSITIVITY** Aspirin is **contra-indicated** in history of hypersensitivity to aspirin or any other NSAID—which includes those in whom attacks of asthma, angioedema, urticaria, or rhinitis have been precipitated by aspirin or any other NSAID.

● **PREGNANCY** Use antiplatelet doses with caution during third trimester; impaired platelet function and risk of haemorrhage; delayed onset and increased duration of labour with increased blood loss; avoid analgesic doses if possible in last few weeks (low doses probably not harmful); high doses may be related to intra-uterine growth restriction, teratogenic effects, closure of fetal ductus arteriosus in utero and possibly persistent pulmonary hypertension of newborn; kernicterus may occur in jaundiced neonates.

● **BREAST FEEDING** Avoid—possible risk of Reye's syndrome; regular use of high doses could impair platelet function and produce hypoprothrombinaemia in infant if neonatal vitamin K stores low.

● **HEPATIC IMPAIRMENT** Manufacturer advises use with caution in mild-to-moderate impairment; avoid in severe impairment.

● **RENAL IMPAIRMENT** Use with caution; avoid in severe impairment; sodium and water retention; deterioration in renal function; increased risk of gastro-intestinal bleeding.

● **PATIENT AND CARER ADVICE**

Medicines for Children leaflet: Aspirin for prevention of blood clots www.medicinesforchildren.org.uk/aspirin-prevention-blood-clots-0

● **MEDICINAL FORMS** There can be variation in the licensing of different medicines containing the same drug. Forms available from special-order manufacturers include: capsule, oral suspension, oral solution

Gastro-resistant tablet

CAUTIONARY AND ADVISORY LABELS 5, 25, 32

▶ **Aspirin (Non-proprietary)**
Aspirin 75 mg Aspirin 75mg gastro-resistant tablets | 28 tablet P £0.86 DT = £0.86 | 56 tablet P £1.66–£1.72
Aspirin 300 mg Aspirin 300mg gastro-resistant tablets | 100 tablet PoM £25.29 DT = £25.29

▶ **Nu-Seals** (Alliance Pharmaceuticals Ltd)
Aspirin 75 mg Nu-Seals 75 gastro-resistant tablets | 56 tablet P £3.12

Tablet

CAUTIONARY AND ADVISORY LABELS 21, 32

▶ **Aspirin (Non-proprietary)**
Aspirin 75 mg Aspirin 75mg tablets | 28 tablet PoM £3.50 DT = £1.38
Aspirin 300 mg Aspirin 300mg tablets | 100 tablet PoM £1.12–£10.68

Dispersible tablet

CAUTIONARY AND ADVISORY LABELS 13, 21, 32

▶ **Aspirin (Non-proprietary)**
Aspirin 75 mg Aspirin 75mg dispersible tablets | 1000 tablet PoM £27.50–£28.90
Aspirin 300 mg Aspirin 300mg dispersible tablets | 100 tablet PoM £0.94 DT = £3.38

▶ **Danamep** (Ecogen Europe Ltd)
Aspirin 75 mg Danamep 75mg dispersible tablets | 28 tablet PoM £0.50 DT = £0.81

Dipyridamole

14-Feb-2019

● **INDICATIONS AND DOSE**

Kawasaki disease (initiated under specialist supervision)

▶ BY MOUTH USING IMMEDIATE-RELEASE MEDICINES

- Child 1 month–11 years: 1 mg/kg 3 times a day

Prevention of thrombus formation after cardiac surgery
- ▶ BY MOUTH USING IMMEDIATE-RELEASE MEDICINES
- ▸ Child 1 month–11 years: 2.5 mg/kg twice daily
- ▸ Child 12–17 years: 100–200 mg 3 times a day

- ● **UNLICENSED USE** Not licensed for use in children.
- ● **CAUTIONS** Aortic stenosis · coagulation disorders · heart failure · hypotension · left ventricular outflow obstruction · may exacerbate migraine · myasthenia gravis (risk of exacerbation)
- ● **INTERACTIONS** → Appendix 1: dipyridamole
- ● **SIDE-EFFECTS**
- ▶ **Common or very common** Angina pectoris · diarrhoea · dizziness · headache · myalgia · nausea · skin reactions · vomiting
- ▶ **Frequency not known** Angioedema · bronchospasm · haemorrhage · hot flush · hypotension · tachycardia · thrombocytopenia
- ● **PREGNANCY** Not known to be harmful.
- ● **BREAST FEEDING** Manufacturers advise use only if essential—small amount present in milk.
- ● **DIRECTIONS FOR ADMINISTRATION** Injection solution can be given orally.

- ● **MEDICINAL FORMS** There can be variation in the licensing of different medicines containing the same drug. Forms available from special-order manufacturers include: oral suspension, oral solution

Oral suspension
- ▸ Dipyridamole (Non-proprietary)
  Dipyridamole 10 mg per 1 ml Dipyridamole 50mg/5ml oral suspension sugar-free | 150 ml PoM £39.40 DT = £39.40
  Dipyridamole 40 mg per 1 ml Dipyridamole 200mg/5ml oral suspension sugar-free | 150 ml PoM £133.53 DT = £133.53

Tablet
CAUTIONARY AND ADVISORY LABELS 22
- ▸ Dipyridamole (Non-proprietary)
  Dipyridamole 25 mg Dipyridamole 25mg tablets | 84 tablet PoM £9.20 DT = £8.96
  Dipyridamole 100 mg Dipyridamole 100mg tablets | 84 tablet PoM £12.50 DT = £5.58

ANTITHROMBOTIC DRUGS › HEPARINOIDS

Danaparoid sodium

21-Jun-2019

- ● **INDICATIONS AND DOSE**

Thromboembolic disease in patients with history of heparin-induced thrombocytopenia
- ▶ INITIALLY BY INTRAVENOUS INJECTION
- ▸ Neonate: Initially 30 units/kg, then (by continuous intravenous infusion) 1.2–2 units/kg/hour, infusion dose to be adjusted according to coagulation activity.
- ▸ Child 1 month–15 years (body-weight up to 55 kg): Initially 30 units/kg (max. per dose 1250 units), then (by continuous intravenous infusion) 1.2–2 units/kg/hour, infusion dose to be adjusted according to coagulation activity
- ▸ Child 1 month–15 years (body-weight 55 kg and above): Initially 30 units/kg (max. per dose 2500 units), then (by continuous intravenous infusion) 1.2–2 units/kg/hour, infusion dose to be adjusted according to coagulation activity
- ▸ Child 16–17 years (body-weight up to 55 kg): Initially 1250 units, then (by continuous intravenous infusion) 400 units/hour for 2 hours, then (by continuous intravenous infusion) 300 units/hour for 2 hours, then (by continuous intravenous infusion) 200 units/hour for 5 days, infusion dose to be adjusted according to coagulation activity
- ▸ Child 16–17 years (body-weight 55–90 kg): Initially 2500 units, then (by continuous intravenous infusion) 400 units/hour for 2 hours, then (by continuous intravenous infusion) 300 units/hour for 2 hours, then (by continuous intravenous infusion) 200 units/hour for 5 days, infusion dose to be adjusted according to coagulation activity
- ▸ Child 16–17 years (body-weight 91 kg and above): Initially 3750 units, then (by continuous intravenous infusion) 400 units/hour for 2 hours, then (by continuous intravenous infusion) 300 units/hour for 2 hours, then (by continuous intravenous infusion) 200 units/hour for 5 days, infusion dose to be adjusted according to coagulation activity

- ● **UNLICENSED USE** Not licensed for use in children.
- ● **CONTRA-INDICATIONS** Active peptic ulcer (unless this is the reason for operation) · acute bacterial endocarditis · diabetic retinopathy · epidural anaesthesia (with treatment doses) · haemophilia and other haemorrhagic disorders · recent cerebral haemorrhage · severe uncontrolled hypertension · spinal anaesthesia (with treatment doses) · thrombocytopenia (unless patient has heparin-induced thrombocytopenia)
- ● **CAUTIONS** Antibodies to heparins (risk of antibody-induced thrombocytopenia) · body-weight over 90 kg · recent bleeding · risk of bleeding
- ● **INTERACTIONS** → Appendix 1: danaparoid
- ● **SIDE-EFFECTS**
- ▶ **Common or very common** Haemorrhage · heparin-induced thrombocytopenia · skin reactions · thrombocytopenia
- ▶ **Uncommon** Post procedural haematoma
- ▶ **Rare or very rare** Anastomotic haemorrhage
- ● **PREGNANCY** Manufacturer advises avoid—limited information available but not known to be harmful.
- ● **BREAST FEEDING** Amount probably too small to be harmful but manufacturer advises avoid.
- ● **HEPATIC IMPAIRMENT** Manufacturer advises caution in moderate impairment with impaired haemostasis—increased risk of bleeding; avoid in severe hepatic failure unless patient has heparin-induced thrombocytopenia and no alternative available.
- ● **RENAL IMPAIRMENT** Use with caution in moderate impairment. Avoid in severe impairment unless patient has heparin-induced thrombocytopenia and no alternative available.
  Monitoring Increased risk of bleeding in renal impairment, monitor anti-Factor Xa activity.
- ● **MONITORING REQUIREMENTS** Monitor anti factor Xa activity in patients with body-weight over 90 kg.
- ● **DIRECTIONS FOR ADMINISTRATION** For *intravenous infusion*, dilute with Glucose 5% or Sodium Chloride 0.9%.

- ● **MEDICINAL FORMS** There can be variation in the licensing of different medicines containing the same drug.

Solution for injection
- ▸ Danaparoid sodium (Non-proprietary)
  Danaparoid sodium 1250 unit per 1 ml Danaparoid sodium 750units/0.6ml solution for injection ampoules | 10 ampoule PoM £599.99 | 10 ampoule PoM £599.99 (Hospital only)

ANTITHROMBOTIC DRUGS › HEPARINS

Heparins

- ● **CONTRA-INDICATIONS** Acute bacterial endocarditis · after major trauma · Avoid injections containing benzyl alcohol in neonates · epidural anaesthesia with treatment doses · haemophilia or other haemorrhagic disorders · peptic ulcer · recent cerebral haemorrhage · recent surgery to eye · recent surgery to nervous system · spinal anaesthesia with treatment doses · thrombocytopenia (including history of heparin-induced thrombocytopenia)

- **CAUTIONS** Severe hypertension
- **SIDE-EFFECTS**
  - **Common or very common** Haemorrhage · heparin-induced thrombocytopenia · skin reactions · thrombocytopenia · thrombocytosis
  - **Uncommon** CNS haemorrhage
  - **Rare or very rare** Alopecia · hyperkalaemia · osteoporosis (following long term use) · priapism
  - **Frequency not known** Hypoaldosteronism

SIDE-EFFECTS, FURTHER INFORMATION **Haemorrhage** If haemorrhage occurs it is usually sufficient to withdraw unfractionated or low molecular weight heparin, but if rapid reversal of the effects of the heparin is required, protamine sulfate is a specific antidote (but only partially reverses the effects of low molecular weight heparins).

Heparin-induced thrombocytopenia Clinically important heparin-induced thrombocytopenia is immune-mediated and can be complicated by thrombosis. Signs of heparin-induced thrombocytopenia include a 30% reduction of platelet count, thrombosis, or skin allergy. If heparin-induced thrombocytopenia is strongly suspected or confirmed, the heparin should be stopped and an alternative anticoagulant, such as danaparoid, should be given. Ensure platelet counts return to normal range in those who require warfarin.

Hyperkalaemia Inhibition of aldosterone secretion by unfractionated or low molecular weight heparin can result in hyperkalaemia; patients with diabetes mellitus, chronic renal failure, acidosis, raised plasma potassium or those taking potassium-sparing drugs seem to be more susceptible. The risk appears to increase with duration of therapy.

- **ALLERGY AND CROSS-SENSITIVITY** Hypersensitivity to unfractionated or low molecular weight heparin.
- **MONITORING REQUIREMENTS**
  - Heparin-induced thrombocytopenia Platelet counts should be measured just before treatment with unfractionated or low molecular weight heparin, and regular monitoring of platelet counts may be required if given for longer than 4 days. See the British Society for Haematology's Guidelines on the diagnosis and management of heparin-induced thrombocytopenia: second edition. *Br J Haematol* 2012; **159**: 528–540.
  - Hyperkalaemia Plasma-potassium concentration should be measured in patients at risk of hyperkalaemia before starting the heparin and monitored regularly thereafter, particularly if treatment is to be continued for longer than 7 days.

F 99

Dalteparin sodium

08-Feb-2019

- **INDICATIONS AND DOSE**

Treatment of thrombotic episodes

- BY SUBCUTANEOUS INJECTION
  - Neonate: 100 units/kg twice daily.
  - Child 1 month–11 years: 100 units/kg twice daily
  - Child 12–17 years: 200 units/kg once daily (max. per dose 18 000 units); reduced to 100 units/kg twice daily, dose reduced if increased risk of bleeding

Treatment of venous thromboembolism in pregnancy

- BY SUBCUTANEOUS INJECTION
  - Child 12–17 years (body-weight up to 50 kg): 5000 units twice daily, use body-weight in early pregnancy to calculate the dose
  - Child 12–17 years (body-weight 50–69 kg): 6000 units twice daily, use body-weight in early pregnancy to calculate the dose
  - Child 12–17 years (body-weight 70–89 kg): 8000 units twice daily, use body-weight in early pregnancy to calculate the dose
  - Child 12–17 years (body-weight 90 kg and above): 10 000 units twice daily, use body-weight in early pregnancy to calculate the dose

Prophylaxis of thrombotic episodes

- BY SUBCUTANEOUS INJECTION
  - Neonate: 100 units/kg once daily.
  - Child 1 month–11 years: 100 units/kg once daily
  - Child 12–17 years: 2500–5000 units once daily

- **UNLICENSED USE** Not licensed for treatment of venous thromboembolism in pregnancy.
  Not licensed for use in children.
- **INTERACTIONS** → Appendix 1: low molecular-weight heparins
- **SIDE-EFFECTS** Epidural haematoma · prosthetic cardiac valve thrombosis
- **PREGNANCY** Not known to be harmful, low molecular weight heparins do not cross the placenta. Multidose vial contains benzyl alcohol—manufacturer advises avoid.
- **BREAST FEEDING** Due to the relatively high molecular weight and inactivation in the gastro-intestinal tract, passage into breast-milk and absorption by the nursing infant are likely to be negligible, however manufacturers advise avoid.
- **HEPATIC IMPAIRMENT** Manufacturer advises caution in severe impairment (increased risk of bleeding complications).
  Dose adjustments Manufacturer advises consider dose reduction in severe impairment.
- **RENAL IMPAIRMENT** Use of unfractionated heparin may be preferable.
  Dose adjustments Risk of bleeding may be increased—dose reduction may be required.
- **MONITORING REQUIREMENTS** Routine monitoring of anti-Factor Xa activity is not usually required during treatment with dalteparin, except in neonates; monitoring may also be necessary in severely ill children and those with renal or hepatic impairment.

- **MEDICINAL FORMS** There can be variation in the licensing of different medicines containing the same drug.

Solution for injection

EXCIPIENTS: May contain Benzyl alcohol

- Fragmin (Pfizer Ltd)

Dalteparin sodium 2500 unit per 1 ml Fragmin 10,000units/4ml solution for injection ampoules | 10 ampoule PoM £51.22 DT = £51.22

Dalteparin sodium 10000 unit per 1 ml Fragmin 10,000units/1ml solution for injection pre-filled syringes | 5 pre-filled disposable injection PoM £28.23 DT = £28.23
Fragmin 10,000units/1ml solution for injection ampoules | 10 ampoule PoM £51.22 DT = £51.22

Dalteparin sodium 12500 unit per 1 ml Fragmin 2,500units/0.2ml solution for injection pre-filled syringes | 10 pre-filled disposable injection PoM £18.58 DT = £18.58

Dalteparin sodium 25000 unit per 1 ml Fragmin 18,000units/0.72ml solution for injection pre-filled syringes | 5 pre-filled disposable injection PoM £50.82 DT = £50.82
Fragmin 15,000units/0.6ml solution for injection pre-filled syringes | 5 pre-filled disposable injection PoM £42.34 DT = £42.34
Fragmin 5,000units/0.2ml solution for injection pre-filled syringes | 10 pre-filled disposable injection PoM £28.23 DT = £28.23
Fragmin 12,500units/0.5ml solution for injection pre-filled syringes | 5 pre-filled disposable injection PoM £35.29 DT = £35.29
Fragmin 7,500units/0.3ml solution for injection pre-filled syringes | 10 pre-filled disposable injection PoM £42.34 DT = £42.34

Fragmin 100,000units/4ml solution for injection vials | 1 vial PoM £48.66 DT = £48.66
Fragmin 10,000units/0.4ml solution for injection pre-filled syringes | 5 pre-filled disposable injection PoM £28.23 DT = £28.23

F 99

Enoxaparin sodium

25-Oct-2019

- **INDICATIONS AND DOSE**

Treatment of thrombotic episodes

▸ BY SUBCUTANEOUS INJECTION

- Neonate: 1.5–2 mg/kg twice daily.
- Child 1 month: 1.5 mg/kg twice daily
- Child 2 months–17 years: 1 mg/kg twice daily

Treatment of venous thromboembolism in pregnancy

▸ BY SUBCUTANEOUS INJECTION

- Child 12–17 years (body-weight up to 50 kg): 40 mg twice daily, dose based on early pregnancy body-weight
- Child 12–17 years (body-weight 50–69 kg): 60 mg twice daily, dose based on early pregnancy body-weight
- Child 12–17 years (body-weight 70–89 kg): 80 mg twice daily, dose based on early pregnancy body-weight
- Child 12–17 years (body-weight 90 kg and above): 100 mg twice daily, dose based on early pregnancy body-weight

Prophylaxis of thrombotic episodes

▸ BY SUBCUTANEOUS INJECTION

- Neonate: 750 micrograms/kg twice daily.
- Child 1 month: 750 micrograms/kg twice daily
- Child 2 months–17 years: 500 micrograms/kg twice daily; maximum 40 mg per day

DOSE EQUIVALENCE AND CONVERSION

- 1 mg equivalent to 100 units.

- **UNLICENSED USE** Not licensed for treatment of venous thromboembolism in pregnancy.
  Not licensed for use in children.
- **INTERACTIONS** → Appendix 1: low molecular-weight heparins
- **SIDE-EFFECTS**
  - **Common or very common** Haemorrhagic anaemia · headache · hypersensitivity
  - **Uncommon** Hepatic disorders · injection site necrosis
  - **Rare or very rare** Cutaneous vasculitis · eosinophilia
- **PREGNANCY** Not known to be harmful, low molecular weight heparins do not cross the placenta. Multidose vial contains benzyl alcohol—avoid.
- **BREAST FEEDING** Manufacturer advises suitable for use during breast feeding—passage into breast milk and absorption by the nursing infant considered to be negligible due to the relatively high molecular weight of enoxaparin and inactivation in the gastro-intestinal tract.
- **HEPATIC IMPAIRMENT**
  Dose adjustments Reduce dose in severe impairment—risk of bleeding may be increased.
- **RENAL IMPAIRMENT** Risk of bleeding increased; use of unfractionated heparin may be preferable. Consult specialist sources.
- **MONITORING REQUIREMENTS** Routine monitoring of anti-Factor Xa activity is not usually required during treatment with enoxaparin, except in neonates; monitoring may also be necessary in severely ill children and those with renal or hepatic impairment.
- **PRESCRIBING AND DISPENSING INFORMATION** Enoxaparin sodium is a biological medicine. Biological medicines must be prescribed and dispensed by brand name, see *Biological medicines* and *Biosimilar medicines*, under Guidance on prescribing p. 1.
- **MEDICINAL FORMS** There can be variation in the licensing of different medicines containing the same drug.

Solution for injection

EXCIPIENTS: May contain Benzyl alcohol

▸ Arovi (ROVI Biotech Ltd) ▼

Enoxaparin sodium 100 mg per 1 ml Arovi 20mg/0.2ml solution for injection pre-filled syringes | 10 pre-filled disposable injection PoM £15.65 DT = £20.86
Arovi 60mg/0.6ml solution for injection pre-filled syringes | 10 pre-filled disposable injection PoM £29.45 DT = £39.26
Arovi 40mg/0.4ml solution for injection pre-filled syringes | 10 pre-filled disposable injection PoM £22.70 DT = £30.27
Arovi 80mg/0.8ml solution for injection pre-filled syringes | 10 pre-filled disposable injection PoM £41.35 DT = £55.13
Arovi 100mg/1ml solution for injection pre-filled syringes | 10 pre-filled disposable injection PoM £54.23 DT = £72.30

Enoxaparin sodium 150 mg per 1 ml Arovi 150mg/1ml solution for injection pre-filled syringes | 10 pre-filled disposable injection PoM £74.93 DT = £99.91
Arovi 120mg/0.8ml solution for injection pre-filled syringes | 10 pre-filled disposable injection PoM £65.95 DT = £87.93

▸ Clexane (Sanofi)

Enoxaparin sodium 100 mg per 1 ml Clexane 60mg/0.6ml solution for injection pre-filled syringes | 10 pre-filled disposable injection PoM £39.26 DT = £39.26
Clexane 300mg/3ml solution for injection multidose vials | 1 vial PoM £21.33 DT = £21.33
Clexane 80mg/0.8ml solution for injection pre-filled syringes | 10 pre-filled disposable injection PoM £55.13 DT = £55.13
Clexane 40mg/0.4ml solution for injection pre-filled syringes | 10 pre-filled disposable injection PoM £30.27 DT = £30.27
Clexane 100mg/1ml solution for injection pre-filled syringes | 10 pre-filled disposable injection PoM £72.30 DT = £72.30
Clexane 20mg/0.2ml solution for injection pre-filled syringes | 10 pre-filled disposable injection PoM £20.86 DT = £20.86

Enoxaparin sodium 150 mg per 1 ml Clexane Forte 120mg/0.8ml solution for injection pre-filled syringes | 10 pre-filled disposable injection PoM £87.93 DT = £87.93
Clexane Forte 150mg/1ml solution for injection pre-filled syringes | 10 pre-filled disposable injection PoM £99.91 DT = £99.91

▸ Inhixa (Techdow Pharma England Ltd) ▼

Enoxaparin sodium 100 mg per 1 ml Inhixa 40mg/0.4ml solution for injection pre-filled syringes | 10 pre-filled disposable injection PoM £30.27 DT = £30.27
Inhixa 80mg/0.8ml solution for injection pre-filled syringes | 10 pre-filled disposable injection PoM £55.13 DT = £55.13
Inhixa 60mg/0.6ml solution for injection pre-filled syringes | 10 pre-filled disposable injection PoM £39.26 DT = £39.26
Inhixa 100mg/1ml solution for injection pre-filled syringes | 10 pre-filled disposable injection PoM £72.30 DT = £72.30
Inhixa 20mg/0.2ml solution for injection pre-filled syringes | 10 pre-filled disposable injection PoM £20.86 DT = £20.86

Enoxaparin sodium 150 mg per 1 ml Inhixa 120mg/0.8ml solution for injection pre-filled syringes | 10 pre-filled disposable injection PoM £87.93 DT = £87.93
Inhixa 150mg/1ml solution for injection pre-filled syringes | 10 pre-filled disposable injection PoM £99.91 DT = £99.91

F 99

Heparin (unfractionated)

05-May-2017

- **INDICATIONS AND DOSE**

Prevention of clotting in extracorporeal circuits

▸ TO THE DEVICE AS A FLUSH

- Child: (consult product literature)

Maintenance of neonatal umbilical arterial catheter

▸ BY INTRAVENOUS INFUSION

- Neonate: 0.5 unit/hour.

Treatment of thombotic episodes

▸ INITIALLY BY INTRAVENOUS INJECTION

- Neonate up to 35 weeks corrected gestational age: Initially 50 units/kg, then (by continuous intravenous infusion) 25 units/kg/hour, adjusted according to APTT.
- Neonate: Initially 75 units/kg, then (by continuous intravenous infusion) 25 units/kg/hour, adjusted according to APTT.

continued →

- Child 1–11 months: Initially 75 units/kg, then (by continuous intravenous infusion) 25 units/kg/hour, adjusted according to APTT
- Child 1–17 years: Initially 75 units/kg, then (by continuous intravenous infusion) 20 units/kg/hour, adjusted according to APTT

▶ BY SUBCUTANEOUS INJECTION
- Child: 250 units/kg twice daily, adjusted according to APTT

Prophylaxis of thrombotic episodes

▶ BY SUBCUTANEOUS INJECTION
- Child: 100 units/kg twice daily (max. per dose 5000 units), adjusted according to APTT

Maintenance of cardiac shunts and critical stents

▶ TO THE DEVICE AS A FLUSH
- Child: (consult local protocol)

- **UNLICENSED USE** Check product literature for licensed use in children.
- **INTERACTIONS** → Appendix 1: heparin (unfractionated)
- **SIDE-EFFECTS** Adrenal insufficiency · hypokalaemia · rebound hyperlipidaemia
- **PREGNANCY** Does not cross the placenta; maternal osteoporosis reported after prolonged use; multidose vials may contain benzyl alcohol—some manufacturers advise avoid.
- **BREAST FEEDING** Not excreted into milk due to high molecular weight.
- **HEPATIC IMPAIRMENT** Manufacturer advises caution; consider avoiding in severe impairment (increased risk of bleeding complications).
  Dose adjustments Manufacturer advises consider dose reduction if used in severe impairment.
- **RENAL IMPAIRMENT**
  Dose adjustments Risk of bleeding increased in severe impairment—dose may need to be reduced.
- **DIRECTIONS FOR ADMINISTRATION** For *continuous intravenous infusion*, dilute with Glucose 5% or Sodium chloride 0.9%.
- In neonates For *maintenance of neonatal umbilical arterial catheter*, dilute 50 units to a final volume of 50 mL with Sodium Chloride 0.45% or use ready-made bag containing 500 units in 500 mL Sodium Chloride 0.9%; infuse at 0.5 mL/hour. For *neonatal intensive care (treatment of thrombosis)*, dilute 1250 units/kg body-weight to a final volume of 50 mL with infusion fluid; an intravenous infusion rate of 1 mL/hour provides a dose of 25 units/kg/hour.

- **MEDICINAL FORMS** There can be variation in the licensing of different medicines containing the same drug. Forms available from special-order manufacturers include: solution for injection, solution for infusion

Solution for injection

EXCIPIENTS: May contain Benzyl alcohol

- Heparin (unfractionated) (Non-proprietary)
  Heparin sodium 1000 unit per 1 ml Heparin sodium 1,000units/1ml solution for injection ampoules | 10 ampoule PoM £14.85 DT = £14.85
  Heparin sodium 5,000units/5ml solution for injection vials | 10 vial PoM £16.50–£37.41 DT = £16.50
  Heparin sodium 20,000units/20ml solution for injection ampoules | 10 ampoule PoM £70.88 DT = £70.88
  Heparin sodium 5,000units/5ml solution for injection ampoules | 10 ampoule PoM £37.47 DT = £37.47
  Heparin sodium 10,000units/10ml solution for injection ampoules | 10 ampoule PoM £64.59 DT = £64.59
  Heparin sodium 5000 unit per 1 ml Heparin sodium 5,000units/1ml solution for injection ampoules | 10 ampoule PoM £29.04 DT = £29.04
  Heparin sodium 25,000units/5ml solution for injection vials | 10 vial PoM £45.00–£84.60 DT = £45.00
  Heparin sodium 25,000units/5ml solution for injection ampoules | 10 ampoule PoM £75.78 DT = £75.78
  Heparin calcium 25000 unit per 1 ml Heparin calcium 5,000units/0.2ml solution for injection ampoules | 10 ampoule PoM £44.70 DT = £44.70
  Heparin sodium 25000 unit per 1 ml Heparin sodium 25,000units/1ml solution for injection ampoules | 10 ampoule PoM £76.95 DT = £76.95
  Heparin sodium 5,000units/0.2ml solution for injection ampoules | 10 ampoule PoM £37.35 DT = £37.35

Intravenous flush

EXCIPIENTS: May contain Benzyl alcohol

- Heparin (unfractionated) (Non-proprietary)
  Heparin sodium 10 unit per 1 ml Heparin sodium 50units/5ml patency solution ampoules | 10 ampoule PoM £14.96 DT = £14.96
  Heparin sodium 50units/5ml I.V. flush solution ampoules | 10 ampoule PoM £14.96 DT = £14.96
  Heparin sodium 100 unit per 1 ml Heparin sodium 200units/2ml I.V. flush solution ampoules | 10 ampoule PoM £15.68 DT = £15.68
  Heparin sodium 200units/2ml patency solution ampoules | 10 ampoule PoM £15.68 DT = £15.68

Infusion

- Heparin (unfractionated) (Non-proprietary)
  Heparin sodium 2 unit per 1 ml Heparin sodium 1,000units/500ml infusion Viaflex bags | 1 bag PoM ⊠
  Heparin sodium 2,000units/1litre infusion Viaflex bags | 1 bag PoM ⊠
  Heparin sodium 5 unit per 1 ml Heparin sodium 5,000units/1litre infusion Viaflex bags | 1 bag PoM ⊠

99

Tinzaparin sodium

06-Aug-2018

- **INDICATIONS AND DOSE**

Treatment of thrombotic episodes

▶ BY SUBCUTANEOUS INJECTION
- Child 1 month: 275 units/kg once daily
- Child 2–11 months: 250 units/kg once daily
- Child 1–4 years: 240 units/kg once daily
- Child 5–9 years: 200 units/kg once daily
- Child 10–17 years: 175 units/kg once daily

Treatment of venous thromboembolism in pregnancy

▶ BY SUBCUTANEOUS INJECTION
- Child 12–17 years: 175 units/kg once daily, dose based on early pregnancy body-weight

Prophylaxis of thrombotic episodes

▶ BY SUBCUTANEOUS INJECTION
- Child: 50 units/kg once daily

- **UNLICENSED USE** Not licensed for the treatment of venous thromboembolism in pregnancy.
  Not licensed for use in children.
- **INTERACTIONS** → Appendix 1: low molecular-weight heparins
- **SIDE-EFFECTS**
  - **Common or very common** Anaemia
  - **Rare or very rare** Angioedema · Stevens-Johnson syndrome
- **PREGNANCY** Not known to be harmful, low molecular weight heparins do not cross the placenta. Vials contain benzyl alcohol—manufacturer advises avoid.
- **BREAST FEEDING** Due to the relatively high molecular weight of tinzaparin and inactivation in the gastro-intestinal tract, passage into breast-milk and absorption by the nursing infant are likely to be negligible; however manufacturer advise avoid.
- **RENAL IMPAIRMENT** Risk of bleeding may be increased. Unfractionated heparin may be preferable. Manufacturer advises caution if estimated glomerular filtration rate less than 30 mL/minute/1.73 m^2.
  Monitoring In renal impairment monitoring of anti-Factor Xa may be required if estimated glomerular filtration rate less than 30 mL/minute/1.73 m^2.
- **MONITORING REQUIREMENTS** Routine monitoring of anti-Factor Xa activity is not usually required except in

neonates; monitoring may also be necessary in severely ill children and those with renal or hepatic impairment.

- **MEDICINAL FORMS** There can be variation in the licensing of different medicines containing the same drug.

Solution for injection

EXCIPIENTS: May contain Benzyl alcohol, sulfites

- Tinzaparin sodium (Non-proprietary)
  Tinzaparin sodium 10000 unit per 1 ml Tinzaparin sodium 3,500units/0.35ml solution for injection pre-filled syringes | 10 pre-filled disposable injection PoM £27.71 DT = £27.71
  Tinzaparin sodium 4,500units/0.45ml solution for injection pre-filled syringes | 10 pre-filled disposable injection PoM £35.63 DT = £35.63
  Tinzaparin sodium 2,500units/0.25ml solution for injection pre-filled syringes | 10 pre-filled disposable injection PoM £19.80 DT = £19.80
- Innohep (LEO Pharma)
  Tinzaparin sodium 10000 unit per 1 ml Innohep 20,000units/2ml solution for injection vials | 10 vial PoM £105.66 DT = £105.66
  Tinzaparin sodium 20000 unit per 1 ml Innohep 18,000units/0.9ml solution for injection pre-filled syringes | 6 pre-filled disposable injection PoM £64.25 | 10 pre-filled disposable injection PoM £107.08 DT = £107.08
  Innohep 8,000units/0.4ml solution for injection pre-filled syringes | 6 pre-filled disposable injection PoM £28.56 | 10 pre-filled disposable injection PoM £47.60 DT = £47.60
  Innohep 40,000units/2ml solution for injection vials | 1 vial PoM £34.20 DT = £34.20
  Innohep 16,000units/0.8ml solution for injection pre-filled syringes | 6 pre-filled disposable injection PoM £57.12 | 10 pre-filled disposable injection PoM £95.20 DT = £95.20
  Innohep 12,000units/0.6ml solution for injection pre-filled syringes | 6 pre-filled disposable injection PoM £42.84 | 10 pre-filled disposable injection PoM £71.40 DT = £71.40
  Innohep 14,000units/0.7ml solution for injection pre-filled syringes | 6 pre-filled disposable injection PoM £49.98 | 10 pre-filled disposable injection PoM £83.30 DT = £83.30
  Innohep 10,000units/0.5ml solution for injection pre-filled syringes | 6 pre-filled disposable injection PoM £35.70 | 10 pre-filled disposable injection PoM £59.50 DT = £59.50

ANTITHROMBOTIC DRUGS > VITAMIN K ANTAGONISTS

Vitamin K antagonists

IMPORTANT SAFETY INFORMATION

MHRA/CHM ADVICE: DIRECT-ACTING ANTIVIRALS TO TREAT CHRONIC HEPATITIS C: RISK OF INTERACTION WITH VITAMIN K ANTAGONISTS AND CHANGES IN INR (JANUARY 2017)

A EU-wide review has identified that changes in liver function, secondary to hepatitis C treatment with direct-acting antivirals, may affect the efficacy of vitamin K antagonists; the MHRA has advised that INR should be monitored closely in patients receiving concomitant treatment.

- **CONTRA-INDICATIONS** Avoid use within 48 hours postpartum · haemorrhagic stroke · significant bleeding
- **CAUTIONS** Bacterial endocarditis (use only if warfarin otherwise indicated) · conditions in which risk of bleeding is increased · history of gastrointestinal bleeding · hyperthyroidism · hypothyroidism · peptic ulcer · postpartum (delay warfarin until risk of haemorrhage is low—usually 5–7 days after delivery) · recent ischaemic stroke · recent surgery · uncontrolled hypertension
- **SIDE-EFFECTS**
  - **Common or very common** Haemorrhage
  - **Rare or very rare** Alopecia · nausea · vomiting
  - **Frequency not known** Blue toe syndrome · CNS haemorrhage · diarrhoea · fever · haemothorax · jaundice · pancreatitis · skin necrosis (increased risk in patients with protein C or protein S deficiency) · skin reactions
- **CONCEPTION AND CONTRACEPTION** Women of child-bearing age should be warned of the danger of teratogenicity.
- **PREGNANCY** Should not be given in the first trimester of pregnancy. Warfarin, acenocoumarol, and phenindione cross the placenta with risk of congenital malformations, and placental, fetal, or neonatal haemorrhage, especially during the last few weeks of pregnancy and at delivery. Therefore, if at all possible, they should be avoided in pregnancy, especially in the first and third trimesters (difficult decisions may have to be made, particularly in women with prosthetic heart valves, atrial fibrillation, or with a history of recurrent venous thrombosis or pulmonary embolism). Stopping these drugs before the sixth week of gestation may largely avoid the risk of fetal abnormality.
- **HEPATIC IMPAIRMENT** In general, manufacturers advise caution in mild to moderate impairment; avoid in severe impairment.
- **MONITORING REQUIREMENTS**
  - The base-line prothrombin time should be determined but the initial dose should not be delayed whilst awaiting the result.
  - It is essential that the INR be determined daily or on alternate days in early days of treatment, *then* at longer intervals (depending on response), *then* up to every 12 weeks.
  - Change in patient's clinical condition, particularly associated with liver disease, intercurrent illness, or drug administration, necessitates more frequent testing.
- **PATIENT AND CARER ADVICE** Anticoagulant treatment booklets should be issued to all patients or their carers; these booklets include advice for patients on anticoagulant treatment, an alert card to be carried by the patient at all times, and a section for recording of INR results and dosage information. In **England**, **Wales**, and **Northern Ireland**, they are available for purchase from:
  3M Security Print and Systems Limited
  Gorse Street, Chadderton
  Oldham
  OL9 9QH
  Tel: 0845 610 1112
  GP practices can obtain supplies through their Local Area Team stores. NHS Trusts can order supplies from www.nhsforms.co.uk or by emailing nhsforms@spsl.uk.com.
  In **Scotland**, treatment booklets and starter information packs can be obtained by emailing stockorders.DPPAS@apsgroup.co.uk or by fax on (0131) 6299 967
  Electronic copies of the booklets and further advice are also available at www.npsa.nhs.uk/nrls/alerts-and-directives/alerts/anticoagulant.

above

Warfarin sodium

10-Oct-2016

- **INDICATIONS AND DOSE**

Treatment and prophylaxis of thrombotic episodes (induction)

- BY MOUTH
  - Neonate (initiated under specialist supervision): Initially 200 micrograms/kg for 1 dose on day 1, then reduced to 100 micrograms/kg once daily for the following 3 days, subsequent doses dependent on INR levels, induction dose may need to be altered according to condition (e.g. abnormal liver function tests, cardiac failure), concomitant interacting drugs, and if baseline INR above 1.3.
  - Child: Initially 200 micrograms/kg (max. per dose 10 mg) for 1 dose on day 1, then reduced to 100 micrograms/kg once daily (max. per dose 5 mg) for the following 3 days, subsequent doses adjusted according to INR levels, induction dose may continued →

need to be altered according to condition (e.g. abnormal liver function tests, cardiac failure), concomitant interacting drugs, and if baseline INR above 1.3

Treatment and prophylaxis of thrombotic episodes following induction dose (if INR still below 1.4)

▶ BY MOUTH

- Neonate (under expert supervision): 200 micrograms/kg once daily.
- Child: 200 micrograms/kg once daily (max. per dose 10 mg)

Treatment and prophylaxis of thrombotic episodes following induction dose (if INR above 3.0)

▶ BY MOUTH

- Neonate (under expert supervision): 50 micrograms/kg once daily.
- Child: 50 micrograms/kg once daily (max. per dose 2.5 mg)

Treatment and prophylaxis of thrombotic episodes following induction dose (if INR above 3.5)

▶ BY MOUTH

- Neonate (under expert supervision): Dose to be omitted.
- Child: Dose to be omitted

Treatment and prophylaxis of thrombotic episodes (usual maintenance)

▶ BY MOUTH

- Neonate (under expert supervision): Maintenance 100–300 micrograms/kg once daily, doses up to 400 micrograms/kg once daily may be required especially if bottle fed, to be adjusted according to INR.
- Child: Maintenance 100–300 micrograms/kg once daily, doses up to 400 micrograms/kg once daily may be required especially if bottle fed, to be adjusted according to INR

- UNLICENSED USE Not licensed for use in children.

> **IMPORTANT SAFETY INFORMATION**
>
> MHRA/CHM ADVICE: WARFARIN: REPORTS OF CALCIPHYLAXIS (JULY 2016)
>
> An EU-wide review has concluded that on rare occasions, warfarin use may lead to calciphylaxis—patients should be advised to consult their doctor if they develop a painful skin rash; if calciphylaxis is diagnosed, appropriate treatment should be started and consideration should be given to stopping treatment with warfarin. The MHRA has advised that calciphylaxis is most commonly observed in patients with known risk factors such as end-stage renal disease, however cases have also been reported in patients with normal renal function.

- INTERACTIONS → Appendix 1: coumarins
- SIDE-EFFECTS Calciphylaxis · hepatic function abnormal
- PREGNANCY Babies of mothers taking warfarin at the time of delivery need to be offered immediate prophylaxis with intramuscular phytomenadione (vitamin K_1).
- BREAST FEEDING Not present in milk in significant amounts and appears safe. Risk of haemorrhage which is increased by vitamin K deficiency.
- RENAL IMPAIRMENT Use with caution in mild to moderate impairment.
  Monitoring In severe renal impairment, monitor INR more frequently.
- PRESCRIBING AND DISPENSING INFORMATION
  Dietary differences Infant formula is supplemented with vitamin K, which makes formula-fed infants resistant to warfarin; they may therefore need higher doses. In contrast breast milk contains low concentrations of vitamin K making breast-fed infants more sensitive to warfarin.
- PATIENT AND CARER ADVICE Anticoagulant card to be provided.
  Medicines for Children leaflet: Warfarin for the treatment and prevention of thrombosis www.medicinesforchildren.org.uk/warfarin-treatment-and-prevention-thrombosis

- MEDICINAL FORMS There can be variation in the licensing of different medicines containing the same drug. Forms available from special-order manufacturers include: oral suspension, oral solution

Oral suspension

CAUTIONARY AND ADVISORY LABELS 10

▸ Warfarin sodium (Non-proprietary)
Warfarin sodium 1 mg per 1 ml Warfarin 1mg/ml oral suspension sugar-free | 150 ml PoM £110.53 DT = £108.00

Tablet

CAUTIONARY AND ADVISORY LABELS 10

▸ Warfarin sodium (Non-proprietary)
Warfarin sodium 500 microgram Warfarin 500microgram tablets | 28 tablet PoM £1.70 DT = £1.41
Warfarin sodium 1 mg Warfarin 1mg tablets | 28 tablet PoM £1.16 DT = £0.82 | 500 tablet PoM £9.46
Warfarin sodium 3 mg Warfarin 3mg tablets | 28 tablet PoM £1.20 DT = £0.86 | 500 tablet PoM £11.07
Warfarin sodium 5 mg Warfarin 5mg tablets | 28 tablet PoM £1.29 DT = £0.97 | 500 tablet PoM £26.79

▸ Coumadin (Imported (Canada))
Warfarin sodium 4 mg Coumadin 4mg tablets | 100 tablet PoM

4 Blood pressure conditions

4.1 Hypertension

Hypertension

Overview

Hypertension in children and adolescents can have a substantial effect on long-term health. Possible causes of hypertension (e.g. congenital heart disease, renal disease and endocrine disorders) and the presence of any complications (e.g. left ventricular hypertrophy) should be established. Treatment should take account of contributory factors and any factors that increase the risk of cardiovascular complications.

Serious hypertension is rare in *neonates* but it can present with signs of congestive heart failure; the cause is often renal and can follow embolic arterial damage.

Children (or their parents or carers) should be given advice on lifestyle changes to reduce blood pressure or cardiovascular risk; these include weight reduction (in obese children), reduction of dietary salt, reduction of total and saturated fat, increasing exercise, increasing fruit and vegetable intake, and not smoking.

Indications for antihypertensive therapy in children include symptomatic hypertension, secondary hypertension, hypertensive target-organ damage, diabetes mellitus, persistent hypertension despite lifestyle measures, and pulmonary hypertension. The effect of antihypertensive treatment on growth and development is not known; treatment should be started only if benefits are clear.

Antihypertensive therapy should be initiated with a single drug at the lowest recommended dose; the dose can be increased until the target blood pressure is achieved. Once the highest recommended dose is reached, or sooner if the patient begins to experience side-effects, a second drug may be added if blood pressure is not controlled. If more than one drug is required, these should be given as separate products to allow dose adjustment of individual drugs, but fixed-dose combination products may be useful in adolescents if compliance is a problem.

Acceptable drug classes for use in children with hypertension include **ACE inhibitors**, **alpha-blockers**, **beta-blockers**, **calcium-channel blockers**, and **thiazide diuretics**. There is limited information on the use of **angiotensin-II receptor antagonists** in children. Diuretics and beta-blockers have a long history of safety and efficacy in children. The newer classes of antihypertensive drugs, including ACE inhibitors and calcium-channel blockers have been shown to be safe and effective in short-term studies in children. Refractory hypertension may require additional treatment with agents such as minoxidil p. 124 or clonidine hydrochloride p. 108.

Cardiovascular risk reduction

Aspirin p. 98 may be used to reduce the risk of cardiovascular events; however, concerns about an increased risk of bleeding and Reye's syndrome need to be considered.

A **statin** can be of benefit in older children who have a high risk of cardiovascular disease and have hypercholesterolaemia.

Hypertension in diabetes

Hypertension can occur in type 2 diabetes and treatment prevents both macrovascular and microvascular complications. ACE inhibitors may be considered in children with diabetes and microalbuminaemia or proteinuric renal disease. Beta-blockers are best avoided in children with, or at a high risk of developing, diabetes, especially when combined with a thiazide diuretic.

Hypertension in renal disease

ACE inhibitors may be considered in children with micro-albuminuria or proteinuric renal disease. High doses of loop diuretics may be required. Specific cautions apply to the use of ACE inhibitors in renal impairment, but ACE inhibitors may be effective. Dihydropyridine calcium-channel blockers may be added.

Hypertension in pregnancy

High blood pressure in pregnancy may usually be due to pre-existing essential hypertension or to pre-eclampsia. Methyldopa is safe in pregnancy. Beta-blockers are effective and safe in the third trimester. Modified-release preparations of nifedipine [unlicensed] p. 115 are also used for hypertension in pregnancy. Intravenous administration of labetalol hydrochloride p. 110 can be used to control hypertensive crises; alternatively hydralazine hydrochloride p. 123 can be given by the intravenous route.

Hypertensive emergencies

Hypertensive emergencies in children may be accompanied by signs of hypertensive encephalopathy, including seizures. Controlled reduction in blood pressure over 72–96 hours is essential; rapid reduction can reduce perfusion leading to organ damage. Treatment should be initiated with intravenous drugs; once blood pressure is controlled, oral therapy can be started. It may be necessary to infuse fluids particularly during the first 12 hours to expand plasma volume should the blood pressure drop too rapidly.

Controlled reduction of blood pressure is achieved by intravenous administration of labetalol hydrochloride or sodium nitroprusside p. 124. Esmolol hydrochloride p. 113 is useful for short-term use and has a short duration of action. Nicardipine hydrochloride p. 115 can be administered as a continuous intravenous infusion for life-threatening hypertension in paediatric intensive care settings. In less severe cases, nifedipine capsules can be used.

Other antihypertensive drugs which can be given intravenously include hydralazine hydrochloride and clonidine hydrochloride.

Hypertension in acute nephritis occurs as a result of sodium and water retention; it should be treated with sodium and fluid restriction, and with furosemide p. 148; antihypertensive drugs may be added if necessary.

Also see advice on short-term management of hypertensive episodes in phaeochromocytoma.

Phaeochromocytoma

Long-term management of phaeochromocytoma involves surgery. However, surgery should not take place until there is adequate blockade of both alpha- and beta-adrenoceptors. Alpha-blockers are used in the short-term management of hypertensive episodes in phaeochromocytoma. Once alpha blockade is established, tachycardia can be controlled by the cautious addition of a beta-blocker; a cardioselective beta-blocker is preferred. There is no nationwide consensus on the optimal drug regimen or doses used for the management of phaeochromocytoma.

Phenoxybenzamine hydrochloride p. 124, a powerful alpha-blocker, is effective in the management of phaeochromocytoma but it has many side-effects.

Pulmonary hypertension

Only pulmonary *arterial* hypertension is currently suitable for drug treatment. Pulmonary arterial hypertension includes persistent pulmonary hypertension of the newborn, idiopathic pulmonary arterial hypertension in children, and pulmonary hypertension related to congenital heart disease and cardiac surgery.

Some types of pulmonary hypertension are treated with vasodilator antihypertensive therapy and oxygen. Diuretics may also have a role in children with right-sided heart failure.

Initial treatment of *persistent pulmonary hypertension of the newborn* involves the administration of **nitric oxide**; epoprostenol p. 126 can be used until nitric oxide is available. Oral sildenafil p. 125 may be helpful in less severe cases. Epoprostenol and sildenafil can cause profound systemic hypotension. In rare circumstances either tolazoline p. 128 or magnesium sulfate p. 646 can be given by intravenous infusion when nitric oxide and epoprostenol have failed.

Treatment of *idiopathic pulmonary arterial hypertension* is determined by acute vasodilator testing; drugs used for treatment include calcium-channel blockers (usually nifedipine), long-term intravenous epoprostenol, nebulised iloprost p. 127, bosentan p. 125, or sildenafil. Anticoagulation (usually with warfarin sodium p. 103) may also be required to prevent secondary thrombosis.

Inhaled nitric oxide is a potent and selective pulmonary vasodilator. It acts on cyclic guanosine monophosphate (cGMP) resulting in smooth muscle relaxation. Inhaled nitric oxide is used in the treatment of persistent pulmonary hypertension of the newborn, and may also be useful in other forms of arterial pulmonary hypertension. Dependency can occur with high doses and prolonged use; to avoid rebound pulmonary hypertension the drug should be withdrawn gradually, often with the aid of sildenafil p. 125.

Excess nitric oxide can cause methaemoglobinaemia; therefore, methaemoglobin concentration should be measured regularly, particularly in neonates.

Nitric oxide increases the risk of haemorrhage by inhibiting platelet aggregation, but it does not usually cause bleeding.

Epoprostenol (prostacyclin) p. 126 is a prostaglandin and a potent vasodilator. It is used in the treatment of persistent pulmonary hypertension of the newborn, idiopathic pulmonary arterial hypertension, and in the acute phase following cardiac surgery. It is given by continuous 24-hour intravenous infusion.

Epoprostenol is a powerful inhibitor of platelet aggregation and there is a possible risk of haemorrhage. It is sometimes used as an antiplatelet in renal dialysis when heparins are unsuitable or contra-indicated. It can also cause serious systemic hypotension and, if withdrawn suddenly, can cause pulmonary hypertensive crisis.

Children on prolonged treatment can become tolerant to epoprostenol, and therefore require an increase in dose.

Iloprost p. 127 is a synthetic analogue of epoprostenol and is efficacious when nebulised in adults with pulmonary arterial hypertension, but experience in children is limited. It is more stable than epoprostenol and has a longer half-life.

Bosentan p. 125 is a dual endothelin receptor antagonist used orally in the treatment of pulmonary arterial hypertension. The concentration of endothelin, a potent vasoconstrictor, is raised in sustained pulmonary hypertension.

Sildenafil, a vasodilator developed for the treatment of erectile dysfunction, is also used for pulmonary arterial hypertension. It is used either alone or as an adjunct to other drugs.

Sildenafil is a selective phosphodiesterase type-5 inhibitor. Inhibition of this enzyme in the lungs enhances the vasodilatory effects of nitric oxide and promotes relaxation of vascular smooth muscle.

Sildenafil has also been used in pulmonary hypertension for weaning children off inhaled nitric oxide following cardiac surgery, and less successfully in idiopathic pulmonary arterial hypertension.

Tolazoline p. 128 is now rarely used to correct pulmonary artery vasospasm in pulmonary hypertension of the newborn as better alternatives are available. Tolazoline is an alpha-blocker and produces both pulmonary and systemic vasodilation.

Advanced Pharmacy Services

Children with hypertension may be eligible for the New Medicines Service / Medicines Use Review service provided by a community pharmacist. For further information, see *Advanced Pharmacy Services* in Medicines optimisation p. 25.

Antihypertensive drugs

Vasodilator antihypertensive drugs

Vasodilators have a potent hypotensive effect, especially when used in combination with a beta-blocker and a thiazide. **Important:** see Hypertension (hypertensive emergencies) for a warning on the hazards of a very rapid fall in blood pressure.

Hydralazine hydrochloride p. 123 is given by mouth as an adjunct to other antihypertensives for the treatment of resistant hypertension but is rarely used; when used alone it causes tachycardia and fluid retention.

Sodium nitroprusside p. 124 is given by intravenous infusion to control severe hypertensive crisis when parenteral treatment is necessary. At low doses it reduces systemic vascular resistance and increases cardiac output; at high doses it can produce profound systemic hypotension—continuous blood pressure monitoring is therefore essential. Sodium nitroprusside may also be used to control paradoxical hypertension after surgery for coarctation of the aorta.

Minoxidil p. 124 should be reserved for the treatment of severe hypertension resistant to other drugs. Vasodilatation is accompanied by increased cardiac output and tachycardia and children develop fluid retention. For this reason the addition of a beta-blocker and a diuretic (usually furosemide p. 148, in high dosage) are mandatory. Hypertrichosis is troublesome and renders this drug unsuitable for females.

Prazosin p. 107 and doxazosin p. 529 have alpha-blocking and vasodilator properties.

Centrally acting antihypertensive drugs

Methyldopa, a centrally acting antihypertensive, is of little value in the management of refractory sustained hypertension in infants and children. On prolonged use it is associated with fluid retention (which may be alleviated by concomitant use of diuretics).

Methyldopa is also effective for the management of hypertension in pregnancy.

Clonidine hydrochloride p. 108 is also a centrally acting antihypertensive but has the disadvantage that sudden withdrawal may cause a hypertensive crisis. Clonidine hydrochloride is also used under specialist supervision for pain management, sedation, and opioid withdrawal, attention deficit hyperactivity disorder, and Tourette syndrome.

Adrenergic neurone blocking drugs

Adrenergic neurone blocking drugs prevent the release of noradrenaline from postganglionic adrenergic neurones. These drugs do not control supine blood pressure and may cause postural hypotension. For this reason they have largely fallen from use in adults and are rarely used in children.

Alpha-adrenoceptor blocking drugs

Doxazosin and prazosin have post-synaptic alpha-blocking and vasodilator properties and rarely cause tachycardia. They can, however, reduce blood pressure rapidly after the first dose and should be introduced with caution.

Alpha-blockers can be used with other antihypertensive drugs in the treatment of resistant hypertension.

Drugs affecting the renin-angiotensin system

Angiotensin-converting enzyme inhibitors

Angiotensin-converting enzyme inhibitors (ACE inhibitors) inhibit the conversion of angiotensin I to angiotensin II. The main indications of ACE inhibitors in children are shown below. In infants and young children, captopril p. 118 is often considered first.

Initiation under specialist supervision

Treatment with ACE inhibitors should be initiated under specialist supervision and with careful clinical monitoring in children.

Heart failure

ACE inhibitors have a valuable role in all grades of heart failure, usually combined with a loop diuretic. Potassium supplements and potassium-sparing diuretics should be discontinued before introducing an ACE inhibitor because of the risk of hyperkalaemia. Profound first-dose hypotension can occur when ACE inhibitors are introduced to children with heart failure who are already taking a high dose of a loop diuretic. Temporary withdrawal of the loop diuretic reduces the risk, but can cause severe rebound pulmonary oedema.

Hypertension

ACE inhibitors may be considered for hypertension when thiazides and beta-blockers are contra-indicated, not tolerated, or fail to control blood pressure; they may be considered for hypertension in children with type 1 diabetes with nephropathy. ACE inhibitors can reduce blood pressure very rapidly in some patients particularly in those receiving diuretic therapy.

Diabetic nephropathy
ACE inhibitors also have a role in the management of diabetic nephropathy.

Renal effects
Renal function and electrolytes should be checked before starting ACE inhibitors (or increasing the dose) and monitored during treatment (more frequently if features mentioned below are present). Hyperkalaemia and other side-effects of ACE inhibitors are more common in children with impaired renal function and the dose may need to be reduced.

Concomitant treatment with NSAIDs increases the risk of renal damage, and potassium-sparing diuretics (or potassium-containing salt substitutes) increase the risk of hyperkalaemia.

In children with severe bilateral renal artery stenosis (or severe stenosis of the artery supplying a single functioning kidney), ACE inhibitors reduce or abolish glomerular filtration and are likely to cause severe and progressive renal failure. They are therefore contra-indicated in children known to have these forms of critical renovascular disease.

ACE inhibitor treatment is unlikely to have an adverse effect on overall renal function in children with severe unilateral renal artery stenosis and a normal contralateral kidney, but glomerular filtration is likely to be reduced (or even abolished) in the affected kidney and the long-term consequences are unknown.

ACE inhibitors are therefore best avoided in those with known or suspected renovascular disease, unless the blood pressure cannot be controlled by other drugs. If they are used in these circumstances renal function needs to be monitored.

ACE inhibitors should also be used with particular caution in children who may have undiagnosed and clinically silent renovascular disease. ACE inhibitors are useful for the management of hypertension and proteinuria in children with nephritis. They are thought to have a beneficial effect by reducing intra-glomerular hypertension and protecting the glomerular capillaries and membrane.

ACE inhibitors in combination with other drugs
Concomitant diuretics
ACE inhibitors can cause a very rapid fall in blood pressure in volume-depleted children; treatment should therefore be initiated with very low doses. In some children the diuretic dose may need to be reduced or the diuretic discontinued at least 24 hours beforehand (may not be possible in heart failure—risk of pulmonary oedema). If high-dose diuretic therapy cannot be stopped, close observation is recommended after administration of the first dose of ACE inhibitor, for at least 2 hours or until the blood pressure has stabilised.

Angiotensin-II receptor antagonists

Candesartan cilexetil p. 121, losartan potassium p. 122 and valsartan p. 122 are specific angiotensin-II receptor antagonists with many properties similar to those of the ACE inhibitors. However, unlike ACE inhibitors, they do not inhibit the breakdown of bradykinin and other kinins, and thus are less likely to cause the persistent dry cough which can complicate ACE inhibitor therapy. They are therefore a useful alternative for children who have to discontinue an ACE inhibitor because of persistent cough.

Candesartan cilexetil, losartan potassium or valsartan can be used as an alternative to an ACE inhibitor in the management of hypertension.

Renal effects
Angiotensin-II receptor antagonists should be used with caution in renal artery stenosis (see also Renal effects under ACE Inhibitors, above).

Neonates

The neonatal response to treatment with ACE inhibitors is very variable, and some neonates develop profound hypotension with even small doses; a test-dose should be used initially and increased cautiously. Adverse effects such as apnoea, seizures, renal failure, and severe unpredictable hypotension are very common in the first month of life and it is therefore recommended that ACE inhibitors are avoided whenever possible, particularly in preterm neonates.

Other drugs used for Hypertension Amiloride hydrochloride, p. 149 · Chlortalidone, p. 150 · Metolazone, p. 150

ALPHA-ADRENOCEPTOR BLOCKERS

Prazosin 09-Feb-2020

● **INDICATIONS AND DOSE**

Hypertension
▶ BY MOUTH
▸ Child 1 month–11 years: Initially 10–15 micrograms/kg 2–4 times a day, initial dose to be taken at bedtime, then increased to 500 micrograms/kg daily in divided doses, dose to be increased gradually; maximum 20 mg per day
▸ Child 12–17 years: Initially 500 micrograms 2–3 times a day for 3-7 days, initial dose to be taken at bedtime, then increased to 1 mg 2–3 times a day for a further 3–7 days, then increased if necessary up to 20 mg daily in divided doses, dose should be increased gradually

Congestive heart failure (rarely used)
▶ BY MOUTH
▸ Child 1 month–11 years: 5 micrograms/kg twice daily, initial dose to be taken at bedtime, then increased to 100 micrograms/kg daily in divided doses, doses should be increased gradually
▸ Child 12–17 years: 500 micrograms 2–4 times a day, initial dose to be taken at bedtime, then increased to 4 mg daily in divided doses; maintenance 4–20 mg daily in divided doses

● **UNLICENSED USE** Not licensed for use in children under 12 years.

● **CONTRA-INDICATIONS** History of postural hypotension · not recommended for congestive heart failure due to mechanical obstruction (e.g. aortic stenosis)

● **CAUTIONS** Cataract surgery (risk of intra-operative floppy iris syndrome) · first dose hypotension

● **INTERACTIONS** → Appendix 1: alpha blockers

● **SIDE-EFFECTS**
▶ **Common or very common** Asthenia · constipation · depression · diarrhoea · dizziness · drowsiness · dry mouth · dyspnoea · headache · nasal congestion · nausea · nervousness · oedema · palpitations · postural hypotension · sexual dysfunction · skin reactions · syncope · urinary disorders · vertigo · vision blurred · vomiting
▶ **Uncommon** Angina pectoris · arrhythmias · arthralgia · epistaxis · eye pain · eye redness · gastrointestinal discomfort · hyperhidrosis · paraesthesia · sleep disorders · tinnitus
▶ **Rare or very rare** Alopecia · fever · flushing · gynaecomastia · hallucination · hepatic function abnormal · pain · pancreatitis · vasculitis

● **PREGNANCY** No evidence of teratogenicity; manufacturers advise use only when potential benefit outweighs risk.

● **BREAST FEEDING** Present in milk, amount probably too small to be harmful; manufacturer advises use with caution.

- **HEPATIC IMPAIRMENT** Manufacturer advises caution (no information available).
  Dose adjustments In children 12 years and above, manufacturer advises initial dose reduction to 500 micrograms daily; increased with caution.
- **RENAL IMPAIRMENT**
  Dose adjustments Start with low doses in moderate to severe impairment; increase with caution.
- **DIRECTIONS FOR ADMINISTRATION** For administration *by mouth*, tablets may be dispersed in water.
- **PATIENT AND CARER ADVICE**
  First dose effect First dose may cause collapse due to hypotensive effect (therefore should be taken on retiring to bed).
  Driving and skilled tasks May affect performance of skilled tasks e.g. driving.

- **MEDICINAL FORMS** There can be variation in the licensing of different medicines containing the same drug. Forms available from special-order manufacturers include: tablet, oral suspension, oral solution

Tablet

- Minipress (Imported (Australia))
  Prazosin (as Prazosin hydrochloride) 2 mg Minipress 2mg tablets | 100 tablet PoM
  Prazosin (as Prazosin hydrochloride) 5 mg Minipress 5mg tablets | 100 tablet PoM
- Hypovase (Pfizer Ltd)
  Prazosin (as Prazosin hydrochloride) 500 microgram Hypovase 500microgram tablets | 60 tablet PoM £2.69 DT = £2.69
  Prazosin (as Prazosin hydrochloride) 1 mg Hypovase 1mg tablets | 60 tablet PoM £3.46 DT = £3.46

ANTIHYPERTENSIVES, CENTRALLY ACTING

Clonidine hydrochloride

15-Jan-2020

- **INDICATIONS AND DOSE**

Severe hypertension

- BY MOUTH
- Child 2–17 years: Initially 0.5–1 microgram/kg 3 times a day, then increased if necessary up to 25 micrograms/kg daily in divided doses, increase dose gradually; maximum 1.2 mg per day
- BY SLOW INTRAVENOUS INJECTION
- Child 2–17 years: 2–6 micrograms/kg (max. per dose 300 micrograms) for 1 dose

- **UNLICENSED USE** Not licensed for use in children.
- **CONTRA-INDICATIONS** Severe bradyarrhythmia secondary to second- or third-degree AV block or sick sinus syndrome
- **CAUTIONS** Cerebrovascular disease · constipation · heart failure · history of depression · mild to moderate bradyarrhythmia · polyneuropathy · Raynaud's syndrome or other occlusive peripheral vascular disease
- **INTERACTIONS** → Appendix 1: clonidine
- **SIDE-EFFECTS**
- **Common or very common** Constipation · depression · dizziness · dry mouth · fatigue · headache · nausea · postural hypotension · salivary gland pain · sedation · sexual dysfunction · sleep disorders · vomiting
- **Uncommon** Delusions · hallucination · malaise · paraesthesia · Raynaud's phenomenon · skin reactions
- **Rare or very rare** Alopecia · atrioventricular block · dry eye · gynaecomastia · intestinal pseudo-obstruction · nasal dryness
- **Frequency not known** Accommodation disorder · arrhythmias · confusion
- **PREGNANCY** May lower fetal heart rate. Avoid oral use unless potential benefit outweighs risk. Avoid using injection.
- **BREAST FEEDING** Avoid—present in milk.
- **RENAL IMPAIRMENT** Use with caution.
- **TREATMENT CESSATION** Must be withdrawn gradually to avoid hypertensive crisis.
- **DIRECTIONS FOR ADMINISTRATION**
- With intravenous use For *intravenous injection*, give over 10–15 minutes; compatible with Sodium Chloride 0.9% *or* Glucose 5%.
- With oral use For administration *by mouth*, tablets may be crushed and dissolved in water.
- **PATIENT AND CARER ADVICE**
  Medicines for Children leaflet: Clonidine for Tourette's syndrome, ADHD and sleep-onset disorder www.medicinesforchildren.org.uk/clonidine-tourettes-syndrome-adhd-and-sleep-onset-disorder
  Driving and skilled tasks Drowsiness may affect performance of skilled tasks (e.g. driving); effects of alcohol may be enhanced.
- **LESS SUITABLE FOR PRESCRIBING** Clonidine is less suitable for prescribing.

- **MEDICINAL FORMS** There can be variation in the licensing of different medicines containing the same drug. Forms available from special-order manufacturers include: oral suspension, oral solution, solution for injection

Tablet

CAUTIONARY AND ADVISORY LABELS 3, 8

- Clonidine hydrochloride (Non-proprietary)
  Clonidine hydrochloride 25 microgram Clonidine 25microgram tablets | 112 tablet PoM £14.44 DT = £4.58
- Catapres (Boehringer Ingelheim Ltd)
  Clonidine hydrochloride 100 microgram Catapres 100microgram tablets | 100 tablet PoM £8.04 DT = £8.04

Solution for injection

- Catapres (Boehringer Ingelheim Ltd)
  Clonidine hydrochloride 150 microgram per 1 ml Catapres 150micrograms/1ml solution for injection ampoules | 5 ampoule PoM £2.09

Oral solution

- Clonidine hydrochloride (Non-proprietary)
  Clonidine hydrochloride 10 microgram per 1 ml Clonidine 50micrograms/5ml oral solution sugar-free | 100 ml PoM £86.69 DT = £85.73

BETA-ADRENOCEPTOR BLOCKERS

Beta-adrenoceptor blocking drugs

Overview

Beta-adrenoceptor blocking drugs (beta-blockers) block the beta-adrenoceptors in the heart, peripheral vasculature, bronchi, pancreas, and liver.

Many beta-blockers are available but experience in children is limited to the use of only a few.

Differences between beta-blockers may affect choice. Water-soluble beta-blockers (such as atenolol p. 112 and sotalol hydrochloride p. 85) are less likely to enter the brain and may therefore cause less sleep disturbance and nightmares. Water-soluble beta-blockers are excreted by the kidneys and dosage reduction is often necessary in renal impairment.

Some beta-blockers, such as atenolol, have an intrinsically longer duration of action and need to be given only once daily. Carvedilol p. 132 and labetalol hydrochloride p. 110 are beta-blockers which have, in addition, an arteriolar vasodilating action and thus lower peripheral resistance. Although carvedilol and labetalol hydrochloride possess both alpha- and beta-blocking properties, these drugs have no important advantages over other beta-blockers in the treatment of hypertension.

Beta-blockers slow the heart and can depress the myocardium; they are contra-indicated in children with second- or third-degree heart block.

Beta-blockers can precipitate asthma and should usually be avoided in children with a history of asthma or bronchospasm. If there is no alternative, a child with well-controlled asthma can be treated for a co-existing condition (e.g. arrhythmia) with a cardioselective beta-blocker, which should be initiated with caution at a low dose by a specialist and the child monitored closely for adverse effects. Atenolol and metoprolol tartrate p. 113 have less effect on the $beta_2$ (bronchial) receptors and are, therefore, relatively *cardioselective*, but they are not *cardiospecific*; they have a lesser effect on airways resistance but are not free of this side-effect.

Beta-blockers are also associated with fatigue, coldness of the extremities, and sleep disturbances with nightmares (may be less common with the water-soluble beta-blockers).

Beta-blockers can affect carbohydrate metabolism causing hypoglycaemia or hyperglycaemia in children with or without diabetes; they can also interfere with metabolic and autonomic responses to hypoglycaemia thereby masking symptoms such as tachycardia. However, beta-blockers are not contra-indicated in diabetes, although the cardioselective beta-blockers (e.g. atenolol and metoprolol tartrate) may be preferred. Beta-blockers should be avoided altogether in those with frequent episodes of hypoglycaemia.

Hypertension

Beta-blockers are effective for reducing blood pressure, but their mode of action is not understood; they reduce cardiac output, alter baroceptor reflex sensitivity, and block peripheral adrenoceptors. Some beta-blockers depress plasma renin secretion. It is possible that a central effect may also partly explain their mode of action. Blood pressure can usually be controlled with relatively few side-effects. In general the dose of beta-blocker does not have to be high.

Labetalol hydrochloride may be given intravenously for *hypertensive emergencies* in children; however, care is needed to avoid dangerous hypotension or beta-blockade, particularly in neonates. Esmolol hydrochloride p. 113 is also used intravenously for the treatment of hypertension particularly in the peri-operative period.

Beta-blockers can be used to control the pulse rate in children with *phaeochromocytoma*. However, they should never be used alone as beta-blockade without concurrent alpha-blockade may lead to a hypertensive crisis; phenoxybenzamine hydrochloride p. 124 should always be used together with the beta-blocker.

Arrhythmias

In arrhythmias, beta-blockers act principally by attenuating the effects of the sympathetic system on automaticity and conductivity within the heart. They can be used alone or in conjunction with digoxin p. 86 to control the ventricular rate in *atrial fibrillation*. Beta-blockers are also useful in the management of *supraventricular tachycardias* and *ventricular tachycardias* particularly to prevent recurrence of the tachycardia.

Esmolol hydrochloride is a relatively cardioselective beta-blocker with a very short duration of action, used intravenously for the short-term treatment of supraventricular arrhythmias and sinus tachycardia, particularly in the peri-operative period.

Sotalol hydrochloride is a non-cardioselective beta-blocker with additional class III anti-arrhythmic activity. Atenolol and sotalol hydrochloride suppress ventricular ectopic beats and non-sustained ventricular tachycardia. However, the pro-arrhythmic effects of sotalol hydrochloride, particularly in children with sick sinus syndrome, may prolong the QT interval and induce torsade de pointes.

Heart failure

Beta-blockers may produce benefit in heart failure by blocking sympathetic activity and the addition of a beta-blocker such as carvedilol to other treatment for heart failure may be beneficial. Treatment should be initiated by those experienced in the management of heart failure.

Thyrotoxicosis

Beta-blockers are used in the management of *thyrotoxicosis* including neonatal thyrotoxicosis; propranolol hydrochloride p. 111 can reverse clinical symptoms within 4 days. Beta-blockers are also used for the pre-operative preparation for thyroidectomy; the thyroid gland is rendered less vascular, thus facilitating surgery.

Other uses

In tetralogy of Fallot, esmolol hydrochloride or propranolol hydrochloride may be given intravenously in the initial management of *cyanotic spells*; propranolol hydrochloride is given by mouth for preventing cyanotic spells. If a severe cyanotic spell in a child with congenital heart disease persists despite optimal use of 100% oxygen, propranolol hydrochloride is given by intravenous infusion. If cyanosis is still present after 10 minutes, sodium bicarbonate intravenous infusion p. 634 is given in a dose to correct acidosis (or dose calculated according to arterial blood gas results); sodium bicarbonate 4.2% intravenous infusion is appropriate for a child under 1 year and sodium bicarbonate 8.4% intravenous infusion in children over 1 year. If blood-glucose concentration is less than 3 mmol/litre, glucose 10% intravenous infusion is given, followed by intravenous or intramuscular injection of morphine p. 299.

Beta-blockers are also used in the *prophylaxis of migraine*. Betaxolol p. 734, levobunolol hydrochloride p. 734, and timolol maleate p. 735 are used topically in *glaucoma*.

Beta-adrenoceptor blockers (systemic)

- **CONTRA-INDICATIONS** Asthma · cardiogenic shock · hypotension · marked bradycardia · metabolic acidosis · phaeochromocytoma (apart from specific use with alpha-blockers) · second-degree AV block · severe peripheral arterial disease · sick sinus syndrome · third-degree AV block · uncontrolled heart failure

  CONTRA-INDICATIONS, FURTHER INFORMATION

  ▸ **Bronchospasm** Beta-blockers, including those considered to be cardioselective, should usually be avoided in patients with a history of asthma, bronchospasm or a history of obstructive airways disease. However, when there is no alternative, a cardioselective beta-blocker can be given to these patients with caution and under specialist supervision. In such cases the risk of inducing bronchospasm should be appreciated and appropriate precautions taken.
- **CAUTIONS** Diabetes · first-degree AV block · history of obstructive airways disease (introduce cautiously) · myasthenia gravis · portal hypertension (risk of deterioration in liver function) · psoriasis · symptoms of thyrotoxicosis may be masked
- **SIDE-EFFECTS**

  ▸ **Common or very common** Abdominal discomfort · bradycardia · confusion · depression · diarrhoea · dizziness · dry eye (reversible on discontinuation) · dyspnoea · erectile dysfunction · fatigue · headache · heart failure · nausea · paraesthesia · peripheral coldness · peripheral vascular disease · rash (reversible on discontinuation) · sleep disorders · syncope · visual impairment · vomiting

  ▸ **Uncommon** Atrioventricular block · bronchospasm

  ▸ **Rare or very rare** Hallucination

SIDE-EFFECTS, FURTHER INFORMATION With administration by intravenous injection, excessive bradycardia can occur and may be countered with **intravenous injection** of atropine sulfate.

Overdose Therapeutic overdosages with beta-blockers may cause lightheadedness, dizziness, and possibly syncope as a result of bradycardia and hypotension; heart failure may be precipitated or exacerbated. With administration by intravenous injection, excessive bradycardia can occur and may be countered with intravenous injection of atropine sulfate.

For details on the management of poisoning, see Beta-blockers, under Emergency treatment of poisoning p. 891.

- ALLERGY AND CROSS-SENSITIVITY Caution is advised in patients with a history of hypersensitivity—may increase sensitivity to allergens and result in more serious hypersensitivity response. Furthermore beta-adrenoceptor blockers may reduce response to adrenaline (epinephrine).
- PREGNANCY Beta-blockers may cause intra-uterine growth restriction, neonatal hypoglycaemia, and bradycardia; the risk is greater in severe hypertension.
- BREAST FEEDING With systemic use in the mother, infants should be monitored as there is a risk of possible toxicity due to beta-blockade. However, the amount of most beta-blockers present in milk is too small to affect infants.
- MONITORING REQUIREMENTS Monitor lung function (in patients with a history of obstructive airway disease).
- TREATMENT CESSATION Avoid abrupt withdrawal.

BETA-ADRENOCEPTOR BLOCKERS ›
ALPHA- AND BETA-ADRENOCEPTOR BLOCKERS

F 109

Labetalol hydrochloride

10-Mar-2020

- INDICATIONS AND DOSE

Hypertensive emergencies

▶ BY INTRAVENOUS INFUSION

- Neonate: Initially 0.5 mg/kg/hour (max. per dose 4 mg/kg/hour), dose to be adjusted according to response at intervals of at least 15 minutes.
- Child 1 month–11 years: Initially 0.5–1 mg/kg/hour (max. per dose 3 mg/kg/hour), dose to be adjusted according to response at intervals of at least 15 minutes
- Child 12–17 years: Initially 30–120 mg/hour, dose to be adjusted according to response at intervals of at least 15 minutes

Hypertension

▶ BY MOUTH

- Child 1 month–11 years: 1–2 mg/kg 3–4 times a day
- Child 12–17 years: Initially 50–100 mg twice daily, dose to be increased if required at intervals of 3–14 days; usual dose 200–400 mg twice daily, higher doses to be given in 3–4 divided doses; maximum 2.4 g per day

▶ BY INTRAVENOUS INJECTION

- Child 1 month–11 years: 250–500 micrograms/kg (max. per dose 20 mg) for 1 dose
- Child 12–17 years: 50 mg, dose to be given over at least 1 minute, then 50 mg after 5 minutes if required; maximum 200 mg per course

- UNLICENSED USE Not licensed for use in children.

IMPORTANT SAFETY INFORMATION

▶ With intravenous use

Consult local guidelines. In hypertensive encephalopathy reduce blood pressure to normotensive level over 24–48 hours (more rapid reduction may lead to cerebral infarction, blindness, and death). If child fitting, reduce blood pressure rapidly, but not to normal levels.

- CAUTIONS Liver damage
- INTERACTIONS → Appendix 1: beta blockers, non-selective
- SIDE-EFFECTS

GENERAL SIDE-EFFECTS

▶ **Common or very common** Drug fever · ejaculation failure · hypersensitivity · urinary disorders
▶ **Rare or very rare** Hepatic disorders · systemic lupus erythematosus (SLE) · toxic myopathy · tremor
▶ **Frequency not known** Alopecia · cyanosis · hyperhidrosis · hyperkalaemia · interstitial lung disease · lethargy · muscle cramps · nasal congestion · peripheral oedema · postural hypotension · psychosis · skin reactions · thrombocytopenia

SPECIFIC SIDE-EFFECTS

▶ With intravenous use Fever · hypoglycaemia masked · thyrotoxicosis masked
▶ With oral use Photosensitivity reaction

- PREGNANCY The use of labetalol in maternal hypertension is not known to be harmful, except possibly in the first trimester. If labetalol is used close to delivery, infants should be monitored for signs of alpha-blockade (as well as beta blockade).
- BREAST FEEDING Infants should be monitored as there is a risk of possible toxicity due to alpha-blockade (in addition to beta-blockade).
- HEPATIC IMPAIRMENT Manufacturer advises caution (risk of slow metabolism).

Dose adjustments Manufacturer advises consider dose reduction.

- RENAL IMPAIRMENT

Dose adjustments Dose reduction may be required.

- MONITORING REQUIREMENTS

▶ Liver damage Severe hepatocellular damage reported after both short-term and long-term treatment. Appropriate laboratory testing needed at first symptom of liver dysfunction and if laboratory evidence of damage (or if jaundice) labetalol should be stopped and not restarted.

- EFFECT ON LABORATORY TESTS Interferes with laboratory tests for catecholamines.
- DIRECTIONS FOR ADMINISTRATION

▶ With intravenous use For *intravenous infusion*, dilute to a concentration of 1 mg/mL in Glucose 5% or Sodium Chloride and Glucose 5%; if fluid restricted may be given undiluted, preferably through a central venous catheter. Avoid upright position during and for 3 hours after intravenous administration.
▶ With oral use For administration *by mouth*, injection may be given orally with squash or juice.

- PATIENT AND CARER ADVICE

Medicines for Children leaflet: Labetalol hydrochloride for hypertension www.medicinesforchildren.org.uk/labetalol-hydrochloride-hypertension

- MEDICINAL FORMS There can be variation in the licensing of different medicines containing the same drug. Forms available from special-order manufacturers include: oral suspension, oral solution

Solution for injection

▶ Labetalol hydrochloride (Non-proprietary)

Labetalol hydrochloride 5 mg per 1 ml Labetalol 100mg/20ml solution for injection ampoules | 5 ampoule PoM £99.34 DT = £98.68 | 5 ampoule PoM £69.00 DT = £98.68 (Hospital only)
Labetalol 50mg/10ml solution for injection ampoules | 10 ampoule PoM [no price] (Hospital only)

Tablet

CAUTIONARY AND ADVISORY LABELS 8, 21

▸ Labetalol hydrochloride (Non-proprietary)

Labetalol hydrochloride 100 mg Labetalol 100mg tablets | 56 tablet PoM £8.56 DT = £6.59

Labetalol hydrochloride 200 mg Labetalol 200mg tablets | 56 tablet PoM £12.68 DT = £9.74

Labetalol hydrochloride 400 mg Labetalol 400mg tablets | 56 tablet PoM £21.12 DT = £19.52

▸ Trandate (RPH Pharmaceuticals AB)

Labetalol hydrochloride 50 mg Trandate 50mg tablets | 56 tablet PoM £3.79 DT = £3.79

Labetalol hydrochloride 100 mg Trandate 100mg tablets | 56 tablet PoM £4.64 DT = £6.59 | 250 tablet PoM £15.62

Labetalol hydrochloride 200 mg Trandate 200mg tablets | 56 tablet PoM £7.41 DT = £9.74 | 250 tablet PoM £24.76

Labetalol hydrochloride 400 mg Trandate 400mg tablets | 56 tablet PoM £10.15 DT = £19.52

BETA-ADRENOCEPTOR BLOCKERS › NON-SELECTIVE

F 109

Propranolol hydrochloride

07-Feb-2018

● **INDICATIONS AND DOSE**

Hyperthyroidism with autonomic symptoms

▶ BY MOUTH

▸ Neonate: Initially 250–500 micrograms/kg every 6–8 hours, adjusted according to response.

▸ Child: Initially 250–500 micrograms/kg every 8 hours, adjusted according to response; increased if necessary up to 1 mg/kg every 8 hours (max. per dose 40 mg every 8 hours)

▶ BY INTRAVENOUS INJECTION

▸ Neonate: Initially 20–50 micrograms/kg every 6–8 hours, adjusted according to response, to be given over 10 minutes.

▸ Child: Initially 25–50 micrograms/kg every 6–8 hours (max. per dose 5 mg), adjusted according to response, to be given over 10 minutes

Thyrotoxicosis (adjunct)

▶ BY MOUTH

▸ Neonate: Initially 250–500 micrograms/kg every 6–8 hours, adjusted according to response.

▸ Child: Initially 250–500 micrograms/kg every 8 hours, adjusted according to response; increased if necessary up to 1 mg/kg every 8 hours (max. per dose 40 mg every 8 hours)

▶ BY INTRAVENOUS INJECTION

▸ Neonate: Initially 20–50 micrograms/kg every 6–8 hours, adjusted according to response, to be given over 10 minutes.

▸ Child: Initially 25–50 micrograms/kg every 6–8 hours (max. per dose 5 mg), adjusted according to response, to be given over 10 minutes

Thyrotoxic crisis

▶ BY MOUTH

▸ Neonate: Initially 250–500 micrograms/kg every 6–8 hours, adjusted according to response.

▸ Child: Initially 250–500 micrograms/kg every 8 hours, adjusted according to response; increased if necessary up to 1 mg/kg every 8 hours (max. per dose 40 mg every 8 hours)

▶ BY INTRAVENOUS INJECTION

▸ Neonate: Initially 20–50 micrograms/kg every 6–8 hours, adjusted according to response, to be given over 10 minutes.

▸ Child: Initially 25–50 micrograms/kg every 6–8 hours (max. per dose 5 mg), adjusted according to response, to be given over 10 minutes

Hypertension

▶ BY MOUTH

▸ Neonate: Initially 250 micrograms/kg 3 times a day, then increased if necessary up to 2 mg/kg 3 times a day.

▸ Child 1 month–11 years: Initially 0.25–1 mg/kg 3 times a day, then increased to 5 mg/kg daily in divided doses, dose should be increased at weekly intervals

▸ Child 12–17 years: Initially 80 mg twice daily, then increased if necessary up to 160–320 mg daily, dose should be increased at weekly intervals, slow-release preparations may be used for once daily administration

Migraine prophylaxis

▶ BY MOUTH

▸ Child 2–11 years: Initially 200–500 micrograms/kg twice daily; usual dose 10–20 mg twice daily (max. per dose 2 mg/kg twice daily)

▸ Child 12–17 years: Initially 20–40 mg twice daily; usual dose 40–80 mg twice daily (max. per dose 120 mg); maximum 4 mg/kg per day

Arrhythmias

▶ BY MOUTH

▸ Neonate: 250–500 micrograms/kg 3 times a day, adjusted according to response.

▸ Child: 250–500 micrograms/kg 3–4 times a day (max. per dose 1 mg/kg 4 times a day), adjusted according to response; maximum 160 mg per day

▶ BY SLOW INTRAVENOUS INJECTION

▸ Neonate: 20–50 micrograms/kg, then 20–50 micrograms/kg every 6–8 hours if required, eCG monitoring required.

▸ Child: 25–50 micrograms/kg, then 25–50 micrograms/kg every 6–8 hours if required, eCG monitoring required

Tetralogy of Fallot

▶ BY MOUTH

▸ Neonate: 0.25–1 mg/kg 2–3 times a day (max. per dose 2 mg/kg 3 times a day).

▸ Child 1 month–11 years: 0.25–1 mg/kg 3–4 times a day, maximum dose to be given in divided doses; maximum 5 mg/kg per day

▶ BY SLOW INTRAVENOUS INJECTION

▸ Neonate: Initially 15–20 micrograms/kg (max. per dose 100 micrograms/kg), then 15–20 micrograms/kg every 12 hours if required, eCG monitoring is required with administration.

▸ Child 1 month–11 years: Initially 15–20 micrograms/kg (max. per dose 100 micrograms/kg), higher doses are rarely necessary, then 15–20 micrograms/kg every 6–8 hours if required, eCG monitoring is required with administration

● **UNLICENSED USE** Not licensed for treatment of hypertension in children under 12 years.

IMPORTANT SAFETY INFORMATION

SAFE PRACTICE

Propranolol has been confused with prednisolone; care must be taken to ensure the correct drug is prescribed and dispensed.

● **INTERACTIONS** → Appendix 1: beta blockers, non-selective

- **SIDE-EFFECTS**
- ▸ **Rare or very rare** Alopecia · memory loss · mood altered · neuromuscular dysfunction · postural hypotension · psychosis · skin reactions · thrombocytopenia
- ▸ **Frequency not known** Hypoglycaemia

Overdose Severe overdosages with propranolol may cause cardiovascular collapse, CNS depression, and convulsions.

- **HEPATIC IMPAIRMENT** Manufacturer advises caution (increased risk of hepatic encephalopathy; risk of increased half-life).

Dose adjustments ▸ With oral use Manufacturer advises consider dose reduction.

- **RENAL IMPAIRMENT**

Dose adjustments Manufacturer advises caution; dose reduction may be required.

- **DIRECTIONS FOR ADMINISTRATION** For *slow intravenous injection*, give over at least 3–5 minutes; rate of administration should not exceed 1 mg/minute. May be diluted with Sodium Chloride 0.9% or Glucose 5%. Incompatible with bicarbonate.
- **PRESCRIBING AND DISPENSING INFORMATION** Modified-release preparations can be used for once daily administration.

- **MEDICINAL FORMS** There can be variation in the licensing of different medicines containing the same drug. Forms available from special-order manufacturers include: oral suspension, oral solution

Oral solution

CAUTIONARY AND ADVISORY LABELS 8

▸ Propranolol hydrochloride (Non-proprietary)

Propranolol hydrochloride 1 mg per 1 ml Propranolol 5mg/5ml oral solution sugar-free | 150 ml [PoM] £23.51 DT = £23.51

Propranolol hydrochloride 2 mg per 1 ml Propranolol 10mg/5ml oral solution sugar-free | 150 ml [PoM] £28.45 DT = £28.45

Propranolol hydrochloride 8 mg per 1 ml Propranolol 40mg/5ml oral solution sugar-free | 150 ml [PoM] £36.51 DT = £36.51

Propranolol hydrochloride 10 mg per 1 ml Propranolol 50mg/5ml oral solution sugar-free | 150 ml [PoM] £38.51 DT = £38.51

Modified-release capsule

CAUTIONARY AND ADVISORY LABELS 8, 25

▸ Bedranol SR (Sandoz Ltd, Almus Pharmaceuticals Ltd)

Propranolol hydrochloride 80 mg Bedranol SR 80mg capsules | 28 capsule [PoM] £4.16 DT = £4.95

Propranolol hydrochloride 160 mg Bedranol SR 160mg capsules | 28 capsule [PoM] £4.59–£5.09 DT = £4.88

▸ Beta-Prograne (Actavis UK Ltd, Teva UK Ltd, Tillomed Laboratories Ltd)

Propranolol hydrochloride 160 mg Beta-Prograne 160mg modified-release capsules | 28 capsule [PoM] £4.88–£6.11 DT = £4.88

▸ Half Beta-Prograne (Actavis UK Ltd, Tillomed Laboratories Ltd, Teva UK Ltd)

Propranolol hydrochloride 80 mg Half Beta-Prograne 80mg modified-release capsules | 28 capsule [PoM] £4.95 DT = £4.95

Tablet

CAUTIONARY AND ADVISORY LABELS 8

▸ Propranolol hydrochloride (Non-proprietary)

Propranolol hydrochloride 10 mg Propranolol 10mg tablets | 28 tablet [PoM] £7.00 DT = £1.97

Propranolol hydrochloride 40 mg Propranolol 40mg tablets | 28 tablet [PoM] £7.00 DT = £2.07

Propranolol hydrochloride 80 mg Propranolol 80mg tablets | 56 tablet [PoM] £5.23 DT = £2.54

Propranolol hydrochloride 160 mg Propranolol 160mg tablets | 56 tablet [PoM] £5.88 DT = £5.88

▸ Bedranol (Ennogen Pharma Ltd)

Propranolol hydrochloride 10 mg Bedranol 10mg tablets | 28 tablet [PoM] £1.54 DT = £1.97

Propranolol hydrochloride 40 mg Bedranol 40mg tablets | 28 tablet [PoM] £1.38 DT = £2.07

Propranolol hydrochloride 80 mg Bedranol 80mg tablets | 56 tablet [PoM] £0.95 DT = £2.54

Propranolol hydrochloride 160 mg Bedranol 160mg tablets | 56 tablet [PoM] £4.70 DT = £5.88

BETA-ADRENOCEPTOR BLOCKERS › SELECTIVE

F 109

Atenolol

03-Mar-2020

- **INDICATIONS AND DOSE**

Hypertension

▸ BY MOUTH

- ▸ Neonate: 0.5–2 mg/kg once daily, dose may be given in 2 divided doses.
- ▸ Child 1 month–11 years: 0.5–2 mg/kg once daily, dose may be given in 2 divided doses, doses higher than 50 mg daily are rarely necessary
- ▸ Child 12–17 years: 25–50 mg once daily, dose may be given in 2 divided doses, higher doses are rarely necessary

Arrhythmias

▸ BY MOUTH

- ▸ Neonate: 0.5–2 mg/kg once daily, dose may be given in 2 divided doses.
- ▸ Child 1 month–11 years: 0.5–2 mg/kg once daily, dose may be given in 2 divided doses; maximum 100 mg per day
- ▸ Child 12–17 years: 50–100 mg once daily, dose may be given in 2 divided doses

- **UNLICENSED USE** Not licensed for use in children under 12 years.

IMPORTANT SAFETY INFORMATION

SAFE PRACTICE

Atenolol has been confused with amlodipine; care must be taken to ensure the correct drug is prescribed and dispensed.

- **INTERACTIONS** → Appendix 1: beta blockers, selective
- **SIDE-EFFECTS**
- ▸ **Common or very common** Gastrointestinal disorder
- ▸ **Rare or very rare** Alopecia · dry mouth · hepatic disorders · mood altered · postural hypotension · psychosis · skin reactions · thrombocytopenia
- ▸ **Frequency not known** Hypersensitivity · lupus-like syndrome
- **BREAST FEEDING** Water soluble beta-blockers such as atenolol are present in breast milk in greater amounts than other beta blockers.
- **RENAL IMPAIRMENT**

Dose adjustments Initially use 50% of usual dose if estimated glomerular filtration rate 10–35 mL/minute/1.73 m^2; initially use 30–50% of usual dose if estimated glomerular filtration rate less than 10 mL/minute/1.73 m^2.

- **PATIENT AND CARER ADVICE**

Medicines for Children leaflet: Atenolol for hypertension www.medicinesforchildren.org.uk/atenolol-hypertension-0

- **MEDICINAL FORMS** There can be variation in the licensing of different medicines containing the same drug. Forms available from special-order manufacturers include: oral suspension, oral solution

Oral solution

CAUTIONARY AND ADVISORY LABELS 8

▸ Atenolol (Non-proprietary)

Atenolol 5 mg per 1 ml Atenolol 25mg/5ml oral solution sugar-free | 300 ml [PoM] £73.00 DT = £5.60

Tablet

CAUTIONARY AND ADVISORY LABELS 8

▸ Atenolol (Non-proprietary)

Atenolol 25 mg Atenolol 25mg tablets | 28 tablet [PoM] £1.39 DT = £0.71

Atenolol 50 mg Atenolol 50mg tablets | 28 tablet PoM £4.09 DT = £0.75
Atenolol 100 mg Atenolol 100mg tablets | 28 tablet PoM £5.19 DT = £0.84
- Tenormin (AstraZeneca UK Ltd)
Atenolol 50 mg Tenormin LS 50mg tablets | 28 tablet PoM £10.22 DT = £0.75

F 109

Esmolol hydrochloride

● **INDICATIONS AND DOSE**

Arrhythmias | Hypertensive emergencies

▸ INITIALLY BY INTRAVENOUS INJECTION

- Child: Loading dose 500 micrograms/kg, to be given over 1 minute, then (by intravenous infusion) maintenance 50 micrograms/kg/minute for 4 minutes (rate reduced if low blood pressure or low heart rate), if inadequate response, repeat loading dose and increase maintenance infusion, (by intravenous injection) loading dose 500 micrograms/kg, given over 1 minute, then (by intravenous infusion) maintenance 100 micrograms/kg/minute for 4 minutes, if response still inadequate, repeat loading dose and increase maintenance infusion, (by intravenous injection) loading dose 500 micrograms/kg, given over 1 minute, then (by intravenous infusion) maintenance 150 micrograms/kg/minute for 4 minutes, if response still inadequate, repeat loading dose and increase maintenance infusion, (by intravenous injection) loading dose 500 micrograms/kg, given over 1 minute, then (by intravenous infusion) maintenance 200 micrograms/kg/minute for 4 minutes, doses over 300 micrograms/kg/minute not recommended

Tetralogy of Fallot

▸ INITIALLY BY INTRAVENOUS INJECTION

- Neonate: Initially 600 micrograms/kg, dose to be given over 1–2 minutes, then (by intravenous infusion) 300–900 micrograms/kg/minute if required.

● **UNLICENSED USE** Not licensed for use in children.

● **INTERACTIONS** → Appendix 1: beta blockers, selective

● **SIDE-EFFECTS**

- **Common or very common** Anxiety · appetite decreased · concentration impaired · drowsiness · hyperhidrosis
- **Uncommon** Arrhythmias · chills · constipation · costochondritis · dry mouth · dyspepsia · fever · flushing · nasal congestion · oedema · pain · pallor · pulmonary oedema · respiratory disorders · seizure · skin reactions · speech disorder · taste altered · thinking abnormal · urinary retention
- **Rare or very rare** Cardiac arrest · extravasation necrosis · thrombophlebitis
- **Frequency not known** Angioedema · coronary vasospasm · hyperkalaemia · metabolic acidosis

● **BREAST FEEDING** Manufacturer advises avoidance.

● **RENAL IMPAIRMENT** Manufacturer advises caution.

● **DIRECTIONS FOR ADMINISTRATION** Give through a central venous catheter; incompatible with bicarbonate.

● **MEDICINAL FORMS** There can be variation in the licensing of different medicines containing the same drug.

Solution for injection

- Esmolol hydrochloride (Non-proprietary)
Esmolol hydrochloride 10 mg per 1 ml Esmolol hydrochloride 100mg/10ml solution for injection vials | 5 vial PoM £38.95 (Hospital only)
Esmolol 100mg/10ml solution for injection vials | 10 vial PoM £100.00 (Hospital only)
- Brevibloc (Baxter Healthcare Ltd)
Esmolol hydrochloride 10 mg per 1 ml Brevibloc Premixed 100mg/10ml solution for injection vials | 5 vial PoM

Solution for infusion

- Brevibloc (Baxter Healthcare Ltd)
Esmolol hydrochloride 10 mg per 1 ml Brevibloc Premixed 2.5g/250ml infusion bags | 1 bag PoM £89.69

F 109

Metoprolol tartrate

● **INDICATIONS AND DOSE**

Hypertension

▸ BY MOUTH USING IMMEDIATE-RELEASE MEDICINES

- Child 1 month–11 years: Initially 1 mg/kg twice daily, increased if necessary up to 8 mg/kg daily in 2–4 divided doses (max. per dose 400 mg)
- Child 12–17 years: Initially 50–100 mg daily, increased if necessary to 200 mg daily in 1–2 divided doses, high doses are rarely necessary; maximum 400 mg per day

▸ BY MOUTH USING MODIFIED-RELEASE MEDICINES

- Child 12–17 years: 200 mg once daily

Arrhythmias

▸ BY MOUTH USING IMMEDIATE-RELEASE MEDICINES

- Child 12–17 years: Usual dose 50 mg 2–3 times a day, then increased if necessary up to 300 mg daily in divided doses

● **UNLICENSED USE** Not licensed for use in children.

● **INTERACTIONS** → Appendix 1: beta blockers, selective

● **SIDE-EFFECTS**

- **Common or very common** Postural disorders
- **Rare or very rare** Alertness decreased · alopecia · arrhythmia · arthritis · auditory disorder · chest pain · constipation · drowsiness · dry mouth · dystrophic skin lesion · eye irritation · gangrene · hyperhidrosis · muscle cramps · oedema · palpitations · personality disorder · rhinitis · sexual dysfunction · skin reactions · thrombocytopenia · weight increased
- **Frequency not known** Conjunctivitis · hepatitis · Peyronie's disease · retroperitoneal fibrosis

● **HEPATIC IMPAIRMENT** Manufacturer advises caution in severe impairment (bioavailability may be increased in patients with liver cirrhosis).
Dose adjustments In adults, manufacturer advises consider dose reduction in severe impairment.

● **MEDICINAL FORMS** There can be variation in the licensing of different medicines containing the same drug. Forms available from special-order manufacturers include: capsule, oral suspension, oral solution

Tablet

CAUTIONARY AND ADVISORY LABELS 8

- Metoprolol tartrate (Non-proprietary)
Metoprolol tartrate 50 mg Metoprolol 50mg tablets | 28 tablet PoM £4.35 DT = £3.63 | 56 tablet PoM £7.26
Metoprolol tartrate 100 mg Metoprolol 100mg tablets | 28 tablet PoM £4.62 DT = £3.46 | 56 tablet PoM £6.92

CALCIUM-CHANNEL BLOCKERS

Calcium-channel blockers

Overview

Calcium-channel blockers differ in their predilection for the various possible sites of action and, therefore, their therapeutic effects are disparate, with much greater variation than those of beta-blockers. There are important differences between verapamil hydrochloride p. 116, diltiazem hydrochloride p. 152, and the dihydropyridine calcium-channel blockers (amlodipine p. 114, nicardipine hydrochloride p. 115, nifedipine p. 115, and nimodipine p. 92). Verapamil hydrochloride and diltiazem hydrochloride should usually be **avoided** in heart failure because they may further depress cardiac function and cause clinically significant deterioration.

Verapamil hydrochloride is used for the treatment of hypertension and arrhythmias. However, it is no longer first-line treatment for arrhythmias in children because it has been associated with fatal collapse especially in infants under 1 year; adenosine p. 84 is now recommended for first-line use.

Verapamil hydrochloride is a highly negatively inotropic calcium channel-blocker and it reduces cardiac output, slows the heart rate, and may impair atrioventricular conduction. It may precipitate heart failure, exacerbate conduction disorders, and cause hypotension at high doses and should **not** be used with beta-blockers. Constipation is the most common side-effect.

Nifedipine relaxes vascular smooth muscle and dilates coronary and peripheral arteries. It has more influence on vessels and less on the myocardium than does verapamil hydrochloride and unlike verapamil hydrochloride has no anti-arrhythmic activity. It rarely precipitates heart failure because any negative inotropic effect is offset by a reduction in left ventricular work. Short-acting formulations of nifedipine may be used if a modified-release preparation delivering the appropriate dose is not available or if a child is unable to swallow (a liquid preparation may be prepared using capsules). Nifedipine may also be used for the management of angina due to coronary artery disease in Kawasaki disease or progeria and in the management of Raynaud's syndrome.

Nicardipine hydrochloride has similar effects to those of nifedipine and may produce less reduction of myocardial contractility; it should only be used for the treatment of life-threatening hypertension in paediatric intensive care settings and in postoperative hypertension.

Amlodipine also resembles nifedipine and nicardipine hydrochloride in its effects and does not reduce myocardial contractility or produce clinical deterioration in heart failure. It has a longer duration of action and can be given once daily. Nifedipine and amlodipine are used for the treatment of hypertension. Side-effects associated with vasodilatation such as flushing and headache (which become less obtrusive after a few days), and ankle swelling (which may respond only partially to diuretics) are common.

Nimodipine is related to nifedipine but the smooth muscle relaxant effect preferentially acts on cerebral arteries. Its use is confined to prevention and treatment of vascular spasm following aneurysmal subarachnoid haemorrhage.

Diltiazem hydrochloride is a peripheral vasodilator and also has mild depressor effects on the myocardium. It is used in the treatment of Raynaud's syndrome.

Calcium-channel blockers

- **DRUG ACTION** Calcium-channel blockers (less correctly called 'calcium-antagonists') interfere with the inward displacement of calcium ions through the slow channels of active cell membranes. They influence the myocardial cells, the cells within the specialised conducting system of the heart, and the cells of vascular smooth muscle. Thus, myocardial contractility may be reduced, the formation and propagation of electrical impulses within the heart may be depressed, and coronary or systemic vascular tone may be diminished.
- **SIDE-EFFECTS**
  - **Common or very common** Abdominal pain · dizziness · drowsiness · flushing · headache · nausea · palpitations · peripheral oedema · skin reactions · tachycardia · vomiting
  - **Uncommon** Angioedema · depression · erectile dysfunction · gingival hyperplasia · myalgia · paraesthesia · syncope

  Overdose Features of calcium-channel blocker poisoning include nausea, vomiting, dizziness, agitation, confusion, and coma in severe poisoning. Metabolic acidosis and hyperglycaemia may occur. In overdose, the dihydropyridine calcium-channel blockers cause severe hypotension secondary to profound peripheral vasodilatation.For details on the management of poisoning, see Calcium-channel blockers, under Emergency treatment of poisoning p. 891.
- **HEPATIC IMPAIRMENT** In general, manufacturers advise caution (risk of increased exposure).
- **TREATMENT CESSATION** There is some evidence that sudden withdrawal of calcium-channel blockers may be associated with an exacerbation of myocardial ischaemia.

F above

Amlodipine

03-Mar-2020

- **DRUG ACTION** Amlodipine is a dihydropyridine calcium-channel blocker.

- **INDICATIONS AND DOSE**

Hypertension
- BY MOUTH
  - Child 1 month–11 years: Initially 100–200 micrograms/kg once daily; increased if necessary up to 400 micrograms/kg once daily, adjusted at intervals of 1–2 weeks; maximum 10 mg per day
  - Child 12–17 years: Initially 5 mg once daily, then increased if necessary up to 10 mg once daily, adjusted at intervals of 1–2 weeks

DOSE EQUIVALENCE AND CONVERSION
- Tablets from various suppliers may contain different salts (e.g. amlodipine besilate, amlodipine maleate, and amlodipine mesilate) but the strength is expressed in terms of amlodipine (base); tablets containing different salts are considered interchangeable.

- **UNLICENSED USE** Not licensed for use in children under 6 years.

IMPORTANT SAFETY INFORMATION

SAFE PRACTICE

Amlodipine has been confused with nimodipine and atenolol; care must be taken to ensure the correct drug is prescribed and dispensed.

- **CONTRA-INDICATIONS** Cardiogenic shock · significant aortic stenosis · unstable angina
- **INTERACTIONS** → Appendix 1: calcium channel blockers
- **SIDE-EFFECTS**
  - **Common or very common** Asthenia · constipation · diarrhoea · dyspepsia · dyspnoea · gastrointestinal disorders · joint disorders · muscle cramps · oedema · vision disorders
  - **Uncommon** Alopecia · anxiety · arrhythmias · chest pain · cough · dry mouth · gynaecomastia · hyperhidrosis · hypotension · insomnia · malaise · mood altered · numbness · pain · rhinitis · taste altered · tinnitus · tremor · urinary disorders · weight changes
  - **Rare or very rare** Confusion · hepatic disorders · hyperglycaemia · hypersensitivity · leucopenia · muscle tone increased · myocardial infarction · pancreatitis · peripheral neuropathy · photosensitivity reaction · Stevens-Johnson syndrome · thrombocytopenia · vasculitis
  - **Frequency not known** Extrapyramidal symptoms · pulmonary oedema
- **PREGNANCY** No information available—manufacturer advises avoid, but risk to fetus should be balanced against risk of uncontrolled maternal hypertension.
- **BREAST FEEDING** Manufacturer advises avoid—no information available.

- **HEPATIC IMPAIRMENT**
Dose adjustments Manufacturer advises initiate at low dose and titrate slowly (limited information available).
- **DIRECTIONS FOR ADMINISTRATION** Tablets may be dispersed in water.
- **PATIENT AND CARER ADVICE**
Medicines for Children leaflet: Amlodipine for high blood pressure www.medicinesforchildren.org.uk/amlodipine-high-blood-pressure

---

- **MEDICINAL FORMS** There can be variation in the licensing of different medicines containing the same drug. Forms available from special-order manufacturers include: oral suspension, oral solution

Oral solution
- Amlodipine (Non-proprietary)
Amlodipine 1 mg per 1 ml Amlodipine 5mg/5ml oral solution sugar-free | 150 ml [PoM] £75.78 DT = £75.78
Amlodipine 2 mg per 1 ml Amlodipine 10mg/5ml oral solution sugar-free | 150 ml [PoM] £115.73 DT = £115.73

Oral suspension
- Amlodipine (Non-proprietary)
Amlodipine 1 mg per 1 ml Amlodipine 5mg/5ml oral suspension sugar-free | 150 ml [PoM] £70.00 DT = £70.00

Tablet
- Amlodipine (Non-proprietary)
Amlodipine 2.5 mg Amlodipine 2.5mg tablets | 28 tablet [PoM] £4.50
Amlodipine 5 mg Amlodipine 5mg tablets | 28 tablet [PoM] £9.99 DT = £0.84 | 500 tablet [PoM] £9.87–£14.82
Amlodipine 10 mg Amlodipine 10mg tablets | 28 tablet [PoM] £14.07 DT = £0.86 | 500 tablet [PoM] £10.17–£15.54
- Istin (Upjohn UK Ltd)
Amlodipine 5 mg Istin 5mg tablets | 28 tablet [PoM] £11.08 DT = £0.84
Amlodipine 10 mg Istin 10mg tablets | 28 tablet [PoM] £16.55 DT = £0.86

F 114

Nicardipine hydrochloride

14-Feb-2020

- **DRUG ACTION** Nicardipine is a dihydropyridine calcium-channel blocker.

- **INDICATIONS AND DOSE**

Life-threatening hypertension (specialist use only) | Post-operative hypertension (specialist use only)

▶ BY CONTINUOUS INTRAVENOUS INFUSION

- Neonate: Initially 500 nanograms/kg/minute (max. per dose 5 micrograms/kg/minute), adjusted according to response; maintenance 1–4 micrograms/kg/minute.
- Child: Initially 500 nanograms/kg/minute (max. per dose 5 micrograms/kg/minute), adjusted according to response; maintenance 1–4 micrograms/kg/minute (max. per dose 250 micrograms/minute)

- **CONTRA-INDICATIONS** Acute porphyrias p. 652 · avoid within 8 days of myocardial infarction · cardiogenic shock · compensatory hypertension · significant or advanced aortic stenosis · unstable or acute attacks of angina
- **CAUTIONS** Congestive heart failure · elevated intracranial pressure · increased risk of serious hypotension · ischaemic heart disease · portal hypertension · pulmonary oedema · significantly impaired left ventricular function · stroke
- **INTERACTIONS** → Appendix 1: calcium channel blockers
- **SIDE-EFFECTS**
▶ **Common or very common** Hypotension
▶ **Frequency not known** Atrioventricular block · hepatic disorders · ischaemic heart disease · paralytic ileus · pulmonary oedema · thrombocytopenia

SIDE-EFFECTS, FURTHER INFORMATION Systemic hypotension and reflex tachycardia with rapid reduction of blood pressure may occur — during intravenous use consider stopping infusion or decreasing dose by half.
- **PREGNANCY** May inhibit labour. Not to be used in multiple pregnancy (twins or more) unless there is no other acceptable alternative. Toxicity in *animal* studies. Risk of severe maternal hypotension and fatal fetal hypoxia—avoid excessive decrease in blood pressure.
- **BREAST FEEDING** Manufacturer advises avoid—present in breast milk.
- **HEPATIC IMPAIRMENT**
Dose adjustments In adults, manufacturer advises dose reduction—consult product literature.
- **RENAL IMPAIRMENT**
Dose adjustments Use with caution—increased risk of serious hypotension; consider using low initial dose.
- **MONITORING REQUIREMENTS** Monitor blood pressure and heart rate at least every 5 minutes during intravenous infusion, and then until stable, and continue monitoring for at least 12 hours after end of infusion.
- **DIRECTIONS FOR ADMINISTRATION** Intravenous nicardipine should only be administered under the supervision of a specialist and in a hospital or intensive care setting in which patients can be closely monitored.

For *continuous intravenous infusion*, dilute to a concentration of 100–200 micrograms/mL with Glucose 5% and give *via* volumetric infusion pump or syringe driver; protect from light; to minimise peripheral venous irritation, change site of infusion every 12 hours; risk of adsorption on to plastic in the presence of saline solutions; incompatible with bicarbonate or alkaline solutions—consult product literature.

- **MEDICINAL FORMS** There can be variation in the licensing of different medicines containing the same drug.

Solution for infusion
- Nicardipine hydrochloride (Non-proprietary)
Nicardipine hydrochloride 1 mg per 1 ml Nicardipine 10mg/10ml solution for injection ampoules | 5 ampoule [PoM] £50.00
Nicardipine hydrochloride 2.5 mg per 1 ml Cardene I.V. 25mg/10ml solution for infusion ampoules | 10 ampoule [PoM] [X]

F 114

Nifedipine

10-Mar-2020

- **INDICATIONS AND DOSE**

Hypertensive crisis | Acute angina in Kawasaki disease or progeria

▶ BY MOUTH USING IMMEDIATE-RELEASE MEDICINES

- Child: Initially 250–500 micrograms/kg (max. per dose 10 mg), then repeat once if necessary, may cause unpredictable and severe reduction of blood pressure—monitor closely following administration; if ineffective consider alternative treatment and seek specialist advice

Hypertension | Angina in Kawasaki disease or progeria

▶ BY MOUTH USING IMMEDIATE-RELEASE MEDICINES

- Child 1 month–11 years: 200–300 micrograms/kg 3 times a day, dose frequency depends on preparation used; maximum 3 mg/kg per day; maximum 90 mg per day
- Child 12–17 years: 5–20 mg 3 times a day, dose frequency depends on preparation used; maximum 90 mg per day

Raynaud's syndrome

▶ BY MOUTH USING IMMEDIATE-RELEASE MEDICINES

- Child 2–17 years: 2.5–10 mg 2–4 times a day, start with low doses at night and increase gradually to avoid postural hypotension, dose frequency depends on preparation used

continued →

Persistent hyperinsulinaemic hypoglycaemia
- ▸ BY MOUTH USING IMMEDIATE-RELEASE MEDICINES
- ▸ Neonate: 100–200 micrograms/kg 4 times a day (max. per dose 600 micrograms/kg).

- **UNLICENSED USE** Not licensed for use in children.
- **CONTRA-INDICATIONS** Cardiogenic shock · significant aortic stenosis · within 1 month of myocardial infarction
- **CAUTIONS** Diabetes mellitus · heart failure · poor cardiac reserve · severe hypotension · short-acting formulations are not recommended for angina or long-term management of hypertension (their use may be associated with large variations in blood pressure and reflex tachycardia) · significantly impaired left ventricular function (heart failure deterioration observed)
- **INTERACTIONS** → Appendix 1: calcium channel blockers
- **SIDE-EFFECTS**
- ▸ **Common or very common** Constipation · malaise · oedema · vasodilation
- ▸ **Uncommon** Allergic oedema · anxiety · chills · diarrhoea · dry mouth · epistaxis · gastrointestinal discomfort · gastrointestinal disorders · hypotension · joint disorders · laryngeal oedema · migraine · muscle complaints · nasal congestion · pain · sleep disorders · tremor · urinary disorders · vertigo · vision disorders
- ▸ **Rare or very rare** Appetite decreased · burping · cardiovascular disorder · fever · hyperhidrosis · mood altered · sensation abnormal
- ▸ **Frequency not known** Agranulocytosis · bezoar · cerebral ischaemia · chest pain · dysphagia · dyspnoea · eye pain · gingival disorder · gynaecomastia (following long term use) · hepatic disorders · hyperglycaemia · ischaemic heart disease · leucopenia · myasthenia gravis aggravated · photoallergic reaction · pulmonary oedema · telangiectasia · toxic epidermal necrolysis · weight decreased
- **PREGNANCY** May inhibit labour; manufacturer advises avoid before week 20, but risk to fetus should be balanced against risk of uncontrolled maternal hypertension. Use only if other treatment options are not indicated or have failed.
- **BREAST FEEDING** Amount too small to be harmful but manufacturers advise avoid.
- **HEPATIC IMPAIRMENT**

  Dose adjustments In adults, manufacturer advises consider dose reduction—consult product literature.
- **DIRECTIONS FOR ADMINISTRATION** For rapid effect in *hypertensive crisis* or *acute angina*, bite capsules and swallow liquid or use liquid preparation if 5 mg or 10 mg dose inappropriate. If liquid unavailable, extract contents of capsule via a syringe and use immediately—cover syringe with foil to protect contents from light; capsule contents may be diluted with water if necessary.
- **PATIENT AND CARER ADVICE**

  Medicines for Children leaflet: Nifedipine for high blood pressure www.medicinesforchildren.org.uk/nifedipine-high-blood-pressure

---

- **MEDICINAL FORMS** There can be variation in the licensing of different medicines containing the same drug. Forms available from special-order manufacturers include: oral suspension, oral drops

Oral drops
- ▸ Nifedipine (Non-proprietary)

  Nifedipine 20 mg per 1 ml Nifedipin-ratiopharm 20mg/ml oral drops | 30 ml [PoM] [unlicensed]

Capsule
- ▸ Nifedipine (Non-proprietary)

  Nifedipine 5 mg Nifedipine 5mg capsules | 90 capsule [PoM] £51.95 DT = £51.95

  Nifedipine 10 mg Nifedipine 10mg capsules | 90 capsule [PoM] £65.63 DT = £65.63

F 114

Verapamil hydrochloride

14-Feb-2020

- **INDICATIONS AND DOSE**

Treatment of supraventricular arrhythmias
- ▸ BY SLOW INTRAVENOUS INJECTION
- ▸ Child 1–17 years (administered on expert advice): 100–300 micrograms/kg (max. per dose 5 mg) for 1 dose, to be given over 2–3 minutes (with ECG and blood-pressure monitoring), dose can be repeated after 30 minutes if necessary

Hypertension
- ▸ BY MOUTH USING IMMEDIATE-RELEASE MEDICINES
- ▸ Child 12–23 months (administered on expert advice): 20 mg 2–3 times a day
- ▸ Child 2–17 years (administered on expert advice): 40–120 mg 2–3 times a day

Prophylaxis of supraventricular arrhythmias (administered on expert advice)
- ▸ BY MOUTH USING IMMEDIATE-RELEASE MEDICINES
- ▸ Child 12–23 months: 20 mg 2–3 times a day
- ▸ Child 2–17 years: 40–120 mg 2–3 times a day

- **CONTRA-INDICATIONS** Acute porphyrias p. 652 · atrial flutter or fibrillation associated with accessory conducting pathways (e.g. Wolff-Parkinson-White-syndrome) · bradycardia · cardiogenic shock · heart failure (with reduced ejection fraction) · history of significantly impaired left ventricular function (even if controlled by therapy) · hypotension · second- and third-degree AV block · sick sinus syndrome · sino-atrial block
- **CAUTIONS** Acute phase of myocardial infarction (avoid if bradycardia, hypotension, left ventricular failure) · first-degree AV block · neuromuscular disorders
- **INTERACTIONS** → Appendix 1: calcium channel blockers
- **SIDE-EFFECTS**

  GENERAL SIDE-EFFECTS
- ▸ **Common or very common** Hypotension
- ▸ **Frequency not known** Atrioventricular block · extrapyramidal symptoms · Stevens-Johnson syndrome · vertigo

  SPECIFIC SIDE-EFFECTS
- ▸ **Common or very common**
- ▸ With intravenous use Bradycardia
- ▸ **Frequency not known**
- ▸ With intravenous use Cardiac arrest · hepatic impairment · hyperhidrosis · myocardial contractility decreased · nervousness · seizure
- ▸ With oral use Abdominal discomfort · alopecia · arrhythmias · arthralgia · constipation · erythromelalgia · fatigue · galactorrhoea · heart failure · ileus · muscle weakness · tinnitus · tremor

  Overdose In overdose, verapamil has a profound cardiac depressant effect causing hypotension and arrhythmias, including complete heart block and asystole.
- **PREGNANCY** May reduce uterine blood flow with fetal hypoxia. Manufacturer advises avoid in first trimester unless absolutely necessary. May inhibit labour.
- **BREAST FEEDING** Amount too small to be harmful.
- **HEPATIC IMPAIRMENT**

  Dose adjustments ▸ With oral use Manufacturer advises dose reduction.
- **DIRECTIONS FOR ADMINISTRATION** For *intravenous injection*, may be diluted with Glucose 5% *or* Sodium Chloride 0.9%. Incompatible with solutions of pH greater than 6.

- **MEDICINAL FORMS** There can be variation in the licensing of different medicines containing the same drug. Forms available from special-order manufacturers include: oral suspension, oral solution

Tablet

- Verapamil hydrochloride (Non-proprietary)
  Verapamil hydrochloride 40 mg Verapamil 40mg tablets | 84 tablet PoM £2.24 DT = £1.89
  Verapamil hydrochloride 80 mg Verapamil 80mg tablets | 84 tablet PoM £2.63 DT = £2.36
  Verapamil hydrochloride 120 mg Verapamil 120mg tablets | 28 tablet PoM £4.43 DT = £4.02
  Verapamil hydrochloride 160 mg Verapamil 160mg tablets | 56 tablet PoM £33.84 DT = £29.47

Solution for injection

- Securon (Mylan)
  Verapamil hydrochloride 2.5 mg per 1 ml Securon IV 5mg/2ml solution for injection ampoules | 5 ampoule PoM £5.41

Oral solution

- Verapamil hydrochloride (Non-proprietary)
  Verapamil hydrochloride 8 mg per 1 ml Verapamil 40mg/5ml oral solution sugar-free | 150 ml PoM £44.92 DT = £41.00

DIURETICS > THIAZIDES AND RELATED DIURETICS

Thiazides and related diuretics

- **CONTRA-INDICATIONS** Addison's disease · hypercalcaemia · hyponatraemia · refractory hypokalaemia · symptomatic hyperuricaemia
- **CAUTIONS** Diabetes · gout · hyperaldosteronism · malnourishment · nephrotic syndrome · systemic lupus erythematosus

CAUTIONS, FURTHER INFORMATION

- Existing conditions Thiazides and related diuretics can exacerbate diabetes, gout, and systemic lupus erythematosus.
- Potassium loss Hypokalaemia can occur with both thiazide and loop diuretics. The risk of hypokalaemia depends on the duration of action as well as the potency and is thus greater with thiazides than with an equipotent dose of a loop diuretic.

  Hypokalaemia is particularly dangerous in children being treated with cardiac glycosides. In hepatic failure hypokalaemia caused by diuretics can precipitate encephalopathy.

  The use of potassium-sparing diuretics avoids the need to take potassium supplements.

- **SIDE-EFFECTS**
  - **Common or very common** Alkalosis hypochloraemic · constipation · diarrhoea · dizziness · dry mouth · electrolyte imbalance · erectile dysfunction · fatigue · headache · hyperglycaemia · hyperuricaemia · nausea · postural hypotension · skin reactions
  - **Uncommon** Agranulocytosis · aplastic anaemia · leucopenia · pancreatitis · photosensitivity reaction · thrombocytopenia · vomiting
  - **Rare or very rare** Paraesthesia
- **PREGNANCY** Thiazides and related diuretics should not be used to treat gestational hypertension. They may cause neonatal thrombocytopenia, bone marrow suppression, jaundice, electrolyte disturbances, and hypoglycaemia; placental perfusion may also be reduced. Stimulation of labour, uterine inertia, and meconium staining have also been reported.
- **HEPATIC IMPAIRMENT** In general, manufacturer advises caution in mild to moderate impairment; avoid in severe impairment.
- **RENAL IMPAIRMENT** Thiazides and related diuretics should be used with caution because they can further reduce renal function. They are ineffective if estimated glomerular filtration rate is less than 30 mL/minute/1.73 m^2 and should be avoided. Metolazone remains effective if estimated glomerular filtration rate is less than 30 mL/minute/1.73 m^2 but is associated with a risk of excessive diuresis.

  Monitoring Electrolytes should be monitored in renal impairment.
- **MONITORING REQUIREMENTS** Electrolytes should be monitored, particularly with high doses and long-term use.

above

Bendroflumethiazide

(Bendrofluazide)

- **INDICATIONS AND DOSE**

Hypertension

- BY MOUTH
  - Child 1 month–1 year: 50–100 micrograms/kg daily, adjusted according to response
  - Child 2–11 years: Initially 50–400 micrograms/kg daily (max. per dose 10 mg), then maintenance 50–100 micrograms/kg daily, adjusted according to response; maximum 10 mg per day
  - Child 12–17 years: 2.5 mg once daily, dose to be taken as a single dose in the morning, higher doses are rarely necessary

Oedema in heart failure, renal disease and hepatic disease | Pulmonary oedema

- BY MOUTH
  - Child 1 month–1 year: 50–100 micrograms/kg daily, adjusted according to response
  - Child 2–11 years: Initially 50–400 micrograms/kg daily (max. per dose 10 mg), then maintenance 50–100 micrograms/kg daily, adjusted according to response; maximum 10 mg per day
  - Child 12–17 years: Initially 5–10 mg once daily or on alternate days, adjusted according to response, dose to be taken as a single dose in the morning; maximum 10 mg per day

- **INTERACTIONS** → Appendix 1: thiazide diuretics
- **SIDE-EFFECTS** Blood disorder · cholestasis · gastrointestinal disorder · gout · neutropenia · pneumonitis · pulmonary oedema · severe cutaneous adverse reactions (SCARs)
- **BREAST FEEDING** The amount present in milk is too small to be harmful. Large doses may suppress lactation.
- **MEDICINAL FORMS** There can be variation in the licensing of different medicines containing the same drug. Forms available from special-order manufacturers include: oral suspension, oral solution

Tablet

- Bendroflumethiazide (Non-proprietary)
  Bendroflumethiazide 2.5 mg Bendroflumethiazide 2.5mg tablets | 28 tablet PoM £0.76 DT = £0.76 | 500 tablet PoM £21.85
  Bendroflumethiazide 5 mg Bendroflumethiazide 5mg tablets | 28 tablet PoM £1.54 DT = £0.88
- Neo-Naclex (Advanz Pharma)
  Bendroflumethiazide 2.5 mg Neo-Naclex 2.5mg tablets | 28 tablet PoM £0.33 DT = £0.76

above

Chlorothiazide

- **INDICATIONS AND DOSE**

Heart failure | Hypertension | Ascites

- BY MOUTH
  - Neonate: 10–20 mg/kg twice daily.
  - Child 1–5 months: 10–20 mg/kg twice daily

continued →

- Child 6 months–11 years: 10 mg/kg twice daily; maximum 1 g per day
- Child 12–17 years: 0.25–1 g once daily, alternatively 125–500 mg twice daily

Reduction of diazoxide-induced sodium and water retention in the management of chronic hypoglycaemia | Potentiating the glyacaemic effect of diazoxide in the management of chronic hypoglycaemia

▶ BY MOUTH
- Child: 3–5 mg/kg twice daily

Nephrogenic and partial pituitary diabetes insipidus

▶ BY MOUTH
- Child: 10–20 mg/kg twice daily (max. per dose 500 mg)

- UNLICENSED USE Not licensed.
- CAUTIONS Neonate (theoretical risk of kernicterus if very jaundiced)
- INTERACTIONS → Appendix 1: thiazide diuretics
- BREAST FEEDING The amount present in milk is too small to be harmful. Large doses may suppress lactation.

- MEDICINAL FORMS There can be variation in the licensing of different medicines containing the same drug. Forms available from special-order manufacturers include: tablet, oral suspension, oral solution

Tablet
- Diuril (Imported (United States))
  Chlorothiazide 250 mg Diuril 250mg tablets | 100 tablet PoM ⊠

DRUGS ACTING ON THE RENIN-ANGIOTENSIN SYSTEM > ACE INHIBITORS

Angiotensin-converting enzyme inhibitors

- CONTRA-INDICATIONS Bilateral renovascular disease
- CAUTIONS Afro-Caribbean patients (may respond less well to ACE inhibitors) · concomitant diuretics · diabetes (may lower blood glucose) · first dose hypotension (especially in patients taking high doses of diuretics, on a low-sodium diet, on dialysis, dehydrated, or with heart failure) · neonates · primary aldosteronism (patients may respond less well to ACE inhibitors) · the risk of agranulocytosis is possibly increased in collagen vascular disease (blood counts recommended) · use with care (or avoid) in those with a history of idiopathic or hereditary angioedema · use with care in patients with hypertrophic cardiomyopathy · use with care in patients with severe or symptomatic aortic stenosis (risk of hypotension)

CAUTIONS, FURTHER INFORMATION
- Anaphylactoid reactions To prevent anaphylactoid reactions, ACE inhibitors should be avoided during dialysis with high-flux polyacrylonitrile membranes and during low-density lipoprotein apheresis with dextran sulfate; they should also be withheld before desensitisation with wasp or bee venom.

- SIDE-EFFECTS
- **Common or very common** Alopecia · angina pectoris · angioedema (may be delayed; more common in Afro-Caribbean patients) · arrhythmias · asthenia · chest pain · constipation · cough · diarrhoea · dizziness · drowsiness · dry mouth · dyspnoea · electrolyte imbalance · gastrointestinal discomfort · headache · hypotension · myalgia · nausea · palpitations · paraesthesia · renal impairment · rhinitis · skin reactions · sleep disorder · syncope · taste altered · tinnitus · vertigo · vomiting
- **Uncommon** Arthralgia · confusion · eosinophilia · erectile dysfunction · fever · haemolytic anaemia · hyperhidrosis · myocardial infarction · pancreatitis · peripheral oedema · photosensitivity reaction · respiratory disorders · stroke
- **Rare or very rare** Agranulocytosis · hepatitis · leucopenia · neutropenia · pancytopenia · Stevens-Johnson syndrome · thrombocytopenia

SIDE-EFFECTS, FURTHER INFORMATION In light of reports of cholestatic jaundice, hepatitis, fulminant hepatic necrosis, and hepatic failure, ACE inhibitors should be discontinued if marked elevation of hepatic enzymes or jaundice occur.

- ALLERGY AND CROSS-SENSITIVITY ACE inhibitors are contra-indicated in patients with hypersensitivity to ACE inhibitors (including angioedema).
- PREGNANCY ACE inhibitors should be avoided in pregnancy unless essential. They may adversely affect fetal and neonatal blood pressure control and renal function; skull defects and oligohydramnios have also been reported.
- BREAST FEEDING Information on the use of ACE inhibitors in breast-feeding is limited.
- RENAL IMPAIRMENT
  Dose adjustments Use with caution, starting with low dose, and adjust according to response. Hyperkalaemia and other side-effects of ACE inhibitors are more common in those with impaired renal function and the dose may need to be reduced.
- MONITORING REQUIREMENTS Renal function and electrolytes should be checked before starting ACE inhibitors (or increasing the dose) and monitored during treatment (more frequently if side effects mentioned are present).
- DIRECTIONS FOR ADMINISTRATION For hypertension the first dose should preferably be given at bedtime.

F above

Captopril

10-Mar-2020

- INDICATIONS AND DOSE

Hypertension

▶ BY MOUTH
- Preterm neonate (initiated under specialist supervision): Test dose 10 micrograms/kg, monitor blood pressure carefully for 1–2 hours; usual dose 10–50 micrograms/kg 2–3 times a day, then increased if necessary up to 300 micrograms/kg daily in divided doses, ongoing doses should only be given if test dose tolerated.
- Neonate (initiated under specialist supervision): Test dose 10–50 micrograms/kg, monitor blood pressure carefully for 1–2 hours; usual dose 10–50 micrograms/kg 2–3 times a day, then increased if necessary up to 2 mg/kg daily in divided doses, ongoing doses should only be given if test dose tolerated.
- Child 1–11 months (initiated under specialist supervision): Test dose 100 micrograms/kg (max. per dose 6.25 mg), monitor blood pressure carefully for 1–2 hours; usual dose 100–300 micrograms/kg 2–3 times a day, then increased if necessary up to 4 mg/kg daily in divided doses, ongoing doses should only be given if test dose tolerated
- Child 1–11 years (initiated under specialist supervision): Test dose 100 micrograms/kg (max. per dose 6.25 mg), monitor blood pressure carefully for 1–2 hours; usual dose 100–300 micrograms/kg 2–3 times a day, then increased if necessary up to 6 mg/kg daily in divided doses, ongoing doses should only be given if test dose tolerated
- Child 12–17 years (initiated under specialist supervision): Test dose 100 micrograms/kg, alternatively test dose 6.25 mg, monitor blood pressure carefully for

1–2 hours; usual dose 12.5–25 mg 2–3 times a day, then increased if necessary up to 150 mg daily in divided doses, ongoing doses should only be given if test dose tolerated

Heart failure

▶ BY MOUTH

- Preterm neonate (initiated under specialist supervision): Test dose 10 micrograms/kg, monitor blood pressure carefully for 1–2 hours; usual dose 10–50 micrograms/kg 2–3 times a day, then increased if necessary up to 300 micrograms/kg daily in divided doses, ongoing doses should only be given if test dose tolerated.
- Neonate (initiated under specialist supervision): Test dose 10–50 micrograms/kg, monitor blood pressure carefully for 1–2 hours; usual dose 10–50 micrograms/kg 2–3 times a day, then increased if necessary up to 2 mg/kg daily in divided doses, ongoing doses should only be given if test dose tolerated.
- Child 1–11 months (initiated under specialist supervision): Test dose 100 micrograms/kg (max. per dose 6.25 mg), monitor blood pressure carefully for 1–2 hours; usual dose 100–300 micrograms/kg 2–3 times a day, then increased if necessary up to 4 mg/kg daily in divided doses, ongoing doses should only be given if test dose tolerated
- Child 1–11 years (initiated under specialist supervision): Test dose 100 micrograms/kg (max. per dose 6.25 mg), monitor blood pressure carefully for 1–2 hours; usual dose 100–300 micrograms/kg 2–3 times a day, then increased if necessary up to 6 mg/kg daily in divided doses, ongoing doses should only be given if test dose tolerated
- Child 12–17 years (initiated under specialist supervision): Test dose 100 micrograms/kg, alternatively test dose 6.25 mg, monitor blood pressure carefully for 1–2 hours; usual dose 12.5–25 mg 2–3 times a day, then increased if necessary up to 150 mg daily in divided doses, ongoing doses should only be given if test dose tolerated

Proteinuria in nephritis (under expert supervision)

▶ BY MOUTH

- Preterm neonate: Test dose 10 micrograms/kg, monitor blood pressure carefully for 1–2 hours; usual dose 10–50 micrograms/kg 2–3 times a day, then increased if necessary up to 300 micrograms/kg daily in divided doses, ongoing doses should only be given if test dose tolerated.
- Neonate: Test dose 10–50 micrograms/kg, monitor blood pressure carefully for 1–2 hours; usual dose 10–50 micrograms/kg 2–3 times a day, then increased if necessary up to 2 mg/kg daily in divided doses, ongoing doses should only be given if test dose tolerated.
- Child 1–11 months: Test dose 100 micrograms/kg (max. per dose 6.25 mg), monitor blood pressure carefully for 1–2 hours; usual dose 100–300 micrograms/kg 2–3 times a day, then increased if necessary up to 4 mg/kg daily in divided doses, ongoing doses should only be given if test dose tolerated
- Child 1–11 years: Test dose 100 micrograms/kg (max. per dose 6.25 mg), monitor blood pressure carefully for 1–2 hours; usual dose 100–300 micrograms/kg 2–3 times a day, then increased if necessary up to 6 mg/kg daily in divided doses, ongoing doses should only be given if test dose tolerated
- Child 12–17 years: Test dose 100 micrograms/kg, alternatively test dose 6.25 mg, monitor blood pressure carefully for 1–2 hours; usual dose 12.5–25 mg 2–3 times a day, then increased if necessary up to 150 mg daily in divided doses, ongoing doses should only be given if test dose tolerated

Diabetic nephropathy in type 1 diabetes mellitus

▶ BY MOUTH

- Child 12–17 years (under expert supervision): Test dose 100 micrograms/kg, alternatively test dose 6.25 mg, monitor blood pressure carefully for 1– 2 hours; usual dose 12.5–25 mg 2–3 times a day, increased if necessary up to 100 mg daily in divided doses, ongoing doses should only be given if test dose tolerated

- **UNLICENSED USE** Not licensed for proteinuria in nephritis. Captopril doses in BNF Publications differs from product licence.
- **CAUTIONS** Children (efficacy and safety not fully established)
- **INTERACTIONS** → Appendix 1: ACE inhibitors
- **SIDE-EFFECTS**
  - ▶ **Common or very common** Insomnia · peptic ulcer
  - ▶ **Uncommon** Appetite decreased · flushing · malaise · pallor · Raynaud's phenomenon
  - ▶ **Rare or very rare** Anaemia · aplastic anaemia · autoimmune disorder · cardiac arrest · cardiogenic shock · cerebrovascular insufficiency · depression · gynaecomastia · hepatic disorders · hypoglycaemia · lymphadenopathy · nephrotic syndrome · oral disorders · proteinuria · urinary disorders · vision blurred
- **BREAST FEEDING** Avoid in first few weeks after delivery, particularly in preterm infants—risk of profound neonatal hypotension; can be used in mothers breast-feeding older infants if essential but monitor infant's blood pressure.
- **DIRECTIONS FOR ADMINISTRATION** Administer under close supervision. Give test dose whilst child supine. Tablets can be dispersed in water.
- **PATIENT AND CARER ADVICE**
  Medicines for Children leaflet: Captopril for heart failure www.medicinesforchildren.org.uk/captopril-heart-failure-0

- **MEDICINAL FORMS** There can be variation in the licensing of different medicines containing the same drug. Forms available from special-order manufacturers include: tablet, capsule, oral suspension, oral solution

Tablet

▸ Captopril (Non-proprietary)
 Captopril 12.5 mg Captopril 12.5mg tablets | 56 tablet PoM £1.54 DT = £1.53
 Captopril 25 mg Captopril 25mg tablets | 56 tablet PoM £1.76 DT = £1.75
 Captopril 50 mg Captopril 50mg tablets | 56 tablet PoM £1.51 DT = £1.51

Oral solution

ELECTROLYTES: May contain Sodium

▸ Captopril (Non-proprietary)
 Captopril 1 mg per 1 ml Captopril 5mg/5ml oral solution sugar-free | 100 ml PoM £98.21 DT = £94.20
 Captopril 5 mg per 1 ml Captopril 25mg/5ml oral solution sugar-free | 100 ml PoM £108.94 DT = £104.51

▸ Noyada (Martindale Pharmaceuticals Ltd)
 Captopril 1 mg per 1 ml Noyada 5mg/5ml oral solution sugar-free | 100 ml PoM £98.21 DT = £94.20
 Captopril 5 mg per 1 ml Noyada 25mg/5ml oral solution sugar-free | 100 ml PoM £108.94 DT = £104.51

118

Enalapril maleate

10-Mar-2020

- **INDICATIONS AND DOSE**

Hypertension

▶ BY MOUTH

- Neonate (under expert supervision): Initially 10 micrograms/kg once daily, monitor blood pressure carefully for 1–2 hours, increased if necessary up to 500 micrograms/kg daily in 1–3 divided doses, limited information.
- Child 1 month–11 years (under expert supervision): Initially 100 micrograms/kg once daily, monitor blood pressure carefully for 1–2 hours, then increased if necessary up to 1 mg/kg daily in 1–2 divided doses
- Child 12–17 years (under expert supervision) (body-weight up to 50 kg): Initially 2.5 mg once daily, monitor blood pressure carefully for 1–2 hours, maintenance 10–20 mg daily in 1–2 divided doses
- Child 12–17 years (under expert supervision) (body-weight 50 kg and above): Initially 2.5 mg once daily, monitor blood pressure carefully for 1–2 hours, maintenance 10–20 mg daily in 1–2 divided doses; maximum 40 mg per day

Heart failure

▶ BY MOUTH

- Neonate (under expert supervision): Initially 10 micrograms/kg once daily, monitor blood pressure carefully for 1–2 hours, increased if necessary up to 500 micrograms/kg daily in 1–3 divided doses, limited information.
- Child 1 month–11 years (under expert supervision): Initially 100 micrograms/kg once daily, monitor blood pressure carefully for 1–2 hours, then increased if necessary up to 1 mg/kg daily in 1–2 divided doses
- Child 12–17 years (under expert supervision) (body-weight up to 50 kg): Initially 2.5 mg once daily, monitor blood pressure carefully for 1–2 hours, maintenance 10–20 mg daily in 1–2 divided doses
- Child 12–17 years (under expert supervision) (body-weight 50 kg and above): Initially 2.5 mg once daily, monitor blood pressure carefully for 1–2 hours, maintenance 10–20 mg daily in 1–2 divided doses; maximum 40 mg per day

Proteinuria in nephritis (under expert supervision)

▶ BY MOUTH

- Neonate: Initially 10 micrograms/kg once daily, monitor blood pressure carefully for 1–2 hours, increased if necessary up to 500 micrograms/kg daily in 1–3 divided doses, limited information.
- Child 1 month–11 years: Initially 100 micrograms/kg once daily, monitor blood pressure carefully for 1–2 hours, then increased if necessary up to 1 mg/kg daily in 1–2 divided doses
- Child 12–17 years (body-weight up to 50 kg): Initially 2.5 mg once daily, monitor blood pressure carefully for 1–2 hours, maintenance 10–20 mg daily in 1–2 divided doses
- Child 12–17 years (body-weight 50 kg and above): Initially 2.5 mg once daily, monitor blood pressure carefully for 1–2 hours, maintenance 10–20 mg daily in 1–2 divided doses; maximum 40 mg per day

Diabetic nephropathy (under expert supervision)

▶ BY MOUTH

- Child 12–17 years (body-weight up to 50 kg): Initially 2.5 mg once daily, monitor blood pressure carefully for 1–2 hours; maintenance 10–20 mg daily in 1–2 divided doses
- Child 12–17 years (body-weight 50 kg and above): Initially 2.5 mg once daily, monitor blood pressure carefully for 1–2 hours; maintenance 10–20 mg daily in 1–2 divided doses; maximum 40 mg per day

- **UNLICENSED USE** Not licensed for use in children for congestive heart failure, proteinuria in nephritis or diabetic nephropathy; not licensed for use in children less than 20 kg for hypertension.
- **INTERACTIONS** → Appendix 1: ACE inhibitors
- **SIDE-EFFECTS**

▶ **Common or very common** Depression · hypersensitivity · vision blurred

▶ **Uncommon** Anaemia · appetite decreased · asthma · bone marrow disorders · flushing · gastrointestinal disorders · hoarseness · hypoglycaemia · malaise · muscle cramps · nervousness · proteinuria · rhinorrhoea · sleep disorders · throat pain

▶ **Rare or very rare** Autoimmune disorder · gynaecomastia · hepatic disorders · lymphadenopathy · oral disorders · Raynaud's phenomenon · toxic epidermal necrolysis

▶ **Frequency not known** Arthritis · leucocytosis · myositis · serositis · SIADH · vasculitis

- **BREAST FEEDING** Avoid in first few weeks after delivery, particularly in preterm infants—risk of profound neonatal hypotension; can be used in mothers breast-feeding older infants if essential but monitor infant's blood pressure.
- **HEPATIC IMPAIRMENT** Enalapril is a prodrug.
- **DIRECTIONS FOR ADMINISTRATION** Tablets may be crushed and suspended in water immediately before use.
- **PATIENT AND CARER ADVICE**

Medicines for Children leaflet: Enalapril for high blood pressure www.medicinesforchildren.org.uk/enalapril-high-blood-pressure

---

- **MEDICINAL FORMS** There can be variation in the licensing of different medicines containing the same drug. Forms available from special-order manufacturers include: oral suspension, oral solution

Tablet

▶ Enalapril maleate (Non-proprietary)

Enalapril maleate 2.5 mg Enalapril 2.5mg tablets | 28 tablet PoM £7.39 DT = £5.73

Enalapril maleate 5 mg Enalapril 5mg tablets | 28 tablet PoM £4.13 DT = £1.52

Enalapril maleate 10 mg Enalapril 10mg tablets | 28 tablet PoM £5.64 DT = £1.79

Enalapril maleate 20 mg Enalapril 20mg tablets | 28 tablet PoM £6.63 DT = £1.96

▶ Innovace (Merck Sharp & Dohme Ltd)

Enalapril maleate 2.5 mg Innovace 2.5mg tablets | 28 tablet PoM £5.35 DT = £5.73

Enalapril maleate 5 mg Innovace 5mg tablets | 28 tablet PoM £7.51 DT = £1.52

Enalapril maleate 10 mg Innovace 10mg tablets | 28 tablet PoM £10.53 DT = £1.79

Enalapril maleate 20 mg Innovace 20mg tablets | 28 tablet PoM £12.51 DT = £1.96

118

Lisinopril

10-Mar-2020

- **INDICATIONS AND DOSE**

Hypertension

▶ BY MOUTH

- Child 6–11 years (under expert supervision): Initially 70 micrograms/kg once daily (max. per dose 5 mg), increased to up to 600 micrograms/kg once daily, alternatively increased to up to 40 mg once daily, dose to be increased in intervals of 1–2 weeks
- Child 12–17 years (under expert supervision): Initially 5 mg once daily; usual maintenance 10–20 mg once daily; maximum 80 mg per day

Proteinuria in nephritis (under expert supervision)
- ▶ BY MOUTH
- ▸ Child 6–11 years: Initially 70 micrograms/kg once daily (max. per dose 5 mg), increased to up to 600 micrograms/kg once daily, alternatively increased to up to 40 mg once daily, dose to be increased in intervals of 1–2 weeks
- ▸ Child 12–17 years: Initially 5 mg once daily; usual maintenance 10–20 mg once daily; maximum 80 mg per day

Diabetic nephropathy (under expert supervision)
- ▶ BY MOUTH
- ▸ Child 12–17 years: Initially 5 mg once daily; usual maintenance 10–20 mg once daily; maximum 80 mg per day

Heart failure (adjunct) (under close medical supervision)
- ▶ BY MOUTH
- ▸ Child 12–17 years: Initially 2.5 mg once daily; increased in steps of up to 10 mg at least every 2 weeks; maximum 35 mg per day

- **UNLICENSED USE** Not licensed for use in children.
- **INTERACTIONS** → Appendix 1: ACE inhibitors
- **SIDE-EFFECTS**
- ▶ **Common or very common** Postural disorders
- ▶ **Uncommon** Hallucination · mood altered · Raynaud's phenomenon
- ▶ **Rare or very rare** Anaemia · autoimmune disorder · azotaemia · bone marrow depression · gynaecomastia · hepatic disorders · hypersensitivity · hypoglycaemia · lymphadenopathy · olfactory nerve disorder · SIADH · sinusitis · toxic epidermal necrolysis
- ▶ **Frequency not known** Depressive symptom · leucocytosis · vasculitis
- **BREAST FEEDING** Not recommended; alternative treatment options, with better established safety information during breast-feeding, are available.
- **PRESCRIBING AND DISPENSING INFORMATION** The RCPCH and NPPG recommend that, when a liquid special of lisinopril is required, the following strength is used: 20 mg/5 mL.
- **PATIENT AND CARER ADVICE**
  Medicines for Children leaflet: Lisinopril for high blood pressure www.medicinesforchildren.org.uk/lisinopril-high-blood-pressure

---

- **MEDICINAL FORMS** There can be variation in the licensing of different medicines containing the same drug. Forms available from special-order manufacturers include: oral suspension, oral solution

Oral solution
- ▸ Lisinopril (Non-proprietary)
  Lisinopril 1 mg per 1 ml Lisinopril 5mg/5ml oral solution sugar-free | 150 ml [PoM] £154.11 DT = £154.11

Tablet
- ▸ Lisinopril (Non-proprietary)
  Lisinopril 2.5 mg Lisinopril 2.5mg tablets | 28 tablet [PoM] £4.81 DT = £0.74 | 500 tablet [PoM] £11.84–£13.75
  Lisinopril 5 mg Lisinopril 5mg tablets | 28 tablet [PoM] £7.54 DT = £0.90 | 500 tablet [PoM] £10.93–£16.07
  Lisinopril 10 mg Lisinopril 10mg tablets | 28 tablet [PoM] £11.81 DT = £0.90 | 500 tablet [PoM] £10.78–£16.43
  Lisinopril 20 mg Lisinopril 20mg tablets | 28 tablet [PoM] £10.42 DT = £0.95 | 500 tablet [PoM] £12.75–£17.86
- ▸ Zestril (AstraZeneca UK Ltd)
  Lisinopril 5 mg Zestril 5mg tablets | 28 tablet [PoM] £9.42 DT = £0.90
  Lisinopril 10 mg Zestril 10mg tablets | 28 tablet [PoM] £14.76 DT = £0.90
  Lisinopril 20 mg Zestril 20mg tablets | 28 tablet [PoM] £13.02 DT = £0.95

DRUGS ACTING ON THE RENIN-ANGIOTENSIN SYSTEM > ANGIOTENSIN II RECEPTOR ANTAGONISTS

Angiotensin II receptor antagonists

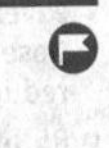

- **CAUTIONS** Afro-Caribbean patients—particularly those with left ventricular hypertrophy (may not benefit from an angiotensin-II receptor antagonist) · aortic or mitral valve stenosis · hypertrophic cardiomyopathy · patients with a history of angioedema · patients with primary aldosteronism (may not benefit from an angiotensin-II receptor antagonist) · renal artery stenosis
- **SIDE-EFFECTS**
- ▶ **Common or very common** Abdominal pain · asthenia · back pain · cough · diarrhoea · dizziness · headache · hyperkalaemia · hypotension · nausea · postural hypotension (more common in patients with intravascular volume depletion, e.g. those taking high-dose diuretics) · renal impairment · skin reactions · vertigo · vomiting
- ▶ **Uncommon** Angioedema · hepatic function abnormal · myalgia · thrombocytopenia
- ▶ **Rare or very rare** Arthralgia
- **PREGNANCY** Angiotensin-II receptor antagonists should be avoided in pregnancy unless essential. They may adversely affect fetal and neonatal blood pressure control and renal function; neonatal skull defects and oligohydramnios have also been reported.
- **BREAST FEEDING** Information on the use of angiotensin-II receptor antagonists in breast-feeding is limited. They are not recommended in breast-feeding and alternative treatment options, with better established safety information during breast-feeding, are available.
- **HEPATIC IMPAIRMENT** In general, manufacturers advise caution in mild to moderate impairment (limited information available); avoid in severe impairment (no information available).
- **RENAL IMPAIRMENT**
  Dose adjustments Use with caution, starting with low dose, and adjust according to response.
- **MONITORING REQUIREMENTS** Monitor plasma-potassium concentration, particularly in children with renal impairment.

F above

Candesartan cilexetil

29-Jul-2019

- **INDICATIONS AND DOSE**

Hypertension
- ▶ BY MOUTH
- ▸ Child 6–17 years (under expert supervision) (body-weight up to 50 kg): Initially 4 mg once daily, adjusted according to response, lower dose may be used in intravascular volume depletion; maximum 8 mg per day
- ▸ Child 6–17 years (under expert supervision) (body-weight 50 kg and above): Initially 4 mg once daily, adjusted according to response, lower dose may be used in intravascular volume depletion; maximum 16 mg per day

- **UNLICENSED USE** [EvGr] Candesartan is used for migraine prophylaxis, ⟨A⟩ but is not licensed for this indication.
- **CONTRA-INDICATIONS** Cholestasis
- **INTERACTIONS** → Appendix 1: angiotensin-II receptor antagonists
- **SIDE-EFFECTS**
- ▶ **Common or very common** Fever · increased risk of infection · oropharyngeal pain · sinus arrhythmia

- **Uncommon** Hyponatraemia
- **Rare or very rare** Agranulocytosis · hepatitis · leucopenia · neutropenia

● **HEPATIC IMPAIRMENT** Manufacturer advises avoid in severe impairment or cholestasis.

Dose adjustments In adults, manufacturer advises dose reduction—consult product literature.

● **RENAL IMPAIRMENT** Use with caution if estimated glomerular filtration rate is less than 30 mL/minute/1.73 m^2—no information available.

Dose adjustments Reduce initial dose.

● **MEDICINAL FORMS** There can be variation in the licensing of different medicines containing the same drug. Forms available from special-order manufacturers include: oral suspension, oral solution

Tablet

- Candesartan cilexetil (Non-proprietary)
  - **Candesartan cilexetil 2 mg** Candesartan 2mg tablets | 7 tablet PoM £16.13 DT = £1.23
  - **Candesartan cilexetil 4 mg** Candesartan 4mg tablets | 7 tablet PoM £3.88 DT = £0.79 | 28 tablet PoM £0.49–£9.78
  - **Candesartan cilexetil 8 mg** Candesartan 8mg tablets | 28 tablet PoM £9.89 DT = £1.68
  - **Candesartan cilexetil 16 mg** Candesartan 16mg tablets | 28 tablet PoM £12.72 DT = £1.71
  - **Candesartan cilexetil 32 mg** Candesartan 32mg tablets | 28 tablet PoM £16.13 DT = £1.94
- Amias (Takeda UK Ltd)
  - **Candesartan cilexetil 2 mg** Amias 2mg tablets | 7 tablet PoM £3.58 DT = £1.23
  - **Candesartan cilexetil 4 mg** Amias 4mg tablets | 7 tablet PoM £3.88 DT = £0.79 | 28 tablet PoM £9.78
  - **Candesartan cilexetil 8 mg** Amias 8mg tablets | 28 tablet PoM £9.89 DT = £1.68
  - **Candesartan cilexetil 16 mg** Amias 16mg tablets | 28 tablet PoM £12.72 DT = £1.71
  - **Candesartan cilexetil 32 mg** Amias 32mg tablets | 28 tablet PoM £16.13 DT = £1.94

F 121

Losartan potassium

03-Aug-2018

● **INDICATIONS AND DOSE**

Hypertension

▶ BY MOUTH

- Child 6–17 years (under expert supervision) (body-weight 20–49 kg): Initially 700 micrograms/kg once daily (max. per dose 25 mg), adjusted according to response to 50 mg daily, lower initial dose may be used in intravascular volume depletion; maximum 50 mg per day
- Child 6–17 years (under expert supervision) (body-weight 50 kg and above): Initially 50 mg once daily, adjusted according to response to 1.4 mg/kg once daily; maximum 100 mg per day

Hypertension with intravascular volume depletion

▶ BY MOUTH

- Child 6–17 years (under expert supervision) (body-weight 50 kg and above): Initially 25 mg once daily; adjusted according to response to 1.4 mg/kg once daily; maximum 100 mg per day

● **CAUTIONS** Severe heart failure

● **INTERACTIONS** → Appendix 1: angiotensin-II receptor antagonists

● **SIDE-EFFECTS**

- **Common or very common** Anaemia · hypoglycaemia · postural disorders
- **Uncommon** Angina pectoris · constipation · drowsiness · dyspnoea · oedema · palpitations · sleep disorder
- **Rare or very rare** Atrial fibrillation · hepatitis · hypersensitivity · paraesthesia · stroke · syncope · vasculitis
- **Frequency not known** Depression · erectile dysfunction · hyponatraemia · influenza like illness · malaise · migraine · pancreatitis · photosensitivity reaction · rhabdomyolysis · taste altered · tinnitus · urinary tract infection

● **HEPATIC IMPAIRMENT** Manufacturer advises avoid in all degrees of impairment (no information available).

● **RENAL IMPAIRMENT** Avoid if estimated glomerular filtration rate is less than 30 mL/minute/1.73 m^2—no information available.

● **PRESCRIBING AND DISPENSING INFORMATION** Flavours of oral liquid formulations may include berry-citrus.

● **MEDICINAL FORMS** There can be variation in the licensing of different medicines containing the same drug. Forms available from special-order manufacturers include: oral suspension, oral solution

Tablet

- Losartan potassium (Non-proprietary)
  - **Losartan potassium 12.5 mg** Losartan 12.5mg tablets | 28 tablet PoM £30.00 DT = £5.19
  - **Losartan potassium 25 mg** Losartan 25mg tablets | 28 tablet PoM £16.18 DT = £1.81
  - **Losartan potassium 50 mg** Losartan 50mg tablets | 28 tablet PoM £12.80 DT = £2.07
  - **Losartan potassium 100 mg** Losartan 100mg tablets | 28 tablet PoM £16.18 DT = £2.60
- Cozaar (Merck Sharp & Dohme Ltd)
  - **Losartan potassium 12.5 mg** Cozaar 12.5mg tablets | 28 tablet PoM £9.70 DT = £5.19
  - **Losartan potassium 25 mg** Cozaar 25mg tablets | 28 tablet PoM £16.18 DT = £1.81
  - **Losartan potassium 50 mg** Cozaar 50mg tablets | 28 tablet PoM £12.80 DT = £2.07
  - **Losartan potassium 100 mg** Cozaar 100mg tablets | 28 tablet PoM £16.18 DT = £2.60

F 121

Valsartan

● **INDICATIONS AND DOSE**

Hypertension

▶ BY MOUTH

- Child 6–17 years (under expert supervision) (body-weight 18–34 kg): Initially 40 mg once daily, adjusted according to response; maximum 80 mg per day
- Child 6–17 years (under expert supervision) (body-weight 35–79 kg): Initially 80 mg once daily, adjusted according to response; maximum 160 mg per day
- Child 6–17 years (under expert supervision) (body-weight 80 kg and above): Initially 80 mg once daily, adjusted according to response; maximum 320 mg per day

● **UNLICENSED USE** Capsules not licensed for use in children.

● **CONTRA-INDICATIONS** Biliary cirrhosis · cholestasis

● **INTERACTIONS** → Appendix 1: angiotensin-II receptor antagonists

● **SIDE-EFFECTS**

- **Uncommon** Heart failure · syncope
- **Frequency not known** Neutropenia · serum sickness · vasculitis

● **HEPATIC IMPAIRMENT**

Dose adjustments Manufacturer advises maximum 80 mg daily in mild to moderate impairment.

● **RENAL IMPAIRMENT** Avoid if estimated glomerular filtration rate is less than 30 mL/minute/1.73 m^2—no information available.

● MEDICINAL FORMS There can be variation in the licensing of different medicines containing the same drug. Forms available from special-order manufacturers include: oral suspension, oral solution

Oral solution

▸ Diovan (Novartis Pharmaceuticals UK Ltd)
Valsartan 3 mg per 1 ml Diovan 3mg/1ml oral solution | 160 ml [PoM] £7.20 DT = £7.20

Tablet

▸ Valsartan (Non-proprietary)
Valsartan 40 mg Valsartan 40mg tablets | 7 tablet [PoM] £7.87 DT = £7.84
Valsartan 160 mg Valsartan 160mg tablets | 28 tablet [PoM] £14.69 DT = £14.69
Valsartan 320 mg Valsartan 320mg tablets | 28 tablet [PoM] £20.23 DT = £18.18

Capsule

▸ Valsartan (Non-proprietary)
Valsartan 40 mg Valsartan 40mg capsules | 28 capsule [PoM] £13.97 DT = £5.54
Valsartan 80 mg Valsartan 80mg capsules | 28 capsule [PoM] £14.35 DT = £9.48
Valsartan 160 mg Valsartan 160mg capsules | 28 capsule [PoM] £18.41 DT = £12.76

VASODILATORS › VASODILATOR ANTIHYPERTENSIVES

Hydralazine hydrochloride

04-Feb-2020

● **INDICATIONS AND DOSE**

Resistant hypertension (adjunct)

▸ BY MOUTH

▸ Neonate: 250–500 micrograms/kg every 8–12 hours, increased if necessary to 2–3 mg/kg every 8 hours.

▸ Child 1 month–11 years: 250–500 micrograms/kg every 8–12 hours, increased if necessary to 7.5 mg/kg daily; maximum 200 mg per day

▸ Child 12–17 years: 25 mg twice daily, increased to 50–100 mg twice daily

▸ BY SLOW INTRAVENOUS INJECTION

▸ Neonate: 100–500 micrograms/kg, dose may be repeated if necessary every 4–6 hours; maximum 3 mg/kg per day.

▸ Child 1 month–11 years: 100–500 micrograms/kg, dose may be repeated if necessary every 4–6 hours; maximum 3 mg/kg per day; maximum 60 mg per day

▸ Child 12–17 years: 5–10 mg, dose may be repeated if necessary every 4–6 hours

▸ BY CONTINUOUS INTRAVENOUS INFUSION

▸ Neonate: 12.5–50 micrograms/kg/hour, continuous intravenous infusion is the preferred route in cardiac patients; maximum 2 mg/kg per day.

▸ Child 1 month–11 years: 12.5–50 micrograms/kg/hour, continuous intravenous infusion is the preferred route in cardiac patients; maximum 3 mg/kg per day

▸ Child 12–17 years: 3–9 mg/hour, continuous intravenous infusion is the preferred route in cardiac patients; maximum 3 mg/kg per day

● UNLICENSED USE Not licensed for use in children.

● CONTRA-INDICATIONS Acute porphyrias p. 652 · cor pulmonale · dissecting aortic aneurysm · high output heart failure · idiopathic systemic lupus erythematosus · myocardial insufficiency due to mechanical obstruction · severe tachycardia

● CAUTIONS Cerebrovascular disease · coronary artery disease (may provoke angina, avoid after myocardial infarction until stabilised) · occasionally blood pressure reduction too rapid even with low parenteral doses

● INTERACTIONS → Appendix 1: hydralazine

● SIDE-EFFECTS

▸ **Common or very common** Angina pectoris · diarrhoea · dizziness · flushing · gastrointestinal disorders · headache · hypotension · joint disorders · lupus-like syndrome (after long-term therapy (more common in slow acetylator individuals)) · myalgia · nasal congestion · nausea · palpitations · tachycardia · vomiting

▸ **Rare or very rare** Acute kidney injury · agranulocytosis · anaemia · anxiety · appetite decreased · conjunctivitis · depression · dyspnoea · eosinophilia · eye disorders · fever · glomerulonephritis · haematuria · haemolytic anaemia · hallucination · heart failure · hepatic disorders · leucocytosis · leucopenia · lymphadenopathy · malaise · nerve disorders · neutropenia · oedema · pancytopenia · paradoxical pressor response · paraesthesia · pleuritic pain · proteinuria · skin reactions · splenomegaly · thrombocytopenia · urinary retention · vasculitis · weight decreased

SIDE-EFFECTS, FURTHER INFORMATION The incidence of side-effects is lower if the dose is kept low, but systemic lupus erythematosus should be suspected if there is unexplained weight loss, arthritis, or any other unexplained ill health.

● PREGNANCY Neonatal thrombocytopenia reported, but risk should be balanced against risk of uncontrolled maternal hypertension. Manufacturer advises avoid before third trimester.

● BREAST FEEDING Present in milk but not known to be harmful.
Monitoring Monitor infant in breast-feeding.

● HEPATIC IMPAIRMENT Manufacturer advises caution (risk of accumulation).
Dose adjustments Manufacturer advises adjust dose or dosing interval according to clinical response.

● RENAL IMPAIRMENT
Dose adjustments Reduce dose if estimated glomerular filtration rate less than 30 mL/minute/1.73 m^2.

● MONITORING REQUIREMENTS Manufacturer advises test for antinuclear factor and for proteinuria every 6 months and check acetylator status before increasing dose, but evidence of clinical value unsatisfactory.

● DIRECTIONS FOR ADMINISTRATION

▸ With oral use For administration *by mouth*, diluted injection may be given orally.

▸ With intravenous use For *continuous intravenous infusion*, initially reconstitute 20 mg with 1 mL Water for Injections, then dilute with Sodium Chloride 0.9%. Incompatible with Glucose intravenous infusion. For *intravenous injection*, initially reconstitute 20 mg with 1 mL Water for Injections, then dilute to a concentration of 0.5–1 mg/mL with Sodium Chloride 0.9% and administer over 5–20 minutes.

● MEDICINAL FORMS There can be variation in the licensing of different medicines containing the same drug. Forms available from special-order manufacturers include: tablet, oral suspension, oral solution

Tablet

EXCIPIENTS: May contain Gluten, propylene glycol

▸ Hydralazine hydrochloride (Non-proprietary)
Hydralazine hydrochloride 25 mg Hydralazine 25mg tablets | 56 tablet [PoM] £7.37 DT = £5.64 | 84 tablet [PoM] £14.00
Hydralazine hydrochloride 50 mg Hydralazine 50mg tablets | 56 tablet [PoM] £15.46 DT = £8.11

▸ Apresoline (Advanz Pharma)
Hydralazine hydrochloride 25 mg Apresoline 25mg tablets | 84 tablet [PoM] £3.38

▸ Apo-Hydralazine (Imported (United States))
Hydralazine hydrochloride 10 mg Apo-Hydralazine 10mg tablets | 100 tablet [PoM] [X]

Powder for solution for injection

▸ Hydralazine hydrochloride (Non-proprietary)

Hydralazine hydrochloride 20 mg Hydralazine 20mg powder for concentrate for solution for injection ampoules | 5 ampoule PoM £74.17

Minoxidil

01-May-2020

● **INDICATIONS AND DOSE**

Severe hypertension

▶ BY MOUTH

▸ Child 1 month–11 years: Initially 200 micrograms/kg daily in 1–2 divided doses, then increased in steps of 100–200 micrograms/kg, increased at intervals of at least 3 days; maximum 1 mg/kg per day

▸ Child 12–17 years: Initially 5 mg daily in 1–2 divided doses, then increased in steps of 5–10 mg daily, increased at intervals of at least 3 days; maximum 100 mg per day

● **CONTRA-INDICATIONS** Phaeochromocytoma

● **CAUTIONS** Acute porphyrias p. 652 · after myocardial infarction (until stabilised) · angina

● **INTERACTIONS** → Appendix 1: minoxidil

● **SIDE-EFFECTS**

▶ **Common or very common** Fluid retention · hair changes · oedema · pericardial disorders · pericarditis · tachycardia

▶ **Rare or very rare** Leucopenia · skin reactions · Stevens-Johnson syndrome · thrombocytopenia

▶ **Frequency not known** Angina pectoris · breast tenderness · gastrointestinal disorder · pleural effusion · sodium retention · weight increased

● **PREGNANCY** Avoid—possible toxicity including reduced placental perfusion. Neonatal hirsutism reported.

● **BREAST FEEDING** Present in milk but not known to be harmful.

● **RENAL IMPAIRMENT** Use with caution in significant impairment.

● **MEDICINAL FORMS** There can be variation in the licensing of different medicines containing the same drug.

Tablet

▸ Loniten (Pfizer Ltd)

Minoxidil 2.5 mg Loniten 2.5mg tablets | 60 tablet PoM £8.88 DT = £8.88

Minoxidil 5 mg Loniten 5mg tablets | 60 tablet PoM £15.83 DT = £15.83

Minoxidil 10 mg Loniten 10mg tablets | 60 tablet PoM £30.68 DT = £30.68

4.1a Hypertension associated with phaeochromocytoma

Other drugs used for Hypertension associated with phaeochromocytoma Propranolol hydrochloride, p. 111

VASODILATORS > PERIPHERAL VASODILATORS

Phenoxybenzamine hydrochloride

01-Apr-2020

● **INDICATIONS AND DOSE**

Hypertension in phaeochromocytoma

▶ BY MOUTH

▸ Child: 0.5–1 mg/kg twice daily, adjusted according to response

● **UNLICENSED USE** Not licensed for use in children.

● **CONTRA-INDICATIONS** During recovery period after myocardial infarction (usually 3–4 weeks) · history of cerebrovascular accident

● **CAUTIONS** Avoid in Acute porphyrias p. 652 · carcinogenic in *animals* · cerebrovascular disease · congestive heart failure · severe ischaemic heart disease

● **SIDE-EFFECTS** Abdominal distress · dizziness · ejaculation failure · fatigue · miosis · nasal congestion · postural hypotension · reflex tachycardia

● **PREGNANCY** Hypotension may occur in newborn.

● **BREAST FEEDING** May be present in milk.

● **RENAL IMPAIRMENT** Use with caution.

● **DIRECTIONS FOR ADMINISTRATION** For administration *by mouth*, capsules may be opened.

● **HANDLING AND STORAGE** Owing to risk of contact sensitisation healthcare professionals should avoid contamination of hands.

● **MEDICINAL FORMS** There can be variation in the licensing of different medicines containing the same drug. Forms available from special-order manufacturers include: oral suspension, oral solution

Capsule

▸ Phenoxybenzamine hydrochloride (Non-proprietary)

Phenoxybenzamine hydrochloride 10 mg Phenoxybenzamine 10mg capsules | 30 capsule PoM £118.00 DT = £118.00

4.1b Hypertensive crises

Other drugs used for Hypertensive crises Hydralazine hydrochloride, p. 123 · Labetalol hydrochloride, p. 110

VASODILATORS > VASODILATOR ANTIHYPERTENSIVES

Sodium nitroprusside

06-Feb-2020

● **INDICATIONS AND DOSE**

Hypertensive emergencies

▶ BY CONTINUOUS INTRAVENOUS INFUSION

▸ Neonate: Initially 500 nanograms/kg/minute, then increased in steps of 200 nanograms/kg/minute (max. per dose 8 micrograms/kg/minute) as required, max. 4 micrograms/kg/minute if used for longer than 24 hours.

▸ Child: Initially 500 nanograms/kg/minute, then increased in steps of 200 nanograms/kg/minute (max. per dose 8 micrograms/kg/minute) as required, max. 4 micrograms/kg/minute if used for longer than 24 hours

● **UNLICENSED USE** Not licensed for use in the UK.

● **CONTRA-INDICATIONS** Compensatory hypertension · impaired cerebral circulation · Leber's optic atrophy · severe vitamin B_{12} deficiency

● **CAUTIONS** Hyponatraemia · hypothermia · hypothyroidism · ischaemic heart disease

● **INTERACTIONS** → Appendix 1: nitroprusside

● **SIDE-EFFECTS** Abdominal pain · anaemia · arrhythmias · chest discomfort · cyanide toxicity · dizziness · flushing · headache · hyperhidrosis · hypothyroidism · hypovolaemia · ileus · intracranial pressure increased · methaemoglobinaemia · muscle twitching · nausea · palpitations · rash · thiocyanate toxicity

SIDE-EFFECTS, FURTHER INFORMATION Side-effects associated with over rapid reduction in blood pressure: Headache, dizziness, nausea, retching, abdominal pain, perspiration, palpitation, anxiety, retrosternal discomfort—reduce infusion rate if any of these side-effects occur.

Overdose Side-effects caused by excessive plasma concentration of the cyanide metabolite include tachycardia, sweating, hyperventilation, arrhythmias, marked metabolic acidosis (discontinue and give antidote, see cyanide in Emergency treatment of poisoning p. 891).

- **PREGNANCY** Avoid prolonged use—potential for accumulation of cyanide in fetus.
- **BREAST FEEDING** No information available. Caution advised due to thiocyanate metabolite.
- **HEPATIC IMPAIRMENT** Use with caution. Avoid in hepatic failure—cyanide or thiocyanate metabolites may accumulate.
- **RENAL IMPAIRMENT** Avoid prolonged use—cyanide or thiocyanate metabolites may accumulate.
- **MONITORING REQUIREMENTS** Monitor blood pressure (including intra-arterial blood pressure) and blood-cyanide concentration, and if treatment exceeds 3 days, also blood thiocyanate concentration.
- **TREATMENT CESSATION** Avoid sudden withdrawal—terminate infusion over 15–30 minutes.
- **DIRECTIONS FOR ADMINISTRATION** For *continuous intravenous infusion* in Glucose 5%, infuse *via* infusion device to allow precise control. For further details, consult product literature. Protect infusion from light.

- **MEDICINAL FORMS** There can be variation in the licensing of different medicines containing the same drug.

Powder and solvent for solution for infusion

- Sodium nitroprusside (Non-proprietary)
  Sodium nitroprusside dihydrate 50 mg Sodium nitroprusside 50mg powder and solvent for solution for infusion vials | 1 vial PoM

4.1c Pulmonary hypertension

ENDOTHELIN RECEPTOR ANTAGONISTS

Bosentan

05-Feb-2020

- **INDICATIONS AND DOSE**

Pulmonary arterial hypertension (initiated under specialist supervision)

- BY MOUTH
- Child 2–17 years (body-weight 10–20 kg): Initially 31.25 mg once daily for 4 weeks, then increased to 31.25 mg twice daily
- Child 2–17 years (body-weight 20–40 kg): Initially 31.25 mg twice daily for 4 weeks, then increased to 62.5 mg twice daily
- Child 12–17 years (body-weight 40 kg and above): Initially 62.5 mg twice daily for 4 weeks, then increased to 125 mg twice daily (max. per dose 250 mg)

- **CONTRA-INDICATIONS** Acute porphyrias p. 652
- **CAUTIONS** Not to be initiated if systemic systolic blood pressure is below 85 mmHg · pulmonary veno-occlusive disease
- **INTERACTIONS** → Appendix 1: bosentan
- **SIDE-EFFECTS**
- **Common or very common** Anaemia · diarrhoea · flushing · gastrooesophageal reflux disease · headache · nasal congestion · palpitations · skin reactions · syncope
- **Uncommon** Hepatic disorders · leucopenia · neutropenia · thrombocytopenia
- **Rare or very rare** Angioedema
- **Frequency not known** Vision blurred
- **CONCEPTION AND CONTRACEPTION** Effective contraception required during administration (hormonal contraception not considered effective). Monthly pregnancy tests advised.
- **PREGNANCY** Avoid (teratogenic in *animal* studies).
- **BREAST FEEDING** Manufacturer advises avoid—no information available.
- **HEPATIC IMPAIRMENT** Manufacturer advises avoid in moderate-to-severe impairment or if baseline serum transaminases exceed 3 times the upper limit of normal.
- **MONITORING REQUIREMENTS**
- Monitor haemoglobin before and during treatment (monthly for first 4 months, then 3-monthly).
- Monitor liver function before treatment, at monthly intervals during treatment, and 2 weeks after dose increase (reduce dose or suspend treatment if liver enzymes raised significantly)—discontinue if symptoms of liver impairment.
- **TREATMENT CESSATION** Avoid abrupt withdrawal—withdraw treatment gradually.

- **MEDICINAL FORMS** There can be variation in the licensing of different medicines containing the same drug.

Tablet

- Bosentan (Non-proprietary)
  Bosentan (as Bosentan monohydrate) 62.5 mg Bosentan 62.5mg tablets | 56 tablet PoM £112.50 (Hospital only) | 56 tablet PoM £1,359.19–£1,510.21
  Bosentan (as Bosentan monohydrate) 125 mg Bosentan 125mg tablets | 56 tablet PoM £112.50 (Hospital only) | 56 tablet PoM £1,359.19–£1,510.21
- Stayveer (Advanz Pharma)
  Bosentan (as Bosentan monohydrate) 62.5 mg Stayveer 62.5mg tablets | 56 tablet PoM £208.34
  Bosentan (as Bosentan monohydrate) 125 mg Stayveer 125mg tablets | 56 tablet PoM £208.34
- Tracleer (Actelion Pharmaceuticals UK Ltd)
  Bosentan (as Bosentan monohydrate) 62.5 mg Tracleer 62.5mg tablets | 56 tablet PoM £1,510.21
  Bosentan (as Bosentan monohydrate) 125 mg Tracleer 125mg tablets | 56 tablet PoM £1,510.21

PHOSPHODIESTERASE TYPE-5 INHIBITORS

Sildenafil

14-Jan-2020

- **INDICATIONS AND DOSE**

Pulmonary arterial hypertension (initiated under specialist supervision)

- BY MOUTH
- Neonate: Initially 250–500 micrograms/kg every 4–8 hours, adjusted according to response, start with the lower dose and frequency, especially if used with other vasodilators; maximum 30 mg per day.
- Child 1–11 months: Initially 250–500 micrograms/kg every 4–8 hours, adjusted according to response, start with the lower dose and frequency, especially if used with other vasodilators; maximum 30 mg per day
- Child 1–17 years (body-weight up to 20 kg): 10 mg 3 times a day
- Child 1–17 years (body-weight 20 kg and above): 20 mg 3 times a day

DOSE ADJUSTMENTS DUE TO INTERACTIONS

- Manufacturer advises reduce dose with concurrent use of moderate and potent inhibitors of CYP3A4 (avoid with ketoconazole, itraconazole and ritonavir)—no specific recommendation made for children.

- **UNLICENSED USE** Not licensed for use in children under 1 year.
- **CONTRA-INDICATIONS** Hereditary degenerative retinal disorders · history of non-arteritic anterior ischaemic optic

neuropathy · recent history of myocardial infarction · recent history of stroke · sickle-cell anaemia

- **CAUTIONS** Active peptic ulceration · anatomical deformation of the penis (e.g. angulation, cavernosal fibrosis, Peyronie's disease) · autonomic dysfunction · bleeding disorders · cardiovascular disease · hypotension (avoid if severe) · intravascular volume depletion · left ventricular outflow obstruction · predisposition to priapism (e.g. in sickle-cell disease, multiple myeloma, or leukaemia) · pulmonary veno-occlusive disease
- **INTERACTIONS** → Appendix 1: phosphodiesterase type-5 inhibitors
- **SIDE-EFFECTS**
  - **Common or very common** Alopecia · anaemia · anxiety · cough · diarrhoea · dizziness · fluid retention · gastrointestinal discomfort · gastrointestinal disorders · headaches · increased risk of infection · insomnia · nasal complaints · nausea · night sweats · pain · skin reactions · tremor · vasodilation · vision disorders
  - **Uncommon** Arrhythmias · chest pain · drowsiness · dry eye · dry mouth · eye discomfort · eye disorders · eye inflammation · fatigue · feeling hot · gynaecomastia · haemorrhage · hypertension · hypotension · myalgia · numbness · palpitations · sinus congestion · tinnitus · vertigo · vomiting
  - **Rare or very rare** Acute coronary syndrome · arteriosclerotic retinopathy · cerebrovascular insufficiency · glaucoma · haematospermia · hearing impairment · irritability · optic neuropathy (discontinue if sudden visual impairment occurs) · oral hypoaesthesia · priapism · retinal occlusion · scleral discolouration · seizure · severe cutaneous adverse reactions (SCARs) · sudden cardiac death · syncope · throat tightness
- **PREGNANCY** Use only if potential benefit outweighs risk—no evidence of harm in *animal* studies.
- **BREAST FEEDING** Manufacturer advises avoid—no information available.
- **HEPATIC IMPAIRMENT** Manufacturer advises caution in mild to moderate impairment; avoid in severe impairment (no information available).
  Dose adjustments Manufacturer advises if not tolerated, consider dose reduction in mild to moderate impairment—consult product literature.
- **RENAL IMPAIRMENT**
  Dose adjustments Reduce dose if not tolerated
- **TREATMENT CESSATION** Avoid abrupt withdrawal.
- **PATIENT AND CARER ADVICE**
  Medicines for Children leaflet: Sildenafil for pulmonary hypertension www.medicinesforchildren.org.uk/sildenafil-pulmonary-hypertension
- **NATIONAL FUNDING/ACCESS DECISIONS**
  Scottish Medicines Consortium (SMC) decisions
  The *Scottish Medicines Consortium* has advised (December 2012) that sildenafil (*Revatio*®) is accepted for restricted use within NHS Scotland for pulmonary arterial hypertension in children aged 1–17 years; sildenafil should only be prescribed on the advice of specialists in the Scottish Pulmonary Vascular Unit or the Scottish Adult Congenital Cardiac Service.

- **MEDICINAL FORMS** There can be variation in the licensing of different medicines containing the same drug. Forms available from special-order manufacturers include: oral suspension, oral solution, pessary

Tablet

- Sildenafil (Non-proprietary)
  Sildenafil (as Sildenafil citrate) 20 mg Sildenafil 20mg tablets | 90 tablet PoM £424.01–£446.33 DT = £446.33
  Sildenafil (as Sildenafil citrate) 25 mg Sildenafil 25mg tablets | 4 tablet PoM £16.59 DT = £0.90 | 8 tablet PoM £1.73–£33.19
  Sildenafil (as Sildenafil citrate) 50 mg Sildenafil 50mg tablets | 4 tablet PoM £21.27 DT = £1.02 | 8 tablet PoM £1.26–£42.54
  Sildenafil (as Sildenafil citrate) 100 mg Sildenafil 100mg tablets | 4 tablet PoM £23.50 DT = £1.09 | 8 tablet PoM £1.44–£46.99
- Granpidam (Accord Healthcare Ltd)
  Sildenafil (as Sildenafil citrate) 20 mg Granpidam 20mg tablets | 90 tablet PoM £424.01 DT = £446.33
- Mysildecard (Mylan)
  Sildenafil (as Sildenafil citrate) 20 mg Mysildecard 20mg tablets | 90 tablet PoM £379.38 DT = £446.33
- Revatio (Upjohn UK Ltd)
  Sildenafil (as Sildenafil citrate) 20 mg Revatio 20mg tablets | 90 tablet PoM £446.33 DT = £446.33

Oral suspension

- Revatio (Upjohn UK Ltd)
  Sildenafil (as Sildenafil citrate) 10 mg per 1 ml Revatio 10mg/ml oral suspension sugar-free | 112 ml PoM £186.75 DT = £186.75

PROSTAGLANDINS AND ANALOGUES

Epoprostenol

20-Apr-2020

(Prostacyclin)

- **DRUG ACTION** Epoprostenol is a prostaglandin and a potent vasodilator. It is also a powerful inhibitor of platelet aggregation.

- **INDICATIONS AND DOSE**

Persistent pulmonary hypertension of the newborn

- BY CONTINUOUS INTRAVENOUS INFUSION
  - Neonate: Initially 2 nanograms/kg/minute (max. per dose 20 nanograms/kg/minute), adjusted according to response, rarely doses up to 40 nanograms/kg/minute are used.

Idiopathic pulmonary arterial hypertension

- BY CONTINUOUS INTRAVENOUS INFUSION
  - Child: Initially 2 nanograms/kg/minute, increased if necessary up to 40 nanograms/kg/minute

PHARMACOKINETICS

- Short half-life of approximately 3 minutes, therefore it must be administered by continuous intravenous infusion.

- **UNLICENSED USE** Not licensed for use in children.
- **CONTRA-INDICATIONS** Pulmonary veno-occlusive disease · severe left ventricular dysfunction
- **CAUTIONS** Avoid abrupt withdrawal (risk of rebound pulmonary hypertension/pulmonary hypertensive crisis) · haemorrhagic diathesis
- **INTERACTIONS** → Appendix 1: epoprostenol
- **SIDE-EFFECTS**
  - **Common or very common** Abdominal pain · anxiety · arrhythmias · arthralgia · chest discomfort · diarrhoea · flushing · haemorrhage · headache · intracranial haemorrhage · nausea · pain · rash · sepsis · vomiting
  - **Uncommon** Dry mouth · hyperhidrosis
  - **Rare or very rare** Fatigue · hyperthyroidism · intravenous catheter occlusion · local infection · pallor
  - **Frequency not known** Ascites · pulmonary oedema (avoid chronic use if occurs during dose titration) · spleen abnormalities
- **PREGNANCY** Manufacturer advises caution—no information available.
- **BREAST FEEDING** Manufacturer advises avoid—no information available.
- **MONITORING REQUIREMENTS**
  - Anticoagulant monitoring required when given with anticoagulants.
  - Monitor blood pressure.

- **TREATMENT CESSATION** Avoid abrupt withdrawal (risk of rebound pulmonary hypertension and pulmonary hypertensive crisis).
- **DIRECTIONS FOR ADMINISTRATION** Directions for administration vary depending on the preparation used—for instructions *in adults*, consult product literature. For *neonatal intensive care*—consult local protocols.

- **MEDICINAL FORMS** There can be variation in the licensing of different medicines containing the same drug.

Powder for solution for infusion

▸ Epoprostenol (Non-proprietary)

Epoprostenol (as Epoprostenol sodium) 500 microgram Epoprostenol 500microgram powder (pH12) for solution for infusion vials | 1 vial PoM (Hospital only)

Epoprostenol (as Epoprostenol sodium) 1.5 mg Epoprostenol 1.5mg powder (pH12) for solution for infusion vials | 1 vial PoM (Hospital only)

▸ Veletri (Actelion Pharmaceuticals UK Ltd)

Epoprostenol (as Epoprostenol sodium) 500 microgram Veletri 500microgram powder for solution for infusion vials | 1 vial PoM £24.44

Epoprostenol (as Epoprostenol sodium) 1.5 mg Veletri 1.5mg powder for solution for infusion vials | 1 vial PoM £49.24

Powder and solvent for solution for infusion

ELECTROLYTES: May contain Sodium

▸ Epoprostenol (Non-proprietary)

Epoprostenol (as Epoprostenol sodium) 500 microgram Epoprostenol 500microgram powder and solvent (pH10.5) for solution for infusion vials | 1 vial PoM £58.95

Epoprostenol (as Epoprostenol sodium) 1.5 mg Epoprostenol 1.5mg powder and solvent (pH10.5) for solution for infusion vials | 1 vial PoM £118.75

▸ Flolan (GlaxoSmithKline UK Ltd)

Epoprostenol (as Epoprostenol sodium) 500 microgram Flolan 500microgram powder and solvent (pH12) for solution for infusion vials | 1 vial PoM £22.22

Epoprostenol (as Epoprostenol sodium) 1.5 mg Flolan 1.5mg powder and solvent (pH12) for solution for infusion vials | 1 vial PoM £44.76

Iloprost

20-Apr-2020

- **INDICATIONS AND DOSE**

Idiopathic or familial pulmonary arterial hypertension (initiated under specialist supervision)

▸ BY INHALATION OF NEBULISED SOLUTION

▸ Child 8–17 years: Initially 2.5 micrograms for 1 dose, increased to 5 micrograms for 1 dose, increased if tolerated to 5 micrograms 6–9 times a day, adjusted according to response; reduced if not tolerated to 2.5 micrograms 6–9 times a day, reduce to lower maintenance dose if high dose not tolerated

Raynaud's syndrome

▸ BY INTRAVENOUS INFUSION

▸ Child 12–17 years: Initially 0.5 nanogram/kg/minute, increased to 1–2 nanograms/kg/minute given over 6 hours daily for 3–5 days, dose increase should be performed gradually

- **UNLICENSED USE** Not licensed for use in children.
- **CONTRA-INDICATIONS**

GENERAL CONTRA-INDICATIONS Conditions which increase risk of haemorrhage · congenital or acquired valvular defects with myocardial function disorders (not related to pulmonary hypertension) · decompensated heart failure (unless under close medical supervision) · severe arrhythmias · severe coronary heart disease · unstable angina · within 3 months of cerebrovascular events · within 6 months of myocardial infarction

SPECIFIC CONTRA-INDICATIONS

▸ When used by inhalation Pulmonary veno-occlusive disease · systolic blood pressure below 85 mmHg · unstable pulmonary hypertension with advanced right heart failure

▸ With intravenous use acute or chronic congestive heart failure (NYHA II-IV) · pulmonary oedema

- **CAUTIONS**

GENERAL CAUTIONS Hypotension

SPECIFIC CAUTIONS

▸ When used by inhalation Acute pulmonary infection · severe asthma

▸ With intravenous use Significant heart disease

- **INTERACTIONS** → Appendix 1: iloprost
- **SIDE-EFFECTS**

GENERAL SIDE-EFFECTS

▸ **Common or very common** Cough · diarrhoea · dizziness · dyspnoea · haemorrhage · hypotension · nausea · pain · palpitations · syncope · vomiting

▸ **Uncommon** Taste altered · thrombocytopenia

SPECIFIC SIDE-EFFECTS

▸ **Common or very common**

▸ When used by inhalation Chest discomfort · headache · oral disorders · rash · tachycardia · throat complaints · vasodilation

▸ With intravenous use Angina pectoris · anxiety · appetite decreased · arrhythmias · arthralgia · asthenia · bradyphrenia · chills · confusion · drowsiness · feeling hot · fever · flushing · gastrointestinal discomfort · headaches · hyperhidrosis · muscle complaints · sensation abnormal · thirst · vertigo

▸ **Uncommon**

▸ With intravenous use Asthma · cerebrovascular insufficiency · constipation · depression · dry mouth · dysphagia · dysuria · embolism and thrombosis · eye discomfort · hallucination · heart failure · hepatic impairment · myocardial infarction · pruritus · pulmonary oedema · renal pain · seizure · tetany · tremor · vision blurred

▸ **Frequency not known**

▸ When used by inhalation Respiratory disorders

- **PREGNANCY**

▸ When used by inhalation Use if potential benefit outweighs risk.

▸ With intravenous use Manufacturer advises avoid–toxicity in *animal* studies.

- **BREAST FEEDING** Manufacturer advises avoid—no information available.
- **HEPATIC IMPAIRMENT** Manufacturer advises caution (risk of increased exposure).

Dose adjustments In adults, manufacturer advises initial dose reduction—consult product literature.

- **MONITORING REQUIREMENTS**

▸ With intravenous use Manufacturer advises monitor blood pressure and heart rate at the start of the infusion and at every dose increase.

- **DIRECTIONS FOR ADMINISTRATION**

▸ With intravenous use For *intravenous infusion* dilute to a concentration of 200 nanograms/mL with Glucose 5% or Sodium Chloride 0.9%; alternatively, may be diluted to a concentration of 2 micrograms/mL and given via syringe driver.

▸ When used by inhalation For *inhaled treatment*, to minimise accidental exposure use only with nebulisers listed in product literature in a well ventilated room.

- **PRESCRIBING AND DISPENSING INFORMATION**

▸ When used by inhalation Delivery characteristics of nebuliser devices may vary—only switch devices under medical supervision.

▸ With intravenous use Concentrate for infusion available on a named patient basis from Bayer Schering in 0.5 mL and 1 mL ampoules.

- **HANDLING AND STORAGE** Manufacturer advises avoid contact with skin and eyes.
- **PATIENT AND CARER ADVICE**
Driving and skilled tasks Manufacturer advises patients and carers should be counselled on the effects on driving and performance of skilled tasks—increased risk of dizziness.

- **MEDICINAL FORMS** There can be variation in the licensing of different medicines containing the same drug.

Solution for infusion
EXCIPIENTS: May contain Ethanol
▸ **Iloprost (Non-proprietary)**
Iloprost (as Iloprost trometamol) 100 microgram per 1 ml Iloprost 100micrograms/1ml solution for infusion ampoules | 1 ampoule PoM
Iloprost 50micrograms/0.5ml concentrate for solution for infusion ampoules | 1 ampoule PoM £75.00 (Hospital only) | 5 ampoule PoM £300.00 (Hospital only)

Nebuliser liquid
EXCIPIENTS: May contain Ethanol
▸ **Iloprost (Non-proprietary)**
Iloprost (as Iloprost trometamol) 10 microgram per 1 ml Iloprost 10micrograms/1ml nebuliser liquid ampoules | 30 ampoule PoM £300.00 | 160 ampoule PoM £1,700.00
Ventavis 10micrograms/ml nebuliser solution 1ml ampoules with Breelib | 168 ampoule PoM £2,241.08
Iloprost (as Iloprost trometamol) 20 microgram per 1 ml Ventavis 20micrograms/ml nebuliser solution 1ml ampoules with Breelib | 168 ampoule PoM £2,241.08
▸ **Ventavis** (Bayer Plc)
Iloprost (as Iloprost trometamol) 10 microgram per 1 ml Ventavis 10micrograms/ml nebuliser solution 1ml ampoules | 42 ampoule PoM £560.27 | 168 ampoule PoM £2,241.08
Iloprost (as Iloprost trometamol) 20 microgram per 1 ml Ventavis 20micrograms/ml nebuliser solution 1ml ampoules | 42 ampoule PoM £560.27

VASODILATORS › PERIPHERAL VASODILATORS

Tolazoline

- **DRUG ACTION** Tolazoline is an alpha-blocker and produces both pulmonary and systemic vasodilation.

- **INDICATIONS AND DOSE**

Correction of pulmonary vasospasm in neonates
▸ INITIALLY BY INTRAVENOUS INJECTION
▸ Neonate: Initially 1 mg/kg, to be given over 2–5 minutes, followed by (by continuous intravenous infusion) maintenance 200 micrograms/kg/hour if required, careful blood pressure monitoring should be carried out, doses above 300 micrograms/kg/hour associated with cardiotoxicity and renal failure.
▸ BY ENDOTRACHEAL TUBE
▸ Neonate: 200 micrograms/kg.

- **UNLICENSED USE** Not licensed for use in children.
- **CONTRA-INDICATIONS** Peptic ulcer disease
- **CAUTIONS** Cardiotoxic accumulation may occur with continuous infusion (particularly in renal impairment) · mitral stenosis
- **SIDE-EFFECTS** Arrhythmias · blood disorder · chills · diarrhoea · epigastric pain · flushing · haematuria · haemorrhage (with high doses) · headache · hyperhidrosis · hypertension (with high doses) · hypotension (severe; with high doses) · metabolic alkalosis · nausea · oliguria · rash macular · renal failure (with high doses) · thrombocytopenia · vomiting
- **RENAL IMPAIRMENT**
Dose adjustments Lower doses may be necessary.
Accumulates in renal impairment. Risk of cardiotoxicity.
- **MONITORING REQUIREMENTS** Monitor blood pressure regularly for sustained systemic hypotension.
- **DIRECTIONS FOR ADMINISTRATION** For *continuous intravenous infusion*, dilute with Glucose 5% or Sodium Chloride 0.9%. Prepare a fresh solution every 24 hours. For *endotracheal administration*, dilute with 0.5–1 mL of Sodium Chloride 0.9%.

- **MEDICINAL FORMS** Forms available from special-order manufacturers include: solution for injection

4.2 Hypotension and shock

Sympathomimetics

Overview

The properties of sympathomimetics vary according to whether they act on alpha or on beta adrenergic receptors. Response to sympathomimetics can also vary considerably in children, particularly neonates. It is important to titrate the dose to the desired effect and to monitor the child closely.

Inotropic sympathomimetics

Dopamine hydrochloride p. 130 has a variable, unpredictable, and dose dependent impact on vascular tone. Low dose infusion normally causes vasodilatation, but there is little evidence that this is clinically beneficial; moderate doses increase myocardial contractility and cardiac output in older children, but in neonates moderate doses may cause a reduction in cardiac output. High doses cause vasoconstriction and increase vascular resistance, and should therefore be used with caution following cardiac surgery, or where there is co-existing neonatal pulmonary hypertension.

In neonates the response to inotropic sympathomimetics varies considerably, particularly in those born prematurely; careful dose titration and monitoring are necessary.

Isoprenaline injection is available from 'special-order' manufacturers or specialist importing companies.

Shock

Shock is a medical emergency associated with a high mortality. The underlying causes of shock such as haemorrhage, sepsis or myocardial insufficiency should be corrected. Additional treatment is dependent on the type of shock.

Septic shock is associated with severe hypovolaemia (due to vasodilation and capillary leak) which should be corrected with crystalloids or colloids. If hypotension persists despite volume replacement, dopamine hydrochloride should be started. For shock refractory to treatment with dopamine hydrochloride, if cardiac output is high and peripheral vascular resistance is low (warm shock), noradrenaline/norepinephrine p. 131 should be added *or* if cardiac output is low and peripheral vascular resistance is high (cold shock), adrenaline/epinephrine p. 143 should be added. Additionally, in cold shock, a vasodilator such as milrinone p. 134, glyceryl trinitrate p. 142, or sodium nitroprusside p. 124 (on specialist advice only) can be used to reduce vascular resistance.

If the shock is resistant to volume expansion and catecholamines, and there is suspected or proven adrenal insufficiency, low dose hydrocortisone p. 476 can be used. ACTH-stimulated plasma-cortisol concentration should be measured; however, hydrocortisone can be started without such information. Alternatively, if the child is resistant to catecholamines, and vascular resistance is low, vasopressin p. 72 can be added.

Neonatal septic shock can be complicated by the transition from fetal to neonatal circulation. Treatment to reverse right ventricular failure, by decreasing pulmonary artery pressures, is commonly needed in neonates with fluid-refractory shock and persistent pulmonary hypertension of the newborn. Rapid administration of fluid in neonates with patent ductus arteriosus may cause left-to-right shunting and congestive heart failure induced by ventricular overload.

In *cardiogenic shock*, the aim is to improve cardiac output and to reduce the afterload on the heart. If central venous pressure is low, cautious volume expansion with a colloid or crystalloid can be used. An inotrope such as adrenaline/epinephrine or dopamine hydrochloride should be given to increase cardiac output. Dobutamine below is a peripheral vasodilator and is an alternative if hypotension is not significant.

Milrinone has both inotropic and vasodilatory effects and can be used when vascular resistance is high. Alternatively, glyceryl trinitrate or sodium nitroprusside (on specialist advice only) can be used to reduce vasoconstriction.

Hypovolaemic shock should be treated with a crystalloid or colloid solution (or whole or reconstituted blood if source of hypovolaemia is haemorrhage) and further steps to improve cardiac output and decrease vascular resistance can be taken, as in cardiogenic shock.

The use of sympathomimetic inotropes and vasoconstrictors should preferably be confined to the intensive care setting and undertaken with invasive haemodynamic monitoring.

See also advice on the management of anaphylactic shock in Antihistamines, allergen immunotherapy and allergic emergencies p. 180.

Vasoconstrictor sympathomimetics

Vasoconstrictor sympathomimetics raise blood pressure transiently by acting on alpha-adrenergic receptors to constrict peripheral vessels. They are sometimes used as an emergency method of elevating blood pressure where other measures have failed.

The danger of vasoconstrictors is that although they raise blood pressure they also reduce perfusion of vital organs such as the kidney.

Ephedrine hydrochloride p. 130 is used to reverse hypotension caused by spinal and epidural anaesthesia.

Metaraminol p. 130 is used as a vasopressor during cardiopulmonary bypass.

Phenylephrine hydrochloride p. 132 causes peripheral vasoconstriction and increases arterial pressure.

Ephedrine hydrochloride, metaraminol and phenylephrine hydrochloride are rarely needed in children and should be used under specialist supervision.

Noradrenaline/norepinephrine is reserved for children with low systemic vascular resistance that is unresponsive to fluid resuscitation following septic shock, spinal shock, and anaphylaxis.

Adrenaline/epinephrine is mainly used for its inotropic action. Low doses (acting on beta receptors) cause systemic and pulmonary vasodilation, with some increase in heart rate and stroke volume and also an increase in contractility; high doses act predominantly on alpha receptors causing intense systemic vasoconstriction.

SYMPATHOMIMETICS › INOTROPIC

Dobutamine

- **DRUG ACTION** Dobutamine is a cardiac stimulant which acts on beta$_1$ receptors in cardiac muscle, and increases contractility.

- **INDICATIONS AND DOSE**

Inotropic support in low cardiac output states, after cardiac surgery, cardiomyopathies, shock

▶ BY CONTINUOUS INTRAVENOUS INFUSION

▶ Neonate: Initially 5 micrograms/kg/minute, then adjusted according to response to 2–20 micrograms/kg/minute, doses as low as 0.5–1 microgram/kg/minute have been used.

▶ Child: Initially 5 micrograms/kg/minute, then adjusted according to response to 2–20 micrograms/kg/minute, doses as low as 0.5–1 microgram/kg/minute have been used

- **CONTRA-INDICATIONS** Phaeochromocytoma
- **CAUTIONS** Acute heart failure · acute myocardial infarction · arrhythmias · correct hypercapnia before starting and during treatment · correct hypovolaemia before starting and during treatment · correct hypoxia before starting and during treatment · correct metabolic acidosis before starting and during treatment · diabetes mellitus · extravasation may cause tissue necrosis · extreme caution or avoid in marked obstruction of cardiac ejection (such as idiopathic hypertrophic subaortic stenosis) · hyperthyroidism · ischaemic heart disease · occlusive vascular disease · severe hypotension · susceptibility to angle-closure glaucoma · tachycardia · tolerance may develop with continuous infusions longer than 72 hours
- **INTERACTIONS** → Appendix 1: sympathomimetics, inotropic
- **SIDE-EFFECTS**

▶ **Common or very common** Arrhythmias · bronchospasm · chest pain · dyspnoea · eosinophilia · fever · inflammation localised · ischaemic heart disease · nausea · palpitations · platelet aggregation inhibition (on prolonged administration) · skin reactions · urinary urgency · vasoconstriction

▶ **Uncommon** Myocardial infarction

▶ **Rare or very rare** Atrioventricular block · cardiac arrest · coronary vasospasm · hypertension · hypokalaemia · hypotension

▶ **Frequency not known** Anxiety · cardiomyopathy · feeling hot · headache · myoclonus · paraesthesia · tremor

- **PREGNANCY** No evidence of harm in *animal* studies—manufacturers advise use only if potential benefit outweighs risk.
- **BREAST FEEDING** Manufacturers advise avoid—no information available.
- **DIRECTIONS FOR ADMINISTRATION** Dobutamine injection should be diluted before use or given undiluted with syringe pump. Dobutamine concentrate for intravenous infusion should be diluted before use.

For *continuous intravenous infusion*, using infusion pump, dilute to a concentration of 0.5–1 mg/mL (max. 5 mg/mL if fluid restricted) with Glucose 5% *or* Sodium Chloride 0.9%; infuse higher concentration solutions through central venous catheter only. Incompatible with bicarbonate and other strong alkaline solutions.

▶ **In neonates** *Neonatal intensive care*, dilute 30 mg/kg body-weight to a final volume of 50 mL with infusion fluid; an intravenous infusion rate of 0.5 mL/hour provides a dose of 5 micrograms/kg/minute; max. concentration of 5 mg/mL; infuse higher concentration solutions through central venous catheter only. Incompatible with bicarbonate and other strong alkaline solutions.

- **MEDICINAL FORMS** There can be variation in the licensing of different medicines containing the same drug. Forms available from special-order manufacturers include: solution for infusion

Solution for infusion

EXCIPIENTS: May contain Sulfites

▶ **Dobutamine (Non-proprietary)**

Dobutamine (as Dobutamine hydrochloride) 5 mg per 1 ml Dobutamine 250mg/50ml solution for infusion vials | 1 vial PoM £7.50

Dobutamine (as Dobutamine hydrochloride) 12.5 mg per 1 ml Dobutamine 250mg/20ml concentrate for solution for infusion ampoules | 5 ampoule PoM £12.00–£29.25 | 10 ampoule PoM £52.50

Dopamine hydrochloride

- **DRUG ACTION** Dopamine is a cardiac stimulant which acts on $beta_1$ receptors in cardiac muscle, and increases contractility with little effect on rate.

- **INDICATIONS AND DOSE**

To correct the haemodynamic imbalance due to acute hypotension, shock, cardiac failure, adjunct following cardiac surgery

▶ BY CONTINUOUS INTRAVENOUS INFUSION

▶ Neonate: Initially 3 micrograms/kg/minute (max. per dose 20 micrograms/kg/minute), adjusted according to response.

▶ Child: Initially 5 micrograms/kg/minute (max. per dose 20 micrograms/kg/minute), adjusted according to response

- **UNLICENSED USE** Not licensed for use in children under 12 years.
- **CONTRA-INDICATIONS** Phaeochromocytoma · tachyarrhythmia
- **CAUTIONS** Correct hypovolaemia · hypertension (may raise blood pressure) · hyperthyroidism
- **INTERACTIONS** → Appendix 1: sympathomimetics, inotropic
- **SIDE-EFFECTS** Angina pectoris · anxiety · arrhythmias · azotaemia · cardiac conduction disorder · dyspnoea · gangrene · headache · hypertension · mydriasis · nausea · palpitations · piloerection · polyuria · tremor · vasoconstriction · vomiting
- **PREGNANCY** No evidence of harm in *animal* studies—manufacturer advises use only if potential benefit outweighs risk.
- **BREAST FEEDING** May suppress lactation—not known to be harmful.
- **DIRECTIONS FOR ADMINISTRATION** Dopamine concentrate for intravenous infusion to be diluted before use.

For *continuous intravenous infusion*, dilute to a max. concentration of 3.2 mg/mL with Glucose 5% *or* Sodium Chloride 0.9%. Infuse higher concentrations through central venous catheter using a syringe pump to avoid extravasation and fluid overload. Incompatible with bicarbonate and other alkaline solutions.

▶ In neonates *Neonatal intensive care*, dilute 30 mg/kg body-weight to a final volume of 50 mL with infusion fluid; an intravenous infusion rate of 0.3 mL/hour provides a dose of 3 micrograms/kg/minute; max. concentration of 3.2 mg/mL; infuse higher concentrations through central venous catheter. Incompatible with bicarbonate and other alkaline solutions.

- **MEDICINAL FORMS** There can be variation in the licensing of different medicines containing the same drug. Forms available from special-order manufacturers include: solution for infusion

Solution for infusion

▶ Dopamine hydrochloride (Non-proprietary)

Dopamine hydrochloride 40 mg per 1 ml Dopamine 200mg/5ml solution for infusion ampoules | 5 ampoule PoM £20.00 (Hospital only) | 5 ampoule PoM £20.00 | 10 ampoule PoM £9.04

Dopamine 200mg/5ml concentrate for solution for infusion ampoules | 10 ampoule PoM [X]

Dopamine hydrochloride 160 mg per 1 ml Dopamine 800mg/5ml solution for infusion ampoules | 10 ampoule PoM [X]

SYMPATHOMIMETICS › VASOCONSTRICTOR

Ephedrine hydrochloride

04-Dec-2019

- **INDICATIONS AND DOSE**

Reversal of hypotension from spinal or epidural anaesthesia

▶ BY SLOW INTRAVENOUS INJECTION

▶ Child 1–11 years: 500–750 micrograms/kg every 3–4 minutes, adjusted according to response, alternatively 17–25 mg/m^2 every 3–4 minutes, adjusted according to response, injection solution to contain ephedrine hydrochloride 3 mg/ml; maximum 30 mg per course

▶ Child 12–17 years: 3–7.5 mg every 3–4 minutes (max. per dose 9 mg), adjusted according to response, injection solution to contain ephedrine hydrochloride 3 mg/ml; maximum 30 mg per course

- **CAUTIONS** Diabetes mellitus · hypertension · hyperthyroidism · susceptibility to angle-closure glaucoma
- **INTERACTIONS** → Appendix 1: sympathomimetics, vasoconstrictor
- **SIDE-EFFECTS**

▶ **Common or very common** Anxiety · arrhythmias · asthenia · confusion · depression · dyspnoea · headache · hyperhidrosis · insomnia · irritability · nausea · palpitations · vomiting

▶ **Rare or very rare** Acute urinary retention

▶ **Frequency not known** Acute angle closure glaucoma · angina pectoris · appetite decreased · cardiac arrest · dizziness · hypokalaemia · intracranial haemorrhage · psychotic disorder · pulmonary oedema · tremor

- **PREGNANCY** Increased fetal heart rate reported with parenteral ephedrine.
- **BREAST FEEDING** Present in milk; manufacturer advises avoid—irritability and disturbed sleep reported.
- **RENAL IMPAIRMENT** Use with caution.
- **DIRECTIONS FOR ADMINISTRATION** For *slow intravenous injection*, give via central venous catheter using a solution containing ephedrine hydrochloride 3 mg/ml.

- **MEDICINAL FORMS** There can be variation in the licensing of different medicines containing the same drug. Forms available from special-order manufacturers include: oral suspension, oral solution, solution for injection, nasal drops

Solution for injection

▶ Ephedrine hydrochloride (Non-proprietary)

Ephedrine hydrochloride 3 mg per 1 ml Ephedrine 30mg/10ml solution for injection ampoules | 10 ampoule PoM £107.44

Ephedrine 30mg/10ml solution for injection pre-filled syringes | 1 pre-filled disposable injection PoM £7.59–£9.50 | 12 pre-filled disposable injection PoM £114.00

Ephedrine hydrochloride 30 mg per 1 ml Ephedrine 30mg/1ml solution for injection ampoules | 10 ampoule PoM £52.50–£69.62 DT = £69.62

Metaraminol

28-Apr-2020

- **INDICATIONS AND DOSE**

Emergency treatment of acute hypotension

▶ INITIALLY BY INTRAVENOUS INJECTION

▶ Child 12–17 years: Initially 0.5–5 mg, then (by intravenous infusion) 15–100 mg, adjusted according to response

Acute hypotension

▶ BY INTRAVENOUS INFUSION

▶ Child 12–17 years: 15–100 mg, adjusted according to response

- **CAUTIONS** Cirrhosis · coronary vascular thrombosis · diabetes mellitus · extravasation at injection site may cause necrosis · following myocardial infarction · hypercapnia · hypertension · hyperthyroidism · hypoxia · mesenteric vascular thrombosis · peripheral vascular thrombosis · Prinzmetal's variant angina · susceptibility to angle-closure glaucoma · uncorrected hypovolaemia

CAUTIONS, FURTHER INFORMATION

- **Hypertensive response** Metaraminol has a longer duration of action than noradrenaline, and an excessive vasopressor response may cause a prolonged rise in blood pressure.

- **INTERACTIONS** → Appendix 1: sympathomimetics, vasoconstrictor
- **SIDE-EFFECTS**
  - **Common or very common** Headache · hypertension
  - **Rare or very rare** Skin exfoliation · soft tissue necrosis
  - **Frequency not known** Abscess · arrhythmias · nausea · palpitations · peripheral ischaemia
- **PREGNANCY** May reduce placental perfusion—manufacturer advises use only if potential benefit outweighs risk.
- **BREAST FEEDING** Manufacturer advises caution—no information available.
- **MONITORING REQUIREMENTS** Monitor blood pressure and rate of flow frequently.
- **DIRECTIONS FOR ADMINISTRATION** For *intravenous infusion*, dilute to a concentration of 30–200 micrograms/mL with Glucose 5% or Sodium Chloride 0.9% and give through a central venous catheter.

- **MEDICINAL FORMS** There can be variation in the licensing of different medicines containing the same drug. Forms available from special-order manufacturers include: solution for injection

Solution for injection

- Metaraminol (Non-proprietary)
  Metaraminol (as Metaraminol tartrate) 10 mg per 1 ml Metaraminol 10mg/1ml solution for injection ampoules | 10 ampoule PoM £30.45

Noradrenaline/norepinephrine

13-May-2020

- **INDICATIONS AND DOSE**

Acute hypotension (septic shock) | Shock secondary to excessive vasodilation

- BY CONTINUOUS INTRAVENOUS INFUSION
  - Neonate: 20–100 nanograms/kg/minute (max. per dose 1 microgram/kg/minute), adjusted according to response, dilute the 1 mg/mL concentrate for infusion for this dose.
  - Child: 20–100 nanograms/kg/minute (max. per dose 1 microgram/kg/minute), adjusted according to response, dilute the 1 mg/mL concentrate for infusion for this dose

DOSE EQUIVALENCE AND CONVERSION

- 1 mg of noradrenaline base is equivalent to 2 mg of noradrenaline acid tartrate. **Doses expressed as the base.**

- **UNLICENSED USE** Not licensed for use in children.

IMPORTANT SAFETY INFORMATION

ASSOCIATION OF NORADRENALINE/NOREPINEPHRINE 0.08 MG/ML (4 MG IN 50 ML) AND 0.16 MG/ML (8 MG IN 50 ML) SOLUTION FOR INFUSION WITH POTENTIAL RISK OF MEDICATION ERRORS

Healthcare professionals should be aware of the differences in strength and presentation between noradrenaline/norepinephrine products—manufacturer advises noradrenaline 0.08 mg/mL solution for infusion and noradrenaline 0.16 mg/mL solution for infusion must **not** be diluted before use and should only be used for the on-going treatment of patients already established on noradrenaline therapy, whose dose requirements are clinically confirmed to be escalating.

- **CONTRA-INDICATIONS** Hypertension
- **CAUTIONS** Coronary vascular thrombosis · diabetes mellitus · extravasation at injection site may cause necrosis · following myocardial infarction · hypercapnia · hyperthyroidism · hypoxia · mesenteric vascular thrombosis · peripheral vascular thrombosis · Prinzmetal's variant angina · susceptibility to angle-closure glaucoma · uncorrected hypovolaemia
- **INTERACTIONS** → Appendix 1: sympathomimetics, vasoconstrictor
- **SIDE-EFFECTS** Acute glaucoma · anxiety · arrhythmias · asthenia · cardiomyopathy · confusion · dyspnoea · extravasation necrosis · gangrene · headache · heart failure · hypovolaemia · hypoxia · injection site necrosis · insomnia · ischaemia · myocardial contractility increased · nausea · palpitations · peripheral ischaemia · psychotic disorder · respiratory failure · tremor · urinary retention · vomiting
- **PREGNANCY** Manufacturer advises use if potential benefit outweighs risk—may reduce placental perfusion and induce fetal bradycardia.
- **MONITORING REQUIREMENTS** Monitor blood pressure and rate of flow frequently.
- **DIRECTIONS FOR ADMINISTRATION** For *continuous intravenous infusion*, using 1 mg/mL concentrate for infusion, dilute to a max. concentration of noradrenaline (base) 40 micrograms/mL (higher concentrations can be used if fluid-restricted) with Glucose 5% or Sodium Chloride and Glucose. Infuse through central venous catheter; discard if discoloured. Incompatible with bicarbonate or alkaline solutions.
  - In neonates For *neonatal intensive care*, using 1 mg/mL concentrate for infusion, dilute 600 micrograms (base)/kg body-weight to a final volume of 50 mL with infusion fluid; an intravenous infusion rate of 0.1 mL/hour provides a dose of 20 nanograms (base)/kg/minute; infuse through central venous catheter; max. concentration of noradrenaline (base) 40 micrograms/mL (higher concentrations can be used if fluid-restricted). Discard if discoloured. Incompatible with bicarbonate or alkaline solutions.
- **PRESCRIBING AND DISPENSING INFORMATION** For a period of time, preparations on the UK market may be described as either noradrenaline base or noradrenaline acid tartrate; doses in the BNF are expressed as the base.

- **MEDICINAL FORMS** There can be variation in the licensing of different medicines containing the same drug. Forms available from special-order manufacturers include: infusion, solution for infusion

Solution for infusion

- Noradrenaline/norepinephrine (Non-proprietary)
  Noradrenaline (as Noradrenaline acid tartrate) 80 microgram per 1 ml Noradrenaline (base) 4mg/50ml solution for infusion vials | 10 vial PoM [CD symbol]
  Noradrenaline (as Noradrenaline acid tartrate) 160 microgram per 1 ml Sinora 8mg/50ml solution for infusion vials | 1 vial PoM £14.22
  Noradrenaline (as Noradrenaline acid tartrate) 1 mg per 1 ml Noradrenaline (base) 4mg/4ml concentrate for solution for infusion ampoules | 10 ampoule PoM £58.00
  Noradrenaline (base) 4mg/4ml solution for infusion ampoules | 5 ampoule PoM £22.00 (Hospital only)
  Noradrenaline (base) 2mg/2ml solution for infusion ampoules | 5 ampoule PoM £12.00 (Hospital only)
  Noradrenaline (base) 8mg/8ml concentrate for solution for infusion ampoules | 10 ampoule PoM £116.00

Phenylephrine hydrochloride

● **INDICATIONS AND DOSE**

Acute hypotension

▸ BY SUBCUTANEOUS INJECTION, OR BY INTRAMUSCULAR INJECTION

▸ Child 1–11 years: 100 micrograms/kg every 1–2 hours (max. per dose 5 mg) as required

▸ Child 12–17 years: Initially 2–5 mg (max. per dose 5 mg), followed by 1–10 mg, after at least 15 minutes if required

▸ BY SLOW INTRAVENOUS INJECTION

▸ Child 1–11 years: Initially 5–20 micrograms/kg (max. per dose 500 micrograms), repeated as necessary after at least 15 minutes

▸ Child 12–17 years: 100–500 micrograms, repeated as necessary after at least 15 minutes

▸ BY INTRAVENOUS INFUSION

▸ Child 1–15 years: Initially 100–500 nanograms/kg/minute, adjusted according to response

▸ Child 16–17 years: Initially up to 180 micrograms/minute, reduced to 30–60 micrograms/minute, adjusted according to response

● **UNLICENSED USE** Not licensed for use in children by intravenous infusion or injection.

● **CONTRA-INDICATIONS** Hypertension · severe hyperthyroidism

● **CAUTIONS** Coronary disease · coronary vascular thrombosis · diabetes · extravasation at injection site may cause necrosis · following myocardial infarction · hypercapnia · hyperthyroidism · hypoxia · mesenteric vascular thrombosis · peripheral vascular thrombosis · Prinzmetal's variant angina · susceptibility to angle-closure glaucoma · uncorrected hypovolaemia

CAUTIONS, FURTHER INFORMATION

▸ Hypertensive response Phenylephrine has a longer duration of action than noradrenaline (norepinephrine), and an excessive vasopressor response may cause a prolonged rise in blood pressure.

● **INTERACTIONS** → Appendix 1: sympathomimetics, vasoconstrictor

● **SIDE-EFFECTS** Angina pectoris · arrhythmias · cardiac arrest · dizziness · dyspnoea · flushing · glucose tolerance impaired · headache · hyperhidrosis · hypersalivation · hypotension · intracranial haemorrhage · metabolic change · mydriasis · palpitations · paraesthesia · peripheral coldness · pulmonary oedema · soft tissue necrosis · syncope · urinary disorders · vomiting

● **PREGNANCY** Avoid if possible; malformations reported following use in first trimester; fetal hypoxia and bradycardia reported in late pregnancy and labour.

● **MONITORING REQUIREMENTS** Contra-indicated in hypertension—monitor blood pressure and rate of flow frequently.

● **DIRECTIONS FOR ADMINISTRATION** For *intravenous injection*, dilute to a concentration of 1 mg/mL with Water for Injections and administer slowly. For *intravenous infusion*, dilute to a concentration of 20 micrograms/mL with Glucose 5% or Sodium Chloride 0.9% and administer as a continuous infusion via a central venous catheter using a controlled infusion device.

● **PRESCRIBING AND DISPENSING INFORMATION** Intravenous administration preferred when managing acute hypotension in children.

● **MEDICINAL FORMS** There can be variation in the licensing of different medicines containing the same drug. Forms available from special-order manufacturers include: solution for injection

Solution for injection

▸ **Phenylephrine hydrochloride (Non-proprietary)**

Phenylephrine (as Phenylephrine hydrochloride) 50 microgram per 1 ml Phenylephrine 500micrograms/10ml solution for injection pre-filled syringes | 1 pre-filled disposable injection PoM £15.00 | 10 pre-filled disposable injection PoM £150.00

Phenylephrine hydrochloride 100 microgram per 1 ml Phenylephrine 1mg/10ml solution for injection ampoules | 10 ampoule PoM £40.00

Phenylephrine hydrochloride 10 mg per 1 ml Phenylephrine 10mg/1ml solution for injection ampoules | 10 ampoule PoM £99.12 Phenylephrine 10mg/1ml concentrate for solution for injection ampoules | 10 ampoule PoM £99.12

5 Heart failure

Other drugs used for Heart failure Bendroflumethiazide, p. 117 · Candesartan cilexetil, p. 121 · Captopril, p. 118 · Chlorothiazide, p. 117 · Chlortalidone, p. 150 · Digoxin, p. 86 · Enalapril maleate, p. 120 · Glyceryl trinitrate, p. 142 · Hydralazine hydrochloride, p. 123 · Lisinopril, p. 120 · Losartan potassium, p. 122 · Metoprolol tartrate, p. 113 · Prazosin, p. 107 · Sodium nitroprusside, p. 124 · Valsartan, p. 122

BETA-ADRENOCEPTOR BLOCKERS ›
ALPHA- AND BETA-ADRENOCEPTOR BLOCKERS

F 109

Carvedilol

10-Mar-2020

● **INDICATIONS AND DOSE**

Adjunct in heart failure (limited information available)

▸ BY MOUTH

▸ Child 2–17 years: Initially 50 micrograms/kg twice daily (max. per dose 3.125 mg) for at least 2 weeks, then increased to 100 micrograms/kg twice daily for at least 2 weeks, then increased to 200 micrograms/kg twice daily, then increased if necessary up to 350 micrograms/kg twice daily (max. per dose 25 mg)

● **UNLICENSED USE** Not licensed for use in children under 18 years.

● **CONTRA-INDICATIONS** Acute or decompensated heart failure requiring intravenous inotropes

● **INTERACTIONS** → Appendix 1: beta blockers, non-selective

● **SIDE-EFFECTS**

▸ **Common or very common** Anaemia · asthma · dyspepsia · eye irritation · fluid imbalance · genital oedema · hypercholesterolaemia · hyperglycaemia · hypoglycaemia · increased risk of infection · oedema · postural hypotension · pulmonary oedema · renal impairment · urinary disorders · weight increased

▸ **Uncommon** Alopecia · angina pectoris · constipation · hyperhidrosis · skin reactions

▸ **Rare or very rare** Dry mouth · hypersensitivity · leucopenia · nasal congestion · severe cutaneous adverse reactions (SCARs) · thrombocytopenia

● **PREGNANCY** Information on the safety of carvedilol during pregnancy is lacking. If carvedilol is used close to delivery, infants should be monitored for signs of alpha-blockade (as well as beta-blockade).

● **BREAST FEEDING** Infants should be monitored as there is a risk of possible toxicity due to alpha-blockade (in addition to beta-blockade).

- **HEPATIC IMPAIRMENT** Manufacturer advises avoid in severe impairment.
  Dose adjustments Manufacturer advises dose adjustment may be required in moderate impairment.
- **MONITORING REQUIREMENTS** Monitor renal function during dose titration in patients with heart failure who also have renal impairment, low blood pressure, ischaemic heart disease, or diffuse vascular disease.
- **PATIENT AND CARER ADVICE**
  Medicines for Children leaflet: Carvedilol for heart failure www.medicinesforchildren.org.uk/carvedilol-heart-failure-0

- **MEDICINAL FORMS** There can be variation in the licensing of different medicines containing the same drug. Forms available from special-order manufacturers include: oral suspension

Tablet

CAUTIONARY AND ADVISORY LABELS 8

- Carvedilol (Non-proprietary)
  - **Carvedilol 3.125 mg** Carvedilol 3.125mg tablets | 28 tablet PoM £3.00 DT = £1.17
  - **Carvedilol 6.25 mg** Carvedilol 6.25mg tablets | 28 tablet PoM £2.20 DT = £1.28
  - **Carvedilol 12.5 mg** Carvedilol 12.5mg tablets | 28 tablet PoM £4.55 DT = £1.75
  - **Carvedilol 25 mg** Carvedilol 25mg tablets | 28 tablet PoM £5.99 DT = £2.11

DIURETICS > POTASSIUM-SPARING DIURETICS > ALDOSTERONE ANTAGONISTS

Potassium canrenoate

- **INDICATIONS AND DOSE**

Short-term diuresis for oedema in heart failure and in ascites

- BY INTRAVENOUS INJECTION, OR BY INTRAVENOUS INFUSION
  - Neonate: 1–2 mg/kg twice daily.
  - Child 1 month–11 years: 1–2 mg/kg twice daily
  - Child 12–17 years: 1–2 mg/kg twice daily (max. per dose 200 mg)

DOSE EQUIVALENCE AND CONVERSION

- To convert to equivalent oral spironolactone dose, multiply potassium canrenoate dose by 0.7.

- **UNLICENSED USE** Not licensed for use in the UK.
- **CONTRA-INDICATIONS** Hyperkalaemia · hyponatraemia
- **CAUTIONS** Acute porphyrias p. 652 · hypotension · potential metabolic products carcinogenic in *rodents*
- **INTERACTIONS** → Appendix 1: potassium canrenoate
- **SIDE-EFFECTS**
  - **Common or very common** Ataxia · drowsiness · headache · hyperuricaemia · menstruation irregular
  - **Uncommon** Electrolyte imbalance · eosinophilia · thrombocytopenia
  - **Rare or very rare** Agranulocytosis · alopecia · hepatotoxicity · hypersensitivity · osteomalacia · skin reactions · voice alteration
  - **Frequency not known** Acidosis hyperchloraemic · breast pain · confusion (transient; with high doses) · gastrointestinal disorder · gynaecomastia · hirsutism · hypotension
- **PREGNANCY** Crosses placenta. Feminisation and undescended testes in male fetus in *animal* studies—manufacturer advises avoid.
- **BREAST FEEDING** Present in breast milk—manufacturer advises avoid.
- **RENAL IMPAIRMENT** Use with caution if estimated glomerular filtration rate 30–60 mL/minute/1.73 m^2. Avoid if estimated glomerular filtration rate less than 30 mL/minute/1.73 m^2.
  Monitoring Monitor plasma-potassium concentration if estimated glomerular filtration rate 30–60 mL/minute/1.73 m^2.
- **MONITORING REQUIREMENTS** Monitor electrolytes (discontinue if hyperkalaemia occurs).
- **DIRECTIONS FOR ADMINISTRATION** Consult product literature. Intravenous injection to be given over at least 3 minutes.
- **PRESCRIBING AND DISPENSING INFORMATION** Potassium canrenoate injection is available from 'special-order' manufacturers or specialist importing companies.

- **MEDICINAL FORMS** There can be variation in the licensing of different medicines containing the same drug.

Solution for injection

- Aldactone (Imported (Germany))
  - **Potassium canrenoate 20 mg per 1 ml** Aldactone 200mg/10ml solution for injection ampoules | 10 ampoule PoM

Spironolactone

10-Mar-2020

- **INDICATIONS AND DOSE**

Oedema in heart failure and in ascites | Nephrotic syndrome | Reduction of hypokalaemia induced by diuretics or amphotericin

- BY MOUTH
  - Neonate: Initially 1–2 mg/kg daily in 1–2 divided doses; increased if necessary up to 7 mg/kg daily, in resistant ascites.
  - Child 1 month–11 years: Initially 1–3 mg/kg daily in 1–2 divided doses; increased if necessary up to 9 mg/kg daily, in resistant ascites
  - Child 12–17 years: Initially 50–100 mg daily in 1–2 divided doses; increased if necessary up to 9 mg/kg daily, in resistant ascites; maximum 400 mg per day

- **UNLICENSED USE** Not licensed for reduction of hypokalaemia induced by diuretics or amphotericin.
- **CONTRA-INDICATIONS** Addison's disease · anuria · hyperkalaemia
- **CAUTIONS** Acute porphyrias p. 652 · potential metabolic products carcinogenic in *rodents*
- **INTERACTIONS** → Appendix 1: aldosterone antagonists
- **SIDE-EFFECTS** Acidosis hyperchloraemic · acute kidney injury · agranulocytosis · alopecia · breast neoplasm benign · breast pain · confusion · dizziness · electrolyte imbalance · gastrointestinal disorder · gynaecomastia · hepatic function abnormal · hyperkalaemia (discontinue) · hypertrichosis · leg cramps · leucopenia · libido disorder · malaise · menstrual disorder · nausea · severe cutaneous adverse reactions (SCARs) · skin reactions · thrombocytopenia
- **PREGNANCY** Use only if potential benefit outweighs risk—feminisation of male fetus in *animal* studies.
- **BREAST FEEDING** Metabolites present in milk, but amount probably too small to be harmful.
- **RENAL IMPAIRMENT** Avoid in acute renal insufficiency or severe impairment.
  Monitoring Monitor plasma-potassium concentration (high risk of hyperkalaemia in renal impairment).
- **MONITORING REQUIREMENTS** Monitor electrolytes—discontinue if hyperkalaemia occurs.
- **PRESCRIBING AND DISPENSING INFORMATION** The RCPCH and NPPG recommend that, when a liquid special of spironolactone is required, the following strength is used: 50 mg/5 mL.

- **PATIENT AND CARER ADVICE**
Medicines for Children leaflet: Spironolactone for heart failure
www.medicinesforchildren.org.uk/spironolactone-heart-failure

- **MEDICINAL FORMS** There can be variation in the licensing of different medicines containing the same drug. Forms available from special-order manufacturers include: oral suspension, oral solution

Tablet

CAUTIONARY AND ADVISORY LABELS 21

▸ Spironolactone (Non-proprietary)
Spironolactone 25 mg Spironolactone 25mg tablets | 28 tablet [PoM] £1.95 DT = £1.24 | 500 tablet [PoM] £26.79
Spironolactone 50 mg Spironolactone 50mg tablets | 28 tablet [PoM] £9.99 DT = £4.68 | 250 tablet [PoM] £46.88
Spironolactone 100 mg Spironolactone 100mg tablets | 28 tablet [PoM] £2.96 DT = £2.22 | 250 tablet [PoM] £19.29

▸ Aldactone (Pfizer Ltd)
Spironolactone 25 mg Aldactone 25mg tablets | 100 tablet [PoM] £8.89
Spironolactone 50 mg Aldactone 50mg tablets | 100 tablet [PoM] £17.78
Spironolactone 100 mg Aldactone 100mg tablets | 28 tablet [PoM] £9.96 DT = £2.22 | 100 tablet [PoM] £35.56

PHOSPHODIESTERASE TYPE-3 INHIBITORS

Enoximone

10-Mar-2020

- **DRUG ACTION** Enoximone is a phosphodiesterase type-3 inhibitor that exerts most effect on the myocardium; it has positive inotropic properties and vasodilator activity.

- **INDICATIONS AND DOSE**

Congestive heart failure, low cardiac output following cardiac surgery

▸ INITIALLY BY SLOW INTRAVENOUS INJECTION

▸ Neonate: Loading dose 500 micrograms/kg, followed by (by continuous intravenous infusion) 5–20 micrograms/kg/minute, adjusted according to response, infusion to be given over 24 hours; maximum 24 mg/kg per day.

▸ Child: Loading dose 500 micrograms/kg, followed by (by continuous intravenous infusion) 5–20 micrograms/kg/minute, adjusted according to response, infusion dose to be given over 24 hours; maximum 24 mg/kg per day

- **UNLICENSED USE** Not licensed for use in children.
- **CAUTIONS** Heart failure associated with hypertrophic cardiomyopathy, stenotic or obstructive valvular disease or other outlet obstruction
- **SIDE-EFFECTS**
▸ **Common or very common** Headache · hypotension · insomnia
▸ **Uncommon** Arrhythmias · diarrhoea · dizziness · nausea · vomiting
▸ **Rare or very rare** Chills · fever · fluid retention · myalgia · oliguria · urinary retention
- **PREGNANCY** Manufacturer advises use only if potential benefit outweighs risk.
- **BREAST FEEDING** Manufacturer advises caution—no information available.
- **RENAL IMPAIRMENT**
Dose adjustments Consider dose reduction.
- **MONITORING REQUIREMENTS** Monitor blood pressure, heart rate, ECG, central venous pressure, fluid and electrolyte status, renal function, platelet count and hepatic enzymes.
- **DIRECTIONS FOR ADMINISTRATION** Incompatible with glucose solutions. Use only plastic containers or syringes; crystal formation if glass used. Avoid extravasation.
For *intravenous administration*, dilute to concentration of 2.5 mg/mL with Sodium Chloride 0.9% or Water for Injections; the initial loading dose should be given by slow intravenous injection over at least 15 minutes.
- **PRESCRIBING AND DISPENSING INFORMATION** Phosphodiesterase type-3 inhibitors possess positive inotropic and vasodilator activity and are useful in infants and children with low cardiac output especially after cardiac surgery. Phosphodiesterase type-3 inhibitors should be limited to short-term use because long-term oral administration has been associated with increased mortality in adults with congestive heart failure.
- **PATIENT AND CARER ADVICE**
Medicines for Children leaflet: Enoximone for pulmonary hypertension www.medicinesforchildren.org.uk/enoximone-pulmonary-hypertension

- **MEDICINAL FORMS** There can be variation in the licensing of different medicines containing the same drug.

Solution for injection

EXCIPIENTS: May contain Alcohol, propylene glycol

▸ Perfan (Carinopharm GmbH)
Enoximone 5 mg per 1 ml Perfan 100mg/20ml solution for injection ampoules | 10 ampoule [PoM] [X] (Hospital only)

Milrinone

27-Jan-2020

- **DRUG ACTION** Milrinone is a phosphodiesterase type-3 inhibitor that exerts most effect on the myocardium; it has positive inotropic properties and vasodilator activity.

- **INDICATIONS AND DOSE**

Congestive heart failure, low cardiac output following cardiac surgery, shock

▸ INITIALLY BY INTRAVENOUS INFUSION

▸ Neonate: Initially 50–75 micrograms/kg, given over 30-60 minutes, reduce or omit initial dose if at risk of hypotension, then (by continuous intravenous infusion) 30–45 micrograms/kg/hour for 2–3 days (usually for 12 hours after cardiac surgery).

▸ Child: Initially 50–75 micrograms/kg, given over 30-60 minutes, reduce or omit initial dose if at risk of hypotension, then (by continuous intravenous infusion) 30–45 micrograms/kg/hour for 2–3 days (usually for 12 hours after cardiac surgery)

- **UNLICENSED USE** Not licensed for use in children under 18 years.
- **CONTRA-INDICATIONS** Severe hypovolaemia
- **CAUTIONS** Correct hypokalaemia · heart failure associated with hypertrophic cardiomyopathy, stenotic or obstructive valvular disease or other outlet obstruction
- **SIDE-EFFECTS**
▸ **Common or very common** Arrhythmia supraventricular (increased risk in patients with pre-existing arrhythmias) · arrhythmias · headache · hypotension
▸ **Uncommon** Angina pectoris · chest pain · hypokalaemia · thrombocytopenia · tremor
▸ **Rare or very rare** Anaphylactic shock · bronchospasm · skin eruption
▸ **Frequency not known** Intraventricular haemorrhage · renal failure
- **PREGNANCY** Manufacturer advises use only if potential benefit outweighs risk.
- **BREAST FEEDING** Manufacturer advises avoid—no information available.
- **RENAL IMPAIRMENT**
Dose adjustments Use half to three-quarters normal dose and monitor response if estimated glomerular filtration rate less than 50 mL/minute/1.73 m^2.

- **MONITORING REQUIREMENTS**
  - Monitor blood pressure, heart rate, ECG, central venous pressure, fluid and electrolyte status, renal function, platelet count and hepatic enzymes.
  - Monitor renal function.
- **DIRECTIONS FOR ADMINISTRATION** Avoid extravasation. For *intravenous infusion* dilute with Glucose 5% or Sodium Chloride 0.9% *or* Sodium Chloride and Glucose intravenous infusion to a concentration of 200 micrograms/mL (higher concentrations of 400 micrograms/mL have been used).

  Loading dose may be given undiluted if fluid-restricted.
- **PRESCRIBING AND DISPENSING INFORMATION** Phosphodiesterase type-3 inhibitors possess positive inotropic and vasodilator activity and are useful in infants and children with low cardiac output especially after cardiac surgery. Phosphodiesterase type-3 inhibitors should be limited to short-term use because long-term oral administration has been associated with increased mortality in adults with congestive heart failure.

- **MEDICINAL FORMS** There can be variation in the licensing of different medicines containing the same drug. Forms available from special-order manufacturers include: solution for infusion

Solution for infusion

- Milrinone (Non-proprietary)

  Milrinone 1 mg per 1 ml Milrinone 10mg/10ml solution for infusion ampoules | 5 ampoule [PoM] £35.00 | 10 ampoule [PoM] £199.06

  Milrinone 10mg/10ml concentrate for solution for infusion ampoules | 10 ampoule [PoM] [X]
- Primacor (Sanofi)

  Milrinone 1 mg per 1 ml Primacor 10mg/10ml solution for injection ampoules | 10 ampoule [PoM] £199.06

6 Hyperlipidaemia

Dyslipidaemias

23-Mar-2018

Cardiovascular disease risk factors

Atherosclerosis begins in childhood and raised serum cholesterol in children is associated with cardiovascular disease in adulthood. Lowering the cholesterol, without hindering growth and development in children and adolescents, should reduce the risk of cardiovascular disease in later life.

The risk factors for developing cardiovascular disease include raised serum cholesterol concentration, smoking, hypertension, impaired glucose tolerance, male sex, ethnicity, obesity, triglyceride concentration, chronic kidney disease, and a family history of cardiovascular disease. Heterozygous familial hypercholesterolaemia is the most common cause of raised serum cholesterol in children; homozygous familial hypercholesterolaemia is very rare and its specialised management is not covered in *BNF for Children*. [EvGr] Familial hypercholesterolaemia can lead to a greater risk of early coronary heart disease and should be managed by a specialist. ⟨A⟩

Secondary causes of hypercholesterolaemia should be addressed, these include obesity, diet, diabetes mellitus, hypothyroidism, nephrotic syndrome, obstructive biliary disease, glycogen storage disease, and drugs such as corticosteroids.

Management

The aim of management of hypercholesterolaemia is to reduce the risk of atherosclerosis while ensuring adequate growth and development. Children with hypercholesterolaemia (or their carers) should receive advice on appropriate lifestyle changes such as improved diet, increased exercise, weight reduction, and Smoking cessation p. 313; Hypertension p. 104 should also be managed appropriately. Drug therapy may also be necessary.

Hypothyroidism

Children with hypothyroidism should receive adequate thyroid replacement therapy before their requirement for lipid-regulating treatment is assessed because correction of hypothyroidism itself may resolve the lipid abnormality. Untreated hypothyroidism increases the risk of myositis with lipid-regulating drugs.

Heterozygous familial hypercholesterolaemia

In heterozygous familial hypercholesterolaemia, drug treatment is often required as lifestyle modifications alone are unlikely to sufficiently lower cholesterol concentration. [EvGr] Treatment with lipid-regulating drugs should be considered by the age of 10 years, although the decision to initiate or defer treatment will depend on the child's age, the age of onset of coronary heart disease within the family, and the presence of other cardiovascular risk factors. Lipid-regulating drug treatment before the age of 10 years, or a higher dose of statin than licensed for use in the appropriate age group, or a combination of lipid-regulating drugs should be considered in children with a family history of coronary heart disease in early adulthood.

Statins are the lipid-regulating drug of choice and treatment should be life-long. In children who are intolerant to statins, ezetimibe p. 137, fibrates, or bile acid sequestrants should be considered as alternative options. Vitamins A, D and K, and folic acid supplementation can be given to patients on long-term bile acid sequestrants. ⟨A⟩

Secondary hypercholesterolaemia

Drug treatment may be indicated in children 10 years and older (rarely necessary in younger children) who are at a high risk of developing cardiovascular disease if 6–12 months of dietary and other lifestyle interventions have failed to lower cholesterol concentration adequately.

Lipid-regulating drugs

Experience in the use of lipid-regulating drugs in children is limited and they should be initiated on specialist advice.

Statins are more effective than other classes of drugs in lowering LDL-cholesterol but less effective than the fibrates in reducing triglycerides. Statins also increase concentrations of HDL-cholesterol. Statins reduce cardiovascular disease events and total mortality in adults, irrespective of the initial cholesterol concentration. They are the drugs of first choice in children and are generally well tolerated; atorvastatin p. 139 and simvastatin p. 141 are the preferred statins. Other lipid-regulating drugs can be used if statins are ineffective or are not tolerated.

Ezetimibe can be used alone when statins are not tolerated, or in combination with a statin when a high dose statin fails to control cholesterol concentration adequately.

Bile acid sequestrants are also available but tolerability of and compliance with these drugs is poor, and their use is declining.

Fibrates may reduce the risk of coronary heart disease in those with low HDL-cholesterol or with raised triglycerides. Evidence for the use of a fibrate (bezafibrate p. 137 or fenofibrate p. 138) in children is limited; fibrates should be considered only if dietary intervention and treatment with a statin and a bile acid sequestrant is unsuccessful or contra-indicated.

Evolocumab p. 142 is licensed for the treatment of homozygous familial hypercholesterolaemia; it is used in combination with other lipid-lowering therapies.

In hypertriglyceridaemia which cannot be controlled by very strict diet, omega-3 fatty acid compounds can be considered.

LIPID MODIFYING DRUGS > BILE ACID SEQUESTRANTS

Bile acid sequestrants

- **DRUG ACTION** Bile acid sequestrants act by binding bile acids, preventing their reabsorption; this promotes hepatic conversion of cholesterol into bile acids; the resultant increased LDL-receptor activity of liver cells increases the clearance of LDL-cholesterol from the plasma.
- **CAUTIONS** Interference with the absorption of fat-soluble vitamins (supplements of vitamins A, D, K, and folic acid may be required when treatment is prolonged).
- **SIDE-EFFECTS**
  - **Common or very common** Constipation · gastrointestinal discomfort · headache · nausea · vomiting
  - **Uncommon** Appetite decreased · diarrhoea · gastrointestinal disorders
- **PREGNANCY** Bile acid sequestrants should be used with caution as although the drugs are not absorbed, they may cause fat-soluble vitamin deficiency on prolonged use.
- **BREAST FEEDING** Bile acid sequestrants should be used with caution as although the drugs are not absorbed, they may cause fat-soluble vitamin deficiency on prolonged use.
- **MONITORING REQUIREMENTS** A child's growth and development should be monitored.

above

Colestipol hydrochloride

- **INDICATIONS AND DOSE**

Familial hypercholesterolaemia

- BY MOUTH
  - Child 12–17 years: Initially 5 g 1–2 times a day, then increased in steps of 5 g every month, total daily dose may be given in 1–2 divided doses or as a single dose if tolerated; maximum 30 g per day

- **UNLICENSED USE** Not licensed for use in children.
- **INTERACTIONS** → Appendix 1: colestipol
- **SIDE-EFFECTS** Angina pectoris · arthralgia · arthritis · asthenia · burping · chest pain · dizziness · dyspnoea · gallbladder disorders · headaches · inflammation · insomnia · pain · peptic ulcer haemorrhage · tachycardia
- **DIRECTIONS FOR ADMINISTRATION** The contents of each sachet should be mixed with at least 100 mL of water or other suitable liquid such as fruit juice or skimmed milk; alternatively it can be mixed with thin soups, cereals, yoghurt, or pulpy fruits ensuring at least 100 mL of liquid is provided.
- **PATIENT AND CARER ADVICE** Patient counselling on administration is advised for colestipol hydrochloride granules (avoid other drugs at same time).

- **MEDICINAL FORMS** There can be variation in the licensing of different medicines containing the same drug. Forms available from special-order manufacturers include: tablet

Granules

CAUTIONARY AND ADVISORY LABELS 13

- Colestid (Pfizer Ltd)
  Colestipol hydrochloride 5 gram Colestid 5g granules sachets plain sugar-free | 30 sachet [PoM] £15.05 DT = £15.05
  Colestid Orange 5g granules sachets sugar-free | 30 sachet [PoM] £15.05 DT = £15.05

Tablet

- Colestid (Imported (Canada))
  Colestipol hydrochloride 1 gram Colestid 1g tablets | 120 tablet [PoM] [X]

above

Colestyramine
(Cholestyramine)

- **INDICATIONS AND DOSE**

Familial hypercholesterolaemia

- BY MOUTH
  - Child 6–11 years: Initially 4 g once daily, then increased to 4 g up to 3 times a day, adjusted according to response
  - Child 12–17 years: Initially 4 g once daily, then increased in steps of 4 g every week; increased to 12–24 g daily in 1–4 divided doses, adjusted according to response; maximum 36 g per day

Pruritus associated with partial biliary obstruction and primary biliary cirrhosis

- BY MOUTH
  - Child 1–11 months: 1 g once daily, adjusted according to response, total daily dose may alternatively be given in 2–4 divided doses; maximum 9 g per day
  - Child 1–5 years: 2 g once daily, adjusted according to response, total daily dose may alternatively be given in 2–4 divided doses; maximum 18 g per day
  - Child 6–11 years: 4 g once daily, adjusted according to response, total daily dose may alternatively be given in 2–4 divided doses; maximum 24 g per day
  - Child 12–17 years: 4–8 g once daily, adjusted according to response, total daily dose may alternatively be given in 2–4 divided doses; maximum 36 g per day

Diarrhoea associated with Crohn's disease, ileal resection, vagotomy, diabetic vagal neuropathy, and radiation

- BY MOUTH
  - Child 1–11 months: 1 g once daily, adjusted according to response, total daily dose may alternatively be given in 2–4 divided doses, if no response within 3 days an alternative therapy should be initiated; maximum 9 g per day
  - Child 1–5 years: 2 g once daily, adjusted according to response, total daily dose may alternatively be given in 2–4 divided doses, if no response within 3 days an alternative therapy should be initiated; maximum 18 g per day
  - Child 6–11 years: 4 g once daily, adjusted according to response, total daily dose may alternatively be given in 2–4 divided doses, if no response within 3 days an alternative therapy should be initiated; maximum 24 g per day
  - Child 12–17 years: 4–8 g once daily, adjusted according to response, total daily dose may alternatively be given in 2–4 divided doses, if no response within 3 days an alternative therapy should be initiated; maximum 36 g per day

- **UNLICENSED USE** Not licensed for use in children under 6 years to reduce cholesterol.
- **CONTRA-INDICATIONS** Complete biliary obstruction (not likely to be effective)
- **INTERACTIONS** → Appendix 1: colestyramine
- **SIDE-EFFECTS**
  - **Uncommon** Acidosis hyperchloraemic · bleeding tendency · hypoprothrombinaemia · night blindness · osteoporosis · skin reactions · tongue irritation · vitamin deficiencies
- **DIRECTIONS FOR ADMINISTRATION** The contents of each sachet should be mixed with at least 150 mL of water or other suitable liquid such as fruit juice, skimmed milk, thin soups, and pulpy fruits with a high moisture content.
- **PATIENT AND CARER ADVICE** Patient counselling on administration is advised for colestyramine powder (avoid other drugs at same time).

- **MEDICINAL FORMS** There can be variation in the licensing of different medicines containing the same drug. Forms available from special-order manufacturers include: oral suspension, oral solution

Powder

CAUTIONARY AND ADVISORY LABELS 13

EXCIPIENTS: May contain Aspartame, sucrose

- Colestyramine (Non-proprietary)
  Colestyramine anhydrous 4 gram Colestyramine 4g oral powder sachets sugar-free | 50 sachet PoM £33.30 DT = £30.34
- Questran (Cheplapharm Arzneimittel GmbH)
  Colestyramine anhydrous 4 gram Questran 4g oral powder sachets | 50 sachet PoM £10.76 DT = £10.76
- Questran Light (Cheplapharm Arzneimittel GmbH)
  Colestyramine anhydrous 4 gram Questran Light 4g oral powder sachets sugar-free | 50 sachet PoM £16.15 DT = £30.34

LIPID MODIFYING DRUGS > CHOLESTEROL ABSORPTION INHIBITORS

Ezetimibe

08-Feb-2019

- **DRUG ACTION** Ezetimibe inhibits the intestinal absorption of cholesterol.

- **INDICATIONS AND DOSE**

Adjunct to dietary measures and statin treatment in primary hypercholesterolaemia | Adjunct to dietary measures and statin in homozygous familial hypercholesterolaemia | Primary hypercholesterolaemia (if statin inappropriate or not tolerated) | Adjunct to dietary measures in homozygous sitosterolaemia

- BY MOUTH
- Child 10–17 years: 10 mg daily

- **INTERACTIONS** → Appendix 1: ezetimibe
- **SIDE-EFFECTS**
- **Common or very common** Asthenia · diarrhoea · gastrointestinal discomfort · gastrointestinal disorders
- **Uncommon** Appetite decreased · arthralgia · chest pain · cough · hot flush · hypertension · muscle complaints · nausea · pain
- **Frequency not known** Constipation · depression · dizziness · dyspnoea · hepatitis · myopathy · pancreatitis · paraesthesia · skin reactions · thrombocytopenia
- **PREGNANCY** Manufacturer advises use only if potential benefit outweighs risk—no information available.
- **BREAST FEEDING** Manufacturer advises avoid—present in milk in *animal* studies.
- **HEPATIC IMPAIRMENT** Manufacturer advises avoid in moderate to severe impairment.

- **MEDICINAL FORMS** There can be variation in the licensing of different medicines containing the same drug.

Tablet

- Ezetimibe (Non-proprietary)
  Ezetimibe 10 mg Ezetimibe 10mg tablets | 28 tablet PoM £26.31 DT = £1.65
- Ezetrol (Merck Sharp & Dohme Ltd)
  Ezetimibe 10 mg Ezetrol 10mg tablets | 28 tablet PoM £26.31 DT = £1.65

Combinations available: *Simvastatin with ezetimibe*, p. 141

LIPID MODIFYING DRUGS > FIBRATES

Bezafibrate

15-Jan-2020

- **DRUG ACTION** Fibrates act by decreasing serum triglycerides; they have variable effect on LDL-cholestrol.

- **INDICATIONS AND DOSE**

Hyperlipidaemia including familial hypercholesterolaemia (administered on expert advice)

- BY MOUTH USING IMMEDIATE-RELEASE MEDICINES
- Child 10–17 years: 200 mg once daily (max. per dose 200 mg 3 times a day), adjusted according to response

- **UNLICENSED USE** Not licensed for use in children.
- **CONTRA-INDICATIONS** Gall bladder disease · hypoalbuminaemia · nephrotic syndrome · photosensitivity to fibrates
- **CAUTIONS** Correct hypothyroidism before initiating treatment · risk factors for myopathy
- **INTERACTIONS** → Appendix 1: fibrates
- **SIDE-EFFECTS**
- **Common or very common** Appetite decreased · gastrointestinal disorder
- **Uncommon** Acute kidney injury · alopecia · cholestasis · constipation · diarrhoea · dizziness · erectile dysfunction · gastrointestinal discomfort · headache · muscle complaints · muscle weakness · nausea · photosensitivity reaction · skin reactions
- **Rare or very rare** Cholelithiasis · depression · insomnia · interstitial lung disease · pancreatitis · pancytopenia · paraesthesia · peripheral neuropathy · rhabdomyolysis (increased risk in renal impairment) · severe cutaneous adverse reactions (SCARs) · thrombocytopenic purpura
- **PREGNANCY** Manufacturers advise avoid—no information available.
- **BREAST FEEDING** Manufacturer advises avoid—no information available.
- **HEPATIC IMPAIRMENT** Manufacturer advises avoid in significant impairment (except in fatty liver disease).
- **RENAL IMPAIRMENT** Avoid *immediate-release* preparations if eGFR less than 15 mL/minute/1.73 m^2. Avoid *modified-release* preparations if eGFR less than 60 mL/minute/1.73 m^2.
  Myotoxicity Special care needed in patients with renal disease, as progressive increases in serum creatinine concentration or failure to follow dosage guidelines may result in myotoxicity (rhabdomyolysis); discontinue if myotoxicity suspected or creatine kinase concentration increases significantly.
  Avoid if estimated glomerular filtration rate less than 15 mL/minute/1.73 m^2.
  Dose adjustments Reduce dose if estimated glomerular filtration rate 15–60 mL/minute/1.73 m^2.
- **MONITORING REQUIREMENTS** Consider monitoring of liver function and creatine kinase when fibrates used in combination with a statin.
- **PRESCRIBING AND DISPENSING INFORMATION** Fibrates are mainly used in those whose serum-triglyceride concentration is greater than 10 mmol/litre or in those who cannot tolerate a statin (specialist use).

- **MEDICINAL FORMS** There can be variation in the licensing of different medicines containing the same drug. Forms available from special-order manufacturers include: oral suspension

Tablet

CAUTIONARY AND ADVISORY LABELS 21

- Bezalip (Teva UK Ltd)
  Bezafibrate 200 mg Bezalip 200mg tablets | 100 tablet PoM £8.63 DT = £8.63

Fenofibrate

15-Jan-2020

- **DRUG ACTION** Fibrates act by decreasing serum triglycerides; they have variable effect on LDL-cholesterol.

- **INDICATIONS AND DOSE**

Hyperlipidaemias including familial hypercholesterolaemia (administered on expert advice)

▶ BY MOUTH USING CAPSULES

- ▶ Child 4–14 years: One 67 mg (micronised) capsule per 20 kg body-weight daily, maximum four 67 mg capsules daily, or max. three 67 mg capsules daily with concomitant statin
- ▶ Child 15–17 years: Initially 3 capsules daily, then increased if necessary to 4 capsules daily, max. 3 capsules daily with concomitant statin, dose relates to 67 mg (micronised) capsules

DOSE ADJUSTMENTS DUE TO INTERACTIONS

- ▶ Manufacturer advises max. dose 200 mg daily with concurrent use of a statin—no specific recommendation made for children.

- **UNLICENSED USE** 200 mg and 267 mg capsules not licensed in children. Tablets not licensed in children.
- **CONTRA-INDICATIONS** Gall bladder disease · pancreatitis (unless due to severe hypertriglyceridaemia) · photosensitivity to fibrates · photosensitivity to ketoprofen
- **CAUTIONS** Correct hypothyroidism before initiating treatment · risk factors for myopathy
- **INTERACTIONS** → Appendix 1: fibrates
- **SIDE-EFFECTS**
- ▶ **Common or very common** Abdominal pain · diarrhoea · flatulence · nausea · vomiting
- ▶ **Uncommon** Cholelithiasis · embolism and thrombosis · headache · muscle complaints · muscle weakness · myopathy · pancreatitis · sexual dysfunction · skin reactions
- ▶ **Rare or very rare** Alopecia · hepatic disorders · photosensitivity reaction
- ▶ **Frequency not known** Fatigue · interstitial lung disease · rhabdomyolysis (increased risk in renal impairment) · severe cutaneous adverse reactions (SCARs)
- **PREGNANCY** Avoid—embryotoxicity in *animal* studies.
- **BREAST FEEDING** Manufacturers advise avoid—no information available.
- **HEPATIC IMPAIRMENT** Manufacturer advises avoid —no information available.
- **RENAL IMPAIRMENT** Manufacturer advises use with caution in mild-to-moderate impairment; avoid if estimated glomerular filtration rate less than 30 mL/minute/1.73 m^2.

Myotoxicity Special care needed in patients with renal disease, as progressive increases in serum creatinine concentration or failure to follow dosage guidelines may result in myotoxicity (rhabdomyolysis); discontinue if myotoxicity suspected or creatine kinase concentration increases significantly.

Dose adjustments Manufacturer advises max. 67 mg daily if estimated glomerular filtration rate 30–59 mL/minute/1.73 m^2.

- **MONITORING REQUIREMENTS** Manufacturer advises monitor hepatic transaminases every 3 months during the first 12 months of treatment and periodically thereafter—discontinue treatment if levels increase to more than 3 times the upper limit of normal; monitor serum creatinine levels during the first 3 months of treatment and periodically thereafter—interrupt treatment if creatinine level is 50% above the upper limit of normal.
- **PRESCRIBING AND DISPENSING INFORMATION** Fibrates are mainly used in those whose serum-triglyceride concentration is greater than 10 mmol/litre or in those who cannot tolerate a statin (specialist use).
- **MEDICINAL FORMS** There can be variation in the licensing of different medicines containing the same drug.

Capsule

CAUTIONARY AND ADVISORY LABELS 21

▶ Fenofibrate (Non-proprietary)

Fenofibrate micronised 67 mg Fenofibrate micronised 67mg capsules | 90 capsule PoM £23.30 DT = £23.23

Fenofibrate micronised 200 mg Fenofibrate micronised 200mg capsules | 28 capsule PoM £11.98 DT = £3.29

Fenofibrate micronised 267 mg Fenofibrate micronised 267mg capsules | 28 capsule PoM £21.75 DT = £2.84

▶ Lipantil Micro (Mylan)

Fenofibrate micronised 67 mg Lipantil Micro 67 capsules | 90 capsule PoM £23.30 DT = £23.23

Fenofibrate micronised 200 mg Lipantil Micro 200 capsules | 28 capsule PoM £14.23 DT = £3.29

Fenofibrate micronised 267 mg Lipantil Micro 267 capsules | 28 capsule PoM £21.75 DT = £2.84

LIPID MODIFYING DRUGS > STATINS

Statins

- **DRUG ACTION** Statins competitively inhibit 3-hydroxy-3-methylglutaryl coenzyme A (HMG CoA) reductase, an enzyme involved in cholesterol synthesis, especially in the liver.
- **CAUTIONS** High alcohol intake · history of liver disease · hypothyroidism · known genetic polymorphisms—consult product literature · patients at increased risk of muscle toxicity, including myopathy or rhabdomyolysis (e.g. those with a personal or family history of muscular disorders, previous history of muscular toxicity and a high alcohol intake)

CAUTIONS, FURTHER INFORMATION

▶ **Muscle effects** Muscle toxicity can occur with all statins, however the likelihood increases with higher doses and in certain patients (see below). Statins should be used with caution in patients at increased risk of muscle toxicity, including those with a personal or family history of muscular disorders, previous history of muscular toxicity, a high alcohol intake, renal impairment or hypothyroidism.

In patients at increased risk of muscle effects, a statin should not usually be started if the baseline creatine kinase concentration is more than 5 times the upper limit of normal (some patients may present with an extremely elevated baseline creatine kinase concentration, for example because of a physical occupation or rigorous exercise—specialist advice should be sought regarding consideration of statin therapy in these patients).

▶ **Hypothyroidism** Hypothyroidism should be managed adequately before starting treatment with a statin.

- **SIDE-EFFECTS**
- ▶ **Common or very common** Asthenia · constipation · diarrhoea · dizziness · flatulence · gastrointestinal discomfort · headache · myalgia · nausea · sleep disorders · thrombocytopenia
- ▶ **Uncommon** Alopecia · hepatic disorders · memory loss · pancreatitis · paraesthesia · sexual dysfunction · skin reactions · vomiting
- ▶ **Rare or very rare** Myopathy · peripheral neuropathy · tendinopathy
- ▶ **Frequency not known** Depression · diabetes mellitus (in those at risk) · interstitial lung disease

SIDE-EFFECTS, FURTHER INFORMATION **Muscle effects**

The risk of myopathy, myositis, and rhabdomyolysis associated with statin use is rare. Although myalgia has been reported commonly in patients receiving statins, muscle toxicity truly attributable to statin use is rare. When a statin is suspected to be the cause of myopathy, and creatine kinase concentration is markedly elevated or if muscular symptoms are severe, treatment should be discontinued. If symptoms resolve and creatine kinase concentrations return to normal, the statin should be reintroduced at a lower dose and the patient monitored closely.

Interstitial lung disease If patients develop symptoms such as dyspnoea, cough, and weight loss, they should seek medical attention.

- **CONCEPTION AND CONTRACEPTION** Adequate contraception is required during treatment and for 1 month afterwards.
- **PREGNANCY** Statins should be avoided in pregnancy (discontinue 3 months before attempting to conceive) as congenital anomalies have been reported and the decreased synthesis of cholesterol possibly affects fetal development.
- **HEPATIC IMPAIRMENT** In general, manufacturers advise caution (risk of increased exposure); avoid in active disease or unexplained persistent elevations in serum transaminases.
- **MONITORING REQUIREMENTS**
  - Before starting treatment with statins, at least one full lipid profile (non-fasting) should be measured, including total cholesterol, HDL-cholesterol, non-HDL-cholesterol (calculated as total cholesterol minus HDL-cholesterol), and triglyceride concentrations, thyroid-stimulating hormone, and renal function should also be assessed.
  - Liver function There is little information available on a rational approach to liver-function monitoring; however, NICE suggests that liver enzymes should be measured before treatment, and repeated within 3 months and at 12 months of starting treatment, unless indicated at other times by signs or symptoms suggestive of hepatotoxicity (NICE clinical guideline 181 (July 2014). Lipid Modification—Cardiovascular risk assessment and the modification of blood lipids for the primary and secondary prevention of cardiovascular disease).
    Those with serum transaminases that are raised, but less than 3 times the upper limit of the reference range, should **not** be routinely excluded from statin therapy. Those with serum transaminases of more than 3 times the upper limit of the reference range should discontinue statin therapy.
  - Creatine kinase Creatine kinase concentration should be measured in children before treatment and if unexplained muscle pain occurs.
- **PATIENT AND CARER ADVICE** Advise patients to report promptly unexplained muscle pain, tenderness, or weakness.

138

Atorvastatin

05-Feb-2020

- **INDICATIONS AND DOSE**

Hyperlipidaemia including familial hypercholesterolaemia
- BY MOUTH
  - Child 10–17 years: Initially 10 mg once daily, then increased if necessary up to 20 mg once daily, dose to be adjusted at intervals of at least 4 weeks

Homozygous familial hypercholestrolaemia
- BY MOUTH
  - Child 10–17 years: Initially 10 mg once daily, then increased if necessary up to 80 mg once daily, dose to be adjusted at intervals of at least 4 weeks

DOSE ADJUSTMENTS DUE TO INTERACTIONS
- Manufacturer advises if concurrent use of ciclosporin is unavoidable, max. dose cannot exceed 10 mg daily.

- **CAUTIONS** Haemorrhagic stroke
- **INTERACTIONS** → Appendix 1: statins
- **SIDE-EFFECTS**
  - **Common or very common** Epistaxis · hyperglycaemia · hypersensitivity · joint disorders · laryngeal pain · muscle complaints · nasopharyngitis · pain
  - **Uncommon** Appetite decreased · burping · chest pain · fever · hypoglycaemia · malaise · numbness · peripheral oedema · taste altered · tinnitus · vision disorders · weight increased
  - **Rare or very rare** Angioedema · gynaecomastia · hearing loss · severe cutaneous adverse reactions (SCARs)
- **BREAST FEEDING** Manufacturer advises avoid—no information available.
- **PATIENT AND CARER ADVICE** Patient counselling is advised for atorvastatin tablets (muscle effects).
  Medicines for Children leaflet: Atorvastatin for high cholesterol www.medicinesforchildren.org.uk/atorvastatin-high-cholesterol-0

- **MEDICINAL FORMS** There can be variation in the licensing of different medicines containing the same drug. Forms available from special-order manufacturers include: oral suspension, oral solution

Tablet
- Atorvastatin (Non-proprietary)
  Atorvastatin (as Atorvastatin calcium trihydrate) 10 mg Atorvastatin 10mg tablets | 28 tablet [PoM] £13.00 DT = £0.89 | 90 tablet [PoM] £41.78 | 500 tablet [PoM] £9.72
  Atorvastatin (as Atorvastatin calcium trihydrate) 20 mg Atorvastatin 20mg tablets | 28 tablet [PoM] £24.64 DT = £1.03 | 90 tablet [PoM] £79.20 | 500 tablet [PoM] £11.69
  Atorvastatin (as Atorvastatin calcium trihydrate) 30 mg Atorvastatin 30mg tablets | 28 tablet [PoM] £24.51 DT = £24.51
  Atorvastatin (as Atorvastatin calcium trihydrate) 40 mg Atorvastatin 40mg tablets | 28 tablet [PoM] £24.64 DT = £1.29 | 90 tablet [PoM] £79.20 | 500 tablet [PoM] £14.42
  Atorvastatin (as Atorvastatin calcium trihydrate) 60 mg Atorvastatin 60mg tablets | 28 tablet [PoM] £28.01 DT = £28.01
  Atorvastatin (as Atorvastatin calcium trihydrate) 80 mg Atorvastatin 80mg tablets | 28 tablet [PoM] £28.21 DT = £1.90 | 90 tablet [PoM] £90.67
- Lipitor (Upjohn UK Ltd)
  Atorvastatin (as Atorvastatin calcium trihydrate) 10 mg Lipitor 10mg tablets | 28 tablet [PoM] £13.00 DT = £0.89
  Atorvastatin (as Atorvastatin calcium trihydrate) 20 mg Lipitor 20mg tablets | 28 tablet [PoM] £24.64 DT = £1.03
  Atorvastatin (as Atorvastatin calcium trihydrate) 40 mg Lipitor 40mg tablets | 28 tablet [PoM] £24.64 DT = £1.29
  Atorvastatin (as Atorvastatin calcium trihydrate) 80 mg Lipitor 80mg tablets | 28 tablet [PoM] £28.21 DT = £1.90

Chewable tablet

CAUTIONARY AND ADVISORY LABELS 24
- Lipitor (Upjohn UK Ltd)
  Atorvastatin (as Atorvastatin calcium trihydrate) 10 mg Lipitor 10mg chewable tablets sugar-free | 30 tablet [PoM] £13.80 DT = £13.80
  Atorvastatin (as Atorvastatin calcium trihydrate) 20 mg Lipitor 20mg chewable tablets sugar-free | 30 tablet [PoM] £26.40 DT = £26.40

138

Fluvastatin

08-Feb-2019

- **INDICATIONS AND DOSE**

Heterozygous familial hypercholesterolaemia
- INITIALLY BY MOUTH USING IMMEDIATE-RELEASE MEDICINES
  - Child 9–17 years: Initially 20 mg daily, dose to be taken in the evening, then (by mouth) adjusted in steps of 20 mg daily (max. per dose 40 mg twice daily), adjusted at intervals of at least 6 weeks; maximum 80 mg per day

continued →

▸ BY MOUTH USING MODIFIED-RELEASE MEDICINES
▸ Child 9–17 years: 80 mg daily, dose form is not appropriate for initial dose titration

- INTERACTIONS → Appendix 1: statins
- SIDE-EFFECTS
▸ **Rare or very rare** Angioedema · face oedema · lupus-like syndrome · muscle weakness · sensation abnormal · vasculitis
- BREAST FEEDING Manufacturer advises avoid—no information available.
- RENAL IMPAIRMENT
Dose adjustments Manufacturer advises doses above 40 mg daily should be initiated with caution if estimated glomerular filtration rate less than 30 mL/minute/1.73 m^2.
- PATIENT AND CARER ADVICE Patient counselling is advised for fluvastatin tablets/capsules (muscle effects).
- NATIONAL FUNDING/ACCESS DECISIONS

Scottish Medicines Consortium (SMC) decisions
SMC No. 76/04
The *Scottish Medicines Consortium* has advised (February 2004) that fluvastatin (*Lescol*®) is accepted for restricted use for the secondary prevention of coronary events after percutaneous coronary angioplasty; if the patient has previously been receiving another statin, then there is no need to change the statin.

- MEDICINAL FORMS There can be variation in the licensing of different medicines containing the same drug.

Modified-release tablet
CAUTIONARY AND ADVISORY LABELS 25
▸ Cadaff XL (Torrent Pharma (UK) Ltd)
Fluvastatin (as Fluvastatin sodium) 80 mg Cadaff XL 80mg tablets | 28 tablet PoM £19.20 DT = £19.20
▸ Dorisin XL (Aspire Pharma Ltd)
Fluvastatin (as Fluvastatin sodium) 80 mg Dorisin XL 80mg tablets | 28 tablet PoM £19.20 DT = £19.20
▸ Lescol XL (Novartis Pharmaceuticals UK Ltd)
Fluvastatin (as Fluvastatin sodium) 80 mg Lescol XL 80mg tablets | 28 tablet PoM £19.20 DT = £19.20
▸ Nandovar XL (Sandoz Ltd)
Fluvastatin (as Fluvastatin sodium) 80 mg Nandovar XL 80mg tablets | 28 tablet PoM £16.32 DT = £19.20

Capsule
▸ Fluvastatin (Non-proprietary)
Fluvastatin (as Fluvastatin sodium) 20 mg Fluvastatin 20mg capsules | 28 capsule PoM £6.96 DT = £2.21
Fluvastatin (as Fluvastatin sodium) 40 mg Fluvastatin 40mg capsules | 28 capsule PoM £7.42 DT = £2.64

⚑ 138

Pravastatin sodium

04-Jun-2017

- INDICATIONS AND DOSE

Hyperlipidaemia including familial hypercholesterolaemia
▸ BY MOUTH
▸ Child 8–13 years: 10 mg daily, then increased if necessary up to 20 mg daily, dose to be taken at night, dose to be adjusted at intervals of at least 4 weeks
▸ Child 14–17 years: 10 mg daily, then increased if necessary up to 40 mg daily, dose to be taken at night, dose to be adjusted at intervals of at least 4 weeks

DOSE ADJUSTMENTS DUE TO INTERACTIONS
▸ Manufacturer advises reduce maximum daily dose with concurrent use of glecaprevir with pibrentasvir—consult product literature.

- INTERACTIONS → Appendix 1: statins
- SIDE-EFFECTS
▸ **Uncommon** Hair abnormal · scalp abnormal · urinary disorders · vision disorders
- BREAST FEEDING Manufacturer advises avoid—small amount of drug present in breast milk.
- HEPATIC IMPAIRMENT
Dose adjustments Manufacturer advises initial dose reduction to 10 mg daily; adjust according to response.
- RENAL IMPAIRMENT
Dose adjustments Start with lower doses in moderate to severe impairment.
- PATIENT AND CARER ADVICE Patient counselling is advised for pravastatin tablets (muscle effects).

- MEDICINAL FORMS There can be variation in the licensing of different medicines containing the same drug. Forms available from special-order manufacturers include: oral suspension, oral solution

Tablet
▸ Pravastatin sodium (Non-proprietary)
Pravastatin sodium 10 mg Pravastatin 10mg tablets | 28 tablet PoM £2.68 DT = £0.95
Pravastatin sodium 20 mg Pravastatin 20mg tablets | 28 tablet PoM £3.05 DT = £1.17
Pravastatin sodium 40 mg Pravastatin 40mg tablets | 28 tablet PoM £3.82 DT = £1.43

⚑ 138

Rosuvastatin

05-Feb-2020

- INDICATIONS AND DOSE

Heterozygous familial hypercholesterolaemia (specialist use only)
▸ BY MOUTH
▸ Child 6–9 years: Initially 5 mg once daily, then increased if necessary up to 10 mg once daily, dose to be increased gradually at intervals of at least 4 weeks
▸ Child 10–17 years: Initially 5 mg once daily, then increased if necessary up to 20 mg once daily, dose to be increased gradually at intervals of at least 4 weeks, use lower max. dose in children with risk factors for myopathy or rhabdomyolysis (including personal or family history of muscular disorders or toxicity)

Homozygous familial hypercholesterolaemia (specialist use only)
▸ BY MOUTH
▸ Child 6–17 years: Initially 5–10 mg once daily, then increased if necessary up to 20 mg once daily, dose to be increased gradually at intervals of at least 4 weeks, use lower max. dose in children with risk factors for myopathy or rhabdomyolysis (including personal or family history of muscular disorders or toxicity)
▸ Child 6–17 years (patients of Asian origin): Initially 5 mg once daily, then increased if necessary up to 20 mg once daily, dose to be increased gradually at intervals of at least 4 weeks, use lower max. dose in children with risk factors for myopathy or rhabdomyolysis (including personal or family history of muscular disorders or toxicity).

DOSE ADJUSTMENTS DUE TO INTERACTIONS
▸ Manufacturer advises max. 5 mg daily with concurrent use of glecaprevir with pibrentasvir.

- INTERACTIONS → Appendix 1: statins
- SIDE-EFFECTS
▸ **Rare or very rare** Arthralgia · gynaecomastia · haematuria · polyneuropathy
▸ **Frequency not known** Cough · dyspnoea · oedema · proteinuria · Stevens-Johnson syndrome · tendon disorders
- BREAST FEEDING Manufacturer advises avoid—no information available.
- RENAL IMPAIRMENT Avoid if estimated glomerular filtration rate less than 30 mL/minute/1.73 m^2.
Dose adjustments Reduce dose if estimated glomerular filtration rate less than 60 mL/minute/1.73 m^2.

- **MONITORING REQUIREMENTS** Manufacturer advises consider routine monitoring of renal function when using 40 mg daily dose.
- **PATIENT AND CARER ADVICE** Patient counselling is advised for rosuvastatin tablets (muscle effects).

- **MEDICINAL FORMS** There can be variation in the licensing of different medicines containing the same drug. Forms available from special-order manufacturers include: oral suspension

Tablet

- Rosuvastatin (Non-proprietary)
  - **Rosuvastatin (as Rosuvastatin calcium) 5 mg** Rosuvastatin 5mg tablets | 28 tablet PoM £18.03 DT = £1.35
  - **Rosuvastatin (as Rosuvastatin calcium) 10 mg** Rosuvastatin 10mg tablets | 28 tablet PoM £18.03 DT = £1.44
  - **Rosuvastatin (as Rosuvastatin calcium) 20 mg** Rosuvastatin 20mg tablets | 28 tablet PoM £26.02 DT = £1.92
  - **Rosuvastatin (as Rosuvastatin calcium) 40 mg** Rosuvastatin 40mg tablets | 28 tablet PoM £29.69 DT = £1.93
- Crestor (AstraZeneca UK Ltd)
  - **Rosuvastatin (as Rosuvastatin calcium) 5 mg** Crestor 5mg tablets | 28 tablet PoM £18.03 DT = £1.35
  - **Rosuvastatin (as Rosuvastatin calcium) 10 mg** Crestor 10mg tablets | 28 tablet PoM £18.03 DT = £1.44
  - **Rosuvastatin (as Rosuvastatin calcium) 20 mg** Crestor 20mg tablets | 28 tablet PoM £26.02 DT = £1.92
  - **Rosuvastatin (as Rosuvastatin calcium) 40 mg** Crestor 40mg tablets | 28 tablet PoM £29.69 DT = £1.93

138

Simvastatin

- **INDICATIONS AND DOSE**

Hyperlipidaemia including familial hypercholesterolaemia

- BY MOUTH
  - Child 5–9 years: Initially 10 mg once daily, then increased if necessary up to 20 mg once daily, dose to be taken at night, increased at intervals of at least 4 weeks
  - Child 10–17 years: Initially 10 mg once daily, then increased if necessary up to 40 mg once daily, dose to be taken at night, increased at intervals of at least 4 weeks

DOSE ADJUSTMENTS DUE TO INTERACTIONS

- Manufacturer advises max. dose 10 mg daily with concurrent use of bezafibrate—no specific recommendation made for children.
- Manufacturer advises max. dose 20 mg daily with concurrent use of amiodarone or amlodipine—no specific recommendation made for children.
- Manufacturer advises reduce dose with concurrent use of some moderate inhibitors of CYP3A4 (max. 20 mg daily with verapamil and diltiazem)—no specific recommendation made for children.

- **UNLICENSED USE** Not licensed for use in children under 10 years.
- **INTERACTIONS** → Appendix 1: statins
- **SIDE-EFFECTS**
  - **Rare or very rare** Acute kidney injury · anaemia · muscle cramps
  - **Frequency not known** Cognitive impairment
- **BREAST FEEDING** Manufacturer advises avoid—no information available.
- **RENAL IMPAIRMENT** Doses above 10 mg daily should be used with caution if estimated glomerular filtration rate less than 30 mL/minute/1.73 m^2.
- **PATIENT AND CARER ADVICE** Patient counselling is advised for simvastatin tablets/oral suspension (muscle effects).

- **MEDICINAL FORMS** There can be variation in the licensing of different medicines containing the same drug. Forms available from special-order manufacturers include: oral suspension, oral solution

Oral suspension

EXCIPIENTS: May contain Propylene glycol

- Simvastatin (Non-proprietary)
  - **Simvastatin 4 mg per 1 ml** Simvastatin 20mg/5ml oral suspension sugar-free | 150 ml PoM £153.04 DT = £152.98
  - **Simvastatin 8 mg per 1 ml** Simvastatin 40mg/5ml oral suspension sugar-free | 150 ml PoM £233.78 DT = £233.68

Tablet

- Simvastatin (Non-proprietary)
  - **Simvastatin 10 mg** Simvastatin 10mg tablets | 28 tablet PoM £14.42 DT = £0.80
  - **Simvastatin 20 mg** Simvastatin 20mg tablets | 28 tablet PoM £23.75 DT = £0.95
  - **Simvastatin 40 mg** Simvastatin 40mg tablets | 28 tablet PoM £23.75 DT = £1.01
  - **Simvastatin 80 mg** Simvastatin 80mg tablets | 28 tablet PoM £6.00 DT = £1.66
- Simvador (Dexcel-Pharma Ltd)
  - **Simvastatin 10 mg** Simvador 10mg tablets | 28 tablet PoM £0.65 DT = £0.80
  - **Simvastatin 20 mg** Simvador 20mg tablets | 28 tablet PoM £0.77 DT = £0.95
  - **Simvastatin 40 mg** Simvador 40mg tablets | 28 tablet PoM £0.88 DT = £1.01
  - **Simvastatin 80 mg** Simvador 80mg tablets | 28 tablet PoM £1.38 DT = £1.66
- Zocor (Merck Sharp & Dohme Ltd)
  - **Simvastatin 10 mg** Zocor 10mg tablets | 28 tablet PoM £18.03 DT = £0.80
  - **Simvastatin 20 mg** Zocor 20mg tablets | 28 tablet PoM £29.69 DT = £0.95
  - **Simvastatin 40 mg** Zocor 40mg tablets | 28 tablet PoM £29.69 DT = £1.01
  - **Simvastatin 80 mg** Zocor 80mg tablets | 28 tablet PoM £29.69 DT = £1.66

Simvastatin with ezetimibe

The properties listed below are those particular to the combination only. For the properties of the components please consider, simvastatin above, ezetimibe p. 137.

- **INDICATIONS AND DOSE**

Homozygous familial hypercholesterolaemia, primary hypercholesterolaemia, and mixed hyperlipidaemia in patients over 10 years stabilised on the individual components in the same proportions, or for patients not adequately controlled by statin alone

- BY MOUTH
  - Child (initiated by a specialist): (consult product literature)

- **INTERACTIONS** → Appendix 1: ezetimibe · statins

- **MEDICINAL FORMS** There can be variation in the licensing of different medicines containing the same drug.

Tablet

- Inegy (Merck Sharp & Dohme Ltd)
  - **Ezetimibe 10 mg, Simvastatin 20 mg** Inegy 10mg/20mg tablets | 28 tablet PoM £33.42 DT = £33.42
  - **Ezetimibe 10 mg, Simvastatin 40 mg** Inegy 10mg/40mg tablets | 28 tablet PoM £38.98 DT = £38.98
  - **Ezetimibe 10 mg, Simvastatin 80 mg** Inegy 10mg/80mg tablets | 28 tablet PoM £41.21 DT = £41.21

LIPID MODIFYING DRUGS > OTHER

Evolocumab

08-Feb-2019

● **DRUG ACTION** Evolocumab binds to a pro-protein involved in the regulation of LDL receptors on liver cells; receptor numbers are increased, which results in increased uptake of LDL-cholesterol from the blood.

● **INDICATIONS AND DOSE**

Homozygous familial hypercholesterolaemia (in combination with other lipid-lowering therapies)

▶ BY SUBCUTANEOUS INJECTION

▸ Child 12–17 years: Initially 420 mg every month; increased if necessary to 420 mg every 2 weeks, if inadequate response after 12 weeks of treatment, to be administered into the thigh, abdomen or upper arm

Homozygous familial hypercholesterolaemia in patients on apheresis (in combination with other lipid-lowering therapies)

▶ BY SUBCUTANEOUS INJECTION

▸ Child 12–17 years: 420 mg every 2 weeks, to correspond with apheresis schedule, to be administered into the thigh, abdomen or upper arm

● **SIDE-EFFECTS**

▶ **Common or very common** Arthralgia · back pain · increased risk of infection · nausea · skin reactions

▶ **Rare or very rare** Angioedema

● **PREGNANCY** Manufacturer advises avoid unless essential—limited information available.

● **BREAST FEEDING** Manufacturer advises avoid—no information available.

● **HEPATIC IMPAIRMENT** Manufacturer advises caution in moderate to severe impairment (risk of reduced efficacy; no information available in severe impairment).

● **RENAL IMPAIRMENT** Manufacturer advises caution if estimated glomerular filtration rate less than 30 mL/minute/1.73 m^2—no information available.

● **HANDLING AND STORAGE** Manufacturer advises store in a refrigerator (2–8°C)—consult product literature for further information regarding storage outside refrigerator.

● **PATIENT AND CARER ADVICE** Patients and their carers should be given training in subcutaneous injection technique.

● **MEDICINAL FORMS** There can be variation in the licensing of different medicines containing the same drug.

Solution for injection

▸ Repatha SureClick (Amgen Ltd) ▼

Evolocumab 140 mg per 1 ml Repatha SureClick 140mg/1ml solution for injection pre-filled pens | 2 pre-filled disposable injection PoM £340.20 DT = £340.20

7 Myocardial ischaemia

NITRATES

Nitrates

Overview

Nitrates are potent coronary vasodilators, but their principal benefit follows from a reduction in venous return which reduces left ventricular work. Unwanted effects such as flushing, headache, and postural hypotension may limit therapy, especially if the child is unusually sensitive to the effects of nitrates or is hypovolaemic. Glyceryl trinitrate below is also used in extravasation.

Nitrates

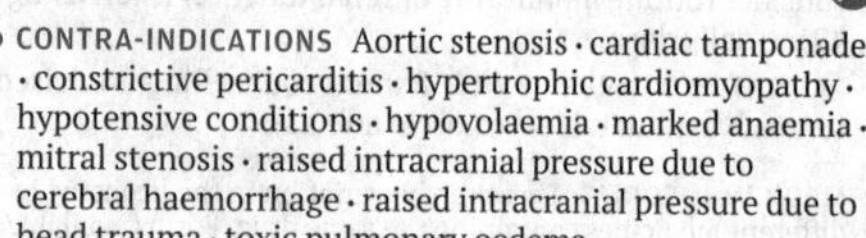

● **CONTRA-INDICATIONS** Aortic stenosis · cardiac tamponade · constrictive pericarditis · hypertrophic cardiomyopathy · hypotensive conditions · hypovolaemia · marked anaemia · mitral stenosis · raised intracranial pressure due to cerebral haemorrhage · raised intracranial pressure due to head trauma · toxic pulmonary oedema

● **CAUTIONS** Heart failure due to obstruction · hypothermia · hypothyroidism · hypoxaemia · malnutrition · metal-containing transdermal systems should be removed before magnetic resonance imaging procedures, cardioversion, or diathermy · recent history of myocardial infarction · susceptibility to angle-closure glaucoma · tolerance · ventilation and perfusion abnormalities

CAUTIONS, FURTHER INFORMATION

▸ Tolerance Children receiving nitrates continuously throughout the day can develop tolerance (with reduced therapeutic effects). Reduction of blood-nitrate concentrations to low levels for 4 to 8 hours each day usually maintains effectiveness in such patients.

● **SIDE-EFFECTS**

▶ **Common or very common** Arrhythmias · asthenia · cerebral ischaemia · dizziness · drowsiness · flushing · headache · hypotension · nausea · vomiting

▶ **Uncommon** Circulatory collapse · diarrhoea · skin reactions · syncope

● **ALLERGY AND CROSS-SENSITIVITY** Contra-indicated in nitrate hypersensitivity.

● **BREAST FEEDING** No information available—manufacturers advise use only if potential benefit outweighs risk.

● **HEPATIC IMPAIRMENT** In general, manufacturers advise caution in severe impairment.

● **RENAL IMPAIRMENT** Manufacturers advise use with caution in severe impairment.

● **MONITORING REQUIREMENTS** Monitor blood pressure and heart rate during intravenous infusion.

● **TREATMENT CESSATION** Avoid abrupt withdrawal.

F above

Glyceryl trinitrate

27-Jul-2018

● **INDICATIONS AND DOSE**

Hypertension during and after cardiac surgery | Heart failure after cardiac surgery | Coronary vasoconstriction in myocardial ischaemia | Vasoconstriction in shock

▶ BY CONTINUOUS INTRAVENOUS INFUSION

▸ Neonate: 0.2–0.5 microgram/kg/minute, adjusted according to response, maintenance 1–3 micrograms/kg/minute (max. per dose 10 micrograms/kg/minute).

▸ Child: Initially 0.2–0.5 microgram/kg/minute, adjusted according to response, maintenance 1–3 micrograms/kg/minute (max. per dose 10 micrograms/kg/minute); maximum 200 micrograms/minute

● **UNLICENSED USE** Not licensed for use in children.

● **INTERACTIONS** → Appendix 1: nitrates

● **SIDE-EFFECTS**

▶ **Uncommon** Cardiac disorder · cyanosis

▶ **Rare or very rare** Methaemoglobinaemia · respiratory disorder · restlessness

▶ **Frequency not known** Hyperhidrosis

● **PREGNANCY** Not known to be harmful.

● **DIRECTIONS FOR ADMINISTRATION**

▸ With intravenous use For *continuous intravenous infusion*, dilute to max. concentration of 400 micrograms/mL (but concentration of 1 mg/mL has been used via a central venous catheter) with Glucose 5% or Sodium Chloride 0.9%. *Neonatal intensive care*, dilute 3 mg/kg body-weight to a final volume of 50 mL with Glucose 5% or Sodium Chloride 0.9%; an intravenous infusion rate of 1 mL/hour provides a dose of 1 microgram/kg/minute; max. concentration of 400 micrograms/mL (but concentration of 1 mg/mL has been used via a central venous catheter). Glass or polyethylene apparatus is preferable; loss of potency will occur if PVC is used. Glyceryl trinitrate 1 mg/ml to be diluted before use or given undiluted with syringe pump. Glyceryl trinitrate 5 mg/ml to be diluted before use.

- **MEDICINAL FORMS** There can be variation in the licensing of different medicines containing the same drug. Forms available from special-order manufacturers include: solution for infusion

Solution for infusion

EXCIPIENTS: May contain Ethanol, propylene glycol

- Glyceryl trinitrate (Non-proprietary)
  Glyceryl trinitrate 1 mg per 1 ml Glyceryl trinitrate 50mg/50ml solution for infusion vials | 1 vial PoM £15.90
  Glyceryl trinitrate 5 mg per 1 ml Glyceryl trinitrate 50mg/10ml solution for infusion ampoules | 5 ampoule PoM £64.90 (Hospital only)
  Glyceryl trinitrate 25mg/5ml solution for infusion ampoules | 5 ampoule PoM £32.45 (Hospital only)
- Nitrocine (Forum Health Products Ltd)
  Glyceryl trinitrate 1 mg per 1 ml Nitrocine 10mg/10ml solution for infusion ampoules | 10 ampoule PoM £58.75 (Hospital only)
- Nitronal (Intrapharm Laboratories Ltd)
  Glyceryl trinitrate 1 mg per 1 ml Nitronal 5mg/5ml solution for infusion ampoules | 10 ampoule PoM £18.04
  Nitronal 50mg/50ml solution for infusion vials | 1 vial PoM £14.76

7.1 Cardiac arrest

Cardiopulmonary resuscitation

Overview

The algorithms for cardiopulmonary resuscitation (Life support algorithm (image), inside back pages) reflect the recommendations of the Resuscitation Council (UK) and cover paediatric basic life support, paediatric advanced life support, and newborn life support; these have been reproduced with the kind permission of the Resuscitation Council (UK). The guidelines are available at www.resus.org.uk.

Paediatric advanced life support

Cardiopulmonary (cardiac) arrest in children is rare and frequently represents the terminal event of progressive shock or respiratory failure.

During cardiopulmonary arrest in children without intravenous access, the intraosseous route is chosen because it provides rapid and effective response; if circulatory access cannot be gained, the endotracheal tube can be used. When the endotracheal route is used ten times the intravenous dose should be used; the drug should be injected quickly down a narrow bore suction catheter beyond the tracheal end of the tube and then flushed in with 1 or 2 mL of sodium chloride 0.9%. The endotracheal route is useful for lipid-soluble drugs, including lidocaine hydrochloride p. 81, adrenaline/epinephrine below, atropine sulfate p. 869, and naloxone hydrochloride p. 901. Drugs that are not lipid-soluble (e.g. sodium bicarbonate p. 634 and calcium chloride p. 642) should **not** be administered by this route because they will injure the airways.

For the management of acute anaphylaxis, see allergic emergencies under Antihistamines, allergen immunotherapy and allergic emergencies p. 180.

SYMPATHOMIMETICS > VASOCONSTRICTOR

Adrenaline/epinephrine

21-May-2020

- **DRUG ACTION** Acts on both alpha and beta receptors and increases both heart rate and contractility (beta$_1$ effects); it can cause peripheral vasodilation (a beta$_2$ effect) or vasoconstriction (an alpha effect).

- **INDICATIONS AND DOSE**

Acute hypotension

▶ BY CONTINUOUS INTRAVENOUS INFUSION

- Neonate: Initially 100 nanograms/kg/minute, adjusted according to response, higher doses up to 1.5 micrograms/kg/minute have been used in acute hypotension.
- Child: Initially 100 nanograms/kg/minute, adjusted according to response, higher doses up to 1.5 micrograms/kg/minute have been used in acute hypotension

Croup (when not effectively controlled with corticosteroid treatment)

▶ BY INHALATION OF NEBULISED SOLUTION

- Child 1 month–11 years: 400 micrograms/kg (max. per dose 5 mg), dose to be repeated after 30 minutes if necessary

PHARMACOKINETICS

- The effects of nebulised adrenaline for the treatment of croup lasts for 2–3 hours.

Emergency treatment of acute anaphylaxis (under expert supervision) | Angioedema (if laryngeal oedema is present) (under expert supervision)

▶ BY INTRAMUSCULAR INJECTION

- Child 1 month–5 years: 150 micrograms, doses may be repeated several times if necessary at 5 minute intervals according to blood pressure, pulse, and respiratory function, suitable syringe to be used for measuring small volume; injected preferably into the anterolateral aspect of the middle third of the thigh
- Child 6–11 years: 300 micrograms, doses may be repeated several times if necessary at 5 minute intervals according to blood pressure, pulse, and respiratory function, to be injected preferably into the anterolateral aspect of the middle third of the thigh
- Child 12–17 years: 500 micrograms, to be injected preferably into the anterolateral aspect of the middle third of the thigh, doses may be repeated several times if necessary at 5 minute intervals according to blood pressure, pulse, and respiratory function, 300 micrograms (0.3 mL) to be administered if child small or prepubertal

Acute anaphylaxis when there is doubt as to the adequacy of the circulation (specialist use only) | Angioedema (if laryngeal oedema is present) (specialist use only)

▶ BY SLOW INTRAVENOUS INJECTION

- Child: 1 microgram/kg (max. per dose 50 micrograms), using dilute 1 in 10 000 adrenaline injection, dose to be repeated according to response, if multiple doses required, adrenaline should be given as a slow intravenous infusion stopping when a response has been obtained

EMERADE® 150 MICROGRAMS

Acute anaphylaxis (for self-administration)—product recalled, see Important Safety Information

▶ BY INTRAMUSCULAR INJECTION

- Child (body-weight up to 15 kg): 150 micrograms, then 150 micrograms after 5–15 minutes as required
- Child (body-weight 15–30 kg): 150 micrograms, then 150 micrograms after 5–15 minutes as required, on the basis of a dose of 10 micrograms/kg,

continued →

300 micrograms may be more appropriate for some children

EMERADE® 300 MICROGRAMS

Acute anaphylaxis (for self-administration)—product recalled, see Important Safety Information
- BY INTRAMUSCULAR INJECTION
- Child (body-weight 30 kg and above): 300 micrograms, then 300 micrograms after 5–15 minutes as required

EMERADE® 500 MICROGRAMS

Acute anaphylaxis (for self-administration)—product recalled, see Important Safety Information
- BY INTRAMUSCULAR INJECTION
- Child 12–17 years: 500 micrograms, then 500 micrograms after 5–15 minutes as required

EPIPEN® AUTO-INJECTOR 0.3MG

Acute anaphylaxis (for self-administration)
- BY INTRAMUSCULAR INJECTION
- Child (body-weight 26 kg and above): 300 micrograms, then 300 micrograms after 5–15 minutes as required

EPIPEN® JR AUTO-INJECTOR 0.15MG

Acute anaphylaxis (for self-administration)
- BY INTRAMUSCULAR INJECTION
- Child (body-weight up to 15 kg): 150 micrograms, then 150 micrograms after 5–15 minutes as required
- Child (body-weight 15–25 kg): 150 micrograms, then 150 micrograms after 5–15 minutes as required, on the basis of a dose of 10 micrograms/kg, 300 micrograms may be more appropriate for some children

JEXT® 150 MICROGRAMS

Acute anaphylaxis (for self-administration)
- BY INTRAMUSCULAR INJECTION
- Child (body-weight up to 15 kg): 150 micrograms, then 150 micrograms after 5–15 minutes as required
- Child (body-weight 15–30 kg): 150 micrograms, then 150 micrograms after 5–15 minutes as required, on the basis of a dose of 10 micrograms/kg, 300 micrograms may be more appropriate for some children

JEXT® 300 MICROGRAMS

Acute anaphylaxis (for self-administration)
- BY INTRAMUSCULAR INJECTION
- Child (body-weight 31 kg and above): 300 micrograms, then 300 micrograms after 5–15 minutes as required

● **UNLICENSED USE**
- With intramuscular use for acute anaphylaxis Auto-injectors delivering 150-microgram dose of adrenaline may not be licensed for use in children with body-weight under 15 kg.
- With intravenous use for acute hypotension Adrenaline 1 in 1000 (1 mg/mL) solution is not licensed for intravenous administration.

IMPORTANT SAFETY INFORMATION

SAFE PRACTICE
- With intravenous use

Intravenous route should be used with **extreme care** by specialists only.

MHRA/CHM ADVICE: ADRENALINE AUTO-INJECTORS: UPDATED ADVICE AFTER EUROPEAN REVIEW (AUGUST 2017)
- With intramuscular use

Following a European review of all adrenaline auto-injectors approved in the EU, the MHRA recommend that 2 adrenaline auto-injectors are prescribed, which patients should carry at all times. This is particularly important for patients with allergic asthma, who are at increased risk of a severe anaphylactic reaction. Patients with allergies and their carers should be trained to use the particular auto-injector they have been prescribed and encouraged to practise using a trainer device. Patients are advised to check the expiry date of the adrenaline auto-injectors and obtain replacements before they expire.

MHRA/CHM ADVICE: CLASS 2 MEDICINES RECALL: *EMERADE®* 150 MICROGRAMS (MARCH 2020); *EMERADE®* 300 MICROGRAMS (APRIL 2020); *EMERADE®* 500 MICROGRAMS (MAY 2020) SOLUTION FOR INJECTION IN PRE-FILLED SYRINGES
- With intramuscular use

The MHRA has advised that all unexpired batches of *Emerade®* 150 microgram, 300 microgram, and 500 microgram auto-injector pens are being recalled from patients due to an error in one component of the auto-injector believed to cause the failure of some pens to activate. Healthcare professionals are advised to identify these patients and review their adrenaline prescription. Patients and their carers should immediately be informed that a prescription for a suitable alternative brand of adrenaline auto-injector is required. They should be advised to return their current *Emerade®* pen(s) to a pharmacy once they have two pens of an alternative brand in their possession. Returned pens should be quarantined in pharmacies and returned to the supplier using the supplier's approved process. This advice also applies to *Emerade®* auto-injector pens that are kept in emergency anaphylaxis kits (e.g. in dental surgeries or schools). For patients who have been prescribed *Emerade®* **500 microgram** auto-injector pens, the MHRA advises that *EpiPen®* or *Jext®* **300 microgram** (maximum strength) pens will be a suitable replacement, based on results from a bioavailability study. The MHRA has produced a Patient Letter on the *Emerade®* recall for each strength of auto-injector which should be provided to patients and their carers. Healthcare professionals are reminded to follow existing advice on the use of adrenaline auto-injectors—see *Prescribing and dispensing information*. For the latest safety alerts, see the MHRA website.

● **CAUTIONS** Arrhythmias · cerebrovascular disease · cor pulmonale · diabetes mellitus · hypercalcaemia · hyperreflexia · hypertension · hyperthyroidism · hypokalaemia · ischaemic heart disease · obstructive cardiomyopathy · occlusive vascular disease · organic brain damage · phaeochromocytoma · prostate disorders · psychoneurosis · severe angina · susceptibility to angle-closure glaucoma

CAUTIONS, FURTHER INFORMATION Cautions listed are only for non-life-threatening situations.

● **INTERACTIONS** → Appendix 1: sympathomimetics, vasoconstrictor

● **SIDE-EFFECTS**

GENERAL SIDE-EFFECTS
- **Rare or very rare** Cardiomyopathy
- **Frequency not known** Angina pectoris · angle closure glaucoma · anxiety · appetite decreased · arrhythmias · asthenia · CNS haemorrhage · confusion · dizziness · dry mouth · dyspnoea · headache · hepatic necrosis · hyperglycaemia · hyperhidrosis · hypersalivation · hypertension (increased risk of cerebral haemorrhage) · hypokalaemia · injection site necrosis · insomnia · intestinal necrosis · metabolic acidosis · mydriasis · myocardial infarction · nausea · pallor · palpitations · peripheral coldness · psychosis · pulmonary oedema (on excessive dosage or extreme sensitivity) · renal necrosis · soft tissue necrosis · tremor · urinary disorders · vomiting

SPECIFIC SIDE-EFFECTS
- With intramuscular use Muscle necrosis · necrotising fasciitis · peripheral ischaemia
- With intravenous use Hemiplegia · muscle rigidity

● **PREGNANCY**
- With intramuscular use or intravenous use May reduce placental perfusion and cause tachycardia, cardiac

irregularities, and extrasystoles in fetus. Can delay second stage of labour. Manufacturers advise use only if benefit outweighs risk.

- **BREAST FEEDING**
  - With intramuscular use or intravenous use Present in milk but unlikely to be harmful as poor oral bioavailability.
- **RENAL IMPAIRMENT** Manufacturers advise use with caution in severe impairment.
- **MONITORING REQUIREMENTS** Monitor blood pressure and ECG.
- **DIRECTIONS FOR ADMINISTRATION**

Acute hypotension

- With intravenous use For *continuous intravenous infusion*, dilute with Glucose 5% or Sodium Chloride 0.9% and give through a central venous catheter. Incompatible with bicarbonate and alkaline solutions. *Neonatal intensive care*, dilute 3 mg/kg body-weight to a final volume of 50 mL with infusion fluid; an intravenous infusion rate of 0.1 mL/hour provides a dose of 100 nanograms/kg/minute; infuse through a central venous catheter. Incompatible with bicarbonate and alkaline solutions. These infusions are usually made up with adrenaline 1 in 1000 (1 mg/mL) solution.
- When used by inhalation For nebulisation in croup, adrenaline 1 in 1000 solution may be diluted with sterile sodium chloride 0.9% solution.

- **PRESCRIBING AND DISPENSING INFORMATION**
  - With intramuscular use It is important, in acute anaphylaxis where intramuscular injection might still succeed, time should not be wasted seeking intravenous access. Great vigilance is needed to ensure that the *correct strength* of adrenaline injection is used; anaphylactic shock kits need to make a *very clear distinction* between the 1 in 10 000 strength and the 1 in 1000 strength. Patients with severe allergy should be instructed in the self-administration of adrenaline by intramuscular injection. Packs for self-administration need to be **clearly labelled with instructions** on how to administer adrenaline (intramuscularly, preferably at the midpoint of the outer thigh, through light clothing if necessary) so that in the case of rapid collapse someone else is able to give it. It is important to ensure individuals at risk and their carers understand that:
    - two injection devices should be carried at all times to treat symptoms until medical assistance is available; if, after the first injection, the individual does not start to feel better, the second injection should be given 5 to 15 minutes after the first;
    - an ambulance should be called after every administration, even if symptoms improve;
    - the individual should lie down with their legs raised (unless they have breathing difficulties, in which case they should sit up) and should not be left alone.

Adrenaline for administration by intramuscular injection is available in 'auto-injectors' (e.g. *Emerade*®—product recalled, see *Important Safety Information, EpiPen*®, or *Jext*®), pre-assembled syringes fitted with a needle suitable for very rapid administration (if necessary by a bystander or a healthcare provider if it is the only preparation available); injection technique is device specific.

To ensure patients receive the auto-injector device that they have been trained to use, prescribers should specify the brand to be dispensed. If switching between brands, patients should receive full training in use of the new auto-injector device.

Licensed doses differ between brands of adrenaline auto-injectors. Adrenaline bioavailability has the potential to be influenced by a number of factors including formulation, propulsive force of the device and needle length—consult product literature for further information.

- **PATIENT AND CARER ADVICE**
  - With intramuscular use Individuals at considerable risk of anaphylaxis need to carry (or have available) adrenaline at all times and the patient, or their carers, need to be *instructed in advance* when and how to inject it.
  - With intramuscular use The MHRA has produced an advice sheet on the use of adrenaline auto-injectors, which should be provided to patients and their carers.

Medicines for Children leaflet: Adrenaline auto-injector for anaphylaxis www.medicinesforchildren.org.uk/adrenaline-auto-injector-anaphylaxis-0

JEXT ® 300 MICROGRAMS 1.1 mL of the solution remains in the auto-injector device after use.

JEXT ® 150 MICROGRAMS 1.25 mL of the solution remains in the auto-injector device after use.

EPIPEN ® JR AUTO-INJECTOR 0.15MG 1.7 mL of the solution remains in the auto-injector device after use.

EMERADE ® 150 MICROGRAMS 0.35 mL of the solution remains in the auto-injector device after use.

EPIPEN ® AUTO-INJECTOR 0.3MG 1.7 mL of the solution remains in the auto-injector device after use.

EMERADE ® 500 MICROGRAMS No solution remains in the auto-injector device after use.

EMERADE ® 300 MICROGRAMS 0.2 mL of the solution remains in the auto-injector device after use.

- **EXCEPTIONS TO LEGAL CATEGORY**
  - With intramuscular use POM restriction does not apply to the intramuscular administration of up to 1 mg of adrenaline injection 1 in 1000 (1 mg/mL) for the emergency treatment of anaphylaxis.

- **MEDICINAL FORMS** There can be variation in the licensing of different medicines containing the same drug. Forms available from special-order manufacturers include: solution for injection

Solution for injection

EXCIPIENTS: May contain Sulfites

- Adrenaline/epinephrine (Non-proprietary)

Adrenaline 100 microgram per 1 ml Adrenaline (base) 100micrograms/1ml (1 in 10,000) dilute solution for injection ampoules | 10 ampoule PoM £88.18
Adrenaline (base) 1mg/10ml (1 in 10,000) dilute solution for injection pre-filled syringes | 1 pre-filled disposable injection PoM £6.87 | 1 pre-filled disposable injection PoM £18.00 (Hospital only) | 10 pre-filled disposable injection PoM £180.00 (Hospital only)

Adrenaline (as Adrenaline acid tartrate) 100 microgram per 1 ml Adrenaline (base) 1mg/10ml (1 in 10,000) dilute solution for injection ampoules | 10 ampoule PoM £102.19
Adrenaline (base) 500micrograms/5ml (1 in 10,000) dilute solution for injection ampoules | 10 ampoule PoM £93.94

Adrenaline 1 mg per 1 ml Adrenaline (base) 10mg/10ml (1 in 1,000) solution for injection ampoules | 10 ampoule PoM £106.02
Adrenaline (base) for anaphylaxis 1mg/1ml (1 in 1,000) solution for injection pre-filled syringes | 1 pre-filled disposable injection PoM £11.88 DT = £11.88
Adrenaline (base) 1mg/1ml (1 in 1,000) solution for injection pre-filled syringes | 1 pre-filled disposable injection PoM £11.88 DT = £11.88

Adrenaline (as Adrenaline acid tartrate) 1 mg per 1 ml Adrenaline (base) 5mg/5ml (1 in 1,000) solution for injection ampoules | 10 ampoule PoM £108.09
Adrenaline (base) 500micrograms/0.5ml (1 in 1,000) solution for injection ampoules | 10 ampoule PoM £88.63 DT = £88.63
Adrenaline (base) 1mg/1ml (1 in 1,000) solution for injection ampoules | 10 ampoule PoM £6.00–£11.01 DT = £9.98

- Emerade (Bausch & Lomb UK Ltd)

Adrenaline 1 mg per 1 ml Emerade 300micrograms/0.3ml (1 in 1,000) solution for injection auto-injectors | 1 pre-filled disposable injection PoM £25.99 DT = £34.30

Adrenaline (as Adrenaline acid tartrate) 1 mg per 1 ml Emerade 150micrograms/0.15ml (1 in 1,000) solution for injection auto-injectors | 1 pre-filled disposable injection PoM £25.99 DT = £23.99
Emerade 500micrograms/0.5ml (1 in 1,000) solution for injection auto-injectors | 1 pre-filled disposable injection PoM £26.99 DT = £26.99

- EpiPen (Mylan)

Adrenaline 500 microgram per 1 ml EpiPen Jr. 150micrograms/0.3ml (1 in 2,000) solution for injection auto-injectors

2 Cardiovascular system

| 1 pre-filled disposable injection PoM £34.30 DT = £34.30 | 2 pre-filled disposable injection PoM £68.60 DT = £68.60

Adrenaline 1 mg per 1 ml EpiPen 300micrograms/0.3ml (1 in 1,000) solution for injection auto-injectors | 1 pre-filled disposable injection PoM £34.30 DT = £34.30 | 2 pre-filled disposable injection PoM £68.60

▸ Jext (ALK-Abello Ltd)

Adrenaline 1 mg per 1 ml Jext 300micrograms/0.3ml (1 in 1,000) solution for injection auto-injectors | 1 pre-filled disposable injection PoM £23.99 DT = £34.30

Adrenaline (as Adrenaline acid tartrate) 1 mg per 1 ml Jext 150micrograms/0.15ml (1 in 1,000) solution for injection auto-injectors | 1 pre-filled disposable injection PoM £23.99 DT = £23.99

8 Oedema

Diuretics

Overview

Diuretics are used for a variety of conditions in children including pulmonary oedema (caused by conditions such as respiratory distress syndrome and bronchopulmonary dysplasia), congestive heart failure, and hypertension. Hypertension in children is often resistant to therapy and may require the use of several drugs in combination. Maintenance of fluid and electrolyte balance can be difficult in children on diuretics, particularly neonates whose renal function may be immature.

Loop diuretics are used for pulmonary oedema, congestive heart failure, and in renal disease.

Thiazides are used less commonly than loop diuretics but are often used in combination with loop diuretics or spironolactone p. 133 in the management of pulmonary oedema and, in lower doses, for hypertension associated with cardiac disease.

Aminophylline **infusion** p. 176 has been used with intravenous furosemide p. 148 to relieve fluid overload in critically ill children.

Heart failure

Heart failure is less common in children than in adults; it can occur as a result of congenital heart disease (e.g. septal defects), dilated cardiomyopathy, myocarditis, or cardiac surgery. Drug treatment of heart failure due to left ventricular systolic dysfunction is covered below; optimal management of heart failure with preserved left ventricular function has not been established.

Acute heart failure can occur after cardiac surgery or as a complication in severe acute infections with or without myocarditis. Therapy consists of volume loading, vasodilator or inotropic drugs.

Chronic heart failure is initially treated with a **loop diuretic**, usually furosemide supplemented with spironolactone, amiloride hydrochloride p. 149, or potassium chloride p. 651.

If diuresis with furosemide is insufficient, the addition of metolazone p. 150 or a **thiazide diuretic** can be considered. With metolazone the resulting diuresis can be profound and care is needed to avoid potentially dangerous electrolyte disturbance.

If diuretics are insufficient an ACE inhibitor, titrated to the maximum tolerated dose, can be used. **ACE inhibitors** are used for the treatment of all grades of heart failure in adults and can also be useful for children with heart failure. Addition of digoxin p. 86 can be considered in children who remain symptomatic despite treatment with a diuretic and an ACE inhibitor.

Some beta-blockers improve outcome in adults with heart failure, but data on beta-blockers in children are limited. Carvedilol p. 132 has vasodilatory properties and therefore (like ACE inhibitors) also lowers afterload.

In children receiving specialist cardiology care, the phosphodiesterase type-3 inhibitor enoximone p. 134 is sometimes used by mouth for its inotropic and vasodilator effects. Spironolactone is usually used as a potassium-sparing drug with a loop diuretic; in adults low doses of spironolactone are effective in the treatment of heart failure. Careful monitoring of serum potassium is necessary if spironolactone is used in combination with an ACE inhibitor.

Thiazides and related diuretics

Thiazides and related compounds are moderately potent diuretics; they inhibit sodium reabsorption at the beginning of the distal convoluted tubule. They are usually administered early in the day so that the diuresis does not interfere with sleep.

In the management of *hypertension* a low dose of a thiazide produces a maximal or near-maximal blood pressure lowering effect, with very little biochemical disturbance. Higher doses cause more marked changes in plasma potassium, sodium, uric acid, glucose, and lipids, with little advantage in blood pressure control. Thiazides also have a role in chronic heart failure.

Bendroflumethiazide p. 117 is licensed for use in children; chlorothiazide p. 117 is also used.

Chlortalidone p. 150, a thiazide-related compound, has a longer duration of action than the thiazides and may be given on alternate days in younger children.

Metolazone is particularly effective when combined with a loop diuretic (even in renal failure) and is most effective when given 30–60 minutes before furosemide profound diuresis can occur and the child should therefore be monitored carefully.

Loop diuretics

Loop diuretics inhibit reabsorption of sodium, potassium, and chloride from the ascending limb of the loop of Henlé in the renal tubule and are powerful diuretics.

Furosemide and bumetanide p. 147 are similar in activity; they produce dose-related diuresis. Furosemide is used extensively in children. It can be used for pulmonary oedema (e.g. in respiratory distress syndrome and bronchopulmonary dysplasia), congestive heart failure, and in renal disease.

Potassium-sparing diuretics and aldosterone antagonists

Spironolactone is the most commonly used potassium sparing diuretic in children; it is an aldosterone antagonist and enhances potassium retention and sodium excretion in the distal tubule. Spironolactone is combined with other diuretics to reduce urinary potassium loss. It is also used in nephrotic syndrome, the long-term management of Bartter's syndrome, and high doses can help to control ascites in babies with chronic neonatal hepatitis. The clinical value of spironolactone in the management of pulmonary oedema in preterm neonates with chronic lung disease is uncertain.

Potassium canrenoate p. 133 given intravenously, is an alternative aldosterone antagonist that may be useful if a potassium-sparing diuretic is required and the child is unable to take oral medication. It is metabolised to canrenone, which is also a metabolite of spironolactone.

Amiloride hydrochloride on its own is a weak diuretic. It causes retention of potassium and is therefore given with thiazide or loop diuretics as an alternative to giving potassium supplements.

A potassium-sparing diuretic such as spironolactone or amiloride hydrochloride may also be used in the management of amphotericin-induced hypokalaemia.

Potassium supplements must **not** be given with potassium-sparing diuretics. Administration of a potassium-sparing diuretic to a child receiving an ACE inhibitor or an angiotensin-II receptor antagonist can also cause severe hyperkalaemia.

Potassium-sparing diuretics with other diuretics

Although it is preferable to prescribe diuretics separately in children, the use of fixed combinations may be justified in older children if compliance is a problem. (Some preparations may not be licensed for use in children—consult product literature).

Other diuretics

Mannitol p. 149 is used to treat cerebral oedema, raised intraocular pressure, peripheral oedema, and acites.

The carbonic anhydrase inhibitor acetazolamide p. 735 is a weak diuretic although it is little used for its diuretic effect. Eye drops of dorzolamide p. 737 and brinzolamide p. 736 inhibit the formation of aqueous humour and are used in glaucoma. Acetazolamide is used in the treatment of epilepsy, and raised intracranial pressure.

Diuretics with potassium

Diuretics and potassium supplements should be prescribed separately.

Advanced Pharmacy Services

Children taking diuretics may be eligible for the New Medicines Service / Medicines Use Review service provided by a community pharmacist. For further information, see *Advanced Pharmacy Services* in Medicines optimisation p. 25.

Other drugs used for Oedema Diamorphine hydrochloride, p. 294

DIURETICS > LOOP DIURETICS

Loop diuretics

- **DRUG ACTION** Loop diuretics inhibit reabsorption from the ascending limb of the loop of Henlé in the renal tubule and are powerful diuretics.
- **CONTRA-INDICATIONS** Anuria · renal failure due to nephrotoxic or hepatotoxic drugs · severe hypokalaemia · severe hyponatraemia
- **CAUTIONS** Can cause acute urinary retention in children with obstruction of urinary outflow · can exacerbate diabetes (but hyperglycaemia less likely than with thiazides) · can exacerbate gout · comatose and precomatose states associated with liver cirrhosis · hypotension should be corrected before initiation of treatment · hypovolaemia should be corrected before initiation of treatment

 CAUTIONS, FURTHER INFORMATION
 - Potassium loss Hypokalaemia can occur with both thiazide and loop diuretics. The risk of hypokalaemia depends on the duration of action as well as the potency and is thus greater with thiazides than with an equipotent dose of a loop diuretic.

 Hypokalaemia is particularly dangerous in children being treated with cardiac glycosides. In hepatic failure hypokalaemia caused by diuretics can precipitate encephalopathy.

 The use of potassium-sparing diuretics avoids the need to take potassium supplements.
 - Urinary retention Loop diuretics can cause acute urinary retention in children with obstruction of urinary outflow, therefore adequate urinary output should be established before initiating treatment.
- **SIDE-EFFECTS**
 - **Common or very common** Dizziness · electrolyte imbalance · fatigue · headache · metabolic alkalosis · muscle spasms · nausea
 - **Uncommon** Diarrhoea
 - **Rare or very rare** Bone marrow depression · photosensitivity reaction
 - **Frequency not known** Deafness (more common in renal impairment) · leucopenia · paraesthesia · rash · severe cutaneous adverse reactions (SCARs) · thrombocytopenia · tinnitus (more common with rapid intravenous administration, and in renal impairment) · vomiting
- **HEPATIC IMPAIRMENT** Hypokalaemia induced by loop diuretics may precipitate hepatic encephalopathy and coma—potassium-sparing diuretics can be used to prevent this.
- **RENAL IMPAIRMENT** High doses or rapid intravenous administration can cause tinnitus and deafness.
 Dose adjustments High doses of loop diuretics may occasionally be needed in renal impairment.
- **MONITORING REQUIREMENTS** Monitor electrolytes during treatment.

above

Bumetanide

- **INDICATIONS AND DOSE**

Oedema in heart failure, renal disease, and hepatic disease | Pulmonary oedema

- BY MOUTH
 - Child 1 month–11 years: 15–50 micrograms/kg 1–4 times a day (max. per dose 2 mg); maximum 5 mg per day
 - Child 12–17 years: Initially 1 mg, dose to be taken in the morning, then 1 mg after 6–8 hours if required

Oedema in heart failure, renal disease, and hepatic disease (severe cases) | Pulmonary oedema (severe cases)

- BY MOUTH
 - Child 12–17 years: Initially 5 mg daily, increased in steps of 5 mg every 12–24 hours, adjusted according to response

- **UNLICENSED USE** Not licensed for use in children under 12 years.
- **INTERACTIONS** → Appendix 1: loop diuretics
- **SIDE-EFFECTS**
 - **Common or very common** Dehydration · hypotension · skin reactions
 - **Uncommon** Breast pain · chest discomfort · ear pain · vertigo
 - **Rare or very rare** Hearing impairment
 - **Frequency not known** Arthralgia · encephalopathy · gastrointestinal discomfort · gynaecomastia · hyperglycaemia · hyperuricaemia · muscle cramps · musculoskeletal pain (with high doses in renal failure)
- **PREGNANCY** Bumetanide should not be used to treat gestational hypertension because of the maternal hypovolaemia associated with this condition.
- **BREAST FEEDING** No information available. May inhibit lactation.

- **MEDICINAL FORMS** There can be variation in the licensing of different medicines containing the same drug. Forms available from special-order manufacturers include: oral suspension

Oral solution

- Bumetanide (Non-proprietary)
 Bumetanide 200 microgram per 1 ml Bumetanide 1mg/5ml oral solution sugar-free | 150 ml PoM £198.00 DT = £198.00

Tablet

- Bumetanide (Non-proprietary)
 Bumetanide 1 mg Bumetanide 1mg tablets | 28 tablet PoM £7.35 DT = £2.45
 Bumetanide 5 mg Bumetanide 5mg tablets | 28 tablet PoM £9.81 DT = £9.76

F 147

Cardiovascular system 2

Furosemide
10-Mar-2020

(Frusemide)

● **INDICATIONS AND DOSE**

Oedema in heart failure, renal disease, and hepatic disease | Pulmonary oedema

▶ BY MOUTH

▶ Neonate: 0.5–2 mg/kg every 12–24 hours, alternatively 0.5–2 mg/kg every 24 hours, if corrected gestational age under 31 weeks.

▶ Child 1 month–11 years: 0.5–2 mg/kg 2–3 times a day, alternatively 0.5–2 mg/kg every 24 hours, if corrected gestational age of under 31 weeks, higher doses may be required in resistant oedema; maximum 80 mg per day; maximum 12 mg/kg per day

▶ Child 12–17 years: 20–40 mg daily; increased to 80–120 mg daily, in resistant oedema

▶ BY SLOW INTRAVENOUS INJECTION

▶ Neonate: 0.5–1 mg/kg every 12–24 hours, alternatively 0.5–1 mg/kg every 24 hours, if corrected gestational age under 31 weeks.

▶ Child 1 month–11 years: 0.5–1 mg/kg every 8 hours (max. per dose 40 mg every 8 hours) as required; maximum 6 mg/kg per day

▶ Child 12–17 years: 20–40 mg every 8 hours as required, higher doses may be required in resistant cases

▶ BY CONTINUOUS INTRAVENOUS INFUSION

▶ Child: 0.1–2 mg/kg/hour

Oedema in heart failure, renal disease, and hepatic disease following cardiac surgery | Pulmonary oedema following cardiac surgery

▶ BY CONTINUOUS INTRAVENOUS INFUSION

▶ Child: Initially 100 micrograms/kg/hour, dose to be doubled every 2 hours until urine output exceeds 1 mL/kg/hour

Oliguria due to acute or chronic renal insufficiency [GFR below 20 mL/minute]

▶ BY MOUTH

▶ Child 12–17 years: Initially 250 mg daily, then increased in steps of 250 mg every 4–6 hours (max. per dose 2 g) if required

▶ BY INTRAVENOUS INFUSION

▶ Child 1 month–11 years: 2–5 mg/kg up to 4 times a day; maximum 1 g per day

▶ Child 12–17 years: Initially 250 mg, dose to be administered over 1 hour, increased to 500 mg, increased dose is given if satisfactory urine output not obtained; dose administered over 2 hours, then increased to 1 g, increased dose given if satisfactory response not obtained within subsequent hour; dose to be administered over 4 hours. If no response obtained dialysis probably required;, effective dose of up to 1 g given at a maximum rate of 4 mg/minute can be repeated every 24 hours

● **CAUTIONS** Effect may be prolonged in neonates · hepatorenal syndrome · hypoproteinaemia may reduce diuretic effect and increase risk of side-effects

● **INTERACTIONS** → Appendix 1: loop diuretics

● **SIDE-EFFECTS**

GENERAL SIDE-EFFECTS Agranulocytosis · aplastic anaemia · auditory disorder (more common with rapid intravenous administration, and in renal impairment) · diabetes mellitus · eosinophilia · fever · gout · haemolytic anaemia · hepatic encephalopathy · malaise · mucosal reaction · nephritis tubulointerstitial · pancreatitis acute · shock · skin eruption · tetany · urolithiases · vasculitis

SPECIFIC SIDE-EFFECTS

▶ With oral use Acute kidney injury · hepatic disorders · metabolic acidosis · psychiatric disorder · urinary disorders

▶ With parenteral use Acute urinary retention · cholestasis

● **PREGNANCY** Furosemide should not be used to treat gestational hypertension because of the maternal hypovolaemia associated with this condition.

● **BREAST FEEDING** Amount too small to be harmful. May inhibit lactation.

● **DIRECTIONS FOR ADMINISTRATION**

▶ With intravenous use For *intravenous injection*, give over 5–10 minutes at a usual rate of 100 micrograms/kg/minute (not exceeding 500 micrograms/kg/minute), max. 4 mg/minute; lower rate of infusion may be necessary in renal impairment. For *intravenous infusion*, dilute with Sodium Chloride 0.9% to a concentration of 1–2 mg/mL. Glucose solutions unsuitable (infusion pH must be above 5.5).

▶ With oral use For administration by *mouth*, tablets can be crushed and mixed with water or injection solution diluted and given by mouth. Risk of ototoxicity may be reduced by giving high oral doses in 2 or more divided doses.

● **PRESCRIBING AND DISPENSING INFORMATION**

▶ With oral use Some liquid preparations contain alcohol, caution especially in neonates.

● **MEDICINAL FORMS** There can be variation in the licensing of different medicines containing the same drug. Forms available from special-order manufacturers include: oral suspension, oral solution

Tablet

▶ Furosemide (Non-proprietary)

Furosemide 20 mg Furosemide 20mg tablets | 28 tablet PoM £5.69 DT = £0.77 | 250 tablet PoM £5.08–£6.88

Furosemide 40 mg Furosemide 40mg tablets | 28 tablet PoM £7.55 DT = £0.80 | 250 tablet PoM £3.50–£7.14 | 1000 tablet PoM £28.21–£48.77

Furosemide 500 mg Furosemide 500mg tablets | 28 tablet PoM £39.02 DT = £39.02

▶ Diuresal (Ennogen Pharma Ltd)

Furosemide 500 mg Diuresal 500mg tablets | 28 tablet PoM £39.02 DT = £39.02

Solution for injection

▶ Furosemide (Non-proprietary)

Furosemide 10 mg per 1 ml Furosemide 250mg/25ml solution for injection ampoules | 10 ampoule PoM £30.00–£40.00

Furosemide 50mg/5ml solution for injection ampoules | 10 ampoule PoM £9.00–£50.00 | 10 ampoule PoM £2.38 (Hospital only)

Furosemide 20mg/2ml solution for injection ampoules | 10 ampoule PoM £4.58 DT = £21.19 (Hospital only) | 10 ampoule PoM £3.50–£40.00 DT = £21.19

Oral solution

EXCIPIENTS: May contain Alcohol

▶ Furosemide (Non-proprietary)

Furosemide 4 mg per 1 ml Furosemide 20mg/5ml oral solution sugar-free | 150 ml PoM £14.81 DT = £14.81

Furosemide 8 mg per 1 ml Furosemide 40mg/5ml oral solution sugar-free | 150 ml PoM £19.53 DT = £19.53

Furosemide 10 mg per 1 ml Furosemide 50mg/5ml oral solution sugar-free | 150 ml PoM £20.21 DT = £20.21

▶ Frusol (Rosemont Pharmaceuticals Ltd)

Furosemide 4 mg per 1 ml Frusol 20mg/5ml oral solution sugar-free | 150 ml PoM £12.07 DT = £14.81

Furosemide 8 mg per 1 ml Frusol 40mg/5ml oral solution sugar-free | 150 ml PoM £15.58 DT = £19.53

Furosemide 10 mg per 1 ml Frusol 50mg/5ml oral solution sugar-free | 150 ml PoM £16.84 DT = £20.21

DIURETICS > OSMOTIC DIURETICS

Mannitol

21-Feb-2019

- **INDICATIONS AND DOSE**

Cerebral oedema

▸ BY INTRAVENOUS INFUSION

▸ Child 1 month–11 years: 0.25–1.5 g/kg, repeated if necessary, to be administered over 30–60 minutes, dose may be repeated 1–2 times after 4–8 hours

▸ Child 12-17 years: 0.25–2 g/kg, repeated if necessary, to be administered over 30-60 minutes, dose may be repeated 1–2 times after 4–8 hours

Peripheral oedema and ascites

▸ BY INTRAVENOUS INFUSION

▸ Child: 1–2 g/kg, to be given over 2–6 hours

- **UNLICENSED USE** Not licensed for use in children under 12 years.
- **CONTRA-INDICATIONS** Anuria · intracranial bleeding (except during craniotomy) · severe cardiac failure · severe dehydration · severe pulmonary oedema
- **CAUTIONS** Extravasation causes inflammation and thrombophlebitis
- **SIDE-EFFECTS**

▸ **Common or very common** Cough · headache · vomiting

▸ **Uncommon** Dizziness · fever · malaise · nausea · pain · skin reactions

▸ **Frequency not known** Arrhythmia · asthenia · azotaemia · chest pain · chills · coma · compartment syndrome · confusion · congestive heart failure · dry mouth · electrolyte imbalance · fluid imbalance · hyperhidrosis · hypersensitivity · hypertension · lethargy · metabolic acidosis · muscle complaints · musculoskeletal stiffness · nephrotic syndrome · neurotoxicity · peripheral oedema · pulmonary oedema · rebound intracranial pressure increase · renal impairment · rhinitis · seizure · thirst · urinary disorders · vision blurred

- **PREGNANCY** Manufacturer advises avoid unless essential— no information available.
- **BREAST FEEDING** Manufacturer advises avoid unless essential—no information available.
- **RENAL IMPAIRMENT** Use with caution in severe impairment.
- **PRE-TREATMENT SCREENING** Assess cardiac function before treatment.
- **MONITORING REQUIREMENTS** Monitor fluid and electrolyte balance, serum osmolality, and cardiac, pulmonary and renal function.
- **DIRECTIONS FOR ADMINISTRATION** Examine infusion for crystals. If crystals present, dissolve by warming infusion fluid (allow to cool to body temperature before administration).

For mannitol 20%, an in-line filter is recommended (15-micron filters have been used).

- **MEDICINAL FORMS** There can be variation in the licensing of different medicines containing the same drug. Forms available from special-order manufacturers include: infusion, solution for infusion

Infusion

▸ **Mannitol (Non-proprietary)**

Mannitol 100 mg per 1 ml Mannitol 50g/500ml (10%) infusion Viaflo bags | 1 bag PoM

Polyfusor K mannitol 10% infusion 500ml bottles | 1 bottle PoM £5.43

Mannitol 150 mg per 1 ml Mannitol 75g/500ml (15%) infusion Viaflo bags | 20 bag PoM

Mannitol 200 mg per 1 ml Mannitol 50g/250ml (20%) infusion Viaflex bags | 1 bag PoM

Polyfusor M mannitol 20% infusion 500ml bottles | 1 bottle PoM £7.12

Mannitol 100g/500ml (20%) infusion Viaflex bags | 1 bag PoM

DIURETICS > POTASSIUM-SPARING DIURETICS

Amiloride hydrochloride

21-Jun-2019

- **INDICATIONS AND DOSE**

Adjunct to thiazide or loop diuretics for oedema in heart failure, and hepatic disease (where potassium conservation desirable)

▸ BY MOUTH

▸ Neonate: 100–200 micrograms/kg twice daily.

▸ Child 1 month–11 years: 100–200 micrograms/kg twice daily; maximum 20 mg per day

▸ Child 12-17 years: 5–10 mg twice daily

- **UNLICENSED USE** Not licensed for use in children.
- **CONTRA-INDICATIONS** Addison's disease · anuria · hyperkalaemia
- **CAUTIONS** Diabetes mellitus
- **INTERACTIONS** → Appendix 1: potassium-sparing diuretics
- **SIDE-EFFECTS** Alopecia · angina pectoris · aplastic anaemia · appetite decreased · arrhythmia · arthralgia · asthenia · atrioventricular block exacerbated · bladder spasm · chest pain · confusion · constipation · cough · depression · diarrhoea · dizziness · drowsiness · dry mouth · dyspnoea · dysuria · electrolyte imbalance · encephalopathy · gastrointestinal discomfort · gastrointestinal disorders · gastrointestinal haemorrhage · gout · headache · insomnia · jaundice · muscle cramps · nasal congestion · nausea · nervousness · neutropenia · pain · palpitations · paraesthesia · postural hypotension · sexual dysfunction · skin reactions · tinnitus · tremor · vertigo · visual impairment · vomiting
- **PREGNANCY** Not to be used to treat gestational hypertension.
- **BREAST FEEDING** Manufacturer advises avoid—no information available.
- **RENAL IMPAIRMENT** Manufacturers advise avoid in severe impairment.

Monitoring Monitor plasma-potassium concentration (high risk of hyperkalaemia in renal impairment).

- **MONITORING REQUIREMENTS** Monitor electrolytes.
- **MEDICINAL FORMS** There can be variation in the licensing of different medicines containing the same drug. Forms available from special-order manufacturers include: oral suspension, oral solution

Oral solution

EXCIPIENTS: May contain Propylene glycol

▸ **Amiloride hydrochloride (Non-proprietary)**

Amiloride hydrochloride 1 mg per 1 ml Amiloride 5mg/5ml oral solution sugar-free | 150 ml PoM £46.45 DT = £42.35

Tablet

▸ **Amiloride hydrochloride (Non-proprietary)**

Amiloride hydrochloride 5 mg Amiloride 5mg tablets | 28 tablet PoM £34.50 DT = £16.69

DIURETICS › THIAZIDES AND RELATED DIURETICS

2 Cardiovascular system

F 117

Chlortalidone

(Chlorthalidone)

● **INDICATIONS AND DOSE**

Ascites | Oedema in nephrotic syndrome

▶ BY MOUTH

▸ Child 5–11 years: 0.5–1 mg/kg every 48 hours (max. per dose 1.7 mg/kg every 48 hours), dose to be taken in the morning

▸ Child 12–17 years: Up to 50 mg daily

Hypertension

▶ BY MOUTH

▸ Child 5–11 years: 0.5–1 mg/kg every 48 hours (max. per dose 1.7 mg/kg every 48 hours), dose to be taken in the morning

▸ Child 12–17 years: 25 mg daily, dose to be taken in the morning, then increased if necessary to 50 mg daily

Stable heart failure

▶ BY MOUTH

▸ Child 5–11 years: 0.5–1 mg/kg every 48 hours (max. per dose 1.7 mg/kg every 48 hours), dose to be taken in the morning

▸ Child 12–17 years: 25–50 mg daily, dose to be taken in the morning, then increased if necessary to 100–200 mg daily, reduce to lowest effective dose for maintenance

● **INTERACTIONS** → Appendix 1: thiazide diuretics

● **SIDE-EFFECTS**

▶ **Common or very common** Appetite decreased · gastrointestinal discomfort

▶ **Uncommon** Gout

▶ **Rare or very rare** Arrhythmia · diabetes mellitus exacerbated · eosinophilia · glycosuria · hepatic disorders · nephritis tubulointerstitial · pulmonary oedema · respiratory disorder

● **BREAST FEEDING** The amount present in milk is too small to be harmful. Large doses may suppress lactation.

● **MEDICINAL FORMS** There can be variation in the licensing of different medicines containing the same drug. Forms available from special-order manufacturers include: oral suspension

Tablet

▸ Chlortalidone (Non-proprietary)

Chlortalidone 25 mg Chlortalidone 25mg tablets | 100 tablet PoM

Chlortalidone 50 mg Chlortalidone 50mg tablets | 30 tablet PoM £90.55 DT = £88.04

F 117

Metolazone

● **INDICATIONS AND DOSE**

Oedema resistant to loop diuretics in heart failure, renal disease and hepatic disease | Pulmonary oedema | Adjunct to loop diuretics to induce diuresis

▶ BY MOUTH

▸ Child 1 month–11 years: 100–200 micrograms/kg 1–2 times a day

▸ Child 12–17 years: 5–10 mg once daily, dose to be taken in the morning; increased if necessary to 5–10 mg twice daily, dose increased in resistant oedema

● **UNLICENSED USE** Not licensed for use in children.

● **CAUTIONS** Acute porphyrias p. 652

● **INTERACTIONS** → Appendix 1: thiazide diuretics

● **SIDE-EFFECTS** Appetite decreased · arthralgia · asthenia · chest discomfort · chills · drowsiness · gastrointestinal discomfort · glycosuria · gout aggravated · haemoconcentration · hepatic disorders · hypoplastic anaemia · hypovolaemia · muscle complaints · palpitations · peripheral neuropathy · psychotic depression · severe cutaneous adverse reactions (SCARs) · syncope · vasculitis · venous thrombosis · vertigo · vision blurred

● **BREAST FEEDING** The amount present in milk is too small to be harmful. Large doses may suppress lactation.

● **DIRECTIONS FOR ADMINISTRATION** Tablets may be crushed and mixed with water immediately before use.

● **MEDICINAL FORMS** There can be variation in the licensing of different medicines containing the same drug. Forms available from special-order manufacturers include: tablet, oral suspension, oral solution

Tablet

▸ Zaroxolyn (Imported (Canada))

Metolazone 2.5 mg Zaroxolyn 2.5mg tablets | 100 tablet PoM

Metolazone 5 mg Zaroxolyn 5mg tablets | 50 tablet PoM

9 Patent ductus arteriosus

Drugs affecting the ductus arteriosus

Closure of the ductus arteriosus

Patent ductus arteriosus is a frequent problem in premature neonates with respiratory distress syndrome. Substantial left-to-right shunting through the ductus arteriosus may increase the risk of intraventricular haemorrhage, necrotising enterocolitis, bronchopulmonary dysplasia, and possibly death.

Indometacin p. 710 or ibuprofen p. 707 can be used to close the ductus arteriosus. Indometacin has been used for many years and is effective but it reduces cerebral blood flow, and causes a transient fall in renal and gastro-intestinal blood flow. Ibuprofen may also be used; it has little effect on renal function (there may be a small reduction in sodium excretion) when used in doses for closure of the ductus arteriosus; gastro-intestinal problems are uncommon.

If drug treatment fails to close the ductus arteriosus, surgery may be indicated.

Maintenance of patency

In the newborn with duct-dependent congenital heart disease it is often necessary to maintain the patency of the ductus arteriosus whilst awaiting surgery. Alprostadil (prostaglandin E1) p. 151 and dinoprostone (prostaglandin E2) p. 151 are potent vasodilators that are effective for maintaining the patency of the ductus arteriosus. They are usually given by continuous intravenous infusion, but oral dosing of dinoprostone is still used in some centres. During the infusion of a prostaglandin, the newborn requires careful monitoring of heart rate, blood pressure, respiratory rate, and core body temperature. In the event of complications such as apnoea, profound bradycardia, or severe hypotension, the infusion should be temporarily stopped and the complication dealt with; the infusion should be restarted at a lower dose. Recurrent or prolonged apnoea may require ventilatory support in order for the prostaglandin infusion to continue.

PROSTAGLANDINS AND ANALOGUES

Alprostadil

20-Apr-2020

- **INDICATIONS AND DOSE**

Maintaining patency of the ductus arteriosus

▸ BY CONTINUOUS INTRAVENOUS INFUSION

▸ **Neonate:** Initially 5 nanograms/kg/minute, adjusted according to response, adjusted in steps of 5 nanograms/kg/minute (max. per dose 100 nanograms/kg/minute), maximum dose associated with increased side-effects.

- **UNLICENSED USE** Alprostadil doses in BNFC may differ from those in product literature.
- **CONTRA-INDICATIONS** Avoid in hyaline membrane disease
- **CAUTIONS** History of haemorrhage
- **INTERACTIONS** → Appendix 1: alprostadil
- **SIDE-EFFECTS**

▸ **Common or very common** Apnoea (more common in neonates under 2 kg) · arrhythmias · diarrhoea · fever · hypotension · seizure · vasodilation

▸ **Uncommon** Exostosis · gastrointestinal disorders · vascular fragility

▸ **Frequency not known** Cardiac arrest · disseminated intravascular coagulation · hypokalaemia · oedema · sepsis

- **MONITORING REQUIREMENTS** During the infusion of a prostaglandin, the newborn requires careful monitoring of heart rate, blood pressure, respiratory rate, and core body temperature.

▸ Monitor arterial pressure, respiratory rate, heart rate, temperature, and venous blood pressure in arm and leg; facilities for intubation and ventilation must be immediately available

- **DIRECTIONS FOR ADMINISTRATION** Dilute 150 micrograms/kg body-weight to a final volume of 50 mL with Glucose 5% or Sodium Chloride 0.9%; an intravenous infusion rate of 0.1 mL/hour provides a dose of 5 nanograms/kg/minute. Undiluted solution must not come into contact with the barrel of the plastic syringe; add the required volume of alprostadil to a volume of infusion fluid in the syringe and then make up to final volume.

- **MEDICINAL FORMS** There can be variation in the licensing of different medicines containing the same drug.

Solution for infusion

▸ Prostin VR (Pfizer Ltd)

Alprostadil 500 microgram per 1 ml Prostin VR 500micrograms/1ml concentrate for solution for infusion ampoules | 5 ampoule [PoM] £375.96 (Hospital only)

Dinoprostone

20-Apr-2020

- **INDICATIONS AND DOSE**

Maintaining patency of the ductus arteriosus

▸ BY CONTINUOUS INTRAVENOUS INFUSION

▸ **Neonate:** Initially 5 nanograms/kg/minute, then increased in steps of 5 nanograms/kg/minute as required; increased to 20 nanograms/kg/minute, doses up to 100 nanogram/kg/minute have been used but are associated with increased side-effects.

▸ BY MOUTH

▸ **Neonate:** 20–25 micrograms/kg every 1–2 hours, then increased if necessary to 40–50 micrograms/kg every 1–2 hours, if treatment continues for more than 1 week gradually reduce the dose.

- **UNLICENSED USE** Not licensed for use in children.
- **CONTRA-INDICATIONS** Avoid in hyaline membrane disease
- **CAUTIONS** History of haemorrhage
- **SIDE-EFFECTS**

▸ **Rare or very rare** Disseminated intravascular coagulation

▸ **Frequency not known** Asthma · back pain · bronchospasm · cardiac arrest · chills · diarrhoea · dizziness · fever · flushing · headache · hypertension · infection · nausea · uterine rupture · vomiting

- **HEPATIC IMPAIRMENT** Manufacturer advises avoid.
- **RENAL IMPAIRMENT** Manufacturers advise avoid.
- **MONITORING REQUIREMENTS** Monitor arterial oxygenation, heart rate, temperature, and blood pressure in arm and leg; facilities for intubation and ventilation must be immediately available. During infusion of dinoprostone, the newborn requires careful monitoring of heart rate, blood pressure, respiratory rate and core body temperature.
- **DIRECTIONS FOR ADMINISTRATION**

▸ **With intravenous use** For *continuous intravenous infusion*, dilute to a concentration of 1 microgram/mL with Glucose 5% or Sodium Chloride 0.9%.

▸ **With oral use** For administration by *mouth*, injection solution can be given orally; dilute with water.

- **MEDICINAL FORMS** There can be variation in the licensing of different medicines containing the same drug.

Solution for infusion

▸ Prostin E2 (Pfizer Ltd)

Dinoprostone 1 mg per 1 ml Prostin E2 750micrograms/0.75ml solution for infusion ampoules | 1 ampoule [PoM] £8.52 (Hospital only)

Dinoprostone 10 mg per 1 ml Prostin E2 5mg/0.5ml solution for infusion ampoules | 1 ampoule [PoM] £18.40 (Hospital only)

10 Vascular disease

Peripheral vascular disease

Classification and management

Raynaud's syndrome, a vasospastic peripheral vascular disease, consists of recurrent, long-lasting, and episodic vasospasm of the fingers and toes often associated with exposure to cold. Management includes avoidance of exposure to cold and Smoking cessation p. 313 (if appropriate). More severe symptoms may require vasodilator treatment, which is most often successful in primary Raynaud's syndrome. Nifedipine p. 115 and diltiazem hydrochloride p. 152 are useful for reducing the frequency and severity of vasospastic attacks. In very severe cases, where digital infarction is likely, intravenous infusion of the prostacyclin analogue iloprost p. 127 may be helpful.

Vasodilator therapy is not established as being effective for *chilblains*.

Advanced Pharmacy Services

Children with peripheral vascular disease may be eligible for the Medicines Use Review service provided by a community pharmacist. For further information, see *Advanced Pharmacy Services* in Medicines optimisation p. 25.

CALCIUM-CHANNEL BLOCKERS

114

Diltiazem hydrochloride

14-Feb-2020

- **INDICATIONS AND DOSE**

Raynaud's syndrome

- BY MOUTH
- Child 12–17 years: 30–60 mg 2–3 times a day

- **UNLICENSED USE** Not licensed for use in Raynaud's syndrome.
- **CONTRA-INDICATIONS** Acute porphyrias p. 652 · cardiogenic shock · heart failure (with reduced ejection fraction) · left ventricular failure with pulmonary congestion · second- or third-degree AV block (unless pacemaker fitted) · severe bradycardia · sick sinus syndrome · significant aortic stenosis
- **CAUTIONS** Bradycardia (avoid if severe) · first degree AV block · prolonged PR interval · significantly impaired left ventricular function
- **INTERACTIONS** → Appendix 1: calcium channel blockers
- **SIDE-EFFECTS**
  - **Common or very common** Cardiac conduction disorders · constipation · gastrointestinal discomfort · malaise
  - **Uncommon** Arrhythmias · diarrhoea · insomnia · nervousness · postural hypotension
  - **Rare or very rare** Dry mouth
  - **Frequency not known** Cardiac arrest · congestive heart failure · extrapyramidal symptoms · fever · gynaecomastia · hepatitis · hyperglycaemia · hyperhidrosis · mood altered · photosensitivity reaction · severe cutaneous adverse reactions (SCARs) · thrombocytopenia · vasculitis

  Overdose In overdose, diltiazem has a profound cardiac depressant effect causing hypotension and arrhythmias, including complete heart block and asystole.
- **PREGNANCY** Avoid.
- **BREAST FEEDING** Significant amount present in milk—no evidence of harm but avoid unless no safer alternative.
- **HEPATIC IMPAIRMENT**

  Dose adjustments In adults, manufacturers advise dose reduction—consult product literature.
- **RENAL IMPAIRMENT**

  Dose adjustments Start with smaller dose.

- **MEDICINAL FORMS** There can be variation in the licensing of different medicines containing the same drug. Forms available from special-order manufacturers include: oral suspension, oral solution

Modified-release tablet

CAUTIONARY AND ADVISORY LABELS 25

- Diltiazem hydrochloride (Non-proprietary)
  Diltiazem hydrochloride 60 mg Diltiazem 60mg modified-release tablets | 84 tablet PoM £42.93 DT = £42.93 | 100 tablet PoM £51.10–£51.11
- Retalzem (Kent Pharmaceuticals Ltd)
  Diltiazem hydrochloride 60 mg Retalzem 60 modified-release tablets | 84 tablet PoM £7.43 DT = £42.93
- Tildiem (Sanofi)
  Diltiazem hydrochloride 60 mg Tildiem 60mg modified-release tablets | 90 tablet PoM £7.96

Chapter 3
Respiratory system

CONTENTS

Respiratory system, drug delivery

13-Nov-2019

Inhalation

This route delivers the drug directly to the airways; the dose required is smaller than when given by mouth and side-effects are reduced.

Children and their carers should be advised to follow manufacturers' instructions on the care and cleansing of inhaler devices.

Inhaler devices

EvGr In young children, a pressurised metered-dose inhaler should be used with a spacer; use of a facemask is required until the child can breathe reproducibly without it. A nebuliser may be required when these methods are ineffective.

In children over the age of 5 years with chronic asthma, a *pressurised metered-dose inhaler* used with a spacer (with or without a spacer for children over 12 years) is as effective as any other hand-held inhaler. A spacer should always be used if the patient is on a high dose of inhaled corticosteroid.

In children over the age of 5 years with mild and moderate acute asthma attacks, a pressurised metered-dose inhaler with a spacer is at least as effective as nebulisation. ⟨A⟩

By the age of 3 years, a child can usually be taught to use a spacer device without a mask. As soon as a child is able to use the mouthpiece, then this is the preferred delivery system. When a pressurised metered-does inhaler with a spacer is unsuitable or inconvenient, a *dry-powder inhaler* or *breath-actuated inhaler* may be used instead if the child is able to use the device effectively.

Dry powder inhalers may be useful in children over 5 years, who are unwilling or unable to use a pressurised metered-dose inhaler with a spacer device; *breath-actuated inhalers* may be useful in older children if they are able to use the device effectively. The child or child's carer should be instructed carefully on the use of the inhaler. It is important to check that the inhaler is being used correctly; poor inhalation technique may be mistaken for a lack of response to the drug.

On changing from a pressurised metered-dose inhaler to a dry powder inhaler, the child may notice a lack of sensation in the mouth and throat previously associated with each actuation; coughing may occur more frequently following use of a dry-powder inhaler.

CFC-free metered-dose inhalers should be cleaned **weekly** according to the manufacturer's instructions.

EvGr Children, and their parents or carers should be instructed carefully on the use of the inhaler. It is important to check that the inhaler continues to be used correctly because inadequate inhalation technique may be mistaken for a lack of response to the drug. The number and different types of inhalers given to a child should be minimised. To help reduce confusion and ensure children receive inhalers they have been given training for, specify brand and inhaler when prescribing. ⟨A⟩

MHRA/CHM advice: Pressurised metered dose inhalers (pMDI): risk of airway obstruction from aspiration of loose objects (July 2018)

The MHRA have received reports of patients who have inhaled objects into the back of the throat—in some cases objects were aspirated, causing airway obstruction. Patients should be reminded to remove the mouthpiece cover fully, shake the device and check that both the outside and inside of the mouthpiece are clear and undamaged before inhaling a dose, and to store the inhaler with the mouthpiece cover on.

Spacer devices

Spacer devices are particularly useful for infants, for children with poor inhalation technique, or for nocturnal asthma, because the device reduces the need for coordination between actuation of a pressurised metered-dose inhaler and inhalation. The spacer device reduces the velocity of the aerosol and subsequent impaction on the oropharynx and allows more time for evaporation of the propellant so that a larger proportion of the particles can be inhaled and deposited in the lungs. Smaller-volume spacers may be more manageable for pre-school children and infants. The spacer device used must be compatible with the prescribed metered-dose inhaler.

Use and care of spacer devices

The suitability of the spacer device should be carefully assessed; opening the one-way valve is dependent on the child's inspiratory flow. Some devices can be tipped to 45° to open the valve during inhaler actuation and inspiration to assist the child.

Inhalation from the spacer device should follow the actuation as soon as possible because the drug aerosol is very short-lived. The total dose (which may be more than a single puff) should be administered as single actuations (with tidal breathing for 10–20 seconds or 5 breaths for each actuation) for children with good inspiratory flow. Larger doses may be necessary for a child with acute bronchospasm.

The device should be cleansed once a month by washing in mild detergent and then allowed to dry in air without rinsing; the mouthpiece should be wiped clean of detergent before use. Some manufacturers recommend more frequent cleaning, but this should be avoided since any electrostatic charge may affect drug delivery. Spacer devices should be replaced every 6–12 months.

Nebulisers

Solutions for nebulisation used in severe and life-threatening asthma attacks are administered over 5–10 minutes from a nebuliser, usually driven by oxygen.

EvGr Children with a severe acute or life-threatening attack of asthma should preferably have oxygen during nebulisation since beta$_2$ agonists can increase arterial hypoxaemia. ⟨A⟩

A nebuliser converts a solution of a drug into an aerosol for inhalation. It is used to deliver higher doses of drug to the airways than is usual with standard inhalers. The main indications for use of a nebuliser are:

- to deliver a beta$_2$ agonist or ipratropium bromide p. 161 to a child with an *acute exacerbation* of asthma or of airways obstruction;
- to deliver *prophylactic medication* to a child unable to use other conventional devices;
- to deliver an antibacterial (such as colistimethate sodium p. 375 or tobramycin p. 334) to a child with chronic purulent infection (as in cystic fibrosis or bronchiectasis);
- to deliver budesonide p. 168 to a child with severe croup.

The proportion of a nebuliser solution that reaches the lungs depends on the type of nebuliser and although it can be as high as 30% it is more frequently close to 10% and sometimes below 10%. The remaining solution is left in the nebuliser as residual volume or it is deposited in the mouthpiece and tubing. The extent to which the nebulised solution is deposited in the airways or alveoli depends on particle size. Particles with a median diameter of 1–5 microns are deposited in the airways and are therefore appropriate for asthma whereas a particle size of 1–2 microns is needed for alveolar deposition. The type of nebuliser is therefore chosen according to the deposition required and according to the viscosity of the solution.

When a nebuliser is prescribed, the child or child's carer must:

- have clear instructions from a doctor, specialist nurse, physiotherapist, or pharmacist on the use of the nebuliser (and on peak-flow monitoring);
- be instructed not to treat acute attacks without also seeking medical help;
- have regular follow up with doctor or specialist nurse.

Jet nebulisers

Jet nebulisers are more widely used than ultrasonic nebulisers. Most jet nebulisers require an optimum flow rate of 6–8 litres/minute and in hospital can be driven by piped air or oxygen; in acute asthma the nebuliser should always be driven by oxygen. Domiciliary oxygen cylinders do not provide an adequate flow rate therefore an electrical compressor is required for domiciliary use.

Some jet nebulisers are able to increase drug output during inspiration and hence increase efficiency.

Safe practice

The Department of Health has reminded users of the need to use the correct grade of tubing when connecting a nebuliser to a medical gas supply or compressor.

Nebuliser diluent

Nebulisation may be carried out using an undiluted nebuliser solution or it may require dilution beforehand. The usual diluent is sterile sodium chloride 0.9% (physiological saline).

In England and Wales nebulisers and compressors are not available on the NHS (but they are free of VAT); some nebulisers (but not compressors) are available on form GP10A in Scotland (for details consult Scottish Drug Tariff).

Oral

Systemic side-effects occur more frequently when a drug is given orally rather than by inhalation. Oral corticosteroids, theophylline p. 178, and leukotriene receptor antagonists are sometimes required for the management of asthma.

Parenteral

Drugs such as beta$_2$ agonists, corticosteroids, and aminophylline p. 176 can be given by injection in acute severe asthma when drug administration by nebulisation is inadequate or inappropriate; in these circumstances the child should generally be treated in a high dependency or intensive care unit.

Peak flow meters

Peak flow meters may be used to assess lung function in children over 5 years with asthma, but symptom monitoring is the most reliable assessment of asthma control. They are best used for short periods to assess the severity of asthma and to monitor response to treatment; continuous use of peak flow meters may detract from compliance with inhalers.

Peak flow charts should be issued to patients where appropriate, and are available to purchase from:

3M Security Print and Systems Limited. Gorse Street, Chadderton, Oldham, OL9 9QH. Tel: 0845 610 1112

GP practices can obtain supplies through their Area Team stores.

NHS Hospitals can order supplies from www.nhsforms.co.uk/ or by emailing nhsforms@mmm.com.

In Scotland, peak flow charts can be obtained by emailing stockorders.dppas@apsgroup.co.uk.

NICE decisions

Inhaler devices for children under 5 years with chronic asthma (August 2000) NICE TA10

When selecting inhaler devices for children under 5 years with chronic asthma, a child's needs and likelihood of good compliance should govern the choice of inhaler and spacer device; only then should cost be considered.

- corticosteroid and bronchodilator therapy should be delivered by pressurised metered-dose inhaler and spacer device, with a facemask if necessary;
- if this is not effective, and depending on the child's condition, nebulised therapy may be considered and, in children over 3 years, a dry powder inhaler may also be considered.

www.nice.org.uk/TA10

Inhaler devices for children 5–15 years with chronic asthma (March 2002) NICE TA38

When selecting inhaler devices for children between 5–15 years with chronic asthma, a child's needs, ability to develop and maintain effective technique, and likelihood of good compliance should govern the choice of inhaler and spacer device; only then should cost be considered.

- corticosteroid therapy should be routinely delivered by a pressurised metered-dose inhaler and spacer device;
- for other inhaled drugs, particularly bronchodilators, choice should be made from a wider range of devices after careful consideration;
- children and their carers should be trained in the use of the chosen device; suitability of the device should be reviewed at least annually. Inhaler technique and compliance should be monitored.

www.nice.org.uk/TA38

1 Airways disease, obstructive

Asthma, chronic

06-May-2020

Description of condition

Asthma is a common chronic inflammatory condition of the airways, associated with airway hyperresponsiveness and variable airflow obstruction. The most frequent symptoms of asthma are cough, wheeze, chest tightness, and breathlessness. Asthma symptoms vary over time and in intensity and can gradually or suddenly worsen, provoking an acute asthma attack that, if severe, may require hospitalisation.

Aims of treatment

The aim of treatment is to achieve control of asthma. Complete control of asthma is defined as no daytime symptoms, no night-time awakening due to asthma, no asthma attacks, no need for rescue medication, no limitations on activity including exercise, normal lung function (in practical terms forced expiratory volume in 1 second (FEV_1) and/or peak expiratory flow (PEF) > 80% predicted or best), and minimal side-effects from treatment. In clinical practice, patients may choose to balance the aims of asthma management against the potential side-effects or inconvenience of taking medication necessary to achieve perfect control.

Lifestyle changes

EvGr Weight loss in overweight patients may lead to an improvement in asthma symptoms. Patients with asthma and parents of children with asthma should be advised about the dangers of smoking, to themselves and to their children, and be offered appropriate support to stop smoking. Ⓐ For further information, see Smoking cessation p. 313.

Management

EvGr A stepwise approach aims to stop symptoms quickly and to improve peak flow. Treatment should be started at the level most appropriate to initial severity of asthma. The aim is to achieve early control and to maintain it by stepping up treatment as necessary and decreasing treatment when control is good. Before initiating a new drug or adjusting treatment, consider whether the diagnosis is correct, check adherence and inhaler technique, and eliminate trigger factors for acute attacks.

A self-management programme comprising of a written personalised action plan and education should be offered to all patients with asthma (and/or their family or carers), and should be supported with regular review from a healthcare professional. Ⓐ

For information on devices used in the management of asthma, see Respiratory system, drug delivery p. 153.

Recommendations on the management of chronic asthma from the *National Institute for Health and Care Excellence (NICE)—Asthma: diagnosis, monitoring and chronic asthma management guidelines (NG80, November 2017), and British Thoracic Society (BTS) and Scottish Intercollegiate Guidelines Network (SIGN)—British guideline on the management of asthma (SIGN 158, July 2019)* differ significantly. Recommendations in BNF publications are based on NICE guidelines, and differences with BTS/SIGN (2019) have been highlighted.

For information on the management of patients during the COVID-19 pandemic, see COVID-19 p. 433.

Child aged over 16 years

NICE (2017) treatment recommendations for child aged over 16 years apply to patients aged 17 years and over. BTS/SIGN (2019) treatment recommendations for child aged over 16 years are the same as those for patients aged over 12 years (see child aged over 5 years section).

Intermittent reliever therapy

EvGr Start an inhaled short-acting $beta_2$ agonist (such as salbutamol p. 164 or terbutaline sulfate p. 166), to be used as required in all patients with asthma. For those with infrequent short-lived wheeze, occasional use of reliever therapy may be the only treatment required. Patients using more than one short-acting $beta_2$ agonist inhaler device a month should have their asthma urgently assessed and action taken to improve poorly controlled asthma. Ⓐ

Regular preventer (maintenance) therapy

NICE (2017) define inhaled corticosteroid (ICS) doses for children aged over 16 years as low, moderate, or high. BTS/SIGN (2019) instead define ICS doses for children aged over 16 years as low, medium or high (refer to individual guidelines for ICS dosing information).

EvGr A low-dose of ICS should be started as maintenance therapy in patients who present with any one of the following features: using an inhaled short-acting $beta_2$ agonist three times a week or more, symptomatic three times a week or more, or waking at night due to asthma symptoms at least once a week. BTS/SIGN (2019) also recommend initiation in patients who have had an asthma attack in the last 2 years, and starting an ICS at a dose appropriate to the severity of asthma.

BTS/SIGN (2019) recommend that inhaled corticosteroids (except ciclesonide p. 170) should initially be taken twice daily, however the same total daily dose taken once a day, can be considered in patients with milder disease if good or complete control of asthma is established. The dose of ICS should be adjusted over time to the lowest effective dose at which control of asthma is maintained.

BTS/SIGN (2019) recommend the prescribing of inhalers by brand. Ⓐ

Initial add-on therapy

EvGr If asthma is uncontrolled on a low-dose of ICS as maintenance therapy, a leukotriene receptor antagonist (LTRA— such as montelukast p. 174) should be offered in addition to the ICS, and the response to treatment reviewed in 4 to 8 weeks.

BTS/SIGN (2019) instead recommend a long-acting $beta_2$ agonist (LABA—such as salmeterol p. 163 or formoterol fumarate p. 162) as initial add-on therapy to low-dose ICS if asthma is uncontrolled. This can be given as either a fixed-dose ICS and LABA regimen, or a MART regimen (Maintenance And Reliever Therapy—a combination of an ICS and a fast-acting LABA such as formoterol in a single inhaler, see budesonide with formoterol p. 169). Combination inhalers containing both a LABA and an ICS are recommended to improve adherence, and ensure that the LABA is not taken alone without the ICS.

BTS/SIGN (2019) also recommend that a MART regimen should be considered in children with a history of asthma attacks on a medium-dose ICS alone, or on a fixed-dose ICS and LABA regimen. Ⓐ

Additional controller therapies

EvGr If asthma is uncontrolled on a low-dose of ICS and a LTRA as maintenance therapy, a LABA in combination with the ICS should be offered with or without continued LTRA treatment, depending on the response achieved from the LTRA.

If asthma remains uncontrolled, offer to change the ICS and LABA maintenance therapy to a MART regimen with a low-dose of ICS as maintenance. See budesonide with formoterol p. 169.

If asthma remains uncontrolled on a MART regimen with a low-dose of ICS as maintenance with or without a LTRA, consider increasing to a moderate-dose of ICS (either continuing a MART regimen, or changing to a fixed-dose regimen of an ICS and a LABA with a short-acting $beta_2$ agonist as reliever therapy).

If asthma is still uncontrolled in patients on a moderate-dose of ICS as maintenance with a LABA (either as a MART or a fixed-dose regimen), with or without a LTRA, consider the following options:

- Increasing the ICS dose to a high-dose as maintenance (this should only be offered as part of a fixed-dose regimen with a short-acting $beta_2$ agonist used as reliever therapy), or
- A trial of an additional drug, for example, a long-acting muscarinic receptor antagonist (such as tiotropium) or modified-release theophylline p. 178, or
- Seeking advice from an asthma specialist.

BTS/SIGN (2019) instead recommend that if the patient is gaining some benefit from addition of a LABA but control remains inadequate, the LABA should be continued and *either* the dose of ICS be increased to a medium-dose (if not already on this dose), or a LTRA be added.

If there is no response to the LABA, consider discontinuing it and either increasing the dose of the ICS to a medium-dose (if not already on this dose), or adding a LTRA.

BTS/SIGN (2019) recommend that all patients whose asthma is not adequately controlled on recommended initial add-on therapy or additional controller therapies, should be referred for specialist asthma care. Ⓐ

High-dose ICS and further add-on treatment (specialist therapies)

EvGr Under specialist care, BTS/SIGN (2019) recommend that if asthma control remains inadequate on a medium-dose of ICS, plus a LABA or LTRA, the following interventions can be considered:

- Increasing the ICS to a high-dose—with high doses of ICS via a pressurised metered dose inhaler (pMDI) a spacer should be used, or
- Adding a LTRA (if not already tried), or modified-release theophylline p. 178, or tiotropium p. 161.

If a trial of a further add-on treatment is ineffective, stop the drug (or in the case of increased dose of ICS, reduce to the original dose). Ⓐ

Continuous or frequent use of oral corticosteroids (specialist therapies)

EvGr Under specialist care, BTS/SIGN (2019) recommend adding a regular oral corticosteroid (prednisolone p. 478) at the lowest dose to provide adequate control in patients with very severe asthma uncontrolled on a high-dose ICS, and who have also tried (or are still receiving) a LABA, LTRA, tiotropium p. 161, or modified-release theophylline p. 178. Ⓐ

For information on the general use and side effects of corticosteroids, see Corticosteroids, general use p. 470. For information on the cessation of oral corticosteroid treatment, see *Treatment cessation* for systemic corticosteroids (such as prednisolone).

Monoclonal antibodies and immunosuppressants (specialist therapies)

EvGr Under specialist initiation, BTS/SIGN (2019) recommend that monoclonal antibodies such as omalizumab p. 174 (for severe persistent allergic asthma), and immunosuppressants such as methotrexate p. 588 [unlicensed] may be considered in children with severe asthma to achieve control and reduce the use of oral corticosteroids. Ⓐ See *National funding/access decisions* for omalizumab p. 174.

Child aged over 5 years

For children aged over 5 years, NICE (2017) treatment recommendations for children apply to children aged 5–16 years, and child over 16 years treatment recommendations apply to those aged 17 years and over. Whereas, for children aged over 5 years, BTS/SIGN (2019) treatment recommendations for children apply to children aged 5–12 years, and child over 16 years treatment recommendations apply to those aged over 12 years.

Intermittent reliever therapy

EvGr Start an inhaled short-acting $beta_2$ agonist (such as salbutamol p. 164 or terbutaline sulfate p. 166), to be used as required in all children with asthma. For those with infrequent short-lived wheeze, occasional use of reliever therapy may be the only treatment required. Children using more than one short-acting $beta_2$ agonist inhaler device a month should have their asthma urgently assessed and action taken to improve poorly controlled asthma. Ⓐ

Regular preventer (maintenance) therapy

NICE (2017) define inhaled corticosteroid (ICS) doses for children (aged 5–16 years) as paediatric low, moderate, or high. BTS/SIGN (2019) instead define ICS doses for children (aged 5–12 years) as very low, low, or medium, and for children over 12 years as low, medium or high (refer to individual guidelines for ICS dosing information).

EvGr A paediatric low-dose of ICS should be started as maintenance therapy in children who present with any one of the following features: using an inhaled short-acting $beta_2$ agonist three times a week or more, symptomatic three times a week or more, or waking at night due to asthma symptoms at least once a week.

BTS/SIGN (2019) instead recommend starting a very low-dose (child aged 5–12 years) or a low-dose (child aged over 12 years) of ICS in children presenting with any one of the following features: using an inhaled short-acting $beta_2$ agonist three times a week or more, symptomatic three times a week or more, waking at night due to asthma symptoms at least once a week, or have had an asthma attack in the last 2 years, and starting an ICS at a dose appropriate to the severity of asthma.

BTS/SIGN (2019) recommend that inhaled corticosteroids (except ciclesonide p. 170) should initially be taken twice daily, however the same total daily dose taken once a day, can be considered in patients with milder disease if good or complete control of asthma is established. The dose of ICS should be adjusted over time to the lowest effective dose at which control of asthma is maintained.

BTS/SIGN (2019) recommend the prescribing of inhalers by brand. Ⓐ

Initial add-on therapy

EvGr If asthma is uncontrolled on a paediatric low-dose of ICS as maintenance therapy, consider a leukotriene receptor antagonist (LTRA—such as montelukast p. 174) in addition to the ICS, and review the response to treatment in 4 to 8 weeks.

BTS/SIGN (2019) instead recommend a long-acting $beta_2$ agonist (LABA—such as salmeterol p. 163 or formoterol fumarate p. 162) as initial add-on therapy to low-dose ICS if asthma is uncontrolled in children aged over 12 years. This can be given as either a fixed-dose ICS and LABA regimen, or a MART regimen (Maintenance And Reliever Therapy—a combination of an ICS and a fast-acting LABA such as formoterol in a single inhaler, see budesonide with formoterol p. 169). Combination inhalers containing both a LABA and an ICS are recommended to improve adherence, and ensure that the LABA is not taken alone without the ICS.

BTS/SIGN (2019) also recommend that a MART regimen should be considered in children aged over 12 years with a history of asthma attacks on a medium-dose ICS alone, or on a fixed-dose ICS and LABA regimen.

In children aged 5–12 years, BTS/SIGN (2019) recommend the addition of a LABA or a LTRA, as an initial add-on therapy to very low-dose ICS if asthma is uncontrolled. Ⓐ

Additional controller therapies

EvGr If asthma is uncontrolled on a paediatric low-dose of ICS and a LTRA as maintenance therapy, consider discontinuation of the LTRA and initiation of a LABA in combination with the ICS.

If asthma remains uncontrolled on a paediatric low-dose of ICS and a LABA as maintenance therapy, consider changing to a MART regimen (Maintenance And Reliever Therapy—a combination of an ICS and fast-acting LABA such as formoterol in a single inhaler) with a paediatric low-dose of ICS as maintenance. See budesonide with formoterol p. 169 [not licensed in all age groups].

If asthma remains uncontrolled on a MART regimen with a paediatric low-dose of ICS as maintenance, consider increasing to a paediatric moderate-dose of ICS (either continuing a MART regimen, or changing to a fixed-dose regimen of an ICS and a LABA with a short-acting $beta_2$ agonist as reliever therapy).

If asthma is still uncontrolled on a paediatric moderate-dose of ICS as maintenance with a LABA (either as a MART or a fixed-dose regimen), consider seeking advice from an asthma specialist and the following options:

- Increasing the ICS dose to a paediatric high-dose as maintenance (this should only be offered as part of a fixed-dose regimen with a short-acting beta$_2$ agonist as reliever therapy), or
- A trial of an additional drug, such as modified-release theophylline p. 178.

BTS/SIGN (2019) instead recommend that in children aged 5-12 years who are gaining some benefit from the addition of a LABA or a LTRA but control remains inadequate, to continue the LABA or LTRA and *either* increase the dose of the ICS to a low-dose (if not already on this dose), or adding a LTRA or LABA (whichever is not being used).

In children aged over 12 years, BTS/SIGN (2019) recommend continuing the LABA and *either* increasing the ICS to a medium-dose (if not already on this dose), or adding a LTRA.

If there is no response to the LABA, consider discontinuing it and *either* increasing the dose of ICS to a low-dose (child 5–12 years) or medium-dose (child over 12 years) if not already on this dose, or adding a LTRA.

BTS/SIGN (2019) recommend that all children whose asthma is not adequately controlled on recommended initial add-on therapy or additional controller therapies, should be referred for specialist asthma care. (A)

High-dose ICS and further add-on treatment (specialist therapies)

EvGr Under specialist care, BTS/SIGN (2019) recommend that if control remains inadequate on a low-dose (child aged 5–12 years) or medium-dose (child aged over 12 years) of ICS, plus a LABA or LTRA, the following interventions can be considered:

- Increasing the ICS dose to a medium-dose (child aged 5–12 years) or high-dose (child aged over 12 years)—with ICS via a pressurised metered dose inhaler (pMDI), a spacer should be used, or
- Adding a LTRA (if not already tried), or modified-release theophylline p. 178, or tiotropium p. 161 (in children over 12 years).

If a trial of a further add-on treatment is ineffective, stop the drug (or in the case of increased dose of ICS, reduce to the original dose). (A)

Continuous or frequent use of oral corticosteroids (specialist therapies)

EvGr Under specialist care, BTS/SIGN (2019) recommend adding a regular oral corticosteroid (prednisolone p. 478) at the lowest dose to provide adequate control in children with very severe asthma uncontrolled on a high-dose ICS, and who have also tried (or are still receiving) a LABA, LTRA, tiotropium p. 161 (child aged over 12 years), or modified-release theophylline p. 178. (A)

For information on the general use and side effects of corticosteroids, see Corticosteroids, general use p. 470. For information on the cessation of oral corticosteroid treatment, see *Treatment cessation* for systemic corticosteroids (such as prednisolone).

Monoclonal antibodies and immunosuppressants (specialist therapies)

EvGr Under specialist initiation, BTS/SIGN (2019) recommend that monoclonal antibodies such as omalizumab p. 174 (child over 6 years for severe persistent allergic asthma), and immunosuppressants such as methotrexate p. 588 [unlicensed] can be considered in children with severe asthma to achieve control and reduce the use of oral corticosteroids. (A) See *National funding/access decisions* for omalizumab p. 174.

Child aged under 5 years

Intermittent reliever therapy

EvGr A short-acting beta$_2$ agonist (such as salbutamol p. 164) as reliever therapy should be offered to children aged under 5 years with suspected asthma. A short-acting beta$_2$ agonist should be used for symptom relief alongside maintenance treatment.

Children using more than one short-acting beta$_2$ agonist inhaler device a month should have their asthma urgently assessed and action taken to improve poorly controlled asthma. (A)

Regular preventer (maintenance) therapy

NICE (2017) define inhaled corticosteroid (ICS) doses for children aged under 5 years as paediatric low or moderate. BTS/SIGN (2019) instead define ICS doses for children aged under 5 years as very low (refer to individual guidelines for ICS dosing information).

EvGr Consider an 8-week trial of a paediatric moderate-dose of ICS in children presenting with any of the following features: asthma-related symptoms three times a week or more, experiencing night-time awakening at least once a week, or suspected asthma that is uncontrolled with a short-acting beta$_2$ agonist alone.

After 8 weeks, stop ICS treatment and continue to monitor the child's symptoms:

- If symptoms did not resolve during the trial period, review whether an alternative diagnosis is likely;
- If symptoms resolved then reoccurred within 4 weeks of stopping ICS treatment, restart the ICS at a paediatric low-dose as first-line maintenance therapy;
- If symptoms resolved but reoccurred beyond 4 weeks after stopping ICS treatment, repeat the 8-week trial of a paediatric moderate-dose of ICS.

BTS/SIGN (2019) instead recommend starting a very low-dose of ICS as initial regular preventer therapy in children presenting with any one of the following features: using an inhaled short-acting beta$_2$ agonist three times a week or more, symptomatic three times a week or more, or waking at night due to asthma symptoms at least once a week. In children unable to take an ICS, a leukotriene receptor antagonist (LTRA, such as montelukast p. 174) may be used as an alternative.

BTS/SIGN (2019) recommend the prescribing of inhalers by brand. (A)

Initial add-on therapy

EvGr If suspected asthma is uncontrolled in children aged under 5 years on a paediatric low-dose of ICS as maintenance therapy, consider a LTRA in addition to the ICS.

If suspected asthma is uncontrolled in children aged under 5 years on a paediatric low-dose of ICS and a LTRA as maintenance therapy, stop the LTRA and refer the child to an asthma specialist. (A)

Decreasing treatment

EvGr Consider decreasing maintenance therapy when a patient's asthma has been controlled with their current maintenance therapy for at least three months. When deciding which drug to decrease first and at what rate, the severity of asthma, the side-effects of treatment, duration on current dose, the beneficial effect achieved, and the patient's preference should be considered. Patients should be regularly reviewed when decreasing treatment.

Patients should be maintained at the lowest possible dose of ICS. Reductions should be considered every three months, decreasing the dose by approximately 25–50% each time. Reduce the dose slowly as patients deteriorate at different rates. Only consider stopping ICS treatment completely for people who are using a paediatric or adult low-dose ICS alone as maintenance therapy and are symptom-free. (A)

Exercise-induced asthma

EvGr For most patients, exercise-induced asthma is an illustration of poorly controlled asthma and regular treatment including an ICS should therefore be reviewed. If exercise is a specific problem in patients already taking an ICS who are otherwise well controlled, consider adding either a LTRA, a long-acting $beta_2$ agonist, sodium cromoglicate p. 176 or nedocromil sodium p. 175, or theophylline p. 178. An inhaled short-acting $beta_2$ agonist used immediately before exercise is the drug of choice. Ⓐ

Pregnancy

EvGr Women with asthma should be closely monitored during pregnancy. It is particularly important that asthma is well controlled during pregnancy; when this is achieved there is little or no increased risk of adverse maternal or fetal complications.

Women should be counselled about the importance and safety of taking their asthma medication during pregnancy to maintain good control. Women who smoke should be advised about the dangers to themselves and to their baby and be offered appropriate support to stop smoking. Ⓐ For further information, see Smoking cessation p. 313.

EvGr Short-acting $beta_2$ agonists, LABAs, oral and inhaled corticosteroids, sodium cromoglicate p. 176 and nedocromil sodium p. 175, and oral and intravenous theophylline p. 178 (with appropriate monitoring) can be used as normal during pregnancy. There is limited information on use of a LTRA during pregnancy, however, where indicated to achieve adequate control, they should not be withheld. Ⓐ

Advanced Pharmacy Services

Patients with asthma may be eligible for the New Medicines Service / Medicines Use Review service provided by a community pharmacist. For further information, see *Advanced Pharmacy Services* in Medicines optimisation p. 25.

Useful Resources

Asthma: diagnosis, monitoring and chronic asthma management. National Institute for Health and Care Excellence. NICE guideline 80. November 2017.
www.nice.org.uk/guidance/ng80

British guideline on the management of asthma. British Thoracic Society and Scottish Intercollegiate Guidelines Network. Full guidance - A national clinical guideline 158. July 2019.
www.sign.ac.uk/assets/sign158.pdf

Patient decision aid: Inhalers for asthma for use by people aged 17 years and over. National Institute for Health and Care Excellence. May 2019.
www.nice.org.uk/about/what-we-do/our-programmes/nice-guidance/nice-guidelines/shared-decision-making

Asthma, acute

07-Oct-2019

Description of condition

Acute asthma is the progressive worsening of asthma symptoms, including breathlessness, wheeze, cough, and chest tightness. An acute exacerbation is marked by a reduction in baseline objective measures of pulmonary function, such as peak expiratory flow rate and FEV_1.

Most asthma attacks severe enough to require hospitalisation develop relatively slowly over a period of six hours or more. In children, intermittent wheezing attacks are usually triggered by viral infections and response to asthma medication may be inconsistent. Low birth weight and/or prematurity may be risk factors for recurrent wheeze.

Aims of treatment

The aim of treatment is to relieve airflow obstruction and prevent future relapses. Early treatment is most advantageous.

Levels of severity

Children

EvGr An acute exacerbation of asthma should be correctly differentiated from poor asthma control and it's severity categorised in order to be appropriately treated. The categories are described as follows: Ⓐ

Moderate acute asthma

- Able to talk in sentences;
- Arterial oxygen saturation (SpO_2) $\geq 92\%$;
- Peak flow $\geq 50\%$ best or predicted;
- Heart rate ≤ 140/minute in children aged 1–5 years; heart rate ≤ 125/minute in children aged over 5 years;
- Respiratory rate ≤ 40/minute in children aged 1–5 years; respiratory rate ≤ 30/minute in children aged over 5 years.

Severe acute asthma

- Can't complete sentences in one breath or too breathless to talk or feed;
- $SpO_2 < 92\%$;
- Peak flow 33–50% best or predicted;
- Heart rate > 140/minute in children aged 1–5 years; heart rate > 125/minute in children aged over 5 years;
- Respiratory rate > 40/minute in children aged 1–5 years; respiratory rate > 30/minute in children aged over 5 years.

Life-threatening acute asthma

Any one of the following in a child with severe asthma:

- $SpO_2 < 92\%$;
- Peak flow $< 33\%$ best or predicted;
- Silent chest;
- Cyanosis;
- Poor respiratory effort;
- Hypotension;
- Exhaustion;
- Confusion.

Management in children aged 2 years and over

EvGr Children with **severe** or **life-threatening** acute asthma should start treatment as soon as possible and be referred to hospital immediately following initial assessment. Supplementary high flow oxygen (via a tight-fitting face mask or nasal cannula) should be given to all children with life-threatening acute asthma or $SpO_2 < 94\%$ to achieve normal saturations of 94–98%.

First-line treatment for acute asthma is an inhaled short-acting $beta_2$ agonist (salbutamol p. 164 or terbutaline sulfate p. 166) given as soon as possible. The dose given should be individualised according to severity and adjusted based on response. Discontinue long-acting $beta_2$ agonist use if a short-acting $beta_2$ agonist is given more than 4 hourly. Seek medical attention if symptoms are not controlled with 10 puffs of salbutamol via a spacer; give additional bronchodilator doses whilst awaiting medical attention if symptoms are severe.

In all cases of acute asthma, children should be prescribed an adequate dose of oral prednisolone p. 478. Treatment for up to 3 days is usually sufficient, but the length of the course should be tailored to the number of days necessary to bring about recovery. Repeat the dose in children who vomit and consider the intravenous route in those who are unable to retain oral medication. It is considered good practice that inhaled corticosteroids are continued at their usual maintenance dose whilst receiving additional treatment for the attack, but they should not be used as a replacement for the oral corticosteroid. Ⓐ

For information on the general use and side effects of corticosteroids, see Corticosteroids, general use p. 470. For information on the cessation of oral corticosteroid treatment, see *Treatment cessation* for systemic corticosteroids (such as prednisolone).

EvGr Nebulised ipratropium bromide p. 161 can be combined with $beta_2$ agonist treatment for children with a poor initial response to $beta_2$ agonist therapy to provide greater bronchodilation. Consider adding magnesium sulfate p. 646 [unlicensed use] to each nebulised salbutamol and ipratropium bromide in the first hour in children with a short duration of severe acute asthma symptoms presenting with an oxygen saturation less than 92%.

Children with continuing severe acute asthma despite frequent nebulised beta$_2$ agonists and ipratropium bromide plus oral corticosteroids, and those with life-threatening features, need urgent review by a specialist with a view to transfer to a high dependency unit or paediatric intensive care unit (PICU) to receive second-line intravenous therapies.

In children who respond poorly to first-line treatments, intravenous magnesium sulfate [unlicensed use] may be considered as first-line intravenous treatment. In a severe asthma attack where the child has not responded to initial inhaled therapy, early addition of a single bolus dose of intravenous salbutamol may be an option. Continuous intravenous infusion of salbutamol, administered under specialist supervision with continuous ECG and electrolyte monitoring, should be considered in children with unreliable inhalation or severe refractory asthma. Aminophylline p. 176 may be considered in children with severe or life-threatening acute asthma unresponsive to maximal doses of bronchodilators and corticosteroids. (A)

Children aged under 2 years

[EvGr] Acute asthma treatment for all children aged under 2 years should be given in the hospital setting. Treatment of children aged under 1 year should be under the direct guidance of a respiratory paediatrician.

For moderate and severe acute asthma attacks, immediate treatment with oxygen via a tight-fitting face mask or nasal prongs should be given to achieve normal SpO_2 saturations of 94-98%. Trial an inhaled short-acting beta$_2$ agonist and if response is poor, combine nebulised ipratropium bromide to each nebulised beta$_2$ agonist dose. Consider oral prednisolone daily for up to 3 days, early in the management of severe asthma attacks.

In children not responsive to first-line treatments or have life-threatening features, discuss management with a senior paediatrician or the PICU team. (A)

Follow up in all cases

[EvGr] Episodes of acute asthma may be a failure of preventative therapy, review is required to prevent further episodes. A careful history should be taken to establish the reason for the asthma attack. Inhaler technique should be checked and regular treatment should be reviewed. Children and their parents or carers should be given a written asthma action plan aimed at preventing relapse, optimising treatment, and preventing delay in seeking assistance in future attacks. It is essential that the child's GP practice is informed within 24 hours of discharge from the emergency department or hospital following an asthma attack, and the child be reviewed by their GP within 2 working days. Children who have had a near-fatal asthma attack should be kept under specialist supervision indefinitely. A respiratory specialist should follow up all children admitted with a severe asthma attack for at least one year after the admission. (A)

Advanced Pharmacy Services

Children with asthma may be eligible for the New Medicines Service / Medicines Use Review service provided by a community pharmacist. For further information, see *Advanced Pharmacy Services* in Medicines optimisation p. 25.

Useful Resources

British guideline on the management of asthma. British Thoracic Society and Scottish Intercollegiate Guidelines Network. Full guidance - A national clinical guideline 158. July 2019.
www.sign.ac.uk/assets/sign158.pdf

Oxygen

Overview

Oxygen should be regarded as a drug. It is prescribed for hypoxaemic patients to increase alveolar oxygen tension and decrease the work of breathing. The concentration of oxygen required depends on the condition being treated; administration of an inappropriate concentration of oxygen may have serious or even fatal consequences. High concentrations of oxygen can cause pulmonary epithelial damage (bronchopulmonary dysplasia), convulsions, and retinal damage, especially in preterm neonates.

Oxygen is probably the most common drug used in medical emergencies. It should be prescribed initially to achieve a normal or near-normal oxygen saturation. In most acutely ill children with an expected or known normal or low arterial carbon dioxide (P_a CO_2), oxygen saturation should be maintained above 92%; some clinicians may aim for a target of 94–98%. In some clinical situations, such as carbon monoxide poisoning, it is more appropriate to aim for the highest possible oxygen saturation until the child is stable. Hypercapnic respiratory failure is rare in children; in those children at risk, a lower oxygen saturation target of 88–92% is indicated.

High concentration oxygen therapy is safe in uncomplicated cases of conditions such as pneumonia, pulmonary thromboembolism, pulmonary fibrosis, shock, severe trauma, sepsis, or anaphylaxis. In such conditions low arterial oxygen (P_a O_2) is usually associated with low or normal arterial carbon dioxide (P_a CO_2), and therefore there is little risk of hypoventilation and carbon dioxide retention.

In severe acute asthma, the arterial carbon dioxide (P_a CO_2) is usually subnormal but as asthma deteriorates it may rise steeply (particularly in children). These patients usually require high concentrations of oxygen and if the arterial carbon dioxide (P_a CO_2) remains high despite other treatment, intermittent positive-pressure ventilation needs to be considered urgently.

Oxygen should not be given to neonates except under expert supervision. Particular care is required in preterm neonates because of the risk of hyperoxia.

Low concentration oxygen therapy (controlled oxygen therapy) is reserved for children at risk of hypercapnic respiratory failure, which is more likely in children with:

- advanced cystic fibrosis;
- advanced non-cystic fibrosis bronchiectasis;
- severe kyphoscoliosis or severe ankylosing spondylitis;
- severe lung scarring caused by tuberculosis;
- musculoskeletal disorders with respiratory weakness, especially if on home ventilation;
- an overdose of opioids, benzodiazepines, or other drugs causing respiratory depression.

Until blood gases can be measured, initial oxygen should be given using a controlled concentration of 28% or less, titrated towards a target concentration of 88–92%. The aim is to provide the child with enough oxygen to achieve an acceptable arterial oxygen tension without worsening carbon dioxide retention and respiratory acidosis. Patients may carry an *oxygen alert card*.

The oxygen alert card template is available at www.brit-thoracic.org.uk.

Domiciliary oxygen

Oxygen should only be prescribed for use in the home after careful evaluation in hospital by a respiratory care specialist. Carers and children who smoke should be advised of the risks of smoking when receiving oxygen, including the risk of fire. Smoking cessation p. 313 therapy should be recommended before home oxygen prescription.

Long-term oxygen therapy

The aim of long-term oxygen therapy is to maintain oxygen saturation of at least 92%. Children (especially those with chronic neonatal lung disease) often require supplemental oxygen, either for 24-hours a day or during periods of sleep; many children are eventually weaned off long-term oxygen therapy as their condition improves.

Long-term oxygen therapy should be considered for children with conditions such as:

- bronchopulmonary dysplasia (chronic neonatal lung disease);
- congenital heart disease with pulmonary hypertension;
- pulmonary hypertension secondary to pulmonary disease;
- idiopathic pulmonary hypertension;
- sickle-cell disease with persistent nocturnal hypoxia;
- interstitial lung disease and obliterative bronchiolitis;
- cystic fibrosis;
- obstructive sleep apnoea syndrome;
- neuromuscular or skeletal disease requiring non-invasive ventilation;
- pulmonary malignancy or other terminal disease with disabling dyspnoea.

Increased respiratory depression is seldom a problem in children with stable respiratory failure treated with low concentrations of oxygen although it may occur during exacerbations; children and their carers should be warned to call for medical help if drowsiness or confusion occurs.

Short-burst oxygen therapy

Oxygen is occasionally prescribed for short-burst (intermittent) use for episodes of breathlessness.

Ambulatory oxygen therapy

Ambulatory oxygen is prescribed for children on long-term oxygen therapy who need to be away from home on a regular basis.

Oxygen therapy equipment

Under the NHS oxygen may be supplied as **oxygen cylinders**. Oxygen flow can be adjusted as the cylinders are equipped with an oxygen flow meter. Oxygen delivered from a cylinder should be passed through a humidifier if used for long periods.

Oxygen concentrators are more economical for children who require oxygen for long periods, and in England and Wales can be ordered on the NHS on a regional tendering basis. A concentrator is recommended for a child who requires oxygen for more than 8 hours a day (or 21 cylinders per month). Exceptionally, if a higher concentration of oxygen is required the output of 2 oxygen concentrators can be combined using a 'Y' connection.

A nasal cannula is usually preferred to a face mask for long-term oxygen therapy from an oxygen concentrator. Nasal cannulas can, however, cause dermatitis and mucosal drying in sensitive individuals.

Giving oxygen by nasal cannula allows the child to talk, eat, and drink, but the concentration of oxygen is not controlled and the method may not be appropriate for acute respiratory failure. When oxygen is given through a nasal cannula at a rate of 1–2 litres/minute the inspiratory oxygen concentration is usually low, but it varies with ventilation and can be high if the patient is underventilating.

Arrangements for supplying oxygen

The following oxygen services may be ordered in England and Wales:

- emergency oxygen;
- short-burst (intermittent) oxygen therapy;
- long-term oxygen therapy;
- ambulatory oxygen.

The type of oxygen service (or combination of services) should be ordered on a Home Oxygen Order Form (HOOF); the amount of oxygen required (hours per day) and flow rate should be specified. The clinician will determine the appropriate equipment to be provided. Special needs or preferences should be specified on the HOOF.

The clinician should obtain the consent of the child or carers to pass on the child's details to the supplier, the fire brigade, and other relevant organisations. The supplier will contact the child or carer to make arrangements for delivery, installation, and maintenance of the equipment. The supplier will also train the child or carer to use the equipment.

The clinician should send the HOOF to the supplier who will continue to provide the service until a revised HOOF is received, or until notified that the child no longer requires the home oxygen service.

- East of England, North East: BOC Medical: Tel: 0800 136 603 Fax: 0800 169 9989
- South West: Air Liquide: Tel: 0808 202 2229 Fax: 0191 497 4340
- London East, Midlands, North West:Air Liquide: Tel: 0500 823 773 Fax: 0800 781 4610
- Yorkshire and Humberside, West Midlands, Wales: Air Products: Tel: 0800 373 580 Fax: 0800 214 709
- South East Coast, South Central: Dolby Vivisol: Tel: 08443 814 402 Fax: 0800 781 4610

In **Scotland** refer the child for assessment by a paediatric respiratory consultant. If the need for a concentrator is confirmed the consultant will arrange for the provision of a concentrator through the Common Services Agency. Prescribers should complete a Scottish Home Oxygen Order Form (SHOOF) and email it to Health Facilities Scotland. Health Facilities Scotland will then liaise with their contractor to arrange the supply of oxygen. Further information can be obtained at www.dolbyvivisol.com/services/healthcare-professionals/.

In **Northern Ireland** oxygen concentrators and cylinders should be prescribed on form HS21; oxygen concentrators are supplied by a local contractor. Prescriptions for oxygen cylinders and accessories can be dispensed by pharmacists contracted to provide domiciliary oxygen services.

Croup

Management

Mild croup is largely self-limiting, but treatment with a single dose of a corticosteroid (e.g. dexamethasone p. 475) by mouth may be of benefit.

More severe croup (or mild croup that might cause complications) calls for hospital admission; a single dose of a corticosteroid (e.g. dexamethasone or prednisolone p. 478 by mouth) should be administered before transfer to hospital. In hospital, dexamethasone (by mouth or by injection) or budesonide p. 168 (by nebulisation) will often reduce symptoms; the dose may need to be repeated after 12 hours if necessary.

For severe croup not effectively controlled with corticosteroid treatment, nebulised adrenaline/epinephrine solution 1 in 1000 (1 mg/mL) p. 143 should be given with close clinical monitoring; the effects of nebulised adrenaline/epinephrine last 2–3 hours and the child needs to be monitored carefully for recurrence of the obstruction.

Other drugs used for Airways disease, obstructive
Dupilumab, p. 799 · Glycopyrronium bromide, p. 870

ANTIMUSCARINICS

Antimuscarinics (inhaled)

09-Feb-2016

- **CAUTIONS** Bladder outflow obstruction · paradoxical bronchospasm · prostatic hyperplasia · susceptibility to angle-closure glaucoma
- **SIDE-EFFECTS**
  - **Common or very common** Arrhythmias · cough · dizziness · dry mouth · headache · nausea
  - **Uncommon** Constipation · dysphonia · glaucoma · palpitations · skin reactions · stomatitis · urinary disorders · vision blurred

above

Ipratropium bromide

25-Jul-2018

- **INDICATIONS AND DOSE**

Reversible airways obstruction

- BY INHALATION OF AEROSOL
  - Child 1 month–5 years: 20 micrograms 3 times a day
  - Child 6–11 years: 20–40 micrograms 3 times a day
  - Child 12–17 years: 20–40 micrograms 3–4 times a day

Acute bronchospasm

- BY INHALATION OF NEBULISED SOLUTION
  - Child 1 month–5 years: 125–250 micrograms as required; maximum 1 mg per day
  - Child 6–11 years: 250 micrograms as required; maximum 1 mg per day
  - Child 12–17 years: 500 micrograms as required, doses higher than max. can be given under medical supervision; maximum 2 mg per day

Severe or life-threatening acute asthma

- BY INHALATION OF NEBULISED SOLUTION
  - Child 1 month–11 years: 250 micrograms every 20–30 minutes for the first 2 hours, then 250 micrograms every 4–6 hours as required
  - Child 12–17 years: 500 micrograms every 4–6 hours as required

PHARMACOKINETICS

- The maximal effect of inhaled ipratropium occurs 30–60 minutes after use; its duration of action is 3 to 6 hours and bronchodilation can usually be maintained with treatment 3 times a day.

- **UNLICENSED USE** EvGr The dose of ipratropium for severe or life-threatening acute asthma is unlicensed. (A)
  Inhalvent® not licensed for use in children under 6 years.

> **IMPORTANT SAFETY INFORMATION**
>
> MHRA/CHM ADVICE: PRESSURISED METERED DOSE INHALERS (PMDI): RISK OF AIRWAY OBSTRUCTION FROM ASPIRATION OF LOOSE OBJECTS (JULY 2018)
>
> See Respiratory system, drug delivery p. 153.

- **CAUTIONS** Avoid spraying near eyes · cystic fibrosis

CAUTIONS, FURTHER INFORMATION

- Glaucoma *Acute angle-closure glaucoma* has been reported with nebulised ipratropium, particularly when given with nebulised salbutamol (and possibly other $beta_2$ agonists); care needed to protect the patient's eyes from nebulised drug or from drug powder.

- **INTERACTIONS** → Appendix 1: ipratropium
- **SIDE-EFFECTS**
  - **Common or very common** Gastrointestinal motility disorder · throat complaints
  - **Uncommon** Corneal oedema · diarrhoea · eye disorders · eye pain · respiratory disorders · vision disorders · vomiting
- **ALLERGY AND CROSS-SENSITIVITY** Contra-indicated in patients with hypersensitivity to atropine or its derivatives.
- **PREGNANCY** Manufacturer advises only use if potential benefit outweighs the risk.
- **BREAST FEEDING** No information available—manufacturer advises only use if potential benefit outweighs risk.
- **DIRECTIONS FOR ADMINISTRATION** If dilution of ipratropium bromide nebuliser solution is necessary use only sterile sodium chloride 0.9%.
- **PATIENT AND CARER ADVICE** Patients or carers should be counselled on appropriate administration technique and warned against accidental contact with the eye (due to risk of ocular complications).

Driving and skilled tasks Manufacturer advises patients and carers should be counselled on the effects on driving and performance of skilled tasks—increased risk of dizziness and vision disorders.

- **MEDICINAL FORMS** There can be variation in the licensing of different medicines containing the same drug.

Nebuliser liquid

- Ipratropium bromide (Non-proprietary)
  Ipratropium bromide 250 microgram per 1 ml Ipratropium bromide 500micrograms/2ml nebuliser liquid unit dose vials | 20 unit dose PoM £3.76 DT = £3.16
  Ipratropium bromide 250micrograms/1ml nebuliser liquid unit dose vials | 20 unit dose PoM £5.71 DT = £5.71
  Ipratropium 250micrograms/1ml nebuliser liquid Steri-Neb unit dose vials | 20 unit dose PoM £6.99 DT = £5.71
  Ipratropium 500micrograms/2ml nebuliser liquid Steri-Neb unit dose vials | 20 unit dose PoM £15.99 DT = £3.16
- Atrovent UDV (Boehringer Ingelheim Ltd)
  Ipratropium bromide 250 microgram per 1 ml Atrovent 500micrograms/2ml nebuliser liquid UDVs | 20 unit dose PoM £4.87 DT = £3.16
  Atrovent 250micrograms/1ml nebuliser liquid UDVs | 20 unit dose PoM £4.14 DT = £5.71

Pressurised inhalation

- Ipratropium bromide (Non-proprietary)
  Ipratropium bromide 20 microgram per 1 dose Ipravent 20micrograms/dose inhaler CFC free | 200 dose PoM £4.99 DT = £5.56
- Atrovent (Boehringer Ingelheim Ltd)
  Ipratropium bromide 20 microgram per 1 dose Atrovent 20micrograms/dose inhaler CFC free | 200 dose PoM £5.56 DT = £5.56
- Inhalvent (Alissa Healthcare Research Ltd)
  Ipratropium bromide 20 microgram per 1 dose Inhalvent 20micrograms/dose inhaler | 200 dose PoM £5.56 DT = £5.56

above

Tiotropium

12-Jun-2018

- **INDICATIONS AND DOSE**

SPIRIVA RESPIMAT®

Severe asthma [add-on to inhaled corticosteroid (over 400 micrograms budesonide daily or equivalent) and 1 controller, or inhaled corticosteroid (200–400 micrograms budesonide daily or equivalent) and 2 controllers, in patients who have suffered one or more severe exacerbations in the last year]

- BY INHALATION
  - Child 6–11 years: 5 micrograms once daily

Severe asthma [add-on to inhaled corticosteroid (over 800 micrograms budesonide daily or equivalent) and 1 controller, or inhaled corticosteroid (400–800 micrograms budesonide daily or equivalent) and 2 controllers, in patients who have suffered one or more severe exacerbations in the last year]

- BY INHALATION
  - Child 12–17 years: 5 micrograms once daily

continued →

DOSE EQUIVALENCE AND CONVERSION
- 2 puffs of inhalation solution is equivalent to 5 micrograms tiotropium.

IMPORTANT SAFETY INFORMATION

MHRA/CHM ADVICE: PRESSURISED METERED DOSE INHALERS (PMDI): RISK OF AIRWAY OBSTRUCTION FROM ASPIRATION OF LOOSE OBJECTS (JULY 2018)

See Respiratory system, drug delivery p. 153.

- **CAUTIONS** Arrhythmia (unstable, life-threatening or requiring intervention in the previous 12 months) · heart failure (hospitalisation for moderate to severe heart failure in the previous 12 months) · myocardial infarction in the previous 6 months
- **INTERACTIONS** → Appendix 1: tiotropium
- **SIDE-EFFECTS**
  - **Uncommon** Gastrointestinal disorders · increased risk of infection · taste altered
  - **Rare or very rare** Bronchospasm · dysphagia · epistaxis · insomnia · oral disorders
  - **Frequency not known** Dehydration · joint swelling · skin ulcer
- **PREGNANCY** Manufacturer advises avoid—limited data available.
- **BREAST FEEDING** Manufacturer advises avoid—no information available.
- **RENAL IMPAIRMENT** Manufacturer advises use only if potential benefit outweighs risk if creatinine clearance less than or equal to 50 mL/minute—plasma-tiotropium concentration raised.
- **PATIENT AND CARER ADVICE** Patients or carers should be given advice on appropriate inhaler technique.
- **NATIONAL FUNDING/ACCESS DECISIONS**

Scottish Medicines Consortium (SMC) decisions

SMC No. SMC2118

The *Scottish Medicines Consortium* has advised (January 2019) that tiotropium (*Spiriva Respimat*®) is accepted for use within NHS Scotland as add-on maintenance bronchodilator treatment in patients aged 6 years and older with severe asthma who experienced one or more severe asthma exacerbations in the preceding year.

All Wales Medicines Strategy Group (AWMSG) decisions

AWMSG No. 1882

The *All Wales Medicines Strategy Group* has advised (December 2018) that tiotropium (*Spiriva Respimat*®) is recommended as an option for use within NHS Wales as add-on maintenance bronchodilator treatment in patients aged 6 years and older with severe asthma who experienced one or more severe asthma exacerbations in the preceding year.

- **MEDICINAL FORMS** There can be variation in the licensing of different medicines containing the same drug.

Inhalation solution

- Spiriva Respimat (Boehringer Ingelheim Ltd)
  Tiotropium (as Tiotropium bromide) 2.5 microgram per 1 dose Spiriva Respimat 2.5micrograms/dose inhalation solution cartridge with device | 60 dose PoM £23.00 DT = £23.00
  Spiriva Respimat 2.5micrograms/dose inhalation solution refill cartridge | 60 dose PoM £23.00

BETA$_2$-ADRENOCEPTOR AGONISTS, SELECTIVE

Beta$_2$- adrenoceptor agonists, selective

12-Feb-2016

- **CAUTIONS** Arrhythmias · cardiovascular disease · diabetes (risk of hyperglycaemia and ketoacidosis, especially with intravenous use) · hypertension · hyperthyroidism · hypokalaemia · susceptibility to QT-interval prolongation

CAUTIONS, FURTHER INFORMATION
- **Hypokalaemia** Potentially serious hypokalaemia may result from beta$_2$ agonist therapy. Particular caution is required in severe asthma, because this effect may be potentiated by concomitant treatment with theophylline and its derivatives, corticosteroids, diuretics, and by hypoxia.
- **SIDE-EFFECTS**
  - **Common or very common** Arrhythmias · dizziness · headache · hypokalaemia (with high doses) · nausea · palpitations · tremor
  - **Uncommon** Hyperglycaemia · myocardial ischaemia
  - **Rare or very rare** Bronchospasm paradoxical (sometimes severe)
- **PREGNANCY** Women planning to become pregnant should be counselled about the importance of taking their asthma medication regularly to maintain good control.
- **MONITORING REQUIREMENTS**
  - In severe asthma, plasma-potassium concentration should be monitored (risk of hypokalaemia).
  - In patients with diabetes, monitor blood glucose (risk of hyperglycaemia and ketoacidosis, especially when beta$_2$ agonist given intravenously).
- **PATIENT AND CARER ADVICE** The **dose**, the frequency, and the maximum number of inhalations in 24 hours of the beta$_2$ agonist should be **stated explicitly** to the patient or their carer. The patient or their carer should be advised to seek medical advice when the prescribed dose of beta$_2$ agonist fails to provide the usual degree of symptomatic relief because this usually indicates a worsening of the asthma and the patient may require a prophylactic drug. Patients or their carers should be advised to follow manufacturers' instructions on the care and cleansing of inhaler devices.

BETA$_2$-ADRENOCEPTOR AGONISTS, SELECTIVE › LONG-ACTING

above

Formoterol fumarate

25-Nov-2019

(Eformoterol fumarate)

- **INDICATIONS AND DOSE**

Reversible airways obstruction in patients requiring long-term regular bronchodilator therapy | Nocturnal asthma in patients requiring long-term regular bronchodilator therapy | Prophylaxis of exercise-induced bronchospasm in patients requiring long-term regular bronchodilator therapy | Chronic asthma in patients who regularly use an inhaled corticosteroid

- BY INHALATION OF POWDER
  - Child 6–11 years: 12 micrograms twice daily, a daily dose of 24 micrograms of formoterol should be sufficient for the majority of children, particularly for younger age-groups; higher doses should be used rarely, and only when control is not maintained on the lower dose
  - Child 12–17 years: 12 micrograms twice daily, dose may be increased in more severe airway obstruction; increased to 24 micrograms twice daily, a daily dose of 24 micrograms of formoterol should be sufficient for the majority of children, particularly for younger age-groups; higher doses should be used rarely, and only when control is not maintained on the lower dose
- BY INHALATION OF AEROSOL
  - Child 12–17 years: 12 micrograms twice daily, dose may be increased in more severe airway obstruction; increased to 24 micrograms twice daily, a daily dose of 24 micrograms of formoterol should be sufficient for the majority of children, particularly for younger age-

groups; higher doses should be used rarely, and only when control is not maintained on the lower dose

OXIS ®

Chronic asthma

▶ BY INHALATION OF POWDER

▸ Child 6–17 years: 6–12 micrograms 1–2 times a day (max. per dose 12 micrograms), occasionally doses up to the maximum daily may be needed, reassess treatment if additional doses required on more than 2 days a week; maximum 48 micrograms per day

Relief of bronchospasm

▶ BY INHALATION OF POWDER

▸ Child 6–17 years: 6–12 micrograms

Prophylaxis of exercise-induced bronchospasm

▶ BY INHALATION OF POWDER

▸ Child 6–17 years: 6–12 micrograms, dose to be taken before exercise

PHARMACOKINETICS

▸ At recommended inhaled doses, the duration of action of formoterol is about 12 hours.

IMPORTANT SAFETY INFORMATION

CHM ADVICE

To ensure safe use, the CHM has advised that for the management of chronic asthma, long-acting beta$_2$ agonist (formoterol) should:

- be added only if regular use of standard-dose inhaled corticosteroids has failed to control asthma adequately;
- not be initiated in patients with rapidly deteriorating asthma;
- be introduced at a low dose and the effect properly monitored before considering dose increase;
- be discontinued in the absence of benefit;
- not be used for the relief of exercise-induced asthma symptoms unless regular inhaled corticosteroids are also used;
- be reviewed as clinically appropriate: stepping down therapy should be considered when good long-term asthma control has been achieved.

MHRA/CHM ADVICE: PRESSURISED METERED DOSE INHALERS (PMDI): RISK OF AIRWAY OBSTRUCTION FROM ASPIRATION OF LOOSE OBJECTS (JULY 2018)

See Respiratory system, drug delivery p. 153.

● **CAUTIONS** High doses of beta$_2$ agonists can be dangerous in some children

● **INTERACTIONS** → Appendix 1: beta$_2$ agonists

● **SIDE-EFFECTS**

▶ **Common or very common** Muscle cramps

▶ **Uncommon** Angina pectoris · bronchospasm · skin reactions · sleep disorder · taste altered

▶ **Rare or very rare** Anxiety · QT interval prolongation

● **PREGNANCY** Inhaled drugs for asthma can be taken as normal during pregnancy.

● **BREAST FEEDING** Inhaled drugs for asthma can be taken as normal during breast-feeding.

● **PATIENT AND CARER ADVICE** Advise patients not to exceed prescribed dose, and to follow manufacturer's directions; if a previously effective dose of inhaled formoterol fails to provide adequate relief, a doctor's advice should be obtained as soon as possible. Patients should be advised to report any deterioration in symptoms following initiation of treatment with a long-acting beta$_2$ agonist. Patient or carer should be given advice on how to administer formoterol fumarate inhalers.

● **MEDICINAL FORMS** There can be variation in the licensing of different medicines containing the same drug.

Inhalation powder

▸ Easyhaler (formoterol) (Orion Pharma (UK) Ltd)

Formoterol fumarate dihydrate 12 microgram per 1 dose Formoterol Easyhaler 12micrograms/dose dry powder inhaler | 120 dose PoM £23.75 DT = £23.75

▸ Foradil (Novartis Pharmaceuticals UK Ltd)

Formoterol fumarate dihydrate 12 microgram Foradil 12microgram inhalation powder capsules with device | 60 capsule PoM £28.06 DT = £28.06

▸ Oxis Turbohaler (AstraZeneca UK Ltd)

Formoterol fumarate dihydrate 6 microgram per 1 dose Oxis 6 Turbohaler | 60 dose PoM £24.80 DT = £24.80

Formoterol fumarate dihydrate 12 microgram per 1 dose Oxis 12 Turbohaler | 60 dose PoM £24.80 DT = £24.80

Pressurised inhalation

EXCIPIENTS: May contain Alcohol

▸ Atimos Modulite (Chiesi Ltd)

Formoterol fumarate dihydrate 12 microgram per 1 dose Atimos Modulite 12micrograms/dose inhaler | 100 dose PoM £30.06 DT = £30.06

Combinations available: ***Budesonide with formoterol***, p. 169 · ***Fluticasone with formoterol***, p. 171

162

Salmeterol

25-Nov-2019

● **INDICATIONS AND DOSE**

Reversible airways obstruction in patients requiring long-term regular bronchodilator therapy | Nocturnal asthma in patients requiring long-term regular bronchodilator therapy | Prevention of exercise-induced bronchospasm in patients requiring long-term regular bronchodilator therapy | Chronic asthma only in patients who regularly use an inhaled corticosteroid (not for immediate relief of acute asthma)

▶ BY INHALATION OF AEROSOL, OR BY INHALATION OF POWDER

▸ Child 5–11 years: 50 micrograms twice daily

▸ Child 12–17 years: 50 micrograms twice daily, dose may be increased in more severe airway obstruction; increased to 100 micrograms twice daily

PHARMACOKINETICS

▸ At recommended inhaled doses, the duration of action of salmeterol is about 12 hours.

● **UNLICENSED USE** *Neovent*® not licensed for use in children under 12 years.

IMPORTANT SAFETY INFORMATION

CHM ADVICE

To ensure safe use, the CHM has advised that for the management of chronic asthma, long-acting beta$_2$ agonist (salmeterol) should:

- be added only if regular use of standard-dose inhaled corticosteroids has failed to control asthma adequately;
- not be initiated in patients with rapidly deteriorating asthma;
- be introduced at a low dose and the effect properly monitored before considering dose increase;
- be discontinued in the absence of benefit;
- not be used for the relief of exercise-induced asthma symptoms unless regular inhaled corticosteroids are also used;
- be reviewed as clinically appropriate: stepping down therapy should be considered when good long-term asthma control has been achieved.

MHRA/CHM ADVICE: PRESSURISED METERED DOSE INHALERS (PMDI): RISK OF AIRWAY OBSTRUCTION FROM ASPIRATION OF LOOSE OBJECTS (JULY 2018)

See Respiratory system, drug delivery p. 153.

- **CAUTIONS** High doses of beta$_2$ agonists can be dangerous in some children
- **INTERACTIONS** → Appendix 1: beta$_2$ agonists
- **SIDE-EFFECTS**
  - **Common or very common** Muscle cramps
  - **Uncommon** Nervousness · skin reactions
  - **Rare or very rare** Arthralgia · bronchospasm · chest pain · insomnia · oedema · oropharyngeal irritation
- **PREGNANCY** Inhaled drugs for asthma can be taken as normal during pregnancy.
- **BREAST FEEDING** Inhaled drugs for asthma can be taken as normal during breast-feeding.
- **PATIENT AND CARER ADVICE** Advise patients that salmeterol should **not** be used for relief of acute attacks, not to exceed prescribed dose, and to follow manufacturer's directions; if a previously effective dose of inhaled salmeterol fails to provide adequate relief, a doctor's advice should be obtained as soon as possible. Patients should be advised to report any deterioration in symptoms following initiation of treatment with a long-acting beta$_2$ agonist.
  Medicines for Children leaflet: Salmeterol inhaler for asthma www.medicinesforchildren.org.uk/salmeterol-inhaler-asthma

- **MEDICINAL FORMS** There can be variation in the licensing of different medicines containing the same drug.

Inhalation powder

- Serevent Accuhaler (GlaxoSmithKline UK Ltd)
  Salmeterol (as Salmeterol xinafoate) 50 microgram per 1 dose Serevent 50micrograms/dose Accuhaler | 60 dose PoM £35.11 DT = £35.11

Pressurised inhalation

- Neovent (Kent Pharmaceuticals Ltd)
  Salmeterol (as Salmeterol xinafoate) 25 microgram per 1 dose Neovent 25micrograms/dose inhaler CFC free | 120 dose PoM £29.26 DT = £29.26
- Serevent Evohaler (GlaxoSmithKline UK Ltd)
  Salmeterol (as Salmeterol xinafoate) 25 microgram per 1 dose Serevent 25micrograms/dose Evohaler | 120 dose PoM £29.26 DT = £29.26
- Soltel (Cipla EU Ltd)
  Salmeterol (as Salmeterol xinafoate) 25 microgram per 1 dose Soltel 25micrograms/dose inhaler CFC free | 120 dose PoM £19.95 DT = £29.26

Combinations available: ***Fluticasone with salmeterol,*** p. 171

BETA$_2$-ADRENOCEPTOR AGONISTS, SELECTIVE › SHORT-ACTING

162

Salbutamol

25-Jul-2018

(Albuterol)

- **INDICATIONS AND DOSE**

Acute asthma

▶ BY INTRAVENOUS INJECTION

- Child 1–23 months: 5 micrograms/kg for 1 dose, dose to be administered over 5 minutes, reserve intravenous beta$_2$ agonists for those in whom inhaled therapy cannot be used reliably or there is no current effect
- Child 2–17 years: 15 micrograms/kg (max. per dose 250 micrograms) for 1 dose, dose to be administered over 5 minutes, reserve intravenous beta$_2$ agonists for those in whom inhaled therapy cannot be used reliably or there is no current effect

▶ BY CONTINUOUS INTRAVENOUS INFUSION

- Child: 1–2 micrograms/kg/minute, adjusted according to response and heart rate, increased if necessary up to 5 micrograms/kg/minute, doses above 2 micrograms/kg/minute should be given in an intensive care setting, reserve intravenous beta$_2$ agonists for those in whom inhaled therapy cannot be used reliably or there is no current effect

Moderate, severe, or life-threatening acute asthma

▶ BY INHALATION OF NEBULISED SOLUTION

- Child 1 month–4 years: 2.5 mg, repeat every 20–30 minutes or when required, give via oxygen-driven nebuliser if available
- Child 5–11 years: 2.5–5 mg, repeat every 20–30 minutes or when required, give via oxygen-driven nebuliser if available
- Child 12–17 years: 5 mg, repeat every 20–30 minutes or when required, give via oxygen-driven nebuliser if available

Moderate and severe acute asthma

▶ BY INHALATION OF AEROSOL

- Child: 2–10 puffs, each puff is to be inhaled separately, repeat every 10–20 minutes or when required, give via large volume spacer (and a close-fitting face mask in children under 3 years), each puff is equivalent to 100 micrograms

Exacerbation of reversible airways obstruction (including nocturnal asthma) | Prophylaxis of allergen- or exercise-induced bronchospasm

▶ BY INHALATION OF AEROSOL

- Child: 100–200 micrograms, up to 4 times a day for persistent symptoms

▶ BY MOUTH USING IMMEDIATE-RELEASE MEDICINES

- Child 1 month–1 year: 100 micrograms/kg 3–4 times a day (max. per dose 2 mg), inhalation route preferred over oral route
- Child 2–5 years: 1–2 mg 3–4 times a day, inhalation route preferred over oral route
- Child 6–11 years: 2 mg 3–4 times a day, inhalation route preferred over oral route
- Child 12–17 years: 2–4 mg 3–4 times a day, inhalation route preferred over oral route

Severe hyperkalaemia

▶ BY INTRAVENOUS INJECTION

- Neonate: 4 micrograms/kg, repeated if necessary, to be administered over 5 minutes.
- Child: 4 micrograms/kg, repeated if necessary, to be administered over 5 minutes

▶ BY INHALATION OF NEBULISED SOLUTION

- Neonate: 2.5–5 mg, repeated if necessary, intravenous injection route preferred over inhalation of nebulised solution.
- Child: 2.5–5 mg, repeated if necessary, intravenous injection route preferred over inhalation of nebulised solution

EASYHALER® SALBUTAMOL

Acute bronchospasm

▶ BY INHALATION OF POWDER

- Child 5–11 years: 100–200 micrograms; maximum 800 micrograms per day
- Child 12–17 years: Initially 100–200 micrograms, increased if necessary to 400 micrograms; maximum 800 micrograms per day

Prophylaxis of allergen- or exercise-induced bronchospasm

▶ BY INHALATION OF POWDER

- Child 5–11 years: 100–200 micrograms
- Child 12–17 years: 200 micrograms

SALBULIN NOVOLIZER®

Acute bronchospasm

▶ BY INHALATION OF POWDER

- Child 6–11 years: 100–200 micrograms, up to 400 micrograms daily for persistent symptoms

- Child 12–17 years: Initially 100–200 micrograms, up to 800 micrograms daily for persistent symptoms

Prophylaxis of allergen- or exercise-induced bronchospasm

- BY INHALATION OF POWDER
- Child 6–11 years: 100–200 micrograms
- Child 12–17 years: 200 micrograms

VENTOLIN ACCUHALER®

Acute bronchospasm

- BY INHALATION OF POWDER
- Child 5–17 years: Initially 200 micrograms, up to 4 times daily for persistent symptoms

Prophylaxis of allergen- or exercise-induced bronchospasm

- BY INHALATION OF POWDER
- Child 5–17 years: 200 micrograms

PHARMACOKINETICS

- At recommended inhaled doses, the duration of action of salbutamol is about 3 to 5 hours.

● **UNLICENSED USE** Not licensed for use in hyperkalaemia.
- With oral use Syrup and tablets not licensed for use in children under 2 years.
- With intravenous use Injection and solution for intravenous infusion not licensed for use in children under 12 years. Administration of undiluted salbutamol injection through a central venous catheter is not licensed.

> **IMPORTANT SAFETY INFORMATION**
>
> MHRA/CHM ADVICE: PRESSURISED METERED DOSE INHALERS (PMDI): RISK OF AIRWAY OBSTRUCTION FROM ASPIRATION OF LOOSE OBJECTS (JULY 2018)
>
> - When used by inhalation
>
> See Respiratory system, drug delivery p. 153.

● **CAUTIONS** High doses of $beta_2$ agonists can be dangerous in some children

● **INTERACTIONS** → Appendix 1: $beta_2$ agonists

● **SIDE-EFFECTS**

GENERAL SIDE-EFFECTS
- **Common or very common** Muscle cramps
- **Rare or very rare** Akathisia · vasodilation
- **Frequency not known** Metabolic change

SPECIFIC SIDE-EFFECTS
- **Uncommon**
- When used by inhalation Oral irritation · throat irritation
- With parenteral use Pulmonary oedema
- **Frequency not known**
- With parenteral use Lactic acidosis (with high doses) · vomiting

● **BREAST FEEDING** Inhaled drugs for asthma can be taken as normal during breast-feeding.

● **DIRECTIONS FOR ADMINISTRATION**
- With intravenous use For *continuous intravenous infusion*, dilute to a concentration of 200 micrograms/mL with Glucose 5% *or* Sodium Chloride 0.9%. If fluid-restricted, can be given undiluted through central venous catheter [unlicensed]. For *intravenous injection*, dilute to a concentration of 50 micrograms/mL with Glucose 5%, Sodium Chloride 0.9%, *or* Water for injections.
- When used by inhalation For *nebulisation*, dilute nebuliser solution with a suitable volume of sterile Sodium Chloride 0.9% solution according to nebuliser type and duration of administration; salbutamol and ipratropium bromide solutions are compatible and can be mixed for nebulisation.

● **PATIENT AND CARER ADVICE**
- When used by inhalation *For inhalation by aerosol or dry powder*, advise patients and carers not to exceed prescribed dose and to follow manufacturer's directions; if a previously effective dose of inhaled salbutamol fails to provide at least 3 hours relief, a doctor's advice should be obtained as soon as possible. *For inhalation by nebuliser*, the dose given by nebuliser is substantially higher than that given by inhaler. Patients should therefore be warned that it is dangerous to exceed the prescribed dose and they should seek medical advice if they fail to respond to the usual dose of the respirator solution.

Medicines for Children leaflet: Salbutamol inhaler for asthma and wheeze www.medicinesforchildren.org.uk/salbutamol-inhaler-asthma-and-wheeze

● **MEDICINAL FORMS** There can be variation in the licensing of different medicines containing the same drug.

Tablet
- Salbutamol (Non-proprietary)
  Salbutamol (as Salbutamol sulfate) 2 mg Salbutamol 2mg tablets | 28 tablet PoM £111.21 DT = £105.03
  Salbutamol (as Salbutamol sulfate) 4 mg Salbutamol 4mg tablets | 28 tablet PoM £113.85 DT = £107.52

Inhalation powder
- Easyhaler (salbutamol) (Orion Pharma (UK) Ltd)
  Salbutamol 100 microgram per 1 dose Easyhaler Salbutamol sulfate 100micrograms/dose dry powder inhaler | 200 dose PoM £3.31 DT = £3.31
  Salbutamol 200 microgram per 1 dose Easyhaler Salbutamol sulfate 200micrograms/dose dry powder inhaler | 200 dose PoM £6.63 DT = £6.63
- Salbulin Novolizer (Mylan)
  Salbutamol (as Salbutamol sulfate) 100 microgram per 1 dose Salbulin Novolizer 100micrograms/dose inhalation powder | 200 dose PoM £4.95 DT = £4.95
  Salbulin Novolizer 100micrograms/dose inhalation powder refill | 200 dose PoM £2.75
- Ventolin Accuhaler (GlaxoSmithKline UK Ltd)
  Salbutamol 200 microgram per 1 dose Ventolin 200micrograms/dose Accuhaler | 60 dose PoM £3.60 DT = £3.60

Solution for injection
- Ventolin (GlaxoSmithKline UK Ltd)
  Salbutamol (as Salbutamol sulfate) 500 microgram per 1 ml Ventolin 500micrograms/1ml solution for injection ampoules | 5 ampoule PoM £1.91

Solution for infusion
- Ventolin (GlaxoSmithKline UK Ltd)
  Salbutamol (as Salbutamol sulfate) 1 mg per 1 ml Ventolin 5mg/5ml solution for infusion ampoules | 10 ampoule PoM £24.81 DT = £24.81

Oral solution
- Salbutamol (Non-proprietary)
  Salbutamol (as Salbutamol sulfate) 400 microgram per 1 ml Salbutamol 2mg/5ml oral solution sugar free sugar-free | 150 ml PoM DT = £1.15
- Ventolin (GlaxoSmithKline UK Ltd)
  Salbutamol (as Salbutamol sulfate) 400 microgram per 1 ml Ventolin 2mg/5ml syrup sugar-free | 150 ml PoM £1.15 DT = £1.15

Pressurised inhalation
- Airomir (Teva UK Ltd)
  Salbutamol (as Salbutamol sulfate) 100 microgram per 1 dose Airomir 100micrograms/dose inhaler | 200 dose PoM £1.97 DT = £1.50
- Airomir Autohaler (Teva UK Ltd)
  Salbutamol (as Salbutamol sulfate) 100 microgram per 1 dose Airomir 100micrograms/dose Autohaler | 200 dose PoM £6.02 DT = £6.30
- Salamol (Teva UK Ltd)
  Salbutamol (as Salbutamol sulfate) 100 microgram per 1 dose Salamol 100micrograms/dose inhaler CFC free | 200 dose PoM £1.46 DT = £1.50
- Salamol Easi-Breathe (Teva UK Ltd)
  Salbutamol (as Salbutamol sulfate) 100 microgram per 1 dose Salamol 100micrograms/dose Easi-Breathe inhaler | 200 dose PoM £6.30 DT = £6.30
- Ventolin Evohaler (GlaxoSmithKline UK Ltd)
  Salbutamol (as Salbutamol sulfate) 100 microgram per 1 dose Ventolin 100micrograms/dose Evohaler | 200 dose PoM £1.50 DT = £1.50

Nebuliser liquid

- Salbutamol (Non-proprietary)
  Salbutamol (as Salbutamol sulfate) 1 mg per 1 ml Salbutamol 2.5mg/2.5ml nebuliser liquid unit dose vials | 20 unit dose PoM £4.94 DT = £3.77
  Salbutamol (as Salbutamol sulfate) 2 mg per 1 ml Salbutamol 5mg/2.5ml nebuliser liquid unit dose vials | 20 unit dose PoM £7.78 DT = £5.94
- Salamol Steri-Neb (Teva UK Ltd)
  Salbutamol (as Salbutamol sulfate) 2 mg per 1 ml Salamol 5mg/2.5ml nebuliser liquid Steri-Neb unit dose vials | 20 unit dose PoM £3.82 DT = £5.94
- Ventolin (GlaxoSmithKline UK Ltd)
  Salbutamol (as Salbutamol sulfate) 5 mg per 1 ml Ventolin 5mg/ml respirator solution | 20 ml PoM £2.18 DT = £2.18
- Ventolin Nebules (GlaxoSmithKline UK Ltd)
  Salbutamol (as Salbutamol sulfate) 1 mg per 1 ml Ventolin 2.5mg Nebules | 20 unit dose PoM £1.65 DT = £3.77
  Salbutamol (as Salbutamol sulfate) 2 mg per 1 ml Ventolin 5mg Nebules | 20 unit dose PoM £2.78 DT = £5.94

162

Terbutaline sulfate

● **INDICATIONS AND DOSE**

Acute asthma

▶ BY SUBCUTANEOUS INJECTION, OR BY SLOW INTRAVENOUS INJECTION
- Child 2–14 years: 10 micrograms/kg up to 4 times a day (max. per dose 300 micrograms), reserve intravenous beta$_2$ agonists for those in whom inhaled therapy cannot be used reliably or there is no current effect
- Child 15–17 years: 250–500 micrograms up to 4 times a day, reserve intravenous beta$_2$ agonists for those in whom inhaled therapy cannot be used reliably or there is no current effect

▶ BY CONTINUOUS INTRAVENOUS INFUSION
- Child: Loading dose 2–4 micrograms/kg, then 1–10 micrograms/kg/hour, dose to be adjusted according to response and heart rate, close monitoring is required for doses above 10 micrograms/kg/hour, reserve intravenous beta$_2$ agonists for those in whom inhaled therapy cannot be used reliably or there is no current effect

Moderate, severe, or life-threatening acute asthma

▶ BY INHALATION OF NEBULISED SOLUTION
- Child 1 month–4 years: 5 mg, repeat every 20–30 minutes or when required, give via oxygen-driven nebuliser if available
- Child 5–11 years: 5–10 mg, repeat every 20–30 minutes or when required, give via oxygen-driven nebuliser if available
- Child 12–17 years: 10 mg, repeat every 20–30 minutes or when required, give via oxygen-driven nebuliser if available

Exacerbation of reversible airways obstruction (including nocturnal asthma) | Prevention of exercise-induced bronchospasm

▶ BY INHALATION OF POWDER
- Child 5–17 years: 500 micrograms up to 4 times a day, for occasional use only

▶ BY MOUTH
- Child 1 month–6 years: 75 micrograms/kg 3 times a day (max. per dose 2.5 mg), administration by mouth is not recommended
- Child 7–14 years: 2.5 mg 2–3 times a day, administration by mouth is not recommended
- Child 15–17 years: Initially 2.5 mg 3 times a day, then increased if necessary to 5 mg 3 times a day, administration by mouth is not recommended

PHARMACOKINETICS
- At recommended inhaled doses, the duration of action of terbutaline is about 3 to 5 hours.

● **UNLICENSED USE**
- With oral use Tablets not licensed for use in children under 7 years.
- With intravenous use or subcutaneous use Injection not licensed for use in children under 2 years.

● **CAUTIONS** High doses of beta$_2$ agonists can be dangerous in some children

● **INTERACTIONS** → Appendix 1: beta$_2$ agonists

● **SIDE-EFFECTS**

GENERAL SIDE-EFFECTS
- **Common or very common** Hypotension · muscle spasms
- **Rare or very rare** Vasodilation
- **Frequency not known** Angioedema · anxiety · behaviour abnormal · bronchospasm · circulatory collapse · oral irritation · skin reactions · sleep disorder · throat irritation

SPECIFIC SIDE-EFFECTS
- **Uncommon**
- With parenteral use Pulmonary oedema
- **Rare or very rare**
- With parenteral use Lactic acidosis
- **Frequency not known**
- With parenteral use Akathisia · bleeding tendency

● **PREGNANCY** Inhaled drugs for asthma can be taken as normal during pregnancy.

● **BREAST FEEDING** Inhaled drugs for asthma can be taken as normal during breast-feeding.

● **DIRECTIONS FOR ADMINISTRATION**
- With intravenous use For *continuous intravenous infusion*, dilute to a concentration of 5 micrograms/mL with Glucose 5% *or* Sodium Chloride 0.9%; if fluid-restricted, dilute to a concentration of 100 micrograms/mL.
- When used by inhalation For *nebulisation*, dilute nebuliser solution with sterile Sodium Chloride 0.9% solution according to nebuliser type and duration of administration; terbutaline and ipratropium bromide solutions are compatible and may be mixed for nebulisation.

● **PATIENT AND CARER ADVICE**
- When used by inhalation *For inhalation by dry powder*, advise patients and carers not to exceed prescribed dose and to follow manufacturer's directions; if a previously effective dose of inhaled terbutaline fails to provide at least 3 hours relief, a doctor's advice should be obtained as soon as possible. *For inhalation by nebuliser*, the dose given by nebuliser is substantially higher than that given by inhaler. Patients should therefore be warned that it is dangerous to exceed the prescribed dose and they should seek medical advice if they fail to respond to the usual dose of the respirator solution.

● **MEDICINAL FORMS** There can be variation in the licensing of different medicines containing the same drug.

Tablet
- Bricanyl (AstraZeneca UK Ltd)
  Terbutaline sulfate 5 mg Bricanyl 5mg tablets | 100 tablet PoM £14.73 DT = £14.73

Inhalation powder
- Bricanyl Turbohaler (AstraZeneca UK Ltd)
  Terbutaline sulfate 500 microgram per 1 dose Bricanyl 500micrograms/dose Turbohaler | 120 dose PoM £8.30 DT = £8.30

Solution for injection
- Bricanyl (AstraZeneca UK Ltd)
  Terbutaline sulfate 500 microgram per 1 ml Bricanyl 2.5mg/5ml solution for injection ampoules | 10 ampoule PoM £20.09 DT = £20.09
  Bricanyl 500micrograms/1ml solution for injection ampoules | 5 ampoule PoM £6.48 DT = £6.48

Nebuliser liquid
- Terbutaline sulfate (Non-proprietary)
  Terbutaline sulfate 2.5 mg per 1 ml Terbutaline 5mg/2ml nebuliser liquid unit dose vials | 20 unit dose PoM £4.26–£5.13 DT = £4.75

▸ Bricanyl Respules (AstraZeneca UK Ltd)
Terbutaline sulfate 2.5 mg per 1 ml Bricanyl 5mg/2ml Respules | 20 unit dose PoM £11.64 DT = £4.75

CORTICOSTEROIDS

Corticosteroids (inhaled)

IMPORTANT SAFETY INFORMATION

MHRA/CHM ADVICE: CORTICOSTEROIDS: RARE RISK OF CENTRAL SEROUS CHORIORETINOPATHY WITH LOCAL AS WELL AS SYSTEMIC ADMINISTRATION (AUGUST 2017)

Central serous chorioretinopathy is a retinal disorder that has been linked to the systemic use of corticosteroids. Recently, it has also been reported after local administration of corticosteroids via inhaled and intranasal, epidural, intra-articular, topical dermal, and periocular routes. The MHRA recommends that patients should be advised to report any blurred vision or other visual disturbances with corticosteroid treatment given by any route; consider referral to an ophthalmologist for evaluation of possible causes if a patient presents with vision problems.

● **SIDE-EFFECTS**

▸ **Common or very common** Headache · oral candidiasis · taste altered · voice alteration
▸ **Uncommon** Anxiety · bronchospasm paradoxical · cataract · vision blurred
▸ **Rare or very rare** Adrenal suppression · behaviour abnormal · glaucoma · growth retardation · sleep disorder
▸ **Frequency not known** Pneumonia (in patients with COPD)

SIDE-EFFECTS, FURTHER INFORMATION Systemic absorption may follow inhaled administration particularly if high doses are used or if treatment is prolonged. Therefore also consider the side-effects of systemic corticosteroids.

Candidiasis The risk of oral candidiasis can be reduced by using a spacer device with the corticosteroid inhaler; rinsing the mouth with water after inhalation of a dose may also be helpful. An anti-fungal oral suspension or oral gel can be used to treat oral candidiasis without discontinuing corticosteroid therapy.

Paradoxical bronchospasm The potential for paradoxical bronchospasm (calling for discontinuation and alternative therapy) should be borne in mind. Mild bronchospasm may be prevented by inhalation of a short-acting $beta_2$ agonist beforehand (or by transfer from an aerosol inhalation to a dry powder inhalation).

● **PREGNANCY** Inhaled drugs for asthma can be taken as normal during pregnancy.

● **BREAST FEEDING** Inhaled corticosteroids for asthma can be taken as normal during breast-feeding.

● **MONITORING REQUIREMENTS** The height and weight of children receiving prolonged treatment with inhaled corticosteroids should be monitored annually; if growth is slowed, referral to a paediatrician should be considered.

● **NATIONAL FUNDING/ACCESS DECISIONS**

NICE decisions

▸ **Inhaled corticosteroids for the treatment of chronic asthma in children under 12 years (November 2007)** NICE TA131

▸ When used by inhalation For children under 12 years with chronic asthma in whom treatment with an inhaled corticosteroid is considered appropriate, the least costly product that is suitable for an individual child (taking into consideration NICE TAs 38 and 10), within its marketing authorisation, is recommended. For children under 12 years with chronic asthma in whom treatment with an inhaled corticosteroid and a long-acting $beta_2$ agonist is considered appropriate, the following apply:
- the use of a combination inhaler within its marketing authorisation is recommended as an option;
- the decision to use a combination inhaler or two agents in separate inhalers should be made on an individual basis, taking into consideration therapeutic need and the likelihood of treatment adherence;
- if a combination inhaler is chosen, then the least costly inhaler that is suitable for the individual child is recommended.

www.nice.org.uk/guidance/ta131

▸ **Inhaled corticosteroids for the treatment of chronic asthma in adults and children over 12 years (March 2008)** NICE TA138

▸ When used by inhalation For adults and children over 12 years with chronic asthma in whom treatment with an inhaled corticosteroid is considered appropriate, the least costly product that is suitable for an individual (taking into consideration NICE TAs 38 and 10), within its marketing authorisation is recommended. For adults and children over 12 years with chronic asthma in whom treatment with an inhaled corticosteroid and a long-acting $beta_2$ agonist is considered appropriate, the following apply:
- the use of a combination inhaler within its marketing authorisation is recommended as an option;
- the decision to use a combination inhaler or two agents in separate inhalers should be made on an individual basis, taking into consideration therapeutic need, and the likelihood of treatment adherence;
- if a combination inhaler is chosen, then the least costly inhaler that is suitable for the individual is recommended.

www.nice.org.uk/guidance/ta138

F above

Beclometasone dipropionate

15-May-2020

(Beclomethasone dipropionate)

● **INDICATIONS AND DOSE**

Prophylaxis of asthma

▸ BY INHALATION OF POWDER
▸ Child 5–11 years: 100–200 micrograms twice daily, dose to be adjusted as necessary
▸ Child 12–17 years: 200–400 micrograms twice daily; increased if necessary up to 800 micrograms twice daily, dose to be adjusted as necessary

CLENIL MODULITE®

Prophylaxis of asthma

▸ BY INHALATION OF AEROSOL
▸ Child 2–11 years: 100–200 micrograms twice daily
▸ Child 12–17 years: 200–400 micrograms twice daily, adjusted according to response; increased if necessary up to 1 mg twice daily

QVAR® PREPARATIONS

Prophylaxis of asthma

▸ BY INHALATION OF AEROSOL
▸ Child 5–11 years: 50–100 micrograms twice daily
▸ Child 12–17 years: 50–200 micrograms twice daily; increased if necessary up to 400 micrograms twice daily

POTENCY

▸ *Qvar*® has extra-fine particles, is more potent than traditional beclometasone dipropionate CFC-containing inhalers and is approximately twice as potent as *Clenil Modulite*®.

SOPROBEC®

Prophylaxis of asthma

▸ BY INHALATION OF AEROSOL
▸ Child: 100 micrograms twice daily; increased if necessary up to 400 micrograms daily in 2–4 divided doses

continued →

DOSE EQUIVALENCE AND CONVERSION
- Dose adjustments may be required for some inhaler devices, see under individual preparations.

- **UNLICENSED USE** *Easyhaler® Beclometasone Dipropionate* is not licensed for use in children. *Clenil Modulite®* 200 and 250 are not licensed for use in children.

IMPORTANT SAFETY INFORMATION

MHRA/CHM ADVICE (JULY 2008)

Beclometasone dipropionate CFC-free pressurised metered-dose inhalers (*Qvar®* and *Clenil Modulite®*) are **not** interchangeable and should be prescribed by brand name; *Qvar®* has extra-fine particles, is more potent than traditional beclometasone dipropionate CFC-containing inhalers, and is approximately twice as potent as *Clenil Modulite®*.

MHRA/CHM ADVICE: PRESSURISED METERED DOSE INHALERS (PMDI): RISK OF AIRWAY OBSTRUCTION FROM ASPIRATION OF LOOSE OBJECTS (JULY 2018)

See Respiratory system, drug delivery p. 153.

- **INTERACTIONS** → Appendix 1: corticosteroids
- **SIDE-EFFECTS**
  - **Common or very common** Throat irritation
  - **Rare or very rare** Wheezing
- **PRESCRIBING AND DISPENSING INFORMATION** The MHRA has advised (July 2008) that beclometasone dipropionate CFC-free inhalers should be prescribed by brand name. Pressurised metered-doses inhalers with extra-fine particles (*Qvar®* and *Kelhale®*) are more potent than, and not interchangeable with, traditional CFC-containing and CFC-free inhalers (*Clenil Modulite®* and *Soprobec®*).

  QVAR® PREPARATIONS When switching a patient with well-controlled asthma from another corticosteroid inhaler, initially a 100-microgram metered dose of *Qvar®* should be prescribed for 200–250 micrograms of beclometasone dipropionate or budesonide and for 100 micrograms of fluticasone propionate. When switching a patient with poorly controlled asthma from another corticosteroid inhaler, initially a 100-microgram metered dose of *Qvar®* should be prescribed for 100 micrograms of beclometasone dipropionate, budesonide, or fluticasone propionate; the dose of *Qvar®* should be adjusted according to response.
- **PATIENT AND CARER ADVICE** Steroid card should be issued with high doses of inhaled beclometasone dipropionate. Medicines for Children leaflet: Beclometasone inhaler for asthma prevention (prophylaxis) www.medicinesforchildren.org.uk/beclometasone-inhaler-asthma-prevention-prophylaxis-0
- **PROFESSION SPECIFIC INFORMATION**

  Dental practitioners' formulary

  Clenil Modulite® 50 micrograms/metered inhalation may be prescribed.

- **MEDICINAL FORMS** There can be variation in the licensing of different medicines containing the same drug. Forms available from special-order manufacturers include: cream, ointment

Inhalation powder

CAUTIONARY AND ADVISORY LABELS 8, 10

- Easyhaler (beclometasone) (Orion Pharma (UK) Ltd)
  - **Beclometasone dipropionate 200 microgram per 1 dose** Easyhaler Beclometasone 200micrograms/dose dry powder inhaler | 200 dose PoM £14.93 DT = £14.93

Pressurised inhalation

CAUTIONARY AND ADVISORY LABELS 8, 10

- Clenil Modulite (Chiesi Ltd)
  - **Beclometasone dipropionate 50 microgram per 1 dose** Clenil Modulite 50micrograms/dose inhaler | 200 dose PoM £3.70 DT = £3.70
  - **Beclometasone dipropionate 100 microgram per 1 dose** Clenil Modulite 100micrograms/dose inhaler | 200 dose PoM £7.42 DT = £7.42
  - **Beclometasone dipropionate 200 microgram per 1 dose** Clenil Modulite 200micrograms/dose inhaler | 200 dose PoM £16.17 DT = £16.17
  - **Beclometasone dipropionate 250 microgram per 1 dose** Clenil Modulite 250micrograms/dose inhaler | 200 dose PoM £16.29 DT = £16.29
- Kelhale (Cipla EU Ltd)
  - **Beclometasone dipropionate 50 microgram per 1 dose** Kelhale 50micrograms/dose inhaler | 200 dose PoM £5.20 DT = £3.70
  - **Beclometasone dipropionate 100 microgram per 1 dose** Kelhale 100micrograms/dose inhaler | 200 dose PoM £5.20 DT = £7.42
- Qvar (Teva UK Ltd)
  - **Beclometasone dipropionate 50 microgram per 1 dose** Qvar 50 inhaler | 200 dose PoM £7.87 DT = £3.70
  - **Beclometasone dipropionate 100 microgram per 1 dose** Qvar 100 inhaler | 200 dose PoM £17.21 DT = £7.42
- Qvar Autohaler (Teva UK Ltd)
  - **Beclometasone dipropionate 50 microgram per 1 dose** Qvar 50 Autohaler | 200 dose PoM £7.87 DT = £7.87
  - **Beclometasone dipropionate 100 microgram per 1 dose** Qvar 100 Autohaler | 200 dose PoM £17.21 DT = £17.21
- Qvar Easi-Breathe (Teva UK Ltd)
  - **Beclometasone dipropionate 50 microgram per 1 dose** Qvar 50micrograms/dose Easi-Breathe inhaler | 200 dose PoM £7.74 DT = £7.87
  - **Beclometasone dipropionate 100 microgram per 1 dose** Qvar 100micrograms/dose Easi-Breathe inhaler | 200 dose PoM £16.95 DT = £17.21
- Soprobec (Glenmark Pharmaceuticals Europe Ltd)
  - **Beclometasone dipropionate 50 microgram per 1 dose** Soprobec 50micrograms/dose inhaler | 200 dose PoM £2.78 DT = £3.70
  - **Beclometasone dipropionate 100 microgram per 1 dose** Soprobec 100micrograms/dose inhaler | 200 dose PoM £5.57 DT = £7.42
  - **Beclometasone dipropionate 200 microgram per 1 dose** Soprobec 200micrograms/dose inhaler | 200 dose PoM £12.13 DT = £16.17
  - **Beclometasone dipropionate 250 microgram per 1 dose** Soprobec 250micrograms/dose inhaler | 200 dose PoM £12.22 DT = £16.29

F 167

Budesonide

21-Dec-2017

- **DRUG ACTION** Budesonide is a glucocorticoid, which exerts significant local anti-inflammatory effects.

- **INDICATIONS AND DOSE**

Bronchopulmonary dysplasia with spontaneous respiration

- BY INHALATION OF NEBULISED SUSPENSION
  - Neonate: 500 micrograms twice daily.
  - Child 1–4 months: 500 micrograms twice daily

Bronchopulmonary dysplasia with spontaneous respiration (severe symptoms)

- BY INHALATION OF NEBULISED SUSPENSION
  - Child 1–4 months (body-weight 2.5 kg and above): 1 mg twice daily

Prophylaxis of mild to moderate asthma (in patients stabilised on twice daily dose)

- BY INHALATION OF POWDER
  - Child 6–11 years: 200–400 micrograms once daily, dose to be given in the evening
  - Child 12–17 years: 200–400 micrograms once daily (max. per dose 800 micrograms), dose to be given in the evening

Prophylaxis of asthma

- BY INHALATION OF POWDER
  - Child 6–11 years: 100–400 micrograms twice daily, dose to be adjusted as necessary
  - Child 12–17 years: 100–800 micrograms twice daily, dose to be adjusted as necessary
- BY INHALATION OF NEBULISED SUSPENSION
  - Child 6 months–11 years: 125–500 micrograms twice daily, adjusted according to response; maximum 2 mg per day

- Child 12–17 years: Initially 0.25–1 mg twice daily, adjusted according to response, doses higher than recommended max. may be used in severe disease; maximum 2 mg per day

BUDELIN NOVOLIZER ®

Prophylaxis of asthma

▶ BY INHALATION OF POWDER

- Child 6–11 years: 200–400 micrograms twice daily, dose is adjusted as necessary
- Child 12–17 years: 200–800 micrograms twice daily, dose is adjusted as necessary

Alternative in mild to moderate asthma, for patients previously stabilised on a twice daily dose

▶ BY INHALATION OF POWDER

- Child 6–11 years: 200–400 micrograms once daily, to be taken in the evening
- Child 12–17 years: 200–400 micrograms once daily (max. per dose 800 micrograms), to be taken in the evening

PULMICORT ® RESPULES

Prophylaxis of asthma

▶ BY INHALATION OF NEBULISED SUSPENSION

- Child 3 months–11 years: Initially 0.5–1 mg twice daily, reduced to 250–500 micrograms twice daily
- Child 12–17 years: Initially 1–2 mg twice daily, reduced to 0.5–1 mg twice daily

Croup

▶ BY INHALATION OF NEBULISED SUSPENSION

- Child: 2 mg for 1 dose, alternatively 1 mg for 2 doses separated by a 30 minute interval, dose may be repeated every 12 hours until clinical improvement

PULMICORT ® TURBOHALER

Prophylaxis of asthma

▶ BY INHALATION OF POWDER

- Child 5–11 years: 100–400 micrograms twice daily, dose to be adjusted as necessary
- Child 12–17 years: 100–800 micrograms twice daily, dose to be adjusted as necessary

Alternative in mild to moderate asthma, for patients previously stabilised on a twice daily dose

▶ BY INHALATION OF POWDER

- Child 5–11 years: 200–400 micrograms once daily, to be taken in the evening
- Child 12–17 years: 200–400 micrograms once daily (max. per dose 800 micrograms), to be taken in the evening

POTENCY

- Dose adjustments may be required for some inhaler devices, see under individual preparations.

● UNLICENSED USE *Pulmicort® nebuliser solution* not licensed for use in children under 3 months; not licensed for use in bronchopulmonary dysplasia.

● INTERACTIONS → Appendix 1: corticosteroids

● DIRECTIONS FOR ADMINISTRATION Budesonide nebuliser suspension is not suitable for use in ultrasonic nebulisers.

● PATIENT AND CARER ADVICE With high doses, a steroid card should be supplied. Patients or carers should be given advice on how to administer budesonide dry powder inhaler and nebuliser suspension.

Medicines for Children leaflet: Budesonide inhaler for asthma prevention (prophylaxis) www.medicinesforchildren.org.uk/budesonide-inhaler-asthma-prevention-prophylaxis

BUDELIN NOVOLIZER ® Patients or carers should be given advice on administration of *Budelin Novolizer®*.

● MEDICINAL FORMS There can be variation in the licensing of different medicines containing the same drug.

Inhalation powder

CAUTIONARY AND ADVISORY LABELS 8, 10

▶ Budelin Novolizer (Mylan)

Budesonide 200 microgram per 1 dose Budelin Novolizer 200micrograms/dose inhalation powder | 100 dose PoM £14.86 DT = £14.86

Budelin Novolizer 200micrograms/dose inhalation powder refill | 100 dose PoM £9.59 DT = £9.59

▶ Easyhaler (budesonide) (Orion Pharma (UK) Ltd)

Budesonide 100 microgram per 1 dose Easyhaler Budesonide 100micrograms/dose dry powder inhaler | 200 dose PoM £8.86 DT = £14.25

Budesonide 200 microgram per 1 dose Easyhaler Budesonide 200micrograms/dose dry powder inhaler | 200 dose PoM £17.71

Budesonide 400 microgram per 1 dose Easyhaler Budesonide 400micrograms/dose dry powder inhaler | 100 dose PoM £17.71

▶ Pulmicort Turbohaler (AstraZeneca UK Ltd)

Budesonide 100 microgram per 1 dose Pulmicort 100 Turbohaler | 200 dose PoM £14.25 DT = £14.25

Budesonide 200 microgram per 1 dose Pulmicort 200 Turbohaler | 100 dose PoM £14.25 DT = £14.25

Budesonide 400 microgram per 1 dose Pulmicort 400 Turbohaler | 50 dose PoM £14.25 DT = £14.25

Nebuliser liquid

CAUTIONARY AND ADVISORY LABELS 8, 10

▶ Budesonide (Non-proprietary)

Budesonide 250 microgram per 1 ml Budesonide 500micrograms/2ml nebuliser liquid unit dose vials | 20 unit dose PoM £26.03 DT = £25.94

Budesonide 500 microgram per 1 ml Budesonide 1mg/2ml nebuliser liquid unit dose vials | 20 unit dose PoM £39.47 DT = £39.47

▶ Pulmicort Respules (AstraZeneca UK Ltd)

Budesonide 250 microgram per 1 ml Pulmicort 0.5mg Respules | 20 unit dose PoM £31.70 DT = £25.94

Budesonide 500 microgram per 1 ml Pulmicort 1mg Respules | 20 unit dose PoM £48.00 DT = £39.47

Budesonide with formoterol

08-Feb-2018

The properties listed below are those particular to the combination only. For the properties of the components please consider, budesonide p. 168, formoterol fumarate p. 162.

● INDICATIONS AND DOSE

SYMBICORT 100/6 TURBOHALER ®

Asthma, maintenance therapy

▶ BY INHALATION OF POWDER

- Child 6–17 years: Initially 1–2 puffs twice daily; reduced to 1 puff daily, dose reduced only if control is maintained

Asthma, maintenance and reliever therapy

▶ BY INHALATION OF POWDER

- Child 12–17 years: Maintenance 2 puffs daily in 1–2 divided doses; 1 puff as required for relief of symptoms, increased if necessary up to 6 puffs as required, max. 8 puffs per day; up to 12 puffs daily can be used for a limited time but medical assessment is recommended

SYMBICORT 200/6 TURBOHALER ®

Asthma, maintenance therapy

▶ BY INHALATION OF POWDER

- Child 12–17 years: Initially 1–2 puffs twice daily; reduced to 1 puff daily, dose reduced only if control is maintained

Asthma, maintenance and reliever therapy

▶ BY INHALATION OF POWDER

- Child 12–17 years: Maintenance 2 puffs daily in 1–2 divided doses, increased if necessary to 2 puffs twice daily; 1 puff as required for relief of

continued →

symptoms, increased if necessary up to 6 puffs as required, max. 8 puffs per day; up to 12 puffs daily can be used for a limited time but medical assessment is recommended

SYMBICORT 400/12 TURBOHALER ®

Asthma, maintenance therapy

▶ BY INHALATION OF POWDER

▸ Child 12–17 years: Initially 1 puff twice daily; reduced to 1 puff daily, dose reduced only if control is maintained

- **INTERACTIONS** → Appendix 1: beta$_2$ agonists · corticosteroids
- **PATIENT AND CARER ADVICE** Patient counselling is advised for budesonide with formoterol inhalation (administration).
  With high doses, a steroid card should be supplied.
- **NATIONAL FUNDING/ACCESS DECISIONS**

Scottish Medicines Consortium (SMC) decisions

The *Scottish Medicines Consortium* has advised (June 2017) that budesonide/formoterol 100 micrograms/6 micrograms and 200 micrograms/6 micrograms (*Symbicort*® SMART ®) is accepted for use within NHS Scotland for regular treatment of asthma where use of a combination (inhaled corticosteroid and a long-acting β_2 adrenoceptor agonist) is appropriate: patients already adequately controlled on both or patients not adequately controlled with inhaled corticosteroids and "as needed" short-acting β_2 adrenoceptor agonists. This advice relates to the extension of the license for *Symbicort* maintenance and reliever therapy (SMART ®) to adolescents aged 12 years and over.

- **MEDICINAL FORMS** There can be variation in the licensing of different medicines containing the same drug.

Inhalation powder

CAUTIONARY AND ADVISORY LABELS 8, 10 (high doses)

▸ Symbicort Turbohaler (AstraZeneca UK Ltd)

Formoterol fumarate dihydrate 6 microgram per 1 dose, Budesonide 100 microgram per 1 dose Symbicort 100/6 Turbohaler | 120 dose [PoM] £28.00 DT = £28.00

Formoterol fumarate dihydrate 6 microgram per 1 dose, Budesonide 200 microgram per 1 dose Symbicort 200/6 Turbohaler | 120 dose [PoM] £28.00 DT = £28.00

Formoterol fumarate dihydrate 12 microgram per 1 dose, Budesonide 400 microgram per 1 dose Symbicort 400/12 Turbohaler | 60 dose [PoM] £28.00 DT = £28.00

F 167

Ciclesonide

01-Feb-2019

- **INDICATIONS AND DOSE**

Prophylaxis of asthma

▶ BY INHALATION OF AEROSOL

▸ Child 12–17 years: 160 micrograms once daily; reduced to 80 micrograms once daily, if control maintained; increased if necessary up to 320 micrograms twice daily, in severe asthma

> **IMPORTANT SAFETY INFORMATION**
>
> MHRA/CHM ADVICE: PRESSURISED METERED DOSE INHALERS (PMDI): RISK OF AIRWAY OBSTRUCTION FROM ASPIRATION OF LOOSE OBJECTS (JULY 2018)
>
> See Respiratory system, drug delivery p. 153.

- **INTERACTIONS** → Appendix 1: corticosteroids
- **SIDE-EFFECTS** Cushing's syndrome
- **HEPATIC IMPAIRMENT** Manufacturer advises caution in severe impairment (risk of increased exposure, no information available).
- **PATIENT AND CARER ADVICE** Patients or carers should be given advice on how to administer ciclesonide aerosol inhaler.
- **MEDICINAL FORMS** There can be variation in the licensing of different medicines containing the same drug.

Pressurised inhalation

CAUTIONARY AND ADVISORY LABELS 8

▸ Alvesco (AstraZeneca UK Ltd)

Ciclesonide 80 microgram per 1 dose Alvesco 80 inhaler | 120 dose [PoM] £32.83 DT = £32.83

Ciclesonide 160 microgram per 1 dose Alvesco 160 inhaler | 60 dose [PoM] £19.31 DT = £19.31 | 120 dose [PoM] £38.62 DT = £38.62

F 167

Fluticasone

21-Dec-2017

- **INDICATIONS AND DOSE**

Prophylaxis of asthma

▶ BY INHALATION OF POWDER

▸ Child 5–15 years: Initially 50–100 micrograms twice daily (max. per dose 200 micrograms twice daily), dose to be adjusted as necessary

▸ Child 16–17 years: Initially 100–500 micrograms twice daily (max. per dose 1 mg twice daily), dose may be increased according to severity of asthma. Doses above 500 micrograms twice daily initiated by a specialist

▶ BY INHALATION OF AEROSOL

▸ Child 4–15 years: Initially 50–100 micrograms twice daily (max. per dose 200 micrograms twice daily), dose to be adjusted as necessary

▸ Child 16–17 years: Initially 100–500 micrograms twice daily (max. per dose 1 mg twice daily), dose may be increased according to severity of asthma. Doses above 500 micrograms twice daily initiated by a specialist

▶ BY INHALATION OF NEBULISED SUSPENSION

▸ Child 4–15 years: 1 mg twice daily

▸ Child 16–17 years: 0.5–2 mg twice daily

> **IMPORTANT SAFETY INFORMATION**
>
> MHRA/CHM ADVICE: PRESSURISED METERED DOSE INHALERS (PMDI): RISK OF AIRWAY OBSTRUCTION FROM ASPIRATION OF LOOSE OBJECTS (JULY 2018)
>
> See Respiratory system, drug delivery p. 153.

- **INTERACTIONS** → Appendix 1: corticosteroids
- **SIDE-EFFECTS**

▶ **Rare or very rare** Dyspepsia

- **DIRECTIONS FOR ADMINISTRATION** Fluticasone nebuliser liquid may be diluted with sterile sodium chloride 0.9%. It is not suitable for use in ultrasonic nebulisers.
- **PATIENT AND CARER ADVICE** Patients or carers should be given advice on how to administer all fluticasone inhalation preparations.
  With high doses, a steroid card should be supplied.
  Medicines for Children leaflet: Fluticasone inhaler for asthma prevention (prophylaxis) www.medicinesforchildren.org.uk/fluticasone-inhaler-asthma-prevention-prophylaxis
- **MEDICINAL FORMS** There can be variation in the licensing of different medicines containing the same drug.

Inhalation powder

CAUTIONARY AND ADVISORY LABELS 8, 10

▸ Flixotide Accuhaler (GlaxoSmithKline UK Ltd)

Fluticasone propionate 50 microgram per 1 dose Flixotide 50micrograms/dose Accuhaler | 60 dose [PoM] £4.00 DT = £4.00

Fluticasone propionate 100 microgram per 1 dose Flixotide 100micrograms/dose Accuhaler | 60 dose [PoM] £8.00 DT = £8.00

Fluticasone propionate 250 microgram per 1 dose Flixotide 250micrograms/dose Accuhaler | 60 dose [PoM] £25.51 DT = £25.51

Fluticasone propionate 500 microgram per 1 dose Flixotide 500micrograms/dose Accuhaler | 60 dose [PoM] £43.37 DT = £43.37

Pressurised inhalation

CAUTIONARY AND ADVISORY LABELS 8, 10

▸ Flixotide Evohaler (GlaxoSmithKline UK Ltd)

Fluticasone propionate 50 microgram per 1 dose Flixotide 50micrograms/dose Evohaler | 120 dose PoM £6.53 DT = £6.53

Fluticasone propionate 125 microgram per 1 dose Flixotide 125micrograms/dose Evohaler | 120 dose PoM £21.26 DT = £21.26

Fluticasone propionate 250 microgram per 1 dose Flixotide 250micrograms/dose Evohaler | 120 dose PoM £36.14 DT = £36.14

Nebuliser liquid

CAUTIONARY AND ADVISORY LABELS 8, 10

▸ Flixotide Nebule (GlaxoSmithKline UK Ltd)

Fluticasone propionate 250 microgram per 1 ml Flixotide 0.5mg/2ml Nebules | 10 unit dose PoM £9.34 DT = £9.34

Fluticasone propionate 1 mg per 1 ml Flixotide 2mg/2ml Nebules | 10 unit dose PoM £37.35 DT = £37.35

Fluticasone with formoterol

16-Mar-2020

The properties listed below are those particular to the combination only. For the properties of the components please consider, fluticasone p. 170, formoterol fumarate p. 162.

● **INDICATIONS AND DOSE**

FLUTIFORM ® 125

Prophylaxis of asthma

▸ BY INHALATION OF AEROSOL

▸ Child 12–17 years: 2 puffs twice daily

FLUTIFORM ® 50

Prophylaxis of asthma

▸ BY INHALATION OF AEROSOL

▸ Child 5–17 years: 2 puffs twice daily

FLUTIFORM ® K-HALER 125

Prophylaxis of asthma

▸ BY INHALATION OF AEROSOL

▸ Child 12–17 years: 2 puffs twice daily

FLUTIFORM ® K-HALER 50

Prophylaxis of asthma

▸ BY INHALATION OF AEROSOL

▸ Child 12–17 years: 2 puffs twice daily

● **INTERACTIONS** → Appendix 1: $beta_2$ agonists · corticosteroids

● **SIDE-EFFECTS**

▸ **Uncommon** Dry mouth · rash · sleep disorders

▸ **Rare or very rare** Asthenia · cough · diarrhoea · dyspepsia · hypertension · muscle spasms · oral fungal infection · peripheral oedema · vertigo

● **PATIENT AND CARER ADVICE** Patients or carers should be given advice on how to administer fluticasone with formoterol aerosol inhalation.

With high doses, a steroid card should be provided.

● **NATIONAL FUNDING/ACCESS DECISIONS**

Scottish Medicines Consortium (SMC) decisions

SMC No. 736/11

The *Scottish Medicines Consortium* has advised (October 2012) that fluticasone propionate with formoterol fumarate metered dose inhaler (*Flutiform* ®) is accepted for use within NHS Scotland for the regular treatment of asthma where the use of a combination product (an inhaled corticosteroid and a long-acting $beta_2$ agonist) is appropriate:

- for patients not adequately controlled with inhaled corticosteroids and 'as required' inhaled short-acting $beta_2$ agonist, **or**
- for patients already adequately controlled on both an inhaled corticosteroid and a long-acting $beta_2$ agonist.

SMC No. SMC2178

The *Scottish Medicines Consortium* has advised (June 2019) that fluticasone propionate with formoterol fumarate (*Flutiform* ®) is accepted for use within NHS Scotland for the regular treatment of asthma in children aged 5 to 12 years where the use of a combination product (an inhaled corticosteroid and a long-acting $beta_2$ agonist) is appropriate:

- for patients not adequately controlled with inhaled corticosteroids and 'as required' inhaled short-acting $beta_2$ agonist, **or**
- for patients already adequately controlled on both an inhaled corticosteroid and a long-acting $beta_2$ agonist.

● **MEDICINAL FORMS** There can be variation in the licensing of different medicines containing the same drug.

Pressurised inhalation

CAUTIONARY AND ADVISORY LABELS 8, 10 (high doses)

▸ Flutiform (Napp Pharmaceuticals Ltd)

Formoterol fumarate dihydrate 5 microgram per 1 dose, Fluticasone propionate 50 microgram per 1 dose Flutiform 50micrograms/dose / 5micrograms/dose inhaler | 120 dose PoM £14.40 DT = £14.40

Formoterol fumarate dihydrate 5 microgram per 1 dose, Fluticasone propionate 125 microgram per 1 dose Flutiform 125micrograms/dose / 5micrograms/dose inhaler | 120 dose PoM £28.00 DT = £28.00

▸ Flutiform K-haler (Napp Pharmaceuticals Ltd)

Formoterol fumarate dihydrate 5 microgram per 1 dose, Fluticasone propionate 50 microgram per 1 dose Flutiform K-haler 50micrograms/dose / 5micrograms/dose breath actuated inhaler | 120 dose PoM £14.40 DT = £14.40

Formoterol fumarate dihydrate 5 microgram per 1 dose, Fluticasone propionate 125 microgram per 1 dose Flutiform K-haler 125micrograms/dose / 5micrograms/dose breath actuated inhaler | 120 dose PoM £28.00 DT = £28.00

Fluticasone with salmeterol

05-May-2020

The properties listed below are those particular to the combination only. For the properties of the components please consider, fluticasone p. 170, salmeterol p. 163.

● **INDICATIONS AND DOSE**

COMBISAL ® 25/125

Prophylaxis of asthma

▸ BY INHALATION OF AEROSOL

▸ Child 12–17 years: 2 inhalations twice daily

COMBISAL ® 25/250

Prophylaxis of asthma

▸ BY INHALATION OF AEROSOL

▸ Child 12–17 years: 2 inhalations twice daily

COMBISAL ® 25/50

Prophylaxis of asthma

▸ BY INHALATION OF AEROSOL

▸ Child 4–17 years: 2 inhalations twice daily, reduced to 2 inhalations once daily, use reduced dose only if control maintained

FUSACOMB 50/250 EASYHALER ®

Prophylaxis of asthma

▸ BY INHALATION OF POWDER

▸ Child 12–17 years: 1 inhalation twice daily, reduced to 1 inhalation once daily, use reduced dose only if control maintained

FUSACOMB 50/500 EASYHALER ®

Prophylaxis of asthma

▸ BY INHALATION OF POWDER

▸ Child 12–17 years: 1 inhalation twice daily

continued →

3 Respiratory system

SERETIDE 100 ACCUHALER ®

Prophylaxis of asthma

▶ BY INHALATION OF POWDER

▸ Child 4–17 years: 1 inhalation twice daily, reduced to 1 inhalation once daily, use reduced dose only if control maintained

SERETIDE 125 EVOHALER ®

Prophylaxis of asthma

▶ BY INHALATION OF AEROSOL

▸ Child 12–17 years: 2 puffs twice daily

SERETIDE 250 ACCUHALER ®

Prophylaxis of asthma

▶ BY INHALATION OF POWDER

▸ Child 12–17 years: 1 inhalation twice daily

SERETIDE 250 EVOHALER ®

Prophylaxis of asthma

▶ BY INHALATION OF AEROSOL

▸ Child 12–17 years: 2 puffs twice daily

SERETIDE 50 EVOHALER ®

Prophylaxis of asthma

▶ BY INHALATION OF AEROSOL

▸ Child 4–17 years: 2 puffs twice daily, reduced to 2 puffs once daily, use reduced dose only if control maintained

SERETIDE 500 ACCUHALER ®

Prophylaxis of asthma

▶ BY INHALATION OF POWDER

▸ Child 12–17 years: 1 inhalation twice daily

● INTERACTIONS → Appendix 1: $beta_2$ agonists · corticosteroids

● PRESCRIBING AND DISPENSING INFORMATION

SEREFLO ® 125 Manufacturer advises spacer devices are not compatible—if spacer device required, switch to alternative fixed-dose combination preparation.

COMBISAL ® 25/50 Manufacturer advises only AeroChamber Plus ® spacer devices are compatible.

COMBISAL ® 25/125 Manufacturer advises only AeroChamber Plus ® spacer devices are compatible.

COMBISAL ® 25/250 Manufacturer advises only AeroChamber Plus ® spacer devices are compatible.

● PATIENT AND CARER ADVICE Patients or carers should be given advice on how to administer fluticasone with salmeterol dry powder inhalation and aerosol inhalation.

With preparations containing greater than 100 micrograms fluticasone, a steroid card should be provided.

● MEDICINAL FORMS There can be variation in the licensing of different medicines containing the same drug.

Inhalation powder

CAUTIONARY AND ADVISORY LABELS 8, 10 (excluding Seretide 100 Accuhaler ®)

▸ Fusacomb Easyhaler (Orion Pharma (UK) Ltd)

Salmeterol (as Salmeterol xinafoate) 50 microgram per 1 dose, Fluticasone propionate 250 microgram per 1 dose Fusacomb Easyhaler 50micrograms/dose / 250micrograms/dose dry powder inhaler | 60 dose PoM £21.50 DT = £33.95

Salmeterol (as Salmeterol xinafoate) 50 microgram per 1 dose, Fluticasone propionate 500 microgram per 1 dose Fusacomb Easyhaler 50micrograms/dose / 500micrograms/dose dry powder inhaler | 60 dose PoM £26.99 DT = £32.74

▸ Seretide Accuhaler (GlaxoSmithKline UK Ltd)

Salmeterol (as Salmeterol xinafoate) 50 microgram per 1 dose, Fluticasone propionate 100 microgram per 1 dose Seretide 100 Accuhaler | 60 dose PoM £17.46 DT = £17.46

Salmeterol (as Salmeterol xinafoate) 50 microgram per 1 dose, Fluticasone propionate 250 microgram per 1 dose Seretide 250 Accuhaler | 60 dose PoM £33.95 DT = £33.95

Salmeterol (as Salmeterol xinafoate) 50 microgram per 1 dose, Fluticasone propionate 500 microgram per 1 dose Seretide 500 Accuhaler | 60 dose PoM £32.74 DT = £32.74

Pressurised inhalation

CAUTIONARY AND ADVISORY LABELS 8, 10 (excluding Seretide 50 Evohaler ®)

▸ Combisal (Aspire Pharma Ltd)

Salmeterol (as Salmeterol xinafoate) 25 microgram per 1 dose, Fluticasone propionate 50 microgram per 1 dose Combisal 25micrograms/dose / 50micrograms/dose inhaler | 120 dose PoM £13.50 DT = £17.46

Salmeterol (as Salmeterol xinafoate) 25 microgram per 1 dose, Fluticasone propionate 125 microgram per 1 dose Combisal 25micrograms/dose / 125micrograms/dose inhaler | 120 dose PoM £17.59 DT = £23.45

Salmeterol (as Salmeterol xinafoate) 25 microgram per 1 dose, Fluticasone propionate 250 microgram per 1 dose Combisal 25micrograms/dose / 250micrograms/dose inhaler | 120 dose PoM £27.99 DT = £29.32

▸ Seretide Evohaler (GlaxoSmithKline UK Ltd)

Salmeterol (as Salmeterol xinafoate) 25 microgram per 1 dose, Fluticasone propionate 50 microgram per 1 dose Seretide 50 Evohaler | 120 dose PoM £17.46 DT = £17.46

Salmeterol (as Salmeterol xinafoate) 25 microgram per 1 dose, Fluticasone propionate 125 microgram per 1 dose Seretide 125 Evohaler | 120 dose PoM £23.45 DT = £23.45

Salmeterol (as Salmeterol xinafoate) 25 microgram per 1 dose, Fluticasone propionate 250 microgram per 1 dose Seretide 250 Evohaler | 120 dose PoM £29.32 DT = £29.32

162

Fluticasone with vilanterol

27-Jul-2018

The properties listed below are those particular to the combination only. For the properties of the components please consider, fluticasone p. 170.

● INDICATIONS AND DOSE

RELVAR ELLIPTA ® 184 MICROGRAMS/22 MICROGRAMS

Prophylaxis of asthma

▶ BY INHALATION OF POWDER

▸ Child 12–17 years: 1 inhalation once daily

RELVAR ELLIPTA ® 92 MICROGRAMS/22 MICROGRAMS

Prophylaxis of asthma

▶ BY INHALATION OF POWDER

▸ Child 12–17 years: 1 inhalation once daily

● INTERACTIONS → Appendix 1: $beta_2$ agonists · corticosteroids

● SIDE-EFFECTS

▶ **Common or very common** Abdominal pain · arthralgia · back pain · bone fracture · cough · dysphonia · fever · increased risk of infection · muscle spasms · oropharyngeal pain

▶ **Uncommon** Vision blurred

▶ **Rare or very rare** Angioedema · anxiety

● PREGNANCY Manufacturer advises use only if potential benefit outweighs risk.

● BREAST FEEDING Manufacturer advises avoid—no information available.

● HEPATIC IMPAIRMENT Manufacturer advises caution.

Dose adjustments Manufacturer advises maximum dose of 92 microgram/22 microgram once daily in moderate to severe impairment.

● PATIENT AND CARER ADVICE Patients or carers should be given advice on how to administer fluticasone with vilanterol powder for inhalation.

A steroid card should be provided.

● MEDICINAL FORMS There can be variation in the licensing of different medicines containing the same drug.

Inhalation powder

CAUTIONARY AND ADVISORY LABELS 8, 10

▸ Relvar Ellipta (GlaxoSmithKline UK Ltd)

Vilanterol 22 microgram per 1 dose, Fluticasone furoate 92 microgram per 1 dose Relvar Ellipta 92micrograms/dose / 22micrograms/dose dry powder inhaler | 30 dose PoM £22.00 DT = £22.00

Vilanterol 22 microgram per 1 dose, Fluticasone furoate 184 microgram per 1 dose Relvar Ellipta 184micrograms/dose / 22micrograms/dose dry powder inhaler | 30 dose PoM £29.50 DT = £29.50

F 167

Mometasone furoate

21-Dec-2017

● **INDICATIONS AND DOSE**

Prophylaxis of asthma

▶ BY INHALATION OF POWDER

▸ Child 12-17 years: Initially 400 micrograms daily in 1–2 divided doses, single dose to be inhaled in the evening, reduced to 200 micrograms once daily, if control maintained

Prophylaxis of severe asthma

▶ BY INHALATION OF POWDER

▸ Child 12-17 years: Increased if necessary up to 400 micrograms twice daily

● **INTERACTIONS** → Appendix 1: corticosteroids

● **SIDE-EFFECTS**

▶ **Common or very common** Candida infection

● **PATIENT AND CARER ADVICE** Patients or carers should be given advice on how to administer mometasone by inhaler. With high doses, a steroid card should be supplied.

Medicines for Children leaflet: Mometasone furoate inhaler for asthma prevention (prophylaxis) www.medicinesforchildren.org.uk/mometasone-furoate-inhaler-asthma-prevention-prophylaxis

● **NATIONAL FUNDING/ACCESS DECISIONS**

Scottish Medicines Consortium (SMC) decisions

The *Scottish Medicines Consortium* has advised (November 2003) that *Asmanex*® is restricted for use following failure of first-line inhaled corticosteroids.

● **MEDICINAL FORMS** There can be variation in the licensing of different medicines containing the same drug. Forms available from special-order manufacturers include: ointment

Inhalation powder

CAUTIONARY AND ADVISORY LABELS 8, 10

▸ Asmanex Twisthaler (Merck Sharp & Dohme Ltd)

Mometasone furoate 200 microgram per 1 dose Asmanex 200micrograms/dose Twisthaler | 30 dose PoM £15.70 DT = £15.70 | 60 dose PoM £23.54 DT = £23.54

Mometasone furoate 400 microgram per 1 dose Asmanex 400micrograms/dose Twisthaler | 30 dose PoM £21.78 DT = £21.78 | 60 dose PoM £36.05 DT = £36.05

IMMUNOSUPPRESSANTS › MONOCLONAL ANTIBODIES

Mepolizumab

09-Oct-2019

● **DRUG ACTION** Mepolizumab is a humanised anti-interleukin-5 (anti-IL-5) monoclonal antibody; it reduces the production and survival of eosinophils.

● **INDICATIONS AND DOSE**

Add on treatment for severe refractory eosinophilic asthma (under expert supervision)

▶ BY SUBCUTANEOUS INJECTION

▸ Child 6-11 years: 40 mg every 4 weeks

▸ Child 12-17 years: 100 mg every 4 weeks

● **CAUTIONS** Helminth infection

CAUTIONS, FURTHER INFORMATION

▸ Helminth infections Manufacturer advises pre-existing helminth infections should be treated before initiation of therapy; if patients become infected during treatment and do not respond to anti-helminth treatment, consider treatment interruption.

● **SIDE-EFFECTS**

▶ **Common or very common** Abdominal pain upper · administration related reaction · back pain · eczema · fever · headache · hypersensitivity · increased risk of infection · nasal congestion

● **PREGNANCY** Manufacturer advises avoid unless potential benefit outweighs risk—limited data available.

● **BREAST FEEDING** Manufacturer advises avoid—present in milk in *animal* studies.

● **DIRECTIONS FOR ADMINISTRATION** Manufacturer advises injection is given into the thigh, abdomen, or upper arm. Patients may self-administer *Nucala*® pre-filled devices into the thigh or abdomen after appropriate training in preparation and administration.

● **PRESCRIBING AND DISPENSING INFORMATION** Mepolizumab is a biological medicine. Biological medicines must be prescribed and dispensed by brand name, see *Biological medicines* and *Biosimilar medicines*, under Guidance on prescribing p. 1; manufacturer advises to record the brand name and batch number after each administration.

● **PATIENT AND CARER ADVICE**

Asthma Patients and their carers should be advised to seek medical advice if their asthma remains uncontrolled or worsens after initiation of treatment.

● **NATIONAL FUNDING/ACCESS DECISIONS**

Scottish Medicines Consortium (SMC) decisions

SMC No. SMC2139

The *Scottish Medicines Consortium* has advised (April 2019) that mepolizumab (*Nucala*®) is accepted for restricted use within NHS Scotland as an add-on treatment for severe refractory eosinophilic asthma in patients aged 6 years and older who have eosinophils of at least 150 cells per microlitre (0.15×10^9/L) at initiation of treatment and have had at least four asthma exacerbations in the preceding year or are receiving maintenance treatment with oral corticosteroids. This advice is contingent upon the continuing availability of the patient access scheme in NHS Scotland or a list price that is equivalent or lower.

All Wales Medicines Strategy Group (AWMSG) decisions

AWMSG No. 3750

The *All Wales Medicines Strategy Group* has advised (April 2019) that mepolizumab (*Nucala*®) is recommended as an option for restricted use within NHS Wales as an add-on treatment for severe refractory eosinophilic asthma in patients aged 6 years and older. It is restricted for use in a subpopulation of the licensed indication in line with NICE TA431 and is not recommended for use within NHS Wales outside of this subpopulation. This recommendation applies only in circumstances where the approved Patient Access Scheme (PAS) is utilised or where the list/contract price is equivalent or lower than the PAS price.

● **MEDICINAL FORMS** There can be variation in the licensing of different medicines containing the same drug.

Solution for injection

EXCIPIENTS: May contain Edetic acid (edta), polysorbates

▸ Mepolizumab (non-proprietary) ▼

Mepolizumab 100 mg per 1 ml Nucala 100mg/1ml solution for injection pre-filled pens | 1 pre-filled disposable injection PoM £840.00

Nucala 100mg/1ml solution for injection pre-filled syringes | 1 pre-filled disposable injection PoM £840.00

Powder for solution for injection

EXCIPIENTS: May contain Polysorbates

▸ Nucala (GlaxoSmithKline UK Ltd) ▼

Mepolizumab 100 mg Nucala 100mg powder for solution for injection vials | 1 vial PoM £840.00 (Hospital only)

3

Respiratory system

Omalizumab

27-Mar-2020

- **INDICATIONS AND DOSE**

Prophylaxis of severe persistent allergic asthma

▶ BY SUBCUTANEOUS INJECTION

▶ Child 6–17 years: Dose according to immunoglobulin E concentration and body-weight (consult product literature)

Add-on therapy for chronic spontaneous urticaria in patients who have had an inadequate response to H_1 antihistamine treatment

▶ BY SUBCUTANEOUS INJECTION

▶ Child 12–17 years: 300 mg every 4 weeks

- **CAUTIONS** Autoimmune disease · susceptibility to helminth infection—discontinue if infection does not respond to anthelmintic
- **SIDE-EFFECTS**

▶ **Common or very common** Fever · gastrointestinal discomfort · headache · skin reactions

▶ **Uncommon** Cough · diarrhoea · dizziness · drowsiness · fatigue · flushing · increased risk of infection · influenza like illness · limb swelling · nausea · paraesthesia · photosensitivity reaction · postural hypotension · respiratory disorders · syncope · weight increased

▶ **Rare or very rare** Angioedema · hypersensitivity · systemic lupus erythematosus (SLE)

▶ **Frequency not known** Alopecia · eosinophilic granulomatosis with polyangiitis · immune thrombocytopenic purpura · joint disorders · lymphadenopathy · myalgia

SIDE-EFFECTS, FURTHER INFORMATION

Eosinophilic granulomatosis with polyangiitis (Churg-Strauss syndrome) Churg-Strauss syndrome has occurred rarely in patients given omalizumab; the reaction is usually associated with the reduction of oral corticosteroid therapy. Churg-Strauss syndrome can present as eosinophilia, vasculitic rash, cardiac complications, worsening pulmonary symptoms, or peripheral neuropathy.

Hypersensitivity reactions Hypersensitivity reactions can also occur immediately following treatment with omalizumab or sometimes more than 24 hours after the first injection.

- **PREGNANCY** Manufacturer advises avoid unless essential—crosses the placenta.
- **BREAST FEEDING** Manufacturer advises avoid—present in milk in *animal* studies.
- **HEPATIC IMPAIRMENT** Manufacturer advises caution (no information available).
- **RENAL IMPAIRMENT** Manufacturer advises caution—no information available.
- **NATIONAL FUNDING/ACCESS DECISIONS**

NICE decisions

▶ **Omalizumab for severe persistent allergic asthma (April 2013)** NICE TA278

Omalizumab is recommended as an option for treating severe persistent confirmed allergic IgE-mediated asthma as an add-on to optimised standard therapy in patients aged 6 years and over:

- who need continuous or frequent treatment with oral corticosteroids (defined as 4 or more courses in the previous year), **and**
- only if the manufacturer makes omalizumab available with the discount agreed in the patient access scheme.

Optimised standard therapy is defined as a full trial of and, if tolerated, documented compliance with inhaled high-dose corticosteroids, long-acting $beta_2$ agonists, leukotriene receptor antagonists, theophyllines, oral corticosteroids, and smoking cessation if clinically appropriate.

Patients currently receiving omalizumab whose disease does not meet the criteria should be able to continue treatment until they and their clinician consider it appropriate to stop.

www.nice.org.uk/guidance/ta278

▶ **Omalizumab for previously treated chronic spontaneous urticaria (June 2015)** NICE TA339

Omalizumab is an option as add-on therapy for the treatment of severe chronic spontaneous urticaria in patients 12 years and over, only if:

- the severity of the condition is assessed objectively, for example, using a weekly urticaria activity score of 28 or more,
- the patient's condition has not responded to standard treatment with H_1-antihistamines and leukotriene receptor antagonists,
- omalizumab is stopped at or before the fourth dose if the condition has not responded,
- omalizumab is stopped at the end of a course of treatment (6 doses) if the condition has responded and is restarted only if the condition relapses,
- omalizumab is administered under the management of a secondary care specialist in dermatology, immunology or allergy,
- the manufacturer provides omalizumab with the discount agreed in the patient access scheme.

Patients currently receiving omalizumab whose disease does not meet the above criteria should have the option to continue treatment until they and their clinician consider it appropriate to stop.

www.nice.org.uk/guidance/ta339

Scottish Medicines Consortium (SMC) decisions

The *Scottish Medicines Consortium* has advised (January 2015) that omalizumab (*Xolair*®) is accepted for restricted use within NHS Scotland for the treatment of chronic spontaneous urticaria in patients aged 12 years and over, who have had an inadequate response to combination therapy with H_1-antihistamines, leukotriene receptor antagonists and H_2-antihistamines, used according to current treatment guidelines.

- **MEDICINAL FORMS** There can be variation in the licensing of different medicines containing the same drug.

Solution for injection

▶ Xolair (Novartis Pharmaceuticals UK Ltd)

Omalizumab 150 mg per 1 ml Xolair 150mg/1ml solution for injection pre-filled syringes | 1 pre-filled disposable injection PoM £256.15 DT = £256.15

Xolair 75mg/0.5ml solution for injection pre-filled syringes | 1 pre-filled disposable injection PoM £128.07 DT = £128.07

LEUKOTRIENE RECEPTOR ANTAGONISTS

Montelukast

18-Mar-2020

- **INDICATIONS AND DOSE**

Prophylaxis of asthma

▶ BY MOUTH

▶ Child 6 months–5 years: 4 mg once daily, dose to be taken in the evening

▶ Child 6–14 years: 5 mg once daily, dose to be taken in the evening

▶ Child 15–17 years: 10 mg once daily, dose to be taken in the evening

Symptomatic relief of seasonal allergic rhinitis in patients with asthma
- ▸ BY MOUTH
- ▸ Child 15-17 years: 10 mg once daily, dose to be taken in the evening

IMPORTANT SAFETY INFORMATION

MHRA/CHM ADVICE: MONTELUKAST (*SINGULAIR*®): REMINDER OF THE RISK OF NEUROPSYCHIATRIC REACTIONS (SEPTEMBER 2019)

Healthcare professionals are advised to be alert for neuropsychiatric reactions, including speech impairment and obsessive-compulsive symptoms, in adults, adolescents, and children taking montelukast. The risks and benefits of continuing treatment should be evaluated if these reactions occur. Patients should be advised to read the list of neuropsychiatric reactions in the information leaflet and seek immediate medical attention if they occur.

- **INTERACTIONS** → Appendix 1: montelukast
- **SIDE-EFFECTS**
- ▸ **Common or very common** Diarrhoea · fever · gastrointestinal discomfort · headache · nausea · skin reactions · upper respiratory tract infection · vomiting
- ▸ **Uncommon** Akathisia · anxiety · arthralgia · asthenia · behaviour abnormal · depression · dizziness · drowsiness · dry mouth · haemorrhage · irritability · malaise · muscle complaints · oedema · seizure · sensation abnormal · sleep disorders
- ▸ **Rare or very rare** Angioedema · concentration impaired · disorientation · eosinophilic granulomatosis with polyangiitis · erythema nodosum · hallucination · hepatic disorders · memory loss · palpitations · psychiatric disorders · pulmonary eosinophilia · speech disorder · suicidal tendencies · tremor

SIDE-EFFECTS, FURTHER INFORMATION Eosinophilic granulomatosis with polyangiitis (Churg-Strauss syndrome) has occurred very rarely in association with the use of montelukast; in many of the reported cases the reaction followed the reduction or withdrawal of oral corticosteroid therapy. Prescribers should be alert to the development of eosinophilia, vasculitic rash, worsening pulmonary symptoms, cardiac complications, or peripheral neuropathy.

- **PREGNANCY** Manufacturer advises avoid unless essential. There is limited evidence for the safe use of montelukast during pregnancy; however, it can be taken as normal in women who have shown a significant improvement in asthma not achievable with other drugs before becoming pregnant.
- **BREAST FEEDING** Manufacturer advises avoid unless essential.
- **DIRECTIONS FOR ADMINISTRATION** Granules may be swallowed or mixed with cold, soft food (not liquid) and taken immediately.
- **PRESCRIBING AND DISPENSING INFORMATION** Flavours of chewable tablet formulations may include cherry.
- **PATIENT AND CARER ADVICE**

Administration Patients or carers should be given advice on how to administer montelukast granules.

Risk of neuropsychiatric reactions The MHRA advises patients and carers to seek medical attention if changes in speech or behaviour occur—see also *Important safety information*.

Medicines for Children leaflet: Montelukast for asthma www.medicinesforchildren.org.uk/montelukast-asthma

- **NATIONAL FUNDING/ACCESS DECISIONS**

SINGULAIR ® GRANULES

Scottish Medicines Consortium (SMC) decisions
- ▸ With oral use The *Scottish Medicines Consortium* has advised (June 2007) that *Singulair*® granules are restricted for use as an alternative to low-dose inhaled corticosteroids for children 2–14 years with mild persistent asthma who have not recently had serious asthma attacks that required oral corticosteroid use and who are not capable of using inhaled corticosteroids; *Singulair*® granules should be initiated by a specialist in paediatric asthma.

SINGULAIR ® CHEWABLE TABLETS

Scottish Medicines Consortium (SMC) decisions
- ▸ With oral use The *Scottish Medicines Consortium* has advised (June 2007) that *Singulair*® chewable tablets are restricted for use as an alternative to low-dose inhaled corticosteroids for children 2–14 years with mild persistent asthma who have not recently had serious asthma attacks that required oral corticosteroid use and who are not capable of using inhaled corticosteroids; *Singulair*® chewable tablets should be initiated by a specialist in paediatric asthma.

- **MEDICINAL FORMS** There can be variation in the licensing of different medicines containing the same drug.

Granules
- ▸ Montelukast (Non-proprietary)
  Montelukast (as Montelukast sodium) 4 mg Montelukast 4mg granules sachets sugar free sugar-free | 28 sachet PoM £19.99 DT = £5.18
- ▸ Singulair (Merck Sharp & Dohme Ltd)
  Montelukast (as Montelukast sodium) 4 mg Singulair Paediatric 4mg granules sachets sugar-free | 28 sachet PoM £25.69 DT = £5.18

Tablet
- ▸ Montelukast (Non-proprietary)
  Montelukast (as Montelukast sodium) 10 mg Montelukast 10mg tablets | 28 tablet PoM £26.97 DT = £2.30
- ▸ Singulair (Merck Sharp & Dohme Ltd)
  Montelukast (as Montelukast sodium) 10 mg Singulair 10mg tablets | 28 tablet PoM £26.97 DT = £2.30

Chewable tablet

CAUTIONARY AND ADVISORY LABELS 23, 24

EXCIPIENTS: May contain Aspartame
- ▸ Montelukast (Non-proprietary)
  Montelukast (as Montelukast sodium) 4 mg Montelukast 4mg chewable tablets sugar free sugar-free | 28 tablet PoM £25.69 DT = £1.51
  Montelukast (as Montelukast sodium) 5 mg Montelukast 5mg chewable tablets sugar free sugar-free | 28 tablet PoM £25.69 DT = £1.91
- ▸ Singulair (Merck Sharp & Dohme Ltd)
  Montelukast (as Montelukast sodium) 4 mg Singulair Paediatric 4mg chewable tablets sugar-free | 28 tablet PoM £25.69 DT = £1.51
  Montelukast (as Montelukast sodium) 5 mg Singulair Paediatric 5mg chewable tablets sugar-free | 28 tablet PoM £25.69 DT = £1.91

MAST-CELL STABILISERS

Nedocromil sodium

25-Jul-2018

- **INDICATIONS AND DOSE**

Prophylaxis of asthma
- ▸ BY INHALATION OF AEROSOL
- ▸ Child 5-17 years: Initially 4 mg 4 times a day, when control achieved may be possible to reduce to twice daily

DOSE EQUIVALENCE AND CONVERSION
- ▸ 2 puffs = 4 mg.

- **UNLICENSED USE** Not licensed for use in children under 6 years.

IMPORTANT SAFETY INFORMATION

MHRA/CHM ADVICE: PRESSURISED METERED DOSE INHALERS (PMDI): RISK OF AIRWAY OBSTRUCTION FROM ASPIRATION OF LOOSE OBJECTS (JULY 2018)

See Respiratory system, drug delivery p. 153.

● SIDE-EFFECTS
▸ **Common or very common** Bronchospasm · cough · gastrointestinal discomfort · headache · nausea · taste altered · vomiting
▸ **Frequency not known** Pharyngitis · throat irritation
SIDE-EFFECTS, FURTHER INFORMATION If paradoxical bronchospasm occurs, a fast-acting inhaled bronchodilator such as salbutamol or terbutaline should be used to control symptoms; treatment with nedocromil should be discontinued.

● PREGNANCY Inhaled drugs can be taken as normal during pregnancy.

● BREAST FEEDING Inhaled drugs can be taken as normal during breast-feeding.

● TREATMENT CESSATION Withdrawal should be done gradually over a period of one week—symptoms of asthma may recur.

● PRESCRIBING AND DISPENSING INFORMATION Flavours of inhalers may include mint.

● PATIENT AND CARER ADVICE Regular use is necessary. Patient counselling is advised for Nedocromil aerosol for inhalation (administration).

● MEDICINAL FORMS There can be variation in the licensing of different medicines containing the same drug.

Pressurised inhalation
CAUTIONARY AND ADVISORY LABELS 8
▸ Tilade (Sanofi)
Nedocromil sodium 2 mg per 1 dose Tilade 2mg/dose inhaler CFC free | 112 dose [PoM] £39.94 DT = £39.94

Sodium cromoglicate

21-May-2020

(Sodium cromoglycate)

● INDICATIONS AND DOSE

Prophylaxis of asthma
▸ BY INHALATION OF AEROSOL
▸ Child 5–17 years: Initially 10 mg 4 times a day, additional dose may also be taken before exercise, increased if necessary to 10 mg 6–8 times a day; maintenance 5 mg 4 times a day, 5 mg is equivalent to 1 puff

Food allergy (in conjunction with dietary restriction)
▸ BY MOUTH
▸ Child 2–13 years: Initially 100 mg 4 times a day for 2–3 weeks, then increased if necessary up to 40 mg/kg daily, then reduced according to response, to be taken before meals
▸ Child 14–17 years: Initially 200 mg 4 times a day for 2–3 weeks, then increased if necessary up to 40 mg/kg daily, then reduced according to response, to be taken before meals

IMPORTANT SAFETY INFORMATION
MHRA/CHM ADVICE: PRESSURISED METERED DOSE INHALERS (PMDI): RISK OF AIRWAY OBSTRUCTION FROM ASPIRATION OF LOOSE OBJECTS (JULY 2018)
▸ When used by inhalation
See Respiratory system, drug delivery p. 153.

● CAUTIONS
▸ When used by inhalation Discontinue if eosinophilic pneumonia occurs

● SIDE-EFFECTS
▸ When used by inhalation Cough · headache · pneumonia eosinophilic · rhinitis · throat irritation
▸ With oral use Arthralgia · nausea · rash
SIDE-EFFECTS, FURTHER INFORMATION When used by inhalation, if paradoxical bronchospasm occurs, a short-acting beta$_2$-agonist should be used to control symptoms; treatment with sodium cromoglicate should be discontinued.

● PREGNANCY Not known to be harmful.
▸ When used by inhalation Can be taken as normal during pregnancy.

● BREAST FEEDING Unlikely to be present in milk.
▸ When used by inhalation Can be taken as normal during breast-feeding.

● TREATMENT CESSATION
▸ When used by inhalation Withdrawal of sodium cromoglicate should be done gradually over a period of one week—symptoms of asthma may recur.

● DIRECTIONS FOR ADMINISTRATION Capsules may be swallowed whole or the contents dissolved in hot water and diluted with cold water before taking.

● PATIENT AND CARER ADVICE
▸ With oral use Patient counselling is advised for sodium cromoglicate capsules (administration).
▸ When used by inhalation Patient counselling is advised for sodium cromoglicate pressurised inhalation (administration).

● MEDICINAL FORMS There can be variation in the licensing of different medicines containing the same drug. Forms available from special-order manufacturers include: oral solution

Capsule
CAUTIONARY AND ADVISORY LABELS 22
▸ Nalcrom (Sanofi)
Sodium cromoglicate 100 mg Nalcrom 100mg capsules | 100 capsule [PoM] £41.14 DT = £41.14

Pressurised inhalation
CAUTIONARY AND ADVISORY LABELS 8
▸ Intal (Sanofi)
Sodium cromoglicate 5 mg per 1 dose Intal 5mg/dose inhaler CFC free | 112 dose [PoM] £18.33 DT = £18.33

XANTHINES

Aminophylline

18-Mar-2020

● INDICATIONS AND DOSE

Severe acute asthma in patients not previously treated with theophylline
▸ BY SLOW INTRAVENOUS INJECTION
▸ Child: 5 mg/kg (max. per dose 500 mg), to be followed by intravenous infusion

Severe acute asthma
▸ BY INTRAVENOUS INFUSION
▸ Child 1 month–11 years: 1 mg/kg/hour, adjusted according to plasma-theophylline concentration
▸ Child 12–17 years: 500–700 micrograms/kg/hour, adjusted according to plasma-theophylline concentration

Chronic asthma
▸ BY MOUTH USING MODIFIED-RELEASE MEDICINES
▸ Child (body-weight 40 kg and above): Initially 225 mg twice daily for 1 week, then increased if necessary to 450 mg twice daily, adjusted according to plasma-theophylline concentration

DOSE ADJUSTMENTS DUE TO INTERACTIONS
▸ Dose adjustment may be necessary if smoking started or stopped during treatment.

DOSES AT EXTREMES OF BODY-WEIGHT
▸ To avoid excessive dosage in obese patients, dose should be calculated on the basis of ideal weight for height.

PHARMACOKINETICS
- Aminophylline is a stable mixture or combination of theophylline and ethylenediamine; the ethylenediamine confers greater solubility in water.
- Theophylline is metabolised in the liver. The plasma-theophylline concentration is increased in heart failure, hepatic impairment, and in viral infections. The plasma-theophylline concentration is decreased in smokers, and by alcohol consumption. Differences in the half-life of aminophylline are important because the toxic dose is close to the therapeutic dose.

- **UNLICENSED USE** Aminophylline injection not licensed for use in children under 6 months.

PHYLLOCONTIN CONTINUS® FORTE
- With oral use *Phyllocontin Continus® Forte* tablets are not licensed for use in children.

- **CAUTIONS** Arrhythmias following rapid intravenous injection · cardiac arrhythmias or other cardiac disease · epilepsy · fever · hypertension · peptic ulcer · risk of hypokalaemia · thyroid disorder
- **INTERACTIONS** → Appendix 1: aminophylline
- **SIDE-EFFECTS**

GENERAL SIDE-EFFECTS
Headache · nausea · palpitations · seizure (more common when given too rapidly by intravenous injection)

SPECIFIC SIDE-EFFECTS
- With intravenous use Abdominal pain · anxiety · arrhythmia (more common when given too rapidly by intravenous injection) · confusion · delirium · diarrhoea · dizziness · electrolyte imbalance · gastrointestinal haemorrhage · gastrooesophageal reflux disease · hyperthermia · hyperventilation · hypotension (more common when given too rapidly by intravenous injection) · insomnia · mania · metabolic disorder · pain · skin reactions · tachycardia (more common when given too rapidly by intravenous injection) · thirst · tremor · vertigo · visual impairment · vomiting
- With oral use Arrhythmias · central nervous system stimulation · epigastric discomfort

SIDE-EFFECTS, FURTHER INFORMATION Potentially serious hypokalaemia may result from beta$_2$-agonist therapy. Particular caution is required in severe asthma, because this effect may be potentiated by concomitant treatment with theophylline and its derivatives, corticosteroids, and diuretics, and by hypoxia. Plasma-potassium concentration should therefore be monitored in severe asthma.

Overdose Theophylline and related drugs are often prescribed as modified-release formulations and toxicity can therefore be delayed. They cause vomiting (which may be severe and intractable), agitation, restlessness, dilated pupils, sinus tachycardia, and hyperglycaemia. More serious effects are haematemesis, convulsions, and supraventricular and ventricular arrhythmias. Severe hypokalaemia may develop rapidly.

For specific details on the management of poisoning, see *Theophylline*, under Emergency treatment of poisoning p. 891.

- **ALLERGY AND CROSS-SENSITIVITY** Allergy to ethylenediamine can cause urticaria, erythema, and exfoliative dermatitis.
- **PREGNANCY** Neonatal irritability and apnoea have been reported. Theophylline can be taken as normal during pregnancy as it is particularly important that asthma should be well controlled during pregnancy.
- **BREAST FEEDING** Present in milk—irritability in infant reported; modified-release preparations preferable. Theophylline can be taken as normal during breast-feeding.
- **HEPATIC IMPAIRMENT** Manufacturer advises caution (risk of reduced clearance).

Dose adjustments ▸ With oral use Manufacturer advises consider dose reduction.
▸ With intravenous use Manufacturer advises maintenance dose reduction—consult product literature.

- **MONITORING REQUIREMENTS**
- Aminophylline is monitored therapeutically in terms of plasma-theophylline concentrations.
- Measurement of plasma-theophylline concentration may be helpful and is **essential** if a loading dose of intravenous aminophylline is to be given to patients who are already taking theophylline, because serious side-effects such as convulsions and arrhythmias can occasionally precede other symptoms of toxicity.
- In most individuals, a plasma-theophylline concentration of 10–20 mg/litre (55–110 micromol/litre) is required for satisfactory bronchodilation, although a lower plasma-theophylline concentration of 5–15 mg/litre may be effective. Adverse effects can occur within the range 10–20 mg/litre and both the frequency and severity increase at concentrations above 20 mg/litre.
- If aminophylline is given intravenously, a blood sample should be taken 4–6 hours after starting treatment.
- With oral use Plasma-theophylline concentration is measured 5 days after starting oral treatment and at least 3 days after any dose adjustment. A blood sample should usually be taken 4–6 hours after an oral dose of a modified-release preparation (sampling times may vary—consult local guidelines).

- **DIRECTIONS FOR ADMINISTRATION**
- With intravenous use For *intravenous injection*, give **very slowly** over at least 20 minutes (with close monitoring). For *intravenous infusion*, dilute to a concentration of 1 mg/mL with Glucose 5% *or* Sodium Chloride 0.9%.
- With intramuscular use Aminophylline is too irritant for intramuscular use.

- **PRESCRIBING AND DISPENSING INFORMATION** Patients taking oral theophylline or aminophylline should not normally receive a loading dose of intravenous aminophylline.

Consider intravenous aminophylline for treatment of severe and life-threatening acute asthma only after consultation with senior medical staff.

Modified release The rate of absorption from modified-release preparations can vary between brands. If a prescription for a modified-release oral aminophylline preparation does not specify a brand name, the pharmacist should contact the prescriber and agree the brand to be dispensed. Additionally, it is essential that a patient discharged from hospital should be maintained on the brand on which that patient was stabilised as an in-patient.

- **MEDICINAL FORMS** There can be variation in the licensing of different medicines containing the same drug. Forms available from special-order manufacturers include: solution for infusion, suppository

Solution for injection

▸ Aminophylline (Non-proprietary)

Aminophylline 25 mg per 1 ml Aminophylline 250mg/10ml solution for injection ampoules | 10 ampoule PoM £8.50 DT = £8.50

Modified-release tablet

CAUTIONARY AND ADVISORY LABELS 25

▸ Phyllocontin Continus (Napp Pharmaceuticals Ltd)

Aminophylline hydrate 225 mg Phyllocontin Continus 225mg tablets | 56 tablet P £2.40 DT = £2.40

Aminophylline hydrate 350 mg Phyllocontin Forte Continus 350mg tablets | 56 tablet P £4.22 DT = £4.22

Theophylline

27-Apr-2020

● **INDICATIONS AND DOSE**

UNIPHYLLIN CONTINUS ®

Chronic asthma

▶ BY MOUTH USING MODIFIED-RELEASE MEDICINES

▸ Child 2–11 years: 9 mg/kg every 12 hours (max. per dose 200 mg), dose may be increased in some children with chronic asthma; increased to 10–16 mg/kg every 12 hours (max. per dose 400 mg), may be appropriate to give larger evening or morning dose to achieve optimum therapeutic effect when symptoms most severe; in patients whose night or daytime symptoms persist despite other therapy, who are not currently receiving theophylline, total daily requirement may be added as single evening or morning dose

▸ Child 12–17 years: 200 mg every 12 hours, adjusted according to response to 400 mg every 12 hours, may be appropriate to give larger evening or morning dose to achieve optimum therapeutic effect when symptoms most severe; in patients whose night or daytime symptoms persist despite other therapy, who are not currently receiving theophylline, total daily requirement may be added as single evening or morning dose

DOSE ADJUSTMENTS DUE TO INTERACTIONS

▸ Dose adjustment may be necessary if smoking started or stopped during treatment.

PHARMACOKINETICS

▸ Theophylline is metabolised in the liver. The plasma-theophylline concentration is increased in heart failure, hepatic impairment, and in viral infections. The plasma-theophylline concentration is decreased in smokers, and by alcohol consumption. Differences in the half-life of theophylline are important because the toxic dose is close to the therapeutic dose.

● **CAUTIONS** Cardiac arrhythmias or other cardiac disease · epilepsy · fever · hypertension · peptic ulcer · risk of hypokalaemia · thyroid disorder

● **INTERACTIONS** → Appendix 1: theophylline

● **SIDE-EFFECTS** Anxiety · arrhythmias · diarrhoea · dizziness · gastrointestinal discomfort · gastrooesophageal reflux disease · headache · hyperuricaemia · nausea · palpitations · seizure · skin reactions · sleep disorders · tremor · urinary disorders · vomiting

SIDE-EFFECTS, FURTHER INFORMATION Potentially serious hypokalaemia may result from beta$_2$-agonist therapy. Particular caution is required in severe asthma, because this effect may be potentiated by concomitant treatment with theophylline and its derivatives, corticosteroids, and diuretics, and by hypoxia. Plasma-potassium concentration should therefore be monitored in severe asthma.

Overdose Theophylline in overdose can cause vomiting (which may be severe and intractable), agitation, restlessness, dilated pupils, sinus tachycardia, and hyperglycaemia. More serious effects are haematemesis, convulsions, and supraventricular and ventricular arrhythmias. Severe hypokalaemia may develop rapidly.

For details on the management of poisoning, see Theophylline, under Emergency treatment of poisoning p. 891.

● **PREGNANCY** Neonatal irritability and apnoea have been reported. Theophylline can be taken as normal during pregnancy as it is particularly important that asthma should be well controlled during pregnancy.

● **BREAST FEEDING** Present in milk—irritability in infant reported; modified-release preparations preferable. Theophylline can be taken as normal during breast-feeding.

● **HEPATIC IMPAIRMENT** Manufacturer advises caution (risk of increased exposure).

Dose adjustments Manufacturer advises consider dose reduction.

● **MONITORING REQUIREMENTS**

▸ In most individuals, a plasma-theophylline concentration of 10–20 mg/litre (55–110 micromol/litre) is required for satisfactory bronchodilation, although a lower plasma-theophylline concentration of 5–15 mg/litre may be effective. Adverse effects can occur within the range 10–20 mg/litre and both the frequency and severity increase at concentrations above 20 mg/litre.

▸ Plasma-theophylline concentration is measured 5 days after starting oral treatment and at least 3 days after any dose adjustment. A blood sample should usually be taken 4–6 hours after an oral dose of a modified-release preparation (sampling times may vary—consult local guidelines).

● **PRESCRIBING AND DISPENSING INFORMATION** The rate of absorption from modified-release preparations can vary between brands. If a prescription for a modified-release oral theophylline preparation does not specify a brand name, the pharmacist should contact the prescriber and agree the brand to be dispensed. Additionally, it is essential that a patient discharged from hospital should be maintained on the brand on which that patient was stabilised as an in-patient.

● **MEDICINAL FORMS** There can be variation in the licensing of different medicines containing the same drug.

Modified-release tablet

CAUTIONARY AND ADVISORY LABELS 21, 25

▸ **Uniphyllin Continus** (Napp Pharmaceuticals Ltd)

Theophylline 200 mg Uniphyllin Continus 200mg tablets | 56 tablet [P] £2.96 DT = £2.96

Theophylline 300 mg Uniphyllin Continus 300mg tablets | 56 tablet [P] £4.77 DT = £4.77

Theophylline 400 mg Uniphyllin Continus 400mg tablets | 56 tablet [P] £5.65 DT = £5.65

Nebuliser solutions

● **HYPERTONIC SODIUM CHLORIDE SOLUTIONS**

● **INDICATIONS AND DOSE**

MUCOCLEAR ® 3%

Mobilise lower respiratory tract secretions in mucous consolidation (e.g. cystic fibrosis) | Mild to moderate acute viral bronchiolitis in infants

▶ BY INHALATION OF NEBULISED SOLUTION

▸ Child: 4 mL 2–4 times a day, temporary irritation, such as coughing, hoarseness, or reversible bronchoconstriction may occur; an inhaled bronchodilator can be used before treatment with hypertonic sodium chloride to reduce the risk of these adverse effects

MucoClear 3% inhalation solution 4ml ampoules (Pari Medical Ltd) **Sodium chloride 30 mg per 1 ml** | 20 ampoule · NHS indicative price = £12.98 · Drug Tariff (Part IXa) | 60 ampoule · NHS indicative price = £27.00 · Drug Tariff (Part IXa)

● **INDICATIONS AND DOSE**

MUCOCLEAR ® 6%

Mobilise lower respiratory tract secretions in mucous consolidation (e.g. cystic fibrosis)

▶ BY INHALATION OF NEBULISED SOLUTION

▸ Child: 4 mL twice daily, temporary irritation, such as coughing, hoarseness, or reversible bronchoconstriction may occur; an inhaled bronchodilator can be used before treatment with hypertonic sodium chloride to reduce the risk of these adverse effects

MucoClear 6% inhalation solution 4ml ampoules (Pari Medical Ltd) **Sodium chloride 60 mg per 1 ml** | 20 ampoule • NHS indicative price = £12.98 • Drug Tariff (Part IXa) | 60 ampoule • NHS indicative price = £27.00 • Drug Tariff (Part IXa)

● **INDICATIONS AND DOSE**

NEBUSAL®

Mobilise lower respiratory tract secretions in mucous consolidation (e.g. cystic fibrosis)

▸ BY INHALATION OF NEBULISED SOLUTION

▸ Child: 4 mL up to twice daily, temporary irritation, such as coughing, hoarseness, or reversible bronchoconstriction may occur; an inhaled bronchodilator can be used before treatment with hypertonic sodium chloride to reduce the risk of these adverse effects

Nebusal 7% inhalation solution 4ml vials (Forest Laboratories UK Ltd) **Sodium chloride 70 mg per 1 ml** | 60 vial • NHS indicative price = £27.00 • Drug Tariff (Part IXa)

● **INDICATIONS AND DOSE**

PULMOCLEAR®

Mobilise lower respiratory tract secretions and prevent drying of bronchial mucous.

▸ BY INHALATION OF NEBULISED SOLUTION

▸ Child: (consult product literature)

PulmoClear 6% inhalation solution 4ml vials (TriOn Pharma Ltd) | 60 vial • NHS indicative price = £18.94 • Drug Tariff (Part IXa)

PulmoClear 3% inhalation solution 4ml vials (TriOn Pharma Ltd) **Sodium chloride 30 mg per 1 ml** | 60 vial • NHS indicative price = £18.94 • Drug Tariff (Part IXa)

PulmoClear 7% inhalation solution 4ml vials (TriOn Pharma Ltd) **Sodium chloride 70 mg per 1 ml** | 60 vial • NHS indicative price = £18.94 • Drug Tariff (Part IXa)

● **INDICATIONS AND DOSE**

RESP-EASE

Mobilise lower respiratory tract secretions and prevent drying of bronchial mucous.

▸ BY INHALATION OF NEBULISED SOLUTION

▸ Child: (consult product literature)

Resp-Ease 7% inhalation solution 4ml vials (Venture Healthcare Ltd) **Sodium chloride 70 mg per 1 ml** | 60 vial • NHS indicative price = £21.60 • Drug Tariff (Part IXa)

Peak flow meters: low range

● LOW RANGE PEAK FLOW METERS

MEDI® LOW RANGE

Range 40–420 litres/minute.

Compliant to standard EN ISO 23747:2007 except for scale range.

Medi peak flow meter low range (Medicareplus International Ltd)
1 device • NHS indicative price = £6.50 • Drug Tariff (Part IXa) price = £6.50

MINI-WRIGHT® LOW RANGE

Range 30–400 litres/minute.

Compliant to standard EN ISO 23747:2007 except for scale range.

Mini-Wright peak flow meter low range (Clement Clarke International Ltd)
1 device • NHS indicative price = £7.14 • Drug Tariff (Part IXa) price = £6.50

POCKETPEAK® LOW RANGE

Range 50–400 litres/minute.

Compliant to standard EN ISO 23747:2007 except for scale range.

nSpire Pocket Peak peak flow meter low range (nSpire Health Ltd)
1 device • NHS indicative price = £6.53 • Drug Tariff (Part IXa) price = £6.50

Peak flow meters: standard range

● STANDARD RANGE PEAK FLOW METERS

AIRZONE®

Range 60–720 litres/minute.

Conforms to standard EN ISO 23747:2007.

AirZone peak flow meter standard range (Clement Clarke International Ltd)
1 device • NHS indicative price = £4.69 • Drug Tariff (Part IXa) price = £4.50

MEDI® STANDARD RANGE

Range 60–800 litres/minute.

Conforms to standard EN ISO 23747:2007.

Medi peak flow meter standard range (Medicareplus International Ltd)
1 device • NHS indicative price = £4.50 • Drug Tariff (Part IXa) price = £4.50

MICROPEAK®

Range 60–900 litres/minute.

Conforms to standard EN ISO 23747:2007.

MicroPeak peak flow meter standard range (Micro Medical Ltd)
1 device • NHS indicative price = £6.50 • Drug Tariff (Part IXa) price = £4.50

MINI-WRIGHT® STANDARD RANGE

Range 60–800 litres/minute.

Conforms to standard EN ISO 23747:2007.

Mini-Wright peak flow meter standard range (Clement Clarke International Ltd)
1 device • NHS indicative price = £7.08 • Drug Tariff (Part IXa) price = £4.50

PIKO-1®

Range 15–999 litres/minute.

Conforms to standard EN ISO 23747:2007.

nSpire PiKo-1 peak flow meter standard range (nSpire Health Ltd)
1 device • NHS indicative price = £9.50 • Drug Tariff (Part IXa) price = £4.50

PINNACLE®

Range 60–900 litres/minute.

Conforms to standard EN ISO 23747:2007.

Fyne Dynamics Pinnacle peak flow meter standard range (Fyne Dynamics Ltd)
1 device • NHS indicative price = £6.50 • Drug Tariff (Part IXa) price = £4.50

POCKETPEAK® STANDARD RANGE

Range 60–800 litres/minute.

Conforms to standard EN ISO 23747:2007.

nSpire Pocket Peak peak flow meter standard range (nSpire Health Ltd)
1 device • NHS indicative price = £6.53 • Drug Tariff (Part IXa) price = £4.50

VITALOGRAPH®

Range 50–800 litres/minute.

Conforms to standard EN ISO 23747:2007.

Vitalograph peak flow meter standard range (Vitalograph Ltd)
1 device • NHS indicative price = £4.83 • Drug Tariff (Part IXa) price = £4.50

Spacers

● SPACERS

A2A SPACER®

For use with all pressurised (aerosol) inhalers.

A2A Spacer (Clement Clarke International Ltd)
1 device • NHS indicative price = £4.15 • Drug Tariff (Part IXa)

A2A Spacer with medium mask (Clement Clarke International Ltd)
1 device • NHS indicative price = £6.68 • Drug Tariff (Part IXa)

A2A Spacer with small mask (Clement Clarke International Ltd)
1 device • NHS indicative price = £6.68 • Drug Tariff (Part IXa)

ABLE SPACER ®

Small-volume device. For use with all pressurised (aerosol) inhalers.

Able Spacer (Clement Clarke International Ltd)
1 device • NHS indicative price = £4.39 • Drug Tariff (Part IXa)

Able Spacer with medium mask (Clement Clarke International Ltd)
1 device • NHS indicative price = £7.16 • Drug Tariff (Part IXa)

Able Spacer with small mask (Clement Clarke International Ltd)
1 device • NHS indicative price = £7.16 • Drug Tariff (Part IXa)

AEROCHAMBER PLUS ®

Medium-volume device. For use with all pressurised (aerosol) inhalers.

AeroChamber Plus (Trudell Medical UK Ltd)
1 device • NHS indicative price = £4.99 • Drug Tariff (Part IXa)

AeroChamber Plus with adult mask (Trudell Medical UK Ltd)
1 device • NHS indicative price = £8.33 • Drug Tariff (Part IXa)

AeroChamber Plus with child mask (Trudell Medical UK Ltd)
1 device • NHS indicative price = £8.33 • Drug Tariff (Part IXa)

AeroChamber Plus with infant mask (Trudell Medical UK Ltd)
1 device • NHS indicative price = £8.33 • Drug Tariff (Part IXa)

BABYHALER ®

For paediatric use with *Flixotide*®, and *Ventolin*® inhalers.

- PRESCRIBING AND DISPENSING INFORMATION

Not available for NHS prescription.

Babyhaler (GlaxoSmithKline UK Ltd)
1 device • No NHS indicative price available • Drug Tariff (Part IXa)

HALERAID ®

Device to place over pressurised (aerosol) inhalers to aid when strength in hands is impaired (e.g. in arthritis). For use with *Flixotide*®, *Seretide*®, *Serevent*®, and *Ventolin*® inhalers.

- PRESCRIBING AND DISPENSING INFORMATION

Not available for NHS prescription.

Haleraid-120 (GlaxoSmithKline UK Ltd)
1 device • No NHS indicative price available • Drug Tariff (Part IXa)

Haleraid-200 (GlaxoSmithKline UK Ltd)
1 device • No NHS indicative price available • Drug Tariff (Part IXa)

OPTICHAMBER ®

For use with all pressurised (aerosol) inhalers.

OptiChamber (Respironics (UK) Ltd)
1 device • NHS indicative price = £4.28 • Drug Tariff (Part IXa)

OPTICHAMBER ® DIAMOND

For use with all pressurised (aerosol) inhalers.

OptiChamber Diamond (Respironics (UK) Ltd)
1 device • NHS indicative price = £4.49 • Drug Tariff (Part IXa)

OptiChamber Diamond with large LiteTouch mask 5 years-adult (Respironics (UK) Ltd)
1 device • NHS indicative price = £7.49 • Drug Tariff (Part IXa)

OptiChamber Diamond with medium LiteTouch mask 1-5 years (Respironics (UK) Ltd)
1 device • NHS indicative price = £7.49 • Drug Tariff (Part IXa)

OptiChamber Diamond with small LiteTouch mask 0-18 months (Respironics (UK) Ltd)
1 device • NHS indicative price = £7.49 • Drug Tariff (Part IXa)

POCKET CHAMBER ®

Small volume device. For use with all pressurised (aerosol) inhalers.

Pocket Chamber (nSpire Health Ltd)
1 device • NHS indicative price = £4.18 • Drug Tariff (Part IXa)

Pocket Chamber with adult mask (nSpire Health Ltd)
1 device • NHS indicative price = £9.75 • Drug Tariff (Part IXa)

Pocket Chamber with child mask (nSpire Health Ltd)
1 device • NHS indicative price = £9.75 • Drug Tariff (Part IXa)

Pocket Chamber with infant mask (nSpire Health Ltd)
1 device • NHS indicative price = £9.75 • Drug Tariff (Part IXa)

Pocket Chamber with teenager mask (nSpire Health Ltd)
1 device • NHS indicative price = £9.75 • Drug Tariff (Part IXa)

SPACE CHAMBER PLUS ®

For use with all pressurised (aerosol) inhalers.

Space Chamber Plus (Medical Developments International Ltd)
1 device • NHS indicative price = £4.26 • Drug Tariff (Part IXa)

Space Chamber Plus with large mask (Medical Developments International Ltd)
1 device • NHS indicative price = £6.98 • Drug Tariff (Part IXa)

Space Chamber Plus with medium mask (Medical Developments International Ltd)
1 device • NHS indicative price = £6.98 • Drug Tariff (Part IXa)

Space Chamber Plus with small mask (Medical Developments International Ltd)
1 device • NHS indicative price = £6.98 • Drug Tariff (Part IXa)

VOLUMATIC ®

Large-volume device. For use with *Clenil Modulite*®, *Flixotide*®, *Seretide*®, *Serevent*®, and *Ventolin*® inhalers.

Volumatic (GlaxoSmithKline UK Ltd)
1 device • NHS indicative price = £3.88 • Drug Tariff (Part IXa)

Volumatic with paediatric mask (GlaxoSmithKline UK Ltd)
1 device • NHS indicative price = £6.83 • Drug Tariff (Part IXa)

VORTEX ®

Medium-volume device. For use with all pressurised (aerosol) inhalers.

2 Allergic conditions

Antihistamines, allergen immunotherapy and allergic emergencies

28-Feb-2020

Antihistamines

Antihistamines (histamine H_1-receptor antagonists) are classified as *sedating* or *non-sedating*, according to their relative potential for CNS depression. Antihistamines differ in their duration of action, incidence of drowsiness, and antimuscarinic effects; the response to an antihistamine may vary from child to child. Either a sedating or a non-sedating antihistamine may be used to treat an acute allergic reaction; for conditions with more persistent symptoms which require regular treatment, a non-sedating anti-histamine should be used to minimise the risk of sedation and psychomotor impairment associated with sedating antihistamines.

Oral antihistamines are used in the treatment of nasal allergies, particularly seasonal allergic rhinitis (hay fever), and may be of some value in vasomotor rhinitis; rhinorrhoea and sneezing is reduced, but antihistamines are usually less effective for nasal congestion. Antihistamines are used topically to treat allergic reactions in the eye and in the nose. Topical application of antihistamines to the skin is not recommended.

An oral antihistamine may be used to prevent urticaria, and for the treatment of acute urticarial rashes, pruritus, insect bites, and stings. Antihistamines are also used in the management of nausea and vomiting, of migraine, and the adjunctive management of anaphylaxis and angioedema.

The *non-sedating* antihistamine cetirizine hydrochloride p. 183 is safe and effective in children. Other non-sedating antihistamines that are used include acrivastine p. 182, bilastine p. 182, desloratadine p. 183 (an active metabolite of loratadine p. 185), fexofenadine hydrochloride p. 184 (an active metabolite of terfenadine), levocetirizine hydrochloride p. 184 (an isomer of cetirizine hydrochloride), loratadine, and mizolastine p. 185. Most non-sedating antihistamines are long-acting (usually 12–24 hours). There is little evidence that desloratadine or levocetirizine hydrochloride confer any additional benefit—they should be reserved for children who cannot tolerate other therapies.

Sedating antihistamines are occasionally useful when insomnia is associated with urticaria and pruritus. Most of the sedating antihistamines are relatively short-acting, but promethazine may be effective for up to 12 hours. Alimemazine tartrate p. 186 and **promethazine** have a more sedative effect than chlorphenamine maleate p. 186 and cyclizine p. 276. Chlorphenamine maleate is used as an adjunct to adrenaline/epinephrine p. 143 in the emergency treatment of anaphylaxis and angioedema.

Allergen immunotherapy

Immunotherapy using allergen vaccines containing house dust mite, animal dander (cat or dog), or extracts of grass and tree pollen can improve symptoms of asthma and allergic rhinoconjunctivitis in children. A vaccine containing extracts of wasp and bee venom is used to reduce the risk of severe anaphylaxis and systemic reactions in children with hypersensitivity to wasp and bee stings. An oral preparation of grass pollen extract (*Grazax*®) is also licensed for disease-modifying treatment of grass pollen-induced rhinitis and conjunctivitis. Children requiring immunotherapy must be referred to a hospital specialist for accurate diagnosis, assessment, and treatment.

Omalizumab p. 174 is a monoclonal antibody that binds to immunoglobulin E (IgE). It is licensed for use as additional therapy in children over 6 years with proven IgE-mediated sensitivity to inhaled allergens, whose severe persistent allergic asthma cannot be controlled adequately with high-dose inhaled corticosteroid together with a long-acting beta$_2$ agonist. Omalizumab should be initiated by physicians experienced in the treatment of severe persistent asthma. Omalizumab is also indicated as add-on therapy for the treatment of chronic spontaneous urticaria in patients who have had an inadequate response to H_1 antihistamine treatment.

Anaphylaxis and allergic emergencies

Anaphylaxis

Anaphylaxis is a severe, life-threatening, generalised or systemic hypersensitivity reaction. It is characterised by the rapid onset of respiratory and/or circulatory problems and is usually associated with skin and mucosal changes; prompt treatment is required. Children with pre-existing asthma, especially poorly controlled asthma, are at particular risk of life-threatening reactions. Insect stings are a recognised risk (in particular wasp and bee stings). Latex and certain foods, including eggs, fish, cow's milk protein, peanuts, sesame, shellfish, soy, and tree nuts may also precipitate anaphylaxis (see Food allergy p. 66). Medicinal products particularly associated with anaphylaxis include blood products, vaccines, allergen immunotherapy preparations, antibacterials, aspirin p. 98 and other NSAIDs, and neuromuscular blocking drugs. In the case of drugs, anaphylaxis is more likely after parenteral administration; resuscitation facilities must always be available for injections associated with special risk. Refined arachis (peanut) oil, which may be present in some medicinal products, is unlikely to cause an allergic reaction—nevertheless it is wise to check the full formula of preparations which may contain allergens.

Treatment of anaphylaxis

Adrenaline/epinephrine provides physiological reversal of the immediate symptoms associated with hypersensitivity reactions such as *anaphylaxis* and *angioedema*.

First-line treatment includes:

- securing the airway, restoration of blood pressure (laying the child flat and raising the legs, or in the recovery position if unconscious or nauseous and at risk of vomiting);
- administering adrenaline/epinephrine by **intramuscular** injection; the dose should be repeated if necessary at 5-minute intervals according to blood pressure, pulse, and respiratory function;
- administering high-flow **oxygen** and **intravenous fluids**;
- administering an antihistamine, such as chlorphenamine maleate, by slow intravenous injection or intramuscular injection as adjunctive treatment given after adrenaline.
- Administering an intravenous corticosteroid such as hydrocortisone p. 476 (preferably as sodium succinate) is of secondary value in the initial management of anaphylaxis because the onset of action is delayed for several hours, but should be given to prevent further deterioration in severely affected children.

Continuing respiratory deterioration requires further treatment with **bronchodilators** including inhaled or intravenous salbutamol p. 164, inhaled ipratropium bromide p. 161, intravenous aminophylline p. 176, or intravenous magnesium sulfate p. 646 [unlicensed indication] (as for acute severe asthma); in addition to oxygen, assisted respiration and possibly emergency tracheotomy may be necessary.

When a child is so ill that there is doubt about the adequacy of the circulation, the initial injection of adrenaline/epinephrine may need to be given as a *dilute solution by the intravenous route*, or by the *intraosseous route* if venous access is difficult; for details see adrenaline/epinephrine.

On discharge, child should be considered for further treatment with an oral antihistamine and an oral corticosteroid for up to 3 days to reduce the risk of further reaction. The child, or carer, should be instructed to return to hospital if symptoms recur and to contact their general practitioner for follow-up.

Children who are suspected of having had an anaphylactic reaction should be referred to a specialist for specific allergy diagnosis. Avoidance of the allergen is the principal treatment; if appropriate, an adrenaline/epinephrine auto-injector should be given for self-administration or a replacement supplied.

Intramuscular adrenaline (epinephrine)

The *intramuscular route is the first choice route* for the administration of adrenaline/epinephrine p. 143 in the management of anaphylaxis. Adrenaline/epinephrine is best given as an intramuscular injection into the anterolateral aspect of the middle third of the thigh; it has a rapid onset of action after intramuscular administration and in the shocked patient its absorption from the intramuscular site is faster and more reliable than from the subcutaneous site.

Children with severe allergy, and their carers, should ideally be instructed in the self-administration of adrenaline/epinephrine by intramuscular injection.

Prompt injection of adrenaline/epinephrine is of paramount importance. The adrenaline/epinephrine doses recommended for the emergency treatment of anaphylaxis by appropriately trained healthcare professionals are based on the revised recommendations of the Working Group of the Resuscitation Council (UK).

The MHRA/CHM have released important safety information regarding the use of auto-injectors. For further information, see *Important safety information* for adrenaline/epinephrine.

Intravenous adrenaline (epinephrine)

Intravenous adrenaline/epinephrine should be given only by those experienced in its use, in a setting where patients can be carefully monitored.

Where the child is severely ill and there is real doubt about adequacy of the circulation and absorption from the intramuscular injection site, adrenaline/epinephrine may be given by **slow***intravenous injection*, repeated according to response; if multiple doses are required consider giving adrenaline by slow intravenous infusion.

It is also important that, where intramuscular injection might still succeed, time should not be wasted seeking intravenous access.

Adrenaline/epinephrine is also given by the intravenous route for *acute hypotension*.

Angioedema

Angioedema is dangerous if *laryngeal oedema* is present. In this circumstance adrenaline/epinephrine injection, oxygen, antihistamines and corticosteroids should be given as described under **Anaphylaxis**. Tracheal intubation may be necessary. In some children with laryngeal oedema, adrenaline 1 in 1000 (1 mg/mL) solution may be given by nebuliser. However, nebulised adrenaline/epinephrine cannot be relied upon for a systemic effect—intramuscular adrenaline/epinephrine should be used.

Hereditary angioedema

The treatment of hereditary angioedema should be under specialist supervision. Unlike allergic angioedema, adrenaline/epinephrine, corticosteroids, and antihistamines should not be used for the treatment of acute attacks, including attacks involving laryngeal oedema, as they are ineffective and may delay appropriate treatment—intubation may be necessary. The administration of C1-esterase inhibitor p. 192 (in fresh frozen plasma or in partially purified form) can terminate acute attacks of *hereditary angioedema*; it can also be used for short-term prophylaxis before dental, medical, or surgical procedures. Tranexamic acid p. 87 is used for short-term or long-term prophylaxis of hereditary angioedema; short-term prophylaxis is started several days before planned procedures which may trigger an acute attack of hereditary angioedema (e.g. dental work) and continued for 2–5 days afterwards. Danazol [unlicensed indication] is best avoided in children because of its androgenic effects, but it can be used for short-term prophylaxis of hereditary angioedema.

Dose of intramuscular injection of adrenaline (epinephrine) for the emergency treatment of anaphylaxis by healthcare professionals

Age	Dose	Volume of adrenaline
▸ Child 1 month-5 years	150 micrograms	0.15 mL 1 in 1000 (1 mg/mL) adrenaline[1]
▸ Child 6-11 years	300 micrograms	0.3 mL 1 in 1000 (1 mg/mL) adrenaline
▸ Child 12-17 years	500 micrograms	0.5 mL 1 in 1000 (1 mg/mL) adrenaline[2]

These doses may be repeated several times if necessary at 5-minute intervals according to blood pressure, pulse and respiratory function.

1. Use suitable syringe for measuring small volume
2. 300 micrograms (0.3 mL) if child is small or prepubertal

ANTIHISTAMINES > NON-SEDATING

Acrivastine

19-Mar-2020

- **INDICATIONS AND DOSE**

Symptomatic relief of allergy such as hayfever, chronic idiopathic urticaria

▸ BY MOUTH

▸ Child 12-17 years: 8 mg 3 times a day

- **CONTRA-INDICATIONS** Avoid in Acute porphyrias p. 652
- **INTERACTIONS** → Appendix 1: antihistamines, non-sedating
- **SIDE-EFFECTS**

▸ **Common or very common** Drowsiness · dry mouth

▸ **Frequency not known** Dizziness · rash

SIDE-EFFECTS, FURTHER INFORMATION Non-sedating antihistamines such as acrivastine cause less sedation and psychomotor impairment than the older antihistamines, but can still occur; sedation is generally minimal. This is because non-sedating antihistamines penetrate the blood brain barrier to a much lesser extent.

- **ALLERGY AND CROSS-SENSITIVITY** Contra-indicated if history of hypersensitivity to triprolidine.
- **PREGNANCY** Most manufacturers of antihistamines advise avoiding their use during pregnancy; however, there is no evidence of teratogenicity.
- **BREAST FEEDING** Most antihistamines are present in breast milk in varying amounts; although not known to be harmful, most manufacturers advise avoiding their use in mothers who are breast-feeding.
- **RENAL IMPAIRMENT** Avoid in severe impairment.
- **PATIENT AND CARER ADVICE**

Driving and skilled tasks Although drowsiness is rare, nevertheless patients should be advised that it can occur and may affect performance of skilled tasks (e.g. cycling or driving); alcohol should be avoided.

- **MEDICINAL FORMS** There can be variation in the licensing of different medicines containing the same drug.

Capsule

▸ Benadryl Allergy Relief (McNeil Products Ltd)

Acrivastine 8 mg Benadryl Allergy Relief 8mg capsules | 24 capsule [P] £5.45 | 48 capsule [P] £9.91

Bilastine

12-Mar-2020

- **INDICATIONS AND DOSE**

Symptomatic relief of allergic rhinoconjunctivitis and urticaria

▸ BY MOUTH

▸ Child 12-17 years: 20 mg once daily

- **CONTRA-INDICATIONS** Avoid in Acute porphyrias p. 652
- **INTERACTIONS** → Appendix 1: antihistamines, non-sedating
- **SIDE-EFFECTS**

▸ **Common or very common** Drowsiness · headache

▸ **Uncommon** Anxiety · appetite increased · asthenia · bundle branch block · diarrhoea · dry mouth · dyspnoea · fever · gastritis · gastrointestinal discomfort · insomnia · nasal complaints · nausea · oral herpes · pre-existing condition improved · pruritus · QT interval prolongation · sinus arrhythmia · thirst · tinnitus · vertigo · weight increased

SIDE-EFFECTS, FURTHER INFORMATION Non-sedating antihistamines such as bilastine cause less sedation and psychomotor impairment than the older antihistamines, but can still occur; sedation is generally minimal. This is because non-sedating antihistamines penetrate the blood brain barrier to a much lesser extent.

- **PREGNANCY** Avoid—limited information available. Most manufacturers of antihistamines advise avoiding their use during pregnancy; however, there is no evidence of teratogenicity.
- **BREAST FEEDING** Avoid—no information available. Most antihistamines are present in breast milk in varying amounts; although not known to be harmful, most manufacturers advise avoiding their use in mothers who are breast-feeding.
- **DIRECTIONS FOR ADMINISTRATION** Take tablet 1 hour before or 2 hours after food or fruit juice.
- **PATIENT AND CARER ADVICE** Patients or carers should be given advice on how to administer bilastine tablets.

Driving and skilled tasks Although drowsiness is rare, nevertheless patients should be advised that it can occur and may affect performance of skilled tasks (e.g. cycling or driving); alcohol should be avoided.

● **MEDICINAL FORMS** There can be variation in the licensing of different medicines containing the same drug.

Tablet

CAUTIONARY AND ADVISORY LABELS 23

▸ Ilaxten (A. Menarini Farmaceutica Internazionale SRL)
Bilastine 20 mg Ilaxten 20mg tablets | 30 tablet PoM £6.00 DT = £6.00

Cetirizine hydrochloride

● **INDICATIONS AND DOSE**

Symptomatic relief of allergy such as hay fever, chronic idiopathic urticaria, atopic dermatitis

▸ BY MOUTH

▸ Child 1 year: 250 micrograms/kg twice daily
▸ Child 2–5 years: 2.5 mg twice daily
▸ Child 6–11 years: 5 mg twice daily
▸ Child 12–17 years: 10 mg once daily

● **UNLICENSED USE** Not licensed for use in children under 2 years.

● **CAUTIONS** Epilepsy

● **INTERACTIONS** → Appendix 1: antihistamines, non-sedating

● **SIDE-EFFECTS**

▸ **Uncommon** Agitation · asthenia · diarrhoea · malaise · paraesthesia · skin reactions

▸ **Rare or very rare** Aggression · angioedema · confusion · depression · hallucination · hepatic function abnormal · insomnia · movement disorders · oculogyration · oedema · seizure · syncope · tachycardia · taste altered · thrombocytopenia · tic · tremor · urinary disorders · vision disorders · weight increased

▸ **Frequency not known** Abdominal pain · appetite increased · dizziness · drowsiness · dry mouth · headache · memory loss · nausea · pharyngitis · suicidal ideation · vertigo

SIDE-EFFECTS, FURTHER INFORMATION Non-sedating antihistamines such as certirizine hydrochloride cause less sedation and psychomotor impairment than the older antihistamines, but can still occur; sedation is generally minimal. This is because non-sedating antihistamines penetrate the blood brain barrier to a much lesser extent.

● **PREGNANCY** Most manufacturers of antihistamines advise avoiding their use during pregnancy; however, there is no evidence of teratogenicity.

● **BREAST FEEDING** Most antihistamines are present in breast milk in varying amounts; although not known to be harmful, most manufacturers advise avoiding their use in mothers who are breast-feeding.

● **RENAL IMPAIRMENT** Avoid if estimated glomerular filtration rate less than 10 mL/minute/1.73 m^2.

Dose adjustments Use half normal dose if estimated glomerular filtration rate 30–50 mL/minute/1.73 m^2.

Use half normal dose and reduce dose frequency to alternate days if estimated glomerular filtration rate 10–30 mL/minute/1.73 m^2.

● **PATIENT AND CARER ADVICE**

Medicines for Children leaflet: Cetirizine for hay fever www.medicinesforchildren.org.uk/cetirizine-hay-fever-0

Driving and skilled tasks Although drowsiness is rare, nevertheless patients should be advised that it can occur and may affect performance of skilled tasks (e.g. cycling or driving); alcohol should be avoided.

● **PROFESSION SPECIFIC INFORMATION**

Dental practitioners' formulary

Cetirizine Tablets 10 mg may be prescribed.
Cetirizine Oral Solution 5 mg/5 mL may be prescribed.

● **MEDICINAL FORMS** There can be variation in the licensing of different medicines containing the same drug.

Oral solution

EXCIPIENTS: May contain Propylene glycol

▸ Cetirizine hydrochloride (Non-proprietary)
Cetirizine hydrochloride 1 mg per 1 ml Cetirizine 1mg/ml oral solution sugar free | 200 ml P DT = £1.55

Tablet

▸ Cetirizine hydrochloride (Non-proprietary)
Cetirizine hydrochloride 10 mg Cetirizine 10mg tablets | 30 tablet PoM £0.79–£1.01 DT = £0.98

Capsule

▸ Benadryl Allergy (McNeil Products Ltd)
Cetirizine hydrochloride 10 mg Benadryl Allergy Liquid Release 10mg capsules | 7 capsule GSL £3.09 DT = £3.09

Desloratadine

12-Mar-2020

● **INDICATIONS AND DOSE**

Symptomatic relief of allergy such as allergic rhinitis, urticaria, chronic idiopathic urticaria

▸ BY MOUTH

▸ Child 1–5 years: 1.25 mg once daily
▸ Child 6–11 years: 2.5 mg once daily
▸ Child 12–17 years: 5 mg once daily

PHARMACOKINETICS

▸ Desloratadine is a metabolite of loratadine.

● **INTERACTIONS** → Appendix 1: antihistamines, non-sedating

● **SIDE-EFFECTS**

▸ **Common or very common** Asthenia · dry mouth · headache

▸ **Rare or very rare** Akathisia · arrhythmias · diarrhoea · dizziness · drowsiness · gastrointestinal discomfort · hallucination · hepatic disorders · insomnia · myalgia · nausea · palpitations · seizure · vomiting

▸ **Frequency not known** Behaviour abnormal · photosensitivity reaction · QT interval prolongation

SIDE-EFFECTS, FURTHER INFORMATION Non-sedating antihistamines such as desloratadine cause less sedation and psychomotor impairment than the older antihistamines, but can still occur; sedation is generally minimal. This is because non-sedating antihistamines penetrate the blood brain barrier to a much lesser extent.

● **ALLERGY AND CROSS-SENSITIVITY** Contra-indicated if history of hypersensitivity to loratadine.

● **PREGNANCY** Most manufacturers of antihistamines advise avoiding their use during pregnancy; however, there is no evidence of teratogenicity.

● **BREAST FEEDING** Most antihistamines are present in breast milk in varying amounts; although not known to be harmful, most manufacturers advise avoiding their use in mothers who are breast-feeding.

● **RENAL IMPAIRMENT** Use with caution in severe impairment.

● **PRESCRIBING AND DISPENSING INFORMATION** Flavours of oral liquid formulations may include bubblegum.

● **PATIENT AND CARER ADVICE**

Driving and skilled tasks Although drowsiness is rare, nevertheless patients should be advised that it can occur and may affect performance of skilled tasks (e.g. cycling or driving); excess alcohol should be avoided.

● **MEDICINAL FORMS** There can be variation in the licensing of different medicines containing the same drug.

Oral solution

EXCIPIENTS: May contain Propylene glycol, sorbitol

▸ Desloratadine (Non-proprietary)
Desloratadine 500 microgram per 1 ml Desloratadine 2.5mg/5ml oral solution sugar free sugar-free | 100 ml PoM £6.57 sugar-free | 150 ml PoM £8.12–£9.86 DT = £9.86

3 Respiratory system

- ▸ Neoclarityn (Merck Sharp & Dohme Ltd)
  Desloratadine 500 microgram per 1 ml Neoclarityn 2.5mg/5ml oral solution sugar-free | 100 ml PoM £6.77 sugar-free | 150 ml PoM £10.15 DT = £9.86

Tablet

- ▸ Desloratadine (Non-proprietary)
  Desloratadine 5 mg Desloratadine 5mg tablets | 30 tablet PoM £6.77 DT = £1.32
- ▸ Neoclarityn (Merck Sharp & Dohme Ltd)
  Desloratadine 5 mg Neoclarityn 5mg tablets | 30 tablet PoM £6.77 DT = £1.32

Fexofenadine hydrochloride

13-Mar-2020

● **INDICATIONS AND DOSE**

Symptomatic relief of seasonal allergic rhinitis

▶ BY MOUTH

- ▸ Child 6–11 years: 30 mg twice daily
- ▸ Child 12–17 years: 120 mg once daily

Symptomatic relief of chronic idiopathic urticaria

▶ BY MOUTH

- ▸ Child 12–17 years: 180 mg once daily

PHARMACOKINETICS

- ▸ Fexofenadine is a metabolite of terfenadine.

● **INTERACTIONS** → Appendix 1: antihistamines, non-sedating

● **SIDE-EFFECTS**

▶ **Common or very common** Dizziness · drowsiness · headache · nausea

▶ **Uncommon** Fatigue

▶ **Frequency not known** Diarrhoea · nervousness · palpitations · skin reactions · sleep disorders · tachycardia

SIDE-EFFECTS, FURTHER INFORMATION Non-sedating antihistamines such as fexofenadine cause less sedation and psychomotor impairment than the older antihistamines, but can still occur; sedation is generally minimal. This is because non-sedating antihistamines penetrate the blood brain barrier to a much lesser extent.

● **PREGNANCY** Most manufacturers of antihistamines advise avoiding their use during pregnancy; however, there is no evidence of teratogenicity.

● **BREAST FEEDING** Most antihistamines are present in breast milk in varying amounts; although not known to be harmful, most manufacturers advise avoiding their use in mothers who are breast-feeding.

● **PATIENT AND CARER ADVICE**

Driving and skilled tasks Although drowsiness is rare, nevertheless patients should be advised that it can occur and may affect performance of skilled tasks (e.g. cycling or driving); alcohol should be avoided.

● **MEDICINAL FORMS** There can be variation in the licensing of different medicines containing the same drug. Forms available from special-order manufacturers include: oral suspension, oral solution

Tablet

CAUTIONARY AND ADVISORY LABELS 5

- ▸ Fexofenadine hydrochloride (Non-proprietary)
  Fexofenadine hydrochloride 120 mg Fexofenadine 120mg tablets | 30 tablet PoM £6.23 DT = £2.12
  Fexofenadine hydrochloride 180 mg Fexofenadine 180mg tablets | 30 tablet PoM £7.89 DT = £3.18
- ▸ Telfast (Sanofi)
  Fexofenadine hydrochloride 30 mg Telfast 30mg tablets | 60 tablet PoM £5.46 DT = £5.46
  Fexofenadine hydrochloride 120 mg Telfast 120mg tablets | 30 tablet PoM £5.99 DT = £2.12
  Fexofenadine hydrochloride 180 mg Telfast 180mg tablets | 30 tablet PoM £7.58 DT = £3.18

Levocetirizine hydrochloride

24-May-2017

● **INDICATIONS AND DOSE**

Symptomatic relief of allergy such as hay fever, urticaria

▶ BY MOUTH

- ▸ Child 2–5 years: 1.25 mg twice daily
- ▸ Child 6–17 years: 5 mg once daily

PHARMACOKINETICS

- ▸ Levocetirizine is an isomer of cetirizine.

● **UNLICENSED USE** Tablets not licensed for use in children under 6 years.

● **CONTRA-INDICATIONS** Avoid in Acute porphyrias p. 652

● **INTERACTIONS** → Appendix 1: antihistamines, non-sedating

● **SIDE-EFFECTS**

▶ **Common or very common** Asthenia · constipation · diarrhoea · drowsiness · dry mouth · sleep disorders

▶ **Uncommon** Abdominal pain

▶ **Frequency not known** Aggression · agitation · angioedema · appetite increased · arthralgia · depression · dizziness · dyspnoea · hallucination · hepatitis · myalgia · nausea · oedema · palpitations · paraesthesia · seizure · skin reactions · suicidal ideation · syncope · tachycardia · taste altered · tremor · urinary disorders · vertigo · vision disorders · vomiting · weight increased

SIDE-EFFECTS, FURTHER INFORMATION Non-sedating antihistamines such as levocetirizine cause less sedation and psychomotor impairment than the older antihistamines, but can still occur; sedation is generally minimal. This is because non-sedating antihistamines penetrate the blood brain barrier to a much lesser extent.

● **PREGNANCY** Most manufacturers of antihistamines advise avoiding their use during pregnancy; however, there is no evidence of teratogenicity.

● **BREAST FEEDING** Most antihistamines are present in breast milk in varying amounts; although not known to be harmful, most manufacturers advise avoiding their use in mothers who are breast-feeding.

● **RENAL IMPAIRMENT** Avoid if estimated glomerular filtration rate less than 10 mL/minute/1.73 m^2.

Dose adjustments Reduce dose frequency to alternate days if estimated glomerular filtration rate 30–50 mL/minute/1.73 m^2.

Reduce dose frequency to every 3 days if estimated glomerular filtration rate 10–30 mL/minute/1.73 m^2.

● **PATIENT AND CARER ADVICE**

Driving and skilled tasks Although drowsiness is rare, nevertheless patients should be advised that it can occur and may affect performance of skilled tasks (e.g. cycling or driving); alcohol should be avoided.

● **MEDICINAL FORMS** There can be variation in the licensing of different medicines containing the same drug.

Oral solution

- ▸ Xyzal (UCB Pharma Ltd)
  Levocetirizine dihydrochloride 500 microgram per 1 ml Xyzal 0.5mg/ml oral solution sugar-free | 200 ml PoM £6.00 DT = £6.00

Tablet

- ▸ Levocetirizine hydrochloride (Non-proprietary)
  Levocetirizine dihydrochloride 5 mg Levocetirizine 5mg tablets | 30 tablet PoM £4.39 DT = £4.21
- ▸ Xyzal (UCB Pharma Ltd)
  Levocetirizine dihydrochloride 5 mg Xyzal 5mg tablets | 30 tablet PoM £4.39 DT = £4.21

Loratadine

25-Mar-2020

● **INDICATIONS AND DOSE**

Symptomatic relief of allergy such as hay fever, chronic idiopathic urticaria

▶ BY MOUTH
- ▶ Child 2–11 years (body-weight up to 31 kg): 5 mg once daily
- ▶ Child 2–11 years (body-weight 31 kg and above): 10 mg once daily
- ▶ Child 12–17 years: 10 mg once daily

● **INTERACTIONS** → Appendix 1: antihistamines, non-sedating

● **SIDE-EFFECTS**
- ▶ **Common or very common** Drowsiness · fatigue · headache · nervousness
- ▶ **Uncommon** Appetite increased · insomnia
- ▶ **Rare or very rare** Alopecia · angioedema · dizziness · dry mouth · gastritis · hepatic function abnormal · nausea · palpitations · rash · seizure · tachycardia

SIDE-EFFECTS, FURTHER INFORMATION Non-sedating antihistamines such as loratadine cause less sedation and psychomotor impairment than the older antihistamines, but can still occur; sedation is generally minimal. This is because non-sedating antihistamines penetrate the blood brain barrier to a much lesser extent.

● **PREGNANCY** Most manufacturers of antihistamines advise avoiding their use during pregnancy; however, there is no evidence of teratogenicity.

● **BREAST FEEDING** Most antihistamines are present in breast milk in varying amounts; although not known to be harmful, most manufacturers advise avoiding their use in mothers who are breast-feeding.

● **HEPATIC IMPAIRMENT** Manufacturer advises caution in severe impairment (risk of increased exposure).

Dose adjustments Manufacturer advises initial dose reduction to alternate days in severe impairment.

● **PATIENT AND CARER ADVICE**

Medicines for Children leaflet: Loratadine for allergy symptoms www.medicinesforchildren.org.uk/loratadine-allergy-symptoms

Driving and skilled tasks Although drowsiness is rare, nevertheless patients and their carers should be advised that it can occur and may affect performance of skilled tasks (e.g. cycling or driving); alcohol should be avoided.

● **PROFESSION SPECIFIC INFORMATION**

Dental practitioners' formulary

Loratadine 10 mg tablets may be prescribed.
Loratadine syrup 5 mg/5 mL may be prescribed.

● **MEDICINAL FORMS** There can be variation in the licensing of different medicines containing the same drug.

Oral solution

EXCIPIENTS: May contain Propylene glycol

▶ Loratadine (Non-proprietary)
Loratadine 1 mg per 1 ml Loratadine 5mg/5ml oral solution | 100 ml [PoM] £1.90 DT = £1.90
Loratadine 5mg/5ml oral solution sugar free | 100 ml [PoM] £2.85

Tablet

▶ Loratadine (Non-proprietary)
Loratadine 10 mg Loratadine 10mg tablets | 30 tablet [PoM] [DPF] DT = £0.95

▶ Clarityn (Loratadine) (Bayer Plc)
Loratadine 10 mg Clarityn Allergy 10mg tablets | 60 tablet [P] £8.85

Mizolastine

12-Mar-2020

● **INDICATIONS AND DOSE**

Symptomatic relief of allergy such as hay fever, urticaria

▶ BY MOUTH
- ▶ Child 12–17 years: 10 mg once daily

● **CONTRA-INDICATIONS** Cardiac disease · susceptibility to QT-interval prolongation

● **INTERACTIONS** → Appendix 1: antihistamines, non-sedating

● **SIDE-EFFECTS**
- ▶ **Common or very common** Appetite increased · asthenia · diarrhoea · dizziness · drowsiness · dry mouth · gastrointestinal discomfort · headache · nausea · weight increased
- ▶ **Uncommon** Anxiety · arrhythmias · arthralgia · depression · myalgia · palpitations
- ▶ **Rare or very rare** Hypersensitivity
- ▶ **Frequency not known** Asthma exacerbated · bronchospasm · QT interval prolongation

SIDE-EFFECTS, FURTHER INFORMATION Non-sedating antihistamines such as mizolastine cause less sedation and psychomotor impairment than the older antihistamines, but can still occur; sedation is generally minimal. This is because non-sedating antihistamines penetrate the blood brain barrier to a much lesser extent.

● **PREGNANCY** Most manufacturers of antihistamines advise avoiding their use during pregnancy; however, there is no evidence of teratogenicity.

● **BREAST FEEDING** Most antihistamines are present in breast milk in varying amounts; although not known to be harmful, most manufacturers advise avoiding their use in mothers who are breast-feeding.

● **HEPATIC IMPAIRMENT** Manufacturer advises avoid in significant impairment.

● **PATIENT AND CARER ADVICE**

Driving and skilled tasks Although drowsiness is rare, nevertheless patients and their carers should be advised that it can occur and may affect performance of skilled tasks (e.g. cycling or driving); alcohol should be avoided.

● **MEDICINAL FORMS** There can be variation in the licensing of different medicines containing the same drug.

Modified-release tablet

CAUTIONARY AND ADVISORY LABELS 25

▶ Mizollen (Sanofi)
Mizolastine 10 mg Mizollen 10mg modified-release tablets | 30 tablet [PoM] £6.92 DT = £6.92

Rupatadine

29-Apr-2019

● **DRUG ACTION** Rupatadine is a second generation non-sedating antihistamine.

● **INDICATIONS AND DOSE**

Symptomatic relief of allergic rhinitis and urticaria

▶ BY MOUTH USING TABLETS
- ▶ Child 12–17 years: 10 mg once daily

▶ BY MOUTH USING ORAL SOLUTION
- ▶ Child 2–11 years (body-weight 10–24 kg): 2.5 mg once daily
- ▶ Child 2–11 years (body-weight 25 kg and above): 5 mg once daily

● **CAUTIONS** History of QT-interval prolongation · predisposition to arrhythmia · uncorrected hypokalaemia

● **INTERACTIONS** → Appendix 1: antihistamines, non-sedating

● **SIDE-EFFECTS**
- ▶ **Common or very common** Asthenia · dizziness · drowsiness · dry mouth · headache
- ▶ **Uncommon** Appetite increased · arthralgia · back pain · concentration impaired · constipation · cough · diarrhoea · dry throat · eosinophilia · epistaxis · fever · gastrointestinal discomfort · increased risk of infection · irritability · malaise · myalgia · nasal dryness · nausea · neutropenia · night sweats · oropharyngeal pain · skin reactions · thirst · vomiting · weight increased

▸ **Rare or very rare** Palpitations · tachycardia

SIDE-EFFECTS, FURTHER INFORMATION Non-sedating antihistamines such as rupatadine cause less sedation and psychomotor impairment than the older antihistamines, but can still occur; sedation is generally minimal. This is because non-sedating antihistamines penetrate the blood brain barrier to a much lesser extent.

- **PREGNANCY** Most manufacturers of antihistamines advise avoiding their use during pregnancy; however, there is no evidence of teratogenicity.
- **BREAST FEEDING** Most antihistamines are present in breast milk in varying amounts; although not known to be harmful, most manufacturers advise avoiding their use in mothers who are breast-feeding.
- **HEPATIC IMPAIRMENT** Manufacturer advises avoid (no information available).
- **RENAL IMPAIRMENT** Manufacturer advises avoid—no information available.

- **MEDICINAL FORMS** There can be variation in the licensing of different medicines containing the same drug.

Oral solution

▸ Rupatadine (Non-proprietary)

Rupatadine (as Rupatadine fumarate) 1 mg per 1 ml Rupatadine 1mg/ml oral solution | 120 ml [PoM] £9.95–£11.94 DT = £11.45

Tablet

▸ Rupatadine (Non-proprietary)

Rupatadine (as Rupatadine fumarate) 10 mg Rupatadine 10mg tablets | 30 tablet [PoM] £36.00 DT = £35.25

ANTIHISTAMINES › SEDATING

Alimemazine tartrate

25-Oct-2019

(Trimeprazine tartrate)

- **INDICATIONS AND DOSE**

Urticaria | Pruritus

▸ BY MOUTH

- Child 6 months–1 year (specialist use only): 250 micrograms/kg 3–4 times a day (max. per dose 2.5 mg)
- Child 2–4 years: 2.5 mg 3–4 times a day
- Child 5–11 years: 5 mg 3–4 times a day
- Child 12–17 years: 10 mg 2–3 times a day, in severe cases up to maximum daily dose has been used; maximum 100 mg per day

Premedication to anaesthesia

▸ BY MOUTH

- Child 2–6 years: Up to 2 mg/kg, to be given 1–2 hours before operation

- **UNLICENSED USE** Not licensed for use in children under 2 years.
- **CONTRA-INDICATIONS** Children under 2 years except on specialist advice (risk of respiratory depression) · epilepsy · hepatic dysfunction · history of narrow angle glaucoma · hypothyroidism · myasthenia gravis · neonate (due to significant antimuscarinic activity) · Parkinson's disease · phaeochromocytoma · renal dysfunction
- **CAUTIONS** Cardiovascular diseases (due to tachycardia-inducing and hypotensive effects of phenothiazines) · exposure to sunlight should be avoided during treatment with high doses · pyloroduodenal obstruction · urinary retention · volume depleted patients who are more susceptible to orthostatic hypotension
- **INTERACTIONS** → Appendix 1: antihistamines, sedating
- **SIDE-EFFECTS** Agitation · agranulocytosis · amenorrhoea · atrioventricular block · autonomic dysfunction · bile thrombus · consciousness impaired · drug fever · dry mouth · eosinophilia · erectile dysfunction · eye disorder · galactorrhoea · gynaecomastia · hepatic disorders · hyperprolactinaemia · hyperthermia · hypotension · insomnia · leucopenia (on prolonged high dose) · movement disorders · muscle rigidity · nasal congestion · neuroleptic malignant syndrome · pallor · parkinsonism · photosensitivity reaction · postural hypotension (more common in the elderly or in volume depletion) · QT interval prolongation · respiratory depression · seizure · skin reactions · tardive dyskinesia (more common after long term high doses) · tremor · ventricular fibrillation (increased risk with hypokalamia and cardiac disease) · ventricular tachycardia (increased risk with hypokalamia and cardiac disease)

SIDE-EFFECTS, FURTHER INFORMATION Drowsiness may diminish after a few days.

Patients on high dosage may develop photosensitivity and should avoid exposure to direct sunlight.

Children are more susceptible to side-effects.

- **PREGNANCY** Most manufacturers of antihistamines advise avoiding their use during pregnancy; however, there is no evidence of teratogenicity. Use in the latter part of the third trimester may cause adverse effects in neonates such as irritability, paradoxical excitability, and tremor.
- **BREAST FEEDING** Most antihistamines are present in breast milk in varying amounts; although not known to be harmful, most manufacturers advise avoiding their use in mothers who are breast-feeding.
- **HEPATIC IMPAIRMENT** Manufacturer advises avoid—no information available.
- **RENAL IMPAIRMENT** Avoid.
- **PATIENT AND CARER ADVICE**

Driving and skilled tasks Drowsiness may affect performance of skilled tasks (e.g. cycling or driving); sedating effects enhanced by alcohol.

- **MEDICINAL FORMS** There can be variation in the licensing of different medicines containing the same drug. Forms available from special-order manufacturers include: oral solution

Oral solution

CAUTIONARY AND ADVISORY LABELS 2

▸ Alimemazine tartrate (Non-proprietary)

Alimemazine tartrate 1.5 mg per 1 ml Alimemazine 7.5mg/5ml oral solution | 100 ml [PoM] £179.58 DT = £179.58

Alimemazine tartrate 6 mg per 1 ml Alimemazine 30mg/5ml oral solution | 100 ml [PoM] £243.51 DT = £243.51

Tablet

CAUTIONARY AND ADVISORY LABELS 2

▸ Alimemazine tartrate (Non-proprietary)

Alimemazine tartrate 10 mg Alimemazine 10mg tablets | 28 tablet [PoM] £112.88 DT = £112.88

Chlorphenamine maleate

28-Nov-2019

(Chlorpheniramine maleate)

- **INDICATIONS AND DOSE**

Symptomatic relief of allergy such as hay fever, urticaria, food allergy, drug reactions | Relief of itch associated with chickenpox

▸ BY MOUTH

- Child 1–23 months: 1 mg twice daily
- Child 2–5 years: 1 mg every 4–6 hours; maximum 6 mg per day
- Child 6–11 years: 2 mg every 4–6 hours; maximum 12 mg per day
- Child 12–17 years: 4 mg every 4–6 hours; maximum 24 mg per day

- ▶ BY INTRAMUSCULAR INJECTION, OR BY INTRAVENOUS INJECTION
- ▶ Child 1–5 months: 250 micrograms/kg (max. per dose 2.5 mg), repeated if necessary; maximum 4 doses per day
- ▶ Child 6 months–5 years: 2.5 mg, repeated if necessary; maximum 4 doses per day
- ▶ Child 6–11 years: 5 mg, repeated if necessary; maximum 4 doses per day
- ▶ Child 12–17 years: 10 mg, repeated if necessary; maximum 4 doses per day

Emergency treatment of anaphylactic reactions

- ▶ BY INTRAMUSCULAR INJECTION, OR BY INTRAVENOUS INJECTION
- ▶ Child 1–5 months: 250 micrograms/kg (max. per dose 2.5 mg), repeated if necessary; maximum 4 doses per day
- ▶ Child 6 months–5 years: 2.5 mg, repeated if necessary; maximum 4 doses per day
- ▶ Child 6–11 years: 5 mg, repeated if necessary; maximum 4 doses per day
- ▶ Child 12–17 years: 10 mg, repeated if necessary; maximum 4 doses per day

● UNLICENSED USE *Injection* not licensed for use in neonates. *Tablets* not licensed for use in children under 6 years. *Syrup* not licensed for use in children under 1 year.

IMPORTANT SAFETY INFORMATION

MHRA/CHM ADVICE: OVER-THE-COUNTER COUGH AND COLD MEDICINES FOR CHILDREN (APRIL 2009)

Children under 6 years should not be given over-the-counter cough and cold medicines containing chlorphenamine.

● CONTRA-INDICATIONS Neonate (due to significant antimuscarinic activity)

● CAUTIONS Epilepsy · pyloroduodenal obstruction · susceptibility to angle-closure glaucoma · urinary retention

● INTERACTIONS → Appendix 1: antihistamines, sedating

● SIDE-EFFECTS

GENERAL SIDE-EFFECTS

- ▶ **Common or very common** Concentration impaired · coordination abnormal · dizziness · dry mouth · fatigue · headache · nausea · vision blurred
- ▶ **Frequency not known** Agitation · appetite decreased · blood disorder · bronchial secretion viscosity increased · depression · diarrhoea · haemolytic anaemia · hypotension · irritability · muscle twitching · muscle weakness · nightmare · palpitations · photosensitivity reaction · skin reactions · tinnitus · urinary retention · vomiting

SPECIFIC SIDE-EFFECTS

- ▶ **Common or very common**
- ▶ With oral use Drowsiness
- ▶ **Frequency not known**
- ▶ With oral use Angioedema · arrhythmias · chest tightness · confusion · gastrointestinal discomfort · hepatic disorders
- ▶ With parenteral use Central nervous system stimulation · dyspepsia · gastrointestinal disorder · hepatitis · sedation

SIDE-EFFECTS, FURTHER INFORMATION Children are more susceptible to side-effects.

● PREGNANCY Most manufacturers of antihistamines advise avoiding their use during pregnancy; however, there is no evidence of teratogenicity. Use in the latter part of the third trimester may cause adverse effects in neonates such as irritability, paradoxical excitability, and tremor.

● BREAST FEEDING Most antihistamines are present in breast milk in varying amounts; although not known to be harmful, most manufacturers advise avoiding their use in mothers who are breast-feeding.

● HEPATIC IMPAIRMENT Manufacturer advises caution.

● DIRECTIONS FOR ADMINISTRATION For *intravenous injection*, give over 1 minute; if small dose required, dilute with Sodium Chloride 0.9%.

● PATIENT AND CARER ADVICE
Medicines for Children leaflet: Chlorphenamine maleate for allergy symptoms www.medicinesforchildren.org.uk/chlorphenamine-maleate-allergy-symptoms-0

Driving and skilled tasks Drowsiness may affect performance of skilled tasks (e.g. cycling or driving); sedating effects enhanced by alcohol.

● PROFESSION SPECIFIC INFORMATION

Dental practitioners' formulary
Chlorphenamine tablets may be prescribed.
Chlorphenamine oral solution may be prescribed.

● EXCEPTIONS TO LEGAL CATEGORY

- ▶ With intramuscular use or intravenous use Prescription only medicine restriction does not apply to chlorphenamine injection where administration is for saving life in emergency.

● MEDICINAL FORMS There can be variation in the licensing of different medicines containing the same drug. Forms available from special-order manufacturers include: oral solution

Solution for injection

- ▶ **Chlorphenamine maleate (Non-proprietary)**
  Chlorphenamine maleate 10 mg per 1 ml Chlorphenamine 10mg/1ml solution for injection ampoules | 5 ampoule [PoM] £22.50 DT = £22.50 | 5 ampoule [PoM] [CD] DT = £22.50 (Hospital only)

Oral solution

CAUTIONARY AND ADVISORY LABELS 2

- ▶ **Chlorphenamine maleate (Non-proprietary)**
  Chlorphenamine maleate 400 microgram per 1 ml Chlorphenamine 2mg/5ml oral solution sugar free sugar-free | 150 ml [P] £2.78 DT = £2.21
- ▶ **Allerief** (Crescent Pharma Ltd)
  Chlorphenamine maleate 400 microgram per 1 ml Allerief 2mg/5ml oral solution sugar-free | 150 ml [P] £2.21 DT = £2.21
- ▶ **Piriton** (GlaxoSmithKline Consumer Healthcare)
  Chlorphenamine maleate 400 microgram per 1 ml Piriton 2mg/5ml syrup | 150 ml [P] £2.78 DT = £2.78

Tablet

CAUTIONARY AND ADVISORY LABELS 2

- ▶ **Chlorphenamine maleate (Non-proprietary)**
  Chlorphenamine maleate 4 mg Chlorphenamine 4mg tablets | 28 tablet [P] £1.00 DT = £0.78
- ▶ **Allerief** (Crescent Pharma Ltd)
  Chlorphenamine maleate 4 mg Allerief 4mg tablets | 28 tablet [P] £1.74 DT = £0.78
- ▶ **Hayleve** (Genesis Pharmaceuticals Ltd)
  Chlorphenamine maleate 4 mg Hayleve 4mg tablets | 28 tablet [P] £0.76 DT = £0.78
- ▶ **Piriton** (GlaxoSmithKline Consumer Healthcare)
  Chlorphenamine maleate 4 mg Piriton 4mg tablets | 500 tablet [P] £6.96
  Piriton Allergy 4mg tablets | 30 tablet [P] £2.23 | 60 tablet [P] £3.90
- ▶ **Pollenase (chlorphenamine)** (East Midlands Pharma Ltd)
  Chlorphenamine maleate 4 mg Pollenase Antihistamine 4mg tablets | 30 tablet [P] £1.00

Hydroxyzine hydrochloride

19-Mar-2020

● DRUG ACTION Hydroxyzine is a sedating antihistamine which exerts its actions by antagonising the effects of histamine.

● INDICATIONS AND DOSE

Pruritus

- ▶ BY MOUTH
- ▶ Child 6 months–5 years: 5–15 mg daily in divided doses, dose adjusted according to weight; maximum 2 mg/kg per day

continued →

- Child 6–17 years (body-weight up to 40 kg): Initially 15–25 mg daily in divided doses, dose increased as necessary, adjusted according to weight; maximum 2 mg/kg per day
- Child 6–17 years (body-weight 40 kg and above): Initially 15–25 mg daily in divided doses, increased if necessary to 50–100 mg daily in divided doses, dose adjusted according to weight

IMPORTANT SAFETY INFORMATION

MHRA/CHM ADVICE: RISK OF QT-INTERVAL PROLONGATION AND TORSADE DE POINTES (APRIL 2015)

Following concerns of heart rhythm abnormalities, the safety and efficacy of hydroxyzine has been reviewed by the European Medicines Agency. The review concludes that hydroxyzine is associated with a small risk of QT-interval prolongation and torsade de pointes; these events are most likely to occur in patients who have risk factors for QT prolongation, e.g. concomitant use of drugs that prolong the QT-interval, cardiovascular disease, family history of sudden cardiac death, significant electrolyte imbalance (low plasma-potassium or plasma-magnesium concentrations), or significant bradycardia.

To minimise the risk of such adverse effects, the following dose restrictions have been made and new cautions and contra-indications added:

- Hydroxyzine is contra-indicated in patients with prolonged QT-interval or who have risk factors for QT-interval prolongation;
- Consider the risks of QT-interval prolongation and torsade de pointes before prescribing to patients taking drugs that lower heart rate or plasma-potassium concentration;
- In children with body-weight up to 40 kg, the maximum daily dose is 2 mg/kg;
- The lowest effective dose for the shortest period of time should be prescribed.

- **CONTRA-INDICATIONS** Acquired or congenital QT interval prolongation · predisposition to QT interval prolongation

CONTRA-INDICATIONS, FURTHER INFORMATION

- **QT interval prolongation** Risk factors for QT interval prolongation include significant electrolyte imbalance, bradycardia, cardiovascular disease, and family history of sudden cardiac death.

- **CAUTIONS** Bladder outflow obstruction · breathing problems · cardiovascular disease · children · decreased gastrointestinal motility · dementia · epilepsy · hypertension · hyperthyroidism · myasthenia gravis · pyloroduodenal obstruction · stenosing peptic ulcer · susceptibility to angle-closure glaucoma · urinary retention

CAUTIONS, FURTHER INFORMATION Children have an increased susceptibility to side-effects, particularly CNS effects.

- **INTERACTIONS** → Appendix 1: antihistamines, sedating
- **SIDE-EFFECTS**
- **Rare or very rare** Severe cutaneous adverse reactions (SCARs) · skin reactions
- **Frequency not known** Agranulocytosis · alopecia · anticholinergic syndrome · anxiety · appetite decreased · arrhythmias · asthenia · blood disorder · bronchial secretion viscosity increased · chest tightness · chills · coma · concentration impaired · confusion · constipation · depression · diarrhoea · dizziness · drowsiness · dry mouth · dry throat · dyskinesia (on discontinuation) · epigastric pain · fever · flushing · gastrointestinal disorders · haemolytic anaemia · hallucination · headache · hepatic function abnormal · hyperhidrosis · hypotension · irritability · labyrinthitis · leucopenia · malaise · menstruation irregular · movement disorders · myalgia · nasal congestion · nausea · palpitations · paraesthesia · QT interval prolongation · respiratory disorders · respiratory tract dryness · seizure (with high doses) · sexual dysfunction · sleep disorders · speech slurred · taste bitter · thrombocytopenia · tinnitus · tremor (with high doses) · urinary disorders · vertigo · vision disorders · vomiting

SIDE-EFFECTS, FURTHER INFORMATION Paradoxical stimulation may occur rarely, especially with high doses. Drowsiness may diminish after a few days of treatment.

- **ALLERGY AND CROSS-SENSITIVITY** Manufacturer advises hydroxyzine should be avoided in patients with previous hypersensitivity to cetirizine or other piperazine derivatives, and aminophylline.
- **PREGNANCY** Manufacturers advise avoid—toxicity in *animal* studies with higher doses. Use in the latter part of the third trimester may cause irritability, paradoxical excitability, and tremor in the neonate.
- **BREAST FEEDING** Manufacturer advises avoid—expected to be present in milk but effect unknown.
- **HEPATIC IMPAIRMENT** Manufacturer advises caution in mild to moderate impairment (increased risk of accumulation); avoid in severe impairment.

Dose adjustments Manufacturer advises dose reduction of 33% in mild to moderate impairment.

- **RENAL IMPAIRMENT**

Dose adjustments Manufacturers advise reduce daily dose by half in moderate to severe renal impairment.

- **EFFECT ON LABORATORY TESTS** May interfere with methacholine test—manufacturer advises stop treatment 96 hours prior to test. May interfere with skin testing for allergy—manufacturer advises stop treatment one week prior to test.
- **PATIENT AND CARER ADVICE**

Driving and skilled tasks Drowsiness may affect performance of skilled tasks (e.g. cycling or driving); sedating effects enhanced by alcohol.

- **MEDICINAL FORMS** There can be variation in the licensing of different medicines containing the same drug. Forms available from special-order manufacturers include: oral suspension, oral solution

Tablet

CAUTIONARY AND ADVISORY LABELS 2

- **Hydroxyzine hydrochloride (Non-proprietary)**

Hydroxyzine hydrochloride 10 mg Hydroxyzine 10mg tablets | 84 tablet PoM £2.10 DT = £1.20

Hydroxyzine hydrochloride 25 mg Hydroxyzine 25mg tablets | 28 tablet PoM £1.91 DT = £1.71

- **Atarax** (Alliance Pharmaceuticals Ltd)

Hydroxyzine hydrochloride 10 mg Atarax 10mg tablets | 84 tablet PoM £1.20 DT = £1.20

Hydroxyzine hydrochloride 25 mg Atarax 25mg tablets | 28 tablet PoM £0.62 DT = £1.71

Ketotifen

13-May-2020

- **INDICATIONS AND DOSE**

Allergic rhinitis

- BY MOUTH
- Child 3–17 years: 1 mg twice daily

- **CONTRA-INDICATIONS** Avoid in Acute porphyrias p. 652 · neonate (due to significant antimuscarinic activity)
- **CAUTIONS** Epilepsy · pyloroduodenal obstruction · susceptibility to angle-closure glaucoma · urinary retention
- **INTERACTIONS** → Appendix 1: antihistamines, sedating
- **SIDE-EFFECTS**
- **Common or very common** Anxiety · insomnia · irritability
- **Uncommon** Cystitis · dizziness · dry mouth · skin reactions

- ▸ **Rare or very rare** Hepatitis · sedation · seizure · Stevens-Johnson syndrome · weight increased

SIDE-EFFECTS, FURTHER INFORMATION Drowsiness is a significant side-effect with most of the older antihistamines although paradoxical stimulation may occur rarely, especially with high doses. Drowsiness may diminish after a few days of treatment and is considerably less of a problem with the newer antihistamines.

- **PREGNANCY** Most manufacturers of antihistamines advise avoiding their use during pregnancy; however, there is no evidence of teratogenicity. Use in the latter part of the third trimester may cause adverse effects in neonates such as irritability, paradoxical excitability, and tremor.
- **BREAST FEEDING** Most antihistamines are present in breast milk in varying amounts; although not known to be harmful, most manufacturers advise avoiding their use in mothers who are breast-feeding.
- **PATIENT AND CARER ADVICE**

Driving and skilled tasks Drowsiness may affect performance of skilled tasks (e.g. driving or cycling); sedating effects enhanced by alcohol.

- **MEDICINAL FORMS** There can be variation in the licensing of different medicines containing the same drug. Forms available from special-order manufacturers include: oral solution

Oral solution

CAUTIONARY AND ADVISORY LABELS 2, 21

▸ Zaditen (CD Pharma Srl)

Ketotifen (as Ketotifen fumarate) 200 microgram per 1 ml Zaditen 1mg/5ml elixir sugar-free | 300 ml [PoM] £8.91 DT = £8.91

Tablet

CAUTIONARY AND ADVISORY LABELS 2, 21

▸ Zaditen (CD Pharma Srl)

Ketotifen (as Ketotifen fumarate) 1 mg Zaditen 1mg tablets | 60 tablet [PoM] £7.53 DT = £7.53

Promethazine hydrochloride

28-Nov-2019

- **INDICATIONS AND DOSE**

Symptomatic relief of allergy such as hay fever and urticaria | Insomnia associated with urticaria and pruritus

▶ BY MOUTH

- ▸ Child 2-4 years: 5 mg twice daily, alternatively 5–15 mg once daily, dose to be taken at night
- ▸ Child 5-9 years: 5–10 mg twice daily, alternatively 10–25 mg once daily, dose to be taken at night
- ▸ Child 10-17 years: 10–20 mg 2–3 times a day, alternatively 25 mg once daily, dose to be taken at night, increased if necessary to 25 mg twice daily

Sedation (short-term use)

▶ BY MOUTH

- ▸ Child 2-4 years: 15–20 mg
- ▸ Child 5-9 years: 20–25 mg
- ▸ Child 10-17 years: 25–50 mg

Sedation in intensive care

▶ BY MOUTH, OR BY SLOW INTRAVENOUS INJECTION, OR BY DEEP INTRAMUSCULAR INJECTION

- ▸ Child 1 month-11 years: 0.5–1 mg/kg 4 times a day (max. per dose 25 mg), adjusted according to response
- ▸ Child 12-17 years: 25–50 mg 4 times a day, adjusted according to response

Nausea | Vomiting | Vertigo | Labyrinthine disorders | Motion sickness

▶ BY MOUTH

- ▸ Child 2-4 years: 5 mg, to be taken at bedtime on night before travel, repeat following morning if necessary
- ▸ Child 5-9 years: 10 mg, to be taken at bedtime on night before travel, repeat following morning if necessary
- ▸ Child 10-17 years: 20–25 mg, to be taken at bedtime on night before travel, repeat following morning if necessary

- **UNLICENSED USE** Not licensed for use for sedation in children under 2 years.

IMPORTANT SAFETY INFORMATION

MHRA/CHM ADVICE: OVER-THE-COUNTER COUGH AND COLD MEDICINES FOR CHILDREN (APRIL 2009)

Children under 6 years should not be given over-the-counter cough and cold medicines containing promethazine.

- **CONTRA-INDICATIONS** Neonate (due to significant antimuscarinic activity) · should not be given to children under 2 years, except on specialist advice, due to the potential for fatal respiratory depression
- **CAUTIONS**

GENERAL CAUTIONS Epilepsy · pyloroduodenal obstruction · severe coronary artery disease · susceptibility to angle-closure glaucoma · urinary retention

SPECIFIC CAUTIONS

- ▸ With intravenous use Avoid extravasation with intravenous injection

- **INTERACTIONS** → Appendix 1: antihistamines, sedating
- **SIDE-EFFECTS**

GENERAL SIDE-EFFECTS

Arrhythmia · blood disorder · confusion · dizziness · drowsiness · dry mouth · headache · hypotension · jaundice · movement disorders · palpitations · photosensitivity reaction · urinary retention · vision blurred

SPECIFIC SIDE-EFFECTS

- ▸ With oral use Agranulocytosis · angle closure glaucoma · anticholinergic syndrome · anxiety · insomnia · leucopenia · nasal congestion · nausea · rash · seizure · thrombocytopenia · tinnitus · tremor · vomiting
- ▸ With parenteral use Appetite decreased · epigastric discomfort · fatigue · haemolytic anaemia · hypersensitivity · muscle spasms · nightmare · restlessness · skin reactions

- **PREGNANCY** Most manufacturers of antihistamines advise avoiding their use during pregnancy; however, there is no evidence of teratogenicity. Use in the latter part of the third trimester may cause adverse effects in neonates such as irritability, paradoxical excitability, and tremor.
- **BREAST FEEDING** Most antihistamines are present in breast milk in varying amounts; although not known to be harmful, most manufacturers advise avoiding their use in mothers who are breast-feeding.
- **HEPATIC IMPAIRMENT** Manufacturer advises caution.
- **RENAL IMPAIRMENT** Use with caution.
- **PATIENT AND CARER ADVICE**

Driving and skilled tasks Drowsiness may affect the performance of skilled tasks (e.g. cycling or driving); sedating effects enhanced by alcohol.

- **PROFESSION SPECIFIC INFORMATION**

Dental practitioners' formulary

Promethazine Hydrochloride Tablets 10 mg or 25 mg may be prescribed.

Promethazine Hydrochloride Oral Solution (elixir) 5 mg/5 mL may be prescribed.

- **LESS SUITABLE FOR PRESCRIBING** Promethazine is less suitable for prescribing for sedation.
- **EXCEPTIONS TO LEGAL CATEGORY** Prescription only medicine restriction does not apply to promethazine hydrochloride injection where administration is for saving life in emergency.

- **MEDICINAL FORMS** There can be variation in the licensing of different medicines containing the same drug. Forms available from special-order manufacturers include: oral suspension, oral solution

Solution for injection
EXCIPIENTS: May contain Sulfites
▸ Phenergan (Sanofi)
Promethazine hydrochloride 25 mg per 1 ml Phenergan 25mg/1ml solution for injection ampoules | 10 ampoule PoM £6.74 DT = £6.74

Oral solution
CAUTIONARY AND ADVISORY LABELS 2
EXCIPIENTS: May contain Sulfites
ELECTROLYTES: May contain Sodium
▸ Phenergan (Sanofi)
Promethazine hydrochloride 1 mg per 1 ml Phenergan 5mg/5ml elixir sugar-free | 100 ml P £2.85 DT = £2.85

Tablet
CAUTIONARY AND ADVISORY LABELS 2
▸ Promethazine hydrochloride (Non-proprietary)
Promethazine hydrochloride 10 mg Promethazine hydrochloride 10mg tablets | 56 tablet PoM £3.67 DT = £3.67
Promethazine hydrochloride 25 mg Promethazine hydrochloride 25mg tablets | 56 tablet P £4.65–£4.91 DT = £4.85
▸ Phenergan (Sanofi)
Promethazine hydrochloride 10 mg Phenergan 10mg tablets | 56 tablet P £2.96 DT = £3.67
Promethazine hydrochloride 25 mg Phenergan Nightime 25mg tablets | 14 tablet P £2.79
Phenergan 25mg tablets | 56 tablet P £4.65 DT = £4.85
▸ Sominex (Teva UK Ltd)
Promethazine hydrochloride 20 mg Sominex 20mg tablets | 8 tablet P £1.89 DT = £1.89 | 16 tablet P £2.69 DT = £2.69

VACCINES > ALLERGEN-TYPE

Bee venom extract

28-Apr-2020

- **INDICATIONS AND DOSE**

Hypersensitivity to bee venom
▸ BY SUBCUTANEOUS INJECTION
▸ Child: (consult product literature)

> **IMPORTANT SAFETY INFORMATION**
> DESENSITISING VACCINES
> In view of concerns about the safety of desensitising vaccines, it is recommended that they are used by specialists and only for the following indications:
> - seasonal allergic hay fever (caused by pollen) that has not responded to anti-allergic drugs;
> - hypersensitivity to wasp and bee venoms.
>
> Manufacturer advises desensitising vaccines should generally be avoided or used with particular care in patients with asthma.

- **CONTRA-INDICATIONS** Consult product literature
- **CAUTIONS** Consult product literature
- **INTERACTIONS** → Appendix 1: bee venom extract
- **SIDE-EFFECTS**

SIDE-EFFECTS, FURTHER INFORMATION Life-threatening hypersensitivity reactions can occur. Cardiopulmonary resuscitation must be immediately available. Manufacturer advises monitoring for at least 1 hour after injection.

- **PREGNANCY** Avoid.
- **PRESCRIBING AND DISPENSING INFORMATION** Each set of allergen extracts usually contains vials for the administration of graded amounts of allergen to patients undergoing hyposensitisation. Maintenance sets containing vials at the highest strength are also available. Product literature must be consulted for details of allergens, vial strengths, and administration.
- **NATIONAL FUNDING/ACCESS DECISIONS**

NICE decisions
▸ ***Pharmalgen®* for the treatment of bee and wasp venom allergy (February 2012)** NICE TA246
Pharmalgen® is an option for the treatment of IgE-mediated bee and wasp venom allergy in those who have had:
- a severe systemic reaction to bee or wasp venom, **or**
- a moderate systemic reaction to bee or wasp venom and who have a raised baseline serum-tryptase concentration, a high risk of future stings, or anxiety about future stings.

Treatment with *Pharmalgen®* should be initiated and monitored in a specialist centre experienced in venom immunotherapy.
www.nice.org.uk/guidance/ta246

- **MEDICINAL FORMS** There can be variation in the licensing of different medicines containing the same drug.

Powder and solvent for solution for injection
▸ Bee Venom (ALK-Abello Ltd)
Bee venom 120 nanogram Pharmalgen Bee Venom 120nanogram powder and solvent for solution for injection vials | 1 vial PoM ✗
Bee venom 1.2 microgram Pharmalgen Bee Venom 1.2microgram powder and solvent for solution for injection vials | 1 vial PoM ✗
Bee venom 12 microgram Pharmalgen Bee Venom 12microgram powder and solvent for solution for injection vials | 1 vial PoM ✗
Bee venom 120 microgram Pharmalgen Bee Venom maintenance set 120microgram powder and solvent for solution for injection vials | 4 vial PoM £150.00

Grass pollen extract

28-Apr-2020

- **INDICATIONS AND DOSE**

Treatment of seasonal allergic hay fever due to grass pollen in patients who have failed to respond to anti-allergy drugs
▸ BY SUBCUTANEOUS INJECTION
▸ Child: (consult product literature)

Treatment of seasonal allergic hay fever due to grass pollen in patients who have failed to respond to anti-allergy drugs (initiated under specialist supervision)
▸ BY MOUTH
▸ Child 5–17 years: 1 tablet daily, treatment to be started at least 4 months before start of pollen season and continue for up to 3 years

> **IMPORTANT SAFETY INFORMATION**
> DESENSITISING VACCINES
> In view of concerns about the safety of desensitising vaccines, it is recommended that they are used by specialists and only for the following indications:
> - seasonal allergic hay fever (caused by pollen) that has not responded to anti-allergic drugs;
> - hypersensitivity to wasp and bee venoms.
>
> Manufacturer advises desensitising vaccines should generally be avoided or used with particular care in patients with asthma.

- **CONTRA-INDICATIONS** Consult product literature
- **CAUTIONS** Consult product literature
- **INTERACTIONS** → Appendix 1: grass pollen extract
- **SIDE-EFFECTS**

SIDE-EFFECTS, FURTHER INFORMATION Hypersensitivity reactions to immunotherapy can be life-threatening; bronchospasm usually develops within 1 hour and anaphylaxis within 30 minutes of injection. Therefore, cardiopulmonary resuscitation must be immediately available and patients need to be monitored for at least 1 hour after injection. If symptoms or signs of hypersensitivity develop (e.g. rash, urticaria, bronchospasm, faintness), **even when mild**, the patient should be observed until these have resolved completely.

- **PREGNANCY** Should be avoided in pregnant women—consult product literature.
- **MONITORING REQUIREMENTS** The first dose of grass pollen extract (*Grazax*®) should be taken under medical supervision and the patient should be monitored for 20–30 minutes.
- **DIRECTIONS FOR ADMINISTRATION** Oral lyophylisates should be placed under the tongue and allowed to disperse. Advise patient not to swallow for 1 minute, or eat or drink for 5 minutes after taking the tablet. The first should be taken under medical supervision and the patient should be monitored for 20–30 minutes.
- **PRESCRIBING AND DISPENSING INFORMATION** Each set of allergen extracts usually contains vials for the administration of graded amounts of allergen to patients undergoing hyposensitisation. Maintenance sets containing vials at the highest strength are also available. Product literature must be consulted for details of allergens, vial strengths, and administration.
- **PATIENT AND CARER ADVICE** Patients or carers should be given advice on how to administer oral lyophilisates.

- **MEDICINAL FORMS** There can be variation in the licensing of different medicines containing the same drug.

Suspension for injection

▸ **Pollinex Grasses + Rye** (Allergy Therapeutics (UK) Ltd)
Pollinex Grasses + Rye suspension for injection treatment and extension course vials | 4 vial PoM £450.00

Oral lyophilisate

▸ **Grazax** (ALK-Abello Ltd)
Phleum pratense 75000 SQ-T Grazax 75,000 SQ-T oral lyophilisates sugar-free | 30 tablet PoM £80.12 DT = £80.12

Tree pollen extract

28-Apr-2020

- **INDICATIONS AND DOSE**

Treatment of seasonal allergic hay fever due to tree pollen in patients who have failed to respond to anti-allergy drugs

▸ BY SUBCUTANEOUS INJECTION
▸ Child: (consult product literature)

IMPORTANT SAFETY INFORMATION

DESENSITISING VACCINES

In view of concerns about the safety of desensitising vaccines, it is recommended that they are used by specialists and only for the following indications:
- seasonal allergic hay fever (caused by pollen) that has not responded to anti-allergic drugs;
- hypersensitivity to wasp and bee venoms.

Manufacturer advises desensitising vaccines should generally be avoided or used with particular care in patients with asthma.

- **CONTRA-INDICATIONS** Consult product literature
- **CAUTIONS** Consult product literature
- **INTERACTIONS** → Appendix 1: tree pollen extract
- **SIDE-EFFECTS**

SIDE-EFFECTS, FURTHER INFORMATION Hypersensitivity reactions to immunotherapy can be life-threatening. Cardiopulmonary resuscitation must be immediately available and patients need to be monitored for at least 1 hour after injection. If symptoms or signs of hypersensitivity develop (e.g. rash, urticaria, bronchospasm, faintness), **even when mild**, the patient should be observed until these have resolved completely.

- **PREGNANCY** Should be avoided in pregnant women—consult product literature.
- **PRESCRIBING AND DISPENSING INFORMATION** Each set of allergen extracts usually contains vials for the administration of graded amounts of allergen to patients undergoing hyposensitisation. Maintenance sets containing vials at the highest strength are also available. Product literature must be consulted for details of allergens, vial strengths, and administration.

- **MEDICINAL FORMS** There can be variation in the licensing of different medicines containing the same drug.

Suspension for injection

▸ **Pollinex Trees** (Allergy Therapeutics (UK) Ltd)
Pollinex Trees No 3 suspension for injection 1ml vials | 1 vial PoM
Pollinex Trees No 2 suspension for injection 1ml vials | 1 vial PoM
Pollinex Trees No 1 suspension for injection 1ml vials | 1 vial PoM
Pollinex Trees suspension for injection treatment and extension course vials | 4 vial PoM £450.00

Wasp venom extract

28-Apr-2020

- **INDICATIONS AND DOSE**

Hypersensitivity to wasp venom

▸ BY SUBCUTANEOUS INJECTION
▸ Child: (consult product literature)

IMPORTANT SAFETY INFORMATION

DESENSITISING VACCINES

In view of concerns about the safety of desensitising vaccines, it is recommended that they are used by specialists and only for the following indications:
- seasonal allergic hay fever (caused by pollen) that has not responded to anti-allergic drugs;
- hypersensitivity to wasp and bee venoms.

Manufacturer advises desensitising vaccines should generally be avoided or used with particular care in patients with asthma.

- **CONTRA-INDICATIONS** Consult product literature
- **CAUTIONS** Consult product literature
- **INTERACTIONS** → Appendix 1: wasp venom extract
- **SIDE-EFFECTS**

SIDE-EFFECTS, FURTHER INFORMATION Hypersensitivity reactions to wasp venom extracts can be life-threatening; cardiopulmonary resuscitation must be immediately available and patients need to be monitored for at least 1 hour after injection. If symptoms or signs of hypersensitivity develop (e.g. rash, urticaria, bronchospasm, faintness), **even when mild,** the patient should be observed until these have resolved completely.

- **PREGNANCY** Avoid.
- **PRESCRIBING AND DISPENSING INFORMATION** Each set of allergen extracts usually contains vials for the administration of graded amounts of allergen to patients undergoing hyposensitisation. Maintenance sets containing vials at the highest strength are also available. Product literature must be consulted for details of allergens, vial strengths, and administration.
- **NATIONAL FUNDING/ACCESS DECISIONS**

NICE decisions

▸ ***Pharmalgen*® for bee and wasp venom allergy (February 2012) NICE TA246**
Pharmalgen® is an option for the treatment of IgE-mediated bee and wasp venom allergy in those who have had:
- a severe systemic reaction to bee or wasp venom;
- a moderate systemic reaction to bee or wasp venom and who have a raised baseline serum-tryptase concentration, a high risk of future stings, or anxiety about future stings.

3 Respiratory system

Treatment with *Pharmalgen®* should be initiated and monitored in a specialist centre experienced in venom immunotherapy.
www.nice.org.uk/guidance/ta246

● **MEDICINAL FORMS** There can be variation in the licensing of different medicines containing the same drug.

Powder and solvent for solution for injection

▸ Wasp Venom (ALK-Abello Ltd)
Wasp venom 120 nanogram Pharmalgen Wasp Venom 120nanogram powder and solvent for solution for injection vials | 1 vial PoM
Wasp venom 1.2 microgram Pharmalgen Wasp Venom 1.2microgram powder and solvent for solution for injection vials | 1 vial PoM
Wasp venom 12 microgram Pharmalgen Wasp Venom 12microgram powder and solvent for solution for injection vials | 1 vial PoM
Wasp venom 120 microgram Pharmalgen Wasp Venom maintenance set 120microgram vaccine powder and solvent for solution for injection vials | 4 vial PoM £150.00

2.1 Angioedema

Other drugs used for Angioedema Adrenaline/epinephrine, p. 143

DRUGS USED IN HEREDITARY ANGIOEDEMA › COMPLEMENT REGULATORY PROTEINS

C1-esterase inhibitor

19-Mar-2020

● **INDICATIONS AND DOSE**

BERINERT®

Acute attacks of hereditary angioedema (under expert supervision)

▸ BY SLOW INTRAVENOUS INJECTION, OR BY INTRAVENOUS INFUSION
▸ Child: 20 units/kg

Short-term prophylaxis of hereditary angioedema before dental, medical, or surgical procedures (under expert supervision)

▸ BY SLOW INTRAVENOUS INJECTION, OR BY INTRAVENOUS INFUSION
▸ Child: 15–30 units/kg (max. per dose 1000 units) for 1 dose, to be administered less than 6 hours before procedure

CINRYZE®

Acute attacks of hereditary angioedema (under expert supervision)

▸ BY SLOW INTRAVENOUS INJECTION
▸ Child 2–11 years (body-weight 10–25 kg): 500 units for 1 dose, dose may be repeated if necessary after 60 minutes
▸ Child 2–11 years (body-weight 26 kg and above): 1000 units for 1 dose, dose may be repeated if necessary after 60 minutes
▸ Child 12–17 years: 1000 units for 1 dose, dose may be repeated if necessary after 60 minutes (or sooner for patients experiencing laryngeal attacks or if treatment initiation is delayed)

Short-term prophylaxis of hereditary angioedema before dental, medical, or surgical procedures (under expert supervision)

▸ BY SLOW INTRAVENOUS INJECTION
▸ Child 2–11 years (body-weight 10–25 kg): 500 units for 1 dose, to be administered up to 24 hours before procedure
▸ Child 2–11 years (body-weight 26 kg and above): 1000 units for 1 dose, to be administered up to 24 hours before procedure
▸ Child 12–17 years: 1000 units for 1 dose, to be administered up to 24 hours before procedure

Long-term prophylaxis of severe, recurrent attacks of hereditary angioedema where acute treatment is inadequate, or when oral prophylaxis is inadequate or not tolerated (under expert supervision)

▸ BY SLOW INTRAVENOUS INJECTION
▸ Child 6–11 years: 500 units every 3–4 days, dose and dosing interval to be adjusted according to response
▸ Child 12–17 years: 1000 units every 3–4 days, interval between doses to be adjusted according to response

● **CAUTIONS** Vaccination against hepatitis A and hepatitis B may be required

● **SIDE-EFFECTS**

▸ **Rare or very rare** Dizziness · dyspnoea · flushing · headache · hypersensitivity · hypertension · hypotension · nausea · tachycardia · thrombosis (with high doses) · urticaria

● **PREGNANCY** Manufacturer advises avoid unless essential.

● **DIRECTIONS FOR ADMINISTRATION**

CINRYZE® For *slow intravenous injection*, reconstitute (with solvent provided) to a concentration of 100 units/mL; give at a rate of 1 mL/minute.

● **PRESCRIBING AND DISPENSING INFORMATION** C1-esterase inhibitor is prepared from human plasma.

● **NATIONAL FUNDING/ACCESS DECISIONS**

CINRYZE®

All Wales Medicines Strategy Group (AWMSG) decisions

The *All Wales Medicines Strategy Group* has advised (October 2017) that C1-esterase inhibitor (*Cinryze®*) is recommended as an option for use within NHS Wales for the treatment and pre-procedure prevention of angioedema attacks in patients 2 years old and above, with hereditary angioedema (HAE); routine prevention of angioedema attacks in patients 6 years old and above, with severe and recurrent attacks of HAE, who are intolerant to or insufficiently protected by oral prevention treatments, or patients who are inadequately managed with repeated acute treatment.

● **MEDICINAL FORMS** There can be variation in the licensing of different medicines containing the same drug.

Powder and solvent for solution for injection

ELECTROLYTES: May contain Sodium

▸ **Berinert P** (CSL Behring UK Ltd)
C1-esterase inhibitor 500 unit Berinert 500unit powder and solvent for solution for injection vials | 1 vial PoM £550.00 DT = £550.00
C1-esterase inhibitor 1500 unit Berinert 1,500unit powder and solvent for solution for injection vials | 1 vial PoM £1,650.00 DT = £1,650.00

▸ **Cinryze** (Shire Pharmaceuticals Ltd) ▼
C1-esterase inhibitor 500 unit Cinryze 500unit powder and solvent for solution for injection vials | 2 vial PoM £1,336.00

DRUGS USED IN HEREDITARY ANGIOEDEMA › KALLIKREIN INHIBITORS

Lanadelumab

05-Nov-2019

- **DRUG ACTION** Lanadelumab is a humanised monoclonal antibody which inhibits plasma kallikrein activity, thereby limiting the production of bradykinin, a potent vasodilator associated with angioedema attacks in patients with hereditary angioedema.

- **INDICATIONS AND DOSE**

Prevention of recurrent attacks of hereditary angioedema (initiated under specialist supervision)

▸ BY SUBCUTANEOUS INJECTION

▸ Child 12–17 years: 300 mg every 2 weeks, reduced to 300 mg every 4 weeks, in those stable and attack free—consult product literature

- **CONTRA-INDICATIONS** Not a treatment for acute attacks of angioedema—initiate individualised treatment for breakthrough attacks
- **SIDE-EFFECTS**

▸ **Common or very common** Dizziness · hypersensitivity · myalgia · oral disorders · skin reactions

- **PREGNANCY** Manufacturer advises preferable to avoid—limited or no information available; *animal* studies do not indicate toxicity.
- **BREAST FEEDING** Manufacturer advises avoid during first few days after birth—possible risk from transfer of antibodies to infant. After this time, use during breast-feeding only if clinically needed.
- **EFFECT ON LABORATORY TESTS** Manufacturer advises may increase activated partial thromboplastin time (aPTT) due to an interaction with the aPTT assay—consult product literature.
- **DIRECTIONS FOR ADMINISTRATION** Manufacturer advises to withdraw dose from the vial into a syringe with an 18 gauge needle and inject, using a suitable gauge needle, into the abdomen, thigh, or upper outer arm within 2 hours—consult product literature for further information. *Takhzyro*® may be self-administered or administered by a carer after appropriate training in subcutaneous injection technique.
- **PRESCRIBING AND DISPENSING INFORMATION** Lanadelumab is a biological medicine. Biological medicines must be prescribed and dispensed by brand name, see *Biological medicines* and *Biosimilar medicines*, under Guidance on prescribing p. 1; manufacturer advises to record the brand name and batch number after each administration.
- **HANDLING AND STORAGE** Manufacturer advises store in a refrigerator (2–8°C) and protect from light—consult product literature for further information regarding storage outside refrigerator.
- **PATIENT AND CARER ADVICE**

Self-administration Manufacturer advises patients and their carers should be given training in subcutaneous injection technique if appropriate.

Missed doses Manufacturer advises if a dose is missed, it should be taken as soon as possible ensuring at least 10 days between doses.

- **NATIONAL FUNDING/ACCESS DECISIONS**

NICE decisions

▸ **Lanadelumab for preventing recurrent attacks of hereditary angioedema (October 2019)** NICE TA606

Lanadelumab (*Takhzyro*®) is recommended as an option for preventing recurrent attacks of hereditary angioedema in patients aged 12 years and older, only if:

- they are eligible for preventive C1-esterase inhibitor treatment, in line with NHS England's commissioning policy, that is, they are having 2 or more clinically significant attacks per week over 8 weeks despite oral preventive therapy, or oral therapy is contra-indicated or not tolerated, **and**
- the lowest dosing frequency of lanadelumab is used in line with the summary of product characteristics, that is, when the condition is in a stable, attack-free phase, **and**
- the manufacturer provides it according to the commercial arrangement.

Patients whose treatment was started within the NHS before this guidance was published should have the option to continue treatment, without change to their funding arrangements, until they (or their carers) and their NHS clinician consider it appropriate to stop.

www.nice.org.uk/guidance/ta606

Scottish Medicines Consortium (SMC) decisions

SMC No. SMC2206

The *Scottish Medicines Consortium* has advised (December 2019) that lanadelumab (*Takhzyro*®) is accepted for restricted use within NHS Scotland for the routine prevention of recurrent attacks of hereditary angioedema (HAE) in patients aged 12 years and older with HAE type I or II, who would otherwise be considered for long-term prophylaxis treatment with C1-esterase inhibitor.This advice is contingent upon the continuing availability of the patient access scheme in NHS Scotland or a list price that is equivalent or lower.

- **MEDICINAL FORMS** There can be variation in the licensing of different medicines containing the same drug.

Solution for injection

EXCIPIENTS: May contain Polysorbates

▸ Takhzyro (Shire Pharmaceuticals Ltd) ▼

Lanadelumab 150 mg per 1 ml Takhzyro 300mg/2ml solution for injection vials | 1 vial [PoM] £12,420.00 (Hospital only)

DRUGS USED IN HEREDITARY ANGIOEDEMA › SELECTIVE BRADYKININ B_2 ANTAGONISTS

Icatibant

13-Jun-2018

- **INDICATIONS AND DOSE**

Acute attacks of hereditary angioedema in patients with C1-esterase inhibitor deficiency

▸ BY SUBCUTANEOUS INJECTION

▸ Child 2–17 years (body-weight 12 kg and above): (consult product literature)

- **CAUTIONS** Ischaemic heart disease · stroke
- **INTERACTIONS** → Appendix 1: icatibant
- **SIDE-EFFECTS**

▸ **Common or very common** Dizziness · fever · headache · nausea · skin reactions

- **PREGNANCY** Manufacturer advises use only if potential benefit outweighs risk—toxicity in *animal* studies.
- **BREAST FEEDING** Manufacturer advises avoid for 12 hours after administration.
- **NATIONAL FUNDING/ACCESS DECISIONS**

Scottish Medicines Consortium (SMC) decisions

SMC No. 1332/18

The *Scottish Medicines Consortium* has advised (May 2018) that icatibant (*Firazyr*®) is accepted for use within NHS Scotland for the symptomatic treatment of acute attacks of hereditary angioedema (HAE) in adolescents and children aged 2 years and older, with C1-esterase-inhibitor deficiency. This advice is contingent upon the continuing availability of the patient access scheme in NHS Scotland.

All Wales Medicines Strategy Group (AWMSG) decisions
AWMSG No. 3293
The *All Wales Medicines Strategy Group* has advised (June 2018) that icatibant acetate (*Firazyr*®) is recommended as an option for use within NHS Wales for the symptomatic treatment of acute attacks of hereditary angioedema (HAE) in adults, adolescents and children aged 2 years and older, with C1 esterase-inhibitor deficiency. This recommendation applies only in circumstances where the approved Wales Patient Access Scheme (WPAS) is utilised or where the list/contract price is equivalent or lower than the WPAS price.

- **MEDICINAL FORMS** There can be variation in the licensing of different medicines containing the same drug.

Solution for injection
- Firazyr (Shire Pharmaceuticals Ltd)
  Icatibant (as Icatibant acetate) 10 mg per 1 ml Firazyr 30mg/3ml solution for injection pre-filled syringes | 1 pre-filled disposable injection PoM £1,395.00

3 Conditions affecting sputum viscosity

MUCOLYTICS

Carbocisteine

18-Mar-2020

- **INDICATIONS AND DOSE**

Reduction of sputum viscosity
- BY MOUTH
  - Child 2–4 years: 62.5–125 mg 4 times a day
  - Child 5–11 years: 250 mg 3 times a day
  - Child 12–17 years: Initially 2.25 g daily in divided doses, then reduced to 1.5 g daily in divided doses, as condition improves

> **IMPORTANT SAFETY INFORMATION**
> *Mucodyne Paediatric*® syrup 250 mg/5 mL has replaced the 125 mg/5 mL formulation—take care to ensure the appropriate dose is administered.

- **CONTRA-INDICATIONS** Active peptic ulceration
- **CAUTIONS** History of peptic ulceration (may disrupt the gastric mucosal barrier)
- **SIDE-EFFECTS** Gastrointestinal haemorrhage · skin reactions · Stevens-Johnson syndrome · vomiting
- **PREGNANCY** Manufacturer advises avoid in first trimester.
- **BREAST FEEDING** No information available.
- **PRESCRIBING AND DISPENSING INFORMATION** Flavours of oral liquid formulations may include cherry, raspberry, cinnamon, or rum.

- **MEDICINAL FORMS** There can be variation in the licensing of different medicines containing the same drug.

Oral solution
- Carbocisteine (Non-proprietary)
  Carbocisteine 50 mg per 1 ml Carbocisteine 250mg/5ml oral solution | 300 ml PoM £8.55 DT = £6.83
  Carbocisteine 75 mg per 1 ml Carbocisteine 750mg/10ml oral solution 10ml sachets sugar free sugar-free | 15 sachet PoM £3.85 DT = £3.85
- Mucodyne (Sanofi)
  Carbocisteine 50 mg per 1 ml Mucodyne Paediatric 250mg/5ml syrup | 125 ml PoM £12.60
  Mucodyne 250mg/5ml syrup | 300 ml PoM £8.39 DT = £6.83

Capsule
- Carbocisteine (Non-proprietary)
  Carbocisteine 375 mg Carbocisteine 375mg capsules | 120 capsule PoM £18.98 DT = £4.78
- Mucodyne (Sanofi)
  Carbocisteine 375 mg Mucodyne 375mg capsules | 120 capsule PoM £18.98 DT = £4.78

3.1 Cystic fibrosis

Cystic fibrosis

06-May-2020

Description of condition

Cystic fibrosis is a genetic disorder affecting the lungs, pancreas, liver, intestine, and reproductive organs. The main clinical signs are pulmonary disease, with recurrent infections and the production of copious viscous sputum, and malabsorption due to pancreatic insufficiency. Other complications include hepatobiliary disease, osteoporosis, cystic fibrosis-related diabetes, and distal intestinal obstruction syndrome.

Aims of treatment

The aim of treatment includes preventing and managing lung infections, loosening and removing thick, sticky mucus from the lungs, preventing or treating intestinal obstruction, and providing sufficient nutrition and hydration.

Lung function is a key predictor of life expectancy in people with cystic fibrosis and optimising lung function is a major aim of care.

Non-drug treatment

Specialist physiotherapists should assess patients with cystic fibrosis and provide advice on airway clearance, nebuliser use, musculoskeletal disorders, physical activity, and urinary incontinence. The importance of airway clearance techniques should be discussed with patients and their parents or carers and appropriate training provided. Patients should be advised that regular exercise improves both lung function and overall fitness.

Drug treatment

Treatment for cystic fibrosis lung disease is based on the prevention of lung infection and the maintenance of lung function. EvGr In patients with cystic fibrosis, who have clinical evidence of lung disease, the frequency of routine review should be based on their clinical condition, but children should be reviewed at least every 8 weeks. More frequent review is required immediately after diagnosis and during early life. ⟨A⟩

For information on the management of patients during the COVID-19 pandemic, see COVID-19 p. 433.

Mucolytics

EvGr Patients with cystic fibrosis who have evidence of lung disease should be offered a mucolytic. Dornase alfa p. 196 is the first choice mucolytic [unlicensed in children under 5 years of age]. If there is an inadequate response, dornase alfa p. 196 and hypertonic sodium chloride p. 178, or hypertonic sodium chloride p. 178 alone should be considered.

Mannitol dry powder for inhalation p. 149 should be considered for children [unlicensed indication] who cannot use dornase alfa p. 196 and hypertonic sodium chloride p. 178 because of ineligibility, intolerance, or inadequate response. ⟨A⟩

Lumacaftor with ivacaftor p. 197 is not recommended for treating cystic fibrosis within its marketing authorisation (see lumacaftor with ivacaftor National funding/access decisions p. 197).

Pulmonary infection

Staphylococcus aureus

EvGr Flucloxacillin p. 373 [unlicensed indication] should be offered for prophylaxis against respiratory *Staphylococcus aureus* infection in children from the point of diagnosis up to 3 years of age. Continuing prophylaxis in children up to 6 years of age should also be considered. An alternative oral antibacterial should be given in children allergic to penicillin.

In children who are already taking prophylaxis and have a respiratory sample culture that is positive for *Staph. aureus*, prophylaxis adherence should be reviewed and antibacterial treatment started. A prophylactic antibacterial should be restarted after treatment (consult local protocol).

Patients who are not taking prophylaxis and have a new *Staph. aureus* infection can be given an oral anti- *Staph. aureus* antibacterial, if they are clinically well. If they are clinically unwell and have pulmonary disease, oral or intravenous (depending on infection severity) broad-spectrum antibacterials with activity against *Staph. aureus* should be given (consult local protocol).

A long-term antibacterial should be considered to suppress **chronic** *Staph. aureus* respiratory infection in patients whose pulmonary disease is stable. In patients with chronic *Staph. aureus* respiratory infection who become clinically unwell with pulmonary disease, oral or intravenous (depending on infection severity) broad-spectrum antibacterials with activity against *Staph. aureus* should be given. In those patients with new evidence of **meticillin-resistant *Staphylococcus aureus*(MRSA)** respiratory infection (with or without pulmonary exacerbation), specialist microbiological advice should be sought.

Antibacterials should not be routinely used to suppress chronic MRSA in patients with stable pulmonary disease.

If a patient with cystic fibrosis and chronic MRSA respiratory infection becomes unwell with a pulmonary exacerbation or shows a decline in pulmonary function, specialist microbiological advice should be sought. Ⓐ

Pseudomonas aeruginosa

EvGr If a patient with cystic fibrosis develops a new *Pseudomonas aeruginosa* infection, eradication therapy with a course of oral antibacterial should be started (by intravenous injection, if they are clinically unwell), in combination with an inhaled antibacterial. An extended course of oral and inhaled antibacterial should follow (consult local protocol).

If eradication therapy is not successful, sustained treatment with an inhaled antibacterial should be offered. Nebulised colistimethate sodium p. 375 should be considered as first-line treatment (but see also colistimethate sodium p. 375 by dry powder inhalation National funding/access decisions).

In patients with **chronic** *Ps. aeruginosa* infection (when treatment has not eradicated the infection) who become clinically unwell with pulmonary exacerbations, an oral antibacterial or a combination of two intravenous antibacterial drugs of different classes (depending on infection severity) should be used. Changing antibacterial regimens should be considered to treat exacerbations (consult local protocol).

Nebulised aztreonam p. 357, nebulised tobramycin p. 334, or tobramycin dry powder for inhalation p. 334 [unlicensed indication in child under 6 years] (see tobramycin National funding/access decisions p. 334) should be considered for those who are deteriorating despite regular inhaled colistimethate sodium p. 375. Ⓐ

Burkholderia cepacia **complex**

EvGr Patients who develop a new *Burkholderia cepacia* complex infection, should be given eradication therapy with a combination of intravenous antibacterial drugs (specialist microbiological advice should be sought on the choice of antibacterials). Ⓐ There is no evidence to support using antibacterials to suppress **chronic** *Burkholderia cepacia* complex infection in patients with cystic fibrosis who have stable pulmonary status.

EvGr Specialist microbiological advice should be sought for patients with chronic *Burkholderia cepacia* complex infection (when treatment has not eradicated the infection) and who become clinically unwell with a pulmonary disease exacerbation.

An inhaled antibacterial should be considered for those who have chronic *Burkholderia cepacia* complex infection and declining pulmonary status; treatment should be stopped if there is no observed benefit. Ⓐ

Haemophilus influenzae

EvGr *Haemophilus influenzae* infection in the absence of clinical evidence of pulmonary infection should be treated with an appropriate oral antibacterial drug. In those who are unwell with clinical evidence of pulmonary infection, an appropriate antibacterial should be given by mouth or intravenously depending on the severity of the illness (consult local protocol). Ⓐ

Non-tuberculous mycobacteria

EvGr Non-tuberculous mycobacterial eradication therapy should be considered for patients with cystic fibrosis who are clinically unwell and whose pulmonary disease has not responded to other recommended treatments. Specialist microbiological advice should be sought on the choice of antibacterial and on the duration of treatment. Ⓐ

Aspergillus fumigatus **complex**

EvGr Treatment with an antifungal drug should only be considered to suppress **chronic** *Aspergillus fumigatus* complex respiratory infection in patients with declining pulmonary status. Specialist microbiological advice should be sought on the choice of antifungal drug. Ⓐ

Unidentified infections

EvGr An oral or intravenous (depending on the exacerbation severity) broad-spectrum antibacterial should be used for patients who have a pulmonary disease exacerbation and no clear cause. If a causative pathogen is identified, an appropriate treatment should be selected (consult local protocol). Ⓐ

Immunomodulatory drugs

EvGr Long-term treatment with azithromycin p. 352 [unlicensed indication], at an immunomodulatory dose, should be offered to patients with deteriorating lung function or repeated pulmonary exacerbations. In those patients with continued deterioration in lung function or continuing pulmonary exacerbations, azithromycin p. 352 should be discontinued and the use of an oral corticosteroid considered. Ⓐ

Nutrition and exocrine pancreatic insufficiency

EvGr A cystic fibrosis specialist dietitian should offer advice on optimal nutrition.

Pancreatin p. 77 should be offered to patients with exocrine pancreatic insufficiency. Dose should be adjusted as needed to minimise any symptoms or signs of malabsorption (see Exocrine pancreatic insufficiency p. 76). An acid-suppressing drug, such as an H_2 receptor antagonist or a proton pump inhibitor [unlicensed indications] can be considered for patients who have persistent symptoms or signs of malabsorption. Ⓐ

Distal intestinal obstruction syndrome

EvGr Oral or intravenous fluids should be offered to ensure adequate hydration for patients with distal intestinal obstruction syndrome. Meglumine amidotrizoate with sodium amidotrizoate solution p. 41 (orally or via an enteral tube) should be considered as first-line treatment for distal intestinal obstruction syndrome. An iso-osmotic polyethylene glycol and electrolyte solution (macrogols) (orally or via an enteral tube) can be considered as a second-line treatment. Surgery is a last resort, if prolonged treatment with a polyethylene glycol solution is not effective. Suspected distal intestinal obstruction syndrome should be managed in a specialist cystic fibrosis centre. Ⓐ

Liver disease

EvGr If liver function blood tests are abnormal in patients with cystic fibrosis, ursodeoxycholic acid p. 71 [unlicensed indication] can be given until liver function is restored. (A)

Bone mineral density

EvGr Patients should be monitored for cystic fibrosis-related low bone mineral density. (A)

Cystic fibrosis-related diabetes

EvGr Patients should be monitored for cystic fibrosis-related diabetes. (A)

Useful Resources

Cystic fibrosis: diagnosis and management. National Institute for Health and Care Excellence. NICE guideline 78. October 2017
www.nice.org.uk/guidance/NG78

MUCOLYTICS

Dornase alfa

18-Mar-2020

(Phosphorylated glycosylated recombinant human deoxyribonuclease 1 (rhDNase))

- **DRUG ACTION** Dornase alfa is a genetically engineered version of a naturally occurring human enzyme which cleaves extracellular deoxyribonucleic acid (DNA).

- **INDICATIONS AND DOSE**

Management of cystic fibrosis patients with a forced vital capacity (FVC) of greater than 40% of predicted to improve pulmonary function

▶ BY INHALATION OF NEBULISED SOLUTION
- Child 5–17 years: 2500 units once daily, administered by jet nebuliser

DOSE EQUIVALENCE AND CONVERSION
- Dornase alfa 1000 units is equivalent to 1 mg

- **SIDE-EFFECTS** Chest pain · conjunctivitis · dyspepsia · dysphonia · dyspnoea · fever · increased risk of infection · skin reactions
- **PREGNANCY** No evidence of teratogenicity; manufacturer advises use only if potential benefit outweighs risk.
- **BREAST FEEDING** Amount probably too small to be harmful—manufacturer advises caution.
- **DIRECTIONS FOR ADMINISTRATION** Dornase alfa is administered by inhalation using a jet nebuliser, usually once daily at least 1 hour before physiotherapy; however, alternate-day therapy may be as effective as daily treatment.

  For use undiluted with jet nebulisers only; ultrasonic nebulisers are unsuitable.
- **PRESCRIBING AND DISPENSING INFORMATION** Not all children benefit from treatment with dornase alfa; improvement occurs within 2 weeks, but in more severely affected children a trial of 6–12 weeks may be required.
- **PATIENT AND CARER ADVICE**

  Medicines for Children leaflet: Dornase alfa for cystic fibrosis
  www.medicinesforchildren.org.uk/dornase-alfa-cystic-fibrosis

- **MEDICINAL FORMS** There can be variation in the licensing of different medicines containing the same drug.

Nebuliser liquid

▶ Pulmozyme (Roche Products Ltd)

Dornase alfa 1 mg per 1 ml Pulmozyme 2.5mg nebuliser liquid 2.5ml ampoules | 30 ampoule PoM £496.43 DT = £496.43

Ivacaftor

20-Mar-2020

- **DRUG ACTION** Ivacaftor is a cystic fibrosis transmembrane conductance regulator (CFTR) protein potentiator that increases chloride transport in the abnormal CFTR protein.

- **INDICATIONS AND DOSE**

Cystic fibrosis (specialist use only)

▶ BY MOUTH
- Child 6–17 years (body-weight 25 kg and above): 150 mg every 12 hours

DOSE ADJUSTMENTS DUE TO INTERACTIONS
- Manufacturer advises reduce dose to 150 mg twice a week with concurrent use of potent inhibitors of CYP3A4.
- Manufacturer advises reduce dose to 150 mg once daily with concurrent use of moderate inhibitors of CYP3A4.

- **CONTRA-INDICATIONS** Organ transplantation (no information available)
- **INTERACTIONS** → Appendix 1: ivacaftor
- **SIDE-EFFECTS**
  - ▶ **Common or very common** Breast abnormalities · diarrhoea · dizziness · ear discomfort · headache · ototoxicity · rash · tympanic membrane hyperaemia
  - ▶ **Uncommon** Gynaecomastia
  - ▶ **Frequency not known** Cataract · hepatic function abnormal

  SIDE-EFFECTS, FURTHER INFORMATION Manufacturer advises interrupt treatment if transaminase levels more than 5 times the upper limit of normal *or* transaminase levels more than 3 times the upper limit of normal **and** blood bilirubin more than twice the upper limit of normal—consult product literature.
- **PREGNANCY** Manufacturer advises use only if potential benefit outweighs risk—limited information available.
- **BREAST FEEDING** Manufacturer advises avoid—present in milk in *animal* studies.
- **HEPATIC IMPAIRMENT** Manufacturer advises caution in moderate to severe impairment (limited information available).

  Dose adjustments Manufacturer advises reduce dose to 150 mg once daily in moderate impairment; in severe impairment reduce starting dose to 150 mg on alternate days, adjust dosing interval according to clinical response and tolerability.
- **RENAL IMPAIRMENT** Caution in severe impairment.
- **MONITORING REQUIREMENTS**
  - ▶ Manufacturer advises monitor liver function before treatment, every 3 months during the first year of treatment, then annually thereafter (more frequent monitoring should be considered in patients with a history of transaminase elevations).
  - ▶ Manufacturer advises baseline and follow-up ophthalmic examinations in children.
- **DIRECTIONS FOR ADMINISTRATION** Tablets should be taken with fat-containing food.
- **PRESCRIBING AND DISPENSING INFORMATION** Ivacaftor should be prescribed by a physician experienced in the treatment of cystic fibrosis.
- **PATIENT AND CARER ADVICE** Patients or carers should be given advice on how to administer ivacaftor tablets.

  Driving and skilled tasks Manufacturer advises that patients and their carers should be counselled on the effects on driving and skilled tasks—increased risk of dizziness.

- **MEDICINAL FORMS** There can be variation in the licensing of different medicines containing the same drug.

Tablet

CAUTIONARY AND ADVISORY LABELS 25

- Kalydeco (Vertex Pharmaceuticals (UK) Ltd)
  Ivacaftor 150 mg Kalydeco 150mg tablets | 28 tablet PoM £7,000.00 | 56 tablet PoM £14,000.00

Lumacaftor with ivacaftor

19-Mar-2020

The properties listed below are those particular to the combination only. For the properties of the components please consider, ivacaftor p. 196.

- **INDICATIONS AND DOSE**

Cystic fibrosis (specialist use only)

- BY MOUTH USING GRANULES
- Child 2-5 years (body-weight up to 14 kg): 100/125 mg every 12 hours
- Child 2-5 years (body-weight 14 kg and above): 150/188 mg every 12 hours
- BY MOUTH USING TABLETS
- Child 6-11 years: 200/250 mg every 12 hours
- Child 12-17 years: 400/250 mg every 12 hours

DOSE ADJUSTMENTS DUE TO INTERACTIONS

- *For children aged* 2–5 *years (body-weight up to* 14 *kg),* manufacturer advises reduce initial dose to 100/125 mg on alternate days for the first week in those also taking a potent inhibitor of CYP3A4.
- *For children aged* 2–5 *years (body-weight* 14 *kg and above),* manufacturer advises reduce initial dose to 150/188 mg on alternate days for the first week in those also taking a potent inhibitor of CYP3A4.
- *For children aged* 6–11 *years,* manufacturer advises reduce initial dose to 100/125 mg daily for the first week in those also taking a potent inhibitor of CYP3A4.
- *For children aged* 12–17 *years,* manufacturer advises reduce initial dose to 200/125 mg daily for the first week in those also taking a potent inhibitor of CYP3A4.

DOSE EQUIVALENCE AND CONVERSION

- Dose expressed as x/y mg of lumacaftor/ivacaftor.

- **CAUTIONS** Forced expiratory volume in 1 second (FEV_1) less than 40% of the predicted normal value—additional monitoring recommended at initiation of treatment · pulmonary exacerbation—no information available
- **INTERACTIONS** → Appendix 1: ivacaftor · lumacaftor
- **SIDE-EFFECTS**
  - **Common or very common** Breast abnormalities · diarrhoea · dizziness · ear discomfort · flatulence · gastrointestinal discomfort · headache · menstrual cycle irregularities · nausea · ototoxicity · rash · tympanic membrane hyperaemia · vomiting
  - **Uncommon** Gynaecomastia · hepatic encephalopathy · hepatitis cholestatic · hypertension
  - **Frequency not known** Cataract

  SIDE-EFFECTS, FURTHER INFORMATION Manufacturer advises interrupt treatment if transaminase levels more than 5 times the upper limit of normal *or* transaminase levels more than 3 times the upper limit of normal **and** blood bilirubin more than twice the upper limit of normal—consult product literature.
- **HEPATIC IMPAIRMENT** Manufacturer advises caution in moderate to severe impairment (risk of increased exposure).

  Dose adjustments *For children aged* 2–5 *years (body-weight up to* 14 *kg),* manufacturer advises omit evening dose on alternate days in moderate impairment; in severe impairment, dose reduction to 100/125 mg every 24 hours is advised.

  For children aged 2–5 *years (body-weight* 14 *kg and above),* manufacturer advises omit evening dose on alternate days in moderate impairment; in severe impairment, dose reduction to 150/188 mg every 24 hours is advised.

  For children aged 6–11 *years,* manufacturer advises dose reduction of evening dose to 100/125 mg in moderate impairment; in severe impairment, dose reduction to 100/125 mg every 12 hours is advised.

  For children aged 12–17 *years,* manufacturer advises dose reduction of evening dose to 200/125 mg in moderate impairment; in severe impairment, dose reduction to 200/125 mg every 12 hours is advised.
- **PRE-TREATMENT SCREENING** If the patient's genotype is unknown, a validated genotyping method should be performed to confirm the presence of the F508del mutation on both alleles of the CFTR gene before starting treatment.
- **MONITORING REQUIREMENTS** Manufacturer advises monitor blood pressure periodically during treatment.
- **EFFECT ON LABORATORY TESTS** False positive urine screening tests for tetrahydrocannabinol have been reported—manufacturer advises consider alternative confirmatory method.
- **DIRECTIONS FOR ADMINISTRATION** Tablets and granules should be taken with fat-containing food. The contents of each sachet of granules should be mixed with 1 teaspoon (5 mL) of soft food or liquid (e.g. puréed fruits, yoghurt, milk, or juice), at room temperature or below, and consumed within an hour.
- **PATIENT AND CARER ADVICE** Patients or carers should be given advice on how to administer tablets.

  Missed doses Manufacturer advises if a dose is more than 6 hours late, the missed dose should not be taken and the next dose should be taken at the normal time.
- **NATIONAL FUNDING/ACCESS DECISIONS**

NICE decisions

- **Lumacaftor with ivacaftor for treating cystic fibrosis homozygous for the F508del mutation (July 2016)** NICE TA398
  Lumacaftor with ivacaftor (*Orkambi*®) is **not** recommended, within its marketing authorisation, for treating cystic fibrosis in patients aged 12 years and older who are homozygous for the F508del mutation in the cystic fibrosis transmembrane conductance regulator (CFTR) gene.

  Patients whose treatment was started within the NHS before this guidance was published should have the option to continue treatment, without change to their funding arrangements, until they (or their carers) and their NHS clinician consider it appropriate to stop.
  www.nice.org.uk/guidance/ta398

Scottish Medicines Consortium (SMC) decisions

SMC No. 1136/16

The *Scottish Medicines Consortium* has advised (May 2016) that lumacaftor with ivacaftor (*Orkambi*®) is **not** recommended within NHS Scotland for the treatment of cystic fibrosis in patients aged 12 years and older who are homozygous for the F508del mutation in the cystic fibrosis transmembrane conductance regulator (CFTR) gene, as the economic case was not demonstrated.

SMC No. SMC2182

The *Scottish Medicines Consortium* has advised (August 2019) that lumacaftor with ivacaftor (*Orkambi*®) is **not** recommended for use within NHS Scotland for the treatment of cystic fibrosis in patients aged 2 years and older who are homozygous for the F508del mutation in the cystic fibrosis transmembrane conductance regulator (CFTR) gene, as the clinical and economic case was not demonstrated.

- **MEDICINAL FORMS** There can be variation in the licensing of different medicines containing the same drug.

Granules

- Orkambi (Vertex Pharmaceuticals (UK) Ltd) ▼
  Lumacaftor 100 mg, Ivacaftor 125 mg Orkambi 100mg/125mg granules sachets | 56 sachet PoM £8,000.00
  Lumacaftor 150 mg, Ivacaftor 188 mg Orkambi 150mg/188mg granules sachets | 56 sachet PoM £8,000.00

Tablet

CAUTIONARY AND ADVISORY LABELS 25

EXCIPIENTS: May contain Propylene glycol

- Orkambi (Vertex Pharmaceuticals (UK) Ltd) ▼
  Lumacaftor 100 mg, Ivacaftor 125 mg Orkambi 100mg/125mg tablets | 112 tablet PoM £8,000.00 (Hospital only)
  Lumacaftor 200 mg, Ivacaftor 125 mg Orkambi 200mg/125mg tablets | 112 tablet PoM £8,000.00 (Hospital only)

Tezacaftor with ivacaftor

19-Mar-2019

The properties listed below are those particular to the combination only. For the properties of the components please consider, ivacaftor p. 196.

- **INDICATIONS AND DOSE**

Cystic fibrosis (in combination with ivacaftor) (specialist use only)

- BY MOUTH
- Child 12–17 years: 100/150 mg, to be taken in the morning and, *Ivacaftor* 150 mg to be taken in the evening

DOSE ADJUSTMENTS DUE TO INTERACTIONS

- With concurrent use of potent CYP3A4 inhibitors, manufacturer advises reduce dose to 100/150 mg tezacaftor/ivacaftor twice a week, taken approximately 3–4 days apart; the evening dose of ivacaftor should not be taken.
- With concurrent use of moderate CYP3A4 inhibitors, manufacturer advises reduce dose to 100/150 mg tezacaftor/ivacaftor every other morning, with ivacaftor 150 mg taken in the mornings alternate to tezacaftor/ivacaftor; the evening dose of ivacaftor should not be taken.

DOSE EQUIVALENCE AND CONVERSION

- Combination dose expressed as x/y mg of tezacaftor/ivacaftor.

- **INTERACTIONS** → Appendix 1: ivacaftor · tezacaftor
- **SIDE-EFFECTS**
- **Common or very common** Abdominal pain · breast abnormalities · diarrhoea · dizziness · ear discomfort · headache · nausea · ototoxicity · rash · tympanic membrane hyperaemia
- **Uncommon** Gynaecomastia
- **Frequency not known** Hepatic function abnormal · lens opacity

SIDE-EFFECTS, FURTHER INFORMATION Manufacturer advises interrupt treatment if transaminase levels more than 5 times the upper limit of normal *or* transaminase levels more than 3 times the upper limit of normal **and** blood bilirubin more than twice the upper limit of normal—consult product literature.

- **HEPATIC IMPAIRMENT** Manufacturer advises caution in moderate to severe impairment (risk of increased exposure).

Dose adjustments Manufacturer advises omit evening dose of ivacaftor in moderate to severe impairment; in severe impairment, adjust dosing interval according to clinical response and tolerability.

- **PATIENT AND CARER ADVICE**

Missed doses Manufacturer advises if a dose is more than 6 hours late, the missed dose should not be taken and the next dose should be taken at the normal time.

- **NATIONAL FUNDING/ACCESS DECISIONS**

Scottish Medicines Consortium (SMC) decisions

SMC No. SMC2183

The *Scottish Medicines Consortium* has advised (August 2019) that tezacaftor with ivacaftor (*Symkevi*®) is **not** recommended for use within NHS Scotland for the treatment of cystic fibrosis in patients aged 12 years and older who are homozygous for the F508del mutation or who are heterozygous for the F508del mutation and have one of the following mutations in the cystic fibrosis transmembrane conductance regulator (CFTR) gene: P67L, R117C, L206W, R352Q, A455E, D579G, 711+3A→G, S945L, S977F, R1070W, D1152H, 2789+5G→A, 3272-26A→G, and 3849+10kbC→T, as the clinical and economic case was not demonstrated.

- **MEDICINAL FORMS** There can be variation in the licensing of different medicines containing the same drug.

Tablet

CAUTIONARY AND ADVISORY LABELS 25

- Symkevi (Vertex Pharmaceuticals (UK) Ltd) ▼
  Tezacaftor 100 mg, Ivacaftor 150 mg Symkevi 100mg/150mg tablets | 28 tablet PoM £6,293.91 (Hospital only)

4 Cough and congestion

Aromatic inhalations, cough preparations and systemic nasal decongestants

Aromatic inhalations

Inhalations containing volatile substances such as eucalyptus oil are traditionally used to relieve congestion and ease breathing. Although the vapour may contain little of the additive it encourages deliberate inspiration of warm moist air which is often comforting. Boiling water should not be used owing to the risk of scalding.

Strong aromatic decongestants (applied as rubs or to pillows) are not recommended for infants under the age of 3 months. Sodium chloride 0.9% solution p. 636 given as nasal drops can be used to liquefy mucous secretions and relieve nasal congestion in infants and young children; administration before feeds may ease feeding difficulties caused by nasal congestion.

Cough preparations

Cough suppressants

Cough may be a symptom of an underlying disorder such as asthma, gastro-oesophageal reflux disease, or rhinitis, which should be addressed before prescribing cough suppressants. Cough may be associated with smoking or environmental pollutants. Cough can also result from bronchiectasis including that associated with cystic fibrosis; cough can also have a significant habit component. There is little evidence of any significant benefit from the use of cough suppressants in children with acute cough in ambulatory settings. Cough suppressants may cause sputum retention and this can be harmful in children with bronchiectasis.

The use of cough suppressants containing pholcodine p. 199 or similar opioid analgesics is not generally recommended in children and should be avoided in children under 6 years; the use of over-the-counter cough suppressants containing codeine phosphate p. 293 should be avoided in children under 12 years and in children of any age known to be CYP2D6 ultra-rapid metabolisers.

Sedating antihistamines are used as the cough suppressant component of many compound cough preparations on sale to the public; all tend to cause drowsiness which may reflect their main mode of action.

Demulcent and expectorant cough preparations
Simple linctus and other demulcent cough preparations containing soothing substances, such as syrup or glycerol, may temporarily relieve a dry irritating cough. These preparations have the advantage of being harmless and inexpensive and sugar-free versions are available.

Expectorants are claimed to promote expulsion of bronchial secretions, but there is no evidence that any drug can specifically facilitate expectoration.

EvGr An over-the-counter cough medicine containing the expectorant guaifenesin may be used for acute cough in children aged over 12 years; there is some evidence to suggest it may reduce symptoms. (A)

Compound cough preparations for children are on sale to the public but should not be used in children under 6 years; the rationale for some is dubious. Care should be taken to give the correct dose and to not use more than one preparation at a time.

MHRA/CHM advice (March 2008 and February 2009)
Children under 6 years should not be given over-the-counter cough and cold medicines containing the following ingredients:
- brompheniramine, chlorphenamine maleate p. 186, diphenhydramine, doxylamine, promethazine, or triprolidine (antihistamines);
- dextromethorphan or pholcodine (cough suppressants);
- guaifenesin or ipecacuanha (expectorants);
- Phenylephrine hydrochloride p. 132, pseudoephedrine hydrochloride p. 749, ephedrine hydrochloride p. 748, oxymetazoline, or xylometazoline hydrochloride p. 749 (decongestants).

Over-the-counter cough and cold medicines can be considered for children aged 6–12 years after basic principles of best care have been tried, but treatment should be restricted to five days or less. Children should not be given more than 1 cough or cold preparation at a time because different brands may contain the same active ingredient; care should be taken to give the correct dose.

Nasal decongestants, systemic

Nasal congestion in children due to allergic or vasomotor rhinitis should be treated with oral antihistamines, topical nasal preparations containing corticosteroids, or topical decongestants.

There is little evidence to support the use of systemic decongestants in children.

Pseudoephedrine hydrochloride has few sympathomimetic effects, and is commonly combined with other ingredients (including antihistamines) in preparations intended for the relief of cough and cold symptoms.

COUGH AND COLD PREPARATIONS > COUGH SUPPRESSANTS

Pholcodine

18-Mar-2020

● **INDICATIONS AND DOSE**

Dry cough
▶ BY MOUTH USING LINCTUS
▸ Child 6-11 years: 2–5 mg 3–4 times a day
▸ Child 12-17 years: 5–10 mg 3–4 times a day

IMPORTANT SAFETY INFORMATION
MHRA/CHM ADVICE (MARCH 2008 AND FEBRUARY 2009) OVER-THE-COUNTER COUGH AND COLD MEDICINES FOR CHILDREN
Children under 6 years should not be given over-the-counter cough and cold medicines containing pholcodine (cough suppressant).

Over-the-counter cough and cold medicines can be considered for children aged 6–12 years after basic principles of best care have been tried, but treatment should be restricted to 5 days or less. Children should not be given more than 1 cough or cold preparation at a time because different brands may contain the same active ingredient; care should be taken to give the correct dose.

● **CONTRA-INDICATIONS** Bronchiectasis · bronchiolitis · chronic bronchitis · patients at risk of respiratory failure
● **CAUTIONS** Asthma · chronic cough · persistent cough · productive cough
● **INTERACTIONS** → Appendix 1: pholcodine
● **SIDE-EFFECTS** Agitation · confusion · constipation · dizziness · drowsiness · gastrointestinal disorder · nausea · skin reactions · sputum retention · vomiting
● **PREGNANCY** Manufacturer advises avoid unless potential benefit outweighs risk.
● **BREAST FEEDING** Manufacturer advises avoid unless potential benefit outweighs risk—no information available.
● **HEPATIC IMPAIRMENT** Manufacturer advises caution; avoid in hepatic failure.
● **RENAL IMPAIRMENT** Use with caution in renal impairment. Avoid in severe renal impairment.
● **PRESCRIBING AND DISPENSING INFORMATION** Pholcodine is not generally recommended for children.
Flavours of oral liquid formulations may include orange.
When prepared extemporaneously, the BP states Pholcodine Linctus, BP consists of pholcodine 5 mg/5 mL in a suitable flavoured vehicle, containing citric acid monohydrate 1% and Pholcodine Linctus, Strong, BP consists of pholcodine 10 mg/5 mL in a suitable flavoured vehicle, containing citric acid monohydrate 2%

● **MEDICINAL FORMS** There can be variation in the licensing of different medicines containing the same drug.

Oral solution
▸ Pholcodine (Non-proprietary)
Pholcodine 1 mg per 1 ml Pholcodine 5mg/5ml linctus | 200 ml P £1.23–£1.32 DT = £1.32 CD5
Pholcodine 5mg/5ml linctus sugar free sugar-free | 200 ml P £1.34 DT = £1.34 CD5 sugar-free | 2000 ml P £13.40 CD5
Pholcodine 2 mg per 1 ml Pholcodine 10mg/5ml linctus strong sugar free sugar-free | 2000 ml P £11.25 DT = £9.88 CD5
Pholcodine 10mg/5ml linctus strong | 200 ml P £1.67 DT = £1.67 CD5
▸ Covonia Dry Cough (Thornton & Ross Ltd)
Pholcodine 1 mg per 1 ml Covonia Dry Cough Sugar Free Formula 5mg/5ml oral solution sugar-free | 150 ml P £3.30 CD5
▸ Galenphol (Thornton & Ross Ltd)
Pholcodine 1 mg per 1 ml Galenphol 5mg/5ml linctus sugar-free | 2000 ml P £8.50 CD5
Pholcodine 2 mg per 1 ml Galenphol Strong 10mg/5ml linctus sugar-free | 2000 ml P £9.88 DT = £9.88 CD5

COUGH AND COLD PREPARATIONS > OTHER

Citric acid

18-Mar-2020

(Formulated as Simple Linctus)

● **INDICATIONS AND DOSE**

Cough
▶ BY MOUTH
▸ Child 1 month-11 years: 5–10 mL 3–4 times a day, this dose is for Simple Linctus, Paediatric, BP (0.625%)

Cough
▶ BY MOUTH
▸ Child 12-17 years: 5 mL 3–4 times a day, this dose is for Simple Linctus, BP (2.5%)

● **PRESCRIBING AND DISPENSING INFORMATION** Flavours of oral liquid formulations may include anise.

When prepared extemporaneously, the BP states Simple Linctus, Paediatric, BP consists of citric acid monohydrate 0.625% and Simple Linctus, BP consists of citric acid monohydrate 2.5%, both in a suitable vehicle with an anise flavour.

- **PATIENT AND CARER ADVICE**
Medicines for Children leaflet: Simple linctus for cough www.medicinesforchildren.org.uk/simple-linctus-cough

- **MEDICINAL FORMS** There can be variation in the licensing of different medicines containing the same drug.

Oral solution

- Citric acid (Non-proprietary)
Citric acid monohydrate 6.25 mg per 1 ml Simple linctus paediatric sugar free sugar-free | 2000 ml GSL
Care Simple linctus paediatric sugar free sugar-free | 200 ml GSL £1.29 DT = £1.29
Simple linctus paediatric | 200 ml GSL £1.05–£1.06 DT = £1.05
Citric acid monohydrate 25 mg per 1 ml Simple linctus sugar free sugar-free | 200 ml GSL £1.25 DT = £0.92 sugar-free | 2000 ml GSL £9.20
Simple linctus | 200 ml GSL £0.93–£1.06 DT = £0.93
Citric acid 100 mg per 1 ml Carbex oral solution 10ml sachets | 10 sachet P

MENTHOL AND DERIVATIVES

Eucalyptus with menthol

18-Mar-2020

- **INDICATIONS AND DOSE**

Aromatic inhalation for relief of nasal congestion

▶ BY INHALATION

- Child 3 months–17 years: Add one teaspoonful to a pint of hot, **not** boiling, water and inhale the vapour; repeat after 4 hours if necessary

- **PRESCRIBING AND DISPENSING INFORMATION** When prepared extemporaneously, the BP states Menthol and Eucalyptus Inhalation, BP 1980 consists of racementhol or levomenthol 2 g, eucalyptus oil 10 mL, light magnesium carbonate 7 g, water to 100 mL.
Not recommended (applied as a rub or to pillows) for infants under the age of 3 months.

- **PROFESSION SPECIFIC INFORMATION**
Dental practitioners' formulary
Menthol and Eucalyptus Inhalation BP, 1980 may be prescribed.

- **MEDICINAL FORMS** There can be variation in the licensing of different medicines containing the same drug.

Inhalation vapour

- Eucalyptus with menthol (Non-proprietary)
Menthol 20 mg per 1 ml, Magnesium carbonate light 70 mg per 1 ml, Eucalyptus oil 100 microlitre per 1 ml Menthol and Eucalyptus inhalation | 100 ml GSL £2.40 DT = £2.40

RESINS

Benzoin tincture, compound

18-Mar-2020

(Friars' Balsam)

- **INDICATIONS AND DOSE**

Aromatic inhalation for relief of nasal congestion

▶ BY INHALATION

- Child 3 months–17 years: Add 5 mL to a pint of hot, **not** boiling, water and inhale the vapour; repeat after 4 hours if necessary

- **SIDE-EFFECTS** Skin sensitisation
- **PRESCRIBING AND DISPENSING INFORMATION** Not recommended (applied as a rub or to pillows) for infants under 3 months.
When prepared extemporaneously, the BP states Benzoin Tincture, Compound, BP consists of balsamic acids approx. 4.5%.

- **MEDICINAL FORMS** There can be variation in the licensing of different medicines containing the same drug.

Liquid

CAUTIONARY AND ADVISORY LABELS 15

- Benzoin tincture, compound (Non-proprietary)
Benzoin sumatra 100 mg per 1 ml, Storax prepared 100 mg per 1 ml Benzoin compound tincture | 500 ml £12.35 DT = £12.11
Friars' Balsam | 50 ml GSL £2.11

5 Respiratory depression, respiratory distress syndrome and apnoea

Respiratory stimulants

Respiratory stimulants

Respiratory stimulants (analeptic drugs), such as caffeine citrate p. 201, reduce the frequency of neonatal apnoea, and the need for mechanical ventilation during the first 7 days of treatment. They are typically used in the management of very preterm neonates, and continued until a corrected gestational age of 34 to 35 weeks is reached (or longer if necessary). They should only be given under **expert supervision** in hospital; it is important to rule out any underlying disorder, such as seizures, hypoglycaemia, or infection, causing respiratory exhaustion before starting treatment with a respiratory stimulant.

Pulmonary surfactants

Pulmonary surfactants derived from animal lungs, beractant below and poractant alfa p. 201 are used to prevent and treat respiratory distress syndrome (hyaline membrane disease) in neonates and preterm neonates. Prophylactic use of a pulmonary surfactant may reduce the need for mechanical ventilation and is more effective than 'rescue treatment' in preterm neonates of 29 weeks or less corrected gestational age. Pulmonary surfactants may also be of benefit in neonates with meconium aspiration syndrome or intrapartum streptococcal infection. Pulmonary immaturity with surfactant deficit is the commonest reason for respiratory failure in the neonate, especially in those of less than 30 weeks corrected gestational age. Betamethasone p. 474 given to the mother (at least 12 hours but preferably 48 hours) before delivery substantially enhances pulmonary maturity in the neonate.

PULMONARY SURFACTANTS

Beractant

29-Apr-2020

- **INDICATIONS AND DOSE**

Treatment of respiratory distress syndrome in preterm neonates, birth-weight over 700 g (specialist use only)

▶ BY ENDOTRACHEAL TUBE

- Preterm neonate: 100 mg/kg, preferably administer within 8 hours of birth; dose may be repeated within 48 hours at intervals of at least 6 hours for up to 4 doses.

Prophylaxis of respiratory distress syndrome in preterm neonates (specialist use only)

▸ BY ENDOTRACHEAL TUBE

▸ Neonate up to 32 weeks corrected gestational age: 100 mg/kg, preferably administer within 15 minutes of birth; dose may be repeated within 48 hours at intervals of at least 6 hours for up to 4 doses.

DOSE EQUIVALENCE AND CONVERSION

▸ Phospholipid 100 mg/kg is equivalent to a volume of 4 mL/kg.

● CAUTIONS Consult product literature

● SIDE-EFFECTS

▸ **Uncommon** Endotracheal tube obstruction

▸ **Frequency not known** Bradycardia · hypoxia

● MEDICINAL FORMS There can be variation in the licensing of different medicines containing the same drug.

Liquid

▸ Survanta (AbbVie Ltd)

Phospholipids (as Beractant) 25 mg per 1 ml Survanta 200mg/8ml endotracheopulmonary suspension bottles | 1 bottle PoM £306.43

Poractant alfa 29-Apr-2020

● INDICATIONS AND DOSE

Treatment of respiratory distress syndrome in neonates, birth weight over 700 g (specialist use only)

▸ BY ENDOTRACHEAL TUBE

▸ Neonate: 100–200 mg/kg, then 100 mg/kg every 12 hours if required, maximum 300–400 mg/kg per course.

Prophylaxis of respiratory distress syndrome (specialist use only)

▸ BY ENDOTRACHEAL TUBE

▸ Neonate 24 weeks to 31 weeks corrected gestational age: 100–200 mg/kg, administer soon after birth, preferably within 15 minutes, then 100 mg/kg after 6–12 hours if required, then 100 mg/kg after 12 hours if required, and if neonate still intubated. Max 300–400 mg/kg per course.

● CAUTIONS Consult product literature

● SIDE-EFFECTS

▸ **Rare or very rare** Bradycardia · hypotension

▸ **Frequency not known** Hyperoxia

● MEDICINAL FORMS There can be variation in the licensing of different medicines containing the same drug.

Liquid

▸ Curosurf (Chiesi Ltd)

Poractant alfa 80 mg per 1 ml Curosurf 240mg/3ml endotracheopulmonary suspension vials | 1 vial PoM £547.40 (Hospital only)

Curosurf 120mg/1.5ml endotracheopulmonary suspension vials | 1 vial PoM £281.64 (Hospital only)

5.1 Neonatal apnoea

XANTHINES

Caffeine citrate 03-Mar-2020

● INDICATIONS AND DOSE

Neonatal apnoea (specialist supervision in hospital)

▸ BY MOUTH, OR BY INTRAVENOUS INFUSION

▸ Neonate: Loading dose 20 mg/kg, then maintenance 5 mg/kg once daily, started 24 hours after the loading dose; increased if necessary up to 20 mg/kg daily, a maintenance dose above 20 mg/kg daily can be considered if therapeutic efficacy is not achieved—the plasma-caffeine concentration should be monitored to ensure that a safe level is maintained.

DOSE EQUIVALENCE AND CONVERSION

▸ Caffeine citrate 2 mg ≡ caffeine base 1 mg

PHARMACOKINETICS

▸ Caffeine citrate is well absorbed when given orally.

● UNLICENSED USE EvGr Higher maintenance doses differ from product literature and adhere to national guidelines (A).

IMPORTANT SAFETY INFORMATION

MHRA/CHM ADVICE: SAFE PRACTICE

From August 2013, all licensed preparations of caffeine are required to be labelled as caffeine citrate. To minimise the risk of dosing errors, **always state dose in terms of caffeine citrate when prescribing caffeine**.

Some stock packaged as caffeine base.

● CAUTIONS Cardiovascular disease · gastro-oesophageal reflux · rhythm disorder · seizure disorders

● INTERACTIONS → Appendix 1: caffeine citrate

● SIDE-EFFECTS

▸ **Common or very common** Arrhythmias · hyperglycaemia

▸ **Uncommon** Seizure

▸ **Frequency not known** Brain injury · deafness · failure to thrive · feeding intolerance · feeling jittery · gastrointestinal disorders · hypoglycaemia · increased cardiac output · irritability · regurgitation · restlessness

● HEPATIC IMPAIRMENT Manufacturer advises caution (risk of increased frequency of side-effects).

Dose adjustments Manufacturer advises consider dose adjustment according to plasma-caffeine concentration.

● RENAL IMPAIRMENT Manufacturer advises caution with impaired renal function—potential for accumulation of caffeine.

Dose adjustments Reduced daily maintenance dose required—consult product literature.

● MONITORING REQUIREMENTS

▸ EvGr The therapeutic range for plasma-caffeine concentration is usually 10–20 mg/litre (50–100 micromol/litre), but a concentration of 25–35 mg/litre (130–180 micromol/litre) may be required. Signs of toxicity only normally occur at concentrations greater than 50 mg/litre (260 micromol/litre). (D)

▸ Monitor for recurrence of apnoea for 1 week after stopping treatment.

● DIRECTIONS FOR ADMINISTRATION Caffeine citrate injection may be administered *by mouth* or *by intravenous infusion*. For *intravenous infusion*, manufacturer advises give loading dose over 30 minutes and maintenance doses over 10 minutes.

● **NATIONAL FUNDING/ACCESS DECISIONS**

Scottish Medicines Consortium (SMC) decisions

SMC No. 814/12

The *Scottish Medicines Consortium* has advised (September 2013) that *Peyona*® is accepted for use within NHS Scotland for the treatment of primary apnoea of premature newborns only whilst *Peyona*® is available at the price agreed in the patient access scheme.

● **MEDICINAL FORMS** There can be variation in the licensing of different medicines containing the same drug. Forms available from special-order manufacturers include: oral suspension, oral solution

Solution for injection

▸ Caffeine citrate (Non-proprietary)

Caffeine citrate 10 mg per 1 ml Caffeine citrate 10mg/1ml solution for injection ampoules | 10 ampoule PoM £48.82

Solution for infusion

▸ Peyona (Chiesi Ltd)

Caffeine citrate 20 mg per 1 ml Peyona 20mg/ml solution for infusion ampoules | 10 ampoule PoM £172.50 (Hospital only)

Oral solution

▸ Caffeine citrate (Non-proprietary)

Caffeine citrate 10 mg per 1 ml Caffeine citrate 50mg/5ml oral solution | 5 ml PoM £25.99 DT = £25.99

Chapter 4 Nervous system

CONTENTS

1 Epilepsy and other seizure disorders

Epilepsy

26-May-2017

Epilepsy control

The object of treatment is to prevent the occurrence of seizures by maintaining an effective dose of one or more antiepileptic drugs. Careful adjustment of doses is necessary, starting with low doses and increasing gradually until seizures are controlled or there are significant adverse effects.

When choosing an antiepileptic drug, the presenting epilepsy syndrome should first be considered. If the syndrome is not clear, the seizure type should determine the choice of treatment. Concomitant medication, co-morbidity, age, and sex should also be taken into account.

The frequency of administration is often determined by the plasma-drug half-life, and should be kept as low as possible to encourage better adherence. Most antiepileptics, when used in usual dosage, can be given twice daily. Lamotrigine p. 216, perampanel p. 219, phenobarbital p. 232 and phenytoin p. 220, which have long half-lives, can be given as a daily dose at bedtime. However, with large doses, some antiepileptics may need to be given three times daily to avoid adverse effects associated with high peak plasma-drug concentrations. Young children metabolise some antiepileptics more rapidly than adults and therefore may require more frequent doses and a higher amount per kilogram body-weight.

Management

When monotherapy with a first-line antiepileptic drug has failed, monotherapy with a second drug should be tried; the diagnosis should be checked before starting an alternative drug if the first drug showed lack of efficacy. The change from one antiepileptic drug to another should be cautious, slowly withdrawing the first drug only when the new regimen has been established. Combination therapy with two or more antiepileptic drugs may be necessary, but the concurrent use of antiepileptic drugs increases the risk of adverse effects and drug interactions. If combination therapy does not bring about worthwhile benefits, revert to the regimen (monotherapy or combination therapy) that provided the best balance between tolerability and efficacy. A single antiepileptic drug should be prescribed wherever possible and will achieve seizure control for the majority of children.

MHRA/CHM advice: Antiepileptic drugs: updated advice on switching between different manufacturers' products (November 2017)

The CHM has reviewed spontaneous adverse reactions received by the MHRA and publications that reported potential harm arising from switching of antiepileptic drugs in patients previously stabilised on a branded product to a generic. The CHM concluded that reports of loss of seizure control and/or worsening of side-effects around the time of switching between products could be explained as chance associations, but that a causal role of switching could not be ruled out in all cases. The following guidance has been issued to help minimise risk:

- Different antiepileptic drugs vary considerably in their characteristics, which influences the risk of whether switching between different manufacturers' products of a particular drug may cause adverse effects or loss of seizure control;
- Antiepileptic drugs have been divided into three risk-based categories to help healthcare professionals decide whether it is necessary to maintain continuity of supply of a specific manufacturer's product. These categories are listed below;
- If it is felt desirable for a patient to be maintained on a specific manufacturer's product this should be prescribed either by specifying a brand name, or by using the generic drug name and name of the manufacturer (otherwise known as the Marketing Authorisation Holder);
- This advice relates only to antiepileptic drug use for treatment of epilepsy; it does not apply to their use in other indications (e.g. mood stabilisation, neuropathic pain);
- Please report on a Yellow Card any suspected adverse reactions to antiepileptic drugs;
- Dispensing pharmacists should ensure the continuity of supply of a particular product when the prescription specifies it. If the prescribed product is unavailable, it may be necessary to dispense a product from a different manufacturer to maintain continuity of treatment of that antiepileptic drug. Such cases should be discussed and agreed with both the prescriber and patient (or carer);
- Usual dispensing practice can be followed when a specific product is not stated.

Category 1
Carbamazepine p. 209, phenobarbital, phenytoin, primidone p. 233. For these drugs, doctors are advised to ensure that their patient is maintained on a specific manufacturer's product.

Category 2
Clobazam p. 234, clonazepam p. 235, eslicarbazepine acetate p. 211, lamotrigine, oxcarbazepine p. 218, perampanel, rufinamide p. 222, topiramate p. 227, valproate, zonisamide p. 231. For these drugs, the need for continued supply of a particular manufacturer's product should be based on clinical judgement and consultation with the patient and/or carer taking into account factors such as seizure frequency, treatment history, and potential implications to the patient of having a breakthrough seizure. Non-clinical factors as for Category 3 drugs should also be considered.

Category 3
Brivaracetam p. 208, ethosuximide p. 212, gabapentin p. 213, lacosamide p. 215, levetiracetam p. 217, pregabalin, tiagabine p. 227, vigabatrin p. 230. For these drugs, it is usually unnecessary to ensure that patients are maintained on a specific manufacturer's product as therapeutic equivalence can be assumed, however, other factors are important when considering whether switching is appropriate. Differences between alternative products (e.g. product name, packaging, appearance, and taste) may be perceived negatively by patients and/or carers, and may lead to dissatisfaction, anxiety, confusion, dosing errors, and reduced adherence. In addition, difficulties for patients with co-morbid autism, mental health problems, or learning disability should also be considered.

Antiepileptic hypersensitivity syndrome

Antiepileptic hypersensitivity syndrome is a rare but potentially fatal syndrome associated with some antiepileptic drugs (carbamazepine, lacosamide, lamotrigine, oxcarbazepine, phenobarbital, phenytoin, primidone, and rufinamide); rarely cross-sensitivity occurs between some of these antiepileptic drugs. Some other antiepileptics (eslicarbazepine acetate, stiripentol p. 226, and zonisamide) have a theoretical risk. The symptoms usually start between 1 and 8 weeks of exposure; fever, rash, and lymphadenopathy are most commonly seen. Other systemic signs include liver dysfunction, haematological, renal, and pulmonary abnormalities, vasculitis, and multi-organ failure. If signs or symptoms of hypersensitivity syndrome occur, the drug should be withdrawn immediately, the child should not be re-exposed, and expert advice should be sought.

Risk of suicidal thoughts and behaviour

The MHRA has advised (August 2008) that all antiepileptic drugs are associated with a small increased risk of suicidal thoughts and behaviour. Symptoms may occur as early as one week after starting treatment. Children and their parents or carers should be advised to seek medical advice if the child develops any mood changes, distressing thoughts, or feelings about suicide or harming themselves, and should be referred for appropriate treatment if necessary.

Interactions

Interactions between antiepileptics are complex and may increase toxicity without a corresponding increase in antiepileptic effect. Interactions are usually caused by hepatic enzyme induction or inhibition; displacement from protein binding sites is not usually a problem. These interactions are highly variable and unpredictable.

Withdrawal

Antiepileptic drugs should be withdrawn under specialist supervision. Avoid abrupt withdrawal, particularly of barbiturates and benzodiazepines, because this can precipitate severe rebound seizures. Reduction in dosage should be gradual and, in the case of barbiturates, withdrawal of the drug may take months.

The decision to withdraw antiepileptic drugs from a seizure-free child, and its timing, is often difficult and depends on individual circumstances. Even in children who have been seizure-free for several years, there is a significant risk of seizure recurrence on drug withdrawal.

Drugs should be gradually withdrawn over at least 2–3 months by reducing the daily dose by 10–25% at intervals of 1–2 weeks. Benzodiazepines may need to be withdrawn over 6 months or longer.

In children receiving several antiepileptic drugs, only one drug should be withdrawn at a time.

Monitoring

Routine measurement of plasma concentrations of antiepileptic drugs is not usually justified, because the target concentration ranges are arbitrary and often vary between individuals. However, plasma-drug concentrations may be measured in children with worsening seizures, status epilepticus, suspected non-compliance, or suspected toxicity. Similarly, haematological and biochemical monitoring should not be undertaken unless clinically indicated.

Plasma concentration of some medications may change during pregnancy and monitoring may be required (see under *Pregnancy*).

Driving

If a driver has a seizure (of any type) they must stop driving immediately and inform the Driver and Vehicle Licensing Agency (DVLA).

Patients who have had a first unprovoked epileptic seizure or a single isolated seizure must not drive for 6 months; driving may then be resumed, provided the patient has been assessed by a specialist as fit to drive and investigations do not suggest a risk of further seizures.

Patients with established epilepsy may drive a motor vehicle provided they are not a danger to the public and are compliant with treatment and follow up. To continue driving, these patients must be seizure-free for at least one year (or have a pattern of seizures established for one year where there is no influence on their level of consciousness or the ability to act); also, they must not have a history of unprovoked seizures.

Patients who have had a *seizure while asleep* are not permitted to drive for one year from the date of each seizure unless:

- a history or pattern of sleep seizures occurring **only** ever while asleep has been established over the course of at least one year from the date of the first sleep seizure; or
- an established pattern of purely asleep seizures can be demonstrated over the course of three years if the patient has previously had seizures whilst awake (or awake and asleep).

The DVLA recommends that patients should not drive during medication changes or withdrawal of antiepileptic drugs, and for 6 months after their last dose. If a seizure occurs due to a prescribed change or withdrawal of epilepsy treatment, the patient will have their driving license revoked for 1 year; relicensing may be considered earlier if treatment has been reinstated for 6 months and no further seizures have occurred.

Pregnancy

Young women of child-bearing potential should discuss with a specialist the impact of both epilepsy, and its treatment, on the outcome of pregnancy.

There is an increased risk of teratogenicity associated with the use of antiepileptic drugs (especially if used during the first trimester and particularly if the patient takes two or more antiepileptic drugs). Valproate is associated with the highest risk of serious developmental disorders (up to 30–40% risk) and congenital malformations (approx. 10%

risk). Valproate must **not** be used in females of childbearing potential unless the conditions of the Pregnancy Prevention Programme are met and alternative treatments are ineffective or not tolerated; during pregnancy, it must not be used for epilepsy, unless it is the only possible treatment. There is also an increased risk of teratogenicity with phenytoin, primidone, phenobarbital, lamotrigine, and carbamazepine. Topiramate carries an increased risk of congenital malformations (including cleft palate, hypospadias, and anomalies involving various body systems) if taken in the first trimester of pregnancy. There is not enough evidence to establish the risk of teratogenicity with other antiepileptic drugs.

Prescribers should also consider carefully the choice of antiepileptic therapy in pre-pubescent girls who may later become pregnant. Young women of child-bearing potential who take antiepileptic drugs should be given advice about the need for an effective contraception method to avoid unplanned pregnancy—for further information, see *Conception and contraception* in the individual drug monographs. Some antiepileptic drugs can reduce the efficacy of hormonal contraceptives, and the efficacy of some antiepileptics may be affected by hormonal contraceptives.

Young women who want to become pregnant should be referred to a specialist for advice in advance of conception. For some women, the severity of seizure or the seizure type may not pose a serious threat, and drug withdrawal may be considered; therapy may be resumed after the first trimester. If treatment with antiepileptic drugs must continue throughout pregnancy, then monotherapy is preferable at the lowest effective dose.

Once an unplanned pregnancy is discovered it is usually too late for changes to be made to the treatment regimen; the risk of harm to the mother and fetus from convulsive seizures outweighs the risk of continued therapy. The likelihood of a woman who is taking antiepileptic drugs having a baby with no malformations is at least 90%, and it is important that women do not stop taking essential treatment because of concern over harm to the fetus. To reduce the risk of neural tube defects, folate supplementation is advised before conception and throughout the first trimester. In the case of sodium valproate p. 223 and valproic acid p. 228 an urgent consultation is required to reconsider the benefits and risks of valproate therapy.

The concentration of antiepileptic drugs in the plasma can change during pregnancy. Doses of phenytoin, carbamazepine, and lamotrigine should be adjusted on the basis of plasma-drug concentration monitoring; the dose of other antiepileptic drugs should be monitored carefully during pregnancy and after birth, and adjustments made on a clinical basis. Plasma-drug concentration monitoring during pregnancy is also useful to check compliance. Additionally, in patients taking topiramate or levetiracetam, it is recommended that fetal growth should be monitored. Women who have seizures in the second half of pregnancy should be assessed for eclampsia before any change is made to antiepileptic treatment. Status epilepticus should be treated according to the standard protocol.

Routine injection of vitamin K at birth minimises the risk of neonatal haemorrhage associated with antiepileptics.

Withdrawal effects in the newborn may occur with some antiepileptic drugs, in particular benzodiazepines and phenobarbital, and can take several days to diminish.

Epilepsy and Pregnancy Register

All pregnant women with epilepsy, whether taking medication or not, should be encouraged to notify the UK Epilepsy and Pregnancy Register (Tel: 0800 389 1248).

Breast-feeding

Young women taking antiepileptic monotherapy should generally be encouraged to breast-feed; if a woman is on combination therapy or if there are other risk factors, such as premature birth, specialist advice should be sought.

All infants should be monitored for sedation, feeding difficulties, adequate weight gain, and developmental milestones. Infants should also be monitored for adverse effects associated with the antiepileptic drug particularly with newer antiepileptics, if the antiepileptic is readily transferred into breast-milk causing high infant serum-drug concentrations (e.g. ethosuximide, lamotrigine, primidone, and zonisamide), or if slower metabolism in the infant causes drugs to accumulate (e.g. phenobarbital and lamotrigine). Serum-drug concentration monitoring should be undertaken in breast-fed infants if suspected adverse reactions develop; if toxicity develops it may be necessary to introduce formula feeds to limit the infant's drug exposure, or to wean the infant off breast-milk altogether.

Primidone, phenobarbital, and the benzodiazepines are associated with an established risk of drowsiness in breast-fed babies and caution is required.

Withdrawal effects may occur in infants if a mother suddenly stops breast-feeding, particularly if she is taking phenobarbital, primidone, or lamotrigine.

Focal seizures with or without secondary generalisation

Carbamazepine p. 209 and lamotrigine p. 216 are the drugs of choice for focal seizures; levetiracetam p. 217, oxcarbazepine p. 218 and sodium valproate p. 223 can be considered if these are unsuitable. These drugs may also be used as adjunctive treatment. Other adjunctive options include clobazam p. 234, gabapentin p. 213, and topiramate p. 227. If adjunctive treatment is ineffective or not tolerated, a tertiary specialist should be consulted who may consider eslicarbazepine acetate p. 211, lacosamide p. 215, phenobarbital p. 232, phenytoin p. 220, pregabalin [unlicensed], tiagabine p. 227, vigabatrin p. 230, and zonisamide p. 231.

Generalised seizures

Tonic-clonic seizures

The drug of choice for newly diagnosed tonic-clonic seizures in children is sodium valproate (except in female patients, see *Valproate* below), or lamotrigine where sodium valproate is unsuitable (but may exacerbate myoclonic seizures). In children with established epilepsy with generalised tonic-clonic seizures only, lamotrigine may be prescribed as the first-line choice. Carbamazepine or oxcarbazepine can also be considered but may exacerbate myoclonic or absence seizures. Clobazam, lamotrigine, levetiracetam, sodium valproate, or topiramate may be used as adjunctive treatment if monotherapy is ineffective or not tolerated.

Absence seizures

Ethosuximide p. 212 and sodium valproate (except in female patients, see *Valproate* below) are the drugs of choice for absence seizures and syndromes; lamotrigine can be used if these are unsuitable, ineffective or not tolerated. Sodium valproate should be used as the first choice if there is a high risk of generalised tonic-clonic seizures. A combination of any two of these drugs may be used if monotherapy is ineffective. Second-line therapy includes clobazam, clonazepam p. 235, levetiracetam, topiramate or zonisamide which may be considered by a tertiary specialist if adjunctive treatment fails. Carbamazepine, gabapentin, oxcarbazepine, phenytoin, pregabalin, tiagabine, and vigabatrin are not recommended in absence seizures or syndromes.

Myoclonic seizures

Myoclonic seizures (myoclonic jerks) occur in a variety of syndromes, and response to treatment varies considerably. Sodium valproate is the drug of choice (except in female patients, see *Valproate* below); consider levetiracetam or topiramate if sodium valproate is unsuitable (but consider the less favourable side-effect profile of topiramate). A combination of two of these drugs may be used if monotherapy is ineffective or poorly tolerated. Second-line therapy includes clobazam, clonazepam, piracetam or zonisamide which should be prescribed under the supervision of a tertiary specialist. Carbamazepine, gabapentin, oxcarbazepine, phenytoin, pregabalin, tiagabine, and vigabatrin are not recommended for the treatment of myoclonic seizures.

Tonic and atonic seizures

Tonic or atonic seizures are treated with sodium valproate (except in female patients, see *Valproate* below); lamotrigine can be considered as adjunctive treatment if sodium valproate is ineffective or not tolerated. If adjunctive treatment fails, a tertiary specialist should be consulted who may consider rufinamide p. 222 or topiramate. Carbamazepine, gabapentin, oxcarbazepine, pregabalin, tiagabine, and vigabatrin are not recommended in atonic or tonic seizures.

Epilepsy syndromes

Infantile spasms

Vigabatrin is the drug of choice for infantile spasms associated with tuberous sclerosis. Corticosteroids, such as prednisolone p. 478 or tetracosactide p. 511, are second-line options if vigabatrin is ineffective. In spasms of other causes, vigabatrin, prednisolone or tetracosactide can be considered as first-line options. A tertiary specialist should be consulted before treating infantile spasms.

Dravet syndrome

A tertiary specialist should be involved in decisions regarding treatment of Dravet syndrome. Sodium valproate (except in pregnancy or females of childbearing potential, see *Valproate* below) or topiramate are first-line treatment options in Dravet syndrome. Clobazam or stiripentol p. 226 may be considered as adjunctive treatment if first-line treatments are ineffective or not tolerated. Carbamazepine, gabapentin, lamotrigine, oxcarbazepine, phenytoin, pregabalin, tiagabine, and vigabatrin should not be used as they may exacerbate myoclonic seizures.

Lennox-Gastaut syndrome

A tertiary specialist should be involved in decisions regarding treatment of Lennox-Gastaut syndrome. Sodium valproate is the first-line drug for treating Lennox-Gastaut syndrome (except in pregnancy or females of childbearing potential, see *Valproate* below); lamotrigine can be used as adjunctive treatment if sodium valproate is unsuitable, ineffective or not tolerated. If adjunctive treatment is ineffective or not tolerated, rufinamide and topiramate may be considered by tertiary specialists. Carbamazepine, gabapentin, oxcarbazepine, pregabalin, tiagabine, and vigabatrin should not be used. Felbamate [unlicensed] may be used in tertiary specialist centres when all other treatment options have failed.

Landau-Kleffner syndrome

Always discuss with or refer to tertiary epilepsy specialists.

Neonatal seizures

Seizures can occur before delivery, but they are most common up to 24 hours after birth. Seizures in neonates occur as a result of biochemical disturbances, inborn errors of metabolism, hypoxic ischaemic encephalopathy, drug withdrawal, meningitis, stroke, cerebral haemorrhage or malformation, or severe jaundice (kernicterus).

Seizures caused by biochemical imbalance and those in neonates with inherited abnormal pyridoxine or biotin metabolism should be corrected by treating the underlying cause. Seizures caused by drug withdrawal following intra-uterine exposure are treated with a drug withdrawal regimen.

Phenobarbital can be used to manage neonatal seizures where there is a risk of recurrence; phenytoin is an alternative. Midazolam p. 239 and **rectal** paraldehyde p. 237 may also be useful in the management of acute neonatal seizures. Lidocaine hydrochloride p. 81 may be used if other treatments are unsuccessful; lidocaine hydrochloride should not be given to neonates who have received phenytoin infusion because of the risk of cardiac toxicity.

Antiepileptic drugs

Carbamazepine and related antiepileptics

Carbamazepine p. 209 is a drug of choice for simple and complex focal seizures and is a first-line treatment option for generalised tonic-clonic seizures. It can be used as adjunctive treatment for focal seizures when monotherapy has been ineffective. It is essential to initiate carbamazepine therapy at a low dose and build this up slowly in small increments every 3–7 days. Carbamazepine may exacerbate tonic, atonic, myoclonic and absence seizures and is therefore not recommended if these seizures are present.

Oxcarbazepine p. 218 is not recommended in tonic, atonic, absence or myoclonic seizures due to the risk of seizure exacerbation.

Ethosuximide

Ethosuximide is a first-line treatment option for absence seizures, and may be used as adjunctive treatment when monotherapy has failed.

Gabapentin

Gabapentin p. 213 is used as adjunctive therapy for the treatment of focal seizures with or without secondary generalisation; it is licensed as monotherapy in children over 12 years. It is not recommended if tonic, atonic, absence or myoclonic seizures are present.

Lamotrigine

Lamotrigine p. 216 is an antiepileptic drug recommended as a first-line treatment for focal seizures and primary and secondary generalised tonic-clonic seizures. It is also licensed as monotherapy for typical absence seizures in children (but efficacy may not be maintained in all children). It may be tried as an adjunctive treatment for atonic and tonic seizures if first-line treatment has failed [unlicensed]. Myoclonic seizures may be exacerbated by lamotrigine and it can cause serious rashes; dose recommendations should be adhered to closely.

Lamotrigine is used either as sole treatment or as an adjunct to treatment with other antiepileptic drugs. Valproate increases plasma-lamotrigine concentration, whereas the enzyme-inducing antiepileptics reduce it; care is therefore required in choosing the appropriate initial dose and subsequent titration. When the potential for interaction is not known, treatment should be initiated with lower doses, such as those used with valproate.

Levetiracetam and brivaracetam

Levetiracetam p. 217 is used for monotherapy and adjunctive treatment of focal seizures with or without secondary generalisation, and for adjunctive treatment of myoclonic seizures in children with juvenile myoclonic epilepsy and primary generalised tonic-clonic seizures. Levetiracetam may be prescribed alone and in combination for the treatment of myoclonic seizures, and under specialist supervision for absence seizures [both unlicensed].

Brivaracetam p. 208 is used as adjunctive therapy in the treatment of partial-onset seizures with or without secondary generalisation.

Phenobarbital and primidone

Phenobarbital p. 232 is effective for tonic-clonic, focal seizures and neonatal seizures but may cause behavioural disturbances and hyperkinesia. It may be tried for atypical absence, atonic, and tonic seizures. For therapeutic purposes phenobarbital and *phenobarbital sodium* should be considered equivalent in effect. Rebound seizures may be a problem on withdrawal.

Primidone p. 233 is largely converted to phenobarbital and this is probably responsible for its antiepileptic action. It is used rarely in children. A low initial dose of primidone is essential.

Phenytoin
Phenytoin p. 220 is licensed for tonic-clonic and focal seizures but may exacerbate absence or myoclonic seizures and should be avoided if theses seizures are present. It has a narrow therapeutic index and the relationship between dose and plasma-drug concentration is non-linear; small dosage increases in some patients may produce large increases in plasma concentration with acute toxic side-effects. Similarly, a few missed doses or a small change in drug absorption may result in a marked change in plasma-drug concentration. Monitoring of plasma-drug concentration improves dosage adjustment.

When only parenteral administration is possible, fosphenytoin sodium p. 213, a pro-drug of phenytoin, may be convenient to give. Whereas phenytoin should be given intravenously only, fosphenytoin sodium may also be given by intramuscular injection.

Rufinamide
Rufinamide p. 222 is licensed for the adjunctive treatment of seizures in Lennox-Gastaut syndrome. It may be considered by a tertiary specialist for the treatment of refractory tonic or atonic seizures [unlicensed].

Topiramate
Topiramate p. 227 can be given alone or as adjunctive treatment in generalised tonic-clonic seizures or focal seizures. It can also be used for absence, tonic and atonic seizures under specialist supervision and as an option in myoclonic seizures [all unlicensed]. Female patients should be fully informed of the risks related to the use of topiramate during pregnancy and the need to use effective contraception—for further information, see *Conception and contraception* and *Pregnancy* in the topiramate drug monograph.

Valproate
Valproate (as either sodium valproate p. 223 or valproic acid p. 228) is effective in controlling tonic-clonic seizures, particularly in primary generalised epilepsy. It is a drug of choice in primary generalised tonic-clonic seizures, focal seizures, generalised absences and myoclonic seizures, and can be tried in atypical absence seizures. It is recommended as a first-line option in atonic and tonic seizures. Valproate should generally be avoided in children under 2 years especially with other antiepileptics, but it may be required in infants with continuing epileptic tendency. Sodium valproate has widespread metabolic effects, and monitoring of liver function tests and full blood count is essential. Because of its high teratogenic potential, valproate must not be used in females of childbearing potential unless the conditions of the Pregnancy Prevention Programme are met and alternative treatments are ineffective or not tolerated. During pregnancy, it must not be used for epilepsy unless it is the only possible treatment. For further information see *Important safety information*, *Conception and contraception*, and *Pregnancy* in the sodium valproate and valproic acid drug monographs. Plasma-valproate concentrations are not a useful index of efficacy, therefore routine monitoring is unhelpful.

Zonisamide
Zonisamide p. 231 can be used as an adjunctive treatment for refractory focal seizures with or without secondary generalisation in children and adolescents aged 6 years and above. It can also be used under the supervision of a specialist for refractory absence and myoclonic seizures [unlicensed indications].

Benzodiazepines
Clobazam p. 234 may be used as adjunctive therapy in the treatment of generalised tonic-clonic and refractory focal seizures. It may be prescribed under the care of a specialist for refractory absence and myoclonic seizures. Clonazepam p. 235 may be prescribed by a specialist for refractory absence and myoclonic seizures, but its sedative side-effects may be prominent.

Other drugs
Acetazolamide p. 735, a carbonic anhydrase inhibitor, has a specific role in treating epilepsy associated with menstruation. Piracetam is used as adjunctive treatment for cortical myoclonus.

Status epilepticus

Convulsive status epilepticus
Immediate measures to manage status epilepticus include positioning the child to avoid injury, supporting respiration including the provision of oxygen, maintaining blood pressure, and the correction of any hypoglycaemia. Pyridoxine hydrochloride p. 678 should be administered if the status epilepticus is caused by pyridoxine deficiency.

Seizures lasting 5 minutes should be treated urgently with buccal midazolam p. 239 or intravenous lorazepam p. 238 (repeated once after 10 minutes if seizures recur or fail to respond). Intravenous diazepam p. 236 is effective but it carries a high risk of venous thrombophlebitis (reduced by using an emulsion formulation of diazepam injection). Patients should be monitored for respiratory depression and hypotension.

Important
If, after initial treatment with benzodiazepines, seizures recur or fail to respond 25 minutes after onset, phenytoin sodium should be used, or if the child is on regular phenytoin p. 220, give phenobarbital sodium intravenously over 5 minutes; the paediatric intensive care unit should be contacted. Paraldehyde p. 237 can be given after starting phenytoin infusion.

If these measures fail to control seizures 45 minutes after onset, anaesthesia with thiopental sodium p. 237 should be instituted with full intensive care support.

Phenytoin sodium can be given by intravenous infusion over 20 minutes, followed by the maintenance dosage if appropriate.

Paraldehyde given rectally causes little respiratory depression and is therefore useful where facilities for resuscitation are poor.

Non-convulsive status epilepticus
The urgency to treat non-convulsive status epilepticus depends on the severity of the child's condition. If there is incomplete loss of awareness, oral antiepileptic therapy should be continued or restarted. Children who fail to respond to oral antiepileptic therapy or have complete lack of awareness can be treated in the same way as for convulsive status epilepticus, although anaesthesia is rarely needed.

Febrile convulsions

Brief febrile convulsions need no specific treatment; antipyretic medication (e.g. paracetamol p. 288), is commonly used to reduce fever and prevent further convulsions but evidence to support this practice is lacking. *Prolonged febrile convulsions* (those lasting 5 minutes or longer), or *recurrent febrile convulsions* without recovery must be treated actively (as for convulsive status epilepticus).

Long-term anticonvulsant prophylaxis for febrile convulsions is rarely indicated.

ANTIEPILEPTICS

Brivaracetam

19-Jul-2018

● **INDICATIONS AND DOSE**

Adjunctive therapy of focal seizures with or without secondary generalisation

▸ BY MOUTH, OR BY INTRAVENOUS INJECTION, OR BY INTRAVENOUS INFUSION

▸ Child 4–17 years (body-weight up to 50 kg): Initially 0.5–1 mg/kg twice daily, adjusted according to response; usual maintenance 1 mg/kg twice daily (max. per dose 2 mg/kg twice daily)

▸ Child 4–17 years (body-weight 50 kg and above): Initially 25–50 mg twice daily, adjusted according to response; usual maintenance 50 mg twice daily (max. per dose 100 mg twice daily)

● **INTERACTIONS** → Appendix 1: antiepileptics

● **SIDE-EFFECTS**

▸ **Common or very common** Anxiety · appetite decreased · constipation · cough · depression · dizziness · drowsiness · fatigue · increased risk of infection · insomnia · irritability · nausea · vertigo · vomiting

▸ **Uncommon** Aggression · psychotic disorder

● **PREGNANCY** Manufacturer advises avoid unless potential benefit outweighs risk—limited information available. See also *Pregnancy* in Epilepsy p. 203.

● **BREAST FEEDING** Manufacturer advises avoid—present in milk in *animal* studies.

● **HEPATIC IMPAIRMENT** Manufacturer advises caution (risk of increased exposure).

Dose adjustments Manufacturer advises initial dose of 25 mg twice daily, max. maintenance dose of 75 mg twice daily in children body-weight 50 kg and above.

Manufacturer advises initial dose of 0.5 mg/kg twice daily, max. maintenance dose of 1.5 mg/kg twice daily in children with body-weight up to 50 kg (no information available).

● **TREATMENT CESSATION** Manufacturer advises avoid abrupt withdrawal—reduce daily dose in steps of 50 mg at weekly intervals, then reduce to 20 mg daily for a final week.

● **DIRECTIONS FOR ADMINISTRATION**

▸ With intravenous use For intermittent *intravenous infusion*, manufacturer advises dilute in Glucose 5% *or* Sodium Chloride 0.9% *or* Lactated Ringer's solution; give over 15 minutes.

▸ With oral use Manufacturer advises oral solution can be diluted in water or juice shortly before swallowing.

● **PRESCRIBING AND DISPENSING INFORMATION** Manufacturer advises if switching between oral therapy and intravenous therapy (for those temporarily unable to take oral medication), the total daily dose and the frequency of administration should be maintained.

● **PATIENT AND CARER ADVICE**

Missed doses Manufacturer advises if one or more doses are missed, a single dose should be taken as soon as possible and the next dose should be taken at the usual time.

Driving and skilled tasks Manufacturer advises patients and carers should be cautioned on the effects on driving and performance of skilled tasks—increased risk of dizziness.

● **NATIONAL FUNDING/ACCESS DECISIONS**

Scottish Medicines Consortium (SMC) decisions

SMC No. 1160/16

The *Scottish Medicines Consortium* has advised (July 2016) that brivaracetam (*Briviact*®) is accepted for restricted use within NHS Scotland as adjunctive therapy in the treatment of partial-onset seizures with or without secondary generalisation in patients from 16 years of age with refractory epilepsy. Treatment should be initiated by physicians who have appropriate experience in the treatment of epilepsy.

SMC No. SMC2113

The *Scottish Medicines Consortium* has advised (December 2018) that brivaracetam (*Briviact*®) is accepted for restricted use within NHS Scotland as adjunctive therapy in the treatment of partial-onset seizures with or without secondary generalisation in patients from 4 to 15 years of age with refractory epilepsy. Treatment should be initiated by physicians who have appropriate experience in the treatment of epilepsy.

All Wales Medicines Strategy Group (AWMSG) decisions

AWMSG No. 3387

The *All Wales Medicines Strategy Group* has advised (December 2018) that brivaracetam (*Briviact*®) is recommended as an option for restricted use within NHS Wales. Brivaracetam (*Briviact*®) should be restricted for use in the treatment of patients with refractory epilepsy, who remain uncontrolled with, or are intolerant to, other adjunctive anti-epileptic medicines, within its licensed indication as adjunctive therapy in the treatment of partial-onset seizures with or without secondary generalisation in patients from 4 years of age with epilepsy. Brivaracetam (*Briviact*®) is not recommended for use within NHS Wales outside of this subpopulation.

● **MEDICINAL FORMS** There can be variation in the licensing of different medicines containing the same drug.

Solution for injection

CAUTIONARY AND ADVISORY LABELS 2

ELECTROLYTES: May contain Sodium

▸ Briviact (UCB Pharma Ltd) ▼

Brivaracetam 10 mg per 1 ml Briviact 50mg/5ml solution for injection vials | 10 vial PoM £222.75

Oral solution

CAUTIONARY AND ADVISORY LABELS 2, 8

EXCIPIENTS: May contain Sorbitol

ELECTROLYTES: May contain Sodium

▸ Briviact (UCB Pharma Ltd) ▼

Brivaracetam 10 mg per 1 ml Briviact 10mg/ml oral solution sugar-free | 300 ml PoM £115.83 DT = £115.83

Tablet

CAUTIONARY AND ADVISORY LABELS 2, 8, 25

▸ Briviact (UCB Pharma Ltd) ▼

Brivaracetam 10 mg Briviact 10mg tablets | 14 tablet PoM £34.64 DT = £34.64

Brivaracetam 25 mg Briviact 25mg tablets | 56 tablet PoM £129.64 DT = £129.64

Brivaracetam 50 mg Briviact 50mg tablets | 56 tablet PoM £129.64 DT = £129.64

Brivaracetam 75 mg Briviact 75mg tablets | 56 tablet PoM £129.64 DT = £129.64

Brivaracetam 100 mg Briviact 100mg tablets | 56 tablet PoM £129.64 DT = £129.64

Cannabidiol

16-Jan-2020

● **INDICATIONS AND DOSE**

Seizures associated with Lennox-Gastaut syndrome [adjunctive treatment with clobazam] (specialist use only)

▸ BY MOUTH

▸ Child 2–17 years: Initially 2.5 mg/kg twice daily for 1 week, then increased to 5 mg/kg twice daily, then increased in steps of 2.5 mg/kg twice daily, adjusted according to response, dose to be increased at weekly intervals, food may affect absorption (take at the same time with respect to food); maximum 20 mg/kg per day

Seizures associated with Dravet syndrome [adjunctive treatment with clobazam] (specialist use only)

▸ BY MOUTH

▸ Child 2–17 years: Initially 2.5 mg/kg twice daily for 1 week, then increased to 5 mg/kg twice daily, then increased in steps of 2.5 mg/kg twice daily, adjusted according to response, dose to be increased at weekly intervals, food may affect absorption (take at the same time with respect to food); maximum 20 mg/kg per day

- **INTERACTIONS** → Appendix 1: cannabidiol
- **SIDE-EFFECTS**

▸ **Common or very common** Agitation · appetite abnormal · behaviour abnormal · cough · diarrhoea · drooling · drowsiness · fatigue · fever · increased risk of infection · insomnia · irritability · rash · tremor · vomiting · weight decreased

▸ **Frequency not known** Anaemia · seizure · suicidal tendencies

- **PREGNANCY** Manufacturer advises avoid unless potential benefit outweighs risk—toxicity in *animal* studies.
- **BREAST FEEDING** Manufacturer advises avoid—limited information available.
- **HEPATIC IMPAIRMENT** Manufacturer advises caution in moderate to severe impairment (risk of increased exposure).

Dose adjustments Manufacturer advises dose reduction in moderate to severe impairment—consult product literature.

- **MONITORING REQUIREMENTS** Manufacturer advises monitor liver function at baseline, at 1 month, 3 months, and 6 months of treatment, then periodically thereafter; more frequent monitoring is recommended in patients with raised baseline ALT or AST or taking valproate. Restart monitoring schedule if dose increased above 10 mg/kg/day. If transaminase or bilirubin levels increase significantly or symptoms of hepatic dysfunction occur, treatment should be withheld or permanently discontinued based on severity—consult product literature.
- **TREATMENT CESSATION** Manufacturer advises avoid abrupt withdrawal—withdraw treatment gradually.
- **PATIENT AND CARER ADVICE**

Missed doses Manufacturer advises if more than 7 doses are missed, dose titration should be re-started.

Driving and skilled tasks Manufacturer advises patients and carers should be counselled on the effects on driving and performance of skilled tasks—increased risk of somnolence and sedation. Effects of alcohol increased.

For information on 2015 legislation regarding driving whilst taking certain controlled drugs, including cannabis, see *Drugs and skilled tasks* under Guidance on prescribing p. 1.

- **NATIONAL FUNDING/ACCESS DECISIONS**

NICE decisions

▸ **Cannabidiol with clobazam for treating seizures associated with Dravet syndrome (December 2019)** NICE TA614

Cannabidiol (*Epidyolex*®) with clobazam is recommended as an option for treating seizures associated with Dravet syndrome in patients aged 2 years and older, only if:

- the frequency of convulsive seizures is checked every 6 months, and cannabidiol is stopped if the frequency has not fallen by at least 30% compared with the 6 months before starting treatment
- the manufacturer provides cannabidiol according to the commercial arrangement.

Patients whose treatment was started within the NHS before this guidance was published should have the option to continue treatment, without change to their funding arrangements, until they and their NHS clinician consider it appropriate to stop.

www.nice.org.uk/guidance/ta614

▸ **Cannabidiol with clobazam for treating seizures associated with Lennox-Gastaut syndrome (December 2019)** NICE TA615

Cannabidiol (*Epidyolex*®) with clobazam is recommended as an option for treating seizures associated with Lennox-Gastaut syndrome in patients aged 2 years and older, only if:

- the frequency of drop seizures is checked every 6 months, and cannabidiol is stopped if the frequency has not fallen by at least 30% compared with the 6 months before starting treatment,
- the manufacturer provides cannabidiol according to the commercial arrangement.

Patients whose treatment was started within the NHS before this guidance was published should have the option to continue treatment, without change to their funding arrangements, until they and their NHS clinician consider it appropriate to stop.

www.nice.org.uk/guidance/ta615

- **MEDICINAL FORMS** There can be variation in the licensing of different medicines containing the same drug. Forms available from special-order manufacturers include: oral solution

Oral solution

CAUTIONARY AND ADVISORY LABELS 2, 8

EXCIPIENTS: May contain Ethanol, sesame oil

▸ Epidyolex (GW Pharma Ltd)

Cannabidiol 100 mg per 1 ml Epidyolex 100mg/ml oral solution sugar-free | 100 ml [PoM] [CD2]

Carbamazepine

26-Jun-2018

- **INDICATIONS AND DOSE**

Trigeminal neuralgia

▸ BY MOUTH USING IMMEDIATE-RELEASE MEDICINES

▸ Child 1 month–11 years: Initially 5 mg/kg once daily, dose to be taken at night, alternatively initially 2.5 mg/kg twice daily, then increased in steps of 2.5–5 mg/kg every 3–7 days as required; maintenance 5 mg/kg 2–3 times a day, increased if necessary up to 20 mg/kg daily

▸ Child 12–17 years: Initially 100–200 mg 1–2 times a day, then increased to 200–400 mg 2–3 times a day, increased if necessary up to 1.8 g daily, dose should be increased slowly

Prophylaxis of bipolar disorder

▸ BY MOUTH USING IMMEDIATE-RELEASE MEDICINES

▸ Child 1 month–11 years: Initially 5 mg/kg once daily, dose to be taken at night, alternatively initially 2.5 mg/kg twice daily, then increased in steps of 2.5–5 mg/kg every 3–7 days as required; maintenance 5 mg/kg 2–3 times a day, increased if necessary up to 20 mg/kg daily

▸ Child 12–17 years: Initially 100–200 mg 1–2 times a day, then increased to 200–400 mg 2–3 times a day, increased if necessary up to 1.8 g daily, dose should be increased slowly

Focal and generalised tonic-clonic seizures

▸ BY MOUTH USING IMMEDIATE-RELEASE MEDICINES

▸ Child 1 month–11 years: Initially 5 mg/kg once daily, dose to be taken at night, alternatively initially 2.5 mg/kg twice daily, then increased in steps of 2.5–5 mg/kg every 3–7 days as required; maintenance 5 mg/kg 2–3 times a day, increased if necessary up to 20 mg/kg daily

▸ Child 12–17 years: Initially 100–200 mg 1–2 times a day, then increased to 200–400 mg 2–3 times a day, increased if necessary up to 1.8 g daily, dose should be increased slowly

continued →

▶ BY RECTUM
- Child: Up to 250 mg up to 4 times a day, to be used for short-term use (max. 7 days) when oral therapy temporarily not possible, use approx. 25% more than the oral dose

DOSE EQUIVALENCE AND CONVERSION
- Suppositories of 125 mg may be considered to be approximately equivalent in therapeutic effect to tablets of 100 mg but final adjustment should always depend on clinical response (plasma concentration monitoring recommended).

CARBAGEN® SR

Trigeminal neuralgia

▶ BY MOUTH
- Child 5–11 years: Initially 5 mg/kg daily in 1–2 divided doses, then increased in steps of 2.5–5 mg/kg every 3–7 days as required; maintenance 10–15 mg/kg daily in 1–2 divided doses, increased if necessary up to 20 mg/kg daily in 1–2 divided doses
- Child 12–17 years: Initially 100–400 mg daily in 1–2 divided doses, then increased to 400–1200 mg daily in 1–2 divided doses, increased if necessary up to 1.8 g daily in 1–2 divided doses, dose should be increased slowly

Focal and generalised tonic-clonic seizures | Prophylaxis of bipolar disorder

▶ BY MOUTH
- Child 5–11 years: Initially 5 mg/kg daily in 1–2 divided doses, then increased in steps of 2.5–5 mg/kg every 3–7 days as required, dose should be increased slowly; maintenance 10–15 mg/kg daily in 1–2 divided doses, increased if necessary up to 20 mg/kg daily in 1–2 divided doses
- Child 12–17 years: Initially 100–400 mg daily in 1–2 divided doses, then increased to 400–1200 mg daily in 1–2 divided doses, increased if necessary up to 1.8 g daily in 1–2 divided doses, dose should be increased slowly

TEGRETOL® PROLONGED RELEASE

Focal and generalised tonic-clonic seizures | Prophylaxis of bipolar disorder

▶ BY MOUTH
- Child 5–11 years: Initially 5 mg/kg daily in 2 divided doses, then increased in steps of 2.5–5 mg/kg every 3–7 days as required; maintenance 10–15 mg/kg daily in 2 divided doses, increased if necessary up to 20 mg/kg daily in 2 divided doses
- Child 12–17 years: Initially 100–400 mg daily in 2 divided doses, dose should be increased slowly; maintenance 400–1200 mg daily in 2 divided doses, increased if necessary up to 1.8 g daily in 2 divided doses

Trigeminal neuralgia

▶ BY MOUTH
- Child 5–11 years: Initially 5 mg/kg daily in 2 divided doses, then increased in steps of 2.5–5 mg/kg every 3–7 days as required; maintenance 10–15 mg/kg daily in 2 divided doses, increased if necessary up to 20 mg/kg daily in 2 divided doses
- Child 12–17 years: Initially 100–400 mg daily in 2 divided doses, dose should be increased slowly; maintenance 400–1200 mg daily in 2 divided doses, increased if necessary up to 1.8 g daily in 2 divided doses, dose should be increased slowly

- **UNLICENSED USE** Not licensed for use in trigeminal neuralgia or prophylaxis of bipolar disorder.
- **CONTRA-INDICATIONS** Acute porphyrias p. 652 · AV conduction abnormalities (unless paced) · history of bone-marrow depression
- **CAUTIONS** Cardiac disease · history of haematological reactions to other drugs · may exacerbate absence and myoclonic seizures · skin reactions · susceptibility to angle-closure glaucoma

CAUTIONS, FURTHER INFORMATION Consider vitamin D supplementation in patients who are immobilised for long periods or who have inadequate sun exposure or dietary intake of calcium.

▶ **Blood, hepatic, or skin disorders** Carbamazepine should be withdrawn immediately in cases of aggravated liver dysfunction or acute liver disease. Leucopenia that is severe, progressive, or associated with clinical symptoms requires withdrawal (if necessary under cover of a suitable alternative).

- **INTERACTIONS** → Appendix 1: antiepileptics
- **SIDE-EFFECTS**

▶ **Common or very common** Dizziness · drowsiness · dry mouth · eosinophilia · fatigue · fluid imbalance · gastrointestinal discomfort · headache · hyponatraemia · leucopenia · movement disorders · nausea · oedema · skin reactions · thrombocytopenia · vision disorders · vomiting · weight increased

▶ **Uncommon** Constipation · diarrhoea · eye disorders · tic · tremor

▶ **Rare or very rare** Aggression · agranulocytosis · albuminuria · alopecia · anaemia · angioedema · anxiety · appetite decreased · arrhythmias · arthralgia · azotaemia · bone disorders · bone marrow disorders · cardiac conduction disorders · circulatory collapse · confusion · congestive heart failure · conjunctivitis · coronary artery disease aggravated · depression · dyspnoea · embolism and thrombosis · erythema nodosum · fever · folate deficiency · galactorrhoea · gynaecomastia · haematuria · haemolytic anaemia · hallucinations · hearing impairment · hepatic disorders · hirsutism · hyperacusia · hyperhidrosis · hypersensitivity · hypertension · hypogammaglobulinaemia · hypotension · lens opacity · leucocytosis · lymphadenopathy · meningitis aseptic · muscle complaints · muscle weakness · nephritis tubulointerstitial · nervous system disorder · neuroleptic malignant syndrome · oral disorders · pancreatitis · paraesthesia · paresis · peripheral neuropathy · photosensitivity reaction · pneumonia · pneumonitis · pseudolymphoma · psychosis · red blood cell abnormalities · renal impairment · severe cutaneous adverse reactions (SCARs) · sexual dysfunction · speech impairment · spermatogenesis abnormal · syncope · systemic lupus erythematosus (SLE) · taste altered · tinnitus · urinary disorders · vanishing bile duct syndrome · vasculitis

▶ **Frequency not known** Bone fracture · colitis · human herpesvirus 6 infection reactivation · memory loss · nail loss

SIDE-EFFECTS, FURTHER INFORMATION Some side-effects (such as headache, ataxia, drowsiness, nausea, vomiting, blurring of vision, dizziness and allergic skin reactions) are dose-related, and may be dose-limiting. These side-effects are more common at the start of treatment.

Overdose For details on the management of poisoning, see Active elimination techniques, under Emergency treatment of poisoning p. 891.

- **ALLERGY AND CROSS-SENSITIVITY** Antiepileptic hypersensitivity syndrome associated with carbamazepine. See under Epilepsy p. 203 for more information. Caution—cross-sensitivity reported with oxcarbazepine and with phenytoin.
- **PREGNANCY** See *Pregnancy* in Epilepsy p. 203.

Monitoring Doses should be adjusted on the basis of plasma-drug concentration monitoring.

- **BREAST FEEDING** Amount probably too small to be harmful.

Monitoring Monitor infant for possible adverse reactions.

- **HEPATIC IMPAIRMENT** Manufacturer advises caution and close monitoring—no information available.
- **RENAL IMPAIRMENT** Use with caution.
- **PRE-TREATMENT SCREENING** Test for HLA-B*1502 allele in individuals of Han Chinese or Thai origin (avoid unless no alternative—risk of Stevens-Johnson syndrome in presence of HLA-B*1502 allele).
- **MONITORING REQUIREMENTS**
  - Plasma concentration for optimum response 4–12 mg/litre (20–50 micromol/litre) measured after 1–2 weeks.
  - Manufacturer recommends blood counts and hepatic and renal function tests (but evidence of practical value uncertain).
- **TREATMENT CESSATION** When stopping treatment with carbamazepine for bipolar disorder, reduce the dose gradually over a period of at least 4 weeks.
- **DIRECTIONS FOR ADMINISTRATION** Oral liquid has been used rectally—should be retained for at least 2 hours (but may have laxative effect).

  TEGRETOL® PROLONGED RELEASE *Tegretol® Prolonged Release* tablets can be halved but should not be chewed.
- **PRESCRIBING AND DISPENSING INFORMATION**

  Switching between formulations Different formulations of oral preparations may vary in bioavailability. Patients being treated for epilepsy should be maintained on a specific manufacturer's product.
- **PATIENT AND CARER ADVICE**

  Blood, hepatic, or skin disorders Patients or their carers should be told how to recognise signs of blood, liver, or skin disorders, and advised to seek immediate medical attention if symptoms such as fever, rash, mouth ulcers, bruising, or bleeding develop.

  Medicines for Children leaflet: Carbamazepine (oral) for preventing seizures www.medicinesforchildren.org.uk/carbamazepine-oral-preventing-seizures-0
- **PROFESSION SPECIFIC INFORMATION**

  Dental practitioners' formulary

  Carbamazepine Tablets may be prescribed.

- **MEDICINAL FORMS** There can be variation in the licensing of different medicines containing the same drug. Forms available from special-order manufacturers include: oral suspension, oral solution

Modified-release tablet

CAUTIONARY AND ADVISORY LABELS 3, 8, 25

- Carbagen SR (Mylan)

  Carbamazepine 200 mg Carbagen SR 200mg tablets | 56 tablet [PoM] £4.16 DT = £5.20

  Carbamazepine 400 mg Carbagen SR 400mg tablets | 56 tablet [PoM] £8.20 DT = £10.24
- Tegretol Retard (Novartis Pharmaceuticals UK Ltd)

  Carbamazepine 200 mg Tegretol Prolonged Release 200mg tablets | 56 tablet [PoM] £5.20 DT = £5.20

  Carbamazepine 400 mg Tegretol Prolonged Release 400mg tablets | 56 tablet [PoM] £10.24 DT = £10.24

Tablet

CAUTIONARY AND ADVISORY LABELS 3, 8

- Carbamazepine (Non-proprietary)

  Carbamazepine 100 mg Carbamazepine 100mg tablets | 84 tablet [PoM] £2.07 DT = £2.07

  Carbamazepine 200 mg Carbamazepine 200mg tablets | 84 tablet [PoM] £3.83–£4.65 DT = £3.83

  Carbamazepine 400 mg Carbamazepine 400mg tablets | 56 tablet [PoM] £5.02 DT = £5.02
- Carbagen (Mylan)

  Carbamazepine 100 mg Carbagen 100mg tablets | 28 tablet [PoM] £5.74 | 84 tablet [PoM] [X] DT = £2.07 (Hospital only)

  Carbamazepine 200 mg Carbagen 200mg tablets | 28 tablet [PoM] £4.99 | 84 tablet [PoM] [X] DT = £3.83 (Hospital only)

  Carbamazepine 400 mg Carbagen 400mg tablets | 28 tablet [PoM] £4.27 | 56 tablet [PoM] [X] DT = £5.02 (Hospital only)
- Tegretol (Novartis Pharmaceuticals UK Ltd)

  Carbamazepine 100 mg Tegretol 100mg tablets | 84 tablet [PoM] £2.07 DT = £2.07

  Carbamazepine 200 mg Tegretol 200mg tablets | 84 tablet [PoM] £3.83 DT = £3.83

  Carbamazepine 400 mg Tegretol 400mg tablets | 56 tablet [PoM] £5.02 DT = £5.02

Suppository

CAUTIONARY AND ADVISORY LABELS 3, 8

- Carbamazepine (Non-proprietary)

  Carbamazepine 125 mg Carbamazepine 125mg suppositories | 5 suppository [PoM] £120.00 DT = £120.00

  Carbamazepine 250 mg Carbamazepine 250mg suppositories | 5 suppository [PoM] £140.00 DT = £140.00

Oral suspension

CAUTIONARY AND ADVISORY LABELS 3, 8

- Carbamazepine (Non-proprietary)

  Carbamazepine 20 mg per 1 ml Carbamazepine 100mg/5ml oral suspension sugar-free | 300 ml [PoM] £9.30 DT = £8.99
- Tegretol (Novartis Pharmaceuticals UK Ltd)

  Carbamazepine 20 mg per 1 ml Tegretol 100mg/5ml liquid sugar-free | 300 ml [PoM] £6.12 DT = £8.99

Eslicarbazepine acetate

20-Nov-2018

- **INDICATIONS AND DOSE**

Adjunctive therapy of focal seizures with or without secondary generalisation

- BY MOUTH
  - Child 6–17 years (body-weight up to 60 kg): Initially 10 mg/kg once daily, then increased in steps of 10 mg/kg daily, every 1–2 weeks, increased if necessary up to 30 mg/kg daily (max. per dose 1.2 g)
  - Child 6–17 years (body-weight 60 kg and above): Initially 400 mg once daily for 1–2 weeks, then increased to 800 mg once daily (max. per dose 1.2 g)

- **CONTRA-INDICATIONS** Second- or third-degree AV block
- **CAUTIONS** Hyponatraemia · PR-interval prolongation
- **INTERACTIONS** → Appendix 1: antiepileptics
- **SIDE-EFFECTS**
  - **Common or very common** Anxiety · appetite decreased · asthenia · concentration impaired · diarrhoea · dizziness · drowsiness · gait abnormal · gastrointestinal discomfort · headaches · movement disorders · nausea · skin reactions · sleep disorders · vertigo · vision disorders · vomiting
  - **Uncommon** Alopecia · anaemia · bradycardia · chest pain · chills · confusion · constipation · depression · dry mouth · electrolyte imbalance · eye disorders · flushing · gastritis · haemorrhage · hearing impairment · hyperhidrosis · hypertension · hypotension · hypothyroidism · increased risk of infection · liver disorder · malaise · mood altered · muscle weakness · myalgia · pain in extremity · palpitations · peripheral coldness · peripheral neuropathy · peripheral oedema · psychomotor retardation · psychotic disorder · sensation abnormal · speech impairment · tinnitus · toothache · weight decreased
  - **Frequency not known** Angioedema · leucopenia · pancreatitis · severe cutaneous adverse reactions (SCARs) · thrombocytopenia
- **ALLERGY AND CROSS-SENSITIVITY** Antiepileptic hypersensitivity syndrome theoretically associated with eslicarbazepine. See under Epilepsy p. 203 for more information.
- **PREGNANCY** Manufacturer advises minimum effective doses and monotherapy if possible—reproductive toxicity in *animal* studies.

  Monitoring The dose should be monitored carefully during pregnancy and after birth, and adjustments made on a clinical basis.
- **BREAST FEEDING** Manufacturer advises avoid—present in milk in *animal* studies.

4 Nervous system

- **HEPATIC IMPAIRMENT** Manufacturer advises caution in mild to moderate impairment—limited information; avoid in severe impairment—no information available.
- **RENAL IMPAIRMENT** Manufacturer advises avoid if creatinine creatinine clearance less than 30 mL/minute.
  Dose adjustments Manufacturer advises reduce initial dose to 5 mg/kg once daily or 10 mg/kg every other day for 2 weeks, then increase to 10 mg/kg once daily if creatinine clearance 30–60 mL/minute. The dose may be further increased based on individual response.
- **PRE-TREATMENT SCREENING** Test for HLA-B*1502 allele in individuals of Han Chinese or Thai origin (avoid unless no alternative— risk of Stevens-Johnson syndrome in presence of HLA-B*1502 allele).
- **MONITORING REQUIREMENTS** Monitor plasma-sodium concentration in patients at risk of hyponatraemia and discontinue treatment if hyponatraemia occurs.
- **PRESCRIBING AND DISPENSING INFORMATION**
  Switching between formulations Care should be taken when switching between oral formulations. The need for continued supply of a particular manufacturer's product should be based on clinical judgement and consultation with the patient or their carer, taking into account factors such as seizure frequency and treatment history.
- **PATIENT AND CARER ADVICE**
  Driving and skilled tasks Manufacturer advises patients and carers should be cautioned on the effects on driving and performance of skilled tasks—increased risk of dizziness, somnolence and visual disorders.
- **NATIONAL FUNDING/ACCESS DECISIONS**
  Scottish Medicines Consortium (SMC) decisions
  SMC No. SMC2087
  The *Scottish Medicines Consortium* has advised (February 2019) that eslicarbazepine acetate (*Zebinix*®) is accepted for restricted use within NHS Scotland as adjunctive therapy in patients aged above 6 years with focal seizures with or without secondary generalisation. It is restricted for use in refractory epilepsy in patients who have been heavily pre-treated and remain uncontrolled with existing anti-epileptic drugs.
  All Wales Medicines Strategy Group (AWMSG) decisions
  AWMSG No. 1214
  The *All Wales Medicines Strategy Group* has advised (June 2019) that eslicarbazepine acetate (*Zebinix*®) is recommended as an option for restricted use within NHS Wales for the treatment of highly refractory patients who remain uncontrolled with, or are intolerant to, other anti-epileptic medicine combinations, within its licensed indication as adjunctive therapy in adults, adolescents and children aged above six years, with partial onset seizures, with or without secondary generalisation. It is not recommended for use within NHS Wales outside of this subpopulation.

- **MEDICINAL FORMS** There can be variation in the licensing of different medicines containing the same drug.

Oral suspension

CAUTIONARY AND ADVISORY LABELS 8

▸ Zebinix (Eisai Ltd)
  Eslicarbazepine acetate 50 mg per 1 ml Zebinix 50mg/1ml oral suspension sugar-free | 200 ml PoM £56.67 DT = £56.67

Tablet

CAUTIONARY AND ADVISORY LABELS 8

▸ Zebinix (Eisai Ltd)
  Eslicarbazepine acetate 200 mg Zebinix 200mg tablets | 60 tablet PoM £68.00 DT = £68.00
  Eslicarbazepine acetate 800 mg Zebinix 800mg tablets | 30 tablet PoM £136.00 DT = £136.00

Ethosuximide

- **INDICATIONS AND DOSE**

Absence seizures | Atypical absence seizures (adjunct) | Myoclonic seizures

▸ BY MOUTH
▸ Child 1 month–5 years: Initially 5 mg/kg twice daily (max. per dose 125 mg), dose to be increased every 5–7 days; maintenance 10–20 mg/kg twice daily (max. per dose 500 mg), total daily dose may rarely be given in 3 divided doses
▸ Child 6–17 years: Initially 250 mg twice daily, then increased in steps of 250 mg every 5–7 days; usual dose 500–750 mg twice daily, increased if necessary up to 1 g twice daily

- **CAUTIONS** Avoid in Acute porphyrias p. 652
- **INTERACTIONS** → Appendix 1: antiepileptics
- **SIDE-EFFECTS** Aggression · agranulocytosis · appetite decreased · blood disorder · bone marrow disorders · concentration impaired · depression · diarrhoea · dizziness · drowsiness · erythema nodosum · fatigue · gastrointestinal discomfort · generalised tonic-clonic seizure · headache · hiccups · leucopenia · libido increased · lupus-like syndrome · mood altered · movement disorders · nausea · nephrotic syndrome · oral disorders · psychosis · rash · sleep disorders · Stevens-Johnson syndrome · vaginal haemorrhage · vision disorders · vomiting · weight decreased
  SIDE-EFFECTS, FURTHER INFORMATION Blood counts required if features of fever, sore throat, mouth ulcers, bruising or bleeding.
- **PREGNANCY** See also *Pregnancy* in Epilepsy p. 203.
  Monitoring The dose should be monitored carefully during pregnancy and after birth, and adjustments made on a clinical basis.
- **BREAST FEEDING** Present in milk. Hyperexcitability and sedation reported.
- **HEPATIC IMPAIRMENT** Use with caution.
- **RENAL IMPAIRMENT** Use with caution.
- **PATIENT AND CARER ADVICE**
  Blood disorders Patients or their carers should be told how to recognise signs of blood disorders, and advised to seek immediate medical attention if symptoms such as fever, mouth ulcers, bruising, or bleeding develop.
  Medicines for Children leaflet: Ethosuximide for preventing seizures www.medicinesforchildren.org.uk/ethosuximide-preventing-seizures

---

- **MEDICINAL FORMS** There can be variation in the licensing of different medicines containing the same drug.

Oral solution

CAUTIONARY AND ADVISORY LABELS 8

▸ Ethosuximide (Non-proprietary)
  Ethosuximide 50 mg per 1 ml Ethosuximide 250mg/5ml syrup | 200 ml PoM £173.00 DT = £173.00
  Ethosuximide 250mg/5ml oral solution sugar-free | 125 ml PoM £86.50–£108.13 sugar-free | 200 ml PoM £173.00–£205.17 sugar-free | 250 ml PoM £216.25 DT = £216.25

Capsule

CAUTIONARY AND ADVISORY LABELS 8

▸ Ethosuximide (Non-proprietary)
  Ethosuximide 250 mg Ethosuximide 250mg capsules | 56 capsule PoM £192.26 DT = £192.26

Fosphenytoin sodium
23-Jul-2018

- **DRUG ACTION** Fosphenytoin is a pro-drug of phenytoin.

- **INDICATIONS AND DOSE**

Status epilepticus

▶ BY INTRAVENOUS INFUSION

▶ Child 5-17 years: Initially 20 mg(PE)/kg, dose to be administered at a rate of 2–3 mg(PE)/kg/minute, maximum 150 mg(PE)/minute, then 4–5 mg(PE)/kg daily in 1–4 divided doses, dose to be administered at a rate of 1–2 mg(PE)/kg/minute, maximum 100 mg (PE)/minute, dose to be adjusted according to response and trough plasma-phenytoin concentration

Prophylaxis or treatment of seizures associated with neurosurgery or head injury

▶ BY INTRAVENOUS INFUSION

▶ Child 5-17 years: Initially 10–15 mg(PE)/kg, then 4–5 mg(PE)/kg daily in 1–4 divided doses, dose to be administered at a rate of 1–2 mg(PE)/kg/minute, maximum 100 mg(PE)/minute, dose to be adjusted according to response and trough plasma-phenytoin concentration

Temporary substitution for oral phenytoin

▶ BY INTRAVENOUS INFUSION

▶ Child 5-17 years: Same dose and same dosing frequency as oral phenytoin therapy, intravenous infusion to be administered at a rate of 1–2 mg(PE)/kg/minute, maximum 100 mg(PE)/minute

DOSE EQUIVALENCE AND CONVERSION

▶ Doses are expressed as phenytoin sodium equivalent (PE); fosphenytoin sodium 1.5 mg ≡ phenytoin sodium 1 mg.

- **UNLICENSED USE** Fosphenytoin sodium doses in BNFC may differ from those in product literature.
- **CONTRA-INDICATIONS** Acute porphyrias p. 652 · second-degree heart block · sino-atrial block · sinus bradycardia · Stokes-Adams syndrome · third-degree heart block
- **CAUTIONS** Heart failure · hypotension · injection solutions alkaline (irritant to tissues) · respiratory depression · resuscitation facilities must be available
- **INTERACTIONS** → Appendix 1: antiepileptics
- **SIDE-EFFECTS**

▶ **Common or very common** Asthenia · chills · dizziness · drowsiness · dry mouth · dysarthria · euphoric mood · headache · hypotension · movement disorders · nausea · nystagmus · sensation abnormal · skin reactions · stupor · taste altered · tinnitus · tremor · vasodilation · vertigo · vision disorders · vomiting

▶ **Uncommon** Cardiac arrest · confusion · hearing impairment · muscle complaints · muscle weakness · nervousness · oral disorders · reflexes abnormal · severe cutaneous adverse reactions (SCARs) · systemic lupus erythematosus (SLE) · thinking abnormal

▶ **Frequency not known** Acute psychosis · agranulocytosis · appetite disorder · atrial conduction depression (more common if injection too rapid) · atrioventricular block · bone disorders · bone fracture · bone marrow disorders · bradycardia · cardiotoxicity · cerebrovascular insufficiency · circulatory collapse (more common if injection too rapid) · coarsening of the facial features · constipation · delirium · Dupuytren's contracture · encephalopathy · granulocytopenia · groin tingling · hair changes · hepatic disorders · hyperglycaemia · hypersensitivity · insomnia · leucopenia · lymphadenopathy · nephritis tubulointerstitial · Peyronie's disease · polyarteritis nodosa · polyarthritis · purple glove syndrome · respiratory disorders · sensory peripheral polyneuropathy · thrombocytopenia · tonic seizure · ventricular conduction depression (more common if injection too rapid) · ventricular fibrillation (more common if injection too rapid)

SIDE-EFFECTS, FURTHER INFORMATION Fosphenytoin has been associated with severe cardiovascular reactions including asystole, ventricular fibrillation, and cardiac arrest. Hypotension, bradycardia, and heart block have also been reported. The following are recommended: monitor heart rate, blood pressure, and respiratory function for duration of infusion; observe patient for at least 30 minutes after infusion; if hypotension occurs, reduce infusion rate or discontinue; reduce dose or infusion rate in renal or hepatic impairment.

- **ALLERGY AND CROSS-SENSITIVITY** Cross-sensitivity reported with carbamazepine.
- **PREGNANCY** See also *Pregnancy* in Epilepsy p. 203.

Monitoring Changes in plasma-protein binding make interpretation of plasma-phenytoin concentrations difficult—monitor unbound fraction.

The dose should be monitored carefully during pregnancy and after birth, and adjustments made on a clinical basis.

- **BREAST FEEDING** Small amounts present in milk, but not known to be harmful.
- **HEPATIC IMPAIRMENT** Manufacturer advises caution—monitor free plasma-phenytoin concentration (rather than total plasma-phenytoin concentration) in hepatic impairment or hypoalbuminaemia and in hyperbilirubinaemia.

Dose adjustments Manufacturer advises consider a 10–25% reduction in dose or infusion rate (except in the treatment of status epilepticus) in hepatic impairment or hypoalbuminaemia.

- **RENAL IMPAIRMENT**

Dose adjustments Consider 10–25% reduction in dose or infusion rate (except initial dose for status epilepticus).

- **PRE-TREATMENT SCREENING** HLA-B* 1502 allele in individuals of Han Chinese or Thai origin—avoid unless essential (increased risk of Stevens-Johnson syndrome).
- **MONITORING REQUIREMENTS**

▶ Manufacturer recommends blood counts (but evidence of practical value uncertain).

▶ With intravenous use Monitor heart rate, blood pressure, ECG, and respiratory function for during infusion.

- **DIRECTIONS FOR ADMINISTRATION** For *intermittent intravenous infusion* (*Pro-Epanutin*®), give *in* Glucose 5% *or* Sodium chloride 0.9%; dilute to a concentration of 1.5–25 mg (phenytoin sodium equivalent (PE))/mL.
- **PRESCRIBING AND DISPENSING INFORMATION** Prescriptions for fosphenytoin sodium should state the dose in terms of phenytoin sodium equivalent (PE); fosphenytoin sodium 1.5 mg ≡ phenytoin sodium 1 mg.

- **MEDICINAL FORMS** There can be variation in the licensing of different medicines containing the same drug.

Solution for injection

ELECTROLYTES: May contain Phosphate

▶ Pro-Epanutin (Pfizer Ltd)

Fosphenytoin sodium 75 mg per 1 ml Pro-Epanutin 750mg/10ml concentrate for solution for injection vials | 10 vial [PoM] £400.00 (Hospital only)

Gabapentin
02-Dec-2019

- **INDICATIONS AND DOSE**

Adjunctive treatment of focal seizures with or without secondary generalisation

▶ BY MOUTH

▶ Child 2-5 years: 10 mg/kg once daily on day 1, then 10 mg/kg twice daily on day 2, then 10 mg/kg 3 times a day on day 3, then increased

continued →

to 30–70 mg/kg daily in 3 divided doses, adjusted according to response, some children may not tolerate daily increments; longer intervals (up to weekly) may be more appropriate

- Child 6–11 years: 10 mg/kg once daily (max. per dose 300 mg) on day 1, then 10 mg/kg twice daily (max. per dose 300 mg) on day 2, then 10 mg/kg 3 times a day (max. per dose 300 mg) on day 3; usual dose 25–35 mg/kg daily in 3 divided doses, some children may not tolerate daily increments; longer intervals (up to weekly) may be more appropriate, daily dose maximum to be given in 3 divided doses; maximum 70 mg/kg per day
- Child 12–17 years: Initially 300 mg once daily on day 1, then 300 mg twice daily on day 2, then 300 mg 3 times a day on day 3, alternatively initially 300 mg 3 times a day on day 1, then increased in steps of 300 mg every 2–3 days in 3 divided doses, adjusted according to response; usual dose 0.9–3.6 g daily in 3 divided doses (max. per dose 1.6 g 3 times a day), some children may not tolerate daily increments; longer intervals (up to weekly) may be more appropriate

Monotherapy for focal seizures with or without secondary generalisation

- BY MOUTH
- Child 12–17 years: Initially 300 mg once daily on day 1, then 300 mg twice daily on day 2, then 300 mg 3 times a day on day 3, alternatively initially 300 mg 3 times a day on day 1, then increased in steps of 300 mg every 2–3 days in 3 divided doses, adjusted according to response; usual dose 0.9–3.6 g daily in 3 divided doses (max. per dose 1.6 g 3 times a day), some children may not tolerate daily increments; longer intervals (up to weekly) may be more appropriate

- **UNLICENSED USE** Not licensed for use in children under 6 years. Not licensed at doses over 50 mg/kg daily in children under 12 years.

IMPORTANT SAFETY INFORMATION

The levels of propylene glycol, acesulfame K and saccharin sodium may exceed the recommended WHO daily intake limits if high doses of gabapentin oral solution (Rosemont brand) are given to adolescents or adults with low body-weight (39–50 kg)—consult product literature.

MHRA/CHM ADVICE: GABAPENTIN (*NEURONTIN*®): RISK OF SEVERE RESPIRATORY DEPRESSION (OCTOBER 2017)

Gabapentin has been associated with a rare risk of severe respiratory depression even without concomitant opioid medicines. Patients with compromised respiratory function, respiratory or neurological disease, renal impairment, and concomitant use of central nervous system (CNS) depressants might be at higher risk of experiencing severe respiratory depression and dose adjustments may be necessary in these patients.

MHRA/CHM ADVICE: GABAPENTIN (*NEURONTIN*®) AND RISK OF ABUSE AND DEPENDENCE: NEW SCHEDULING REQUIREMENTS FROM 1 APRIL (APRIL 2019)

Following concerns about abuse, gabapentin has been reclassified as a Class C controlled substance and is now a Schedule 3 drug, but is exempt from safe custody requirements. Healthcare professionals should evaluate patients carefully for a history of drug abuse before prescribing gabapentin, and observe patients for signs of abuse and dependence. Patients should be informed of the potentially fatal risks of interactions between gabapentin and alcohol, and with other medicines that cause CNS depression, particularly opioids.

- **CAUTIONS** Diabetes mellitus · high doses of oral solution in adolescents and adults with low body-weight · history of psychotic illness · history of substance abuse · mixed seizures (including absences)
- **INTERACTIONS** → Appendix 1: antiepileptics
- **SIDE-EFFECTS**
  - **Common or very common** Anxiety · appetite abnormal · arthralgia · asthenia · behaviour abnormal · confusion · constipation · cough · depression · diarrhoea · dizziness · drowsiness · dry mouth · dysarthria · dyspnoea · emotional lability · flatulence · gait abnormal · gastrointestinal discomfort · headache · hypertension · increased risk of infection · insomnia · leucopenia · malaise · movement disorders · muscle complaints · nausea · nystagmus · oedema · pain · reflexes abnormal · seizure · sensation abnormal · sexual dysfunction · skin reactions · thinking abnormal · tooth disorder · tremor · vasodilation · vertigo · visual impairment · vomiting
  - **Uncommon** Cognitive impairment · palpitations
  - **Frequency not known** Acute kidney injury · alopecia · angioedema · breast enlargement · drug use disorders · gynaecomastia · hallucination · hepatic disorders · hyponatraemia · pancreatitis · rhabdomyolysis · severe cutaneous adverse reactions (SCARs) · thrombocytopenia · tinnitus · urinary incontinence
- **PREGNANCY** Manufacturer advises avoid unless benefit outweighs risk — toxicity reported. See also *Pregnancy* in Epilepsy p. 203.
- **BREAST FEEDING** Present in milk—manufacturer advises use only if potential benefit outweighs risk. See also *Breast-feeding* in Epilepsy p. 203.
- **RENAL IMPAIRMENT**
  Dose adjustments Reduce dose if estimated glomerular filtration rate less than 80 mL/minute/1.73 m^2; consult product literature.
- **MONITORING REQUIREMENTS** Monitor for signs of gabapentin abuse.
- **EFFECT ON LABORATORY TESTS** False positive readings with some urinary protein tests.
- **DIRECTIONS FOR ADMINISTRATION** Capsules can be opened but the bitter taste is difficult to mask.
- **PATIENT AND CARER ADVICE**
  Medicines for Children leaflet: Gabapentin for neuropathic pain www.medicinesforchildren.org.uk/gabapentin-neuropathic-pain
  Medicines for Children leaflet: Gabapentin for preventing seizures www.medicinesforchildren.org.uk/gabapentin-preventing-seizures
  Patient leaflet NHS England has produced a patient leaflet with information on the reclassification of gabapentin.

- **MEDICINAL FORMS** There can be variation in the licensing of different medicines containing the same drug. Forms available from special-order manufacturers include: oral suspension, oral solution

Tablet

CAUTIONARY AND ADVISORY LABELS 3, 5, 8, 25

- **Gabapentin (Non-proprietary)**
  Gabapentin 600 mg Gabapentin 600mg tablets | 100 tablet PoM £106.00 DT = £8.44 CD3
  Gabapentin 800 mg Gabapentin 800mg tablets | 100 tablet PoM £78.00 DT = £28.27 CD3
- **Neurontin** (Upjohn UK Ltd)
  Gabapentin 600 mg Neurontin 600mg tablets | 100 tablet PoM £84.80 DT = £8.44 CD3
  Gabapentin 800 mg Neurontin 800mg tablets | 100 tablet PoM £98.13 DT = £28.27 CD3

Oral solution

CAUTIONARY AND ADVISORY LABELS 3, 5, 8
EXCIPIENTS: May contain Propylene glycol
ELECTROLYTES: May contain Potassium, sodium

- **Gabapentin (Non-proprietary)**
  Gabapentin 50 mg per 1 ml Gabapentin 50mg/ml oral solution sugar-free | 150 ml PoM £68.09 DT = £67.52 CD3

Capsule

CAUTIONARY AND ADVISORY LABELS 3, 5, 8, 25

▸ Gabapentin (Non-proprietary)

Gabapentin 100 mg Gabapentin 100mg capsules | 100 capsule PoM £18.29 DT = £2.00 CD3

Gabapentin 300 mg Gabapentin 300mg capsules | 100 capsule PoM £42.40 DT = £3.18 CD3

Gabapentin 400 mg Gabapentin 400mg capsules | 100 capsule PoM £49.06 DT = £3.70 CD3

▸ Neurontin (Upjohn UK Ltd)

Gabapentin 100 mg Neurontin 100mg capsules | 100 capsule PoM £18.29 DT = £2.00 CD3

Gabapentin 300 mg Neurontin 300mg capsules | 100 capsule PoM £42.40 DT = £3.18 CD3

Gabapentin 400 mg Neurontin 400mg capsules | 100 capsule PoM £49.06 DT = £3.70 CD3

Lacosamide

10-Mar-2020

● **INDICATIONS AND DOSE**

Monotherapy of focal seizures with or without secondary generalisation

▸ BY MOUTH, OR BY INTRAVENOUS INFUSION

▸ Child (body-weight 50 kg and above): Initially 50 mg twice daily, then increased to 100 mg twice daily, after one week, alternatively initially 100 mg twice daily; increased in steps of 50 mg twice daily (max. per dose 300 mg twice daily) if necessary and if tolerated, dose to be increased at weekly intervals

▸ Child 4–17 years (body-weight up to 50 kg): (consult product literature)

Monotherapy of focal seizures with or without secondary generalisation (alternative loading dose regimen when it is necessary to rapidly attain therapeutic plasma concentrations) (under close medical supervision)

▸ BY MOUTH, OR BY INTRAVENOUS INFUSION

▸ Child (body-weight 50 kg and above): Loading dose 200 mg, followed by 100 mg twice daily, to be given 12 hours after initial dose; increased in steps of 50 mg twice daily (max. per dose 300 mg twice daily) if necessary and if tolerated, dose to be increased at weekly intervals

Adjunctive treatment of focal seizures with or without secondary generalisation

▸ BY MOUTH, OR BY INTRAVENOUS INFUSION

▸ Child (body-weight 50 kg and above): Initially 50 mg twice daily, then increased to 100 mg twice daily, after one week; increased in steps of 50 mg twice daily (max. per dose 200 mg twice daily) if necessary and if tolerated, dose to be increased at weekly intervals

▸ Child 4–17 years (body-weight up to 50 kg): (consult product literature)

Adjunctive treatment of focal seizures with or without secondary generalisation (alternative loading dose regimen when it is necessary to rapidly attain therapeutic plasma concentrations) (under close medical supervision)

▸ BY MOUTH, OR BY INTRAVENOUS INFUSION

▸ Child (body-weight 50 kg and above): Loading dose 200 mg, followed by 100 mg twice daily, to be given 12 hours after initial dose; increased in steps of 50 mg twice daily (max. per dose 200 mg twice daily) if necessary and if tolerated, dose to be increased at weekly intervals

● **CONTRA-INDICATIONS** Second- or third-degree AV block

● **CAUTIONS** Conduction problems · risk of PR-interval prolongation · severe cardiac disease

● **INTERACTIONS** → Appendix 1: antiepileptics

● **SIDE-EFFECTS**

▸ **Common or very common** Asthenia · concentration impaired · confusion · constipation · depression · diarrhoea · dizziness · drowsiness · dry mouth · dysarthria · dyspepsia · flatulence · gait abnormal · headache · insomnia · mood altered · movement disorders · muscle spasms · nausea · nystagmus · sensation abnormal · skin reactions · tinnitus · vertigo · vision disorders · vomiting

▸ **Uncommon** Aggression · agitation · angioedema · arrhythmias · atrioventricular block · hallucination · psychotic disorder · suicidal tendencies · syncope

▸ **Frequency not known** Agranulocytosis

● **ALLERGY AND CROSS-SENSITIVITY** Antiepileptic hypersensitivity syndrome associated with lacosamide. See under Epilepsy p. 203 for more information.

● **PREGNANCY** See also *Pregnancy* in Epilepsy p. 203.

Monitoring The dose should be monitored carefully during pregnancy and after birth, and adjustments made on a clinical basis.

● **BREAST FEEDING** Manufacturer advises avoid—present in milk in *animal* studies.

● **HEPATIC IMPAIRMENT** Manufacturer advises caution (risk of increased exposure), particularly in severe impairment (no information available).

Dose adjustments Manufacturer advises consider dose reduction—consult product literature.

● **RENAL IMPAIRMENT** Consult product literature.

● **DIRECTIONS FOR ADMINISTRATION**

▸ With intravenous use For *intermittent intravenous infusion*, manufacturer advises give undiluted or dilute with Glucose 5% *or* Sodium Chloride 0.9% *or* Lactated Ringer's Solution; give over 15–60 minutes—give doses greater than 200 mg over at least 30 minutes.

● **PRESCRIBING AND DISPENSING INFORMATION** Flavours of syrup may include strawberry.

● **PATIENT AND CARER ADVICE**

Medicines for Children leaflet: Lacosamide for preventing seizures www.medicinesforchildren.org.uk/lacosamide-preventing-seizures

● **NATIONAL FUNDING/ACCESS DECISIONS**

Scottish Medicines Consortium (SMC) decisions

SMC No. 532/09

The *Scottish Medicines Consortium* has advised (February 2009) that lacosamide (*Vimpat*®) is accepted for restricted use within NHS Scotland as adjunctive treatment for focal seizures with or without secondary generalisation in patients from 16 years. It is restricted for specialist use in refractory epilepsy.

SMC No. 1301/18

The *Scottish Medicines Consortium* has advised (February 2018) that lacosamide (*Vimpat*®) is accepted for restricted use within NHS Scotland as adjunctive treatment for focal seizures with or without secondary generalisation in adolescents and children from 4 years of age with epilepsy. It is restricted for specialist use in refractory epilepsy.

All Wales Medicines Strategy Group (AWMSG) decisions

AWMSG No. 3343

The *All Wales Medicines Strategy Group* has advised (March 2018) that lacosamide (*Vimpat*®) is recommended as an option for use within NHS Wales as adjunctive therapy in the treatment of focal seizures with or without secondary generalisation in children from 4 years of age up to 15 years of age with epilepsy.

● **MEDICINAL FORMS** There can be variation in the licensing of different medicines containing the same drug.

Solution for infusion

ELECTROLYTES: May contain Sodium

▸ Vimpat (UCB Pharma Ltd)

Lacosamide 10 mg per 1 ml Vimpat 200mg/20ml solution for infusion vials | 1 vial PoM £29.70

Oral solution

CAUTIONARY AND ADVISORY LABELS 8

EXCIPIENTS: May contain Aspartame, propylene glycol

ELECTROLYTES: May contain Sodium

▸ Vimpat (UCB Pharma Ltd)
 Lacosamide 10 mg per 1 ml Vimpat 10mg/ml syrup sugar-free | 200 ml PoM £25.74 DT = £25.74

Tablet

CAUTIONARY AND ADVISORY LABELS 8

▸ Vimpat (UCB Pharma Ltd)
 Lacosamide 50 mg Vimpat 50mg tablets | 14 tablet PoM £10.81 DT = £10.81
 Lacosamide 100 mg Vimpat 100mg tablets | 14 tablet PoM £21.62 | 56 tablet PoM £86.50 DT = £86.50
 Lacosamide 150 mg Vimpat 150mg tablets | 14 tablet PoM £32.44 | 56 tablet PoM £129.74 DT = £129.74
 Lacosamide 200 mg Vimpat 200mg tablets | 56 tablet PoM £144.16 DT = £144.16

Lamotrigine

04-Dec-2019

● **INDICATIONS AND DOSE**

Monotherapy of focal seizures | Monotherapy of primary and secondary generalised tonic-clonic seizures | Monotherapy of seizures associated with Lennox-Gastaut syndrome

▶ BY MOUTH

▸ Child 12–17 years: Initially 25 mg once daily for 14 days, then increased to 50 mg once daily for further 14 days, then increased in steps of up to 100 mg every 7–14 days; maintenance 100–200 mg daily in 1–2 divided doses; increased if necessary up to 500 mg daily, dose titration should be repeated if restarting after interval of more than 5 days

Monotherapy of typical absence seizures

▶ BY MOUTH

▸ Child 2–11 years: Initially 300 micrograms/kg daily in 1–2 divided doses, for 14 days, then 600 micrograms/kg daily in 1–2 divided doses, for further 14 days, then increased in steps of up to 600 micrograms/kg every 7–14 days; maintenance 1–10 mg/kg daily in 1–2 divided doses, increased if necessary up to 15 mg/kg daily, dose titration should be repeated if restarting after interval of more than 5 days

Adjunctive therapy of focal seizures with valproate | Adjunctive therapy of primary and secondary generalised tonic-clonic seizures with valproate | Adjunctive therapy of seizures associated with Lennox-Gastaut syndrome with valproate

▶ BY MOUTH

▸ Child 2–11 years (body-weight up to 13 kg): Initially 2 mg once daily on alternate days for first 14 days, then 300 micrograms/kg once daily for further 14 days, then increased in steps of up to 300 micrograms/kg every 7–14 days; maintenance 1–5 mg/kg daily in 1–2 divided doses, dose titration should be repeated if restarting after interval of more than 5 days; maximum 200 mg per day

▸ Child 2–11 years (body-weight 13 kg and above): Initially 150 micrograms/kg once daily for 14 days, then 300 micrograms/kg once daily for further 14 days, then increased in steps of up to 300 micrograms/kg every 7–14 days; maintenance 1–5 mg/kg daily in 1–2 divided doses, dose titration should be repeated if restarting after interval of more than 5 days; maximum 200 mg per day

▸ Child 12–17 years: Initially 25 mg once daily on alternate days for 14 days, then 25 mg once daily for further 14 days, then increased in steps of up to 50 mg every 7–14 days; maintenance 100–200 mg daily in 1–2 divided doses, dose titration should be repeated if restarting after interval of more than 5 days

Adjunctive therapy of focal seizures (with enzyme inducing drugs) without valproate | Adjunctive therapy of primary and secondary generalised tonic-clonic seizures (with enzyme inducing drugs) without valproate | Adjunctive therapy of seizures associated with Lennox-Gastaut syndromes (with enzyme inducing drugs) without valproate

▶ BY MOUTH

▸ Child 2–11 years: Initially 300 micrograms/kg twice daily for 14 days, then 600 micrograms/kg twice daily for further 14 days, then increased in steps of up to 1.2 mg/kg every 7–14 days; maintenance 5–15 mg/kg daily in 1–2 divided doses, dose titration should be repeated if restarting after interval of more than 5 days; maximum 400 mg per day

▸ Child 12–17 years: Initially 50 mg once daily for 14 days, then 50 mg twice daily for further 14 days, then increased in steps of up to 100 mg every 7–14 days; maintenance 200–400 mg daily in 2 divided doses, increased if necessary up to 700 mg daily, dose titration should be repeated if restarting after interval of more than 5 days

Adjunctive therapy of focal seizures (without enzyme inducing drugs) without valproate | Adjunctive therapy of primary and secondary generalised tonic-clonic seizures (without enzyme inducing drugs) without valproate | Adjunctive therapy of seizures associated with Lennox-Gastaut syndromes (without enzyme inducing drugs) without valproate

▶ BY MOUTH

▸ Child 2–11 years: Initially 300 micrograms/kg daily in 1–2 divided doses for 14 days, then 600 micrograms/kg daily in 1–2 divided doses for further 14 days, then increased in steps of up to 600 micrograms/kg every 7–14 days; maintenance 1–10 mg/kg daily in 1–2 divided doses, dose titration should be repeated if restarting after interval of more than 5 days; maximum 200 mg per day

▸ Child 12–17 years: Initially 25 mg once daily for 14 days, then increased to 50 mg once daily for further 14 days, then increased in steps of up to 100 mg every 7–14 days; maintenance 100–200 mg daily in 1–2 divided doses, dose titration should be repeated if restarting after interval of more than 5 days

● **CAUTIONS** Myoclonic seizures (may be exacerbated)

● **INTERACTIONS** → Appendix 1: antiepileptics

● **SIDE-EFFECTS**

▶ **Common or very common** Aggression · agitation · arthralgia · diarrhoea · dizziness · drowsiness · dry mouth · fatigue · headache · irritability · nausea · pain · rash · sleep disorders · tremor · vomiting

▶ **Uncommon** Alopecia · movement disorders · vision disorders

▶ **Rare or very rare** Confusion · conjunctivitis · disseminated intravascular coagulation · face oedema · fever · hallucination · hepatic disorders · lupus-like syndrome · lymphadenopathy · meningitis aseptic · multi organ failure · nystagmus · seizure · severe cutaneous adverse reactions (SCARs) · tic

SIDE-EFFECTS, FURTHER INFORMATION Serious skin reactions including Stevens-Johnson syndrome and toxic epidermal necrolysis have developed; most rashes occur in the first 8 weeks. Rash is sometimes associated with hypersensitivity syndrome and is more common in patients with history of allergy or rash from other antiepileptic drugs. Consider withdrawal if rash or signs of hypersensitivity syndrome develop. Factors associated with increased risk of serious skin reactions include concomitant use of valproate, initial lamotrigine dosing higher than recommended, and more rapid dose escalation than recommended.

- **ALLERGY AND CROSS-SENSITIVITY** Antiepileptic hypersensitivity syndrome associated with lamotrigine. See under Epilepsy p. 203 for more information.
- **PREGNANCY** See also *Pregnancy* in Epilepsy p. 203.
  Monitoring Doses should be adjusted on the basis of plasma-drug concentration monitoring.
- **BREAST FEEDING** Present in milk, but limited data suggest no harmful effect on infant.
- **HEPATIC IMPAIRMENT** Manufacturer advises caution in moderate to severe impairment.
  Dose adjustments Manufacturer advises dose reduction of approx. 50% in moderate impairment, and approx. 75% in severe impairment; adjust according to response.
- **RENAL IMPAIRMENT** Caution in renal failure; metabolite may accumulate.
  Dose adjustments Consider reducing maintenance dose in significant impairment.
- **TREATMENT CESSATION** Avoid abrupt withdrawal (taper off over 2 weeks or longer) unless serious skin reaction occurs.
- **PRESCRIBING AND DISPENSING INFORMATION** Patients being treated for epilepsy may need to be maintained on a specific manufacturer's branded or generic lamotrigine product.
  Switching between formulations Care should be taken when switching between oral formulations in the treatment of epilepsy. The need for continued supply of a particular manufacturer's product should be based on clinical judgement and consultation with the patient or their carer, taking into account factors such as seizure frequency and treatment history.
- **PATIENT AND CARER ADVICE**
  Skin reactions Warn patients and carers to see their doctor immediately if rash or signs or symptoms of hypersensitivity syndrome develop.
  Blood disorders Patients and their carers should be alert for symptoms and signs suggestive of bone-marrow failure, such as anaemia, bruising, or infection. Aplastic anaemia, bone-marrow depression, and pancytopenia have been associated rarely with lamotrigine.
  Medicines for Children leaflet: Lamotrigine for preventing seizures www.medicinesforchildren.org.uk/lamotrigine-preventing-seizures

- **MEDICINAL FORMS** There can be variation in the licensing of different medicines containing the same drug. Forms available from special-order manufacturers include: oral suspension, oral solution

Dispersible tablet

CAUTIONARY AND ADVISORY LABELS 8, 13

- Lamotrigine (Non-proprietary)
  Lamotrigine 5 mg Lamotrigine 5mg dispersible tablets sugar free sugar-free | 28 tablet PoM £15.00 DT = £6.87
  Lamotrigine 25 mg Lamotrigine 25mg dispersible tablets sugar free sugar-free | 56 tablet PoM £20.00 DT = £4.21
  Lamotrigine 100 mg Lamotrigine 100mg dispersible tablets sugar free sugar-free | 56 tablet PoM £58.68 DT = £5.63
- Lamictal (GlaxoSmithKline UK Ltd)
  Lamotrigine 2 mg Lamictal 2mg dispersible tablets sugar-free | 30 tablet PoM £18.81 DT = £18.81
  Lamotrigine 5 mg Lamictal 5mg dispersible tablets sugar-free | 28 tablet PoM £9.38 DT = £6.87
  Lamotrigine 25 mg Lamictal 25mg dispersible tablets sugar-free | 56 tablet PoM £23.53 DT = £4.21
  Lamotrigine 100 mg Lamictal 100mg dispersible tablets sugar-free | 56 tablet PoM £69.04 DT = £5.63

Tablet

CAUTIONARY AND ADVISORY LABELS 8

- Lamotrigine (Non-proprietary)
  Lamotrigine 25 mg Lamotrigine 25mg tablets | 56 tablet PoM £23.53 DT = £1.70
  Lamotrigine 50 mg Lamotrigine 50mg tablets | 56 tablet PoM £40.02 DT = £2.21
  Lamotrigine 100 mg Lamotrigine 100mg tablets | 56 tablet PoM £69.04 DT = £3.12
  Lamotrigine 200 mg Lamotrigine 200mg tablets | 56 tablet PoM £117.35 DT = £3.92
- Lamictal (GlaxoSmithKline UK Ltd)
  Lamotrigine 25 mg Lamictal 25mg tablets | 56 tablet PoM £23.53 DT = £1.70
  Lamotrigine 50 mg Lamictal 50mg tablets | 56 tablet PoM £40.02 DT = £2.21
  Lamotrigine 100 mg Lamictal 100mg tablets | 56 tablet PoM £69.04 DT = £3.12
  Lamotrigine 200 mg Lamictal 200mg tablets | 56 tablet PoM £117.35 DT = £3.92

Levetiracetam

10-Mar-2020

- **INDICATIONS AND DOSE**

Monotherapy of focal seizures with or without secondary generalisation

▶ BY MOUTH, OR BY INTRAVENOUS INFUSION

- Child 16–17 years: Initially 250 mg once daily for 1 week, then increased to 250 mg twice daily, then increased in steps of 250 mg twice daily (max. per dose 1.5 g twice daily), adjusted according to response, dose to be increased every 2 weeks

Adjunctive therapy of focal seizures with or without secondary generalisation

▶ BY MOUTH

- Child 1–5 months: Initially 7 mg/kg once daily, then increased in steps of up to 7 mg/kg twice daily (max. per dose 21 mg/kg twice daily), dose to be increased every 2 weeks
- Child 6 months–17 years (body-weight up to 50 kg): Initially 10 mg/kg once daily, then increased in steps of up to 10 mg/kg twice daily (max. per dose 30 mg/kg twice daily), dose to be increased every 2 weeks
- Child 12–17 years (body-weight 50 kg and above): Initially 250 mg twice daily, then increased in steps of 500 mg twice daily (max. per dose 1.5 g twice daily), dose to be increased every 2–4 weeks

▶ BY INTRAVENOUS INFUSION

- Child 4–17 years (body-weight up to 50 kg): Initially 10 mg/kg once daily, then increased in steps of up to 10 mg/kg twice daily (max. per dose 30 mg/kg twice daily), dose to be increased every 2 weeks
- Child 12–17 years (body-weight 50 kg and above): Initially 250 mg twice daily, then increased in steps of 500 mg twice daily (max. per dose 1.5 g twice daily), dose to be increased every 2 weeks

Adjunctive therapy of myoclonic seizures and tonic-clonic seizures

▶ BY MOUTH, OR BY INTRAVENOUS INFUSION

- Child 12–17 years (body-weight up to 50 kg): Initially 10 mg/kg once daily, then increased in steps of up to 10 mg/kg twice daily (max. per dose 30 mg/kg twice daily), dose to be increased every 2 weeks
- Child 12–17 years (body-weight 50 kg and above): Initially 250 mg twice daily, then increased in steps of 500 mg twice daily (max. per dose 1.5 g twice daily), dose to be increased every 2 weeks

- **UNLICENSED USE** EvGr Initial dosing recommendations for levetiracetam ⟨E⟩ in BNF Publications differ from product licence.
- ▶ With oral use Manufacturer advises *granules* not licensed for use in children under 6 years, for initial treatment in children with body-weight less than 25 kg, or for the administration of doses below 250 mg—oral solution should be used.
- **INTERACTIONS** → Appendix 1: antiepileptics

- **SIDE-EFFECTS**
- **Common or very common** Anxiety · appetite decreased · asthenia · behaviour abnormal · cough · depression · diarrhoea · dizziness · drowsiness · gastrointestinal discomfort · headache · increased risk of infection · insomnia · mood altered · movement disorders · nausea · skin reactions · vertigo · vomiting
- **Uncommon** Alopecia · concentration impaired · confusion · hallucination · leucopenia · muscle weakness · myalgia · paraesthesia · psychotic disorder · suicidal tendencies · thrombocytopenia · vision disorders · weight changes
- **Rare or very rare** Acute kidney injury · agranulocytosis · hepatic disorders · hyponatraemia · neutropenia · pancreatitis · pancytopenia · personality disorder · rhabdomyolysis · severe cutaneous adverse reactions (SCARs) · thinking abnormal

- **PREGNANCY** See also *Pregnancy* in Epilepsy p. 203.
Monitoring The dose should be monitored carefully during pregnancy and after birth, and adjustments made on a clinical basis. It is recommended that the fetal growth should be monitored.
- **BREAST FEEDING** Present in milk—manufacturer advises avoid.
- **HEPATIC IMPAIRMENT** Manufacturer advises caution in severe impairment.
Dose adjustments Manufacturer advises maintenance dose reduction of 50% in severe impairment if creatinine clearance is less than 60 mL/minute/1.73 m^2—consult product literature.
- **RENAL IMPAIRMENT**
Dose adjustments Reduce dose if estimated glomerular filtration rate less than 80 mL/minute/1.73 m^2 (consult product literature).
- **DIRECTIONS FOR ADMINISTRATION**
- With intravenous use For *intravenous infusion* (*Keppra®*), dilute requisite dose with at least 100 mL Glucose 5% or Sodium Chloride 0.9%; give over 15 minutes.
- With oral use For administration of *oral solution*, requisite dose may be diluted in a glass of water.
- **PRESCRIBING AND DISPENSING INFORMATION** If switching between oral therapy and intravenous therapy (for those temporarily unable to take oral medication), the intravenous dose should be the same as the established oral dose.
- **PATIENT AND CARER ADVICE**
Medicines for Children leaflet: Levetiracetam for preventing seizures www.medicinesforchildren.org.uk/levetiracetam-preventing-seizures

---

- **MEDICINAL FORMS** There can be variation in the licensing of different medicines containing the same drug. Forms available from special-order manufacturers include: oral suspension, oral solution

Granules

CAUTIONARY AND ADVISORY LABELS 8

- Desitrend (Desitin Pharma Ltd)
Levetiracetam 250 mg Desitrend 250mg granules sachets sugar-free | 60 sachet PoM £22.41 DT = £22.41
Levetiracetam 500 mg Desitrend 500mg granules sachets sugar-free | 60 sachet PoM £39.46 DT = £39.46
Levetiracetam 1 gram Desitrend 1000mg granules sachets sugar-free | 60 sachet PoM £76.27 DT = £76.27

Tablet

CAUTIONARY AND ADVISORY LABELS 8

- **Levetiracetam (Non-proprietary)**
Levetiracetam 250 mg Levetiracetam 250mg tablets | 60 tablet PoM £28.01 DT = £5.12
Levetiracetam 500 mg Levetiracetam 500mg tablets | 60 tablet PoM £49.32 DT = £8.93
Levetiracetam 750 mg Levetiracetam 750mg tablets | 60 tablet PoM £84.02 DT = £8.02
Levetiracetam 1 gram Levetiracetam 1g tablets | 60 tablet PoM £95.34 DT = £13.40
- Keppra (UCB Pharma Ltd)
Levetiracetam 250 mg Keppra 250mg tablets | 60 tablet PoM £28.01 DT = £5.12
Levetiracetam 500 mg Keppra 500mg tablets | 60 tablet PoM £49.32 DT = £8.93
Levetiracetam 750 mg Keppra 750mg tablets | 60 tablet PoM £84.02 DT = £8.02
Levetiracetam 1 gram Keppra 1g tablets | 60 tablet PoM £95.34 DT = £13.40

Solution for infusion

ELECTROLYTES: May contain Sodium

- **Levetiracetam (Non-proprietary)**
Levetiracetam 100 mg per 1 ml Levetiracetam 500mg/5ml concentrate for solution for infusion vials | 10 vial PoM £127.31 DT = £127.31 | 10 vial PoM £127.31 DT = £127.31 (Hospital only)
- **Desitrend** (Desitin Pharma Ltd)
Levetiracetam 100 mg per 1 ml Desitrend 500mg/5ml concentrate for solution for infusion ampoules | 10 ampoule PoM £127.31 DT = £127.31
- Keppra (UCB Pharma Ltd)
Levetiracetam 100 mg per 1 ml Keppra 500mg/5ml concentrate for solution for infusion vials | 10 vial PoM £127.31 DT = £127.31

Oral solution

CAUTIONARY AND ADVISORY LABELS 8

- **Levetiracetam (Non-proprietary)**
Levetiracetam 100 mg per 1 ml Levetiracetam 100mg/ml oral solution sugar-free | 150 ml PoM £27.00 | 300 ml PoM £60.26 DT = £6.89
- Keppra (UCB Pharma Ltd)
Levetiracetam 100 mg per 1 ml Keppra 100mg/ml oral solution sugar-free | 150 ml PoM £33.48 | 300 ml PoM £66.95 DT = £6.89

Oxcarbazepine

- **INDICATIONS AND DOSE**

Monotherapy for the treatment of focal seizures with or without secondary generalised tonic-clonic seizures

- BY MOUTH
- Child 6–17 years: Initially 4–5 mg/kg twice daily (max. per dose 300 mg), then increased in steps of up to 5 mg/kg twice daily, adjusted according to response, dose to be adjusted at weekly intervals; maximum 46 mg/kg per day

Adjunctive therapy for the treatment of focal seizures with or without secondary generalised tonic-clonic seizures

- BY MOUTH
- Child 6–17 years: Initially 4–5 mg/kg twice daily (max. per dose 300 mg), then increased in steps of up to 5 mg/kg twice daily, adjusted according to response, dose to be adjusted at weekly intervals; maintenance 15 mg/kg twice daily; maximum 46 mg/kg per day

DOSE ADJUSTMENTS DUE TO INTERACTIONS

- In adjunctive therapy, the dose of concomitant antiepileptics may need to be reduced when using high doses of oxcarbazepine.

- **CAUTIONS** Avoid in Acute porphyrias p. 652 · cardiac conduction disorders · heart failure · hyponatraemia
- **INTERACTIONS** → Appendix 1: antiepileptics
- **SIDE-EFFECTS**
- **Common or very common** Abdominal pain · agitation · alopecia · asthenia · ataxia · concentration impaired · constipation · depression · diarrhoea · dizziness · drowsiness · emotional lability · headache · hyponatraemia · nausea · nystagmus · skin reactions · vertigo · vision disorders · vomiting
- **Uncommon** Leucopenia
- **Rare or very rare** Angioedema · arrhythmia · atrioventricular block · hepatitis · hypothyroidism · pancreatitis · severe cutaneous adverse reactions (SCARs) · systemic lupus erythematosus (SLE) · thrombocytopenia

- ▸ **Frequency not known** Agranulocytosis · bone disorders · bone marrow disorders · hypertension · inappropriate antidiuretic hormone secretion like-syndrome · neutropenia · speech impairment
- **ALLERGY AND CROSS-SENSITIVITY** Caution in patients with hypersensitivity to carbamazepine. Antiepileptic hypersensitivity syndrome associated with oxcarbazepine. See under Epilepsy p. 203 for more information.
- **PREGNANCY** See also *Pregnancy* in Epilepsy p. 203.
  Monitoring The dose should be monitored carefully during pregnancy and after birth, and adjustments made on a clinical basis.
- **BREAST FEEDING** Amount probably too small to be harmful but manufacturer advises avoid.
- **HEPATIC IMPAIRMENT** Manufacturer advises caution in severe impairment (no information available).
- **RENAL IMPAIRMENT**
  Dose adjustments Halve initial dose if estimated glomerular filtration rate less than 30 mL/minute/1.73 m^2, increase according to response at intervals of at least 1 week.
- **PRE-TREATMENT SCREENING** Test for HLA-B*1502 allele in individuals of Han Chinese or Thai origin (avoid unless no alternative—risk of Stevens-Johnson syndrome in presence of HLA-B*1502 allele).
- **MONITORING REQUIREMENTS**
- ▸ Monitor plasma-sodium concentration in patients at risk of hyponatraemia.
- ▸ Monitor body-weight in patients with heart failure.
- **PRESCRIBING AND DISPENSING INFORMATION** Patients may need to be maintained on a specific manufacturer's branded or generic oxcarbazepine product.
  Switching between formulations Care should be taken when switching between oral formulations. The need for continued supply of a particular manufacturer's product should be based on clinical judgement and consultation with the patient or their carer, taking into account factors such as seizure frequency and treatment history.
- **PATIENT AND CARER ADVICE**
  Blood, hepatic, or skin disorders Patients or their carers should be told how to recognise signs of blood, liver, or skin disorders, and advised to seek immediate medical attention if symptoms such as lethargy, confusion, muscular twitching, fever, rash, blistering, mouth ulcers, bruising, or bleeding develop.
  Medicines for Children: Oxcarbazepine for preventing seizures www.medicinesforchildren.org.uk/oxcarbazepine-preventing-seizures

---

- **MEDICINAL FORMS** There can be variation in the licensing of different medicines containing the same drug. Forms available from special-order manufacturers include: oral suspension

Oral suspension

CAUTIONARY AND ADVISORY LABELS 3, 8
EXCIPIENTS: May contain Propylene glycol

▸ Trileptal (Novartis Pharmaceuticals UK Ltd)
Oxcarbazepine 60 mg per 1 ml Trileptal 60mg/ml oral suspension sugar-free | 250 ml [PoM] £48.96 DT = £48.96

Tablet

CAUTIONARY AND ADVISORY LABELS 3, 8

▸ Oxcarbazepine (Non-proprietary)
Oxcarbazepine 150 mg Oxcarbazepine 150mg tablets | 50 tablet [PoM] £11.14 DT = £8.37
Oxcarbazepine 300 mg Oxcarbazepine 300mg tablets | 50 tablet [PoM] £22.61 DT = £7.09
Oxcarbazepine 600 mg Oxcarbazepine 600mg tablets | 50 tablet [PoM] £45.19 DT = £38.71

▸ Trileptal (Novartis Pharmaceuticals UK Ltd)
Oxcarbazepine 150 mg Trileptal 150mg tablets | 50 tablet [PoM] £12.24 DT = £8.37
Oxcarbazepine 300 mg Trileptal 300mg tablets | 50 tablet [PoM] £24.48 DT = £7.09
Oxcarbazepine 600 mg Trileptal 600mg tablets | 50 tablet [PoM] £48.96 DT = £38.71

Perampanel

12-Sep-2019

- **INDICATIONS AND DOSE**

Adjunctive treatment of focal seizures with or without secondary generalised seizures

▸ BY MOUTH
▸ Child 12–17 years: Initially 2 mg once daily, dose to be taken before bedtime, then increased, if tolerated, in steps of 2 mg at intervals of at least every 2 weeks, adjusted according to response; maintenance 4–8 mg once daily; maximum 12 mg per day

Adjunctive treatment of primary generalised tonic-clonic seizures

▸ BY MOUTH
▸ Child 12–17 years: Initially 2 mg once daily, dose to be taken before bedtime, then increased, if tolerated, in steps of 2 mg at intervals of at least every 2 weeks, adjusted according to response, maintenance up to 8 mg once daily; maximum 12 mg per day

DOSE ADJUSTMENTS DUE TO INTERACTIONS
▸ Titrate at intervals of at least 1 week with concomitant carbamazepine, fosphenytoin, oxcarbazepine, or phenytoin.

- **INTERACTIONS** → Appendix 1: antiepileptics
- **SIDE-EFFECTS**
- ▸ **Common or very common** Anxiety · appetite abnormal · back pain · behaviour abnormal · confusion · dizziness · drowsiness · dysarthria · fatigue · gait abnormal · irritability · movement disorders · nausea · vertigo · vision disorders · weight increased
- ▸ **Frequency not known** Severe cutaneous adverse reactions (SCARs)
- **PREGNANCY** Manufacturer advises avoid. See also *Pregnancy* in Epilepsy p. 203.
  Monitoring The dose should be monitored carefully during pregnancy and after birth, and adjustments made on a clinical basis.
- **BREAST FEEDING** Avoid—present in milk in *animal* studies.
- **HEPATIC IMPAIRMENT** Manufacturer advises caution in mild to moderate impairment; avoid in severe impairment.
  Dose adjustments Manufacturer advises maximum 8 mg per day in mild to moderate impairment.
- **RENAL IMPAIRMENT** Avoid in moderate or severe impairment.
- **PRESCRIBING AND DISPENSING INFORMATION**
  Switching between formulations Care should be taken when switching between oral formulations. The need for continued supply of a particular manufacturer's product should be based on clinical judgement and consultation with the patient or their carer, taking into account factors such as seizure frequency and treatment history.
  Patients may need to be maintained on a specific manufacturer's branded or generic perampanel product.
- **PATIENT AND CARER ADVICE**
  Driving and skilled tasks Manufacturer advises patients and carers should be cautioned on the effects on driving and performance of skilled tasks—increased risk of dizziness and drowsiness.
- **NATIONAL FUNDING/ACCESS DECISIONS**

Scottish Medicines Consortium (SMC) decisions

SMC No. 819/12
The *Scottish Medicines Consortium* has advised (December 2012) that perampanel (*Fycompa*®) is accepted for restricted use within NHS Scotland as a second-line adjunctive treatment in patients with refractory focal seizures, with or without secondary generalised seizures.

Treatment should be initiated only by physicians who have appropriate experience in the treatment of epilepsy. This advice is contingent upon the continuing availability of the patient access scheme or a list price that is equivalent or lower.
SMC No. SMC2172
The *Scottish Medicines Consortium* has advised (August 2019) that perampanel (*Fycompa*®) oral suspension is accepted for restricted use within NHS Scotland as a second-line adjunctive treatment in patients with refractory focal seizures, with or without secondary generalised seizures, who are unable to swallow perampanel tablets. Treatment should be initiated only by physicians who have appropriate experience in the treatment of epilepsy.

- **MEDICINAL FORMS** There can be variation in the licensing of different medicines containing the same drug. Forms available from special-order manufacturers include: oral suspension

Oral suspension
CAUTIONARY AND ADVISORY LABELS 3, 8
EXCIPIENTS: May contain Sorbitol
▸ Fycompa (Eisai Ltd)
Perampanel 500 microgram per 1 ml Fycompa 0.5mg/ml oral suspension sugar-free | 340 ml [PoM] £127.50 DT = £127.50

Tablet
CAUTIONARY AND ADVISORY LABELS 3, 8, 25
▸ Fycompa (Eisai Ltd)
Perampanel 2 mg Fycompa 2mg tablets | 7 tablet [PoM] £35.00 DT = £35.00 | 28 tablet [PoM] £140.00 DT = £140.00
Perampanel 4 mg Fycompa 4mg tablets | 28 tablet [PoM] £140.00 DT = £140.00
Perampanel 6 mg Fycompa 6mg tablets | 28 tablet [PoM] £140.00 DT = £140.00
Perampanel 8 mg Fycompa 8mg tablets | 28 tablet [PoM] £140.00 DT = £140.00
Perampanel 10 mg Fycompa 10mg tablets | 28 tablet [PoM] £140.00 DT = £140.00
Perampanel 12 mg Fycompa 12mg tablets | 28 tablet [PoM] £140.00 DT = £140.00

Phenytoin

02-Dec-2019

- **INDICATIONS AND DOSE**

Tonic-clonic seizures | Focal seizures
▸ BY MOUTH
▸ Child 1 month–11 years: Initially 1.5–2.5 mg/kg twice daily, then adjusted according to response to 2.5–5 mg/kg twice daily (max. per dose 7.5 mg/kg twice daily), dose also adjusted according to plasma-phenytoin concentration; maximum 300 mg per day
▸ Child 12–17 years: Initially 75–150 mg twice daily, then adjusted according to response to 150–200 mg twice daily (max. per dose 300 mg twice daily), dose also adjusted according to plasma-phenytoin concentration
▸ INITIALLY BY SLOW INTRAVENOUS INJECTION
▸ Neonate: Loading dose 18 mg/kg, dose to be administered over 20–30 minutes, then (by mouth) 2.5–5 mg/kg twice daily (max. per dose 7.5 mg/kg twice daily), adjusted according to response, dose also adjusted according to plasma-phenytoin concentration.

Prevention and treatment of seizures during or following neurosurgery or severe head injury
▸ BY MOUTH
▸ Child: Initially 2.5 mg/kg twice daily, then adjusted according to response to 4–8 mg/kg daily, dose also adjusted according to plasma-phenytoin concentration; maximum 300 mg per day

Status epilepticus | Acute symptomatic seizures associated with head trauma or neurosurgery
▸ INITIALLY BY SLOW INTRAVENOUS INJECTION, OR BY INTRAVENOUS INFUSION
▸ Neonate: Loading dose 20 mg/kg, then (by slow intravenous injection or by intravenous infusion) 2.5–5 mg/kg twice daily.
▸ Child 1 month–11 years: Loading dose 20 mg/kg, then (by slow intravenous injection or by intravenous infusion) 2.5–5 mg/kg twice daily
▸ Child 12–17 years: Loading dose 20 mg/kg, then (by intravenous infusion or by slow intravenous injection) up to 100 mg 3–4 times a day

DOSE EQUIVALENCE AND CONVERSION
▸ Preparations containing phenytoin sodium are **not** bioequivalent to those containing phenytoin base (such as *Epanutin Infatabs*® and *Epanutin*® suspension); 100 mg of phenytoin sodium is approximately equivalent in therapeutic effect to 92 mg phenytoin base. The dose is the same for all phenytoin products when initiating therapy. However, if switching between these products the difference in phenytoin content may be clinically significant. Care is needed when making changes between formulations and plasma-phenytoin concentration monitoring is recommended.

- **UNLICENSED USE**

▸ With oral use Licensed for use in children (age range not specified by manufacturer).
▸ With intravenous use Phenytoin doses in BNF publications may differ from those in product literature.

IMPORTANT SAFETY INFORMATION
NHS IMPROVEMENT PATIENT SAFETY ALERT: RISK OF DEATH AND SEVERE HARM FROM ERROR WITH INJECTABLE PHENYTOIN (NOVEMBER 2016)
Use of injectable phenytoin is error-prone throughout the prescribing, preparation, administration and monitoring processes; all relevant staff should be made aware of appropriate guidance on the safe use of injectable phenytoin to reduce the risk of error.

- **CONTRA-INDICATIONS**

GENERAL CONTRA-INDICATIONS Acute porphyrias p. 652
SPECIFIC CONTRA-INDICATIONS
▸ With intravenous use Second- and third-degree heart block · sino-atrial block · sinus bradycardia · Stokes-Adams syndrome

- **CAUTIONS**

GENERAL CAUTIONS Enteral feeding (interrupt feeding for 2 hours before and after dose; more frequent monitoring may be necessary)
SPECIFIC CAUTIONS
▸ With intravenous use Heart failure · hypotension · injection solutions alkaline (irritant to tissues) · respiratory depression · resuscitation facilities must be available
CAUTIONS, FURTHER INFORMATION Consider vitamin D supplementation in patients who are immobilised for long periods or who have inadequate sun exposure or dietary intake of calcium.
Intramuscular phenytoin should not be used (absorption is slow and erratic).

- **INTERACTIONS** → Appendix 1: antiepileptics
- **SIDE-EFFECTS**

GENERAL SIDE-EFFECTS Agranulocytosis · bone disorders · bone fracture · bone marrow disorders · cerebrovascular insufficiency · coarsening of the facial features · confusion · constipation · dizziness · drowsiness · Dupuytren's contracture · dysarthria · eosinophilia · fever · gingival hyperplasia (maintain good oral hygiene) · granulocytopenia · hair changes · headache · hepatic disorders · hypersensitivity · insomnia · joint disorders · leucopenia · lip swelling · lymphatic abnormalities · macrocytosis · megaloblastic anaemia · movement disorders · muscle twitching · nausea · neoplasms · nephritis tubulointerstitial · nervousness · nystagmus · paraesthesia · Peyronie's disease · polyarteritis nodosa · pseudolymphoma · sensory peripheral polyneuropathy · severe cutaneous adverse reactions (SCARs) · skin reactions · systemic lupus erythematosus (SLE) · taste altered · thrombocytopenia · tremor · vertigo · vomiting

SPECIFIC SIDE-EFFECTS

- With oral use Electrolyte imbalance · pneumonitis · vitamin D deficiency
- With parenteral use Arrhythmias · atrial conduction depression (more common if injection too rapid) · cardiac arrest · extravasation necrosis · hypotension · injection site necrosis · purple glove syndrome · respiratory arrest (more common if injection too rapid) · respiratory disorders · tonic seizure (more common if injection too rapid) · ventricular conduction depression (more common if injection too rapid) · ventricular fibrillation (more common if injection too rapid)

SIDE-EFFECTS, FURTHER INFORMATION **Rash** Discontinue; if mild re-introduce cautiously but discontinue immediately if recurrence.

Bradycardia and hypotension With intravenous use; reduce rate of administration if bradycardia or hypotension occurs.

Overdose Symptoms of phenytoin toxicity include nystagmus, diplopia, slurred speech, ataxia, confusion, and hyperglycaemia.

- **ALLERGY AND CROSS-SENSITIVITY** Cross-sensitivity reported with carbamazepine. Antiepileptic hypersensitivity syndrome associated with phenytoin. See under Epilepsy p. 203 for more information.
- **PREGNANCY** See also *Pregnancy* in Epilepsy p. 203.
  Monitoring Changes in plasma-protein binding make interpretation of plasma-phenytoin concentrations difficult—monitor unbound fraction.
  Doses should be adjusted on the basis of plasma-drug concentration monitoring.
- **BREAST FEEDING** Small amounts present in milk, but not known to be harmful.
- **HEPATIC IMPAIRMENT** Manufacturer advises caution (increased risk of accumulation and toxicity due to decreased protein binding in hepatic impairment, hypoalbuminaemia, or hyperbilirubinaemia).
  Dose adjustments ▸ With oral use Manufacturer advises consider dose reduction.
  ▸ With intravenous use Manufacturer advises consider maintenance dose reduction.
- **PRE-TREATMENT SCREENING** HLAB* 1502 allele in individuals of Han Chinese or Thai origin—avoid unless essential (increased risk of Stevens- Johnson syndrome).
- **MONITORING REQUIREMENTS**
  - Therapeutic plasma-phenytoin concentrations reduced in first 3 months of life because of reduced protein binding.
  - Trough plasma concentration for optimum response: neonate–3 months, 6–15 mg/litre (25–60 micromol/litre); child 3 months–18 years, 10–20 mg/litre (40–80 micromol/litre).
  - Manufacturer recommends blood counts (but evidence of practical value uncertain).
  - With intravenous use Monitor ECG and blood pressure.
- **DIRECTIONS FOR ADMINISTRATION** Manufacturer advises each injection or infusion should be preceded and followed by an injection of Sodium Chloride 0.9% through the same needle or catheter to avoid local venous irritation.
  - With intravenous use [EvGr] For *intravenous injection*, give into a large vein at a rate not exceeding 1 mg/kg/minute (max. 50 mg/minute). ⟨D⟩ Manufacturer advises for *intravenous infusion*, dilute to a concentration not exceeding 10 mg/mL with Sodium Chloride 0.9% and give into a large vein through an in-line filter (0.22–0.50 micron). [EvGr] Give at a rate not exceeding 1 mg/kg/minute (max. 50 mg/minute). ⟨D⟩ Complete administration within 1 hour of preparation.
- **PRESCRIBING AND DISPENSING INFORMATION**
  Switching between formulations Different formulations of oral preparations may vary in bioavailability. Patients being treated for epilepsy should be maintained on a specific manufacturer's product.
- **PATIENT AND CARER ADVICE**
  Blood or skin disorders Patients or their carers should be told how to recognise signs of blood or skin disorders, and advised to seek immediate medical attention if symptoms such as fever, rash, mouth ulcers, bruising, or bleeding develop. Leucopenia that is severe, progressive, or associated with clinical symptoms requires withdrawal (if necessary under cover of a suitable alternative).
  Medicines for Children leaflet: Phenytoin for preventing seizures www.medicinesforchildren.org.uk/phenytoin-preventing-seizures

---

- **MEDICINAL FORMS** There can be variation in the licensing of different medicines containing the same drug. Forms available from special-order manufacturers include: chewable tablet, oral suspension, oral solution

Tablet

CAUTIONARY AND ADVISORY LABELS 8

▸ Phenytoin (Non-proprietary)
Phenytoin sodium 100 mg Phenytoin sodium 100mg tablets | 28 tablet [PoM] £30.00 DT = £10.07

Solution for injection

EXCIPIENTS: May contain Alcohol, propylene glycol
ELECTROLYTES: May contain Sodium

▸ Phenytoin (Non-proprietary)
Phenytoin sodium 50 mg per 1 ml Phenytoin sodium 250mg/5ml solution for injection ampoules | 5 ampoule [PoM] £24.40 (Hospital only)

▸ Epanutin (Upjohn UK Ltd)
Phenytoin sodium 50 mg per 1 ml Epanutin Ready-Mixed Parenteral 250mg/5ml solution for injection ampoules | 10 ampoule [PoM] £48.79 (Hospital only)

Oral suspension

CAUTIONARY AND ADVISORY LABELS 8

▸ Epanutin (Upjohn UK Ltd)
Phenytoin 6 mg per 1 ml Epanutin 30mg/5ml oral suspension | 500 ml [PoM] £4.27 DT = £4.27

Chewable tablet

CAUTIONARY AND ADVISORY LABELS 8, 24

▸ Epanutin (Upjohn UK Ltd)
Phenytoin 50 mg Epanutin Infatabs 50mg chewable tablets | 200 tablet [PoM] £13.18 DT = £13.18

Capsule

CAUTIONARY AND ADVISORY LABELS 8

▸ Phenytoin (Non-proprietary)
Phenytoin sodium 25 mg Phenytoin sodium 25mg capsules | 28 capsule [PoM] £7.24 DT = £7.24
Phenytoin sodium 50 mg Phenytoin sodium 50mg capsules | 28 capsule [PoM] £7.07 DT = £7.07
Phenytoin sodium 100 mg Phenytoin sodium 100mg capsules | 84 capsule [PoM] £67.50 DT = £11.32
Phenytoin sodium 300 mg Phenytoin sodium 300mg capsules | 28 capsule [PoM] £9.11 DT = £9.11

Rufinamide

15-May-2019

● **INDICATIONS AND DOSE**

Adjunctive treatment of seizures in Lennox-Gastaut syndrome without valproate (initiated by a specialist)

▶ BY MOUTH

- Child 1–3 years: Initially 5 mg/kg twice daily, then increased in steps of up to 5 mg/kg twice daily (max. per dose 22.5 mg/kg twice daily), adjusted according to response, dose to be increased at intervals of not less than 3 days to the target dose (maximum dose), each dose should be given to the nearest 0.5 mL
- Child 4–17 years (body-weight up to 30 kg): Initially 100 mg twice daily, then increased in steps of 100 mg twice daily (max. per dose 500 mg twice daily), adjusted according to response, dose to be increased at intervals of not less than 3 days
- Child 4–17 years (body-weight 30–50 kg): Initially 200 mg twice daily, then increased in steps of 200 mg twice daily (max. per dose 900 mg twice daily), adjusted according to response, dose to be increased at intervals of not less than 2 days
- Child 4–17 years (body-weight 50.1–70 kg): Initially 200 mg twice daily, then increased in steps of 200 mg twice daily (max. per dose 1.2 g twice daily), adjusted according to response, dose to be increased at intervals of not less than 2 days
- Child 4–17 years (body-weight 70.1 kg and above): Initially 200 mg twice daily, then increased in steps of 200 mg twice daily (max. per dose 1.6 g twice daily), adjusted according to response, dose to be increased at intervals of not less than 2 days

Adjunctive treatment of seizures in Lennox-Gastaut syndrome with valproate (initiated by a specialist)

▶ BY MOUTH

- Child 1–3 years: Initially 5 mg/kg twice daily, then increased in steps of up to 5 mg/kg twice daily (max. per dose 15 mg/kg twice daily), adjusted according to response, dose to be increased at intervals of not less than 3 days to the target dose (maximum dose), each dose should be given to the nearest 0.5 mL
- Child 4–17 years (body-weight up to 30 kg): Initially 100 mg twice daily, then increased in steps of 100 mg twice daily (max. per dose 300 mg twice daily), adjusted according to response, dose to be increased at intervals of not less than 2 days
- Child 4–17 years (body-weight 30–50 kg): Initially 200 mg twice daily, then increased in steps of 200 mg twice daily (max. per dose 600 mg twice daily), adjusted according to response, dose to be increased at intervals of not less than 2 days
- Child 4–17 years (body-weight 50.1–70 kg): Initially 200 mg twice daily, then increased in steps of 200 mg twice daily (max. per dose 800 mg twice daily), adjusted according to response, dose to be increased at intervals of not less than 2 days
- Child 4–17 years (body-weight 70.1 kg and above): Initially 200 mg twice daily, then increased in steps of 200 mg twice daily (max. per dose 1.1 g twice daily), adjusted according to response, dose to be increased at intervals of not less than 2 days

● **CAUTIONS** Patients at risk of further shortening of QTc interval

● **INTERACTIONS** → Appendix 1: antiepileptics

● **SIDE-EFFECTS**

▶ **Common or very common** Anxiety · appetite decreased · back pain · constipation · diarrhoea · dizziness · drowsiness · eating disorder · epistaxis · fatigue · gait abnormal · gastrointestinal discomfort · headache · increased risk of infection · insomnia · movement disorders · nausea · nystagmus · oligomenorrhoea · seizures · skin reactions · tremor · vertigo · vision disorders · vomiting · weight decreased

▶ **Uncommon** Hypersensitivity

● **ALLERGY AND CROSS-SENSITIVITY** Antiepileptic hypersensitivity syndrome associated with rufinamide. See under Epilepsy p. 203 for more information.

● **PREGNANCY** Manufacturer advises avoid unless essential—toxicity in *animal* studies. See also *Pregnancy* in Epilepsy p. 203.

● **BREAST FEEDING** Manufacturer advises avoid—no information available.

● **HEPATIC IMPAIRMENT** Manufacturer advises caution in mild to moderate impairment; avoid in severe impairment (no information available).

Dose adjustments Manufacturer advises cautious dose titration in mild to moderate impairment.

● **DIRECTIONS FOR ADMINISTRATION** Manufacturer advises tablets may be crushed and given in half a glass of water.

● **PRESCRIBING AND DISPENSING INFORMATION**

Switching between formulations Care should be taken when switching between oral formulations. The need for continued supply of a particular manufacturer's product should be based on clinical judgement and consultation with the patient or their carer, taking into account factors such as seizure frequency and treatment history.

Patients may need to be maintained on a specific manufacturer's branded or generic rufinamide product.

● **PATIENT AND CARER ADVICE** Counselling on antiepileptic hypersensitivity syndrome is advised.

Medicines for Children leaflet: Rufinamide for preventing seizures www.medicinesforchildren.org.uk/rufinamide-preventing-seizures

Driving and skilled tasks Manufacturer advises patients and carers should be cautioned on the effects on driving and performance of skilled tasks—increased risk of dizziness, somnolence and blurred vision.

● **NATIONAL FUNDING/ACCESS DECISIONS**

Scottish Medicines Consortium (SMC) decisions

SMC No. 416/07

The *Scottish Medicines Consortium* has advised (November 2008) that rufinamide (*Inovelon*®) is accepted for restricted use within NHS Scotland as adjunctive therapy in the treatment of seizures associated with Lennox-Gastaut syndrome in patients 4 years and above. It is restricted for use when alternative traditional antiepileptic drugs are unsatisfactory.

SMC No. 795/12

The *Scottish Medicines Consortium* has advised (July 2012) that rufinamide 40 mg/mL oral suspension (*Inovelon*®) is accepted for restricted use within NHS Scotland as adjunctive therapy in the treatment of seizures associated with Lennox-Gastaut syndrome in patients 4 years and above. It is restricted for use when alternative traditional antiepileptic drugs are unsatisfactory.

SMC No. SMC2146

The *Scottish Medicines Consortium* has advised (April 2019) that rufinamide (*Inovelon*®) is accepted for restricted use within NHS Scotland as adjunctive therapy in the treatment of seizures associated with Lennox-Gastaut syndrome in patients aged 1 year up to 4 years. It is restricted for use when alternative traditional antiepileptic drugs are unsatisfactory.

All Wales Medicines Strategy Group (AWMSG) decisions

AWMSG No. 991

The *All Wales Medicines Strategy Group* has advised (June 2019) that rufinamide 40 mg/mL oral suspension (*Inovelon*®) is recommended as an option for restricted use within NHS Wales as adjunctive therapy in the treatment of seizures associated with Lennox-Gastaut syndrome in patients aged one year and older where other adjunctive treatments have proved sub-optimal or have not been tolerated. It is not recommended for use within NHS Wales outside of this subpopulation.

● **MEDICINAL FORMS** There can be variation in the licensing of different medicines containing the same drug.

Oral suspension

CAUTIONARY AND ADVISORY LABELS 8, 21

EXCIPIENTS: May contain Propylene glycol

▸ Inovelon (Eisai Ltd)

Rufinamide 40 mg per 1 ml Inovelon 40mg/ml oral suspension sugar-free | 460 ml PoM £94.71 DT = £94.71

Tablet

CAUTIONARY AND ADVISORY LABELS 8, 21

▸ Inovelon (Eisai Ltd)

Rufinamide 100 mg Inovelon 100mg tablets | 10 tablet PoM £5.15 DT = £5.15

Rufinamide 200 mg Inovelon 200mg tablets | 60 tablet PoM £61.77 DT = £61.77

Rufinamide 400 mg Inovelon 400mg tablets | 60 tablet PoM £102.96 DT = £102.96

Sodium valproate

14-Feb-2020

● **INDICATIONS AND DOSE**

All forms of epilepsy

▸ BY MOUTH USING IMMEDIATE-RELEASE MEDICINES

▸ Neonate: Initially 20 mg/kg once daily; maintenance 10 mg/kg twice daily.

▸ Child 1 month–11 years: Initially 10–15 mg/kg daily in 1–2 divided doses (max. per dose 600 mg); maintenance 25–30 mg/kg daily in 2 divided doses, doses up to 60 mg/kg daily in 2 divided doses may be used in infantile spasms; monitor clinical chemistry and haematological parameters if dose exceeds 40 mg/kg daily

▸ Child 12–17 years: Initially 600 mg daily in 1–2 divided doses, increased in steps of 150–300 mg every 3 days; maintenance 1–2 g daily in 2 divided doses; maximum 2.5 g per day

▸ BY RECTUM

▸ Neonate: Initially 20 mg/kg once daily; maintenance 10 mg/kg twice daily.

▸ Child 1 month–11 years: Initially 10–15 mg/kg daily in 1–2 divided doses (max. per dose 600 mg); maintenance 25–30 mg/kg daily in 2 divided doses, doses up to 60 mg/kg daily in 2 divided doses may be used in infantile spasms; monitor clinical chemistry and haematological parameters if dose exceeds 40 mg/kg daily

▸ Child 12–17 years: Initially 600 mg daily in 1–2 divided doses, increased in steps of 150–300 mg every 3 days; maintenance 1–2 g daily in 2 divided doses; maximum 2.5 g per day

Initiation of valproate treatment

▸ INITIALLY BY INTRAVENOUS INJECTION

▸ Neonate: 10 mg/kg twice daily.

▸ Child 1 month–11 years: Initially 10 mg/kg, then (by intravenous infusion or by intravenous injection) increased to 20–40 mg/kg daily in 2–4 divided doses, alternatively (by continuous intravenous infusion) increased to 20–40 mg/kg daily, monitor clinical chemistry and haematological parameters if dose exceeds 40 mg/kg daily

▸ Child 12–17 years: Initially 10 mg/kg, followed by (by intravenous infusion or by intravenous injection) up to 2.5 g daily in 2–4 divided doses, alternatively (by continuous intravenous infusion) up to 2.5 g daily; (by intravenous injection or by intravenous infusion or by continuous intravenous infusion) usual dose 1–2 g daily, alternatively (by intravenous injection or by intravenous infusion or by continuous intravenous infusion) usual dose 20–30 mg/kg daily, intravenous injection to be administered over 3–5 minutes

Continuation of valproate treatment

▸ BY INTRAVENOUS INJECTION, OR BY INTRAVENOUS INFUSION, OR BY CONTINUOUS INTRAVENOUS INFUSION

▸ Child: If switching from oral therapy to intravenous therapy give the same dose as current oral daily dose, give over 3–5 minutes by intravenous injection *or* in 2–4 divided doses by intravenous infusion

EPILIM CHRONOSPHERE ®

All forms of epilepsy

▸ BY MOUTH

▸ Child: Total daily dose to be given in 1–2 divided doses (consult product literature)

EPILIM CHRONO ®

All forms of epilepsy

▸ BY MOUTH

▸ Child (body-weight 20 kg and above): Total daily dose to be given in 1–2 divided doses (consult product literature)

EPISENTA ® CAPSULES

All forms of epilepsy

▸ BY MOUTH

▸ Child: Total daily dose to be given in 1–2 divided doses (consult product literature)

EPISENTA ® GRANULES

All forms of epilepsy

▸ BY MOUTH

▸ Child: Total daily dose to be given in 1–2 divided doses (consult product literature)

EPIVAL ®

All forms of epilepsy

▸ BY MOUTH

▸ Child: Total daily dose to be given in 1–2 divided doses (consult product literature)

IMPORTANT SAFETY INFORMATION

MHRA/CHM ADVICE: VALPROATE MEDICINES: CONTRA-INDICATED IN WOMEN AND GIRLS OF CHILDBEARING POTENTIAL UNLESS CONDITIONS OF PREGNANCY PREVENTION PROGRAMME ARE MET (APRIL 2018)

Valproate is highly teratogenic and evidence supports that use in pregnancy leads to neurodevelopmental disorders (approx. 30–40% risk) and congenital malformations (approx. 10% risk).

Valproate must not be used in women and girls of childbearing potential unless the conditions of the Pregnancy Prevention Programme are met (see *Conception and contraception*) and only if other treatments are ineffective or not tolerated, as judged by an experienced specialist.

Use of valproate in pregnancy is contra-indicated for migraine prophylaxis [unlicensed] and bipolar disorder; it must only be considered for epilepsy if there is no suitable alternative treatment (see *Pregnancy*).

Women and girls (and their carers) must be fully informed of the risks and the need to avoid exposure to valproate medicines in pregnancy; supporting materials have been provided to use in the implementation of the Pregnancy Prevention Programme (see *Prescribing and dispensing Information*). The MHRA advises that:

- GPs must recall all women and girls who may be of childbearing potential, provide the Patient Guide, check they have been reviewed by a specialist in the last year and are on highly effective contraception;

- Specialists must book in review appointments at least annually with women and girls under the Pregnancy Prevention Programme, re-evaluate treatment as necessary, explain clearly the conditions as outlined in the supporting materials and complete and sign the Risk Acknowledgement Form—copies of the form must be given to the patient or carer and sent to their GP;
- Pharmacists must ensure valproate medicines are dispensed in whole packs whenever possible—all packs dispensed to women and girls of childbearing potential should have a warning label either on the carton or via a sticker. They must also discuss risks in pregnancy with female patients each time valproate medicines are dispensed, ensure they have the Patient Guide and have seen their GP or specialist to discuss their treatment and the need for contraception.

MHRA/CHM ADVICE: VALPROATE MEDICINES: ARE YOU ACTING IN COMPLIANCE WITH THE PREGNANCY PREVENTION MEASURES? (DECEMBER 2018)

The MHRA advises that all healthcare professionals must continue to identify and review all female patients on valproate, including when used outside licensed indications (off-label use) and provide them with the patient information materials every time they attend appointments or receive their medicines.

Guidance for psychiatrists on the withdrawal of, and alternatives to, valproate in women of childbearing potential who have a psychiatric illness is available from the Royal College of Psychiatrists.

MHRA/CHM ADVICE: VALPROATE MEDICINES AND SERIOUS HARMS IN PREGNANCY: NEW ANNUAL RISK ACKNOWLEDGEMENT FORM AND CLINICAL GUIDANCE FROM PROFESSIONAL BODIES TO SUPPORT COMPLIANCE WITH THE PREGNANCY PREVENTION PROGRAMME (APRIL 2019)

The Annual Risk Acknowledgement Form has been updated and should be used for all future reviews of female patients on valproate. Specialists should comply with guidance given on the form if they consider the patient is not at risk of pregnancy, including the need for review in case her risk status changes.

Guidance has been published to support healthcare professionals with the use of valproate. These include a summary by NICE of their guidance and safety advice, pan-college guidance by national healthcare bodies, and paediatric guidance by the British Paediatric Neurology Association and the Royal College of Paediatrics and Child Health.

MHRA/CHM ADVICE (UPDATED JANUARY 2020): VALPROATE PREGNANCY PREVENTION PROGRAMME

The Guide for Healthcare Professionals has been updated and should be used for all future reviews of female patients on valproate medicines, in conjunction with other supporting materials (see *Prescribing and dispensing Information*).

- **CONTRA-INDICATIONS** Acute porphyrias p. 652 · known or suspected mitochondrial disorders (higher rate of acute liver failure and liver-related deaths) · personal or family history of severe hepatic dysfunction · urea cycle disorders (risk of hyperammonaemia)
- **CAUTIONS** Systemic lupus erythematosus

CAUTIONS, FURTHER INFORMATION Consider vitamin D supplementation in patients that are immobilised for long periods or who have inadequate sun exposure or dietary intake of calcium.

▸ Liver toxicity Liver dysfunction (including fatal hepatic failure) has occurred in association with valproate (especially in children under 3 years and in those with metabolic or degenerative disorders, organic brain disease or severe seizure disorders associated with mental retardation) usually in first 6 months and usually involving multiple antiepileptic therapy. Raised liver enzymes during valproate treatment are usually transient but patients should be reassessed clinically and liver function (including prothrombin time) monitored until return to normal—discontinue if abnormally prolonged prothrombin time (particularly in association with other relevant abnormalities).

- **INTERACTIONS** → Appendix 1: antiepileptics
- **SIDE-EFFECTS**

GENERAL SIDE-EFFECTS

▸ **Common or very common** Abdominal pain · agitation · alopecia (regrowth may be curly) · anaemia · behaviour abnormal · concentration impaired · confusion · deafness · diarrhoea · drowsiness · haemorrhage · hallucination · headache · hepatic disorders · hypersensitivity · hyponatraemia · memory loss · menstrual cycle irregularities · movement disorders · nail disorder · nausea · nystagmus · oral disorders · seizures · stupor · thrombocytopenia · tremor · urinary disorders · vomiting · weight increased

▸ **Uncommon** Androgenetic alopecia · angioedema · bone disorders · bone fracture · bone marrow disorders · coma · encephalopathy · hair changes · hypothermia · leucopenia · pancreatitis · paraesthesia · parkinsonism · peripheral oedema · pleural effusion · renal failure · SIADH · skin reactions · vasculitis · virilism

▸ **Rare or very rare** Agranulocytosis · cerebral atrophy · cognitive disorder · dementia · diplopia · gynaecomastia · hyperammonaemia · hypothyroidism · infertility male · learning disability · myelodysplastic syndrome · nephritis tubulointerstitial · polycystic ovaries · red blood cell abnormalities · rhabdomyolysis · severe cutaneous adverse reactions (SCARs) · systemic lupus erythematosus (SLE) · urine abnormalities

▸ **Frequency not known** Alertness increased

SPECIFIC SIDE-EFFECTS

▸ **Common or very common**

▸ With intravenous use Dizziness

SIDE-EFFECTS, FURTHER INFORMATION **Hepatic dysfunction** Withdraw treatment immediately if persistent vomiting and abdominal pain, anorexia, jaundice, oedema, malaise, drowsiness, or loss of seizure control.

Pancreatitis Discontinue treatment if symptoms of pancreatitis develop.

- **CONCEPTION AND CONTRACEPTION** The MHRA advises that all women and girls of childbearing potential being treated with valproate medicines must be supported on a Pregnancy Prevention Programme—pregnancy should be excluded before treatment initiation and highly effective contraception must be used during treatment.
- **PREGNANCY** For *migraine prophylaxis* [unlicensed] and *bipolar disorder*, the MHRA advises that valproate must not be used. For *epilepsy*, the MHRA advises valproate must not be used unless there is no suitable alternative treatment; in such cases, access to counselling about the risks should be provided (see Healthcare Professional Guide for more information) and a Risk Acknowledgement Form signed by both specialist and patient. If valproate is to be used during pregnancy, the lowest effective dose should be prescribed in divided doses or as modified-release tablets to avoid peaks in plasma-valproate concentrations; doses greater than 1 g daily are associated with an increased risk of teratogenicity. Neonatal bleeding (related to hypofibrinaemia) reported. Neonatal hepatotoxicity also reported. See also *Pregnancy* in Epilepsy p. 203.

Monitoring Specialist prenatal monitoring should be instigated when valproate has been taken in pregnancy.

The dose should be monitored carefully during pregnancy and after birth, and adjustments made on a clinical basis.

- **BREAST FEEDING** Present in milk—risk of haematological disorders in breast-fed newborns and infants.
- **HEPATIC IMPAIRMENT** Manufacturer advises avoid.
- **RENAL IMPAIRMENT**

Dose adjustments Reduce dose.

- **MONITORING REQUIREMENTS**
  - Plasma-valproate concentrations are not a useful index of efficacy, therefore routine monitoring is unhelpful.
  - Monitor liver function before therapy and during first 6 months especially in patients most at risk.
  - Measure full blood count and ensure no undue potential for bleeding before starting and before surgery.
- **EFFECT ON LABORATORY TESTS** False-positive urine tests for ketones.
- **TREATMENT CESSATION** [EvGr] Avoid abrupt withdrawal; if treatment with valproate is stopped, reduce the dose gradually over at least 4 weeks. ⟨A⟩
- **DIRECTIONS FOR ADMINISTRATION**
  - With intravenous use Manufacturer advises for *intravenous injection*, give over 3–5 minutes. For *intravenous infusion*, dilute with Glucose 5% *or* Sodium Chloride 0.9%. Reconstitute *Epilim*® with solvent provided then dilute with infusion fluid if required. Displacement value may be significant, consult local guidelines.
  - With rectal use For *rectal administration*, sodium valproate oral solution may be given rectally and retained for 15 minutes (may require dilution with water to prevent rapid expulsion).

EPIVAL® Tablets may be halved but not crushed or chewed.

EPISENTA® CAPSULES Contents of capsule may be mixed with cold soft food or drink and swallowed immediately without chewing.

EPILIM® SYRUP May be diluted, preferably in Syrup BP; use within 14 days.

EPISENTA® GRANULES Granules may be mixed with cold soft food or drink and swallowed immediately without chewing.

EPILIM CHRONOSPHERE® Granules may be mixed with soft food or drink that is cold or at room temperature, and swallowed immediately without chewing.

- **PRESCRIBING AND DISPENSING INFORMATION** The Pregnancy Prevention Programme is supported by the following materials provided by the manufacturer: *Patient Guide, Guide for Healthcare Professionals, Risk Acknowledgement Form*, and for pharmacists, *Patient Cards* and *Stickers with warning symbols*; the MHRA has also produced a patient information sheet providing advice for women and girls taking valproate medicines.

The Royal Pharmaceutical Society has also produced a safe supply algorithm, available at: www.rpharms.com/safesupplyvalproate

Switching between formulations Care should be taken when switching between oral formulations in the treatment of epilepsy. The need for continued supply of a particular manufacturer's product should be based on clinical judgement and consultation with the patient or their carer, taking into account factors such as seizure frequency and treatment history.

Patients being treated for epilepsy may need to be maintained on a specific manufacturer's branded or generic oral sodium valproate product.

EPILIM CHRONOSPHERE® Prescribe dose to the nearest whole 50-mg sachet.

- **PATIENT AND CARER ADVICE**

Valproate use by women and girls The MHRA advises women and girls should **not** stop taking valproate without first discussing it with their doctor.

Blood or hepatic disorders Patients or their carers should be told how to recognise signs and symptoms of blood or liver disorders and advised to seek immediate medical attention if symptoms develop.

Pancreatitis Patients or their carers should be told how to recognise signs and symptoms of pancreatitis and advised to seek immediate medical attention if symptoms such as abdominal pain, nausea, or vomiting develop.

Pregnancy Prevention Programme Pharmacists must ensure that female patients have a patient card—see also *Important safety information*.

Medicines for Children leaflet: Sodium valproate for preventing seizures www.medicinesforchildren.org.uk/sodium-valproate-preventing-seizures

Medicines for Children leaflet: Sodium valproate and pregnancy - information for girls and young women www.medicinesforchildren.org.uk/sodium-valproate-and-pregnancy-information-girls-and-young-women

Medicines for Children leaflet: Sodium valproate and pregnancy - information for parents and carers www.medicinesforchildren.org.uk/sodium-valproate-and-pregnancy-information-parents-and-carers

EPISENTA® CAPSULES Patients and carers should be counselled on the administration of capsules.

EPISENTA® GRANULES, EPILIM CHRONOSPHERE® Patients and carers should be counselled on the administration of granules.

- **MEDICINAL FORMS** There can be variation in the licensing of different medicines containing the same drug. Forms available from special-order manufacturers include: oral suspension, oral solution, suppository

Modified-release tablet

CAUTIONARY AND ADVISORY LABELS 8, 10, 21, 25

- Epilim Chrono (Sanofi) ▼

Sodium valproate 200 mg Epilim Chrono 200 tablets | 30 tablet [PoM] £3.50 | 100 tablet [PoM] £11.65 DT = £11.65

Sodium valproate 300 mg Epilim Chrono 300 tablets | 30 tablet [PoM] £5.24 | 100 tablet [PoM] £17.47 DT = £17.47

Sodium valproate 500 mg Epilim Chrono 500 tablets | 30 tablet [PoM] £8.73 | 100 tablet [PoM] £29.10 DT = £29.10

- Epival CR (Healthcare Pharma Ltd) ▼

Sodium valproate 300 mg Epival CR 300mg tablets | 30 tablet [PoM] £5.24 | 100 tablet [PoM] £17.47 DT = £17.47

Sodium valproate 500 mg Epival CR 500mg tablets | 30 tablet [PoM] £8.73 | 100 tablet [PoM] £29.10 DT = £29.10

Gastro-resistant tablet

CAUTIONARY AND ADVISORY LABELS 5, 8, 10, 25

- Sodium valproate (non-proprietary) ▼

Sodium valproate 200 mg Sodium valproate 200mg gastro-resistant tablets | 30 tablet [PoM] £2.77 | 100 tablet [PoM] £9.45-£14.51 DT = £9.45

Sodium valproate 500 mg Sodium valproate 500mg gastro-resistant tablets | 30 tablet [PoM] £6.93 | 100 tablet [PoM] £22.76-£34.95 DT = £22.76

- Epilim (Sanofi) ▼

Sodium valproate 200 mg Epilim 200 gastro-resistant tablets | 30 tablet [PoM] £2.31 | 100 tablet [PoM] £7.70 DT = £9.45

Sodium valproate 500 mg Epilim 500 gastro-resistant tablets | 30 tablet [PoM] £5.78 | 100 tablet [PoM] £19.25 DT = £22.76

Tablet

CAUTIONARY AND ADVISORY LABELS 8, 10, 21

- Epilim (Sanofi) ▼

Sodium valproate 100 mg Epilim 100mg crushable tablets | 30 tablet [PoM] £1.68 | 100 tablet [PoM] £5.60 DT = £5.60

Powder and solvent for solution for injection

- Sodium valproate (non-proprietary) ▼

Sodium valproate 400 mg Sodium valproate 400mg powder and solvent for solution for injection vials | 4 vial [PoM] £49.00

- Epilim (Sanofi) ▼

Sodium valproate 400 mg Epilim Intravenous 400mg powder and solvent for solution for injection vials | 1 vial [PoM] £13.32 DT = £13.32

Solution for injection

- Sodium valproate (non-proprietary) ▼

Sodium valproate 100 mg per 1 ml Sodium valproate 400mg/4ml solution for injection ampoules | 5 ampoule [PoM] £57.90 DT = £57.90

▸ Episenta (Desitin Pharma Ltd) ▼
Sodium valproate 100 mg per 1 ml Episenta 300mg/3ml solution for injection ampoules | 5 ampoule PoM £35.00 DT = £35.00

Modified-release capsule

CAUTIONARY AND ADVISORY LABELS 8, 10, 21, 25

▸ Episenta (Desitin Pharma Ltd) ▼
Sodium valproate 150 mg Episenta 150mg modified-release capsules | 100 capsule PoM £7.00 DT = £7.00
Sodium valproate 300 mg Episenta 300mg modified-release capsules | 100 capsule PoM £13.00 DT = £13.00

Oral solution

CAUTIONARY AND ADVISORY LABELS 8, 10, 21

▸ Sodium valproate (non-proprietary) ▼
Sodium valproate 40 mg per 1 ml Sodium valproate 200mg/5ml oral solution sugar-free | 300 ml PoM £14.66 DT = £9.52

▸ Epilim (Sanofi) ▼
Sodium valproate 40 mg per 1 ml Epilim 200mg/5ml liquid sugar-free | 300 ml PoM £7.78 DT = £9.52
Epilim 200mg/5ml syrup | 300 ml PoM £9.33 DT = £9.33

Modified-release granules

CAUTIONARY AND ADVISORY LABELS 8, 10, 21, 25

▸ Epilim Chronosphere MR (Sanofi) ▼
Sodium valproate 50 mg Epilim Chronosphere MR 50mg granules sachets sugar-free | 30 sachet PoM £30.00 DT = £30.00
Sodium valproate 100 mg Epilim Chronosphere MR 100mg granules sachets sugar-free | 30 sachet PoM £30.00 DT = £30.00
Sodium valproate 250 mg Epilim Chronosphere MR 250mg granules sachets sugar-free | 30 sachet PoM £30.00 DT = £30.00
Sodium valproate 500 mg Epilim Chronosphere MR 500mg granules sachets sugar-free | 30 sachet PoM £30.00 DT = £30.00
Sodium valproate 750 mg Epilim Chronosphere MR 750mg granules sachets sugar-free | 30 sachet PoM £30.00 DT = £30.00
Sodium valproate 1 gram Epilim Chronosphere MR 1000mg granules sachets sugar-free | 30 sachet PoM £30.00 DT = £30.00

▸ Episenta (Desitin Pharma Ltd) ▼
Sodium valproate 500 mg Episenta 500mg modified-release granules sachets sugar-free | 100 sachet PoM £21.00 DT = £21.00
Sodium valproate 1 gram Episenta 1000mg modified-release granules sachets sugar-free | 100 sachet PoM £41.00 DT = £41.00

Stiripentol

10-Mar-2020

● **INDICATIONS AND DOSE**

Adjunctive therapy of refractory generalised tonic-clonic seizures in patients with severe myoclonic epilepsy in infancy (Dravet syndrome) in combination with clobazam and valproate (under expert supervision)

▸ BY MOUTH

▸ Child 3–5 years: Initially 20 mg/kg daily in 2–3 divided doses for 1 week, then increased to 30 mg/kg daily in 2–3 divided doses for 1 week, then increased to 50 mg/kg daily in 2–3 divided doses
▸ Child 6–11 years: Initially 20 mg/kg daily in 2–3 divided doses for 1 week, then increased in steps of 10 mg/kg daily in 2–3 divided doses, dose to be increased at intervals of 1 week to 50 mg/kg daily in 2–3 divided doses
▸ Child 12–17 years: Initially 20 mg/kg daily in 2–3 divided doses for 1 week, then increased to 30 mg/kg daily in 2–3 divided doses for 1 week, then increased in steps of 5 mg/kg daily in 2–3 divided doses, dose to be increased at intervals of 1 week, until the optimum dose is reached based on clinical judgement; maximum 50 mg/kg per day

DOSE EQUIVALENCE AND CONVERSION

▸ Stiripentol capsules and oral powder sachets are **not** bioequivalent. If a switch of formulation is required, manufacturer advises this is done under clinical supervision in case of intolerance.

● **CONTRA-INDICATIONS** History of psychosis in the form of episodes of delirium

● **INTERACTIONS** → Appendix 1: antiepileptics

● **SIDE-EFFECTS**

▸ **Common or very common** Agitation · appetite decreased · behaviour abnormal · drowsiness · irritability · movement disorders · muscle tone decreased · nausea · neutropenia · sleep disorders · vomiting · weight decreased
▸ **Uncommon** Diplopia · fatigue · photosensitivity reaction · skin reactions
▸ **Rare or very rare** Thrombocytopenia

● **ALLERGY AND CROSS-SENSITIVITY** Antiepileptic hypersensitivity syndrome theoretically associated with stiripentol. See under Epilepsy p. 203 for more information.

● **PREGNANCY** See also *Pregnancy* in Epilepsy p. 203.
Monitoring The dose should be monitored carefully during pregnancy and after birth, and adjustments made on a clinical basis.

● **BREAST FEEDING** Present in milk in *animal* studies.

● **HEPATIC IMPAIRMENT** Manufacturer advises avoid (no information available).

● **RENAL IMPAIRMENT** Avoid—no information available.

● **MONITORING REQUIREMENTS**

▸ Perform full blood count and liver function tests prior to initiating treatment and every 6 months thereafter.
▸ Manufacturer advises monitor growth.

● **PATIENT AND CARER ADVICE**
Medicines for Children leaflet: Stiripentol for preventing seizures www.medicinesforchildren.org.uk/stiripentol-preventing-seizures

● **NATIONAL FUNDING/ACCESS DECISIONS**

Scottish Medicines Consortium (SMC) decisions
The *Scottish Medicines Consortium* has advised (September 2017) that stiripentol (*Diacomit*®) is accepted for use within NHS Scotland in conjunction with clobazam and valproate as adjunctive therapy of refractory generalised tonic-clonic seizures in patients with severe myoclonic epilepsy in infancy whose seizures are not adequately controlled with clobazam and valproate.

All Wales Medicines Strategy Group (AWMSG) decisions
The *All Wales Medicines Strategy Group* has advised (November 2017) that stiripentol (*Diacomit*®) is recommended for use within NHS Wales for use in conjunction with clobazam and valproate as adjunctive therapy of refractory generalized tonic-clonic seizures in patients with severe myoclonic epilepsy in infancy (SMEI, Dravet syndrome) whose seizures are not adequately controlled with clobazam and valproate.

● **MEDICINAL FORMS** There can be variation in the licensing of different medicines containing the same drug.

Powder

CAUTIONARY AND ADVISORY LABELS 1, 8, 13, 21
EXCIPIENTS: May contain Aspartame

▸ Diacomit (Alan Pharmaceuticals)
Stiripentol 250 mg Diacomit 250mg oral powder sachets | 60 sachet PoM £284.00 DT = £284.00
Stiripentol 500 mg Diacomit 500mg oral powder sachets | 60 sachet PoM £493.00 DT = £493.00

Capsule

CAUTIONARY AND ADVISORY LABELS 1, 8, 21

▸ Diacomit (Alan Pharmaceuticals)
Stiripentol 250 mg Diacomit 250mg capsules | 60 capsule PoM £284.00 DT = £284.00
Stiripentol 500 mg Diacomit 500mg capsules | 60 capsule PoM £493.00 DT = £493.00

Tiagabine

● **INDICATIONS AND DOSE**

Adjunctive treatment for focal seizures with or without secondary generalisation that are not satisfactorily controlled by other antiepileptics (with enzyme-inducing drugs)

▶ BY MOUTH

▸ Child 12–17 years: Initially 5–10 mg daily in 1–2 divided doses, then increased in steps of 5–10 mg/24 hours every week; maintenance 30–45 mg daily in 2–3 divided doses

Adjunctive treatment for focal seizures with or without secondary generalisation that are not satisfactorily controlled by other antiepileptics (without enzyme-inducing drugs)

▶ BY MOUTH

▸ Child 12–17 years: Initially 5–10 mg daily in 1–2 divided doses, then increased in steps of 5–10 mg/24 hours every week; maintenance 15–30 mg daily in 2–3 divided doses

● **CAUTIONS** Avoid in Acute porphyrias p. 652

CAUTIONS, FURTHER INFORMATION Tiagabine should be avoided in absence, myoclonic, tonic and atonic seizures due to risk of seizure exacerbation.

● **INTERACTIONS** → Appendix 1: antiepileptics

● **SIDE-EFFECTS**

▶ **Common or very common** Abdominal pain · behaviour abnormal · concentration impaired · depression · diarrhoea · dizziness · emotional lability · fatigue · gait abnormal · insomnia · nausea · nervousness · speech disorder · tremor · vision disorders · vomiting

▶ **Uncommon** Drowsiness · psychosis · skin reactions

▶ **Rare or very rare** Delusions · hallucination

● **PREGNANCY** See also *Pregnancy* in Epilepsy p. 203.

Monitoring The dose should be monitored carefully during pregnancy and after birth, and adjustments made on a clinical basis.

● **HEPATIC IMPAIRMENT** Manufacturer advises caution in mild to moderate impairment (risk of increased exposure); avoid in severe impairment.

Dose adjustments Manufacturer advises dose reduction and/or longer dose interval with careful titration in mild to moderate impairment.

● **PATIENT AND CARER ADVICE**

Medicines for Children leaflet: Tiagibine for preventing seizures www.medicinesforchildren.org.uk/tiagabine-preventing-seizures

Driving and skilled tasks May impair performance of skilled tasks (e.g. driving).

● **MEDICINAL FORMS** There can be variation in the licensing of different medicines containing the same drug. Forms available from special-order manufacturers include: oral suspension

Tablet

CAUTIONARY AND ADVISORY LABELS 21

▸ Gabitril (Teva UK Ltd)

Tiagabine (as Tiagabine hydrochloride monohydrate)
5 mg Gabitril 5mg tablets | 100 tablet [PoM] £52.04 DT = £52.04

Tiagabine (as Tiagabine hydrochloride monohydrate)
10 mg Gabitril 10mg tablets | 100 tablet [PoM] £104.09 DT = £104.09

Tiagabine (as Tiagabine hydrochloride monohydrate)
15 mg Gabitril 15mg tablets | 100 tablet [PoM] £156.13 DT = £156.13

Topiramate

10-Mar-2020

● **INDICATIONS AND DOSE**

Monotherapy of generalised tonic-clonic seizures or focal seizures with or without secondary generalisation

▶ BY MOUTH

▸ Child 6–17 years: Initially 0.5–1 mg/kg once daily (max. per dose 25 mg) for 1 week, dose to be taken at night, then increased in steps of 250–500 micrograms/kg twice daily, dose to be increased by a maximum of 25 mg twice daily at intervals of 1–2 weeks; usual dose 50 mg twice daily (max. per dose 7.5 mg/kg twice daily), if child cannot tolerate titration regimens recommended above then smaller steps or longer interval between steps may be used; maximum 500 mg per day

Adjunctive treatment of generalised tonic-clonic seizures or focal seizures with or without secondary generalisation | Adjunctive treatment for seizures associated with Lennox-Gastaut syndrome

▶ BY MOUTH

▸ Child 2–17 years: Initially 1–3 mg/kg once daily (max. per dose 25 mg) for 1 week, dose to be taken at night, then increased in steps of 0.5–1.5 mg/kg twice daily, dose to be increased by a maximum of 25 mg twice daily at intervals of 1–2 weeks; usual dose 2.5–4.5 mg/kg twice daily (max. per dose 7.5 mg/kg twice daily), if child cannot tolerate recommended titration regimen then smaller steps or longer interval between steps may be used; maximum 400 mg per day

Migraine prophylaxis

▶ BY MOUTH

▸ Child 16–17 years: Initially 25 mg once daily for 1 week, dose to be taken at night, then increased in steps of 25 mg every week; usual dose 50–100 mg daily in 2 divided doses, if child cannot tolerate recommended titration regimen then smaller steps or longer interval between steps may be used; maximum 200 mg per day

● **UNLICENSED USE** Not licensed for use in children for migraine prophylaxis.

● **CAUTIONS** Avoid in Acute porphyrias p. 652 · risk of metabolic acidosis · risk of nephrolithiasis—ensure adequate hydration (especially in strenuous activity or warm environment)

● **INTERACTIONS** → Appendix 1: antiepileptics

● **SIDE-EFFECTS**

▶ **Common or very common** Alopecia · anaemia · anxiety · appetite abnormal · asthenia · behaviour abnormal · cognitive impairment · concentration impaired · confusion · constipation · cough · depression · diarrhoea · dizziness · drowsiness · dry mouth · dyspnoea · ear discomfort · eye disorders · feeling abnormal · fever · gait abnormal · gastrointestinal discomfort · gastrointestinal disorders · haemorrhage · hypersensitivity · joint disorders · malaise · memory loss · mood altered · movement disorders · muscle complaints · muscle weakness · nasal complaints · nasopharyngitis · nausea · oral disorders · pain · seizures · sensation abnormal · skin reactions · sleep disorders · speech impairment · taste altered · tinnitus · tremor · urinary disorders · urolithiases · vertigo · vision disorders · vomiting · weight changes

▶ **Uncommon** Abnormal sensation in eye · anhidrosis · arrhythmias · aura · cerebellar syndrome · consciousness impaired · crying · drooling · dry eye · dysgraphia · dysphonia · eosinophilia · facial swelling · hallucinations · hearing impairment · hyperthermia · hypokalaemia · hypotension · influenza like illness · learning disability · leucopenia · lymphadenopathy · metabolic acidosis · musculoskeletal stiffness · palpitations · pancreatitis · paranasal sinus hypersecretion · peripheral coldness ·

4 Nervous system

peripheral neuropathy · polydipsia · psychotic disorder · renal pain · sexual dysfunction · smell altered · suicidal tendencies · syncope · thinking abnormal · thirst · thrombocytopenia · vasodilation

- **Rare or very rare** Eye inflammation · face oedema · glaucoma · hepatic disorders · limb discomfort · neutropenia · Raynaud's phenomenon · renal tubular acidosis · severe cutaneous adverse reactions (SCARs) · unresponsive to stimuli

SIDE-EFFECTS, FURTHER INFORMATION Topiramate has been associated with acute myopia with secondary angle-closure glaucoma, typically occurring within 1 month of starting treatment. Choroidal effusions resulting in anterior displacement of the lens and iris have also been reported. If raised intra-ocular pressure occurs: seek specialist ophthalmological advice; use appropriate measures to reduce intra-ocular pressure and stop topiramate as rapidly as feasible.

- **CONCEPTION AND CONTRACEPTION** Manufacturer advises perform pregnancy test before the initiation of treatment—a highly effective contraceptive method is advised in women of child-bearing potential; patients should be fully informed of the risks related to the use of topiramate during pregnancy.
- **PREGNANCY** Increased risk of major congenital malformations following exposure during the first trimester. *For migraine prophylaxis* manufacturer advises avoid. *For epilepsy* manufacturer advises consider alternative treatment options. See also *Pregnancy* in Epilepsy p. 203.

Monitoring Manufacturer advises in case of administration during first trimester, careful prenatal monitoring should be performed.

It is recommended that the fetal growth should be monitored.

The dose should be monitored carefully during pregnancy and after birth, and adjustments made on a clinical basis.

- **BREAST FEEDING** Manufacturer advises avoid—present in milk.
- **HEPATIC IMPAIRMENT** Manufacturer advises caution (risk of decreased clearance).
- **RENAL IMPAIRMENT** Use with caution.

Dose adjustments Half usual starting and maintenance dose if estimated glomerular filtration less than 70 mL/minute/1.73 m^2—reduced clearance and longer time to steady-state plasma concentration.

- **DIRECTIONS FOR ADMINISTRATION**

TOPAMAX® CAPSULES Swallow whole or sprinkle contents of capsule on soft food and swallow immediately without chewing.

- **PRESCRIBING AND DISPENSING INFORMATION**

Switching between formulations Care should be taken when switching between oral formulations in the treatment of epilepsy. The need for continued supply of a particular manufacturer's product should be based on clinical judgement and consultation with the patient or their carer, taking into account factors such as seizure frequency and treatment history.

Patients being treated for epilepsy may need to be maintained on a specific manufacturer's branded or generic topiramate product.

- **PATIENT AND CARER ADVICE**

Medicines for Children leaflet: Topiramate for preventing seizures www.medicinesforchildren.org.uk/topiramate-preventing-seizures

TOPAMAX® CAPSULES Patients or carers should be given advice on how to administer *Topamax® Sprinkle* capsules.

- **MEDICINAL FORMS** There can be variation in the licensing of different medicines containing the same drug. Forms available from special-order manufacturers include: oral suspension, oral solution

Oral suspension

- Topiramate (Non-proprietary)

Topiramate 10 mg per 1 ml Topiramate 50mg/5ml oral suspension sugar-free | 150 ml PoM £129.00 DT = £129.00

Topiramate 20 mg per 1 ml Topiramate 100mg/5ml oral suspension sugar-free | 280 ml PoM £195.69 DT = £195.69

Tablet

CAUTIONARY AND ADVISORY LABELS 3, 8

- Topiramate (Non-proprietary)

Topiramate 25 mg Topiramate 25 mg tablets | 60 tablet PoM £15.43 DT = £5.11

Topiramate 25mg tablets | 60 tablet PoM £10.00 DT = £5.11

Topiramate 50 mg Topiramate 50mg tablets | 60 tablet PoM £36.75 DT = £9.48

Topiramate 100 mg Topiramate 100mg tablets | 60 tablet PoM £45.41 DT = £15.63

Topiramate 200 mg Topiramate 200mg tablets | 60 tablet PoM £88.18 DT = £44.38

- Topamax (Janssen-Cilag Ltd)

Topiramate 25 mg Topamax 25mg tablets | 60 tablet PoM £19.29 DT = £5.11

Topiramate 50 mg Topamax 50mg tablets | 60 tablet PoM £31.69 DT = £9.48

Topiramate 100 mg Topamax 100mg tablets | 60 tablet PoM £56.76 DT = £15.63

Topiramate 200 mg Topamax 200mg tablets | 60 tablet PoM £110.23 DT = £44.38

Capsule

CAUTIONARY AND ADVISORY LABELS 3, 8

- Topamax (Janssen-Cilag Ltd)

Topiramate 15 mg Topamax 15mg sprinkle capsules | 60 capsule PoM £14.79 DT = £14.79

Topiramate 25 mg Topamax 25mg sprinkle capsules | 60 capsule PoM £22.18 DT = £13.33

Topiramate 50 mg Topamax 50mg sprinkle capsules | 60 capsule PoM £36.45 DT = £36.45

Valproic acid

14-Feb-2020

- **INDICATIONS AND DOSE**

CONVULEX®

Epilepsy

- BY MOUTH
- Child 1 month–11 years: Initially 10–15 mg/kg daily in 2–4 divided doses, max. 600 mg daily; usual maintenance 25–30 mg/kg daily in 2–4 divided doses, doses up to 60 mg/kg daily in 2–4 divided doses in infantile spasms; monitor clinical chemistry and haematological parameters if dose exceeds 40 mg/kg daily
- Child 12–17 years: Initially 600 mg daily in 2–4 divided doses, increased in steps of 150–300 mg every 3 days; usual maintenance 1–2 g daily in 2–4 divided doses, max. 2.5 g daily in 2–4 divided doses

DOSE EQUIVALENCE AND CONVERSION

- *Convulex®* has a 1:1 dose relationship with products containing sodium valproate, but nevertheless care is needed if switching or making changes.

IMPORTANT SAFETY INFORMATION

MHRA/CHM ADVICE: VALPROATE MEDICINES: CONTRA-INDICATED IN WOMEN AND GIRLS OF CHILDBEARING POTENTIAL UNLESS CONDITIONS OF PREGNANCY PREVENTION PROGRAMME ARE MET (APRIL 2018)

Valproate is highly teratogenic and evidence supports that use in pregnancy leads to neurodevelopmental disorders (approx. 30–40% risk) and congenital malformations (approx. 10% risk).

Valproate must not be used in women and girls of childbearing potential unless the conditions of the

Pregnancy Prevention Programme are met (see *Conception and contraception*) and only if other treatments are ineffective or not tolerated, as judged by an experienced specialist.

Use of valproate in pregnancy is contra-indicated for migraine prophylaxis [unlicensed] and bipolar disorder; it must only be considered for epilepsy if there is no suitable alternative treatment (see *Pregnancy*).

Women and girls (and their carers) must be fully informed of the risks and the need to avoid exposure to valproate medicines in pregnancy; supporting materials have been provided to use in the implementation of the Pregnancy Prevention Programme (see *Prescribing and dispensing information*). The MHRA advises that:

- GPs must recall all women and girls who may be of childbearing potential, provide the Patient Guide, check they have been reviewed by a specialist in the last year and are on highly effective contraception;
- Specialists must book in review appointments at least annually with women and girls under the Pregnancy Prevention Programme, re-evaluate treatment as necessary, explain clearly the conditions as outlined in the supporting materials and complete and sign the Risk Acknowledgement Form—copies of the form must be given to the patient or carer and sent to their GP;
- Pharmacists must ensure valproate medicines are dispensed in whole packs whenever possible—all packs dispensed to women and girls of childbearing potential should have a warning label either on the carton or via a sticker. They must also discuss risks in pregnancy with female patients each time valproate medicines are dispensed, ensure they have the Patient Guide and have seen their GP or specialist to discuss their treatment and the need for contraception.

MHRA/CHM ADVICE: VALPROATE MEDICINES: ARE YOU ACTING IN COMPLIANCE WITH THE PREGNANCY PREVENTION MEASURES? (DECEMBER 2018)

The MHRA advises that all healthcare professionals must continue to identify and review all female patients on valproate, including when used outside licensed indications (off-label use) and provide them with the patient information materials every time they attend appointments or receive their medicines.

Guidance for psychiatrists on the withdrawal of, and alternatives to, valproate in women of childbearing potential who have a psychiatric illness is available from the Royal College of Psychiatrists.

MHRA/CHM ADVICE: VALPROATE MEDICINES AND SERIOUS HARMS IN PREGNANCY: NEW ANNUAL RISK ACKNOWLEDGEMENT FORM AND CLINICAL GUIDANCE FROM PROFESSIONAL BODIES TO SUPPORT COMPLIANCE WITH THE PREGNANCY PREVENTION PROGRAMME (APRIL 2019)

The Annual Risk Acknowledgement Form has been updated and should be used for all future reviews of female patients on valproate. Specialists should comply with guidance given on the form if they consider the patient is not at risk of pregnancy, including the need for review in case her risk status changes.

Guidance has been published to support healthcare professionals with the use of valproate. These include a summary by NICE of their guidance and safety advice, pan-college guidance by national healthcare bodies, and paediatric guidance by the British Paediatric Neurology Association and the Royal College of Paediatrics and Child Health.

MHRA/CHM ADVICE (UPDATED JANUARY 2020): VALPROATE PREGNANCY PREVENTION PROGRAMME

The Guide for Healthcare Professionals has been updated and should be used for all future reviews of female patients on valproate medicines, in conjunction with other supporting materials (see *Prescribing and dispensing Information*).

- **CONTRA-INDICATIONS** Acute porphyrias p. 652 · known or suspected mitochondrial disorders (higher rate of acute liver failure and liver-related deaths) · personal or family history of severe hepatic dysfunction
- **CAUTIONS** Systemic lupus erythematosus

CAUTIONS, FURTHER INFORMATION

- Liver toxicity Liver dysfunction (including fatal hepatic failure) has occurred in association with valproate (especially in children under 3 years and in those with metabolic or degenerative disorders, organic brain disease or severe seizure disorders associated with mental retardation) usually in first 6 months and usually involving multiple antiepileptic therapy. Raised liver enzymes during valproate treatment are usually transient but patients should be reassessed clinically and liver function (including prothrombin time) monitored until return to normal—discontinue if abnormally prolonged prothrombin time (particularly in association with other relevant abnormalities).

Consider vitamin D supplementation in patients who are immobilised for long periods or who have inadequate sun exposure or dietary intake of calcium.

- **INTERACTIONS** → Appendix 1: antiepileptics
- **SIDE-EFFECTS** Abdominal pain · alertness increased · alopecia (regrowth may be curly) · anaemia · behaviour abnormal · bone disorders · bone fracture · cerebral atrophy · coma · confusion · consciousness impaired · dementia · diarrhoea · diplopia · drowsiness · encephalopathy · fine postural tremor · gastrointestinal disorder · gynaecomastia · haemorrhage · hallucination · hearing loss · hepatic disorders · hirsutism · hyperammonaemia · leucopenia · menstrual cycle irregularities · movement disorders · nail disorder · nausea · obesity · pancreatitis · pancytopenia · parkinsonism · peripheral oedema · seizure · severe cutaneous adverse reactions (SCARs) · skin reactions · thrombocytopenia · urine abnormalities · vasculitis · vomiting · weight increased

SIDE-EFFECTS, FURTHER INFORMATION **Hepatic dysfunction** Withdraw treatment immediately if persistent vomiting and abdominal pain, anorexia, jaundice, oedema, malaise, drowsiness, or loss of seizure control.

Pancreatitis Discontinue treatment if symptoms of pancreatitis develop.

- **CONCEPTION AND CONTRACEPTION** The MHRA advises that all women and girls of childbearing potential being treated with valproate medicines must be supported on a Pregnancy Prevention Programme—pregnancy should be excluded before treatment initiation and highly effective contraception must be used during treatment.
- **PREGNANCY** For *migraine prophylaxis* [unlicensed] and *bipolar disorder*, the MHRA advises that valproate must not be used. For *epilepsy*, the MHRA advises valproate must not be used unless there is no suitable alternative treatment; in such cases, access to counselling about the risks should be provided (see Healthcare Professional Guide for more information) and a Risk Acknowledgement Form signed by both specialist and patient. If valproate is to be used during pregnancy, the lowest effective dose should be prescribed in divided doses to avoid peaks in plasma-valproate concentrations; doses greater than 1 g daily are associated with an increased risk of teratogenicity. Neonatal bleeding (related to hypofibrinaemia). Neonatal hepatotoxicity also reported. See also *Pregnancy* in Epilepsy p. 203.

Monitoring Specialist prenatal monitoring should be instigated when valproate has been taken in pregnancy.

The dose should be monitored carefully during pregnancy and after birth, and adjustments made on a clinical basis.

- **BREAST FEEDING** Present in milk—risk of haematological disorders in breast-fed newborns and infants.
- **HEPATIC IMPAIRMENT** Manufacturer advises avoid.
- **RENAL IMPAIRMENT**

Dose adjustments Reduce dose.
- **MONITORING REQUIREMENTS**
  - Monitor closely if dose greater than 45 mg/kg daily.
  - Monitor liver function before therapy and during first 6 months especially in patients most at risk.
  - Measure full blood count and ensure no undue potential for bleeding before starting and before surgery.
- **EFFECT ON LABORATORY TESTS** False-positive urine tests for ketones.
- **TREATMENT CESSATION** [EvGr] In bipolar disorder, avoid abrupt withdrawal; if treatment with valproate is stopped, reduce the dose gradually over at least 4 weeks. (A)
- **PRESCRIBING AND DISPENSING INFORMATION** The Pregnancy Prevention Programme is supported by the following materials provided by the manufacturer: *Patient Guide, Guide for Healthcare Professionals, Risk Acknowledgement Form*, and for pharmacists, *Patient Cards* and *Stickers with warning symbols*; the MHRA has also produced a patient information sheet providing advice for women and girls taking valproate medicines.

The Royal Pharmaceutical Society has also produced a safe supply algorithm, available at: www.rpharms.com/safesupplyvalproate

CONVULEX® Patients being treated for epilepsy may need to be maintained on a specific manufacturer's branded or generic oral valproic acid product.
- **PATIENT AND CARER ADVICE**

Valproate use by women and girls The MHRA advises women and girls should **not** stop taking valproate without first discussing it with their doctor.

Blood or hepatic disorders Patients or their carers should be told how to recognise signs and symptoms of blood or liver disorders and advised to seek immediate medical attention if symptoms develop.

Pancreatitis Patients or their carers should be told how to recognise signs and symptoms of pancreatitis and advised to seek immediate medical attention if symptoms such as abdominal pain, nausea, or vomiting develop.

Pregnancy Prevention Programme Pharmacists must ensure that female patients have a patient card—see also *Important safety information*.

- **MEDICINAL FORMS** There can be variation in the licensing of different medicines containing the same drug. Forms available from special-order manufacturers include: oral suspension, oral solution

Gastro-resistant capsule

CAUTIONARY AND ADVISORY LABELS 8, 10, 21, 25

- Convulex (G.L. Pharma UK Ltd) ▼

Valproic acid 150 mg Convulex 150mg gastro-resistant capsules | 100 capsule [PoM] £3.68 DT = £3.68

Valproic acid 300 mg Convulex 300mg gastro-resistant capsules | 100 capsule [PoM] £7.35 DT = £7.35

Valproic acid 500 mg Convulex 500mg gastro-resistant capsules | 100 capsule [PoM] £12.25 DT = £12.25

Vigabatrin

- **INDICATIONS AND DOSE**

Adjunctive treatment of focal seizures with or without secondary generalisation not satisfactorily controlled with other antiepileptics (under expert supervision)

- BY MOUTH
  - Neonate: Initially 15–20 mg/kg twice daily, to be increased over 2–3 weeks to usual maintenance dose, usual maintenance 30–40 mg/kg twice daily (max. per dose 75 mg/kg).
  - Child 1-23 months: Initially 15–20 mg/kg twice daily (max. per dose 250 mg), to be increased over 2–3 weeks to usual maintenance dose, usual maintenance 30–40 mg/kg twice daily (max. per dose 75 mg/kg)
  - Child 2-11 years: Initially 15–20 mg/kg twice daily (max. per dose 250 mg), to be increased over 2–3 weeks to usual maintenance dose, usual maintenance 30–40 mg/kg twice daily (max. per dose 1.5 g)
  - Child 12-17 years: Initially 250 mg twice daily, to be increased over 2–3 weeks to usual maintenance dose, usual maintenance 1–1.5 g twice daily
- BY RECTUM
  - Child 1-23 months: Initially 15–20 mg/kg twice daily (max. per dose 250 mg), to be increased over 2–3 weeks to usual maintenance dose, usual maintenance 30–40 mg/kg twice daily (max. per dose 75 mg/kg)
  - Child 2-11 years: Initially 15–20 mg/kg twice daily (max. per dose 250 mg), to be increased over 2–3 weeks to usual maintenance dose, usual maintenance 30–40 mg/kg twice daily (max. per dose 1.5 g)
  - Child 12-17 years: Initially 250 mg twice daily, to be increased over 2–3 weeks to usual maintenance dose, usual maintenance 1–1.5 g twice daily

Monotherapy in the management of infantile spasms in West's syndrome (under expert supervision)

- BY MOUTH
  - Neonate: Initially 15–25 mg/kg twice daily, to be adjusted according to response over 7 days to usual maintenance dose; usual maintenance 40–50 mg/kg twice daily (max. per dose 75 mg/kg).
  - Child 1 month-1 year: Initially 15–25 mg/kg twice daily, to be adjusted according to response over 7 days to usual maintenance dose; usual maintenance 40–50 mg/kg twice daily (max. per dose 75 mg/kg)

- **UNLICENSED USE** Granules not licensed for rectal use. Tablets not licensed to be crushed and dispersed in liquid. Vigabatrin doses in BNF publications may differ from those in product literature.
- **CONTRA-INDICATIONS** Visual field defects
- **CAUTIONS** History of behavioural problems · history of depression · history of psychosis

CAUTIONS, FURTHER INFORMATION Vigabatrin may worsen absence, myoclonic, tonic and atonic seizures.
  - Visual field defects Vigabatrin is associated with visual field defects. The onset of symptoms varies from 1 month to several years after starting. In most cases, visual field defects have persisted despite discontinuation, and further deterioration after discontinuation cannot be excluded. Product literature advises visual field testing before treatment and at 6-month intervals. Patients and their carers should be warned to report any new visual symptoms that develop and those with symptoms should be referred for an urgent ophthalmological opinion. Gradual withdrawal of vigabatrin should be considered.
- **INTERACTIONS** → Appendix 1: antiepileptics
- **SIDE-EFFECTS**
  - **Common or very common** Abdominal pain · anaemia · anxiety · arthralgia · behaviour abnormal · concentration impaired · depression · dizziness · drowsiness · eye disorders · fatigue · headache · memory loss · mood altered · nausea · oedema · paraesthesia · speech disorder · thinking abnormal · tremor · vision disorders · vomiting · weight increased
  - **Uncommon** Movement disorders · psychotic disorder · seizure (patients with myoclonic seizures at greater risk) · skin reactions
  - **Rare or very rare** Angioedema · encephalopathy · hallucination · hepatitis · optic neuritis · suicide attempt

- **Frequency not known** Movement disorder (in infantile spasms) · muscle tone increased

SIDE-EFFECTS, FURTHER INFORMATION **Encephalopathic symptoms** Encephalopathic symptoms including marked sedation, stupor, and confusion with non-specific slow wave EEG can occur rarely -reduce dose or withdraw.
Visual field defects About one-third of patients treated with vigabatrin have suffered visual field defects; counselling and careful monitoring for this side-effect are required.

- **PREGNANCY** See also *Pregnancy* in Epilepsy p. 203.
Monitoring The dose should be monitored carefully during pregnancy and after birth, and adjustments made on a clinical basis.
- **BREAST FEEDING** Present in milk—manufacturer advises avoid.
- **RENAL IMPAIRMENT**
Dose adjustments Consider reduced dose or increased dose interval if estimated glomerular filtration rate less than 60 mL/minute/1.73 m^2.
- **MONITORING REQUIREMENTS** Closely monitor neurological function.
- **DIRECTIONS FOR ADMINISTRATION**
- **With oral use** The contents of a sachet should be dissolved in water or a soft drink immediately before taking. Tablets may be crushed and dispersed in liquid.
- **With rectal use** Dissolve contents of sachet in small amount of water and administer rectally [unlicensed use].
- **PATIENT AND CARER ADVICE** Patients and their carers should be warned to report any new visual symptoms that develop.
Medicines for Children leaflet: Vigabatrin for preventing seizures www.medicinesforchildren.org.uk/vigabatrin-preventing-seizures

---

- **MEDICINAL FORMS** There can be variation in the licensing of different medicines containing the same drug. Forms available from special-order manufacturers include: oral solution

Powder

CAUTIONARY AND ADVISORY LABELS 3, 8, 13

- Sabril (Sanofi)
Vigabatrin 500 mg Sabril 500mg oral powder sachets sugar-free | 50 sachet [PoM] £24.60 DT = £24.60

Tablet

CAUTIONARY AND ADVISORY LABELS 3, 8

- Sabril (Sanofi)
Vigabatrin 500 mg Sabril 500mg tablets | 100 tablet [PoM] £44.41 DT = £44.41

Zonisamide

20-Feb-2019

- **INDICATIONS AND DOSE**

Adjunctive treatment for refractory focal seizures with or without secondary generalisation

- BY MOUTH
- Child 6–17 years (body-weight 20–54 kg): Initially 1 mg/kg once daily for 7 days, then increased in steps of 1 mg/kg every 7 days, usual maintenance 6–8 mg/kg once daily (max. per dose 500 mg once daily), dose to be increased at 2-week intervals in patients who are **not** receiving concomitant carbamazepine, phenytoin, phenobarbital or other potent inducers of cytochrome P450 enzyme CYP3A4
- Child 6–17 years (body-weight 55 kg and above): Initially 1 mg/kg once daily for 7 days, then increased in steps of 1 mg/kg every 7 days, usual maintenance 300–500 mg once daily, dose to be increased at 2-week intervals in patients who are **not** receiving concomitant carbamazepine, phenytoin, phenobarbital or other potent inducers of cytochrome P450 enzyme CYP3A4

- **CAUTIONS** Low body-weight or poor appetite—monitor weight throughout treatment (fatal cases of weight loss reported in children) · metabolic acidosis—monitor serum bicarbonate concentration in children and those with other risk factors (consider dose reduction or discontinuation if metabolic acidosis develops) · risk factors for renal stone formation (particularly predisposition to nephrolithiasis)

CAUTIONS, FURTHER INFORMATION Avoid overheating and ensure adequate hydration especially in children, during strenuous activity or if in warm environment (fatal cases of heat stroke reported in children).

- **INTERACTIONS** → Appendix 1: antiepileptics
- **SIDE-EFFECTS**
- **Common or very common** Alopecia · anxiety · appetite decreased · ataxia · bradyphrenia · concentration impaired · confusion · constipation · depression · diarrhoea · dizziness · drowsiness · fatigue · fever · gastrointestinal discomfort · hypersensitivity · influenza like illness · insomnia · memory loss · mood altered · nausea · nystagmus · paraesthesia · peripheral oedema · psychosis · rash (consider discontinuation) · skin reactions · speech disorder · tremor · urolithiases · vision disorders · vomiting · weight decreased
- **Uncommon** Behaviour abnormal · gallbladder disorders · hallucination · hypokalaemia · increased risk of infection · leucopenia · respiratory disorders · seizures · suicidal tendencies · thrombocytopenia
- **Rare or very rare** Agranulocytosis · angle closure glaucoma · anhidrosis · bone marrow disorders · coma · dyspnoea · eye pain · heat stroke · hepatocellular injury · hydronephrosis · leucocytosis · lymphadenopathy · metabolic acidosis · myasthenic syndrome · neuroleptic malignant syndrome · pancreatitis · renal failure · renal tubular acidosis · rhabdomyolysis · severe cutaneous adverse reactions (SCARs) · urine abnormal
- **Frequency not known** Sudden unexplained death in epilepsy
- **ALLERGY AND CROSS-SENSITIVITY** Contra-indicated in sulfonamide hypersensitivity.
Antiepileptic hypersensitivity syndrome theoretically associated with zonisamide. See under Epilepsy p. 203 for more information.
- **CONCEPTION AND CONTRACEPTION** Manufacturer advises women of childbearing potential should use effective contraception during treatment and for one month after last dose—avoid in women of childbearing potential not using effective contraception unless clearly necessary and the potential benefit outweighs risk; patients should be fully informed of the risks related to the use of zonisamide during pregnancy.
- **PREGNANCY** Manufacturer advises use only if clearly necessary and the potential benefit outweighs risk—toxicity in *animal* studies; patients should be fully informed of the risks related to the use of zonisamide during pregnancy. See also *Pregnancy* in Epilepsy p. 203.
Monitoring The dose should be monitored carefully during pregnancy and after birth, and adjustments made on a clinical basis.
- **BREAST FEEDING** Manufacturer advises avoid for 4 weeks after last dose.
- **HEPATIC IMPAIRMENT** Avoid in severe impairment.
Dose adjustments Initially increase dose at 2-week intervals if mild or moderate impairment.
- **RENAL IMPAIRMENT**
Dose adjustments Initially increase dose at 2-week intervals; discontinue if renal function deteriorates.
- **TREATMENT CESSATION** Avoid abrupt withdrawal (consult product literature for recommended withdrawal regimens in children).

- **PRESCRIBING AND DISPENSING INFORMATION**
Switching between formulations Care should be taken when switching between oral formulations. The need for continued supply of a particular manufacturer's product should be based on clinical judgement and consultation with the patient or their carer, taking into account factors such as seizure frequency and treatment history.
Patients may need to be maintained on a specific manufacturer's branded or generic zonisamide product.
- **PATIENT AND CARER ADVICE** Children and their carers should be made aware of how to prevent and recognise overheating and dehydration.
Medicines for Children leaflet: Zonisamide for preventing seizures www.medicinesforchildren.org.uk/zonisamide-preventing-seizures
- **NATIONAL FUNDING/ACCESS DECISIONS**

Scottish Medicines Consortium (SMC) decisions
SMC No. 949/14
The *Scottish Medicines Consortium* has advised (March 2014) that zonisamide (*Zonegran®*) is accepted for restricted use within NHS Scotland as adjunctive treatment of focal seizures, with or without secondary generalisation, in adolescents and children aged 6 years and above. It is restricted to use on advice from specialists in paediatric neurology or epilepsy.

- **MEDICINAL FORMS** There can be variation in the licensing of different medicines containing the same drug. Forms available from special-order manufacturers include: oral suspension, oral solution

Capsule
CAUTIONARY AND ADVISORY LABELS 3, 8, 10
- Zonisamide (Non-proprietary)
Zonisamide 25 mg Zonisamide 25mg capsules | 14 capsule PoM £8.82 DT = £7.50
Zonisamide 50 mg Zonisamide 50mg capsules | 56 capsule PoM £47.04 DT = £39.77
Zonisamide 100 mg Zonisamide 100mg capsules | 56 capsule PoM £62.72 DT = £4.72
- Zonegran (Eisai Ltd)
Zonisamide 25 mg Zonegran 25mg capsules | 14 capsule PoM £8.82 DT = £7.50
Zonisamide 50 mg Zonegran 50mg capsules | 56 capsule PoM £47.04 DT = £39.77
Zonisamide 100 mg Zonegran 100mg capsules | 56 capsule PoM £62.72 DT = £4.72

ANTIEPILEPTICS > BARBITURATES

Phenobarbital

10-Mar-2020

(Phenobarbitone)

- **INDICATIONS AND DOSE**

All forms of epilepsy except typical absence seizures
- BY MOUTH
- Child 1 month–11 years: Initially 1–1.5 mg/kg twice daily, then increased in steps of 2 mg/kg daily as required; maintenance 2.5–4 mg/kg 1–2 times a day
- Child 12–17 years: 60–180 mg once daily
- INITIALLY BY SLOW INTRAVENOUS INJECTION
- Neonate: Initially 20 mg/kg, then (by slow intravenous injection or by mouth) 2.5–5 mg/kg once daily, adjusted according to response.

Status epilepticus
- BY SLOW INTRAVENOUS INJECTION
- Neonate: Initially 20 mg/kg, dose to be administered at a rate no faster than 1 mg/kg/minute, then 2.5–5 mg/kg 1–2 times a day.
- Child 1 month–11 years: Initially 20 mg/kg, dose to be administered at a rate no faster than 1 mg/kg/minute, then 2.5–5 mg/kg 1–2 times a day
- Child 12–17 years: Initially 20 mg/kg (max. per dose 1 g), dose to be administered at a rate no faster than 1 mg/kg/minute, then 300 mg twice daily

DOSE EQUIVALENCE AND CONVERSION
- For therapeutic purposes phenobarbital and phenobarbital sodium may be considered equivalent in effect.

- **CAUTIONS** Avoid in Acute porphyrias p. 652 · children · debilitated · history of alcohol abuse · history of drug abuse · respiratory depression (avoid if severe)
CAUTIONS, FURTHER INFORMATION Consider vitamin D supplementation in patients who are immobilised for long periods or who have inadequate sun exposure or dietary intake of calcium.
- **INTERACTIONS** → Appendix 1: antiepileptics
- **SIDE-EFFECTS**
GENERAL SIDE-EFFECTS
Agitation · agranulocytosis · anticonvulsant hypersensitivity syndrome · behaviour abnormal · bone disorders · bone fracture · cognitive impairment · confusion · depression · drowsiness · folate deficiency · hepatic disorders · memory loss · movement disorders · nystagmus · respiratory depression · skin reactions
SPECIFIC SIDE-EFFECTS
- With oral use Hallucination · hypotension · megaloblastic anaemia · severe cutaneous adverse reactions (SCARs) · thrombocytopenia
- With parenteral use Anaemia · aplastic anaemia · Dupuytren's contracture · hypocalcaemia · irritability · toxic epidermal necrolysis

Overdose For details on the management of poisoning, see Active elimination techniques, under Emergency treatment of poisoning p. 891.
- **ALLERGY AND CROSS-SENSITIVITY** Antiepileptic hypersensitivity syndrome associated with phenobarbital. See under Epilepsy p. 203 for more information.
- **PREGNANCY**
Monitoring The dose should be monitored carefully during pregnancy and after birth, and adjustments made on a clinical basis.
- **BREAST FEEDING** Avoid if possible; drowsiness may occur.
- **HEPATIC IMPAIRMENT** Manufacturer advises caution in mild to moderate impairment; avoid in severe impairment.
- **RENAL IMPAIRMENT** Use with caution.
- **MONITORING REQUIREMENTS**
- Plasma-phenobarbital concentration for optimum response is 15–40 mg/litre (60–180 micromol/litre); however, monitoring the plasma-drug concentration is less useful than with other drugs because tolerance occurs.
- **TREATMENT CESSATION** Avoid abrupt withdrawal (dependence with prolonged use).
- **DIRECTIONS FOR ADMINISTRATION**
- With oral use For administration by *mouth*, tablets may be crushed.
- With intravenous use For *intravenous injection*, dilute to a concentration of 20 mg/mL with Water for Injections; give over 20 minutes (no faster than 1 mg/kg/minute).
- **PRESCRIBING AND DISPENSING INFORMATION** The RCPCH and NPPG recommend that, when a liquid special of phenobarbital is required, it is alcohol-free and the following strength is used: 50 mg/5 mL.
Switching between formulations Different formulations of oral preparations may vary in bioavailability. Patients should be maintained on a specific manufacturer's product.

- **PATIENT AND CARER ADVICE**
Medicines for Children leaflet: Phenobarbital for preventing seizures www.medicinesforchildren.org.uk/phenobarbital-preventing-seizures

- **MEDICINAL FORMS** There can be variation in the licensing of different medicines containing the same drug. Forms available from special-order manufacturers include: tablet, capsule, oral suspension, oral solution

Tablet

CAUTIONARY AND ADVISORY LABELS 2, 8

▸ Phenobarbital (Non-proprietary)

Phenobarbital 15 mg Phenobarbital 15mg tablets | 28 tablet PoM £24.95 DT = £21.13 CD3

Phenobarbital 30 mg Phenobarbital 30mg tablets | 28 tablet PoM £5.99 DT = £1.01 CD3

Phenobarbital 60 mg Phenobarbital 60mg tablets | 28 tablet PoM £7.99 DT = £7.35 CD3

Solution for injection

EXCIPIENTS: May contain Propylene glycol

▸ Phenobarbital (Non-proprietary)

Phenobarbital sodium 30 mg per 1 ml Phenobarbital 30mg/1ml solution for injection ampoules | 10 ampoule PoM £113.67 DT = £113.67 CD3

Phenobarbital sodium 60 mg per 1 ml Phenobarbital 60mg/1ml solution for injection ampoules | 10 ampoule PoM £119.93 DT = £119.93 CD3

Phenobarbital sodium 200 mg per 1 ml Phenobarbital 200mg/1ml solution for injection ampoules | 10 ampoule PoM £97.78 DT = £97.78 CD3

Oral solution

CAUTIONARY AND ADVISORY LABELS 2, 8

EXCIPIENTS: May contain Alcohol

▸ Phenobarbital (Non-proprietary)

Phenobarbital 3 mg per 1 ml Phenobarbital 15mg/5ml elixir | 500 ml PoM £83.00–£83.01 DT = £83.01 CD3

Primidone

- **INDICATIONS AND DOSE**

All forms of epilepsy except typical absence seizures

▸ BY MOUTH

▸ Child 1 month–1 year: Initially 125 mg daily, dose to be taken at bedtime, then increased in steps of 125 mg every 3 days, adjusted according to response; maintenance 125–250 mg twice daily

▸ Child 2–4 years: Initially 125 mg once daily, dose to be taken at bedtime, then increased in steps of 125 mg every 3 days, adjusted according to response; maintenance 250–375 mg twice daily

▸ Child 5–8 years: Initially 125 mg once daily, dose to be taken at bedtime, then increased in steps of 125 mg every 3 days, adjusted according to response; maintenance 375–500 mg twice daily

▸ Child 9–17 years: Initially 125 mg once daily, dose to be taken at bedtime, then increased in steps of 125 mg every 3 days, increased to 250 mg twice daily, then increased in steps of 250 mg every 3 days (max. per dose 750 mg twice daily), adjusted according to response

- **CAUTIONS** Avoid in Acute porphyrias p. 652 · children · debilitated · history of alcohol abuse · history of drug abuse · respiratory depression (avoid if severe)

CAUTIONS, FURTHER INFORMATION Consider vitamin D supplementation in patients who are immobilised for long periods or who have inadequate sun exposure or dietary intake of calcium.

- **INTERACTIONS** → Appendix 1: antiepileptics
- **SIDE-EFFECTS**

▸ **Common or very common** Apathy · ataxia · drowsiness · nausea · nystagmus · visual impairment

▸ **Uncommon** Dizziness · headache · hypersensitivity · skin reactions · vomiting

▸ **Rare or very rare** Arthralgia · blood disorder · bone disorders · Dupuytren's contracture · megaloblastic anaemia (may be treated with folic acid) · personality change · psychotic disorder · severe cutaneous adverse reactions (SCARs) · systemic lupus erythematosus (SLE)

▸ **Frequency not known** Bone fracture

- **ALLERGY AND CROSS-SENSITIVITY** Antiepileptic hypersensitivity syndrome associated with primidone. See under Epilepsy p. 203 for more information.
- **PREGNANCY**

Monitoring The dose should be monitored carefully during pregnancy and after birth, and adjustments made on a clinical basis.

- **HEPATIC IMPAIRMENT** Manufacturer advises caution.

Dose adjustments Manufacturer advises consider dose reduction.

- **RENAL IMPAIRMENT** Use with caution.
- **MONITORING REQUIREMENTS**

▸ Monitor plasma concentrations of derived phenobarbital; plasma concentration for optimum response is 15–40 mg/litre (60–180 micromol/litre).

- **TREATMENT CESSATION** Avoid abrupt withdrawal (dependence with prolonged use).
- **PRESCRIBING AND DISPENSING INFORMATION**

Switching between formulations Different formulations of oral preparations may vary in bioavailability. Patients being treated for epilepsy should be maintained on a specific manufacturer's product.

- **MEDICINAL FORMS** There can be variation in the licensing of different medicines containing the same drug. Forms available from special-order manufacturers include: capsule, oral suspension

Tablet

CAUTIONARY AND ADVISORY LABELS 2, 8

▸ Primidone (Non-proprietary)

Primidone 50 mg Primidone 50mg tablets | 100 tablet PoM £112.50 DT = £111.66

Primidone 250 mg Primidone 250mg tablets | 100 tablet PoM £99.65–£123.00 DT = £111.12

HYPNOTICS, SEDATIVES AND ANXIOLYTICS > BENZODIAZEPINES

Benzodiazepines

IMPORTANT SAFETY INFORMATION

MHRA/CHM ADVICE: BENZODIAZEPINES AND OPIOIDS: REMINDER OF RISK OF POTENTIALLY FATAL RESPIRATORY DEPRESSION (MARCH 2020)

The MHRA reminds healthcare professionals that benzodiazepines and benzodiazepine-like drugs co-prescribed with opioids can produce additive CNS depressant effects, thereby increasing the risk of sedation, respiratory depression, coma, and death. Healthcare professionals are advised to only co-prescribe if there is no alternative and, if necessary, the lowest possible doses should be given for the shortest duration. Patients should be closely monitored for signs of respiratory depression at initiation of treatment and when there is any change in prescribing, such as dose adjustments or new interactions. If methadone is co-prescribed with a benzodiazepine or benzodiazepine-like drug, the respiratory depressant effect of methadone may be delayed; patients should be monitored for at least 2 weeks after initiation or changes in prescribing. Patients should be informed of the signs and symptoms of respiratory depression and sedation, and advised to seek urgent medical attention should these occur.

- **CONTRA-INDICATIONS** Acute pulmonary insufficiency · marked neuromuscular respiratory weakness · obsessional states · phobic states · sleep apnoea syndrome · unstable myasthenia gravis
- **CAUTIONS** Avoid prolonged use (and abrupt withdrawal thereafter) · history of alcohol dependence or abuse · history of drug dependence or abuse · myasthenia gravis · personality disorder (within the fearful group—dependent, avoidant, obsessive-compulsive) may increase risk of dependence · respiratory disease

CAUTIONS, FURTHER INFORMATION

- Paradoxical effects A paradoxical increase in hostility and aggression may be reported by patients taking benzodiazepines. The effects range from talkativeness and excitement to aggressive and antisocial acts. Adjustment of the dose (up or down) sometimes attenuates the impulses. Increased anxiety and perceptual disorders are other paradoxical effects.

- **SIDE-EFFECTS**
  - **Common or very common** Alertness decreased · anxiety · ataxia · confusion · depression · dizziness · drowsiness · dysarthria · fatigue · gastrointestinal disorder · headache · hypotension · mood altered · muscle weakness · nausea · respiratory depression (particularly with high dose and intravenous use—facilities for its treatment are essential) · sleep disorders · suicidal ideation · tremor · vertigo · vision disorders · withdrawal syndrome
  - **Uncommon** Agitation (more common in children and elderly) · anterograde amnesia · behaviour abnormal · hallucination · libido disorder · rash · urinary disorders
  - **Rare or very rare** Aggression (more common in children and elderly) · blood disorder · delusions · jaundice · paradoxical drug reaction · psychosis · restlessness (with sedative and peri-operative use)
  - **Frequency not known** Drug dependence

Overdose Benzodiazepines taken alone cause drowsiness, ataxia, dysarthria, nystagmus, and occasionally respiratory depression, and coma. For details on the management of poisoning, see Benzodiazepines, under Emergency treatment of poisoning p. 891.

- **PREGNANCY** Risk of neonatal withdrawal symptoms when used during pregnancy. Avoid regular use and use only if there is a clear indication such as seizure control. High doses administered during late pregnancy or labour may cause neonatal hypothermia, hypotonia, and respiratory depression.
- **HEPATIC IMPAIRMENT** In general, manufacturers advise caution in mild to moderate impairment; avoid in severe impairment. Benzodiazepines with a shorter half-life are considered safer.

  Dose adjustments In general, manufacturers advise dose reduction in mild to moderate impairment, adjust dose according to response.
- **RENAL IMPAIRMENT** Increased cerebral sensitivity to benzodiazepines.
- **PATIENT AND CARER ADVICE**

  Driving and skilled tasks May cause drowsiness, impair judgement and increase reaction time, and so affect ability to drive or perform skilled tasks; effects of alcohol increased. Moreover the hangover effects of a night dose may impair performance on the following day.

  For information on 2015 legislation regarding driving whilst taking certain controlled drugs, including benzodiazepines, see *Drugs and skilled tasks* under Guidance on prescribing p. 1.

F 233

Clobazam

10-Mar-2020

- **INDICATIONS AND DOSE**

Adjunct in epilepsy

- BY MOUTH
  - Child 1 month–5 years: Initially 125 micrograms/kg twice daily, dose to be increased if necessary every 5 days, maintenance 250 micrograms/kg twice daily (max. per dose 500 micrograms/kg twice daily); maximum 30 mg per day
  - Child 6–17 years: Initially 5 mg daily, dose to be increased if necessary at intervals of 5 days, maintenance 0.3–1 mg/kg daily, daily doses of up to 30 mg may be given as a single dose at bedtime, higher doses should be divided; maximum 60 mg per day

Monotherapy for catamenial (menstruation) seizures (usually for 7–10 days each month, just before and during menstruation) (under expert supervision) | Cluster seizures

- BY MOUTH
  - Child 1 month–5 years: Initially 125 micrograms/kg twice daily, dose to be increased if necessary every 5 days, maintenance 250 micrograms/kg twice daily (max. per dose 500 micrograms/kg twice daily); maximum 30 mg per day
  - Child 6–17 years: Initially 5 mg daily, dose to be increased if necessary at intervals of 5 days, maintenance 0.3–1 mg/kg daily, daily doses of up to 30 mg may be given as a single dose at bedtime, higher doses should be divided; maximum 60 mg per day

- **UNLICENSED USE** Not licensed for use in children under 6 years. Not licensed as monotherapy.

> IMPORTANT SAFETY INFORMATION
>
> SAFE PRACTICE
>
> Clobazam has been confused with clonazepam; care must be taken to ensure the correct drug is prescribed and dispensed.

- **CONTRA-INDICATIONS** Respiratory depression
- **CAUTIONS** Muscle weakness · organic brain changes

  CAUTIONS, FURTHER INFORMATION The effectiveness of clobazam may decrease significantly after weeks or months of continuous therapy.
- **INTERACTIONS** → Appendix 1: clobazam
- **SIDE-EFFECTS** Appetite decreased · consciousness impaired · constipation · drug abuse · dry mouth · fall · gait unsteady · libido loss · movement disorders · muscle spasms · nystagmus · respiratory disorder · severe cutaneous adverse reactions (SCARs) · skin reactions · speech impairment · weight increased
- **BREAST FEEDING** Benzodiazepines are present in milk, and should be avoided if possible during breast-feeding.

  Monitoring All infants should be monitored for sedation, feeding difficulties, adequate weight gain, and developmental milestones.
- **RENAL IMPAIRMENT**

  Dose adjustments Start with small doses in severe impairment.
- **MONITORING REQUIREMENTS** Routine measurement of plasma concentrations of antiepileptic drugs is not usually justified, because the target concentration ranges are arbitrary and often vary between individuals. However, plasma drug concentrations may be measured in children with worsening seizures, status epilepticus, suspected noncompliance, or suspected toxicity. Similarly, haematological and biochemical monitoring should not be undertaken unless clinically indicated.

- **PRESCRIBING AND DISPENSING INFORMATION**
Switching between formulations Care should be taken when switching between oral formulations in the treatment of epilepsy. The need for continued supply of a particular manufacturer's product should be based on clinical judgement and consultation with the patient or their carer, taking into account factors such as seizure frequency and treatment history.
Patients being treated for epilepsy may need to be maintained on a specific manufacturer's branded or generic clobazam product.
- **PATIENT AND CARER ADVICE**
Medicines for Children leaflet: Clobazam for preventing seizures www.medicinesforchildren.org.uk/clobazam-preventing-seizures-0
- **NATIONAL FUNDING/ACCESS DECISIONS**
NHS restrictions Clobazam is not prescribable in NHS primary care except for the treatment of epilepsy; endorse prescription 'SLS'.

- **MEDICINAL FORMS** There can be variation in the licensing of different medicines containing the same drug. Forms available from special-order manufacturers include: capsule, oral suspension

Oral suspension

CAUTIONARY AND ADVISORY LABELS 2, 8, 19

- Clobazam (Non-proprietary)
Clobazam 1 mg per 1 ml Clobazam 5mg/5ml oral suspension sugar-free | 150 ml PoM £90.00 DT = £90.00 CD4-1 sugar-free | 250 ml PoM £150.00 CD4-1
Clobazam 2 mg per 1 ml Clobazam 10mg/5ml oral suspension sugar-free | 150 ml PoM £95.00 DT = £95.00 CD4-1 sugar-free | 250 ml PoM £158.33 CD4-1
- Perizam (Rosemont Pharmaceuticals Ltd)
Clobazam 1 mg per 1 ml Perizam 1mg/ml oral suspension sugar-free | 150 ml PoM £90.00 DT = £90.00 CD4-1
Clobazam 2 mg per 1 ml Perizam 2mg/ml oral suspension sugar-free | 150 ml PoM £95.00 DT = £95.00 CD4-1
- Tapclob (Martindale Pharmaceuticals Ltd)
Clobazam 1 mg per 1 ml Tapclob 5mg/5ml oral suspension sugar-free | 150 ml PoM £90.00 DT = £90.00 CD4-1 | 250 ml PoM £150.00 CD4-1
Clobazam 2 mg per 1 ml Tapclob 10mg/5ml oral suspension sugar-free | 150 ml PoM £95.00 DT = £95.00 CD4-1 | 250 ml PoM £158.34 CD4-1
- Zacco (Thame Laboratories Ltd)
Clobazam 1 mg per 1 ml Zacco 5mg/5ml oral suspension sugar-free | 150 ml PoM £82.00 DT = £90.00 CD4-1
Clobazam 2 mg per 1 ml Zacco 10mg/5ml oral suspension sugar-free | 150 ml PoM £87.00 DT = £95.00 CD4-1

Tablet

CAUTIONARY AND ADVISORY LABELS 2, 8, 19

- Clobazam (Non-proprietary)
Clobazam 10 mg Clobazam 10mg tablets | 30 tablet PoM £3.78 DT = £3.76 CD4-1
- Frisium (Sanofi)
Clobazam 10 mg Frisium 10mg tablets | 30 tablet PoM £2.51 DT = £3.76 CD4-1

F 233

Clonazepam

10-Mar-2020

- **INDICATIONS AND DOSE**

All forms of epilepsy

▶ BY MOUTH

- Child 1–11 months: Initially 250 micrograms once daily for 4 nights, dose to be increased over 2–4 weeks, usual dose 0.5–1 mg daily, dose to be taken at night; may be given in 3 divided doses if necessary
- Child 1–4 years: Initially 250 micrograms once daily for 4 nights, dose to be increased over 2–4 weeks, usual dose 1–3 mg daily, dose to be taken at night; may be given in 3 divided doses if necessary
- Child 5–11 years: Initially 500 micrograms once daily for 4 nights, dose to be increased over 2–4 weeks, usual dose 3–6 mg daily, dose to be taken at night; may be given in 3 divided doses if necessary
- Child 12–17 years: Initially 1 mg once daily for 4 nights, dose to be increased over 2–4 weeks, usual dose 4–8 mg daily, dose usually taken at night; may be given in 3–4 divided doses if necessary

- **UNLICENSED USE** Clonazepam doses in BNFC may differ from those in product literature.

IMPORTANT SAFETY INFORMATION

SAFE PRACTICE

Clonazepam has been confused with clobazam; care must be taken to ensure the correct drug is prescribed and dispensed.

- **CONTRA-INDICATIONS** Coma · current alcohol abuse · current drug abuse · respiratory depression
- **CAUTIONS** Acute porphyrias p. 652 · airways obstruction · brain damage · cerebellar ataxia · depression · spinal ataxia · suicidal ideation
CAUTIONS, FURTHER INFORMATION The effectiveness of clonazepam may decrease significantly after weeks or months of continuous therapy.
- **INTERACTIONS** → Appendix 1: clonazepam
- **SIDE-EFFECTS** Alopecia · bronchial secretion increased · concentration impaired · coordination abnormal · drooling · hypersalivation · incomplete precocious puberty · muscle tone decreased · nystagmus · seizures · sexual dysfunction · skin reactions · speech impairment
- **BREAST FEEDING** Present in milk, and should be avoided if possible during breast-feeding.
Monitoring All infants should be monitored for sedation, feeding difficulties, adequate weight gain, and developmental milestones.
- **RENAL IMPAIRMENT**
Dose adjustments Start with small doses in severe impairment.
- **MONITORING REQUIREMENTS** Routine measurement of plasma concentrations of antiepileptic drugs is not usually justified, because the target concentration ranges are arbitrary and often vary between individuals. However, plasma drug concentrations may be measured in children with worsening seizures, status epilepticus, suspected noncompliance, or suspected toxicity. Similarly, haematological and biochemical monitoring should not be undertaken unless clinically indicated.
- **PRESCRIBING AND DISPENSING INFORMATION** The RCPCH and NPPG recommend that, when a liquid special of clonazepam is required, the following strength is used: 2 mg/5 mL.
Switching between formulations Care should be taken when switching between oral formulations in the treatment of epilepsy. The need for continued supply of a particular manufacturer's product should be based on clinical judgement and consultation with the patient or their carer, taking into account factors such as seizure frequency and treatment history.
Patients being treated for epilepsy may need to be maintained on a specific manufacturer's branded or generic oral clonazepam product.
- **PATIENT AND CARER ADVICE**
Medicines for Children leaflet: Clonazepam for preventing seizures www.medicinesforchildren.org.uk/clonazepam-preventing-seizures-0

- **MEDICINAL FORMS** There can be variation in the licensing of different medicines containing the same drug. Forms available from special-order manufacturers include: orodispersible tablet, oral suspension, oral solution

Tablet

CAUTIONARY AND ADVISORY LABELS 2, 8

- Clonazepam (Non-proprietary)
  Clonazepam 500 microgram Clonazepam 500microgram tablets | 100 tablet [PoM] £31.82 DT = £31.67 [CD4-1]
  Clonazepam 2 mg Clonazepam 2mg tablets | 100 tablet [PoM] £34.50 DT = £34.33 [CD4-1]

Oral solution

CAUTIONARY AND ADVISORY LABELS 2, 8
EXCIPIENTS: May contain Ethanol

- Clonazepam (Non-proprietary)
  Clonazepam 100 microgram per 1 ml Clonazepam 500micrograms/5ml oral solution sugar free sugar-free | 150 ml [PoM] £77.09 DT = £77.09 [CD4-1]
  Clonazepam 400 microgram per 1 ml Clonazepam 2mg/5ml oral solution sugar free sugar-free | 150 ml [PoM] £108.38 DT = £108.38 [CD4-1]

233

Diazepam

21-Oct-2019

- **INDICATIONS AND DOSE**

Tetanus

- BY INTRAVENOUS INJECTION
- Child: 100–300 micrograms/kg every 1–4 hours
- BY INTRAVENOUS INFUSION, OR BY NASODUODENAL TUBE
- Child: 3–10 mg/kg, adjusted according to response, to be given over 24 hours

Muscle spasm in cerebral spasticity or in postoperative skeletal muscle spasm

- BY MOUTH
- Child 1–11 months: Initially 250 micrograms/kg twice daily
- Child 1–4 years: Initially 2.5 mg twice daily
- Child 5–11 years: Initially 5 mg twice daily
- Child 12–17 years: Initially 10 mg twice daily; maximum 40 mg per day

Status epilepticus | Febrile convulsions | Convulsions due to poisoning

- BY INTRAVENOUS INJECTION
- Neonate: 300–400 micrograms/kg, then 300–400 micrograms/kg after 10 minutes if required, to be given over 3–5 minutes.
- Child 1 month–11 years: 300–400 micrograms/kg (max. per dose 10 mg), then 300–400 micrograms/kg after 10 minutes if required, to be given over 3–5 minutes
- Child 12–17 years: 10 mg, then 10 mg after 10 minutes if required, to be given over 3–5 minutes
- BY RECTUM
- Neonate: 1.25–2.5 mg, then 1.25–2.5 mg after 10 minutes if required.
- Child 1 month–1 year: 5 mg, then 5 mg after 10 minutes if required
- Child 2–11 years: 5–10 mg, then 5–10 mg after 10 minutes if required
- Child 12–17 years: 10–20 mg, then 10–20 mg after 10 minutes if required

Life-threatening acute drug-induced dystonic reactions

- BY INTRAVENOUS INJECTION
- Child 1 month–11 years: 100 micrograms/kg, repeated if necessary, to be given over 3–5 minutes
- Child 12–17 years: 5–10 mg, repeated if necessary, to be given over 3–5 minutes

- **UNLICENSED USE**
- With rectal use *Diazepam Desitin®*, *Diazepam Rectubes®*, and *Stesolid Rectal Tubes®* not licensed for use in children under 1 year.

IMPORTANT SAFETY INFORMATION

ANAESTHESIA

Benzodiazepines should only be administered for anaesthesia by, or under the direct supervision of, personnel experienced in their use, with adequate training in anaesthesia and airway management.

- **CONTRA-INDICATIONS** Avoid injections containing benzyl alcohol in neonates · CNS depression · compromised airway · hyperkinesis · respiratory depression
- **CAUTIONS**

GENERAL CAUTIONS Muscle weakness · organic brain changes · parenteral administration (close observation required until full recovery from sedation)

SPECIFIC CAUTIONS

- With intravenous use High risk of venous thrombophlebitis with intravenous use (reduced by using an emulsion formulation)

CAUTIONS, FURTHER INFORMATION

- Special precautions for intravenous injection When given intravenously facilities for reversing respiratory depression with mechanical ventilation must be immediately available.

- **INTERACTIONS** → Appendix 1: diazepam
- **SIDE-EFFECTS**

GENERAL SIDE-EFFECTS

- **Common or very common** Appetite abnormal · movement disorders · muscle spasms · palpitations · sensory disorder
- **Uncommon** Concentration impaired · constipation · diarrhoea · hypersalivation · skin reactions · speech slurred · vomiting
- **Rare or very rare** Bradycardia · bronchial secretion increased · cardiac arrest · dry mouth · gynaecomastia · heart failure · leucopenia · loss of consciousness · memory loss · respiratory arrest · sexual dysfunction · syncope
- **Frequency not known** Apnoea · nystagmus

SPECIFIC SIDE-EFFECTS

- **Rare or very rare**
- With intravenous or oral use Psychiatric disorder

- **PREGNANCY** Women who have seizures in the second half of pregnancy should be assessed for eclampsia before any change is made to antiepileptic treatment. Status epilepticus should be treated according to the standard protocol.
  Epilepsy and Pregnancy Register All pregnant women with epilepsy, whether taking medication or not, should be encouraged to notify the UK Epilepsy and Pregnancy Register (Tel: 0800 389 1248).
- **BREAST FEEDING** Present in milk, and should be avoided if possible during breast-feeding.
- **RENAL IMPAIRMENT**
  Dose adjustments Start with small doses in severe impairment.
- **DIRECTIONS FOR ADMINISTRATION**
- With intravenous use Diazepam is adsorbed by plastics of infusion bags and giving sets. Emulsion formulation preferred for intravenous injection.
  For *continuous intravenous infusion* of diazepam emulsion, dilute to a concentration of max. 400 micrograms/mL with Glucose 5% or 10%; max. 6 hours between addition and completion of infusion. For *continuous intravenous infusion* of diazepam solution, dilute to a concentration of max. 50 micrograms/mL with Glucose 5% or Sodium Chloride 0.9%.

- **PATIENT AND CARER ADVICE** Patients or carers should be given advice on how and when to administer rectal diazepam. Patients given sedatives and analgesics during minor outpatient procedures should be very carefully warned about the risks of undertaking skilled tasks (e.g. driving) afterwards. For intravenous benzodiazepines the risk extends to **at least 24 hours** after administration. Responsible persons should be available to take patients home afterwards. The dangers of taking **alcohol** should be emphasised.
Medicines for Children leaflet: Diazepam (rectal) for stopping seizures www.medicinesforchildren.org.uk/diazepam-rectal-stopping-seizures-0
Medicines for Children leaflet: Diazepam for muscle spasm www.medicinesforchildren.org.uk/diazepam-muscle-spasm-0
- **PROFESSION SPECIFIC INFORMATION**
Dental practitioners' formulary
Diazepam Tablets may be prescribed.
Diazepam Oral Solution 2 mg/5 mL may be prescribed.

- **MEDICINAL FORMS** There can be variation in the licensing of different medicines containing the same drug. Forms available from special-order manufacturers include: oral suspension, oral solution, suppository

Tablet
CAUTIONARY AND ADVISORY LABELS 2, 19
- Diazepam (Non-proprietary)
Diazepam 2 mg Diazepam 2mg tablets | 28 tablet PoM £1.10 DT = £0.80 CD4-1
Diazepam 5 mg Diazepam 5mg tablets | 28 tablet PoM £1.12 DT = £0.82 CD4-1
Diazepam 10 mg Diazepam 10mg tablets | 28 tablet PoM £4.99 DT = £0.92 CD4-1

Emulsion for injection
- Diazemuls (Accord Healthcare Ltd)
Diazepam 5 mg per 1 ml Diazemuls 10mg/2ml emulsion for injection ampoules | 10 ampoule PoM £9.05 CD4-1

Solution for injection
EXCIPIENTS: May contain Benzyl alcohol, ethanol, propylene glycol
- Diazepam (Non-proprietary)
Diazepam 5 mg per 1 ml Diazepam 10mg/2ml solution for injection ampoules | 10 ampoule PoM £5.50–£6.50 DT = £5.50 CD4-1

Oral suspension
CAUTIONARY AND ADVISORY LABELS 2, 19
- Diazepam (Non-proprietary)
Diazepam 400 microgram per 1 ml Diazepam 2mg/5ml oral suspension | 100 ml PoM £31.75–£48.84 DT = £38.32 CD4-1

Oral solution
CAUTIONARY AND ADVISORY LABELS 2, 19
- Diazepam (Non-proprietary)
Diazepam 400 microgram per 1 ml Diazepam 2mg/5ml oral solution sugar-free | 100 ml PoM £58.35 DT = £54.14 CD4-1

Enema
CAUTIONARY AND ADVISORY LABELS 2, 19
- Diazepam (Non-proprietary)
Diazepam 2 mg per 1 ml Diazepam 5mg RecTubes | 5 tube PoM £5.85 DT = £6.49 CD4-1
Diazepam 2.5mg RecTubes | 5 tube PoM £5.65 DT = £5.65 CD4-1
Diazepam 5mg/2.5ml rectal solution tube | 5 tube PoM £5.85–£6.55 DT = £6.49 CD4-1
Diazepam 4 mg per 1 ml Diazepam 10mg RecTubes | 5 tube PoM £7.35 DT = £7.40 CD4-1
Diazepam 10mg/2.5ml rectal solution tube | 5 tube PoM £7.40 DT = £7.40 CD4-1
- Stesolid (Accord Healthcare Ltd)
Diazepam 2 mg per 1 ml Stesolid 5mg rectal tube | 5 tube PoM £6.89 DT = £6.49 CD4-1
Diazepam 4 mg per 1 ml Stesolid 10mg rectal tube | 5 tube PoM £8.78 DT = £7.40 CD4-1

1.1 Status epilepticus

Other drugs used for Status epilepticus Diazepam, p. 236 · Fosphenytoin sodium, p. 213 · Phenobarbital, p. 232 · Phenytoin, p. 220

ANTIEPILEPTICS

Paraldehyde

10-Mar-2020

- **INDICATIONS AND DOSE**

Status epilepticus
- BY RECTUM
  - Neonate: 0.8 mL/kilogram for 1 dose, the dose is based on the use of a premixed solution of paraldehyde in olive oil in equal volumes.
  - Child: 0.8 mL/kilogram (max. per dose 20 mL) for 1 dose, the dose is based on the use of a premixed solution of paraldehyde in olive oil in equal volumes

- **UNLICENSED USE** Not licensed for use in children as an enema.
- **CONTRA-INDICATIONS** Gastric disorders · rectal administration in colitis
- **CAUTIONS** Bronchopulmonary disease
- **INTERACTIONS** → Appendix 1: antiepileptics
- **SIDE-EFFECTS** Rash
- **PREGNANCY** Avoid unless essential—crosses placenta. See also *Pregnancy* in Epilepsy p. 203.
- **BREAST FEEDING** Avoid unless essential—present in milk.
- **HEPATIC IMPAIRMENT** Manufacturer advises caution.
- **PATIENT AND CARER ADVICE**
Medicines for Children leaflet: Paraldehyde for seizures www.medicinesforchildren.org.uk/paraldehyde-seizures

- **MEDICINAL FORMS** Forms available from special-order manufacturers include: enema

ANTIEPILEPTICS > BARBITURATES

Thiopental sodium

02-Dec-2019

(Thiopentone sodium)

- **INDICATIONS AND DOSE**

Prolonged status epilepticus
- INITIALLY BY SLOW INTRAVENOUS INJECTION
  - Neonate: Initially up to 2 mg/kg, then (by continuous intravenous infusion) up to 8 mg/kg/hour, adjusted according to response.
  - Child: Initially up to 4 mg/kg, then (by continuous intravenous infusion) up to 8 mg/kg/hour, adjusted according to response

Induction of anaesthesia
- BY SLOW INTRAVENOUS INJECTION
  - Neonate: Initially up to 2 mg/kg, then 1 mg/kg, repeated if necessary; maximum 4 mg/kg per course.
  - Child: Initially up to 4 mg/kg, then 1 mg/kg, repeated if necessary; maximum 7 mg/kg per course

- **UNLICENSED USE** Not licensed for use in status epilepticus. Not licensed for use by intravenous infusion.

IMPORTANT SAFETY INFORMATION
Thiopental sodium should only be administered by, or under the direct supervision of, personnel experienced

4 Nervous system

in its use, with adequate training in anaesthesia and airway management, and when resuscitation equipment is available.

- **CONTRA-INDICATIONS** Acute porphyrias p. 652 · myotonic dystrophy
- **CAUTIONS** Acute circulatory failure (shock) · avoid intra-arterial injection · cardiovascular disease · fixed cardiac output · hypovolaemia · reconstituted solution is highly alkaline (extravasation causes tissue necrosis and severe pain)
- **INTERACTIONS** → Appendix 1: thiopental
- **SIDE-EFFECTS**
  - **Common or very common** Arrhythmia · myocardial contractility decreased
  - **Frequency not known** Appetite decreased · circulatory collapse · cough · electrolyte imbalance · extravasation necrosis · hypotension · respiratory disorders · skin eruption · sneezing
- **PREGNANCY** May depress neonatal respiration when used during delivery.
- **BREAST FEEDING** Breast-feeding can be resumed as soon as mother has recovered sufficiently from anaesthesia.
- **HEPATIC IMPAIRMENT** Manufacturer advises caution.
  Dose adjustments Manufacturer advises dose reduction.
- **RENAL IMPAIRMENT** Caution in severe impairment.
- **DIRECTIONS FOR ADMINISTRATION** For *intravenous injection*, reconstitute 500-mg vial with 20 mL Water for Injections to give 25 mg/mL solution; give over at least 10–15 seconds; for *intravenous infusion* reconstituted solution may be further diluted with Sodium Chloride 0.9%.
- **PATIENT AND CARER ADVICE**
  Driving and skilled tasks Patients given sedatives and analgesics during minor outpatient procedures should be very carefully warned about the risk of driving or undertaking skilled tasks afterwards. For a short general anaesthetic the risk extends to **at least 24 hours** after administration. Responsible persons should be available to take patients home. The dangers of taking **alcohol** should also be emphasised.
- **MEDICINAL FORMS** There can be variation in the licensing of different medicines containing the same drug. Forms available from special-order manufacturers include: solution for injection

Powder for solution for injection

- Thiopental sodium (Non-proprietary)
  Thiopental sodium 500 mg Thiopental 500mg powder for solution for injection vials | 10 vial [PoM] £57.60-£69.00 | 25 vial [PoM] £172.50

HYPNOTICS, SEDATIVES AND ANXIOLYTICS > BENZODIAZEPINES

233

Lorazepam

21-Oct-2019

- **INDICATIONS AND DOSE**

Premedication

▶ BY MOUTH

- Child 1 month–11 years: 50–100 micrograms/kg (max. per dose 4 mg), to be given at least 1 hour before procedure, same dose may be given the night before procedure in addition to, or to replace, dose before procedure
- Child 12–17 years: 1–4 mg, to be given at least 1 hour before procedure, same dose may be given the night before procedure in addition to, or to replace, dose before procedure

▶ BY INTRAVENOUS INJECTION

- Child: 50–100 micrograms/kg (max. per dose 4 mg), to be administered 30–45 minutes before procedure

Status epilepticus | Febrile convulsions | Convulsions caused by poisoning

▶ BY SLOW INTRAVENOUS INJECTION

- Neonate: 100 micrograms/kg for 1 dose, then 100 micrograms/kg after 10 minutes if required for 1 dose, to be administered into a large vein.
- Child 1 month–11 years: 100 micrograms/kg (max. per dose 4 mg) for 1 dose, then 100 micrograms/kg after 10 minutes (max. per dose 4 mg) if required for 1 dose, to be administered into a large vein
- Child 12–17 years: 4 mg for 1 dose, then 4 mg after 10 minutes if required for 1 dose, to be administered into a large vein

- **UNLICENSED USE** Not licensed for use in febrile convulsions. Not licensed for use in convulsions caused by poisoning. Not licensed for use as intravenous premedication in children under 12 years. Not licensed for use as oral premedication in children under 5 years.

IMPORTANT SAFETY INFORMATION

ANAESTHESIA

Benzodiazepines should only be administered for anaesthesia by, or under the direct supervision of, personnel experienced in their use, with adequate training in anaesthesia and airway management.

- **CONTRA-INDICATIONS** Avoid injections containing benzyl alcohol in neonates · CNS depression · compromised airway · respiratory depression
- **CAUTIONS** Muscle weakness · organic brain changes · parenteral administration

  CAUTIONS, FURTHER INFORMATION
  - Paradoxical effects A paradoxical increase in hostility and aggression may be reported by patients taking benzodiazepines. The effects range from talkativeness and excitement to aggressive and antisocial acts. Adjustment of the dose (up or down) sometimes attenuates the impulses. Increased anxiety and perceptual disorders are other paradoxical effects.
  - Special precautions for parenteral administration When given parenterally, facilities for managing respiratory depression with mechanical ventilation must be available. Close observation required until full recovery from sedation.
- **INTERACTIONS** → Appendix 1: lorazepam
- **SIDE-EFFECTS**

  GENERAL SIDE-EFFECTS
  - **Common or very common** Apnoea · asthenia · coma · disinhibition · extrapyramidal symptoms · hypothermia · memory loss · speech slurred · suicide attempt
  - **Uncommon** Allergic dermatitis · constipation · sexual dysfunction
  - **Rare or very rare** Agranulocytosis · hyponatraemia · pancytopenia · SIADH · thrombocytopenia

  SPECIFIC SIDE-EFFECTS
  - **Rare or very rare**
    - With oral use Saliva altered
  - **Frequency not known**
    - With parenteral use Leucopenia
- **BREAST FEEDING** Benzodiazepines are present in milk, and should be avoided if possible during breast-feeding.
- **RENAL IMPAIRMENT**
  Dose adjustments Start with small doses in severe impairment.
- **DIRECTIONS FOR ADMINISTRATION** For *intravenous injection*, dilute with an equal volume of Sodium Chloride

0.9% (for neonates, dilute injection solution to a concentration of 100 micrograms/mL). Give over 3–5 minutes; max. rate 50 micrograms/kg over 3 minutes.

- **PATIENT AND CARER ADVICE**

Driving and skilled tasks Patients given sedatives and analgesics during minor outpatient procedures should be very carefully warned about the risks of undertaking skilled tasks (e.g. driving) afterwards. For intravenous benzodiazepines the risk extends to **at least 24 hours** after administration. Responsible persons should be available to take patients home afterwards. The dangers of taking **alcohol** should be emphasised.

- **MEDICINAL FORMS** There can be variation in the licensing of different medicines containing the same drug. Forms available from special-order manufacturers include: oral suspension, oral solution, solution for injection

Solution for injection

EXCIPIENTS: May contain Benzyl alcohol, propylene glycol

▸ Lorazepam (Non-proprietary)

Lorazepam 2 mg per 1 ml Lorazepam 2mg/1ml solution for injection vials | 10 vial PoM ⊠ CD4-1

▸ Ativan (Pfizer Ltd)

Lorazepam 4 mg per 1 ml Ativan 4mg/1ml solution for injection ampoules | 10 ampoule PoM £3.54 CD4-1

Tablet

CAUTIONARY AND ADVISORY LABELS 2, 19

▸ Lorazepam (Non-proprietary)

Lorazepam 500 microgram Lorazepam 500microgram tablets | 28 tablet PoM £10.00–£12.75 DT = £11.00 CD4-1

Lorazepam 1 mg Lorazepam 1mg tablets | 28 tablet PoM £6.59 DT = £3.29 CD4-1

Lorazepam 2.5 mg Lorazepam 2.5mg tablets | 28 tablet PoM £11.43 DT = £7.25 CD4-1

233

Midazolam

21-Mar-2018

- **INDICATIONS AND DOSE**

Status epilepticus | Febrile convulsions

▸ BY BUCCAL ADMINISTRATION

- Neonate: 300 micrograms/kg, then 300 micrograms/kg after 10 minutes if required.
- Child 1–2 months: 300 micrograms/kg (max. per dose 2.5 mg), then 300 micrograms/kg after 10 minutes (max. per dose 2.5 mg) if required
- Child 3–11 months: 2.5 mg, then 2.5 mg after 10 minutes if required
- Child 1–4 years: 5 mg, then 5 mg after 10 minutes if required
- Child 5–9 years: 7.5 mg, then 7.5 mg after 10 minutes if required
- Child 10–17 years: 10 mg, then 10 mg after 10 minutes if required

▸ INITIALLY BY INTRAVENOUS INJECTION

- Neonate: Initially 150–200 micrograms/kg, followed by (by continuous intravenous infusion) 60 micrograms/kg/hour, (by continuous intravenous infusion) increased in steps of 60 micrograms/kg/hour every 15 minutes (max. per dose 300 micrograms/kg/hour) until seizure controlled.
- Child: Initially 150–200 micrograms/kg, followed by (by continuous intravenous infusion) 60 micrograms/kg/hour, (by continuous intravenous infusion) increased in steps of 60 micrograms/kg/hour every 15 minutes (max. per dose 300 micrograms/kg/hour) until seizure controlled

Conscious sedation for procedures

▸ BY MOUTH

- Child: 500 micrograms/kg (max. per dose 20 mg), to be administered 30–60 minutes before procedure

▸ BY BUCCAL ADMINISTRATION

- Child 6 months–9 years: 200–300 micrograms/kg (max. per dose 5 mg)
- Child 10–17 years (body-weight up to 70 kg): 6–7 mg
- Child 10–17 years (body-weight 70 kg and above): 6–7 mg (max. per dose 8 mg)

▸ BY RECTUM

- Child 6 months–11 years: 300–500 micrograms/kg, to be administered 15–30 minutes before procedure

▸ BY INTRAVENOUS INJECTION

- Child 1 month–5 years: Initially 25–50 micrograms/kg, to be administered over 2–3 minutes, 5–10 minutes before procedure, dose can be increased if necessary in small steps to maximum total dose per course; maximum 6 mg per course
- Child 6–11 years: Initially 25–50 micrograms/kg, to be administered over 2–3 minutes, 5–10 minutes before procedure, dose can be increased if necessary in small steps to maximum total dose per course; maximum 10 mg per course
- Child 12–17 years: Initially 25–50 micrograms/kg, to be administered over 2–3 minutes, 5–10 minutes before procedure, dose can be increased if necessary in small steps to maximum total dose per course; maximum 7.5 mg per course

Premedication

▸ BY MOUTH

- Child: 500 micrograms/kg (max. per dose 20 mg), to be taken 15–30 minutes before the procedure

▸ BY RECTUM

- Child 6 months–11 years: 300–500 micrograms/kg, to be administered 15–30 minutes before induction

Induction of anaesthesia (but rarely used)

▸ BY SLOW INTRAVENOUS INJECTION

- Child 7–17 years: Initially 150 micrograms/kg (max. per dose 7.5 mg), dose to be given in steps of 50 micrograms/kg (max. 2.5 mg) over 2–5 minutes; wait for 2–5 minutes before subsequent dosing, then 50 micrograms/kg every 2 minutes (max. per dose 2.5 mg) if required; maximum 500 micrograms/kg per course; maximum 25 mg per course

Sedation of patient receiving intensive care

▸ INITIALLY BY SLOW INTRAVENOUS INJECTION

- Child 6 months–11 years: Initially 50–200 micrograms/kg, to be administered over at least 3 minutes, followed by (by continuous intravenous infusion) 30–120 micrograms/kg/hour, adjusted according to response, initial dose may not be required and lower maintenance doses needed if opioid analgesics also used; reduce dose (or reduce or omit initial dose) in hypovolaemia, vasoconstriction, or hypothermia
- Child 12–17 years: Initially 30–300 micrograms/kg, dose to be given in steps of 1–2.5 mg every 2 minutes, followed by (by continuous intravenous infusion) 30–200 micrograms/kg/hour, adjusted according to response, initial dose may not be required and lower maintenance doses needed if opioid analgesics also used; reduce dose (or reduce or omit initial dose) in hypovolaemia, vasoconstriction, or hypothermia

▸ BY CONTINUOUS INTRAVENOUS INFUSION

- Neonate up to 32 weeks corrected gestational age: 60 micrograms/kg/hour for 24 hours, then reduced to 30 micrograms/kg/hour, adjusted according to response for maximum treatment duration of 4 days.
- Neonate 32 weeks corrected gestational age and above: 60 micrograms/kg/hour, adjusted according to response for maximum treatment duration of 4 days.
- Child 1–5 months: 60 micrograms/kg/hour, adjusted according to response

- **UNLICENSED USE** Oromucosal solution not licensed for use in children under 3 months. Unlicensed oromucosal formulations are also available and may have different doses—refer to product literature.

  Injection not licensed for use in status epilepticus or febrile convulsions.

  Not licensed for use in children under 6 months for premedication and conscious sedation.

  Not licensed for use by mouth.

  Not licensed for use by buccal administration for conscious sedation.

IMPORTANT SAFETY INFORMATION

ANAESTHESIA

Benzodiazepines should only be administered for anaesthesia by, or under the direct supervision of, personnel experienced in their use, with adequate training in anaesthesia and airway management.

NHS NEVER EVENT: MIS-SELECTION OF HIGH-STRENGTH MIDAZOLAM DURING CONSCIOUS SEDATION (JANUARY 2018).

In clinical areas performing conscious sedation, high-strength preparations (5 mg/mL in 2 mL and 10 mL ampoules, or 2 mg/mL in 5 mL ampoules) should **not** be selected in place of the 1 mg/mL preparation.

The areas where high-strength midazolam is used should be restricted to those performing general anaesthesia, intensive care, palliative care, or areas where its use has been formally risk-assessed in the organisation. In these situations the higher strength may be more appropriate to administer the prescribed dose.

It is advised that flumazenil is available when midazolam is used, to reverse the effects if necessary.

- **CONTRA-INDICATIONS** CNS depression · compromised airway · severe respiratory depression
- **CAUTIONS** Cardiac disease · children (particularly if cardiovascular impairment) · concentration of midazolam in children under 15 kg not to exceed 1 mg/mL · debilitated patients (reduce dose) · hypothermia · hypovolaemia (risk of severe hypotension) · neonates · risk of airways obstruction and hypoventilation in children under 6 months (monitor respiratory rate and oxygen saturation) · vasoconstriction

  CAUTIONS, FURTHER INFORMATION

  - Recovery when used for sedation Midazolam has a fast onset of action, recovery is faster than for other benzodiazepines such as diazepam, but may be significantly longer in the elderly, in patients with a low cardiac output, or after repeated dosing.
- **INTERACTIONS** → Appendix 1: midazolam
- **SIDE-EFFECTS**

  GENERAL SIDE-EFFECTS

  - **Common or very common** Vomiting
  - **Uncommon** Skin reactions
  - **Rare or very rare** Dry mouth · dyspnoea · hiccups · movement disorders · respiratory disorders
  - **Frequency not known** Disinhibition (severe; with sedative and peri-operative use)

  SPECIFIC SIDE-EFFECTS

  - **Common or very common**
  - With buccal use Level of consciousness decreased
  - **Rare or very rare**
  - With buccal use Apnoea · bradycardia · cardiac arrest · constipation · physical assault · vasodilation
  - **Frequency not known**
  - With buccal use Appetite increased · fall · saliva altered · thrombosis
  - With oral use Angioedema · arrhythmias · asthenia · gait instability · hypersalivation · hypoxia · myopathy
  - With parenteral use Angioedema · apnoea · appetite increased · bradycardia · cardiac arrest · constipation · drug abuse · drug withdrawal seizure · embolism and thrombosis · fall · level of consciousness decreased · physical assault · saliva altered · vasodilation
  - With rectal use Angioedema · apnoea · appetite increased · bradycardia · cardiac arrest · constipation · drug abuse · drug withdrawal seizure · embolism and thrombosis · fall · level of consciousness decreased · physical assault · respiratory arrest (more common with high doses) · saliva altered · vasodilation

  SIDE-EFFECTS, FURTHER INFORMATION Higher doses are associated with prolonged sedation and risk of hypoventilation. The co-administration of midazolam with other sedative, hypnotic, or CNS-depressant drugs results in increased sedation. Midazolam accumulates in adipose tissue, which can significantly prolong sedation, especially in patients with obesity, hepatic impairment or renal impairment.

  Overdose There have been reports of overdosage when high strength midazolam has been used for conscious sedation. The use of high-strength midazolam (5mg/mL in 2mL and 10mL ampoules, or 2mg/mL in 5mL ampoules) should be restricted to general anaesthesia, intensive care, palliative care, or other situations where the risk has been assessed. It is advised that flumazenil is available when midazolam is used, to reverse the effects if necessary.
- **BREAST FEEDING** Small amount present in milk—avoid breast-feeding for 24 hours after administration (although amount probably too small to be harmful after single doses).
- **HEPATIC IMPAIRMENT** For *parenteral preparations* manufacturer advises caution in all degrees of impairment.

  Dose adjustments For *parenteral preparations* manufacturer advises consider dose reduction in all degrees of impairment.
- **RENAL IMPAIRMENT** Use with caution in chronic renal failure.
- **DIRECTIONS FOR ADMINISTRATION**
  - With intravenous use For *intravenous infusion* (*Hypnovel®*), give continuously *in* Glucose 5% *or* Sodium chloride 0.9%. For *intravenous injection* in status epilepticus and febrile convulsions, dilute with Glucose 5% or Sodium Chloride 0.9%; rapid intravenous injection (less than 2 minutes) may cause seizure-like myoclonus in preterm neonate. For neonate and children under 15 kg dilute to a max. concentration of 1 mg/mL. *Neonatal intensive care*, dilute 15 mg/kg body-weight to a final volume of 50 mL with infusion fluid; an intravenous infusion rate of 0.1 mL/hour provides a dose of 30 micrograms/kg/hour.
  - With oral use For administration *by mouth* for sedation and premedication, injection solution may be diluted with apple or black currant juice, chocolate sauce, or cola.
- **PRESCRIBING AND DISPENSING INFORMATION** The RCPCH and NPPG recommend that, when a liquid special of midazolam is required, the following strength is used: 10 mg/5 mL.
- **PATIENT AND CARER ADVICE** Patients or carers should be given advice on how and when to administer midazolam oromucosal solution.

  Patients given sedatives and analgesics during minor outpatient procedures should be very carefully warned about the risks of undertaking skilled tasks (e.g. driving) afterwards. For intravenous benzodiazepines the risk extends to **at least 24 hours** after administration. Responsible persons should be available to take patients home afterwards. The dangers of taking **alcohol** should be emphasised.

  Medicines for Children leaflet: Midazolam for stopping seizures www.medicinesforchildren.org.uk/midazolam-stopping-seizures

● **NATIONAL FUNDING/ACCESS DECISIONS**

EPISTATUS OROMUCOSAL SOLUTION

Scottish Medicines Consortium (SMC) decisions

The *Scottish Medicines Consortium* has advised (November 2017) that midazolam oromucosal solution (*Epistatus*®) is accepted for use within NHS Scotland for the treatment of prolonged, acute, convulsive seizures in patients aged 10 years to less than 18 years.

● **MEDICINAL FORMS** There can be variation in the licensing of different medicines containing the same drug. Forms available from special-order manufacturers include: oromucosal solution, solution for injection, infusion, solution for infusion

Solution for injection

▸ Midazolam (Non-proprietary)

Midazolam (as Midazolam hydrochloride) 1 mg per 1 ml Midazolam 5mg/5ml solution for injection ampoules | 10 ampoule PoM £10.29 DT = £10.29 CD3 | 10 ampoule PoM £16.89 DT = £10.29 (Hospital only) CD3

Midazolam 2mg/2ml solution for injection ampoules | 10 ampoule PoM £4.50–£6.00 DT = £6.00 CD3

Midazolam (as Midazolam hydrochloride) 2 mg per 1 ml Midazolam 10mg/5ml solution for injection ampoules | 10 ampoule PoM £7.51 DT = £7.26 CD3 | 10 ampoule PoM £6.75 DT = £7.26 (Hospital only) CD3

Midazolam (as Midazolam hydrochloride) 5 mg per 1 ml Midazolam 50mg/10ml solution for injection ampoules | 10 ampoule PoM £33.77 DT = £29.25 (Hospital only) CD3 | 10 ampoule PoM £29.25 DT = £29.25 CD3

Midazolam 10mg/2ml solution for injection ampoules | 10 ampoule PoM £7.65 DT = £7.04 CD3 | 10 ampoule PoM £6.75 DT = £7.04 (Hospital only) CD3

▸ Hypnovel (Cheplapharm Arzneimittel GmbH)

Midazolam (as Midazolam hydrochloride) 5 mg per 1 ml Hypnovel 10mg/2ml solution for injection ampoules | 10 ampoule PoM £7.11 DT = £7.04 CD3

Solution for infusion

▸ Midazolam (Non-proprietary)

Midazolam (as Midazolam hydrochloride) 1 mg per 1 ml Midazolam 50mg/50ml solution for infusion pre-filled syringes | 1 pre-filled disposable injection PoM ⊠ (Hospital only) CD3

Midazolam 50mg/50ml solution for infusion vials | 1 vial PoM £9.56–£12.00 CD3

Midazolam (as Midazolam hydrochloride) 2 mg per 1 ml Midazolam 100mg/50ml solution for infusion vials | 1 vial PoM £9.96–£13.50 CD3

Midazolam 100mg/50ml solution for infusion pre-filled syringes | 1 pre-filled disposable injection PoM ⊠ (Hospital only) CD3

Oromucosal solution

CAUTIONARY AND ADVISORY LABELS 2

EXCIPIENTS: May contain Ethanol

▸ Buccolam (Shire Pharmaceuticals Ltd)

Midazolam (as Midazolam hydrochloride) 5 mg per 1 ml Buccolam 10mg/2ml oromucosal solution pre-filled oral syringes sugar-free | 4 unit dose PoM £91.50 DT = £91.50 CD3

Buccolam 7.5mg/1.5ml oromucosal solution pre-filled oral syringes sugar-free | 4 unit dose PoM £89.00 DT = £89.00 CD3

Buccolam 5mg/1ml oromucosal solution pre-filled oral syringes sugar-free | 4 unit dose PoM £85.50 DT = £85.50 CD3

Buccolam 2.5mg/0.5ml oromucosal solution pre-filled oral syringes sugar-free | 4 unit dose PoM £82.00 DT = £82.00 CD3

▸ Epistatus (Veriton Pharma Ltd)

Midazolam (as Midazolam maleate) 10 mg per 1 ml Epistatus 10mg/1ml oromucosal solution pre-filled oral syringes sugar-free | 1 unit dose PoM £45.76 DT = £45.76 CD3

2 Mental health disorders

2.1 Attention deficit hyperactivity disorder

Attention deficit hyperactivity disorder

04-Aug-2018

Description of condition

Attention deficit hyperactivity disorder (ADHD) is a behavioural disorder characterised by hyperactivity, impulsivity and inattention, which can lead to functional impairment such as psychological, social, educational or occupational difficulties. While these symptoms tend to co-exist, some patients are predominantly hyperactive and impulsive, while others are principally inattentive. Symptoms typically appear in children aged 3–7 years, but may not be recognised until after 7 years of age, especially if hyperactivity is not present. ADHD is more commonly diagnosed in males than in females.

ADHD is usually a persisting disorder and some children continue to have symptoms throughout adolescence and into adulthood, where inattentive symptoms tend to persist, and hyperactive-impulsive symptoms tend to recede over time. ADHD is also associated with an increased risk of disorders such as oppositional defiant disorder (ODD), conduct disorder, and possibly mood disorders such as depression, mania, and anxiety, as well as substance misuse.

Aims of treatment

The aims of treatment are to reduce functional impairment, severity of symptoms, and to improve quality of life.

Non-drug treatment

EvGr Children and their parents, or carers should be advised about the importance of a balanced diet, good nutrition and regular exercise. If hyperactivity appears to be influenced by certain foods or drinks, parents or carers should be advised to keep a diary of food or drinks consumed and the associated behaviour. A referral to a dietician should be made where appropriate. ⟨A⟩

Environmental modifications are changes made to the physical environment that can help reduce the impact of ADHD symptoms on a child's day-to-day life. EvGr The modifications should be specific to the child's circumstances, and may involve changes to seating arrangements, lighting and noise, reducing distractions, optimising education by having shorter periods of focus with movement breaks, and the appropriate use of teaching assistants at school. These changes should form part of the discussion at the time of diagnosis of ADHD and be trialled and reviewed for effectiveness before drug treatment is started.

In children aged under 5 years, an ADHD-focused parent-training programme that teaches parents or carers behaviour therapy techniques is recommended as first-line treatment. Specialist advice should be sought if symptoms are still causing significant impairment after completion of the programme and implementation of environmental modifications.

In children aged 5 years and over, advice about ADHD and ADHD-focused support should be given to all parents or carers. In children with ADHD and symptoms of oppositional defiant disorder or conduct disorder, a training programme specific for the coexisting condition, involving either the parent or carer with or without the child is also recommended. Drug treatment should be reserved for children whose symptoms are causing persistent and significant impairment of at least one area of function (such as interpersonal relationships, education attainment, and risk awareness) despite environmental modifications.

In adolescents, a course of cognitive behavioural therapy (CBT) in combination with drug treatment should be considered for those who have had some benefit from drug treatment, but still have symptoms causing significant impairment in at least one area of function (such as social skills with peers, problem-solving, self-control, active listening skills, or dealing with and expressing feelings). (A)

Drug treatment

Child aged under 5 years

EvGr Drug treatment should only be considered in children under 5 years of age on advice from a specialist ADHD service. (A)

Child aged 5 years and over

EvGr Drug treatment should be initiated by a specialist trained in the diagnosis and management of ADHD. Following dose stabilisation, continuation and monitoring of drug treatment can be undertaken by the child's general practitioner under a shared care arrangement. Children with ADHD and anxiety disorder, tic disorder, or autism spectrum disorder should be offered the same treatment options as other children with ADHD. (A) Treatment options for ADHD are not licensed for use in children under 6 years of age.

EvGr Methylphenidate hydrochloride p. 243 is recommended as first-line treatment. If a 6-week trial of methylphenidate hydrochloride p. 243 at the maximum tolerated dose does not reduce symptoms and associated impairment, consider switching to lisdexamfetamine mesilate p. 246. Dexamfetamine sulfate p. 245 can be given to children who are having a beneficial response to lisdexamfetamine mesilate but cannot tolerate its longer duration of effect.

Modified-release preparations of stimulants are preferred because of their pharmacokinetic profile, convenience, improved adherence, reduced risk of drug diversion (drugs being forwarded to others for non-prescription use or misuse), and the lack of need to be taken to school. Immediate-release preparations can be given when more flexible dosing regimens are required, or during initial dose titration. A combination of a modified-release and immediate-release preparation taken at different times of the day can be used to extend the duration of effect. The magnitude, duration of effect, and side-effects of stimulants vary between patients.

Atomoxetine below or guanfacine p. 247 can be given to children who are intolerant of both methylphenidate hydrochloride p. 243 and lisdexamfetamine mesilate, or if symptoms have not responded to separate 6-week trials of both drugs following adequate dose titration and consideration of alternative preparations. If sustained orthostatic hypotension or fainting episodes occur with guanfacine p. 247 treatment, the dose should be reduced or an alternative treatment offered.

Advice from, or referral to a tertiary specialist ADHD service should be considered if the child is unresponsive to one or more stimulant drugs (e.g. methylphenidate hydrochloride p. 243 and lisdexamfetamine mesilate) and one non-stimulant drug (e.g. atomoxetine below and guanfacine p. 247). A specialist service should also be consulted for advice before starting clonidine hydrochloride p. 108 [unlicensed] in children with ADHD and sleep disturbances, rages or tics, and before starting atypical antipsychotics in addition to stimulants in children with ADHD and co-existing pervasive aggression, rages or irritability. (A)

Other treatment options such as bupropion hydrochloride, modafinil, and tricyclic antidepressants [all unlicensed] have been used in the management of ADHD, but due to limited evidence their use is not recommended without specialist advice.

EvGr Children should be monitored for effectiveness of treatment and side-effects, in addition to changes in sleep pattern, and the potential for stimulant diversion or misuse. If the child develops new, or has worsening of existing seizures, review drug treatment and stop any drug that might be contributing to the seizures; treatment can be cautiously reintroduced if it is unlikely to be the cause. Monitor children for the development of tics associated with stimulant use. If tics are stimulant related, consider a dose reduction, stopping treatment, or changing to a non-stimulant drug. If there is worsening of behaviour, consider adjusting drug treatment and reviewing the diagnosis.

Treatment should be reviewed by a specialist at least once a year and trials of treatment-free periods, or dose reductions considered where appropriate. (A)

Useful Resources

Attention deficit hyperactivity disorder: diagnosis and management. National Institute for Health and Care Excellence. Clinical guideline 87. March 2018.
www.nice.org.uk/guidance/ng87

CNS STIMULANTS > CENTRALLY ACTING SYMPATHOMIMETICS

Atomoxetine

30-Jul-2018

- **INDICATIONS AND DOSE**

Attention deficit hyperactivity disorder (initiated by a specialist)

▶ BY MOUTH

▶ Child 6–17 years (body-weight up to 70 kg): Initially 500 micrograms/kg daily for 7 days, dose is increased according to response; maintenance 1.2 mg/kg daily, total daily dose may be given either as a single dose in the morning or in 2 divided doses with last dose no later than early evening, high daily doses to be given under the direction of a specialist; maximum 1.8 mg/kg per day; maximum 120 mg per day

▶ Child 6–17 years (body-weight 70 kg and above): Initially 40 mg daily for 7 days, dose is increased according to response; maintenance 80 mg daily, total daily dose may be given either as a single dose in the morning or in 2 divided doses with last dose no later than early evening, high daily doses to be given under the direction of a specialist; maximum 120 mg per day

- **UNLICENSED USE** Atomoxetine doses in BNF may differ from those in product literature. Doses above 100 mg daily not licensed.
- **CONTRA-INDICATIONS** Phaeochromocytoma · severe cardiovascular disease · severe cerebrovascular disease
- **CAUTIONS** Aggressive behaviour · cardiovascular disease · cerebrovascular disease · emotional lability · history of seizures · hostility · hypertension · mania · psychosis · QT-interval prolongation · structural cardiac abnormalities · susceptibility to angle-closure glaucoma · tachycardia
- **INTERACTIONS** → Appendix 1: atomoxetine
- **SIDE-EFFECTS**

▶ **Common or very common** Anxiety · appetite decreased · asthenia · chest pain · constipation · depression · dizziness · drowsiness · gastrointestinal discomfort · headaches · insomnia · mood altered · mydriasis · nausea · skin reactions · tic · vomiting · weight decreased

▶ **Uncommon** Behaviour abnormal · dyspnoea · hallucination · hyperhidrosis · hypersensitivity · palpitations · psychosis · QT interval prolongation · seizure · sensation abnormal · sinus tachycardia · suicidal behaviour · syncope · tremor · vision blurred

▶ **Rare or very rare** Genital pain · hepatic disorders · priapism · Raynaud's phenomenon · urinary disorders

- **Frequency not known** Sudden cardiac death

- **PREGNANCY** Manufacturer advises avoid unless potential benefit outweighs risk.
- **BREAST FEEDING** Avoid–present in milk in *animal* studies.
- **HEPATIC IMPAIRMENT**

Dose adjustments Manufacturer advises halve dose in moderate impairment and quarter dose in severe impairment.

- **MONITORING REQUIREMENTS**
  - Monitor for appearance or worsening of anxiety, depression or tics.
  - Pulse, blood pressure, psychiatric symptoms, appetite, weight and height should be recorded at initiation of therapy, following each dose adjustment, and at least every 6 months thereafter.
- **PATIENT AND CARER ADVICE**

Suicidal ideation Following reports of suicidal thoughts and behaviour, patients and their carers should be informed about the risk and told to report clinical worsening, suicidal thoughts or behaviour, irritability, agitation, or depression.

Hepatic impairment Following rare reports of hepatic disorders, patients and carers should be advised of the risk and be told how to recognise symptoms; prompt medical attention should be sought in case of abdominal pain, unexplained nausea, malaise, darkening of the urine, or jaundice.

Medicines for Children leaflet: Atomoxetine for attention deficit hyperactivity disorder (ADHD) www.medicinesforchildren.org.uk/atomoxetine-attention-deficit-hyperactivity-disorder-adhd

- **NATIONAL FUNDING/ACCESS DECISIONS**

Scottish Medicines Consortium (SMC) decisions

SMC No. 1107/15

The *Scottish Medicines Consortium* has advised (December 2015) that atomoxetine oral solution (*Strattera®*) is accepted for restricted use within NHS Scotland for the treatment of attention deficit hyperactivity disorder (ADHD) in children of 6 years and older, in adolescents and in adults. It is restricted to patients who are unable to swallow capsules.

- **MEDICINAL FORMS** There can be variation in the licensing of different medicines containing the same drug. Forms available from special-order manufacturers include: oral suspension, oral solution

Oral solution

CAUTIONARY AND ADVISORY LABELS 3

- Strattera (Eli Lilly and Company Ltd)

Atomoxetine (as Atomoxetine hydrochloride) 4 mg per 1 ml Strattera 4mg/1ml oral solution sugar-free | 300 ml PoM £85.00 DT = £85.00

Capsule

CAUTIONARY AND ADVISORY LABELS 3

- Atomoxetine (Non-proprietary)

Atomoxetine (as Atomoxetine hydrochloride) 10 mg Atomoxetine 10mg capsules | 7 capsule PoM £11.94–£13.28 | 28 capsule PoM £53.09 DT = £49.74

Atomoxetine (as Atomoxetine hydrochloride) 18 mg Atomoxetine 18mg capsules | 7 capsule PoM £11.94–£13.28 | 28 capsule PoM £53.09 DT = £49.74

Atomoxetine (as Atomoxetine hydrochloride) 25 mg Atomoxetine 25mg capsules | 7 capsule PoM £11.94–£13.28 | 28 capsule PoM £53.09 DT = £48.88

Atomoxetine (as Atomoxetine hydrochloride) 40 mg Atomoxetine 40mg capsules | 7 capsule PoM £11.94–£13.28 | 28 capsule PoM £53.09 DT = £48.88

Atomoxetine (as Atomoxetine hydrochloride) 60 mg Atomoxetine 60mg capsules | 28 capsule PoM £53.09 DT = £49.63

Atomoxetine (as Atomoxetine hydrochloride) 80 mg Atomoxetine 80mg capsules | 28 capsule PoM £70.79 DT = £66.17

Atomoxetine (as Atomoxetine hydrochloride) 100 mg Atomoxetine 100mg capsules | 28 capsule PoM £70.79 DT = £66.17

- Strattera (Eli Lilly and Company Ltd)

Atomoxetine (as Atomoxetine hydrochloride) 10 mg Strattera 10mg capsules | 7 capsule PoM £13.28 | 28 capsule PoM £53.09 DT = £49.74

Atomoxetine (as Atomoxetine hydrochloride) 18 mg Strattera 18mg capsules | 7 capsule PoM £13.28 | 28 capsule PoM £53.09 DT = £49.74

Atomoxetine (as Atomoxetine hydrochloride) 25 mg Strattera 25mg capsules | 7 capsule PoM £13.28 | 28 capsule PoM £53.09 DT = £48.88

Atomoxetine (as Atomoxetine hydrochloride) 40 mg Strattera 40mg capsules | 7 capsule PoM £13.28 | 28 capsule PoM £53.09 DT = £48.88

Atomoxetine (as Atomoxetine hydrochloride) 60 mg Strattera 60mg capsules | 28 capsule PoM £53.09 DT = £49.63

Atomoxetine (as Atomoxetine hydrochloride) 80 mg Strattera 80mg capsules | 28 capsule PoM £70.79 DT = £66.17

Atomoxetine (as Atomoxetine hydrochloride) 100 mg Strattera 100mg capsules | 28 capsule PoM £70.79 DT = £66.17

Methylphenidate hydrochloride 01-Oct-2019

- **INDICATIONS AND DOSE**

Attention deficit hyperactivity disorder (initiated under specialist supervision)

▶ BY MOUTH USING IMMEDIATE-RELEASE MEDICINES

- Child 4–5 years: Initially 2.5 mg twice daily, increased in steps of 2.5 mg daily if required, at weekly intervals, increased if necessary up to 1.4 mg/kg daily in 2–3 divided doses, discontinue if no response after 1 month, if effect wears off in evening (with rebound hyperactivity) a dose at bedtime may be appropriate (establish need with trial bedtime dose). Treatment may be started using a modified-release preparation
- Child 6–17 years: Initially 5 mg 1–2 times a day, increased in steps of 5–10 mg daily if required, at weekly intervals, increased if necessary up to 60 mg daily in 2–3 divided doses, increased if necessary up to 2.1 mg/kg daily in 2–3 divided doses, the licensed maximum dose is 60 mg daily in 2–3 doses, higher dose (up to a maximum of 90 mg daily) under the direction of a specialist, discontinue if no response after 1 month, if effect wears off in evening (with rebound hyperactivity) a dose at bedtime may be appropriate (establish need with trial bedtime dose). Treatment may be started using a modified-release preparation

DOSE EQUIVALENCE AND CONVERSION

- When switching from *immediate-release* preparations to *modified-release* preparations—consult product literature.

CONCERTA ® XL

Attention deficit hyperactivity disorder

▶ BY MOUTH

- Child 6–17 years: Initially 18 mg once daily, dose to be taken in the morning, increased in steps of 18 mg every week, adjusted according to response; increased if necessary up to 2.1 mg/kg daily, licensed max. dose is 54 mg once daily, to be increased to higher dose only under direction of specialist; discontinue if no response after 1 month; maximum 108 mg per day

DOSE EQUIVALENCE AND CONVERSION

- Total daily dose of 15 mg of standard-release formulation is considered equivalent to *Concerta®* XL 18 mg once daily.

DELMOSART ® PROLONGED-RELEASE TABLET

Attention deficit hyperactivity disorder (under expert supervision)

▶ BY MOUTH

- Child 6–17 years: Initially 18 mg once daily, dose to be taken in the morning, then increased in steps of 18 mg every week if required, discontinue if no response after 1 month; maximum 54 mg per day

continued →

DOSE EQUIVALENCE AND CONVERSION
- Total daily dose of 15 mg of standard-release formulation is considered equivalent to *Delmosart*® 18 mg once daily.

EQUASYM® XL

Attention deficit hyperactivity disorder

- BY MOUTH
- Child 6–17 years: Initially 10 mg once daily, dose to be taken in the morning before breakfast; increased gradually at weekly intervals if necessary; increased if necessary up to 2.1 mg/kg daily, licensed max. dose is 60 mg daily, to be increased to higher dose only under direction of specialist; discontinue if no response after 1 month; maximum 90 mg per day

MEDIKINET® XL

Attention deficit hyperactivity disorder

- BY MOUTH
- Child 6–17 years: Initially 10 mg once daily, dose to be taken in the morning with breakfast; adjusted at weekly intervals according to response; increased if necessary up to 2.1 mg/kg daily, licensed max. dose is 60 mg daily, to be increased to higher dose only under direction of specialist; discontinue if no response after 1 month; maximum 90 mg per day

XAGGITIN® XL

Attention deficit hyperactivity disorder (under expert supervision)

- BY MOUTH
- Child 6–17 years: Initially 18 mg once daily, dose to be taken in the morning, increased in steps of 18 mg every week, adjusted according to response, discontinue if no response after 1 month; maximum 54 mg per day

DOSE EQUIVALENCE AND CONVERSION
- Total daily dose of 15 mg of standard-release formulation is considered equivalent to *Xaggitin*® XL 18 mg once daily.

- **UNLICENSED USE** Doses over 60 mg daily not licensed; doses of *Concerta XL* over 54 mg daily not licensed. Not licensed for use in children under 6 years.
- **CONTRA-INDICATIONS** Anorexia nervosa · arrhythmias · cardiomyopathy · cardiovascular disease · cerebrovascular disorders · heart failure · hyperthyroidism · mania · phaeochromocytoma · psychosis · severe depression · severe hypertension · structural cardiac abnormalities · suicidal tendencies · uncontrolled bipolar disorder · vasculitis
- **CAUTIONS** Agitation · alcohol dependence · anxiety · drug dependence · epilepsy (discontinue if increased seizure frequency) · family history of Tourette syndrome · susceptibility to angle-closure glaucoma · tics

CONCERTA® XL, DELMOSART® PROLONGED-RELEASE TABLET Dysphagia (dose form not appropriate) · restricted gastro-intestinal lumen (dose form not appropriate)

XAGGITIN® XL Dysphagia (dose form not appropriate)

- **INTERACTIONS** → Appendix 1: methylphenidate
- **SIDE-EFFECTS**
- **Common or very common** Alopecia · anxiety · appetite decreased · arrhythmias · arthralgia · behaviour abnormal · cough · depression · diarrhoea · dizziness · drowsiness · dry mouth · fever · gastrointestinal discomfort · growth retardation · headaches · hypertension · laryngeal pain · mood altered · movement disorders · nasopharyngitis · nausea · palpitations · sleep disorders · vomiting · weight decreased
- **Uncommon** Chest discomfort · constipation · dyspnoea · fatigue · haematuria · hallucinations · muscle complaints · psychotic disorder · suicidal tendencies · tic · tremor · vision disorders
- **Rare or very rare** Anaemia · angina pectoris · cardiac arrest · cerebrovascular insufficiency · confusion · gynaecomastia · hepatic coma · hyperfocus · hyperhidrosis · leucopenia · mydriasis · myocardial infarction · neuroleptic malignant syndrome · peripheral coldness · Raynaud's phenomenon · seizures · sexual dysfunction · skin reactions · sudden cardiac death · thinking abnormal · thrombocytopenia
- **Frequency not known** Delusions · drug dependence · hyperpyrexia · intracranial haemorrhage · logorrhea · pancytopenia · vasculitis

- **PREGNANCY** Limited experience—avoid unless potential benefit outweighs risk.
- **BREAST FEEDING** Limited information available—avoid.
- **MONITORING REQUIREMENTS**
  - Monitor for psychiatric disorders.
  - Pulse, blood pressure, psychiatric symptoms, appetite, weight and height should be recorded at initiation of therapy, following each dose adjustment, and at least every 6 months thereafter.
- **TREATMENT CESSATION** Avoid abrupt withdrawal.
- **DIRECTIONS FOR ADMINISTRATION**

MEDIKINET® XL Contents of capsule can be sprinkled on a tablespoon of apple sauce or yoghurt (then swallowed immediately without chewing).

EQUASYM® XL Contents of capsule can be sprinkled on a tablespoon of apple sauce (then swallowed immediately without chewing).

- **PRESCRIBING AND DISPENSING INFORMATION** Different versions of modified-release preparations may not have the same clinical effect. To avoid confusion between these different formulations of methylphenidate, prescribers should specify the brand to be dispensed.

CONCERTA® XL Consists of an immediate-release component (22% of the dose) and a modified-release component (78% of the dose).

MEDIKINET® XL Consists of an immediate-release component (50% of the dose) and a modified-release component (50% of the dose).

EQUASYM® XL Consists of an immediate-release component (30% of the dose) and a modified-release component (70% of the dose).

- **PATIENT AND CARER ADVICE**

Medicines for Children leaflet: Methylphenidate for attention deficit hyperactivity disorder (ADHD) www.medicinesforchildren.org.uk/methylphenidate-attention-deficit-hyperactivity-disorder-adhd

Driving and skilled tasks **Drugs and Driving** Prescribers and other healthcare professionals should advise patients if treatment is likely to affect their ability to perform skilled tasks (e.g. driving). This applies especially to drugs with sedative effects; patients should be warned that these effects are increased by alcohol. General information about a patient's fitness to drive is available from the Driver and Vehicle Licensing Agency at www.gov.uk/government/organisations/driver-and-vehicle-licensing-agency.

2015 legislation regarding driving whilst taking certain drugs, may also apply to methylphenidate, see *Drugs and skilled tasks* under Guidance on prescribing p. 1.

CONCERTA® XL Tablet membrane may pass through gastro-intestinal tract unchanged.

DELMOSART® PROLONGED-RELEASE TABLET Manufacturer advises tablet membrane may pass through gastro-intestinal tract unchanged.

- **MEDICINAL FORMS** There can be variation in the licensing of different medicines containing the same drug. Forms available from special-order manufacturers include: modified-release tablet, oral suspension, oral solution

Modified-release tablet

CAUTIONARY AND ADVISORY LABELS 25

▸ Concerta XL (Janssen-Cilag Ltd)
Methylphenidate hydrochloride 18 mg Concerta XL 18mg tablets | 30 tablet PoM £31.19 DT = £31.19 CD2
Methylphenidate hydrochloride 27 mg Concerta XL 27mg tablets | 30 tablet PoM £36.81 DT = £36.81 CD2
Methylphenidate hydrochloride 36 mg Concerta XL 36mg tablets | 30 tablet PoM £42.45 DT = £42.45 CD2
Methylphenidate hydrochloride 54 mg Concerta XL 54mg tablets | 30 tablet PoM £73.62 DT = £36.80 CD2

▸ Delmosart (Actavis UK Ltd)
Methylphenidate hydrochloride 18 mg Delmosart 18mg modified-release tablets | 30 tablet PoM £15.57 DT = £31.19 CD2
Methylphenidate hydrochloride 27 mg Delmosart 27mg modified-release tablets | 30 tablet PoM £18.39 DT = £36.81 CD2
Methylphenidate hydrochloride 36 mg Delmosart 36mg modified-release tablets | 30 tablet PoM £21.21 DT = £42.45 CD2
Methylphenidate hydrochloride 54 mg Delmosart 54mg modified-release tablets | 30 tablet PoM £36.79 DT = £36.80 CD2

▸ Xaggitin XL (Ethypharm UK Ltd)
Methylphenidate hydrochloride 18 mg Xaggitin XL 18mg tablets | 30 tablet PoM £15.58 DT = £31.19 CD2
Methylphenidate hydrochloride 27 mg Xaggitin XL 27mg tablets | 30 tablet PoM £18.40 DT = £36.81 CD2
Methylphenidate hydrochloride 36 mg Xaggitin XL 36mg tablets | 30 tablet PoM £21.22 DT = £42.45 CD2
Methylphenidate hydrochloride 54 mg Xaggitin XL 54mg tablets | 30 tablet PoM £36.80 DT = £36.80 CD2

Tablet

▸ Methylphenidate hydrochloride (Non-proprietary)
Methylphenidate hydrochloride 5 mg Methylphenidate 5mg tablets | 30 tablet PoM £3.82 DT = £3.03 CD2
Methylphenidate hydrochloride 10 mg Methylphenidate 10mg tablets | 30 tablet PoM £5.29 DT = £3.80 CD2
Methylphenidate hydrochloride 20 mg Methylphenidate 20mg tablets | 30 tablet PoM £12.88 DT = £10.92 CD2

▸ Medikinet (Flynn Pharma Ltd)
Methylphenidate hydrochloride 5 mg Medikinet 5mg tablets | 30 tablet PoM £3.03 DT = £3.03 CD2
Methylphenidate hydrochloride 10 mg Medikinet 10mg tablets | 30 tablet PoM £5.49 DT = £3.80 CD2
Methylphenidate hydrochloride 20 mg Medikinet 20mg tablets | 30 tablet PoM £10.92 DT = £10.92 CD2

▸ Ritalin (Novartis Pharmaceuticals UK Ltd)
Methylphenidate hydrochloride 10 mg Ritalin 10mg tablets | 30 tablet PoM £6.68 DT = £3.80 CD2

▸ Tranquilyn (Genesis Pharmaceuticals Ltd)
Methylphenidate hydrochloride 5 mg Tranquilyn 5mg tablets | 30 tablet PoM £3.03 DT = £3.03 CD2
Methylphenidate hydrochloride 10 mg Tranquilyn 10mg tablets | 30 tablet PoM £4.27 DT = £3.80 CD2
Methylphenidate hydrochloride 20 mg Tranquilyn 20mg tablets | 30 tablet PoM £10.92 DT = £10.92 CD2

Modified-release capsule

CAUTIONARY AND ADVISORY LABELS 25

▸ Methylphenidate hydrochloride (Non-proprietary)
Methylphenidate hydrochloride 10 mg Ritalin XL 10mg capsules | 30 capsule PoM £23.92 DT = £25.00 CD2
Methylphenidate hydrochloride 20 mg Ritalin XL 20mg capsules | 30 capsule PoM £28.72 DT = £30.00 CD2
Methylphenidate hydrochloride 30 mg Ritalin XL 30mg capsules | 30 capsule PoM £33.49 DT = £35.00 CD2
Methylphenidate hydrochloride 40 mg Ritalin XL 40mg capsules | 30 capsule PoM £57.43 DT = £57.72 CD2
Methylphenidate hydrochloride 60 mg Ritalin XL 60mg capsules | 30 capsule PoM £66.98 DT = £67.32 CD2

▸ Equasym XL (Shire Pharmaceuticals Ltd)
Methylphenidate hydrochloride 10 mg Equasym XL 10mg capsules | 30 capsule PoM £25.00 DT = £25.00 CD2
Methylphenidate hydrochloride 20 mg Equasym XL 20mg capsules | 30 capsule PoM £30.00 DT = £30.00 CD2
Methylphenidate hydrochloride 30 mg Equasym XL 30mg capsules | 30 capsule PoM £35.00 DT = £35.00 CD2

▸ Medikinet XL (Flynn Pharma Ltd) ▼
Methylphenidate hydrochloride 5 mg Medikinet XL 5mg capsules | 30 capsule PoM £24.04 DT = £24.04 CD2
Methylphenidate hydrochloride 10 mg Medikinet XL 10mg capsules | 30 capsule PoM £24.04 DT = £25.00 CD2
Methylphenidate hydrochloride 20 mg Medikinet XL 20mg capsules | 30 capsule PoM £28.86 DT = £30.00 CD2
Methylphenidate hydrochloride 30 mg Medikinet XL 30mg capsules | 30 capsule PoM £33.66 DT = £35.00 CD2
Methylphenidate hydrochloride 40 mg Medikinet XL 40mg capsules | 30 capsule PoM £57.72 DT = £57.72 CD2
Methylphenidate hydrochloride 50 mg Medikinet XL 50mg capsules | 30 capsule PoM £62.52 DT = £62.52 CD2
Methylphenidate hydrochloride 60 mg Medikinet XL 60mg capsules | 30 capsule PoM £67.32 DT = £67.32 CD2

CNS STIMULANTS › CENTRALLY ACTING SYMPATHOMIMETICS › AMFETAMINES

Dexamfetamine sulfate

13-Dec-2019

(Dexamphetamine sulfate)

- **INDICATIONS AND DOSE**

Refractory attention deficit hyperactivity disorder (initiated under specialist supervision)

▸ BY MOUTH

▸ Child 6–17 years: Initially 2.5 mg 2–3 times a day, increased in steps of 5 mg once weekly if required; usual maximum 1 mg/kg daily, up to 20 mg daily (40 mg daily has been required in some children); maintenance dose to be given in 2–4 divided doses

- **CONTRA-INDICATIONS** Advanced arteriosclerosis · anorexia · arrhythmias (life-threatening) · cardiomyopathies · cardiovascular disease · cerebrovascular disorders · heart failure · history of alcohol abuse · history of drug abuse · hyperexcitability · hyperthyroidism · moderate hypertension · psychiatric disorders · psychosis · severe hypertension · structural cardiac abnormalities · suicidal tendencies

CONTRA-INDICATIONS, FURTHER INFORMATION

▸ Psychiatric disorders Psychiatric disorders include severe depression, schizophrenia, borderline personality disorder and uncontrolled bipolar disorder. Co-morbidity with psychiatric disorders is common in attention deficit hyperactivity disorder. Manufacturer advises if new psychiatric symptoms develop or exacerbation of psychiatric disorders occurs, continue use only if benefits outweigh risks.

- **CAUTIONS** History of epilepsy (discontinue if seizures occur) · mild hypertension · susceptibility to angle-closure glaucoma · tics · Tourette syndrome

CAUTIONS, FURTHER INFORMATION

▸ Tics and Tourette syndrome Discontinue use if tics occur.

▸ Growth restriction in children Monitor height and weight as growth restriction may occur during prolonged therapy (drug-free periods may allow catch-up in growth but withdraw slowly to avoid inducing depression or renewed hyperactivity).

- **INTERACTIONS** → Appendix 1: amfetamines
- **SIDE-EFFECTS**

▸ **Common or very common** Abdominal pain · anxiety · appetite decreased · arrhythmias · arthralgia · behaviour abnormal · depression · dry mouth · headache · mood altered · movement disorders · muscle cramps · nausea · palpitations · poor weight gain · sleep disorders · vertigo · vomiting · weight decreased

▸ **Rare or very rare** Anaemia · angina pectoris · cardiac arrest · cerebrovascular insufficiency · fatigue · growth retardation · hallucination · hepatic coma · hepatic function abnormal · intracranial haemorrhage · leucopenia · mydriasis · psychosis · seizure · skin reactions · suicidal

tendencies · thrombocytopenia · tic (in those at risk) · vasculitis cerebral · vision disorders
- **Frequency not known** Acidosis · alopecia · cardiomyopathy · chest pain · circulatory collapse · colitis ischaemic · concentration impaired · confusion · diarrhoea · dizziness · drug dependence · hyperhidrosis · hypermetabolism · hyperpyrexia · kidney injury · myocardial infarction · neuroleptic malignant syndrome · obsessive-compulsive disorder · reflexes increased · rhabdomyolysis · sexual dysfunction · sudden death · taste altered · tremor

Overdose Amfetamines cause wakefulness, excessive activity, paranoia, hallucinations, and hypertension followed by exhaustion, convulsions, hyperthermia, and coma. See Stimulants under Emergency treatment of poisoning p. 891.

- **PREGNANCY** Avoid (retrospective evidence of uncertain significance suggesting possible embryotoxicity).
- **BREAST FEEDING** Significant amount in milk—avoid.
- **RENAL IMPAIRMENT** Use with caution.
- **MONITORING REQUIREMENTS**
  - Monitor growth in children.
  - Monitor for aggressive behaviour or hostility during initial treatment.
  - Pulse, blood pressure, psychiatric symptoms, appetite, weight and height should be recorded at initiation of therapy, following each dose adjustment, and at least every 6 months thereafter.
- **TREATMENT CESSATION** Avoid abrupt withdrawal.
- **DIRECTIONS FOR ADMINISTRATION** Tablets can be halved.
- **PRESCRIBING AND DISPENSING INFORMATION** Data on safety and efficacy of long-term use not complete.
- **PATIENT AND CARER ADVICE**

Driving and skilled tasks **Drugs and Driving** Prescribers and other healthcare professionals should advise patients if treatment is likely to affect their ability to perform skilled tasks (e.g. driving). This applies especially to drugs with sedative effects; patients should be warned that these effects are increased by alcohol. General information about a patient's fitness to drive is available from the Driver and Vehicle Licensing Agency at www.dvla.gov.uk.

For information on 2015 legislation regarding driving whilst taking certain controlled drugs, including amfetamines, see *Drugs and skilled tasks* under Guidance on prescribing p. 1.

- **MEDICINAL FORMS** There can be variation in the licensing of different medicines containing the same drug. Forms available from special-order manufacturers include: modified-release capsule, oral suspension, oral solution

Oral solution
- Dexamfetamine sulfate (Non-proprietary)
  Dexamfetamine sulfate 1 mg per 1 ml Dexamfetamine 5mg/5ml oral solution sugar-free | 150 ml [PoM] £114.49 DT = £114.49 [CD2]

Modified-release capsule
- Dexedrine Spansules (Imported (United States))
  Dexamfetamine sulfate 5 mg Dexedrine 5mg Spansules | 100 capsule [PoM] [X] [CD2]
  Dexamfetamine sulfate 10 mg Dexedrine 10mg Spansules | 100 capsule [PoM] [X] [CD2]
  Dexamfetamine sulfate 15 mg Dexedrine 15mg Spansules | 100 capsule [PoM] [X] [CD2]

Tablet
- Dexamfetamine sulfate (Non-proprietary)
  Dexamfetamine sulfate 5 mg Dexamfetamine 5mg tablets | 28 tablet [PoM] £24.75 DT = £24.72 [CD2]
- Amfexa (Flynn Pharma Ltd)
  Dexamfetamine sulfate 5 mg Amfexa 5mg tablets | 30 tablet [PoM] £19.89 [CD2]
  Dexamfetamine sulfate 10 mg Amfexa 10mg tablets | 30 tablet [PoM] £39.78 DT = £39.78 [CD2]
  Dexamfetamine sulfate 20 mg Amfexa 20mg tablets | 30 tablet [PoM] £79.56 DT = £79.56 [CD2]

Lisdexamfetamine mesilate

14-Jan-2020

- **DRUG ACTION** Lisdexamfetamine is a prodrug of dexamfetamine.
- **INDICATIONS AND DOSE**

Attention deficit hyperactivity disorder (initiated by a specialist)
- BY MOUTH
  - Child 6–17 years: Initially 30 mg once daily, alternatively initially 20 mg once daily, increased in steps of 10–20 mg every week if required, dose to be taken in the morning, discontinue if response insufficient after 1 month; maximum 70 mg per day

- **CONTRA-INDICATIONS** Advanced arteriosclerosis · agitated states · hyperthyroidism · moderate hypertension · severe hypertension · symptomatic cardiovascular disease
- **CAUTIONS** Bipolar disorder · history of cardiovascular disease · history of substance abuse · may lower seizure threshold (discontinue if seizures occur) · psychotic disorders · susceptibility to angle-closure glaucoma · tics · Tourette syndrome

CAUTIONS, FURTHER INFORMATION
- Cardiovascular disease Manufacturer advises caution in patients with underlying conditions that might be compromised by increases in blood pressure or heart rate; see also *Contra-indications*.

- **INTERACTIONS** → Appendix 1: amfetamines
- **SIDE-EFFECTS**
  - **Common or very common** Abdominal pain upper · anxiety · appetite decreased · behaviour abnormal · constipation · depression · diarrhoea · dizziness · drowsiness · dry mouth · dyspnoea · fatigue · feeling jittery · fever · headache · insomnia · mood altered · nausea · palpitations · psychiatric disorders · skin reactions · tachycardia · tremor · vomiting · weight decreased
  - **Uncommon** Cardiomyopathy · erectile dysfunction · hallucination · hyperhidrosis · logorrhea · movement disorders · mydriasis · Raynaud's phenomenon · taste altered · vision blurred
  - **Frequency not known** Angioedema · drug dependence · hepatitis allergic · psychotic disorder · seizure · Stevens-Johnson syndrome

Overdose Amfetamines cause wakefulness, excessive activity, paranoia, hallucinations, and hypertension followed by exhaustion, convulsions, hyperthermia, and coma. See Stimulants under Emergency treatment of poisoning p. 891.

- **PREGNANCY** Manufacturer advises use only if potential benefit outweighs risk.
- **BREAST FEEDING** Manufacturer advises avoid—present in human milk.
- **RENAL IMPAIRMENT**

Dose adjustments Manufacturer advises max. dose 50 mg daily in severe impairment.

- **MONITORING REQUIREMENTS**
  - Manufacturer advises monitor for aggressive behaviour or hostility during initial treatment.
  - Manufacturer advises monitor pulse, blood pressure, and for psychiatric symptoms before treatment initiation, following each dose adjustment, and at least every 6 months thereafter. Monitor weight in adults before treatment initiation and during treatment; in children, height and weight should be recorded before treatment initiation, and height, weight and appetite monitored at least every 6 months during treatment.
- **TREATMENT CESSATION** Avoid abrupt withdrawal.
- **DIRECTIONS FOR ADMINISTRATION** Manufacturer advises swallow whole or mix contents of capsule with soft food

such as yoghurt or in a glass of water or orange juice; contents should be dispersed completely and consumed immediately.

- **PATIENT AND CARER ADVICE** Patients and carers should be counselled on the administration of capsules.

Driving and skilled tasks **Drugs and Driving** Prescribers and other healthcare professionals should advise patients if treatment is likely to affect their ability to perform skilled tasks (e.g. driving). This applies especially to drugs with sedative effects; patients should be warned that these effects are increased by alcohol. General information about a patient's fitness to drive is available from the Driver and Vehicle Licensing Agency at www.gov.uk/government/organisations/driver-and-vehicle-licensing-agency.

For information on 2015 legislation regarding driving whilst taking certain controlled drugs, including amfetamines, see *Drugs and skilled tasks* under Guidance on prescribing p. 1.

- **NATIONAL FUNDING/ACCESS DECISIONS**

Scottish Medicines Consortium (SMC) decisions

The *Scottish Medicines Consortium* has advised (May 2013) that lisdexamfetamine dimesylate (*Elvanse*®) is accepted for use within NHS Scotland as part of a comprehensive treatment programme for attention deficit hyperactivity disorder (ADHD) in children aged 6 years and over when response to previous methylphenidate treatment is considered clinically inadequate.

All Wales Medicines Strategy Group (AWMSG) decisions

The *All Wales Medicines Strategy Group* has advised (December 2013) that lisdexamfetamine dimesylate (*Elvanse*®) is recommended as an option for use within NHS Wales as part of a comprehensive treatment programme for attention deficit hyperactivity disorder (ADHD) in children aged six years and over when response to previous methylphenidate treatment is considered clinically inadequate. Treatment must be under the supervision of a specialist in childhood and/or adolescent behavioural disorders.

- **MEDICINAL FORMS** There can be variation in the licensing of different medicines containing the same drug.

Capsule

CAUTIONARY AND ADVISORY LABELS 3, 25

- Elvanse (Shire Pharmaceuticals Ltd)
  - **Lisdexamfetamine dimesylate 20 mg** Elvanse 20mg capsules | 28 capsule PoM £54.62 DT = £54.62 CD2
  - **Lisdexamfetamine dimesylate 30 mg** Elvanse Adult 30mg capsules | 28 capsule PoM £58.24 DT = £58.24 CD2
  - Elvanse 30mg capsules | 28 capsule PoM £58.24 DT = £58.24 CD2
  - **Lisdexamfetamine dimesylate 40 mg** Elvanse 40mg capsules | 28 capsule PoM £62.82 DT = £62.82 CD2
  - **Lisdexamfetamine dimesylate 50 mg** Elvanse Adult 50mg capsules | 28 capsule PoM £68.60 DT = £68.60 CD2
  - Elvanse 50mg capsules | 28 capsule PoM £68.60 DT = £68.60 CD2
  - **Lisdexamfetamine dimesylate 60 mg** Elvanse 60mg capsules | 28 capsule PoM £75.18 DT = £75.18 CD2
  - **Lisdexamfetamine dimesylate 70 mg** Elvanse 70mg capsules | 28 capsule PoM £83.16 DT = £83.16 CD2
  - Elvanse Adult 70mg capsules | 28 capsule PoM £83.16 DT = £83.16 CD2

SYMPATHOMIMETICS > ALPHA$_2$-ADRENOCEPTOR AGONISTS

Guanfacine

03-Apr-2020

- **INDICATIONS AND DOSE**

Attention deficit hyperactivity disorder in children for whom stimulants are not suitable, not tolerated or ineffective (initiated under specialist supervision)

- BY MOUTH
  - Child 6–12 years (body-weight 25 kg and above): Initially 1 mg once daily; adjusted in steps of 1 mg every week if necessary and if tolerated; maintenance 0.05–0.12 mg/kg once daily (max. per dose 4 mg), for optimal weight-adjusted dose titrations, consult product literature
  - Child 13–17 years (body-weight 34–41.4 kg): Initially 1 mg once daily; adjusted in steps of 1 mg every week if necessary and if tolerated; maintenance 0.05–0.12 mg/kg once daily (max. per dose 4 mg), for optimal weight-adjusted dose titrations, consult product literature
  - Child 13–17 years (body-weight 41.5–49.4 kg): Initially 1 mg once daily; adjusted in steps of 1 mg every week if necessary and if tolerated; maintenance 0.05–0.12 mg/kg once daily (max. per dose 5 mg), for optimal weight-adjusted dose titrations, consult product literature
  - Child 13–17 years (body-weight 49.5–58.4 kg): Initially 1 mg once daily; adjusted in steps of 1 mg every week if necessary and if tolerated; maintenance 0.05–0.12 mg/kg once daily (max. per dose 6 mg), for optimal weight-adjusted dose titrations, consult product literature
  - Child 13–17 years (body-weight 58.5 kg and above): Initially 1 mg once daily; adjusted in steps of 1 mg every week if necessary and if tolerated; maintenance 0.05–0.12 mg/kg once daily (max. per dose 7 mg), for optimal weight-adjusted dose titrations, consult product literature

DOSE ADJUSTMENTS DUE TO INTERACTIONS

- Manufacturer advises reduce dose by half with concurrent use of moderate and potent inhibitors of CYP3A4.
- Manufacturer advises increase dose up to max. 7 mg daily with concurrent use of potent inducers of CYP3A4—no specific recommendation made for children.

- **CAUTIONS** Bradycardia (risk of torsade de pointes) · heart block (risk of torsade de pointes) · history of cardiovascular disease · history of QT-interval prolongation · hypokalaemia (risk of torsade de pointes)
- **INTERACTIONS** → Appendix 1: guanfacine
- **SIDE-EFFECTS**
  - **Common or very common** Anxiety · appetite decreased · arrhythmias · asthenia · constipation · depression · diarrhoea · dizziness · drowsiness · dry mouth · gastrointestinal discomfort · headache · hypotension · mood altered · nausea · skin reactions · sleep disorders · urinary disorders · vomiting · weight increased
  - **Uncommon** Asthma · atrioventricular block · chest pain · hallucination · loss of consciousness · pallor · seizure · syncope
  - **Rare or very rare** Hypertension · hypertensive encephalopathy · malaise
  - **Frequency not known** Erectile dysfunction

SIDE-EFFECTS, FURTHER INFORMATION Somnolence and sedation may occur, predominantly during the first 2-3 weeks of treatment and with dose increases; manufacturer advises to consider dose reduction or discontinuation of treatment if symptoms are clinically significant or persistent.

Overdose Features may include hypotension, initial hypertension, bradycardia, lethargy, and respiratory depression. Manufacturer advises that patients who develop lethargy should be observed for development of more serious toxicity for up to 24 hours.

- **CONCEPTION AND CONTRACEPTION** Manufacturer recommends effective contraception in females of childbearing potential.
- **PREGNANCY** Manufacturer advises avoid—toxicity in *animal* studies.

- **BREAST FEEDING** Manufacturer advises avoid—present in milk in *animal* studies.
- **HEPATIC IMPAIRMENT** Manufacturer advises caution (pharmacokinetics have not been assessed in paediatric patients with hepatic impairment).
  Dose adjustments Manufacturer advises consider dose reduction.
- **RENAL IMPAIRMENT**
  Dose adjustments Manufacturer advises consider dose reduction in severe impairment and end-stage renal disease.
- **MONITORING REQUIREMENTS**
  - Manufacturer advises to conduct a baseline evaluation to identify patients at risk of somnolence, sedation, hypotension, bradycardia, QT-prolongation, and arrhythmia; this should include assessment of cardiovascular status. Monitor for signs of these adverse effects weekly during dose titration and then every 3 months during the first year of treatment, and every 6 months thereafter. Monitor BMI prior to treatment and then every 3 months for the first year of treatment, and every 6 months thereafter. More frequent monitoring is advised following dose adjustments.
  - Monitor blood pressure and pulse during dose downward titration and following discontinuation of treatment.
- **TREATMENT CESSATION** Manufacturer advises avoid abrupt withdrawal; consider dose tapering to minimise potential withdrawal effects.
- **DIRECTIONS FOR ADMINISTRATION** Manufacturer advises avoid administration with high fat meals (may increase absorption).
- **PATIENT AND CARER ADVICE** Patients or carers should be counselled on administration of guanfacine modified-release tablets.
  Missed doses Manufacturer advises that patients and carers should inform their prescriber if more than one dose is missed; consider dose re-titration.
  Driving and skilled tasks Manufacturer advises patients and carers should be counselled about the effects on driving and performance of skilled tasks—increased risk of dizziness and syncope.

- **MEDICINAL FORMS** There can be variation in the licensing of different medicines containing the same drug.

Modified-release tablet

CAUTIONARY AND ADVISORY LABELS 2, 25

- Intuniv (Shire Pharmaceuticals Ltd) ▼
  Guanfacine (as Guanfacine hydrochloride) 1 mg Intuniv 1mg modified-release tablets | 28 tablet PoM £56.00 DT = £56.00
  Guanfacine (as Guanfacine hydrochloride) 2 mg Intuniv 2mg modified-release tablets | 28 tablet PoM £58.52 DT = £58.52
  Guanfacine (as Guanfacine hydrochloride) 3 mg Intuniv 3mg modified-release tablets | 28 tablet PoM £65.52 DT = £65.52
  Guanfacine (as Guanfacine hydrochloride) 4 mg Intuniv 4mg modified-release tablets | 28 tablet PoM £76.16 DT = £76.16

2.2 Bipolar disorder and mania

Mania and hypomania

21-Feb-2020

Overview

Antimanic drugs are used to control acute attacks and to prevent recurrence of episodes of mania or hypomania.

An antidepressant drug may also be required for the treatment of co-existing depression, but should be avoided in patients with rapid-cycling bipolar disorder, a recent history of hypomania, or with rapid mood fluctuations.

Benzodiazepines

Use of benzodiazepines may be helpful in the initial stages of treatment for behavioural disturbance or agitation; they should not be used for long periods because of the risk of dependence.

Antipsychotic drugs

Antipsychotic drugs (normally olanzapine p. 267, quetiapine p. 268, or risperidone p. 270) are useful in acute episodes of mania and hypomania; if the response to antipsychotic drugs is inadequate, lithium or valproate may be added. An antipsychotic drug may be used concomitantly with lithium or valproate in the initial treatment of severe acute mania. See *Important safety information*, *Conception and contraception*, and *Pregnancy* in the valproic acid p. 228 and sodium valproate p. 223 monographs.

Atypical antipsychotics are the treatment of choice for the long-term management of bipolar disorder in children and adolescents; if the patient has frequent relapses or continuing functional impairment, consider concomitant therapy with lithium or valproate. An atypical antipsychotic that causes less weight gain and does not increase prolactin levels is preferred.

When discontinuing antipsychotics, the dose should be reduced gradually over at least 4 weeks if the child is continuing on other antimanic drugs; if the child is not continuing on other antimanic drugs, or has a history of manic relapse, a withdrawal period of up to 3 months is required.

Carbamazepine

Carbamazepine p. 209 may be used under specialist supervision for the prophylaxis of bipolar disorder (manic-depressive disorder) in children unresponsive to a combination of other prophylactic drugs; it is used in patients with rapid-cycling manic-depressive illness (4 or more affective episodes per year). The dose of carbamazepine should not normally be increased if an acute episode of mania occurs.

Valproate

Valproic acid (as the semisodium salt) is licensed in adults for the treatment of manic episodes associated with bipolar disorder. Sodium valproate is unlicensed for the treatment of bipolar disorder. Valproate (valproic acid and sodium valproate) can also be used for the prophylaxis of bipolar disorder [unlicensed use]. It must be started and supervised by a specialist experienced in managing bipolar disorder. Because of its teratogenic risk, valproate must not be used in females of childbearing potential unless the conditions of the Pregnancy Prevention Programme are met and alternative treatments are ineffective or not tolerated. Valproic acid and sodium valproate must not be used during pregnancy in bipolar disorder. The benefit and risk of valproate therapy should be carefully reconsidered at regular treatment reviews. For further information, see *Important safety information*, *Conception and contraception*, and *Pregnancy* in the valproic acid and sodium valproate monographs.

In patients with frequent relapse or continuing functional impairment, consider switching therapy to lithium or an atypical antipsychotic, or adding lithium or an atypical antipsychotic to valproate. If a patient taking valproate experiences an acute episode of mania that is not ameliorated by increasing the valproate dose, consider concomitant therapy with olanzapine, quetiapine, or risperidone.

Lithium

Lithium salts are used in the prophylaxis and treatment of mania, in the prophylaxis of bipolar disorder (manic-depressive disorder), and bipolar depression, and as concomitant therapy with antidepressant medication in children who have had an incomplete response to treatment for acute depression in bipolar disorder [unlicensed indication]. It is also used for the treatment of aggressive or self-harming behaviour [unlicensed indication].

The decision to give prophylactic lithium requires specialist advice, and must be based on careful consideration of the likelihood of recurrence in the individual child, and the benefit of treatment weighed against the risks. The full prophylactic effect of lithium may not occur for six to twelve months after the initiation of therapy. An atypical antipsychotic or valproate (given alone or as adjunctive therapy with lithium) are alternative prophylactic treatments in patients who experience frequent relapses or continued functional impairment.

Other drugs used for Bipolar disorder and mania
Aripiprazole, p. 265 · Chlorpromazine hydrochloride, p. 261 · Haloperidol, p. 261 · Lamotrigine, p. 216 · Prochlorperazine, p. 285

ANTIPSYCHOTICS > LITHIUM SALTS

Lithium salts

- **CONTRA-INDICATIONS** Addison's disease · cardiac disease associated with rhythm disorder · cardiac insufficiency · dehydration · family history of Brugada syndrome · low sodium diets · personal history of Brugada syndrome · untreated hypothyroidism
- **CAUTIONS** Avoid abrupt withdrawal · cardiac disease · concurrent ECT (may lower seizure threshold) · diuretic treatment (risk of toxicity) · epilepsy (may lower seizure threshold) · myasthenia gravis · psoriasis (risk of exacerbation) · QT interval prolongation · review dose as necessary in diarrhoea · review dose as necessary in intercurrent infection (especially if sweating profusely) · review dose as necessary in vomiting · surgery

  CAUTIONS, FURTHER INFORMATION

  ▸ Long-term use Long-term use of lithium has been associated with thyroid disorders and mild cognitive and memory impairment. Long-term treatment should therefore be undertaken only with careful assessment of risk and benefit, and with monitoring of thyroid function every 6 months (more often if there is evidence of deterioration).

  The need for continued therapy should be assessed regularly and patients should be maintained on lithium after 3–5 years only if benefit persists.
- **SIDE-EFFECTS**

  ▸ **Rare or very rare** Nephropathy

  ▸ **Frequency not known** Abdominal discomfort · alopecia · angioedema · appetite decreased · arrhythmias · atrioventricular block · cardiomyopathy · cerebellar syndrome · circulatory collapse · coma · delirium · diarrhoea · dizziness · dry mouth · electrolyte imbalance · encephalopathy · folliculitis · gastritis · goitre · hyperglycaemia · hyperparathyroidism · hypersalivation · hypotension · hypothyroidism · idiopathic intracranial hypertension · leucocytosis · memory loss · movement disorders · muscle weakness · myasthenia gravis · nausea · neoplasms · nystagmus · peripheral neuropathy · peripheral oedema · polyuria · QT interval prolongation · reflexes abnormal · renal disorders · renal impairment · rhabdomyolysis · seizure · sexual dysfunction · skin reactions · skin ulcer · speech impairment · taste altered · thyrotoxicosis · tremor · vertigo · vision disorders · vomiting · weight increased

  Overdose Signs of intoxication require withdrawal of treatment and include increasing gastro-intestinal disturbances (vomiting, diarrhoea), visual disturbances, polyuria, muscle weakness, fine tremor increasing to coarse tremor, CNS disturbances (confusion and drowsiness increasing to lack of coordination, restlessness, stupor); abnormal reflexes, myoclonus, incontinence, hypernatraemia. With severe overdosage seizures, cardiac arrhythmias (including sino-atrial block, bradycardia and first-degree heart block), blood pressure changes, circulatory failure, renal failure, coma and sudden death reported.

  For details on the management of poisoning, see Lithium, under Emergency treatment of poisoning p. 891.
- **CONCEPTION AND CONTRACEPTION** Manufacturer advises effective contraception during treatment for women of child bearing potential.
- **PREGNANCY** Avoid if possible, particularly in the first trimester (risk of teratogenicity, including cardiac abnormalities).

  Dose adjustments Dose requirements increased during the second and third trimesters (but on delivery return abruptly to normal).

  Monitoring Close monitoring of serum-lithium concentration advised in pregnancy (risk of toxicity in neonate).
- **BREAST FEEDING** Present in milk and risk of toxicity in infant—avoid.
- **RENAL IMPAIRMENT** Caution in mild to moderate impairment. Avoid in severe impairment.

  Monitoring In renal impairment monitor serum-lithium concentration closely and adjust dose accordingly.
- **MONITORING REQUIREMENTS**

  ▸ Serum concentrations Lithium salts have a narrow therapeutic/toxic ratio and should therefore not be prescribed unless facilities for monitoring serum-lithium concentrations are available.

  Samples should be taken 12 hours after the dose to achieve a serum-lithium concentration of 0.4–1 mmol/litre (lower end of the range for maintenance therapy).

  A target serum-lithium concentration of 0.8–1 mmol/litre is recommended for acute episodes of mania, and for patients who have previously relapsed or have sub-syndromal symptoms. It is important to determine the optimum range for each individual patient.

  [EvGr] Routine serum-lithium monitoring should be performed weekly after initiation and after each dose change until concentrations are stable, then every 3 months for the first year, and every 6 months thereafter. Patients who are taking drugs that interact with lithium, at risk of impaired renal or thyroid function, raised calcium levels or other complications, have poor symptom control or poor adherence, or whose last serum-lithium concentration was 0.8 mmol/litre or higher, should be monitored every 3 months. ⟨A⟩ Additional serum-lithium measurements should be made if a patient develops significant intercurrent disease or if there is a significant change in a patient's sodium or fluid intake.

  ▸ Manufacturer advises to assess renal, cardiac, and thyroid function before treatment initiation. [EvGr] An ECG is recommended in patients with cardiovascular disease or risk factors for it. Body-weight or BMI, serum electrolytes, and a full blood count should also be measured before treatment initiation.

  ▸ Monitor body-weight or BMI, serum electrolytes, eGFR, and thyroid function every 6 months during treatment, and more often if there is evidence of impaired renal or thyroid function, or raised calcium levels. ⟨A⟩

  Manufacturer also advises to monitor cardiac function regularly.
- **TREATMENT CESSATION** While there is no clear evidence of withdrawal or rebound psychosis, abrupt discontinuation of lithium increases the risk of relapse. If lithium is to be discontinued, the dose should be reduced gradually over a period of at least 4 weeks (preferably over a period of up to 3 months). Patients and their carers should be warned of the risk of relapse if lithium is discontinued abruptly. If

lithium is stopped or is to be discontinued abruptly, consider changing therapy to an atypical antipsychotic or valproate.

- **PATIENT AND CARER ADVICE** Patients should be advised to report signs and symptoms of lithium toxicity, hypothyroidism, renal dysfunction (including polyuria and polydipsia), and benign intracranial hypertension (persistent headache and visual disturbance). Maintain adequate fluid intake and avoid dietary changes which reduce or increase sodium intake.
Lithium treatment packs A lithium treatment pack should be given to patients on initiation of treatment with lithium. The pack consists of a patient information booklet, lithium alert card, and a record book for tracking serum-lithium concentration. Packs may be purchased from
3M
0845 610 1112
nhsforms@mmm.uk.com
Driving and skilled tasks May impair performance of skilled tasks (e.g. driving, operating machinery).

F 249

Lithium carbonate

- **INDICATIONS AND DOSE**

Treatment and prophylaxis of mania | Treatment and prophylaxis of bipolar disorder | Treatment and prophylaxis of recurrent depression | Treatment and prophylaxis of aggressive or self-harming behaviour

▶ BY MOUTH

▸ Child 12–17 years: Dose adjusted according to serum-lithium concentration, doses are initially divided throughout the day, but once daily administration is preferred when serum-lithium concentration stabilised

DOSE EQUIVALENCE AND CONVERSION

▸ **Preparations vary widely in bioavailability;** changing the preparation requires the same precautions as initiation of treatment.

CAMCOLIT ® IMMEDIATE-RELEASE TABLET

Treatment of mania | Treatment of bipolar disorder | Treatment of recurrent depression | Treatment of aggressive or self-harming behaviour

▶ BY MOUTH

▸ Child 12–17 years: Initially 1–1.5 g daily, dose adjusted according to serum-lithium concentration, doses are initially divided throughout the day, but once daily administration is preferred when serum-lithium concentration stabilised

Prophylaxis of mania | Prophylaxis of bipolar disorder | Prophylaxis of recurrent depression | Prophylaxis of aggressive or self-harming behaviour

▶ BY MOUTH

▸ Child 12–17 years: Initially 300–400 mg daily, dose adjusted according to serum-lithium concentration, doses are initially divided throughout the day, but once daily administration is preferred when serum-lithium concentration stabilised

CAMCOLIT ® MODIFIED-RELEASE TABLET

Treatment of mania | Treatment of bipolar disorder | Treatment of recurrent depression | Treatment of aggressive or self-harming behaviour

▶ BY MOUTH

▸ Child 12–17 years: Initially 1–1.5 g daily, dose adjusted according to serum-lithium concentration, doses are initially divided throughout the day, but once daily administration is preferred when serum-lithium concentration stabilised

Prophylaxis of mania | Prophylaxis of bipolar disorder | Prophylaxis of recurrent depression | Prophylaxis of aggressive or self-harming behaviour

▶ BY MOUTH

▸ Child 12–17 years: Initially 300–400 mg daily, dose adjusted according to serum-lithium concentration, doses are initially divided throughout the day, but once daily administration is preferred when serum-lithium concentration stabilised

LISKONUM ®

Treatment of mania | Treatment of bipolar disorder | Treatment of recurrent depression | Treatment of aggressive or self-harming behaviour

▶ BY MOUTH

▸ Child 12–17 years: Initially 225–675 mg twice daily, dose adjusted according to serum-lithium concentration, doses are initially divided throughout the day, but once daily administration is preferred when serum-lithium concentration stabilised

Prophylaxis of mania | Prophylaxis of bipolar disorder | Prophylaxis of recurrent depression | Prophylaxis of aggressive or self-harming behaviour

▶ BY MOUTH

▸ Child 12–17 years: Initially 225–450 mg twice daily, dose adjusted according to serum-lithium concentration, doses are initially divided throughout the day, but once daily administration is preferred when serum-lithium concentration stabilised

- **UNLICENSED USE** Not licensed for aggressive or self-harming behaviour. Not licensed for concomitant therapy with antidepressant medication in children who have had an incomplete response to treatment for acute depression in bipolar disorder. *Camcolit* ® brand not licensed for use in children.
- **INTERACTIONS** → Appendix 1: lithium

- **MEDICINAL FORMS** There can be variation in the licensing of different medicines containing the same drug. Forms available from special-order manufacturers include: oral suspension

Modified-release tablet

CAUTIONARY AND ADVISORY LABELS 10, 25

▸ Camcolit (Essential Pharma Ltd)
Lithium carbonate 400 mg Camcolit 400 modified-release tablets | 100 tablet PoM £48.18 DT = £4.02

▸ Liskonum (Teofarma)
Lithium carbonate 450 mg Liskonum 450mg modified-release tablets | 60 tablet PoM £11.84 DT = £11.84

▸ Priadel (lithium carbonate) (Essential Pharma M)
Lithium carbonate 200 mg Priadel 200mg modified-release tablets | 100 tablet PoM £2.76 DT = £2.76
Lithium carbonate 400 mg Priadel 400mg modified-release tablets | 100 tablet PoM £4.02 DT = £4.02

Tablet

CAUTIONARY AND ADVISORY LABELS 10

▸ Lithium carbonate (Non-proprietary)
Lithium carbonate 250 mg Lithium carbonate 250mg tablets | 100 tablet PoM £87.00 DT = £87.00

F 249

Lithium citrate

- **INDICATIONS AND DOSE**

Treatment and prophylaxis of mania | Treatment and prophylaxis of bipolar disorder | Treatment and prophylaxis of recurrent depression | Treatment and prophylaxis of aggressive or self-harming behaviour

▶ BY MOUTH

▸ Child: Dose adjusted according to serum-lithium concentration; doses are initially divided throughout the day, but once daily administration is preferred when serum-lithium concentration stabilised

DOSE EQUIVALENCE AND CONVERSION
- **Preparations vary widely in bioavailability**; changing the preparation requires the same precautions as initiation of treatment.

LI-LIQUID ®

Treatment and prophylaxis of mania | Treatment and prophylaxis of bipolar disorder | Treatment and prophylaxis of recurrent depression | Treatment and prophylaxis of aggressive or self-harming behaviour
- BY MOUTH
- Child: Dose adjusted according to serum-lithium concentration

DOSE EQUIVALENCE AND CONVERSION
- For *Li-Liquid*®: Lithium citrate tetrahydrate 509 mg is equivalent to lithium carbonate 200 mg.

PRIADEL ® LIQUID

Treatment and prophylaxis of mania | Treatment and prophylaxis of bipolar disorder | Treatment and prophylaxis of recurrent depression | Treatment and prophylaxis of aggressive or self-harming behaviour
- BY MOUTH
- Child: Dose adjusted according to serum-lithium concentration, doses are initially divided throughout the day, but once daily administration is preferred when serum-lithium concentration stabilised

DOSE EQUIVALENCE AND CONVERSION
- For *Priadel® liquid* : Lithium citrate tetrahydrate 520 mg is equivalent to lithium carbonate 204 mg.

- UNLICENSED USE Not licensed for use in children.
- INTERACTIONS → Appendix 1: lithium
- SIDE-EFFECTS Polydipsia

- MEDICINAL FORMS There can be variation in the licensing of different medicines containing the same drug.

Oral solution

CAUTIONARY AND ADVISORY LABELS 10
- Li-Liquid (Rosemont Pharmaceuticals Ltd)
  Lithium citrate 101.8 mg per 1 ml Li-Liquid 509mg/5ml oral solution | 150 ml PoM £5.79 DT = £5.79
  Lithium citrate 203.6 mg per 1 ml Li-Liquid 1.018g/5ml oral solution | 150 ml PoM £17.49 DT = £11.58
- Priadel (lithium citrate) (Essential Pharma M)
  Lithium citrate 104 mg per 1 ml Priadel 520mg/5ml liquid sugar-free | 150 ml PoM £6.73 DT = £6.73

2.3 Depression

Depression

10-Jul-2019

Description of condition

Depression is characterised by persistent low mood which can present as irritability, fatigue, and/or a loss of interest or pleasure in most activities and may be accompanied by symptoms of anxiety.

Associated symptoms, which determine disease severity, are sleep and appetite disturbance, lack of concentration, low self-confidence, agitation, guilt or self-blame and suicidal thoughts or acts.

Based on the International Statistical Classification of Diseases (ICD-10), depression can be classified as mild (four symptoms), moderate (five to six symptoms) or severe (seven or more symptoms, with or without psychotic symptoms).

Depression in childhood is not common and can have a more gradual onset than in adults. Affecting twice as many adolescent females than males, depression often occurs with other behavioural disorders. In almost half of the cases it resolves spontaneously within the first year.

Non-drug treatment

EvGr When assessing a child or young person with depression, take into account family history of mood disorders, experience of bullying or abuse, any alcohol and drug misuse and the possibility of parental substance misuse as this may impact on disease severity or treatment efficacy.

Any co-morbid diagnoses and developmental, social and educational problems should be assessed and managed, either in sequence or in parallel with the treatment for depression.

St John's wort is a herbal remedy available without prescription for treating mild depression in adults. It should not be used for the treatment of depression in children. Ⓐ

Lifestyle changes

EvGr Regular exercise (45 minutes to 1 hour per session, up to three times a week) following a structured programme for 10 to 12 weeks, should be encouraged. Give children, and their parents or carers, advice about good sleep hygiene, anxiety management, nutrition and the benefits of a balanced diet. Ⓐ

Psychological therapy

EvGr Offer three months of psychological therapy as first-line treatment from a therapist trained in child and adolescent mental health, or a healthcare practitioner specifically trained in the psychological therapy. Therapy options include cognitive behavioural therapy (CBT), interpersonal psychotherapy (IPT), IPT for adolescents (IPT-A), non-directive supportive therapy (NDST), psychodynamic psychotherapy, family therapy, brief psychosocial interventions, and intensive psychological therapy.

In mild depression, for those who do not meet referral criteria or who do not want an intervention, a period of watchful waiting and re-assessment of symptoms within two weeks should be arranged. Ⓐ For further information on criteria for referral to Child and Adolescent Mental Health Services (CAMHS) see NICE clinical guideline **Depression in children and young people** (see *Useful resources*).

Drug treatment

Child aged 5 years and over

EvGr Antidepressants should not be used for the initial treatment of children with mild depression. For cases refractory to psychological treatment, antidepressant therapy may be considered under specialist advice.

Drug treatment should only be prescribed following assessment and diagnosis by a child and adolescent psychiatrist.

When an antidepressant is prescribed, the selective serotonin re-uptake inhibitor (SSRI) fluoxetine p. 253 is the first-line treatment in children.

The use of fluoxetine in children aged 5 to 11 years should be cautiously considered as effectiveness in this age group is not established.

For moderate to severe depression, antidepressants should only be offered to children in combination with concurrent psychological therapy.

In children aged 12 years and over, following multidisciplinary review, combination therapy can be considered as an alternative to psychological monotherapy, or in cases refractory to psychological therapy.

Children should be carefully monitored at the start of treatment (for example weekly contact for the first four weeks or according to individual needs). Following remission (no symptoms and full functioning for at least eight weeks), antidepressant treatment should be continued at the same dose for at least six months.

For children unresponsive to treatment with fluoxetine in combination with a psychological therapy, it is

4 Nervous system

recommended to consider an alternative psychological therapy.

In children who present with severe depression and recurrent depressive episodes who do not respond to or cannot tolerate fluoxetine, citalopram p. 253 [unlicensed indication] or sertraline p. 254 [unlicensed indication] can be used as an alternative under specialist supervision.

Paroxetine, venlafaxine and tricyclic antidepressants should not be used for the treatment of depression in children and young people.

In children aged 12 years and over with very severe depression and life-threatening symptoms (such as suicidal behaviour), or who have not responded to other treatments, electroconvulsive therapy can be considered under specialist care. ⟨A⟩

Psychotic depression

EvGr Augmenting existing antidepressant treatment with second generation antipsychotics (under specialist supervision) should be considered for children with psychotic depression, although the optimum dose and duration of treatment are unknown. ⟨A⟩

Suicidal behaviour and antidepressant therapy

EvGr The use of antidepressant drugs has been linked with suicidal thoughts and behaviour, mainly in the early stages of treatment. Children should be monitored for suicidal behaviour, self-harm or hostility, particularly at the beginning of treatment, with medication changes and at times of increased personal stress. ⟨A⟩ For further information on SSRI use and safety, see MHRA/CHM guidance **Selective serotonin reuptake inhibitors (SSRIs) and serotonin and noradrenaline reuptake inhibitors (SNRIs)** (see *Useful resources*).

Useful Resources

Depression in children and young people: identification and management. National Institute for Health and Care Excellence. National Guideline 134. September 2005 (updated June 2019)
www.nice.org.uk/guidance/ng134

Depression in children. National Institute for Health and Care Excellence. Clinical Knowledge Summary. March 2016
cks.nice.org.uk/depression-in-children

Selective serotonin reuptake inhibitors (SSRIs) and serotonin and noradrenaline reuptake inhibitors (SNRIs): use and safety. Medicines and Healthcare products Regulatory Agency. Guidance. December 2014.
www.gov.uk/government/publications/ssris-and-snris-use-and-safety/selective-serotonin-reuptake-inhibitors-ssris-and-serotonin-and-noradrenaline-reuptake-inhibitors-snris-use-and-safety

Other drugs used for Depression Lithium carbonate, p. 250 · Lithium citrate, p. 250 · Quetiapine, p. 268

ANTIDEPRESSANTS › SELECTIVE SEROTONIN RE-UPTAKE INHIBITORS

Selective serotonin re-uptake inhibitors

- **DRUG ACTION** Selectively inhibit the re-uptake of serotonin (5-hydroxytryptamine, 5-HT).
- **CONTRA-INDICATIONS** Poorly controlled epilepsy · SSRIs should not be used if the patient enters a manic phase
- **CAUTIONS** Cardiac disease · concurrent electroconvulsive therapy · diabetes mellitus · epilepsy (discontinue if convulsions develop) · history of bleeding disorders (especially gastro-intestinal bleeding) · history of mania · susceptibility to angle-closure glaucoma
- **SIDE-EFFECTS**
  - ▶ **Common or very common** Anxiety · appetite abnormal · arrhythmias · arthralgia · asthenia · concentration impaired · confusion · constipation · depersonalisation · diarrhoea · dizziness · drowsiness · dry mouth · fever · gastrointestinal discomfort · haemorrhage · headache · hyperhidrosis · malaise · mania · memory loss · menstrual cycle irregularities · myalgia · mydriasis · nausea (dose-related) · palpitations · paraesthesia · QT interval prolongation · sexual dysfunction · skin reactions · sleep disorders · taste altered · tinnitus · tremor · urinary disorders · visual impairment · vomiting · weight changes · yawning
  - ▶ **Uncommon** Alopecia · angioedema · behaviour abnormal · hallucination · movement disorders · photosensitivity reaction · postural hypotension · seizure · suicidal tendencies · syncope
  - ▶ **Rare or very rare** Galactorrhoea · hepatitis · hyperprolactinaemia · hyponatraemia · serotonin syndrome · severe cutaneous adverse reactions (SCARs) · SIADH · thrombocytopenia
  - ▶ **Frequency not known** Withdrawal syndrome

  SIDE-EFFECTS, FURTHER INFORMATION Symptoms of sexual dysfunction may persist after treatment has stopped.

  Overdose Symptoms of poisoning by selective serotonin re-uptake inhibitors include nausea, vomiting, agitation, tremor, nystagmus, drowsiness, and sinus tachycardia; convulsions may occur. Rarely, severe poisoning results in the serotonin syndrome, with marked neuropsychiatric effects, neuromuscular hyperactivity, and autonomic instability; hyperthermia, rhabdomyolysis, renal failure, and coagulopathies may develop.

  For details on the management of poisoning, see Selective serotonin re-uptake inhibitors, under Emergency treatment of poisoning p. 891.
- **PREGNANCY** Manufacturers advise avoid during pregnancy unless the potential benefit outweighs the risk. There is a small increased risk of congenital heart defects when taken during early pregnancy. If used during the third trimester there is a risk of neonatal withdrawal symptoms, and persistent pulmonary hypertension in the newborn has been reported.
- **HEPATIC IMPAIRMENT** In general, manufacturers advise caution (prolonged half-life).
- **TREATMENT CESSATION** Gastro-intestinal disturbances, headache, anxiety, dizziness, paraesthesia, electric shock sensation in the head, neck, and spine, tinnitus, sleep disturbances, fatigue, influenza-like symptoms, and sweating are the most common features of abrupt withdrawal of an SSRI or marked reduction of the dose; palpitation and visual disturbances can occur less commonly. The dose should be tapered over at least a few weeks to avoid these effects. For some patients, it may be necessary to withdraw treatment over a longer period; consider obtaining specialist advice if symptoms persist.

  Withdrawal effects may occur within 5 days of stopping treatment with antidepressant drugs; they are usually mild and self-limiting, but in some cases may be severe. The risk of withdrawal symptoms is increased if the antidepressant is stopped suddenly after regular administration for 8 weeks or more.
- **PATIENT AND CARER ADVICE**

  Driving and skilled tasks May also impair performance of skilled tasks (e.g. driving, operating machinery).

252

Citalopram

31-Jul-2018

● **INDICATIONS AND DOSE**

Major depression

▸ BY MOUTH USING TABLETS

▸ Child 12-17 years: Initially 10 mg once daily, increased if necessary to 20 mg once daily, dose to be increased over 2–4 weeks; maximum 40 mg per day

▸ BY MOUTH USING ORAL DROPS

▸ Child 12-17 years: Initially 8 mg once daily, increased if necessary to 16 mg once daily, dose to be increased over 2–4 weeks; maximum 32 mg per day

DOSE EQUIVALENCE AND CONVERSION

▸ 4 oral drops (8 mg) is equivalent in therapeutic effect to 10 mg tablet.

● **UNLICENSED USE** Not licensed for use in children.

● **CONTRA-INDICATIONS** QT-interval prolongation

● **CAUTIONS** Susceptibility to QT-interval prolongation

● **INTERACTIONS** → Appendix 1: SSRIs

● **SIDE-EFFECTS**

▸ **Common or very common** Acute angle closure glaucoma · apathy · flatulence · hypersalivation · migraine · rhinitis

▸ **Uncommon** Oedema

▸ **Rare or very rare** Cough · generalised tonic-clonic seizure

▸ **Frequency not known** Hypokalaemia

● **BREAST FEEDING** Present in milk—use with caution.

● **HEPATIC IMPAIRMENT**

Dose adjustments For *tablets* manufacturer advises lower initial doses, may be increased to max. 20 mg daily; use with extra caution and careful dose titration in severe impairment.

For *oral drops* manufacturer advises lower initial dose, may be increased to max. 16 mg daily; use with extra caution and careful dose titration in severe impairment.

● **RENAL IMPAIRMENT** No information available for estimated glomerular filtration rate less than 20 mL/minute/1.73 m^2.

● **TREATMENT CESSATION** The dose should preferably be reduced gradually over about 4 weeks, or longer if withdrawal symptoms emerge (6 months in patients who have been on long-term maintenance treatment).

● **DIRECTIONS FOR ADMINISTRATION** *Cipramil®* oral drops should be mixed with water, orange juice, or apple juice before taking.

● **PATIENT AND CARER ADVICE** Counselling on administration of oral drops is advised.

Driving and skilled tasks Patients should be advised of the effects of citalopram on driving and skilled tasks.

● **MEDICINAL FORMS** There can be variation in the licensing of different medicines containing the same drug.

Oral drops

EXCIPIENTS: May contain Alcohol

▸ **Citalopram (Non-proprietary)**

Citalopram (as Citalopram hydrochloride) 40 mg per 1 ml Citalopram 40mg/ml oral drops sugar-free | 15 ml PoM £18.17 DT = £15.16

▸ **Cipramil** (Lundbeck Ltd)

Citalopram (as Citalopram hydrochloride) 40 mg per 1 ml Cipramil 40mg/ml drops sugar-free | 15 ml PoM £10.08 DT = £15.16

Tablet

▸ **Citalopram (Non-proprietary)**

Citalopram (as Citalopram hydrobromide) 10 mg Citalopram 10mg tablets | 28 tablet PoM £12.36 DT = £0.90

Citalopram (as Citalopram hydrobromide) 20 mg Citalopram 20mg tablets | 28 tablet PoM £14.66 DT = £0.95

Citalopram (as Citalopram hydrobromide) 40 mg Citalopram 40mg tablets | 28 tablet PoM £16.47 DT = £1.11

▸ **Cipramil** (Lundbeck Ltd)

Citalopram (as Citalopram hydrobromide) 20 mg Cipramil 20mg tablets | 28 tablet PoM £8.95 DT = £0.95

252

Fluoxetine

23-Jul-2018

● **INDICATIONS AND DOSE**

Major depression

▸ BY MOUTH

▸ Child 8-17 years: Initially 10 mg daily, increased if necessary up to 20 mg daily, dose to be increased after 1–2 weeks of initial dose, daily dose may be administered as a single or divided dose

PHARMACOKINETICS

▸ Consider the long half-life of fluoxetine when adjusting dosage (or in overdosage).

● **INTERACTIONS** → Appendix 1: SSRIs

● **SIDE-EFFECTS**

▸ **Common or very common** Chills · feeling abnormal · postmenopausal haemorrhage · uterine disorder · vasodilation · vision blurred

▸ **Uncommon** Cold sweat · dysphagia · dyspnoea · hypotension · mood altered · muscle twitching · self-injurious behaviour · temperature sensation altered · thinking abnormal

▸ **Rare or very rare** Buccoglossal syndrome · leucopenia · neutropenia · oesophageal pain · pharyngitis · respiratory disorders · serum sickness · speech disorder · vasculitis

▸ **Frequency not known** Growth retardation

● **BREAST FEEDING** Present in milk—avoid.

● **HEPATIC IMPAIRMENT**

Dose adjustments Manufacturer advises dose reduction or increasing dose interval.

● **DIRECTIONS FOR ADMINISTRATION** Dispersible tablets can be dispersed in water for administration or swallowed whole with plenty of water.

● **PATIENT AND CARER ADVICE** Patients and carers should be counselled on the administration of dispersible tablets.

Medicines for Children leaflet: Fluoxetine for depression, obsessive compulsive disorder and bulimia nervosa www.medicinesforchildren.org.uk/fluoxetine-depression-obsessive-compulsive-disorder-and-bulimia-nervosa

Driving and skilled tasks Patients should be counselled about the effects on driving and skilled tasks.

● **MEDICINAL FORMS** There can be variation in the licensing of different medicines containing the same drug. Forms available from special-order manufacturers include: oral suspension, oral solution

Tablet

▸ **Fluoxetine (Non-proprietary)**

Fluoxetine (as Fluoxetine hydrochloride) 10 mg Fluoxetine 10mg tablets | 30 tablet PoM £64.66 DT = £56.09

Dispersible tablet

CAUTIONARY AND ADVISORY LABELS 10

▸ **Olena** (Advanz Pharma)

Fluoxetine (as Fluoxetine hydrochloride) 20 mg Olena 20mg dispersible tablets sugar-free | 28 tablet PoM £3.44 DT = £3.44

Oral solution

▸ **Fluoxetine (Non-proprietary)**

Fluoxetine (as Fluoxetine hydrochloride) 4 mg per 1 ml Fluoxetine 20mg/5ml oral solution | 70 ml PoM £12.75 DT = £4.53
Fluoxetine 20mg/5ml oral solution sugar-free | 70 ml PoM £12.95 DT = £12.95

▸ **Prozep** (Chemidex Pharma Ltd)

Fluoxetine (as Fluoxetine hydrochloride) 4 mg per 1 ml Prozep 20mg/5ml oral solution sugar-free | 70 ml PoM £12.95 DT = £12.95

Capsule

▸ **Fluoxetine (Non-proprietary)**

Fluoxetine (as Fluoxetine hydrochloride) 10 mg Fluoxetine 10mg capsules | 30 capsule PoM £63.00 DT = £60.59

Fluoxetine (as Fluoxetine hydrochloride) 20 mg Fluoxetine 20mg capsules | 30 capsule PoM £5.00 DT = £1.15 | 100 capsule PoM £4.70

Fluoxetine (as Fluoxetine hydrochloride) 30 mg Fluoxetine 30mg capsules | 30 capsule PoM £1.80 DT = £1.80

Fluoxetine (as Fluoxetine hydrochloride) 40 mg Fluoxetine 40mg capsules | 30 capsule PoM £1.80 DT = £1.80

Fluoxetine (as Fluoxetine hydrochloride) 60 mg Fluoxetine 60mg capsules | 30 capsule PoM £54.36 DT = £4.98

252

Fluvoxamine maleate

23-Jul-2018

● **INDICATIONS AND DOSE**

Obsessive-compulsive disorder

▶ BY MOUTH

▸ Child 8–17 years: Initially 25 mg daily, then increased in steps of 25 mg every 4–7 days (max. per dose 100 mg twice daily) if required, dose to be increased according to response, doses above 50 mg should be given in 2 divided doses, if no improvement in obsessive-compulsive disorder within 10 weeks, treatment should be reconsidered

● **INTERACTIONS** → Appendix 1: SSRIs

● **SIDE-EFFECTS**

▶ **Rare or very rare** Hepatic function abnormal (discontinue)

▶ **Frequency not known** Bone fracture · glaucoma · hypomania · neuroleptic malignant-like syndrome · withdrawal syndrome neonatal

● **BREAST FEEDING** Present in milk—avoid.

● **HEPATIC IMPAIRMENT**

Dose adjustments Manufacturer advises low initial dose.

● **RENAL IMPAIRMENT**

Dose adjustments Start with low dose.

● **TREATMENT CESSATION** The dose should preferably be reduced gradually over about 4 weeks, or longer if withdrawal symptoms emerge (6 months in patients who have been on long-term maintenance treatment).

● **PATIENT AND CARER ADVICE**

Driving and skilled tasks Patients should be counselled about the effects on driving and skilled tasks.

● **MEDICINAL FORMS** There can be variation in the licensing of different medicines containing the same drug. Forms available from special-order manufacturers include: oral suspension

Tablet

▸ Fluvoxamine maleate (Non-proprietary)

Fluvoxamine maleate 50 mg Fluvoxamine 50mg tablets | 60 tablet PoM £20.98 DT = £17.53

Fluvoxamine maleate 100 mg Fluvoxamine 100mg tablets | 30 tablet PoM £20.98 DT = £17.70

▸ Faverin (Mylan)

Fluvoxamine maleate 50 mg Faverin 50mg tablets | 60 tablet PoM £17.10 DT = £17.53

Fluvoxamine maleate 100 mg Faverin 100mg tablets | 30 tablet PoM £17.10 DT = £17.70

252

Sertraline

19-Mar-2018

● **INDICATIONS AND DOSE**

Obsessive-compulsive disorder

▶ BY MOUTH

▸ Child 6–11 years: Initially 25 mg daily for 1 week, then increased to 50 mg daily, then increased in steps of 50 mg at intervals of at least 1 week if required; maximum 200 mg per day

▸ Child 12–17 years: Initially 50 mg daily, then increased in steps of 50 mg at intervals of at least 1 week if required; maximum 200 mg per day

Major depression

▶ BY MOUTH

▸ Child 12–17 years: Initially 50 mg once daily, then increased in steps of 50 mg at intervals of at least 1 week if required; maximum 200 mg per day

● **UNLICENSED USE** Not licensed for use in children for depression.

● **INTERACTIONS** → Appendix 1: SSRIs

● **SIDE-EFFECTS**

▶ **Common or very common** Chest pain · depression · gastrointestinal disorders · increased risk of infection · mood altered · neuromuscular dysfunction · vasodilation

▶ **Uncommon** Albuminuria · anaemia · back pain · breast pain · burping · chills · cold sweat · cystitis · dysphagia · dyspnoea · ear pain · eye pain · hypertension · hypothyroidism · migraine · muscle complaints · muscle weakness · oedema · oral disorders · osteoarthritis · periorbital oedema · respiratory disorders · sensation abnormal · speech disorder · thinking abnormal · thirst

▶ **Rare or very rare** Balanoposthitis · bone disorder · cardiac disorder · coma · conversion disorder · diabetes mellitus · drug dependence · dysphonia · eye disorders · gait abnormal · genital discharge · glaucoma · hair texture abnormal · hepatic disorders · hiccups · hypercholesterolaemia · hypoglycaemia · injury · lymphadenopathy · myocardial infarction · neoplasms · oliguria · peripheral ischaemia · psychotic disorder · vasodilation procedure · vision disorders · vulvovaginal atrophy

▶ **Frequency not known** Cerebrovascular insufficiency · gynaecomastia · hyperglycaemia · leucopenia · neuroleptic malignant syndrome · pancreatitis

● **BREAST FEEDING** Not known to be harmful but consider discontinuing breast-feeding.

● **HEPATIC IMPAIRMENT** Manufacturer advises avoid in severe impairment (no information available).

Dose adjustments Manufacturer advises dose reduction or increasing dose interval in mild to moderate impairment.

● **RENAL IMPAIRMENT** Use with caution.

● **TREATMENT CESSATION** The dose should preferably be reduced gradually over about 4 weeks, or longer if withdrawal symptoms emerge (6 months in patients who have been on long-term maintenance treatment).

● **PRESCRIBING AND DISPENSING INFORMATION** The RCPCH and NPPG recommend that, when a liquid special of sertraline is required, the following strength is used: 50 mg/5 mL.

● **PATIENT AND CARER ADVICE**

Medicines for Children leaflet: Sertraline for OCD (obsessive compulsive disorder) and depression www.medicinesforchildren.org.uk/sertraline-ocd-obsessive-compulsive-disorder-and-depression

Driving and skilled tasks Patients should be counselled on the effects on driving and skilled tasks.

● **MEDICINAL FORMS** There can be variation in the licensing of different medicines containing the same drug. Forms available from special-order manufacturers include: tablet, oral suspension

Tablet

▸ Sertraline (Non-proprietary)

Sertraline (as Sertraline hydrochloride) 50 mg Sertraline 50mg tablets | 28 tablet PoM £17.00 DT = £1.27 | 500 tablet PoM £12.45–£23.57

Sertraline (as Sertraline hydrochloride) 100 mg Sertraline 100mg tablets | 28 tablet PoM £28.00 DT = £1.55 | 500 tablet PoM £16.39–£27.86

▸ Lustral (Upjohn UK Ltd)

Sertraline (as Sertraline hydrochloride) 50 mg Lustral 50mg tablets | 28 tablet PoM £17.82 DT = £1.27

Sertraline (as Sertraline hydrochloride) 100 mg Lustral 100mg tablets | 28 tablet [PoM] £29.16 DT = £1.55

ANTIDEPRESSANTS > TRICYCLIC ANTIDEPRESSANTS

Amitriptyline hydrochloride

16-Jul-2019

- **INDICATIONS AND DOSE**

Neuropathic pain

▶ BY MOUTH

▶ **Child 2-11 years:** Initially 200–500 micrograms/kg once daily (max. per dose 10 mg), dose to be taken at night, increased if necessary; maximum 1 mg/kg twice daily on specialist advice

▶ **Child 12-17 years:** Initially 10 mg once daily, increased if necessary to 75 mg once daily, dose to be taken at night, dose to be increased gradually, higher doses to be given on specialist advice

- **UNLICENSED USE** Not licensed for use in neuropathic pain.
- **CONTRA-INDICATIONS** Arrhythmias · during manic phase of bipolar disorder · heart block · immediate recovery period after myocardial infarction
- **CAUTIONS** Cardiovascular disease · chronic constipation · diabetes · epilepsy · history of bipolar disorder · history of psychosis · hyperthyroidism (risk of arrhythmias) · patients with a significant risk of suicide · phaeochromocytoma (risk of arrhythmias) · susceptibility to angle-closure glaucoma · urinary retention

  CAUTIONS, FURTHER INFORMATION Treatment should be stopped if the patient enters a manic phase.
- **INTERACTIONS** → Appendix 1: tricyclic antidepressants
- **SIDE-EFFECTS**

▶ **Common or very common** Anticholinergic syndrome · drowsiness · QT interval prolongation

▶ **Frequency not known** Agranulocytosis · alopecia · anxiety · appetite abnormal · arrhythmias · asthenia · bone marrow depression · breast enlargement · cardiac conduction disorders · coma · concentration impaired · confusion · constipation · delirium · delusions · diarrhoea · dizziness · dry mouth · dysarthria · eosinophilia · epigastric distress · face oedema · galactorrhoea · gynaecomastia · hallucination · headache · hepatic disorders · hyperhidrosis · hyperpyrexia · hypertension · hyponatraemia · hypotension · leucopenia · mood altered · movement disorders · mydriasis · myocardial infarction · nausea · neuroleptic malignant syndrome · oral disorders · palpitations · paralytic ileus · peripheral neuropathy · photosensitivity reaction · seizure · sensation abnormal · sexual dysfunction · SIADH · skin reactions · sleep disorders · stroke · sudden cardiac death · suicidal tendencies · syncope · taste altered · testicular swelling · thrombocytopenia · tinnitus · tremor · urinary disorders · urinary tract dilation · vision disorders · vomiting · weight changes · withdrawal syndrome

Overdose Overdosage with amitriptyline is associated with a relatively high rate of fatality. Symptoms of overdosage may include dry mouth, coma of varying degree, hypotension, hypothermia, hyperreflexia, extensor plantar responses, convulsions, respiratory failure, cardiac conduction defects, and arrhythmias. Dilated pupils and urinary retention also occur. For details on the management of poisoning, see Tricyclic and related antidepressants, under Emergency treatment of poisoning p. 891.

- **PREGNANCY** Use only if potential benefit outweighs risk.
- **BREAST FEEDING** The amount secreted into breast milk is too small to be harmful.
- **HEPATIC IMPAIRMENT** Manufacturer advises use with caution in mild-to-moderate impairment; avoid in severe impairment.
- **TREATMENT CESSATION** Withdrawal effects may occur within 5 days of stopping treatment with antidepressant drugs; they are usually mild and self-limiting, but in some cases may be severe. The risk of withdrawal symptoms is increased if the antidepressant is stopped suddenly after regular administration for 8 weeks or more. The dose should preferably be reduced gradually over about 4 weeks, or longer if withdrawal symptoms emerge (6 months in patients who have been on long-term maintenance treatment). If possible tricyclic and related antidepressants should be withdrawn slowly.
- **PRESCRIBING AND DISPENSING INFORMATION** Limited quantities of tricyclic antidepressants should be prescribed at any one time because their cardiovascular and epileptogenic effects are dangerous in overdosage.
- **PATIENT AND CARER ADVICE**

  Medicines for Children leaflet: Amitriptyline for neuropathic pain www.medicinesforchildren.org.uk/amitriptyline-neuropathic-pain-0

  Driving and skilled tasks Drowsiness may affect the performance of skilled tasks (e.g. driving). Effects of alcohol enhanced.

- **MEDICINAL FORMS** There can be variation in the licensing of different medicines containing the same drug. Forms available from special-order manufacturers include: oral suspension, oral solution

Oral solution

CAUTIONARY AND ADVISORY LABELS 2

▶ **Amitriptyline hydrochloride (Non-proprietary)**

Amitriptyline hydrochloride 2 mg per 1 ml Amitriptyline 10mg/5ml oral solution sugar-free | 150 ml [PoM] £136.47 DT = £136.47

Amitriptyline hydrochloride 5 mg per 1 ml Amitriptyline 25mg/5ml oral solution sugar-free | 150 ml [PoM] £18.00 DT = £18.00

Amitriptyline hydrochloride 10 mg per 1 ml Amitriptyline 50mg/5ml oral solution sugar-free | 150 ml [PoM] £24.00 DT = £19.20

Tablet

CAUTIONARY AND ADVISORY LABELS 2

▶ **Amitriptyline hydrochloride (Non-proprietary)**

Amitriptyline hydrochloride 10 mg Amitriptyline 10mg tablets | 28 tablet [PoM] £1.50 DT = £1.00

Amitriptyline hydrochloride 25 mg Amitriptyline 25mg tablets | 28 tablet [PoM] £1.75 DT = £0.86

Amitriptyline hydrochloride 50 mg Amitriptyline 50mg tablets | 28 tablet [PoM] £5.99 DT = £1.83

Doxepin

05-Jul-2019

- **INDICATIONS AND DOSE**

Depressive illness (particularly where sedation is required)

▶ BY MOUTH

▶ **Child 12-17 years:** Initially 75 mg daily in divided doses, alternatively 75 mg once daily, adjusted according to response, dose to taken at bedtime; maintenance 25–300 mg daily, doses above 100 mg given in 3 divided doses

- **CONTRA-INDICATIONS** Acute porphyrias p. 652 · during manic phase of bipolar disorder
- **CAUTIONS** Arrhythmias · cardiovascular disease · chronic constipation · diabetes · epilepsy · heart block · history of bipolar disorder · history of psychosis · hyperthyroidism (risk of arrhythmias) · immediate recovery period after myocardial infarction · patients with significant risk of suicide · phaeochromocytoma (risk of arrhythmias) · susceptibility to angle-closure glaucoma · urinary retention

CAUTIONS, FURTHER INFORMATION Treatment should be stopped if the patient enters a manic phase.

- INTERACTIONS → Appendix 1: tricyclic antidepressants
- SIDE-EFFECTS Agitation · agranulocytosis · alopecia · anticholinergic syndrome · appetite decreased · asthenia · asthma exacerbated · bone marrow depression · breast enlargement · cardiovascular effects · chills · confusion · constipation · diarrhoea · dizziness · drowsiness · dry mouth · dyspepsia · eosinophilia · face oedema · flushing · galactorrhoea · gynaecomastia · haemolytic anaemia · hallucination · headache · hyperhidrosis · hyperpyrexia · increased risk of fracture · jaundice · leucopenia · mania · movement disorders · nausea · oral ulceration · paranoid delusions · photosensitivity reaction · postural hypotension · psychosis · seizure · sensation abnormal · sexual dysfunction · SIADH · skin reactions · sleep disorders · suicidal tendencies · tachycardia · taste altered · testicular swelling · thrombocytopenia · tinnitus · tremor · urinary retention · vision blurred · vomiting · weight increased · withdrawal syndrome (in neonates)

Overdose Tricyclic and related antidepressants cause dry mouth, coma of varying degree, hypotension, hypothermia, hyperreflexia, extensor plantar responses, convulsions, respiratory failure, cardiac conduction defects, and arrhythmias. Dilated pupils and urinary retention also occur. For details on the management of poisoning see Tricyclic and related antidepressants under Emergency treatment of poisoning p. 891.

- PREGNANCY Use with caution—limited information available.
- BREAST FEEDING The amount secreted into breast milk is too small to be harmful. Accumulation of metabolite may cause sedation and respiratory depression in neonate.
- HEPATIC IMPAIRMENT Manufacturer advises caution in mild to moderate impairment; avoid in severe impairment.

Dose adjustments Manufacturer advises consider dose reduction in mild to moderate impairment.

- RENAL IMPAIRMENT Use with caution.
- TREATMENT CESSATION Withdrawal effects may occur within 5 days of stopping treatment with antidepressant drugs; they are usually mild and self-limiting, but in some cases may be severe. The risk of withdrawal symptoms is increased if the antidepressant is stopped suddenly after regular administration for 8 weeks or more. The dose should preferably be reduced gradually over about 4 weeks, or longer if withdrawal symptoms emerge (6 months in patients who have been on long-term maintenance treatment). If possible tricyclic and related antidepressants should be withdrawn slowly.
- PRESCRIBING AND DISPENSING INFORMATION Limited quantities of tricyclic antidepressants should be prescribed at any one time because their cardiovascular and epileptogenic effects are dangerous in overdosage.
- PATIENT AND CARER ADVICE

Driving and skilled tasks Drowsiness may affect performance of skilled tasks (e.g. driving). Effects of alcohol enhanced.

- MEDICINAL FORMS There can be variation in the licensing of different medicines containing the same drug. Forms available from special-order manufacturers include: capsule, oral suspension, oral solution

Capsule

CAUTIONARY AND ADVISORY LABELS 2

- Doxepin (Non-proprietary)

Doxepin (as Doxepin hydrochloride) 25 mg Doxepin 25mg capsules | 28 capsule PoM £97.00 DT = £97.00

Doxepin (as Doxepin hydrochloride) 50 mg Doxepin 50mg capsules | 28 capsule PoM £154.00 DT = £154.00

Imipramine hydrochloride

30-Mar-2017

- INDICATIONS AND DOSE

Nocturnal enuresis

- BY MOUTH
  - Child 6–7 years: 25 mg once daily, to be taken at bedtime, initial period of treatment (including gradual withdrawal) 3 months—full physical examination before further course
  - Child 8–10 years: 25–50 mg once daily, to be taken at bedtime, initial period of treatment (including gradual withdrawal) 3 months—full physical examination before further course
  - Child 11–17 years: 50–75 mg once daily, to be taken at bedtime, initial period of treatment (including gradual withdrawal) 3 months—full physical examination before further course

Attention deficit hyperactivity disorder (under expert supervision)

- BY MOUTH
  - Child 6–17 years: 10–30 mg twice daily

- UNLICENSED USE Not licensed for use for attention deficit hyperactivity disorder.
- CONTRA-INDICATIONS Immediate recovery period after myocardial infarction · Acute porphyrias p. 652 · arrhythmia · during the manic phase of bipolar disorder · heart block
- CAUTIONS Cardiovascular disease · chronic constipation · diabetes · epilepsy · history of bipolar disorder · history of psychosis · hyperthyroidism (risk of arrhythmias) · patients with a significant risk of suicide · phaeochromocytoma (risk of arrhythmias) · susceptibility to angle-closure glaucoma · urinary retention

CAUTIONS, FURTHER INFORMATION Treatment should be stopped if the patient enters a manic phase.

- INTERACTIONS → Appendix 1: tricyclic antidepressants
- SIDE-EFFECTS
  - **Common or very common** Anxiety · appetite decreased · arrhythmias · asthenia · cardiac conduction disorders · confusion · delirium · depression · dizziness · drowsiness · epilepsy · hallucination · headache · hepatic disorders · hypotension · mood altered · nausea · palpitations · paraesthesia · sexual dysfunction · skin reactions · sleep disorder · tremor · vomiting · weight changes
  - **Uncommon** Psychosis
  - **Rare or very rare** Aggression · agranulocytosis · alopecia · bone marrow depression · enlarged mammary gland · eosinophilia · fever · galactorrhoea · gastrointestinal disorders · glaucoma · heart failure · leucopenia · movement disorders · mydriasis · oedema · oral disorders · peripheral vasospastic reaction · photosensitivity reaction · respiratory disorders (frequency not known in neonates) · SIADH · speech disorder · thrombocytopenia
  - **Frequency not known** Anticholinergic syndrome · cardiovascular effects · drug fever · hyponatraemia · increased risk of fracture · neurological effects · paranoid delusions exacerbated · psychiatric disorder · suicidal tendencies · tinnitus · urinary disorder · withdrawal symptoms

Overdose Tricyclic and related antidepressants cause dry mouth, coma of varying degree, hypotension, hypothermia, hyperreflexia, extensor plantar responses, convulsions, respiratory failure, cardiac conduction defects, and arrhythmias. Dilated pupils and urinary retention also occur. For details on the management of poisoning see Tricyclic and related antidepressants under Emergency treatment of poisoning p. 891.

- PREGNANCY Colic, tachycardia, dyspnoea, irritability, muscle spasms, respiratory depression and withdrawal symptoms reported in neonates when used in the third trimester.

- **BREAST FEEDING** The amount secreted into breast milk is too small to be harmful.
- **HEPATIC IMPAIRMENT** Manufacturer advises caution in mild to moderate impairment; avoid in severe impairment.
- **RENAL IMPAIRMENT** Use with caution in severe impairment.
- **TREATMENT CESSATION** Withdrawal effects may occur within 5 days of stopping treatment with antidepressant drugs; they are usually mild and self-limiting, but in some cases may be severe. The risk of withdrawal symptoms is increased if the antidepressant is stopped suddenly after regular administration for 8 weeks or more. The dose should preferably be reduced gradually over about 4 weeks, or longer if withdrawal symptoms emerge (6 months in patients who have been on long-term maintenance treatment). If possible tricyclic antidepressants should be withdrawn slowly.
- **PRESCRIBING AND DISPENSING INFORMATION** Limited quantities of tricyclic antidepressants should be prescribed at any one time because their cardiovascular and epileptogenic effects are dangerous in overdosage.
- **PATIENT AND CARER ADVICE**
Medicines for Children leaflet: Imipramine for various conditions www.medicinesforchildren.org.uk/imipramine-various-conditions
Driving and skilled tasks Drowsiness may affect the performance of skilled tasks (e.g. driving). Effects of alcohol enhanced.

- **MEDICINAL FORMS** There can be variation in the licensing of different medicines containing the same drug. Forms available from special-order manufacturers include: oral suspension, oral solution

Oral solution

CAUTIONARY AND ADVISORY LABELS 2

- Imipramine hydrochloride (Non-proprietary)
Imipramine hydrochloride 5 mg per 1 ml Imipramine 25mg/5ml oral solution sugar-free | 150 ml [PoM] £49.09 DT = £45.00

Tablet

CAUTIONARY AND ADVISORY LABELS 2

- Imipramine hydrochloride (Non-proprietary)
Imipramine hydrochloride 10 mg Imipramine 10mg tablets | 28 tablet [PoM] £2.10 DT = £1.32
Imipramine hydrochloride 25 mg Imipramine 25mg tablets | 28 tablet [PoM] £8.25 DT = £1.93

Nortriptyline

- **INDICATIONS AND DOSE**

Depressive illness

- BY MOUTH
- Child 12–17 years: To be initiated at a low dose, then increased if necessary to 30–50 mg daily in divided doses, alternatively increased if necessary to 30–50 mg once daily; maximum 150 mg per day

- **CONTRA-INDICATIONS** Arrhythmias · during the manic phase of bipolar disorder · heart block · immediate recovery period after myocardial infarction
- **CAUTIONS** Cardiovascular disease · chronic constipation · diabetes · epilepsy · history of bipolar disorder · history of psychosis · hyperthyroidism (risk of arrhythmias) · patients with a significant risk of suicide · phaeochromocytoma (risk of arrhythmias) · susceptibility to angle-closure glaucoma · urinary retention
CAUTIONS, FURTHER INFORMATION Treatment should be stopped if the patient enters a manic phase.
- **INTERACTIONS** → Appendix 1: tricyclic antidepressants
- **SIDE-EFFECTS** Agranulocytosis · alopecia · anxiety · appetite decreased · arrhythmias · asthenia · atrioventricular block · bone marrow disorders · breast enlargement · confusion · constipation · delusions · diarrhoea · dizziness · drowsiness · drug cross-reactivity · drug fever · dry mouth · eosinophilia · fever · flushing · galactorrhoea · gastrointestinal discomfort · gynaecomastia · hallucination · headache · hepatic disorders · hyperhidrosis · hypertension · hypomania · hypotension · increased risk of fracture · increased risk of infection · malaise · movement disorders · mydriasis · myocardial infarction · nausea · oedema · oral disorders · palpitations · paralytic ileus · peripheral neuropathy · photosensitivity reaction · psychosis exacerbated · seizure · sensation abnormal · sexual dysfunction · SIADH · skin reactions · sleep disorders · stroke · suicidal tendencies · taste altered · testicular swelling · thrombocytopenia · tinnitus · tremor · urinary disorders · urinary tract dilation · vision disorders · vomiting · weight changes
Overdose Tricyclic and related antidepressants cause dry mouth, coma of varying degree, hypotension, hypothermia, hyperreflexia, extensor plantar responses, convulsions, respiratory failure, cardiac conduction defects, and arrhythmias. Dilated pupils and urinary retention also occur. For details on the management of poisoning see Tricyclic and related antidepressants under Emergency treatment of poisoning p. 891.
- **PREGNANCY** Use only if potential benefit outweighs risk.
- **BREAST FEEDING** The amount secreted into breast milk is too small to be harmful.
- **HEPATIC IMPAIRMENT** Manufacture advises avoid in severe impairment.
- **MONITORING REQUIREMENTS**
- Manufacturer advises plasma-nortriptyline concentration monitoring if dose above 100 mg daily, but evidence of practical value uncertain.
- **TREATMENT CESSATION** Withdrawal effects may occur within 5 days of stopping treatment with antidepressant drugs; they are usually mild and self-limiting, but in some cases may be severe. The risk of withdrawal symptoms is increased if the antidepressant is stopped suddenly after regular administration for 8 weeks or more. The dose should preferably be reduced gradually over about 4 weeks, or longer if withdrawal symptoms emerge (6 months in patients who have been on long-term maintenance treatment). If possible tricyclic and related antidepressants should be withdrawn slowly.
- **PRESCRIBING AND DISPENSING INFORMATION** Limited quantities of tricyclic antidepressants should be prescribed at any one time because their cardiovascular and epileptogenic effects are dangerous in overdosage.
- **PATIENT AND CARER ADVICE** Drowsiness may affect the performance of skilled tasks (e.g. driving). Effects of alcohol enhanced.

- **MEDICINAL FORMS** There can be variation in the licensing of different medicines containing the same drug. Forms available from special-order manufacturers include: oral suspension, oral solution

Oral solution

- Nortriptyline (Non-proprietary)
Nortriptyline (as Nortriptyline hydrochloride) 2 mg per 1 ml Nortriptyline 10mg/5ml oral solution sugar-free | 250 ml [PoM] £246.00
Nortriptyline (as Nortriptyline hydrochloride) 5 mg per 1 ml Nortriptyline 25mg/5ml oral solution sugar-free | 250 ml [PoM] £324.00

Tablet

CAUTIONARY AND ADVISORY LABELS 2

- Nortriptyline (Non-proprietary)
Nortriptyline (as Nortriptyline hydrochloride) 10 mg Nortriptyline 10mg tablets | 28 tablet [PoM] £1.85–£2.14 | 30 tablet [PoM] £6.87–

4 Nervous system

£11.79 | 84 tablet PoM £5.54–£6.42 | 100 tablet PoM £39.30 DT = £6.60

Nortriptyline (as Nortriptyline hydrochloride) 25 mg Nortriptyline 25mg tablets | 28 tablet PoM £2.27–£2.46 | 30 tablet PoM £6.81–£12.43 | 84 tablet PoM £6.80–£7.38 | 100 tablet PoM £41.44 DT = £8.09

Nortriptyline (as Nortriptyline hydrochloride) 50 mg Nortriptyline 50mg tablets | 30 tablet PoM £42.00 DT = £33.75

2.4 Psychoses and schizophrenia

Psychoses and related disorders

06-Mar-2017

Advice on doses of antipsychotic drugs above BNF *for Children* upper limit

- Consider alternative approaches including adjuvant therapy.
- Bear in mind risk factors, including obesity. Consider potential for drug interactions—see interactions: Appendix 1 (antipsychotics).
- Carry out ECG to exclude untoward abnormalities such as prolonged QT interval; repeat ECG periodically **and** reduce dose if prolonged QT interval or other adverse abnormality develops.
- Increase dose slowly and not more often than once weekly.
- Carry out regular pulse, blood pressure, and temperature checks; ensure that patient maintains adequate fluid intake.
- Consider high-dose therapy to be for limited period and review regularly; abandon if no improvement after 3 months (return to standard dosage).

Important: When prescribing an antipsychotic for administration on an emergency basis, the intramuscular dose should be **lower** than the corresponding oral dose (owing to absence of first-pass effect), particularly if the child is very active (increased blood flow to muscle considerably increases the rate of absorption). The prescription should specify the dose for **each route** and should not imply that the same dose can be given by mouth or by intramuscular injection. The dose of antipsychotic for emergency use should be reviewed at least **daily**.

Antipsychotic drugs

There is little information on the efficacy and safety of antipsychotic drugs in children and adolescents and much of the information available has been extrapolated from adult data; in particular, little is known about the long-term effects of antipsychotic drugs on the developing nervous system. Antipsychotic drugs should be initiated and managed under the close supervision of an appropriate specialist.

Antipsychotic drugs are also known as 'neuroleptics' and (misleadingly) as 'major tranquillisers'.

In the short term they are used to calm disturbed children whatever the underlying psychopathology, which may be schizophrenia, brain damage, mania, toxic delirium, or agitated depression. Antipsychotic drugs are used to alleviate severe anxiety but this too should be a short-term measure.

Schizophrenia

The aim of treatment is to alleviate the suffering of the child (and carer) and to improve social and cognitive functioning. Many children require life-long treatment with antipsychotic medication. Antipsychotic drugs relieve positive psychotic symptoms such as thought disorder, hallucinations, and delusions, and prevent relapse; they are usually less effective on negative symptoms such as apathy and social withdrawal. In many patients, negative symptoms persist between episodes of treated positive symptoms, but earlier treatment of psychotic illness may protect against the development of negative symptoms over time. Children with acute schizophrenia generally respond better than those with chronic symptoms.

Long-term treatment of a child with a definitive diagnosis of schizophrenia is usually required after the first episode of illness in order to prevent relapses. Doses that are effective in acute episodes should generally be continued as prophylaxis.

First-generation antipsychotic drugs

The first-generation antipsychotic drugs act predominantly by blocking dopamine D_2 receptors in the brain. First-generation antipsychotic drugs are not selective for any of the four dopamine pathways in the brain and so can cause a range of side-effects, particularly extrapyramidal symptoms and elevated prolactin. The **phenothiazine** derivatives can be divided into 3 main groups:

- *Group* 1: chlorpromazine hydrochloride p. 261, levomepromazine p. 285, and promazine hydrochloride, generally characterised by pronounced sedative effects and moderate antimuscarinic and extrapyramidal side-effects.
- *Group* 2: pericyazine p. 262, generally characterised by moderate sedative effects, but fewer extrapyramidal side-effects than groups 1 or 3.
- *Group* 3: perphenazine, prochlorperazine p. 285, and trifluoperazine p. 264, generally characterised by fewer sedative and antimuscarinic effects, but more pronounced extrapyramidal side-effects than groups 1 and 2.

Butyrophenones (e.g. haloperidol p. 261) resemble the group 3 phenothiazines in their clinical properties. **Diphenylbutylpiperidines** (pimozide p. 263) and the **substituted benzamides** (sulpiride p. 263) have reduced sedative, antimuscarinic, and extrapyramidal effects.

Second-generation antipsychotic drugs

The second-generation antipsychotic drugs (also referred to as atypical antipsychotic drugs) act on a range of receptors in comparison to first-generation antipsychotic drugs and have more distinct clinical profiles, particularly with regard to side-effects.

Prescribing of antipsychotic drugs in children with learning disabilities

EvGr When prescribing for children with learning disabilities who are prescribed antipsychotic drugs and who are not experiencing psychotic symptoms, the following considerations should be taken into account:

- a reduction in dose or the discontinuation of long-term antipsychotic treatment;
- review of the child's condition after dose reduction or discontinuation of an antipsychotic agent;
- referral to a psychiatrist experienced in working with children who have learning disabilities and mental health problems;
- annual documentation of the reasons for continuing a prescription if the antipsychotic is not reduced in dose or discontinued ⟨A⟩.

Side effects of antipsychotic drugs

Side-effects caused by antipsychotic drugs are common and contribute significantly to non-adherence to therapy.

Extrapyramidal symptoms

Extrapyramidal symptoms occur most frequently with the piperazine phenothiazines (fluphenazine, perphenazine, prochlorperazine, and trifluoperazine), the butyrophenones (benperidol and haloperidol), and the first-generation depot preparations. They are easy to recognise but cannot be predicted accurately because they depend on the dose, the type of drug, and on individual susceptibility.

Extrapyramidal symptoms consist of:

- *parkinsonian symptoms* (including tremor), which may occur more commonly in adults or the elderly and may appear gradually;
- *dystonia* (abnormal face and body movements) and dyskinesia, which occur more commonly in children or young adults and appear after only a few doses;
- *akathisia* (restlessness), which characteristically occurs after large initial doses and may resemble an exacerbation of the condition being treated;
- *tardive dyskinesia* (rhythmic, involuntary movements of tongue, face, and jaw), which usually develops on long-term therapy or with high dosage, but it may develop on short-term treatment with low doses—short-lived tardive dyskinesia may occur after withdrawal of the drug.

Parkinsonian symptoms remit if the drug is withdrawn and may be suppressed by the administration of antimuscarinic drugs. However, routine administration of such drugs is not justified because not all patients are affected and they may unmask or worsen tardive dyskinesia.

Tardive dyskinesia is the most serious manifestation of extrapyramidal symptoms; it is of particular concern because it may be irreversible on withdrawing therapy and treatment is usually ineffective. In children, tardive dyskinesia is more likely to occur when the antipsychotic drug is withdrawn. However, some manufacturers suggest that drug withdrawal at the earliest signs of tardive dyskinesia (fine vermicular movements of the tongue) may halt its full development. Tardive dyskinesia occurs fairly frequently, especially in the elderly, and treatment must be carefully and regularly reviewed.

Hyperprolactinaemia

Most antipsychotic drugs, both first- and second-generation, increase prolactin concentration to some extent because dopamine inhibits prolactin release. Aripiprazole reduces prolactin because it is a dopamine-receptor partial agonist. Risperidone, amisulpride, and first-generation antipsychotic drugs are most likely to cause symptomatic hyperprolactinaemia. The clinical symptoms of hyperprolactinaemia include sexual dysfunction, reduced bone mineral density, menstrual disturbances, breast enlargement, and galactorrhoea.

Sexual dysfunction

Sexual dysfunction is one of the main causes of non-adherence to antipsychotic medication; physical illness, psychiatric illness, and substance misuse are contributing factors. Antipsychotic-induced sexual dysfunction is caused by more than one mechanism. Reduced dopamine transmission and hyperprolactinaemia decrease libido; antimuscarinic effects can cause disorders of arousal; and $alpha_1$-adrenoceptor antagonists are associated with erection and ejaculation problems in men. Risperidone and haloperidol commonly cause sexual dysfunction. If sexual dysfunction is thought to be antipsychotic-induced, dose reduction or switching medication should be considered.

Cardiovascular side-effects

Antipsychotic drugs have been associated with cardiovascular side-effects such as tachycardia, arrhythmias, and hypotension. QT-interval prolongation is a particular concern with pimozide and haloperidol. There is also a higher probability of QT-interval prolongation in patients using any intravenous antipsychotic drug, or any antipsychotic drug or combination of antipsychotic drugs with doses exceeding the recommended maximum. Cases of sudden death have occurred.

Hyperglycaemia and weight gain

Hyperglycaemia, and sometimes diabetes, can occur with antipsychotic drugs, particularly clozapine, olanzapine, quetiapine, and risperidone. All antipsychotic drugs may cause weight gain, but the risk and extent varies. Clozapine and olanzapine commonly cause weight gain. Olanzapine is associated with more weight gain than other second generation antipsychotic drugs. Weight gain happens soon after treatment with olanzapine has started.

Hypotension and interference with temperature regulation

Hypotension and interference with temperature regulation are dose-related side-effects. Clozapine, chlorpromazine, and quetiapine can cause postural hypotension (especially during initial dose titration) which may be associated with syncope or reflex tachycardia in some children.

Neuroleptic malignant syndrome

Neuroleptic malignant syndrome (hyperthermia, fluctuating level of consciousness, muscle rigidity, and autonomic dysfunction with pallor, tachycardia, labile blood pressure, sweating, and urinary incontinence) is a rare but potentially fatal side-effect of all antipsychotic drugs. Discontinuation of the antipsychotic drug is essential because there is no proven effective treatment, but bromocriptine and dantrolene have been used. The syndrome, which usually lasts for 5–7 days after drug discontinuation, may be unduly prolonged if depot preparations have been used.

Blood dyscrasias

Perform blood counts if unexplained infection or fever develops.

Choice

The antipsychotic drugs most commonly used in children are haloperidol p. 261, risperidone p. 270, and olanzapine p. 267. There is little meaningful difference in efficacy between each of the antipsychotic drugs (other than clozapine p. 266), and response and tolerability to each antipsychotic drug varies. There is no first-line antipsychotic drug which is suitable for all children. Choice of antipsychotic medication is influenced by the child's medication history, the degree of sedation required (although tolerance to this usually develops), and consideration of individual patient factors such as risk of extrapyramidal side-effects, weight gain, impaired glucose tolerance, QT-interval prolongation, or the presence of negative symptoms.

Negative symptoms

Second generation antipsychotic drugs may be better at treating the negative symptoms of schizophrenia.

Extrapyramidal side-effects

Second-generation antipsychotic drugs may be prescribed if extrapyramidal side-effects are a particular concern. Of these, aripiprazole p. 265, clozapine, olanzapine, and quetiapine p. 268 are least likely to cause extrapyramidal side-effects. Although amisulpride p. 264 is a dopamine-receptor antagonist, extrapyramidal side-effects are less common than with the first-generation antipsychotic drugs because amisulpride selectively blocks mesolimbic dopamine receptors, and extrapyramidal symptoms are caused by blockade of the striatal dopamine pathway.

QT interval

Aripiprazole has negligible effect on the QT interval. Other antipsychotic drugs with a reduced tendency to prolong QT interval include amisulpride, clozapine, olanzapine, perphenazine, risperidone, and sulpiride p. 263.

Diabetes

Schizophrenia is associated with insulin resistance and diabetes; the risk of diabetes is increased in children with schizophrenia who take antipsychotic drugs. First-generation antipsychotic drugs are less likely to cause diabetes than second-generation antipsychotic drugs, and of the first-generation antipsychotic drugs, haloperidol has the lowest risk. Amisulpride and aripiprazole have the lowest risk of diabetes of the second-generation antipsychotic drugs. Amisulpride, aripiprazole, haloperidol, sulpiride, and trifluoperazine p. 264 are least likely to cause weight gain.

Sexual dysfunction and prolactin

The antipsychotic drugs with the lowest risk of sexual dysfunction are aripiprazole and quetiapine. Olanzapine may be considered if sexual dysfunction is judged to be secondary to hyperprolactinaemia. Hyperprolactinaemia is usually not clinically significant with aripiprazole, clozapine, olanzapine, and quetiapine treatment. When changing from other antipsychotic drugs, a reduction in prolactin concentration may increase fertility.

Children should receive an antipsychotic drug for 4–6 weeks before it is deemed ineffective. Prescribing more than one antipsychotic drug at a time should be avoided except in exceptional circumstances (e.g. clozapine augmentation or when changing medication during titration) because of the increased risk of adverse effects such as extrapyramidal symptoms, QT-interval prolongation, and sudden cardiac death.

Clozapine is used for the treatment of schizophrenia in children unresponsive to, or intolerant of, other antipsychotic drugs. Clozapine should be introduced if schizophrenia is not controlled despite the sequential use of two or more antipsychotic drugs (one of which should be a second-generation antipsychotic drug), each for at least 6–8 weeks. If symptoms do not respond adequately to an optimised dose of clozapine, plasma-clozapine concentration should be checked before adding a second antipsychotic drug to augment clozapine; allow 8–10 weeks' treatment to assess response. Children must be registered with a clozapine patient monitoring service.

Monitoring

Full blood count, urea and electrolytes, and liver function test monitoring is required at the start of therapy with antipsychotic drugs, and then annually thereafter.

Blood lipids and weight should be measured at baseline, at 3 months (weight should be measured at frequent intervals during the first 3 months), and then yearly.

Fasting blood glucose should be measured at baseline, at 4–6 months, and then yearly.

Before initiating antipsychotic drugs, an ECG may be required, particularly if physical examination identifies cardiovascular risk factors, if there is a personal history of cardiovascular disease, or if the child is being admitted as an inpatient.

Blood pressure monitoring is advised before starting therapy and frequently during dose titration of antipsychotic drugs.

Other uses

Nausea and vomiting, choreas, motor tics, and intractable hiccup.

Dosage

After an initial period of stabilisation, the total daily oral dose of antipsychotic drugs can be given as a single dose in most children.

Antipsychotic depot injections

There is limited information on the use of antipsychotic depot injections in children and use should be restricted to specialist centres.

ANTIPSYCHOTICS

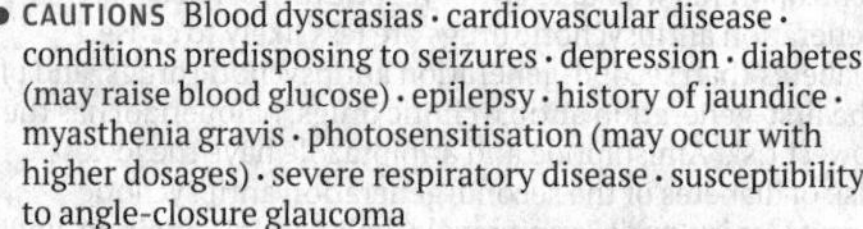

Antipsychotic drugs

- **CAUTIONS** Blood dyscrasias · cardiovascular disease · conditions predisposing to seizures · depression · diabetes (may raise blood glucose) · epilepsy · history of jaundice · myasthenia gravis · photosensitisation (may occur with higher dosages) · severe respiratory disease · susceptibility to angle-closure glaucoma

  CAUTIONS, FURTHER INFORMATION

  ▸ **Cardiovascular disease** An ECG may be required, particularly if physical examination identifies cardiovascular risk factors, personal history of cardiovascular disease, or if the patient is being admitted as an inpatient.

- **SIDE-EFFECTS**

  ▸ **Common or very common** Agitation · amenorrhoea · arrhythmias · constipation · dizziness · drowsiness · dry mouth · erectile dysfunction · galactorrhoea · gynaecomastia · hyperprolactinaemia · hypotension (dose-related) · insomnia · leucopenia · movement disorders · neutropenia · parkinsonism · QT interval prolongation · rash · seizure · tremor · urinary retention · vomiting · weight increased

  ▸ **Uncommon** Agranulocytosis · embolism and thrombosis · neuroleptic malignant syndrome (discontinue—potentially fatal)

  ▸ **Rare or very rare** Sudden death · withdrawal syndrome neonatal

  Overdose Phenothiazines cause less depression of consciousness and respiration than other sedatives. Hypotension, hypothermia, sinus tachycardia, and arrhythmias may complicate poisoning. For details on the management of poisoning see Antipsychotics under Emergency treatment of poisoning p. 891.

- **PREGNANCY** Extrapyramidal effects and withdrawal syndrome have been reported occasionally in the neonate when antipsychotic drugs are taken during the third trimester of pregnancy. Following maternal use of antipsychotic drugs in the third trimester, neonates should be monitored for symptoms including agitation, hypertonia, hypotonia, tremor, drowsiness, feeding problems, and respiratory distress.

- **BREAST FEEDING** There is limited information available on the short- and long-term effects of antipsychotic drugs on the breast-fed infant. *Animal studies* indicate possible adverse effects of antipsychotic medicines on the developing nervous system. Chronic treatment with antipsychotic drugs whilst breast-feeding should be avoided unless absolutely necessary. Phenothiazine derivatives are sometimes used in breast-feeding women for short-term treatment of nausea and vomiting.

- **MONITORING REQUIREMENTS**

  ▸ It is advisable to monitor prolactin concentration at the start of therapy, at 6 months, and then yearly. Patients taking antipsychotic drugs not normally associated with symptomatic hyperprolactinaemia should be considered for prolactin monitoring if they show symptoms of hyperprolactinaemia (such as breast enlargement and galactorrhoea).

  ▸ Patients with schizophrenia should have physical health monitoring (including cardiovascular disease risk assessment) at least once per year.

  ▸ Regular clinical monitoring of endocrine function should be considered when children are taking an antipsychotic drug known to increase prolactin levels; this includes measuring weight and height, assessing sexual maturation, and monitoring menstrual function.

- **TREATMENT CESSATION** There is a high risk of relapse if medication is stopped after 1–2 years. Withdrawal of antipsychotic drugs after long-term therapy should always be gradual and closely monitored to avoid the risk of acute withdrawal syndromes or rapid relapse. Patients should be monitored for 2 years after withdrawal of antipsychotic medication for signs and symptoms of relapse.

- **PATIENT AND CARER ADVICE** As photosensitisation may occur with higher dosages, patients should avoid direct sunlight.

  Driving and skilled tasks Drowsiness may affect performance of skilled tasks (e.g. driving or operating machinery), especially at start of treatment; effects of alcohol are enhanced.

ANTIPSYCHOTICS > FIRST-GENERATION

F 260

Chlorpromazine hydrochloride 13-Mar-2020

● **INDICATIONS AND DOSE**

Childhood schizophrenia and other psychoses (under expert supervision)

▶ BY MOUTH

- Child 1-5 years: 500 micrograms/kg every 4–6 hours, adjusted according to response; maximum 40 mg per day
- Child 6-11 years: 10 mg 3 times a day, adjusted according to response; maximum 75 mg per day
- Child 12-17 years: Initially 25 mg 3 times a day, adjusted according to response, alternatively initially 75 mg once daily, adjusted according to response, dose to be taken at night; maintenance 75–300 mg daily, increased if necessary up to 1 g daily

Relief of acute symptoms of psychoses (under expert supervision)

▶ BY DEEP INTRAMUSCULAR INJECTION

- Child 1-5 years: 500 micrograms/kg every 6–8 hours; maximum 40 mg per day
- Child 6-11 years: 500 micrograms/kg every 6–8 hours; maximum 75 mg per day
- Child 12-17 years: 25–50 mg every 6–8 hours

Nausea and vomiting in palliative care (where other drugs have failed or are not available)

▶ BY MOUTH

- Child 1-5 years: 500 micrograms/kg every 4–6 hours; maximum 40 mg per day
- Child 6-11 years: 500 micrograms/kg every 4–6 hours; maximum 75 mg per day
- Child 12-17 years: 10–25 mg every 4–6 hours

▶ BY DEEP INTRAMUSCULAR INJECTION

- Child 1-5 years: 500 micrograms/kg every 6–8 hours; maximum 40 mg per day
- Child 6-11 years: 500 micrograms/kg every 6–8 hours; maximum 75 mg per day
- Child 12-17 years: Initially 25 mg, then 25–50 mg every 3–4 hours until vomiting stops

DOSE EQUIVALENCE AND CONVERSION

- For equivalent therapeutic effect 100 mg chlorpromazine base given *rectally* as a suppository ≡ 20–25 mg chlorpromazine hydrochloride *by intramuscular injection* ≡ 40–50 mg of chlorpromazine base or hydrochloride given *by mouth*.

● **CONTRA-INDICATIONS** CNS depression · comatose states · hypothyroidism · phaeochromocytoma

● **INTERACTIONS** → Appendix 1: phenothiazines

● **SIDE-EFFECTS**

GENERAL SIDE-EFFECTS

▶ **Common or very common** Anxiety · glucose tolerance impaired · mood altered · muscle tone increased

▶ **Frequency not known** Accommodation disorder · angioedema · atrioventricular block · cardiac arrest · eye deposit · eye disorders · gastrointestinal disorders · hepatic disorders · hyperglycaemia · hypertriglyceridaemia · hyponatraemia · photosensitivity reaction · respiratory disorders · sexual dysfunction · SIADH · skin reactions · systemic lupus erythematosus (SLE) · temperature regulation disorder · trismus

SPECIFIC SIDE-EFFECTS

▶ With intramuscular use Muscle rigidity · nasal congestion

SIDE-EFFECTS, FURTHER INFORMATION Acute dystonic reactions may occur; children are particularly susceptible.

● **HEPATIC IMPAIRMENT** Manufacturer advises caution in severe hepatic failure (increased risk of accumulation).

● **RENAL IMPAIRMENT**

Dose adjustments Start with small doses in severe renal impairment because of increased cerebral sensitivity.

● **MONITORING REQUIREMENTS**

▶ With intramuscular use Patients should remain supine, with blood pressure monitoring for 30 minutes after intramuscular injection.

● **PRESCRIBING AND DISPENSING INFORMATION**

Palliative care For further information on the use of chlorpromazine hydrochloride in palliative care, see www.medicinescomplete.com/#/content/palliative/antipsychotics.

● **HANDLING AND STORAGE** Owing to the risk of contact sensitisation, pharmacists, nurses, and other health workers should avoid direct contact with chlorpromazine; tablets should not be crushed and solutions should be handled with care.

● **MEDICINAL FORMS** There can be variation in the licensing of different medicines containing the same drug. Forms available from special-order manufacturers include: tablet, capsule, oral suspension, oral solution

Tablet

CAUTIONARY AND ADVISORY LABELS 2, 11

▶ Chlorpromazine hydrochloride (Non-proprietary)

Chlorpromazine hydrochloride 25 mg Chlorpromazine 25mg tablets | 28 tablet PoM £37.13 DT = £26.46

Chlorpromazine hydrochloride 50 mg Chlorpromazine 50mg tablets | 28 tablet PoM £37.50 DT = £26.23

Chlorpromazine hydrochloride 100 mg Chlorpromazine 100mg tablets | 28 tablet PoM £39.99 DT = £26.79

Solution for injection

▶ Largactil (Sanofi)

Chlorpromazine hydrochloride 25 mg per 1 ml Largactil 50mg/2ml solution for injection ampoules | 10 ampoule PoM £7.51

Oral solution

CAUTIONARY AND ADVISORY LABELS 2, 11

▶ Chlorpromazine hydrochloride (Non-proprietary)

Chlorpromazine hydrochloride 5 mg per 1 ml Chlorpromazine 25mg/5ml syrup | 150 ml PoM £2.35 DT = £2.35

Chlorpromazine 25mg/5ml oral solution sugar-free | 150 ml PoM £2.66 DT = £2.40

Chlorpromazine 25mg/5ml oral solution | 150 ml PoM £2.35 DT = £2.35

Chlorpromazine hydrochloride 20 mg per 1 ml Chlorpromazine 100mg/5ml oral solution | 150 ml PoM £5.50 DT = £5.50

F 260

Haloperidol 20-Nov-2019

● **INDICATIONS AND DOSE**

Nausea and vomiting in palliative care

▶ BY MOUTH

- Child 12-17 years: 1.5 mg once daily, dose to be taken at night, increased if necessary to 1.5 mg twice daily (max. per dose 5 mg twice daily)

▶ BY CONTINUOUS INTRAVENOUS INFUSION, OR BY CONTINUOUS SUBCUTANEOUS INFUSION

- Child 1 month–11 years: 25–85 micrograms/kg, to be administered over 24 hours
- Child 12-17 years: 1.5–5 mg, to be administered over 24 hours

Schizophrenia [when alternatives ineffective or not tolerated] (under expert supervision)

▶ BY MOUTH

- Child 13-17 years: 0.25–1.5 mg twice daily, alternatively 0.16–1 mg 3 times a day, individual benefit-risk should be assessed when considering doses above 3 mg daily; maximum 5 mg per day

continued →

4 Nervous system

Persistent, severe aggression in autism or pervasive developmental disorders [when other treatments ineffective or not tolerated] (under expert supervision)
- BY MOUTH
- Child 6–11 years: 0.25–1.5 mg twice daily, alternatively 0.16–1 mg 3 times a day, the need for continued treatment must be reassessed after a maximum of 6 weeks and regularly thereafter
- Child 12–17 years: 0.25–2.5 mg twice daily, alternatively 0.16–1.6 mg 3 times a day, the need for continued treatment must be reassessed after a maximum of 6 weeks and regularly thereafter

Severe tic disorders, including Tourette's syndrome [when educational, psychological and other pharmacological treatments ineffective] (under expert supervision)
- BY MOUTH
- Child 10–17 years: 0.25–1.5 mg twice daily, alternatively 0.16–1 mg 3 times a day, the need for continued treatment must be reassessed every 6–12 months

Restlessness and confusion in palliative care
- BY MOUTH
- Child 1–17 years: 10–20 micrograms/kg every 8–12 hours

- UNLICENSED USE Not licensed for use in palliative care.
- CONTRA-INDICATIONS CNS depression · comatose states · congenital long QT syndrome · history of torsade de pointes · history of ventricular arrhythmia · QTc-interval prolongation · recent acute myocardial infarction · uncompensated heart failure · uncorrected hypokalaemia
- CAUTIONS Bradycardia · electrolyte disturbances (correct before treatment initiation) · family history of QTc-interval prolongation · history of heavy alcohol exposure · hyperthyroidism · hypotension (including orthostatic hypotension) · prolactin-dependent tumours · prolactinaemia
- INTERACTIONS → Appendix 1: haloperidol
- SIDE-EFFECTS

GENERAL SIDE-EFFECTS
- **Common or very common** Depression · eye disorders · headache · hypersalivation · nausea · neuromuscular dysfunction · psychotic disorder · vision disorders · weight decreased
- **Uncommon** Breast abnormalities · confusion · dyspnoea · gait abnormal · hepatic disorders · hyperhidrosis · menstrual cycle irregularities · muscle complaints · musculoskeletal stiffness · oedema · photosensitivity reaction · restlessness · sexual dysfunction · skin reactions · temperature regulation disorders
- **Rare or very rare** Hypoglycaemia · respiratory disorders · SIADH · trismus
- **Frequency not known** Hypersensitivity vasculitis · pancytopenia · rhabdomyolysis · thrombocytopenia

SPECIFIC SIDE-EFFECTS
- With oral use Angioedema
- With parenteral use Severe cutaneous adverse reactions (SCARs)

SIDE-EFFECTS, FURTHER INFORMATION Haloperidol is a less sedating antipsychotic.

- PREGNANCY Manufacturer advises it is preferable to avoid—moderate amount of data indicate no malformative or fetal/neonatal toxicity, however there are isolated case reports of birth defects following fetal exposure, mostly in combination with other drugs; reproductive toxicity shown in *animal* studies.
- HEPATIC IMPAIRMENT Manufacturer advises caution.
Dose adjustments Manufacturer advises halve initial dose and then adjust if necessary with smaller increments and at longer intervals.
- RENAL IMPAIRMENT Manufacturer advises use with caution.
Dose adjustments Manufacturer advises consider lower initial dose in severe impairment and then adjust if necessary with smaller increments and at longer intervals.
- MONITORING REQUIREMENTS
  - Manufacturer advises monitor electrolytes before treatment initiation and periodically during treatment.
  - Manufacturer advises perform ECG before treatment initiation and assess need for further ECGs during treatment on an individual basis.
- PRESCRIBING AND DISPENSING INFORMATION
Palliative care For further information on the use of haloperidol in palliative care, see www.medicinescomplete.com/#/content/palliative/haloperidol.
- MEDICINAL FORMS There can be variation in the licensing of different medicines containing the same drug. Forms available from special-order manufacturers include: oral suspension, oral solution

Solution for injection
- Haloperidol (Non-proprietary)
Haloperidol 5 mg per 1 ml Haloperidol 5mg/1ml solution for injection ampoules | 10 ampoule PoM £35.00 DT = £35.00

Oral solution
CAUTIONARY AND ADVISORY LABELS 2
- Haloperidol (Non-proprietary)
Haloperidol 1 mg per 1 ml Haloperidol 5mg/5ml oral solution sugar-free | 100 ml PoM £35.99 DT = £6.48 sugar-free | 500 ml PoM £32.40
Haloperidol 2 mg per 1 ml Haloperidol 10mg/5ml oral solution sugar-free | 100 ml PoM £46.75 DT = £7.10
- Haldol (Janssen-Cilag Ltd)
Haloperidol 2 mg per 1 ml Haldol 2mg/ml oral solution sugar-free | 100 ml PoM £4.45 DT = £7.10
- Halkid (Thame Laboratories Ltd)
Haloperidol 200 microgram per 1 ml Halkid 200micrograms/ml oral solution sugar-free | 100 ml PoM £89.90 DT = £89.90

Tablet
CAUTIONARY AND ADVISORY LABELS 2
- Haloperidol (Non-proprietary)
Haloperidol 500 microgram Haloperidol 500microgram tablets | 28 tablet PoM £22.05–£55.14 DT = £45.26
Haloperidol 1.5 mg Haloperidol 1.5mg tablets | 28 tablet PoM £14.00 DT = £4.63
Haloperidol 5 mg Haloperidol 5mg tablets | 28 tablet PoM £16.00 DT = £5.90
Haloperidol 10 mg Haloperidol 10mg tablets | 28 tablet PoM £18.00 DT = £17.73

F 260

Pericyazine

(Periciazine)

- INDICATIONS AND DOSE

Schizophrenia (under expert supervision) | Psychoses (severe mental or behavioural disorders only) (under expert supervision)
- BY MOUTH
- Child 1–11 years: Initially 500 micrograms daily for 10-kg child, increased by 1 mg for each additional 5 kg; dose may be gradually increased according to response but maintenance should not exceed twice initial dose; maximum 10 mg per day
- Child 12–17 years: Initially 25 mg 3 times a day, increased in steps of 25 mg every week, adjusted according to response, increased if necessary up to 100 mg 3 times a day, total daily dose may alternatively be given in 2 divided doses

- UNLICENSED USE Tablets not licensed for use in children.
- CONTRA-INDICATIONS CNS depression · comatose states · phaeochromocytoma
- CAUTIONS Hypothyroidism

- **INTERACTIONS** → Appendix 1: phenothiazines
- **SIDE-EFFECTS** Atrioventricular block · cardiac arrest · consciousness impaired · contact dermatitis · glucose tolerance impaired · hepatic disorders · hyperglycaemia · hyperthermia · nasal congestion · priapism · respiratory depression
- **HEPATIC IMPAIRMENT** Can precipitate coma; phenothiazines are hepatotoxic.
- **RENAL IMPAIRMENT** Avoid in renal impairment.

- **MEDICINAL FORMS** There can be variation in the licensing of different medicines containing the same drug. Forms available from special-order manufacturers include: oral suspension, oral solution

Oral solution

CAUTIONARY AND ADVISORY LABELS 2

- Pericyazine (Non-proprietary)
  Pericyazine 2 mg per 1 ml Pericyazine 10mg/5ml oral solution | 100 ml [PoM] £82.80 DT = £82.80

Tablet

CAUTIONARY AND ADVISORY LABELS 2

- Pericyazine (Non-proprietary)
  Pericyazine 2.5 mg Pericyazine 2.5mg tablets | 84 tablet [PoM] £27.90 DT = £27.90
  Pericyazine 10 mg Pericyazine 10mg tablets | 84 tablet [PoM] £72.00 DT = £72.00

F 260

Pimozide

- **INDICATIONS AND DOSE**

Schizophrenia

▶ BY MOUTH

- Child 12–17 years (under expert supervision): Initially 1 mg daily, adjusted according to response, then increased in steps of 2–4 mg at intervals of not less than 1 week; usual dose 2–20 mg daily

Tourette syndrome (under expert supervision)

▶ BY MOUTH

- Child 2–11 years: 1–4 mg daily
- Child 12–17 years: 2–10 mg daily

- **UNLICENSED USE** Not licensed for use in Tourette syndrome.
- **CONTRA-INDICATIONS** CNS depression · comatose states · history of arrhythmias · history or family history of congenital QT prolongation · phaeochromocytoma
- **INTERACTIONS** → Appendix 1: pimozide
- **SIDE-EFFECTS**
  - **Common or very common** Appetite decreased · depression · fatigue · headache · hyperhidrosis · hypersalivation · muscle complaints · restlessness · sebaceous gland overactivity · urinary disorders · vision blurred
  - **Uncommon** Dysarthria · face oedema · oculogyric crisis · skin reactions
  - **Frequency not known** Cardiac arrest · generalised tonic-clonic seizure · glycosuria · hyperglycaemia · hyponatraemia · libido decreased · neck stiffness · temperature regulation disorders
- **HEPATIC IMPAIRMENT** Manufacturer advises caution.
- **RENAL IMPAIRMENT**
  Dose adjustments Start with small doses in severe renal impairment because of increased cerebral sensitivity.
- **MONITORING REQUIREMENTS**
  - **ECG monitoring** Following reports of sudden unexplained death, an ECG is recommended before treatment. It is also recommended that patients taking pimozide should have an annual ECG (if the QT interval is prolonged, treatment should be reviewed and either withdrawn or dose reduced under close supervision) and that pimozide should not be given with other antipsychotic drugs (including depot preparations), tricyclic antidepressants or other drugs which prolong the QT interval, such as certain antimalarials, antiarrhythmic drugs and certain antihistamines and should not be given with drugs which cause electrolyte disturbances (especially diuretics).

- **MEDICINAL FORMS** There can be variation in the licensing of different medicines containing the same drug. Forms available from special-order manufacturers include: oral suspension

Tablet

CAUTIONARY AND ADVISORY LABELS 2

- Orap (Imported (United States))
  Pimozide 1 mg Orap 1mg tablets | 100 tablet [PoM] [X]
- Orap (Eumedica Pharmaceuticals)
  Pimozide 4 mg Orap 4mg tablets | 100 tablet [PoM] £40.31 DT = £40.31

F 260

Sulpiride

10-Mar-2020

- **INDICATIONS AND DOSE**

Schizophrenia with predominantly negative symptoms

▶ BY MOUTH

- Child 14–17 years (under expert supervision): 200–400 mg twice daily; maximum 800 mg per day

Schizophrenia with mainly positive symptoms

▶ BY MOUTH

- Child 14–17 years (under expert supervision): 200–400 mg twice daily; maximum 2.4 g per day

Tourette syndrome (under expert supervision)

▶ BY MOUTH

- Child 2–11 years: 50–400 mg twice daily
- Child 12–17 years: 100–400 mg twice daily

- **UNLICENSED USE** Not licensed for use in Tourette syndrome.
- **CONTRA-INDICATIONS** CNS depression · comatose states · phaeochromocytoma
- **CAUTIONS** Aggressive patients (even low doses may aggravate symptoms) · agitated patients (even low doses may aggravate symptoms) · excited patients (even low doses may aggravate symptoms)
- **INTERACTIONS** → Appendix 1: sulpiride
- **SIDE-EFFECTS**
  - **Common or very common** Breast abnormalities
  - **Uncommon** Hypersalivation · muscle tone increased · orgasm abnormal
  - **Rare or very rare** Oculogyric crisis
  - **Frequency not known** Cardiac arrest · confusion · dyspnoea · hyponatraemia · SIADH · trismus · urticaria
- **RENAL IMPAIRMENT**
  Dose adjustments Start with small doses in severe renal impairment because of increased cerebral sensitivity.
- **MONITORING REQUIREMENTS** Sulpiride does not affect blood pressure to the same extent as other antipsychotic drugs and so blood pressure monitoring is not mandatory for this drug.
- **PRESCRIBING AND DISPENSING INFORMATION** Flavours of oral liquid formulations may include lemon and aniseed.
- **PATIENT AND CARER ADVICE**
  Medicines for Children leaflet: Sulpiride for schizophrenia and Tourette's syndrome www.medicinesforchildren.org.uk/sulpiride-schizophrenia-and-tourettes-syndrome

- **MEDICINAL FORMS** There can be variation in the licensing of different medicines containing the same drug. Forms available from special-order manufacturers include: oral suspension, oral solution

Oral solution

CAUTIONARY AND ADVISORY LABELS 2

- Sulpiride (Non-proprietary)
  Sulpiride 40 mg per 1 ml Sulpiride 200mg/5ml oral solution sugar-free | 150 ml [PoM] £36.32 DT = £31.00

Tablet

CAUTIONARY AND ADVISORY LABELS 2

- Sulpiride (Non-proprietary)
  Sulpiride 200 mg Sulpiride 200mg tablets | 30 tablet [PoM] £9.00 DT = £6.35
  Sulpiride 400 mg Sulpiride 400mg tablets | 30 tablet [PoM] £23.50 DT = £20.65

F 260

Trifluoperazine

● **INDICATIONS AND DOSE**

Schizophrenia and other psychoses | Short-term adjunctive management of psychomotor agitation, excitement, and violent or dangerously impulsive behaviour

▶ BY MOUTH

- Child 12–17 years (under expert supervision): Initially 5 mg twice daily, daily dose may be increased by 5 mg after 1 week. If necessary, dose may be further increased in steps of 5 mg at intervals of 3 days. When satisfactory control has been achieved, reduce gradually until an effective maintenance level has been established

Short-term adjunctive management of severe anxiety

▶ BY MOUTH

- Child 3–5 years (under expert supervision): Up to 500 micrograms twice daily
- Child 6–11 years (under expert supervision): Up to 2 mg twice daily
- Child 12–17 years (under expert supervision): 1–2 mg twice daily, increased if necessary to 3 mg twice daily

Severe nausea and vomiting unresponsive to other antiemetics

▶ BY MOUTH

- Child 3–5 years: Up to 500 micrograms twice daily
- Child 6–11 years: Up to 2 mg twice daily
- Child 12–17 years: 1–2 mg twice daily (max. per dose 3 mg twice daily)

● **CONTRA-INDICATIONS** CNS depression · comatose states · phaeochromocytoma

● **INTERACTIONS** → Appendix 1: phenothiazines

● **SIDE-EFFECTS** Alertness decreased · anxiety · appetite decreased · blood disorder · cardiac arrest · confusion · fatigue · hyperpyrexia · jaundice cholestatic · lens opacity · muscle weakness · oedema · pancytopenia · photosensitivity reaction · postural hypotension (dose-related) · skin reactions · thrombocytopenia · urinary hesitation · vision blurred · withdrawal syndrome

SIDE-EFFECTS, FURTHER INFORMATION Extrapyramidal symptoms are more frequent at doses exceeding 6mg daily. Acute dystonias are more common with potent first generation antipsychotics. The risk is increased in men, young adults, children, antipsychotic-naïve patients, rapid dose escalation, and abrupt treatment discontinuation.

● **HEPATIC IMPAIRMENT** Manufacturer advises avoid.

● **RENAL IMPAIRMENT**

Dose adjustments Start with small doses in severe renal impairment because of increased cerebral sensitivity.

● **MONITORING REQUIREMENTS** Trifluoperazine does not affect blood pressure to the same extent as other antipsychotic drugs and so blood pressure monitoring is not mandatory for this drug.

● **MEDICINAL FORMS** There can be variation in the licensing of different medicines containing the same drug.

Oral solution

CAUTIONARY AND ADVISORY LABELS 2

- Trifluoperazine (Non-proprietary)
  Trifluoperazine (as Trifluoperazine hydrochloride) 200 microgram per 1 ml Trifluoperazine 1mg/5ml oral solution sugar-free | 200 ml [PoM] £125.00 DT = £125.00
  Trifluoperazine (as Trifluoperazine hydrochloride) 1 mg per 1 ml Trifluoperazine 5mg/5ml oral solution sugar-free | 150 ml [PoM] £30.00 DT = £29.25

Tablet

CAUTIONARY AND ADVISORY LABELS 2

- Trifluoperazine (Non-proprietary)
  Trifluoperazine (as Trifluoperazine hydrochloride) 1 mg Trifluoperazine 1mg tablets | 112 tablet [PoM] £59.12–£99.80 DT = £59.12
  Trifluoperazine (as Trifluoperazine hydrochloride) 5 mg Trifluoperazine 5mg tablets | 112 tablet [PoM] £134.89–£165.00 DT = £134.89

ANTIPSYCHOTICS > SECOND-GENERATION

F 260

Amisulpride

● **DRUG ACTION** Amisulpride is a selective dopamine receptor antagonist with high affinity for mesolimbic D_2 and D_3 receptors.

● **INDICATIONS AND DOSE**

Acute psychotic episode in schizophrenia

▶ BY MOUTH

- Child 15–17 years (under expert supervision): 200–400 mg twice daily, adjusted according to response; maximum 1.2 g per day

Schizophrenia with predominantly negative symptoms

▶ BY MOUTH

- Child 15–17 years (under expert supervision): 50–300 mg daily

● **UNLICENSED USE** Not licensed for use in children under 18 years.

● **CONTRA-INDICATIONS** CNS depression · comatose states · phaeochromocytoma · pre-pubertal children · prolactin-dependent tumours

● **INTERACTIONS** → Appendix 1: amisulpride

● **SIDE-EFFECTS**

▶ **Common or very common** Anxiety · breast pain · hypersalivation · muscle rigidity · nausea · oculogyric crisis · orgasm abnormal · trismus

▶ **Uncommon** Hyperglycaemia

▶ **Frequency not known** Angioedema · bone disorders · cardiac arrest · confusion · dyslipidaemia · hyponatraemia · nasal congestion · neoplasms · SIADH · urticaria · vision blurred

● **PREGNANCY** Avoid.

● **BREAST FEEDING** Avoid—no information available.

● **RENAL IMPAIRMENT** No information available if estimated glomerular filtration rate less than 10 mL/minute/1.73 m^2.

Dose adjustments Halve dose if estimated glomerular filtration rate 30–60 mL/minute/1.73 m^2.

Use one-third dose if estimated glomerular filtration rate 10–30 mL/minute/1.73 m^2.

● **MONITORING REQUIREMENTS** Amisulpride does not affect blood pressure to the same extent as other antipsychotic drugs and so blood pressure monitoring is not mandatory for this drug.

● **PRESCRIBING AND DISPENSING INFORMATION** Flavours of oral liquid formulations may include caramel.

● **MEDICINAL FORMS** There can be variation in the licensing of different medicines containing the same drug. Forms available from special-order manufacturers include: oral suspension, oral solution

Oral solution

CAUTIONARY AND ADVISORY LABELS 2

- Amisulpride (Non-proprietary)
  Amisulpride 100 mg per 1 ml Amisulpride 100mg/ml oral solution sugar-free | 60 ml [PoM] £88.50 DT = £77.13

▸ Solian (Sanofi)
Amisulpride 100 mg per 1 ml Solian 100mg/ml oral solution sugar-free | 60 ml PoM £33.76 DT = £77.13

Tablet

CAUTIONARY AND ADVISORY LABELS 2

▸ Amisulpride (Non-proprietary)
Amisulpride 50 mg Amisulpride 50mg tablets | 60 tablet PoM £19.74 DT = £5.39
Amisulpride 100 mg Amisulpride 100mg tablets | 60 tablet PoM £39.48 DT = £9.10
Amisulpride 200 mg Amisulpride 200mg tablets | 60 tablet PoM £66.00 DT = £12.85
Amisulpride 400 mg Amisulpride 400mg tablets | 60 tablet PoM £132.00 DT = £42.08

▸ Solian (Sanofi)
Amisulpride 50 mg Solian 50 tablets | 60 tablet PoM £22.76 DT = £5.39
Amisulpride 100 mg Solian 100 tablets | 60 tablet PoM £35.29 DT = £9.10
Amisulpride 200 mg Solian 200 tablets | 60 tablet PoM £58.99 DT = £12.85
Amisulpride 400 mg Solian 400 tablets | 60 tablet PoM £117.97 DT = £42.08

260

Aripiprazole

20-Nov-2019

● DRUG ACTION Aripiprazole is a dopamine D_2 partial agonist with weak $5\text{-}HT_{1a}$ partial agonism and $5\text{-}HT_{2A}$ receptor antagonism.

● **INDICATIONS AND DOSE**

Schizophrenia

▸ BY MOUTH

▸ Child 15–17 years (under expert supervision): Initially 2 mg once daily for 2 days, increased to 5 mg once daily for 2 days, then increased to 10 mg once daily, then increased in steps of 5 mg if required; maximum 30 mg per day

Treatment of mania (under expert supervision)

▸ BY MOUTH

▸ Child 13–17 years: Initially 2 mg once daily for 2 days, increased to 5 mg once daily for 2 days, then increased to 10 mg once daily, increased in steps of 5 mg if required, maximum duration of treatment 12 weeks, doses above 10 mg daily should only be used in exceptional cases; maximum 30 mg per day

DOSE ADJUSTMENTS DUE TO INTERACTIONS
Manufacturer advises double the dose with concurrent use of potent inducers of CYP3A4—no specific recommendation made for children. Manufacturer advises reduce dose by half with concurrent use of potent inhibitors of CYP3A4 or CYP2D6—no specific recommendation made for children.

IMPORTANT SAFETY INFORMATION
When prescribing, dispensing, or administering, check that the correct preparation is used—the preparation usually used in hospital for the rapid control of an *acute episode* (solution for injection containing aripiprazole 7.5 mg/mL) should **not** be confused with depot preparations (aripiprazole 400-mg vial with solvent), which are usually used in the community or clinics for *maintenance treatment*.

● CONTRA-INDICATIONS CNS depression · comatose state · phaeochromocytoma

● CAUTIONS Cerebrovascular disease

● INTERACTIONS → Appendix 1: aripiprazole

● SIDE-EFFECTS

▸ **Common or very common** Anxiety · appetite abnormal · diabetes mellitus · fatigue · gastrointestinal discomfort · headache · hypersalivation · nausea · vision disorders

▸ **Uncommon** Depression · hiccups · hyperglycaemia · sexual dysfunction

▸ **Frequency not known** Aggression · alopecia · cardiac arrest · chest pain · diabetic hyperosmolar coma · diabetic ketoacidosis · diarrhoea · dysphagia · generalised tonic-clonic seizure · hepatic disorders · hyperhidrosis · hypertension · hyponatraemia · laryngospasm · musculoskeletal stiffness · myalgia · oropharyngeal spasm · pancreatitis · pathological gambling · peripheral oedema · photosensitivity reaction · pneumonia aspiration · rhabdomyolysis · serotonin syndrome · speech disorder · suicidal tendencies · syncope · temperature regulation disorder · thrombocytopenia · urinary incontinence · weight decreased

SIDE-EFFECTS, FURTHER INFORMATION Increased incidence of side-effects associated with doses of 30 mg daily; doses above 10 mg daily should only be used in exceptional cases and with close clinical monitoring.

● PREGNANCY Use only if potential benefit outweighs risk.

● BREAST FEEDING Manufacturer advises avoid—present in milk.

● HEPATIC IMPAIRMENT Manufacturer advises caution in severe impairment (oral treatment preferred to intramuscular administration; limited information available).

● MONITORING REQUIREMENTS Aripiprazole does not affect blood pressure to the same extent as other antipsychotic drugs and so blood pressure monitoring is not mandatory for this drug.

● DIRECTIONS FOR ADMINISTRATION Orodispersible tablets should be placed on the tongue and allowed to dissolve, or be dispersed in water and swallowed.

● PATIENT AND CARER ADVICE Patients or carers should be given advice on how to administer aripiprazole orodispersible tablets.
Medicines for Children leaflet: Aripiprazole for schizophrenia, bipolar disorder and tics www.medicinesforchildren.org.uk/aripiprazole-schizophrenia-bipolar-disorder-and-tics

● NATIONAL FUNDING/ACCESS DECISIONS

NICE decisions

▸ **Aripiprazole for the treatment of schizophrenia in people aged 15 to 17 years (January 2011)** NICE TA213
Aripiprazole is recommended as an option for the treatment of schizophrenia in adolescents aged 15 to 17 years who have not responded adequately to, or who are intolerant of, risperidone, or for whom risperidone is contra-indicated.
Patients whose treatment was started within the NHS before this guidance was published should have the option to continue treatment until they and their NHS clinician consider it appropriate to stop.
www.nice.org.uk/guidance/ta213

▸ **Aripiprazole for treating moderate to severe manic episodes in adolescents with bipolar I disorder (July 2013)** NICE TA292
Aripiprazole is recommended as an option for the treatment of moderate to severe manic episodes for up to 12 weeks in adolescents aged 13 years and older with bipolar I disorder.
www.nice.org.uk/guidance/ta292

ABILIFY® ORAL SOLUTION

Scottish Medicines Consortium (SMC) decisions

The *Scottish Medicines Consortium*, has advised (August 2013) that oral aripiprazole (*Abilify®*) is accepted for restricted use within NHS Scotland for the treatment of moderate to severe manic episodes in Bipolar I Disorder in adolescents aged 13 years and older for a period of up to 12 weeks. It is restricted to initiation and management under the supervision of a child/adolescent psychiatrist.

- **MEDICINAL FORMS** There can be variation in the licensing of different medicines containing the same drug. Forms available from special-order manufacturers include: oral solution

Tablet

CAUTIONARY AND ADVISORY LABELS 2

- ▸ Aripiprazole (Non-proprietary)
  - **Aripiprazole 5 mg** Aripiprazole 5mg tablets | 28 tablet PoM £96.04 DT = £1.36
  - **Aripiprazole 10 mg** Aripiprazole 10mg tablets | 28 tablet PoM £96.04 DT = £1.36
  - **Aripiprazole 15 mg** Aripiprazole 15mg tablets | 28 tablet PoM £96.04 DT = £1.57
  - **Aripiprazole 30 mg** Aripiprazole 30mg tablets | 28 tablet PoM £192.08 DT = £13.94
- ▸ Arpoya (Torrent Pharma (UK) Ltd)
  - **Aripiprazole 5 mg** Arpoya 5mg tablets | 28 tablet PoM £96.04 DT = £1.36
  - **Aripiprazole 10 mg** Arpoya 10mg tablets | 28 tablet PoM £96.04 DT = £1.36
  - **Aripiprazole 15 mg** Arpoya 15mg tablets | 28 tablet PoM £96.04 DT = £1.57
  - **Aripiprazole 30 mg** Arpoya 30mg tablets | 28 tablet PoM £192.08 DT = £13.94

Oral solution

CAUTIONARY AND ADVISORY LABELS 2

- ▸ Aripiprazole (Non-proprietary)
  - **Aripiprazole 1 mg per 1 ml** Aripiprazole 1mg/ml oral solution sugar-free | 150 ml PoM £101.20
  - Aripiprazole 1mg/ml oral solution | 150 ml PoM £102.90 DT = £99.55
- ▸ Abilify (Otsuka Pharmaceuticals (U.K.) Ltd)
  - **Aripiprazole 1 mg per 1 ml** Abilify 1mg/ml oral solution | 150 ml PoM £102.90 DT = £99.55

Orodispersible tablet

CAUTIONARY AND ADVISORY LABELS 2

EXCIPIENTS: May contain Aspartame

- ▸ Aripiprazole (Non-proprietary)
  - **Aripiprazole 10 mg** Aripiprazole 10mg orodispersible tablets sugar-free | 28 tablet PoM £96.04 DT = £65.69
  - **Aripiprazole 15 mg** Aripiprazole 15mg orodispersible tablets sugar-free | 28 tablet PoM £96.04 DT = £65.69

F 260

Clozapine

02-Jul-2018

- **DRUG ACTION** Clozapine is a dopamine D_1, dopamine D_2, 5-HT_{2A}, alpha$_1$-adrenoceptor, and muscarinic-receptor antagonist.

- **INDICATIONS AND DOSE**

Schizophrenia in patients unresponsive to, or intolerant of, conventional antipsychotic drugs

▸ BY MOUTH

▸ Child 12–17 years (under expert supervision): 12.5 mg 1–2 times a day for day 1, then 25–50 mg for day 2, then increased, if tolerated, in steps of 25–50 mg daily, dose to be increased gradually over 14–21 days, increased to up to 300 mg daily in divided doses, larger dose to be taken at night, up to 200 mg daily may be taken as a single dose at bedtime; increased in steps of 50–100 mg 1–2 times a week if required, it is preferable to increase once a week; usual dose 200–450 mg daily, max. 900 mg per day, if restarting after interval of more than 48 hours, 12.5 mg once or twice on first day (but may be feasible to increase more quickly than on initiation)—extreme caution if previous respiratory or cardiac arrest with initial dosing

- **UNLICENSED USE** Not licensed for use in children under 16 years.

IMPORTANT SAFETY INFORMATION

MHRA/CHM ADVICE: CLOZAPINE: REMINDER OF POTENTIALLY FATAL RISK OF INTESTINAL OBSTRUCTION, FAECAL IMPACTION, AND PARALYTIC ILEUS (OCTOBER 2017)

Clozapine has been associated with varying degrees of impairment of intestinal peristalsis—see Cautions and Contra-indications for further information. Patients and their carers should be advised to seek immediate medical advice before taking the next dose of clozapine if constipation develops.

- **CONTRA-INDICATIONS** Alcoholic and toxic psychoses · bone-marrow disorders · coma · drug intoxication · history of agranulocytosis · history of circulatory collapse · history of neutropenia · paralytic ileus · severe cardiac disorders (e.g. myocarditis) · severe CNS depression · uncontrolled epilepsy
- **CAUTIONS** Susceptibility to angle-closure glaucoma · taper off other antipsychotics before starting

CAUTIONS, FURTHER INFORMATION

▸ Agranulocytosis Neutropenia and potentially fatal agranulocytosis reported. Leucocyte and differential blood counts must be normal before starting; monitor counts every week for 18 weeks then at least every 2 weeks and if clozapine continued and blood count stable after 1 year at least every 4 weeks (and 4 weeks after discontinuation); if leucocyte count below 3000 /mm^3 or if absolute neutrophil count below 1500 /mm^3 discontinue permanently and refer to haematologist. Patients who have a low white blood cell count because of benign ethnic neutropenia may be started on clozapine with the agreement of a haematologist. Avoid drugs which depress leucopoiesis; patients should report immediately symptoms of infection, especially influenza-like illness.

▸ Myocarditis and cardiomyopathy Fatal myocarditis (most commonly in first 2 months) and cardiomyopathy reported.
- Perform physical examination and take full medical history before starting
- Specialist examination required if cardiac abnormalities or history of heart disease found—clozapine initiated only in absence of severe heart disease and if benefit outweighs risk
- Persistent tachycardia especially in first 2 months should prompt observation for other indicators for myocarditis or cardiomyopathy
- If myocarditis or cardiomyopathy suspected clozapine should be stopped and patient evaluated urgently by cardiologist
- Discontinue permanently in clozapine-induced myocarditis or cardiomyopathy

▸ Intestinal obstruction Impairment of intestinal peristalsis, including constipation, intestinal obstruction, faecal impaction, and paralytic ileus, (including fatal cases) reported. Clozapine should be used with caution in patients receiving drugs that may cause constipation (e.g. antimuscarinic drugs) or in those with a history of colonic disease or lower abdominal surgery. It is essential that constipation is recognised and actively treated.

- **INTERACTIONS** → Appendix 1: clozapine
- **SIDE-EFFECTS**

▸ **Common or very common** Appetite decreased · eosinophilia · fatigue · fever · headache · hypertension · leucocytosis · muscle complaints · nausea · oral disorders · postural hypotension (dose-related) · speech impairment · sweating abnormal · syncope · temperature regulation disorders · urinary disorders · vision blurred

▸ **Uncommon** Fall

▸ **Rare or very rare** Anaemia · cardiac arrest · cardiac inflammation · cardiomyopathy · circulatory collapse · confusion · delirium · diabetes mellitus · dyslipidaemia · dysphagia · gastrointestinal disorders · glucose tolerance impaired · hepatic disorders · hyperglycaemia · increased risk of infection · intestinal obstruction (including fatal cases) · ketoacidosis · nephritis tubulointerstitial · obsessive-compulsive disorder · pancreatitis · pericardial effusion · respiratory disorders · restlessness · sexual

dysfunction · skin reactions · sleep apnoea · thrombocytopenia · thrombocytosis
- **Frequency not known** Angina pectoris · angioedema · chest pain · cholinergic syndrome · diarrhoea · gastrointestinal discomfort · hypersensitivity vasculitis · mitral valve incompetence · muscle weakness · myocardial infarction · nasal congestion · palpitations · polyserositis · pseudophaeochromocytoma · renal failure · rhabdomyolysis · sepsis · systemic lupus erythematosus (SLE)

SIDE-EFFECTS, FURTHER INFORMATION Hypersalivation associated with clozapine therapy can be treated with hyoscine hydrobromide [unlicensed indication], provided that the patient is not at particular risk from the additive antimuscarinic side-effects of hyoscine and clozapine.

- **PREGNANCY** Use with caution.
- **BREAST FEEDING** Avoid.
- **HEPATIC IMPAIRMENT** Manufacturer advises caution—monitor liver function (discontinue if liver enzymes are greater than 3 times the upper limit of normal or jaundice occurs); avoid in symptomatic or progressive impairment and in hepatic failure.
- **RENAL IMPAIRMENT** Avoid in severe impairment.
- **MONITORING REQUIREMENTS**
  - Monitor leucocyte and differential blood counts. Clozapine requires differential white blood cell monitoring weekly for 18 weeks, then fortnightly for up to one year, and then monthly as part of the clozapine patient monitoring service.
  - Close medical supervision during initiation (risk of collapse because of hypotension and convulsions).
  - Blood lipids and weight should be measured at baseline, at 3 months (weight should be measured at frequent intervals during the first 3 months), and then yearly with antipsychotics. Patients taking clozapine require more frequent monitoring of these parameters: every 3 months for the first year, then yearly.
  - Fasting blood glucose should be measured at baseline, at 4–6 months, and then yearly. Patients taking clozapine should have fasting blood glucose tested at baseline, after one months' treatment, then every 4–6 months.
  - Patient, prescriber, and supplying pharmacist must be registered with the appropriate Patient Monitoring Service—it takes several days to do this.
- **TREATMENT CESSATION** On planned withdrawal reduce dose over 1–2 weeks to avoid risk of rebound psychosis. If abrupt withdrawal necessary observe patient carefully.
- **DIRECTIONS FOR ADMINISTRATION** Shake oral suspension well for 90 seconds when dispensing or if visibly settled and stand for 24 hours before use; otherwise shake well for 10 seconds before use. May be diluted with water. Orodispersible tablets should be placed on the tongue, allowed to dissolve and swallowed.
- **PRESCRIBING AND DISPENSING INFORMATION** Clozapine has been used for psychosis in Parkinson's disease in children aged 16 years and over.
- **PATIENT AND CARER ADVICE** Patients or carers should be given advice on how to administer clozapine oral suspension and orodispersible tablets.

- **MEDICINAL FORMS** There can be variation in the licensing of different medicines containing the same drug. Forms available from special-order manufacturers include: oral suspension, oral solution

Tablet

CAUTIONARY AND ADVISORY LABELS 2, 10

- Clozaril (Mylan)
  - **Clozapine 25 mg** Clozaril 25mg tablets | 28 tablet PoM £3.02 (Hospital only) | 84 tablet PoM £8.40 DT = £16.64 (Hospital only) | 100 tablet PoM £10.00 (Hospital only)
  - **Clozapine 100 mg** Clozaril 100mg tablets | 28 tablet PoM £12.07 (Hospital only) | 84 tablet PoM £33.60 DT = £66.53 (Hospital only) | 100 tablet PoM £39.00 (Hospital only)
- Denzapine (Britannia Pharmaceuticals Ltd)
  - **Clozapine 25 mg** Denzapine 25mg tablets | 84 tablet PoM £16.64 DT = £16.64 | 100 tablet PoM £19.80
  - **Clozapine 50 mg** Denzapine 50mg tablets | 100 tablet PoM £39.60 DT = £39.60
  - **Clozapine 100 mg** Denzapine 100mg tablets | 84 tablet PoM £66.53 DT = £66.53 | 100 tablet PoM £79.20
  - **Clozapine 200 mg** Denzapine 200mg tablets | 100 tablet PoM £158.40 DT = £158.40
- Zaponex (Leyden Delta B.V.)
  - **Clozapine 25 mg** Zaponex 25mg tablets | 84 tablet PoM £8.28 DT = £16.64 | 500 tablet PoM £48.39
  - **Clozapine 100 mg** Zaponex 100mg tablets | 84 tablet PoM £33.88 DT = £66.53 | 500 tablet PoM £196.43

Oral suspension

CAUTIONARY AND ADVISORY LABELS 2, 10

- Denzapine (Britannia Pharmaceuticals Ltd)
  - **Clozapine 50 mg per 1 ml** Denzapine 50mg/ml oral suspension sugar-free | 100 ml PoM £39.60 DT = £39.60

Orodispersible tablet

CAUTIONARY AND ADVISORY LABELS 2, 10

EXCIPIENTS: May contain Aspartame

- Clozapine (Non-proprietary)
  - **Clozapine 12.5 mg** Zaponex 12.5mg orodispersible tablets sugar-free | 28 tablet PoM £3.38
  - **Clozapine 25 mg** Zaponex 25mg orodispersible tablets sugar-free | 28 tablet PoM £6.77
  - **Clozapine 50 mg** Zaponex 50mg orodispersible tablets sugar-free | 28 tablet PoM £13.53
  - **Clozapine 100 mg** Zaponex 100mg orodispersible tablets sugar-free | 28 tablet PoM £27.06
  - **Clozapine 200 mg** Zaponex 200mg orodispersible tablets sugar-free | 28 tablet PoM £54.11

F 260

Olanzapine

- **DRUG ACTION** Olanzapine is a dopamine D_1, D_2, D_4, 5-HT_2, histamine- 1-, and muscarinic-receptor antagonist.

- **INDICATIONS AND DOSE**

Schizophrenia | Combination therapy for mania

- BY MOUTH
  - Child 12–17 years (under expert supervision): Initially 5–10 mg daily, adjusted according to response, usual dose 5–20 mg daily, doses greater than 10 mg daily only after reassessment, when one or more factors present that might result in slower metabolism (e.g. female gender, non-smoker) consider lower initial dose and more gradual dose increase; maximum 20 mg per day

Monotherapy for mania

- BY MOUTH
  - Child 12–17 years (under expert supervision): 15 mg daily, adjusted according to response, usual dose 5–20 mg daily, doses greater than 15 mg daily only after reassessment, when one or more factors present that might result in slower metabolism (e.g. female gender, non-smoker) consider lower initial dose and more gradual dose increase; maximum 20 mg per day

- **UNLICENSED USE** Not licensed for use in children.
- **CAUTIONS** Bone-marrow depression · hypereosinophilic disorders · low leucocyte count · low neutrophil count · myeloproliferative disease · paralytic ileus
- **INTERACTIONS** → Appendix 1: olanzapine
- **SIDE-EFFECTS**
  - **Common or very common** Anticholinergic syndrome · appetite increased · arthralgia · asthenia · eosinophilia · fever · glycosuria · hypersomnia · oedema · sexual dysfunction

- **Uncommon** Abdominal distension · alopecia · breast enlargement · diabetes mellitus · diabetic coma · dysarthria · epistaxis · ketoacidosis · memory loss · oculogyration · photosensitivity reaction · urinary disorders
- **Rare or very rare** Hepatic disorders · hypothermia · pancreatitis · rhabdomyolysis · thrombocytopenia

- **PREGNANCY** Use only if potential benefit outweighs risk; neonatal lethargy, tremor, and hypertonia reported when used in third trimester.
- **BREAST FEEDING** Avoid—present in milk.
- **HEPATIC IMPAIRMENT** Manufacturer advises caution. **Dose adjustments** In adults, manufacturer advises consider initial dose reduction—consult product literature.
- **RENAL IMPAIRMENT**
Dose adjustments Consider initial dose of 5 mg daily.
- **MONITORING REQUIREMENTS**
  - Blood lipids and weight should be measured at baseline, at 3 months (weight should be measured at frequent intervals during the first 3 months), and then yearly with antipsychotic drugs. Patients taking olanzapine require more frequent monitoring of these parameters: every 3 months for the first year, then yearly.
  - Fasting blood glucose should be measured at baseline, at 4–6 months, and then yearly. Patients taking olanzapine should have fasting blood glucose tested at baseline, after one months' treatment, then every 4–6 months.
- **DIRECTIONS FOR ADMINISTRATION** Olanzapine orodispersible tablet may be placed on the tongue and allowed to dissolve, or dispersed in water, orange juice, apple juice, milk, or coffee.
- **PATIENT AND CARER ADVICE** Patients or carers should be given advice on how to administer orodispersible tablets. Medicines for Children leaflet: Olanzapine for schizophrenia, bipolar disorder, mania and agitation www.medicinesforchildren.org.uk/olanzapine-schizophrenia-bipolar-disorder-mania-and-agitation

---

- **MEDICINAL FORMS** There can be variation in the licensing of different medicines containing the same drug. Forms available from special-order manufacturers include: oral suspension, oral solution

Tablet

CAUTIONARY AND ADVISORY LABELS 2

- Olanzapine (Non-proprietary)
  Olanzapine 2.5 mg Olanzapine 2.5mg tablets | 28 tablet [PoM] £21.85 DT = £1.36
  Olanzapine 5 mg Olanzapine 5mg tablets | 28 tablet [PoM] £43.70 DT = £1.55
  Olanzapine 7.5 mg Olanzapine 7.5mg tablets | 28 tablet [PoM] £62.27 DT = £1.97 | 56 tablet [PoM] £3.96–£131.10
  Olanzapine 10 mg Olanzapine 10mg tablets | 28 tablet [PoM] £87.40 DT = £1.53
  Olanzapine 15 mg Olanzapine 15mg tablets | 28 tablet [PoM] £119.18 DT = £1.95
  Olanzapine 20 mg Olanzapine 20mg tablets | 28 tablet [PoM] £158.90 DT = £2.28
- Zalasta (Consilient Health Ltd)
  Olanzapine 2.5 mg Zalasta 2.5mg tablets | 28 tablet [PoM] £18.57 DT = £1.36
  Olanzapine 5 mg Zalasta 5mg tablets | 28 tablet [PoM] £37.14 DT = £1.55
  Olanzapine 7.5 mg Zalasta 7.5mg tablets | 56 tablet [PoM] £111.43
  Olanzapine 10 mg Zalasta 10mg tablets | 28 tablet [PoM] £74.29 DT = £1.53
  Olanzapine 15 mg Zalasta 15mg tablets | 28 tablet [PoM] £101.30 DT = £1.95
  Olanzapine 20 mg Zalasta 20mg tablets | 28 tablet [PoM] £135.06 DT = £2.28
- Zyprexa (Eli Lilly and Company Ltd)
  Olanzapine 2.5 mg Zyprexa 2.5mg tablets | 28 tablet [PoM] £21.85 DT = £1.36
  Olanzapine 5 mg Zyprexa 5mg tablets | 28 tablet [PoM] £43.70 DT = £1.55
  Olanzapine 7.5 mg Zyprexa 7.5mg tablets | 56 tablet [PoM] £131.10
  Olanzapine 10 mg Zyprexa 10mg tablets | 28 tablet [PoM] £87.40 DT = £1.53
  Olanzapine 15 mg Zyprexa 15mg tablets | 28 tablet [PoM] £119.18 DT = £1.95
  Olanzapine 20 mg Zyprexa 20mg tablets | 28 tablet [PoM] £158.90 DT = £2.28

Oral lyophilisate

- Zyprexa (Eli Lilly and Company Ltd)
  Olanzapine 5 mg Zyprexa 5mg Velotabs sugar-free | 28 tablet [PoM] £48.07 DT = £48.07
  Olanzapine 10 mg Zyprexa 10mg Velotabs sugar-free | 28 tablet [PoM] £87.40 DT = £87.40
  Olanzapine 15 mg Zyprexa 15mg Velotabs sugar-free | 28 tablet [PoM] £131.10 DT = £131.10
  Olanzapine 20 mg Zyprexa 20mg Velotabs sugar-free | 28 tablet [PoM] £174.79 DT = £174.79

Orodispersible tablet

CAUTIONARY AND ADVISORY LABELS 2
EXCIPIENTS: May contain Aspartame

- Olanzapine (Non-proprietary)
  Olanzapine 5 mg Olanzapine 5mg orodispersible tablets sugar-free | 28 tablet [PoM] £6.86–£40.85 DT = £6.86
  Olanzapine 5mg orodispersible tablets | 28 tablet [PoM] £30.00 DT = £29.35
  Olanzapine 10 mg Olanzapine 10mg orodispersible tablets | 28 tablet [PoM] £50.00 DT = £49.00
  Olanzapine 10mg orodispersible tablets sugar-free | 28 tablet [PoM] £11.50–£74.29 DT = £11.50
  Olanzapine 15 mg Olanzapine 15mg orodispersible tablets sugar-free | 28 tablet [PoM] £11.65–£66.76 DT = £11.65
  Olanzapine 15mg orodispersible tablets | 28 tablet [PoM] £48.82 DT = £48.82
  Olanzapine 20 mg Olanzapine 20mg orodispersible tablets sugar-free | 28 tablet [PoM] £18.93–£96.14 DT = £18.93
  Olanzapine 20mg orodispersible tablets | 28 tablet [PoM] £80.00 DT = £78.93
- Zalasta (Consilient Health Ltd)
  Olanzapine 5 mg Zalasta 5mg orodispersible tablets sugar-free | 28 tablet [PoM] £40.85 DT = £6.86
  Olanzapine 10 mg Zalasta 10mg orodispersible tablets sugar-free | 28 tablet [PoM] £74.20 DT = £11.50
  Olanzapine 15 mg Zalasta 15mg orodispersible tablets sugar-free | 28 tablet [PoM] £111.43 DT = £11.65
  Olanzapine 20 mg Zalasta 20mg orodispersible tablets sugar-free | 28 tablet [PoM] £148.57 DT = £18.93

F 260

Quetiapine

- **DRUG ACTION** Quetiapine is a dopamine D_1, dopamine D_2, 5-HT_2, alpha$_1$-adrenoceptor, and histamine-1 receptor antagonist.

- **INDICATIONS AND DOSE**

Schizophrenia

- BY MOUTH USING IMMEDIATE-RELEASE MEDICINES
- Child 12–17 years (under expert supervision): Initially 25 mg twice daily, adjusted according to response. adjusted in steps of 25–50 mg; maximum 750 mg per day
- BY MOUTH USING MODIFIED-RELEASE MEDICINES
- Child 12–17 years (under expert supervision): Initially 50 mg once daily, adjusted according to response. adjusted in steps of 50 mg daily, usual dose 400–800 mg once daily; maximum 800 mg per day

Treatment of mania in bipolar disorder

- BY MOUTH USING IMMEDIATE-RELEASE MEDICINES
- Child 12–17 years (under expert supervision): 25 mg twice daily for day 1, then 50 mg twice daily for day 2, then 100 mg twice daily for day 3, then 150 mg twice daily for day 4, then 200 mg twice daily for day 5, then adjusted in steps of up to 100 mg daily, adjusted according to response, usual dose 400–600 mg daily in 2 divided doses

DOSE EQUIVALENCE AND CONVERSION
- Patients can be switched from immediate-release to modified-release tablets at the equivalent daily dose; to maintain clinical response, dose titration may be required.

- **UNLICENSED USE** Not licensed for use in children.
- **CAUTIONS** Cerebrovascular disease · patients at risk of aspiration pneumonia · treatment of depression in patients under 25 years (increased risk of suicide)
- **INTERACTIONS** → Appendix 1: quetiapine
- **SIDE-EFFECTS**
- **Common or very common** Appetite increased · asthenia · dysarthria · dyspepsia · dyspnoea · fever · headache · hyperglycaemia · irritability · palpitations · peripheral oedema · rhinitis · sleep disorders · suicidal behaviour (particularly on initiation) · suicidal ideation (particularly on initiation) · syncope · vision blurred · withdrawal syndrome
- **Uncommon** Anaemia · diabetes mellitus · dysphagia · hyponatraemia · hypothyroidism · sexual dysfunction · skin reactions · thrombocytopenia
- **Rare or very rare** Angioedema · breast swelling · gastrointestinal disorders · hepatic disorders · hypothermia · menstrual disorder · metabolic syndrome · pancreatitis · rhabdomyolysis · severe cutaneous adverse reactions (SCARs) · SIADH
- **PREGNANCY** Use only if potential benefit outweighs risk.
- **BREAST FEEDING** Manufacturer advises avoid.
- **HEPATIC IMPAIRMENT** Manufacturer advises caution (risk of increased plasma concentrations).
  Dose adjustments In adults, manufacturer advises dose reduction—consult product literature.

- **MEDICINAL FORMS** There can be variation in the licensing of different medicines containing the same drug. Forms available from special-order manufacturers include: oral suspension, oral solution, powder

Modified-release tablet

CAUTIONARY AND ADVISORY LABELS 2, 23, 25

- **Atrolak XL** (Accord Healthcare Ltd)
  Quetiapine (as Quetiapine fumarate) 50 mg Atrolak XL 50mg tablets | 60 tablet PoM £67.65 DT = £67.66
  Quetiapine (as Quetiapine fumarate) 150 mg Atrolak XL 150mg tablets | 60 tablet PoM £107.45 DT = £113.10
  Quetiapine (as Quetiapine fumarate) 200 mg Atrolak XL 200mg tablets | 60 tablet PoM £113.09 DT = £113.10
  Quetiapine (as Quetiapine fumarate) 300 mg Atrolak XL 300mg tablets | 60 tablet PoM £169.99 DT = £170.00
  Quetiapine (as Quetiapine fumarate) 400 mg Atrolak XL 400mg tablets | 60 tablet PoM £226.19 DT = £226.20
- **Biquelle XL** (Aspire Pharma Ltd)
  Quetiapine (as Quetiapine fumarate) 50 mg Biquelle XL 50mg tablets | 60 tablet PoM £29.45 DT = £67.66
  Quetiapine (as Quetiapine fumarate) 150 mg Biquelle XL 150mg tablets | 60 tablet PoM £49.45 DT = £113.10
  Quetiapine (as Quetiapine fumarate) 200 mg Biquelle XL 200mg tablets | 60 tablet PoM £49.45 DT = £113.10
  Quetiapine (as Quetiapine fumarate) 300 mg Biquelle XL 300mg tablets | 60 tablet PoM £74.45 DT = £170.00
  Quetiapine (as Quetiapine fumarate) 400 mg Biquelle XL 400mg tablets | 60 tablet PoM £98.95 DT = £226.20
- **Brancico XL** (Zentiva)
  Quetiapine (as Quetiapine fumarate) 50 mg Brancico XL 50mg tablets | 60 tablet PoM £8.99 DT = £67.66
  Quetiapine (as Quetiapine fumarate) 150 mg Brancico XL 150mg tablets | 60 tablet PoM £19.49 DT = £113.10
  Quetiapine (as Quetiapine fumarate) 200 mg Brancico XL 200mg tablets | 60 tablet PoM £19.49 DT = £113.10
  Quetiapine (as Quetiapine fumarate) 300 mg Brancico XL 300mg tablets | 60 tablet PoM £33.74 DT = £170.00
  Quetiapine (as Quetiapine fumarate) 400 mg Brancico XL 400mg tablets | 60 tablet PoM £44.99 DT = £226.20
- **Mintreleq XL** (Aristo Pharma Ltd)
  Quetiapine (as Quetiapine fumarate) 50 mg Mintreleq XL 50mg tablets | 60 tablet PoM £14.99 DT = £67.66
  Quetiapine (as Quetiapine fumarate) 150 mg Mintreleq XL 150mg tablets | 60 tablet PoM £29.99 DT = £113.10
  Quetiapine (as Quetiapine fumarate) 200 mg Mintreleq XL 200mg tablets | 60 tablet PoM £29.99 DT = £113.10
  Quetiapine (as Quetiapine fumarate) 300 mg Mintreleq XL 300mg tablets | 60 tablet PoM £49.99 DT = £170.00
  Quetiapine (as Quetiapine fumarate) 400 mg Mintreleq XL 400mg tablets | 60 tablet PoM £64.99 DT = £226.20
- **Seroquel XL** (AstraZeneca UK Ltd)
  Quetiapine (as Quetiapine fumarate) 50 mg Seroquel XL 50mg tablets | 60 tablet PoM £67.66 DT = £67.66
  Quetiapine (as Quetiapine fumarate) 150 mg Seroquel XL 150mg tablets | 60 tablet PoM £113.10 DT = £113.10
  Quetiapine (as Quetiapine fumarate) 200 mg Seroquel XL 200mg tablets | 60 tablet PoM £113.10 DT = £113.10
  Quetiapine (as Quetiapine fumarate) 300 mg Seroquel XL 300mg tablets | 60 tablet PoM £170.00 DT = £170.00
  Quetiapine (as Quetiapine fumarate) 400 mg Seroquel XL 400mg tablets | 60 tablet PoM £226.20 DT = £226.20
- **Sondate XL** (Teva UK Ltd)
  Quetiapine (as Quetiapine fumarate) 50 mg Sondate XL 50mg tablets | 60 tablet PoM £11.99 DT = £67.66
  Quetiapine (as Quetiapine fumarate) 150 mg Sondate XL 150mg tablets | 60 tablet PoM £25.99 DT = £113.10
  Quetiapine (as Quetiapine fumarate) 200 mg Sondate XL 200mg tablets | 60 tablet PoM £25.99 DT = £113.10
  Quetiapine (as Quetiapine fumarate) 300 mg Sondate XL 300mg tablets | 60 tablet PoM £44.99 DT = £170.00
  Quetiapine (as Quetiapine fumarate) 400 mg Sondate XL 400mg tablets | 60 tablet PoM £59.99 DT = £226.20
- **Zaluron XL** (Fontus Health Ltd)
  Quetiapine (as Quetiapine fumarate) 50 mg Zaluron XL 50mg tablets | 60 tablet PoM £27.96 DT = £67.66
  Quetiapine (as Quetiapine fumarate) 150 mg Zaluron XL 150mg tablets | 60 tablet PoM £46.96 DT = £113.10
  Quetiapine (as Quetiapine fumarate) 200 mg Zaluron XL 200mg tablets | 60 tablet PoM £46.96 DT = £113.10
  Quetiapine (as Quetiapine fumarate) 300 mg Zaluron XL 300mg tablets | 60 tablet PoM £70.71 DT = £170.00
  Quetiapine (as Quetiapine fumarate) 400 mg Zaluron XL 400mg tablets | 60 tablet PoM £93.98 DT = £226.20

Tablet

CAUTIONARY AND ADVISORY LABELS 2

- **Quetiapine (Non-proprietary)**
  Quetiapine (as Quetiapine fumarate) 25 mg Quetiapine 25mg tablets | 60 tablet PoM £38.05 DT = £2.68
  Quetiapine (as Quetiapine fumarate) 100 mg Quetiapine 100mg tablets | 60 tablet PoM £113.10 DT = £4.10
  Quetiapine (as Quetiapine fumarate) 150 mg Quetiapine 150mg tablets | 60 tablet PoM £113.10 DT = £4.51
  Quetiapine (as Quetiapine fumarate) 200 mg Quetiapine 200mg tablets | 60 tablet PoM £133.10 DT = £5.82
  Quetiapine (as Quetiapine fumarate) 300 mg Quetiapine 300mg tablets | 60 tablet PoM £170.00 DT = £6.37
- **Seroquel** (AstraZeneca UK Ltd)
  Quetiapine (as Quetiapine fumarate) 25 mg Seroquel 25mg tablets | 60 tablet PoM £48.60 DT = £2.68
  Quetiapine (as Quetiapine fumarate) 100 mg Seroquel 100mg tablets | 60 tablet PoM £135.72 DT = £4.10
  Quetiapine (as Quetiapine fumarate) 200 mg Seroquel 200mg tablets | 60 tablet PoM £135.72 DT = £5.82
  Quetiapine (as Quetiapine fumarate) 300 mg Seroquel 300mg tablets | 60 tablet PoM £204.00 DT = £6.37

Oral suspension

CAUTIONARY AND ADVISORY LABELS 2

- **Quetiapine (Non-proprietary)**
  Quetiapine (as Quetiapine fumarate) 20 mg per 1 ml Quetiapine 20mg/ml oral suspension sugar-free | 150 ml PoM £99.28 DT = £99.28

260

Risperidone

07-Feb-2018

- **DRUG ACTION** Risperidone is a dopamine D_2, $5\text{-}HT_{2A}$, $alpha_1$-adrenoceptor, and histamine-1 receptor antagonist.

- **INDICATIONS AND DOSE**

Acute and chronic psychosis

▶ BY MOUTH

▸ Child 12–17 years (under expert supervision): 2 mg daily in 1–2 divided doses for day 1, then 4 mg daily in 1–2 divided doses for day 2, slower titration is appropriate in some patients; usual dose 4–6 mg daily, doses above 10 mg daily only if benefit considered to outweigh risk; maximum 16 mg per day

Short-term monotherapy of mania in bipolar disorder (under expert supervision)

▶ BY MOUTH

▸ Child 12–17 years: Initially 500 micrograms once daily, then adjusted in steps of 0.5–1 mg daily, adjusted according to response; usual dose 2.5 mg daily in 1–2 divided doses; maximum 6 mg per day

Short-term treatment (up to 6 weeks) of persistent aggression in conduct disorder (under expert supervision)

▶ BY MOUTH

▸ Child 5–17 years (body-weight up to 50 kg): Initially 250 micrograms once daily, then increased in steps of 250 micrograms once daily on alternate days, adjusted according to response; usual dose 500 micrograms once daily; maximum 750 micrograms per day

▸ Child 5–17 years (body-weight 50 kg and above): Initially 500 micrograms once daily, then increased in steps of 500 micrograms once daily on alternate days, adjusted according to response; usual dose 1 mg once daily; maximum 1.5 mg per day

Short-term treatment of severe aggression in autism (under expert supervision)

▶ BY MOUTH

▸ Child 5–17 years (body-weight 15–20 kg): Initially 250 micrograms daily for at least 4 days, then increased if necessary to 500 micrograms daily, then increased in steps of 250 micrograms daily, dose to be increased at intervals of 2 weeks, review effectiveness and any side-effects after 3–4 weeks; stop if no response at 6 weeks; maximum 1 mg per day

▸ Child 5–17 years (body-weight 20–45 kg): Initially 500 micrograms daily for at least 4 days, then increased if necessary to 1 mg daily, then increased in steps of 500 micrograms daily, dose to be increased at intervals of 2 weeks, review effectiveness and any side-effects after 3–4 weeks; stop if no response at 6 weeks; maximum 2.5 mg per day

▸ Child 5–17 years (body-weight 45 kg and above): Initially 500 micrograms daily for at least 4 days, then increased if necessary to 1 mg daily, then increased in steps of 500 micrograms daily, dose to be increased at intervals of 2 weeks, review effectiveness and any side-effects after 3–4 weeks; stop if no response at 6 weeks; maximum 3 mg per day

- **UNLICENSED USE** Not licensed for use in children for psychosis, mania, or autism.

IMPORTANT SAFETY INFORMATION

SAFE PRACTICE

Risperidone has been confused with ropinirole; care must be taken to ensure the correct drug is prescribed and dispensed.

- **CAUTIONS** Avoid in Acute porphyrias p. 652 · cataract surgery (risk of intra-operative floppy iris syndrome) · dehydration · family history of sudden cardiac death (perform ECG) · prolactin-dependent tumours
- **INTERACTIONS** → Appendix 1: risperidone
- **SIDE-EFFECTS**

▶ **Common or very common** Anxiety · appetite abnormal · asthenia · chest discomfort · conjunctivitis · cough · depression · diarrhoea · dyspnoea · epistaxis · fall · fever · gastrointestinal discomfort · headache · hypertension · increased risk of infection · joint disorders · laryngeal pain · muscle spasms · nasal congestion · nausea · oedema · oral disorders · pain · skin reactions · sleep disorders · urinary disorders · vision disorders

▶ **Uncommon** Alopecia · anaemia · breast abnormalities · cardiac conduction disorders · cerebrovascular insufficiency · chills · coma · concentration impaired · confusion · consciousness impaired · cystitis · diabetes mellitus · dry eye · dysarthria · dysphagia · dysphonia · ear pain · eye disorders · feeling abnormal · flushing · gait abnormal · gastrointestinal disorders · hyperglycaemia · malaise · menstrual cycle irregularities · mood altered · muscle weakness · palpitations · polydipsia · posture abnormal · procedural pain · respiratory disorders · sensation abnormal · sexual dysfunction · syncope · taste altered · thirst · thrombocytopenia · tinnitus · vaginal discharge · vertigo · weight decreased

▶ **Rare or very rare** Angioedema · dandruff · diabetic ketoacidosis · eyelid crusting · glaucoma · hypoglycaemia · hypothermia · induration · jaundice · pancreatitis · peripheral coldness · rhabdomyolysis · SIADH · sleep apnoea · water intoxication · withdrawal syndrome

▶ **Frequency not known** Cardiac arrest

- **PREGNANCY** Use only if potential benefit outweighs risk.
- **BREAST FEEDING** Use only if potential benefit outweighs risk—small amount present in milk.
- **HEPATIC IMPAIRMENT** Manufacturer advises caution.
Dose adjustments Manufacturer advises dose reduction to half the usual dose, and slower dose titration.
- **RENAL IMPAIRMENT**
Dose adjustments Initial and subsequent oral doses should be halved.
- **DIRECTIONS FOR ADMINISTRATION** Orodispersible tablets should be placed on the tongue, allowed to dissolve and swallowed. Oral liquid may be diluted with any non-alcoholic drink, except tea.
- **PATIENT AND CARER ADVICE** Patients or carers should be given advice on how to administer risperidone orodispersible tablets and oral liquid (counselling on use of dose syringe advised).
Medicines for Children leaflet: Risperidone for psychological disorders www.medicinesforchildren.org.uk/risperidone-psychological-disorders

- **MEDICINAL FORMS** There can be variation in the licensing of different medicines containing the same drug. Forms available from special-order manufacturers include: oral solution

Tablet

CAUTIONARY AND ADVISORY LABELS 2

▸ Risperidone (Non-proprietary)

Risperidone 500 microgram Risperidone 500microgram tablets | 20 tablet [PoM] £6.95 DT = £1.68

Risperidone 1 mg Risperidone 1mg tablets | 20 tablet [PoM] £10.16 DT = £1.98 | 60 tablet [PoM] £5.94–£17.56

Risperidone 2 mg Risperidone 2mg tablets | 60 tablet [PoM] £60.10 DT = £5.97

Risperidone 3 mg Risperidone 3mg tablets | 60 tablet [PoM] £88.38 DT = £10.87

Risperidone 4 mg Risperidone 4mg tablets | 60 tablet [PoM] £116.67 DT = £8.95

Risperidone 6 mg Risperidone 6mg tablets | 28 tablet [PoM] £82.50 DT = £49.21

- ▸ Risperdal (Janssen-Cilag Ltd)
  Risperidone 500 microgram Risperdal 500microgram tablets | 20 tablet PoM £5.08 DT = £1.68
  Risperidone 1 mg Risperdal 1mg tablets | 20 tablet PoM £8.36 DT = £1.98 | 60 tablet PoM £17.56
  Risperidone 2 mg Risperdal 2mg tablets | 60 tablet PoM £34.62 DT = £5.97
  Risperidone 3 mg Risperdal 3mg tablets | 60 tablet PoM £50.91 DT = £10.87
  Risperidone 4 mg Risperdal 4mg tablets | 60 tablet PoM £67.20 DT = £8.95
  Risperidone 6 mg Risperdal 6mg tablets | 28 tablet PoM £67.88 DT = £49.21

Oral solution

CAUTIONARY AND ADVISORY LABELS 2

- ▸ Risperidone (Non-proprietary)
  Risperidone 1 mg per 1 ml Risperidone 1mg/ml oral solution sugar-free | 100 ml PoM £58.22 DT = £4.04
- ▸ Risperdal (Janssen-Cilag Ltd)
  Risperidone 1 mg per 1 ml Risperdal 1mg/ml oral solution sugar-free | 100 ml PoM £37.01 DT = £4.04

Orodispersible tablet

CAUTIONARY AND ADVISORY LABELS 2

EXCIPIENTS: May contain Aspartame

- ▸ Risperidone (Non-proprietary)
  Risperidone 500 microgram Risperidone 500microgram orodispersible tablets sugar-free | 28 tablet PoM £18.64 DT = £18.28
  Risperidone 1 mg Risperidone 1mg orodispersible tablets sugar-free | 28 tablet PoM £22.50 DT = £22.07
  Risperidone 2 mg Risperidone 2mg orodispersible tablets sugar-free | 28 tablet PoM £39.03 DT = £39.03
  Risperidone 3 mg Risperidone 3mg orodispersible tablets sugar-free | 28 tablet PoM £43.50 DT = £43.50
  Risperidone 4 mg Risperidone 4mg orodispersible tablets sugar-free | 28 tablet PoM £50.29 DT = £50.29

3 Movement disorders

Cerebral palsy and spasticity

27-Feb-2017

Description of condition

Cerebral palsy is a group of permanent, non-progressive abnormalities of the developing fetal or neonatal brain that lead to movement and posture disorders, causing activity limitation and functional impact. There can be accompanying clinical and developmental comorbidities. These include disturbances of sensation, perception, cognition, communication and behaviour, epilepsy, and secondary musculoskeletal problems (such as muscle contracture and abnormal torsion). Cerebral palsy is not curable and the comorbidities can impact on many areas of participation and quality of life, particularly eating, drinking, comfort, and sleep.

Spasticity

Spasticity in children is most commonly associated with cerebral palsy, but can also be associated with other non-progressive brain disorders.

Aims of treatment

Treatment involves managing spasticity to optimise movement and posture, while minimising potential secondary musculoskeletal deformity, as well as managing developmental and clinical comorbidities.

Non-drug treatment

EvGr All children with spasticity should be offered physiotherapy and, where necessary, occupational therapy. They can also benefit from orthoses.

Orthopaedic surgery can be used, as an adjunct to other interventions, to prevent deterioration and improve function. ⟨A⟩

Drug treatment

Spasticity

EvGr Oral diazepam p. 236 or oral baclofen p. 701 can be used to treat discomfort, pain, muscle spasm and functional disability. If oral diazepam is initially used because of its rapid onset of action, consider changing to oral baclofen if a sustained, longer duration of effect is required or if long-term treatment is necessary. If the response to diazepam or baclofen after 4–6 weeks is unsatisfactory, a trial of combined treatment using both drugs can be considered. Consider reducing the dose if adverse effects such as drowsiness occur. Treatment cessation should be considered when management is reviewed and at least every six months.

If **dystonia** is considered to contribute significantly to problems with posture, function and pain, a trial of treatment with oral trihexyphenidyl hydrochloride p. 273, levodopa, or baclofen [unlicensed indications] can be considered.

Treatment with botulinum toxin type A p. 275 [unlicensed under 2 years] should be considered for those in whom focal spasticity of the upper or lower limbs is inhibiting fine motor function, affecting care and hygiene, causing pain or disturbing sleep, impeding tolerance of other treatments (such as orthoses), or causing cosmetic concerns. A trial of botulinum toxin type A treatment can also be considered in those with spasticity when *focal dystonia* is causing problems, such as postural or functional difficulties or pain. Ongoing assessment of muscle tone, range of movement and motor function is required. Botulinum toxin type A treatment should **not** be offered to children receiving treatment with Aminoglycosides p. 331.

Treatment with intrathecal baclofen [unlicensed under 4 years] (administered by continuous pump) can be considered in children with spasticity if (despite the use of non-invasive treatments) spasticity or dystonia are causing difficulties with pain, muscle spasm, posture, function or self-care. Before deciding to implant the intrathecal baclofen pump, an intrathecal baclofen test should be performed to assess the therapeutic effect and to check for adverse effects. ⟨A⟩

Developmental and clinical comorbidities

EvGr Regular assessment and appropriate nutritional support should be provided, especially if there are concerns about oral intake, growth or nutritional status. Enteral tube feeding can be provided if oral intake is insufficient to provide adequate nutrition. ⟨A⟩

Children with cerebral palsy are likely to have risk factors for low bone mineral density and can have an increased risk of low-impact fractures. EvGr Calcium and vitamin D supplementation (such as colecalciferol with calcium carbonate p. 683) may be required. Children with reduced bone density and a history of low-impact fracture can be considered for bisphosphonate therapy (under specialist guidance). ⟨A⟩

Pain is common in children with cerebral palsy, especially those with more severe motor impairment. Condition-specific causes of pain and discomfort include musculoskeletal problems (for example, scoliosis, hip subluxation and dislocation), increased muscle tone (including dystonia and spasticity), muscle fatigue and immobility, constipation, vomiting, and gastro-oesophageal reflux disease. Reversible causes of pain should be treated as appropriate, see *Spasticity* (above), Constipation p. 44, Gastro-oesophageal reflux disease p. 64, Urinary frequency, enuresis and incontinence p. 526, Nocturnal enuresis in children p. 526, and Urinary-tract infections p. 400.

Other types of pain include non-specific back pain, headache, non-specific abdominal pain, dental pain and dysmenorrhoea. EvGr Initially, a 'stepped approach' trial of simple analgesia (such as paracetamol p. 288, ibuprofen p. 707, or both) for mild-to-moderate pain can be considered. If such a trial is unsuccessful, the child should be referred to a specialist pain team. Ⓐ

In children with cerebral palsy, sleep disturbances are common. EvGr If no treatable cause is found, a trial of melatonin p. 312 [unlicensed] can be considered to manage sleep disturbances, particularly for problems with falling asleep. Regular sedative medication should **not** be used to manage primary sleep disorders in children with cerebral palsy without seeking specialist advice. Ⓐ

Epilepsy can be associated with cerebral palsy; for its management, see Epilepsy p. 203.

Children with cerebral palsy are at greater risk of mental health problems, in comparison with the general age comparison population. For management of these conditions, see Depression p. 251, Anxiety (Hypnotics and anxiolytics p. 311), and Attention deficit hyperactivity disorder p. 241.

Drooling

EvGr Drooling can be managed with an antimuscarinic drug, such as glycopyrronium bromide p. 870 [unlicensed in under 3 years] (oral or by enteral tube) or hyoscine hydrobromide p. 283 [unlicensed] (transdermal). For children with dyskinetic cerebral palsy, trihexyphenidyl hydrochloride [unlicensed] can be used (on specialist advice). If antimuscarinic drugs provide insufficient benefit or are not tolerated, botulinum toxin type A [unlicensed indication] injections to the salivary glands can be considered. High-dose botulinum toxin type A [unlicensed indication] injections to the salivary glands can, rarely, cause breathing and swallowing difficulties, which requires urgent hospital admission. Surgery can be an option in cases resistant to drug treatment. Ⓐ

Related drugs

Other drugs used for Cerebral palsy and spasticity: co-careldopa p. 274, dantrolene sodium p. 880.

Transition planning

For guidance on the patient's transition from paediatric to adult services, see *Transitional services for chronic conditions* in Guidance on prescribing p. 1.

Useful Resources

Cerebral palsy in under 25s: assessment and management. National Institute for Health and Care Excellence. Clinical guideline 62. January 2017.
www.nice.org.uk/guidance/ng62

Spasticity in under 19s: management. National Institute for Health and Care Excellence. Clinical guideline 145. July 2012 (updated November 2016).
www.nice.org.uk/guidance/cg145

3.1 Dystonias and other involuntary movements

Dystonias and related disorders

Dystonias

Dystonias may result from conditions such as cerebral palsy or may be related to a deficiency of the neurotransmitter dopamine as in Segawa syndrome.

Dopaminergic drugs used in dystonias

Levodopa, the amino-acid precursor of dopamine, acts by replenishing depleted striatal dopamine. It is given with an extracerebral **dopa-decarboxylase inhibitor**, which reduces the peripheral conversion of levodopa to dopamine, thereby limiting side-effects such as nausea, vomiting, and cardiovascular effects; additionally, effective brain-dopamine concentrations are achieved with lower doses of levodopa. The extracerebral dopa-decarboxylase inhibitor most commonly used in children is carbidopa (in co-careldopa p. 274).

Levodopa therapy should be initiated at a low dose and increased in small steps; the final dose should be as low as possible. Intervals between doses should be chosen to suit the needs of the individual child.

In severe dystonias related to cerebral palsy, improvement can be expected within 2 weeks. Children with Segawa syndrome are particularly sensitive to levodopa; they may even become symptom free on small doses. Levodopa also has a role in treating metabolic disorders such as defects in tetrahydrobiopterin synthesis and dihydrobiopterin reductase deficiency. Tetrahydrobiopterin may have a role in metabolic disorders.

Children may experience nausea within 2 hours of taking a dose; nausea and vomiting with co-careldopa is rarely dose-limiting.

In dystonic cerebral palsy, treatment with larger doses of levodopa is associated with the development of potentially troublesome motor complications (including response fluctuations and dyskinesias). Response fluctuations are characterised by large variations in motor performance, with normal function during the 'on' period, and weakness and restricted mobility during the 'off' period.

Antimuscarinic drugs used in dystonias

The antimuscarinic drugs procyclidine hydrochloride p. 273 and trihexyphenidyl hydrochloride p. 273 reduce the symptoms of dystonias, including those induced by antipsychotic drugs; there is no justification for giving them routinely in the absence of dystonic symptoms. Tardive dyskinesia is not improved by antimuscarinic drugs and may be made worse.

There are no important differences between the antimuscarinic drugs, but some children tolerate one better than another.

Procyclidine hydrochloride can be given parenterally and is effective emergency treatment for acute drug-induced dystonic reactions.

If treatment with an antimuscarinic is ineffective, intravenous diazepam p. 236 can be given for life-threatening acute drug-induced dystonic reactions.

Drugs used in essential tremor, chorea, tics, and related disorders

Haloperidol p. 261 can also improve motor tics and symptoms of Tourette syndrome and related choreas. Other treatments for Tourette syndrome include pimozide p. 263 [unlicensed indication] (**important**: ECG monitoring required), and sulpiride p. 263 [unlicensed indication].

Propranolol hydrochloride p. 111 or another beta-adrenoceptor blocking drug may be useful in treating essential tremor or tremor associated with anxiety or thyrotoxicosis.

Botulinum toxin type A p. 275 should be used under specialist supervision. Treatment with botulinum toxin type A can be considered after an acquired non-progressive brain injury if rapid-onset spasticity causes postural or functional difficulties, and in children with spasticity in whom focal dystonia causes postural or functional difficulties or pain.

Other drugs used for Dystonias and other involuntary movements Chlorpromazine hydrochloride, p. 261 · Clonidine hydrochloride, p. 108 · Clozapine, p. 266 · Pericyazine, p. 262 · Prochlorperazine, p. 285 · Trifluoperazine, p. 264

ANTIMUSCARINICS

Procyclidine hydrochloride

31-Oct-2019

- **DRUG ACTION** Procyclidine exerts its antiparkinsonian action by reducing the effects of the relative central cholinergic excess that occurs as a result of dopamine deficiency.

- **INDICATIONS AND DOSE**

Acute dystonia

▶ BY INTRAMUSCULAR INJECTION, OR BY INTRAVENOUS INJECTION

- Child 1 month–1 year: 0.5–2 mg for 1 dose, dose usually effective in 5–10 minutes but may need 30 minutes for relief
- Child 2–9 years: 2–5 mg for 1 dose, dose usually effective in 5–10 minutes but may need 30 minutes for relief
- Child 10–17 years: 5–10 mg, occasionally, more than 10 mg, dose usually effective in 5–10 minutes but may need 30 minutes for relief

Dystonia

▶ BY MOUTH

- Child 7–11 years: 1.25 mg 3 times a day
- Child 12–17 years: 2.5 mg 3 times a day

- **UNLICENSED USE** Not licensed for use in children.
- **CONTRA-INDICATIONS** Gastro-intestinal obstruction
- **CAUTIONS** Cardiovascular disease · hypertension · liable to abuse · psychotic disorders · pyrexia · those susceptible to angle-closure glaucoma
- **INTERACTIONS** → Appendix 1: procyclidine
- **SIDE-EFFECTS**

▶ **Common or very common** Constipation · dry mouth · urinary retention · vision blurred

▶ **Uncommon** Anxiety · cognitive impairment · confusion · dizziness · gingivitis · hallucination · memory loss · nausea · rash · vomiting

▶ **Rare or very rare** Psychotic disorder

- **PREGNANCY** Use only if potential benefit outweighs risk.
- **BREAST FEEDING** No information available.
- **HEPATIC IMPAIRMENT** Manufacturer advises caution.
- **RENAL IMPAIRMENT** Use with caution.
- **TREATMENT CESSATION** Avoid abrupt withdrawal in patients taking long-term treatment.
- **PATIENT AND CARER ADVICE**

Driving and skilled tasks May affect performance of skilled tasks (e.g. driving).

- **MEDICINAL FORMS** There can be variation in the licensing of different medicines containing the same drug. Forms available from special-order manufacturers include: oral suspension, oral solution

Solution for injection

▶ Procyclidine hydrochloride (Non-proprietary)

Procyclidine hydrochloride 5 mg per 1 ml Procyclidine 10mg/2ml solution for injection ampoules | 5 ampoule PoM £72.50–£73.16 DT = £73.16

Oral solution

▶ Procyclidine hydrochloride (Non-proprietary)

Procyclidine hydrochloride 500 microgram per 1 ml Procyclidine 2.5mg/5ml oral solution sugar-free | 150 ml PoM £17.10 DT = £14.02

Procyclidine hydrochloride 1 mg per 1 ml Procyclidine 5mg/5ml oral solution sugar-free | 150 ml PoM £24.63 DT = £21.67

Tablet

▶ Procyclidine hydrochloride (Non-proprietary)

Procyclidine hydrochloride 5 mg Procyclidine 5mg tablets | 28 tablet PoM £12.65 DT = £1.62 | 100 tablet PoM £5.79–£8.94 | 500 tablet PoM £28.93–£44.63

▶ Kemadrin (Aspen Pharma Trading Ltd)

Procyclidine hydrochloride 5 mg Kemadrin 5mg tablets | 100 tablet PoM £4.72 | 500 tablet PoM £23.62

Trihexyphenidyl hydrochloride

10-Jul-2019

(Benzhexol hydrochloride)

- **DRUG ACTION** Trihexyphenidyl exerts its effects by reducing the effects of the relative central cholinergic excess that occurs as a result of dopamine deficiency.

- **INDICATIONS AND DOSE**

Dystonia

▶ BY MOUTH

- Child 3 months–17 years: Initially 1–2 mg daily in 1–2 divided doses, then increased in steps of 1 mg every 3–7 days, dose to be adjusted according to response and side-effects; maximum 2 mg/kg per day

- **UNLICENSED USE** Not licensed for use in children.
- **CONTRA-INDICATIONS** Myasthenia gravis
- **CAUTIONS** Cardiovascular disease · gastro-intestinal obstruction · hypertension · liable to abuse · psychotic disorders · pyrexia · those susceptible to angle-closure glaucoma
- **INTERACTIONS** → Appendix 1: trihexyphenidyl
- **SIDE-EFFECTS** Anxiety · bronchial secretion decreased · confusion · constipation · delusions · dizziness · dry mouth · dysphagia · euphoric mood · fever · flushing · hallucination · insomnia · memory loss · myasthenia gravis aggravated · mydriasis · nausea · skin reactions · tachycardia · thirst · urinary disorders · vision disorders · vomiting
- **PREGNANCY** Use only if potential benefit outweighs risk.
- **BREAST FEEDING** Avoid.
- **HEPATIC IMPAIRMENT** Manufacturer advises caution.
- **RENAL IMPAIRMENT** Use with caution.
- **TREATMENT CESSATION** Avoid abrupt withdrawal in patients taking long-term treatment.
- **DIRECTIONS FOR ADMINISTRATION** Tablets should be taken with or after food.
- **PATIENT AND CARER ADVICE**

Medicines for Children leaflet: Trihexyphenidyl hydrochloride for dystonia www.medicinesforchildren.org.uk/trihexyphenidyl-hydrochloride-dystonia

Driving and skilled tasks May affect performance of skilled tasks (e.g. driving).

- **MEDICINAL FORMS** There can be variation in the licensing of different medicines containing the same drug. Forms available from special-order manufacturers include: oral suspension, oral solution

Oral solution

EXCIPIENTS: May contain Propylene glycol

▶ Trihexyphenidyl hydrochloride (Non-proprietary)

Trihexyphenidyl hydrochloride 1 mg per 1 ml Trihexyphenidyl 5mg/5ml oral solution | 200 ml PoM £31.60 DT = £27.47

Tablet

▶ Trihexyphenidyl hydrochloride (Non-proprietary)

Trihexyphenidyl hydrochloride 2 mg Trihexyphenidyl 2mg tablets | 84 tablet PoM £13.50 DT = £4.65

Trihexyphenidyl hydrochloride 5 mg Trihexyphenidyl 5mg tablets | 84 tablet PoM £21.00 DT = £19.48

DOPAMINERGIC DRUGS › DOPAMINE PRECURSORS

Co-careldopa

20-Dec-2019

- **INDICATIONS AND DOSE**

Dopamine-sensitive dystonias including Segawa syndrome and dystonias related to cerebral palsy (dose expressed as levodopa)

▶ BY MOUTH

▶ Child 3 months–17 years: Initially 250 micrograms/kg 2–3 times a day, dose to be increased according to response every 2–3 days, increased if necessary up to 1 mg/kg 3 times a day, preparation containing 1:4 ratio of carbidopa:levodopa is to be used

Treatment of defects in tetrahydrobiopterin synthesis and dihydrobiopterin reductase deficiency (dose expressed as levodopa)

▶ BY MOUTH

▶ Neonate: Initially 250–500 micrograms/kg 4 times a day, dose to be increased every 4–5 days according to response, a preparation containing 1:4 carbidopa: levodopa to be administered; maintenance 2.5–3 mg/kg 4 times a day, at higher doses consider preparation containing 1:10 carbidopa:levodopa, review regularly (every 3–6 months).

▶ Child: Initially 250–500 micrograms/kg 4 times a day, dose to be increased every 4–5 days according to response, a preparation containing 1:4 carbidopa: levodopa to be administered; maintenance 2.5–3 mg/kg 4 times a day, at higher doses consider preparation containing 1:10 carbidopa:levodopa, review regularly (every 3–6 months in early childhood)

DOSE EQUIVALENCE AND CONVERSION

▶ The proportions are expressed in the form x/y where x and y are the strengths in milligrams of carbidopa and levodopa respectively.

▶ 2 tablets *Sinemet*® 12.5 mg/50 mg is equivalent to 1 tablet *Sinemet*® Plus 25 mg/100 mg.

- **UNLICENSED USE** Not licensed for use in children.
- **CAUTIONS** Cardiovascular disease · diabetes mellitus · history of myocardial infarction with residual arrhythmia · history of peptic ulcer · history of skin melanoma (risk of activation) · osteomalacia · psychiatric illness (avoid if severe and discontinue if deterioration) · pulmonary disease · susceptibility to angle-closure glaucoma
- **INTERACTIONS** → Appendix 1: carbidopa · levodopa
- **SIDE-EFFECTS**

▶ **Rare or very rare** Drowsiness · seizure · sleep disorders

▶ **Frequency not known** Agranulocytosis · alertness decreased · alopecia · anaemia · angioedema · anxiety · appetite decreased · asthenia · cardiac disorder · chest pain · compulsions · confusion · constipation · delusions · depression · diarrhoea · dizziness · dry mouth · dyskinesia (may be dose-limiting) · dysphagia · dyspnoea · eating disorders · euphoric mood · eye disorders · fall · focal tremor · gait abnormal · gastrointestinal discomfort · gastrointestinal disorders · gastrointestinal haemorrhage · haemolytic anaemia · hallucination · headache · Henoch-Schönlein purpura · hiccups · hoarseness · Horner's syndrome exacerbated · hypertension · hypotension · leucopenia · malaise · malignant melanoma · movement disorders · muscle complaints · nausea · neuroleptic malignant syndrome (on abrupt discontinuation) · oedema · oral disorders · palpitations · pathological gambling · postural disorders · psychotic disorder · respiration abnormal · sensation abnormal · sexual dysfunction · skin reactions · suicidal ideation · sweat changes · syncope · taste bitter · teeth grinding · thrombocytopenia · trismus · urinary disorders · urine dark · vasodilation · vision disorders · vomiting · weight changes

- **PREGNANCY** Use with caution—toxicity has occurred in *animal* studies.
- **BREAST FEEDING** May suppress lactation; present in milk—avoid.
- **HEPATIC IMPAIRMENT** Manufacturer advises use with caution in hepatic disease.

DUODOPA® **Dose adjustments** Manufacturer advises titrate dose with caution in severe impairment.

- **MONITORING REQUIREMENTS** In prolonged therapy, psychiatric, hepatic, haematological, renal, and cardiovascular monitoring is advisable; warn patients to resume normal activities gradually.
- **EFFECT ON LABORATORY TESTS** False positive tests for urinary ketones have been reported.
- **TREATMENT CESSATION** Avoid abrupt withdrawal.
- **PRESCRIBING AND DISPENSING INFORMATION** Co-careldopa is a mixture of carbidopa and levodopa; the proportions are expressed in the form x/y where x and y are the strengths in milligrams of carbidopa and levodopa respectively.
- **PATIENT AND CARER ADVICE** Warn patients to resume normal activity gradually.

Driving and skilled tasks **Sudden onset of sleep** Excessive daytime sleepiness and sudden onset of sleep can occur with co-careldopa.

Patients starting treatment with these drugs should be warned of the risk and of the need to exercise caution when driving or operating machinery. Those who have experienced excessive sedation or sudden onset of sleep should refrain from driving or operating machines until these effects have stopped occurring.

Management of excessive daytime sleepiness should focus on the identification of an underlying cause, such as depression or concomitant medication. Patients should be counselled on improving sleep behaviour.

- **MEDICINAL FORMS** There can be variation in the licensing of different medicines containing the same drug. Forms available from special-order manufacturers include: oral suspension, oral solution

Tablet

CAUTIONARY AND ADVISORY LABELS 10, 14

▶ **Co-careldopa (Non-proprietary)**

Carbidopa (as Carbidopa monohydrate) 12.5 mg, Levodopa 50 mg Co-careldopa 12.5mg/50mg tablets | 90 tablet [PoM] £18.57 DT = £18.56

Carbidopa (as Carbidopa monohydrate) 25 mg, Levodopa 100 mg Co-careldopa 25mg/100mg tablets | 90 tablet [PoM] £5.71 | 100 tablet [PoM] £26.99 DT = £11.01

Carbidopa (as Carbidopa monohydrate) 10 mg, Levodopa 100 mg Co-careldopa 10mg/100mg tablets | 100 tablet [PoM] £14.00 DT = £13.88

Carbidopa (as Carbidopa monohydrate) 25 mg, Levodopa 250 mg Co-careldopa 25mg/250mg tablets | 100 tablet [PoM] £35.00 DT = £34.99

▶ **Sinemet 110** (Merck Sharp & Dohme Ltd)

Carbidopa (as Carbidopa monohydrate) 10 mg, Levodopa 100 mg Sinemet 10mg/100mg tablets | 100 tablet [PoM] £7.30 DT = £13.88

▶ **Sinemet 275** (Merck Sharp & Dohme Ltd)

Carbidopa (as Carbidopa monohydrate) 25 mg, Levodopa 250 mg Sinemet 25mg/250mg tablets | 100 tablet [PoM] £18.29 DT = £34.99

▶ **Sinemet 62.5** (Merck Sharp & Dohme Ltd)

Carbidopa (as Carbidopa monohydrate) 12.5 mg, Levodopa 50 mg Sinemet 12.5mg/50mg tablets | 90 tablet [PoM] £6.28 DT = £18.56

▶ **Sinemet Plus** (Merck Sharp & Dohme Ltd)

Carbidopa (as Carbidopa monohydrate) 25 mg, Levodopa 100 mg Sinemet Plus 25mg/100mg tablets | 100 tablet [PoM] £12.88 DT = £11.01

MUSCLE RELAXANTS > PERIPHERALLY ACTING > NEUROTOXINS (BOTULINUM TOXINS)

Botulinum toxin type A

27-Nov-2019

● **INDICATIONS AND DOSE**

Dynamic equinus foot deformity caused by spasticity in ambulant paediatric cerebral palsy

▸ BY INTRAMUSCULAR INJECTION

▸ Child 2–17 years: (consult product literature)

DOSE EQUIVALENCE AND CONVERSION

▸ **Important**: information is specific to each individual preparation.

● **CONTRA-INDICATIONS** Infection at injection site

● **CAUTIONS** Atrophy in target muscle · chronic respiratory disorder · excessive weakness in target muscle · history of aspiration · history of dysphagia · inflammation in target muscle · neurological disorders · neuromuscular disorders · off-label use (fatal adverse events reported)

CAUTIONS, FURTHER INFORMATION Neuromuscular or neurological disorders can lead to increased sensitivity and exaggerated muscle weakness including dysphagia and respiratory compromise.

● **INTERACTIONS** → Appendix 1: botulinum toxins

● **SIDE-EFFECTS**

▸ **Common or very common** Alopecia · asthenia · autonomic dysreflexia · bladder diverticulum · constipation · dizziness · drowsiness · dry eye · dry mouth · dysphagia (most common after injection into sternocleidomastoid muscle and salivary gland) · ecchymosis (minimised by applying gentle pressure at injection site immediately after injection) · eye discomfort · eye disorders · eye inflammation · fall · fever · gait abnormal · haematuria · headaches · hot flush · increased risk of infection · influenza like illness · insomnia · joint disorders · leukocyturia · malaise · muscle complaints · muscle weakness · musculoskeletal stiffness · nausea · neuromuscular dysfunction · oedema · pain · paresis · sensation abnormal · skin reactions · subcutaneous nodule · urinary disorders · vision disorders

▸ **Uncommon** Anxiety · coordination abnormal · depression · dysphonia · dyspnoea · facial paralysis · memory loss · oral paraesthesia · photosensitivity reaction · postural hypotension · speech impairment · taste altered · vertigo

▸ **Frequency not known** Abdominal pain · angioedema · angle closure glaucoma · appetite decreased · arrhythmia · diarrhoea · hearing impairment · hypersensitivity · myocardial infarction · myopathy · nerve disorders · respiratory disorders · seizure · syncope · tinnitus · vomiting

● **CONCEPTION AND CONTRACEPTION** Avoid in women of child-bearing age unless using effective contraception.

● **PREGNANCY** Avoid unless essential—toxicity in *animal* studies (manufacturer of *Botox*® advise avoid).

● **BREAST FEEDING** Low risk of systemic absorption but avoid unless essential.

● **PRESCRIBING AND DISPENSING INFORMATION** Preparations are not interchangeable.

● **PATIENT AND CARER ADVICE** Patients and carers should be warned of the signs and symptoms of toxin spread, such as muscle weakness and breathing difficulties; they should be advised to seek immediate medical attention if swallowing, speech or breathing difficulties occur.

Medicines for Children leaflet: Botulinum toxin for muscle spasticity www.medicinesforchildren.org.uk/botulinum-toxin-muscle-spasticity-0

● **MEDICINAL FORMS** There can be variation in the licensing of different medicines containing the same drug.

Powder for solution for injection

▸ **Azzalure** (Galderma (UK) Ltd)

Botulinum toxin type A 125 unit Azzalure 125unit powder for solution for injection vials | 1 vial PoM £64.00 | 2 vial PoM £128.00

▸ **Bocouture** (Merz Pharma UK Ltd)

Botulinum toxin type A 50 unit Bocouture 50unit powder for solution for injection vials | 1 vial PoM £72.00

Botulinum toxin type A 100 unit Bocouture 100unit powder for solution for injection vials | 1 vial PoM £229.90

▸ **Botox** (Allergan Ltd)

Botulinum toxin type A 50 unit Botox 50unit powder for solution for injection vials | 1 vial PoM £77.50 (Hospital only)

Botulinum toxin type A 100 unit Botox 100unit powder for solution for injection vials | 1 vial PoM £138.20 (Hospital only)

Botulinum toxin type A 200 unit Botox 200unit powder for solution for injection vials | 1 vial PoM £276.40 (Hospital only)

▸ **Dysport** (Ipsen Ltd)

Botulinum toxin type A 300 unit Dysport 300unit powder for solution for injection vials | 1 vial PoM £92.40

Botulinum toxin type A 500 unit Dysport 500unit powder for solution for injection vials | 2 vial PoM £308.00

▸ **Xeomin** (Merz Pharma UK Ltd)

Botulinum toxin type A 50 unit Xeomin 50unit powder for solution for injection vials | 1 vial PoM £72.00

Botulinum toxin type A 100 unit Xeomin 100unit powder for solution for injection vials | 1 vial PoM £129.90

Botulinum toxin type A 200 unit Xeomin 200unit powder for solution for injection vials | 1 vial PoM £259.80 (Hospital only)

4 Nausea and labyrinth disorders

Nausea and labyrinth disorders

19-Feb-2020

Drug treatment

Antiemetics should be prescribed only when the cause of vomiting is known because otherwise they may delay diagnosis, particularly in children. Antiemetics are unnecessary and sometimes harmful when the cause can be treated, such as in diabetic ketoacidosis, or in digoxin p. 86 or antiepileptic overdose.

If antiemetic drug treatment is indicated, the drug is chosen according to the aetiology of vomiting.

Antihistamines are effective against nausea and vomiting resulting from many underlying conditions. There is no evidence that any one antihistamine is superior to another but their duration of action and incidence of adverse effects (drowsiness and antimuscarinic effects) differ.

The **phenothiazines** are dopamine antagonists and act centrally by blocking the chemoreceptor trigger zone. They are of considerable value for the prophylaxis and treatment of nausea and vomiting associated with diffuse neoplastic disease, radiation sickness, and the emesis caused by drugs such as opioids, general anaesthetics, and cytotoxics. Prochlorperazine p. 285, perphenazine, and trifluoperazine p. 264 are less sedating than chlorpromazine hydrochloride p. 261; severe dystonic reactions sometimes occur with phenothiazines. Some phenothiazines are available as rectal suppositories, which can be useful in children with persistent vomiting or with severe nausea; for children over 12 years prochlorperazine can also be administered as a buccal tablet which is placed between the upper lip and the gum.

Other antipsychotic drugs including haloperidol p. 261 and levomepromazine p. 285 are used for the relief of nausea in palliative care.

Metoclopramide hydrochloride p. 278 is an effective antiemetic and its activity closely resembles that of the phenothiazines. Metoclopramide hydrochloride also acts directly on the gastro-intestinal tract and it may be superior to the phenothiazines for emesis associated with gastroduodenal, hepatic, and biliary disease. Due to the risk of neurological side effects, metoclopramide hydrochloride should only be used in children as second line therapy in postoperative and cytotoxic induced nausea and vomiting.

Domperidone p. 278 acts at the chemoreceptor trigger zone; it has the advantage over metoclopramide hydrochloride and the phenothiazines of being less likely to cause central effects such as sedation and dystonic reactions because it does not readily cross the blood-brain barrier. The MHRA and CHM have released important safety information and restrictions regarding the use of domperidone for nausea and vomiting in children aged under 12 years or those weighing less than 35 kg, and a reminder of contra-indications. For further information, see *Important safety information* for domperidone.

Granisetron p. 281 and ondansetron p. 281 are specific $5HT_3$-receptor antagonists which block $5HT_3$ receptors in the gastro-intestinal tract and in the CNS. They are of value in the management of nausea and vomiting in children receiving cytotoxics and in postoperative nausea and vomiting.

Aprepitant p. 279 is a neurokinin 1-receptor antagonist, licensed for the prevention of nausea and vomiting associated with highly and moderately emetogenic cancer chemotherapy; it is given in combination with a $5HT_3$-receptor antagonist (with or without a corticosteroid). For further information on the prevention of nausea and vomiting caused by chemotherapy, see Cytotoxic drugs p. 575.

Dexamethasone p. 475 has antiemetic effects. Dexamethasone may also have a role in cytotoxic-induced nausea and vomiting.

Nabilone p. 277 is a synthetic cannabinoid with antiemetic properties. There is limited evidence for nabilone use in children for nausea and vomiting caused by cytotoxic chemotherapy unresponsive to conventional antiemetics [unlicensed].

Vomiting during pregnancy

Nausea in the first trimester of pregnancy is generally mild and does not require drug therapy. On rare occasions if vomiting is severe, short-term treatment with an antihistamine, such as **promethazine**, may be required. Prochlorperazine or metoclopramide hydrochloride are alternatives. If symptoms do not settle in 24 to 48 hours then specialist opinion should be sought. Hyperemesis gravidarum is a more serious condition, which requires regular antiemetic therapy, intravenous fluid and electrolyte replacement and sometimes nutritional support. Supplementation with thiamine p. 678 must be considered in order to reduce the risk of Wernicke's encephalopathy.

Postoperative nausea and vomiting

The incidence of postoperative nausea and vomiting depends on many factors including the anaesthetic used, and the type and duration of surgery. Other risk factors include female sex, non-smokers, a history of postoperative nausea and vomiting or motion sickness, and intraoperative and postoperative use of opioids. Therapy to prevent postoperative nausea and vomiting should be based on the assessed risk. Drugs used include **$5HT_3$-receptor antagonists**, droperidol p. 285, dexamethasone, some **phenothiazines** (e.g. prochlorperazine), and **antihistamines** (e.g. cyclizine below). A combination of two or more antiemetic drugs that have different mechanisms of action is often indicated in those at high risk of postoperative nausea and vomiting or where postoperative vomiting presents a particular danger (e.g. in some types of surgery). When a prophylactic antiemetic drug has failed, postoperative nausea and vomiting should be treated with one or more drugs from a different class.

Opioid-induced nausea and vomiting

Cyclizine, ondansetron, and prochlorperazine are used to relieve opioid-induced nausea and vomiting; ondansetron has the advantage of not producing sedation.

Motion sickness

Antiemetics should be given to prevent motion sickness rather than after nausea or vomiting develop. The most effective drug for the prevention of motion sickness is hyoscine hydrobromide p. 283. For children over 10 years old, a transdermal hyoscine patch provides prolonged activity but it needs to be applied several hours before travelling. The sedating antihistamines are slightly less effective against motion sickness, but are generally better tolerated than hyoscine. If a sedative effect is desired **promethazine** is useful, but generally a slightly less sedating antihistamine such as cyclizine or cinnarizine p. 282 is preferred. Domperidone, metoclopramide hydrochloride, $5HT_3$-receptor antagonists, and the phenothiazines (except the antihistamine phenothiazine promethazine) are **ineffective** in motion sickness.

Other vestibular disorders

Management of vestibular diseases is aimed at treating the underlying cause as well as treating symptoms of the balance disturbance and associated nausea and vomiting. **Antihistamines** (such as cinnarizine), and **phenothiazines** (such as prochlorperazine) are effective for prophylaxis and treatment of nausea and vertigo resulting from vestibular disorders; however, when nausea and vertigo are associated with middle ear surgery, treatment can be difficult.

Nausea and vomiting associated with migraine

For information on antiemetic use in migraine attacks, see Migraine p. 307.

Other drugs used for Nausea and labyrinth disorders
Promethazine hydrochloride, p. 189

ANTIEMETICS AND ANTINAUSEANTS › ANTIHISTAMINES

Cyclizine

30-Jun-2018

● **INDICATIONS AND DOSE**

Nausea and vomiting of known cause | Nausea and vomiting associated with vestibular disorders

- ▶ BY MOUTH, OR BY INTRAVENOUS INJECTION
- ▶ Child 1 month–5 years: 0.5–1 mg/kg up to 3 times a day (max. per dose 25 mg), intravenous injection to be given over 3–5 minutes, for motion sickness, take 1–2 hours before departure
- ▶ Child 6–11 years: 25 mg up to 3 times a day, intravenous injection to be given over 3–5 minutes, for motion sickness, take 1–2 hours before departure
- ▶ Child 12–17 years: 50 mg up to 3 times a day, intravenous injection to be given over 3–5 minutes, for motion sickness, take 1–2 hours before departure
- ▶ BY RECTUM
- ▶ Child 2–5 years: 12.5 mg up to 3 times a day
- ▶ Child 6–11 years: 25 mg up to 3 times a day
- ▶ Child 12–17 years: 50 mg up to 3 times a day
- ▶ BY CONTINUOUS INTRAVENOUS INFUSION, OR BY SUBCUTANEOUS INFUSION
- ▶ Child 1–23 months: 3 mg/kg, dose to be given over 24 hours

- ▸ Child 2-5 years: 50 mg, dose to be given over 24 hours
- ▸ Child 6-11 years: 75 mg, dose to be given over 24 hours
- ▸ Child 12-17 years: 150 mg, dose to be given over 24 hours

Nausea and vomiting in palliative care

▶ BY SUBCUTANEOUS INFUSION
- ▸ Child 1-23 months: 3 mg/kg, dose to be given over 24 hours
- ▸ Child 2-5 years: 50 mg, dose to be given over 24 hours
- ▸ Child 6-11 years: 75 mg, dose to be given over 24 hours
- ▸ Child 12-17 years: 150 mg, dose to be given over 24 hours

▶ BY MOUTH
- ▸ Child 1 month-5 years: 0.5–1 mg/kg up to 3 times a day (max. per dose 25 mg)
- ▸ Child 6-11 years: 25 mg up to 3 times a day
- ▸ Child 12-17 years: 50 mg up to 3 times a day

▶ BY INTRAVENOUS INJECTION
- ▸ Child 1 month-5 years: 0.5–1 mg/kg up to 3 times a day (max. per dose 25 mg), intravenous injection to be given over 3–5 minutes
- ▸ Child 6-11 years: 25 mg up to 3 times a day, intravenous injection to be given over 3–5 minutes
- ▸ Child 12-17 years: 50 mg up to 3 times a day, intravenous injection to be given over 3–5 minutes

▶ BY CONTINUOUS INTRAVENOUS INFUSION
- ▸ Child 1-23 months: 3 mg/kg, dose to be given over 24 hours
- ▸ Child 2-5 years: 50 mg, dose to be given over 24 hours
- ▸ Child 6-11 years: 75 mg, dose to be given over 24 hours
- ▸ Child 12-17 years: 150 mg, dose to be given over 24 hours

▶ BY RECTUM
- ▸ Child 2-5 years: 12.5 mg up to 3 times a day
- ▸ Child 6-11 years: 25 mg up to 3 times a day
- ▸ Child 12-17 years: 50 mg up to 3 times a day

- **UNLICENSED USE** Tablets not licensed for use in children under 6 years. Injection not licensed for use in children.
- **CONTRA-INDICATIONS** Neonate (due to significant antimuscarinic activity)
- **CAUTIONS** Epilepsy · glaucoma · may counteract haemodynamic benefits of opioids · neuromuscular disorders—increased risk of transient paralysis with intravenous use · pyloroduodenal obstruction · severe heart failure—may cause fall in cardiac output and associated increase in heart rate, mean arterial pressure and pulmonary wedge pressure · urinary retention
- **INTERACTIONS** → Appendix 1: antihistamines, sedating
- **SIDE-EFFECTS**

GENERAL SIDE-EFFECTS
- ▶ **Rare or very rare** Agitation (more common at high doses) · angle closure glaucoma · depression
- ▶ **Frequency not known** Abdominal pain · agranulocytosis · angioedema · anxiety · apnoea · appetite decreased · arrhythmias · asthenia · bronchospasm · constipation · diarrhoea · disorientation · dizziness · drowsiness · dry mouth · dry throat · euphoric mood · haemolytic anaemia · hallucinations · headache · hepatic disorders · hypertension · hypotension · increased gastric reflux · insomnia · leucopenia · movement disorders · muscle complaints · nasal dryness · nausea · oculogyric crisis · palpitations · paraesthesia · photosensitivity reaction · seizure · skin reactions · speech disorder · thrombocytopenia · tinnitus · tremor · urinary retention · vision blurred · vomiting

SPECIFIC SIDE-EFFECTS
- ▸ With oral use Level of consciousness decreased
- ▸ With parenteral use Chills · consciousness impaired · injection site necrosis · pain · paralysis · sensation of pressure · thrombophlebitis

- **PREGNANCY** Manufacturer advises avoid; however, there is no evidence of teratogenicity. The use of sedating antihistamines in the latter part of the third trimester may cause adverse effects in neonates such as irritability, paradoxical excitability, and tremor.
- **BREAST FEEDING** No information available. Most antihistamines are present in breast milk in varying amounts; although not known to be harmful, most manufacturers advise avoiding their use in mothers who are breast-feeding.
- **HEPATIC IMPAIRMENT** Manufacturer advises caution.
- **DIRECTIONS FOR ADMINISTRATION** For administration *by mouth*, tablets may be crushed.

Mixing and compatibility for the use of syringe drivers in palliative care Cyclizine may precipitate at concentrations above 10 mg/mL or in the presence of sodium chloride 0.9% *or* as the concentration of diamorphine relative to cyclizine increases; mixtures of diamorphine and cyclizine are also likely to precipitate after 24 hours.
- **PRESCRIBING AND DISPENSING INFORMATION**

Palliative care For further information on the use of cyclizine in palliative care, see www.medicinescomplete.com/#/content/palliative/antihistaminic-antimuscarinic-anti-emetics.
- **PATIENT AND CARER ADVICE**

Driving and skilled tasks Drowsiness may affect performance of skilled tasks (e.g. cycling, driving); effects of alcohol enhanced.

- **MEDICINAL FORMS** There can be variation in the licensing of different medicines containing the same drug. Forms available from special-order manufacturers include: oral suspension, oral solution, suppository

Tablet

CAUTIONARY AND ADVISORY LABELS 2

▸ Cyclizine (Non-proprietary)

Cyclizine hydrochloride 50 mg Cyclizine 50mg tablets | 30 tablet [P] £2.95–£5.00 | 100 tablet [P] £12.15 DT = £7.04

Solution for injection

▸ Cyclizine (Non-proprietary)

Cyclizine lactate 50 mg per 1 ml Cyclizine 50mg/1ml solution for injection ampoules | 5 ampoule [PoM] £17.42 DT = £18.58 | 10 ampoule [PoM] £25.00–£37.16

ANTIEMETICS AND ANTINAUSEANTS › CANNABINOIDS

Nabilone

21-Jan-2020

- **INDICATIONS AND DOSE**

Nausea and vomiting caused by cytotoxic chemotherapy, unresponsive to conventional antiemetics (preferably in hospital setting) (under close medical supervision)

▶ BY MOUTH
- ▸ Child: (consult local protocol)

- **UNLICENSED USE** Not licensed for use in children.
- **CAUTIONS** Adverse effects on mental state can persist for 48–72 hours after stopping · heart disease · history of psychiatric disorder · hypertension
- **INTERACTIONS** → Appendix 1: nabilone
- **SIDE-EFFECTS** Abdominal pain · appetite decreased · concentration impaired · confusion · depression · dizziness · drowsiness · drug use disorders · dry mouth · euphoric mood · feeling of relaxation · hallucination · headache · hypotension · movement disorders · nausea · psychosis · sleep disorder · tachycardia · tremor · vertigo · visual impairment

SIDE-EFFECTS, FURTHER INFORMATION Drowsiness and dizziness occur frequently with standard doses.
- **PREGNANCY** Avoid unless essential.

- **BREAST FEEDING** Avoid—no information available.
- **HEPATIC IMPAIRMENT** Manufacturer advises avoid in severe impairment (primarily biliary excretion).
- **PATIENT AND CARER ADVICE**
Behavioural effects Patients should be made aware of possible changes of mood and other adverse behavioural effects.
Driving and skilled tasks Drowsiness may affect performance of skilled tasks (e.g. driving). Effects of alcohol enhanced. For information on 2015 legislation regarding driving whilst taking certain controlled drugs, including nabilone, see *Drugs and skilled tasks* under Guidance on prescribing p. 1.

- **MEDICINAL FORMS** There can be variation in the licensing of different medicines containing the same drug. Forms available from special-order manufacturers include: capsule

Capsule
CAUTIONARY AND ADVISORY LABELS 2
- Nabilone (Brown & Burk UK Ltd)
Nabilone 250 microgram Nabilone 250microgram capsules | 20 capsule [PoM] £150.00 DT = £150.00 [CD2]
Nabilone 1 mg Nabilone 1mg capsules | 20 capsule [PoM] £196.00 DT = £196.00 [CD2]

ANTIEMETICS AND ANTINAUSEANTS › DOPAMINE RECEPTOR ANTAGONISTS

Domperidone

21-Jan-2020

- **INDICATIONS AND DOSE**

Relief of nausea and vomiting
- BY MOUTH
- Child 12–17 years (body-weight 35 kg and above): 10 mg up to 3 times a day for a usual maximum of 1 week; maximum 30 mg per day

Gastro-oesophageal reflux disease (but efficacy not proven) (specialist use only)
- BY MOUTH
- Neonate: 250 micrograms/kg 3 times a day, dose can be increased if response inadequate, increased if necessary up to 400 micrograms/kg 3 times a day, interrupt treatment occasionally to assess recurrence—consider restarting if symptoms recur, discontinue if response inadequate at higher dose.
- Child: 250 micrograms/kg 3 times a day (max. per dose 10 mg), dose can be increased if response inadequate, increased if necessary up to 400 micrograms/kg 3 times a day (max. per dose 20 mg), interrupt treatment occasionally to assess recurrence—consider restarting if symptoms recur, discontinue if response inadequate at higher dose

- **UNLICENSED USE** Not licensed for use in children for gastro-oesophageal reflux disease.

IMPORTANT SAFETY INFORMATION

MHRA/CHM ADVICE (UPDATED DECEMBER 2019): DOMPERIDONE FOR NAUSEA AND VOMITING: LACK OF EFFICACY IN CHILDREN; REMINDER OF CONTRA-INDICATIONS IN ADULTS AND ADOLESCENTS

Domperidone is no longer indicated for the relief of nausea and vomiting in children aged under 12 years or those weighing less than 35 kg. A European review concluded that domperidone is not as effective in this population as previously thought and alternative treatments should be considered. Healthcare professionals are advised to adhere to the licensed dose and to use the lowest effective dose for the shortest possible duration (max. treatment duration should not usually exceed 1 week).

Healthcare professionals are also reminded of the existing contra-indications for use of domperidone (see *Contra-indications*, *Hepatic impairment*, and *Interactions*).

- **CONTRA-INDICATIONS** Cardiac disease · conditions where cardiac conduction is, or could be, impaired · gastro-intestinal haemorrhage · gastro-intestinal mechanical obstruction · gastro-intestinal mechanical perforation · if increased gastro-intestinal motility harmful · prolactinoma
- **INTERACTIONS** → Appendix 1: domperidone
- **SIDE-EFFECTS**
  - **Common or very common** Dry mouth
  - **Uncommon** Anxiety · asthenia · breast abnormalities · diarrhoea · drowsiness · headache · lactation disorders · libido loss
  - **Frequency not known** Arrhythmias · depression · gynaecomastia · menstrual cycle irregularities · movement disorders · oculogyric crisis · QT interval prolongation · seizure · sudden cardiac death · urinary retention
- **PREGNANCY** Use only if potential benefit outweighs risk.
- **BREAST FEEDING** Amount too small to be harmful.
- **HEPATIC IMPAIRMENT** Manufacturer advises avoid in moderate to severe impairment.
- **RENAL IMPAIRMENT**
Dose adjustments Reduce frequency.
- **PATIENT AND CARER ADVICE**
Arrhythmia Patients and their carers should be told how to recognise signs of arrhythmia and advised to seek medical attention if symptoms such as palpitation or syncope develop.
Medicines for Children leaflet: Domperidone for gastro-oesophageal reflux www.medicinesforchildren.org.uk/domperidone-gastro-oesophageal-reflux

- **MEDICINAL FORMS** There can be variation in the licensing of different medicines containing the same drug. Forms available from special-order manufacturers include: oral suspension

Oral suspension
CAUTIONARY AND ADVISORY LABELS 22
- Domperidone (Non-proprietary)
Domperidone 1 mg per 1 ml Domperidone 1mg/ml oral suspension sugar-free | 200 ml [PoM] £24.85 DT = £24.85

Tablet
CAUTIONARY AND ADVISORY LABELS 22
- Domperidone (Non-proprietary)
Domperidone (as Domperidone maleate) 10 mg Domperidone 10mg tablets | 30 tablet [PoM] £2.71 DT = £0.89 | 100 tablet [PoM] £9.04 DT = £2.97
- Motilium (Zentiva)
Domperidone (as Domperidone maleate) 10 mg Motilium 10mg tablets | 30 tablet [PoM] £2.71 DT = £0.89 | 100 tablet [PoM] £9.04 DT = £2.97

Metoclopramide hydrochloride

03-Feb-2020

- **INDICATIONS AND DOSE**

Second-line option for treatment of established postoperative nausea and vomiting | Prevention of delayed chemotherapy-induced nausea and vomiting
- BY MOUTH, OR BY INTRAMUSCULAR INJECTION, OR BY INTRAVENOUS INJECTION
- Child: 100–150 micrograms/kg up to 3 times a day (max. per dose 10 mg), when administered by slow intravenous injection, to be given over at least 3 minutes

- **UNLICENSED USE** *Maxolon*® tablets not licensed for use in children.

> **IMPORTANT SAFETY INFORMATION**
>
> MHRA/CHM ADVICE—METOCLOPRAMIDE: RISK OF NEUROLOGICAL ADVERSE EFFECTS—RESTRICTED DOSE AND DURATION OF USE (AUGUST 2013)
>
> The benefits and risks of metoclopramide have been reviewed by the European Medicines Agency's Committee on Medicinal Products for Human Use, which concluded that the risk of neurological effects such as extrapyramidal disorders and tardive dyskinesia outweigh the benefits in long-term or high-dose treatment. To help minimise the risk of potentially serious neurological adverse effects, the following restrictions to indications, dose and duration of use have been made:
>
> - In children aged 1–18 years, metoclopramide should only be used as a second-line option for prevention of delayed chemotherapy-induced nausea and vomiting and for treatment of established postoperative nausea and vomiting;
> - Use of metoclopramide is contra-indicated in children aged under 1 year;
> - Metoclopramide should only be prescribed for short-term use (up to 5 days);
> - Recommended dose is 100–150 micrograms/kg (max. 10 mg), repeated up to 3 times daily;
> - Intravenous doses should be administered as a slow bolus over at least 3 minutes;
> - Oral liquid formulations should be given via an appropriately designed, graduated oral syringe to ensure dose accuracy.
>
> This advice does not apply to unlicensed uses of metoclopramide (e.g. palliative care).

- **CONTRA-INDICATIONS** 3–4 days after gastrointestinal surgery · epilepsy · gastro-intestinal haemorrhage · gastro-intestinal obstruction · gastro-intestinal perforation · phaeochromocytoma
- **CAUTIONS** Asthma · atopic allergy · bradycardia · cardiac conduction disturbances · children · may mask underlying disorders such as cerebral irritation · uncorrected electrolyte imbalance · young adults
- **INTERACTIONS** → Appendix 1: metoclopramide
- **SIDE-EFFECTS**

GENERAL SIDE-EFFECTS

- **Common or very common** Asthenia · depression · diarrhoea · drowsiness · hypotension · menstrual cycle irregularities · movement disorders · parkinsonism
- **Uncommon** Arrhythmias · hallucination · hyperprolactinaemia · level of consciousness decreased
- **Rare or very rare** Confusion · galactorrhoea · seizure
- **Frequency not known** Atrioventricular block · blood disorders · cardiac arrest · gynaecomastia · hypertension · neuroleptic malignant syndrome · QT interval prolongation · shock · syncope · tremor

SPECIFIC SIDE-EFFECTS

- **With parenteral use** Anxiety · dizziness · dyspnoea · oedema · skin reactions · visual impairment

SIDE-EFFECTS, FURTHER INFORMATION Metoclopramide can induce acute dystonic reactions involving facial and skeletal muscle spasms and oculogyric crises. These dystonic effects are more common in the young, especially girls and young women; they usually occur shortly after starting treatment with metoclopramide and subside within 24 hours of stopping it. Use of an antimuscarinic drug such as procyclidine will abort dystonic attacks.

- **PREGNANCY** Not known to be harmful.
- **BREAST FEEDING** Small amount present in milk; avoid.
- **HEPATIC IMPAIRMENT** Manufacturer advises caution in severe impairment (risk of accumulation).
  Dose adjustments Manufacturer advises dose reduction of 50% in severe impairment.
- **RENAL IMPAIRMENT**
  Dose adjustments Avoid or use small dose in severe impairment; increased risk of extrapyramidal reactions.
- **DIRECTIONS FOR ADMINISTRATION** Oral liquid preparation to be given via a graduated oral dosing syringe.
- **PATIENT AND CARER ADVICE** Counselling on use of pipette advised with oral solution.

- **MEDICINAL FORMS** There can be variation in the licensing of different medicines containing the same drug. Forms available from special-order manufacturers include: oral solution

Solution for injection

- Metoclopramide hydrochloride (Non-proprietary)
  Metoclopramide hydrochloride 5 mg per 1 ml Metoclopramide 10mg/2ml solution for injection ampoules | 5 ampoule PoM £1.31–£15.00 | 10 ampoule PoM £25.00 DT = £2.88
- Maxolon (Advanz Pharma)
  Metoclopramide hydrochloride 5 mg per 1 ml Maxolon High Dose 100mg/20ml solution for injection ampoules | 10 ampoule PoM £26.68

Oral solution

- Metoclopramide hydrochloride (Non-proprietary)
  Metoclopramide hydrochloride 1 mg per 1 ml Metoclopramide 5mg/5ml oral solution sugar-free | 150 ml PoM £19.79 DT = £19.79

Tablet

- Metoclopramide hydrochloride (Non-proprietary)
  Metoclopramide hydrochloride 10 mg Metoclopramide 10mg tablets | 28 tablet PoM £1.80 DT = £0.88
- Maxolon (Advanz Pharma)
  Metoclopramide hydrochloride 10 mg Maxolon 10mg tablets | 84 tablet PoM £5.24

ANTIEMETICS AND ANTINAUSEANTS > NEUROKININ RECEPTOR ANTAGONISTS

Aprepitant

11-Sep-2018

- **INDICATIONS AND DOSE**

Adjunct treatment to prevent nausea and vomiting associated with moderately and highly emetogenic chemotherapy

- BY MOUTH
- Child 6 months–11 years (body-weight 6 kg and above): (consult product literature)
- Child 12–17 years: Initially 125 mg, dose to be taken 1 hour before chemotherapy, then 80 mg once daily for 2 days, dose to be taken 1 hour before chemotherapy *or* in the morning if no chemotherapy is given, consult product literature for dose of concomitant $5HT_3$-antagonist (and corticosteroid if required)

- **CONTRA-INDICATIONS** Acute porphyrias p. 652
- **INTERACTIONS** → Appendix 1: aprepitant
- **SIDE-EFFECTS**
- **Common or very common** Appetite decreased · asthenia · constipation · gastrointestinal discomfort · headache · hiccups
- **Uncommon** Anaemia · anxiety · burping · dizziness · drowsiness · dry mouth · febrile neutropenia · gastrointestinal disorders · hot flush · malaise · nausea · palpitations · skin reactions · urinary disorders · vomiting
- **Rare or very rare** Bradycardia · cardiovascular disorder · chest discomfort · cognitive disorder · conjunctivitis · cough · disorientation · euphoric mood · gait abnormal · hyperhidrosis · increased risk of infection · muscle spasms · muscle weakness · oedema · oropharyngeal pain · photosensitivity reaction · polydipsia · seborrhoea · severe cutaneous adverse reactions (SCARs) · sneezing ·

stomatitis · taste altered · throat irritation · tinnitus · weight decreased
- **Frequency not known** Dysarthria · dyspnoea · insomnia · miosis · sensation abnormal · visual acuity decreased · wheezing

- **CONCEPTION AND CONTRACEPTION** Manufacturer advises effectiveness of hormonal contraceptives may be reduced—alternative non-hormonal methods of contraception necessary during treatment and for 2 months after stopping aprepitant.
- **PREGNANCY** Manufacturer advises avoid unless clearly necessary—no information available.
- **BREAST FEEDING** Manufacturer advises avoid—present in milk in *animal* studies.
- **HEPATIC IMPAIRMENT** Manufacturer advises caution in moderate to severe impairment—limited information available.
- **NATIONAL FUNDING/ACCESS DECISIONS**

Scottish Medicines Consortium (SMC) decisions

The *Scottish Medicines Consortium* has advised (June 2017) that aprepitant (*Emend*®) is accepted for use within NHS Scotland as part of combination therapy, for the prevention of nausea and vomiting associated with moderately emetogenic cancer chemotherapy in infants, toddlers and children from the age of six months to less than 12 years (powder for oral suspension) and adolescents from the age of 12 years to 17 years (hard capsules).

The *Scottish Medicines Consortium* has advised (July 2017) that aprepitant (*Emend*®) is accepted for use within NHS Scotland as part of combination therapy, for the prevention of nausea and vomiting associated with highly emetogenic cancer chemotherapy in children from the age of six months to under 12 years (powder for oral suspension), and adolescents from the age of 12 years to 17 years (hard capsules).

- **MEDICINAL FORMS** There can be variation in the licensing of different medicines containing the same drug. Forms available from special-order manufacturers include: oral suspension

Powder

- Emend (Merck Sharp & Dohme Ltd)
  Aprepitant 125 mg Emend 125mg oral powder sachets | 1 sachet PoM £15.81

Capsule

- Aprepitant (Non-proprietary)
  Aprepitant 80 mg Aprepitant 80mg capsules | 2 capsule PoM £26.87–£31.61 DT = £31.61 | 2 capsule PoM £31.61 DT = £31.61 (Hospital only)
  Aprepitant 125 mg Aprepitant 125mg capsules | 5 capsule PoM £67.18–£79.03 DT = £79.03 | 5 capsule PoM £79.03 DT = £79.03 (Hospital only)
- Emend (Merck Sharp & Dohme Ltd)
  Aprepitant 80 mg Emend 80mg capsules | 2 capsule PoM £31.61 DT = £31.61
  Aprepitant 125 mg Emend 125mg capsules | 5 capsule PoM £79.03 DT = £79.03

Fosaprepitant

29-Aug-2018

- **DRUG ACTION** Fosaprepitant is a prodrug of aprepitant.

- **INDICATIONS AND DOSE**

Adjunct to $5HT_3$-receptor antagonist (with or without dexamethasone) in preventing nausea and vomiting associated with moderately and highly emetogenic chemotherapy

- BY INTRAVENOUS INFUSION
- Child 6 months–11 years (body-weight 6 kg and above): Initially 3 mg/kg (max. per dose 115 mg) on day 1 of cycle, then 2 mg/kg (max. per dose 80 mg) on days 2 and 3 of cycle, dose to be administered over 60 minutes and completed 30 minutes before chemotherapy, consult product literature for dose of concomitant corticosteroid and $5HT_3$-receptor antagonist and for information on alternative dosing for single and multi-day regimens
- Child 12–17 years: Initially 115 mg on day 1 of cycle, then 80 mg on days 2 and 3 of cycle, dose to be administered over 30 minutes and completed 30 minutes before chemotherapy, consult product literature for dose of concomitant corticosteroid and $5HT_3$-receptor antagonist and for information on alternative dosing for single and multi-day regimens

- **CONTRA-INDICATIONS** Acute porphyrias p. 652
- **INTERACTIONS** → Appendix 1: fosaprepitant
- **SIDE-EFFECTS**
- **Common or very common** Appetite decreased · asthenia · constipation · flushing · gastrointestinal discomfort · headache · hiccups
- **Uncommon** Anaemia · anxiety · burping · dizziness · drowsiness · dry mouth · febrile neutropenia · gastrointestinal disorders · malaise · nausea · palpitations · skin reactions · thrombophlebitis · urinary disorders · vomiting
- **Rare or very rare** Bradycardia · cardiovascular disorder · chest discomfort · cognitive disorder · conjunctivitis · cough · disorientation · euphoric mood · gait abnormal · hyperhidrosis · increased risk of infection · muscle spasms · muscle weakness · oedema · oropharyngeal pain · photosensitivity reaction · polydipsia · seborrhoea · severe cutaneous adverse reactions (SCARs) · sneezing · stomatitis · taste altered · throat irritation · tinnitus · weight decreased
- **Frequency not known** Dysarthria · dyspnoea · insomnia · miosis · sensation abnormal · visual acuity decreased · wheezing

- **CONCEPTION AND CONTRACEPTION** Effectiveness of hormonal contraceptives reduced—effective non-hormonal methods of contraception necessary during treatment and for 2 months after stopping fosaprepitant.
- **PREGNANCY** Avoid unless potential benefit outweighs risk—no information available.
- **BREAST FEEDING** Avoid—present in milk in *animal* studies.
- **HEPATIC IMPAIRMENT** Manufacturer advises caution in moderate to severe impairment—limited information available.
- **DIRECTIONS FOR ADMINISTRATION** For *intravenous infusion* (*Ivemend*®), manufacturer advises give intermittently *in* Sodium chloride 0.9%; reconstitute each 150 mg vial with 5 mL sodium chloride 0.9% gently without shaking to avoid foaming, then dilute in 145 mL infusion fluid; for volumes less than 150 ml, transfer the required volume to a bag or syringe prior to infusion; infuse through central venous catheter.
- **NATIONAL FUNDING/ACCESS DECISIONS**

Scottish Medicines Consortium (SMC) decisions

SMC No. SMC2108

The *Scottish Medicines Consortium* has advised (November 2018) that fosaprepitant (*Ivemend*®) is accepted for use within NHS Scotland for the prevention of nausea and vomiting associated with highly and moderately emetogenic chemotherapy in children aged 6 months to 17 years.

All Wales Medicines Strategy Group (AWMSG) decisions

AWMSG No. 3789

The *All Wales Medicines Strategy Group* has advised (December 2018) that fosaprepitant (*Ivemend*®) is recommended as an option for use within NHS Wales for the prevention of nausea and vomiting associated with highly and moderately emetogenic cancer chemotherapy in patients aged from 6 months to 17 years.

- **MEDICINAL FORMS** There can be variation in the licensing of different medicines containing the same drug.

Powder for solution for infusion

- Ivemend (Merck Sharp & Dohme Ltd)
  Fosaprepitant (as Fosaprepitant dimeglumine) 150 mg Ivemend 150mg powder for solution for infusion vials | 1 vial PoM £47.42

ANTIEMETICS AND ANTINAUSEANTS > SEROTONIN (5HT3) RECEPTOR ANTAGONISTS

Granisetron

21-Jan-2020

- **DRUG ACTION** Granisetron is a specific $5HT_3$-receptor antagonist which blocks $5HT_3$ receptors in the gastro-intestinal tract and in the CNS.

- **INDICATIONS AND DOSE**

Management of nausea and vomiting induced by cytotoxic chemotherapy

- BY MOUTH
- Child 12–17 years: 1–2 mg, to be taken within 1 hour before start of treatment, then 2 mg daily in 1–2 divided doses for up to 1 week following chemotherapy
- BY INTRAVENOUS INFUSION
- Child 2–17 years: 10–40 micrograms/kg (max. per dose 3 mg), repeated if necessary, to be given before start of chemotherapy, for treatment, dose may be repeated within 24 hours if necessary, not less than 10 minutes after initial dose; maximum 2 doses per day

- **UNLICENSED USE** Tablets not licensed in children (age range not specified by manufacturer).
- **CAUTIONS** Subacute intestinal obstruction · susceptibility to QT-interval prolongation (including electrolyte disturbances)
- **INTERACTIONS** → Appendix 1: granisetron
- **SIDE-EFFECTS**
- **Common or very common** Constipation · diarrhoea · headache · insomnia
- **Uncommon** Extrapyramidal symptoms · QT interval prolongation · serotonin syndrome
- **PREGNANCY** Manufacturer advises avoid.
- **BREAST FEEDING** Avoid—no information available.
- **HEPATIC IMPAIRMENT** Manufacturer advises caution.
- **DIRECTIONS FOR ADMINISTRATION** For *intravenous infusion*, dilute up to 3 mL of granisetron injection in Glucose 5% or Sodium Chloride 0.9% to a total volume of 10–30 mL; give over 5 minutes.

- **MEDICINAL FORMS** There can be variation in the licensing of different medicines containing the same drug.

Solution for injection

- Granisetron (Non-proprietary)
  Granisetron (as Granisetron hydrochloride) 1 mg per 1 ml Granisetron 3mg/3ml concentrate for solution for injection ampoules | 10 ampoule PoM £60.00
  Granisetron 1mg/1ml concentrate for solution for injection ampoules | 5 ampoule PoM £10.00–£20.00 | 10 ampoule PoM £20.00

Tablet

- Granisetron (Non-proprietary)
  Granisetron (as Granisetron hydrochloride) 1 mg Granisetron 1mg tablets | 10 tablet PoM £51.20 DT = £40.80
  Granisetron (as Granisetron hydrochloride) 2 mg Granisetron 2mg tablets | 5 tablet PoM ☒ DT = £52.39
- Kytril (Atnahs Pharma UK Ltd)
  Granisetron (as Granisetron hydrochloride) 1 mg Kytril 1mg tablets | 10 tablet PoM £52.39 DT = £40.80
  Granisetron (as Granisetron hydrochloride) 2 mg Kytril 2mg tablets | 5 tablet PoM £52.39 DT = £52.39

Ondansetron

22-Apr-2020

- **DRUG ACTION** Ondansetron is a specific $5HT_3$-receptor antagonist which blocks $5HT_3$ receptors in the gastro-intestinal tract and in the CNS.

- **INDICATIONS AND DOSE**

Prevention of postoperative nausea and vomiting

- BY SLOW INTRAVENOUS INJECTION
- Child: 100 micrograms/kg (max. per dose 4 mg) for 1 dose, dose to be given over at least 30 seconds before, during, or after induction of anaesthesia

Treatment of postoperative nausea and vomiting

- BY SLOW INTRAVENOUS INJECTION
- Child: 100 micrograms/kg (max. per dose 4 mg) for 1 dose, dose to be given over at least 30 seconds

Prevention and treatment of chemotherapy- and radiotherapy-induced nausea and vomiting—initial dose

- BY INTRAVENOUS INFUSION
- Child 6 months–17 years (body surface area up to 1.3 m^2): 5 mg/m^2 for 1 dose then give orally, alternatively 150 micrograms/kg (max. per dose 8 mg), dose to be administered immediately before chemotherapy, then 150 micrograms/kg every 4 hours (max. per dose 8 mg) for 2 further doses then give orally; maximum 32 mg per day
- Child 6 months–17 years (body surface area 1.3 m^2 and above): 8 mg for 1 dose then give orally, alternatively 150 micrograms/kg (max. per dose 8 mg), dose to be administered immediately before chemotherapy, then 150 micrograms/kg every 4 hours (max. per dose 8 mg) for 2 further doses then give orally, intravenous infusion to be administered over at least 15 minutes; maximum 32 mg per day

Prevention and treatment of chemotherapy- and radiotherapy-induced nausea and vomiting—(follow-on dose based on body surface area)

- BY MOUTH
- Child 6 months–17 years (body surface area up to 0.6 m^2): 2 mg every 12 hours for up to 5 days (dose can be started 12 hours after intravenous administration); maximum 32 mg per day
- Child 6 months–17 years (body surface area 0.6–1.2 m^2): 4 mg every 12 hours for up to 5 days (dose can be started 12 hours after intravenous administration); maximum 32 mg per day
- Child 6 months–17 years (body surface area 1.3 m^2 and above): 8 mg every 12 hours for up to 5 days (dose can be started 12 hours after intravenous administration); maximum 32 mg per day

Prevention and treatment of chemotherapy- and radiotherapy-induced nausea and vomiting—(follow-on dose based on body-weight)

- BY MOUTH
- Child 6 months–17 years (body-weight up to 10.1 kg): 2 mg every 12 hours for up to 5 days (dose can be started 12 hours after intravenous administration); maximum 32 mg per day
- Child 6 months–17 years (body-weight 10.1–40 kg): 4 mg every 12 hours for up to 5 days (dose can be started 12 hours after intravenous administration); maximum 32 mg per day
- Child 6 months–17 years (body-weight 41 kg and above): 8 mg every 12 hours for up to 5 days (dose can be started 12 hours after intravenous administration); maximum 32 mg per day

- **UNLICENSED USE** Not licensed for radiotherapy-induced nausea and vomiting in children.

> **IMPORTANT SAFETY INFORMATION**
> MHRA/CHM ADVICE: ONDANSETRON: SMALL INCREASED RISK OF ORAL CLEFTS FOLLOWING USE IN THE FIRST 12 WEEKS OF PREGNANCY (JANUARY 2020)
> Epidemiological studies have identified a small increased risk of cleft lip and/or cleft palate in babies born to women who used oral ondansetron during the first trimester of pregnancy. Healthcare professionals are advised that if there is a clinical need for ondansetron in pregnancy, patients should be counselled on the potential benefits and risks, and the final decision made jointly.

- **CONTRA-INDICATIONS** Congenital long QT syndrome
- **CAUTIONS** Adenotonsillar surgery · subacute intestinal obstruction · susceptibility to QT-interval prolongation (including electrolyte disturbances)
- **INTERACTIONS** → Appendix 1: ondansetron
- **SIDE-EFFECTS**
  - **Common or very common** Constipation · feeling hot · headache · sensation abnormal
  - **Uncommon** Arrhythmias · chest pain · hiccups · hypotension · movement disorders · oculogyric crisis · seizure
  - **Rare or very rare** Dizziness · QT interval prolongation · vision disorders
- **PREGNANCY** Manufacturer advises avoid in first trimester—small increased risk of congenital abnormalities such as orofacial clefts, see *Important safety information*.
- **BREAST FEEDING** Present in milk in *animal* studies—avoid.
- **HEPATIC IMPAIRMENT** Manufacturer advises caution in moderate to severe impairment (decreased clearance).
  Dose adjustments Manufacturer advises a reduced maximum daily dose in moderate to severe impairment—consult product literature.
- **DIRECTIONS FOR ADMINISTRATION**
  - With intravenous use For *intravenous infusion*, dilute to a concentration of 320–640 micrograms/mL with Glucose 5% or Sodium Chloride 0.9%; give over at least 15 minutes.
  - With oral use Orodispersible films and lyophilisates should be placed on the tongue, allowed to disperse and swallowed.
- **PRESCRIBING AND DISPENSING INFORMATION** Flavours of oral liquid formulations may include strawberry.
- **PATIENT AND CARER ADVICE** Patients or carers should be given advice on how to administer orodispersible films and lyophilisates.

- **MEDICINAL FORMS** There can be variation in the licensing of different medicines containing the same drug. Forms available from special-order manufacturers include: oral suspension, oral solution

Tablet

- Ondansetron (Non-proprietary)
  Ondansetron (as Ondansetron hydrochloride) 4 mg Ondansetron 4mg tablets | 10 tablet PoM £25.46 DT = £1.55 | 30 tablet PoM £4.65–£86.33
  Ondansetron (as Ondansetron hydrochloride) 8 mg Ondansetron 8mg tablets | 10 tablet PoM £57.55 DT = £1.57
- Ondemet (Alliance Pharmaceuticals Ltd)
  Ondansetron (as Ondansetron hydrochloride) 8 mg Ondemet 8mg tablets | 10 tablet PoM £54.36 DT = £1.57 (Hospital only)
- Zofran (Novartis Pharmaceuticals UK Ltd)
  Ondansetron (as Ondansetron hydrochloride) 4 mg Zofran 4mg tablets | 30 tablet PoM £107.91
  Ondansetron (as Ondansetron hydrochloride) 8 mg Zofran 8mg tablets | 10 tablet PoM £71.94 DT = £1.57

Solution for injection

- Ondansetron (Non-proprietary)
  Ondansetron (as Ondansetron hydrochloride) 2 mg per 1 ml Ondansetron 8mg/4ml solution for injection ampoules | 5 ampoule PoM £56.95 DT = £59.95 (Hospital only) | 5 ampoule PoM £11.80–£58.45 DT = £59.95
  Ondansetron 4mg/2ml solution for injection ampoules | 5 ampoule PoM £28.47 DT = £29.97 (Hospital only) | 5 ampoule PoM £5.80–£34.44 DT = £29.97 | 10 ampoule PoM £15.00 DT = £15.00
- Zofran Flexi-amp (Novartis Pharmaceuticals UK Ltd)
  Ondansetron (as Ondansetron hydrochloride) 2 mg per 1 ml Zofran Flexi-amp 4mg/2ml solution for injection ampoules | 5 ampoule PoM £29.97 DT = £29.97
  Zofran Flexi-amp 8mg/4ml solution for injection ampoules | 5 ampoule PoM £59.95 DT = £59.95

Oral solution

- Ondansetron (Non-proprietary)
  Ondansetron (as Ondansetron hydrochloride) 800 microgram per 1 ml Ondansetron 4mg/5ml oral solution sugar-free | 50 ml PoM £42.68 DT = £42.28
- Zofran (Novartis Pharmaceuticals UK Ltd)
  Ondansetron (as Ondansetron hydrochloride) 800 microgram per 1 ml Zofran 4mg/5ml syrup sugar-free | 50 ml PoM £35.97 DT = £42.28

Orodispersible film

- Setofilm (Norgine Pharmaceuticals Ltd)
  Ondansetron 4 mg Setofilm 4mg orodispersible films sugar-free | 10 film PoM £28.50 DT = £28.50
  Ondansetron 8 mg Setofilm 8mg orodispersible films sugar-free | 10 film PoM £57.00 DT = £57.00

Oral lyophilisate

EXCIPIENTS: May contain Aspartame

- Zofran Melt (Novartis Pharmaceuticals UK Ltd)
  Ondansetron 4 mg Zofran Melt 4mg oral lyophilisates sugar-free | 10 tablet PoM £35.97 DT = £35.97
  Ondansetron 8 mg Zofran Melt 8mg oral lyophilisates sugar-free | 10 tablet PoM £71.94 DT = £71.94

Orodispersible tablet

- Ondansetron (Non-proprietary)
  Ondansetron 4 mg Ondansetron 4mg orodispersible tablets | 10 tablet PoM £43.48 DT = £43.48
  Ondansetron 8 mg Ondansetron 8mg orodispersible tablets | 10 tablet PoM £85.43 DT = £85.43

ANTIHISTAMINES › SEDATING

Cinnarizine

20-Mar-2020

- **INDICATIONS AND DOSE**

Relief of symptoms of vestibular disorders, such as vertigo, tinnitus, nausea, and vomiting in Ménière's disease

- BY MOUTH
  - Child 5–11 years: 15 mg 3 times a day
  - Child 12–17 years: 30 mg 3 times a day

Motion sickness

- BY MOUTH
  - Child 5–11 years: Initially 15 mg, dose to be taken 2 hours before travel, then 7.5 mg every 8 hours if required, dose to be taken during journey
  - Child 12–17 years: Initially 30 mg, dose to be taken 2 hours before travel, then 15 mg every 8 hours if required, dose to be taken during journey

- **CONTRA-INDICATIONS** Avoid in Acute porphyrias p. 652 · neonate (due to significant antimuscarinic activity)
- **CAUTIONS** Epilepsy · glaucoma · pyloroduodenal obstruction · urinary retention
- **INTERACTIONS** → Appendix 1: antihistamines, sedating
- **SIDE-EFFECTS**
  - **Common or very common** Drowsiness · gastrointestinal discomfort · nausea · weight increased
  - **Uncommon** Fatigue · hyperhidrosis · vomiting

- ▶ **Frequency not known** Dry mouth · gastrointestinal disorder · headache · jaundice cholestatic · movement disorders · muscle rigidity · parkinsonism · skin reactions · subacute cutaneous lupus erythematosus · tremor
- **PREGNANCY** Manufacturer advises avoid; however, there is no evidence of teratogenicity. The use of sedating antihistamines in the latter part of the third trimester may cause adverse effects in neonates such as irritability, paradoxical excitability, and tremor.
- **BREAST FEEDING** Most antihistamines are present in breast milk in varying amounts; although not known to be harmful, most manufacturers advise avoiding their use in mothers who are breast-feeding.
- **HEPATIC IMPAIRMENT** Manufacturer advises caution in hepatic insufficiency—no information available.
- **RENAL IMPAIRMENT** Use with caution—no information available.
- **PATIENT AND CARER ADVICE**
  Driving and skilled tasks Drowsiness may affect performance of skilled tasks (e.g. cycling, driving); sedating effects enhanced by alcohol.

- **MEDICINAL FORMS** There can be variation in the licensing of different medicines containing the same drug. Forms available from special-order manufacturers include: oral suspension

Tablet

CAUTIONARY AND ADVISORY LABELS 2

- ▸ Cinnarizine (Non-proprietary)
  Cinnarizine 15 mg Cinnarizine 15mg tablets | 84 tablet [PoM] £6.88 DT = £4.75 | 84 tablet [P] £15.40 DT = £4.75
- ▸ Stugeron (Johnson & Johnson Ltd, Janssen-Cilag Ltd)
  Cinnarizine 15 mg Stugeron 15mg tablets | 15 tablet [P] £2.36 | 100 tablet [P] £4.18

Promethazine teoclate

28-Nov-2019

- **INDICATIONS AND DOSE**

Nausea | Vomiting | Labyrinthine disorders

▶ BY MOUTH
- ▸ Child 5–9 years: 12.5–37.5 mg daily
- ▸ Child 10–17 years: 25–75 mg daily; maximum 100 mg per day

Motion sickness prevention (acts longer than promethazine hydrochloride)

▶ BY MOUTH
- ▸ Child 5–9 years: 12.5 mg once daily, dose to be taken at bedtime on night before travel or 1–2 hours before travel
- ▸ Child 10–17 years: 25 mg once daily, dose to be taken at bedtime on night before travel or 1–2 hours before travel

Motion sickness treatment (acts longer than promethazine hydrochloride)

▶ BY MOUTH
- ▸ Child 5–9 years: 12.5 mg, dose to be taken at onset of motion sickness, then 12.5 mg daily for 2 days, dose to be taken at bedtime
- ▸ Child 10–17 years: 25 mg, dose to be taken at onset of motion sickness, then 25 mg once daily for 2 days, dose to be taken at bedtime

IMPORTANT SAFETY INFORMATION

MHRA/CHM ADVICE: OVER-THE-COUNTER COUGH AND COLD MEDICINES FOR CHILDREN (APRIL 2009)

Children under 6 years should not be given over-the-counter cough and cold medicines containing promethazine.

- **CONTRA-INDICATIONS** Neonate (due to significant antimuscarinic activity) · should not be given to children under 2 years, except on specialist advice (potential for fatal respiratory depression)
- **CAUTIONS** Asthma · bronchiectasis · bronchitis · epilepsy · pyloroduodenal obstruction · Reye's syndrome · severe coronary artery disease · susceptibility to angle-closure glaucoma · urinary retention
- **INTERACTIONS** → Appendix 1: antihistamines, sedating
- **SIDE-EFFECTS** Anticholinergic syndrome · anxiety · appetite decreased · arrhythmia · blood disorder · bronchial secretion viscosity increased · confusion · dizziness · drowsiness · dry mouth · epigastric discomfort · fatigue · haemolytic anaemia · headache · hypotension · jaundice · movement disorders · muscle spasms · nightmare · palpitations · photosensitivity reaction · urinary retention · vision blurred
  SIDE-EFFECTS, FURTHER INFORMATION Paradoxical stimulation may occur, especially with high doses.
- **PREGNANCY** Most manufacturers of antihistamines advise avoiding their use during pregnancy; however, there is no evidence of teratogenicity. Use in the latter part of the third trimester may cause adverse effects in neonates such as irritability, paradoxical excitability, and tremor.
- **BREAST FEEDING** Most antihistamines are present in breast milk in varying amounts; although not known to be harmful, most manufacturers advise avoiding their use in mothers who are breast-feeding.
- **HEPATIC IMPAIRMENT** Manufacturer advises caution.
- **RENAL IMPAIRMENT** Use with caution.
- **PATIENT AND CARER ADVICE**
  Driving and skilled tasks Drowsiness may affect performance of skilled tasks (e.g. cycling or driving); sedating effects enhanced by alcohol.

- **MEDICINAL FORMS** There can be variation in the licensing of different medicines containing the same drug.

Tablet

CAUTIONARY AND ADVISORY LABELS 2

- ▸ Avomine (Manx Healthcare Ltd)
  Promethazine teoclate 25 mg Avomine 25mg tablets | 10 tablet [P] £1.13 | 28 tablet [P] £3.13 DT = £3.13
- ▸ Vertigon (Manx Healthcare Ltd)
  Promethazine teoclate 25 mg Vertigon 25mg tablets | 28 tablet [P] [X] DT = £3.13

ANTIMUSCARINICS

527

Hyoscine hydrobromide

06-Dec-2019

(Scopolamine hydrobromide)

- **INDICATIONS AND DOSE**

Motion sickness

▶ BY MOUTH
- ▸ Child 4–9 years: 75–150 micrograms, dose to be taken up to 30 minutes before the start of journey, then 75–150 micrograms every 6 hours if required; maximum 450 micrograms per day
- ▸ Child 10–17 years: 150–300 micrograms, dose to be taken up to 30 minutes before the start of journey, then 150–300 micrograms every 6 hours if required; maximum 900 micrograms per day

▶ BY TRANSDERMAL APPLICATION
- ▸ Child 10–17 years: Apply 1 patch, apply behind ear 5–6 hours before journey, then apply 1 patch after 72 hours if required, remove old patch and site replacement patch behind the other ear

Hypersalivation associated with clozapine therapy

▶ BY MOUTH
- ▸ Child 12–17 years: 300 micrograms up to 3 times a day; maximum 900 micrograms per day

continued →

Excessive respiratory secretions
- ▶ BY MOUTH, OR BY SUBLINGUAL ADMINISTRATION
- ▶ Child 2–11 years: 10 micrograms/kg 4 times a day (max. per dose 300 micrograms)
- ▶ Child 12–17 years: 300 micrograms 4 times a day
- ▶ BY TRANSDERMAL APPLICATION
- ▶ Child 1 month–2 years: 250 micrograms every 72 hours, dose equates to a quarter patch
- ▶ Child 3–9 years: 500 micrograms every 72 hours, dose equates to a half patch
- ▶ Child 10–17 years: 1 mg every 72 hours, dose equates to one patch

Excessive respiratory secretion in palliative care
- ▶ BY SUBCUTANEOUS INJECTION, OR BY INTRAVENOUS INJECTION
- ▶ Child: 10 micrograms/kg every 4–8 hours (max. per dose 600 micrograms)
- ▶ BY CONTINUOUS SUBCUTANEOUS INFUSION, OR BY INTRAVENOUS INFUSION
- ▶ Child: 40–60 micrograms/kg over 24 hours

Bowel colic pain in palliative care
- ▶ BY MOUTH USING SUBLINGUAL TABLETS
- ▶ Child: 10 micrograms/kg 3 times a day (max. per dose 300 micrograms), as *Kwells®*.

Premedication
- ▶ BY SUBCUTANEOUS INJECTION, OR BY INTRAMUSCULAR INJECTION
- ▶ Child 1–11 years: 15 micrograms/kg (max. per dose 600 micrograms), to be administered 30–60 minutes before induction of anaesthesia
- ▶ Child 12–17 years: 200–600 micrograms, to be administered 30–60 minutes before induction of anaesthesia
- ▶ BY INTRAVENOUS INJECTION
- ▶ Child 1–11 years: 15 micrograms/kg (max. per dose 600 micrograms), to be administered immediately before induction of anaesthesia
- ▶ Child 12–17 years: 200–600 micrograms, to be administered immediately before induction of anaesthesia

● **UNLICENSED USE** Not licensed for use in excessive respiratory secretions or hypersalivation associated with clozapine therapy.

> **IMPORTANT SAFETY INFORMATION**
> Antimuscarinic drugs used for premedication to general anaesthesia should only be administered by, or under the direct supervision of, personnel experienced in their use.

● **CAUTIONS** Epilepsy

CAUTIONS, FURTHER INFORMATION
- ▶ Anticholinergic syndrome
- ▶ With systemic use In some children hyoscine may cause the central anticholinergic syndrome (excitement, ataxia, hallucinations, behavioural abnormalities, and drowsiness).

● **INTERACTIONS** → Appendix 1: hyoscine

● **SIDE-EFFECTS**
- ▶ **Common or very common**
- ▶ With transdermal use Eye disorders · eyelid irritation
- ▶ **Rare or very rare**
- ▶ With transdermal use Concentration impaired · glaucoma · hallucinations · memory loss · restlessness
- ▶ **Frequency not known**
- ▶ With oral use Asthma · cardiovascular disorders · central nervous system stimulation · gastrointestinal disorder · hallucination · hypersensitivity · hyperthermia · hypohidrosis · mydriasis · oedema · respiratory tract reaction · restlessness · seizure
- ▶ With parenteral use Agitation · angle closure glaucoma · arrhythmias · delirium · dysphagia · dyspnoea · epilepsy exacerbated · hallucination · hypersensitivity · idiosyncratic drug reaction · loss of consciousness · mydriasis · neuroleptic malignant syndrome · psychotic disorder · thirst
- ▶ With transdermal use Balance impaired

● **PREGNANCY** Use only if potential benefit outweighs risk. Injection may depress neonatal respiration.

● **BREAST FEEDING** Amount too small to be harmful.

● **HEPATIC IMPAIRMENT** Manufacturer advises caution.

● **RENAL IMPAIRMENT** Use with caution.

● **DIRECTIONS FOR ADMINISTRATION**
- ▶ With transdermal use *Patch* applied to hairless area of skin behind ear; if less than whole patch required **either** cut with scissors along full thickness ensuring membrane is not peeled away **or** cover portion to prevent contact with skin.
- ▶ With oral use For administration by *mouth*, injection solution may be given orally.

● **PRESCRIBING AND DISPENSING INFORMATION** Flavours of chewable tablet formulations may include raspberry.

Palliative care For further information on the use of hyoscine hydrobromide in palliative care, see www.medicinescomplete.com/#/content/palliative/hyoscine-hydrobromide.

● **PATIENT AND CARER ADVICE**
- ▶ With transdermal use Explain accompanying instructions to patient and in particular emphasise advice to wash hands after handling and to wash application site after removing, and to use one patch at a time.

Driving and skilled tasks ▶ With transdermal use Drowsiness may persist for up to 24 hours or longer after removal of patch; effects of alcohol enhanced.

● **MEDICINAL FORMS** There can be variation in the licensing of different medicines containing the same drug. Forms available from special-order manufacturers include: oral suspension, oral solution

Tablet

CAUTIONARY AND ADVISORY LABELS 2
- ▶ **Kwells** (Bayer Plc)
  Hyoscine hydrobromide 150 microgram Kwells Kids 150microgram tablets | 12 tablet [P] £1.84 DT = £1.84
  Hyoscine hydrobromide 300 microgram Kwells 300microgram tablets | 12 tablet [P] £1.84 DT = £1.84
- ▶ **Travel Calm** (The Boots Company Plc)
  Hyoscine hydrobromide 300 microgram Travel Calm 300microgram tablets | 12 tablet [P] [X] DT = £1.84

Solution for injection
- ▶ **Hyoscine hydrobromide (Non-proprietary)**
  Hyoscine hydrobromide 400 microgram per 1 ml Hyoscine hydrobromide 400micrograms/1ml solution for injection ampoules | 10 ampoule [PoM] £47.21 DT = £47.21
  Hyoscine hydrobromide 600 microgram per 1 ml Hyoscine hydrobromide 600micrograms/1ml solution for injection ampoules | 10 ampoule [PoM] £59.32 DT = £59.32

Transdermal patch

CAUTIONARY AND ADVISORY LABELS 19
- ▶ **Scopoderm** (GlaxoSmithKline Consumer Healthcare)
  Hyoscine 1 mg per 72 hour Scopoderm 1.5mg patches | 2 patch [P] £12.87 DT = £12.87

Chewable tablet

CAUTIONARY AND ADVISORY LABELS 2, 24
- ▶ **Joy-Rides** (Teva UK Ltd)
  Hyoscine hydrobromide 150 microgram Joy-rides 150microgram chewable tablets sugar-free | 12 tablet [P] £1.99 DT = £1.99

ANTIPSYCHOTICS > FIRST-GENERATION

F 260

Droperidol

06-Aug-2019

- **DRUG ACTION** Droperidol is a butyrophenone, structurally related to haloperidol, which blocks dopamine receptors in the chemoreceptor trigger zone.

- **INDICATIONS AND DOSE**

Prevention and treatment of postoperative nausea and vomiting

▶ BY INTRAVENOUS INJECTION

▸ Child 2-17 years: 20–50 micrograms/kg (max. per dose 1.25 mg), dose to be given 30 minutes before end of surgery, then 20–50 micrograms/kg every 6 hours (max. per dose 1.25 mg) if required

- **CONTRA-INDICATIONS** Bradycardia · comatose states · hypokalaemia · hypomagnesaemia · phaeochromocytoma · QT-interval prolongation
- **CAUTIONS** Chronic obstructive pulmonary disease · CNS depression · electrolyte disturbances · history of alcohol abuse · respiratory failure
- **INTERACTIONS** → Appendix 1: droperidol
- **SIDE-EFFECTS**
- ▶ **Uncommon** Anxiety · oculogyration
- ▶ **Rare or very rare** Blood disorder · cardiac arrest · confusion · dysphoria
- ▶ **Frequency not known** Coma · epilepsy · hallucination · oligomenorrhoea · respiratory disorders · SIADH · syncope
- **BREAST FEEDING** Limited information available—avoid repeated administration.
- **HEPATIC IMPAIRMENT** Manufacturer advises caution.
  Dose adjustments Manufacturer advises maximum 625 micrograms repeated every 6 hours as required.
- **RENAL IMPAIRMENT**
  Dose adjustments In postoperative nausea and vomiting, max. 625 micrograms repeated every 6 hours as required.
- **MONITORING REQUIREMENTS** Continuous pulse oximetry required if risk of ventricular arrhythmia—continue for 30 minutes following administration.

- **MEDICINAL FORMS** There can be variation in the licensing of different medicines containing the same drug.

Solution for injection

▸ Droperidol (Non-proprietary)
Droperidol 2.5 mg per 1 ml Droperidol 2.5mg/1ml solution for injection ampoules | 10 ampoule PoM [CD]

▸ Xomolix (Kyowa Kirin Ltd)
Droperidol 2.5 mg per 1 ml Xomolix 2.5mg/1ml solution for injection ampoules | 10 ampoule PoM £39.40

F 260

Levomepromazine (Methotrimeprazine)

25-Oct-2019

- **INDICATIONS AND DOSE**

Restlessness and confusion in palliative care

▶ BY CONTINUOUS SUBCUTANEOUS INFUSION

▸ Child 1-11 years: 0.35–3 mg/kg, to be administered over 24 hours

▸ Child 12-17 years: 12.5–200 mg, to be administered over 24 hours

Nausea and vomiting in palliative care

▶ BY CONTINUOUS INTRAVENOUS INFUSION, OR BY SUBCUTANEOUS INFUSION

▸ Child 1 month–11 years: 100–400 micrograms/kg, to be administered over 24 hours

▸ Child 12-17 years: 5–25 mg, to be administered over 24 hours

- **CONTRA-INDICATIONS** CNS depression · comatose states · phaeochromocytoma
- **CAUTIONS** Patients receiving large initial doses should remain supine
- **INTERACTIONS** → Appendix 1: phenothiazines
- **SIDE-EFFECTS**
- ▶ **Common or very common** Asthenia · heat stroke
- ▶ **Rare or very rare** Cardiac arrest · hepatic disorders
- ▶ **Frequency not known** Allergic dermatitis · confusion · delirium · gastrointestinal disorders · glucose tolerance impaired · hyperglycaemia · hyponatraemia · photosensitivity reaction · priapism · SIADH
- **HEPATIC IMPAIRMENT** Manufacturer advises consider avoiding.
- **RENAL IMPAIRMENT**
  Dose adjustments Start with small doses in severe renal impairment because of increased cerebral sensitivity.
- **DIRECTIONS FOR ADMINISTRATION** For administration by *subcutaneous infusion* dilute with a suitable volume of Sodium Chloride 0.9%.
- **PRESCRIBING AND DISPENSING INFORMATION**
  Palliative care For further information on the use of levomepromazine in palliative care, see www.medicinescomplete.com/#/content/palliative/levomepromazine.

- **MEDICINAL FORMS** There can be variation in the licensing of different medicines containing the same drug.

Solution for injection

▸ Levomepromazine (Non-proprietary)
Levomepromazine hydrochloride 25 mg per 1 ml Levomepromazine 25mg/1ml solution for injection ampoules | 10 ampoule PoM £20.13 DT = £20.13

▸ Nozinan (Sanofi)
Levomepromazine hydrochloride 25 mg per 1 ml Nozinan 25mg/1ml solution for injection ampoules | 10 ampoule PoM £20.13 DT = £20.13

F 260

Prochlorperazine

31-Oct-2019

- **INDICATIONS AND DOSE**

Prevention and treatment of nausea and vomiting

▶ BY MOUTH

▸ Child 1-11 years (body-weight 10 kg and above): 250 micrograms/kg 2–3 times a day

▸ Child 12-17 years: 5–10 mg up to 3 times a day if required

▶ BY INTRAMUSCULAR INJECTION

▸ Child 2-4 years: 1.25–2.5 mg up to 3 times a day if required

▸ Child 5-11 years: 5–6.25 mg up to 3 times a day if required

▸ Child 12-17 years: 12.5 mg up to 3 times a day if required

Nausea and vomiting in previously diagnosed migraine

▶ BY MOUTH USING BUCCAL TABLET

▸ Child 12-17 years: 3–6 mg twice daily, tablets to be placed high between upper lip and gum and left to dissolve

DOSE EQUIVALENCE AND CONVERSION

▸ Doses are expressed as prochlorperazine maleate or mesilate; 1 mg prochlorperazine maleate ≡ 1 mg prochlorperazine mesilate.

- **UNLICENSED USE** Injection not licensed for use in children. *Buccastem M*® tablets not licensed for use in children.
- **CONTRA-INDICATIONS** Avoid oral route in child under 10 kg · CNS depression · comatose states · phaeochromocytoma
- **CAUTIONS** Hypotension (more likely after intramuscular injection)

- **INTERACTIONS** → Appendix 1: phenothiazines
- **SIDE-EFFECTS**

GENERAL SIDE-EFFECTS
- **Rare or very rare** Glucose tolerance impaired · hyperglycaemia · hyponatraemia · SIADH
- **Frequency not known** Photosensitivity reaction

SPECIFIC SIDE-EFFECTS
- **Rare or very rare**
- With buccal use Blood disorder · hepatic disorders
- **Frequency not known**
- With buccal use Oral disorders · skin eruption
- With intramuscular use Atrioventricular block · cardiac arrest · eye disorders · jaundice · muscle rigidity · nasal congestion · respiratory depression · skin reactions
- With oral use Atrioventricular block · autonomic dysfunction · cardiac arrest · consciousness impaired · hyperthermia · jaundice · muscle rigidity · nasal congestion · oculogyric crisis · respiratory depression · skin reactions

SIDE-EFFECTS, FURTHER INFORMATION Acute dytonias are more common with potent first-generation antipsychotics. The risk is increased in men, young adults, children, antipsychotic-naïve patients, rapid dose escalation, and abrupt treatment discontinuation.

- **HEPATIC IMPAIRMENT** Manufacturer advises avoid.
- **RENAL IMPAIRMENT**

Dose adjustments Start with small doses in severe renal impairment because of increased cerebral sensitivity.

- **DIRECTIONS FOR ADMINISTRATION**
- With buccal use Buccal tablets are placed high between upper lip and gum and left to dissolve.
- **PATIENT AND CARER ADVICE**
- With buccal use Patients or carers should be given advice on how to administer prochlorperazine buccal tablets.

- **MEDICINAL FORMS** There can be variation in the licensing of different medicines containing the same drug.

Tablet

CAUTIONARY AND ADVISORY LABELS 2
- Prochlorperazine (Non-proprietary)
  Prochlorperazine maleate 5 mg Prochlorperazine 5mg tablets | 28 tablet PoM £1.98 DT = £1.11 | 84 tablet PoM £1.96–£3.33
- Stemetil (Sanofi)
  Prochlorperazine maleate 5 mg Stemetil 5mg tablets | 28 tablet PoM £1.98 DT = £1.11 | 84 tablet PoM £5.94

Solution for injection
- Stemetil (Sanofi)
  Prochlorperazine mesilate 12.5 mg per 1 ml Stemetil 12.5mg/1ml solution for injection ampoules | 10 ampoule PoM £5.23 DT = £5.23

Buccal tablet

CAUTIONARY AND ADVISORY LABELS 2
- Prochlorperazine (Non-proprietary)
  Prochlorperazine maleate 3 mg Prochlorperazine 3mg buccal tablets | 50 tablet PoM £50.27 DT = £27.61
- Buccastem (Alliance Pharmaceuticals Ltd)
  Prochlorperazine maleate 3 mg Buccastem M 3mg tablets | 8 tablet P £4.01

Oral solution

CAUTIONARY AND ADVISORY LABELS 2
- Stemetil (Sanofi)
  Prochlorperazine mesilate 1 mg per 1 ml Stemetil 5mg/5ml syrup | 100 ml PoM £3.34 DT = £3.34

5 Pain

Analgesics

Pain relief

The non-opioid drugs, paracetamol p. 288 and ibuprofen p. 707 (and other NSAIDs), are particularly suitable for pain in musculoskeletal conditions, whereas the opioid analgesics are more suitable for moderate to severe pain, particularly of visceral origin.

Pain in sickle-cell disease

The pain of mild sickle-cell crises is managed with paracetamol, an NSAID, codeine phosphate p. 293, or dihydrocodeine tartrate p. 295. Severe crises may require the use of morphine p. 299 or diamorphine hydrochloride p. 294; concomitant use of an NSAID may potentiate analgesia and allow lower doses of the opioid to be used. A mixture of nitrous oxide and oxygen (*Entonox*®, *Equanox*®) may also be used.

Dental and orofacial pain

Analgesics should be used judiciously in dental care as a **temporary** measure until the cause of the pain has been dealt with.

Dental pain of inflammatory origin, such as that associated with pulpitis, apical infection, localised osteitis or pericoronitis is usually best managed by treating the infection, providing drainage, restorative procedures, and other local measures. Analgesics provide temporary relief of pain (usually for about 1 to 7 days) until the causative factors have been brought under control. In the case of pulpitis, intra-osseous infection or abscess, reliance on analgesics alone is usually inappropriate.

Similarly the pain and discomfort associated with acute problems of the oral mucosa (e.g. acute herpetic gingivostomatitis, erythema multiforme) may be relieved by benzydamine hydrochloride p. 759 or topical anaesthetics until the cause of the mucosal disorder has been dealt with. However, where a child is febrile, the antipyretic action of paracetamol or ibuprofen is often helpful.

The *choice* of an analgesic for dental purposes should be based on its suitability for the child. Most dental pain is relieved effectively by non-steroidal anti-inflammatory drugs (NSAIDs) e.g. ibuprofen. Paracetamol has analgesic and antipyretic effects but no anti-inflammatory effect.

Opioid analgesics such as dihydrocodeine tartrate act on the central nervous system and are traditionally used for *moderate to severe pain*. However, opioid analgesics are relatively ineffective in dental pain and their side-effects can be unpleasant.

Combining a non-opioid with an opioid analgesic can provide greater relief of pain than either analgesic given alone. However, this applies only when an adequate dose of each analgesic is used. Most combination analgesic preparations have not been shown to provide greater relief of pain than an adequate dose of the non-opioid component given alone. Moreover, combination preparations have the disadvantage of an increased number of side-effects.

Any analgesic given before a dental procedure should have a low risk of increasing postoperative bleeding. In the case of pain after the dental procedure, taking an analgesic before the effect of the local anaesthetic has worn off can improve control. Postoperative analgesia with ibuprofen is usually continued for about 24 to 72 hours.

Dysmenorrhoea

Paracetamol or a NSAID will generally provide adequate relief of pain from dysmenorrhoea. Alternatively use of a combined hormonal contraceptive in adolescent girls may prevent the pain.

Non-opioid analgesics and compound analgesic preparations

Paracetamol has analgesic and antipyretic properties but no demonstrable anti-inflammatory activity; unlike opioid analgesics, it does not cause respiratory depression and is less irritant to the stomach than the NSAIDs. **Overdosage** with paracetamol is particularly dangerous as it may cause hepatic damage which is sometimes not apparent for 4 to 6 days.

Non-steroidal anti-inflammatory analgesics (NSAIDs) are particularly useful for the treatment of children with chronic disease accompanied by pain and inflammation. Some of them are also used in the short-term treatment of mild to moderate pain including transient musculoskeletal pain but paracetamol is now often preferred. They are also suitable for the relief of pain in *dysmenorrhoea* and to treat pain caused by *secondary bone tumours*, many of which produce lysis of bone and release prostaglandins. Due to an association with Reye's syndrome, aspirin p. 98 should be avoided in children under 16 years except in Kawasaki disease or for its antiplatelet action. Several NSAIDs are also used for postoperative analgesia.

Compound analgesic preparations

Compound analgesic preparations that contain a simple analgesic (such as paracetamol) with an opioid component reduce the scope for effective titration of the individual components in the management of pain of varying intensity.

Compound analgesic preparations containing paracetamol with a *low dose* of an opioid analgesic (e.g. 8 mg of codeine phosphate per compound tablet) may be used in older children but the advantages have not been substantiated. The low dose of the opioid may be enough to cause opioid side-effects (in particular, constipation) and can complicate the treatment of **overdosage** yet may not provide significant additional relief of pain.

A *full dose* of the opioid component (e.g. 60 mg codeine phosphate) in compound analgesic preparations effectively augments the analgesic activity but is associated with the full range of opioid side-effects (including nausea, vomiting, severe constipation, drowsiness, respiratory depression, and risk of dependence on long-term administration).

In general, when assessing pain, it is necessary to weigh up carefully whether there is a need for a non-opioid and an opioid analgesic to be taken simultaneously.

Opioid analgesics and dependence

Opioid analgesics are usually used to relieve moderate to severe pain particularly of visceral origin. Repeated administration may cause tolerance, but this is no deterrent in the control of pain in terminal illness. Regular use of a potent opioid may be appropriate for certain cases of chronic non-malignant pain.

Strong opioids

Morphine remains the most valuable opioid analgesic for severe pain although it frequently causes nausea and vomiting. It is the standard against which other opioid analgesics are compared. In addition to relief of pain, morphine also confers a state of euphoria and mental detachment.

Morphine is the opioid of choice for the oral treatment of *severe pain in palliative care*. It is given regularly every 4 hours (or every 12 or 24 hours as modified-release preparations).

Buprenorphine p. 291 has both opioid agonist and antagonist properties and may precipitate withdrawal symptoms, including pain, in children dependent on other opioids. It has abuse potential and may itself cause dependence. It has a much longer duration of action than morphine and sublingually is an effective analgesic for 6 to 8 hours. Unlike most opioid analgesics, the effects of buprenorphine p. 291 are only partially reversed by naloxone hydrochloride p. 901. It is rarely used in children.

Diamorphine hydrochloride p. 294 (heroin) is a powerful opioid analgesic. It may cause less nausea and hypotension than morphine p. 299. In *palliative care* the greater solubility of diamorphine hydrochloride allows effective doses to be injected in smaller volumes and this is important in the emaciated child. Diamorphine hydrochloride is sometimes given by the intranasal route to treat acute pain in children and is available as a nasal spray; intranasal administration of diamorphine injection has been used [unlicensed].

Alfentanil p. 877, fentanyl p. 296 and remifentanil p. 878 are used by injection for intra-operative analgesia. Fentanyl is available in a transdermal drug delivery system as a self-adhesive patch which is changed every 72 hours.

Methadone hydrochloride p. 317 is less sedating than morphine and acts for longer periods. In prolonged use, methadone hydrochloride should not be administered more often than twice daily to avoid the risk of accumulation and opioid overdosage. Methadone hydrochloride may be used instead of morphine when excitation (or exacerbation of pain) occurs with morphine. Methadone hydrochloride may also be used to treat children with neonatal abstinence syndrome.

Papaveretum should not be used in children; morphine is easier to prescribe and less prone to error with regard to the strength and dose.

Pethidine hydrochloride p. 304 produces prompt but short-lasting analgesia; it is less constipating than morphine, but even in high doses is a less potent analgesic. Its use in children is not recommended. Pethidine hydrochloride is used for analgesia in labour; however, other opioids, such as morphine or diamorphine hydrochloride, are often preferred for obstetric pain.

Tramadol hydrochloride p. 305 is used in older children and produces analgesia by two mechanisms: an opioid effect and an enhancement of serotonergic and adrenergic pathways. It has fewer of the typical opioid side-effects (notably, less respiratory depression, less constipation and less addiction potential); psychiatric reactions have been reported.

Weak opioids

Codeine phosphate p. 293 can be used for the relief of short-term acute moderate pain in children older than 12 years where other painkillers such as paracetamol p. 288 or ibuprofen p. 707 have proved ineffective.

Dihydrocodeine tartrate p. 295 has an analgesic efficacy similar to that of codeine phosphate.

Postoperative analgesia

A combination of opioid and non-opioid analgesics is used to treat postoperative pain. The use of intra-operative opioids affects the prescribing of postoperative analgesics. A postoperative opioid analgesic should be given with care since it may potentiate any residual respiratory depression.

Morphine is used most widely. Tramadol hydrochloride is not as effective in severe pain as other opioid analgesics. Buprenorphine may antagonise the analgesic effect of previously administered opioids and is generally not recommended. Pethidine hydrochloride is generally not recommended for postoperative pain because it is metabolised to norpethidine which may accumulate, particularly in neonates and in renal impairment; norpethidine stimulates the central nervous system and may cause convulsions.

Opioids are also given epidurally [unlicensed route] in the postoperative period but are associated with side- effects such as pruritus, urinary retention, nausea and vomiting; respiratory depression can be delayed, particularly with morphine.

Patient-controlled analgesia (PCA) and nurse-controlled analgesia (NCA) can be used to relieve postoperative pain—consult hospital protocols.

Pain management and opioid dependence

Although caution is necessary, patients who are dependent on opioids or have a history of drug dependence may be treated with opioid analgesics when there is a clinical need. Treatment with opioid analgesics in this patient group should normally be carried out with the advice of specialists. However, doctors do not require a special licence to prescribe opioid analgesics to patients with opioid dependence for relief of pain due to organic disease or injury.

Other drugs used for Pain Diclofenac potassium, p. 704 · Levomepromazine, p. 285 · Mefenamic acid, p. 711

ANALGESICS > NON-OPIOID

Paracetamol

10-Mar-2020

(Acetaminophen

● INDICATIONS AND DOSE

Pain | Pyrexia with discomfort

▶ BY MOUTH

- Neonate 28 weeks to 32 weeks corrected gestational age: 20 mg/kg for 1 dose, then 10–15 mg/kg every 8–12 hours as required, maximum daily dose to be given in divided doses; maximum 30 mg/kg per day.
- Neonate 32 weeks corrected gestational age and above: 20 mg/kg for 1 dose, then 10–15 mg/kg every 6–8 hours as required, maximum daily dose to be given in divided doses; maximum 60 mg/kg per day.
- Child 1-2 months: 30–60 mg every 8 hours as required, maximum daily dose to be given in divided doses; maximum 60 mg/kg per day
- Child 3-5 months: 60 mg every 4–6 hours; maximum 4 doses per day
- Child 6-23 months: 120 mg every 4–6 hours; maximum 4 doses per day
- Child 2-3 years: 180 mg every 4–6 hours; maximum 4 doses per day
- Child 4-5 years: 240 mg every 4–6 hours; maximum 4 doses per day
- Child 6-7 years: 240–250 mg every 4–6 hours; maximum 4 doses per day
- Child 8-9 years: 360–375 mg every 4–6 hours; maximum 4 doses per day
- Child 10-11 years: 480–500 mg every 4–6 hours; maximum 4 doses per day
- Child 12-15 years: 480–750 mg every 4–6 hours; maximum 4 doses per day
- Child 16-17 years: 0.5–1 g every 4–6 hours; maximum 4 doses per day

▶ BY RECTUM

- Neonate 28 weeks to 32 weeks corrected gestational age: 20 mg/kg for 1 dose, then 10–15 mg/kg every 12 hours as required, maximum daily dose to be given in divided doses; maximum 30 mg/kg per day.
- Neonate 32 weeks corrected gestational age and above: 30 mg/kg for 1 dose, then 15–20 mg/kg every 8 hours as required, maximum daily dose to be given in divided doses; maximum 60 mg/kg per day.
- Child 1-2 months: 30–60 mg every 8 hours as required, maximum daily dose to be given in divided doses; maximum 60 mg/kg per day
- Child 3-11 months: 60–125 mg every 4–6 hours as required; maximum 4 doses per day
- Child 1-4 years: 125–250 mg every 4–6 hours as required; maximum 4 doses per day
- Child 5-11 years: 250–500 mg every 4–6 hours as required; maximum 4 doses per day
- Child 12-17 years: 500 mg every 4–6 hours

▶ BY INTRAVENOUS INFUSION

- Neonate 32 weeks corrected gestational age and above: 7.5 mg/kg every 8 hours, dose to be administered over 15 minutes.
- Neonate: 10 mg/kg every 4–6 hours, dose to be administered over 15 minutes; maximum 30 mg/kg per day.
- Child (body-weight up to 10 kg): 10 mg/kg every 4–6 hours, dose to be administered over 15 minutes; maximum 30 mg/kg per day
- Child (body-weight 10-50 kg): 15 mg/kg every 4–6 hours, dose to be administered over 15 minutes; maximum 60 mg/kg per day
- Child (body-weight 50 kg and above): 1 g every 4–6 hours, dose to be administered over 15 minutes; maximum 4 g per day

Pain in children with risk factors for hepatotoxicity | Pyrexia with discomfort in children with risk factors for hepatotoxicity

▶ BY INTRAVENOUS INFUSION

- Neonate 32 weeks corrected gestational age and above: 7.5 mg/kg every 8 hours, dose to be administered over 15 minutes.
- Neonate: 10 mg/kg every 4–6 hours, dose to be administered over 15 minutes; maximum 30 mg/kg per day.
- Child (body-weight up to 10 kg): 10 mg/kg every 4–6 hours, dose to be administered over 15 minutes; maximum 30 mg/kg per day
- Child (body-weight 10-50 kg): 15 mg/kg every 4–6 hours, dose to be administered over 15 minutes; maximum 60 mg/kg per day
- Child (body-weight 50 kg and above): 1 g every 4–6 hours, dose to be administered over 15 minutes; maximum 3 g per day

Post-operative pain

▶ BY MOUTH

- Child 1 month-5 years: 20–30 mg/kg for 1 dose, then 15–20 mg/kg every 4–6 hours, maximum daily dose to be given in divided doses; maximum 75 mg/kg per day
- Child 6-11 years: 20–30 mg/kg (max. per dose 1 g) for 1 dose, then 15–20 mg/kg every 4–6 hours, maximum daily dose to be given in divided doses; maximum 75 mg/kg per day; maximum 4 g per day
- Child 12-17 years: 1 g every 4–6 hours; maximum 4 doses per day

▶ BY RECTUM

- Child 1-2 months: 30 mg/kg for 1 dose, then 15–20 mg/kg every 4–6 hours, maximum daily dose to be given in divided doses; maximum 75 mg/kg per day
- Child 3 months-5 years: 30–40 mg/kg for 1 dose, then 15–20 mg/kg every 4–6 hours, maximum daily dose to be given in divided doses; maximum 75 mg/kg per day
- Child 6-11 years: 30–40 mg/kg (max. per dose 1 g) for 1 dose, then 15–20 mg/kg every 4–6 hours, maximum daily dose to be given in divided doses; maximum 75 mg/kg per day; maximum 4 g per day
- Child 12-17 years: 1 g every 4–6 hours; maximum 4 doses per day

Prophylaxis of post-immunisation pyrexia following immunisation with meningococcal group B vaccine (Bexsero®) given as part of the routine immunisation schedule

▶ BY MOUTH

- Child 2 months: 60 mg, first dose to be given at the time of vaccination, then 60 mg after 4–6 hours, then 60 mg after 4–6 hours, use weight-based doses for preterm infants born at less than 32 weeks gestation and currently weighing less than 4 kg—see oral doses for pain and pyrexia with discomfort
- Child 4 months: 60 mg, first dose to be given at the time of vaccination, then 60 mg after 4–6 hours, then 60 mg after 4–6 hours, use weight-based doses for preterm infants born at less than 32 weeks gestation and currently weighing less than 4 kg—see oral doses for pain and pyrexia with discomfort

Post-immunisation pyrexia in infants

- ▸ BY MOUTH
- ▸ Child 2–3 months: 60 mg for 1 dose, then 60 mg after 4–6 hours if required
- ▸ Child 4 months: 60 mg for 1 dose, then 60 mg after 4–6 hours; maximum 4 doses per day

- **UNLICENSED USE** Paracetamol oral suspension 500 mg/5 mL not licensed for use in children under 16 years. Not licensed for use in children under 2 months by mouth; under 3 months by rectum. EvGr Not licensed for use as prophylaxis of post-immunisation pyrexia following immunisation with meningococcal group B vaccine. ⟨E⟩ Intravenous infusion not licensed in pre-term neonates. Intravenous infusion dose not licensed in children and neonates with body-weight under 10 kg.
- **CAUTIONS** Before administering, check when paracetamol last administered and cumulative paracetamol dose over previous 24 hours · body-weight under 50 kg · chronic alcohol consumption · chronic dehydration · chronic malnutrition · hepatocellular insufficiency · long-term use (especially in those who are malnourished)

  CAUTIONS, FURTHER INFORMATION EvGr Some patients may be at increased risk of experiencing toxicity at therapeutic doses, particularly those with a body-weight under 50 kg and those with risk factors for hepatotoxicity. Clinical judgement should be used to adjust the dose of oral and intravenous paracetamol in these patients.

  Co-administration of enzyme-inducing antiepileptic medications may increase toxicity; doses should be reduced. ⟨E⟩
- **INTERACTIONS** → Appendix 1: paracetamol
- **SIDE-EFFECTS**

  GENERAL SIDE-EFFECTS
  - ▸ **Rare or very rare** Thrombocytopenia

  SPECIFIC SIDE-EFFECTS
  - ▸ **Common or very common**
  - ▸ With rectal use Anorectal erythema
  - ▸ **Rare or very rare**
  - ▸ With intravenous use Hypersensitivity · hypotension · leucopenia · malaise · neutropenia
  - ▸ With rectal use Angioedema · liver injury · skin reactions
  - ▸ **Frequency not known**
  - ▸ With intravenous use Flushing · skin reactions · tachycardia
  - ▸ With oral use Agranulocytosis · bronchospasm · hepatic function abnormal · rash · severe cutaneous adverse reactions (SCARs)
  - ▸ With rectal use Agranulocytosis · blood disorder · severe cutaneous adverse reactions (SCARs)

  Overdose Liver damage and less frequently renal damage can occur following overdose.

  Nausea and vomiting, the only early features of poisoning, usually settle within 24 hours. Persistence beyond this time, often associated with the onset of right subcostal pain and tenderness, usually indicates development of hepatic necrosis.

  For specific details on the management of poisoning, see Paracetamol, under Emergency treatment of poisoning p. 891.
- **PREGNANCY** Not known to be harmful.
- **BREAST FEEDING** Amount too small to be harmful.
- **HEPATIC IMPAIRMENT** Manufacturer advises caution (increased risk of toxicity).
- **RENAL IMPAIRMENT**

  Dose adjustments Increase infusion dose interval to every 6 hours if estimated glomerular filtration rate less than 30 mL/minute/1.73 m^2.
- **DIRECTIONS FOR ADMINISTRATION** For *intravenous infusion* (*Perfalgan®*), give in Glucose 5% *or* Sodium Chloride 0.9%; dilute to a concentration of not less than 1 mg/mL and use within an hour; may also be given undiluted. For children under 33 kg, use 50 mL-vial.
- **PRESCRIBING AND DISPENSING INFORMATION** BP directs that when Paediatric Paracetamol Oral Suspension or Paediatric Paracetamol Mixture is prescribed Paracetamol Oral Suspension 120 mg/5 mL should be dispensed.
- **PATIENT AND CARER ADVICE**

  Medicines for Children leaflet: Paracetamol for mild-to-moderate pain www.medicinesforchildren.org.uk/paracetamol-mild-moderate-pain
- **PROFESSION SPECIFIC INFORMATION**

  Dental practitioners' formulary

  Paracetamol Tablets may be prescribed.

  Paracetamol Soluble Tablets 500 mg may be prescribed.

  Paracetamol Oral Suspension may be prescribed.
- **EXCEPTIONS TO LEGAL CATEGORY** Paracetamol capsules or tablets can be sold to the public provided packs contain no more than 32 capsules or tablets; pharmacists can sell multiple packs up to a total quantity of 100 capsules or tablets in justifiable circumstances.

- **MEDICINAL FORMS** There can be variation in the licensing of different medicines containing the same drug. Forms available from special-order manufacturers include: oral suspension, oral solution, suppository, powder

Tablet

CAUTIONARY AND ADVISORY LABELS 29 (500 mg tablets in adults), 30

▸ Paracetamol (Non-proprietary)

Paracetamol 500 mg Paracetamol 500mg caplets | 100 tablet PoM £3.05 DT = £2.41

Paracetamol 500mg tablets | 100 tablet PoM £2.41 DT = £2.41 | 1000 tablet PoM £24.10

Paracetamol 1 gram Paracetamol 1g tablets | 100 tablet PoM £2.49 DT = £2.49

▸ Mandanol (M & A Pharmachem Ltd)

Paracetamol 500 mg Mandanol 500mg caplets | 100 tablet PoM £1.34 DT = £2.41

Mandanol 500mg tablets | 100 tablet PoM £1.34 DT = £2.41

▸ Paravict (Ecogen Europe Ltd)

Paracetamol 500 mg Paravict 500mg tablets | 100 tablet PoM £1.62 DT = £2.41

Suppository

CAUTIONARY AND ADVISORY LABELS 30

▸ Paracetamol (Non-proprietary)

Paracetamol 80 mg Paracetamol 80mg suppositories | 10 suppository P £10.00 DT = £10.00

Paracetamol 120 mg Paracetamol 120mg suppositories | 10 suppository P £12.39 DT = £12.39

Paracetamol 125 mg Paracetamol 125mg suppositories | 10 suppository P £15.00 DT = £13.80

Paracetamol 240 mg Paracetamol 240mg suppositories | 10 suppository P £22.01 DT = £22.01

Paracetamol 250 mg Paracetamol 250mg suppositories | 10 suppository P £33.38 DT = £27.60

Paracetamol 500 mg Paracetamol 500mg suppositories | 10 suppository P £36.50 DT = £36.50

Paracetamol 1 gram Paracetamol 1g suppositories | 10 suppository P £60.00 DT = £59.50

▸ Alvedon (Intrapharm Laboratories Ltd)

Paracetamol 60 mg Alvedon 60mg suppositories | 10 suppository P £11.95 DT = £11.95

Paracetamol 125 mg Alvedon 125mg suppositories | 10 suppository P £13.80 DT = £13.80

Paracetamol 250 mg Alvedon 250mg suppositories | 10 suppository P £27.60 DT = £27.60

Oral suspension

CAUTIONARY AND ADVISORY LABELS 30

▸ Paracetamol (Non-proprietary)

Paracetamol 24 mg per 1 ml Paracetamol 120mg/5ml oral suspension paediatric | 100 ml P £1.25–£1.70 | 500 ml P £6.23 DT = £6.23

Paracetamol 120mg/5ml oral suspension paediatric sugar-free | 100 ml P £1.83 DT = £1.37 sugar-free | 200 ml P £2.72–£3.20 sugar-free | 500 ml P £8.00 sugar-free | 1000 ml P £10.48

4 Nervous system

Paracetamol 50 mg per 1 ml Paracetamol 250mg/5ml oral suspension | 100 ml [P] £2.00–£2.40 DT = £2.06 | 500 ml [P] £10.00–£12.00
Paracetamol 250mg/5ml oral suspension sugar-free | 100 ml [P] £1.35–£1.89 sugar-free | 200 ml [P] £2.96 DT = £2.69 sugar-free | 500 ml [P] £6.67–£6.73 sugar-free | 1000 ml [P] £13.35
Paracetamol 100 mg per 1 ml Paracetamol 500mg/5ml oral suspension sugar-free | 150 ml [PoM] £24.00 DT = £24.00

▸ **Calpol** (McNeil Products Ltd)
Paracetamol 24 mg per 1 ml Calpol Infant 120mg/5ml oral suspension | 200 ml [P] £3.78
Calpol Infant 120mg/5ml oral suspension sugar-free | 200 ml [P] £3.78
Paracetamol 50 mg per 1 ml Calpol Six Plus 250mg/5ml oral suspension 5ml sachets sugar-free | 12 sachet [GSL] £2.93 DT = £2.93
Calpol Six Plus 250mg/5ml oral suspension | 200 ml [P] £4.40
Calpol Six Plus 250mg/5ml oral suspension sugar-free | 100 ml [P] £2.64 sugar-free | 200 ml [P] £4.40 DT = £2.69

Effervescent tablet

CAUTIONARY AND ADVISORY LABELS 13, 29 (500 mg tablets in adults), 30

▸ **Paracetamol (Non-proprietary)**
Paracetamol 500 mg Paracetamol 500mg soluble tablets | 60 tablet [P] £26.56 | 100 tablet [PoM] [CD] DT = £6.25
Paracetamol 500mg effervescent tablets | 24 tablet [PoM] £1.64–£2.18 | 60 tablet [PoM] £4.10 | 100 tablet [PoM] £6.83 DT = £6.83

▸ **Altridexamol** (TriOn Pharma Ltd)
Paracetamol 1 gram Altridexamol 1000mg effervescent tablets sugar-free | 50 tablet [PoM] £6.59 DT = £6.59

Solution for infusion

▸ **Paracetamol (Non-proprietary)**
Paracetamol 10 mg per 1 ml Paracetamol 500mg/50ml solution for infusion bottles | 10 bottle [PoM] £11.00 (Hospital only)
Paracetamol 500mg/50ml solution for infusion vials | 10 vial [PoM] £15.10
Paracetamol 1g/100ml solution for infusion bottles | 10 bottle [PoM] [CD]
Paracetamol 1g/100ml solution for infusion vials | 10 vial [PoM] £12.00 DT = £12.00 (Hospital only) | 10 vial [PoM] £16.40 DT = £12.00 | 20 vial [PoM] £24.00 (Hospital only)
Paracetamol 100mg/10ml solution for infusion ampoules | 20 ampoule [PoM] £12.00

▸ **Perfalgan** (Bristol-Myers Squibb Pharmaceuticals Ltd)
Paracetamol 10 mg per 1 ml Perfalgan 1g/100ml solution for infusion vials | 12 vial [PoM] £14.96
Perfalgan 500mg/50ml solution for infusion vials | 12 vial [PoM] £13.60

Oral solution

CAUTIONARY AND ADVISORY LABELS 30

▸ **Paracetamol (Non-proprietary)**
Paracetamol 24 mg per 1 ml Paracetamol 120mg/5ml oral solution paediatric sugar-free | 2000 ml [P] £23.80 DT = £23.80
Paracetamol 100 mg per 1 ml Paracetamol 500mg/5ml oral solution sugar-free | 150 ml [PoM] £24.00 sugar-free | 200 ml [PoM] £18.00 DT = £18.00

Powder

▸ **Paracetamol (Non-proprietary)**
Paracetamol 650 mg 650mg oral powder sachets | 5 sachet [GSL] [CD] | 10 sachet [GSL] [CD]

Capsule

CAUTIONARY AND ADVISORY LABELS 29, 30

▸ **Paracetamol (Non-proprietary)**
Paracetamol 500 mg Paracetamol 500mg capsules | 100 capsule [PoM] £3.85 DT = £3.16

Orodispersible tablet

CAUTIONARY AND ADVISORY LABELS 30

▸ **Calpol Fastmelts** (McNeil Products Ltd)
Paracetamol 250 mg Calpol Six Plus Fastmelts 250mg tablets sugar-free | 24 tablet [P] £4.12 DT = £4.12

Combinations available: *Co-codamol,* p. 292 · *Dihydrocodeine with paracetamol,* p. 296 · *Tramadol with paracetamol,* p. 307

ANALGESICS › OPIOIDS

Opioids

IMPORTANT SAFETY INFORMATION

MHRA/CHM ADVICE: BENZODIAZEPINES AND OPIOIDS: REMINDER OF RISK OF POTENTIALLY FATAL RESPIRATORY DEPRESSION (MARCH 2020)

The MHRA reminds healthcare professionals that opioids co-prescribed with benzodiazepines and benzodiazepine-like drugs can produce additive CNS depressant effects, thereby increasing the risk of sedation, respiratory depression, coma, and death. Healthcare professionals are advised to only co-prescribe if there is no alternative and, if necessary, the lowest possible doses should be given for the shortest duration. Patients should be closely monitored for signs of respiratory depression at initiation of treatment and when there is any change in prescribing, such as dose adjustments or new interactions. If methadone is co-prescribed with a benzodiazepine or benzodiazepine-like drug, the respiratory depressant effect of methadone may be delayed; patients should be monitored for at least 2 weeks after initiation or changes in prescribing. Patients should be informed of the signs and symptoms of respiratory depression and sedation, and advised to seek urgent medical attention should these occur.

● **CONTRA-INDICATIONS** Acute respiratory depression · comatose patients · head injury (opioid analgesics interfere with pupillary responses vital for neurological assessment) · raised intracranial pressure (opioid analgesics interfere with pupillary responses vital for neurological assessment) · risk of paralytic ileus

● **CAUTIONS** Adrenocortical insufficiency (reduced dose is recommended) · asthma (avoid during an acute attack) · convulsive disorders · diseases of the biliary tract · hypotension · hypothyroidism (reduced dose is recommended) · impaired respiratory function (avoid in chronic obstructive pulmonary disease) · inflammatory bowel disorders · myasthenia gravis · obstructive bowel disorders · shock

CAUTIONS, FURTHER INFORMATION

▸ **Dependence** Repeated use of opioid analgesics is associated with the development of psychological and physical dependence; although this is rarely a problem with therapeutic use, caution is advised if prescribing for patients with a history of drug dependence.

▸ **Palliative care** In the control of pain in terminal illness, the cautions listed should not necessarily be a deterrent to the use of opioid analgesics.

● **SIDE-EFFECTS**

▸ **Common or very common** Arrhythmias · confusion · constipation · dizziness · drowsiness · dry mouth · euphoric mood · flushing · hallucination · headache · hyperhidrosis · hypotension (with high doses) · miosis · nausea (more common on initiation) · palpitations · respiratory depression (with high doses) · skin reactions · urinary retention · vertigo · visual impairment · vomiting (more common on initiation)

▸ **Uncommon** Drug dependence · dysphoria · withdrawal syndrome

SIDE-EFFECTS, FURTHER INFORMATION **Respiratory depression** Respiratory depression is a major concern with opioid analgesics and it may be treated by artificial ventilation or be reversed by naloxone. Neonates (particularly if pre-term) may be more susceptible.
Dependence and withdrawal Psychological dependence rarely occurs when opioids are used therapeutically (e.g. for pain relief), but tolerance can develop during long-term treatment.

Overdose Opioids (narcotic analgesics) cause coma, respiratory depression, and pinpoint pupils. For details on the management of poisoning, see Opioids, under Emergency treatment of poisoning p. 891 and consider the specific antidote, naloxone hydrochloride.

- **PREGNANCY** Respiratory depression and withdrawal symptoms can occur in the neonate if opioid analgesics are used during delivery; also gastric stasis and inhalation pneumonia has been reported in the mother if opioid analgesics are used during labour.
- **TREATMENT CESSATION** Avoid abrupt withdrawal after long-term treatment; they should be withdrawn gradually to avoid abstinence symptoms.
- **PRESCRIBING AND DISPENSING INFORMATION** The *Faculty of Pain Medicine* has produced resources for healthcare professionals around opioid prescribing: www.fpm.ac.uk/faculty-of-pain-medicine/opioids-aware
- **PATIENT AND CARER ADVICE**

Driving and skilled tasks Drowsiness may affect performance of skilled tasks (e.g. driving); effects of alcohol enhanced. Driving at the start of therapy with opioid analgesics, and following dose changes, should be avoided.

For information on 2015 legislation regarding driving whilst taking certain controlled drugs, including opioids, see *Drugs and skilled tasks* under Guidance on prescribing p. 1.

F 290

Buprenorphine

02-Dec-2019

- **DRUG ACTION** Buprenorphine is an opioid-receptor partial agonist (it has opioid agonist and antagonist properties).

- **INDICATIONS AND DOSE**

Moderate to severe pain

▶ BY SUBLINGUAL ADMINISTRATION
- Child (body-weight 16-25 kg): 100 micrograms every 6–8 hours
- Child (body-weight 25-37.5 kg): 100–200 micrograms every 6–8 hours
- Child (body-weight 37.5-50 kg): 200–300 micrograms every 6–8 hours
- Child (body-weight 50 kg and above): 200–400 micrograms every 6–8 hours

▶ BY INTRAMUSCULAR INJECTION, OR BY SLOW INTRAVENOUS INJECTION
- Child 6 months-11 years: 3–6 micrograms/kg every 6–8 hours (max. per dose 9 micrograms/kg)
- Child 12-17 years: 300–600 micrograms every 6–8 hours

- **UNLICENSED USE**
  - With oral use Sublingual tablets not licensed for use in children under 6 years.
  - With intramuscular use or intravenous use Injection not licensed for use in children under 6 months.
- **CAUTIONS** Impaired consciousness

BUVIDAL® Susceptibility to QT-interval prolongation

- **INTERACTIONS** → Appendix 1: opioids
- **SIDE-EFFECTS**

GENERAL SIDE-EFFECTS
- **Rare or very rare** Angioedema · bronchospasm
- **Frequency not known** Hepatic disorders

SPECIFIC SIDE-EFFECTS
- **Common or very common**
  - With parenteral use Hypersensitivity · withdrawal syndrome neonatal
  - With sublingual use Fatigue · sleep disorders
- **Uncommon**
  - With sublingual use Anxiety · apnoea · appetite decreased · atrioventricular block · coma · conjunctivitis · coordination abnormal · cyanosis · depersonalisation · depression · diarrhoea · diplopia · dyspepsia · dyspnoea · hypertension · pallor · paraesthesia · psychosis · seizure · speech slurred · tinnitus · tremor · urinary disorder
- **Frequency not known**
  - With parenteral use Psychotic disorder · vision blurred
  - With sublingual use Cerebrospinal fluid pressure increased · circulation impaired · haemorrhagic diathesis · oral disorders · syncope

Overdose The effects of buprenorphine are only partially reversed by naloxone.

- **BREAST FEEDING** Present in low levels in breast milk.

Monitoring Neonates should be monitored for drowsiness, adequate weight gain, and developmental milestones.

- **HEPATIC IMPAIRMENT** Manufacturer advises caution; avoid in severe impairment (limited information available).
- **RENAL IMPAIRMENT** Avoid use or reduce dose; opioid effects increased and prolonged; increased cerebral sensitivity.
- **PRE-TREATMENT SCREENING** Documentation of viral hepatitis status is recommended before commencing therapy for opioid dependence.
- **MONITORING REQUIREMENTS** Monitor liver function; when used in opioid dependence baseline liver function test is recommended before commencing therapy, and regular liver function tests should be performed throughout treatment.
- **DIRECTIONS FOR ADMINISTRATION** *Sublingual tablets* may be halved.
- **PATIENT AND CARER ADVICE** Patients or carers should be given advice on how to administer buprenorphine products.

- **MEDICINAL FORMS** There can be variation in the licensing of different medicines containing the same drug.

Solution for injection

▶ **Temgesic** (Indivior UK Ltd)

Buprenorphine (as Buprenorphine hydrochloride) 300 microgram per 1 ml Temgesic 300micrograms/1ml solution for injection ampoules | 5 ampoule [PoM] £2.46 [CD3]

Sublingual tablet

CAUTIONARY AND ADVISORY LABELS 2, 26

▶ **Buprenorphine (Non-proprietary)**

Buprenorphine (as Buprenorphine hydrochloride) 400 microgram Buprenorphine 400microgram sublingual tablets sugar-free | 7 tablet [PoM] £1.72 DT = £1.36 [CD3] sugar-free | 50 tablet [PoM] £12.09 DT = £10.07 [CD3]

Buprenorphine (as Buprenorphine hydrochloride) 2 mg Buprenorphine 2mg sublingual tablets sugar-free | 7 tablet [PoM] £8.35 DT = £4.61 [CD3]

Buprenorphine (as Buprenorphine hydrochloride) 8 mg Buprenorphine 8mg sublingual tablets sugar-free | 7 tablet [PoM] £22.50 DT = £16.93 [CD3]

▶ **Natzon** (Morningside Healthcare Ltd)

Buprenorphine (as Buprenorphine hydrochloride) 400 microgram Natzon 0.4mg sublingual tablets sugar-free | 7 tablet [PoM] £1.60 DT = £1.36 [CD3]

Buprenorphine (as Buprenorphine hydrochloride) 2 mg Natzon 2mg sublingual tablets sugar-free | 7 tablet [PoM] £6.35 DT = £4.61 [CD3]

Buprenorphine (as Buprenorphine hydrochloride) 8 mg Natzon 8mg sublingual tablets sugar-free | 7 tablet [PoM] £19.05 DT = £16.93 [CD3]

▶ **Prefibin** (Sandoz Ltd)

Buprenorphine (as Buprenorphine hydrochloride) 400 microgram Prefibin 0.4mg sublingual tablets sugar-free | 7 tablet [PoM] £1.60 DT = £1.36 [CD3]

Buprenorphine (as Buprenorphine hydrochloride) 2 mg Prefibin 2mg sublingual tablets sugar-free | 7 tablet [PoM] £5.38 DT = £4.61 [CD3]

Buprenorphine (as Buprenorphine hydrochloride) 8 mg Prefibin 8mg sublingual tablets sugar-free | 7 tablet [PoM] £16.15 DT = £16.93 [CD3]

▸ **Subutex** (Indivior UK Ltd)
Buprenorphine (as Buprenorphine hydrochloride) 400 microgram Subutex 0.4mg sublingual tablets sugar-free | 7 tablet [PoM] £1.36 DT = £1.36 [CD3]
Buprenorphine (as Buprenorphine hydrochloride) 2 mg Subutex 2mg sublingual tablets sugar-free | 7 tablet [PoM] £4.45 DT = £4.61 [CD3]
Buprenorphine (as Buprenorphine hydrochloride) 8 mg Subutex 8mg sublingual tablets sugar-free | 7 tablet [PoM] £13.34 DT = £16.93 [CD3]

▸ **Temgesic** (Indivior UK Ltd)
Buprenorphine (as Buprenorphine hydrochloride) 200 microgram Temgesic 200microgram sublingual tablets sugar-free | 50 tablet [PoM] £5.04 DT = £5.04 [CD3]
Buprenorphine (as Buprenorphine hydrochloride) 400 microgram Temgesic 400microgram sublingual tablets sugar-free | 50 tablet [PoM] £10.07 DT = £10.07 [CD3]

▸ **Tephine** (Sandoz Ltd)
Buprenorphine (as Buprenorphine hydrochloride) 200 microgram Tephine 200microgram sublingual tablets sugar-free | 50 tablet [PoM] £4.27 DT = £5.04 [CD3]
Buprenorphine (as Buprenorphine hydrochloride) 400 microgram Tephine 400microgram sublingual tablets sugar-free | 50 tablet [PoM] £8.54 DT = £10.07 [CD3]

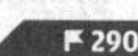

Co-codamol

26-May-2020

The properties listed below are those particular to the combination only. For the properties of the components please consider, paracetamol p. 288.

● **INDICATIONS AND DOSE**

Short-term treatment of acute moderate pain (using co-codamol 8/500 preparations only)

▶ BY MOUTH

▸ Child 12–15 years: 8/500 mg every 6 hours as required for maximum 3 days; maximum 32/2000 mg per day
▸ Child 16–17 years: 8/500–16/1000 mg every 6 hours as required for maximum 3 days; maximum 64/4000 mg per day

Short-term treatment of acute moderate pain (using co-codamol 15/500 preparations only)

▶ BY MOUTH

▸ Child 12–15 years: 15/500 mg every 6 hours as required for maximum 3 days; maximum 60/2000 mg per day
▸ Child 16–17 years: 15/500–30/1000 mg every 6 hours as required for maximum 3 days; maximum 120/4000 mg per day

Short-term treatment of acute moderate pain (using co-codamol 30/500 preparations only)

▶ BY MOUTH

▸ Child 12–15 years: 30/500 mg every 6 hours as required for maximum 3 days; maximum 120/2000 mg per day
▸ Child 16–17 years: 30/500–60/1000 mg every 6 hours as required for maximum 3 days; maximum 240/4000 mg per day

KAPAKE® 15/500

Short-term treatment of acute pain

▶ BY MOUTH

▸ Child 12–15 years: 1 tablet every 6 hours as required for maximum 3 days; maximum 4 tablets per day
▸ Child 16–17 years: 2 tablets every 6 hours as required for maximum 3 days; maximum 8 tablets per day

IMPORTANT SAFETY INFORMATION

See codeine phosphate p. 293 for MHRA/CHM advice for restrictions on the use of codeine as an analgesic in children.

● **CONTRA-INDICATIONS** Acute ulcerative colitis · antibiotic-associated colitis · children who undergo the removal of tonsils or adenoids for the treatment of obstructive sleep apnoea · conditions where abdominal distention develops · conditions where inhibition of peristalsis should be avoided · known ultra-rapid codeine metabolisers

● **CAUTIONS** Acute abdomen · alcohol dependence · avoid abrupt withdrawal after long-term treatment · cardiac arrhythmias · chronic alcoholism · chronic dehydration · chronic malnutrition · convulsive disorders · gallstones · hepatocellular insufficiency

CAUTIONS, FURTHER INFORMATION

▸ Variation in metabolism The capacity to metabolise codeine to morphine can vary considerably between individuals; there is a marked increase in morphine toxicity in patients who are ultra-rapid codeine metabolisers (CYP2D6 ultra-rapid metabolisers) and a reduced therapeutic effect in poor codeine metabolisers.

● **INTERACTIONS** → Appendix 1: opioids · paracetamol

● **SIDE-EFFECTS** Abdominal pain · addiction · agranulocytosis · blood disorder · irritability · pancreatitis · restlessness · severe cutaneous adverse reactions (SCARs) · thrombocytopenia

Overdose Liver damage (and less frequently renal damage) following overdosage with paracetamol.

● **BREAST FEEDING** Manufacturer advises avoid (recommendation also supported by MHRA and specialist sources). Present in milk and mothers vary considerably in their capacity to metabolise codeine; risk of opioid toxicity in infant.

● **HEPATIC IMPAIRMENT** Manufacturer advises caution in mild to moderate impairment; avoid in severe impairment.

Dose adjustments Manufacturer advises consider dose reduction in mild to moderate impairment.

● **RENAL IMPAIRMENT** Reduce dose or avoid codeine; increased and prolonged effect; increased cerebral sensitivity.

● **PRESCRIBING AND DISPENSING INFORMATION** Co-codamol is a mixture of codeine phosphate and paracetamol; the proportions are expressed in the form x/y, where x and y are the strengths in milligrams of codeine phosphate and paracetamol respectively.

When co-codamol tablets, dispersible (or effervescent) tablets, or capsules are prescribed and **no strength is stated**, tablets, dispersible (or effervescent) tablets, or capsules, respectively, containing codeine phosphate 8 mg and paracetamol 500 mg should be dispensed.

The Drug Tariff allows tablets of co-codamol labelled 'dispersible' to be dispensed against an order for 'effervescent' and *vice versa*.

● **LESS SUITABLE FOR PRESCRIBING** Co-codamol is less suitable for prescribing.

● **EXCEPTIONS TO LEGAL CATEGORY** Co-codamol 8/500 can be sold to the public in certain circumstances; for exemptions see *Medicines, Ethics and Practice,* London, Pharmaceutical Press (always consult latest edition).

● **MEDICINAL FORMS** There can be variation in the licensing of different medicines containing the same drug. Forms available from special-order manufacturers include: oral suspension, oral solution

Tablet

CAUTIONARY AND ADVISORY LABELS 2 (does not apply to the 8/500 tablet), 29, 30

▸ **Co-codamol (Non-proprietary)**
Codeine phosphate 8 mg, Paracetamol 500 mg Co-codamol 8mg/500mg tablets | 100 tablet [PoM] £5.75 DT = £3.40 [CD5] | 500 tablet [PoM] £17.00 [CD5] | 1000 tablet [PoM] £34.00 [CD5]
Co-codamol 8mg/500mg caplets | 32 tablet [P] £0.95–£2.32 [CD5]
Codeine phosphate 15 mg, Paracetamol 500 mg Co-codamol 15mg/500mg tablets | 100 tablet [PoM] £15.00 DT = £3.68 [CD5]
Codeine phosphate 30 mg, Paracetamol 500 mg Co-codamol 30mg/500mg caplets | 100 tablet [PoM] £4.60 DT = £4.47 [CD5]
Co-codamol 30mg/500mg tablets | 30 tablet [PoM] £1.38 DT = £1.34 [CD5] | 100 tablet [PoM] £7.53 DT = £4.47 [CD5]

▸ Codipar (Advanz Pharma)
Codeine phosphate 15 mg, Paracetamol 500 mg Codipar 15mg/500mg tablets | 100 tablet PoM £8.25 DT = £3.68 CD5

▸ Emcozin (M & A Pharmachem Ltd)
Codeine phosphate 30 mg, Paracetamol 500 mg Emcozin 30mg/500mg tablets | 100 tablet PoM £2.94 DT = £4.47 CD5

▸ Kapake (Galen Ltd)
Codeine phosphate 30 mg, Paracetamol 500 mg Kapake 30mg/500mg tablets | 100 tablet PoM £7.10 DT = £4.47 CD5

▸ Migraleve Yellow (McNeil Products Ltd)
Codeine phosphate 8 mg, Paracetamol 500 mg Migraleve Yellow tablets | 16 tablet PoM ⊠ CD5

▸ Panadol Ultra (GlaxoSmithKline Consumer Healthcare)
Codeine phosphate 12.8 mg, Paracetamol 500 mg Panadol Ultra 12.8mg/500mg tablets | 20 tablet P £2.61 DT = £3.81 CD5

▸ Solpadeine Max (Omega Pharma Ltd)
Codeine phosphate 12.8 mg, Paracetamol 500 mg Solpadeine Max 12.8mg/500mg tablets | 20 tablet P £3.81 DT = £3.81 CD5 | 30 tablet P £4.91 DT = £4.91 CD5

▸ Solpadol (Sanofi)
Codeine phosphate 30 mg, Paracetamol 500 mg Solpadol 30mg/500mg caplets | 30 tablet PoM £2.02 DT = £1.34 CD5 | 100 tablet PoM £6.74 DT = £4.47 CD5

▸ Zapain (Advanz Pharma)
Codeine phosphate 30 mg, Paracetamol 500 mg Zapain 30mg/500mg tablets | 100 tablet PoM £3.11 DT = £4.47 CD5

Effervescent tablet

CAUTIONARY AND ADVISORY LABELS 2 (does not apply to the 8/500 tablet), 13, 29, 30
EXCIPIENTS: May contain Aspartame
ELECTROLYTES: May contain Sodium

▸ Co-codamol (Non-proprietary)
Codeine phosphate 8 mg, Paracetamol 500 mg Co-codamol 8mg/500mg effervescent tablets | 100 tablet PoM £8.75 DT = £8.03 CD5
Codeine phosphate 30 mg, Paracetamol 500 mg Co-codamol 30mg/500mg effervescent tablets | 32 tablet PoM £5.40 DT = £2.53 CD5 | 100 tablet PoM £19.20 DT = £7.91 CD5

▸ Codipar (Advanz Pharma)
Codeine phosphate 15 mg, Paracetamol 500 mg Codipar 15mg/500mg effervescent tablets sugar-free | 100 tablet PoM £8.25 DT = £8.25 CD5

▸ Paracodol (Bayer Plc)
Codeine phosphate 8 mg, Paracetamol 500 mg Paracodol 8mg/500mg effervescent tablets | 32 tablet P £3.02 DT = £2.57 CD5

▸ Solpadol (Sanofi)
Codeine phosphate 30 mg, Paracetamol 500 mg Solpadol 30mg/500mg effervescent tablets | 32 tablet PoM £2.59 DT = £2.53 CD5 | 100 tablet PoM £8.90 DT = £7.91 CD5

Oral solution

▸ Co-codamol (Non-proprietary)
Codeine phosphate 6 mg per 1 ml, Paracetamol 100 mg per 1 ml Co-codamol 30mg/500mg/5ml oral solution sugar-free | 150 ml PoM £11.99 CD5

Capsule

CAUTIONARY AND ADVISORY LABELS 2 (does not apply to the 8/500 capsule), 29, 30
EXCIPIENTS: May contain Sulfites

▸ Co-codamol (Non-proprietary)
Codeine phosphate 8 mg, Paracetamol 500 mg Co-codamol 8mg/500mg capsules | 32 capsule PoM ⊠ DT = £6.69 CD5 | 100 capsule PoM £20.90 DT = £20.90 CD5
Codeine phosphate 15 mg, Paracetamol 500 mg Co-codamol 15mg/500mg capsules | 100 capsule PoM £9.05 DT = £9.05 CD5
Codeine phosphate 30 mg, Paracetamol 500 mg Co-codamol 30mg/500mg capsules | 100 capsule PoM £7.01 DT = £5.46 CD5

▸ Codipar (Advanz Pharma)
Codeine phosphate 15 mg, Paracetamol 500 mg Codipar 15mg/500mg capsules | 100 capsule PoM £7.25 DT = £9.05 CD5

▸ Kapake (Galen Ltd)
Codeine phosphate 30 mg, Paracetamol 500 mg Kapake 30mg/500mg capsules | 100 capsule PoM £7.10 DT = £5.46 CD5

▸ Solpadol (Sanofi)
Codeine phosphate 30 mg, Paracetamol 500 mg Solpadol 30mg/500mg capsules | 100 capsule PoM £6.74 DT = £5.46 CD5

▸ Tylex (UCB Pharma Ltd)
Codeine phosphate 30 mg, Paracetamol 500 mg Tylex 30mg/500mg capsules | 100 capsule PoM £7.93 DT = £5.46 CD5

▸ Zapain (Advanz Pharma)
Codeine phosphate 30 mg, Paracetamol 500 mg Zapain 30mg/500mg capsules | 100 capsule PoM £3.85 DT = £5.46 CD5

F 290

Codeine phosphate

26-May-2020

● **INDICATIONS AND DOSE**

Acute diarrhoea

▸ BY MOUTH

▸ Child 12-17 years: 30 mg 3–4 times a day; usual dose 15–60 mg 3–4 times a day

Short-term treatment of acute moderate pain

▸ BY MOUTH, OR BY INTRAMUSCULAR INJECTION

▸ Child 12-17 years: 30–60 mg every 6 hours if required for maximum 3 days; maximum 240 mg per day

IMPORTANT SAFETY INFORMATION

MHRA/CHM ADVICE (JULY 2013) CODEINE FOR ANALGESIA: RESTRICTED USE IN CHILDREN DUE TO REPORTS OF MORPHINE TOXICITY

Codeine should only be used to relieve acute moderate pain in children older than 12 years and only if it cannot be relieved by other painkillers such as paracetamol or ibuprofen alone. A significant risk of serious and life-threatening adverse reactions has been identified in children with obstructive sleep apnoea who received codeine after tonsillectomy or adenoidectomy:

- in children aged 12–18 years, the maximum daily dose of codeine should not exceed 240 mg. Doses may be taken up to four times a day at intervals of no less than 6 hours. The lowest effective dose should be used and duration of treatment should be limited to 3 days
- codeine is contra-indicated in all children (under 18 years) who undergo the removal of tonsils or adenoids for the treatment of obstructive sleep apnoea
- codeine is not recommended for use in children whose breathing may be compromised, including those with neuromuscular disorders, severe cardiac or respiratory conditions, respiratory infections, multiple trauma or extensive surgical procedures
- codeine is contra-indicated in patients of any age who are known to be ultra-rapid metabolisers of codeine (CYP2D6 ultra-rapid metabolisers)
- codeine should not be used in breast-feeding mothers because it can pass to the baby through breast milk
- parents and carers should be advised on how to recognise signs and symptoms of morphine toxicity, and to stop treatment and seek medical attention if signs or symptoms of toxicity occur (including reduced consciousness, lack of appetite, somnolence, constipation, respiratory depression, 'pin-point' pupils, nausea, vomiting)

MHRA/CHM ADVICE (APRIL 2015) CODEINE FOR COUGH AND COLD: RESTRICTED USE IN CHILDREN

Do not use codeine in children under 12 years as it is associated with a risk of respiratory side effects. Codeine is not recommended for adolescents (12–18 years) who have problems with breathing. When prescribing or dispensing codeine-containing medicines for cough and cold, consider that codeine is contra-indicated in:

- children younger than 12 years old
- patients of any age known to be CYP2D6 ultra-rapid metabolisers
- breastfeeding mothers

● **CONTRA-INDICATIONS** Acute ulcerative colitis · antibiotic-associated colitis · children under 18 years who undergo the removal of tonsils or adenoids for the treatment of obstructive sleep apnoea · conditions where abdominal distension develops · conditions where inhibition of peristalsis should be avoided · known ultra-rapid codeine metabolisers

- **CAUTIONS** Acute abdomen · cardiac arrhythmias · gallstones · not recommended for adolescents aged 12–18 years with breathing problems

CAUTIONS, FURTHER INFORMATION

- Variation in metabolism The capacity to metabolise codeine to morphine can vary considerably between individuals; there is a marked increase in morphine toxicity in patients who are ultra-rapid codeine metabolisers (CYP2D6 ultra-rapid metabolisers) and a reduced therapeutic effect in poor codeine metabolisers.

- **INTERACTIONS** → Appendix 1: opioids
- **SIDE-EFFECTS**

GENERAL SIDE-EFFECTS

Biliary spasm · hypothermia · mood altered · sexual dysfunction · ureteral spasm

SPECIFIC SIDE-EFFECTS

- With oral use Abdominal cramps · addiction · appetite decreased · depression · drug reaction with eosinophilia and systemic symptoms (DRESS) · dyskinesia · dyspnoea · face oedema · fatigue · fever · hyperglycaemia · hypersensitivity · intracranial pressure increased · lymphadenopathy · malaise · muscle rigidity (with high doses) · nightmare · pancreatitis · restlessness · seizure · splenomegaly · urinary disorders · vision disorders
- With parenteral use Dysuria

- **BREAST FEEDING** Manufacturer advises avoid (recommendation also supported by MHRA and specialist sources). Present in milk and mothers vary considerably in their capacity to metabolise codeine; risk of opioid toxicity in infant.
- **HEPATIC IMPAIRMENT**
  - With oral use Manufacturer advises caution in mild to moderate impairment; avoid in severe impairment.
  - With intravenous use Manufacturer advises avoid.

Dose adjustments ▸ With oral use Manufacturer advises dose reduction in mild to moderate impairment.

- **RENAL IMPAIRMENT** Avoid use or reduce dose; opioid effects increased and prolonged and increased cerebral sensitivity occurs.
- **PRESCRIBING AND DISPENSING INFORMATION** BP directs that when Diabetic Codeine Linctus is prescribed, Codeine Linctus formulated with a vehicle appropriate for administration to diabetics, whether or not labelled 'Diabetic Codeine Linctus', shall be dispensed or supplied.
- **PATIENT AND CARER ADVICE**

Medicines for Children leaflet: Codeine phosphate for pain www.medicinesforchildren.org.uk/codeine-phosphate-pain-0

- **MEDICINAL FORMS** There can be variation in the licensing of different medicines containing the same drug. Forms available from special-order manufacturers include: oral suspension, oral solution, solution for injection

Tablet

CAUTIONARY AND ADVISORY LABELS 2

- Codeine phosphate (Non-proprietary)

Codeine phosphate 15 mg Codeine 15mg tablets | 28 tablet [PoM] £1.50 DT = £1.02 [CD5] | 100 tablet [PoM] £3.64 DT = £3.64 [CD5]

Codeine phosphate 30 mg Codeine 30mg tablets | 28 tablet [PoM] £1.79 DT = £1.25 [CD5] | 100 tablet [PoM] £5.68 DT = £4.46 [CD5] | 500 tablet [PoM] £22.30 [CD5]

Codeine phosphate 60 mg Codeine 60mg tablets | 28 tablet [PoM] £3.39 DT = £2.88 [CD5]

Solution for injection

- Codeine phosphate (Non-proprietary)

Codeine phosphate 60 mg per 1 ml Codeine 60mg/1ml solution for injection ampoules | 10 ampoule [PoM] £25.90 DT = £24.19 [CD2]

Oral solution

CAUTIONARY AND ADVISORY LABELS 2

- Codeine phosphate (Non-proprietary)

Codeine phosphate 3 mg per 1 ml Codeine 15mg/5ml linctus sugar-free | 200 ml [P] £1.90 DT = £1.63 [CD5] sugar-free | 2000 ml [P] £16.30 [CD5]

Codeine 15mg/5ml linctus | 200 ml [P] £1.73–£1.90 DT = £1.90 [CD5]

Codeine phosphate 5 mg per 1 ml Codeine 25mg/5ml oral solution | 500 ml [PoM] £6.64 DT = £6.64 [CD5]

- Galcodine (Thornton & Ross Ltd)

Codeine phosphate 3 mg per 1 ml Galcodine 15mg/5ml linctus sugar-free | 2000 ml [P] £9.90 [CD5]

F 290

Diamorphine hydrochloride

12-Dec-2019

(Heroin hydrochloride)

- **INDICATIONS AND DOSE**

Acute or chronic pain

▶ BY MOUTH

- Child 1 month–11 years: 100–200 micrograms/kg every 4 hours (max. per dose 10 mg), adjusted according to response
- Child 12–17 years: 5–10 mg every 4 hours, adjusted according to response

▶ BY CONTINUOUS INTRAVENOUS INFUSION

- Child 1 month–11 years: 12.5–25 micrograms/kg/hour, adjusted according to response

▶ BY INTRAVENOUS INJECTION

- Child 1–2 months: 20 micrograms/kg every 6 hours, adjusted according to response
- Child 3–5 months: 25–50 micrograms/kg every 6 hours, adjusted according to response
- Child 6–11 months: 75 micrograms/kg every 4 hours, adjusted according to response
- Child 1–11 years: 75–100 micrograms/kg every 4 hours (max. per dose 5 mg), adjusted according to response
- Child 12–17 years: 2.5–5 mg every 4 hours, adjusted according to response

▶ BY INTRAMUSCULAR INJECTION, OR BY SUBCUTANEOUS INJECTION

- Child 12–17 years: 5 mg every 4 hours, adjusted according to response

Acute or chronic pain in ventilated neonates

▶ INITIALLY BY INTRAVENOUS INJECTION

- Neonate: Initially 50 micrograms/kg, dose to be administered over 30 minutes, followed by (by continuous intravenous infusion) 15 micrograms/kg/hour, adjusted according to response.

Acute or chronic pain in non-ventilated neonates

▶ BY CONTINUOUS INTRAVENOUS INFUSION

- Neonate: 2.5–7 micrograms/kg/hour, adjusted according to response.

Acute severe nociceptive pain in an emergency setting (specialist supervision in hospital)

▶ BY INTRANASAL ADMINISTRATION

- Child 2–15 years (body-weight 12–17 kg): 1.44 mg for 1 dose, spray into alternate nostrils
- Child 2–15 years (body-weight 18–23 kg): 2.16 mg for 1 dose, spray into alternate nostrils
- Child 2–15 years (body-weight 24–29 kg): 2.88 mg for 1 dose, spray into alternate nostrils
- Child 2–15 years (body-weight 30–39 kg): 3.2 mg for 1 dose, spray into alternate nostrils
- Child 2–15 years (body-weight 40–50 kg): 4.8 mg for 1 dose, spray into alternate nostrils

- **CONTRA-INDICATIONS** Delayed gastric emptying · phaeochromocytoma

- **CAUTIONS** CNS depression · severe cor pulmonale · severe diarrhoea · toxic psychosis
- **INTERACTIONS** → Appendix 1: opioids
- **SIDE-EFFECTS**
  - **Common or very common**
  - With intranasal use Haemorrhage · laryngitis · nasal complaints · procedural pain · taste altered
  - **Uncommon**
  - With intranasal use Abdominal pain · anxiety · conjunctivitis · drug toxicity · eye pruritus · feeling hot · fever · hiccups · hypoxia · level of consciousness decreased · pallor · paraesthesia
  - **Frequency not known**
  - With parenteral use Biliary spasm · circulatory depression · intracranial pressure increased · mood altered
- **BREAST FEEDING** Therapeutic doses unlikely to affect infant; withdrawal symptoms in infants of dependent mothers; breast-feeding not best method of treating dependence in offspring.
- **HEPATIC IMPAIRMENT** Manufacturer advises caution.
  Dose adjustments Manufacturer advises dose reduction.
- **RENAL IMPAIRMENT** Avoid use or reduce dose; opioid effects increased and prolonged; increased cerebral sensitivity.
- **MONITORING REQUIREMENTS**
  - With intranasal use Manufacturer advises monitor for at least 30 minutes following administration.
- **DIRECTIONS FOR ADMINISTRATION**
  - With intravenous use For *intravenous infusion*, dilute in Glucose 5% or Sodium Chloride 0.9%; Glucose 5% is preferable as an infusion fluid.
  - With intranasal use Manufacturer advises spray should be directed at the nasal side wall whilst the patient is in a semi-recumbent position.
- **PRESCRIBING AND DISPENSING INFORMATION** Intranasal administration of diamorphine hydrochloride injection has been used [unlicensed]—no dose recommendation.
- **NATIONAL FUNDING/ACCESS DECISIONS**
  All Wales Medicines Strategy Group (AWMSG) decisions
  AWMSG No. 2406
  - With intranasal use The *All Wales Medicines Strategy Group* has advised (November 2019) that diamorphine hydrochloride (*Ayendi*®) is recommended as an option for use within NHS Wales for the treatment of acute severe nociceptive pain in patients aged 2 to15 years in a hospital setting. It should be administered in the emergency setting by practitioners experienced in the administration of opioids in children and with the appropriate monitoring.

- **MEDICINAL FORMS** There can be variation in the licensing of different medicines containing the same drug. Forms available from special-order manufacturers include: capsule, oral solution, solution for injection, powder for solution for injection

Tablet

CAUTIONARY AND ADVISORY LABELS 2

- Diamorphine hydrochloride (Non-proprietary)
  Diamorphine hydrochloride 10 mg Diamorphine 10mg tablets | 100 tablet PoM £37.13 DT = £37.13 CD2

Powder for solution for injection

- Diamorphine hydrochloride (Non-proprietary)
  Diamorphine hydrochloride 5 mg Diamorphine 5mg powder for solution for injection ampoules | 5 ampoule PoM £12.81 DT = £12.81 CD2
  Diamorphine hydrochloride 10 mg Diamorphine 10mg powder for solution for injection ampoules | 5 ampoule PoM £16.56 DT = £15.02 CD2
  Diamorphine hydrochloride 30 mg Diamorphine 30mg powder for solution for injection ampoules | 5 ampoule PoM £16.91 DT = £15.66 CD2
  Diamorphine hydrochloride 100 mg Diamorphine 100mg powder for solution for injection ampoules | 5 ampoule PoM £43.50 DT = £43.10 CD2
  Diamorphine hydrochloride 500 mg Diamorphine 500mg powder for solution for injection ampoules | 5 ampoule PoM £189.72 DT = £188.99 CD2

Spray

EXCIPIENTS: May contain Benzalkonium chloride, disodium edetate

- Ayendi (Wockhardt UK Ltd)
  Diamorphine (as Diamorphine hydrochloride) 720 microgram per 1 dose Ayendi 720micrograms/actuation nasal spray | 68 dose PoM £107.90 (Hospital only) CD2 | 160 dose PoM £112.50 (Hospital only) CD2
  Diamorphine (as Diamorphine hydrochloride) 1.6 mg per 1 dose Ayendi 1600micrograms/actuation nasal spray | 68 dose PoM £113.52 (Hospital only) CD2 | 160 dose PoM £123.75 (Hospital only) CD2

F 290

Dihydrocodeine tartrate

- **INDICATIONS AND DOSE**

Moderate to severe pain

- BY MOUTH USING IMMEDIATE-RELEASE MEDICINES
  - Child 1–3 years: 500 micrograms/kg every 4–6 hours
  - Child 4–11 years: 0.5–1 mg/kg every 4–6 hours (max. per dose 30 mg)
  - Child 12–17 years: 30 mg every 4–6 hours
- BY INTRAMUSCULAR INJECTION, OR BY SUBCUTANEOUS INJECTION
  - Child 1–3 years: 500 micrograms/kg every 4–6 hours
  - Child 4–11 years: 0.5–1 mg/kg every 4–6 hours (max. per dose 30 mg)
  - Child 12–17 years: 30 mg every 4–6 hours (max. per dose 50 mg)

Chronic severe pain

- BY MOUTH USING MODIFIED-RELEASE MEDICINES
  - Child 12–17 years: 60–120 mg every 12 hours

DF118 FORTE®

Severe pain

- BY MOUTH
  - Child 12–17 years: 40–80 mg 3 times a day; maximum 240 mg per day

- **UNLICENSED USE** Most preparations not licensed for use in children under 4 years.
- **CAUTIONS** Pancreatitis · severe cor pulmonale
- **INTERACTIONS** → Appendix 1: opioids
- **SIDE-EFFECTS**
  GENERAL SIDE-EFFECTS
  Dysuria · mood altered
  SPECIFIC SIDE-EFFECTS
  - With oral use Biliary spasm · bronchospasm · hypothermia · sexual dysfunction · ureteral spasm
- **BREAST FEEDING** Use only if potential benefit outweighs risk.
- **HEPATIC IMPAIRMENT** Manufacturer advises caution; consider avoiding.
  Dose adjustments Manufacturer advises dose reduction, if used.
- **RENAL IMPAIRMENT** Avoid use or reduce dose; opioid effects increased and prolonged and increased cerebral sensitivity occurs.
- **PROFESSION SPECIFIC INFORMATION**
  Dental practitioners' formulary
  Dihydrocodeine tablets 30 mg may be prescribed.

- **MEDICINAL FORMS** There can be variation in the licensing of different medicines containing the same drug. Forms available from special-order manufacturers include: oral suspension, oral solution

Modified-release tablet

CAUTIONARY AND ADVISORY LABELS 2, 25

- DHC Continus (Napp Pharmaceuticals Ltd)
  Dihydrocodeine tartrate 60 mg DHC Continus 60mg tablets | 56 tablet PoM £5.20 DT = £5.20 CD5
  Dihydrocodeine tartrate 90 mg DHC Continus 90mg tablets | 56 tablet PoM £8.66 DT = £8.66 CD5
  Dihydrocodeine tartrate 120 mg DHC Continus 120mg tablets | 56 tablet PoM £10.95 DT = £10.95 CD5

Tablet

CAUTIONARY AND ADVISORY LABELS 2

- Dihydrocodeine tartrate (Non-proprietary)
  Dihydrocodeine tartrate 30 mg Dihydrocodeine 30mg tablets | 28 tablet PoM £1.21 DT = £1.21 CD5 | 30 tablet PoM £1.17–£1.56 CD5 | 100 tablet PoM £4.32 DT = £4.32 CD5
- DF 118 (Martindale Pharmaceuticals Ltd)
  Dihydrocodeine tartrate 40 mg DF 118 Forte 40mg tablets | 100 tablet PoM £11.51 DT = £11.51 CD5

Solution for injection

- Dihydrocodeine tartrate (Non-proprietary)
  Dihydrocodeine tartrate 50 mg per 1 ml Dihydrocodeine 50mg/1ml solution for injection ampoules | 10 ampoule PoM £133.75 DT = £133.75 CD2

Oral solution

CAUTIONARY AND ADVISORY LABELS 2

- Dihydrocodeine tartrate (Non-proprietary)
  Dihydrocodeine tartrate 2 mg per 1 ml Dihydrocodeine 10mg/5ml oral solution | 150 ml PoM £9.83 DT = £9.83 CD5

F 290

Dihydrocodeine with paracetamol

18-Jan-2018

The properties listed below are those particular to the combination only. For the properties of the components please consider, paracetamol p. 288.

- **INDICATIONS AND DOSE**

Mild to moderate pain (using 10/500 preparations only)

- BY MOUTH
- Child 12–17 years: 10/500–20/1000 mg every 4–6 hours as required; maximum 80/4000 mg per day

Severe pain (using 20/500 preparations only)

- BY MOUTH
- Child 12–17 years: 20/500–40/1000 mg every 4–6 hours as required; maximum 160/4000 mg per day

Severe pain (using 30/500 preparations only)

- BY MOUTH
- Child 12–17 years: 30/500–60/1000 mg every 4–6 hours as required; maximum 240/4000 mg per day

DOSE EQUIVALENCE AND CONVERSION

- A mixture of dihydrocodeine tartrate and paracetamol; the proportions are expressed in the form x/y, where x and y are the strengths in milligrams of dihydrocodeine and paracetamol respectively.

IMPORTANT SAFETY INFORMATION

MHRA/CHM ADVICE: DIHYDROCODEINE WITH PARACETAMOL (CO-DYDRAMOL): PRESCRIBE AND DISPENSE BY STRENGTH TO MINIMISE RISK OF MEDICATION ERROR (JANUARY 2018)

The MHRA has advised that dihydrocodeine with paracetamol preparations are prescribed and dispensed by strength to minimise dispensing errors and the risk of accidental opioid overdose—see Prescribing and dispensing information.

- **CAUTIONS** Alcohol dependence · before administering, check when paracetamol last administered and cumulative paracetamol dose over previous 24 hours · chronic alcoholism · chronic dehydration · chronic malnutrition · hepatocellular insufficiency · pancreatitis · severe cor pulmonale
- **INTERACTIONS** → Appendix 1: opioids · paracetamol
- **SIDE-EFFECTS** Abdominal pain · blood disorder · leucopenia · malaise · neutropenia · pancreatitis · paraesthesia · paralytic ileus · severe cutaneous adverse reactions (SCARs) · thrombocytopenia

  Overdose Liver damage (and less frequently renal damage) following overdosage with paracetamol.
- **BREAST FEEDING** Amount of dihydrocodeine too small to be harmful but use only if potential benefit outweighs risk.
- **HEPATIC IMPAIRMENT** Manufacturer advises consider avoiding in mild to moderate impairment; avoid in severe impairment.

  Dose adjustments Manufacturer advises dose reduction in mild to moderate impairment, if used.
- **RENAL IMPAIRMENT** Reduce dose or avoid dihydrocodeine; increased and prolonged effect; increased cerebral sensitivity.
- **PRESCRIBING AND DISPENSING INFORMATION** The MHRA advises when prescribing dihydrocodeine with paracetamol, the tablet strength and dose must be clearly indicated; when dispensing dihydrocodeine with paracetamol, ensure the prescribed strength is supplied—contact the prescriber if in doubt.

  The BP defines *Co-dydramol* Tablets as containing dihydrocodeine tartrate 10 mg and paracetamol 500 mg.
- **LESS SUITABLE FOR PRESCRIBING** Dihydrocodeine with paracetamol is less suitable for prescribing.
- **MEDICINAL FORMS** There can be variation in the licensing of different medicines containing the same drug. Forms available from special-order manufacturers include: oral suspension, oral solution

Tablet

CAUTIONARY AND ADVISORY LABELS 2, 29, 30

- Dihydrocodeine with paracetamol (Non-proprietary)
  Dihydrocodeine tartrate 10 mg, Paracetamol 500 mg Co-dydramol 10mg/500mg tablets | 30 tablet PoM £2.40 DT = £1.21 CD5 | 100 tablet PoM £8.00 DT = £4.03 CD5 | 500 tablet PoM £20.15 CD5
  Dihydrocodeine tartrate 20 mg, Paracetamol 500 mg Co-dydramol 20mg/500mg tablets | 56 tablet PoM £5.87–£6.55 CD5 | 112 tablet PoM £13.10 DT = £13.10 CD5
  Dihydrocodeine tartrate 30 mg, Paracetamol 500 mg Co-dydramol 30mg/500mg tablets | 56 tablet PoM £12.46 DT = £12.46 CD5
- Eroset (M & A Pharmachem Ltd)
  Dihydrocodeine tartrate 10 mg, Paracetamol 500 mg Eroset 500mg/10mg tablets | 30 tablet PoM £0.68 DT = £1.21 CD5 | 100 tablet PoM £1.91 DT = £4.03 CD5
- Paramol (SSL International Plc)
  Dihydrocodeine tartrate 7.46 mg, Paracetamol 500 mg Paramol tablets | 12 tablet P £2.45 CD5 | 24 tablet P £4.20 CD5 | 32 tablet P £4.85 CD5
- Remedeine (Crescent Pharma Ltd)
  Dihydrocodeine tartrate 20 mg, Paracetamol 500 mg Remedeine tablets | 56 tablet PoM £5.87 CD5 | 112 tablet PoM £11.13 DT = £13.10 CD5
  Dihydrocodeine tartrate 30 mg, Paracetamol 500 mg Remedeine Forte tablets | 56 tablet PoM £6.82 DT = £12.46 CD5

F 290

Fentanyl

25-Oct-2018

- **INDICATIONS AND DOSE**

Chronic intractable pain not currently treated with a strong opioid analgesic

- BY TRANSDERMAL APPLICATION
- Child 16–17 years: Initially 12 micrograms/hour every 72 hours, alternatively initially 25 micrograms/hour every 72 hours, when starting, evaluation of the analgesic effect should not be made before the system

has been worn for 24 hours (to allow for the gradual increase in plasma-fentanyl concentration)—previous analgesic therapy should be phased out gradually from time of first patch application, dose should be adjusted at 48–72 hour intervals in steps of 12–25 micrograms/hour if necessary, more than one patch may be used at a time (but applied at the same time to avoid confusion)—consider additional or alternative analgesic therapy if dose required exceeds 300 micrograms/hour (important: it takes 17 hours or more for the plasma-fentanyl concentration to decrease by 50%— replacement opioid therapy should be initiated at a low dose and increased gradually)

Chronic intractable pain currently treated with a strong opioid analgesic

▶ BY TRANSDERMAL APPLICATION

▸ Child 2-17 years: Initial dose based on previous 24-hour opioid requirement (consult product literature), for evaluating analgesic efficacy and dose increments, see under *Chronic intractable pain not currently treated with a strong opioid analgesic*, for conversion from long term oral morphine to transdermal fentanyl, see *Pain management with opioids* under Prescribing in palliative care p. 21.

Spontaneous respiration: analgesia and enhancement of anaesthesia, during operation

▶ BY INTRAVENOUS INJECTION

▸ Child 1 month–11 years: Initially 1–3 micrograms/kg, then 1 microgram/kg as required, dose to be administered over at least 30 seconds
▸ Child 12–17 years: Initially 50–100 micrograms (max. per dose 200 micrograms), dose maximum on specialist advice, then 25–50 micrograms as required, dose to be administered over at least 30 seconds

Assisted ventilation: analgesia and enhancement of anaesthesia during operation

▶ BY INTRAVENOUS INJECTION

▸ Neonate: Initially 1–5 micrograms/kg, then 1–3 micrograms/kg as required, dose to be administered over at least 30 seconds.

▸ Child 1 month–11 years: Initially 1–5 micrograms/kg, then 1–3 micrograms/kg as required, dose to be administered over at least 30 seconds
▸ Child 12–17 years: Initially 1–5 micrograms/kg, then 50–200 micrograms as required, dose to be administered over at least 30 seconds

Assisted ventilation: analgesia and respiratory depression in intensive care

▶ INITIALLY BY INTRAVENOUS INJECTION

▸ Neonate: Initially 1–5 micrograms/kg, then (by intravenous infusion) 1.5 micrograms/kg/hour, adjusted according to response.

▸ Child: Initially 1–5 micrograms/kg, then (by intravenous infusion) 1–6 micrograms/kg/hour, adjusted according to response

Breakthrough pain in patients receiving opioid therapy for chronic cancer pain

▶ BY BUCCAL ADMINISTRATION USING LOZENGES

▸ Child 16–17 years: Initially 200 micrograms, dose to be given over 15 minutes, then 200 micrograms after 15 minutes if required, no more than 2 dose units for each pain episode; if adequate pain relief not achieved with 1 dose unit for consecutive breakthrough pain episodes, increase the strength of the dose unit until adequate pain relief achieved with 4 lozenges or less daily, if more than 4 episodes of breakthrough pain each day, adjust background analgesia

DOSE EQUIVALENCE AND CONVERSION

▸ Fentanyl films are **not bioequivalent** to other fentanyl preparations.
▸ Fentanyl preparations for the treatment of breakthrough pain are not interchangeable; if patients are switched from another fentanyl-containing preparation, a new dose titration is required.

DOSES AT EXTREMES OF BODY-WEIGHT

▸ To avoid excessive dosage in obese patients, weight-based doses may need to be calculated on the basis of ideal bodyweight.

● **UNLICENSED USE**

▸ With intravenous use Not licensed for use in children under 2 years; infusion not licensed for use in children under 12 years.

IMPORTANT SAFETY INFORMATION

MHRA/CHM ADVICE: TRANSDERMAL FENTANYL PATCHES: LIFE-THREATENING AND FATAL OPIOID TOXICITY FROM ACCIDENTAL EXPOSURE, PARTICULARLY IN CHILDREN (OCTOBER 2018)

Accidental exposure to transdermal fentanyl can occur if a patch is swallowed or transferred to another individual. Always fully inform patients and their carers about directions for safe use of fentanyl patches, including the importance of:

- not exceeding the prescribed dose;
- following the correct frequency of patch application, avoiding touching the adhesive side of patches, and washing hands after application;
- not cutting patches and avoiding exposure of patches to heat including via hot water;
- ensuring that old patches are removed before applying a new one;
- following instructions for safe storage and properly disposing of used patches or those which are not needed.

Patients and carers should be advised to seek immediate medical attention if overdose is suspected—see *Side-effects* and *Patient and carer advice* for further information.

● **CAUTIONS** Cerebral tumour · diabetes mellitus (with *Actiq*® and *Cynril*® lozenges) · impaired consciousness

CAUTIONS, FURTHER INFORMATION

▸ With transdermal use Transdermal fentanyl patches are not suitable for acute pain or in those patients whose analgesic requirements are changing rapidly because the long time to steady state prevents rapid titration of the dose. Risk of fatal respiratory depression, particularly in patients not previously treated with a strong opioid analgesic; manufacturer recommends use only in opioid tolerant patients.
▸ With intravenous use Repeated intra-operative doses should be given with care since the resulting respiratory depression can persist postoperatively and occasionally it may become apparent for the first time postoperatively when monitoring of the patient might be less intensive.

● **INTERACTIONS** → Appendix 1: opioids

● **SIDE-EFFECTS**

▶ **Common or very common**

▸ With parenteral use Apnoea · hypertension · movement disorders · muscle rigidity · post procedural complications · respiratory disorders · vascular pain
▸ With transdermal use Anxiety · appetite decreased · asthenia · depression · diarrhoea · dyspnoea · gastrointestinal discomfort · hypertension · insomnia · malaise · muscle complaints · peripheral oedema · sensation abnormal · temperature sensation altered · tremor

▶ **Uncommon**

▸ With parenteral use Airway complication of anaesthesia · chills · hiccups · hypothermia

4 Nervous system

- ▸ With transdermal use Consciousness impaired · cyanosis · fever · gastrointestinal disorders · influenza like illness · memory loss · respiratory disorders · seizures · sexual dysfunction · vision blurred
- ▸ **Rare or very rare**
- ▸ With transdermal use Apnoea
- ▸ **Frequency not known**
- ▸ With buccal use Adrenal insufficiency · androgen deficiency · anxiety · appetite decreased · asthenia · coma · depersonalisation · depression · diarrhoea · dyspnoea · emotional lability · fever · gait abnormal · gastrointestinal discomfort · gastrointestinal disorders · gingival haemorrhage · gingivitis · injury · loss of consciousness · malaise · myoclonus · oral disorders · peripheral oedema · seizure · sensation abnormal · sleep disorders · speech slurred · taste altered · thinking abnormal · throat oedema · vasodilation · vision disorders · weight decreased · withdrawal syndrome neonatal
- ▸ With parenteral use Biliary spasm · cardiac arrest · cough · hyperalgesia · loss of consciousness · seizure
- ▸ With transdermal use Myoclonus · withdrawal syndrome neonatal

SIDE-EFFECTS, FURTHER INFORMATION **Muscle rigidity** Intravenous administration of fentanyl can cause muscle rigidity, which may involve the thoracic muscles. Manufacturer advises administration by slow intravenous injection to avoid; higher doses may require premedication with benzodiazepines and muscle relaxants.

Transdermal use Monitor patients using patches for increased side-effects if fever is present (increased absorption possible); avoid exposing application site to external heat, for example a hot bath or sauna (may also increase absorption).

● **BREAST FEEDING**
- ▸ With buccal use Manufacturer advises avoid during treatment and for 5 days after last administration—present in milk.
- ▸ With intravenous use Manufacturer advises avoid during treatment and for 24 hours after last administration—present in milk.
- ▸ With transdermal use Manufacturer advises avoid during treatment and for 72 hours after removal of patch—present in milk.

● **HEPATIC IMPAIRMENT** Manufacturer advises caution (risk of accumulation).

Dose adjustments Manufacturer advises cautious dose titration.

● **RENAL IMPAIRMENT** Avoid use or reduce dose; opioid effects increased and prolonged and increased cerebral sensitivity occurs.

● **DIRECTIONS FOR ADMINISTRATION**
- ▸ With transdermal use For *patches*, apply to dry, non-irritated, non-irradiated, non-hairy skin on torso or upper arm, removing after 72 hours and siting replacement patch on a different area (avoid using the same area for several days).
- ▸ With intravenous use For *intravenous infusion*, injection solution may be diluted in Glucose 5% or Sodium Chloride 0.9%.
- ▸ With buccal use Patients should be advised to place the lozenge in the mouth against the cheek and move it around the mouth using the applicator; each lozenge should be sucked over a 15 minute period. In patients with a dry mouth, water may be used to moisten the buccal mucosa. Patients with diabetes should be advised each lozenge contains approximately 2 g glucose.

● **PRESCRIBING AND DISPENSING INFORMATION**
- ▸ With transdermal use Prescriptions for fentanyl patches can be written to show the strength in terms of the release rate and it is acceptable to write *'Fentanyl 25 patches'* to prescribe patches that release fentanyl 25 micrograms per hour. The dosage should be expressed in terms of the interval between applying a patch and replacing it with a new one, e.g. *'one patch to be applied every 72 hours'*. The total quantity of patches to be supplied should be written in words and figures.

● **PATIENT AND CARER ADVICE**
- ▸ With transdermal use Patients and carers should be informed about safe use, including correct administration and disposal, strict adherence to dosage instructions, and the symptoms and signs of opioid overdosage. Patches should be removed immediately in case of breathing difficulties, marked drowsiness, confusion, dizziness, or impaired speech, and patients and carers should seek prompt medical attention.

Medicines for Children leaflet: Fentanyl lozenges for pain www.medicinesforchildren.org.uk/fentanyl-lozenges-pain
Medicines for Children leaflet: Fentanyl patches for pain www.medicinesforchildren.org.uk/fentanyl-patches-pain

---

● **MEDICINAL FORMS** There can be variation in the licensing of different medicines containing the same drug. Forms available from special-order manufacturers include: solution for injection, infusion, solution for infusion

Solution for injection

▸ **Fentanyl (Non-proprietary)**

Fentanyl (as Fentanyl citrate) 50 microgram per 1 ml Fentanyl 100micrograms/2ml solution for injection ampoules | 10 ampoule PoM £11.50–£14.33 DT = £14.33 CD2
Fentanyl 500micrograms/10ml solution for injection ampoules | 10 ampoule PoM £14.50–£16.15 CD2

▸ **Sublimaze** (Piramal Critical Care Ltd)

Fentanyl (as Fentanyl citrate) 50 microgram per 1 ml Sublimaze 500micrograms/10ml solution for injection ampoules | 5 ampoule PoM £15.00 CD2

Solution for infusion

▸ **Fentanyl (Non-proprietary)**

Fentanyl (as Fentanyl citrate) 50 microgram per 1 ml Fentanyl 2.5mg/50ml solution for infusion vials | 1 vial PoM £5.50 CD2

Transdermal patch

CAUTIONARY AND ADVISORY LABELS 2

▸ **Durogesic DTrans** (Janssen-Cilag Ltd)

Fentanyl 12 microgram per 1 hour Durogesic DTrans 12micrograms/hour transdermal patches | 5 patch PoM £12.59 DT = £12.59 CD2
Fentanyl 25 microgram per 1 hour Durogesic DTrans 25micrograms/hour transdermal patches | 5 patch PoM £17.99 DT = £17.99 CD2
Fentanyl 50 microgram per 1 hour Durogesic DTrans 50micrograms/hour transdermal patches | 5 patch PoM £33.66 DT = £33.66 CD2
Fentanyl 75 microgram per 1 hour Durogesic DTrans 75micrograms/hour transdermal patches | 5 patch PoM £46.99 DT = £46.99 CD2
Fentanyl 100 microgram per 1 hour Durogesic DTrans 100micrograms/hour transdermal patches | 5 patch PoM £57.86 DT = £57.86 CD2

▸ **Fencino** (Ethypharm UK Ltd)

Fentanyl 12 microgram per 1 hour Fencino 12micrograms/hour transdermal patches | 5 patch PoM £8.46 DT = £12.59 CD2
Fentanyl 25 microgram per 1 hour Fencino 25micrograms/hour transdermal patches | 5 patch PoM £12.10 DT = £17.99 CD2
Fentanyl 50 microgram per 1 hour Fencino 50micrograms/hour transdermal patches | 5 patch PoM £22.62 DT = £33.66 CD2
Fentanyl 75 microgram per 1 hour Fencino 75micrograms/hour transdermal patches | 5 patch PoM £31.54 DT = £46.99 CD2
Fentanyl 100 microgram per 1 hour Fencino 100micrograms/hour transdermal patches | 5 patch PoM £38.88 DT = £57.86 CD2

▸ **Fentalis** (Sandoz Ltd)

Fentanyl 25 microgram per 1 hour Fentalis Reservoir 25micrograms/hour transdermal patches | 5 patch PoM £22.89 DT = £17.99 CD2
Fentanyl 50 microgram per 1 hour Fentalis Reservoir 50micrograms/hour transdermal patches | 5 patch PoM £42.77 DT = £33.66 CD2
Fentanyl 75 microgram per 1 hour Fentalis Reservoir 75micrograms/hour transdermal patches | 5 patch PoM £59.62 DT = £46.99 CD2

Fentanyl 100 microgram per 1 hour Fentalis Reservoir 100micrograms/hour transdermal patches | 5 patch PoM £73.49 DT = £57.86 CD2

▸ **Matrifen** (Teva UK Ltd)

Fentanyl 12 microgram per 1 hour Matrifen 12micrograms/hour transdermal patches | 5 patch PoM £7.52 DT = £12.59 CD2

Fentanyl 25 microgram per 1 hour Matrifen 25micrograms/hour transdermal patches | 5 patch PoM £10.76 DT = £17.99 CD2

Fentanyl 50 microgram per 1 hour Matrifen 50micrograms/hour transdermal patches | 5 patch PoM £20.12 DT = £33.66 CD2

Fentanyl 75 microgram per 1 hour Matrifen 75micrograms/hour transdermal patches | 5 patch PoM £28.06 DT = £46.99 CD2

Fentanyl 100 microgram per 1 hour Matrifen 100micrograms/hour transdermal patches | 5 patch PoM £34.59 DT = £57.86 CD2

▸ **Mezolar Matrix** (Sandoz Ltd)

Fentanyl 12 microgram per 1 hour Mezolar Matrix 12micrograms/hour transdermal patches | 5 patch PoM £7.53 DT = £12.59 CD2

Fentanyl 25 microgram per 1 hour Mezolar Matrix 25micrograms/hour transdermal patches | 5 patch PoM £10.77 DT = £17.99 CD2

Fentanyl 37.5 microgram per 1 hour Mezolar Matrix 37.5microgram/hour transdermal patches | 5 patch PoM £15.46 DT = £15.46 CD2

Fentanyl 50 microgram per 1 hour Mezolar Matrix 50micrograms/hour transdermal patches | 5 patch PoM £20.13 DT = £33.66 CD2

Fentanyl 75 microgram per 1 hour Mezolar Matrix 75micrograms/hour transdermal patches | 5 patch PoM £28.07 DT = £46.99 CD2

Fentanyl 100 microgram per 1 hour Mezolar Matrix 100micrograms/hour transdermal patches | 5 patch PoM £34.60 DT = £57.86 CD2

▸ **Victanyl** (Accord Healthcare Ltd)

Fentanyl 12 microgram per 1 hour Victanyl 12micrograms/hour transdermal patches | 5 patch PoM £12.58 DT = £12.59 CD2

Fentanyl 25 microgram per 1 hour Victanyl 25micrograms/hour transdermal patches | 5 patch PoM £25.89 DT = £17.99 CD2

Fentanyl 50 microgram per 1 hour Victanyl 50micrograms/hour transdermal patches | 5 patch PoM £48.36 DT = £33.66 CD2

Fentanyl 75 microgram per 1 hour Victanyl 75micrograms/hour transdermal patches | 5 patch PoM £67.41 DT = £46.99 CD2

Fentanyl 100 microgram per 1 hour Victanyl 100micrograms/hour transdermal patches | 5 patch PoM £83.09 DT = £57.86 CD2

▸ **Yemex** (Sandoz Ltd)

Fentanyl 12 microgram per 1 hour Yemex 12micrograms/hour transdermal patches | 5 patch PoM £12.59 DT = £12.59 CD2

Fentanyl 25 microgram per 1 hour Yemex 25micrograms/hour transdermal patches | 5 patch PoM £17.99 DT = £17.99 CD2

Fentanyl 50 microgram per 1 hour Yemex 50micrograms/hour transdermal patches | 5 patch PoM £33.66 DT = £33.66 CD2

Fentanyl 75 microgram per 1 hour Yemex 75micrograms/hour transdermal patches | 5 patch PoM £46.99 DT = £46.99 CD2

Fentanyl 100 microgram per 1 hour Yemex 100micrograms/hour transdermal patches | 5 patch PoM £57.86 DT = £57.86 CD2

Lozenge

CAUTIONARY AND ADVISORY LABELS 2

EXCIPIENTS: May contain Propylene glycol

▸ **Actiq** (Teva UK Ltd)

Fentanyl (as Fentanyl citrate) 200 microgram Actiq 200microgram lozenges with integral oromucosal applicator | 3 lozenge PoM £21.05 DT = £21.05 CD2 | 30 lozenge PoM £210.41 DT = £210.41 CD2

Fentanyl (as Fentanyl citrate) 400 microgram Actiq 400microgram lozenges with integral oromucosal applicator | 3 lozenge PoM £21.05 DT = £21.05 CD2 | 30 lozenge PoM £210.41 DT = £210.41 CD2

Fentanyl (as Fentanyl citrate) 600 microgram Actiq 600microgram lozenges with integral oromucosal applicator | 3 lozenge PoM £21.05 DT = £21.05 CD2 | 30 lozenge PoM £210.41 DT = £210.41 CD2

Fentanyl (as Fentanyl citrate) 800 microgram Actiq 800microgram lozenges with integral oromucosal applicator | 3 lozenge PoM £21.05 DT = £21.05 CD2 | 30 lozenge PoM £210.41 DT = £210.41 CD2

Fentanyl (as Fentanyl citrate) 1.2 mg Actiq 1.2mg lozenges with integral oromucosal applicator | 3 lozenge PoM £21.05 DT = £21.05 CD2 | 30 lozenge PoM £210.41 DT = £210.41 CD2

Fentanyl (as Fentanyl citrate) 1.6 mg Actiq 1.6mg lozenges with integral oromucosal applicator | 3 lozenge PoM £21.05 DT = £21.05 CD2 | 30 lozenge PoM £210.41 DT = £210.41 CD2

⚑ 290

Hydromorphone hydrochloride

● **INDICATIONS AND DOSE**

Severe pain in cancer

▸ BY MOUTH USING IMMEDIATE-RELEASE MEDICINES

▸ Child 12–17 years: 1.3 mg every 4 hours, dose to be increased if necessary according to severity of pain

▸ BY MOUTH USING MODIFIED-RELEASE MEDICINES

▸ Child 12–17 years: 4 mg every 12 hours, dose to be increased if necessary according to severity of pain

● **CONTRA-INDICATIONS** Acute abdomen

● **CAUTIONS** Pancreatitis · toxic psychosis

● **INTERACTIONS** → Appendix 1: opioids

● **SIDE-EFFECTS**

▸ **Common or very common** Abdominal pain · anxiety · appetite decreased · asthenia · sleep disorders

▸ **Uncommon** Depression · diarrhoea · dyspnoea · erectile dysfunction · malaise · movement disorders · paraesthesia · peripheral oedema · taste altered · tremor

▸ **Frequency not known** Hyperalgesia · paralytic ileus · seizure · withdrawal syndrome neonatal

● **BREAST FEEDING** Avoid—no information available.

● **HEPATIC IMPAIRMENT** Manufacturer advises avoid.

● **RENAL IMPAIRMENT** Avoid use or reduce dose; opioid effects increased and prolonged and increased cerebral sensitivity occurs.

● **DIRECTIONS FOR ADMINISTRATION** For *immediate-release* capsules, swallow whole capsule or sprinkle contents on soft food. For *modified-release* capsules, swallow whole or open capsule and sprinkle contents on soft cold food (swallow the pellets within the capsule whole; do not crush or chew).

● **PATIENT AND CARER ADVICE** Patients or carers should be given advice on how to administer hydromorphone hydrochloride capsules and modified-release capsules.

● **MEDICINAL FORMS** There can be variation in the licensing of different medicines containing the same drug. Forms available from special-order manufacturers include: oral solution

Modified-release capsule

CAUTIONARY AND ADVISORY LABELS 2

▸ **Palladone SR** (Napp Pharmaceuticals Ltd)

Hydromorphone hydrochloride 2 mg Palladone SR 2mg capsules | 56 capsule PoM £20.98 DT = £20.98 CD2

Hydromorphone hydrochloride 4 mg Palladone SR 4mg capsules | 56 capsule PoM £28.75 DT = £28.75 CD2

Hydromorphone hydrochloride 8 mg Palladone SR 8mg capsules | 56 capsule PoM £56.08 DT = £56.08 CD2

Hydromorphone hydrochloride 16 mg Palladone SR 16mg capsules | 56 capsule PoM £106.53 DT = £106.53 CD2

Hydromorphone hydrochloride 24 mg Palladone SR 24mg capsules | 56 capsule PoM £159.82 DT = £159.82 CD2

Capsule

CAUTIONARY AND ADVISORY LABELS 2

▸ **Palladone** (Napp Pharmaceuticals Ltd)

Hydromorphone hydrochloride 1.3 mg Palladone 1.3mg capsules | 56 capsule PoM £8.82 DT = £8.82 CD2

Hydromorphone hydrochloride 2.6 mg Palladone 2.6mg capsules | 56 capsule PoM £17.64 DT = £17.64 CD2

⚑ 290

Morphine

02-Dec-2019

● **INDICATIONS AND DOSE**

Pain

▸ BY SUBCUTANEOUS INJECTION

▸ Neonate: Initially 100 micrograms/kg every 6 hours, adjusted according to response.

continued →

- Child 1–5 months: Initially 100–200 micrograms/kg every 6 hours, adjusted according to response
- Child 6 months–1 year: Initially 100–200 micrograms/kg every 4 hours, adjusted according to response
- Child 2–11 years: Initially 200 micrograms/kg every 4 hours, adjusted according to response
- Child 12–17 years: Initially 2.5–10 mg every 4 hours, adjusted according to response

▶ INITIALLY BY INTRAVENOUS INJECTION

- Neonate: 50 micrograms/kg every 6 hours, adjusted according to response, dose to be administered over at least 5 minutes, alternatively (by intravenous injection) initially 50 micrograms/kg, dose to be administered over at least 5 minutes, followed by (by continuous intravenous infusion) 5–20 micrograms/kg/hour, adjusted according to response.
- Child 1–5 months: 100 micrograms/kg every 6 hours, adjusted according to response, dose to be administered over at least 5 minutes, alternatively (by intravenous injection) initially 100 micrograms/kg, dose to be administered over at least 5 minutes, followed by (by continuous intravenous infusion) 10–30 micrograms/kg/hour, adjusted according to response
- Child 6 months–11 years: 100 micrograms/kg every 4 hours, adjusted according to response, dose to be administered over at least 5 minutes, alternatively (by intravenous injection) initially 100 micrograms/kg, dose to be administered over at least 5 minutes, followed by (by continuous intravenous infusion) 20–30 micrograms/kg/hour, adjusted according to response
- Child 12–17 years: 5 mg every 4 hours, adjusted according to response, dose to be administered over at least 5 minutes, alternatively (by intravenous injection) initially 5 mg, dose to be administered over at least 5 minutes, followed by (by continuous intravenous infusion) 20–30 micrograms/kg/hour, adjusted according to response

▶ BY MOUTH, OR BY RECTUM

- Child 1–2 months: Initially 50–100 micrograms/kg every 4 hours, adjusted according to response
- Child 3–5 months: 100–150 micrograms/kg every 4 hours, adjusted according to response
- Child 6–11 months: 200 micrograms/kg every 4 hours, adjusted according to response
- Child 1 year: Initially 200–300 micrograms/kg every 4 hours, adjusted according to response
- Child 2–11 years: Initially 200–300 micrograms/kg every 4 hours (max. per dose 10 mg), adjusted according to response
- Child 12–17 years: Initially 5–10 mg every 4 hours, adjusted according to response

▶ BY CONTINUOUS SUBCUTANEOUS INFUSION

- Child 1–2 months: 10 micrograms/kg/hour, adjusted according to response
- Child 3 months–17 years: 20 micrograms/kg/hour, adjusted according to response

Pain (with modified-release 12-hourly preparations)

▶ BY MOUTH USING MODIFIED-RELEASE MEDICINES

- Child: Every 12 hours, dose adjusted according to daily morphine requirements, dosage requirements should be reviewed if the brand is altered

Pain (with modified-release 24-hourly preparations)

▶ BY MOUTH USING MODIFIED-RELEASE MEDICINES

- Child: Every 24 hours, dose adjusted according to daily morphine requirements, dosage requirements should be reviewed if the brand is altered

Neonatal opioid withdrawal (under expert supervision)

▶ BY MOUTH

- Neonate: Initially 40 micrograms/kg every 4 hours until symptoms controlled, dose to be increased if necessary; reduce frequency gradually over 6–10 days, stop when 40 micrograms/kg once daily achieved, dose may vary—consult local guidelines.

Persistent cyanosis in congenital heart disease when blood glucose less than 3 mmol/litre (following glucose)

▶ BY INTRAVENOUS INJECTION, OR BY INTRAMUSCULAR INJECTION

- Child: 100 micrograms/kg

DOSE EQUIVALENCE AND CONVERSION

- The doses stated refer equally to morphine hydrochloride and sulfate.

● **UNLICENSED USE**

- With oral use *Oramorph®* solution and *MXL®* capsules not licensed for use in children under 1 year. *Sevredol®* tablets not licensed for use in children under 3 years. *Oramorph®* unit dose vials and *Filnarine®* SR tablets not licensed for use in children under 6 years. *MST Continus®* preparations licensed to treat children with cancer pain (age-range not specified by manufacturer).
- With rectal use Suppositories are not licensed for use in children.

> IMPORTANT SAFETY INFORMATION
> Do not confuse modified-release 12-hourly preparations with 24-hourly preparations, see *Prescribing and dispensing information*.

● **CONTRA-INDICATIONS** Acute abdomen · delayed gastric emptying · heart failure secondary to chronic lung disease · phaeochromocytoma

● **CAUTIONS** Cardiac arrhythmias · pancreatitis · severe cor pulmonale

● **INTERACTIONS** → Appendix 1: opioids

● **SIDE-EFFECTS**

▶ **Common or very common**

- With oral use Appetite decreased · asthenic conditions · gastrointestinal discomfort · insomnia · neuromuscular dysfunction

▶ **Uncommon**

- With oral use Agitation · bronchospasm · ileus · mood altered · myoclonus · peripheral oedema · pulmonary oedema · seizure · sensation abnormal · syncope · taste altered

▶ **Frequency not known**

- With oral use Amenorrhoea · biliary pain · cough decreased · hyperalgesia · hypertension · pancreatitis exacerbated · sexual dysfunction · thinking abnormal · ureteral spasm
- With parenteral use Alertness decreased · bile duct disorders · mood altered · myoclonus · sexual dysfunction · ureteral spasm · urinary disorders · vision disorders

● **BREAST FEEDING** Therapeutic doses unlikely to affect infant.

● **HEPATIC IMPAIRMENT** Manufacturer advises caution. Avoid *oral preparations* in acute impairment; for *injectable preparations*—consult product literature.
Dose adjustments Manufacturer advises consider dose reduction—consult product literature.

● **RENAL IMPAIRMENT** Avoid use or reduce dose; opioid effects increased and prolonged; increased cerebral sensitivity.

● **MONITORING REQUIREMENTS** Possible association between acute chest syndrome in patients with sickle cell disease treated with morphine during a vaso-occlusive crisis—manufacturer advises close monitoring for acute chest syndrome symptoms during treatment.

● **DIRECTIONS FOR ADMINISTRATION**

▸ With intravenous use For *continuous intravenous infusion*, dilute with Glucose 5% or 10% or Sodium Chloride 0.9%.

▸ With intravenous use in neonates *Neonatal intensive care*, dilute 2.5 mg/kg body-weight to a final volume of 50 mL with infusion fluid; an intravenous infusion rate of 0.1 mL/hour provides a dose of 5 micrograms/kg/hour.

▸ With oral use For *modified release capsules*—swallow whole or open capsule and sprinkle contents on soft food.

● **PRESCRIBING AND DISPENSING INFORMATION** Modified-release preparations are available as 12-hourly or 24-hourly formulations; prescribers must ensure that the correct preparation is prescribed. Preparations that should be given 12-hourly include *Filnarine® SR*, *MST Continus®*, *Morphgesic® SR* and *Zomorph®*. Preparations that should be given 24-hourly include *MXL®*.

Prescriptions must specify the 'form'.

▸ With rectal use Both the strength of the suppositories and the morphine salt contained in them must be specified by the prescriber.

● **PATIENT AND CARER ADVICE**

▸ With oral use Patients or carers should be given advice on how to administer morphine modified-release capsules.

Medicines for Children leaflet: Morphine for pain www.medicinesforchildren.org.uk/morphine-pain

● **EXCEPTIONS TO LEGAL CATEGORY**

Morphine Oral Solutions Prescription-only medicines or schedule 2 controlled drug. The proportion of morphine hydrochloride may be altered when specified by the prescriber; if above 13 mg per 5 mL the solution becomes a schedule 2 controlled drug. It is usual to adjust the strength so that the dose volume is 5 or 10 mL.

Oral solutions of morphine can be prescribed by writing the formula:

Morphine hydrochloride 5 mg
Chloroform water to 5 mL

● **MEDICINAL FORMS** There can be variation in the licensing of different medicines containing the same drug. Forms available from special-order manufacturers include: capsule, oral solution, solution for injection, infusion, solution for infusion, suppository

Modified-release tablet

CAUTIONARY AND ADVISORY LABELS 2, 25

▸ **MST Continus** (Napp Pharmaceuticals Ltd)

Morphine sulfate 5 mg MST Continus 5mg tablets | 60 tablet [PoM] £3.29 DT = £3.29 [CD2]

Morphine sulfate 10 mg MST Continus 10mg tablets | 60 tablet [PoM] £5.20 DT = £5.20 [CD2]

Morphine sulfate 15 mg MST Continus 15mg tablets | 60 tablet [PoM] £9.10 DT = £9.10 [CD2]

Morphine sulfate 30 mg MST Continus 30mg tablets | 60 tablet [PoM] £12.47 DT = £12.47 [CD2]

Morphine sulfate 60 mg MST Continus 60mg tablets | 60 tablet [PoM] £24.32 DT = £24.32 [CD2]

Morphine sulfate 100 mg MST Continus 100mg tablets | 60 tablet [PoM] £38.50 DT = £38.50 [CD2]

Morphine sulfate 200 mg MST Continus 200mg tablets | 60 tablet [PoM] £81.34 DT = £81.34 [CD2]

▸ **Morphgesic SR** (Advanz Pharma)

Morphine sulfate 10 mg Morphgesic SR 10mg tablets | 60 tablet [PoM] £3.85 DT = £5.20 [CD2]

Morphine sulfate 30 mg Morphgesic SR 30mg tablets | 60 tablet [PoM] £9.24 DT = £12.47 [CD2]

Morphine sulfate 60 mg Morphgesic SR 60mg tablets | 60 tablet [PoM] £18.04 DT = £24.32 [CD2]

Morphine sulfate 100 mg Morphgesic SR 100mg tablets | 60 tablet [PoM] £28.54 DT = £38.50 [CD2]

Tablet

CAUTIONARY AND ADVISORY LABELS 2

▸ **Sevredol** (Napp Pharmaceuticals Ltd)

Morphine sulfate 10 mg Sevredol 10mg tablets | 56 tablet [PoM] £5.31 DT = £5.31 [CD2]

Morphine sulfate 20 mg Sevredol 20mg tablets | 56 tablet [PoM] £10.61 DT = £10.61 [CD2]

Morphine sulfate 50 mg Sevredol 50mg tablets | 56 tablet [PoM] £28.02 DT = £28.02 [CD2]

Solution for injection

▸ **Morphine (Non-proprietary)**

Morphine sulfate 1 mg per 1 ml Morphine sulfate 5mg/5ml solution for injection ampoules | 10 ampoule [PoM] £47.30 DT = £47.30 [CD2]
Morphine sulfate 1mg/1ml solution for injection ampoules | 10 ampoule [PoM] £37.50 [CD2]
Morphine sulfate 10mg/10ml solution for injection ampoules | 10 ampoule [PoM] £15.00–£49.30 [CD2]

Morphine sulfate 10 mg per 1 ml Morphine sulfate 10mg/1ml solution for injection ampoules | 10 ampoule [PoM] £11.87 DT = £11.47 [CD2]

Morphine sulfate 15 mg per 1 ml Morphine sulfate 15mg/1ml solution for injection ampoules | 10 ampoule [PoM] £10.74–£13.10 DT = £10.74 [CD2]

Morphine sulfate 20 mg per 1 ml Morphine sulfate 20mg/1ml solution for injection ampoules | 10 ampoule [PoM] £75.85 DT = £75.85 [CD2]

Morphine sulfate 30 mg per 1 ml Morphine sulfate 30mg/1ml solution for injection ampoules | 10 ampoule [PoM] £14.02 DT = £11.49 [CD2]
Morphine sulfate 60mg/2ml solution for injection ampoules | 5 ampoule [PoM] £10.07 DT = £10.07 [CD2]

Modified-release capsule

CAUTIONARY AND ADVISORY LABELS 2

▸ **MXL** (Napp Pharmaceuticals Ltd)

Morphine sulfate 30 mg MXL 30mg capsules | 28 capsule [PoM] £10.91 [CD2]

Morphine sulfate 60 mg MXL 60mg capsules | 28 capsule [PoM] £14.95 [CD2]

Morphine sulfate 90 mg MXL 90mg capsules | 28 capsule [PoM] £22.04 DT = £22.04 [CD2]

Morphine sulfate 120 mg MXL 120mg capsules | 28 capsule [PoM] £29.15 DT = £29.15 [CD2]

Morphine sulfate 150 mg MXL 150mg capsules | 28 capsule [PoM] £36.43 DT = £36.43 [CD2]

Morphine sulfate 200 mg MXL 200mg capsules | 28 capsule [PoM] £46.15 [CD2]

▸ **Zomorph** (Ethypharm UK Ltd)

Morphine sulfate 10 mg Zomorph 10mg modified-release capsules | 60 capsule [PoM] £3.47 DT = £3.47 [CD2]

Morphine sulfate 30 mg Zomorph 30mg modified-release capsules | 60 capsule [PoM] £8.30 DT = £8.30 [CD2]

Morphine sulfate 60 mg Zomorph 60mg modified-release capsules | 60 capsule [PoM] £16.20 DT = £16.20 [CD2]

Morphine sulfate 100 mg Zomorph 100mg modified-release capsules | 60 capsule [PoM] £21.80 DT = £21.80 [CD2]

Morphine sulfate 200 mg Zomorph 200mg modified-release capsules | 60 capsule [PoM] £43.60 DT = £43.60 [CD2]

Solution for infusion

▸ **Morphine (Non-proprietary)**

Morphine sulfate 1 mg per 1 ml Morphine sulfate 50mg/50ml solution for infusion vials | 1 vial [PoM] £5.78 DT = £5.78 [CD2] | 10 vial [PoM] £43.90 [CD2]

Morphine sulfate 2 mg per 1 ml Morphine sulfate 100mg/50ml solution for infusion vials | 1 vial [PoM] £6.48 [CD2] | 10 vial [PoM] £69.70 [CD2]

Oral solution

CAUTIONARY AND ADVISORY LABELS 2

▸ **Morphine (Non-proprietary)**

Morphine sulfate 2 mg per 1 ml Morphine sulfate 10mg/5ml oral solution | 100 ml [PoM] £1.68–£3.00 [CD5] | 300 ml [PoM] £9.00 DT = £6.21 [CD5] | 500 ml [PoM] £7.10–£15.00 [CD5]

▸ **Oramorph** (Boehringer Ingelheim Ltd)

Morphine sulfate 2 mg per 1 ml Oramorph 10mg/5ml oral solution | 100 ml [PoM] £1.89 [CD5] | 300 ml [PoM] £5.45 DT = £6.21 [CD5] | 500 ml [PoM] £8.50 [CD5]

Morphine sulfate 20 mg per 1 ml Oramorph 20mg/ml concentrated oral solution sugar-free | 120 ml [PoM] £19.50 DT = £19.50 [CD2]

Modified-release granules

CAUTIONARY AND ADVISORY LABELS 2, 13

▸ **MST Continus** (Napp Pharmaceuticals Ltd)

Morphine sulfate 20 mg MST Continus suspension 20mg granules sachets sugar-free | 30 sachet [PoM] £24.58 DT = £24.58 [CD2]

Morphine sulfate 30 mg MST Continus suspension 30mg granules sachets sugar-free | 30 sachet [PoM] £25.54 DT = £25.54 [CD2]

Morphine sulfate 60 mg MST Continus suspension 60mg granules sachets sugar-free | 30 sachet [PoM] £51.09 DT = £51.09 [CD2]

Morphine sulfate 100 mg MST Continus suspension 100mg granules sachets sugar-free | 30 sachet PoM £85.15 DT = £85.15 CD2
Morphine sulfate 200 mg MST Continus suspension 200mg granules sachets sugar-free | 30 sachet PoM £170.30 DT = £170.30 CD2

Morphine with cyclizine

The properties listed below are those particular to the combination only. For the properties of the components please consider, morphine p. 299, cyclizine p. 276.

- **INDICATIONS AND DOSE**

CYCLIMORPH-10®

Moderate to severe pain (short-term use only)

- BY SUBCUTANEOUS INJECTION, OR BY INTRAMUSCULAR INJECTION, OR BY INTRAVENOUS INJECTION
- Child 12–17 years: 1 mL, do not repeat dose more often than every 4 hours; maximum 3 doses per day

CYCLIMORPH-15®

Moderate to severe pain (short-term use only)

- BY SUBCUTANEOUS INJECTION, OR BY INTRAMUSCULAR INJECTION, OR BY INTRAVENOUS INJECTION
- Child 12–17 years: 1 mL, do not repeat dose more often than every 4 hours; maximum 3 doses per day

- **CAUTIONS** Myocardial infarction (cyclizine may aggravate severe heart failure and counteract the haemodynamic benefits of opioids) · not recommended in palliative care
- **INTERACTIONS** → Appendix 1: antihistamines, sedating · opioids

- **MEDICINAL FORMS** There can be variation in the licensing of different medicines containing the same drug.

Solution for injection

- Cyclimorph (Advanz Pharma)
  Morphine tartrate 15 mg per 1 ml, Cyclizine tartrate 50 mg per 1 ml Cyclimorph 15 solution for injection 1ml ampoules | 5 ampoule PoM £9.12 DT = £9.12 CD2
  Morphine tartrate 10 mg per 1 ml, Cyclizine tartrate 50 mg per 1 ml Cyclimorph 10 solution for injection 1ml ampoules | 5 ampoule PoM £8.77 DT = £8.77 CD2

F 290

Oxycodone hydrochloride

12-Apr-2019

- **INDICATIONS AND DOSE**

Moderate to severe pain in palliative care

- BY MOUTH USING IMMEDIATE-RELEASE MEDICINES
- Child 1 month–11 years: Initially 200 micrograms/kg every 4–6 hours (max. per dose 5 mg), dose to be increased if necessary according to severity of pain
- Child 12–17 years: Initially 5 mg every 4–6 hours, dose to be increased if necessary according to severity of pain
- BY MOUTH USING MODIFIED-RELEASE MEDICINES
- Child 8–11 years: Initially 5 mg every 12 hours, dose to be increased if necessary according to severity of pain, use 12-hourly modified-release preparations for this dose; see *Prescribing and dispensing information*
- Child 12–17 years: Initially 10 mg every 12 hours, dose to be increased if necessary according to severity of pain, use 12-hourly modified-release preparations for this dose; see *Prescribing and dispensing information*

DOSE EQUIVALENCE AND CONVERSION

- 2 mg oral oxycodone is approximately equivalent to 1 mg parenteral oxycodone.

ONEXILA XL®

Severe pain

- BY MOUTH
- Child 12–17 years: Initially 10 mg every 24 hours, dose to be increased if necessary according to severity of pain, some patients may require higher doses than the maximum daily dose; maximum 400 mg per day

- **UNLICENSED USE** Oxycodone preparations are not licensed for use in children under 12 years and some may not be licensed for use in children—further information can be found in the product literature of the individual preparations.

> **IMPORTANT SAFETY INFORMATION**
> Do not confuse modified-release 12-hourly preparations with 24-hourly preparations, see *Prescribing and dispensing information.*

- **CONTRA-INDICATIONS** Acute abdomen · chronic constipation · cor pulmonale · delayed gastric emptying
- **CAUTIONS** Pancreatitis · toxic psychosis
- **INTERACTIONS** → Appendix 1: opioids
- **SIDE-EFFECTS**
  - **Common or very common** Anxiety · appetite abnormal · asthenic conditions · bronchospasm · cognitive impairment · depression · diarrhoea · dyspnoea · gastrointestinal discomfort · hiccups · insomnia · mood altered · movement disorders · perception altered · psychiatric disorders · tremor · urinary frequency increased
  - **Uncommon** Biliary colic · burping · chest pain · chills · cough · dehydration · dysphagia · gastrointestinal disorders · hyperacusia · increased risk of infection · injury · lacrimation disorder · malaise · memory loss · migraine · neuromuscular dysfunction · oedema · oral disorders · pain · seizure · sensation abnormal · sexual dysfunction · SIADH · speech disorder · syncope · taste altered · thirst · vasodilation · voice alteration
  - **Rare or very rare** Haemorrhage · lymphadenopathy · muscle spasms · photosensitivity reaction · tooth discolouration · weight changes
  - **Frequency not known** Aggression · amenorrhoea · cholestasis
- **BREAST FEEDING** Present in milk—avoid.
- **HEPATIC IMPAIRMENT** Manufacturer advises caution in mild impairment; avoid in moderate to severe impairment.
  Dose adjustments In adults, manufacturer advises initial dose reduction in mild impairment—consult product literature.
- **RENAL IMPAIRMENT** Opioid effects increased and prolonged and increased cerebral sensitivity occurs. Avoid if estimated glomerular filtration rate less than 10 mL/minute/1.73 m^2.
  Dose adjustments Max. initial dose 2.5 mg every 6 hours in patients not currently treated with an opioid with mild to moderate impairment.
- **PRESCRIBING AND DISPENSING INFORMATION** Modified-release preparations are available as 12-hourly or 24-hourly formulations. Preparations that should be given 12-hourly include *Abtard®*, *Carexil®*, *Ixyldone®*, *Leveraxo®*, *Longtec®*, *Oxeltra®*, *OxyContin®*, *Oxypro®*, *Oxylan®*, *Reltebon®*, and *Renocontin®*. Preparations that should be given 24-hourly include *Onexila® XL*.
  Palliative care For further information on the use of oxycodone in palliative care, see www.medicinescomplete.com/#/content/palliative/oxycodone.

- **MEDICINAL FORMS** There can be variation in the licensing of different medicines containing the same drug. Forms available from special-order manufacturers include: oral solution, solution for infusion

Modified-release tablet

CAUTIONARY AND ADVISORY LABELS 2, 25

- Abtard (Ethypharm UK Ltd)
  Oxycodone hydrochloride 5 mg Abtard 5mg modified-release tablets | 28 tablet PoM £6.26 DT = £12.52 CD2
  Oxycodone hydrochloride 10 mg Abtard 10mg modified-release tablets | 56 tablet PoM £12.52 DT = £25.04 CD2
  Oxycodone hydrochloride 15 mg Abtard 15mg modified-release tablets | 56 tablet PoM £19.06 DT = £38.12 CD2

Oxycodone hydrochloride 20 mg Abtard 20mg modified-release tablets | 56 tablet PoM £25.04 DT = £50.08 CD2
Oxycodone hydrochloride 30 mg Abtard 30mg modified-release tablets | 56 tablet PoM £38.11 DT = £76.23 CD2
Oxycodone hydrochloride 40 mg Abtard 40mg modified-release tablets | 56 tablet PoM £50.09 DT = £100.19 CD2
Oxycodone hydrochloride 60 mg Abtard 60mg modified-release tablets | 56 tablet PoM £76.24 DT = £152.49 CD2
Oxycodone hydrochloride 80 mg Abtard 80mg modified-release tablets | 56 tablet PoM £100.19 DT = £200.39 CD2

▸ **Carexil** (Sandoz Ltd)
Oxycodone hydrochloride 5 mg Carexil 5mg modified-release tablets | 28 tablet PoM £6.26 DT = £12.52 CD2
Oxycodone hydrochloride 10 mg Carexil 10mg modified-release tablets | 56 tablet PoM £12.52 DT = £25.04 CD2
Oxycodone hydrochloride 20 mg Carexil 20mg modified-release tablets | 56 tablet PoM £25.04 DT = £50.08 CD2
Oxycodone hydrochloride 40 mg Carexil 40mg modified-release tablets | 56 tablet PoM £60.11 DT = £100.19 CD2
Oxycodone hydrochloride 80 mg Carexil 80mg modified-release tablets | 56 tablet PoM £120.23 DT = £200.39 CD2

▸ **Ixyldone** (Morningside Healthcare Ltd)
Oxycodone hydrochloride 5 mg Ixyldone 5mg modified-release tablets | 28 tablet PoM £2.96 DT = £12.52 CD2
Oxycodone hydrochloride 10 mg Ixyldone 10mg modified-release tablets | 56 tablet PoM £5.94 DT = £25.04 CD2
Oxycodone hydrochloride 15 mg Ixyldone 15mg modified-release tablets | 56 tablet PoM £9.05 DT = £38.12 CD2
Oxycodone hydrochloride 20 mg Ixyldone 20mg modified-release tablets | 56 tablet PoM £11.88 DT = £50.08 CD2
Oxycodone hydrochloride 30 mg Ixyldone 30mg modified-release tablets | 56 tablet PoM £18.10 DT = £76.23 CD2
Oxycodone hydrochloride 40 mg Ixyldone 40mg modified-release tablets | 56 tablet PoM £23.79 DT = £100.19 CD2
Oxycodone hydrochloride 60 mg Ixyldone 60mg modified-release tablets | 56 tablet PoM £36.19 DT = £152.49 CD2
Oxycodone hydrochloride 80 mg Ixyldone 80mg modified-release tablets | 56 tablet PoM £47.58 DT = £200.39 CD2

▸ **Leveraxo** (Mylan)
Oxycodone hydrochloride 30 mg Leveraxo 30mg modified-release tablets | 56 tablet PoM £75.47 DT = £76.23 CD2
Oxycodone hydrochloride 60 mg Leveraxo 60mg modified-release tablets | 56 tablet PoM £150.97 DT = £152.49 CD2

▸ **Longtec** (Qdem Pharmaceuticals Ltd)
Oxycodone hydrochloride 5 mg Longtec 5mg modified-release tablets | 28 tablet PoM £6.26 DT = £12.52 CD2
Oxycodone hydrochloride 10 mg Longtec 10mg modified-release tablets | 56 tablet PoM £12.52 DT = £25.04 CD2
Oxycodone hydrochloride 15 mg Longtec 15mg modified-release tablets | 56 tablet PoM £19.06 DT = £38.12 CD2
Oxycodone hydrochloride 20 mg Longtec 20mg modified-release tablets | 56 tablet PoM £25.04 DT = £50.08 CD2
Oxycodone hydrochloride 30 mg Longtec 30mg modified-release tablets | 56 tablet PoM £38.11 DT = £76.23 CD2
Oxycodone hydrochloride 40 mg Longtec 40mg modified-release tablets | 56 tablet PoM £50.09 DT = £100.19 CD2
Oxycodone hydrochloride 60 mg Longtec 60mg modified-release tablets | 56 tablet PoM £76.24 DT = £152.49 CD2
Oxycodone hydrochloride 80 mg Longtec 80mg modified-release tablets | 56 tablet PoM £100.19 DT = £200.39 CD2
Oxycodone hydrochloride 120 mg Longtec 120mg modified-release tablets | 56 tablet PoM £152.51 DT = £305.02 CD2

▸ **Onexila XL** (Aspire Pharma Ltd)
Oxycodone hydrochloride 10 mg Onexila XL 10mg tablets | 28 tablet PoM £12.52 CD2
Oxycodone hydrochloride 20 mg Onexila XL 20mg tablets | 28 tablet PoM £12.52 CD2
Oxycodone hydrochloride 40 mg Onexila XL 40mg tablets | 28 tablet PoM £25.04 CD2
Oxycodone hydrochloride 80 mg Onexila XL 80mg tablets | 28 tablet PoM £50.09 CD2

▸ **Oxeltra** (Wockhardt UK Ltd)
Oxycodone hydrochloride 5 mg Oxeltra 5mg modified-release tablets | 28 tablet PoM £3.13 DT = £12.52 CD2
Oxycodone hydrochloride 10 mg Oxeltra 10mg modified-release tablets | 56 tablet PoM £6.26 DT = £25.04 CD2
Oxycodone hydrochloride 15 mg Oxeltra 15mg modified-release tablets | 56 tablet PoM £9.53 DT = £38.12 CD2
Oxycodone hydrochloride 20 mg Oxeltra 20mg modified-release tablets | 56 tablet PoM £12.52 DT = £50.08 CD2
Oxycodone hydrochloride 30 mg Oxeltra 30mg modified-release tablets | 56 tablet PoM £19.06 DT = £76.23 CD2
Oxycodone hydrochloride 40 mg Oxeltra 40mg modified-release tablets | 56 tablet PoM £25.05 DT = £100.19 CD2
Oxycodone hydrochloride 60 mg Oxeltra 60mg modified-release tablets | 56 tablet PoM £38.12 DT = £152.49 CD2
Oxycodone hydrochloride 80 mg Oxeltra 80mg modified-release tablets | 56 tablet PoM £50.10 DT = £200.39 CD2

▸ **OxyContin** (Napp Pharmaceuticals Ltd)
Oxycodone hydrochloride 5 mg OxyContin 5mg modified-release tablets | 28 tablet PoM £12.52 DT = £12.52 CD2
Oxycodone hydrochloride 10 mg OxyContin 10mg modified-release tablets | 56 tablet PoM £25.04 DT = £25.04 CD2
Oxycodone hydrochloride 15 mg OxyContin 15mg modified-release tablets | 56 tablet PoM £38.12 DT = £38.12 CD2
Oxycodone hydrochloride 20 mg OxyContin 20mg modified-release tablets | 56 tablet PoM £50.08 DT = £50.08 CD2
Oxycodone hydrochloride 30 mg OxyContin 30mg modified-release tablets | 56 tablet PoM £76.23 DT = £76.23 CD2
Oxycodone hydrochloride 40 mg OxyContin 40mg modified-release tablets | 56 tablet PoM £100.19 DT = £100.19 CD2
Oxycodone hydrochloride 60 mg OxyContin 60mg modified-release tablets | 56 tablet PoM £152.49 DT = £152.49 CD2
Oxycodone hydrochloride 80 mg OxyContin 80mg modified-release tablets | 56 tablet PoM £200.39 DT = £200.39 CD2
Oxycodone hydrochloride 120 mg OxyContin 120mg modified-release tablets | 56 tablet PoM £305.02 DT = £305.02 CD2

▸ **Oxylan** (Healthcare Pharma Ltd)
Oxycodone hydrochloride 5 mg Oxylan 5mg modified-release tablets | 28 tablet PoM £12.50 DT = £12.52 CD2
Oxycodone hydrochloride 10 mg Oxylan 10mg modified-release tablets | 56 tablet PoM £24.99 DT = £25.04 CD2
Oxycodone hydrochloride 20 mg Oxylan 20mg modified-release tablets | 56 tablet PoM £49.98 DT = £50.08 CD2
Oxycodone hydrochloride 40 mg Oxylan 40mg modified-release tablets | 56 tablet PoM £99.98 DT = £100.19 CD2
Oxycodone hydrochloride 80 mg Oxylan 80mg modified-release tablets | 56 tablet PoM £199.97 DT = £200.39 CD2

▸ **Oxypro** (Ridge Pharma Ltd)
Oxycodone hydrochloride 5 mg Oxypro 5mg modified-release tablets | 28 tablet PoM £3.13 DT = £12.52 CD2
Oxycodone hydrochloride 10 mg Oxypro 10mg modified-release tablets | 56 tablet PoM £6.26 DT = £25.04 CD2
Oxycodone hydrochloride 15 mg Oxypro 15mg modified-release tablets | 56 tablet PoM £9.53 DT = £38.12 CD2
Oxycodone hydrochloride 20 mg Oxypro 20mg modified-release tablets | 56 tablet PoM £12.52 DT = £50.08 CD2
Oxycodone hydrochloride 30 mg Oxypro 30mg modified-release tablets | 56 tablet PoM £19.06 DT = £76.23 CD2
Oxycodone hydrochloride 40 mg Oxypro 40mg modified-release tablets | 56 tablet PoM £25.05 DT = £100.19 CD2
Oxycodone hydrochloride 60 mg Oxypro 60mg modified-release tablets | 56 tablet PoM £38.12 DT = £152.49 CD2
Oxycodone hydrochloride 80 mg Oxypro 80mg modified-release tablets | 56 tablet PoM £50.10 DT = £200.39 CD2

▸ **Reltebon** (Accord Healthcare Ltd)
Oxycodone hydrochloride 5 mg Reltebon 5mg modified-release tablets | 28 tablet PoM £6.26 DT = £12.52 CD2
Oxycodone hydrochloride 10 mg Reltebon 10mg modified-release tablets | 56 tablet PoM £12.52 DT = £25.04 CD2
Oxycodone hydrochloride 15 mg Reltebon 15mg modified-release tablets | 56 tablet PoM £19.06 DT = £38.12 CD2
Oxycodone hydrochloride 20 mg Reltebon 20mg modified-release tablets | 56 tablet PoM £25.04 DT = £50.08 CD2
Oxycodone hydrochloride 30 mg Reltebon 30mg modified-release tablets | 56 tablet PoM £38.11 DT = £76.23 CD2
Oxycodone hydrochloride 40 mg Reltebon 40mg modified-release tablets | 56 tablet PoM £50.09 DT = £100.19 CD2
Oxycodone hydrochloride 60 mg Reltebon 60mg modified-release tablets | 56 tablet PoM £76.24 DT = £152.49 CD2
Oxycodone hydrochloride 80 mg Reltebon 80mg modified-release tablets | 56 tablet PoM £100.19 DT = £200.39 CD2

▸ **Renocontin** (Glenmark Pharmaceuticals Europe Ltd)
Oxycodone hydrochloride 5 mg Renocontin 5mg modified-release tablets | 28 tablet PoM £2.97 DT = £12.52 CD2
Oxycodone hydrochloride 10 mg Renocontin 10mg modified-release tablets | 56 tablet PoM £5.95 DT = £25.04 CD2
Oxycodone hydrochloride 15 mg Renocontin 15mg modified-release tablets | 56 tablet PoM £9.05 DT = £38.12 CD2

Oxycodone hydrochloride 20 mg Renocontin 20mg modified-release tablets | 56 tablet PoM £11.89 DT = £50.08 CD2
Oxycodone hydrochloride 30 mg Renocontin 30mg modified-release tablets | 56 tablet PoM £18.11 DT = £76.23 CD2
Oxycodone hydrochloride 40 mg Renocontin 40mg modified-release tablets | 56 tablet PoM £23.80 DT = £100.19 CD2
Oxycodone hydrochloride 60 mg Renocontin 60mg modified-release tablets | 56 tablet PoM £36.20 DT = £152.49 CD2

Solution for injection

- Oxycodone hydrochloride (Non-proprietary)

Oxycodone hydrochloride 10 mg per 1 ml Oxycodone 10mg/1ml solution for injection ampoules | 5 ampoule PoM £8.00 DT = £8.00 (Hospital only) CD2 | 5 ampoule PoM £8.00 DT = £8.00 CD2 | 10 ampoule PoM £15.00 CD2
Oxycodone 20mg/2ml solution for injection ampoules | 5 ampoule PoM £16.00 DT = £16.00 CD2 | 5 ampoule PoM £16.00 DT = £16.00 (Hospital only) CD2 | 10 ampoule PoM £30.00 CD2
Oxycodone hydrochloride 50 mg per 1 ml Oxycodone 50mg/1ml solution for injection ampoules | 5 ampoule PoM £70.10 DT = £70.10 (Hospital only) CD2 | 5 ampoule PoM £70.10 DT = £70.10 CD2 | 10 ampoule PoM £135.00 CD2

- OxyNorm (Napp Pharmaceuticals Ltd)

Oxycodone hydrochloride 10 mg per 1 ml OxyNorm 10mg/1ml solution for injection ampoules | 5 ampoule PoM £8.00 DT = £8.00 CD2
OxyNorm 20mg/2ml solution for injection ampoules | 5 ampoule PoM £16.00 DT = £16.00 CD2
Oxycodone hydrochloride 50 mg per 1 ml OxyNorm 50mg/1ml solution for injection ampoules | 5 ampoule PoM £70.10 DT = £70.10 CD2

- Shortec (Qdem Pharmaceuticals Ltd)

Oxycodone hydrochloride 10 mg per 1 ml Shortec 20mg/2ml solution for injection ampoules | 5 ampoule PoM £13.60 DT = £16.00 CD2
Shortec 10mg/1ml solution for injection ampoules | 5 ampoule PoM £6.80 DT = £8.00 CD2
Oxycodone hydrochloride 50 mg per 1 ml Shortec 50mg/1ml solution for injection ampoules | 5 ampoule PoM £59.59 DT = £70.10 CD2

Oral solution

CAUTIONARY AND ADVISORY LABELS 2

- Oxycodone hydrochloride (Non-proprietary)

Oxycodone hydrochloride 1 mg per 1 ml Oxycodone 5mg/5ml oral solution sugar-free | 250 ml PoM £11.63 DT = £9.71 CD2
Oxycodone hydrochloride 10 mg per 1 ml Oxycodone 10mg/ml oral solution sugar-free | 120 ml PoM £55.95 DT = £46.63 CD2

- OxyNorm (Napp Pharmaceuticals Ltd)

Oxycodone hydrochloride 1 mg per 1 ml OxyNorm liquid 1mg/ml oral solution sugar-free | 250 ml PoM £9.71 DT = £9.71 CD2
Oxycodone hydrochloride 10 mg per 1 ml OxyNorm 10mg/ml concentrate oral solution sugar-free | 120 ml PoM £46.63 DT = £46.63 CD2

- Shortec (Qdem Pharmaceuticals Ltd)

Oxycodone hydrochloride 1 mg per 1 ml Shortec liquid 5mg/5ml oral solution sugar-free | 250 ml PoM £8.25 DT = £9.71 CD2
Oxycodone hydrochloride 10 mg per 1 ml Shortec 10mg/ml concentrate oral solution sugar-free | 120 ml PoM £39.64 DT = £46.63 CD2

Capsule

CAUTIONARY AND ADVISORY LABELS 2

- Lynlor (Accord Healthcare Ltd)

Oxycodone hydrochloride 5 mg Lynlor 5mg capsules | 56 capsule PoM £6.86 DT = £11.43 CD2
Oxycodone hydrochloride 10 mg Lynlor 10mg capsules | 56 capsule PoM £13.72 DT = £22.86 CD2
Oxycodone hydrochloride 20 mg Lynlor 20mg capsules | 56 capsule PoM £27.43 DT = £45.71 CD2

- OxyNorm (Napp Pharmaceuticals Ltd)

Oxycodone hydrochloride 5 mg OxyNorm 5mg capsules | 56 capsule PoM £11.43 DT = £11.43 CD2
Oxycodone hydrochloride 10 mg OxyNorm 10mg capsules | 56 capsule PoM £22.86 DT = £22.86 CD2
Oxycodone hydrochloride 20 mg OxyNorm 20mg capsules | 56 capsule PoM £45.71 DT = £45.71 CD2

- Shortec (Qdem Pharmaceuticals Ltd)

Oxycodone hydrochloride 5 mg Shortec 5mg capsules | 56 capsule PoM £6.86 DT = £11.43 CD2
Oxycodone hydrochloride 10 mg Shortec 10mg capsules | 56 capsule PoM £13.72 DT = £22.86 CD2
Oxycodone hydrochloride 20 mg Shortec 20mg capsules | 56 capsule PoM £27.43 DT = £45.71 CD2

F 290

Pethidine hydrochloride

(Meperidine)

- **INDICATIONS AND DOSE**

Obstetric analgesia

- BY SUBCUTANEOUS INJECTION, OR BY INTRAMUSCULAR INJECTION
  - Child 12–17 years: 1 mg/kg (max. per dose 100 mg), then 1 mg/kg after 1–3 hours if required; maximum 400 mg per day

- **CONTRA-INDICATIONS** Phaeochromocytoma
- **CAUTIONS** Accumulation of metabolites may result in neurotoxicity · cardiac arrhythmias · not suitable for severe continuing pain · severe cor pulmonale
- **INTERACTIONS** → Appendix 1: opioids
- **SIDE-EFFECTS** Anxiety · asthenia · biliary spasm · coordination abnormal · delirium · dysuria · hypothermia · seizure · syncope · tremor
  Overdose Convulsions reported in overdosage.
- **BREAST FEEDING** Present in milk but not known to be harmful.
- **HEPATIC IMPAIRMENT** Manufacturer advises caution in mild to moderate impairment; avoid in severe impairment.
  Dose adjustments Manufacturer advises dose reduction in mild to moderate impairment.
- **RENAL IMPAIRMENT** Avoid use or reduce dose; opioid effects increased and prolonged and increased cerebral sensitivity occurs.

- **MEDICINAL FORMS** There can be variation in the licensing of different medicines containing the same drug. Forms available from special-order manufacturers include: solution for injection

Solution for injection

- Pethidine hydrochloride (Non-proprietary)

Pethidine hydrochloride 50 mg per 1 ml Pethidine 50mg/1ml solution for injection ampoules | 10 ampoule PoM £5.11 DT = £5.11 CD2
Pethidine 100mg/2ml solution for injection ampoules | 10 ampoule PoM £4.66 DT = £4.66 CD2

F 290

Tapentadol

20-Feb-2019

- **INDICATIONS AND DOSE**

Moderate to severe acute pain which can be managed only with opioid analgesics

- BY MOUTH USING ORAL SOLUTION
  - Child 2–17 years (specialist supervision in hospital): 1.25 mg/kg every 4 hours (max. per dose 100 mg) for up to 3 days, the dose for children with a high BMI must not exceed the calculated dose for a body-weight at the 97.5 percentile for the given age

IMPORTANT SAFETY INFORMATION

MHRA/CHM ADVICE: TAPENTADOL (*PALEXIA*®): RISK OF SEIZURES AND REPORTS OF SEROTONIN SYNDROME WHEN CO-ADMINISTERED WITH OTHER MEDICINES (JANUARY 2019)

Tapentadol can induce seizures and should be prescribed with caution in patients with a history of seizure disorders or epilepsy. Seizure risk may be increased in patients taking other medicines that lower seizure threshold, for example, antidepressants such as selective serotonin reuptake inhibitors (SSRIs), serotonin-noradrenaline reuptake inhibitors (SNRIs), tricyclic antidepressants, and antipsychotics.

Serotonin syndrome has been reported when tapentadol is used in combination with serotonergic antidepressants—withdrawal of the serotonergic medicine, together with supportive symptomatic care, usually brings about a rapid improvement in serotonin syndrome.

- **CAUTIONS** Obesity
- **INTERACTIONS** → Appendix 1: opioids
- **SIDE-EFFECTS**
  - **Common or very common** Anxiety · appetite decreased · asthenia · diarrhoea · feeling of body temperature change · gastrointestinal discomfort · muscle spasms · sleep disorders · tremor
  - **Uncommon** Concentration impaired · depressed mood · dysarthria · dyspnoea · feeling abnormal · irritability · memory loss · movement disorders · muscle contractions involuntary · oedema · sensation abnormal · urinary disorders
  - **Rare or very rare** Angioedema · impaired gastric emptying · level of consciousness decreased · seizure · thinking abnormal
- **BREAST FEEDING** Avoid—no information available.
- **HEPATIC IMPAIRMENT** Manufacturer advises avoid (no information available).
- **RENAL IMPAIRMENT** Manufacturer advises avoid (no information available).

- **MEDICINAL FORMS** There can be variation in the licensing of different medicines containing the same drug.

Oral solution

CAUTIONARY AND ADVISORY LABELS 2

EXCIPIENTS: May contain Propylene glycol

- Palexia (Grunenthal Ltd)

Tapentadol (as Tapentadol hydrochloride) 20 mg per 1 ml Palexia 20mg/ml oral solution sugar-free | 100 ml PoM £17.80 DT = £17.80 CD2

290

Tramadol hydrochloride

27-Jan-2020

- **INDICATIONS AND DOSE**

Moderate to severe pain

- BY INTRAMUSCULAR INJECTION, OR BY INTRAVENOUS INJECTION, OR BY INTRAVENOUS INFUSION, OR BY SUBCUTANEOUS INJECTION
  - Child 12–17 years: 50–100 mg every 4–6 hours, intravenous injection to be given over 2–3 minutes; Usual maximum 400 mg/24 hours

Moderate to severe acute pain

- BY MOUTH USING IMMEDIATE-RELEASE MEDICINES
  - Child 12–17 years: Initially 100 mg, then 50–100 mg every 4–6 hours; Usual maximum 400 mg/24 hours

Moderate to severe chronic pain

- BY MOUTH USING IMMEDIATE-RELEASE MEDICINES
  - Child 12–17 years: Initially 50 mg, then, adjusted according to response; Usual maximum 400 mg/24 hours

Postoperative pain

- BY INTRAVENOUS INJECTION, OR BY INTRAMUSCULAR INJECTION, OR BY INTRAVENOUS INFUSION, OR BY SUBCUTANEOUS INJECTION
  - Child 12–17 years: Initially 100 mg, then 50 mg every 10–20 minutes if required up to total maximum 250 mg (including initial dose) in first hour, then 50–100 mg every 4–6 hours, intravenous injection to be given over 2–3 minutes; Usual maximum 400 mg/24 hours

Moderate to severe pain (with modified-release 12-hourly preparations)

- BY MOUTH USING MODIFIED-RELEASE MEDICINES
  - Child 12–17 years: 50–100 mg twice daily, increased if necessary to 150–200 mg twice daily, doses exceeding the usual maximum not generally required; Usual maximum 400 mg/24 hours

Moderate to severe pain (with modified-release 24-hourly preparations)

- BY MOUTH USING MODIFIED-RELEASE MEDICINES
  - Child 12–17 years: Initially 100–150 mg once daily, increased if necessary up to 400 mg once daily; Usual maximum 400 mg/24 hours

ZYDOL® XL

Moderate to severe pain

- BY MOUTH USING MODIFIED-RELEASE TABLETS
  - Child 12–17 years: Initially 150 mg once daily, increased if necessary up to 400 mg once daily

IMPORTANT SAFETY INFORMATION

Do not confuse modified-release 12-hourly preparations with 24-hourly preparations, see *Prescribing and dispensing information.*

- **CONTRA-INDICATIONS** Acute intoxication with alcohol · acute intoxication with analgesics · acute intoxication with hypnotics · acute intoxication with opioids · compromised respiratory function · not suitable for narcotic withdrawal treatment · uncontrolled epilepsy
- **CAUTIONS** Excessive bronchial secretions · history of epilepsy—use tramadol only if compelling reasons · impaired consciousness · not suitable as a substitute in opioid-dependent patients · not suitable in some types of general anaesthesia · postoperative use · susceptibility to seizures—use tramadol only if compelling reasons · variation in metabolism

CAUTIONS, FURTHER INFORMATION

- General anaesthesia Not recommended for analgesia during potentially light planes of general anaesthesia (possibly increased intra-operative recall reported).
- Variation in metabolism The capacity to metabolise tramadol can vary considerably between individuals; there is a risk of developing side-effects of opioid toxicity in patients who are ultra-rapid tramadol metabolisers (CYP2D6 ultra-rapid metabolisers) and the therapeutic effect may be reduced in poor tramadol metabolisers.
- Postoperative use Manufacturer advises extreme caution when used for postoperative pain relief in children—reports of rare, but life threatening adverse events after tonsillectomy and/or adenoidectomy for obstructive sleep apnoea; if used, monitor closely for symptoms of opioid toxicity.

- **INTERACTIONS** → Appendix 1: opioids
- **SIDE-EFFECTS**

GENERAL SIDE-EFFECTS

- **Common or very common** Fatigue
- **Rare or very rare** Dyspnoea · epileptiform seizure · respiratory disorders · sleep disorders · vision blurred
- **Frequency not known** Asthma exacerbated · hypoglycaemia

SPECIFIC SIDE-EFFECTS

- **Uncommon**
  - With parenteral use Circulatory collapse · gastrointestinal discomfort
- **Rare or very rare**
  - With parenteral use Angioedema · appetite change · behaviour abnormal · cognitive disorder · dysuria · hypersensitivity · mood altered · movement disorders · muscle weakness · perception disorders · psychiatric disorder · sensation abnormal

- ▸ **Frequency not known**
- ▸ With oral use Anxiety · blood disorder · gastrointestinal disorder · hyperkinesia · hypertension · paraesthesia · syncope · tremor · urinary disorder

- **PREGNANCY** Embryotoxic in *animal* studies—manufacturers advise avoid.
- **BREAST FEEDING** Amount probably too small to be harmful, but manufacturer advises avoid.
- **HEPATIC IMPAIRMENT** Manufacturers advise caution (risk of delayed elimination); some *oral preparations* should be avoided in severe impairment—consult product literature.
  Dose adjustments Manufacturers advise consider increasing dosage interval.
- **RENAL IMPAIRMENT** Avoid use or reduce dose; opioid effects increased and prolonged and increased cerebral sensitivity occurs. Caution (avoid for *oral drops*) in severe impairment.
- **TREATMENT CESSATION** Manufacturer advises consider tapering the dose gradually to prevent withdrawal symptoms.
- **DIRECTIONS FOR ADMINISTRATION** Tramadol hydrochloride *orodispersible tablets* should be sucked and then swallowed. May also be dispersed in water. Some tramadol hydrochloride modified-release capsule preparations may be opened and the contents swallowed immediately without chewing—check individual preparations.
  For *intravenous infusion*, dilute in Glucose 5% or Sodium Chloride 0.9%.
- **PRESCRIBING AND DISPENSING INFORMATION** Modified-release preparations are available as 12-hourly or 24-hourly formulations. Non-proprietary preparations of modified-release tramadol may be available as either 12-hourly or 24-hourly formulations; prescribers and dispensers must ensure that the correct formulation is prescribed and dispensed. Branded preparations that should be given 12-hourly include *Invodol® SR*, *Mabron®*, *Maneo®*, *Marol®*, *Maxitram® SR*, *Oldaram®*, *Tilodol® SR*, *Tramquel® SR*, *Tramulief® SR*, *Zamadol® SR*, *Zeridame® SR* and *Zydol SR®*. Preparations that should be given 24-hourly include *Tradorec XL®*, *Zamadol® 24hr*, and *Zydol XL®*.
- **PATIENT AND CARER ADVICE** Patients or carers should be given advice on how to administer tramadol hydrochloride orodispersible tablets.
  Medicines for Children leaflet: Tramadol for pain www.medicinesforchildren.org.uk/tramadol-pain

- **MEDICINAL FORMS** There can be variation in the licensing of different medicines containing the same drug. Forms available from special-order manufacturers include: oral suspension

Modified-release tablet

CAUTIONARY AND ADVISORY LABELS 2, 25

- ▸ **Brimisol PR** (Bristol Laboratories Ltd)
  Tramadol hydrochloride 100 mg Brimisol PR 100mg tablets | 60 tablet [PoM] [NHS] [CD3]
- ▸ **Invodol SR** (Ennogen Healthcare Ltd)
  Tramadol hydrochloride 100 mg Invodol SR 100mg tablets | 60 tablet [PoM] £5.55 [CD3]
  Tramadol hydrochloride 150 mg Invodol SR 150mg tablets | 60 tablet [PoM] £8.31 [CD3]
  Tramadol hydrochloride 200 mg Invodol SR 200mg tablets | 60 tablet [PoM] £11.35 [CD3]
- ▸ **Mabron** (Teva UK Ltd)
  Tramadol hydrochloride 100 mg Mabron 100mg modified-release tablets | 60 tablet [PoM] £15.52 [CD3]
  Tramadol hydrochloride 150 mg Mabron 150mg modified-release tablets | 60 tablet [PoM] £23.28 [CD3]
  Tramadol hydrochloride 200 mg Mabron 200mg modified-release tablets | 60 tablet [PoM] £31.04 [CD3]
- ▸ **Maneo** (Mylan)
  Tramadol hydrochloride 100 mg Maneo 100mg modified-release tablets | 60 tablet [PoM] £6.95 [CD3]
  Tramadol hydrochloride 150 mg Maneo 150mg modified-release tablets | 60 tablet [PoM] £10.40 [CD3]
  Tramadol hydrochloride 200 mg Maneo 200mg modified-release tablets | 60 tablet [PoM] £14.20 [CD3]
- ▸ **Marol** (Teva UK Ltd)
  Tramadol hydrochloride 100 mg Marol 100mg modified-release tablets | 60 tablet [PoM] £6.94 [CD3]
  Tramadol hydrochloride 150 mg Marol 150mg modified-release tablets | 60 tablet [PoM] £10.39 [CD3]
  Tramadol hydrochloride 200 mg Marol 200mg modified-release tablets | 60 tablet [PoM] £14.19 [CD3]
- ▸ **Tilodol SR** (Sandoz Ltd)
  Tramadol hydrochloride 100 mg Tilodol SR 100mg tablets | 60 tablet [PoM] £15.52 [CD3]
  Tramadol hydrochloride 150 mg Tilodol SR 150mg tablets | 60 tablet [PoM] £23.28 [CD3]
  Tramadol hydrochloride 200 mg Tilodol SR 200mg tablets | 60 tablet [PoM] £31.04 [CD3]
- ▸ **Tradorec XL** (Endo Ventures Ltd)
  Tramadol hydrochloride 100 mg Tradorec XL 100mg tablets | 30 tablet [PoM] £14.10 [CD3]
  Tramadol hydrochloride 200 mg Tradorec XL 200mg tablets | 30 tablet [PoM] £14.98 [CD3]
  Tramadol hydrochloride 300 mg Tradorec XL 300mg tablets | 30 tablet [PoM] £22.47 [CD3]
- ▸ **Tramulief SR** (Advanz Pharma)
  Tramadol hydrochloride 100 mg Tramulief SR 100mg tablets | 60 tablet [PoM] £6.98 [CD3]
  Tramadol hydrochloride 150 mg Tramulief SR 150mg tablets | 60 tablet [PoM] £10.48 [CD3]
  Tramadol hydrochloride 200 mg Tramulief SR 200mg tablets | 60 tablet [PoM] £14.28 [CD3]
- ▸ **Zamadol 24hr** (Mylan)
  Tramadol hydrochloride 150 mg Zamadol 24hr 150mg modified-release tablets | 28 tablet [PoM] £10.70 [CD3]
  Tramadol hydrochloride 200 mg Zamadol 24hr 200mg modified-release tablets | 28 tablet [PoM] £14.26 [CD3]
  Tramadol hydrochloride 300 mg Zamadol 24hr 300mg modified-release tablets | 28 tablet [PoM] £21.39 [CD3]
  Tramadol hydrochloride 400 mg Zamadol 24hr 400mg modified-release tablets | 28 tablet [PoM] £28.51 DT = £28.51 [CD3]
- ▸ **Zydol SR** (Grunenthal Ltd)
  Tramadol hydrochloride 50 mg Zydol SR 50mg tablets | 60 tablet [PoM] £4.60 DT = £4.60 [CD3]
  Tramadol hydrochloride 100 mg Zydol SR 100mg tablets | 60 tablet [PoM] £17.22 [CD3]
  Tramadol hydrochloride 150 mg Zydol SR 150mg tablets | 60 tablet [PoM] £25.83 [CD3]
  Tramadol hydrochloride 200 mg Zydol SR 200mg tablets | 60 tablet [PoM] £34.40 [CD3]
- ▸ **Zydol XL** (Grunenthal Ltd)
  Tramadol hydrochloride 150 mg Zydol XL 150mg tablets | 30 tablet [PoM] £12.18 [CD3]
  Tramadol hydrochloride 200 mg Zydol XL 200mg tablets | 30 tablet [PoM] £17.98 [CD3]
  Tramadol hydrochloride 300 mg Zydol XL 300mg tablets | 30 tablet [PoM] £24.94 [CD3]
  Tramadol hydrochloride 400 mg Zydol XL 400mg tablets | 30 tablet [PoM] £32.47 [CD3]

Soluble tablet

CAUTIONARY AND ADVISORY LABELS 2, 13

- ▸ **Zydol** (Grunenthal Ltd)
  Tramadol hydrochloride 50 mg Zydol 50mg soluble tablets sugar-free | 20 tablet [PoM] £2.79 Schedule 3 (CD No Register Exempt Safe Custody) sugar-free | 100 tablet [PoM] £13.33 DT = £13.33 [CD3]

Solution for injection

- ▸ **Tramadol hydrochloride (Non-proprietary)**
  Tramadol hydrochloride 50 mg per 1 ml Tramadol 100mg/2ml solution for injection ampoules | 5 ampoule [PoM] £4.90 DT = £4.00 [CD3] | 10 ampoule [PoM] £10.00 [CD3]
- ▸ **Zamadol** (Mylan)
  Tramadol hydrochloride 50 mg per 1 ml Zamadol 100mg/2ml solution for injection ampoules | 5 ampoule [PoM] £5.49 DT = £4.00 [CD3]
- ▸ **Zydol** (Grunenthal Ltd)
  Tramadol hydrochloride 50 mg per 1 ml Zydol 100mg/2ml solution for injection ampoules | 5 ampoule [PoM] £4.00 DT = £4.00 [CD3]

Modified-release capsule

CAUTIONARY AND ADVISORY LABELS 2, 25

▸ Maxitram SR (Chiesi Ltd)

Tramadol hydrochloride 50 mg Maxitram SR 50mg capsules | 60 capsule PoM £4.55 DT = £7.24 CD3

Tramadol hydrochloride 100 mg Maxitram SR 100mg capsules | 60 capsule PoM £12.14 DT = £14.47 CD3

Tramadol hydrochloride 150 mg Maxitram SR 150mg capsules | 60 capsule PoM £18.21 DT = £21.71 CD3

Tramadol hydrochloride 200 mg Maxitram SR 200mg capsules | 60 capsule PoM £24.28 DT = £28.93 CD3

▸ Tramquel SR (Mylan)

Tramadol hydrochloride 50 mg Tramquel SR 50mg capsules | 60 capsule PoM £7.24 DT = £7.24 CD3

Tramadol hydrochloride 100 mg Tramquel SR 100mg capsules | 60 capsule PoM £14.47 DT = £14.47 CD3

Tramadol hydrochloride 150 mg Tramquel SR 150mg capsules | 60 capsule PoM £21.71 DT = £21.71 CD3

Tramadol hydrochloride 200 mg Tramquel SR 200mg capsules | 60 capsule PoM £28.93 DT = £28.93 CD3

▸ Zamadol SR (Mylan)

Tramadol hydrochloride 50 mg Zamadol SR 50mg capsules | 60 capsule PoM £7.24 DT = £7.24 CD3

Tramadol hydrochloride 100 mg Zamadol SR 100mg capsules | 60 capsule PoM £14.47 DT = £14.47 CD3

Tramadol hydrochloride 150 mg Zamadol SR 150mg capsules | 60 capsule PoM £21.71 DT = £21.71 CD3

Tramadol hydrochloride 200 mg Zamadol SR 200mg capsules | 60 capsule PoM £28.93 DT = £28.93 CD3

Oral drops

CAUTIONARY AND ADVISORY LABELS 2, 13

▸ Tramadol hydrochloride (Non-proprietary)

Tramadol (as Tramadol hydrochloride) 100 mg per 1 ml Tramadol 100mg/ml oral drops | 10 ml PoM £25.00 DT = £25.00 CD3

Capsule

CAUTIONARY AND ADVISORY LABELS 2

▸ Tramadol hydrochloride (Non-proprietary)

Tramadol hydrochloride 50 mg Tramadol 50mg capsules | 30 capsule PoM £0.98 DT = £0.87 CD3 | 100 capsule PoM £14.40 DT = £2.90 CD3

▸ Zamadol (Mylan)

Tramadol hydrochloride 50 mg Zamadol 50mg capsules | 100 capsule PoM £8.00 DT = £2.90 CD3

▸ Zydol (Grunenthal Ltd)

Tramadol hydrochloride 50 mg Zydol 50mg capsules | 30 capsule PoM £2.29 DT = £0.87 CD3 | 100 capsule PoM £7.63 DT = £2.90 CD3

Orodispersible tablet

CAUTIONARY AND ADVISORY LABELS 2

▸ Zamadol Melt (Mylan)

Tramadol hydrochloride 50 mg Zamadol Melt 50mg tablets sugar-free | 60 tablet PoM £7.12 DT = £7.12 CD3

Tramadol with paracetamol

22-Feb-2018

The properties listed below are those particular to the combination only. For the properties of the components please consider, paracetamol p. 288, tramadol hydrochloride p. 305.

● **INDICATIONS AND DOSE**

Moderate to severe pain

▸ BY MOUTH

▸ Child 12–17 years: 75/650 mg every 6 hours as required

DOSE EQUIVALENCE AND CONVERSION

▸ The proportions are expressed in the form x/y, where x and y are the strengths in milligrams of tramadol and paracetamol respectively.

● **INTERACTIONS** → Appendix 1: opioids · paracetamol

● **MEDICINAL FORMS** There can be variation in the licensing of different medicines containing the same drug.

Effervescent tablet

CAUTIONARY AND ADVISORY LABELS 2, 13, 29, 30

ELECTROLYTES: May contain Sodium

▸ Tramacet (Grunenthal Ltd)

Tramadol hydrochloride 37.5 mg, Paracetamol 325 mg Tramacet 37.5mg/325mg effervescent tablets sugar-free | 60 tablet PoM £9.68 DT = £9.68 CD3

Tablet

CAUTIONARY AND ADVISORY LABELS 2, 25, 29, 30

▸ Tramadol with paracetamol (Non-proprietary)

Tramadol hydrochloride 37.5 mg, Paracetamol 325 mg Tramadol 37.5mg / Paracetamol 325mg tablets | 60 tablet PoM £9.68 DT = £2.31 CD3

Tramadol hydrochloride 75 mg, Paracetamol 650 mg Tramadol 75mg / Paracetamol 650mg tablets | 30 tablet PoM £19.50 CD3

▸ Tramacet (Grunenthal Ltd)

Tramadol hydrochloride 37.5 mg, Paracetamol 325 mg Tramacet 37.5mg/325mg tablets | 60 tablet PoM £9.68 DT = £2.31 CD3

▸ Trapadex (Noumed Life Sciences Ltd)

Tramadol hydrochloride 37.5 mg, Paracetamol 325 mg Trapadex 37.5mg/325mg tablets | 60 tablet PoM ☒ DT = £2.31 CD3

5.1 Migraine

Migraine

19-Feb-2020

Treatment of acute migraine

Treatment of a migraine attack should be guided by response to previous treatment and the severity of the attacks. A **simple analgesic** such as paracetamol p. 288 (preferably in a soluble or dispersible form) or an NSAID, usually ibuprofen p. 707, is often effective; concomitant antiemetic treatment may be required. If treatment with an analgesic is inadequate, an attack may be treated with a specific antimigraine compound such as the $5HT_1$- receptor agonist sumatriptan p. 309. **Ergot alkaloids** are associated with many side-effects and should be avoided.

Excessive use of acute treatments for migraine (opioid and non-opioid analgesics, $5HT_1$-receptor agonists, and ergotamine) is associated with medication-overuse headache (analgesic-induced headache); therefore, increasing consumption of these medicines needs careful management.

$5HT_1$-receptor agonists

$5HT_1$-receptor agonists are used in the treatment of acute migraine attacks; treatment of children should be initiated by a specialist. A $5HT_1$-receptor agonist may be used during the established headache phase of an attack and is the preferred treatment in those who fail to respond to conventional analgesics. $5HT_1$-receptor agonists are **not** indicated for the treatment of hemiplegic, basilar, or ophthalmoplegic migraine.

If a child does not respond to one $5HT_1$-receptor agonist, an alternative $5HT_1$-receptor agonist should be tried. For children who have prolonged attacks that frequently recur despite treatment with a $5HT_1$-receptor agonist, combination therapy with an NSAID such as naproxen p. 712 can be considered. Sumatriptan and zolmitriptan p. 310 are used for migraine in children. They may also be of value in cluster headache.

Antiemetics

Antiemetics, including domperidone p. 278 [unlicensed in children aged under 12 years or those weighing less than 35 kg], phenothiazines, and antihistamines, relieve the nausea associated with migraine attacks. Antiemetics may be given by intramuscular injection or rectally if vomiting is a problem. Domperidone has the added advantage of promoting gastric emptying and normal peristalsis; a single dose should be given at the onset of symptoms. The MHRA and CHM have released important safety information and restrictions regarding the use of domperidone for nausea and vomiting in children aged under 12 years or those weighing less than 35 kg, and a reminder of contra-indications. For further information, see *Important safety information* for domperidone.

Prophylaxis of migraine

Where migraine attacks are frequent, possible provoking factors such as stress should be sought; combined oral contraceptives may also provoke migraine. Preventive treatment should be considered if migraine attacks interfere with school and social life, particularly for children who:

- suffer at least two attacks a month;
- suffer an increasing frequency of headaches;
- suffer significant disability despite suitable treatment for migraine attacks;
- cannot take suitable treatment for migraine attacks.

In children it is often possible to stop prophylaxis after a period of treatment.

Propranolol hydrochloride p. 111 may be effective in preventing migraine in children but it is contra-indicated in those with asthma. Side-effects such as depression and postural hypotension can further limit its use.

Pizotifen below, an antihistamine and a serotonin-receptor antagonist, may also be used but its efficacy in children has not been clearly established. Common side-effects include drowsiness and weight gain.

Topiramate p. 227 is licensed for migraine prophylaxis; see *Conception and contraception*, and *Pregnancy* in the topiramate drug monograph for information on use in females of childbearing potential and pregnancy.

Cluster headache and other trigeminal autonomic cephalalgias

Management

Cluster headache rarely responds to standard analgesics. Sumatriptan p. 309 given by subcutaneous injection is the drug of choice for the treatment of cluster headache. If an injection is unsuitable, sumatriptan nasal spray or zolmitriptan p. 310 nasal spray may be used. Treatment should be initiated by a specialist. Alternatively, 100% oxygen at a rate of 10–15 litres/minute for 10–20 minutes is useful in aborting an attack.

The other trigeminal autonomic cephalalgias, paroxysmal hemicrania (sensitive to indometacin p. 710), and short-lasting unilateral neuralgiform headache attacks with conjunctival injection and tearing, are seen rarely and are best managed by a specialist.

Other drugs used for Migraine Clonidine hydrochloride, p. 108 · Cyclizine, p. 276 · Trifluoperazine, p. 264 · Valproic acid, p. 228

ANTIHISTAMINES › SEDATING

Paracetamol with buclizine hydrochloride and codeine phosphate

22-Nov-2019

The properties listed below are those particular to the combination only. For the properties of the components please consider, paracetamol p. 288, codeine phosphate p. 293.

- **INDICATIONS AND DOSE**

MIGRALEVE®

Acute migraine

▶ BY MOUTH

- ▶ Child 12–15 years: Initially 1 tablet, (pink tablet) to be taken at onset of attack, or if it is imminent, followed by 1 tablet every 4 hours if required, (yellow tablet) to be taken following initial dose; maximum 1 pink and 3 yellow tablets in 24 hours
- ▶ Child 16–17 years: Initially 2 tablets, (pink tablets) to be taken at onset of attack or if it is imminent, followed by 2 tablets every 4 hours if required, (yellow tablets) to be taken following initial dose; maximum 2 pink and 6 yellow tablets in 24 hours

- **INTERACTIONS** → Appendix 1: antihistamines, sedating · opioids · paracetamol
- **PRESCRIBING AND DISPENSING INFORMATION** See co-codamol p. 292 for Migraleve Yellow preparations.
- **LESS SUITABLE FOR PRESCRIBING**

MIGRALEVE® *Migraleve®* is less suitable for prescribing.

- **MEDICINAL FORMS** There can be variation in the licensing of different medicines containing the same drug.

Tablet

CAUTIONARY AND ADVISORY LABELS 2, 17, 30

▶ Migraleve Pink (McNeil Products Ltd)
Buclizine hydrochloride 6.25 mg, Codeine phosphate 8 mg, Paracetamol 500 mg Migraleve Pink tablets | 12 tablet [P] £3.79 [CD5] | 24 tablet [P] £6.08 [CD5] | 48 tablet [PoM] £3.97 [CD5]

Pizotifen

- **INDICATIONS AND DOSE**

Prophylaxis of migraine

▶ BY MOUTH

- ▶ Child 5–17 years: Initially 500 micrograms once daily, dose to be taken at night, then increased to up to 1.5 mg daily in divided doses, dose to be increased gradually, max. single dose (at night) 1 mg

- **UNLICENSED USE** 1.5 mg tablets not licensed for use in children.
- **CONTRA-INDICATIONS** Acute porphyrias p. 652
- **CAUTIONS** Avoid abrupt withdrawal · history of epilepsy · susceptibility to angle-closure glaucoma · urinary retention
- **INTERACTIONS** → Appendix 1: antihistamines, sedating
- **SIDE-EFFECTS**
  - ▶ **Common or very common** Appetite increased · dizziness · drowsiness · dry mouth · fatigue · nausea · weight increased
  - ▶ **Uncommon** Constipation
  - ▶ **Rare or very rare** Aggression · anxiety · arthralgia · central nervous system stimulation · depression · hallucination · muscle complaints · paraesthesia · seizure · skin reactions · sleep disorders
  - ▶ **Frequency not known** Hepatic disorders
- **PREGNANCY** Avoid unless potential benefit outweighs risk.

- **BREAST FEEDING** Amount probably too small to be harmful, but manufacturer advises avoid.
- **HEPATIC IMPAIRMENT** Manufacturer advises caution.
  Dose adjustments Manufacturer advises consider dose reduction.
- **RENAL IMPAIRMENT** Use with caution.
- **PATIENT AND CARER ADVICE**
  Medicines for Children leaflet: Pizotifen to prevent migraine headaches www.medicinesforchildren.org.uk/pizotifen-prevent-migraine-headaches
  Driving and skilled tasks Drowsiness may affect performance of skilled tasks (e.g. driving); effects of alcohol enhanced.

- **MEDICINAL FORMS** There can be variation in the licensing of different medicines containing the same drug. Forms available from special-order manufacturers include: oral solution

Tablet

CAUTIONARY AND ADVISORY LABELS 2

- Pizotifen (Non-proprietary)
  Pizotifen (as Pizotifen hydrogen malate)
  500 microgram Pizotifen 500microgram tablets | 28 tablet PoM £16.25 DT = £1.73
  Pizotifen (as Pizotifen hydrogen malate) 1.5 mg Pizotifen 1.5mg tablets | 28 tablet PoM £16.25 DT = £4.85

TRIPTANS

Sumatriptan

05-Mar-2020

- **INDICATIONS AND DOSE**

Treatment of acute migraine

- BY MOUTH
  - Child 6–9 years: Initially 25 mg for 1 dose, followed by 25 mg after at least 2 hours if required, to be taken only if migraine recurs (patient not responding to initial dose should not take second dose for same attack)
  - Child 10–11 years: Initially 50 mg for 1 dose, followed by 50 mg after at least 2 hours, to be taken only if migraine recurs (patient not responding to initial dose should not take second dose for same attack)
  - Child 12–17 years: Initially 50–100 mg for 1 dose, followed by 50–100 mg after at least 2 hours if required, to be taken only if migraine recurs (patient not responding to initial dose should not take second dose for same attack)
- BY SUBCUTANEOUS INJECTION
  - Child 10–17 years: Initially 6 mg for 1 dose, followed by 6 mg after at least 1 hour if required, to be taken only if migraine recurs (patient not responding to initial dose should not take second dose for same attack), dose to be administered using an auto-injector; maximum 12 mg per day
- BY INTRANASAL ADMINISTRATION
  - Child 12–17 years: Initially 10–20 mg for 1 dose, followed by 10–20 mg after at least 2 hours if required, to be taken only if migraine recurs (patient not responding to initial dose should not take second dose for same attack); maximum 40 mg per day

Treatment of acute cluster headache

- BY SUBCUTANEOUS INJECTION
  - Child 10–17 years (under expert supervision): Initially 6 mg for 1 dose, followed by 6 mg after at least 1 hour if required, to be taken only if headache recurs (patient not responding to initial dose should not take second dose for same attack), dose to be administered using auto-injector; maximum 12 mg per day
- BY INTRANASAL ADMINISTRATION
  - Child 12–17 years (under expert supervision): Initially 10–20 mg for 1 dose, followed by 10–20 mg after at least 2 hours if required, to be taken only if headache recurs (patient not responding to initial dose should not take second dose for same attack); maximum 40 mg per day

- **UNLICENSED USE** Tablets and injection not licensed for use in children. Not licensed for treating cluster headache in children. Intranasal doses for treating acute migraine in children may differ from those in product literature.
- **CONTRA-INDICATIONS** Coronary vasospasm · ischaemic heart disease · mild uncontrolled hypertension · moderate and severe hypertension · peripheral vascular disease · previous cerebrovascular accident · previous myocardial infarction · previous transient ischaemic attack · Prinzmetal's angina
- **CAUTIONS** Conditions which predispose to coronary artery disease · history of seizures · mild, controlled hypertension · risk factors for seizures
- **INTERACTIONS** → Appendix 1: sumatriptan
- **SIDE-EFFECTS**
  GENERAL SIDE-EFFECTS
  - **Common or very common** Asthenia · dizziness · drowsiness · dyspnoea · feeling abnormal · flushing · myalgia · nausea · pain · sensation abnormal · skin reactions · temperature sensation altered · vomiting
  - **Rare or very rare** Hypersensitivity
  - **Frequency not known** Angina pectoris · anxiety · arrhythmias · arthralgia · colitis ischaemic · coronary vasospasm · diarrhoea · dystonia · hyperhidrosis · hypotension · myocardial infarction · nystagmus · palpitations · Raynaud's phenomenon · seizure · tremor · vision disorders

  SPECIFIC SIDE-EFFECTS
  - **Common or very common**
    - With intranasal use Epistaxis · nasal irritation · taste altered · throat irritation
    - With subcutaneous use Haemorrhage · swelling

  SIDE-EFFECTS, FURTHER INFORMATION Discontinue if symptoms of heat, heaviness, pressure or tightness (including throat and chest) occur.
- **ALLERGY AND CROSS-SENSITIVITY** Caution in patients with sensitivity to sulfonamides.
- **PREGNANCY** There is limited experience of using $5HT_1$-receptor agonists during pregnancy; manufacturers advise that they should be avoided unless the potential benefit outweighs the risk.
- **BREAST FEEDING** Present in milk but amount probably too small to be harmful; withhold breast-feeding for 12 hours after treatment.
- **HEPATIC IMPAIRMENT** Manufacturer advises caution (reduced pre-systemic clearance increases exposure); avoid in severe impairment (no information available).
  Dose adjustments ▸ With oral use In adults, manufacturer advises consider dose reduction—consult product literature.
- **RENAL IMPAIRMENT** Use with caution.
- **PATIENT AND CARER ADVICE**
  Medicines for Children leaflet: Sumatriptan for migraine headaches www.medicinesforchildren.org.uk/sumatriptan-migraine-headaches
  Driving and skilled tasks Drowsiness may affect performance of skilled tasks (e.g. driving).

- **MEDICINAL FORMS** There can be variation in the licensing of different medicines containing the same drug.

Solution for injection

CAUTIONARY AND ADVISORY LABELS 3, 10

- Sumatriptan (Non-proprietary)
  Sumatriptan (as Sumatriptan succinate) 12 mg per 1 ml Sumatriptan 6mg/0.5ml solution for injection pre-filled pens | 2 pre-filled disposable injection PoM £60.00 DT = £52.07

4 Nervous system

- ▸ Imigran Subject (GlaxoSmithKline UK Ltd)
  Sumatriptan (as Sumatriptan succinate) 12 mg per 1 ml Imigran Subject 6mg/0.5ml solution for injection syringe refill pack | 2 pre-filled disposable injection [PoM] £48.49 DT = £48.49
  Imigran Subject 6mg/0.5ml solution for injection pre-filled syringes with device | 2 pre-filled disposable injection [PoM] £50.96 DT = £50.96

Spray

CAUTIONARY AND ADVISORY LABELS 3, 10

- ▸ Imigran (GlaxoSmithKline UK Ltd)
  Sumatriptan 100 mg per 1 ml Imigran 10mg nasal spray | 2 unit dose [PoM] £14.16 DT = £14.16
  Sumatriptan 200 mg per 1 ml Imigran 20mg nasal spray | 2 unit dose [PoM] £14.16 | 6 unit dose [PoM] £42.47 DT = £42.47

Tablet

CAUTIONARY AND ADVISORY LABELS 3, 10

- ▸ Sumatriptan (Non-proprietary)
  Sumatriptan (as Sumatriptan succinate) 50 mg Sumatriptan 50mg tablets | 6 tablet [PoM] £31.85 DT = £1.36
  Sumatriptan (as Sumatriptan succinate) 100 mg Sumatriptan 100mg tablets | 6 tablet [PoM] £51.48 DT = £1.70
- ▸ Imigran (GlaxoSmithKline UK Ltd)
  Sumatriptan (as Sumatriptan succinate) 50 mg Imigran Radis 50mg tablets | 6 tablet [PoM] £23.90 DT = £1.36
  Imigran 50mg tablets | 6 tablet [PoM] £31.85 DT = £1.36
  Sumatriptan (as Sumatriptan succinate) 100 mg Imigran 100mg tablets | 6 tablet [PoM] £51.48 DT = £1.70
  Imigran Radis 100mg tablets | 6 tablet [PoM] £42.90 DT = £1.70
- ▸ Migraitan (Bristol Laboratories Ltd)
  Sumatriptan (as Sumatriptan succinate) 50 mg Migraitan 50mg tablets | 2 tablet [P] £4.44

Zolmitriptan

05-Mar-2020

● **INDICATIONS AND DOSE**

Treatment of acute migraine

▸ BY MOUTH

- ▸ Child 12–17 years: 2.5 mg, followed by 2.5 mg after at least 2 hours if required, dose to be taken only if migraine recurs, if response unsatisfactory after 3 attacks consider increasing dose to 5 mg or switching to alternative treatment; maximum 10 mg per day

▸ BY INTRANASAL ADMINISTRATION

- ▸ Child 12–17 years: 5 mg, dose to be administered as soon as possible after onset into one nostril only, followed by 5 mg after at least 2 hours if required, dose to be administered only if migraine recurs; maximum 10 mg per day

Treatment of acute cluster headache

▸ BY INTRANASAL ADMINISTRATION

- ▸ Child 12–17 years: 5 mg, dose to be administered as soon as possible after onset into one nostril only, followed by 5 mg after at least 2 hours if required, dose to be administered only if migraine recurs; maximum 10 mg per day

DOSE ADJUSTMENTS DUE TO INTERACTIONS

- ▸ Manufacturer advises max. dose 5 mg in 24 hours with concurrent use of moderate and potent inhibitors of CYP1A2, cimetidine and moclobemide.

DOSE EQUIVALENCE AND CONVERSION

- ▸ 1 spray of *Zomig®* nasal spray = 5 mg zolmitriptan.

● **UNLICENSED USE** Not licensed for use in children.

● **CONTRA-INDICATIONS** Arrhythmias associated with accessory cardiac conduction pathways · coronary vasospasm · ischaemic heart disease · moderate to severe hypertension · peripheral vascular disease · previous cerebrovascular accident · previous myocardial infarction · Prinzmetal's angina · transient ischaemic attack · uncontrolled hypertension · Wolff-Parkinson-White syndrome

● **CAUTIONS** Conditions which predispose to coronary artery disease

● **INTERACTIONS** → Appendix 1: zolmitriptan

● **SIDE-EFFECTS**

GENERAL SIDE-EFFECTS

- ▸ **Common or very common** Abdominal pain · asthenia · chest discomfort · dizziness · drowsiness · dry mouth · dysphagia · feeling hot · headache · limb discomfort · muscle weakness · nausea · pain · palpitations · sensation abnormal · vomiting
- ▸ **Uncommon** Tachycardia · urinary disorders
- ▸ **Rare or very rare** Angina pectoris · angioedema · coronary vasospasm · gastrointestinal disorders · gastrointestinal infarction · hypersensitivity · myocardial infarction · splenic infarction · urticaria

SPECIFIC SIDE-EFFECTS

- ▸ **Common or very common**
- ▸ With intranasal use Feeling abnormal · haemorrhage · myalgia · nasal discomfort · taste altered · throat pain
- ▸ With oral use Muscle complaints · sensation of pressure · throat complaints
- ▸ **Rare or very rare**
- ▸ With oral use Diarrhoea

SIDE-EFFECTS, FURTHER INFORMATION Discontinue if symptoms of heat, heaviness, pressure or tightness (including throat and chest) occur.

● **PREGNANCY** There is limited experience of using $5HT_1$-receptor agonists during pregnancy; manufacturers advise that they should be avoided unless the potential benefit outweighs the risk.

● **BREAST FEEDING** Use with caution—present in milk in *animal* studies.

● **HEPATIC IMPAIRMENT** Manufacturer advises caution in moderate to severe impairment (risk of increased exposure).

Dose adjustments In adults, manufacturer advises maximum 5 mg in 24 hours in moderate to severe impairment.

● **DIRECTIONS FOR ADMINISTRATION** Zolmitriptan orodispersible tablets should be placed on the tongue, allowed to disperse and swallowed.

● **PATIENT AND CARER ADVICE** Patients or carers should be given advice on how to administer zolmitriptan orodispersible tablets.

● **MEDICINAL FORMS** There can be variation in the licensing of different medicines containing the same drug.

Spray

- ▸ Zomig (Grunenthal Ltd)
  Zolmitriptan 50 mg per 1 ml Zomig 5mg/0.1ml nasal spray 0.1ml unit dose | 6 unit dose [PoM] £36.50 DT = £36.50

Orodispersible tablet

EXCIPIENTS: May contain Aspartame

- ▸ Zolmitriptan (Non-proprietary)
  Zolmitriptan 2.5 mg Zolmitriptan 2.5mg orodispersible tablets sugar-free | 6 tablet [PoM] £20.35 DT = £11.50
  Zolmitriptan 5 mg Zolmitriptan 5mg orodispersible tablets sugar-free | 6 tablet [PoM] £20.35 DT = £13.41
- ▸ Zomig Rapimelt (Grunenthal Ltd)
  Zolmitriptan 2.5 mg Zomig Rapimelt 2.5mg orodispersible tablets sugar-free | 6 tablet [PoM] £23.99 DT = £11.50
  Zolmitriptan 5 mg Zomig Rapimelt 5mg orodispersible tablets sugar-free | 6 tablet [PoM] £23.94 DT = £13.41

Tablet

- ▸ Zolmitriptan (Non-proprietary)
  Zolmitriptan 2.5 mg Zolmitriptan 2.5mg tablets | 6 tablet [PoM] £23.94 DT = £6.20 | 12 tablet [PoM] £18.16–£28.00
  Zolmitriptan 5 mg Zolmitriptan 5mg tablets | 6 tablet [PoM] £4.27 DT = £3.60 | 12 tablet [PoM] £7.20
- ▸ Zomig (Grunenthal Ltd)
  Zolmitriptan 2.5 mg Zomig 2.5mg tablets | 6 tablet [PoM] £23.94 DT = £6.20

5.2 Neuropathic pain

Neuropathic pain

Overview and management

Neuropathic pain, which occurs as a result of damage to neural tissue, includes *compression neuropathies*, *peripheral neuropathies* (e.g. due to Diabetic complications p. 486, HIV infection p. 445, chemotherapy), *trauma*, *idiopathic neuropathy*, *central pain* (e.g. pain following spinal cord injury and syringomyelia), *postherpetic neuralgia*, and *phantom limb pain*. The pain may occur in an area of sensory deficit and may be described as burning, shooting or scalding; it may be accompanied by pain that is evoked by a nonnoxious stimulus (allodynia).

Children with chronic neuropathic pain require multidisciplinary management, which may include physiotherapy and psychological support. Neuropathic pain is generally managed with a **tricyclic antidepressant** such as amitriptyline hydrochloride p. 255 or **antiepileptic drugs** such as carbamazepine p. 209. Children with localised pain may benefit from **topical local anaesthetic** preparations, particularly while awaiting specialist review. Neuropathic pain may respond only partially to **opioid analgesics**. A corticosteroid may help to relieve pressure in compression neuropathy and thereby reduce pain.

Chronic facial pain

Chronic oral and facial pain including *persistent idiopathic facial pain* (also termed 'atypical facial pain') and *temporomandibular dysfunction* (previously termed temporomandibular joint pain dysfunction syndrome) may call for prolonged use of analgesics or for other drugs. **Tricyclic antidepressants** may be useful for facial pain [unlicensed indication], but are not on the Dental Practitioners' List. Disorders of this type require specialist referral and psychological support to accompany drug treatment. Children on long-term therapy need to be monitored both for progress and for side-effects.

6 Sleep disorders

6.1 Insomnia

Hypnotics and anxiolytics

Overview

Most anxiolytics ('sedatives') will induce sleep when given at night and most hypnotics will sedate when given during the day. Hypnotics and anxiolytics should be reserved for short courses to alleviate acute conditions after causal factors have been established.

The role of drug therapy in the management of anxiety disorders in children and adolescents is uncertain; drug therapy should be initiated only by specialists after psychosocial interventions have failed. Benzodiazepines and tricyclic antidepressants have been used but adverse effects may be problematic.

Hypnotics

The prescribing of hypnotics to children, except for occasional use such as for sedation for procedures is not justified. There is a risk of habituation with prolonged use. Problems settling children at night should be managed with behavioural therapy.

Dental procedures

Some anxious children may benefit from the use of a hypnotic the night before a dental appointment.

Chloral and derivatives

Chloral hydrate below and derivatives were formerly popular hypnotics for children. Chloral hydrate is now mainly used for sedation during diagnostic procedures.

Antihistamines

Some **antihistamines** such as promethazine hydrochloride p. 189 are used for occasional insomnia in adults; their prolonged duration of action can often cause drowsiness the following day. The sedative effect of antihistamines may diminish after a few days of continued treatment; antihistamines are associated with headache, psychomotor impairment and antimuscarinic effects. The use of hypnotics in children is not usually justified.

Melatonin

Melatonin p. 312 is a pineal hormone that may affect sleep pattern. Clinical experience suggests that when appropriate behavioural sleep interventions fail, melatonin may be of value for treating sleep onset insomnia and delayed sleep phase syndrome in children with conditions such as visual impairment, cerebral palsy, autism, and learning difficulties. It is also sometimes used before magnetic resonance imaging (MRI), computed tomography (CT), or EEG investigations. Little is known about its long-term effects in children, and there is uncertainty as to the effect on other circadian rhythms including endocrine or reproductive hormone secretion. The need to continue melatonin therapy should be reviewed every 6 months.

Anxiolytics

Anxiolytic treatment should be used in children only to relieve acute anxiety (and related insomnia) caused by fear (e.g. before surgery). Anxiolytic treatment should be limited to the lowest possible dose for the shortest possible time.

Buspirone

Buspirone hydrochloride is thought to act at specific serotonin ($5HT_{1A}$) receptors; safety and efficacy in children have yet to be determined.

HYPNOTICS, SEDATIVES AND ANXIOLYTICS › NON-BENZODIAZEPINE

Chloral hydrate

20-May-2020

● **INDICATIONS AND DOSE**

Sedation for painless procedures

▶ BY MOUTH, OR BY RECTUM

- Neonate: 30–50 mg/kg, to be given 45–60 minutes before procedure, doses up to 100 mg/kg may be used with respiratory monitoring, administration by rectum only if oral route not available.
- Child 1 month–11 years: 30–50 mg/kg (max. per dose 1 g), to be given 45–60 minutes before procedure, administration by rectum only if oral route not available, increased if necessary up to 100 mg/kg (max. per dose 2 g)
- Child 12–17 years: 1–2 g, to be given 45–60 minutes before procedure, administration by rectum only if oral route not available

Insomnia (short-term use), using chloral hydrate 143.3 mg/5 mL oral solution

▶ BY MOUTH USING ORAL SOLUTION

- Child 2–11 years: 30–50 mg/kg once daily (max. per dose 1 g), dose to be taken with water or milk at bedtime
- Child 12–17 years: 430–860 mg once daily (max. per dose 2 g), dose to be taken with water or milk at bedtime

continued →

Insomnia (short-term use), using chloral betaine 707 mg (≡ 414 mg chloral hydrate) tablets

▶ BY MOUTH USING TABLETS

▸ Child 12–17 years: 1–2 tablets, alternatively 414–828 mg once daily, dose to be taken with water or milk at bedtime; maximum 4 tablets per day; maximum 2 g per day

- **UNLICENSED USE** Not licensed for sedation for painless procedures.
- **CONTRA-INDICATIONS** Acute porphyrias p. 652 · gastritis · severe cardiac disease
- **CAUTIONS** Avoid contact with mucous membranes · avoid contact with skin · avoid prolonged use (and abrupt withdrawal thereafter)
- **INTERACTIONS** → Appendix 1: chloral hydrate
- **SIDE-EFFECTS** Agitation · allergic dermatitis · ataxia · confusion · delirium (more common on abrupt discontinuation) · drug use disorders · gastrointestinal discomfort · gastrointestinal disorders · headache · injury · ketonuria · kidney injury
- **PREGNANCY** Avoid.
- **BREAST FEEDING** Risk of sedation in infant—avoid.
- **HEPATIC IMPAIRMENT** Manufacturer advises avoid in marked impairment.
- **RENAL IMPAIRMENT** Avoid in severe impairment.
- **DIRECTIONS FOR ADMINISTRATION**

▸ With oral use For administration *by mouth* dilute liquid with plenty of water or juice to mask unpleasant taste.

- **PRESCRIBING AND DISPENSING INFORMATION** Flavours of oral liquid formulations may include black currant.

  The RCPCH and NPPG recommend that, when a liquid special of chloral hydrate is required, the following strength is used: 500 mg/5 mL.
- **PATIENT AND CARER ADVICE**

Driving and skilled tasks Drowsiness may persist the next day and affect performance of skilled tasks (e.g. driving); effects of alcohol enhanced.

- **MEDICINAL FORMS** There can be variation in the licensing of different medicines containing the same drug. Forms available from special-order manufacturers include: oral suspension, oral solution, suppository, enema

Tablet

CAUTIONARY AND ADVISORY LABELS 19, 27

▸ **Chloral hydrate (Non-proprietary)**

Cloral betaine 707 mg Cloral betaine 707mg tablets | 30 tablet [PoM] £138.59 DT = £138.59

Oral solution

CAUTIONARY AND ADVISORY LABELS 1(paediatric solution only), 19 (solution other than paediatric only), 27

▸ **Chloral hydrate (Non-proprietary)**

Chloral hydrate 28.66 mg per 1 ml Chloral hydrate 143.3mg/5ml oral solution BP | 150 ml [PoM] £244.25 DT = £244.25

Melatonin

10-Mar-2020

- **INDICATIONS AND DOSE**

Sleep onset insomnia (initiated under specialist supervision) | Delayed sleep phase syndrome (initiated under specialist supervision)

▶ BY MOUTH USING MODIFIED-RELEASE TABLETS

▸ Child: Initially 2–3 mg daily for 1–2 weeks, then increased if necessary to 4–6 mg daily, dose to be taken before bedtime; maximum 10 mg per day

Insomnia in patients with learning disabilities [where sleep hygiene measures have been insufficient] (initiated under specialist supervision)

▶ BY MOUTH USING MODIFIED-RELEASE TABLETS

▸ Child: Initially 2 mg once daily, increased if necessary to 4–6 mg once daily, dose to be taken 30–60 minutes before bedtime; maximum 10 mg per day

SLENYTO®

Insomnia with autism spectrum disorder [where sleep hygiene measures have been insufficient] | Insomnia with Smith-Magenis syndrome [where sleep hygiene measures have been insufficient]

▶ BY MOUTH USING MODIFIED-RELEASE TABLETS

▸ Child 2–17 years: Initially 2 mg once daily, increased if necessary to 5 mg once daily, dose to be taken 30-60 minutes before bedtime; maximum 10 mg per day

- **UNLICENSED USE** [EvGr] Melatonin is used for insomnia in patients with learning disabilities, ⟨E⟩ but is not licensed for this indication.

  Melatonin is used for sleep onset insomnia and delayed sleep phase syndrome, but is not licensed for these indications.
- **CAUTIONS** Autoimmune disease (manufacturer advises avoid—no information available)
- **INTERACTIONS** → Appendix 1: melatonin
- **SIDE-EFFECTS**

▸ **Common or very common** Arthralgia · behaviour abnormal · drowsiness · feeling abnormal · headaches · increased risk of infection · mood altered · pain · sleep disorders

▸ **Uncommon** Anxiety · asthenia · chest pain · dizziness · dry mouth · gastrointestinal discomfort · hyperbilirubinaemia · hypertension · menopausal symptoms · movement disorders · nausea · night sweats · oral disorders · skin reactions · urine abnormalities · weight increased

▸ **Rare or very rare** Angina pectoris · arthritis · concentration impaired · crying · depression · disorientation · electrolyte imbalance · excessive tearing · gastrointestinal disorders · haemorrhage · hot flush · hypertriglyceridaemia · leucopenia · memory loss · muscle complaints · nail disorder · palpitations · paraesthesia · prostatitis · seizures · sexual dysfunction · syncope · thirst · thrombocytopenia · urinary disorders · vertigo · vision disorders · vomiting

▸ **Frequency not known** Angioedema · appetite decreased · constipation · dyspnoea · galactorrhoea · hyperglycaemia · neutropenia

- **PREGNANCY** No information available—avoid.
- **BREAST FEEDING** Present in milk—avoid.
- **HEPATIC IMPAIRMENT** Manufacturer advises avoid (risk of decreased clearance; limited information available).
- **RENAL IMPAIRMENT** No information available—use with caution.
- **DIRECTIONS FOR ADMINISTRATION** Manufacturers advise that modified-release tablets should be taken with or after food. Licensed immediate-release formulations should be taken on an empty stomach, 2 hours before or 2 hours after food—intake with carbohydrate-rich meals may impair blood glucose control.
- **PRESCRIBING AND DISPENSING INFORMATION** Treatment with melatonin should be initiated and supervised by a specialist, but may be continued by general practitioners. The need to continue melatonin therapy should be reviewed every 6 months.

  Melatonin is available as a modified-release tablet (*Circadin*® and *Slenyto*®) and also as immediate-release formulations. *Circadin*® is licensed for the short-term treatment of primary insomnia in adults aged over 55 years, and some immediate-release formulations are licensed for the short-term treatment of jet lag in adults.

Unlicensed preparations are also available, however, there is variability in clinical effect of unlicensed formulations.

The RCPCH and NPPG recommend that, when a liquid special of melatonin is required, the following strength is used: 1 mg/mL.

- **PATIENT AND CARER ADVICE**
Medicines for Children leaflet: Melatonin for sleep disorders www.medicinesforchildren.org.uk/melatonin-sleep-disorders
- **NATIONAL FUNDING/ACCESS DECISIONS**

Scottish Medicines Consortium (SMC) decisions

SMC No. SMC2168

The *Scottish Medicines Consortium* has advised (September 2019) that melatonin prolonged-release (*Slenyto®*) is **not** recommended for use within NHS Scotland for the treatment of insomnia in children aged 2 years and over with autism spectrum disorder and/or Smith-Magenis syndrome, where sleep hygiene measures have been insufficient, as the clinical and economic case was not demonstrated.

All Wales Medicines Strategy Group (AWMSG) decisions

AWMSG No. 3947

The *All Wales Medicines Strategy Group* has advised (November 2019) that melatonin prolonged-release (*Slenyto®*) is **not** recommended for use within NHS Wales for the treatment of insomnia in children aged 2 years and older with autism spectrum disorder and/or Smith Magenis syndrome, where sleep hygiene measures have been insufficient. The case for cost-effectiveness has not been proven.

- **MEDICINAL FORMS** There can be variation in the licensing of different medicines containing the same drug. Forms available from special-order manufacturers include: tablet, modified-release tablet, oral solution

Modified-release tablet

CAUTIONARY AND ADVISORY LABELS 2, 21, 25

- **Melatonin (Non-proprietary)**
Melatonin 3 mg Melatonin 3mg modified-release tablets | 120 tablet PoM
- **Circadin** (Flynn Pharma Ltd)
Melatonin 2 mg Circadin 2mg modified-release tablets | 30 tablet PoM £15.39 DT = £15.39
- **Slenyto** (Flynn Pharma Ltd)
Melatonin 1 mg Slenyto 1mg modified-release tablets | 60 tablet PoM £41.20 DT = £41.20
Melatonin 5 mg Slenyto 5mg modified-release tablets | 30 tablet PoM £103.00 DT = £103.00

7 Substance dependence

Substance dependence

Guidance on treatment of drug misuse

Treatment of alcohol or opioid dependence in children requires specialist management. The UK health departments have produced guidance on the treatment of drug misuse in the UK. *Drug Misuse and Dependence: UK Guidelines on Clinical Management (*2017*)* is available at www.gov.uk/government/publications/drug-misuse-and-dependence-uk-guidelines-on-clinical-management.

Nicotine dependence

See Smoking cessation below.

Neonatal abstinence syndrome

Neonatal abstinence syndrome occurs at birth as a result of intra-uterine exposure to opioids or high-dose benzodiazepines. Treatment is usually initiated if:

- feeding becomes a problem and tube feeding is required;
- there is profuse vomiting or watery diarrhoea;
- the baby remains very unsettled after two consecutive feeds despite gentle swaddling and the use of a pacifier.

Treatment involves weaning the baby from the drug on which it is dependent. Morphine p. 299 or methadone hydrochloride p. 317 can be used in babies of mothers who have been taking opioids. Morphine p. 299 is widely used because the dose can be easily adjusted, but methadone hydrochloride p. 317 may provide smoother control of symptoms. Weaning babies from opioids usually takes 7–10 days.

Weaning babies from benzodiazepines that have a long half-life is difficult to manage; chlorpromazine hydrochloride p. 261 may be used in these situations but excessive sedation may occur. For babies who are dependent on barbiturates, phenobarbital p. 232 may be tried, although it does not control gastro-intestinal symptoms.

7.1 Nicotine dependence

Smoking cessation

14-Aug-2018

Overview

Smoking tobacco is the main cause of preventable illness and premature death in the UK. It is linked to a number of diseases such as cancer (primarily lung cancer), chronic obstructive pulmonary disease, and cardiovascular disease, and can lead to complications during pregnancy. Smoking cessation reduces the risk of developing or worsening of smoking-related illnesses, and the benefits begin as soon as a person stops smoking.

Smoking cessation may be associated with temporary withdrawal symptoms caused by nicotine dependence, making it difficult for people to stop. These symptoms include nicotine cravings, irritability, depression, restlessness, poor concentration, light-headedness, sleep disturbances, and increased appetite. Weight gain is a concern for many people who stop smoking, however it is less likely to occur when drug treatment is used to aid smoking cessation.

Non-drug treatment

EvGr All smokers, including those who smoke e-cigarettes, should be advised to stop smoking and be offered support to facilitate smoking cessation. They should also be advised that stopping in one step ('abrupt quitting') offers the best chance of lasting success, and that a combination of drug treatment and behavioural support is likely to be the most effective approach. ⟨A⟩ 'Abrupt quitting' is when a smoker makes a commitment to stop smoking on or before a particular date (the quit date), rather than by gradually reducing their smoking.

EvGr Smokers who wish to stop smoking should be referred to their local NHS Stop Smoking Services, where they will be provided with advice, drug treatment, and behavioural support options such as individual counselling or group meetings. Smokers who decline to attend their local NHS Stop Smoking Services should be referred to a suitable healthcare professional who can also offer drug treatment and practical advice. ⟨A⟩

Child aged over 12 years

EvGr Nicotine replacement therapy (NRT) is the only drug treatment recommended to aid smoking cessation in children over 12 years of age. A combination of long-acting NRT (transdermal patch) and short-acting NRT (lozenges, gum, sublingual tablets, inhalator, nasal spray and oral spray) may be beneficial in children with a high-level of nicotine dependence, or in those who have previously failed to stop smoking despite NRT treatment. ⟨A⟩ Nicotine transdermal patches are generally applied for 16 hours, with

4 Nervous system

the patch removed overnight; if the child experiences strong nicotine cravings upon waking, a 24 hour patch can be used instead. Short-acting nicotine preparations are used whenever the urge to smoke occurs or to prevent cravings. EvGr As all NRT preparations appear to be equally effective, the choice of preparation for each child should take into consideration the child's likely adherence, preferences, and previous experience of smoking-cessation aids, as well as contra-indications, side-effects, and license of each preparation. Ⓐ Some preparations are not licensed in children under 18 years of age.

EvGr A quit date should be agreed when NRT is prescribed for smoking cessation, and treatment should be available before the child stops smoking. Children should be prescribed enough treatment to last 2 weeks after their agreed quit date, and be re-assessed shortly before the prescription ends.

Children who are unwilling or not ready to stop smoking may also benefit from the use of NRT as part of a 'harm reduction approach', because the amount of nicotine in NRT is much lower and less addictive than in smoking tobacco. Harm reduction approaches include stopping smoking whilst using NRT to prevent relapse, and smoking reduction or temporary abstinence, with or without the use of NRT. These children should be advised that NRT will make it easier to reduce how much they smoke and improve their chance of stopping in the long-term. Ⓐ In the UK, sale of e-cigarettes is prohibited in children under 18 years of age.

Pregnancy

EvGr Pregnant females should be advised to stop smoking completely, and be informed about the risks to the unborn child of smoking during pregnancy, and the harmful effects of exposure to second-hand smoke for both mother and baby. All pregnant females who smoke or have stopped smoking in the last 2 weeks should be referred to their local NHS Stop Smoking Services, and ongoing support should be offered during and following pregnancy. Smoking cessation should also be encouraged for all members of the household. Pregnant females who smoke should be advised to contact the NHS Pregnancy Smoking Helpline for further information (Tel: 0800 169 9169).

NRT should only be used in pregnant females if non-drug treatment options have failed. Clinical judgement should be used when deciding whether to prescribe NRT following a discussion about its risks and benefits. Subsequent prescriptions should only be given to pregnant females who have demonstrated they are still not smoking. Ⓐ

Concomitant drugs

Polycyclic aromatic hydrocarbons found in tobacco smoke increase the metabolism of some drugs by inducing hepatic enzymes, often requiring an increase in dose. Information about drugs interacting with tobacco smoke can be found under *Interactions* of the relevant drug monograph.

Useful Resources

Stop smoking interventions and services. National Institute for Health and Care Excellence. NICE guideline 92. March 2018.
www.nice.org.uk/guidance/ng92

Smoking: harm reduction. National Institute for Health and Care Excellence. Public health guidance 45. June 2013.
www.nice.org.uk/guidance/ph45

National Centre for Smoking Cessation and Training.
www.ncsct.co.uk

NICOTINIC RECEPTOR AGONISTS

Nicotine

● **INDICATIONS AND DOSE**

Nicotine replacement therapy in individuals who smoke fewer than 20 cigarettes each day

▶ BY MOUTH USING CHEWING GUM
▶ Child 12–17 years: 2 mg as required, chew 1 piece of gum when the urge to smoke occurs or to prevent cravings, if attempting smoking cessation, treatment should continue for 3 months before reducing the dose

▶ BY SUBLINGUAL ADMINISTRATION USING SUBLINGUAL TABLETS
▶ Child 12–17 years: 1 tablet every 1 hour, increased to 2 tablets every 1 hour if required, if attempting smoking cessation, treatment should continue for up to 3 months before reducing the dose; maximum 40 tablets per day

Nicotine replacement therapy in individuals who smoke more than 20 cigarettes each day or who require more than 15 pieces of 2-mg strength gum each day

▶ BY MOUTH USING CHEWING GUM
▶ Child 12–17 years: 4 mg as required, chew 1 piece of gum when the urge to smoke occurs or to prevent cravings, individuals should not exceed 15 pieces of 4-mg strength gum daily, if attempting smoking cessation, treatment should continue for 3 months before reducing the dose

Nicotine replacement therapy in individuals who smoke more than 20 cigarettes each day

▶ BY SUBLINGUAL ADMINISTRATION USING SUBLINGUAL TABLETS
▶ Child 12–17 years: 2 tablets every 1 hour, if attempting smoking cessation, treatment should continue for up to 3 months before reducing the dose; maximum 40 tablets per day

Nicotine replacement therapy

▶ BY INHALATION USING INHALATOR
▶ Child 12–17 years: As required, the cartridges can be used when the urge to smoke occurs or to prevent cravings, individuals should not exceed 12 cartridges of the 10-mg strength daily, or 6 cartridges of the 15-mg strength daily

▶ BY MOUTH USING LOZENGES
▶ Child 12–17 years: 1 lozenge every 1–2 hours as required, one lozenge should be used when the urge to smoke occurs, individuals who smoke less than 20 cigarettes each day should usually use the lower-strength lozenges; individuals who smoke more than 20 cigarettes each day and those who fail to stop smoking with the low-strength lozenges should use the higher-strength lozenges; If attempting smoking cessation, treatment should continue for 6–12 weeks before attempting a reduction in dose; maximum 15 lozenges per day

▶ BY MOUTH USING OROMUCOSAL SPRAY
▶ Child 12–17 years: 1–2 sprays as required, individuals can spray in the mouth when the urge to smoke occurs or to prevent cravings, individuals should not exceed 2 sprays per episode (up to 4 sprays every hour); maximum 64 sprays per day

▶ BY INTRANASAL ADMINISTRATION USING NASAL SPRAY
▶ Child 12–17 years: 1 spray as required, individuals can spray into each nostril when the urge to smoke occurs, up to twice every hour for 16 hours daily, if attempting smoking cessation, treatment should continue for 8 weeks before reducing the dose; maximum 64 sprays per day

▶ BY TRANSDERMAL APPLICATION USING PATCHES
▶ Child 12–17 years: Individuals who smoke more than 10 cigarettes daily should apply a high-strength patch daily for 6–8 weeks, followed by the medium-strength

patch for 2 weeks, and then the low-strength patch for the final 2 weeks; individuals who smoke fewer than 10 cigarettes daily can usually start with the medium-strength patch for 6–8 weeks, followed by the low-strength patch for 2–4 weeks; a slower titration schedule can be used in individuals who are not ready to quit but want to reduce cigarette consumption before a quit attempt; if abstinence is not achieved, or if withdrawal symptoms are experienced, the strength of the patch used should be maintained or increased until the patient is stabilised; individuals using the high-strength patch who experience excessive side-effects, that do not resolve within a few days, should change to a medium-strength patch for the remainder of the initial period and then use the low-strength patch for 2–4 weeks

- **UNLICENSED USE** All preparations are licensed for children over 12 years (with the exception of *Nicotinell®* lozenges which are licensed for children under 18 years only when recommended by a doctor).
- **CAUTIONS**

GENERAL CAUTIONS Diabetes mellitus—blood-glucose concentration should be monitored closely when initiating treatment · haemodynamically unstable patients hospitalised with cerebrovascular accident · haemodynamically unstable patients hospitalised with myocardial infarction · haemodynamically unstable patients hospitalised with severe arrhythmias · phaeochromocytoma · uncontrolled hyperthyroidism

SPECIFIC CAUTIONS

- When used by inhalation Bronchospastic disease · chronic throat disease · obstructive lung disease
- With intranasal use Bronchial asthma (may exacerbate)
- With oral use Gastritis (can be aggravated by swallowed nicotine) · *gum* may also stick to and damage dentures · oesophagitis (can be aggravated by swallowed nicotine) · peptic ulcers (can be aggravated by swallowed nicotine)
- With transdermal use *Patches* should not be placed on broken skin · patients with skin disorders

CAUTIONS, FURTHER INFORMATION Most warnings for nicotine replacement therapy also apply to continued cigarette smoking, but the risk of continued smoking outweighs any risks of using nicotine preparations.

Specific cautions for individual preparations are usually related to the local effect of nicotine.

- **SIDE-EFFECTS**

GENERAL SIDE-EFFECTS

- **Common or very common** Dizziness · headache · hyperhidrosis · nausea · palpitations · skin reactions · vomiting
- **Uncommon** Flushing

SPECIFIC SIDE-EFFECTS

- **Common or very common**
- When used by inhalation Asthenia · cough · dry mouth · flatulence · gastrointestinal discomfort · hiccups · hypersensitivity · nasal complaints · oral disorders · taste altered · throat complaints
- With intranasal use Chest discomfort · cough · dyspnoea · epistaxis · nasal complaints · paraesthesia · throat irritation
- With oral use Anxiety · appetite abnormal · burping · diarrhoea · dyspepsia (may be caused by swallowed nicotine) · gastrointestinal disorders · hiccups · increased risk of infection · mood altered · oral disorders · sleep disorders
- With sublingual use Asthenia · cough · dry mouth · flatulence · gastrointestinal discomfort · hiccups · hypersensitivity · oral disorders · rhinitis · taste altered · throat complaints
- **Uncommon**
- When used by inhalation Abnormal dreams · arrhythmias · bronchospasm · burping · chest discomfort · dysphonia · dyspnoea · hypertension · malaise
- With intranasal use Abnormal dreams · asthenia · hypertension · malaise
- With oral use Anger · asthma exacerbated · cough · dyspepsia aggravated · dysphagia · haemorrhage · laryngospasm · nasal complaints · nocturia · numbness · overdose · pain · palpitations exacerbated · peripheral oedema · tachycardia · taste altered · throat complaints · vascular disorders
- With sublingual use Abnormal dreams · arrhythmias · bronchospasm · burping · chest discomfort · dysphonia · dyspnoea · hypertension · malaise · nasal complaints
- With transdermal use Arrhythmias · asthenia · chest discomfort · dyspnoea · hypertension · malaise · myalgia · paraesthesia
- **Rare or very rare**
- When used by inhalation Dysphagia
- With intranasal use Arrhythmias
- With oral use Coagulation disorder · platelet disorder
- With sublingual use Dysphagia
- With transdermal use Abdominal discomfort · angioedema · pain in extremity
- **Frequency not known**
- When used by inhalation Angioedema · excessive tearing · vision blurred
- With intranasal use Abdominal discomfort · angioedema · excessive tearing · oropharyngeal complaints
- With sublingual use Excessive tearing · muscle tightness · vision blurred

SIDE-EFFECTS, FURTHER INFORMATION Some systemic effects occur on initiation of therapy, particularly if the patient is using high-strength preparations; however, the patient may confuse side-effects of the nicotine-replacement preparation with nicotine withdrawal symptoms. Common symptoms of nicotine withdrawal include malaise, headache, dizziness, sleep disturbance, coughing, influenza–like symptoms, depression, irritability, increased appetite, weight gain, restlessness, anxiety, drowsiness, aphthous ulcers, decreased heart rate, and impaired concentration.

- **PREGNANCY** The use of nicotine replacement therapy in pregnancy is preferable to the continuation of smoking, but should be used only if smoking cessation without nicotine replacement fails. Intermittent therapy is preferable to patches but avoid liquorice-flavoured nicotine products. Patches are useful, however, if the patient is experiencing pregnancy-related nausea and vomiting. If patches are used, they should be removed before bed.
- **BREAST FEEDING** Nicotine is present in milk; however, the amount to which the infant is exposed is small and less hazardous than second-hand smoke. Intermittent therapy is preferred.
- **HEPATIC IMPAIRMENT** Manufacturer advises caution in moderate to severe impairment (risk of decreased clearance).
- **RENAL IMPAIRMENT** Use with caution in severe renal impairment.
- **DIRECTIONS FOR ADMINISTRATION** Acidic beverages, such as coffee or fruit juice, may decrease the absorption of nicotine through the buccal mucosa and should be avoided for 15 minutes before the use of oral nicotine replacement therapy.

Administration by transdermal patch Patches should be applied on waking to dry, non-hairy skin on the hip, trunk, or upper arm and held in position for 10–20 seconds to ensure adhesion; place next patch on a different area and avoid using the same site for several days.

Administration by nasal spray Initially 1 spray should be used in both nostrils but when withdrawing from therapy, the dose can be gradually reduced to 1 spray in 1 nostril.
Administration by oral spray The oral spray should be released into the mouth, holding the spray as close to the mouth as possible and avoiding the lips. The patient should not inhale while spraying and avoid swallowing for a few seconds after use. If using the oral spray for the first time, or if unit not used for 2 or more days, prime the unit before administration.
Administration by sublingual tablet Each tablet should be placed under the tongue and allowed to dissolve.
Administration by lozenge Slowly allow each lozenge to dissolve in the mouth; periodically move the lozenge from one side of the mouth to the other. Lozenges last for 10–30 minutes, depending on their size.
Administration by inhalation Insert the cartridge into the device and draw in air through the mouthpiece; each session can last for approximately 5 minutes. The amount of nicotine from 1 puff of the cartridge is less than that from a cigarette, therefore it is necessary to inhale more often than when smoking a cigarette. A single 10 mg cartridge lasts for approximately 20 minutes of intense use; a single 15 mg cartridge lasts for approximately 40 minutes of intense use.
Administration by medicated chewing gum Chew the gum until the taste becomes strong, then rest it between the cheek and gum; when the taste starts to fade, repeat this process. One piece of gum lasts for approximately 30 minutes.

- **PRESCRIBING AND DISPENSING INFORMATION** Flavours of chewing gum and lozenges may include mint, freshfruit, freshmint, icy white, or cherry.
- **PATIENT AND CARER ADVICE** Patient or carers should be given advice on how to administer nicotine chewing gum, inhalators, lozenges, sublingual tablets, oral spray, nasal spray and patches.

- **MEDICINAL FORMS** There can be variation in the licensing of different medicines containing the same drug.

Spray
EXCIPIENTS: May contain Ethanol
▸ Nicorette QuickMist (McNeil Products Ltd)
Nicotine 1 mg per 1 actuation Nicorette QuickMist SmartTrack 1mg/dose mouthspray sugar-free | 13.2 ml [GSL] £11.48 DT = £13.03 sugar-free | 26.4 ml [GSL] £18.50
▸ Brands may include Nicorette, Nicorette QuickMist

Sublingual tablet
CAUTIONARY AND ADVISORY LABELS 26
▸ Nicorette Microtab (McNeil Products Ltd)
Nicotine (as Nicotine cyclodextrin complex) 2 mg Nicorette Microtab 2mg sublingual tablets sugar-free | 100 tablet [GSL] £15.23 DT = £15.23

Transdermal patch
▸ NiQuitin (Omega Pharma Ltd)
Nicotine 7 mg per 24 hour NiQuitin 7mg patches | 7 patch [GSL] £11.48 DT = £9.12
Nicotine 14 mg per 24 hour NiQuitin 14mg patches | 7 patch [GSL] £11.48 DT = £9.40
Nicotine 21 mg per 24 hour NiQuitin 21mg patches | 7 patch [GSL] £11.48 DT = £9.97 | 14 patch [GSL] £18.79
▸ NiQuitin Clear (Omega Pharma Ltd)
Nicotine 7 mg per 24 hour NiQuitin Clear 7mg patches | 7 patch [GSL] £11.48 DT = £9.12
Nicotine 14 mg per 24 hour NiQuitin Clear 14mg patches | 7 patch [GSL] £11.48 DT = £9.40
Nicotine 21 mg per 24 hour NiQuitin Clear 21mg patches | 7 patch [GSL] £11.48 DT = £9.97 | 14 patch [GSL] £18.79
NiQuitin Pre-Quit Clear 21mg patches | 7 patch [GSL] £11.48 DT = £9.97
▸ Nicorette invisi (McNeil Products Ltd)
Nicotine 10 mg per 16 hour Nicorette invisi 10mg/16hours patches | 7 patch [GSL] £10.99 DT = £10.99
Nicotine 15 mg per 16 hour Nicorette invisi 15mg/16hours patches | 7 patch [GSL] £11.10 DT = £11.10
Nicotine 25 mg per 16 hour Nicorette invisi 25mg/16hours patches | 7 patch [GSL] £11.15 DT = £11.15 | 14 patch [GSL] £18.28
▸ Nicotinell TTS (GlaxoSmithKline Consumer Healthcare)
Nicotine 7 mg per 24 hour Nicotinell TTS 10 patches | 7 patch [GSL] £9.12 DT = £9.12
Nicotine 14 mg per 24 hour Nicotinell TTS 20 patches | 7 patch [GSL] £9.40 DT = £9.40
Nicotine 21 mg per 24 hour Nicotinell TTS 30 patches | 7 patch [GSL] £9.97 DT = £9.97 | 21 patch [GSL] £24.51

Medicated chewing-gum
▸ Nicorette (McNeil Products Ltd)
Nicotine 2 mg Nicorette Freshmint 2mg medicated chewing gum sugar-free | 25 piece [GSL] £3.52 sugar-free | 105 piece [GSL] £10.27 sugar-free | 210 piece [GSL] £16.42
Nicorette Fruitfusion 2mg medicated chewing gum sugar-free | 105 piece [GSL] £10.27
Nicorette Original 2mg medicated chewing gum sugar-free | 105 piece [GSL] £10.27 sugar-free | 210 piece [GSL] £16.42
Nicotine 4 mg Nicorette Fruitfusion 4mg medicated chewing gum sugar-free | 105 piece [GSL] £12.57
Nicorette Original 4mg medicated chewing gum sugar-free | 105 piece [GSL] £12.56 sugar-free | 210 piece [GSL] £20.28
Nicorette Freshmint 4mg medicated chewing gum sugar-free | 25 piece [GSL] £3.53 sugar-free | 105 piece [GSL] £12.56 sugar-free | 210 piece [GSL] £20.28
▸ Nicorette Icy White (McNeil Products Ltd)
Nicotine 2 mg Nicorette Icy White 2mg medicated chewing gum sugar-free | 25 piece [GSL] £3.52 sugar-free | 105 piece [GSL] £10.26 sugar-free | 210 piece [GSL] £16.41
Nicotine 4 mg Nicorette Icy White 4mg medicated chewing gum sugar-free | 105 piece [GSL] £12.55
▸ Nicotinell (GlaxoSmithKline Consumer Healthcare)
Nicotine 2 mg Nicotinell Mint 2mg medicated chewing gum sugar-free | 96 piece [GSL] £8.26 DT = £8.26 sugar-free | 204 piece [GSL] £14.23
Nicotinell Fruit 2mg medicated chewing gum sugar-free | 96 piece [GSL] £8.26 DT = £8.26 sugar-free | 204 piece [GSL] £14.23
Nicotine 4 mg Nicotinell Mint 4mg medicated chewing gum sugar-free | 96 piece [GSL] £10.26 DT = £10.26
Nicotinell Fruit 4mg medicated chewing gum sugar-free | 96 piece [GSL] £10.26 DT = £10.26

Lozenge
EXCIPIENTS: May contain Aspartame
ELECTROLYTES: May contain Sodium
▸ NiQuitin (Omega Pharma Ltd)
Nicotine 1.5 mg NiQuitin Minis Mint 1.5mg lozenges sugar-free | 20 lozenge [GSL] £4.14 sugar-free | 60 lozenge [GSL] £10.85 DT = £10.85 sugar-free | 100 lozenge [GSL] £14.04
Nicotine 2 mg NiQuitin Mint 2mg lozenges sugar-free | 72 lozenge [GSL] £7.40 DT = £7.40
Nicotine 4 mg NiQuitin Mint 4mg lozenges sugar-free | 36 lozenge [GSL] £5.91 sugar-free | 72 lozenge [GSL] £7.40 DT = £7.40
NiQuitin Minis Mint 4mg lozenges sugar-free | 20 lozenge [GSL] £4.14 sugar-free | 60 lozenge [GSL] £10.85 sugar-free | 100 lozenge [GSL] £14.04
▸ Nicorette (McNeil Products Ltd)
Nicotine 2 mg Nicorette Fruit 2mg lozenges sugar-free | 80 lozenge [GSL] £12.05
Nicorette Cools 2mg lozenges sugar-free | 20 lozenge [GSL] £3.34 sugar-free | 80 lozenge [GSL] £12.05
Nicotine 4 mg Nicorette Cools 4mg lozenges sugar-free | 80 lozenge [GSL] £12.17
▸ Nicotinell (GlaxoSmithKline Consumer Healthcare)
Nicotine (as Nicotine bitartrate) 1 mg Nicotinell 1mg lozenges sugar-free | 12 lozenge [GSL] £1.59 sugar-free | 96 lozenge [GSL] £9.12 DT = £9.12 sugar-free | 144 lozenge [GSL] £11.48 sugar-free | 204 lozenge [GSL] £12.77
Nicotine (as Nicotine bitartrate) 2 mg Nicotinell 2mg lozenges sugar-free | 96 lozenge [GSL] £10.60 sugar-free | 144 lozenge [GSL] £13.50 sugar-free | 204 lozenge [GSL] £14.94

Inhalation vapour
▸ Nicorette (McNeil Products Ltd)
Nicotine 15 mg Nicorette 15mg Inhalator | 4 cartridge [GSL] £4.87 DT = £4.87 | 20 cartridge [GSL] £17.78 DT = £17.78 | 36 cartridge [GSL] £28.28 DT = £28.28

7.2 Opioid dependence

ANALGESICS > OPIOIDS

F 290

Methadone hydrochloride 04-Dec-2019

- **INDICATIONS AND DOSE**

Neonatal opioid withdrawal

▶ BY MOUTH

▶ Neonate: Initially 100 micrograms/kg, then increased in steps of 50 micrograms/kg every 6 hours until symptoms are controlled, doses may vary, consult local guidelines, for maintenance, total daily dose that controls symptoms to be given in 2 divided doses.

DOSE EQUIVALENCE AND CONVERSION

▶ See buprenorphine p. 291 for dose adjustments in opioid substitution therapy, for patients taking methadone who want to switch to buprenorphine.

- **UNLICENSED USE** Not licensed for use in children.

IMPORTANT SAFETY INFORMATION

Many preparations of Methadone oral solution are licensed for opioid drug addiction only but some are also licensed for analgesia in severe pain.

- **CONTRA-INDICATIONS** Phaeochromocytoma
- **CAUTIONS** Family history of sudden death (ECG monitoring recommended) · history of cardiac conduction abnormalities

CAUTIONS, FURTHER INFORMATION

▶ QT-interval prolongation Patients with the following risk factors for QT-interval prolongation should be carefully monitored while taking methadone: heart or liver disease, electrolyte abnormalities, or concomitant treatment with drugs that can prolong QT interval; patients requiring more than 100 mg daily should also be monitored.

- **INTERACTIONS** → Appendix 1: opioids
- **SIDE-EFFECTS** Dry eye · dysuria · hyperprolactinaemia · hypothermia · intracranial pressure increased · mood altered · nasal dryness · QT interval prolongation

SIDE-EFFECTS, FURTHER INFORMATION Methadone is a long-acting opioid therefore effects may be cumulative.

Methadone, even in low doses is a special hazard for children; non-dependent adults are also at risk of toxicity; dependent adults are at risk if tolerance is incorrectly assessed during induction.

Overdose Methadone has a very long duration of action; patients may need to be monitored for long periods following large overdoses.

- **BREAST FEEDING** Withdrawal symptoms in infant; breast-feeding permissible during maintenance but dose should be as low as possible and infant monitored to avoid sedation (high doses of methadone carry an increased risk of sedation and respiratory depression in the neonate).
- **HEPATIC IMPAIRMENT** Manufacturer advises caution; consider avoiding in severe impairment (risk of increased exposure).

Dose adjustments Manufacturer advises consider dose reduction.

- **RENAL IMPAIRMENT** Avoid use or reduce dose; opioid effects increased and prolonged and increased cerebral sensitivity occurs.
- **TREATMENT CESSATION** Avoid abrupt withdrawal.

▶ In neonates When used for neonatal opioid withdraw, reduce dose over 7–10 days.

- **DIRECTIONS FOR ADMINISTRATION** Syrup preserved with hydroxybenzoate (parabens) esters may be incompatible with methadone hydrochloride.
- **PRESCRIBING AND DISPENSING INFORMATION** Flavours of oral liquid formulations may include tolu.

METHADOSE® The final strength of the methadone mixture to be dispensed to the patient must be specified on the prescription.

Important—care is required in prescribing and dispensing the **correct strength** since any confusion could lead to an overdose; this preparation should be dispensed only **after dilution** as appropriate with *Methadose®* Diluent (life of diluted solution 3 months) and is for drug dependent persons.

- **MEDICINAL FORMS** There can be variation in the licensing of different medicines containing the same drug. Forms available from special-order manufacturers include: tablet, capsule, oral suspension, oral solution

Tablet

CAUTIONARY AND ADVISORY LABELS 2

▶ **Physeptone** (Martindale Pharmaceuticals Ltd)

Methadone hydrochloride 5 mg Physeptone 5mg tablets | 50 tablet PoM £2.84 DT = £2.84 CD2

Oral solution

CAUTIONARY AND ADVISORY LABELS 2

▶ **Methadone hydrochloride (Non-proprietary)**

Methadone hydrochloride 1 mg per 1 ml Methadone 1mg/ml oral solution | 100 ml PoM £1.08–£1.20 DT = £1.08 CD2 | 500 ml PoM £4.30–£7.11 DT = £5.40 CD2 | 2500 ml PoM £27.00–£32.10 CD2

Methadone 1mg/ml oral solution sugar free sugar-free | 50 ml PoM £1.00 CD2 sugar-free | 100 ml PoM £1.20 DT = £1.09 CD2 sugar-free | 500 ml PoM £4.30–£7.14 DT = £5.45 CD2 sugar-free | 2500 ml PoM £27.25–£32.10 CD2

▶ **Methadose** (Rosemont Pharmaceuticals Ltd)

Methadone hydrochloride 10 mg per 1 ml Methadose 10mg/ml oral solution concentrate sugar-free | 150 ml PoM £12.01 DT = £12.01 CD2 sugar-free | 500 ml PoM £30.75 CD2

Methadone hydrochloride 20 mg per 1 ml Methadose 20mg/ml oral solution concentrate sugar-free | 150 ml PoM £24.02 DT = £24.02 CD2

▶ **Metharose** (Rosemont Pharmaceuticals Ltd)

Methadone hydrochloride 1 mg per 1 ml Metharose 1mg/ml oral solution sugar free sugar-free | 500 ml PoM £6.82 DT = £5.45 CD2

▶ **Physeptone** (Martindale Pharmaceuticals Ltd)

Methadone hydrochloride 1 mg per 1 ml Physeptone 1mg/ml oral solution sugar free sugar-free | 100 ml PoM £1.27 DT = £1.09 CD2 sugar-free | 500 ml PoM £6.42 DT = £5.45 CD2 sugar-free | 2500 ml PoM £32.10 CD2

Physeptone 1mg/ml mixture | 100 ml PoM £1.27 DT = £1.08 CD2 | 500 ml PoM £6.42 DT = £5.40 CD2 | 2500 ml PoM £32.10 CD2

Chapter 5 Infection

CONTENTS

1 Bacterial infection

Antibacterials, principles of therapy

25-Mar-2020

Antibacterial drug choice

Before selecting an antibacterial the clinician must first consider three factors— the patient, the known or likely causative organism, and the risk of bacterial resistance with repeated courses.

Factors related to the patient which must be considered include history of allergy, renal and hepatic function, susceptibility to infection (i.e. whether immunocompromised), ability to tolerate drugs by mouth, severity of illness, risk of complications, ethnic origin, age, whether taking other medication and, if female, whether pregnant, breast-feeding or taking an oral contraceptive.

The known or likely organism and its antibacterial sensitivity, in association with the factors above, will provide one or more antibacterial option. [EvGr] In children receiving antibacterial prophylaxis, an antibacterial from a different class should be used. ⟨A⟩

Some children may be at higher risk of treatment failure. They include those who have had repeated antibacterial courses, a previous or current culture with resistant bacteria, or those at higher risk of developing complications.

Antibacterials, considerations before starting therapy

The following precepts should be considered before starting:

- Viral infections should not be treated with antibacterials. However, antibacterials may be used to treat secondary bacterial infection (e.g. bacterial pneumonia secondary to influenza);
- Samples should be taken for culture and sensitivity testing as appropriate; '**blind**' antibacterial prescribing for unexplained pyrexia usually leads to further difficulty in establishing the diagnosis;
- Knowledge of **prevalent organisms** and their current sensitivity is of great help in choosing an antibacterial before bacteriological confirmation is available. Generally, narrow-spectrum antibacterials are preferred to broad-spectrum antibacterials unless there is a clear clinical indication (e.g. life-threatening sepsis);
- The **dose** of an antibacterial varies according to a number of factors including age, weight, hepatic function, renal function, and severity of infection. The prescribing of the so-called 'standard' dose in serious infections may result in failure of treatment or even death of the patient; therefore it is important to prescribe a dose appropriate to the condition. An inadequate dose may also increase the likelihood of antibacterial resistance. On the other hand, for an antibacterial with a narrow margin between the toxic and therapeutic dose (e.g. an aminoglycoside) it is also important to avoid an excessive dose and the concentration of the drug in the plasma may need to be monitored;
- The **route** of administration of an antibacterial often depends on the severity of the infection. Life-threatening infections often require intravenous therapy. Antibacterials that are well absorbed may be given by mouth even for some serious infections. Parenteral administration is also appropriate when the oral route cannot be used (e.g. because of vomiting) or if absorption is inadequate (e.g. in neonates and young children). Whenever possible, painful intramuscular injections should be avoided in children;
- **Duration** of therapy depends on the nature of the infection and the response to treatment. Courses should not be unduly prolonged because they encourage resistance, they may lead to side-effects and they are costly. However, in certain infections such as tuberculosis or osteomyelitis it may be necessary to treat for prolonged periods. The prescription for an antibacterial should specify the duration of treatment or the date when treatment is to be reviewed.

For further guidance on the appropriate and effective use of antibacterials, see Antimicrobial stewardship p. 27

Advice to be given to children and their parents and/or carers

If an antibacterial is given, advice should be given about directions for correct use and possible side-effects using verbal and written information.

If an antibacterial is **not** given, advice should be given about an antibacterial not being needed currently—discuss alternative options as appropriate, such as self-care with over-the-counter preparations, back-up (delayed) prescribing, or other non-pharmacological interventions.

Children and their parents, or carers should be advised to seek medical help if symptoms worsen rapidly or significantly at any time, if symptoms do not start to improve within an agreed time, if problems arise as a result of treatment, or if the child becomes systemically very unwell.

For information on advice for children and their family and/or carers when deciding if antibacterial treatment is necessary, see *Advice for patients and their family and/or carers* in Antimicrobial stewardship p. 27.

Antibacterials, considerations during therapy

EvGr Review choice of antibacterial if susceptibility results indicate bacterial resistance and symptoms are not improving—consult local microbiologist as needed. (A) If no bacterium is cultured, the antibacterial can be continued or stopped on clinical grounds.

Superinfection

In general, broad-spectrum antibacterial drugs such as the cephalosporins are more likely to be associated with adverse reactions related to the selection of resistant organisms e.g. *fungal infections* or *antibiotic-associated colitis* (pseudomembranous colitis); other problems associated with superinfection include vaginitis and pruritus ani.

Antibacterials, switching from parenteral to oral treatment

EvGr The ongoing parenteral administration of an antibacterial should be reviewed within 48 hours of treatment initiation and a switch to oral treatment considered if appropriate. (A) In older children it may be possible to switch to an oral antibacterial; in neonates and infants this should be done more cautiously because of the relatively high incidence of bacteraemia and the possibility of variable oral absorption.

Antibacterials for prophylaxis

In most situations, only a short course of prophylactic antibacterial is needed. Longer-term antibacterial prophylaxis is appropriate in specific indications such as vesico-ureteric reflux.

Notifiable diseases

Registered medical practitioners must notify the Proper Officer at their local council or local health protection team of any patient(s) suspected of suffering from any of the diseases listed below; a notification form should be completed immediately. For further information on reporting notifiable diseases, see **Public Health England** guidance at: www.gov.uk/guidance/notifiable-diseases-and-causative-organisms-how-to-report.

Anthrax	Mumps
Botulism	Paratyphoid fever
Brucellosis	Plague
Cholera	Poliomyelitis, acute
Diarrhoea (infectious bloody)	Rabies
Diphtheria	Rubella
Encephalitis, acute	SARS
Food poisoning	Scarlet fever
Haemolytic uraemic syndrome	Smallpox
Haemorrhagic fever (viral)	Streptococcal disease (Group A, invasive)
Hepatitis, viral	
Legionnaires' disease	Tetanus
Leprosy	Tuberculosis
Malaria	Typhoid fever
Measles	Typhus
Meningitis	Whooping cough
Meningococcal septicaemia	Yellow fever

Note It is good practice for registered medical practitioners to also report other diseases that may present a significant risk to human health. These should be done under the category 'other significant disease'.

Sepsis, early management

EvGr Children identified as being at high risk of severe illness or death due to suspected sepsis should be given a broad-spectrum antibacterial at the maximum recommended dose without delay (ideally within one hour). Microbiological samples and blood cultures must be taken prior to administration of antibiotics; the prescription should be adjusted subsequently according to susceptibility results.

A thorough clinical examination should be carried out to identify sources of infection. If the cause of infection is identified, treat in line with local antibacterial guidance or susceptibility results.

Children aged up to 17 years with suspected community-acquired sepsis of any cause should be treated with ceftriaxone p. 343. If the child is already in hospital or is known to have previously been infected or colonised with ceftriaxone-resistant bacteria, an alternative antibiotic should be chosen following local guidelines. Children younger than 3 months should also receive an additional antibiotic that is active against *listeria* (such as ampicillin p. 368 or amoxicillin p. 366).

Neonates who are in hospital with suspected sepsis within 72 hours of birth, should be treated with intravenous benzylpenicillin sodium p. 364 and gentamicin p. 333. Community-acquired sepsis in neonates (who are more than 40 weeks corrected gestational age) should be treated with ceftriaxone, unless already receiving an intravenous calcium infusion. Neonates aged 40 weeks corrected gestational age or below, or receiving an intravenous calcium infusion, should receive cefotaxime p. 342, dosed according to age.

The need for intravenous fluids, inotropes, vasopressors and oxygen should also be assessed without delay, taking into consideration the child's lactate concentration, systolic blood pressure (in children over 12 years) and their risk of severe illness or death. Children at high risk should be monitored continuously if possible, and no less than every 30 minutes.

Children with suspected sepsis who are not immediately deemed to be at high risk of severe illness or death, should be re-assessed regularly for the need for empirical treatment, taking into consideration all risk factors including lactate concentration and evidence of acute kidney injury. (A)

Antibacterials, use for prophylaxis

16-Mar-2017

Rheumatic fever: prevention of reccurence

- Phenoxymethylpenicillin p. 365 by mouth *or* erythromycin p. 355 by mouth.

Invasive group A streptococcal infection: prevention of secondary cases

- Phenoxymethylpenicillin by mouth.

If child penicillin allergic, *either* erythromycin by mouth or azithromycin p. 352 by mouth [unlicensed indication].

For details of those who should receive chemoprophylaxis contact a consultant in communicable disease control (or a consultant in infectious diseases or the local Public Health England Laboratory).

Meningococcal meningitis: prevention of secondary cases

- Ciprofloxacin p. 377 by mouth [unlicensed indication] *or* rifampicin p. 396 by mouth *or* ceftriaxone p. 343 by intramuscular injection [unlicensed indication].

For details of those who should receive chemoprophylaxis contact a consultant in communicable disease control (or a consultant in infectious diseases or the local Public Health England laboratory). Unless there has been direct exposure of the mouth or nose to infectious droplets from a patient with meningococcal disease who has received less than 24 hours of antibacterial treatment, healthcare workers do not generally require chemoprophylaxis.

Haemophilus influenzae type b disease: prevention of secondary cases

- Rifampicin by mouth *or* (if rifampicin cannot be used) ceftriaxone by intramuscular injection, or by intravenous injection, or by intravenous infusion [unlicensed indication].

For details of those who should receive chemoprophylaxis contact a consultant in communicable disease control (or a consultant in infectious diseases or the local Public Health England laboratory). Unless there has been direct exposure of the mouth or nose to infectious droplets from a patient with meningococcal disease who has received less than 24 hours of antibacterial treatment, healthcare workers do not generally require chemoprophylaxis.

Within 4 weeks of illness onset in an index case with confirmed or suspected invasive *Haemophilus influenzae* type b disease, give antibacterial prophylaxis to all household contacts if there is a vulnerable individual in the household. Also, give antibacterial prophylaxis to the index case if they are in contact with vulnerable household contacts or if they are under 10 years of age. Vulnerable individuals include the immunocompromised, those with asplenia, or children under 10 years of age. If there are 2 or more cases of invasive *Haemophilus influenzae* type b disease within 120 days in a pre-school or primary school, antibacterial prophylaxis should also be given to all room contacts (including staff). Also see immunisation against *Haemophilus influenzae* type b disease.

Diphtheria in non-immune patients: prevention of secondary cases

- Erythromycin (*or* another macrolide e.g. azithromycin *or* clarithromycin p. 353) by mouth.

Treat for further 10 days if nasopharyngeal swabs positive after first 7 days' treatment.

Pertussis, antibacterial prophylaxis

- Clarithromycin (*or* azithromycin *or* erythromycin) by mouth.

Within 3 weeks of onset of cough in the index case, give antibacterial prophylaxis to all close contacts if amongst them there is at least one unimmunised or partially immunised child under 1 year of age, *or* if there is at least one individual who has not received a pertussis-containing vaccine more than 1 week and less than 5 years ago (so long as that individual lives or works with children under 4 months of age, is pregnant at over 32 weeks gestation, or is a healthcare worker who works with children under 1 year of age or with pregnant women).

Pneumococcal infection in asplenia or in patients with sickle-cell disease, antibacterial prophylaxis

- Phenoxymethylpenicillin by mouth.

If cover also needed for *H. influenzae* in child give amoxicillin p. 366 instead.

If penicillin-allergic, erythromycin by mouth.

Antibacterial prophylaxis is not fully reliable. Antibacterial prophylaxis may be discontinued in children over 5 years of age with sickle-cell disease who have received pneumococcal immunisation and who do not have a history of severe pneumococcal infection.

Staphylococcus aureus lung infection in cystic fibrosis, antibacterial prophylaxis

- *Primary prevention*, flucloxacillin p. 373 by mouth.
  Secondary prevention, flucloxacillin by mouth.

Tuberculosis antibacterial prophylaxis in susceptible close contacts or those who have become tuberculin positive

- See *Close contacts* and *Treatment of latent tuberculosis* under Tuberculosis p. 392.

Animal and human bites, antibacterial prophylaxis

- Co-amoxiclav p. 370 alone (*or* clindamycin p. 351 if penicillin-allergic).

Cleanse wound thoroughly. For tetanus-prone wound, give human tetanus immunoglobulin p. 826 (with a tetanus-containing vaccine if necessary, according to immunisation history and risk of infection).

Consider rabies prophylaxis for bites from animals in endemic countries. Assess risk of blood-borne viruses (including HIV, hepatitis B and C) and give appropriate prophylaxis to prevent viral spread. Antibacterial prophylaxis recommended for wounds less than 48–72 hours old when the risk of infection is high (e.g. bites from humans or cats; bites to the hand, foot, face, or genital area; bites involving oedema, crush or puncture injury, or other moderate to severe injury; wounds that cannot be debrided adequately; patients with diabetes mellitus, cirrhosis, asplenia, prosthetic joints or valves, or those who are immunocompromised). Give antibacterial prophylaxis for up to 5 days.

Gastro-intestinal procedures, antibacterial prophylaxis

Operations on stomach or oesophagus

- Single dose of i/v gentamicin p. 333 *or* i/v cefuroxime p. 341 *or* i/v co-amoxiclav (additional intra-operative or postoperative doses may be given for prolonged procedures or if there is major blood loss).

Intravenous antibacterial prophylaxis should be given up to 30 minutes before the procedure.

Add i/v teicoplanin p. 348 (*or* vancomycin p. 349) if high risk of meticillin-resistant *Staphylococcus aureus*.

Open biliary surgery

- Single dose of i/v cefuroxime + i/v metronidazole p. 358 *or* i/v gentamicin + i/v metronidazole *or* i/v co-amoxiclav alone (additional intra-operative or postoperative doses may be given for prolonged procedures or if there is major blood loss).

Intravenous antibacterial prophylaxis should be given up to 30 minutes before the procedure.

Where i/v metronidazole is suggested, it may alternatively be given by suppository but to allow adequate absorption, it should be given 2 hours before surgery.

Add i/v teicoplanin (*or* vancomycin) if high risk of meticillin-resistant *Staphylococcus aureus*.

Resections of colon and rectum, and resections in inflammatory bowel disease, and appendicectomy

- Single dose of i/v gentamicin + i/v metronidazole *or* i/v cefuroxime + i/v metronidazole *or* i/v co-amoxiclav alone (additional intra-operative or postoperative doses may be given for prolonged procedures or if there is major blood loss).

Intravenous antibacterial prophylaxis should be given up to 30 minutes before the procedure.

Where i/v metronidazole is suggested, it may alternatively be given by suppository but to allow adequate absorption, it should be given 2 hours before surgery.

Add i/v teicoplanin (*or* vancomycin) if high risk of meticillin-resistant *Staphylococcus aureus*.

Endoscopic retrograde cholangiopancreatography

- Single dose of i/v gentamicin p. 333 *or* oral *or* i/v ciprofloxacin p. 377.

Intravenous antibacterial prophylaxis should be given up to 30 minutes before the procedure.

Prophylaxis recommended if pancreatic pseudocyst, immunocompromised, history of liver transplantation, or risk of incomplete biliary drainage. For biliary complications following liver transplantation, add i/v amoxicillin p. 366 or i/v teicoplanin p. 348 (*or* vancomycin p. 349).

Percutaneous endoscopic gastrostomy or jejunostomy

- Single dose of i/v co-amoxiclav p. 370 or i/v cefuroxime p. 341.

Intravenous antibacterial prophylaxis should be given up to 30 minutes before the procedure.

Use single dose of i/v teicoplanin (*or* vancomycin) if history of allergy to penicillins or cephalosporins, or if high risk of meticillin-resistant *Staphylococcus aureus*.

Orthopaedic surgery, antibacterial prophylaxis

Closed fractures

- Single dose of i/v cefuroxime *or* i/v flucloxacillin p. 373 (additional intra-operative or postoperative doses may be given for prolonged procedures or if there is major blood loss).

Intravenous antibacterial prophylaxis should be given up to 30 minutes before the procedure.

If history of allergy to penicillins or to cephalosporins or if high risk of meticillin-resistant *Staphylococcus aureus*, use single dose of i/v teicoplanin (*or* vancomycin) (additional intra-operative or postoperative doses may be given for prolonged procedures or if there is major blood loss).

Open fractures

- Use i/v co-amoxiclav alone *or* i/v cefuroxime + i/v metronidazole p. 358 (*or* i/v clindamycin p. 351 alone if history of allergy to penicillins or to cephalosporins).

Add i/v teicoplanin (*or* vancomycin) if high risk of meticillin-resistant *Staphylococcus aureus*. Start prophylaxis within 3 hours of injury and continue until soft tissue closure (max. 72 hours).

At first debridement also use a single dose of i/v cefuroxime + i/v metronidazole + i/v gentamicin *or* i/v co-amoxiclav + i/v gentamicin (*or* i/v clindamycin + i/v gentamicin if history of allergy to penicillins or to cephalosporins).

At time of skeletal stabilisation and definitive soft tissue closure use a single dose of i/v gentamicin and i/v teicoplanin (*or* vancomycin) (intravenous antibacterial prophylaxis should be given up to 30 minutes before the procedure.

High lower-limb amputation

- Use i/v co-amoxiclav alone *or* i/v cefuroxime + i/v metronidazole.

Intravenous antibacterial prophylaxis should be given up to 30 minutes before the procedure.

Continue antibacterial prophylaxis for at least 2 doses after procedure (max. duration of prophylaxis 5 days). If history of allergy to penicillin or to cephalosporins, or if high risk of meticillin-resistant *Staphylococcus aureus*, use i/v teicoplanin (*or* vancomycin) + i/v gentamicin + i/v metronidazole.

Where i/v metronidazole is suggested, it may alternatively be given by suppository but to allow adequate absorption, it should be given 2 hours before surgery.

Obstetric surgery, antibacterial prophylaxis

Termination of pregnancy

- Single dose of oral metronidazole (additional intra-operative or postoperative doses may be given for prolonged procedures or if there is major blood loss).

If genital chlamydial infection cannot be ruled out, give doxycycline p. 381 postoperatively.

Infective endocarditis, antibacterial prophylaxis

NICE guidance: Antimicrobial prophylaxis against infective endocarditis in adults and children undergoing interventional procedures (March 2008, updated 2016)

- Chlorhexidine mouthwash is **not** recommended for the prevention of infective endocarditis in at risk children undergoing dental procedures.

Antibacterial prophylaxis is **not***routinely* recommended for the prevention of infective endocarditis in children undergoing the following procedures:

- dental;
- upper and lower respiratory tract (including ear, nose, and throat procedures and bronchoscopy);
- genito-urinary tract (including urological, gynaecological, and obstetric procedures);
- upper and lower gastro-intestinal tract.

While these procedures can cause bacteraemia, there is no clear association with the development of infective endocarditis. Prophylaxis may expose children to the adverse effects of antimicrobials when the evidence of benefit has not been proven.

Any infection in children at risk of endocarditis should be investigated promptly and treated appropriately to reduce the risk of endocarditis.

If children at risk of infective endocarditis are undergoing a gastro-intestinal or genito-urinary tract procedure at a site where infection is suspected, they should receive appropriate antibacterial therapy that includes cover against organisms that cause endocarditis.

Children at risk of infective endocarditis should be:

- advised to maintain good oral hygiene;
- told how to recognise signs of infective endocarditis, and advised when to seek expert advice.

Patients at risk of infective endocarditis include those with valve replacement, acquired valvular heart disease with stenosis or regurgitation, structural congenital heart disease (including surgically corrected or palliated structural conditions, but excluding isolated atrial septal defect, fully repaired ventricular septal defect, fully repaired patent ductus arteriosus, and closure devices considered to be endothelialised), hypertrophic cardiomyopathy, or a previous episode of infective endocarditis.

Dermatological procedures

Advice of a Working Party of the British Society for Antimicrobial Chemotherapy is that patients who undergo dermatological procedures do not require antibacterial prophylaxis against endocarditis.

The British Association of Dermatologists Therapy Guidelines and Audit Subcommittee advise that such dermatological procedures include skin biopsies and excision of moles or of malignant lesions.

Joint prostheses and dental treatment, antibacterial prophylaxis

Advice of a Working Party of the British Society for Antimicrobial Chemotherapy is that patients with prosthetic joint implants (including total hip replacements) do not require antibacterial prophylaxis for dental treatment. The Working Party considers that it is unacceptable to expose patients to the adverse effects of antibacterials when there is no evidence that such prophylaxis is of any benefit, but that those who develop any intercurrent infection require prompt treatment with antibacterials to which the infecting organisms are sensitive.

The Working Party has commented that joint infections have rarely been shown to follow dental procedures and are even more rarely caused by oral streptococci.

Immunosuppression and indwelling intraperitoneal catheters

Advice of a Working Party of the British Society for Antimicrobial Chemotherapy is that patients who are immunosuppressed (including transplant patients) and patients with indwelling intraperitoneal catheters do not require antibacterial prophylaxis for dental treatment provided there is no other indication for prophylaxis.

The Working Party has commented that there is little evidence that dental treatment is followed by infection in immunosuppressed and immunodeficient patients nor is there evidence that dental treatment is followed by infection in patients with indwelling intraperitoneal catheters.

Blood infections, antibacterial therapy

Septicaemia (community-acquired)

- *Child 1 month–18 years*, aminoglycoside + amoxicillin p. 366 (*or* ampicillin p. 368) *or* cefotaxime p. 342 (*or* ceftriaxone p. 343) alone
- ▸ If pseudomonas or resistant micro-organisms suspected, use a broad-spectrum antipseudomonal beta-lactam antibacterial.
- ▸ If anaerobic infection suspected, add metronidazole p. 358.
- ▸ If Gram-positive infection suspected, add flucloxacillin p. 373 *or* vancomycin p. 349 (*or* teicoplanin p. 348).
- ▸ *Suggested duration of treatment* at least 5 days.

Septicaemia (hospital-acquired)

- *Child 1 month–18 years*, a broad-spectrum antipseudomonal beta-lactam antibacterial (e.g. piperacillin with tazobactam p. 362, ticarcillin with clavulanic acid p. 363, imipenem with cilastatin p. 336, *or* meropenem p. 337)
- ▸ If pseudomonas suspected, or if multiple-resistant organisms suspected, or if severe sepsis, add aminoglycoside.
- ▸ If meticillin-resistant *Staphylococcus aureus* suspected, add vancomycin (*or* teicoplanin).
- ▸ If anaerobic infection suspected, add metronidazole to a broad-spectrum cephalosporin.
- ▸ *Suggested duration of treatment* at least 5 days.

Septicaemia related to vascular catheter

- Vancomycin (*or* teicoplanin)
- ▸ If Gram-negative sepsis suspected, especially in the immunocompromised, add a broad-spectrum antipseudomonal beta-lactam.
- ▸ Consider removing vascular catheter, particularly if infection caused by *Staphylococcus aureus*, pseudomonas, or *Candida* species.

Meningococcal septicaemia

If meningococcal disease suspected, a single dose of benzylpenicillin sodium p. 364 should be given before urgent transfer to hospital, so long as this does not delay the transfer; cefotaxime may be an alternative in penicillin allergy; chloramphenicol p. 385 may be used if history of immediate hypersensitivity reaction to penicillin or to cephalosporins.

- Benzylpenicillin sodium or cefotaxime (*or* ceftriaxone)
- *If history of immediate hypersensitivity reaction to penicillin or to cephalosporins*, chloramphenicol

To eliminate nasopharyngeal carriage, ciprofloxacin p. 377, or rifampicin p. 396, or ceftriaxone may be used.

Septicaemia in neonates

- *Neonate less than 72 hours old*, benzylpenicillin sodium + gentamicin p. 333
- ▸ If Gram-negative septicaemia suspected, use benzylpenicillin sodium + gentamicin + cefotaxime; stop benzylpenicillin sodium if Gram-negative infection confirmed.
- ▸ *Suggested duration of treatment* usually 7 days.
- *Neonate more than 72 hours old*, flucloxacillin + gentamicin *or* amoxicillin (*or* ampicillin) + cefotaxime
- ▸ *Suggested duration of treatment* usually 7 days.

Cardiovascular system infections, antibacterial therapy

Endocarditis: initial 'blind' therapy

- Flucloxacillin p. 373 (*or* benzylpenicillin sodium p. 364 if symptoms less severe) + gentamicin p. 333
- *If cardiac prostheses present, or if penicillin-allergic, or if meticillin-resistant Staphylococcus aureus suspected*, vancomycin p. 349 + rifampicin p. 396 + gentamicin

Endocarditis caused by staphylococci

- Flucloxacillin
- ▸ Add rifampicin for at least 2 weeks in prosthetic valve endocarditis
- ▸ *Suggested duration of treatment* at least 4 weeks (at least 6 weeks for prosthetic valve endocarditis)
- *If penicillin-allergic or if meticillin-resistantStaphylococcus aureus*, vancomycin + rifampicin
- ▸ *Suggested duration of treatment* at least 4 weeks (at least 6 weeks for prosthetic valve endocarditis)

Endocarditis (native valve) caused by fully-sensitive streptococci e.g. viridans streptococci

- Benzylpenicillin sodium
- ▸ *Suggested duration of treatment* 4 weeks
- *Alternative if a large vegetation, intracardial abscess, or infected emboli are absent*, benzylpenicillin sodium + gentamicin
- ▸ *Suggested duration of treatment* 2 weeks
- *If penicillin-allergic*, vancomycin
- ▸ *Suggested duration of treatment* 4 weeks

Endocarditis (native valve) caused by less-sensitive streptococci

- Benzylpenicillin sodium + gentamicin
- ▸ *Suggested duration of treatment* 4–6 weeks (stop gentamicin after 2 weeks for micro-organisms moderately sensitive to penicillin)
- *If aminoglycoside cannot be used and if streptococci moderately sensitive to penicillin*, benzylpenicillin sodium
- ▸ *Suggested duration of treatment* 4 weeks
- *If penicillin-allergic or highly penicillin-resistant*, vancomycin (*or* teicoplanin p. 348) + gentamicin
- ▸ *Suggested duration of treatment* 4–6 weeks (stop gentamicin after 2 weeks for micro-organisms moderately sensitive to penicillin)

Endocarditis (prosthetic valve) caused by streptococci

- Benzylpenicillin sodium + gentamicin
- ▸ *Suggested duration of treatment* at least 6 weeks (stop gentamicin after 2 weeks if micro-organisms fully sensitive to penicillin)
- *If penicillin-allergic or highly penicillin-resistant*, vancomycin (*or* teicoplanin) + gentamicin
- ▸ *Suggested duration of treatment* at least 6 weeks (stop gentamicin after 2 weeks if micro-organisms fully sensitive to penicillin)

Endocarditis caused by enterococci (e.g. *Enterococcus faecalis*)

- Amoxicillin p. 366 (*or* ampicillin p. 368) + gentamicin
- ▸ If gentamicin-resistant, substitute gentamicin with streptomycin p. 334
- ▸ *Suggested duration of treatment* at least 4 weeks (at least 6 weeks for prosthetic valve endocarditis)
- *If penicillin-allergic or penicillin-resistant*, vancomycin (*or* teicoplanin) + gentamicin
- ▸ If gentamicin-resistant, substitute gentamicin with streptomycin
- ▸ *Suggested duration of treatment* at least 4 weeks (at least 6 weeks for prosthetic valve endocarditis)

Endocarditis caused by *Haemophilus*, *Actinobacillus*, *Cardiobacterium*, *Eikenella*, and *Kingella*species ('HACEK' micro-organisms)

- Amoxicillin (*or* ampicillin) + gentamicin
- ▸ *Suggested duration of treatment* 4 weeks (6 weeks for prosthetic valve endocarditis); stop gentamicin after 2 weeks
- *If amoxicillin-resistant*, ceftriaxone p. 343 + gentamicin
- ▸ *Suggested duration of treatment* 4 weeks (6 weeks for prosthetic valve endocarditis); stop gentamicin after 2 weeks

Central nervous system infections, antibacterial therapy

Meningitis: initial empirical therapy

- Transfer patient to hospital urgently.
- If *meningococcal disease* (meningitis with non-blanching rash or meningococcal septicaemia) suspected, benzylpenicillin sodium p. 364 should be given before transfer to hospital, so long as this does not delay the transfer. If a patient with suspected bacterial meningitis without non-blanching rash cannot be transferred to hospital urgently, benzylpenicillin sodium should be given before the transfer. Cefotaxime p. 342 may be an alternative in penicillin allergy; chloramphenicol p. 385 may be used if history of immediate hypersensitivity reaction to penicillin or to cephalosporins.
- In hospital, consider adjunctive treatment with dexamethasone p. 475, preferably starting before or with first dose of antibacterial, but no later than 12 hours after starting antibacterial; avoid dexamethasone in septic shock, meningococcal septicaemia, or if immunocompromised, or in meningitis following surgery.

In hospital, if aetiology unknown:

- *Neonate and child 1–3 months*, cefotaxime (*or* ceftriaxone p. 343) + amoxicillin p. 366 (*or* ampicillin p. 368)
- ▸ Consider adding vancomycin p. 349 if prolonged or multiple use of other antibacterials in the last 3 months, or if travelled, in the last 3 months, to areas outside the UK with highly penicillin- and cephalosporin-resistant pneumococci
- ▸ *Suggested duration of treatment* at least 14 days
- *Child 3 months–18 years* cefotaxime (*or* ceftriaxone)
- ▸ Consider adding vancomycin if prolonged or multiple use of other antibacterials in the last 3 months, or if travelled, in the last 3 months, to areas outside the UK with highly penicillin- and cephalosporin-resistant pneumococci
- ▸ *Suggested duration of treatment* at least 10 days

Meningitis caused by group B streptococcus

- Benzylpenicillin sodium + gentamicin p. 333 *or* cefotaxime (*or* ceftriaxone) alone
- ▸ *Suggested duration of treatment* at least 14 days; stop gentamicin after 5 days

Meningitis caused by meningococci

- Benzylpenicillin sodium *or* cefotaxime (*or* ceftriaxone)
- ▸ *Suggested duration of treatment* 7 days.
- *If history of immediate hypersensitivity reaction to penicillin or to cephalosporins*, chloramphenicol
- ▸ *Suggested duration of treatment* 7 days.

Meningitis caused by pneumococci

- Cefotaxime (*or* ceftriaxone)
- ▸ Consider adjunctive treatment with dexamethasone, preferably starting before or with first dose of antibacterial, but no later than 12 hours after starting antibacterial (may reduce penetration of vancomycin into cerebrospinal fluid).
- ▸ If micro-organism penicillin-sensitive, replace cefotaxime with benzylpenicillin sodium.
- ▸ If micro-organism highly penicillin- and cephalosporin-resistant, add vancomycin and if necessary rifampicin p. 396.
- ▸ *Suggested duration of antibacterial treatment* 14 days.

Meningitis caused by *Haemophilus influenzae*

- Cefotaxime (*or* ceftriaxone)
- ▸ Consider adjunctive treatment with dexamethasone, preferably starting before or with first dose of antibacterial, but no later than 12 hours after starting antibacterial.
- ▸ *Suggested duration of antibacterial treatment* 10 days.
- ▸ For *H. influenzae* type b give rifampicin for 4 days before hospital discharge to those under 10 years of age or to those in contact with vulnerable household contacts
- *If history of immediate hypersensitivity reaction to penicillin or to cephalosporins, or if micro-organism resistant to cefotaxime* , chloramphenicol
- ▸ Consider adjunctive treatment with dexamethasone, preferably starting before or with first dose of antibacterial, but no later than 12 hours after starting antibacterial.
- ▸ *Suggested duration of antibacterial treatment* 10 days.
- ▸ For *H. influenzae* type b give rifampicin for 4 days before hospital discharge to those under 10 years of age or to those in contact with vulnerable household contacts

Meningitis caused by Listeria

- Amoxicillin (*or* ampicillin) + gentamicin
- ▸ *Suggested duration of treatment* 21 days.
- ▸ Consider stopping gentamicin after 7 days
- *If history of immediate hypersensitivity reaction to penicillin*, co-trimoxazole p. 378
- ▸ *Suggested duration of treatment* 21 days.

Diabetic foot infections, antibacterial therapy

13-Nov-2019

Diabetic foot infection

Diabetic foot infection is defined as any type of skin, soft tissue or bone infection below the ankle in children with diabetes. It includes cellulitis, paronychia, abscesses, myositis, tendonitis, necrotising fasciitis, osteomyelitis, and septic arthritis. It is defined clinically by the presence of at least 2 of the following: local swelling or induration, erythema, local tenderness or pain, local warmth, or purulent discharge.

For guidance on classification of infection severity, see NICE guideline: **Diabetic foot problems** (see *Useful resources*).

Treatment

EvGr Refer children immediately to acute services and inform the multidisciplinary foot care service if they have a limb-threatening or life-threatening diabetic foot problem, such as ulceration with fever or any signs of sepsis, ulceration with limb ischaemia, or gangrene.

Antibacterial treatment should be started as soon as possible if diabetic foot infection is suspected. Samples (such as soft tissue, bone sample, or deep swab) should be taken for microbiological testing before, or as close as possible to, the start of antibacterial treatment.

Offer an antibacterial taking into account the severity of infection, risk of complications, previous microbiological results, recent antibacterial use, and patient preferences. Ⓐ

For other considerations such as switching from intravenous to oral antibacterials, and for advice to be given to children and their parents, or carers, see Antibacterials, principles of therapy p. 318.

Reassessment

EvGr Reassess if symptoms worsen rapidly or significantly at any time, do not start to improve within 1–2 days of starting antibacterial treatment, or the patient becomes systemically very unwell or has severe pain out of proportion to the infection. Take into account other diagnoses (such as pressure sores, gout, or non-infected ulcers), signs and symptoms of a more serious illness (such as limb ischaemia, osteomyelitis, necrotising fasciitis, or sepsis), and previous antibacterial use.

Review the choice of antibacterial when microbiological results are available and change according to the results, using a narrower-spectrum antibacterial if appropriate. Ⓐ

Choice of antibacterial therapy

EvGr Seek specialist advice if a diabetic foot infection is suspected or confirmed in children. Ⓐ

Useful Resources

Diabetic foot problems: prevention and management. National Institute for Health and Care Excellence. NICE guideline 19. August 2015, updated October 2019.
www.nice.org.uk/guidance/ng19

Ear infections, antibacterial therapy

03-Sep-2018

Otitis externa

Otitis externa can be triggered by a bacterial infection caused by *Pseudomonas aeruginosa* or *Staphylococcus aureus*. Consider systemic antibacterial if spreading cellulitis or patient systemically unwell.

Choice of antibacterial therapy

No penicillin allergy

- Flucloxacillin p. 373

Penicillin allergy or intolerance

- Clarithromycin p. 353 (*or* azithromycin p. 352 *or* erythromycin p. 355)

If pseudomonas suspected

- Ciprofloxacin p. 377 (*or* an aminoglycoside)

For topical treatments, see *Otitis externa*, under Ear p. 741.

Otitis media

Acute otitis media is an inflammation in the middle ear associated with effusion and accompanied by an ear infection. Acute otitis media is commonly seen in children and is generally caused by viruses (respiratory syncytial virus and rhinovirus) or bacteria (*Haemophilus influenzae, Streptococcus pneumoniae, Streptococcus pyogenes*, and *Moraxella catarrhalis*); both virus and bacteria often co-exist. For further information see *Acute otitis media* in Ear p. 741.

EvGr Antibacterial therapy should be offered to children with acute otitis media who are systemically very unwell, have signs and symptoms of a more serious illness, or those who are at high-risk of serious complications due to pre-existing comorbidities. Antibacterial therapy should also be considered if otorrhoea (discharge following perforation of the eardrum) is present, or in children under 2 years of age with bilateral otitis media. Ⓐ

Choice of antibacterial therapy in children

No penicillin allergy

- *First line*: EvGr amoxicillin p. 366. Ⓐ
- *Second line* (worsening symptoms despite 2 to 3 days of antibacterial treatment): EvGr co-amoxiclav p. 370. Ⓐ

Penicillin allergy or intolerance

- *First line*: EvGr clarithromycin p. 353 or erythromycin p. 355 (preferred in pregnancy). Ⓐ
- *Second line* (worsening symptoms despite 2 to 3 days of antibacterial treatment): EvGr Consult local microbiologist. Ⓐ

Eye infections, antibacterial therapy

Purulent conjunctivitis

- Chloramphenicol p. 729 eye drops.

Congenital chlamydial conjunctivitis

- Erythromycin p. 355 (by mouth)
- ▸ *Suggested duration of treatment* 14 days

Congenital gonococcal conjunctivitis

- Cefotaxime p. 342 (*or* ceftriaxone p. 343)
- ▸ *Suggested duration of treatment* single dose.

Gastro-intestinal system infections, antibacterial therapy

Gastro-enteritis

Frequently self-limiting and may not be bacterial.

- Antibacterial not usually indicated.

Campylobacter enteritis

Frequently self-limiting; treat if immunocompromised or if severe infection.

- Clarithromycin p. 353 (*or* azithromycin p. 352 *or* erythromycin p. 355)
- *Alternative*, ciprofloxacin p. 377
  - Strains with decreased sensitivity to ciprofloxacin isolated frequently

Salmonella (non-typhoid)

Treat invasive or severe infection. Do not treat less severe infection unless there is a risk of developing invasive infection (e.g. immunocompromised children, those with haemoglobinopathy, or children under 6 months of age).

- Ciprofloxacin *or* cefotaxime p. 342

Shigellosis

Antibacterial not indicated for mild cases.

- Azithromycin *or* ciprofloxacin
- *Alternatives if micro-organism sensitive*, amoxicillin p. 366 *or* trimethoprim p. 390

Typhoid fever

Infections from Middle-East, South Asia, and South-East Asia may be multiple-antibacterial-resistant and sensitivity should be tested.

- Cefotaxime (*or* ceftriaxone p. 343)
  - azithromycin may be an alternative in mild or moderate disease caused by multiple-antibacterial-resistant micro-organisms
- *Alternative if micro-organism sensitive*, ciprofloxacin *or* chloramphenicol p. 385

Clostridioides difficile infection

Clostridioides difficile infection is caused by colonisation of the colon with *Clostridioides difficile* and production of toxin. It often follows antibiotic therapy and is usually of acute onset, but may become chronic. It is a particular hazard of ampicillin p. 368, amoxicillin, co-amoxiclav p. 370, second- and third-generation cephalosporins, clindamycin p. 351, and quinolones, but few antibacterials are free of this side-effect. Oral metronidazole p. 358 or oral vancomycin p. 349 are used as specific treatment; vancomycin may be preferred for very sick patients. Metronidazole can be given by intravenous infusion if oral treatment is inappropriate.

- *For first episode of mild to moderate infection*, oral metronidazole
  - *Suggested duration of treatment* 10–14 days
- *For second or subsequent episode of infection, for severe infection, for infection not responding to metronidazole, or in children intolerant of metronidazole*, oral vancomycin
  - *Suggested duration of treatment* 10–14 days
- *For infection not responding to vancomycin, or for life-threatening infection, or in patients with ileus*, oral vancomycin + i/v metronidazole
  - *Suggested duration of treatment* 10–14 days

Peritonitis

- A cephalosporin + metronidazole *or* amoxicillin + gentamicin p. 333 + metronidazole *or* piperacillin with tazobactam p. 362 alone

Peritonitis: peritoneal dialysis-associated

- Vancomycin (*or* teicoplanin p. 348) + ceftazidime p. 343 added to dialysis fluid *or* vancomycin added to dialysis fluid + ciprofloxacin by mouth
  - *Suggested duration of treatment* 14 days or longer

Necrotising enterocolitis in neonates

- Benzylpenicillin sodium p. 364 + gentamicin + metronidazole *or* amoxicillin (*or* ampicillin) + gentamicin + metronidazole *or* amoxicillin (*or* ampicillin) + cefotaxime + metronidazole

Genital system infections, antibacterial therapy

Uncomplicated genital chlamydial infection, non-gonococcal urethritis, and non-specific genital infection

Contact tracing recommended.

- *Child under* 12 *years*, erythromycin p. 355
  - *Suggested duration of treatment* 14 days
- *Child* 12–17 *years*, azithromycin p. 352 as a single dose *or* doxycycline p. 381 for 7 days
- *Alternatively*, erythromycin for 14 days

Gonorrhoea: uncomplicated

Contact tracing recommended. Consider chlamydia co-infection. Choice of antibacterial depends on locality where infection acquired.

- *Child under* 12 *years*, single-dose of ceftriaxone p. 343
- *Child* 12–17 *years*, single-dose of cefixime p. 342
- *Alternatively, if micro-organism sensitive*, single-dose of ciprofloxacin p. 377
- *Child* 12–17 *years with pharyngeal infection*, single-dose of ceftriaxone

Pelvic inflammatory disease

Contact tracing recommended.

- *Child* 2–11 *years*, erythromycin + metronidazole p. 358 + single-dose of i/m ceftriaxone
  - *Suggested duration of treatment* 14 days (except i/m ceftriaxone)
- *Child* 12–17 *years*, doxycycline + metronidazole + single-dose of i/m ceftriaxone
  - If severely ill, seek specialist advice.
  - *Suggested duration of treatment* 14 days (except i/m ceftriaxone)

Syphilis

Contact tracing recommended.

- *Child under* 12 *years*, benzylpenicillin sodium p. 364 *or* procaine benzylpenicillin [unlicensed]
  - *Suggested duration of treatment* 10 days

Early syphilis (infection of less than 2 years)

- *Child* 12–17 *years*, benzathine benzylpenicillin p. 363
  - *Suggested duration of treatment* single-dose (repeat dose after 7 days for females in the third trimester of pregnancy)
- *Alternatively*, doxycycline or erythromycin
  - *Suggested duration of treatment* 14 days

Late latent syphilis (asymptomatic infection of more than 2 years)

- *Child* 12–17 *years*, benzathine benzylpenicillin.
  - *Suggested duration of treatment* once weekly for 2 weeks
- *Alternatively*, doxycycline
  - *Suggested duration of treatment* 28 days

Asymptomatic contacts of patients with infectious syphilis

- *Child* 12–17 *years*, doxycycline
- ▸ *Suggested duration of treatment* 14 days

Neonatal congenital syphilis

- Benzylpenicillin sodium
- ▸ Also consider treating neonates with suspected congenital syphilis whose mothers were treated inadequately for syphilis, or whose mothers were treated for syphilis in the 4 weeks before delivery, or whose mothers were treated with non-penicillin antibacterials for syphilis.
- ▸ *Suggested duration of treatment* 10 days.

Musculoskeletal system infections, antibacterial therapy

Osteomyelitis

For management of osteomyelitis below the ankle in individuals with diabetes mellitus, see Diabetic foot infections, antibacterial therapy p. 324.

Seek specialist advice if chronic infection or prostheses present.

- Flucloxacillin p. 373
- ▸ Consider adding fusidic acid p. 387 or rifampicin p. 396 for initial 2 weeks.
- ▸ *Suggested duration of treatment* 6 weeks for acute infection
- *If penicillin-allergic*, clindamycin p. 351
- ▸ Consider adding fusidic acid or rifampicin for initial 2 weeks.
- ▸ *Suggested duration of treatment* 6 weeks for acute infection
- *If meticillin-resistant Staphylococcus aureus suspected*, vancomycin p. 349 (*or* teicoplanin p. 348)
- ▸ Consider adding fusidic acid or rifampicin for initial 2 weeks.
- ▸ *Suggested duration of treatment* 6 weeks for acute infection

Septic arthritis

For management of septic arthritis below the ankle in individuals with diabetes mellitus, see Diabetic foot infections, antibacterial therapy p. 324.

Seek specialist advice if prostheses present.

- Flucloxacillin
- ▸ *Suggested duration of treatment* 4–6 weeks (longer if infection complicated).
- *If penicillin-allergic*, clindamycin
- ▸ *Suggested duration of treatment* 4–6 weeks (longer if infection complicated).
- *If meticillin-resistant Staphylococcus aureus suspected*, vancomycin (*or* teicoplanin)
- ▸ *Suggested duration of treatment* 4–6 weeks (longer if infection complicated).
- *If gonococcal arthritis or Gram-negative infection suspected*, cefotaxime p. 342 (*or* ceftriaxone p. 343)
- ▸ *Suggested duration of treatment* 4–6 weeks (longer if infection complicated; treat gonococcal infection for 2 weeks).

Nose infections, antibacterial therapy

31-Oct-2017

Sinusitis (acute)

Acute sinusitis is generally triggered by a viral infection, although occasionally it may become complicated by a bacterial infection caused by *Streptococcus pneumoniae*, *Haemophylus influenzae*, *Moraxella catharrhalis*, or *Staphylococcus aureus*. For further information *see* Sinusitis (acute) p. 750.

Treatment

EvGr Antibacterial therapy should *only* be offered to children with acute sinusitis who are systemically very unwell, have signs and symptoms of a more serious illness, those who are at high-risk of complications due to pre-existing comorbidities, or whenever bacterial sinusitis is suspected. (A) For further information *see* Sinusitis (acute) p. 750.

Choice of antibacterial therapy

No penicillin allergy

- *First line*:
- ▸ EvGr Non-life threatening symptoms: phenoxymethylpenicillin p. 365.
- ▸ Systemically very unwell, signs and symptoms of a more serious illness, or at high-risk of complications: co-amoxiclav p. 370. (A)
- *Second line* (worsening symptoms despite 2 or 3 days of antibiotic treatment):
- ▸ EvGr Non-life threatening symptoms: co-amoxiclav.
- ▸ Systemically very unwell, signs and symptoms of a more serious illness or at high-risk of complications: consult local microbiologist. (A)

Penicillin allergy or intolerance

- *First line*: EvGr clarithromycin p. 353, or doxycycline p. 381 (for children above 12 years old). (A)
- *Second line* (worsening symptoms despite 2 or 3 days of antibiotic treatment): EvGr Consult local microbiologist. (A)

Useful Resources

Sinusitis (acute): antimicrobial prescribing. National Institute for Health and Care Excellence. NICE guideline 79. October 2017.
www.nice.org.uk/guidance/ng79

Oral bacterial infections

Antibacterial drugs

Antibacterial drugs should only be prescribed for the *treatment* of oral infections on the basis of defined need. They may be used in conjunction with (but not as an alternative to) other appropriate measures, such as providing drainage or extracting a tooth.

The 'blind' prescribing of an antibacterial for unexplained pyrexia, cervical lymphadenopathy, or facial swelling can lead to difficulty in establishing the diagnosis. In severe oral infections, a sample should always be taken for bacteriology.

Oral infections which may require antibacterial treatment include acute periapical or periodontal abscess, cellulitis, acutely created oral-antral communication (and acute sinusitis), severe pericoronitis, localised osteitis, acute necrotising ulcerative gingivitis, and destructive forms of chronic periodontal disease. Most of these infections are readily resolved by the early establishment of drainage and removal of the cause (typically an infected necrotic pulp). Antibacterials may be required if treatment has to be delayed, in immunocompromised patients, or in those with conditions such as diabetes. Certain rarer infections including bacterial sialadenitis, osteomyelitis, actinomycosis, and infections involving fascial spaces such as Ludwig's angina, require antibiotics and specialist hospital care.

Antibacterial drugs may also be useful after dental surgery in some cases of spreading infection. Infection may spread to involve local lymph nodes, to fascial spaces (where it can cause airway obstruction), or into the bloodstream (where it can lead to cavernous sinus thrombosis and other serious complications). Extension of an infection can also lead to maxillary sinusitis; osteomyelitis is a complication, which usually arises when host resistance is reduced.

If the oral infection fails to respond to antibacterial treatment within 48 hours the antibacterial should be changed, preferably on the basis of bacteriological investigation. Failure to respond may also suggest an incorrect diagnosis, lack of essential additional measures (such as drainage), poor host resistance, or poor patient compliance.

Combination of a penicillin (or a macrolide) with metronidazole p. 358 may sometimes be helpful for the treatment of severe oral infections or oral infections.

Penicillins

Phenoxymethylpenicillin p. 365 is effective for dentoalveolar abscess.

Broad-spectrum penicillins

Amoxicillin p. 366 is as effective as phenoxymethylpenicillin but is better absorbed; however, it may encourage emergence of resistant organisms.

Like phenoxymethylpenicillin, amoxicillin is ineffective against bacteria that produce beta-lactamases.

Co-amoxiclav p. 370 is active against beta-lactamase-producing bacteria that are resistant to amoxicillin. Co-amoxiclav may be used for severe dental infection with spreading cellulitis or dental infection not responding to first-line antibacterial treatment.

Cephalosporins

The cephalosporins offer little advantage over the penicillins in dental infections, often being less active against anaerobes. Infections due to oral streptococci (often termed viridans streptococci) which become resistant to penicillin are usually also resistant to cephalosporins. This is of importance in the case of patients who have had rheumatic fever and are on long-term penicillin therapy. Cefalexin p. 339 and cefradine p. 339 have been used in the treatment of oral infections.

Tetracyclines

In children over 12 years of age, tetracyclines can be effective against oral anaerobes but the development of resistance (especially by oral streptococci) has reduced their usefulness for the treatment of acute oral infections; they may still have a role in the treatment of destructive (refractory) forms of periodontal disease. Doxycycline p. 381 has a longer duration of action than tetracycline p. 384 or oxytetracycline p. 383 and need only be given once daily; it is reported to be more active against anaerobes than some other tetracyclines.

Doxycycline may have a role in the treatment of recurrent aphthous ulceration, or as an adjunct to gingival scaling and root planing for periodontitis.

Macrolides

The macrolides are an alternative for oral infections in penicillin-allergic patients or where a beta-lactamase producing organism is involved. However, many organisms are now resistant to macrolides or rapidly develop resistance; their use should therefore be limited to short courses.

Clindamycin

Clindamycin p. 351 should not be used routinely for the treatment of oral infections because it may be no more effective than penicillins against anaerobes and there may be cross-resistance with erythromycin p. 355-resistant bacteria. Clindamycin can be used for the treatment of dentoalveolar abscess that has not responded to penicillin or to metronidazole.

Metronidazole and tinidazole

Metronidazole is an alternative to a penicillin for the treatment of many oral infections where the patient is allergic to penicillin or the infection is due to beta-lactamase-producing anaerobes. It is the drug of first choice for the treatment of acute necrotising ulcerative gingivitis (Vincent's infection) and pericoronitis; amoxicillin is a suitable alternative. For these purposes metronidazole for 3 days is sufficient, but the duration of treatment may need to be longer in pericoronitis. Tinidazole p. 360 is licensed for the treatment of acute ulcerative gingivitis.

Respiratory system infections, antibacterial therapy

22-Oct-2019

Epiglottitis (*Haemophilus influenzae*)

- Cefotaxime p. 342 (*or* ceftriaxone p. 343)
- *If history of immediate hypersensitivity reaction to penicillin or to cephalosporins*, chloramphenicol p. 385

Bronchiectasis (non-cystic fibrosis), acute exacerbation

Bronchiectasis is a persistent or progressive condition, caused by chronic inflammatory damage to the airways and is characterised by thick-walled, dilated bronchi. Signs and symptoms may range from intermittent expectoration and infection, to chronic cough, persistent daily production of sputum, bacterial colonisation, and recurrent infections. An acute exacerbation is defined as sustained deterioration of the child's signs and symptoms from their baseline and presents with worsening local symptoms, with or without increased wheeze, breathlessness or haemoptysis and may be accompanied by fever or pleurisy.

Treatment

EvGr Obtain a sputum sample and send for culture and susceptibility testing. Antibacterial therapy should be given to all children with an acute exacerbation. (A)

For children receiving prophylactic antibacterial therapy, switching from intravenous to oral antibacterials, and for advice to be given to children and their parents, or carers, see Antibacterials, principles of therapy p. 318.

EvGr Refer children to hospital if they have signs or symptoms suggestive of a more serious illness such as cardiorespiratory failure or sepsis. (A)

Reassessment

EvGr Reassess if symptoms worsen rapidly or significantly at any time and consider:

- Other diagnoses such as pneumonia, or signs and symptoms of a more serious illness such as cardiorespiratory failure, or sepsis;
- Previous antibacterial use that may have led to resistance.

Review choice of antibacterial if susceptibility results indicate bacterial resistance and symptoms are not improving—consult local microbiologist as needed. (A)

Choice of antibacterial therapy

EvGr The recommended total duration of treatment is 7–14 days.

Treatment should be guided by the most recent sputum culture and susceptibility results when available.

Seek specialist advice for children whose symptoms are not improving with repeated courses, or who are resistant to, or cannot take oral antibacterials. (A)

- ***Oral** first line* :
  - EvGr Amoxicillin p. 366, clarithromycin p. 353, or doxycycline p. 381 (child over 12 years).
  - Alternative if at high risk of treatment failure (repeated courses of antibacterials, previous culture with resistant or

5 Infection

atypical bacteria, or high risk of complications): co-amoxiclav p. 370, or ciprofloxacin p. 377 (on specialist advice). Ⓐ

- ***Intravenous** first line* (severely unwell or unable to take oral treatment):
  - ▸ EvGr Co-amoxiclav, piperacillin with tazobactam p. 362, or ciprofloxacin (on specialist advice). Ⓐ

Antibacterial prophylaxis

EvGr For children with repeated acute exacerbations, a trial of antibacterial prophylaxis may be given on specialist advice only. Ⓐ

Cough, acute

Acute cough is usually self-limiting and often resolves within 3–4 weeks without antibacterials. It is most commonly caused by a viral upper respiratory tract infection, but can have other infective causes such as acute bronchitis or pneumonia, or non-infective causes such as interstitial lung disease or gastro-oesophageal reflux disease.

Treatment

EvGr Children and their parents, or carers should be advised that an acute cough is usually self-limiting and to manage symptoms using self-care treatments. These include honey (for children over the age of 1 year) and over-the-counter cough medicines containing expectorants or cough suppressants, however there is limited evidence to support the use of such products. For more information, see Aromatic inhalations, cough preparations and systemic nasal decongestants p. 198.

Children with an acute cough who are systemically very unwell should be offered immediate antibacterial treatment.

Do not routinely offer an antibacterial to treat an acute cough associated with an upper respiratory tract infection or acute bronchitis in children who are not systemically very unwell or at higher risk of complications.

Children with a pre-existing co-morbidity or young children who were born prematurely are considered to be at a higher risk of complications if they present with an acute cough. In these patients, the need for immediate antibacterial treatment should be considered based on the face-to-face clinical examination. Ⓐ

For general advice to give to children and their parents, or carers, see Antibacterials, principles of therapy p. 318.

EvGr Seek specialist advice, or refer children with an acute cough to hospital if they have signs or symptoms of a more serious illness or condition. Ⓐ

Reassessment

EvGr Reassess if symptoms worsen rapidly or significantly taking into account alternative diagnoses, signs or symptoms suggestive of a more serious condition, and previous antibacterial use which may have led to resistant bacteria. Ⓐ

Choice of antibacterial therapy

EvGr The recommended duration of oral treatment is 5 days. Ⓐ

- *First line*:
  - ▸ EvGr Amoxicillin. Ⓐ
  - ▸ EvGr Alternative *first line* choices: clarithromycin, erythromycin p. 355, or doxycycline (child over 12 years). Ⓐ
- Choice during pregnancy:
  - ▸ EvGr Amoxicillin or erythromycin. Ⓐ

Pneumonia, community-acquired

Pneumonia is an acute infection of the lung parenchyma that presents with symptoms such as cough, chest pain, dyspnoea, and fever. It is classified as community-acquired if acquired outside of hospital.

Treatment

EvGr Offer an antibacterial taking into account the severity of signs or symptoms based on clinical judgement, risk of complications, local antimicrobial resistance and surveillance data, recent antibacterial use, and recent microbiological test results.

Antibacterial treatment should be started as soon as possible and within 4 hours of establishing a diagnosis (within 1 hour if the child has suspected sepsis and meets any of the high risk criteria for this — see NICE guideline on sepsis at: www.nice.org.uk/guidance/ng51).

Consider referring children to hospital or seeking specialist paediatric advice on further investigation and management.

For children in hospital with community-acquired pneumonia, and severe signs or symptoms or a comorbidity, consider sending a sample for microbiological testing. Ⓐ

For other considerations such as switching from intravenous to oral antibacterials, and for advice to be given to children and their parents, or carers, see Antibacterials, principles of therapy p. 318.

Reassessment

EvGr Reassess if signs or symptoms do not improve or worsen rapidly or significantly, and consider other possible non-bacterial causes such as influenza.

If a sample has been sent for microbiological testing, review the choice of antibacterial and consider changing according to the results, using a narrower-spectrum antibacterial if appropriate.

Send a sample (such as a sputum sample) for testing if there is no improvement after antibacterial therapy and this has not already been done. Ⓐ

Choice of antibacterial therapy

EvGr Treatment should be based on clinical judgement, suspected micro-organism, and if severe signs or symptoms guided by microbiological results when available.

Offer oral antibacterials to children who are able to take oral treatment and the severity of their condition does not require intravenous treatment.

Children under 1 month should be referred to a paediatric specialist. Ⓐ

Non-severe

- ***Oral** first line* in children aged 1 month and over:
  - ▸ EvGr Amoxicillin p. 366.
  - ▸ Alternative in penicillin allergy or amoxicillin unsuitable (e.g. atypical pathogens suspected): clarithromycin p. 353, doxycycline p. 381 (child over 12 years), or erythromycin p. 355 (in pregnancy). Ⓐ

Severe

- ***Oral** or **Intravenous** first line* in children aged 1 month and over:
  - ▸ EvGr Co-amoxiclav p. 370.
  - ▸ If atypical pathogens suspected: co-amoxiclav **with** clarithromycin **or** oral erythromycin (in pregnancy).
  - ▸ For alternative in penicillin allergy consult local microbiologist. Ⓐ

Pneumonia, hospital-acquired

Pneumonia is an acute infection of the lung parenchyma that presents with symptoms such as cough, chest pain, dyspnoea, and fever. It is classified as hospital-acquired when it develops 48 hours or more after hospital admission.

Treatment

EvGr In children with signs or symptoms of pneumonia starting within 48 hours of hospital admission, follow the recommendations for children with community-acquired pneumonia. Ⓐ

Offer an antibacterial taking into account:

- EvGr The severity of signs or symptoms;
- The number of days in hospital before onset of symptoms;
- The risk of complications;

- Local hospital and ward-based antimicrobial resistance data;
- Recentantibacterial use;
- Recent microbiological test results;
- Recent contact with health or social care settings;
- Risk of adverse effects such as *Clostridioides difficile* infection.

Antibacterial treatment should be started as soon as possible and within 4 hours of establishing a diagnosis (within 1 hour if the child has suspected sepsis and meets any of the high risk criteria for this — see NICE guideline on sepsis at: www.nice.org.uk/guidance/ng51).

A sample (for example, sputum sample, nasopharyngeal swab or tracheal aspirate) should be taken for microbiological testing. Ⓐ

For other considerations such as switching from intravenous to oral antibacterials, and for advice to be given to children and their parents, or carers see Antibacterials, principles of therapy p. 318.

Reassessment

EvGr Reassess if symptoms do not improve or worsen rapidly or significantly.

When microbiological results are available, review the choice of antibacterial and change according to the results, using a narrower-spectrum antibacterial if appropriate.

Seek advice from a microbiologist if symptoms do not improve as expected with treatment, or multidrug-resistant bacteria are present. Ⓐ

Choice of antibacterial therapy

EvGr For children with non-severe signs or symptoms and not at higher risk of resistance, treatment should be guided by microbiological results when available. For children with severe signs or symptoms or at higher risk of resistance, treatment should be based on specialist microbiological advice and local resistance data.

Higher risk of resistance includes signs or symptoms starting more than 5 days after hospital admission, relevant comorbidity, recent use of broad-spectrum antibacterials, colonisation with multidrug-resistant bacteria, and recent contact with a health or social care setting before the current admission.

In children with signs or symptoms of pneumonia starting within 3 to 5 days of hospital admission and not at higher risk of resistance, consider following the recommendations for community-acquired pneumonia for choice of antibacterial.

In children under 1 month obtain specialist microbiological advice and consider local resistance data. Ⓐ

Non-severe signs or symptoms and not at higher risk of resistance

- ***Oral** first line* in children aged 1 month and over:
  - ▸ EvGr Co-amoxiclav.
  - ▸ Alternative in penicillin allergy or co-amoxiclav unsuitable: clarithromycin. Other options can be considered based on specialist microbiological advice and local resistance data. Ⓐ

Severe signs or symptoms or at higher risk of resistance

- ***Intravenous** first line* in children aged 1 month and over:
  - ▸ EvGr Piperacillin with tazobactam p. 362, ceftazidime p. 343, or ceftriaxone p. 343.
  - ▸ If meticillin-resistant *Staphylococcus aureus* confirmed or suspected, **add** teicoplanin p. 348, or vancomycin p. 349, or linezolid p. 389 [unlicensed] (child over 3 months under specialist advice only if vancomycin cannot be used). Ⓐ

Lung infection in cystic fibrosis (*Staphylococcus* spp.)

- Flucloxacillin p. 373
  - ▸ If child already taking flucloxacillin prophylaxis or if severe exacerbation, add fusidic acid p. 387 or rifampicin p. 396; use flucloxacillin at treatment dose
- *If penicillin-allergic*, clarithromycin (*or* azithromycin p. 352 *or* erythromycin) or clindamycin p. 351
  - ▸ Use clarithromycin only if micro-organism sensitive

Lung infection in cystic fibrosis (*Haemophilus influenzae*)

- Amoxicillin *or* a broad-spectrum cephalosporin
  - ▸ In severe exacerbation use a third-generation cephalosporin (e.g. cefotaxime p. 342)

Lung infection in cystic fibrosis (*Pseudomonas* spp.)

- Ciprofloxacin p. 377 + *nebulised* colistimethate sodium p. 375
  - ▸ *For severe exacerbation*, an antipseudomonal beta-lactam antibacterial + parenteral tobramycin p. 334

Useful resources

Bronchiectasis (non-cystic fibrosis), acute exacerbation: antimicrobial prescribing. National Institute for Health and Care Excellence. NICE guideline 117. December 2018.

www.nice.org.uk/guidance/ng117

Cough (acute): antimicrobial prescribing. National Institute for Health and Care Excellence. NICE guideline 120. February 2019.

www.nice.org.uk/guidance/ng120

Pneumonia (community-acquired): antimicrobial prescribing. National Institute for Health and Care Excellence. NICE guideline 138. September 2019.

www.nice.org.uk/guidance/ng138

Pneumonia (hospital-acquired): antimicrobial prescribing. National Institute for Health and Care Excellence. NICE guideline 139. September 2019.

www.nice.org.uk/guidance/ng139

Skin infections, antibacterial therapy

22-Mar-2020

Impetigo

Impetigo is a contagious, superficial bacterial infection of the skin that affects all age groups, but it is more common in young children. Transmission occurs directly through close contact with an infected individual or indirectly via contaminated objects such as toys, clothing, or towels.

Impetigo can develop as a primary infection or as a secondary complication of pre-existing skin conditions such as eczema, scabies, or chickenpox. The two main clinical forms are non-bullous impetigo (most common form) and bullous impetigo. Non-bullous impetigo is characterised by thin-walled vesicles or pustules that rupture quickly, forming a golden-brown crust, while bullous impetigo is characterised by the presence of fluid-filled vesicles and blisters that rupture, leaving a thin, flat, yellow-brown crust.

Initial treatment

EvGr Patients, and if appropriate their family or carers, should be advised on good hygiene measures to reduce the spread of impetigo to other body areas and to other people.

In patients with **localised non-bullous impetigo** who are not systemically unwell or at high risk of complications, consider hydrogen peroxide 1% cream p. 814; if unsuitable (e.g. if impetigo is around the eyes), offer a topical antibacterial.

In patients with **widespread non-bullous impetigo** who are not systemically unwell or at high risk of complications, offer a topical **or** oral antibacterial. Take into account that both routes of administration are effective; any previous use of topical antibacterials that could have led to resistance; and the preferences of the patient and, their family or carers (if appropriate), including the practicalities of administration (particularly to large areas).

In patients with **non-bullous impetigo** who are systemically unwell or at high risk of complications and in all patients with **bullous impetigo**, offer an oral antibacterial.

Combination treatment with a topical and oral antibacterial is not recommended. ⟨A⟩

For other considerations such as advice to be given to patients, and if appropriate their family or carers, see Antibacterials, principles of therapy p. 318.

EvGr Refer patients to hospital if they have any signs or symptoms suggestive of a more serious condition or illness, or if they have widespread impetigo and are immunocompromised.

Consider referral to hospital or seeking specialist advice for patients who are systemically unwell, have a higher risk of complications, or if impetigo is difficult to treat (such as bullous impetigo (particularly in children aged under 1 year) or frequently recurrent impetigo). ⟨A⟩

Reassessment and further treatment

EvGr Reassess if symptoms worsen rapidly or significantly at any time, or do not improve after completion of the treatment course. Take into consideration other possible diagnoses (such as herpes simplex infection), signs or symptoms suggesting a more serious illness or condition (such as cellulitis), and previous antibacterial use that might have led to resistance.

For patients whose impetigo is worsening or has not improved after treatment with hydrogen peroxide 1% cream, offer a topical antibacterial if the infection remains localised, or a topical **or** oral antibacterial if infection has become widespread.

Offer an oral antibacterial to patients whose impetigo is worsening or has not improved after completing a course of topical antibacterial.

For patients whose impetigo is worsening or has not improved after completing a course of topical or oral antibacterials, consider sending a skin swab for microbiological testing.

For patients with impetigo that recurs frequently, send a skin swab for microbiological testing and consider taking a nasal swab and starting treatment for decolonisation (using topical treatments and personal hygiene measures).

If a skin swab has been sent for microbiological testing, review the choice of antibacterial and change according to the results if symptoms are not improving, using a narrower-spectrum antibacterial if possible. ⟨A⟩

Choice of antibacterial therapy

EvGr Treatment should be based on infection severity and number of lesions, suspected micro-organism, local antibacterial resistance data, and be guided by microbiological results if available. ⟨A⟩

- ***Topical** first line* if hydrogen peroxide unsuitable or ineffective:
  - ▸ EvGr fusidic acid p. 387.
  - ▸ Alternative if fusidic acid resistance suspected or confirmed: mupirocin p. 776. ⟨A⟩
- ***Oral** first line*:
  - ▸ EvGr Flucloxacillin p. 373.
  - ▸ Alternative if penicillin allergy or flucloxacillin unsuitable: clarithromycin p. 353 or erythromycin p. 355 (in pregnancy). ⟨A⟩
- If meticillin-resistant *Staphylococcus aureus* (MRSA) infection suspected or confirmed: EvGr Consult local microbiologist. ⟨A⟩

Cellulitis and erysipelas

Cellulitis and erysipelas are infections of the subcutaneous tissues, which usually result from contamination of a break in the skin. Both conditions are characterised by acute localised inflammation and oedema. Lesions are more superficial in erysipelas and have a well-defined, raised margin.

For management of infection below the ankle in children with diabetes, see Diabetic foot infections, antibacterial therapy p. 324.

Treatment

EvGr Consider taking a swab for microbiological testing **only** if the skin is broken and there is risk of infection by an uncommon pathogen (for example, after a penetrating injury, exposure to water-born organisms, or an infection acquired outside the UK).

Drawing around the extent of the infection to monitor progress prior to initiating antibacterial treatment can also be considered, taking into account that redness may be less visible on darker skin tones.

Offer an antibacterial taking into account the severity of symptoms, site of infection, risk of uncommon pathogens, previous microbiological results from a swab, and the patient's meticillin-resistant *Staphylococcus aureus* (MRSA) status if known. ⟨A⟩

For other considerations such as switching from intravenous to oral antibacterials, and for advice to be given to children and their parents, or carers, see Antibacterials, principles of therapy p. 318.

EvGr Manage any underlying condition that may predispose to cellulitis or erysipelas, such as diabetes mellitus, venous insufficiency, eczema, and oedema.

Refer children to hospital if they have signs or symptoms suggestive of a more serious illness, such as orbital cellulitis, osteomyelitis, septic arthritis, necrotising fasciitis, or sepsis.

Consider referral to hospital or seeking specialist advice for patients who have lymphangitis, are severely unwell, are unable to take oral antibacterials, have infection near the eyes or nose, or that could be caused by an uncommon pathogen. ⟨A⟩

Reassessment

EvGr Reassess if symptoms worsen rapidly or significantly at any time, do not improve within 2–3 days of starting an antibacterial, or the child becomes systemically very unwell, has severe pain out of proportion to the infection, or has redness or swelling spreading beyond the initial presentation (taking into account that some initial spreading may occur). Take into consideration other possible diagnoses (such as an inflammatory reaction to an insect bite or deep vein thrombosis), any underlying condition that may predispose to cellulitis or erysipelas, signs or symptoms suggesting a more serious illness, results from microbiological tests, and previous antibacterial use that might have led to resistance.

Consider taking a swab for testing if the skin is broken and this has not already been done.

If a swab has been sent for microbiological testing, review the choice of antibacterial and change according to the results if signs or symptoms are not improving, using a narrower-spectrum antibacterial if possible.

Consider referral to hospital or seeking specialist advice if the infection has spread and is not responding to oral antibacterials. ⟨A⟩

Choice of antibacterial therapy

EvGr Treatment should be based on clinical assessment, infection severity, suspected micro-organism, and site of infection.

Offer oral antibacterials to children who are able to take oral treatment and the severity of their condition does not require intravenous treatment.

Consider referral to hospital or seeking specialist advice if bacteria are resistant to oral antibacterials, patients cannot take oral treatment, or have infection near the eyes or nose.

Antibacterial choice for children under 1 month should be based on specialist advice. ⟨A⟩

First choice antibacterials in children aged 1 month and over

- ***Oral** or **Intravenous** first line* :
  - EvGr Flucloxacillin p. 373.
  - Alternative in penicillin allergy or if flucloxacillin unsuitable: co-amoxiclav p. 370 (**not** in penicillin allergy), clarithromycin p. 353, or oral erythromycin p. 355 (in pregnancy). Ⓐ
- ***Oral** or **Intravenous** first line if infection near the eyes or nose* :
  - EvGr Co-amoxiclav.
  - Alternative in penicillin allergy or co-amoxiclav unsuitable: clarithromycin. If anaerobes suspected, **add** metronidazole p. 358. Ⓐ

Alternative choice antibacterials for severe infection in children aged 1 month and over

- ***Oral** or **Intravenous***:
  - EvGr Co-amoxiclav, clindamycin p. 351, or intravenous cefuroxime p. 341.
  - If meticillin-resistant *Staphylococcus aureus* confirmed or suspected, **add** intravenous vancomycin p. 349, intravenous teicoplanin p. 348, or linezolid p. 389 (specialist use only if vancomycin or teicoplanin cannot be used).
  - Other antibacterials may be appropriate based on microbiological results and specialist advice. Ⓐ

Staphylococcal scalded skin syndrome

- Flucloxacillin
  - *Suggested duration of treatment* 7–10 days.
- *If penicillin-allergic*, clarithromycin (*or* azithromycin p. 352 *or* erythromycin)
  - *Suggested duration of treatment* 7–10 days.

Animal and human bites

Cleanse wound thoroughly. For tetanus-prone wound, give human tetanus immunoglobulin p. 826 (with a tetanus-containing vaccine if necessary, according to immunisation history and risk of infection). Consider rabies prophylaxis for bites from animals in endemic countries; assess risk of blood-borne viruses (including HIV, hepatitis B and C) and give appropriate prophylaxis to prevent viral spread.

- Co-amoxiclav
  - *If penicillin-allergic*, clindamycin

Surgical wound infection

- Flucloxacillin *or* co-amoxiclav

Paronychia or 'septic spots' in neonate

- Flucloxacillin
  - If systemically unwell, add an aminoglycoside.

Useful Resources

Cellulitis and erysipelas: antimicrobial prescribing. National Institute for Health and Care Excellence. NICE guideline 141. September 2019.
www.nice.org.uk/guidance/ng141

Impetigo: antimicrobial prescribing. National Institute for Health and Care Excellence. NICE guideline 153. February 2020.
www.nice.org.uk/guidance/ng153

ANTIBACTERIALS > AMINOGLYCOSIDES

Aminoglycosides

Overview

These include amikacin p. 332, gentamicin p. 333, neomycin sulfate p. 774, streptomycin p. 334, and tobramycin p. 334. All are bactericidal and active against some Gram-positive and many Gram-negative organisms. Amikacin, gentamicin, and tobramycin are also active against *Pseudomonas aeruginosa*; streptomycin is active against *Mycobacterium tuberculosis* and is now almost entirely reserved for tuberculosis.

The aminoglycosides are not absorbed from the gut (although there is a risk of absorption in inflammatory bowel disease and liver failure) and must therefore be given by injection for systemic infections.

Gentamicin is the aminoglycoside of choice in the UK and is used widely for the treatment of serious infections. It has a broad spectrum but is inactive against anaerobes and has poor activity against haemolytic streptococci and pneumococci. When used for the 'blind' therapy of undiagnosed serious infections it is usually given in conjunction with a penicillin or metronidazole p. 358 (or both). Gentamicin is used together with another antibiotic for the treatment of endocarditis. Streptomycin may be used as an alternative in gentamicin-resistant enterococcal endocarditis.

Loading and maintenance doses of gentamicin may be calculated on the basis of the patient's weight and renal function (e.g. using a nomogram); adjustments are then made according to serum-gentamicin concentrations. High doses are occasionally indicated for serious infections, especially in the neonate, in the patient with cystic fibrosis, or in the immunocompromised patient. Whenever possible treatment should not exceed 7 days.

Amikacin is more stable than gentamicin to enzyme inactivation. Amikacin is used in the treatment of serious infections caused by gentamicin-resistant Gram-negative bacilli.

Tobramycin has similar activity to gentamicin. It is slightly more active against *Ps. aeruginosa* but shows less activity against certain other Gram-negative bacteria.

Neomycin sulfate is too toxic for parenteral administration and can only be used for infections of the skin or mucous membranes or to reduce the bacterial population of the colon prior to bowel surgery or in hepatic failure. Oral administration may lead to malabsorption. Small amounts of neomycin sulfate may be absorbed from the gut in patients with hepatic failure and, as these patients may also be uraemic, cumulation may occur with resultant ototoxicity.

Cystic fibrosis

A higher dose of parenteral aminoglycoside is often required in children with cystic fibrosis because renal clearance of the aminoglycoside is increased. Aminoglycosides have a role in the treatment of pseudomonal lung infections in cystic fibrosis. Tobramycin can be administered by nebuliser or by inhalation of powder on a cyclical basis (28 days of tobramycin followed by a 28-day tobramycin-free interval) for the treatment of chronic pulmonary *Ps. aeruginosa* infection in cystic fibrosis; however, resistance may develop and some patients do not respond to treatment.

Once daily dosage

Once daily administration of aminoglycosides is more convenient, provides adequate serum concentrations, and has largely superseded *multiple-daily dose regimens* (given in 2–3 divided doses during the 24 hours). Local guidelines on dosage and serum concentrations should be consulted. A once-daily, high-dose regimen of an aminoglycoside should be avoided in children with endocarditis or burns of more than 20% of the total body surface area. There is insufficient evidence to recommend a once daily, high-dose regimen of an aminoglycoside in pregnancy.

Serum concentrations

Serum concentration monitoring avoids both excessive and subtherapeutic concentrations thus preventing toxicity and ensuring efficacy. Serum-aminoglycoside concentrations should be monitored in patients receiving parenteral aminoglycosides and **must** be determined in obesity, and in cystic fibrois, or if high doses are being given, or if there is renal impairment.

Neonates

As aminoglycosides are eliminated principally via the kidney, neonatal treatment must reflect the changes in glomerular filtration that occur with increasing gestational and postnatal age. The *extended interval dose regimen* is used in neonates, and serum-aminoglycoside concentrations **must** be measured. In patients on single daily dose regimens it may become necessary to prolong the dose interval to more than 24 hours if the trough concentration is high.

Aminoglycosides (by injection)

- **CONTRA-INDICATIONS** Myasthenia gravis (aminoglycosides may impair neuromuscular transmission)
- **CAUTIONS** Auditory disorder · care must be taken with dosage (the main side-effects of the aminoglycosides are dose-related) · conditions characterised by muscular weakness (aminoglycosides may impair neuromuscular transmission) · if possible, dehydration should be corrected before starting an aminoglycoside · vestibular disorder · whenever possible, parenteral treatment should not exceed 7 days
- **SIDE-EFFECTS**
  - **Common or very common** Tinnitus
  - **Uncommon** Nausea · skin reactions · vomiting
  - **Rare or very rare** Anaemia · azotaemia · bronchospasm · eosinophilia · fever · headache · hearing impairment · hypomagnesaemia · paraesthesia · renal impairment
  - **Frequency not known** Confusion · lethargy · leucopenia · nephrotoxicity · thrombocytopenia · vertigo

  SIDE-EFFECTS, FURTHER INFORMATION Ototoxicity and nephrotoxicity are important side-effects to consider with aminoglycoside therapy. Nephrotoxicity occurs most commonly in patients with renal impairment
- **PREGNANCY** There is a risk of auditory or vestibular nerve damage in the infant when aminoglycosides are used in the second and third trimesters of pregnancy. The risk is greatest with streptomycin. The risk is probably very small with gentamicin and tobramycin, but their use should be avoided unless essential.

  Monitoring If given during pregnancy, serum-aminoglycoside concentration monitoring is essential.
- **RENAL IMPAIRMENT** Excretion of aminoglycosides is principally via the kidney and accumulation occurs in renal impairment. Ototoxicity and nephrotoxicity occur commonly in patients with renal failure. A once-daily, high-dose regimen of an aminoglycoside should be avoided in children over 1 month of age with a creatinine clearance less than 20 mL/minute/1.73 m^2.

  Dose adjustments If there is impairment of renal function, the interval between doses must be increased; if the renal impairment is severe, the dose itself should be reduced as well.

  Monitoring Serum-aminoglycoside concentrations **must** be monitored in patients with renal impairment; earlier and more frequent measurement of aminoglycoside concentration may be required.
- **MONITORING REQUIREMENTS**
  - Serum concentrations Serum concentration monitoring avoids both excessive and subtherapeutic concentrations thus preventing toxicity and ensuring efficacy.

    Serum-aminoglycoside concentrations should be measured in all patients receiving parenteral aminoglycosides and **must** be determined in obesity, if high doses are being given and in cystic fibrosis.

    Serum aminoglycoside concentrations **must** be determined in neonates.

    In children with normal renal function, aminoglycoside concentrations should be measured after 3 or 4 doses of a multiple daily dose regimen.

    Blood samples should be taken just before the next dose is administered ('trough' concentration). If the pre-dose ('trough') concentration is high, the interval between doses must be increased. For multiple daily dose regimens, blood samples should also be taken approximately 1 hour after intramuscular or intravenous administration ('peak' concentration). If the post-dose ('peak') concentration is high, the dose must be decreased.
  - Renal function should be assessed before starting an aminoglycoside and during treatment.
  - Auditory and vestibular function should also be monitored during treatment.

above

Amikacin

- **INDICATIONS AND DOSE**

Serious Gram-negative infections resistant to gentamicin (multiple daily dose regimen)

- BY SLOW INTRAVENOUS INJECTION
  - Child 1 month–11 years: 7.5 mg/kg every 12 hours, to be administered over 3–5 minutes
  - Child 12–17 years: 7.5 mg/kg every 12 hours; increased to 7.5 mg/kg every 8 hours (max. per dose 500 mg every 8 hours) for up to 10 days, higher dose to be used in severe infection, to be administered over 3–5 minutes; maximum 15 g per course

Serious Gram-negative infections resistant to gentamicin (once daily dose regimen)

- BY INTRAVENOUS INFUSION, OR BY INTRAVENOUS INJECTION
  - Child: Initially 15 mg/kg once daily adjusted according to plasma-concentration monitoring, not to be used for endocarditis or meningitis, dose to be adjusted according to serum-amikacin concentration, intravenous injection to be administered over 3–5 minutes

Neonatal sepsis (extended interval dose regimen)

- BY SLOW INTRAVENOUS INJECTION, OR BY INTRAVENOUS INFUSION
  - Neonate: 15 mg/kg every 24 hours, intravenous injection to be administered over 3–5 minutes.

Neonatal sepsis (multiple daily dose regimen)

- BY INTRAMUSCULAR INJECTION, OR BY SLOW INTRAVENOUS INJECTION, OR BY INTRAVENOUS INFUSION
  - Neonate: Loading dose 10 mg/kg, then 7.5 mg/kg every 12 hours, intravenous injection to be administered over 3–5 minutes.

Pseudomonal lung infection in cystic fibrosis

- BY SLOW INTRAVENOUS INJECTION, OR BY INTRAVENOUS INFUSION
  - Child: 10 mg/kg every 8 hours (max. per dose 500 mg every 8 hours), intravenous injection to be administered over 3–5 minutes

Acute pyelonephritis (once daily dose regimen) | Urinary tract infection (catheter-associated, once daily dose regimen)

- BY INTRAVENOUS INFUSION, OR BY SLOW INTRAVENOUS INJECTION
  - Child 3 months–15 years: Initially 15 mg/kg once daily, dose to be adjusted according to serum-amikacin concentration
  - Child 16–17 years: Initially 15 mg/kg once daily (max. per dose 1.5 g once daily), dose to be adjusted

according to serum-amikacin concentration; maximum 15 g per course

DOSES AT EXTREMES OF BODY-WEIGHT

- To avoid excessive dosage in obese patients, use ideal weight for height to calculate dose and monitor serum-amikacin concentration closely

- **UNLICENSED USE**
  - With intravenous use Dose for cystic fibrosis not licensed.
- **INTERACTIONS** → Appendix 1: aminoglycosides
- **SIDE-EFFECTS**
  - **Uncommon** Superinfection
  - **Rare or very rare** Albuminuria · arthralgia · balance impaired · hypotension · muscle twitching · tremor
  - **Frequency not known** Apnoea · neuromuscular blockade · paralysis
- **MONITORING REQUIREMENTS**
  - With intravenous use *Multiple daily dose regimen*: one-hour ('peak') serum concentration should not exceed 30 mg/litre; pre-dose ('trough') concentration should be less than 10 mg/litre. *Once daily dose regimen*: pre-dose ('trough') concentration should be less than 5 mg/litre.
- **DIRECTIONS FOR ADMINISTRATION**
  - With intravenous use For *intravenous infusion*, dilute with Glucose 5% *or* Sodium Chloride 0.9%; give over 30–60 minutes.
- **PRESCRIBING AND DISPENSING INFORMATION** Local guidelines may vary in the dosing advice provided.

- **MEDICINAL FORMS** There can be variation in the licensing of different medicines containing the same drug. Forms available from special-order manufacturers include: solution for injection

Solution for injection

- Amikacin (Non-proprietary)
  Amikacin (as Amikacin sulfate) 250 mg per 1 ml Amikacin 500mg/2ml solution for injection vials | 5 vial [PoM] £60.00 (Hospital only)
- Amikin (Vianex S.A.)
  Amikacin (as Amikacin sulfate) 50 mg per 1 ml Amikin 100mg/2ml solution for injection vials | 5 vial [PoM] £10.33

332

Gentamicin

19-Mar-2020

- **INDICATIONS AND DOSE**

Septicaemia | Meningitis and other CNS infections | Biliary-tract infection | Endocarditis | Pneumonia in hospital patients | Adjunct in listerial meningitis

- BY INTRAVENOUS INFUSION
  - Child: Initially 7 mg/kg, to be given in a once daily regimen (not suitable for endocarditis or meningitis), subsequent doses adjusted according to serum-gentamicin concentration
- BY INTRAMUSCULAR INJECTION, OR BY SLOW INTRAVENOUS INJECTION
  - Child 1 month–11 years: 2.5 mg/kg every 8 hours, to be given in a multiple daily dose regimen, intravenous injection to be administered over at least 3 minutes
  - Child 12–17 years: 2 mg/kg every 8 hours, to be given in a multiple daily dose regimen, intravenous injection to be administered over at least 3 minutes

Neonatal sepsis

- BY SLOW INTRAVENOUS INJECTION, OR BY INTRAVENOUS INFUSION
  - Neonate up to 7 days: 5 mg/kg every 36 hours, to be given in an extended interval dose regimen.
  - Neonate 7 days to 28 days: 5 mg/kg every 24 hours, to be given in an extended interval dose regimen.

Pseudomonal lung infection in cystic fibrosis

- BY SLOW INTRAVENOUS INJECTION, OR BY INTRAVENOUS INFUSION
  - Child: 3 mg/kg every 8 hours, to be given in a multiple daily dose regimen, intravenous injection to be administered over at least 3 minutes

Bacterial ventriculitis and CNS infection (supplement to systemic therapy) (administered on expert advice)

- BY INTRATHECAL INJECTION, OR BY INTRAVENTRICULAR INJECTION
  - Neonate: (consult local protocol).
  - Child: Initially 1 mg daily, then increased if necessary to 5 mg daily, seek specialist advice

Acute pyelonephritis (once daily dose regimen) | Urinary tract infection (catheter-associated, once daily dose regimen)

- BY INTRAVENOUS INFUSION
  - Child 3 months–15 years: Initially 7 mg/kg once daily, subsequent doses adjusted according to serum-gentamicin concentration
  - Child 16–17 years: Initially 5–7 mg/kg once daily, subsequent doses adjusted according to serum-gentamicin concentration

DOSES AT EXTREMES OF BODY-WEIGHT

- With intramuscular use or intravenous use To avoid excessive dosage in obese patients, use ideal weight for height to calculate parenteral dose and monitor serum-gentamicin concentration closely.

- **UNLICENSED USE** Gentamicin doses in BNF publications may differ from those in product literature.

> **IMPORTANT SAFETY INFORMATION**
> MHRA/CHM ADVICE: POTENTIAL FOR HISTAMINE-RELATED ADVERSE DRUG REACTIONS WITH SOME BATCHES (NOVEMBER 2017)
> - With intramuscular use or intrathecal use or intravenous use Following reports that some batches of gentamicin sulphate active pharmaceutical ingredient (API) used to manufacture gentamicin may contain higher than expected levels of histamine, which is a residual from the manufacturing process, the MHRA advise to monitor patients for signs of histamine-related adverse reactions; particular caution is required in patients taking concomitant drugs known to cause histamine release, in children, and in patients with severe renal impairment.

- **INTERACTIONS** → Appendix 1: aminoglycosides
- **SIDE-EFFECTS** Antibiotic associated colitis · blood disorder · depression · encephalopathy · hallucination · hepatic reaction · neurotoxicity · peripheral neuropathy · seizure · stomatitis · vestibular damage
- **MONITORING REQUIREMENTS**
  - With intravenous use in neonates Extended interval dose regimen in neonates: pre-dose ('trough') concentration should be less than 2 mg/litre (less than 1 mg/litre if more than 3 doses administered); consider monitoring one hour ('peak') concentration in neonates with poor response to treatment, with oedema, with Gram-negative infection, or with birth-weight greater than 4.5 kg (consider increasing dose if 'peak' concentration less than 8 mg/litre in severe sepsis).
  - With intravenous use Once daily dose regimen: pre-dose ('trough') concentration should be less than 1 mg/litre.
  - With intramuscular use or intravenous use Multiple daily dose regimen: one hour ('peak') serum concentration should be 5–10 mg/litre; pre-dose ('trough') concentration should be less than 2 mg/litre. Multiple daily dose regimen for endocarditis: one hour ('peak') serum concentration should be 3–5 mg/litre; pre-dose ('trough') concentration should be less than 1 mg/litre. Serum-gentamicin

concentration should be determined twice each week (more often in renal impairment). Multiple daily dose regimen for cystic fibrosis: one hour ('peak') serum concentration should be 8–12 mg/litre; pre-dose ('trough') concentration should be less than 2 mg/litre.
- With intrathecal use or intraventricular use Intrathecal/intraventricular injection: cerebrospinal fluid concentration should not exceed 10 mg/litre.

- **DIRECTIONS FOR ADMINISTRATION**
- With intrathecal use or intraventricular use For *intrathecal* or *intraventricular* injection, use preservative-free intrathecal preparations only.
- With intravenous use For *intravenous infusion*, dilute in Glucose 5% or Sodium Chloride 0.9%; give over 30 minutes.
- When used by inhalation For *nebulisation*, dilute preservative-free preparation in 3 mL sodium chloride 0.9%. Administer after physiotherapy and bronchodilators.
- **PRESCRIBING AND DISPENSING INFORMATION** Local guidelines may vary in the dosing advice provided.
- With intrathecal use Only preservative-free intrathecal preparation should be used.

- **MEDICINAL FORMS** There can be variation in the licensing of different medicines containing the same drug.

Solution for injection

- Gentamicin (Non-proprietary)
  Gentamicin (as Gentamicin sulfate) 5 mg per 1 ml Gentamicin Intrathecal 5mg/1ml solution for injection ampoules | 5 ampoule PoM £36.28 DT = £36.28 (Hospital only)
  Gentamicin (as Gentamicin sulfate) 10 mg per 1 ml Gentamicin 20mg/2ml solution for injection ampoules | 5 ampoule PoM £11.25 DT = £11.25
  Gentamicin Paediatric 20mg/2ml solution for injection vials | 5 vial PoM £11.25 DT = £11.25
  Gentamicin (as Gentamicin sulfate) 40 mg per 1 ml Gentamicin 80mg/2ml solution for injection vials | 5 vial PoM £20.00 DT = £6.88 (Hospital only)
  Gentamicin 80mg/2ml solution for injection ampoules | 5 ampoule PoM £6.88 DT = £6.88 | 10 ampoule PoM £12.00
- Cidomycin (Sanofi)
  Gentamicin (as Gentamicin sulfate) 40 mg per 1 ml Cidomycin 80mg/2ml solution for injection vials | 5 vial PoM £6.88 DT = £6.88
  Cidomycin 80mg/2ml solution for injection ampoules | 5 ampoule PoM £6.88 DT = £6.88

Infusion

- Gentamicin (Non-proprietary)
  Gentamicin (as Gentamicin sulfate) 1 mg per 1 ml Gentamicin 80mg/80ml infusion bags | 20 bag PoM £40.17–£44.19
  Gentamicin (as Gentamicin sulfate) 3 mg per 1 ml Gentamicin 240mg/80ml infusion bags | 20 bag PoM £122.58–£134.83
  Gentamicin 360mg/120ml infusion bags | 20 bag PoM £174.07–£191.48

F 332

Streptomycin

- **INDICATIONS AND DOSE**

Tuberculosis, resistant to other treatment, in combination with other drugs

- BY DEEP INTRAMUSCULAR INJECTION
- Child: 15 mg/kg once daily (max. per dose 1 g)

Adjunct to doxycycline in brucellosis (administered on expert advice)

- BY DEEP INTRAMUSCULAR INJECTION
- Child: 5–10 mg/kg every 6 hours, total daily dose may alternatively be given in 2–3 divided doses

- **UNLICENSED USE** Not licensed for use in children.

IMPORTANT SAFETY INFORMATION
Side-effects increase after a cumulative dose of 100 g, which should only be exceeded in exceptional circumstances.

- **INTERACTIONS** → Appendix 1: aminoglycosides
- **SIDE-EFFECTS** Amblyopia · angioedema · Clostridioides difficile colitis · haemolytic anaemia · muscle weakness · ototoxicity · pancytopenia
- **RENAL IMPAIRMENT**
  Dose adjustments Should preferably be avoided. If essential, use with great care and consider dose reduction.
- **MONITORING REQUIREMENTS**
- One-hour ('peak') concentration should be 15–40 mg/litre; pre-dose ('trough') concentration should be less than 5 mg/litre (less than 1 mg/litre in renal impairment).

- **MEDICINAL FORMS** Forms available from special-order manufacturers include: powder for solution for injection

F 332

Tobramycin

16-Mar-2020

- **INDICATIONS AND DOSE**

Chronic *Pseudomonas aeruginosa* infection in patients with cystic fibrosis

- BY INHALATION OF NEBULISED SOLUTION
- Child 6–17 years: 300 mg every 12 hours for 28 days, subsequent courses repeated after 28-day interval without tobramycin nebuliser solution
- BY INHALATION OF POWDER
- Child 6–17 years: 112 mg every 12 hours for 28 days, subsequent courses repeated after 28-day interval without tobramycin inhalation powder

Pseudomonal lung infection in cystic fibrosis

- BY SLOW INTRAVENOUS INJECTION
- Child: 8–10 mg/kg daily in 3 divided doses, to be given as a multiple daily dose regimen over 3–5 minutes
- BY INTRAVENOUS INFUSION
- Child: Initially 10 mg/kg once daily (max. per dose 660 mg), to be given over 30 minutes, subsequent doses adjusted according to serum-tobramycin concentration

Septicaemia | Meningitis and other CNS infections | Biliary-tract infection | Acute pyelonephritis | Pneumonia in hospital patients

- BY SLOW INTRAVENOUS INJECTION
- Child 1 month–11 years: 2–2.5 mg/kg every 8 hours, to be given as a multiple daily dose regimen over 3–5 minutes
- Child 12–17 years: 1 mg/kg every 8 hours, to be given as a multiple daily dose regimen over 3–5 minutes; increased if necessary up to 5 mg/kg daily in 3–4 divided doses, to be given in severe infections as a multiple daily dose regimen over 3–5 minutes, dose to be reduced back to 3 mg/kg as soon as clinically indicated
- BY INTRAVENOUS INFUSION
- Child: Initially 7 mg/kg, to be given as a once daily dose regimen, subsequent doses adjusted according to serum-tobramycin concentration

Neonatal sepsis

- BY INTRAVENOUS INJECTION, OR BY INTRAVENOUS INFUSION
- Neonate up to 32 weeks corrected gestational age: 4–5 mg/kg every 36 hours, to be given as an extended interval dose regimen, intravenous injection to be given over 3–5 minutes.
- Neonate 32 weeks corrected gestational age and above: 4–5 mg/kg every 24 hours, to be given as an extended interval dose regimen, intravenous injection to be given over 3–5 minutes.

▶ BY SLOW INTRAVENOUS INJECTION, OR BY INTRAVENOUS INFUSION

▶ Neonate up to 7 days: 2 mg/kg every 12 hours, to be given as a multiple daily dose regimen.

▶ Neonate 7 days to 28 days: 2–2.5 mg/kg every 8 hours, to be given as a multiple daily dose regimen.

DOSES AT EXTREMES OF BODY-WEIGHT

▶ With intravenous use To avoid excessive dosage in obese patients, use ideal weight for height to calculate parenteral dose and monitor serum-tobramycin concentration closely.

VANTOBRA ® NEBULISER SOLUTION

Chronic pulmonary *Pseudomonas aeruginosa* infection in patients with cystic fibrosis

▶ BY INHALATION OF NEBULISED SOLUTION

▶ Child 6-17 years: 170 mg every 12 hours for 28 days, subsequent courses repeated after 28-day interval without tobramycin nebuliser solution

● CAUTIONS

▶ When used by inhalation Auditory disorder · conditions characterised by muscular weakness (may impair neuromuscular transmission) · history of prolonged previous or concomitant intravenous aminoglycosides (increased risk of ototoxicity) · renal impairment (limited information available) · severe haemoptysis (risk of further haemorrhage) · vestibular disorder

● INTERACTIONS → Appendix 1: aminoglycosides

● SIDE-EFFECTS

GENERAL SIDE-EFFECTS

▶ **Rare or very rare** Diarrhoea · dizziness

SPECIFIC SIDE-EFFECTS

▶ **Common or very common**

▶ When used by inhalation Dysphonia · malaise · respiratory disorder · sputum discolouration

▶ **Uncommon**

▶ When used by inhalation Cough

▶ **Rare or very rare**

▶ When used by inhalation Abdominal pain · aphonia · appetite decreased · asthenia · asthma · chest discomfort · drowsiness · ear disorder · ear pain · haemorrhage · hypoxia · increased risk of infection · lymphadenopathy · oral ulceration · pain · taste altered

▶ **Frequency not known**

▶ When used by inhalation Oropharyngeal pain

▶ With parenteral use Granulocytopenia · leucocytosis · nerve disorders · urine abnormalities

SIDE-EFFECTS, FURTHER INFORMATION Manufacturer advises to monitor serum-tobramycin concentration in patients with known or suspected signs of auditory dysfunction; if ototoxicity develops — discontinue treatment until serum concentration falls below 2 mg/litre.

● RENAL IMPAIRMENT

▶ When used by inhalation Manufacturer advises monitor serum-tobramycin concentration; if nephrotoxicity develops—discontinue treatment until serum concentration falls below 2 mg/litre.

● MONITORING REQUIREMENTS

▶ With intravenous use in neonates *Extended interval dose regimen in neonates*: pre-dose ('trough') concentration should be less than 2 mg/litre.

▶ With intravenous use *Once daily dose regimen*: pre-dose ('trough') concentration should be less than 1 mg/litre. *Multiple daily dose regimen*: one-hour ('peak') serum concentration should not exceed 10 mg/litre (8–12 mg/litre in cystic fibrosis); pre-dose ('trough') concentration should be less than 2 mg/litre.

▶ When used by inhalation Measure lung function before and after initial dose of tobramycin and monitor for bronchospasm; if bronchospasm occurs in a patient not using a bronchodilator, repeat test using bronchodilator. Manufacturer advises monitor renal function before treatment and then annually.

● DIRECTIONS FOR ADMINISTRATION

▶ With intravenous use For *intravenous infusion*, dilute with Glucose 5% or Sodium Chloride 0.9%; give over 20–60 minutes.

▶ When used by inhalation Other inhaled drugs should be administered before tobramycin.

● PRESCRIBING AND DISPENSING INFORMATION Local guidelines may vary in dosing advice provided.

● PATIENT AND CARER ADVICE

▶ When used by inhalation Patient counselling is advised for Tobramycin dry powder for inhalation (administration).

VANTOBRA ® NEBULISER SOLUTION

Missed doses ▶ When used by inhalation Manufacturer advises if a dose is more than 6 hours late, the missed dose should not be taken and the next dose should be taken at the normal time.

● NATIONAL FUNDING/ACCESS DECISIONS

NICE decisions

▶ **Tobramycin by dry powder inhalation for pseudomonal lung infection in cystic fibrosis (March 2013)** NICE TA276
Tobramycin dry powder for inhalation is recommended for chronic pulmonary infection caused by *Pseudomonas aeruginosa* in patients with cystic fibrosis only if there is an inadequate response to colistimethate sodium, or if colistimethate sodium cannot be used because of contra-indications or intolerance. The manufacturer must provide tobramycin dry powder for inhalation at the discount agreed as part of the patient access scheme to primary, secondary and tertiary care in the NHS. Patients currently receiving tobramycin dry powder for inhalation can continue treatment until they and their clinician consider it appropriate to stop.
www.nice.org.uk/guidance/ta276

● MEDICINAL FORMS There can be variation in the licensing of different medicines containing the same drug.

Solution for injection

▶ Tobramycin (Non-proprietary)
Tobramycin 40 mg per 1 ml Tobramycin 80mg/2ml solution for injection vials | 1 vial PoM £5.37 DT = £5.37 | 5 vial PoM £20.80 DT = £20.80
Tobramycin 240mg/6ml solution for injection vials | 1 vial PoM £19.20 DT = £19.20

▶ **Nebcin** (Flynn Pharma Ltd)
Tobramycin 40 mg per 1 ml Nebcin 80mg/2ml solution for injection vials | 1 vial PoM £5.37 DT = £5.37

Inhalation powder

▶ **Tobi Podhaler** (Mylan)
Tobramycin 28 mg Tobi Podhaler 28mg inhalation powder capsules with device | 224 capsule PoM £1,790.00 DT = £1,790.00

Nebuliser liquid

▶ Tobramycin (Non-proprietary)
Tobramycin 60 mg per 1 ml Tobramycin 300mg/5ml nebuliser liquid ampoules | 56 ampoule PoM £1,187.00–£1,305.92 DT = £780.00
Munuza 300mg/5ml nebuliser solution 5ml ampoules | 56 ampoule PoM £779.99 DT = £780.00

▶ **Bramitob** (Chiesi Ltd)
Tobramycin 75 mg per 1 ml Bramitob 300mg/4ml nebuliser solution 4ml ampoules | 56 ampoule PoM £1,187.00 DT = £1,187.00

▶ **TOBI** (Mylan)
Tobramycin 60 mg per 1 ml Tobi 300mg/5ml nebuliser solution 5ml ampoules | 56 ampoule PoM £1,305.92 DT = £780.00

▶ **Tymbrineb** (Teva UK Ltd)
Tobramycin 60 mg per 1 ml Tymbrineb 300mg/5ml nebuliser solution 5ml ampoules | 56 ampoule PoM £780.00 DT = £780.00

▶ **Vantobra** (Pari Medical Ltd)
Tobramycin 100 mg per 1 ml Vantobra 170mg/1.7ml nebuliser solution 1.7ml ampoules | 56 ampoule PoM £1,305.00

ANTIBACTERIALS > CARBAPENEMS

Carbapenems

Overview

The carbapenems are beta-lactam antibacterials with a broad-spectrum of activity which includes many Gram-positive and Gram-negative bacteria, and anaerobes; **imipenem** (imipenem with cilastatin below) and meropenem p. 337 have good activity against *Pseudomonas aeruginosa*. The carbapenems are not active against meticillin-resistant *Staphylococcus aureus* and *Enterococcus faecium*.

Imipenem (imipenem with cilastatin) and meropenem are used for the treatment of severe hospital-acquired infections and polymicrobial infections caused by multiple-antibacterial resistant organisms (including septicaemia, hospital-acquired pneumonia, intra-abdominal infections, skin and soft-tissue infections, and complicated urinary-tract infections).

Ertapenem below is licensed for treating abdominal and gynaecological infections and for community-acquired pneumonia, but it is not active against atypical respiratory pathogens and it has limited activity against penicillin-resistant pneumococci. Unlike the other carbapenems, ertapenem is not active against *Pseudomonas* or against *Acinetobacter spp*.

Imipenem is partially inactivated in the kidney by enzymatic activity and is therefore administered in combination with **cilastatin** (imipenem with cilastatin), a specific enzyme inhibitor, which blocks its renal metabolism. Meropenem and ertapenem are stable to the renal enzyme which inactivates imipenem and therefore can be given without cilastatin.

Side-effects of imipenem with cilastatin are similar to those of other beta-lactam antibiotics. Meropenem has less seizure-inducing potential and can be used to treat central nervous system infection.

Ertapenem

29-Apr-2020

- **INDICATIONS AND DOSE**

Abdominal infections | Acute gynaecological infections | Community-acquired pneumonia

▸ BY INTRAVENOUS INFUSION

- Child 3 months–12 years: 15 mg/kg every 12 hours; maximum 1 g per day
- Child 13–17 years: 1 g once daily

Diabetic foot infections of the skin and soft-tissue

▸ BY INTRAVENOUS INFUSION

- Child 13–17 years: 1 g once daily

- **CAUTIONS** CNS disorders—risk of seizures
- **INTERACTIONS** → Appendix 1: carbapenems
- **SIDE-EFFECTS**

▸ **Common or very common** Diarrhoea · skin reactions

▸ **Uncommon** Faeces discoloured · headache · hot flush · hypertension · melaena

▸ **Frequency not known** Aggression · hallucination · psychiatric disorder

- **ALLERGY AND CROSS-SENSITIVITY** Avoid if history of **immediate hypersensitivity** reaction to beta-lactam antibacterials.

  Use with caution in patients with sensitivity to beta-lactam antibacterials.
- **PREGNANCY** Manufacturer advises avoid unless potential benefit outweighs risk.
- **BREAST FEEDING** Present in milk—manufacturer advises avoid.
- **RENAL IMPAIRMENT** Use with caution (risk of seizures); avoid if estimated glomerular filtration rate less than 30 mL/minute/1.73 m^2.
- **DIRECTIONS FOR ADMINISTRATION** For *intravenous infusion* (*Invanz*®), give intermittently *in* Sodium chloride 0.9%. Reconstitute 1 g with 10 mL Water for injections *or* Sodium chloride 0.9%; dilute requisite dose in infusion fluid to a final concentration not exceeding 20 mg/mL; give over 30 minutes; incompatible with glucose solutions.
- **PRESCRIBING AND DISPENSING INFORMATION** For choice of antibacterial therapy, see Diabetic foot infections, antibacterial therapy p. 324, Gastro-intestinal system infections, antibacterial therapy p. 324, Respiratory system infections, antibacterial therapy p. 327.

- **MEDICINAL FORMS** There can be variation in the licensing of different medicines containing the same drug.

Powder for solution for infusion

ELECTROLYTES: May contain Sodium

▸ **Ertapenem (Non-proprietary)**

Ertapenem (as Ertapenem sodium) 1 gram Ertapenem 1g powder for concentrate for solution for infusion vials | 10 vial PoM ⓗ (Hospital only)

▸ **Invanz (Merck Sharp & Dohme Ltd)**

Ertapenem (as Ertapenem sodium) 1 gram Invanz 1g powder for solution for infusion vials | 1 vial PoM £31.65 DT = £31.65

Imipenem with cilastatin

29-Apr-2020

- **INDICATIONS AND DOSE**

Aerobic and anaerobic Gram-positive and Gram-negative infections (not indicated for CNS infections) | Hospital-acquired septicaemia

▸ BY INTRAVENOUS INFUSION

- Neonate up to 7 days: 20 mg/kg every 12 hours.
- Neonate 7 days to 20 days: 20 mg/kg every 8 hours.
- Neonate 21 days to 28 days: 20 mg/kg every 6 hours.
- Child 1–2 months: 20 mg/kg every 6 hours
- Child 3 months–17 years: 15 mg/kg every 6 hours (max. per dose 500 mg)

Infection caused by *Pseudomonas* or other less sensitive organisms | Empirical treatment of infection in febrile patients with neutropenia | Life-threatening infection

▸ BY INTRAVENOUS INFUSION

- Child 3 months–17 years: 25 mg/kg every 6 hours (max. per dose 1 g)

Cystic fibrosis

▸ BY INTRAVENOUS INFUSION

- Child: 25 mg/kg every 6 hours (max. per dose 1 g)

DOSE EQUIVALENCE AND CONVERSION

- Dose expressed in terms of imipenem.

- **UNLICENSED USE** Not licensed for use in children under 1 year.
- **CAUTIONS** CNS disorders · epilepsy
- **INTERACTIONS** → Appendix 1: carbapenems
- **SIDE-EFFECTS**

▸ **Common or very common** Diarrhoea · eosinophilia · nausea · skin reactions · thrombophlebitis · vomiting

▸ **Uncommon** Bone marrow disorders · confusion · dizziness · drowsiness · hallucination · hypotension · leucopenia · movement disorders · psychiatric disorder · seizure · thrombocytopenia · thrombocytosis

▸ **Rare or very rare** Agranulocytosis · anaphylactic reaction · angioedema · chest discomfort · colitis haemorrhagic · cyanosis · dyspnoea · encephalopathy · flushing · focal tremor · gastrointestinal discomfort · haemolytic anaemia · headache · hearing loss · hepatic disorders · hyperhidrosis ·

hyperventilation · increased risk of infection · myasthenia gravis aggravated · oral disorders · palpitations · paraesthesia · polyarthralgia · polyuria · pseudomembranous enterocolitis · renal impairment · severe cutaneous adverse reactions (SCARs) · spinal pain · tachycardia · taste altered · tinnitus · tongue discolouration · tooth discolouration · urine discolouration · vertigo

▸ **Frequency not known** Agitation

● ALLERGY AND CROSS-SENSITIVITY Avoid if history of **immediate hypersensitivity** reaction to beta-lactam antibacterials.

Use with caution in patients with sensitivity to beta-lactam antibacterials.

● PREGNANCY Manufacturer advises avoid unless potential benefit outweighs risk (toxicity in *animal* studies).

● BREAST FEEDING Present in milk but unlikely to be absorbed.

● RENAL IMPAIRMENT Clinical data are insufficient to recommend dosing for children with impairment (serum creatinine greater than 2 mg/dl)—in *adults*, manufacturer advises reduce dose (consult product literature).

● EFFECT ON LABORATORY TESTS Positive Coombs' test.

● DIRECTIONS FOR ADMINISTRATION For *intravenous infusion* dilute to a concentration of 5 mg (as imipenem)/mL in Sodium chloride 0.9%; give up to 500 mg (as imipenem) over 20–30 minutes, give dose greater than 500 mg (as imipenem) over 40–60 minutes.

● MEDICINAL FORMS There can be variation in the licensing of different medicines containing the same drug.

Powder for solution for infusion

ELECTROLYTES: May contain Sodium

▸ Imipenem with cilastatin (Non-proprietary)
Cilastatin (as Cilastatin sodium) 500 mg, Imipenem (as Imipenem monohydrate) 500 mg Imipenem 500mg / Cilastatin 500mg powder for solution for infusion vials | 10 vial PoM £130.30

▸ Primaxin I.V. (Merck Sharp & Dohme Ltd)
Cilastatin (as Cilastatin sodium) 500 mg, Imipenem (as Imipenem monohydrate) 500 mg Primaxin IV 500mg powder for solution for infusion vials | 1 vial PoM £12.00

Meropenem

06-Aug-2018

● INDICATIONS AND DOSE

Aerobic and anaerobic Gram-positive and Gram-negative infections | Hospital-acquired septicaemia

▶ BY INTRAVENOUS INFUSION, OR BY INTRAVENOUS INJECTION

▸ Neonate up to 7 days: 20 mg/kg every 12 hours.

▸ Neonate 7 days to 28 days: 20 mg/kg every 8 hours.

▸ Child 1 month–11 years (body-weight up to 50 kg): 10–20 mg/kg every 8 hours

▸ Child 1 month–11 years (body-weight 50 kg and above): 0.5–1 g every 8 hours

▸ Child 12–17 years: 0.5–1 g every 8 hours

Severe aerobic and anaerobic Gram-positive and Gram-negative infections

▶ BY INTRAVENOUS INFUSION, OR BY INTRAVENOUS INJECTION

▸ Neonate up to 7 days: 40 mg/kg every 12 hours.

▸ Neonate 7 days to 28 days: 40 mg/kg every 8 hours.

Exacerbations of chronic lower respiratory-tract infection in cystic fibrosis

▶ BY INTRAVENOUS INFUSION

▸ Child 1 month–11 years (body-weight up to 50 kg): 40 mg/kg every 8 hours

▸ Child 1 month–11 years (body-weight 50 kg and above): 2 g every 8 hours

▸ Child 12–17 years: 2 g every 8 hours

Meningitis

▶ BY INTRAVENOUS INFUSION

▸ Neonate up to 7 days: 40 mg/kg every 12 hours.

▸ Neonate 7 days to 28 days: 40 mg/kg every 8 hours.

▸ Child 1 month–11 years (body-weight up to 50 kg): 40 mg/kg every 8 hours

▸ Child 1 month–11 years (body-weight 50 kg and above): 2 g every 8 hours

▸ Child 12–17 years: 2 g every 8 hours

● UNLICENSED USE Not licensed for use in children under 3 months.

● INTERACTIONS → Appendix 1: carbapenems

● SIDE-EFFECTS

▸ **Common or very common** Abdominal pain · diarrhoea · headache · inflammation · nausea · pain · skin reactions · thrombocytosis · vomiting

▸ **Uncommon** Agranulocytosis · antibiotic associated colitis · eosinophilia · haemolytic anaemia · increased risk of infection · leucopenia · neutropenia · paraesthesia · severe cutaneous adverse reactions (SCARs) · thrombocytopenia · thrombophlebitis

▸ **Rare or very rare** Seizure

● ALLERGY AND CROSS-SENSITIVITY Avoid if history of **immediate hypersensitivity** reaction to beta-lactam antibacterials.

Use with caution in patients with sensitivity to beta-lactam antibacterials.

● PREGNANCY Use only if potential benefit outweighs risk—no information available.

● BREAST FEEDING Unlikely to be absorbed (however, manufacturer advises avoid).

● RENAL IMPAIRMENT

Dose adjustments Use normal dose every 12 hours if estimated glomerular filtration rate 26–50 mL/minute/1.73 m^2.

Use half normal dose every 12 hours if estimated glomerular filtration rate 10–25 mL/minute/1.73 m^2.

Use half normal dose every 24 hours if estimated glomerular filtration rate less than 10 mL/minute/1.73 m^2.

● MONITORING REQUIREMENTS Manufacturer advises monitor liver function—risk of hepatotoxicity.

● EFFECT ON LABORATORY TESTS Positive Coombs' test.

● DIRECTIONS FOR ADMINISTRATION *Intravenous injection* to be administered over 5 minutes.

Displacement value may be significant when reconstituting injection, consult local guidelines. For *intravenous infusion*, dilute reconstituted solution further to a concentration of 1–20 mg/mL *in* Glucose 5% *or* Sodium Chloride 0.9%; give over 15–30 minutes.

● MEDICINAL FORMS There can be variation in the licensing of different medicines containing the same drug.

Powder for solution for injection

ELECTROLYTES: May contain Sodium

▸ Meropenem (Non-proprietary)
Meropenem (as Meropenem trihydrate) 500 mg Meropenem 500mg powder for solution for injection vials | 10 vial PoM £103.14 DT = £93.30 (Hospital only) | 10 vial PoM £90.00–£103.14 DT = £93.30
Meropenem (as Meropenem trihydrate) 1 gram Meropenem 1g powder for solution for injection vials | 10 vial PoM £186.70–£206.30 DT = £186.70 | 10 vial PoM £206.28 DT = £186.70 (Hospital only)

▸ Meronem (Pfizer Ltd)
Meropenem (as Meropenem trihydrate) 500 mg Meronem 500mg powder for solution for injection vials | 10 vial PoM £103.14 DT = £93.30
Meropenem (as Meropenem trihydrate) 1 gram Meronem 1g powder for solution for injection vials | 10 vial PoM £206.28 DT = £186.70

ANTIBACTERIALS > CEPHALOSPORINS

Cephalosporins

Overview

The cephalosporins are broad-spectrum antibiotics which are used for the treatment of septicaemia, pneumonia, meningitis, biliary-tract infections, peritonitis, and urinary-tract infections. The pharmacology of the cephalosporins is similar to that of the penicillins, excretion being principally renal. Cephalosporins penetrate the cerebrospinal fluid poorly unless the meninges are inflamed; cefotaxime p. 342 and ceftriaxone p. 343 are suitable cephalosporins for infections of the CNS (e.g meningitis).

The principal side-effect of the cephalosporins is hypersensitivity and about 0.5–6.5% of penicillin-sensitive patients will also be allergic to the cephalosporins. If a cephalosporin is essential in patients with a history of immediate hypersensitivity to penicillin, because a suitable alternative antibacterial is not available, then cefixime p. 342, cefotaxime, ceftazidime p. 343, ceftriaxone, or cefuroxime p. 341 can be used with caution; cefaclor p. 340, cefadroxil below, cefalexin p. 339, and cefradine p. 339 should be avoided.

The orally active 'first generation' cephalosporins, cefalexin, cefradine, and cefadroxil and the 'second generation' cephalosporin, cefaclor have a similar antimicrobial spectrum. They are useful for urinary-tract infections, respiratory-tract infections, otitis media, and skin and soft-tissue infections. Cefaclor has good activity against *H. influenzae*. Cefadroxil has a long duration of action and can be given twice daily; it has poor activity against *H. influenzae*. **Cefuroxime axetil**, an ester of the 'second generation' cephalosporin cefuroxime, has the same antibacterial spectrum as the parent compound; it is poorly absorbed and needs to be given with food to maximise absorption.

Cefixime is an orally active 'third generation' cephalosporin. It has a longer duration of action than the other cephalosporins that are active by mouth. It is only licensed for acute infections.

Cefuroxime is a 'second generation' cephalosporin that is less susceptible than the earlier cephalosporins to inactivation by beta-lactamases. It is, therefore, active against certain bacteria which are resistant to the other drugs and has greater activity against *Haemophilus influenzae*.

Cefotaxime, ceftazidime and ceftriaxone are 'third generation' cephalosporins with greater activity than the 'second generation' cephalosporins against certain Gram-negative bacteria. However, they are less active than cefuroxime against Gram-positive bacteria, most notably *Staphylococcus aureus*. Their broad antibacterial spectrum may encourage superinfection with resistant bacteria or fungi.

Ceftazidime has good activity against pseudomonas. It is also active against other Gram-negative bacteria.

Ceftriaxone has a longer half-life and therefore needs to be given only once daily. Indications include serious infections such as septicaemia, pneumonia, and meningitis. The calcium salt of ceftriaxone forms a precipitate in the gall bladder which may rarely cause symptoms but these usually resolve when the antibacterial is stopped. In neonates, ceftriaxone may displace bilirubin from plasma-albumin and should be avoided in neonates with unconjugated hyperbilirubinaemia, hypoalbuminaemia, acidosis or impaired bilirubin binding.

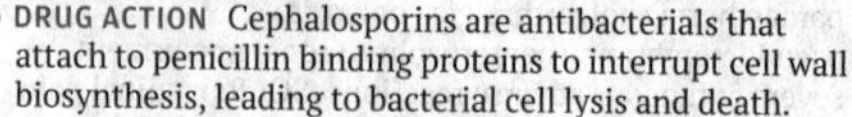

Cephalosporins

- **DRUG ACTION** Cephalosporins are antibacterials that attach to penicillin binding proteins to interrupt cell wall biosynthesis, leading to bacterial cell lysis and death.
- **SIDE-EFFECTS**
  - **Common or very common** Abdominal pain · diarrhoea · dizziness · eosinophilia · headache · leucopenia · nausea · neutropenia · skin reactions · thrombocytopenia · vomiting · vulvovaginal candidiasis
  - **Uncommon** Anaphylactic reaction · pseudomembranous enterocolitis
  - **Rare or very rare** Agranulocytosis · angioedema · nephritis tubulointerstitial (reversible) · severe cutaneous adverse reactions (SCARs)
  - **Frequency not known** Haemolytic anaemia
- **ALLERGY AND CROSS-SENSITIVITY** Contra-indicated in patients with cephalosporin hypersensitivity.
  - **Cross-sensitivity with other beta-lactam antibacterials** About 0.5–6.5% of penicillin-sensitive patients will also be allergic to the cephalosporins. Patients with a history of **immediate hypersensitivity** to penicillin and other beta-lactams should not receive a cephalosporin. Cephalosporins should be used with caution in patients with sensitivity to penicillin and other beta-lactams.
- **EFFECT ON LABORATORY TESTS** False positive urinary glucose (if tested for reducing substances). False positive Coombs' test.

ANTIBACTERIALS > CEPHALOSPORINS, FIRST-GENERATION

above

Cefadroxil

- **INDICATIONS AND DOSE**

Susceptible infections due to sensitive Gram-positive and Gram-negative bacteria

- BY MOUTH
  - Child 6–17 years (body-weight up to 40 kg): 0.5 g twice daily
  - Child 6–17 years (body-weight 40 kg and above): 0.5–1 g twice daily

Skin infections | Soft-tissue infections | Uncomplicated urinary-tract infections

- BY MOUTH
  - Child 6–17 years (body-weight 40 kg and above): 1 g once daily

- **INTERACTIONS** → Appendix 1: cephalosporins
- **SIDE-EFFECTS**
  - **Common or very common** Dyspepsia · glossitis
  - **Uncommon** Fungal infection
  - **Rare or very rare** Arthralgia · drug fever · fatigue · hepatic disorders · insomnia · nervousness · serum sickness-like reaction
- **PREGNANCY** Not known to be harmful.
- **BREAST FEEDING** Present in milk in low concentration, but appropriate to use.
- **RENAL IMPAIRMENT**

  Dose adjustments Reduce dose if estimated glomerular filtration rate less than 50 mL/minute/1.73 m^2.

- **MEDICINAL FORMS** There can be variation in the licensing of different medicines containing the same drug.

Capsule

CAUTIONARY AND ADVISORY LABELS 9

- Cefadroxil (Non-proprietary)

  Cefadroxil (as Cefadroxil monohydrate) 500 mg Cefadroxil 500mg capsules | 20 capsule [PoM] £22.38 DT = £6.45

338

Cefalexin

26-Mar-2020

(Cephalexin)

- **INDICATIONS AND DOSE**

Susceptible infections due to sensitive Gram-positive and Gram-negative bacteria

▶ BY MOUTH

- ▶ Neonate up to 7 days: 25 mg/kg twice daily (max. per dose 125 mg).
- ▶ Neonate 7 days to 20 days: 25 mg/kg 3 times a day (max. per dose 125 mg).
- ▶ Neonate 21 days to 28 days: 25 mg/kg 4 times a day (max. per dose 125 mg).
- ▶ Child 1–11 months: 12.5 mg/kg twice daily, alternatively 125 mg twice daily
- ▶ Child 1–4 years: 12.5 mg/kg twice daily, alternatively 125 mg 3 times a day
- ▶ Child 5–11 years: 12.5 mg/kg twice daily, alternatively 250 mg 3 times a day
- ▶ Child 12–17 years: 500 mg 2–3 times a day

Serious susceptible infections due to sensitive Gram-positive and Gram-negative bacteria

▶ BY MOUTH

- ▶ Child 1 month–11 years: 25 mg/kg 2–4 times a day (max. per dose 1 g 4 times a day)
- ▶ Child 12–17 years: 1–1.5 g 3–4 times a day

Prophylaxis of recurrent urinary-tract infection

▶ BY MOUTH

- ▶ Child 3 months–15 years: 12.5 mg/kg once daily (max. per dose 125 mg), dose to be taken at night
- ▶ Child 16–17 years: 125 mg once daily, dose to be taken at night, alternatively 500 mg for 1 dose, following exposure to a trigger

Acute pyelonephritis | Urinary-tract infection (catheter-associated)

▶ BY MOUTH

- ▶ Child 3–11 months: 12.5 mg/kg twice daily for 7 to 10 days, alternatively 125 mg twice daily; increased if necessary to 25 mg/kg 2–4 times a day (max. per dose 1 g 4 times a day), increased dose used in severe infections
- ▶ Child 1–4 years: 12.5 mg/kg twice daily, alternatively 125 mg 3 times a day for 7 to 10 days; increased if necessary to 25 mg/kg 2–4 times a day (max. per dose 1 g 4 times a day), increased dose used in severe infections
- ▶ Child 5–11 years: 12.5 mg/kg twice daily, alternatively 250 mg 3 times a day for 7 to 10 days; increased if necessary to 25 mg/kg 2–4 times a day (max. per dose 1 g 4 times a day), increased dose used in severe infections
- ▶ Child 12–17 years: 500 mg 2–3 times a day for 7 to 10 days; increased to 1–1.5 g 3–4 times a day, increased dose used in severe infections

Lower urinary-tract infection in pregnancy

▶ BY MOUTH

- ▶ Child 12–17 years: 500 mg twice daily for 7 days

Lower urinary-tract infection

▶ BY MOUTH

- ▶ Child 3–11 months: 12.5 mg/kg twice daily, alternatively 125 mg twice daily for 3 days
- ▶ Child 1–4 years: 12.5 mg/kg twice daily, alternatively 125 mg 3 times a day for 3 days
- ▶ Child 5–11 years: 12.5 mg/kg twice daily, alternatively 250 mg 3 times a day for 3 days
- ▶ Child 12–15 years: 500 mg twice daily for 3 days

- **UNLICENSED USE** EvGr Cefalexin is used for prophylaxis of recurrent urinary-tract infection, ⟨A⟩ but is not licensed for this indication.
- **INTERACTIONS** → Appendix 1: cephalosporins
- **SIDE-EFFECTS** Agitation · arthritis · confusion · fatigue · fungal infection · gastrointestinal discomfort · genital pruritus · hallucination · hepatitis (transient) · hypersensitivity · jaundice cholestatic (transient) · joint disorders · vaginal discharge
- **PREGNANCY** Not known to be harmful.
- **BREAST FEEDING** Present in milk in low concentration, but appropriate to use.
- **RENAL IMPAIRMENT**

Dose adjustments Reduce dose in moderate impairment.

- **PRESCRIBING AND DISPENSING INFORMATION** For choice of antibacterial therapy, see Urinary-tract infections p. 400.
- **PATIENT AND CARER ADVICE**

Medicines for Children leaflet: Cefalexin for bacterial infections www.medicinesforchildren.org.uk/cefalexin-bacterial-infections-0

- **PROFESSION SPECIFIC INFORMATION**

Dental practitioners' formulary

Cefalexin Capsules may be prescribed. Cefalexin Tablets may be prescribed. Cefalexin Oral Suspension may be prescribed.

- **MEDICINAL FORMS** There can be variation in the licensing of different medicines containing the same drug.

Oral suspension

CAUTIONARY AND ADVISORY LABELS 9

▶ Cefalexin (Non-proprietary)

Cefalexin 25 mg per 1 ml Cefalexin 125mg/5ml oral suspension sugar-free | 100 ml PoM £0.84–£2.92 DT = £2.74

Cefalexin 125mg/5ml oral suspension | 100 ml PoM £1.95 DT = £1.95

Cefalexin 50 mg per 1 ml Cefalexin 250mg/5ml oral suspension sugar-free | 100 ml PoM £1.72–£3.38 DT = £3.19

Cefalexin 250mg/5ml oral suspension | 100 ml PoM £2.25 DT = £2.25

Tablet

CAUTIONARY AND ADVISORY LABELS 9

▶ Cefalexin (Non-proprietary)

Cefalexin 250 mg Cefalexin 250mg tablets | 28 tablet PoM £2.59 DT = £2.59

Cefalexin 500 mg Cefalexin 500mg tablets | 21 tablet PoM £5.35 DT = £2.90

▶ Keflex (Flynn Pharma Ltd)

Cefalexin 500 mg Keflex 500mg tablets | 21 tablet PoM £2.08 DT = £2.90

Capsule

CAUTIONARY AND ADVISORY LABELS 9

▶ Cefalexin (Non-proprietary)

Cefalexin 250 mg Cefalexin 250mg capsules | 28 capsule PoM £2.03 DT = £1.90

Cefalexin 500 mg Cefalexin 500mg capsules | 21 capsule PoM £2.45 DT = £2.15

338

Cefradine

(Cephradine)

- **INDICATIONS AND DOSE**

Susceptible infections due to sensitive Gram-positive and Gram-negative bacteria | Surgical prophylaxis

▶ BY MOUTH

- ▶ Child 7–11 years: 25–50 mg/kg daily in 2–4 divided doses
- ▶ Child 12–17 years: 250–500 mg 4 times a day, alternatively 0.5–1 g twice daily; increased if necessary up to 1 g 4 times a day, increased dose may be used in severe infections

continued →

Prevention of *Staphylococcus aureus* lung infection in cystic fibrosis
▶ BY MOUTH
▸ Child 7–17 years: 2 g twice daily

- **UNLICENSED USE** Not licensed for use in children for prevention of *Staphylococcus aureus* lung infection in cystic fibrosis.
- **INTERACTIONS** → Appendix 1: cephalosporins
- **SIDE-EFFECTS** Akathisia · antibiotic associated colitis · aplastic anaemia · arthralgia · blood disorder · chest tightness · confusion · gastrointestinal discomfort · glossitis · hepatitis (transient) · hypersensitivity · increased risk of infection · jaundice cholestatic · muscle tone increased · nervousness · oedema · sleep disorder
- **PREGNANCY** Not known to be harmful.
- **BREAST FEEDING** Present in milk in low concentration, but appropriate to use.
- **RENAL IMPAIRMENT**
Dose adjustments Reduce dose if estimated glomerular filtration rate less than 20 mL/minute/1.73 m^2.
- **PROFESSION SPECIFIC INFORMATION**
Dental practitioners' formulary
Cefradine Capsules may be prescribed.

- **MEDICINAL FORMS** There can be variation in the licensing of different medicines containing the same drug.

Capsule
CAUTIONARY AND ADVISORY LABELS 9
▸ Cefradine (Non-proprietary)
Cefradine 250 mg Cefradine 250mg capsules | 20 capsule [PoM] £6.00 DT = £3.92
Cefradine 500 mg Cefradine 500mg capsules | 20 capsule [PoM] £8.75 DT = £4.88

ANTIBACTERIALS > CEPHALOSPORINS, SECOND-GENERATION

338

Cefaclor

- **INDICATIONS AND DOSE**

Susceptible infections due to sensitive Gram-positive and Gram-negative bacteria
▶ BY MOUTH USING IMMEDIATE-RELEASE MEDICINES
▸ Child 1–11 months: 20 mg/kg daily in 3 divided doses, alternatively 62.5 mg 3 times a day
▸ Child 1–4 years: 20 mg/kg daily in 3 divided doses, alternatively 125 mg 3 times a day
▸ Child 5–11 years: 20 mg/kg daily in 3 divided doses, usual max. 1 g daily, alternatively 250 mg 3 times a day
▸ Child 12–17 years: 250 mg 3 times a day; maximum 4 g per day
▶ BY MOUTH USING MODIFIED-RELEASE MEDICINES
▸ Child 12–17 years: 375 mg every 12 hours, dose to be taken with food

Severe susceptible infections due to sensitive Gram-positive and Gram-negative bacteria
▶ BY MOUTH USING IMMEDIATE-RELEASE MEDICINES
▸ Child 1–11 months: 40 mg/kg daily in 3 divided doses, usual max. 1 g daily, alternatively 125 mg 3 times a day
▸ Child 1–4 years: 40 mg/kg daily in 3 divided doses, usual max. 1 g daily, alternatively 250 mg 3 times a day
▸ Child 5–11 years: 40 mg/kg daily in 3 divided doses, usual max. 1 g daily
▸ Child 12–17 years: 500 mg 3 times a day; maximum 4 g per day

Pneumonia
▶ BY MOUTH USING MODIFIED-RELEASE TABLETS
▸ Child 12–17 years: 750 mg every 12 hours, dose to be taken with food

Lower urinary-tract infections
▶ BY MOUTH USING MODIFIED-RELEASE MEDICINES
▸ Child 12–17 years: 375 mg every 12 hours, dose to be taken with food

Asymptomatic carriage of *Haemophilus influenzae* or mild exacerbations in cystic fibrosis
▶ BY MOUTH USING IMMEDIATE-RELEASE MEDICINES
▸ Child 1–11 months: 125 mg every 8 hours
▸ Child 1–6 years: 250 mg 3 times a day
▸ Child 7–17 years: 500 mg 3 times a day

- **INTERACTIONS** → Appendix 1: cephalosporins
- **SIDE-EFFECTS** Akathisia · anxiety · aplastic anaemia · arthralgia · arthritis · asthenia · colitis · confusion · drowsiness · dyspnoea · fever · fungal infection · genital pruritus · hallucination · hepatitis (transient) · hypersensitivity · insomnia · jaundice cholestatic (transient) · lymphadenopathy · lymphocytosis · muscle tone increased · oedema · paraesthesia · proteinuria · syncope · vasodilation
SIDE-EFFECTS, FURTHER INFORMATION Cefaclor is associated with protracted skin reactions, especially in children.
- **PREGNANCY** Not known to be harmful.
- **BREAST FEEDING** Present in milk in low concentration, but appropriate to use.
- **RENAL IMPAIRMENT** Manufacturer advises caution.
Dose adjustments No dose adjustment required.

- **MEDICINAL FORMS** There can be variation in the licensing of different medicines containing the same drug.

Oral suspension
CAUTIONARY AND ADVISORY LABELS 9
▸ Distaclor (Flynn Pharma Ltd)
Cefaclor (as Cefaclor monohydrate) 25 mg per 1 ml Distaclor 125mg/5ml oral suspension | 100 ml [PoM] £4.13 DT = £4.13
Cefaclor (as Cefaclor monohydrate) 50 mg per 1 ml Distaclor 250mg/5ml oral suspension | 100 ml [PoM] £8.26 DT = £8.26

Modified-release tablet
CAUTIONARY AND ADVISORY LABELS 9, 21, 25
▸ Distaclor MR (Flynn Pharma Ltd)
Cefaclor (as Cefaclor monohydrate) 375 mg Distaclor MR 375mg tablets | 14 tablet [PoM] £9.10 DT = £9.10

Capsule
CAUTIONARY AND ADVISORY LABELS 9
▸ Distaclor (Flynn Pharma Ltd)
Cefaclor (as Cefaclor monohydrate) 500 mg Distaclor 500mg capsules | 21 capsule [PoM] £7.50 DT = £7.50

338

Cefoxitin

21-Aug-2019

- **INDICATIONS AND DOSE**

Complicated urinary tract infection | Pyelonephritis
▶ BY SLOW INTRAVENOUS INJECTION
▸ Child 12–17 years: 2 g every 4–6 hours; maximum 12 g per day

- **INTERACTIONS** → Appendix 1: cephalosporins
- **SIDE-EFFECTS** Anaemia · bone marrow failure · encephalopathy · fever · hypersensitivity · local reaction · myasthenia gravis aggravated · overgrowth of nonsusceptible organisms · renal impairment · thrombophlebitis
- **PREGNANCY** Manufacturer advises not known to be harmful.
- **BREAST FEEDING** [EvGr] Specialist sources indicate present in milk in low concentrations, but appropriate to use. ⟨D⟩
- **RENAL IMPAIRMENT**
Dose adjustments Manufacturer advises increase dosing interval to every 8-12 hours if creatinine clearance 30-50 mL/minute, or every 12-24 hours if creatinine clearance

10-29 mL/minute. Consult product literature if creatinine clearance less than 10 mL/minute.

- **DIRECTIONS FOR ADMINISTRATION** For *slow intravenous injection*, reconstitute with 10 mL water for injections; give over 3 to 5 minutes.

- **MEDICINAL FORMS** There can be variation in the licensing of different medicines containing the same drug. Forms available from special-order manufacturers include: powder for solution for injection

Powder for solution for injection

ELECTROLYTES: May contain Sodium

- Cefoxitin (Non-proprietary)
  Cefoxitin (as Cefoxitin sodium) 1 gram Cefoxitin 1g powder for solution for injection vials | 10 vial PoM
  Renoxitin 1g powder for solution for injection vials | 10 vial PoM £156.00 (Hospital only)
  Cefoxitin (as Cefoxitin sodium) 2 gram Renoxitin 2g powder for solution for injection vials | 10 vial PoM £269.00 (Hospital only)
  Cefoxitin 2g powder for solution for injection vials | 10 vial PoM

F 338

Cefuroxime

21-May-2020

- **INDICATIONS AND DOSE**

Susceptible infections due to Gram-positive and Gram-negative bacteria

- BY MOUTH
- Child 3 months–1 year: 10 mg/kg twice daily (max. per dose 125 mg)
- Child 2–11 years: 15 mg/kg twice daily (max. per dose 250 mg)
- Child 12–17 years: 250 mg twice daily, dose may be doubled in severe lower respiratory-tract infections or if pneumonia is suspected
- BY INTRAVENOUS INFUSION, OR BY INTRAVENOUS INJECTION
- Neonate up to 7 days: 25 mg/kg every 12 hours, increased if necessary to 50 mg/kg every 12 hours, increased dose used in severe infection.
- Neonate 7 days to 20 days: 25 mg/kg every 8 hours, increased if necessary to 50 mg/kg every 8 hours, increased dose used in severe infection.
- Neonate 21 days to 28 days: 25 mg/kg every 6 hours, increased if necessary to 50 mg/kg every 6 hours, increased dose used in severe infection.
- BY INTRAVENOUS INFUSION, OR BY INTRAVENOUS INJECTION, OR BY INTRAMUSCULAR INJECTION
- Child: 20 mg/kg every 8 hours (max. per dose 750 mg); increased to 50–60 mg/kg every 6–8 hours (max. per dose 1.5 g), increased dose used for severe infection and cystic fibrosis

Cellulitis | Erysipelas

- BY INTRAVENOUS INJECTION, OR BY INTRAVENOUS INFUSION
- Child: 20 mg/kg every 8 hours (max. per dose 750 mg); increased if necessary up to 50–60 mg/kg every 6–8 hours (max. per dose 1.5 g)

Lyme disease

- BY MOUTH
- Child 3 months–11 years: 15 mg/kg twice daily (max. per dose 500 mg) for 14–21 days (for 28 days in Lyme arthritis)
- Child 12–17 years: 500 mg twice daily for 14–21 days (for 28 days in Lyme arthritis)

Surgical prophylaxis

- INITIALLY BY INTRAVENOUS INJECTION
- Child: 50 mg/kg (max. per dose 1.5 g), to be administered up to 30 minutes before the procedure, then (by intravenous injection or by intramuscular injection) 30 mg/kg every 8 hours (max. per dose 750 mg) if required for up to 3 doses (for high-risk procedures)

Urinary-tract infection (lower)

- BY MOUTH
- Child (body-weight up to 40 kg): 15 mg/kg twice daily (max. per dose 250 mg)
- Child (body-weight 40 kg and above): 250 mg twice daily

Urinary tract infection (catheter-associated)

- BY INTRAVENOUS INFUSION, OR BY INTRAVENOUS INJECTION
- Child 3 months–15 years: 20 mg/kg every 8 hours (max. per dose 750 mg); increased to 50–60 mg/kg every 6–8 hours (max. per dose 1.5 g), increased dose used for severe infection
- Child 16–17 years: 0.75–1.5 g every 6–8 hours

Acute pyelonephritis

- BY MOUTH
- Child (body-weight up to 40 kg): 15 mg/kg twice daily (max. per dose 250 mg)
- Child (body-weight 40 kg and above): 250 mg twice daily
- BY INTRAVENOUS INFUSION, OR BY INTRAVENOUS INJECTION
- Child 3 months–15 years: 20 mg/kg every 8 hours (max. per dose 750 mg); increased to 50–60 mg/kg every 6–8 hours (max. per dose 1.5 g), increased dose used for severe infection
- Child 16–17 years: 0.75–1.5 g every 6–8 hours

- **UNLICENSED USE** EvGr Cefuroxime is used for the treatment of cellulitis, (A) but the dose increase is not licensed for this indication.
  EvGr Cefuroxime is used for the treatment of erysipelas, (A) but the dose increase is not licensed for this indication.
  Not licensed for treatment of Lyme disease in children under 12 years. Duration of treatment in Lyme disease is unlicensed.
- **INTERACTIONS** → Appendix 1: cephalosporins
- **SIDE-EFFECTS**
  GENERAL SIDE-EFFECTS
  - **Common or very common** Increased risk of infection
  - **Frequency not known** Drug fever

  SPECIFIC SIDE-EFFECTS
  - **Uncommon**
    - With parenteral use Gastrointestinal disorder
  - **Frequency not known**
    - With oral use Hepatic disorders · Jarisch-Herxheimer reaction · serum sickness
    - With parenteral use Cutaneous vasculitis
- **PREGNANCY** Not known to be harmful.
- **BREAST FEEDING** Present in milk in low concentration, but appropriate to use.
- **RENAL IMPAIRMENT**
  Dose adjustments Reduce parenteral dose if estimated glomerular filtration rate less than 20 mL/minute/1.73 m^2.
- **DIRECTIONS FOR ADMINISTRATION**
  - With intramuscular use or intravenous use Single doses over 750 mg should be administered by the intravenous route only.
  - With intravenous use Displacement value may be significant when reconstituting injection, consult local guidelines. For intermittent intravenous infusion, dilute reconstituted solution further in glucose 5% or sodium chloride 0.9%; give over 30 minutes.
- **PRESCRIBING AND DISPENSING INFORMATION** For choice of antibacterial therapy, see Antibacterials, use for prophylaxis p. 319, Lyme disease p. 391, Skin infections, antibacterial therapy p. 329, Urinary-tract infections p. 400.

5 Infection

- **MEDICINAL FORMS** There can be variation in the licensing of different medicines containing the same drug. Forms available from special-order manufacturers include: solution for injection, infusion

Tablet

CAUTIONARY AND ADVISORY LABELS 9, 21, 25

- Cefuroxime (Non-proprietary)
  - **Cefuroxime (as Cefuroxime axetil) 250 mg** Cefuroxime 250mg tablets | 14 tablet PoM £17.72 DT = £17.72
- Zinnat (GlaxoSmithKline UK Ltd)
  - **Cefuroxime (as Cefuroxime axetil) 125 mg** Zinnat 125mg tablets | 14 tablet PoM £4.56 DT = £4.56
  - **Cefuroxime (as Cefuroxime axetil) 250 mg** Zinnat 250mg tablets | 14 tablet PoM £9.11 DT = £17.72

Powder for injection

ELECTROLYTES: May contain Sodium

- Cefuroxime (Non-proprietary)
  - **Cefuroxime (as Cefuroxime sodium) 250 mg** Cefuroxime 250mg powder for injection vials | 10 vial PoM £9.25 (Hospital only)
  - **Cefuroxime (as Cefuroxime sodium) 750 mg** Cefuroxime 750mg powder for injection vials | 1 vial PoM £2.52 | 10 vial PoM £25.20 | 10 vial PoM £26.10 (Hospital only)
  - **Cefuroxime (as Cefuroxime sodium) 1.5 gram** Cefuroxime 1.5g powder for injection vials | 1 vial PoM £5.05 | 10 vial PoM £50.50 | 10 vial PoM £53.00 (Hospital only)
- Zinacef (GlaxoSmithKline UK Ltd)
  - **Cefuroxime (as Cefuroxime sodium) 250 mg** Zinacef 250mg powder for injection vials | 5 vial PoM £4.70
  - **Cefuroxime (as Cefuroxime sodium) 750 mg** Zinacef 750mg powder for injection vials | 5 vial PoM £11.72 (Hospital only)
  - **Cefuroxime (as Cefuroxime sodium) 1.5 gram** Zinacef 1.5g powder for injection vials | 1 vial PoM £4.70

Oral suspension

CAUTIONARY AND ADVISORY LABELS 9, 21

EXCIPIENTS: May contain Aspartame, sucrose

- Zinnat (GlaxoSmithKline UK Ltd)
  - **Cefuroxime (as Cefuroxime axetil) 25 mg per 1 ml** Zinnat 125mg/5ml oral suspension | 70 ml PoM £5.20 DT = £5.20

ANTIBACTERIALS > CEPHALOSPORINS, THIRD-GENERATION

F 338

Cefixime

- **INDICATIONS AND DOSE**

Acute infections due to sensitive Gram-positive and Gram-negative bacteria

- BY MOUTH
  - Child 6–11 months: 75 mg daily
  - Child 1–4 years: 100 mg daily
  - Child 5–9 years: 200 mg daily
  - Child 10–17 years: 200–400 mg daily, alternatively 100–200 mg twice daily

Uncomplicated gonorrhoea

- BY MOUTH
  - Child 12–17 years: 400 mg for 1 dose

- **UNLICENSED USE** Use of cefixime for uncomplicated gonorrhoea is an unlicensed indication.
- **INTERACTIONS** → Appendix 1: cephalosporins
- **SIDE-EFFECTS** Acute kidney injury · arthralgia · drug fever · dyspepsia · dyspnoea · face oedema · flatulence · genital pruritus · hypereosinophilia · jaundice · serum sickness-like reaction · thrombocytosis
- **PREGNANCY** Not known to be harmful.
- **BREAST FEEDING** Manufacturer advises avoid unless essential—no information available.
- **RENAL IMPAIRMENT**

Dose adjustments Reduce dose if estimated glomerular filtration rate less than 20 mL/minute/1.73 m^2.

- **MEDICINAL FORMS** There can be variation in the licensing of different medicines containing the same drug.

Tablet

CAUTIONARY AND ADVISORY LABELS 9

- Suprax (Sanofi)
  - **Cefixime 200 mg** Suprax 200mg tablets | 7 tablet PoM £13.23 DT = £13.23

F 338

Cefotaxime

- **INDICATIONS AND DOSE**

Uncomplicated gonorrhoea

- BY INTRAMUSCULAR INJECTION
  - Child 12–17 years: 500 mg for 1 dose

Severe exacerbations of *Haemophilus influenzae* infection in cystic fibrosis

- BY INTRAVENOUS INJECTION, OR BY INTRAVENOUS INFUSION
  - Child: 50 mg/kg every 6–8 hours; maximum 12 g per day

Congenital gonococcal conjunctivitis

- BY INTRAMUSCULAR INJECTION
  - Neonate: 100 mg/kg (max. per dose 1 g) for 1 dose.

Infections due to sensitive Gram-positive and Gram-negative bacteria | Surgical prophylaxis | Haemophilus epiglottitis

- BY INTRAMUSCULAR INJECTION, OR BY INTRAVENOUS INJECTION, OR BY INTRAVENOUS INFUSION
  - Neonate up to 7 days: 25 mg/kg every 12 hours.
  - Neonate 7 days to 20 days: 25 mg/kg every 8 hours.
  - Neonate 21 days to 28 days: 25 mg/kg every 6–8 hours.
  - Child: 50 mg/kg every 8–12 hours

Severe susceptible infections due to sensitive Gram-positive and Gram-negative bacteria | Meningitis

- BY INTRAMUSCULAR INJECTION, OR BY INTRAVENOUS INJECTION, OR BY INTRAVENOUS INFUSION
  - Neonate up to 7 days: 50 mg/kg every 12 hours.
  - Neonate 7 days to 20 days: 50 mg/kg every 8 hours.
  - Neonate 21 days to 28 days: 50 mg/kg every 6–8 hours.
  - Child: 50 mg/kg every 6 hours; maximum 12 g per day

Emergency treatment of suspected bacterial meningitis or meningococcal disease, before urgent transfer to hospital, in patients who cannot be given benzylpenicillin (e.g. because of an allergy)

- BY INTRAVENOUS INJECTION, OR BY INTRAMUSCULAR INJECTION
  - Child 1 month–11 years: 50 mg/kg for 1 dose
  - Child 12–17 years: 1 g for 1 dose

- **INTERACTIONS** → Appendix 1: cephalosporins
- **SIDE-EFFECTS**
  - **Uncommon** Drug fever · Jarisch-Herxheimer reaction · renal impairment · seizure
  - **Frequency not known** Arrhythmia (following rapid injection) · bronchospasm · encephalopathy · fungal infection · hepatic disorders
- **PREGNANCY** Not known to be harmful.
- **BREAST FEEDING** Present in milk in low concentration, but appropriate to use.
- **RENAL IMPAIRMENT**

Dose adjustments Usual initial dose, then use half normal dose if estimated glomerular filtration rate less than 5 mL/minute/1.73 m^2.

- **DIRECTIONS FOR ADMINISTRATION**
- ▸ With intravenous use Displacement value may be significant, consult local guidelines. For intermittent *intravenous infusion* dilute in glucose 5% *or* sodium chloride 0.9%; administer over 20–60 minutes; incompatible with alkaline solutions.

- **MEDICINAL FORMS** There can be variation in the licensing of different medicines containing the same drug.

Powder for solution for injection

▸ Cefotaxime (Non-proprietary)

Cefotaxime (as Cefotaxime sodium) 500 mg Cefotaxime 500mg powder for solution for injection vials | 10 vial PoM £30.00 | 10 vial PoM £21.00 (Hospital only)

Cefotaxime (as Cefotaxime sodium) 1 gram Cefotaxime 1g powder for solution for injection vials | 10 vial PoM £35.00 | 10 vial PoM £42.00 (Hospital only)

Cefotaxime (as Cefotaxime sodium) 2 gram Cefotaxime 2g powder for solution for injection vials | 10 vial PoM £37.50

F 338

Ceftazidime

15-Jun-2018

- **INDICATIONS AND DOSE**

Pseudomonal lung infection in cystic fibrosis

▸ BY INTRAVENOUS INFUSION, OR BY INTRAVENOUS INJECTION, OR BY DEEP INTRAMUSCULAR INJECTION

▸ Child: 50 mg/kg every 8 hours; maximum 9 g per day

Febrile neutropenia

▸ BY INTRAVENOUS INFUSION, OR BY INTRAVENOUS INJECTION

▸ Child: 50 mg/kg every 8 hours; maximum 6 g per day

Meningitis

▸ BY INTRAVENOUS INJECTION, OR BY INTRAVENOUS INFUSION

▸ Neonate up to 7 days: 50 mg/kg every 24 hours.

▸ Neonate 7 days to 20 days: 50 mg/kg every 12 hours.

▸ Neonate 21 days to 28 days: 50 mg/kg every 8 hours.

▸ Child: 50 mg/kg every 8 hours; maximum 6 g per day

Susceptible infections due to sensitive Gram-positive and Gram-negative bacteria

▸ BY INTRAVENOUS INJECTION, OR BY INTRAVENOUS INFUSION

▸ Neonate up to 7 days: 25 mg/kg every 24 hours.

▸ Neonate 7 days to 20 days: 25 mg/kg every 12 hours.

▸ Neonate 21 days to 28 days: 25 mg/kg every 8 hours.

▸ Child: 25 mg/kg every 8 hours; maximum 6 g per day

Severe susceptible infections due to sensitive Gram-positive and Gram-negative bacteria

▸ BY INTRAVENOUS INJECTION, OR BY INTRAVENOUS INFUSION

▸ Neonate up to 7 days: 50 mg/kg every 24 hours.

▸ Neonate 7 days to 20 days: 50 mg/kg every 12 hours.

▸ Neonate 21 days to 28 days: 50 mg/kg every 8 hours.

▸ Child: 50 mg/kg every 8 hours; maximum 6 g per day

Chronic *Burkholderia cepacia* infection in cystic fibrosis

▸ BY INHALATION OF NEBULISED SOLUTION

▸ Child: 1 g twice daily

- **UNLICENSED USE** Nebulised route unlicensed.
- **INTERACTIONS** → Appendix 1: cephalosporins
- **SIDE-EFFECTS**
- ▸ **Common or very common** Thrombocytosis · thrombophlebitis
- ▸ **Uncommon** Antibiotic associated colitis · fungal infection
- ▸ **Rare or very rare** Acute kidney injury
- ▸ **Frequency not known** Coma · encephalopathy · jaundice · lymphocytosis · myoclonus · neurological effects · paraesthesia · seizure · taste altered · tremor

- **PREGNANCY** Not known to be harmful.
- **BREAST FEEDING** Present in milk in low concentration, but appropriate to use.
- **HEPATIC IMPAIRMENT** Manufacturer advises caution in severe impairment (no information available).
- **RENAL IMPAIRMENT**

Dose adjustments Manufacturer advises reduce dose if creatinine clearance 50 mL/minute or less—consult product literature.

- **DIRECTIONS FOR ADMINISTRATION** Intramuscular administration used when intravenous administration not possible; single doses over 1 g by intravenous route only.
- ▸ With intravenous use Displacement value may be significant, consult local guidelines. For intermittent intravenous infusion dilute reconstituted solution further to a concentration of not more than 40 mg/mL in Glucose 5% or Glucose 10% *or* Sodium chloride 0.9%; give over 20–30 minutes.
- ▸ When used by inhalation For nebulisation, dissolve dose in 3 mL of water for injection.

- **MEDICINAL FORMS** There can be variation in the licensing of different medicines containing the same drug. Forms available from special-order manufacturers include: infusion, solution for infusion

Powder for solution for injection

ELECTROLYTES: May contain Sodium

▸ Ceftazidime (Non-proprietary)

Ceftazidime (as Ceftazidime pentahydrate) 500 mg Ceftazidime 500mg powder for solution for injection vials | 1 vial PoM £4.25-£4.91 (Hospital only)

Ceftazidime (as Ceftazidime pentahydrate) 1 gram Ceftazidime 1g powder for solution for injection vials | 1 vial PoM £9.51 (Hospital only) | 10 vial PoM £13.90-£79.00 | 10 vial PoM £79.10 (Hospital only)

Ceftazidime (as Ceftazidime pentahydrate) 2 gram Ceftazidime 2g powder for solution for injection vials | 1 vial PoM £20.04 (Hospital only) | 5 vial PoM £79.15 (Hospital only) | 10 vial PoM £27.70-£176.00

Ceftazidime (as Ceftazidime pentahydrate) 3 gram Ceftazidime 3g powder for solution for injection vials | 10 vial PoM £257.60 (Hospital only)

▸ Fortum (GlaxoSmithKline UK Ltd)

Ceftazidime (as Ceftazidime pentahydrate) 500 mg Fortum 500mg powder for solution for injection vials | 1 vial PoM £4.40 (Hospital only)

Ceftazidime (as Ceftazidime pentahydrate) 1 gram Fortum 1g powder for solution for injection vials | 1 vial PoM £8.79 (Hospital only)

Ceftazidime (as Ceftazidime pentahydrate) 2 gram Fortum 2g powder for solution for injection vials | 1 vial PoM £17.59 (Hospital only)

Ceftazidime (as Ceftazidime pentahydrate) 3 gram Fortum 3g powder for solution for injection vials | 1 vial PoM £25.76 (Hospital only)

F 338

Ceftriaxone

22-May-2020

- **INDICATIONS AND DOSE**

Community-acquired pneumonia | Hospital-acquired pneumonia | Intra-abdominal infections | Complicated urinary-tract infections

▸ BY INTRAVENOUS INFUSION

▸ Neonate up to 15 days: 20–50 mg/kg once daily, doses at the higher end of the recommended range used in severe cases.

▸ Neonate 15 days to 28 days: 50–80 mg/kg once daily, doses at the higher end of the recommended range used in severe cases.

continued →

- Child 1 month–11 years (body-weight up to 50 kg): 50–80 mg/kg once daily, doses at the higher end of the recommended range used in severe cases; maximum 4 g per day
- Child 9–11 years (body-weight 50 kg and above): 1–2 g once daily, 2 g dose to be used for hospital-acquired pneumonia and severe cases
- Child 12–17 years: 1–2 g once daily, 2 g dose to be used for hospital-acquired pneumonia and severe cases

▶ BY INTRAVENOUS INJECTION
- Child 9–11 years (body-weight 50 kg and above): 1–2 g once daily, 2 g dose to be used for hospital-acquired pneumonia and severe cases
- Child 12–17 years: 1–2 g once daily, 2 g dose to be used for hospital-acquired pneumonia and severe cases

▶ BY DEEP INTRAMUSCULAR INJECTION
- Child 1 month–11 years (body-weight up to 50 kg): 50–80 mg/kg daily, doses at the higher end of the recommended range used in severe cases; maximum 4 g per day
- Child 9–11 years (body-weight 50 kg and above): 1–2 g once daily, 2 g dose to be used for hospital-acquired pneumonia and severe cases
- Child 12–17 years: 1–2 g once daily, 2 g dose to be used for hospital-acquired pneumonia and severe cases

Complicated skin and soft tissue infections | Infections of bones and joints

▶ BY INTRAVENOUS INFUSION
- Neonate up to 15 days: 20–50 mg/kg once daily, doses at the higher end of the recommended range used in severe cases.
- Neonate 15 days to 28 days: 50–100 mg/kg once daily, doses at the higher end of the recommended range used in severe cases.
- Child 1 month–11 years (body-weight up to 50 kg): 50–100 mg/kg once daily, doses at the higher end of the recommended range used in severe cases; maximum 4 g per day
- Child 9–11 years (body-weight 50 kg and above): 2 g once daily
- Child 12–17 years: 2 g once daily

▶ BY INTRAVENOUS INJECTION
- Child 9–11 years (body-weight 50 kg and above): 2 g once daily
- Child 12–17 years: 2 g once daily

▶ BY DEEP INTRAMUSCULAR INJECTION
- Child 1 month–11 years (body-weight up to 50 kg): 50–100 mg/kg daily, doses at the higher end of the recommended range used in severe cases; maximum 4 g per day
- Child 9–11 years (body-weight 50 kg and above): 2 g once daily
- Child 12–17 years: 2 g once daily

Suspected bacterial infection in neutropenic patients

▶ BY INTRAVENOUS INFUSION
- Neonate up to 15 days: 20–50 mg/kg once daily, doses at the higher end of the recommended range used in severe cases.
- Neonate 15 days to 28 days: 50–100 mg/kg once daily, doses at the higher end of the recommended range used in severe cases.
- Child 1 month–11 years (body-weight up to 50 kg): 50–100 mg/kg once daily, doses at the higher end of the recommended range used in severe cases; maximum 4 g per day
- Child 9–11 years (body-weight 50 kg and above): 2–4 g once daily, doses at the higher end of the recommended range used in severe cases
- Child 12–17 years: 2–4 g once daily, doses at the higher end of the recommended range used in severe cases

▶ BY INTRAVENOUS INJECTION
- Child 9–11 years (body-weight 50 kg and above): 2–4 g once daily, doses at the higher end of the recommended range used in severe cases; doses of 50 mg/kg or more should be given by infusion
- Child 12–17 years: 2–4 g once daily, doses at the higher end of the recommended range used in severe cases

▶ BY DEEP INTRAMUSCULAR INJECTION
- Child 1 month–11 years (body-weight up to 50 kg): 50–100 mg/kg daily, doses at the higher end of the recommended range used in severe cases; maximum 4 g per day
- Child 9–11 years (body-weight 50 kg and above): 2–4 g daily, doses at the higher end of the recommended range used in severe cases
- Child 12–17 years: 2–4 g daily, doses at the higher end of the recommended range used in severe cases

Bacterial meningitis | Bacterial endocarditis

▶ BY INTRAVENOUS INFUSION
- Neonate up to 15 days: 50 mg/kg once daily.
- Neonate 15 days to 28 days: 80–100 mg/kg once daily, 100 mg/kg once daily dose should be used for bacterial endocarditis.
- Child 1 month–11 years (body-weight up to 50 kg): 80–100 mg/kg once daily, 100 mg/kg once daily dose should be used for bacterial endocarditis; maximum 4 g per day
- Child 9–11 years (body-weight 50 kg and above): 2–4 g once daily, doses at the higher end of the recommended range used in severe cases
- Child 12–17 years: 2–4 g once daily, doses at the higher end of the recommended range used in severe cases

▶ BY INTRAVENOUS INJECTION
- Child 9–11 years (body-weight 50 kg and above): 2–4 g once daily, doses at the higher end of the recommended range used in severe cases; doses of 50 mg/kg or more should be given by infusion
- Child 12–17 years: 2–4 g once daily, doses at the higher end of the recommended range used in severe cases

▶ BY DEEP INTRAMUSCULAR INJECTION
- Child 1 month–11 years (body-weight up to 50 kg): 80–100 mg/kg daily, 100 mg/kg daily dose should be used for bacterial endocarditis; maximum 4 g per day
- Child 9–11 years (body-weight 50 kg and above): 2–4 g daily, doses at the higher end of the recommended range used in severe cases
- Child 12–17 years: 2–4 g daily, doses at the higher end of the recommended range used in severe cases

Surgical prophylaxis

▶ BY INTRAVENOUS INFUSION
- Neonate up to 15 days: 20–50 mg/kg for 1 dose, dose to be administered 30–90 minutes before procedure.
- Neonate 15 days to 28 days: 50–80 mg/kg for 1 dose, dose to be administered 30–90 minutes before procedure.
- Child 1 month–11 years (body-weight up to 50 kg): 50–80 mg/kg (max. per dose 2 g) for 1 dose, dose to be administered 30–90 minutes before procedure
- Child 9–11 years (body-weight 50 kg and above): 2 g for 1 dose, dose to be administered 30–90 minutes before procedure
- Child 12–17 years: 2 g for 1 dose, dose to be administered 30–90 minutes before procedure

▸ BY INTRAVENOUS INJECTION
▸ Child 9–11 years (body-weight 50 kg and above): 2 g for 1 dose, dose to be administered 30–90 minutes before procedure
▸ Child 12–17 years: 2 g for 1 dose, dose to be administered 30–90 minutes before procedure
▸ BY DEEP INTRAMUSCULAR INJECTION
▸ Child 1 month–11 years (body-weight up to 50 kg): 50–80 mg/kg (max. per dose 2 g) for 1 dose, dose to be administered 30–90 minutes before procedure
▸ Child 9–11 years (body-weight 50 kg and above): 2 g for 1 dose, dose to be administered 30–90 minutes before procedure
▸ Child 12–17 years: 2 g for 1 dose, dose to be administered 30–90 minutes before procedure

Uncomplicated gonorrhoea | Pelvic inflammatory disease
▸ BY DEEP INTRAMUSCULAR INJECTION
▸ Child 1 month–11 years (body-weight up to 45 kg): 125 mg for 1 dose
▸ Child 9–11 years (body-weight 45 kg and above): 250 mg for 1 dose
▸ Child 12–17 years: 500 mg for 1 dose

Syphilis
▸ BY INTRAVENOUS INFUSION
▸ Neonate up to 15 days: 50 mg/kg once daily for 10–14 days.
▸ Neonate 15 days to 28 days: 75–100 mg/kg once daily for 10–14 days.
▸ Child 1 month–11 years (body-weight up to 50 kg): 75–100 mg/kg once daily for 10–14 days; maximum 4 g per day
▸ Child 9–11 years (body-weight 50 kg and above): 0.5–1 g once daily for 10–14 days, dose increased to 2 g once daily for neurosyphilis
▸ Child 12–17 years: 0.5–1 g once daily for 10–14 days, dose increased to 2 g once daily for neurosyphilis
▸ BY INTRAVENOUS INJECTION
▸ Child 9–11 years (body-weight 50 kg and above): 0.5–1 g once daily for 10–14 days, dose increased to 2 g once daily for neurosyphilis
▸ Child 12–17 years: 0.5–1 g once daily for 10–14 days, dose increased to 2 g once daily for neurosyphilis
▸ BY DEEP INTRAMUSCULAR INJECTION
▸ Child 1 month–11 years (body-weight up to 50 kg): 75–100 mg/kg daily for 10–14 days; maximum 4 g per day
▸ Child 9–11 years (body-weight 50 kg and above): 0.5–1 g once daily for 10–14 days, dose increased to 2 g once daily for neurosyphilis
▸ Child 12–17 years: 0.5–1 g once daily for 10–14 days, dose increased to 2 g once daily for neurosyphilis

Disseminated Lyme borreliosis (early [Stage II] and late [Stage III]) (administered on expert advice)
▸ BY INTRAVENOUS INFUSION
▸ Neonate 15 days to 28 days: 50–80 mg/kg once daily for 14–21 days, the recommended treatment durations vary and national or local guidelines should be taken into consideration.

Lyme disease [affecting central nervous system]
▸ BY INTRAVENOUS INFUSION
▸ Child 1 month–11 years (administered on expert advice) (body-weight up to 50 kg): 80 mg/kg once daily (max. per dose 4 g) for 21 days
▸ Child 1 month–11 years (administered on expert advice) (body-weight 50 kg and above): 2 g twice daily for 21 days, alternatively 4 g once daily for 21 days
▸ Child 12–17 years (administered on expert advice): 2 g twice daily for 21 days, alternatively 4 g once daily for 21 days
▸ BY INTRAVENOUS INJECTION
▸ Child 1 month–11 years (administered on expert advice) (body-weight 50 kg and above): 2 g twice daily for 21 days
▸ Child 12–17 years (administered on expert advice): 2 g twice daily for 21 days, alternatively 4 g once daily for 21 days

Lyme arthritis | Acrodermatitis chronica atrophicans
▸ BY INTRAVENOUS INFUSION
▸ Child 1 month–11 years (administered on expert advice) (body-weight up to 50 kg): 80 mg/kg once daily (max. per dose 2 g) for 28 days
▸ BY INTRAVENOUS INFUSION, OR BY INTRAVENOUS INJECTION
▸ Child 1 month–11 years (administered on expert advice) (body-weight 50 kg and above): 2 g once daily for 28 days
▸ Child 12–17 years (administered on expert advice): 2 g once daily for 28 days

Lyme carditis
▸ BY INTRAVENOUS INFUSION
▸ Child 1 month–11 years (administered on expert advice) (body-weight up to 50 kg): 80 mg/kg once daily (max. per dose 2 g) for 21 days
▸ BY INTRAVENOUS INFUSION, OR BY INTRAVENOUS INJECTION
▸ Child 1 month–11 years (administered on expert advice) (body-weight 50 kg and above): 2 g once daily for 21 days
▸ Child 12–17 years (administered on expert advice): 2 g once daily for 21 days

Congenital gonococcal conjunctivitis
▸ BY DEEP INTRAMUSCULAR INJECTION, OR BY INTRAVENOUS INFUSION
▸ Neonate: 25–50 mg/kg (max. per dose 125 mg) for 1 dose, intravenous infusion to be administered over 60 minutes.

Prevention of secondary case of meningococcal meningitis
▸ BY INTRAMUSCULAR INJECTION
▸ Child 1 month–11 years: 125 mg for 1 dose
▸ Child 12–17 years: 250 mg for 1 dose

Prevention of secondary case of *Haemophilus influenzae* type b disease
▸ BY INTRAVENOUS INFUSION
▸ Child 1 month–11 years: 50 mg/kg daily (max. per dose 1 g) for 2 days
▸ BY INTRAMUSCULAR INJECTION, OR BY INTRAVENOUS INJECTION, OR BY INTRAVENOUS INFUSION
▸ Child 12–17 years: 1 g daily for 2 days

Acute otitis media
▸ BY DEEP INTRAMUSCULAR INJECTION
▸ Child 1 month–11 years (body-weight up to 50 kg): 50 mg/kg (max. per dose 2 g) for 1 dose, dose can be given for 3 days if severely ill or previous therapy failed
▸ Child 9–11 years (body-weight 50 kg and above): 1–2 g for 1 dose, dose can be given for 3 days if severely ill or previous therapy failed
▸ Child 12–17 years: 1–2 g for 1 dose, dose can be given for 3 days if severely ill or previous therapy failed

● **UNLICENSED USE** EvGr Not licensed for prophylaxis of *Haemophilus influenzae* type b disease. ⟨E⟩ Not licensed for prophylaxis of meningococcal meningitis.

EvGr Not licensed for congenital gonococcal conjunctivitis. Not licensed for use in children under 12 years of age for uncomplicated gonorrhoea. Not licensed for use in children for pelvic inflammatory disease. ⟨E⟩

EvGr Ceftriaxone is used for Lyme disease affecting the central nervous system in children with body-weight 50 kg and over and in children aged 12 years and over, (A) but the dose is not licensed for this indication.

- **CONTRA-INDICATIONS** Concomitant treatment with intravenous calcium (including total parenteral nutrition containing calcium) in premature and full-term neonates—risk of precipitation in urine and lungs (fatal reactions) · full-term neonates with jaundice, hypoalbuminaemia, acidosis, unconjugated hyperbilirubinaemia, or impaired bilirubin binding—risk of developing bilirubin encephalopathy · premature neonates less than 41 weeks corrected gestational age
- **CAUTIONS**

GENERAL CAUTIONS History of hypercalciuria · history of kidney stones · use with caution in neonates

SPECIFIC CAUTIONS
- With intravenous use Concomitant treatment with intravenous calcium (including total parenteral nutrition containing calcium)
- **INTERACTIONS** → Appendix 1: cephalosporins
- **SIDE-EFFECTS**
- **Uncommon** Anaemia · coagulation disorder · fungal infection
- **Rare or very rare** Bronchospasm · glycosuria · haematuria · oedema
- **Frequency not known** Antibiotic associated colitis · cholelithiasis · hypersensitivity · kernicterus (in neonates) · nephrolithiasis · oral disorders · pancreatitis · seizure · vertigo

SIDE-EFFECTS, FURTHER INFORMATION Precipitates of calcium ceftriaxone can occur in the gall bladder and urine (particularly in very young, dehydrated or those who are immobilised)—consider discontinuation if symptomatic.
- **PREGNANCY** Manufacturer advises use only if benefit outweighs risk—limited data available but not known to be harmful in *animal* studies. [EvGr] Specialist sources indicate suitable for use in pregnancy. (D)
- **BREAST FEEDING** [EvGr] Specialist sources advise ceftriaxone is compatible with breastfeeding—present in milk in low concentration but limited effects to breast-fed infant. (D)
- **HEPATIC IMPAIRMENT** Manufacturer advises caution in severe impairment (no information available).
- **RENAL IMPAIRMENT**

Dose adjustments Manufacturer advises reduce dose and monitor efficacy in patients with severe renal impairment in combination with hepatic impairment—no information available.

Manufacturer advises reduce dose if estimated glomeruler filtration rate less than 10 mL/minute/1.73 m^2 max. 50 mg/kg daily or max. 2 g daily).
- **MONITORING REQUIREMENTS** Manufacturer advises to monitor full blood count regularly during prolonged treatment.
- **DIRECTIONS FOR ADMINISTRATION**
- With intramuscular use or intravenous use Twice daily dosing may be considered for doses greater than 2 g daily.
- With intravenous use For *intravenous infusion* (preferred route), dilute reconstituted solution with Glucose 5% (or 10% in neonates) *or* Sodium Chloride 0.9%; give over at least 30 minutes (60 minutes in neonates—may displace bilirubin from serum albumin). Not to be given simultaneously with parenteral nutrition or infusion fluids containing calcium, even by different infusion lines; in children, may be infused sequentially with infusion fluids containing calcium if infusion lines at different sites are used, or if the infusion lines are replaced or thoroughly flushed between infusions with Sodium Chloride 0.9% to avoid precipitation—consult product literature. Displacement value may be significant, consult local guidelines. For *intravenous injection*, give over 5 minutes.
- With intramuscular use For *intramuscular injection*, may be mixed with 1% Lidocaine Hydrochloride Injection to reduce pain at intramuscular injection site. Intramuscular injection should only be considered when the intravenous route is not possible or less appropriate. If administered by intramuscular injection, the lower end of the dose range should be used for the shortest time possible; volume depends on the age and size of the child, but doses over 1 g must be divided between more than one site. Displacement value may be significant, consult local guidelines. The maximum single intramuscular dose is 2 g, doses greater than 2 g must be given in divided doses *or* by intravenous administration (see above).
- **PRESCRIBING AND DISPENSING INFORMATION** For choice of antibacterial therapy, see Antibacterials, use for prophylaxis p. 319, Cardiovascular system infections, antibacterial therapy p. 322, Central nervous system infections, antibacterial therapy p. 323, Ear infections, antibacterial therapy p. 324, Eye infections, antibacterial therapy p. 324, Gastro-intestinal system infections, antibacterial therapy p. 324, Genital system infections, antibacterial therapy p. 325, Lyme disease p. 391, Musculoskeletal system infections, antibacterial therapy p. 326, Respiratory system infections, antibacterial therapy p. 327, Skin infections, antibacterial therapy p. 329, Urinary-tract infections p. 400.

- **MEDICINAL FORMS** There can be variation in the licensing of different medicines containing the same drug. Forms available from special-order manufacturers include: infusion

Powder for solution for injection

ELECTROLYTES: May contain Sodium

- Ceftriaxone (Non-proprietary)

Ceftriaxone (as Ceftriaxone sodium) 250 mg Ceftriaxone 250mg powder for solution for injection vials | 1 vial [PoM] £2.30 DT = £2.40 (Hospital only)

Ceftriaxone (as Ceftriaxone sodium) 1 gram Ceftriaxone 1g powder for solution for injection vials | 1 vial [PoM] £3.62 DT = £9.58 (Hospital only) | 1 vial [PoM] [X] DT = £9.58 | 10 vial [PoM] £95.80 | 10 vial [PoM] £91.50 (Hospital only)

Ceftriaxone (as Ceftriaxone sodium) 2 gram Ceftriaxone 2g powder for solution for injection vials | 1 vial [PoM] £18.30 DT = £19.18 (Hospital only) | 1 vial [PoM] [X] DT = £19.18 | 10 vial [PoM] £191.80

Ceftriaxone 2g powder for solution for infusion vials | 1 vial [PoM] £19.18 DT = £19.18 | 10 vial [PoM] £191.80

- Rocephin (Roche Products Ltd)

Ceftriaxone (as Ceftriaxone sodium) 250 mg Rocephin 250mg powder for solution for injection vials | 1 vial [PoM] £2.40 DT = £2.40

Ceftriaxone (as Ceftriaxone sodium) 1 gram Rocephin 1g powder for solution for injection vials | 1 vial [PoM] £9.58 DT = £9.58

Ceftriaxone (as Ceftriaxone sodium) 2 gram Rocephin 2g powder for solution for injection vials | 1 vial [PoM] £19.18 DT = £19.18

ANTIBACTERIALS > CEPHALOSPORINS, OTHER

F 338

Cefepime

12-Dec-2019

- **INDICATIONS AND DOSE**

Infections due to sensitive Gram-positive and Gram-negative bacteria

- BY INTRAVENOUS INJECTION, OR BY INTRAVENOUS INFUSION, OR BY INTRAMUSCULAR INJECTION
- Child 1 month: 30 mg/kg every 8–12 hours, experience in children aged less than 2 months is limited—consult product literature; intravenous route preferred in severe infections
- Child 2 months–17 years (body-weight up to 41 kg): 50 mg/kg every 12 hours (max. per dose 2 g), increased if necessary to 50 mg/kg every 8 hours (max. per dose 2 g), increased dose used for severe infections, experience of intramuscular use is limited; intravenous route preferred in severe infections

Mild to moderate urinary tract infections
▸ BY INTRAVENOUS INJECTION, OR BY INTRAVENOUS INFUSION, OR BY INTRAMUSCULAR INJECTION
▸ Child (body-weight 41 kg and above): 0.5–1 g every 12 hours, experience of intramuscular use is limited

Mild to moderate infections due to sensitive Gram-positive and Gram-negative bacteria
▸ BY INTRAVENOUS INJECTION, OR BY INTRAVENOUS INFUSION, OR BY INTRAMUSCULAR INJECTION
▸ Child (body-weight 41 kg and above): 1 g every 12 hours, experience of intramuscular use is limited

Severe infections due to sensitive Gram-positive and Gram-negative bacteria
▸ BY INTRAVENOUS INJECTION, OR BY INTRAVENOUS INFUSION
▸ Child (body-weight 41 kg and above): 2 g every 12 hours, increased if necessary to 2 g every 8 hours, increased dose used for very severe infections

● **INTERACTIONS** → Appendix 1: cephalosporins

● **SIDE-EFFECTS**
▸ **Common or very common** Anaemia
▸ **Uncommon** Gastrointestinal disorders · increased risk of infection
▸ **Rare or very rare** Constipation · dyspnoea · genital pruritus · paraesthesia · seizure · taste altered · vasodilation
▸ **Frequency not known** Anaphylactic shock · aplastic anaemia · coma · confusion · consciousness impaired · encephalopathy · haemorrhage · hallucination · myoclonus · nephrotoxicity · renal failure

● **PREGNANCY** Manufacturer advises caution—no data available but not known to be harmful in *animal* studies.

● **BREAST FEEDING** Manufacturer advises caution—present in milk in very low quantities.

● **RENAL IMPAIRMENT** Manufacturer advises use with caution.
Dose adjustments Manufacturer advises reduce dose—consult product literature.

● **DIRECTIONS FOR ADMINISTRATION** After reconstitution the solution is yellow to yellow-brown. Displacement value may be significant when reconstituting injection, consult local guidelines. For *intravenous infusion*, manufacturer advises reconstitute with 50 mL Glucose 5% or 10% *or* Sodium Chloride 0.9%; give over 30 minutes. For *intravenous injection*, manufacturer advises reconstitute with 10 mL Glucose 5% or 10% *or* Sodium Chloride 0.9%. For *intramuscular injection*, manufacturer advises reconstitute with 3 mL Water for Injection.

● **NATIONAL FUNDING/ACCESS DECISIONS**
All Wales Medicines Strategy Group (AWMSG) decisions
AWMSG No. 4129
The *All Wales Medicines Strategy Group* has advised (November 2019) that cefepime (*Renapime*®) is recommended as an option for restricted use within NHS Wales. It should be restricted to use in the treatment of resistant pseudomonas infections where first-line agents are not effective or contra-indicated. It is not recommended for use within NHS Wales outside of this subpopulation.

● **MEDICINAL FORMS** There can be variation in the licensing of different medicines containing the same drug.
Powder for solution for injection
▸ Renapime (Renascience Pharma Ltd)
Cefepime (as Cefepime dihydrochloride monohydrate)
1 gram Renapime 1g powder for solution for injection vials | 10 vial PoM £70.00
Cefepime (as Cefepime dihydrochloride monohydrate)
2 gram Renapime 2g powder for solution for injection vials | 10 vial PoM £110.00

F 338

Ceftaroline fosamil

21-May-2020

● **INDICATIONS AND DOSE**
Community-acquired pneumonia
▸ BY INTRAVENOUS INFUSION
▸ Neonate: 6 mg/kg every 8 hours for 5–7 days.
▸ Child up to 2 months: 6 mg/kg every 8 hours for 5–7 days
▸ Child 2–23 months: 8 mg/kg every 8 hours for 5–7 days
▸ Child 2–11 years: 12 mg/kg every 8 hours (max. per dose 400 mg) for 5–7 days
▸ Child 12–17 years (body-weight up to 33 kg): 12 mg/kg every 8 hours (max. per dose 400 mg) for 5–7 days
▸ Child 12–17 years (body-weight 33 kg and above): 600 mg every 12 hours for 5–7 days

Complicated skin infections | Complicated soft-tissue infections
▸ BY INTRAVENOUS INFUSION
▸ Neonate: 6 mg/kg every 8 hours for 5–14 days.
▸ Child up to 2 months: 6 mg/kg every 8 hours for 5–14 days
▸ Child 2–23 months: 8 mg/kg every 8 hours for 5–14 days, for high dose regimen consult product literature
▸ Child 2–11 years: 12 mg/kg every 8 hours (max. per dose 400 mg) for 5–14 days, for high dose regimen consult product literature
▸ Child 12–17 years (body-weight up to 33 kg): 12 mg/kg every 8 hours (max. per dose 400 mg) for 5–14 days, for high dose regimen consult product literature
▸ Child 12–17 years (body-weight 33 kg and above): 600 mg every 12 hours for 5–14 days, for high dose regimen consult product literature

● **CAUTIONS** Seizure disorders

● **INTERACTIONS** → Appendix 1: cephalosporins

● **SIDE-EFFECTS**
▸ **Uncommon** Anaemia · antibiotic associated colitis · hypersensitivity

● **PREGNANCY** Manufacturer advises avoid unless essential—limited information; *animal* studies do not indicate toxicity.

● **BREAST FEEDING** Manufacturer advises avoid—no information available.

● **RENAL IMPAIRMENT**
Dose adjustments Manufacturer advises reduce dose if creatinine clearance less than 51 mL/minute—consult product literature.

● **DIRECTIONS FOR ADMINISTRATION** For *intravenous infusion*, give intermittently *in* Glucose 5% *or* Sodium chloride 0.9%. Dilute reconstituted solution to 50, 100, or 250 mL with infusion fluid; give over 5 to 60 minutes. Consult product literature for administration of high-dose regimen.

● **NATIONAL FUNDING/ACCESS DECISIONS**
Scottish Medicines Consortium (SMC) decisions
The *Scottish Medicines Consortium*, has advised (Dec 2012) that ceftaroline fosamil (*Zinforo*®) is accepted for restricted use within NHS Scotland when meticillin-resistant *S. aureus* is suspected in complicated skin and soft-tissue infection and vancomycin cannot be used.

● **MEDICINAL FORMS** There can be variation in the licensing of different medicines containing the same drug.
Powder for solution for infusion
▸ Zinforo (Pfizer Ltd)
Ceftaroline fosamil (as Ceftaroline fosamil acetic acid solvate monohydrate) 600 mg Zinforo 600mg powder for concentrate for solution for infusion vials | 10 vial PoM £375.00 (Hospital only)

5 Infection

ANTIBACTERIALS > GLYCOPEPTIDE

Teicoplanin

18-May-2020

- **DRUG ACTION** The glycopeptide antibiotic teicoplanin has bactericidal activity against aerobic and anaerobic Gram-positive bacteria including multi-resistant staphylococci. However, there are reports of *Staphylococcus aureus* with reduced susceptibility to glycopeptides and increasing reports of glycopeptide-resistant enterococci. Teicoplanin is similar to vancomycin, but has a significantly longer duration of action, allowing once daily administration after the loading dose.

- **INDICATIONS AND DOSE**

***Clostridioides difficile* infection**

▸ BY MOUTH

▸ Child 12–17 years: 100–200 mg twice daily for 7–14 days

Cellulitis | Erysipelas

▸ BY INTRAVENOUS INJECTION, OR BY INTRAVENOUS INFUSION

▸ Child 1 month: Initially 16 mg/kg for 1 dose, followed by 8 mg/kg once daily, subsequent dose to be administered 24 hours after initial dose, doses to be given by intravenous infusion

▸ Child 2 months–11 years: Initially 10 mg/kg every 12 hours for 3 doses, then 6–10 mg/kg once daily

▸ Child 12–17 years: Initially 6 mg/kg every 12 hours for 3 doses, then 6 mg/kg once daily

Serious infections caused by Gram-positive bacteria (e.g. complicated skin and soft-tissue infections, pneumonia, complicated urinary tract infections)

▸ BY INTRAVENOUS INJECTION, OR BY INTRAVENOUS INFUSION, OR BY INTRAMUSCULAR INJECTION

▸ Child 12–17 years: Initially 6 mg/kg every 12 hours for 3 doses, then 6 mg/kg once daily

Streptococcal or enterococcal endocarditis (in combination with another antibacterial) | Bone and joint infections

▸ INITIALLY BY INTRAVENOUS INJECTION, OR BY INTRAVENOUS INFUSION

▸ Child 12–17 years: 12 mg/kg every 12 hours for 3–5 doses, then (by intravenous injection or by intravenous infusion or by intramuscular injection) 12 mg/kg once daily

Surgical prophylaxis

▸ BY INTRAVENOUS INJECTION

▸ Child: (consult local protocol)

Serious infections caused by Gram-positive bacteria (including endocarditis, complicated skin and soft-tissue infections, pneumonia, complicated urinary tract infections, bone and joint infections)

▸ BY INTRAVENOUS INJECTION, OR BY INTRAVENOUS INFUSION

▸ Neonate: Initially 16 mg/kg for 1 dose, followed by 8 mg/kg once daily, subsequent dose to be administered 24 hours after initial dose, doses to be given by intravenous infusion.

▸ Child 1 month: Initially 16 mg/kg for 1 dose, followed by 8 mg/kg once daily, subsequent dose to be administered 24 hours after initial dose, doses to be given by intravenous infusion

▸ Child 2 months–11 years: Initially 10 mg/kg every 12 hours for 3 doses, then 6–10 mg/kg once daily

Peritonitis associated with peritoneal dialysis (added to dialysis fluid)

▸ BY INTRAPERITONEAL INFUSION

▸ Child 12–17 years: (consult local protocol)

PHARMACOKINETICS

▸ Teicoplanin should **not** be given by mouth for systemic infections because it is not absorbed significantly.

- **UNLICENSED USE** Not licensed for surgical prophylaxis.
- **INTERACTIONS** → Appendix 1: teicoplanin
- **SIDE-EFFECTS**

▸ **Common or very common** Fever · pain · skin reactions

▸ **Uncommon** Bronchospasm · diarrhoea · dizziness · eosinophilia · headache · hearing impairment · hypersensitivity · leucopenia · nausea · ototoxicity · thrombocytopenia · vomiting

▸ **Rare or very rare** Abscess · red man syndrome

▸ **Frequency not known** Agranulocytosis · angioedema · chills · neutropenia · overgrowth of nonsusceptible organisms · renal impairment · seizure · severe cutaneous adverse reactions (SCARs) · thrombophlebitis

SIDE-EFFECTS, FURTHER INFORMATION Teicoplanin is associated with a lower incidence of nephrotoxicity than vancomycin.

- **ALLERGY AND CROSS-SENSITIVITY** Caution if history of vancomycin sensitivity.
- **PREGNANCY** Manufacturer advises use only if potential benefit outweighs risk.
- **BREAST FEEDING** No information available.
- **RENAL IMPAIRMENT**

Dose adjustments Use normal dose regimen on days 1–4, then use normal maintenance dose every 48 hours if estimated glomerular filtration rate 30–80 mL/minute/1.73 m^2 and use normal maintenance dose every 72 hours if estimated glomerular filtration rate less than 30 mL/minute/1.73 m^2.

Monitoring Monitor renal and auditory function during prolonged treatment in renal impairment.

- **MONITORING REQUIREMENTS**

▸ With intramuscular use or intravenous use Manufacturer advises monitor serum-teicoplanin trough concentration at steady state after completion of loading dose and during maintenance treatment—consult product literature.

▸ Blood counts and liver and kidney function tests required.

▸ Manufacturer advises monitoring for adverse reactions when doses of 12 mg/kg twice daily are administered.

- **DIRECTIONS FOR ADMINISTRATION**

▸ With intravenous use For intermittent intravenous infusion, dilute reconstituted solution further in sodium chloride 0.9% *or* glucose 5%; give over 30 minutes.

▸ With oral use Injection can be used to prepare solution for oral administration.

- **PRESCRIBING AND DISPENSING INFORMATION** For choice of antibacterial therapy, see Antibacterials, use for prophylaxis p. 319, Cardiovascular system infections, antibacterial therapy p. 322, Gastro-intestinal system infections, antibacterial therapy p. 324, Musculoskeletal system infections, antibacterial therapy p. 326, Respiratory system infections, antibacterial therapy p. 327, Skin infections, antibacterial therapy p. 329, Urinary-tract infections p. 400.

- **MEDICINAL FORMS** There can be variation in the licensing of different medicines containing the same drug. Forms available from special-order manufacturers include: solution for injection

Powder and solvent for solution for injection

ELECTROLYTES: May contain Sodium

▸ **Teicoplanin (non-proprietary)** ▼

Teicoplanin 200 mg Teicoplanin 200mg powder and solvent for solution for injection vials | 1 vial [PoM] £4.45 DT = £3.93

Teicoplanin 400 mg Teicoplanin 400mg powder and solvent for solution for injection vials | 1 vial [PoM] £7.57 DT = £7.32

▸ **Targocid** (Sanofi) ▼

Teicoplanin 200 mg Targocid 200mg powder and solvent for solution for injection vials | 1 vial [PoM] £3.93 DT = £3.93

Teicoplanin 400 mg Targocid 400mg powder and solvent for solution for injection vials | 1 vial [PoM] £7.32 DT = £7.32

Vancomycin
18-May-2020

- **DRUG ACTION** The glycopeptide antibiotic vancomycin has bactericidal activity against aerobic and anaerobic Gram-positive bacteria including multi-resistant staphylococci. However, there are reports of *Staphylococcus aureus* with reduced susceptibility to glycopeptides. There are increasing reports of glycopeptide-resistant enterococci. Penetration into cerebrospinal fluid is poor.

- **INDICATIONS AND DOSE**

***Clostridioides difficile* infection**

▶ BY MOUTH

▸ Neonate: 10 mg/kg every 6 hours for 10 days, treatment duration may need to be tailored to the clinical course of individual patients.

▸ Child 1 month–11 years: 10 mg/kg every 6 hours for 10 days, treatment duration may need to be tailored to the clinical course of individual patients; maximum 2 g per day

***Clostridioides difficile* infection [first episode]**

▶ BY MOUTH

▸ Child 12–17 years: 125 mg every 6 hours for 10 days; increased if necessary to 500 mg every 6 hours for 10 days, increased dose if severe or complicated infection

***Clostridioides difficile* infection [multiple recurrences]**

▶ BY MOUTH

▸ Child 12–17 years: 125 mg every 6 hours for 10 days, followed by, either tapering the dose (gradually reducing until 125 mg daily) or a pulse regimen (125–500 mg every 2–3 days for at least 3 weeks)

Cellulitis | Erysipelas

▶ BY INTRAVENOUS INFUSION

▸ Child 1 month–11 years: 10–15 mg/kg every 6 hours adjusted according to plasma-concentration monitoring

▸ Child 12–17 years: 15–20 mg/kg every 8–12 hours (max. per dose 2 g) adjusted according to plasma-concentration monitoring

Complicated skin and soft tissue infections | Bone infections | Joint infections | Community-acquired pneumonia | Hospital-acquired pneumonia [including ventilator-associated pneumonia] | Infective endocarditis | Acute bacterial meningitis | Bacteraemia [occurring in association with or suspected to be associated with the licensed indications]

▶ BY INTRAVENOUS INFUSION

▸ Neonate up to 29 weeks corrected gestational age (administered on expert advice): 15 mg/kg every 24 hours adjusted according to plasma-concentration monitoring, duration should be tailored to type and severity of infection and the individual clinical response—consult product literature for further information.

▸ Neonate 29 weeks to 35 weeks corrected gestational age (administered on expert advice): 15 mg/kg every 12 hours adjusted according to plasma-concentration monitoring, duration should be tailored to type and severity of infection and the individual clinical response—consult product literature for further information.

▸ Neonate 35 weeks corrected gestational age and above (administered on expert advice): 15 mg/kg every 8 hours adjusted according to plasma-concentration monitoring, duration should be tailored to type and severity of infection and the individual clinical response—consult product literature for further information.

▸ Child 1 month–11 years: 10–15 mg/kg every 6 hours adjusted according to plasma-concentration monitoring, duration should be tailored to type and severity of infection and the individual clinical response—consult product literature for further information, doses higher than 60 mg/kg/day cannot be generally recommended as the safety of increased dosing has not been fully assessed

▸ Child 12–17 years: 15–20 mg/kg every 8–12 hours (max. per dose 2 g) adjusted according to plasma-concentration monitoring, duration should be tailored to type and severity of infection and the individual clinical response—consult product literature for further information, in seriously ill patients, a loading dose of 25–30 mg/kg (usual max. 2 g) can be used to facilitate rapid attainment of the target trough serum-vancomycin concentration

Perioperative prophylaxis of bacterial endocarditis [in patients at high risk of developing bacterial endocarditis when undergoing major surgical procedures]

▶ BY INTRAVENOUS INFUSION

▸ Neonate: 15 mg/kg, to be given prior to induction of anaesthesia, a second dose may be required depending on duration of surgery.

▸ Child: 15 mg/kg, to be given prior to induction of anaesthesia, a second dose may be required depending on duration of surgery

Surgical prophylaxis (when high risk of MRSA)

▶ BY INTRAVENOUS INFUSION

▸ Child: (consult local protocol)

CNS infection e.g. ventriculitis (administered on expert advice)

▶ BY INTRAVENTRICULAR ADMINISTRATION

▸ Neonate: 10 mg every 24 hours.

▸ Child: 10 mg every 24 hours, for all children reduce to 5 mg daily if ventricular size reduced or increase to 15–20 mg once daily if ventricular size increased, adjust dose according to CSF concentration after 3–4 days; aim for pre-dose ('trough') concentration less than 10 mg/litre. If CSF not draining free reduce dose frequency to once every 2–3 days

Peritonitis associated with peritoneal dialysis

▶ BY INTRAPERITONEAL ADMINISTRATION

▸ Child: Add to each bag of dialysis fluid to achieve a concentration of 20–25 mg/litre

Eradication of meticillin-resistant *Staphylococcus aureus* from the respiratory tract in cystic fibrosis

▶ BY INHALATION OF NEBULISED SOLUTION

▸ Child: 4 mg/kg twice daily (max. per dose 250 mg) for 5 days, alternatively 4 mg/kg 4 times a day (max. per dose 250 mg) for 5 days

PHARMACOKINETICS

▸ Vancomycin should **not** be given by mouth for systemic infections because it is not absorbed significantly.

- **UNLICENSED USE** Vancomycin doses in BNF publications may differ from those in product literature. Use of vancomycin (added to dialysis fluid) for the treatment of peritonitis associated with peritoneal dialysis is an unlicensed route. Not licensed for intraventricular use or inhalation. Not licensed for use by the *intrathecal* route for the treatment of meningitis.

- **CONTRA-INDICATIONS**

▸ With intravenous use Previous hearing loss

- **CAUTIONS**
- ▸ With intravenous use Premature neonates (monitor serum-concentration carefully) · young infants (monitor serum-concentration carefully)
- ▸ With oral use Systemic absorption may be enhanced in patients with inflammatory disorders of the intestinal mucosa or with *Clostridioides difficile*-induced pseudomembranous colitis (increased risk of adverse reactions)
- **INTERACTIONS** → Appendix 1: vancomycin
- **SIDE-EFFECTS**

GENERAL SIDE-EFFECTS
Agranulocytosis · dizziness · drug fever · eosinophilia · hypersensitivity · nausea · nephritis tubulointerstitial · neutropenia (more common after 1 week or cumulative dose of 25g) · renal failure · severe cutaneous adverse reactions (SCARs) · skin reactions · thrombocytopenia · tinnitus (discontinue) · vasculitis · vertigo

SPECIFIC SIDE-EFFECTS
- ▸ With intravenous use Back pain · bradycardia · cardiac arrest (on rapid intravenous injection) · cardiogenic shock (on rapid intravenous injection) · chest pain · dyspnoea · hearing loss · hypotension · muscle complaints · pseudomembranous enterocolitis · red man syndrome · wheezing

SIDE-EFFECTS, FURTHER INFORMATION Vancomycin is associated with a higher incidence of nephrotoxicity than teicoplanin.
- **ALLERGY AND CROSS-SENSITIVITY** Caution if teicoplanin sensitivity.
- **PREGNANCY** Manufacturer advises use only if potential benefit outweighs risk.
  Monitoring Plasma-vancomycin concentration monitoring essential to reduce risk of fetal toxicity.
- **BREAST FEEDING** Present in milk—significant absorption following oral administration unlikely.
- **RENAL IMPAIRMENT** Manufacturer advises serial monitoring of renal function.
- ▸ With intravenous use Manufacturer advises use with caution—increased risk of toxic effects with prolonged high blood concentration.

Dose adjustments
- ▸ With oral use Manufacturer advises dose adjustment is unlikely to be required unless substantial oral absorption occurs in inflammatory disorders of the intestinal mucosa or with *Clostridioides difficile*-induced pseudomembranous colitis, see *Monitoring*.
- ▸ With intravenous use Manufacturer advises initial dose must not be reduced—consult product literature.
- **MONITORING REQUIREMENTS**
- ▸ With intravenous use Manufacturer advises initial doses should be based on body-weight; subsequent dose adjustments should be based on serum-vancomycin concentrations to achieve targeted therapeutic concentrations. All patients require serum-vancomycin measurement (on the second day of treatment, immediately before the next dose if renal function normal, earlier if renal impairment—consult product literature). Frequency of monitoring depends on the clinical situation and response to treatment; regular monitoring indicated in high-dose therapy and longer-term use, particularly in patients with impaired renal function, impaired hearing, or concurrent use of nephrotoxic or ototoxic drugs. Manufacturer advises pre-dose ('trough') concentration should normally be 10–20 mg/litre depending on the site of infection and the susceptibility of the pathogen; trough concentration of 15–20 mg/litre is usually recommended to cover susceptible pathogens with MIC greater than or equal to 1 mg/litre—consult product literature.

  Manufacturer advises periodic testing of auditory function. Manufacturer advises monitor blood counts, urinalysis, hepatic and renal function periodically in all patients; monitor leucocyte count regularly in patients receiving long-term vancomycin or if given concurrently with other drugs that may cause neutropenia or agranulocytosis.
- ▸ With oral use Manufacturer advises monitoring serum-vancomycin concentration in inflammatory intestinal disorders.

  Manufacturer advises serial tests of auditory function may be helpful to minimise the risk of ototoxicity in patients with an underlying hearing loss, or who are receiving concomitant therapy with other ototoxic drugs.
- ▸ With intraventricular use Aim for pre-dose ('trough') concentration less than 10 mg/litre.
- ▸ When used by inhalation Measure lung function before and after initial dose of vancomycin and monitor for bronchospasm.
- **DIRECTIONS FOR ADMINISTRATION**
- ▸ With intravenous use Avoid rapid infusion (risk of anaphylactoid reactions) and rotate infusion sites.

  Displacement value may be significant, consult product literature and local guidelines. For intermittent intravenous infusion, the reconstituted preparation should be further diluted in sodium chloride 0.9% *or* glucose 5% to a concentration of up to 5 mg/mL; give over at least 60 minutes (rate not to exceed 10 mg/minute for doses over 500 mg); use continuous infusion only if intermittent not available (limited evidence); 10 mg/mL can be used if infused via a central venous line over at least 1 hour.
- ▸ With oral use Injection can be used to prepare solution for oral administration—consult product literature.
- ▸ When used by inhalation *For nebulisation* administer required dose in 4 mL of sodium chloride 0.9% (or water for injections). Administer inhaled bronchodilator before vancomycin.
- **PRESCRIBING AND DISPENSING INFORMATION** For choice of antibacterial therapy, see Antibacterials, use for prophylaxis p. 319, Blood infections, antibacterial therapy p. 322, Cardiovascular system infections, antibacterial therapy p. 322, Central nervous system infections, antibacterial therapy p. 323, Gastro-intestinal system infections, antibacterial therapy p. 324, Musculoskeletal system infections, antibacterial therapy p. 326, Respiratory system infections, antibacterial therapy p. 327, Skin infections, antibacterial therapy p. 329.

- **MEDICINAL FORMS** There can be variation in the licensing of different medicines containing the same drug. Forms available from special-order manufacturers include: oral suspension, oral solution, solution for injection, infusion

Powder for solution for infusion

▸ Vancomycin (Non-proprietary)

Vancomycin (as Vancomycin hydrochloride) 500 mg Vancomycin 500mg powder for solution for infusion vials | 1 vial PoM £7.25 DT = £5.49 | 10 vial PoM £62.50 DT = £62.50
Vancomycin 500mg powder for concentrate for solution for infusion vials | 1 vial PoM £5.49–£8.50 DT = £5.49 (Hospital only) | 10 vial PoM £62.50 DT = £62.50 (Hospital only) | 10 vial PoM £62.50–£72.50 DT = £62.50

Vancomycin (as Vancomycin hydrochloride) 1 gram Vancomycin 1g powder for solution for infusion vials | 1 vial PoM £14.50 DT = £11.25 | 10 vial PoM £125.00 DT = £125.00
Vancomycin 1g powder for concentrate for solution for infusion vials | 1 vial PoM £11.25–£17.25 DT = £11.25 (Hospital only) | 10 vial PoM £125.00 DT = £125.00 (Hospital only) | 10 vial PoM £125.00 DT = £125.00

▸ Vancocin (Flynn Pharma Ltd)

Vancomycin (as Vancomycin hydrochloride) 500 mg Vancocin 500mg powder for solution for infusion vials | 1 vial PoM £6.25 DT = £5.49

Vancomycin (as Vancomycin hydrochloride) 1 gram Vancocin 1g powder for solution for infusion vials | 1 vial PoM £12.50 DT = £11.25

Capsule

CAUTIONARY AND ADVISORY LABELS 9

▸ Vancomycin (Non-proprietary)

Vancomycin (as Vancomycin hydrochloride) 125 mg Vancomycin 125mg capsules | 28 capsule PoM DT = £132.49 (Hospital only) | 28 capsule PoM £132.49 DT = £132.49

Vancomycin (as Vancomycin hydrochloride) 250 mg Vancomycin 250mg capsules | 28 capsule PoM DT = £146.38 (Hospital only) | 28 capsule PoM £146.38 DT = £146.38

▸ Vancocin Matrigel (Flynn Pharma Ltd)

Vancomycin (as Vancomycin hydrochloride) 125 mg Vancocin Matrigel 125mg capsules | 28 capsule PoM £88.31 DT = £132.49

ANTIBACTERIALS › LINCOSAMIDES

Clindamycin

18-May-2020

● DRUG ACTION Clindamycin is active against Gram-positive cocci, including streptococci and penicillin-resistant staphylococci, and also against many anaerobes, especially *Bacteroides fragilis*. It is well concentrated in bone and excreted in bile and urine.

● **INDICATIONS AND DOSE**

Staphylococcal bone and joint infections such as osteomyelitis | Peritonitis | Intra-abdominal sepsis | Meticillin-resistant *Staphylococcus aureus* (MRSA) in bronchiectasis, bone and joint infections, and skin and soft-tissue infections

▸ BY MOUTH

▸ Neonate up to 14 days: 3–6 mg/kg 3 times a day.

▸ Neonate 14 days to 28 days: 3–6 mg/kg 4 times a day.

▸ Child: 3–6 mg/kg 4 times a day (max. per dose 450 mg)

▸ BY DEEP INTRAMUSCULAR INJECTION, OR BY INTRAVENOUS INFUSION

▸ Child: 3.75–6.25 mg/kg 4 times a day; increased if necessary up to 10 mg/kg 4 times a day (max. per dose 1.2 g), increased dose used for severe infections, total daily dose may alternatively be given in 3 divided doses, single doses above 600 mg to be administered by intravenous infusion only, single doses by intravenous infusion not to exceed 1.2 g

Cellulitis | Erysipelas

▸ BY MOUTH

▸ Child: 3–6 mg/kg 4 times a day (max. per dose 450 mg) for 7 days then review

▸ BY INTRAVENOUS INFUSION

▸ Child: 3.75–6.25 mg/kg 4 times a day; increased if necessary up to 10 mg/kg 4 times a day (max. per dose 1.2 g), increased dose used in life-threatening infection, total daily dose may alternatively be given in 3 divided doses

Staphylococcal lung infection in cystic fibrosis

▸ BY MOUTH

▸ Child: 5–7 mg/kg 4 times a day (max. per dose 600 mg)

Treatment of falciparum malaria (to be given with or following quinine)

▸ BY MOUTH

▸ Child: 7–13 mg/kg every 8 hours (max. per dose 450 mg) for 7 days

● UNLICENSED USE Not licensed for treatment of falciparum malaria.

● CONTRA-INDICATIONS Avoid injections containing benzyl alcohol in neonates (in neonates) · diarrhoeal states

● CAUTIONS Avoid in Acute porphyrias p. 652

● INTERACTIONS → Appendix 1: clindamycin

● SIDE-EFFECTS

GENERAL SIDE-EFFECTS

▸ **Common or very common** Skin reactions

SPECIFIC SIDE-EFFECTS

▸ **Common or very common**

▸ With oral use Abdominal pain · antibiotic associated colitis · diarrhoea (discontinue)

▸ **Uncommon**

▸ With oral use Nausea · vomiting

▸ **Frequency not known**

▸ With oral use Agranulocytosis · angioedema · eosinophilia · gastrointestinal disorders · jaundice · leucopenia · neutropenia · severe cutaneous adverse reactions (SCARs) · taste altered · thrombocytopenia · vulvovaginal infection

▸ With parenteral use Abdominal pain · agranulocytosis · antibiotic associated colitis · cardiac arrest · diarrhoea (discontinue) · eosinophilia · hypotension · jaundice · leucopenia · nausea · neutropenia · severe cutaneous adverse reactions (SCARs) · taste altered · thrombocytopenia · thrombophlebitis · vomiting · vulvovaginal infection

SIDE-EFFECTS, FURTHER INFORMATION Clindamycin has been associated with antibiotic-associated colitis, which may be fatal. Although antibiotic-associated colitis can occur with most antibacterials, it occurs more frequently with clindamycin. If *C difficile* infection is suspected or confirmed, discontinue the antibiotic if appropriate. Seek specialist advice if the antibiotic cannot be stopped and the diarrhoea is severe.

● PREGNANCY Manufacturer advises not known to be harmful in the second and third trimesters; use with caution in the first trimester—limited data.

● BREAST FEEDING EvGr Specialist sources indicate use with caution—present in milk. Monitor infant for effects on the gastrointestinal flora such as diarrhoea, candidiasis, or rarely, blood in the stool indicating possible antibiotic-associated colitis. ⟨D⟩

● MONITORING REQUIREMENTS Monitor liver and renal function if treatment exceeds 10 days. Monitor liver and renal function in neonates and infants.

● DIRECTIONS FOR ADMINISTRATION

▸ With intravenous use Avoid rapid intravenous administration. For *intravenous infusion*, dilute to a concentration of not more than 18 mg/mL with Glucose 5% *or* Sodium Chloride 0.9%; give over 10–60 minutes at a max. rate of 20 mg/kg/hour.

● PRESCRIBING AND DISPENSING INFORMATION For choice of antibacterial therapy, see Gastro-intestinal system infections, antibacterial therapy p. 324, Malaria, treatment p. 426, MRSA p. 392, Musculoskeletal system infections, antibacterial therapy p. 326, Skin infections, antibacterial therapy p. 329.

● PATIENT AND CARER ADVICE Patients and their carers should be advised to discontinue and contact a doctor immediately if severe, prolonged or bloody diarrhoea develops.

▸ With oral use Capsules should be swallowed with a glass of water.

● PROFESSION SPECIFIC INFORMATION

Dental practitioners' formulary

▸ With oral use Clindamycin capsules may be prescribed.

- **MEDICINAL FORMS** There can be variation in the licensing of different medicines containing the same drug. Forms available from special-order manufacturers include: oral suspension, oral solution

Solution for injection

EXCIPIENTS: May contain Benzyl alcohol

- Clindamycin (Non-proprietary)
  Clindamycin (as Clindamycin phosphate) 150 mg per 1 ml Clindamycin 600mg/4ml solution for injection ampoules | 5 ampoule PoM £59.00 (Hospital only) | 5 ampoule PoM £61.75
  Clindamycin 300mg/2ml solution for injection ampoules | 5 ampoule PoM £29.50 (Hospital only) | 5 ampoule PoM £31.01
- Dalacin C (Pfizer Ltd)
  Clindamycin (as Clindamycin phosphate) 150 mg per 1 ml Dalacin C Phosphate 300mg/2ml solution for injection ampoules | 5 ampoule PoM £31.01 (Hospital only)
  Dalacin C Phosphate 600mg/4ml solution for injection ampoules | 5 ampoule PoM £61.75 (Hospital only)

Capsule

CAUTIONARY AND ADVISORY LABELS 9, 27

- Clindamycin (Non-proprietary)
  Clindamycin (as Clindamycin hydrochloride) 75 mg Clindamycin 75mg capsules | 24 capsule PoM £7.45 DT = £7.45
  Clindamycin (as Clindamycin hydrochloride) 150 mg Clindamycin 150mg capsules | 24 capsule PoM £13.72 DT = £2.51 | 100 capsule PoM £4.26–£55.08
  Clindamycin (as Clindamycin hydrochloride) 300 mg Clindamycin 300mg capsules | 30 capsule PoM £42.00 DT = £38.23
- Dalacin C (Pfizer Ltd)
  Clindamycin (as Clindamycin hydrochloride) 75 mg Dalacin C 75mg capsules | 24 capsule PoM £7.45 DT = £7.45
  Clindamycin (as Clindamycin hydrochloride) 150 mg Dalacin C 150mg capsules | 24 capsule PoM £13.72 DT = £2.51 | 100 capsule PoM £55.08

ANTIBACTERIALS > MACROLIDES

Macrolides

18-Jun-2018

Overview

The macrolides have an antibacterial spectrum that is similar but not identical to that of penicillin; they are thus an alternative in penicillin-allergic patients. They are active against many-penicillin-resistant staphylococci, but some are now also resistant to the macrolides.

Indications for the macrolides include campylobacter enteritis, respiratory infections (including pneumonia, whooping cough, Legionella, chlamydia, and mycoplasma infection), and skin infections.

Erythromycin p. 355 is also used in the treatment of early syphilis, uncomplicated genital chlamydial infection, and non-gonococcal urethritis. Erythromycin has poor activity against *Haemophilus influenzae*. Erythromycin causes nausea, vomiting, and diarrhoea in some patients; in mild to moderate infections this can be avoided by giving a lower dose or the total dose in 4 divided doses, but if a more serious infection, such as Legionella pneumonia, is suspected higher doses are needed.

Azithromycin below is a macrolide with slightly less activity than erythromycin against Gram-positive bacteria, but enhanced activity against some Gram-negative organisms including *H. influenzae*. Plasma concentrations are very low, but tissue concentrations are much higher. It has a long tissue half-life and once daily dosage is recommended. Azithromycin is also used in the treatment of uncomplicated genital chlamydial infection, non-gonococcal urethritis, typhoid [unlicensed indication], trachoma [unlicensed indication], and Lyme disease [unlicensed indication].

Clarithromycin p. 353 is an erythromycin derivative with slightly greater activity than the parent compound. Tissue concentrations are higher than with erythromycin. Clarithromycin is also used in regimens for *Helicobacter pylori* eradication.

Spiramycin is also a macrolide which is used for the treatment of toxoplasmosis.

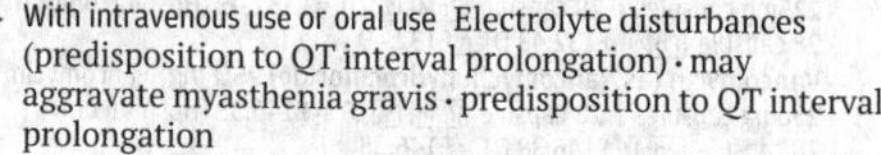

Macrolides

- **CAUTIONS**
  - **With intravenous use or oral use** Electrolyte disturbances (predisposition to QT interval prolongation) · may aggravate myasthenia gravis · predisposition to QT interval prolongation
- **SIDE-EFFECTS**
  - **Common or very common** Appetite decreased · diarrhoea · dizziness · gastrointestinal discomfort · gastrointestinal disorders · headache · hearing impairment · insomnia · nausea · pancreatitis · paraesthesia · skin reactions · taste altered · vasodilation · vision disorders · vomiting
  - **Uncommon** Angioedema · anxiety · arrhythmias · candida infection · chest pain · constipation · drowsiness · eosinophilia · hepatic disorders · leucopenia · neutropenia · palpitations · QT interval prolongation · severe cutaneous adverse reactions (SCARs) · tinnitus · vertigo
  - **Rare or very rare** Antibiotic associated colitis · myasthenia gravis · nephritis tubulointerstitial
  - **Frequency not known** Hallucination · hypotension · seizure · smell altered · thrombocytopenia · tongue discolouration

F above

Azithromycin

03-Mar-2020

- **INDICATIONS AND DOSE**

Prevention of secondary case of invasive group A streptococcal infection in patients who are allergic to penicillin

▶ BY MOUTH

- Child 6 months–11 years: 12 mg/kg once daily (max. per dose 500 mg) for 5 days
- Child 12–17 years: 500 mg once daily for 5 days

Respiratory-tract infections, otitis media, skin and soft-tissue infections

▶ BY MOUTH

- Child 6 months–17 years: 10 mg/kg once daily (max. per dose 500 mg) for 3 days
- Child 6 months–17 years (body-weight 15–25 kg): 200 mg once daily for 3 days
- Child 6 months–17 years (body-weight 26–35 kg): 300 mg once daily for 3 days
- Child 6 months–17 years (body-weight 36–45 kg): 400 mg once daily for 3 days
- Child 6 months–17 years (body-weight 46 kg and above): 500 mg once daily for 3 days

Infection in cystic fibrosis

▶ BY MOUTH

- Child 6 months–17 years: 10 mg/kg once daily (max. per dose 500 mg) for 3 days, repeated after 1 week to complete course, treatment may be repeated as necessary

Chronic *Pseudomonas aeruginosa* infection in cystic fibrosis

▶ BY MOUTH

- Child 6–17 years (body-weight 25–40 kg): 250 mg 3 times a week
- Child 6–17 years (body-weight 41 kg and above): 500 mg 3 times a week

Uncomplicated genital chlamydial infections | Non-gonococcal urethritis

▶ BY MOUTH

- Child 12–17 years: 1 g for 1 dose

Lyme disease [erythema migrans and/or non-focal symptoms]
- ▶ BY MOUTH
- ▶ Child 1 month–11 years (administered on expert advice) (body-weight up to 51 kg): 10 mg/kg daily for 17 days
- ▶ Child 1 month–11 years (administered on expert advice) (body-weight 51 kg and above): 500 mg daily for 17 days
- ▶ Child 12–17 years (administered on expert advice): 500 mg daily for 17 days

Mild to moderate typhoid due to multiple-antibacterial resistant organisms
- ▶ BY MOUTH
- ▶ Child 6 months–17 years: 10 mg/kg once daily (max. per dose 500 mg) for 7 days

- UNLICENSED USE Azithromycin may be used as detailed below, although these situations are considered outside the scope of its licence:
  - prevention of group A streptococcal infection;
  - chronic *Pseudomonas aeruginosa* infection in cystic fibrosis;
  - EvGr Lyme disease (A);
  - mild to moderate typhoid due to multiple-antibacterial resistant organisms.
- INTERACTIONS → Appendix 1: macrolides
- SIDE-EFFECTS
- ▶ **Common or very common** Arthralgia
- ▶ **Uncommon** Numbness · oedema · photosensitivity reaction
- ▶ **Frequency not known** Acute kidney injury · aggression · akathisia · haemolytic anaemia · syncope
- PREGNANCY Manufacturers advise use only if adequate alternatives not available.
- BREAST FEEDING Present in milk; use only if no suitable alternatives.
- HEPATIC IMPAIRMENT Manufacturer advises caution; consider avoiding in severe impairment (no information available).
- RENAL IMPAIRMENT Use with caution if estimated glomerular filtration rate less than 10 mL/minute/1.73 m^2.
- PRESCRIBING AND DISPENSING INFORMATION See Lyme disease p. 391 for place in therapy and further information on treatment. Flavours of oral liquid formulations may include cherry or banana.
- PATIENT AND CARER ADVICE
  Medicines for Children leaflet: Azithromycin for bacterial infections www.medicinesforchildren.org.uk/azithromycin-bacterial-infections-0
- PROFESSION SPECIFIC INFORMATION

Dental practitioners' formulary
Azithromycin Capsules may be prescribed. Azithromycin Tablets may be prescribed. Azithromycin Oral Suspension 200 mg/5 mL may be prescribed.

- EXCEPTIONS TO LEGAL CATEGORY Azithromycin tablets can be sold to the public for the treatment of confirmed, asymptomatic *Chlamydia trachomatis* genital infection in those over 16 years of age, and for the epidemiological treatment of their sexual partners, subject to maximum single dose of 1 g, maximum daily dose 1 g, and a pack size of 1 g.

- MEDICINAL FORMS There can be variation in the licensing of different medicines containing the same drug. Forms available from special-order manufacturers include: oral suspension

Tablet
CAUTIONARY AND ADVISORY LABELS 5, 9
- ▶ Azithromycin (Non-proprietary)
  Azithromycin 250 mg Azithromycin 250mg tablets | 4 tablet PoM £10.11 DT = £1.29 | 6 tablet PoM £1.94–£2.67
  Azithromycin 500 mg Azithromycin 500mg tablets | 3 tablet PoM £9.80 DT = £1.29

Oral suspension
CAUTIONARY AND ADVISORY LABELS 5, 9
- ▶ Azithromycin (Non-proprietary)
  Azithromycin 40 mg per 1 ml Azithromycin 200mg/5ml oral suspension | 15 ml PoM £6.18 DT = £4.06 | 30 ml PoM £11.04 DT = £11.04
- ▶ Zithromax (Pfizer Ltd)
  Azithromycin 40 mg per 1 ml Zithromax 200mg/5ml oral suspension | 15 ml PoM £4.06 DT = £4.06 | 22.5 ml PoM £6.10 DT = £6.10 | 30 ml PoM £11.04 DT = £11.04

Capsule
CAUTIONARY AND ADVISORY LABELS 5, 9, 23
- ▶ Azithromycin (Non-proprietary)
  Azithromycin (as Azithromycin dihydrate) 250 mg Azithromycin 250mg capsules | 4 capsule PoM £1.55–£10.10 | 6 capsule PoM £15.15 DT = £2.33
- ▶ Zithromax (Pfizer Ltd)
  Azithromycin (as Azithromycin dihydrate) 250 mg Zithromax 250mg capsules | 4 capsule PoM £7.16 | 6 capsule PoM £10.74 DT = £2.33

F 352

Clarithromycin

18-May-2020

- INDICATIONS AND DOSE

Cellulitis | Erysipelas
- ▶ BY MOUTH USING IMMEDIATE-RELEASE MEDICINES
- ▶ Child 1 month–11 years (body-weight up to 8 kg): 7.5 mg/kg twice daily for 5–7 days then review (review after 7 days if infection near the eyes or nose)
- ▶ Child 1 month–11 years (body-weight 8–11 kg): 62.5 mg twice daily for 5–7 days then review (review after 7 days if infection near the eyes or nose)
- ▶ Child 1 month–11 years (body-weight 12–19 kg): 125 mg twice daily for 5–7 days then review (review after 7 days if infection near the eyes or nose)
- ▶ Child 1 month–11 years (body-weight 20–29 kg): 187.5 mg twice daily for 5–7 days then review (review after 7 days if infection near the eyes or nose)
- ▶ Child 1 month–11 years (body-weight 30–40 kg): 250 mg twice daily for 5–7 days then review (review after 7 days if infection near the eyes or nose)
- ▶ Child 12–17 years: 250–500 mg twice daily for 5–7 days then review (review after 7 days if infection near the eyes or nose)
- ▶ BY INTRAVENOUS INFUSION
- ▶ Child 1 month–11 years: 7.5 mg/kg every 12 hours (max. per dose 500 mg every 12 hours)
- ▶ Child 12–17 years: 500 mg every 12 hours

Impetigo
- ▶ BY MOUTH USING IMMEDIATE-RELEASE MEDICINES
- ▶ Child 1 month–11 years (body-weight up to 8 kg): 7.5 mg/kg twice daily for 5–7 days
- ▶ Child 1 month–11 years (body-weight 8–11 kg): 62.5 mg twice daily for 5–7 days
- ▶ Child 1 month–11 years (body-weight 12–19 kg): 125 mg twice daily for 5–7 days
- ▶ Child 1 month–11 years (body-weight 20–29 kg): 187.5 mg twice daily for 5–7 days
- ▶ Child 1 month–11 years (body-weight 30–40 kg): 250 mg twice daily for 5–7 days
- ▶ Child 12–17 years: 250 mg twice daily for 5–7 days, increased if necessary to 500 mg twice daily, increased dose used in severe infections

Community-acquired pneumonia
- ▶ BY MOUTH USING IMMEDIATE-RELEASE MEDICINES
- ▶ Child 1 month–11 years (body-weight up to 8 kg): 7.5 mg/kg twice daily for 5 days
- ▶ Child 1 month–11 years (body-weight 8–11 kg): 62.5 mg twice daily for 5 days
- ▶ Child 1 month–11 years (body-weight 12–19 kg): 125 mg twice daily for 5 days

continued →

- Child 1 month–11 years (body-weight 20–29 kg): 187.5 mg twice daily for 5 days
- Child 1 month–11 years (body-weight 30–40 kg): 250 mg twice daily for 5 days
- Child 12–17 years: 250–500 mg twice daily for 5 days

▶ BY INTRAVENOUS INFUSION
- Child 1 month–11 years: 7.5 mg/kg every 12 hours (max. per dose 500 mg every 12 hours)
- Child 12–17 years: 500 mg every 12 hours

Hospital-acquired pneumonia

▶ BY MOUTH USING IMMEDIATE-RELEASE MEDICINES
- Child 1 month–11 years (body-weight up to 8 kg): 7.5 mg/kg twice daily for 5 days then review
- Child 1 month–11 years (body-weight 8–11 kg): 62.5 mg twice daily for 5 days then review
- Child 1 month–11 years (body-weight 12–19 kg): 125 mg twice daily for 5 days then review
- Child 1 month–11 years (body-weight 20–29 kg): 187.5 mg twice daily for 5 days then review
- Child 1 month–11 years (body-weight 30–40 kg): 250 mg twice daily for 5 days then review
- Child 12–17 years: 500 mg twice daily for 5 days then review

Respiratory-tract infections | Mild to moderate skin and soft-tissue infections

▶ BY MOUTH USING IMMEDIATE-RELEASE MEDICINES
- Neonate: 7.5 mg/kg twice daily.

- Child 1 month–11 years (body-weight up to 8 kg): 7.5 mg/kg twice daily
- Child 1 month–11 years (body-weight 8–11 kg): 62.5 mg twice daily
- Child 1 month–11 years (body-weight 12–19 kg): 125 mg twice daily
- Child 1 month–11 years (body-weight 20–29 kg): 187.5 mg twice daily
- Child 1 month–11 years (body-weight 30–40 kg): 250 mg twice daily
- Child 12–17 years: 250 mg twice daily usually for 7–14 days, increased to 500 mg twice daily, if required in severe infections

▶ BY MOUTH USING MODIFIED-RELEASE MEDICINES
- Child 12–17 years: 500 mg once daily usually for 7–14 days, increased to 1 g once daily, if required in severe infections

▶ BY INTRAVENOUS INFUSION
- Child 1 month–11 years: 7.5 mg/kg every 12 hours (max. per dose 500 mg every 12 hours) maximum duration 5 days, switch to oral route when appropriate, to be administered into a large proximal vein
- Child 12–17 years: 500 mg every 12 hours maximum duration 5 days, switch to oral route when appropriate, to be administered into a large proximal vein

Acute exacerbation of bronchiectasis

▶ BY MOUTH USING IMMEDIATE-RELEASE MEDICINES
- Child 1 month–11 years (body-weight up to 8 kg): 7.5 mg/kg twice daily for 7–14 days
- Child 1 month–11 years (body-weight 8–11 kg): 62.5 mg twice daily for 7–14 days
- Child 1 month–11 years (body-weight 12–19 kg): 125 mg twice daily for 7–14 days
- Child 1 month–11 years (body-weight 20–29 kg): 187.5 mg twice daily for 7–14 days
- Child 1 month–11 years (body-weight 30–40 kg): 250 mg twice daily for 7–14 days
- Child 12–17 years: 250–500 mg twice daily for 7–14 days

Acute cough [if systemically very unwell or at higher risk of complications] | Acute sore throat

▶ BY MOUTH USING IMMEDIATE-RELEASE MEDICINES
- Child 1 month–11 years (body-weight up to 8 kg): 7.5 mg/kg twice daily for 5 days
- Child 1 month–11 years (body-weight 8–11 kg): 62.5 mg twice daily for 5 days
- Child 1 month–11 years (body-weight 12–19 kg): 125 mg twice daily for 5 days
- Child 1 month–11 years (body-weight 20–29 kg): 187.5 mg twice daily for 5 days
- Child 1 month–11 years (body-weight 30–40 kg): 250 mg twice daily for 5 days
- Child 12–17 years: 250–500 mg twice daily for 5 days

Acute otitis media

▶ BY MOUTH USING IMMEDIATE-RELEASE MEDICINES
- Neonate: 7.5 mg/kg twice daily.

- Child 1 month–11 years (body-weight up to 8 kg): 7.5 mg/kg twice daily for 5–7 days
- Child 1 month–11 years (body-weight 8–11 kg): 62.5 mg twice daily for 5–7 days
- Child 1 month–11 years (body-weight 12–19 kg): 125 mg twice daily for 5–7 days
- Child 1 month–11 years (body-weight 20–29 kg): 187.5 mg twice daily for 5–7 days
- Child 1 month–11 years (body-weight 30–40 kg): 250 mg twice daily for 5–7 days
- Child 12–17 years: 250–500 mg twice daily for 5–7 days

▶ BY INTRAVENOUS INFUSION
- Child 1 month–11 years: 7.5 mg/kg every 12 hours (max. per dose 500 mg every 12 hours) maximum duration 5 days, switch to oral route when appropriate, to be administered into a large proximal vein
- Child 12–17 years: 500 mg every 12 hours maximum duration 5 days, switch to oral route when appropriate, to be administered into a large proximal vein

Prevention of pertussis

▶ BY MOUTH USING IMMEDIATE-RELEASE MEDICINES
- Neonate: 7.5 mg/kg twice daily for 7 days.

- Child 1 month–11 years (body-weight up to 8 kg): 7.5 mg/kg twice daily for 7 days
- Child 1 month–11 years (body-weight 8–11 kg): 62.5 mg twice daily for 7 days
- Child 1 month–11 years (body-weight 12–19 kg): 125 mg twice daily for 7 days
- Child 1 month–11 years (body-weight 20–29 kg): 187.5 mg twice daily for 7 days
- Child 1 month–11 years (body-weight 30–40 kg): 250 mg twice daily for 7 days
- Child 12–17 years: 500 mg twice daily for 7 days

***Helicobacter pylori* eradication in combination with omeprazole, and amoxicillin or metronidazole**

▶ BY MOUTH
- Child 1–5 years: 7.5 mg/kg twice daily (max. per dose 500 mg)
- Child 6–11 years: 7.5 mg/kg twice daily (max. per dose 500 mg)
- Child 12–17 years: 500 mg twice daily

Acute sinusitis

▶ BY MOUTH USING IMMEDIATE-RELEASE MEDICINES
- Child 1 month–11 years (body-weight up to 8 kg): 7.5 mg/kg twice daily for 5 days
- Child 1 month–11 years (body-weight 8–11 kg): 62.5 mg twice daily for 5 days
- Child 1 month–11 years (body-weight 12–19 kg): 125 mg twice daily for 5 days
- Child 1 month–11 years (body-weight 20–29 kg): 187.5 mg twice daily for 5 days
- Child 1 month–11 years (body-weight 30–40 kg): 250 mg twice daily for 5 days
- Child 12–17 years: 250 mg twice daily for 5 days, alternatively 500 mg twice daily for 5 days

- **UNLICENSED USE** EvGr Duration of treatment for acute sinusitis differs from product literature and adheres to national guidelines. ⟨A⟩
- With oral use EvGr Duration of treatment for acute otitis media differs from product literature and adheres to national guidelines. ⟨A⟩ Tablets not licensed for use in children under 12 years; oral suspension not licensed for use in infants under 6 months.
- With intravenous use Intravenous infusion not licensed for use in children under 12 years.
- **INTERACTIONS** → Appendix 1: macrolides
- **SIDE-EFFECTS**

GENERAL SIDE-EFFECTS
- **Uncommon** Burping · dry mouth · muscle complaints · oral disorders · thrombocytosis · tremor
- **Frequency not known** Abnormal dreams · agranulocytosis · depersonalisation · depression · mania · myopathy · psychotic disorder · renal failure · tooth discolouration · urine discolouration

SPECIFIC SIDE-EFFECTS
- **Uncommon**
- With oral use Epistaxis
- With parenteral use Cardiac arrest · dyskinesia · haemorrhage · loss of consciousness · pulmonary embolism

- **PREGNANCY** Manufacturer advises avoid, particularly in the first trimester, unless potential benefit outweighs risk.
- **BREAST FEEDING** Manufacturer advises avoid unless potential benefit outweighs risk—present in milk.
- **HEPATIC IMPAIRMENT** Manufacturer advises caution; avoid in severe failure if renal impairment also present.
- **RENAL IMPAIRMENT** Avoid if severe hepatic impairment also present.
- With oral use Avoid *Klaricid XL*® or clarithromyin m/r preparations if estimated glomerular filtration rate less than 30 mL/minute/1.73 m^2.

Dose adjustments Use half normal dose if estimated glomerular filtration rate less than 30 mL/minute/1.73 m^2, max. duration 14 days.

- **DIRECTIONS FOR ADMINISTRATION**
- With intravenous use For intermittent intravenous infusion dilute reconstituted solution further in Glucose 5% *or* Sodium chloride 0.9% to a concentration of 2 mg/mL; give into large proximal vein over 60 minutes.
- **PRESCRIBING AND DISPENSING INFORMATION** For choice of antibacterial therapy, see Antibacterials, use for prophylaxis p. 319, Ear infections, antibacterial therapy p. 324, Nose infections, antibacterial therapy p. 326, Oropharyngeal infections, antibacterial therapy p. 761, Peptic ulceration p. 58, Respiratory system infections, antibacterial therapy p. 327, Skin infections, antibacterial therapy p. 329.
- **PATIENT AND CARER ADVICE**

Medicines for Children leaflet: Clarithromycin for bacterial infections www.medicinesforchildren.org.uk/clarithromycin-bacterial-infections

- **PROFESSION SPECIFIC INFORMATION**

Dental practitioners' formulary

Clarithromycin Tablets may be prescribed.

Clarithromycin Oral Suspension may be prescribed.

- **MEDICINAL FORMS** There can be variation in the licensing of different medicines containing the same drug. Forms available from special-order manufacturers include: infusion

Modified-release tablet

CAUTIONARY AND ADVISORY LABELS 9, 21, 25
- Klaricid XL (Mylan)

Clarithromycin 500 mg Klaricid XL 500mg tablets | 7 tablet PoM £6.72 DT = £6.72 | 14 tablet PoM £13.23
- Xetinin XL (Morningside Healthcare Ltd)

Clarithromycin 500 mg Xetinin XL 500mg tablets | 7 tablet PoM £6.72 DT = £6.72 | 14 tablet PoM £13.23

Granules

CAUTIONARY AND ADVISORY LABELS 9, 13
- Klaricid (Mylan)

Clarithromycin 250 mg Klaricid Adult 250mg granules sachets | 14 sachet PoM £11.68 DT = £11.68

Tablet

CAUTIONARY AND ADVISORY LABELS 9
- Clarithromycin (Non-proprietary)

Clarithromycin 250 mg Clarithromycin 250mg tablets | 14 tablet PoM £10.50 DT = £1.49

Clarithromycin 500 mg Clarithromycin 500mg tablets | 14 tablet PoM £21.50 DT = £2.44

Oral suspension

CAUTIONARY AND ADVISORY LABELS 9
- Clarithromycin (Non-proprietary)

Clarithromycin 25 mg per 1 ml Clarithromycin 125mg/5ml oral suspension | 70 ml PoM £4.91 DT = £3.59

Clarithromycin 50 mg per 1 ml Clarithromycin 250mg/5ml oral suspension | 70 ml PoM £9.88 DT = £4.94
- Klaricid (Mylan)

Clarithromycin 25 mg per 1 ml Klaricid Paediatric 125mg/5ml oral suspension | 70 ml PoM £5.26 DT = £3.59 | 100 ml PoM £9.04

Clarithromycin 50 mg per 1 ml Klaricid Paediatric 250mg/5ml oral suspension | 70 ml PoM £10.51 DT = £4.94

Powder for solution for infusion

ELECTROLYTES: May contain Sodium
- Clarithromycin (Non-proprietary)

Clarithromycin 500 mg Clarithromycin 500mg powder for solution for infusion vials | 1 vial PoM £11.25 DT = £9.45 (Hospital only) Clarithromycin 500mg powder for concentrate for solution for infusion vials | 1 vial PoM £11.15 DT = £9.45 | 10 vial PoM £111.50
- Klaricid (Mylan)

Clarithromycin 500 mg Klaricid IV 500mg powder for solution for infusion vials | 1 vial PoM £9.45 DT = £9.45

F 352

Erythromycin

18-May-2020

- **INDICATIONS AND DOSE**

Susceptible infections in patients with penicillin hypersensitivity (e.g. respiratory-tract infections (including Legionella infection), skin and oral infections, and campylobacter enteritis)

- BY MOUTH
- Neonate: 12.5 mg/kg every 6 hours.
- Child 1–23 months: 125 mg 4 times a day, total daily dose may alternatively be given in two divided doses, increased to 250 mg 4 times a day, dose increase may be used in severe infections
- Child 2–7 years: 250 mg 4 times a day, total daily dose may alternatively be given in two divided doses, increased to 500 mg 4 times a day, dose increase may be used in severe infections
- Child 8–17 years: 250–500 mg 4 times a day, total daily dose may alternatively be given in two divided doses, increased to 500–1000 mg 4 times a day, dose increase may be used in severe infections
- BY INTRAVENOUS INFUSION
- Neonate: 10–12.5 mg/kg every 6 hours.
- Child: 12.5 mg/kg every 6 hours (max. per dose 1 g)

Impetigo
- BY MOUTH
- Child 8–17 years: 250–500 mg 4 times a day for 5–7 days

Cellulitis | Erysipelas
- BY MOUTH
- Child 8–17 years: 250–500 mg 4 times a day for 5–7 days then review

Community-acquired pneumonia
- BY MOUTH
- Child 8–17 years: 250–500 mg 4 times a day for 5 days

continued →

Acute cough [if systemically very unwell or at higher risk of complications] | Acute sore throat
- ▶ BY MOUTH
- ▶ Child 1–23 months: 125 mg 4 times a day for 5 days, alternatively 250 mg twice daily for 5 days
- ▶ Child 2–7 years: 250 mg 4 times a day for 5 days, alternatively 500 mg twice daily for 5 days
- ▶ Child 8–17 years: 250–500 mg 4 times a day for 5 days, alternatively 500–1000 mg twice daily for 5 days

Acute otitis media
- ▶ BY MOUTH
- ▶ Child 1–23 months: 125 mg 4 times a day for 5–7 days, alternatively 250 mg twice daily for 5–7 days
- ▶ Child 2–7 years: 250 mg 4 times a day for 5–7 days, alternatively 500 mg twice daily for 5–7 days
- ▶ Child 8–17 years: 250–500 mg 4 times a day for 5–7 days, alternatively 500–1000 mg twice daily for 5–7 days

Chlamydial ophthalmia
- ▶ BY MOUTH
- ▶ Neonate: 12.5 mg/kg every 6 hours.
- ▶ Child 1–23 months: 125 mg 4 times a day, increased to 250 mg every 6 hours, dose increase for severe infections, total daily dose may alternatively be given in two divided doses
- ▶ Child 2–7 years: 250 mg 4 times a day, increased to 500 mg every 6 hours, dose increase for severe infections, total daily dose may alternatively be given in two divided doses
- ▶ Child 8–17 years: 250–500 mg 4 times a day, increased to 500–1000 mg every 6 hours, dose increase for severe infections, total daily dose may alternatively be given in two divided doses
- ▶ BY INTRAVENOUS INFUSION
- ▶ Neonate: 10–12.5 mg/kg every 6 hours.
- ▶ Child: 12.5 mg/kg every 6 hours (max. per dose 1 g)

Early syphilis
- ▶ BY MOUTH
- ▶ Child 12–17 years: 500 mg 4 times a day for 14 days

Uncomplicated genital chlamydia | Non-gonococcal urethritis
- ▶ BY MOUTH
- ▶ Child 1–23 months: 12.5 mg/kg 4 times a day for 14 days
- ▶ Child 2–11 years: 250 mg twice daily for 14 days
- ▶ Child 12–17 years: 500 mg twice daily for 14 days

Pelvic inflammatory disease
- ▶ BY MOUTH
- ▶ Child 1–23 months: 12.5 mg/kg 4 times a day for 14 days
- ▶ Child 2–11 years: 250 mg twice daily for 14 days
- ▶ Child 12–17 years: 500 mg twice daily for 14 days

Prevention and treatment of pertussis
- ▶ BY MOUTH
- ▶ Neonate: 12.5 mg/kg every 6 hours.
- ▶ Child 1–23 months: 125 mg 4 times a day, total daily dose may alternatively be given in two divided doses, increased to 250 mg 4 times a day, dose increase may be used in severe infections
- ▶ Child 2–7 years: 250 mg 4 times a day, total daily dose may alternatively be given in two divided doses, increased to 500 mg 4 times a day, dose increase may be used in severe infections
- ▶ Child 8–17 years: 250–500 mg 4 times a day, total daily dose may alternatively be given in two divided doses, increased to 500–1000 mg 4 times a day, dose increase may be used in severe infections
- ▶ BY INTRAVENOUS INFUSION
- ▶ Neonate: 10–12.5 mg/kg every 6 hours.
- ▶ Child: 12.5 mg/kg every 6 hours (max. per dose 1 g)

Prevention of secondary case of diphtheria in non-immune patient
- ▶ BY MOUTH
- ▶ Child 1–23 months: 125 mg every 6 hours for 7 days, treat for further 10 days if nasopharyngeal swabs positive after first 7 days' treatment
- ▶ Child 2–7 years: 250 mg every 6 hours for 7 days, treat for further 10 days if nasopharyngeal swabs positive after first 7 days' treatment
- ▶ Child 8–17 years: 500 mg every 6 hours for 7 days, treat for further 10 days if nasopharyngeal swabs positive after first 7 days' treatment

Prevention of secondary case of invasive group A streptococcal infection in penicillin allergic patients
- ▶ BY MOUTH
- ▶ Child 1–23 months: 125 mg every 6 hours for 10 days
- ▶ Child 2–7 years: 250 mg every 6 hours for 10 days
- ▶ Child 8–17 years: 250–500 mg every 6 hours for 10 days

Prevention of pneumococcal infection in asplenia or in patients with sickle-cell disease (if penicillin-allergic)
- ▶ BY MOUTH
- ▶ Child 1–23 months: 125 mg twice daily, antibiotic prophylaxis is not fully reliable
- ▶ Child 2–7 years: 250 mg twice daily, antibiotic prophylaxis is not fully reliable. It may be discontinued in those over 5 years of age with sickle-cell disease who have received pneumococcal immunisation and who do not have a history of severe pneumococcal infection
- ▶ Child 8–17 years: 500 mg twice daily, antibiotic prophylaxis is not fully reliable. It may be discontinued in those with sickle-cell disease who have received pneumococcal immunisation and who do not have a history of severe pneumococcal infection

Prevention of recurrence of rheumatic fever
- ▶ BY MOUTH
- ▶ Child 1–23 months: 125 mg twice daily
- ▶ Child 2–17 years: 250 mg twice daily

Acne
- ▶ BY MOUTH
- ▶ Child 1–23 months: 250 mg once daily, alternatively 125 mg twice daily
- ▶ Child 12–17 years: 500 mg twice daily

Gastro-intestinal stasis
- ▶ BY MOUTH
- ▶ Neonate: 3 mg/kg 4 times a day.
- ▶ Child: 3 mg/kg 4 times a day
- ▶ BY INTRAVENOUS INFUSION
- ▶ Neonate: 3 mg/kg 4 times a day.
- ▶ Child 1–11 months: 3 mg/kg 4 times a day

- **UNLICENSED USE** EvGr Duration of treatment for acute otitis media differs from product literature and adheres to national guidelines. Ⓐ

  Erythromycin may be used for gastro-intestinal stasis, but it is not licensed for this indication.
- **CAUTIONS** Avoid in Acute porphyrias p. 652 · neonate under 2 weeks (risk of hypertrophic pyloric stenosis)
- **INTERACTIONS** → Appendix 1: macrolides
- **SIDE-EFFECTS**

  GENERAL SIDE-EFFECTS
  - ▶ **Rare or very rare** Hearing loss (can occur after large doses)

  SPECIFIC SIDE-EFFECTS
  - ▶ **With oral use** Cerebral impairment
  - ▶ **With parenteral use** Atrioventricular block

- **PREGNANCY** Not known to be harmful.
- **BREAST FEEDING** Only small amounts in milk—not known to be harmful.
- **HEPATIC IMPAIRMENT** Manufacturer advises caution.
- **RENAL IMPAIRMENT**

Dose adjustments Reduce dose in severe renal impairment (ototoxicity).

- **DIRECTIONS FOR ADMINISTRATION**
- ▸ With intravenous use Dilute reconstituted solution further in glucose 5% (neutralised with Sodium bicarbonate) or sodium chloride 0.9% to a concentration of 1–5 mg/mL; give over 20–60 minutes. Concentration of up to 10 mg/mL may be used in fluid-restriction if administered via a central venous catheter.
- **PRESCRIBING AND DISPENSING INFORMATION** For choice of antibacterial therapy, see Antibacterials, use for prophylaxis p. 319, Ear infections, antibacterial therapy p. 324, Eye infections, antibacterial therapy p. 324, Gastro-intestinal system infections, antibacterial therapy p. 324, Genital system infections, antibacterial therapy p. 325, Oropharyngeal infections, antibacterial therapy p. 761, Respiratory system infections, antibacterial therapy p. 327, Skin infections, antibacterial therapy p. 329.
- **PATIENT AND CARER ADVICE**

Medicines for Children leaflet: Erythromycin for bacterial infections www.medicinesforchildren.org.uk/erythromycin-bacterial-infections

- **PROFESSION SPECIFIC INFORMATION**

Dental practitioners' formulary

▸ With oral use Erythromycin tablets e/c may be prescribed. Erythromycin ethyl succinate oral suspension may be prescribed. Erythromycin stearate tablets may be prescribed. Erythromycin ethyl succinate tablets may be prescribed.

- **MEDICINAL FORMS** There can be variation in the licensing of different medicines containing the same drug.

Gastro-resistant tablet

CAUTIONARY AND ADVISORY LABELS 5, 9, 25

▸ Erythromycin (Non-proprietary)

Erythromycin 250 mg Erythromycin 250mg gastro-resistant tablets | 28 tablet [PoM] £11.23 DT = £1.73 | 500 tablet [PoM] £158.04

Tablet

CAUTIONARY AND ADVISORY LABELS 9

▸ Erythromycin (Non-proprietary)

Erythromycin (as Erythromycin stearate) 250 mg Erythromycin stearate 250mg tablets | 28 tablet [PoM] £5.10

Erythromycin (as Erythromycin ethyl succinate) 500 mg Erythromycin ethyl succinate 500mg tablets | 28 tablet [PoM] £15.95 DT = £10.78

Erythromycin (as Erythromycin stearate) 500 mg Erythromycin stearate 500mg tablets | 28 tablet [PoM] £10.19

▸ Erythrocin (Advanz Pharma)

Erythromycin (as Erythromycin stearate) 250 mg Erythrocin 250 tablets | 100 tablet [PoM] £18.20 DT = £18.20

Erythromycin (as Erythromycin stearate) 500 mg Erythrocin 500 tablets | 100 tablet [PoM] £36.40 DT = £36.40

▸ Erythrolar (Ennogen Pharma Ltd)

Erythromycin (as Erythromycin stearate) 250 mg Erythrolar 250mg tablets | 100 tablet [PoM] £22.80 DT = £18.20

Erythromycin (as Erythromycin stearate) 500 mg Erythrolar 500mg tablets | 100 tablet [PoM] £45.60 DT = £36.40

▸ Erythroped A (Advanz Pharma)

Erythromycin (as Erythromycin ethyl succinate) 500 mg Erythroped A 500mg tablets | 28 tablet [PoM] £10.78 DT = £10.78

Oral suspension

CAUTIONARY AND ADVISORY LABELS 9

▸ Erythromycin (Non-proprietary)

Erythromycin (as Erythromycin ethyl succinate) 25 mg per 1 ml Erythromycin ethyl succinate 125mg/5ml oral suspension | 100 ml [PoM] £5.37 DT = £5.37

Erythromycin ethyl succinate 125mg/5ml oral suspension sugar free sugar-free | 100 ml [PoM] £5.35 DT = £5.35

Erythromycin (as Erythromycin ethyl succinate) 50 mg per 1 ml Erythromycin ethyl succinate 250mg/5ml oral suspension | 100 ml [PoM] £8.89 DT = £8.80

Erythromycin ethyl succinate 250mg/5ml oral suspension sugar free sugar-free | 100 ml [PoM] £8.89 DT = £8.48

Erythromycin (as Erythromycin ethyl succinate) 100 mg per 1 ml Erythromycin ethyl succinate 500mg/5ml oral suspension | 100 ml [PoM] £15.73 DT = £15.00

Erythromycin ethyl succinate 500mg/5ml oral suspension sugar free sugar-free | 100 ml [PoM] [NHS]

▸ Erythroped (Advanz Pharma)

Erythromycin (as Erythromycin ethyl succinate) 25 mg per 1 ml Erythroped PI SF 125mg/5ml oral suspension sugar-free | 140 ml [PoM] £3.06

Erythromycin (as Erythromycin ethyl succinate) 50 mg per 1 ml Erythroped SF 250mg/5ml oral suspension sugar-free | 140 ml [PoM] £5.95

Erythromycin (as Erythromycin ethyl succinate) 100 mg per 1 ml Erythroped Forte SF 500mg/5ml oral suspension sugar-free | 140 ml [PoM] £10.56 DT = £10.56

Powder for solution for infusion

▸ Erythromycin (Non-proprietary)

Erythromycin (as Erythromycin lactobionate) 1 gram Erythromycin 1g powder for solution for infusion vials | 1 vial [PoM] £22.00 (Hospital only) | 1 vial [PoM] £22.92

ANTIBACTERIALS > MONOBACTAMS

Aztreonam

11-May-2020

- **DRUG ACTION** Aztreonam is a monocyclic beta-lactam ('monobactam') antibiotic with an antibacterial spectrum limited to Gram-negative aerobic bacteria including *Pseudomonas aeruginosa*, *Neisseria meningitidis*, and *Haemophilus influenzae*; it should not be used alone for 'blind' treatment since it is not active against Gram-positive organisms. Aztreonam is also effective against *Neisseria gonorrhoeae* (but not against concurrent chlamydial infection).

- **INDICATIONS AND DOSE**

Gram-negative infections including *Pseudomonas aeruginosa*, *Haemophilus influenzae*, and *Neisseria meningitidis*

▸ BY INTRAVENOUS INJECTION, OR BY INTRAVENOUS INFUSION

- ▸ Neonate up to 7 days: 30 mg/kg every 12 hours.
- ▸ Neonate 7 days to 28 days: 30 mg/kg every 6–8 hours.
- ▸ Child 1 month–11 years: 30 mg/kg every 6–8 hours
- ▸ Child 12–17 years: 1 g every 8 hours, alternatively 2 g every 12 hours

Severe gram-negative infections including *Pseudomonas aeruginosa*, *Haemophilus influenzae*, *Neisseria meningitidis*, and lung infections in cystic fibrosis

▸ BY INTRAVENOUS INFUSION, OR BY INTRAVENOUS INJECTION

- ▸ Child 2–11 years: 50 mg/kg every 6–8 hours (max. per dose 2 g 4 times a day)
- ▸ Child 12–17 years: 2 g every 6–8 hours

Chronic pulmonary *Pseudomonas aeruginosa* infection in patients with cystic fibrosis

▸ BY INHALATION OF NEBULISED SOLUTION

- ▸ Child 6–17 years: 75 mg 3 times a day for 28 days, doses to be administered at least 4 hours apart, subsequent courses repeated after 28-day interval without aztreonam nebuliser solution

- **UNLICENSED USE**
- ▸ With systemic use Injection not licensed for use in children under 7 days.
- **CAUTIONS**
- ▸ When used by inhalation Haemoptysis— risk of further haemorrhage

5 Infection

● **SIDE-EFFECTS**

GENERAL SIDE-EFFECTS

▶ **Common or very common** Dyspnoea · respiratory disorders

SPECIFIC SIDE-EFFECTS

▶ **Common or very common**

▸ When used by inhalation Cough · haemoptysis · joint disorders · laryngeal pain · nasal complaints · rash

▶ **Rare or very rare**

▸ With parenteral use Anaemia · asthenia · breast tenderness · chest pain · confusion · diplopia · dizziness · eosinophilia · haemorrhage · headache · hepatic disorders · hypotension · insomnia · leucocytosis · myalgia · nasal congestion · neutropenia · oral disorders · pancytopenia · paraesthesia · pseudomembranous enterocolitis · seizure · thrombocytopenia · thrombocytosis · tinnitus · vertigo · vulvovaginal candidiasis

▶ **Frequency not known**

▸ With parenteral use Abdominal pain · angioedema · diarrhoea · nausea · skin reactions · taste altered · toxic epidermal necrolysis · vomiting

● **ALLERGY AND CROSS-SENSITIVITY** Contra-indicated in aztreonam hypersensitivity.

Use with caution in patients with hypersensitivity to other beta-lactam antibiotics (although aztreonam may be less likely than other beta-lactams to cause hypersensitivity in penicillin-sensitive patients).

● **PREGNANCY**

▸ With systemic use No information available; manufacturer of injection advises avoid.

▸ When used by inhalation No information available; manufacturer of powder for nebuliser solution advises avoid unless essential.

● **BREAST FEEDING** Amount in milk probably too small to be harmful.

● **HEPATIC IMPAIRMENT**

▸ With systemic use Manufacturer advises caution in chronic impairment with cirrhosis.

Dose adjustments ▸ With systemic use Manufacturer advises dose reduction of 20—25% for long term treatment of patients with chronic impairment with cirrhosis, especially in alcoholic cirrhosis and concomitant renal impairment.

● **RENAL IMPAIRMENT**

Dose adjustments ▸ With systemic use If estimated glomerular filtration rate 10–30 mL/minute/1.73 m^2, usual initial dose of injection, then half normal dose. If estimated glomerular filtration rate less than 10 mL/minute/1.73 m^2, usual initial dose of injection, then one-quarter normal dose.

● **MONITORING REQUIREMENTS**

▸ When used by inhalation Measure lung function before and after initial dose of aztreonam and monitor for bronchospasm.

● **DIRECTIONS FOR ADMINISTRATION**

▸ With intravenous use For *intravenous injection*, give over 3–5 minutes. Displacement value of injection may be significant, consult local guidelines. For intermittent *intravenous infusion*, dilute reconstituted solution further in Glucose 5% *or* Sodium chloride 0.9% to a concentration of less than 20 mg/mL; to be given over 20–60 minutes.

▸ When used by inhalation Other inhaled drugs should be administered before aztreonam; a bronchodilator should be administered before each dose.

● **NATIONAL FUNDING/ACCESS DECISIONS**

Scottish Medicines Consortium (SMC) decisions

SMC No. 753/12

The *Scottish Medicines Consortium* has advised (January 2015) that aztreonam powder for nebuliser solution (*Cayston*®) is accepted for restricted use within NHS Scotland when inhaled colistimethate sodium and inhaled tobramycin are not tolerated or are not providing satisfactory therapeutic benefit (measured as ≥2% decline in forced expiratory volume in 1 second). This advice is contingent upon the continuing availability of the Patient Access Scheme in NHS Scotland or a list price that is equivalent or lower.

● **MEDICINAL FORMS** There can be variation in the licensing of different medicines containing the same drug.

Powder and solvent for nebuliser solution

▸ Cayston (Gilead Sciences International Ltd)

Aztreonam (as Aztreonam lysine) 75 mg Cayston 75mg powder and solvent for nebuliser solution vials with Altera Nebuliser Handset | 84 vial PoM £2,181.53 DT = £2,181.53

Powder for solution for injection

▸ Azactam (Bristol-Myers Squibb Pharmaceuticals Ltd)

Aztreonam 1 gram Azactam 1g powder for solution for injection vials | 1 vial PoM £9.40 (Hospital only)

Aztreonam 2 gram Azactam 2g powder for solution for injection vials | 1 vial PoM £18.82 (Hospital only)

ANTIBACTERIALS > NITROIMIDAZOLE DERIVATIVES

Metronidazole

18-May-2020

● **DRUG ACTION** Metronidazole is an antimicrobial drug with high activity against anaerobic bacteria and protozoa.

● **INDICATIONS AND DOSE**

Anaerobic infections

▶ BY MOUTH

▸ Child 1 month: 7.5 mg/kg every 12 hours usually treated for 7 days (for 10–14 days in *Clostridioides difficile* infection)

▸ Child 2 months–11 years: 7.5 mg/kg every 8 hours (max. per dose 400 mg) usually treated for 7 days (for 10–14 days in *Clostridioides difficile* infection)

▸ Child 12–17 years: 400 mg every 8 hours usually treated for 7 days (for 10–14 days in *Clostridioides difficile* infection)

▶ BY RECTUM

▸ Child 1–11 months: 125 mg 3 times a day for 3 days, then 125 mg twice daily, for usual total treatment duration of 7 days

▸ Child 1–4 years: 250 mg 3 times a day for 3 days, then 250 mg twice daily, for usual total treatment duration of 7 days

▸ Child 5–9 years: 500 mg 3 times a day for 3 days, then 500 mg twice daily, for usual total treatment duration of 7 days

▸ Child 10–17 years: 1 g 3 times a day for 3 days, then 1 g twice daily, for usual total treatment duration of 7 days

▶ BY INTRAVENOUS INFUSION

▸ Neonate up to 26 weeks corrected gestational age: Loading dose 15 mg/kg, followed by 7.5 mg/kg after 24 hours, then 7.5 mg/kg daily usually treated for a total duration of 7 days (for 10–14 days in *Clostridioides difficile* infection).

▸ Neonate 26 weeks to 34 weeks corrected gestational age: Loading dose 15 mg/kg, followed by 7.5 mg/kg after 12 hours, then 7.5 mg/kg every 12 hours usually treated for a total duration of 7 days (for 10–14 days in *Clostridioides difficile* infection).

▸ Neonate 34 weeks corrected gestational age and above: Loading dose 15 mg/kg, followed by 7.5 mg/kg after 8 hours, then 7.5 mg/kg every 8 hours usually treated for a total duration of 7 days (for 10–14 days in *Clostridioides difficile* infection).

▸ Child 1 month: Loading dose 15 mg/kg, followed by 7.5 mg/kg after 8 hours, then 7.5 mg/kg every 8 hours

usually treated for a total duration of 7 days (for 10–14 days in *Clostridioides difficile* infection)
- Child 2 months–17 years: 7.5 mg/kg every 8 hours (max. per dose 500 mg) usually treated for 7 days (for 10–14 days in *Clostridioides difficile* infection)

Cellulitis | Erysipelas
- BY MOUTH
- Child 1 month: 7.5 mg/kg every 12 hours for 7 days then review
- Child 2 months–11 years: 7.5 mg/kg every 8 hours (max. per dose 400 mg) for 7 days then review
- Child 12–17 years: 400 mg every 8 hours for 7 days then review
- BY INTRAVENOUS INFUSION
- Child 1 month: Loading dose 15 mg/kg, followed by 7.5 mg/kg after 8 hours, then 7.5 mg/kg every 8 hours
- Child 2 months–17 years: 7.5 mg/kg every 8 hours (max. per dose 500 mg)

***Helicobacter pylori* eradication; in combination with clarithromycin and omeprazole**
- BY MOUTH
- Child 1–5 years: 100 mg twice daily
- Child 6–11 years: 200 mg twice daily
- Child 12–17 years: 400 mg twice daily

***Helicobacter pylori* eradication; in combination with amoxicillin and omeprazole**
- BY MOUTH
- Child 1–5 years: 100 mg 3 times a day
- Child 6–11 years: 200 mg 3 times a day
- Child 12–17 years: 400 mg 3 times a day

Fistulating Crohn's disease
- BY MOUTH
- Child: 7.5 mg/kg 3 times a day usually given for 1 month but should not be used for longer than 3 months because of concerns about peripheral neuropathy

Bacterial vaginosis
- BY VAGINA USING VAGINAL GEL
- Child: 1 applicatorful daily for 5 days, dose to be administered at night

DOSE EQUIVALENCE AND CONVERSION
- 1 applicatorful of vaginal gel delivers a 5 g dose of metronidazole 0.75%.

Pelvic inflammatory disease
- BY MOUTH
- Child 12–17 years: 400 mg twice daily for 14 days

Acute ulcerative gingivitis
- BY MOUTH
- Child 1–2 years: 50 mg every 8 hours for 3 days
- Child 3–6 years: 100 mg every 12 hours for 3 days
- Child 7–9 years: 100 mg every 8 hours for 3 days
- Child 10–17 years: 200–250 mg every 8 hours for 3 days

Acute oral infections
- BY MOUTH
- Child 1–2 years: 50 mg every 8 hours for 3–7 days
- Child 3–6 years: 100 mg every 12 hours for 3–7 days
- Child 7–9 years: 100 mg every 8 hours for 3–7 days
- Child 10–17 years: 200–250 mg every 8 hours for 3–7 days

Surgical prophylaxis
- BY MOUTH
- Child 1 month–11 years: 30 mg/kg (max. per dose 500 mg), to be administered 2 hours before surgery
- Child 12–17 years: 400–500 mg, to be administered 2 hours before surgery, then 400–500 mg every 8 hours if required for up to 3 doses (in high-risk procedures)
- BY RECTUM
- Child 5–9 years: 500 mg, to be administered 2 hours before surgery, then 500 mg every 8 hours if required for up to 3 doses (in high-risk procedures)
- Child 10–17 years: 1 g, to be administered 2 hours before surgery, then 1 g every 8 hours if required for up to 3 doses (in high-risk procedures)
- BY INTRAVENOUS INFUSION
- Neonate up to 40 weeks corrected gestational age: 10 mg/kg, to be administered up to 30 minutes before the procedure.
- Neonate 40 weeks corrected gestational age and above: 20–30 mg/kg, to be administered up to 30 minutes before the procedure.
- Child 1 month–11 years: 30 mg/kg (max. per dose 500 mg), to be administered up to 30 minutes before the procedure
- Child 12–17 years: 500 mg, to be administered up to 30 minutes before the procedure, then 500 mg every 8 hours if required for up to 3 further doses (in high-risk procedures)

Invasive intestinal amoebiasis | Extra-intestinal amoebiasis (including liver abscess)
- BY MOUTH
- Child 1–2 years: 200 mg 3 times a day for 5 days in intestinal infection (for 5–10 days in extra-intestinal infection)
- Child 3–6 years: 200 mg 4 times a day for 5 days in intestinal infection (for 5–10 days in extra-intestinal infection)
- Child 7–9 years: 400 mg 3 times a day for 5 days in intestinal infection (for 5–10 days in extra-intestinal infection)
- Child 10–17 years: 800 mg 3 times a day for 5 days in intestinal infection (for 5–10 days in extra-intestinal infection)

Urogenital trichomoniasis
- BY MOUTH
- Child 1–2 years: 50 mg 3 times a day for 7 days
- Child 3–6 years: 100 mg twice daily for 7 days
- Child 7–9 years: 100 mg 3 times a day for 7 days
- Child 10–17 years: 200 mg 3 times a day for 7 days, alternatively 400–500 mg twice daily for 5–7 days, alternatively 2 g for 1 dose

Giardiasis
- BY MOUTH
- Child 1–2 years: 500 mg once daily for 3 days
- Child 3–6 years: 600–800 mg once daily for 3 days
- Child 7–9 years: 1 g once daily for 3 days
- Child 10–17 years: 2 g once daily for 3 days, alternatively 400 mg 3 times a day for 5 days, alternatively 500 mg twice daily for 7–10 days

Established case of tetanus
- BY INTRAVENOUS INFUSION
- Child: (consult product literature)

- **UNLICENSED USE** EvGr Metronidazole is used for the treatment of cellulitis, Ⓐ but is not licensed for this indication.

  EvGr Metronidazole is used for the treatment of erysipelas, Ⓐ but is not licensed for this indication.
- With vaginal use Metronidazole vaginal gel not licensed for use in children under 18 years.

- **CAUTIONS**
- With vaginal use Avoid intravaginal preparations (particularly those that require the use of an applicator) in young girls who are not sexually active, unless there is no alternative • not recommended during menstruation • some systemic absorption may occur with vaginal gel

- **INTERACTIONS** → Appendix 1: metronidazole

5 Infection

● **SIDE-EFFECTS**
▸ **Common or very common**
▸ With systemic use Dry mouth · myalgia · nausea · oral disorders · taste altered · vomiting
▸ With vaginal use Pelvic discomfort · vulvovaginal candidiasis · vulvovaginal disorders
▸ **Uncommon**
▸ With systemic use Asthenia · headache · leucopenia (with long term or intensive therapy)
▸ With vaginal use Menstrual cycle irregularities · vaginal haemorrhage
▸ **Rare or very rare**
▸ With systemic use Agranulocytosis · angioedema · appetite decreased · ataxia · cerebellar syndrome · confusion · diarrhoea · dizziness · drowsiness · encephalopathy · epigastric pain · epileptiform seizure (with long term or intensive therapy) · flushing · hallucination · hepatic disorders · meningitis aseptic · mucositis · nerve disorders · neutropenia · pancreatitis · pancytopenia · peripheral neuropathy (with long term or intensive therapy) · psychotic disorder · seizure · severe cutaneous adverse reactions (SCARs) · skin reactions · thrombocytopenia · urine dark · vision disorders
▸ **Frequency not known**
▸ With systemic use Depressed mood · gastrointestinal disorder · hearing impairment · tinnitus

● **PREGNANCY**
▸ With systemic use Manufacturer advises avoidance of high-dose regimens; use only if potential benefit outweighs risk.

● **BREAST FEEDING**
▸ With systemic use Significant amount in milk; manufacturer advises avoid large single doses though otherwise compatible; may give milk a bitter taste.

● **HEPATIC IMPAIRMENT**
▸ With oral use or rectal use Manufacturer advises caution in hepatic encephalopathy (risk of decreased clearance).
▸ With intravenous use Manufacturer advises caution in severe impairment (risk of decreased clearance).
Dose adjustments ▸ With oral use or rectal use Manufacturer advises dose reduction to one-third of the daily dose in hepatic encephalopathy (dose may be given once daily).
▸ With intravenous use Manufacturer advises consider dose reduction in severe impairment.

● **MONITORING REQUIREMENTS**
▸ With systemic use Clinical and laboratory monitoring advised if treatment exceeds 10 days.

● **DIRECTIONS FOR ADMINISTRATION**
▸ With intravenous use For *intravenous infusion*, give over 20–30 minutes.

● **PRESCRIBING AND DISPENSING INFORMATION** For choice of antibacterial therapy, see Antibacterials, use for prophylaxis p. 319, Antiprotozoal drugs p. 418, Gastro-intestinal system infections, antibacterial therapy p. 324, Genital system infections, antibacterial therapy p. 325, Oropharyngeal infections, antibacterial therapy p. 761, Peptic ulceration p. 58, Skin infections, antibacterial therapy p. 329.
▸ With systemic use Metronidazole is well absorbed orally and the intravenous route is normally reserved for severe infections. Metronidazole by the rectal route is an effective alternative to the intravenous route when oral administration is not possible.

● **PATIENT AND CARER ADVICE**
Medicines for Children leaflet: Metronidazole for bacterial infections www.medicinesforchildren.org.uk/metronidazole-bacterial-infections

● **PROFESSION SPECIFIC INFORMATION**
Dental practitioners' formulary
▸ With oral use Metronidazole Tablets may be prescribed. Metronidazole Oral Suspension may be prescribed.

● **MEDICINAL FORMS** There can be variation in the licensing of different medicines containing the same drug. Forms available from special-order manufacturers include: oral suspension, oral solution, suppository

Tablet
CAUTIONARY AND ADVISORY LABELS 4, 9, 21, 25, 27
▸ **Metronidazole (Non-proprietary)**
Metronidazole 200 mg Metronidazole 200mg tablets | 21 tablet PoM £4.03 DT = £4.03
Metronidazole 400 mg Metronidazole 400mg tablets | 21 tablet PoM £5.75 DT = £3.75
Metronidazole 500 mg Metronidazole 500mg tablets | 21 tablet PoM £39.29 DT = £39.29
▸ **Flagyl** (Sanofi)
Metronidazole 200 mg Flagyl 200mg tablets | 21 tablet PoM £4.49 DT = £4.03
Metronidazole 400 mg Flagyl 400mg tablets | 14 tablet PoM £6.34

Suppository
CAUTIONARY AND ADVISORY LABELS 4, 9
▸ **Flagyl** (Sanofi)
Metronidazole 500 mg Flagyl 500mg suppositories | 10 suppository PoM £15.18 DT = £15.18
Metronidazole 1 gram Flagyl 1g suppositories | 10 suppository PoM £23.06 DT = £23.06

Oral suspension
CAUTIONARY AND ADVISORY LABELS 4, 9
▸ **Metronidazole (Non-proprietary)**
Metronidazole (as Metronidazole benzoate) 40 mg per 1 ml Metronidazole 200mg/5ml oral suspension | 100 ml PoM £37.29 DT = £37.29

Vaginal gel
EXCIPIENTS: May contain Disodium edetate, hydroxybenzoates (parabens), propylene glycol
▸ **Zidoval** (Mylan)
Metronidazole 7.5 mg per 1 gram Zidoval 0.75% vaginal gel | 40 gram PoM £4.31 DT = £4.31

Infusion
ELECTROLYTES: May contain Sodium
▸ **Metronidazole (Non-proprietary)**
Metronidazole 5 mg per 1 ml Metronidazole 500mg/100ml infusion 100ml bags | 20 bag PoM £67.05 DT = £67.05

Tinidazole

● **DRUG ACTION** Tinidazole is an antimicrobial drug with high activity against anaerobic bacteria and protozoa; it has a longer duration of action than metronidazole.

● **INDICATIONS AND DOSE**

Intestinal amoebiasis
▸ BY MOUTH
▸ Child 1 month–11 years: 50–60 mg/kg once daily (max. per dose 2 g) for 3 days
▸ Child 12–17 years: 2 g once daily for 2–3 days

Amoebic involvement of liver
▸ BY MOUTH
▸ Child 1 month–11 years: 50–60 mg/kg once daily (max. per dose 2 g) for 5 days
▸ Child 12–17 years: 1.5–2 g once daily for 3–6 days

Urogenital trichomoniasis | Giardiasis
▸ BY MOUTH
▸ Child 1 month–11 years: 50–75 mg/kg (max. per dose 2 g) for 1 single dose, dose may be repeated once if necessary
▸ Child 12–17 years: 2 g for 1 single dose, dose may be repeated once if necessary

● **INTERACTIONS** → Appendix 1: tinidazole

● **SIDE-EFFECTS**
▸ **Common or very common** Abdominal pain · appetite decreased · diarrhoea · headache · nausea · skin reactions · vertigo · vomiting
▸ **Frequency not known** Angioedema · ataxia · dizziness · fatigue · flushing · leucopenia · oral disorders · peripheral

neuropathy · seizure · sensation abnormal · taste altered · tongue discolouration · urine discolouration

- **PREGNANCY** Manufacturer advises avoid in first trimester.
- **BREAST FEEDING** Present in milk—manufacturer advises avoid breast-feeding during and for 3 days after stopping treatment.
- **MONITORING REQUIREMENTS** Clinical and laboratory monitoring advised if treatment exceeds 10 days.

- **MEDICINAL FORMS** There can be variation in the licensing of different medicines containing the same drug.

Tablet

CAUTIONARY AND ADVISORY LABELS 4, 9, 21, 25

▸ Fasigyn (Pfizer Ltd)

Tinidazole 500 mg Fasigyn 500mg tablets | 16 tablet [PoM] £11.04 DT = £11.04

ANTIBACTERIALS > PENICILLINS

Penicillins

Benzylpenicillin and phenoxymethylpenicillin

Benzylpenicillin sodium p. 364 (Penicillin G) remains an important and useful antibiotic but is inactivated by bacterial beta-lactamases. It is effective for many streptococcal (including pneumococcal), gonococcal, and meningococcal infections and also for anthrax, diphtheria, gas-gangrene, and leptospirosis. It is also used in combination with gentamicin p. 333 for the empirical treatment of sepsis in neonates less than 48 hours old. Pneumococci, meningococci, and gonococci which have decreased sensitivity to penicillin have been isolated; benzylpenicillin sodium **is no longer the drug of first choice for pneumococcal meningitis**. Although benzylpenicillin sodium is effective in the treatment of tetanus, metronidazole p. 358 is preferred. Benzylpenicillin sodium is inactivated by gastric acid and absorption from the gastro-intestinal tract is low; therefore it must be given by injection.

Benzathine benzylpenicillin p. 363 or **procaine benzylpenicillin** are used in the treatment of syphilis.

Phenoxymethylpenicillin p. 365 (Penicillin V) has a similar antibacterial spectrum to benzylpenicillin sodium, but is less active. It is gastric acid-stable, so is suitable for oral administration. It should not be used for serious infections because absorption can be unpredictable and plasma concentrations variable. It is indicated principally for respiratory-tract infections in children, for streptococcal tonsillitis, and for continuing treatment after one or more injections of benzylpenicillin sodium when clinical response has begun. It should not be used for meningococcal or gonococcal infections. Phenoxymethylpenicillin is used for prophylaxis against streptococcal infections following rheumatic fever and against pneumococcal infections following splenectomy or in sickle cell disease.

Penicillinase-resistant penicillins

Most staphylococci are now resistant to benzylpenicillin sodium because they produce penicillinases. Flucloxacillin p. 373, however, is not inactivated by these enzymes and is thus effective in infections caused by penicillin-resistant staphylococci, which is the main indication for its use. Flucloxacillin is acid-stable and can, therefore, be given by mouth as well as by injection. Flucloxacillin is well absorbed from the gut.

Broad-spectrum penicillins

Ampicillin p. 368 is active against certain Gram-positive and Gram-negative organisms but is inactivated by penicillinases including those produced by *Staphylococcus aureus* and by common Gram-negative bacilli such as *Escherichia coli*. Ampicillin is also active against *Listeria* spp. and enterococci. Almost all staphylococci, approx. 60% of *E. coli* strains and approx. 20% of *Haemophilus influenzae* strains are now resistant. The likelihood of resistance should therefore be considered before using ampicillin for the 'blind' treatment of infections; in particular, it should not be used for hospital patients without checking sensitivity.

Ampicillin can be given by mouth, but less than half the dose is absorbed and absorption is further decreased by the presence of food in the gut. Ampicillin is well excreted in the bile and urine.

Amoxicillin p. 366 is a derivative of ampicillin and has a similar antibacterial spectrum. It is better absorbed than ampicillin when given by mouth, producing higher plasma and tissue concentrations; unlike ampicillin, absorption is not affected by the presence of food in the stomach.

Amoxicillin or ampicillin are principally indicated for the treatment of community-acquired pneumonia and middle ear infections, both of which may be due to *Streptococcus pneumoniae* and *H. influenzae*, and for urinary-tract infections. They are also used in the treatment of endocarditis and listerial meningitis. Amoxicillin is also used for the treatment of Lyme disease.

Maculopapular rashes occur commonly with ampicillin (and amoxicillin) but are not usually related to true penicillin allergy. They often occur in children with glandular fever; broad-spectrum penicillins should not therefore be used for 'blind' treatment of a sore throat. The risk of rash is also increased in children with acute or chronic lymphocytic leukaemia or in cytomegalovirus infection.

Co-amoxiclav p. 370 consists of amoxicillin with the beta-lactamase inhibitor clavulanic acid. Clavulanic acid itself has no significant antibacterial activity but, by inactivating beta-lactamases, it makes the combination active against beta-lactamase-producing bacteria that are resistant to amoxicillin. These include resistant strains of *Staph. aureus*, *E. coli*, and *H. influenzae*, as well as many *Bacteroides* and *Klebsiella* spp. Co-amoxiclav should be reserved for infections likely, or known, to be caused by amoxicillin-resistant beta-lactamase-producing strains.

A combination of ampicillin with flucloxacillin (as co-fluampicil p. 369) is available to treat infections involving either streptococci or staphylococci.

Antipseudomonal penicillins

Piperacillin, a ureidopenicillin, is only available in combination with the beta-lactamase inhibitor tazobactam. **Ticarcillin**, a carboxypenicillin, is only available in combination with the beta-lactamase inhibitor clavulanic acid. Both preparations have a broad spectrum of activity against a range of Gram-positive and Gram-negative bacteria, and anaerobes. Piperacillin with tazobactam p. 362 has activity against a wider range of Gram-negative organisms than ticarcillin with clavulanic acid p. 363 and it is more active against *Pseudomonas aeruginosa*. These antibacterials are not active against MRSA. They are used in the treatment of septicaemia, hospital-acquired pneumonia, and complicated infections involving the urinary-tract, skin and soft tissue, or intra-abdomen. They may be used for the empirical treatment of septicaemia in immunocompromised children but otherwise should generally be reserved for serious infections resistant to other antibacterials. For severe pseudomonas infections these antipseudomonal penicillins can be given with an aminoglycoside (e.g. gentamicin) since they have a synergistic effect.

Piperacillin with tazobactam is used in cystic fibrosis for the treatment of *Ps. aeruginosa* colonisation when ciprofloxacin p. 377 and nebulised colistimethate sodium p. 375 have been ineffective; it can also be used in infective exacerbations, when it is combined with an aminoglycoside.

Mecillinams

Pivmecillinam hydrochloride p. 373 has significant activity against many Gram-negative bacteria including *Escherichia coli*, klebsiella, enterobacter, and salmonellae. It is not active against *Pseudomonas aeruginosa* or enterococci. Pivmecillinam hydrochloride is hydrolysed to mecillinam, which is the active drug.

Penicillins

- DRUG ACTION The penicillins are bactericidal and act by interfering with bacterial cell wall synthesis. They diffuse well into body tissues and fluids, but penetration into the cerebrospinal fluid is poor except when the meninges are inflamed. They are excreted in the urine in therapeutic concentrations.
- CAUTIONS History of allergy
- SIDE-EFFECTS
  - **Common or very common** Diarrhoea · hypersensitivity · nausea · skin reactions · thrombocytopenia · vomiting
  - **Uncommon** Antibiotic associated colitis · leucopenia
  - **Rare or very rare** Agranulocytosis · angioedema · haemolytic anaemia · hepatic disorders · nephritis tubulointerstitial · seizure · severe cutaneous adverse reactions (SCARs)

  SIDE-EFFECTS, FURTHER INFORMATION Diarrhoea frequently occurs during oral penicillin therapy. It is most common with broad-spectrum penicillins, which can cause antibiotic-associated colitis.
- ALLERGY AND CROSS-SENSITIVITY The most important side-effect of the penicillins is hypersensitivity which causes rashes and anaphylaxis and can be fatal. Allergic reactions to penicillins occur in 1–10% of exposed individuals; anaphylactic reactions occur in fewer than 0.05% of treated patients. Patients with a history of atopic allergy (e.g. asthma, eczema, hay fever) are at a higher risk of anaphylactic reactions to penicillins. Individuals with a history of anaphylaxis, urticaria, or rash immediately after penicillin administration are at risk of immediate hypersensitivity to a penicillin; these individuals should not receive a penicillin. Individuals with a history of a minor rash (i.e. non-confluent, non-pruritic rash restricted to a small area of the body) or a rash that occurs more than 72 hours after penicillin administration are probably not allergic to penicillin and in these individuals a penicillin should not be withheld unnecessarily for serious infections; the possibility of an allergic reaction should, however, be borne in mind. Other beta-lactam antibiotics (including cephalosporins) can be used in these patients.

  Patients who are allergic to one penicillin will be allergic to all because the hypersensitivity is related to the basic penicillin structure. Patients with a history of immediate hypersensitivity to penicillins may also react to the cephalosporins and other beta-lactam antibiotics, they should not receive these antibiotics. If a penicillin (or another beta-lactam antibiotic) is essential in an individual with immediate hypersensitivity to penicillin then specialist advice should be sought on hypersensitivity testing or using a beta-lactam antibiotic with a different structure to the penicillin that caused the hypersensitivity.

ANTIBACTERIALS › PENICILLINS, ANTIPSEUDOMONAL WITH BETA-LACTAMASE INHIBITOR

above

Piperacillin with tazobactam

22-May-2020

- INDICATIONS AND DOSE

Hospital-acquired pneumonia | Septicaemia | Complicated infections involving the urinary-tract | Complicated infections involving the skin | Complicated infections involving the soft-tissues

▶ BY INTRAVENOUS INFUSION
- Neonate: 90 mg/kg every 8 hours.
- Child 1 month–11 years: 90 mg/kg every 6–8 hours (max. per dose 4.5 g every 6 hours)
- Child 12–17 years: 4.5 g every 8 hours; increased if necessary to 4.5 g every 6 hours, increased frequency may be used for severe infections

Complicated intra-abdominal infections

▶ BY INTRAVENOUS INFUSION
- Child 2–11 years: 112.5 mg/kg every 8 hours (max. per dose 4.5 g)
- Child 12–17 years: 4.5 g every 8 hours; increased if necessary to 4.5 g every 6 hours, increased frequency may be used for severe infections

Acute exacerbation of bronchiectasis

▶ BY INTRAVENOUS INFUSION
- Child 1 month–11 years: 90 mg/kg every 6–8 hours (max. per dose 4.5 g every 6 hours)
- Child 12–17 years: 4.5 g every 8 hours; increased if necessary to 4.5 g every 6 hours, increased frequency may be used for severe infections

Infections in neutropenic patients

▶ BY INTRAVENOUS INFUSION
- Child: 90 mg/kg every 6 hours (max. per dose 4.5 g)

- UNLICENSED USE Not licensed for use in children under 12 years (except for children 2–12 years with neutropenia and complicated intra-abdominal infections).

  EvGr Piperacillin with tazobactam is used for the treatment of acute exacerbation of bronchiectasis, (A) but is not licensed for this indication.
- CAUTIONS High doses may lead to hypernatraemia (owing to sodium content of preparations)
- INTERACTIONS → Appendix 1: penicillins
- SIDE-EFFECTS
  - **Common or very common** Anaemia · candida infection · constipation · gastrointestinal discomfort · headache · insomnia
  - **Uncommon** Arthralgia · flushing · hypokalaemia · hypotension · myalgia · thrombophlebitis
  - **Rare or very rare** Epistaxis · stomatitis
  - **Frequency not known** Eosinophilia · neutropenia · pancytopenia · pneumonia eosinophilic · renal failure · thrombocytosis
- PREGNANCY Manufacturers advise use only if potential benefit outweighs risk.
- BREAST FEEDING Trace amount in milk, but appropriate to use.
- RENAL IMPAIRMENT

  Dose adjustments *Child under 12 years* 78.75 mg/kg (max. 4.5 g) every 8 hours if estimated glomerular filtration rate less than 50 mL/minute/1.73 m^2.

  Child 12–18 years max. 4.5 g every 8 hours if estimated glomerular filtration rate 20–40 mL/minute/1.73 m^2; max. 4.5 g every 12 hours if estimated glomerular filtration rate less than 20 mL/minute/1.73 m^2.

- **EFFECT ON LABORATORY TESTS** False-positive urinary glucose (if tested for reducing substances).
- **DIRECTIONS FOR ADMINISTRATION** Displacement value may be significant when reconstituting injection, consult local guidelines. For *intravenous infusion*, dilute reconstituted solution to a concentration of 15–90 mg/mL with Glucose 5% *or* Sodium Chloride 0.9%; give over 30 minutes.
- **PRESCRIBING AND DISPENSING INFORMATION** Dose expressed as a combination of piperacillin and tazobactam (both as sodium salts) in a ratio of 8:1.

  For choice of antibacterial therapy, see Blood infections, antibacterial therapy p. 322, Gastro-intestinal system infections, antibacterial therapy p. 324, Respiratory system infections, antibacterial therapy p. 327, Skin infections, antibacterial therapy p. 329, Urinary-tract infections p. 400.

- **MEDICINAL FORMS** There can be variation in the licensing of different medicines containing the same drug. Forms available from special-order manufacturers include: infusion, powder for solution for infusion

Powder for solution for infusion

ELECTROLYTES: May contain Sodium

- Piperacillin with tazobactam (Non-proprietary)
  Tazobactam (as Tazobactam sodium) 250 mg, Piperacillin (as Piperacillin sodium) 2 gram Piperacillin 2g / Tazobactam 250mg powder for solution for infusion vials | 1 vial PoM £9.55 DT = £7.65 (Hospital only) | 10 vial PoM £86.40 (Hospital only)
  Tazobactam (as Tazobactam sodium) 500 mg, Piperacillin (as Piperacillin sodium) 4 gram Piperacillin 4g / Tazobactam 500mg powder for solution for infusion vials | 1 vial PoM £15.75–£19.97 (Hospital only) | 1 vial PoM £12.90 | 10 vial PoM £48.00–£76.50 | 10 vial PoM £99.00 (Hospital only)
- Tazocin (Pfizer Ltd)
  Tazobactam (as Tazobactam sodium) 250 mg, Piperacillin (as Piperacillin sodium) 2 gram Tazocin 2g/0.25g powder for solution for infusion vials | 1 vial PoM £7.65 DT = £7.65
  Tazobactam (as Tazobactam sodium) 500 mg, Piperacillin (as Piperacillin sodium) 4 gram Tazocin 4g/0.5g powder for solution for infusion vials | 1 vial PoM £15.17

362

Ticarcillin with clavulanic acid

22-May-2020

- **INDICATIONS AND DOSE**

Infections due to *Pseudomonas* and *Proteus* spp.

▶ BY INTRAVENOUS INFUSION

- Preterm neonate (body-weight up to 2 kg): 80 mg/kg every 12 hours.
- Preterm neonate (body-weight 2 kg and above): 80 mg/kg every 8 hours; increased if necessary to 80 mg/kg every 6 hours, increased frequency used for more severe infections.
- Neonate: 80 mg/kg every 8 hours; increased if necessary to 80 mg/kg every 6 hours, increased frequency used for more severe infections.
- Child (body-weight up to 40 kg): 80 mg/kg every 8 hours; increased if necessary to 80 mg/kg every 6 hours, increased frequency used for more severe infections
- Child (body-weight 40 kg and above): 3.2 g every 6–8 hours; increased if necessary to 3.2 g every 4 hours, increased frequency used for more severe infections

- **CAUTIONS** High doses may lead to hypernatraemia (owing to sodium content of preparations)
- **INTERACTIONS** → Appendix 1: clavulanate · penicillins
- **SIDE-EFFECTS** Eosinophilia · haemorrhage · hypokalaemia · thrombophlebitis
- **PREGNANCY** Not known to be harmful.
- **BREAST FEEDING** Trace amounts in milk, but appropriate to use.
- **HEPATIC IMPAIRMENT** Manufacturer advises caution in severe impairment.
- **RENAL IMPAIRMENT** Accumulation of electrolytes contained in preparation can occur in patients with renal failure.

  Dose adjustments In neonates, reduce dose if estimated glomerular filtration rate less than 60 mL/minute/1.73 m^2.

  In children aged 1 month–17 years, use normal dose every 8 hours if estimated glomerular filtration rate 30–60 mL/minute/1.73 m^2; use half normal dose every 8 hours if estimated glomerular filtration rate 10–30 mL/minute/1.73 m^2; use half normal dose every 12 hours if estimated glomerular filtration rate less than 10 mL/minute/1.73 m^2.
- **EFFECT ON LABORATORY TESTS** False-positive urinary glucose (if tested for reducing substances).
- **DIRECTIONS FOR ADMINISTRATION** Displacement value may be important, consult local guidelines. For intermittent infusion, dilute reconstituted solution further to a concentration of 16–32 mg/mL with glucose 5%; infuse over 30–40 minutes.
- **PRESCRIBING AND DISPENSING INFORMATION** Dose is expressed as a combination of ticarcillin (as sodium salt) and clavulanic acid (as potassium salt) in a ratio of 15:1.

- **MEDICINAL FORMS** There can be variation in the licensing of different medicines containing the same drug.

Powder for solution for infusion

ELECTROLYTES: May contain Potassium, sodium

- Timentin (GlaxoSmithKline UK Ltd)
  Clavulanic acid (as Potassium clavulanate) 200 mg, Ticarcillin (as Ticarcillin sodium) 3 gram Timentin 3.2g powder for solution for infusion vials | 4 vial PoM £21.32

ANTIBACTERIALS > PENICILLINS, BETA-LACTAMASE SENSITIVE

362

Benzathine benzylpenicillin

24-Apr-2020

(Benzathine penicillin G)

- **INDICATIONS AND DOSE**

Erysipelas | Yaws | Pinta

▶ BY DEEP INTRAMUSCULAR INJECTION

- Child (body-weight up to 30 kg): 0.6 million units as a single dose, mid-lateral thigh muscle is the preferred site of injection
- Child (body-weight 30 kg and above): 1.2 million units as a single dose, mid-lateral thigh muscle is the preferred site of injection

Syphilis [primary and secondary stage]

▶ BY DEEP INTRAMUSCULAR INJECTION

- Child 1 month–11 years: 50 000 units/kg (max. per dose 2.4 million units) as a single dose, mid-lateral thigh muscle is the preferred site of injection, if clinical symptoms recur or laboratory findings remain strongly positive—repeat treatment
- Child 12–17 years: 2.4 million units as a single dose, outer quadrant of the gluteus maximus or Hochstetter's ventrogluteal field is the preferred site of injection, if clinical symptoms recur or laboratory findings remain strongly positive—repeat treatment

Syphilis [late-stage (latent seropositive)]

▶ BY DEEP INTRAMUSCULAR INJECTION

- Child 1 month–11 years: 50 000 units/kg once weekly (max. per dose 2.4 million units) for 3 weeks, mid-lateral thigh muscle is the preferred site of injection
- Child 12–17 years: 2.4 million units once weekly for 3 weeks, outer quadrant of the gluteus

continued →

maximus or Hochstetter's ventrogluteal field is the preferred site of injection

Congenital syphilis [without neurological involvement]

▶ BY DEEP INTRAMUSCULAR INJECTION

▸ Neonate: 50 000 units/kg as a single dose, mid-lateral thigh muscle is the preferred site of injection.

▸ Child 1–24 months: 50 000 units/kg as a single dose, mid-lateral thigh muscle is the preferred site of injection

Prophylaxis of rheumatic fever [without cardiac involvement] | Prophylaxis of poststreptococcal glomerulonephritis [without cardiac involvement] | Prophylaxis of erysipelas [without cardiac involvement]

▶ BY DEEP INTRAMUSCULAR INJECTION

▸ Child (body-weight up to 30 kg): 0.6 million units every 3–4 weeks for at least 5 years or up to 21 years of age (whichever is longer), mid-lateral thigh muscle is the preferred site of injection in children

▸ Child (body-weight 30 kg and above): 1.2 million units every 3–4 weeks for at least 5 years or up to 21 years of age (whichever is longer), mid-lateral thigh muscle is the preferred site of injection in children

Prophylaxis of rheumatic fever [transient cardiac involvement] | Prophylaxis of poststreptococcal glomerulonephritis [transient cardiac involvement] | Prophylaxis of erysipelas [transient cardiac involvement]

▶ BY DEEP INTRAMUSCULAR INJECTION

▸ Child (body-weight up to 30 kg): 0.6 million units every 3–4 weeks for at least 10 years or up to 21 years of age (whichever is longer), mid-lateral thigh muscle is the preferred site of injection in children

▸ Child (body-weight 30 kg and above): 1.2 million units every 3–4 weeks for at least 10 years or up to 21 years of age (whichever is longer), mid-lateral thigh muscle is the preferred site of injection in children

Prophylaxis of rheumatic fever [persistent cardiac involvement] | Prophylaxis of poststreptococcal glomerulonephritis [persistent cardiac involvement] | Prophylaxis of erysipelas [persistent cardiac involvement]

▶ BY DEEP INTRAMUSCULAR INJECTION

▸ Child (body-weight up to 30 kg): 0.6 million units every 3–4 weeks for at least 10 years or up to 40 years of age (whichever is longer); life-long prophylaxis may be necessary, mid-lateral thigh muscle is the preferred site of injection in children

▸ Child (body-weight 30 kg and above): 1.2 million units every 3–4 weeks for at least 10 years or up to 40 years of age (whichever is longer); life-long prophylaxis may be necessary, mid-lateral thigh muscle is the preferred site of injection in children

● **INTERACTIONS** → Appendix 1: penicillins

● **SIDE-EFFECTS**

▶ **Common or very common** Increased risk of infection

▶ **Uncommon** Oral disorders

▶ **Rare or very rare** Arthralgia · nephropathy

▶ **Frequency not known** Encephalopathy · Hoigne's syndrome · Jarisch-Herxheimer reaction · local reaction (in infants)

● **ALLERGY AND CROSS-SENSITIVITY** Contra-indicated in patients allergic to peanuts or soya (contains phospholipids from soya lecithin).

● **PREGNANCY** Manufacturer advises not known to be harmful.

● **BREAST FEEDING** Manufacturer advises present in milk in small amounts but not known to be harmful. Monitor infant for effects on the gastrointestinal flora; discontinue breast feeding if diarrhoea, candidiasis or rash in the infant occur.

● **HEPATIC IMPAIRMENT** Manufacturer advises caution in impairment (possible risk of delayed metabolism and excretion in severe impairment).

● **RENAL IMPAIRMENT** Manufacturer advises caution in impairment (possible risk of delayed metabolism and excretion in severe impairment).

Dose adjustments Manufacturer advises reduce daily dose by 25% and give as a single dose if creatinine clearance 15–59 mL/minute; reduce daily dose by 50–80% and give in 2–3 divided doses if creatinine clearance less than 15 mL/minute (maximum 1–3 million units per day).

● **MONITORING REQUIREMENTS**

▶ Manufacturer advises observe the patient for hypersensitivity reactions for at least 30 minutes after the injection.

▶ Manufacturer advises monitor renal, hepatic and haematopoietic function periodically in patients on long-term treatment.

● **EFFECT ON LABORATORY TESTS** False-positive direct Coombs' test. False-positive urinary glucose. False-positive urobilinogen. False-positive urinary protein using precipitation techniques, the Folin-Ciocalteu-Lowry method, or the biuret method. False-positive urinary amino acids using the ninhydrin method. Increased levels of urinary 17-ketosteriods using the Zimmermann reaction.

● **DIRECTIONS FOR ADMINISTRATION** For *deep intramuscular injection*, manufacturer advises reconstitute with water for injection and inject slowly with low pressure. No more than 5 mL should be administered per injection site and do not administer into tissues with reduced perfusion. Avoid rubbing the injection site after the injection.

● **MEDICINAL FORMS** There can be variation in the licensing of different medicines containing the same drug.

Powder and solvent for suspension for injection

EXCIPIENTS: May contain Lecithin, polysorbates

▸ **Benzathine benzylpenicillin (Non-proprietary)**

Benzathine benzylpenicillin 1.2 mega unit Benzathine benzylpenicillin 1.2million unit powder and solvent for suspension for injection vials | 1 vial PoM £9.50

Benzathine benzylpenicillin 2.4 mega unit Benzathine benzylpenicillin 2.4million unit powder and solvent for suspension for injection vials | 1 vial PoM £9.50

▸ **Extencilline (Imported (France))**

Benzathine benzylpenicillin 600000 unit Extencilline 600,000units powder and solvent for suspension for injection vials | 50 vial PoM

362

Benzylpenicillin sodium

21-May-2020

(Penicillin G)

● **INDICATIONS AND DOSE**

Mild to moderate susceptible infections | Throat infections | Otitis media | Pneumonia | Cellulitis

▶ BY INTRAMUSCULAR INJECTION, OR BY SLOW INTRAVENOUS INJECTION, OR BY INTRAVENOUS INFUSION

▸ Neonate up to 7 days: 25 mg/kg every 12 hours; increased if necessary to 25 mg/kg every 8 hours, intravenous route recommended in neonates.

▸ Neonate 7 days to 28 days: 25 mg/kg every 8 hours; increased if necessary to 50 mg/kg every 8 hours in severe infection, intravenous route recommended in neonates.

▸ Child: 25 mg/kg every 6 hours; increased if necessary to 50 mg/kg every 4–6 hours (max. per dose 2.4 g every 4 hours) in severe infection, intravenous route recommended in infants

Endocarditis (in combination with other antibacterial if necessary)

▶ BY SLOW INTRAVENOUS INJECTION, OR BY INTRAVENOUS INFUSION

▸ Child: 25 mg/kg every 4 hours; increased if necessary to 50 mg/kg every 4 hours (max. per dose 2.4 g every 4 hours)

Meningitis | Meningococcal disease

▶ BY INTRAVENOUS INFUSION

▸ Neonate up to 7 days: 50 mg/kg every 12 hours.

▸ Neonate 7 days to 28 days: 50 mg/kg every 8 hours.

▸ Child: 50 mg/kg every 4–6 hours (max. per dose 2.4 g every 4 hours)

Suspected meningococcal disease (meningitis with non-blanching rash or meningococcal septicaemia) prior to urgent transfer to hospital

▶ BY INTRAVENOUS INJECTION, OR BY INTRAMUSCULAR INJECTION

▸ Child 1-11 months: 300 mg, administer as single dose prior to urgent transfer to hospital so long as does not delay transfer
▸ Child 1-9 years: 600 mg, administer as single dose prior to urgent transfer to hospital so long as does not delay transfer
▸ Child 10-17 years: 1.2 g, administer as single dose prior to urgent transfer to hospital so long as does not delay transfer

Suspected bacterial meningitis without non-blanching rash where patient cannot be transferred to hospital urgently

▶ BY INTRAVENOUS INJECTION, OR BY INTRAMUSCULAR INJECTION

▸ Child 1-11 months: 300 mg, administer as single dose prior to transfer to hospital
▸ Child 1-9 years: 600 mg, administer as single dose prior to transfer to hospital
▸ Child 10-17 years: 1.2 g, administer as single dose prior to transfer to hospital

Neonatal sepsis

▶ BY INTRAMUSCULAR INJECTION, OR BY SLOW INTRAVENOUS INJECTION, OR BY INTRAVENOUS INFUSION

▸ Neonate up to 7 days: 25 mg/kg every 12 hours; increased if necessary to 25 mg/kg every 8 hours, intravenous route recommended in neonates.

▸ Neonate 7 days to 28 days: 25 mg/kg every 8 hours; increased if necessary to 50 mg/kg every 8 hours in severe infection, intravenous route recommended in neonates.

> IMPORTANT SAFETY INFORMATION
> Intrathecal injection of benzylpenicillin is **not** recommended.

- CAUTIONS Accumulation of sodium from injection can occur with high doses
- INTERACTIONS → Appendix 1: penicillins
- SIDE-EFFECTS

▸ **Common or very common** Fever · Jarisch-Herxheimer reaction
▸ **Rare or very rare** Neurotoxicity · neutropenia
▸ **Frequency not known** Coma

- PREGNANCY Not known to be harmful.
- BREAST FEEDING Trace amounts in milk, but appropriate to use.
- RENAL IMPAIRMENT Accumulation of sodium from injection can occur in renal failure. High doses may cause neurotoxicity, including cerebral irritation, convulsions, or coma.

Dose adjustments Estimated glomerular filtration rate 10–50 mL/minute/1.73 m^2, use normal dose every 8–12 hours.

Estimated glomerular filtration rate less than 10 mL/minute/1.73 m^2 use normal dose every 12 hours.

- EFFECT ON LABORATORY TESTS False-positive urinary glucose (if tested for reducing substances).
- DIRECTIONS FOR ADMINISTRATION

▸ With intravenous use Intravenous route recommended in neonates and infants. For *intravenous infusion*, dilute with Glucose 5% *or* Sodium Chloride 0.9%; give over 15–30 minutes. Longer administration time is particularly important when using doses of 50 mg/kg (or greater) to avoid CNS toxicity.

- PRESCRIBING AND DISPENSING INFORMATION For choice of antibacterial therapy, see Blood infections, antibacterial therapy p. 322, Cardiovascular system infections, antibacterial therapy p. 322, Central nervous system infections, antibacterial therapy p. 323, Ear infections, antibacterial therapy p. 324, Oropharyngeal infections, antibacterial therapy p. 761, Respiratory system infections, antibacterial therapy p. 327, Skin infections, antibacterial therapy p. 329.

- MEDICINAL FORMS There can be variation in the licensing of different medicines containing the same drug. Forms available from special-order manufacturers include: infusion

Powder for solution for injection

ELECTROLYTES: May contain Sodium

▸ **Benzylpenicillin sodium (Non-proprietary)**
Benzylpenicillin sodium 600 mg Benzylpenicillin 600mg powder for solution for injection vials | 2 vial PoM £6.01-£6.02 DT = £6.02 | 25 vial PoM £75.12-£75.25
Benzylpenicillin sodium 1.2 gram Benzylpenicillin 1.2g powder for solution for injection vials | 25 vial PoM £109.49-£109.51 DT = £109.51

F 362

Phenoxymethylpenicillin (Penicillin V)

18-May-2020

- **INDICATIONS AND DOSE**

Oral infections | Otitis media

▶ BY MOUTH

▸ Child 1-11 months: 62.5 mg 4 times a day; increased if necessary up to 12.5 mg/kg 4 times a day
▸ Child 1-5 years: 125 mg 4 times a day; increased if necessary up to 12.5 mg/kg 4 times a day
▸ Child 6-11 years: 250 mg 4 times a day; increased if necessary up to 12.5 mg/kg 4 times a day
▸ Child 12-17 years: 500 mg 4 times a day; increased if necessary up to 1 g 4 times a day

Acute sore throat

▶ BY MOUTH

▸ Child 1-11 months: 62.5 mg 4 times a day, alternatively 125 mg twice daily for 5–10 days
▸ Child 1-5 years: 125 mg 4 times a day, alternatively 250 mg twice daily for 5–10 days
▸ Child 6-11 years: 250 mg 4 times a day, alternatively 500 mg twice daily for 5–10 days
▸ Child 12-17 years: 500 mg 4 times a day, alternatively 1000 mg twice daily for 5–10 days

Prevention of recurrence of rheumatic fever

▶ BY MOUTH

▸ Child 1 month-5 years: 125 mg twice daily
▸ Child 6-17 years: 250 mg twice daily

continued →

Prevention of secondary case of invasive group A streptococcal infection

▶ BY MOUTH

- Neonate: 12.5 mg/kg every 6 hours (max. per dose 62.5 mg) for 10 days.

- Child 1–11 months: 62.5 mg every 6 hours for 10 days
- Child 1–5 years: 125 mg every 6 hours for 10 days
- Child 6–11 years: 250 mg every 6 hours for 10 days
- Child 12–17 years: 250–500 mg every 6 hours for 10 days

Prevention of pneumococcal infection in asplenia or in patients with sickle-cell disease

▶ BY MOUTH

- Child 1–11 months: 62.5 mg twice daily
- Child 1–4 years: 125 mg twice daily
- Child 5–17 years: 250 mg twice daily

Acute sinusitis

▶ BY MOUTH

- Child 1–11 months: 62.5 mg 4 times a day for 5 days
- Child 1–5 years: 125 mg 4 times a day for 5 days
- Child 6–11 years: 250 mg 4 times a day for 5 days
- Child 12–17 years: 500 mg 4 times a day for 5 days

- **UNLICENSED USE** EvGr Duration of treatment for acute sinusitis adheres to national guidelines. (A) See Sinusitis (acute) p. 750 for further information.

  Phenoxymethylpenicillin doses in the BNF may differ from product literature.
- **INTERACTIONS** → Appendix 1: penicillins
- **SIDE-EFFECTS** Arthralgia · circulatory collapse · coagulation disorder · eosinophilia · faeces soft · fever · increased risk of infection · neurotoxicity · neutropenia · oral disorders · paraesthesia
- **PREGNANCY** Not known to be harmful.
- **BREAST FEEDING** Trace amounts in milk, but appropriate to use.
- **EFFECT ON LABORATORY TESTS** False-positive urinary glucose (if tested for reducing substances).
- **PRESCRIBING AND DISPENSING INFORMATION** For choice of antibacterial therapy, see Antibacterials, use for prophylaxis p. 319, Ear infections, antibacterial therapy p. 324, Nose infections, antibacterial therapy p. 326, Oral bacterial infections p. 326, Oropharyngeal infections, antibacterial therapy p. 761.
- **PATIENT AND CARER ADVICE**

  Medicines for Children leaflet: Penicillin V for bacterial infections www.medicinesforchildren.org.uk/penicillin-v-bacterial-infections

  Medicines for Children leaflet: Penicillin V for prevention of pneumococcal infection www.medicinesforchildren.org.uk/penicillin-v-prevention-pneumococcal-infection
- **PROFESSION SPECIFIC INFORMATION**

  Dental practitioners' formulary

  Phenoxymethylpenicillin Tablets may be prescribed. Phenoxymethylpenicillin Oral Solution may be prescribed.

- **MEDICINAL FORMS** There can be variation in the licensing of different medicines containing the same drug.

Oral solution

CAUTIONARY AND ADVISORY LABELS 9, 23

- Phenoxymethylpenicillin (Non-proprietary)

  Phenoxymethylpenicillin (as Phenoxymethylpenicillin potassium) 25 mg per 1 ml Phenoxymethylpenicillin 125mg/5ml oral solution | 100 ml PoM £34.00 DT = £2.53

  Phenoxymethylpenicillin 125mg/5ml oral solution sugar free sugar-free | 100 ml PoM £25.00 DT = £7.10

  Phenoxymethylpenicillin (as Phenoxymethylpenicillin potassium) 50 mg per 1 ml Phenoxymethylpenicillin 250mg/5ml oral solution | 100 ml PoM £35.00 DT = £5.81

  Phenoxymethylpenicillin 250mg/5ml oral solution sugar free sugar-free | 100 ml PoM £35.00 DT = £7.47

Tablet

CAUTIONARY AND ADVISORY LABELS 9, 23

- Phenoxymethylpenicillin (Non-proprietary)

  Phenoxymethylpenicillin (as Phenoxymethylpenicillin potassium) 250 mg Phenoxymethylpenicillin 250mg tablets | 28 tablet PoM £5.00 DT = £1.14

ANTIBACTERIALS > PENICILLINS, BROAD-SPECTRUM

362

Amoxicillin

21-May-2020

(Amoxycillin)

- **INDICATIONS AND DOSE**

Susceptible infections (e.g. sinusitis, salmonellosis, oral infections)

▶ BY MOUTH

- Neonate 7 days to 28 days: 30 mg/kg 3 times a day (max. per dose 125 mg).

- Child 1–11 months: 125 mg 3 times a day; increased if necessary up to 30 mg/kg 3 times a day
- Child 1–4 years: 250 mg 3 times a day; increased if necessary up to 30 mg/kg 3 times a day
- Child 5–11 years: 500 mg 3 times a day; increased if necessary up to 30 mg/kg 3 times a day (max. per dose 1 g)
- Child 12–17 years: 500 mg 3 times a day; increased if necessary up to 1 g 3 times a day, use increased dose in severe infections

▶ BY INTRAVENOUS INJECTION, OR BY INTRAVENOUS INFUSION

- Neonate up to 7 days: 30 mg/kg every 12 hours, increased if necessary to 60 mg/kg every 12 hours, increased dose used in severe infection.

- Neonate 7 days to 28 days: 30 mg/kg every 8 hours, increased if necessary to 60 mg/kg every 8 hours, increased dose used in severe infection.

- Child: 20–30 mg/kg every 8 hours (max. per dose 500 mg), increased if necessary to 40–60 mg/kg every 8 hours (max. per dose 1 g every 8 hours), increased dose used in severe infection

Community-acquired pneumonia

▶ BY MOUTH

- Child 1–11 months: 125 mg 3 times a day for 5 days; increased if necessary up to 30 mg/kg 3 times a day
- Child 1–4 years: 250 mg 3 times a day for 5 days; increased if necessary up to 30 mg/kg 3 times a day
- Child 5–11 years: 500 mg 3 times a day for 5 days; increased if necessary up to 30 mg/kg 3 times a day (max. per dose 1 g 3 times a day)
- Child 12–17 years: 500 mg 3 times a day for 5 days; increased if necessary up to 1 g 3 times a day

Acute exacerbation of bronchiectasis

▶ BY MOUTH

- Child 1–11 months: 125 mg 3 times a day for 7–14 days
- Child 1–4 years: 250 mg 3 times a day for 7–14 days
- Child 5–17 years: 500 mg 3 times a day for 7–14 days

Acute cough [if systemically very unwell or at higher risk of complications]

▶ BY MOUTH

- Child 1–11 months: 125 mg 3 times a day for 5 days
- Child 1–4 years: 250 mg 3 times a day for 5 days
- Child 5–17 years: 500 mg 3 times a day for 5 days

Acute otitis media

▶ BY MOUTH

- Child 1–11 months: 125 mg 3 times a day for 5–7 days
- Child 1–4 years: 250 mg 3 times a day for 5–7 days
- Child 5–17 years: 500 mg 3 times a day for 5–7 days

Cystic fibrosis (treatment of asymptomatic *Haemophilus influenzae* carriage or mild exacerbation)

▶ BY MOUTH

- ▶ Neonate 7 days to 28 days: 30 mg/kg 3 times a day (max. per dose 125 mg).
- ▶ Child 1–11 months: 125 mg 3 times a day; increased if necessary up to 30 mg/kg 3 times a day
- ▶ Child 1–4 years: 250 mg 3 times a day; increased if necessary up to 30 mg/kg 3 times a day
- ▶ Child 5–11 years: 500 mg 3 times a day; increased if necessary up to 30 mg/kg 3 times a day (max. per dose 1 g)
- ▶ Child 12–17 years: 500 mg 3 times a day; increased if necessary up to 1 g 3 times a day, use increased dose in severe infections

▶ BY INTRAVENOUS INJECTION, OR BY INTRAVENOUS INFUSION

- ▶ Neonate up to 7 days: 30 mg/kg every 12 hours, increased if necessary to 60 mg/kg every 12 hours, increased dose used in severe infection.
- ▶ Neonate 7 days to 28 days: 30 mg/kg every 8 hours, increased if necessary to 60 mg/kg every 8 hours, increased dose used in severe infection.
- ▶ Child: 20–30 mg/kg every 8 hours (max. per dose 500 mg), increased if necessary to 40–60 mg/kg every 8 hours (max. per dose 1 g every 8 hours), increased dose used in severe infection

Lyme disease (under expert supervision)

▶ BY MOUTH

- ▶ Neonate 7 days to 28 days: 30 mg/kg 3 times a day (max. per dose 125 mg 3 times a day) usual duration 2–4 weeks.

Lyme disease [erythema migrans and/or non-focal symptoms] | Lyme disease [affecting cranial nerves or peripheral nervous system]

▶ BY MOUTH

- ▶ Child 1 month–11 years (administered on expert advice) (body-weight up to 34 kg): 30 mg/kg 3 times a day for 21 days
- ▶ Child 1 month–11 years (administered on expert advice) (body-weight 34 kg and above): 1 g 3 times a day for 21 days
- ▶ Child 12–17 years (administered on expert advice): 1 g 3 times a day for 21 days

Lyme arthritis | Acrodermatitis chronica atrophicans

▶ BY MOUTH

- ▶ Child 1 month–11 years (administered on expert advice) (body-weight up to 34 kg): 30 mg/kg 3 times a day for 28 days
- ▶ Child 1 month–11 years (administered on expert advice) (body-weight 34 kg and above): 1 g 3 times a day for 28 days
- ▶ Child 12–17 years (administered on expert advice): 1 g 3 times a day for 28 days

Anthrax (treatment and post-exposure prophylaxis)

▶ BY MOUTH

- ▶ Child (body-weight up to 20 kg): 80 mg/kg daily in 3 divided doses
- ▶ Child (body-weight 20 kg and above): 500 mg 3 times a day

Listerial meningitis (in combination with another antibiotic)

▶ BY INTRAVENOUS INFUSION

- ▶ Neonate up to 7 days: 50–100 mg/kg every 12 hours.
- ▶ Neonate 7 days to 28 days: 50–100 mg/kg every 8 hours.
- ▶ Child: 50 mg/kg every 4–6 hours (max. per dose 2 g every 4 hours)

Group B streptococcal infection | Enterococcal endocarditis (in combination with another antibiotic)

▶ BY INTRAVENOUS INFUSION

- ▶ Neonate up to 7 days: 50 mg/kg every 12 hours.
- ▶ Neonate 7 days to 28 days: 50 mg/kg every 8 hours.
- ▶ Child: 50 mg/kg every 4–6 hours (max. per dose 2 g every 4 hours)

Prevention of pneumococcal infection in asplenia or in patients with sickle-cell disease—if cover also needed for *Haemophilus influenzae*

▶ BY MOUTH

- ▶ Child 1 month–4 years: 125 mg twice daily
- ▶ Child 5–11 years: 250 mg twice daily
- ▶ Child 12–17 years: 500 mg twice daily

***Helicobacter pylori* eradication in combination with clarithromycin and omeprazole**

▶ BY MOUTH

- ▶ Child 1–5 years: 250 mg twice daily
- ▶ Child 6–11 years: 500 mg twice daily
- ▶ Child 12–17 years: 1 g twice daily

***Helicobacter pylori* eradication in combination with metronidazole and omeprazole**

▶ BY MOUTH

- ▶ Child 1–5 years: 125 mg 3 times a day
- ▶ Child 6–11 years: 250 mg 3 times a day
- ▶ Child 12–17 years: 500 mg 3 times a day

Prophylaxis of recurrent urinary-tract infection

▶ BY MOUTH

- ▶ Child 16–17 years: 250 mg once daily, dose to be taken at night, alternatively 500 mg for 1 dose, following exposure to a trigger

Prophylaxis of recurrent urinary-tract infection (initiated under specialist supervision)

▶ BY MOUTH

- ▶ Child 3–11 months: 62.5 mg once daily, dose to be taken at night
- ▶ Child 1–4 years: 125 mg once daily, dose to be taken at night
- ▶ Child 5–15 years: 250 mg once daily, dose to be taken at night

Lower urinary-tract infection in pregnancy

▶ BY MOUTH

- ▶ Child 12–17 years: 500 mg 3 times a day for 7 days

Lower urinary-tract infection

▶ BY MOUTH

- ▶ Child 3–11 months: 125 mg 3 times a day for 3 days
- ▶ Child 1–4 years: 250 mg 3 times a day for 3 days
- ▶ Child 5–15 years: 500 mg 3 times a day for 3 days

Asymptomatic bacteriuria in pregnancy

▶ BY MOUTH

- ▶ Child (body-weight 40 kg and above): 250–500 mg 3 times a day, alternatively 750–1000 mg twice daily

Urinary-tract infection (catheter-associated)

▶ BY MOUTH

- ▶ Child 3–11 months: 125 mg 3 times a day for 7 to 10 days
- ▶ Child 1–4 years: 250 mg 3 times a day for 7 to 10 days
- ▶ Child 5–15 years: 500 mg 3 times a day for 7 to 10 days
- ▶ Child 16–17 years: 500 mg 3 times a day for 7 days

● **UNLICENSED USE** Amoxicillin doses in BNF Publications may differ from those in product literature.

EvGr Duration of treatment for acute otitis media differs from product literature and adheres to national guidelines. Ⓐ

[EvGr] Amoxicillin is used for the treatment of acute exacerbation of bronchiectasis, ⟨A⟩ but is not licensed for this indication.

[EvGr] Amoxicillin is used for prophylaxis of recurrent urinary-tract infection, ⟨A⟩ but is not licensed for this indication.

- **CAUTIONS**

GENERAL CAUTIONS Acute lymphocytic leukaemia (increased risk of erythematous rashes) · chronic lymphocytic leukaemia (increased risk of erythematous rashes) · cytomegalovirus infection (increased risk of erythematous rashes) · glandular fever (erythematous rashes common) · maintain adequate hydration with high doses (particularly during parenteral therapy)

SPECIFIC CAUTIONS
- With intravenous use Accumulation of sodium can occur with high parenteral doses

- **INTERACTIONS** → Appendix 1: penicillins
- **SIDE-EFFECTS**

GENERAL SIDE-EFFECTS
- **Rare or very rare** Colitis haemorrhagic · crystalluria · dizziness · hyperkinesia · hypersensitivity vasculitis · mucocutaneous candidiasis · neutropenia
- **Frequency not known** Jarisch-Herxheimer reaction

SPECIFIC SIDE-EFFECTS
- **Rare or very rare**
- With oral use Black hairy tongue

- **PREGNANCY** Not known to be harmful.
- **BREAST FEEDING** Trace amount in milk, but appropriate to use.
- **HEPATIC IMPAIRMENT** Manufacturer advises caution.
- **RENAL IMPAIRMENT** Risk of crystalluria with high doses (particularly during parenteral therapy).
- With intravenous use Accumulation of sodium from injection can occur in patients with renal failure.

Dose adjustments Reduce dose in severe impairment; rashes more common.

- **DIRECTIONS FOR ADMINISTRATION**
- With intravenous use Displacement value may be significant when reconstituting injection, consult local guidelines. Dilute intravenous injection to a concentration of 50 mg/mL (100 mg/mL for neonates). May be further diluted with Glucose 5% *or* Glucose 10% *or* Sodium chloride 0.9% *or* 0.45% for intravenous infusion. Give intravenous infusion over 30 minutes when using doses over 30 mg/kg.

- **PRESCRIBING AND DISPENSING INFORMATION** For choice of antibacterial therapy, see Anthrax p. 391, Antibacterials, use for prophylaxis p. 319, Cardiovascular system infections, antibacterial therapy p. 322, Central nervous system infections, antibacterial therapy p. 323, Ear infections, antibacterial therapy p. 324, Gastro-intestinal system infections, antibacterial therapy p. 324, Lyme disease p. 391, Nose infections, antibacterial therapy p. 326, Oral bacterial infections p. 326, Peptic ulceration p. 58, Respiratory system infections, antibacterial therapy p. 327, Urinary-tract infections p. 400.
- **PATIENT AND CARER ADVICE** Patient counselling is advised for Amoxicillin (*Amoxil*®) paediatric suspension (use of pipette).

Medicines for Children leaflet: Amoxicillin for bacterial infections www.medicinesforchildren.org.uk/amoxicillin-bacterial-infections-0

- **PROFESSION SPECIFIC INFORMATION**

Dental practitioners' formulary

Amoxicillin capsules may be prescribed. Amoxicillin sachets may be prescribed as Amoxicillin Oral Powder. Amoxicillin Oral Suspension may be prescribed.

- **MEDICINAL FORMS** There can be variation in the licensing of different medicines containing the same drug.

Powder for solution for injection

ELECTROLYTES: May contain Sodium

- Amoxicillin (Non-proprietary)

Amoxicillin (as Amoxicillin sodium) 250 mg Amoxicillin 250mg powder for solution for injection vials | 10 vial [PoM] £4.80 | 10 vial [PoM] £4.50 (Hospital only)

Amoxicillin (as Amoxicillin sodium) 500 mg Amoxicillin 500mg powder for solution for injection vials | 10 vial [PoM] £9.60 DT = £5.48 | 10 vial [PoM] £12.00 DT = £5.48 (Hospital only)

Amoxicillin (as Amoxicillin sodium) 1 gram Amoxicillin 1g powder for solution for injection vials | 1 vial [PoM] £1.92 | 10 vial [PoM] £16.50 DT = £10.96 (Hospital only)

- Amoxil (GlaxoSmithKline UK Ltd)

Amoxicillin (as Amoxicillin sodium) 500 mg Amoxil 500mg powder for solution for injection vials | 10 vial [PoM] £5.48 DT = £5.48

Amoxicillin (as Amoxicillin sodium) 1 gram Amoxil 1g powder for solution for injection vials | 10 vial [PoM] £10.96 DT = £10.96

Oral suspension

CAUTIONARY AND ADVISORY LABELS 9

EXCIPIENTS: May contain Sucrose

- Amoxicillin (Non-proprietary)

Amoxicillin (as Amoxicillin trihydrate) 25 mg per 1 ml Amoxicillin 125mg/5ml oral suspension sugar free sugar-free | 100 ml [PoM] £25.00 DT = £1.40

Amoxicillin 125mg/5ml oral suspension | 100 ml [PoM] £25.00 DT = £1.74

Amoxicillin (as Amoxicillin trihydrate) 50 mg per 1 ml Amoxicillin 250mg/5ml oral suspension sugar free sugar-free | 100 ml [PoM] £35.00 DT = £1.65

Amoxicillin 250mg/5ml oral suspension | 100 ml [PoM] £35.00 DT = £1.93

- Amoxil (GlaxoSmithKline UK Ltd)

Amoxicillin (as Amoxicillin trihydrate) 100 mg per 1 ml Amoxil 125mg/1.25ml paediatric oral suspension | 20 ml [PoM] £3.18 DT = £3.18

Powder

CAUTIONARY AND ADVISORY LABELS 9, 13

- Amoxicillin (Non-proprietary)

Amoxicillin (as Amoxicillin trihydrate) 3 gram Amoxicillin 3g oral powder sachets sugar free sugar-free | 2 sachet [PoM] £15.00 DT = £10.36

Capsule

CAUTIONARY AND ADVISORY LABELS 9

- Amoxicillin (Non-proprietary)

Amoxicillin (as Amoxicillin trihydrate) 250 mg Amoxicillin 250mg capsules | 15 capsule [PoM] £5.00 DT = £1.02 | 21 capsule [PoM] £8.99 DT = £1.43 | 500 capsule [PoM] £31.00-£120.00

Amoxicillin (as Amoxicillin trihydrate) 500 mg Amoxicillin 500mg capsules | 15 capsule [PoM] £7.50 DT = £1.12 | 21 capsule [PoM] £15.00 DT = £1.57 | 100 capsule [PoM] £7.00-£75.00

Combinations available: *Co-amoxiclav*, p. 370

362

Ampicillin

21-May-2020

- **INDICATIONS AND DOSE**

Susceptible infections (including bronchitis, urinary-tract infections, otitis media, sinusitis, uncomplicated community-acquired pneumonia, salmonellosis)

- BY MOUTH
- Neonate 7 days to 20 days: 30 mg/kg 3 times a day (max. per dose 125 mg).
- Neonate 21 days to 28 days: 30 mg/kg 4 times a day (max. per dose 125 mg).
- Child 1–11 months: 125 mg 4 times a day; increased if necessary up to 30 mg/kg 4 times a day
- Child 1–4 years: 250 mg 4 times a day; increased if necessary up to 30 mg/kg 4 times a day
- Child 5–11 years: 500 mg 4 times a day; increased if necessary up to 30 mg/kg 4 times a day (max. per dose 1 g)

- ▸ Child 12–17 years: 500 mg 4 times a day; increased if necessary to 1 g 4 times a day, use increased dose in severe infection

▶ BY INTRAVENOUS INJECTION, OR BY INTRAVENOUS INFUSION

- ▸ Neonate up to 7 days: 30 mg/kg every 12 hours, increased if necessary to 60 mg/kg every 12 hours, increased dose used in severe infection, community-acquired pneumonia or salmonellosis.
- ▸ Neonate 7 days to 20 days: 30 mg/kg every 8 hours, increased if necessary to 60 mg/kg every 8 hours, increased dose used in severe infection, community-acquired pneumonia or salmonellosis.
- ▸ Neonate 21 days to 28 days: 30 mg/kg every 6 hours, increased if necessary to 60 mg/kg every 6 hours, increased dose used in severe infection, community-acquired pneumonia or salmonellosis.
- ▸ Child: 25 mg/kg every 6 hours (max. per dose 500 mg every 6 hours), increased if necessary to 50 mg/kg every 6 hours (max. per dose 1 g every 6 hours), increased dose used in severe infection

Group B streptococcal infection | Enterococcal endocarditis (in combination with another antibacterial)

▶ BY INTRAVENOUS INFUSION

- ▸ Neonate up to 7 days: 50 mg/kg every 12 hours.
- ▸ Neonate 7 days to 20 days: 50 mg/kg every 8 hours.
- ▸ Neonate 21 days to 28 days: 50 mg/kg every 6 hours.
- ▸ Child: 50 mg/kg every 4–6 hours (max. per dose 2 g every 4 hours)

Listerial meningitis

▶ BY INTRAVENOUS INFUSION

- ▸ Neonate up to 7 days: 100 mg/kg every 12 hours.
- ▸ Neonate 7 days to 20 days: 100 mg/kg every 8 hours.
- ▸ Neonate 21 days to 28 days: 100 mg/kg every 6 hours.
- ▸ Child: 50 mg/kg every 4–6 hours (max. per dose 2 g every 4 hours)

● **CAUTIONS**

GENERAL CAUTIONS Acute lymphocytic leukaemia (increased risk of erythematous rashes) · chronic lymphocytic leukaemia (increased risk of erythematous rashes) · cytomegalovirus infection (increased risk of erythematous rashes) · glandular fever (erythematous rashes common)

SPECIFIC CAUTIONS

- ▸ With intravenous use Accumulation of electrolytes contained in parenteral preparations can occur with high doses

● **INTERACTIONS** → Appendix 1: penicillins

● **SIDE-EFFECTS** Colitis haemorrhagic

● **PREGNANCY** Not known to be harmful.

● **BREAST FEEDING** Trace amounts in milk, but appropriate to use.

● **RENAL IMPAIRMENT**

- ▸ With intravenous use Accumulation of electrolytes contained in parenteral preparations can occur in patients with renal failure.

Dose adjustments If estimated glomerular filtration rate less than 10 mL/minute/1.73 m^2 reduce dose or frequency; rashes more common.

● **DIRECTIONS FOR ADMINISTRATION**

- ▸ With oral use Administer at least 30 minutes before food.
- ▸ With intravenous use Displacement value may be significant when reconstituting injection, consult local guidelines. Dilute intravenous injection to a concentration of 50–100 mg/mL. May be further diluted with glucose 5% or 10% *or* sodium chloride 0.9% or 0.45% for infusion. Give over 30 minutes when using doses of greater than 50 mg/kg to avoid CNS toxicity including convulsions.

● **PATIENT AND CARER ADVICE**

Medicines for Children leaflet: Ampicillin for bacterial infection www.medicinesforchildren.org.uk/ampicillin-bacterial-infection

● **MEDICINAL FORMS** There can be variation in the licensing of different medicines containing the same drug.

Oral suspension

CAUTIONARY AND ADVISORY LABELS 9, 23

▸ Ampicillin (Non-proprietary)

Ampicillin 25 mg per 1 ml Ampicillin 125mg/5ml oral suspension | 100 ml [PoM] £29.86 DT = £29.86

Ampicillin 50 mg per 1 ml Ampicillin 250mg/5ml oral suspension | 100 ml [PoM] £38.86 DT = £38.86

Capsule

CAUTIONARY AND ADVISORY LABELS 9, 23

▸ Ampicillin (Non-proprietary)

Ampicillin 250 mg Ampicillin 250mg capsules | 28 capsule [PoM] £20.50 DT = £20.50

Ampicillin 500 mg Ampicillin 500mg capsules | 28 capsule [PoM] £40.30 DT = £40.30

Powder for solution for injection

▸ Ampicillin (Non-proprietary)

Ampicillin (as Ampicillin sodium) 500 mg Ampicillin 500mg powder for solution for injection vials | 10 vial [PoM] £78.30 DT = £78.30

362

Co-fluampicil

26-May-2020

● **INDICATIONS AND DOSE**

Mixed infections involving beta-lactamase-producing staphylococci

▶ BY MOUTH

- ▸ Child 10–17 years: 250/250 mg every 6 hours

Severe mixed infections involving beta-lactamase-producing staphylococci

▶ BY MOUTH

- ▸ Child 10–17 years: 500/500 mg every 6 hours

IMPORTANT SAFETY INFORMATION

HEPATIC DISORDERS

Cholestatic jaundice and hepatitis may occur very rarely, up to two months after treatment with flucloxacillin has been stopped. Administration for more than 2 weeks and increasing age are risk factors. Manufacturer advises:

- flucloxacillin should not be used in patients with a history of hepatic dysfunction associated with flucloxacillin;
- flucloxacillin should be used with caution in patients with hepatic impairment;
- careful enquiry should be made about hypersensitivity reactions to beta-lactam antibacterials.

● **CAUTIONS** Acute lymphocytic leukaemia (increased risk of erythematous rashes) · chronic lymphocytic leukaemia (increased risk of erythematous rashes) · cytomegalovirus infection (increased risk of erythematous rashes) · glandular fever (erythematous rashes common)

● **INTERACTIONS** → Appendix 1: penicillins

● **SIDE-EFFECTS** Arthralgia · bronchospasm · coma · dyspnoea · electrolyte imbalance · eosinophilia · erythema nodosum · gastrointestinal disorder · hallucination · Jarisch-Herxheimer reaction · myalgia · purpura non-thrombocytopenic · vasculitis

● **PREGNANCY** Not known to be harmful.

- **BREAST FEEDING** Trace amount in milk, but appropriate to use.
- **HEPATIC IMPAIRMENT** Manufacturer advises caution.
- **RENAL IMPAIRMENT**
  Dose adjustments Reduce dose or frequency if estimated glomerular filtration rate less than 10 mL/minute/1.73 m^2; rashes more common.
- **EFFECT ON LABORATORY TESTS** False-positive urinary glucose (if tested for reducing substances).
- **PRESCRIBING AND DISPENSING INFORMATION** Dose expressed as a combination of equal parts by mass of flucloxacillin and ampicillin.

- **MEDICINAL FORMS** There can be variation in the licensing of different medicines containing the same drug.

Capsule

CAUTIONARY AND ADVISORY LABELS 9, 22

▸ Co-fluampicil (Non-proprietary)
Ampicillin (as Ampicillin trihydrate) 250 mg, Flucloxacillin (as Flucloxacillin sodium) 250 mg Co-fluampicil 250mg/250mg capsules | 28 capsule [PoM] £28.71 DT = £2.61 | 100 capsule [PoM] £9.32

ANTIBACTERIALS › PENICILLINS, BROAD-SPECTRUM WITH BETA-LACTAMASE INHIBITOR

362

Co-amoxiclav

21-May-2020

- **INDICATIONS AND DOSE**

Infections due to beta-lactamase-producing strains (where amoxicillin alone not appropriate), including respiratory tract infections, bone and joint infections, genito-urinary and abdominal infections, and animal bites

▶ BY MOUTH USING TABLETS

▸ Child 12–17 years: 250/125 mg every 8 hours; increased to 500/125 mg every 8 hours, increased dose used for severe infection

▶ BY INTRAVENOUS INJECTION, OR BY INTRAVENOUS INFUSION

▸ Neonate: 30 mg/kg every 12 hours, intravenous infusion recommended in children less than 3 months.

▸ Child 1–2 months: 30 mg/kg every 12 hours, intravenous infusion recommended in children less than 3 months

▸ Child 3 months–17 years: 30 mg/kg every 8 hours (max. per dose 1.2 g every 8 hours)

Infections due to beta-lactamase-producing strains (where amoxicillin alone not appropriate) including respiratory-tract infections, bone and joint infections, genito-urinary and abdominal infections, and animal bites (doses for 125/31 suspension)

▶ BY MOUTH USING ORAL SUSPENSION

▸ Neonate: 0.25 mL/kilogram 3 times a day.

▸ Child 1–11 months: 0.25 mL/kilogram 3 times a day, dose doubled in severe infection

▸ Child 1–5 years: 0.25 mL/kilogram 3 times a day, alternatively 5 mL 3 times a day, dose doubled in severe infection

Infections due to beta-lactamase-producing strains (where amoxicillin alone not appropriate) including respiratory-tract infections, bone and joint infections, genito-urinary and abdominal infections, and animal bites (doses for 250/62 suspension)

▶ BY MOUTH USING ORAL SUSPENSION

▸ Child 6–11 years: 0.15 mL/kilogram 3 times a day, alternatively 5 mL 3 times a day, dose doubled in severe infection

Infections due to beta-lactamase-producing strains (where amoxicillin alone not appropriate) including respiratory-tract infections, bone and joint infections, genito-urinary and abdominal infections, and animal bites (doses for 400/57 suspension)

▶ BY MOUTH USING ORAL SUSPENSION

▸ Child 2–23 months: 0.15 mL/kilogram twice daily, doubled in severe infection

▸ Child 2–6 years (body-weight 13–21 kg): 2.5 mL twice daily, doubled in severe infection

▸ Child 7–12 years (body-weight 22–40 kg): 5 mL twice daily, doubled in severe infection

▸ Child 12–17 years (body-weight 41 kg and above): 10 mL twice daily; increased if necessary to 10 mL 3 times a day, increased frequency to be used in severe infection

Cellulitis | Erysipelas

▶ BY MOUTH USING TABLETS

▸ Child 12–17 years: 250/125 mg every 8 hours, alternatively 500/125 mg every 8 hours for 5–7 days then review (review after 7 days in severe infection or if infection near the eyes or nose)

▶ BY INTRAVENOUS INJECTION, OR BY INTRAVENOUS INFUSION

▸ Child 1–2 months: 30 mg/kg every 12 hours, intravenous infusion recommended in children less than 3 months

▸ Child 3 months–17 years: 30 mg/kg every 8 hours (max. per dose 1.2 g every 8 hours)

Cellulitis (doses for 125/31 suspension) | Erysipelas (doses for 125/31 suspension)

▶ BY MOUTH USING ORAL SUSPENSION

▸ Child 1–11 months: 0.25 mL/kilogram 3 times a day for 5–7 days then review (review after 7 days in severe infection or if infection near the eyes or nose), dose doubled in severe infection

▸ Child 1–5 years: 0.25 mL/kilogram 3 times a day, alternatively 5 mL 3 times a day for 5–7 days then review (review after 7 days in severe infection or if infection near the eyes or nose), dose doubled in severe infection

Cellulitis (doses for 250/62 suspension) | Erysipelas (doses for 250/62 suspension)

▶ BY MOUTH USING ORAL SUSPENSION

▸ Child 6–11 years: 0.15 mL/kilogram 3 times a day, alternatively 5 mL 3 times a day for 5–7 days then review (review after 7 days in severe infection or if infection near the eyes or nose), dose doubled in severe infection

Severe dental infection with spreading cellulitis | Dental infection not responding to first-line antibacterial

▶ BY MOUTH USING TABLETS

▸ Child 12–17 years: 250/125 mg every 8 hours for 5 days

Community-acquired pneumonia (doses for 125/31 suspension)

▶ BY MOUTH USING ORAL SUSPENSION

▸ Child 1–11 months: 0.5 mL/kilogram 3 times a day for 5 days

▸ Child 1–5 years: 0.5 mL/kilogram 3 times a day for 5 days, alternatively 10 mL 3 times a day for 5 days

Community-acquired pneumonia (doses for 250/62 suspension)

▶ BY MOUTH USING ORAL SUSPENSION

▸ Child 6–11 years: 0.3 mL/kilogram 3 times a day for 5 days, alternatively 10 mL 3 times a day for 5 days

Community-acquired pneumonia

▶ BY MOUTH USING TABLETS

▸ Child 12–17 years: 500/125 mg 3 times a day for 5 days

▶ BY INTRAVENOUS INJECTION, OR BY INTRAVENOUS INFUSION

▸ Child 1–2 months: 30 mg/kg every 12 hours, intravenous infusion recommended in children less than 3 months

▸ Child 3 months–17 years: 30 mg/kg every 8 hours (max. per dose 1.2 g every 8 hours)

Hospital-acquired pneumonia (doses for 125/31 suspension)
- ▸ BY MOUTH USING ORAL SUSPENSION
- ▸ Child 1–11 months: 0.5 mL/kilogram 3 times a day for 5 days then review
- ▸ Child 1–5 years: 0.5 mL/kilogram 3 times a day for 5 days then review, alternatively 10 mL 3 times a day for 5 days then review

Hospital-acquired pneumonia (doses for 250/62 suspension)
- ▸ BY MOUTH USING ORAL SUSPENSION
- ▸ Child 6–11 years: 0.3 mL/kilogram 3 times a day for 5 days then review, alternatively 10 mL 3 times a day for 5 days then review

Hospital-acquired pneumonia
- ▸ BY MOUTH USING TABLETS
- ▸ Child 12–17 years: 500/125 mg 3 times a day for 5 days then review

Acute exacerbation of bronchiectasis (doses for 125/31 suspension)
- ▸ BY MOUTH USING ORAL SUSPENSION
- ▸ Child 1–11 months: 0.25 mL/kilogram 3 times a day for 7–14 days
- ▸ Child 1–5 years: 5 mL 3 times a day for 7–14 days, alternatively 0.25 mL/kilogram 3 times a day for 7–14 days

Acute exacerbation of bronchiectasis (doses for 250/62 suspension)
- ▸ BY MOUTH USING ORAL SUSPENSION
- ▸ Child 6–11 years: 5 mL 3 times a day for 7–14 days, alternatively 0.15 mL/kilogram 3 times a day for 7–14 days

Acute exacerbation of bronchiectasis
- ▸ BY MOUTH USING TABLETS
- ▸ Child 12–17 years: 250/125 mg 3 times a day for 7–14 days, alternatively 500/125 mg 3 times a day for 7–14 days
- ▸ BY INTRAVENOUS INFUSION, OR BY INTRAVENOUS INJECTION
- ▸ Child 1–2 months: 30 mg/kg every 12 hours, intravenous infusion is recommended in children less than 3 months
- ▸ Child 3 months–17 years: 30 mg/kg every 8 hours (max. per dose 1.2 g every 8 hours)

Acute sinusitis (doses for 125/31 suspension)
- ▸ BY MOUTH USING ORAL SUSPENSION
- ▸ Child 1–11 months: 0.25 mL/kilogram 3 times a day for 5 days
- ▸ Child 1–5 years: 5 mL 3 times a day for 5 days, alternatively 0.25 mL/kilogram 3 times a day for 5 days

Acute sinusitis (doses for 250/62 suspension)
- ▸ BY MOUTH USING ORAL SUSPENSION
- ▸ Child 6–11 years: 5 mL 3 times a day for 5 days, alternatively 0.15 mL/kilogram 3 times a day for 5 days

Acute sinusitis
- ▸ BY MOUTH USING TABLETS
- ▸ Child 12–17 years: 250/125 mg 3 times a day for 5 days, alternatively 500/125 mg 3 times a day for 5 days

Acute otitis media (doses for 125/31 suspension)
- ▸ BY MOUTH USING ORAL SUSPENSION
- ▸ Child 1–11 months: 0.25 mL/kilogram 3 times a day for 5–7 days
- ▸ Child 1–5 years: 5 mL 3 times a day for 5–7 days, alternatively 0.25 mL/kilogram 3 times a day for 5–7 days

Acute otitis media (doses for 250/62 suspension)
- ▸ BY MOUTH USING ORAL SUSPENSION
- ▸ Child 6–11 years: 5 mL 3 times a day for 5–7 days, alternatively 0.15 mL/kilogram 3 times a day for 5–7 days

Acute otitis media
- ▸ BY MOUTH USING TABLETS
- ▸ Child 12–17 years: 250/125 mg 3 times a day for 5–7 days, alternatively 500/125 mg 3 times a day for 5–7 days

Acute pyelonephritis (doses for 125/31 suspension) | Urinary-tract infection (catheter-associated) (doses for 125/31 suspension)
- ▸ BY MOUTH USING ORAL SUSPENSION
- ▸ Child 3–11 months: 0.25 mL/kilogram 3 times a day for 7 to 10 days, dose doubled in severe infection
- ▸ Child 1–5 years: 0.25 mL/kilogram 3 times a day, alternatively 5 mL 3 times a day for 7 to 10 days, dose doubled in severe infection

Acute pyelonephritis (doses for 250/62 suspension) | Urinary-tract infection (catheter-associated) (doses for 250/62 suspension)
- ▸ BY MOUTH USING ORAL SUSPENSION
- ▸ Child 6–11 years: 0.15 mL/kilogram 3 times a day, alternatively 5 mL 3 times a day for 7 to 10 days, dose doubled in severe infection

Acute pyelonephritis | Urinary-tract infection (catheter-associated)
- ▸ BY MOUTH USING TABLETS
- ▸ Child 12–15 years: 250/125 mg 3 times a day for 7–10 days, alternatively 500/125 mg 3 times a day for 7–10 days
- ▸ Child 16–17 years: 500/125 mg 3 times a day for 7–10 days
- ▸ BY SLOW INTRAVENOUS INJECTION, OR BY INTRAVENOUS INFUSION
- ▸ Child 3 months–15 years: 30 mg/kg every 8 hours (max. per dose 1.2 g)
- ▸ Child 16–17 years: 1.2 g every 8 hours

DOSE EQUIVALENCE AND CONVERSION
- ▸ Doses are expressed as co-amoxiclav.
- ▸ A mixture of amoxicillin (as the trihydrate or as the sodium salt) and clavulanic acid (as potassium clavulanate); the proportions are expressed in the form x/y where x and y are the strengths in milligrams of amoxicillin and clavulanic acid respectively.

- **UNLICENSED USE** Co-amoxiclav may be used as detailed below, although these situations are considered unlicensed:
  - EvGr treatment of acute exacerbation of bronchiectasis
  - treatment of hospital-acquired pneumonia
  - duration of treatment for acute sinusitis
  - duration of treatment for acute otitis media (A)
- **CONTRA-INDICATIONS** History of co-amoxiclav-associated jaundice or hepatic dysfunction · history of penicillin-associated jaundice or hepatic dysfunction
- **CAUTIONS**

GENERAL CAUTIONS Acute lymphocytic leukaemia (increased risk of erythematous rashes) · chronic lymphocytic leukaemia (increased risk of erythematous rashes) · cytomegalovirus infection (increased risk of erythematous rashes) · glandular fever (erythematous rashes common) · maintain adequate hydration with high doses (particularly during parental therapy)

SPECIFIC CAUTIONS
- ▸ With intravenous use Accumulation of electrolytes contained in parenteral preparations can occur with high doses

- **INTERACTIONS** → Appendix 1: clavulanate · penicillins
- **SIDE-EFFECTS**

GENERAL SIDE-EFFECTS
- ▸ **Common or very common** Increased risk of infection
- ▸ **Uncommon** Dizziness · dyspepsia · headache
- ▸ **Rare or very rare** Neutropenia

▸ **Frequency not known** Colitis haemorrhagic · crystalluria · hypersensitivity vasculitis · meningitis aseptic

SPECIFIC SIDE-EFFECTS

▸ With oral use Akathisia · black hairy tongue · cholangitis · Kounis syndrome

SIDE-EFFECTS, FURTHER INFORMATION Hepatic events have been rarely reported in children.

Signs and symptoms usually occur during or shortly after treatment but in some cases may occur several weeks after discontinuation.

- **PREGNANCY** Manufacturer advises avoid unless essential—may be associated with an increased risk of necrotising enterocolitis in neonates.
- **BREAST FEEDING** Trace amount in milk, but appropriate to use.
- **HEPATIC IMPAIRMENT** Manufacturer advises caution. **Monitoring** Monitor liver function in liver disease.
- **RENAL IMPAIRMENT** Risk of crystalluria with high doses (particularly during parenteral therapy).

▸ With intravenous use Accumulation of electrolytes contained in parenteral preparations can occur in patients with renal failure.

Dose adjustments ▸ With oral use *Co-amoxiclav* 125/31 *suspension*, 250/62 *suspension*, 250/125 *tablets, or* 500/125 *tablets*: use normal dose every 12 hours if estimated glomerular filtration rate 10–30 mL/minute/1.73 m^2. Use the normal dose recommended for mild or moderate infections every 12 hours if estimated glomerular filtration rate less than 10 mL/minute/1.73 m^2. *Co-amoxiclav* 400/57 *suspension*: avoid if estimated glomerular filtration rate less than 30 mL/minute/1.73 m^2.

▸ With intravenous use *Co-amoxiclav injection*: use normal initial dose and then use half normal dose every 12 hours if estimated glomerular filtration rate 10–30 mL/minute/1.73 m^2; use normal initial dose and then use half normal dose every 24 hours if estimated glomerular filtration rate less than 10 mL/minute/1.73 m^2.

- **DIRECTIONS FOR ADMINISTRATION**

▸ With intravenous use For *intravenous infusion*, dilute reconstituted solution to a concentration of 10 mg/mL with Sodium Chloride 0.9%; give intermittently over 30–40 minutes. For *intravenous injection*, administer over 3–4 minutes.

- **PRESCRIBING AND DISPENSING INFORMATION** Doses are expressed as co-amoxiclav: a mixture of amoxicillin (as the trihydrate or as the sodium salt) and clavulanic acid (as potassium clavulanate); the proportions are expressed in the form x/y where x and y are the strengths in milligrams of amoxicillin and clavulanic acid respectively.

For choice of antibacterial therapy, see Antibacterials, use for prophylaxis p. 319, Ear infections, antibacterial therapy p. 324, Gastro-intestinal system infections, antibacterial therapy p. 324, Musculoskeletal system infections, antibacterial therapy p. 326, Nose infections, antibacterial therapy p. 326, Oropharyngeal infections, antibacterial therapy p. 761, Respiratory system infections, antibacterial therapy p. 327, Skin infections, antibacterial therapy p. 329, Urinary-tract infections p. 400.

- **PATIENT AND CARER ADVICE**

Medicines for Children leaflet: Co-amoxiclav for bacterial infections www.medicinesforchildren.org.uk/co-amoxiclav-bacterial-infections-0

- **PROFESSION SPECIFIC INFORMATION**

Dental practitioners' formulary

Co-amoxiclav 250/125 Tablets may be prescribed.
Co-amoxiclav 125/31 Suspension may be prescribed.
Co-amoxiclav 250/62 Suspension may be prescribed.

- **MEDICINAL FORMS** There can be variation in the licensing of different medicines containing the same drug. Forms available from special-order manufacturers include: infusion

Oral suspension

CAUTIONARY AND ADVISORY LABELS 9

EXCIPIENTS: May contain Aspartame

▸ Co-amoxiclav (Non-proprietary)

Clavulanic acid (as Potassium clavulanate) 6.25 mg per 1 ml, Amoxicillin (as Amoxicillin trihydrate) 25 mg per 1 ml Co-amoxiclav 125mg/31mg/5ml oral suspension | 100 ml PoM £5.00 DT = £5.00

Co-amoxiclav 125mg/31mg/5ml oral suspension sugar free sugar-free | 100 ml PoM £2.14 DT = £2.14

Clavulanic acid (as Potassium clavulanate) 12.5 mg per 1 ml, Amoxicillin (as Amoxicillin trihydrate) 50 mg per 1 ml Co-amoxiclav 250mg/62mg/5ml oral suspension | 100 ml PoM £5.00 DT = £5.00

Co-amoxiclav 250mg/62mg/5ml oral suspension sugar free sugar-free | 70 ml PoM £2.05 sugar-free | 100 ml PoM £2.59 DT = £1.59

Clavulanic acid (as Potassium clavulanate) 11.4 mg per 1 ml, Amoxicillin (as Amoxicillin trihydrate) 80 mg per 1 ml Co-amoxiclav 400mg/57mg/5ml oral suspension sugar free sugar-free | 35 ml PoM £4.13 DT = £4.13 sugar-free | 70 ml PoM £6.97 DT = £5.79

▸ Augmentin (GlaxoSmithKline UK Ltd)

Clavulanic acid (as Potassium clavulanate) 6.25 mg per 1 ml, Amoxicillin (as Amoxicillin trihydrate) 25 mg per 1 ml Augmentin 125/31 SF oral suspension sugar-free | 100 ml PoM £3.54 DT = £2.14

Clavulanic acid (as Potassium clavulanate) 12.5 mg per 1 ml, Amoxicillin (as Amoxicillin trihydrate) 50 mg per 1 ml Augmentin 250/62 SF oral suspension sugar-free | 100 ml PoM £3.60 DT = £1.59

▸ Augmentin-Duo (GlaxoSmithKline UK Ltd)

Clavulanic acid (as Potassium clavulanate) 11.4 mg per 1 ml, Amoxicillin (as Amoxicillin trihydrate) 80 mg per 1 ml Augmentin-Duo 400/57 oral suspension sugar-free | 35 ml PoM £4.13 DT = £4.13 sugar-free | 70 ml PoM £5.79 DT = £5.79

Tablet

CAUTIONARY AND ADVISORY LABELS 9

▸ Co-amoxiclav (Non-proprietary)

Clavulanic acid (as Potassium clavulanate) 125 mg, Amoxicillin (as Amoxicillin trihydrate) 250 mg Co-amoxiclav 250mg/125mg tablets | 21 tablet PoM £6.00 DT = £1.88

Clavulanic acid (as Potassium clavulanate) 125 mg, Amoxicillin (as Amoxicillin trihydrate) 500 mg Co-amoxiclav 500mg/125mg tablets | 21 tablet PoM £15.00 DT = £2.36

Clavulanic acid (as Potassium clavulanate) 125 mg, Amoxicillin (as Amoxicillin trihydrate) 875 mg Co-amoxiclav 875mg/125mg tablets | 14 tablet PoM £18.00 DT = £18.00

▸ Augmentin (GlaxoSmithKline UK Ltd)

Clavulanic acid (as Potassium clavulanate) 125 mg, Amoxicillin (as Amoxicillin trihydrate) 250 mg Augmentin 375mg tablets | 21 tablet PoM £5.03 DT = £1.88

Clavulanic acid (as Potassium clavulanate) 125 mg, Amoxicillin (as Amoxicillin trihydrate) 500 mg Augmentin 625mg tablets | 21 tablet PoM £9.60 DT = £2.36

Powder for solution for injection

ELECTROLYTES: May contain Potassium, sodium

▸ Co-amoxiclav (Non-proprietary)

Clavulanic acid (as Potassium clavulanate) 100 mg, Amoxicillin (as Amoxicillin sodium) 500 mg Co-amoxiclav 500mg/100mg powder for solution for injection vials | 10 vial PoM £10.60–£14.90 | 10 vial PoM £13.50 (Hospital only)

Clavulanic acid (as Potassium clavulanate) 200 mg, Amoxicillin (as Amoxicillin sodium) 1000 mg Co-amoxiclav 1000mg/200mg powder for solution for injection vials | 10 vial PoM £10.60–£39.70 | 10 vial PoM £27.50 (Hospital only)

▸ Augmentin Intravenous (GlaxoSmithKline UK Ltd)

Clavulanic acid (as Potassium clavulanate) 100 mg, Amoxicillin (as Amoxicillin sodium) 500 mg Augmentin Intravenous 600mg powder for solution for injection vials | 10 vial PoM £10.60

Clavulanic acid (as Potassium clavulanate) 200 mg, Amoxicillin (as Amoxicillin sodium) 1000 mg Augmentin Intravenous 1.2g powder for solution for injection vials | 10 vial PoM £10.60

ANTIBACTERIALS › PENICILLINS, MECILLINAM-TYPE

F 362

Pivmecillinam hydrochloride

22-May-2020

- **INDICATIONS AND DOSE**

Acute uncomplicated cystitis

▶ BY MOUTH

▸ Child (body-weight 40 kg and above): Initially 400 mg for 1 dose, then 200 mg every 8 hours to a total of 10 tablets

Chronic or recurrent bacteriuria

▶ BY MOUTH

▸ Child (body-weight 40 kg and above): 400 mg every 6–8 hours

Urinary-tract infections

▶ BY MOUTH

▸ Child (body-weight up to 40 kg): 5–10 mg/kg every 6 hours, alternatively 20–40 mg/kg daily in 3 divided doses

- **UNLICENSED USE** Not licensed for use in children under 3 months.
- **CONTRA-INDICATIONS** Carnitine deficiency · gastro-intestinal obstruction · oesophageal strictures
- **CAUTIONS** Avoid in Acute porphyrias p. 652
- **INTERACTIONS** → Appendix 1: penicillins
- **SIDE-EFFECTS**

▶ **Common or very common** Vulvovaginal fungal infection

▶ **Uncommon** Dizziness · fatigue · gastrointestinal discomfort · gastrointestinal disorders · headache · oral ulceration · vertigo

- **PREGNANCY** Not known to be harmful, but manufacturer advises avoid.
- **BREAST FEEDING** Trace amount in milk, but appropriate to use.
- **MONITORING REQUIREMENTS** Liver and renal function tests required in long-term use.
- **EFFECT ON LABORATORY TESTS** False positive urinary glucose (if tested for reducing substances). False positive newborn screening results for isovaleric acidaemia may occur in neonates born to mothers receiving pivmecillinam during late pregnancy.
- **DIRECTIONS FOR ADMINISTRATION** Tablets should be swallowed whole with plenty of fluid during meals while sitting or standing.
- **PATIENT AND CARER ADVICE** Patient counselling is advised on administration of pivmecillinam hydrochloride tablets (posture).

- **MEDICINAL FORMS** There can be variation in the licensing of different medicines containing the same drug.

Tablet

CAUTIONARY AND ADVISORY LABELS 9, 21, 27

▸ Pivmecillinam hydrochloride (Non-proprietary)

Pivmecillinam hydrochloride 200 mg Pivmecillinam 200mg tablets | 10 tablet [PoM] £5.40 DT = £5.40

▸ Selexid (Karo Pharma)

Pivmecillinam hydrochloride 200 mg Selexid 200mg tablets | 10 tablet [PoM] £5.40 DT = £5.40 | 18 tablet [PoM] £9.72

ANTIBACTERIALS › PENICILLINS, PENICILLINASE-RESISTANT

F 362

Flucloxacillin

21-May-2020

- **INDICATIONS AND DOSE**

Infections due to beta-lactamase-producing staphylococci including otitis externa | Adjunct in pneumonia

▶ BY MOUTH

▸ Neonate up to 7 days: 25 mg/kg twice daily.

▸ Neonate 7 days to 20 days: 25 mg/kg 3 times a day.

▸ Neonate 21 days to 28 days: 25 mg/kg 4 times a day.

▸ Child 1 month–1 year: 62.5–125 mg 4 times a day

▸ Child 2–9 years: 125–250 mg 4 times a day

▸ Child 10–17 years: 250–500 mg 4 times a day

▶ BY INTRAMUSCULAR INJECTION

▸ Child: 12.5–25 mg/kg every 6 hours (max. per dose 500 mg every 6 hours)

▶ BY SLOW INTRAVENOUS INJECTION, OR BY INTRAVENOUS INFUSION

▸ Neonate up to 7 days: 25 mg/kg every 12 hours.

▸ Neonate 7 days to 20 days: 25 mg/kg every 8 hours.

▸ Neonate 21 days to 28 days: 25 mg/kg every 6 hours.

▸ Child: 12.5–25 mg/kg every 6 hours (max. per dose 1 g every 6 hours)

Impetigo

▶ BY MOUTH

▸ Neonate up to 7 days: 25 mg/kg twice daily.

▸ Neonate 7 days to 20 days: 25 mg/kg 3 times a day.

▸ Neonate 21 days to 28 days: 25 mg/kg 4 times a day.

▸ Child 1 month–1 year: 62.5–125 mg 4 times a day for 5–7 days

▸ Child 2–9 years: 125–250 mg 4 times a day for 5–7 days

▸ Child 10–17 years: 250–500 mg 4 times a day for 5–7 days

▶ BY INTRAMUSCULAR INJECTION

▸ Child: 12.5–25 mg/kg every 6 hours (max. per dose 500 mg every 6 hours)

▶ BY SLOW INTRAVENOUS INJECTION, OR BY INTRAVENOUS INFUSION

▸ Neonate up to 7 days: 25 mg/kg every 12 hours.

▸ Neonate 7 days to 20 days: 25 mg/kg every 8 hours.

▸ Neonate 21 days to 28 days: 25 mg/kg every 6 hours.

▸ Child: 12.5–25 mg/kg every 6 hours (max. per dose 1 g every 6 hours)

Severe infections due to beta-lactamase-producing staphylococci including otitis externa | Adjunct in pneumonia (severe infection) | Adjunct in impetigo (severe infection)

▶ BY SLOW INTRAVENOUS INJECTION, OR BY INTRAVENOUS INFUSION

▸ Neonate up to 7 days: 50 mg/kg every 12 hours.

▸ Neonate 7 days to 20 days: 50 mg/kg every 8 hours.

▸ Neonate 21 days to 28 days: 50 mg/kg every 6 hours.

▸ Child: 25–50 mg/kg every 6 hours (max. per dose 2 g every 6 hours)

continued →

Cellulitis | Erysipelas
- ▶ BY MOUTH
- ▸ Child 1 month–1 year: 62.5–125 mg 4 times a day for 5–7 days then review
- ▸ Child 2–9 years: 125–250 mg 4 times a day for 5–7 days then review
- ▸ Child 10–17 years: 250–500 mg 4 times a day for 5–7 days then review
- ▶ BY SLOW INTRAVENOUS INJECTION, OR BY INTRAVENOUS INFUSION
- ▸ Child: 12.5–25 mg/kg every 6 hours (max. per dose 1 g every 6 hours)

Endocarditis (in combination with other antibacterial if necessary)
- ▶ BY SLOW INTRAVENOUS INJECTION, OR BY INTRAVENOUS INFUSION
- ▸ Child: 50 mg/kg every 6 hours (max. per dose 2 g every 6 hours)

Osteomyelitis
- ▶ BY SLOW INTRAVENOUS INJECTION, OR BY INTRAVENOUS INFUSION
- ▸ Neonate up to 7 days: 50–100 mg/kg every 12 hours.
- ▸ Neonate 7 days to 20 days: 50–100 mg/kg every 8 hours.
- ▸ Neonate 21 days to 28 days: 50–100 mg/kg every 6 hours.
- ▸ Child: 50 mg/kg every 6 hours (max. per dose 2 g every 6 hours)

Cerebral abscess | Staphylococcal meningitis
- ▶ BY SLOW INTRAVENOUS INJECTION, OR BY INTRAVENOUS INFUSION
- ▸ Neonate up to 7 days: 50–100 mg/kg every 12 hours.
- ▸ Neonate 7 days to 20 days: 50–100 mg/kg every 8 hours.
- ▸ Neonate 21 days to 28 days: 50–100 mg/kg every 6 hours.
- ▸ Child: 50 mg/kg every 6 hours (max. per dose 2 g every 6 hours)

Staphylococcal lung infection in cystic fibrosis
- ▶ BY MOUTH
- ▸ Child: 25 mg/kg 4 times a day (max. per dose 1 g), alternatively 100 mg/kg daily in 3 divided doses; maximum 4 g per day
- ▶ BY SLOW INTRAVENOUS INJECTION, OR BY INTRAVENOUS INFUSION
- ▸ Child: 50 mg/kg every 6 hours (max. per dose 2 g every 6 hours)

Prevention of *Staphylococcus aureus* lung infection in cystic fibrosis—primary prevention
- ▶ BY MOUTH
- ▸ Neonate: 125 mg twice daily.
- ▸ Child 1 month–3 years: 125 mg twice daily

Prevention of *Staphylococcus aureus* lung infection in cystic fibrosis—secondary prevention
- ▶ BY MOUTH
- ▸ Child: 50 mg/kg twice daily (max. per dose 1 g twice daily)

- ● **UNLICENSED USE** Flucloxacillin doses in the BNF may differ from those in product literature.

IMPORTANT SAFETY INFORMATION

HEPATIC DISORDERS

Cholestatic jaundice and hepatitis may occur very rarely, up to two months after treatment with flucloxacillin has been stopped. Administration for more than 2 weeks and increasing age are risk factors. Manufacturer advises:
- flucloxacillin should not be used in patients with a history of hepatic dysfunction associated with flucloxacillin
- flucloxacillin should be used with caution in patients with hepatic impairment
- careful enquiry should be made about hypersensitivity reactions to beta-lactam antibacterials

- ● **CAUTIONS**
  - ▸ With intravenous use accumulation of electrolytes can occur with high doses · risk of kernicterus in jaundiced neonates when high doses given parenterally
- ● **INTERACTIONS** → Appendix 1: penicillins
- ● **SIDE-EFFECTS**

GENERAL SIDE-EFFECTS
- ▶ **Rare or very rare** Arthralgia · fever · neutropenia

SPECIFIC SIDE-EFFECTS
- ▶ **Common or very common**
  - ▸ With oral use Gastrointestinal disorder
- ▶ **Rare or very rare**
  - ▸ With oral use Eosinophilia · myalgia
- ▶ **Frequency not known**
  - ▸ With parenteral use Bronchospasm · coma · dyspnoea · electrolyte imbalance · erythema nodosum · hallucination · Jarisch-Herxheimer reaction · nephropathy · neurotoxicity · oral candidiasis · platelet dysfunction · purpura non-thrombocytopenic · vasculitis

- ● **PREGNANCY** Not known to be harmful.
- ● **BREAST FEEDING** Trace amounts in milk, but appropriate to use.
- ● **HEPATIC IMPAIRMENT** Manufacturer advises caution; including in those with risk factors for hepatic reactions.
- ● **RENAL IMPAIRMENT**
  - ▸ With intravenous use Accumulation of electrolytes can occur in patients with renal failure.

  Dose adjustments Use normal dose every 8 hours if estimated glomerular filtration rate less than 10 mL/minute/1.73 m^2.
- ● **EFFECT ON LABORATORY TESTS** False-positive urinary glucose (if tested for reducing substances).
- ● **DIRECTIONS FOR ADMINISTRATION**
  - ▸ With intravenous use For *intravenous infusion*, dilute reconstituted solution *in* Glucose 5% *or* Sodium Chloride 0.9% and give intermittently over 30–60 minutes.
- ● **PRESCRIBING AND DISPENSING INFORMATION** For choice of antibacterial therapy, see Antibacterials, use for prophylaxis p. 319, Cardiovascular system infections, antibacterial therapy p. 322, Ear infections, antibacterial therapy p. 324, Musculoskeletal system infections, antibacterial therapy p. 326, Respiratory system infections, antibacterial therapy p. 327, Skin infections, antibacterial therapy p. 329.
- ● **PATIENT AND CARER ADVICE**

  Medicines for Children leaflet: Flucloxacillin for bacterial infections www.medicinesforchildren.org.uk/flucloxacillin-bacterial-infections

---

- ● **MEDICINAL FORMS** There can be variation in the licensing of different medicines containing the same drug. Forms available from special-order manufacturers include: infusion

Oral solution

CAUTIONARY AND ADVISORY LABELS 9, 23
- ▸ Flucloxacillin (Non-proprietary)

  Flucloxacillin (as Flucloxacillin sodium) 25 mg per 1 ml Flucloxacillin 125mg/5ml oral solution | 100 ml PoM £20.99 DT = £2.67

  Flucloxacillin 125mg/5ml oral solution sugar free sugar-free | 100 ml PoM £25.90 DT = £17.04

  Flucloxacillin (as Flucloxacillin sodium) 50 mg per 1 ml Flucloxacillin 250mg/5ml oral solution sugar free sugar-free | 100 ml PoM £27.39 DT = £20.55

Flucloxacillin 250mg/5ml oral solution | 100 ml PoM £47.10 DT = £8.24

Capsule

CAUTIONARY AND ADVISORY LABELS 9, 23

▸ Flucloxacillin (Non-proprietary)

Flucloxacillin (as Flucloxacillin sodium) 250 mg Flucloxacillin 250mg capsules | 28 capsule PoM £1.87 DT = £1.87 | 100 capsule PoM £5.96–£17.80

Flucloxacillin (as Flucloxacillin sodium) 500 mg Flucloxacillin 500mg capsules | 28 capsule PoM £10.50 DT = £2.53 | 100 capsule PoM £9.04–£37.50

Powder for solution for injection

▸ Flucloxacillin (Non-proprietary)

Flucloxacillin (as Flucloxacillin sodium) 250 mg Flucloxacillin 250mg powder for solution for injection vials | 10 vial PoM £8.60 DT = £8.60 (Hospital only) | 10 vial PoM £12.25 DT = £8.60

Flucloxacillin (as Flucloxacillin sodium) 500 mg Flucloxacillin 500mg powder for solution for injection vials | 10 vial PoM £24.50–£35.00 DT = £17.20 | 10 vial PoM £17.20 DT = £17.20 (Hospital only)

Flucloxacillin (as Flucloxacillin sodium) 1 gram Flucloxacillin 1g powder for solution for injection vials | 10 vial PoM £34.50 DT = £34.50 (Hospital only) | 10 vial PoM £45.00–£49.00 DT = £34.50

Flucloxacillin (as Flucloxacillin sodium) 2 gram Flucloxacillin 2g powder for solution for injection vials | 1 vial PoM £6.00 DT = £6.00 (Hospital only)

Combinations available: ***Co-fluampicil***, p. 369

ANTIBACTERIALS › POLYMYXINS

Colistimethate sodium

01-May-2020

(Colistin sulfomethate sodium)

● **DRUG ACTION** The polymyxin antibiotic, colistimethate sodium (colistin sulfomethate sodium), is active against Gram-negative organisms including *Pseudomonas aeruginosa*, *Acinetobacter baumanii*, and *Klebsiella pneumoniae*. It is not absorbed by mouth and thus needs to be given by injection for a systemic effect.

● **INDICATIONS AND DOSE**

Serious infections due to selected aerobic Gram-negative bacteria in patients with limited treatment options

▸ BY INTRAVENOUS INFUSION

▸ Child (body-weight up to 41 kg): 75 000–150 000 units/kg daily in 3 divided doses, the data supporting the dose regimen are very limited—consult product literature for available information, including recommendation to use lean body-weight for dosing

▸ Child (body-weight 41 kg and above): 9 million units daily in 2–3 divided doses, the data supporting the dose regimen are very limited—consult product literature for available information, including recommendation to use lean body-weight for dosing

Management of chronic pulmonary infections due to *Pseudomonas aeruginosa* in patients with cystic fibrosis

▸ BY INHALATION OF NEBULISED SOLUTION

▸ Child 1–23 months: 0.5–1 million units twice daily, for specific advice on administration using nebulisers—consult product literature; maximum 2 million units per day

▸ Child 2–17 years: 1–2 million units 2–3 times a day, for specific advice on administration using nebulisers—consult product literature; maximum 6 million units per day

▸ BY INHALATION OF POWDER

▸ Child 6–17 years: 1.66 million units twice daily

● **CONTRA-INDICATIONS** Myasthenia gravis

● **CAUTIONS**

GENERAL CAUTIONS Children under 1 year of age (effects of immature renal and metabolic function on conversion to active colistin not known)

SPECIFIC CAUTIONS

▸ When used by inhalation Severe haemoptysis—risk of further haemorrhage

● **INTERACTIONS** → Appendix 1: colistimethate

● **SIDE-EFFECTS**

▸ **Common or very common**

▸ When used by inhalation Arthralgia · asthenia · asthma · balance impaired · chest discomfort · cough · dysphonia · dyspnoea · fever · haemorrhage · headache · lower respiratory tract infection · nausea · respiratory disorders · taste altered · throat complaints · tinnitus · vomiting

▸ **Uncommon**

▸ When used by inhalation Anxiety · appetite decreased · diarrhoea · drowsiness · ear congestion · flatulence · oral disorders · proteinuria · seizure · sputum purulent · thirst · weight change

▸ **Rare or very rare**

▸ With parenteral use Confusion · nephrotoxicity · presyncope · psychosis · speech slurred · visual impairment

▸ **Frequency not known**

▸ With parenteral use Apnoea · neurological effects · neurotoxicity · renal disorder · sensory disorder

SIDE-EFFECTS, FURTHER INFORMATION Neurotoxicity and nephrotoxicity are dose-related.

● **PREGNANCY**

▸ When used by inhalation Clinical use suggests probably safe.

▸ With intravenous use Manufacturer advises use only if potential benefit outweighs risk.

● **BREAST FEEDING** Present in milk but poorly absorbed from gut; manufacturers advise avoid (or use only if potential benefit outweighs risk).

● **HEPATIC IMPAIRMENT**

▸ With intravenous use Manufacturer advises caution (no information available).

● **RENAL IMPAIRMENT**

▸ When used by inhalation Manufacturer advises caution.

▸ With intravenous use Consult product literature.

Monitoring ▸ With intravenous use In renal impairment, monitor plasma colistimethate sodium concentration during parenteral treatment—consult product literature. Recommended 'peak' plasma colistimethate sodium concentration (approx. 1 hour after intravenous injection or infusion) 5–15 mg/litre; pre-dose ('trough') concentration 2–6 mg/litre.

● **MONITORING REQUIREMENTS**

▸ With intravenous use Monitor renal function.

▸ When used by inhalation Measure lung function before and after initial dose of colistimethate sodium and monitor for bronchospasm; if bronchospasm occurs in a patient not using a bronchodilator, repeat test using a bronchodilator before the dose of colistimethate sodium.

● **DIRECTIONS FOR ADMINISTRATION**

▸ When used by inhalation Manufacturer advises if other treatments are being administered, they should be taken in the order recommended by the physician. For *nebulisation*, consult product literature for information on reconstitution and dilution.

▸ With intravenous use For *intravenous infusion*, dilute to a concentration of 40 000 units/mL with Sodium Chloride 0.9%; give over 30–60 minutes. Patients fitted with a totally implantable venous access device may tolerate an injection. For *slow intravenous injection* into a totally implantable venous access device, dilute to a concentration of 90 000 units/mL with Sodium Chloride 0.9% for child under 12 years (200 000 units/mL for child over 12 years); give over at least 5 minutes.

● **PRESCRIBING AND DISPENSING INFORMATION** Colistimethate sodium is included in some preparations for topical application.

- **PATIENT AND CARER ADVICE**
- When used by inhalation Patient should be advised to rinse mouth with water after each dose of dry powder inhalation. Patients or carers should be given advice on how to administer colistimethate sodium; first dose should be given under medical supervision.
Driving and skilled tasks Manufacturer advises patients and carers should be counselled on the effects on driving and performance of skilled tasks—increased risk of dizziness, confusion and visual disturbances.

- **NATIONAL FUNDING/ACCESS DECISIONS**

NICE decisions

- **Colistimethate sodium and tobramycin dry powders for inhalation for treating pseudomonas lung infection in cystic fibrosis (March 2013)** NICE TA276
Colistimethate sodium dry powder for inhalation is recommended for chronic pulmonary infection caused by *Pseudomonas aeruginosa* in patients with cystic fibrosis who would benefit from continued treatment, but do not tolerate the drug in its nebulised form. The manufacturer must provide colistimethate sodium dry powder for inhalation at the discount agreed as part of the patient access scheme to primary, secondary and tertiary care in the NHS. Patients currently receiving colistimethate sodium dry powder for inhalation can continue treatment until they and their NHS clinician consider it appropriate to stop.
www.nice.org.uk/guidance/ta276

- **MEDICINAL FORMS** There can be variation in the licensing of different medicines containing the same drug.

Powder for solution for injection

ELECTROLYTES: May contain Sodium

- **Colistimethate sodium (Non-proprietary)**
Colistimethate sodium 1000000 unit Colistimethate 1million unit powder for solution for injection vials | 10 vial PoM £30.00 DT = £18.00 (Hospital only)
- **Colomycin** (Teva UK Ltd)
Colistimethate sodium 1000000 unit Colomycin 1million unit powder for solution for injection vials | 10 vial PoM £18.00 DT = £18.00
Colistimethate sodium 2000000 unit Colomycin 2million unit powder for solution for injection vials | 10 vial PoM £32.40 DT = £32.40
- **Promixin** (Profile Pharma Ltd)
Colistimethate sodium 1000000 unit Promixin 1million unit powder for solution for injection vials | 10 vial PoM £37.50 DT = £18.00 (Hospital only)

Inhalation powder

- **Colobreathe** (Teva UK Ltd)
Colistimethate sodium 1662500 unit Colobreathe 1,662,500unit inhalation powder capsules | 56 capsule PoM £968.80 DT = £968.80

Powder for nebuliser solution

- **Promixin** (Profile Pharma Ltd)
Colistimethate sodium 1000000 unit Promixin 1million unit powder for nebuliser solution unit dose vials | 30 unit dose PoM £204.00 DT = £204.00

ANTIBACTERIALS > QUINOLONES

Quinolones

31-Oct-2017

MHRA/CHM advice: Systemic and inhaled fluoroquinolones (November 2018, and March 2019)

The MHRA and CHM have released important safety information regarding the use of systemic and inhaled fluoroquinolones. For restrictions and precautions, see *Important safety information* for all quinolones (ciprofloxacin p. 377).

Overview

In the UK, only fluoroquinolones are available; the recommendations below therefore refer to the use of fluoroquinolones.

Ciprofloxacin is active against both Gram-positive and Gram-negative bacteria. It is particularly active against Gram-negative bacteria, including *Salmonella*, *Shigella*, *Campylobacter*, *Neisseria*, and *Pseudomonas*. Ciprofloxacin has only moderate activity against Gram-positive bacteria such as *Streptococcus pneumoniae* and *Enterococcus faecalis*; it should not be used for pneumococcal pneumonia. It is active against *Chlamydia* and some mycobacteria. Most anaerobic organisms are not susceptible.

Many *Staphylococci* are resistant to quinolones and their use should be avoided in MRSA infections.

Ofloxacin p. 729 eye drops are used in ophthalmic infections.

There is much less experience of the other quinolones in children; expert advice should be sought.

Quinolones

IMPORTANT SAFETY INFORMATION

- With intravenous use or oral use or when used by inhalation

The CSM has warned that quinolones may induce **convulsions** in patients with or without a history of convulsions; taking NSAIDs at the same time may also induce them.

TENDON DAMAGE

- With intravenous use or oral use

Tendon damage (including rupture) has been reported rarely in patients receiving quinolones. Tendon rupture may occur within 48 hours of starting treatment; cases have also been reported several months after stopping a quinolone. Healthcare professionals are reminded that:

- quinolones are contra-indicated in patients with a history of tendon disorders related to quinolone use;
- the risk of tendon damage is increased by the concomitant use of corticosteroids;
- if tendinitis is suspected, the quinolone should be discontinued immediately.

MHRA/CHM ADVICE: SYSTEMIC AND INHALED FLUOROQUINOLONES: SMALL INCREASED RISK OF AORTIC ANEURYSM AND DISSECTION; ADVICE FOR PRESCRIBING IN HIGH-RISK PATIENTS (NOVEMBER 2018)

- With intravenous use or oral use

The MHRA advises that benefit-risk should be assessed and other therapeutic options considered before using fluoroquinolones in patients at risk of aortic aneurysm and dissection. Patients (particularly those at risk) and their carers should be informed about rare events of aortic aneurysm and dissection, and advised to seek immediate medical attention if sudden-onset severe abdominal, chest, or back pain develops.

MHRA/CHM ADVICE: FLUOROQUINOLONE ANTIBIOTICS: NEW RESTRICTIONS AND PRECAUTIONS FOR USE DUE TO VERY RARE REPORTS OF DISABLING AND POTENTIALLY LONG-LASTING OR IRREVERSIBLE SIDE EFFECTS (MARCH 2019)

- With intravenous use or oral use

Disabling, long-lasting or potentially irreversible adverse reactions affecting musculoskeletal and nervous systems have been reported very rarely with fluoroquinolone antibiotics. Healthcare professionals are advised to inform patients to stop treatment at the first signs of a serious adverse reaction, such as tendinitis or tendon rupture, muscle pain, muscle weakness, joint pain, joint swelling, peripheral neuropathy, and CNS effects, and to contact their doctor immediately. Fluoroquinolones should not be prescribed for non-severe or self-limiting infections, or non-bacterial conditions. Unless other commonly recommended antibiotics are inappropriate, fluoroquinolones should not be prescribed for mild to moderate infections. Fluoroquinolones should be avoided in patients who have previously had serious adverse reactions. Use of fluoroquinolones with corticosteroids should also be avoided as it may exacerbate fluoroquinolone-induced tendinitis and tendon rupture. Fluoroquinolones should be prescribed with caution in patients with renal impairment or solid-organ transplants as they are at a higher risk of tendon injury.

- **CONTRA-INDICATIONS**
- ▸ With intravenous use or oral use or when used by inhalation History of tendon disorders related to quinolone use
- **CAUTIONS**
- ▸ With intravenous use or oral use or when used by inhalation Can prolong the QT interval · conditions that predispose to seizures · diabetes (may affect blood glucose) · exposure to excessive sunlight and UV radiation should be avoided during treatment and for 48 hours after stopping treatment · G6PD deficiency · history of epilepsy · myasthenia gravis (risk of exacerbation) · psychiatric disorders
- ▸ With intravenous use or oral use children or adolescents (arthropathy has developed in weight-bearing joints in young *animals*)

CAUTIONS, FURTHER INFORMATION
- ▸ With intravenous use or oral use Quinolones cause arthropathy in the weight-bearing joints of immature *animals* and are therefore generally not recommended in children and growing adolescents. However, the significance of this effect in humans is uncertain and in some specific circumstances use of ciprofloxacin may be justified in children.
- **SIDE-EFFECTS**
- ▸ **Common or very common** Diarrhoea · eye discomfort · eye disorders · nausea · skin reactions · taste altered · vision disorders · vomiting
- ▸ **Uncommon** Anxiety · appetite decreased · arrhythmias · arthralgia · asthenia · chest pain · confusion · dizziness · dry eye · eosinophilia · eye inflammation · fever · flatulence · gastrointestinal discomfort · hallucination · headache · hearing impairment · hepatic disorders · hypotension · movement disorders · oedema · pain · renal impairment · rhinitis · seizure · sensation abnormal · sleep disorders · thrombocytopenia · thrombocytosis · tinnitus · vasodilation · vertigo
- ▸ **Rare or very rare** Agranulocytosis · anaemia · angioedema · antibiotic associated colitis · arthritis · asthma · depression · dyspnoea · gait abnormal · haemolytic anaemia · hyperglycaemia · hyperhidrosis · hypersensitivity · hypoglycaemia · idiopathic intracranial hypertension · laryngeal oedema · leucopenia · muscle complaints · muscle weakness · myasthenia gravis aggravated · nephritis tubulointerstitial · neutropenia · pancreatitis · pancytopenia · photosensitivity reaction · psychotic disorder · severe cutaneous adverse reactions (SCARs) · suicidal tendencies · syncope · tendon disorders · tremor · vasculitis
- ▸ **Frequency not known** Corneal deposits (reversible after completion of treatment) · drowsiness · increased risk of aortic aneurysm · increased risk of aortic dissection · palpitations · peripheral neuropathy (sometimes irreversible) · polyneuropathy · QT interval prolongation · self-injurious behaviour

SIDE-EFFECTS, FURTHER INFORMATION The drug should be discontinued if neurological, psychiatric, tendon disorders or hypersensitivity reactions (including severe rash) occur. For more information regarding the safety of fluoroquinolones, please see Important Safety Information.

- **ALLERGY AND CROSS-SENSITIVITY** Use of quinolones contra-indicated in quinolone hypersensitivity.
- **PREGNANCY**
- ▸ With intravenous use or oral use or when used by inhalation Avoid in pregnancy—shown to cause arthropathy in *animal* studies; safer alternatives are available.
- **PATIENT AND CARER ADVICE**
- ▸ With intravenous use or oral use The MHRA has produced an advice sheet on serious adverse reactions affecting musculoskeletal and nervous systems associated with fluoroquinolone use, which should be provided to patients and their carers.

F 376

Ciprofloxacin

17-Apr-2020

- **INDICATIONS AND DOSE**

Fistulating Crohn's disease
- ▸ BY MOUTH
- ▸ Child: 5 mg/kg twice daily

Severe respiratory-tract infections, gastro-intestinal infection
- ▸ BY MOUTH
- ▸ Neonate: 15 mg/kg twice daily.
- ▸ Child: 20 mg/kg twice daily (max. per dose 750 mg)
- ▸ BY INTRAVENOUS INFUSION
- ▸ Neonate: 10 mg/kg every 12 hours, to be given over 60 minutes.
- ▸ Child: 10 mg/kg every 8 hours (max. per dose 400 mg), to be given over 60 minutes

Acute exacerbation of bronchiectasis (administered on expert advice)
- ▸ BY MOUTH
- ▸ Child 1–17 years: 20 mg/kg twice daily (max. per dose 750 mg) for 7–14 days
- ▸ BY INTRAVENOUS INFUSION
- ▸ Child 1–17 years: 10 mg/kg every 8 hours (max. per dose 400 mg), to be given over 60 minutes

Pseudomonal lower respiratory-tract infection in cystic fibrosis
- ▸ BY MOUTH
- ▸ Child: 20 mg/kg twice daily (max. per dose 750 mg)
- ▸ BY INTRAVENOUS INFUSION
- ▸ Child: 10 mg/kg every 8 hours (max. per dose 400 mg), to be given over 60 minutes

Complicated urinary-tract infections
- ▸ BY MOUTH
- ▸ Neonate: 10 mg/kg twice daily.
- ▸ Child: 10 mg/kg twice daily, dose to be doubled in severe infection (max. 750 mg twice daily)
- ▸ BY INTRAVENOUS INFUSION
- ▸ Neonate: 6 mg/kg every 12 hours, to be given over 60 minutes.
- ▸ Child: 6 mg/kg every 8 hours; increased to 10 mg/kg every 8 hours (max. per dose 400 mg), in severe infection

Gonorrhoea
- ▸ BY MOUTH
- ▸ Child 12–17 years: 500 mg for 1 dose

Anthrax (treatment and post-exposure prophylaxis)
- ▸ BY MOUTH
- ▸ Child: 15 mg/kg twice daily (max. per dose 500 mg)

continued →

▶ BY INTRAVENOUS INFUSION
- Child: 10 mg/kg every 12 hours (max. per dose 400 mg)

Prevention of secondary case of meningococcal meningitis

▶ BY MOUTH
- Neonate: 30 mg/kg (max. per dose 125 mg) for 1 dose.
- Child 1 month–4 years: 30 mg/kg (max. per dose 125 mg) for 1 dose
- Child 5–11 years: 250 mg for 1 dose
- Child 12–17 years: 500 mg for 1 dose

Acute pyelonephritis | Urinary tract infection (catheter-associated)

▶ BY MOUTH
- Child 16–17 years: 500 mg twice daily for 7 days

▶ BY INTRAVENOUS INFUSION
- Child 16–17 years: 400 mg every 8–12 hours

● UNLICENSED USE Not licensed for use in children under 1 year of age. Licensed for use in children over 1 year for complicated urinary-tract infections, for pseudomonal lower respiratory-tract infections in cystic fibrosis, for prophylaxis and treatment of inhalational anthrax. Licensed for use in children over 1 year for other infections where the benefit is considered to outweigh the potential risks. Not licensed for use in children for gastro-intestinal anthrax. Not licensed for use in children for prophylaxis of meningococcal meningitis.

● CAUTIONS Acute myocardial infarction (risk factor for QT interval prolongation) · avoid excessive alkalinity of urine (risk of crystalluria) · bradycardia (risk factor for QT interval prolongation) · congenital long QT syndrome (risk factor for QT interval prolongation) · electrolyte disturbances (risk factor for QT interval prolongation) · ensure adequate fluid intake (risk of crystalluria) · heart failure with reduced left ventricular ejection fraction (risk factor for QT interval prolongation) · history of symptomatic arrhythmias (risk factor for QT interval prolongation)

● INTERACTIONS → Appendix 1: quinolones

● SIDE-EFFECTS
- **Common or very common** Arthropathy
- **Uncommon** Fungal superinfection
- **Rare or very rare** Bone marrow depression · crystalluria · erythema nodosum · haematuria · intracranial pressure increased · leucocytosis · migraine · muscle tone increased · olfactory nerve disorder · status epilepticus
- **Frequency not known** Mood altered

● PREGNANCY A single dose of ciprofloxacin may be used for the prevention of a secondary case of meningococcal meningitis.

● BREAST FEEDING Amount too small to be harmful but manufacturer advises avoid.

● RENAL IMPAIRMENT
Dose adjustments Reduce dose if estimated glomerular filtration rate less than 30 mL/minute/1.73 m^2—consult product literature.

● PRESCRIBING AND DISPENSING INFORMATION For choice of antibacterial therapy, see Antibacterials, use for prophylaxis p. 319, Anthrax p. 391, Gastro-intestinal system infections, antibacterial therapy p. 324, Genital system infections, antibacterial therapy p. 325, Respiratory system infections, antibacterial therapy p. 327, Urinary-tract infections p. 400.

● PATIENT AND CARER ADVICE
Medicines for Children leaflet: Ciprofloxacin for bacterial infections www.medicinesforchildren.org.uk/ciprofloxacin-bacterial-infection
Driving and skilled tasks May impair performance of skilled tasks (e.g. driving); effects enhanced by alcohol.

● MEDICINAL FORMS There can be variation in the licensing of different medicines containing the same drug. Forms available from special-order manufacturers include: oral suspension

Tablet

CAUTIONARY AND ADVISORY LABELS 7, 9, 25
- Ciprofloxacin (Non-proprietary)
  Ciprofloxacin (as Ciprofloxacin hydrochloride) 100 mg Ciprofloxacin 100mg tablets | 6 tablet PoM £4.50 DT = £2.11
  Ciprofloxacin (as Ciprofloxacin hydrochloride) 250 mg Ciprofloxacin 250mg tablets | 10 tablet PoM £7.21 DT = £0.79 | 20 tablet PoM £1.39–£14.42 | 100 tablet PoM £7.90
  Ciprofloxacin (as Ciprofloxacin hydrochloride) 500 mg Ciprofloxacin 500mg tablets | 10 tablet PoM £12.49 DT = £1.05 | 20 tablet PoM £1.56–£27.29 | 100 tablet PoM £9.10
  Ciprofloxacin (as Ciprofloxacin hydrochloride) 750 mg Ciprofloxacin 750mg tablets | 10 tablet PoM £17.78 DT = £8.00 | 20 tablet PoM £15.99
- Ciproxin (Bayer Plc)
  Ciprofloxacin (as Ciprofloxacin hydrochloride) 500 mg Ciproxin 500mg tablets | 10 tablet PoM £12.49 DT = £1.05

Oral suspension

CAUTIONARY AND ADVISORY LABELS 7, 9, 25
- Ciproxin (Bayer Plc)
  Ciprofloxacin 50 mg per 1 ml Ciproxin 250mg/5ml oral suspension | 100 ml PoM £21.29 DT = £21.29

Solution for infusion

ELECTROLYTES: May contain Sodium
- Ciprofloxacin (Non-proprietary)
  Ciprofloxacin (as Ciprofloxacin lactate) 2 mg per 1 ml Ciprofloxacin 200mg/100ml solution for infusion vials | 1 vial PoM £10.00
  Ciprofloxacin 200mg/100ml solution for infusion bottles | 10 bottle PoM £131.00–£144.50
  Ciprofloxacin 100mg/50ml solution for infusion vials | 1 vial PoM £10.00–£13.00
  Ciprofloxacin 400mg/200ml solution for infusion bottles | 1 bottle PoM £10.00 | 10 bottle PoM £195.90–£199.20
  Ciprofloxacin 400mg/200ml solution for infusion vials | 1 vial PoM £10.00
- Ciproxin (Bayer Plc)
  Ciprofloxacin (as Ciprofloxacin lactate) 2 mg per 1 ml Ciproxin 100mg/50ml solution for infusion bottles | 1 bottle PoM £7.61 (Hospital only)
  Ciproxin 200mg/100ml solution for infusion bottles | 1 bottle PoM £15.01 (Hospital only) | 5 bottle PoM £75.06 (Hospital only)
  Ciproxin 400mg/200ml solution for infusion bottles | 1 bottle PoM £22.85 (Hospital only) | 5 bottle PoM £114.23 (Hospital only)

Infusion
- Ciprofloxacin (Non-proprietary)
  Ciprofloxacin (as Ciprofloxacin lactate) 2 mg per 1 ml Ciprofloxacin 200mg/100ml infusion bags | 5 bag PoM £60.00 (Hospital only) | 10 bag PoM £120.00 (Hospital only)
  Ciprofloxacin 400mg/200ml infusion bags | 5 bag PoM £85.00 (Hospital only) | 10 bag PoM £170.00–£228.46 (Hospital only)

ANTIBACTERIALS > SULFONAMIDES

Co-trimoxazole

26-May-2020

● DRUG ACTION Sulfamethoxazole and trimethoprim are used in combination (as co-trimoxazole) because of their synergistic activity (the importance of the sulfonamides has decreased as a result of increasing bacterial resistance and their replacement by antibacterials which are generally more active and less toxic).

● INDICATIONS AND DOSE

Treatment of susceptible infections

▶ BY MOUTH
- Child 6 weeks–5 months: 120 mg twice daily, alternatively 24 mg/kg twice daily
- Child 6 months–5 years: 240 mg twice daily, alternatively 24 mg/kg twice daily
- Child 6–11 years: 480 mg twice daily, alternatively 24 mg/kg twice daily
- Child 12–17 years: 960 mg twice daily

▶ BY INTRAVENOUS INFUSION
▸ Child 6 weeks–17 years: 18 mg/kg every 12 hours; increased to 27 mg/kg every 12 hours (max. per dose 1.44 g), increased dose used in severe infection

Treatment of *Pneumocystis jirovecii* (*Pneumocystis carinii*) infections (undertaken where facilities for appropriate monitoring available—consult microbiologist and product literature)

▶ BY MOUTH, OR BY INTRAVENOUS INFUSION
▸ Child: 120 mg/kg daily in 2–4 divided doses for 14–21 days, oral route preferred for children

Prophylaxis of *Pneumocystis jirovecii* (*Pneumocystis carinii*) infections

▶ BY MOUTH
▸ Child: 450 mg/m^2 twice daily (max. per dose 960 mg twice daily) for 3 days of the week (either consecutively or on alternate days), dose regimens may vary, consult local guidelines

DOSE EQUIVALENCE AND CONVERSION
▸ 480 mg of co-trimoxazole consists of sulfamethoxazole 400 mg and trimethoprim 80 mg.

- **UNLICENSED USE** Co-trimoxazole may be used as detailed below, although these situations are considered unlicensed:
  - Treatment of *Burkholderia cepacia* infections in cystic fibrosis;
  - Treatment of *Stenotrophomonas maltophilia* infections; Not licensed for use in children under 6 weeks.

> **IMPORTANT SAFETY INFORMATION**
> RESTRICTIONS ON THE USE OF CO-TRIMOXAZOLE
> Co-trimoxazole is the drug of choice in the prophylaxis and treatment of *Pneumocystis jirovecii* (*Pneumocystis carinii*) pneumonia; it is also indicated for nocardiasis, *Stenotrophomonas maltophilia* infection [unlicensed indication], and toxoplasmosis. It should only be considered for use in acute exacerbations of chronic bronchitis and infections of the urinary tract when there is bacteriological evidence of sensitivity to co-trimoxazole and good reason to prefer this combination to a single antibacterial; similarly it should only be used in acute otitis media in children when there is good reason to prefer it. Co-trimoxazole is also used for the treatment of infections caused by *Burkholderia cepacia* in cystic fibrosis [unlicensed indication].

- **CONTRA-INDICATIONS** Acute porphyrias p. 652
- **CAUTIONS** Asthma · avoid in blood disorders (unless under specialist supervision) · avoid in infants under 6 weeks (except for treatment or prophylaxis of pneumocystis pneumonia) because of the risk of kernicterus · G6PD deficiency (risk of haemolytic anaemia) · maintain adequate fluid intake · predisposition to folate deficiency · predisposition to hyperkalaemia
- **INTERACTIONS** → Appendix 1: sulfonamides · trimethoprim
- **SIDE-EFFECTS**
▸ **Common or very common** Diarrhoea · electrolyte imbalance · fungal overgrowth · headache · nausea · skin reactions
▸ **Uncommon** Vomiting
▸ **Rare or very rare** Agranulocytosis · angioedema · aplastic anaemia · appetite decreased · arthralgia · ataxia · cough · depression · dizziness · dyspnoea · eosinophilia · fever · haemolysis · haemolytic anaemia · hallucination · hepatic disorders · hypoglycaemia · leucopenia · lung infiltration · megaloblastic anaemia · meningitis aseptic · metabolic acidosis · methaemoglobinaemia · myalgia · myocarditis allergic · nephritis tubulointerstitial · neutropenia · oral disorders · pancreatitis · peripheral neuritis · photosensitivity reaction · pseudomembranous enterocolitis · renal impairment · renal tubular acidosis · seizure · serum sickness · severe cutaneous adverse reactions (SCARs) · systemic lupus erythematosus (SLE) · thrombocytopenia · tinnitus · uveitis · vasculitis · vertigo

SIDE-EFFECTS, FURTHER INFORMATION Co-trimoxazole is associated with rare but serious side effects. Discontinue immediately if blood disorders (including leucopenia, thrombocytopenia, megaloblastic anaemia, eosinophilia) or rash (including Stevens-Johnson syndrome or toxic epidermal necrolysis) develop.

- **PREGNANCY** Teratogenic risk in first trimester (trimethoprim a folate antagonist). Neonatal haemolysis and methaemoglobinaemia in third trimester; fear of increased risk of kernicterus in neonates appears to be unfounded.
- **BREAST FEEDING** Small risk of kernicterus in jaundiced infants and of haemolysis in G6PD-deficient infants (due to sulfamethoxazole).
- **HEPATIC IMPAIRMENT** Manufacturer advises avoid in severe liver disease.
- **RENAL IMPAIRMENT** Avoid if estimated glomerular filtration rate less than 15 mL/minute/1.73 m^2 and if plasma-sulfamethoxazole concentration cannot be monitored.
Dose adjustments Use half normal dose if estimated glomerular filtration rate 15–30 mL/minute/1.73 m^2.
Monitoring Plasma concentration monitoring may be required in patients with moderate to severe renal impairment; seek expert advice.
- **MONITORING REQUIREMENTS**
▸ Monitor blood counts on prolonged treatment.
▸ Plasma concentration monitoring may be required with high doses; seek expert advice.
- **DIRECTIONS FOR ADMINISTRATION**
▸ With intravenous use For intermittent *intravenous infusion*, may be further diluted in glucose 5% and 10% or sodium chloride 0.9%. Dilute contents of 1 ampoule (5 mL) to 125 mL, 2 ampoules (10 mL) to 250 mL or 3 ampoules (15 mL) to 500 mL; suggested duration of infusion 60–90 minutes (but may be adjusted according to fluid requirements); if fluid restriction necessary, 1 ampoule (5 mL) may be diluted with 75 mL glucose 5% and the required dose infused over max. 60 minutes; check container for haze or precipitant during administration. In severe fluid restriction may be given undiluted via a central venous line.
- **PRESCRIBING AND DISPENSING INFORMATION** Co-trimoxazole is a mixture of trimethoprim and sulfamethoxazole (sulphamethoxazole) in the proportions of 1 part to 5 parts.
For choice of antibacterial therapy, see Pneumocystis pneumonia p. 413.

- **MEDICINAL FORMS** There can be variation in the licensing of different medicines containing the same drug.

Solution for infusion

EXCIPIENTS: May contain Alcohol, propylene glycol, sulfites
ELECTROLYTES: May contain Sodium

▸ **Co-trimoxazole (Non-proprietary)**
Trimethoprim 16 mg per 1 ml, Sulfamethoxazole 80 mg per 1 ml Co-trimoxazole 80mg/400mg/5ml solution for infusion ampoules | 10 ampoule PoM £47.15 DT = £47.15

Oral suspension

CAUTIONARY AND ADVISORY LABELS 9

▸ **Co-trimoxazole (Non-proprietary)**
Trimethoprim 8 mg per 1 ml, Sulfamethoxazole 40 mg per 1 ml Co-trimoxazole 40mg/200mg/5ml oral suspension sugar free sugar-free | 100 ml PoM £9.96 DT = £9.96
Trimethoprim 16 mg per 1 ml, Sulfamethoxazole 80 mg per 1 ml Co-trimoxazole 80mg/400mg/5ml oral suspension | 100 ml PoM £10.95–£10.96 DT = £10.96

Tablet

CAUTIONARY AND ADVISORY LABELS 9

▸ Co-trimoxazole (Non-proprietary)

Trimethoprim 80 mg, Sulfamethoxazole 400 mg Co-trimoxazole 80mg/400mg tablets | 28 tablet PoM £15.50 DT = £1.96 | 100 tablet PoM £7.00–£10.91

Trimethoprim 160 mg, Sulfamethoxazole 800 mg Co-trimoxazole 160mg/800mg tablets | 100 tablet PoM £23.48 DT = £23.48

Sulfadiazine

26-May-2020

(Sulphadiazine)

- **DRUG ACTION** Sulfadiazine is a short-acting sulphonamide with bacteriostatic activity against a broad spectrum of organisms. The importance of the sulfonamides has decreased as a result of increasing bacterial resistance and their replacement by antibacterials which are generally more active and less toxic.

- **INDICATIONS AND DOSE**

Toxoplasmosis in pregnancy (in combination with pyrimethamine and folinic acid)

▸ BY MOUTH

▸ Child 12–17 years: 1 g 3 times a day until delivery

Congenital toxoplasmosis (in combination with pyrimethamine and folinic acid)

▸ BY MOUTH

▸ Neonate: 50 mg/kg twice daily for 12 months.

- **UNLICENSED USE** Not licensed for use in toxoplasmosis.

> **IMPORTANT SAFETY INFORMATION**
> SAFE PRACTICE
> Sulfadiazine has been confused with sulfasalazine; care must be taken to ensure the correct drug is prescribed and dispensed.

- **CONTRA-INDICATIONS** Acute porphyrias p. 652
- **CAUTIONS** Asthma · avoid in blood disorders · G6PD deficiency (risk of haemolytic anaemia) · maintain adequate fluid intake · neonates (risk of kernicterus) · predisposition to folate deficiency
- **INTERACTIONS** → Appendix 1: sulfonamides
- **SIDE-EFFECTS**

▸ **Rare or very rare** Haemolytic anaemia

▸ **Frequency not known** Agranulocytosis · aplastic anaemia · appetite decreased · ataxia · back pain · blood disorders · cough · crystalluria · cyanosis · depression · diarrhoea · dizziness · drowsiness · dyspnoea · eosinophilia · erythema nodosum · fatigue · fever · haematuria · hallucination · headache · hepatic disorders · hypoglycaemia · hypoprothrombinaemia · hypothyroidism · idiopathic intracranial hypertension · insomnia · kernicterus (in neonates) · leucopenia · meningitis aseptic · myocarditis · nausea · nephritis tubulointerstitial · nephrotoxicity · nerve disorders · neurological effects · neutropenia · oral disorders · pancreatitis · photosensitivity reaction · pseudomembranous enterocolitis · psychosis · renal impairment · renal tubular necrosis · respiratory disorders · seizure · serum sickness-like reaction · severe cutaneous adverse reactions (SCARs) · skin reactions · systemic lupus erythematosus (SLE) · thrombocytopenia · tinnitus · vasculitis · vertigo · vomiting

SIDE-EFFECTS, FURTHER INFORMATION Discontinue immediately if blood disorders (including leucopenia, thrombocytopenia, megaloblastic anaemia, eosinophilia) or rash (including Stevens-Johnson syndrome, toxic epidermal necrolysis) develop.

- **PREGNANCY** Risk of neonatal haemolysis and methaemoglobinaemia in third trimester; fear of increased risk of kernicterus in neonates appears to be unfounded.
- **BREAST FEEDING** Small risk of kernicterus in jaundiced infants and of haemolysis in G6PD-deficient infants.
- **HEPATIC IMPAIRMENT** Manufacturer advises caution in mild to moderate impairment; avoid in severe impairment or jaundice.
- **RENAL IMPAIRMENT** Use with caution in mild to moderate impairment; avoid in severe impairment; high risk of crystalluria.
- **MONITORING REQUIREMENTS** Monitor blood counts on prolonged treatment.

- **MEDICINAL FORMS** There can be variation in the licensing of different medicines containing the same drug. Forms available from special-order manufacturers include: oral suspension

Tablet

CAUTIONARY AND ADVISORY LABELS 9, 27

▸ Sulfadiazine (Non-proprietary)

Sulfadiazine 500 mg Sulfadiazine 500mg tablets | 56 tablet PoM £275.84 DT = £242.18

ANTIBACTERIALS › TETRACYCLINES AND RELATED DRUGS

Tetracyclines

Overview

The tetracyclines are broad-spectrum antibiotics whose value has decreased owing to increasing bacterial resistance. In children over 12 years of age they are useful for infections caused by chlamydia (trachoma, psittacosis, salpingitis, urethritis, and lymphogranuloma venereum), rickettsia (including Q-fever), brucella (doxycycline p. 381 with either streptomycin p. 334 or rifampicin p. 396), and the spirochaete, *Borrelia burgdorferi* (See Lyme disease). They are also used in respiratory and genital mycoplasma infections, in acne, in destructive (refractory) periodontal disease, in exacerbations of chronic respiratory diseases (because of their activity against *Haemophilus influenzae*), and for leptospirosis in penicillin hypersensitivity (as an alternative to erythromycin p. 355).

Microbiologically, there is little to choose between the various tetracyclines, the only exception being minocycline p. 383 which has a broader spectrum; it is active against *Neisseria meningitidis* and has been used for meningococcal prophylaxis but is no longer recommended because of side-effects including dizziness and vertigo. Compared to other tetracyclines, minocycline is associated with a greater risk of lupus-erythematosus-like syndrome. Minocycline sometimes causes irreversible pigmentation.

Tetracyclines have a role in the management of meticillin-resistant *Staphylococcus aureus* (MRSA) infections.

Tetracyclines

- **CAUTIONS** Myasthenia gravis (muscle weakness may be increased) · systemic lupus erythematosus (may be exacerbated)
- **SIDE-EFFECTS**

▸ **Common or very common** Angioedema · diarrhoea · headache · Henoch-Schönlein purpura · hypersensitivity · nausea · pericarditis · photosensitivity reaction · skin reactions · systemic lupus erythematosus exacerbated · vomiting

▸ **Rare or very rare** Appetite decreased · discolouration of thyroid gland · dysphagia · eosinophilia · fontanelle bulging (in infants) · gastrointestinal disorders · haemolytic anaemia · hepatic disorders · idiopathic

intracranial hypertension · increased risk of infection · neutropenia · oral disorders · pancreatitis · pseudomembranous enterocolitis · Stevens-Johnson syndrome · thrombocytopenia
- ▶ **Frequency not known** Dizziness · tooth discolouration

SIDE-EFFECTS, FURTHER INFORMATION Headache and visual disturbances may indicate benign intracranial hypertension (discontinue treatment if raised intracranial pressure develops).

- **PREGNANCY** Should **not** be given to pregnant women; effects on skeletal development have been documented in the first trimester in *animal* studies. Administration during the second or third trimester may cause discoloration of the child's teeth, and maternal hepatotoxicity has been reported with large parenteral doses.
- **BREAST FEEDING** Should **not** be given to women who are breast-feeding (although absorption and therefore discoloration of teeth in the infant is probably usually prevented by chelation with calcium in milk).
- **HEPATIC IMPAIRMENT** In general, manufacturers advise caution.

▸ 380

Demeclocycline hydrochloride

09-Apr-2020

- **INDICATIONS AND DOSE**

Susceptible infections (e.g. chlamydia, rickettsia and mycoplasma)

▶ BY MOUTH
- ▶ Child 12–17 years: 150 mg 4 times a day, alternatively 300 mg twice daily

- **CONTRA-INDICATIONS** Children under 12 years (deposition in growing bone and teeth, by binding to calcium, causes staining and occasionally dental hypoplasia)
- **CAUTIONS** Photosensitivity more common than with other tetracyclines
- **INTERACTIONS** → Appendix 1: tetracyclines
- **SIDE-EFFECTS**
- ▶ **Rare or very rare** Agranulocytosis · aplastic anaemia · hearing impairment · nephritis · severe cutaneous adverse reactions (SCARs)
- ▶ **Frequency not known** Intracranial pressure increased · muscle weakness · nephrogenic diabetes insipidus · vision disorders
- **HEPATIC IMPAIRMENT**

Dose adjustments Manufacturer advises maximum 1 g daily in divided doses.

- **RENAL IMPAIRMENT** May exacerbate renal failure and should **not** be given to patients with renal impairment.
- **PATIENT AND CARER ADVICE** Patients should be advised to avoid exposure to sunlight or sun lamps.

- **MEDICINAL FORMS** There can be variation in the licensing of different medicines containing the same drug. Forms available from special-order manufacturers include: tablet, oral suspension, oral solution

Tablet

- ▶ Demeclocycline hydrochloride (Non-proprietary)
  Demeclocycline hydrochloride 150 mg Demeclocycline 150mg tablets | 100 tablet [PoM] [X]

Capsule

CAUTIONARY AND ADVISORY LABELS 7, 9, 11, 23

- ▶ Demeclocycline hydrochloride (Non-proprietary)
  Demeclocycline hydrochloride 150 mg Demeclocycline 150mg capsules | 28 capsule [PoM] £200.66 DT = £200.66
- ▶ Ledermycin (Imported (Netherlands))
  Demeclocycline hydrochloride 300 mg Ledermycin 300mg capsules | 16 capsule [PoM] [X]

▸ 380

Doxycycline

18-May-2020

- **INDICATIONS AND DOSE**

Susceptible infections (e.g. chlamydia, rickettsia and mycoplasma)

▶ BY MOUTH USING IMMEDIATE-RELEASE MEDICINES
- ▶ Child 8–11 years (administered on expert advice) (body-weight up to 45 kg): Initially 4.4 mg/kg daily in 1–2 divided doses for 1 day, then maintenance 2.2 mg/kg daily in 1–2 divided doses
- ▶ Child 8–11 years (administered on expert advice) (body-weight 45 kg and above): Initially 200 mg daily in 1–2 divided doses for 1 day, then maintenance 100 mg daily
- ▶ Child 12–17 years: Initially 200 mg daily in 1–2 divided doses for 1 day, then maintenance 100 mg daily

Severe infections (including refractory urinary-tract infections)

▶ BY MOUTH USING IMMEDIATE-RELEASE MEDICINES
- ▶ Child 8–11 years (administered on expert advice) (body-weight up to 45 kg): Initially 4.4 mg/kg daily in 1–2 divided doses for 1 day, then maintenance 2.2–4.4 mg/kg daily in 1–2 divided doses
- ▶ Child 8–11 years (administered on expert advice) (body-weight 45 kg and above): 200 mg daily
- ▶ Child 12–17 years: 200 mg daily

Acute sinusitis | Acute cough [if systemically very unwell or at higher risk of complications] | Community-acquired pneumonia

▶ BY MOUTH USING IMMEDIATE-RELEASE MEDICINES
- ▶ Child 12–17 years: Initially 200 mg daily for 1 dose, then maintenance 100 mg once daily for 5 days in total

Acute exacerbation of bronchiectasis

▶ BY MOUTH USING IMMEDIATE-RELEASE MEDICINES
- ▶ Child 12–17 years: Initially 200 mg daily for 1 dose, then maintenance 100 mg once daily for 7–14 days in total

Acne

▶ BY MOUTH USING IMMEDIATE-RELEASE MEDICINES
- ▶ Child 12–17 years: 100 mg once daily

Early syphilis

▶ BY MOUTH USING IMMEDIATE-RELEASE MEDICINES
- ▶ Child 12–17 years: 100 mg twice daily for 14 days

Late latent syphilis

▶ BY MOUTH USING IMMEDIATE-RELEASE MEDICINES
- ▶ Child 12–17 years: 100 mg twice daily for 28 days

Uncomplicated genital chlamydia | Non-gonococcal urethritis

▶ BY MOUTH USING IMMEDIATE-RELEASE MEDICINES
- ▶ Child 12–17 years: 100 mg twice daily for 7 days

Pelvic inflammatory disease

▶ BY MOUTH USING IMMEDIATE-RELEASE MEDICINES
- ▶ Child 12–17 years: 100 mg twice daily for 14 days

Lyme disease [erythema migrans and/or non-focal symptoms] | Lyme disease [affecting cranial nerves or peripheral nervous system] | Lyme carditis

▶ BY MOUTH USING IMMEDIATE-RELEASE MEDICINES
- ▶ Child 9–11 years (administered on expert advice) (body-weight up to 45 kg): Initially 5 mg/kg in 2 divided doses on day 1, then 2.5 mg/kg daily in 1–2 divided doses for a total of 21 days, increased if necessary up to 5 mg/kg daily for 21 days, increased dose used in severe infections; maximum 200 mg per day
- ▶ Child 9–11 years (administered on expert advice) (body-weight 45 kg and above): 200 mg daily in 1–2 divided doses for 21 days
- ▶ Child 12–17 years (administered on expert advice): 200 mg daily in 1–2 divided doses for 21 days

continued →

Lyme disease [affecting central nervous system]

▶ BY MOUTH USING IMMEDIATE-RELEASE MEDICINES

▸ Child 9-11 years (administered on expert advice) (body-weight up to 45 kg): Initially 5 mg/kg in 2 divided doses on day 1, then 2.5 mg/kg daily in 1–2 divided doses for a total of 21 days, increased if necessary up to 5 mg/kg daily, increased dose used in severe infections

▸ Child 9-11 years (administered on expert advice) (body-weight 45 kg and above): 400 mg daily in 1–2 divided doses for 21 days

▸ Child 12-17 years (administered on expert advice): 400 mg daily in 1–2 divided doses for 21 days

Lyme arthritis | Acrodermatitis chronica atrophicans

▶ BY MOUTH USING IMMEDIATE-RELEASE MEDICINES

▸ Child 9-11 years (administered on expert advice) (body-weight up to 45 kg): Initially 5 mg/kg in 2 divided doses on day 1, then 2.5 mg/kg daily in 1–2 divided doses for a total of 28 days, increased if necessary up to 5 mg/kg daily for 28 days, increased dose used in severe infections; maximum 200 mg per day

▸ Child 9-11 years (administered on expert advice) (body-weight 45 kg and above): 200 mg daily in 1–2 divided doses for 28 days

▸ Child 12-17 years (administered on expert advice): 200 mg daily in 1–2 divided doses for 28 days

Anthrax (treatment or post-exposure prophylaxis)

▶ BY MOUTH USING IMMEDIATE-RELEASE MEDICINES

▸ Child 1 month–11 years: 2.5 mg/kg twice daily (max. per dose 100 mg twice daily), only to be used in children under 12 years if alternative antibacterial cannot be given

▸ Child 12-17 years: 100 mg twice daily

Prophylaxis of malaria

▶ BY MOUTH USING IMMEDIATE-RELEASE MEDICINES

▸ Child 12-17 years: 100 mg once daily, to be started 1–2 days before entering endemic area and continued for 4 weeks after leaving, can be used for up to 2 years

Adjunct to quinine in treatment of *Plasmodium falciparum* malaria

▶ BY MOUTH USING IMMEDIATE-RELEASE MEDICINES

▸ Child 12-17 years: 200 mg daily for 7 days

Periodontitis (as an adjunct to gingival scaling and root planing)

▶ BY MOUTH USING IMMEDIATE-RELEASE MEDICINES

▸ Child 12-17 years: 20 mg twice daily for 3 months

Rocky Mountain spotted fever

▶ BY MOUTH USING DISPERSIBLE TABLETS

▸ Child (administered on expert advice) (body-weight up to 45 kg): 2.2 mg/kg twice daily, continue treatment for at least 3 days after fever subsides, minimum treatment duration is 5–7 days

▸ Child (administered on expert advice) (body-weight 45 kg and above): 100 mg twice daily, continue treatment for at least 3 days after fever subsides, minimum treatment duration is 5–7 days

● UNLICENSED USE Doxycycline may be used as detailed below, although these situations are considered outside the scope of its licence:

- [EvGr] Duration of treatment for acute sinusitis;
- Lyme disease ⟨A⟩;
- treatment or post-exposure prophylaxis of anthrax;
- malaria prophylaxis during pregnancy;
- recurrent aphthous ulceration.

● CAUTIONS Alcohol dependence · children 8–11 years—use only in acute or severe infections when there are no adequate alternatives (deposition in growing bone and teeth, by binding to calcium, causes staining and occasionally dental hypoplasia) · children under 8 years—use only in severe or life-threatening conditions (e.g. Rocky Mountain spotted fever) when there are no adequate alternatives (deposition in growing bone and teeth, by binding to calcium, causes staining and occasionally dental hypoplasia)

● INTERACTIONS → Appendix 1: tetracyclines

● SIDE-EFFECTS

▶ **Common or very common** Dyspnoea · hypotension · peripheral oedema · tachycardia

▶ **Uncommon** Gastrointestinal discomfort

▶ **Rare or very rare** Antibiotic associated colitis · anxiety · arthralgia · flushing · intracranial pressure increased with papilloedema · Jarisch-Herxheimer reaction · myalgia · photoonycholysis · severe cutaneous adverse reactions (SCARs) · skin hyperpigmentation (long term use) · tinnitus · vision disorders

● PREGNANCY When travel to malarious areas is unavoidable during pregnancy, doxycycline can be used for malaria prophylaxis if other regimens are unsuitable, and if the entire course of doxycycline can be completed before 15 weeks' gestation.

● RENAL IMPAIRMENT Use with caution (avoid excessive doses).

● MONITORING REQUIREMENTS When used for periodontitis, monitor for superficial fungal infection, particularly if predisposition to oral candidiasis.

● DIRECTIONS FOR ADMINISTRATION Capsules and Tablets should be swallowed whole with plenty of fluid, while sitting or standing. Capsules should be taken during meals.

● PRESCRIBING AND DISPENSING INFORMATION For choice of antibacterial therapy, see Anthrax p. 391, Genital system infections, antibacterial therapy p. 325, Lyme disease p. 391, Malaria, prophylaxis p. 420, Malaria, treatment p. 426, Nose infections, antibacterial therapy p. 326, Oropharyngeal infections, antibacterial therapy p. 761, Respiratory system infections, antibacterial therapy p. 327, Urinary-tract infections p. 400.

● PATIENT AND CARER ADVICE Counselling on administration advised.

Photosensitivity Patients should be advised to avoid exposure to sunlight or sun lamps.

● PROFESSION SPECIFIC INFORMATION

Dental practitioners' formulary

Doxycycline Capsules 100 mg may be prescribed. Dispersible tablets may be prescribed as Dispersible Doxycycline Tablets. Tablets may be prescribed as Doxycycline Tablets 20 mg.

● MEDICINAL FORMS There can be variation in the licensing of different medicines containing the same drug. Forms available from special-order manufacturers include: oral suspension, oral solution

Tablet

CAUTIONARY AND ADVISORY LABELS 6, 11, 27

▸ **Doxycycline (Non-proprietary)**

Doxycycline (as Doxycycline hyclate) 100 mg Doxycycline 100mg tablets | 10 tablet [PoM] £1.64

▸ **Periostat** (Alliance Pharmaceuticals Ltd)

Doxycycline (as Doxycycline hyclate) 20 mg Periostat 20mg tablets | 56 tablet [PoM] £17.30 DT = £17.30

Dispersible tablet

CAUTIONARY AND ADVISORY LABELS 6, 9, 11, 13

▸ **Vibramycin-D** (Pfizer Ltd)

Doxycycline (as Doxycycline monohydrate) 100 mg Vibramycin-D 100mg dispersible tablets sugar-free | 8 tablet [PoM] £4.91 DT = £4.91

Capsule

CAUTIONARY AND ADVISORY LABELS 6, 9, 11, 27

▸ **Doxycycline (Non-proprietary)**

Doxycycline (as Doxycycline hyclate) 50 mg Doxycycline 50mg capsules | 28 capsule [PoM] £4.00 DT = £2.09

Doxycycline (as Doxycycline hyclate) 100 mg Doxycycline 100mg capsules | 8 capsule [PoM] £3.00 DT = £1.43 | 14 capsule [PoM] £5.25 | 50 capsule [PoM] £8.94–£19.00

380

Lymecycline

14-Nov-2018

- **INDICATIONS AND DOSE**

Susceptible infections (e.g. chlamydia, rickettsia and mycoplasma)

▶ BY MOUTH

▶ Child 12–17 years: 408 mg twice daily, increased to 1.224–1.632 g daily, (in severe infection)

Acne

▶ BY MOUTH

▶ Child 12–17 years: 408 mg daily for at least 8 weeks

- **CONTRA-INDICATIONS** Children under 8 years (deposition in growing bone and teeth, by binding to calcium, causes staining and occasionally dental hypoplasia)
- **INTERACTIONS** → Appendix 1: tetracyclines
- **SIDE-EFFECTS**

▶ **Common or very common** Gastrointestinal discomfort

▶ **Frequency not known** Visual impairment

- **RENAL IMPAIRMENT** May exacerbate renal failure and should **not** be given to patients with renal impairment.

- **MEDICINAL FORMS** There can be variation in the licensing of different medicines containing the same drug.

Capsule

CAUTIONARY AND ADVISORY LABELS 6, 9

▶ Lymecycline (Non-proprietary)

Lymecycline 408 mg Lymecycline 408mg capsules | 28 capsule PoM £8.25 DT = £4.57 | 56 capsule PoM £11.53–£13.80

▶ Tetralysal (Galderma (UK) Ltd)

Lymecycline 408 mg Tetralysal 300 capsules | 28 capsule PoM £6.95 DT = £4.57 | 56 capsule PoM £11.53

380

Minocycline

09-Apr-2020

- **INDICATIONS AND DOSE**

Susceptible infections (e.g. chlamydia, rickettsia and mycoplasma)

▶ BY MOUTH USING IMMEDIATE-RELEASE MEDICINES

▶ Child 12–17 years: 100 mg twice daily

Acne

▶ BY MOUTH USING IMMEDIATE-RELEASE MEDICINES

▶ Child 12–17 years: 100 mg once daily, alternatively 50 mg twice daily

▶ BY MOUTH USING MODIFIED-RELEASE MEDICINES

▶ Child 12–17 years: 100 mg daily

- **CONTRA-INDICATIONS** Children under 12 years (deposition in growing bone and teeth, by binding to calcium, causes staining and occasionally dental hypoplasia)
- **CAUTIONS** Systemic lupus erythematosus
- **INTERACTIONS** → Appendix 1: tetracyclines
- **SIDE-EFFECTS**

▶ **Rare or very rare** Acute kidney injury · hearing impairment · respiratory disorders · tinnitus

▶ **Frequency not known** Alopecia · antibiotic associated colitis · arthralgia · ataxia · breast secretion · conjunctival discolouration · drug reaction with eosinophilia and systemic symptoms (DRESS) · dyspepsia · hyperbilirubinaemia · hyperhidrosis · polyarteritis nodosa · sensation abnormal · tear discolouration · tongue discolouration · vertigo

- **RENAL IMPAIRMENT** Use with caution (avoid excessive doses).
- **MONITORING REQUIREMENTS** If treatment continued for longer than 6 months, monitor every 3 months for hepatotoxicity, pigmentation and for systemic lupus erythematosus—discontinue if these develop or if pre-existing systemic lupus erythematosus worsens.
- **DIRECTIONS FOR ADMINISTRATION** Tablets or capsules should be swallowed whole with plenty of fluid while sitting or standing.
- **PATIENT AND CARER ADVICE** Counselling on administration advised (posture).
- **LESS SUITABLE FOR PRESCRIBING** Less suitable for prescribing (compared with other tetracyclines, minocycline is associated with a greater risk of lupus-erythematosus-like syndrome; it sometimes causes irreversible pigmentation).

- **MEDICINAL FORMS** There can be variation in the licensing of different medicines containing the same drug. Forms available from special-order manufacturers include: oral suspension, oral solution

Tablet

CAUTIONARY AND ADVISORY LABELS 6, 9

▶ Minocycline (Non-proprietary)

Minocycline (as Minocycline hydrochloride) 50 mg Minocycline 50mg tablets | 28 tablet PoM £8.50 DT = £6.19

Minocycline (as Minocycline hydrochloride) 100 mg Minocycline 100mg tablets | 28 tablet PoM £14.50 DT = £14.18

Modified-release capsule

CAUTIONARY AND ADVISORY LABELS 6, 25

▶ Acnamino MR (Dexcel-Pharma Ltd)

Minocycline (as Minocycline hydrochloride) 100 mg Acnamino MR 100mg capsules | 56 capsule PoM £21.14 DT = £20.08

▶ Minocin MR (Mylan)

Minocycline (as Minocycline hydrochloride) 100 mg Minocin MR 100mg capsules | 56 capsule PoM £20.08 DT = £20.08

Capsule

CAUTIONARY AND ADVISORY LABELS 6, 9

▶ Aknemin (Almirall Ltd)

Minocycline (as Minocycline hydrochloride) 100 mg Aknemin 100mg capsules | 28 capsule PoM £13.09 DT = £13.09

380

Oxytetracycline

14-Nov-2018

- **INDICATIONS AND DOSE**

Susceptible infections (e.g. chlamydia, rickettsia and mycoplasma)

▶ BY MOUTH

▶ Child 12–17 years: 250–500 mg 4 times a day

Acne

▶ BY MOUTH

▶ Child 12–17 years: 500 mg twice daily for at least 3 months, if there is no improvement after the first 3 months another oral antibacterial should be used, maximum improvement usually occurs after 4 to 6 months but in more severe cases treatment may need to be continued for 2 years or longer

- **CONTRA-INDICATIONS** Children under 12 years (deposition in growing bone and teeth, by binding to calcium, causes staining and occasionally dental hypoplasia)
- **INTERACTIONS** → Appendix 1: tetracyclines
- **SIDE-EFFECTS** Gastrointestinal discomfort · renal impairment
- **HEPATIC IMPAIRMENT**

Dose adjustments Manufacturer advises avoid in high doses.

- **RENAL IMPAIRMENT** May exacerbate renal failure and should **not** be given to patients with renal impairment.
- **PROFESSION SPECIFIC INFORMATION**

Dental practitioners' formulary

Oxytetracycline Tablets may be prescribed.

- **MEDICINAL FORMS** There can be variation in the licensing of different medicines containing the same drug. Forms available from special-order manufacturers include: oral suspension

Tablet

CAUTIONARY AND ADVISORY LABELS 7, 9, 23

▸ Oxytetracycline (Non-proprietary)
Oxytetracycline (as Oxytetracycline dihydrate)
250 mg Oxytetracycline 250mg tablets | 28 tablet PoM £6.00 DT = £3.48

F 380

Tetracycline

17-Dec-2019

- **INDICATIONS AND DOSE**

Susceptible infections (e.g. chlamydia, rickettsia, mycoplasma)

▸ BY MOUTH

▸ Child 12–17 years: 250 mg 4 times a day, increased if necessary to 500 mg 3–4 times a day, increased dose used in severe infections

Acne

▸ BY MOUTH

▸ Child 12–17 years: 500 mg twice daily for at least 3 months, if there is no improvement after the first 3 months another oral antibacterial should be used, maximum improvement usually occurs after 4 to 6 months but in more severe cases treatment may need to be continued for 2 years or longer

Non-gonococcal urethritis

▸ BY MOUTH

▸ Child 12–17 years: 500 mg 4 times a day for 7–14 days (21 days if failure or relapse after first course)

- **CONTRA-INDICATIONS** Children under 12 years (deposition in growing bone and teeth, by binding to calcium, causes staining and occasionally dental hypoplasia)
- **INTERACTIONS** → Appendix 1: tetracyclines
- **SIDE-EFFECTS**

▸ **Rare or very rare** Agranulocytosis · aplastic anaemia · nephritis · renal impairment

▸ **Frequency not known** Gastrointestinal discomfort · toxic epidermal necrolysis

- **HEPATIC IMPAIRMENT**

Dose adjustments Manufacturer advises avoid in high doses.

- **RENAL IMPAIRMENT** May exacerbate renal failure and should **not** be given to patients with renal impairment.
- **DIRECTIONS FOR ADMINISTRATION** Tablets should be swallowed whole with plenty of fluid while sitting or standing.
- **PATIENT AND CARER ADVICE** Counselling on administration advised.
- **PROFESSION SPECIFIC INFORMATION**

Dental practitioners' formulary
Tetracycline Tablets may be prescribed.

- **MEDICINAL FORMS** There can be variation in the licensing of different medicines containing the same drug. Forms available from special-order manufacturers include: capsule, oral solution

Tablet

CAUTIONARY AND ADVISORY LABELS 7, 9, 23

▸ Tetracycline (Non-proprietary)
Tetracycline hydrochloride 250 mg Tetracycline 250mg tablets | 28 tablet PoM £6.75 DT = £4.15

Tigecycline

06-Apr-2020

- **DRUG ACTION** Tigecycline is a glycylcycline antibacterial structurally related to the tetracyclines. Tigecycline is active against Gram-positive and Gram-negative bacteria, including tetracycline-resistant organisms, and some anaerobes. It is also active against meticillin-resistant *Staphylococcus aureus* and vancomycin-resistant enterococci, but *Pseudomonas aeruginosa* and many strains of *Proteus spp* are resistant to tigecycline.

- **INDICATIONS AND DOSE**

Complicated skin and soft tissue infections (when other antibiotics are not suitable) | Complicated intra-abdominal infections (when other antibiotics are not suitable)

▸ BY INTRAVENOUS INFUSION

▸ Child 8–11 years (under expert supervision): 1.2 mg/kg every 12 hours (max. per dose 50 mg) for 5–14 days

▸ Child 12–17 years (under expert supervision): 50 mg every 12 hours for 5–14 days

- **CONTRA-INDICATIONS** Children under 8 years (deposition in growing bone and teeth, by binding to calcium, causes staining and occasionally dental hypoplasia) · Diabetic foot infections
- **CAUTIONS** Cholestasis
- **INTERACTIONS** → Appendix 1: tigecycline
- **SIDE-EFFECTS**

▸ **Common or very common** Abscess · appetite decreased · diarrhoea · dizziness · gastrointestinal discomfort · headache · healing impaired · hyperbilirubinaemia · hypoglycaemia · hypoproteinaemia · increased risk of infection · nausea · sepsis · skin reactions · vomiting

▸ **Uncommon** Hepatic disorders · pancreatitis · thrombocytopenia · thrombophlebitis

▸ **Frequency not known** Acidosis · azotaemia · hyperphosphataemia · hypofibrinogenaemia · idiopathic intracranial hypertension · photosensitivity reaction · pseudomembranous enterocolitis · severe cutaneous adverse reactions (SCARs) · tooth discolouration

SIDE-EFFECTS, FURTHER INFORMATION Side-effects similar to those of the tetracyclines can potentially occur.

- **ALLERGY AND CROSS-SENSITIVITY** Contra-indicated in patients hypersensitive to tetracyclines.
- **PREGNANCY** Tetracyclines should **not** be given to pregnant women; effects on skeletal development have been documented in the first trimester in *animal* studies. Administration during the second or third trimester may cause discoloration of the child's teeth, and maternal hepatotoxicity has been reported with large parenteral doses.
- **BREAST FEEDING** Manufacturer advises avoid—present in milk in *animal* studies.
- **HEPATIC IMPAIRMENT** Manufacturer advises caution in severe impairment.

Dose adjustments Manufacturer advises dose reduction of 50% in severe impairment.

- **MONITORING REQUIREMENTS** Manufacturer advises monitor liver function tests, amylase, lipase, coagulation and haematology parameters before starting treatment, and regularly during treatment.
- **DIRECTIONS FOR ADMINISTRATION** For *intravenous infusion* (*Tygacil*®), give intermittently *in* Glucose 5% *or* Sodium Chloride 0.9%. Reconstitute each vial with 5.3 mL infusion fluid to produce a 10 mg/mL solution; dilute requisite dose in 100 mL infusion fluid; give over 30–60 minutes (preferably 60 minutes).

- **PATIENT AND CARER ADVICE**
Driving and skilled tasks Manufacturer advises patients and carers should be cautioned on the effects on driving and performance of skilled tasks—increased risk of dizziness.

- **MEDICINAL FORMS** There can be variation in the licensing of different medicines containing the same drug.

Powder for solution for infusion

- Tigecycline (Non-proprietary)
Tigecycline 50 mg Tigecycline 50mg powder for solution for infusion vials | 10 vial PoM £290.79 (Hospital only)
- Tygacil (Pfizer Ltd)
Tigecycline 50 mg Tygacil 50mg powder for solution for infusion vials | 10 vial PoM £323.10 (Hospital only)

ANTIBACTERIALS > OTHER

Chloramphenicol

13-May-2020

- **DRUG ACTION** Chloramphenicol is a potent broad-spectrum antibiotic.

- **INDICATIONS AND DOSE**

Life threatening infections particularly those caused by *Haemophilus influenzae* | Typhoid fever

- BY MOUTH, OR BY INTRAVENOUS INJECTION, OR BY INTRAVENOUS INFUSION
- Child: 12.5 mg/kg every 6 hours, dose may be doubled in severe infections such as septicaemia, meningitis and epiglottitis providing plasma-chloramphenicol concentrations are measured and high doses reduced as soon as indicated
- BY INTRAVENOUS INJECTION
- Neonate up to 14 days: 12.5 mg/kg twice daily, doses should be checked carefully as overdosage can be fatal.
- Neonate 14 days to 28 days: 12.5 mg/kg 2–4 times a day, doses should be checked carefully as overdosage can be fatal.

Cystic fibrosis for the treatment of respiratory *Burkholderia cepacia* infection resistant to other antibacterials

- BY MOUTH, OR BY INTRAVENOUS INFUSION, OR BY INTRAVENOUS INJECTION
- Child: (consult product literature)

- **CONTRA-INDICATIONS** Acute porphyrias p. 652
- **CAUTIONS** Avoid repeated courses and prolonged treatment
- **INTERACTIONS** → Appendix 1: chloramphenicol
- **SIDE-EFFECTS**
- **Rare or very rare**
- With parenteral use Aplastic anaemia (reversible or irreversible, with reports of resulting leukaemia)
- **Frequency not known**
- With oral use Bone marrow disorders · circulatory collapse · diarrhoea · enterocolitis · nausea · optic neuritis · oral disorders · ototoxicity · vomiting
- With parenteral use Agranulocytosis · bone marrow disorders · depression · diarrhoea · dry mouth · fungal superinfection · headache · nausea · nerve disorders · thrombocytopenic purpura · urticaria · vision disorders · vomiting

SIDE-EFFECTS, FURTHER INFORMATION Associated with serious haematological side-effects when given systemically and should therefore be reserved for the treatment of life-threatening infections.

Grey syndrome Grey baby syndrome (abdominal distension, pallid cyanosis, circulatory collapse) may follow excessive doses in neonates with immature hepatic metabolism.

- **PREGNANCY** Manufacturer advises avoid; neonatal 'grey-baby syndrome' if used in third trimester.
- **BREAST FEEDING** Manufacturer advises avoid; use another antibiotic; may cause bone-marrow toxicity in infant; concentration in milk usually insufficient to cause 'grey syndrome'.
- **HEPATIC IMPAIRMENT** Manufacturer advises caution (increased risk of bone-marrow depression)—monitor plasma-chloramphenicol concentration.
Dose adjustments Manufacturer advises consider dose reduction.
Monitoring Monitor plasma-chloramphenicol concentration in hepatic impairment.
- **RENAL IMPAIRMENT** Avoid in severe renal impairment unless no alternative; dose-related depression of haematopoiesis.
- **MONITORING REQUIREMENTS**
- Plasma concentration monitoring preferred in those under 4 years of age.
- Recommended peak plasma concentration (approx. 2 hours after administration by mouth, intravenous injection or infusion) 10–25 mg/litre; pre-dose ('trough') concentration should not exceed 15 mg/litre. Blood counts required before and periodically during treatment.
- In neonates Plasma concentration monitoring required in neonates. Grey baby syndrome may follow excessive doses in neonates with immature hepatic metabolism.
- **DIRECTIONS FOR ADMINISTRATION**
- With intravenous use Displacement value may be significant for injection, consult local guidelines. For intermittent intravenous infusion, dilute reconstituted solution further in glucose 5% *or* sodium chloride 0.9%.

- **MEDICINAL FORMS** There can be variation in the licensing of different medicines containing the same drug.

Powder for solution for injection

ELECTROLYTES: May contain Sodium

- **Chloramphenicol (Non-proprietary)**
Chloramphenicol (as Chloramphenicol sodium succinate)
1 gram Chloramphenicol 1g powder for solution for injection vials | 1 vial PoM £88.00 DT = £88.00

Capsule

- **Chloramphenicol (Non-proprietary)**
Chloramphenicol 250 mg Chloramphenicol 250mg capsules | 60 capsule PoM £377.00 DT = £377.00

Daptomycin

21-Feb-2019

- **DRUG ACTION** Daptomycin is a lipopeptide antibacterial with a spectrum of activity similar to vancomycin but its efficacy against enterococci has not been established. It needs to be given with other antibacterials for mixed infections involving Gram-negative bacteria and some anaerobes.

- **INDICATIONS AND DOSE**

Complicated skin and soft-tissue infections caused by Gram-positive bacteria

- BY INTRAVENOUS INFUSION
- Child 12–23 months: 10 mg/kg once daily for up to 14 days, alternatively 12 mg/kg once daily, higher dose only if associated with *Staphylococcus aureus* bacteraemia—duration of treatment in accordance with risk of complications in individual patients
- Child 2–6 years: 9 mg/kg once daily for up to 14 days, alternatively 12 mg/kg once daily, higher dose only if associated with *Staphylococcus aureus* bacteraemia—duration of treatment in accordance with risk of complications in individual patients
- Child 7–11 years: 7 mg/kg once daily for up to 14 days, alternatively 9 mg/kg once daily, higher

continued →

5 Infection

dose only if associated with *Staphylococcus aureus* bacteraemia—duration of treatment in accordance with risk of complications in individual patients
- Child 12–17 years: 5 mg/kg once daily for up to 14 days, alternatively 7 mg/kg once daily, higher dose only if associated with *Staphylococcus aureus* bacteraemia—duration of treatment in accordance with risk of complications in individual patients

- **CAUTIONS** Obesity (limited information on safety and efficacy)
- **INTERACTIONS** → Appendix 1: daptomycin
- **SIDE-EFFECTS**
- **Common or very common** Anaemia · anxiety · asthenia · constipation · diarrhoea · dizziness · fever · flatulence · gastrointestinal discomfort · headache · hypertension · hypotension · increased risk of infection · insomnia · nausea · pain · skin reactions · vomiting
- **Uncommon** Appetite decreased · arrhythmias · arthralgia · electrolyte imbalance · eosinophilia · flushing · glossitis · hyperglycaemia · muscle weakness · myalgia · myopathy · paraesthesia · renal impairment · taste altered · thrombocytosis · tremor · vertigo
- **Rare or very rare** Jaundice
- **Frequency not known** Acute generalised exanthematous pustulosis (AGEP) · antibiotic associated colitis · chills · cough · infusion related reaction · peripheral neuropathy · respiratory disorders · syncope

SIDE-EFFECTS, FURTHER INFORMATION If unexplained muscle pain, tenderness, weakness, or cramps develop during treatment, measure creatine kinase every 2 days; discontinue if unexplained muscular symptoms and creatine elevated markedly.

- **PREGNANCY** Manufacturer advises use only if potential benefit outweighs risk—no information available.
- **BREAST FEEDING** Present in milk in small amounts, but absorption from gastrointestinal tract negligible.
- **HEPATIC IMPAIRMENT** Manufacturer advises caution in severe impairment—no information available.
- **RENAL IMPAIRMENT** Manufacturer advises the dosage regimen has not been established—use with caution and monitor renal function regularly.
- **MONITORING REQUIREMENTS**
- Manufacturer advises monitor plasma creatine phosphokinase (CPK) before treatment and then at least weekly during treatment; monitor CPK more frequently in patients at higher risk of developing myopathy, including those with renal impairment, taking other drugs associated with myopathy, or if CPK elevated more than 5 times upper limit of normal before treatment.
- Manufacturer advises monitor renal function regularly during concomitant administration of potentially nephrotoxic drugs.
- **EFFECT ON LABORATORY TESTS** Interference with assay for prothrombin time and INR—take blood sample immediately before daptomycin dose.
- **DIRECTIONS FOR ADMINISTRATION** For *intravenous infusion*, manufacturer advises give intermittently in Sodium Chloride 0.9%; reconstitute with Sodium Chloride 0.9% (350 mg in 7 mL, 500 mg in 10 mL); gently rotate vial without shaking; allow to stand for at least 10 minutes then rotate gently to dissolve; dilute requisite dose in 50 mL infusion fluid and give over 60 minutes for children aged 1–6 years and over 30 minutes for children aged 7–17 years.
- **HANDLING AND STORAGE** Manufacturer advises store in a refrigerator (2–8 °C)—consult product literature for further information regarding storage after reconstitution and dilution.

- **MEDICINAL FORMS** There can be variation in the licensing of different medicines containing the same drug.

Powder for solution for infusion

- Daptomycin (Non-proprietary)
  Daptomycin 350 mg Daptomycin 350mg powder for solution for infusion vials | 1 vial PoM £60.00–£62.00 (Hospital only)
  Daptomycin 500 mg Daptomycin 500mg powder for solution for infusion vials | 1 vial PoM £88.00–£88.57 (Hospital only)
- Cubicin (Merck Sharp & Dohme Ltd)
  Daptomycin 350 mg Cubicin 350mg powder for concentrate for solution for infusion vials | 1 vial PoM £62.00 (Hospital only)
  Daptomycin 500 mg Cubicin 500mg powder for concentrate for solution for infusion vials | 1 vial PoM £88.57 (Hospital only)

Fosfomycin

11-May-2020

- **DRUG ACTION** Fosfomycin, a phosphonic acid antibacterial, is active against a range of Gram-positive and Gram-negative bacteria including *Staphylococcus aureus* and Enterobacteriaceae.

- **INDICATIONS AND DOSE**

Acute uncomplicated lower urinary-tract infections (in females)

▶ BY MOUTH USING GRANULES
- Child 12–17 years (female): 3 g for 1 dose.

Osteomyelitis when first-line treatments are inappropriate or ineffective | Hospital-acquired lower respiratory-tract infections when first-line treatments are inappropriate or ineffective

▶ BY INTRAVENOUS INFUSION
- Neonate up to 40 weeks corrected gestational age: 100 mg/kg daily in 2 divided doses.
- Neonate 40 weeks to 44 weeks corrected gestational age: 200 mg/kg daily in 3 divided doses.
- Child 1–11 months (body-weight up to 10 kg): 200–300 mg/kg daily in 3 divided doses, consider using the high-dose regimen in severe infection, particularly when suspected or known to be caused by less sensitive organisms
- Child 1–11 years (body-weight 10–39 kg): 200–400 mg/kg daily in 3–4 divided doses, consider using the high-dose regimen in severe infection, particularly when suspected or known to be caused by less sensitive organisms
- Child 12–17 years (body-weight 40 kg and above): 12–24 g daily in 2–3 divided doses (max. per dose 8 g), use the high-dose regimen in severe infection, particularly when suspected or known to be caused by less sensitive organisms

Complicated urinary-tract infections when first-line treatment ineffective or inappropriate

▶ BY INTRAVENOUS INFUSION
- Neonate up to 40 weeks corrected gestational age: 100 mg/kg daily in 2 divided doses.
- Neonate 40 weeks to 44 weeks corrected gestational age: 200 mg/kg daily in 3 divided doses.
- Child 1–11 months (body-weight up to 10 kg): 200–300 mg/kg daily in 3 divided doses, consider using the high-dose regimen in severe infection, particularly when suspected or known to be caused by less sensitive organisms
- Child 1–11 years (body-weight 10–39 kg): 200–400 mg/kg daily in 3–4 divided doses, consider using the high-dose regimen in severe infection, particularly when suspected or known to be caused by less sensitive organisms

- Child 12-17 years (body-weight 40 kg and above): 12–16 g daily in 2–3 divided doses (max. per dose 8 g), use the high-dose regimen in severe infection, particularly when suspected or known to be caused by less sensitive organisms

Bacterial meningitis when first-line treatment ineffective or inappropriate

▶ BY INTRAVENOUS INFUSION

- Neonate up to 40 weeks corrected gestational age: 100 mg/kg daily in 2 divided doses.
- Neonate 40 weeks to 44 weeks corrected gestational age: 200 mg/kg daily in 3 divided doses.
- Child 1-11 months (body-weight up to 10 kg): 200–300 mg/kg daily in 3 divided doses, consider using the high-dose regimen in severe infection, particularly when suspected or known to be caused by less sensitive organisms
- Child 1-11 years (body-weight 10-39 kg): 200–400 mg/kg daily in 3–4 divided doses, consider using the high-dose regimen in severe infection, particularly when suspected or known to be caused by less sensitive organisms
- Child 12-17 years (body-weight 40 kg and above): 16–24 g daily in 3–4 divided doses (max. per dose 8 g), use the high-dose regimen in severe infection suspected or known to be caused by less sensitive organisms

● CAUTIONS

- With intravenous use Cardiac insufficiency · hyperaldosteronism · hypernatraemia · hypertension · pulmonary oedema

● SIDE-EFFECTS

GENERAL SIDE-EFFECTS

- **Common or very common** Abdominal pain · diarrhoea · headache · nausea · vomiting
- **Uncommon** Skin reactions
- **Frequency not known** Antibiotic associated colitis

SPECIFIC SIDE-EFFECTS

- **Common or very common**
  - With oral use Dizziness · vulvovaginal infection
- **Uncommon**
  - With parenteral use Appetite decreased · dyspnoea · electrolyte imbalance · fatigue · oedema · taste altered · vertigo
- **Rare or very rare**
  - With parenteral use Bone marrow disorders · eosinophilia · hepatic disorders · visual impairment
- **Frequency not known**
  - With parenteral use Agranulocytosis · asthmatic attack · confusion · leucopenia · neutropenia · tachycardia · thrombocytopenia

● PREGNANCY Manufacturer advises use only if potential benefit outweighs risk.

● BREAST FEEDING Manufacturer advises use only if potential benefit outweighs risk—present in milk.

● RENAL IMPAIRMENT

- With oral use Avoid *oral* treatment if estimated glomerular filtration rate less than 10 mL/minute/1.73 m^2.
- With intravenous use Age under 12 years (body-weight under 40 kg)—no information available. Age 12–18 years (body-weight over 40 kg)—use with caution if estimated glomerular filtration rate 40–80 mL/minute/1.73 m^2, and consult product literature for dose if estimated glomerular filtration rate less than 40 mL/minute/1.73 m^2.

● MONITORING REQUIREMENTS

- With intravenous use Monitor electrolytes and fluid balance.

● DIRECTIONS FOR ADMINISTRATION

- With intravenous use Displacement value may be significant when reconstituting injection, consult local guidelines. Reconstitute each 2-g vial with 50 mL Glucose 5% *or* Glucose 10% *or* Water for Injections; do not exceed infusion rate of 133 mg/minute.
- With oral use Manufacturer advises granules should be taken on an empty stomach (about 2–3 hours before or after a meal), preferably before bedtime and after emptying the bladder. The granules should be dissolved into a glass of water and taken immediately.

● PRESCRIBING AND DISPENSING INFORMATION Doses expressed as fosfomycin base.

● NATIONAL FUNDING/ACCESS DECISIONS

Scottish Medicines Consortium (SMC) decisions

SMC No. 1033/15

The *Scottish Medicines Consortium* has advised (March 2015) that fosfomycin (*Fomicyt*®) is accepted for restricted use within NHS Scotland; initiation should be restricted to microbiologists or infectious disease specialists.

SMC No. 1163/16

The *Scottish Medicines Consortium* has advised (September 2016) that fosfomycin trometamol (*Monuril*®) is accepted for use within NHS Scotland for the treatment of acute lower uncomplicated urinary tract infections, caused by pathogens sensitive to fosfomycin in adult and adolescent females and for prophylaxis in diagnostic and surgical transurethral procedures.

● MEDICINAL FORMS There can be variation in the licensing of different medicines containing the same drug.

Powder for solution for infusion

ELECTROLYTES: May contain Sodium

- Fosfomycin (Non-proprietary)
  Fosfomycin (as Fosfomycin sodium) 5 gram Infectofos 5g powder for solution for infusion vials | 10 vial PoM ⊠
- Fomicyt (Kent Pharmaceuticals Ltd)
  Fosfomycin (as Fosfomycin sodium) 2 gram Fomicyt 2g powder for solution for infusion vials | 10 vial PoM £150.00
  Fosfomycin (as Fosfomycin sodium) 4 gram Fomicyt 4g powder for solution for infusion vials | 10 vial PoM £300.00

Granules

CAUTIONARY AND ADVISORY LABELS 9, 13, 23

EXCIPIENTS: May contain Sucrose

- Fosfomycin (Non-proprietary)
  Fosfomycin (as Fosfomycin trometamol) 3 gram Fosfomycin 3g granules sachets | 1 sachet PoM £75.45 DT = £4.86
- Monuril (Profile Pharma Ltd)
  Fosfomycin (as Fosfomycin trometamol) 3 gram Monuril 3g granules sachets | 1 sachet PoM £4.86 DT = £4.86

Fusidic acid

30-Apr-2020

● DRUG ACTION Fusidic acid and its salts are narrow-spectrum antibiotics used for staphylococcal infections.

● INDICATIONS AND DOSE

Staphylococcal skin infection

▶ TO THE SKIN

- Child: Apply 3–4 times a day usually for 7 days

▶ BY MOUTH USING TABLETS

- Child 12-17 years: 250 mg every 12 hours for 5-10 days, dose expressed as sodium fusidate

Non-bullous impetigo [in patients who are not systemically unwell or at high risk of complications]

▶ TO THE SKIN

- Child: Apply 3 times a day for 5–7 days

Penicillin-resistant staphylococcal infection including osteomyelitis | Staphylococcal endocarditis in combination with other antibacterials

▶ BY MOUTH USING ORAL SUSPENSION

- Neonate: 15 mg/kg 3 times a day.
- Child 1-11 months: 15 mg/kg 3 times a day
- Child 1-4 years: 250 mg 3 times a day

continued →

- ▸ Child 5–11 years: 500 mg 3 times a day
- ▸ Child 12–17 years: 750 mg 3 times a day

▶ BY MOUTH USING TABLETS

- ▸ Child 12–17 years: 500 mg every 8 hours, increased to 1 g every 8 hours, increased dose can be used for severe infections, dose expressed as sodium fusidate

Staphylococcal infections due to susceptible organisms

▶ BY INTRAVENOUS INFUSION

- ▸ Child (body-weight up to 50 kg): 6–7 mg/kg 3 times a day, dose expressed as sodium fusidate
- ▸ Child (body-weight 50 kg and above): 500 mg 3 times a day, dose expressed as sodium fusidate

DOSE EQUIVALENCE AND CONVERSION

- ▸ Fusidic acid is incompletely absorbed and doses recommended for suspension are proportionately higher than those for sodium fusidate tablets.

● **CAUTIONS**

- ▸ With systemic use Impaired transport and metabolism of bilirubin
- ▸ With topical use Avoid contact of cream or ointment with eyes

CAUTIONS, FURTHER INFORMATION

- ▸ Avoiding resistance
- ▸ With topical use To avoid the development of resistance, fusidic acid should not be used for longer than 10 days and local microbiology advice should be sought before using it in hospital.

● **INTERACTIONS** → Appendix 1: fusidate

● **SIDE-EFFECTS**

GENERAL SIDE-EFFECTS

▶ **Uncommon** Skin reactions

SPECIFIC SIDE-EFFECTS

▶ **Common or very common**

- ▸ With intravenous use Dizziness · drowsiness · hepatic disorders · hyperbilirubinaemia · thrombophlebitis · vascular pain (reduced if given via central vein)
- ▸ With oral use Diarrhoea · dizziness · drowsiness · gastrointestinal discomfort · nausea · vomiting

▶ **Uncommon**

- ▸ With intravenous use Appetite decreased · asthenia · headache · malaise
- ▸ With oral use Appetite decreased · asthenia · headache · malaise · rash pustular

▶ **Rare or very rare**

- ▸ With topical use Angioedema · conjunctivitis

▶ **Frequency not known**

- ▸ With intravenous use Agranulocytosis · anaemia · leucopenia · neutropenia · pancytopenia · renal failure · rhabdomyolysis · thrombocytopenia
- ▸ With oral use Agranulocytosis · anaemia · hepatic disorders · hyperbilirubinaemia · leucopenia · neutropenia · pancytopenia · renal failure · rhabdomyolysis · thrombocytopenia

SIDE-EFFECTS, FURTHER INFORMATION Elevated liver enzymes, hyperbilirubinaemia and jaundice can occur with systemic use—these effects are usually reversible following withdrawal of therapy.

● **PREGNANCY**

- ▸ With systemic use Not known to be harmful; manufacturer advises use only if potential benefit outweighs risk.

● **BREAST FEEDING**

- ▸ With systemic use Present in milk—manufacturer advises caution.

● **HEPATIC IMPAIRMENT**

- ▸ With systemic use Manufacturer advises caution.

● **MONITORING REQUIREMENTS**

- ▸ With systemic use Manufacturer advises monitor liver function with high doses or on prolonged therapy; monitoring also advised for patients with biliary tract obstruction, those taking potentially hepatotoxic medication, or those taking concurrent medication with a similar excretion pathway.

● **DIRECTIONS FOR ADMINISTRATION**

- ▸ With intravenous use Manufacturer advises *for intravenous infusion*, give intermittently in Sodium chloride 0.9% or Glucose 5%; reconstitute each vial with 10 mL buffer solution, then add contents of vial to 500 mL infusion fluid to give a solution containing approximately 1 mg/mL. Give requisite dose via a central line over 2 hours (give over at least 6 hours if administered via a large peripheral vein).

● **PRESCRIBING AND DISPENSING INFORMATION** For choice of antibacterial therapy, see Cardiovascular system infections, antibacterial therapy p. 322, Musculoskeletal system infections, antibacterial therapy p. 326, Skin infections, antibacterial therapy p. 329.

● **PROFESSION SPECIFIC INFORMATION**

Dental practitioners' formulary

May be prescribed as Sodium Fusidate ointment.

● **MEDICINAL FORMS** There can be variation in the licensing of different medicines containing the same drug.

Tablet

CAUTIONARY AND ADVISORY LABELS 9

▸ Fucidin (LEO Pharma)

Sodium fusidate 250 mg Fucidin 250mg tablets | 10 tablet PoM £6.02 DT = £6.02 | 100 tablet PoM £54.99

Oral suspension

CAUTIONARY AND ADVISORY LABELS 9

▸ Fucidin (LEO Pharma)

Fusidic acid 50 mg per 1 ml Fucidin 250mg/5ml oral suspension | 90 ml PoM £12.11

Cream

EXCIPIENTS: May contain Butylated hydroxyanisole, cetostearyl alcohol (including cetyl and stearyl alcohol)

▸ Fusidic acid (Non-proprietary)

Fusidic acid 20 mg per 1 gram Fusidic acid 2% cream | 15 gram PoM £3.00 DT = £2.64 | 30 gram PoM £5.28 DT = £5.28

▸ Fucidin (LEO Pharma)

Fusidic acid 20 mg per 1 gram Fucidin 20mg/g cream | 15 gram PoM £1.92 DT = £2.64 | 30 gram PoM £3.59 DT = £5.28

Ointment

EXCIPIENTS: May contain Cetostearyl alcohol (including cetyl and stearyl alcohol), woolfat and related substances (including lanolin)

▸ Fucidin (LEO Pharma)

Sodium fusidate 20 mg per 1 gram Fucidin 20mg/g ointment | 15 gram PoM £2.68 DT = £2.68 | 30 gram PoM £4.55 DT = £4.55

Powder and solvent for solution for infusion

ELECTROLYTES: May contain Sodium

▸ Fusidic acid (Non-proprietary)

Sodium fusidate 500 mg Sodium fusidate 500mg powder and solvent for solution for infusion vials | 1 vial PoM £20.50–£20.90 DT = £20.70

Linezolid

18-May-2020

- **DRUG ACTION** Linezolid, an oxazolidinone antibacterial, is active against Gram-positive bacteria including meticillin-resistant *Staphylococcus aureus* (MRSA), and glycopeptide-resistant enterococci. Resistance to linezolid can develop with prolonged treatment or if the dose is less than that recommended. Linezolid is **not** active against common Gram-negative organisms; it must be given in combination with other antibacterials for mixed infections that also involve Gram-negative organisms.

- **INDICATIONS AND DOSE**

Pneumonia (when other antibacterials e.g. a glycopetide, such as vancomycin, cannot be used) (initiated under specialist supervision) | Complicated skin and soft-tissue infections caused by Gram-positive bacteria, when other antibacterials cannot be used (initiated under specialist supervision)

▶ BY MOUTH, OR BY INTRAVENOUS INFUSION

▸ Neonate up to 7 days: 10 mg/kg every 12 hours, increased if necessary to 10 mg/kg every 8 hours, increased dose can be used if poor response.

▸ Neonate 7 days to 28 days: 10 mg/kg every 8 hours.

▸ Child 1 month–11 years: 10 mg/kg every 8 hours (max. per dose 600 mg)

▸ Child 12–17 years: 600 mg every 12 hours

Cellulitis (specialist use only) | Erysipelas (specialist use only)

▶ BY MOUTH, OR BY INTRAVENOUS INFUSION

▸ Child 1 month–11 years: 10 mg/kg every 8 hours (max. per dose 600 mg)

▸ Child 12–17 years: 600 mg every 12 hours

- **UNLICENSED USE** Not licensed for use in children.

> IMPORTANT SAFETY INFORMATION
>
> CHM ADVICE (OPTIC NEUROPATHY)
>
> Severe optic neuropathy may occur rarely, particularly if linezolid is used for longer than 28 days. The CHM recommends that:
>
> - patients should be warned to report symptoms of visual impairment (including blurred vision, visual field defect, changes in visual acuity and colour vision) immediately;
> - patients experiencing new visual symptoms (regardless of treatment duration) should be evaluated promptly, and referred to an ophthalmologist if necessary;
> - visual function should be monitored regularly if treatment is required for longer than 28 days.
>
> BLOOD DISORDERS
>
> Haematopoietic disorders (including thrombocytopenia, anaemia, leucopenia, and pancytopenia) have been reported in patients receiving linezolid. It is recommended that full blood counts are monitored weekly. Close monitoring is recommended in patients who:
>
> - receive treatment for more than 10–14 days;
> - have pre-existing myelosuppression;
> - are receiving drugs that may have adverse effects on haemoglobin, blood counts, or platelet function;
> - have severe renal impairment.
>
> If significant myelosuppression occurs, treatment should be stopped unless it is considered essential, in which case intensive monitoring of blood counts and appropriate management should be implemented.

- **CAUTIONS** Acute confusional states · bipolar depression · carcinoid tumour · history of seizures · phaeochromocytoma · schizophrenia · thyrotoxicosis · uncontrolled hypertension

CAUTIONS, FURTHER INFORMATION

▶ Close observation Unless close observation and blood pressure monitoring possible, linezolid should be avoided in uncontrolled hypertension, phaeochromocytoma, carcinoid tumour, thyrotoxicosis, bipolar depression, schizophrenia, or acute confusional states.

- **INTERACTIONS** → Appendix 1: linezolid

- **SIDE-EFFECTS**

▶ **Common or very common** Anaemia · constipation · diarrhoea · dizziness · gastrointestinal discomfort · headache · hypertension · increased risk of infection · insomnia · localised pain · nausea · skin reactions · taste altered · vomiting

▶ **Uncommon** Arrhythmia · chills · dry mouth · eosinophilia · fatigue · gastritis · hyperhidrosis · hyponatraemia · leucopenia · neutropenia · oral disorders · pancreatitis · polyuria · renal failure · seizure · sensation abnormal · thirst · thrombocytopenia · thrombophlebitis · tinnitus · tongue discolouration · transient ischaemic attack · vision disorders · vulvovaginal disorder

▶ **Rare or very rare** Antibiotic associated colitis · bone marrow disorders · tooth discolouration

▶ **Frequency not known** Alopecia · angioedema · lactic acidosis · nerve disorders · serotonin syndrome · severe cutaneous adverse reactions (SCARs)

- **PREGNANCY** Manufacturer advises use only if potential benefit outweighs risk—no information available.
- **BREAST FEEDING** Manufacturer advises avoid—present in milk in *animal* studies.
- **HEPATIC IMPAIRMENT** Manufacturer advises caution in severe impairment (no information available).
- **RENAL IMPAIRMENT** No dose adjustment necessary but metabolites may accumulate if estimated glomerular filtration rate less than 30 mL/minute/1.73 m^2.
- **MONITORING REQUIREMENTS** Monitor full blood count (including platelet count) weekly.
- **DIRECTIONS FOR ADMINISTRATION**

▶ With intravenous use Infusion to be administered over 30–120 minutes.

- **PRESCRIBING AND DISPENSING INFORMATION** For choice of antibacterial therapy, see Respiratory system infections, antibacterial therapy p. 327, Skin infections, antibacterial therapy p. 329.

There is limited information on use in children and expert advice should be sought.

- **PATIENT AND CARER ADVICE** Patients should be advised to read the patient information leaflet given with linezolid.

- **MEDICINAL FORMS** There can be variation in the licensing of different medicines containing the same drug.

Infusion

EXCIPIENTS: May contain Glucose

ELECTROLYTES: May contain Sodium

▸ Linezolid (Non-proprietary)

Linezolid 2 mg per 1 ml Linezolid 600mg/300ml infusion bags | 10 bag [PoM] £445.00–£541.00 (Hospital only)

▸ Zyvox (Pfizer Ltd)

Linezolid 2 mg per 1 ml Zyvox 600mg/300ml infusion bags | 10 bag [PoM] £445.00

Oral suspension

CAUTIONARY AND ADVISORY LABELS 9, 10

EXCIPIENTS: May contain Aspartame

▸ Zyvox (Pfizer Ltd)

Linezolid 20 mg per 1 ml Zyvox 100mg/5ml granules for oral suspension | 150 ml [PoM] £222.50 DT = £222.50

Tablet

CAUTIONARY AND ADVISORY LABELS 9, 10

- Linezolid (Non-proprietary)
  Linezolid 600 mg Linezolid 600mg tablets | 10 tablet PoM £239.16 DT = £327.24 (Hospital only) | 10 tablet PoM £82.12–£445.00 DT = £327.24
- Zyvox (Pfizer Ltd)
  Linezolid 600 mg Zyvox 600mg tablets | 10 tablet PoM £445.00 DT = £327.24

Trimethoprim

26-May-2020

● **INDICATIONS AND DOSE**

Respiratory-tract infections

▶ BY MOUTH

- Neonate: Initially 3 mg/kg for 1 dose, then 1–2 mg/kg twice daily.

- Child 4–5 weeks: 4 mg/kg twice daily (max. per dose 200 mg)
- Child 6 weeks–5 months: 4 mg/kg twice daily (max. per dose 200 mg), alternatively 25 mg twice daily
- Child 6 months–5 years: 4 mg/kg twice daily (max. per dose 200 mg), alternatively 50 mg twice daily
- Child 6–11 years: 4 mg/kg twice daily (max. per dose 200 mg), alternatively 100 mg twice daily
- Child 12–17 years: 200 mg twice daily

Prophylaxis of recurrent urinary-tract infection

▶ BY MOUTH

- Neonate: 2 mg/kg once daily, dose to be taken at night.

- Child 4–5 weeks: 2 mg/kg once daily, dose to be taken at night
- Child 6 weeks–5 months: 2 mg/kg once daily, alternatively 12.5 mg once daily, dose to be taken at night
- Child 6 months–5 years: 2 mg/kg once daily (max. per dose 100 mg), alternatively 25 mg once daily, dose to be taken at night
- Child 6–11 years: 2 mg/kg once daily (max. per dose 100 mg), alternatively 50 mg once daily, dose to be taken at night
- Child 12–15 years: 100 mg once daily, dose to be taken at night
- Child 16–17 years: 100 mg once daily, dose to be taken at night, alternatively 200 mg for 1 dose, following exposure to a trigger

Treatment of mild to moderate *Pneumocystis jirovecii* (*Pneumocystis carinii*) pneumonia in patients who cannot tolerate co-trimoxazole (in combination with dapsone)

▶ BY MOUTH

- Child: 5 mg/kg every 6–8 hours

Shigellosis | Invasive salmonella infection

▶ BY MOUTH

- Child: (consult product literature)

Acute pyelonephritis

▶ BY MOUTH

- Child 16–17 years: 200 mg twice daily for 14 days

Urinary-tract infection (catheter-associated)

▶ BY MOUTH

- Child 3–5 months: 4 mg/kg twice daily (max. per dose 200 mg) for 7–10 days, alternatively 25 mg twice daily for 7–10 days
- Child 6 months–5 years: 4 mg/kg twice daily (max. per dose 200 mg) for 7–10 days, alternatively 50 mg twice daily for 7–10 days
- Child 6–11 years: 4 mg/kg twice daily (max. per dose 200 mg) for 7–10 days, alternatively 100 mg twice daily for 7–10 days
- Child 12–15 years: 200 mg twice daily for 7–10 days
- Child 16–17 years: 200 mg twice daily for 7 days (14 days if upper urinary-tract symptoms are present)

Lower urinary-tract infection

▶ BY MOUTH

- Neonate: Initially 3 mg/kg for 1 dose, then 1–2 mg/kg twice daily.

- Child 4–5 weeks: 4 mg/kg twice daily (max. per dose 200 mg)
- Child 6 weeks–2 months: 4 mg/kg twice daily (max. per dose 200 mg), alternatively 25 mg twice daily
- Child 3–5 months: 4 mg/kg twice daily (max. per dose 200 mg) for 3 days, alternatively 25 mg twice daily for 3 days
- Child 6 months–5 years: 4 mg/kg twice daily (max. per dose 200 mg) for 3 days, alternatively 50 mg twice daily for 3 days
- Child 6–11 years: 4 mg/kg twice daily (max. per dose 200 mg) for 3 days, alternatively 100 mg twice daily for 3 days
- Child 12–15 years: 200 mg twice daily for 3 days
- Child 16–17 years: 200 mg twice daily for 3 days (7 days in males)

● **UNLICENSED USE** EvGr Trimethoprim can be given as a single dose for the prophylaxis of recurrent urinary-tract infection following exposure to a trigger, Ⓐ but this dosing regimen is not licensed. Not licensed for treatment of pneumocystis pneumonia.

Not licensed for use in children under 6 months for the prophylaxis of recurrent urinary-tract infection.

Not licensed for use in children under 6 weeks.

● **CONTRA-INDICATIONS** Blood dyscrasias

● **CAUTIONS** Acute porphyrias p. 652 · neonates (specialist supervision required) · predisposition to folate deficiency

● **INTERACTIONS** → Appendix 1: trimethoprim

● **SIDE-EFFECTS**

▶ **Common or very common** Diarrhoea · electrolyte imbalance · fungal overgrowth · headache · nausea · skin reactions · vomiting

▶ **Rare or very rare** Agranulocytosis · angioedema · anxiety · appetite decreased · arthralgia · behaviour abnormal · bone marrow disorders · confusion · constipation · cough · depression · dizziness · dyspnoea · eosinophilia · erythema nodosum · fever · haemolysis · haemolytic anaemia · haemorrhage · hallucination · hepatic disorders · hypoglycaemia · lethargy · leucopenia · meningitis aseptic · movement disorders · myalgia · neutropenia · oral disorders · pancreatitis · paraesthesia · peripheral neuritis · photosensitivity reaction · pseudomembranous enterocolitis · renal impairment · seizure · severe cutaneous adverse reactions (SCARs) · sleep disorders · syncope · systemic lupus erythematosus (SLE) · thrombocytopenia · tinnitus · tremor · uveitis · vasculitis · vertigo · wheezing

▶ **Frequency not known** Gastrointestinal disorder · megaloblastic anaemia · methaemoglobinaemia

● **PREGNANCY** Teratogenic risk in first trimester (folate antagonist). Manufacturers advise avoid during pregnancy.

● **BREAST FEEDING** Present in milk—short-term use not known to be harmful.

● **RENAL IMPAIRMENT** Manufacturer advises caution in impairment.

Dose adjustments Manufacturer advises dose reduction to half normal dose after 3 days if estimated glomerular filtration rate 15–30 mL/minute/1.73 m^2.

Manufacturer advises dose reduction to half normal dose if estimated glomerular filtration rate less than 15 mL/minute/1.73 m^2.

- **MONITORING REQUIREMENTS**
- ▸ Manufacturer advises monitor blood counts with long-term use and in those with, or at risk of, folate deficiency.
- ▸ Manufacturer advises monitor serum electrolytes in patients at risk of developing hyperkalaemia, and consider monitoring in other patients, particularly with long-term use.
- ▸ Manufacturer advises consider monitoring renal function, particularly with long-term use.
- ▸ Manufacturer advises monitoring of plasma-trimethoprim concentration may be considered with long-term use and under specialist advice.
- **PRESCRIBING AND DISPENSING INFORMATION** For choice of antibacterial therapy, see Gastro-intestinal system infections, antibacterial therapy p. 324, Pneumocystis pneumonia p. 413, Respiratory system infections, antibacterial therapy p. 327, Urinary-tract infections p. 400.
- **PATIENT AND CARER ADVICE**

Blood disorders On long-term treatment, patients and their carers should be told how to recognise signs of blood disorders and advised to seek immediate medical attention if symptoms such as fever, sore throat, rash, mouth ulcers, purpura, bruising or bleeding develop.

Medicines for Children leaflet: Trimethoprim for bacterial infections www.medicinesforchildren.org.uk/trimethoprim-bacterial-infections

- **MEDICINAL FORMS** There can be variation in the licensing of different medicines containing the same drug. Forms available from special-order manufacturers include: oral suspension, oral solution

Oral suspension

CAUTIONARY AND ADVISORY LABELS 9

- ▸ Trimethoprim (Non-proprietary)

Trimethoprim 10 mg per 1 ml Trimethoprim 50mg/5ml oral suspension sugar free sugar-free | 100 ml PoM £6.82 DT = £4.89

- ▸ Monotrim (Chemidex Pharma Ltd)

Trimethoprim 10 mg per 1 ml Monotrim 50mg/5ml oral suspension sugar-free | 100 ml PoM £1.77 DT = £4.89

Tablet

CAUTIONARY AND ADVISORY LABELS 9

- ▸ Trimethoprim (Non-proprietary)

Trimethoprim 100 mg Trimogal 100mg tablets | 28 tablet PoM £0.89 DT = £0.88
Trimethoprim 100mg tablets | 28 tablet PoM £1.39 DT = £0.88
Trimethoprim 200 mg Trimogal 200mg tablets | 14 tablet PoM £0.91 DT = £0.91
Trimethoprim 200mg tablets | 6 tablet PoM £2.15 DT = £0.39 | 14 tablet PoM £5.00 DT = £0.91

Combinations available: *Co-trimoxazole*, p. 378

1.1 Anthrax

Anthrax

Treatment and post-exposure prophylaxis

Inhalation or *gastro-intestinal anthrax* should be treated initially with either ciprofloxacin p. 377 or, in patients over 12 years, doxycycline p. 381 [unlicensed indication] combined with one or two other antibacterials (such as amoxicillin p. 366, benzylpenicillin sodium p. 364, chloramphenicol p. 385, clarithromycin p. 353, clindamycin p. 351, imipenem with cilastatin p. 336, rifampicin p. 396 [unlicensed indication], and vancomycin p. 349). When the condition improves and the sensitivity of the *Bacillus anthracis* strain is known, treatment may be switched to a single antibacterial. Treatment should continue for 60 days because germination may be delayed.

Cutaneous anthrax should be treated with either ciprofloxacin [unlicensed indication] or doxycycline [unlicensed indication] for 7 days. Treatment may be switched to amoxicillin if the infecting strain is susceptible. Treatment may need to be extended to 60 days if exposure is due to aerosol. A combination of antibacterials for 14 days is recommended for cutaneous anthrax with systemic features, extensive oedema, or lesions of the head or neck.

Ciprofloxacin or doxycycline may be given for *post-exposure prophylaxis*. If exposure is confirmed, antibacterial prophylaxis should continue for 60 days. Antibacterial prophylaxis may be switched to amoxicillin after 10–14 days if the strain of *B. anthracis* is susceptible. Vaccination against anthrax may allow the duration of antibacterial prophylaxis to be shortened.

1.2 Lyme disease

Lyme disease

14-Nov-2018

Description of condition

Lyme disease, also known as Lyme borreliosis, is an infection caused by bacteria called *Borrelia burgdorferi*. It is transmitted to humans by the bite of an infected tick. Ticks are mainly found in grassy and wooded areas including urban gardens and parks. Most tick bites do not cause Lyme disease, and the prompt and correct removal of the tick reduces the risk of infection.

Lyme disease usually presents with a characteristic erythema migrans rash. This usually becomes visible 1–4 weeks after a tick bite, but can appear from 3 days to 3 months, and last for several weeks. It may be accompanied by non-focal (non-organ related) symptoms, such as fever, swollen glands, malaise, fatigue, neck pain or stiffness, joint or muscle pain, headache, cognitive impairment, or paraesthesia.

Other signs and symptoms of Lyme disease may also appear months or years after the initial infection and are typically characterised by focal symptoms (relating to at least 1 organ system). These include neurological (affecting cranial nerves, peripheral and central nervous systems), joint (Lyme arthritis), cardiac (Lyme carditis), or skin (acrodermatitis chronica atrophicans) manifestations.

Drug treatment

EvGr The diagnosis and management of Lyme disease in children should be discussed with a specialist unless the child presents with a single erythema migrans lesion and no other symptoms. Children diagnosed with Lyme disease should be given treatment with an antibacterial drug; the choice of drug should be based on presenting symptoms. (A)

Child aged 9 years and over

EvGr In children presenting with *erythema migrans rash with or without non-focal symptoms* oral doxycycline p. 381 [unlicensed] is recommended as first-line treatment. If doxycycline p. 381 cannot be given, oral amoxicillin p. 366 should be used as an alternative. Oral azithromycin p. 352 [unlicensed] should be given if both doxycycline p. 381 and amoxicillin p. 366 are unsuitable.

In children presenting with focal symptoms of *cranial nerve or peripheral nervous system* involvement, oral doxycycline p. 381 [unlicensed] is recommended as first-line treatment. If doxycycline p. 381 cannot be given, oral amoxicillin p. 366 should be used as an alternative.

In children presenting with symptoms of *central nervous system* involvement, intravenous ceftriaxone p. 343 is recommended as first-line treatment. Oral doxycycline p. 381 [unlicensed] should be used as an alternative if ceftriaxone p. 343 cannot be given, or when switching to oral antibacterial treatment.

In children with symptoms of *Lyme arthritis or acrodermatitis chronica atrophicans*, oral doxycycline p. 381 [unlicensed] is recommended as first-line treatment. If doxycycline p. 381 cannot be given, oral amoxicillin p. 366 should be used as an alternative. Intravenous ceftriaxone p. 343 should be used if both doxycycline p. 381 and amoxicillin p. 366 are unsuitable.

In children with symptoms of *Lyme carditis* who are *haemodynamically stable*, oral doxycycline p. 381 [unlicensed] is recommended as first-line treatment. If doxycycline p. 381 cannot be given, intravenous ceftriaxone p. 343 should be used as an alternative.

In children with symptoms of *Lyme carditis who are haemodynamically unstable*, intravenous ceftriaxone p. 343 is recommended. If ceftriaxone p. 343 cannot be given, oral doxycycline p. 381 [unlicensed] should be used as an alternative. ⟨A⟩

Child aged under 9 years

EvGr In children presenting with *erythema migrans rash with or without non-focal symptoms*, oral amoxicillin p. 366 is recommended as first-line treatment. If oral amoxicillin p. 366 cannot be given, oral azithromycin p. 352 [unlicensed] should be used as an alternative.

In children presenting with focal symptoms of *cranial nerve or peripheral nervous system* involvement, oral amoxicillin p. 366 is recommended.

In children presenting with symptoms of *central nervous system* involvement, intravenous ceftriaxone p. 343 is recommended.

In children with symptoms of *Lyme arthritis or acrodermatitis chronica atrophicans*, oral amoxicillin p. 366 is recommended as first-line treatment. If amoxicillin p. 366 cannot be given, intravenous ceftriaxone p. 343 should be used as an alternative.

In children with symptoms of *Lyme carditis* (*both haemodynamically stable and unstable*), intravenous ceftriaxone p. 343 is recommended. ⟨A⟩

Ongoing symptom management

EvGr If symptoms continue to persist or worsen after antibacterial treatment, patients should be assessed for possible alternative causes, re-infection with Lyme disease, treatment failure or non-adherence to previous antibacterial treatment, or progression to organ damage caused by Lyme disease (such as nerve palsy).

A second course of antibacterial treatment should be given to patients presenting with signs and symptoms of re-infection. In patients presenting with ongoing symptoms due to possible treatment failure, treatment with an alternative antibacterial drug should be considered. A third course of antibacterial treatment is not recommended, and further management should be discussed with a national reference laboratory or suitable specialist depending on symptoms (for example, a rheumatologist or neurologist). ⟨A⟩

Useful Resources

Lyme disease. National Institute for Health and Care Excellence. NICE guideline 95. April 2018.
www.nice.org.uk/guidance/ng95

'Be tick aware'–Toolkit for raising awareness of the potential risk posed by ticks and tick-borne disease in England. Public Health England. March 2018.
www.gov.uk/government/publications/tick-bite-risks-and-prevention-of-lyme-disease

1.3 Methicillin-resistant staphylococcus aureus

MRSA

Management

Infection from *Staphylococcus aureus* strains resistant to meticillin [now discontinued] (meticillin-resistant *Staph. aureus*, MRSA) and to flucloxacillin p. 373 can be difficult to manage. Treatment is guided by the sensitivity of the infecting strain.

Rifampicin p. 396 or fusidic acid p. 387 should **not** be used alone because resistance may develop rapidly. Clindamycin p. 351 alone or a combination of rifampicin and fusidic acid can be used for *skin* and *soft-tissue infections* caused by MRSA; a **tetracycline** is an alternative in children over 12 years of age. A **glycopeptide** (e.g. vancomycin p. 349) can be used for severe skin and soft-tissue infections associated with MRSA. A combination of a glycopeptide and fusidic acid or a glycopeptide and rifampicin can be considered for skin and soft-tissue infections that have failed to respond to a single antibacterial. Linezolid p. 389 should be reserved for skin and soft-tissue infections that have not responded to other antibacterials or for children who cannot tolerate other antibacterials.

A **glycopeptide** can be used for *pneumonia* associated with MRSA. Linezolid should be reserved for hospital-acquired pneumonia that has not responded to other antibacterials or for children who cannot tolerate other antibacterials.

Trimethoprim p. 390 or nitrofurantoin p. 403 can be used for *urinary-tract infections* caused by MRSA; a **tetracycline** is an alternative in children over 12 years of age. A **glycopeptide** can be used for urinary-tract infections that are severe or resistant to other antibacterials.

A **glycopeptide** can be used for septicaemia associated with MRSA.

See the management of endocarditis, osteomyelitis, or septic arthritis associated with MRSA.

Prophylaxis with vancomycin or teicoplanin p. 348 (alone or in combination with another antibacterial active against other pathogens) is appropriate for patients undergoing surgery if:

- there is a history of MRSA colonisation or infection without documented eradication;
- there is a risk that the patient's MRSA carriage has recurred;
- the patient comes from an area with a high prevalence of MRSA.

It is important that hospitals have infection control guidelines to minimise MRSA transmission, including policies on isolation and treatment of MRSA carriers and on hand hygiene. See eradication of nasal carriage of MRSA in Nose p. 747.

1.4 Tuberculosis

Tuberculosis

24-Oct-2019

Overview

Tuberculosis is a curable infectious disease caused by bacteria of the *Mycobacterium tuberculosis* complex (*M. tuberculosis*, *M. africanum*, *M. bovis* or *M. microti*) and is spread by breathing in infected respiratory droplets from a person with infectious tuberculosis. The most common form of tuberculosis infection is in the lungs (**pulmonary**) but infection can also spread and develop in other parts of the body (**extrapulmonary**).

The initial infection with tuberculosis clears in the majority of individuals. However, in some cases the bacteria may become dormant and remain in the body with no symptoms (**latent** tuberculosis) or progress to being symptomatic (**active** tuberculosis) over the following weeks or months. In individuals with latent tuberculosis only a small proportion will develop active tuberculosis.

Many cases of tuberculosis can be prevented by public health measures and when clinical disease does occur most individuals can be cured if treated properly with the correct dose, combination and duration of treatment. Drug-resistant strains of tuberculosis are much harder to treat and significantly increase an individual's risk of long-term complications or death.

Treatment phases, overview

The standard treatment of active tuberculosis is completed in two phases—an **initial phase** using four drugs and a **continuation phase** using two drugs, in fully sensitive cases. EvGr The management and investigation of tuberculosis in children should be undertaken by either a paediatrician with experience and training in tuberculosis or a general paediatrician with advice from a specialist clinician. This tuberculosis service should include specialised nurses and health visitors. (A)

Within the UK there are two regimens recommended for the treatment of tuberculosis: **unsupervised** or **supervised**; with the choice of either regimen dependent on a risk assessment to identify if a child needs enhanced case management.

EvGr In all phases of treatment for tuberculosis, fixed-dose combination tablets should be used, and a daily dosing schedule should be considered. (A)

Initial phase

EvGr As standard treatment for children with active tuberculosis, offer rifampicin p. 396, ethambutol hydrochloride p. 398, pyrazinamide p. 400 and isoniazid p. 399 (with pyridoxine hydrochloride p. 678) in the initial phase of treatment; modified according to drug susceptibility testing; and continued for 2 months.

Treatment should be started without waiting for culture results if clinical signs and symptoms are consistent with a tuberculosis diagnosis; consider completing the standard treatment even if subsequent culture results are negative. (A)

Continuation phase

EvGr After the initial phase, offer standard continuation treatment with rifampicin and isoniazid (with pyridoxine hydrochloride) for a further 4 months in children with active tuberculosis without central nervous system involvement. Longer treatment of 10 months should be offered to children with active tuberculosis of the central nervous system, with or without spinal involvement.

Treatment should be modified according to drug susceptibility testing. (A)

Unsupervised treatment

The unsupervised treatment regimen is for children who are likely to take antituberculosis drugs (or have treatment administered by a parent or carer) reliably and willingly without supervision by a healthcare worker.

Supervised treatment

For children or families requiring supervised treatment (directly observed therapy, DOT), this is offered as part of enhanced case management. EvGr A 3 times weekly dosing schedule can be considered in children with active tuberculosis if they require enhanced case management and daily directly observed therapy is not available.
Antituberculosis treatment dosing regimens of fewer than 3 times a week are not recommended.

Directly observed therapy should be offered to children or to children whose carers:

- have a current risk or history of non-adherence;
- have previously been treated for tuberculosis;
- have a history of homelessness, drug or alcohol misuse;
- are in a young offender institution, or have been in the past 5 years;
- have a major psychiatric, memory or cognitive disorder;
- are in denial of the tuberculosis diagnosis;
- have multi-drug resistant tuberculosis;
- request directly observed therapy after discussion with the clinical team;
- are too ill to self-administer treatment.

Advice and support should be offered to those children and their carers to assist with treatment completion. (A)

Individuals with comorbidities or coexisting conditions, including the immunocompromised

EvGr Children with comorbidities or coexisting conditions (such as HIV, severe liver disease or diabetes) should be managed by a specialist multidisciplinary team with experience in managing tuberculosis and the comorbidity or coexisting condition.

In children who are HIV-positive with active tuberculosis, treatment with the standard regimen should not routinely exceed 6 months, unless the tuberculosis has central nervous system involvement, in which case treatment should not routinely extend beyond 12 months.

Care should be taken to avoid drug interactions when co-prescribing antiretroviral and antituberculosis drugs. (A) For further information on the **management of tuberculosis in HIV infection** consult the Children's HIV Association of UK and Ireland (www.chiva.org.uk/guidelines/).

Extrapulmonary tuberculosis

Central nervous system tuberculosis

EvGr Children with central nervous system tuberculosis should be offered standard treatment with **initial phase** drugs for 2 months (see *Initial phase* for specific drugs). After completion of the initial treatment phase, standard treatment with **continuation phase** drugs should then be offered (see *Continuation phase* for specific drugs); and continued for a further 10 months. Treatment for tuberculosis meningitis should be offered if clinical signs and other laboratory findings are consistent with the diagnosis, even if a rapid diagnostic test is negative.

An initial high dose of *dexamethasone* or *prednisolone* should be offered at the same time as antituberculosis treatment, then slowly withdrawn over 4–8 weeks.

Referral for surgery should only be considered in children who have raised intracranial pressure; or have spinal TB with spinal instability or evidence of spinal cord compression. (A)

Pericardial tuberculosis

EvGr An initial high dose of oral *prednisolone* should be offered to children with active pericardial tuberculosis, at the same time as antituberculosis treatment, then slowly withdrawn over 2–3 weeks. (A)

Latent tuberculosis

Some children with latent tuberculosis are at increased risk of developing active tuberculosis (such as children who are HIV-positive, diabetic or receiving treatment with an anti-tumor necrosis factor alpha inhibitor). EvGr These children and their carers should be informed of the risks and symptoms of active tuberculosis. (A)

Close contacts

EvGr Children who are a close contact (prolonged, frequent or intense contact, for example household contacts) of a person with pulmonary or laryngeal tuberculosis should be tested for latent tuberculosis. Children aged under 2 years should be assessed by a specialist. (A)

5 Infection

Recommended dosage for standard unsupervised 6-month treatment

Isoniazid	Child: 10 mg/kg once daily (max. per dose 300 mg) for 6 months (initial and continuation phases)
Rifampicin	Child: ▸ body-weight up to 50 kg 15 mg/kg once daily for 6 months (initial and continuation phases); maximum 450 mg per day ; ▸ body-weight 50 kg and above 15 mg/kg once daily for 6 months (initial and continuation phases); maximum 600 mg per day
Pyrazinamide	Child: ▸ body-weight up to 50 kg 35 mg/kg once daily for 2 months (initial phase); maximum 1.5 g per day ; ▸ body-weight 50 kg and above 35 mg/kg once daily for 2 months (initial phase); maximum 2 g per day
Ethambutol hydrochloride	Child: 20 mg/kg once daily for 2 months (initial phase)

In general, doses should be rounded up to facilitate administration of suitable volumes of liquid or an appropriate strength of tablet. The exception is ethambutol hydrochloride p. 398 due to the risk of toxicity. Doses may also need to be recalculated to allow for weight gain in younger children.
The fixed-dose combination preparations (*Rifater*®, *Rifinah*®) are unlicensed for use in children. Consideration may be given to use of these preparations in older children, provided the respective dose of each drug is appropriate for the weight of the child.

Recommended dosage for intermittent supervised 6-month treatment

Isoniazid	Child: 15 mg/kg 3 times a week (max. per dose 900 mg) for 6 months (initial and continuation phases)
Rifampicin	Child: 15 mg/kg 3 times a week (max. per dose 900 mg) for 6 months (initial and continuation phases)
Pyrazinamide	Child: ▸ body-weight up to 50 kg 50 mg/kg 3 times a week (max. per dose 2 g 3 times a week) for 2 months (initial phase) ; ▸ body-weight 50 kg and above 50 mg/kg 3 times a week (max. per dose 2.5 g 3 times a week) for 2 months (initial phase)
Ethambutol hydrochloride	Child: 30 mg/kg 3 times a week for 2 months (initial phase)

In general, doses should be rounded up to facilitate administration of suitable volumes of liquid or an appropriate strength of tablet. The exception is ethambutol hydrochloride due to the risk of toxicity. Doses may also need to be recalculated to allow for weight gain in younger children.
The fixed-dose combination preparations (*Rifater*®, *Rifinah*®) are unlicensed for use in children. Consideration may be given to use of these preparations in older children, provided the respective dose of each drug is appropriate for the weight of the child.

Immunocompromised

EvGr Children who are anticipated to be, or who are currently immunocompromised should be referred to a specialist if latent tuberculosis is suspected (for example if they are from a high incidence country or have been in close contact with people with *suspected infectious* or *confirmed* pulmonary or laryngeal tuberculosis). Ⓐ

Treatment of latent tuberculosis

EvGr **Neonates** who have been in close contact with a person with tuberculosis which has not yet been treated for at least two weeks, should start treatment with isoniazid p. 399 (with pyridoxine hydrochloride p. 678) followed by a Mantoux test after 6 weeks of treatment.

If the Mantoux test is positive (and active tuberculosis is not present) treatment should be continued for 6 months; if negative (and confirmed by a negative interferon-gamma release assay), the treatment should be stopped and a BCG vaccination given. If the interferon-gamma release assay result is positive (and active tuberculosis is not present) treatment should be continued for 6 months.

Childrenaged 4 weeks to 2 years who have been in close contact with a person with tuberculosis which has not been treated for at least two weeks, should start treatment for latent tuberculosis and have a Mantoux test. Treatment is either isoniazid (with pyridoxine hydrochloride) alone for 6 months (preferred regimen if interactions with rifamycins are a concern) or rifampicin p. 396 and isoniazid (with pyridoxine hydrochloride) for 3 months (recommended when hepatotoxicity is a concern).

If the Mantoux test is positive (and active tuberculosis is not present), the treatment course should be completed. If the test is negative, treatment should be continued and the child should be re-assessed for active tuberculosis after 6 weeks. If the results are then negative (and confirmed by a negative interferon-gamma release assay), the treatment should be stopped and a BCG vaccination given (if the child has not already had one). If the result is positive (and active tuberculosis is not present), the course of treatment should be continued.

Childrenaged over 2 years should be offered a Mantoux test, and if positive (and active tuberculosis is not present), then treat as above for children aged 4 weeks to 2 years. If the test is negative, then offer an interferon-gamma release assay after 6 weeks and repeat the Mantoux test. Ⓐ

The choice of regimen is dependent on clinical factors, including age, risk of hepatotoxicity and possible drug interactions. EvGr Testing for HIV, hepatitis B and hepatitis C should be offered before starting antituberculosis treatment as this may affect choice of therapy.

Children with severe liver disease should be treated under the care of a specialist team. Careful monitoring of liver function is necessary in children with non-severe liver disease, abnormal liver function, or who misuse alcohol or drugs. Ⓐ

For advice on tuberculin testing and immunisation against tuberculosis, see Bacillus Calmette-Guérin vaccine p. 831.

Treatment failure

Major causes of treatment failure include incorrect prescribing by the clinician and inadequate compliance by the child or carer. EvGr All children diagnosed with tuberculosis should have an allocated case manager to help with the development of a health and social care plan, supervision of treatment, and support with the completion of treatment. Multidisciplinary tuberculosis teams should implement strategies (such as random urine tests, pill counts, home visits, health education counselling, and language appropriate reminder services) to help with adherence to, and successful completion of treatment. Ⓐ

Treatment interruptions

A break in antituberculosis treatment of at least 2 weeks (during the initial phase) or missing more than 20% of prescribed doses is classified as treatment interruption. Re-establishing treatment appropriately following interruptions is key to ensuring treatment success without relapse, drug resistance or further adverse events. EvGr If an adverse reaction recurs upon re-introducing a particular drug, do not give that drug in future regimens and consider extending the total regimen accordingly. ⟨A⟩

Treatment interruptions due to drug-induced hepatotoxicity

EvGr Following treatment interruption due to drug-induced hepatotoxicty, all potential causes of hepatotoxicity should be investigated. Once aspartate or alanine transaminase levels fall below twice the upper limit of normal, bilirubin levels have returned to the normal range, and hepatotoxic symptoms have resolved, antituberculosis therapy should be sequentially re-introduced at previous full doses over a period of no more than 10 days. Start with ethambutol hydrochloride p. 398 and either isoniazid (with pyridoxine hydrochloride) or rifampicin.

In children with severe or highly infectious tuberculosis who need to interrupt the standard regimen, consider continuing treatment with at least 2 drugs with low risk of hepatotoxicity, such as ethambutol hydrochloride and streptomycin p. 334 (with or without a fluoroquinolone antibiotic, such as levofloxacin p. 728 or moxifloxacin p. 729), with ongoing monitoring by a liver specialist. ⟨A⟩

Treatment interruptions due to cutaneous reactions

EvGr If a child with severe or highly infectious tuberculosis has a cutaneous reaction, consider continuing treatment with a combination of at least 2 drugs with low risk for causing cutaneous reactions, such as ethambutol hydrochloride and streptomycin, with monitoring by a dermatologist. ⟨A⟩

Drug-resistant tuberculosis

EvGr Treatment of drug-resistant tuberculosis should be managed by a multidisciplinary team with experience in such cases, and where appropriate facilities for infection-control exist. ⟨A⟩ The risk of resistance is minimised by ensuring therapy is administered in the correct dose and combination for the prescribed duration.

Single drug-resistant tuberculosis

EvGr For single drug-resistance in individuals with tuberculosis with central nervous system involvement, refer to a specialist with experience in managing drug-resistant tuberculosis. ⟨A⟩ For those without central nervous system involvement, the following treatment regimens are recommended:

Resistance to isoniazid:

- EvGr First 2 months (initial phase): rifampicin, pyrazinamide p. 400 and ethambutol hydrochloride;
- Continue with (continuation phase): rifampicin and ethambutol hydrochloride for 7 months (up to 10 months for extensive disease). ⟨A⟩

Resistance to pyrazinamide:

- EvGr First 2 months (initial phase): rifampicin, ethambutol hydrochloride and isoniazid (with pyridoxine hydrochloride);
- Continue with (continuation phase): rifampicin and isoniazid (with pyridoxine hydrochloride) for 7 months. ⟨A⟩

Resistance to ethambutol hydrochloride:

- EvGr First 2 months (initial phase): rifampicin, pyrazinamide and isoniazid (with pyridoxine hydrochloride);
- Continue with (continuation phase): rifampicin and isoniazid (with pyridoxine hydrochloride) for 4 months. ⟨A⟩

Resistance to rifampicin:

- EvGr Offer treatment with at least 6 antituberculosis drugs to which the mycobacterium is likely to be sensitive. ⟨A⟩

Multi-drug resistant tuberculosis

EvGr In multidrug-resistant tuberculosis (*resistance to isoniazid and rifampicin, with or without any other resistance*), positive cases of rifampicin resistance require treatment with at least 6 antituberculosis drugs to which the mycobacterium is likely to be sensitive. Testing for resistance to second-line drugs is recommended and treatment should be modified according to susceptibility. ⟨A⟩

Useful Resources

Tuberculosis. National Institute for Health and Care Excellence. NICE guideline 33. September 2019.
www.nice.org.uk/guidance/ng33

Other drugs used for Tuberculosis Rifabutin, below

ANTIMYCOBACTERIALS › RIFAMYCINS

Rifabutin

09-May-2020

- **INDICATIONS AND DOSE**

Prophylaxis of *Mycobacterium avium* complex infections in immunosuppressed patients with low CD4 count

▶ BY MOUTH

- Child 1 month–11 years: 5 mg/kg once daily (max. per dose 300 mg), also consult product literature
- Child 12–17 years: 300 mg once daily, also consult product literature

Treatment of non-tuberculous mycobacterial disease, in combination with other drugs

▶ BY MOUTH

- Child 1 month–11 years: 5 mg/kg once daily for up to 6 months after cultures negative
- Child 12–17 years: 450–600 mg once daily for up to 6 months after cultures negative

Treatment of pulmonary tuberculosis, in combination with other drugs

▶ BY MOUTH

- Child 12–17 years: 150–450 mg once daily for at least 6 months

- **UNLICENSED USE** Not licensed for use in children.
- **CAUTIONS** Acute porphyrias p. 652 · discolours soft contact lenses
- **INTERACTIONS** → Appendix 1: rifabutin
- **SIDE-EFFECTS** Agranulocytosis · anaemia · arthralgia · bronchospasm · chest pain · corneal deposits · decreased leucocytes · dyspnoea · eosinophilia · fever · haemolysis · hepatic disorders · influenza like illness · myalgia · nausea · neutropenia · pancytopenia · skin reactions · thrombocytopenia · urine discolouration · uveitis (more common following high doses or concomitant use with drugs that increase plasma concentration) · vomiting
- **ALLERGY AND CROSS-SENSITIVITY** Contra-indicated in patients with rifamycin hypersensitivity.
- **CONCEPTION AND CONTRACEPTION**
Important Rifabutin induces hepatic enzymes and the effectiveness of hormonal contraceptives is reduced; alternative family planning advice should be offered.
- **PREGNANCY** Manufacturer advises avoid—no information available.
- **BREAST FEEDING** Manufacturer advises avoid—no information available.
- **HEPATIC IMPAIRMENT** Manufacturer advises caution in severe impairment.
- **RENAL IMPAIRMENT**
Dose adjustments Use half normal dose if estimated glomerular filtration rate less than 30 mL/minute/1.73 m^2.

- **MONITORING REQUIREMENTS**
  - *Renal function* should be checked before treatment.
  - *Hepatic function* should be checked before treatment. If there is no evidence of liver disease (and pre-treatment liver function is normal), further checks are only necessary if the patient develops fever, malaise, vomiting, jaundice or unexplained deterioration during treatment. However, hepatic function should be monitored on prolonged therapy.
  - Blood counts should be monitored on prolonged therapy.
- **PRESCRIBING AND DISPENSING INFORMATION** If treatment interruption occurs, re-introduce with low dosage and increase gradually.
- **PATIENT AND CARER ADVICE**

  Soft contact lenses Patients or their carers should be advised that rifabutin discolours soft contact lenses.

  Hepatic disorders Patients or their carers should be told how to recognise signs of liver disorder, and advised to discontinue treatment and seek immediate medical attention if symptoms such as persistent nausea, vomiting, malaise or jaundice develop.

- **MEDICINAL FORMS** There can be variation in the licensing of different medicines containing the same drug. Forms available from special-order manufacturers include: oral suspension, oral solution

Capsule

CAUTIONARY AND ADVISORY LABELS 8, 14

- Mycobutin (Pfizer Ltd)

  Rifabutin 150 mg Mycobutin 150mg capsules | 30 capsule PoM £90.38 DT = £90.38

Rifampicin

09-May-2020

- **INDICATIONS AND DOSE**

Brucellosis in combination with other antibacterials | Legionnaires disease in combination with other antibacterials | Serious staphylococcal infections in combination with other antibacterials

- BY MOUTH, OR BY INTRAVENOUS INFUSION
  - Neonate: 5–10 mg/kg twice daily.
  - Child 1–11 months: 5–10 mg/kg twice daily
  - Child 1–17 years: 10 mg/kg twice daily (max. per dose 600 mg)

Tuberculosis, in combination with other drugs (intermittent supervised 6-month treatment) (under expert supervision)

- BY MOUTH
  - Child: 15 mg/kg 3 times a week (max. per dose 900 mg) for 6 months (initial and continuation phases)

Tuberculosis, in combination with other drugs (standard unsupervised 6-month treatment)

- BY MOUTH
  - Child (body-weight up to 50 kg): 15 mg/kg once daily for 6 months (initial and continuation phases); maximum 450 mg per day
  - Child (body-weight 50 kg and above): 15 mg/kg once daily for 6 months (initial and continuation phases); maximum 600 mg per day

Congenital tuberculosis

- BY MOUTH
  - Neonate: 15 mg/kg once daily for 6 months (initial and continuation phases).

Prevention of tuberculosis in susceptible close contacts or those who have become tuberculin positive, in combination with isoniazid

- BY MOUTH
  - Child 1 month–11 years (body-weight up to 50 kg): 15 mg/kg daily for 3 months; maximum 450 mg per day
  - Child 1 month–11 years (body-weight 50 kg and above): 15 mg/kg daily for 3 months; maximum 600 mg per day
  - Child 12–17 years (body-weight up to 50 kg): 450 mg daily for 3 months
  - Child 12–17 years (body-weight 50 kg and above): 600 mg daily for 3 months

Prevention of tuberculosis in susceptible close contacts or those who have become tuberculin positive, who are isoniazid-resistant

- BY MOUTH
  - Child 1 month–11 years (body-weight up to 50 kg): 15 mg/kg daily for 6 months; maximum 450 mg per day
  - Child 1 month–11 years (body-weight 50 kg and above): 15 mg/kg daily for 6 months; maximum 600 mg per day
  - Child 12–17 years (body-weight up to 50 kg): 450 mg daily for 6 months
  - Child 12–17 years (body-weight 50 kg and above): 600 mg daily for 6 months

Prevention of secondary case of *Haemophilus influenzae* type b disease

- BY MOUTH
  - Child 1–2 months: 10 mg/kg once daily for 4 days
  - Child 3 months–11 years: 20 mg/kg once daily (max. per dose 600 mg) for 4 days
  - Child 12–17 years: 600 mg once daily for 4 days

Prevention of secondary case of meningococcal meningitis

- BY MOUTH
  - Neonate: 5 mg/kg every 12 hours for 2 days.
  - Child 1–11 months: 5 mg/kg every 12 hours for 2 days
  - Child 1–11 years: 10 mg/kg every 12 hours (max. per dose 600 mg), for 2 days
  - Child 12–17 years: 600 mg every 12 hours for 2 days

Pruritus due to cholestasis

- BY MOUTH
  - Child: 5–10 mg/kg once daily (max. per dose 600 mg)

- **UNLICENSED USE** Not licensed for use in children for pruritus due to cholestasis.
- **CONTRA-INDICATIONS** Acute porphyrias p. 652 · jaundice
- **CAUTIONS** Discolours soft contact lenses
- **INTERACTIONS** → Appendix 1: rifampicin
- **SIDE-EFFECTS**

  GENERAL SIDE-EFFECTS
  - **Common or very common** Nausea · thrombocytopenia · vomiting
  - **Uncommon** Diarrhoea · leucopenia
  - **Frequency not known** Abdominal discomfort · acute kidney injury · adrenal insufficiency · agranulocytosis · appetite decreased · disseminated intravascular coagulation · dyspnoea · eosinophilia · flushing · haemolytic anaemia · hepatitis · hypersensitivity · influenza · intracranial haemorrhage · menstrual disorder · muscle weakness · myopathy · oedema · pseudomembranous enterocolitis · severe cutaneous adverse reactions (SCARs) · shock · skin reactions · sputum discolouration · sweat discolouration · tear discolouration · urine discolouration · vasculitis · wheezing

  SPECIFIC SIDE-EFFECTS
  - With intravenous use Bone pain · gastrointestinal disorder · hyperbilirubinaemia · psychotic disorder
  - With oral use Psychosis

  SIDE-EFFECTS, FURTHER INFORMATION Side-effects that mainly occur with intermittent therapy include influenza-like symptoms (with chills, fever, dizziness, bone pain), respiratory symptoms (including shortness of breath), collapse and shock, haemolytic anaemia, thrombocytopenic purpura, and acute renal failure.

Discontinue if serious side-effects develop.

- **ALLERGY AND CROSS-SENSITIVITY** Contra-indicated in patients with rifamycin hypersensitivity.
- **CONCEPTION AND CONTRACEPTION**
  Important Effectiveness of hormonal contraceptives is reduced and alternative family planning advice should be offered.
- **PREGNANCY** Manufacturers advise very high doses teratogenic in *animal* studies in first trimester; risk of neonatal bleeding may be increased in third trimester.
- **BREAST FEEDING** Amount too small to be harmful.
- **HEPATIC IMPAIRMENT** Manufacturer advises caution—monitor liver function weekly for two weeks, then every two weeks for the next six weeks.
  Dose adjustments Manufacturer advises maximum 8 mg/kg per day.
- **RENAL IMPAIRMENT** Use with caution if doses above 10 mg/kg daily.
- **MONITORING REQUIREMENTS**
  - *Renal function* should be checked before treatment.
  - *Hepatic function* should be checked before treatment. If there is no evidence of liver disease (and pre-treatment liver function is normal), further checks are only necessary if the patient develops fever, malaise, vomiting, jaundice or unexplained deterioration during treatment. However, liver function should be monitored on prolonged therapy.
  - Blood counts should be monitored in patients on prolonged therapy.
- **DIRECTIONS FOR ADMINISTRATION**
  - With intravenous use Displacement value may be significant, consult local reconstitution guidelines; reconstitute with solvent provided. May be further diluted with Glucose 5% *or* Sodium chloride 0.9% to a final concentration of 1.2 mg/mL. Infuse over 2–3 hours.
- **PRESCRIBING AND DISPENSING INFORMATION** If treatment interruption occurs, re-introduce with low dosage and increase gradually.
  Flavours of syrup may include raspberry.
  - With oral use In general, doses should be rounded up to facilitate administration of suitable volumes of liquid or an appropriate strength of tablet. Doses may also need to be recalculated to allow for weight gain in younger children.
- **PATIENT AND CARER ADVICE**
  Soft contact lenses Patients or their carers should be advised that rifampicin discolours soft contact lenses.
  Hepatic disorders Patients or their carers should be told how to recognise signs of liver disorder, and advised to discontinue treatment and seek immediate medical attention if symptoms such as persistent nausea, vomiting, malaise or jaundice develop.
  Medicines for Children leaflet: Rifampicin for meningococcal prophylaxis www.medicinesforchildren.org.uk/rifampicin-meningococcal-prophylaxis
  Medicines for Children leaflet: Rifampicin for the treatment of tuberculosis www.medicinesforchildren.org.uk/rifampicin-treatment-tuberculosis
- **MEDICINAL FORMS** There can be variation in the licensing of different medicines containing the same drug. Forms available from special-order manufacturers include: oral suspension, oral solution

Oral suspension

CAUTIONARY AND ADVISORY LABELS 8, 14, 23
EXCIPIENTS: May contain Sucrose

- Rifadin (Sanofi)
  Rifampicin 20 mg per 1 ml Rifadin 100mg/5ml syrup | 120 ml PoM £4.27 DT = £4.27

Capsule

CAUTIONARY AND ADVISORY LABELS 8, 14, 23

- Rifampicin (Non-proprietary)
  Rifampicin 150 mg Rifampicin 150mg capsules | 100 capsule PoM £54.85 DT = £54.85
  Rifampicin 300 mg Rifampicin 300mg capsules | 100 capsule PoM £123.90 DT = £123.90
- Rifadin (Sanofi)
  Rifampicin 150 mg Rifadin 150mg capsules | 100 capsule PoM £18.32 DT = £54.85
  Rifampicin 300 mg Rifadin 300mg capsules | 100 capsule PoM £36.63 DT = £123.90
- Rimactane (Sandoz Ltd)
  Rifampicin 300 mg Rimactane 300mg capsules | 60 capsule PoM £21.98

Powder and solvent for solution for infusion

ELECTROLYTES: May contain Sodium

- Rifadin (Sanofi)
  Rifampicin 600 mg Rifadin 600mg powder and solvent for solution for infusion vials | 1 vial PoM £9.20

Rifampicin with isoniazid

10-Mar-2020

The properties listed below are those particular to the combination only. For the properties of the components please consider, rifampicin p. 396, isoniazid p. 399.

- **INDICATIONS AND DOSE**

Treatment of tuberculosis (continuation phase)

- BY MOUTH
  - Child: Although not licensed in children, consideration may be given to use of *Rifinah*® in older children, provided the respective dose of each drug is appropriate for the weight of the child (consult local protocol).

DOSE EQUIVALENCE AND CONVERSION

- *Rifinah*® Tablets contain rifampicin and isoniazid; the proportions are expressed in the form x/y where x and y are the strengths in milligrams of rifampicin and isoniazid respectively.
- Each *Rifinah*® 150/100 Tablet contains rifampicin 150 mg and isoniazid 100 mg.
- Each *Rifinah*® 300/150 Tablet contains rifampicin 300 mg and isoniazid 150 mg.

- **UNLICENSED USE** Not licensed for use in children.
- **INTERACTIONS** → Appendix 1: isoniazid · rifampicin
- **PATIENT AND CARER ADVICE**
  Medicines for Children leaflet: Isoniazid and rifampicin combination for latent tuberculosis www.medicinesforchildren.org.uk/isoniazid-and-rifampicin-combination-latent-tuberculosis
- **MEDICINAL FORMS** There can be variation in the licensing of different medicines containing the same drug.

Tablet

CAUTIONARY AND ADVISORY LABELS 8, 14, 23

- Rifinah (Sanofi)
  Isoniazid 100 mg, Rifampicin 150 mg Rifinah 150mg/100mg tablets | 84 tablet PoM £19.09 DT = £19.09
  Isoniazid 150 mg, Rifampicin 300 mg Rifinah 300mg/150mg tablets | 56 tablet PoM £25.22 DT = £25.22

Rifampicin with isoniazid and pyrazinamide

The properties listed below are those particular to the combination only. For the properties of the components please consider, rifampicin p. 396, isoniazid p. 399, pyrazinamide p. 400.

- **INDICATIONS AND DOSE**

Initial treatment of tuberculosis (in combination with ethambutol)

- Child: Although not licensed in children, consideration may be given to use of *Rifater*® in older children, provided the respective dose of each drug is appropriate for the weight of the child (consult local protocol).

DOSE EQUIVALENCE AND CONVERSION

- Tablet quantities refer to the number of *Rifater*® Tablets which should be taken. Each *Rifater*® Tablet contains isoniazid 50 mg, pyrazinamide 300 mg and rifampicin 120 mg.

- **UNLICENSED USE** Not licensed for use in children.
- **INTERACTIONS** → Appendix 1: isoniazid · pyrazinamide · rifampicin

- **MEDICINAL FORMS** There can be variation in the licensing of different medicines containing the same drug.

Tablet

CAUTIONARY AND ADVISORY LABELS 8, 14, 22

- Rifater (Sanofi)
  Isoniazid 50 mg, Rifampicin 120 mg, Pyrazinamide 300 mg Rifater tablets | 100 tablet PoM £26.34

ANTIMYCOBACTERIALS › OTHER

Cycloserine

- **INDICATIONS AND DOSE**

Tuberculosis resistant to first-line drugs, in combination with other drugs

▶ BY MOUTH

- Child 2–11 years: Initially 5 mg/kg twice daily (max. per dose 250 mg), then increased if necessary up to 10 mg/kg twice daily (max. per dose 500 mg), dose to be increased according to blood concentration and response
- Child 12–17 years: Initially 250 mg every 12 hours for 2 weeks, then increased if necessary up to 500 mg every 12 hours, dose to be increased according to blood concentration and response

PHARMACOKINETICS

- Cycloserine penetrates the CNS.

- **UNLICENSED USE** Licensed for use in children (age range not specified by manufacturer).
- **CONTRA-INDICATIONS** Alcohol dependence · depression · epilepsy · psychotic states · severe anxiety
- **INTERACTIONS** → Appendix 1: cycloserine
- **SIDE-EFFECTS** Behaviour abnormal · coma · confusion · congestive heart failure · drowsiness · dysarthria · headache · hyperirritability · megaloblastic anaemia · memory loss · neurological effects · paraesthesia · paresis · psychosis · rash · reflexes increased · seizures · suicidal ideation · tremor · vertigo

SIDE-EFFECTS, FURTHER INFORMATION **CNS toxicity** Discontinue or reduce dose if symptoms of CNS toxicity occur.

Rashes or allergic dermatitis Discontinue or reduce dose if rashes or allergic dermatitis develop.

- **PREGNANCY** Manufacturer advises use only if potential benefit outweighs risk—crosses the placenta.
- **BREAST FEEDING** Present in milk—amount too small to be harmful.
- **RENAL IMPAIRMENT**

Dose adjustments Increase interval between doses if creatinine clearance less than 50 mL/minute/1.73 m^2.
Monitoring Monitor blood-cycloserine concentration if creatinine clearance less than 50 mL/minute/1.73 m^2.

- **MONITORING REQUIREMENTS**

- Blood concentration should not exceed a peak concentration of 30 mg/litre (measured 3–4 hours after the dose).
- Monitor haematological, renal, and hepatic function.

- **MEDICINAL FORMS** There can be variation in the licensing of different medicines containing the same drug.

Capsule

CAUTIONARY AND ADVISORY LABELS 2, 8

- **Cycloserine (Non-proprietary)**
  Cycloserine 250 mg Cycloserine 250mg capsules | 100 capsule PoM £442.89 DT = £442.89

Ethambutol hydrochloride

11-May-2020

- **INDICATIONS AND DOSE**

Tuberculosis, in combination with other drugs (standard unsupervised 6-month treatment)

▶ BY MOUTH

- Child: 20 mg/kg once daily for 2 months (initial phase)

Tuberculosis, in combination with other drugs (intermittent supervised 6-month treatment) (under expert supervision)

▶ BY MOUTH

- Child: 30 mg/kg 3 times a week for 2 months (initial phase)

Congenital tuberculosis, in combination with other drugs

▶ BY MOUTH

- Neonate: 20 mg/kg once daily for 2 months (initial phase).

- **CONTRA-INDICATIONS** Optic neuritis · poor vision
- **CAUTIONS** Young children

CAUTIONS, FURTHER INFORMATION

- Understanding warnings Patients who cannot understand warnings about visual side-effects should, if possible, be given an alternative drug. In particular, ethambutol should be used with caution in children until they are at least 5 years old and capable of reporting symptomatic visual changes accurately.

- **INTERACTIONS** → Appendix 1: ethambutol
- **SIDE-EFFECTS**

- **Common or very common** Hyperuricaemia · nerve disorders · visual impairment
- **Rare or very rare** Nephritis tubulointerstitial
- **Frequency not known** Alveolitis allergic · appetite decreased · asthenia · confusion · dizziness · eosinophilia · fever · flatulence · gastrointestinal discomfort · gout · hallucination · headache · jaundice · leucopenia · nausea · nephrotoxicity · neutropenia · photosensitive lichenoid eruption · sensation abnormal · severe cutaneous adverse reactions (SCARs) · skin reactions · taste metallic · thrombocytopenia · tremor · vomiting

SIDE-EFFECTS, FURTHER INFORMATION Ocular toxicity is more common where excessive dosage is used or if the patient's renal function is impaired. Early discontinuation of the drug is almost always followed by recovery of eyesight.

- **PREGNANCY** Not known to be harmful.

- **BREAST FEEDING** Amount too small to be harmful.
- **RENAL IMPAIRMENT** Risk of optic nerve damage. Should preferably be avoided in patients with renal impairment.
  Dose adjustments If creatinine clearance less than 30 mL/minute/1.73 m^2, use 15–25 mg/kg (max. 2.5 g) 3 times a week.
  Monitoring If creatinine clearance less than 30 mL/minute/1.73 m^2, monitor plasma-ethambutol concentration.
- **MONITORING REQUIREMENTS**
  - 'Peak' concentration (2–2.5 hours after dose) should be 2–6 mg/litre (7–22 micromol/litre); 'trough' (pre-dose) concentration should be less than 1 mg/litre (4 micromol/litre).
  - Renal function should be checked before treatment.
  - Visual acuity should be tested by Snellen chart before treatment with ethambutol.
  - In young children, routine ophthalmological monitoring recommended.
- **PRESCRIBING AND DISPENSING INFORMATION** The RCPCH and NPPG recommend that, when a liquid special of ethambutol is required, the following strength is used: 400 mg/5 mL.
- **PATIENT AND CARER ADVICE**
  Ocular toxicity The earliest features of ocular toxicity are subjective and patients should be advised to discontinue therapy immediately if they develop deterioration in vision and promptly seek further advice.
  Medicines for Children leaflet: Ethambutol for the treatment of tuberculosis www.medicinesforchildren.org.uk/ethambutol-treatment-tuberculosis

- **MEDICINAL FORMS** There can be variation in the licensing of different medicines containing the same drug. Forms available from special-order manufacturers include: oral suspension, oral solution

Tablet

CAUTIONARY AND ADVISORY LABELS 8

- Ethambutol hydrochloride (Non-proprietary)
  Ethambutol hydrochloride 100 mg Ethambutol 100mg tablets | 56 tablet [PoM] £17.00 DT = £11.51
  Ethambutol hydrochloride 400 mg Ethambutol 400mg tablets | 56 tablet [PoM] £42.74 DT = £42.74

Isoniazid

08-May-2020

- **INDICATIONS AND DOSE**

Tuberculosis, in combination with other drugs (standard unsupervised 6-month treatment)

- BY MOUTH, OR BY INTRAMUSCULAR INJECTION, OR BY INTRAVENOUS INJECTION
  - Child: 10 mg/kg once daily (max. per dose 300 mg) for 6 months (initial and continuation phases)

Tuberculosis, in combination with other drugs (intermittent supervised 6-month treatment) (under expert supervision)

- BY MOUTH, OR BY INTRAMUSCULAR INJECTION, OR BY INTRAVENOUS INJECTION
  - Child: 15 mg/kg 3 times a week (max. per dose 900 mg) for 6 months (initial and continuation phases)

Congenital tuberculosis, in combination with other drugs

- BY MOUTH, OR BY INTRAMUSCULAR INJECTION, OR BY INTRAVENOUS INJECTION
  - Neonate: 10 mg/kg daily for 6 months (initial and continuation phases).

Prevention of tuberculosis in susceptible close contacts or those who have become tuberculin positive

- INITIALLY BY MOUTH, OR BY INTRAMUSCULAR INJECTION, OR BY INTRAVENOUS INJECTION
  - Neonate: 10 mg/kg daily for 6 months.
  - Child 1 month–11 years: 10 mg/kg daily (max. per dose 300 mg) for 6 months, alternatively (by mouth) 10 mg/kg daily (max. per dose 300 mg) for 3 months, to be taken in combination with rifampicin
  - Child 12–17 years: 300 mg daily for 6 months, alternatively (by mouth) 300 mg daily for 3 months, to be taken in combination with rifampicin

- **CONTRA-INDICATIONS** Drug-induced liver disease
- **CAUTIONS** Acute porphyrias p. 652 · alcohol dependence · diabetes mellitus · epilepsy · history of psychosis · HIV infection · malnutrition · slow acetylator status (increased risk of side-effects)
  CAUTIONS, FURTHER INFORMATION
  - Peripheral neuropathy Pyridoxine hydrochloride p. 678 should be given prophylactically in all patients from the start of treatment. Peripheral neuropathy is more likely to occur where there are pre-existing risk factors such as diabetes, alcohol dependence, chronic renal failure, pregnancy, malnutrition and HIV infection.
- **INTERACTIONS** → Appendix 1: isoniazid
- **SIDE-EFFECTS**
  - **Uncommon** Hepatic disorders
  - **Rare or very rare** Severe cutaneous adverse reactions (SCARs)
  - **Frequency not known** Agranulocytosis · alopecia · anaemia · aplastic anaemia · eosinophilia · fever · gynaecomastia · haemolytic anaemia · hyperglycaemia · lupus-like syndrome · nerve disorders · optic atrophy · pancreatitis · pellagra · psychosis · seizure · skin reactions · thrombocytopenia · vasculitis
- **PREGNANCY** Not known to be harmful; prophylactic pyridoxine recommended.
- **BREAST FEEDING** Theoretical risk of convulsions and neuropathy; prophylactic pyridoxine advisable in mother.
  Monitoring In breast-feeding, monitor infant for possible toxicity.
- **HEPATIC IMPAIRMENT** Manufacturer advises caution (increased risk of hepatotoxicity).
  Monitoring In patients with pre-existing liver disease or hepatic impairment monitor liver function regularly and particularly frequently in the first 2 months.
- **RENAL IMPAIRMENT** Risk of ototoxicity and peripheral neuropathy; prophylactic pyridoxine hydrochloride p. 678 recommended.
- **MONITORING REQUIREMENTS**
  - *Renal function* should be checked before treatment.
  - *Hepatic function* should be checked before treatment. If there is no evidence of liver disease (and pre-treatment liver function is normal), further checks are only necessary if the patient develops fever, malaise, vomiting, jaundice or unexplained deterioration during treatment.
- **PRESCRIBING AND DISPENSING INFORMATION**
  - With oral use In general, doses should be rounded up to facilitate administration of suitable volumes of liquid or an appropriate strength of tablet. The RCPCH and NPPG recommend that, when a liquid special of isoniazid is required, the following strength is used: 50 mg/5 mL.
    Doses may need to be recalculated to allow for weight gain in younger children.
- **PATIENT AND CARER ADVICE**
  Hepatic disorders Patients or their carers should be told how to recognise signs of liver disorder, and advised to discontinue treatment and seek immediate medical

attention if symptoms such as persistent nausea, vomiting, malaise or jaundice develop.
Medicines for Children leaflet: Isoniazid for latent tuberculosis www.medicinesforchildren.org.uk/isoniazid-latent-tuberculosis
Medicines for Children leaflet: Isoniazid for the treatment of tuberculosis www.medicinesforchildren.org.uk/isoniazid-treatment-tuberculosis

- **MEDICINAL FORMS** There can be variation in the licensing of different medicines containing the same drug. Forms available from special-order manufacturers include: oral suspension, oral solution

Solution for injection

- **Isoniazid (Non-proprietary)**
  Isoniazid 25 mg per 1 ml Isoniazid 50mg/2ml solution for injection ampoules | 10 ampoule PoM £387.32

Tablet
CAUTIONARY AND ADVISORY LABELS 8, 22

- **Isoniazid (Non-proprietary)**
  Isoniazid 50 mg Isoniazid 50mg tablets | 56 tablet PoM £19.25 DT = £19.25
  Isoniazid 100 mg Isoniazid 100mg tablets | 28 tablet PoM £25.13 DT = £24.85
  Isoniazid 300 mg Isoniazid 300mg tablets | 30 tablet PoM ⊠

Combinations available: ***Rifampicin with isoniazid,*** **p. 397 ·** ***Rifampicin with isoniazid and pyrazinamide,*** **p. 398**

Pyrazinamide

12-May-2020

- **INDICATIONS AND DOSE**

Tuberculosis, in combination with other drugs (standard unsupervised 6-month treatment)

▶ BY MOUTH

- Child (body-weight up to 50 kg): 35 mg/kg once daily for 2 months (initial phase); maximum 1.5 g per day
- Child (body-weight 50 kg and above): 35 mg/kg once daily for 2 months (initial phase); maximum 2 g per day

Tuberculosis, in combination with other drugs (intermittent supervised 6-month treatment) (under expert supervision)

▶ BY MOUTH

- Child (body-weight up to 50 kg): 50 mg/kg 3 times a week (max. per dose 2 g 3 times a week) for 2 months (initial phase)
- Child (body-weight 50 kg and above): 50 mg/kg 3 times a week (max. per dose 2.5 g 3 times a week) for 2 months (initial phase)

Congenital tuberculosis, in combination with other drugs

▶ BY MOUTH

- Neonate: 35 mg/kg once daily for 2 months (initial phase).

- **CAUTIONS** Diabetes
- **INTERACTIONS** → Appendix 1: pyrazinamide
- **SIDE-EFFECTS** Appetite decreased · arthralgia · dysuria · flushing · gout aggravated · hepatic disorders · malaise · nausea · peptic ulcer aggravated · photosensitivity reaction · sideroblastic anaemia · skin reactions · splenomegaly · vomiting
- **PREGNANCY** Manufacturer advises use only if potential benefit outweighs risk.
- **BREAST FEEDING** Amount too small to be harmful.
- **HEPATIC IMPAIRMENT** Manufacturer advises avoid in severe impairment, acute hepatic disease and for up to 6 months after occurrence of hepatitis (risk of increased exposure).
- **RENAL IMPAIRMENT**
  Dose adjustments If estimated glomerular filtration rate less than 30 mL/minute/1.73 m^2, use 25–30 mg/kg 3 times a week.
- **MONITORING REQUIREMENTS**
  - *Renal function* should be checked before treatment.
  - *Hepatic function* should be checked before treatment. If there is no evidence of liver disease (and pre-treatment liver function is normal), further checks are only necessary if the patient develops fever, malaise, vomiting, jaundice or unexplained deterioration during treatment.
- **PRESCRIBING AND DISPENSING INFORMATION** In general, doses should be rounded up to facilitate administration of suitable volumes of liquid or an appropriate strength of tablet. Doses may also need to be recalculated to allow for weight gain in younger children.
  The RCPCH and NPPG recommend that, when a liquid special of pyrazinamide is required, the following strength is used: 500 mg/5 mL.
- **PATIENT AND CARER ADVICE**
  Hepatic disorders Patients or their carers should be told how to recognise signs of liver disorder, and advised to discontinue treatment and seek immediate medical attention if symptoms such as persistent nausea, vomiting, malaise or jaundice develop.
  Medicines for Children leaflet: Pyrazinamide for treatment of tuberculosis www.medicinesforchildren.org.uk/pyrazinamide-treatment-tuberculosis

- **MEDICINAL FORMS** There can be variation in the licensing of different medicines containing the same drug. Forms available from special-order manufacturers include: oral suspension, oral solution

Tablet
CAUTIONARY AND ADVISORY LABELS 8

- **Pyrazinamide (Non-proprietary)**
  Pyrazinamide 500 mg Pyrazinamide 500mg tablets | 30 tablet PoM £40.06 DT = £40.06
- **Zinamide** (Genus Pharmaceuticals Ltd)
  Pyrazinamide 500 mg Zinamide 500mg tablets | 30 tablet PoM £31.35 DT = £40.06

Combinations available: ***Rifampicin with isoniazid and pyrazinamide,*** **p. 398**

1.5 Urinary tract infections

Urinary-tract infections

12-Feb-2019

Description of condition

Urinary-tract infections (UTIs) are common infections that can affect any part of the urinary tract. They occur more frequently in females, and are usually independent of any risk factor. The risk of a UTI is greater in children aged under 1 year, in those with functional and structural abnormalities that may cause urinary retention, and in those who are sexually active. UTIs are predominantly caused by bacteria from the gastrointestinal tract entering the urinary tract with *Escherichia coli* being the most common cause.

Lower UTIs are associated with inflammation of the bladder (cystitis) and urethra (urethritis). In some children the infection can ascend the urinary tract and lead to an upper UTI. Upper UTIs affect the proximal part of the ureters (pyelitis) or the proximal part of the ureters and the kidneys (pyelonephritis). Acute pyelonephritis, especially in children with vesicoureteric reflux, may lead to renal scarring, hypertension or failure, and sepsis. The most common UTI symptoms in children younger than 3 months of age are fever, vomiting, lethargy, and irritability. Children older than 3 months of age usually present with fever, dysuria, or increased urinary frequency, that may be accompanied by vomiting, poor feeding, lethargy, irritability and abdominal pain or tenderness.

In pregnant females, asymptomatic bacteriuria is a risk factor for pyelonephritis and premature labour. UTIs in pregnant females have been associated with developmental delay and cerebral palsy in the infant, as well as fetal death.

Insertion of a catheter into the urinary tract also increases the risk of developing a UTI, and the longer the catheter is in place for, further increases the risk of bacteriuria.

UTIs are considered recurrent after at least two episodes of acute pyelonephritis, three episodes of a lower UTI, or one episode of acute pyelonephritis in addition to one or more episodes of a lower UTI.

Aims of treatment

The aims of treatment are to relieve symptoms, treat the underlying infection, prevent systemic infection, and to reduce the risk of complications.

Non-drug treatment

EvGr Parents or carers of children with a UTI should be advised to ensure their child drinks plenty of fluids to avoid dehydration, and to use self-care strategies to reduce the risk of recurrent infections. These include wiping from front to back after defaecation, not delaying urination, and not wearing occlusive underwear.

Cranberry products may be used for the prevention of recurrent UTIs on the advice of a specialist, however the benefit of these products is uncertain. Children and their parents or carers should be advised to consider the sugar content of these products. (A)

Drug treatment

EvGr When prescribing antibacterial therapy the severity of symptoms, risk of developing complications, previous urine culture and susceptibility results, and previous antibacterial use should be taken into consideration.

With the exception of pregnant females, asymptomatic bacteriuria is not routinely treated with antibacterials. (A)

For other considerations such as for children receiving prophylactic antibacterial therapy, switching from *intravenous* to *oral* antibacterials, and for advice to give to children and their parents, or carers, see Antibacterials, principles of therapy p. 318.

EvGr Reassess children if symptoms worsen at any time, or do not start to improve within 48 hours of starting treatment.

Refer children to hospital if they have any symptoms or signs suggestive of a more serious illness or condition.

Review choice of antibacterial when microbiological results are available, and change treatment as appropriate if susceptibility results indicate bacterial resistance.

Advise parents or carers that paracetamol or ibuprofen can be used for pain relief as appropriate. In acute pyelonephritis, codeine may also be considered (child aged 12 years and over). (A)

Child under 3 months of age

EvGr Children under 3 months of age with a possible UTI should be referred to a paediatric specialist. (A)

Lower urinary-tract infection

Non-pregnant females aged 16 years and over

EvGr Consider a back-up antibacterial prescription for use if symptoms worsen or do not improve within 48 hours **or** an immediate antibacterial prescription. (A)

Choice of antibacterial therapy

- ***Oral*** *first line*:
  - ▸ EvGr Nitrofurantoin p. 403, or trimethoprim p. 390 (if low risk of resistance). (A)
- ***Oral*** *second line* (if no improvement after at least 48 hours **or** first line not suitable):
  - ▸ EvGr Nitrofurantoin (if not used first line), fosfomycin p. 386, or pivmecillinam hydrochloride p. 373. (A)

Males aged 16 years and over

EvGr An immediate antibacterial prescription should be given and a midstream urine sample obtained before treatment is taken and sent for culture and susceptibility testing. (A)

Choice of antibacterial therapy

- ***Oral*** *first line*:
  - ▸ EvGr Nitrofurantoin, or trimethoprim. (A)
- ***Oral*** *second line* (if no improvement after at least 48 hours, or first line not suitable):
  - ▸ Consider pyelonephritis or prostatitis. See *pyelonephritis, acute*, or *prostatitis, acute* below for guidance.

Pregnant females aged 12 years and over

EvGr An immediate antibacterial prescription should be given and a urine sample obtained before treatment is taken and sent for culture and susceptibility testing. (A)

Choice of antibacterial therapy

- ***Oral*** *first line*:
  - ▸ EvGr Nitrofurantoin. (A)
- ***Oral*** *second line* (if no improvement after at least 48 hours, **or** first line not suitable):
  - ▸ EvGr Amoxicillin p. 366 (only if culture susceptible), or cefalexin p. 339. (A)
- ***Alternative*** *second line*:
  - ▸ EvGr Consult local microbiologist. (A)
- ***Asymptomatic bacteriuria***:
  - ▸ EvGr Amoxicillin, cefalexin, or nitrofurantoin. (A)

Children aged 3 months to under 16 years of age

EvGr An immediate antibacterial prescription should be given and a urine sample obtained before treatment is taken and sent for culture and susceptibility testing. In children aged 3 months and over a dipstick urine test may be used. (A)

Choice of antibacterial therapy

- ***Oral*** *first line*:
  - ▸ EvGr Nitrofurantoin, or trimethoprim (if low risk of resistance). (A)
- ***Oral*** *second line* (if no improvement after at least 48 hours **or** first line not suitable):
  - ▸ EvGr Nitrofurantoin (if not used first line), or amoxicillin (if culture susceptible), or cefalexin. (A)

Pyelonephritis, acute

EvGr An immediate antibacterial prescription should be given and a urine sample obtained before treatment is taken and sent for culture and susceptibility testing.

Consider referring or seeking specialist advice for children with pyelonephritis who are significantly dehydrated or are unable to take oral fluids and medicines, are pregnant, or have a higher risk of developing complications. (A)

Non-pregnant females and males aged 16 years and over

Choice of antibacterial therapy

- ***Oral*** *first line*:
  - ▸ EvGr Cefalexin, or ciprofloxacin p. 377. If sensitivity known: co-amoxiclav p. 370, or trimethoprim p. 390. (A)
- ***Intravenous*** *first line* (if severely unwell or unable to take oral treatment). EvGr Antibacterials may be combined if concerned about susceptibility or sepsis.
  - ▸ Amikacin p. 332, ceftriaxone p. 343, cefuroxime p. 341, ciprofloxacin p. 377, or gentamicin p. 333. Co-amoxiclav p. 370 may be used if given in combination or sensitivity known. (A)
- ***Intravenous*** *second line*:
  - ▸ EvGr Consult local microbiologist. (A)

Pregnant females aged 12 years and over

Choice of antibacterial therapy

- ***Oral*** *first line*:
  - ▸ EvGr Cefalexin p. 339. (A)
- ***Intravenous*** *first line* (if severely unwell or unable to take oral treatment):
  - ▸ EvGr Cefuroxime. (A)
- *Second line* or combining antibacterials if concerned about susceptibility or sepsis:
  - ▸ EvGr Consult local microbiologist. (A)

Children aged 3 months to under 16 years

Choice of antibacterial therapy

- ***Oral*** *first line*:
- ▸ EvGr Cefalexin, or co-amoxiclav (if sensitivity known). Ⓐ
- ***Intravenous*** *first line* (if severely unwell or unable to take oral treatment). EvGr Antibacterials may be combined if concerned about susceptibility or sepsis.
- ▸ Amikacin, ceftriaxone, cefuroxime, gentamicin, or co-amoxiclav (if given in combination or sensitivity known). Ⓐ
- ***Intravenous*** *second line*:
- ▸ EvGr Consult local microbiologist. Ⓐ

Recurrent urinary-tract infection

EvGr For children with recurrent UTIs, refer or seek specialist advice for those at high risk of serious illness, males aged 16 years and over, pregnant females, children with suspected cancer, those presenting with recurrent upper UTI, and those with recurrent lower UTI with an unknown cause.

Consider a trial of antibacterial prophylaxis in non-pregnant females if behavioural and personal hygiene measures have not been effective or appropriate.

In non-pregnant females aged 16 years and over, single-dose antibacterial prophylaxis [unlicensed indication] should be considered for use when exposed to an identifiable trigger. Daily antibacterial prophylaxis should be considered in non-pregnant females aged 16 years and over who have had no improvement after single-dose antibacterial prophylaxis, or have no identifiable triggers.

With specialist advice, daily antibacterial prophylaxis should be considered in males, pregnant females, and children under 16 years of age if behavioural and personal hygiene measures alone are not effective or appropriate.

Advise parents or carers about the risk of resistance with long-term antibacterial use, seeking medical help if the child develops symptoms of an acute UTI, and to return for review within 6 months.

Review the success, and ongoing need of prophylaxis at least every 6 months. If antibacterial prophylaxis is stopped ensure the child has rapid access to treatment if they develop an acute UTI. Ⓐ

Females and males

Choice of antibacterial therapy

- ***Oral*** *first line*:
- ▸ EvGr Trimethoprim, or nitrofurantoin p. 403.
- ***Oral*** *second line*:
- ▸ EvGr Amoxicillin p. 366 [unlicensed indication], or cefalexin. Ⓐ

Catheter-associated urinary-tract infection

EvGr For children with a catheter-associated urinary-tract infection, consider removing or changing the catheter as soon as possible if it has been in place for longer than 7 days, without delaying antibacterial treatment. An immediate antibacterial prescription should be given and a urine sample obtained before treatment is taken and sent for culture and susceptibility testing.

Consider referring or seeking specialist advice for children with a catheter-associated UTI who are significantly dehydrated or unable to take oral fluids and medicines, are pregnant, have a higher risk of developing complications, have recurrent catheter-associated UTIs, or have bacteria resistant to oral antibacterials. Ⓐ

Non-pregnant females and males aged 16 years and over

Choice of antibacterial therapy

- ***Oral*** *first line* (if **no** upper UTI symptoms):
- ▸ EvGr Amoxicillin (only if culture susceptible), nitrofurantoin, or trimethoprim (if low risk of resistance). Ⓐ
- ***Oral*** *second line* (if **no** upper UTI symptoms and first line not suitable):
- ▸ EvGr Pivmecillinam hydrochloride p. 373. Ⓐ
- ***Oral*** *first line* (upper UTI symptoms):
- ▸ EvGr Cefalexin, ciprofloxacin, co-amoxiclav (only if culture susceptible), or trimethoprim (only if culture susceptible). Ⓐ
- ***Intravenous*** *first line* (if severely unwell or unable to take oral treatment). EvGr Antibacterials may be combined if concerned about susceptibility or sepsis.
- ▸ Amikacin, ceftriaxone, cefuroxime, ciprofloxacin, gentamicin, or co-amoxiclav (only in combination, unless culture results confirm susceptibility). Ⓐ
- ***Intravenous*** *second line*:
- ▸ EvGr Consult local microbiologist. Ⓐ

Pregnant females aged 12 years and over

Choice of antibacterial therapy

- ***Oral*** *first line*:
- ▸ EvGr Cefalexin. Ⓐ
- ***Intravenous*** *first line* (if severely unwell or unable to take oral treatment)
- ▸ EvGr Cefuroxime. Ⓐ
- *Second line or combining if concerned about susceptibility or sepsis*:
- ▸ EvGr Consult local microbiologist. Ⓐ

Children aged 3 months to under 16 years

Choice of antibacterial therapy

- ***Oral*** *first line*:
- ▸ EvGr Cefalexin or trimethoprim (if low risk of resistance), amoxicillin (if culture susceptible), or co-amoxiclav (if culture susceptible). Ⓐ
- ***Intravenous*** *first line* (if severely unwell or unable to take oral treatment). EvGr Antibacterials may be combined if concerned about susceptibility or sepsis.
- ▸ Amikacin, ceftriaxone, cefuroxime, gentamicin, or co-amoxiclav (only in combination, unless culture results confirm susceptibility). Ⓐ
- ***Intravenous*** *second line*:
- ▸ EvGr Consult local microbiologist. Ⓐ

Useful Resources

Urinary tract infection (lower): antimicrobial prescribing. National Institute for Health and Care Excellence. Clinical Guideline 109. October 2018.
www.nice.org.uk/guidance/ng109

Pyelonephritis (acute): antimicrobial prescribing. National Institute for Health and Care Excellence. Clinical Guideline 111. October 2018.
www.nice.org.uk/guidance/ng111

Urinary tract infection (recurrent): antimicrobial prescribing. National Institute for Health and Care Excellence. Clinical Guideline 112. October 2018.
www.nice.org.uk/guidance/ng112

Urinary tract infection (catheter-associated): antimicrobial prescribing. National Institute for Health and Care Excellence. Clinical Guideline 113. November 2018.
www.nice.org.uk/guidance/ng113

Patient decision aids: Urinary tract infection (lower); Urinary tract infection (recurrent) National Institute for Health and Care Excellence. November 2018.
www.nice.org.uk/about/what-we-do/our-programmes/nice-guidance/nice-guidelines/shared-decision-making

ANTIBACTERIALS > OTHER

Nitrofurantoin

11-May-2020

● **INDICATIONS AND DOSE**

Lower urinary-tract infections

▶ BY MOUTH USING IMMEDIATE-RELEASE MEDICINES
- Child 3 months–11 years: 750 micrograms/kg 4 times a day for 3 days
- Child 12–15 years: 50 mg 4 times a day for 3 days (7 days in pregnant women)
- Child 16–17 years: 50 mg 4 times a day for 3 days (7 days in males and pregnant women)

▶ BY MOUTH USING MODIFIED-RELEASE MEDICINES
- Child 12–15 years: 100 mg twice daily for 3 days (7 days in pregnant women)
- Child 16–17 years: 100 mg twice daily for 3 days (7 days in males and pregnant women)

Urinary-tract infections (catheter-associated)

▶ BY MOUTH USING IMMEDIATE-RELEASE MEDICINES
- Child 16–17 years: 50 mg 4 times a day for 7 days, to be used if modified-release preparations are unavailable

▶ BY MOUTH USING MODIFIED-RELEASE MEDICINES
- Child 16–17 years: 100 mg twice daily for 7 days

Severe chronic recurrent urinary-tract infections

▶ BY MOUTH USING IMMEDIATE-RELEASE MEDICINES
- Child 12–17 years: 100 mg 4 times a day for 3–7 days

Prophylaxis of recurrent urinary-tract infection

▶ BY MOUTH USING IMMEDIATE-RELEASE MEDICINES
- Child 3 months–11 years: 1 mg/kg once daily, dose to be taken at night
- Child 12–15 years: 50–100 mg once daily, dose to be taken at night
- Child 16–17 years: 50–100 mg once daily, dose to be taken at night, alternatively 100 mg for 1 dose, following exposure to a trigger

Genito-urinary surgical prophylaxis

▶ BY MOUTH USING MODIFIED-RELEASE MEDICINES
- Child 12–17 years: 100 mg twice daily on day of procedure and for 3 days after

● **UNLICENSED USE** EvGr Duration of treatment for lower urinary-tract infection differs from product literature and adheres to national guidelines. (A) See Urinary-tract infections p. 400 for further information. EvGr Nitrofurantoin can be given as a single dose for the prophylaxis of recurrent urinary tract infection following exposure to a trigger, (A) but this dosing regimen is not licensed. See Urinary-tract infections p. 400 for further information.

● **CONTRA-INDICATIONS** Acute porphyrias p. 652 · G6PD deficiency · infants less than 3 months old

● **CAUTIONS** Anaemia · diabetes mellitus · electrolyte imbalance · folate deficiency · pulmonary disease · susceptibility to peripheral neuropathy · urine may be coloured yellow or brown · vitamin B deficiency

● **INTERACTIONS** → Appendix 1: nitrofurantoin

● **SIDE-EFFECTS** Agranulocytosis · alopecia · anaemia · angioedema · aplastic anaemia · appetite decreased · arthralgia · asthenia · chest pain · chills · circulatory collapse · confusion · cough · cyanosis · depression · diarrhoea · dizziness · drowsiness · dyspnoea · eosinophilia · euphoric mood · fever · granulocytopenia · haemolytic anaemia · headache · hepatic disorders · idiopathic intracranial hypertension · increased risk of infection · leucopenia · lupus-like syndrome · nausea · nerve disorders · nystagmus · pancreatitis · psychotic disorder · pulmonary hypersensitivity · pulmonary reaction (possible association with lupus erythematosus-like syndrome) · respiratory disorders · skin reactions · Stevens-Johnson syndrome · thrombocytopenia · urine discolouration · vertigo · vomiting

● **PREGNANCY** Avoid at term—may produce neonatal haemolysis.

● **BREAST FEEDING** Avoid; only small amounts in milk but enough to produce haemolysis in G6PD-deficient infants.

● **HEPATIC IMPAIRMENT** Manufacturer advises caution.

● **RENAL IMPAIRMENT** Risk of peripheral neuropathy; antibacterial efficacy depends on renal secretion of the drug into urinary tract. Avoid if estimated glomerular filtration rate less than 45 mL/minute/1.73 m^2; may be used with caution if estimated glomerular filtration rate 30–44 mL/minute/1.73 m^2 as a short-course only (3 to 7 days), to treat uncomplicated lower urinary-tract infection caused by suspected or proven multidrug resistant bacteria and only if potential benefit outweighs risk.

● **MONITORING REQUIREMENTS** On long-term therapy, monitor liver function and monitor for pulmonary symptoms (discontinue if deterioration in lung function).

● **EFFECT ON LABORATORY TESTS** False positive urinary glucose (if tested for reducing substances).

● **PATIENT AND CARER ADVICE**
Medicines for Children leaflet: Nitrofurantoin for urinary tract infections www.medicinesforchildren.org.uk/nitrofurantoin-urinary-tract-infections

● **MEDICINAL FORMS** There can be variation in the licensing of different medicines containing the same drug. Forms available from special-order manufacturers include: oral suspension, oral solution

Tablet

CAUTIONARY AND ADVISORY LABELS 9, 14, 21

▶ Nitrofurantoin (Non-proprietary)
Nitrofurantoin 50 mg Nitrofurantoin 50mg tablets | 28 tablet PoM £31.33 DT = £10.41 | 100 tablet PoM £28.21–£111.89
Nitrofurantoin 100 mg Nitrofurantoin 100mg tablets | 28 tablet PoM £12.99 DT = £8.66 | 100 tablet PoM £21.07–£38.14

▶ Genfura (Genesis Pharmaceuticals Ltd)
Nitrofurantoin 50 mg Genfura 50mg tablets | 28 tablet PoM £8.00 DT = £10.41 | 100 tablet PoM £28.57
Nitrofurantoin 100 mg Genfura 100mg tablets | 100 tablet PoM £30.36

Oral suspension

CAUTIONARY AND ADVISORY LABELS 9, 14, 21

▶ Nitrofurantoin (Non-proprietary)
Nitrofurantoin 5 mg per 1 ml Nitrofurantoin 25mg/5ml oral suspension sugar free sugar-free | 300 ml PoM £446.95–£603.38 DT = £525.17

Modified-release capsule

CAUTIONARY AND ADVISORY LABELS 9, 14, 21, 25

▶ Macrobid (Advanz Pharma)
Nitrofurantoin 100 mg Macrobid 100mg modified-release capsules | 14 capsule PoM £9.50 DT = £9.50

Capsule

CAUTIONARY AND ADVISORY LABELS 9, 14, 21

▶ Nitrofurantoin (Non-proprietary)
Nitrofurantoin 50 mg Nitrofurantoin 50mg capsules | 30 capsule PoM £16.47 DT = £12.20
Nitrofurantoin 100 mg Nitrofurantoin 100mg capsules | 30 capsule PoM £10.43 DT = £10.43

2 Fungal infection

Antifungals, systemic use

Fungal infections

The systemic treatment of common fungal infections is outlined below; specialist treatment is required in most forms of systemic or disseminated fungal infections. Local treatment is suitable for a number of fungal infections (genital, bladder, eye, ear, oropharynx, and skin).

Aspergillosis

Aspergillosis most commonly affects the respiratory tract but in severely immunocompromised patients, invasive forms can affect the heart, brain, and skin. Voriconazole p. 410 is the treatment of choice for aspergillosis; liposomal amphotericin p. 406 is an alternative first-line treatment when voriconazole cannot be used. Caspofungin p. 405 or itraconazole p. 409 can be used in patients who are refractory to, or intolerant of voriconazole and liposomal amphotericin. Itraconazole is also used for the treatment of chronic pulmonary aspergillosis or as an adjunct in the treatment of allergic bronchopulmonary aspergillosis [unlicensed indication].

Candidiasis

Many superficial candidal infections, including infections of the skin, are treated locally. Systemic antifungal treatment is required in widespread or intractable infection. Vaginal candidiasis can be treated with locally acting antifungals; alternatively, fluconazole p. 407 can be given by mouth.

Oropharyngeal candidiasis generally responds to topical therapy. Fluconazole is given by mouth for unresponsive infections; it is reliably absorbed and is effective. Itraconazole may be used for infections that do not respond to fluconazole. Topical therapy may not be adequate in immunocompromised children and an oral triazole antifungal is preferred.

For *invasive or disseminated candidiasis*, either amphotericin by intravenous infusion or an **echinocandin** can be used. Fluconazole is an alternative for *Candida albicans* infection in clinically stable children who have not received an azole antifungal recently. Amphotericin should be considered for the initial treatment of CNS candidiasis. Voriconazole can be used for infections caused by fluconazole-resistant *Candida* spp. when oral therapy is required, or in children intolerant of amphotericin or an echinocandin. In refractory cases, flucytosine p. 412 can be used with intravenous amphotericin.

Cryptococcosis

Cryptococcosis is uncommon but infection in the immunocompromised, especially in HIV-positive patients, can be life-threatening; cryptococcal meningitis is the most common form of fungal meningitis. The treatment of choice in cryptococcal meningitis is amphotericin by intravenous infusion and flucytosine by intravenous infusion for 2 weeks, followed by fluconazole by mouth for 8 weeks or until cultures are negative. In cryptococcosis, fluconazole is sometimes given alone as an alternative in HIV-positive patients with mild, localised infections or in those who cannot tolerate amphotericin. Following successful treatment, fluconazole can be used for prophylaxis against relapse until immunity recovers.

Histoplasmosis

Histoplasmosis is rare in temperate climates; it can be life-threatening, particularly in HIV-infected persons. Itraconazole can be used for the treatment of immunocompetent patients with indolent non-meningeal infection, including chronic pulmonary histoplasmosis. Amphotericin by intravenous infusion is used for the initial treatment of fulminant or severe infections, followed by a course of itraconazole by mouth. Following successful treatment, itraconazole can be used for prophylaxis against relapse until immunity recovers.

Skin and nail infections

Mild localised fungal infections of the skin (including tinea corporis, tinea cruris, and tinea pedis) respond to topical therapy. Systemic therapy is appropriate if topical therapy fails, if many areas are affected, or if the site of infection is difficult to treat such as in infections of the nails (onychomycosis) and of the scalp (tinea capitis).

Oral imidazole or triazole antifungals (particularly itraconazole) and terbinafine p. 778 are used more frequently than griseofulvin p. 412 because they have a broader spectrum of activity and require a shorter duration of treatment.

Tinea capitis is treated systemically; additional topical application of an antifungal may reduce transmission. Griseofulvin is used for tinea capitis in adults and children; it is effective against infections caused by *Trichophyton tonsurans* and *Microsporum* spp. Terbinafine is used for tinea capitis caused by *T. tonsurans*[unlicensed indication]. The role of terbinafine in the management of *Microsporum* infections is uncertain. Fluconazole or itraconazole are alternatives in the treatment of tinea capitis caused by *T. tonsurans* or *Microsporum* spp. [both unlicensed indications].

Pityriasis versicolor may be treated with itraconazole by mouth if topical therapy is ineffective; fluconazole by mouth is an alternative. Oral terbinafine is **not** effective for pityriasis versicolor.

Antifungal treatment may not be necessary in asymptomatic patients with tinea infection of the nails. If treatment is necessary, a systemic antifungal is more effective than topical therapy. Terbinafine and itraconazole have largely replaced griseofulvin for the systemic treatment of *onychomycosis*, particularly of the toenail; they should be used under specialist advice in children. Although terbinafine is not licensed for use in children, it is considered to be the drug of choice for onychomycosis. Itraconazole can be administered as intermittent 'pulse' therapy. Topical antifungals also have a role in the treatment of onychomycosis.

Immunocompromised children

Immunocompromised children are at particular risk of fungal infections and may receive antifungal drugs prophylactically; oral triazole antifungals are the drugs of choice for prophylaxis. Fluconazole is more reliably absorbed than itraconazole, but fluconazole is not effective against *Aspergillus* spp. Itraconazole is preferred in patients at risk of invasive aspergillosis. Micafungin p. 405 can be used for prophylaxis of candidiasis in patients undergoing haematopoietic stem cell transplantation when fluconazole or itraconazole cannot be used.

Amphotericin by intravenous infusion or caspofungin is used for the empirical *treatment* of serious fungal infections in immunocompromised children; caspofungin is not effective against fungal infections of the CNS.

Triazole antifungals

Triazole antifungal drugs have a role in the prevention and systemic treatment of fungal infections.

Fluconazole is very well absorbed after oral administration. It also achieves good penetration into the cerebrospinal fluid to treat fungal meningitis. Fluconazole is excreted largely unchanged in the urine and can be used to treat candiduria.

Itraconazole is active against a wide range of dermatophytes. There is limited information available on use in children. Itraconazole capsules require an acid environment in the stomach for optimal absorption. Itraconazole has been associated with liver damage and should be avoided or used with caution in patients with liver disease; fluconazole is less frequently associated with hepatotoxicity.

Voriconazole is a broad-spectrum antifungal drug which is licensed in adults for use in life-threatening infections.

Imidazole antifungals

The imidazole antifungals include clotrimazole p. 555, econazole nitrate p. 555, ketoconazole p. 777, and tioconazole p. 777. They are used for the local treatment of vaginal candidiasis and for dermatophyte infections. Miconazole p. 762 can be used locally for oral infections; it is also effective in intestinal infections. Systemic absorption may follow use of miconazole oral gel and may result in significant drug interactions.

Polyene antifungals

The polyene antifungals include amphotericin p. 406 and nystatin p. 763; neither drug is absorbed when given by mouth. Nystatin is used for oral, oropharyngeal, and perioral infections by local application in the mouth. Nystatin is also used for *Candida albicans* infection of the skin.

Amphotericin by intravenous infusion is used for the treatment of systemic fungal infections and is active against most fungi and yeasts. It is highly protein bound and penetrates poorly into body fluids and tissues. When given parenterally amphotericin is toxic and side-effects are common. Lipid formulations of amphotericin (*Abelcet®* and *AmBisome®*) are significantly less toxic and are recommended when the conventional formulation of amphotericin is contra-indicated because of toxicity, especially nephrotoxicity or when response to conventional amphotericin is inadequate; lipid formulations are more expensive.

Echinocandin antifungals

The echinocandin antifungals include caspofungin below and micafungin below. They are only active against *Aspergillus* spp. and *Candida* spp.; however, micafungin is not used for the treatment of aspergillosis. Echinocandins are not effective against fungal infections of the CNS. Echinocandin antifungals have a role in the prevention and systemic treatment of fungal infections.

Other antifungals

Flucytosine p. 412 is used with amphotericin in a synergistic combination. Bone marrow depression can occur which limits its use, particularly in HIV-positive patients; weekly blood counts are necessary during prolonged therapy. Resistance to flucytosine can develop during therapy and sensitivity testing is essential before and during treatment. Flucytosine has a role in the treatment of systemic candidiasis and cryptococcal meningitis.

Griseofulvin p. 412 is effective for widespread or intractable dermatophyte infections but has been superseded by newer antifungals, particularly for nail infections. Griseofulvin is used in the treatment of tinea capitis. It is the drug of choice for trichophyton infections in children. Duration of therapy is dependent on the site of the infection and may extend to a number of months.

Terbinafine p. 778 is the drug of choice for fungal nail infections and is also used for ringworm infections where oral treatment is considered appropriate.

ANTIFUNGALS › ECHINOCANDIN ANTIFUNGALS

Caspofungin

● **INDICATIONS AND DOSE**

Invasive aspergillosis | Invasive candidiasis | Empirical treatment of systemic fungal infections in patients with neutropenia

▶ BY INTRAVENOUS INFUSION

- Neonate: 25 mg/m² once daily.

- Child 1–2 months: 25 mg/m² once daily
- Child 3–11 months: 50 mg/m² once daily
- Child 1–17 years: 70 mg/m² once daily (max. per dose 70 mg) for 1 day, then 50 mg/m² once daily (max. per dose 70 mg); increased to 70 mg/m² once daily (max. per dose 70 mg), dose may be increased if lower dose tolerated but inadequate response

DOSE ADJUSTMENTS DUE TO INTERACTIONS

- Manufacturer advises increase dose to 70 mg/m² daily (max. 70 mg daily) with concurrent use of some enzyme inducers (such as carbamazepine, dexamethasone, phenytoin, and rifampicin).

● **INTERACTIONS** → Appendix 1: caspofungin

● **SIDE-EFFECTS**

▶ **Common or very common** Arrhythmias · arthralgia · diarrhoea · dyspnoea · electrolyte imbalance · fever · flushing · headache · hyperhidrosis · hypotension · nausea · skin reactions · vomiting

▶ **Uncommon** Anaemia · anxiety · appetite decreased · ascites · chest discomfort · coagulation disorder · congestive heart failure · constipation · cough · disorientation · dizziness · drowsiness · dry mouth · dysphagia · excessive tearing · eyelid oedema · fatigue · flatulence · fluid overload · gastrointestinal discomfort · haematuria · hepatic disorders · hyperbilirubinaemia · hyperglycaemia · hypertension · hypoxia · induration · insomnia · laryngeal pain · leucopenia · malaise · metabolic acidosis · muscle weakness · myalgia · nasal congestion · oedema · pain · palpitations · renal impairment · respiratory disorders · sensation abnormal · taste altered · thrombocytopenia · thrombophlebitis · tremor · vision blurred

▶ **Frequency not known** Severe cutaneous adverse reactions (SCARs)

● **PREGNANCY** Manufacturer advises avoid unless essential—toxicity in *animal* studies.

● **BREAST FEEDING** Present in milk in *animal* studies—manufacturer advises avoid.

● **HEPATIC IMPAIRMENT** No information available for severe impairment.

Dose adjustments Usual initial dose, then use 70% of normal maintenance dose in moderate impairment.

● **DIRECTIONS FOR ADMINISTRATION** For *intravenous infusion* (*Cancidas®*), allow vial to reach room temperature; initially reconstitute 50 mg with 10.5 mL Water for Injections to produce a 5.2 mg/mL solution, or reconstitute 70 mg with 10.5 mL Water for Injections to produce a 7.2 mg/mL solution; mix gently to dissolve; dilute requisite dose to a final concentration not exceeding 500 micrograms/mL with Sodium Chloride 0.9%; give over 60 minutes; incompatible with glucose solutions.

● **MEDICINAL FORMS** There can be variation in the licensing of different medicines containing the same drug.

Powder for solution for infusion

▶ Caspofungin (Non-proprietary)

Caspofungin (as Caspofungin acetate) 50 mg Caspofungin 50mg powder for concentrate for solution for infusion vials | 1 vial [PoM] £50.25–£327.67

Caspofungin (as Caspofungin acetate) 70 mg Caspofungin 70mg powder for concentrate for solution for infusion vials | 1 vial [PoM] £52.91–£416.78

▶ Cancidas (Merck Sharp & Dohme Ltd)

Caspofungin (as Caspofungin acetate) 50 mg Cancidas 50mg powder for solution for infusion vials | 1 vial [PoM] £327.67

Caspofungin (as Caspofungin acetate) 70 mg Cancidas 70mg powder for solution for infusion vials | 1 vial [PoM] £416.78

Micafungin

● **INDICATIONS AND DOSE**

Invasive candidiasis

▶ BY INTRAVENOUS INFUSION

- Neonate (administered on expert advice): 2 mg/kg once daily for at least 14 days; increased if necessary to 4 mg/kg once daily, increase dose if response inadequate.

continued →

- Child (body-weight up to 40 kg): 2 mg/kg once daily for at least 14 days; increased if necessary to 4 mg/kg once daily, increase dose if response inadequate
- Child (body-weight 40 kg and above): 100 mg once daily for at least 14 days; increased if necessary to 200 mg once daily, increase dose if response inadequate

Oesophageal candidiasis

▶ BY INTRAVENOUS INFUSION

- Child 16–17 years (body-weight up to 40 kg): 3 mg/kg once daily
- Child 16–17 years (body-weight 40 kg and above): 150 mg once daily

Prophylaxis of candidiasis in patients undergoing bone-marrow transplantation or who are expected to become neutropenic for over 10 days

▶ BY INTRAVENOUS INFUSION

- Neonate: 1 mg/kg once daily continue for at least 7 days after neutrophil count is in desirable range.
- Child (body-weight up to 40 kg): 1 mg/kg once daily continue for at least 7 days after neutrophil count is in desirable range
- Child (body-weight 40 kg and above): 50 mg once daily continue for at least 7 days after neutrophil count is in desirable range

● **INTERACTIONS** → Appendix 1: micafungin

● **SIDE-EFFECTS** Anaemia · anxiety · appetite decreased · arrhythmias · confusion · constipation · diarrhoea · disseminated intravascular coagulation · dizziness · drowsiness · dyspnoea · electrolyte imbalance · eosinophilia · flushing · gastrointestinal discomfort · haemolysis · haemolytic anaemia · headache · hepatic disorders · hepatic failure (potentially life-threatening) · hyperbilirubinaemia · hyperhidrosis · hypersensitivity · hypertension · hypoalbuminaemia · hypotension · insomnia · leucopenia · nausea · neutropenia · palpitations · pancytopenia · peripheral oedema · renal impairment · severe cutaneous adverse reactions (SCARs) · shock · skin reactions · taste altered · thrombocytopenia · tremor · vomiting

● **PREGNANCY** Manufacturer advises avoid unless essential—toxicity in *animal* studies.

● **BREAST FEEDING** Manufacturer advises use only if potential benefit outweighs risk—present in milk in *animal* studies.

● **HEPATIC IMPAIRMENT** Manufacturer advises caution in chronic impairment; avoid in severe impairment (limited information available).

● **RENAL IMPAIRMENT** Use with caution; renal function may deteriorate.

● **MONITORING REQUIREMENTS**

- Monitor renal function.
- Monitor liver function—discontinue if significant and persistent abnormalities in liver function tests develop.

● **DIRECTIONS FOR ADMINISTRATION** For *intravenous infusion* reconstitute each vial with 5 mL Glucose 5% *or* Sodium Chloride 0.9%; gently rotate vial, without shaking, to dissolve; dilute requisite dose to a concentration of 0.5–2 mg/mL with Glucose 5% *or* Sodium Chloride 0.9%; protect infusion from light; give over 60 minutes.

● **MEDICINAL FORMS** There can be variation in the licensing of different medicines containing the same drug.

Powder for solution for infusion

- Mycamine (Astellas Pharma Ltd)
  Micafungin (as Micafungin sodium) 50 mg Mycamine 50mg powder for solution for infusion vials | 1 vial PoM £196.08
  Micafungin (as Micafungin sodium) 100 mg Mycamine 100mg powder for solution for infusion vials | 1 vial PoM £341.00

ANTIFUNGALS > POLYENE ANTIFUNGALS

Amphotericin (Amphotericin B)

21-Nov-2019

● **INDICATIONS AND DOSE**

ABELCET®

Severe invasive candidiasis | Severe systemic fungal infections in patients not responding to conventional amphotericin or to other antifungal drugs or where toxicity or renal impairment precludes conventional amphotericin, including invasive aspergillosis, cryptococcal meningitis and disseminated cryptococcosis in HIV patients

▶ BY INTRAVENOUS INFUSION

- Child: Test dose 100 micrograms/kg (max. per dose 1 mg), then 5 mg/kg once daily

AMBISOME®

Severe systemic or deep mycoses where toxicity (particularly nephrotoxicity) precludes use of conventional amphotericin | Suspected or proven infection in febrile neutropenic patients unresponsive to broad-spectrum antibacterials

▶ BY INTRAVENOUS INFUSION

- Neonate: 1 mg/kg once daily, increased if necessary to 3 mg/kg once daily; maximum 5 mg/kg per day.
- Child: Test dose 100 micrograms/kg (max. per dose 1 mg), to be given over 10 minutes, then 3 mg/kg once daily; maximum 5 mg/kg per day

Visceral leishmaniasis (unresponsive to the antimonial alone)

▶ BY INTRAVENOUS INFUSION

- Child: 1–3 mg/kg daily for 10–21 days to a cumulative dose of 21–30 mg/kg, alternatively 3 mg/kg for 5 consecutive days, followed by 3 mg/kg after 6 days for 1 dose

FUNGIZONE®

Systemic fungal infections

▶ BY INTRAVENOUS INFUSION

- Neonate: 1 mg/kg once daily, increased if necessary to 1.5 mg/kg daily for 7 days, then reduced to 1–1.5 mg/kg once daily on alternate days if required.
- Child: Test dose 100 micrograms/kg (max. per dose 1 mg), included as part of first dose of 250 micrograms/kg daily, then increased if tolerated to 1 mg/kg daily, dose is gradually increased over 2–4 days; in severe infection max. 1.5 mg/kg daily or on alternate days. Prolonged treatment usually necessary; if interrupted for longer than 7 days recommence at 250 micrograms/kg daily and increase gradually

● **UNLICENSED USE**

AMBISOME® *Ambisome®* not licensed for use in children under 1 month.

FUNGIZONE® Intravenous conventional formulation amphotericin (*Fungizone®*) is licensed for use in children (age range not specified by manufacturer).

IMPORTANT SAFETY INFORMATION

MHRA/CHM ADVICE: PARENTERAL AMPHOTERICIN B: REMINDER OF RISK OF POTENTIALLY FATAL ADVERSE REACTION IF FORMULATIONS CONFUSED (JULY 2018)

The MHRA is aware of three fatal overdoses which were caused by medication error in which *Fungizone®* was administered (a non-lipid-based formulation of amphotericin B) instead of a lipid-based formulation. Healthcare professionals are advised:

- when prescribing and dispensing amphotericin products, both the complete generic name and the proprietary name should be used;
- the product name and dose should be verified before administration, especially if the dose prescribed exceeds the maximum recommended dose for *Fungizone®*.

- **CAUTIONS** Avoid rapid infusion (risk of arrhythmias) · when given parenterally, toxicity common (close supervision necessary and close observation required for at least 30 minutes after test dose)

CAUTIONS, FURTHER INFORMATION

▸ Anaphylaxis Anaphylaxis can occur with any intravenous amphotericin product and a test dose is advisable before the first infusion in children over 1 month of age; the patient should be carefully observed for at least 30 minutes after the test dose. Prophylactic antipyretics or hydrocortisone should only be used in patients who have previously experienced acute adverse reactions (in whom continued treatment with amphotericin is essential).

- **INTERACTIONS** → Appendix 1: amphotericin
- **SIDE-EFFECTS**

▸ **Common or very common** Anaemia · appetite decreased · azotaemia · chills · diarrhoea · dyspnoea · electrolyte imbalance · fever · headache · hepatic function abnormal (discontinue) · hyposthenuria · hypotension · nausea · nephrocalcinosis · renal impairment · renal tubular acidosis · skin reactions · vomiting

▸ **Uncommon** Agranulocytosis · arrhythmias · flushing · gastrointestinal discomfort · hepatic disorders · leucopenia · myalgia · peripheral neuropathy · respiratory disorders · thrombocytopenia

▸ **Rare or very rare** Arthralgia · cardiac arrest · coagulation disorder · deafness · encephalopathy · eosinophilia · haemorrhage · heart failure · hypersensitivity · hypertension · malaise · nephrogenic diabetes insipidus · pain · pulmonary oedema non-cardiogenic · seizure · severe cutaneous adverse reactions (SCARs) · shock · tinnitus · vertigo · vision disorders · weight decreased

- **PREGNANCY** Not known to be harmful but manufacturers advise avoid unless potential benefit outweighs risk.
- **BREAST FEEDING** No information available.
- **RENAL IMPAIRMENT** Use only if no alternative; nephrotoxicity may be reduced with use of lipid formulation.
- **MONITORING REQUIREMENTS** Hepatic and renal function tests, blood counts, and plasma electrolyte (including plasma-potassium and magnesium concentration) monitoring required.
- **DIRECTIONS FOR ADMINISTRATION**

ABELCET® **Amphotericin (lipid complex)**

For *intravenous infusion*, allow suspension to reach room temperature, shake gently to ensure no yellow settlement, withdraw requisite dose (using 17–19 gauge needle) into one or more 20-mL syringes; replace needle on syringe with a 5-micron filter needle provided (fresh needle for each syringe) and dilute in Glucose 5% to a concentration of 2 mg/mL; preferably give *via* an infusion pump at a rate of 2.5 mg/kg/hour (initial test dose given over 15 minutes); an in-line filter (pore size no less than 15 micron) may be used; do not use sodium chloride or other electrolyte solutions—flush existing intravenous line with Glucose 5% or use separate line.

AMBISOME® **Amphotericin (liposomal)**

For *intravenous infusion*, reconstitute each vial with 12 mL Water for Injections and shake vigorously to produce a preparation containing 4 mg/mL; withdraw requisite dose from vial and introduce into Glucose 5% or 10% through the 5-micron filter provided, to produce a final concentration of 0.2–2 mg/mL; infuse over 30–60 minutes, or if non-anaphylactic infusion-related reactions occur infuse over 2 hours (initial test dose given over 10 minutes); an in-line filter (pore size no less than 1 micron) may be used; incompatible with sodium chloride solutions—flush existing intravenous line with Glucose 5% or 10%, or use separate line.

FUNGIZONE® **Amphotericin (as sodium deoxycholate complex)**

For *intravenous infusion*, reconstitute each vial with 10 mL Water for Injections and shake immediately to produce a 5 mg/mL colloidal solution; dilute further in Glucose 5% to a concentration of 100 micrograms/mL (in fluid-restricted children, up to 400 micrograms/mL given via a central line); pH of glucose solution must not be below 4.2 (check each container—consult product literature for details of buffer); infuse over 4–6 hours, or if tolerated over a minimum of 2 hours (initial test dose given over 20–30 minutes); begin infusion immediately after dilution and protect from light; incompatible with Sodium Chloride solutions—flush existing intravenous line with Glucose 5% or use separate line; an in-line filter (pore size no less than 1 micron) may be used.

- **PRESCRIBING AND DISPENSING INFORMATION** Amphotericin is available as *conventional, liposomal* and *lipid complex* formulations. These different formulations vary in their licensed indications, pharmacokinetics, dosage and administration, and are **not** interchangeable.

- **MEDICINAL FORMS** There can be variation in the licensing of different medicines containing the same drug.

Suspension for infusion

ELECTROLYTES: May contain Sodium

▸ Abelcet (Teva UK Ltd)

Amphotericin B (as Amphotericin B phospholipid complex) 5 mg per 1 ml Abelcet 100mg/20ml concentrate for suspension for infusion vials | 10 vial PoM £775.04 (Hospital only)

Powder for solution for infusion

EXCIPIENTS: May contain Sucrose

ELECTROLYTES: May contain Sodium

▸ Fungizone (Cheplapharm Arzneimittel GmbH)

Amphotericin B 50 mg Fungizone 50mg powder for concentrate for solution for infusion vials | 1 vial PoM £3.88 DT = £3.88

ANTIFUNGALS › TRIAZOLE ANTIFUNGALS

Fluconazole

10-Mar-2020

- **INDICATIONS AND DOSE**

Candidal balanitis

▸ BY MOUTH

▸ Child 16–17 years: 150 mg for 1 dose

Vaginal candidiasis

▸ BY MOUTH

▸ Child: 150 mg for 1 dose, for use in patients who are post-puberty

Vulvovaginal candidiasis (recurrent)

▸ BY MOUTH

▸ Child: Initially 150 mg every 72 hours for 3 doses, then 150 mg once weekly for 6 months, for use in patients who are post-puberty

Mucosal candidiasis (except genital)

▸ BY MOUTH, OR BY INTRAVENOUS INFUSION

▸ Neonate up to 14 days: 3–6 mg/kg, dose to be given on first day, then 3 mg/kg every 72 hours.

▸ Neonate 14 days to 28 days: 3–6 mg/kg, dose to be given on first day, then 3 mg/kg every 48 hours.

▸ Child 1 month–11 years: 3–6 mg/kg, dose to be given on first day, then 3 mg/kg daily (max. per dose 100 mg) for

continued →

5 Infection

7–14 days in oropharyngeal candidiasis (max. 14 days except in severely immunocompromised patients); for 14–30 days in other mucosal infections (e.g. oesophagitis, candiduria, non-invasive bronchopulmonary infections)
- Child 12–17 years: 50 mg daily for 7–14 days in oropharyngeal candidiasis (max. 14 days except in severely immunocompromised patients); for 14–30 days in other mucosal infections (e.g. oesophagitis, candiduria, non-invasive bronchopulmonary infections); increased to 100 mg daily, increased dose only for unusually difficult infections

Tinea capitis
- ▶ BY MOUTH
- Child 1–17 years: 6 mg/kg daily (max. per dose 300 mg) for 2–4 weeks

Tinea pedis, corporis, cruris, pityriasis versicolor | Dermal candidiasis
- ▶ BY MOUTH
- Child: 3 mg/kg daily (max. per dose 50 mg) for 2–4 weeks (for up to 6 weeks in tinea pedis); max. duration of treatment 6 weeks

Invasive candidal infections (including candidaemia and disseminated candidiasis) and cryptococcal infections (including meningitis)
- ▶ BY MOUTH, OR BY INTRAVENOUS INFUSION
- Neonate up to 14 days: 6–12 mg/kg every 72 hours, treatment continued according to response (at least 8 weeks for cryptococcal meningitis).
- Neonate 14 days to 28 days: 6–12 mg/kg every 48 hours, treatment continued according to response (at least 8 weeks for cryptococcal meningitis).
- Child: 6–12 mg/kg daily (max. per dose 800 mg), treatment continued according to response (at least 8 weeks for cryptococcal meningitis)

Prevention of fungal infections in immunocompromised patients
- ▶ BY MOUTH, OR BY INTRAVENOUS INFUSION
- Neonate up to 14 days: 3–12 mg/kg every 72 hours, dose given according to extent and duration of neutropenia.
- Neonate 14 days to 28 days: 3–12 mg/kg every 48 hours, dose given according to extent and duration of neutropenia.
- Child: 3–12 mg/kg daily (max. per dose 400 mg), commence treatment before anticipated onset of neutropenia and continue for 7 days after neutrophil count in desirable range, dose given according to extent and duration of neutropenia

Prevention of fungal infections in immunocompromised patients (for patients with high risk of systemic infections e.g. following bone-marrow transplantation)
- ▶ BY MOUTH, OR BY INTRAVENOUS INFUSION
- Child: 12 mg/kg daily (max. per dose 400 mg), commence treatment before anticipated onset of neutropenia and continue for 7 days after neutrophil count in desirable range

Prevention of relapse of cryptococcal meningitis in HIV-infected patients after completion of primary therapy
- ▶ BY MOUTH, OR BY INTRAVENOUS INFUSION
- Child: 6 mg/kg daily (max. per dose 200 mg)

- **UNLICENSED USE** Not licensed for tinea infections in children, or for vaginal candidiasis in girls under 16 years, or for prevention of relapse of cryptococcal meningitis after completion of primary therapy in children with AIDS.
- **CONTRA-INDICATIONS** Acute porphyrias p. 652
- **CAUTIONS** Susceptibility to QT interval prolongation
- **INTERACTIONS** → Appendix 1: antifungals, azoles
- **SIDE-EFFECTS**

GENERAL SIDE-EFFECTS
- ▶ **Common or very common** Diarrhoea · gastrointestinal discomfort · headache · nausea · skin reactions · vomiting
- ▶ **Uncommon** Dizziness · flatulence · hepatic disorders · seizure · taste altered
- ▶ **Rare or very rare** Agranulocytosis · alopecia · dyslipidaemia · hypokalaemia · leucopenia · neutropenia · QT interval prolongation · severe cutaneous adverse reactions (SCARs) · thrombocytopenia · torsade de pointes

SPECIFIC SIDE-EFFECTS
- ▶ **Uncommon**
- With parenteral use Anaemia · appetite decreased · asthenia · constipation · drowsiness · dry mouth · fever · hyperhidrosis · insomnia · malaise · myalgia · paraesthesia · vertigo
- ▶ **Rare or very rare**
- With parenteral use Angioedema · face oedema · tremor
- ▶ **Frequency not known**
- With oral use Cardio-respiratory distress · oedema

SIDE-EFFECTS, FURTHER INFORMATION If rash occurs, discontinue treatment (or monitor closely if infection invasive or systemic); severe cutaneous reactions are more likely in patients with AIDS.

- **PREGNANCY** Manufacturer advises avoid—multiple congenital abnormalities reported with long-term high doses.
- **BREAST FEEDING** Present in milk but amount probably too small to be harmful.
- **HEPATIC IMPAIRMENT** Manufacturer advises caution—limited information available.
- **RENAL IMPAIRMENT**

Dose adjustments Usual initial dose then halve subsequent doses if estimated glomerular filtration rate less than 50 mL/minute/1.73 m^2.

- **MONITORING REQUIREMENTS** Monitor liver function with high doses or extended courses—discontinue if signs or symptoms of hepatic disease (risk of hepatic necrosis).
- **DIRECTIONS FOR ADMINISTRATION**
- With intravenous use For *intravenous infusion*, give over 10–30 minutes; do not exceed an infusion rate of 5–10 mL/minute.
- **PRESCRIBING AND DISPENSING INFORMATION** Flavours of oral liquid formulations may include orange.
- **PATIENT AND CARER ADVICE**

Medicines for Children leaflet: Fluconazole for yeast and fungal infections www.medicinesforchildren.org.uk/fluconazole-yeast-and-fungal-infections

- **PROFESSION SPECIFIC INFORMATION**

Dental practitioners' formulary
Fluconazole Capsules 50 mg may be prescribed.

Fluconazole Oral Suspension 50 mg/5 mL may be prescribed.

- **EXCEPTIONS TO LEGAL CATEGORY** Fluconazole capsules can be sold to the public for vaginal candidiasis and associated candidal balanitis in those aged 16–60 years, in a container or packaging containing not more than 150 mg and labelled to show a max. dose of 150 mg.

- **MEDICINAL FORMS** There can be variation in the licensing of different medicines containing the same drug.

Infusion
- ▶ Fluconazole (Non-proprietary)

Fluconazole 2 mg per 1 ml Fluconazole 200mg/100ml infusion bags | 5 bag PoM £19.45 (Hospital only) | 10 bag PoM £65.00 (Hospital only)
Fluconazole 400mg/200ml infusion bags | 5 bag PoM £72.50 (Hospital only)

Solution for infusion

ELECTROLYTES: May contain Sodium

▸ **Fluconazole (Non-proprietary)**

Fluconazole 2 mg per 1 ml Fluconazole 200mg/100ml solution for infusion vials | 1 vial PoM £15.00–£29.28 DT = £29.28
Fluconazole 100mg/50ml solution for infusion vials | 5 vial PoM £12.60 (Hospital only)
Fluconazole 50mg/25ml solution for infusion vials | 1 vial PoM £20.00
Fluconazole 200mg/100ml solution for infusion bottles | 10 bottle PoM £392.30 | 20 bottle PoM £603.17

Oral suspension

CAUTIONARY AND ADVISORY LABELS 9

▸ **Fluconazole (Non-proprietary)**

Fluconazole 10 mg per 1 ml Fluconazole 50mg/5ml oral suspension | 35 ml PoM £25.85 DT = £25.85

▸ **Diflucan** (Pfizer Ltd)

Fluconazole 10 mg per 1 ml Diflucan 50mg/5ml oral suspension | 35 ml PoM £16.61 DT = £25.85
Fluconazole 40 mg per 1 ml Diflucan 200mg/5ml oral suspension | 35 ml PoM £66.42 DT = £66.42

Capsule

CAUTIONARY AND ADVISORY LABELS 9 (50 mg and 200 mg strengths only)

▸ **Fluconazole (Non-proprietary)**

Fluconazole 50 mg Fluconazole 50mg capsules | 7 capsule PoM £5.00 DT = £0.94
Azocan 50mg capsules | 7 capsule PoM ⊠ DT = £0.94
Fluconazole 150 mg Azocan 150mg capsules | 1 capsule PoM ⊠ DT = £0.90
Fluconazole 150mg capsules | 1 capsule PoM £8.50 DT = £0.90
Fluconazole 200 mg Fluconazole 200mg capsules | 7 capsule PoM £6.02 DT = £4.88
Azocan 200mg capsules | 7 capsule PoM ⊠ DT = £4.88

▸ **Diflucan** (Pfizer Ltd)

Fluconazole 50 mg Diflucan 50mg capsules | 7 capsule PoM £16.61 DT = £0.94
Fluconazole 150 mg Diflucan 150mg capsules | 1 capsule PoM £7.12 DT = £0.90
Fluconazole 200 mg Diflucan 200mg capsules | 7 capsule PoM £66.42 DT = £4.88

Itraconazole

19-Feb-2020

● **INDICATIONS AND DOSE**

Oropharyngeal candidiasis

▸ BY MOUTH

▸ Child 1 month–11 years: 3–5 mg/kg once daily for 15 days; maximum 100 mg per day
▸ Child 12–17 years: 100 mg once daily for 15 days

Oropharyngeal candidiasis in patients with AIDS or neutropenia

▸ BY MOUTH

▸ Child 1 month–11 years: 3–5 mg/kg once daily for 15 days; maximum 200 mg per day
▸ Child 12–17 years: 200 mg once daily for 15 days

Systemic candidiasis where other antifungal drugs inappropriate or ineffective

▸ BY MOUTH

▸ Child: 5 mg/kg once daily (max. per dose 200 mg), dose increased in invasive or disseminated disease and in cryptococcal meningitis, increased to 5 mg/kg twice daily (max. per dose 200 mg)

▸ BY INTRAVENOUS INFUSION

▸ Child: 2.5 mg/kg every 12 hours (max. per dose 200 mg) for 2 days, then 2.5 mg/kg once daily (max. per dose 200 mg) for max. 12 days

Pityriasis versicolor

▸ BY MOUTH

▸ Child 1 month–11 years: 3–5 mg/kg once daily (max. per dose 200 mg) for 7 days
▸ Child 12–17 years: 200 mg once daily for 7 days

Tinea pedis | Tinea manuum

▸ BY MOUTH

▸ Child 1 month–11 years: 3–5 mg/kg once daily (max. per dose 100 mg) for 30 days
▸ Child 12–17 years: 100 mg once daily for 30 days, alternatively 200 mg twice daily for 7 days

Tinea corporis | Tinea cruris

▸ BY MOUTH

▸ Child 1 month–11 years: 3–5 mg/kg once daily (max. per dose 100 mg) for 15 days
▸ Child 12–17 years: 100 mg once daily for 15 days, alternatively 200 mg once daily for 7 days

Tinea capitis

▸ BY MOUTH

▸ Child 1–17 years: 3–5 mg/kg once daily (max. per dose 200 mg) for 2–6 weeks

Onychomycosis

▸ BY MOUTH

▸ Child 1–11 years: 5 mg/kg daily (max. per dose 200 mg) for 7 days, subsequent courses repeated after 21-day intervals; fingernails 2 courses, toenails 3 courses
▸ Child 12–17 years: 200 mg once daily for 3 months, alternatively 200 mg twice daily for 7 days, subsequent courses repeated after 21-day intervals; fingernails 2 courses, toenails 3 courses

Systemic aspergillosis where other antifungal drugs inappropriate or ineffective

▸ BY INTRAVENOUS INFUSION

▸ Child: 2.5 mg/kg every 12 hours (max. per dose 200 mg) for 2 days, then 2.5 mg/kg once daily (max. per dose 200 mg) for max. 12 days

▸ BY MOUTH

▸ Child: 5 mg/kg once daily (max. per dose 200 mg), increased to 5 mg/kg twice daily (max. per dose 200 mg), dose increased in invasive or disseminated disease and in cryptococcal meningitis

Histoplasmosis

▸ BY MOUTH

▸ Child: 5 mg/kg 1–2 times a day (max. per dose 200 mg)

Systemic cryptococcosis including cryptococcal meningitis where other antifungal drugs inappropriate or ineffective

▸ BY MOUTH

▸ Child: 5 mg/kg once daily (max. per dose 200 mg), dose increased in invasive or disseminated disease and in cryptococcal meningitis, increased to 5 mg/kg twice daily (max. per dose 200 mg)

▸ BY INTRAVENOUS INFUSION

▸ Child: 2.5 mg/kg every 12 hours (max. per dose 200 mg) for 2 days, then 2.5 mg/kg once daily (max. per dose 200 mg) for max. 12 days

Maintenance in HIV-infected patients to prevent relapse of underlying fungal infection and prophylaxis in neutropenia when standard therapy inappropriate

▸ BY MOUTH

▸ Child: 5 mg/kg once daily (max. per dose 200 mg), then increased to 5 mg/kg twice daily (max. per dose 200 mg), dose increased only if low plasma-itraconazole concentration

Prophylaxis of deep fungal infections (when standard therapy inappropriate) in patients with haematological malignancy or undergoing bone-marrow transplantation who are expected to become neutropenic

▸ BY MOUTH USING ORAL SOLUTION

▸ Child: 2.5 mg/kg twice daily, to be started before transplantation or before chemotherapy (taking care to avoid interaction with cytotoxic drugs) and continued until neutrophil count recovers, safety and efficacy not established

- **UNLICENSED USE** Not licensed for use in children (age range not specified by manufacturer).
- **CONTRA-INDICATIONS** Acute porphyrias p. 652
- **CAUTIONS** Active liver disease · history of hepatotoxicity with other drugs · susceptibility to congestive heart failure

CAUTIONS, FURTHER INFORMATION

- Susceptibility to congestive heart failure There have been reports of heart failure associated with itraconazole. Those at risk may include patients receiving higher daily doses and longer courses, patients with cardiac disease, patients with chronic lung disease, and patients receiving treatment with calcium channel blockers. Manufacturer advises avoid in patients with ventricular dysfunction, such as history of congestive heart failure, unless the infection is serious.

- **INTERACTIONS** → Appendix 1: antifungals, azoles
- **SIDE-EFFECTS**

GENERAL SIDE-EFFECTS

- **Common or very common** Alopecia · constipation · diarrhoea · dyspnoea · gastrointestinal discomfort · headache · heart failure · hepatic disorders · hyperbilirubinaemia · hypotension · nausea · oedema · pulmonary oedema · skin reactions · vision disorders · vomiting
- **Uncommon** Hearing loss · taste altered
- **Rare or very rare** Angioedema · hypersensitivity vasculitis · hypertriglyceridaemia · pancreatitis · photosensitivity reaction · severe cutaneous adverse reactions (SCARs)
- **Frequency not known** Peripheral neuropathy (discontinue)

SPECIFIC SIDE-EFFECTS

- **Common or very common**
- With intravenous use Chest pain · confusion · cough · dizziness · drowsiness · electrolyte imbalance · fatigue · gastrointestinal disorder · granulocytopenia · hyperglycaemia · hyperhidrosis · hypersensitivity · hypertension · myalgia · pain · renal impairment · tachycardia · tremor · urinary incontinence
- **Uncommon**
- With intravenous use Dysphonia · numbness · thrombocytopenia
- With oral use Flatulence · increased risk of infection · menstrual disorder
- **Rare or very rare**
- With oral use Erectile dysfunction · leucopenia · sensation abnormal · serum sickness · tinnitus · urinary frequency increased

SIDE-EFFECTS, FURTHER INFORMATION Potentially life-threatening hepatotoxicity reported very rarely — discontinue if signs of hepatitis develop.

- **CONCEPTION AND CONTRACEPTION** Ensure effective contraception during treatment and until the next menstrual period following end of treatment.
- **PREGNANCY** Manufacturer advises use only in life-threatening situations (toxicity at high doses in *animal* studies).
- **BREAST FEEDING** Small amounts present in milk—may accumulate; manufacturer advises avoid.
- **HEPATIC IMPAIRMENT** Manufacturer advises use only in serious or life-saving situations where potential benefit outweighs risk of hepatotoxicity.
- **RENAL IMPAIRMENT** Risk of congestive heart failure.
- With oral use Bioavailability of oral formulations possibly reduced.
- With intravenous use Use intravenous infusion with caution if estimated glomerular filtration rate 30–80 mL/minute/1.73 m^2 (monitor renal function); avoid intravenous infusion if estimated golmerular filtration rate less than 30 mL/minute/1.73 m^2.
- **MONITORING REQUIREMENTS**
- Absorption reduced in AIDS and neutropenia (monitor plasma-itraconazole concentration and increase dose if necessary).
- Monitor liver function if treatment continues for longer than one month, if receiving other hepatotoxic drugs, or if history of hepatotoxicity with other drugs.
- **DIRECTIONS FOR ADMINISTRATION**
- With intravenous use For *intravenous infusion*, dilute 250 mg with 50 mL Sodium Chloride 0.9% and give requisite dose through an in-line filter (0.2 micron) over 60 minutes.
- With oral use For *oral liquid*, do not take with food; swish around mouth and swallow, do not rinse afterwards.
- **PRESCRIBING AND DISPENSING INFORMATION** Flavours of oral liquid formulations may include cherry.
- **PATIENT AND CARER ADVICE** Patients should be told how to recognise signs of liver disorder and advised to seek prompt medical attention if symptoms such as anorexia, nausea, vomiting, fatigue, abdominal pain or dark urine develop.
- With oral use Patients or carers should be given advice on how to administer itraconazole oral liquid.

- **MEDICINAL FORMS** There can be variation in the licensing of different medicines containing the same drug. Forms available from special-order manufacturers include: oral suspension, oral solution

Solution for infusion

EXCIPIENTS: May contain Propylene glycol

- Sporanox (Janssen-Cilag Ltd)
  Itraconazole 10 mg per 1 ml Sporanox I.V. 250mg/25ml solution for infusion ampoules and diluent | 1 ampoule PoM £79.71

Oral solution

CAUTIONARY AND ADVISORY LABELS 9, 23

- Itraconazole (Non-proprietary)
  Itraconazole 10 mg per 1 ml Itraconazole 50mg/5ml oral solution sugar free sugar-free | 150 ml PoM £59.28 DT = £59.28
- Sporanox (Janssen-Cilag Ltd)
  Itraconazole 10 mg per 1 ml Sporanox 50mg/5ml oral solution sugar-free | 150 ml PoM £58.34 DT = £59.28

Capsule

CAUTIONARY AND ADVISORY LABELS 5, 9, 21, 25

- Itraconazole (Non-proprietary)
  Itraconazole 100 mg Itraconazole 100mg capsules | 15 capsule PoM £13.77 DT = £3.55 | 60 capsule PoM £14.20–£55.10
- Sporanox (Janssen-Cilag Ltd)
  Itraconazole 100 mg Sporanox-Pulse 100mg capsules | 28 capsule PoM £25.72
  Sporanox 100mg capsules | 4 capsule PoM £3.67 | 15 capsule PoM £13.77 DT = £3.55 | 60 capsule PoM £55.10

Voriconazole

24-Jan-2020

- **INDICATIONS AND DOSE**

Invasive aspergillosis | Serious infections caused by *Scedosporium* spp., *Fusarium* spp., or invasive fluconazole-resistant *Candida* spp. (including *C. krusei*)

▶ BY MOUTH

- Child 2–11 years: Treatment should be initiated with intravenous regimen, and oral regimen should be considered only after there is a significant clinical improvement; maintenance 9 mg/kg every 12 hours, adjusted in steps of 1 mg/kg and increased if necessary up to 350 mg every 12 hours, then adjusted in steps of 50 mg as required
- Child 12–14 years (body-weight up to 50 kg): Treatment should be initiated with intravenous regimen, and oral regimen should be considered only after there is a significant clinical improvement; maintenance 9 mg/kg every 12 hours, adjusted in steps of 1 mg/kg and increased if necessary up to 350 mg every 12 hours, then adjusted in steps of 50 mg as required

- Child 12–14 years (body-weight 50 kg and above): Initially 400 mg every 12 hours for 2 doses, then 200 mg every 12 hours, increased if necessary to 300 mg every 12 hours
- Child 15–17 years (body-weight up to 40 kg): Initially 200 mg every 12 hours for 2 doses, then 100 mg every 12 hours, increased if necessary to 150 mg every 12 hours
- Child 15–17 years (body-weight 40 kg and above): Initially 400 mg every 12 hours for 2 doses, then 200 mg every 12 hours, increased if necessary to 300 mg every 12 hours

- BY INTRAVENOUS INFUSION
- Child 2–11 years: Initially 9 mg/kg every 12 hours for 2 doses, then 8 mg/kg every 12 hours; adjusted in steps of 1 mg/kg as required; for max. 6 months
- Child 12–14 years (body-weight up to 50 kg): Initially 9 mg/kg every 12 hours for 2 doses, then 8 mg/kg every 12 hours; adjusted in steps of 1 mg/kg as required; for max. 6 months
- Child 12–14 years (body-weight 50 kg and above): Initially 6 mg/kg every 12 hours for 2 doses, then 4 mg/kg every 12 hours; reduced if not tolerated to 3 mg/kg every 12 hours; for max. 6 months
- Child 15–17 years: Initially 6 mg/kg every 12 hours for 2 doses, then 4 mg/kg every 12 hours; reduced if not tolerated to 3 mg/kg every 12 hours; for max. 6 months

DOSE ADJUSTMENTS DUE TO INTERACTIONS
- Manufacturer advises increasing the maintenance dose with concurrent use of fosphenytoin, phenytoin, or rifabutin—no specific recommendations made for children.

- **CONTRA-INDICATIONS** Acute porphyrias p. 652
- **CAUTIONS** Avoid exposure to sunlight · bradycardia · cardiomyopathy · electrolyte disturbances · history of QT interval prolongation · patients at risk of pancreatitis · symptomatic arrhythmias
- **INTERACTIONS** → Appendix 1: antifungals, azoles
- **SIDE-EFFECTS**

GENERAL SIDE-EFFECTS
- **Common or very common** Acute kidney injury · agranulocytosis · alopecia · anaemia · anxiety · arrhythmias · asthenia · bone marrow disorders · chest pain · chills · confusion · constipation · depression · diarrhoea · dizziness · drowsiness · dyspnoea · electrolyte imbalance · eye disorders · eye inflammation · fever · gastrointestinal discomfort · haemorrhage · hallucination · headache · hepatic disorders · hypoglycaemia · hypotension · increased risk of infection · insomnia · leucopenia · muscle tone increased · nausea · neutropenia · oedema · oral disorders · pain · pulmonary oedema · respiratory disorders · seizure · sensation abnormal · skin reactions · syncope · tetany · thrombocytopenia · tremor · vision disorders · vomiting
- **Uncommon** Adrenal insufficiency · arthritis · brain oedema · duodenitis · encephalopathy · eosinophilia · gallbladder disorders · hearing impairment · hypothyroidism · influenza like illness · lymphadenopathy · lymphangitis · movement disorders · nephritis · nerve disorders · pancreatitis · parkinsonism · phototoxicity · proteinuria · pseudomembranous enterocolitis · QT interval prolongation · renal tubular necrosis · severe cutaneous adverse reactions (SCARs) · taste altered · thrombophlebitis · tinnitus · vertigo
- **Rare or very rare** Angioedema · cardiac conduction disorders · disseminated intravascular coagulation · hyperthyroidism
- **Frequency not known** Cutaneous lupus erythematosus · periostitis (more common in transplant patients) · squamous cell carcinoma (more common in presence of phototoxicity)

SPECIFIC SIDE-EFFECTS
- With intravenous use Infusion related reaction

SIDE-EFFECTS, FURTHER INFORMATION **Hepatotoxicity** Hepatitis, cholestasis, and acute hepatic failure have been reported; risk of hepatotoxicity increased in patients with haematological malignancy. Consider treatment discontinuation if severe abnormalities in liver function tests.

Phototoxicity Phototoxicity occurs uncommonly. If phototoxicity occurs, consider treatment discontinuation; if treatment is continued, monitor for pre-malignant skin lesions and squamous cell carcinoma, and discontinue treatment if they occur.

- **CONCEPTION AND CONTRACEPTION** Effective contraception required during treatment.
- **PREGNANCY** Toxicity in *animal* studies—manufacturer advises avoid unless potential benefit outweighs risk.
- **BREAST FEEDING** Manufacturer advises avoid—no information available.
- **HEPATIC IMPAIRMENT** Manufacturer advises caution, particularly in severe impairment (no information available).

Dose adjustments **Child 12–17 years** Manufacturer advises use usual initial loading dose then halve maintenance doses in mild to moderate cirrhosis.

- **RENAL IMPAIRMENT**

Child 2–12 years No information available.

Child 12–17 years Intravenous vehicle may accumulate if estimated glomerular filtration rate less than 50 mL/minute/1.73 m^2—use intravenous infusion only if potential benefit outweighs risk, and monitor renal function; alternatively, use tablets or oral suspension (no dose adjustment required).

- **MONITORING REQUIREMENTS**
- Monitor renal function.
- Monitor liver function before starting treatment, then at least weekly for 1 month, and then monthly during treatment.

- **DIRECTIONS FOR ADMINISTRATION**
- With intravenous use For *intravenous infusion*, reconstitute each 200 mg with 19 mL Water for Injections *or* Sodium Chloride 0.9% to produce a 10 mg/mL solution; dilute dose to concentration of 0.5–5 mg/mL with Glucose 5% or Sodium Chloride 0.9% and give intermittently at a rate not exceeding 3 mg/kg/hour.

- **PRESCRIBING AND DISPENSING INFORMATION** Flavours of oral liquid formulations may include orange.
- **PATIENT AND CARER ADVICE** Patients and their carers should be told how to recognise symptoms of liver disorder, and advised to seek immediate medical attention if symptoms such as persistent nausea, vomiting, malaise or jaundice develop.

Patients and their carers should be advised that patients should avoid intense or prolonged exposure to direct sunlight, and to avoid the use of sunbeds. In sunlight, patients should cover sun-exposed areas of skin and use a sunscreen with a high sun protection factor. Patients should seek medical attention if they experience sunburn or a severe skin reaction following exposure to light or sun.

Patients and their carers should be advised to keep the alert card with them at all times.

5 Infection

- **MEDICINAL FORMS** There can be variation in the licensing of different medicines containing the same drug.

Powder for solution for infusion

EXCIPIENTS: May contain Sulfobutylether beta cyclodextrin sodium

ELECTROLYTES: May contain Sodium

- Voriconazole (Non-proprietary)
  Voriconazole 200 mg Voriconazole 200mg powder for solution for infusion vials | 1 vial [PoM] £51.43–£77.14 (Hospital only)
- VFEND (Pfizer Ltd)
  Voriconazole 200 mg VFEND 200mg powder for solution for infusion vials | 1 vial [PoM] £77.14 (Hospital only)

Oral suspension

CAUTIONARY AND ADVISORY LABELS 9, 11, 23

- VFEND (Pfizer Ltd)
  Voriconazole 40 mg per 1 ml VFEND 40mg/ml oral suspension | 75 ml [PoM] £551.37 DT = £551.37

Tablet

CAUTIONARY AND ADVISORY LABELS 9, 11, 23

- Voriconazole (Non-proprietary)
  Voriconazole 50 mg Voriconazole 50mg tablets | 28 tablet [PoM] £275.68 DT = £162.68 | 28 tablet [PoM] £47.47 DT = £162.68 (Hospital only)
  Voriconazole 100 mg Voriconazole 100mg tablets | 28 tablet [PoM] £275.68
  Voriconazole 200 mg Voriconazole 200mg tablets | 28 tablet [PoM] £164.58 DT = £635.34 (Hospital only) | 28 tablet [PoM] £1,102.74 DT = £635.34
- VFEND (Pfizer Ltd)
  Voriconazole 50 mg VFEND 50mg tablets | 28 tablet [PoM] £275.68 DT = £162.68
  Voriconazole 200 mg VFEND 200mg tablets | 28 tablet [PoM] £1,102.74 DT = £635.34

ANTIFUNGALS > OTHER

Flucytosine

20-Jan-2020

- **INDICATIONS AND DOSE**

Systemic yeast and fungal infections | Adjunct to amphotericin in severe systemic candidiasis and in other severe or long-standing infections

▶ BY INTRAVENOUS INFUSION, OR BY MOUTH

- Neonate: 50 mg/kg every 12 hours.
- Child: Usual dose 50 mg/kg every 6 hours usually for not more than 7 days, alternatively 25–37.5 mg/kg every 6 hours usually for not more than 7 days, lower dose may be sufficient for sensitive organisms

Cryptococcal meningitis (adjunct to amphotericin)

▶ BY INTRAVENOUS INFUSION, OR BY MOUTH

- Neonate: 50 mg/kg every 12 hours.
- Child: 25 mg/kg every 6 hours for 2 weeks

- **UNLICENSED USE** Tablets not licensed.
- **CAUTIONS** Blood disorders
- **INTERACTIONS** → Appendix 1: flucytosine
- **SIDE-EFFECTS** Agranulocytosis · aplastic anaemia · blood disorder · cardiotoxicity · confusion · diarrhoea · hallucination · headache · hepatic disorders · leucopenia · nausea · rash · sedation · seizure · thrombocytopenia · toxic epidermal necrolysis · ventricular dysfunction · vertigo · vomiting
- **PREGNANCY** Teratogenic in *animal* studies; manufacturer advises use only if potential benefit outweighs risk.
- **BREAST FEEDING** Manufacturer advises avoid.
- **RENAL IMPAIRMENT**

Dose adjustments Use normal dose every 12 hours if creatinine clearance 20–40 mL/minute; use normal dose every 24 hours if creatinine clearance 10–20 mL/minute; use initial normal dose if creatinine clearance less than 10 mL/minute and then adjust dose according to plasma-flucytosine concentration.

Monitoring In renal impairment liver- and kidney-function tests and blood counts required weekly.

- **MONITORING REQUIREMENTS**
  - For plasma concentration monitoring, blood should be taken shortly before starting the next infusion; plasma concentration for optimum response 25–50 mg/litre (200–400 micromol/litre)—should not be allowed to exceed 80 mg/litre (620 micromol/litre).
  - Liver- and kidney-function tests and blood counts required (weekly in blood disorders).
- **DIRECTIONS FOR ADMINISTRATION** For *intravenous infusion*, give over 20–40 minutes.

- **MEDICINAL FORMS** There can be variation in the licensing of different medicines containing the same drug. Forms available from special-order manufacturers include: oral solution

Solution for infusion

ELECTROLYTES: May contain Sodium

- Ancotil (Mylan)
  Flucytosine 10 mg per 1 ml Ancotil 2.5g/250ml solution for infusion bottles | 5 bottle [PoM] £151.67 (Hospital only)

Tablet

- Ancotil (ICN Pharmaceuticals France S.A.)
  Flucytosine 500 mg Ancotil 500mg tablets | 100 tablet [PoM] [not NHS]

Griseofulvin

16-Jan-2020

- **INDICATIONS AND DOSE**

Dermatophyte infections of the skin, scalp, hair and nails where topical therapy has failed or is inappropriate

▶ BY MOUTH

- Child 1 month–11 years: Usual dose 10 mg/kg daily (max. per dose 500 mg), increased if necessary to 20 mg/kg daily (max. per dose 1 g), for severe infections; reduce dose when response occurs, daily dose may be taken once daily or in divided doses
- Child 12–17 years: 500 mg daily, increased if necessary to 1 g daily, for severe infections; reduce dose when response occurs, daily dose may be taken once daily or in divided doses

Tinea capitis caused by *Trichophyton tonsurans*

▶ BY MOUTH

- Child 1 month–11 years: 15–20 mg/kg once daily (max. per dose 1 g), alternatively 15–20 mg/kg daily in divided doses (max. per dose 1 g)
- Child 12–17 years: 1 g once daily, alternatively 1 g daily in divided doses

- **UNLICENSED USE** Licensed for use in children (age range not specified by manufacturer).
- **CONTRA-INDICATIONS** Acute porphyrias p. 652 · systemic lupus erythematosus (risk of exacerbation)
- **INTERACTIONS** → Appendix 1: griseofulvin
- **SIDE-EFFECTS**
  - **Common or very common** Diarrhoea · epigastric discomfort · headache · nausea · vomiting
  - **Uncommon** Appetite decreased · confusion · coordination abnormal · dizziness · drowsiness · insomnia · irritability · peripheral neuropathy · photosensitivity reaction · skin reactions · taste altered · toxic epidermal necrolysis
  - **Rare or very rare** Anaemia · hepatic disorders · leucopenia · neutropenia · systemic lupus erythematosus (SLE)
- **CONCEPTION AND CONTRACEPTION** Effective contraception required during and for at least 1 month after administration to women (important: effectiveness of oral contraceptives may be reduced, additional contraceptive precautions e.g. barrier method, required). Men should avoid fathering a child during and for at least 6 months after administration
- **PREGNANCY** Avoid (fetotoxicity and teratogenicity in *animals*).

- **BREAST FEEDING** Avoid—no information available.
- **HEPATIC IMPAIRMENT** Manufacturer advises caution in mild to moderate impairment (risk of deterioration); avoid in severe impairment.
- **PATIENT AND CARER ADVICE**
Medicines for Children leaflet: Griseofulvin for fungal infections www.medicinesforchildren.org.uk/griseofulvin-fungal-infections
Driving and skilled tasks May impair performance of skilled tasks (e.g. driving); effects of alcohol enhanced.

- **MEDICINAL FORMS** There can be variation in the licensing of different medicines containing the same drug. Forms available from special-order manufacturers include: oral suspension

Tablet

CAUTIONARY AND ADVISORY LABELS 9, 21

▸ Griseofulvin (Non-proprietary)
Griseofulvin 125 mg Griseofulvin 125mg tablets | 100 tablet PoM £96.67 DT = £96.67
Griseofulvin 500 mg Griseofulvin 500mg tablets | 90 tablet PoM £81.32 | 100 tablet PoM £90.34 DT = £90.35

2.1 Pneumocystis pneumonia

Pneumocystis pneumonia

Overview

Pneumonia caused by *Pneumocystis jirovecii* (*Pneumocystis carinii*) occurs in immunosuppressed patients; it is a common cause of pneumonia in AIDS. Pneumocystis pneumonia should generally be treated by those experienced in its management. Blood gas measurement is used to assess disease severity.

Treatment

The recommended duration of treatment is generally 14–21 days.

Mild to moderate disease

Co-trimoxazole p. 378 in high dosage is the drug of choice for the treatment of mild to moderate pneumocystis pneumonia.

Atovaquone below or a combination of dapsone p. 414 with trimethoprim p. 390 is given by mouth for the treatment of mild to moderate disease [unlicensed indication] in children who cannot tolerate co-trimoxazole.

A combination of clindamycin p. 351 and primaquine p. 430 may be used in the treatment of mild to moderate disease [unlicensed indication]; this combination is associated with considerable toxicity.

Severe disease

Co-trimoxazole in high dosage, given by mouth or by intravenous infusion, is the drug of choice for the treatment of severe pneumocystis pneumonia. Pentamidine isetionate p. 414 given by intravenous infusion is an alternative for children who cannot tolerate co-trimoxazole, or who have not responded to it. Pentamidine isetionate is a potentially toxic drug that can cause severe hypotension during or immediately after infusion. If there is clinical improvement after 7–10 days of intravenous therapy with pentamidine isetionate, patients can be switched to oral treatment (e.g. atovaquone) to complete 21 days treatment.

Corticosteroid treatment can be lifesaving in those with severe pneumocystis pneumonia.

Adjunctive therapy

In moderate to severe pneumocystis infections associated with HIV infection, prednisolone p. 478 is given by mouth for 5 days (alternatively, hydrocortisone p. 476 may be given parenterally); the dose is then reduced over the next 16 days and then stopped. Corticosteroid treatment should ideally be started at the same time as the anti-pneumocystis therapy and certainly no later than 24–72 hours afterwards. The corticosteroid should be withdrawn before anti-pneumocystis treatment is complete.

Prophylaxis

Prophylaxis against pneumocystis pneumonia should be given to all children with a history of this infection, and to all HIV-infected infants aged 1 month–1 year. Prophylaxis against pneumocystis pneumonia should also be considered for severely immunocompromised children. Prophylaxis should continue until immunity recovers sufficiently. It should not be discontinued if the child has oral candidiasis, continues to lose weight, or is receiving cytotoxic therapy or long-term immunosuppressant therapy.

Prophylaxis should also be given to infants aged 1 month–1 year who are suspected to be HIV-positive, *or* whose mothers had a viral load greater than 1000 HIV RNA copies/mL between 36 weeks' gestation and delivery; prophylaxis should be continued until HIV infection is excluded or until immunity recovers.

Co-trimoxazole by mouth is the drug of choice for prophylaxis against pneumocystis pneumonia. Co-trimoxazole may be used in infants born to mothers with a high risk of transmission of infection.

Inhaled pentamidine isetionate is better tolerated than parenteral pentamidine isetionate. Intermittent inhalation of pentamidine isetionate is used for prophylaxis against pneumocystis pneumonia in children unable to tolerate co-trimoxazole. It is effective but children may be prone to extrapulmonary infection. Alternatively, dapsone can be used.

ANTIPROTOZOALS › OTHER

Atovaquone

27-May-2020

- **INDICATIONS AND DOSE**

Treatment of mild to moderate *Pneumocystis jirovecii* (*Pneumocystis carinii*) pneumonia in patients intolerant of co-trimoxazole

▸ BY MOUTH
▸ Child 1-2 months: 15–20 mg/kg twice daily for 14–21 days, dose to be taken with food, particularly high fat food
▸ Child 3 months-1 year: 22.5 mg/kg twice daily for 14–21 days, dose to be taken with food, particularly high fat food
▸ Child 2-17 years: 15–20 mg/kg twice daily (max. per dose 750 mg) for 14–21 days, dose to be taken with food, particularly high fat food

- **UNLICENSED USE** Not licensed for use in children.
- **CAUTIONS** Initial diarrhoea and difficulty in taking with food may reduce absorption (and require alternative therapy) · other causes of pulmonary disease should be sought and treated
- **INTERACTIONS** → Appendix 1: antimalarials
- **SIDE-EFFECTS**
▸ **Common or very common** Anaemia · angioedema · bronchospasm · diarrhoea · headache · hypersensitivity · hyponatraemia · insomnia · nausea · neutropenia · skin reactions · throat tightness · vomiting
▸ **Frequency not known** Stevens-Johnson syndrome
- **PREGNANCY** Manufacturer advises avoid unless potential benefit outweighs risk—no information available.
- **BREAST FEEDING** Manufacturer advises avoid.
- **HEPATIC IMPAIRMENT** Manufacturer advises use with caution in significant impairment and monitor closely—no information available.
- **RENAL IMPAIRMENT** Manufacturer advises caution.
Monitoring Monitor more closely in renal impairment.

5 Infection

- **PRESCRIBING AND DISPENSING INFORMATION** Flavours of oral liquid formulations may include tutti-frutti.

- **MEDICINAL FORMS** There can be variation in the licensing of different medicines containing the same drug.

Oral suspension

CAUTIONARY AND ADVISORY LABELS 21

- Atovaquone (Non-proprietary)
  Atovaquone 150 mg per 1 ml Atovaquone 750mg/5ml oral suspension sugar free sugar-free | 250 ml PoM £470.60
- Wellvone (GlaxoSmithKline UK Ltd)
  Atovaquone 150 mg per 1 ml Wellvone 750mg/5ml oral suspension sugar-free | 226 ml PoM £486.37 DT = £486.37

Dapsone

05-May-2020

- **INDICATIONS AND DOSE**

Treatment of mild to moderate *Pneumocystis jirovecii* (*Pneumocystis carinii*) pneumonia (in combination with trimethoprim)

- BY MOUTH
- Child 1 month–11 years: 2 mg/kg once daily (max. per dose 100 mg)
- Child 12–17 years: 100 mg once daily

Prophylaxis of *Pneumocystis jirovecii* (*Pneumocystis carinii*) pneumonia

- BY MOUTH
- Child: 2 mg/kg once daily (max. per dose 100 mg)

- **UNLICENSED USE** Not licensed for treatment of pneumocystis (*P. jirovecii*) pneumonia. Monotherapy not licensed for children for prophylaxis of *P. jirovecii* pneumonia.
- **CAUTIONS** Anaemia (treat severe anaemia before starting) · avoid in Acute porphyrias p. 652 · cardiac disease · G6PD deficiency · pulmonary disease · susceptibility to haemolysis
- **INTERACTIONS** → Appendix 1: dapsone
- **SIDE-EFFECTS** Agranulocytosis · appetite decreased · haemolysis · haemolytic anaemia · headache · hepatic disorders · hypoalbuminaemia · insomnia · lepra reaction · methaemoglobinaemia · motor loss · nausea · peripheral neuropathy · photosensitivity reaction · psychosis · severe cutaneous adverse reactions (SCARs) · skin reactions · tachycardia · vomiting

  SIDE-EFFECTS, FURTHER INFORMATION Side-effects are dose-related. If dapsone syndrome occurs (rash with fever and eosinophilia)—discontinue immediately (may progress to exfoliative dermatitis, hepatitis, hypoalbuminaemia, psychosis and death).
- **PREGNANCY** Folic acid p. 620 (higher dose) should be given to mother throughout pregnancy; neonatal haemolysis and methaemoglobinaemia reported in third trimester.
- **BREAST FEEDING** Haemolytic anaemia; although significant amount in milk, risk to infant very small unless infant is G6PD deficient.
- **PATIENT AND CARER ADVICE**

  Blood disorders On long-term treatment, patients and their carers should be told how to recognise signs of blood disorders and advised to seek immediate medical attention if symptoms such as fever, sore throat, rash, mouth ulcers, purpura, bruising or bleeding develop.

- **MEDICINAL FORMS** There can be variation in the licensing of different medicines containing the same drug. Forms available from special-order manufacturers include: oral suspension, oral solution

Tablet

CAUTIONARY AND ADVISORY LABELS 8

- Dapsone (Non-proprietary)
  Dapsone 50 mg Dapsone 50mg tablets | 28 tablet PoM £36.22 DT = £11.56
  Dapsone 100 mg Dapsone 100mg tablets | 28 tablet PoM £97.39 DT = £57.37

Pentamidine isetionate

16-Mar-2020

- **INDICATIONS AND DOSE**

Treatment of *Pneumocystis jirovecii* (*Pneumocystis carinii*) pneumonia (specialist use only)

- BY INTRAVENOUS INFUSION
- Child: 4 mg/kg once daily for at least 7–10 days

Prophylaxis of *Pneumocystis jirovecii* (*Pneumocystis carinii*) pneumonia (specialist use only)

- BY INHALATION OF NEBULISED SOLUTION
- Child 5–17 years: 300 mg every 4 weeks, alternatively 150 mg every 2 weeks, using suitable equipment—consult product literature

Visceral leishmaniasis (specialist use only)

- BY DEEP INTRAMUSCULAR INJECTION
- Child 1–17 years: 3–4 mg/kg once daily on alternate days, maximum total of 10 injections, course may be repeated if necessary

Cutaneous leishmaniasis (specialist use only)

- BY DEEP INTRAMUSCULAR INJECTION
- Child 1–17 years: 3–4 mg/kg 1–2 times a week until condition resolves

Trypanosomiasis (specialist use only)

- BY DEEP INTRAMUSCULAR INJECTION, OR BY INTRAVENOUS INFUSION
- Child 1–17 years: 4 mg/kg once daily or on alternate days for a total of 7–10 injections

- **UNLICENSED USE** Not licensed for prevention of pneumocystis pneumonia in children.
- **CAUTIONS** Anaemia · bradycardia · coronary heart disease · history of ventricular arrhythmias · hyperglycaemia · hypertension · hypoglycaemia · hypokalaemia · hypomagnesaemia · hypotension · leucopenia · risk of severe hypotension following administration · thrombocytopenia
- **INTERACTIONS** → Appendix 1: pentamidine
- **SIDE-EFFECTS**

  GENERAL SIDE-EFFECTS
  - **Common or very common** Dizziness · hypoglycaemia (can be severe and sometimes fatal) · hypotension (can be severe and sometimes fatal) · local reaction · nausea · rash · taste altered
  - **Rare or very rare** QT interval prolongation
  - **Frequency not known** Pancreatitis acute (can be severe and sometimes fatal)

  SPECIFIC SIDE-EFFECTS
  - **Common or very common**
  - When used by inhalation Cough · dyspnoea · respiratory disorders
  - With parenteral use Acute kidney injury · anaemia · azotaemia · electrolyte imbalance · flushing · haematuria · hyperglycaemia · induration · leucopenia · localised pain · myopathy · syncope · thrombocytopenia · vomiting
  - **Rare or very rare**
  - With parenteral use Arrhythmia (can be severe and sometimes fatal) · pancreatitis (can be severe and sometimes fatal)

- **Frequency not known**
   - When used by inhalation Angioedema · appetite decreased · bradycardia · fatigue · renal failure
   - With parenteral use Arrhythmias · perioral hypoaesthesia · sensation abnormal · Stevens-Johnson syndrome

- **PREGNANCY** Manufacturer advises avoid unless essential.
- **BREAST FEEDING** Manufacturer advises avoid unless essential—no information available.
- **HEPATIC IMPAIRMENT** Manufacturer advises caution.
- **RENAL IMPAIRMENT**
Dose adjustments Reduce intravenous dose for pneumocystis pneumonia if creatinine clearance less than 10 mL/minute: in *life-threatening infection*, use 4 mg/kg once daily for 7–10 days, then 4 mg/kg on alternate days to complete course of at least 14 doses; in *less severe infection*, use 4 mg/kg on alternate days for at least 14 doses.
- **MONITORING REQUIREMENTS**
   - Monitor blood pressure before starting treatment, during administration, and at regular intervals, until treatment concluded.
   - Carry out laboratory monitoring according to product literature.
- **DIRECTIONS FOR ADMINISTRATION** Patient should be lying down when receiving drug parenterally. Direct intravenous injection should be avoided whenever possible and **never** given rapidly; intramuscular injections should be deep and preferably given into the buttock. For *intravenous infusion*, reconstitute 300 mg with 3–5 mL Water for Injections (displacement value may be significant), then dilute required dose with 50–250 mL Glucose 5% *or* Sodium Chloride 0.9%; give over at least 60 minutes.
Powder for injection (dissolved in water for injection) may be used for nebulisation.
- **HANDLING AND STORAGE** Pentamidine isetionate is toxic and personnel should be adequately protected during handling and administration—consult product literature.

- **MEDICINAL FORMS** There can be variation in the licensing of different medicines containing the same drug.

Powder for solution for injection

- Pentacarinat (Sanofi)
Pentamidine isetionate 300 mg Pentacarinat 300mg powder for solution for injection vials | 5 vial PoM £158.86

3 Helminth infection

Helminth infections

Specialist centres

Advice on prophylaxis and treatment of helminth infections is available from the following specialist centres:

Birmingham	(0121) 424 0357
Scotland	Contact local Infectious Diseases Unit
Liverpool	(0151) 705 3100
London	0845 155 5000 (treatment)

Threadworms

Anthelmintics are effective in threadworm (pinworms, *Enterobius vermicularis*) infections, but their use needs to be combined with hygienic measures to break the cycle of auto-infection. All members of the family require treatment.

Adult threadworms do not live for longer than 6 weeks and for development of fresh worms, ova must be swallowed and exposed to the action of digestive juices in the upper intestinal tract. Direct multiplication of worms does not take place in the large bowel. Adult female worms lay ova on the perianal skin which causes pruritus; scratching the area then leads to ova being transmitted on fingers to the mouth, often via food eaten with unwashed hands. Washing hands and scrubbing nails before each meal and after each visit to the toilet is essential. A bath taken immediately after rising will remove ova laid during the night.

Mebendazole p. 417 is the drug of choice for treating threadworm infection in patients of all ages over 6 months. It is given as a single dose; as reinfection is very common, a second dose may be given after 2 weeks.

Ascaricides (common roundworm infections)

Mebendazole is effective against *Ascaris lumbricoides* and is generally considered to be the drug of choice.

Levamisole p. 417 [unlicensed] (available from 'special-order' manufacturers or specialist importing companies) is an alternative when mebendazole cannot be used. It is very well tolerated.

Tapeworm infections

Taenicides

Niclosamide [unlicensed] (available from 'special-order' manufacturers or specialist importing companies) is the most widely used drug for tapeworm infections and side-effects are limited to occasional gastro-intestinal upset, lightheadedness, and pruritus; it is not effective against larval worms. Fears of developing cysticercosis in *Taenia solium* infections have proved unfounded. All the same, an antiemetic can be given before treatment and a laxative can be given 2 hours after niclosamide.

Praziquantel p. 417 [unlicensed] (available from 'special-order' manufacturers or specialist importing companies) is as effective as niclosamide.

Hydatid disease

Cysts caused by *Echinococcus granulosus* grow slowly and asymptomatic patients do not always require treatment. Surgical treatment remains the method of choice in many situations. Albendazole p. 416 [unlicensed] (available from 'special-order' manufacturers or specialist importing companies) is used in conjunction with surgery to reduce the risk of recurrence or as primary treatment in inoperable cases. Alveolar echinococcosis due to *E. multilocularis* is usually fatal if untreated. Surgical removal with albendazole cover is the treatment of choice, but where effective surgery is impossible, repeated cycles of albendazole (for a year or more) may help. Careful monitoring of liver function is particularly important during drug treatment.

Hookworms

Hookworms (ancylostomiasis, necatoriasis) live in the upper small intestine and draw blood from the point of their attachment to their host. An iron-deficiency anaemia may occur and, if present, effective treatment of the infection requires not only expulsion of the worms but treatment of the anaemia.

Mebendazole has a useful broad-spectrum activity, and is effective against hookworms. Albendazole [unlicensed] (available from 'special-order' manufacturers or specialist importing companies) is an alternative. Levamisole is also is also effective in children.

Schistosomicides (bilharziasis)

Adult *Schistosoma haematobium* worms live in the genito-urinary veins and adult *S. mansoni* in those of the colon and mesentery. *S. japonicum* is more widely distributed in veins of the alimentary tract and portal system.

Praziquantel [unlicensed] is available from Merck Serono (*Cysticide*®) and is effective against all human schistosomes. No serious adverse effects have been reported. Of all the available schistosomicides, it has the most attractive combination of effectiveness, broad-spectrum activity, and low toxicity.

Filaricides

Diethylcarbamazine [unlicensed] (available from 'special-order' manufacturers or specialist importing companies) is effective against microfilariae and adults of *Loa loa*, *Wuchereria bancrofti*, and *Brugia malayi*. To minimise reactions, treatment in adults and children over 1 month, is commenced with a dose of diethylcarbamazine citrate on the first day and increased gradually over 3 days. Length of treatment varies according to infection type, and usually gives a radical cure for these infections. Close medical supervision is necessary particularly in the early phase of treatment.

In heavy infections there may be a febrile reaction, and in heavy *Loa loa* infection there is a small risk of encephalopathy. In such cases specialist advice should be sought, and treatment must be given under careful in-patient supervision and stopped at the first sign of cerebral involvement.

Ivermectin below [unlicensed] (available from 'special-order' manufacturers or specialist importing companies) is very effective in *onchocerciasis* and it is now the drug of choice; reactions are usually slight. Diethylcarbamazine or suramin should no longer be used for *onchocerciasis* because of their toxicity.

Cutaneous larva migrans (creeping eruption)

Dog and cat hookworm larvae may enter human skin where they produce slowly extending itching tracks usually on the foot. Single tracks can be treated with topical tiabendazole (no commercial preparation available). Multiple infections respond to ivermectin, albendazole or **tiabendazole** (thiabendazole) by mouth [all unlicensed] (available from 'special-order' manufacturers or specialist importing companies).

Strongyloidiasis

Adult *Strongyloides stercoralis* live in the gut and produce larvae which penetrate the gut wall and invade the tissues, setting up a cycle of auto-infection. Ivermectin [unlicensed] (available from 'special-order' manufacturers or specialist importing companies) is the treatment of choice for chronic *Strongyloides* infection in adults and children over 5 years. Albendazole [unlicensed] (available from 'special order' manufacturers or specialist importing companies) is an alternative given to adults and children over 2 years.

ANTHELMINTICS

Albendazole

- **INDICATIONS AND DOSE**

Chronic *Strongyloides* infection

▶ BY MOUTH

▸ Child 2–17 years: 400 mg twice daily for 3 days, dose may be repeated after 3 weeks if necessary

Hydatid disease, in conjunction with surgery to reduce the risk of recurrence or as primary treatment in inoperable cases

▶ BY MOUTH

▸ Child 2–17 years: 7.5 mg/kg twice daily (max. per dose 400 mg twice daily) for 28 days followed by 14-day break, repeated for up to 2–3 cycles

Hookworm infections

▶ BY MOUTH

▸ Child 2–17 years: 400 mg for 1 dose

- **UNLICENSED USE** Albendazole is an unlicensed drug.
- **INTERACTIONS** → Appendix 1: albendazole
- **MEDICINAL FORMS** There can be variation in the licensing of different medicines containing the same drug. Forms available from special-order manufacturers include: tablet, chewable tablet, oral suspension

Tablet

CAUTIONARY AND ADVISORY LABELS 9

▸ Eskazole (Imported (France))

Albendazole 400 mg Eskazole 400mg tablets | 60 tablet [PoM] [X]

Chewable tablet

CAUTIONARY AND ADVISORY LABELS 9

▸ Zentel (Imported)

Albendazole 200 mg Zentel 200mg chewable tablets | 6 tablet [PoM] [X]

Albendazole 400 mg Zentel 400mg chewable tablets | 1 tablet [PoM] [X]

Diethylcarbamazine

- **INDICATIONS AND DOSE**

***Wuchereria bancrofti* infections | *Brugia malayi* infections**

▶ BY MOUTH

▸ Child 1 month–9 years: Initially 1 mg/kg daily in divided doses on the first day, then increased to 3 mg/kg daily in divided doses, dose to be increased gradually over 3 days

▸ Child 10–17 years: Initially 1 mg/kg daily in divided doses on the first day, then increased to 6 mg/kg daily in divided doses, dose to be increased gradually over 3 days

***Loa loa* infections**

▶ BY MOUTH

▸ Child 1 month–9 years: Initially 1 mg/kg daily in divided doses on the first day, then increased to 3 mg/kg daily in divided doses, dose to be increased gradually over 3 days

▸ Child 10–17 years: Initially 1 mg/kg daily in divided doses on the first day, then increased to 6 mg/kg daily in divided doses, dose to be increased gradually over 3 days

- **UNLICENSED USE** Diethylcarbamazine is an unlicensed drug.
- **MEDICINAL FORMS** No licensed medicines listed.

Ivermectin

17-May-2017

- **INDICATIONS AND DOSE**

Chronic *Strongyloides* infection

▶ BY MOUTH

▸ Child 5–17 years: 200 micrograms/kg daily for 2 days

Onchocerciasis

▶ BY MOUTH

▸ Child 5–17 years: 150 micrograms/kg for 1 dose, retreatment at intervals of 6 to12 months, depending on symptoms, must be given until adult worms die out

Scabies, in combination with topical drugs, for the treatment of hyperkeratotic (crusted or 'Norwegian') scabies that does not respond to topical treatment alone

▶ BY MOUTH

▸ Child: (consult product literature)

- **UNLICENSED USE** Ivermectin is unlicensed.
- **INTERACTIONS** → Appendix 1: ivermectin
- **SIDE-EFFECTS**

▶ **Common or very common** Skin reactions

▶ **Frequency not known** Abnormal sensation in eye · anaemia · appetite decreased · asthenia · asthma exacerbated · chest discomfort · coma · confusion · conjunctival haemorrhage · constipation · diarrhoea · difficulty standing · difficulty walking · dizziness · drowsiness · dyspnoea ·

encephalopathy · eosinophilia · eye inflammation · faecal incontinence · fever · gastrointestinal discomfort · headache · hepatitis · hypotension · joint disorders · leucopenia · lymphatic abnormalities · Mazzotti reaction aggravated · myalgia · nausea · oedema · pain · psychiatric disorder · seizure · severe cutaneous adverse reactions (SCARs) · stupor · tachycardia · tremor · urinary incontinence · vertigo · vomiting

- **MEDICINAL FORMS** There can be variation in the licensing of different medicines containing the same drug. Forms available from special-order manufacturers include: tablet

Tablet

- Ivermectin (Non-proprietary)
  Ivermectin 3 mg Stromectol 3mg tablets | 4 tablet PoM

Levamisole

10-Mar-2020

- **INDICATIONS AND DOSE**

Roundworm infections

- BY MOUTH
- Child: 2.5–3 mg/kg (max. per dose 150 mg) for 1 dose

Hookworm infections

- BY MOUTH
- Child: 2.5 mg/kg (max. per dose 150 mg) for 1 dose, dose to be repeated after 7 days if severe

Nephrotic syndrome (initiated under specialist supervision)

- BY MOUTH
- Child: 2.5 mg/kg once daily on alternate days (max. per dose 150 mg)

- **UNLICENSED USE** Not licensed.
- **CONTRA-INDICATIONS** Blood disorders
- **CAUTIONS** Epilepsy · juvenile idiopathic arthritis · Sjögren's syndrome
- **INTERACTIONS** → Appendix 1: levamisole
- **SIDE-EFFECTS** Arthralgia (long term use) · blood disorder (long term use) · diarrhoea · dizziness · headache · influenza like illness (long term use) · insomnia (long term use) · myalgia (long term use) · nausea · rash (long term use) · seizure (long term use) · taste altered (long term use) · vasculitis (long term use) · vomiting
- **PREGNANCY** Embryotoxic in *animal* studies, avoid if possible.
- **BREAST FEEDING** No information available.
- **HEPATIC IMPAIRMENT**
  Dose adjustments Use with caution—dose adjustment may be necessary.
- **PATIENT AND CARER ADVICE**
  Medicines for Children leaflet: Levamisole for nephrotic syndrome www.medicinesforchildren.org.uk/levamisole-nephrotic-syndrome
- **MEDICINAL FORMS** There can be variation in the licensing of different medicines containing the same drug. Forms available from special-order manufacturers include: tablet

Tablet

CAUTIONARY AND ADVISORY LABELS 4

- **Ergamisol** (Imported (Belgium))
  Levamisole (as Levamisole hydrochloride) 50 mg Ergamisol 50mg tablets | 20 tablet PoM

Mebendazole

10-Mar-2020

- **INDICATIONS AND DOSE**

Threadworm infections

- BY MOUTH
- Child 6 months–17 years: 100 mg for 1 dose, if reinfection occurs, second dose may be needed after 2 weeks

Whipworm infections | Hookworm infections

- BY MOUTH
- Child 1–17 years: 100 mg twice daily for 3 days

Roundworm infections

- BY MOUTH
- Child 1 year: 100 mg twice daily for 3 days
- Child 2–17 years: 100 mg twice daily for 3 days, alternatively 500 mg for 1 dose

Threadworm infections (dose approved for use by community practitioner nurse prescribers)

- BY MOUTH
- Child 2–17 years: 100 mg for 1 dose, if reinfection occurs, second dose may be needed after 2 weeks

- **UNLICENSED USE** Not licensed for use as a single dose of 500 mg in roundworm infections. Not licensed for use in children under 2 years.
- **INTERACTIONS** → Appendix 1: mebendazole
- **SIDE-EFFECTS**
  - **Common or very common** Gastrointestinal discomfort
  - **Uncommon** Diarrhoea · flatulence
  - **Rare or very rare** Alopecia · dizziness · hepatitis · neutropenia · seizure · severe cutaneous adverse reactions (SCARs) · skin reactions
- **PREGNANCY** Manufacturer advises avoid—toxicity in *animal* studies.
- **BREAST FEEDING** Amount present in milk too small to be harmful but manufacturer advises avoid.
- **PRESCRIBING AND DISPENSING INFORMATION** Flavours of oral liquid formulations may include banana.
- **PATIENT AND CARER ADVICE**
  Medicines for Children leaflet: Mebendazole for worm infections www.medicinesforchildren.org.uk/mebendazole-worm-infections
- **EXCEPTIONS TO LEGAL CATEGORY** Mebendazole tablets can be sold to the public if supplied for oral use in the treatment of enterobiasis in adults and children over 2 years provided its container or package is labelled to show a max. single dose of 100 mg and it is supplied in a container or package containing not more than 800 mg.
- **MEDICINAL FORMS** There can be variation in the licensing of different medicines containing the same drug.

Oral suspension

- Vermox (Janssen-Cilag Ltd)
  Mebendazole 20 mg per 1 ml Vermox 100mg/5ml oral suspension | 30 ml PoM £1.55 DT = £1.55

Chewable tablet

- Vermox (Janssen-Cilag Ltd)
  Mebendazole 100 mg Vermox 100mg chewable tablets sugar-free | 6 tablet PoM £1.34 DT = £1.34

Praziquantel

- **INDICATIONS AND DOSE**

Tapeworm infections (*Taenia solium*)

- BY MOUTH
- Child 4–17 years: 5–10 mg/kg for 1 dose, to be taken after a light breakfast

continued →

Tapeworm infections (*Hymenolepis nana*)
▶ BY MOUTH
▸ Child 4–17 years: 25 mg/kg for 1 dose, to be taken after a light breakfast

***Schistosoma haematobium* worm infections | *Schistosoma mansoni* worm infections**
▶ BY MOUTH
▸ Child 4–17 years: 20 mg/kg, followed by 20 mg/kg after 4–6 hours

***Schistosoma japonicum* worm infections**
▶ BY MOUTH
▸ Child 4–17 years: 20 mg/kg 3 times a day for 1 day

- **UNLICENSED USE** Praziquantel is an unlicensed drug.
- **INTERACTIONS** → Appendix 1: praziquantel

- **MEDICINAL FORMS** There can be variation in the licensing of different medicines containing the same drug. Forms available from special-order manufacturers include: tablet

Tablet
▸ Praziquantel (Imported)
Praziquantel 150 mg Cesol 150mg tablets | 6 tablet [PoM]
Praziquantel 600 mg Biltricide 600mg tablets | 6 tablet [PoM]
▸ Cysticide (Imported (Germany))
Praziquantel 500 mg Cysticide 500mg tablets | 90 tablet [PoM]

4 Protozoal infection

Antiprotozoal drugs

Amoebicides

Metronidazole p. 358 is the drug of choice for *acute invasive amoebic dysentery* since it is very effective against vegetative forms of *Entamoeba histolytica* in ulcers. Tinidazole p. 360 is also effective. Metronidazole and tinidazole are also active against amoebae which may have migrated to the liver. Treatment with metronidazole (or tinidazole) is followed by a 10-day course of diloxanide furoate.

Diloxanide furoate is the drug of choice for asymptomatic patients with *E. histolytica* cysts in the faeces; metronidazole and tinidazole are relatively ineffective. Diloxanide furoate is relatively free from toxic effects and the usual course is of 10 days, given alone for chronic infections or following metronidazole or tinidazole treatment.

For *amoebic abscesses* of the liver metronidazole is effective; tinidazole is an alternative. Aspiration of the abscess is indicated where it is suspected that it may rupture or where there is no improvement after 72 hours of metronidazole; the aspiration may need to be repeated. Aspiration aids penetration of metronidazole and, for abscesses with large volumes of pus, if carried out in conjunction with drug therapy, may reduce the period of disability.

Diloxanide furoate is not effective against hepatic amoebiasis, but a 10-day course should be given at the completion of metronidazole or tinidazole treatment to destroy any amoebae in the gut.

Trichomonacides

Metronidazole is the treatment of choice for *Trichomonas vaginalis* infection. Contact tracing is recommended and sexual contacts should be treated simultaneously. If metronidazole is ineffective, tinidazole may be tried.

Antigiardial drugs

Metronidazole is the treatment of choice for *Giardia lamblia* infections. Tinidazole may be used as an alternative to metronidazole.

Leishmaniacides

Cutaneous leishmaniasis frequently heals spontaneously but if skin lesions are extensive or unsightly, treatment is indicated, as it is in visceral leishmaniasis (kala-azar). Leishmaniasis should be treated under specialist supervision.

Sodium stibogluconate p. 419, an organic pentavalent antimony compound, is used for visceral leishmaniasis. The dosage varies with different geographical regions and expert advice should be obtained. Skin lesions can also be treated with sodium stibogluconate.

Amphotericin p. 406 is used with or after an antimony compound for visceral leishmaniasis unresponsive to the antimonial alone; side-effects may be reduced by using liposomal amphotericin (*AmBisome*®). *Abelcet*®, a lipid formulation of amphotericin, is also likely to be effective but less information is available.

Pentamidine isetionate p. 414 (pentamidine isethionate) has been used in antimony-resistant visceral leishmaniasis, but although the initial response is often good, the relapse rate is high; it is associated with serious side-effects. Other treatments include paromomycin [unlicensed] (available from 'special-order' manufacturers or specialist importing companies).

Trypanocides

The prophylaxis and treatment of trypanosomiasis is difficult and differs according to the strain of organism. Expert advice should therefore be obtained.

Toxoplasmosis

Most infections caused by *Toxoplasma gondii* are self-limiting, and treatment is not necessary. Exceptions are patients with eye involvement (toxoplasma choroidoretinitis), and those who are immunosuppressed. Toxoplasmic encephalitis is a common complication of AIDS. The treatment of choice is a combination of pyrimethamine p. 431 and sulfadiazine p. 380, given for several weeks (expert advice **essential**). Pyrimethamine is a folate antagonist, and adverse reactions to this combination are relatively common (folinic acid supplements and weekly blood counts needed). Alternative regimens use combinations of pyrimethamine with clindamycin p. 351 or clarithromycin p. 353 or azithromycin p. 352. Long-term secondary prophylaxis is required after treatment of toxoplasmosis in immunocompromised patients; prophylaxis should continue until immunity recovers.

If toxoplasmosis is acquired in pregnancy, transplacental infection may lead to severe disease in the fetus; specialist advice should be sought on management. Spiramycin [unlicensed] (available from 'special-order' manufacturers or specialist importing companies) may reduce the risk of transmission of maternal infection to the fetus. When there is evidence of placental or fetal infection, pyrimethamine may be given with sulfadiazine and folinic acid p. 600 after the first trimester.

In neonates without signs of toxoplasmosis, but born to mothers known to have become infected, spiramycin is given while awaiting laboratory results. If toxoplasmosis is confirmed in the infant, pyrimethamine and sulfadiazine are given for 12 months, together with folinic acid.

4.1 Leishmaniasis

Other drugs used for Leishmaniasis Amphotericin, p. 406 · Pentamidine isetionate, p. 414

5 Infection

ANTIPROTOZOALS › OTHER

Sodium stibogluconate

● **INDICATIONS AND DOSE**

Visceral leishmaniasis (specialist use only)

▶ BY INTRAVENOUS INJECTION, OR BY INTRAMUSCULAR INJECTION

▶ Child: 20 mg/kg daily for at least 20 days

● **UNLICENSED USE**

▶ With intravenous use Licensed for use in children (age range not specified by manufacturer).

● **CAUTIONS** Heart disease (withdraw if conduction disturbances occur) · mucocutaneous disease · predisposition to QT interval prolongation · treat intercurrent infection (e.g. pneumonia)

CAUTIONS, FURTHER INFORMATION

▶ Mucocutaneous disease Successful treatment of mucocutaneous leishmaniasis may induce severe inflammation around the lesions (may be life-threatening if pharyngeal or tracheal involvement)—may require corticosteroid.

● **INTERACTIONS** → Appendix 1: sodium stibogluconate

● **SIDE-EFFECTS**

▶ **Common or very common** Abdominal pain · appetite decreased · arthralgia · diarrhoea · headache · lethargy · malaise · myalgia · nausea · vomiting

▶ **Rare or very rare** Chest pain · chills · fever · flushing · haemorrhage · hyperhidrosis · jaundice · skin reactions · vertigo

▶ **Frequency not known** Arrhythmias · cough · pain · pancreatitis · pneumonia · QT interval prolongation · thrombosis

● **PREGNANCY** Manufacturer advises use only if potential benefit outweighs risk.

● **BREAST FEEDING** Amount probably too small to be harmful.

● **HEPATIC IMPAIRMENT** Manufacturer advises caution (limited information available; abnormalities in hepatic function may be expected in visceral leishmaniasis).

● **RENAL IMPAIRMENT** Avoid in significant impairment.

● **MONITORING REQUIREMENTS** Monitor ECG before and during treatment.

● **DIRECTIONS FOR ADMINISTRATION** Intravenous injections must be given slowly over 5 minutes (to reduce risk of local thrombosis) and stopped if coughing or substernal pain occur. Injection should be filtered immediately before administration using a filter of 5 microns or less.

● **MEDICINAL FORMS** There can be variation in the licensing of different medicines containing the same drug.

Solution for injection

▶ Pentostam (GlaxoSmithKline UK Ltd)
Antimony pentavalent (as Sodium stibogluconate) 100 mg per 1 ml Pentostam 10g/100ml solution for injection vials | 1 vial PoM £66.43

4.2 Malaria

Antimalarials

20-Nov-2019

Artemether with lumefantrine

Artemether with lumefantrine p. 427 is licensed for the *treatment of acute uncomplicated falciparum malaria.*

Artenimol with piperaquine

Artenimol with piperaquine phosphate p. 427 is not recommended for the first-line treatment of acute uncomplicated falciparum malaria because there is limited experience of its use in travellers who usually reside in areas where malaria is not endemic. Piperaquine has a long half-life.

Atovaquone with proguanil

Atovaquone with proguanil hydrochloride p. 428 is licensed for the *prophylaxis of falciparum malaria* (for details, see Recommended regimens for prophylaxis against malaria p. 421) and for the treatment of *acute, uncomplicated falciparum malaria.*

Chloroquine

Chloroquine p. 429 is usually used with proguanil hydrochloride p. 431 for the *prophylaxis of malaria* in areas of the world where there is little chloroquine resistance (for details, see Recommended regimens for prophylaxis against malaria p. 421).

Guidelines for malaria prevention in travellers from the United Kingdom (2019) published by Public Health England state that patients already taking hydroxychloroquine sulfate p. 690 for another indication, and for whom chloroquine would be an appropriate antimalarial, can remain on hydroxychloroquine sulfate.

Chloroquine is **no longer recommended** for the *treatment of falciparum malaria* owing to widespread resistance, nor is it recommended if the infective species is *not known* or if the infection is *mixed*; in these cases treatment should be with quinine p. 432, atovaquone with proguanil hydrochloride p. 428, or artemether with lumefantrine. It is still recommended for the *treatment of non-falciparum malaria.*

Doxycycline

Doxycycline p. 381 is used in adults and children over 12 years as an option for the *prophylaxis of malaria* in areas of *chloroquine resistance*. Doxycycline is also used as an alternative to mefloquine p. 430 or atovaquone with proguanil hydrochloride p. 428 (for details, see Recommended regimens for prophylaxis against malaria p. 421).

Mefloquine

Mefloquine is used for the *prophylaxis of malaria* in areas of *chloroquine resistance*. Mefloquine is also used as an alternative to doxycycline or atovaquone with proguanil hydrochloride p. 428, (for details, see Recommended regimens for prophylaxis against malaria p. 421).

Mefloquine is now rarely used for the *treatment of falciparum malaria* because of increased resistance. It is rarely used for the *treatment of non-falciparum malaria* because better tolerated alternatives are available. Mefloquine should not be used for treatment if it has been used for prophylaxis.

Primaquine

Primaquine p. 430 is used to eliminate the liver stages of *P. vivax* or *P. ovale* following chloroquine treatment.

Proguanil

Proguanil hydrochloride is usually used in combination with chloroquine or atovaquone for the *prophylaxis of malaria*, (for details, see Recommended regimens for prophylaxis against malaria p. 421).

Proguanil hydrochloride used alone is not suitable for the *treatment of malaria*; however atovaquone with proguanil hydrochloride is licensed for the treatment of acute uncomplicated falciparum malaria. Atovaquone with proguanil hydrochloride is also used for the *prophylaxis of falciparum malaria* in areas of *chloroquine resistance.*

Atovaquone with proguanil hydrochloride is also used as an alternative to mefloquine or doxycycline. Atovaquone with proguanil hydrochloride is particularly suitable for short trips to chloroquine-resistant areas because it needs to be taken only for 7 days after leaving an endemic area.

Pyrimethamine

Pyrimethamine p. 431 should not be used alone, but is used with sulfadoxine.

Pyrimethamine with sulfadoxine can be used in the *treatment of falciparum malaria with (or following) quinine*.

Quinine

Quinine is used for the *treatment of falciparum malaria*, if the infective species is *not known*, or if the infection is mixed (for details see Malaria, treatment p. 426).

Useful resources

Recommendations on prophylaxis against malaria reflect guidelines agreed by the Advisory Committee on Malaria Prevention (ACMP), published in the Public Health England (PHE) Guidelines for malaria prevention in travellers from the United Kingdom, 2019. The advice is aimed at residents of the UK who travel to endemic areas. www.gov.uk/government/publications/malaria-prevention-guidelines-for-travellers-from-the-uk

Malaria, prophylaxis

20-Nov-2019

Prophylaxis against malaria

The recommendations on prophylaxis reflect guidelines agreed by the Advisory Committee on Malaria Prevention (ACMP), published in the Public Health England (PHE) Guidelines for malaria prevention in travellers from the United Kingdom, 2019. The advice is aimed at residents of the UK who travel to endemic areas.

For specialist centres offering advice on specific malaria-related problems, see Malaria, treatment p. 426. The choice of drug for a particular individual should take into account:

- risk of exposure to malaria
- extent of drug resistance
- efficacy of the recommended drugs
- side-effects of the drugs
- patient-related factors (e.g. age, pregnancy, renal or hepatic impairment, compliance with prophylactic regimen)

For more information on choice of drug, see also Antimalarials p. 419. Prophylactic doses are based on guidelines agreed by UK malaria experts and may differ from advice in product literature. **Weight is a better guide than age**. If in doubt obtain advice from a specialist centre, see Malaria, treatment p. 426.

Protection against bites

Prophylaxis is not absolute, and breakthrough infection can occur with any of the drugs recommended. Personal protection against being bitten is very important and is recommended even in malaria-free areas as a preventive measure against other insect vector-borne diseases. Mosquito nets impregnated with a pyrethroid insecticide, such as permethrin p. 780, improves protection against insects and should be used if sleeping outdoors or in unscreened lodging; vaporised insecticides are also useful. Long sleeves and trousers worn after dusk also provide protection against bites.

Insect repellents give protection against bites also, but attention to the correct application of product is required. Diethyltoluamide (DEET) 20–50% (available in various preparations including sprays and modified-release polymer formulations) is safe and effective when applied to the skin of adults and children over 2 months of age. It can also be used during pregnancy and breast-feeding. However, ingestion should be avoided, therefore breast-feeding mothers should wash their hands and breast tissue before handling infants. The duration of protection varies according to the concentration of DEET and is longest for DEET 50%. When sunscreen is also required, DEET should be applied after the sunscreen. DEET reduces the SPF of sunscreen, so a sunscreen of SPF 30–50 should be applied. If DEET is not tolerated or is unavailable, for alternative options see Public Health England Guidelines for malaria prevention in travellers from the United Kingdom (see *Useful resources*).

Length of prophylaxis

Prophylaxis should generally be started before travel into an endemic area; 1 week before travel for chloroquine p. 429 and proguanil hydrochloride p. 431; 2–3 weeks before travel for mefloquine p. 430; and 1–2 days before travel for atovaquone with proguanil hydrochloride p. 428 or doxycycline p. 381 (children aged 12 years and over). Prophylaxis should be continued for **4 weeks after leaving the area** (except for atovaquone with proguanil hydrochloride prophylaxis which should be stopped 1 week after leaving). For extensive journeys across different regions, the traveller must be protected in all areas of risk.

In those requiring long-term prophylaxis, chloroquine and proguanil hydrochloride may be used. However, there is considerable concern over the protective efficacy of the combination of chloroquine and proguanil hydrochloride in certain areas where it was previously useful. Mefloquine is licensed for use up to 1 year (although, if it is tolerated in the short term, there is no evidence of harm when it is used for up to 3 years). Doxycycline (children aged 12 years and over) can be used for up to 2 years, and atovaquone with proguanil hydrochloride for up to 1 year. Prophylaxis with mefloquine, doxycycline, or atovaquone with proguanil hydrochloride may be considered for longer durations if it is justified by the risk of exposure to malaria. Specialist advice may be sought for long-term prophylaxis.

Return from malarial region

It is important to consider that any illness that occurs within 1 year and **especially within 3 months of return might be malaria** even if all recommended precautions against malaria were taken. Travellers should be warned of this and told that if they develop any illness after their return they should see a doctor early, and specifically mention their risk of exposure to malaria.

Epilepsy

Both chloroquine and mefloquine are unsuitable for malaria prophylaxis in individuals with a history of epilepsy. In these patients, doxycycline (children aged 12 years and over) or atovaquone with proguanil hydrochloride may be used. However doxycycline may interact with some antiepileptics and its dose may need to be adjusted, see *interactions* information for doxycycline.

Asplenia

Asplenic individuals (or those with severe splenic dysfunction) are at particular risk of severe malaria. If travel to malarious areas is unavoidable, rigorous precautions are required against contracting the disease.

Pregnancy

Travel to malarious areas should be avoided during pregnancy; if travel is unavoidable, pregnant individuals must be informed about the risks and benefits of effective prophylaxis. Chloroquine and proguanil hydrochloride can be given in the usual doses during pregnancy, but these drugs are not appropriate for most areas because their effectiveness has declined; in the case of proguanil hydrochloride, folic acid p. 620 (dosed as a pregnancy at 'high-risk' of neural tube defects) should be given for the length of time that it is used during pregnancy. If travelling to high risk areas or there is resistance to other drugs,

Key to recommended regimens for prophylaxis against malaria

Codes for regimens	Details of regimens for prophylaxis against malaria
-	No risk
1	Chemoprophylaxis not recommended, but avoid mosquito bites and consider malaria if fever presents
2	Chloroquine only
3	Chloroquine with proguanil
4	Atovaquone with proguanil hydrochloride or doxycycline or mefloquine

Specific recommendations

Country	Comments on risk of malaria and regional or seasonal variation	Codes for regimens
Afghanistan	Low risk below 2000 m from May–November	1
	Very low risk below 2000 m from December–April	1
Algeria	No risk	1
Andaman and Nicobar Islands (India)	Low risk	1
Angola	High risk	4
Argentina	No risk	1
Armenia	No risk	1
Azerbaijan	Very low risk	1
Bangladesh	High risk in Chittagong Hill Tract districts (but not Chittagong city)	4
	Very low risk in Chittagong city and other areas, except Chittagong Hill Tract districts	1
Belize	Low risk in rural areas	1
	No risk in Belize district (including Belize city and islands)	-
Benin	High risk	4
Bhutan	Low risk in southern belt districts, along border with India: Chukha, Geyleg-phug, Samchi, Samdrup Jonkhar, and Shemgang	1
	No risk in areas other than those above	-
Bolivia	Low risk in Amazon basin	1
	Low risk in rural areas below 2500 m (other than above)	1
	No risk above 2500 m	-
Botswana	High risk from November–June in northern half, including Okavango Delta area	4
	Low risk from July–October in northern half, including Okavango Delta area	1
	Very low risk in southern half	1
Brazil	Low risk in Amazon basin, including city of Manaus	1
	Very low risk in areas other than those above	1
	No risk in Iguaçu Falls	-
Brunei Darussalam	Very low risk	1
Burkina Faso	High risk	4
Burundi	High risk	4
Cambodia	Low risk. Mefloquine resistance widespread in western provinces bordering Thailand	1
	Very low risk in Angkor Wat and Lake Tonle Sap, including Siem Reap	1
	No risk in Phnom Penh	-
Cameroon	High risk	4
Cape Verde	Individuals travelling to Praia who are at increased risk of malaria (such as long-term travellers and those at risk of severe complications from malaria including pregnant women, infants and young children, the elderly, and asplenic individuals) should consider taking antimalarials, seek advice from a travel health advisor. Very low risk on island of Santiago (Sao Tiago) and Boa Vista	1
Central African Republic	High risk	4
Chad	High risk	4

Country	Comments on risk of malaria and regional or seasonal variation	Codes for regimens
China	Low risk in Yunnan and Hainan provinces	1
	Very low risk in southern and some central provinces, including Anhui, Ghuizhou, Hena, Hubei, and Jiangsu below 1500 m	1
	Very low risk in areas other than those above and below	1
	No risk in Hong Kong	-
Colombia	Low risk in rural areas below 1600 m	1
	Very low risk above 1600 m and in Cartagena	1
Comoros	High risk	4
Congo	High risk	4
Costa Rica	Low risk in Limon province, but not city of Limon (Puerto Limon)	1
	Very low risk in areas other than those above	1
Cote d'Ivoire (Ivory Coast)	High risk	4
Democratic Republic of the Congo	High risk	4
Djibouti	High risk	4
Dominican Republic	Low risk	1
	No risk in cities of Santiago and Santo Domingo	-
East Timor (Timor-Leste)	Risk present	4
Ecuador	Low risk in areas below 1500 m including coastal provinces and Amazon basin	1
	No risk in Galapagos islands or city of Guayaquil	-
Egypt	No risk	1
El Salvador	Low risk in rural areas of Santa Ana, Ahuachapán, and La Unión provinces in western part of country	1
	Very low risk in areas other than those above	1
Equatorial Guinea	High risk	4
Eritrea	High risk below 2200 m	4
	No risk in Asmara or in areas above 2200 m	-
Ethiopia	High risk below 2000 m	4
	No risk in Addis Ababa or in areas above 2000 m	-
French Guiana	Risk present (particularly in border areas) except city of Cayenne or Devil's Island (Ile du Diable)	4
	Low risk in city of Cayenne or Devil's Island (Ile du Diable)	1
Gabon	High risk	4
Gambia	High risk	4
Georgia	Very low risk from June–October in rural south east	1
	No risk from November-May in rural south east	-
Ghana	High risk	4
Guatemala	Low risk below 1500 m	1
	No risk in Guatemala City, Antigua, or Lake Atitlan and above 1500 m	-
Guinea	High risk	4
Guinea-Bissau	High risk	4
Guyana	Risk present in all interior regions	4
	Very low risk in Georgetown and coastal region	1
Haiti	Risk present	3
Honduras	Low risk below 1000 m and in Roatán and other Bay Islands	1
	No risk in San Pedro Sula or Tegucigalpa and areas above 1000 m	-
India	Risk present in states of Assam and Orissa, districts of East Godavari, Srikakulam, Vishakhapatnam, and Vizianagaram in the state of Andhra Pradesh, and districts of Balaghat, Dindori, Mandla, and Seoni in the state of Madhya Pradesh	4
	Low risk in areas other than those above or below (including Goa, Andaman and Nicobar islands)	1
	Exceptional circumstances in low risk areas (dependent on individual risk assessment)	3
	No risk in Lakshadweep islands	-

Key to recommended regimens for prophylaxis against malaria

Codes for regimens	Details of regimens for prophylaxis against malaria
-	No risk
1	Chemoprophylaxis not recommended, but avoid mosquito bites and consider malaria if fever presents
2	Chloroquine only
3	Chloroquine with proguanil
4	Atovaquone with proguanil hydrochloride or doxycycline or mefloquine

Specific recommendations

Country	Comments on risk of malaria and regional or seasonal variation	Codes for regimens
Indonesia	High risk in Irian Jaya (Papua)	4
	Low risk in Bali, Lombok and islands of Java and Sumatra	1
	No risk in city of Jakarta	-
Indonesia (Borneo)	Low risk	1
Iran	Low risk from March–November in rural south eastern provinces and in north, along Azerbaijan border in Ardabil, and near Turkmenistan border in North Khorasan	1
	Very low risk in areas other than those above	1
Iraq	Very low risk from May–November in rural northern area below 1500 m	1
	No risk in areas other than those above	-
Kenya	High risk (except city of Nairobi)	4
	Very low risk in the highlands above 2500 m and in city of Nairobi	1
Kyrgyzstan	No risk	-
Lao People's Democratic Republic (Laos)	Low risk	1
	Very low risk in city of Vientiane	1
Liberia	High risk	4
Libya	No risk	1
Madagascar	High risk	4
Malawi	High risk	4
Malaysia	Low risk in mainland Malaysia	1
Malaysia (Borneo)	Low risk in inland areas of Sabah and in inland, forested areas of Sarawak	1
	Very low risk in areas other than those above, including coastal areas of Sabah and Sarawak	1
Mali	High risk	4
Mauritania	High risk all year in southern provinces, and from July–October in the northern provinces	4
	Low risk from November–June in the northern provinces	1
Mauritius	No risk	1
Mayotte	Risk present	4
Mexico	Very low risk	1
Mozambique	High risk	4
Myanmar	Low risk	1
Namibia	High risk all year in regions of Caprivi Strip, Kavango, and Kunene river, and from November–June in northern third of country	4
	Low risk from July–October in northern third of country, except as above in regions of Caprivi Strip, Kavango, and Kunene river	1
	Very low risk in areas other than those above	1
Nepal	Low risk below 1500 m, including the Terai district	1
	No risk in city of Kathmandu and on typical Himalayan treks	-
Nicaragua	Low risk (except Managua)	1
	Very low risk in Managua	1
Niger	High risk	4
Nigeria	High risk	4
North Korea	Very low risk in some southern areas	1
Pakistan	Low risk below 2000 m	1
	Very low risk above 2000 m	1

Country	Comments on risk of malaria and regional or seasonal variation	Codes for regimens
Panama	Low risk east of Canal Zone	1
	Very low risk west of Canal Zone	1
	No risk in Panama City or Canal Zone itself	-
Papua New Guinea	High risk below 1800 m	4
	Very low risk above 1800 m	1
Paraguay	No risk	1
Peru	Low risk in Amazon basin along border with Brazil, particularly in Loreto province and in rural areas below 2000 m including the Amazon basin bordering Bolivia	1
	No risk in city of Lima and coastal region south of Chiclayo	-
Philippines	Low risk in rural areas below 600 m and on islands of Luzon, Mindanao, Mindoro, and Palawan	1
	No risk in cities or on islands of Boracay, Bohol, Catanduanes, Cebu, or Leyte	-
Rwanda	High risk	4
São Tomé and Principe	High risk	4
Saudi Arabia	Low risk in south-western provinces along border with Yemen, including below 2000 m in Asir province	1
	No risk in cities of Jeddah, Makkah (Mecca), Medina, Riyadh, or Ta'if, or above 2000 m in Asir province	-
Senegal	High risk	4
Sierra Leone	High risk	4
Singapore	No risk	1
Solomon Islands	High risk	4
Somalia	High risk	4
South Africa	Risk from September–May in low altitude areas of Mpumalanga and Limpopo, particularly those bordering Mozambique, Swaziland (Estwatini), and Zimbabwe (including Kruger National Park)	4
	Low risk in north-east KwaZulu-Natal and in designated areas of Mpumalanga and Limpopo	1
	Very low risk in North West Province (adjacent to Molopo river) and Northern Cape Province (adjacent to Orange river)	1
South Korea	Very low risk in northern areas, in Gangwon-do and Gyeonggi-do provinces, and Incheon city (towards Demilitarized Zone)	1
South Sudan	High risk	4
Sri Lanka	No risk	1
Sudan	High risk in central and southern areas; risk also present in rest of country (except Khartoum)	4
	Very low risk in Khartoum	1
Suriname	Risk present on the French Guiana border	4
	Low risk in areas other than above and below	1
	No risk in city of Paramaribo	-
Swaziland	Risk in northern and eastern regions bordering Mozambique and South Africa, including all of Lubombo district and Big Bend, Mhlume, Simunye, and Tshaneni regions	4
	Very low risk in the areas other than those above	1
Syria	Very low risk in small, remote foci of El Hasakah	1
Tajikistan	Very low risk	1
	No risk above 2000 m	-
Tanzania	High risk below 1800 m; risk also in Zanzibar	4
	No risk above 1800 m	-
Thailand	Mefloquine resistance present. Low risk in rural forested borders with Cambodia, Laos, and Myanmar	1
	Very low risk in areas other than those above, including Kanchanaburi (Kwai Bridge)	1
	No risk in cities of Bangkok, Chiang Mai, Chiang Rai, Koh Phangan, Koh Samui, and Pattaya	-
Togo	High risk	4
Turkey	Very low risk	1
Uganda	High risk	4

Key to recommended regimens for prophylaxis against malaria

Codes for regimens	Details of regimens for prophylaxis against malaria
-	No risk
1	Chemoprophylaxis not recommended, but avoid mosquito bites and consider malaria if fever presents
2	Chloroquine only
3	Chloroquine with proguanil
4	Atovaquone with proguanil hydrochloride or doxycycline or mefloquine

Specific recommendations

Country	Comments on risk of malaria and regional or seasonal variation	Codes for regimens
Uzbekistan	No risk	1
Vanuatu	Risk present	4
Venezuela	Risk in all areas south of, and including, the Orinoco river and Angel Falls, rural areas of Apure, Monagas, Sucre, and Zulia states	1
	Increase in reported malaria cases between 2010 and 2017, mainly in the Bolivar state	1
	No risk in city of Caracas or on Margarita Island	
Vietnam	Low risk in rural areas, and in southern provinces of Tay Ninh, Lam Dong, Dac Lac, Gia Lai, and Kon Tum	1
	No risk in large cities (including Ho Chi Minh City (Saigon) and Hanoi), the Red River delta, coastal areas north of Nha Trang and Phu Quoc Island	1
Western Sahara	No risk	1
Yemen	Risk below 2000 m	3
	Very low risk on Socrota Island	1
	No risk above 2000 m, including Sana'a city	1
Zambia	High risk	4
Zimbabwe	High risk all year in Zambezi valley, and from November–June in areas below 1200 m	4
	Low risk from July–October in areas below 1200 m	1
	Very low risk all year in Harare and Bulawayo	1

mefloquine may be considered during the second or third trimester of pregnancy. Mefloquine can be used in the first trimester with caution if the benefits outweigh the risks. Doxycycline is contra-indicated during pregnancy; however, it can be used for malaria prophylaxis if other regimens are unsuitable, and if the entire course of doxycycline can be completed before 15 weeks' gestation [unlicensed]. Atovaquone with proguanil hydrochloride should be avoided during pregnancy, however, it can be considered during the second and third trimesters if there is no suitable alternative. Folic acid (dosed as a pregnancy at 'high-risk' of neural tube defects) should be given if atovaquone with proguanil hydrochloride is used during pregnancy.

Breast-feeding
Some antimalarials should be avoided when breast feeding, see individual drugs for details.

Prophylaxis is required in **breast-fed infants**; although antimalarials are present in milk, the amounts are too variable to give reliable protection.

Anticoagulants
Travellers taking warfarin sodium p. 103 should begin chemoprophylaxis 2–3 weeks before departure and the INR should be stable before departure. It should be measured before starting chemoprophylaxis, 7 days after starting, and after completing the course. For prolonged stays, the INR should be checked at regular intervals.

Other medical conditions
For additional information on malaria prophylaxis in patients with other medical conditions, see Public Health England Guidelines for malaria prevention in travellers from the United Kingdom (see *Useful resources*).

Emergency standby treatment
Children and their parents or carers on prophylaxis visiting remote, malarious areas should carry standby emergency treatment if they are likely to be more than 24 hours away from medical care. Standby emergency treatment should also be considered in long-term travellers living in or visiting remote, malarious areas that may be far from appropriate medical attention; this does not replace the need to consider prophylaxis. Self-medication should be **avoided** if medical help is accessible.

In order to use standby treatment appropriately, children and their parents or carers should be provided with **written instructions** which include seeking urgent medical attention if fever (38°C or more) develops 7 days (or more) after arriving in a malarious area and that self-treatment is indicated if medical help is not available within 24 hours of fever onset.

In view of the continuing emergence of resistant strains and of the different regimens required for different areas expert advice should be sought on the best treatment course for an individual traveller. A drug used for chemoprophylaxis should not be considered for standby treatment for the same traveller due to concerns over drug resistance and to minimise drug toxicity.

Malaria prophylaxis, specific recommendations

Travellers planning journeys across continents can travel into areas that have different malaria prophylaxis recommendations. The choice of prophylaxis medication must reflect overall risk to ensure protection in all areas; it may be possible to change from one regimen to another. Those travelling to remote or little-visited areas may require expert advice. For further information see *Recommended regimens for prophylaxis against malaria*, and Public Health England Guidelines for malaria prevention in travellers from the United Kingdom (see *Useful resources*).

Important

Settled immigrants (or long-term visitors) to the UK may be unaware that **any immunity they may have acquired while living in malarious areas is lost rapidly** after migration to the UK, or that any non-malarious areas where they lived previously **may now be malarious.**

Useful resources

Public Health England guideline: Guidelines for malaria prevention in travellers from the United Kingdom. September 2019.

www.gov.uk/government/publications/malaria-prevention-guidelines-for-travellers-from-the-uk

Malaria, treatment

20-Nov-2019

Advice for healthcare professionals

A number of specialist centres are able to provide advice on specific problems.

Public Health England (PHE) Malaria Reference Laboratory (prophylaxis) www.gov.uk/government/collections/malaria-reference-laboratory-mrl

National Travel Health Network and Centre (NaTHNaC) 0845 602 6712 www.travelhealthpro.org.uk/

TRAVAX (Health Protection Scotland) 0141 300 1130 www.travax.nhs.uk (for registered users of the NHS Travax website only)

Hospital for Tropical Diseases (HTD) (treatment) www.thehtd.org/

Liverpool School of Tropical Medicine (LSTM) (treatment) 0151 705 3100 Monday to Friday: 9 a.m.–5 p.m. and via Royal Liverpool Hospital switchboard at all other times 0151 706 2000 www.lstmed.ac.uk/

Birmingham 0121 424 2358

Your local infectious diseases unit

Advice for travellers

Hospital for Tropical Diseases Travel Healthline 020 7950 7799 www.fitfortravel.nhs.uk/home

WHO advice on international travel and health www.who.int/ith/en/

National Travel Health Network and Centre (NaTHNaC) www.travelhealthpro.org.uk/

Treatment

Recommendations on the prophylaxis and treatment of malaria reflect guidelines agreed by UK malaria specialists. Choice will depend on the age of the child.

If the infective species is **not known**, or if the infection is **mixed**, initial treatment should be as for *falciparum malaria* with quinine p. 432, *Malarone*® (atovaquone with proguanil hydrochloride p. 428), or *Riamet*® (artemether with lumefantrine p. 427). Falciparum malaria can progress rapidly in unprotected individuals and antimalarial treatment should be considered in those with features of severe malaria and possible exposure, even if the initial blood tests for the organism are negative.

Falciparum malaria (treatment)

Falciparum malaria (malignant malaria) is caused by *Plasmodium falciparum*. In most parts of the world *P. falciparum* is now resistant to chloroquine p. 429 which should not therefore be given for treatment. Quinine, ***Malarone***® (atovaquone with proguanil hydrochloride), or ***Riamet***® (artemether with lumefantrine) can be given by mouth if the child can swallow and retain tablets and there are no serious manifestations (e.g. impaired consciousness); quinine should be given by intravenous infusion if the child is seriously ill or unable to take tablets. Mefloquine p. 430 is now rarely used for treatment because of concerns about resistance.

Oral quinine is well tolerated by children although the salts are bitter. Quinine is given by mouth together with or followed by clindamycin p. 351 [unlicensed indication] or, in children over 12 doxycycline p. 381.

If the parasite is likely to be sensitive, pyrimethamine with sulfadoxine as a single dose [unlicensed] may be given (instead of either clindamycin or doxycycline) together with, or after, a course of quinine.

Alternatively, ***Malarone***®, or ***Riamet***® may be given instead of quinine. It is not necessary to give clindamycin, doxycycline, or pyrimethamine with sulfadoxine after *Malarone*® or *Riamet*® treatment.

If the child is seriously ill or unable to swallow tablets, or if more than 2% of red blood cell are parasitized, quinine should be given by *intravenous infusion*[unlicensed] (until patient can swallow tablets to complete the 7-day course *together with* or *followed by either* doxycycline in children over 12 years, or clindamycin).

Specialist advice should be sought in difficult cases (e.g. very high parasite count, deterioration on optimal doses of quinine, infection acquired in quinine-resistant areas of south east Asia) because intravenous **artesunate** may be available for 'named-patient' use.

Pregnancy

Falciparum malaria is particularly dangerous in pregnancy, especially in the last trimester. The treatment doses of oral and intravenous quinine (including the loading dose) can safely be given in pregnancy. Clindamycin [unlicensed indication] should be given for 7 days with or after quinine. Doxycycline should be avoided in pregnancy (affects teeth and skeletal development in fetus); pyrimethamine with sulfadoxine, Malarone®, and Riamet® are also best avoided until more information is available. Specialist advice should be sought in difficult cases (e.g. very high parasite count, deterioration on optimal doses of quinine, infection acquired in quinine-resistant areas of south east Asia) because intravenous artesunate may be available for 'named patient' use.

Non-falciparum malaria (treatment)

Non-falciparum malaria is usually caused by *Plasmodium vivax* and less commonly by *P. ovale* and *P. malariae*. *P. knowlesi* is also present in the Asia-Pacific region. Chloroquine is the drug of choice for the treatment of non-falciparum malaria (but chloroquine-resistant *P. vivax* has been reported in the Indonesian archipelago, the Malay Peninsula, including Myanmar, and eastward to Southern Vietnam).

For the treatment of chloroquine-resistant non-falciparum malaria, *Malarone*®[unlicensed indication], quinine, or *Riamet*®[unlicensed indication] can be used; as with chloroquine, primaquine p. 430 should be given for radical cure.

Chloroquine alone is adequate for *P. malariae* and *P. knowlesi* infections but in the case of *P. vivax* and *P. ovale*, a *radical cure* (to destroy parasites in the liver and thus prevent relapses) is required. This is achieved with primaquine [unlicensed] given after chloroquine.

For a radical cure, primaquine [unlicensed] is then given to children over 6 months of age; specialist advice should be sought for children under 6 months of age.

Parenteral

If the child is unable to take oral therapy, quinine can be given by intravenous infusion, changed to oral chloroquine as soon as the patient's condition permits.

Pregnancy
Treatment doses of chloroquine can be given for non-falciparum malaria. In the case of *P. vivax* or *P. ovale*, however, the radical cure with primaquine should be **postponed** until the pregnancy is over; instead chloroquine should be continued, given weekly, during the pregnancy.

ANTIPROTOZOALS › ANTIMALARIALS

Artemether with lumefantrine

28-May-2018

● **INDICATIONS AND DOSE**

Treatment of acute uncomplicated falciparum malaria | Treatment of chloroquine-resistant non-falciparum malaria

▶ BY MOUTH

▶ Child (body-weight 5–14 kg): Initially 1 tablet, followed by 1 tablet for 5 doses each given at 8, 24, 36, 48, and 60 hours (total 6 tablets over 60 hours)
▶ Child (body-weight 15–24 kg): Initially 2 tablets, followed by 2 tablets for 5 doses each given at 8, 24, 36, 48, and 60 hours (total 12 tablets over 60 hours)
▶ Child (body-weight 25–34 kg): Initially 3 tablets, followed by 3 tablets for 5 doses each given at 8, 24, 36, 48, and 60 hours (total 18 tablets over 60 hours)
▶ Child 12–17 years (body-weight 35 kg and above): Initially 4 tablets, followed by 4 tablets for 5 doses each given at 8, 24, 36, 48, and 60 hours (total 24 tablets over 60 hours)

● **UNLICENSED USE** Use in treatment of non-falciparum malaria is an unlicensed indication.

● **CONTRA-INDICATIONS** Family history of congenital QT interval prolongation · family history of sudden death · history of arrhythmias · history of clinically relevant bradycardia · history of congestive heart failure accompanied by reduced left ventricular ejection fraction

● **CAUTIONS** Avoid in Acute porphyrias p. 652 · electrolyte disturbances

● **INTERACTIONS** → Appendix 1: antimalarials

● **SIDE-EFFECTS**

▶ **Common or very common** Abdominal pain · appetite decreased · arthralgia · asthenia · cough · diarrhoea · dizziness · headache · myalgia · nausea · palpitations · QT interval prolongation · skin reactions · sleep disorders · vomiting
▶ **Uncommon** Clonus · drowsiness
▶ **Frequency not known** Angioedema

● **PREGNANCY** Toxicity in *animal* studies with artemether. Manufacturer advises use only if potential benefit outweighs risk.

● **BREAST FEEDING** Manufacturer advises avoid breastfeeding for at least 1 week after last dose. Present in milk in *animal* studies.

● **HEPATIC IMPAIRMENT** Manufacturer advises caution in severe impairment (no information available)—monitor ECG and plasma potassium concentration.

● **RENAL IMPAIRMENT** Manufacturer advises caution in severe impairment.
Monitoring In severe renal impairment monitor ECG and plasma potassium concentration.

● **MONITORING REQUIREMENTS** Monitor patients unable to take food (greater risk of recrudescence).

● **DIRECTIONS FOR ADMINISTRATION** Tablets may be crushed just before administration.

● **PATIENT AND CARER ADVICE**
Driving and skilled tasks Dizziness may affect performance of skilled tasks (e.g. driving).

● **MEDICINAL FORMS** There can be variation in the licensing of different medicines containing the same drug.

Tablet

CAUTIONARY AND ADVISORY LABELS 21

▶ Riamet (Novartis Pharmaceuticals UK Ltd)
Artemether 20 mg, Lumefantrine 120 mg Riamet tablets | 24 tablet [PoM] £22.50

Artenimol with piperaquine phosphate

18-Jun-2018

(Piperaquine tetraphosphate with dihydroartemisinin)

● **INDICATIONS AND DOSE**

Treatment of uncomplicated falciparum malaria

▶ BY MOUTH

▶ Child 6 months–17 years (body-weight 7–12 kg): 0.5 tablet once daily for 3 days, max. 2 courses in 12 months; second course given at least 2 months after first course
▶ Child 6 months–17 years (body-weight 13–23 kg): 1 tablet once daily for 3 days, max. 2 courses in 12 months; second course given at least 2 months after first course
▶ Child 6 months–17 years (body-weight 24–35 kg): 2 tablets once daily for 3 days, max. 2 courses in 12 months; second course given at least 2 months after first course
▶ Child 6 months–17 years (body-weight 36–74 kg): 3 tablets once daily for 3 days, max. 2 courses in 12 months; second course given at least 2 months after first course
▶ Child 6 months–17 years (body-weight 75–99 kg): 4 tablets once daily for 3 days, max. 2 courses in 12 months; second course given at least 2 months after first course

● **CONTRA-INDICATIONS** Acute myocardial infarction · bradycardia · congenital long QT syndrome · electrolyte disturbances · family history of sudden death · heart failure with reduced left ventricular ejection fraction · history of symptomatic arrhythmias · left ventricular hypertrophy · risk factors for QT interval prolongation · severe hypertension

● **INTERACTIONS** → Appendix 1: antimalarials

● **SIDE-EFFECTS**

▶ **Common or very common** Abdominal pain · anaemia · appetite decreased · asthenia · conjunctivitis · cough · diarrhoea · eosinophilia · fever · increased risk of infection · leucocytosis · leucopenia · neutropenia · QT interval prolongation · skin reactions · thrombocytopenia · vomiting
▶ **Uncommon** Arthralgia · cardiac conduction disorder · epistaxis · headache · hepatic disorders · hypochromia · lymphadenopathy · nausea · rhinorrhoea · seizure · splenomegaly · stomatitis · thrombocytosis

● **PREGNANCY** Teratogenic in *animal* studies—manufacturer advises use only if other antimalarials cannot be used.

● **BREAST FEEDING** Manufacturer advises avoid—present in milk in *animal* studies.

● **HEPATIC IMPAIRMENT** Manufacturer advises caution in jaundice or in moderate to severe failure (no information available)—monitor ECG and plasma potassium concentration.
Monitoring Manufacturer advises monitor ECG and plasma-potassium concentration in moderate to severe hepatic impairment.

● **RENAL IMPAIRMENT** No information available in moderate to severe impairment.
Monitoring Manufacturer advises monitor ECG and plasma-potassium concentration in moderate to severe renal impairment.

- **MONITORING REQUIREMENTS**
- ▶ Consider obtaining ECG in all patients before third dose and 4–6 hours after third dose. If QT_C interval more than 500 milliseconds, discontinue treatment and monitor ECG for a further 24–48 hours.
- ▶ Obtain ECG as soon as possible after starting treatment then continue monitoring in those taking medicines that increase plasma-piperaquine concentration, in children who are vomiting or in females.
- **DIRECTIONS FOR ADMINISTRATION** Tablets to be taken at least 3 hours before and at least 3 hours after food. Tablets may be crushed and mixed with water immediately before administration.
- **PATIENT AND CARER ADVICE** Patients or carers should be given advice on how to administer tablets containing piperaquine phosphate with artenimol.

- **MEDICINAL FORMS** There can be variation in the licensing of different medicines containing the same drug.

Tablet

▸ Eurartesim (Logixx Pharma Solutions Ltd)
Artenimol 40 mg, Piperaquine phosphate 320 mg Eurartesim 320mg/40mg tablets | 12 tablet [PoM] £40.00

Atovaquone with proguanil hydrochloride

28-May-2019

- **INDICATIONS AND DOSE**

MALARONE ® 250MG/100MG

Prophylaxis of falciparum malaria, particularly where resistance to other antimalarial drugs suspected

▶ BY MOUTH
- ▸ Child (body-weight 40 kg and above): 1 tablet once daily, to be started 1–2 days before entering endemic area and continued for 1 week after leaving

Treatment of acute uncomplicated falciparum malaria | Treatment of non-falciparum malaria

▶ BY MOUTH
- ▸ Child (body-weight 11–20 kg): 1 tablet once daily for 3 days
- ▸ Child (body-weight 21–30 kg): 2 tablets once daily for 3 days
- ▸ Child (body-weight 31–40 kg): 3 tablets once daily for 3 days
- ▸ Child (body-weight 41 kg and above): 4 tablets once daily for 3 days

DOSE EQUIVALENCE AND CONVERSION
- ▸ Each tablet of *Malarone*® contains 250 mg of atovaquone and 100 mg of proguanil hydrochloride.

MALARONE ® PAEDIATRIC

Prophylaxis of falciparum malaria, particularly where resistance to other antimalarial drugs suspected

▶ BY MOUTH
- ▸ Child (body-weight 5–7 kg): 0.5 tablet once daily, to be started 1–2 days before entering endemic area and continued for 1 week after leaving
- ▸ Child (body-weight 8–9 kg): 0.75 tablet once daily, to be started 1–2 days before entering endemic area and continued for 1 week after leaving
- ▸ Child (body-weight 10–19 kg): 1 tablet once daily, to be started 1–2 days before entering endemic area and continued for 1 week after leaving
- ▸ Child (body-weight 20–29 kg): 2 tablets once daily, to be started 1–2 days before entering endemic area and continued for 1 week after leaving
- ▸ Child (body-weight 30–39 kg): 3 tablets once daily, to be started 1–2 days before entering endemic area and continued for 1 week after leaving
- ▸ Child (body-weight 40 kg and above): Use *Malarone*® (standard) tablets.

Treatment of acute uncomplicated falciparum malaria | Treatment of non-falciparum malaria

▶ BY MOUTH
- ▸ Child (body-weight 5–8 kg): 2 tablets once daily for 3 days
- ▸ Child (body-weight 9–10 kg): 3 tablets once daily for 3 days
- ▸ Child (body-weight 11 kg and above): Use *Malarone*® (standard) tablets.

DOSE EQUIVALENCE AND CONVERSION
- ▸ Each tablet of *Malarone*® paediatric contains 62.5 mg atovaquone and 25 mg proguanil hydrochloride.

- **UNLICENSED USE** Not licensed for treatment of non-falciparum malaria. Not licensed for prophylaxis of malaria in children under 11 kg.

  Dosing for prophylaxis of malaria differs from product literature and adheres to Public Health England guidelines.
- **CAUTIONS** Diarrhoea or vomiting (reduced absorption of atovaquone) · efficacy not evaluated in cerebral or complicated malaria (including hyperparasitaemia, pulmonary oedema or renal failure)
- **INTERACTIONS** → Appendix 1: antimalarials
- **SIDE-EFFECTS**
- ▶ **Common or very common** Abdominal pain · appetite decreased · cough · depression · diarrhoea · dizziness · fever · headache · nausea · skin reactions · sleep disorders · vomiting
- ▶ **Uncommon** Alopecia · anxiety · blood disorder · hyponatraemia · oral disorders · palpitations
- ▶ **Frequency not known** Hallucination · hepatic disorders · photosensitivity reaction · seizure · Stevens-Johnson syndrome · tachycardia · vasculitis
- **PREGNANCY** Manufacturer advises use only if potential benefit outweighs risk. See also *Pregnancy* in Malaria, prophylaxis p. 420.
- **BREAST FEEDING** Use only if no suitable alternative available.
- **RENAL IMPAIRMENT** Avoid for malaria prophylaxis and, if possible, for treatment if estimated glomerular filtration rate less than 30 mL/minute/1.73 m^2.
- **DIRECTIONS FOR ADMINISTRATION**

  MALARONE ® PAEDIATRIC Tablets may be crushed and mixed with food or milky drink just before administration.
- **PATIENT AND CARER ADVICE** Warn travellers about **importance** of avoiding mosquito bites, **importance** of taking prophylaxis regularly, and **importance** of immediate visit to doctor if ill within 1 year and **especially** within 3 months of return.

  Medicines for Children leaflet: Malarone for prevention of malaria www.medicinesforchildren.org.uk/malarone-prevention-malaria
- **NATIONAL FUNDING/ACCESS DECISIONS**

  NHS restrictions Drugs for malaria prophylaxis are not prescribable in NHS primary care; health authorities may investigate circumstances under which antimalarials are prescribed.

- **MEDICINAL FORMS** There can be variation in the licensing of different medicines containing the same drug.

Tablet

CAUTIONARY AND ADVISORY LABELS 21

▸ Malarone (GlaxoSmithKline UK Ltd)
Proguanil hydrochloride 25 mg, Atovaquone 62.5 mg Malarone Paediatric 62.5mg/25mg tablets | 12 tablet [PoM] £6.26 DT = £6.26
Proguanil hydrochloride 100 mg, Atovaquone 250 mg Malarone 250mg/100mg tablets | 12 tablet [PoM] £25.21 DT = £31.69

Chloroquine

11-May-2020

● **INDICATIONS AND DOSE**

Prophylaxis of malaria

▶ INITIALLY BY MOUTH USING SYRUP

▸ Child 4–5 weeks (body-weight up to 4.5 kg): 25 mg once weekly, started 1 week before entering endemic area and continued for 4 weeks after leaving

▸ Child 6 weeks–5 months (body-weight 4.5–7 kg): 50 mg once weekly, started 1 week before entering endemic area and continued for 4 weeks after leaving

▸ Child 6–11 months (body-weight 8–10 kg): 75 mg once weekly, started 1 week before entering endemic area and continued for 4 weeks after leaving

▸ Child 1–2 years (body-weight 11–14 kg): 100 mg once weekly, started 1 week before entering endemic area and continued for 4 weeks after leaving

▸ Child 3–4 years (body-weight 15–16.4 kg): 125 mg once weekly, started 1 week before entering endemic area and continued for 4 weeks after leaving

▸ Child 5–7 years (body-weight 16.5–24 kg): 150 mg once weekly, alternatively (by mouth using tablets) 155 mg once weekly, started 1 week before entering endemic area and continued for 4 weeks after leaving

▸ Child 8–13 years (body-weight 25–44 kg): 225 mg once weekly, alternatively (by mouth using tablets) 232.5 mg once weekly, started 1 week before entering endemic area and continued for 4 weeks after leaving

▶ INITIALLY BY MOUTH USING TABLETS

▸ Child 14–17 years (body-weight 45 kg and above): 310 mg once weekly, alternatively (by mouth using syrup) 300 mg once weekly, started 1 week before entering endemic area and continued for 4 weeks after leaving

Treatment of non-falciparum malaria

▶ BY MOUTH

▸ Child: Initially 10 mg/kg (max. per dose 620 mg), then 5 mg/kg after 6–8 hours (max. per dose 310 mg), then 5 mg/kg daily (max. per dose 310 mg) for 2 days

***P. vivax* or *P. ovale* infection during pregnancy while radical cure is postponed**

▶ BY MOUTH

▸ Child: 10 mg/kg once weekly (max. per dose 310 mg)

DOSE EQUIVALENCE AND CONVERSION

▸ Doses expressed as chloroquine base.

▸ Each tablet contains 155 mg of chloroquine base (equivalent to 250 mg of chloroquine phosphate). Syrup contains 50 mg/5 mL of chloroquine base (equivalent to 80 mg/5 mL of chloroquine phosphate).

● **UNLICENSED USE** Chloroquine doses for the treatment and prophylaxis of malaria in BNF publications may differ from those in product literature.

● **CAUTIONS** Acute porphyrias p. 652 · diabetes (may lower blood glucose) · G6PD deficiency · long-term therapy (risk of retinopathy and cardiomyopathy) · may aggravate myasthenia gravis · may exacerbate psoriasis · neurological disorders, especially epilepsy (may lower seizure threshold)—avoid for prophylaxis of malaria if history of epilepsy · severe gastro-intestinal disorders

● **INTERACTIONS** → Appendix 1: antimalarials

● **SIDE-EFFECTS**

▶ **Rare or very rare** Cardiomyopathy · hallucination · hepatitis

▶ **Frequency not known** Abdominal pain · agranulocytosis · alopecia · anxiety · atrioventricular block · bone marrow disorders · confusion · corneal deposits · depression · diarrhoea · eye disorders · gastrointestinal disorder · headache · hearing impairment · hypoglycaemia · hypotension · insomnia · interstitial lung disease · movement disorders · myopathy · nausea · neuromyopathy · neutropenia · personality change · photosensitivity reaction · psychotic disorder · QT interval prolongation · seizure · severe cutaneous adverse reactions (SCARs) · skin reactions · thrombocytopenia · tinnitus · tongue protrusion · vision disorders · vomiting

SIDE-EFFECTS, FURTHER INFORMATION Side-effects which occur at doses used in the prophylaxis or treatment of malaria are generally not serious.

Overdose Chloroquine is very toxic in overdosage; overdosage is extremely hazardous and difficult to treat. Urgent advice from the National Poisons Information Service is essential. Life-threatening features include arrhythmias (which can have a very rapid onset) and convulsions (which can be intractable).

● **PREGNANCY** Benefit of use in prophylaxis and treatment in malaria outweighs risk. For rheumatoid disease, it is not necessary to withdraw an antimalarial drug during pregnancy if the disease is well controlled.

● **BREAST FEEDING** Present in breast milk and breast-feeding should be avoided when used to treat rheumatic disease. Amount in milk probably too small to be harmful when used for malaria.

● **HEPATIC IMPAIRMENT** Manufacturer advises caution, particularly in cirrhosis.

● **RENAL IMPAIRMENT** Manufacturers advise caution.

Dose adjustments Only partially excreted by the kidneys and reduction of the dose is not required for prophylaxis of malaria except in severe impairment.

For rheumatoid arthritis and lupus erythematosus, reduce dose.

● **MONITORING REQUIREMENTS** Expert sources advise ophthalmic examination with long-term therapy.

● **PATIENT AND CARER ADVICE** Warn travellers going to malarious areas about **importance** of avoiding mosquito bites, **importance** of taking prophylaxis regularly, and **importance** of immediate visit to doctor if ill within 1 year and **especially** within 3 months of return.

● **NATIONAL FUNDING/ACCESS DECISIONS**

NHS restrictions Drugs for malaria prophylaxis are not prescribable in NHS primary care; health authorities may investigate circumstances under which antimalarials are prescribed.

● **EXCEPTIONS TO LEGAL CATEGORY** *Tablets* can be sold to the public provided it is licensed and labelled for the prophylaxis of malaria.

● **MEDICINAL FORMS** There can be variation in the licensing of different medicines containing the same drug. Forms available from special-order manufacturers include: oral solution

Oral solution

CAUTIONARY AND ADVISORY LABELS 5

▸ **Malarivon** (Wallace Manufacturing Chemists Ltd)

Chloroquine phosphate 16 mg per 1 ml Malarivon 80mg/5ml syrup | 75 ml [PoM] £30.00 DT = £30.00

Tablet

CAUTIONARY AND ADVISORY LABELS 5

▸ **Avloclor** (Alliance Pharmaceuticals Ltd)

Chloroquine phosphate 250 mg Avloclor 250mg tablets | 20 tablet [P] £8.59 DT = £8.59

Chloroquine with proguanil

The properties listed below are those particular to the combination only. For the properties of the components please consider, chloroquine above, proguanil hydrochloride p. 431.

● **INDICATIONS AND DOSE**

Prophylaxis of malaria

▶ BY MOUTH

▸ Child: (consult product literature)

- **INTERACTIONS** → Appendix 1: antimalarials
- **EXCEPTIONS TO LEGAL CATEGORY** Can be sold to the public provided it is licensed and labelled for the prophylaxis of malaria.

- **MEDICINAL FORMS** There can be variation in the licensing of different medicines containing the same drug.

Form unstated

- Paludrine/Avloclor (Alliance Pharmaceuticals Ltd)
  Paludrine/Avloclor tablets anti-malarial travel pack | 112 tablet [P] £13.50

Mefloquine

05-Aug-2018

- **INDICATIONS AND DOSE**

Treatment of malaria

- BY MOUTH
- Child: (consult product literature)

Prophylaxis of malaria

- BY MOUTH
- Child (body-weight 5-15 kg): 62.5 mg once weekly, dose to be started 2–3 weeks before entering endemic area and continued for 4 weeks after leaving
- Child (body-weight 16-24 kg): 125 mg once weekly, dose to be started 2–3 weeks before entering endemic area and continued for 4 weeks after leaving
- Child (body-weight 25-44 kg): 187.5 mg once weekly, dose to be started 2–3 weeks before entering endemic area and continued for 4 weeks after leaving
- Child (body-weight 45 kg and above): 250 mg once weekly, dose to be started 2–3 weeks before entering endemic area and continued for 4 weeks after leaving

- **UNLICENSED USE** Mefloquine doses in BNF Publications may differ from those in product literature.
  Not licensed for use in children under 5 kg body-weight and under 3 months.
- **CONTRA-INDICATIONS** Avoid for prophylaxis if history of psychiatric disorders (including depression) or convulsions · avoid for standby treatment if history of convulsions · history of blackwater fever
- **CAUTIONS** Cardiac conduction disorders · epilepsy (avoid for prophylaxis) · not recommended in infants under 3 months (5 kg) · traumatic brain injury

CAUTIONS, FURTHER INFORMATION

- Neuropsychiatric reactions Mefloquine is associated with potentially serious neuropsychiatric reactions. Abnormal dreams, insomnia, anxiety, and depression occur commonly. Psychosis, suicidal ideation, and suicide have also been reported. Psychiatric symptoms such as insomnia, nightmares, acute anxiety, depression, restlessness, or confusion should be regarded as potentially prodromal for a more serious event. Adverse reactions may occur and persist up to several months after discontinuation because mefloquine has a long half-life. For a prescribing checklist, and further information on side-effects, particularly neuropsychiatric side-effects, which may be associated with the use of mefloquine for malaria prophylaxis, see the *Guide for Healthcare Professionals* provided by the manufacturer.

- **INTERACTIONS** → Appendix 1: antimalarials
- **SIDE-EFFECTS**
- **Common or very common** Anxiety · depression · diarrhoea · dizziness · gastrointestinal discomfort · headache · nausea · skin reactions · sleep disorders · vision disorders · vomiting
- **Frequency not known** Acute kidney injury · agranulocytosis · alopecia · aplastic anaemia · appetite decreased · arrhythmias · arthralgia · asthenia · behaviour abnormal · cardiac conduction disorders · cataract · chest pain · chills · concentration impaired · confusion · cranial nerve paralysis · delusional disorder · depersonalisation · drowsiness · dyspnoea · encephalopathy · eye disorder · fever · flushing · gait abnormal · hallucination · hearing impairment · hepatic disorders · hyperacusia · hyperhidrosis · hypertension · hypotension · leucocytosis · leucopenia · malaise · memory loss · mood altered · movement disorders · muscle complaints · muscle weakness · nephritis · nerve disorders · oedema · palpitations · pancreatitis · paraesthesia · pneumonia · pneumonitis · psychosis · seizure · self-endangering behaviour · speech disorder · Stevens-Johnson syndrome · suicidal tendencies · syncope · thrombocytopenia · tinnitus · tremor · vertigo

- **ALLERGY AND CROSS-SENSITIVITY** Contra-indicated in patients with hypersensitivity to quinine.
- **CONCEPTION AND CONTRACEPTION** Manufacturer advises adequate contraception during prophylaxis and for 3 months after stopping (teratogenicity in *animal* studies).
- **PREGNANCY** Manufacturer advises avoid (particularly in the first trimester) unless the potential benefit outweighs the risk; however, studies of mefloquine in pregnancy (including use in the first trimester) indicate that it can be considered for travel to chloroquine-resistant areas.
- **BREAST FEEDING** Present in milk but risk to infant minimal.
- **HEPATIC IMPAIRMENT** Manufacturer advises avoid in severe impairment—elimination may be prolonged.
- **RENAL IMPAIRMENT** Manufacturer advises caution.
- **DIRECTIONS FOR ADMINISTRATION** Tablet may be crushed and mixed with food such as jam or honey just before administration.
- **PATIENT AND CARER ADVICE** Manufacturer advises that patients receiving mefloquine for malaria prophylaxis should be informed to discontinue its use if neuropsychiatric symptoms occur and seek immediate medical advice so that mefloquine can be replaced with an alternative antimalarial. Travellers should also be warned about **importance** of avoiding mosquito bites, **importance** of taking prophylaxis regularly, and **importance** of immediate visit to doctor if ill within 1 year and especially within 3 months of return.
  A patient alert card should be provided.
  Driving and skilled tasks Dizziness or a disturbed sense of balance may affect performance of skilled tasks (e.g. driving); effects may occur and persist up to several months after stopping mefloquine.
- **NATIONAL FUNDING/ACCESS DECISIONS**
  NHS restrictions Drugs for malaria prophylaxis are not prescribable in NHS primary care; health authorities may investigate circumstances under which antimalarials are prescribed.

- **MEDICINAL FORMS** There can be variation in the licensing of different medicines containing the same drug.

Tablet

CAUTIONARY AND ADVISORY LABELS 10, 21, 27

- Lariam (Cheplapharm Arzneimittel GmbH)
  Mefloquine (as Mefloquine hydrochloride) 250 mg Lariam 250mg tablets | 8 tablet [PoM] £14.53 DT = £14.53

Primaquine

- **INDICATIONS AND DOSE**

Adjunct in the treatment of non-falciparum malaria caused by *P. vivax* infection

- BY MOUTH
- Child 6 months–17 years: 500 micrograms/kg daily (max. per dose 30 mg) for 14 days

Adjunct in the treatment of non-falciparum malaria caused by *P. ovale* infection

- ▶ BY MOUTH
  - ▸ Child 6 months–17 years: 250 micrograms/kg daily (max. per dose 15 mg) for 14 days

Adjunct in the treatment of non-falciparum malaria caused by *P. vivax* infection in patients with mild G6PD deficiency (administered on expert advice) | Adjunct in the treatment of non-falciparum malaria caused by *P. ovale* infection in patients with mild G6PD deficiency (administered on expert advice)

- ▶ BY MOUTH
  - ▸ Child: 750 micrograms/kg once weekly for 8 weeks; maximum 45 mg per week

Treatment of mild to moderate pneumocystis infection (in combination with clindamycin)

- ▶ BY MOUTH
  - ▸ Child: This combination is associated with considerable toxicity (consult product literature)

- **UNLICENSED USE** Not licensed.
- **CAUTIONS** G6PD deficiency · systemic diseases associated with granulocytopenia (e.g. juvenile idiopathic arthritis, rheumatoid arthritis, lupus erythematosus)
- **INTERACTIONS** → Appendix 1: antimalarials
- **SIDE-EFFECTS** Arrhythmia · dizziness · gastrointestinal discomfort · haemolytic anaemia (in G6PD deficiency) · leucopenia · methaemoglobinaemia (in NADH methaemoglobin reductase deficiency) · nausea · QT interval prolongation · skin reactions · vomiting
- **PREGNANCY** Risk of neonatal haemolysis and methaemoglobinaemia in third trimester.
- **BREAST FEEDING** No information available; theoretical risk of haemolysis in G6PD-deficient infants.
- **PRE-TREATMENT SCREENING** Before starting primaquine, blood should be tested for glucose-6-phosphate dehydrogenase (G6PD) activity since the drug can cause haemolysis in G6PD-deficient patients. Specialist advice should be obtained in G6PD deficiency.

- **MEDICINAL FORMS** There can be variation in the licensing of different medicines containing the same drug. Forms available from special-order manufacturers include: oral suspension

Tablet

- ▸ Primaquine (Non-proprietary)
  Primaquine (as Primaquine phosphate) 7.5 mg Primaquine 7.5mg tablets | 100 tablet £199.70
  Primaquine (as Primaquine phosphate) 15 mg Primaquine 15mg tablets | 100 tablet [PoM] [CD-exempt symbol]

Proguanil hydrochloride

03-Aug-2018

- **INDICATIONS AND DOSE**

Prophylaxis of malaria

- ▶ BY MOUTH
  - ▸ Child 4–11 weeks (body-weight up to 6 kg): 25 mg once daily, dose to be started 1 week before entering endemic area and continued for 4 weeks after leaving
  - ▸ Child 3–11 months (body-weight 6–9 kg): 50 mg once daily, dose to be started 1 week before entering endemic area and continued for 4 weeks after leaving
  - ▸ Child 1–3 years (body-weight 10–15 kg): 75 mg once daily, dose to be started 1 week before entering endemic area and continued for 4 weeks after leaving
  - ▸ Child 4–7 years (body-weight 16–24 kg): 100 mg once daily, dose to be started 1 week before entering endemic area and continued for 4 weeks after leaving
  - ▸ Child 8–12 years (body-weight 25–44 kg): 150 mg once daily, dose to be started 1 week before entering endemic area and continued for 4 weeks after leaving
  - ▸ Child 13–17 years (body-weight 45 kg and above): 200 mg once daily, dose to be started 1 week before entering endemic area and continued for 4 weeks after leaving

- **UNLICENSED USE** Proguanil doses in BNF Publications may differ from those in product literature.
- **INTERACTIONS** → Appendix 1: antimalarials
- **SIDE-EFFECTS** Alopecia · angioedema · bone marrow disorders · cholestasis · constipation · diarrhoea · fever · gastric disorder · megaloblastic anaemia · oral disorders · skin reactions · vasculitis
- **PREGNANCY** Benefit of prophylaxis in malaria outweighs risk. Adequate folate supplements should be given to mother.
- **BREAST FEEDING** Amount in milk probably too small to be harmful when used for malaria prophylaxis.
- **RENAL IMPAIRMENT**
  Dose adjustments Use half normal dose if estimated glomerular filtration rate 20–60 mL/minute/1.73m^2.
  Use one-quarter normal dose on alternate days if estimated glomerular filtration rate 10–20 mL/minute/1.73m^2.
  Use one-quarter normal dose once weekly if estimated glomerular filtration rate less than 10 mL/minute/1.73m^2; increased risk of haematological toxicity in severe impairment.
- **DIRECTIONS FOR ADMINISTRATION** Tablet may be crushed and mixed with food such as milk, jam, or honey just before administration.
- **PATIENT AND CARER ADVICE** Warn travellers about **importance** of avoiding mosquito bites, **importance** of taking prophylaxis regularly, and **importance** of immediate visit to doctor if ill within 1 year and **especially** within 3 months of return.
- **NATIONAL FUNDING/ACCESS DECISIONS**
  NHS restrictions Drugs for malaria prophylaxis are not prescribable in NHS primary care; health authorities may investigate circumstances under which antimalarials are prescribed.
- **EXCEPTIONS TO LEGAL CATEGORY** Can be sold to the public provided it is licensed and labelled for the prophylaxis of malaria.

- **MEDICINAL FORMS** There can be variation in the licensing of different medicines containing the same drug. Forms available from special-order manufacturers include: oral suspension, oral solution

Tablet

CAUTIONARY AND ADVISORY LABELS 21

- ▸ Paludrine (Alliance Pharmaceuticals Ltd)
  Proguanil hydrochloride 100 mg Paludrine 100mg tablets | 98 tablet [P] £11.95 DT = £11.95

Pyrimethamine

- **INDICATIONS AND DOSE**

Toxoplasmosis in pregnancy (in combination with sulfadiazine and folinic acid)

- ▶ BY MOUTH
  - ▸ Child 12–17 years: 50 mg once daily until delivery

Congenital toxoplasmosis (in combination with sulfadiazine and folinic acid)

- ▶ BY MOUTH
  - ▸ Neonate: 1 mg/kg twice daily for 2 days, then 1 mg/kg once daily for 6 months, then 1 mg/kg 3 times a week for 6 months.

- **UNLICENSED USE** Not licensed for use in children under 5 years.

- **CAUTIONS** History of seizures—avoid large loading doses · predisposition to folate deficiency
- **INTERACTIONS** → Appendix 1: antimalarials
- **SIDE-EFFECTS**
- ▶ **Common or very common** Anaemia · diarrhoea · dizziness · headache · leucopenia · nausea · skin reactions · thrombocytopenia · vomiting
- ▶ **Uncommon** Fever
- ▶ **Rare or very rare** Abdominal pain · oral ulceration · pancytopenia · pneumonia eosinophilic · seizure
- **PREGNANCY** Theoretical teratogenic risk in *first trimester* (folate antagonist). Adequate folate supplements should be given to the mother.
- **BREAST FEEDING** Significant amount in milk—avoid administration of other folate antagonists to infant. Avoid breast-feeding during toxoplasmosis treatment.
- **HEPATIC IMPAIRMENT** Manufacturer advises caution.
- **RENAL IMPAIRMENT** Manufacturer advises caution.
- **MONITORING REQUIREMENTS** Blood counts required with prolonged treatment.

- **MEDICINAL FORMS** There can be variation in the licensing of different medicines containing the same drug. Forms available from special-order manufacturers include: oral suspension

Tablet

▶ Daraprim (GlaxoSmithKline UK Ltd)

Pyrimethamine 25 mg Daraprim 25mg tablets | 30 tablet PoM £13.00

Quinine

04-Dec-2017

- **INDICATIONS AND DOSE**

Non-falciparum malaria

▶ BY INTRAVENOUS INFUSION

▶ Child: 10 mg/kg every 8 hours (max. per dose 700 mg), infused over 4 hours, given if patient is unable to take oral therapy. Change to oral chloroquine as soon as the patient's condition permits, reduce dose to 5–7 mg/kg if parenteral treatment is required for more than 48 hours

Falciparum malaria

▶ BY MOUTH

▶ Child: 10 mg/kg every 8 hours (max. per dose 600 mg) for 7 days, to be given together with or followed by either doxycycline (in children over 12 years), or clindamycin

▶ BY INTRAVENOUS INFUSION

▶ Neonate: Loading dose 20 mg/kg, infused over 4 hours, the loading dose of 20 mg/kg should **not** be used if the patient has received quinine or mefloquine during the previous 12 hours, then maintenance 10 mg/kg every 8 hours until patient can swallow oral medication to complete the 7-day course, maintenance dose to be given 8 hours after the start of the loading dose and infused over 4 hours, to be given together with or followed by clindamycin, reduce maintenance dose to 5–7 mg/kg if parenteral treatment is required for more than 48 hours.

▶ Child: Loading dose 20 mg/kg (max. per dose 1.4 g), infused over 4 hours, the loading dose of 20 mg/kg should **not** be used if the patient has received quinine or mefloquine during the previous 12 hours, then maintenance 10 mg/kg every 8 hours (max. per dose 700 mg) until patient can swallow tablets to complete the 7-day course, maintenance dose to be given 8 hours after the start of the loading dose and infused over 4 hours, to be given together with or followed by either doxycycline (in children over 12 years), or clindamycin, reduce maintenance dose to 5–7 mg/kg if parenteral treatment is required for more than 48 hours

Falciparum malaria (in intensive care unit)

▶ BY INTRAVENOUS INFUSION

▶ Neonate: Loading dose 7 mg/kg, infused over 30 minutes, followed immediately by 10 mg/kg, infused over 4 hours, then maintenance 10 mg/kg every 8 hours until patient can swallow oral medication to complete the 7-day course, maintenance dose to be given 8 hours after the start of the loading dose and infused over 4 hours, to be given together with or followed by clindamycin, reduce maintenance dose to 5–7 mg/kg if parenteral treatment is required for more than 48 hours.

▶ Child: Loading dose 7 mg/kg, infused over 30 minutes, followed immediately by 10 mg/kg, infused over 4 hours, then maintenance 10 mg/kg every 8 hours (max. per dose 700 mg) until patient can swallow tablets to complete the 7-day course, maintenance dose to be given 8 hours after the start of the loading dose and infused over 4 hours, to be given together with or followed by either doxycycline (in children over 12 years), or clindamycin, reduce maintenance dose to 5–7 mg/kg if parenteral treatment is required for more than 48 hours

DOSE EQUIVALENCE AND CONVERSION

- ▶ When using quinine for malaria, doses are valid for quinine hydrochloride, dihydrochloride, and sulfate; they are **not valid** for quinine bisulfate which contains a correspondingly smaller amount of quinine.
- ▶ Quinine (anhydrous base) 100 mg = quinine bisulfate 169 mg; quinine dihydrochloride 122 mg; quinine hydrochloride 122 mg; and quinine sulfate 121 mg. Quinine bisulfate 300 mg tablets are available but provide less quinine than 300 mg of the dihydrochloride, hydrochloride, or sulfate.

- **UNLICENSED USE** Injection not licensed.

IMPORTANT SAFETY INFORMATION

MHRA/CHM ADVICE: REMINDER OF DOSE-DEPENDENT QT-PROLONGING EFFECTS (NOVEMBER 2017)

Quinine has been associated with dose-dependent QT-interval-prolonging effects and should be used with caution in patients with risk factors for QT prolongation or in those with atrioventricular block—see Cautions for further information.

- **CONTRA-INDICATIONS** Haemoglobinuria · myasthenia gravis · optic neuritis · tinnitus
- **CAUTIONS** Atrial fibrillation (monitor ECG during parenteral treatment) · cardiac disease (monitor ECG during parenteral treatment) · conduction defects (monitor ECG during parenteral treatment) · electrolyte disturbance · G6PD deficiency · heart block (monitor ECG during parenteral treatment)
- **INTERACTIONS** → Appendix 1: antimalarials
- **SIDE-EFFECTS** Abdominal pain · agitation · agranulocytosis · angioedema · asthma · atrioventricular conduction changes · bronchospasm · cardiotoxicity · cerebral impairment · coagulation disorders · coma · confusion · death · diarrhoea · dyspnoea · fever · flushing · gastrointestinal disorder · haemoglobinuria · haemolysis · haemolytic uraemic syndrome · headache · hearing impairment · hypersensitivity · loss of consciousness · muscle weakness · myasthenia gravis aggravated · nausea · ocular toxicity · oedema · pancytopenia · photosensitivity reaction · QT interval prolongation · renal impairment · skin reactions · thrombocytopenia · tinnitus · vertigo · vision disorders · vomiting

Overdose Quinine is very toxic in overdosage; life-threatening features include arrhythmias (which can have a very rapid onset) and convulsions (which can be intractable).

For details on the management of poisoning, see Emergency treatment of poisoning p. 891.

- **PREGNANCY** High doses are teratogenic in *first trimester*, but in malaria benefit of treatment outweighs risk.
- **BREAST FEEDING** Present in milk but not known to be harmful.
- **HEPATIC IMPAIRMENT**
  - ▶ With oral use Manufacturer advises caution (risk of prolonged half-life).

  Dose adjustments ▶ With intravenous use For treatment of malaria in severe impairment, reduce parenteral maintenance dose to 5–7 mg/kg of quinine salt.

  ▶ With oral use Manufacturer advises dose reduction or increased dose interval.
- **RENAL IMPAIRMENT**

  Dose adjustments ▶ With intravenous use For treatment of malaria in severe impairment, reduce parenteral maintenance dose to 5–7 mg/kg of quinine salt.
- **MONITORING REQUIREMENTS**
  - ▶ With intravenous use Monitor blood glucose and electrolyte concentration during parenteral treatment.
- **DIRECTIONS FOR ADMINISTRATION**
  - ▶ With intravenous use For *intravenous infusion*, dilute to a concentration of 2 mg/mL (max. 30 mg/mL in fluid restriction) with Glucose 5% *or* Sodium Chloride 0.9% and give over 4 hours.
- **PRESCRIBING AND DISPENSING INFORMATION**
  - ▶ With intravenous use Intravenous injection of quinine is so hazardous that it has been superseded by infusion.

- **MEDICINAL FORMS** There can be variation in the licensing of different medicines containing the same drug. Forms available from special-order manufacturers include: capsule, oral suspension, oral solution, solution for infusion

Tablet

▶ Quinine (Non-proprietary)

Quinine sulfate 200 mg Quinine sulfate 200mg tablets | 28 tablet PoM £4.65 DT = £2.25

Quinine bisulfate 300 mg Quinine bisulfate 300mg tablets | 28 tablet PoM £5.50 DT = £4.55

Quinine sulfate 300 mg Quinine sulfate 300mg tablets | 28 tablet PoM £9.09 DT = £5.33

4.3 Toxoplasmosis

Other drugs used for Toxoplasmosis Pyrimethamine, p. 431

ANTIBACTERIALS › MACROLIDES

Spiramycin

20-Apr-2020

- **INDICATIONS AND DOSE**

Toxoplasmosis in pregnancy

▶ BY MOUTH

▶ Child 12-17 years: 1.5 g twice daily until delivery

Chemoprophylaxis of congenital toxoplasmosis

▶ BY MOUTH

▶ Neonate: 50 mg/kg twice daily.

DOSE EQUIVALENCE AND CONVERSION

▶ 3000 units ≡ 1 mg spiramycin.

- **UNLICENSED USE** Not licensed.
- **CAUTIONS** Arrhythmias · cardiac disease · G6PD deficiency · predisposition to QT interval prolongation
- **SIDE-EFFECTS**
  - ▶ **Rare or very rare** Vasculitis
  - ▶ **Frequency not known** Angioedema · diarrhoea · haemolysis · nausea · paraesthesia · pseudomembranous enterocolitis · skin reactions · vomiting
- **ALLERGY AND CROSS-SENSITIVITY** Sensitivity to other macrolides.
- **BREAST FEEDING** Present in breast milk.
- **HEPATIC IMPAIRMENT** Manufacturer advises caution.
- **MEDICINAL FORMS** There can be variation in the licensing of different medicines containing the same drug.

Tablet

▶ Rovamycine (Imported (France))

Spiramycin 1.5 mega unit Rovamycine 1.5million unit tablets | 16 tablet PoM

Spiramycin 3 mega unit Rovamycine 3million unit tablets | 10 tablet PoM

5 Viral infection

5.1 Coronavirus

COVID-19

06-May-2020

Description of condition

COVID-19 is the syndrome caused by a novel coronavirus, SARS-CoV-2, which was originally detected late 2019 in Wuhan, Hubei Province, China. Primary transmission between people is through respiratory droplets generated by coughing and sneezing, and through contact with contaminated surfaces.

COVID-19 is predominantly a respiratory illness with early non-specific symptoms that can last 2–10 days before more specific signs or symptoms develop. The most common symptoms are fever, cough, and shortness of breath. Other symptoms, such as anxiety, delirium, agitation, fatigue, muscle aches, headache, and a loss of sense of smell may also be present. The illness varies in severity from no symptoms present in some individuals to severe pneumonia in others. Children with co-morbidities (such as cystic fibrosis, asthma, cardiovascular disease, and diabetes), frailty, impaired immunity, or a reduced ability to cough and clear secretions are more likely to develop severe pneumonia. Children with severe symptoms of COVID-19 may deteriorate rapidly.

Management

Medical practitioners must notify the Proper Officer at their local council or local health protection team of all suspected cases of COVID-19. For further information, see *Notifiable diseases* in Antibacterials, principles of therapy p. 318.

NICE have developed rapid guidelines to maximise patient safety, optimise treatment management, protect staff from infection, and make the best use of NHS resources. These guidelines provide recommendations around the provision of care during the pandemic (such as systemic anticancer treatments) and managing symptoms (including at the end of life). They also include recommendations for patients with conditions that increase the risk of developing COVID-19 (such as in immunocompromised patients, those with severe asthma; cystic fibrosis; rheumatological autoimmune, inflammatory and metabolic bone disorders; or conditions treated with drugs that affect the immune response). NICE are also developing rapid evidence summaries focusing on whether certain medications (such as non-steroidal anti-inflammatory drugs) may increase the severity/length of the COVID-19 illness, and advice on the safety and efficacy of COVID-19 treatments. For further information, see NICE rapid guidelines and evidence summaries: **Coronavirus (COVID-19)**(see *Useful resources*).

NHS England and NHS Improvement have produced guidance for clinicians and NHS managers working in primary and secondary care, and community-based health, social care, mental health trusts and ambulance services. For further information, see NHS England: **Coronavirus guidance for clinicians and NHS managers** (see *Useful resources*).

PHE have also produced guidance for health professionals, the public, and non-clinical settings; on infection prevention and control; and sampling and diagnostics. For further information, see the PHE collection: **Coronavirus (COVID-19): guidance** (see *Useful resources*).

The MHRA have issued COVID-19 guidance for industry, in addition to information about medications and COVID-19, and guidance on medical devices (such as COVID-19 tests and testing kits). For further information, see the MHRA collection: **MHRA guidance on coronavirus (COVID-19)** (see *Useful resources*).

The UKTIS have produced an information page summarising the fetal and neonatal risks of exposure to COVID-19 treatments that have either been identified as possible options or listed as investigational medicinal products. For further information, see UKTIS: **Medications used to treat COVID-19 in pregnancy** (see *Useful resources*).

The Joint Committee on Vaccination and Immunisation have issued a statement on immunisation prioritisation during the COVID-19 pandemic (available at: www.gov.uk/government/publications/jcvi-statement-on-immunisation-prioritisation/statement-from-jcvi-on-immunisation-prioritisation).

Additional country-specific guidance is available for Northern Ireland, Scotland, and Wales (see *Useful resources*).

Useful Resources

Medicines and Healthcare products Regulatory Agency (MHRA). MHRA guidance on coronavirus (COVID-19) collection.
www.gov.uk/government/collections/mhra-guidance-on-coronavirus-covid-19

National Health Service England (NHSE) and National Health Service Improvement (NHSI). Coronavirus guidance for clinicians and NHS managers.
www.england.nhs.uk/coronavirus/

National Institute for Health and Care Excellence (NICE). Coronavirus (COVID-19) rapid guidelines and evidence summaries.
www.nice.org.uk/covid-19

Public Health England (PHE). Coronavirus (COVID-19) collection.
www.gov.uk/government/collections/coronavirus-covid-19-list-of-guidance

UK Teratology Information Service (UKTIS). Medications used to treat COVID-19 in pregnancy.
www.medicinesinpregnancy.org/bumps/monographs/MEDICATIONS-USED-TO-TREAT-COVID-19-IN-PREGNANCY/

Northern Ireland Government Services. Coronavirus (COVID-19).
www.nidirect.gov.uk/campaigns/coronavirus-covid-19

Public Health Agency in Northern Ireland. Coronavirus (COVID-19).
www.publichealth.hscni.net/news/covid-19-coronavirus

Scottish Government. Coronavirus in Scotland.
www.gov.scot/coronavirus-covid-19/

Health Protection Scotland. Coronavirus (COVID-19).
www.hps.scot.nhs.uk/a-to-z-of-topics/wuhan-novel-coronavirus/

Welsh Government. Coronavirus (COVID-19).
gov.wales/coronavirus

Public Health Wales. Novel Coronavirus (COVID-19).
phw.nhs.wales/topics/latest-information-on-novel-coronavirus-covid-19/

5.2 Hepatitis

Hepatitis

Overview

Treatment for viral hepatitis should be initiated by a specialist in hepatology or infectious diseases. The management of uncomplicated acute viral hepatitis is largely symptomatic. Hepatitis B and hepatitis C viruses are major causes of chronic hepatitis. Active or passive immunisation against hepatitis A and B infections can be given.

Chronic hepatitis B

Interferon alfa p. 602, **peginterferon alfa-2a**, lamivudine p. 455, adefovir dipivoxil, entecavir, and tenofovir disoproxil p. 456 have a role in the treatment of chronic hepatitis B in adults, but their role in children has not been well established. Specialist supervision is required for the management of chronic hepatitis B.

Tenofovir disoproxil, or a combination of tenofovir disoproxil with either emtricitabine p. 453 or lamivudine, may be used with other antiretrovirals, as part of 'highly active antiretroviral therapy' in children who require treatment for both HIV and chronic hepatitis B. If children infected with both HIV and chronic hepatitis B only require treatment for chronic hepatitis B, they should receive antivirals that are not active against HIV. Management of these children should be co-ordinated between HIV and hepatology specialists.

Chronic hepatitis C

Treatment should be considered for children with moderate or severe liver disease. Specialist supervision is required and the regimen is chosen according to the genotype of the infecting virus and the viral load. A combination of ribavirin p. 435 with either interferon alfa or **peginterferon alfa-2b** is licensed for use in children over 3 years with chronic hepatitis C. A combination of peginterferon alfa p. 438 and ribavirin is preferred.

5.3 Hepatitis infections

5.3a Chronic hepatitis B

Other drugs used for Chronic hepatitis B Interferon alfa, p. 602 · Lamivudine, p. 455 · Tenofovir disoproxil, p. 456

ANTIVIRALS › NUCLEOSIDE REVERSE TRANSCRIPTASE INHIBITORS

F 451

Tenofovir alafenamide

26-Feb-2018

● **INDICATIONS AND DOSE**

Chronic hepatitis B (initiated by a specialist)

▸ BY MOUTH

▸ Child 12–17 years (body-weight 35 kg and above): 25 mg once daily (for duration of treatment consult product literature)

● **CAUTIONS** Decompensated liver disease · HIV co-infection

● **INTERACTIONS** → Appendix 1: tenofovir alafenamide

- **SIDE-EFFECTS**
- ▶ **Common or very common** Abdominal distension · arthralgia · flatulence
- ▶ **Frequency not known** Hepatitis aggravated (during or following treatment) · nephrotoxicity
- **BREAST FEEDING** Manufacturer advises avoid—present in milk in *animal* studies.
- **HEPATIC IMPAIRMENT** Manufacturer advises caution in decompensated hepatic disease (no information available).
- **PRE-TREATMENT SCREENING** Manufacturer advises HIV antibody testing should be offered to those with unknown HIV-1 status before initiation of treatment.
- **MONITORING REQUIREMENTS** Manufacturer advises monitor liver function tests at repeated intervals during treatment and for at least 6 months after last dose—recurrent hepatitis may occur on discontinuation.
- **PATIENT AND CARER ADVICE**

Missed doses Manufacturer advises if a dose is more than 18 hours late, the missed dose should not be taken and the next dose should be taken at the normal time.

- **MEDICINAL FORMS** There can be variation in the licensing of different medicines containing the same drug.

Tablet

CAUTIONARY AND ADVISORY LABELS 21

▸ Vemlidy (Gilead Sciences International Ltd) ▼
Tenofovir alafenamide (as Tenofovir alafenamide fumarate)
25 mg Vemlidy 25mg tablets | 30 tablet PoM £325.73

5.3b Chronic hepatitis C

Other drugs used for Chronic hepatitis C Interferon alfa, p. 602 · Peginterferon alfa, p. 438

ANTIVIRALS > NUCLEOSIDE ANALOGUES

Ribavirin

27-Aug-2019

(Tribavirin)

- **INDICATIONS AND DOSE**

Bronchiolitis

▶ BY INHALATION OF AEROSOL, OR BY INHALATION OF NEBULISED SOLUTION

- ▸ Child 1–23 months: Inhale a solution containing 20 mg/mL for 12–18 hours for at least 3 days, maximum of 7 days, to be administered via small particle aerosol generator

Life-threatening RSV, parainfluenza virus, and adenovirus infection in immunocompromised children (administered on expert advice)

▶ BY INTRAVENOUS INFUSION

- ▸ Child: 33 mg/kg for 1 dose, to be administered over 15 minutes, then 16 mg/kg every 6 hours for 4 days, then 8 mg/kg every 8 hours for 3 days

REBETOL ® CAPSULES

Chronic hepatitis C (in combination with interferon alfa or peginterferon alfa) in previously untreated children without liver decompensation

▶ BY MOUTH

- ▸ Child 3–17 years (body-weight up to 47 kg): 15 mg/kg daily in 2 divided doses
- ▸ Child 3–17 years (body-weight 47–49 kg): 200 mg, dose to be given in the morning and 400 mg, dose to be given in the evening
- ▸ Child 3–17 years (body-weight 50–64 kg): 400 mg twice daily
- ▸ Child 3–17 years (body-weight 65–80 kg): 400 mg, dose to be given in the morning and 600 mg, dose to be given in the evening
- ▸ Child 3–17 years (body-weight 81–104 kg): 600 mg twice daily
- ▸ Child 3–17 years (body-weight 105 kg and above): 600 mg, dose to be given in the morning and 800 mg, dose to be given in the evening

REBETOL ® ORAL SOLUTION

Chronic hepatitis C (in combination with interferon alfa or peginterferon alfa) in previously untreated children without liver decompensation

▶ BY MOUTH

- ▸ Child 3–17 years (body-weight up to 47 kg): 15 mg/kg daily in 2 divided doses
- ▸ Child 3–17 years (body-weight 47–49 kg): 200 mg, dose to be given in the morning and 400 mg, dose to be given in the evening
- ▸ Child 3–17 years (body-weight 50–64 kg): 400 mg twice daily
- ▸ Child 3–17 years (body-weight 65–80 kg): 400 mg, dose to be given in the morning and 600 mg, dose to be given in the evening
- ▸ Child 3–17 years (body-weight 81–104 kg): 600 mg twice daily
- ▸ Child 3–17 years (body-weight 105 kg and above): 600 mg, dose to be given in the morning and 800 mg, dose to be given in the evening

- **UNLICENSED USE**
- ▸ When used by inhalation Inhalation licensed for use in children (age range not specified by manufacturer).
- ▸ With intravenous use Intravenous preparation not licensed.
- **CONTRA-INDICATIONS**
- ▸ With systemic use Consult product literature for specific contra-indications when ribavirin used in combination with other medicinal products · haemoglobinopathies · severe, uncontrolled cardiac disease in children with chronic hepatitis C
- **CAUTIONS**
- ▸ When used by inhalation Maintain standard supportive respiratory and fluid management therapy
- ▸ With systemic use Cardiac disease (assessment including ECG recommended before and during treatment—discontinue if deterioration) · consult product literature for specific cautions when ribavirin used in combination with other medicinal products · patients with a transplant—risk of rejection · risk of growth retardation in children, the reversibility of which is uncertain—if possible, consider starting treatment after pubertal growth spurt
- **INTERACTIONS** → Appendix 1: ribavirin
- **SIDE-EFFECTS**
- ▶ **Common or very common** Alopecia · anaemia · anxiety · appetite decreased · arrhythmias · arthralgia · arthritis · asthenia · behaviour abnormal · chest pain · chills · concentration impaired · constipation · cough · depression · diarrhoea · dizziness · drowsiness · dry mouth · dysphagia · dyspnoea · ear pain · eye disorders · eye inflammation · eye pain · fever · gastrointestinal discomfort · gastrointestinal disorders · haemorrhage · headaches · hyperthyroidism · hypotension · hypothyroidism · increased risk of infection · influenza like illness · lymphadenopathy · malaise · memory loss · mood altered · muscle complaints · muscle weakness · nasal congestion · nausea · neutropenia · oral disorders · pain · palpitations · peripheral oedema · photosensitivity reaction · respiratory disorders · sensation abnormal · sexual dysfunction · skin reactions · sleep disorders · sweat changes · syncope · taste altered · thirst · throat pain · thrombocytopenia · tinnitus · tremor ·

5 Infection

vasodilation · vertigo · vision disorders · vomiting · weight decreased

- **Uncommon** Dehydration · diabetes mellitus · hallucination · hearing loss · hepatic disorders · hypertension · nerve disorders · sarcoidosis · suicidal tendencies · thyroiditis
- **Rare or very rare** Angina pectoris · angioedema · bone marrow disorders · cardiac inflammation · cerebral ischaemia · cholangitis · coma · congestive heart failure · facial paralysis · hepatic failure (discontinue) · hypersensitivity · intracranial haemorrhage · myocardial infarction · myopathy · pancreatitis · psychotic disorder · pulmonary embolism · retinopathy · seizure · severe cutaneous adverse reactions (SCARs) · systemic lupus erythematosus (SLE) · vasculitis
- **Frequency not known** Haemolytic anaemia · homicidal ideation · nephrotic syndrome · pure red cell aplasia · renal failure · solid organ transplant rejection · tongue discolouration · ulcerative colitis

SIDE-EFFECTS, FURTHER INFORMATION Side effects listed are reported when oral ribavirin is used in combination with peginterferon alfa or interferon alfa, consult product literature for details.

- **CONCEPTION AND CONTRACEPTION**
  - With systemic use Exclude pregnancy before treatment in females of childbearing age. Effective contraception essential during treatment and for 4 months after treatment in females and for 7 months after treatment in males of childbearing age. Routine monthly pregnancy tests recommended. Condoms must be used if partner of male patient is pregnant (ribavirin excreted in semen).
  - When used by inhalation Women planning pregnancy should avoid exposure to aerosol.
- **PREGNANCY** Avoid; teratogenicity in *animal* studies.
  - When used by inhalation Pregnant women should avoid exposure to aerosol.
- **BREAST FEEDING** Avoid—no information available.
- **RENAL IMPAIRMENT** Plasma-ribavirin concentration increased. Manufacturer advises avoid oral ribavirin if estimated glomerular filtration rate less than 50 mL/minute/1.73 m^2—monitor haemoglobin concentration closely.

  Manufacturer advises use intravenous preparation with caution if estimated glomerular filtration rate less than 30 mL/minute/1.73 m^2.
- **MONITORING REQUIREMENTS**
  - When used by inhalation Monitor electrolytes closely. Monitor equipment for precipitation.
  - With systemic use Determine full blood count, platelets, electrolytes, serum creatinine, liver function tests and uric acid before starting treatment and then on weeks 2 and 4 of treatment, then as indicated clinically—adjust dose if adverse reactions or laboratory abnormalities develop (consult product literature). Test thyroid function before treatment and then every 3 months.
  - With oral use Eye examination recommended before treatment. Eye examination also recommended during treatment if pre-existing ophthalmological disorder or if decrease in vision reported—discontinue treatment if ophthalmological disorder deteriorates or if new ophthalmological disorder develops.
- **PRESCRIBING AND DISPENSING INFORMATION** Flavours of oral liquid formulations may include bubble-gum.
- **NATIONAL FUNDING/ACCESS DECISIONS**

NICE decisions

- **Peginterferon alfa and ribavirin for chronic hepatitis C (November 2013)** NICE TA300

Peginterferon alfa in combination with ribavirin is recommended (within the marketing authorisation) as an option for treating chronic hepatitis C in children. www.nice.org.uk/guidance/ta300

- **LESS SUITABLE FOR PRESCRIBING** Ribavirin inhalation is less suitable for prescribing.

- **MEDICINAL FORMS** There can be variation in the licensing of different medicines containing the same drug.

Solution for injection

- Virazole (Mylan)

  Ribavirin 100 mg per 1 ml Virazole 1.2g/12ml solution for injection vials | 5 vial [PoM] £3,600.00

Oral solution

CAUTIONARY AND ADVISORY LABELS 21

- Rebetol (Merck Sharp & Dohme Ltd)

  Ribavirin 40 mg per 1 ml Rebetol 40mg/ml oral solution | 100 ml [PoM] £67.08

Capsule

CAUTIONARY AND ADVISORY LABELS 21

- Ribavirin (Non-proprietary)

  Ribavirin 200 mg Ribavirin 200mg capsules | 84 capsule [PoM] £160.69 | 140 capsule [PoM] £267.81 | 168 capsule [PoM] £321.38
- Rebetol (Merck Sharp & Dohme Ltd)

  Ribavirin 200 mg Rebetol 200mg capsules | 168 capsule [PoM] £321.38

ANTIVIRALS > NUCLEOTIDE ANALOGUES

Ledipasvir with sofosbuvir

11-Jul-2018

The properties listed below are those particular to the combination only. For the properties of the components please consider, sofosbuvir p. 437.

- **DRUG ACTION** Sofosbuvir is a nucleotide analogue inhibitor and ledipasvir is an HCV inhibitor; they reduce viral load by inhibiting hepatitis C virus RNA replication.

- **INDICATIONS AND DOSE**

Chronic hepatitis C infection (initiated by a specialist)

- BY MOUTH
  - Child 12–17 years: 90/400 mg once daily, for duration of treatment consult product literature

DOSE ADJUSTMENTS DUE TO INTERACTIONS

- Manufacturer advises reduce dose of concurrent H_2-receptor antagonist if above a dose comparable to famotidine 40 mg twice daily.
- Manufacturer advises reduce dose of concurrent proton pump inhibitor if above a dose comparable to omeprazole 20 mg; take at the same time as sofosbuvir with ledipasvir.

DOSE EQUIVALENCE AND CONVERSION

- Dose expressed as x/y mg ledipasvir/sofosbuvir.

- **CAUTIONS** Retreatment following treatment failure—efficacy not established
- **INTERACTIONS** → Appendix 1: ledipasvir · sofosbuvir
- **SIDE-EFFECTS**
  - **Common or very common** Fatigue · headache · rash
  - **Frequency not known** Angioedema · arrhythmia
- **PRESCRIBING AND DISPENSING INFORMATION** Dispense in original container (contains desiccant).
- **PATIENT AND CARER ADVICE**

  Vomiting If vomiting occurs within 5 hours of administration, an additional dose should be taken.

  Missed doses If a dose is more than 18 hours late, the missed dose should not be taken and the next dose should be taken at the normal time.
- **NATIONAL FUNDING/ACCESS DECISIONS**

Scottish Medicines Consortium (SMC) decisions

SMC No. 1343/18

The *Scottish Medicines Consortium* has advised (June 2018) that ledipasvir with sofosbuvir (*Harvoni*®) is accepted for restricted use within NHS Scotland for the treatment of chronic hepatitis C infection of genotypes 1 and 4 only in patients aged 12 years up to 18 years.

- **MEDICINAL FORMS** There can be variation in the licensing of different medicines containing the same drug.

Tablet

CAUTIONARY AND ADVISORY LABELS 25

▸ Harvoni (Gilead Sciences International Ltd) ▼
Ledipasvir 90 mg, Sofosbuvir 400 mg Harvoni 90mg/400mg tablets | 28 tablet PoM £12,993.33

Sofosbuvir

26-Mar-2019

- **INDICATIONS AND DOSE**

Chronic hepatitis C infection

▸ BY MOUTH

▸ Child 12-17 years: 400 mg once daily, for duration of treatment consult product literature

> **IMPORTANT SAFETY INFORMATION**
>
> MHRA/CHM ADVICE: DIRECT-ACTING ANTIVIRALS TO TREAT CHRONIC HEPATITIS C: RISK OF INTERACTION WITH VITAMIN K ANTAGONISTS AND CHANGES IN INR (JANUARY 2017)
>
> An EU-wide review has identified that changes in liver function, secondary to hepatitis C treatment with direct-acting antivirals, may affect the efficacy of vitamin K antagonists; the MHRA has advised that INR should be monitored closely in patients receiving concomitant treatment.
>
> MHRA/CHM ADVICE: DIRECT-ACTING ANTIVIRAL INTERFERON-FREE REGIMENS TO TREAT CHRONIC HEPATITIS C: RISK OF HEPATITIS B REACTIVATION (JANUARY 2017)
>
> An EU-wide review has concluded that direct-acting antiviral interferon-free regimens for chronic hepatitis C can cause hepatitis B reactivation in patients co-infected with hepatitis B and C viruses; the MHRA recommends to screen patients for hepatitis B before starting treatment—patients infected with both hepatitis B and C viruses must be monitored and managed according to current clinical guidelines.
>
> MHRA/CHM ADVICE: DIRECT-ACTING ANTIVIRALS FOR CHRONIC HEPATITIS C: RISK OF HYPOGLYCAEMIA IN PATIENTS WITH DIABETES (DECEMBER 2018)
>
> Rapid reduction in hepatitis C viral load during direct-acting antiviral therapy for hepatitis C may improve glucose metabolism in patients with diabetes and result in symptomatic hypoglycaemia if diabetic treatment is continued at the same dose.
>
> The MHRA advises healthcare professionals:
>
> - to monitor glucose levels closely in patients with diabetes during direct-acting antiviral therapy for hepatitis C, especially within the first 3 months of treatment and modify diabetic medication or doses when necessary;
> - to be vigilant for changes in glucose tolerance and advise patients of the risk of hypoglycaemia;
> - to inform the healthcare professional in charge of the diabetic care of the patient when direct-acting antiviral therapy is initiated.

- **CAUTIONS**

CAUTIONS, FURTHER INFORMATION Manufacturer advises in chronic hepatitis C of genotype 1, 4, 5, or 6, only use sofosbuvir with ribavirin dual therapy in those with intolerance or contra-indications to peginterferon alfa who require urgent treatment.

- **INTERACTIONS** → Appendix 1: sofosbuvir
- **SIDE-EFFECTS**

▸ **Common or very common** Alopecia · anaemia · anxiety · appetite decreased · arthralgia · asthenia · chest pain · chills · concentration impaired · constipation · cough · depression · diarrhoea · dizziness · dry mouth · dyspnoea · fever · gastrointestinal discomfort · gastrooesophageal reflux disease · headaches · influenza like illness · insomnia · irritability · memory loss · muscle complaints · nasopharyngitis · nausea · neutropenia · pain · skin reactions · vision blurred · vomiting · weight decreased

▸ **Frequency not known** Arrhythmia

SIDE-EFFECTS, FURTHER INFORMATION Side-effects listed are reported when sofosbuvir is used in combination with ribavirin or with ribavirin and peginterferon alfa.

- **PREGNANCY** Manufacturer advises avoid—limited information available.
- **BREAST FEEDING** Manufacturer advises avoid—present in milk in *animal* studies.
- **RENAL IMPAIRMENT** Safety and efficacy not established if eGFR less than 30 mL/minute/1.73 m^2—accumulation may occur.
- **PRESCRIBING AND DISPENSING INFORMATION** Dispense in original container (contains desiccant).
- **PATIENT AND CARER ADVICE**

Missed doses Manufacturer advises if a dose is more than 18 hours late, the missed dose should not be taken and the next dose should be taken at the normal time.

- **NATIONAL FUNDING/ACCESS DECISIONS**

NICE decisions

▸ **Sofosbuvir for treating chronic hepatitis C (February 2015)**
NICE TA330

Sofosbuvir (*Sovaldi*®) in combination with peginterferon alfa and ribavirin is an option for treating adults with chronic hepatitis C infection:

- of genotype 1
- of genotype 3 with cirrhosis (treatment naive patients)
- of genotype 3 that has not adequately responded to interferon-based treatment
- of genotype 4, 5, or 6 with cirrhosis.

Sofosbuvir (*Sovaldi*®) in combination with ribavirin is an option for treating adults with chronic hepatitis C infection:

- of genotype 2 who are intolerant to *or* ineligible for interferon (treatment naive patients)
- of genotype 2 that has not adequately responded to interferon-based treatment
- of genotype 3 with cirrhosis who are intolerant to *or* ineligible for interferon (treatment naive patients)
- of genotype 3 with cirrhosis that has not adequately responded to interferon-based treatment

Patients whose treatment was started within the NHS before this guidance was published should have the option to continue treatment, without change to their funding arrangements, until they and their NHS clinician consider it appropriate to stop.
www.nice.org.uk/guidance/ta330

▸ **Sofosbuvir for treating chronic hepatitis C (February 2015)**
NICE TA330

Sofosbuvir (*Sovaldi*®) in combination with ribavirin is not recommended for the treatment of adults with chronic hepatitis C infection of genotypes 1, 4, 5, or 6.

Patients whose treatment was started within the NHS before this guidance was published should have the option to continue treatment, without change to their funding arrangements, until they and their NHS clinician consider it appropriate to stop.
www.nice.org.uk/guidance/ta330

Scottish Medicines Consortium (SMC) decisions

SMC No. 964/14

The *Scottish Medicines Consortium* has advised (June 2014) that sofosbuvir (*Sovaldi*®) is accepted for restricted use within NHS Scotland for the treatment of chronic hepatitis C infection of genotypes 1 to 6; its use in combination with ribavirin as dual therapy for chronic hepatitis C infection of either genotype 2 (in treatment naive patients) or genotype 3 is restricted to those who cannot use peginterferon alfa because of intolerance or contra-indications.

- **MEDICINAL FORMS** There can be variation in the licensing of different medicines containing the same drug.

Tablet

CAUTIONARY AND ADVISORY LABELS 21, 25

- **Sovaldi** (Gilead Sciences International Ltd) ▼
  Sofosbuvir 400 mg Sovaldi 400mg tablets | 28 tablet PoM £11,660.98

ANTIVIRALS > PROTEASE INHIBITORS, HEPATITIS

Glecaprevir with pibrentasvir

25-Oct-2017

- **INDICATIONS AND DOSE**

Chronic hepatitis C (specialist use only)

- BY MOUTH
- Child 12–17 years: 300/120 mg once daily, for duration of treatment, consult product literature

DOSE EQUIVALENCE AND CONVERSION

- Dose expressed as x/y mg glecaprevir/pibrentasvir.

IMPORTANT SAFETY INFORMATION

HEPATITIS B INFECTION

Cases of hepatitis B reactivation, sometimes fatal, have been reported in patients co-infected with hepatitis B and C viruses; manufacturer advises to assess patients for hepatitis B prior to initiation of therapy and manage according to current clinical guidelines.

MHRA/CHM ADVICE: DIRECT-ACTING ANTIVIRALS TO TREAT CHRONIC HEPATITIS C: RISK OF INTERACTION WITH VITAMIN K ANTAGONISTS AND CHANGES IN INR (JANUARY 2017)

An EU-wide review has identified that changes in liver function, secondary to hepatitis C treatment with direct-acting antivirals, may affect the efficacy of vitamin K antagonists; the MHRA has advised that INR should be monitored closely in patients receiving concomitant treatment.

MHRA/CHM ADVICE: DIRECT-ACTING ANTIVIRALS FOR CHRONIC HEPATITIS C: RISK OF HYPOGLYCAEMIA IN PATIENTS WITH DIABETES (DECEMBER 2018)

Rapid reduction in hepatitis C viral load during direct-acting antiviral therapy for hepatitis C may improve glucose metabolism in patients with diabetes and result in symptomatic hypoglycaemia if diabetic treatment is continued at the same dose.

The MHRA advises healthcare professionals:

- to monitor glucose levels closely in patients with diabetes during direct-acting antiviral therapy for hepatitis C, especially within the first 3 months of treatment and modify diabetic medication or doses when necessary;
- to be vigilant for changes in glucose tolerance and advise patients of the risk of hypoglycaemia;
- to inform the healthcare professional in charge of the diabetic care of the patient when direct-acting antiviral therapy is initiated.

- **CAUTIONS** Hepatitis B infection · post-liver transplant patients · re-treatment of patients with prior exposure to NS3/4A- or NS5A-inhibitors—efficacy not established
- **INTERACTIONS** → Appendix 1: glecaprevir · pibrentasvir
- **SIDE-EFFECTS**
- **Common or very common** Asthenia · diarrhoea · headache · nausea
- **Frequency not known** Pruritus · transient ischaemic attack
- **PREGNANCY** Manufacturer advises avoid—limited information available.
- **BREAST FEEDING** Manufacturer advises avoid—present in milk in *animal* studies.
- **HEPATIC IMPAIRMENT** Manufacturer advises avoid in moderate to severe impairment (risk of increased exposure).
- **PATIENT AND CARER ADVICE**

Missed doses Manufacturer advises if a dose is more than 18 hours late, the missed dose should not be taken and the next dose should be taken at the normal time.

- **NATIONAL FUNDING/ACCESS DECISIONS**

Scottish Medicines Consortium (SMC) decisions

SMC No. SMC2214

The *Scottish Medicines Consortium* has advised (November 2019) that glecaprevir with pibrentasvir (*Maviret*®) is accepted for use within NHS Scotland for the treatment of chronic hepatitis C virus (HCV) infection in patients aged 12 years up to 18 years. This advice is contingent upon the continuing availability of the patient access scheme in NHS Scotland or a list price that is equivalent or lower.

All Wales Medicines Strategy Group (AWMSG) decisions

AWMSG No. 3917

The *All Wales Medicines Strategy Group* has advised (October 2019) that glecaprevir/pibrentasvir (*Maviret*®) is recommended as an option for use within NHS Wales for the treatment of chronic hepatitis C virus (HCV) infection in adolescents aged 12 years or older. This recommendation applies only in circumstances where the approved Wales Patient Access Scheme (WPAS) is utilised or where the list/contract price is equivalent or lower than the WPAS price.

- **MEDICINAL FORMS** There can be variation in the licensing of different medicines containing the same drug.

Tablet

CAUTIONARY AND ADVISORY LABELS 21, 25

- **Maviret** (AbbVie Ltd) ▼
  Pibrentasvir 40 mg, Glecaprevir 100 mg Maviret 100mg/40mg tablets | 84 tablet PoM £12,993.66

IMMUNOSTIMULANTS > INTERFERONS

Peginterferon alfa

- **DRUG ACTION** Polyethylene glycol-conjugated ('pegylated') derivatives of interferon alfa (**peginterferon alfa-2a** and **peginterferon alfa-2b**) are available; pegylation increases the persistence of the interferon in the blood.
- **INDICATIONS AND DOSE**

PEGASYS®

Chronic hepatitis C (in combination with ribavirin) in previously untreated children without liver decompensation

- BY SUBCUTANEOUS INJECTION
- Child 5–17 years: (consult product literature)

- **CONTRA-INDICATIONS** Severe psychiatric illness

CONTRA-INDICATIONS, FURTHER INFORMATION

For contra-indications consult product literature.

- **CAUTIONS**

CAUTIONS, FURTHER INFORMATION For cautions consult product literature.

- **INTERACTIONS** → Appendix 1: interferons
- **SIDE-EFFECTS**
- **Common or very common** Alopecia · anaemia · anxiety · appetite decreased · arthralgia · asthenia · behaviour abnormal · chills · concentration impaired · cough · depression · diabetes mellitus · diarrhoea · dizziness · drowsiness · dyspnoea · ear pain · eye discomfort · face oedema · feeling cold · fever · flushing · gastrointestinal discomfort · growth retardation · haemorrhage · headaches · hypotension · hypothyroidism · increased risk of infection

· influenza like illness · laryngeal pain · leucopenia · lymphadenopathy · malaise · mood altered · muscle complaints · nausea · neutropenia · oral disorders · pain · palpitations · skin reactions · sleep disorders · syncope · tachycardia · taste altered · thrombocytopenia · urinary disorders · urinary tract disorder · vertigo · vision disorders · vomiting
- **Uncommon** Akathisia · chest discomfort · dysmenorrhoea · hallucination · hypersensitivity · keratitis · muscle contractions involuntary · nasal complaints · pallor · photosensitivity reaction · proteinuria · retinal exudate · sensation abnormal · tremor · vaginal discharge · wheezing

SIDE-EFFECTS, FURTHER INFORMATION Respiratory symptoms should be investigated and if pulmonary infiltrates are suspected or lung function is impaired the discontinuation of peginterferon alfa should be considered.

- **CONCEPTION AND CONTRACEPTION** Effective contraception required during treatment—consult product literature.
- **PREGNANCY** Manufacturers recommend avoid unless potential benefit outweighs risk (toxicity in *animal* studies).
- **BREAST FEEDING** Manufacturers advise avoid—no information available.
- **HEPATIC IMPAIRMENT** Manufacturer advises avoid in severe impairment and decompensated cirrhosis.
- **RENAL IMPAIRMENT** For further information on peginterferon alfa use in renal impairment consult product literature.
  Dose adjustments Reduce dose in moderate to severe impairment.
  Monitoring Close monitoring required in renal impairment.
- **MONITORING REQUIREMENTS**
  - Monitoring of lipid concentration is recommended.
  - Monitoring of hepatic function is recommended.
- **NATIONAL FUNDING/ACCESS DECISIONS**

NICE decisions

- **Peginterferon alfa and ribavirin for chronic hepatitis C (November 2013)** NICE TA300
  Peginterferon alfa in combination with ribavirin is recommended (within the marketing authorisation) as an option for treating chronic hepatitis C in children.
  www.nice.org.uk/guidance/ta300

- **MEDICINAL FORMS** There can be variation in the licensing of different medicines containing the same drug.

Solution for injection

EXCIPIENTS: May contain Benzyl alcohol

- Pegasys (Roche Products Ltd)
  Interferon alfa-2a (as Peginterferon alfa-2a) 180 microgram per 1 ml Pegasys 90micrograms/0.5ml solution for injection pre-filled syringes | 1 pre-filled disposable injection PoM £76.51
  Interferon alfa-2a (as Peginterferon alfa-2a) 270 microgram per 1 ml Pegasys 135micrograms/0.5ml solution for injection pre-filled syringes | 1 pre-filled disposable injection PoM £107.76 DT = £107.76
  Interferon alfa-2a (as Peginterferon alfa-2a) 360 microgram per 1 ml Pegasys 180micrograms/0.5ml solution for injection pre-filled syringes | 4 pre-filled disposable injection PoM £497.60

5.4 Herpesvirus infections

Herpesvirus infections

Herpes simplex and varicella–zoster infection

The two most important herpesvirus pathogens are herpes simplex virus (herpesvirus hominis) and varicella–zoster virus.

Herpes simplex infections

Herpes infection of the mouth and lips and in the eye is generally associated with herpes simplex virus serotype 1 (HSV-1); other areas of the skin may also be infected, especially in immunodeficiency. Genital infection is most often associated with HSV-2 and also HSV-1. Treatment of herpes simplex infection should start as early as possible and usually within 5 days of the appearance of the infection.

In individuals with good immune function, mild infection of the eye (ocular herpes) and of the lips (herpes labialis or cold sores) is treated with a topical antiviral drug. Primary herpetic gingivostomatitis is managed by changes to diet and with analgesics. Severe infection, neonatal herpes infection or infection in immunocompromised individuals requires treatment with a systemic antiviral drug. After completing parenteral treatment of neonatal herpes simplex encephalitis, oral suppression therapy with aciclovir p. 440 for 6 months can be considered on specialist advice. Primary or recurrent genital herpes simplex infection is treated with an antiviral drug given by mouth. Persistence of a lesion or recurrence in an immunocompromised patient may signal the development of resistance.

Specialist advice should be sought for systemic treatment of herpes simplex infection in pregnancy.

Varicella-zoster infections

Regardless of immune function and the use of any immunoglobulins, neonates with *chickenpox* should be treated with a parenteral antiviral to reduce the risk of severe disease. Oral therapy in children is not recommended as absorption is variable. Chickenpox in otherwise healthy children between 1 month and 12 years is usually mild and antiviral treatment is not usually required.

Chickenpox is more severe in adolescents than in children; antiviral treatment started within 24 hours of the onset of rash may reduce the duration and severity of symptoms in otherwise healthy adolescents. Antiviral treatment is generally recommended in immunocompromised patients and those at special risk (e.g. because of severe cardiovascular or respiratory disease or chronic skin disorder); in such cases, an antiviral is given for 10 days with at least 7 days of parenteral treatment.

In pregnancy severe chickenpox may cause complications, especially varicella pneumonia. Specialist advice should be sought for the treatment of chickenpox during pregnancy.

Neonates and children who have been exposed to chickenpox and are at special risk of complications may require prophylaxis with varicella-zoster immunoglobulin (see under Disease-specific Immunoglobulins). Prophylactic intravenous aciclovir should be considered for neonates whose mothers develop chickenpox 4 days before to 2 days after delivery.

In *herpes zoster* (shingles) systemic antiviral treatment can reduce the severity and duration of pain, reduce complications, and reduce viral shedding. Treatment with the antiviral should be started within 72 hours of the onset of rash and is usually continued for 7–10 days. Immunocompromised patients at high risk of disseminated or severe infection should be treated with a parenteral antiviral drug.

Chronic pain which persists after the rash has healed (postherpetic neuralgia) requires specific management.

Choice

Aciclovir is active against herpesviruses but does not eradicate them. Uses of aciclovir include systemic treatment of varicella–zoster and the systemic and topical treatment of herpes simplex infections of the skin and mucous membranes. It is used by mouth for severe herpetic stomatitis. Aciclovir eye ointment is used for herpes simplex infections of the eye; it is combined with systemic treatment for ophthalmic zoster.

Famciclovir, a prodrug of penciclovir, is similar to aciclovir and is licensed in adults for use in herpes zoster and genital

5 Infection

herpes; there is limited information available on use in children.

Valaciclovir p. 442 is an ester of aciclovir, licensed in adults for herpes zoster and herpes simplex infections of the skin and mucous membranes (including genital herpes); it is also licensed in children over 12 years for preventing cytomegalovirus disease following solid organ transplantation. Valaciclovir may be used for the treatment of mild herpes zoster in immunocompromised children over 12 years; treatment should be initiated under specialist supervision.

Cytomegalovirus infection

Ganciclovir p. 443 is related to aciclovir but it is more active against cytomegalovirus (CMV); it is also much more toxic than aciclovir and should therefore be prescribed under specialist supervision and only when the potential benefit outweighs the risks. Ganciclovir is administered by intravenous infusion for the *initial treatment* of CMV infection. The use of ganciclovir may also be considered for symptomatic congenital CMV infection. Ganciclovir causes profound myelosuppression when given with zidovudine p. 457; the two should not normally be given together particularly during initial ganciclovir therapy. The likelihood of ganciclovir resistance increases in patients with a high viral load or in those who receive the drug over a long duration.

Valaciclovir is licensed for use in children over 12 years for prevention of cytomegalovirus disease following renal transplantation.

Foscarnet sodium p. 444 is also active against cytomegalovirus; it is toxic and can cause renal impairment. It is deposited in teeth, bone and cartilage, and *animal* studies have shown that deposition is greater in young animals. Its effect on skeletal development in children is not known. Foscarnet sodium should be prescribed under specialist supervision.

ANTIVIRALS › NUCLEOSIDE ANALOGUES

Aciclovir 10-Mar-2020

(Acyclovir)

● **INDICATIONS AND DOSE**

Herpes simplex, suppression

▶ BY MOUTH

- Child 12–17 years: 400 mg twice daily, alternatively 200 mg 4 times a day; increased to 400 mg 3 times a day, dose may be increased if recurrences occur on standard suppressive therapy or for suppression of genital herpes during late pregnancy (from 36 weeks gestation), therapy interrupted every 6–12 months to reassess recurrence frequency—consider restarting after two or more recurrences

Herpes simplex, prophylaxis in the immunocompromised

▶ BY MOUTH

- Child 1–23 months: 100–200 mg 4 times a day
- Child 2–17 years: 200–400 mg 4 times a day

Herpes simplex, treatment

▶ BY MOUTH

- Child 1–23 months: 100 mg 5 times a day usually for 5 days (longer if new lesions appear during treatment or if healing incomplete)
- Child 2–17 years: 200 mg 5 times a day usually for 5 days (longer if new lesions appear during treatment or if healing incomplete)

▶ BY INTRAVENOUS INFUSION

- Neonate: 20 mg/kg every 8 hours for 14 days (for at least 21 days if CNS involvement—confirm cerebrospinal fluid negative for herpes simplex virus before stopping treatment).
- Child 1–2 months: 20 mg/kg every 8 hours for 14 days (for at least 21 days if CNS involvement—confirm cerebrospinal fluid negative for herpes simplex virus before stopping treatment)
- Child 3 months–11 years: 250 mg/m^2 every 8 hours usually for 5 days
- Child 12–17 years: 5 mg/kg every 8 hours usually for 5 days

Herpes simplex, treatment, in immunocompromised or if absorption impaired

▶ BY MOUTH

- Child 1–23 months: 200 mg 5 times a day usually for 5 days (longer if new lesions appear during treatment or if healing incomplete)
- Child 2–17 years: 400 mg 5 times a day usually for 5 days (longer if new lesions appear during treatment or if healing incomplete)

Herpes simplex, treatment, in immunocompromised or in simplex encephalitis

▶ BY INTRAVENOUS INFUSION

- Child 3 months–11 years: 500 mg/m^2 every 8 hours usually for 5 days (given for at least 21 days in encephalitis—confirm cerebrospinal fluid negative for herpes simplex virus before stopping treatment)
- Child 12–17 years: 10 mg/kg every 8 hours usually for 5 days (given for at least 14 days in encephalitis and for at least 21 days if also immunocompromised—confirm cerebrospinal fluid negative for herpes simplex virus before stopping treatment)

Varicella zoster (chickenpox), treatment | Herpes zoster (shingles), treatment

▶ BY MOUTH

- Child 1–23 months: 200 mg 4 times a day for 5 days
- Child 2–5 years: 400 mg 4 times a day for 5 days
- Child 6–11 years: 800 mg 4 times a day for 5 days
- Child 12–17 years: 800 mg 5 times a day for 7 days

▶ BY INTRAVENOUS INFUSION

- Neonate: 10–20 mg/kg every 8 hours for at least 7 days.
- Child 1–2 months: 10–20 mg/kg every 8 hours for at least 7 days
- Child 3 months–11 years: 250 mg/m^2 every 8 hours usually for 5 days
- Child 12–17 years: 5 mg/kg every 8 hours usually for 5 days

Varicella zoster (chickenpox), treatment in immunocompromised | Herpes zoster (shingles), treatment in immunocompromised

▶ BY INTRAVENOUS INFUSION

- Child 3 months–11 years: 500 mg/m^2 every 8 hours usually for 5 days
- Child 12–17 years: 10 mg/kg every 8 hours usually for 5 days

Herpes zoster (shingles), treatment in immunocompromised

▶ BY MOUTH

- Child 1–23 months: 200 mg 4 times a day continued for 2 days after crusting of lesions
- Child 2–5 years: 400 mg 4 times a day continued for 2 days after crusting of lesions
- Child 6–11 years: 800 mg 4 times a day continued for 2 days after crusting of lesions
- Child 12–17 years: 800 mg 5 times a day continued for 2 days after crusting of lesions

Herpes zoster, treatment in encephalitis | Varicella zoster, treatment in encephalitis

▶ BY INTRAVENOUS INFUSION

▸ Neonate: 10–20 mg/kg every 8 hours given for 10–14 days in encephalitis, possibly longer if also immunocompromised.

▸ Child 1-2 months: 10–20 mg/kg every 8 hours given for 10–14 days in encephalitis, possibly longer if also immunocompromised

▸ Child 3 months-11 years: 500 mg/m^2 every 8 hours given for 10–14 days in encephalitis, possibly longer if also immunocompromised

▸ Child 12-17 years: 10 mg/kg every 8 hours given for 10–14 days in encephalitis, possibly longer if also immunocompromised

Varicella zoster (chickenpox), attenuation of infection if varicella–zoster immunoglobulin not indicated

▶ BY MOUTH

▸ Child: 10 mg/kg 4 times a day for 7 days, to be started 1 week after exposure

Varicella zoster (chickenpox), prophylaxis after delivery

▶ BY INTRAVENOUS INFUSION

▸ Neonate: 10 mg/kg every 8 hours continued until serological tests confirm absence of virus.

DOSES AT EXTREMES OF BODY-WEIGHT

▸ With intravenous use To avoid excessive dosage in obese patients parenteral dose should be calculated on the basis of ideal weight for height.

- **UNLICENSED USE**

▸ With oral use Tablets and suspension not licensed for suppression of herpes simplex or for treatment of herpes zoster in children (age range not specified by manufacturer).

▸ With intravenous use Intravenous infusion not licensed for herpes zoster in children under 18 years.

▸ With oral use Aciclovir doses in BNF may differ from those in product literature. Attenuation of chickenpox is an unlicensed indication.

- **CAUTIONS** Maintain adequate hydration (especially with infusion or high doses)
- **INTERACTIONS** → Appendix 1: aciclovir
- **SIDE-EFFECTS**

▶ **Common or very common**

▸ With intravenous use Nausea · photosensitivity reaction · skin reactions · vomiting

▸ With oral use Abdominal pain · diarrhoea · dizziness · fatigue · fever · headache · nausea · photosensitivity reaction · skin reactions · vomiting

▶ **Uncommon**

▸ With intravenous use Anaemia · leucopenia · thrombocytopenia

▶ **Rare or very rare**

▸ With intravenous use Abdominal pain · agitation · angioedema · ataxia · coma · confusion · diarrhoea · dizziness · drowsiness · dysarthria · dyspnoea · encephalopathy · fatigue · fever · hallucination · headache · hepatic disorders · inflammation localised · psychosis · renal impairment · renal pain · seizure · tremor

▸ With oral use Agitation · anaemia · angioedema · ataxia · coma · confusion · drowsiness · dysarthria · dyspnoea · encephalopathy · hallucination · hepatic disorders · leucopenia · psychosis · renal impairment · renal pain · seizure · thrombocytopenia · tremor

▶ **Frequency not known**

▸ With intravenous use Crystalluria

▸ With oral use Alopecia · crystalluria

- **PREGNANCY** Not known to be harmful—manufacturers advise use only when potential benefit outweighs risk.
- **BREAST FEEDING** Significant amount in milk after systemic administration—not known to be harmful but manufacturer advises caution.
- **RENAL IMPAIRMENT** Risk of neurological reactions increased. Maintain adequate hydration (especially during renal impairment).

Dose adjustments ▸ With intravenous use Use *normal intravenous dose* every 12 hours if estimated glomerular filtration rate 25–50 mL/minute/1.73 m^2 (every 24 hours if estimated glomerular filtration rate 10–25 mL/minute/1.73 m^2. Consult product literature for intravenous dose if estimated glomerular filtration rate less than 10 mL/minute/1.73 m^2.

▸ With oral use For *herpes zoster*, use normal oral dose every 8 hours if estimated glomerular filtration rate 10–25 mL/minute/1.73 m^2 (every 12 hours if estimated glomerular filtration rate less than 10 mL/minute/1.73 m^2. For *herpes simplex*, use normal dose every 12 hours if estimated glomerular filtration rate less than 10 mL/minute/1.73 m^2.

- **DIRECTIONS FOR ADMINISTRATION**

▸ With intravenous use For *intravenous infusion*, reconstitute to 25 mg/mL with Water for Injections or Sodium Chloride 0.9% then dilute to concentration of 5 mg/mL with Sodium Chloride 0.9% or Sodium Chloride and Glucose and give over 1 hour; alternatively, may be administered in a concentration of 25 mg/mL using a suitable infusion pump and central venous access and given over 1 hour.

- **PRESCRIBING AND DISPENSING INFORMATION** Flavours of oral liquid preparations may include banana, or orange.
- **PATIENT AND CARER ADVICE**

Medicines for Children leaflet: Aciclovir (oral) for viral infections

▸ With oral use www.medicinesforchildren.org.uk/aciclovir-oral-viral-infections-0

- **PROFESSION SPECIFIC INFORMATION**

Dental practitioners' formulary

Aciclovir Tablets 200 mg or 800 mg may be prescribed.
Aciclovir Oral Suspension 200 mg/5mL may be prescribed.

- **MEDICINAL FORMS** There can be variation in the licensing of different medicines containing the same drug.

Tablet

CAUTIONARY AND ADVISORY LABELS 9

▸ Aciclovir (Non-proprietary)

Aciclovir 200 mg Aciclovir 200mg tablets | 25 tablet PoM £2.03 DT = £1.40

Aciclovir 400 mg Aciclovir 400mg tablets | 56 tablet PoM £4.62 DT = £2.94

Aciclovir 800 mg Aciclovir 800mg tablets | 35 tablet PoM £6.41 DT = £4.13

Dispersible tablet

CAUTIONARY AND ADVISORY LABELS 9

▸ Aciclovir (Non-proprietary)

Aciclovir 200 mg Aciclovir 200mg dispersible tablets | 25 tablet PoM £1.47 DT = £1.47

Aciclovir 400 mg Aciclovir 400mg dispersible tablets | 56 tablet PoM £11.99 DT = £11.99

Aciclovir 800 mg Aciclovir 800mg dispersible tablets | 35 tablet PoM £10.99 DT = £10.99

▸ Zovirax (GlaxoSmithKline UK Ltd)

Aciclovir 200 mg Zovirax 200mg dispersible tablets | 25 tablet PoM £2.85 DT = £1.47

Aciclovir 800 mg Zovirax 800mg dispersible tablets | 35 tablet PoM £10.50 DT = £10.99

Oral suspension

CAUTIONARY AND ADVISORY LABELS 9

▸ Aciclovir (Non-proprietary)

Aciclovir 40 mg per 1 ml Aciclovir 200mg/5ml oral suspension sugar free sugar-free | 125 ml PoM £35.78 DT = £35.78

Aciclovir 80 mg per 1 ml Aciclovir 400mg/5ml oral suspension sugar free sugar-free | 100 ml PoM £39.49 DT = £39.49

▸ Zovirax (GlaxoSmithKline UK Ltd)

Aciclovir 40 mg per 1 ml Zovirax 200mg/5ml oral suspension sugar-free | 125 ml PoM £29.56 DT = £35.78

Aciclovir 80 mg per 1 ml Zovirax Double Strength 400mg/5ml oral suspension sugar-free | 100 ml PoM £33.02 DT = £39.49

Solution for infusion

ELECTROLYTES: May contain Sodium

▸ Aciclovir (Non-proprietary)

Aciclovir (as Aciclovir sodium) 25 mg per 1 ml Aciclovir 1g/40ml solution for infusion vials | 1 vial PoM £40.00 (Hospital only)
Aciclovir 250mg/10ml concentrate for solution for infusion vials | 5 vial PoM £50.00 (Hospital only) | 5 vial PoM £30.00–£40.00
Aciclovir 500mg/20ml solution for infusion vials | 5 vial PoM £100.00 (Hospital only) | 5 vial PoM £50.00
Aciclovir 500mg/20ml concentrate for solution for infusion vials | 5 vial PoM £40.00 (Hospital only)

Powder for solution for infusion

ELECTROLYTES: May contain Sodium

▸ Aciclovir (Non-proprietary)

Aciclovir (as Aciclovir sodium) 250 mg Aciclovir 250mg powder for solution for infusion vials | 5 vial PoM £16.50 (Hospital only)
Aciclovir 250mg powder for solution for infusion vials | 5 vial PoM £49.30 | 10 vial PoM £91.30 (Hospital only)

Aciclovir (as Aciclovir sodium) 500 mg Aciclovir 500mg powder for solution for infusion vials | 10 vial PoM £182.00 (Hospital only)

▸ Zovirax I.V. (GlaxoSmithKline UK Ltd)

Aciclovir (as Aciclovir sodium) 250 mg Zovirax I.V. 250mg powder for solution for infusion vials | 5 vial PoM £16.70

Aciclovir (as Aciclovir sodium) 500 mg Zovirax I.V. 500mg powder for solution for infusion vials | 5 vial PoM £17.00

Valaciclovir

● **INDICATIONS AND DOSE**

Herpes zoster infection, treatment in immunocompromised patients

▸ BY MOUTH

▸ Child 12–17 years: 1 g 3 times a day for at least 7 days and continued for 2 days after crusting of lesions

Herpes simplex, treatment of first infective episode

▸ BY MOUTH

▸ Child 12–17 years: 500 mg twice daily for 5 days (longer if new lesions appear during treatment or healing is incomplete)

Herpes simplex infections treatment of first episode in immunocompromised or HIV-positive patients

▸ BY MOUTH

▸ Child 12–17 years: 1 g twice daily for 10 days

Herpes simplex, treatment of recurrent infections

▸ BY MOUTH

▸ Child 12–17 years: 500 mg twice daily for 3–5 days

Treatment of recurrent herpes simplex infections in immunocompromised or HIV-positive patients

▸ BY MOUTH

▸ Child 12–17 years: 1 g twice daily for 5–10 days

Herpes labialis treatment

▸ BY MOUTH

▸ Child 12–17 years: Initially 2 g, then 2 g after 12 hours

Herpes simplex, suppression of infections

▸ BY MOUTH

▸ Child 12–17 years: 500 mg daily in 1–2 divided doses, therapy to be interrupted every 6–12 months to reassess recurrence frequency—consider restarting after two or more recurrences

Herpes simplex, suppression of infections in immunocompromised or HIV-positive patients

▸ BY MOUTH

▸ Child 12–17 years: 500 mg twice daily, therapy to be interrupted every 6–12 months to reassess recurrence frequency—consider restarting after two or more recurrences

Prevention of cytomegalovirus disease following solid organ transplantation when valganciclovir or ganciclovir cannot be used

▸ BY MOUTH

▸ Child 12–17 years: 2 g 4 times a day usually for 90 days, preferably starting within 72 hours of transplantation

● **UNLICENSED USE** Not licensed for treatment of herpes zoster in children. Not licensed for treatment or suppression of herpes simplex infection in immunocompromised or HIV-positive children.

● **CAUTIONS** Maintain adequate hydration (especially with high doses)

● **INTERACTIONS** → Appendix 1: valaciclovir

● **SIDE-EFFECTS**

▸ **Common or very common** Diarrhoea · dizziness · headache · nausea · photosensitivity reaction · skin reactions · vomiting

▸ **Uncommon** Abdominal discomfort · agitation · confusion · dyspnoea · haematuria · hallucination · leucopenia · level of consciousness decreased · renal pain · thrombocytopenia · tremor

▸ **Rare or very rare** Angioedema · ataxia · coma · delirium · dysarthria · encephalopathy · nephrolithiasis · psychosis · renal impairment · seizure

▸ **Frequency not known** Microangiopathic haemolytic anaemia

SIDE-EFFECTS, FURTHER INFORMATION Neurological reactions more frequent with higher doses.

● **PREGNANCY** Not known to be harmful—manufacturers advise use only when potential benefit outweighs risk.

● **BREAST FEEDING** Significant amount in milk after systemic administration—not known to be harmful but manufacturer advises caution.

● **HEPATIC IMPAIRMENT** Manufacturer advises caution with doses of 4 g or more per day (no information available).

● **RENAL IMPAIRMENT** Maintain adequate hydration.

Dose adjustments For *herpes zoster*, 1 g every 12 hours if estimated glomerular filtration rate 30–50 mL/minute/1.73 m^2 (1 g every 24 hours if estimated glomerular filtration rate 10–30 mL/minute/1.73 m^2; 500 mg every 24 hours if estimated glomerular filtration rate less than 10 mL/minute/1.73 m^2).

For *treatment of herpes simplex*, 500 mg (1 g in immunocompromised or HIV-positive children) every 24 hours if estimated glomerular filtration rate less than 30 mL/minute/1.73 m^2.

For *treatment of herpes labialis*, if estimated glomerular filtration rate 30–50 mL/minute/1.73 m^2, initially 1 g, then 1 g 12 hours after initial dose (if estimated glomerular filtration rate 10–30 mL/minute/1.73 m^2, initially 500 mg, then 500 mg 12 hours after initial dose; if estimated glomerular filtration rate less than 10 mL/minute/1.73 m^2, 500 mg as a single dose).

For *suppression of herpes simplex*, 250 mg (500 mg in immunocompromised or HIV-positive children) every 24 hours if estimated glomerular filtration rate less than 30 mL/minute/1.73 m^2.

Reduce dose according to estimated glomerular filtration rate for *cytomegalovirus prophylaxis* following solid organ transplantation (consult product literature).

● **PRESCRIBING AND DISPENSING INFORMATION** Valaciclovir is a pro-drug of aciclovir.

● **MEDICINAL FORMS** There can be variation in the licensing of different medicines containing the same drug. Forms available from special-order manufacturers include: oral suspension

Tablet

CAUTIONARY AND ADVISORY LABELS 9

▸ **Valaciclovir (Non-proprietary)**
Valaciclovir (as Valaciclovir hydrochloride) 500 mg Valaciclovir 500mg tablets | 10 tablet PoM £22.05 DT = £2.55 | 42 tablet PoM £78.83

▸ **Valtrex** (GlaxoSmithKline UK Ltd)
Valaciclovir (as Valaciclovir hydrochloride) 250 mg Valtrex 250mg tablets | 60 tablet PoM £123.28 DT = £123.28
Valaciclovir (as Valaciclovir hydrochloride) 500 mg Valtrex 500mg tablets | 10 tablet PoM £20.59 DT = £2.55 | 42 tablet PoM £86.30

5.4a Cytomegalovirus infections

ANTIVIRALS > NUCLEOSIDE ANALOGUES

Ganciclovir

31-May-2018

● **INDICATIONS AND DOSE**

Prevention of cytomegalovirus disease [pre-emptive therapy in patients with drug-induced immunosuppression]

▸ BY INTRAVENOUS INFUSION

▸ Child 12–17 years: Initially 5 mg/kg every 12 hours for 7–14 days, then maintenance 6 mg/kg once daily, on 5 days of the week, alternatively maintenance 5 mg/kg once daily

Prevention of cytomegalovirus disease [universal prophylaxis in patients with drug-induced immunosuppression]

▸ BY INTRAVENOUS INFUSION

▸ Neonate: (consult product literature).

▸ Child 1 month–16 years: (consult product literature)

▸ Child 17 years: 6 mg/kg once daily, on 5 days of the week, alternatively 5 mg/kg once daily

Treatment of cytomegalovirus disease [in immunocompromised patients]

▸ BY INTRAVENOUS INFUSION

▸ Child: Initially 5 mg/kg every 12 hours for 14–21 days, then maintenance 6 mg/kg once daily, on 5 days of the week, alternatively maintenance 5 mg/kg once daily, maintenance only for patients at risk of relapse; if disease progresses initial induction treatment may be repeated

Congenital cytomegalovirus infection of the CNS

▸ BY INTRAVENOUS INFUSION

▸ Neonate: 6 mg/kg every 12 hours for 6 weeks.

● **UNLICENSED USE** Not licensed for use in children under 12 years for the treatment of cytomegalovirus disease in immunocompromised patients. Not licensed for congenital cytomegalovirus infection of the CNS.

● **CONTRA-INDICATIONS** Abnormally low haemoglobin count (consult product literature) · abnormally low neutrophil count (consult product literature) · abnormally low platelet count (consult product literature)

● **CAUTIONS** History of cytopenia · potential carcinogen (including long-term carcinogenicity) · potential teratogen (including long-term teratogenicity) · radiotherapy

● **INTERACTIONS** → Appendix 1: ganciclovir

● **SIDE-EFFECTS**

▸ **Common or very common** Anaemia · anxiety · appetite decreased · arthralgia · asthenia · bone marrow disorders · chest pain · chills · confusion · constipation · cough · depression · diarrhoea · dizziness · dysphagia · dyspnoea · ear pain · eye disorders · eye inflammation · eye pain · fever · flatulence · gastrointestinal discomfort · headache · hepatic function abnormal · increased risk of infection · insomnia · leucopenia · malaise · muscle complaints · nausea · neutropenia · night sweats · pain · peripheral neuropathy · renal impairment · seizure · sensation abnormal · sepsis · skin reactions · taste altered · thinking abnormal · thrombocytopenia · vomiting · weight decreased

▸ **Uncommon** Alopecia · arrhythmia · deafness · haematuria · hypotension · infertility male · oral ulceration · pancreatitis · psychotic disorder · tremor · visual impairment

▸ **Rare or very rare** Agranulocytosis · hallucination

● **ALLERGY AND CROSS-SENSITIVITY** Contra-indicated in patients hypersensitive to valganciclovir, aciclovir, or valaciclovir.

● **CONCEPTION AND CONTRACEPTION** Manufacturer advises women of childbearing potential should use effective contraception during and for at least 30 days after treatment; men with partners of childbearing potential should be advised to use barrier contraception during and for at least 90 days after treatment. Ganciclovir may cause temporary or permanent inhibition of spermatogenesis—impaired fertility observed in *animal* studies.

● **PREGNANCY** Manufacturer advises avoid unless potential benefit outweighs risk—teratogenicity in *animal* studies.

● **BREAST FEEDING** Manufacturer advises avoid—present in milk in *animal* studies.

● **RENAL IMPAIRMENT**

Dose adjustments Manufacturer advises reduce dose for patients receiving mg/kg dosing if creatinine clearance less than 70 mL/minute—consult product literature.

● **MONITORING REQUIREMENTS** Monitor full blood count closely (severe deterioration may require correction and possibly treatment interruption).

● **DIRECTIONS FOR ADMINISTRATION** Manufacturer advises, for *intravenous infusion*, give intermittently in Glucose 5% or Sodium Chloride 0.9%. Reconstitute with Water for Injections (500 mg/10 mL) then dilute requisite dose to a concentration of not more than 10 mg/mL with infusion fluid; give over 1 hour into a vein with adequate flow, preferably using a plastic cannula.

● **HANDLING AND STORAGE**

Caution in handling Ganciclovir is a potential teratogen and carcinogen. Manufacturer advises avoid inhalation of the powder or direct contact of the powder or reconstituted solution with the skin or mucous membranes; if contact occurs, wash thoroughly with soap and water; rinse eyes thoroughly with plain water.

● **MEDICINAL FORMS** There can be variation in the licensing of different medicines containing the same drug.

Powder for solution for infusion

ELECTROLYTES: May contain Sodium

▸ **Ganciclovir (Non-proprietary)**
Ganciclovir (as Ganciclovir sodium) 500 mg Ganciclovir 500mg powder for concentrate for solution for infusion vials | 5 vial PoM £115.00 (Hospital only) | 5 vial PoM £125.95

▸ **Cymevene** (Cheplapharm Arzneimittel GmbH)
Ganciclovir (as Ganciclovir sodium) 500 mg Cymevene 500mg powder for concentrate for solution for infusion vials | 5 vial PoM £148.83

Valganciclovir

31-May-2018

● **INDICATIONS AND DOSE**

Prevention of cytomegalovirus disease [following solid organ transplantation from a cytomegalovirus positive donor]

▶ BY MOUTH

▶ Neonate: (consult product literature).

▶ Child: (consult product literature)

DOSE EQUIVALENCE AND CONVERSION

▶ Oral valganciclovir 900 mg twice daily is equivalent to intravenous ganciclovir 5 mg/kg twice daily.

● **CONTRA-INDICATIONS** Abnormally low haemoglobin count (consult product literature) · abnormally low neutrophil count (consult product literature) · abnormally low platelet count (consult product literature)

● **CAUTIONS** History of cytopenia · potential carcinogen (including long-term carcinogenicity) · potential teratogen (including long-term teratogenicity) · radiotherapy

● **INTERACTIONS** → Appendix 1: valganciclovir

● **SIDE-EFFECTS**

▶ **Common or very common** Anaemia · anxiety · appetite decreased · arthralgia · asthenia · bone marrow disorders · chest pain · confusion · constipation · cough · depression · diarrhoea · dizziness · dysphagia · dyspnoea · ear pain · eye disorders · eye inflammation · eye pain · flatulence · gastrointestinal discomfort · headache · hepatic function abnormal · increased risk of infection · insomnia · leucopenia · malaise · muscle complaints · nausea · neutropenia · night sweats · pain · peripheral neuropathy · renal impairment · seizure · sensation abnormal · sepsis · skin reactions · taste altered · thinking abnormal · thrombocytopenia · vomiting · weight decreased

▶ **Uncommon** Alopecia · arrhythmia · deafness · haematuria · hallucination · hypotension · infertility male · oral ulceration · pancreatitis · psychotic disorder · tremor · visual impairment

● **ALLERGY AND CROSS-SENSITIVITY** Contra-indicated in patients hypersensitive to ganciclovir, aciclovir, or valaciclovir.

● **CONCEPTION AND CONTRACEPTION** Manufacturer advises women of childbearing potential should use effective contraception during and for at least 30 days after treatment; men with partners of childbearing potential should be advised to use barrier contraception during and for at least 90 days after treatment. *Ganciclovir* may cause temporary or permanent inhibition of spermatogenesis—impaired fertility observed in *animal* studies.

● **PREGNANCY** Manufacturer advises avoid unless potential benefit outweighs risk—teratogenicity observed with *ganciclovir* in *animal* studies.

● **BREAST FEEDING** Manufacturer advises avoid— *ganciclovir* present in milk in *animal* studies.

● **MONITORING REQUIREMENTS** Monitor full blood count closely (severe deterioration may require correction and possibly treatment interruption).

● **PRESCRIBING AND DISPENSING INFORMATION** Valganciclovir is a pro-drug of ganciclovir.

Flavours of oral liquid formulations may include tutti-frutti.

● **HANDLING AND STORAGE** Manufacturer advises reconstituted powder for oral solution should be stored in a refrigerator (2–8°C) for up to 49 days.

Caution in handling Valganciclovir is a potential teratogen and carcinogen. Manufacturer advises caution when handling the powder, reconstituted solution, or broken tablets and avoid inhalation of powder; if contact with skin or mucous membranes occurs, wash thoroughly with soap and water; rinse eyes thoroughly with plain water.

● **MEDICINAL FORMS** There can be variation in the licensing of different medicines containing the same drug. Forms available from special-order manufacturers include: oral solution

Oral solution

CAUTIONARY AND ADVISORY LABELS 21

▶ Valcyte (Roche Products Ltd)

Valganciclovir (as Valganciclovir hydrochloride) 50 mg per 1 ml Valcyte 50mg/ml oral solution sugar-free | 100 ml PoM £230.32 DT = £230.32

Tablet

CAUTIONARY AND ADVISORY LABELS 21

▶ **Valganciclovir (Non-proprietary)**

Valganciclovir (as Valganciclovir hydrochloride) 450 mg Valganciclovir 450mg tablets | 60 tablet PoM £865.17–£1,081.46 DT = £1,027.40

▶ Valcyte (Roche Products Ltd)

Valganciclovir (as Valganciclovir hydrochloride) 450 mg Valcyte 450mg tablets | 60 tablet PoM £1,081.46 DT = £1,027.40

ANTIVIRALS › OTHER

Foscarnet sodium

26-May-2020

● **INDICATIONS AND DOSE**

Cytomegalovirus disease

▶ BY INTRAVENOUS INFUSION

▶ Child (under expert supervision): Initially 60 mg/kg every 8 hours 2–3 weeks, then maintenance 60 mg/kg daily, increased if tolerated to 90–120 mg/kg daily, if disease progresses on maintenance dose, repeat induction regimen

Mucocutaneous herpes simplex virus infections unresponsive to aciclovir in immunocompromised patients

▶ BY INTRAVENOUS INFUSION

▶ Child (under expert supervision): 40 mg/kg every 8 hours for 2–3 weeks or until lesions heal

● **UNLICENSED USE** Not licensed for use in children.

● **CAUTIONS** Conditions where excess sodium should be avoided · ensure adequate hydration

● **INTERACTIONS** → Appendix 1: foscarnet

● **SIDE-EFFECTS**

▶ **Common or very common** Aggression · anaemia · anxiety · appetite decreased · arrhythmias · asthenia · chest pain · chills · confusion · constipation · coordination abnormal · dehydration · depression · diarrhoea · dizziness · electrolyte imbalance · fever · gastrointestinal discomfort · genital discomfort (due to high concentrations excreted in urine) · genital ulceration (due to high concentrations excreted in urine) · haemorrhage · headache · hepatic function abnormal · hypertension · hypotension · leucopenia · malaise · muscle contractions involuntary · myalgia · nausea (reduce infusion rate) · neutropenia · numbness · oedema · palpitations · pancreatitis · paraesthesia (reduce infusion rate) · peripheral neuropathy · proteinuria · renal impairment · seizure · sepsis · skin reactions · thrombocytopenia · thrombophlebitis · tremor · urinary disorders · vomiting

▶ **Uncommon** Acidosis · angioedema · glomerulonephritis · nephropathy · pancytopenia

▶ **Frequency not known** Anaphylactoid reaction · diabetes insipidus · muscle weakness · myopathy · oesophageal ulcer · QT interval prolongation · renal pain · renal tubular acidosis · severe cutaneous adverse reactions (SCARs)

● **CONCEPTION AND CONTRACEPTION** Men should avoid fathering a child during and for 6 months after treatment.

● **PREGNANCY** Manufacturer advises avoid.

● **BREAST FEEDING** Avoid—present in milk in *animal* studies.

- **RENAL IMPAIRMENT**
  Dose adjustments Reduce dose; consult product literature.
- **MONITORING REQUIREMENTS**
  - Monitor electrolytes, particularly calcium and magnesium.
  - Monitor serum creatinine every second day during induction and every week during maintenance.
- **DIRECTIONS FOR ADMINISTRATION** Avoid rapid infusion. For *intravenous infusion*, give undiluted solution via a central venous catheter; alternatively dilute to a concentration of 12 mg/mL with Glucose 5% *or* Sodium Chloride 0.9% for administration via a peripheral vein; give over at least 1 hour (give doses greater than 60 mg/kg over 2 hours).

- **MEDICINAL FORMS** There can be variation in the licensing of different medicines containing the same drug.

Solution for infusion

ELECTROLYTES: May contain Sodium

- Foscavir (Clinigen Healthcare Ltd)
  Foscarnet sodium 24 mg per 1 ml Foscavir 6g/250ml solution for infusion bottles | 1 bottle [PoM] £119.85 (Hospital only)

5.5 HIV infection

HIV infection

19-Apr-2020

Overview

The human immunodeficiency virus (HIV) is a retrovirus that causes immunodeficiency by infecting and destroying cells of the immune system, particularly the CD4 cells. The prognosis of HIV has greatly improved due to more effective and better tolerated antiretroviral therapy (ART). The greatest risk to excess mortality and morbidity is delayed HIV diagnosis and treatment.

Drug treatment should only be prescribed by specialists within a paediatric HIV clinical network.

Further information on the management of children with HIV can be obtained from the Children's HIV Association (CHIVA) www.chiva.org.uk. For further information on antiretroviral use and toxicity in children see Paediatric European Network for Treatment of AIDS (PENTA) guidelines for treatment of paediatric HIV-1 infection available at penta-id.org/ and the British HIV Association guidelines available at www.bhiva.org/guidelines.

Aims of treatment

Treatment aims to achieve an undetectable viral load, to preserve immune function, and to reduce the mortality and morbidity associated with chronic HIV infection whilst minimising drug toxicity. Treatment with a combination of ART aims to improve the physical and psychological well-being of infected children and optimise general health for a full and productive adult life.

Initiation of treatment

[EvGr] Antiretroviral therapy (ART) should be started in all children diagnosed with HIV irrespective of age, CD4 count and viral load. Infants born to women living with HIV require urgent diagnosis and treatment. The choice of antiviral treatment for children should take into account the method and frequency of administration, risk of side-effects, compatibility of drugs with food, palatability, and the appropriateness of the formulation. Additionally, potential transmitted resistance and resistance resulting from maternal or infant antiretroviral exposure during failed vertical transmission treatment should also be considered. ⟨A⟩ Commitment to treatment and strict adherence over many years are required.

[EvGr] In children, treatment of HIV infection is initiated with a combination of two nucleoside reverse transcriptase inhibitors (NRTI) as a backbone regimen plus *one* of the following as a third drug: an integrase inhibitor (INI), a non-nucleoside reverse transcriptase inhibitor (NNRTI), *or* a boosted protease inhibitor (PI).

Abacavir p. 451 with lamivudine p. 455 is the NRTI backbone combination of choice for initial therapy however, abacavir should not be given to children who are positive for the HLA-B*5701 allele. Alternative NRTI backbones regimens and third drug options, depending on the age of the child, can be found at penta-id.org/.

The metabolism of many antiretroviral drugs varies in young children, it may therefore be necessary to adjust the dose according to the plasma-drug concentration. Children who require treatment for both HIV and chronic hepatitis B should be treated with antivirals active against both diseases. ⟨A⟩

Switching therapy

[EvGr] Deterioration of the condition (including clinical, virological, and CD4 cell count changes) may require a change in therapy. The choice of an alternative regimen should be guided by factors such as the response to previous treatment, tolerability, drug-drug interactions, and the possibility of drug resistance. ⟨A⟩ For further information see Paediatric European Network for Treatment of AIDS (PENTA) HIV first and second line antiretroviral treatment guidelines available at www.chiva.org.uk.

HIV infection and pregnancy

[EvGr] Management of HIV infection in pregnancy should focus on the well-being of the women living with HIV, by ensuring that their ART regimen maximally suppresses viral replication as early as possible (if possible before conception) in order to minimise vertical transmission of HIV. Information on the teratogenic potential of most antiretroviral drugs is limited, however, all pregnant women living with HIV who conceive whilst on effective ART should continue this treatment throughout their pregnancy. All other women should start ART during their pregnancy. The recommended regimen is a NRTI backbone of either tenofovir disoproxil p. 456 or abacavir, with either emtricitabine p. 453 or lamivudine; the third drug should be efavirenz p. 448 or ritonavir-boosted p. 461 atazanavir p. 458. All treatment options require careful assessment by a specialist. ⟨A⟩ For further information, including alternative ART options, see British HIV Association guidelines for the management of HIV in pregnancy and postpartum available at www.bhiva.org/guidelines.

[EvGr] Pregnancies in women with HIV and babies born to them should be reported prospectively to the National Study of HIV in Pregnancy and Childhood at www.ucl.ac.uk/nshpc/ and to the Antiretroviral Pregnancy Registry at www.apregistry.com. ⟨A⟩

HIV infection and breast-feeding

[EvGr] Breast-feeding by HIV-positive mothers may cause HIV infection in the infant and should be avoided. ⟨A⟩ For further information see British HIV Association guidelines for the management of HIV in pregnancy and postpartum available at www.bhiva.org/guidelines.

HIV infection, post-exposure prophylaxis

[EvGr] Children exposed to HIV infection through needlestick injury or by another route should be sent immediately to an accident and emergency department for post-exposure prophylaxis [unlicensed indication]. ⟨A⟩ For further information see recommendations produced by the Children's HIV Association available at www.chiva.org.uk.

Drug treatment

Drugs that are licensed for the treatment of HIV/AIDS in children are listed below according to drug class.

Nucleoside reverse transcriptase inhibitors (NRTI or 'nucleoside analogue'): abacavir (ABC); emtricitabine (FTC), lamivudine (3TC); stavudine p. 456 (d4T), tenofovir alafenamide p. 434 fumarate (TAF), tenofovir disoproxil fumarate (TDF), and zidovudine p. 457 (AZT).

Non-nucleoside reverse transcriptase inhibitors (NNRTI):efavirenz (EFV), etravirine p. 449 (ETR), nevirapine p. 449 (NVP), and rilpivirine p. 450 (RPV).

Protease inhibitors (PI): atazanavir (ATZ), darunavir p. 459 (DRV), fosamprenavir p. 460 (FOS-APV), lopinavir (LPV), ritonavir (RTV), and tipranavir p. 462 (TPV).

CCR5 antagonist: maraviroc p. 462 (MVC).

Integrase inhibitors (INI): dolutegravir below (DTG), elvitegravir (EVG), and raltegravir p. 447 (RAL).

Fusion inhibitor: enfuvirtide below (T-20).

Pharmacokinetic enhancers: cobicistat (c), and low-dose ritonavir (r). They boost the concentrations of other antiretrovirals metabolised by CYP3A4, but have no antiretroviral activity themselves.

HIV infection in neonates

EvGr In order to prevent transmission of infection, neonates born to HIV-positive mothers should be given post-exposure prophylaxis as soon as possible (within 4 hours) after birth and starting no later than 72 hours after birth. Zidovudine monotherapy can be given where there is a very low or low risk of HIV transmission. Risk is determined by the mother's viral load at the time of delivery and whether the mother has been on combination ART for more than 10 weeks. Combination ART should be given to neonates at high risk of infection or whose mothers are found to be HIV positive after delivery. The preferred treatment regimen is zidovudine and lamivudine as the NRTI backbone and nevirapine as the third drug. Prophylaxis is given for 2–4 weeks depending on the risk of infection. ⟨A⟩ For further information see British HIV Association guidelines for the management of HIV in pregnancy and postpartum available at www.bhiva.org/guidelines.

ANTIVIRALS › HIV-FUSION INHIBITORS

Enfuvirtide

14-Jul-2018

- **DRUG ACTION** Enfuvirtide inhibits the fusion of HIV to the host cell.

- **INDICATIONS AND DOSE**

HIV infection in combination with other antiretroviral drugs for resistant infection or for patients intolerant to other antiretroviral regimens

▶ BY SUBCUTANEOUS INJECTION

▶ Child 6–15 years: 2 mg/kg twice daily (max. per dose 90 mg)

▶ Child 16–17 years: 90 mg twice daily

- **SIDE-EFFECTS**

▶ **Common or very common** Anxiety · appetite decreased · asthenia · concentration impaired · conjunctivitis · diabetes mellitus · gastrooesophageal reflux disease · haematuria · hypertriglyceridaemia · increased risk of infection · influenza like illness · irritability · lymphadenopathy · myalgia · nasal congestion · nephrolithiasis · nightmare · numbness · pancreatitis · peripheral neuropathy · skin papilloma · skin reactions · tremor · vertigo · weight decreased

▶ **Frequency not known** Diarrhoea · hypersensitivity · immune reconstitution inflammatory syndrome · nausea · osteonecrosis

SIDE-EFFECTS, FURTHER INFORMATION **Hypersensitivity** Hypersensitivity reactions including rash, fever, nausea, vomiting, chills, rigors, low blood pressure, respiratory distress, glomerulonephritis, and raised liver enzymes reported; discontinue immediately if any signs or symptoms of systemic hypersensitivity develop and do not rechallenge.

Osteonecrosis Osteonecrosis has been reported in patients with advanced HIV disease or following long-term exposure to combination antiretroviral therapy.

- **PREGNANCY** Manufacturer advises use only if potential benefit outweighs risk.
- **HEPATIC IMPAIRMENT** Manufacturer advises caution (no information available); increased risk of hepatic side effects in patients with chronic hepatitis B or C.
- **DIRECTIONS FOR ADMINISTRATION** For *subcutaneous injection*, reconstitute with 1.1 mL Water for Injections and allow to stand (for up to 45 minutes) to dissolve; do **not** shake or invert vial.
- **PATIENT AND CARER ADVICE**

Hypersensitivity reactions Patients or carers should be told how to recognise signs of hypersensitivity, and advised to discontinue treatment and seek immediate medical attention if symptoms develop.

- **MEDICINAL FORMS** There can be variation in the licensing of different medicines containing the same drug.

Powder and solvent for solution for injection

ELECTROLYTES: May contain Sodium

▶ Fuzeon (Roche Products Ltd)

Enfuvirtide 108 mg Fuzeon 108mg powder and solvent for solution for injection vials | 60 vial PoM £1,081.57

ANTIVIRALS › HIV-INTEGRASE INHIBITORS

Dolutegravir

11-Jul-2018

- **DRUG ACTION** Dolutegravir is an inhibitor of HIV integrase.

- **INDICATIONS AND DOSE**

HIV infection without resistance to other inhibitors of HIV integrase, in combination with other antiretroviral drugs

▶ BY MOUTH

▶ Child 12–17 years (body-weight 40 kg and above): 50 mg once daily

HIV infection in combination with other antiretroviral drugs (with concomitant carbamazepine, efavirenz, etravirine (without boosted protease inhibitors, but see also Interactions), fosphenytoin, phenobarbital, phenytoin, primidone, nevirapine, oxcarbazepine, St John's wort, rifampicin, or tipranavir)

▶ BY MOUTH

▶ Child 12–17 years (body-weight 40 kg and above): 50 mg twice daily, avoid concomitant use with these drugs if resistance to other inhibitors of HIV integrase suspected

IMPORTANT SAFETY INFORMATION

MHRA/CHM ADVICE: DOLUTEGRAVIR (*TIVICAY*®, *TRIUMEQ*®, *JULUCA*®): SIGNAL OF INCREASED RISK OF NEURAL TUBE DEFECTS; DO NOT PRESCRIBE TO WOMEN SEEKING TO BECOME PREGNANT; EXCLUDE PREGNANCY BEFORE INITIATION AND ADVISE USE OF EFFECTIVE CONTRACEPTION (JUNE 2018)

New safety recommendations have been issued while an EU review evaluates cases of neural tube defects in babies born to mothers who became pregnant while taking dolutegravir. The MHRA advises:

- dolutegravir should not be prescribed to women who are trying to become pregnant;
- pregnancy should be excluded in women of childbearing potential with pregnancy testing before starting dolutegravir;
- women of childbearing potential should be advised to use effective contraception throughout treatment with dolutegravir;

- if pregnancy is confirmed in the first trimester while a woman is taking dolutegravir, switch to an alternative treatment unless there is no suitable alternative;
- women taking dolutegravir for HIV should be advised not to stop taking their medicine without first consulting their doctor.

● **INTERACTIONS** → Appendix 1: dolutegravir

● **SIDE-EFFECTS**

▸ **Common or very common** Anxiety · depression · diarrhoea · dizziness · fatigue · flatulence · gastrointestinal discomfort · headache · nausea · skin reactions · sleep disorders · vomiting

▸ **Uncommon** Arthralgia · hepatic disorders · hypersensitivity · immune reconstitution inflammatory syndrome · myalgia · suicidal tendencies

SIDE-EFFECTS, FURTHER INFORMATION **Hypersensitivity** Hypersensitivity reactions (including severe rash, or rash accompanied by fever, malaise, arthralgia, myalgia, blistering, oral lesions, conjunctivitis, angioedema, eosinophilia, or raised liver enzymes) reported uncommonly. Discontinue immediately if any sign or symptoms of hypersensitivity reactions develop.

Osteonecrosis Osteonecrosis has been reported in patients with advanced HIV disease or following long-term exposure to combination antiretroviral therapy.

● **PREGNANCY** Manufacturer advises avoid, see *Important Safety Information*.

● **HEPATIC IMPAIRMENT** Manufacturer advises caution in severe impairment—no information available.

● **PATIENT AND CARER ADVICE** Patients or carers should be given advice on how to administer dolutegravir tablets.
Missed doses If a dose is more than 20 hours late on the once daily regimen (or more than 8 hours late on the twice daily regimen), the missed dose should not be taken and the next dose should be taken at the normal time.

● **NATIONAL FUNDING/ACCESS DECISIONS**

Scottish Medicines Consortium (SMC) decisions

The *Scottish Medicines Consortium* has advised (May 2014) that dolutegravir (*Tivicay*®) is accepted for use within NHS Scotland when used in combination with other anti-retroviral medicines for the treatment of HIV infected adolescents above 12 years. This advice is contingent upon the continuing availability of the patient access scheme in NHS Scotland or a list price that is equivalent or lower.

The *Scottish Medicines Consortium* has advised (July 2017) that dolutegravir (*Tivicay*®) is accepted for use within NHS Scotland when used in combination with other anti-retroviral medicines for the treatment of HIV infected children aged 6 to 12 years of age. This advice is contingent upon the continuing availability of the patient access scheme in NHS Scotland or a list price that is equivalent or lower.

All Wales Medicines Strategy Group (AWMSG) decisions

The *All Wales Medicines Strategy Group* has advised (October 2017) that dolutegravir (*Tivicay*®) is recommended as an option for use within NHS Wales in combination with other anti-retroviral medicinal products for the treatment of HIV infected patients above 6 years of age. This recommendation applies only in circumstances where the approved Wales Patient Access Scheme (WPAS) is utilised or where the list/contract price is equivalent or lower than the WPAS price.

● **MEDICINAL FORMS** There can be variation in the licensing of different medicines containing the same drug.

Tablet

▸ Tivicay (ViiV Healthcare UK Ltd)

Dolutegravir (as Dolutegravir sodium) 10 mg Tivicay 10mg tablets | 30 tablet PoM £99.75 DT = £99.75

Dolutegravir (as Dolutegravir sodium) 25 mg Tivicay 25mg tablets | 30 tablet PoM £249.38 DT = £249.38

Dolutegravir (as Dolutegravir sodium) 50 mg Tivicay 50mg tablets | 30 tablet PoM £498.75 DT = £498.75

Combinations available: ***Abacavir with dolutegravir and lamivudine***, p. 452 · ***Lamivudine with dolutegravir***, p. 456

5 Infection

Raltegravir

08-Feb-2019

● **DRUG ACTION** Raltegravir is an inhibitor of HIV integrase.

● **INDICATIONS AND DOSE**

HIV-1 infection (initiated by a specialist)

▸ BY MOUTH USING TABLETS

- Child (body-weight 25 kg and above): 400 mg twice daily
- Child (body-weight 40 kg and above): 1200 mg once daily, once daily dosing for use in patients who are treatment naive or virologically suppressed on an initial regimen of 400 mg twice daily—use 600 mg tablets only

▸ BY MOUTH USING CHEWABLE TABLETS

- Child (body-weight 11–13 kg): 75 mg twice daily
- Child (body-weight 14–19 kg): 100 mg twice daily
- Child (body-weight 20–27 kg): 150 mg twice daily
- Child (body-weight 28–39 kg): 200 mg twice daily
- Child (body-weight 40 kg and above): 300 mg twice daily

▸ BY MOUTH USING ORAL SUSPENSION

- Neonate up to 7 days (body-weight 2–2 kg): 4 mg once daily.
- Neonate up to 7 days (body-weight 3–3 kg): 5 mg once daily.
- Neonate up to 7 days (body-weight 4–4 kg): 7 mg once daily.
- Neonate 7 days to 28 days (body-weight 2–2 kg): 8 mg twice daily.
- Neonate 7 days to 28 days (body-weight 3–3 kg): 10 mg twice daily.
- Neonate 7 days to 28 days (body-weight 4–4 kg): 15 mg twice daily.
- Child (body-weight 3–3 kg): 25 mg twice daily
- Child (body-weight 4–5 kg): 30 mg twice daily
- Child (body-weight 6–7 kg): 40 mg twice daily
- Child (body-weight 8–10 kg): 60 mg twice daily
- Child (body-weight 11–13 kg): 80 mg twice daily
- Child (body-weight 14–19 kg): 100 mg twice daily

DOSE EQUIVALENCE AND CONVERSION

- Raltegravir granules for oral suspension and chewable tablets are **not** bioequivalent or interchangeable with the 400 mg and 600 mg *standard* tablets.

● **CONTRA-INDICATIONS** Pre-term neonates—no information available

● **CAUTIONS** Psychiatric illness (may exacerbate underlying illness including depression) · risk factors for myopathy · risk factors for rhabdomyolysis

● **INTERACTIONS** → Appendix 1: raltegravir

● **SIDE-EFFECTS**

▸ **Common or very common** Akathisia · appetite abnormal · asthenia · behaviour abnormal · depression · diarrhoea · dizziness · fever · gastrointestinal discomfort · gastrointestinal disorders · headaches · nausea · skin reactions · sleep disorders · vertigo · vomiting

▸ **Uncommon** Alopecia · anaemia · anxiety · arrhythmias · arthralgia · arthritis · body fat disorder · burping · cachexia · chest discomfort · chills · cognitive disorder · concentration impaired · confusion · constipation · diabetes mellitus · drowsiness · dry mouth · dyslipidaemia · dysphonia · erectile dysfunction · feeling jittery · glossitis ·

gynaecomastia · haemorrhage · hepatic disorders · hot flush · hyperglycaemia · hypersensitivity · hypertension · immune reconstitution inflammatory syndrome · increased risk of infection · lipodystrophy · lymph node abscess · lymphatic abnormalities · malaise · memory loss · menopausal symptoms · mood altered · myalgia · myopathy · nasal congestion · nephritis · nephrolithiasis · nerve disorders · neutropenia · nocturia · odynophagia · oedema · osteopenia · pain · palpitations · pancreatitis acute · polydipsia · psychiatric disorder · renal cyst · renal impairment · sensation abnormal · severe cutaneous adverse reactions (SCARs) · skin papilloma · submandibular mass · suicidal tendencies · sweat changes · taste altered · tendinitis · thrombocytopenia · tinnitus · tremor · visual impairment · weight increased

- **Frequency not known** Osteonecrosis

SIDE-EFFECTS, FURTHER INFORMATION Rash occurs commonly. Discontinue if severe rash or rash accompanied by fever, malaise, arthralgia, myalgia, blistering, mouth ulceration, conjunctivitis, angioedema, hepatitis, or eosinophilia.

- **PREGNANCY** Manufacturer advises avoid—toxicity in *animal* studies.
- **HEPATIC IMPAIRMENT** Manufacturer advises caution in severe impairment (no information available), and in patients with chronic hepatitis B or C (consider interrupting or discontinuing treatment if impairment worsens; increased risk of hepatic side-effects).
- **DIRECTIONS FOR ADMINISTRATION** Manufacturer advises for *chewable tablets*, the 100 mg strength can be divided into equal 50 mg doses.
- **PRESCRIBING AND DISPENSING INFORMATION** Dispense raltegravir chewable tablets in original container (contains desiccant).
- **NATIONAL FUNDING/ACCESS DECISIONS**

Scottish Medicines Consortium (SMC) decisions

SMC No. 902/13

The *Scottish Medicines Consortium* has advised (September 2013) that raltegravir (*Isentress*®) is accepted for restricted use within NHS Scotland for the treatment of HIV-1 infection in adolescents and children aged 2 to 17 years when non-nucleoside reverse transcriptase inhibitors or protease inhibitors cannot be used because of intolerance, drug interactions, or resistance; raltegravir should be prescribed under the supervision of specialists in paediatric HIV.

SMC No. 1102/15

The *Scottish Medicines Consortium* has advised (November 2015) that raltegravir granules for oral suspension (*Isentress*®) are accepted for restricted use within NHS Scotland for the treatment of HIV-1 infection in adults, adolescents, children, toddlers and infants from the age of 4 weeks when non-nucleoside reverse transcriptase inhibitors or protease inhibitors cannot be used because of intolerance, drug interactions, or resistance; raltegravir granules should be prescribed under the supervision of specialists in paediatric HIV.

SMC No. 1113/15

The *Scottish Medicines Consortium* has advised (November 2015) that raltegravir chewable tablets (*Isentress*®) are accepted for restricted use within NHS Scotland for the treatment of HIV-1 infection in children from the age of 4 weeks to <2 years when non-nucleoside reverse transcriptase inhibitors or protease inhibitors cannot be used because of intolerance, drug interactions, or resistance; raltegravir chewable tablets should be prescribed under the supervision of specialists in paediatric HIV.

SMC No. 1280/17

The *Scottish Medicines Consortium* has advised (November 2017) that raltegravir 600 mg film-coated tablets (*Isentress*®) are accepted for restricted use within NHS Scotland for the treatment of HIV-1 infection in adults and paediatric patients weighing at least 40 kg when non-nucleoside reverse transcriptase inhibitors or protease inhibitors cannot be used because of intolerance, drug interactions, or resistance.

- **MEDICINAL FORMS** There can be variation in the licensing of different medicines containing the same drug.

Granules

EXCIPIENTS: May contain Sorbitol

- Isentress (Merck Sharp & Dohme Ltd)
  Raltegravir 100 mg Isentress 100mg granules sachets | 60 sachet PoM £213.02 DT = £213.02

Tablet

CAUTIONARY AND ADVISORY LABELS 25

- Isentress (Merck Sharp & Dohme Ltd)
  Raltegravir 400 mg Isentress 400mg tablets | 60 tablet PoM £471.41 DT = £471.41
  Raltegravir 600 mg Isentress 600mg tablets | 60 tablet PoM £471.41 DT = £471.41

Chewable tablet

CAUTIONARY AND ADVISORY LABELS 24

EXCIPIENTS: May contain Aspartame

- Isentress (Merck Sharp & Dohme Ltd)
  Raltegravir 25 mg Isentress 25mg chewable tablets | 60 tablet PoM £29.46 DT = £29.46
  Raltegravir 100 mg Isentress 100mg chewable tablets | 60 tablet PoM £117.85 DT = £117.85

ANTIVIRALS > NON-NUCLEOSIDE REVERSE TRANSCRIPTASE INHIBITORS

Efavirenz

- **INDICATIONS AND DOSE**

HIV infection in combination with other antiretroviral drugs

- BY MOUTH USING CAPSULES
- Child 3 months–17 years (body-weight 3.5–4 kg): 100 mg once daily
- Child 3 months–17 years (body-weight 5–7.4 kg): 150 mg once daily
- Child 3 months–17 years (body-weight 7.5–14 kg): 200 mg once daily
- Child 3 months–17 years (body-weight 15–19 kg): 250 mg once daily
- Child 3 months–17 years (body-weight 20–24 kg): 300 mg once daily
- Child 3 months–17 years (body-weight 25–32.4 kg): 350 mg once daily
- Child 3 months–17 years (body-weight 32.5–39 kg): 400 mg once daily
- Child 3 months–17 years (body-weight 40 kg and above): 600 mg once daily
- BY MOUTH USING TABLETS
- Child (body-weight 40 kg and above): 600 mg once daily

- **CAUTIONS** Acute porphyrias p. 652 · history of psychiatric disorders · history of seizures
- **INTERACTIONS** → Appendix 1: efavirenz
- **SIDE-EFFECTS**
- **Common or very common** Abdominal pain · anxiety · concentration impaired · depression · diarrhoea · dizziness · drowsiness · dyslipidaemia · fatigue · headache · movement disorders · nausea · skin reactions · sleep disorders · vomiting
- **Uncommon** Behaviour abnormal · confusion · flushing · gynaecomastia · hallucination · hepatic disorders · memory loss · mood altered · pancreatitis · psychosis · seizure · Stevens-Johnson syndrome · suicidal tendencies · thinking abnormal · tinnitus · tremor · vertigo · vision blurred
- **Rare or very rare** Delusions · photosensitivity reaction

- **Frequency not known** Immune reconstitution inflammatory syndrome · osteonecrosis

SIDE-EFFECTS, FURTHER INFORMATION **Rash** Rash, usually in the first 2 weeks, is the most common side-effect; discontinue if severe rash with blistering, desquamation, mucosal involvement or fever; if rash mild or moderate, may continue without interruption—usually resolves within 1 month.

CNS effects Administration at bedtime especially in first 2–4 weeks reduces CNS effects.

Abnormal hepatic function Manufacturer advises interrupt or discontinue treatment if transaminases more than 5 times the upper limit of normal.

- PREGNANCY Reports of neural tube defects when used in first trimester.
- HEPATIC IMPAIRMENT Greater risk of hepatic side-effects in chronic hepatitis B or C. Manufacturer advises avoid in severe impairment (limited information available).
- RENAL IMPAIRMENT Manufacturer advises caution in severe renal failure—no information available.
- MONITORING REQUIREMENTS Monitor liver function if receiving other hepatotoxic drugs.
- DIRECTIONS FOR ADMINISTRATION For patients who cannot swallow capsules, the capsule may be opened and contents added to a small amount of food—consult product literature. No additional food should be consumed for up to 2 hours after administration of efavirenz.
- PATIENT AND CARER ADVICE

Psychiatric disorders Patients or their carers should be advised to seek immediate medical attention if symptoms such as severe depression, psychosis or suicidal ideation occur.

- MEDICINAL FORMS There can be variation in the licensing of different medicines containing the same drug.

Tablet

CAUTIONARY AND ADVISORY LABELS 23

- Efavirenz (Non-proprietary)

Efavirenz 600 mg Efavirenz 600mg tablets | 30 tablet PoM £31.35–£452.94 | 30 tablet PoM £31.41 (Hospital only)

- Sustiva (Bristol-Myers Squibb Pharmaceuticals Ltd)

Efavirenz 600 mg Sustiva 600mg tablets | 30 tablet PoM £200.27 (Hospital only)

Capsule

CAUTIONARY AND ADVISORY LABELS 23

- Sustiva (Bristol-Myers Squibb Pharmaceuticals Ltd)

Efavirenz 50 mg Sustiva 50mg capsules | 30 capsule PoM £16.73 (Hospital only)

Efavirenz 100 mg Sustiva 100mg capsules | 30 capsule PoM £33.41 (Hospital only)

Efavirenz 200 mg Sustiva 200mg capsules | 90 capsule PoM £200.27 (Hospital only)

Etravirine

12-Jul-2018

- **INDICATIONS AND DOSE**

HIV infection resistant to other non-nucleoside reverse transcriptase inhibitor and protease inhibitors in combination with other antiretroviral drugs (including a boosted protease inhibitor)

- BY MOUTH
- Child 6–17 years (body-weight 16–19 kg): 100 mg twice daily
- Child 6–17 years (body-weight 20–24 kg): 125 mg twice daily
- Child 6–17 years (body-weight 25–29 kg): 150 mg twice daily
- Child 6–17 years (body-weight 30 kg and above): 200 mg twice daily

- CONTRA-INDICATIONS Acute porphyrias p. 652
- INTERACTIONS → Appendix 1: etravirine
- SIDE-EFFECTS
- **Common or very common** Diabetes mellitus · diarrhoea · headache · hyperglycaemia · myocardial infarction · nausea · skin reactions · vomiting
- **Uncommon** Angioedema · bronchospasm · dry mouth · dyslipidaemia · gynaecomastia · haematemesis · hepatic disorders · hyperhidrosis · hypersensitivity · hypersomnia · numbness · pancreatitis · sluggishness · vision blurred
- **Rare or very rare** Severe cutaneous adverse reactions (SCARs)
- **Frequency not known** Haemorrhagic stroke · osteonecrosis · weight increased

SIDE-EFFECTS, FURTHER INFORMATION **Hypersensitivity reactions** Rash, usually in the second week, is the most common side-effect and appears more frequently in females. Life-threatening hypersensitivity reactions reported usually during week 3–6 of treatment and characterised by rash, eosinophilia, and systemic symptoms (including fever, general malaise, myalgia, arthralgia, blistering, oral lesions, conjunctivitis, and hepatitis). Discontinue permanently if hypersensitivity reaction or severe rash develop. If rash mild or moderate (without signs of hypersensitivity reaction), may continue without interruption—usually resolves within 2 weeks.

- HEPATIC IMPAIRMENT Manufacturer advises caution in moderate impairment and in patients with hepatitis B or C (increased risk of hepatic side effects); avoid in severe impairment (no information available).
- DIRECTIONS FOR ADMINISTRATION Patients with swallowing difficulties may disperse tablets in a glass of water just before administration.
- PRESCRIBING AND DISPENSING INFORMATION Dispense in original container (contains desiccant).
- PATIENT AND CARER ADVICE

Hypersensitivity reactions Patients or carers should be told how to recognise hypersensitivity reactions and advised to seek immediate medical attention if hypersensitivity reaction or severe rash develop.

Missed doses If a dose is more than 6 hours late, the missed dose should not be taken and the next dose should be taken at the normal time.

- MEDICINAL FORMS There can be variation in the licensing of different medicines containing the same drug.

Tablet

CAUTIONARY AND ADVISORY LABELS 21

- Intelence (Janssen-Cilag Ltd)

Etravirine 100 mg Intelence 100mg tablets | 120 tablet PoM £301.27

Etravirine 200 mg Intelence 200mg tablets | 60 tablet PoM £301.27

Nevirapine

- **INDICATIONS AND DOSE**

HIV infection in combination with other antiretroviral drugs (initial dose)

- BY MOUTH USING IMMEDIATE-RELEASE MEDICINES
- Child: Initially 150–200 mg/m^2 once daily (max. per dose 200 mg) for first 14 days, initial dose titration using 'immediate-release' preparation should not exceed 28 days; if rash occurs and is not resolved within 28 days, alternative treatment should be sought. If treatment interrupted for more than 7 days, restart using the lower dose of the 'immediate-release' preparation for the first 14 days as for new treatment

continued →

5 Infection

HIV infection in combination with other antiretroviral drugs (maintenance dose following initial dose titration if no rash present)
- ▶ BY MOUTH USING IMMEDIATE-RELEASE MEDICINES
- ▶ Child 1 month–2 years: 150–200 mg/m^2 twice daily (max. per dose 200 mg), alternatively 300–400 mg/m^2 once daily (max. per dose 400 mg)
- ▶ Child 3–17 years: 150–200 mg/m^2 twice daily (max. per dose 200 mg)

HIV infection in combination with other antiretroviral drugs (maintenance dose following initial dose titration if no rash present)
- ▶ BY MOUTH USING IMMEDIATE-RELEASE MEDICINES
- ▶ Child 3–17 years (body surface area 0.58–0.83 m^2): 200 mg once daily
- ▶ Child 3–17 years (body surface area 0.84–1.17 m^2): 300 mg once daily
- ▶ Child 3–17 years (body surface area 1.18 m^2 and above): 400 mg once daily
- ▶ BY MOUTH USING MODIFIED-RELEASE MEDICINES
- ▶ Child 3–17 years (body surface area 0.58–0.83 m^2): 200 mg once daily
- ▶ Child 3–17 years (body surface area 0.84–1.17 m^2): 300 mg once daily
- ▶ Child 3–17 years (body surface area 1.18 m^2 and above): 400 mg once daily

- **UNLICENSED USE** 'Immediate-release' tablets not licensed for use in children weighing less than 50 kg or with body surface area less than 1.25 m^2; 'immediate-release' tablets and suspension not licensed for once daily dose after the initial dose titration.
- **CONTRA-INDICATIONS** Acute porphyrias p. 652 · post-exposure prophylaxis
- **CAUTIONS** Females (at greater risk of hepatic side effects) · high CD4 cell count (at greater risk of hepatic side effects)
- **INTERACTIONS** → Appendix 1: nevirapine
- **SIDE-EFFECTS**
- ▶ **Common or very common** Abdominal pain · angioedema · diarrhoea · fatigue · fever · headache · hepatic disorders · hypersensitivity · hypertransaminasaemia · nausea · skin reactions · vomiting
- ▶ **Uncommon** Anaemia · arthralgia · myalgia · severe cutaneous adverse reactions (SCARs)
- ▶ **Frequency not known** Eosinophilia · osteonecrosis · weight increased

SIDE-EFFECTS, FURTHER INFORMATION **Hepatic effects** Potentially life-threatening hepatotoxicity including fatal fulminant hepatitis reported usually in first 6 weeks; discontinue permanently if abnormalities in liver function tests accompanied by hypersensitivity reaction (rash, fever, arthralgia, myalgia, lymphadenopathy, hepatitis, renal impairment, eosinophilia, granulocytopenia); suspend if severe abnormalities in liver function tests but no hypersensitivity reaction—discontinue permanently if significant liver function abnormalities recur; monitor patient closely if mild to moderate abnormalities in liver function tests with no hypersensitivity reaction.

Rash Rash, usually in first 6 weeks, is most common side-effect; incidence reduced if introduced at low dose and dose increased gradually (after 14 days); Discontinue permanently if severe rash or if rash accompanied by blistering, oral lesions, conjunctivitis, facial oedema, general malaise or hypersensitivity reactions; if rash mild or moderate may continue without interruption but dose should not be increased until rash resolves.

Osteonecrosis Osteonecrosis has been reported in patients with advanced HIV disease or following long-term exposure to combination antiretroviral therapy.

- **HEPATIC IMPAIRMENT** For *modified-release* preparations, manufacturer advises avoid (no information available). For *immediate-release* preparations, manufacturer advises caution in moderate impairment and chronic hepatitis (increased risk of hepatic side effects; consider interrupting or discontinuing treatment if hepatic function worsens); avoid in severe impairment (no information available).
- **RENAL IMPAIRMENT** Manufacturer advises avoid modified-release preparation—no information available.
- **MONITORING REQUIREMENTS**
- ▶ Hepatic disease Close monitoring of liver function required during first 18 weeks; monitor liver function before treatment then every 2 weeks for 2 months then after 1 month and then regularly.
- ▶ Rash Monitor closely for skin reactions during first 18 weeks.
- **PATIENT AND CARER ADVICE**

Hypersensitivity reactions Patients or carers should be told how to recognise hypersensitivity reactions and advised to discontinue treatment and seek immediate medical attention if severe skin reaction, hypersensitivity reactions, or symptoms of hepatitis develop.

- **MEDICINAL FORMS** There can be variation in the licensing of different medicines containing the same drug.

Oral suspension
- ▶ Viramune (Boehringer Ingelheim Ltd)
  Nevirapine (as Nevirapine hemihydrate) 10 mg per 1 ml Viramune 50mg/5ml oral suspension | 240 ml PoM £50.40

Modified-release tablet

CAUTIONARY AND ADVISORY LABELS 25
- ▶ Nevirapine (Non-proprietary)
  Nevirapine 400 mg Nevirapine 400mg modified-release tablets | 30 tablet PoM £52.13–£170.00 DT = £81.75
- ▶ Viramune (Boehringer Ingelheim Ltd)
  Nevirapine 100 mg Viramune 100mg modified-release tablets | 90 tablet PoM £127.50 (Hospital only)

Tablet
- ▶ Nevirapine (Non-proprietary)
  Nevirapine 200 mg Nevirapine 200mg tablets | 60 tablet PoM £21.45–£170.00

Rilpivirine

07-Feb-2019

- **INDICATIONS AND DOSE**

HIV infection in combination with other antiretroviral drugs in patients not previously treated with antiretroviral therapy and if plasma HIV-1 RNA concentration less than or equal to 100 000 copies/mL
- ▶ BY MOUTH
- ▶ Child 12–17 years: 25 mg once daily

- **CAUTIONS** Acute porphyrias p. 652
- **INTERACTIONS** → Appendix 1: rilpivirine
- **SIDE-EFFECTS**
- ▶ **Common or very common** Appetite decreased · depression · dizziness · drowsiness · dry mouth · fatigue · gastrointestinal discomfort · headache · nausea · rash · sleep disorders · vomiting
- ▶ **Uncommon** Immune reconstitution inflammatory syndrome
- **PREGNANCY** Manufacturer advises avoid unless essential— no information available.
- **HEPATIC IMPAIRMENT** Manufacturer advises caution in moderate impairment (limited information available); avoid in severe impairment (no information available).
- **RENAL IMPAIRMENT** Manufacturer advises caution in severe impairment.
- **PATIENT AND CARER ADVICE** Patients or carers should be given advice on how to administer rilpivirine tablets.

Missed doses If a dose is more than 12 hours late, the missed dose should not be taken and the next dose should be taken at the normal time.

- **NATIONAL FUNDING/ACCESS DECISIONS**

All Wales Medicines Strategy Group (AWMSG) decisions

AWMSG No. 2936

The *All Wales Medicines Strategy Group* has advised (October 2016) that rilpivirine (*Edurant*®) is recommended as an option for use within NHS Wales in combination with other antiretroviral medicinal products for the treatment of human immunodeficiency virus type 1 (HIV-1) infection in antiretroviral treatment-naive patients from 12 years old to < 18 years old with a viral load ≤ 100,000 HIV-1 RNA copies/ml.

- **MEDICINAL FORMS** There can be variation in the licensing of different medicines containing the same drug.

Tablet

CAUTIONARY AND ADVISORY LABELS 3, 21, 25

- Edurant (Janssen-Cilag Ltd)
  Rilpivirine (as Rilpivirine hydrochloride) 25 mg Edurant 25mg tablets | 30 tablet PoM £200.27

Combinations available: *Emtricitabine with rilpivirine and tenofovir alafenamide*, p. 453

ANTIVIRALS > NUCLEOSIDE REVERSE TRANSCRIPTASE INHIBITORS

Nucleoside reverse transcriptase inhibitors

- **SIDE-EFFECTS**
- **Common or very common** Abdominal pain · anaemia (may require transfusion) · asthenia · diarrhoea · dizziness · headache · insomnia · nausea · neutropenia · skin reactions · vomiting
- **Uncommon** Angioedema · lactic acidosis · pancreatitis
- **Frequency not known** Immune reconstitution inflammatory syndrome · osteonecrosis

SIDE-EFFECTS, FURTHER INFORMATION Osteonecrosis has been reported in patients with advanced HIV disease or following long-term exposure to combination antiretroviral therapy.

- **PREGNANCY**

Monitoring Mitochondrial dysfunction has been reported in infants exposed to nucleoside reverse transcriptase inhibitors in utero; the main effects include haematological, metabolic, and neurological disorders; all infants whose mothers received nucleoside reverse transcriptase inhibitors during pregnancy should be monitored for relevant signs or symptoms.

- **HEPATIC IMPAIRMENT** In general, manufacturers advise caution in patients with chronic hepatitis B or C (increased risk of hepatic side-effects).

above

Abacavir

10-Sep-2018

- **INDICATIONS AND DOSE**

HIV infection in combination with other antiretroviral drugs

- BY MOUTH
- Child 3 months–11 years: 8 mg/kg twice daily (max. per dose 300 mg), alternatively 16 mg/kg once daily (max. per dose 600 mg)
- Child 3 months–11 years (body-weight 14–20 kg): 150 mg twice daily, alternatively 300 mg once daily
- Child 3 months–11 years (body-weight 21–29 kg): 150 mg, taken in the morning and 300 mg, taken in the evening, alternatively 450 mg once daily
- Child 3 months–11 years (body-weight 30 kg and above): 300 mg twice daily, alternatively 600 mg once daily
- Child 12–17 years: 300 mg twice daily, alternatively 600 mg once daily

- **INTERACTIONS** → Appendix 1: abacavir
- **SIDE-EFFECTS**
- **Common or very common** Appetite decreased · fever · lethargy
- **Rare or very rare** Severe cutaneous adverse reactions (SCARs)
- **Frequency not known** Hypersensitivity · weight increased

SIDE-EFFECTS, FURTHER INFORMATION Life-threatening hypersensitivity reactions have been reported-characterised by fever or rash and possibly nausea, vomiting, diarrhoea, abdominal pain, dyspnoea, cough, lethargy, malaise, headache, and myalgia; less frequently mouth ulceration, oedema, hypotension, sore throat, acute respiratory distress syndrome, anaphylaxis, paraesthesia, arthralgia, conjunctivitis, lymphadenopathy, lymphocytopenia and renal failure; rarely myolysis. Laboratory abnormalities may include raised liver function tests and creatine kinase; symptoms usually appear in the first 6 weeks, but may occur at any time. Discontinue immediately if any symptom of hypersensitivity develops and do not rechallenge (risk of more severe hypersensitivity reaction).

- **ALLERGY AND CROSS-SENSITIVITY** Caution—increased risk of hypersensitivity reaction in presence of HLA-B*5701 allele.
- **HEPATIC IMPAIRMENT** Manufacturer advises caution in mild impairment; consider avoiding in moderate to severe impairment (no information available).
- **RENAL IMPAIRMENT** Manufacturer advises avoid in end-stage renal disease.
- **PRE-TREATMENT SCREENING** Test for HLA-B*5701 allele before treatment or if restarting treatment and HLA-B*5701 status not known.
- **MONITORING REQUIREMENTS** Monitor for symptoms of hypersensitivity reaction every 2 weeks for 2 months.
- **PRESCRIBING AND DISPENSING INFORMATION** Flavours of oral liquid formulations may include banana, or strawberry.
- **PATIENT AND CARER ADVICE** Patients and their carers should be told the importance of regular dosing (intermittent therapy may increase the risk of sensitisation), how to recognise signs of hypersensitivity, and advised to seek immediate medical attention if symptoms develop or before re-starting treatment.

Patients should be provided with an alert card and advised to keep it with them at all times.

- **MEDICINAL FORMS** There can be variation in the licensing of different medicines containing the same drug.

Oral solution

EXCIPIENTS: May contain Propylene glycol

- Ziagen (ViiV Healthcare UK Ltd)
  Abacavir (as Abacavir sulfate) 20 mg per 1 ml Ziagen 20mg/ml oral solution sugar-free | 240 ml PoM £55.72

Tablet

- Abacavir (Non-proprietary)
  Abacavir (as Abacavir sulfate) 300 mg Abacavir 300mg tablets | 60 tablet PoM £177.60–£177.61
- Ziagen (ViiV Healthcare UK Ltd)
  Abacavir (as Abacavir sulfate) 300 mg Ziagen 300mg tablets | 60 tablet PoM £208.95

Abacavir with dolutegravir and lamivudine

The properties listed below are those particular to the combination only. For the properties of the components please consider, abacavir p. 451, lamivudine p. 455, dolutegravir p. 446.

- **INDICATIONS AND DOSE**

HIV infection

▶ BY MOUTH

▶ Child 12–17 years (body-weight 40 kg and above): 1 tablet once daily

- **INTERACTIONS** → Appendix 1: abacavir · dolutegravir · lamivudine
- **RENAL IMPAIRMENT** Avoid *Triumeq®* if estimated glomerular filtration rate less than 50 mL/minute/1.73 m^2.
- **PATIENT AND CARER ADVICE**
Missed doses If a dose is more than 20 hours late, the missed dose should not be taken and the next dose should be taken at the normal time.

- **MEDICINAL FORMS** There can be variation in the licensing of different medicines containing the same drug.

Tablet

▶ Triumeq (ViiV Healthcare UK Ltd)
Dolutegravir (as Dolutegravir sodium) 50 mg, Lamivudine 300 mg, Abacavir (as Abacavir sulfate) 600 mg Triumeq 50mg/600mg/300mg tablets | 30 tablet PoM £798.16

Abacavir with lamivudine

The properties listed below are those particular to the combination only. For the properties of the components please consider, abacavir p. 451, lamivudine p. 455.

- **INDICATIONS AND DOSE**

HIV infection in combination with other antiretrovirals

▶ BY MOUTH

▶ Child 12–17 years (body-weight 40 kg and above): 1 tablet once daily

- **INTERACTIONS** → Appendix 1: abacavir · lamivudine
- **RENAL IMPAIRMENT** Avoid *Kivexa®* if estimated glomerular filtration rate less than 50 mL/minute/1.73 m^2.

- **MEDICINAL FORMS** There can be variation in the licensing of different medicines containing the same drug.

Tablet

▶ Abacavir with lamivudine (Non-proprietary)
Lamivudine 300 mg, Abacavir 600 mg Abacavir 600mg / Lamivudine 300mg tablets | 30 tablet PoM £352.25 DT = £190.00 | 30 tablet PoM £224.56 DT = £190.00 (Hospital only)

▶ Kivexa (ViiV Healthcare UK Ltd)
Lamivudine 300 mg, Abacavir 600 mg Kivexa 600mg/300mg tablets | 30 tablet PoM £352.25 DT = £190.00

Abacavir with lamivudine and zidovudine

The properties listed below are those particular to the combination only. For the properties of the components please consider, abacavir p. 451, lamivudine p. 455, zidovudine p. 457.

- **INDICATIONS AND DOSE**

HIV infection (use only if patient is stabilised for 6–8 weeks on the individual components in the same proportions)

▶ BY MOUTH

▶ Child (body-weight 30 kg and above): 1 tablet twice daily

- **UNLICENSED USE** *Trizivir®* not licensed for use in children.
- **INTERACTIONS** → Appendix 1: abacavir · lamivudine · zidovudine
- **RENAL IMPAIRMENT** Avoid *Trizivir®* if estimated glomerular filtration rate less than 50 mL/minute/1.73 m^2.

- **MEDICINAL FORMS** There can be variation in the licensing of different medicines containing the same drug.

Tablet

▶ Trizivir (ViiV Healthcare UK Ltd)
Lamivudine 150 mg, Abacavir (as Abacavir sulfate) 300 mg, Zidovudine 300 mg Trizivir tablets | 60 tablet PoM £509.06

Elvitegravir with cobicistat, emtricitabine and tenofovir alafenamide

22-May-2019

The properties listed below are those particular to the combination only. For the properties of the components please consider, emtricitabine p. 453, elvitegravir, cobicistat, tenofovir alafenamide p. 434.

- **INDICATIONS AND DOSE**

HIV-1 infection (specialist use only)

▶ BY MOUTH

▶ Child 6–11 years (body-weight 25 kg and above): 1 tablet once daily

▶ Child 12–17 years (body-weight 35 kg and above): 1 tablet once daily

IMPORTANT SAFETY INFORMATION

MHRA/CHM ADVICE: ELVITEGRAVIR BOOSTED WITH COBICISTAT: AVOID USE IN PREGNANCY DUE TO RISK OF TREATMENT FAILURE AND MATERNAL-TO-CHILD TRANSMISSION OF HIV-1 (APRIL 2019)

Pharmacokinetic data show mean exposure of elvitegravir boosted with cobicistat (available in combination in *Genvoya®* and *Stribild®*) to be lower during the second and third trimesters of pregnancy than postpartum. Low elvitegravir exposure may be associated with an increased risk of treatment failure and an increased risk of HIV-1 transmission to the unborn child. For further information, see *Pregnancy*.

- **INTERACTIONS** → Appendix 1: cobicistat · elvitegravir · tenofovir alafenamide
- **SIDE-EFFECTS**

▶ **Common or very common** Abnormal dreams · diarrhoea · dizziness · fatigue · flatulence · gastrointestinal discomfort · headache · nausea · skin reactions · vomiting

▶ **Uncommon** Anaemia · angioedema · depression

▶ **Frequency not known** Nephrotoxicity · osteonecrosis · weight increased

- **CONCEPTION AND CONTRACEPTION** Manufacturer advises effective contraception in women of childbearing potential; if using a hormonal contraceptive, it must contain drospirenone or norgestimate as the progestogen and at least 30 micrograms ethinylestradiol.
- **PREGNANCY** Manufacturer advises not to be initiated during pregnancy due to low elvitegravir exposure; women who become pregnant during therapy should be switched to an alternative regimen.
- **HEPATIC IMPAIRMENT** Manufacturer advises caution (increased risk of hepatic side-effects); avoid in severe impairment (no information available).
- **RENAL IMPAIRMENT** Manufacturer advises avoid if creatinine clearance less than 30 mL/minute—limited information available. Manufacturer advises caution in children under 12 years with renal impairment—no information available.

- **PRESCRIBING AND DISPENSING INFORMATION** Dispense in original container—contains desiccant.
- **PATIENT AND CARER ADVICE**

Missed doses Manufacturer advises if a dose is more than 18 hours late, the missed dose should not be taken and the next dose should be taken at the normal time.

Driving and skilled tasks Manufacturer advises patients and carers should be counselled on the effects on driving and performance of skilled tasks—increased risk of dizziness.

- **NATIONAL FUNDING/ACCESS DECISIONS**

Scottish Medicines Consortium (SMC) decisions

SMC No. 1142/16

The *Scottish Medicines Consortium* has advised (May 2016) that elvitegravir with cobicistat, emtricitabine and tenofovir alafenamide (*Genvoya®*) is accepted for use within NHS Scotland for the treatment of adults and adolescents (aged 12 years and older with body weight at least 35 kg) infected with human immunodeficiency virus-1 (HIV-1), without known mutations associated with resistance to the integrase inhibitor class, emtricitabine or tenofovir. This advice is contingent upon the continuing availability of the patient access scheme in NHS Scotland or a list price that is equivalent or lower.

All Wales Medicines Strategy Group (AWMSG) decisions

AWMSG No. 2248

The *All Wales Medicines Strategy Group* has advised (July 2016) that elvitegravir with cobicistat, emtricitabine and tenofovir alafenamide (*Genvoya®*) is recommended as an option for use within NHS Wales for the treatment of adults and adolescents (aged 12 years and older with body weight at least 35 kg) infected with human immunodeficiency virus-1 (HIV-1), without known mutations associated with resistance to the integrase inhibitor class, emtricitabine or tenofovir. The recommendation applies only if the approved Wales Patient Access Scheme (WPAS) is used or where the list price is equivalent or lower.

- **MEDICINAL FORMS** There can be variation in the licensing of different medicines containing the same drug.

Tablet

CAUTIONARY AND ADVISORY LABELS 21

- Genvoya (Gilead Sciences International Ltd) ▼

Tenofovir alafenamide 10 mg, Cobicistat 150 mg, Elvitegravir 150 mg, Emtricitabine 200 mg Genvoya 150mg/150mg/200mg/10mg tablets | 30 tablet PoM £879.51

451

Emtricitabine

(FTC)

- **INDICATIONS AND DOSE**

HIV infection in combination with other antiretroviral drugs

- BY MOUTH USING CAPSULES
  - Child (body-weight 33 kg and above): 200 mg once daily
- BY MOUTH USING ORAL SOLUTION
  - Child 4 months–17 years (body-weight up to 33 kg): 6 mg/kg once daily
  - Child 4 months–17 years (body-weight 33 kg and above): 240 mg once daily

DOSE EQUIVALENCE AND CONVERSION

- 240 mg oral solution ≡ 200 mg capsule; where appropriate the capsule may be used instead of the oral solution.

- **SIDE-EFFECTS**
  - **Common or very common** Abnormal dreams · dyspepsia · hyperbilirubinaemia · hyperglycaemia · hypersensitivity · hypertriglyceridaemia · pain · rash pustular
  - **Frequency not known** Weight increased
- **HEPATIC IMPAIRMENT**

Monitoring On discontinuation, monitor patients with hepatitis B (risk of exacerbation of hepatitis).

- **RENAL IMPAIRMENT**

Dose adjustments Reduce dose or increase dosage interval if estimated glomerular filtration rate less than 50 mL/minute/1.73 m^2; consult product literature.

- **PRESCRIBING AND DISPENSING INFORMATION** Flavours of oral liquid formulations may include candy.
- **PATIENT AND CARER ADVICE**

Missed doses If a dose is more than 12 hours late, the missed dose should not be taken and the next dose should be taken at the normal time.

- **MEDICINAL FORMS** There can be variation in the licensing of different medicines containing the same drug.

Oral solution

ELECTROLYTES: May contain Sodium

- Emtriva (Gilead Sciences International Ltd)

Emtricitabine 10 mg per 1 ml Emtriva 10mg/ml oral solution sugar-free | 170 ml PoM £39.53

Capsule

- Emtriva (Gilead Sciences International Ltd)

Emtricitabine 200 mg Emtriva 200mg capsules | 30 capsule PoM £138.98

Combinations available: *Darunavir with cobicistat, emtricitabine and tenofovir alafenamide,* p. 460

Emtricitabine with rilpivirine and tenofovir alafenamide

05-Jun-2017

The properties listed below are those particular to the combination only. For the properties of the components please consider, emtricitabine above, rilpivirine p. 450, tenofovir alafenamide p. 434.

- **INDICATIONS AND DOSE**

HIV infection in patients with plasma HIV-1 RNA concentration of 100 000 copies/mL or less (specialist use only)

- BY MOUTH
  - Child 12–17 years (body-weight 35 kg and above): 1 tablet once daily

- **INTERACTIONS** → Appendix 1: rilpivirine · tenofovir alafenamide
- **SIDE-EFFECTS**
  - **Common or very common** Appetite decreased · depression · diarrhoea · dizziness · drowsiness · dry mouth · fatigue · flatulence · gastrointestinal discomfort · headache · nausea · skin reactions · sleep disorders · vomiting
  - **Uncommon** Anaemia · angioedema · arthralgia · immune reconstitution inflammatory syndrome
  - **Frequency not known** Conjunctivitis · drug reaction with eosinophilia and systemic symptoms (DRESS) · eosinophilia · fever · osteonecrosis · QT interval prolongation · weight increased

SIDE-EFFECTS, FURTHER INFORMATION Systemic symptoms reported with severe skin reactions include fever, blisters, conjunctivitis, angioedema, elevated liver function tests, and eosinophilia.

- **HEPATIC IMPAIRMENT** Manufacturer advises caution in moderate impairment (increased risk of hepatic side-effects); avoid in severe impairment (no information available).
- **RENAL IMPAIRMENT** Manufacturer advises avoid if creatinine clearance less than 30 mL/minute—no information available.

- **PATIENT AND CARER ADVICE**
Vomiting Manufacturer advises if vomiting occurs within 4 hours of taking a dose, a replacement dose should be taken.
Driving and skilled tasks Manufacturer advises patients and carers should be counselled on the effects on driving and performance of skilled tasks—increased risk of dizziness.
- **NATIONAL FUNDING/ACCESS DECISIONS**
Scottish Medicines Consortium (SMC) decisions
The *Scottish Medicines Consortium* has advised (October 2016) that emtricitabine with rilpivirine and tenofovir alafenamide (*Odefsey*®) is accepted for use within NHS Scotland for the treatment of human immunodeficiency virus type 1 (HIV-1), without known mutations associated with resistance to the non-nucleoside reverse transcriptase inhibitor (NNRTI) class, tenofovir or emtricitabine, and with viral load HIV-1 RNA of 100 000 copies/mL or less.
All Wales Medicines Strategy Group (AWMSG) decisions
The *All Wales Medicines Strategy Group* has advised (November 2016) that emtricitabine with rilpivirine and tenofovir alafenamide (*Odefsey*®) is recommended as an option for use within NHS Wales for the treatment of human immunodeficiency virus type 1, without known mutations associated with resistance to the non-nucleoside reverse transcriptase inhibitor (NNRTI) class, tenofovir or emtricitabine, and with viral load HIV-1 RNA of 100 000 copies/mL or less.

- **MEDICINAL FORMS** There can be variation in the licensing of different medicines containing the same drug.
Tablet
CAUTIONARY AND ADVISORY LABELS 3, 21
▸ Odefsey (Gilead Sciences International Ltd) ▼
Rilpivirine (as Rilpivirine hydrochloride) 25 mg, Tenofovir alafenamide (as Tenofovir alafenamide fumarate) 25 mg, Emtricitabine 200 mg Odefsey 200mg/25mg/25mg tablets | 30 tablet PoM £525.95

Emtricitabine with tenofovir alafenamide

05-Jun-2017

The properties listed below are those particular to the combination only. For the properties of the components please consider, emtricitabine p. 453, tenofovir alafenamide p. 434.

- **INDICATIONS AND DOSE**
HIV infection in combination with other antiretroviral drugs (specialist use only)
▸ BY MOUTH
▸ Child 12–17 years (body-weight 35 kg and above): 200/10–200/25 mg once daily, dose is dependent on drug regimen—consult product literature
DOSE EQUIVALENCE AND CONVERSION
▸ Dose expressed as x/y mg emtricitabine/tenofovir alafenamide.
- **INTERACTIONS** → Appendix 1: tenofovir alafenamide
- **SIDE-EFFECTS**
▸ **Common or very common** Abnormal dreams · diarrhoea · dizziness · fatigue · flatulence · gastrointestinal discomfort · headache · nausea · skin reactions · vomiting
▸ **Uncommon** Anaemia · arthralgia
▸ **Frequency not known** Angioedema · osteonecrosis
- **HEPATIC IMPAIRMENT** Manufacturer advises caution (increased risk of hepatic side-effects).
- **RENAL IMPAIRMENT** Manufacturer advises avoid if creatinine clearance less than 30 mL/minute—limited information available.
- **PATIENT AND CARER ADVICE**
Driving and skilled tasks Manufacturer advises patients and carers should be counselled on the effects on driving and performance of skilled tasks—increased risk of dizziness.
- **NATIONAL FUNDING/ACCESS DECISIONS**
Scottish Medicines Consortium (SMC) decisions
The *Scottish Medicines Consortium* has advised (August 2016) that emtricitabine with tenofovir alafenamide (*Descovy*®) is accepted for use within NHS Scotland for the treatment of human immunodeficiency virus type 1 in combination with other antiretroviral agents.
All Wales Medicines Strategy Group (AWMSG) decisions
The *All Wales Medicines Strategy Group* has advised (September 2016) that emtricitabine with tenofovir alafenamide (*Descovy*®) is recommended as an option for use within NHS Wales for the treatment of human immunodeficiency virus type 1 in combination with other antiretroviral agents.

- **MEDICINAL FORMS** There can be variation in the licensing of different medicines containing the same drug.
Tablet
▸ Descovy (Gilead Sciences International Ltd) ▼
Tenofovir alafenamide (as Tenofovir alafenamide fumarate) 25 mg, Emtricitabine 200 mg Descovy 200mg/25mg tablets | 30 tablet PoM £355.73
Tenofovir alafenamide (as Tenofovir alafenamide fumarate) 10 mg, Emtricitabine 200 mg Descovy 200mg/10mg tablets | 30 tablet PoM £355.73

Emtricitabine with tenofovir disoproxil

15-Nov-2018

The properties listed below are those particular to the combination only. For the properties of the components please consider, tenofovir disoproxil p. 456, emtricitabine p. 453.

- **INDICATIONS AND DOSE**
HIV-1 infection (initiated by a specialist)
▸ BY MOUTH
▸ Child 12–17 years (body-weight 35 kg and above): 200/245 mg once daily
Pre-exposure prophylaxis of HIV-1 infection (initiated by a specialist)
▸ BY MOUTH
▸ Child 12–17 years (body-weight 35 kg and above): 200/245 mg once daily
DOSE EQUIVALENCE AND CONVERSION
▸ Dose expressed as x/y mg emtricitabine/tenofovir disoproxil.
- **INTERACTIONS** → Appendix 1: tenofovir disoproxil
- **HEPATIC IMPAIRMENT** Manufacturer advises caution (increased risk of hepatic side-effects).
- **RENAL IMPAIRMENT** Manufacturer advises avoid.
- **DIRECTIONS FOR ADMINISTRATION** Patients with swallowing difficulties may disperse tablet in half a glass of water, orange juice, or grape juice (but bitter taste).
- **PATIENT AND CARER ADVICE** Patients or carers should be given advice on how to administer emtricitabine with tenofovir tablets.
Missed doses If a dose is more than 12 hours late, the missed dose should not be taken and the next dose should be taken at the normal time.

- **MEDICINAL FORMS** There can be variation in the licensing of different medicines containing the same drug.

Tablet

CAUTIONARY AND ADVISORY LABELS 21

- Emtricitabine with tenofovir disoproxil (Non-proprietary)
  Emtricitabine 200 mg, Tenofovir disoproxil (as Tenofovir disoproxil fumarate) 245 mg Emtricitabine 200mg / Tenofovir 245mg tablets | 30 tablet PoM £355.73 DT = £355.73 (Hospital only) | 30 tablet PoM £106.72–£355.73 DT = £355.73
- Ictastan (Actavis UK Ltd)
  Emtricitabine 200 mg, Tenofovir disoproxil (as Tenofovir disoproxil fumarate) 245 mg Ictastan 200mg/245mg tablets | 30 tablet PoM £355.72 DT = £355.73
- Truvada (Gilead Sciences International Ltd)
  Emtricitabine 200 mg, Tenofovir disoproxil (as Tenofovir disoproxil fumarate) 245 mg Truvada 200mg/245mg tablets | 30 tablet PoM £355.73 DT = £355.73

F 451

Lamivudine

(3TC)

- **INDICATIONS AND DOSE**

EPIVIR ® ORAL SOLUTION

HIV infection in combination with other antiretroviral drugs

- BY MOUTH
- Child 1–2 months: 4 mg/kg twice daily
- Child 3 months–11 years (body-weight up to 14 kg): 4 mg/kg twice daily (max. per dose 150 mg), alternatively 8 mg/kg once daily (max. per dose 300 mg)
- Child 3 months–11 years (body-weight 14–20 kg): 4 mg/kg twice daily (max. per dose 150 mg), alternatively 8 mg/kg once daily (max. per dose 300 mg), alternatively 75 mg twice daily, alternatively 150 mg once daily
- Child 3 months–11 years (body-weight 21–29 kg): 4 mg/kg twice daily (max. per dose 150 mg), alternatively 8 mg/kg once daily (max. per dose 300 mg), alternatively 75 mg daily, dose to be taken in the morning and 150 mg daily, dose to be taken in the evening, alternatively 225 mg once daily
- Child 3 months–11 years (body-weight 30 kg and above): 4 mg/kg twice daily (max. per dose 150 mg), alternatively 8 mg/kg once daily (max. per dose 300 mg), alternatively 150 mg twice daily, alternatively 300 mg once daily
- Child 12–17 years: 150 mg twice daily, alternatively 300 mg once daily

EPIVIR ® TABLETS

HIV infection in combination with other antiretroviral drugs

- BY MOUTH
- Child 1–2 months: 4 mg/kg twice daily
- Child 3 months–11 years (body-weight up to 14 kg): 4 mg/kg twice daily, alternatively 8 mg/kg once daily
- Child 3 months–11 years (body-weight 14–20 kg): 4 mg/kg twice daily (max. per dose 150 mg), alternatively 8 mg/kg once daily (max. per dose 300 mg), alternatively 75 mg twice daily, alternatively 150 mg once daily
- Child 3 months–11 years (body-weight 21–29 kg): 4 mg/kg twice daily (max. per dose 150 mg), alternatively 8 mg/kg once daily (max. per dose 300 mg), alternatively 75 mg daily, dose to be taken in the morning and 150 mg daily, dose to be taken in the evening, alternatively 225 mg once daily
- Child 3 months–11 years (body-weight 30 kg and above): 4 mg/kg twice daily (max. per dose 150 mg), alternatively 8 mg/kg once daily (max. per dose 300 mg), alternatively 150 mg twice daily, alternatively 300 mg once daily
- Child 12–17 years: 150 mg twice daily, alternatively 300 mg once daily

ZEFFIX ®

Chronic hepatitis B infection either with compensated liver disease (with evidence of viral replication and histology of active liver inflammation or fibrosis) when first-line treatments cannot be used, or (in combination with another antiviral drug without cross-resistance to lamivudine) with decompensated liver disease

- BY MOUTH
- Child 2–11 years: 3 mg/kg once daily (max. per dose 100 mg), children receiving lamivudine for concomitant HIV infection should continue to receive lamivudine in a dose appropriate for HIV infection
- Child 12–17 years: 100 mg once daily, patients receiving lamivudine for concomitant HIV infection should continue to receive lamivudine in a dose appropriate for HIV infection

- **UNLICENSED USE**

EPIVIR ® ORAL SOLUTION Not licensed for use in children under 3 months.

EPIVIR ® TABLETS Not licensed for use in children under 3 months.

ZEFFIX ® Not licensed for use in children.

- **CAUTIONS** Recurrent hepatitis in patients with chronic hepatitis B may occur on discontinuation of lamivudine
- **INTERACTIONS** → Appendix 1: lamivudine
- **SIDE-EFFECTS**
  - **Common or very common** Alopecia · arthralgia · cough · fever · gastrointestinal discomfort · hepatic disorders · malaise · muscle complaints · myopathy · nasal disorder
  - **Uncommon** Thrombocytopenia
  - **Rare or very rare** Paraesthesia · peripheral neuropathy · pure red cell aplasia
  - **Frequency not known** Respiratory tract infection · throat complaints
- **BREAST FEEDING** Can be used with caution in women infected with chronic hepatitis B alone, providing that adequate measures are taken to prevent hepatitis B infection in infants.
- **RENAL IMPAIRMENT**
  Dose adjustments Reduce dose if estimated glomerular filtration rate less than 50 mL/minute/1.73 m^2; consult product literature.
- **MONITORING REQUIREMENTS** When treating chronic hepatitis B with lamivudine, monitor liver function tests every 3 months, and viral markers of hepatitis B every 3–6 months, more frequently in patients with advanced liver disease or following transplantation (monitoring to continue for at least 1 year after discontinuation—recurrent hepatitis may occur on discontinuation).
- **PRESCRIBING AND DISPENSING INFORMATION** Flavours of oral liquid formulations may include banana and strawberry.

- **MEDICINAL FORMS** There can be variation in the licensing of different medicines containing the same drug.

Oral solution

EXCIPIENTS: May contain Sucrose

- Epivir (ViiV Healthcare UK Ltd)
  Lamivudine 10 mg per 1 ml Epivir 50mg/5ml oral solution | 240 ml PoM £39.01

Tablet

- Epivir (ViiV Healthcare UK Ltd)
  Lamivudine 150 mg Epivir 150mg tablets | 60 tablet PoM £143.32 DT = £143.32
  Lamivudine 300 mg Epivir 300mg tablets | 30 tablet PoM £157.51 DT = £157.51

5 Infection

▸ Zeffix (GlaxoSmithKline UK Ltd)
Lamivudine 100 mg Zeffix 100mg tablets | 28 tablet PoM £78.09 DT = £74.17

Lamivudine with dolutegravir

30-Sep-2019

The properties listed below are those particular to the combination only. For the properties of the components please consider, lamivudine p. 455, dolutegravir p. 446.

● **INDICATIONS AND DOSE**

HIV-1 infection

▸ BY MOUTH

▸ Child 12–17 years (body-weight 40 kg and above): 300/50 mg once daily

DOSE EQUIVALENCE AND CONVERSION

▸ Dose expressed as x/y mg lamivudine/dolutegravir.

● **INTERACTIONS** → Appendix 1: dolutegravir · lamivudine

● **RENAL IMPAIRMENT** Manufacturer advises avoid if creatinine clearance less than 50 mL/minute.

● **PATIENT AND CARER ADVICE**

Missed doses Manufacturer advises if a dose is more than 20 hours late, the missed dose should not be taken and the next dose should be taken at the normal time.

● **NATIONAL FUNDING/ACCESS DECISIONS**

Scottish Medicines Consortium (SMC) decisions

SMC No. SMC2205

The *Scottish Medicines Consortium* has advised (September 2019) that lamivudine with dolutegravir (*Dovato*®) is accepted for use within NHS Scotland for the treatment of HIV-1 infection in adults and adolescents aged 12 years or older, weighing at least 40 kg, with no known or suspected resistance to the integrase inhibitor class, or lamivudine. This advice is contingent upon the continuing availability of the patient access scheme in NHS Scotland or a list price that is equivalent or lower.

All Wales Medicines Strategy Group (AWMSG) decisions

AWMSG No. 3659

The *All Wales Medicines Strategy Group* has advised (February 2020) that lamivudine with dolutegravir (*Dovato*®) is recommended as an option for use within NHS Wales for the treatment of HIV-1 infection in adults and adolescents above 12 years of age weighing at least 40 kg, with no known or suspected resistance to the integrase inhibitor class, or lamivudine. This recommendation applies only in circumstances where the approved Wales Patient Access Scheme (WPAS) is utilised or where the list/contract price is equivalent or lower than the WPAS price.

● **MEDICINAL FORMS** There can be variation in the licensing of different medicines containing the same drug.

Tablet

▸ Dovato (ViiV Healthcare UK Ltd) ▼
Dolutegravir (as Dolutegravir sodium) 50 mg, Lamivudine 300 mg Dovato 50mg/300mg tablets | 30 tablet PoM £656.26

F 451

Stavudine

01-Sep-2016

(d4T)

● **INDICATIONS AND DOSE**

HIV infection in combination with other antiretroviral drugs when no suitable alternative available and when prescribed for shortest period possible

▸ BY MOUTH

▸ Child (body-weight up to 30 kg): 1 mg/kg twice daily, to be taken preferably at least 1 hour before food

▸ Child (body-weight 30–59 kg): 30 mg twice daily, to be taken preferably at least 1 hour before food

▸ Child (body-weight 60 kg and above): 40 mg twice daily, to be taken preferably at least 1 hour before food

● **UNLICENSED USE** Capsules not licensed for use in children under 3 months.

● **CAUTIONS** Excessive alcohol intake · history of pancreatitis · history of peripheral neuropathy · lactic acidosis (especially when used in combination with didanosine)—use only if alternative regimens are not suitable

CAUTIONS, FURTHER INFORMATION

▸ Lactic acidosis Lactic acidosis associated with hepatomegaly and hepatic steatosis has been reported with stavudine. Use with caution in patients with hepatomegaly, hepatitis, or other risk factors for liver disease and hepatic steatosis (including obesity and alcohol abuse). Discontinue treatment if symptoms of hyperlactataemia, lactic acidosis, progressive hepatomegaly or rapid deterioration of liver function become apparent.

● **INTERACTIONS** → Appendix 1: stavudine

● **SIDE-EFFECTS**

▸ **Common or very common** Abnormal dreams · depression · drowsiness · dyspepsia · hyperlactacidaemia · lipoatrophy · nerve disorders · paraesthesia · peripheral neuropathy (switch to another antiretroviral if peripheral neuropathy develops) · thinking abnormal

▸ **Uncommon** Anxiety · appetite decreased · arthralgia · emotional lability · gynaecomastia · hepatic disorders · myalgia

▸ **Rare or very rare** Diabetes mellitus · hyperglycaemia · muscle weakness · thrombocytopenia

SIDE-EFFECTS, FURTHER INFORMATION Metabolic effects may occur with stavudine; plasma lipids and blood glucose concentrations should be measured routinely.

● **PREGNANCY** Manufacturer advises use only if potential benefit outweighs risk.

● **RENAL IMPAIRMENT** Risk of peripheral neuropathy.

Dose adjustments Reduce dose to 50% if estimated glomerular filtration rate 25–50 mL/minute/1.73 m^2; reduce dose to 25% if estimated glomerular filtration rate less than 25 mL/minute/1.73 m^2.

● **PRESCRIBING AND DISPENSING INFORMATION** Flavours of oral liquid formulations may include cherry.

● **LESS SUITABLE FOR PRESCRIBING** Stavudine (especially in combination with didanosine) is associated with a higher risk of lipoatrophy and should be used only if alternative regimens are not suitable; it is considered to be less suitable for prescribing.

● **MEDICINAL FORMS** No licensed medicines listed.

F 451

Tenofovir disoproxil

● **INDICATIONS AND DOSE**

HIV infection in combination with other antiretroviral drugs when first-line nucleoside reverse transcriptase inhibitors cannot be used because of resistance or contra-indications

▸ BY MOUTH

▸ Child 2–17 years: 6.5 mg/kg once daily (max. per dose 245 mg)

▸ Child 6–17 years (body-weight 17–21 kg): 123 mg once daily

▸ Child 6–17 years (body-weight 22–27 kg): 163 mg once daily

▸ Child 6–17 years (body-weight 28–34 kg): 204 mg once daily

- Child 6-17 years (body-weight 35 kg and above): 245 mg once daily

Chronic hepatitis B infection with compensated liver disease (with evidence of viral replication, and histology of active liver inflammation or fibrosis)

- BY MOUTH
- Child 12-17 years (body-weight 35 kg and above): 245 mg once daily

DOSE EQUIVALENCE AND CONVERSION
- 7.5 scoops of granules contains approx. 245 mg tenofovir disoproxil (as fumarate).

- **INTERACTIONS** → Appendix 1: tenofovir disoproxil
- **SIDE-EFFECTS**
- **Common or very common** Abdominal distension · flatulence
- **Uncommon** Proximal renal tubulopathy
- **Rare or very rare** Acute tubular necrosis · hepatic disorders · nephritis · nephrogenic diabetes insipidus · renal impairment
- **HEPATIC IMPAIRMENT** Manufacturer advises caution in decompensated hepatic disease (limited information available).
- **RENAL IMPAIRMENT** Manufacturer advises avoid—no information available.
- **MONITORING REQUIREMENTS**
- Test renal function and serum phosphate before treatment, then every 4 weeks (more frequently if at increased risk of renal impairment) for 1 year and then every 3 months, interrupt treatment if renal function deteriorates or serum phosphate decreases.
- When treating chronic hepatitis B with tenofovir, monitor liver function tests every 3 months and viral markers for hepatitis B every 3–6 months during treatment (continue monitoring for at least 1 year after discontinuation—recurrent hepatitis may occur on discontinuation).
- **DIRECTIONS FOR ADMINISTRATION** *Granules*: mix 1 scoop of granules with 1 tablespoon of soft food (e.g. yoghurt, apple sauce) and take immediately without chewing. Do **not** mix granules with liquids.
- **PATIENT AND CARER ADVICE** Patients or carers should be given advice on how to administer tenofovir granules.
Missed doses If a dose is more than 12 hours late, the missed dose should not be taken and the next dose should be taken at the normal time.

- **MEDICINAL FORMS** There can be variation in the licensing of different medicines containing the same drug.

Granules

CAUTIONARY AND ADVISORY LABELS 21
- **Viread** (Gilead Sciences International Ltd)
Tenofovir disoproxil (as Tenofovir disoproxil fumarate) 33 mg per 1 gram Viread 33mg/g granules | 60 gram PoM £54.50

Tablet

CAUTIONARY AND ADVISORY LABELS 21
- **Tenofovir disoproxil (Non-proprietary)**
Tenofovir disoproxil 245 mg Tenofovir 245mg tablets | 30 tablet PoM £64.08 DT = £39.05 (Hospital only) | 30 tablet PoM £16.84–£204.39 DT = £39.05 | 168 tablet PoM £36.36
- **Viread** (Gilead Sciences International Ltd)
Tenofovir disoproxil (as Tenofovir disoproxil fumarate) 123 mg Viread 123mg tablets | 30 tablet PoM £102.60 DT = £102.60
Tenofovir disoproxil (as Tenofovir disoproxil fumarate) 163 mg Viread 163mg tablets | 30 tablet PoM £135.98 DT = £135.98
Tenofovir disoproxil (as Tenofovir disoproxil fumarate) 204 mg Viread 204mg tablets | 30 tablet PoM £170.19 DT = £170.19
Tenofovir disoproxil 245 mg Viread 245mg tablets | 30 tablet PoM £204.39 DT = £39.05

451

Zidovudine

10-Mar-2020

(Azidothymidine; AZT)

- **INDICATIONS AND DOSE**

HIV infection in combination with other antiretroviral drugs

- BY MOUTH
- Child: 180 mg/m^2 twice daily (max. per dose 300 mg)
- Child (body-weight 8-13 kg): 100 mg twice daily
- Child (body-weight 14-20 kg): 100 mg, to be taken in the morning and 200 mg, to be taken in the evening
- Child (body-weight 21-27 kg): 200 mg twice daily
- Child (body-weight 28-29 kg): 200–250 mg twice daily
- Child (body-weight 30 kg and above): 250–300 mg twice daily

HIV infection in combination with other antiretroviral drugs (dose expressed in mg/kg)

- BY MOUTH
- Child (body-weight 4-8 kg): 12 mg/kg twice daily
- Child (body-weight 9-29 kg): 9 mg/kg twice daily

Prevention of maternal-fetal HIV transmission

- BY MOUTH, OR BY INTRAVENOUS INFUSION
- Child: Seek specialist advice (combination therapy preferred) (consult local protocol)

HIV infection in combination with other antiretroviral drugs in patients temporarily unable to take zidovudine by mouth

- BY INTRAVENOUS INFUSION
- Child 3 months-11 years: 60–80 mg/m^2 every 6 hours usually for not more than 2 weeks, dose approximating to 9–12 mg/kg twice daily by mouth
- Child 12-17 years: 0.8–1 mg/kg every 4 hours usually for not more than 2 weeks, dose approximating to 1.2–1.5 mg/kg every 4 hours by mouth

- **CONTRA-INDICATIONS** Abnormally low haemoglobin concentration (consult product literature) · abnormally low neutrophil counts (consult product literature) · neonates with hyperbilirubinaemia requiring treatment other than phototherapy, or with raised transaminase (consult product literature)
- **CAUTIONS** Lactic acidosis · risk of haematological toxicity particularly with high dose and advanced disease · vitamin B_{12} deficiency (increased risk of neutropenia)

CAUTIONS, FURTHER INFORMATION
- Lactic acidosis Lactic acidosis associated with hepatomegaly and hepatic steatosis has been reported with zidovudine. Use with caution in patients with hepatomegaly, hepatitis, or other risk factors for liver disease and hepatic steatosis (including obesity and alcohol abuse). Discontinue treatment if symptoms of hyperlactataemia, lactic acidosis, progressive hepatomegaly or rapid deterioration of liver function become apparent.

- **INTERACTIONS** → Appendix 1: zidovudine
- **SIDE-EFFECTS**

GENERAL SIDE-EFFECTS
- **Common or very common** Leucopenia · malaise · myalgia
- **Uncommon** Bone marrow disorders · dyspnoea · fever · flatulence · generalised pain · myopathy · thrombocytopenia
- **Rare or very rare** Alertness decreased · anxiety · appetite decreased · cardiomyopathy · chest pain · chills · cough · depression · drowsiness · dyspepsia · gynaecomastia · hepatic disorders · hyperhidrosis · influenza like illness · nail discolouration · oral discolouration · paraesthesia · pure red cell aplasia · seizure · taste altered · urinary frequency increased
- **Frequency not known** Lipoatrophy

SPECIFIC SIDE-EFFECTS
▸ With intravenous use Weight increased

SIDE-EFFECTS, FURTHER INFORMATION **Anaemia and myelosuppression** If anaemia or myelosuppression occur, reduce dose or interrupt treatment according to product literature, or consider other treatment.

Lipodystrophy syndrome Metabolic effects may occur with zidovudine; plasma lipids and blood glucose concentrations should be measured routinely.

● HEPATIC IMPAIRMENT Manufacturer advises caution in moderate to severe impairment (increased risk of accumulation).

Dose adjustments Manufacturer advises consider dose reduction in moderate to severe impairment—consult product literature.

● RENAL IMPAIRMENT

Dose adjustments Reduce dose if estimated glomerular filtration rate less than 10 mL/minute/1.73 m^2—consult product literature.

● MONITORING REQUIREMENTS Monitor full blood count after 4 weeks of treatment, then every 3 months.

● DIRECTIONS FOR ADMINISTRATION
▸ With intravenous use For *intermittent intravenous infusion*, dilute to a concentration of 2 mg/mL or 4 mg/mL with Glucose 5% and give over 1 hour.

● PRESCRIBING AND DISPENSING INFORMATION The abbreviation AZT which is sometimes used for zidovudine has also been used for another drug.

● PATIENT AND CARER ADVICE
Medicines for Children leaflet: Zidovudine for treatment of HIV infection www.medicinesforchildren.org.uk/zidovudine-treatment-hiv-infection

● MEDICINAL FORMS There can be variation in the licensing of different medicines containing the same drug.

Solution for infusion
▸ Retrovir (ViiV Healthcare UK Ltd)
Zidovudine 10 mg per 1 ml Retrovir IV 200mg/20ml concentrate for solution for infusion vials | 5 vial [PoM] £52.48

Oral solution
▸ Retrovir (ViiV Healthcare UK Ltd)
Zidovudine 10 mg per 1 ml Retrovir 100mg/10ml oral solution sugar-free | 200 ml [PoM] £20.91

Capsule
▸ Zidovudine (Non-proprietary)
Zidovudine 100 mg Zidovudine 100mg capsules | 60 capsule [PoM] £53.31
Zidovudine 250 mg Zidovudine 250mg capsules | 60 capsule [PoM] £13.32
▸ Retrovir (ViiV Healthcare UK Ltd)
Zidovudine 100 mg Retrovir 100mg capsules | 100 capsule [PoM] £104.54
Zidovudine 250 mg Retrovir 250mg capsules | 40 capsule [PoM] £104.54

Zidovudine with lamivudine

The properties listed below are those particular to the combination only. For the properties of the components please consider, zidovudine p. 457, lamivudine p. 455.

● INDICATIONS AND DOSE

HIV infection in combination with other antiretroviral drugs
▸ BY MOUTH
▸ Child (body-weight 14–20 kg): 0.5 tablet twice daily
▸ Child (body-weight 21–29 kg): 0.5 tablet daily, to be given in the morning and 1 tablet daily, to be given in the evening
▸ Child (body-weight 30 kg and above): 1 tablet twice daily

● INTERACTIONS → Appendix 1: lamivudine · zidovudine

● RENAL IMPAIRMENT Avoid if estimated glomerular filtration rate less than 50 mL/minute/1.73 m^2.

● DIRECTIONS FOR ADMINISTRATION
COMBIVIR ® TABLETS Tablets may be crushed and mixed with semi-solid food or liquid just before administration.

● MEDICINAL FORMS There can be variation in the licensing of different medicines containing the same drug.

Tablet
▸ Zidovudine with lamivudine (Non-proprietary)
Lamivudine 150 mg, Zidovudine 300 mg Zidovudine 300mg / Lamivudine 150mg tablets | 60 tablet [PoM] £240.10–£255.10 DT = £300.12
▸ Combivir (ViiV Healthcare UK Ltd)
Lamivudine 150 mg, Zidovudine 300 mg Combivir 150mg/300mg tablets | 60 tablet [PoM] £300.12 DT = £300.12

ANTIVIRALS > PROTEASE INHIBITORS, HIV

Protease inhibitors

● CONTRA-INDICATIONS Acute porphyrias p. 652

● CAUTIONS Haemophilia (increased risk of bleeding)

● SIDE-EFFECTS
▸ **Common or very common** Alopecia · anaemia · angioedema · anxiety · appetite abnormal · arthralgia · asthenia · diabetes mellitus · diarrhoea · dizziness · dry mouth · dyslipidaemia · dyspnoea · fever · gastrointestinal discomfort · gastrointestinal disorders · headache · hepatic disorders · hypersensitivity · hypertension · malaise · muscle complaints · nausea · neutropenia · oral ulceration · pancreatitis · peripheral neuropathy · seizure · skin reactions · sleep disorders · taste altered · vomiting
▸ **Uncommon** Drowsiness · immune reconstitution inflammatory syndrome · osteonecrosis · Stevens-Johnson syndrome · weight increased

● HEPATIC IMPAIRMENT In general, manufacturers advise use with caution in patients with chronic hepatitis B or C (increased risk of hepatic side-effects).

above

Atazanavir

06-May-2020

● INDICATIONS AND DOSE

HIV infection in combination with other antiretroviral drugs—with low-dose ritonavir
▸ BY MOUTH
▸ Child 6–17 years (body-weight 15–19 kg): 150 mg once daily
▸ Child 6–17 years (body-weight 20–39 kg): 200 mg once daily
▸ Child 6–17 years (body-weight 40 kg and above): 300 mg once daily

● CAUTIONS Cardiac conduction disorders · electrolyte disturbances · predisposition to QT interval prolongation

● INTERACTIONS → Appendix 1: HIV-protease inhibitors

● SIDE-EFFECTS
▸ **Uncommon** Chest pain · chronic kidney disease · depression · disorientation · drug reaction with eosinophilia and systemic symptoms (DRESS) · gallbladder disorders · gynaecomastia · haematuria · memory loss · myopathy · nephritis tubulointerstitial · nephrolithiasis · proteinuria · syncope · torsade de pointes · urinary frequency increased
▸ **Rare or very rare** Gait abnormal · oedema · palpitations · QT interval prolongation · renal pain · vasodilation

SIDE-EFFECTS, FURTHER INFORMATION Mild to moderate rash occurs commonly, usually within the first 3 weeks of therapy. Severe rash occurs less frequently and may be accompanied by systemic symptoms. Discontinue if severe rash develops.

- **PREGNANCY** Theoretical risk of hyperbilirubinaemia in neonate if used at term.
Monitoring In pregnancy, monitor viral load and plasma-atazanavir concentration during third trimester.
- **HEPATIC IMPAIRMENT** Manufacturer advises caution in mild impairment; avoid in moderate to severe impairment (no information available).

- **MEDICINAL FORMS** There can be variation in the licensing of different medicines containing the same drug.

Capsule

CAUTIONARY AND ADVISORY LABELS 5, 21

▸ Atazanavir (Non-proprietary)
Atazanavir (as Atazanavir sulfate) 150 mg Atazanavir 150mg capsules | 60 capsule PoM £303.38
Atazanavir (as Atazanavir sulfate) 200 mg Atazanavir 200mg capsules | 60 capsule PoM £303.37-£303.38 | 60 capsule PoM £303.37 (Hospital only)
Atazanavir (as Atazanavir sulfate) 300 mg Atazanavir 300mg capsules | 30 capsule PoM £303.37 (Hospital only) | 30 capsule PoM £257.87-£303.38

▸ Reyataz (Bristol-Myers Squibb Pharmaceuticals Ltd)
Atazanavir (as Atazanavir sulfate) 150 mg Reyataz 150mg capsules | 60 capsule PoM £303.38 (Hospital only)
Atazanavir (as Atazanavir sulfate) 200 mg Reyataz 200mg capsules | 60 capsule PoM £303.38 (Hospital only)
Atazanavir (as Atazanavir sulfate) 300 mg Reyataz 300mg capsules | 30 capsule PoM £303.38 (Hospital only)

F 458

Darunavir

31-Jul-2018

- **INDICATIONS AND DOSE**

HIV infection in combination with other antiretroviral drugs in patients previously treated with antiretroviral therapy—with low-dose ritonavir

▸ BY MOUTH

▸ Child 3–17 years (body-weight 15–29 kg): 375 mg twice daily

▸ Child 3–17 years (body-weight 30–39 kg): 450 mg twice daily

▸ Child 3–17 years (body-weight 40 kg and above): 600 mg twice daily

▸ Child 12–17 years: 800 mg once daily, once daily dose only to be used if no resistance to darunavir, if plasma HIV-RNA concentration less than 100 000 copies/mL, and if CD4 cell count greater than 100 cells × 10^6/ litre

HIV infection in combination with other antiretroviral drugs in patients not previously treated with antiretroviral therapy—with low-dose ritonavir

▸ BY MOUTH

▸ Child 12–17 years (body-weight 40 kg and above): 800 mg once daily

- **INTERACTIONS** → Appendix 1: HIV-protease inhibitors
- **SIDE-EFFECTS**

▸ **Uncommon** Angina pectoris · arrhythmias · burping · chest pain · concentration impaired · confusion · constipation · cough · depression · dry eye · eye erythema · feeling hot · flushing · gout · gynaecomastia · haemorrhage · herpes simplex · hyperglycaemia · hypothyroidism · leucopenia · memory loss · mood altered · muscle weakness · myocardial infarction · nail discolouration · nephrolithiasis · oral disorders · osteoporosis · pain · peripheral oedema · polydipsia · QT interval prolongation · renal impairment · sensation abnormal · sexual dysfunction · sweat changes · throat irritation · thrombocytopenia · urinary disorders · urine abnormalities · vertigo

▸ **Rare or very rare** Arthritis · chills · feeling abnormal · joint stiffness · musculoskeletal stiffness · palpitations · rhinorrhoea · severe cutaneous adverse reactions (SCARs) · syncope · visual impairment

SIDE-EFFECTS, FURTHER INFORMATION Mild to moderate rash occurs commonly, usually within the first 4 weeks of therapy and resolves without stopping treatment. Severe skin rash (including Stevens-Johnson syndrome and toxic epidermal necrolysis) occurs less frequently and may be accompanied by fever, malaise, arthralgia, myalgia, oral lesions, conjunctivitis, hepatitis, or eosinophilia; treatment should be stopped if this develops.

- **ALLERGY AND CROSS-SENSITIVITY** Use with caution in patients with sulfonamide sensitivity.
- **PREGNANCY** Manufacturer advises use only if potential benefit outweighs risk; if required, use the twice daily dose regimen.
- **HEPATIC IMPAIRMENT** Manufacturer advises caution in mild to moderate impairment; avoid in severe impairment (no information available).
- **MONITORING REQUIREMENTS** Monitor liver function before and during treatment.
- **PRESCRIBING AND DISPENSING INFORMATION** Flavours of oral liquid formulations may include strawberry.
- **PATIENT AND CARER ADVICE**
Missed doses If a dose is more than 6 hours late on the twice daily regimen (or more than 12 hours late on the once daily regimen), the missed dose should not be taken and the next dose should be taken at the normal time.

- **MEDICINAL FORMS** There can be variation in the licensing of different medicines containing the same drug.

Oral suspension

CAUTIONARY AND ADVISORY LABELS 21

▸ Prezista (Janssen-Cilag Ltd)
Darunavir (as Darunavir ethanolate) 100 mg per 1 ml Prezista 100mg/ml oral suspension sugar-free | 200 ml PoM £248.17

Tablet

CAUTIONARY AND ADVISORY LABELS 21

▸ Darunavir (Non-proprietary)
Darunavir (as Darunavir ethanolate) 400 mg Darunavir 400mg tablets | 60 tablet PoM £297.80
Darunavir (as Darunavir ethanolate) 600 mg Darunavir 600mg tablets | 60 tablet PoM £402.02 (Hospital only) | 60 tablet PoM £379.67-£446.70
Darunavir (as Darunavir ethanolate) 800 mg Darunavir 800mg tablets | 30 tablet PoM £268.02 DT = £268.02 (Hospital only) | 30 tablet PoM £253.13-£297.80 DT = £268.02

▸ Prezista (Janssen-Cilag Ltd)
Darunavir (as Darunavir ethanolate) 75 mg Prezista 75mg tablets | 480 tablet PoM £446.70
Darunavir (as Darunavir ethanolate) 150 mg Prezista 150mg tablets | 240 tablet PoM £446.70
Darunavir (as Darunavir ethanolate) 400 mg Prezista 400mg tablets | 60 tablet PoM £297.80
Darunavir (as Darunavir ethanolate) 600 mg Prezista 600mg tablets | 60 tablet PoM £446.70
Darunavir (as Darunavir ethanolate) 800 mg Prezista 800mg tablets | 30 tablet PoM £297.80 DT = £268.02

5 Infection

Darunavir with cobicistat, emtricitabine and tenofovir alafenamide

25-Jul-2018

The properties listed below are those particular to the combination only. For the properties of the components please consider, darunavir p. 459, cobicistat, emtricitabine p. 453, tenofovir alafenamide p. 434.

- **INDICATIONS AND DOSE**

HIV infection (initiated by a specialist)

▶ BY MOUTH

- Child 12–17 years (body-weight 40 kg and above): 1 tablet once daily

> **IMPORTANT SAFETY INFORMATION**
>
> MHRA/CHM ADVICE: DARUNAVIR BOOSTED WITH COBICISTAT: AVOID USE IN PREGNANCY DUE TO RISK OF TREATMENT FAILURE AND MATERNAL-TO-CHILD TRANSMISSION OF HIV-1 (JULY 2018)
>
> Pharmacokinetic data show mean exposure of darunavir boosted with cobicistat (available in combination in *Rezolsta®* and *Symtuza®*) to be lower during the second and third trimesters of pregnancy than during 6–12 weeks postpartum. Low darunavir exposure may be associated with an increased risk of treatment failure and an increased risk of HIV-1 transmission to the unborn child. For further information, see *Pregnancy*.

- **INTERACTIONS** → Appendix 1: cobicistat · HIV-protease inhibitors · tenofovir alafenamide
- **PREGNANCY** Manufacturer advises not to be initiated during pregnancy due to low darunavir exposure; women who become pregnant during therapy should be switched to an alternative regimen.
- **RENAL IMPAIRMENT** Manufacturer advises avoid if estimated glomerular filtration rate less than 30 mL/minute/1.73 m^2—no information available.
- **PATIENT AND CARER ADVICE**

Driving and skilled tasks Manufacturer advises patients and carers should be counselled on the effects on driving and performance of skilled tasks—increased risk of dizziness.

- **NATIONAL FUNDING/ACCESS DECISIONS**

Scottish Medicines Consortium (SMC) decisions

SMC No. 1290/18

The *Scottish Medicines Consortium* has advised (January 2018) that darunavir with cobicistat, emtricitabine and tenofovir alafenamide (*Symtuza®*) is accepted for use within NHS Scotland for the treatment of human immunodeficiency virus type 1 (HIV-1) infection in adults and adolescents (aged 12 years and older with body weight at least 40 kg).

All Wales Medicines Strategy Group (AWMSG) decisions

AWMSG No. 2418

The *All Wales Medicines Strategy Group* has advised (March 2018) that darunavir with cobicistat, emtricitabine and tenofovir alafenamide (*Symtuza®*) is recommended as an option for use within NHS Wales for the treatment of human immunodeficiency virus type 1 (HIV-1) infection in adults and adolescents (aged 12 years and older with body weight at least 40 kg).

- **MEDICINAL FORMS** There can be variation in the licensing of different medicines containing the same drug.

Tablet

CAUTIONARY AND ADVISORY LABELS 21

- Symtuza (Janssen-Cilag Ltd) ▼

Tenofovir alafenamide (as Tenofovir alafenamide fumarate) 10 mg, Cobicistat 150 mg, Emtricitabine 200 mg, Darunavir (as Darunavir ethanolate) 800 mg Symtuza 800mg/150mg/200mg/10mg tablets | 30 tablet PoM £672.97

F 458

Fosamprenavir

- **DRUG ACTION** Fosamprenavir is a pro-drug of amprenavir.

- **INDICATIONS AND DOSE**

HIV infection in combination with other antiretroviral drugs—with low-dose ritonavir

▶ BY MOUTH

- Child 6–17 years (body-weight 25–39 kg): 18 mg/kg twice daily (max. per dose 700 mg)
- Child 6–17 years (body-weight 40 kg and above): 700 mg twice daily

DOSE EQUIVALENCE AND CONVERSION

- 700 mg fosamprenavir is equivalent to approximately 600 mg amprenavir.

- **INTERACTIONS** → Appendix 1: HIV-protease inhibitors
- **SIDE-EFFECTS**

▶ **Common or very common** Oral paraesthesia

SIDE-EFFECTS, FURTHER INFORMATION Rash may occur, usually in the second week of therapy; discontinue permanently if severe rash with systemic or allergic symptoms or, mucosal involvement; if rash mild or moderate, may continue without interruption—usually resolves and may respond to antihistamines.

- **PREGNANCY** Toxicity in *animal* studies; manufacturer advises use only if potential benefit outweighs risk.
- **HEPATIC IMPAIRMENT** Manufacturer advises caution.

Dose adjustments In adults, manufacturer advises dose reduction—consult product literature.

- **DIRECTIONS FOR ADMINISTRATION** In children, oral suspension should be taken with food.
- **PRESCRIBING AND DISPENSING INFORMATION** Flavours of oral liquid formulations may include grape, bubblegum, or peppermint.
- **PATIENT AND CARER ADVICE** Patients or carers should be given advice on how to administer fosamprenavir oral suspension.

- **MEDICINAL FORMS** There can be variation in the licensing of different medicines containing the same drug.

Oral suspension

EXCIPIENTS: May contain Propylene glycol

- Telzir (ViiV Healthcare UK Ltd)

Fosamprenavir (as Fosamprenavir calcium) 50 mg per 1 ml Telzir 50mg/ml oral suspension | 225 ml PoM £69.06

Tablet

- Telzir (ViiV Healthcare UK Ltd)

Fosamprenavir (as Fosamprenavir calcium) 700 mg Telzir 700mg tablets | 60 tablet PoM £258.97

F 458

Lopinavir with ritonavir

06-May-2020

- **INDICATIONS AND DOSE**

HIV infection in combination with other antiretroviral drugs

▶ BY MOUTH USING TABLETS

- Child 2–17 years (body-weight up to 40 kg and body surface area 0.5–0.7 m^2): 200/50 mg twice daily
- Child 2–17 years (body-weight up to 40 kg and body surface area 0.8–1.1 m^2): 300/75 mg twice daily
- Child 2–17 years (body-weight 40 kg and above and body surface area 1.2 m^2 and above): 400/100 mg twice daily

▶ BY MOUTH USING ORAL SOLUTION

- Child 14 days–5 months: 3.75 mL/m^2 twice daily
- Child 6 months–17 years: 2.9 mL/m^2 twice daily (max. per dose 5 mL)

DOSE EQUIVALENCE AND CONVERSION

- Oral solution contains 400 mg lopinavir, 100 mg ritonavir/5 mL (or 80 mg lopinavir, 20 mg ritonavir/mL).

- **CAUTIONS** Cardiac conduction disorders · pancreatitis · patients at high risk of cardiovascular disease · structural heart disease
- **INTERACTIONS** → Appendix 1: HIV-protease inhibitors
- **SIDE-EFFECTS**
- ▸ **Common or very common** Increased risk of infection · leucopenia · lymphadenopathy · menstrual cycle irregularities · migraine · muscle weakness · myopathy · night sweats · pain · sexual dysfunction
- ▸ **Uncommon** Atherosclerosis · atrioventricular block · cholangitis · constipation · deep vein thrombosis · haemorrhage · hyperbilirubinaemia · hypogonadism · myocardial infarction · nephritis · stomatitis · stroke · tinnitus · tremor · tricuspid valve incompetence · vasculitis · vertigo · visual impairment

SIDE-EFFECTS, FURTHER INFORMATION Signs and symptoms suggestive of pancreatitis (including raised serum lipase) should be evaluated—discontinue if pancreatitis diagnosed.

- **PREGNANCY** For *tablets*, manufacturer advises only use if potential benefit outweighs risk—toxicity in *animal* studies (recommendation also supported by specialist sources). Avoid *oral solution* due to high alcohol and propylene glycol content.
- **HEPATIC IMPAIRMENT** For *oral solution*, manufacturer advises avoid due to propylene glycol content (risk of toxicity). For *tablets*, manufacturer advises avoid in severe impairment (no information available).
- **RENAL IMPAIRMENT** Avoid *oral solution* due to high propylene glycol content.
- **MONITORING REQUIREMENTS**
- ▸ Manufacturer advises monitor liver function before and during treatment.
- ▸ For *oral solution*, manufacturer advises monitor for signs of alcohol and propylene glycol toxicity (particularly in infants).
- **PRESCRIBING AND DISPENSING INFORMATION** For *oral solution*, manufacturer advises high alcohol (42 % v/v) and propylene glycol content—consider total amounts from all medicines that are to be given to infants in order to avoid toxicity; caution in patients for which consumption may be harmful.
- **PATIENT AND CARER ADVICE** Oral solution tastes bitter.
- **NATIONAL FUNDING/ACCESS DECISIONS**

Scottish Medicines Consortium (SMC) decisions

SMC No. 1302/18

The *Scottish Medicines Consortium* has advised (February 2018) that lopinavir with ritonavir oral solution (*Kaletra*®) is accepted for use within NHS Scotland in combination with other antiretrovirals for the treatment of HIV-1 infected children aged from 14 days up to 2 years.

SMC No. 326/06

The *Scottish Medicines Consortium* has advised (November 2006) that lopinavir with ritonavir tablet (*Kaletra*®) is accepted for use within NHS Scotland in combination with other antiretrovirals for the treatment of HIV-1 infected adults and children above the age of 2 years.

All Wales Medicines Strategy Group (AWMSG) decisions

AWMSG No. 3557

The *All Wales Medicines Strategy Group* has advised (March 2018) that lopinavir with ritonavir oral solution (*Kaletra*®) is recommended as an option for use within NHS Wales in combination with other antiretroviral medicinal products for the treatment of human immunodeficiency virus (HIV-1) infected children aged from 14 days to less than 2 years old.

- **MEDICINAL FORMS** There can be variation in the licensing of different medicines containing the same drug.

Oral solution

CAUTIONARY AND ADVISORY LABELS 21

EXCIPIENTS: May contain Alcohol, propylene glycol

- ▸ Kaletra (AbbVie Ltd)
  Ritonavir 20 mg per 1 ml, Lopinavir 80 mg per 1 ml Kaletra 80mg/20mg/1ml oral solution | 120 ml PoM £122.96 | 300 ml PoM £307.39

Tablet

CAUTIONARY AND ADVISORY LABELS 25

- ▸ **Lopinavir with ritonavir (Non-proprietary)**
  Ritonavir 50 mg, Lopinavir 200 mg Lopinavir 200mg / Ritonavir 50mg tablets | 120 tablet PoM £285.40 (Hospital only) | 120 tablet PoM £242.60–£285.40
- ▸ Kaletra (AbbVie Ltd)
  Ritonavir 25 mg, Lopinavir 100 mg Kaletra 100mg/25mg tablets | 60 tablet PoM £76.85
  Ritonavir 50 mg, Lopinavir 200 mg Kaletra 200mg/50mg tablets | 120 tablet PoM £285.41

F 458

Ritonavir

06-May-2020

- **INDICATIONS AND DOSE**

HIV infection in combination with other antiretroviral drugs (high-dose ritonavir)

▸ BY MOUTH

- ▸ Child 2–17 years: Initially 250 mg/m² twice daily, increased in steps of 50 mg/m² every 2–3 days; increased to 350 mg/m² twice daily (max. per dose 600 mg twice daily), tolerability of this regimen is poor

Low-dose ritonavir to increase the effect of atazanavir

▸ BY MOUTH

- ▸ Child 6–17 years (body-weight 15–19 kg): 80–100 mg once daily
- ▸ Child 6–17 years (body-weight 20 kg and above): 100 mg once daily

Low-dose ritonavir to increase the effect of darunavir

▸ BY MOUTH

- ▸ Child 3–17 years (body-weight 15–29 kg): 50 mg twice daily
- ▸ Child 3–17 years (body-weight 30–39 kg): 60 mg twice daily
- ▸ Child 3–17 years (body-weight 40 kg and above): 100 mg twice daily
- ▸ Child 12–17 years (body-weight 40 kg and above): 100 mg once daily for use in patients taking darunavir once daily

Low-dose ritonavir to increase the effect of fosamprenavir

▸ BY MOUTH

- ▸ Child 6–17 years (body-weight 25–32 kg): 3 mg/kg twice daily
- ▸ Child 6–17 years (body-weight 33 kg and above): 100 mg twice daily

Low-dose ritonavir to increase the effect of tipranavir

▸ BY MOUTH

- ▸ Child 2–11 years: 150 mg/m² twice daily (max. per dose 200 mg)
- ▸ Child 12–17 years: 200 mg twice daily

- **CAUTIONS** Cardiac conduction disorders · pancreatitis · structural heart disease
- **INTERACTIONS** → Appendix 1: HIV-protease inhibitors
- **SIDE-EFFECTS**
- ▸ **Common or very common** Back pain · concentration impaired · confusion · cough · dehydration · feeling hot · flushing · gastrointestinal haemorrhage · gout · hypotension · menorrhagia · myopathy · oedema · oral paraesthesia · oropharyngeal pain · paraesthesia · peripheral coldness · pharyngitis · renal impairment · syncope · thrombocytopenia · urinary frequency increased · vision blurred
- ▸ **Uncommon** Myocardial infarction

- **Rare or very rare** Hyperglycaemia · toxic epidermal necrolysis

SIDE-EFFECTS, FURTHER INFORMATION Signs and symptoms suggestive of pancreatitis (including raised serum lipase) should be evaluated — discontinue if pancreatitis diagnosed.

- **PREGNANCY**

Dose adjustments Only use low-dose booster to increase the effect of other protease inhibitors.

- **HEPATIC IMPAIRMENT** When used as a *low-dose booster*, manufacturer advises caution in severe impairment; avoid in decompensated liver disease. When used in *high-doses*, manufacturer advises avoid in severe impairment.

Dose adjustments Manufacturer advises consult product literature of co-administered protease inhibitor.

- **MEDICINAL FORMS** There can be variation in the licensing of different medicines containing the same drug.

Tablet

CAUTIONARY AND ADVISORY LABELS 21, 25

- Ritonavir (Non-proprietary)

Ritonavir 100 mg Ritonavir 100mg tablets | 30 tablet PoM £16.52-£19.44 | 30 tablet PoM £19.44 (Hospital only)

- Norvir (AbbVie Ltd)

Ritonavir 100 mg Norvir 100mg tablets | 30 tablet PoM £19.44

F 458

Tipranavir

06-May-2020

- **INDICATIONS AND DOSE**

HIV infection resistant to other protease inhibitors, in combination with other antiretroviral drugs in patients previously treated with antiretrovirals–with low-dose ritonavir

- BY MOUTH USING CAPSULES
- Child 12–17 years: 500 mg twice daily
- BY MOUTH USING ORAL SOLUTION
- Child 2–11 years: 375 mg/m^2 twice daily (max. per dose 500 mg)

DOSE EQUIVALENCE AND CONVERSION

- The bioavailability of tipranavir oral solution is higher than that of the capsules; the oral solution is not interchangeable with the capsules on a milligram-for-milligram basis.

- **CAUTIONS** Abnormal liver function tests and/or signs or symptoms of liver injury (consider delaying treatment if serum transaminases are greater than 5 times the upper limit of normal—consult product literature) · patients at risk of increased bleeding from trauma, surgery or other pathological conditions
- **INTERACTIONS** → Appendix 1: HIV-protease inhibitors
- **SIDE-EFFECTS**
- **Uncommon** Hyperamylasaemia · hyperglycaemia · influenza like illness · renal failure · thrombocytopenia
- **Rare or very rare** Dehydration · hyperbilirubinaemia · intracranial haemorrhage
- **Frequency not known** Bleeding tendency

SIDE-EFFECTS, FURTHER INFORMATION Potentially life-threatening hepatotoxicity reported. Discontinue if signs or symptoms of hepatitis develop or if liver-function abnormality develops (consult product literature).

- **PREGNANCY** Manufacturer advises use only if potential benefit outweighs risk—toxicity in *animal* studies.
- **HEPATIC IMPAIRMENT** Manufacturer advises caution in mild impairment (risk of increased exposure)—monitor liver function before treatment, then every two weeks for 3 months, then monthly until 48 weeks, then every 8 to 12 weeks thereafter, and discontinue if liver function worsens; avoid in moderate to severe impairment.
- **MONITORING REQUIREMENTS** Monitor liver function before treatment, then every 2 weeks for 1 month, then every 4 weeks until 24 weeks, then every 8 to 12 weeks thereafter.
- **PRESCRIBING AND DISPENSING INFORMATION** Flavours of oral liquid formulations may include toffee and mint.
- **PATIENT AND CARER ADVICE** Patients or carers should be told to observe the oral solution for crystallisation; the bottle should be replaced if more than a thin layer of crystals form (doses should continue to be taken at the normal time until the bottle is replaced).

- **MEDICINAL FORMS** There can be variation in the licensing of different medicines containing the same drug.

Capsule

CAUTIONARY AND ADVISORY LABELS 5, 21

EXCIPIENTS: May contain Ethanol

- Aptivus (Boehringer Ingelheim Ltd)

Tipranavir 250 mg Aptivus 250mg capsules | 120 capsule PoM £441.00

ANTIVIRALS > OTHER

Maraviroc

20-May-2020

- **DRUG ACTION** Maraviroc is an antagonist of the CCR5 chemokine receptor.

- **INDICATIONS AND DOSE**

CCR5-tropic HIV infection in combination with other antiretroviral drugs in patients previously treated with antiretrovirals

- BY MOUTH
- Child: (consult local protocol)

- **UNLICENSED USE** Not licensed for use in children.
- **CAUTIONS** Cardiovascular disease
- **INTERACTIONS** → Appendix 1: maraviroc
- **SIDE-EFFECTS**
- **Common or very common** Abdominal pain · anaemia · appetite decreased · asthenia · depression · diarrhoea · flatulence · headache · insomnia · nausea · rash
- **Uncommon** Hyperbilirubinaemia · increased risk of infection · myopathy · postural hypotension · proteinuria · renal failure · seizure
- **Rare or very rare** Angina pectoris · granulocytopenia · hepatic disorders · metastases · neoplasms · pancytopenia · severe cutaneous adverse reactions (SCARs)
- **Frequency not known** Fever · hypersensitivity · immune reconstitution inflammatory syndrome · organ dysfunction · osteonecrosis

SIDE-EFFECTS, FURTHER INFORMATION **Osteonecrosis** Osteonecrosis has been reported in patients with advanced HIV disease or following long-term exposure to combination antiretroviral therapy.

Hepatotoxicity Manufacturer advises consider discontinuation if signs or symptoms of acute hepatitis, or increased liver transaminases with systemic symptoms of hypersensitivity occur.

- **PREGNANCY** Manufacturer advises use only if potential benefit outweighs risk—toxicity in *animal* studies.
- **HEPATIC IMPAIRMENT** Manufacturer advises caution in impairment and in patients with chronic hepatitis (increased risk of hepatic side-effects; limited information available).
- **RENAL IMPAIRMENT** If estimated glomerular filtration rate less than 80 mL/minute/1.73 m^2, consult product literature.

- **MEDICINAL FORMS** There can be variation in the licensing of different medicines containing the same drug.

Tablet

▸ Celsentri (ViiV Healthcare UK Ltd)

Maraviroc 25 mg Celsentri 25mg tablets | 120 tablet PoM £147.09 DT = £147.09

Maraviroc 75 mg Celsentri 75mg tablets | 120 tablet PoM £441.27 DT = £441.27

Maraviroc 150 mg Celsentri 150mg tablets | 60 tablet PoM £519.14 DT = £519.14

Maraviroc 300 mg Celsentri 300mg tablets | 60 tablet PoM £519.14 DT = £519.14

5.6 Influenza

Influenza

Management

Oseltamivir below and zanamivir p. 464 are most effective for the treatment of influenza if started within a few hours of the onset of symptoms; oseltamivir is licensed for use within 48 hours of the first symptoms while zanamivir is licensed for use within 36 hours of the first symptoms. In otherwise healthy individuals they reduce the duration of symptoms by about 1–1.5 days.

Oseltamivir and zanamivir are licensed for post-exposure prophylaxis of influenza when influenza is circulating in the community. Oseltamivir should be given within 48 hours of exposure to influenza while zanamivir should be given within 36 hours of exposure to influenza. However, in children with severe influenza or in those who are immunocompromised, antivirals may still be effective after this time if viral shedding continues [unlicensed use]. Oseltamivir and zanamivir are also licensed for use in exceptional circumstances (e.g. when vaccination does not cover the infecting strain) to prevent influenza in an epidemic.

There is evidence that some strains of influenza A virus have reduced susceptibility to oseltamivir, but may retain susceptibility to zanamivir. Resistance to oseltamivir may be greater in severely immunocompromised children.

Zanamivir should be reserved for patients who are severely immunocompromised, or when oseltamivir cannot be used, or when resistance to oseltamivir is suspected. For those unable to use the dry powder for inhalation, zanamivir is available as a solution that can be administered by nebuliser [unlicensed] or intravenously.

Information on pandemic influenza, avian influenza, and swine influenza may be found at www.gov.uk/phe.

Immunisation against influenza is recommended for persons at high risk, and to reduce transmission of infection.

Oseltamivir in children under 1 year of age

Data on the use of oseltamivir in children under 1 year of age is limited. Furthermore, oseltamivir may be ineffective in neonates because they may not be able to metabolise oseltamivir to its active form. However, oseltamivir can be used (under specialist supervision) for the treatment or post-exposure prophylaxis of influenza in children under 1 year of age. The Department of Health has advised (May 2009) that during a pandemic, treatment with oseltamivir can be overseen by healthcare professionals experienced in assessing children.

Amantadine hydrochloride is licensed for prophylaxis and treatment of influenza A in children over 10 years of age, but it is no longer recommended.

ANTIVIRALS > NEURAMINIDASE INHIBITORS

Oseltamivir

10-Mar-2020

- **DRUG ACTION** Reduces replication of influenza A and B viruses by inhibiting viral neuraminidase.

- **INDICATIONS AND DOSE**

Prevention of influenza

▸ BY MOUTH

▸ Neonate: 3 mg/kg once daily for 10 days for post-exposure prophylaxis.

▸ Child 1–11 months: 3 mg/kg once daily for 10 days for post-exposure prophylaxis

▸ Child 1–12 years (body-weight 10–15 kg): 30 mg once daily for 10 days for post-exposure prophylaxis; for up to 6 weeks during an epidemic

▸ Child 1–12 years (body-weight 15–23 kg): 45 mg once daily for 10 days for post-exposure prophylaxis; for up to 6 weeks during an epidemic

▸ Child 1–12 years (body-weight 23–40 kg): 60 mg once daily for 10 days for post-exposure prophylaxis; for up to 6 weeks during an epidemic

▸ Child 1–12 years (body-weight 40 kg and above): 75 mg once daily for 10 days for post-exposure prophylaxis; for up to 6 weeks during an epidemic

▸ Child 13–17 years: 75 mg once daily for 10 days for post-exposure prophylaxis; for up to 6 weeks during an epidemic

Treatment of influenza

▸ BY MOUTH

▸ Neonate: 3 mg/kg twice daily for 5 days.

▸ Child 1–11 months: 3 mg/kg twice daily for 5 days

▸ Child 1–12 years (body-weight 10–15 kg): 30 mg twice daily for 5 days

▸ Child 1–12 years (body-weight 15–23 kg): 45 mg twice daily for 5 days

▸ Child 1–12 years (body-weight 23–40 kg): 60 mg twice daily for 5 days

▸ Child 1–12 years (body-weight 40 kg and above): 75 mg twice daily for 5 days

▸ Child 13–17 years: 75 mg twice daily for 5 days

- **UNLICENSED USE** Not licensed for use in premature infants.
- **INTERACTIONS** → Appendix 1: oseltamivir
- **SIDE-EFFECTS**

▸ **Common or very common** Dizziness · gastrointestinal discomfort · herpes simplex · nausea · sleep disorders · vertigo · vomiting

▸ **Uncommon** Arrhythmia · seizure · skin reactions

▸ **Rare or very rare** Angioedema · anxiety · behaviour abnormal · confusion · delirium · delusions · gastrointestinal haemorrhage · hallucination · hepatic disorders · self-injurious behaviour · severe cutaneous adverse reactions (SCARs) · thrombocytopenia · visual impairment

- **PREGNANCY** Although safety data are limited, oseltamivir can be used in women who are pregnant when the potential benefit outweighs the risk (e.g. during a pandemic).
- **BREAST FEEDING** Although safety data are limited, oseltamivir can be used in women who are breast-feeding when the potential benefit outweighs the risk (e.g. during a pandemic). Oseltamivir is the preferred drug in women who are breast-feeding.
- **RENAL IMPAIRMENT** Avoid for *treatment* and *prevention* if estimated glomerular filtration rate less than 10 mL/minute/1.73 m^2.

5 Infection

Dose adjustments For *treatment*, use 40% of normal dose twice daily if estimated glomerular filtration rate 30–60 mL/minute/1.73 m^2 (40% of normal dose once daily if estimated glomerular filtration rate 10–30 mL/minute/1.73 m^2).

For *prevention*, use 40% of normal dose once daily if estimated glomerular filtration rate 30–60 mL/minute/1.73 m^2 (40% of normal dose every 48 hours if estimated glomerular filtration rate 10–30 mL/minute/1.73 m^2).

- **DIRECTIONS FOR ADMINISTRATION** If suspension not available, capsules can be opened and the contents mixed with a small amount of sweetened food, such as sugar water or chocolate syrup, just before administration.
- **PRESCRIBING AND DISPENSING INFORMATION** Flavours of oral liquid formulations may include tutti-frutti.
- **PATIENT AND CARER ADVICE**
Medicines for Children leaflet: Oseltamivir for influenza (flu) www.medicinesforchildren.org.uk/oseltamivir-influenza-flu
- **NATIONAL FUNDING/ACCESS DECISIONS**

NICE decisions

▸ **Oseltamivir, zanamivir, and amantadine for prophylaxis of influenza (September 2008)** NICE TA158

Oseltamivir is **not** a substitute for vaccination, which remains the most effective way of preventing illness from influenza.

- Oseltamivir is **not** recommended for seasonal prophylaxis against influenza.
- When influenza is circulating in the community, oseltamivir is an option recommended (in accordance with UK licensing) for post-exposure prophylaxis in at-risk patients who are not effectively protected by influenza vaccine, and who have been in close contact with someone suffering from influenza-like illness in the same household or residential setting. Oseltamivir should be given within 48 hours of exposure to influenza. (National surveillance schemes, including those run by Public Health England, should be used to indicate when influenza is circulating in the community.)
- During local outbreaks of influenza-like illness, when there is a high level of certainty that influenza is present, oseltamivir may be used for post-exposure prophylaxis in at-risk patients (regardless of influenza vaccination) living in long-term residential or nursing homes.

At risk patients include those aged 65 years or older *or* those who have one or more of the following conditions:

- chronic respiratory disease (including asthma and chronic obstructive pulmonary disease);
- chronic heart disease;
- chronic renal disease;
- chronic liver disease;
- chronic neurological disease;
- immunosuppression;
- diabetes mellitus.

The Department of Health in England has advised (November 2010 and April 2011) that 'at risk patients' also includes patients under 65 years of age who are at risk of developing medical complications from influenza (treatment only) or women who are pregnant.

This guidance does not cover the circumstances of a pandemic, an impending pandemic, or a widespread epidemic of a new strain of influenza to which there is little or no immunity in the community.
www.nice.org.uk/guidance/ta158

▸ **Oseltamivir, zanamivir, and amantadine for treatment of influenza (February 2009)** NICE TA168

Oseltamivir is **not** a substitute for vaccination, which remains the most effective way of preventing illness from influenza.

- When influenza is circulating in the community, oseltamivir is an option recommended (in accordance with UK licensing) for the treatment of influenza in at-risk patients who can start treatment within 48 hours of the onset of symptoms. (National surveillance schemes, including those run by Public Health England, should be used to indicate when influenza is circulating in the community.)
- During local outbreaks of influenza-like illness, when there is a high level of certainty that influenza is present, oseltamivir may be used for treatment in at-risk patients living in long-term residential or nursing homes.

At risk patients include those aged over 65 years *or* those who have one or more of the following conditions:

- chronic respiratory disease (including asthma and chronic obstructive pulmonary disease);
- chronic heart disease;
- chronic renal disease;
- chronic liver disease;
- chronic neurological disease;
- immunosuppression;
- diabetes mellitus.

The Department of Health in England has advised (November 2010 and April 2011) that 'at risk patients' also includes patients under 65 years of age who are at risk of developing medical complications from influenza (treatment only) or women who are pregnant.

This guidance does not cover the circumstances of a pandemic, an impending pandemic, or a widespread epidemic of a new strain of influenza to which there is little or no immunity in the community.
www.nice.org.uk/guidance/ta168

NHS restrictions *Tamiflu*® is not prescribable in NHS primary care except for the treatment and prophylaxis of influenza as indicated in the NICE guidance; endorse prescription 'SLS'.

- **MEDICINAL FORMS** There can be variation in the licensing of different medicines containing the same drug. Forms available from special-order manufacturers include: oral suspension, oral solution

Oral suspension

CAUTIONARY AND ADVISORY LABELS 9
EXCIPIENTS: May contain Sorbitol

▸ **Tamiflu** (Roche Products Ltd)
Oseltamivir (as Oseltamivir phosphate) 6 mg per 1 ml Tamiflu 6mg/ml oral suspension sugar-free | 65 ml PoM £10.27 DT = £10.27

Capsule

CAUTIONARY AND ADVISORY LABELS 9

▸ **Tamiflu** (Roche Products Ltd)
Oseltamivir (as Oseltamivir phosphate) 30 mg Tamiflu 30mg capsules | 10 capsule PoM £7.71 DT = £7.71
Oseltamivir (as Oseltamivir phosphate) 45 mg Tamiflu 45mg capsules | 10 capsule PoM £15.41 DT = £15.41
Oseltamivir (as Oseltamivir phosphate) 75 mg Tamiflu 75mg capsules | 10 capsule PoM £15.41 DT = £15.41

Zanamivir

20-May-2020

- **DRUG ACTION** Reduces replication of influenza A and B viruses by inhibiting viral neuraminidase.

- **INDICATIONS AND DOSE**

Post-exposure prophylaxis of influenza

▸ BY INHALATION OF POWDER
▸ Child 5–17 years: 10 mg once daily for 10 days

Prevention of influenza during an epidemic

▸ BY INHALATION OF POWDER
▸ Child 5–17 years: 10 mg once daily for up to 28 days

Treatment of influenza
- ▶ BY INHALATION OF POWDER
- ▶ Child 5–17 years: 10 mg twice daily for 5 days (for up to 10 days if resistance to oseltamivir suspected)

Treatment of influenza [complicated and potentially life-threatening, resistant to other anti-influenza medicinal products and/or other treatments, including inhaled zanamivir]
- ▶ BY INTRAVENOUS INFUSION
- ▶ Child 6 months–5 years: 14 mg/kg twice daily for 5 to 10 days
- ▶ Child 6–17 years: 12 mg/kg twice daily (max. per dose 600 mg) for 5 to 10 days

● **UNLICENSED USE**
- ▶ When used by inhalation Use of zanamivir for up to 10 days if resistance to oseltamivir suspected is an unlicensed duration.

● **CAUTIONS**
- ▶ When used by inhalation Asthma · chronic pulmonary disease · uncontrolled chronic illness

CAUTIONS, FURTHER INFORMATION
- ▶ Asthma and chronic pulmonary disease Risk of bronchospasm—short-acting bronchodilator should be available. Avoid in severe asthma unless close monitoring possible and appropriate facilities available to treat bronchospasm.

● **SIDE-EFFECTS**

GENERAL SIDE-EFFECTS
- ▶ **Common or very common** Skin reactions
- ▶ **Uncommon** Oropharyngeal oedema · severe cutaneous adverse reactions (SCARs)
- ▶ **Rare or very rare** Face oedema
- ▶ **Frequency not known** Behaviour abnormal · delirium · hallucination · level of consciousness decreased · seizure

SPECIFIC SIDE-EFFECTS
- ▶ **Common or very common**
- ▶ With intravenous use Diarrhoea · hepatocellular injury
- ▶ **Uncommon**
- ▶ When used by inhalation Bronchospasm · dehydration · dyspnoea · presyncope · throat tightness
- ▶ **Frequency not known**
- ▶ When used by inhalation Psychiatric disorder

SIDE-EFFECTS, FURTHER INFORMATION Neurological and psychiatric disorders occur more commonly in children and adolescents.

● **PREGNANCY** Manufacturer advises avoid unless potential benefit outweighs risk (e.g. during a pandemic).—limited information available; *animal* studies do not indicate toxicity.

● **BREAST FEEDING** Manufacturer advises use only if potential benefit outweighs risk (e.g. during a pandemic)—limited information available; present in low levels in milk in *animal* studies.

● **RENAL IMPAIRMENT**

Dose adjustments ▶ With intravenous use Manufacturer advises reduce dose if creatinine clearance less than 80 mL/minute—consult product literature for details.

● **DIRECTIONS FOR ADMINISTRATION**
- ▶ When used by inhalation Other inhaled drugs should be administered before zanamivir.
- ▶ With intravenous use Manufacturer advises for *intermittent intravenous infusion*, give undiluted or dilute to a concentration of not less than 200 micrograms/mL with Sodium Chloride 0.9%; give over 30 minutes.

● **PRESCRIBING AND DISPENSING INFORMATION**
- ▶ When used by inhalation Except for the treatment and prophylaxis of influenza as indicated in the NICE guidance; endorse prescription 'SLS'.

● **NATIONAL FUNDING/ACCESS DECISIONS**

NICE decisions

▶ **Oseltamivir, zanamivir, and amantadine for prophylaxis of influenza (September 2008)** NICE TA158

Zanamivir is **not** a substitute for vaccination, which remains the most effective way of preventing illness from influenza.
- Zanamivir is **not** recommended for seasonal prophylaxis against influenza.
- When influenza is circulating in the community, zanamivir is an option recommended (in accordance with UK licensing) for post-exposure prophylaxis in at-risk patients who are not effectively protected by influenza vaccine, and who have been in close contact with someone suffering from influenza-like illness in the same household or residential setting. Zanamivir should be given within 36 hours of exposure to influenza. (National surveillance schemes, including those run by Public Health England, should be used to indicate when influenza is circulating in the community).
- During local outbreaks of influenza-like illness, when there is a high level of certainty that influenza is present, zanamivir may be used for post-exposure prophylaxis in at-risk patients (regardless of influenza vaccination) living in long-term residential or nursing homes.

At risk patients include those aged over 65 years *or* those who have one or more of the following conditions:
- chronic respiratory disease (including asthma and chronic obstructive pulmonary disease);
- chronic heart disease;
- chronic renal disease;
- chronic liver disease;
- chronic neurological disease;
- immunosuppression;
- diabetes mellitus.

The Department of Health in England has advised (November 2010 and April 2011) that 'at risk patients' also includes patients under 65 years of age who are at risk of developing medical complications from influenza (treatment only) or women who are pregnant.

This guidance does not cover the circumstances of a pandemic, an impending pandemic, or a widespread epidemic of a new strain of influenza to which there is little or no immunity in the community.

www.nice.org.uk/guidance/ta158

▶ **Oseltamivir, zanamivir, and amantadine for treatment of influenza (February 2009)** NICE TA168
- ▶ When used by inhalation Zanamivir is **not** a substitute for vaccination, which remains the most effective way of preventing illness from influenza.
  - When influenza is circulating in the community, zanamivir is an option recommended (in accordance with UK licensing) for the treatment of influenza in at-risk patients who can start treatment within 48 hours (within 36 hours for zanamivir in children) of the onset of symptoms. (National surveillance schemes, including those run by Public Health England, should be used to indicate when influenza is circulating in the community.)
  - During local outbreaks of influenza-like illness, when there is a high level of certainty that influenza is present, zanamivir may be used for treatment in at-risk patients living in long-term residential or nursing homes.

  At risk patients include those aged over 65 years *or* those who have one or more of the following conditions:
  - chronic respiratory disease (including asthma and chronic obstructive pulmonary disease);
  - chronic heart disease;
  - chronic renal disease;
  - chronic liver disease;

- chronic neurological disease;
- immunosuppression;
- diabetes mellitus.

The Department of Health in England has advised (November 2010 and April 2011) that 'at risk patients' also includes patients under 65 years of age who are at risk of developing medical complications from influenza (treatment only) or women who are pregnant.

This guidance does not cover the circumstances of a pandemic, an impending pandemic, or a widespread epidemic of a new strain of influenza to which there is little or no immunity in the community.
www.nice.org.uk/guidance/TA168

Scottish Medicines Consortium (SMC) decisions
SMC No. SMC2204

- With intravenous use The *Scottish Medicines Consortium* has advised (December 2019) that zanamivir (*Dectova*®) is accepted for use within NHS Scotland for the treatment of complicated and potentially life-threatening influenza A or B virus infection in adult and paediatric patients aged 6 months and older when: the patient's influenza virus is known or suspected to be resistant to anti-influenza medicinal products other than zanamivir, and/or other anti-viral medicinal products for treatment of influenza, including inhaled zanamivir, are not suitable for the individual patient. Zanamivir (*Dectova*®) should be used in accordance with official guidance.

All Wales Medicines Strategy Group (AWMSG) decisions
AWMSG No. 4130

- With intravenous use The *All Wales Medicines Strategy Group* has advised (October 2019) that zanamivir (*Dectova*®) is recommended as an option for use within NHS Wales for the treatment of complicated and potentially life-threatening influenza A or B virus infection in adults and children (aged 6 months and older), when: the patient's influenza virus is known or suspected to be resistant to anti-influenza medicinal products other than zanamivir, and/or other anti-viral medicinal products for treatment of influenza, including inhaled zanamivir, are not suitable for the individual patient. Zanamivir (*Dectova*®) should be used in accordance with official guidance.

- **MEDICINAL FORMS** There can be variation in the licensing of different medicines containing the same drug.

Solution for infusion
ELECTROLYTES: May contain Sodium

- **Dectova** (GlaxoSmithKline UK Ltd) ▼
  Zanamivir 10 mg per 1 ml Dectova 200mg/20ml solution for infusion vials | 1 vial PoM £27.83

Inhalation powder

- **Relenza** (GlaxoSmithKline UK Ltd)
  Zanamivir 5 mg Relenza 5mg inhalation powder blisters with Diskhaler | 20 blister PoM £16.36

5.7 Respiratory syncytial virus

Respiratory syncytial virus

Management

Ribavirin p. 435 inhibits a wide range of DNA and RNA viruses. It is licensed for administration by inhalation for the treatment of severe bronchiolitis caused by the respiratory syncytial virus (RSV) in infants, especially when they have other serious diseases. However, there is no evidence that ribavirin produces clinically relevant benefit in RSV bronchiolitis. Ribavirin is effective in Lassa fever and has also been used parenterally in the treatment of life-threatening RSV, parainfluenza virus, and adenovirus infections in immunocompromised children [unlicensed indications].

Palivizumab below is a monoclonal antibody licensed for preventing serious lower respiratory-tract disease caused by respiratory syncytial virus in children at high risk of the disease; it should be prescribed under specialist supervision and on the basis of the likelihood of hospitalisation.
Palivizumab is recommended for:

- children under 9 months of age with chronic lung disease (defined as requiring oxygen for at least 28 days from birth) and who were born preterm;
- children under 6 months of age with haemodynamically significant, acyanotic congenital heart disease who were born preterm.

Palivizumab should be considered for:

- children under 2 years of age with severe combined immunodeficiency syndrome;
- children under 1 year of age who require long-term ventilation;
- children 1–2 years of age who require long-term ventilation and have an additional co-morbidity (including cardiac disease or pulmonary hypertension).

For details of the preterm age groups included in the recommendations, see *Immunisation against Infectious Disease* (2006), available at www.gov.uk/dh.

DRUGS FOR RESPIRATORY DISEASES › MONOCLONAL ANTIBODIES

Palivizumab

- **INDICATIONS AND DOSE**

Prevention of serious lower respiratory-tract disease caused by respiratory syncytial virus in children at high risk of the disease (under expert supervision)

- BY INTRAMUSCULAR INJECTION
- Neonate: 15 mg/kg once a month, preferably injected in the anterolateral thigh, to be administered during season of RSV risk.
- Child 1–23 months: 15 mg/kg once a month, preferably injected in the anterolateral thigh, to be administered during season of RSV risk, injection volume over 1 mL should be divided between 2 or more sites

Prevention of serious lower respiratory-tract disease caused by respiratory syncytial virus in children at high risk of the disease and undergoing cardiac bypass surgery (under expert supervision)

- BY INTRAMUSCULAR INJECTION
- Child 1–23 months: Initially 15 mg/kg, to be administered as soon as stable after surgery, preferably in the anterolateral thigh, then 15 mg/kg once a month, preferably injected in the anterolateral thigh, to be administered during season of RSV risk, injection volume over 1 mL should be divided between 2 or more sites

- **UNLICENSED USE** Licensed for the prevention of serious lower respiratory-tract disease caused by respiratory syncytial virus (RSV) in children under 6 months of age (at the start of the RSV season) and born at less than 35 weeks corrected gestational age, or in children under 2 years of age who have received treatment for bronchopulmonary dysplasia in the last 6 months, or in children under 2 years of age with haemodynamically significant congenital heart disease.
- **CAUTIONS** Moderate to severe acute infection · moderate to severe febrile illness · serum-palivizumab concentration may be reduced after cardiac surgery · thrombocytopenia
- **SIDE-EFFECTS**
  - **Common or very common** Apnoea
  - **Uncommon** Seizure · thrombocytopenia · urticaria
  - **Frequency not known** Hypersensitivity

● **ALLERGY AND CROSS-SENSITIVITY** Hypersensitivity to humanised monoclonal antibodies.

● **MEDICINAL FORMS** There can be variation in the licensing of different medicines containing the same drug.

Solution for injection

▸ Synagis (AbbVie Ltd)

Palivizumab 100 mg per 1 ml Synagis 100mg/1ml solution for injection vials | 1 vial PoM £563.64

Synagis 50mg/0.5ml solution for injection vials | 1 vial PoM £306.34

Chapter 6 Endocrine system

CONTENTS

1 Antidiuretic hormone disorders

Posterior pituitary hormones and antagonists

Posterior pituitary hormones

Diabetes insipidus

Diabetes insipidus is caused by either a deficiency of antidiuretic hormone (ADH, vasopressin p. 72) secretion (cranial, neurogenic, or pituitary diabetes insipidus) or by failure of the renal tubules to react to secreted antidiuretic hormone (nephrogenic diabetes insipidus).

Vasopressin (antidiuretic hormone, ADH) is used in the treatment of *pituitary diabetes insipidus* as is its analogue desmopressin below. Dosage is tailored to produce a regular diuresis every 24 hours to avoid water intoxication. Treatment may be required permanently or for a limited period only in diabetes insipidus following trauma or pituitary surgery.

Desmopressin is more potent and has a longer duration of action than vasopressin; unlike vasopressin it has no vasoconstrictor effect. It is given by mouth or intranasally for maintenance therapy, and by injection in the postoperative period or in unconscious patients. Desmopressin is also used in the differential diagnosis of diabetes insipidus; following an intramuscular or intranasal dose, restoration of the ability to concentrate urine after water deprivation confirms a diagnosis of pituitary diabetes insipidus. Failure to respond suggests nephrogenic diabetes insipidus. Fluid input must be managed carefully to avoid hyponatraemia; this test is not usually recommended in young children.

In *nephrogenic* and *partial pituitary diabetes insipidus* benefit may be gained from the paradoxical antidiuretic effect of thiazides.

Other uses

Desmopressin is also used to boost factor VIII concentration in mild to moderate haemophilia and in von Willebrand's disease; it is also used to test fibrinolytic response. Desmopressin also has a role in nocturnal enuresis.

Vasopressin infusion is used to control variceal bleeding in portal hypertension, before introducing more definitive treatment. Terlipressin acetate, a derivative of vasopressin with reportedly less pressor and antidiuretic activity, and octreotide are used similarly but experience in children is limited.

1.1 Diabetes insipidus

Other drugs used for Diabetes insipidus Chlorothiazide, p. 117 · Chlortalidone, p. 150

PITUITARY AND HYPOTHALAMIC HORMONES AND ANALOGUES › VASOPRESSIN AND ANALOGUES

Desmopressin

02-Dec-2019

- **DRUG ACTION** Desmopressin is an analogue of vasopressin.

- **INDICATIONS AND DOSE**

Diabetes insipidus, treatment

▶ BY MOUTH

- ▶ Neonate: Initially 1–4 micrograms 2–3 times a day, adjusted according to response.
- ▶ Child 1–23 months: Initially 10 micrograms 2–3 times a day, adjusted according to response; usual dose 30–150 micrograms daily
- ▶ Child 2–11 years: Initially 50 micrograms 2–3 times a day, adjusted according to response; usual dose 100–800 micrograms daily
- ▶ Child 12–17 years: Initially 100 micrograms 2–3 times a day, adjusted according to response; usual dose 0.2–1.2 mg daily

▶ BY SUBLINGUAL ADMINISTRATION
▸ Child 2–17 years: Initially 60 micrograms 3 times a day, adjusted according to response; usual dose 40–240 micrograms 3 times a day
▶ BY INTRANASAL ADMINISTRATION
▸ Neonate: Initially 100–500 nanograms, adjusted according to response; usual dose 1.25–10 micrograms daily in 1–2 divided doses.
▸ Child 1–23 months: Initially 2.5–5 micrograms 1–2 times a day, adjusted according to response
▸ Child 2–11 years: Initially 5–20 micrograms 1–2 times a day, adjusted according to response
▸ Child 12–17 years: Initially 10–20 micrograms 1–2 times a day, adjusted according to response
▶ BY INTRAMUSCULAR INJECTION
▸ Neonate: Initially 100 nanograms once daily, adjusted according to response.
▶ BY SUBCUTANEOUS INJECTION, OR BY INTRAMUSCULAR INJECTION
▸ Child 1 month–11 years: Initially 400 nanograms once daily, adjusted according to response
▸ Child 12–17 years: Initially 1–4 micrograms once daily, adjusted according to response

Primary nocturnal enuresis
▶ BY MOUTH
▸ Child 5–17 years: 200 micrograms once daily, only increased to 400 micrograms if lower dose not effective; withdraw for at least 1 week for reassessment after 3 months, dose to be taken at bedtime, limit fluid intake from 1 hour before to 8 hours after administration
▶ BY SUBLINGUAL ADMINISTRATION
▸ Child 5–17 years: 120 micrograms once daily, increased if necessary to 240 micrograms once daily, dose to be taken at bedtime, limit fluid intake from 1 hour before to 8 hours after administration, dose to be increased only if lower dose not effective, reassess after 3 months by withdrawing treatment for at least 1 week

Diabetes insipidus, diagnosis (water deprivation test)
▶ BY INTRANASAL ADMINISTRATION
▸ Neonate: Not recommended, use trial of treatment.
▸ Child 1–23 months: 5–10 micrograms for 1 dose, manage fluid input carefully to avoid hyponatraemia, not usually recommended
▸ Child 2–11 years: 10–20 micrograms for 1 dose, manage fluid input carefully to avoid hyponatraemia
▸ Child 12–17 years: 20 micrograms for 1 dose, manage fluid input carefully to avoid hyponatraemia
▶ BY INTRAMUSCULAR INJECTION, OR BY SUBCUTANEOUS INJECTION
▸ Neonate: Not recommended, use trial of treatment.
▸ Child 1–23 months: 400 nanograms for 1 dose, manage fluid input carefully to avoid hyponatraemia, not usually recommended
▸ Child 2–11 years: 0.5–1 microgram for 1 dose, manage fluid input carefully to avoid hyponatraemia
▸ Child 12–17 years: 1–2 micrograms for 1 dose, manage fluid input carefully to avoid hyponatraemia

Renal function testing
▶ BY INTRANASAL ADMINISTRATION
▸ Child 1–11 months: 10 micrograms, empty bladder at time of administration and restrict fluid intake to 50% at next 2 feeds to avoid fluid overload
▸ Child 1–14 years: 20 micrograms, empty bladder at time of administration and restrict fluid intake to 500 mL from 1 hour before until 8 hours after administration to avoid fluid overload
▸ Child 15–17 years: 40 micrograms, empty bladder at time of administration and limit fluid intake to 500 mL from 1 hour before until 8 hours after administration to avoid fluid overload
▶ BY SUBCUTANEOUS INJECTION, OR BY INTRAMUSCULAR INJECTION
▸ Child 1–11 months: 400 nanograms, empty bladder at time of administration and restrict fluid intake to 50% at next 2 feeds to avoid fluid overload
▸ Child 1–17 years: 2 micrograms, empty bladder at time of administration and restrict fluid intake to 500 mL from 1 hour before until 8 hours after administration to avoid fluid overload

Mild to moderate haemophilia and von Willebrand's disease
▶ BY INTRANASAL ADMINISTRATION
▸ Child 1–17 years: 4 micrograms/kg for 1 dose, for pre-operative use give 2 hours before procedure
▶ BY INTRAVENOUS INFUSION, OR BY SUBCUTANEOUS INJECTION
▸ Child: 300 nanograms/kg for 1 dose, to be administered immediately before surgery or after trauma; may be repeated at intervals of 12 hours if no tachycardia

Fibrinolytic response testing
▶ BY SUBCUTANEOUS INJECTION, OR BY INTRAVENOUS INJECTION
▸ Child 2–17 years: 300 nanograms/kg for 1 dose, blood to be sampled after 20 minutes for fibrinolytic activity

Assessment of antidiuretic hormone secretion (congenital deficiency suspected) (specialist use only)
▶ BY INTRANASAL ADMINISTRATION
▸ Child 1–23 months: Initially 100–500 nanograms for 1 dose

Assessment of antidiuretic hormone secretion (congenital deficiency not suspected) (specialist use only)
▶ BY INTRANASAL ADMINISTRATION
▸ Child 1–23 months: 1–5 micrograms for 1 dose

● UNLICENSED USE Consult product literature for individual preparations. Not licensed for assessment of antidiuretic hormone secretion. Oral use of *DDAVP* intravenous injection is not licensed.

● CONTRA-INDICATIONS Cardiac insufficiency · conditions treated with diuretics · history of hyponatraemia · polydipsia in alcohol dependence · psychogenic polydipsia · syndrome of inappropriate ADH secretion · von Willebrand's Disease Type IIB (may result in pseudothrombocytopenia)

● CAUTIONS
GENERAL CAUTIONS Asthma · avoid fluid overload · cardiovascular disease (not indicated for nocturnal enuresis or nocturia) · conditions which might be aggravated by water retention · cystic fibrosis · epilepsy · heart failure · hypertension (not indicated for nocturnal enuresis or nocturia) · migraine · nocturia—limit fluid intake to minimum from 1 hour before dose until 8 hours afterwards · nocturnal enuresis—limit fluid intake to minimum from 1 hour before dose until 8 hours afterwards
SPECIFIC CAUTIONS
▸ With intranasal use Should not be given intranasally for nocturnal enuresis due to an increased incidence of side-effects

● INTERACTIONS → Appendix 1: desmopressin

● SIDE-EFFECTS
GENERAL SIDE-EFFECTS
▶ **Common or very common** Hyponatraemia (on administration without restricting fluid intake) · nausea
▶ **Frequency not known** Abdominal pain · aggression · allergic dermatitis · emotional disorder · fluid retention · headache · hyponatraemic seizure · vomiting · weight increased
SPECIFIC SIDE-EFFECTS
▸ With intranasal use Epistaxis · nasal congestion · rhinitis

6 Endocrine system

▸ With intravenous use Vasodilation

SIDE-EFFECTS, FURTHER INFORMATION Manufacturer advises avoiding concomitant use of drugs which increase secretion of vasopressin (e.g. tricyclic antidepressants)—increases risk of hyponatraemia.

- **PREGNANCY** Small oxytocic effect in third trimester; increased risk of pre-eclampsia.
- **BREAST FEEDING** Amount too small to be harmful.
- **RENAL IMPAIRMENT** Use with caution; antidiuretic effect may be reduced.
- **MONITORING REQUIREMENTS** In *nocturia*, periodic blood pressure and weight checks are needed to monitor for fluid overload.
- **DIRECTIONS FOR ADMINISTRATION** *DDAVP*® and *Desmotabs*® tablets may be crushed.

DDAVP® intranasal solution may be diluted with Sodium Chloride 0.9% to a concentration of 10 micrograms/mL.

DDAVP® injection may be administered orally.

Desmopressin oral lyophilisates are for sublingual administration.

▸ With intravenous use Higher doses of *DDAVP*® by *intravenous infusion*, used in mild to moderate haemophilia and von Willebrand's disease, may be diluted with 30–50 mL Sodium Chloride 0.9% intravenous infusion. For *intravenous infusion* (*Octim*®), dilute with 50 mL of Sodium Chloride 0.9% and give over 20 minutes.

- **PRESCRIBING AND DISPENSING INFORMATION** Oral, intranasal, intravenous, subcutaneous and intramuscular doses are expressed as desmopressin acetate; sublingual doses are expressed as desmopressin base.

Children requiring an intranasal dose of less than 10 micrograms should be given *DDAVP*® intranasal solution.

- **PATIENT AND CARER ADVICE**

Hyponatraemic convulsions Patients being treated for primary nocturnal enuresis should be warned to avoid fluid overload (including during swimming) and to stop taking desmopressin during an episode of vomiting or diarrhoea (until fluid balance normal).

Medicines for Children leaflet: Desmopressin for bedwetting www.medicinesforchildren.org.uk/desmopressin-bedwetting-0

- **MEDICINAL FORMS** There can be variation in the licensing of different medicines containing the same drug. Forms available from special-order manufacturers include: capsule, oral suspension, oral solution, spray, nasal drops

Tablet

▸ **Desmopressin (Non-proprietary)**

Desmopressin acetate 100 microgram Desmopressin 100microgram tablets | 90 tablet PoM £76.62 DT = £63.09

Desmopressin acetate 200 microgram Desmopressin 200microgram tablets | 30 tablet PoM £28.50 DT = £23.52

▸ **DDAVP** (Ferring Pharmaceuticals Ltd)

Desmopressin acetate 100 microgram DDAVP 0.1mg tablets | 90 tablet PoM £44.12 DT = £63.09

Desmopressin acetate 200 microgram DDAVP 0.2mg tablets | 90 tablet PoM £88.23

▸ **Desmotabs** (Ferring Pharmaceuticals Ltd)

Desmopressin acetate 200 microgram Desmotabs 0.2mg tablets | 30 tablet PoM £29.43 DT = £23.52

Solution for injection

▸ **DDAVP** (Ferring Pharmaceuticals Ltd)

Desmopressin acetate 4 microgram per 1 ml DDAVP 4micrograms/1ml solution for injection ampoules | 10 ampoule PoM £13.16 DT = £13.16

▸ **Octim** (Ferring Pharmaceuticals Ltd)

Desmopressin acetate 15 microgram per 1 ml Octim 15micrograms/1ml solution for injection ampoules | 10 ampoule PoM £192.20

Spray

▸ **Desmopressin (Non-proprietary)**

Desmopressin acetate 10 microgram per 1 dose Desmopressin 10micrograms/dose nasal spray | 60 dose PoM £23.04 DT = £17.85

▸ **Desmospray** (Ferring Pharmaceuticals Ltd)

Desmopressin acetate 2.5 microgram per 1 dose Desmospray 2.5micrograms/dose nasal spray | 50 dose ℞

Desmopressin acetate 10 microgram per 1 dose Desmospray 10micrograms/dose nasal spray | 60 dose PoM £25.02 DT = £17.85

▸ **Octim** (Ferring Pharmaceuticals Ltd)

Desmopressin acetate 150 microgram per 1 dose Octim 150micrograms/dose nasal spray | 25 dose PoM £576.60 DT = £576.60

Oral lyophilisate

CAUTIONARY AND ADVISORY LABELS 26

▸ **DDAVP Melt** (Ferring Pharmaceuticals Ltd)

Desmopressin (as Desmopressin acetate) 60 microgram DDAVP Melt 60microgram oral lyophilisates sugar-free | 100 tablet PoM £50.53 DT = £50.53

Desmopressin (as Desmopressin acetate) 120 microgram DDAVP Melt 120microgram oral lyophilisates sugar-free | 100 tablet PoM £101.07 DT = £101.07

Desmopressin (as Desmopressin acetate) 240 microgram DDAVP Melt 240microgram oral lyophilisates sugar-free | 100 tablet PoM £202.14

▸ **DesmoMelt** (Ferring Pharmaceuticals Ltd)

Desmopressin (as Desmopressin acetate) 120 microgram DesmoMelt 120microgram oral lyophilisates sugar-free | 30 tablet PoM £30.34 DT = £30.34

Desmopressin (as Desmopressin acetate) 240 microgram DesmoMelt 240microgram oral lyophilisates sugar-free | 30 tablet PoM £60.68 DT = £60.68

▸ **Noqdirna** (Ferring Pharmaceuticals Ltd)

Desmopressin (as Desmopressin acetate) 25 microgram Noqdirna 25microgram oral lyophilisates sugar-free | 30 tablet PoM £15.16 DT = £15.16

Desmopressin (as Desmopressin acetate) 50 microgram Noqdirna 50microgram oral lyophilisates sugar-free | 30 tablet PoM £15.16 DT = £15.16

Nasal drops

▸ **DDAVP** (Ferring Pharmaceuticals Ltd)

Desmopressin acetate 100 microgram per 1 ml DDAVP 100micrograms/ml intranasal solution | 2.5 ml PoM £9.72 DT = £9.72

2 Corticosteroid responsive conditions

CORTICOSTEROIDS

Corticosteroids, general use

13-Nov-2019

Overview

Dosages of corticosteroids vary widely in different diseases and in different patients. If the use of a corticosteroid can save or prolong life, as in exfoliative dermatitis, pemphigus, acute leukaemia or acute transplant rejection, high doses may need to be given, because the complications of therapy are likely to be less serious than the effects of the disease itself.

When long-term corticosteroid therapy is used in some chronic diseases, the adverse effects of treatment may become greater than the disabilities caused by the disease. To minimise side-effects the maintenance dose should be kept as low as possible.

When potentially less harmful measures are ineffective corticosteroids are used topically for the treatment of inflammatory conditions of the skin. Corticosteroids should be avoided or used only under specialist supervision in psoriasis.

Corticosteroids are used both topically (by rectum) and systemically (by mouth or intravenously) in the management of ulcerative colitis and Crohn's disease.

Use can be made of the mineralocorticoid activity of fludrocortisone acetate p. 476 to treat postural hypotension in autonomic neuropathy.

High-dose corticosteroids should be avoided for the management of septic shock. However, low-dose hydrocortisone p. 476 can be used in septic shock that is resistant to volume expansion and catecholamines, and is accompanied by suspected or proven adrenal insufficiency.

The suppressive action of glucocorticoids on the hypothalamic-pituitary-adrenal axis is greatest and most prolonged when they are given at night. In most adults a single dose of dexamethasone p. 475 at night is sufficient to inhibit corticotropin secretion for 24 hours. This is the basis of the 'overnight dexamethasone suppression test' for diagnosing Cushing's syndrome.

Betamethasone p. 474 and dexamethasone are also appropriate for conditions where water retention would be a disadvantage.

A corticosteroid may be used in the management of raised intracranial pressure or cerebral oedema that occurs as a result of malignancy (see Prescribing in palliative care p. 21). However, a corticosteroid should **not** be used for the management of head injury or stroke because it is unlikely to be of benefit and may even be harmful.

In acute hypersensitivity reactions, such as angioedema of the upper respiratory tract and anaphylaxis, corticosteroids are indicated as an adjunct to emergency treatment with adrenaline/epinephrine p. 143. In such cases hydrocortisone (as sodium succinate) by intravenous injection may be required.

EvGr In the management of asthma, corticosteroids are preferably used by inhalation. Systemic therapy along with bronchodilators is required for the treatment of acute asthma and in some very severe cases of chronic asthma. (A)

Betamethasone is used in women at risk of preterm delivery to reduce the incidence of neonatal respiratory distress syndrome [unlicensed use].

Dexamethasone should not be used routinely for the prophylaxis and treatment of chronic lung disease in neonates because of an association with adverse neurological effects.

Corticosteroids may be useful in conditions such as autoimmune hepatitis, rheumatoid arthritis, and sarcoidosis; they may also lead to remissions of acquired haemolytic anaemia and thrombocytopenic purpura.

High doses of a corticosteroid (usually prednisolone p. 478) are used in the treatment of *glomerular kidney disease*, including *nephrotic syndrome*. The condition frequently recurs; a corticosteroid given in high doses and for prolonged periods may delay relapse but the higher incidence of adverse effects limits the overall benefit. Those who suffer frequent relapses may be treated with prednisolone given in a low dose (daily or on alternate days) for 3–6 months; the dose should be adjusted to minimise effects on growth and development. Other drugs used in the treatment of glomerular kidney disease include levamisole p. 417, cyclophosphamide p. 579, chlorambucil p. 579, and ciclosporin p. 559. *Congenital nephrotic syndrome* may be resistant to corticosteroids and immunosuppressants; indometacin p. 710 and an ACE inhibitor such as captopril p. 118 have been used.

Corticosteroids can improve the prognosis of serious conditions such as systemic lupus erythematosus and polyarteritis nodosa; the effects of the disease process may be suppressed and symptoms relieved, but the underlying condition is not cured, although it may ultimately remit. It is usual to begin therapy in these conditions at fairly high dose and then to reduce the dose to the lowest commensurate with disease control.

For other references to the use of corticosteroids see: Prescribing in Palliative Care, immunosuppression, rheumatic diseases, eye, otitis externa, allergic rhinitis, and aphthous ulcers.

Side-effects

MHRA/CHM advice: Corticosteroids: rare risk of central serous chorioretinopathy with local as well as systemic administration (August 2017)

Central serous chorioretinopathy is a retinal disorder that has been linked to the systemic use of corticosteroids. Recently, it has also been reported after local administration of corticosteroids via inhaled and intranasal, epidural, intra-articular, topical dermal, and periocular routes. The MHRA recommends that patients should be advised to report any blurred vision or other visual disturbances with corticosteroid treatment given by any route; consider referral to an ophthalmologist for evaluation of possible causes if a patient presents with vision problems.

Overdosage or prolonged use can exaggerate some of the normal physiological actions of corticosteroids leading to mineralocorticoid and glucocorticoid side-effects.

Mineralocorticoid side effects

- hypertension
- sodium retention
- water retention
- potassium loss
- calcium loss

Mineralocorticoid side effects are most marked with fludrocortisone acetate, but are significant with hydrocortisone, corticotropin, and tetracosactide p. 511. Mineralocorticoid actions are negligible with the high potency glucocorticoids, betamethasone and dexamethasone, and occur only slightly with methylprednisolone p. 478, prednisolone, and triamcinolone.

Glucocorticoid side effects

- diabetes
- osteoporosis
- in addition high doses are associated with avascular necrosis of the femoral head.
- Muscle wasting (proximal myopathy) can also occur.
- Corticosteroid therapy is also weakly linked with peptic ulceration and perforation.
- Psychiatric reactions may also occur.

Managing side-effects

Side-effects can be minimised by using lowest effective dose for minimum period possible. The suppressive action of a corticosteroid on cortisol secretion is least when it is given as a single dose in the morning. In an attempt to reduce pituitary-adrenal suppression further, the total dose for two days can sometimes be taken as a single dose on alternate days; alternate-day administration has not been very successful in the management of asthma. Pituitary-adrenal suppression can also be reduced by means of intermittent therapy with short courses. In some conditions it may be possible to reduce the dose of corticosteroid by adding a small dose of an immunosuppressive drug.

For information on the cessation of oral corticosteroid treatment, see *Treatment cessation*, for systemic corticosteroids (e.g. prednisolone p. 478).

Whenever possible *local treatment* with creams, intra-articular injections, inhalations, eye-drops, or enemas should be used in preference to *systemic treatment*.

Inhaled corticosteroids have considerably fewer systemic effects than oral corticosteroids, but adverse effects including adrenal suppression have been reported. Use of other corticosteroid therapy (including topical) or concurrent use of drugs which inhibit corticosteroid metabolism should be taken into account when assessing systemic risk. In children being treated for asthma, administration of medium or high dose inhaled corticosteroids may be associated with systemic side effects such as growth failure, reduced bone mineral density and adrenal suppression, but this risk is likely to be outweighed by their ability to reduce the need for multiple courses of oral corticosteroids for acute asthma attacks.

Corticosteroids, replacement therapy

Overview

The adrenal cortex normally secretes hydrocortisone p. 476 (cortisol) which has glucocorticoid activity and weak mineralocorticoid activity. It also secretes the mineralocorticoid aldosterone.

In deficiency states, physiological replacement is best achieved with a combination of hydrocortisone and the mineralocorticoid fludrocortisone acetate p. 476; hydrocortisone alone does not usually provide sufficient mineralocorticoid activity for complete replacement.

In *Addison's disease* or following adrenalectomy, hydrocortisone by mouth is usually required. This is given in 2–3 divided doses, the larger in the morning and the smaller in the evening, mimicking the normal diurnal rhythm of cortisol secretion. The optimum daily dose is determined on the basis of clinical response. Glucocorticoid therapy is supplemented by fludrocortisone acetate.

In *acute adrenocortical insufficiency*, hydrocortisone is given intravenously (preferably as sodium succinate) every 6 to 8 hours in sodium chloride intravenous infusion 0.9% p. 636.

In *hypopituitarism*, glucocorticoids should be given as in adrenocortical insufficiency, but since production of aldosterone is also regulated by the renin-angiotensin system a mineralocorticoid is not usually required. Additional replacement therapy with levothyroxine sodium p. 524 and sex hormones should be given as indicated by the pattern of hormone deficiency.

In *congenital adrenal hyperplasia*, the pituitary gland increases production of corticotropin to compensate for reduced formation of cortisol; this results in excessive adrenal androgen production. Treatment is aimed at suppressing corticotropin using hydrocortisone. Careful and continual dose titration is required to avoid growth retardation and toxicity; for this reason potent, synthetic glucocorticoids such as dexamethasone are usually reserved for use in adolescents. The dose is adjusted according to clinical response and measurement of adrenal androgens and 17-hydroxyprogesterone. Salt-losing forms of congenital adrenal hyperplasia (where there is a lack of aldosterone production) also require mineralocorticoid replacement and salt supplementation (particularly in early life). The dose of mineralocorticoid is adjusted according to electrolyte concentration and plasma-renin activity.

Glucocorticoid therapy

Glucocorticoid and mineralocorticoid activity

In comparing the relative potencies of corticosteroids in terms of their anti-inflammatory (glucocorticoid) effects it should be borne in mind that high glucocorticoid activity in itself is of no advantage unless it is accompanied by relatively low mineralocorticoid activity (see Disadvantages of Corticosteroids). The mineralocorticoid activity of fludrocortisone acetate p. 476 is so high that its anti-inflammatory activity is of no clinical relevance.

Equivalent anti-inflammatory doses of corticosteroids

This table takes no account of mineralocorticoid effects, nor does it take account of variations in duration of action

Prednisolone 1 mg	≡	Betamethasone 150 micrograms
	≡	Deflazacort 1.2 mg
	≡	Dexamethasone 150 micrograms
	≡	Hydrocortisone 4 mg
	≡	Methylprednisolone 800 micrograms
	≡	Triamcinolone 800 micrograms

The relatively high mineralocorticoid activity of hydrocortisone p. 476, and the resulting fluid retention, makes it unsuitable for disease suppression on a long-term basis. However, hydrocortisone can be used for adrenal replacement therapy. Hydrocortisone is used on a short-term basis by intravenous injection for the emergency management of some conditions. The relatively moderate anti-inflammatory potency of hydrocortisone also makes it a useful topical corticosteroid for the management of inflammatory skin conditions because side-effects (both topical and systemic) are less marked.

Prednisolone p. 478 has predominantly glucocorticoid activity and is the corticosteroid most commonly used by mouth for long-term disease suppression.

Betamethasone p. 474 and dexamethasone p. 475 have very high glucocorticoid activity in conjunction with insignificant mineralocorticoid activity. This makes them particularly suitable for high-dose therapy in conditions where fluid retention would be a disadvantage.

Betamethasone and dexamethasone also have a long duration of action and this, coupled with their lack of mineralocorticoid action makes them particularly suitable for conditions which require suppression of corticotropin (corticotrophin) secretion.

Some esters of betamethasone and of beclometasone dipropionate p. 167 (beclomethasone) exert a considerably more marked topical effect (e.g. on the skin or the lungs) than when given by mouth; use is made of this to obtain topical effects whilst minimising systemic side-effects (e.g. for skin applications and asthma inhalations).

Deflazacort p. 474 has a high glucocorticoid activity; it is derived from prednisolone.

Corticosteroids (systemic) 

IMPORTANT SAFETY INFORMATION

MHRA/CHM ADVICE: CORTICOSTEROIDS: RARE RISK OF CENTRAL SEROUS CHORIORETINOPATHY WITH LOCAL AS WELL AS SYSTEMIC ADMINISTRATION (AUGUST 2017)

Central serous chorioretinopathy is a retinal disorder that has been linked to the systemic use of corticosteroids. Recently, it has also been reported after local administration of corticosteroids via inhaled and intranasal, epidural, intra-articular, topical dermal, and periocular routes. The MHRA recommends that patients should be advised to report any blurred vision or other visual disturbances with corticosteroid treatment given by any route; consider referral to an ophthalmologist for evaluation of possible causes if a patient presents with vision problems.

- **CONTRA-INDICATIONS** Avoid injections containing benzyl alcohol in neonates · avoid live virus vaccines in those receiving immunosuppressive doses (serum antibody response diminished) · systemic infection (unless specific therapy given)

CONTRA-INDICATIONS, FURTHER INFORMATION

▸ **With intra-articular use or intradermal use or intralesional use** For further information on contra-indications associated with intra-articular, intradermal and intralesional preparations, consult product literature.

- **CAUTIONS** Congestive heart failure · diabetes mellitus (including a family history of) · diverticulitis · epilepsy · glaucoma (including a family history of or susceptibility to) · history of steroid myopathy · history of tuberculosis or X-ray changes (frequent monitoring required) · hypertension · hypothyroidism · infection (particularly untreated) · long-term use · myasthenia gravis · ocular herpes simplex (risk of corneal perforation) · osteoporosis · peptic ulcer · psychiatric reactions · recent intestinal anastomoses · recent myocardial infarction (rupture reported) · severe affective disorders (particularly if history of steroid-induced psychosis) · thromboembolic disorders · ulcerative colitis

CAUTIONS, FURTHER INFORMATION

▸ **With intra-articular use or intradermal use or intralesional use** For further information on cautions associated with intra-articular, intradermal and intralesional preparations, consult product literature.

- **SIDE-EFFECTS**

▸ **Common or very common** Anxiety · behaviour abnormal · cataract subcapsular · cognitive impairment · Cushing's syndrome · electrolyte imbalance · fatigue · fluid retention · gastrointestinal discomfort · growth retardation · headache · healing impaired · hirsutism · hypertension · increased risk of infection · menstrual cycle irregularities · mood altered · nausea · osteoporosis · peptic ulcer · psychotic disorder · skin reactions · sleep disorders · weight increased

▸ **Uncommon** Adrenal suppression · alkalosis hypokalaemic · appetite increased · bone fractures · diabetic control impaired · eye disorders · glaucoma · haemorrhage · heart failure · hyperhidrosis · hypotension · leucocytosis · myopathy · osteonecrosis · pancreatitis · papilloedema · seizure · thromboembolism · tuberculosis reactivation · vertigo · vision blurred

▸ **Rare or very rare** Malaise · tendon rupture

▸ **Frequency not known** Chorioretinopathy · intracranial pressure increased with papilloedema (usually after withdrawal) · telangiectasia

SIDE-EFFECTS, FURTHER INFORMATION **Adrenal suppression** During prolonged therapy with corticosteroids, particularly with systemic use, adrenal atrophy develops and can persist for years after stopping. Abrupt withdrawal after a prolonged period can lead to acute adrenal insufficiency, hypotension, or death. To compensate for a diminished adrenocortical response caused by prolonged corticosteroid treatment, any significant intercurrent illness, trauma, or surgical procedure requires a temporary increase in corticosteroid dose, or if already stopped, a temporary reintroduction of corticosteroid treatment. Patients on long-term corticosteroid treatment should carry a steroid treatment card which gives guidance on minimising risk and provides details of prescriber, drug, dosage and duration of treatment.

Infections Prolonged courses of corticosteroids increase susceptibility to infections and severity of infections; clinical presentation of infections may also be atypical. Serious infections e.g. septicaemia and tuberculosis may reach an advanced stage before being recognised, and amoebiasis or strongyloidiasis may be activated or exacerbated (exclude before initiating a corticosteroid in those at risk or with suggestive symptoms). Fungal or viral ocular infections may also be exacerbated.

Chickenpox Unless they have had chickenpox, patients receiving oral or parenteral corticosteroids for purposes other than replacement should be regarded as being at risk of severe chickenpox. Manifestations of fulminant illness include pneumonia, hepatitis and disseminated intravascular coagulation; rash is not necessarily a prominent feature. Passive immunisation with varicella–zoster immunoglobulin is needed for exposed non–immune patients receiving systemic corticosteroids or for those who have used them within the previous 3 months. Confirmed chickenpox warrants specialist care and urgent treatment. Corticosteroids should not be stopped and dosage may need to be increased.

Measles Patients taking corticosteroids should be advised to take particular care to avoid exposure to measles and to seek immediate medical advice if exposure occurs. Prophylaxis with intramuscular normal immunoglobulin may be needed.

Psychiatric reactions Systemic corticosteroids, particularly in high doses, are linked to psychiatric reactions including euphoria, insomnia, irritability, mood lability, suicidal thoughts, psychotic reactions, and behavioural disturbances. These reactions frequently subside on reducing the dose or discontinuing the corticosteroid but they may also require specific management. Patients should be advised to seek medical advice if psychiatric symptoms (especially depression and suicidal thoughts) occur and they should also be alert to the rare possibility of such reactions during withdrawal of corticosteroid treatment. Systemic corticosteroids should be prescribed with care in those predisposed to psychiatric reactions, including those who have previously suffered corticosteroid–induced psychosis, or who have a personal or family history of psychiatric disorders.

- **PREGNANCY** The benefit of treatment with corticosteroids during pregnancy outweighs the risk. Corticosteroid cover is required during labour. Following a review of the data on the safety of systemic corticosteroids used in pregnancy and breast-feeding the CSM (May 1998) concluded that corticosteroids vary in their ability to cross the placenta but there is no convincing evidence that systemic corticosteroids increase the incidence of congenital abnormalities such as cleft palate or lip. When administration is prolonged or repeated during pregnancy, systemic corticosteroids increase the risk of intra-uterine growth restriction; there is no evidence of intra-uterine growth restriction following short-term treatment (e.g. prophylactic treatment for neonatal respiratory distress syndrome). Any adrenal suppression in the neonate following prenatal exposure usually resolves spontaneously after birth and is rarely clinically important.
Monitoring Pregnant women with fluid retention should be monitored closely when given systemic corticosteroids.
- **BREAST FEEDING** The benefit of treatment with corticosteroids during breast-feeding outweighs the risk.
- **HEPATIC IMPAIRMENT** In general, manufacturers advise caution (risk of increased exposure).
- **RENAL IMPAIRMENT** Use by oral and injectable routes should be undertaken with caution.
- **MONITORING REQUIREMENTS** The height and weight of children receiving prolonged treatment with corticosteroids should be monitored annually; if growth is slowed, referral to a paediatrician should be considered.
- **EFFECT ON LABORATORY TESTS** May suppress skin test reactions.
- **TREATMENT CESSATION** The magnitude and speed of dose reduction in corticosteroid withdrawal should be determined on a case-by–case basis, taking into consideration the underlying condition that is being treated, and individual patient factors such as the likelihood of relapse and the duration of corticosteroid treatment. *Gradual* withdrawal of systemic corticosteroids should be considered in those whose disease is unlikely to relapse and have:

6 Endocrine system

- received more than 40 mg prednisolone (or equivalent) daily for more than 1 week *or* 2 mg/kg daily for 1 week *or* 1 mg/kg daily for 1 month;
- been given repeat doses in the evening;
- received more than 3 weeks' treatment;
- recently received repeated courses (particularly if taken for longer than 3 weeks);
- taken a short course within 1 year of stopping long-term therapy;
- other possible causes of adrenal suppression.

Systemic corticosteroids may be stopped abruptly in those whose disease is unlikely to relapse *and* who have received treatment for 3 weeks or less *and* who are not included in the patient groups described above.

During corticosteroid withdrawal the dose may be reduced rapidly down to physiological doses (equivalent to prednisolone 2–2.5 mg/m^2 daily) and then reduced more slowly. Assessment of the disease may be needed during withdrawal to ensure that relapse does not occur.

- **PATIENT AND CARER ADVICE**

Advice for patients Patients on long-term corticosteroid treatment should carry a Steroid Treatment Card which gives guidance on minimising risk and provides details of prescriber, drug, dosage and duration of treatment.

A patient information leaflet should be supplied to every patient when a systemic corticosteroid is prescribed. Patients should especially be advised of the following:

- **Immunosuppression** Prolonged courses of corticosteroids can increase susceptibility to infection and serious infections can go unrecognised. Unless already immune, patients are at risk of severe **chickenpox** and should avoid close contact with people who have chickenpox or shingles. Similarly, precautions should also be taken against contracting **measles**;
- **Adrenal suppression** If the corticosteroid is given for longer than 3 weeks, treatment must not be stopped abruptly. Adrenal suppression can last for a year or more after stopping treatment and the patient must mention the course of corticosteroid when receiving treatment for any illness or injury;
- **Mood and behaviour changes** Corticosteroid treatment, especially with high doses, can alter mood and behaviour early in treatment—the patient can become confused, irritable and suffer from delusion and suicidal thoughts. These effects can also occur when corticosteroid treatment is being withdrawn. Medical advice should be sought if worrying psychological changes occur;
- **Other serious effects** Serious gastro-intestinal, musculoskeletal, and ophthalmic effects which require medical help can also occur.

Steroid treatment cards Steroid treatment cards should be issued where appropriate. Consider giving a 'steroid card' to support communication of the risks associated with treatment, and specific written advice to consider corticosteroid replacement during an episode of stress, such as severe intercurrent illness or an operation, to patients using greater than maximum licensed doses of inhaled corticosteroids. Steroid treatment cards are available for purchase from the NHS Print online ordering portal www.nhsforms.co.uk

GP practices can obtain supplies through Primary Care Support England. NHS Trusts can order supplies via the online ordering portal.

In **Scotland**, steroid treatment cards can be obtained from APS Group Scotland by emailing stockorders.dppas@apsgroup.co.uk or by fax on 0131 629 9967.

472

Betamethasone

28-Nov-2019

- **DRUG ACTION** Betamethasone has very high glucocorticoid activity and insignificant mineralocorticoid activity.

- **INDICATIONS AND DOSE**

Suppression of inflammatory and allergic disorders | Congenital adrenal hyperplasia

▶ BY SLOW INTRAVENOUS INJECTION, OR BY INTRAVENOUS INFUSION

- Child 1–11 months: Initially 1 mg, repeated up to 4 times in 24 hours according to response
- Child 1–5 years: Initially 2 mg, repeated up to 4 times in 24 hours according to response
- Child 6–11 years: Initially 4 mg, repeated up to 4 times in 24 hours according to response
- Child 12–17 years: 4–20 mg, repeated up to 4 times in 24 hours according to response

- **INTERACTIONS** → Appendix 1: corticosteroids
- **SIDE-EFFECTS** Hiccups · myocardial rupture (following recent myocardial infarction) · oedema · Stevens-Johnson syndrome
- **PREGNANCY** Readily crosses the placenta. Transient effect on fetal movements and heart rate.
- **DIRECTIONS FOR ADMINISTRATION** For *intravenous infusion*, dilute with Glucose 5% or Sodium Chloride 0.9%.
- **MEDICINAL FORMS** There can be variation in the licensing of different medicines containing the same drug.

Solution for injection

CAUTIONARY AND ADVISORY LABELS 10

▶ Betamethasone (Non-proprietary)

Betamethasone (as Betamethasone sodium phosphate) 4 mg per 1 ml Betamethasone 4mg/1ml solution for injection ampoules | 5 ampoule PoM £30.46 DT = £30.26

472

Deflazacort

21-Dec-2017

- **DRUG ACTION** Deflazacort is derived from prednisolone; it has predominantly glucocorticoid activity.

- **INDICATIONS AND DOSE**

Inflammatory and allergic disorders

▶ BY MOUTH

- Child 1 month–11 years: 0.25–1.5 mg/kg once daily or on alternate days; increased if necessary up to 2.4 mg/kg daily (max. per dose 120 mg), in emergency situations
- Child 12–17 years: 3–18 mg once daily or on alternate days; increased if necessary up to 2.4 mg/kg daily (max. per dose 120 mg), in emergency situations

Nephrotic syndrome

▶ BY MOUTH

- Child: Initially 1.5 mg/kg once daily (max. per dose 120 mg), reduced to the lowest effective dose for maintenance

- **INTERACTIONS** → Appendix 1: corticosteroids
- **SIDE-EFFECTS**

▶ **Uncommon** Oedema

- **HEPATIC IMPAIRMENT**

Dose adjustments Manufacturer advises adjust to the minimum effective dose.

- **PATIENT AND CARER ADVICE** Patient counselling is advised for deflazacort tablets (steroid card).

● **MEDICINAL FORMS** There can be variation in the licensing of different medicines containing the same drug. Forms available from special-order manufacturers include: tablet

Tablet

CAUTIONARY AND ADVISORY LABELS 5, 10

▸ Calcort (Sanofi)
Deflazacort 6 mg Calcort 6mg tablets | 60 tablet PoM £15.82 DT = £15.82

F 472

Dexamethasone

10-Mar-2020

● **DRUG ACTION** Dexamethasone has very high glucocorticoid activity and insignificant mineralocorticoid activity.

● **INDICATIONS AND DOSE**

Physiological replacement

▸ BY MOUTH, OR BY SLOW INTRAVENOUS INJECTION
▸ Child: 250–500 micrograms/m² every 12 hours, adjusted according to response

Suppression of inflammatory and allergic disorders

▸ BY MOUTH
▸ Child: 10–100 micrograms/kg daily in 1–2 divided doses, adjusted according to response; up to 300 micrograms/kg daily may be required in emergency situations

▸ BY INTRAMUSCULAR INJECTION, OR BY SLOW INTRAVENOUS INJECTION, OR BY INTRAVENOUS INFUSION
▸ Child 1 month–11 years: 83–333 micrograms/kg daily in 1–2 divided doses; maximum 20 mg per day
▸ Child 12–17 years: Initially 0.4–20 mg daily

Mild croup

▸ BY MOUTH
▸ Child: 150 micrograms/kg for 1 dose

Severe croup (or mild croup that might cause complications)

▸ INITIALLY BY MOUTH
▸ Child: Initially 150 micrograms/kg for 1 dose, to be given before transfer to hospital, then (by mouth or by intravenous injection) 150 micrograms/kg, then (by mouth or by intravenous injection) 150 micrograms/kg after 12 hours if required

Adjunctive treatment of bacterial meningitis (starting before or with first dose of antibacterial)

▸ BY SLOW INTRAVENOUS INJECTION
▸ Child 3 months–17 years: 150 micrograms/kg every 6 hours (max. per dose 10 mg) for 4 days

Life-threatening cerebral oedema

▸ BY INTRAVENOUS INJECTION
▸ Child (body-weight up to 35 kg): Initially 16.7 mg, then 3.3 mg every 3 hours for 3 days, then 3.3 mg every 6 hours for 1 day, then 1.7 mg every 6 hours for 4 days, then reduced in steps of 0.8 mg daily
▸ Child (body-weight 35 kg and above): Initially 20.8 mg, then 3.3 mg every 2 hours for 3 days, then 3.3 mg every 4 hours for 1 day, then 3.3 mg every 6 hours for 4 days, then reduced in steps of 1.7 mg daily

● **UNLICENSED USE**
▸ With intravenous use Consult product literature; not licensed for use in bacterial meningitis.

● **INTERACTIONS** → Appendix 1: corticosteroids

● **SIDE-EFFECTS**
▸ With oral use Hiccups · hyperglycaemia · myocardial rupture (following recent myocardial infarction) · protein catabolism
▸ With parenteral use Perineal irritation (may occur following the intravenous injection of large doses of the phosphate ester)

● **PREGNANCY** Dexamethasone readily crosses the placenta.

● **DIRECTIONS FOR ADMINISTRATION**
▸ With oral use For administration *by mouth* tablets may be dispersed in water or injection solution given by mouth.
▸ With intravenous use For *intravenous infusion* dilute with Glucose 5% or Sodium Chloride 0.9%; give over 15–20 minutes.

● **PRESCRIBING AND DISPENSING INFORMATION** Dexamethasone 3.8 mg/mL Injection has replaced dexamethasone 4 mg/mL Injection. All dosage recommendations for intravenous, intramuscular, intrarticular use or local infiltration; are given in units of dexamethasone base.

● **PATIENT AND CARER ADVICE**
Medicines for Children leaflet: Dexamethasone for croup www.medicinesforchildren.org.uk/dexamethasone-croup-0

● **MEDICINAL FORMS** There can be variation in the licensing of different medicines containing the same drug. Forms available from special-order manufacturers include: capsule, oral suspension, oral solution

Soluble tablet

▸ Dexamethasone (Non-proprietary)
Dexamethasone (as Dexamethasone sodium phosphate) 2 mg Dexamethasone 2mg soluble tablets sugar free sugar-free | 50 tablet PoM £30.01 DT = £30.01
Dexamethasone (as Dexamethasone sodium phosphate) 4 mg Dexamethasone 4mg soluble tablets sugar free sugar-free | 50 tablet PoM £60.01 DT = £60.01
Dexamethasone (as Dexamethasone sodium phosphate) 8 mg Dexamethasone 8mg soluble tablets sugar free sugar-free | 50 tablet PoM £120.01 DT = £120.01

▸ Glensoludex (Glenmark Pharmaceuticals Europe Ltd)
Dexamethasone (as Dexamethasone sodium phosphate) 2 mg Glensoludex 2mg soluble tablets sugar-free | 50 tablet PoM £10.00 DT = £30.01
Dexamethasone (as Dexamethasone sodium phosphate) 4 mg Glensoludex 4mg soluble tablets sugar-free | 50 tablet PoM £20.00 DT = £60.01
Dexamethasone (as Dexamethasone sodium phosphate) 8 mg Glensoludex 8mg soluble tablets sugar-free | 50 tablet PoM £40.00 DT = £120.01

Tablet

CAUTIONARY AND ADVISORY LABELS 10, 21

▸ Dexamethasone (Non-proprietary)
Dexamethasone 500 microgram Dexamethasone 500microgram tablets | 28 tablet PoM £54.24 DT = £6.40 | 30 tablet PoM £6.86–£64.82
Dexamethasone 2 mg Dexamethasone 2mg tablets | 50 tablet PoM £49.00 DT = £6.84 | 100 tablet PoM £17.98–£98.00
Dexamethasone 4 mg Dexamethasone 4mg tablets | 50 tablet PoM £85.00 DT = £83.01 | 100 tablet PoM £166.02–£169.40

▸ Neofordex (Aspire Pharma Ltd)
Dexamethasone 40 mg Neofordex 40mg tablets | 10 tablet PoM £200.00 DT = £200.00

Solution for injection

CAUTIONARY AND ADVISORY LABELS 10

▸ Dexamethasone (Non-proprietary)
Dexamethasone (as Dexamethasone sodium phosphate) 3.3 mg per 1 ml Dexamethasone (base) 6.6mg/2ml solution for injection ampoules | 10 ampoule PoM £22.00 DT = £22.00
Dexamethasone (base) 6.6mg/2ml solution for injection vials | 5 vial PoM £24.00 DT = £24.00
Dexamethasone (base) 3.3mg/1ml solution for injection ampoules | 5 ampoule PoM £12.00 | 10 ampoule PoM £15.00–£23.66 DT = £23.66
Dexamethasone (as Dexamethasone sodium phosphate) 3.8 mg per 1 ml Dexamethasone (base) 3.8mg/1ml solution for injection vials | 10 vial PoM £19.99 DT = £20.00 (Hospital only) | 10 vial PoM £19.99–£20.00 DT = £20.00

Oral solution

CAUTIONARY AND ADVISORY LABELS 10, 21

▸ Dexamethasone (Non-proprietary)
Dexamethasone (as Dexamethasone sodium phosphate) 400 microgram per 1 ml Dexamethasone 2mg/5ml oral solution sugar free sugar-free | 150 ml PoM £42.30 DT = £42.30

Dexamethasone (as Dexamethasone sodium phosphate) 2 mg per 1 ml Dexamethasone 10mg/5ml oral solution sugar free sugar-free | 50 ml [PoM] £24.50–£24.95 sugar-free | 150 ml [PoM] £101.40 DT = £94.44

Dexamethasone (as Dexamethasone sodium phosphate) 4 mg per 1 ml Dexamethasone 20mg/5ml oral solution sugar free sugar-free | 50 ml [PoM] £49.50 DT = £49.50

- Dexsol (Rosemont Pharmaceuticals Ltd)
  Dexamethasone (as Dexamethasone sodium phosphate) 400 microgram per 1 ml Dexsol 2mg/5ml oral solution sugar-free | 75 ml [PoM] £21.15 sugar-free | 150 ml [PoM] £42.30 DT = £42.30
- Martapan (Martindale Pharmaceuticals Ltd)
  Dexamethasone (as Dexamethasone sodium phosphate) 400 microgram per 1 ml Martapan 2mg/5ml oral solution sugar-free | 150 ml [PoM] £35.96 DT = £42.30

F 472

Fludrocortisone acetate

10-Mar-2020

- **DRUG ACTION** Fludrocortisone has very high mineralocorticoid activity and insignificant glucocorticoid activity.

- **INDICATIONS AND DOSE**

Mineralocorticoid replacement in adrenocortical insufficiency

▶ BY MOUTH

- Neonate: Initially 50 micrograms once daily, adjusted according to response; usual dose 50–200 micrograms once daily, higher doses may be required, dose adjustment may be required if salt supplements are administered.
- Child: Initially 50–100 micrograms once daily; maintenance 50–300 micrograms once daily, adjusted according to response, dose adjustment may be required if salt supplements are administered

- **INTERACTIONS** → Appendix 1: corticosteroids
- **SIDE-EFFECTS** Conjunctivitis · idiopathic intracranial hypertension · muscle weakness · thrombophlebitis
- **HEPATIC IMPAIRMENT**
  Monitoring Monitor patient closely in hepatic impairment.
- **PATIENT AND CARER ADVICE**
  Medicines for Children leaflet: Fludrocortisone for hormone replacement www.medicinesforchildren.org.uk/fludrocortisone-hormone-replacement

- **MEDICINAL FORMS** There can be variation in the licensing of different medicines containing the same drug. Forms available from special-order manufacturers include: tablet, capsule, oral suspension

Tablet

CAUTIONARY AND ADVISORY LABELS 10

- Fludrocortisone acetate (Non-proprietary)
  Fludrocortisone acetate 100 microgram Fludrocortisone 100microgram tablets | 30 tablet [PoM] £13.60 DT = £13.60

F 472

Hydrocortisone

17-Dec-2019

- **DRUG ACTION** Hydrocortisone has equal glucocorticoid and mineralocorticoid activity.

- **INDICATIONS AND DOSE**

Acute adrenocortical insufficiency (Addisonian crisis)

▶ INITIALLY BY SLOW INTRAVENOUS INJECTION

- Neonate: Initially 10 mg, then (by continuous intravenous infusion) 100 mg/m^2 daily, alternatively (by intravenous infusion) 100 mg/m^2 daily in divided doses, to be given every 6–8 hours; adjusted according to response, when stable reduce over 4–5 days to oral maintenance dose.

▶ BY SLOW INTRAVENOUS INJECTION, OR BY INTRAVENOUS INFUSION

- Child 1 month–11 years: Initially 2–4 mg/kg, then 2–4 mg/kg every 6 hours, adjusted according to response, when stable reduce over 4–5 days to oral maintenance dose
- Child 12–17 years: 100 mg every 6–8 hours

Congenital adrenal hyperplasia

▶ BY MOUTH USING IMMEDIATE-RELEASE MEDICINES

- Neonate: 9–15 mg/m^2 in 3 divided doses, adjusted according to response.
- Child: 9–15 mg/m^2 in 3 divided doses, adjusted according to response

Adrenal hypoplasia | Addison's disease, chronic maintenance or replacement therapy

▶ BY MOUTH USING IMMEDIATE-RELEASE MEDICINES

- Neonate: 8–10 mg/m^2 daily in 3 divided doses, the larger dose to be given in the morning and the smaller in the evening, higher doses may be needed.
- Child: 8–10 mg/m^2 daily in 3 divided doses, the larger dose to be given in the morning and the smaller in the evening, higher doses may be needed

Inflammatory bowel disease—induction of remission

▶ BY INTRAVENOUS INJECTION

- Child 2–17 years: 2.5 mg/kg every 6 hours (max. per dose 100 mg)

▶ BY CONTINUOUS INTRAVENOUS INFUSION

- Child 2–17 years: 10 mg/kg daily; maximum 400 mg per day

Ulcerative colitis | Proctitis | Proctosigmoiditis

▶ BY RECTUM USING RECTAL FOAM

- Child 2–17 years: Initially 1 metered application 1–2 times a day for 2–3 weeks, then reduced to 1 metered application once daily on alternate days, to be inserted into the rectum

Acute hypersensitivity reactions | Angioedema

▶ BY INTRAMUSCULAR INJECTION, OR BY INTRAVENOUS INJECTION

- Child 1–5 months: Initially 25 mg 3 times a day, adjusted according to response
- Child 6 months–5 years: Initially 50 mg 3 times a day, adjusted according to response
- Child 6–11 years: Initially 100 mg 3 times a day, adjusted according to response
- Child 12–17 years: Initially 200 mg 3 times a day, adjusted according to response

Hypotension resistant to inotropic treatment and volume replacement (limited evidence)

▶ BY INTRAVENOUS INJECTION

- Neonate: Initially 2.5 mg/kg, then 2.5 mg/kg after 4 hours if required, followed by 2.5 mg/kg every 6 hours for 48 hours or until blood pressure recovers, dose to then be reduced gradually over at least 48 hours.
- Child: 1 mg/kg every 6 hours (max. per dose 100 mg)

Severe acute asthma | Life-threatening acute asthma

▶ BY INTRAVENOUS INJECTION

- Child 1 month–1 year: 4 mg/kg every 6 hours (max. per dose 100 mg), alternatively 25 mg every 6 hours until conversion to oral prednisolone is possible, dose given, preferably, as sodium succinate
- Child 2–4 years: 4 mg/kg every 6 hours (max. per dose 100 mg), alternatively 50 mg every 6 hours until conversion to oral prednisolone is possible, dose given, preferably, as sodium succinate
- Child 5–11 years: 4 mg/kg every 6 hours (max. per dose 100 mg), alternatively 100 mg every 6 hours until

conversion to oral prednisolone is possible, dose given, preferably, as sodium succinate
- Child 12-17 years: 4 mg/kg every 6 hours (max. per dose 100 mg), alternatively 100 mg every 6 hours until conversion to oral prednisolone is possible, dose given, preferably, as sodium succinate

- **UNLICENSED USE**
- With oral use Use of injection by mouth is unlicensed.

> **IMPORTANT SAFETY INFORMATION**
>
> MHRA/CHM ADVICE: HYDROCORTISONE MUCO-ADHESIVE BUCCAL TABLETS: SHOULD NOT BE USED OFF-LABEL FOR ADRENAL INSUFFICIENCY IN CHILDREN DUE TO SERIOUS RISKS (DECEMBER 2018)
>
> The MHRA has received reports of off-label use of hydrocortisone muco-adhesive buccal tablets for adrenal insufficiency in children.
>
> Healthcare professionals are advised that:
> - hydrocortisone muco-adhesive buccal tablets are indicated only for local use in the mouth for aphthous ulceration and should not be used to treat adrenal insufficiency;
> - substitution of licensed oral hydrocortisone formulations with muco-adhesive buccal tablets can result in insufficient cortisol absorption and, in stress situations, life-threatening adrenal crisis;
> - only hydrocortisone products licensed for adrenal replacement therapy should be used.

- **CONTRA-INDICATIONS**
- With rectal use Abdominal or local infection · abscess · bowel perforation · extensive fistulas · intestinal obstruction · recent intestinal anastomoses
- **CAUTIONS**
- With rectal use Systemic absorption may occur
- **INTERACTIONS** → Appendix 1: corticosteroids
- **SIDE-EFFECTS**
- With oral use Dyslipidaemia · myocardial rupture (following recent myocardial infarction) · oedema
- With parenteral use Hiccups · Kaposi's sarcoma · lipomatosis · myocardial rupture (following recent myocardial infarction)
- **DIRECTIONS FOR ADMINISTRATION**
- With intravenous use For *intravenous administration*, dilute with Glucose 5% or Sodium Chloride 0.9%. For *intermittent infusion* give over 20–30 minutes.
- With oral use For administration *by mouth*, injection solution may be swallowed [unlicensed use] but consider phosphate content. For *Alkindi*®, manufacturer advises capsule should be opened and granules either administered directly into the mouth and then followed immediately with a drink, or sprinkled onto a spoonful of soft food (such as yoghurt) and given immediately. Granules should not be chewed or added to liquid before administration due to the bitter taste, and they should not be given via a nasogastric tube.
- **PRESCRIBING AND DISPENSING INFORMATION** The RCPCH and NPPG recommend that, when a liquid special of hydrocortisone is required, the following strength is used: 5 mg/5 mL.
- **PATIENT AND CARER ADVICE**
- With systemic use Patient counselling is advised for hydrocortisone tablets and injections (steroid card).
- **NATIONAL FUNDING/ACCESS DECISIONS**

Scottish Medicines Consortium (SMC) decisions

SMC No. SMC2088
- With oral use The *Scottish Medicines Consortium* (October 2018) has advised that hydrocortisone (*Alkindi*®) is accepted for restricted use within NHS Scotland for the first-line treatment of patients with adrenal insufficiency aged from birth to less than six years of age for whom hydrocortisone must otherwise be individually prepared by manipulation such as by compounding (or crushing) or by production of special solutions in order to produce age-appropriate doses, or hydrocortisone given as off-label buccal tablets. This advice is contingent upon the continuing availability of the patient access scheme in NHS Scotland or a list price that is equivalent or lower.

- **LESS SUITABLE FOR PRESCRIBING**
- With intravenous use Hydrocortisone as the sodium phosphate is less suitable for prescribing as paraesthesia and pain (particularly in the perineal region) may follow intravenous injection.
- **EXCEPTIONS TO LEGAL CATEGORY**
- With intramuscular use or intravenous use Prescription only medicine restriction does not apply where administration is for saving life in emergency.

- **MEDICINAL FORMS** There can be variation in the licensing of different medicines containing the same drug. Forms available from special-order manufacturers include: capsule, oral suspension, oral solution, liquid

Granules

CAUTIONARY AND ADVISORY LABELS 10
- Alkindi (Diurnal Ltd)
  - **Hydrocortisone 500 microgram** Alkindi 0.5mg granules in capsules for opening | 50 capsule PoM £33.75 DT = £33.75
  - **Hydrocortisone 1 mg** Alkindi 1mg granules in capsules for opening | 50 capsule PoM £67.50 DT = £67.50
  - **Hydrocortisone 2 mg** Alkindi 2mg granules in capsules for opening | 50 capsule PoM £135.00 DT = £135.00
  - **Hydrocortisone 5 mg** Alkindi 5mg granules in capsules for opening | 50 capsule PoM £337.50 DT = £337.50

Soluble tablet
- Hydrocortisone (Non-proprietary)
  - **Hydrocortisone (as Hydrocortisone sodium phosphate) 10 mg** Hydrocortisone 10mg soluble tablets sugar free sugar-free | 30 tablet PoM £37.50 DT = £37.50

Tablet

CAUTIONARY AND ADVISORY LABELS 10, 21
- Hydrocortisone (Non-proprietary)
  - **Hydrocortisone 10 mg** Hydrocortisone 10mg tablets | 30 tablet PoM £84.45 DT = £7.52
  - **Hydrocortisone 20 mg** Hydrocortisone 20mg tablets | 30 tablet PoM £147.26 DT = £7.04
- Hydventia (OcXia)
  - **Hydrocortisone 10 mg** Hydventia 10mg tablets | 30 tablet PoM £10.47 DT = £7.52
  - **Hydrocortisone 20 mg** Hydventia 20mg tablets | 30 tablet PoM £20.94 DT = £7.04

Powder for solution for injection
- Solu-Cortef (Pfizer Ltd)
  - **Hydrocortisone (as Hydrocortisone sodium succinate) 100 mg** Solu-Cortef 100mg powder for solution for injection vials | 10 vial PoM £9.17 DT = £9.17

Suspension for injection
- Hydrocortistab (Advanz Pharma)
  - **Hydrocortisone acetate 25 mg per 1 ml** Hydrocortistab 25mg/1ml suspension for injection ampoules | 10 ampoule PoM £68.72 DT = £68.72

Powder and solvent for solution for injection

CAUTIONARY AND ADVISORY LABELS 10
- Solu-Cortef (Pfizer Ltd)
  - **Hydrocortisone (as Hydrocortisone sodium succinate) 100 mg** Solu-Cortef 100mg powder and solvent for solution for injection vials | 1 vial PoM £1.16 DT = £1.16

Solution for injection

CAUTIONARY AND ADVISORY LABELS 10
- Hydrocortisone (Non-proprietary)
  - **Hydrocortisone (as Hydrocortisone sodium phosphate) 100 mg per 1 ml** Hydrocortisone sodium phosphate 100mg/1ml solution for injection ampoules | 5 ampoule PoM £10.60 DT = £10.60

6 Endocrine system

472

Methylprednisolone

11-Oct-2019

- **DRUG ACTION** Methylprednisolone exerts predominantly glucocorticoid effects with minimal mineralcorticoid effects.

- **INDICATIONS AND DOSE**

Inflammatory and allergic disorders

▶ BY MOUTH, OR BY SLOW INTRAVENOUS INJECTION, OR BY INTRAVENOUS INFUSION

▸ Child: 0.5–1.7 mg/kg daily in 2–4 divided doses, divide doses depending on condition and response

Treatment of graft rejection reactions

▶ BY INTRAVENOUS INJECTION

▸ Child: 10–20 mg/kg once daily for 3 days, alternatively 400–600 mg/m^2 once daily (max. per dose 1 g) for 3 days

Severe erythema multiforme | Lupus nephritis | Systemic onset juvenile idiopathic arthritis

▶ BY INTRAVENOUS INJECTION

▸ Child: 10–30 mg/kg once daily or on alternate days (max. per dose 1 g) for up to 3 doses

DEPO-MEDRONE ®

Suppression of inflammatory and allergic disorders

▶ BY DEEP INTRAMUSCULAR INJECTION

▸ Child: Seek specialist advice, to be injected into the gluteal muscle

IMPORTANT SAFETY INFORMATION

MHRA/CHM ADVICE: METHYLPREDNISOLONE INJECTABLE MEDICINE CONTAINING LACTOSE (*SOLU-MEDRONE®* 40 MG): DO NOT USE IN PATIENTS WITH COWS' MILK ALLERGY (OCTOBER 2017)

▸ With intramuscular use or intravenous use

An EU-wide review has concluded that *Solu-Medrone®* 40 mg may contain trace amounts of milk proteins and should not be used in patients with a known or suspected allergy to cows' milk. Serious allergic reactions, including bronchospasm and anaphylaxis, have been reported in patients allergic to cows' milk proteins. If a patient's symptoms worsen or new allergic symptoms occur, administration should be stopped and the patient treated accordingly.

- **CAUTIONS**

▸ With intravenous use Rapid intravenous administration of large doses associated with cardiovascular collapse

▸ With systemic use Systemic sclerosis (increased incidence of scleroderma renal crisis)

- **INTERACTIONS** → Appendix 1: corticosteroids

- **SIDE-EFFECTS**

▶ **Common or very common**

▸ With oral use Depressed mood

▶ **Frequency not known**

▸ With oral use Confusion · delusions · diarrhoea · dizziness · dyslipidaemia · hallucination · hiccups · Kaposi's sarcoma · lipomatosis · myocardial rupture (following recent myocardial infarction) · oedema · schizophrenia · suicidal ideation · withdrawal syndrome

▸ With parenteral use Confusion · delusions · depressed mood · diarrhoea · dizziness · dyslipidaemia · hallucination · hiccups · Kaposi's sarcoma · lipomatosis · oedema · schizophrenia · suicidal thoughts · vomiting · withdrawal syndrome

- **MONITORING REQUIREMENTS** Manufacturer advises monitor blood pressure and renal function (s-creatinine) routinely in patients with systemic sclerosis—increased incidence of scleroderma renal crisis.

- **DIRECTIONS FOR ADMINISTRATION**

▸ With intravenous use Intravenous injection given over 30 minutes. For intravenous infusion, may be diluted with sodium chloride intravenous infusion 0.9% or 0.45%, or glucose intravenous infusion 5% or 10%.

- **PATIENT AND CARER ADVICE** Patient counselling is advised for methylprednisolone tablets and injections (steroid card).

- **MEDICINAL FORMS** There can be variation in the licensing of different medicines containing the same drug. Forms available from special-order manufacturers include: oral suspension

Powder and solvent for solution for injection

CAUTIONARY AND ADVISORY LABELS 10

▸ Solu-Medrone (Pfizer Ltd)

Methylprednisolone (as Methylprednisolone sodium succinate) 40 mg Solu-Medrone 40mg powder and solvent for solution for injection vials | 1 vial PoM £1.58

Methylprednisolone (as Methylprednisolone sodium succinate) 125 mg Solu-Medrone 125mg powder and solvent for solution for injection vials | 1 vial PoM £4.75

Methylprednisolone (as Methylprednisolone sodium succinate) 500 mg Solu-Medrone 500mg powder and solvent for solution for injection vials | 1 vial PoM £9.60

Methylprednisolone (as Methylprednisolone sodium succinate) 1 gram Solu-Medrone 1g powder and solvent for solution for injection vials | 1 vial PoM £17.30

Tablet

CAUTIONARY AND ADVISORY LABELS 10, 21

▸ Medrone (Pfizer Ltd)

Methylprednisolone 2 mg Medrone 2mg tablets | 30 tablet PoM £3.88 DT = £3.88

Methylprednisolone 4 mg Medrone 4mg tablets | 30 tablet PoM £6.19 DT = £6.19

Methylprednisolone 16 mg Medrone 16mg tablets | 30 tablet PoM £17.17 DT = £17.17

Methylprednisolone 100 mg Medrone 100mg tablets | 20 tablet PoM £48.32 DT = £48.32

Suspension for injection

CAUTIONARY AND ADVISORY LABELS 10

▸ Depo-Medrone (Pfizer Ltd)

Methylprednisolone acetate 40 mg per 1 ml Depo-Medrone 40mg/1ml suspension for injection vials | 1 vial PoM £3.44 DT = £3.44 | 10 vial PoM £34.04

Depo-Medrone 80mg/2ml suspension for injection vials | 1 vial PoM £6.18 DT = £6.18 | 10 vial PoM £61.39

Depo-Medrone 120mg/3ml suspension for injection vials | 1 vial PoM £8.96 DT = £8.96 | 10 vial PoM £88.81

472

Prednisolone

29-Nov-2019

- **DRUG ACTION** Prednisolone exerts predominantly glucocorticoid effects with minimal mineralocorticoid effects.

- **INDICATIONS AND DOSE**

Severe croup (before transfer to hospital) | Mild croup that might cause complications (before transfer to hospital)

▶ BY MOUTH

▸ Child: 1–2 mg/kg

Mild to moderate acute asthma (when oral corticosteroid taken for more than a few days) | Severe or life-threatening acute asthma (when oral corticosteroid taken for more than a few days)

▶ BY MOUTH

▸ Child 1 month-11 years: 2 mg/kg once daily (max. per dose 60 mg) for up to 3 days, longer if necessary

Mild to moderate acute asthma | Severe or life-threatening acute asthma

▶ BY MOUTH

▸ Child 1 month-11 years: 1–2 mg/kg once daily (max. per dose 40 mg) for up to 3 days, longer if necessary

▸ Child 12-17 years: 40–50 mg daily for at least 5 days

Autoimmune inflammatory disorders (including juvenile idiopathic arthritis, connective tissue disorders and systemic lupus erythematosus)
- ▶ BY MOUTH
  - Child: Initially 1–2 mg/kg once daily, to be reduced after a few days if appropriate; maximum 60 mg per day

Autoimmune hepatitis
- ▶ BY MOUTH
  - Child: Initially 2 mg/kg once daily, to then be reduced to minimum effective dose; maximum 40 mg per day

Corticosteroid replacement therapy
- ▶ BY MOUTH
  - Child 12–17 years: 2–2.5 mg/m^2 daily in 1–2 divided doses, adjusted according to response

Infantile spasms
- ▶ BY MOUTH
  - Child 1 month–1 year: Initially 10 mg 4 times a day for 14 days; increased to 20 mg 3 times a day for 7 days if seizures not controlled after initial 7 days, reduce dose gradually over 15 days until stopped

Infantile spasms (dose reduction in patient taking 40 mg daily)
- ▶ BY MOUTH
  - Child 1 month–1 year: Reduced in steps of 10 mg every 5 days, then stop

Infantile spasms (dose reduction in patient taking 60 mg daily)
- ▶ BY MOUTH
  - Child 1 month–1 year: Reduced to 40 mg daily for 5 days, then reduced to 20 mg daily for 5 days, then reduced to 10 mg daily for 5 days and then stop

Idiopathic thrombocytopenic purpura
- ▶ BY MOUTH
  - Child 1–9 years: 1–2 mg/kg daily for maximum of 14 days, alternatively 4 mg/kg daily for a maximum of 4 days

Nephrotic syndrome
- ▶ BY MOUTH
  - Child: Initially 60 mg/m^2 once daily for 4–6 weeks until proteinuria ceases, then reduced to 40 mg/m^2 once daily on alternate days for 4–6 weeks, then withdraw by reducing dose gradually; maximum 80 mg per day

Nephrotic syndrome (prevention of relapse)
- ▶ BY MOUTH
  - Child: 0.5–1 mg/kg once daily or on alternate days for 3–6 months

Ulcerative colitis | Crohn's disease
- ▶ BY MOUTH
  - Child 2–17 years: 2 mg/kg once daily (max. per dose 60 mg) until remission occurs, followed by reducing doses

Pneumocystis pneumonia in moderate to severe infections associated with HIV infection
- ▶ BY MOUTH
  - Child: 2 mg/kg daily for 5 days, the dose is then reduced over the next 16 days and then stopped, corticosteroid treatment should ideally be started at the same time as the anti-pneumocystis therapy and certainly no later than 24–72 hours afterwards, the corticosteroid should be withdrawn before anti-pneumocystis treatment is complete; maximum 80 mg per day

Proctitis
- ▶ BY RECTUM USING RECTAL FOAM
  - Child 12–17 years: 1 metered application 1–2 times a day for 2 weeks, continued for further 2 weeks if good response, to be inserted into the rectum, 1 metered application contains 20 mg prednisolone
- ▶ BY RECTUM USING SUPPOSITORIES
  - Child 2–17 years: 5 mg twice daily, to be inserted in to the rectum morning and night, after a bowel movement

Distal ulcerative colitis
- ▶ BY RECTUM USING RECTAL FOAM
  - Child 12–17 years: 1 metered application 1–2 times a day for 2 weeks, continued for further 2 weeks if good response, to be inserted into the rectum, 1 metered application contains 20 mg prednisolone

Rectal complications of Crohn's disease
- ▶ BY RECTUM USING SUPPOSITORIES
  - Child 2–17 years: 5 mg twice daily, to be inserted in to the rectum morning and night, after a bowel movement

● **UNLICENSED USE**
- With rectal use Prednisolone rectal foam not licensed for use in children (age range not specified by manufacturer).

IMPORTANT SAFETY INFORMATION

SAFE PRACTICE
- With systemic use

Prednisolone has been confused with propranolol; care must be taken to ensure the correct drug is prescribed and dispensed.

● **CONTRA-INDICATIONS**
- With rectal use Abdominal or local infection · bowel perforation · extensive fistulas · intestinal obstruction · recent intestinal anastomoses

● **CAUTIONS**
- With rectal use Systemic absorption may occur with rectal preparations
- With systemic use Duchenne's muscular dystrophy (possible transient rhabdomyolysis and myoglobinuria following strenuous physical activity) · systemic sclerosis (increased incidence of scleroderma renal crisis with a daily dose of 15 mg or more)

● **INTERACTIONS** → Appendix 1: corticosteroids

● **SIDE-EFFECTS**
- With oral use Diarrhoea · dizziness · dyslipidaemia · lipomatosis · protein catabolism · scleroderma renal crisis

● **PREGNANCY** As it crosses the placenta 88% of prednisolone is inactivated.
Monitoring ▸ With systemic use Pregnant women with fluid retention should be monitored closely.

● **BREAST FEEDING** Prednisolone appears in small amounts in breast milk but maternal doses of up to 40 mg daily are unlikely to cause systemic effects in the infant.
Monitoring ▸ With systemic use Infant should be monitored for adrenal suppression if mother is taking a dose higher than 40 mg.

● **MONITORING REQUIREMENTS**
- With systemic use Manufacturer advises monitor blood pressure and renal function (s-creatinine) routinely in patients with systemic sclerosis—increased incidence of scleroderma renal crisis.

● **PATIENT AND CARER ADVICE**
Prednisolone (oral) for nephrotic syndrome
www.medicinesforchildren.org.uk/prednisolone-oral-nephrotic-syndrome
Medicines for Children leaflet: Prednisolone for asthma
www.medicinesforchildren.org.uk/prednisolone-asthma

6 Endocrine system

- **MEDICINAL FORMS** There can be variation in the licensing of different medicines containing the same drug. Forms available from special-order manufacturers include: oral suspension, oral solution

Foam

- Prednisolone (Non-proprietary)
  Prednisolone (as Prednisolone sodium metasulfobenzoate)
  20 mg per 1 application Prednisolone 20mg/application foam enema | 14 dose [PoM] £187.00 DT = £187.00

Gastro-resistant tablet

CAUTIONARY AND ADVISORY LABELS 5, 10, 25

- Prednisolone (Non-proprietary)
  Prednisolone 1 mg Prednisolone 1mg gastro-resistant tablets | 30 tablet [PoM] £2.23 DT = £2.23
  Prednisolone 2.5 mg Prednisolone 2.5mg gastro-resistant tablets | 28 tablet [PoM] £1.29 DT = £1.26 | 30 tablet [PoM] £1.23–£6.15
  Prednisolone 5 mg Prednisolone 5mg gastro-resistant tablets | 28 tablet [PoM] £3.79 DT = £1.68 | 30 tablet [PoM] £1.76–£6.29
- Deltacortril Enteric (Alliance Pharmaceuticals Ltd)
  Prednisolone 2.5 mg Deltacortril 2.5mg gastro-resistant tablets | 30 tablet [PoM] £1.16
  Prednisolone 5 mg Deltacortril 5mg gastro-resistant tablets | 30 tablet [PoM] £1.19
- Dilacort (Crescent Pharma Ltd, Teva UK Ltd)
  Prednisolone 2.5 mg Dilacort 2.5mg gastro-resistant tablets | 28 tablet [PoM] £1.14–£1.85 DT = £1.26
  Prednisolone 5 mg Dilacort 5mg gastro-resistant tablets | 28 tablet [PoM] £1.85 DT = £1.68

Soluble tablet

CAUTIONARY AND ADVISORY LABELS 10, 13, 21

- Prednisolone (Non-proprietary)
  Prednisolone (as Prednisolone sodium phosphate)
  5 mg Prednisolone 5mg soluble tablets | 30 tablet [PoM] £53.48 DT = £12.62

Tablet

CAUTIONARY AND ADVISORY LABELS 10, 21

- Prednisolone (Non-proprietary)
  Prednisolone 1 mg Prednisolone 1mg tablets | 28 tablet [PoM] £4.00 DT = £0.85
  Prednisolone 2.5 mg Prednisolone 2.5mg tablets | 28 tablet [PoM] £3.91
  Prednisolone 5 mg Prednisolone 5mg tablets | 28 tablet [PoM] £9.86 DT = £1.48
  Prednisolone 10 mg Prednisolone 10mg tablets | 28 tablet [PoM] £15.62
  Prednisolone 20 mg Prednisolone 20mg tablets | 28 tablet [PoM] £31.24
  Prednisolone 25 mg Prednisolone 25mg tablets | 56 tablet [PoM] £78.10 DT = £78.09
  Prednisolone 30 mg Prednisolone 30mg tablets | 28 tablet [PoM] £46.86 DT = £46.86
- Pevanti (Advanz Pharma)
  Prednisolone 2.5 mg Pevanti 2.5mg tablets | 30 tablet [PoM] £1.42 DT = £1.42
  Prednisolone 5 mg Pevanti 5mg tablets | 30 tablet [PoM] £0.95
  Prednisolone 10 mg Pevanti 10mg tablets | 30 tablet [PoM] £1.90 DT = £1.90
  Prednisolone 20 mg Pevanti 20mg tablets | 30 tablet [PoM] £3.80 DT = £3.80
  Prednisolone 25 mg Pevanti 25mg tablets | 56 tablet [PoM] £40.00 DT = £78.09

Suppository

- Prednisolone (Non-proprietary)
  Prednisolone (as Prednisolone sodium phosphate)
  5 mg Prednisolone sodium phosphate 5mg suppositories | 10 suppository [PoM] £90.05 DT = £89.45

Oral solution

CAUTIONARY AND ADVISORY LABELS 10

- Prednisolone (Non-proprietary)
  Prednisolone 1 mg per 1 ml Prednisolone 5mg/5ml oral solution unit dose | 10 unit dose [PoM] £11.41 DT = £11.41
  Prednisolone 10 mg per 1 ml Prednisolone 10mg/ml oral solution sugar free sugar-free | 30 ml [PoM] £55.50 DT = £55.50

2.1 Cushing's syndrome and disease

Cushing's Syndrome

Management

Most types of *Cushing's syndrome* are treated surgically. Metyrapone p. 481 may be useful to control the symptoms of the disease or to prepare the child for surgery. The dosages of metyrapone used are either low, and tailored to cortisol production, or high, in which case corticosteroid replacement therapy is also needed.

Ketoconazole below may have a direct effect on corticotropic tumour cells in patients with Cushing's disease. It is used under specialist supervision in children over 12 years for treatment of endogenous Cushing's syndrome.

ENZYME INHIBITORS

Ketoconazole

04-Feb-2020

- **DRUG ACTION** An imidazole derivative which acts as a potent inhibitor of cortisol and aldosterone synthesis by inhibiting the activity of 17α-hydroxylase, 11-hydroxylation steps and at higher doses the cholesterol side-chain cleavage enzyme. It also inhibits the activity of adrenal C17-20 lyase enzymes resulting in androgen synthesis inhibition, and may have a direct effect on corticotropic tumour cells in patients with Cushing's disease.

- **INDICATIONS AND DOSE**

Endogenous Cushing's syndrome (specialist use only)

- BY MOUTH
  - Child 12–17 years: Initially 400–600 mg daily in 2–3 divided doses, increased to 800–1200 mg daily; maintenance 400–800 mg daily in 2–3 divided doses, for dose titrations in patients with established dose, adjustments in adrenal insufficiency, or concomitant corticosteroid replacement therapy, consult product literature; maximum 1200 mg per day

- **CONTRA-INDICATIONS** Acquired QTc prolongation · Acute porphyrias p. 652 · avoid concomitant use of hepatotoxic drugs · congenital QTc prolongation
- **CAUTIONS** Pre-treatment liver enzymes should not exceed 2 times the normal upper limit · risk of adrenal insufficiency
- **INTERACTIONS** → Appendix 1: antifungals, azoles
- **SIDE-EFFECTS**
  - **Common or very common** Adrenal insufficiency · diarrhoea · gastrointestinal discomfort · nausea · skin reactions · vomiting
  - **Uncommon** Allergic conditions · alopecia · angioedema · asthenia · dizziness · drowsiness · headache · thrombocytopenia
  - **Rare or very rare** Fever · hepatic disorders · taste altered
  - **Frequency not known** Alcohol intolerance · appetite abnormal · arthralgia · azoospermia · dry mouth · epistaxis · flatulence · fontanelle bulging · gynaecomastia · hot flush · insomnia · intracranial pressure increased · malaise · menstrual disorder · myalgia · nervousness · papilloedema · paraesthesia · peripheral oedema · photophobia · photosensitivity reaction · tongue discolouration

  SIDE-EFFECTS, FURTHER INFORMATION Potentially life-threatening hepatotoxicity reported rarely with oral use. Manufacturer advises reduce dose if hepatic enzymes increased to less than 3 times the upper limit of normal—

consult product literature; discontinue permanently if hepatic enzymes at least 3 times the upper limit of normal.

- **CONCEPTION AND CONTRACEPTION** Effective contraception must be used in women of child-bearing potential.
- **PREGNANCY** Manufacturer advises avoid—teratogenic in *animal* studies.
- **BREAST FEEDING** Manufacturer advises avoid—present in breast milk.
- **HEPATIC IMPAIRMENT** Manufacturer advises avoid.
- **MONITORING REQUIREMENTS**
  - Monitor ECG before and one week after initiation, and then as clinically indicated thereafter.
  - Adrenal insufficiency Monitor adrenal function within one week of initiation, then regularly thereafter. When cortisol levels are normalised or close to target and effective dose established, monitor every 3–6 months as there is a risk of autoimmune disease development or exacerbation after normalisation of cortisol levels. If symptoms suggestive of adrenal insufficiency such as fatigue, anorexia, nausea, vomiting, hypotension, hyponatraemia, hyperkalaemia, and/or hypoglycaemia occur, measure cortisol levels and discontinue treatment temporarily (can be resumed thereafter at lower dose) or reduce dose and if necessary, initiate corticosteroid substitution.
  - Hepatotoxicity Monitor liver function before initiation of treatment, then weekly for 1 month after initiation, then monthly for 6 months—more frequently if dose adjusted or abnormal liver function detected.
- **PATIENT AND CARER ADVICE** Patients or their carers should be told how to recognise signs of liver disorder, and advised to discontinue treatment and seek prompt medical attention if symptoms such as anorexia, nausea, vomiting, fatigue, jaundice, abdominal pain, or dark urine develop. Patients or their carers should also be told how to recognise signs of adrenal insufficiency.
  Driving and skilled tasks Dizziness and somnolence may affect the performance of skilled tasks (e.g. driving).

- **MEDICINAL FORMS** There can be variation in the licensing of different medicines containing the same drug. Forms available from special-order manufacturers include: oral suspension

Tablet

CAUTIONARY AND ADVISORY LABELS 2, 5, 21

- Ketoconazole (non-proprietary) ▼
  Ketoconazole 200 mg Ketoconazole 200mg tablets | 60 tablet PoM £480.00 DT = £480.00

Metyrapone

- **DRUG ACTION** Metyrapone is a competitive inhibitor of 11β-hydroxylation in the adrenal cortex; the resulting inhibition of cortisol (and to a lesser extent aldosterone) production leads to an increase in ACTH production which, in turn, leads to increased synthesis and release of cortisol precursors. Metyrapone may be used as a test of anterior pituitary function.

- **INDICATIONS AND DOSE**

Differential diagnosis of ACTH-dependent Cushing's syndrome (specialist supervision in hospital)

- BY MOUTH
- Child: 15 mg/kg every 4 hours for 6 doses, alternatively 300 mg/m^2 every 4 hours for 6 doses; usual dose 250–750 mg every 4 hours

Management of Cushing's syndrome (specialist supervision in hospital)

- BY MOUTH
- Child: Usual dose 0.25–6 g daily, dose to be tailored to cortisol production, dose is either low, and tailored to cortisol production, or high, in which case corticosteroid replacement therapy is also needed

- **CONTRA-INDICATIONS** Adrenocortical insufficiency
- **CAUTIONS** Avoid in Acute porphyrias p. 652 · gross hypopituitarism (risk of precipitating acute adrenal failure) · hypertension on long-term administration · hypothyroidism (delayed response)
- **INTERACTIONS** → Appendix 1: metyrapone
- **SIDE-EFFECTS**
  - **Common or very common** Dizziness · headache · hypotension · nausea · sedation · vomiting
  - **Rare or very rare** Abdominal pain · adrenal insufficiency · allergic dermatitis · hirsutism
  - **Frequency not known** Alopecia · bone marrow failure · hypertension
- **PREGNANCY** Avoid (may impair biosynthesis of fetal-placental steroids).
- **BREAST FEEDING** Avoid—no information available.
- **HEPATIC IMPAIRMENT** Manufacturer advises caution (risk of delayed response).
- **PATIENT AND CARER ADVICE**
  Driving and skilled tasks Drowsiness may affect the performance of skilled tasks (e.g. driving).

- **MEDICINAL FORMS** There can be variation in the licensing of different medicines containing the same drug.

Capsule

CAUTIONARY AND ADVISORY LABELS 21

- Metopirone (HRA Pharma UK Ltd)
  Metyrapone 250 mg Metopirone 250mg capsules | 100 capsule PoM £363.66 DT = £363.66

3 Diabetes mellitus and hypoglycaemia

3.1 Diabetes mellitus

Diabetes

05-Jun-2017

Description of condition

Diabetes mellitus is a group of metabolic disorders in which persistent hyperglycaemia is caused by deficient insulin secretion or by resistance to the action of insulin. This leads to the abnormalities of carbohydrate, fat and protein metabolism that are characteristic of diabetes mellitus.

Type 1 diabetes mellitus p. 482 and Type 2 diabetes mellitus p. 485 are the two most common classifications of diabetes. Other common types of diabetes are gestational diabetes (develops during pregnancy and resolves after delivery) and secondary diabetes (may be caused by pancreatic damage, hepatic cirrhosis, or endocrine disease). Treatment with endocrine, antiviral or antipsychotic drugs may also cause secondary diabetes. In children, conditions such as cystic fibrosis can lead to diabetes; monogenic diabetes (previously known as maturity onset diabetes in the young) can also occur due to a single gene defect.

Driving

Information on the requirements for driving vehicles by young people receiving treatment for diabetes is available in the BNF or from the DVLA at www.gov.uk/guidance/diabetes-mellitus-assessing-fitness-to-drive.

Alcohol

Adolescents and their carers should be made aware that alcohol can make the signs of hypoglycaemia less clear, and can cause delayed hypoglycaemia; (note: specialist sources recommend that **adult** patients with diabetes should drink alcohol only in moderation, and when accompanied by food).

Oral glucose tolerance tests

The oral glucose tolerance test is used mainly for diagnosis of impaired glucose tolerance; it is **not** recommended or necessary for routine diagnostic use of diabetes when severe symptoms of hyperglycaemia are present. In children who have less severe symptoms and blood-glucose levels that do not establish or exclude diabetes (e.g. impaired fasting glycaemia), an oral glucose tolerance test may be required. It may be useful for diagnosis of monogenic diabetes or cystic fibrosis related diabetes, and is used to establish the presence of gestational diabetes.

An oral glucose tolerance test involves measuring the blood-glucose concentration after fasting, and then 2 hours after drinking a standard anhydrous glucose drink. Anhydrous glucose may alternatively be given as the appropriate amount of *Polycal*® or as *Rapilose*® OGTT oral solution.

HbA1c measurement

Glycated haemoglobin (HbA1c) forms when red blood cells are exposed to glucose in the plasma. The HbA1c test reflects average plasma glucose over the previous 2 to 3 months and provides a good indicator of glycaemic control. Unlike the oral glucose tolerance test, an HbA1c test can be performed at any time of the day and does not require any special preparation such as fasting.

HbA1c values are expressed in *mmol of glycated haemoglobin per mol of haemoglobin (mmol/mol)*, a standardised unit specific for HbA1c created by the International Federation of Clinical Chemistry and Laboratory Medicine (IFCC). HbA1c values were previously aligned to the assay used in the Diabetes Control and Complications Trial (DCCT) and expressed as a percentage.

Equivalent values

IFCC-HbA1c (mmol/mol)	DCCT-HbA1c (%)
42	6.0
48	6.5
53	7.0
59	7.5
64	8.0
69	8.5
75	9.0

The HbA1c test is used for monitoring glycaemic control in both Type 1 diabetes below and Type 2 diabetes p. 485 in children, and for diagnosis of Type 2 diabetes p. 485 in adults. EvGr HbA1c should not be used to diagnose diabetes in children. Ⓐ

HbA1c is also a reliable predictor of microvascular and macrovascular complications and mortality. Lower HbA1c is associated with a lower risk of long term vascular complications, and children and their carers should be supported to aim for an individualised HbA1c target (see Type 1 diabetes below and Type 2 diabetes p. 485). EvGr HbA1c should usually be measured in children with type 1 and type 2 diabetes every 3 months; and more frequently in children with type 1 diabetes if blood-glucose is poorly controlled. Ⓐ

HbA1c monitoring is invalid in children with disturbed erythrocyte turnover or in children with a lack of, or abnormal haemoglobin (for example, any anaemia, a recent blood transfusion, or an altered red cell lifespan). In these cases, quality-controlled plasma glucose profiles, total glycated haemoglobin estimation (if there is abnormal haemoglobin), or fructosamine estimation can be used.

Laboratory measurement of fructosamine concentration measures the glycated fraction of all plasma proteins over the previous 14 to 21 days but is a less accurate measure of glycaemic control than HbA1c.

Advanced Pharmacy Services

Patients with diabetes may be eligible for the New Medicines Service / Medicines Use Review service provided by a community pharmacist. For further information, see *Advanced Pharmacy Services* in Medicines optimisation p. 25.

Type 1 diabetes

05-Jun-2017

Description of condition

Type 1 diabetes describes an absolute insulin deficiency in which there is little or no endogenous insulin secretory capacity due to destruction of insulin-producing beta-cells in the pancreatic islets of Langerhans. This form of the disease has an auto-immune basis in most cases, and it can occur at any age, but most commonly before adulthood.

Loss of insulin secretion results in hyperglycaemia and other metabolic abnormalities. If poorly managed, the resulting tissue damage has both short-term and long-term adverse effects on health; this can result in retinopathy, nephropathy, premature cardiovascular disease, and peripheral artery disease.

Typical features in children presenting with type 1 diabetes are hyperglycaemia, polyuria, polydipsia, weight loss, and excessive tiredness.

Aims of treatment

Treatment is aimed at using insulin regimens to achieve as optimal a level of blood-glucose control as is feasible, while avoiding or reducing the frequency of hypoglycaemic episodes, in order to minimise the risk of long-term microvascular and macrovascular complications. Disability from complications can often be prevented by early detection and active management of the disease (Diabetic complications p. 486).

EvGr The target for glycaemic control should be individualised for each child, considering factors such as daily activities, aspirations, likelihood of complications, adherence to treatment, comorbidities, and history of hypoglycaemia. Tighter control of blood-glucose is now recommended for children with type 1 diabetes and treatment should attempt to reach near normal HbA1c and blood-glucose concentration. A target HbA1c concentration of 48 mmol/mol (6.5%) or lower is recommended in children to minimise the risk of long-term complications. The optimal plasma glucose targets for children are:

- fasting blood-glucose concentration of 4–7 mmol/litre on waking;
- a blood-glucose concentration of 4–7 mmol/litre before meals at other times of the day;
- a blood-glucose concentration of 5–9 mmol/litre after meals;
- a blood-glucose concentration of at least 5 mmol/litre in young people when driving. Ⓐ

Overview

EvGr Type 1 diabetes requires insulin replacement, supported when necessary by active management of other associated cardiovascular risk factors such as hypertension. Tight glycaemic control may be achieved by intensive insulin management (multiple daily injections or insulin pump therapy) from diagnosis, accompanied by carbohydrate counting.

The effectiveness of metformin in combination with insulin is not yet known in children, and so should not be used; other oral antidiabetic drugs should not be used in combination with insulin as their use may increase the risk of hypoglycaemia.

Dietary control is important in both type 1 and type 2 diabetes and children (with their families) should be encouraged to develop good knowledge of nutrition and how it affects their diabetes and insulin requirements. Healthy eating, regular exercise, and control of body-weight can reduce cardiovascular risk and help improve glycaemic control.

Children with type 1 diabetes over the age of 6 months should receive immunisation against influenza and pneumococcal infection (in children treated with antidiabetic drugs)—see Influenza vaccine p. 835 and Pneumococcal vaccine p. 838. (A)

Insulin therapy in type 1 diabetes

EvGr All children with type 1 diabetes require insulin therapy (**see also Insulin p. 484**). Treatment should be initiated and managed by clinicians with relevant expertise; there are three basic types of insulin regimen, although each regimen should be individualised.

Children should also be offered carbohydrate-counting training as part of a structured education programme. (A)

Multiple daily injection basal-bolus insulin regimens

One or more separate daily injections of intermediate-acting insulin or long-acting insulin analogue as the basal insulin; alongside multiple bolus injections of short-acting insulin before meals. This regimen offers flexibility to tailor insulin therapy with the carbohydrate load of each meal.

Mixed (biphasic) regimen

One, two, or three insulin injections per day of short-acting insulin mixed with intermediate-acting insulin. The insulin preparations may be mixed by the patient at the time of injection, or a premixed product can be used.

Continuous subcutaneous insulin infusion (insulin pump)

A regular or continuous amount of insulin (usually in the form of a rapid-acting insulin analogue or soluble insulin), delivered by a programmable pump and insulin storage reservoir via a subcutaneous needle or cannula.

Recommended insulin regimens

EvGr Children should be offered multiple daily injection basal-bolus regimens initiated at diagnosis, considering personal and family circumstances, and personal preferences. Children and their carers should be encouraged to adjust the insulin dose as appropriate after each blood-glucose measurement, and to inject rapid-acting insulin analogues before eating (rather than after eating); this reduces blood-glucose concentrations after meals and helps to optimise blood-glucose control.

If a multiple daily injection basal-bolus insulin regimen is unsuitable, or the child does not have optimal blood-glucose control, it may be necessary to offer an alternative insulin regimen (either continuous subcutaneous insulin infusion or once-, twice- or three-times daily mixed injections) as well as additional support (such as increased contact with their specialist diabetes team).

Continuous subcutaneous insulin infusion (or insulin pump) therapy may be considered under the care of a specialist team. It should only be offered to children over 12 years who suffer disabling hypoglycaemia, or, who have high HbA1c concentrations (69 mmol/mol [8.5%] or above) with multiple daily injection therapy (including, if appropriate, the use of long-acting insulin analogues) despite a high level of care. Children under 12 years may be offered insulin pump therapy if a multiple daily injection regimen is impractical or inappropriate, but they should undergo a trial of a multiple dose injection regimen between the ages of 12 and 18 years.

If the chosen regimen is a twice daily injection regimen, the insulin dose should be adjusted according to the general trend in pre-meal, bedtime and occasional night-time blood-glucose concentration. (A)

Insulin requirements

EvGr The dosage of insulin must be determined individually for each child and should be adjusted as necessary according to the results of regular monitoring of blood-glucose concentrations.

Prescribers and patients should be aware that initiation of insulin may be followed by a **temporary** partial remission phase or 'honeymoon period' when lower doses of insulin are required than are subsequently necessary to maintain glycaemic control with an HbA1c concentration of less than 48 mmol/mol (6.5%). (A)

EvGr Insulin doses should be reviewed after puberty (around 1 year after menarche or after the growth spurt in boys) as insulin resistance falls after puberty, and maintenance of pubertal doses may increase the risk for excessive weight gain. (E)

Persistent poor glucose control, leading to erratic insulin requirements or episodes of hypoglycaemia, may be due to many factors, including adherence, injection technique, injection site problems, blood-glucose monitoring skills, lifestyle issues (including diet and exercise), psychological issues, and organic causes such as renal disease, thyroid disorders, coeliac disease, Addison's disease or gastroparesis. EvGr A review of the child's injection sites should be offered at each clinic visit. (A)

Infection, stress, accidental or surgical trauma, and puberty may all increase the required insulin dose. Insulin requirements may be decreased (and therefore susceptibility to hypoglycaemia increased) by physical activity, intercurrent illness, reduced food intake, and in certain endocrine disorders, such as anterior pituitary or adrenocortical insufficiency and hypothyroidism.

EvGr Rapid-acting insulin analogues should be supplied for use during intercurrent illness and episodes of hyperglycaemia. (A)

Risks of hypoglycaemia with insulin

EvGr Hypoglycaemia is an inevitable adverse effect of insulin treatment, and children and their carers should be advised of the warning signs and actions to take (for guidance on management, see Hypoglycaemia p. 501). (A)

Impaired awareness of hypoglycaemia can occur, when the ability to recognise usual symptoms is lost, or when the symptoms are blunted or no longer present. EvGr Awareness of hypoglycaemia should be discussed and assessed with the child and their carer approximately every 3 months. (E)

An increase in the frequency of hypoglycaemic episodes may reduce the warning symptoms experienced by the child. Impaired awareness of symptoms below 3 mmol/litre is associated with a significantly increased risk of severe hypoglycaemia. Beta-blockers can also blunt hypoglycaemic awareness, by reducing warning signs such as tremor.

Loss of warning of hypoglycaemia among insulin-treated children can be a serious hazard, especially for adolescents who are drivers, cyclists, or in dangerous occupations. Advice should be given in line with the Driver and Vehicle Licensing Agency (DVLA) guidance (see *Driving*, under Diabetes p. 481).

EvGr To restore the warning signs, episodes of hypoglycaemia must be minimised. Insulin regimens, doses and blood-glucose targets should be reviewed and continuous subcutaneous insulin infusion therapy and real-time continuous glucose monitoring should be considered. (A)

EvGr Children and their carers should receive structured education to ensure they are following the principles of a flexible insulin regimen correctly, with additional education regarding avoiding and treating hypoglycaemia for those who continue to have impaired awareness. If recurrent severe episodes of hypoglycaemia continue despite appropriate interventions, the child should be referred to a specialist centre. ⟨E⟩

Manufacturers advise any switch between brands or formulation of insulin (including switching from animal to human insulin) should be done under strict supervision; a change in dose may be required.

Hypodermic equipment

EvGr Children and their carers should be advised on the safe disposal of lancets, single-use syringes, and needles, and should be provided with suitable disposal containers. Arrangements should be made for the suitable disposal of these containers. ⟨A⟩

Lancets, needles, syringes, and accessories are listed under Hypodermic Equipment in Part IXA of the Drug Tariff (Part III of the Northern Ireland Drug Tariff, Part 3 of the Scottish Drug Tariff). The drug Tariffs can be accessed online at:

- National Health Service Drug Tariff for England and Wales: www.nhsbsa.nhs.uk/pharmacies-gp-practices-and-appliance-contractors/drug-tariff
- Health and Personal Social Services for Northern Ireland Drug Tariff:www.hscbusiness.hscni.net/services/2034.htm
- Scottish Drug Tariff: www.isdscotland.org/Health-Topics/Prescribing-and-Medicines/Scottish-Drug-Tariff

Useful Resources

Diabetes (type 1 and type 2) in children and young people: diagnosis and management. National Institute for Health and Care Excellence. Clinical guideline NG18. August 2015. www.nice.org.uk/guidance/ng18

Insulin

05-Jun-2017

Overview

For recommended insulin regimens see Type 1 diabetes p. 482 and Type 2 diabetes p. 485.

Insulin is a polypeptide hormone secreted by pancreatic beta-cells. Insulin increases glucose uptake by adipose tissue and muscles, and suppresses hepatic glucose release. The role of insulin is to lower blood-glucose concentrations in order to prevent hyperglycaemia and its associated microvascular, macrovascular and metabolic complications.

The natural profile of insulin secretion in the body consists of basal insulin (a low and steady secretion of background insulin that controls the glucose continuously released from the liver) and meal-time bolus insulin (secreted in response to glucose absorbed from food and drink).

Sources of insulin

Three types of insulin are available in the UK: human insulin, human insulin analogues, and animal insulin. Animal insulins are extracted and purified from animal sources (bovine or porcine insulin). Although widely used in the past, animal insulins are no longer initiated in people with diabetes but may still be used by some adult patients who cannot, or do not wish to, change to human insulins.

Human insulins are produced by recombinant DNA technology and have the same amino acid sequence as endogenous human insulin. Human insulin analogues are produced in the same way as human insulins, but the insulin is modified to produce a desired kinetic characteristic, such as an extended duration of action or faster absorption and onset of action.

Immunological resistance to insulin is uncommon and true insulin allergy is rare. Human insulin and insulin analogues are less immunogenic than animal insulins.

Administration of insulin

Insulin is inactivated by gastro-intestinal enzymes and must therefore be given by injection; the subcutaneous route is ideal in most circumstances. Insulin should be injected into a body area with plenty of subcutaneous fat—usually the abdomen (fastest absorption rate) or outer thighs/buttocks (slower absorption compared with the abdomen or inner thighs).

Absorption from a limb site can vary considerably (by as much as 20–40%) day-to-day, particularly in children. Local tissue reactions, changes in insulin sensitivity, injection site, blood flow, depth of injection, and the amount of insulin injected can all affect the rate of absorption. Increased blood flow around the injection site due to exercise can also increase insulin absorption.

EvGr Lipohypertrophy can occur due to repeatedly injecting into the same small area, and can cause erratic absorption of insulin, and contribute to poor glycaemic control. Patients should be advised not to use affected areas for further injection until the skin has recovered. Lipohypertrophy can be minimised by using different injection sites in rotation. Injection sites should be checked for signs of infection, swelling, bruising, and lipohypertrophy before administration. ⟨A⟩

Insulin preparations

Insulin preparations can be broadly categorised into three groups based on their time-action profiles: short-acting insulins (including soluble insulin and rapid-acting insulins), intermediate-acting insulins and long-acting insulins. The duration of action of each particular type of insulin varies considerably from one patient to another, and needs to be assessed individually.

Short-acting insulins

Short-acting insulins have a short duration and a relatively rapid onset of action, to replicate the insulin normally produced by the body in response to glucose absorbed from a meal. These are available as soluble Insulin above (human and, bovine or porcine—both rarely used), and the rapid-acting insulin analogues (insulin aspart p. 492, insulin glulisine p. 493 and insulin lispro p. 493).

Soluble insulin

Soluble insulin is usually given subcutaneously but some preparations can be given intravenously and intramuscularly. For maintenance regimens, it is usual to inject the insulin 15 to 30 minutes before meals, depending on the insulin preparation used.

When injected subcutaneously, soluble insulin has a rapid onset of action (30 to 60 minutes), a peak action between 1 and 4 hours, and a duration of action of up to 9 hours.

When injected intravenously, soluble insulin has a short half-life of only a few minutes and its onset of action is instantaneous.

Soluble insulin administered intravenously is the most appropriate form of insulin for use in diabetic emergencies e.g. Diabetic ketoacidosis p. 486 and peri-operatively.

Rapid-acting insulin

Insulin aspart, insulin glulisine, and insulin lispro have a faster onset of action (within 15 minutes) and shorter duration of action (approximately 2–5 hours) than soluble insulin, and are usually given by subcutaneous injection.

EvGr For maintenance regimens, these insulins should ideally be injected immediately before meals. Rapid-acting insulin, administered before meals, has an advantage over short-acting soluble insulin in terms of improved glucose control, reduction of HbA1c, and reduction in the incidence of severe hypoglycaemia, including nocturnal hypoglycaemia.

The routine use of *post-meal* injections of rapid-acting insulin should be avoided—when given during or after meals, they are associated with poorer glucose control, an increased risk of high postprandial-glucose concentration, and subsequent hypoglycaemia. ⟨A⟩

Intermediate-acting insulin

Intermediate-acting insulins (isophane insulin p. 494) have an intermediate duration of action, designed to mimic the effect of endogenous basal insulin. When given by subcutaneous injection, they have an onset of action of approximately 1–2 hours, a maximal effect at 3–12 hours, and a duration of action of 11–24 hours.

Isophane insulin is a suspension of insulin with protamine; it may be given as one or more daily injections alongside separate meal-time short-acting insulin injections, or mixed with a short-acting (soluble or rapid-acting) insulin in the same syringe—for recommended insulin regimens see Type 1 diabetes p. 482 and Type 2 diabetes below. Isophane insulin may be mixed with a short-acting insulin by the patient, or a pre-mixed biphasic insulin can be supplied (biphasic isophane insulin p. 494, biphasic insulin aspart p. 495 and biphasic insulin lispro p. 495).

Biphasic insulins (biphasic isophane insulin, biphasic insulin aspart, biphasic insulin lispro) are pre-mixed insulin preparations containing various combinations of short-acting insulin (soluble insulin or rapid-acting analogue insulin) and an intermediate-acting insulin.

The percentage of short-acting insulin varies from 15% to 50%. These preparations should be administered by subcutaneous injection immediately before a meal.

Long-acting insulin

Like intermediate-acting insulins, the long-acting insulins (protamine zinc insulin, insulin zinc suspension, insulin detemir p. 496, insulin glargine p. 496, insulin degludec p. 495) mimic endogenous basal insulin secretion, but their duration of action may last up to 36 hours. They achieve a steady-state level after 2–4 days to produce a constant level of insulin.

Insulin glargine and insulin degludec are given once daily and insulin detemir is given once or twice daily according to individual requirements. The older long-acting insulins, (insulin zinc suspension and protamine zinc insulin) are now rarely prescribed.

Type 2 diabetes

05-Jun-2017

Description of condition

Type 2 diabetes is a chronic metabolic condition characterised by insulin resistance. Insufficient pancreatic insulin production also occurs progressively over time, resulting in hyperglycaemia.

Type 2 diabetes in children is associated with increased body-weight, increased risk of renal complications, hypertension, and dyslipidaemia; therefore it increases cardiovascular risk. It is associated with long-term microvascular and macrovascular complications, together with reduced quality of life and life expectancy.

Type 2 diabetes typically develops later in life but is increasingly diagnosed in children, despite previously being considered a disease of adulthood.

Aims of treatment

Treatment is aimed at minimising the risk of long-term microvascular and macrovascular complications by effective blood-glucose control and maintenance of HbA1c at or below the target value set for each individual child.

Overview

EvGr Lifestyle modifications (including weight loss, smoking cessation and regular exercise) can help to reduce both hyperglycaemia and cardiovascular risk and should be encouraged where appropriate. Children and their carers should also receive advice from a paediatric dietitian to help optimise body-weight and blood-glucose control.

Lifestyle modifications alone are often unsuccessful at achieving glycaemic control in children, therefore antidiabetic drugs should be offered and initiated alongside lifestyle interventions such as diet and exercise, from the time of diagnosis.

Children with type 2 diabetes should receive immunisation against influenza (over the age of 6 months) and pneumococcal infection—see Influenza vaccine p. 835 and Pneumococcal vaccine p. 838. (A)

Antidiabetic drugs

In children, type 2 diabetes does not usually occur until adolescence and information on the use of oral antidiabetic drugs in children is limited. For recommended treatment regimens and the place in therapy of each drug, see *Treatment of type 2 diabetes*.

EvGr Treatment with antidiabetic drugs should be initiated under specialist supervision **only**. (E)

Metformin hydrochloride p. 488 is the only oral antidiabetic drug licensed for use in children. It has an anti-hyperglycaemic effect, lowering both basal and postprandial blood-glucose concentrations. Metformin hydrochloride does not stimulate insulin secretion and therefore, when given alone, does not cause hypoglycaemia.

EvGr The dose of standard-release metformin hydrochloride should be increased gradually to minimise the risk of gastro-intestinal side-effects. (A)

There is little experience of the use of other non-insulin antidiabetic drugs in children, with most evidence extrapolated from adult studies.

Several **sulfonylureas** (such as gliclazide p. 490, glibenclamide p. 489 and tolbutamide p. 490) are available but experience in children is limited; they are not the recommended choice of treatment in children; therefore treatment should be initiated by a specialist. The sulfonylureas may cause hypoglycaemia which may be more common in children than in adults. Hypoglycaemia is more likely with long-acting sulfonylureas such as glibenclamide, which has been associated with severe, prolonged and sometimes fatal cases—for this reason sulfonylureas are usually avoided in children.

Treatment of type 2 diabetes

EvGr A target HbA1c concentration of 48 mmol/mol (6.5%) or lower is ideal to minimise the risk of long-term complications, however an individualised lowest achievable target should be agreed with each child and their carers taking into account factors such as daily activities, individual life goals, complications, and comorbidities. HbA1c concentrations should be monitored every 3 months.

Note: Consider relaxing the target HbA1c level on a case-by-case basis, with particular consideration for children where tight blood-glucose control is not appropriate or poses a high risk of the consequences of hypoglycaemia.

Standard-release metformin hydrochloride is the first-line choice for initial treatment in children and should be offered from diagnosis, alongside nutrition and lifestyle advice.

If the combination of lifestyle changes and metformin hydrochloride fails to reduce HbA1c to the agreed target within 3 to 4 months of therapy, addition of a long-acting insulin or once-daily human isophane insulin p. 494 should be considered (see also, Insulin p. 484). (A)

EvGr Initiation of insulin should be under specialist care. (E)

EvGr Metformin hydrochloride should be continued alongside insulin, to improve insulin sensitivity. The combination of metformin hydrochloride and once-daily insulin is usually an effective treatment for maintaining glycaemic control in the majority of children for extended periods of time.

If the combination of basal insulin and metformin does not achieve the HbA1c target (and postprandial hyperglycaemia persists) addition of prandial rapid- or short-acting insulin should be initiated and titrated until the target HbA1c is met. Ⓐ Weight gain may occur and can be particularly problematic in children with type 2 diabetes when insulin therapy is initiated, unless there is careful attention and adherence to dietary measures. EvGr The importance of diet and exercise should be emphasised. Ⓐ

Advanced Pharmacy Services

Children with type 2 diabetes may be eligible for the New Medicines Service / Medicines Use Review service provided by a community pharmacist. For further information, see *Advanced Pharmacy Services* in Medicines optimisation p. 25.

Useful Resources

Diabetes (type 1 and type 2) in children and young people: diagnosis and management. National Institute for Health and Care Excellence. Clinical guideline NG18. August 2015. www.nice.org.uk/guidance/ng18.

Diabetic complications

10-May-2018

See also

Diabetes p. 481
Type 1 diabetes p. 482
Type 2 diabetes p. 485
Diabetic foot infections, antibacterial therapy p. 324. For guidance on other diabetic foot problems, see NICE guideline **Diabetic foot problems** at: https://www.nice.org.uk/guidance/ng19.

Diabetes and cardiovascular disease

Diabetes is a strong risk factor for cardiovascular disease later in life. EvGr Other risk factors for cardiovascular disease that should also be addressed are: smoking, hypertension, obesity and dyslipidaemia. Ⓐ The use of an ACE inhibitor (or an angiotensin-II receptor antagonist) and lipid-regulating drugs can be beneficial in children with diabetes and a high cardiovascular disease risk. ACE inhibitors and angiotensin-II receptor antagonists may also have a role in the management of diabetic nephropathy. For guidance on stopping smoking, see Smoking cessation p. 313.

Diabetic nephropathy

EvGr In diabetic children with nephropathy, blood pressure should be reduced to the lowest achievable level to slow the rate of decline of glomerular filtration rate and reduce proteinuria. Microalbuminuria can occur transiently during puberty. Provided there are no contra-indications, all diabetic children with nephropathy causing proteinuria or with established microalbuminuria should be treated with an ACE inhibitor or an angiotensin-II receptor antagonist, even if the blood pressure is normal. ACE inhibitors or angiotensin-II receptor antagonists should also be given as monotherapy, or combined therapy, in children with chronic kidney disease and proteinuria, to reduce the rate of progression of chronic kidney disease. Ⓐ

ACE inhibitors can potentiate the hypoglycaemic effect of insulin and oral antidiabetic drugs; this effect is more likely during the first weeks of combined treatment and in children with renal impairment.

See also treatment of hypertension in diabetes in Hypertension p. 104.

Diabetic neuropathy

Clinical neuropathy is rare in children whose diabetes is well controlled.

Visual impairment

EvGr Optimal diabetic control (HbA1c ideally around 7% or 53 mmol/mol) and blood pressure control (<130/80 mmHg) should be maintained to prevent onset and progression of diabetic eye disease. Ⓐ

Diabetic ketoacidosis

Management

The management of diabetic ketoacidosis involves the replacement of fluid and electrolytes and the administration of insulin. Guidelines for the Management of Diabetic Ketoacidosis, published by the British Society of Paediatric Endocrinology and Diabetes, (available at www.bsped.org.uk) should be followed. Clinically well children with mild ketoacidosis who are dehydrated up to 5% usually respond to oral rehydration and subcutaneous insulin. For those who do not respond, or are clinically unwell, or are dehydrated by more than 5%, insulin and replacement fluids are best given by intravenous infusion.

- To restore circulating volume for children in *shock*, give 10 mL/kg **sodium chloride 0.9%** as a rapid infusion, repeat as necessary up to a maximum of 30 mL/kg.
- Further fluid should be given by intravenous infusion at a rate that replaces deficit and provides maintenance over 48 hours; initially use **sodium chloride 0.9%**, changing to **sodium chloride 0.45%** and **glucose 5%** after 12 hours if response is adequate and plasma-sodium concentration is stable.
- Include **potassium chloride** in the fluids unless anuria is suspected, adjust according to plasma-potassium concentration.
- Insulin infusion is necessary to switch off ketogenesis and reverse acidosis; it should not be started until at least 1 hour after the start of intravenous rehydration fluids.
- **Soluble insulin** should be diluted (and **mixed thoroughly**) with **sodium chloride 0.9%** intravenous infusion to a concentration of 1 unit/mL and infused at a rate of 0.1 units/kg/hour.
- **Sodium bicarbonate** infusion (1.26% or 2.74%) is rarely necessary and is used only in cases of extreme acidosis (blood pH less than 6.9) and shock, since the acid-base disturbance is normally corrected by treatment with insulin.
- Once blood glucose falls to 14 mmol/litre, **glucose intravenous infusion 5%** *or* **10%** should be added to the fluids.
- The insulin infusion rate can be reduced to no less than 0.05 units/kg/hour when blood-glucose concentration has fallen to 14 mmol/litre *and* blood pH is greater than 7.3 *and* a glucose infusion has been started; it is continued until the child is ready to take food by mouth. Subcutaneous insulin can then be started.
- The insulin infusion should not be stopped until 1 hour after starting subcutaneous soluble or long acting insulin, or 10 minutes after starting subcutaneous insulin aspart p. 492, or insulin glulisine p. 493, or insulin lispro p. 493.

Hyperosmolar hyperglycaemic state or hyperosmolar hyperglycaemic nonketotic coma occurs rarely in children. Treatment is similar to that of diabetic ketoacidosis, although lower rates of insulin infusion and slower rehydration may be required.

Diabetes, surgery and medical illness

05-Jun-2017

Management of diabetes during surgery

EvGr Children with diabetes should undergo surgery in centres with facilities and expertise for the care of children with diabetes. Detailed local protocols should be available to all healthcare professionals involved in the treatment of these children. All surgery requiring general anaesthesia in children with type 1 and type 2 diabetes requires hospital admission. Ⓐ

Note: The following recommendations provide general guidance for the management of diabetes during surgery. **Local protocols and guidelines should be referred to where they exist.**

Use of insulin during surgery

Elective surgery—minor procedures

EvGr *Minor procedures* (procedures of less than 2 hours requiring either general anaesthesia or heavy sedation) in children who have type 1 or type 2 diabetes should not have a major impact on glycaemic control, and a slight modification of the usual regimen may be all that is necessary—adjustments should be made following local protocol; taking into consideration the type of insulin or antidiabetic drugs the child usually takes, whether fasting is required, the time of day of the operation, and requirement for intravenous fluids and glucose. All children who are usually prescribed insulin require intravenous insulin during surgery, to avoid ketoacidosis. Ⓐ

Elective surgery—major procedures

EvGr *Major procedures* (procedures requiring general anaesthesia for more than 2 hours) in children who have type 1 or type 2 diabetes, should ideally be performed when diabetes is under optimal control. If glycaemic control is poor, the procedure should be delayed if possible; otherwise it is advisable to admit the child well in advance of surgery for stabilisation of glycaemic control.

Blood-glucose concentration should be maintained within the usual target range of 5–10 mmol/litre throughout the peri-operative period for all surgical procedures.

Children usually prescribed insulin for type 1 or type 2 diabetes require an intravenous insulin infusion p. 491 during surgery (even if fasting) to avoid ketoacidosis. Detailed local protocols should be consulted. In general, the following steps should be followed:

- on the *evening before surgery*, the usual insulin regimen should be given as normal; the usual bedtime snack should be given and hourly capillary blood-glucose monitoring should be initiated to detect hypoglycaemia or hyperglycaemia before the procedure. Ketones should also be checked if blood-glucose is above 14 mmol/litre, and an appropriate dose of short-acting insulin should be administered to restore blood-glucose to the target range;
- on the *morning of surgery* the **usual** insulin dose should be omitted;
- at least 2 *hours before the procedure*, a maintenance fluid infusion of sodium chloride 0.45 % and glucose 5 % (sodium chloride with glucose p. 638) intravenous infusion should be started. A switch to sodium chloride 0.9 % infusion p. 636 may be required if sodium concentration falls and there is risk of hyponatraemia. After surgery, potassium chloride p. 651 should be added to the intravenous fluid, according to the child's body weight and fluid requirements. Electrolytes must be measured frequently throughout, and adjustments to the infusion made as necessary;
- soluble human insulin 1 unit/mL in sodium chloride 0.9 % intravenous infusion should be started with the maintenance fluids at an infusion rate appropriate to the blood-glucose concentration, to maintain a concentration between 5 and 10 mmol/litre, adjusted according to hourly blood-glucose monitoring;
- if the blood-glucose concentration falls below 6 mmol/litre the insulin infusion should **not** be stopped as this will cause rebound hyperglycaemia; instead the rate should be reduced; however, if blood-glucose concentration drops below 4 mmol/litre the insulin infusion can be stopped temporarily for 10–15 minutes.

After surgery, continue the glucose infusion, and the intravenous insulin infusion or additional short-acting insulin as necessary, until the child can eat and drink normally and their usual treatment regimen can resume. A short-acting insulin can also be given if required to reduce hyperglycaemia. Ⓐ

Emergency surgery

EvGr Children with diabetes (type 1 and 2) requiring emergency surgery, should always have their blood-glucose, blood or urinary ketone concentration, and serum electrolytes checked before surgery. If ketones are high, blood gases should also be checked. If ketoacidosis is present, recommendations for Diabetic ketoacidosis p. 486 should be followed immediately, and surgery delayed if possible. If there is no acidosis, intravenous fluids and an insulin infusion should be started and managed as for *major elective surgery* (above). Ⓐ

Use of antidiabetic drugs during surgery

EvGr If elective *minor surgical procedures* only require a short-fasting period (just one missed meal), it may be possible to adjust antidiabetic drugs to avoid a switch to a variable rate intravenous insulin infusion; normal drug treatment can continue.

Children who usually take **sulfonylureas** should have their medication stopped on the day of surgery. Ⓐ

EvGr **Sulfonylureas** are associated with hypoglycaemia in the fasted state and therefore should not be recommenced until the child is eating and drinking normally. Ⓔ

EvGr Children undergoing *minor procedures* require hourly blood-glucose monitoring and, if blood-glucose concentration rises above 10 mmol/litre, should be treated with subcutaneous rapid-acting insulin no more frequently than every 3 hours.

Children undergoing a *major surgical* procedure expected to last at least 2 hours should be managed on an intravenous insulin infusion following the recommendations for *Elective surgery* (above). Ⓐ

EvGr Insulin is almost always required in medical and surgical emergencies. Ⓔ

EvGr **Metformin hydrochloride p. 488** is renally excreted; renal impairment may lead to accumulation and lactic acidosis during surgery. In children undergoing *major surgery* lasting more than 2 hours, metformin hydrochloride should be discontinued 24 hours before the procedure. Children having minor surgery lasting less than 2 hours may stop their metformin on the day of surgery. Metformin hydrochloride should not be restarted until at least 48 hours after surgery or after the child is eating again, and only once normal renal function has been established. Ⓐ

The manufacturer advises that metformin should also be omitted if contrast medium is administered during surgery to reduce the risk of contrast-induced nephropathy. It should be stopped prior to, or at the time of the test, and not to be restarted until 48 hours afterwards, and only once normal renal function has been established.

Use of antidiabetic drugs during medical illness

Manufacturers of some antidiabetic drugs recommend that they may need to be replaced temporarily with insulin during intercurrent illness when the drug is unlikely to control hyperglycaemia (such as coma, severe infection, trauma and other medical emergencies). Consult individual product literature.

Diabetes, pregnancy and breast-feeding

01-Aug-2017

Description of condition

Diabetes in pregnancy is associated with increased risks to the young woman (such as pre-eclampsia and rapidly

6 Endocrine system

worsening retinopathy), and to the developing fetus, compared with pregnancy in non-diabetic young women. Effective blood-glucose control before conception and throughout pregnancy reduces (but does not eliminate) the risk of adverse outcomes such as miscarriage, congenital malformation, stillbirth, and neonatal death.

Management of pre-existing diabetes

EvGr Young women with pre-existing diabetes who are planning on becoming pregnant should aim to keep their HbA1c concentration below 48 mmol/mol (6.5%) if possible without causing problematic hypoglycaemia. Any reduction towards this target is likely to reduce the risk of congenital malformations in the newborn.

Young women with pre-existing diabetes who are planning to become pregnant should be advised to take folic acid at the dose for young women who are at high-risk of conceiving a child with a neural tube defect, see folic acid p. 620. Ⓐ

Overview

Oral antidiabetic drugs

EvGr All oral antidiabetic drugs, except metformin hydrochloride below, should be discontinued before pregnancy (or as soon as an unplanned pregnancy is identified) and substituted with insulin therapy. Young women with diabetes may be treated with metformin hydrochloride below [unlicensed in pregnancy] as an adjunct or alternative to insulin in the preconception period and during pregnancy, when the likely benefits from improved blood-glucose control outweigh the potential for harm. Metformin hydrochloride below can be continued immediately after birth and during breast-feeding for those with pre-existing Type 2 diabetes p. 485. All other antidiabetic drugs should be avoided while breast-feeding. Ⓐ

Insulin

Limited evidence suggests that the rapid-acting insulin analogues (insulin aspart p. 492 and insulin lispro p. 493) can be associated with fewer episodes of hypoglycaemia, a reduction in postprandial glucose excursions, and an improvement in overall glycaemic control compared with regular human insulin.

EvGr Isophane insulin p. 494 is the first-choice for long-acting insulin during pregnancy, however in young women who have good blood-glucose control before pregnancy with the long-acting insulin analogues (insulin detemir p. 496 or insulin glargine p. 496), it may be appropriate to continue their use throughout pregnancy.

Continuous subcutaneous insulin infusion p. 491 (insulin pump therapy) may be appropriate for young women who have difficulty achieving glycaemic control with multiple daily injections of insulin p. 491 without significant disabling hypoglycaemia.

All young women treated with insulin p. 491 during pregnancy should be aware of the risks of hypoglycaemia, particularly in the first trimester, and should be advised to always carry a fast-acting form of glucose, such as dextrose tablets or a glucose-containing drink. Pregnant young women with Type 1 diabetes p. 482 should also be prescribed glucagon p. 502 for use if needed.

Young women with pre-existing diabetes treated with insulin p. 491 during pregnancy are at increased risk of hypoglycaemia in the postnatal period and should reduce their insulin immediately after birth. Blood-glucose levels should be monitored carefully to establish the appropriate dose. Ⓐ

Medication for diabetic complications

EvGr Angiotensin-converting enzyme inhibitors and angiotensin-II receptor antagonists should be discontinued and replaced with an alternative antihypertensive suitable for use in pregnancy before conception or as soon as pregnancy is confirmed. Statins should not be prescribed during pregnancy and should be discontinued before a planned pregnancy. Ⓐ

Gestational diabetes

EvGr Young women with gestational diabetes who have a fasting plasma glucose below 7 mmol/litre at diagnosis, should first attempt a change in diet and exercise alone in order to reduce blood-glucose. If blood-glucose targets are not met within 1 to 2 weeks, metformin hydrochloride below may be prescribed [unlicensed use]. Insulin p. 491 may be prescribed if metformin is contra-indicated or not acceptable, and may also be added to treatment if metformin is not effective alone.

Young women who have a fasting plasma glucose above 7 mmol/litre at diagnosis should be treated with insulin p. 491 immediately with or without metformin hydrochloride below, in addition to a change in diet and exercise.

Young women who have a fasting plasma glucose between 6 and 6.9 mmol/litre alongside complications, such as macrosomia or hydramnios, should be considered for immediate insulin treatment p. 491, with or without metformin hydrochloride below.

Young women with gestational diabetes should discontinue hypoglycaemic treatment immediately after giving birth. Ⓐ

Useful Resources

Management of diabetes. Scottish Intercollegiate Guidelines Network. Clinical guideline 116. March 2010 (updated November 2017).
www.sign.ac.uk/assets/sign116.pdf

Diabetes in pregnancy: management from preconception to the postnatal period. National Institute for Health and Care Excellence. Clinical guideline NG3. February 2015.
www.nice.org.uk/guidance/ng3

BLOOD GLUCOSE LOWERING DRUGS ›
BIGUANIDES

Metformin hydrochloride

26-Jul-2018

- **DRUG ACTION** Metformin exerts its effect mainly by decreasing gluconeogenesis and by increasing peripheral utilisation of glucose; since it acts only in the presence of endogenous insulin it is effective only if there are some residual functioning pancreatic islet cells.

- **INDICATIONS AND DOSE**

Type 2 diabetes mellitus [monotherapy or in combination with other antidiabetic drugs (including insulin)]

▸ BY MOUTH USING IMMEDIATE-RELEASE MEDICINES
▸ Child 8–9 years (specialist use only): Initially 200 mg once daily, dose to be adjusted according to response at intervals of at least 1 week, maximum daily dose to be given in 2–3 divided doses; maximum 2 g per day
▸ Child 10–17 years (specialist use only): Initially 500 mg once daily, dose to be adjusted according to response at intervals of at least 1 week, maximum daily dose to be given in 2–3 divided doses; maximum 2 g per day

- **UNLICENSED USE** Not licensed for use in children under 10 years.
- **CONTRA-INDICATIONS** Acute metabolic acidosis (including lactic acidosis and diabetic ketoacidosis)
- **CAUTIONS** Risk factors for lactic acidosis

CAUTIONS, FURTHER INFORMATION
▸ Risk factors for lactic acidosis Manufacturer advises caution in chronic stable heart failure (monitor cardiac function), and concomitant use of drugs that can acutely impair renal function; interrupt treatment if dehydration occurs, and avoid in conditions that can acutely worsen renal function, or cause tissue hypoxia.

- **INTERACTIONS** → Appendix 1: metformin
- **SIDE-EFFECTS**
  - **Common or very common** Abdominal pain · appetite decreased · diarrhoea (usually transient) · gastrointestinal disorder · nausea · taste altered · vomiting
  - **Rare or very rare** Hepatitis · lactic acidosis (discontinue) · skin reactions · vitamin B12 absorption decreased

  SIDE-EFFECTS, FURTHER INFORMATION Gastro-intestinal side-effects are initially common with metformin, and may persist in some patients, particularly when very high doses are given. A slow increase in dose may improve tolerability.
- **PREGNANCY** Can be used in pregnancy for both pre-existing and gestational diabetes. Women with gestational diabetes should discontinue treatment after giving birth.
- **BREAST FEEDING** May be used during breast-feeding in women with pre-existing diabetes.
- **HEPATIC IMPAIRMENT** Withdraw if tissue hypoxia likely.
- **RENAL IMPAIRMENT** Manufacturer advises avoid if estimated glomerular filtration rate is less than 30 mL/minute/1.73 m^2.

  Dose adjustments Manufacturer advises consider dose reduction in moderate impairment.
- **MONITORING REQUIREMENTS** Determine renal function before treatment and at least annually (at least twice a year in patients with additional risk factors for renal impairment, or if deterioration suspected).
- **PATIENT AND CARER ADVICE** Manufacturer advises that patients and their carers should be informed of the risk of lactic acidosis and told to seek immediate medical attention if symptoms such as dyspnoea, muscle cramps, abdominal pain, hypothermia, or asthenia occur.

  Medicines for Children leaflet: Metformin for diabetes www.medicinesforchildren.org.uk/metformin-diabetes

---

- **MEDICINAL FORMS** There can be variation in the licensing of different medicines containing the same drug. Forms available from special-order manufacturers include: capsule, oral suspension, oral solution

Tablet

CAUTIONARY AND ADVISORY LABELS 21

- Metformin hydrochloride (Non-proprietary)

  Metformin hydrochloride 500 mg Metformin 500mg tablets | 28 tablet PoM £2.88 DT = £1.36 | 84 tablet PoM £2.30–£4.13 | 500 tablet PoM £18.75–£24.29

  Metformin hydrochloride 850 mg Metformin 850mg tablets | 56 tablet PoM £2.56 DT = £1.34 | 300 tablet PoM £7.18–£8.86
- Glucophage (Merck Serono Ltd)

  Metformin hydrochloride 500 mg Glucophage 500mg tablets | 84 tablet PoM £2.88

  Metformin hydrochloride 850 mg Glucophage 850mg tablets | 56 tablet PoM £3.20 DT = £1.34

Oral solution

CAUTIONARY AND ADVISORY LABELS 21

- Metformin hydrochloride (Non-proprietary)

  Metformin hydrochloride 100 mg per 1 ml Metformin 500mg/5ml oral solution sugar free sugar-free | 100 ml PoM £4.50–£5.74 sugar-free | 150 ml PoM £60.00 DT = £6.75

  Metformin hydrochloride 170 mg per 1 ml Metformin 850mg/5ml oral solution sugar free sugar-free | 150 ml PoM £19.95 DT = £19.95

  Metformin hydrochloride 200 mg per 1 ml Metformin 1g/5ml oral solution sugar free sugar-free | 150 ml PoM £24.00 DT = £24.00

BLOOD GLUCOSE LOWERING DRUGS ›
SULFONYLUREAS

Sulfonylureas

- **DRUG ACTION** The sulfonylureas act mainly by augmenting insulin secretion and consequently are effective only when some residual pancreatic beta-cell activity is present; during long-term administration they also have an extrapancreatic action.
- **CONTRA-INDICATIONS** Presence of ketoacidosis
- **CAUTIONS** Can encourage weight gain · G6PD deficiency
- **SIDE-EFFECTS**
  - **Common or very common** Abdominal pain · diarrhoea · hypoglycaemia · nausea · vomiting
  - **Uncommon** Hepatic disorders
  - **Rare or very rare** Agranulocytosis · erythropenia · granulocytopenia · haemolytic anaemia · leucopenia · pancytopenia · thrombocytopenia
  - **Frequency not known** Allergic dermatitis (usually in the first 6–8 weeks of therapy) · constipation · photosensitivity reaction · skin reactions · visual impairment
- **HEPATIC IMPAIRMENT** In general, manufacturers advise avoid in severe impairment (increased risk of hypoglycaemia).
- **RENAL IMPAIRMENT** Sulfonylureas should be used with care in those with mild to moderate renal impairment, because of the hazard of hypoglycaemia. Care is required to use the lowest dose that adequately controls blood glucose. Avoid where possible in severe renal impairment.
- **PATIENT AND CARER ADVICE**

  Driving and skilled tasks Drivers need to be particularly careful to avoid hypoglycaemia and should be warned of the problems.

F above

Glibenclamide

16-Dec-2019

- **INDICATIONS AND DOSE**

Type 2 diabetes mellitus

- BY MOUTH USING TABLETS
  - Child 12-17 years: Initially 2.5 mg daily, adjusted according to response, dose to be taken with or immediately after breakfast; maximum 15 mg per day

Maturity-onset diabetes of the young (specialist use only)

- BY MOUTH USING TABLETS
  - Child 12-17 years: Initially 2.5 mg daily, adjusted according to response, dose to be taken with or immediately after breakfast; maximum 15 mg per day

Neonatal diabetes mellitus (initiated by a specialist)

- BY MOUTH USING ORAL SUSPENSION
  - Neonate: Initially 0.2 mg/kg daily in 2 divided doses, before feeding, increase dose according to product literature; usual maintenance 0.2–0.5 mg/kg daily in 2–4 divided doses, oral suspension is available in 2 different strengths and contains sodium benzoate—see *Prescribing and dispensing information* for information regarding the maximum volume per day.
  - Child: Initially 0.2 mg/kg daily in 2 divided doses, before feeding, increase dose according to product literature; usual maintenance 0.2–0.5 mg/kg daily in 2–4 divided doses, oral suspension is available in 2 different strengths and contains sodium benzoate—see *Prescribing and dispensing information* for information regarding the maximum volume per day

- **UNLICENSED USE** Not licensed for use in breast feeding women with pre-existing diabetes. Not licensed for use in gestational diabetes.

  Not licensed for use in type 2 diabetes mellitus or maturity-onset diabetes of the young.
- **CONTRA-INDICATIONS** Avoid where possible in Acute porphyrias p. 652
- **INTERACTIONS** → Appendix 1: sulfonylureas
- **SIDE-EFFECTS**
  - **Common or very common** Dyspepsia · neutropenia · tooth discolouration
  - **Frequency not known** Bone marrow depression · hypereosinophilia · vision disorders

- **PREGNANCY** The use of sulfonylureas in pregnancy should generally be avoided because of the risk of neonatal hypoglycaemia; however, glibenclamide can be used during the second and third trimesters of pregnancy in women with gestational diabetes.
- **BREAST FEEDING** Glibenclamide can be used during breast-feeding in women with pre-existing diabetes.
- **PRESCRIBING AND DISPENSING INFORMATION** Manufacturer advises care when prescribing and dispensing glibenclamide oral suspension as 2 different strengths are available. The prescriber must state the strength of the oral suspension to be used. Glibenclamide oral suspension contains sodium benzoate, and the maximum volume that can be given is 1 mL/kg per day, regardless of the strength of the suspension. If the calculated daily dose exceeds this maximum volume using the lower-strength suspension, the higher-strength suspension must be used to administer the dose—consult product literature.

- **MEDICINAL FORMS** There can be variation in the licensing of different medicines containing the same drug. Forms available from special-order manufacturers include: oral suspension

Oral suspension

ELECTROLYTES: May contain Sodium

▸ Amglidia (Amring Pharmaceuticals Ltd)

Glibenclamide 600 microgram per 1 ml Amglidia 0.6mg/ml oral suspension with 5ml oral syringe sugar-free | 30 ml PoM £2,100.00
Amglidia 0.6mg/ml oral suspension with 1ml oral syringe sugar-free | 30 ml PoM £2,100.00

Glibenclamide 6 mg per 1 ml Amglidia 6mg/ml oral suspension with 5ml oral syringe sugar-free | 30 ml PoM £21,000.00
Amglidia 6mg/ml oral suspension with 1ml oral syringe sugar-free | 30 ml PoM £21,000.00

F 489

Gliclazide

10-Mar-2020

- **INDICATIONS AND DOSE**

Type 2 diabetes mellitus

▶ BY MOUTH USING IMMEDIATE-RELEASE MEDICINES

▸ Child 12–17 years: Initially 20 mg once daily, adjusted according to response, increased if necessary up to 160 mg once daily (max. per dose 160 mg twice daily), dose to be taken with breakfast

Maturity-onset diabetes of the young (specialist use only)

▶ BY MOUTH USING IMMEDIATE-RELEASE MEDICINES

▸ Child 12–17 years: Initially 20 mg once daily, adjusted according to response, increased if necessary up to 160 mg once daily (max. per dose 160 mg twice daily), dose to be taken with breakfast

- **UNLICENSED USE** Not licensed for use in children.
- **CONTRA-INDICATIONS** Avoid where possible in Acute porphyrias p. 652
- **INTERACTIONS** → Appendix 1: sulfonylureas
- **SIDE-EFFECTS** Anaemia · angioedema · dyspepsia · gastrointestinal disorder · hypersensitivity vasculitis · hyponatraemia · severe cutaneous adverse reactions (SCARs)
- **PREGNANCY** The use of sulfonylureas in pregnancy should generally be avoided because of the risk of neonatal hypoglycaemia.
- **BREAST FEEDING** Avoid—theoretical possibility of hypoglycaemia in the infant.
- **RENAL IMPAIRMENT** If necessary, gliclazide which is principally metabolised in the liver, can be used in renal impairment but careful monitoring of blood-glucose concentration is essential.
- **PATIENT AND CARER ADVICE** Medicines for Children leaflet: Gliclazide for type 2 diabetes mellitus and maturity-onset diabetes of the young www.medicinesforchildren.org.uk/gliclazide-type-2-diabetes-mellitus-and-maturity-onset-diabetes-young

- **MEDICINAL FORMS** There can be variation in the licensing of different medicines containing the same drug. Forms available from special-order manufacturers include: oral suspension

Tablet

▸ Gliclazide (Non-proprietary)

Gliclazide 40 mg Gliclazide 40mg tablets | 28 tablet PoM £3.19 DT = £1.51

Gliclazide 80 mg Gliclazide 80mg tablets | 28 tablet PoM £1.80 DT = £1.07 | 60 tablet PoM £0.81–£2.29

▸ Diamicron (Servier Laboratories Ltd)

Gliclazide 80 mg Diamicron 80mg tablets | 60 tablet PoM £4.38

▸ Zicron (Bristol Laboratories Ltd)

Gliclazide 40 mg Zicron 40mg tablets | 28 tablet PoM £3.36 DT = £1.51

F 489

Tolbutamide

- **INDICATIONS AND DOSE**

Type 2 diabetes mellitus

▶ BY MOUTH

▸ Child 12–17 years (specialist use only): 0.5–1.5 g daily in divided doses, dose to be taken with or immediately after meals, alternatively 0.5–1.5 g once daily, dose to be taken with or immediately after breakfast; maximum 2 g per day

- **UNLICENSED USE** Not licensed for use in children.
- **CONTRA-INDICATIONS** Avoid where possible in Acute porphyrias p. 652
- **INTERACTIONS** → Appendix 1: sulfonylureas
- **SIDE-EFFECTS**
  - ▶ **Rare or very rare** Aplastic anaemia · blood disorder
  - ▶ **Frequency not known** Alcohol intolerance · appetite abnormal · erythema multiforme (usually in the first 6–8 weeks of therapy) · exfoliative dermatitis (usually in the first 6–8 weeks of therapy) · fever (usually in the first 6–8 weeks of therapy) · headache · hypersensitivity (usually in the first 6–8 weeks of therapy) · paraesthesia · tinnitus · weight increased
- **PREGNANCY** The use of sulfonylureas in pregnancy should generally be avoided because of the risk of neonatal hypoglycaemia.
- **BREAST FEEDING** The use of sulfonylureas in breast-feeding should be avoided because there is a theoretical possibility of hypoglycaemia in the infant.
- **RENAL IMPAIRMENT** If necessary, the short-acting drug tolbutamide can be used in renal impairment but careful monitoring of blood-glucose concentration is essential.

- **MEDICINAL FORMS** There can be variation in the licensing of different medicines containing the same drug. Forms available from special-order manufacturers include: oral suspension

Tablet

▸ Tolbutamide (Non-proprietary)

Tolbutamide 500 mg Tolbutamide 500mg tablets | 28 tablet PoM £34.88 DT = £20.66 | 112 tablet PoM £82.64

INSULINS

Insulins

IMPORTANT SAFETY INFORMATION

NHS NEVER EVENT: OVERDOSE OF INSULIN DUE TO ABBREVIATIONS OR INCORRECT DEVICE (JANUARY 2018)

The words 'unit' or 'international units' should **not** be abbreviated.

Specific insulin administration devices should always be used to measure insulin i.e. Insulin syringes and pens.

Insulin should **not** be withdrawn from an insulin pen or pen refill and then administered using a syringe and needle.

NHS IMPROVEMENT PATIENT SAFETY ALERT: RISK OF SEVERE HARM AND DEATH DUE TO WITHDRAWING INSULIN FROM PEN DEVICES (NOVEMBER 2016)

Insulin should not be extracted from insulin pen devices.

The strength of insulin in pen devices can vary by multiples of 100 units/mL. Insulin syringes have graduations only suitable for calculating doses of standard 100 units/mL. If insulin extracted from a pen or cartridge is of a higher strength, and that is not considered in determining the volume required, it can lead to a significant and potentially fatal overdose.

- **SIDE-EFFECTS**
- ▶ **Common or very common** Oedema
- ▶ **Uncommon** Lipodystrophy

Overdose Overdose causes hypoglycaemia.

- **PREGNANCY**

Dose adjustments During pregnancy, insulin requirements may alter and doses should be assessed frequently by an experienced diabetes physician.

The dose of insulin generally needs to be increased in the second and third trimesters of pregnancy.

- **BREAST FEEDING**

Dose adjustments During breast-feeding, insulin requirements may alter and doses should be assessed frequently by an experienced diabetes physician.

- **HEPATIC IMPAIRMENT** Insulin requirements may be decreased.
- **RENAL IMPAIRMENT** The compensatory response to hypoglycaemia is impaired in renal impairment.

Dose adjustments Insulin requirements may decrease in patients with renal impairment and therefore dose reduction may be necessary.

- **MONITORING REQUIREMENTS**
- ▶ Many patients now monitor their own blood-glucose concentrations; all carers and children need to be trained to do this.
- ▶ Since blood-glucose concentration varies substantially throughout the day, 'normoglycaemia' cannot always be achieved throughout a 24-hour period without causing damaging hypoglycaemia.
- ▶ It is therefore best to recommend that children should maintain a blood-glucose concentration of between 4 and 10 mmol/litre for most of the time (4–8 mmol/litre before meals and less than 10 mmol/litre after meals).
- ▶ While accepting that on occasions, for brief periods, the blood-glucose concentration will be above these values; strenuous efforts should be made to prevent it from falling below 4 mmol/litre. Patients using multiple injection regimens should understand how to adjust their insulin dose according to their carbohydrate intake. With fixed-dose insulin regimens, the carbohydrate intake needs to be regulated, and should be distributed throughout the day to match the insulin regimen. The intake of energy and of simple and complex carbohydrates should be adequate to allow normal growth and development but obesity must be avoided.
- **DIRECTIONS FOR ADMINISTRATION** Insulin is generally given by *subcutaneous injection*; the injection site should be rotated to prevent lipodystrophy. Injection devices ('pens'), which hold the insulin in a cartridge and meter the required dose, are convenient to use. Insulin syringes (for use with needles) are required for insulins not available in cartridge form, but are less popular with children and carers. For intensive insulin regimens multiple subcutaneous injections (3 or more times daily) are usually recommended.
- **PRESCRIBING AND DISPENSING INFORMATION** Show container to patient or carer and confirm the expected version is dispensed.

Units The word 'unit' should **not** be abbreviated.

- **PATIENT AND CARER ADVICE**

Hypoglycaemia Hypoglycaemia is a potential problem with insulin therapy. All patients must be carefully instructed on how to avoid it; this involves appropriate adjustment of insulin type, dose and frequency together with suitable timing and quantity of meals and snacks.

Insulin Passport Insulin Passports and patient information booklets should be offered to patients receiving insulin. The Insulin Passport provides a record of the patient's current insulin preparations and contains a section for emergency information. The patient information booklet provides advice on the safe use of insulin. They are available for purchase from:

3M Security Print and Systems Limited
Gorse Street, Chadderton
Oldham
OL9 9QH
Tel: 0845 610 1112

GP practices can obtain supplies through their Local Area Team stores.

NHS Trusts can order supplies from www.nhsforms.co.uk/ or by emailing nhsforms@mmm.com. Further information is available at www.npsa.nhs.uk.

Driving and skilled tasks Drivers need to be particularly careful to avoid hypoglycaemia and should be warned of the problems.

INSULINS > RAPID-ACTING

F 490

Insulin

(Insulin Injection; Neutral Insulin; Soluble Insulin–short acting)

- **INDICATIONS AND DOSE**

Diabetes mellitus

▶ BY SUBCUTANEOUS INJECTION

- ▶ Child: According to requirements

Hyperglycaemia during illness

▶ BY INTRAVENOUS INFUSION

- ▶ Neonate: 0.02–0.125 unit/kg/hour, dose to be adjusted according to blood-glucose concentration.
- ▶ Child: 0.025–0.1 unit/kg/hour, dose to be adjusted according to blood-glucose concentration

Neonatal hyperglycaemia | Neonatal diabetes

▶ BY INTRAVENOUS INFUSION

- ▶ Neonate: 0.02–0.125 unit/kg/hour, dose to be adjusted according to blood-glucose concentration.

Diabetic ketoacidosis | Diabetes during surgery

▶ BY INTRAVENOUS INFUSION

- ▶ Child: (consult local protocol)

- **INTERACTIONS** → Appendix 1: insulins
- **SIDE-EFFECTS**
- ▶ **Uncommon** Skin reactions
- ▶ **Rare or very rare** Refraction disorder
- **DIRECTIONS FOR ADMINISTRATION** Short-acting injectable insulins can be given by continuous subcutaneous infusion using a portable infusion pump. This device delivers a continuous basal insulin infusion and patient-activated bolus doses at meal times. This technique can be useful for patients who suffer recurrent hypoglycaemia or marked morning rise in blood-glucose concentration despite optimised multiple-injection regimens. Patients on subcutaneous insulin infusion must be highly motivated,

able to monitor their blood-glucose concentration, and have expert training, advice and supervision from an experienced healthcare team. Some insulin preparations are not recommended for use in subcutaneous insulin infusion pumps—may precipitate in catheter or needle—consult product literature.

- With intravenous use For *intravenous infusion*, dilute to a concentration of 1 unit/mL with Sodium Chloride 0.9% and mix thoroughly; insulin may be adsorbed by plastics, flush giving set with 5 mL of infusion fluid containing insulin. *For intravenous infusion in neonatal intensive care*, dilute 5 units to a final volume of 50 mL with Sodium Chloride 0.9% and mix thoroughly; an intravenous infusion rate of 0.1 mL/kg/hour provides a dose of 0.01 units/kg/hour.

● **PRESCRIBING AND DISPENSING INFORMATION** A sterile solution of insulin (i.e. bovine or porcine) or of human insulin; pH 6.6–8.0.

● **NATIONAL FUNDING/ACCESS DECISIONS**

NICE decisions

- **Continuous subcutaneous insulin infusion for the treatment of diabetes mellitus (type 1) (July 2008)** NICE TA151
Continuous subcutaneous insulin infusion is recommended as an option in adults and children 12 years and over with type 1 diabetes:
  - who suffer repeated and unpredictable hypoglycaemia, whilst attempting to achieve optimal glycaemic control with multiple-injection regimens, **or**
  - whose glycaemic control remains inadequate (HbA_{1c} over 8.5% [69 mmol/mol]) despite optimised multiple-injection regimens (including the use of long-acting insulin analogues where appropriate).

Continuous subcutaneous insulin infusion is also recommended as an option for children under 12 years with type 1 diabetes for whom multiple-injection regimens are considered impractical or inappropriate. Children on insulin pumps should undergo a trial of multiple-injection therapy between the ages of 12 and 18 years.
www.nice.org.uk/guidance/TA151

● **MEDICINAL FORMS** There can be variation in the licensing of different medicines containing the same drug. Forms available from special-order manufacturers include: solution for injection, solution for infusion

Solution for injection

- **Humulin R** (Imported (United States))
Insulin human 500 unit per 1 ml Humulin R 500units/ml solution for injection 20ml vials | 1 vial PoM [X]
Humulin R KwikPen 500units/ml solution for injection 3ml pre-filled pens | 2 pre-filled disposable injection PoM [X]
- **Actrapid** (Novo Nordisk Ltd)
Insulin human (as Insulin soluble human) 100 unit per 1 ml Actrapid 100units/ml solution for injection 10ml vials | 1 vial PoM £7.48 DT = £15.68
- **Humulin S** (Eli Lilly and Company Ltd)
Insulin human (as Insulin soluble human) 100 unit per 1 ml Humulin S 100units/ml solution for injection 10ml vials | 1 vial PoM £15.68 DT = £15.68
Humulin S 100units/ml solution for injection 3ml cartridges | 5 cartridge PoM £19.08 DT = £19.08
- **Hypurin Porcine Neutral** (Wockhardt UK Ltd)
Insulin porcine (as Insulin soluble porcine) 100 unit per 1 ml Hypurin Porcine Neutral 100units/ml solution for injection 10ml vials | 1 vial PoM £34.43 DT = £34.43
Hypurin Porcine Neutral 100units/ml solution for injection 3ml cartridges | 5 cartridge PoM £51.64 DT = £51.64
- **Insuman Infusat** (Sanofi)
Insulin human 100 unit per 1 ml Insuman Infusat 100units/ml solution for injection 3.15ml cartridges | 5 cartridge PoM £250.00 DT = £250.00
- **Insuman Rapid** (Sanofi)
Insulin human (as Insulin soluble human) 100 unit per 1 ml Insuman Rapid 100units/ml solution for injection 3ml cartridges | 5 cartridge PoM £17.50 DT = £19.08

F 490

Insulin aspart

16-Dec-2019

(Recombinant human insulin analogue—short acting)

● **INDICATIONS AND DOSE**

FIASP®

Diabetes mellitus

- BY SUBCUTANEOUS INJECTION
- Child 1–17 years: Administer immediately before meals or when necessary shortly after meals, according to requirements
- BY SUBCUTANEOUS INFUSION, OR BY INTRAVENOUS INFUSION, OR BY INTRAVENOUS INJECTION
- Child 1–17 years: According to requirements

NOVORAPID®

Diabetes mellitus

- BY SUBCUTANEOUS INJECTION
- Child: Administer immediately before meals or when necessary shortly after meals, according to requirements
- BY SUBCUTANEOUS INFUSION, OR BY INTRAVENOUS INFUSION, OR BY INTRAVENOUS INJECTION
- Child: According to requirements

● **UNLICENSED USE** Not licensed for use in children under 1 year.

● **INTERACTIONS** → Appendix 1: insulins

● **SIDE-EFFECTS**

- **Common or very common** Skin reactions
- **Uncommon** Refraction disorder

● **PREGNANCY** Not known to be harmful—may be used during pregnancy.

● **BREAST FEEDING** Not known to be harmful—may be used during lactation.

● **DIRECTIONS FOR ADMINISTRATION** Short-acting injectable insulins can be given by continuous subcutaneous infusion using a portable infusion pump. This device delivers a continuous basal insulin infusion and patient-activated bolus doses at meal times. This technique can be useful for patients who suffer recurrent hypoglycaemia or marked morning rise in blood-glucose concentration despite optimised multiple-injection regimens. Patients on subcutaneous insulin infusion must be highly motivated, able to monitor their blood-glucose concentration, and have expert training, advice and supervision from an experienced healthcare team.

- With intravenous use For *intravenous infusion*, dilute to a concentration of 0.05–1 unit/mL with Glucose 5% or Sodium Chloride 0.9% and mix thoroughly; insulin may be adsorbed by plastics, flush giving set with 5 mL of infusion fluid containing insulin.

● **NATIONAL FUNDING/ACCESS DECISIONS**

NICE decisions

- **Continuous subcutaneous insulin infusion for the treatment of diabetes mellitus (type 1) (July 2008)** NICE TA151
Continuous subcutaneous insulin infusion is recommended as an option in adults and children 12 years and over with type 1 diabetes:
  - who suffer repeated and unpredictable hypoglycaemia, whilst attempting to achieve optimal glycaemic control with multiple-injection regimens, **or**
  - whose glycaemic control remains inadequate (HbA_{1c} over 8.5% [69 mmol/mol]) despite optimised multiple-injection regimens (including the use of long-acting insulin analogues where appropriate).

Continuous subcutaneous insulin infusion is also recommended as an option for children under 12 years with type 1 diabetes for whom multiple-injection regimens

are considered impractical or inappropriate. Children on insulin pumps should undergo a trial of multiple-injection therapy between the ages of 12 and 18 years.
www.nice.org.uk/guidance/ta151

● **MEDICINAL FORMS** There can be variation in the licensing of different medicines containing the same drug.

Solution for injection

▸ Fiasp (Novo Nordisk Ltd) ▼
Insulin aspart 100 unit per 1 ml Fiasp 100units/ml solution for injection 10ml vials | 1 vial PoM £14.08 DT = £14.08

▸ Fiasp FlexTouch (Novo Nordisk Ltd) ▼
Insulin aspart 100 unit per 1 ml Fiasp FlexTouch 100units/ml solution for injection 3ml pre-filled pens | 5 pre-filled disposable injection PoM £30.60 DT = £30.60

▸ Fiasp Penfill (Novo Nordisk Ltd) ▼
Insulin aspart 100 unit per 1 ml Fiasp Penfill 100units/ml solution for injection 3ml cartridges | 5 cartridge PoM £28.31 DT = £28.31

▸ NovoRapid (Novo Nordisk Ltd)
Insulin aspart 100 unit per 1 ml NovoRapid 100units/ml solution for injection 10ml vials | 1 vial PoM £14.08 DT = £14.08

▸ NovoRapid FlexPen (Novo Nordisk Ltd)
Insulin aspart 100 unit per 1 ml NovoRapid FlexPen 100units/ml solution for injection 3ml pre-filled pens | 5 pre-filled disposable injection PoM £30.60 DT = £30.60

▸ NovoRapid FlexTouch (Novo Nordisk Ltd)
Insulin aspart 100 unit per 1 ml NovoRapid FlexTouch 100units/ml solution for injection 3ml pre-filled pens | 5 pre-filled disposable injection PoM £32.13 DT = £30.60

▸ NovoRapid Penfill (Novo Nordisk Ltd)
Insulin aspart 100 unit per 1 ml NovoRapid Penfill 100units/ml solution for injection 3ml cartridges | 5 cartridge PoM £28.31 DT = £28.31

▸ NovoRapid PumpCart (Novo Nordisk Ltd)
Insulin aspart 100 unit per 1 ml NovoRapid PumpCart 100units/ml solution for injection 1.6ml cartridges | 5 cartridge PoM £15.10 DT = £15.10

F 490

Insulin glulisine

27-Jul-2018

(Recombinant human insulin analogue—short acting)

● **INDICATIONS AND DOSE**

Diabetes mellitus

▸ BY SUBCUTANEOUS INJECTION
▸ Child: Administer immediately before meals or when necessary shortly after meals, according to requirements

▸ BY SUBCUTANEOUS INFUSION, OR BY INTRAVENOUS INFUSION
▸ Child: According to requirements

● **UNLICENSED USE** Not licensed for children under 6 years.

● **INTERACTIONS** → Appendix 1: insulins

● **DIRECTIONS FOR ADMINISTRATION** Short-acting injectable insulins can be given by continuous subcutaneous infusion using a portable infusion pump. This device delivers a continuous basal insulin infusion and patient-activated bolus doses at meal times. This technique can be useful for patients who suffer recurrent hypoglycaemia or marked morning rise in blood-glucose concentration despite optimised multiple-injection regimens. Patients on subcutaneous insulin infusion must be highly motivated, able to monitor their blood-glucose concentration, and have expert training, advice and supervision from an experienced healthcare team.

● **NATIONAL FUNDING/ACCESS DECISIONS**

NICE decisions

▸ **Continuous subcutaneous insulin infusion for the treatment of diabetes mellitus (type 1) (July 2008)** NICE TA151
Continuous subcutaneous insulin infusion is recommended as an option in adults and children 12 years and over with type 1 diabetes:
- who suffer repeated and unpredictable hypoglycaemia, whilst attempting to achieve optimal glycaemic control with multiple-injection regimens, **or**
- whose glycaemic control remains inadequate (HbA_{1c} over 8.5% [69 mmol/mol]) despite optimised multiple-injection regimens (including the use of long-acting insulin analogues where appropriate).

Continuous subcutaneous insulin infusion is also recommended as an option for children under 12 years with type 1 diabetes for whom multiple-injection regimens are considered impractical or inappropriate. Children on insulin pumps should undergo a trial of multiple-injection therapy between the ages of 12 and 18 years.
www.nice.org.uk/guidance/ta151

Scottish Medicines Consortium (SMC) decisions

The *Scottish Medicines Consortium* has advised (November 2008) that *Apidra*® is accepted for restricted use within NHS Scotland for the treatment of adults and children over 6 years with diabetes mellitus in whom the use of a short-acting insulin analogue is appropriate.

● **MEDICINAL FORMS** There can be variation in the licensing of different medicines containing the same drug.

Solution for injection

▸ Apidra (Sanofi)
Insulin glulisine 100 unit per 1 ml Apidra 100units/ml solution for injection 3ml cartridges | 5 cartridge PoM £28.30 DT = £28.30
Apidra 100units/ml solution for injection 10ml vials | 1 vial PoM £16.00 DT = £16.00

▸ Apidra SoloStar (Sanofi)
Insulin glulisine 100 unit per 1 ml Apidra 100units/ml solution for injection 3ml pre-filled SoloStar pens | 5 pre-filled disposable injection PoM £28.30 DT = £28.30

F 490

Insulin lispro

18-Feb-2020

(Recombinant human insulin analogue—short acting)

● **INDICATIONS AND DOSE**

Diabetes mellitus

▸ BY SUBCUTANEOUS INJECTION
▸ Child 1 month–1 year: Administer shortly before meals or when necessary shortly after meals, according to requirements
▸ Child 2–17 years: Administer shortly before meals or when necessary shortly after meals, according to requirements

▸ BY SUBCUTANEOUS INFUSION, OR BY INTRAVENOUS INFUSION, OR BY INTRAVENOUS INJECTION
▸ Child 1 month–1 year: According to requirements
▸ Child 2–17 years: According to requirements

● **UNLICENSED USE** Not licensed for use in children under 2 years.

● **INTERACTIONS** → Appendix 1: insulins

● **PREGNANCY** Not known to be harmful—may be used during pregnancy.

● **BREAST FEEDING** Not known to be harmful—may be used during lactation.

● **DIRECTIONS FOR ADMINISTRATION** Short-acting injectable insulins can be given by continuous subcutaneous infusion using a portable infusion pump. This device delivers a continuous basal insulin infusion and patient-activated bolus doses at meal times. This technique can be useful for patients who suffer recurrent hypoglycaemia or marked morning rise in blood-glucose concentration despite optimised multiple-injection regimens (see also NICE guidance, below). Patients on subcutaneous insulin infusion must be highly motivated, able to monitor their blood-glucose concentration, and have expert training, advice and supervision from an experienced healthcare team.

▸ With intravenous use For *intravenous infusion*, dilute to a concentration of 0.1–1 unit/mL with Glucose 5% or Sodium Chloride 0.9% and mix thoroughly; insulin may be adsorbed by plastics, flush giving set with 5 mL of infusion fluid containing insulin.

● **PRESCRIBING AND DISPENSING INFORMATION** Insulin lispro is a biological medicine. Biological medicines must be prescribed and dispensed by brand name, see *Biological medicines* and *Biosimilar medicines*, under Guidance on prescribing p. 1.

● **NATIONAL FUNDING/ACCESS DECISIONS**

NICE decisions

▸ **Continuous subcutaneous insulin infusion for the treatment of diabetes mellitus (type 1) (July 2008)** NICE TA151
Continuous subcutaneous insulin infusion is recommended as an option in adults and children 12 years and over with type 1 diabetes:
- who suffer repeated and unpredictable hypoglycaemia, whilst attempting to achieve optimal glycaemic control with multiple-injection regimens, **or**
- whose glycaemic control remains inadequate (HbA_{1c} over 8.5% [69 mmol/mol]) despite optimised multiple-injection regimens (including the use of long-acting insulin analogues where appropriate).

Continuous subcutaneous insulin infusion is also recommended as an option for children under 12 years with type 1 diabetes for whom multiple-injection regimens are considered impractical or inappropriate. Children on insulin pumps should undergo a trial of multiple-injection therapy between the ages of 12 and 18 years.
www.nice.org.uk/guidance/ta151

● **MEDICINAL FORMS** There can be variation in the licensing of different medicines containing the same drug.

Solution for injection

▸ Insulin lispro (non-proprietary) ▼
Insulin lispro 100 unit per 1 ml Insulin lispro Sanofi 100units/ml solution for injection 3ml pre-filled pens | 5 pre-filled disposable injection PoM £25.04 DT = £29.46
Insulin lispro Sanofi 100units/ml solution for injection 3ml cartridges | 5 cartridge PoM £24.06 DT = £28.31
Insulin lispro Sanofi 100units/ml solution for injection 10ml vials | 1 vial PoM £14.12 DT = £16.61

▸ Humalog (Eli Lilly and Company Ltd)
Insulin lispro 100 unit per 1 ml Humalog 100units/ml solution for injection 10ml vials | 1 vial PoM £16.61 DT = £16.61
Humalog 100units/ml solution for injection 3ml cartridges | 5 cartridge PoM £28.31 DT = £28.31

▸ Humalog Junior KwikPen (Eli Lilly and Company Ltd)
Insulin lispro 100 unit per 1 ml Humalog Junior KwikPen 100units/ml solution for injection 3ml pre-filled pens | 5 pre-filled disposable injection PoM £29.46 DT = £29.46

▸ Humalog KwikPen (Eli Lilly and Company Ltd)
Insulin lispro 100 unit per 1 ml Humalog KwikPen 100units/ml solution for injection 3ml pre-filled pens | 5 pre-filled disposable injection PoM £29.46 DT = £29.46
Insulin lispro 200 unit per 1 ml Humalog KwikPen 200units/ml solution for injection 3ml pre-filled pens | 5 pre-filled disposable injection PoM £58.92 DT = £58.92

INSULINS > INTERMEDIATE-ACTING

F 490

Biphasic isophane insulin

(Biphasic Isophane Insulin Injection– intermediate acting)

● **INDICATIONS AND DOSE**

Diabetes mellitus

▸ BY SUBCUTANEOUS INJECTION
▸ Child: According to requirements

● **INTERACTIONS** → Appendix 1: insulins

● **SIDE-EFFECTS**
▸ **Rare or very rare** Angioedema
▸ **Frequency not known** Hypokalaemia · weight increased

● **PRESCRIBING AND DISPENSING INFORMATION** A sterile buffered suspension of either porcine or human insulin complexed with protamine sulfate (or another suitable protamine) in a solution of insulin of the same species.

Check product container—the proportions of the two components should be checked carefully (the order in which the proportions are stated may not be the same in other countries).

● **MEDICINAL FORMS** There can be variation in the licensing of different medicines containing the same drug.

Suspension for injection

▸ Humulin M3 (Eli Lilly and Company Ltd)
Insulin human (as Insulin soluble human) 30 unit per 1 ml, Insulin human (as Insulin isophane human) 70 unit per 1 ml Humulin M3 100units/ml suspension for injection 3ml cartridges | 5 cartridge PoM £19.08 DT = £19.08
Humulin M3 100units/ml suspension for injection 10ml vials | 1 vial PoM £15.68 DT = £15.68

▸ Humulin M3 KwikPen (Eli Lilly and Company Ltd)
Insulin human (as Insulin soluble human) 30 unit per 1 ml, Insulin human (as Insulin isophane human) 70 unit per 1 ml Humulin M3 KwikPen 100units/ml suspension for injection 3ml pre-filled pens | 5 pre-filled disposable injection PoM £21.70 DT = £21.70

▸ Hypurin Porcine 30/70 Mix (Wockhardt UK Ltd)
Insulin porcine (as Insulin soluble porcine) 30 unit per 1 ml, Insulin porcine (as Insulin isophane porcine) 70 unit per 1 ml Hypurin Porcine 30/70 Mix 100units/ml suspension for injection 3ml cartridges | 5 cartridge PoM £51.64 DT = £51.64
Hypurin Porcine 30/70 Mix 100units/ml suspension for injection 10ml vials | 1 vial PoM £34.43 DT = £34.43

▸ Insuman Comb 15 (Sanofi)
Insulin human (as Insulin soluble human) 15 unit per 1 ml, Insulin human (as Insulin isophane human) 85 unit per 1 ml Insuman Comb 15 100units/ml suspension for injection 3ml cartridges | 5 cartridge PoM £17.50 DT = £17.50

▸ Insuman Comb 25 (Sanofi)
Insulin human (as Insulin soluble human) 25 unit per 1 ml, Insulin human (as Insulin isophane human) 75 unit per 1 ml Insuman Comb 25 100units/ml suspension for injection 5ml vials | 1 vial PoM £5.61
Insuman Comb 25 100units/ml suspension for injection 3ml cartridges | 5 cartridge PoM £17.50 DT = £17.50
Insuman Comb 25 100units/ml suspension for injection 3ml pre-filled SoloStar pens | 5 pre-filled disposable injection PoM £19.80 DT = £19.80

▸ Insuman Comb 50 (Sanofi)
Insulin human (as Insulin isophane human) 50 unit per 1 ml, Insulin human (as Insulin soluble human) 50 unit per 1 ml Insuman Comb 50 100units/ml suspension for injection 3ml cartridges | 5 cartridge PoM £17.50 DT = £17.50

F 490

Isophane insulin

(Isophane Insulin Injection; Isophane Protamine Insulin Injection; Isophane Insulin (NPH)– intermediate acting)

● **INDICATIONS AND DOSE**

Diabetes mellitus

▸ BY SUBCUTANEOUS INJECTION
▸ Child: According to requirements

● **INTERACTIONS** → Appendix 1: insulins

● **PREGNANCY** Recommended where longer-acting insulins are needed.

● **PRESCRIBING AND DISPENSING INFORMATION** A sterile suspension of bovine or porcine insulin or of human insulin in the form of a complex obtained by the addition of protamine sulfate or another suitable protamine.

- **MEDICINAL FORMS** There can be variation in the licensing of different medicines containing the same drug.

Suspension for injection

- ▸ **Humulin I** (Eli Lilly and Company Ltd)
  Insulin human (as Insulin isophane human) 100 unit per 1 ml Humulin I 100units/ml suspension for injection 10ml vials | 1 vial PoM £15.68 DT = £15.68
  Humulin I 100units/ml suspension for injection 3ml cartridges | 5 cartridge PoM £19.08 DT = £19.08
- ▸ **Humulin I KwikPen** (Eli Lilly and Company Ltd)
  Insulin human (as Insulin isophane human) 100 unit per 1 ml Humulin I KwikPen 100units/ml suspension for injection 3ml pre-filled pens | 5 pre-filled disposable injection PoM £21.70 DT = £21.70
- ▸ **Hypurin Porcine Isophane** (Wockhardt UK Ltd)
  Insulin porcine (as Insulin isophane porcine) 100 unit per 1 ml Hypurin Porcine Isophane 100units/ml suspension for injection 3ml cartridges | 5 cartridge PoM £51.64 DT = £51.64
  Hypurin Porcine Isophane 100units/ml suspension for injection 10ml vials | 1 vial PoM £34.43 DT = £34.43
- ▸ **Insulatard** (Novo Nordisk Ltd)
  Insulin human (as Insulin isophane human) 100 unit per 1 ml Insulatard 100units/ml suspension for injection 10ml vials | 1 vial PoM £7.48 DT = £15.68
- ▸ **Insulatard InnoLet** (Novo Nordisk Ltd)
  Insulin human (as Insulin isophane human) 100 unit per 1 ml Insulatard InnoLet 100units/ml suspension for injection 3ml pre-filled pens | 5 pre-filled disposable injection PoM £20.40 DT = £21.70
- ▸ **Insulatard Penfill** (Novo Nordisk Ltd)
  Insulin human (as Insulin isophane human) 100 unit per 1 ml Insulatard Penfill 100units/ml suspension for injection 3ml cartridges | 5 cartridge PoM £22.90 DT = £19.08
- ▸ **Insuman Basal** (Sanofi)
  Insulin human (as Insulin isophane human) 100 unit per 1 ml Insuman Basal 100units/ml suspension for injection 5ml vials | 1 vial PoM £5.61
  Insuman Basal 100units/ml suspension for injection 3ml cartridges | 5 cartridge PoM £17.50 DT = £19.08
- ▸ **Insuman Basal SoloStar** (Sanofi)
  Insulin human (as Insulin isophane human) 100 unit per 1 ml Insuman Basal 100units/ml suspension for injection 3ml pre-filled SoloStar pens | 5 pre-filled disposable injection PoM £19.80 DT = £21.70

INSULINS > INTERMEDIATE-ACTING COMBINED WITH RAPID-ACTING

F 490

Biphasic insulin aspart

(Intermediate-acting insulin)

- **INDICATIONS AND DOSE**

Diabetes mellitus

▸ BY SUBCUTANEOUS INJECTION
- ▸ Child: Administer up to 10 minutes before or soon after a meal, according to requirements

- **INTERACTIONS** → Appendix 1: insulins
- **SIDE-EFFECTS**
  ▸ **Uncommon** Skin reactions
- **PRESCRIBING AND DISPENSING INFORMATION** Check product container—the proportions of the two components should be checked carefully (the order in which the proportions are stated may not be the same in other countries).

- **MEDICINAL FORMS** There can be variation in the licensing of different medicines containing the same drug.

Suspension for injection

- ▸ **NovoMix 30 FlexPen** (Novo Nordisk Ltd)
  Insulin aspart 30 unit per 1 ml, Insulin aspart (as Insulin aspart protamine) 70 unit per 1 ml NovoMix 30 FlexPen 100units/ml suspension for injection 3ml pre-filled pens | 5 pre-filled disposable injection PoM £29.89 DT = £29.89
- ▸ **NovoMix 30 Penfill** (Novo Nordisk Ltd)
  Insulin aspart 30 unit per 1 ml, Insulin aspart (as Insulin aspart protamine) 70 unit per 1 ml NovoMix 30 Penfill 100units/ml suspension for injection 3ml cartridges | 5 cartridge PoM £28.79 DT = £28.79

F 490

Biphasic insulin lispro 03-Feb-2020

(Intermediate-acting insulin)

- **INDICATIONS AND DOSE**

Diabetes mellitus

▸ BY SUBCUTANEOUS INJECTION
- ▸ Child: Administer up to 15 minutes before or soon after a meal, according to requirements

- **CAUTIONS** Children under 12 years (use only if benefit likely compared to soluble insulin)
- **INTERACTIONS** → Appendix 1: insulins
- **PRESCRIBING AND DISPENSING INFORMATION** Check product container—the proportions of the two components should be checked carefully (the order in which the proportions are stated may not be the same in other countries).

- **MEDICINAL FORMS** There can be variation in the licensing of different medicines containing the same drug.

Suspension for injection

- ▸ **Humalog Mix25** (Eli Lilly and Company Ltd)
  Insulin lispro 25 unit per 1 ml, Insulin lispro (as Insulin lispro protamine) 75 unit per 1 ml Humalog Mix25 100units/ml suspension for injection 10ml vials | 1 vial PoM £16.61 DT = £16.61
  Humalog Mix25 100units/ml suspension for injection 3ml cartridges | 5 cartridge PoM £29.46 DT = £29.46
- ▸ **Humalog Mix25 KwikPen** (Eli Lilly and Company Ltd)
  Insulin lispro 25 unit per 1 ml, Insulin lispro (as Insulin lispro protamine) 75 unit per 1 ml Humalog Mix25 KwikPen 100units/ml suspension for injection 3ml pre-filled pens | 5 pre-filled disposable injection PoM £30.98 DT = £30.98
- ▸ **Humalog Mix50** (Eli Lilly and Company Ltd)
  Insulin lispro 50 unit per 1 ml, Insulin lispro (as Insulin lispro protamine) 50 unit per 1 ml Humalog Mix50 100units/ml suspension for injection 3ml cartridges | 5 cartridge PoM £29.46 DT = £29.46
- ▸ **Humalog Mix50 KwikPen** (Eli Lilly and Company Ltd)
  Insulin lispro 50 unit per 1 ml, Insulin lispro (as Insulin lispro protamine) 50 unit per 1 ml Humalog Mix50 KwikPen 100units/ml suspension for injection 3ml pre-filled pens | 5 pre-filled disposable injection PoM £30.98 DT = £30.98

INSULINS > LONG-ACTING

F 490

Insulin degludec 08-Feb-2019

(Recombinant human insulin analogue—long acting)

- **INDICATIONS AND DOSE**

Diabetes mellitus

▸ BY SUBCUTANEOUS INJECTION
- ▸ Child 1–17 years: Dose to be given according to requirements

- **INTERACTIONS** → Appendix 1: insulins
- **SIDE-EFFECTS**
  ▸ **Rare or very rare** Urticaria
- **PREGNANCY** Evidence of the safety of long-acting insulin analogues in pregnancy is limited, therefore isophane insulin is recommended where longer-acting insulins are needed; insulin detemir may also be considered.
- **PRESCRIBING AND DISPENSING INFORMATION** Insulin degludec (*Tresiba*®) is available in strengths of 100 units/mL (allows 1-unit dose adjustment) and 200 units/mL (allows 2-unit dose adjustment)—ensure correct strength prescribed.

- **NATIONAL FUNDING/ACCESS DECISIONS**

All Wales Medicines Strategy Group (AWMSG) decisions
AWMSG No. 3158
The *All Wales Medicines Strategy Group* has advised (October 2016) that insulin degludec (*Tresiba*®) is **not** recommended for use within NHS Wales for the treatment of diabetes mellitus in adolescents and children from the age of 1 year.

- **MEDICINAL FORMS** There can be variation in the licensing of different medicines containing the same drug.

Solution for injection
- Tresiba FlexTouch (Novo Nordisk Ltd)
  Insulin degludec 100 unit per 1 ml Tresiba FlexTouch 100units/ml solution for injection 3ml pre-filled pens | 5 pre-filled disposable injection PoM £46.60 DT = £46.60
  Insulin degludec 200 unit per 1 ml Tresiba FlexTouch 200units/ml solution for injection 3ml pre-filled pens | 3 pre-filled disposable injection PoM £55.92 DT = £55.92
- Tresiba Penfill (Novo Nordisk Ltd)
  Insulin degludec 100 unit per 1 ml Tresiba Penfill 100units/ml solution for injection 3ml cartridges | 5 cartridge PoM £46.60 DT = £46.60

490

Insulin detemir

(Recombinant human insulin analogue—long acting)

- **INDICATIONS AND DOSE**

Diabetes mellitus
- BY SUBCUTANEOUS INJECTION
- Child 2–17 years: According to requirements

- **INTERACTIONS** → Appendix 1: insulins
- **SIDE-EFFECTS**
- **Uncommon** Refraction disorder
- **PREGNANCY** Evidence of the safety of long-acting insulin analogues in pregnancy is limited, therefore isophane insulin p. 494 is recommended where longer-acting insulins are needed; insulin detemir may also be considered where longer-acting insulins are needed.
- **MEDICINAL FORMS** There can be variation in the licensing of different medicines containing the same drug.

Solution for injection
- Levemir FlexPen (Novo Nordisk Ltd)
  Insulin detemir 100 unit per 1 ml Levemir FlexPen 100units/ml solution for injection 3ml pre-filled pens | 5 pre-filled disposable injection PoM £42.00 DT = £42.00
- Levemir InnoLet (Novo Nordisk Ltd)
  Insulin detemir 100 unit per 1 ml Levemir InnoLet 100units/ml solution for injection 3ml pre-filled pens | 5 pre-filled disposable injection PoM £44.85 DT = £42.00
- Levemir Penfill (Novo Nordisk Ltd)
  Insulin detemir 100 unit per 1 ml Levemir Penfill 100units/ml solution for injection 3ml cartridges | 5 cartridge PoM £42.00 DT = £42.00

490

Insulin glargine

(Recombinant human insulin analogue—long acting)

- **INDICATIONS AND DOSE**

Diabetes mellitus
- BY SUBCUTANEOUS INJECTION
- Child 2–17 years: According to requirements

- **INTERACTIONS** → Appendix 1: insulins
- **SIDE-EFFECTS**
- **Rare or very rare** Myalgia · sodium retention · taste altered
- **PREGNANCY** Evidence of the safety of long-acting insulin analogues in pregnancy is limited, therefore isophane insulin is recommended where longer-acting insulins are needed; insulin detemir may also be considered.
- **PRESCRIBING AND DISPENSING INFORMATION** Insulin glargine is a biological medicine. Biological medicines must be prescribed and dispensed by brand name, see *Biological medicines* and *Biosimilar medicines*, under Guidance on prescribing p. 1. Dose adjustments and close metabolic monitoring is recommended if switching between insulin glargine preparations.
- **NATIONAL FUNDING/ACCESS DECISIONS**

Scottish Medicines Consortium (SMC) decisions
The *Scottish Medicines Consortium* has advised that *Lantus*® preparations (April 2013) and *Toujeo*® (August 2015) are accepted for restricted use within NHS Scotland for the treatment of type 1 diabetes:
- in those who are at risk of or experience unacceptable frequency or severity of nocturnal hypoglycaemia on attempting to achieve better hypoglycaemic control during treatment with other insulins
- as a once daily insulin therapy for patients who require a carer to administer their insulin

It is **not** recommended for routine use in patients with type 2 diabetes unless they suffer from recurrent episodes of hypoglycaemia or require assistance with their insulin injections.

- **MEDICINAL FORMS** There can be variation in the licensing of different medicines containing the same drug.

Solution for injection
- Abasaglar (Eli Lilly and Company Ltd)
  Insulin glargine 100 unit per 1 ml Abasaglar 100units/ml solution for injection 3ml cartridges | 5 cartridge PoM £35.28 DT = £37.77
- Abasaglar KwikPen (Eli Lilly and Company Ltd)
  Insulin glargine 100 unit per 1 ml Abasaglar KwikPen 100units/ml solution for injection 3ml pre-filled pens | 5 pre-filled disposable injection PoM £35.28 DT = £37.77
- Lantus (Sanofi)
  Insulin glargine 100 unit per 1 ml Lantus 100units/ml solution for injection 3ml cartridges | 5 cartridge PoM £37.77 DT = £37.77
  Lantus 100units/ml solution for injection 3ml pre-filled SoloStar pens | 5 pre-filled disposable injection PoM £37.77 DT = £37.77
  Lantus 100units/ml solution for injection 10ml vials | 1 vial PoM £27.92 DT = £27.92
- Semglee (Mylan) ▼
  Insulin glargine 100 unit per 1 ml Semglee 100units/ml solution for injection 3ml pre-filled pens | 5 pre-filled disposable injection PoM £29.99 DT = £37.77
- Toujeo (Sanofi)
  Insulin glargine 300 unit per 1 ml Toujeo 300units/ml solution for injection 1.5ml pre-filled SoloStar pens | 3 pre-filled disposable injection PoM £32.14 DT = £32.14
- Toujeo DoubleStar (Sanofi)
  Insulin glargine 300 unit per 1 ml Toujeo 300units/ml solution for injection 3ml pre-filled DoubleStar pens | 3 pre-filled disposable injection PoM £64.27 DT = £64.27

3.1a Diabetes, diagnosis and monitoring

Diabetes mellitus, diagnostic and monitoring devices

Urinalysis: urinary glucose

Reagent strips are available for measuring for glucose in the urine. Tests for ketones by patients are rarely required unless they become unwell—see Blood Monitoring.

Microalbuminuria can be detected with *Micral-Test II*® but this should be followed by confirmation in the laboratory, since false positive results are common.

Blood glucose monitoring

Blood glucose monitoring using a meter gives a direct measure of the glucose concentration at the time of the test and can detect hypoglycaemia as well as hyperglycaemia. Carers and children should be properly trained in the use of blood glucose monitoring systems and the appropriate action to take on the results obtained. Inadequate understanding of the normal fluctuations in blood glucose can lead to confusion and inappropriate action.

Children using multiple injection regimens should understand how to adjust their insulin dose according to their carbohydrate intake. With fixed-dose insulin regimens, the carbohydrate intake needs to be regulated, and should be distributed throughout the day to match the insulin regimen.

In the UK blood-glucose concentration is expressed in mmol/litre and Diabetes UK advises that these units should be used for self-monitoring of blood glucose. In other European countries units of mg/100 mL (or mg/dL) are commonly used.

It is advisable to check that the meter is pre-set in the correct units.

If the blood glucose level is high or if the child is unwell, blood **ketones** should be measured according to local guidelines in order to detect diabetic ketoacidosis. Children and their carers should be trained in the use of blood ketone monitoring systems and to take appropriate action on the results obtained, including when to seek medical attention.

Other drugs used for Diabetes, diagnosis and monitoring
Glucose, p. 638

Blood glucose testing strips

● **BLOOD GLUCOSE TESTING STRIPS**

4SURE testing strips (Nipro Diagnostics (UK) Ltd)
50 strip • NHS indicative price = £8.99 • Drug Tariff (Part IXr)

Accu-Chek Inform II testing strips (Roche Diagnostics Ltd)
50 strip • No NHS indicative price available • Drug Tariff (Part IXr)

Active testing strips (Roche Diabetes Care Ltd)
50 strip • NHS indicative price = £10.03 • Drug Tariff (Part IXr)

Advocate Redi-Code+ testing strips (Diabetes Care Technology Ltd)
50 strip • NHS indicative price = £9.95 • Drug Tariff (Part IXr)

AutoSense testing strips (Advance Diagnostic Products (NI) Ltd)
25 strip • NHS indicative price = £4.50 • Drug Tariff (Part IXr)

Aviva testing strips (Roche Diabetes Care Ltd)
50 strip • NHS indicative price = £16.21 • Drug Tariff (Part IXr)

BGStar testing strips (Sanofi)
50 strip • NHS indicative price = £14.73 • Drug Tariff (Part IXr)

Betachek C50 cassette (National Diagnostic Products)
100 device • NHS indicative price = £29.98 • Drug Tariff (Part IXr)

Betachek G5 testing strips (National Diagnostic Products)
50 strip • NHS indicative price = £14.19 • Drug Tariff (Part IXr)

Betachek Visual testing strips (National Diagnostic Products)
50 strip • NHS indicative price = £6.80 • Drug Tariff (Part IXr)

Breeze 2 testing discs (Bayer Plc)
50 strip • NHS indicative price = £15.00 • Drug Tariff (Part IXr)

CareSens N testing strips (Spirit Healthcare Ltd)
50 strip • NHS indicative price = £12.75 • Drug Tariff (Part IXr)

CareSens PRO testing strips (Spirit Healthcare Ltd)
50 strip • NHS indicative price = £9.95 • Drug Tariff (Part IXr)

Contour Next testing strips (Ascensia Diabetes Care UK Ltd)
50 strip • NHS indicative price = £15.16 • Drug Tariff (Part IXr)

Contour Plus testing strips (Ascensia Diabetes Care UK Ltd)
50 strip • NHS indicative price = £8.50 • Drug Tariff (Part IXr)

Contour TS testing strips (Ascensia Diabetes Care UK Ltd)
50 strip • NHS indicative price = £9.60 • Drug Tariff (Part IXr)

Contour testing strips (Ascensia Diabetes Care UK Ltd)
50 strip • NHS indicative price = £9.99 • Drug Tariff (Part IXr)

Dario Lite testing strips (LabStyle Innovations Ltd)
50 strip • NHS indicative price = £9.95 • Drug Tariff (Part IXr)

Dario testing strips (LabStyle Innovations Ltd)
50 strip • NHS indicative price = £14.95 • Drug Tariff (Part IXr)

Element testing strips (Neon Diagnostics Ltd)
50 strip • NHS indicative price = £9.89 • Drug Tariff (Part IXr)

Finetest Lite testing strips (Neon Diagnostics Ltd)
50 strip • NHS indicative price = £5.95 • Drug Tariff (Part IXr)

Fora Advanced pro GD40 testing strips (B.Braun Medical Ltd)
50 strip • NHS indicative price = £9.25 • Drug Tariff (Part IXr)

FreeStyle Lite testing strips (Abbott Laboratories Ltd)
50 strip • NHS indicative price = £16.41 • Drug Tariff (Part IXr)

FreeStyle Optium H testing strips (Abbott Laboratories Ltd)
100 strip • No NHS indicative price available • Drug Tariff (Part IXr)

FreeStyle Optium Neo H testing strips (Abbott Laboratories Ltd)
100 strip • No NHS indicative price available • Drug Tariff (Part IXr)

FreeStyle Optium testing strips (Abbott Laboratories Ltd)
50 strip • NHS indicative price = £16.30 • Drug Tariff (Part IXr)

FreeStyle Precision Pro testing strips (Abbott Laboratories Ltd)
100 strip • No NHS indicative price available • Drug Tariff (Part IXr)

FreeStyle testing strips (Abbott Laboratories Ltd)
50 strip • NHS indicative price = £16.40 • Drug Tariff (Part IXr)

GluNEO testing strips (Neon Diagnostics Ltd)
50 strip • NHS indicative price = £9.89 • Drug Tariff (Part IXr)

GlucoDock testing strips (Medisana Healthcare (UK) Ltd)
50 strip • NHS indicative price = £14.90 • Drug Tariff (Part IXr)

GlucoLab testing strips (Neon Diagnostics Ltd)
50 strip • NHS indicative price = £9.89 • Drug Tariff (Part IXr)

GlucoMen LX Sensor testing strips (A. Menarini Diagnostics Ltd)
50 strip • NHS indicative price = £15.76 • Drug Tariff (Part IXr)

GlucoMen areo Sensor testing strips (A. Menarini Diagnostics Ltd)
50 strip • NHS indicative price = £9.95 • Drug Tariff (Part IXr)

GlucoRx GO Professional testing strips (GlucoRx Ltd)
50 strip • NHS indicative price = £9.95 • Drug Tariff (Part IXr)

GlucoRx GO testing strips (GlucoRx Ltd)
50 strip • NHS indicative price = £9.95 • Drug Tariff (Part IXr)

GlucoRx HCT Glucose testing strips (GlucoRx Ltd)
50 strip • NHS indicative price = £8.95 • Drug Tariff (Part IXr)

GlucoRx Nexus testing strips (GlucoRx Ltd)
50 strip • NHS indicative price = £8.95 • Drug Tariff (Part IXr)

GlucoRx Q testing strips (GlucoRx Ltd)
50 strip • NHS indicative price = £5.45 • Drug Tariff (Part IXr)

GlucoZen.auto testing strips (GlucoZen Ltd)
50 strip • NHS indicative price = £7.64 • Drug Tariff (Part IXr)100 strip • NHS indicative price = £10.85 • Drug Tariff (Part IXr)

Glucoflex-R testing strips (Bio-Diagnostics Ltd)
50 strip • NHS indicative price = £6.75 • Drug Tariff (Part IXr)

Guide testing strips (Roche Diabetes Care Ltd)
50 strip • NHS indicative price = £16.21 • Drug Tariff (Part IXr)

IME-DC testing strips (Arctic Medical Ltd)
50 strip • NHS indicative price = £14.10 • Drug Tariff (Part IXr)

Kinetik Wellbeing testing strips (Kinetik Medical Devices Ltd)
50 strip • NHS indicative price = £8.49 • Drug Tariff (Part IXr)100 strip • NHS indicative price = £13.98 • Drug Tariff (Part IXr)

MODZ testing strips (Modz Oy)
50 strip • NHS indicative price = £14.00 • Drug Tariff (Part IXr)

MediSense SoftSense testing strips (Abbott Laboratories Ltd)
50 strip • NHS indicative price = £15.05 • Drug Tariff (Part IXr)

MediTouch 2 testing strips (Medisana Healthcare (UK) Ltd)
50 strip • NHS indicative price = £12.49 • Drug Tariff (Part IXr)

MediTouch testing strips (Medisana Healthcare (UK) Ltd)
50 strip • NHS indicative price = £14.90 • Drug Tariff (Part IXr)

Mendor Discreet testing strips (SpringMed Solutions Ltd)
50 strip • NHS indicative price = £14.75 • Drug Tariff (Part IXr)

Microdot Max testing strips (Cambridge Sensors Ltd)
50 strip • NHS indicative price = £7.49 • Drug Tariff (Part IXr)

Microdot+ testing strips (Cambridge Sensors Ltd)
50 strip • NHS indicative price = £9.49 • Drug Tariff (Part IXr)

Mobile cassette (Roche Diabetes Care Ltd)
50 device • NHS indicative price = £9.99 • Drug Tariff (Part IXr)

Myglucohealth testing strips (Entra Health Systems Ltd)
50 strip • NHS indicative price = £15.50 • Drug Tariff (Part IXr)

Meters and test strips

Meter (all NHS)	Type of monitoring	Compatible test strips	Test strip net price	Sensitivity range (mmol/litre)	Manufacturer
Accu-Chek® Active	Blood glucose	Active®	50 strip= £10.03	0.6- 33.3 mmol/litre	Roche Diabetes Care Ltd
Accu-Chek® Advantage Meter no longer available	Blood glucose	Advantage Plus®	50 strip= £0.00	0.6- 33.3 mmol/litre	Roche Diabetes Care Ltd
Accu-Chek® Aviva	Blood glucose	Aviva®	50 strip= £16.21	0.6- 33.3 mmol/litre	Roche Diabetes Care Ltd
Accu-Chek® Aviva Expert	Blood glucose	Aviva®	50 strip= £16.21	0.6- 33.3 mmol/litre	Roche Diabetes Care Ltd
Accu-Chek® Compact Plus Meter no longer available	Blood glucose	Compact®	3 × 17 strips= £0.00	0.6- 33.3 mmol/litre	Roche Diabetes Care Ltd
Accu-Chek® Mobile	Blood glucose	Mobile®	100 device= £0.00	0.3- 33.3 mmol/litre	Roche Diabetes Care Ltd
Accu-Chek® Aviva Nano	Blood glucose	Aviva®	50 strip= £16.21	0.6- 33.3 mmol/litre	Roche Diabetes Care Ltd
BGStar® Free of charge from diabetes healthcare professionals	Blood glucose	BGStar®	50 strip= £14.73	1.1- 33.3 mmol/litre	Sanofi
Breeze 2®	Blood glucose	Breeze 2®	50 strip= £15.00	0.6- 33.3 mmol/litre	Bayer Plc
CareSens N® Free of charge from diabetes healthcare professionals	Blood glucose	CareSens N®	50 strip= £12.75	1.1- 33.3 mmol/litre	Spirit Healthcare Ltd
Contour®	Blood glucose	Contour®	50 strip= £9.99	0.6- 33.3 mmol/litre	Ascensia Diabetes Care UK Ltd
Contour® XT	Blood glucose	Contour® Next	50 strip= £15.16	0.6- 33.3 mmol/litre	Ascensia Diabetes Care UK Ltd
Element®	Blood glucose	Element®	50 strip= £9.89	0.55- 33.3 mmol/litre	Neon Diagnostics Ltd
FreeStyle® Meter no longer available	Blood glucose	FreeStyle®	50 strip= £16.40	1.1- 27.8 mmol/litre	Abbott Laboratories Ltd
FreeStyle Freedom® Meter no longer available	Blood glucose	FreeStyle®	50 strip= £16.40	1.1- 27.8 mmol/litre	Abbott Laboratories Ltd
FreeStyle Freedom Lite®	Blood glucose	FreeStyle Lite®	50 strip= £16.41	1.1- 27.8 mmol/litre	Abbott Laboratories Ltd
FreeStyle InsuLinx®	Blood glucose	FreeStyle Lite®	50 strip= £16.41	1.1- 27.8 mmol/litre	Abbott Laboratories Ltd
FreeStyle Lite®	Blood glucose	FreeStyle Lite®	50 strip= £16.41	1.1- 27.8 mmol/litre	Abbott Laboratories Ltd
FreeStyle Mini® Meter no longer available	Blood glucose	FreeStyle®	50 strip= £16.40	1.1- 27.8 mmol/litre	Abbott Laboratories Ltd
FreeStyle Optium®	Blood glucose	FreeStyle Optium®	50 strip= £16.30	1.1- 27.8 mmol/litre	Abbott Laboratories Ltd
FreeStyle Optium®	Blood ketones	FreeStyle Optium® β-ketone	10 strip= £21.94	0- 8.0 mmol/litre	Abbott Laboratories Ltd
FreeStyle Optium Neo®	Blood glucose	FreeStyle Optium®	50 strip= £16.30	1.1- 27.8 mmol/litre	Abbott Laboratories Ltd
FreeStyle Optium Neo®	Blood ketones	FreeStyle Optium® β-ketone	10 strip= £21.94	0- 8.0 mmol/litre	Abbott Laboratories Ltd
GlucoDock® module	Blood glucose	GlucoDock®	50 strip= £14.90	1.1- 33.3 mmol/litre For use with iPhone®, iPod touch®, and iPad®	Medisana Healthcare (UK) Ltd

Meter (all NHS)	Type of monitoring	Compatible test strips	Test strip net price	Sensitivity range (mmol/litre)	Manufacturer
GlucoLab®	Blood glucose	GlucoLab®	50 strip= £9.89	0.55- 33.3 mmol/litre	Neon Diagnostics Ltd
GlucoMen® GM	Blood glucose	GlucoMen® GM	50 strip= £0.00	0.6- 33.3 mmol/litre	A. Menarini Diagnostics Ltd
GlucoMen® LX	Blood glucose	GlucoMen® LX Sensor	50 strip= £15.76	1.1- 33.3 mmol/litre	A. Menarini Diagnostics Ltd
GlucoMen® LX Plus	Blood glucose	GlucoMen® LX Sensor	50 strip= £15.76	1.1- 33.3 mmol/litre	A. Menarini Diagnostics Ltd
GlucoMen® LX Plus	Blood ketones	GlucoMen® LX Ketone	10 strip= £21.06	0- 0.8 mmol/litre	A. Menarini Diagnostics Ltd
GlucoMen® Visio	Blood glucose	GlucoMen® Visio Sensor	50 strip= £0.00	1.1- 33.3 mmol/litre	A. Menarini Diagnostics Ltd
GlucoRx® Free of charge from diabetes healthcare professionals	Blood glucose	GlucoRx®	50 strip= £5.45	1.1- 33.3 mmol/litre	GlucoRx Ltd
GlucoRx Nexus® Free of charge from diabetes healthcare professionals	Blood glucose	GlucoRx Nexus®	50 strip= £8.95	1.1- 33.3 mmol/litre	GlucoRx Ltd
Glucotrend® Meter no longer available	Blood glucose	Active®	50 strip= £10.03	0.6- 33.3 mmol/litre	Roche Diabetes Care Ltd
iBGStar®	Blood glucose	BGStar®	50 strip= £14.73	1.1- 33.3 mmol/litre	Sanofi
IME-DC®	Blood glucose	IME-DC®	50 strip= £14.10	1.1- 33.3 mmol/litre	Arctic Medical Ltd
Mendor Discreet®	Blood glucose	Mendor Discreet®	50 strip= £14.75	1.1- 33.3 mmol/litre	SpringMed Solutions Ltd
Microdot®+ Free of charge from diabetes healthcare professionals	Blood glucose	Microdot®+	50 strip= £9.49	1.1- 29.2 mmol/litre	Cambridge Sensors Ltd
MyGlucoHealth®	Blood glucose	MyGlucoHealth®	50 strip= £15.50	0.6- 33.3 mmol/litre	Entra Health Systems Ltd
Omnitest® 3	Blood glucose	Omnitest® 3	50 strip= £9.89	0.6- 33.3 mmol/litre	B.Braun Medical Ltd
One Touch Ultra® Meter no longer available	Blood glucose	One Touch Ultra®	50 strip= £0.00	1.1- 33.3 mmol/litre	LifeScan
One Touch Ultra 2® Free of charge from diabetes healthcare professionals	Blood glucose	One Touch Ultra®	50 strip= £0.00	1.1- 33.3 mmol/litre	LifeScan
One Touch UltraEasy® Free of charge from diabetes healthcare professionals	Blood glucose	One Touch Ultra®	50 strip= £0.00	1.1- 33.3 mmol/litre	LifeScan
One Touch UltraSmart® Free of charge from diabetes healthcare professionals	Blood glucose	One Touch Ultra®	50 strip= £0.00	1.1- 33.3 mmol/litre	LifeScan
One Touch® VerioPro Free of charge from diabetes healthcare professionals	Blood glucose	One Touch® Verio	50 strip= £15.12	1.1- 33.3 mmol/litre	LifeScan
One Touch® Vita Free of charge from diabetes healthcare professionals	Blood glucose	One Touch® Vita	50 strip= £0.00	1.1- 33.3 mmol/litre	LifeScan
SD CodeFree®	Blood glucose	SD CodeFree®	50 strip= £6.99	0.6- 33.3 mmol/litre	SD Biosensor Inc
Sensocard Plus® Meter no longer available	Blood glucose	Sensocard®	50 strip= £16.30	1.1- 33.3 mmol/litre	BBI Healthcare Ltd

Meter (all NHS)	Type of monitoring	Compatible test strips	Test strip net price	Sensitivity range (mmol/litre)	Manufacturer
SuperCheck2® Free of charge from diabetes healthcare professionals	Blood glucose	SuperCheck2®	50 strip= £0.00	1.1- 33.3 mmol/litre	Apollo Medical Technologies Ltd
TRUEone® All-in-one test strips and meter	Blood glucose	TRUEone®	50 strip= £0.00	1.1- 33.3 mmol/litre	Nipro Diagnostics (UK) Ltd
TRUEresult® Free of charge from diabetes healthcare professionals	Blood glucose	TRUEresult®	50 strip= £0.00	1.1- 33.3 mmol/litre	Nipro Diagnostics (UK) Ltd
TRUEresult twist® Free of charge from diabetes healthcare professionals	Blood glucose	TRUEresult®	50 strip= £0.00	1.1- 33.3 mmol/litre	Nipro Diagnostics (UK) Ltd
TRUEtrack® Free of charge from diabetes healthcare professionals	Blood glucose	TRUEtrack®	50 strip= £0.00	1.1- 33.3 mmol/litre	Nipro Diagnostics (UK) Ltd
TRUEyou mini®	Blood glucose	TRUEyou®	50 strip= £9.92	1.1- 33.3 mmol/litre	Nipro Diagnostics (UK) Ltd
WaveSense JAZZ® Free of charge from diabetes healthcare professionals	Blood glucose	WaveSense JAZZ®	50 strip= £8.74	1.1- 33.3 mmol/litre	AgaMatrix Europe Ltd

Mylife Pura testing strips (Ypsomed Ltd)
50 strip • NHS indicative price = £9.50 • Drug Tariff (Part IXr)

Mylife Unio testing strips (Ypsomed Ltd)
50 strip • NHS indicative price = £9.50 • Drug Tariff (Part IXr)

OKmeter Core testing strips (Syringa UK Ltd)
50 strip • NHS indicative price = £9.90 • Drug Tariff (Part IXr)

Oh'Care Lite testing strips (Neon Diagnostics Ltd)
50 strip • NHS indicative price = £8.88 • Drug Tariff (Part IXr)

Omnitest 3 testing strips (B.Braun Medical Ltd)
50 strip • NHS indicative price = £9.89 • Drug Tariff (Part IXr)

Omnitest 5 testing strips (B.Braun Medical Ltd)
50 strip • NHS indicative price = £9.89 • Drug Tariff (Part IXr)

On Call Extra testing strips (Acon Laboratories, Inc)
50 strip • NHS indicative price = £7.50 • Drug Tariff (Part IXr)

On Call Sure testing strips (Acon Laboratories, Inc)
50 strip • NHS indicative price = £9.20 • Drug Tariff (Part IXr)

On-Call Advanced testing strips (Point Of Care Testing Ltd)
50 strip • NHS indicative price = £13.65 • Drug Tariff (Part IXr)

OneTouch Select Plus testing strips (LifeScan)
50 strip • NHS indicative price = £9.99 • Drug Tariff (Part IXr)

OneTouch Verio testing strips (LifeScan)
50 strip • NHS indicative price = £15.12 • Drug Tariff (Part IXr)

Performa testing strips (Roche Diabetes Care Ltd)
50 strip • NHS indicative price = £7.50 • Drug Tariff (Part IXr)

SD CodeFree testing strips (SD Biosensor Inc)
50 strip • NHS indicative price = £6.99 • Drug Tariff (Part IXr)

SURESIGN Resure testing strips (Ciga Healthcare Ltd)
50 strip • NHS indicative price = £8.49 • Drug Tariff (Part IXr)

Sensocard testing strips (BBI Healthcare Ltd)
50 strip • NHS indicative price = £16.30 • Drug Tariff (Part IXr)

StatStrip testing strips (Nova Biomedical)
50 strip • No NHS indicative price available • Drug Tariff (Part IXr)

TEE2 testing strips (Spirit Healthcare Ltd)
50 strip • NHS indicative price = £7.75 • Drug Tariff (Part IXr)

True Metrix testing strips (Trividia Health UK Ltd)
50 strip • NHS indicative price = £6.95 • Drug Tariff (Part IXr)100 strip • NHS indicative price = £12.50 • Drug Tariff (Part IXr)

VivaChek Ino testing strips (JR Biomedical Ltd)
50 strip • NHS indicative price = £8.99 • Drug Tariff (Part IXr)

WaveSense JAZZ Duo testing strips (AgaMatrix Europe Ltd)
50 strip • NHS indicative price = £8.74 • Drug Tariff (Part IXr)

WaveSense JAZZ testing strips (AgaMatrix Europe Ltd)
50 strip • NHS indicative price = £8.74 • Drug Tariff (Part IXr)

Xceed Precision Pro testing strips (Abbott Laboratories Ltd)
10 strip • No NHS indicative price available50 strip • No NHS indicative price available • Drug Tariff (Part IXr)100 strip • No NHS indicative price available • Drug Tariff (Part IXr)

palmdoc iCare Advanced Solo testing strips (Palmdoc Ltd)
50 strip • NHS indicative price = £13.50 • Drug Tariff (Part IXr)

palmdoc iCare Advanced testing strips (Palmdoc Ltd)
50 strip • NHS indicative price = £9.70 • Drug Tariff (Part IXr)

palmdoc testing strips (Palmdoc Ltd)
50 strip • NHS indicative price = £5.90 • Drug Tariff (Part IXr)

Blood ketones testing strips

● **BLOOD KETONES TESTING STRIPS**

4SURE beta-ketone testing strips (Nipro Diagnostics (UK) Ltd) | 10 strip • NHS indicative price = £9.92 • Drug Tariff (Part IXr)

Fora Advanced pro GD40 Ketone testing strips (B.Braun Medical Ltd) | 10 strip • NHS indicative price = £9.25 • Drug Tariff (Part IXr)

FreeStyle Optium H beta-ketone testing strips (Abbott Laboratories Ltd) | 10 strip • No NHS indicative price available • Drug Tariff (Part IXr)

FreeStyle Optium beta-ketone testing strips (Abbott Laboratories Ltd) | 10 strip • NHS indicative price = £21.94 • Drug Tariff (Part IXr)

FreeStyle Precision Pro beta-ketone testing strips (Abbott Laboratories Ltd) | 50 strip • No NHS indicative price available

GlucoMen LX beta-ketone testing strips (A. Menarini Diagnostics Ltd) | 10 strip • NHS indicative price = £21.06 • Drug Tariff (Part IXr)

GlucoMen areo Ketone Sensor testing strips (A. Menarini Diagnostics Ltd) | 10 strip • NHS indicative price = £9.95 • Drug Tariff (Part IXr)

GlucoRx HCT Ketone testing strips (GlucoRx Ltd) | 10 strip • NHS indicative price = £9.95 • Drug Tariff (Part IXr)

KetoSens testing strips (Spirit Healthcare Ltd) | 10 strip • NHS indicative price = £9.95 • Drug Tariff (Part IXr)

StatStrip beta-ketone testing strips (Nova Biomedical) | 50 strip • No NHS indicative price available

Xceed Precision Pro beta-ketone testing strips (Abbott Laboratories Ltd) | 10 strip • No NHS indicative price available • Drug Tariff (Part IXr) | 50 strip • No NHS indicative price available | 100 strip • No NHS indicative price available

Glucose interstitial fluid detection sensors

● **GLUCOSE INTERSTITIAL FLUID DETECTION SENSORS**

FreeStyle Libre Sensor (Abbott Laboratories Ltd)
1 kit • NHS indicative price = £35.00 • Drug Tariff (Part IXa)

Hypodermic insulin injection pens

● **HYPODERMIC INSULIN INJECTION PENS**

AUTOPEN® 24

Autopen® 24 (for use with Sanofi- Aventis 3-mL insulin cartridges), allowing 1-unit dosage adjustment, max. 21 units (single-unit version) or 2-unit dosage adjustment, max. 42 units (2- unit version).

Autopen 24 hypodermic insulin injection pen reusable for 3ml cartridge 1 unit dial up / range 1-21 units (Owen Mumford Ltd)
1 device • NHS indicative price = £16.89 • Drug Tariff (Part IXa)

Autopen 24 hypodermic insulin injection pen reusable for 3ml cartridge 2 unit dial up / range 2-42 units (Owen Mumford Ltd)
1 device • NHS indicative price = £16.89 • Drug Tariff (Part IXa)

AUTOPEN® CLASSIC

Autopen® Classic (for use with Lilly and Wockhardt 3-mL insulin cartridges), allowing 1-unit dosage adjustment, max. 21 units (single-unit version) or 2-unit dosage adjustment, max. 42 units (2-unit version).

Autopen Classic hypodermic insulin injection pen reusable for 3ml cartridge 1 unit dial up / range 1-21 units (Owen Mumford Ltd)
1 device • NHS indicative price = £17.15 • Drug Tariff (Part IXa)

Autopen Classic hypodermic insulin injection pen reusable for 3ml cartridge 2 unit dial up / range 2-42 units (Owen Mumford Ltd)
1 device • NHS indicative price = £17.15 • Drug Tariff (Part IXa)

CLIKSTAR®

For use with *Lantus®*, *Apidra®*, and *Insuman®* 3-mL insulin cartridges; allowing 1-unit dose adjustment, max. 80 units.

HUMAPEN® LUXURA HD

For use with *Humulin®* and *Humalog®* 3-mL cartridges; allowing 0.5-unit dosage adjustment, max. 30 units.

HumaPen Luxura HD hypodermic insulin injection pen reusable for 3ml cartridge 0.5 unit dial up / range 1-30 units (Eli Lilly and Company Ltd)
1 device • NHS indicative price = £27.01 • Drug Tariff (Part IXa)

NOVOPEN® 4

For use with *Penfill®* 3-mL insulin cartridges; allowing 1-unit dosage adjustment, max. 60 units.

Needle free insulin delivery systems

● **NEEDLE FREE INSULIN DELIVERY SYSTEMS**

INSUJET®

For use with any 10-mL vial or 3-mL cartridge of insulin, allowing 1-unit dosage adjustment, max 40 units. Available as *starter set* (*InsuJet®* device, nozzle cap, nozzle and piston, 1 × 10-mL adaptor, 1 × 3-mL adaptor, 1 cartridge cap removal key), *nozzle pack* (15 nozzles), *cartridge adaptor pack* (15 adaptors), or *vial adaptor pack* (15 adaptors).

InsuJet starter set (Spirit Healthcare Ltd)
1 pack • NHS indicative price = £90.00 • Drug Tariff (Part IXa)

Urine glucose testing strips

● **URINE GLUCOSE TESTING STRIPS**

Diastix testing strips (Ascensia Diabetes Care UK Ltd)
50 strip • NHS indicative price = £2.89 • Drug Tariff (Part IXr)

Medi-Test Glucose testing strips (BHR Pharmaceuticals Ltd)
50 strip • NHS indicative price = £2.36 • Drug Tariff (Part IXr)

Urine ketone testing strips

● **URINE KETONES TESTING STRIPS**

GlucoRx KetoRx Sticks 2GK testing strips (GlucoRx Ltd)
50 strip • NHS indicative price = £2.25 • Drug Tariff (Part IXr)

Ketostix testing strips (Ascensia Diabetes Care UK Ltd)
50 strip • NHS indicative price = £3.06 • Drug Tariff (Part IXr)

Urine protein testing strips

● **URINE PROTEIN TESTING STRIPS**

Albustix testing strips (Siemens Medical Solutions Diagnostics Ltd)
50 strip • NHS indicative price = £4.10 • Drug Tariff (Part IXr)

Medi-Test Protein 2 testing strips (BHR Pharmaceuticals Ltd)
50 strip • NHS indicative price = £3.31 • Drug Tariff (Part IXr)

3.2 Hypoglycaemia

Hypoglycaemia

09-Apr-2020

Description of condition

Hypoglycaemia results from an imbalance between glucose supply, glucose utilisation, and existing insulin concentration. Clinical hypoglycaemia is defined as a blood-glucose concentration low enough to cause symptoms or signs of impaired brain function. In clinical practice, a glucose value of ≤ 3.9 mmol/litre is used as the threshold value to initiate treatment for hypoglycaemia in children with diabetes.

Symptoms of hypoglycaemia in the young include shakiness, pounding heart, sweatiness, headache, drowsiness, and difficulty concentrating. In young children, behavioural changes such as irritability, agitation, quietness, and tantrums, may be prominent.

Short-term complications of severe hypoglycaemia include transient neurological symptoms such as paresis, convulsions, encephalopathy, loss of consciousness, and rarely, subsequent neurological damage and mild intellectual impairment.

Diabetes mellitus, idiopathic ketotic hypoglycaemia, adrenal insufficiency, hyperinsulinism, fatty acid oxidation disorders, and glycogen storage disease (amongst others), may cause acute hypoglycaemia in children. Common clinical precipitants for hypoglycaemia in children with diabetes may include insufficient food consumption (i.e. missed meals, nocturnal hypoglycaemia), excessive insulin dosing, exercise, alcohol ingestion (in adolescents), and sulfonylureas [unlicensed].

Treatment of acute hypoglycaemia

For a quick reference resource with doses for the treatment of hypoglycaemia, see *Hypoglycaemia* in Medical emergencies in the community, inside back pages.

Prompt treatment of hypoglycaemia in children is essential whatever the cause. Hypoglycaemia caused by a sulfonylurea (although rarely used in children) or a long acting insulin, may persist for up to 24–36 hours following the last dose, especially if there is concurrent renal impairment (rare in children). EvGr Close monitoring is required and hospital care should be considered. ⟨E⟩

6 Endocrine system

Severe hypoglycaemia

Intravenous management

Hypoglycaemia which causes unconsciousness or seizures is an emergency. EvGr If the child is in hospital and rapid intravenous access is possible, severe hypoglycaemia should be treated with glucose 10% intravenous infusion p. 638. Ⓐ

EvGr A bolus dose using glucose 10% can be given before the glucose infusion to rapidly increase the plasma-glucose concentration, in order to allow glucose to cross the blood brain barrier and alleviate neuroglycopaenia. Ⓔ

Pain and phlebitis may occur during administration, particularly if infused too quickly. Glucose 50% intravenous infusion is not recommended as it is hypertonic, thus increases the risk of extravasation injury, and is viscous, making administration difficult.

Oral and intramuscular management

EvGr Severe hypoglycaemia outside of hospital or when rapid intravenous access is not available, may be treated with concentrated oral glucose solution, as long as the child is **conscious and able to swallow**. Ⓐ Proprietary products of fast-acting carbohydrate, as glucose 40% gel (e.g. *Glucogel*®, *Dextrogel*®, or *Rapilose gel*®, see glucose) are available for the patient to keep at hand in case of severe hypoglycaemia.

EvGr If the child is **unconscious or unable to swallow**, intramuscular glucagon below should be given and blood-glucose concentration monitored. Ⓐ Glucagon increases blood glucose by mobilising glycogen stored in the liver. The manufacturer advises that it is ineffective in patients whose liver glycogen is depleted, therefore should not be used in anyone who has fasted for a prolonged period, has adrenal insufficiency, chronic hypoglycaemia, or alcohol-induced hypoglycaemia. EvGr Glucagon may also be less effective in children taking a sulfonylurea; in these cases, intravenous glucose will be required. Ⓔ

EvGr As symptoms improve or normoglycaemia is restored, and the child is sufficiently awake, an oral long-acting carbohydrate snack (e.g. two biscuits, one banana) or a meal should be given to maintain normal blood-glucose concentration. The blood-glucose concentration should be checked repeatedly in children and young people who have persistently reduced consciousness after a severe hypoglycaemic episode, to determine whether further glucose is needed. Ⓐ

Advice for parents or carers

EvGr Parents or carers of insulin-treated children should be trained and equipped to give intramuscular glucagon for emergency use in severe hypoglycaemic attacks.

Parents or carers should be advised to seek medical assistance if glucagon is not effective within 10 minutes as intravenous glucose is required. Ⓐ

Non-severe hypoglycaemia

EvGr In children who **are able to swallow**, non-severe hypoglycaemia is treated with 10–20 g of fast-acting carbohydrate by mouth, preferably in liquid form, which may be taken more easily. Oral glucose solutions should not be used if consciousness is reduced as this could be dangerous (risk of choking). 10–20 g is available from approximately 2–4 teaspoonfuls of sugar added to a cup of water, or 3–6 glucose tablets.

Chocolates and biscuits should be avoided if possible, because they have a lower sugar content and their high fat content may delay stomach emptying.

Administration of fast-acting carbohydrates may need to be in frequent small amounts, because hypoglycaemia can cause vomiting. Ⓐ Blood-glucose concentrations should rise within 5–15 minutes; EvGr if hypoglycaemia persists after 15 minutes, repeat the fast-acting glucose.As symptoms improve or normoglycaemia is restored, a long-acting carbohydrate snack (e.g. two biscuits, one banana) or a meal, can be given to prevent blood-glucose concentration from falling again. Ⓐ

Neonatal hypoglycaemia in term babies

Infants at risk of impaired metabolic adaptation and hypoglycaemia include infants of mothers with diabetes (including gestational diabetes), those whose mothers have taken beta-blockers, and those with intra-uterine growth restriction. EvGr Severe or persistent hypoglycaemia may be a presenting feature of an underlying inborn error of metabolism and requires urgent medical review.

Asymptomatic neonatal hypoglycaemia may be treated by increasing breast-feeding frequency, supplementing with a breast milk substitute (i.e. formula), or intravenous glucose therapy. Buccal glucose gel may be used in conjunction with a feeding plan.When feeding interventions are offered, blood-glucose concentrations should be re-checked in 1 hour to ensure there has been a response. If feeding interventions are not effective, glucose 10% intravenous infusion should be given, and blood-glucose re-tested within 15 minutes.

Symptomatic hypoglycaemic neonates should be treated immediately with a glucose intravenous infusion.If there is a delay in obtaining intravenous access, consider either buccal glucose gel or intramuscular glucagon. If blood glucose is <1 mmol/litre, buccal glucose gel should only be used as an interim measure while arranging treatment with intravenous glucose infusion. Neonates requiring 12 mg/kg/minute or more of glucose to maintain normoglycaemia, should be investigated for congenital hyperinsulinism. Ⓔ

GLYCOGENOLYTIC HORMONES

Glucagon

23-Apr-2020

● **INDICATIONS AND DOSE**

Diabetic hypoglycaemia

▶ BY SUBCUTANEOUS INJECTION, OR BY INTRAMUSCULAR INJECTION

▶ Neonate: 20 micrograms/kg.

▶ Child 1 month–8 years (body-weight up to 25 kg): 500 micrograms, if no response within 10 minutes intravenous glucose must be given

▶ Child 9–17 years (body-weight 25 kg and above): 1 mg, if no response within 10 minutes intravenous glucose must be given

Endogenous hyperinsulinism

▶ BY INTRAMUSCULAR INJECTION, OR BY INTRAVENOUS INJECTION

▶ Neonate: 200 micrograms/kg (max. per dose 1 mg) for 1 dose.

▶ Child 1 month–1 year: 1 mg for 1 dose

▶ BY CONTINUOUS INTRAVENOUS INFUSION

▶ Neonate: 1–18 micrograms/kg/hour (max. per dose 50 micrograms/kg/hour), adjusted according to response.

▶ Child 1 month–1 year: 1–10 micrograms/kg/hour, dose to be adjusted as necessary

Diagnosis of growth hormone secretion (specialist use only)

▶ BY INTRAMUSCULAR INJECTION

▶ Child: 100 micrograms/kg (max. per dose 1 mg) for 1 dose, dose may vary, consult local guidelines

Beta-blocker poisoning (cardiogenic shock unresponsive to atropine)

▶ INITIALLY BY INTRAVENOUS INJECTION

▶ Child: 50–150 micrograms/kg (max. per dose 10 mg), to be administered in glucose 5% (with precautions to protect the airway in case of vomiting), followed by (by intravenous infusion) 50 micrograms/kg/hour

DOSE EQUIVALENCE AND CONVERSION

▶ 1 unit of glucagon = 1 mg of glucagon.

- **UNLICENSED USE** Dose and indication for cardiogenic shock unresponsive to atropine in beta-blocker overdose not licensed.

  Unlicensed for growth hormone test and hyperinsulinism.
- **CONTRA-INDICATIONS** Phaeochromocytoma
- **CAUTIONS** Glucagonoma · ineffective in chronic hypoglycaemia, starvation, and adrenal insufficiency · insulinoma · when used in the diagnosis of growth hormone secretion, delayed hypoglycaemia may result—deaths reported (ensure a meal is eaten before discharge)
- **INTERACTIONS** → Appendix 1: glucagon
- **SIDE-EFFECTS**
  - **Common or very common** Nausea
  - **Uncommon** Vomiting
  - **Rare or very rare** Abdominal pain · hypertension · hypotension · tachycardia
- **DIRECTIONS FOR ADMINISTRATION**
  - **With intravenous use** When administered by *continuous intravenous infusion*, do not add to infusion fluids containing calcium—precipitation may occur.
- **PATIENT AND CARER ADVICE**

  Medicines for Children leaflet: Glucagon for hypoglycaemia www.medicinesforchildren.org.uk/glucagon-hypoglycaemia
- **EXCEPTIONS TO LEGAL CATEGORY** Prescription-only medicine restriction does not apply where administration is for saving life in emergency.

- **MEDICINAL FORMS** There can be variation in the licensing of different medicines containing the same drug.

Powder and solvent for solution for injection

- GlucaGen Hypokit (Novo Nordisk Ltd)

  Glucagon hydrochloride 1 mg GlucaGen Hypokit 1mg powder and solvent for solution for injection | 1 vial PoM £11.52 DT = £11.52

3.2a Chronic hypoglycaemia

Other drugs used for Chronic hypoglycaemia
Chlorothiazide, p. 117

GLYCOGENOLYTIC HORMONES

Diazoxide

- **INDICATIONS AND DOSE**

Resistant hypertension

► BY MOUTH

- Neonate: Initially 1.7 mg/kg 3 times a day, adjusted according to response; maximum 15 mg/kg per day.
- Child: Initially 1.7 mg/kg 3 times a day, adjusted according to response; maximum 15 mg/kg per day

Chronic intractable hypoglycaemia

► BY MOUTH

- Neonate: Initially 5 mg/kg twice daily, adjusted according to response, initial dose used to establish response; maintenance 1.5–3 mg/kg 2–3 times a day; increased if necessary up to 7 mg/kg 3 times a day, higher doses are unlikely to be beneficial, but may be required in some cases.
- Child: Initially 1.7 mg/kg 3 times a day, adjusted according to response; maintenance 1.5–3 mg/kg 2–3 times a day, increased if necessary up to 5 mg/kg 3 times a day, doses up to 5 mg/kg may be required in some cases, but higher doses are unlikely to be beneficial

- **UNLICENSED USE** Not licensed for resistant hypertension.
- **CAUTIONS** Aortic coarctation · aortic stenosis · arteriovenous shunt · heart failure · hyperuricaemia · impaired cardiac circulation · impaired cerebral circulation
- **INTERACTIONS** → Appendix 1: diazoxide
- **SIDE-EFFECTS** Abdominal pain · albuminuria · appetite decreased (long term use) · arrhythmia · azotaemia · cardiomegaly · cataract · constipation · diabetic hyperosmolar coma · diarrhoea · dizziness · dyspnoea · eosinophilia · extrapyramidal symptoms · face abnormal · fever · fluid retention · galactorrhoea · haemorrhage · headache · heart failure · hirsutism · hyperglycaemia · hyperuricaemia (long term use) · hypogammaglobulinaemia · hypotension · ileus · ketoacidosis · leucopenia · libido decreased · musculoskeletal pain · nausea · nephritic syndrome · oculogyric crisis · pancreatitis · parkinsonism · pulmonary hypertension · skin reactions · sodium retention · taste altered · thrombocytopenia · tinnitus · vision disorders · voice alteration (long term use) · vomiting
- **PREGNANCY** Use only if essential; alopecia and hypertrichosis reported in neonates with prolonged use; may inhibit uterine activity during labour.
- **BREAST FEEDING** Manufacturer advises avoid—no information available.
- **RENAL IMPAIRMENT**

  Dose adjustments Dose reduction may be required.
- **MONITORING REQUIREMENTS**
  - Monitor blood pressure.
  - Monitor white cell and platelet count during prolonged use.
  - Regularly assess growth, bone, and psychological development during prolonged use.

- **MEDICINAL FORMS** There can be variation in the licensing of different medicines containing the same drug. Forms available from special-order manufacturers include: capsule, oral suspension, oral solution

Tablet

- Eudemine (RPH Pharmaceuticals AB)

  Diazoxide 50 mg Eudemine 50mg tablets | 100 tablet PoM £72.55 DT = £72.55

Capsule

- Proglycem (Imported (Germany))

  Diazoxide 25 mg Proglycem 25 capsules | 100 capsule PoM 

PITUITARY AND HYPOTHALAMIC HORMONES AND ANALOGUES > SOMATOSTATIN ANALOGUES

Somatostatin analogues

- **CAUTIONS** Diabetes mellitus (antidiabetic requirements may be reduced) · insulinoma (increased depth and duration of hypoglycaemia may occur—observe patients and monitor blood glucose levels when initiating treatment and changing doses)
- **SIDE-EFFECTS**
  - **Common or very common** Alopecia · appetite decreased · asthenia · cholecystitis · cholelithiasis (following long term use) · cholestasis · constipation · diabetes mellitus · diarrhoea · dizziness · gastrointestinal discomfort · gastrointestinal disorders · glucose tolerance impaired (following long term use) · headache · hyperglycaemia (long term use) · hypoglycaemia · myalgia · nausea · pruritus · sinus bradycardia · vomiting
- **DIRECTIONS FOR ADMINISTRATION** Injection sites should be rotated.

503

6 Endocrine system

Octreotide

04-Oct-2018

- **INDICATIONS AND DOSE**

Persistent hyperinsulinaemic hypoglycaemia unresponsive to diazoxide and glucose

▸ BY SUBCUTANEOUS INJECTION

▸ Neonate: Initially 2–5 micrograms/kg every 6–8 hours, adjusted according to response; increased if necessary up to 7 micrograms/kg every 4 hours, dosing up to 7 micrograms/kg may rarely be required.

▸ Child: Initially 1–2 micrograms/kg every 4–6 hours, adjusted according to response; increased if necessary up to 7 micrograms/kg every 4 hours, dosing up to 7 micrograms/kg may rarely be required

Bleeding from oesophageal or gastric varices

▸ BY CONTINUOUS INTRAVENOUS INFUSION

▸ Child: 1 microgram/kg/hour, higher doses may be required initially, when no active bleeding reduce dose over 24 hours; Usual maximum 50 micrograms/hour

- **UNLICENSED USE** Not licensed in children.
- **INTERACTIONS** → Appendix 1: octreotide
- **SIDE-EFFECTS**

▸ **Common or very common** Arrhythmias · biliary sludge · dyspnoea · hyperbilirubinaemia · hypothyroidism · skin reactions · thyroid disorder

▸ **Uncommon** Dehydration

▸ **Frequency not known** Hepatic disorders · pancreatitis acute (after administration) · thrombocytopenia

SIDE-EFFECTS, FURTHER INFORMATION Administering non-depot injections of octreotide between meals and at bedtime may reduce gastrointestinal side-effects.

- **CONCEPTION AND CONTRACEPTION** Effective contraception required during treatment.
- **PREGNANCY** Possible effect on fetal growth; manufacturer advises use only if potential benefit outweighs risk.
- **BREAST FEEDING** Manufacturer advises avoid—present in milk in *animal* studies.
- **HEPATIC IMPAIRMENT** Manufacturer advises caution (risk of increased half-life in cirrhosis).

Dose adjustments In adults, manufacturer advises consider dose reduction—consult product literature.

- **MONITORING REQUIREMENTS**

▸ Monitor thyroid function on long-term therapy.

▸ Monitor liver function.

- **TREATMENT CESSATION** Avoid abrupt withdrawal of short-acting subcutaneous octreotide (associated with biliary colic and pancreatitis).
- **DIRECTIONS FOR ADMINISTRATION** For *intravenous injection* or *intravenous infusion*, dilute with Sodium Chloride 0.9% to a concentration of 10–50%.

- **MEDICINAL FORMS** There can be variation in the licensing of different medicines containing the same drug.

Solution for injection

▸ Octreotide (Non-proprietary)

Octreotide (as Octreotide acetate) 50 microgram per 1 ml Octreotide 50micrograms/1ml solution for injection pre-filled syringes | 5 pre-filled disposable injection PoM £18.85–£18.88 DT = £18.88

Octreotide 50micrograms/1ml solution for injection ampoules | 5 ampoule PoM £2.97–£18.60 DT = £14.87

Octreotide 50micrograms/1ml solution for injection vials | 5 vial PoM £22.00

Octreotide (as Octreotide acetate) 100 microgram per 1 ml Octreotide 100micrograms/1ml solution for injection ampoules | 5 ampoule PoM £32.65 DT = £27.97

Octreotide 100micrograms/1ml solution for injection pre-filled syringes | 5 pre-filled disposable injection PoM £30.33–£32.90 DT = £30.33

Octreotide 100micrograms/1ml solution for injection vials | 5 vial PoM £32.65 DT = £32.65

Octreotide (as Octreotide acetate) 200 microgram per 1 ml Octreotide 1mg/5ml solution for injection vials | 1 vial PoM £65.00 DT = £65.00

Octreotide (as Octreotide acetate) 500 microgram per 1 ml Octreotide 500micrograms/1ml solution for injection vials | 5 vial PoM £158.25 DT = £158.25

Octreotide 500micrograms/1ml solution for injection ampoules | 5 ampoule PoM £27.09–£169.35 DT = £135.47

Octreotide 500micrograms/1ml solution for injection pre-filled syringes | 5 pre-filled disposable injection PoM £154.22–£169.00 DT = £154.22

▸ Sandostatin (Novartis Pharmaceuticals UK Ltd)

Octreotide (as Octreotide acetate) 50 microgram per 1 ml Sandostatin 50micrograms/1ml solution for injection ampoules | 5 ampoule PoM £14.87 DT = £14.87

Octreotide (as Octreotide acetate) 100 microgram per 1 ml Sandostatin 100micrograms/1ml solution for injection ampoules | 5 ampoule PoM £27.97 DT = £27.97

Octreotide (as Octreotide acetate) 500 microgram per 1 ml Sandostatin 500micrograms/1ml solution for injection ampoules | 5 ampoule PoM £135.47 DT = £135.47

Powder and solvent for suspension for injection

▸ Octreotide (Non-proprietary)

Octreotide (as Octreotide acetate) 10 mg Olatuton 10mg powder and solvent for prolonged-release suspension for injection vials | 1 vial PoM £494.74 DT = £549.71

Octreotide (as Octreotide acetate) 20 mg Olatuton 20mg powder and solvent for prolonged-release suspension for injection vials | 1 vial PoM £719.40 DT = £799.33

Octreotide (as Octreotide acetate) 30 mg Olatuton 30mg powder and solvent for prolonged-release suspension for injection vials | 1 vial PoM £898.57 DT = £998.41

▸ Sandostatin LAR (Novartis Pharmaceuticals UK Ltd)

Octreotide (as Octreotide acetate) 10 mg Sandostatin LAR 10mg powder and solvent for suspension for injection vials | 1 vial PoM £549.71 DT = £549.71

Octreotide (as Octreotide acetate) 20 mg Sandostatin LAR 20mg powder and solvent for suspension for injection vials | 1 vial PoM £799.33 DT = £799.33

Octreotide (as Octreotide acetate) 30 mg Sandostatin LAR 30mg powder and solvent for suspension for injection vials | 1 vial PoM £998.41 DT = £998.41

4 Disorders of bone metabolism

Bone metabolism

Disorders of bone metabolism

The two main disorders of bone metabolism that occur in children are rickets and osteoporosis. The two most common forms of rickets are Vitamin D deficiency rickets and hypophosphataemic rickets. See also calcium.

Osteoporosis

Osteoporosis in children may be primary (e.g. *osteogenesis imperfecta* and *idiopathic juvenile osteoporosis*), or secondary (e.g. due to inflammatory disorders, immobilisation, or corticosteroids); specialist management is required.

Corticosteroid-induced osteoporosis

To reduce the risk of osteoporosis doses of oral corticosteroids should be as low as possible and courses of treatment as short as possible.

Calcitonin

Calcitonin is involved with parathyroid hormone in the regulation of bone turnover and hence in the maintenance of calcium balance and homoeostasis. Calcitonin (salmon) p. 508 (synthetic or recombinant salmon calcitonin) is used by specialists to lower the plasma-calcium concentration in children with hypercalcaemia associated with malignancy.

Bisphosphonates

A bisphosphonate such as pamidronate disodium p. 506 is used in the management of severe forms of *osteogenesis imperfecta* and other causes of osteoporosis in children to reduce the number of fractures; the long-term effects of bisphosphonates in children has not been established. Single doses of biphosphonates are also used to manage hypercalcaemia. Treatment should be initiated under specialist advice **only**.

Other drugs used for Disorders of bone metabolism
Calcitriol, p. 681

BISPHOSPHONATES

Bisphosphonates

- **DRUG ACTION** Bisphosphonates are adsorbed onto hydroxyapatite crystals in bone, slowing both their rate of growth and dissolution, and therefore reducing the rate of bone turnover.

IMPORTANT SAFETY INFORMATION

MHRA/CHM ADVICE: BISPHOSPHONATES: ATYPICAL FEMORAL FRACTURES (JUNE 2011)

Atypical femoral fractures have been reported rarely with bisphosphonate treatment, mainly in patients receiving long-term treatment for osteoporosis.

The need to continue bisphosphonate treatment for osteoporosis should be re-evaluated periodically based on an assessment of the benefits and risks of treatment for individual patients, particularly after 5 or more years of use.

Patients should be advised to report any thigh, hip, or groin pain during treatment with a bisphosphonate.

Discontinuation of bisphosphonate treatment in patients suspected to have an atypical femoral fracture should be considered after an assessment of the benefits and risks of continued treatment.

MHRA/CHM ADVICE: BISPHOSPHONATES: OSTEONECROSIS OF THE JAW (NOVEMBER 2009) AND INTRAVENOUS BISPHOSPHONATES: OSTEONECROSIS OF THE JAW—FURTHER MEASURES TO MINIMISE RISK (JULY 2015)

The risk of osteonecrosis of the jaw is substantially greater for patients receiving intravenous bisphosphonates in the treatment of cancer than for patients receiving oral bisphosphonates for osteoporosis or Paget's disease.

Risk factors for developing osteonecrosis of the jaw that should be considered are: potency of bisphosphonate (highest for zoledronate), route of administration, cumulative dose, duration and type of malignant disease, concomitant treatment, smoking, comorbid conditions, and history of dental disease.

All patients with cancer and patients with poor dental status should have a dental check-up (and any necessary remedial work should be performed) before bisphosphonate treatment, or as soon as possible after starting treatment. Patients should also maintain good oral hygiene, receive routine dental check-ups, and report any oral symptoms such as dental mobility, pain, or swelling, non-healing sores or discharge to a doctor and dentist during treatment.

Before prescribing an intravenous bisphosphonate, patients should be given a patient reminder card and informed of the risk of osteonecrosis of the jaw. Advise patients to tell their doctor if they have any problems with their mouth or teeth before starting treatment, and if the patient wears dentures, they should make sure their dentures fit properly. Patients should tell their doctor and dentist that they are receiving an intravenous bisphosphonate if they need dental treatment or dental surgery.

Guidance for dentists in primary care is included in *Oral Health Management of Patients Prescribed Bisphosphonates: Dental Clinical Guidance*, Scottish Dental Clinical Effectiveness Programme, April 2011 (available at www.sdcep.org.uk).

MHRA/CHM ADVICE: BISPHOSPHONATES: OSTEONECROSIS OF THE EXTERNAL AUDITORY CANAL (DECEMBER 2015)

Benign idiopathic osteonecrosis of the external auditory canal has been reported very rarely with bisphosphonate treatment, mainly in patients receiving long-term therapy (2 years or longer).

The possibility of osteonecrosis of the external auditory canal should be considered in patients receiving bisphosphonates who present with ear symptoms, including chronic ear infections, or suspected cholesteatoma.

Risk factors for developing osteonecrosis of the external auditory canal include: steroid use, chemotherapy, infection, an ear operation, or cotton-bud use.

Patients should be advised to report any ear pain, discharge from the ear, or an ear infection during treatment with a bisphosphonate.

- **SIDE-EFFECTS**
  - **Common or very common** Alopecia · anaemia · arthralgia · asthenia · constipation · diarrhoea · dizziness · dysphagia · electrolyte imbalance · eye inflammation · fever · gastritis · gastrointestinal discomfort · headache · influenza like illness · malaise · myalgia · nausea · oesophageal ulcer (discontinue) · oesophagitis (discontinue) · pain · peripheral oedema · renal impairment · skin reactions · taste altered · vomiting
  - **Uncommon** Anaphylactic reaction · angioedema · bronchospasm · oesophageal stenosis (discontinue) · osteonecrosis
  - **Rare or very rare** Atypical femur fracture · Stevens-Johnson syndrome
- **PATIENT AND CARER ADVICE**

Atypical femoral fractures Patients should be advised to report any thigh, hip, or groin pain during treatment with a bisphosphonate.

Osteonecrosis of the jaw During bisphosphonate treatment patients should maintain good oral hygiene, receive routine dental check-ups, and report any oral symptoms.

Osteonecrosis of the external auditory canal Patients should be advised to report any ear pain, discharge from ear or an ear infection during treatment with a bisphosphonate.

above

Alendronic acid

20-Mar-2020

(Alendronate)

- **INDICATIONS AND DOSE**

Osteoporosis (due to osteogenesis imperfecta and other causes) (initiated under specialist supervision) | Hypercalcaemia (initiated under specialist supervision)

- BY MOUTH
  - Child: (consult local protocol)

- **UNLICENSED USE** Not licensed for use in children.
- **CONTRA-INDICATIONS** Abnormalities of oesophagus · hypocalcaemia · other factors which delay emptying (e.g. stricture or achalasia)
- **CAUTIONS** Active gastro-intestinal bleeding · atypical femoral fractures · duodenitis · dysphagia · exclude other causes of osteoporosis · gastritis · history (within 1 year) of ulcers · surgery of the upper gastro-intestinal tract ·

symptomatic oesophageal disease · ulcers · upper gastro-intestinal disorders

- **INTERACTIONS** → Appendix 1: bisphosphonates
- **SIDE-EFFECTS**
- ▶ **Common or very common** Gastrointestinal disorders · joint swelling · vertigo
- ▶ **Uncommon** Haemorrhage
- ▶ **Rare or very rare** Femoral stress fracture · oropharyngeal ulceration · photosensitivity reaction · severe cutaneous adverse reactions (SCARs)

SIDE-EFFECTS, FURTHER INFORMATION Severe oesophageal reactions (oesophagitis, oesophageal ulcers, oesophageal stricture and oesophageal erosions) have been reported; patients should be advised to stop taking the tablets and to seek medical attention if they develop symptoms of oesophageal irritation such as dysphagia, new or worsening heartburn, pain on swallowing or retrosternal pain.

- **PREGNANCY** Avoid.
- **BREAST FEEDING** Manufacturer advises avoid—no information available.
- **RENAL IMPAIRMENT** Avoid if estimated glomerular filtration rate is less than 35 mL/minute/1.73 m^2.
- **MONITORING REQUIREMENTS** Correct disturbances of calcium and mineral metabolism (e.g. vitamin-D deficiency, hypocalcaemia) before starting treatment. Monitor serum-calcium concentration during treatment.
- **DIRECTIONS FOR ADMINISTRATION** Tablets should be swallowed whole and oral solution should be swallowed as a single 100 mL dose. Doses should be taken with plenty of water while sitting or standing, on an empty stomach at least 30 minutes before breakfast (or another oral medicine); patient should stand or sit upright for at least 30 minutes after administration.
- **PATIENT AND CARER ADVICE** Patients or their carers should be given advice on how to administer alendronic acid tablets and oral solution.

Oesophageal reactions Patients (or their carers) should be advised to stop taking alendronic acid and to seek medical attention if they develop symptoms of oesophageal irritation such as dysphagia, new or worsening heartburn, pain on swallowing or retrosternal pain.

- **MEDICINAL FORMS** There can be variation in the licensing of different medicines containing the same drug. Forms available from special-order manufacturers include: oral solution

Oral solution

- ▶ Alendronic acid (Non-proprietary)

Alendronic acid 700 microgram per 1 ml Alendronic acid 70mg/100ml oral solution unit dose sugar free sugar-free | 4 unit dose PoM £28.58 DT = £28.58

Effervescent tablet

- ▶ Binosto (Internis Pharmaceuticals Ltd)

Alendronic acid (as Alendronate sodium) 70 mg Binosto 70mg effervescent tablets sugar-free | 4 tablet PoM £22.80 DT = £22.80

Tablet

- ▶ Alendronic acid (Non-proprietary)

Alendronic acid (as Alendronate sodium) 10 mg Alendronic acid 10mg tablets | 28 tablet PoM £7.00 DT = £2.61

Alendronic acid (as Alendronate sodium) 70 mg Alendronic acid 70mg tablets | 4 tablet PoM £22.80 DT = £0.92

- ▶ Fosamax Once Weekly (Merck Sharp & Dohme Ltd)

Alendronic acid (as Alendronate sodium) 70 mg Fosamax Once Weekly 70mg tablets | 4 tablet PoM £22.80 DT = £0.92

505

Pamidronate disodium

23-Mar-2020

(Formerly called aminohydroxypropylidenediphosphonate disodium (APD))

- **INDICATIONS AND DOSE**

Osteoporosis (due to osteogenesis imperfecta and other causes) (specialist use only) | Hypercalcaemia (specialist use only)

▶ BY INTRAVENOUS INFUSION

▶ Child: (consult product literature)

- **UNLICENSED USE** Not licensed for use in children.
- **CAUTIONS** Atypical femoral fractures · cardiac disease · ensure adequate hydration · previous thyroid surgery (risk of hypocalcaemia)
- **INTERACTIONS** → Appendix 1: bisphosphonates
- **SIDE-EFFECTS**
- ▶ **Common or very common** Appetite decreased · chills · decreased leucocytes · drowsiness · flushing · hypertension · insomnia · paraesthesia · tetany · thrombocytopenia
- ▶ **Uncommon** Agitation · dyspnoea · hypotension · muscle cramps · seizure
- ▶ **Rare or very rare** Confusion · glomerulonephritis · haematuria · heart failure · nephritis tubulointerstitial · nephrotic syndrome · oedema · pulmonary oedema · reactivation of infections · renal disorder exacerbated · renal tubular disorder · respiratory disorders · visual hallucinations · xanthopsia
- ▶ **Frequency not known** Atrial fibrillation
- **PREGNANCY** Avoid—toxicity in *animal* studies.
- **BREAST FEEDING** Avoid.
- **HEPATIC IMPAIRMENT** Manufacturer advises caution in severe hepatic impairment (no information available).
- **RENAL IMPAIRMENT**

Monitoring Monitor renal function in renal disease or predisposition to renal impairment (e.g. in tumour-induced hypercalcaemia).

- **DIRECTIONS FOR ADMINISTRATION** For *slow intravenous infusion* (*Pamidronate disodium*, Hospira, Medac, Wockhardt), give intermittently in Glucose 5% or Sodium chloride 0.9%; give at a rate not exceeding 1 mg/minute; not to be given with infusion fluids containing calcium. For *Pamidronate disodium* (Medac, Hospira, Wockhardt) dilute with infusion fluid to a concentration of not more than 90 mg in 250 mL.
- **PATIENT AND CARER ADVICE** A patient reminder card should be provided (risk of osteonecrosis of the jaw).

Driving and skilled tasks Patients should be warned against performing skilled tasks (e.g. cycling, driving or operating machinery) immediately after treatment (somnolence or dizziness can occur).

- **MEDICINAL FORMS** There can be variation in the licensing of different medicines containing the same drug.

Solution for infusion

- ▶ Pamidronate disodium (Non-proprietary)

Pamidronate disodium 3 mg per 1 ml Pamidronate disodium 15mg/5ml solution for infusion vials | 1 vial PoM £27.50 (Hospital only) | 5 vial PoM £149.15 (Hospital only)

Pamidronate disodium 30mg/10ml solution for infusion vials | 1 vial PoM £55.00–£59.66 (Hospital only)

Pamidronate disodium 60mg/20ml solution for infusion vials | 1 vial PoM £110.00 (Hospital only)

Pamidronate disodium 90mg/30ml solution for infusion vials | 1 vial PoM £165.00 (Hospital only)

Pamidronate disodium 9 mg per 1 ml Pamidronate disodium 90mg/10ml solution for infusion vials | 1 vial PoM £170.45 (Hospital only)

Pamidronate disodium 15 mg per 1 ml Pamidronate disodium 60mg/4ml solution for infusion ampoules | 1 ampoule PoM £119.32
Pamidronate disodium 15mg/1ml solution for infusion ampoules | 4 ampoule PoM £119.32
Pamidronate disodium 90mg/6ml solution for infusion ampoules | 1 ampoule PoM £170.46
Pamidronate disodium 30mg/2ml solution for infusion ampoules | 2 ampoule PoM £119.32

F 505

Risedronate sodium

23-Mar-2020

- **INDICATIONS AND DOSE**

Osteoporosis (due to osteogenesis imperfecta and other causes) (specialist use only) | Hypercalcaemia (specialist use only)
- BY MOUTH
- Child: (consult local protocol)

- **UNLICENSED USE** Not licensed for use in children.
- **CONTRA-INDICATIONS** Hypocalcaemia
- **CAUTIONS** Atypical femoral fractures · oesophageal abnormalities · other factors which delay transit or emptying (e.g. stricture or achalasia) · upper gastro-intestinal disorders
- **INTERACTIONS** → Appendix 1: bisphosphonates
- **SIDE-EFFECTS**
  - **Uncommon** Gastrointestinal disorders
  - **Rare or very rare** Glossitis
  - **Frequency not known** Amblyopia · apnoea · chest pain · corneal lesion · dry eye · hypersensitivity · hypersensitivity vasculitis · increased risk of infection · leg cramps · liver disorder · muscle weakness · neoplasms · nocturia · tinnitus · toxic epidermal necrolysis · weight decreased
- **PREGNANCY** Avoid.
- **BREAST FEEDING** Avoid.
- **RENAL IMPAIRMENT** Avoid if estimated glomerular filtration rate is less than 30 mL/minute/1.73 m^2.
- **MONITORING REQUIREMENTS**
  - Correct hypocalcaemia before starting.
  - Correct other disturbances of bone and mineral metabolism (e.g. vitamin-D deficiency) at onset of treatment.
- **DIRECTIONS FOR ADMINISTRATION** Swallow tablets whole with full glass of water; on rising, take on an empty stomach at least 30 minutes before first food or drink of the day **or**, if taking at any other time of the day, avoid food and drink for at least 2 hours before or after risedronate (particularly avoid calcium-containing products e.g. milk; also avoid iron and mineral supplements and antacids); stand or sit upright for at least 30 minutes; do not take tablets at bedtime or before rising.
- **PATIENT AND CARER ADVICE** Patients or carers should be given advice on how to administer risedronate sodium tablets.
  Oesophageal reactions Patients should be advised to stop taking the tablets and seek medical attention if they develop symptoms of oesophageal irritation such as dysphagia, pain on swallowing, retrosternal pain, or heartburn.
  Medicines for Children leaflet: Risedronate for brittle bones www.medicinesforchildren.org.uk/risedronate-brittle-bones

- **MEDICINAL FORMS** There can be variation in the licensing of different medicines containing the same drug. Forms available from special-order manufacturers include: oral suspension, oral solution

Tablet
- Risedronate sodium (Non-proprietary)
  Risedronate sodium 5 mg Risedronate sodium 5mg tablets | 28 tablet PoM £24.78 DT = £18.88
  Risedronate sodium 30 mg Risedronate sodium 30mg tablets | 28 tablet PoM £155.28 DT = £155.28
  Risedronate sodium 35 mg Risedronate sodium 35mg tablets | 4 tablet PoM £19.12 DT = £9.95
- Actonel (Warner Chilcott UK Ltd, Teva UK Ltd)
  Risedronate sodium 5 mg Actonel 5mg tablets | 28 tablet PoM £17.99 DT = £18.88
  Risedronate sodium 30 mg Actonel 30mg tablets | 28 tablet PoM £143.95 DT = £155.28
  Risedronate sodium 35 mg Actonel Once a Week 35mg tablets | 4 tablet PoM £19.12 DT = £9.95
  Actonel 35mg tablets | 4 tablet PoM ☒ DT = £9.95

F 505

Sodium clodronate

24-Mar-2020

- **INDICATIONS AND DOSE**

Osteoporosis (due to osteogenesis imperfecta or other causes) (specialist use only) | Hypercalcaemia (specialist use only)
- BY MOUTH
- Child: (consult local protocol)

- **UNLICENSED USE** Not licensed for use in children.
- **CONTRA-INDICATIONS** Acute severe gastro-intestinal inflammatory conditions
- **CAUTIONS** Atypical femoral fractures · maintain adequate fluid intake during treatment · upper gastro-intestinal disorders
- **INTERACTIONS** → Appendix 1: bisphosphonates
- **SIDE-EFFECTS** Proteinuria · respiratory disorder
- **PREGNANCY** Avoid.
- **BREAST FEEDING** Manufacturer advises avoid—no information available.
- **RENAL IMPAIRMENT** Avoid if estimated glomerular filtration rate less than 10 mL/minute/1.73 m^2.
  Dose adjustments Reduce dose if estimated glomerular filtration rate 30—50 mL/minute/1.73m^2.
  Use half normal dose if estimated glomerular filtration rate 10–30 mL/minute/1.73 m^2.
- **MONITORING REQUIREMENTS** Monitor renal function, serum calcium and serum phosphate before and during treatment.
- **DIRECTIONS FOR ADMINISTRATION** Avoid food for 2 hours before and 1 hour after treatment, particularly calcium-containing products e.g. milk; also avoid iron and mineral supplements and antacids; maintain adequate fluid intake.
- **PATIENT AND CARER ADVICE** Patients or carers should be given advice on how to administer sodium clodronate capsules and tablets.

- **MEDICINAL FORMS** There can be variation in the licensing of different medicines containing the same drug.

Tablet

CAUTIONARY AND ADVISORY LABELS 10
- Bonefos (Bayer Plc)
  Sodium clodronate 800 mg Bonefos 800mg tablets | 60 tablet PoM £146.43 DT = £146.43
- Clasteon (Kent Pharmaceuticals Ltd)
  Sodium clodronate 800 mg Clasteon 800mg tablets | 60 tablet PoM £146.43 DT = £146.43
- Loron (Intrapharm Laboratories Ltd)
  Sodium clodronate 520 mg Loron 520mg tablets | 60 tablet PoM £114.44 DT = £114.44

Capsule
- Sodium clodronate (Non-proprietary)
  Sodium clodronate 400 mg Sodium clodronate 400mg capsules | 30 capsule PoM £34.96 | 120 capsule PoM £139.83 DT = £139.83
- Bonefos (Bayer Plc)
  Sodium clodronate 400 mg Bonefos 400mg capsules | 120 capsule PoM £139.83 DT = £139.83
- Clasteon (Kent Pharmaceuticals Ltd)
  Sodium clodronate 400 mg Clasteon 400mg capsules | 30 capsule PoM £34.96 | 120 capsule PoM £139.83 DT = £139.83

CALCIUM REGULATING DRUGS > BONE RESORPTION INHIBITORS

Calcitonin (salmon) (Salcatonin)

21-Jan-2020

● **INDICATIONS AND DOSE**

Hypercalcaemia (limited experience in children) (specialist use only)

▸ BY SUBCUTANEOUS INJECTION, OR BY INTRAMUSCULAR INJECTION

▸ Child: 2.5–5 units/kg every 12 hours (max. per dose 400 units every 6–8 hours), adjusted according to response, no additional benefit with doses over 8 units/kg every 6 hours

▸ BY INTRAVENOUS INFUSION

▸ Child: 5–10 units/kg, to be administered by slow intravenous infusion over at least 6 hours

Osteoporosis (specialist use only)

▸ BY INTRAMUSCULAR INJECTION, OR BY SUBCUTANEOUS INJECTION

▸ Child: Refer for specialist advice, experience very limited

● **UNLICENSED USE** Not licensed in children.

● **CONTRA-INDICATIONS** Hypocalcaemia

● **CAUTIONS** History of allergy (skin test advised) · risk of malignancy—avoid prolonged use (use lowest effective dose for shortest possible time)

● **INTERACTIONS** → Appendix 1: calcitonins

● **SIDE-EFFECTS**

▸ **Common or very common** Abdominal pain · arthralgia · diarrhoea · dizziness · fatigue · flushing · headache · musculoskeletal pain · nausea · secondary malignancy (long term use) · taste altered · vomiting

▸ **Uncommon** Hypersensitivity · hypertension · influenza like illness · oedema · polyuria · skin reactions · visual impairment

▸ **Rare or very rare** Bronchospasm · throat swelling · tongue swelling

▸ **Frequency not known** Hypocalcaemia · tremor

● **PREGNANCY** Avoid unless potential benefit outweighs risk (toxicity in *animal* studies).

● **BREAST FEEDING** Avoid; inhibits lactation in *animals*.

● **RENAL IMPAIRMENT** Use with caution.

● **MONITORING REQUIREMENTS** Monitor bone growth.

● **DIRECTIONS FOR ADMINISTRATION**

▸ With intravenous use For *intravenous infusion*, dilute injection solution (e.g. 400 units in 500 mL) with Sodium Chloride 0.9% and give over at least 6 hours; glass or hard plastic containers should not be used; some loss of potency on dilution and administration—use diluted solution without delay.

● **MEDICINAL FORMS** There can be variation in the licensing of different medicines containing the same drug.

Solution for injection

▸ Calcitonin (salmon) (Non-proprietary)

Calcitonin (salmon) 50 unit per 1 ml Calcitonin (salmon) 50units/1ml solution for injection ampoules | 5 ampoule PoM £167.50 DT = £167.50

Calcitonin (salmon) 100 unit per 1 ml Calcitonin (salmon) 100units/1ml solution for injection ampoules | 5 ampoule PoM £220.00 DT = £220.00

Calcitonin (salmon) 200 unit per 1 ml Calcitonin (salmon) 400units/2ml solution for injection vials | 1 vial PoM £352.00 DT = £352.00

DRUGS AFFECTING BONE STRUCTURE AND MINERALISATION > MONOCLONAL ANTIBODIES

Denosumab

27-Apr-2020

● **DRUG ACTION** Denosumab is a human monoclonal antibody that inhibits osteoclast formation, function, and survival, thereby decreasing bone resorption.

● **INDICATIONS AND DOSE**

XGEVA®

Giant cell tumour of bone that is unresectable or where surgical resection is likely to result in severe morbidity in skeletally mature adolescents

▸ BY SUBCUTANEOUS INJECTION

▸ Child: 120 mg every 4 weeks, give additional dose on days 8 and 15 of the first month of treatment only, supplementation of at least calcium 500 mg and Vitamin D 400 units daily should also be taken unless hypercalcaemia is present, to be administered into the thigh, abdomen or upper arm

IMPORTANT SAFETY INFORMATION

MHRA/CHM ADVICE: DENOSUMAB: ATYPICAL FEMORAL FRACTURES (FEBRUARY 2013)

Atypical femoral fractures have been reported rarely in patients receiving denosumab for the long-term treatment (2.5 or more years) of postmenopausal osteoporosis.

Patients should be advised to report any new or unusual thigh, hip, or groin pain during treatment with denosumab.

Discontinuation of denosumab in patients suspected to have an atypical femoral fracture should be considered after an assessment of the benefits and risks of continued treatment.

MHRA/CHM ADVICE: DENOSUMAB: MINIMISING THE RISK OF OSTEONECROSIS OF THE JAW; MONITORING FOR HYPOCALCAEMIA—UPDATED RECOMMENDATIONS (SEPTEMBER 2014) AND DENOSUMAB: OSTEONECROSIS OF THE JAW—FURTHER MEASURES TO MINIMISE RISK (JULY 2015)

Denosumab is associated with a risk of osteonecrosis of the jaw (ONJ) and with a risk of hypocalcaemia.

Osteonecrosis of the jaw Osteonecrosis of the jaw is a well-known and common side-effect in patients receiving denosumab 120 mg for cancer. Risk factors include smoking, poor oral hygiene, invasive dental procedures (including tooth extractions, dental implants, oral surgery), comorbidity (including dental disease, anaemia, coagulopathy, infection), advanced cancer, previous treatment with bisphosphonates, and concomitant treatments (including chemotherapy, anti-angiogenic biologics, corticosteroids, and radiotherapy to head and neck). The following precautions are now recommended to reduce the risk of ONJ:

Denosumab 120 mg (cancer indication)

- A dental examination and appropriate preventative dentistry before starting treatment are now recommended for all patients
- Do not start denosumab in patients with a dental or jaw condition requiring surgery, or in patients who have unhealed lesions from dental or oral surgery

All patients should be given a patient reminder card and informed of the risk of ONJ. Advise patients to tell their doctor if they have any problems with their mouth or teeth before starting treatment, if they wear dentures they should make sure their dentures fit properly before starting treatment, to maintain good oral hygiene, receive routine dental check-ups during treatment, and immediately report any oral symptoms such as dental mobility, pain, swelling, non-healing sores or discharge to a doctor and dentist. Patients should tell their doctor and dentist that they are receiving denosumab if they need dental treatment or dental surgery.

Hypocalcaemia Denosumab is associated with a risk of hypocalcaemia. This risk increases with the degree of renal impairment. Hypocalcaemia usually occurs in the first weeks of denosumab treatment, but it can also occur later in treatment.

Plasma-calcium concentration monitoring is recommended for denosumab 120 mg (cancer indication):

- before the first dose
- within two weeks after the initial dose
- if suspected symptoms of hypocalcaemia occur
- consider monitoring more frequently in patients with risk factors for hypocalcaemia (e.g. severe renal impairment, creatinine clearance less than 30 mL/minute)

All patients should be advised to report symptoms of hypocalcaemia to their doctor (e.g. muscle spasms, twitches, cramps, numbness or tingling in the fingers, toes, or around the mouth).

MHRA/CHM ADVICE: DENOSUMAB: REPORTS OF OSTEONECROSIS OF THE EXTERNAL AUDITORY CANAL (JUNE 2017)

Osteonecrosis of the external auditory canal has been reported with denosumab and this should be considered in patients who present with ear symptoms including chronic ear infections or in those with suspected cholesteatoma. Possible risk factors include steroid use and chemotherapy, with or without local risk factors such as infection or trauma. The MHRA recommends advising patients to report any ear pain, discharge from the ear, or an ear infection during denosumab treatment.

MHRA/CHM ADVICE: DENOSUMAB (*XGEVA*®) FOR GIANT CELL TUMOUR OF BONE: RISK OF CLINICALLY SIGNIFICANT HYPERCALCAEMIA FOLLOWING DISCONTINUATION (JUNE 2018)

Cases of clinically significant hypercalcaemia (rebound hypercalcaemia) have been reported up to 9 months after discontinuation of denosumab treatment for giant cell tumour of bone. The MHRA recommends that prescribers should monitor patients for signs and symptoms of hypercalcaemia after discontinuation, consider periodic assessment of serum calcium, re-evaluate the patient's calcium and vitamin D supplementation requirements, and advise patients to report symptoms of hypercalcaemia.

Denosumab is not recommended in patients with growing skeletons.

- **CONTRA-INDICATIONS** Hypocalcaemia

  XGEVA® Unhealed lesions from dental or oral surgery
- **CAUTIONS** Risk factors for osteonecrosis of the external auditory canal · risk factors for osteonecrosis of the jaw—consider temporary interruption of denosumab if occurs during treatment
- **SIDE-EFFECTS**
  - **Common or very common** Abdominal discomfort · cataract · constipation · hypocalcaemia (including fatal cases) · increased risk of infection · pain · sciatica · second primary malignancy · skin reactions
  - **Uncommon** Cellulitis (seek prompt medical attention) · hypercalcaemia (on discontinuation)
  - **Rare or very rare** Atypical femur fracture · hypersensitivity · osteonecrosis
- **CONCEPTION AND CONTRACEPTION** Ensure effective contraception in women of child-bearing potential, during treatment and for at least 5 months after stopping treatment.
- **PREGNANCY** Manufacturer advises avoid—toxicity in *animal* studies; risk of toxicity increases with each trimester.
- **BREAST FEEDING** Manufacturer advises avoid.
- **RENAL IMPAIRMENT** Increased risk of hypocalcaemia if creatinine clearance less than 30 mL/minute.
- **MONITORING REQUIREMENTS** Correct hypocalcaemia and vitamin D deficiency before starting. Monitor plasma-calcium concentration during therapy.
- **PATIENT AND CARER ADVICE**

  Atypical femoral fractures Patients should be advised to report any new or unusual thigh, hip, or groin pain during treatment with denosumab.

  Osteonecrosis of the jaw All patients should be informed to maintain good oral hygiene, receive routine dental check-ups, and immediately report any oral symptoms such as dental mobility, pain, or swelling to a doctor and dentist.

  Hypocalcaemia All patients should be advised to report symptoms of hypocalcaemia to their doctor (e.g. muscle spasms, twitches, cramps, numbness or tingling in the fingers, toes, or around the mouth).

  Patient reminder card A patient reminder card should be provided (risk of osteonecrosis of the jaw).
- **MEDICINAL FORMS** There can be variation in the licensing of different medicines containing the same drug.

Solution for injection

CAUTIONARY AND ADVISORY LABELS 10

EXCIPIENTS: May contain Sorbitol

- Xgeva (Amgen Ltd)

  Denosumab 70 mg per 1 ml Xgeva 120mg/1.7ml solution for injection vials | 1 vial PoM £309.86 DT = £309.86

5 Gonadotrophin responsive conditions

PITUITARY AND HYPOTHALAMIC HORMONES AND ANALOGUES > GONADOTROPHIN-RELEASING HORMONES

Goserelin

- **DRUG ACTION** Administration of gonadorelin analogues produces an initial phase of stimulation; continued administration is followed by down-regulation of gonadotrophin-releasing hormone receptors, thereby reducing the release of gonadotrophins (follicle stimulating hormone and luteinising hormone) which in turn leads to inhibition of androgen and oestrogen production.

- **INDICATIONS AND DOSE**

ZOLADEX LA®

Gonadotrophin-dependent precocious puberty

- BY SUBCUTANEOUS INJECTION
- Child: 10.8 mg every 12 weeks, to be administered into the anterior abdominal wall, injections may be required more frequently in some cases

ZOLADEX®

Gonadotrophin-dependent precocious puberty

- BY SUBCUTANEOUS INJECTION
- Child: 3.6 mg every 28 days, to be administered into the anterior abdominal wall, injections may be required more frequently in some cases

- **UNLICENSED USE** Not licensed for use in children.
- **CONTRA-INDICATIONS** Undiagnosed vaginal bleeding
- **CAUTIONS** Depression · patients with metabolic bone disease (decrease in bone mineral density can occur)
- **SIDE-EFFECTS** Asthma · body hair change · breast abnormalities · depression · headache · hypersensitivity · mood altered · ovarian cyst · paraesthesia · skin reactions ·

vaginal haemorrhage · visual impairment · weight change · withdrawal bleed

- **CONCEPTION AND CONTRACEPTION** Non-hormonal, barrier methods of contraception should be used during entire treatment period. Pregnancy should be excluded before treatment, the first injection should be given during menstruation or shortly afterwards or use barrier contraception for 1 month beforehand.
- **PREGNANCY** Avoid.
- **BREAST FEEDING** Avoid.
- **MONITORING REQUIREMENTS** Monitor bone mineral density.
- **DIRECTIONS FOR ADMINISTRATION** Rotate injection site to prevent atrophy and nodule formation.

- **MEDICINAL FORMS** There can be variation in the licensing of different medicines containing the same drug.

Implant

- ▶ Zoladex (AstraZeneca UK Ltd)
  Goserelin (as Goserelin acetate) 3.6 mg Zoladex 3.6mg implant SafeSystem pre-filled syringes | 1 pre-filled disposable injection PoM £70.00 DT = £70.00
- ▶ Zoladex LA (AstraZeneca UK Ltd)
  Goserelin (as Goserelin acetate) 10.8 mg Zoladex LA 10.8mg implant SafeSystem pre-filled syringes | 1 pre-filled disposable injection PoM £235.00 DT = £235.00

Leuprorelin acetate

26-May-2020

- **DRUG ACTION** Administration of gonadorelin analogues produces an initial phase of stimulation; continued administration is followed by down-regulation of gonadotrophin-releasing hormone receptors, thereby reducing the release of gonadotrophins (follicle stimulating hormone and luteinising hormone) which in turn leads to inhibition of androgen and oestrogen production.

- **INDICATIONS AND DOSE**

PROSTAP 3 DCS®

Gonadotrophin-dependent precocious puberty (specialist use only)

▶ BY SUBCUTANEOUS INJECTION

- ▶ Child (body-weight up to 19 kg): 5.625 mg every 3 months, dose may be increased if necessary. Discontinue when bone maturation consistent with age of 12 years in girls or 13 years in boys
- ▶ Child (body-weight 20 kg and above): 11.25 mg every 3 months, dose may be increased if necessary. Discontinue when bone maturation consistent with age of 12 years in girls or 13 years in boys

PROSTAP SR DCS®

Gonadotrophin-dependent precocious puberty (specialist use only)

▶ BY SUBCUTANEOUS INJECTION

- ▶ Child (body-weight up to 19 kg): 1.88 mg every month, dose may be increased if necessary. Discontinue when bone maturation consistent with age of 12 years in girls or 13 years in boys
- ▶ Child (body-weight 20 kg and above): 3.75 mg every month, dose may be increased if necessary. Discontinue when bone maturation consistent with age of 12 years in girls or 13 years in boys

- **CONTRA-INDICATIONS** Undiagnosed vaginal bleeding
- **CAUTIONS** Patients with metabolic bone disease (decrease in bone mineral density can occur)
- **SIDE-EFFECTS**

▶ **Common or very common** Acne · emotional lability · gastrointestinal discomfort · haemorrhage · headache · metrorrhagia · nausea · vaginal discharge · vomiting

▶ **Frequency not known** Interstitial lung disease · seizure

- **PREGNANCY** Avoid—teratogenic in *animal* studies.
- **BREAST FEEDING** Avoid.
- **MONITORING REQUIREMENTS** Monitor bone mineral density.
- **DIRECTIONS FOR ADMINISTRATION** Rotate injection site to prevent atrophy and nodule formation.

- **MEDICINAL FORMS** There can be variation in the licensing of different medicines containing the same drug.

Powder and solvent for suspension for injection

- ▶ Prostap 3 DCS (Takeda UK Ltd)
  Leuprorelin acetate 11.25 mg Prostap 3 DCS 11.25mg powder and solvent for suspension for injection pre-filled syringes | 1 pre-filled disposable injection PoM £225.72 DT = £225.72
- ▶ Prostap SR DCS (Takeda UK Ltd)
  Leuprorelin acetate 3.75 mg Prostap SR DCS 3.75mg powder and solvent for suspension for injection pre-filled syringes | 1 pre-filled disposable injection PoM £75.24 DT = £75.24

Triptorelin

26-Nov-2019

- **DRUG ACTION** Administration of gonadorelin analogues produces an initial phase of stimulation; continued administration is followed by down-regulation of gonadotrophin-releasing hormone receptors, thereby reducing the release of gonadotrophins (follicle stimulating hormone and luteinising hormone) which in turn leads to inhibition of androgen and oestrogen production.

- **INDICATIONS AND DOSE**

DECAPEPTYL® SR 11.25MG

Gonadotrophin-dependent precocious puberty (specialist use only)

▶ BY INTRAMUSCULAR INJECTION

- ▶ Child: 11.25 mg every 3 months, discontinue when bone maturation consistent with age of 12 years in girls or 13–14 years in boys

DECAPEPTYL® SR 22.5MG

Gonadotrophin-dependent precocious puberty (specialist use only)

▶ BY INTRAMUSCULAR INJECTION

- ▶ Child: 22.5 mg every 6 months, discontinue when bone maturation consistent with age of 12–13 years in girls or 13–14 years in boys

GONAPEPTYL DEPOT®

Gonadotrophin-dependent precocious puberty

▶ BY SUBCUTANEOUS INJECTION, OR BY DEEP INTRAMUSCULAR INJECTION

- ▶ Child (body-weight up to 20 kg): Initially 1.875 mg every 2 weeks for 3 doses, to be administered on days 0, 14, and 28 of treatment, then 1.875 mg every 3–4 weeks, discontinue when bone maturation consistent with age over 12 years in girls and over 13 years in boys
- ▶ Child (body-weight 20-30 kg): Initially 2.5 mg every 2 weeks for 3 doses, to be administered on days 0, 14, and 28 of treatment, then 2.5 mg every 3–4 weeks, discontinue when bone maturation consistent with age over 12 years in girls and over 13 years in boys
- ▶ Child (body-weight 31 kg and above): Initially 3.75 mg every 2 weeks for 3 doses, to be administered on days 0, 14, and 28 of treatment, then 3.75 mg every 3–4 weeks, discontinue when bone maturation consistent with age over 12 years in girls and over 13 years in boys

- **CONTRA-INDICATIONS** Undiagnosed vaginal bleeding
- **SIDE-EFFECTS**

▶ **Common or very common** Depression · mood altered

▶ **Uncommon** Anaphylactic reaction · haemorrhage · nausea · vaginal discharge · vomiting

▸ **Frequency not known** Alopecia · angioedema · epiphysiolysis · gastrointestinal discomfort · headache · hot flush · malaise · myalgia · nervousness · pain · skin reactions · vision disorders · weight increased

- **CONCEPTION AND CONTRACEPTION** Non-hormonal, barrier methods of contraception should be used during entire treatment period. Pregnancy should be excluded before treatment, the first injection should be given during menstruation or shortly afterwards or use barrier contraception for 1 month beforehand.
- **PREGNANCY** Avoid.
- **BREAST FEEDING** Avoid.
- **MONITORING REQUIREMENTS** Monitor bone mineral density.
- **DIRECTIONS FOR ADMINISTRATION** Rotate injection site to prevent atrophy and nodule formation.
- **PRESCRIBING AND DISPENSING INFORMATION**
  DECAPEPTYL® SR 22.5MG Each vial includes an overage to allow accurate administration of a 22.5 mg dose.
  DECAPEPTYL® SR 11.25MG Each vial includes an overage to allow accurate administration of an 11.25 mg dose.

- **MEDICINAL FORMS** There can be variation in the licensing of different medicines containing the same drug.

Powder and solvent for suspension for injection

▸ Decapeptyl SR (Ipsen Ltd)
Triptorelin 11.25 mg Decapeptyl SR 11.25mg powder and solvent for suspension for injection vials | 1 vial PoM £207.00 DT = £207.00
Triptorelin (as Triptorelin embonate) 22.5 mg Decapeptyl SR 22.5mg powder and solvent for suspension for injection vials | 1 vial PoM £414.00 DT = £414.00

▸ Gonapeptyl Depot (Ferring Pharmaceuticals Ltd)
Triptorelin (as Triptorelin acetate) 3.75 mg Gonapeptyl Depot 3.75mg powder and solvent for suspension for injection pre-filled syringes | 1 pre-filled disposable injection PoM £81.69 DT = £81.69

6 Hypothalamic and anterior pituitary hormone related disorders

Hypothalamic and anterior pituitary hormones

Anterior pituitary hormones

Corticotrophins

Tetracosactide below (tetracosactrin), an analogue of corticotropin (adrenocorticotrophic hormone, ACTH), is used to test adrenocortical function; failure of plasma-cortisol concentration to rise after administration of tetracosactide indicates adrenocortical insufficiency. A low-dose test is considered by some clinicians to be more sensitive when used to confirm established, partial adrenal suppression.

Tetracosactide should be given only if no other ACTH preparations have been given previously. Tetracosactide depot injection (*Synacthen Depot*®) is also used in the treatment of infantile spasms but it is contra-indicated in neonates because of the presence of benzyl alcohol in the injection. Corticotropin-releasing factor, corticorelin p. 512, (also known as corticotropin-releasing hormone, CRH) is used to test anterior pituitary function and secretion of corticotropin.

Gonadotrophins

Gonadotrophins are occasionally used in the treatment of hypogonadotrophic hypogonadism and associated oligospermia. There is no justification for their use in primary gonadal failure.

Growth hormone

Growth hormone is used to treat proven deficiency of the hormone, Prader-Willi syndrome, Turner's syndrome, growth disturbance in children born small for corrected gestational age, chronic renal insufficiency, and short stature homeobox-containing gene (SHOX) deficiency. Growth hormone is also used in Noonan syndrome and idiopathic short stature [unlicensed indications] under specialist management. Treatment should be initiated and monitored by a paediatrician with expertise in managing growth-hormone disorders; treatment can be continued under a shared-care protocol by a general practitioner.

Growth hormone of human origin (HGH; somatotrophin) has been replaced by a growth hormone of human sequence, somatropin p. 513, produced using recombinant DNA technology.

Mecasermin p. 515, a human insulin-like growth factor-I (rhIGF-I), is licensed to treat growth failure in children with severe primary insulin-like growth factor-I deficiency.

Hypothalamic hormones

Gonadorelin p. 512 when injected intravenously in post-pubertal girls leads to a rapid rise in plasma concentrations of both luteinising hormone (LH) and follicle-stimulating hormone (FSH). It has not proved to be very helpful, however, in distinguishing hypothalamic from pituitary lesions. It is used in the assessment of delayed or precocious puberty.

Other growth hormone stimulation tests involve the use of insulin, glucagon p. 502, arginine p. 662, and clonidine hydrochloride p. 108 [all unlicensed uses]. The tests should be carried out in specialist centres.

6.1 Adrenocortical function testing

PITUITARY AND HYPOTHALAMIC HORMONES AND ANALOGUES › CORTICOTROPHINS

Tetracosactide

(Tetracosactrin)

- **INDICATIONS AND DOSE**

Diagnosis of adrenocortical insufficiency (diagnostic 30-minute test), standard-dose test

▸ BY INTRAMUSCULAR INJECTION, OR BY INTRAVENOUS INJECTION
▸ Child: 145 micrograms/m^2 (max. per dose 250 micrograms) for 1 dose

Diagnosis of adrenocortical insufficiency (diagnostic 30-minute test), low-dose test

▸ BY INTRAMUSCULAR INJECTION, OR BY INTRAVENOUS INJECTION
▸ Child: 0.3 microgram/m^2 for 1 dose

Infantile spasm

▸ BY INTRAMUSCULAR INJECTION USING DEPOT INJECTION
▸ Child 1–23 months: Initially 500 micrograms once daily on alternate days, adjusted according to response

- **UNLICENSED USE** Not licensed for low-dose test for adrenocortical insufficiency. Not licensed for treatment of infantile spasms.
- **CONTRA-INDICATIONS** Acute psychosis · adrenogenital syndrome · allergic disorders · asthma · avoid injections containing benzyl alcohol in neonates · Cushing's

syndrome · infectious diseases · peptic ulcer · primary adrenocortical insufficiency · refractory heart failure

- CAUTIONS Active infectious diseases (should not be used unless adequate disease-specific therapy is being given) · active systemic diseases (should not be used unless adequate disease-specific therapy is being given) · diabetes mellitus · diverticulitis · history of asthma · history of atopic allergy · history of eczema · history of hayfever · history of hypersensitivity · hypertension · latent amoebiasis (may become activated) · latent tuberculosis (may become activated) · myasthenia gravis · ocular herpes simplex · osteoporosis · predisposition to thromboembolic · pscyhological disturbances may be triggered · recent intestinal anastomosis · reduced immune response (should not be used unless adequate disease-specific therapy is being given) · ulcerative colitis

  CAUTIONS, FURTHER INFORMATION
  - Risk of anaphylaxis Should only be administered under medical supervision. Consult product literature.
  - Hypertension Patients already receiving medication for moderate to severe hypertension must have their dosage adjusted if treatment started.
  - Diabetes mellitus Patients already receiving medication for diabetes mellitus must have their dosage adjusted if treatment started.
- SIDE-EFFECTS Abdominal distension · abscess · adrenocortical unresponsiveness · angioedema · appetite increased · bone fractures · congestive heart failure · Cushing's syndrome · diabetes mellitus exacerbated · dizziness · dyspnoea · electrolyte imbalance · exophthalmos · fluid retention · flushing · gastrointestinal disorders · glaucoma · growth retardation · haemorrhage · headache · healing impaired · hirsutism · hyperglycaemia · hyperhidrosis · hypersensitivity (may be more severe in patients susceptible to allergies, especially asthma) · hypertension · idiopathic intracranial hypertension exacerbated · increased risk of infection · leucocytosis · malaise · menstruation irregular · muscle weakness · myopathy · nausea · osteonecrosis · osteoporosis · pancreatitis · papilloedema · pituitary unresponsiveness · posterior subcapsular cataract · protein catabolism · psychiatric disorder · seizure · skin reactions · tendon rupture · thromboembolism · vasculitis necrotising · ventricular hypertrophy · vertigo · vomiting · weight increased
- ALLERGY AND CROSS-SENSITIVITY Contra-indicated in patients with history of hypersensitivity to tetracosactide/corticotrophins or excipients.
- PREGNANCY Avoid (but may be used diagnostically if essential).
- BREAST FEEDING Avoid (but may be used diagnostically if essential).
- HEPATIC IMPAIRMENT For *depot injection*, manufacturer advises caution in cirrhosis (may enhance effect of tetracosactide therapy).
- RENAL IMPAIRMENT Use with caution in patients with renal impairment.
- EFFECT ON LABORATORY TESTS May suppress skin test reactions.

  Post administration total plasma cortisol levels during 30-minute test for diagnosis of adrenocotical insufficiency might be misleading due to altered cortisol binding globulin levels in some special clinical situations including, patients on oral contraceptives, post-operative patients, critical illness, severe liver disease and nephrotic syndrome.
- DIRECTIONS FOR ADMINISTRATION For *intramuscular* or *intravenous injection*, may be diluted in sodium chloride 0.9% to 250 nanograms/mL.
- MEDICINAL FORMS There can be variation in the licensing of different medicines containing the same drug.

Solution for injection

- Synacthen (Atnahs Pharma UK Ltd)
  - **Tetracosactide acetate 250 microgram per 1 ml** Synacthen 250micrograms/1ml solution for injection ampoules | 1 ampoule [PoM] £38.00 DT = £38.00

Suspension for injection

EXCIPIENTS: May contain Benzyl alcohol

- Synacthen Depot (Atnahs Pharma UK Ltd)
  - **Tetracosactide acetate 1 mg per 1 ml** Synacthen Depot 1mg/1ml suspension for injection ampoules | 1 ampoule [PoM] £346.28 DT = £346.28

6.2 Assessment of pituitary function

DIAGNOSTIC AGENTS

Corticorelin

(Corticotrophin-releasing hormone; CRH)

- INDICATIONS AND DOSE

Test of anterior pituitary function
- BY INTRAVENOUS INJECTION
  - Child: 1 microgram/kg (max. per dose 100 micrograms) for 1 dose, to be administered over 30 seconds

- UNLICENSED USE Not licensed.
- SIDE-EFFECTS Angioedema · cardiac arrest · chest tightness · dyspnoea · flushing · hypersensitivity · hypotension · loss of consciousness · tachycardia · urticaria · wheezing
- PREGNANCY Avoid.
- BREAST FEEDING Avoid.
- MEDICINAL FORMS No licensed medicines listed.

PITUITARY AND HYPOTHALAMIC HORMONES AND ANALOGUES > GONADOTROPHIN-RELEASING HORMONES

Gonadorelin

(Gonadotrophin-releasing hormone; GnRH; LH-RH)

- INDICATIONS AND DOSE

Assessment of anterior pituitary function | Assessment of delayed puberty
- BY INTRAVENOUS INJECTION, OR BY SUBCUTANEOUS INJECTION
  - Child 1–17 years: 2.5 micrograms/kg (max. per dose 100 micrograms) for 1 dose

- CAUTIONS Pituitary adenoma
- SIDE-EFFECTS
  - **Uncommon** Pain · skin reactions · swelling
  - **Rare or very rare** Abdominal discomfort · bronchospasm · dizziness · eye erythema · flushing · headache · nausea · tachycardia
  - **Frequency not known** Menorrhagia · sepsis · thrombophlebitis
- PREGNANCY Avoid.
- BREAST FEEDING Avoid.

- **MEDICINAL FORMS** There can be variation in the licensing of different medicines containing the same drug.

Powder for solution for injection

- Gonadorelin (Non-proprietary)
  Gonadorelin (as Gonadorelin hydrochloride)
  100 microgram Gonadorelin 100microgram powder for solution for injection vials | 1 vial PoM £75.00 (Hospital only)

6.3 Growth hormone disorders

PITUITARY AND HYPOTHALAMIC HORMONES AND ANALOGUES > HUMAN GROWTH HORMONES

Somatropin

25-Jul-2018

(Recombinant Human Growth Hormone)

- **INDICATIONS AND DOSE**

Gonadal dysgenesis (Turner syndrome)

- BY SUBCUTANEOUS INJECTION
- Child: 1.4 mg/m^2 daily, alternatively 45–50 micrograms/kg daily

Deficiency of growth hormone

- BY SUBCUTANEOUS INJECTION, OR BY INTRAMUSCULAR INJECTION
- Child: 23–39 micrograms/kg daily, alternatively 0.7–1 mg/m^2 daily

Growth disturbance in children born small for gestational age whose growth has not caught up by 4 years or later | Noonan syndrome

- BY SUBCUTANEOUS INJECTION
- Child 4–17 years: 35 micrograms/kg daily, alternatively 1 mg/m^2 daily

Prader-Willi syndrome, in children with growth velocity greater than 1 cm/year, in combination with energy-restricted diet

- BY SUBCUTANEOUS INJECTION
- Child: 1 mg/m^2 daily, alternatively 35 micrograms/kg daily; maximum 2.7 mg per day

Chronic renal insufficiency (renal function decreased to less than 50%)

- BY SUBCUTANEOUS INJECTION
- Child: 45–50 micrograms/kg daily, alternatively 1.4 mg/m^2 daily, higher doses may be needed, adjust if necessary after 6 months

SHOX deficiency

- BY SUBCUTANEOUS INJECTION
- Child: 45–50 micrograms/kg daily

DOSE EQUIVALENCE AND CONVERSION

- Dose formerly expressed in units; somatropin 1 mg ≡ 3 units.

- **UNLICENSED USE** Not licensed for use in Noonan syndrome.
- **CONTRA-INDICATIONS** Avoid injections containing benzyl alcohol in neonates · evidence of tumour activity (complete antitumour therapy and ensure intracranial lesions inactive before starting) · not to be used after renal transplantation · not to be used for growth promotion in children with closed epiphyses (or near closure in Prader-Willi syndrome) · severe obesity in Prader-Willi syndrome · severe respiratory impairment in Prader-Willi syndrome
- **CAUTIONS** Diabetes mellitus (adjustment of antidiabetic therapy may be necessary) · disorders of the epiphysis of the hip (monitor for limping) · history of malignant disease · hypoadrenalism (initiation or adjustment of glucocorticoid replacement therapy may be necessary) · hypothyroidism—manufacturers recommend periodic thyroid function tests but limited evidence of clinical value · initiation of treatment close to puberty not recommended in child born small for corrected gestational age · papilloedema · relative deficiencies of other pituitary hormones · resolved intracranial hypertension (monitor closely) · Silver-Russell syndrome
- **INTERACTIONS** → Appendix 1: somatropin
- **SIDE-EFFECTS**
  - **Common or very common** Headache · lipoatrophy
  - **Uncommon** Arthralgia · carpal tunnel syndrome · fluid retention · gynaecomastia · idiopathic intracranial hypertension · musculoskeletal stiffness · myalgia · oedema · paraesthesia
  - **Rare or very rare** Hyperglycaemia · hyperinsulinism · hypothyroidism · osteonecrosis of femur · pancreatitis · slipped capital femoral epiphysis
  - **Frequency not known** Leukaemia

  SIDE-EFFECTS, FURTHER INFORMATION Funduscopy for papilloedema recommended if severe or recurrent headache, visual problems, nausea and vomiting occur—if papilloedema confirmed consider benign intracranial hypertension (rare cases reported).
- **PREGNANCY** Discontinue if pregnancy occurs—no information available.
- **BREAST FEEDING** No information available. Absorption from milk unlikely.
- **DIRECTIONS FOR ADMINISTRATION** Rotate subcutaneous injection sites to prevent lipoatrophy.

  GENOTROPIN®, NORDITROPIN®, NUTROPINAQ®, OMNITROPE®, SAIZEN®, ZOMACTON® For use by subcutaneous injection.

  HUMATROPE® Cartridges for use by subcutaneous injection. Powder for reconstitution for use by subcutaneous or intramuscular injection.
- **PRESCRIBING AND DISPENSING INFORMATION** Somatropin is a biological medicine. Biological medicines must be prescribed and dispensed by brand name, see *Biological medicines* and *Biosimilar medicines*, under Guidance on prescribing p. 1.

  SAIZEN® SOLUTION FOR INJECTION For use with *cool.click®* needle-free autoinjector device or *easypod®* autoinjector device (non-NHS but available free of charge from clinics).

  NORDITROPIN® PREPARATIONS Cartridges are for use with appropriate *NordiPen®* device (non-NHS but available free of charge from clinics).

  Multidose disposable prefilled pens for use with *NovoFine®* or *NovoTwist®* needles.

  OMNITROPE® For use with *Omnitrope Pen 5®* and *Omnitrope Pen 10®* devices (non-NHS but available free of charge from clinics).

  NUTROPINAQ® For use with *NutropinAq®* Pen device (non-NHS but available free of charge from clinics).

  ZOMACTON® 4 mg vial for use with *ZomaJet 2® Vision* needle-free device (non-NHS but available free of charge from clinics) or with needles and syringes.

  10 mg vial for use with *ZomaJet Vision X®* needle-free device (non-NHS but available free of charge from clinics) or with needles and syringes.

  SAIZEN® POWDER AND SOLVENT FOR SOLUTION FOR INJECTION For use with *one. click®* autoinjector device or *cool.click®* needle-free autoinjector device or *easypod®* autoinjector device (non-NHS but available free of charge from clinics).

  GENOTROPIN® PREPARATIONS Cartridges are for use with *Genotropin®* Pen device (non-NHS but available free of charge from clinics).

6 Endocrine system

● **NATIONAL FUNDING/ACCESS DECISIONS**

NICE decisions

▶ **Somatropin for the treatment of growth failure in children (May 2010) NICE TA188**

Somatropin is recommended for children with growth failure who:
- have growth-hormone deficiency
- have Turner syndrome
- have Prader-Willi syndrome
- have chronic renal insufficiency
- are born small for gestational age with subsequent growth failure at 4 years of age or later
- have short stature homeobox-containing gene (SHOX) deficiency.

Treatment should be discontinued if growth velocity increases by less than 50% from baseline in the first year of treatment.
www.nice.org.uk/guidance/ta188

● **MEDICINAL FORMS** There can be variation in the licensing of different medicines containing the same drug.

Solution for injection

EXCIPIENTS: May contain Benzyl alcohol

▶ **Norditropin NordiFlex** (Novo Nordisk Ltd)

Somatropin (epr) 3.3 mg per 1 ml Norditropin NordiFlex 5mg/1.5ml solution for injection pre-filled pens | 1 pre-filled disposable injection PoM £115.90 DT = £115.90 CD4-2

Somatropin (epr) 6.7 mg per 1 ml Norditropin NordiFlex 10mg/1.5ml solution for injection pre-filled pens | 1 pre-filled disposable injection PoM £231.80 DT = £231.80 CD4-2

Somatropin (epr) 10 mg per 1 ml Norditropin NordiFlex 15mg/1.5ml solution for injection pre-filled pens | 1 pre-filled disposable injection PoM £347.70 DT = £347.70 CD4-2

▶ **Norditropin SimpleXx** (Novo Nordisk Ltd)

Somatropin (epr) 3.3 mg per 1 ml Norditropin SimpleXx 5mg/1.5ml solution for injection cartridges | 1 cartridge PoM £106.35 DT = £106.35 CD4-2

Somatropin (epr) 6.7 mg per 1 ml Norditropin SimpleXx 10mg/1.5ml solution for injection cartridges | 1 cartridge PoM £212.70 DT = £212.70 CD4-2

Somatropin (epr) 10 mg per 1 ml Norditropin SimpleXx 15mg/1.5ml solution for injection cartridges | 1 cartridge PoM £319.05 DT = £319.05 CD4-2

▶ **NutropinAq** (Ipsen Ltd)

Somatropin (rbe) 5 mg per 1 ml NutropinAq 10mg/2ml solution for injection cartridges | 1 cartridge PoM £203.00 DT = £203.00 CD4-2 | 3 cartridge PoM £609.00 DT = £609.00 CD4-2

▶ **Omnitrope** (Sandoz Ltd)

Somatropin (rbe) 3.333 mg per 1 ml Omnitrope Pen 5 5mg/1.5ml solution for injection cartridges | 5 cartridge PoM £368.74 DT = £368.74 CD4-2

▶ **Omnitrope SurePal** (Sandoz Ltd)

Somatropin (rbe) 3.333 mg per 1 ml Omnitrope SurePal 5 5mg/1.5ml solution for injection cartridges | 5 cartridge PoM £368.74 DT = £368.74 CD4-2

Somatropin (rbe) 6.667 mg per 1 ml Omnitrope SurePal 10 10mg/1.5ml solution for injection cartridges | 5 cartridge PoM £737.49 DT = £737.49 CD4-2

Somatropin (rbe) 10 mg per 1 ml Omnitrope SurePal 15 15mg/1.5ml solution for injection cartridges | 5 cartridge PoM £1,106.22 DT = £1,106.22 CD4-2

▶ **Saizen** (Merck Serono Ltd)

Somatropin (rmc) 5.825 mg per 1 ml Saizen 6mg/1.03ml solution for injection cartridges | 1 cartridge PoM £139.08 DT = £139.08 CD4-2

Somatropin (rmc) 8 mg per 1 ml Saizen 12mg/1.5ml solution for injection cartridges | 1 cartridge PoM £278.16 DT = £278.16 CD4-2
Saizen 20mg/2.5ml solution for injection cartridges | 1 cartridge PoM £463.60 DT = £463.60 CD4-2

Powder and solvent for solution for injection

EXCIPIENTS: May contain Benzyl alcohol

▶ **Genotropin** (Pfizer Ltd)

Somatropin (rbe) 5.3 mg Genotropin 5.3mg powder and solvent for solution for injection cartridges | 1 cartridge PoM £92.15 DT = £92.15 CD4-2

Somatropin (rbe) 12 mg Genotropin 12mg powder and solvent for solution for injection cartridges | 1 cartridge PoM £208.65 DT = £208.65 CD4-2

▶ **Genotropin GoQuick** (Pfizer Ltd)

Somatropin (rbe) 5.3 mg Genotropin GoQuick 5.3mg powder and solvent for solution for injection pre-filled pens | 1 pre-filled disposable injection PoM £92.15 DT = £92.15 CD4-2

Somatropin (rbe) 12 mg Genotropin GoQuick 12mg powder and solvent for solution for injection pre-filled pens | 1 pre-filled disposable injection PoM £208.65 DT = £208.65 CD4-2

▶ **Genotropin MiniQuick** (Pfizer Ltd)

Somatropin (rbe) 200 microgram Genotropin MiniQuick 200microgram powder and solvent for solution for injection pre-filled disposable devices | 7 pre-filled disposable injection PoM £24.35 DT = £24.35 CD4-2

Somatropin (rbe) 400 microgram Genotropin MiniQuick 400microgram powder and solvent for solution for injection pre-filled disposable devices | 7 pre-filled disposable injection PoM £48.68 DT = £48.68 CD4-2

Somatropin (rbe) 600 microgram Genotropin MiniQuick 600microgram powder and solvent for solution for injection pre-filled disposable devices | 7 pre-filled disposable injection PoM £73.03 DT = £73.03 CD4-2

Somatropin (rbe) 800 microgram Genotropin MiniQuick 800microgram powder and solvent for solution for injection pre-filled disposable devices | 7 pre-filled disposable injection PoM £97.37 DT = £97.37 CD4-2

Somatropin (rbe) 1 mg Genotropin MiniQuick 1mg powder and solvent for solution for injection pre-filled disposable devices | 7 pre-filled disposable injection PoM £121.71 DT = £121.71 CD4-2

Somatropin (rbe) 1.2 mg Genotropin MiniQuick 1.2mg powder and solvent for solution for injection pre-filled disposable devices | 7 pre-filled disposable injection PoM £146.06 DT = £146.06 CD4-2

Somatropin (rbe) 1.4 mg Genotropin MiniQuick 1.4mg powder and solvent for solution for injection pre-filled disposable devices | 7 pre-filled disposable injection PoM £170.39 DT = £170.39 CD4-2

Somatropin (rbe) 1.6 mg Genotropin MiniQuick 1.6mg powder and solvent for solution for injection pre-filled disposable devices | 7 pre-filled disposable injection PoM £194.74 DT = £194.74 CD4-2

Somatropin (rbe) 1.8 mg Genotropin MiniQuick 1.8mg powder and solvent for solution for injection pre-filled disposable devices | 7 pre-filled disposable injection PoM £219.08 DT = £219.08 CD4-2

Somatropin (rbe) 2 mg Genotropin MiniQuick 2mg powder and solvent for solution for injection pre-filled disposable devices | 7 pre-filled disposable injection PoM £243.42 DT = £243.42 CD4-2

▶ **Humatrope** (Eli Lilly and Company Ltd)

Somatropin (rbe) 6 mg Humatrope 6mg powder and solvent for solution for injection cartridges | 1 cartridge PoM £108.00 DT = £108.00 CD4-2

Somatropin (rbe) 12 mg Humatrope 12mg powder and solvent for solution for injection cartridges | 1 cartridge PoM £216.00 DT = £208.65 CD4-2

Somatropin (rbe) 24 mg Humatrope 24mg powder and solvent for solution for injection cartridges | 1 cartridge PoM £432.00 DT = £432.00 CD4-2

▶ **Saizen** (Merck Serono Ltd)

Somatropin (rmc) 8 mg Saizen 8mg click.easy powder and solvent for solution for injection vials | 1 vial PoM £185.44 DT = £185.44 CD4-2

▶ **Zomacton** (Ferring Pharmaceuticals Ltd)

Somatropin (rbe) 4 mg Zomacton 4mg powder and solvent for solution for injection vials | 1 vial PoM £68.28 DT = £68.28 CD4-2

Somatropin (rbe) 10 mg Zomacton 10mg powder and solvent for solution for injection vials | 1 vial PoM £170.70 DT = £170.70 CD4-2

6.3a Insulin-like growth factor-I deficiency

PITUITARY AND HYPOTHALAMIC HORMONES AND ANALOGUES > SOMATOMEDINS

Mecasermin
12-Feb-2020

(Recombinant human insulin-like growth factor-I; rhIGF-I)

- **DRUG ACTION** Somatomedins are a group of polypeptide hormones structurally related to insulin and commonly known as insulin-like growth factors (IGFs). Mecasermin, a human insulin-like growth factor-I (rhIGF-I), is the principal mediator of the somatotropic effects of human growth hormone.

- **INDICATIONS AND DOSE**

Treatment of growth failure in children with severe primary insulin-like growth factor-I deficiency

▸ BY SUBCUTANEOUS INJECTION

▸ Child 2–17 years: Initially 40 micrograms/kg twice daily for 1 week, increased, if tolerated, in steps of 40 micrograms/kg (max. per dose 120 micrograms/kg twice daily), discontinue if no response within 1 year, reduce dose if hypoglycaemia occurs despite adequate food intake; withhold injection if patient unable to eat

IMPORTANT SAFETY INFORMATION

MHRA/CHM ADVICE: MECASERMIN (*INCRELEX*®): RISK OF BENIGN AND MALIGNANT NEOPLASIA (JANUARY 2020)

Cases of benign and malignant tumours have been observed in children and adolescents treated with mecasermin; the risk of neoplasia is higher when used outside the licensed indication or dose. If a physician determines that there is a clinical need for such use, the patient and their carers should be consulted and fully informed of the potential benefits and risks, and the final decision made jointly. Physicians should be vigilant for the development of potential malignancies in such patients.

Healthcare professionals are advised that mecasermin is contra-indicated in children and adolescents with active or suspected neoplasia and in any condition or medical history that increases the risk of benign or malignant neoplasia. If benign or malignant neoplasm develops during treatment, mecasermin should be permanently discontinued.

- **CONTRA-INDICATIONS** Evidence of tumour activity (discontinue treatment)
- **CAUTIONS** Correct hypothyroidism before initiating treatment · diabetes mellitus (adjustment of antidiabetic therapy may be necessary) · papilloedema
- **SIDE-EFFECTS**

▸ **Common or very common** Adenoidal hypertrophy · arthralgia · dizziness · ear discomfort · gastrointestinal discomfort · gynaecomastia · hair texture abnormal · headache · hearing impairment · hyperglycaemia · hypoglycaemia · melanocytic naevus · myalgia · otitis media · pain in extremity · papilloedema · scoliosis · seizures · skin hypertrophy · sleep apnoea · snoring · tachycardia · thymus enlargement · tonsillar hypertrophy · tremor · vomiting

▸ **Uncommon** Cardiac hypertrophy · cardiac valve disorders · depression · idiopathic intracranial hypertension · lipohypertrophy · nervousness · weight increased

▸ **Frequency not known** Alopecia · benign neoplasm (discontinue permanently) · neoplasm malignant (discontinue permanently)

SIDE-EFFECTS, FURTHER INFORMATION Funduscopy for papilloedema recommended regularly during treatment and if severe or recurrent headache, visual problems, nausea and vomiting occur—if papilloedema confirmed consider benign intracranial hypertension.

- **CONCEPTION AND CONTRACEPTION** Contraception advised in women of child-bearing potential.
- **PREGNANCY** Avoid unless essential.
- **BREAST FEEDING** Avoid.
- **MONITORING REQUIREMENTS**

▸ Monitor ECG before and on termination of treatment (and during treatment if ECG abnormal).

▸ Monitor for disorders of the epiphysis of the hip (monitor for limping).

▸ Monitor for signs of tonsillar hypertrophy (snoring, sleep apnoea, and chronic middle ear effusions).

- **DIRECTIONS FOR ADMINISTRATION** Dose should be administered just before or after food.
- **PATIENT AND CARER ADVICE** Patients or carers should be given advice on how to administer mecasermin injection.

Missed doses Patients or carers should be advised not to increase dose if a dose is missed.

- **MEDICINAL FORMS** There can be variation in the licensing of different medicines containing the same drug.

Solution for injection

EXCIPIENTS: May contain Benzyl alcohol

▸ Increlex (Ipsen Ltd) ▼

Mecasermin 10 mg per 1 ml Increlex 40mg/4ml solution for injection vials | 1 vial PoM £605.00

7 Sex hormone responsive conditions

Sex hormones

Hormone replacement therapy

Sex hormone replacement therapy is indicated in children for the treatment of gonadotrophin deficiency, gonadal disorders, or delayed puberty that interferes with quality of life. Indications include constitutional delay in puberty, congenital or acquired hypogonadotrophic hypogonadism, hypergonadotrophic hypogonadism (Turner's syndrome, Klinefelter's syndrome), endocrine disorders (Cushing's syndrome or hyperprolactinaemia), and chronic illnesses, such as cystic fibrosis or sickle-cell disease, that may affect the onset of puberty.

Replacement therapy is generally started at the appropriate age for the development of puberty and should be managed by a paediatric endocrinologist. Patients with constitutional delay, chronic illness, or eating disorders may need only small doses of hormone supplements for 4 to 6 months to induce puberty and endogenous sex hormone production, which is then sustained. Patients with organic causes of hormone deficiency will require life-long replacement, adjusted to allow normal development.

Inadequate treatment may lead to poor bone mineralisation, resulting in fractures and osteoporosis.

Female sex hormones

Oestrogens

Oestrogens are necessary for the development of female secondary sexual characteristics. If onset of puberty is delayed because of organic pathology, puberty can be induced with ethinylestradiol p. 516 in increasing doses, guided by breast staging and uterine scans. Cyclical progestogen replacement is added after 12–18 months of oestrogen treatment. Once the adult dosage of oestrogen has been reached, it may be more convenient to provide replacement either as a low-dose oestrogen containing oral contraceptive formulation [unlicensed indication] or as a combined oestrogen and progestogen hormone replacement therapy preparation [unlicensed indication]. There is limited experience in the use of transdermal patches or gels in children; compliance and skin irritation are sometimes a problem.

Ethinylestradiol is occasionally used, under **specialist supervision**, for the management of hereditary haemorrhagic telangiectasia (but evidence of benefit is limited), for the prevention of tall stature, and in tests of growth hormone secretion.

Topical oestrogen creams are used in the treatment of labial adhesions.

Progestogens

There are two main groups of progestogen, *progesterone and its analogues* (dydrogesterone and medroxyprogesterone acetate p. 553) and *testosterone analogues* (norethisterone p. 517 and norgestrel). The newer progestogens (desogestrel p. 547, norgestimate, and gestodene) are all derivatives of norgestrel; levonorgestrel p. 549 is the active isomer of norgestrel and has twice its potency. Progesterone and its analogues are less androgenic than the testosterone derivatives and neither progesterone nor dydrogesterone causes virilisation.

In delayed puberty cyclical progestogen is added after 12–18 months of oestrogen therapy to establish a menstrual cycle.

Norethisterone is also used to postpone menstruation during a cycle; treatment is started 3 days before the expected onset of menstruation.

Heavy menstrual bleeding

04-Jan-2019

Description of condition

Heavy menstrual bleeding, also known as menorrhagia, is excessive menstrual blood loss of 80 mL or more, or for a duration of more than 7 days, which results in the need to change menstrual products every 1–2 hours. Heavy menstrual bleeding occurs regularly, every 24–35 days.

Drug treatment

EvGr The choice of treatment should be guided by the presence or absence of fibroids (including size, number and location), polyps, endometrial pathology or adenomyosis, other symptoms (such as pressure or pain), co-morbidities, and patient preference.

In females with heavy menstrual bleeding and unidentified pathology, fibroids less than 3 cm in diameter causing no distortion of the uterine cavity, or suspected or diagnosed adenomyosis, a levonorgestrel-releasing intra-uterine system p. 549 is the first-line treatment option. Patients should be advised that irregular menstrual bleeding can occur particularly during the first months of use and that the full benefit of treatment may take at least 6 months.

If a levonorgestrel-releasing intra-uterine system p. 549 is unsuitable, either tranexamic acid p. 87, an NSAID, a combined hormonal contraceptive, or a cyclical oral progestogen should be considered. Progestogen-only contraceptives may suppress menstruation and be beneficial to females with heavy menstrual bleeding. A non-hormonal treatment is recommended in patients actively trying to conceive.

If drug treatment is unsuccessful or declined by the patient, or if symptoms are severe, referral to a specialist for alternative drug treatment or surgery should be considered.

In females with fibroids of 3 cm or more in diameter, referral to a specialist should be considered. Treatment options include tranexamic acid, an NSAID, a levonorgestrel-releasing intra-uterine system p. 549, a combined hormonal contraceptive, a cyclical oral progestogen, uterine artery embolisation, or surgery. Treatment choice depends on the size, number and location of the fibroids, and severity of symptoms. If drug treatment is required while investigations and definitive treatment is being organised, either tranexamic acid, or an NSAID, or both, can be given. ⟨A⟩

The effectiveness of drug treatment for heavy menstrual bleeding may be limited in females with fibroids that are substantially greater than 3 cm in diameter. EvGr Treatment with a gonadotrophin-releasing hormone analogue before hysterectomy and myomectomy should be considered if uterine fibroids are causing an enlarged or distorted uterus. ⟨A⟩

Useful Resources

Heavy menstrual bleeding: assessment and management. National Institute for Health and Care Excellence. NICE guideline 88. November 2018.
www.nice.org.uk/guidance/ng88

7.1 Female sex hormone responsive conditions

Other drugs used for Female sex hormone responsive conditions Clonidine hydrochloride, p. 108 · Ulipristal acetate, p. 547

OESTROGENS

Ethinylestradiol

22-May-2020

(Ethinyloestradiol)

- **INDICATIONS AND DOSE**

Induction of sexual maturation in girls

▶ BY MOUTH

▶ Child (female): Initially 2 micrograms daily for 6 months, then increased to 5 micrograms daily for 6 months, then increased to 10 micrograms daily for 6 months, then increased to 20 micrograms daily, after 12–18 months of treatment give progestogen for 7 days of each 28-day cycle.

Maintenance of sexual maturation in girls

▶ BY MOUTH

▶ Child (female): 20 micrograms daily, to be given with cyclical progestogen for 7 days of each 28-day cycle.

Prevention of tall stature in girls

▶ BY MOUTH

▶ Child 2–11 years (female): 20–50 micrograms daily.

- **UNLICENSED USE** Unlicensed for use in children.
- **CONTRA-INDICATIONS** Active or recent arterial thromboembolic disease (e.g. angina or myocardial infarction) · Acute porphyrias p. 652 · cardiovascular disease (risk of fluid retention) · family history of thromboembolism · history of breast cancer · history of venous thromboembolism · liver disease (where liver function tests have failed to return to normal) · oestrogen-dependent cancer · thrombophilic disorder · undiagnosed vaginal bleeding · untreated endometrial hyperplasia
- **CAUTIONS** Diabetes (increased risk of heart disease) · history of breast nodules or fibrocystic disease—closely monitor breast status (risk of breast cancer) · history of endometrial hyperplasia · history of hypertriglyceridaemia (increased risk of pancreatitis) · hypophyseal tumours ·

increased risk of gall-bladder disease · migraine (migraine-like headaches) · presence of antiphospholipid antibodies (increased risk of thrombotic events) · prolonged exposure to unopposed oestrogens may increase risk of developing endometrial cancer · risk factors for oestrogen-dependent tumours (e.g. breast cancer in first-degree relative) · risk factors for venous thromboembolism · symptoms of endometriosis may be exacerbated · uterine fibroids may increase in size

- **INTERACTIONS** → Appendix 1: hormone replacement therapy
- **SIDE-EFFECTS** Breast abnormalities · cervical mucus increased · cholelithiasis · contact lens intolerance · depression · electrolyte imbalance · embolism and thrombosis · erythema nodosum · feminisation · fluid retention · headaches · hypertension · jaundice cholestatic · metrorrhagia · mood altered · myocardial infarction · nausea · neoplasms · skin reactions · stroke · uterine disorders · vomiting · weight change
- **PREGNANCY** Avoid.
- **BREAST FEEDING** Avoid until weaning or for 6 months after birth (adverse effects on lactation).
- **HEPATIC IMPAIRMENT** Manufacturer advises caution; avoid in acute or active disease.

- **MEDICINAL FORMS** There can be variation in the licensing of different medicines containing the same drug. Forms available from special-order manufacturers include: tablet, capsule, oral suspension

Tablet

- Ethinylestradiol (Non-proprietary)
  - **Ethinylestradiol 2 microgram** Ethinylestradiol 2microgram tablets | 100 tablet PoM £200.00
  - **Ethinylestradiol 10 microgram** Ethinylestradiol 10microgram tablets | 21 tablet PoM £200.00 DT = £200.00
  - **Ethinylestradiol 50 microgram** Ethinylestradiol 50microgram tablets | 21 tablet PoM £200.00 DT = £200.00
  - **Ethinylestradiol 1 mg** Ethinylestradiol 1mg tablets | 28 tablet PoM £200.00 DT = £200.00

PROGESTOGENS

Dienogest

17-Feb-2020

- **DRUG ACTION** Dienogest is a nortestosterone derivative that has a progestogenic effect in the uterus, reducing the production of estradiol and thereby suppressing endometriotic lesions.

- **INDICATIONS AND DOSE**

Endometriosis

- BY MOUTH
  - Females of childbearing potential: 2 mg once daily, can be started on any day of cycle, dose should be taken continuously at the same time each day

- **CONTRA-INDICATIONS** Arterial disease (past or present) · cardiovascular disease (past or present) · diabetes with vascular involvement · liver tumours (past or present) · sex hormone-dependent malignancies (confirmed or suspected) · undiagnosed vaginal bleeding · venous thromboembolism (active)
- **CAUTIONS** Diabetes (progestogens can decrease glucose tolerance—monitor patient closely) · history of depression · history of ectopic pregnancy · history of gestational diabetes · patients at risk of osteoporosis · patients at risk of venous thromboembolism

CAUTIONS, FURTHER INFORMATION

- Immobilisation Manufacturer advises to discontinue treatment during prolonged immobilisation. For elective surgery, treatment should be discontinued at least 4 weeks before surgery; treatment may be restarted 2 weeks after complete remobilisation.

- **INTERACTIONS** → Appendix 1: dienogest
- **SIDE-EFFECTS**
  - **Common or very common** Alopecia · anxiety · asthenic conditions · breast abnormalities · depression · gastrointestinal discomfort · gastrointestinal disorders · haemorrhage · headaches · hot flush · libido loss · mood altered · nausea · ovarian cyst · pain · skin reactions · sleep disorder · vomiting · vulvovaginal disorders · weight changes
  - **Uncommon** Anaemia · appetite increased · autonomic dysfunction · broken nails · circulatory system disorder · concentration impaired · constipation · dandruff · diarrhoea · dry eye · dyspnoea · genital discharge · hair changes · hyperhidrosis · hypotension · increased risk of infection · limb discomfort · muscle spasms · oedema · palpitations · pelvic pain · photosensitivity reaction · tinnitus
  - **Frequency not known** Glucose tolerance impaired · insulin resistance · menstrual cycle irregularities
- **CONCEPTION AND CONTRACEPTION** Manufacturer advises that, if contraception is required, females of childbearing potential should use non-hormonal contraception during treatment. The menstrual cycle usually returns to normal within 2 months after stopping treatment.
- **BREAST FEEDING** Manufacturer advises avoid—present in milk in *animal* studies.
- **HEPATIC IMPAIRMENT** Manufacturer advises avoid in severe impairment (no information available).
- **PATIENT AND CARER ADVICE** Manufacturer advises patients with a history of chloasma gravidarum to avoid sunlight or UV radiation exposure during treatment.
  Missed doses Manufacturer advises if one or more tablets are missed, or if vomiting and/or diarrhoea occurs within 3–4 hours of taking a tablet, another tablet should be taken as soon as possible and the next dose taken at the normal time.

- **MEDICINAL FORMS** There can be variation in the licensing of different medicines containing the same drug.

Tablet

- Zalkya (Stragen UK Ltd)
  - **Dienogest 2 mg** Zalkya 2mg tablets | 28 tablet PoM £20.68

Norethisterone

- **INDICATIONS AND DOSE**

Postponement of menstruation

- BY MOUTH
  - Females of childbearing potential: 5 mg 3 times a day, to be started 3 days before expected onset (menstruation occurs 2–3 days after stopping)

Induction and maintenance of sexual maturation in females (combined with an oestrogen after 12–18 months oestrogen therapy)

- BY MOUTH
  - Child: 5 mg once daily for the last 7 days of 28-day cycle

Short-term contraception

- BY DEEP INTRAMUSCULAR INJECTION
  - Females of childbearing potential: 200 mg, to be administered within first 5 days of cycle or immediately after parturition (duration 8 weeks). To be injected into the gluteal muscle, then 200 mg after 8 weeks if required

Contraception

- BY MOUTH
  - Females of childbearing potential: 350 micrograms daily, dose to be taken at same time each day, starting on day 1 of cycle then continuously, if administration delayed for 3 hours or more it should be regarded as a ‘missed pill’

6 Endocrine system

- **UNLICENSED USE**
  - When used for Induction and maintenance of sexual maturation in females or Postponement of menstruation Not licensed for use in children.
  - When used for Contraception Consult product literature for the licensing status of individual preparations.
- **CONTRA-INDICATIONS**

GENERAL CONTRA-INDICATIONS Avoid in patients with a history of liver tumours · breast cancer (unless progestogens are being used in the management of this condition) · genital cancer (unless progestogens are being used in the management of this condition) · history during pregnancy of idiopathic jaundice · history during pregnancy of pemphigoid gestationis (non-contraceptive indications) · history during pregnancy of severe pruritus (non-contraceptive indications) · when used as a contraceptive, history of breast cancer (can be used after 5 years if no evidence of disease and non-hormonal contraceptive methods unacceptable)

SPECIFIC CONTRA-INDICATIONS
- With oral use Acute porphyrias p. 652 · severe arterial disease · undiagnosed vaginal bleeding

- **CAUTIONS**

GENERAL CAUTIONS Asthma · cardiac dysfunction · conditions that may worsen with fluid retention · diabetes (progestogens can decrease glucose tolerance—monitor patient closely) · epilepsy · history of depression · hypertension · migraine · susceptibility to thromboembolism (particular caution with high dose)

SPECIFIC CAUTIONS
- When used for contraception Active trophoblastic disease (until return to normal of urine- and plasma-gonadotrophin concentration)—seek specialist advice · arterial disease · functional ovarian cysts · history of jaundice in pregnancy · malabsorption syndromes · past ectopic pregnancy · sex-steroid dependent cancer · systemic lupus erythematosus with positive (or unknown) anti-phospholipid antibodies
- With intramuscular use for contraception Disturbances of lipid metabolism · history during pregnancy of deterioration of otosclerosis · history during pregnancy of pruritus · possible risk of breast cancer

CAUTIONS, FURTHER INFORMATION
- Use as a contraceptive in co-morbidities The product literature advises caution in patients with history of thromboembolism, hypertension, diabetes mellitus and migraine; evidence for caution in these conditions is unsatisfactory.
- Breast cancer risk with contraceptive use There is a small increase in the risk of having breast cancer diagnosed in women using, or who have recently used, a progestogen-only contraceptive pill; this relative risk may be due to an earlier diagnosis. The most important risk factor appears to be the age at which the contraceptive is stopped rather than the duration of use; the risk disappears gradually during the 10 years after stopping and there is no excess risk by 10 years. A possible small increase in the risk of breast cancer should be weighed against the benefits.

- **INTERACTIONS** → Appendix 1: norethisterone
- **SIDE-EFFECTS**

GENERAL SIDE-EFFECTS
- **Common or very common** Menstrual cycle irregularities
- **Uncommon** Breast tenderness
- **Frequency not known** Hepatic cancer · thromboembolism

SPECIFIC SIDE-EFFECTS
- **Common or very common**
- With intramuscular use Dizziness · haemorrhage · headache · hypersensitivity · nausea · skin reactions · weight increased
- **Uncommon**
- With intramuscular use Abdominal distension · depressed mood
- **Frequency not known**
- With oral use Appetite change · depression · fatigue · gastrointestinal disorder · headaches · hypertension · libido disorder · nervousness · rash · weight change

- **PREGNANCY** Not known to be harmful in contraceptive doses. Avoid in other indications.
- **BREAST FEEDING** Progestogen-only contraceptives do not affect lactation.
  - With intramuscular use Withhold breast-feeding for neonates with severe or persistent jaundice requiring medical treatment.
- **HEPATIC IMPAIRMENT** Manufacturers advise caution; avoid in severe or active disease.
- **RENAL IMPAIRMENT** Use with caution in non-contraceptive indications.
- **PATIENT AND CARER ADVICE**

Diarrhoea and vomiting with oral contraceptives Vomiting and persistent, severe diarrhoea can interfere with the absorption of oral progestogen-only contraceptives. If vomiting occurs within 2 hours of taking an oral progestogen-only contraceptive, another pill should be taken as soon as possible. If a replacement pill is not taken within 3 hours of the normal time for taking the progestogen-only pill, or in cases of persistent vomiting or very severe diarrhoea, additional precautions should be used during illness and for 2 days after recovery.

Starting routine for oral contraceptives One tablet daily, on a continuous basis, starting on day 1 of cycle and taken at the same time each day (if delayed by longer than 3 hours contraceptive protection may be lost). Additional contraceptive precautions are not required if norethisterone is started up to and including day 5 of the menstrual cycle; if started after this time, additional contraceptive precautions are required for 2 days.

Changing from a combined oral contraceptive Start on the day following completion of the combined oral contraceptive course without a break (or in the case of ED tablets omitting the inactive ones).

After childbirth Oral progestogen-only contraceptives can be started up to and including day 21 postpartum without the need for additional contraceptive precautions. If started more than 21 days postpartum, additional contraceptive precautions are required for 2 days.

Contraceptives by injection Full counselling backed by *patient information leaflet* required before administration—likelihood of menstrual disturbance and the potential for a delay in return to full fertility. Delayed return of fertility and irregular cycles may occur after discontinuation of treatment but there is no evidence of permanent infertility.

Missed oral contraceptive pill The following advice is recommended: 'If you forget a pill, take it as soon as you remember and carry on with the next pill at the right time. If the pill was more than 3 hours overdue you are not protected. Continue normal pill-taking but you must also use another method, such as the condom, for the next 2 days.'

The Faculty of Sexual and Reproductive Healthcare recommends emergency contraception if one or more progestogen-only contraceptive tablets are missed or taken more than 3 hours late and unprotected intercourse has occurred before 2 further tablets have been correctly taken.

- **MEDICINAL FORMS** There can be variation in the licensing of different medicines containing the same drug. Forms available from special-order manufacturers include: oral suspension

Solution for injection

- Noristerat (Bayer Plc)
  Norethisterone enantate 200 mg per 1 ml Noristerat 200mg/1ml solution for injection ampoules | 1 ampoule PoM £4.05

Tablet

- Norethisterone (Non-proprietary)
  Norethisterone 5 mg Norethisterone 5mg tablets | 30 tablet PoM £4.15 DT = £2.70
- Noriday (Pfizer Ltd)
  Norethisterone 350 microgram Noriday 350microgram tablets | 84 tablet PoM £2.10 DT = £2.10
- Primolut N (Bayer Plc)
  Norethisterone 5 mg Primolut N 5mg tablets | 30 tablet PoM £2.26 DT = £2.70
- Utovlan (Pfizer Ltd)
  Norethisterone 5 mg Utovlan 5mg tablets | 30 tablet PoM £1.40 DT = £2.70 | 90 tablet PoM £4.21

7.2 Male sex hormone responsive conditions

Androgens, anti-androgens and anabolic steroids

Androgens

Androgens cause masculinisation; they are used as replacement therapy in androgen deficiency, in delayed puberty, and in those who are hypogonadal due to either pituitary or testicular disease.

When given to patients with hypopituitarism androgens can lead to normal sexual development and potency but not to fertility. If fertility is desired, the usual treatment is with gonadotrophins or pulsatile gonadotrophin-releasing hormone which stimulates spermatogenesis as well as androgen production.

Intramuscular depot preparations of **testosterone esters** are preferred for replacement therapy. Testosterone enantate or propionate or alternatively *Sustanon*®, which consists of a mixture of testosterone esters and has a longer duration of action, can be used. For induction of puberty, depot testosterone injections are given monthly and the doses increased every 6 to 12 months according to response. Single ester testosterone injections may need to be given more frequently.

Oral **testosterone undecanoate** is used for induction of puberty. An alternative approach that promotes growth rather than sexual maturation uses oral oxandrolone below.

Testosterone topical gel is also available but experience of use in children under 15 years is limited. Topical testosterone is applied to the penis in the treatment of microphallus; an extemporaneously prepared cream should be used because the alcohol in proprietary gel formulations causes irritation.

Anti-androgens and precocious puberty

The gonadorelin stimulation test is used to distinguish between *gonadotrophin-dependent (central) precocious puberty* and *gonadotrophin-independent precocious puberty*. Treatment requires specialist management.

Gonadorelin analogues, used in the management of gonadotrophin-dependent precocious puberty, delay development of secondary sexual characteristics and growth velocity.

Testolactone p. 521 and cyproterone acetate p. 520 are used in the management of gonadotrophin-independent precocious puberty, resulting from McCune-Albright syndrome, familial male precocious puberty (testotoxicosis), hormone-secreting tumours, and ovarian and testicular disorders. Testolactone inhibits the aromatisation of testosterone, the rate limiting step in oestrogen synthesis. Cyproterone acetate is a progestogen with anti-androgen properties.

Spironolactone p. 133 is sometimes used in combination with testolactone because it has some androgen receptor blocking properties.

High blood concentration of sex hormones may activate release of gonadotrophin releasing hormone, leading to development of secondary, central gonadotrophin-dependent precocious puberty. This may require the addition of gonadorelin analogues to prevent progression of pubertal development and skeletal maturation.

Anabolic steroids have some androgenic activity but they cause less virilisation than androgens in girls. They are used in the treatment of some *aplastic anaemias*.

Oxandrolone is used to stimulate late pre-pubertal growth prior to induction of sexual maturation in boys with short stature and in girls with Turner's syndrome; specialist management is required.

ANABOLIC STEROIDS › ANDROSTAN DERIVATIVES

Oxandrolone

- **INDICATIONS AND DOSE**

Stimulation of late pre-pubertal growth in boys (of appropriate age) with short stature

- BY MOUTH
- Child 10–17 years (male): 1.25–2.5 mg daily for 3–6 months.

Stimulation of late pre-pubertal growth in girls with Turner's syndrome

- BY MOUTH
- Child (female): 0.625–2.5 mg daily, to be taken in combination with growth hormone.

- **CONTRA-INDICATIONS** History of primary liver tumours · hypercalcaemia · nephrosis
- **CAUTIONS** Cardiac impairment · diabetes mellitus · epilepsy · hypertension · migraine · skeletal metastases (risk of hypercalcaemia)
- **SIDE-EFFECTS**
  - **Common or very common** Androgenetic alopecia · androgenic effects · anxiety · asthenia · bone formation increased · depression · electrolyte imbalance · epiphyses premature fusion (in pre-pubertal males) · gastrointestinal haemorrhage · gynaecomastia · headache · hirsutism · hypertension · jaundice cholestatic · nausea · oedema · paraesthesia · polycythaemia · precocious puberty (in pre-pubertal males) · seborrhoea · sexual dysfunction · skin reactions · spermatogenesis reduced · virilism · weight increased
  - **Rare or very rare** Hepatic neoplasm
  - **Frequency not known** Sleep apnoea
- **PREGNANCY** Avoid—causes masculinisation of female fetus.
- **BREAST FEEDING** Avoid; may cause masculinisation in the female infant or precocious development in the male infant. High doses suppress lactation.
- **HEPATIC IMPAIRMENT** Avoid if possible—fluid retention and dose-related toxicity.
- **RENAL IMPAIRMENT** Use with caution—potential for fluid retention.

- **MEDICINAL FORMS** There can be variation in the licensing of different medicines containing the same drug. Forms available from special-order manufacturers include: tablet

Tablet

▸ Oxandrin (Imported (Australia))

Oxandrolone 2.5 mg Oxandrin 2.5mg tablets | 100 tablet [PoM] [CD4-2]

ANDROGENS

Androgens

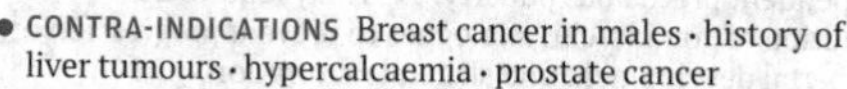

- **CONTRA-INDICATIONS** Breast cancer in males · history of liver tumours · hypercalcaemia · prostate cancer
- **CAUTIONS** Cardiac impairment · diabetes mellitus · epilepsy · hypertension · ischaemic heart disease · migraine · pre-pubertal boys (fusion of epiphyses is hastened and may result in short stature)—statural growth and sexual development should be monitored · risk factors for venous thromboembolism · skeletal metastases—risk of hypercalcaemia or hypercalciuria (if this occurs, treat appropriately and restart treatment once normal serum calcium concentration restored) · sleep apnoea · stop treatment or reduce dose if severe polycythaemia occurs · thrombophilia—increased risk of thrombosis · tumours—risk of hypercalcaemia or hypercalciuria (if this occurs, treat appropriately and restart treatment once normal serum calcium concentration restored)
- **SIDE-EFFECTS**
  - ▸ **Common or very common** Hot flush · hypertension · polycythaemia · prostate abnormalities · skin reactions · weight increased
  - ▸ **Uncommon** Alopecia · asthenia · behaviour abnormal · depression · dizziness · dyspnoea · dysuria · gynaecomastia · headache · hyperhidrosis · insomnia · nausea · sexual dysfunction
  - ▸ **Rare or very rare** Pulmonary oil microembolism
  - ▸ **Frequency not known** Anxiety · epiphyses premature fusion · fluid retention · jaundice · oedema · oligozoospermia · paraesthesia · precocious puberty · prostate cancer · seborrhoea · sleep apnoea · urinary tract obstruction

  SIDE-EFFECTS, FURTHER INFORMATION Stop treatment or reduce dose if severe polycythaemia occurs.
- **PREGNANCY** Avoid—causes masculinisation of female fetus.
- **BREAST FEEDING** Avoid.
- **HEPATIC IMPAIRMENT** In general, manufacturers advise caution (increased risk of fluid retention and heart failure).
- **RENAL IMPAIRMENT** Caution—potential for fluid retention.
- **MONITORING REQUIREMENTS** Monitor haematocrit and haemoglobulin before treatment, every three months for the first year, and yearly thereafter.

above

Testosterone enantate

13-May-2020

- **INDICATIONS AND DOSE**

Induction and maintenance of sexual maturation in males (specialist use only)

▸ BY DEEP INTRAMUSCULAR INJECTION

▸ Child 12–17 years: 25–50 mg/m^2 every month, increase dose every 6–12 months according to response

- **UNLICENSED USE** Not licensed for use in children.
- **SIDE-EFFECTS** Bone formation increased · circulatory system disorder · gastrointestinal disorder · gastrointestinal haemorrhage · hepatomegaly · hypercalcaemia · neoplasms · spermatogenesis abnormal
- **MEDICINAL FORMS** There can be variation in the licensing of different medicines containing the same drug.

Solution for injection

▸ Testosterone enantate (Non-proprietary)

Testosterone enantate 250 mg per 1 ml Testosterone enantate 250mg/1ml solution for injection ampoules | 3 ampoule [PoM] £83.74–£87.73 DT = £85.74 [CD4-2]

above

Testosterone propionate

13-May-2020

- **INDICATIONS AND DOSE**

Delayed puberty in males

▸ BY INTRAMUSCULAR INJECTION

▸ Child: 50 mg once weekly

Treatment of microphallus (specialist use only)

▸ TO THE SKIN USING CREAM

▸ Child: Apply 3 times a day for 3 weeks

- **MEDICINAL FORMS** Forms available from special-order manufacturers include: solution for injection, cream

above

Testosterone undecanoate

13-May-2020

- **INDICATIONS AND DOSE**

Induction and maintenance of sexual maturation in males (specialist use only)

▸ BY MOUTH

▸ Child 12–17 years: 40 mg once daily on alternate days, adjusted according to response to 120 mg daily

- **SIDE-EFFECTS**

  GENERAL SIDE-EFFECTS
  - ▸ **Uncommon** Diarrhoea · mood altered

  SPECIFIC SIDE-EFFECTS
  - ▸ **Frequency not known** Azoospermia · fluid imbalance · gastrointestinal discomfort · hepatic function abnormal · lipid metabolism change · myalgia · penis enlarged
- **MEDICINAL FORMS** There can be variation in the licensing of different medicines containing the same drug.

Capsule

CAUTIONARY AND ADVISORY LABELS 21, 25

▸ Restandol (Merck Sharp & Dohme Ltd)

Testosterone undecanoate 40 mg Restandol 40mg Testocaps | 30 capsule [PoM] £8.55 [CD4-2] | 60 capsule [PoM] £17.10 DT = £17.10 [CD4-2]

7.2a Male sex hormone antagonism

ANTI-ANDROGENS

Cyproterone acetate

18-Oct-2019

- **INDICATIONS AND DOSE**

Gonadotrophin-independent precocious puberty (specialist use only)

▸ BY MOUTH

▸ Child: Initially 25 mg twice daily, adjusted according to response

- **UNLICENSED USE** Unlicensed for use in children.
- **CONTRA-INDICATIONS** Dubin-Johnson syndrome · existing or history of thromboembolic disorders · malignant diseases · meningioma or history of meningioma · previous or existing liver tumours · Rotor syndrome · severe depression · severe diabetes (with vascular changes) · sickle-cell anaemia · wasting diseases · youths under

18 years (may arrest bone maturation and testicular development)

- **CAUTIONS** Diabetes mellitus · in prostate cancer, severe depression · in prostate cancer, sickle-cell anaemia · ineffective for male hypersexuality in chronic alcoholism (relevance to prostate cancer not known)
- **SIDE-EFFECTS**
  - **Common or very common** Depressed mood · dyspnoea · fatigue · gynaecomastia · hepatic disorders · hot flush · hyperhidrosis · nipple pain · restlessness · weight change
  - **Uncommon** Skin reactions
  - **Rare or very rare** Galactorrhoea · neoplasms
  - **Frequency not known** Adrenocortical suppression · anaemia · azoospermia · hair changes · hypotrichosis · osteoporosis · sebaceous gland underactivity (may clear acne) · thromboembolism

  SIDE-EFFECTS, FURTHER INFORMATION Direct hepatic toxicity including jaundice, hepatitis and hepatic failure have been reported (fatalities reported, usually after several months, at dosages of 100 mg and above). If hepatotoxicity is confirmed, cyproterone should normally be withdrawn unless the hepatotoxicity can be explained by another cause such as metastatic disease (in which case cyproterone should be continued only if the perceived benefit exceeds the risk).
- **HEPATIC IMPAIRMENT** Manufacturer advises avoid.
- **MONITORING REQUIREMENTS**
  - Monitor blood counts initially and throughout treatment.
  - Monitor adrenocortical function regularly.
  - Monitor hepatic function regularly—liver function tests should be performed before and regularly during treatment and whenever symptoms suggestive of hepatotoxicity occur.
- **PATIENT AND CARER ADVICE**

  Driving and skilled tasks Fatigue and lassitude may impair performance of skilled tasks (e.g. driving).

- **MEDICINAL FORMS** There can be variation in the licensing of different medicines containing the same drug. Forms available from special-order manufacturers include: tablet, capsule, oral suspension, oral solution

Tablet

CAUTIONARY AND ADVISORY LABELS 21

- Cyproterone acetate (Non-proprietary)

  Cyproterone acetate 50 mg Cyproterone 50mg tablets | 56 tablet [PoM] £48.95 DT = £30.41

  Cyproterone acetate 100 mg Cyproterone 100mg tablets | 84 tablet [PoM] £132.57 DT = £57.89
- Androcur (Bayer Plc)

  Cyproterone acetate 50 mg Androcur 50mg tablets | 60 tablet [PoM] £31.34
- Cyprostat (Bayer Plc)

  Cyproterone acetate 50 mg Cyprostat 50mg tablets | 160 tablet [PoM] £82.86

  Cyproterone acetate 100 mg Cyprostat 100mg tablets | 80 tablet [PoM] £82.86

HORMONE ANTAGONISTS AND RELATED AGENTS > AROMATASE INHIBITORS

Testolactone

- **INDICATIONS AND DOSE**

  Gonadotrophin-independent precocious puberty (specialist use only)
  - BY MOUTH
    - Child: 5 mg/kg 3–4 times a day; increased if necessary up to 10 mg/kg 4 times a day
- **SIDE-EFFECTS**
  - **Common or very common** Appetite decreased · diarrhoea · hair growth abnormal · hypertension · nausea · peripheral neuropathy · vomiting · weight change
  - **Rare or very rare** Hypersensitivity · rash
- **PREGNANCY** Avoid.
- **BREAST FEEDING** No information available.

- **MEDICINAL FORMS** There can be variation in the licensing of different medicines containing the same drug.

Tablet

- Teslac (Imported (United States))

  Testolactone 50 mg Teslac 50mg tablets | 100 tablet [PoM] [X]

6 Endocrine system

8 Thyroid disorders

8.1 Hyperthyroidism

Antithyroid drugs

Overview

Antithyroid drugs are used for hyperthyroidism either to prepare children for thyroidectomy or for long-term management. In the UK carbimazole p. 522 is the most commonly used drug. Propylthiouracil p. 523 should be reserved for children who are intolerant of, or for those who experience sensitivity reactions to carbimazole (sensitivity is not necessarily displayed to both drugs), and for whom other treatments are inappropriate. Both drugs act primarily by interfering with the synthesis of thyroid hormones.

Treatment in children should be undertaken by a specialist.

Carbimazole or propylthiouracil are initially given in large doses to block thyroid function. This dose is continued until the child becomes euthyroid, usually after 4 to 8 weeks, and is then gradually reduced to a maintenance dose of 30–60% of the initial dose. Alternatively high-dose treatment is continued in combination with levothyroxine sodium p. 524 replacement (*blocking-replacement regimen*); this is particularly useful when dose adjustment proves difficult. Treatment is usually continued for 12 to 24 months. The blocking-replacement regimen is **not** suitable during pregnancy. Hypothyroidism should be avoided particularly during pregnancy as it can cause fetal goitre.

Iodine has been used as an adjunct to antithyroid drugs for 10 to 14 days before partial thyroidectomy; however, there is little evidence of a beneficial effect. Iodine should not be used for long-term treatment because its antithyroid action tends to diminish.

Radioactive sodium iodide (^{131}I) solution is used increasingly for the treatment of thyrotoxicosis at all ages, particularly where medical therapy or compliance is a problem, in patients with cardiac disease, and in patients who relapse after thyroidectomy.

Propranolol hydrochloride p. 111 is useful for rapid relief of thyrotoxic symptoms and can be used in conjunction with antithyroid drugs or as an adjunct to radioactive iodine. Beta-blockers are also useful in neonatal thyrotoxicosis and in supraventricular arrhythmias due to hyperthyroidism. Propranolol hydrochloride has been used in conjunction with iodine to prepare mildly thyrotoxic patients for surgery but it is preferable to make the patient euthyroid with carbimazole. Laboratory tests of thyroid function are not altered by beta-blockers. Most experience in treating thyrotoxicosis has been gained with propranolol but atenolol p. 112 is also used.

Thyrotoxic crisis ('thyroid storm') requires emergency treatment with intravenous administration of fluids, propranolol hydrochloride and hydrocortisone p. 476 as sodium succinate, as well as oral iodine solution and carbimazole or propylthiouracil which may need to be administered by nasogastric tube.

Antithyroid drugs in pregnancy

Radioactive iodine therapy is contra-indicated during pregnancy. Propylthiouracil and carbimazole can be given but the blocking-replacement regimen is **not** suitable. Carbimazole is associated with congenital defects, including aplasia cutis of the neonate, therefore propylthiouracil remains the drug of choice during the first trimester of pregnancy. In the second trimester, consider switching to carbimazole because of the potential risk of hepatotoxicity with propylthiouracil. Both propylthiouracil and carbimazole cross the placenta and in high doses may cause fetal goitre and hypothyroidism—the lowest dose that will control the hyperthyroid state should be used (requirements in Graves' disease tend to fall during pregnancy). See also *Important safety information* in the carbimazole below drug monograph.

Antithyroid drugs in neonates

Neonatal hyperthyroidism is treated with carbimazole or propylthiouracil, usually for 8 to 12 weeks. In severe symptomatic disease iodine may be needed to block the thyroid and propranolol required to treat peripheral symptoms.

Other drugs used for Hyperthyroidism Metoprolol tartrate, p. 113

ANTITHYROID DRUGS › SULFUR-CONTAINING IMIDAZOLES

Carbimazole

22-Nov-2019

● **INDICATIONS AND DOSE**

Hyperthyroidism (blocking-replacement regimen) in combination with levothyroxine

▸ BY MOUTH

▸ Child: Therapy usually given for 12 to 24 months (consult product literature or local protocols)

Hyperthyroidism (including Graves' disease)

▸ BY MOUTH

▸ Neonate: Initially 750 micrograms/kg daily until patient is euthyroid, usually after 8 to 12 weeks, then gradually reduce to a maintenance dose of 30–60% of the initial dose; higher initial doses (up to 1 mg/kg daily) are occasionally required, particularly in thyrotoxic crisis, dose may be given in single or divided doses.

▸ Child 1 month–11 years: Initially 750 micrograms/kg daily until patient is euthyroid, usually after 4–8 weeks, then gradually reduce to a maintenance dose of 30–60% of the initial dose; higher initial doses are occasionally required, particularly in thyrotoxic crisis, dose may be given in single or divided doses; maximum 30 mg per day

▸ Child 12–17 years: Initially 30 mg daily until euthyroid, usually after 4–8 weeks, then gradually reduce to a maintenance dose of 30–60% of the initial dose; higher initial doses are occasionally required, particularly in thyrotoxic crisis, dose may be given in single or divided doses

DOSE EQUIVALENCE AND CONVERSION

▸ When substituting, carbimazole 1 mg is considered equivalent to propylthiouracil 10 mg but the dose may need adjusting according to response.

IMPORTANT SAFETY INFORMATION

NEUTROPENIA AND AGRANULOCYTOSIS

Manufacturer advises of the importance of recognising bone marrow suppression induced by carbimazole and the need to stop treatment promptly.

- Patient should be asked to report symptoms and signs suggestive of infection, especially sore throat.
- A white blood cell count should be performed if there is any clinical evidence of infection.
- Carbimazole should be stopped promptly if there is clinical or laboratory evidence of neutropenia.

MHRA/CHM ADVICE: CARBIMAZOLE: INCREASED RISK OF CONGENITAL MALFORMATIONS; STRENGTHENED ADVICE ON CONTRACEPTION (FEBRUARY 2019)

Carbimazole is associated with an increased risk of congenital malformations when used during pregnancy, especially in the first trimester and at high doses (daily dose of 15 mg or more).

Women of childbearing potential should use effective contraception during treatment with carbimazole. It should only be considered in pregnancy after a thorough benefit-risk assessment, and at the lowest effective dose without additional administration of thyroid hormones—close maternal, fetal, and neonatal monitoring is recommended.

MHRA/CHM ADVICE: CARBIMAZOLE: RISK OF ACUTE PANCREATITIS (FEBRUARY 2019)

Cases of acute pancreatitis have been reported during treatment with carbimazole. It should be stopped immediately and permanently if acute pancreatitis occurs.

Carbimazole should not be used in patients with a history of acute pancreatitis associated with previous treatment—re-exposure may result in life-threatening acute pancreatitis with a decreased time to onset.

● **CONTRA-INDICATIONS** Severe blood disorders

● **INTERACTIONS** → Appendix 1: carbimazole

● **SIDE-EFFECTS**

▸ **Rare or very rare** Bone marrow disorders · haemolytic anaemia · severe cutaneous adverse reactions (SCARs) · thrombocytopenia

▸ **Frequency not known** Agranulocytosis · alopecia · angioedema · dyspepsia · eosinophilia · fever · gastrointestinal disorder · generalised lymphadenopathy · haemorrhage · headache · hepatic disorders · insulin autoimmune syndrome · leucopenia · malaise · myopathy · nausea · nerve disorders · neutropenia · pancreatitis acute (discontinue permanently) · salivary gland enlargement · skin reactions · taste loss

● **CONCEPTION AND CONTRACEPTION** The MHRA advises that females of childbearing potential should use effective contraception during treatment.

● **PREGNANCY** The MHRA advises consider use only after a thorough benefit-risk assessment. See *Important Safety Information* and Antithyroid drugs p. 521 for further information.

● **BREAST FEEDING** Present in breast milk but this does not preclude breast-feeding as long as neonatal development is closely monitored and the lowest effective dose is used. Amount in milk may be sufficient to affect neonatal thyroid function therefore lowest effective dose should be used.

● **HEPATIC IMPAIRMENT** Manufacturer advises use with caution in mild to moderate insufficiency—half-life may be prolonged; avoid in severe insufficiency.

● **PATIENT AND CARER ADVICE** Warn patient or carers to tell doctor **immediately** if sore throat, mouth ulcers, bruising, fever, malaise, or non-specific illness develops.

Medicines for Children leaflet: Carbimazole for hyperthyroidism www.medicinesforchildren.org.uk/carbimazole-hyperthyroidism

● **MEDICINAL FORMS** There can be variation in the licensing of different medicines containing the same drug. Forms available from special-order manufacturers include: capsule, oral suspension, oral solution

Tablet

▸ Carbimazole (Non-proprietary)
Carbimazole 5 mg Carbimazole 5mg tablets | 100 tablet PoM £84.80 DT = £6.16
Carbimazole 10 mg Carbimazole 10mg tablets | 100 tablet PoM £104.08 DT = £81.32
Carbimazole 15 mg Carbimazole 15mg tablets | 100 tablet PoM £156.13 DT = £127.03
Carbimazole 20 mg Carbimazole 20mg tablets | 100 tablet PoM £208.17 DT = £30.95

ANTITHYROID DRUGS > THIOURACILS

Propylthiouracil

● **INDICATIONS AND DOSE**

Hyperthyroidism (including Graves' disease)

▸ BY MOUTH

▸ Neonate: Initially 2.5–5 mg/kg twice daily until euthyroid, usually after 8 to 12 weeks, then gradually reduce to a maintenance dose of 30–60% of the initial dose; higher initial doses are occasionally required, particularly in thyrotoxic crisis.

▸ Child 1-11 months: Initially 2.5 mg/kg 3 times a day until euthyroid, usually after 4 to 8 weeks, then gradually reduce to a maintenance dose of 30–60% of the initial dose; higher initial doses are occasionally required, particularly in thyrotoxic crisis
▸ Child 1-4 years: Initially 25 mg 3 times a day until euthyroid, usually after 4 to 8 weeks, then gradually reduce to a maintenance dose of 30–60% of the initial dose; higher initial doses are occasionally required, particularly in thyrotoxic crisis
▸ Child 5-11 years: Initially 50 mg 3 times a day until euthyroid, usually after 4 to 8 weeks, then gradually reduce to a maintenance dose of 30–60% of the initial dose; higher initial doses are occasionally required, particularly in thyrotoxic crisis
▸ Child 12-17 years: Initially 100 mg 3 times a day until euthyroid, usually after 4 to 8 weeks, then gradually reduce to a maintenance dose of 30–60% of the initial dose; higher initial doses are occasionally required, particularly in thyrotoxic crisis

DOSE EQUIVALENCE AND CONVERSION
▸ When substituting, carbimazole 1 mg is considered equivalent to propylthiouracil 10 mg but the dose may need adjusting according to response.

● **UNLICENSED USE** Not licensed for use in children under 6 years of age.

● **INTERACTIONS** → Appendix 1: propylthiouracil

● **SIDE-EFFECTS**
▸ **Rare or very rare** Agranulocytosis · bone marrow disorders · glomerulonephritis acute · hearing impairment · leucopenia · thrombocytopenia · vomiting
▸ **Frequency not known** Alopecia · arthralgia · arthritis · encephalopathy · fever · gastrointestinal disorder · haemorrhage · headache · hepatic disorders · hypoprothrombinaemia · interstitial pneumonitis · lupus-like syndrome · lymphadenopathy · myopathy · nausea · nephritis · skin reactions · taste altered · vasculitis

SIDE-EFFECTS, FURTHER INFORMATION Severe hepatic reactions have been reported, including fatal cases and cases requiring liver transplant—discontinue if significant liver-enzyme abnormalities develop.

● **PREGNANCY** Propylthiouracil can be given but the blocking-replacement regimen is **not** suitable.
Propylthiouracil crosses the placenta and in high doses may cause fetal goitre and hypothyroidism—the lowest dose that will control the hyperthyroid state should be used (requirements in Graves' disease tend to fall during pregnancy).

● **BREAST FEEDING** Present in breast milk but this does not preclude breast-feeding as long as neonatal development is closely monitored and the lowest effective dose is used. Amount in milk probably too small to affect infant; high doses may affect neonatal thyroid function.
Monitoring Monitor infant's thyroid status.

● **HEPATIC IMPAIRMENT** Manufacturer advises caution (risk of increased half life).
Dose adjustments Manufacturer advises consider dose reduction.

● **RENAL IMPAIRMENT**
Dose adjustments Use 75% of normal dose if estimated glomerular filtration rate 10–50 mL/minute/1.73 m^2.
Use 50% of normal dose if estimated glomerular filtration rate less than 10 mL/minute/1.73 m^2.

● **MONITORING REQUIREMENTS** Monitor for hepatotoxicity.

● **PATIENT AND CARER ADVICE** Patients should be told how to recognise signs of liver disorder and advised to seek prompt medical attention if symptoms such as anorexia, nausea, vomiting, fatigue, abdominal pain, jaundice, dark urine, or pruritus develop.

● **MEDICINAL FORMS** There can be variation in the licensing of different medicines containing the same drug. Forms available from special-order manufacturers include: oral suspension, oral solution

Tablet

▸ Propylthiouracil (Non-proprietary)
Propylthiouracil 50 mg Propylthiouracil 50mg tablets | 56 tablet PoM £57.58 DT = £9.67 | 100 tablet PoM £17.27-£115.98

VITAMINS AND TRACE ELEMENTS

Iodide with iodine

(Lugol's Solution; Aqueous Iodine Oral Solution)

● **INDICATIONS AND DOSE**

Thyrotoxicosis (pre-operative)

▸ BY MOUTH USING ORAL SOLUTION

▸ Neonate: 0.1–0.3 mL 3 times a day.

▸ Child: 0.1–0.3 mL 3 times a day

Neonatal thyrotoxicosis

▸ BY MOUTH USING ORAL SOLUTION

▸ Neonate: 0.05–0.1 mL 3 times a day.

Thyrotoxic crisis

▸ BY MOUTH USING ORAL SOLUTION

▸ Child 1 month–1 year: 0.2–0.3 mL 3 times a day

DOSE EQUIVALENCE AND CONVERSION
▸ Doses based on the use of an aqueous oral solution containing iodine 50 mg/mL and potassium iodide 100 mg/mL.

● **CAUTIONS** Children · not for long-term treatment

● **SIDE-EFFECTS** Conjunctivitis · depression (long term use) · erectile dysfunction (long term use) · excessive tearing · headache · hypersensitivity · increased risk of infection · influenza like illness · insomnia (long term use) · rash · salivary gland pain

● **PREGNANCY** Neonatal goitre and hypothyroidism.

● **BREAST FEEDING** Stop breast-feeding. Danger of neonatal hypothyroidism or goitre. Appears to be concentrated in milk.

- **DIRECTIONS FOR ADMINISTRATION** For oral solution, dilute well with milk or water.

- **MEDICINAL FORMS** Forms available from special-order manufacturers include: oral solution

8.2 Hypothyroidism

Thyroid hormones

Overview

Thyroid hormones are used in hypothyroidism (juvenile myxoedema), and also in diffuse non-toxic goitre, congenital or neonatal hypothyroidism, and Hashimoto's thyroiditis (lymphadenoid goitre). Neonatal hypothyroidism requires prompt treatment to facilitate normal development.

Levothyroxine sodium below (thyroxine sodium) is the treatment of choice for *maintenance* therapy.

Doses for congenital hypothyroidism and juvenile myxoedema should be titrated according to clinical response, growth assessment, and measurement of plasma thyroxine and thyroid-stimulating hormone concentrations. In congenital hypothyroidism higher initial doses may normalise metabolism more quickly, with associated beneficial effects on mental development.

Liothyronine sodium p. 525 has a similar action to levothyroxine sodium but is more rapidly metabolised and has a more rapid effect. Its effects develop after a few hours and disappear within 24 to 48 hours of discontinuing treatment. It may be used in *severe hypothyroid states* when a rapid response is desired.

Liothyronine sodium by intravenous injection is the treatment of choice in *hypothyroid coma*. Adjunctive therapy includes intravenous fluids, hydrocortisone p. 476, and treatment of infection; assisted ventilation is often required.

Advanced Pharmacy Services

Children with thyroid disorders may be eligible for the Medicines Use Review service provided by a community pharmacist. For further information, see *Advanced Pharmacy Services* in Medicines optimisation p. 25.

THYROID HORMONES

Levothyroxine sodium

10-Mar-2020

(Thyroxine sodium)

- **INDICATIONS AND DOSE**

Hypothyroidism

▶ BY MOUTH

- ▸ Neonate: Initially 10–15 micrograms/kg once daily (max. per dose 50 micrograms); adjusted in steps of 5 micrograms/kg every 2 weeks, alternatively adjusted in steps of 5 micrograms/kg as required; maintenance 20–50 micrograms daily, levothyroxine should be taken at the same time each day, preferably 30 minutes before meals, caffeine-containing drinks, or other medicines; this could be before breakfast or another more convenient time.
- ▸ Child 1 month–1 year: Initially 5 micrograms/kg once daily (max. per dose 50 micrograms); adjusted in steps of 10–25 micrograms every 2–4 weeks until metabolism normalised; maintenance 25–75 micrograms daily, levothyroxine should be taken at the same time each day, preferably 30 minutes before meals, caffeine-containing drinks, or other medicines; this could be before breakfast or another more convenient time
- ▸ Child 2-11 years: Initially 50 micrograms once daily; adjusted in steps of 25 micrograms every 2–4 weeks until metabolism normalised; maintenance 75–100 micrograms daily, levothyroxine should be taken at the same time each day, preferably 30 minutes before meals, caffeine-containing drinks, or other medicines; this could be before breakfast or another more convenient time
- ▸ Child 12-17 years: Initially 50 micrograms once daily; adjusted in steps of 25–50 micrograms every 3–4 weeks until metabolism normalised; maintenance 100–200 micrograms daily, levothyroxine should be taken at the same time each day, preferably 30 minutes before meals, caffeine-containing drinks, or other medicines; this could be before breakfast or another more convenient time

Hyperthyroidism (blocking-replacement regimen) in combination with carbimazole

▶ BY MOUTH

- ▸ Child: Therapy usually given for 12 to 24 months (consult product literature or local protocols)

- **CONTRA-INDICATIONS** Thyrotoxicosis
- **CAUTIONS** Cardiac disorders (monitor ECG; start at low dose and carefully titrate) · diabetes insipidus · diabetes mellitus (dose of antidiabetic drugs including insulin may need to be increased) · long-standing hypothyroidism · panhypopituitarism (initiate corticosteroid therapy before starting levothyroxine) · predisposition to adrenal insufficiency (initiate corticosteroid therapy before starting levothyroxine)
- **INTERACTIONS** → Appendix 1: thyroid hormones
- **SIDE-EFFECTS** Alopecia · angina pectoris · anxiety · arrhythmias · arthralgia · diarrhoea · dyspnoea · epiphyses premature fusion · fever · flushing · headache · heat intolerance · hyperhidrosis · idiopathic intracranial hypertension · insomnia · malaise · menstruation irregular · muscle spasms · muscle weakness · oedema · palpitations · skin reactions · thyrotoxic crisis · tremor · vomiting · weight decreased
- **PREGNANCY** Levothyroxine may cross the placenta. Excessive or insufficient maternal thyroid hormones can be detrimental to fetus.

  Dose adjustments Levothyroxine requirement may increase during pregnancy.

  Monitoring Assess maternal thyroid function before conception (if possible), at diagnosis of pregnancy, at antenatal booking, during both the second and third trimesters, and after delivery (more frequent monitoring required on initiation or adjustment of levothyroxine).
- **BREAST FEEDING** Amount too small to affect tests for neonatal hypothyroidism.
- **PRESCRIBING AND DISPENSING INFORMATION** Levothyroxine equivalent to 100 micrograms/m^2/day can be used as a guide to the requirements in children.
- **PATIENT AND CARER ADVICE**

  Medicines for Children leaflet: Levothyroxine for hypothyroidism www.medicinesforchildren.org.uk/levothyroxine-hypothyroidism

- **MEDICINAL FORMS** There can be variation in the licensing of different medicines containing the same drug. Forms available from special-order manufacturers include: capsule, oral suspension, oral solution

Tablet

- ▸ **Levothyroxine sodium (Non-proprietary)**

  Levothyroxine sodium anhydrous 12.5 microgram Levothyroxine sodium 12.5microgram tablets | 28 tablet PoM £12.49 DT = £8.19

  Levothyroxine sodium anhydrous 25 microgram Levothyroxine sodium 25microgram tablets | 28 tablet PoM £3.05 DT = £1.50 | 500 tablet PoM £41.61–£54.46

Levothyroxine sodium 25microgram tablets lactose free | 100 tablet PoM ⊠

Levothyroxine sodium anhydrous 50 microgram Levothyroxine sodium 50microgram tablets lactose free | 100 tablet PoM ⊠

Levothyroxine sodium 50microgram tablets | 28 tablet PoM £1.50 DT = £1.19 | 1000 tablet PoM £42.50–£55.71

Levothyroxine sodium anhydrous 75 microgram Levothyroxine sodium 75microgram tablets | 28 tablet PoM £4.00 DT = £3.07

Levothyroxine sodium anhydrous 100 microgram Levothyroxine sodium 100microgram tablets lactose free | 100 tablet PoM ⊠

Levothyroxine sodium 100microgram tablets | 28 tablet PoM £1.77 DT = £1.19 | 1000 tablet PoM £42.50–£56.07

▸ Eltroxin (Advanz Pharma)

Levothyroxine sodium anhydrous 25 microgram Eltroxin 25microgram tablets | 28 tablet PoM £2.54 DT = £1.50

Levothyroxine sodium anhydrous 50 microgram Eltroxin 50microgram tablets | 28 tablet PoM £1.77 DT = £1.19

Levothyroxine sodium anhydrous 100 microgram Eltroxin 100microgram tablets | 28 tablet PoM £1.78 DT = £1.19

Oral solution

▸ Levothyroxine sodium (Non-proprietary)

Levothyroxine sodium anhydrous 5 microgram per 1 ml Levothyroxine sodium 25micrograms/5ml oral solution sugar free sugar-free | 100 ml PoM £118.63 DT = £94.99

Levothyroxine sodium anhydrous 10 microgram per 1 ml Levothyroxine sodium 50micrograms/5ml oral solution sugar free sugar-free | 100 ml PoM £107.93 DT = £96.57

Levothyroxine sodium anhydrous 20 microgram per 1 ml Levothyroxine sodium 100micrograms/5ml oral solution sugar free sugar-free | 100 ml PoM £165.00 DT = £164.99

Levothyroxine sodium anhydrous 25 microgram per 1 ml Levothyroxine sodium 125micrograms/5ml oral solution sugar free sugar-free | 100 ml PoM £185.00 DT = £185.00

Liothyronine sodium

08-Jul-2019

(L-Tri-iodothyronine sodium)

● **INDICATIONS AND DOSE**

Hypothyroidism

▸ BY MOUTH

▸ Child 12–17 years: Initially 10–20 micrograms daily; increased to 60 micrograms daily in 2–3 divided doses

Hypothyroid coma

▸ BY SLOW INTRAVENOUS INJECTION

▸ Child 12–17 years: 5–20 micrograms every 12 hours, increased to 5–20 micrograms every 4 hours if required, alternatively initially 50 micrograms for 1 dose, then 25 micrograms every 8 hours, reduced to 25 micrograms twice daily

Hypothyroidism (replacement for oral levothyroxine)

▸ BY SLOW INTRAVENOUS INJECTION

▸ Child: Convert daily levothyroxine dose to liothyronine and give in 2–3 divided doses, adjusted according to response

DOSE EQUIVALENCE AND CONVERSION

▸ 20–25 micrograms of liothyronine sodium is equivalent to approximately 100 micrograms of levothyroxine sodium.

▸ Brands without a UK licence may not be bioequivalent and dose adjustment may be necessary.

● **CONTRA-INDICATIONS** Thyrotoxicosis

● **CAUTIONS** Cardiac disorders (monitor ECG; start at low dose and carefully titrate) · diabetes insipidus · diabetes mellitus (dose of antidiabetic drugs including insulin may need to be increased) · prolonged hypothyroidism (initiate corticosteroid therapy in adrenal insufficiency) · severe hypothyroidism (initiate corticosteroid therapy in adrenal insufficiency)

● **INTERACTIONS** → Appendix 1: thyroid hormones

● **SIDE-EFFECTS**

GENERAL SIDE-EFFECTS

▸ **Frequency not known**

Alopecia · angina pectoris · anxiety · arrhythmias · diarrhoea · fever · flushing · headache · heat intolerance · hyperhidrosis · insomnia · muscle cramps · muscle weakness · palpitations · tremor · vomiting · weight decreased

SPECIFIC SIDE-EFFECTS

▸ **Rare or very rare**

▸ With intravenous use Idiopathic intracranial hypertension

▸ **Frequency not known**

▸ With intravenous use Epiphyses premature fusion · menstruation irregular

● **PREGNANCY** Does not cross the placenta in significant amounts. Excessive or insufficient maternal thyroid hormones can be detrimental to fetus.

Dose adjustments Liothyronine requirement may increase during pregnancy.

Monitoring Assess maternal thyroid function before conception (if possible), at diagnosis of pregnancy, at antenatal booking, during both the second and third trimesters, and after delivery (more frequent monitoring required on initiation or adjustment of liothyronine).

● **BREAST FEEDING** Amount too small to affect tests for neonatal hypothyroidism.

● **PRESCRIBING AND DISPENSING INFORMATION**

Switching to a different brand Patients switched to a different brand should be monitored (particularly if pregnant or if heart disease present) as brands without a UK licence may not be bioequivalent. Pregnant women or those with heart disease should undergo an early review of thyroid status, and other patients should have thyroid function assessed if experiencing a significant change in symptoms. If liothyronine is continued long-term, thyroid function tests should be repeated 1–2 months after any change in brand.

● **MEDICINAL FORMS** There can be variation in the licensing of different medicines containing the same drug. Forms available from special-order manufacturers include: tablet, capsule, oral suspension, oral solution, solution for injection

Tablet

▸ Liothyronine sodium (Non-proprietary)

Liothyronine sodium 5 microgram Liothyronine 5microgram tablets | 28 tablet PoM £98.00 DT = £98.00

Liothyronine sodium 10 microgram Liothyronine 10microgram tablets | 28 tablet PoM £148.00 DT = £148.00

Liothyronine sodium 20 microgram Liothyronine 20microgram tablets | 28 tablet PoM £245.29 DT = £154.83

▸ Cytomel (Imported (United States))

Liothyronine sodium 25 microgram Cytomel 25microgram tablets | 100 tablet PoM ⊠

Powder for solution for injection

▸ Liothyronine sodium (Non-proprietary)

Liothyronine sodium 20 microgram Liothyronine 20microgram powder for solution for injection vials | 5 vial PoM £1,567.50 DT = £1,567.50

Chapter 7
Genito-urinary system

CONTENTS

1 Bladder and urinary disorders

1.1 Urinary frequency, enuresis, and incontinence

Urinary frequency, enuresis and incontinence

Urinary incontinence

Antimuscarinic drugs reduce symptoms of urgency and urge incontinence and increase bladder capacity; oxybutynin hydrochloride p. 527 also has a direct relaxant effect on urinary smooth muscle. Oxybutynin hydrochloride can be considered first for children under 12 years. Side-effects limit the use of oxybutynin hydrochloride, but they may be reduced by starting at a lower dose and then slowly titrating upwards; alternatively oxybutynin hydrochloride can be given by intravesicular instillation. Tolterodine tartrate p. 528 is also effective for urinary incontinence; it can be considered for children over 12 years, or for younger children who have failed to respond to oxybutynin hydrochloride. Modified-release preparations of oxybutynin hydrochloride and tolterodine tartrate are available; they may have fewer side-effects. Antimuscarinic treatment should be reviewed soon after it is commenced, and then at regular intervals; a response generally occurs within 6 months but occasionally may take longer. Children with nocturnal enuresis may require specific additional measures if night-time symptoms also need to be controlled.

See also Nocturnal enuresis in children below.

Nocturnal enuresis in children

23-May-2017

Description of condition

Nocturnal enuresis is the involuntary discharge of urine during sleep, which is common in young children. Children are generally expected to be dry by a developmental age of 5 years, and historically it has been common practice to consider children for treatment only when they reach 7 years; however, symptoms may still persist in a small proportion by the age of 10 years.

Treatment

Children under 5 years

EvGr For children under 5 years, treatment is usually unnecessary as the condition is likely to resolve spontaneously. Reassurance and advice can be useful for some families. (A)

Non Drug Treatment

EvGr Initially, advice should be given on fluid intake, diet, toileting behaviour, and use of reward systems. For children who do not respond to this advice (more than 1–2 wet beds per week), an enuresis alarm should be the recommended treatment for motivated, well-supported children. Alarms in children under 7 years should be considered depending on the child's maturity, motivation and understanding of the alarm. Alarms have a lower relapse rate than drug treatment when discontinued.

Treatment using an alarm should be reviewed after 4 weeks and continued until a minimum of 2 weeks' uninterrupted dry nights have been achieved. If complete dryness is not achieved after 3 months but the condition is still improving and the child remains motivated to use the alarm, it is recommended to continue the treatment. Combined treatment with desmopressin p. 468, or the use of desmopressin alone, is recommended if the initial alarm treatment is unsuccessful or it is no longer appropriate or desirable. (A)

Drug Treatment

EvGr Treatment with oral or sublingual desmopressin is recommended for children over 5 years of age when alarm use is inappropriate or undesirable, or when rapid or short-term results are the priority (for example, to cover periods away from home). Desmopressin alone can also be used if there has been a partial response to a combination of desmopressin and an alarm following initial treatment with an alarm alone. Treatment should be assessed after 4 weeks and continued for 3 months if there are signs of response. Repeated courses of desmopressin can be used in responsive children who experience repeated recurrences of bedwetting, but should be withdrawn **gradually** at regular intervals (for 1 week every 3 months) for full reassessment.

Under specialist supervision, nocturnal enuresis associated with daytime symptoms (overactive bladder) can be managed with desmopressin alone or in combination with an antimuscarinic drug (such as oxybutynin hydrochloride p. 527 or tolterodine tartrate p. 528 [unlicensed indication]).

Treatment should be continued for 3 months; the course can be repeated if necessary.

The tricyclic antidepressant imipramine hydrochloride p. 256 can be considered for children who have not responded to all other treatments and have undergone specialist assessment, however relapse is common after withdrawal and children and their carers should be aware of the dangers of overdose. Initial treatment should continue for 3 months; further courses can be considered following a medical review every 3 months. Tricyclic antidepressants should be withdrawn gradually. (A)

Useful Resources

Bedwetting in under 19s. National Institute for Health and Care Excellence. Clinical guideline CG111. October 2010. www.nice.org.uk/guidance/cg111

Other drugs used for Urinary frequency, enuresis, and incontinence Propantheline bromide, p. 68

ANTIMUSCARINICS

Antimuscarinics (systemic)

- **CONTRA-INDICATIONS** Angle-closure glaucoma · gastro-intestinal obstruction · intestinal atony · myasthenia gravis (but some antimuscarinics may be used to decrease muscarinic side-effects of anticholinesterases) · paralytic ileus · pyloric stenosis · severe ulcerative colitis · significant bladder outflow obstruction · toxic megacolon · urinary retention
- **CAUTIONS** Arrhythmias (may be worsened) · autonomic neuropathy · cardiac insufficiency (due to association with tachycardia) · cardiac surgery (due to association with tachycardia) · children (increased risk of side-effects) · conditions characterised by tachycardia · congestive heart failure (may be worsened) · coronary artery disease (may be worsened) · diarrhoea · gastro-oesophageal reflux disease · hiatus hernia with reflux oesophagitis · hypertension · hyperthyroidism (due to association with tachycardia) · individuals susceptible to angle-closure glaucoma · pyrexia · ulcerative colitis
- **SIDE-EFFECTS**
  - **Common or very common** Confusion · constipation · dizziness · drowsiness · dry mouth · dyspepsia · flushing · headache · nausea · palpitations · skin reactions · tachycardia · urinary disorders · vision disorders · vomiting
  - **Rare or very rare** Angioedema
- **PATIENT AND CARER ADVICE**
  Driving and skilled tasks Antimuscarinics can affect the performance of skilled tasks (e.g. driving).

ANTIMUSCARINICS > URINARY

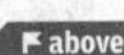

Oxybutynin hydrochloride

24-Jul-2018

- **INDICATIONS AND DOSE**

Urinary frequency | Urinary urgency | Urinary incontinence | Neurogenic bladder instability

- BY MOUTH USING IMMEDIATE-RELEASE MEDICINES
  - Child 2–4 years: 1.25–2.5 mg 2–3 times a day
  - Child 5–11 years: Initially 2.5–3 mg twice daily, increased to 5 mg 2–3 times a day
  - Child 12–17 years: Initially 5 mg 2–3 times a day, increased if necessary up to 5 mg 4 times a day
- BY INTRAVESICAL INSTILLATION
  - Child 2–17 years: 5 mg 2–3 times a day
- BY MOUTH USING MODIFIED-RELEASE TABLETS
  - Child 5–17 years: Initially 5 mg once daily, adjusted in steps of 5 mg every week, adjusted according to response; maximum 15 mg per day

Nocturnal enuresis associated with overactive bladder

- BY MOUTH USING IMMEDIATE-RELEASE MEDICINES
  - Child 5–17 years: 2.5–3 mg twice daily, increased to 5 mg 2–3 times a day, last dose to be taken before bedtime
- BY MOUTH USING MODIFIED-RELEASE TABLETS
  - Child 5–17 years: Initially 5 mg once daily, adjusted in steps of 5 mg every week, adjusted according to response; maximum 15 mg per day

DOSE EQUIVALENCE AND CONVERSION
- Patients taking immediate-release oxybutynin may be transferred to the nearest equivalent daily dose of *Lyrinel® XL*

- **UNLICENSED USE** Not licensed for use in children under 5 years. Intravesical instillation not licensed for use in children.
- **CAUTIONS** Acute porphyrias p. 652
- **INTERACTIONS** → Appendix 1: oxybutynin
- **SIDE-EFFECTS**
  - **Common or very common** Diarrhoea · dry eye
  - **Uncommon** Abdominal discomfort · appetite decreased · dysphagia
  - **Frequency not known** Anxiety · arrhythmia · cognitive disorder · depressive symptom · drug dependence · gastrointestinal disorders · glaucoma · hallucination · heat stroke · hypohidrosis · mydriasis · nightmare · paranoia · photosensitivity reaction · seizure · urinary tract infection
- **PREGNANCY** Manufacturers advise avoid unless essential—toxicity in *animal* studies.
- **BREAST FEEDING** Manufacturers advise avoid—present in milk in *animal* studies.
- **HEPATIC IMPAIRMENT** Manufacturer advises caution.
- **RENAL IMPAIRMENT** Manufacturer advises caution.
- **PRESCRIBING AND DISPENSING INFORMATION** The need for therapy for urinary indications should be reviewed soon after it has been commenced and then at regular intervals; a response usually occurs within 6 months but may take longer.

  Intravesical instillation may be available from 'special-order' manufacturers or specialist importing companies.
- **PATIENT AND CARER ADVICE**
  Medicines for Children leaflet: Oxybutynin for daytime urinary symptoms www.medicinesforchildren.org.uk/oxybutynin-daytime-urinary-symptoms

- **MEDICINAL FORMS** There can be variation in the licensing of different medicines containing the same drug. Forms available from special-order manufacturers include: oral suspension, oral solution, bladder irrigation

Modified-release tablet

CAUTIONARY AND ADVISORY LABELS 3, 25

- Lyrinel XL (Janssen-Cilag Ltd)
  Oxybutynin hydrochloride 5 mg Lyrinel XL 5mg tablets | 30 tablet [PoM] £13.77 DT = £13.77
  Oxybutynin hydrochloride 10 mg Lyrinel XL 10mg tablets | 30 tablet [PoM] £27.54 DT = £27.54

Tablet

CAUTIONARY AND ADVISORY LABELS 3

- Oxybutynin hydrochloride (Non-proprietary)
  Oxybutynin hydrochloride 2.5 mg Oxybutynin 2.5mg tablets | 56 tablet [PoM] £6.58 DT = £2.03 | 84 tablet [PoM] £2.96–£7.71
  Oxybutynin hydrochloride 3 mg Oxybutynin 3mg tablets | 56 tablet [PoM] £17.91 DT = £17.82
  Oxybutynin hydrochloride 5 mg Oxybutynin 5mg tablets | 56 tablet [PoM] £13.85 DT = £2.18 | 84 tablet [PoM] £3.27–£20.77

▸ Cystrin (Sanofi)
Oxybutynin hydrochloride 5 mg Cystrin 5mg tablets | 84 tablet PoM £21.99

▸ Ditropan (Sanofi)
Oxybutynin hydrochloride 2.5 mg Ditropan 2.5mg tablets | 84 tablet PoM £1.60
Oxybutynin hydrochloride 5 mg Ditropan 5mg tablets | 84 tablet PoM £2.90

Oral solution

CAUTIONARY AND ADVISORY LABELS 3

▸ Oxybutynin hydrochloride (Non-proprietary)
Oxybutynin hydrochloride 500 microgram per 1 ml Oxybutynin 2.5mg/5ml oral solution sugar-free | 150 ml PoM £214.84 DT = £214.77
Oxybutynin hydrochloride 1 mg per 1 ml Oxybutynin 5mg/5ml oral solution sugar-free | 150 ml PoM £235.53 DT = £235.53

527

Tolterodine tartrate

20-Jan-2020

● **INDICATIONS AND DOSE**

Urinary frequency | Urinary urgency | Urinary incontinence

▸ BY MOUTH USING IMMEDIATE-RELEASE MEDICINES
▸ Child 2–17 years: 1 mg once daily, then increased if necessary up to 2 mg twice daily, adjusted according to response

▸ BY MOUTH USING MODIFIED-RELEASE CAPSULES
▸ Child 2–17 years: 4 mg once daily

Nocturnal enuresis associated with overactive bladder

▸ BY MOUTH USING IMMEDIATE-RELEASE MEDICINES
▸ Child 5–17 years: 1 mg once daily, dose to be taken at bedtime, then increased if necessary up to 2 mg twice daily, adjusted according to response

DOSE EQUIVALENCE AND CONVERSION
▸ Children stabilised on immediate-release tolterodine tartrate 2 mg twice daily may be transferred to modified-release tolterodine tartrate 4 mg once daily.

● **UNLICENSED USE** Not licensed for use in children.

● **CAUTIONS** History of QT-interval prolongation

● **INTERACTIONS** → Appendix 1: tolterodine

● **SIDE-EFFECTS**

▸ **Common or very common** Abdominal pain · bronchitis · chest pain · diarrhoea · dry eye · fatigue · gastrointestinal disorders · paraesthesia · peripheral oedema · vertigo · weight increased

▸ **Uncommon** Arrhythmia · heart failure · memory loss · nervousness

▸ **Frequency not known** Hallucination

● **PREGNANCY** Manufacturer advises avoid—toxicity in *animal* studies.

● **BREAST FEEDING** Manufacturer advises avoid—no information available.

● **HEPATIC IMPAIRMENT** Manufacturer advises caution (risk of increased exposure).
Dose adjustments In adults, manufacturers advise dose reduction—consult product literature.

● **RENAL IMPAIRMENT** Manufacturer advises caution (risk of increased exposure) Avoid modified-release preparations if estimated glomerular filtration rate less than 30 mL/minute/1.73m^2.
Dose adjustments Reduce dose if estimated glomerular filtration less than 30 mL/minute/1.73m^2.

● **PRESCRIBING AND DISPENSING INFORMATION** The need for therapy for urinary indications should be reviewed soon after it has been commenced and then at regular intervals; a response usually occurs within 6 months but may take longer.

● **MEDICINAL FORMS** There can be variation in the licensing of different medicines containing the same drug. Forms available from special-order manufacturers include: oral suspension, oral solution, powder

Tablet

CAUTIONARY AND ADVISORY LABELS 3

▸ Tolterodine tartrate (Non-proprietary)
Tolterodine tartrate 1 mg Tolterodine 1mg tablets | 56 tablet PoM £29.03 DT = £1.70
Tolterodine tartrate 2 mg Tolterodine 2mg tablets | 56 tablet PoM £30.56 DT = £2.01

▸ Detrusitol (Upjohn UK Ltd)
Tolterodine tartrate 1 mg Detrusitol 1mg tablets | 56 tablet PoM £29.03 DT = £1.70
Tolterodine tartrate 2 mg Detrusitol 2mg tablets | 56 tablet PoM £30.56 DT = £2.01

Modified-release capsule

CAUTIONARY AND ADVISORY LABELS 3, 25

▸ Tolterodine tartrate (Non-proprietary)
Tolterodine tartrate 2 mg Tolthen XL 2mg capsules | 28 capsule PoM £11.60 DT = £11.60
Tolterma XL 2mg capsules | 28 capsule PoM £24.36 DT = £11.60
Tolterodine tartrate 4 mg Tolthen XL 4mg capsules | 28 capsule PoM £12.89 DT = £25.78
Tolterma XL 4mg capsules | 28 capsule PoM £25.78 DT = £25.78

▸ Blerone XL (Zentiva)
Tolterodine tartrate 4 mg Blerone XL 4mg capsules | 28 capsule PoM £12.80 DT = £25.78

▸ Detrusitol XL (Upjohn UK Ltd)
Tolterodine tartrate 4 mg Detrusitol XL 4mg capsules | 28 capsule PoM £25.78 DT = £25.78

▸ Inconex XL (Sandoz Ltd)
Tolterodine tartrate 4 mg Inconex XL 4mg capsules | 28 capsule PoM £21.91 DT = £25.78

▸ Mariosea XL (Teva UK Ltd)
Tolterodine tartrate 2 mg Mariosea XL 2mg capsules | 28 capsule PoM £11.59 DT = £11.60
Tolterodine tartrate 4 mg Mariosea XL 4mg capsules | 28 capsule PoM £12.79 DT = £25.78

▸ Neditol XL (Aspire Pharma Ltd)
Tolterodine tartrate 2 mg Neditol XL 2mg capsules | 28 capsule PoM £11.60 DT = £11.60
Tolterodine tartrate 4 mg Neditol XL 4mg capsules | 28 capsule PoM £12.89 DT = £25.78

▸ Preblacon XL (Accord Healthcare Ltd)
Tolterodine tartrate 4 mg Preblacon XL 4mg capsules | 28 capsule PoM £25.78 DT = £25.78

▸ Santizor XL (Upjohn UK Ltd)
Tolterodine tartrate 4 mg Santizor XL 4mg capsules | 28 capsule PoM £25.78 DT = £25.78

527

Trospium chloride

11-May-2018

● **INDICATIONS AND DOSE**

Urinary frequency | Urinary urgency | Urge incontinence

▸ BY MOUTH USING IMMEDIATE-RELEASE MEDICINES
▸ Child 12–17 years: 20 mg twice daily, to be taken before food

● **INTERACTIONS** → Appendix 1: trospium

● **SIDE-EFFECTS**

▸ **Common or very common** Abdominal pain

▸ **Uncommon** Chest pain · diarrhoea · flatulence

▸ **Rare or very rare** Arthralgia · asthenia · dyspnoea · myalgia

▸ **Frequency not known** Agitation · anaphylactic reaction · hallucination · severe cutaneous adverse reactions (SCARs)

● **PREGNANCY** Manufacturer advises caution.

● **BREAST FEEDING** Manufacturer advises caution.

● **HEPATIC IMPAIRMENT** Manufacturer advises caution in mild to moderate impairment; avoid in severe impairment (no information available).

● **RENAL IMPAIRMENT** Use with caution. Avoid *Regurin® XL.*
Dose adjustments Reduce dose to 20 mg once daily or 20 mg on alternate days if eGFR 10–30 mL/minute/1.73m^2.

- **PRESCRIBING AND DISPENSING INFORMATION** The need for continuing therapy for urinary incontinence should be reviewed every 4–6 weeks until symptoms stabilise, and then every 6–12 months.

- **MEDICINAL FORMS** There can be variation in the licensing of different medicines containing the same drug. Forms available from special-order manufacturers include: oral solution

Tablet

CAUTIONARY AND ADVISORY LABELS 23

- Trospium chloride (Non-proprietary)
  Trospium chloride 20 mg Trospium chloride 20mg tablets | 60 tablet [PoM] £7.42 DT = £5.54
- Flotros (Galen Ltd)
  Trospium chloride 20 mg Flotros 20mg tablets | 60 tablet [PoM] £18.20 DT = £5.54
- Regurin (Mylan)
  Trospium chloride 20 mg Regurin 20mg tablets | 60 tablet [PoM] £26.00 DT = £5.54
- Uraplex (Contura Ltd)
  Trospium chloride 20 mg Uraplex 20mg tablets | 60 tablet [PoM] £26.00 DT = £5.54

1.2 Urinary retention

Urinary retention

31-May-2017

Description of condition

Urinary retention is the inability to voluntarily urinate. Causes in children can include severe voiding dysfunction, urethral blockage, drug treatment (such as opioids and antimuscarinic drugs), conditions that reduce detrusor contractions or interfere with relaxation of the urethra, and neurogenic causes.

Acute urinary retention is a medical emergency characterised by the abrupt (over a period of hours) development of the inability to pass urine, associated with increasing pain and the presence of a distended bladder, which can be palpated on examination.

Chronic urinary retention is the gradual (over months or years) development of the inability to empty the bladder completely, characterised by difficulties with initiating and maintaining urinary stream, urinary overflow, no sensation for needing to void and a post-void residual.

Treatment

[EvGr] Treatment of urinary retention depends on the underlying condition. Catheterisation is used as an effective initial management strategy, which should be followed by diagnostic evaluation and appropriate treatment of the underlying cause. Clean intermittent catheterisation on a long-term basis is effective for children with idiopathic or neurogenic bladder dysfunction.

The selective alpha-adrenoceptor blockers, doxazosin below and tamsulosin hydrochloride p. 530, have been shown to be of use in primary bladder neck dysfunction and dysfunctional voiding; they reduce urethral sphincteric pressure, thereby improving bladder emptying in children. Treatment should be under specialist advice only. ⟨E⟩

ALPHA-ADRENOCEPTOR BLOCKERS

Doxazosin

09-Feb-2020

- **INDICATIONS AND DOSE**

Hypertension

- BY MOUTH USING IMMEDIATE-RELEASE MEDICINES
- Child 6–11 years: Initially 500 micrograms once daily, then increased to 2–4 mg once daily, dose should be increased at intervals of 1 week
- Child 12–17 years: Initially 1 mg once daily for 1–2 weeks, then increased to 2 mg once daily, then increased if necessary to 4 mg once daily, rarely doses of up to 16 mg daily may be required

Dysfunctional voiding (initiated under specialist supervision)

- BY MOUTH USING IMMEDIATE-RELEASE MEDICINES
- Child 4–11 years: Initially 0.5 mg daily, adjusted according to response, dose should be increased at monthly intervals; maximum 2 mg per day
- Child 12–17 years: Initially 1 mg daily, adjusted according to response, dose may be doubled at intervals of 1 month; usual maintenance 2–4 mg daily; maximum 8 mg per day

DOSE EQUIVALENCE AND CONVERSION

- Patients stabilised on immediate-release doxazosin can be transferred to the equivalent dose of modified-release doxazosin.

- **UNLICENSED USE** Not licensed for use in children.
- **CONTRA-INDICATIONS** History of postural hypotension
- **CAUTIONS** Care with initial dose (postural hypotension) · cataract surgery (risk of intra-operative floppy iris syndrome) · heart failure · pulmonary oedema due to aortic or mitral stenosis
- **INTERACTIONS** → Appendix 1: alpha blockers
- **SIDE-EFFECTS**
  - **Common or very common** Arrhythmias · asthenia · chest pain · cough · cystitis · dizziness · drowsiness · dry mouth · dyspnoea · gastrointestinal discomfort · headache · hypotension · increased risk of infection · influenza like illness · muscle complaints · nausea · oedema · pain · palpitations · skin reactions · urinary disorders · vertigo
  - **Uncommon** Angina pectoris · anxiety · appetite abnormal · arthralgia · constipation · depression · diarrhoea · gastrointestinal disorders · gout · haemorrhage · insomnia · myocardial infarction · sensation abnormal · sexual dysfunction · stroke · syncope · tinnitus · tremor · vomiting · weight increased
  - **Rare or very rare** Alopecia · bronchospasm · flushing · gynaecomastia · hepatic disorders · leucopenia · malaise · muscle weakness · thrombocytopenia · vision blurred
  - **Frequency not known** Floppy iris syndrome
- **PREGNANCY** No evidence of teratogenicity; manufacturers advise use only when potential benefit outweighs risk.
- **BREAST FEEDING** Accumulates in milk in *animal* studies—manufacturer advises avoid.
- **HEPATIC IMPAIRMENT** Manufacturer advises caution in mild to moderate impairment (limited information available); avoid in severe impairment (no information available).
- **PATIENT AND CARER ADVICE** Patient counselling is advised for doxazosin tablets (initial dose).
  Driving and skilled tasks May affect performance of skilled tasks e.g. driving.

- **MEDICINAL FORMS** There can be variation in the licensing of different medicines containing the same drug. Forms available from special-order manufacturers include: capsule, oral suspension, oral solution

Modified-release tablet

CAUTIONARY AND ADVISORY LABELS 25

- Cardura XL (Upjohn UK Ltd)
  Doxazosin (as Doxazosin mesilate) 4 mg Cardura XL 4mg tablets | 28 tablet [PoM] £5.00 DT = £5.00
  Doxazosin (as Doxazosin mesilate) 8 mg Cardura XL 8mg tablets | 28 tablet [PoM] £9.98 DT = £9.98
- Doxadura XL (Dexcel-Pharma Ltd)
  Doxazosin (as Doxazosin mesilate) 4 mg Doxadura XL 4mg tablets | 28 tablet [PoM] £4.75 DT = £5.00

- ▸ **Larbex XL** (Teva UK Ltd)
  Doxazosin (as Doxazosin mesilate) 4 mg Larbex XL 4mg tablets | 28 tablet PoM £6.08 DT = £5.00
- ▸ **Raporsin XL** (Actavis UK Ltd)
  Doxazosin (as Doxazosin mesilate) 4 mg Raporsin XL 4mg tablets | 28 tablet PoM £5.70 DT = £5.00
- ▸ **Slocinx XL** (Zentiva)
  Doxazosin (as Doxazosin mesilate) 4 mg Slocinx XL 4mg tablets | 28 tablet PoM £5.96 DT = £5.00

Tablet

- ▸ **Doxazosin (Non-proprietary)**
  Doxazosin (as Doxazosin mesilate) 1 mg Doxazosin 1mg tablets | 28 tablet PoM £10.56 DT = £0.97
  Doxazosin (as Doxazosin mesilate) 2 mg Doxazosin 2mg tablets | 28 tablet PoM £14.08 DT = £0.99
  Doxazosin (as Doxazosin mesilate) 4 mg Doxazosin 4mg tablets | 28 tablet PoM £14.08 DT = £1.17
  Doxazosin (as Doxazosin mesilate) 8 mg Doxazosin 8mg tablets | 28 tablet PoM £6.25–£8.25 DT = £6.25
- ▸ **Cardura** (Upjohn UK Ltd)
  Doxazosin (as Doxazosin mesilate) 1 mg Cardura 1mg tablets | 28 tablet PoM £10.56 DT = £0.97
  Doxazosin (as Doxazosin mesilate) 2 mg Cardura 2mg tablets | 28 tablet PoM £14.08 DT = £0.99
- ▸ **Doxadura** (Dexcel-Pharma Ltd)
  Doxazosin (as Doxazosin mesilate) 4 mg Doxadura 4mg tablets | 28 tablet PoM £1.04 DT = £1.17

7

Genito-urinary system

Tamsulosin hydrochloride

09-Feb-2020

● **INDICATIONS AND DOSE**

Dysfunctional voiding (administered on expert advice)

▸ BY MOUTH USING MODIFIED-RELEASE MEDICINES

▸ Child 12–17 years: 400 micrograms once daily

● **UNLICENSED USE** Not licensed for use in children.

● **CONTRA-INDICATIONS** History of postural hypotension

● **CAUTIONS** Care with initial dose (postural hypotension) · cataract surgery (risk of intra-operative floppy iris syndrome)

● **INTERACTIONS** → Appendix 1: alpha blockers

● **SIDE-EFFECTS**

- ▸ **Common or very common** Dizziness · sexual dysfunction
- ▸ **Uncommon** Asthenia · constipation · diarrhoea · headache · nausea · palpitations · postural hypotension · rhinitis · skin reactions · vomiting
- ▸ **Rare or very rare** Angioedema · Stevens-Johnson syndrome · syncope
- ▸ **Frequency not known** Dry mouth · epistaxis · vision disorders

● **HEPATIC IMPAIRMENT** Manufacturer advises avoid in severe impairment.

● **RENAL IMPAIRMENT** Use with caution if estimated glomerular filtration rate less than 10 mL/minute/1.73 m^2.

● **PATIENT AND CARER ADVICE**

Driving and skilled tasks May affect performance of skilled tasks e.g. driving.

● **MEDICINAL FORMS** There can be variation in the licensing of different medicines containing the same drug.

Modified-release tablet

CAUTIONARY AND ADVISORY LABELS 25

- ▸ **Tamsulosin hydrochloride (Non-proprietary)**
  Tamsulosin hydrochloride 400 microgram Faramsil 400microgram modified-release tablets | 30 tablet PoM £8.89 DT = £10.47
- ▸ **Cositam XL** (Consilient Health Ltd)
  Tamsulosin hydrochloride 400 microgram Cositam XL 400microgram tablets | 30 tablet PoM £8.89 DT = £10.47
- ▸ **Faramsil** (Sandoz Ltd)
  Tamsulosin hydrochloride 400 microgram Faramsil 400microgram modified-release tablets | 30 tablet PoM £8.89 DT = £10.47
- ▸ **Flectone XL** (Teva UK Ltd)
  Tamsulosin hydrochloride 400 microgram Flectone XL 400microgram tablets | 30 tablet PoM £9.95 DT = £10.47
- ▸ **Flomaxtra XL** (Astellas Pharma Ltd)
  Tamsulosin hydrochloride 400 microgram Flomaxtra XL 400microgram tablets | 30 tablet PoM £10.47 DT = £10.47

Modified-release capsule

CAUTIONARY AND ADVISORY LABELS 25

- ▸ **Tamsulosin hydrochloride (Non-proprietary)**
  Tamsulosin hydrochloride 400 microgram Tamsulosin 400microgram modified-release capsules | 30 capsule PoM £3.87–£5.07 DT = £3.87
  Contiflo XL 400microgram capsules | 30 capsule PoM £7.44 DT = £3.87
- ▸ **Contiflo XL** (Ranbaxy (UK) Ltd)
  Tamsulosin hydrochloride 400 microgram Contiflo XL 400microgram capsules | 30 capsule PoM £7.44 DT = £3.87
- ▸ **Flomax MR** (Sanofi)
  Tamsulosin hydrochloride 400 microgram Flomax Relief MR 400microgram capsules | 14 capsule P £5.58 | 28 capsule P £10.55
- ▸ **Losinate MR** (Consilient Health Ltd)
  Tamsulosin hydrochloride 400 microgram Losinate MR 400microgram capsules | 30 capsule PoM £10.14 DT = £3.87 | 200 capsule PoM £67.60
- ▸ **Pamsvax XL** (Actavis UK Ltd, Almus Pharmaceuticals Ltd)
  Tamsulosin hydrochloride 400 microgram Pamsvax XL 400microgram capsules | 30 capsule PoM £1.28 DT = £3.87
- ▸ **Petyme MR** (Teva UK Ltd)
  Tamsulosin hydrochloride 400 microgram Petyme 400microgram MR capsules | 30 capsule PoM £4.06 DT = £3.87
- ▸ **Tabphyn MR** (Genus Pharmaceuticals Ltd)
  Tamsulosin hydrochloride 400 microgram Tabphyn MR 400microgram capsules | 30 capsule PoM £4.45 DT = £3.87
- ▸ **Tamfrex XL** (Milpharm Ltd)
  Tamsulosin hydrochloride 400 microgram Tamfrex XL 400microgram capsules | 30 capsule PoM £28.51 DT = £3.87
- ▸ **Tamsumac** (Macleods Pharma UK Ltd)
  Tamsulosin hydrochloride 400 microgram Tamsumac 0.4mg modified-release capsules | 30 capsule PoM £3.87 DT = £3.87
- ▸ **Tamurex** (Somex Pharma)
  Tamsulosin hydrochloride 400 microgram Tamurex 400microgram modified-release capsules | 30 capsule PoM £3.87 DT = £3.87

1.3 Urolithiasis

Renal and ureteric stones

03-Apr-2019

Description of condition

Renal and ureteric stones are crystalline calculi that may form anywhere in the upper urinary tract. They are often asymptomatic but may cause pain when they move or obstruct the flow of urine. Most stones are composed of calcium salts (calcium oxalate, calcium phosphate or both). The rest are composed of struvite, uric acid, cystine and other substances. Patients are susceptible to stone formation when there is a decrease in urine volume and/or an excess of stone forming substances in the urine.

The following are risk factors that have been associated with stone formation: dehydration, change in urine pH, positive family history, obesity, urinary anatomical abnormalities, and excessive dietary intake of oxalate, urate, sodium, and animal protein. Certain diseases which alter urinary volume, pH, and concentrations of certain ions (such as calcium, phosphate, oxalate, sodium, and uric acid) may also increase the risk of stone formation. Certain drugs such as calcium or vitamin D supplements, protease inhibitors, or diuretics may also increase the risk of stone formation.

Symptoms of acute renal or ureteric stones can include an abrupt onset of severe unilateral abdominal pain radiating to the groin (known as renal colic) that may be accompanied with nausea, vomiting, haematuria, increased urinary frequency, dysuria and fever (if concomitant urinary infection is present).

Stones can pass spontaneously and will depend on a number of factors, including the size of the stone (stones greater than 6 mm have a very low chance of spontaneous passage), the location (distal ureteral stones are more likely to pass than proximal ureteral stones), and the degree of obstruction.

Aims of treatment

EvGr The aim of treatment is to improve the detection, clearance and prevention of renal and ureteric stones thereby reducing pain and improving quality of life. (A)

Non-drug treatment

EvGr Consider watchful waiting for asymptomatic renal stones if they are less than 5mm in diameter. If they are larger than this then the specialist will discuss the risk and benefit of this option with the patient or parents.

Options for surgical stone removal should be discussed by the specialist team in hospital depending on severity of obstruction, patient factors, size and site of stone. Options include shockwave lithotripsy, percutaneous nephrolithotomy and ureteroscopy.

For patients with recurrent calcium stones avoid excessive intake of oxalate-rich products, such as rhubarb, spinach, cocoa, tea, nuts, soy products, strawberries, and wheat bran. For patients with recurrent uric acid stones, avoid excessive dietary intake of urate rich products, such as liver, kidney, calf thymus, poultry skin, and certain fish (herring with skin, sardines and anchovies). (A)

Child aged under 16 years

EvGr Consider referring children and young patients with renal or ureteric stones to a paediatric nephrologist or urologist with expertise in this area for assessment and metabolic investigations.

Advise children to drink or carers to give their children 1–2 litres of water a day (depending on age) with the addition of fresh lemon juice and to avoid carbonated drinks. Advise children or carers to maintain a normal daily calcium intake of 350–1000mg and daily salt intake of 2–6g (depending on age). (A)

Child aged 16 years and over

EvGr Consider stone analysis and measure serum calcium for children with recurring renal or ureteric stones.

Along with maintaining a healthy lifestyle, advise children to drink 2.5–3 litres of water a day with the addition of fresh lemon juice and to avoid carbonated drinks. Maintain a normal daily calcium intake of 700–1,200mg and salt intake of no more than 6g a day. (A)

Pain Management

EvGr Offer NSAIDs as first line treatment for the management of pain associated with suspected renal colic or renal and ureteric stones. If NSAIDs are contra-indicated or not sufficiently controlling the pain, consider intravenous paracetamol. Subsequently, opioids can be used if both paracetamol and NSAIDs are contra-indicated or not sufficiently controlling the pain. Do not offer antispasmodics to patients with suspected renal colic. (A)

Medical Expulsive Therapy

EvGr Consider alpha-adrenoceptor blockers for children with distal ureteric stones less than 10mm in diameter. (A)

Child aged 16 years and over

EvGr Alpha-adrenoceptor blockers may also be considered as adjunctive therapy for children having shockwave lithotripsy for ureteric stones less than 10mm. (A)

Prevention of recurrence of stones

Child aged under 16 years

EvGr Alongside lifestyle advice, consider potassium citrate [unlicensed] in children with recurrent stones composed of at least 50% calcium oxalate, and those with hypercalciuria and hypocitraturia. (A)

Child aged 16 years and over

EvGr Alongside lifestyle advice, consider potassium citrate [unlicensed] in children with recurrent stones composed of at least 50% calcium oxalate. Thiazides [unlicensed] may be given if children also have hypercalciuria after restricting their sodium intake to no more than 6g a day. (A)

1.4 Urological pain

Urological pain

03-Apr-2019

Treatment

Lidocaine hydrochloride gel is a useful topical application in *urethral pain* or to relieve the discomfort of catheterisation.

For information on the management of pain in renal and ureteric stones, see Renal and ureteric stones p. 530.

Alkalinisation of urine

Alkalinisation of urine can be undertaken with potassium citrate. The alkalinising action may relieve the discomfort of *cystitis* caused by lower urinary tract infections.

ALKALISING DRUGS

Citric acid with potassium citrate

12-May-2020

● **INDICATIONS AND DOSE**

Relief of discomfort in mild urinary-tract infections | Alkalinisation of urine

▶ BY MOUTH USING ORAL SOLUTION

▶ Child 1–5 years: 5 mL 3 times a day, diluted well with water

▶ Child 6–17 years: 10 mL 3 times a day, diluted well with water

● **CAUTIONS** Cardiac disease

● **INTERACTIONS** → Appendix 1: potassium citrate

● **SIDE-EFFECTS** Hyperkalaemia · nausea · vomiting

● **RENAL IMPAIRMENT** Avoid in severe impairment.
Monitoring Close monitoring required in renal impairment—high risk of hyperkalaemia.

● **PRESCRIBING AND DISPENSING INFORMATION** When prepared extemporaneously, the BP states Potassium Citrate Mixture BP consists of potassium citrate 30%, citric acid monohydrate 5% in a suitable vehicle with a lemon flavour. Extemporaneous preparations should be recently prepared according to the following formula: potassium citrate 3 g, citric acid monohydrate 500 mg, syrup 2.5 mL, quillaia tincture 0.1 mL, lemon spirit 0.05 mL, double-strength chloroform water 3 mL, water to 10 mL. Contains about 28 mmol K^+/10 mL.

● **EXCEPTIONS TO LEGAL CATEGORY** Proprietary brands of potassium citrate are on sale to the public for the relief of discomfort in mild urinary-tract infections.

● **MEDICINAL FORMS** There can be variation in the licensing of different medicines containing the same drug.

Oral solution

CAUTIONARY AND ADVISORY LABELS 27

▸ **Citric acid with potassium citrate (Non-proprietary)**
Citric acid monohydrate 50 mg per 1 ml, Potassium citrate 300 mg per 1 ml Potassium citrate mixture | 200 ml GSL £1.38 DT = £1.38 | 200 ml P £1.38 DT = £1.38

2 Bladder instillations and urological surgery

Bladder instillations and urological surgery

Bladder infection

Various solutions are available as irrigations or washouts.

Aqueous chlorhexidine p. 756 can be used in the management of common infections of the bladder but it is ineffective against most *Pseudomonas spp*. Solutions containing chlorhexidine 1 in 5000 (0.02%) are used but they may irritate the mucosa and cause burning and haematuria (in which case they should be discontinued); sterile sodium chloride **solution 0.9%** (physiological saline) p. 636 is usually adequate and is preferred as a mechanical irrigant.

Dissolution of blood clots

Clot retention is usually treated by irrigation with sterile sodium chloride solution 0.9% but sterile sodium citrate solution for bladder irrigation 3% may also be helpful.

Maintenance of indwelling urinary catheters

The deposition which occurs in catheterised patients is usually chiefly composed of phosphate and to minimise this the catheter (if latex) should be changed at least as often as every 6 weeks. If the catheter is to be left for longer periods a silicone catheter should be used together with the appropriate use of catheter maintenance solutions. Repeated blockage usually indicates that the catheter needs to be changed.

Catheter maintenance solutions

● **CATHETER MAINTENANCE SOLUTIONS**

OptiFlo G citric acid 3.23% catheter maintenance solution (Bard Ltd)
50 ml · NHS indicative price = £3.70 · Drug Tariff (Part IXa)100 ml · NHS indicative price = £3.70 · Drug Tariff (Part IXa)

OptiFlo R citric acid 6% catheter maintenance solution (Bard Ltd)
50 ml · NHS indicative price = £3.70 · Drug Tariff (Part IXa)100 ml · NHS indicative price = £3.70 · Drug Tariff (Part IXa)

Uro-Tainer PHMB polihexanide 0.02% catheter maintenance solution (B.Braun Medical Ltd)
100 ml · NHS indicative price = £3.49 · Drug Tariff (Part IXa)

Uro-Tainer Twin Solutio R citric acid 6% catheter maintenance solution (B.Braun Medical Ltd)
60 ml · NHS indicative price = £4.94 · Drug Tariff (Part IXa)

Uro-Tainer Twin Suby G citric acid 3.23% catheter maintenance solution (B.Braun Medical Ltd)
60 ml · NHS indicative price = £4.94 · Drug Tariff (Part IXa)

OptiFlo S saline 0.9% catheter maintenance solution (Bard Ltd)
Sodium chloride 9 mg per 1 ml 50 ml · NHS indicative price = £3.49 · Drug Tariff (Part IXa)100 ml · NHS indicative price = £3.49 · Drug Tariff (Part IXa)

Uro-Tainer M sodium chloride 0.9% catheter maintenance solution (B.Braun Medical Ltd) **Sodium chloride 9 mg per 1 ml** 50 ml · No NHS indicative price available · Drug Tariff (Part IXa)100 ml · No NHS indicative price available · Drug Tariff (Part IXa)

Uro-Tainer sodium chloride 0.9% catheter maintenance solution (B.Braun Medical Ltd) **Sodium chloride 9 mg per 1 ml** 50 ml · NHS indicative price = £3.61 · Drug Tariff (Part IXa)100 ml · NHS indicative price = £3.61 · Drug Tariff (Part IXa)

3 Contraception

Contraceptives, hormonal

Overview

Hormonal contraception includes combined hormonal contraception (containing an oestrogen and a progestogen) and progestogen-only contraception.

EvGr When prescribing contraception, information should be given on all available methods taking into consideration medical eligibility. This should include contraceptive effectiveness (including factors that alter efficacy), non-contraceptive benefits, health risks, and side effects to allow an informed decision to be made on the most suitable choice. ⟨A⟩

In adolescents, hormonal contraception is used after menarche. When prescribing contraception for females under 16 years of age, it is considered good practice for health professionals to follow the criteria in the Department of Health Guidance (July 2004), commonly known as the Fraser Guidelines available at tinyurl.com/yy3hl2gt.

The UK Medical Eligibility Criteria for Contraceptive Use (available at www.fsrh.org) is published by the Faculty of Sexual and Reproductive Healthcare (FSRH); it categorises the risks of using contraceptive methods with pre-existing medical conditions.

Contraception in patients taking medication with teratogenic potential: FSRH (February 2018) and MHRA (May 2019) guidance

Females of childbearing potential should be advised to use highly effective contraception if they or their male partners are taking known teratogenic drugs or drugs with potential teratogenic effects. Highly effective contraception should be used both during treatment and for the recommended duration after discontinuation to avoid unintended pregnancy. Pregnancy testing should be performed before treatment initiation to exclude pregnancy and repeat testing may be required.

Methods of contraception considered to be 'highly effective' include the long-acting reversible contraceptives (LARC) copper intra-uterine device (Cu-IUD), levonorgestrel intra-uterine system (LNG-IUS) and progestogen-only implant (IMP), and male and female sterilisation. For more information see the FSRH CEU statement (www.fsrh.org/standards-and-guidance/documents/fsrh-ceu-statement-contraception-for-women-using-known/), MHRA drug safety update (www.gov.uk/drug-safety-update/medicines-with-teratogenic-potential-what-is-effective-contraception-and-how-often-is-pregnancy-testing-needed), and the UK teratogenic information service (www.uktis.org).

Combined hormonal contraceptives

Combined hormonal contraceptives (CHC) are available as tablets (COC), transdermal patches (CTP), and vaginal rings (CVR). They are highly user-dependant methods where the failure rate if used perfectly (i.e. correctly and consistently) is less than 1%. Certain factors such as the person's weight, malabsorption (COC only), and drug interactions may contribute to contraceptive failure. Prescriptions of up to

12 months' supply for CHC initiation or continuation may be appropriate to avoid unwanted discontinuation and increased risk of pregnancy.

EvGr It is recommended that combined hormonal contraceptives are not continued beyond 50 years of age as safer alternatives exist. (A)

CHC use may be associated with some health benefits such as:

- Reduced risk of ovarian, endometrial and colorectal cancer;
- Predictable bleeding patterns
- Reduced dysmenorrhoea and menorrhagia;
- Management of symptoms of polycystic ovary syndrome (PCOS), endometriosis and premenstrual syndrome;
- Improvement of acne;
- Reduced menopausal symptoms;
- Maintaining bone mineral density in peri-menopausal females under the age of 50 years.

The use of CHC is, however also associated with health risks. For information on these risks, and further information on the benefits, see FSRH clinical guideline: **Combined Hormonal Contraception** (see *Useful resources*).

For information on advice to give to patients on switching between CHC and other contraception, and the management of incorrect CHC use, see FSRH clinical guidance: **Combined Hormonal Contraception** and **Incorrect use of Combined Hormonal Contraception** (see *Useful resources*).

Preparation choice

Combined oral contraceptives (COCs) containing a fixed amount of an oestrogen and a progestogen in each active tablet are termed 'monophasic'; those with varying amounts of the two hormones are termed 'multiphasic'.

Combined oral contraceptives usually contain ethinylestradiol as the oestrogen component; mestranol and estradiol are also used. The ethinylestradiol content of COCs range from 20–40 micrograms. EvGr A monophasic preparation containing 30 micrograms or less of ethinylestradiol in combination with levonorgestrel or norethisterone (to minimise cardiovascular risk), is generally used as the first line option. However, choice should be made taking into account the patients medical history, personal preference, previous contraceptive experience, and any age related considerations.

Due to potential reduced efficacy, non-oral CHC should be considered if there are concerns over absorption. In females who weigh 90 kg or more, consider non-topical options or use additional precautions with CTP. (A)

Combined Oral Contraceptives Monophasic 21-day preparations

Oestrogen content	Progestogen content	Brand
Ethinylestradiol 20 micrograms	Desogestrel 150 micrograms	Gedarel® 20/150
Ethinylestradiol 20 micrograms	Desogestrel 150 micrograms	Mercilon®
Ethinylestradiol 20 micrograms	Gestodene 75 micrograms	Femodette®
Ethinylestradiol 20 micrograms	Gestodene 75 micrograms	Millinette® 20/75
Ethinylestradiol 20 micrograms	Gestodene 75 micrograms	Sunya® 20/75
Ethinylestradiol 20 micrograms	Norethisterone acetate 1 mg	Loestrin® 20
Ethinylestradiol 30 micrograms	Desogestrel 150 micrograms	Gedarel® 30/150
Ethinylestradiol 30 micrograms	Desogestrel 150 micrograms	Marvelon®
Ethinylestradiol 30 micrograms	Drospirenone 3 mg	Yasmin®
Ethinylestradiol 30 micrograms	Gestodene 75 micrograms	Femodene®
Ethinylestradiol 30 micrograms	Gestodene 75 micrograms	Katya® 30/75
Ethinylestradiol 30 micrograms	Gestodene 75 micrograms	Millinette® 30/75
Ethinylestradiol 30 micrograms	Levonorgestrel 150 micrograms	Levest®
Ethinylestradiol 30 micrograms	Levonorgestrel 150 micrograms	Microgynon® 30
Ethinylestradiol 30 micrograms	Levonorgestrel 150 micrograms	Ovranette®
Ethinylestradiol 30 micrograms	Levonorgestrel 150 micrograms	Rigevidon®
Ethinylestradiol 30 micrograms	Norethisterone acetate 1.5 mg	Loestrin® 30
Ethinylestradiol 35 micrograms	Norgestimate 250 micrograms	Cilest®
Ethinylestradiol 35 micrograms	Norethisterone 500 micrograms	Brevinor®
Ethinylestradiol 35 micrograms	Norethisterone 1 mg	Norimin®
Mestranol 50 micrograms	Norethisterone 1 mg	Norinyl-1®

Combined Oral Contraceptives Monophasic 28-day preparations

Oestrogen content	Progestogen content	Brand
Ethinylestradiol 30 micrograms	Gestodene 75 micrograms	Femodene® ED
Ethinylestradiol 30 micrograms	Levonorgestrel 150 micrograms	Microgynon® 30 ED
Estradiol (as hemihydrate) 1.5 mg	Nomegestrol acetate 2.5 mg	Zoely®

7 Genito-urinary system

Combined Oral Contraceptives Multiphasic 21-day preparations

Oestrogen content	Progestogen content	Brand
Ethinylestradiol 30 micrograms	Levonorgestrel 50 micrograms	Logynon®
Ethinylestradiol 40 micrograms	Levonorgestrel 75 micrograms	
Ethinylestradiol 30 micrograms	Levonorgestrel 125 micrograms	
Ethinylestradiol 30 micrograms	Levonorgestrel 50 micrograms	TriRegol®
Ethinylestradiol 40 micrograms	Levonorgestrel 75 micrograms	
Ethinylestradiol 30 micrograms	Levonorgestrel 125 micrograms	
Ethinylestradiol 35 micrograms	Norethisterone 500 micrograms	Synphase®
Ethinylestradiol 35 micrograms	Norethisterone 1 mg	
Ethinylestradiol 35 micrograms	Norethisterone 500 micrograms	

Combined Oral Contraceptives Multiphasic 28-day preparations

Oestrogen content	Progestogen content	Brand
Ethinylestradiol 30 micrograms	Levonorgestrel 50 micrograms	Logynon® ED
Ethinylestradiol 40 micrograms	Levonorgestrel 75 micrograms	
Ethinylestradiol 30 micrograms	Levonorgestrel 125 micrograms	
Estradiol valerate 3 mg		Qlaira®
Estradiol valerate 2 mg	Dienogest 2 mg	
Estradiol valerate 2 mg	Dienogest 3 mg	
Estradiol valerate 1 mg		

Regimen choice

EvGr Information should be given to females on both the traditional 21 day CHC regimen with a monthly withdrawal bleed during the 7 day hormone free interval (HFI), and 'tailored' CHC regimens [unlicensed use]. Tailored CHC regimens can only be used with monophasic CHC containing ethinylestradiol [unlicensed use]; they offer the choice of either a shortened, or less frequent, or no hormone free interval based on the person's preference.

The following tailored regimens may be used [unlicensed use]:

- Shortened HFI: 21 days of continuous use followed by a 4 day HFI;
- Extended use (tricycling): 9 weeks of continuous use followed by a 4 or 7 day HFI;
- Flexible extended use: continuous use for 21 days or more followed by a 4 day HFI when breakthrough bleeding occurs;
- Continuous use: continuous CHC use with no HFI. ⟨A⟩

Withdrawal bleeds do not represent physiological menstruation and there is no difference in efficacy or safety of using the traditional 21 day regimen, which mimics the natural menstrual cycle, over using extended or continuous regimens. Use of the traditional regimen may be associated with disadvantages such as heavy or painful withdrawal bleeds, headaches, mood changes, and increased risk of incorrect use with subsequent unplanned pregnancy. EvGr Withdrawal bleeds during traditional CHC use has been reported in women who are pregnant and should therefore not be relied on as reassurance of a person's pregnancy status. ⟨A⟩

Follow up

EvGr A review of continued medical eligibility, satisfaction and adherence, drug interactions, and consideration of alternative contraception should be undertaken annually. Body mass index and blood pressure should also be checked annually. ⟨A⟩

Surgery

The manufacturers of CHC recommend that CHC use should be discontinued at least 4 weeks prior to major elective surgery, any surgery to the legs or pelvis, or surgery that involves prolonged immobilisation of a lower limb. An alternative method of contraception should be used to prevent unintentional pregnancy, and CHC may be recommenced 2 weeks after full remobilisation. When discontinuation is not possible, e.g. after trauma or if a patient admitted for an elective procedure is still on CHC, thromboprophylaxis should be considered.

When to seek further advice

EvGr All females should be advised to seek advice from a healthcare professional if they experience any troublesome side effects, have a significant health event, start any new medication, would like to discontinue CHC, or to discuss alternative methods at any time. For further information, see FSRH guidance **Combined Hormonal Contraception** (refer to *Useful resources* below). ⟨A⟩

Progestogen-only contraceptives

Oral progestogen-only contraceptives

Oral progestogen-only preparations alter cervical mucus to prevent sperm penetration and may inhibit ovulation in some women; oral desogestrel-only preparations consistently inhibit ovulation and this is their primary mechanism of action. There is insufficient clinical trial evidence to compare the efficacy of oral progestogen-only contraceptives with each other or with combined hormonal contraceptives. Progestogen-only contraceptives offer a suitable alternative to combined hormonal contraceptives when oestrogens are contra-indicated (including those with venous thrombosis or a past history or predisposition to venous thrombosis, heavy smokers, those with hypertension above systolic 160 mmHg or diastolic 95 mmHg, valvular heart disease, diabetes mellitus with complications, and migraine with aura).

Parenteral progestogen-only contraceptives

Medroxyprogesterone acetate p. 553 (*Depo-Provera®*, *SAYANA PRESS®*) is a long-acting progestogen given by injection; it is at least as effective as the combined oral preparations but because of its prolonged action it should never be given without *full counselling backed by the patient information leaflet*. It may be used as a short-term or long-term contraceptive for women who have been counselled about the likelihood of menstrual disturbance and the potential for a delay in return to full fertility. Delayed return of fertility and irregular cycles may occur after discontinuation of treatment but there is no evidence of permanent infertility. Troublesome bleeding has been reported in patients given medroxyprogesterone acetate in the immediate puerperium; delaying the first injection until 6 weeks after birth may minimise bleeding problems. If the woman is not breast-feeding, the first injection may be given within 5 days postpartum (she should be warned that the risk of troublesome bleeding may be increased).

- In adolescents, medroxyprogesterone acetate (*Depo-Provera*®, *SAYANA PRESS*®) should be used only when other methods of contraception are inappropriate;
- in all women, the benefits of using medroxyprogesterone acetate beyond 2 years should be evaluated against the risks;
- in women with risk factors for osteoporosis, a method of contraception other than medroxyprogesterone acetate should be considered.

Norethisterone enantate (*Noristerat*®) is a long-acting progestogen given as an oily injection which provides contraception for 8 weeks; it is used as short-term interim contraception e.g. before vasectomy becomes effective.

An **etonogestrel-releasing implant** (*Nexplanon*®) is also available. It is a highly effective long-acting contraceptive, consisting of a single flexible rod that is inserted subdermally into the lower surface of the upper arm and provides contraception for up to 3 years. The manufacturer advises that in heavier women, blood-etonogestrel concentrations are lower and therefore the implant may not provide effective contraception during the third year; they advise that earlier replacement may be considered in such patients—however, evidence to support this recommendation is lacking. Local reactions such as bruising and itching can occur at the insertion site. The contraceptive effect of etonogestrel is rapidly reversed on removal of the implant.

Intra-uterine progestogen-only device

The progestogen-only intra-uterine systems *Mirena*®, *Jaydess*® and *Levosert*® release levonorgestrel p. 549 directly into the uterine cavity. *Mirena*® is licensed for use as a contraceptive, for the treatment of primary menorrhagia and for the prevention of endometrial hyperplasia during oestrogen replacement therapy. *Jaydess*® and *Levosert*® are licensed for contraception, and *Levosert*® is additionally licensed for the treatment of menorrhagia. These may therefore be a contraceptive method of choice for women who have excessively heavy menses.

The effects of the progestogen-only intra-uterine system are mainly local and hormonal including prevention of endometrial proliferation, thickening of cervical mucus, and suppression of ovulation in some women (in some cycles). In addition to the progestogenic activity, the intra-uterine system itself may contribute slightly to the contraceptive effect. Return of fertility after removal is rapid and appears to be complete.

Advantages of the progestogen-only intra-uterine system over copper intra-uterine devices are that there may be an improvement in any dysmenorrhoea and a reduction in blood loss; there is also evidence that the frequency of pelvic inflammatory disease may be reduced (particularly in the youngest age groups who are most at risk).

In primary menorrhagia, menstrual bleeding is reduced significantly within 3–6 months of inserting the progestogen-only intra-uterine system, probably because it prevents endometrial proliferation. Another treatment should be considered if menorrhagia does not improve within this time.

Surgery

All progestogen-only contraceptives (including those given by injection) are suitable for use as an alternative to combined hormonal contraceptives before major elective surgery, before all surgery to the legs, or before surgery which involves prolonged immobilisation of a lower limb.

Useful resources

FSRH guideline: Combined Hormonal Contraception. The Faculty of Sexual & Reproductive Healthcare. February 2019.
www.fsrh.org/standards-and-guidance/documents/combined-hormonal-contraception/

FSRH CEU guidance: Recommended actions after incorrect use of combined hormonal contraception (e.g. late or missed pills, ring and patch). The Faculty of Sexual & Reproductive Healthcare. March 2020.
www.fsrh.org/documents/fsrh-ceu-guidance-recommended-actions-after-incorrect-use-of/

Contraceptives, non-hormonal

Contraception in patients taking medication with teratogenic potential: FSRH (February 2018) and MHRA (May 2019) guidance

Females of childbearing potential should be advised to use highly effective contraception if they or their male partners are taking known teratogenic drugs or drugs with potential teratogenic effects. Highly effective contraception should be used both during treatment and for the recommended duration after discontinuation to avoid unintended pregnancy. Pregnancy testing should be performed before treatment initiation to exclude pregnancy and repeat testing may be required.

Methods of contraception considered to be 'highly effective' include the long-acting reversible contraceptives (LARC) copper intra-uterine device (Cu-IUD), levonorgestrel intra-uterine system (LNG-IUS) and progestogen-only implant (IMP), and male and female sterilisation. For more information see the FSRH CEU statement (www.fsrh.org/standards-and-guidance/documents/fsrh-ceu-statement-contraception-for-women-using-known/), MHRA drug safety update (www.gov.uk/drug-safety-update/medicines-with-teratogenic-potential-what-is-effective-contraception-and-how-often-is-pregnancy-testing-needed), and the UK teratogenic information service (www.uktis.org).

Barrier methods

Barrier methods include condoms, diaphragms and cervical caps. Male condoms are less effective than some other contraception methods but are effective when used consistently and correctly, and provide significant protection against some sexually transmitted infections (STIs). A female condom (*Femidom*®) is also available; it is pre-lubricated with a non-spermicidal lubricant.

There is no evidence that condoms lubricated with spermicide provide additional protection against pregnancy or STIs. Diaphragms and caps must be used in conjunction with a **spermicide** and should not be removed until at least 6 hours after the last episode of intercourse.

Spermicidal contraceptives

Spermicidal contraceptives are useful additional safeguards but do **not** give adequate protection if used alone unless fertility is already significantly diminished. They have two components: a spermicide and a vehicle which itself may have some inhibiting effect on sperm activity. They are suitable for use with barrier methods, such as diaphragms or caps; however, spermicidal contraceptives are not recommended for use with condoms, as there is no evidence of any additional protection compared with non-spermicidal lubricants.

Spermicidal contraceptives are not suitable for use in those with or at high risk of sexually transmitted infections (including HIV); high frequency use of the spermicide nonoxinol '9' p. 553 has been associated with genital lesions, which may increase the risk of acquiring these infections.

Contraceptive devices

Intra-uterine devices

The intra-uterine device (IUD) is a suitable contraceptive for young women irrespective of parity; however, it is less appropriate for those with an increased risk of pelvic inflammatory disease e.g. women under 25 years.

The most effective intra-uterine devices have at least 380 mm^2 of copper and have banded copper on the arms. Smaller devices have been introduced to minimise side-effects; these consist of a plastic carrier wound with copper wire or fitted with copper bands; some also have a central core of silver to prevent fragmentation of the copper.

7 A frameless, copper-bearing intra-uterine device (*Gyne Fix*®) is also available. It consists of a knotted, polypropylene thread with 6 copper sleeves; the device is anchored in the uterus by inserting the knot into the uterine fundus.

Caution with oil-based lubricants

Products such as petroleum jelly (*Vaseline*®), baby oil and oil-based vaginal and rectal preparations are likely to damage condoms and contraceptive diaphragms made from latex rubber, and may render them less effective as a barrier method of contraception and as a protection from sexually transmitted infections (including HIV).

Emergency contraception

31-Aug-2017

Overview

EvGr Emergency contraception is intended for occasional use, to reduce the risk of pregnancy after unprotected sexual intercourse. It does not replace effective regular contraception.

Women who do not wish to conceive should be offered emergency contraception after unprotected sexual intercourse that has taken place on any day of a natural menstrual cycle. Emergency contraception should also be offered after unprotected intercourse from day 21 after childbirth (unless the criteria for lactational amenorrhoea are met), and from day 5 after abortion, miscarriage, ectopic pregnancy or uterine evacuation for gestational trophoblastic disease.

Emergency contraception should also be offered to women if their regular contraception has been compromised or has been used incorrectly. Ⓐ

Emergency contraceptive methods

Copper intra-uterine devices

EvGr Insertion of a copper intra-uterine device (see intra-uterine contraceptive devices (copper) p. 545) is the most effective form of emergency contraception and should be offered (if appropriate) to all women who have had unprotected sexual intercourse and do not want to conceive. A copper intra-uterine contraceptive device can be inserted up to 120 hours (5 days) after unprotected intercourse or up to 5 days after the earliest likely calculated ovulation (i.e. within the minimum period before implantation), regardless of the number of episodes of unprotected intercourse earlier in the cycle. Antibacterial cover should be considered for copper intra-uterine contraceptive device insertion if there is a significant risk of sexually transmitted infection that could be associated with ascending pelvic infection.

A copper intra-uterine device is not known to be affected by body mass index (BMI) or body-weight or by other drugs. Ⓐ

Hormonal methods

EvGr Hormonal emergency contraceptives (includes levonorgestrel p. 549 and ulipristal acetate p. 547) should be offered as soon as possible after unprotected intercourse if a copper intra-uterine device is not appropriate or is not acceptable to the patient; either drug should be taken as soon as possible after unprotected intercourse to increase efficacy. Hormonal emergency contraception administered after ovulation is ineffective.

Levonorgestrel is effective if taken within 72 hours (3 days) of unprotected intercourse and may also be used between 72 and 96 hours after unprotected intercourse [unlicensed use], but efficacy decreases with time. Ulipristal acetate is effective if taken within 120 hours (5 days) of unprotected intercourse. Ulipristal acetate has been demonstrated to be more effective than levonorgestrel for emergency contraception.

It is possible that a higher body-weight or BMI could reduce the effectiveness of oral emergency contraception, particularly levonorgestrel; if BMI is greater than 26 kg/m^2 or body-weight is greater than 70 kg, it is recommended that either ulipristal acetate or a double dose of levonorgestrel [unlicensed indication] (see *Emergency contraception* under levonorgestrel) is given. It is unknown which is more effective.

Ulipristal acetate should be considered as the first-line hormonal emergency contraceptive for a woman who has had unprotected intercourse 96–120 hours ago (even if she has also had unprotected intercourse within the last 96 hours). It should also be considered first line for a woman who has had unprotected sexual intercourse within the last 5 days if it is likely to have taken place during the 5 days before the estimated day of ovulation. Ⓐ

Hormonal emergency contraception interactions

See Contraceptives, interactions below.

Starting hormonal contraception after emergency hormonal contraception

Emergency hormonal contraception methods do **not** provide ongoing contraception. EvGr After taking levonorgestrel, women should start suitable hormonal contraception immediately. They must use condoms reliably or abstain from intercourse until contraception becomes effective.

Women should wait 5 days after taking ulipristal acetate before starting suitable hormonal contraception. Women must use condoms reliably or abstain from intercourse during the 5 day waiting period and also until their contraceptive method is effective. Ⓐ

The copper intra-uterine device immediately provides effective ongoing contraception.

Useful Resources

Emergency Contraception. The Faculty of Sexual and Reproductive Healthcare. Clinical guidance. March 2017. www.fsrh.org/standards-and-guidance/documents/ceu-clinical-guidance-emergency-contraception-march-2017

Contraceptives, interactions

06-Jun-2017

Overview

The effectiveness of *combined* oral contraceptives, *progestogen-only* oral contraceptives, contraceptive patches, vaginal rings, and emergency hormonal contraception can be considerably reduced by interaction with drugs that induce hepatic enzyme activity (e.g. carbamazepine p. 209, eslicarbazepine acetate, nevirapine p. 449, oxcarbazepine p. 218, phenytoin p. 220, phenobarbital p. 232, primidone p. 233, ritonavir p. 461, St John's Wort, topiramate p. 227 and, above all, rifabutin p. 395 and rifampicin p. 396). and possibly also griseofulvin p. 412. A condom together with a long-acting method (such as an injectable contraceptive) may be more suitable for patients with HIV infection or at risk of HIV infection; advice on the possibility of interaction with antiretroviral drugs should be sought from HIV specialists.

For further information on other drug interactions with hormonal contraceptives, see the *Interactions* section of the relevant drug monograph.

Combined hormonal contraceptives interactions

Women using combined hormonal contraceptive patches, vaginal rings or oral tablets who require enzyme-inducing drugs or griseofulvin should be advised to change to a reliable contraceptive method that is unaffected by enzyme-inducers, such as some parenteral progestogen-only contraceptives (medroxyprogesterone acetate p. 553 and norethisterone p. 517) or intra-uterine devices (levonorgestrel p. 549; see also Contraceptives, non-hormonal p. 535). This should be continued for the duration of treatment and for four weeks after stopping. If a change in contraceptive method is undesirable or inappropriate the following options should be discussed:

Short course (2 months or less) of an enzyme-inducing drug

Continuing the combined hormonal contraceptive method may be appropriate if used in combination with consistent and careful use of condoms for the duration of treatment and for four weeks after stopping the enzyme-inducing drug.

Long-term course (over 2 months) of an enzyme-inducing drug (except rifampicin or rifabutin) or a course of griseofulvin

Use a monophasic combined oral contraceptive at a dose of ethinylestradiol 50 micrograms or more daily [unlicensed use] and use either an extended or a 'tricycling' regimen (i.e. taking three packets of monophasic tablets without a break followed by a shortened tablet-free interval of four days [unlicensed use]); continue for the duration of treatment with the interacting drug and for four weeks after stopping.

If breakthrough bleeding occurs (and all other causes are ruled out) it is recommended that the dose of ethinylestradiol is increased by increments of 10 micrograms up to a maximum of 70 micrograms daily [unlicensed use] on specialist advice, or to use additional precautions, or to change to a method unaffected by the interacting drugs.

Use of contraceptive patches and vaginal rings (including concurrent use of two patches or two vaginal rings) is not recommended for women taking enzyme-inducing drugs over a long period.

Long-term course (over 2 months) of rifampicin or rifabutin

An alternative method of contraception (such as an IUD) is **always** recommended because they are such potent enzyme-inducing drugs; the alternative method of contraception should be continued for four weeks after stopping the enzyme-inducing drug.

Antibacterials that do not induce liver enzymes

It is recommended that no additional contraceptive precautions are required when *combined* oral contraceptives, contraceptive patches or vaginal rings are used with antibacterials that do not induce liver enzymes, unless diarrhoea or vomiting occur. These recommendations should be discussed with the woman.

There had been concerns that some antibacterials that do not induce liver enzymes (e.g. ampicillin p. 368, doxycycline p. 381) reduce the efficacy of *combined* oral contraceptives by impairing the bacterial flora responsible for recycling ethinylestradiol from the large bowel. However, there is a lack of evidence to support this interaction.

***Oral* progestogen-only contraceptives interactions**

Effectiveness of oral progestogen-only preparations is not affected by antibacterials that do not induce liver enzymes. The efficacy of oral progestogen-only preparations is, however, reduced by enzyme-inducing drugs or griseofulvin and an alternative contraceptive method, unaffected by the interacting drug, is recommended during treatment with an interacting drug and for at least 4 weeks afterwards.

For a short course of an enzyme-inducing drug (less than two months), continuing the progestogen-only oral method may be appropriate if used in combination with consistent and careful use of condoms for the duration of treatment and for four weeks after stopping the enzyme-inducing drug.

***Parenteral* progestogen-only contraceptives interactions**

Effectiveness of parenteral progestogen-only contraceptives is not affected by antibacterials that do not induce liver enzymes. The effectiveness of intramuscular norethisterone injection and intramuscular and subcutaneous medroxyprogesterone acetate injections is not affected by enzyme-inducing drugs and they may be continued as normal during courses of these drugs.

Effectiveness of the etonogestrel-releasing implant p. 552 may be reduced by enzyme-inducing drugs or griseofulvin and an alternative contraceptive method, unaffected by the interacting drug, is recommended during treatment with the interacting drug and for at least 4 weeks after stopping.

For a short course of an enzyme-inducing drug, if a change in contraceptive method is undesirable or inappropriate, continued contraception with the implant may be appropriate if used in combination with consistent and careful use of condoms for the duration of treatment and for 4 weeks after stopping the enzyme-inducing drug.

Hormonal emergency contraception interactions

The effectiveness of levonorgestrel and ulipristal acetate p. 547 is reduced in women taking enzyme-inducing drugs or griseofulvin (and for at least 4 weeks after stopping). EvGr A copper intra-uterine device can be offered instead. If the copper intra-uterine device is declined or unsuitable, the dose of levonorgestrel should be increased (See *Dose adjustments due to interactions* under levonorgestrel). There is no need to increase the dose for emergency contraception if the patient is taking antibacterials that are not enzyme inducers. Ⓐ

The effectiveness of ulipristal acetate for emergency contraception in women using drugs that increase gastric pH has not been studied. Levonorgestrel or a copper intra-uterine device should be considered as alternatives.

EvGr Hormonal contraception should not be newly initiated in a patient until five days after administration of ulipristal acetate as emergency hormonal contraception—the contraceptive effect of ulipristal acetate will be reduced. Consistent and careful use of condoms is recommended.

Ulipristal acetate can be used as emergency hormonal contraception more than once in the same cycle. Ⓐ Conversely, manufacturer advises that use of levonorgestrel as emergency contraception more than once in the same cycle is not advisable due to increased risk of side-effects (such as menstrual irregularities).

EvGr Levonorgestrel should not be used (as emergency hormonal contraception) within 5 days of administration of ulipristal acetate (as emergency hormonal contraception), as the contraceptive effect of ulipristal acetate may be reduced by progestogens.

Ulipristal acetate is not recommend for use in women who have severe asthma treated by oral corticosteroids, due to the antiglucocorticoid effect of ulipristal acetate. Ⓐ

Useful Resources

Drug interactions with hormonal contraception. The Faculty of Sexual and Reproductive Healthcare. Clinical guidance. January 2018.
www.fsrh.org/standards-and-guidance/current-clinical-guidance/drug-interactions

Emergency Contraception. The Faculty of Sexual and Reproductive Healthcare. FSRH guideline. December 2017.
www.fsrh.org/documents/ceu-clinical-guidance-emergency-contraception-march-2017/

Genito-urinary system 7

3.1 Contraception, combined

OESTROGENS COMBINED WITH PROGESTOGENS

Combined hormonal contraceptives

● **CONTRA-INDICATIONS** Acute porphyrias p. 652 · gallstones · heart disease associated with pulmonary hypertension or risk of embolus · history during pregnancy of cholestatic jaundice · history during pregnancy of chorea · history during pregnancy of pemphigoid gestationis · history during pregnancy of pruritus · history of breast cancer (but can be used after 5 years if no evidence of disease and non-hormonal methods unacceptable) · history of haemolytic uraemic syndrome · migraine with aura · personal history of venous or arterial thrombosis · sclerosing treatment for varicose veins · severe or multiple risk factors for arterial disease · severe or multiple risk factors for venous thromboembolism · systemic lupus erythematosus · transient cerebral ischaemic attacks without headaches · undiagnosed vaginal bleeding

● **CAUTIONS** Active trophoblastic disease (until return to normal of urine- and plasma-gonadotrophin concentration)—seek specialist advice · Crohn's disease · gene mutations associated with breast cancer (e.g. BRCA 1) · history of severe depression especially if induced by hormonal contraceptive · hyperprolactinaemia (seek specialist advice) · inflammatory bowel disease · migraine · personal or family history of hypertriglyceridaemia (increased risk of pancreatitis) · risk factors for arterial disease · risk factors for venous thromboembolism · sickle-cell disease · undiagnosed breast mass

CAUTIONS, FURTHER INFORMATION

▸ **Risk of venous thromboembolism** There is an increased risk of venous thromboembolic disease in users of combined hormonal contraceptives particularly during the first year and possibly after restarting combined hormonal contraceptives following a break of four weeks or more. This risk is considerably smaller than that associated with pregnancy (about 60 cases of venous thromboembolic disease per 100 000 pregnancies). In all cases the risk of venous thromboembolism increases with age and in the presence of other risk factors, such as obesity. The risk also varies depending on the type of progestogen.

Provided that women are informed of the relative risks of venous thromboembolism and accept them, the choice of oral contraceptive is for the woman together with the prescriber jointly to make in light of her individual medical history and any contra-indications.

Combined hormonal contraceptives also slightly increase the risk of *arterial* thromboembolism; however, there is no evidence to suggest that this risk varies between different preparations.

▸ **Risk factors for venous thromboembolism** Use with **caution** if any of following factors present but **avoid** if two or more factors present:

- *family history of venous thromboembolism* in first-degree relative aged under 45 years (avoid contraceptive containing desogestrel or gestodene, *or* avoid if known prothrombotic coagulation abnormality e.g. factor V Leiden or antiphospholipid antibodies (including lupus anticoagulant));
- *obesity*; body mass index $\geq$ 30 kg/m^2 (avoid if body mass index $\geq$ 35 kg/m^2 unless no suitable alternative); (in adolescents, caution if obese according to BMI (adjusted for age and gender); in those who are markedly obese, avoid unless no suitable alternative);
- *long-term immobilisation* e.g. in a wheelchair (avoid if confined to bed or leg in plaster cast);
- *history of superficial thrombophlebitis*;
- *smoking*.

Combined Hormonal Contraception and Risk of Venous Thromboembolism

Progestogen in Combined Hormonal Contraceptive	Estimated incidence per 10 000 women per year of use
Non-pregnant, not using combined hormonal contraception	2
Levonorgesterol[1]	5-7
Norgestimate[1]	5-7
Norethisterone[1]	5-7
Etonogestrel[1]	6-12
Norelgestromin[1]	6-12
Gestodene[1]	9-12
Desogestrel[1]	9-12
Drospirenone[1]	9-12
Dienogest[2]	Not known—insufficient data
Nomegestrol[2]	Not known—insufficient data

[1] Combined with ethinylestradiol [2] Combined with estradiol

▸ **Risk factors for arterial disease** Use with **caution** if any one of following factors present but **avoid** if two or more factors present:

- *family history of arterial disease* in first degree relative aged under 45 years (avoid if atherogenic lipid profile);
- *diabetes mellitus* (avoid if diabetes complications present);
- *hypertension*; blood pressure above *systolic* 140 *mmHg* or *diastolic* 90 *mmHg* (avoid if blood pressure above *systolic* 160 *mmHg* or *diastolic* 95 *mmHg*); (in adolescents, avoid if blood pressure very high);
- *smoking* (avoid if smoking 40 or more cigarettes daily);
- *obesity* (avoid if body mass index $\geq$ 35 kg/m^2 unless no suitable alternative); (in adolescents, caution if obese according to BMI (adjusted for age and gender); in those who are markedly obese, avoid unless no suitable alternative);
- *migraine without aura* (avoid if *migraine with aura* (focal symptoms), *or* severe migraine frequently lasting over 72 hours despite treatment, *or* migraine treated with ergot derivatives).

▸ **Migraine** Women should report any increase in headache frequency or onset of focal symptoms (discontinue immediately and refer urgently to neurology expert if focal neurological symptoms not typical of aura persist for more than 1 hour).

Combined hormonal contraceptives should be stopped (pending investigation and treatment), if serious neurological effects occur, including unusual severe, prolonged headache especially if first time or getting progressively worse *or* sudden partial or complete loss of vision *or* sudden disturbance of hearing or other perceptual disorders *or* dysphasia *or* bad fainting attack or collapse *or* first unexplained epileptic seizure *or* weakness, motor disturbances, very marked numbness suddenly affecting one side or one part of body.

● **SIDE-EFFECTS**

▸ **Common or very common** Acne · fluid retention · headaches · metrorrhagia · nausea · weight increased

▸ **Uncommon** Alopecia · hypertension

▸ **Rare or very rare** Venous thromboembolism

SIDE-EFFECTS, FURTHER INFORMATION **Breast cancer** There is a small increase in the risk of having breast cancer diagnosed in women taking the combined oral contraceptive pill; this relative risk may be due to an earlier diagnosis. In users of combined oral contraceptive pills the cancers are more likely to be localised to the breast. The most important factor for diagnosing breast cancer appears to be the age at which the contraceptive is stopped rather than the duration of use; any increase in the rate of diagnosis diminishes gradually during the 10 years after stopping and disappears by 10 years.

Cervical cancer Use of combined oral contraceptives for 5 years or longer is associated with a small increased risk of cervical cancer; the risk diminishes after stopping and disappears by about 10 years. The possible small increase in the risk of breast cancer and cervical cancer should be weighed against the protective effect against cancers of the ovary and endometrium.

- PREGNANCY Not known to be harmful.
- BREAST FEEDING Avoid until weaning or for 6 months after birth (adverse effects on lactation).
- HEPATIC IMPAIRMENT In general, manufacturer advises caution; avoid in acute disease, severe chronic disease, or liver tumour.
- DIRECTIONS FOR ADMINISTRATION
  - With oral use Each tablet should be taken at approximately same time each day; if delayed, contraceptive protection may be lost. 21-*day combined preparations*, 1 tablet daily for 21 days; subsequent courses repeated after a 7-day interval (during which withdrawal bleeding occurs); if reasonably certain woman is not pregnant, first course can be started on any day of cycle—if starting on day 6 of cycle or later, additional precautions (barrier methods) necessary during first 7 days. *Every day (ED) combined preparations*, 1 *active* tablet daily for 21 days, followed by 1 *inactive* tablet daily for 7 days; subsequent courses repeated without interval (withdrawal bleeding occurs when *inactive* tablets being taken); if reasonably certain woman is not pregnant, first course can be started on any day of cycle—if starting on day 6 of cycle or later, additional precautions (barrier methods) necessary during first 7 days.

  Changing to combined preparation containing different progestogen If previous contraceptive used correctly, or pregnancy can reasonably be excluded, start the first active tablet of new brand immediately. See individual monographs for requirements of specific preparations.

  Changing from progestogen-only tablet If previous contraceptive used correctly, or pregnancy can reasonably be excluded, start new brand immediately, additional precautions (barrier methods) necessary for first 7 days.

  Secondary amenorrhoea (exclude pregnancy) Start any day, additional precautions (barrier methods) necessary during first 7 days (9 days for *Qlaira*®).

  After childbirth (not breast-feeding) Start 3 weeks after birth (increased risk of thrombosis if started earlier); later than 3 weeks postpartum additional precautions (barrier methods) necessary for first 7 days (9 days for *Qlaira*®).

  After abortion or miscarriage Start same day.
- PATIENT AND CARER ADVICE

  Travel Women taking oral contraceptives or using the patch or vaginal ring are at an increased risk of deep vein thrombosis during travel involving long periods of immobility (over 3 hours). The risk may be reduced by appropriate exercise during the journey and possibly by wearing graduated compression hosiery.

  Diarrhoea and vomiting Vomiting and severe diarrhoea can interfere with the absorption of combined oral contraceptives. The FSRH advises following the instructions for missed pills if vomiting occurs within 3 hours of taking a combined oral contraceptive or severe diarrhoea occurs for more than 24 hours. Use of non-oral contraception should be considered if diarrhoea or vomiting persist.

  Missed doses The critical time for loss of contraceptive protection is when a pill is omitted at the *beginning* or *end* of a cycle (which lengthens the pill-free interval). If a woman forgets to take a pill, it should be taken as soon as she remembers, and the next one taken at the normal time (even if this means taking 2 pills together). A missed pill is one that is 24 or more hours late. If a woman misses only one pill, she should take an active pill as soon as she remembers and then resume normal pill-taking. No additional precautions are necessary. If a woman misses 2 or more pills (especially from the first 7 in a packet), she may not be protected. She should take an active pill as soon as she remembers and then resume normal pill-taking. In addition, she must either abstain from sex or use an additional method of contraception such as a condom for the next 7 days. If these 7 days run beyond the end of the packet, the next packet should be started at once, omitting the pill-free interval (or, in the case of *everyday* (ED) pills, omitting the 7 inactive tablets). Emergency contraception is recommended if 2 or more combined oral contraceptive tablets are missed from the first 7 tablets in a packet and unprotected intercourse has occurred since finishing the last packet.

538

Dienogest with estradiol valerate

- **INDICATIONS AND DOSE**

Contraception with 28-day combined preparations | Menstrual symptoms with 28-day combined preparations

- BY MOUTH
  - Females of childbearing potential: 1 active tablet daily for 26 days, followed by 1 inactive tablet daily for 2 days, to be started on day 1 of cycle with first active tablet (withdrawal bleeding may occur during the 2-day interval of inactive tablets); subsequent courses repeated without interval

- UNLICENSED USE Consult product literature for the licensing status.
- INTERACTIONS → Appendix 1: combined hormonal contraceptives
- SIDE-EFFECTS
  - **Common or very common** Breast abnormalities · gastrointestinal discomfort · increased risk of infection · menstrual cycle irregularities
  - **Uncommon** Appetite increased · cervical abnormalities · crying · depression · diarrhoea · dizziness · fatigue · haemorrhage · hot flush · hyperhidrosis · mood altered · muscle spasms · neoplasms · oedema · ovarian and fallopian tube disorders · painful sexual intercourse · pelvic disorders · sexual dysfunction · skin reactions · sleep disorders · uterine cramps · vomiting · vulvovaginal disorders · weight decreased
  - **Rare or very rare** Aggression · anxiety · arterial thromboembolism · asthma · chest pain · cholecystitis chronic · concentration impaired · constipation · contact lens intolerance · dry eye · dry mouth · dyspnoea · eye swelling · fever · galactorrhoea · gastrooesophageal reflux disease · genital discharge · hair changes · hypertriglyceridaemia · hypotension · lymphadenopathy · malaise · myocardial infarction · pain · palpitations · paraesthesia · seborrhoea · sensation of pressure · urinary tract pain · vascular disorders · vertigo
- DIRECTIONS FOR ADMINISTRATION

  Changing to *Qlaira*® Start the first active *Qlaira*® tablet on the day after taking the last active tablet of the previous brand.

● **PATIENT AND CARER ADVICE**
Diarrhoea and vomiting In cases of persistent vomiting or severe diarrhoea lasting more than 12 hours in women taking *Qlaira*®, refer to product literature.
Missed doses A missed pill for a patient taking *Qlaira*® is one that is 12 hours or more late; for information on how to manage missed pills in women taking *Qlaira*®, refer to product literature.

● **MEDICINAL FORMS** There can be variation in the licensing of different medicines containing the same drug.
Tablet
▸ Qlaira (Bayer Plc)
Qlaira tablets | 84 tablet PoM £25.18

538

Estradiol with nomegestrol

● **INDICATIONS AND DOSE**
Contraception
▶ BY MOUTH
▸ Females of childbearing potential: 1 active tablet daily for 24 days, followed by 1 inactive tablet daily for 4 days, to be started on day 1 of cycle with first active tablet (withdrawal bleeding occurs when inactive tablets being taken); subsequent courses repeated without interval

● **INTERACTIONS** → Appendix 1: combined hormonal contraceptives

● **SIDE-EFFECTS**
▶ **Common or very common** Breast abnormalities · depression · menstrual cycle irregularities · mood altered · pelvic pain · sexual dysfunction
▶ **Uncommon** Abdominal distension · appetite abnormal · galactorrhoea · hot flush · hyperhidrosis · oedema · painful sexual intercourse · seborrhoea · sensation of pressure · skin reactions · uterine cramps · vulvovaginal disorders
▶ **Rare or very rare** Cerebrovascular insufficiency · concentration impaired · contact lens intolerance · dry eye · dry mouth · gallbladder disorders · hypertrichosis

● **PREGNANCY** Toxicity in *animal* studies.

● **DIRECTIONS FOR ADMINISTRATION** *Zoely*® *(every day (ED) combined (monophasic) preparation)*, 1 *active* tablet daily for 24 days, followed by 1 *inactive* tablet daily for 4 days, starting on day 1 of cycle with first *active* tablet; subsequent courses repeated without interval (withdrawal bleeding occurs when *inactive* tablets being taken).
Changing to *Zoely*® Start the first active *Zoely*® tablet on the day after taking the last active tablet of the previous brand or, at the latest, the day after the tablet-free or inactive tablet interval of the previous brand.

● **PATIENT AND CARER ADVICE**
Diarrhoea and vomiting In cases of persistent vomiting or severe diarrhoea lasting more than 12 hours in women taking *Zoely*®, refer to product literature.
Missed doses A missed pill for a patient taking *Zoely*® is one that is 12 hours or more late; for information on how to manage missed pills in women taking *Zoely*®, refer to product literature.

● **MEDICINAL FORMS** There can be variation in the licensing of different medicines containing the same drug.
Tablet
▸ Zoely (Merck Sharp & Dohme Ltd) ▼
Estradiol (as Estradiol hemihydrate) 1.5 mg, Nomegestrol acetate 2.5 mg Zoely 2.5mg/1.5mg tablets | 84 tablet PoM £19.80 DT = £19.80

538

Ethinylestradiol with desogestrel

● **INDICATIONS AND DOSE**
Menstrual symptoms with 21-day combined preparations
▶ BY MOUTH
▸ Females of childbearing potential: 1 tablet once daily for 21 days; subsequent courses repeated after 7-day interval, withdrawal bleeding occurs during the 7-day interval, if reasonably certain woman is not pregnant, first course can be started on any day of cycle—if starting on day 6 of cycle or later, additional precautions (barrier methods) necessary during first 7 days, tablets should be taken at approximately the same time each day

Contraception with 21-day combined preparations
▶ BY MOUTH
▸ Females of childbearing potential: 1 tablet once daily for 21 days; subsequent courses repeated after hormone-free interval, withdrawal bleeding occurs during the hormone-free interval, if reasonably certain woman is not pregnant, first course can be started on any day of cycle—if starting on day 6 of cycle or later, additional precautions (barrier methods) necessary during first 7 days, tablets should be taken at approximately the same time each day, see Contraceptives, hormonal p. 532 for recommendations from the FSRH on 'traditional' and 'tailored' regimens in which there is a shortened, less frequent, or no hormone-free interval.

● **UNLICENSED USE** Consult product literature for the licensing status.

● **INTERACTIONS** → Appendix 1: combined hormonal contraceptives

● **MEDICINAL FORMS** There can be variation in the licensing of different medicines containing the same drug.
Tablet
▸ Bimizza (Morningside Healthcare Ltd)
Ethinylestradiol 20 microgram, Desogestrel 150 microgram Bimizza 150microgram/20microgram tablets | 63 tablet PoM £5.04 DT = £5.08
▸ Cimizt (Morningside Healthcare Ltd)
Ethinylestradiol 30 microgram, Desogestrel 150 microgram Cimizt 30microgram/150microgram tablets | 63 tablet PoM £3.80 DT = £4.19
▸ Gedarel (Consilient Health Ltd)
Ethinylestradiol 20 microgram, Desogestrel 150 microgram Gedarel 20microgram/150microgram tablets | 63 tablet PoM £5.08 DT = £5.08
Ethinylestradiol 30 microgram, Desogestrel 150 microgram Gedarel 30microgram/150microgram tablets | 63 tablet PoM £4.19 DT = £4.19
▸ Marvelon (Merck Sharp & Dohme Ltd)
Ethinylestradiol 30 microgram, Desogestrel 150 microgram Marvelon tablets | 63 tablet PoM £7.10 DT = £4.19
▸ Mercilon (Merck Sharp & Dohme Ltd)
Ethinylestradiol 20 microgram, Desogestrel 150 microgram Mercilon 150microgram/20microgram tablets | 63 tablet PoM £8.44 DT = £5.08

538

Ethinylestradiol with drospirenone

● **INDICATIONS AND DOSE**
Menstrual symptoms with 21-day combined preparations
▶ BY MOUTH
▸ Females of childbearing potential: 1 tablet once daily for 21 days; subsequent courses repeated after 7-day interval, withdrawal bleeding occurs during the 7-day interval

Contraception with 21-day combined preparations
- ▶ BY MOUTH
- ▶ Females of childbearing potential: 1 tablet once daily for 21 days; subsequent courses repeated after hormone-free interval, withdrawal bleeding occurs during the hormone-free interval, see Contraceptives, hormonal p. 532 for recommendations from the FSRH on 'traditional' and 'tailored' regimens in which there is a shortened, less frequent, or no hormone-free interval.

Menstrual symptoms with 28-day combined preparations
- ▶ BY MOUTH
- ▶ Females of childbearing potential: 1 active tablet once daily for 24 days, followed by 1 inactive tablet once daily for 4 days, to be started on day 1 of cycle with first active tablet (withdrawal bleeding may occur during the 4-day interval of inactive tablets); subsequent courses repeated without interval

Contraception with 28-day combined preparations
- ▶ BY MOUTH
- ▶ Females of childbearing potential: 1 active tablet once daily for 24 days, followed by 1 inactive tablet once daily for 4 days, to be started on day 1 of cycle with first active tablet (withdrawal bleeding may occur during the 4-day interval of inactive tablets); subsequent courses repeated without interval, see Contraceptives, hormonal p. 532 for recommendations from the FSRH on 'tailored' regimens in which there is a shortened, less frequent, or no interval where *inactive* tablets are taken.

- **UNLICENSED USE** Consult product literature for the licensing status.
- **INTERACTIONS** → Appendix 1: combined hormonal contraceptives
- **SIDE-EFFECTS**
  - ▶ **Common or very common** Breast abnormalities · depressed mood · increased risk of infection · menstrual disorder · vaginal discharge
  - ▶ **Uncommon** Diarrhoea · hypotension · sexual dysfunction · skin reactions · vomiting · weight decreased
  - ▶ **Rare or very rare** Arterial thromboembolism · asthma · erythema nodosum · hearing impairment
- **PATIENT AND CARER ADVICE**
  Pill-free interval Withdrawal bleeding can occur during the 7-day tablet-free interval.

- **MEDICINAL FORMS** There can be variation in the licensing of different medicines containing the same drug.

Tablet
- ▶ Dretine (Theramex HQ UK Ltd)
  Ethinylestradiol 30 microgram, Drospirenone 3 mg Dretine 0.03mg/3mg tablets | 63 tablet [PoM] £8.34 DT = £14.70
- ▶ ELOINE (Bayer Plc)
  Ethinylestradiol 20 microgram, Drospirenone 3 mg Eloine 0.02mg/3mg tablets | 84 tablet [PoM] £14.70 DT = £14.70
- ▶ Lucette (Consilient Health Ltd)
  Ethinylestradiol 30 microgram, Drospirenone 3 mg Lucette 0.03mg/3mg tablets | 63 tablet [PoM] £9.35 DT = £14.70
- ▶ Yacella (Morningside Healthcare Ltd)
  Ethinylestradiol 30 microgram, Drospirenone 3 mg Yacella 0.03mg/3mg tablets | 63 tablet [PoM] £8.30 DT = £14.70
- ▶ Yasmin (Bayer Plc)
  Ethinylestradiol 30 microgram, Drospirenone 3 mg Yasmin tablets | 63 tablet [PoM] £14.70 DT = £14.70
- ▶ Yiznell (Lupin Healthcare (UK) Ltd)
  Ethinylestradiol 30 microgram, Drospirenone 3 mg Yiznell 0.03mg/3mg tablets | 63 tablet [PoM] £8.30 DT = £14.70

538

Ethinylestradiol with etonogestrel

- **INDICATIONS AND DOSE**

Menstrual symptoms
- ▶ BY VAGINA
- ▶ Females of childbearing potential: 1 unit, insert the ring into the vagina on day 1 of cycle and leave in for 3 weeks; remove ring on day 22; subsequent courses repeated after 7-day ring free interval (during which withdrawal bleeding occurs)

Contraception
- ▶ BY VAGINA
- ▶ Females of childbearing potential: 1 unit, insert the ring into the vagina on day 1 of cycle and leave in for 3 weeks; remove ring on day 22; subsequent courses repeated after 7-day ring free interval (during which withdrawal bleeding occurs), see Contraceptives, hormonal p. 532 for recommendations from the FSRH on 'tailored' regimens in which there is a shortened, less frequent, or no ring-free interval.

- **INTERACTIONS** → Appendix 1: combined hormonal contraceptives
- **DIRECTIONS FOR ADMINISTRATION**
  Changing method of contraception to vaginal ring
  Changing from combined hormonal contraception Insert ring at the latest on the day after the usual tablet-free, patch-free, or inactive-tablet interval. If previous contraceptive used correctly, or pregnancy can reasonably be excluded, can switch to ring on any day of cycle.
  Changing from progestogen-only method From an implant or intra-uterine progestogen-only device, insert ring on the day implant or intra-uterine progestogen-only device removed; from an injection, insert ring when next injection due; from oral preparation, first ring may be inserted on any day after stopping pill. For all methods additional precautions (barrier methods) should be used concurrently for first 7 days.
- **PATIENT AND CARER ADVICE** Patients or carers should be given advice on how to administer vaginal ring.
  Counselling The presence of the ring should be checked regularly.
  Missed doses Expulsion, delayed insertion or removal, or broken vaginal ring If the vaginal ring is expelled for *less than* 3 *hours*, rinse the ring with cool water and reinsert immediately; no additional contraception is needed.

  If the ring remains outside the vagina for *more than* 3 *hours* or if the user does not know when the ring was expelled, contraceptive protection may be reduced:
  - If ring expelled during week 1 or 2 of cycle, rinse ring with cool water and reinsert; use additional precautions (barrier methods) for next 7 days;
  - If ring expelled during week 3 of cycle, either insert a new ring to start a new cycle *or* allow a withdrawal bleed and insert a new ring no later than 7 days after ring was expelled; latter option only available if ring was used continuously for at least 7 days before expulsion.

If insertion of a new ring at the start of a new cycle is delayed, contraceptive protection is lost. A new ring should be inserted as soon as possible; additional precautions (barrier methods) should be used for the first 7 days of the new cycle. If intercourse occurred during the extended ring-free interval, pregnancy should be considered.

No additional contraception is required if removal of the ring is delayed by up to 1 week (4 weeks of continuous use). The 7-day ring-free interval should be observed and subsequently a new ring should be inserted. Contraceptive protection may be reduced with continuous use of the ring for more than 4 weeks—pregnancy should be ruled out before inserting a new ring.

If the ring breaks during use, remove it and insert a new ring immediately; additional precautions (barrier methods) should be used for the first 7 days of the new cycle.

- **MEDICINAL FORMS** There can be variation in the licensing of different medicines containing the same drug.

Vaginal delivery system

- NuvaRing (Merck Sharp & Dohme Ltd)
  Ethinylestradiol 2.7 mg, Etonogestrel 11.7 mg NuvaRing 0.12mg/0.015mg per day vaginal delivery system | 3 system PoM £29.70 DT = £29.70
- SyreniRing (Crescent Pharma Ltd)
  Ethinylestradiol 2.7 mg, Etonogestrel 11.7 mg SyreniRing 0.12mg/0.015mg per day vaginal delivery system | 3 system PoM £23.76 DT = £29.70

F 538

Ethinylestradiol with gestodene

- **INDICATIONS AND DOSE**

Menstrual symptoms with 21-day combined preparations

▶ BY MOUTH

- Females of childbearing potential: 1 tablet once daily for 21 days; subsequent courses repeated after 7-day interval, withdrawal bleeding occurs during the 7-day interval, if reasonably certain woman is not pregnant, first course can be started on any day of cycle—if starting on day 6 of cycle or later, additional precautions (barrier methods) necessary during first 7 days, tablets should be taken at approximately the same time each day

Contraception with 21-day combined preparations

▶ BY MOUTH

- Females of childbearing potential: 1 tablet once daily for 21 days; subsequent courses repeated after hormone-free interval, withdrawal bleeding occurs during the hormone-free interval, if reasonably certain woman is not pregnant, first course can be started on any day of cycle—if starting on day 6 of cycle or later, additional precautions (barrier methods) necessary during first 7 days, tablets should be taken at approximately the same time each day, see Contraceptives, hormonal p. 532 for recommendations from the FSRH on 'traditional' and 'tailored' regimens in which there is a shortened, less frequent, or no hormone-free interval.

Menstrual symptoms with 28-day combined preparations

▶ BY MOUTH

- Females of childbearing potential: 1 active tablet once daily for 21 days, followed by 1 inactive tablet daily for 7 days; subsequent courses repeated without interval, withdrawal bleeding occurs during the 7-day interval of *inactive* tablets being taken, if reasonably certain woman is not pregnant, first course can be started on any day of cycle—if starting on day 6 of cycle or later, additional precautions (barrier methods) necessary during first 7 days, tablets should be taken at approximately the same time each day

Contraception with 28-day combined preparations

▶ BY MOUTH

- Females of childbearing potential: 1 active tablet once daily for 21 days, followed by 1 inactive tablet daily for 7 days; subsequent courses repeated without interval, withdrawal bleeding occurs during the interval of *inactive* tablets being taken, if reasonably certain woman is not pregnant, first course can be started on any day of cycle—if starting on day 6 of cycle or later, additional precautions (barrier methods) necessary during first 7 days, tablets should be taken at approximately the same time each day, see Contraceptives, hormonal p. 532 for recommendations from the FSRH on 'tailored' regimens in which *inactive* tablets are taken for a shortened, less frequent, or absent interval.

- **UNLICENSED USE** Consult product literature for the licensing status.
- **INTERACTIONS** → Appendix 1: combined hormonal contraceptives
- **SIDE-EFFECTS**

▶ **Common or very common** Abdominal pain · breast abnormalities · depression · dizziness · increased risk of infection · menstrual cycle irregularities · mood swings · nervousness · vaginal discharge

▶ **Uncommon** Appetite abnormal · diarrhoea · hirsutism · hypertriglyceridaemia · sexual dysfunction · skin reactions · vomiting

▶ **Rare or very rare** Angioedema · chorea exacerbated · ear disorders · embolism and thrombosis · erythema nodosum · eye irritation · gallbladder disorders · gastrointestinal disorders · haemolytic uraemic syndrome · hepatic disorders · hypersensitivity · inflammatory bowel disease · neoplasms · optic neuritis · pancreatitis · systemic lupus erythematosus exacerbated · varicose veins exacerbated · weight decreased

- **MEDICINAL FORMS** There can be variation in the licensing of different medicines containing the same drug.

Tablet

- Ethinylestradiol with gestodene (Non-proprietary)
  Ethinylestradiol 30 microgram, Gestodene 50 microgram Ethinylestradiol 30microgram / Gestodene 50microgram tablets | 18 tablet PoM ⊠
  Ethinylestradiol 40 microgram, Gestodene 70 microgram Ethinylestradiol 40microgram / Gestodene 70microgram tablets | 15 tablet PoM ⊠
  Ethinylestradiol 30 microgram, Gestodene 100 microgram Ethinylestradiol 30microgram / Gestodene 100microgram tablets | 30 tablet PoM ⊠
- Akizza (Morningside Healthcare Ltd)
  Ethinylestradiol 20 microgram, Gestodene 75 microgram Akizza 75microgram/20microgram tablets | 63 tablet PoM ⊠ DT = £8.85
  Ethinylestradiol 30 microgram, Gestodene 75 microgram Akizza 75microgram/30microgram tablets | 63 tablet PoM ⊠ DT = £6.73
- Femodene (Bayer Plc)
  Ethinylestradiol 30 microgram, Gestodene 75 microgram Femodene tablets | 63 tablet PoM £6.73 DT = £6.73
- Femodette (Bayer Plc)
  Ethinylestradiol 20 microgram, Gestodene 75 microgram Femodette tablets | 63 tablet PoM £8.85 DT = £8.85
- Katya (Stragen UK Ltd)
  Ethinylestradiol 30 microgram, Gestodene 75 microgram Katya 30/75 tablets | 63 tablet PoM £5.03 DT = £6.73
- Millinette (Consilient Health Ltd)
  Ethinylestradiol 30 microgram, Gestodene 75 microgram Millinette 30microgram/75microgram tablets | 63 tablet PoM £4.12 DT = £6.73
  Ethinylestradiol 20 microgram, Gestodene 75 microgram Millinette 20microgram/75microgram tablets | 63 tablet PoM £5.41 DT = £8.85
- Sofiperla (Actavis UK Ltd)
  Ethinylestradiol 30 microgram, Gestodene 75 microgram Sofiperla 75microgram/30microgram tablets | 63 tablet PoM £4.12 DT = £6.73
- Sunya (Stragen UK Ltd)
  Ethinylestradiol 20 microgram, Gestodene 75 microgram Sunya 20/75 tablets | 63 tablet PoM £6.62 DT = £8.85

F 538

Ethinylestradiol with levonorgestrel

- **INDICATIONS AND DOSE**

Menstrual symptoms with 21-day combined preparations

▶ BY MOUTH

- Females of childbearing potential: 1 tablet once daily for 21 days; subsequent courses repeated after 7-day interval, withdrawal bleeding occurs during the 7-day interval, if reasonably certain woman is not pregnant, first course can be started on any day of cycle—if starting on day 6 of cycle or later, additional precautions (barrier methods) necessary during first 7 days, tablets should be taken at approximately the same time each day

Contraception with 21-day combined preparations

▶ BY MOUTH

▶ Females of childbearing potential: 1 tablet once daily for 21 days; subsequent courses repeated after hormone-free interval, withdrawal bleeding occurs during the hormone-free interval, if reasonably certain woman is not pregnant, first course can be started on any day of cycle—if starting on day 6 of cycle or later, additional precautions (barrier methods) necessary during first 7 days, tablets should be taken at approximately the same time each day, see Contraceptives, hormonal p. 532 for recommendations from the FSRH on 'traditional' and 'tailored' regimens in which there is a shortened, less frequent, or no hormone-free interval.

Menstrual symptoms with 28-day combined preparations

▶ BY MOUTH

▶ Females of childbearing potential: 1 active tablet once daily for 21 days, followed by 1 inactive tablet once daily for 7 days, withdrawal bleeding occurs during the 7-day interval of *inactive* tablets being taken, if reasonably certain woman is not pregnant, first course can be started on any day of cycle—if starting on day 6 of cycle or later, additional precautions (barrier methods) necessary during first 7 days, tablets should be taken at approximately the same time each day. Subsequent courses repeated without interval

Contraception with 28-day combined preparations

▶ BY MOUTH

▶ Females of childbearing potential: 1 active tablet once daily for 21 days, followed by 1 inactive tablet once daily for 7 days, withdrawal bleeding occurs during the interval of *inactive* tablets being taken, if reasonably certain woman is not pregnant, first course can be started on any day of cycle—if starting on day 6 of cycle or later, additional precautions (barrier methods) necessary during first 7 days, tablets should be taken at approximately the same time each day. Subsequent courses repeated without interval, see Contraceptives, hormonal p. 532 for recommendations from the FSRH on 'tailored' regimens in which there is a shortened, less frequent, or no interval where *inactive* tablets are taken.

● **UNLICENSED USE** Consult product literature for the licensing status of individual preparations.

● **INTERACTIONS** → Appendix 1: combined hormonal contraceptives

● **MEDICINAL FORMS** There can be variation in the licensing of different medicines containing the same drug.

Tablet

▶ Ethinylestradiol with levonorgestrel (Non-proprietary)
Ethinylestradiol 30 microgram, Levonorgestrel 50 microgram Ethinylestradiol 30microgram / Levonorgestrel 50microgram tablets | 6 tablet [PoM] [X]
Ethinylestradiol 40 microgram, Levonorgestrel 75 microgram Ethinylestradiol 40microgram / Levonorgestrel 75microgram tablets | 5 tablet [PoM] [X]
Ethinylestradiol 30 microgram, Levonorgestrel 125 microgram Ethinylestradiol 30microgram / Levonorgestrel 125microgram tablets | 10 tablet [PoM] [X]

▶ Elevin (MedRx Licences Ltd)
Ethinylestradiol 30 microgram, Levonorgestrel 150 microgram Elevin 150microgram/30microgram tablets | 63 tablet [PoM] £29.25 DT = £2.82

▶ Leandra (Genesis Pharmaceuticals Ltd)
Ethinylestradiol 30 microgram, Levonorgestrel 150 microgram Leandra 30microgram/150microgram tablets | 63 tablet [PoM] £2.82 DT = £2.82

▶ Levest (Morningside Healthcare Ltd)
Ethinylestradiol 30 microgram, Levonorgestrel 150 microgram Levest 150/30 tablets | 21 tablet [PoM] £0.85 (Hospital only) | 63 tablet [PoM] £1.80 DT = £2.82

▶ Maexeni (Lupin Healthcare (UK) Ltd)
Ethinylestradiol 30 microgram, Levonorgestrel 150 microgram Maexeni 150microgram/30microgram tablets | 63 tablet [PoM] £1.88 DT = £2.82

▶ Microgynon 30 (Bayer Plc)
Ethinylestradiol 30 microgram, Levonorgestrel 150 microgram Microgynon 30 tablets | 63 tablet [PoM] £2.82 DT = £2.82

▶ Ovranette (Pfizer Ltd)
Ethinylestradiol 30 microgram, Levonorgestrel 150 microgram Ovranette 150microgram/30microgram tablets | 63 tablet [PoM] £2.20 DT = £2.82

▶ Rigevidon (Consilient Health Ltd)
Ethinylestradiol 30 microgram, Levonorgestrel 150 microgram Rigevidon tablets | 63 tablet [PoM] £1.89 DT = £2.82

F 538

Ethinylestradiol with norelgestromin

08-Feb-2019

● **INDICATIONS AND DOSE**

Menstrual symptoms

▶ BY TRANSDERMAL APPLICATION

▶ Females of childbearing potential: Apply 1 patch once weekly for 3 weeks, apply first patch on day 1 of cycle, change patch on days 8 and 15; remove third patch on day 22 and apply new patch after 7-day patch-free interval to start subsequent contraceptive cycle, subsequent courses repeated after a 7-day patch free interval (during which withdrawal bleeding occurs)

Contraception

▶ BY TRANSDERMAL APPLICATION

▶ Females of childbearing potential: Apply 1 patch once weekly for 3 weeks, apply first patch on day 1 of cycle, change patch on days 8 and 15; remove third patch on day 22 and apply new patch after a patch-free interval to start subsequent contraceptive cycle, subsequent courses repeated after a patch-free interval (during which withdrawal bleeding occurs), see Contraceptives, hormonal p. 532 for recommendations from the FSRH on 'traditional' and 'tailored' regimens in which there is a shortened, less frequent, or no patch-free interval.

● **UNLICENSED USE** Consult product literature for the licensing status of individual preparations.

● **INTERACTIONS** → Appendix 1: combined hormonal contraceptives

● **SIDE-EFFECTS**

▶ **Common or very common** Anxiety · breast abnormalities · diarrhoea · dizziness · fatigue · gastrointestinal discomfort · increased risk of infection · malaise · menstrual cycle irregularities · mood altered · muscle spasms · skin reactions · uterine cramps · vaginal haemorrhage · vomiting · vulvovaginal disorders

▶ **Uncommon** Appetite increased · dyslipidaemia · insomnia · lactation disorders · oedema · photosensitivity reaction · sexual dysfunction

▶ **Rare or very rare** Embolism and thrombosis · gallbladder disorders · genital discharge · neoplasms · stroke · swelling

▶ **Frequency not known** Anger · angioedema · cervical dysplasia · colitis · contact lens intolerance · erythema nodosum · hepatic disorders · hyperglycaemia · intracranial haemorrhage · myocardial infarction · pulmonary artery thrombosis · taste altered

- DIRECTIONS FOR ADMINISTRATION Adhesives or bandages should not be used to hold patch in place. If no longer sticky do not reapply but use a new patch.

Changing to a transdermal combined hormonal contraceptive
Changing from combined oral contraception Apply patch on the first day of withdrawal bleeding; if no withdrawal bleeding within 5 days of taking last *active* tablet, rule out pregnancy before applying first patch. Unless patch is applied on first day of withdrawal bleeding, additional precautions (barrier methods) should be used concurrently for first 7 days.

Changing from progestogen-only method
- from an implant, apply first patch on the day implant removed
- from an injection, apply first patch when next injection due
- from oral progestogen, first patch may be applied on any day after stopping pill

For all methods additional precautions (barrier methods) should be used concurrently for first 7 days.

After childbirth (not breast-feeding) Start 4 weeks after birth; if started later than 4 weeks after birth additional precautions (barrier methods) should be used for first 7 days.

After abortion or miscarriage Before 20 weeks' gestation start immediately; no additional contraception required if started immediately. After 20 weeks' gestation start on day 21 after abortion or on the first day of first spontaneous menstruation; additional precautions (barrier methods) should be used for first 7 days after applying the patch.

- PATIENT AND CARER ADVICE Patients and carers should be given advice on how to administer patches.

Travel Women using patches are at an increased risk of deep vein thrombosis during travel involving long periods of immobility (over 3 hours). The risk may be reduced by appropriate exercise during the journey and possibly by wearing graduated compression hosiery.

Missed doses **Delayed application or detached patch** If a patch is partly detached for less than 24 hours, reapply to the same site or replace with a new patch immediately; no additional contraception is needed and the next patch should be applied on the usual 'change day'. If a patch remains detached for more than 24 hours or if the user is not aware when the patch became detached, then stop the current contraceptive cycle and start a new cycle by applying a new patch, giving a new 'Day 1'; an additional non-hormonal contraceptive must be used concurrently for the first 7 days of the new cycle.

If application of a new patch at the start of a new cycle is delayed, contraceptive protection is lost. A new patch should be applied as soon as remembered giving a new 'Day 1'; additional non-hormonal methods of contraception should be used for the first 7 days of the new cycle. If application of a patch in the middle of the cycle is delayed (i.e. the patch is not changed on day 8 or day 15):
- for up to 48 hours, apply a new patch immediately; next patch 'change day' remains the same and no additional contraception is required;
- for more than 48 hours, contraceptive protection may have been lost. Stop the current cycle and start a new 4-week cycle immediately by applying a new patch giving a new 'Day 1'; additional non-hormonal contraception should be used for the first 7 days of the new cycle.

If the patch is not removed at the end of the cycle (day 22), remove it as soon as possible and start the next cycle on the usual 'change day', the day after day 28; no additional contraception is required.

- NATIONAL FUNDING/ACCESS DECISIONS

Scottish Medicines Consortium (SMC) decisions
SMC No. 48/03
The *Scottish Medicines Consortium* has advised (September 2003) that *Evra*® patches should be restricted for use in women who are likely to comply poorly with combined oral contraceptives.

- MEDICINAL FORMS There can be variation in the licensing of different medicines containing the same drug.

Transdermal patch
- Evra (Janssen-Cilag Ltd)
Ethinylestradiol 33.9 microgram per 24 hour, Norelgestromin 203 microgram per 24 hour Evra transdermal patches | 9 patch PoM £19.51 DT = £19.51

538

Ethinylestradiol with norethisterone

- INDICATIONS AND DOSE

Menstrual symptoms with 21-day combined preparations
- BY MOUTH
- Females of childbearing potential: 1 tablet once daily for 21 days; subsequent courses repeated after 7-day interval, withdrawal bleeding occurs during the 7-day interval, if reasonably certain woman is not pregnant, first course can be started on any day of cycle—if starting on day 6 of cycle or later, additional precautions (barrier methods) necessary during first 7 days, tablets should be taken at approximately the same time each day

Contraception with 21-day combined preparations
- BY MOUTH
- Females of childbearing potential: 1 tablet once daily for 21 days; subsequent courses repeated after hormone-free interval, withdrawal bleeding occurs during the hormone-free interval, if reasonably certain woman is not pregnant, first course can be started on any day of cycle—if starting on day 6 of cycle or later, additional precautions (barrier methods) necessary during first 7 days, tablets should be taken at approximately the same time each day, see Contraceptives, hormonal p. 532 for recommendations from the FSRH on 'traditional' and 'tailored' regimens in which there is a shortened, less frequent, or no hormone-free interval.

- UNLICENSED USE Consult product literature for the licensing status.
- INTERACTIONS → Appendix 1: combined hormonal contraceptives

- MEDICINAL FORMS There can be variation in the licensing of different medicines containing the same drug.

Tablet
- Ethinylestradiol with norethisterone (Non-proprietary)
Ethinylestradiol 35 microgram, Norethisterone 500 microgram Ethinylestradiol 35microgram / Norethisterone 500microgram tablets | 5 tablet PoM ⊠
Ethinylestradiol 35 microgram, Norethisterone 750 microgram Ethinylestradiol 35microgram / Norethisterone 750microgram tablets | 21 tablet PoM ⊠
Ethinylestradiol 35 microgram, Norethisterone 1 mg Ethinylestradiol 35microgram / Norethisterone 1mg tablets | 9 tablet PoM ⊠
- Brevinor (Pfizer Ltd)
Ethinylestradiol 35 microgram, Norethisterone 500 microgram Brevinor 500microgram/35microgram tablets | 63 tablet PoM £1.99 DT = £1.99
- Norimin (Pfizer Ltd)
Ethinylestradiol 35 microgram, Norethisterone 1 mg Norimin 1mg/35microgram tablets | 63 tablet PoM £2.28 DT = £2.28

538

Ethinylestradiol with norgestimate

● **INDICATIONS AND DOSE**

Menstrual symptoms with 21-day combined preparations

▶ BY MOUTH

▸ Females of childbearing potential: 1 tablet once daily for 21 days; subsequent courses repeated after 7-day interval, withdrawal bleeding occurs during the 7-day interval, if reasonably certain woman is not pregnant, first course can be started on any day of cycle—if starting on day 6 of cycle or later, additional precautions (barrier methods) necessary during first 7 days, tablets should be taken at approximately the same time each day

Contraception with 21-day combined preparations

▶ BY MOUTH

▸ Females of childbearing potential: 1 tablet once daily for 21 days; subsequent courses repeated after hormone-free interval, withdrawal bleeding occurs during the hormone-free interval, if reasonably certain woman is not pregnant, first course can be started on any day of cycle—if starting on day 6 of cycle or later, additional precautions (barrier methods) necessary during first 7 days, tablets should be taken at approximately the same time each day, see Contraceptives, hormonal p. 532 for recommendations from the FSRH on 'traditional' and 'tailored' regimens in which there is a shortened, less frequent, or no hormone-free interval.

● **UNLICENSED USE** Consult product literature for the licensing status.

● **INTERACTIONS** → Appendix 1: combined hormonal contraceptives

● **SIDE-EFFECTS**

▶ **Common or very common** Anxiety · asthenic conditions · breast abnormalities · chest pain · constipation · depression · diarrhoea · dizziness · gastrointestinal discomfort · gastrointestinal disorders · genital discharge · hypersensitivity · increased risk of infection · insomnia · menstrual cycle irregularities · mood altered · muscle complaints · oedema · pain · skin reactions · vomiting

▶ **Uncommon** Appetite abnormal · cervical dysplasia · dry eye · dyspnoea · embolism and thrombosis · hirsutism · hot flush · libido disorder · ovarian cyst · palpitations · paraesthesia · syncope · visual impairment · vulvovaginal disorders · weight changes

▶ **Rare or very rare** Hepatic disorders · pancreatitis · photosensitivity reaction · sweat changes · tachycardia · vertigo

▶ **Frequency not known** Angioedema · contact lens intolerance · dyslipidaemia · erythema nodosum · neoplasms · seizure · suppressed lactation

● **MEDICINAL FORMS** There can be variation in the licensing of different medicines containing the same drug.

Tablet

▸ Cilique (Consilient Health Ltd)
Ethinylestradiol 35 microgram, Norgestimate 250 microgram Cilique 250microgram/35microgram tablets | 63 tablet [PoM] £4.65 DT = £4.65

▸ Lizinna (Morningside Healthcare Ltd)
Ethinylestradiol 35 microgram, Norgestimate 250 microgram Lizinna 250microgram/35microgram tablets | 63 tablet [PoM] £4.64 DT = £4.65

538

Norethisterone with mestranol

● **INDICATIONS AND DOSE**

Contraception | Menstrual symptoms

▶ BY MOUTH

▸ Females of childbearing potential: 1 tablet once daily for 21 days; subsequent courses repeated after 7-day interval, withdrawal bleeding can occur during the 7-day interval, if reasonably certain woman is not pregnant, first course can be started on any day of cycle—if starting on day 6 of cycle or later, additional precautions (barrier methods) necessary during first 7 days, tablets should be taken at the same time each day

● **UNLICENSED USE** Consult product literature for the licensing status of individual preparations.

● **INTERACTIONS** → Appendix 1: combined hormonal contraceptives

● **SIDE-EFFECTS** Appetite change · breast tenderness · depression · gastrointestinal disorder · libido disorder · metabolic disorders · uterine leiomyoma exacerbated

● **MEDICINAL FORMS** There can be variation in the licensing of different medicines containing the same drug.

Tablet

▸ Norinyl-1 (Pfizer Ltd)
Mestranol 50 microgram, Norethisterone 1 mg Norinyl-1 tablets | 63 tablet [PoM] £2.19 DT = £2.19

3.2 Contraception, devices

Other drugs used for Contraception, devices
Levonorgestrel, p. 549

CONTRACEPTIVE DEVICES

Intra-uterine contraceptive devices (copper)

22-Apr-2020

● **INDICATIONS AND DOSE**

Contraception

▶ BY INTRA-UTERINE ADMINISTRATION

▸ Females of childbearing potential: (consult product literature)

IMPORTANT SAFETY INFORMATION

MHRA/CHM ADVICE (JUNE 2015) INTRA-UTERINE CONTRACEPTION: UTERINE PERFORATION—UPDATED INFORMATION ON RISK FACTORS

Uterine perforation most often occurs during insertion, but might not be detected until sometime later. The risk of uterine perforation is increased when the device is inserted up to 36 weeks postpartum or in patients who are breastfeeding. Before inserting an intra-uterine contraceptive device, inform patients that perforation occurs in approximately 1 in every 1000 insertions and signs and symptoms include:

- severe pelvic pain after insertion (worse than period cramps);
- pain or increased bleeding after insertion which continues for more than a few weeks;
- sudden changes in periods;
- pain during intercourse;
- unable to feel the threads.

Patients should be informed on how to check their threads and to arrange a check-up if threads cannot be felt, especially if they also have significant pain. Partial

7 Genito-urinary system

perforation may occur even if the threads can be seen; consider this if there is severe pain following insertion and perform an ultrasound.

- **CONTRA-INDICATIONS** Active trophoblastic disease (until return to normal of urine and plasma-gonadotrophin concentration) · genital malignancy · medical diathermy · pelvic inflammatory disease · post-abortion sepsis · postpartum sepsis · recent sexually transmitted infection (if not fully investigated and treated) · severe anaemia · unexplained uterine bleeding · Wilson's disease
- **CAUTIONS** Anaemia · anatomical abnormalities—seek specialist advice · anticoagulant therapy · cardiac disease—seek specialist advice · endometriosis · epilepsy (risk of seizure at time of insertion) · immunosuppression (risk of infection)—seek specialist advice · menorrhagia (progestogen intra-uterine system might be preferable) · postpartum—seek specialist advice · risk of sexually transmitted infections · severe primary dysmenorrhoea · young age

 CAUTIONS, FURTHER INFORMATION The Faculty of Sexual and Reproductive Healthcare advises if removal is after day 3 of the menstrual cycle, intercourse should be avoided or another method of contraception used for at least 7 days before removal of device—emergency contraception may need to be considered if recent intercourse has occurred and the intra-uterine device is removed after day 3 of the menstrual cycle.

 ▸ **Sexually transmitted infections and pelvic inflammatory disease** The main excess risk of pelvic infection occurs in the first 20 days after insertion and is believed to be related to existing carriage of a sexually transmitted infection. Women are considered to be at a higher risk of sexually transmitted infections if:
 - they are under 25 years old *or*
 - they are over 25 years old *and*
   - have a new partner *or*
   - have had more than one partner in the past year *or*
   - their regular partner has other partners.

 The Faculty of Sexual and Reproductive Healthcare advises pre-insertion screening (for chlamydia and, depending on sexual history and local prevalence of disease, *Neisseria gonorrhoeae*) be performed in these women. If results are unavailable at the time of fitting an intra-uterine device for emergency contraception, consider appropriate prophylactic antibacterial cover. The woman should be advised to attend *as an emergency* if she experiences sustained pain during the next 20 days.

- **SIDE-EFFECTS** Device complications · epilepsy (on insertion) · haemorrhage (on insertion) · hypersensitivity · menstrual cycle irregularities · pain (on insertion—alleviated by NSAID such as ibuprofen 30 minutes before insertion) · pelvic infection exacerbated · presyncope (on insertion) · uterine injuries

 SIDE-EFFECTS, FURTHER INFORMATION Advise the patient to seek medical attention promptly in case of significant symptoms—very small risk of uterine perforation, ectopic pregnancy and pelvic inflammatory disease.

- **ALLERGY AND CROSS-SENSITIVITY** Contra-indicated if patient has a copper allergy.
- **PREGNANCY** If an intra-uterine device fails and the woman wishes to continue to full-term the device should be removed in the first trimester if possible. Remove device; if pregnancy occurs, increased likelihood that it may be ectopic.
- **BREAST FEEDING** Not known to be harmful.
- **MONITORING REQUIREMENTS** Gynaecological examination before insertion, 6–8 weeks after insertion, then annually.
- **DIRECTIONS FOR ADMINISTRATION** The timing and technique of fitting an intra-uterine device are critical for its subsequent performance. *The healthcare professional inserting (or removing) the device should be fully trained in the technique and should provide full counselling backed, where available, by the patient information leaflet.* Devices should not be fitted during the heavy days of the period; they are best fitted after the end of menstruation and before the calculated time of implantation.
- **PRESCRIBING AND DISPENSING INFORMATION**

 TT380® SLIMLINE For uterine length 6.5–9 cm; replacement every 10 years.

 LOAD® 375 For uterine length over 7 cm; replacement every 5 years.

 NOVAPLUS T 380® AG '*Mini*' size for minimum uterine length 5 cm; '*Normal*' size for uterine length 6.5–9 cm; replacement every 5 years.

 MULTILOAD® CU375 For uterine length 6–9 cm; replacement every 5 years.

 GYNEFIX® Suitable for all uterine sizes; replacement every 5 years.

 IUB BALLERINE MIDI® For uterine length over 6 cm; replacement every 5 years.

 UT380 STANDARD® For uterine length 6.5–9 cm; replacement every 5 years.

 UT380 SHORT® For uterine length 5–7 cm; replacement every 5 years.

 MULTI-SAFE® 375 For uterine length 6–9 cm; replacement every 5 years.

 ANCORA® 375 CU For uterine length over 6.5 cm; replacement every 5 years.

 T-SAFE® 380A QL For uterine length 6.5–9 cm; replacement every 10 years.

 NEO-SAFE® T380 For uterine length 6.5–9 cm; replacement every 5 years.

 MINI TT380® SLIMLINE For minimum uterine length 5 cm; replacement every 5 years.

 COPPER T380 A® For uterine length 6.5–9 cm; replacement every 10 years.

 NOVAPLUS T 380® CU '*Mini*' size for minimum uterine length 5 cm; '*Normal*' size for uterine length 6.5–9 cm; replacement every 5 years.

 NOVA-T® 380 For uterine length 6.5–9 cm; replacement every 5 years.

 FLEXI-T®+ 380 For uterine length over 6 cm; replacement every 5 years.

 FLEXI-T® 300 For uterine length over 5 cm; replacement every 5 years.

- **MEDICINAL FORMS** There can be variation in the licensing of different medicines containing the same drug.

Intra-uterine contraceptive device

▸ **Intra-uterine contraceptive devices (copper) (Non-proprietary)**
IUB Ballerine MIDI intra-uterine contraceptive device | 1 device £25.00

▸ **Intra-uterine contraceptive devices** (R.F. Medical Supplies Ltd, Farla Medical Ltd, Durbin Plc, Williams Medical Supplies Ltd, Bayer Plc, Organon Laboratories Ltd)
Copper T380 A intra-uterine contraceptive device | 1 device £8.95
Steriload intra-uterine contraceptive device | 1 device £9.65
Load 375 intra-uterine contraceptive device | 1 device £8.52
Novaplus T 380 Ag intra-uterine contraceptive device mini | 1 device £12.50
T-Safe 380A QL intra-uterine contraceptive device | 1 device £10.55
UT380 Standard intra-uterine contraceptive device | 1 device £11.22
Nova-T 380 intra-uterine contraceptive device | 1 device £15.20
Flexi-T+ 380 intra-uterine contraceptive device | 1 device £10.06
Mini TT380 Slimline intra-uterine contraceptive device | 1 device £12.46
Flexi-T 300 intra-uterine contraceptive device | 1 device £9.47
Multi-Safe 375 intra-uterine contraceptive device | 1 device £8.96
Multiload Cu375 intra-uterine contraceptive device | 1 device £9.24
Optima TCu 380A intra-uterine contraceptive device | 1 device £9.65
Novaplus T 380 Ag intra-uterine contraceptive device normal | 1 device £12.50

GyneFix intra-uterine contraceptive device | 1 device £27.11
Novaplus T 380 Cu intra-uterine contraceptive device mini | 1 device £10.95
TT380 Slimline intra-uterine contraceptive device | 1 device £12.46
Ancora 375 Cu intra-uterine contraceptive device | 1 device £7.95
Novaplus T 380 Cu intra-uterine contraceptive device normal | 1 device £10.95
Neo-Safe T380 intra-uterine contraceptive device | 1 device £13.40
UT380 Short intra-uterine contraceptive device | 1 device £11.22

Silicone contraceptive pessaries

● **SILICONE CONTRACEPTIVE PESSARIES**

FemCap 22mm (Durbin Plc)
| 1 device · NHS indicative price = £15.29 · Drug Tariff (Part IXa)

FemCap 26mm (Durbin Plc)
| 1 device · NHS indicative price = £15.29 · Drug Tariff (Part IXa)

FemCap 30mm (Durbin Plc)
| 1 device · NHS indicative price = £15.29 · Drug Tariff (Part IXa)

3.3 Contraception, emergency

Other drugs used for Contraception, emergency
Levonorgestrel, p. 549

PROGESTERONE RECEPTOR MODULATORS

Ulipristal acetate

26-May-2020

● **DRUG ACTION** Ulipristal acetate is a progesterone receptor modulator with a partial progesterone antagonist effect.

● **INDICATIONS AND DOSE**

Emergency contraception

▸ BY MOUTH

▸ Females of childbearing potential: 30 mg for 1 dose, to be taken as soon as possible after coitus, but no later than after 120 hours

IMPORTANT SAFETY INFORMATION

MHRA/CHM ADVICE: *ESMYA*® (ULIPRISTAL ACETATE): SUSPENSION OF THE LICENCE DUE TO RISK OF SERIOUS LIVER INJURY (MARCH 2020)

Rare but serious cases of liver injury, including hepatic failure requiring liver transplantation, have been reported worldwide in women treated with *Esmya*® for symptoms of uterine fibroids. The licence of *Esmya*® has been suspended while a safety review is carried out, following a further case of liver injury requiring transplantation despite liver function monitoring. Healthcare professionals are advised not to start *Esmya*® in new patients and to stop treatment in current patients; alternative treatment options for uterine fibroids should be considered. Liver function tests should be performed 2–4 weeks after stopping treatment, and patients advised to be vigilant for the signs and symptoms of liver injury and to seek immediate medical advice if these occur, even if 1–2 months after stopping treatment. There are currently no concerns with the use of the emergency contraceptive *ellaOne*®—see *Indications and Dose*.

● **CAUTIONS** Uncontrolled severe asthma

● **INTERACTIONS** → Appendix 1: ulipristal

● **SIDE-EFFECTS**

▸ **Common or very common** Back pain · breast tenderness · dizziness · fatigue · gastrointestinal discomfort · headaches · menstrual cycle irregularities · mood altered · myalgia · nausea · pelvic pain · vomiting

▸ **Uncommon** Anxiety · appetite disorder · chills · concentration impaired · diarrhoea · drowsiness · dry mouth · fever · flatulence · hot flush · increased risk of infection · insomnia · libido disorder · malaise · skin reactions · vision disorders · vulvovaginal disorders

▸ **Rare or very rare** Abnormal sensation in eye · disorientation · dry throat · eye erythema · genital pruritus · ovarian cyst ruptured · painful sexual intercourse · syncope · taste altered · thirst · tremor · vertigo

● **PREGNANCY** Limited information available—if pregnancy occurs, manufacturer advises report to the *ellaOne*® pregnancy registry.

● **BREAST FEEDING** Manufacturer advises avoid for 1 week after administration—present in milk.

● **HEPATIC IMPAIRMENT** Manufacturer advises avoid in severe impairment (no information available).

● **PRESCRIBING AND DISPENSING INFORMATION** The manufacturer of *Esmya*® has provided a *Physician's Guide to Prescribing Esmya*®.

● **PATIENT AND CARER ADVICE** When prescribing or supplying hormonal emergency contraception, manufacturer advises women should be told:

- if vomiting occurs within 3 hours of taking a dose, a replacement dose should be taken;
- that their next period may be early or late;
- to seek medical attention promptly if any lower abdominal pain occurs because this could signify an ectopic pregnancy.

The Faculty of Sexual and Reproductive Healthcare also advises women should be told:

- that a barrier method of contraception needs to be used—see Emergency contraception p. 536 for further information;
- that a pregnancy test should be performed if the next menstrual period is delayed by more than 7 days, is lighter than usual, or is associated with abdominal pain that is not typical of the woman's usual dysmenorrhoea;
- that a pregnancy test should be performed if hormonal contraception is started soon after use of emergency contraception even if they have bleeding; bleeding associated with the contraceptive method may not represent menstruation.

● **MEDICINAL FORMS** There can be variation in the licensing of different medicines containing the same drug.

Tablet

▸ Ellaone (HRA Pharma UK Ltd)
Ulipristal acetate 30 mg EllaOne 30mg tablets | 1 tablet [P] £14.05 DT = £14.05

▸ Esmya (Gedeon Richter (UK) Ltd)
Ulipristal acetate 5 mg Esmya 5mg tablets | 28 tablet [PoM] £114.13 DT = £114.13

3.4 Contraception, oral progestogen-only

Other drugs used for Contraception, oral progestogen-only Norethisterone, p. 517

PROGESTOGENS

Desogestrel

19-Jul-2018

● **INDICATIONS AND DOSE**

Contraception

▸ BY MOUTH

▸ Females of childbearing potential: 75 micrograms daily, dose to be taken at same time each day, starting on day 1 of cycle then continuously, if continued →

7 Genito-urinary system

administration delayed for 12 hours or more it should be regarded as a 'missed pill'

- **UNLICENSED USE** Consult product literature for the licensing status of individual preparations.
- **CONTRA-INDICATIONS** Acute porphyrias p. 652 · history of breast cancer but can be used after 5 years if no evidence of disease and non-hormonal contraceptive methods unacceptable · severe arterial disease · undiagnosed vaginal bleeding
- **CAUTIONS** Active trophoblastic disease (until return to normal of urine- and plasma-gonadotrophin concentration)—seek specialist advice · arterial disease · functional ovarian cysts · history of jaundice in pregnancy · malabsorption syndromes · past ectopic pregnancy · sex-steroid dependent cancer · systemic lupus erythematosus with positive (or unknown) antiphospholipid antibodies

CAUTIONS, FURTHER INFORMATION

- Other conditions The product literature advises caution in patients with history of thromboembolism, hypertension, diabetes mellitus and migraine; evidence for caution in these conditions is unsatisfactory.

- **INTERACTIONS** → Appendix 1: desogestrel
- **SIDE-EFFECTS**
  - **Common or very common** Breast abnormalities · depressed mood · headache · libido decreased · menstrual cycle irregularities · mood altered · nausea · skin reactions · weight increased
  - **Uncommon** Alopecia · contact lens intolerance · fatigue · ovarian cyst · vomiting · vulvovaginal infection
  - **Rare or very rare** Erythema nodosum
  - **Frequency not known** Angioedema · embolism and thrombosis · neoplasms

SIDE-EFFECTS, FURTHER INFORMATION The benefits of using progestogen-only contraceptives (POCs), such as desogestrel, should be weighed against the possible risks for each individual woman.

There is a small increase in the risk of having breast cancer diagnosed in women using a combined oral contraceptive pill (COC); this relative risk may be due to an earlier diagnosis, biological effects of the pill or a combination of both. This increased risk is related to the age of the woman using the COC rather than the duration of use and disappears gradually within 10 years after discontinuation.

The risk of breast cancer in users of POCs is possibly of similar magnitude as that associated with COCs, however the evidence is less conclusive.

Available evidence does not support an association between the use of a progestegen-only contraceptive pill and breast cancer. Any increased risk is likely to be small and reduces gradually during the 10 years after stopping; there is no excess risk 10 years after stopping. The older age at which the contraceptive is stopped appears to have a greater influence on increased risk rather than the duration of use.

- **PREGNANCY** Not known to be harmful.
- **BREAST FEEDING** Progestogen-only contraceptives do not affect lactation.
- **HEPATIC IMPAIRMENT** Manufacturer advises caution; avoid in severe or active disease.
- **PATIENT AND CARER ADVICE**

Surgery All progestogen-only contraceptives are suitable for use as an alternative to combined hormonal contraceptives before major elective surgery, before all surgery to the legs, or before surgery which involves prolonged immobilisation of a lower limb.

Starting routine One tablet daily, on a continuous basis, starting on day 1 of cycle and taken at the same time each day (if delayed by longer than 12 hours contraceptive protection may be lost). Additional contraceptive precautions are not required if desogestrel is started up to and including day 5 of the menstrual cycle; if started after this time, additional contraceptive precautions are required for 2 days.

Changing from a combined oral contraceptive Start on the day following completion of the combined oral contraceptive course without a break (or in the case of ED tablets omitting the inactive ones).

After childbirth Oral progestogen-only contraceptives can be started up to and including day 21 postpartum without the need for additional contraceptive precautions. If started more than 21 days postpartum, additional contraceptive precautions are required for 2 days.

Diarrhoea and vomiting Vomiting and persistent, severe diarrhoea can interfere with the absorption of oral progestogen-only contraceptives. If vomiting occurs within 2 hours of taking desogestrel, another pill should be taken as soon as possible. If a replacement pill is not taken within 12 hours of the normal time for taking desogestrel, or in cases of persistent vomiting or very severe diarrhoea, additional precautions should be used during illness and for 2 days after recovery.

Missed doses The following advice is recommended: 'If you forget a pill, take it as soon as you remember and carry on with the next pill at the right time. If the pill was more than 12 hours overdue you are not protected. Continue normal pill-taking but you must also use another method, such as the condom, for the next 2 days'.

The Faculty of Sexual and Reproductive Healthcare recommends emergency contraception if one or more tablets are missed or taken more than 12 hours late and unprotected intercourse has occurred before 2 further tablets have been correctly taken.

- **NATIONAL FUNDING/ACCESS DECISIONS**

Scottish Medicines Consortium (SMC) decisions

SMC No. 36/03

The *Scottish Medicines Consortium* has advised (September 2003) that *Cerazette*® should be restricted for use in women who cannot tolerate oestrogen-containing contraceptives or in whom such preparations are contra-indicated.

- **MEDICINAL FORMS** There can be variation in the licensing of different medicines containing the same drug.

Tablet

- **Desogestrel (Non-proprietary)**
  Desogestrel 75 microgram Desogestrel 75microgram tablets | 84 tablet PoM £9.55 DT = £2.87
- **Cerazette** (Merck Sharp & Dohme Ltd)
  Desogestrel 75 microgram Cerazette 75microgram tablets | 84 tablet PoM £9.55 DT = £2.87
- **Cerelle** (Consilient Health Ltd)
  Desogestrel 75 microgram Cerelle 75microgram tablets | 84 tablet PoM £3.50 DT = £2.87
- **Desomono** (MedRx Licences Ltd)
  Desogestrel 75 microgram Desomono 75microgram tablets | 84 tablet PoM £6.50 DT = £2.87
- **Desorex** (Somex Pharma)
  Desogestrel 75 microgram Desorex 75microgram tablets | 84 tablet PoM £2.45 DT = £2.87
- **Feanolla** (Lupin Healthcare (UK) Ltd)
  Desogestrel 75 microgram Feanolla 75microgram tablets | 84 tablet PoM £3.49 DT = £2.87
- **Moonia** (Stragen UK Ltd)
  Desogestrel 75 microgram Moonia 75microgram tablets | 84 tablet PoM ⊠ DT = £2.87
- **Zelleta** (Morningside Healthcare Ltd)
  Desogestrel 75 microgram Zelleta 75microgram tablets | 84 tablet PoM £2.98 DT = £2.87

Levonorgestrel

03-Mar-2020

- **INDICATIONS AND DOSE**

Emergency contraception

▶ BY MOUTH

▶ Females of childbearing potential: 1.5 mg for 1 dose, taken as soon as possible after coitus, preferably within 12 hours and no later than after 72 hours (may also be used between 72–96 hours after coitus but efficacy decreases with time), alternatively 3 mg for 1 dose, taken as soon as possible after coitus, preferably within 12 hours and no later than after 72 hours (may also be used between 72–96 hours after coitus but efficacy decreases with time). Higher dose should be considered for patients with body-weight over 70 kg or BMI over 26 kg/m^2

Contraception

▶ BY MOUTH

▶ Females of childbearing potential: 30 micrograms daily starting on day 1 of the cycle then continuously, dose is to be taken at the same time each day, if administration delayed for 3 hours or more it should be regarded as a "missed pill"

DOSE ADJUSTMENTS DUE TO INTERACTIONS

▶ When used orally as an emergency contraceptive, the effectiveness of levonorgestrel is reduced in women taking enzyme-inducing drugs (and for up to 4 weeks after stopping); a copper intra-uterine device should preferably be used instead. If the copper intra-uterine device is undesirable or inappropriate, the dose of levonorgestrel should be increased to a total of 3 mg taken as a single dose; pregnancy should be excluded following use, and medical advice sought if pregnancy occurs.

▶ There is no need to increase the dose for emergency contraception if the patient is taking antibacterials that are not enzyme inducers.

▶ With the progestogen-only intra-uterine device, levonorgestrel is released close to the site of the main contraceptive action (on cervical mucus and endometrium) and therefore progestogenic side-effects and interactions are less likely; in particular, enzyme-inducing drugs are unlikely to significantly reduce the contraceptive effect of the progestogen-only intra-uterine system and additional contraceptive precautions are not required.

JAYDESS ® 13.5MG INTRA-UTERINE DEVICE

Contraception

▶ BY INTRA-UTERINE ADMINISTRATION

▶ Females of childbearing potential: Insert into uterine cavity within 7 days of onset of menstruation, or any time if replacement (additional precautions (e.g. barrier methods) advised for at least 7 days before), or any time if reasonably certain woman is not pregnant and there is no risk of conception (additional precautions (e.g. barrier methods) necessary for next 7 days), or immediately following termination of pregnancy below 24 weeks' gestation; postpartum insertions should be delayed until at least 4 weeks after delivery; effective for 3 years

KYLEENA ® 19.5MG INTRA-UTERINE DEVICE

Contraception

▶ BY INTRA-UTERINE ADMINISTRATION

▶ Females of childbearing potential: Insert into uterine cavity within 7 days of onset of menstruation, or any time if replacement (additional precautions (e.g. barrier methods) advised for at least 7 days before), or any time if reasonably certain woman is not pregnant and there is no risk of conception (additional precautions (e.g. barrier methods) necessary for next 7 days), or immediately following termination of pregnancy below 24 weeks' gestation; postpartum insertions should be delayed until at least 4 weeks after delivery; effective for 5 years

LEVOSERT ® 20MICROGRAMS/24HOURS INTRA-UTERINE DEVICE

Contraception | Menorrhagia

▶ BY INTRA-UTERINE ADMINISTRATION

▶ Females of childbearing potential: Insert into uterine cavity within 7 days of onset of menstruation, or any time if replacement (additional precautions (e.g. barrier methods) advised for at least 7 days before), or any time if reasonably certain woman is not pregnant and there is no risk of conception (additional precautions (e.g. barrier methods) necessary for next 7 days), or immediately following termination of pregnancy below 24 weeks' gestation; postpartum insertions should be delayed until at least 4 weeks after delivery; effective for 5 years

MIRENA ® 20MICROGRAMS/24HOURS INTRA-UTERINE DEVICE

Contraception | Menorrhagia

▶ BY INTRA-UTERINE ADMINISTRATION

▶ Females of childbearing potential: Insert into uterine cavity within 7 days of onset of menstruation, or any time if replacement (additional precautions (e.g. barrier methods) advised for at least 7 days before), or any time if reasonably certain woman is not pregnant and there is no risk of conception (additional precautions (e.g. barrier methods) necessary for next 7 days), or immediately following termination of pregnancy below 24 weeks' gestation; postpartum insertions should be delayed until at least 4 weeks after delivery; effective for 5 years

Prevention of endometrial hyperplasia during oestrogen replacement therapy

▶ BY INTRA-UTERINE ADMINISTRATION

▶ Females of childbearing potential: Insert during last days of menstruation or withdrawal bleeding or at any time if amenorrhoeic; effective for 4 years

- **UNLICENSED USE**

▶ With intra-uterine use The Faculty of Sexual and Reproductive Healthcare (FSRH) advises levonorgestrel is used as detailed below, although these situations are considered unlicensed:

- Insertion at any time if reasonably certain the woman is not pregnant or at risk of pregnancy;
- Additional precautions (e.g. barrier methods) for at least 7 days before replacement even if immediate replacement is intended;
- Insertion immediately following termination of pregnancy below 24 weeks' gestation;
- Postpartum insertions 4 weeks after delivery.

▶ With oral use The FSRH advises levonorgestrel is used as detailed below, although these situations are considered unlicensed:

- Higher dose option for emergency contraception in patients with body-weight over 70 kg or BMI over 26 kg/m^2;
- Use for emergency contraception between 72–96 hours after coitus.

▶ With intra-uterine use or oral use Consult product literature for licensing status of individual preparations.

IMPORTANT SAFETY INFORMATION

MHRA/CHM ADVICE (JUNE 2015) INTRA-UTERINE CONTRACEPTION: UTERINE PERFORATION—UPDATED INFORMATION ON RISK FACTORS

Uterine perforation most often occurs during insertion, but might not be detected until sometime later. The risk of uterine perforation is increased when the device is inserted up to 36 weeks postpartum or in patients who are breastfeeding. Before inserting an intra-uterine contraceptive device, inform patients that perforation occurs in approximately 1 in every 1000 insertions and signs and symptoms include:

- severe pelvic pain after insertion (worse than period cramps);
- pain or increased bleeding after insertion which continues for more than a few weeks;
- sudden changes in periods;
- pain during intercourse;
- unable to feel the threads.

Patients should be informed on how to check their threads and to arrange a check-up if threads cannot be felt, especially if they also have significant pain. Partial perforation may occur even if the threads can be seen; consider this if there is severe pain following insertion and perform an ultrasound.

- **CONTRA-INDICATIONS**
  - ▸ With intra-uterine use Active trophoblastic disease (until return to normal of urine- and plasma-gonadotrophin concentration · acute cervicitis · acute malignancies affecting the blood (use with caution in remission) · acute vaginitis · distorted uterine cavity · history of breast cancer but can be considered for a woman in long-term remission who has menorrhagia and requires effective contraception · increased risk factors for pelvic infections · infected abortion during the previous three months · not suitable for emergency contraception · pelvic inflammatory disease · postpartum endometritis · unexplained uterine bleeding · unresolved cervical intraepithelial neoplasia · uterine or cervical malignancy
  - ▸ With oral use Acute porphyrias p. 652
  - ▸ With oral use for contraception History of breast cancer but can be used after 5 years if no evidence of disease and non-hormonal contraceptive methods unacceptable · severe arterial disease · undiagnosed vaginal bleeding
- **CAUTIONS**

GENERAL CAUTIONS Risk factors for ectopic pregnancy (including previous ectopic pregnancy, tubal surgery or pelvic infection)

SPECIFIC CAUTIONS
- ▸ With intra-uterine use Disease-induced immunosuppression (risk of infection—avoid if marked immunosuppression) · acute venous thromboembolism (consider removal) · anaemia · anticoagulant therapy (avoid if possible) · diabetes · drug-induced immunosuppression (risk of infection—avoid if marked immunosuppression) · endometriosis · epilepsy (risk of seizure at time of insertion) · fertility problems · history of pelvic inflammatory disease · increased risk of expulsion if inserted before uterine involution · jaundice (consider removal) · marked increase of blood pressure (consider removal) · migraine (consider removal) · nulliparity · severe arterial disease (consider removal) · severe cervical stenosis · severe headache (consider removal) · severe primary dysmenorrhoea · severely scarred uterus (including after endometrial resection) · young age
- ▸ With oral use for contraception Active trophoblastic disease (until return to normal of urine- and plasma-gonadotrophin concentration)—seek specialist advice · arterial disease · functional ovarian cysts · history of jaundice in pregnancy · malabsorption syndromes · past ectopic pregnancy · sex-steroid dependent cancer · systemic lupus erythematosus with positive (or unknown) antiphospholipid antibodies
- ▸ With oral use for emergency contraception Active trophoblastic disease (until return to normal of urine- and plasma-gonadotrophin concentration)—seek specialist advice · past ectopic pregnancy · severe malabsorption syndromes

CAUTIONS, FURTHER INFORMATION
- ▸ With intra-uterine use The Faculty of Sexual and Reproductive Healthcare advises intercourse should be avoided or another method of contraception used for at least 7 days before removal of intra-uterine device—emergency contraception may need to be considered if recent intercourse has occurred and the intra-uterine device is removed.
- ▸ Risk of infection with intra-uterine devices The main excess risk of infection occurs in the first 20 days after insertion and is believed to be related to existing carriage of a sexually transmitted infection. Women are considered to be at a higher risk of sexually transmitted infections if:
  - they are under 25 years old *or*
  - they are over 25 years old *and*
    - have a new partner *or*
    - have had more than one partner in the past year *or*
    - their regular partner has other partners.

  In these women, pre-insertion screening (for chlamydia and, depending on sexual history and local prevalence of disease, *Neisseria gonorrhoeae*) should be performed. If results are unavailable at the time of fitting an intra-uterine device for emergency contraception, appropriate prophylactic antibacterial cover should be given. The woman should be advised to attend *as an emergency* if she experiences sustained pain during the next 20 days.
- ▸ Use as a contraceptive in co-morbidities
- ▸ With oral use The product literature advises caution in patients with history of thromboembolism, hypertension, diabetes mellitus and migraine; evidence for caution in these conditions is unsatisfactory.

MIRENA ® 20MICROGRAMS/24HOURS INTRA-UTERINE DEVICE Advanced uterine atrophy

- **INTERACTIONS** → Appendix 1: levonorgestrel
- **SIDE-EFFECTS**

GENERAL SIDE-EFFECTS
- ▸ **Common or very common** Gastrointestinal discomfort · headaches · menstrual cycle irregularities · nausea · skin reactions

SPECIFIC SIDE-EFFECTS
- ▸ **Common or very common**
  - ▸ With intra-uterine use Back pain · breast abnormalities · depression · device expulsion · hirsutism · increased risk of infection · libido decreased · nervousness · ovarian cyst · pelvic disorders · uterine haemorrhage (on insertion) · vaginal haemorrhage (on insertion) · vulvovaginal disorders · weight increased
  - ▸ With oral use Breast tenderness · diarrhoea · dizziness · fatigue · haemorrhage · vomiting
- ▸ **Uncommon**
  - ▸ With intra-uterine use Alopecia · endometritis · oedema · uterine rupture
- ▸ **Rare or very rare**
  - ▸ With oral use Face oedema · pelvic pain
- ▸ **Frequency not known**
  - ▸ With oral use Cerebrovascular insufficiency · depressed mood · diabetes mellitus · embolism and thrombosis · neoplasms · sexual dysfunction · weight changes

SIDE-EFFECTS, FURTHER INFORMATION **Breast cancer** There is a small increase in the risk of having breast cancer diagnosed in women using, or who have recently used, a progestogen-only contraceptive pill; this relative risk may be due to an earlier diagnosis. The most important risk factor appears to be the age at which the contraceptive is stopped rather than the duration of use; the risk disappears gradually during the 10 years after stopping and there is no excess risk by 10 years. A possible small increase in the risk of breast cancer should be weighed against the benefits.

With intra-uterine use There is no evidence of an association between the levonorgestrel intra-uterine system and breast cancer. The levonorgestrel intra-uterine system should be avoided in patients with a history of breast cancer; any consideration of it's use should be by a specialist in contraception and in consultation with the patients cancer specialist.

Patients should be informed about the device that has been inserted and when it should be removed or replaced (including refering them to a patient information leaflet and other sources of information).

Patients may experience irregular, prolonged or infrequent menstrual bleeding in the 3–6 months following insertion; bleeding pattern improves with time but persists in some patients.

Progestogenic side-effects resolve with time (after the first few months).

- **PREGNANCY**
  - With oral use Not known to be harmful.
  - With intra-uterine use If an intra-uterine device fails and the woman wishes to continue to full-term the device should be removed in the first trimester if possible. Avoid; if pregnancy occurs remove intra-uterine system.
- **BREAST FEEDING** Progestogen-only contraceptives do not affect lactation.
- **HEPATIC IMPAIRMENT**
  - With intra-uterine use or oral use for Contraception Manufacturer advises avoid in liver tumour.
  - With oral use for Contraception or Emergency contraception Manufacturer advises avoid in severe impairment.
  - With intra-uterine use Manufacturer advises avoid in acute hepatic disease or in severe impairment (no information available)—consult product literature.
- **MONITORING REQUIREMENTS**
  - With intra-uterine use Gynaecological examination before insertion, 4–6 weeks after insertion, then annually.
- **DIRECTIONS FOR ADMINISTRATION**
  - With intra-uterine use *The doctor or nurse administering (or removing) the system should be fully trained in the technique and should provide full counselling reinforced by the patient information leaflet.*
- **PRESCRIBING AND DISPENSING INFORMATION**
  - With intra-uterine use Levonorgestrel-releasing intra-uterine devices vary in licensed indication, duration of use and insertion technique—the MHRA recommends to prescribe and dispense by brand name to avoid inadvertent switching.
- **PATIENT AND CARER ADVICE**

Diarrhoea and vomiting with use as an oral contraceptive Vomiting and persistent, severe diarrhoea can interfere with the absorption of oral progestogen-only contraceptives. If vomiting occurs within 2 hours of taking an oral progestogen-only contraceptive, another pill should be taken as soon as possible. If a replacement pill is not taken within 3 hours of the normal time for taking the progestogen-only pill, or in cases of persistent vomiting or very severe diarrhoea, additional precautions should be used during illness and for 2 days after recovery.

Starting routine

- With oral use for Contraception One tablet daily, on a continuous basis, starting on day 1 of cycle and taken at the same time each day (if delayed by longer than 3 hours contraceptive protection may be lost). Additional contraceptive precautions are not required if levonorgestrel is started up to and including day 5 of the menstrual cycle; if started after this time, additional contraceptive precautions are required for 2 days.

Changing from a combined oral contraceptive Start on the day following completion of the combined oral contraceptive course without a break (or in the case of ED tablets omitting the inactive ones).

After childbirth Oral progestogen-only contraceptives can be started up to and including day 21 postpartum without the need for additional contraceptive precautions. If started more than 21 days postpartum, additional contraceptive precautions are required for 2 days.

- With oral use for Emergency contraception When prescribing or supplying hormonal emergency contraception, manufacturer advises women should be told:
  - if vomiting occurs within 3 hours, a replacement dose should be taken;
  - that their next period may be early or late;
  - to seek medical attention promptly if any lower abdominal pain occurs because this could signify an ectopic pregnancy.

  The Faculty of Sexual and Reproductive Healthcare also advises women should be told:
  - that a barrier method of contraception needs to be used—see Emergency contraception p. 536 for further information;
  - that a pregnancy test should be performed if the next menstrual period is delayed by more than 7 days, is lighter than usual, or is associated with abdominal pain that is not typical of the woman's usual dysmenorrhoea;
  - that a pregnancy test should be performed if hormonal contraception is started soon after use of emergency contraception even if they have bleeding; bleeding associated with the contraceptive method may not represent menstruation.
- With intra-uterine use Counsel women on the signs, symptoms and risks of perforation and ectopic pregnancy.

Missed doses When used as an oral contraceptive, the following advice is recommended 'If you forget a pill, take it as soon as you remember and carry on with the next pill at the right time. If the pill was more than 3 hours overdue you are not protected. Continue normal pill-taking but you must also use another method, such as the condom, for the next 2 days'.

The Faculty of Sexual and Reproductive Healthcare recommends emergency contraception if one or more progestogen-only contraceptive tablets are missed or taken more than 3 hours late and unprotected intercourse has occurred before 2 further tablets have been correctly taken.

- **NATIONAL FUNDING/ACCESS DECISIONS**

Scottish Medicines Consortium (SMC) decisions

SMC No. 1299/18

The *Scottish Medicines Consortium* has advised (February 2018) that levonorgestrel (*Kyleena*®) is accepted for use within NHS Scotland as a contraceptive device for up to 5 years.

All Wales Medicines Strategy Group (AWMSG) decisions

AWMSG No. 3582

The *All Wales Medicines Strategy Group* has advised (September 2018) that levonorgestrel (*Kyleena*®) is recommended as an option for use within NHS Wales for contraception for up to five years.

- **EXCEPTIONS TO LEGAL CATEGORY** *Levonelle*® *One Step* can be sold to women over 16 years; when supplying emergency contraception to the public, pharmacists should refer to guidance issued by the Royal Pharmaceutical Society.

- **MEDICINAL FORMS** There can be variation in the licensing of different medicines containing the same drug.

Intra-uterine device

- Jaydess (Bayer Plc) ▼

  Levonorgestrel 13.5 mg Jaydess 13.5mg intra-uterine device | 1 device PoM £69.22 DT = £69.22
- Kyleena (Bayer Plc)

  Levonorgestrel 19.5 mg Kyleena 19.5mg intra-uterine device | 1 device PoM £76.00 DT = £76.00

- Levosert (Gedeon Richter (UK) Ltd)
  Levonorgestrel 20 microgram per 24 hour Levosert 20micrograms/24hours intra-uterine device | 1 device PoM £66.00 DT = £88.00
- Mirena (Bayer Plc)
  Levonorgestrel 20 microgram per 24 hour Mirena 20micrograms/24hours intra-uterine device | 1 device PoM £88.00 DT = £88.00

Tablet

- Levonorgestrel (Non-proprietary)
  Levonorgestrel 1.5 mg Levonorgestrel 1.5mg tablets | 1 tablet PoM £3.74–£5.20 DT = £5.20
- Emerres (Morningside Healthcare Ltd)
  Levonorgestrel 1.5 mg Emerres 1.5mg tablets | 1 tablet PoM £3.65 DT = £5.20
- Levonelle (Bayer Plc)
  Levonorgestrel 1.5 mg Levonelle 1500microgram tablets | 1 tablet PoM £5.20 DT = £5.20
- Melkine (Crescent Pharma Ltd)
  Levonorgestrel 1.5 mg Melkine 1.5mg tablets | 1 tablet PoM £4.16 DT = £5.20
- Norgeston (Bayer Plc)
  Levonorgestrel 30 microgram Norgeston 30microgram tablets | 35 tablet PoM £0.92 DT = £0.92
- Upostelle (Gedeon Richter (UK) Ltd)
  Levonorgestrel 1.5 mg Upostelle 1500microgram tablets | 1 tablet PoM £3.75 DT = £5.20

3.5 Contraception, parenteral progestogen-only

Other drugs used for Contraception, parenteral progestogen-only Norethisterone, p. 517

PROGESTOGENS

Etonogestrel

10-Mar-2020

● **INDICATIONS AND DOSE**

Contraception (no hormonal contraceptive use in previous month)

▶ BY SUBDERMAL IMPLANTATION

- Females of childbearing potential: 1 implant inserted during first 5 days of cycle, implant should be removed within 3 years of insertion

Contraception (postpartum)

▶ BY SUBDERMAL IMPLANTATION

- Females of childbearing potential: 1 implant to be inserted 21–28 days after delivery (delay until 28 days postpartum if breast-feeding), implant should be removed within 3 years of insertion

Contraception following abortion or miscarriage in the second trimester

▶ BY SUBDERMAL IMPLANTATION

- Females of childbearing potential: 1 implant to be inserted 21–28 days after abortion or miscarriage, implant should be removed within 3 years of insertion

Contraception following abortion or miscarriage in the first trimester

▶ BY SUBDERMAL IMPLANTATION

- Females of childbearing potential: 1 implant to be inserted within 5 days after abortion or miscarriage, implant should be removed within 3 years of insertion

Contraception (changing from other hormonal contraceptive)

▶ BY SUBDERMAL IMPLANTATION

- Females of childbearing potential: Implant should be removed within 3 years of insertion (consult product literature)

● **UNLICENSED USE** *Nexplanon*® not licensed for use in females outside of the age range 18–40 years.

IMPORTANT SAFETY INFORMATION

MHRA/CHM ADVICE (UPDATED FEBRUARY 2020): *NEXPLANON*® (ETONOGESTREL) CONTRACEPTIVE IMPLANTS: NEW INSERTION SITE TO REDUCE RARE RISK OF NEUROVASCULAR INJURY AND IMPLANT MIGRATION

There have been reports of neurovascular injury and migration of *Nexplanon*® implants from the insertion site to the vasculature, including the pulmonary artery in rare cases. Correct subdermal insertion by an appropriately trained and accredited healthcare professional is recommended to reduce the risk of these events. Healthcare professionals are advised to review the updated guidance from the manufacturer and the statement from the Faculty of Sexual and Reproductive Healthcare (FSRH) on how to correctly insert the implant. Patients should be advised on how to locate the implant, informed to check this occasionally and report any concerns. An implant that cannot be palpated at its insertion site should be located and removed as soon as possible; if unable to locate implant within the arm, the MHRA recommends using chest imaging. Implants inserted at a previous site that can be palpated should not pose a risk and should only be replaced if there are issues with its location or if a routine replacement is due.

● **CONTRA-INDICATIONS** Acute porphyrias p. 652 · history of breast cancer but can be used after 5 years if no evidence of disease and non-hormonal contraceptive methods unacceptable · severe arterial disease · undiagnosed vaginal bleeding

● **CAUTIONS** Active trophoblastic disease (until return to normal of urine- and plasma-gonadotrophin concentration)—seek specialist advice · arterial disease · disturbances of lipid metabolism · history during pregnancy of deterioration of otosclerosis · history during pregnancy of pruritus · history of jaundice in pregnancy · malabsorption syndromes · possible risk of breast cancer · sex-steroid dependent cancer · systemic lupus erythematosus with positive (or unknown) antiphospholipid antibodies

● **INTERACTIONS** → Appendix 1: etonogestrel

● **SIDE-EFFECTS**

▶ **Common or very common** Abdominal pain · alopecia · anxiety · appetite increased · breast abnormalities · depressed mood · dizziness · emotional lability · fatigue · flatulence · headaches · hot flush · increased risk of infection · influenza like illness · libido decreased · menstrual cycle irregularities · nausea · ovarian cyst · pain · skin reactions · weight changes

▶ **Uncommon** Arthralgia · constipation · diarrhoea · drowsiness · dysuria · fever · galactorrhoea · genital abnormalities · hypertrichosis · insomnia · myalgia · oedema · vomiting · vulvovaginal discomfort

▶ **Frequency not known** Abscess · angioedema · embolism and thrombosis · haemorrhage · insulin resistance · neoplasms · paraesthesia · seborrhoea

SIDE-EFFECTS, FURTHER INFORMATION The benefits of using progestogen-only contraceptives (POCs), such as etonogestrel, should be weighed against the possible risks for each individual woman.

There is a small increase in the risk of having breast cancer diagnosed in women using a combined oral contraceptive pill (COC); this relative risk may be due to an earlier diagnosis, biological effects of the pill or a combination of both. This increased risk is related to the age of the woman using the COC rather than the duration of use and disappears gradually within 10 years after discontinuation.

The risk of breast cancer in users of POCs is possibly of similar magnitude as that associated with COCs, however the evidence is less conclusive.

- **PREGNANCY** Not known to be harmful, remove implant if pregnancy occurs.
- **BREAST FEEDING** Progestogen-only contraceptives do not affect lactation.
- **DIRECTIONS FOR ADMINISTRATION** The doctor or nurse administering (or removing) the system should be fully trained in the technique and should provide full counselling reinforced by the patient information leaflet.
- **PATIENT AND CARER ADVICE** Full counselling backed by patient information leaflet required before administration.

- **MEDICINAL FORMS** There can be variation in the licensing of different medicines containing the same drug.

Implant

- Nexplanon (Merck Sharp & Dohme Ltd)

  Etonogestrel 68 mg Nexplanon 68mg implant | 1 device PoM £83.43 DT = £83.43

Medroxyprogesterone acetate 24-May-2017

- **INDICATIONS AND DOSE**

Contraception

- BY DEEP INTRAMUSCULAR INJECTION
- Females of childbearing potential: 150 mg, to be administered within the first 5 days of cycle or within first 5 days after parturition (delay until 6 weeks after parturition if breast-feeding)
- BY SUBCUTANEOUS INJECTION
- Females of childbearing potential: 104 mg, to be administered within first 5 days of cycle or within 5 days postpartum (delay until 6 weeks postpartum if breast-feeding), injected into anterior thigh or abdomen, dose only suitable if no hormonal contraceptive use in previous month

Long-term contraception

- BY DEEP INTRAMUSCULAR INJECTION
- Females of childbearing potential: 150 mg every 12 weeks, first dose to be administered within the first 5 days of cycle or within first 5 days after parturition (delay until 6 weeks after parturition if breast-feeding)
- BY SUBCUTANEOUS INJECTION
- Females of childbearing potential: 104 mg every 13 weeks, first dose to be administered within first 5 days of cycle or within 5 days postpartum (delay until 6 weeks postpartum if breast-feeding), injected into anterior thigh or abdomen, dose only suitable if no hormonal contraceptive use in previous month

Contraception (when patient changing from other hormonal contraceptive)

- BY SUBCUTANEOUS INJECTION
- Females of childbearing potential: (consult product literature)

- **CONTRA-INDICATIONS**

GENERAL CONTRA-INDICATIONS Acute porphyrias p. 652 · severe arterial disease · undiagnosed vaginal bleeding

SPECIFIC CONTRA-INDICATIONS History of breast cancer but can be used after 5 years if no evidence of disease and non-hormonal contraceptive methods unacceptable

- **CAUTIONS**

GENERAL CAUTIONS Possible risk of breast cancer

SPECIFIC CAUTIONS History during pregnancy in disturbances of lipid metabolism · history during pregnancy of deterioration of otosclerosis · history during pregnancy of pruritus

- **INTERACTIONS** → Appendix 1: medroxyprogesterone
- **SIDE-EFFECTS**
- **Common or very common** Anxiety · asthenia · breast abnormalities · depression · dizziness · gastrointestinal discomfort · headaches · insomnia · menstrual cycle irregularities · mood altered · nausea · pain · sexual dysfunction · skin reactions · vulvovaginal infection · weight changes
- **Uncommon** Alopecia · appetite abnormal · arthralgia · drowsiness · fever · fluid retention · galactorrhoea · hirsutism · hot flush · hypertension · muscle spasms · ovarian cyst · painful sexual intercourse · tachycardia · uterine haemorrhage · varicose veins · vertigo · vulvovaginal disorders
- **Rare or very rare** Breast cancer · lipodystrophy
- **Frequency not known** Embolism and thrombosis · hepatic disorders · osteoporosis · osteoporotic fractures · seizure

SIDE-EFFECTS, FURTHER INFORMATION Reduction in bone mineral density is greater with increasing duration of use. The loss is mostly recovered on discontinuation.

- **CONCEPTION AND CONTRACEPTION**
- With intramuscular use If interval between dose is greater than 12 weeks and 5 days (in long-term contraception), rule out pregnancy before next injection and advise patient to use additional contraceptive measures (e.g. barrier) for 14 days after the injection.
- With subcutaneous use If interval between dose is greater than 13 weeks and 7 days (in long-term contraception), rule out pregnancy before next injection.
- **PREGNANCY** Not known to be harmful.
- **BREAST FEEDING** Present in milk—no adverse effects reported. Progestogen-only contraceptives do not affect lactation. The manufacturers advise that in women who are breast-feeding, the first dose should be delayed until 6 weeks after birth; however, evidence suggests no harmful effect to infant if given earlier. The benefits of using medroxyprogesterone acetate in breast-feeding women outweigh any risks.
- **HEPATIC IMPAIRMENT** Manufacturer advises caution; avoid in severe or active disease.
- **PATIENT AND CARER ADVICE** Full counselling backed by *patient information leaflet* required before administration—likelihood of menstrual disturbance and the potential for a delay in return to full fertility. Delayed return of fertility and irregular cycles may occur after discontinuation of treatment but there is no evidence of permanent infertility.

- **MEDICINAL FORMS** There can be variation in the licensing of different medicines containing the same drug.

Suspension for injection

- Depo-Provera (Pfizer Ltd)

  Medroxyprogesterone acetate 150 mg per 1 ml Depo-Provera 150mg/1ml suspension for injection pre-filled syringes | 1 pre-filled disposable injection PoM £6.01 DT = £6.01
- Sayana Press (Pfizer Ltd)

  Medroxyprogesterone acetate 160 mg per 1 ml Sayana Press 104mg/0.65 ml suspension for injection pre-filled disposable devices | 1 pre-filled disposable injection PoM £6.90 DT = £6.90

3.6 Contraception, spermicidal

SPERMICIDALS

Nonoxinol

- **INDICATIONS AND DOSE**

Spermicidal contraceptive in conjunction with barrier methods of contraception such as diaphragms or caps

- BY VAGINA
- Females of childbearing potential: (consult product literature)

- **SIDE-EFFECTS** Genital erosion · increased risk of HIV infection · pain · paraesthesia · skin reactions · vaginal redness

  SIDE-EFFECTS, FURTHER INFORMATION High frequency use of the spermicide nonoxinol-9 has been associated with genital lesions, which may increase the risk of acquiring sexually transmitted infections.
- **CONCEPTION AND CONTRACEPTION** No evidence of harm to diaphragms.
- **PREGNANCY** Toxicity in *animal* studies.
- **BREAST FEEDING** Present in milk in *animal* studies.

- **MEDICINAL FORMS** There can be variation in the licensing of different medicines containing the same drug.

Gel

EXCIPIENTS: May contain Hydroxybenzoates (parabens), propylene glycol, sorbic acid

▸ Gygel (Marlborough Pharmaceuticals Ltd)
Nonoxinol-9 20 mg per 1 ml Gygel 2% contraceptive jelly | 81 gram [GSL] £11.00 DT = £11.00

4 Vaginal and vulval conditions

Vaginal and vulval conditions

Management

Pre-pubertal girls may be particularly susceptible to vulvovaginitis. Barrier preparations applied after cleansing can be useful when the symptoms are due to non-specific irritation, but systemic drugs are required in the treatment of bacterial infection or threadworm infestation. Intravaginal preparations, particularly those that require the use of an applicator, are not generally suitable for young girls; topical preparations may be useful in some adolescent girls.

In older girls symptoms are often restricted to the vulva, but infections almost invariably involve the vagina, which should also be treated; treatment should be as for adults.

Vaginal and vulval changes

Topical oestrogen creams containing **estriol** 0.01% (*Gynest*®) are used in the treatment of labial adhesions; treatment is usually restricted to symptomatic cases. Estriol cream should be applied to the adhesions once or twice daily for 2–6 weeks; adhesions may recur following treatment.

Vaginal and vulval infections

Effective specific treatments are available for the common vaginal infections.

Fungal infections

Vaginal fungal infections are not normally a problem in younger girls but can occur in adolescents. *Candidal vulvitis* can be treated locally with cream, but is almost invariably associated with vaginal infection which should also be treated. *Vaginal candidiasis*, rare in girls before puberty, can be treated with antifungal pessaries or cream inserted high into the vagina (including during menstruation), however, these are not recommended for pre-pubertal girls and treatment with an external cream may be more appropriate. Single-dose intravaginal preparations offer an advantage when compliance is a problem. Local irritation can occur on application of vaginal antifungal products.

Imidazole drugs (clotrimazole p. 555, econazole nitrate p. 555, fenticonazole nitrate p. 556, and miconazole) are effective against candida in short courses of 1 to 3 days according to the preparation used; treatment can be repeated if initial course fails to control symptoms or if symptoms recur. Vaginal applications may be supplemented with antifungal cream for vulvitis and to treat other superficial sites of infection.

Oral treatment of vaginal infection with fluconazole p. 407 may be considered for girls post-puberty.

Vulvovaginal candidiasis in pregnancy

Vulvovaginal candidiasis is common during pregnancy and can be treated with vaginal application of an imidazole (such as clotrimazole), and a topical imidazole cream for vulvitis. Pregnant women need a longer duration of treatment, usually about 7 days, to clear the infection. There is limited absorption of imidazoles from the skin and vagina. Oral antifungal treatment should be avoided during pregnancy.

Recurrent vulvovaginal candidiasis

Recurrent vulvovaginal candidiasis is very rare in children, but can occur if there are predisposing factors such as antibacterial therapy, pregnancy, diabetes mellitus, or possibly oral contraceptive use. Reservoirs of infection can also lead to recontamination and should be treated; these include other skin sites such as the digits, nail beds, and umbilicus, as well as the gastro-intestinal tract and the bladder. The sexual partner may also be the source of re-infection and, if symptomatic, should be treated with a topical imidazole cream at the same time.

Treatment against candida may need to be extended for 6 months in recurrent vulvovaginal candidiasis.

Other infections

Trichomonal infections commonly involve the lower urinary tract as well as the genital system and need systemic treatment with metronidazole p. 358 or tinidazole p. 360.

Bacterial infections with Gram-negative organisms are particularly common in association with gynaecological operations and trauma. Metronidazole is effective against certain Gram-negative organisms, especially *Bacteroides* spp. and can be used prophylactically in gynaecological surgery.

Clindamycin cream below and metronidazole gel are indicated for bacterial vaginosis.

The antiviral drugs aciclovir p. 440 and valaciclovir p. 442 can be used in the treatment of genital infection due to *herpes simplex virus*, the HSV type 2 being a major cause of genital ulceration. They have a beneficial effect on virus shedding and healing, generally giving relief from pain and other symptoms.

4.1 Vaginal and vulval infections

4.1a Vaginal and vulval bacterial infections

ANTIBACTERIALS › LINCOSAMIDES

Clindamycin

18-May-2020

- **INDICATIONS AND DOSE**

DALACIN® 2% CREAM

Bacterial vaginosis

▸ BY VAGINA

▸ Child: 1 applicatorful daily for 3–7 nights, dose to be administered at night

DOSE EQUIVALENCE AND CONVERSION

▸ 1 applicatorful delivers a 5 g dose of clindamycin 2%.

- **UNLICENSED USE** Not licensed for use in children.
- **CAUTIONS** Avoid intravaginal preparations (particularly those that require the use of an applicator) in young girls who are not sexually active, unless there is no alternative
- **INTERACTIONS** → Appendix 1: clindamycin
- **SIDE-EFFECTS**

▸ **Common or very common** Skin reactions

- **Frequency not known** Constipation · diarrhoea (discontinue) · dizziness · gastrointestinal discomfort · headache · increased risk of infection · nausea · vertigo · vomiting · vulvovaginal irritation

 SIDE-EFFECTS, FURTHER INFORMATION Clindamycin 2% cream is poorly absorbed into the blood—low risk of systemic effects.

- **CONCEPTION AND CONTRACEPTION** Damages latex condoms and diaphragms.
- **PRESCRIBING AND DISPENSING INFORMATION** For choice of antibacterial therapy, see Genital system infections, antibacterial therapy p. 325.
- **PATIENT AND CARER ADVICE** Patients and their carers should be advised to discontinue and contact a doctor immediately if severe, prolonged or bloody diarrhoea develops.

- **MEDICINAL FORMS** There can be variation in the licensing of different medicines containing the same drug.

Cream

EXCIPIENTS: May contain Benzyl alcohol, cetostearyl alcohol (including cetyl and stearyl alcohol), polysorbates, propylene glycol

- Dalacin (Pfizer Ltd)
 Clindamycin (as Clindamycin phosphate) 20 mg per 1 gram Dalacin 2% cream | 40 gram [PoM] £10.86 DT = £10.86

CARBOXYLIC ACIDS

Lactic acid

- **INDICATIONS AND DOSE**

BALANCE ACTIV RX® GEL

Prevention of bacterial vaginosis

- BY VAGINA
- Child: 5 mL 1–2 times a week, insert the content of 1 tube (5 mL)

- **ALLERGY AND CROSS-SENSITIVITY** Contra-indicated in shellfish allergy.

- **MEDICINAL FORMS** There can be variation in the licensing of different medicines containing the same drug.

Vaginal Gel

EXCIPIENTS: May contain Propylene glycol

- Balance Activ (BBI Healthcare Ltd)
 Balance Activ BV vaginal pH correction gel | 7 device £5.25

4.1b Vaginal and vulval fungal infections

Other drugs used for Vaginal and vulval fungal infections
Fluconazole, p. 407

ANTIFUNGALS > IMIDAZOLE

Clotrimazole

10-Mar-2020

- **INDICATIONS AND DOSE**

Superficial sites of infection in vaginal and vulval candidiasis (dose for 1% or 2% cream)

- BY VAGINA USING CREAM
- Child: Apply 2–3 times a day, to be applied to anogenital area

Vaginal candidiasis (dose for 10% intravaginal cream)

- BY VAGINA USING VAGINAL CREAM
- Child: 5 g for 1 dose, one applicatorful to be inserted into the vagina at night, dose can be repeated once if necessary

Vaginal candidiasis

- BY VAGINA USING PESSARIES
- Child: 200 mg for 3 nights, course can be repeated once if necessary, alternatively 500 mg for 1 night, dose can be repeated once if necessary

Recurrent vulvovaginal candidiasis

- BY VAGINA USING PESSARIES
- Child: 500 mg every week for 6 months, dose to be administered following topical imidazole for 10–14 days

- **UNLICENSED USE** Consult product literature for individual preparations.
- **CAUTIONS** Avoid intravaginal preparations (particularly those that require use of an applicator) in young girls who are not sexually active, unless there is no alternative
- **INTERACTIONS** → Appendix 1: antifungals, azoles
- **SIDE-EFFECTS**

 GENERAL SIDE-EFFECTS Oedema · paraesthesia · skin reactions

 SPECIFIC SIDE-EFFECTS Abdominal pain · discomfort · genital peeling · pelvic pain · vaginal haemorrhage
- **CONCEPTION AND CONTRACEPTION** Cream and pessaries may damage latex condoms and diaphragms.
- **PREGNANCY**

 Dose adjustments Pregnant women need a longer duration of treatment, usually about 7 days, to clear the infection. Oral antifungal treatment should be avoided during pregnancy.
- **PATIENT AND CARER ADVICE**

 Medicines for Children leaflet: Clotrimazole for fungal infections www.medicinesforchildren.org.uk/clotrimazole-fungal-infections
- **EXCEPTIONS TO LEGAL CATEGORY** Brands for sale to the public include *Canesten*® Internal Cream.

- **MEDICINAL FORMS** There can be variation in the licensing of different medicines containing the same drug.

Pessary

EXCIPIENTS: May contain Benzyl alcohol, cetostearyl alcohol (including cetyl and stearyl alcohol), polysorbates

- Canesten (clotrimazole) (Bayer Plc)
 Clotrimazole 100 mg Canesten 100mg pessaries | 6 pessary [P] £3.85 DT = £3.85
 Clotrimazole 200 mg Canesten 200mg pessaries | 3 pessary [P] £3.41 DT = £3.41
 Clotrimazole 500 mg Canesten Vaginal 500mg pessaries | 1 pessary [PoM] £2.00 DT = £5.56

Cream

EXCIPIENTS: May contain Benzyl alcohol, cetostearyl alcohol (including cetyl and stearyl alcohol), polysorbates

- Clotrimazole (Non-proprietary)
 Clotrimazole 10 mg per 1 gram Clotrimazole 1% cream | 20 gram [P] £2.06 DT = £1.29 | 50 gram [P] £5.45 DT = £3.23
- Canesten (clotrimazole) (Bayer Plc)
 Clotrimazole 10 mg per 1 gram Canesten 1% cream | 20 gram [P] £2.20 DT = £1.29 | 50 gram [P] £3.64 DT = £3.23
 Clotrimazole 20 mg per 1 gram Canesten 2% thrush cream | 20 gram [P] £4.76 DT = £4.76
 Clotrimazole 100 mg per 1 gram Canesten 10% VC cream | 5 gram [PoM] £4.50 DT = £6.23

Econazole nitrate

08-May-2020

- **INDICATIONS AND DOSE**

GYNO-PEVARYL® ONCE

Vaginal and vulval candidiasis

- BY VAGINA
- Child: 1 pessary for 1 dose, pessary to be inserted at night, dose to be repeated once if necessary continued →

7 Genito-urinary system

GYNO-PEVARYL ® PESSARY

Vaginal and vulval candidiasis

▸ BY VAGINA

▸ Child: 1 pessary daily for 3 days, pessary to be inserted at night, course can be repeated once if necessary

- CAUTIONS Avoid intravaginal preparations (particularly those that require use of an applicator) in young girls who are not sexually active, unless there is no alternative
- SIDE-EFFECTS
  - ▸ **Common or very common** Skin reactions
  - ▸ **Uncommon** Vaginal burning
  - ▸ **Frequency not known** Angioedema
- CONCEPTION AND CONTRACEPTION Cream and pessaries damage latex condoms and diaphragms.
- PREGNANCY Pregnant women need a longer duration of treatment, usually about 7 days, to clear the infection.

- MEDICINAL FORMS There can be variation in the licensing of different medicines containing the same drug.

Pessary

▸ Gyno-Pevaryl (Janssen-Cilag Ltd)
Econazole nitrate 150 mg Gyno-Pevaryl Once 150mg vaginal pessary | 1 pessary PoM £3.69 DT = £3.69
Gyno-Pevaryl 150mg vaginal pessaries | 3 pessary PoM £4.17 DT = £4.17

Fenticonazole nitrate

- INDICATIONS AND DOSE

Vaginal and vulva candidiasis

▸ BY VAGINA USING CAPSULES

▸ Child: 200 mg daily for 3 days, alternatively 600 mg daily for 1 dose, to be inserted at night

▸ BY VAGINA USING CREAM

▸ Child: 1 applicatorful twice daily for 3 days

DOSE EQUIVALENCE AND CONVERSION

▸ 1 applicatorful delivers a 5 g dose of fenticonazole 2 %.

- CAUTIONS Avoid intravaginal preparations (particularly those that require use of an applicator) in young girls who are not sexually active, unless there is no alternative
- SIDE-EFFECTS Paraesthesia
- CONCEPTION AND CONTRACEPTION Intravaginal cream and vaginal capsules damage latex condoms and diaphragms.

- MEDICINAL FORMS There can be variation in the licensing of different medicines containing the same drug.

Cream

EXCIPIENTS: May contain Cetostearyl alcohol (including cetyl and stearyl alcohol), propylene glycol, woolfat and related substances (including lanolin)

▸ Gynoxin (Recordati Pharmaceuticals Ltd)
Fenticonazole nitrate 20 mg per 1 gram Gynoxin 2% vaginal cream | 30 gram PoM £3.74

Capsule

EXCIPIENTS: May contain Hydroxybenzoates (parabens)

▸ Gynoxin (Recordati Pharmaceuticals Ltd)
Fenticonazole nitrate 200 mg Gynoxin 200mg vaginal capsules | 3 capsule PoM £2.42
Fenticonazole nitrate 600 mg Gynoxin 600mg vaginal capsules | 1 capsule PoM £2.62

7 Genito-urinary system

Chapter 8
Immune system and malignant disease

CONTENTS

Immune system

1 Immune system disorders and transplantation

Immune response

Inflammatory bowel disease

Azathioprine p. 558, mercaptopurine p. 587, or once weekly methotrexate p. 588 are used to induce remission in unresponsive or chronically active Crohn's disease. Azathioprine or mercaptopurine may also be helpful for retaining remission in frequently relapsing inflammatory bowel disease; once weekly methotrexate is used in Crohn's disease when azathioprine or mercaptopurine are ineffective or not tolerated. Response to azathioprine or mercaptopurine may not become apparent for several months. Folic acid p. 620 should be given to reduce the possibility of methotrexate toxicity. Folic acid is usually given weekly on a different day to the methotrexate; alternative regimens may be used in some settings.

Ciclosporin (cyclosporin) p. 559 is a potent immunosuppressant and is markedly nephrotoxic. In children with severe ulcerative colitis unresponsive to other treatment, ciclosporin may reduce the need for urgent colorectal surgery.

Immunosuppressant therapy

Immunosuppressants are used to suppress rejection in organ transplant recipients and to treat a variety of chronic inflammatory and autoimmune diseases. Solid organ transplant patients are maintained on drug regimens, which may include antiproliferative drugs (azathioprine or mycophenolate mofetil p. 566), calcineurin inhibitors (ciclosporin or tacrolimus p. 562), corticosteroids, or sirolimus p. 561. Choice is dependent on the type of organ, time after transplant, and clinical condition of the patient. Specialist management is required and other immunomodulators may be used to initiate treatment or to treat rejection.

Impaired immune responsiveness

Infections in the immunocompromised child can be severe and show atypical features. Specific local protocols should be followed for the management of infection. Corticosteroids may suppress clinical signs of infection and allow diseases such as septicaemia or tuberculosis to reach an advanced stage before being recognised. Children should be up-to-date with their childhood vaccinations before initiation of immunosuppressant therapy (e.g. before transplantation); vaccination with varicella-zoster vaccine is also necessary during this period— **important**: normal immunoglobulin administration should be considered as soon as possible after measles exposure, and varicella–zoster immunoglobulin (VZIG) is recommended for individuals who have significant chickenpox (varicella) exposure. Specialist advice should be sought on the use of live vaccines for those being treated with immunosuppressive drugs.

Antiproliferative immunosuppressants

Azathioprine is widely used for transplant recipients and it is also used to treat a number of auto-immune conditions, usually when corticosteroid therapy alone provides inadequate control. It is metabolised to mercaptopurine, and doses should be reduced (to one quarter of the original dose in children) when allopurinol p. 601 is given concurrently.

Mycophenolate mofetil is metabolised to mycophenolic acid which has a more selective mode of action than azathioprine.

There is evidence that compared with similar regimens incorporating azathioprine, mycophenolate mofetil may reduce the risk of acute rejection episodes; the risk of opportunistic infections (particularly due to tissue-invasive cytomegalovirus) and the occurrence of blood disorders such as leucopenia may be higher. Children may suffer a high incidence of side-effects, particularly gastrointestinal effects, calling for temporary reduction in dose or interruption of treatment.

Cyclophosphamide p. 579 is less commonly prescribed as an immunosuppressant.

Corticosteroids and other immunosuppressants

The corticosteroids prednisolone p. 478 and dexamethasone p. 475 are widely used in paediatric oncology; they have a marked antitumour effect. Dexamethasone is preferred for acute lymphoblastic leukaemia whilst prednisolone may be used for Hodgkin's disease, non-Hodgkin's lymphoma, and B-cell lymphoma and leukaemia.

Dexamethasone is the corticosteroid of choice in paediatric supportive and palliative care. For children who are not receiving a corticosteroid as a component of their chemotherapy, dexamethasone may be used to reduce raised intracranial pressure, or to help control emesis when combined with an appropriate anti-emetic.

The corticosteroids are also powerful immunosuppressants. They are used to prevent organ transplant rejection, and in high dose to treat rejection episodes.

Ciclosporin (cyclosporin), a calcineurin inhibitor, is a potent immunosuppressant which is virtually non-myelotoxic but markedly nephrotoxic. It may be used in organ and tissue transplantation, for prevention of graft rejection following bone marrow, kidney, liver, pancreas, heart, lung, and heart-lung transplantation, and for prophylaxis and treatment of graft-versus-host disease. Ciclosporin also has a role in steroid-sensitive and steroid-resistant nephrotic syndrome; in corticosteroid-sensitive nephrotic syndrome it may be given with prednisolone.

Tacrolimus is also a calcineurin inhibitor. Although not chemically related to ciclosporin it has a similar mode of action and side-effects.

Other drugs used for Immune system disorders and transplantation Anakinra, p. 691 · Chloroquine, p. 429 · Everolimus, p. 605 · Hydroxychloroquine sulfate, p. 690 · Rituximab, p. 574

IMMUNE SERA AND IMMUNOGLOBULINS › IMMUNOGLOBULINS

Antithymocyte immunoglobulin (rabbit)

28-Nov-2017

● **INDICATIONS AND DOSE**

Prophylaxis of organ rejection in heart allograft recipients

▶ BY INTRAVENOUS INFUSION

▸ Child: 1–2.5 mg/kg daily for 3–5 days, start treatment on day of transplantation, to be given over at least 6 hours

Prophylaxis of organ rejection in renal allograft recipients

▶ BY INTRAVENOUS INFUSION

▸ Child 1–17 years: 1–1.5 mg/kg daily for 3–9 days, start treatment on day of transplantation, to be given over at least 6 hours

Treatment of corticosteroid-resistant allograft rejection in renal transplantation

▶ BY INTRAVENOUS INFUSION

▸ Child 1–17 years: 1.5 mg/kg daily for 7–14 days, to be given over at least 6 hours

DOSES AT EXTREMES OF BODY-WEIGHT

▸ To avoid excessive dosage in obese patients, calculate dose on the basis of ideal body weight.

● **CONTRA-INDICATIONS** Infection

● **INTERACTIONS** → Appendix 1: immunoglobulins

● **SIDE-EFFECTS**

▶ **Common or very common** Chills · diarrhoea · dysphagia · dyspnoea · fever · hypotension · infection · lymphopenia · myalgia · nausea · neoplasm malignant · neoplasms · neutropenia · reactivation of infection · secondary malignancy · sepsis · skin reactions · thrombocytopenia · vomiting

▶ **Uncommon** Cytokine release syndrome · hepatic disorders · hypersensitivity · infusion related reaction

SIDE-EFFECTS, FURTHER INFORMATION Tolerability is increased by pretreatment with an intravenous corticosteroid and antihistamine; an antipyretic drug such as paracetamol may also be beneficial.

● **PREGNANCY** Manufacturer advises use only if potential benefit outweighs risk—no information available.

● **BREAST FEEDING** Manufacturer advises avoid—no information available.

● **MONITORING REQUIREMENTS** Monitor blood count.

● **DIRECTIONS FOR ADMINISTRATION** For *continuous intravenous infusion* reconstitute each vial with 5 mL water for injections to produce a solution of 5 mg/mL; gently rotate to dissolve. Dilute requisite dose with Glucose 5% *or* Sodium Chloride 0.9% to an approx. concentration of 0.5 mg/mL; begin infusion immediately after dilution; give through an in-line filter (pore size 0.22 micron); incompatible with unfractionated heparin and hydrocortisone in glucose infusion—precipitation reported.

● **NATIONAL FUNDING/ACCESS DECISIONS**

NICE decisions

▶ **Immunosuppressive therapy for kidney transplant in children and young people (October 2017)** NICE TA482
Antithymocyte immunoglobulin (rabbit) is not recommended as an initial treatment to prevent organ rejection in patients having a kidney transplant. Patients whose treatment was started within the NHS before this guidance was published should have the option to continue treatment, without change to their funding arrangements, until they and their NHS clinician consider it appropriate to stop. www.nice.org.uk/guidance/TA482

● **MEDICINAL FORMS** There can be variation in the licensing of different medicines containing the same drug.

Solution for infusion

▸ Grafalon (Imported (Germany))
Antithymocyte immunoglobulin (rabbit) 20 mg per 1 ml Grafalon 100mg/5ml concentrate for solution for infusion vials | 1 vial [PoM] [X]

Powder and solvent for solution for infusion

▸ Thymoglobulin (Sanofi)
Antithymocyte immunoglobulin (rabbit) 25 mg Thymoglobuline 25mg powder and solvent for solution for infusion vials | 1 vial [PoM] £158.77 (Hospital only)

IMMUNOSUPPRESSANTS › ANTIMETABOLITES

Azathioprine

13-Jun-2018

● **DRUG ACTION** Azathioprine is metabolised to mercaptopurine.

● **INDICATIONS AND DOSE**

Severe ulcerative colitis | Severe Crohn's disease

▶ BY MOUTH

▸ Child 2–17 years: Initially 2 mg/kg once daily, then increased if necessary up to 2.5 mg/kg once daily

Systemic lupus erythematosus | Vasculitis | Autoimmune conditions usually when corticosteroid therapy alone has proved inadequate

▶ BY MOUTH

▸ Child: Initially 1 mg/kg daily, then adjusted according to response to 3 mg/kg daily, consider withdrawal if no improvement within 3 months; maximum 3 mg/kg per day

Suppression of transplant rejection

▶ BY MOUTH, OR BY INTRAVENOUS INFUSION

▸ Child: Maintenance 1–3 mg/kg daily, adjusted according to response, consult local treatment protocol for details, oral route preferred, but if oral route is not possible then can be given by intravenous infusion, the total daily dose may alternatively be given in 2 divided doses

DOSE ADJUSTMENTS DUE TO INTERACTIONS

▸ Manufacturer advises reduce dose to one-quarter of the usual dose with concurrent use of allopurinol.

● **CAUTIONS** Reduced thiopurine methyltransferase activity

● **INTERACTIONS** → Appendix 1: azathioprine

● **SIDE-EFFECTS**

GENERAL SIDE-EFFECTS

▶ **Common or very common** Bone marrow depression (dose-related) · increased risk of infection · leucopenia · pancreatitis · thrombocytopenia

▶ **Uncommon** Anaemia · hepatic disorders · hypersensitivity

- **Rare or very rare** Agranulocytosis · alopecia · bone marrow disorders · diarrhoea · gastrointestinal disorders · neoplasms · photosensitivity reaction · pneumonitis · severe cutaneous adverse reactions (SCARs)
- **Frequency not known** Nodular regenerative hyperplasia · sinusoidal obstruction syndrome

SPECIFIC SIDE-EFFECTS

- With oral use Nausea

SIDE-EFFECTS, FURTHER INFORMATION Side-effects may require drug withdrawal.

Hypersensitivity reactions Hypersensitivity reactions (including malaise, dizziness, vomiting, diarrhoea, fever, rigors, myalgia, arthralgia, rash, hypotension and renal dysfunction) call for immediate withdrawal.

Neutropenia and thrombocytopenia Neutropenia is dose-dependent. Management of neutropenia and thrombocytopenia requires careful monitoring and dose adjustment.

- **ALLERGY AND CROSS-SENSITIVITY** Contra-indicated in hypersensitivity to mercaptopurine.
- **PREGNANCY** Transplant patients immunosuppressed with azathioprine should not discontinue it on becoming pregnant. However, there have been reports of premature birth and low birth-weight following exposure to azathioprine, particularly in combination with corticosteroids. Spontaneous abortion has been reported following maternal or paternal exposure. Azathioprine is teratogenic in *animal* studies. The use of azathioprine during pregnancy needs to be supervised in specialist units. Treatment should not generally be initiated during pregnancy.
- **BREAST FEEDING** Present in milk in low concentration. No evidence of harm in small studies—use if potential benefit outweighs risk.
- **HEPATIC IMPAIRMENT** Manufacturer advises caution (impaired metabolism)—monitor liver function and complete blood count more frequently in those with severe impairment.

Dose adjustments Manufacturer advises use doses at lower end of the dose range in hepatic failure; reduce dose if hepatic or haematological toxicity occur.

- **RENAL IMPAIRMENT**

Dose adjustments Reduce dose.

- **PRE-TREATMENT SCREENING**

Thiopurine methyltransferase The enzyme thiopurine methyltransferase (TPMT) metabolises thiopurine drugs (azathioprine, mercaptopurine, tioguanine); the risk of myelosuppression is increased in patients with reduced activity of the enzyme, particularly for the few individuals in whom TPMT activity is undetectable. Consider measuring TPMT activity before starting azathioprine, mercaptopurine, or tioguanine therapy. Patients with absent TPMT activity should not receive thiopurine drugs; those with reduced TPMT activity may be treated under specialist supervision.

- **MONITORING REQUIREMENTS**
  - Monitor for toxicity throughout treatment.
  - Monitor full blood count weekly (more frequently with higher doses or if severe renal impairment) for first 4 weeks (manufacturer advises weekly monitoring for 8 weeks but evidence of practical value unsatisfactory), thereafter reduce frequency of monitoring to at least every 3 months.
  - Blood tests and monitoring for signs of myelosuppression are essential in long-term treatment.
- **DIRECTIONS FOR ADMINISTRATION**
  - With intravenous use Consult local treatment protocol for details. For *intravenous injection*, reconstitute 50 mg with 5–15 mL Water for Injections; give over at least 1 minute. For *intravenous infusion*, reconstitute 50 mg with 5–15 mL Water for Injections; dilute requisite dose to a concentration of 0.25–2.5 mg/mL in Glucose 5% *or* Sodium Chloride 0.9%. Intravenous injection is alkaline and very irritant. Intravenous route should therefore be used **only** if oral route not feasible and discontinued as soon as oral route can be tolerated. To reduce irritation flush line with infusion fluid.
- **PRESCRIBING AND DISPENSING INFORMATION** The RCPCH and NPPG recommend that, when a liquid special of azathioprine is required, the following strength is used: 50 mg/5 mL.
- **PATIENT AND CARER ADVICE**

Bone marrow suppression Patients and their carers should be warned to report immediately any signs or symptoms of bone marrow suppression e.g. inexplicable bruising or bleeding, infection.

Medicines for Children leaflet: Azathioprine for inflammatory bowel disease www.medicinesforchildren.org.uk/azathioprine-inflammatory-bowel-disease-0

Medicines for Children leaflet: Azathioprine for renal (kidney) transplant www.medicinesforchildren.org.uk/azathioprine-renal-kidney-transplant-0

Medicines for Children leaflet: Azathioprine for severe atopic eczema www.medicinesforchildren.org.uk/azathioprine-severe-atopic-eczema-0

- **MEDICINAL FORMS** There can be variation in the licensing of different medicines containing the same drug. Forms available from special-order manufacturers include: capsule, oral suspension, oral solution

Tablet

CAUTIONARY AND ADVISORY LABELS 21

- Azathioprine (Non-proprietary)
  Azathioprine 25 mg Azathioprine 25mg tablets | 28 tablet PoM £6.64 DT = £1.89 | 100 tablet PoM £8.98–£33.26
  Azathioprine 50 mg Azathioprine 50mg tablets | 56 tablet PoM £7.28 DT = £2.57 | 100 tablet PoM £4.65–£16.55
- Azapress (Ennogen Pharma Ltd)
  Azathioprine 50 mg Azapress 50mg tablets | 56 tablet PoM £2.83 DT = £2.57
- Imuran (Aspen Pharma Trading Ltd)
  Azathioprine 25 mg Imuran 25mg tablets | 100 tablet PoM £10.99
  Azathioprine 50 mg Imuran 50mg tablets | 100 tablet PoM £7.99

Powder for solution for injection

- Imuran (Aspen Pharma Trading Ltd)
  Azathioprine 50 mg Imuran 50mg powder for solution for injection vials | 1 vial PoM £15.38

IMMUNOSUPPRESSANTS > CALCINEURIN INHIBITORS AND RELATED DRUGS

Ciclosporin

26-Nov-2019

(Cyclosporin)

- **DRUG ACTION** Ciclosporin inhibits production and release of lymphokines, thereby suppressing cell-mediated immune response.

- **INDICATIONS AND DOSE**

Refractory ulcerative colitis

- BY MOUTH
  - Child 2–17 years: Initially 2 mg/kg twice daily (max. per dose 5 mg/kg twice daily), dose adjusted according to blood-ciclosporin concentration and response
- BY INTRAVENOUS INFUSION
  - Child 3–17 years: Initially 0.5–1 mg/kg twice daily, dose adjusted according to blood-ciclosporin concentration and response

continued →

Short-term treatment of severe atopic dermatitis where conventional therapy ineffective or inappropriate (administered on expert advice)

▸ BY MOUTH

▸ Child: Initially 1.25 mg/kg twice daily (max. per dose 2.5 mg/kg twice daily) usual maximum duration of 8 weeks but may be used for longer under specialist supervision, if good initial response not achieved within 2 weeks, increase dose rapidly up to maximum

Short-term treatment of very severe atopic dermatitis where conventional therapy ineffective or inappropriate (administered on expert advice)

▸ BY MOUTH

▸ Child: 2.5 mg/kg twice daily usual maximum duration of 8 weeks but may be used for longer under specialist supervision

Severe psoriasis where conventional therapy ineffective or inappropriate (administered on expert advice)

▸ BY MOUTH

▸ Child: Initially 1.25 mg/kg twice daily (max. per dose 2.5 mg/kg twice daily), increased gradually to maximum if no improvement within 1 month, initial dose of 2.5 mg/kg twice daily justified if condition requires rapid improvement; discontinue if inadequate response after 3 months at the optimum dose; max. duration of treatment usually 1 year unless other treatments cannot be used

Prevention of graft rejection following bone-marrow, kidney, liver, pancreas, heart, lung, and heart-lung transplantation | Prevention and treatment of graft-versus-host disease

▸ BY MOUTH, OR BY INTRAVENOUS INFUSION

▸ Child: (consult local protocol)

Nephrotic syndrome

▸ BY MOUTH

▸ Child: 3 mg/kg twice daily, dose can be increased if necessary in corticosteroid-resistant disease; for maintenance reduce to lowest effective dose according to whole blood-ciclosporin concentrations, proteinuria, and renal function

DOSE ADJUSTMENTS DUE TO INTERACTIONS

▸ With oral use Manufacturer advises increase dose by 50% or switch to intravenous administration with concurrent use of octreotide.

- UNLICENSED USE Not licensed for use in children under 3 months. Not licensed for use in children under 16 years for atopic eczema (dermatitis) or psoriasis. Not licensed for use in ulcerative colitis.

> IMPORTANT SAFETY INFORMATION
>
> MHRA/CHM ADVICE: CICLOSPORIN MUST BE PRESCRIBED AND DISPENSED BY BRAND NAME (DECEMBER 2009)
>
> Patients should be stabilised on a particular brand of oral ciclosporin because switching between formulations without close monitoring may lead to clinically important changes in blood-ciclosporin concentration.

- CONTRA-INDICATIONS Malignancy (in non-transplant indications) · uncontrolled hypertension (in non-transplant indications) · uncontrolled infections (in non-transplant indications)
- CAUTIONS Hyperuricaemia · in atopic dermatitis, active herpes simplex infections—allow infection to clear before starting (if they occur during treatment withdraw if severe) · in atopic dermatitis, *Staphylococcus aureus* skin infections—not absolute contra-indication providing controlled (but avoid erythromycin unless no other alternative) · in psoriasis treat, patients with malignant or pre-malignant conditions of skin only after appropriate treatment (and if no other option) · in uveitis, Behcet's syndrome (monitor neurological status) · lymphoproliferative disorders (discontinue treatment) · malignancy

CAUTIONS, FURTHER INFORMATION

▸ Malignancy In psoriasis, exclude malignancies (including those of skin and cervix) before starting (biopsy any lesions not typical of psoriasis) and treat patients with malignant or pre-malignant conditions of skin only after appropriate treatment (and if no other option); discontinue if lymphoproliferative disorder develops.

- INTERACTIONS → Appendix 1: ciclosporin
- SIDE-EFFECTS

GENERAL SIDE-EFFECTS

▸ **Common or very common** Eye inflammation

SPECIFIC SIDE-EFFECTS

▸ **Common or very common** Appetite decreased · diarrhoea · electrolyte imbalance · fatigue · fever · flushing · gastrointestinal discomfort · gingival hyperplasia · hair changes · headaches · hepatic disorders · hyperglycaemia · hyperlipidaemia · hypertension · hyperuricaemia · leucopenia · muscle complaints · nausea · paraesthesia · peptic ulcer · renal impairment (renal structural changes on long-term administration) · seizure · skin reactions · tremor · vomiting

▸ **Uncommon** Anaemia · encephalopathy · oedema · thrombocytopenia · weight increased

▸ **Rare or very rare** Gynaecomastia · haemolytic anaemia · idiopathic intracranial hypertension · menstrual disorder · multifocal motor neuropathy · muscle weakness · myopathy · pancreatitis

▸ **Frequency not known** Pain in extremity · thrombotic microangiopathy

- PREGNANCY Crosses placenta; manufacturer advises avoid unless potential benefit outweighs risk—toxicity in *animal* studies.
- BREAST FEEDING Manufacturer advises avoid—present in milk.
- HEPATIC IMPAIRMENT Manufacturer advises caution in severe impairment (risk of increased exposure).

Dose adjustments Manufacturer advises consider dose reduction in severe impairment to maintain blood-ciclosporin concentration in target range—monitor until concentration stable.

- RENAL IMPAIRMENT

Dose adjustments In non-transplant indications, manufacturer advises establishing baseline renal function before initiation of treatment; if baseline function is impaired in non-transplant indications, except nephrotic syndrome—avoid. In nephrotic syndrome, manufacturer advises initial dose should not exceed 2.5 mg/kg daily in patients with baseline renal impairment. *During treatment* for non-transplant indications, manufacturer recommends if the estimated glomerular filtration rate decreases by more than 25% below baseline on more than one measurement, reduce dose by 25–50%. If the estimated glomerular filtration rate decrease from baseline exceeds 35%, further dose reduction should be considered (even if within normal range); discontinue if reduction not successful within 1 month.

- MONITORING REQUIREMENTS

▸ Monitor whole blood ciclosporin concentration (trough level dependent on indication—consult local treatment protocol for details).

▸ In long-term management of nephrotic syndrome, perform renal biopsies every 1–2 years.

- DIRECTIONS FOR ADMINISTRATION

▸ With oral use Mix solution with orange or apple juice, or other soft drink (to improve taste) immediately before taking (and rinse with more to ensure total dose). Do not mix with grapefruit juice. Total daily dose should be taken in 2 divided doses.

▸ With intravenous use For intermittent *intravenous infusion*, dilute to a concentration of 0.5–2.5 mg/mL with Glucose 5% *or* Sodium Chloride 0.9%; give over 2–6 hours; not to be used with PVC equipment. Observe patient for signs of anaphylaxis for at least 30 minutes after starting infusion and at frequent intervals thereafter.

● **PRESCRIBING AND DISPENSING INFORMATION**
Brand name prescribing Prescribing and dispensing of ciclosporin should be by brand name to avoid inadvertent switching. If it is necessary to switch a patient to a different brand of ciclosporin, the patient should be monitored closely for changes in blood-ciclosporin concentration, serum creatinine, blood pressure, and transplant function (for transplant indications).
Sandimmun® capsules and oral solution are available direct from Novartis for patients who cannot be transferred to a different oral preparation.

● **PATIENT AND CARER ADVICE** Patients and carers should be counselled on the administration of different formulations of ciclosporin. Manufacturer advises avoid excessive exposure to UV light, including sunlight. In psoriasis and atopic dermatitis, avoid use of UVB or PUVA.
Medicines for Children leaflet: Ciclosporin for nephrotic syndrome www.medicinesforchildren.org.uk/ciclosporin-nephrotic-syndrome-0

● **MEDICINAL FORMS** There can be variation in the licensing of different medicines containing the same drug.

Solution for infusion
CAUTIONARY AND ADVISORY LABELS 11
EXCIPIENTS: May contain Alcohol, polyoxyl castor oils
▸ Sandimmun (Novartis Pharmaceuticals UK Ltd)
Ciclosporin 50 mg per 1 ml Sandimmun 250mg/5ml concentrate for solution for infusion ampoules | 10 ampoule [PoM] £110.05
Sandimmun 50mg/1ml concentrate for solution for infusion ampoules | 10 ampoule [PoM] £23.23

Oral solution
CAUTIONARY AND ADVISORY LABELS 11
EXCIPIENTS: May contain Alcohol, propylene glycol
▸ Capsorin (Morningside Healthcare Ltd)
Ciclosporin 100 mg per 1 ml Capsorin 100mg/ml oral solution sugar-free | 50 ml [PoM] £86.96 DT = £164.72
▸ Neoral (Novartis Pharmaceuticals UK Ltd)
Ciclosporin 100 mg per 1 ml Neoral 100mg/ml oral solution sugar-free | 50 ml [PoM] £102.30 DT = £164.72
▸ Sandimmun (Novartis Pharmaceuticals UK Ltd)
Ciclosporin 100 mg per 1 ml Sandimmun 100mg/ml oral solution sugar-free | 50 ml [PoM] £164.72 DT = £164.72

Capsule
CAUTIONARY AND ADVISORY LABELS 11
EXCIPIENTS: May contain Ethanol, ethyl lactate, propylene glycol
▸ Ciclosporin (Non-proprietary)
Ciclosporin 25 mg Ciclosporin 25mg capsules | 30 capsule [PoM] [X] DT = £18.37
Ciclosporin 50 mg Ciclosporin 50mg capsules | 30 capsule [PoM] [X] DT = £35.97
Ciclosporin 100 mg Ciclosporin 100mg capsules | 30 capsule [PoM] [X] DT = £68.28
▸ Capimune (Mylan)
Ciclosporin 25 mg Capimune 25mg capsules | 30 capsule [PoM] £13.05 DT = £18.37
Ciclosporin 50 mg Capimune 50mg capsules | 30 capsule [PoM] £25.50 DT = £35.97
Ciclosporin 100 mg Capimune 100mg capsules | 30 capsule [PoM] £48.50 DT = £68.28
▸ Capsorin (Morningside Healthcare Ltd)
Ciclosporin 25 mg Capsorin 25mg capsules | 30 capsule [PoM] £11.14 DT = £18.37
Ciclosporin 50 mg Capsorin 50mg capsules | 30 capsule [PoM] £21.80 DT = £35.97
Ciclosporin 100 mg Capsorin 100mg capsules | 30 capsule [PoM] £41.59 DT = £68.28
▸ Deximune (Dexcel-Pharma Ltd)
Ciclosporin 25 mg Deximune 25mg capsules | 30 capsule [PoM] £13.06 DT = £18.37
Ciclosporin 50 mg Deximune 50mg capsules | 30 capsule [PoM] £25.60 DT = £35.97
Ciclosporin 100 mg Deximune 100mg capsules | 30 capsule [PoM] £48.90 DT = £68.28
▸ Neoral (Novartis Pharmaceuticals UK Ltd)
Ciclosporin 10 mg Neoral 10mg capsules | 60 capsule [PoM] £18.25 DT = £18.25
Ciclosporin 25 mg Neoral 25mg capsules | 30 capsule [PoM] £18.37 DT = £18.37
Ciclosporin 50 mg Neoral 50mg capsules | 30 capsule [PoM] £35.97 DT = £35.97
Ciclosporin 100 mg Neoral 100mg capsules | 30 capsule [PoM] £68.28 DT = £68.28
▸ Sandimmun (Novartis Pharmaceuticals UK Ltd)
Ciclosporin 25 mg Sandimmun 25mg capsules | 30 capsule [PoM] £29.58 DT = £18.37
Ciclosporin 50 mg Sandimmun 50mg capsules | 30 capsule [PoM] £57.92 DT = £35.97
Ciclosporin 100 mg Sandimmun 100mg capsules | 30 capsule [PoM] £109.93 DT = £68.28
▸ Vanquoral (Teva UK Ltd)
Ciclosporin 10 mg Vanquoral 10mg capsules | 60 capsule [PoM] £12.75 DT = £18.25
Ciclosporin 25 mg Vanquoral 25mg capsules | 30 capsule [PoM] £13.05 DT = £18.37
Ciclosporin 50 mg Vanquoral 50mg capsules | 30 capsule [PoM] £25.59 DT = £35.97
Ciclosporin 100 mg Vanquoral 100mg capsules | 30 capsule [PoM] £48.89 DT = £68.28

Sirolimus

16-Nov-2017

● **DRUG ACTION** Sirolimus is a non-calcineurin inhibiting immunosuppressant.

● **INDICATIONS AND DOSE**

As a component of immunosuppressive therapy for renal transplantation in children and adolescents only if intolerance necessitates the withdrawal of a calcineurin inhibitor
▸ BY MOUTH
▸ Child: (consult local protocol)

DOSE EQUIVALENCE AND CONVERSION
▸ The 500 microgram tablet is not bioequivalent to the 1 mg and 2 mg tablets. Multiples of 500 microgram tablets should **not** be used as a substitute for other tablet strengths.

● **UNLICENSED USE** Not licensed for use in children.

● **CAUTIONS** Hyperlipidaemia · increased susceptibility to infection (especially urinary-tract infection) · increased susceptibility to lymphoma and other malignancies, particularly of the skin (limit exposure to UV light)

● **INTERACTIONS** → Appendix 1: sirolimus

● **SIDE-EFFECTS**
▸ **Common or very common** Abdominal pain · anaemia · arthralgia · ascites · constipation · diabetes mellitus · diarrhoea · dyslipidaemia · electrolyte imbalance · embolism and thrombosis · fever · haemolytic uraemic syndrome · haemorrhage · headache · healing impaired · hyperglycaemia · hypertension · increased risk of infection · leucopenia · lymphatic vessel disorders · menstrual cycle irregularities · nausea · neoplasms · neutropenia · oedema · osteonecrosis · ovarian cyst · pain · pancreatitis · pericardial effusion · proteinuria · respiratory disorders · sepsis · skin reactions · stomatitis · tachycardia · thrombocytopenia
▸ **Uncommon** Antibiotic associated colitis · focal segmental glomerulosclerosis · hepatic failure · nephrotic syndrome · pancytopenia · post transplant lymphoproliferative disorder
▸ **Frequency not known** Posterior reversible encephalopathy syndrome (PRES)

- **CONCEPTION AND CONTRACEPTION** Effective contraception must be used during treatment and for 12 weeks after stopping.
- **PREGNANCY** Avoid unless essential—toxicity in *animal* studies.
- **BREAST FEEDING** Discontinue breast-feeding.
- **HEPATIC IMPAIRMENT** Manufacturer advises caution (risk of increased exposure).
  Dose adjustments In adults, manufacturer advises maintenance dose reduction in severe impairment—consult product literature.
- **MONITORING REQUIREMENTS**
  - Monitor whole blood-sirolimus trough concentration (Afro-Caribbean patients may require higher doses).
  - Monitor kidney function when given with ciclosporin; monitor lipids; monitor urine proteins.
- **DIRECTIONS FOR ADMINISTRATION** Food may affect absorption (take at the same time with respect to food). Sirolimus oral solution should be mixed with at least 60 mL water or orange juice in a glass or plastic container immediately before taking; refill container with at least 120 mL of water or orange juice and drink immediately (to ensure total dose). Do not mix with any other liquids.
- **PATIENT AND CARER ADVICE** Patient or carers should be given advice on how to administer sirolimus.
  Patients should be advised to avoid excessive exposure to UV light.
- **NATIONAL FUNDING/ACCESS DECISIONS**
  NICE decisions
  - **Immunosuppressive therapy for kidney transplant in children and young people (October 2017)** NICE TA482
    Sirolimus is not recommended as an initial treatment to prevent organ rejection in patients having a kidney transplant. Patients whose treatment was started within the NHS before this guidance was published should have the option to continue treatment, without change to their funding arrangements, until they and their NHS clinician consider it appropriate to stop. www.nice.org.uk/guidance/TA482

- **MEDICINAL FORMS** There can be variation in the licensing of different medicines containing the same drug.
  Oral solution
  EXCIPIENTS: May contain Ethanol
  - Rapamune (Pfizer Ltd)
    Sirolimus 1 mg per 1 ml Rapamune 1mg/ml oral solution sugar-free | 60 ml [PoM] £162.41 DT = £162.41

  Tablet
  - Rapamune (Pfizer Ltd)
    Sirolimus 500 microgram Rapamune 0.5mg tablets | 30 tablet [PoM] £69.00 DT = £69.00
    Sirolimus 1 mg Rapamune 1mg tablets | 30 tablet [PoM] £86.49 DT = £86.49
    Sirolimus 2 mg Rapamune 2mg tablets | 30 tablet [PoM] £172.98 DT = £172.98

Tacrolimus

16-Apr-2020

- **DRUG ACTION** Tacrolimus is a calcineurin inhibitor.
- **INDICATIONS AND DOSE**

ADOPORT®

Prophylaxis of graft rejection following liver transplantation, starting 12 hours after transplantation
▸ BY MOUTH
- Neonate: Initially 150 micrograms/kg twice daily.
- Child: Initially 150 micrograms/kg twice daily

Prophylaxis of graft rejection following kidney transplantation, starting within 24 hours of transplantation
▸ BY MOUTH
- Neonate: Initially 150 micrograms/kg twice daily.
- Child: Initially 150 micrograms/kg twice daily, a lower initial dose of 100 micrograms/kg twice daily has been used in adolescents to prevent very high 'trough' concentrations

Prophylaxis of graft rejection following heart transplantation following antibody induction, starting within 5 days of transplantation
▸ BY MOUTH
- Neonate: Initially 50–150 micrograms/kg twice daily.
- Child: Initially 50–150 micrograms/kg twice daily

Prophylaxis of graft rejection following heart transplantation without antibody induction, starting within 12 hours of transplantation
▸ BY MOUTH
- Neonate: Initially 150 micrograms/kg twice daily, dose to be given as soon as clinically possible (8–12 hours after discontinuation of intravenous infusion).
- Child: Initially 150 micrograms/kg twice daily, dose to be given as soon as clinically possible (8–12 hours after discontinuation of intravenous infusion)

Allograft rejection resistant to conventional immunosuppressive therapy
▸ BY MOUTH
- Child: Seek specialist advice

MODIGRAF®

Prophylaxis of graft rejection following liver transplantation, starting 12 hours after transplantation
▸ BY MOUTH
- Neonate: Initially 150 micrograms/kg twice daily.
- Child: Initially 150 micrograms/kg twice daily

Prophylaxis of graft rejection following kidney transplantation, starting within 24 hours of transplantation
▸ BY MOUTH
- Neonate: Initially 150 micrograms/kg twice daily.
- Child: Initially 150 micrograms/kg twice daily, a lower initial dose of 100 micrograms/kg twice daily has been used in adolescents to prevent very high 'trough' concentrations

Prophylaxis of graft rejection following heart transplantation following antibody induction, starting within 5 days of transplantation
▸ BY MOUTH
- Neonate: Initially 50–150 micrograms/kg twice daily.
- Child: Initially 50–150 micrograms/kg twice daily

Prophylaxis of graft rejection following heart transplantation without antibody induction, starting within 12 hours of transplantation
▸ BY MOUTH
- Neonate: Initially 150 micrograms/kg twice daily, dose to be given as soon as clinically possible (8–12 hours after discontinuation of intravenous infusion).
- Child: Initially 150 micrograms/kg twice daily, dose to be given as soon as clinically possible (8–12 hours after discontinuation of intravenous infusion)

Allograft rejection resistant to conventional immunosuppressive therapy

▶ BY MOUTH

▶ Child: Seek specialist advice

PROGRAF® CAPSULES

Prophylaxis of graft rejection following liver transplantation, starting 12 hours after transplantation

▶ BY MOUTH

▶ Neonate: Initially 150 micrograms/kg twice daily.

▶ Child: Initially 150 micrograms/kg twice daily

Prophylaxis of graft rejection following kidney transplantation, starting within 24 hours of transplantation

▶ BY MOUTH

▶ Neonate: Initially 150 micrograms/kg twice daily.

▶ Child: Initially 150 micrograms/kg twice daily, a lower initial dose of 100 micrograms/kg twice daily has been used in adolescents to prevent very high 'trough' concentrations

Prophylaxis of graft rejection following heart transplantation following antibody induction, starting within 5 days of transplantation

▶ BY MOUTH

▶ Neonate: Initially 50–150 micrograms/kg twice daily.

▶ Child: Initially 50–150 micrograms/kg twice daily

Prophylaxis of graft rejection following heart transplantation without antibody induction, starting within 12 hours of transplantation

▶ BY MOUTH

▶ Neonate: Initially 150 micrograms/kg twice daily, dose to be given as soon as clinically possible (8–12 hours after discontinuation of intravenous infusion).

▶ Child: Initially 150 micrograms/kg twice daily, dose to be given as soon as clinically possible (8–12 hours after discontinuation of intravenous infusion)

Allograft rejection resistant to conventional immunosuppressive therapy

▶ BY MOUTH

▶ Child: Seek specialist advice

PROGRAF® INFUSION

Prophylaxis of graft rejection following liver transplantation, starting 12 hours after transplantation when oral route not appropriate

▶ BY CONTINUOUS INTRAVENOUS INFUSION

▶ Neonate: Initially 50 micrograms/kg daily for up to 7 days (then transfer to oral therapy), dose to be administered over 24 hours.

▶ Child: Initially 50 micrograms/kg daily for up to 7 days (then transfer to oral therapy), dose to be administered over 24 hours

Prophylaxis of graft rejection following kidney transplantation, starting within 24 hours of transplantation when oral route not appropriate

▶ BY CONTINUOUS INTRAVENOUS INFUSION

▶ Neonate: Initially 75–100 micrograms/kg daily for up to 7 days (then transfer to oral therapy), dose to be administered over 24 hours.

▶ Child: Initially 75–100 micrograms/kg daily for up to 7 days (then transfer to oral therapy), dose to be administered over 24 hours

Prophylaxis of graft rejection following heart transplantation without antibody induction, starting within 12 hours of transplantation

▶ BY CONTINUOUS INTRAVENOUS INFUSION

▶ Neonate: Initially 30–50 micrograms/kg daily for up to 7 days (then transfer to oral therapy), dose to be administered over 24 hours.

▶ Child: Initially 30–50 micrograms/kg daily for up to 7 days (then transfer to oral therapy), dose to be administered over 24 hours

Allograft rejection resistant to conventional immunosuppressive therapy

▶ BY CONTINUOUS INTRAVENOUS INFUSION

▶ Child: Seek specialist advice (consult local protocol)

DOSE EQUIVALENCE AND CONVERSION

▶ For *Prograf*®: Intravenous and oral doses are **not** interchangeable due to differences in bioavailability. Follow correct dosing recommendations for the dosage form when switching formulations.

TACNI®

Prophylaxis of graft rejection following liver transplantation, starting 12 hours after transplantation

▶ BY MOUTH

▶ Neonate: Initially 150 micrograms/kg twice daily.

▶ Child: Initially 150 micrograms/kg twice daily

Prophylaxis of graft rejection following kidney transplantation, starting within 24 hours of transplantation

▶ BY MOUTH

▶ Neonate: Initially 150 micrograms/kg twice daily.

▶ Child: Initially 150 micrograms/kg twice daily, a lower initial dose of 100 micrograms/kg twice daily has been used in adolescents to prevent very high 'trough' concentrations

Prophylaxis of graft rejection following heart transplantation following antibody induction, starting within 5 days of transplantation

▶ BY MOUTH

▶ Neonate: Initially 50–150 micrograms/kg twice daily.

▶ Child: Initially 50–150 micrograms/kg twice daily

Prophylaxis of graft rejection following heart transplantation without antibody induction, starting within 12 hours of transplantation

▶ BY MOUTH

▶ Neonate: Initially 150 micrograms/kg twice daily, dose to be given as soon as clinically possible (8–12 hours after discontinuation of intravenous infusion).

▶ Child: Initially 150 micrograms/kg twice daily, dose to be given as soon as clinically possible (8–12 hours after discontinuation of intravenous infusion)

Allograft rejection resistant to conventional immunosuppressive therapy

▶ BY MOUTH

▶ Child: Seek specialist advice

● **UNLICENSED USE**
ADVAGRAF ® *Advagraf*® not licensed for use in children.

> **IMPORTANT SAFETY INFORMATION**
> MHRA/CHM ADVICE: ORAL TACROLIMUS PRODUCTS: PRESCRIBE AND DISPENSE BY BRAND NAME ONLY, TO MINIMISE THE RISK OF INADVERTENT SWITCHING BETWEEN PRODUCTS, WHICH HAS BEEN ASSOCIATED WITH REPORTS OF TOXICITY AND GRAFT REJECTION (JUNE 2012)
> ▸ With oral use
> Inadvertent switching between oral tacrolimus products has been associated with reports of toxicity and graft rejection. To ensure maintenance of therapeutic response when a patient is stabilised on a particular brand, oral tacrolimus products should be prescribed and dispensed by brand name only.
> - *Adoport*®, *Prograf*®, *Capexion*® and *Tacni*® are immediate-release capsules that are taken twice daily, once in the morning and once in the evening;
> - *Modigraf*® granules are used to prepare an immediate-release oral suspension which is taken twice daily, once in the morning and once in the evening;
> - *Advagraf*® is a prolonged-release capsule that is taken once daily in the morning.
>
> Switching between tacrolimus brands requires careful supervision and therapeutic monitoring by an appropriate specialist.
> Important: *Envarsus*® is not interchangeable with other oral tacrolimus containing products; the MHRA has advised (June 2012) that oral tacrolimus products should be prescribed and dispensed by brand only.

● **CAUTIONS** Increased risk of infections · lymphoproliferative disorders · malignancies · neurotoxicity · QT-interval prolongation · UV light (avoid excessive exposure to sunlight and sunlamps)

● **INTERACTIONS** → Appendix 1: tacrolimus

● **SIDE-EFFECTS**
GENERAL SIDE-EFFECTS
▸ **Common or very common** Alopecia · anaemia · anxiety · appetite decreased · arrhythmias · ascites · asthenic conditions · bile duct disorders · confusion · consciousness impaired · constipation · coronary artery disease · cough · depression · diabetes mellitus · diarrhoea · dizziness · dysgraphia · dyslipidaemia · dyspnoea · electrolyte imbalance · embolism and thrombosis · eye disorder · febrile disorders · fluid imbalance · gastrointestinal discomfort · gastrointestinal disorders · gastrointestinal inflammatory disorders · haemorrhage · hallucination · headache · hepatic disorders · hyperglycaemia · hyperhidrosis · hypertension · hyperuricaemia · hypotension · increased risk of infection · ischaemia · joint disorders · leucocytosis · leucopenia · metabolic acidosis · mood altered · muscle spasms · nasal complaints · nausea · nephropathy · nervous system disorder · oedema · oral disorders · pain · peripheral neuropathy · peripheral vascular disease · primary transplant dysfunction · psychiatric disorder · renal impairment · renal tubular necrosis · respiratory disorders · seizure · sensation abnormal · skin reactions · sleep disorders · temperature sensation altered · thrombocytopenia · tinnitus · tremor · urinary tract disorder · urine abnormal · vision disorders · vomiting · weight changes
▸ **Uncommon** Asthma · cardiac arrest · cardiomyopathy · cataract · central nervous system haemorrhage · chest discomfort · coagulation disorders · coma · dysmenorrhoea · encephalopathy · feeling abnormal · haemolytic anaemia · hearing impairment · heart failure · hypoglycaemia · hypoproteinaemia · influenza like illness · memory loss · multi organ failure · neutropenia · palpitations · pancreatitis · pancytopenia · paralysis · paresis · photosensitivity reaction · psychotic disorder · shock · speech disorder · stroke · ventricular hypertrophy
▸ **Rare or very rare** Fall · hirsutism · mobility decreased · muscle tone increased · muscle weakness · pancreatic pseudocyst · pericardial effusion · QT interval prolongation · severe cutaneous adverse reactions (SCARs) · sinusoidal obstruction syndrome · thirst · ulcer
▸ **Frequency not known** Agranulocytosis · neoplasm malignant · neoplasms · polyomavirus-associated nephropathy · progressive multifocal leukoencephalopathy (PML) · pure red cell aplasia

SPECIFIC SIDE-EFFECTS
▸ With intravenous use Anaphylactoid reaction (due to excipient) · hypersensitivity

SIDE-EFFECTS, FURTHER INFORMATION Cardiomyopathy has been reported to occur primarily in children with tacrolimus blood trough concentrations much higher than the recommended maximum levels. Patients should be monitored by echocardiography for hypertrophic changes—consider dose reduction or discontinuation if these occur.

● **ALLERGY AND CROSS-SENSITIVITY** Contra-indicated if history of hypersensitivity to macrolides.

● **CONCEPTION AND CONTRACEPTION** Exclude pregnancy before treatment.

● **PREGNANCY** Avoid unless potential benefit outweighs risk—crosses the placenta and risk of premature delivery, intra-uterine growth restriction, and hyperkalaemia.

● **BREAST FEEDING** Avoid—present in breast milk (following systemic administration).

● **HEPATIC IMPAIRMENT** Manufacturer advises caution in severe impairment.
Dose adjustments Manufacturer advises consider dose reduction in severe impairment.

● **MONITORING REQUIREMENTS** After initial dosing, and for maintenance treatment, tacrolimus doses should be adjusted according to whole-blood concentration. Monitor whole blood-tacrolimus trough concentration (especially during episodes of diarrhoea)—consult local treatment protocol for details.
▸ Monitor blood pressure, ECG (for hypertrophic changes—risk of cardiomyopathy), fasting blood-glucose concentration, haematological and neurological (including visual) and coagulation parameters, electrolytes, hepatic and renal function.

● **DIRECTIONS FOR ADMINISTRATION**
▸ With intravenous use For *continuous intravenous infusion* over 24 hours, dilute to a concentration of 4–100 micrograms/mL with Glucose 5% *or* Sodium Chloride 0.9%, to a total volume between 20–500mL. Tacrolimus is incompatible with PVC.

● **PRESCRIBING AND DISPENSING INFORMATION** The RCPCH and NPPG recommend that, when a liquid special of tacrolimus is required, the following strength is used: 5 mg/5 mL.
PROGRAF ® INFUSION Intravenous route should only be used if oral route is inappropriate.

● **PATIENT AND CARER ADVICE** Avoid excessive exposure to UV light including sunlight.
Medicines for Children leaflet: Tacrolimus for prevention of transplant rejection www.medicinesforchildren.org.uk/tacrolimus-prevention-transplant-rejection
Driving and skilled tasks May affect performance of skilled tasks (e.g. driving).

● **NATIONAL FUNDING/ACCESS DECISIONS**
NICE decisions
▸ **Immunosuppressive therapy for kidney transplant in children and young people (October 2017)** NICE TA482
Immediate-release tacrolimus, when used as part of an immunosuppressive regimen, is recommended as an initial

option to prevent organ rejection in patients having a kidney transplant. Treatment should be started with the least expensive product, but if this is not suitable, an alternative dosage form may be given. Tacrolimus granules for oral suspension (*Modigraf*®) should be used only if the manufacturer provides it at the same price or lower than that agreed with the Commercial Medicines Unit. Patients whose treatment was started within the NHS before this guidance was published should have the option to continue treatment, without change to their funding arrangements, until they and their NHS clinician consider it appropriate to stop.
www.nice.org.uk/guidance/TA482

▸ **Immunosuppressive therapy for kidney transplant in children and young people (October 2017)** NICE TA482
Prolonged-release tacrolimus is not recommended as an initial treatment to prevent organ rejection in patients having a kidney transplant. Patients whose treatment was started within the NHS before this guidance was published should have the option to continue treatment, without change to their funding arrangements, until they and their NHS clinician consider it appropriate to stop.
www.nice.org.uk/guidance/TA482

Scottish Medicines Consortium (SMC) decisions
The *Scottish Medicines Consortium* has advised (December 2010) that tacrolimus granules for suspension (*Modigraf*®) are accepted for restricted use within NHS Scotland in patients for whom tacrolimus is an appropriate choice of immunosuppressive therapy and where small changes (less than 500 micrograms) in dosing increments are required (such as, in paediatric patients) or in seriously ill patients who are unable to swallow tacrolimus capsules.

● **MEDICINAL FORMS** There can be variation in the licensing of different medicines containing the same drug.

Granules

CAUTIONARY AND ADVISORY LABELS 13, 23

▸ Modigraf (Astellas Pharma Ltd)
Tacrolimus (as Tacrolimus monohydrate) 200 microgram Modigraf 0.2mg granules sachets sugar-free | 50 sachet [PoM] £71.30 DT = £71.30
Tacrolimus (as Tacrolimus monohydrate) 1 mg Modigraf 1mg granules sachets sugar-free | 50 sachet [PoM] £356.65 DT = £356.65

Solution for infusion

EXCIPIENTS: May contain Polyoxyl castor oils

▸ Prograf (Astellas Pharma Ltd)
Tacrolimus 5 mg per 1 ml Prograf 5mg/1ml solution for infusion ampoules | 10 ampoule [PoM] £584.51

Capsule

CAUTIONARY AND ADVISORY LABELS 23

▸ Adoport (Sandoz Ltd)
Tacrolimus 500 microgram Adoport 0.5mg capsules | 50 capsule [PoM] £42.92 DT = £61.88
Tacrolimus 1 mg Adoport 1mg capsules | 50 capsule [PoM] £55.69 DT = £80.28 | 100 capsule [PoM] £111.36
Tacrolimus 5 mg Adoport 5mg capsules | 50 capsule [PoM] £205.74 DT = £296.58

▸ Prograf (Astellas Pharma Ltd)
Tacrolimus 500 microgram Prograf 500microgram capsules | 50 capsule [PoM] £61.88 DT = £61.88
Tacrolimus 1 mg Prograf 1mg capsules | 50 capsule [PoM] £80.28 DT = £80.28 | 100 capsule [PoM] £160.54
Tacrolimus 5 mg Prograf 5mg capsules | 50 capsule [PoM] £296.58 DT = £296.58

IMMUNOSUPPRESSANTS › MONOCLONAL ANTIBODIES

Canakinumab

20-Jun-2019

● **DRUG ACTION** Canakinumab is a recombinant human monoclonal antibody that selectively inhibits interleukin-1 beta receptor binding.

● **INDICATIONS AND DOSE**

Cryopyrin-associated periodic syndromes (specialist use only)

▸ BY SUBCUTANEOUS INJECTION

▸ Child 2–3 years (body-weight 7.5–14 kg): 4 mg/kg every 8 weeks, to be administered to the upper thigh, abdomen, upper arm or buttocks, additional doses may be considered if clinical response not achieved within 7 days—consult product literature
▸ Child 4–17 years (body-weight 7.5–14 kg): 4 mg/kg every 8 weeks, to be administered to the upper thigh, abdomen, upper arm or buttocks, additional doses may be considered if clinical response not achieved within 7 days—consult product literature
▸ Child 4–17 years (body-weight 15–40 kg): 2 mg/kg every 8 weeks, to be administered to the upper thigh, abdomen, upper arm or buttocks, additional doses may be considered if clinical response not achieved within 7 days—consult product literature
▸ Child 4–17 years (body-weight 41 kg and above): 150 mg every 8 weeks, to be administered to the upper thigh, abdomen, upper arm or buttocks, additional doses may be considered if clinical response not achieved within 7 days—consult product literature

Tumour necrosis factor receptor associated periodic syndrome (specialist use only) | Hyperimmunoglobulin D syndrome (specialist use only) | Familial Mediterranean fever (specialist use only)

▸ BY SUBCUTANEOUS INJECTION

▸ Child 2–17 years (body-weight 7.5–40 kg): 2 mg/kg every 4 weeks, to be administered to the upper thigh, abdomen, upper arm or buttocks, a second dose may be considered if clinical response not achieved within 7 days—consult product literature
▸ Child 2–17 years (body-weight 41 kg and above): 150 mg every 4 weeks, to be administered to the upper thigh, abdomen, upper arm or buttocks, a second dose may be considered if clinical response not achieved within 7 days—consult product literature

Still's disease (specialist use only)

▸ BY SUBCUTANEOUS INJECTION

▸ Child 2–17 years (body-weight 7.5 kg and above): 4 mg/kg every 4 weeks (max. per dose 300 mg), to be administered to the upper thigh, abdomen, upper arm or buttocks

● **CONTRA-INDICATIONS** Active severe infection · leucopenia · neutropenia

● **CAUTIONS** History of recurrent infection · latent and active tuberculosis · predisposition to infection

CAUTIONS, FURTHER INFORMATION

▸ Vaccinations Patients should receive all recommended vaccinations (including pneumococcal and inactivated influenza vaccine) before starting treatment; avoid live vaccines unless potential benefit outweighs risk—consult product literature for further information.

● **INTERACTIONS** → Appendix 1: monoclonal antibodies

● **SIDE-EFFECTS**

▸ **Common or very common** Abdominal pain upper · arthralgia · asthenia · dizziness · increased risk of infection · leucopenia · neutropenia · pain · proteinuria · vertigo
▸ **Uncommon** Gastrooesophageal reflux disease

8

Immune system and malignant disease

- **CONCEPTION AND CONTRACEPTION** Effective contraception required during treatment and for up to 3 months after last dose.
- **PREGNANCY** Manufacturer advises avoid unless potential benefit outweighs risk.
- **BREAST FEEDING** Consider if benefit outweighs risk—not known if present in human milk.
- **RENAL IMPAIRMENT** Limited information available but manufacturer advises no dose adjustment required.
- **PRE-TREATMENT SCREENING** Patients should be evaluated for latent and active tuberculosis before starting treatment.
- **MONITORING REQUIREMENTS**
  - ▶ Manufacturer advises monitor full blood count including neutrophil count before starting treatment, 1–2 months after starting treatment, and periodically thereafter.
  - ▶ Manufacturer advises monitor for signs and symptoms of infection (including tuberculosis) during and after treatment.
- **HANDLING AND STORAGE** Manufacturer advises store in a refrigerator (2–8 °C).
- **PATIENT AND CARER ADVICE** Manufacturer advises patients and carers should be instructed to seek medical advice if signs or symptoms suggestive of tuberculosis (including persistent cough, weight loss and subfebrile temperature) occur.

  Driving and skilled tasks Manufacturer advises patients and carers should be counselled on the effects on driving and performance of skilled tasks—increased risk of dizziness and drowsiness.

- **MEDICINAL FORMS** There can be variation in the licensing of different medicines containing the same drug.

  Solution for injection
  - ▶ Ilaris (Novartis Pharmaceuticals UK Ltd)

    Canakinumab 150 mg per 1 ml Ilaris 150mg/1ml solution for injection vials | 1 vial PoM £9,927.80

IMMUNOSUPPRESSANTS › MONOCLONAL ANTIBODIES › ANTI-LYMPHOCYTE

Basiliximab

16-Nov-2017

- **DRUG ACTION** Basiliximab is a monoclonal antibody that acts as an interleukin-2 receptor antagonist and prevents T-lymphocyte proliferation.

- **INDICATIONS AND DOSE**

  Prophylaxis of acute rejection in allogeneic renal transplantation used in combination with ciclosporin and corticosteroid-containing immunosuppression regimens (specialist use only)

  ▶ BY INTRAVENOUS INJECTION, OR BY INTRAVENOUS INFUSION
  - ▶ Child 1–17 years (body-weight up to 35 kg): Initially 10 mg, dose to be administered within 2 hours before transplant surgery, followed by 10 mg after 4 days, dose administered after transplant surgery, withhold second dose if severe hypersensitivity or graft loss occurs
  - ▶ Child 1–17 years (body-weight 35 kg and above): Initially 20 mg, administered within 2 hours before transplant surgery, followed by 20 mg after 4 days, dose to be administered after surgery, withhold second dose if severe hypersensitivity or graft loss occurs

- **CAUTIONS** Off-label use in cardiac transplantation—increased risk of serious cardiac side-effects
- **INTERACTIONS** → Appendix 1: monoclonal antibodies
- **SIDE-EFFECTS** Capillary leak syndrome · constipation · cytokine release syndrome · dyspnoea · fever · heart failure · hypersensitivity · hypertension · hypertrichosis · hypotension · increased risk of infection · myocardial infarction · pulmonary oedema · respiratory disorders · sepsis · skin reactions · sneezing · tachycardia
- **CONCEPTION AND CONTRACEPTION** Adequate contraception must be used during treatment and for 16 weeks after last dose.
- **PREGNANCY** Manufacturer advises avoid—no information available.
- **BREAST FEEDING** Manufacturer advises avoid—no information available.
- **DIRECTIONS FOR ADMINISTRATION** For *intravenous infusion*, dilute reconstituted solution to a concentration not exceeding 400 micrograms/mL, with Glucose 5% *or* Sodium Chloride 0.9%; give over 20–30 minutes.
- **NATIONAL FUNDING/ACCESS DECISIONS**

  NICE decisions
  - ▶ **Immunosuppressive therapy for kidney transplant in children and young people (October 2017)** NICE TA482

    Basiliximab, when used as part of an immunosuppressive regimen that includes a calcineurin inhibitor, is recommended as an initial option to prevent organ rejection in patients having a kidney transplant. The use of basiliximab with tacrolimus is outside the terms of the marketing authorisation. If this combination is prescribed, the prescriber should follow relevant professional guidance, taking full responsibility for the decision. Informed consent should be obtained and documented.

    Patients whose treatment was started within the NHS before this guidance was published should have the option to continue treatment, without change to their funding arrangements, until they and their NHS clinician consider it appropriate to stop. www.nice.org.uk/guidance/TA482

- **MEDICINAL FORMS** There can be variation in the licensing of different medicines containing the same drug.

  Powder and solvent for solution for injection
  - ▶ Simulect (Novartis Pharmaceuticals UK Ltd)

    Basiliximab 10 mg Simulect 10mg powder and solvent for solution for injection vials | 1 vial PoM £758.69 (Hospital only)

    Basiliximab 20 mg Simulect 20mg powder and solvent for solution for injection vials | 1 vial PoM £842.38 (Hospital only)

IMMUNOSUPPRESSANTS › PURINE SYNTHESIS INHIBITORS

Mycophenolate mofetil

09-Mar-2018

- **INDICATIONS AND DOSE**

  Prophylaxis of acute rejection in renal transplantation (in combination with a corticosteroid and ciclosporin) (under expert supervision)

  ▶ BY MOUTH
  - ▶ Child: 600 mg/m^2 twice daily, consult local protocol for details; maximum 2 g per day

  Prophylaxis of acute rejection in renal transplantation (in combination with a corticosteroid and tacrolimus) (under expert supervision)

  ▶ BY MOUTH
  - ▶ Child: 300 mg/m^2 twice daily, consult local protocol for details; maximum 2 g per day

  Prophylaxis of acute rejection in hepatic transplantation (in combination with a corticosteroid and ciclosporin or tacrolimus) (under expert supervision)

  ▶ BY MOUTH
  - ▶ Child: 10 mg/kg twice daily, increased to 20 mg/kg twice daily, consult local protocol for details; maximum 2 g per day

- **UNLICENSED USE** Not licensed for use in children under 2 years for the prophylaxis of acute rejection in renal transplantation. Not licensed for use in children for the prophylaxis of acute rejection in hepatic transplantation.

IMPORTANT SAFETY INFORMATION

MHRA/CHM ADVICE: MYCOPHENOLATE MOFETIL, MYCOPHENOLIC ACID: UPDATED CONTRACEPTION ADVICE FOR MALE PATIENTS (FEBRUARY 2018)

Available clinical evidence does not indicate an increased risk of malformations or miscarriage in pregnancies where the father was taking mycophenolate medicines, however mycophenolate mofetil and mycophenolic acid are genotoxic and a risk cannot be fully excluded; for further information, see Conception and contraception and Patient and carer advice.

- **CAUTIONS** Active serious gastro-intestinal disease (risk of haemorrhage, ulceration and perforation) · children (higher incidence of side-effects may call for temporary reduction of dose or interruption) · delayed graft function · increased susceptibility to skin cancer (avoid exposure to strong sunlight) · risk of hypogammaglobulinaemia or bronchiectasis when used in combination with other immunosuppressants

  CAUTIONS, FURTHER INFORMATION

  - Hypogammaglobulinaemia or bronchiectasis Measure serum immunoglobulin levels if recurrent infections develop, and consider bronchiectasis or pulmonary fibrosis if persistent respiratory symptoms such as cough and dyspnoea develop.
- **INTERACTIONS** → Appendix 1: mycophenolate
- **SIDE-EFFECTS**
  - **Common or very common** Acidosis · alopecia · anaemia · anxiety · appetite decreased · arthralgia · asthenia · bone marrow disorders · burping · chills · confusion · constipation · cough · depression · diarrhoea · dizziness · drowsiness · dyslipidaemia · dyspnoea · electrolyte imbalance · fever · gastrointestinal discomfort · gastrointestinal disorders · gastrointestinal haemorrhage · gout · headache · hepatic disorders · hyperbilirubinaemia · hyperglycaemia · hypertension · hyperuricaemia · hypotension · increased risk of infection · insomnia · leucocytosis · leucopenia · malaise · nausea · neoplasms · neuromuscular dysfunction · oedema · oral disorders · pain · pancreatitis · paraesthesia · renal impairment · respiratory disorders · seizure · sepsis · skin reactions · tachycardia · taste altered · thinking abnormal · thrombocytopenia · tremor · vasodilation · vomiting · weight decreased
  - **Uncommon** Agranulocytosis
  - **Frequency not known** Endocarditis · hypogammaglobulinaemia · malignancy · meningitis · neutropenia · polyomavirus-associated nephropathy · progressive multifocal leukoencephalopathy (PML) · pure red cell aplasia

  SIDE-EFFECTS, FURTHER INFORMATION Cases of pure red cell aplasia have been reported with mycophenolate mofetil; dose reduction or discontinuation should be considered under specialist supervision.
- **CONCEPTION AND CONTRACEPTION**

  Pregnancy prevention The MHRA advises to exclude pregnancy in females of child-bearing potential before treatment—2 pregnancy tests 8–10 days apart are recommended. Women should use at least 1 method of effective contraception before and during treatment, and for 6 weeks after discontinuation—2 methods of effective contraception are preferred. Male patients or their female partner should use effective contraception during treatment and for 90 days after discontinuation.
- **PREGNANCY** Avoid unless no suitable alternative—congenital malformations and spontaneous abortions reported.
- **BREAST FEEDING** Manufacturer advises avoid—present in milk in *animal* studies.
- **RENAL IMPAIRMENT**

  Dose adjustments Manufacturer advises consider dose reduction if estimated glomerular filtration rate less than 25 mL/minute/1.73 m^2.
- **MONITORING REQUIREMENTS** Monitor full blood count every week for 4 weeks then twice a month for 2 months then every month in the first year (consider interrupting treatment if neutropenia develops).
- **PRESCRIBING AND DISPENSING INFORMATION** Tablets and capsules not appropriate for dose titration in children with body surface are less than 1.25 m^2.
- **PATIENT AND CARER ADVICE**

  Pregnancy prevention advice The MHRA advises that prescribers should ensure that female patients understand the need to comply with the pregnancy prevention advice, and they should be informed to seek immediate medical attention if there is a possibility of pregnancy; male patients planning to conceive children should be informed of the implications of both immunosuppression and the effect of the prescribed medications on the pregnancy.

  Bone marrow suppression Patients should be warned to report immediately any signs or symptoms of bone marrow suppression e.g. infection or inexplicable bruising or bleeding.

  Medicines for Children leaflet: Mycophenolate mofetil for nephrotic syndrome www.medicinesforchildren.org.uk/mycophenolate-mofetil-nephrotic-syndrome
- **NATIONAL FUNDING/ACCESS DECISIONS**

  NICE decisions

  - **Immunosuppressive therapy for kidney transplant in children and young people (October 2017)** NICE TA482

    Mycophenolate mofetil, when used as part of an immunosuppressive regimen, is recommended as an initial option to prevent organ rejection in patients having a kidney transplant. Treatment should be started with the least expensive product, but if this is not suitable, an alternative dosage form may be given. The use of mycophenolate mofetil with tacrolimus is outside the terms of the marketing authorisation. If this combination is prescribed, the prescriber should follow relevant professional guidance, taking full responsibility for the decision. Informed consent should be obtained and documented.

    Patients whose treatment was started within the NHS before this guidance was published should have the option to continue treatment, without change to their funding arrangements, until they and their NHS clinician consider it appropriate to stop. www.nice.org.uk/guidance/TA482
- **MEDICINAL FORMS** There can be variation in the licensing of different medicines containing the same drug. Forms available from special-order manufacturers include: oral suspension

Tablet

- Mycophenolate mofetil (Non-proprietary)

  Mycophenolate mofetil 500 mg Mycophenolate mofetil 500mg tablets | 50 tablet PoM £10.44 DT = £6.16
- CellCept (Roche Products Ltd)

  Mycophenolate mofetil 500 mg CellCept 500mg tablets | 50 tablet PoM £82.26 DT = £6.16
- Myfenax (Teva UK Ltd)

  Mycophenolate mofetil 500 mg Myfenax 500mg tablets | 50 tablet PoM £78.15 DT = £6.16

Oral suspension

EXCIPIENTS: May contain Aspartame

- CellCept (Roche Products Ltd)

  Mycophenolate mofetil 200 mg per 1 ml CellCept 1g/5ml oral suspension sugar-free | 175 ml PoM £115.16 DT = £115.16

Capsule

- Mycophenolate mofetil (Non-proprietary)

  Mycophenolate mofetil 250 mg Mycophenolate mofetil 250mg capsules | 100 capsule PoM £33.40 DT = £27.12

- ▸ CellCept (Roche Products Ltd)
  Mycophenolate mofetil 250 mg CellCept 250mg capsules | 100 capsule PoM £82.26 DT = £27.12
- ▸ Myfenax (Teva UK Ltd)
  Mycophenolate mofetil 250 mg Myfenax 250mg capsules | 100 capsule PoM £78.15 DT = £27.12

1.1 Multiple sclerosis

IMMUNOSUPPRESSANTS › IMMUNOMODULATING DRUGS

Fingolimod

23-Mar-2020

● **DRUG ACTION** Fingolimod is a sphingosine-1-phosphate receptor modulator, which prevents movement of lymphocytes out of lymph nodes, thereby limiting inflammation in the central nervous system.

● **INDICATIONS AND DOSE**

Multiple sclerosis (initiated by a specialist)

▸ BY MOUTH

- ▸ Child 10–17 years (body-weight up to 40 kg): 250 micrograms once daily
- ▸ Child 10–17 years (body-weight 40 kg and above): 500 micrograms once daily

IMPORTANT SAFETY INFORMATION

MHRA/CHM ADVICE: FINGOLIMOD—NOT RECOMMENDED FOR PATIENTS AT KNOWN RISK OF CARDIOVASCULAR EVENTS. ADVICE FOR EXTENDED MONITORING FOR THOSE WITH SIGNIFICANT BRADYCARDIA OR HEART BLOCK AFTER THE FIRST DOSE AND FOLLOWING TREATMENT INTERRUPTION (JANUARY 2013)

Fingolimod is known to cause transient bradycardias and heart block after the first dose—see *Cautions*, *Contra-indications*, and *Monitoring* for further information.

MHRA/CHM ADVICE: FINGOLIMOD: NEW CONTRA-INDICATIONS IN RELATION TO CARDIAC RISK (DECEMBER 2017)

Fingolimod can cause persistent bradycardia, which can increase the risk of serious cardiac arrhythmias. New contra-indications have been introduced for patients with pre-existing cardiac disorders—see *Contra-indications* for further information.

MHRA/CHM ADVICE: MULTIPLE SCLEROSIS THERAPIES: SIGNAL OF REBOUND EFFECT AFTER STOPPING OR SWITCHING THERAPY (APRIL 2017)

A signal of rebound syndrome in multiple sclerosis patients whose treatment with fingolimod was stopped or switched to other treatments has been reported in two recently published articles. The MHRA advise to be vigilant for such events and report any suspected adverse effects relating to fingolimod, or other treatments for multiple sclerosis, via the Yellow Card Scheme, while this report is under investigation.

MHRA/CHM ADVICE: FINGOLIMOD: UPDATED ADVICE ABOUT RISK OF CANCERS AND SERIOUS INFECTIONS (DECEMBER 2017)

Fingolimod has an immunosuppressive effect and can increase the risk of skin cancers and lymphoma. Following a recent EU review, the MHRA has recommended the following strengthened warnings:

- re-assess the benefit-risk balance of fingolimod therapy in individual patients, particularly those with additional risk factors for malignancy—either closely monitor for skin cancers or consider discontinuation on a case-by-case basis
- examine all patients for skin lesions before they start fingolimod and then re-examine at least every 6 to 12 months
- advise patients to protect themselves against UV radiation exposure and seek urgent medical advice if they notice any skin lesions
- refer patients with suspicious lesions to a dermatologist

Fingolimod has also been associated with risk of fatal fungal infections and reports of progressive multifocal leukoencephalopathy (PML)—see *Monitoring* and *Side effects* for further information.

MHRA/CHM ADVICE: FINGOLIMOD (*GILENYA*®): INCREASED RISK OF CONGENITAL MALFORMATIONS; NEW CONTRA-INDICATION DURING PREGNANCY AND IN WOMEN OF CHILDBEARING POTENTIAL NOT USING EFFECTIVE CONTRACEPTION (SEPTEMBER 2019)

An increased risk of major congenital malformations, including cardiac, renal, and musculoskeletal defects, has been associated with the use of fingolimod in pregnancy. Females of childbearing potential must use effective contraception during, and for 2 months after stopping, treatment. Healthcare professionals are advised that fingolimod is contra-indicated in pregnancy and that female patients should be informed of the risk of congenital malformations and given a pregnancy-specific patient reminder card. Pregnancy should be excluded before starting treatment, and pregnancy testing repeated at suitable intervals during treatment. Fingolimod should be stopped 2 months before planning a pregnancy. If a female taking fingolimod becomes pregnant, treatment should be stopped immediately, and the patient referred to an obstetrician for close monitoring. Exposed pregnancies should be enrolled on the pregnancy registry.

● **CONTRA-INDICATIONS** Heart failure in the previous 6 months (New York Heart Association class III/IV) · active malignancies · baseline QTc interval 500 milliseconds or greater · cerebrovascular disease (including transient ischaemic attack) in the previous 6 months · decompensated heart failure (requiring inpatient treatment) in the previous 6 months · increased risk for opportunistic infections (including immunosuppression) · myocardial infarction in the previous 6 months · second-degree Mobitz type II atrioventricular block or third-degree AV block, or sick-sinus syndrome, if the patient does not have a pacemaker · severe active infection · severe cardiac arrhythmias requiring treatment with class Ia or class III anti-arrhythmic drugs · unstable angina in the previous 6 months

● **CAUTIONS** Body-weight less than 40 kg (limited information available) · check varicella zoster virus status—consult product literature for further information · children should be brought up-to-date with current immunisation schedule before starting treatment · children under 12 years (limited information available) · chronic obstructive pulmonary disease · history of myocardial infarction · history of symptomatic bradycardia or recurrent syncope · patients receiving anti-arrhythmic or heart-rate lowering drugs, including beta-blockers and heart rate-lowering calcium-channel blockers (seek advice from cardiologist regarding switching to alternative drugs, or appropriate monitoring if unable to switch) · pulmonary fibrosis · severe respiratory disease · severe sleep apnoea · significant QT prolongation (QTc greater than 460 milliseconds in females, or QTc greater than 450 milliseconds in males); if QTc 500 milliseconds or greater—see Contra-indications · susceptibility to QT-interval prolongation (including electrolyte disturbances) · Tanner stage I (limited information available) · uncontrolled hypertension

CAUTIONS, FURTHER INFORMATION

▸ Washout period A washout period is recommended when switching treatment from some disease modifying therapies—consult product literature for further information.

▸ Bradycardia and cardiac rhythm disturbance Fingolimod may cause transient bradycardia, atrioventricular conduction delays and heart block after the first dose. Fingolimod is not recommended in patients with the cardiovascular risks listed above unless the anticipated benefits outweigh the potential risks, and advice from a cardiologist (including monitoring advice) is sought before initiation.

- INTERACTIONS → Appendix 1: fingolimod
- SIDE-EFFECTS
▸ **Common or very common** Alopecia · arthralgia · asthenia · atrioventricular block · back pain · bradycardia · cough · decreased leucocytes · depression · diarrhoea · dizziness · dyspnoea · headaches · hypertension · increased risk of infection · myalgia · neoplasms · skin reactions · vision blurred · weight decreased
▸ **Uncommon** Macular oedema · nausea · seizures · thrombocytopenia
▸ **Rare or very rare** Posterior reversible encephalopathy syndrome (PRES)
▸ **Frequency not known** Anxiety · autoimmune haemolytic anaemia · haemophagocytic lymphohistiocytosis · peripheral oedema · progressive multifocal leukoencephalopathy (PML)

SIDE-EFFECTS, FURTHER INFORMATION **Basal-cell carcinoma** Patients should be advised to seek medical advice if they have any signs of basal-cell carcinoma including skin nodules, patches or open sores that do not heal within weeks.

Progressive multifocal leukoencephalopathy (PML) and other opportunistic infections Patients should be advised to seek medical attention if they have any signs of PML or any other infections. Suspension of treatment should be considered if a patient develops a severe infection, taking into consideration the risk-benefit.

- CONCEPTION AND CONTRACEPTION Manufacturer advises females of childbearing potential should use effective contraception during treatment and for 2 months after last treatment—see *Important safety information* for further information.
- PREGNANCY Manufacturer advises avoid—teratogenic.
- BREAST FEEDING Avoid.
- HEPATIC IMPAIRMENT Manufacturer advises caution when initiating treatment in mild to moderate impairment; avoid in severe impairment.
- MONITORING REQUIREMENTS

▸ **All** patients receiving fingolimod should be monitored at treatment initiation, (first dose monitoring—before, during and after dose), and after treatment interruption (see note below); monitoring should include:
▸ **Pre-treatment**
  - an ECG and blood pressure measurement before starting
▸ **During the first 6 hours of treatment**
  - continuous ECG monitoring for 6 hours
  - blood pressure and heart rate measurement every hour
▸ **After 6 hours of treatment**
  - a further ECG and blood pressure measurement
▸ If heart rate at the end of the 6 hour period is at its lowest since fingolimod was first administered, monitoring should be extended by at least 2 hours and until heart rate increases.
▸ If post-dose bradyarrhythmia-related symptoms occur, appropriate clinical management should be initiated and monitoring should be continued until the symptoms have resolved. If pharmacological intervention is required during the first-dose monitoring, overnight monitoring should follow, and the first-dose monitoring should then be repeated after the second dose.
▸ If after 6 hours, the heart rate is less than 55 beats per minute in children aged 12 years and above, or less than 60 beats per minute in children under 12 years, or the ECG shows new onset second degree or higher grade AV block, or a QTc interval of 500 milliseconds or greater, monitoring should be extended (at least overnight, until side-effect resolution).
▸ The occurrence at any time of third degree AV block requires extended monitoring (at least overnight, until side-effect resolution).
▸ In case of T-wave inversion, ensure there are no associated signs or symptoms of myocardial ischaemia—if suspected seek advice from a cardiologist.
▸ **Note**
▸ First dose monitoring as above **should be repeated** in all patients whose treatment is interrupted for:
  - 1 day or more during the first 2 weeks of treatment
  - more than 7 days during weeks 3 and 4 of treatment
  - more than 2 weeks after one month of treatment
▸ If the treatment interruption is of shorter duration than the above, treatment should be continued with the next dose as planned.
▸ Manufacturer advises eye examination recommended 3–4 months after initiation of treatment (and before initiation of treatment in patients with diabetes or history of uveitis).
▸ Manufacturer advises skin examination for skin lesions before starting treatment and then every 6 to 12 months thereafter or as clinically indicated.
▸ Monitor hepatic transaminases before treatment, then every 3 months for 1 year, then periodically thereafter.
▸ Monitor full blood count before treatment, at 3 months, then at least yearly thereafter and if signs of infection (interrupt treatment if lymphocyte count reduced)—consult product literature.
▸ Monitor for signs and symptoms of haemophagocytic syndrome (including pyrexia, asthenia, hepato-splenomegaly and adenopathy—may be associated with hepatic failure and respiratory distress; also progressive cytopenia, elevated serum-ferritin concentrations, hypertriglyceridaemia, hypofibrinogenaemia, coagulopathy, hepatic cytolysis, hyponatraemia)—initiate treatment immediately.
▸ Manufacturer advises to monitor routine MRI for lesions suggestive of progressive multifocal leukoencephalopathy (PML), particularly in patients considered at increased risk; monitor for signs and symptoms of new neurological dysfunction.

- PRESCRIBING AND DISPENSING INFORMATION The manufacturer of *Gilenya®* has provided a *Prescriber's checklist*.
- PATIENT AND CARER ADVICE

Patient reminder card Patients should be given a patient reminder card.
Female patients of childbearing potential should also be given a pregnancy-specific patient reminder card.

- NATIONAL FUNDING/ACCESS DECISIONS

Scottish Medicines Consortium (SMC) decisions
The *Scottish Medicines Consortium* has advised (September 2012) that fingolimod (*Gilenya®*) is accepted for restricted use within NHS Scotland as single disease-modifying therapy in highly active relapsing-remitting multiple sclerosis despite treatment with interferon beta, with an unchanged or increased relapse rate or ongoing severe relapses, as compared to the previous year. This advice is contingent upon the continuing availability of the patient access scheme in NHS Scotland.
SMC No. SMC2154

The *Scottish Medicines Consortium* has advised (June 2019) that fingolimod (*Gilenya®*) is accepted for use within NHS Scotland as a single disease-modifying therapy in highly active relapsing-remitting multiple sclerosis for patients aged 10 years to less than 18 years with:
- highly active disease despite a full and adequate course of treatment with at least one disease-modifying therapy, **or**

- rapidly-evolving severe relapsing-remitting multiple sclerosis defined by two or more disabling relapses in one year, and with one or more gadolinium-enhancing lesions on brain MRI or a significant increase in T2 lesion load as compared to a previous MRI.

This advice is contingent upon the continuing availability of the patient access scheme in NHS Scotland, or a list price that is equivalent or lower.

All Wales Medicines Strategy Group (AWMSG) decisions
The *All Wales Medicines Strategy Group* has advised (January 2017) that fingolimod (*Gilenya*®) is recommended as an option for use within NHS Wales as a single disease-modifying therapy in highly active relapsing-remitting multiple sclerosis only in patients with rapidly-evolving severe relapsing-remitting multiple sclerosis defined by 2 or more disabling relapses in 1 year and with 1 or more gadolinium-enhancing lesions on brain magnetic resonance imaging (MRI) or a significant increase in T2 lesion load compared with a previous recent MRI, only if the manufacturer provides fingolimod with the discount agreed as part of the patient access scheme or where the list price is equivalent or lower.
AWMSG No. 2777

The *All Wales Medicines Strategy Group* has advised (June 2019) that fingolimod (*Gilenya*®) is recommended as an option for use within NHS Wales as a single disease-modifying therapy in highly active relapsing-remitting multiple sclerosis for patients aged 10 to 17 years with:

- highly active disease despite a full and adequate course of treatment with at least one disease modifying therapy, **or**
- rapidly-evolving severe relapsing-remitting multiple sclerosis defined by two or more disabling relapses in one year, and with one or more gadolinium-enhancing lesions on brain MRI or a significant increase in T2 lesion load as compared to a previous recent MRI.

This recommendation applies only in circumstances where the approved Patient Access Scheme (PAS) is utilised or where the list/contract price is equivalent or lower than the PAS price.

NHS restrictions
NHS England Clinical Commissioning Policy NHS England (May 2014) has provided guidance on the use of fingolimod for the treatment of multiple sclerosis in England. An NHS England Clinical Commissioning Policy outlines the funding arrangements and the criteria for initiating and discontinuing this treatment option, see www.england.nhs.uk/commissioning/spec-services/npc-crg/group-d/d04/.

- **MEDICINAL FORMS** There can be variation in the licensing of different medicines containing the same drug.

Capsule

▸ Gilenya (Novartis Pharmaceuticals UK Ltd) ▼
Fingolimod (as Fingolimod hydrochloride)
250 microgram Gilenya 0.25mg capsules | 28 capsule PoM £1,470.00
Fingolimod (as Fingolimod hydrochloride)
500 microgram Gilenya 0.5mg capsules | 7 capsule PoM £367.50 | 28 capsule PoM £1,470.00 DT = £1,470.00

8 Immune system and malignant disease

Malignant disease

1 Antibody responsive malignancy

ANTINEOPLASTIC DRUGS > MONOCLONAL ANTIBODIES

Blinatumomab

26-Feb-2020

- **DRUG ACTION** The anti-lymphocyte monoclonal antibodies cause lysis of B lymphocytes.

- **INDICATIONS AND DOSE**

Relapsed or refractory Philadelphia chromosome-negative acute lymphoblastic leukaemia (initiated by a specialist)
▸ BY CONTINUOUS INTRAVENOUS INFUSION
▸ Child 1-17 years: (consult product literature)

- **CAUTIONS** Aphasia · brain injuries (severe) · cerebellar disease · dementia · elderly—limited information available · epilepsy · paresis · Parkinson's disease · patients may need pre-medication to minimise adverse reactions · psychosis · seizure · severe hepatic impairment · severe renal impairment · stroke

CAUTIONS, FURTHER INFORMATION
▸ Pre-medication Manufacturer advises pre-medication with a corticosteroid and an anti-pyretic—consult product literature.
▸ Neurological events There is potentially a higher risk of neurological events in patients with clinically relevant CNS pathology—manufacturer advises caution.

- **INTERACTIONS** → Appendix 1: monoclonal antibodies
- **SIDE-EFFECTS**

▸ **Common or very common** Abdominal pain · anaemia · aphasia · appetite decreased · arthralgia · chest pain · chills · cognitive disorder · confusion · constipation · cough · decreased leucocytes · diarrhoea · dizziness · dyspnoea · electrolyte imbalance · encephalopathy · facial swelling · fatigue · fever · flushing · headache · hyperglycaemia · hypersensitivity · hypertension · hypoalbuminaemia · hypotension · immune disorder · increased risk of infection · infusion related reaction · insomnia · leucocytosis · memory loss · nausea · neutropenia · oedema · pain · paraesthesia · rash · respiratory disorders · seizure · sepsis · tachycardia · thrombocytopenia · tremor · tumour lysis syndrome · vomiting · weight increased
▸ **Uncommon** Capillary leak syndrome · cranial nerve disorder · pancreatitis
▸ **Frequency not known** Device related infection · hypoxia · multi organ failure

SIDE-EFFECTS, FURTHER INFORMATION **Pancreatitis** Life-threatening or fatal cases of pancreatitis have been reported; manufacturer advises monitor for signs and symptoms of pancreatitis during treatment—temporary interruption or discontinuation may be required (consult product literature).

Cytokine release syndrome, infusion-reactions and tumour lysis syndrome Life-threatening (including fatal) cases of cytokine release syndrome and tumour lysis syndrome have been reported in patients taking blinatumomab. Manufacturer advises monitor signs and symptoms of cytokine release syndrome and infusion reactions during treatment; temporary interruption or discontinuation may be required—consult product literature.

- **CONCEPTION AND CONTRACEPTION** Manufacturer advises effective contraception during treatment and for at least 48 hours after treatment in women of child-bearing potential. See also Pregnancy and reproductive function in Cytotoxic drugs p. 575.
- **PREGNANCY** Manufacturer advises avoid unless potential benefit outweighs risk—no information available; if exposed during pregnancy, monitor infant for B-cell depletion. See also Pregnancy and reproductive function in Cytotoxic drugs p. 575.
- **BREAST FEEDING** Manufacturer advises avoid during and for at least 48 hours after treatment—no information available.
- **HEPATIC IMPAIRMENT** Manufacturer advises caution in severe impairment (no information available).
- **RENAL IMPAIRMENT** Manufacturer advises caution in severe impairment—no information available.
- **MONITORING REQUIREMENTS** Manufacturer advises neurological examination prior to the initiation of treatment and continued monitoring during treatment—consult product literature.
- **HANDLING AND STORAGE** Manufacturer advises store in a refrigerator (2–8°C); consult product literature for storage conditions after reconstitution and dilution.
- **PATIENT AND CARER ADVICE** A patient alert card should be provided. Educational materials should be provided to patients, carers and healthcare professionals to ensure blinatumomab is used in a safe and effective way, and to prevent the risk of medication errors and neurological events—consult product information.

  Driving and skilled tasks Manufacturer advises patients and carers should be counselled about the effects on driving and performance of skilled tasks—increased risk of confusion, disorientation, co-ordination and balance disorders, seizures and disturbances in consciousness.
- **NATIONAL FUNDING/ACCESS DECISIONS**

  Scottish Medicines Consortium (SMC) decisions

  SMC No. SMC2148

  The *Scottish Medicines Consortium* has advised (April 2019) that blinatumomab (*Blincyto*®) is accepted for use within NHS Scotland as monotherapy for the treatment of paediatric patients aged 1 year or older with Philadelphia chromosome-negative CD19 positive B-cell precursor acute lymphoblastic leukaemia which is refractory or in relapse after receiving at least two prior therapies or in relapse after receiving prior allogeneic hematopoietic stem cell transplantation. This advice is contingent upon the continuing availability of the patient access scheme in NHS Scotland or a list price that is equivalent or lower.

  All Wales Medicines Strategy Group (AWMSG) decisions

  AWMSG No. 3769

  The *All Wales Medicines Strategy Group* has advised (April 2019) that blinatumomab (*Blincyto*®) is recommended as an option for use within NHS Wales as monotherapy for the treatment of paediatric patients aged 1 year or older with Philadelphia chromosome-negative CD19 positive B-cell precursor acute lymphoblastic leukaemia which is refractory or in relapse after receiving at least two prior therapies or in relapse after receiving prior allogeneic haematopoietic stem cell transplantation. This recommendation applies only in circumstances where the approved Patient Access Scheme (PAS) is utilised or where the list/contract price is equivalent or lower than the PAS price.
- **MEDICINAL FORMS** There can be variation in the licensing of different medicines containing the same drug.

  Powder for solution for infusion

  EXCIPIENTS: May contain Polysorbates

  ▸ Blincyto (Amgen Ltd) ▼

  Blinatumomab 38.5 microgram Blincyto 38.5micrograms powder for concentrate and solution for solution for infusion vials | 1 vial PoM £2,017.00

Dinutuximab beta

10-Sep-2018

- **DRUG ACTION** Dinutuximab beta is a chimeric monoclonal antibody; it specifically targets the carbohydrate moiety of disialoganglioside 2, which is overexpressed on neuroblastoma cells.

- **INDICATIONS AND DOSE**

  High-risk neuroblastoma (specialist use only)

  ▸ BY INTRAVENOUS INFUSION

  ▸ Child 1–17 years: (consult product literature)

- **CONTRA-INDICATIONS** Acute grade 3 or 4, or extensive chronic graft-versus-host disease
- **CAUTIONS** Avoid vaccinations during and for at least 10 weeks after treatment cessation (increased risk of immune stimulation and neurological toxicity) · ensure absence of systemic infection—any other infection should be controlled before treatment initiation · pre-medication must be administered to minimise the risk of infusion-related reactions and neuropathic pain

  CAUTIONS, FURTHER INFORMATION

  ▸ Pre-medication Severe infusion-related reactions can occur and dinutuximab beta should only be administered when appropriately trained staff and resuscitation facilities are immediately available; manufacturer advises pre-medication with an antihistamine, and to monitor closely, particularly during the first and second treatment course; discontinue immediately if reaction occurs and treat as indicated—consult product literature.

  Manufacturer advises pre-medication with non-opioid analgesics, gabapentin and opioids—consult product literature.
- **INTERACTIONS** → Appendix 1: monoclonal antibodies
- **SIDE-EFFECTS**

  ▸ **Common or very common** Abdominal distension · anaemia · anxiety · appetite decreased · ascites · capillary leak syndrome · chills · cough · cytokine release syndrome · decreased leucocytes · device related infection · dizziness · dyspnoea · electrolyte imbalance · eye disorders · eye inflammation · fever · fluid imbalance · gastrointestinal disorders · haematuria · headache · heart failure · hyperhidrosis · hypersensitivity · hypertension · hypertriglyceridaemia · hypoalbuminaemia · hypotension · hypoxia · increased risk of infection · left ventricular dysfunction · muscle spasms · nausea · neutropenia · oedema · oral disorders · pain · paraesthesia · pericardial effusion · peripheral neuropathy · photosensitivity reaction · pulmonary oedema · renal impairment · respiratory disorders · seizure · sepsis · skin reactions · tachycardia · thrombocytopenia · tremor · urinary retention · urine abnormalities · vision disorders · vomiting · weight changes

  ▸ **Uncommon** Disseminated intravascular coagulation · eosinophilia · hepatocellular injury · hypovolaemic shock · intracranial pressure increased · peripheral vascular disease · posterior reversible encephalopathy syndrome (PRES)
- **CONCEPTION AND CONTRACEPTION** Manufacturer advises women of childbearing potential should use contraception during and for 6 months after stopping treatment. See also *Pregnancy and reproductive function* in Cytotoxic drugs p. 575.

- **PREGNANCY** Manufacturer advises avoid—no information available. See also *Pregnancy and reproductive function* in Cytotoxic drugs p. 575.
- **BREAST FEEDING** Manufacturer advises avoid during treatment and for 6 months after the last dose—no information available.
- **MONITORING REQUIREMENTS**
- ▸ Manufacturer advises pre-treatment evaluation of pulse oximetry, bone marrow function, liver function and renal function—consult product literature for values required for treatment initiation.
- ▸ Manufacturer advises monitor circulatory and respiratory function—risk of capillary leak syndrome.
- ▸ Manufacturer advises monitor liver function and electrolytes regularly.
- **HANDLING AND STORAGE** Manufacturer advises store in a refrigerator (2–8°C)—consult product literature for further information regarding storage conditions outside refrigerator and after preparation of the infusion.
- **PATIENT AND CARER ADVICE**

Driving and skilled tasks Manufacturer advises patients should not use or drive machines during treatment.

- **NATIONAL FUNDING/ACCESS DECISIONS**

NICE decisions

▸ **Dinutuximab beta for treating neuroblastoma (August 2018)**
NICE TA538

Dinutuximab beta (*Qarziba*®) is recommended as an option for treating high-risk neuroblastoma in people aged 12 months and over whose disease has at least partially responded to induction chemotherapy, followed by myeloablative therapy and stem cell transplant, only if:
- they have not already had anti-GD2 immunotherapy, **and**
- the manufacturer provides dinutuximab beta according to the commercial arrangement.

Patients whose treatment was started within the NHS before this guidance was published should have the option to continue treatment, without change to their funding arrangements, until they and their NHS clinician consider it appropriate to stop. www.nice.org.uk/guidance/ta538

Scottish Medicines Consortium (SMC) decisions

SMC No. SMC2105

The *Scottish Medicines Consortium* has advised (November 2018) that dinutuximab beta (*Qarziba*®) is accepted for use within NHS Scotland for the treatment of high-risk neuroblastoma in patients aged 12 months and over whose disease has at least partially responded to induction chemotherapy, followed by myeloablative therapy and stem cell transplantation, as well as patients with a history of relapsed or refractory neuroblastoma, with or without residual disease.

In patients with a history of relapsed or refractory disease and in patients who have not achieved a complete response after first line therapy, dinutuximab beta should be combined with interleukin-2.

This advice is contingent upon the continuing availability of the patient access scheme in NHS Scotland or a list price that is equivalent or lower.

- **MEDICINAL FORMS** There can be variation in the licensing of different medicines containing the same drug.

Solution for infusion

▸ Qarziba (EUSA Pharma Ltd) ▼
Dinutuximab beta 4.5 mg per 1 ml Qarziba 20mg/4.5ml concentrate for solution for infusion vials | 1 vial PoM £7,610.00 (Hospital only)

Gemtuzumab ozogamicin

17-Oct-2018

- **DRUG ACTION** Gemtuzumab ozogamicin is a monoclonal antibody that binds to CD33-expressing tumour cells to induce cell cycle arrest and apoptotic cell death.
- **INDICATIONS AND DOSE**

CD33-positive acute myeloid leukaemia (specialist use only)

▸ BY INTRAVENOUS INFUSION
▸ Child 15–17 years: (consult product literature)

- **CAUTIONS** Adverse-risk cytogenetics (consider benefits and risks of treatment, consult product literature) · haematopoietic stem cell transplantation (increased risk of hepatotoxicity) · pre-medication recommended to minimise adverse reactions

CAUTIONS, FURTHER INFORMATION

▸ Pre-medication Serious infusion-related reactions can occur and gemtuzumab ozogamicin should only be administered when appropriately trained staff and resuscitation facilities are immediately available; manufacturer advises pre-medication with a corticosteroid, paracetamol and antihistamine 1 hour prior to dosing, and to take appropriate measures to help prevent the development of tumour lysis-related hyperuricaemia—consult product literature.

- **SIDE-EFFECTS**

▸ **Common or very common** Anaemia · appetite decreased · ascites · chills · constipation · decreased leucocytes · diarrhoea · dyspnoea · fatigue · fever · gastrointestinal discomfort · gastrointestinal disorders · haemorrhage · headache · hepatic disorders · hyperbilirubinaemia · hyperglycaemia · hypertension · hypotension · infection · infusion related reaction (including fatal cases) · multi organ failure · nausea · neutropenia · oedema · pancytopenia · sinusoidal obstruction syndrome · skin reactions · stomatitis · tachycardia · thrombocytopenia · tumour lysis syndrome (including fatal cases) · vomiting

▸ **Frequency not known** Interstitial pneumonia

SIDE-EFFECTS, FURTHER INFORMATION Infusion-related reactions (including fatal cases) can occur during the first 24 hours after administration. Manufacturer advises interrupt treatment immediately and treat as clinically indicated (consult product literature); permanent discontinuation should be strongly considered in patients who develop signs and symptoms of anaphylaxis.

- **CONCEPTION AND CONTRACEPTION** Manufacturer advises women of childbearing potential should use 2 methods of effective contraception during treatment and for at least 7 months after the last dose; male patients should use 2 methods of effective contraception during treatment and for at least 4 months after the last dose if their partner is of childbearing potential. See also Pregnancy and reproductive function in Cytotoxic drugs p. 575.
- **PREGNANCY** Manufacturer advises avoid unless potential benefit outweighs risk—toxicity in *animal* studies. See also Pregnancy and reproductive function in Cytotoxic drugs p. 575.
- **BREAST FEEDING** Manufacturer advises avoid during treatment and for at least one month after the last dose—no information available.
- **HEPATIC IMPAIRMENT** Manufacturer advises caution in moderate-to-severe impairment—increased risk of developing hepatotoxicity; postpone treatment if serum transaminases (ALT or AST) greater than 2.5 times the upper limit of normal or total bilirubin greater than 2 times the upper limit of normal.
- **MONITORING REQUIREMENTS**
- ▸ Manufacturer advises monitor complete blood counts prior to each dose as well as signs and symptoms of infection,

bleeding and other effects of myelosuppression during treatment; dose interruption or discontinuation of treatment may be required—consult product literature.
- Manufacturer advises monitor for signs and symptoms of infusion-related reactions—close clinical monitoring, including pulse, blood pressure and temperature, should be performed during infusion; monitor for signs and symptoms of tumour lysis syndrome.
- Manufacturer advises monitor for signs and symptoms of hepatotoxicity (including hepatic veno-occlusive disease); liver tests should be monitored prior to each dose—consult product literature.

- **PRESCRIBING AND DISPENSING INFORMATION** Gemtuzumab ozogamicin is a biological medicine. Biological medicines must be prescribed and dispensed by brand name, see *Biological medicines* and *Biosimilar medicines*, under Guidance on prescribing p. 1.
- **HANDLING AND STORAGE** Manufacturer advises store in a refrigerator (2–8°C) and protect from light—consult product literature for storage conditions after reconstitution and dilution.
- **PATIENT AND CARER ADVICE**

Driving and skilled tasks Manufacturer advises patients and carers should be counselled on the effects on driving and performance of skilled tasks—increased risk of fatigue and headache.

- **NATIONAL FUNDING/ACCESS DECISIONS**

NICE decisions

- **Gemtuzumab ozogamicin for untreated acute myeloid leukaemia (November 2018) NICE TA545**

Gemtuzumab ozogamicin (*Mylotarg*®), with daunorubicin and cytarabine, is recommended as an option for untreated *de novo* CD33-positive acute myeloid leukaemia (AML), except acute promyelocytic leukaemia, in people 15 years and over, only if:

- they start induction therapy when either the cytogenetic test confirms that the disease has favourable, intermediate or unknown cytogenetics (that is, because the test was unsuccessful) or when their cytogenetic test results are not yet available, **and**
- they start consolidation therapy when their cytogenetic test confirms that the disease has favourable, intermediate or unknown cytogenetics (because the test was unsuccessful), **and**
- the manufacturer provides gemtuzumab ozogamicin according to the commercial arrangement.

Patients whose treatment was started within the NHS before this guidance was published should have the option to continue treatment, without change to their funding arrangements, until they and their NHS clinician consider it appropriate to stop. www.nice.org.uk/guidance/ta545

Scottish Medicines Consortium (SMC) decisions

SMC No. SMC2089

The *Scottish Medicines Consortium* has advised (October 2018) that gemtuzumab ozogamicin (*Mylotarg*®) is accepted for restricted use within NHS Scotland as combination therapy with daunorubicin and cytarabine for the treatment of previously untreated, *de novo* CD33-positive acute myeloid leukaemia in patients aged 15 years and above with a favourable, intermediate or unknown cytogenetic profile.

- **MEDICINAL FORMS** There can be variation in the licensing of different medicines containing the same drug.

Powder for solution for infusion

- Mylotarg (Pfizer Ltd) ▼

Gemtuzumab ozogamicin 5 mg Mylotarg 5mg powder for concentrate for solution for infusion vials | 1 vial PoM £6,300.00 (Hospital only)

Ipilimumab

13-Feb-2019

- **DRUG ACTION** Ipilimumab is a monoclonal antibody which causes T-cell activation resulting in tumour cell death.
- **INDICATIONS AND DOSE**

Melanoma (as monotherapy) (specialist use only)

- BY INTRAVENOUS INFUSION
- Child 12–17 years: 3 mg/kg every 3 weeks for 4 doses, for dose interruption or discontinuation of treatment due to immune-related side-effects—consult product literature

IMPORTANT SAFETY INFORMATION

MHRA/CHM ADVICE: IPILIMUMAB (*YERVOY*®): REPORTS OF CYTOMEGALOVIRUS (CMV) GASTROINTESTINAL INFECTION OR REACTIVATION (JANUARY 2019)

There have been post-marketing cases of gastrointestinal CMV infection or reactivation in ipilimumab-treated patients reported to have corticosteroid-refractory immune-related colitis, including fatal cases.

Patients should be advised to contact their healthcare professional immediately at the onset of symptoms of colitis. Possible causes, including infections, should be investigated; a stool infection work-up should be performed and patients screened for CMV. For patients with corticosteroid-refractory immune-related colitis, use of an additional immunosuppressive agent should only be considered if other causes are excluded using viral PCR on biopsy, and eliminating other viral, bacterial, and parasitic causes.

- **CAUTIONS** For full details consult product literature.
- **INTERACTIONS** → Appendix 1: monoclonal antibodies
- **SIDE-EFFECTS**
- **Common or very common** Alopecia · anaemia · appetite decreased · arthralgia · asthenia · cancer pain · chills · confusion · constipation · cough · dehydration · diarrhoea · dizziness · dyspnoea · electrolyte imbalance · eye discomfort · fever · gastrointestinal discomfort · gastrointestinal disorders · haemorrhage · headache · hepatic disorders · hypophysitis · hypopituitarism · hypotension · hypothyroidism · influenza like illness · lethargy · lymphopenia · mucositis · muscle complaints · nausea · nerve disorders · night sweats · oedema · pain · skin reactions · vasodilation · vision disorders · vomiting · weight decreased
- **Uncommon** Adrenal hypofunction · alkalosis · allergic rhinitis · amenorrhoea · arrhythmias · arthritis · brain oedema · depression · dysarthria · eosinophilia · eye inflammation · glomerulonephritis · haemolytic anaemia · hair colour changes · hypersensitivity · hyperthyroidism · hypogonadism · increased risk of infection · infusion related reaction · libido decreased · meningitis · movement disorders · multi organ failure · muscle weakness · myopathy · nephritis autoimmune · neutropenia · pancreatitis · paraneoplastic syndrome · peripheral ischaemia · polymyalgia rheumatica · psychiatric disorder · pulmonary oedema · renal failure · renal tubular acidosis · respiratory disorders · sepsis · severe cutaneous adverse reactions (SCARs) · syncope · systemic inflammatory response syndrome · thrombocytopenia · tremor · tumour lysis syndrome · vascular disorders · vasculitis
- **Rare or very rare** Myasthenia gravis · proteinuria · thyroiditis
- **Frequency not known** Cytomegalovirus infection reactivation

SIDE-EFFECTS, FURTHER INFORMATION A corticosteroid can be used after starting ipilimumab, to treat immune-related reactions.

- **CONCEPTION AND CONTRACEPTION** Use effective contraception.
- **PREGNANCY** Manufacturer advises avoid unless potential benefit outweighs risk—toxicity in *animal* studies.
- **BREAST FEEDING** Manufacturer advises avoid—present in milk in *animal* studies.
- **HEPATIC IMPAIRMENT** Manufacturer advises caution if bilirubin greater than 3 times upper limit of normal range or if transaminases equal to or greater than 5 times upper limit of normal range (limited information available).
- **MONITORING REQUIREMENTS**
  - Manufacturer advises monitor liver function tests and thyroid function prior to initiation of treatment and before each dose.
  - Manufacturer advises monitor for signs or symptoms of immune-related side-effects and gastrointestinal perforation—consult product literature.
- **DIRECTIONS FOR ADMINISTRATION** Manufacturer advises for *intravenous infusion*, give undiluted or dilute to a concentration of 1–4 mg/mL with Glucose 5% *or* Sodium Chloride 0.9%; give over 90 minutes.
- **PRESCRIBING AND DISPENSING INFORMATION** Infusion-related side-effects have been reported; premedication with paracetamol and an antihistamine is recommended.
- **HANDLING AND STORAGE** Manufacturer advises store in a refrigerator (2–8 °C) and protect from light—consult product literature for further information regarding storage conditions outside refrigerator and after preparation of the infusion.
- **NATIONAL FUNDING/ACCESS DECISIONS**

Scottish Medicines Consortium (SMC) decisions

SMC No. SMC2094

The *Scottish Medicines Consortium* has advised (October 2018) that ipilimumab (*Yervoy*®) is accepted for use within NHS Scotland as monotherapy for the treatment of advanced (unresectable or metastatic) melanoma in adolescents 12 years of age and older. This advice is contingent upon the continuing availability of the patient access scheme in NHS Scotland or a list price that is equivalent or lower.

All Wales Medicines Strategy Group (AWMSG) decisions

AWMSG No. 3604

The *All Wales Medicines Strategy Group* has advised (November 2018) that ipilimumab (*Yervoy*®) is recommended as an option for use within NHS Wales as monotherapy for the treatment of advanced (unresectable or metastatic) melanoma in adolescents 12 to 17 years of age. This recommendation applies only in circumstances where the approved Wales Patient Access Scheme (WPAS) is utilised or where the list/contract price is equivalent or lower than the WPAS price.

- **MEDICINAL FORMS** There can be variation in the licensing of different medicines containing the same drug.

Solution for infusion

ELECTROLYTES: May contain Sodium

- Yervoy (Bristol-Myers Squibb Pharmaceuticals Ltd)

  Ipilimumab 5 mg per 1 ml Yervoy 50mg/10ml concentrate for solution for infusion vials | 1 vial PoM £3,750.00 (Hospital only) Yervoy 200mg/40ml concentrate for solution for infusion vials | 1 vial PoM £15,000.00 (Hospital only)

IMMUNOSUPPRESSANTS > MONOCLONAL ANTIBODIES > ANTI-LYMPHOCYTE

Anti-lymphocyte monoclonal antibodies

- **DRUG ACTION** The anti-lymphocyte monoclonal antibodies cause lysis of B lymphocytes.

> **IMPORTANT SAFETY INFORMATION**
> All anti-lymphocyte monoclonal antibodies should be given under the supervision of an experienced specialist, in an environment where full resuscitation facilities are immediately available.

- **SIDE-EFFECTS**
  - **Common or very common** Alopecia · anaemia · anaphylactic reaction · arthralgia · asthenia · conjunctivitis · constipation · cough · depression · diarrhoea · fever · headache · hypersensitivity (discontinue permanently) · increased risk of infection · infusion related reaction · leucopenia · myocardial infarction · neutropenia · night sweats · pain · thrombocytopenia · vomiting
  - **Uncommon** Haemolytic anaemia · progressive multifocal leukoencephalopathy (PML)
  - **Rare or very rare** Hepatitis B reactivation

  SIDE-EFFECTS, FURTHER INFORMATION **Infusion-related side-effects** In rare cases infusion reactions may be fatal. Infusion-related side-effects occur predominantly during the first infusion. Patients should receive premedication before administration of anti-lymphocyte monoclonal antibodies to reduce these effects—consult product literature for details of individual regimens. The infusion may have to be stopped temporarily and the infusion-related effects treated—consult product literature for appropriate management.

  Cytokine release syndrome Fatalities following severe cytokine release syndrome (characterised by severe dyspnoea) and associated with features of tumour lysis syndrome have occurred after infusions of anti-lymphocyte monoclonal antibodies. Patients with a high tumour burden as well as those with pulmonary insufficiency or infiltration are at increased risk and should be monitored very closely (and a slower rate of infusion considered).
- **PRE-TREATMENT SCREENING** All patients should be screened for hepatitis B before treatment.

above

Rituximab

26-Apr-2019

- **INDICATIONS AND DOSE**

Post-transplantation lymphoproliferative disease (under expert supervision) | Non-Hodgkin's lymphoma (under expert supervision) | Hodgkin's lymphoma (under expert supervision) | Severe cases of resistant immune modulated disease including idiopathic thrombocytopenia purpura, haemolytic anaemia, and systemic lupus erythematosus (under expert supervision)

- BY INTRAVENOUS INFUSION
  - Child: Patients should receive premedication before each dose (consult product literature for details) (consult local protocol)

- **UNLICENSED USE** Not licensed for use in children.
- **CAUTIONS** History of cardiovascular disease; in adults exacerbation of angina, arrhythmia, and heart failure have been reported · transient hypotension occurs frequently during infusion (anti-hypertensives may need to be withheld for 12 hours before infusion)

CAUTIONS, FURTHER INFORMATION For full details on cautions, consult product literature or local treatment protocol.

▸ Hepatitis B infection and reactivation Hepatitis B infection and reactivation (including fatal cases) have been reported in patients taking **rituximab**. Patients with positive hepatitis B serology should be referred to a liver specialist for monitoring and initiation of antiviral therapy before treatment initiation; treatment should not be initiated in patients with evidence of current hepatitis B infection until the infection has been adequately treated. Patients should be closely monitored for clinical and laboratory signs of active hepatitis B infection during treatment and for up to a year following the last infusion (consult product literature).

- INTERACTIONS → Appendix 1: monoclonal antibodies
- SIDE-EFFECTS
  - ▸ **Common or very common** Angioedema · anxiety · appetite decreased · arrhythmias · bone marrow disorders · bursitis · cancer pain · cardiac disorder · chest pain · chills · dizziness · dysphagia · dyspnoea · ear pain · electrolyte imbalance · gastrointestinal discomfort · gastrointestinal disorders · hepatitis B · hypercholesterolaemia · hyperglycaemia · hyperhidrosis · hypertension · hypotension · insomnia · lacrimation disorder · malaise · migraine · multi organ failure · muscle complaints · muscle tone increased · nausea · nerve disorders · oedema · oral disorders · osteoarthritis · respiratory disorders · sensation abnormal · sepsis · skin reactions · throat irritation · tinnitus · vasodilation · weight decreased
  - ▸ **Uncommon** Asthma · coagulation disorder · heart failure · hypoxia · ischaemic heart disease · lymphadenopathy · taste altered
  - ▸ **Rare or very rare** Cytokine release syndrome · facial paralysis · renal failure · Stevens-Johnson syndrome (discontinue) · toxic epidermal necrolysis (discontinue) · tumour lysis syndrome · vasculitis · vision disorders
  - ▸ **Frequency not known** Epistaxis · hearing loss · hypogammaglobulinaemia · infective thrombosis · influenza like illness · irritability · muscle weakness · nasal congestion · posterior reversible encephalopathy syndrome (PRES) · psychiatric disorder · seizure · skin papilloma · tremor

  SIDE-EFFECTS, FURTHER INFORMATION Associated with infections, sometimes severe, including tuberculosis, septicaemia, and hepatitis B reactivation.

  Progressive multifocal leucoencephalopathy has been reported in association with rituximab; patients should be monitored for cognitive, neurological, or psychiatric signs and symptoms. If progressive multifocal leucoencephalopathy is suspected, suspend treatment until it has been excluded.
- CONCEPTION AND CONTRACEPTION Effective contraception (in both sexes) required during and for 12 months after treatment.
- PREGNANCY Avoid unless potential benefit to mother outweighs risk of B-lymphocyte depletion in fetus.
- BREAST FEEDING Avoid breast-feeding during and for 12 months after treatment.
- MONITORING REQUIREMENTS For full details on monitoring requirements consult product literature.
- PRESCRIBING AND DISPENSING INFORMATION Rituximab is a biological medicine. Biological medicines must be prescribed and dispensed by brand name, see *Biological medicines* and *Biosimilar medicines*, under Guidance on prescribing p. 1.
- MEDICINAL FORMS There can be variation in the licensing of different medicines containing the same drug.

Solution for infusion

EXCIPIENTS: May contain Polysorbates

ELECTROLYTES: May contain Sodium

▸ **MabThera** (Roche Products Ltd)

Rituximab 10 mg per 1 ml MabThera 100mg/10ml concentrate for solution for infusion vials | 2 vial PoM £349.25

MabThera 500mg/50ml concentrate for solution for infusion vials | 1 vial PoM £873.15

▸ **Rixathon** (Sandoz Ltd) ▼

Rituximab 10 mg per 1 ml Rixathon 100mg/10ml concentrate for solution for infusion vials | 2 vial PoM £314.33 (Hospital only)

Rixathon 500mg/50ml concentrate for solution for infusion vials | 1 vial PoM £785.84 (Hospital only) | 2 vial PoM £1,571.67 (Hospital only)

▸ **Truxima** (Napp Pharmaceuticals Ltd) ▼

Rituximab 10 mg per 1 ml Truxima 100mg/10ml concentrate for solution for infusion vials | 2 vial PoM £314.33 (Hospital only)

Truxima 500mg/50ml concentrate for solution for infusion vials | 1 vial PoM £785.84 (Hospital only)

2 Cytotoxic responsive malignancy

Cytotoxic drugs

Overview

The management of childhood cancer is complex and is generally confined to specialist regional centres and some associated shared-care units.

Cytotoxic drugs have both anti-cancer activity and the potential for damage to normal tissue. In children, chemotherapy is almost always started with curative intent, but may be continued as palliation if the disease is refractory.

Chemotherapy with a combination of two or more cytotoxic drugs aims to reduce the development of resistance and to improve cytotoxic effect. Treatment protocols generally incorporate a series of treatment courses at defined intervals with clear criteria for starting each course, such as adequate bone-marrow recovery and renal or cardiac function. The principal component of treatment for leukaemias in children is cytotoxic therapy, whereas solid tumours may be managed with surgery or radiotherapy in addition to chemotherapy.

Only medical or nursing staff who have received appropriate training should administer parenteral cytotoxics. In most instances central venous access will be required for the intravenous administration of cytotoxics to children; care is required to avoid the risk of extravasation (see Side-effects of Cytotoxic Drugs and their Management).

Cytotoxic drug handling guidelines

- Trained personnel should reconstitute cytotoxics
- Reconstitution should be carried out in designated pharmacy areas
- Protective clothing (including gloves, gowns, and masks) should be worn
- The eyes should be protected and means of first aid should be specified
- Pregnant staff should avoid exposure to cytotoxic drugs (all females of child-bearing age should be informed of the reproductive hazard)
- Use local procedures for dealing with spillages and safe disposal of waste material, including syringes, containers, and absorbent material
- Staff exposure to cytotoxic drugs should be monitored

Intrathecal chemotherapy

A Health Service Circular (HSC 2008/001) provides guidance on the introduction of safe practice in NHS Trusts where intrathecal chemotherapy is administered; written local guidance covering all aspects of national guidance should be available. Support for training programmes is also available.

Copies, and further information may be obtained from the Department of Health and Social Care website (www.gov.uk/government/organisations/department-of-health-and-social-care).

Safe systems for cytotoxic medicines

Safe system requirements for cytotoxic medicines:

- Cytotoxic drugs for the treatment of cancer should be given as part of a wider pathway of care that is co-ordinated by a multi-disciplinary team
- Cytotoxic drugs should be prescribed, dispensed and administered only in the context of a written protocol or treatment plan
- Injectable cytotoxic drugs should only be dispensed if they are prepared for administration
- Oral cytotoxic medicines should be dispensed with clear directions for use

Cytotoxic drugs: important safety information

Risks of incorrect dosing of oral anti-cancer medicines

The National Patient Safety Agency has advised (January 2008) that the prescribing and use of oral cytotoxic medicines should be carried out to the same standard as parenteral cytotoxic therapy. Standards to be followed to achieve this include:

- non-specialists who prescribe or administer on-going oral cytotoxic medication should have access to written protocols and treatment plans, including guidance on the monitoring and treatment of toxicity;
- staff dispensing oral cytotoxic medicines should confirm that the prescribed dose is appropriate for the patient. Patients should have written information that includes details of the intended oral anti-cancer regimen, the treatment plan, and arrangements for monitoring, taken from the original protocol from the initiating hospital. Staff dispensing oral cytotoxic medicines should also have access to this information, and to advice from an experienced cancer pharmacist in the initiating hospital.

Cytotoxic drug doses

Doses of cytotoxic drugs are determined using a variety of different methods including age, body-surface area, or body-weight. Alternatively, doses may be fixed. Doses may be further adjusted following consideration of a patient's neutrophil count, renal and hepatic function, and history of previous adverse effects to the cytotoxic drug. Doses may also differ depending on whether a drug is used alone or in combination.

Because of the complexity of dosage regimens in the treatment of malignant disease, dose statements have been omitted from many of the drug entries in this chapter.

Cytotoxic drugs: effect on pregnancy and reproductive function

Most cytotoxic drugs are teratogenic and should not be administered during pregnancy, especially during the first trimester. Exclude pregnancy before treatment with cytotoxic drugs. Considerable caution is necessary if a pregnant woman presents with cancer requiring chemotherapy, and specialist advice should always be sought.

Contraceptive advice should be given to men and women before cytotoxic therapy begins (and should cover the duration of contraception required after therapy has ended). Alkylating drugs can have an adverse effect on gametogenesis, which may be reversible particularly in females. Regimens that do not contain an alkylating drug or procarbazine may have less effect on fertility, but those with an alkylating drug or procarbazine carry the risk of causing permanent male sterility (there is no effect on potency). Pretreatment counselling and consideration of sperm storage may be appropriate. Women are less severely affected, though the span of reproductive life may be shortened by the onset of a premature menopause. No increase in fetal abnormalities or abortion rate has been recorded in patients who remain fertile after cytotoxic chemotherapy. Amenorrhoea may occur, which also may be reversible.

Management of cytotoxic drug side-effects

Gastro-intestinal effects

Management of gastrointestinal effects of cytotoxic drugs includes the use of antacids, H_2-receptor antagonists, and proton pump inhibitors to protect the gastric mucosa, laxatives to treat constipation, and enteral and parenteral nutritional support.

Oral mucositis

Good oral hygiene keeps the mouth clean and moist and helps to prevent mucositis; prevention is more effective than treatment of the complication. Good oral hygiene measures for children over 6 months include brushing teeth with a soft small brush with fluoride toothpaste 2–3 times daily, and rinsing the mouth frequently. Daily fluoride supplements can be used on the advice of the child's dental team. For children under 6 months or when it is not possible to brush teeth, carers should be instructed how to clean the mouth using an oral sponge moistened with water or with an antimicrobial solution such as diluted chlorhexidine. Mucositis related to chemotherapy can be extremely painful and may, in some circumstances, require opioid analgesia. Secondary infection with candida is frequent; treatment with a systemically absorbed antifungal, such as fluconazole p. 407, is effective.

Nausea and vomiting

Nausea and vomiting cause considerable distress to many children who receive chemotherapy, and to a lesser extent abdominal radiotherapy, and may lead to refusal of further treatment; prophylaxis of nausea and vomiting is therefore extremely important. Symptoms may be acute (occurring within 24 hours of treatment), delayed (first occurring more than 24 hours after treatment), or anticipatory (occurring prior to subsequent doses). Delayed and anticipatory symptoms are more difficult to control than acute symptoms and require different management.

Susceptibility to nausea and vomiting may increase with repeated exposure to the cytotoxic drug.

Drugs may be divided according to their emetogenic potential and some examples are given below, but the symptoms vary according to the dose, to other drugs administered, and to the individual's susceptibility to emetogenic stimuli.

Mildly emetogenic treatment— fluorouracil, etoposide p. 593, low doses of methotrexate p. 588, the vinca alkaloids, and abdominal radiotherapy.

Moderately emetogenic treatment— carboplatin p. 592, doxorubicin hydrochloride p. 583, intermediate and low doses of cyclophosphamide p. 579, mitoxantrone p. 585, and high doses of methotrexate.

Highly emetogenic treatment— cisplatin p. 592, dacarbazine p. 580, and high doses of alkylating drugs.

Anti-emetic drugs, when given regularly, help prevent or ameliorate emesis associated with chemotherapy in children.

Prevention of acute symptoms: For patients at low risk of emesis, pretreatment with a $5HT_3$-receptor antagonist may be of benefit.

For patients at high risk of *emesis* or when other treatment is inadequate, a $5HT_3$-receptor antagonist is often highly effective. The addition of dexamethasone p. 475 and other anti-emetics may also be required.

Prevention of delayed symptoms: dexamethasone, given by mouth, is the drug of choice for preventing delayed symptoms; it is used alone or with metoclopramide hydrochloride p. 278. Due to the risks of neurological side-effects, metoclopramide hydrochloride should only be used in children as a second-line option. The $5HT_3$-receptor antagonists may have a role in preventing uncontrolled symptoms. Aprepitant p. 279 given in combination with a $5HT_3$-receptor antagonist (with or without dexamethasone) is licensed for prevention of nausea and vomiting associated with highly and moderately emetogenic cancer chemotherapy.

Prevention of anticipatory symptoms: Good symptom control is the best way to prevent anticipatory symptoms. Lorazepam p. 238 can be helpful for its amnesiac, sedative, and anxiolytic effects.

For information on the treatment of nausea and vomiting, see Nausea and labyrinth disorders p. 275.

Bone-marrow suppression

All cytotoxic drugs except vincristine sulfate p. 594 and bleomycin p. 591 cause bone-marrow suppression. This commonly occurs 7 to 10 days after administration, but is delayed for certain drugs, such as melphalan p. 581. Peripheral blood counts must be checked before each treatment. The duration and severity of neutropenia can be reduced by the use of granulocyte-colony stimulating factors; their use should be reserved for children who have previously experienced severe neutropenia.

Cytotoxic drugs may be contra-indicated in children with acute infection; any infection should be treated before, or when starting, cytotoxic drugs.

Infection in a child with neutropenia requires immediate broad-spectrum antibacterial treatment that covers all likely pathogens. Appropriate bacteriological investigations should be conducted as soon as possible. Children taking cytotoxic drugs who have signs or symptoms of infection (or their carers) should be advised to seek prompt medical attention. All children should be investigated and treated under the supervision of an appropriate oncology or haematology specialist. Antifungal treatment may be required in a child with prolonged neutropenia or fever lasting longer than 4–5 days. Chickenpox and measles can be particularly hazardous in immunocompromised children. Varicella-zoster immunoglobulin p. 827 is indicated if the child does not have immunity against varicella and has had close contact with infectious chickenpox or herpes zoster. Antiviral prophylaxis can be considered in addition to varicella-zoster immunoglobulin or as an alternative if varicella–zoster immunoglobulin is inappropriate. If an immunocompromised child has come into close contact with an infectious individual with measles, normal immunoglobulin p. 825 should be given.

Alopecia

Reversible hair loss is a common complication, although it varies in degree between drugs and individual patients.

Long-term and delayed toxicity

Cytotoxic drugs may produce specific organ-related toxicity in children (e.g. cardiotoxicity with doxorubicin hydrochloride or nephrotoxicity with cisplatin and ifosfamide p. 580). Manifestations of such toxicity may not appear for several months or even years after cancer treatment. Careful follow-up of survivors of childhood cancer is therefore vital; national and local guidelines have been developed to facilitate this.

Thromboembolism

Venous thromboembolism can be a complication of cancer itself, but chemotherapy increases the risk.

Tumour lysis syndrome

Tumour lysis syndrome occurs secondary to spontaneous or treatment related rapid destruction of malignant cells. Patients at risk of tumour lysis syndrome include those with non- Hodgkin's lymphoma (especially if high grade and bulky disease), Burkitt's lymphoma, acute lymphoblastic leukaemia and acute myeloid leukaemia (particularly if high white blood cell counts or bulky disease), and occasionally those with solid tumours. Pre-existing hyperuricaemia, dehydration and renal impairment are also predisposing factors. Features, include hyperkalaemia, hyperuricaemia, and hyperphosphataemia with hypocalcaemia; renal damage and arrhythmias can follow. Early recognition of patients at risk, and initiation of prophylaxis or therapy for tumour lysis syndrome, is essential.

Treatment of cytotoxic drug side-effects

Hyperuricaemia

Hyperuricaemia, which may be present in high-grade lymphoma and leukaemia, can be markedly worsened by chemotherapy and is associated with acute renal failure.

Allopurinol p. 601 is used routinely in children at low to moderate risk of hyperuricaemia. It should be started 24 hours before treatment; patients should be adequately hydrated (consideration should be given to omitting phosphate and potassium from hydration fluids). The dose of mercaptopurine p. 587 or azathioprine p. 558 should be reduced if allopurinol is given concomitantly.

Rasburicase p. 601 is a recombinant urate oxidase used in children who are at high-risk of developing hyperuricaemia. It rapidly reduces plasma-uric acid concentration and may be of particular value in preventing complications following treatment of leukaemias or bulky lymphomas.

Methotrexate-induced mucositis and myelosuppression

Folinic acid p. 600 (given as calcium folinate) is used to counteract the folate-antagonist action of methotrexate and thus speed recovery from methotrexate-induced mucositis or myelosuppression ('folinic acid rescue').

The calcium salt of levofolinic acid p. 600, a single isomer of folinic acid, is also used following methotrexate administration. The dose of calcium levofolinate is generally half that of calcium folinate.

The disodium salts of folinic acid and levofolinic acid are also used for rescue therapy following methotrexate administration.

The efficacy of high dose methotrexate is enhanced by delaying initiation of folinic acid for at least 24 hours, local protocols define the correct time. Folinic acid p. 600 is normally continued until the plasma-methotrexate concentration falls to 45–90 nanograms/mL (100–200 nanomol/litre).

In the treatment of methotrexate p. 588 overdose, folinate should be administered immediately; other measures to enhance the elimination of methotrexate are also necessary.

Urothelial toxicity

Haemorrhagic cystitis is a common manifestation of urothelial toxicity which occurs with the oxazaphosphorines, cyclophosphamide p. 579 and ifosfamide p. 580; it is caused by the metabolite acrolein. Adequate hydration is essential to reduce the risk of urothelial toxicity. Mesna p. 599 reacts specifically with acrolein in the urinary tract, preventing toxicity. Mesna is given for the same duration as cyclophosphamide or ifosfamide. It is generally given intravenously; the dose of mesna is equal to or greater than that of the oxazaphosphorine.

Cytotoxic antibiotics

Cytotoxic antibiotics are widely used. Many act as radiomimetics and simultaneous use of radiotherapy should be **avoided** because it may markedly increase toxicity.

Daunorubicin p. 583, doxorubicin hydrochloride p. 583, and epirubicin hydrochloride p. 584 are anthracycline antibiotics. Mitoxantrone p. 585 (mitozantrone) is an anthracycline derivative.

Epirubicin hydrochloride and mitoxantrone are considered less toxic than the other anthracycline antibiotics, and may be suitable for children who have received high cumulative doses of other anthracyclines.

Vinca alkaloids

The vinca alkaloids, vinblastine sulfate p. 594 and vincristine sulfate p. 594 are used to treat a variety of cancers including leukaemias, lymphomas, and some solid tumours.

Antimetabolites

Antimetabolites are incorporated into new nuclear material or they combine irreversibly with cellular enzymes and prevent normal cellular division. Cytarabine p. 585, fludarabine phosphate p. 586, mercaptopurine p. 587, methotrexate, and tioguanine p. 590 are commonly used in paediatric chemotherapy.

Other antineoplastic drugs

Asparaginase is used almost exclusively in the treatment of acute lymphoblastic leukaemia. Hypersensitivity reactions may occur and facilities for the management of anaphylaxis should be available. A number of different preparations of asparaginase exist and only the product specified in the treatment protocol should be used.

ANTINEOPLASTIC DRUGS > ALKYLATING AGENTS

Busulfan

12-Jun-2018

(Busulphan)

● **INDICATIONS AND DOSE**

Conditioning treatment before haematopoietic progenitor cell transplantation

▶ BY MOUTH, OR BY INTRAVENOUS INFUSION

▶ Child: (consult local protocol)

DOSES AT EXTREMES OF BODY-WEIGHT

▶ Dose may need to be calculated based on body surface area or adjusted ideal body weight in obese patients—consult product literature.

IMPORTANT SAFETY INFORMATION

RISKS OF INCORRECT DOSING OF ORAL ANTI-CANCER MEDICINES

See Cytotoxic drugs p. 575.

● **CAUTIONS** Avoid in Acute porphyrias p. 652 · high dose (antiepileptic prophylaxis required) · history of seizures (antiepileptic prophylaxis required) · ineffective once in blast crisis phase · previous progenitor cell transplant (increased risk of hepatic veno-occlusive disease) · previous radiation therapy (increased risk of hepatic veno-occlusive disease) · risk of second malignancy · three or more cycles of chemotherapy (increased risk of hepatic veno-occlusive disease)

● **INTERACTIONS** → Appendix 1: alkylating agents

● **SIDE-EFFECTS**

GENERAL SIDE-EFFECTS

▶ **Common or very common** Alopecia · diarrhoea · hepatic disorders · nausea · respiratory disorders · sinusoidal obstruction syndrome · skin reactions · thrombocytopenia · vomiting

▶ **Uncommon** Seizure

▶ **Rare or very rare** Cataract · eye disorders

SPECIFIC SIDE-EFFECTS

▶ **Common or very common**

▶ With intravenous use Anaemia · anxiety · appetite decreased · arrhythmias · arthralgia · ascites · asthenia · asthma · cardiomegaly · chest pain · chills · confusion · constipation · cough · depression · dizziness · dyspnoea · dysuria · electrolyte imbalance · embolism and thrombosis · fever · gastrointestinal discomfort · gastrointestinal disorders · haemorrhage · headache · hiccups · hyperglycaemia · hypersensitivity · hypertension · hypoalbuminaemia · hypotension · increased risk of infection · insomnia · mucositis · myalgia · nervous system disorder · neutropenia · oedema · pain · pancytopenia · pericardial effusion · pericarditis · reactivation of infections · renal disorder · renal impairment · stomatitis · vasodilation · weight increased

▶ With oral use Amenorrhoea (may be reversible) · azoospermia · bone marrow disorders · cardiac tamponade · delayed puberty · hyperbilirubinaemia · infertility male · leucopenia · leukaemia · menopausal symptoms · oral disorders · ovarian and fallopian tube disorders · testicular atrophy

▶ **Uncommon**

▶ With intravenous use Capillary leak syndrome · delirium · encephalopathy · hallucination · hypoxia · intracranial haemorrhage

▶ **Rare or very rare**

▶ With oral use Dry mouth · erythema nodosum · gynaecomastia · myasthenia gravis · radiation injury · Sjögren's syndrome

▶ **Frequency not known**

▶ With intravenous use Hypogonadism · ovarian failure · premature menopause · sepsis

SIDE-EFFECTS, FURTHER INFORMATION **Lung toxicity** Discontinue if lung toxicity develops.

Secondary malignancy Use of busulfan is associated with an increased incidence of secondary malignancy.

Fluid retention Alkylating drugs can cause fluid retention with oedema and dilutional hyponatraemia in younger children; the risk of this complication is higher in the first 2 days and also when given with concomitant vinca alkaloids.

● **CONCEPTION AND CONTRACEPTION** Manufacturers advise effective contraception during and for 6 months after treatment in men or women. See also *Pregnancy and reproductive function* in Cytotoxic drugs p. 575.

● **PREGNANCY** Avoid (teratogenic in *animals*). See also *Pregnancy and reproductive function* in Cytotoxic drugs p. 575.

● **BREAST FEEDING** Discontinue breast-feeding.

● **HEPATIC IMPAIRMENT** Manufacturer advises caution (no information available)—monitor hepatic function, especially following transplant (consult product literature).

● **MONITORING REQUIREMENTS**

▶ Monitor cardiac and liver function.

▶ Monitor full blood count regularly throughout treatment.

● **MEDICINAL FORMS** There can be variation in the licensing of different medicines containing the same drug. Forms available from special-order manufacturers include: capsule, oral suspension, oral solution

Tablet

▶ **Busulfan (Non-proprietary)**

Busulfan 2 mg Busulfan 2mg tablets | 25 tablet PoM £69.02 DT = £69.02

Solution for infusion

▶ **Busulfan (Non-proprietary)**

Busulfan 6 mg per 1 ml Busulfan 60mg/10ml concentrate for solution for infusion vials | 8 vial PoM £1,529.50–£2,157.52 (Hospital only)

▶ **Busilvex** (Pierre Fabre Ltd)

Busulfan 6 mg per 1 ml Busilvex 60mg/10ml concentrate for solution for infusion ampoules | 8 ampoule PoM £1,610.00 (Hospital only)

Chlorambucil

10-Mar-2020

● **INDICATIONS AND DOSE**

Hodgkin's disease | Non-Hodgkin's lymphoma

▶ BY MOUTH

▸ Child: (consult local protocol)

Relapsing steroid-sensitive nephrotic syndrome (initiated in specialist centres)

▶ BY MOUTH

▸ Child 3 months–17 years: 200 micrograms/kg daily for 8 weeks

● **UNLICENSED USE** Not licensed for use in nephrotic syndrome.

> **IMPORTANT SAFETY INFORMATION**
> RISKS OF INCORRECT DOSING OF ORAL ANTI-CANCER MEDICINES
> See Cytotoxic drugs p. 575.

● **CAUTIONS** Children with nephrotic syndrome (increased seizure risk) · history of epilepsy (increased seizure risk)

● **INTERACTIONS** → Appendix 1: alkylating agents

● **SIDE-EFFECTS**

▶ **Common or very common** Anaemia · bone marrow disorders · diarrhoea · gastrointestinal disorder · leucopenia · nausea · neoplasms · neutropenia · oral ulceration · seizures · thrombocytopenia · vomiting

▶ **Uncommon** Skin reactions

▶ **Rare or very rare** Cystitis · fever · hepatic disorders · movement disorders · muscle twitching · peripheral neuropathy · respiratory disorders · severe cutaneous adverse reactions (SCARs) · tremor

▶ **Frequency not known** Amenorrhoea · azoospermia

SIDE-EFFECTS, FURTHER INFORMATION **Secondary malignancy** Use of chlorambucil is associated with an increased incidence of acute leukaemia, particularly with prolonged use.

Skin reactions Manufacturer advises assessing continued use if rash occurs—has been reported to progress to Stevens-Johnson syndrome and toxic epidermal necrolysis.

Fluid retention Alkylating drugs can cause fluid retention with oedema and dilutional hyponatraemia in younger children; the risk of this complication is higher in the first 2 days and also when given with concomitant vinca alkaloids.

● **CONCEPTION AND CONTRACEPTION** Contraceptive advice required, see *Pregnancy and reproductive function* in Cytotoxic drugs p. 575.

● **PREGNANCY** Avoid. See also *Pregnancy and reproductive function* in Cytotoxic drugs p. 575.

● **BREAST FEEDING** Discontinue breast-feeding.

● **HEPATIC IMPAIRMENT** Manufacturer advises caution—monitor for signs and symptoms of toxicity.
Dose adjustments Manufacturer advises consider dose reduction in severe impairment—limited information available.

● **MONITORING REQUIREMENTS** Monitor full blood count regularly throughout treatment.

● **PATIENT AND CARER ADVICE**
Medicines for Children leaflet: Chlorambucil for nephrotic syndrome www.medicinesforchildren.org.uk/chlorambucil-nephrotic-syndrome-0

● **MEDICINAL FORMS** There can be variation in the licensing of different medicines containing the same drug.

Tablet

▸ **Chlorambucil (Non-proprietary)**
Chlorambucil 2 mg Chlorambucil 2mg tablets | 25 tablet PoM £42.87 DT = £42.87

Cyclophosphamide

10-Mar-2020

● **INDICATIONS AND DOSE**

Acute lymphoblastic leukaemia, non-Hodgkin's lymphoma, retinoblastoma, neuroblastoma, rhabdomyosarcoma, soft-tissue sarcomas, Ewing tumour, neuroectodermal tumours (including medulloblastoma), infant brain tumours, ependymona, high-dose conditioning for bone marrow transplantation, lupus nephritis

▶ BY MOUTH, OR BY INTRAVENOUS INFUSION

▸ Child: (consult local protocol)

Steroid-sensitive nephrotic syndrome

▶ BY MOUTH

▸ Child 3 months–17 years: 2–3 mg/kg daily for 8 weeks

▶ BY INTRAVENOUS INFUSION

▸ Child 3 months–17 years: 500 mg/m^2 once a month for 6 months

● **UNLICENSED USE** Not licensed for use in children.

> **IMPORTANT SAFETY INFORMATION**
> RISKS OF INCORRECT DOSING OF ORAL ANTI-CANCER MEDICINES
> See Cytotoxic drugs p. 575.

● **CAUTIONS** Avoid in Acute porphyrias p. 652 · diabetes mellitus · haemorrhagic cystitis · previous or concurrent mediastinal irradiation—risk of cardiotoxicity

● **INTERACTIONS** → Appendix 1: alkylating agents

● **SIDE-EFFECTS**

GENERAL SIDE-EFFECTS

▶ **Common or very common** Agranulocytosis · alopecia · anaemia · asthenia · bone marrow disorders · cystitis · decreased leucocytes · fever · haemolytic uraemic syndrome · haemorrhage · hepatic disorders · immunosuppression · increased risk of infection · mucosal abnormalities · neutropenia · progressive multifocal leukoencephalopathy (PML) · reactivation of infections · sperm abnormalities · thrombocytopenia

▶ **Uncommon** Appetite decreased · embolism and thrombosis · flushing · hypersensitivity · ovarian and fallopian tube disorders · sepsis

▶ **Rare or very rare** Bladder disorders · chest pain · confusion · constipation · diarrhoea · disseminated intravascular coagulation · dizziness · eye inflammation · fluid imbalance · headache · hyponatraemia · menstrual cycle irregularities · nail discolouration · nausea · neoplasms · oral disorders · pancreatitis acute · renal failure · secondary neoplasm · seizure · severe cutaneous adverse reactions (SCARs) · SIADH · skin reactions · visual impairment · vomiting

▶ **Frequency not known** Abdominal pain · altered smell sensation · arrhythmias · arthralgia · ascites · cardiac inflammation · cardiogenic shock · cardiomyopathy · cough · deafness · dyspnoea · encephalopathy · excessive tearing · facial swelling · gastrointestinal disorders · heart failure · hyperhidrosis · hypoxia · infertility · influenza like illness · multi organ failure · muscle complaints · myelopathy · myocardial infarction · nasal complaints · nephropathy · nerve disorders · neuralgia · neurotoxicity · oedema · oropharyngeal pain · palpitations · pericardial effusion · peripheral ischaemia · pulmonary hypertension · pulmonary oedema · QT interval prolongation · radiation injuries · renal tubular disorder · renal tubular necrosis · respiratory disorders · rhabdomyolysis · scleroderma · sensation abnormal · sinusoidal obstruction syndrome · taste altered · testicular atrophy · tinnitus · tremor · tumour lysis syndrome · vasculitis

SPECIFIC SIDE-EFFECTS

▸ **With intravenous use** Infusion site necrosis · injection site necrosis

SIDE-EFFECTS, FURTHER INFORMATION **Haemorrhagic cystitis** A urinary metabolite of cyclophosphamide, acrolein, can cause haemorrhagic cystitis; this is a rare but serious complication that may be prevented by increasing fluid intake for 24–48 hours after intravenous injection. Mesna can also help prevent cystitis.

Secondary malignancy As with all cytotoxic therapy, treatment with cyclophosphamide is associated with an increased incidence of secondary malignancies.

Fluid retention Alkylating drugs can cause fluid retention with oedema and dilutional hyponatraemia in younger children; the risk of this complication is higher in the first 2 days and also when given with concomitant vinca alkaloids.

- **CONCEPTION AND CONTRACEPTION** Manufacturer advises effective contraception during and for at least 3 months after treatment in men or women. See also *Pregnancy and reproductive function* in Cytotoxic drugs p. 575.
- **PREGNANCY** Avoid. See also *Pregnancy and reproductive function* in Cytotoxic drugs p. 575.
- **BREAST FEEDING** Discontinue breast-feeding during and for 36 hours after stopping treatment.
- **HEPATIC IMPAIRMENT** Manufacturer advises caution (risk of decreased cyclophosphamide activation and increased risk of veno-occlusive liver disease).
  Dose adjustments Manufacturer advises consider dose adjustment in severe impairment—consult product literature.
- **RENAL IMPAIRMENT**
  Dose adjustments Reduce dose—consult local treatment protocol for details.
- **DIRECTIONS FOR ADMINISTRATION** Consult local treatment protocol for details.
- **PATIENT AND CARER ADVICE**
  Medicines for Children leaflet: Cyclophosphamide for nephrotic syndrome www.medicinesforchildren.org.uk/cyclophosphamide-nephrotic-syndrome-0

- **MEDICINAL FORMS** There can be variation in the licensing of different medicines containing the same drug. Forms available from special-order manufacturers include: tablet, oral suspension, oral solution, solution for injection, solution for infusion

Tablet

CAUTIONARY AND ADVISORY LABELS 25, 27

▸ Cyclophosphamide (Non-proprietary)
Cyclophosphamide (as Cyclophosphamide monohydrate) 50 mg Cyclophosphamide 50mg tablets | 100 tablet PoM £139.00 DT = £139.00

▸ Cytoxan (Imported (United States))
Cyclophosphamide 25 mg Cytoxan 25mg tablets | 100 tablet PoM [no NHS indicator]

Powder for solution for injection

▸ Cyclophosphamide (Non-proprietary)
Cyclophosphamide (as Cyclophosphamide monohydrate) 500 mg Cyclophosphamide 500mg powder for solution for injection vials | 1 vial PoM £9.20 (Hospital only) | 1 vial PoM £9.66
Cyclophosphamide (as Cyclophosphamide monohydrate) 1 gram Cyclophosphamide 1g powder for solution for injection vials | 1 vial PoM £10.66 (Hospital only) | 1 vial PoM £17.91
Cyclophosphamide (as Cyclophosphamide monohydrate) 2 gram Cyclophosphamide 2g powder for solution for injection vials | 1 vial PoM £31.64 (Hospital only)

Dacarbazine

- **INDICATIONS AND DOSE**

Hodgkin's disease | Paediatric solid tumours

▸ BY INTRAVENOUS INJECTION, OR BY INTRAVENOUS INFUSION
▸ Child: (consult local protocol)

- **CAUTIONS** Caution in handling—irritant to tissues
- **INTERACTIONS** → Appendix 1: alkylating agents
- **SIDE-EFFECTS**
  - ▸ **Common or very common** Anaemia · appetite decreased · leucopenia · nausea · thrombocytopenia · vomiting
  - ▸ **Uncommon** Alopecia · infection · influenza like illness · photosensitivity reaction · skin reactions
  - ▸ **Rare or very rare** Agranulocytosis · confusion · diarrhoea · flushing · headache · hepatic disorders · lethargy · pancytopenia · paraesthesia · renal impairment · seizure · visual impairment
- **CONCEPTION AND CONTRACEPTION** Ensure effective contraception during and for at least 6 months after treatment in men or women. See also *Pregnancy and reproductive function* in Cytotoxic drugs p. 575.
- **PREGNANCY** Avoid (carcinogenic and teratogenic in *animal* studies). See also *Pregnancy and reproductive function* in Cytotoxic drugs p. 575.
- **BREAST FEEDING** Discontinue breast-feeding.
- **HEPATIC IMPAIRMENT** Avoid in severe impairment.
  Dose adjustments Dose reduction may be required in combined renal and hepatic impairment.
- **RENAL IMPAIRMENT** Avoid in severe impairment.
  Dose adjustments Dose reduction may be required in combined renal and hepatic impairment.
- **PRESCRIBING AND DISPENSING INFORMATION** Dacarbazine is a component of a commonly used combination for Hodgkin's disease (ABVD—doxorubicin [previously *Adriamycin*®], bleomycin, vinblastine, and dacarbazine).

- **MEDICINAL FORMS** There can be variation in the licensing of different medicines containing the same drug.

Powder for solution for infusion

▸ Dacarbazine (Non-proprietary)
Dacarbazine (as Dacarbazine citrate) 500 mg Dacarbazine 500mg powder for solution for infusion vials | 1 vial PoM £37.50
Dacarbazine (as Dacarbazine citrate) 1 gram Dacarbazine 1g powder for solution for infusion vials | 1 vial PoM £70.00

Powder for solution for injection

▸ Dacarbazine (Non-proprietary)
Dacarbazine (as Dacarbazine citrate) 100 mg Dacarbazine 100mg powder for solution for injection vials | 10 vial PoM £90.00
Dacarbazine (as Dacarbazine citrate) 200 mg Dacarbazine 200mg powder for solution for injection vials | 10 vial PoM £160.00

Ifosfamide

24-Jul-2019

- **INDICATIONS AND DOSE**

Rhabdomyosarcoma | Soft-tissue sarcomas | Ewing tumour | Germ cell tumour | Osteogenic sarcoma

▸ BY INTRAVENOUS INFUSION
▸ Child: (consult local protocol)

- **CONTRA-INDICATIONS** Acute infection · cystitis · urinary-tract obstruction · urothelial damage
- **CAUTIONS** Avoid in Acute porphyrias p. 652
- **INTERACTIONS** → Appendix 1: alkylating agents
- **SIDE-EFFECTS**
  - ▸ **Common or very common** Alopecia · appetite decreased · bone marrow disorders · haemorrhage · hepatic disorders · infection · leucopenia · nausea · reactivation of infection · renal impairment · thrombocytopenia · vomiting
  - ▸ **Uncommon** Cardiotoxicity · diarrhoea · hypotension · oral disorders
  - ▸ **Rare or very rare** Skin reactions
  - ▸ **Frequency not known** Abdominal pain · agranulocytosis · amenorrhoea · anaemia · angina pectoris · angioedema · arrhythmias · arthralgia · asterixis · behaviour abnormal · blood disorders · bone disorders · cancer progression · capillary leak syndrome · cardiac arrest · cardiomyopathy · chills · conjunctivitis · constipation · cough · deafness · delirium · delusions · disseminated intravascular

coagulation · dysarthria · dyspnoea · electrolyte imbalance · embolism and thrombosis · encephalopathy · eye irritation · fatigue · fever · flushing · gait abnormal · gastrointestinal disorders · growth retardation · haemolytic anaemia · heart failure · hyperglycaemia · hyperhidrosis · hyperphosphaturia · hypertension · hypoxia · immunosuppression · infertility · malaise · mania · memory loss · metabolic acidosis · movement disorders · mucosal ulceration · multi organ failure · muscle complaints · myocardial infarction · nail disorder · neoplasms · nephritis tubulointerstitial · nephrogenic diabetes insipidus · neurotoxicity · oedema · ovarian and fallopian tube disorders · pain · pancreatitis · panic attack · peripheral neuropathy · polydipsia · premature menopause · psychiatric disorders · pulmonary hypertension · pulmonary oedema · radiation recall reaction · respiratory disorders · rhabdomyolysis · secondary malignancy · sensation abnormal · sepsis · severe cutaneous adverse reactions (SCARs) · SIADH · sinusoidal obstruction syndrome · sperm abnormalities · status epilepticus · tinnitus · tumour lysis syndrome · urinary disorders · vasculitis · vertigo · visual impairment

SIDE-EFFECTS, FURTHER INFORMATION **Urothelial toxicity** Mesna is routinely given with ifosfamide to reduce urothelial toxicity.

Secondary malignancy Use of ifosfamide is associated with an increased incidence of acute leukaemia.

Fluid retention Alkylating drugs can cause fluid retention with oedema and dilutional hyponatraemia in younger children; the risk of this complication is higher in the first 2 days and also when given with concomitant vinca alkaloids.

- CONCEPTION AND CONTRACEPTION Manufacturer advises adequate contraception during and for at least 6 months after treatment in men or women. See also *Pregnancy and reproductive function* in Cytotoxic drugs p. 575.
- PREGNANCY Avoid (teratogenic and carcinogenic in *animals*). See also *Pregnancy and reproductive function* in Cytotoxic drugs p. 575.
- BREAST FEEDING Discontinue breast-feeding.
- HEPATIC IMPAIRMENT Manufacturer advises avoid.
- RENAL IMPAIRMENT Avoid.
- MONITORING REQUIREMENTS Ensure satisfactory electrolyte balance and renal function before each course (risk of tubular dysfunction, Fanconi's syndrome or diabetes insipidus if renal toxicity not treated promptly).

- MEDICINAL FORMS There can be variation in the licensing of different medicines containing the same drug.

Powder for solution for injection

- Ifosfamide (Non-proprietary)
  Ifosfamide 1 gram Ifosfamide 1g powder for concentrate for solution for injection vials | 1 vial PoM £115.79–£119.27
  Ifosfamide 2 gram Ifosfamide 2g powder for concentrate for solution for injection vials | 1 vial PoM £228.09–£234.94

Melphalan

- INDICATIONS AND DOSE

High intravenous dose with haematopoietic stem cell transplantation in the treatment of childhood neuroblastoma and some other advanced embryonal tumours

- BY INTRAVENOUS INFUSION
- Child: (consult local protocol)

- UNLICENSED USE Not licensed for use in embryonal tumours.

IMPORTANT SAFETY INFORMATION
RISKS OF INCORRECT DOSING OF ORAL ANTI-CANCER MEDICINES
See Cytotoxic drugs p. 575.

- CAUTIONS Consider use of prophylactic anti-infective agents · for high-dose intravenous administration establish adequate hydration · haematopoietic stem cell transplantation essential for high dose treatment (consult local treatment protocol for details)
- INTERACTIONS → Appendix 1: alkylating agents
- SIDE-EFFECTS
  - **Common or very common** Alopecia · anaemia · bone marrow depression (delayed) · diarrhoea · feeling hot · myalgia · myopathy · nausea · paraesthesia · stomatitis · thrombocytopenia · vomiting
  - **Rare or very rare** Haemolytic anaemia · hepatic disorders · peripheral vascular disease · respiratory disorders · skin reactions

SIDE-EFFECTS, FURTHER INFORMATION **Secondary malignancy** Use of melphalan is associated with an increased incidence of acute leukaemias.

Fluid retention Alkylating drugs can cause fluid retention with oedema and dilutional hyponatraemia in younger children; the risk of this complication is higher in the first 2 days and also when given with concomitant vinca alkaloids.

- CONCEPTION AND CONTRACEPTION Manufacturer advises adequate contraception during treatment in men or women. See also *Pregnancy and reproductive function* in Cytotoxic drugs p. 575.
- PREGNANCY Avoid. See also *Pregnancy and reproductive function* in Cytotoxic drugs p. 575.
- BREAST FEEDING Discontinue breast-feeding.
- RENAL IMPAIRMENT
  Dose adjustments Reduce dose initially (consult product literature).
- MONITORING REQUIREMENTS Monitor full blood count before and throughout treatment.

- MEDICINAL FORMS There can be variation in the licensing of different medicines containing the same drug.

Powder and solvent for solution for injection

- Melphalan (Non-proprietary)
  Melphalan (as Melphalan hydrochloride) 50 mg Melphalan 50mg powder and solvent for solution for injection vials | 1 vial PoM £137.37 (Hospital only) | 1 vial PoM £137.37

Temozolomide

25-Jul-2018

- DRUG ACTION Temozolomide is structurally related to dacarbazine.

- INDICATIONS AND DOSE

Treatment of recurrent or progressive malignant glioma

- BY MOUTH
- Child 3–17 years: (consult local protocol)

IMPORTANT SAFETY INFORMATION
RISKS OF INCORRECT DOSING OF ORAL ANTI-CANCER MEDICINES
See Cytotoxic drugs p. 575.

- CAUTIONS *Pneumocystis jirovecii* pneumonia—consult product literature for monitoring and prophylaxis requirements
- INTERACTIONS → Appendix 1: alkylating agents

- **SIDE-EFFECTS**
- ▸ **Common or very common** Alopecia · anxiety · appetite decreased · arthralgia · asthenia · chills · concentration impaired · confusion · constipation · cough · decreased leucocytes · diarrhoea · dizziness · drowsiness · dysphagia · dyspnoea · emotional lability · fever · gastrointestinal discomfort · haemorrhage · headache · hearing impairment · hemiparesis · hyperglycaemia · hypersensitivity · increased risk of infection · insomnia · level of consciousness decreased · malaise · memory loss · movement disorders · muscle weakness · nausea · neutropenia · oedema · pain · peripheral neuropathy · radiation injury · seizures · sensation abnormal · skin reactions · speech impairment · stomatitis · taste altered · thrombocytopenia · tremor · urinary disorders · vision disorders · vomiting · weight changes
- ▸ **Uncommon** Altered smell sensation · anaemia · behaviour disorder · bone marrow disorders · cognitive impairment · condition aggravated · Cushing's syndrome · depression · diabetes insipidus · ear pain · erectile dysfunction · eye pain · gait abnormal · hallucination · hepatic disorders · hyperacusia · hyperbilirubinaemia · hypertension · hypokalaemia · intracranial haemorrhage · myalgia · myopathy · nasal congestion · nervous system disorder · palpitations · photosensitivity reaction · reactivation of infections · thirst · tinnitus · tongue discolouration · vasodilation
- ▸ **Rare or very rare** Neoplasms · respiratory disorders · secondary malignancy · severe cutaneous adverse reactions (SCARs)
- **CONCEPTION AND CONTRACEPTION** Manufacturer advises adequate contraception during treatment. Men should avoid fathering a child during and for at least 6 months after treatment. See also *Pregnancy and reproductive function* in Cytotoxic drugs p. 575.
- **PREGNANCY** Avoid (teratogenic and embryotoxic in *animal* studies). See also *Pregnancy and reproductive function* in Cytotoxic drugs p. 575.
- **BREAST FEEDING** Discontinue breast-feeding.
- **HEPATIC IMPAIRMENT** Manufacturer advises caution in severe impairment (no information available).
- **RENAL IMPAIRMENT** Manufacturer advises caution—no information available.
- **MONITORING REQUIREMENTS**
- ▸ Monitor liver function before treatment initiation, after each treatment cycle and midway through 42-day treatment cycles—consider the balance of benefits and risks of treatment if results are abnormal at any point (fatal liver injury reported).
- ▸ Monitor for myelodysplastic syndrome.
- ▸ Monitor for secondary malignancies.

- **MEDICINAL FORMS** There can be variation in the licensing of different medicines containing the same drug. Forms available from special-order manufacturers include: oral suspension

Capsule

CAUTIONARY AND ADVISORY LABELS 23, 25

- ▸ Temozolomide (Non-proprietary)

Temozolomide 5 mg Temozolomide 5mg capsules | 5 capsule PoM £16.00 | 5 capsule PoM £10.06 (Hospital only)
Temozolomide 20 mg Temozolomide 20mg capsules | 5 capsule PoM £65.00 | 5 capsule PoM £40.23 (Hospital only)
Temozolomide 100 mg Temozolomide 100mg capsules | 5 capsule PoM £325.00 | 5 capsule PoM £201.18 (Hospital only)
Temozolomide 140 mg Temozolomide 140mg capsules | 5 capsule PoM £465.00 | 5 capsule PoM £296.47 (Hospital only)
Temozolomide 180 mg Temozolomide 180mg capsules | 5 capsule PoM £586.00 | 5 capsule PoM £381.18 (Hospital only)
Temozolomide 250 mg Temozolomide 250mg capsules | 5 capsule PoM £814.00 | 5 capsule PoM £529.42 (Hospital only)

- ▸ Temodal (Merck Sharp & Dohme Ltd)

Temozolomide 5 mg Temodal 5mg capsules | 5 capsule PoM £10.59 (Hospital only)
Temozolomide 20 mg Temodal 20mg capsules | 5 capsule PoM £42.35 (Hospital only)
Temozolomide 100 mg Temodal 100mg capsules | 5 capsule PoM £211.77 (Hospital only)
Temozolomide 140 mg Temodal 140mg capsules | 5 capsule PoM £296.48 (Hospital only)
Temozolomide 180 mg Temodal 180mg capsules | 5 capsule PoM £381.19 (Hospital only)
Temozolomide 250 mg Temodal 250mg capsules | 5 capsule PoM £529.43 (Hospital only)

Thiotepa

07-Feb-2019

- **INDICATIONS AND DOSE**

Conditioning treatment before haematopoietic stem cell transplantation in the treatment of haematological disease or solid tumours, in combination with other chemotherapy

- ▸ BY INTRAVENOUS INFUSION
- ▸ Child: (consult local protocol)

- **CAUTIONS** Avoid in Acute porphyrias p. 652
- **INTERACTIONS** → Appendix 1: alkylating agents
- **SIDE-EFFECTS**
- ▸ **Common or very common** Abdominal pain · anaemia · appetite decreased · ataxia · bladder disorder · cardiac arrest · cardiovascular insufficiency · diarrhoea · encephalopathy · fever · gastrointestinal disorders · graft versus host disease · growth retardation · haemorrhage · headache · hearing impairment · heart failure · hepatic failure · hyperglycaemia · hypertension · hypogonadism · hypopituitarism · hypothyroidism · hypoxia · increased risk of infection · intracranial haemorrhage · memory loss · mucositis · multi organ failure · nausea · neutropenia · pain · pancytopenia · paresis · psychiatric disorder · pulmonary oedema · renal failure · respiratory disorders · secondary malignancy · seizure · sepsis · sinusoidal obstruction syndrome · skin reactions · stomatitis · thrombocytopenia · vomiting
- ▸ **Frequency not known** Pulmonary arterial hypertension · severe cutaneous adverse reactions (SCARs)

SIDE-EFFECTS, FURTHER INFORMATION Alkylating drugs can cause fluid retention with oedema and dilutional hyponatraemia in younger children; the risk of this complication is higher in the first 2 days and also when given with concomitant vinca alkaloids.

- **CONCEPTION AND CONTRACEPTION** Contraceptive advice required, see *Pregnancy and reproductive function* in Cytotoxic drugs p. 575.
- **PREGNANCY** Avoid (teratogenic and embryotoxic in *animals*). See also *Pregnancy and reproductive function* in Cytotoxic drugs p. 575.
- **BREAST FEEDING** Discontinue breast-feeding.
- **NATIONAL FUNDING/ACCESS DECISIONS**

Scottish Medicines Consortium (SMC) decisions

SMC No. 790/12

The *Scottish Medicines Consortium* has advised (June 2012) that thiotepa (*Tepadina*®) is **not** recommended for use within NHS Scotland in combination with other chemotherapy as conditioning treatment in adults or children with haematological diseases, or solid tumours prior to haematopoietic stem cell transplantation.

- **MEDICINAL FORMS** There can be variation in the licensing of different medicines containing the same drug.

Powder for solution for infusion

- ▸ Tepadina (Adienne Pharma & Biotech)

Thiotepa 15 mg Tepadina 15mg powder for concentrate for solution for infusion vials | 1 vial PoM
Thiotepa 100 mg Tepadina 100mg powder for concentrate for solution for infusion vials | 1 vial PoM

ANTINEOPLASTIC DRUGS > ANTHRACYCLINES AND RELATED DRUGS

Daunorubicin

21-Nov-2019

● **INDICATIONS AND DOSE**

Acute myelogenous leukaemia | Acute lymphocytic leukaemia

▸ BY INTRAVENOUS INFUSION

▸ Child: (consult local protocol)

● UNLICENSED USE *DaunoXome®* is not licensed for use in children.

● CONTRA-INDICATIONS Myocardial insufficiency · previous treatment with maximum cumulative doses of daunorubicin or other anthracycline · recent myocardial infarction · severe arrhythmia

● CAUTIONS Caution in handling—irritant to tissues

● INTERACTIONS → Appendix 1: anthracyclines

● SIDE-EFFECTS Abdominal pain · alopecia · amenorrhoea · anaemia · arrhythmias · ascites · atrioventricular block · azoospermia · bone marrow disorders · cardiac inflammation · cardiomyopathy · chills · congestive heart failure · cyanosis · death · dehydration · diarrhoea · dyspnoea · extravasation necrosis · fever · flushing · gastrointestinal disorders · haemorrhage · hepatomegaly · hyperpyrexia · hyperuricaemia · hypoxia · infection · ischaemic heart disease · leucopenia · mucositis · myocardial infarction · nail discolouration · nausea · nephropathy · neutropenia · oedema · pain · paraesthesia · pleural effusion · radiation injuries · shock · skin reactions · stomatitis · thrombocytopenia · thrombophlebitis · urine red · venous sclerosis · vomiting

SIDE-EFFECTS, FURTHER INFORMATION Cardiotoxicity is cumulative and may be irreversible, however responds to treatment if detected early.

● CONCEPTION AND CONTRACEPTION Contraceptive advice required, see *Pregnancy and reproductive function* in Cytotoxic drugs p. 575.

● PREGNANCY Avoid (teratogenic and carcinogenic in *animal* studies). See also *Pregnancy and reproductive function* in Cytotoxic drugs p. 575.

● BREAST FEEDING Discontinue breast-feeding.

● HEPATIC IMPAIRMENT For *solution for infusion* manufacturer advises caution. For *powder for solution for infusion* manufacturer advises caution in mild to moderate impairment; avoid in severe impairment.

Dose adjustments Manufacturer advises dose reduction according to serum bilirubin concentration—consult product literature.

● RENAL IMPAIRMENT Avoid in severe impairment.

Dose adjustments Reduce dose—consult local treatment protocol for details.

● MONITORING REQUIREMENTS

▸ Cardiac monitoring essential.

▸ Cardiac function should be monitored before and at regular intervals throughout treatment and afterwards.

● PRESCRIBING AND DISPENSING INFORMATION

Daunorubicin is available as *conventional* and *liposomal* formulations. These different formulations vary in their licensed indications, pharmacokinetics, dosage and administration, and are **not** interchangeable.

● MEDICINAL FORMS There can be variation in the licensing of different medicines containing the same drug.

Solution for infusion

▸ DaunoXome (Galen Ltd)

Daunorubicin (as Daunorubicin hydrochloride citrate liposomal pegylated) 2 mg per 1 ml DaunoXome 50mg/25ml concentrate for solution for infusion vials | 1 vial PoM £250.00

Powder for solution for infusion

▸ Daunorubicin (Non-proprietary)

Daunorubicin (as Daunorubicin hydrochloride)

20 mg Daunorubicin 20mg powder for solution for infusion vials | 10 vial PoM £715.00 (Hospital only)

Doxorubicin hydrochloride

21-Nov-2019

● **INDICATIONS AND DOSE**

Some paediatric malignancies | Ewing's sarcoma | Osteogenic sarcoma | Wilm's tumour | Neuroblastoma | Retinoblastoma | Some liver tumours | Acute lymphoblastic leukaemia | Hodgkin's lymphoma | Non-Hodgkin's lymphoma

▸ BY INTRAVENOUS INFUSION

▸ Child: (consult local protocol)

● CONTRA-INDICATIONS Acute inflammatory heart disease · increased haemorrhagic tendency · marked persisting myelosuppression induced by previous treatment · marked persisting stomatitis induced by previous treatment · previous myocardial infarction · previous treatment with maximum cumulative doses of doxorubicin · previous treatment with maximum cumulative doses of other anthracycline · severe arrhythmia · severe myocardial insufficiency

● CAUTIONS Caution in handling—irritant to tissues · consult product literature

● INTERACTIONS → Appendix 1: anthracyclines

● SIDE-EFFECTS

▸ **Common or very common** Alopecia · anaemia · anxiety · appetite decreased · arrhythmias · arthralgia · asthenia · bone marrow depression · breast pain · cachexia · cardiovascular disorder · chest discomfort · chills · constipation · cough · decreased leucocytes · dehydration · depression · diarrhoea · dizziness · drowsiness · dry mouth · dysphagia · dyspnoea · dysuria · electrolyte imbalance · epistaxis · eye inflammation · fever · gastrointestinal discomfort · gastrointestinal disorders · headache · hyperhidrosis · hypersensitivity · hypertension · hyperthermia · hypotension · increased risk of infection · influenza like illness · infusion related reaction · insomnia · malaise · mucosal abnormalities · muscle complaints · muscle tone increased · muscle weakness · nail disorder · nausea · nerve disorders · neutropenia · oedema · oral disorders · pain · scrotal erythema · sensation abnormal · sepsis · skin reactions · skin ulcer · syncope · taste altered · thrombocytopenia · vasodilation · vision blurred · vomiting · weight decreased

▸ **Uncommon** Confusion · embolism and thrombosis

▸ **Rare or very rare** Secondary oral neoplasms · severe cutaneous adverse reactions (SCARs)

▸ **Frequency not known** Asthma · congestive heart failure · secondary malignancy · throat tightness

SIDE-EFFECTS, FURTHER INFORMATION Extravasation can cause tissue necrosis.

Cardiotoxicity All anthracycline antibiotics have been associated with varying degrees of cardiac toxicity—this may be idiosyncratic and reversible, but is commonly related to total cumulative dose and is irreversible.

● CONCEPTION AND CONTRACEPTION Manufacturer advises effective contraception during and for at least 6 months after treatment in men or women.

● PREGNANCY Avoid (teratogenic and toxic in *animal* studies). See also *Pregnancy and reproductive function* in Cytotoxic drugs p. 575.

● BREAST FEEDING Discontinue breast-feeding.

- **HEPATIC IMPAIRMENT** For *solution for injection or infusion*, manufacturer advises caution in mild to moderate impairment; avoid in severe impairment.
  Dose adjustments Manufacturer advises dose reduction according to bilirubin concentration.
- **RENAL IMPAIRMENT** Consult product literature in severe impairment.
- **MONITORING REQUIREMENTS** Cardiac function should be monitored before and at regular intervals throughout treatment and afterwards.

- **MEDICINAL FORMS** There can be variation in the licensing of different medicines containing the same drug. Forms available from special-order manufacturers include: solution for injection, solution for infusion

Solution for injection

- Doxorubicin hydrochloride (Non-proprietary)
  Doxorubicin hydrochloride 2 mg per 1 ml Doxorubicin 10mg/5ml solution for injection vials | 1 vial PoM £18.54 (Hospital only)
  Doxorubicin 50mg/25ml solution for injection Cytosafe vials | 1 vial PoM £103.00 (Hospital only)
  Doxorubicin 50mg/25ml solution for infusion vials | 1 vial PoM £103.00 (Hospital only)
  Doxorubicin 10mg/5ml solution for injection Cytosafe vials | 1 vial PoM £20.60 (Hospital only)
  Doxorubicin 10mg/5ml concentrate for solution for infusion vials | 1 vial PoM £11.55–£19.57 (Hospital only)
  Doxorubicin 10mg/5ml solution for infusion vials | 1 vial PoM £20.60 (Hospital only)
  Doxorubicin 50mg/25ml solution for injection vials | 1 vial PoM £92.70 (Hospital only)
  Doxorubicin 50mg/25ml concentrate for solution for infusion vials | 1 vial PoM £54.00–£97.85 (Hospital only)

Solution for infusion

- Doxorubicin hydrochloride (Non-proprietary)
  Doxorubicin hydrochloride 2 mg per 1 ml Doxorubicin 200mg/100ml solution for infusion vials | 1 vial PoM £412.00 (Hospital only)
  Doxorubicin 20mg/10ml concentrate for solution for infusion vials | 1 vial PoM ⊠ (Hospital only)
  Doxorubicin 100mg/50ml concentrate for solution for infusion vials | 1 vial PoM ⊠ (Hospital only)
  Doxorubicin 200mg/100ml solution for injection Cytosafe vials | 1 vial PoM £412.00 (Hospital only)
  Doxorubicin 200mg/100ml concentrate for solution for infusion vials | 1 vial PoM £234.66–£391.40 (Hospital only)
- Caelyx (Janssen-Cilag Ltd)
  Doxorubicin hydrochloride (as Doxorubicin hydrochloride liposomal pegylated) 2 mg per 1 ml Caelyx pegylated liposomal 50mg/25ml concentrate for solution for infusion vials | 1 vial PoM £712.49
  Caelyx pegylated liposomal 20mg/10ml concentrate for solution for infusion vials | 1 vial PoM £360.23

Epirubicin hydrochloride

18-Nov-2019

- **INDICATIONS AND DOSE**

Recurrent acute lymphoblastic leukaemia | Rhabdomyosarcoma | Other soft-tissue tumours of childhood

- BY INTRAVENOUS INFUSION
- Child: (consult local protocol)

- **UNLICENSED USE** Not licensed for use in children.
- **CONTRA-INDICATIONS** Myocardiopathy · previous treatment with maximum cumulative doses of epirubicin or other anthracycline · recent myocardial infarction · severe arrhythmia · severe myocardial insufficiency · unstable angina
- **CAUTIONS** Caution in handling—irritant to tissues
- **INTERACTIONS** → Appendix 1: anthracyclines
- **SIDE-EFFECTS**
- **Common or very common** Alopecia · amenorrhoea · anaemia · appetite decreased · arrhythmias · cardiac conduction disorders · chills · congestive heart failure · dehydration · diarrhoea · eye inflammation · fever · gastrointestinal discomfort · gastrointestinal disorders · haemorrhage · increased risk of infection · leucopenia · malaise · mucositis · nail discolouration · nausea · neutropenia · oral disorders · skin reactions · thrombocytopenia · urine discolouration · vasodilation · vomiting
- **Uncommon** Asthenia · embolism and thrombosis · sepsis
- **Rare or very rare** Hyperuricaemia
- **Frequency not known** Bone marrow depression · cardiomyopathy · cardiotoxicity · photosensitivity reaction · radiation injuries · shock

SIDE-EFFECTS, FURTHER INFORMATION **Cardiotoxicity** All anthracycline antibiotics have been associated with varying degrees of cardiac toxicity—this may be idiosyncratic and reversible, but is commonly related to total cumulative dose and is irreversible.

Cumulative doses of other anthracycline Epirubicin is considered less toxic than other anthracyline antibiotics, and may be suitable for children who have received high cumulative doses of other anthracyclines.

- **CONCEPTION AND CONTRACEPTION** Contraceptive advice required, see *Pregnancy and reproductive function* in Cytotoxic drugs p. 575.
- **PREGNANCY** Avoid (carcinogenic in *animal* studies). See also *Pregnancy and reproductive function* in Cytotoxic drugs p. 575.
- **BREAST FEEDING** Discontinue breast-feeding.
- **HEPATIC IMPAIRMENT** Manufacturer advises caution in mild to moderate impairment; avoid in severe impairment.
  Dose adjustments In adults, manufacturer advises dose reduction according to bilirubin level.
- **RENAL IMPAIRMENT**
  Dose adjustments Dose reduction may be necessary in severe impairment.
- **MONITORING REQUIREMENTS**
- Cardiac toxicity Cardiac function should be monitored before and at regular intervals throughout treatment and afterwards.

- **MEDICINAL FORMS** There can be variation in the licensing of different medicines containing the same drug. Forms available from special-order manufacturers include: solution for injection, solution for infusion

Solution for injection

- Epirubicin hydrochloride (Non-proprietary)
  Epirubicin hydrochloride 2 mg per 1 ml Epirubicin 10mg/5ml solution for injection vials | 1 vial PoM £20.18 (Hospital only) | 1 vial PoM £17.38
  Epirubicin 50mg/25ml solution for injection vials | 1 vial PoM £100.88 (Hospital only) | 1 vial PoM £86.89
- Pharmorubicin (Pfizer Ltd)
  Epirubicin hydrochloride 2 mg per 1 ml Pharmorubicin 50mg/25ml solution for injection Cytosafe vials | 1 vial PoM £106.19 (Hospital only)
  Pharmorubicin 10mg/5ml solution for injection Cytosafe vials | 1 vial PoM £21.24 (Hospital only)

Solution for infusion

- Epirubicin hydrochloride (Non-proprietary)
  Epirubicin hydrochloride 2 mg per 1 ml Epirubicin 200mg/100ml solution for infusion vials | 1 vial PoM £366.85 (Hospital only) | 1 vial PoM £306.20–£347.55
  Epirubicin 100mg/50ml solution for infusion vials | 1 vial PoM £201.76 (Hospital only)
- Pharmorubicin (Pfizer Ltd)
  Epirubicin hydrochloride 2 mg per 1 ml Pharmorubicin 200mg/100ml solution for infusion Cytosafe vials | 1 vial PoM £386.16 (Hospital only)

Mitoxantrone

18-Nov-2019

(Mitozantrone)

- **INDICATIONS AND DOSE**

Acute myeloid leukaemia | Recurrent acute lymphoblastic leukaemia

▸ BY INTRAVENOUS INFUSION

▸ Child: (consult local protocol)

- **UNLICENSED USE** Not licensed for use in children.
- **INTERACTIONS** → Appendix 1: anthracyclines
- **SIDE-EFFECTS** Abdominal pain · acute leukaemia · alopecia · amenorrhoea · anxiety · appetite decreased · arrhythmia · asthenia · bone marrow depression · confusion · constipation · diarrhoea · drowsiness · dyspnoea · fever · gastrointestinal haemorrhage · heart failure · mucositis · nail discolouration · nail dystrophy · nausea · neurological effects · paraesthesia · scleral discolouration · skin discolouration · stomatitis · thrombocytopenia · urine blue · vomiting

SIDE-EFFECTS, FURTHER INFORMATION All anthracycline antibiotics have been associated with varying degrees of cardiac toxicity—this may be idiosyncratic and reversible, but is commonly related to total cumulative dose and is irreversible.

- **CONCEPTION AND CONTRACEPTION** Manufacturer advises effective contraception during and for at least 6 months after treatment in men or women.
- **PREGNANCY** Avoid. See also *Pregnancy and reproductive function* in Cytotoxic drugs p. 575.
- **BREAST FEEDING** Discontinue breast-feeding.
- **HEPATIC IMPAIRMENT** Manufacturer advises caution (limited information available).

Dose adjustments Manufacturer advises consider dose reduction.

- **MONITORING REQUIREMENTS**

▸ Cardiac toxicity Cardiac function should be monitored before and at regular intervals throughout treatment and afterwards.

- **MEDICINAL FORMS** There can be variation in the licensing of different medicines containing the same drug.

Solution for infusion

▸ Mitoxantrone (Non-proprietary)

Mitoxantrone (as Mitoxantrone hydrochloride) 2 mg per 1 ml Mitoxantrone 20mg/10ml concentrate for solution for infusion vials | 1 vial PoM £51.43–£121.85 (Hospital only) | 1 vial PoM £51.43

▸ Onkotrone (Baxter Healthcare Ltd)

Mitoxantrone (as Mitoxantrone hydrochloride) 2 mg per 1 ml Onkotrone 20mg/10ml solution for infusion vials | 1 vial PoM £103.57

Onkotrone 25mg/12.5ml solution for infusion vials | 1 vial PoM £129.48

ANTINEOPLASTIC DRUGS > ANTIMETABOLITES

Clofarabine

02-Jul-2018

- **INDICATIONS AND DOSE**

Relapsed or refractory acute lymphoblastic leukaemia in patients who have received at least two previous regimens

▸ BY INTRAVENOUS INFUSION

▸ Child 1–17 years: (consult local protocol)

- **UNLICENSED USE** Not licensed for use in children under 1 year.
- **CAUTIONS** Cardiac disease
- **INTERACTIONS** → Appendix 1: clofarabine
- **SIDE-EFFECTS**

▸ **Common or very common** Alopecia · anxiety · appetite decreased · arthralgia · capillary leak syndrome · chills · cough · dehydration · diarrhoea · dizziness · drowsiness · dyspnoea · fatigue · feeling abnormal · feeling hot · fever · flushing · gastrointestinal discomfort · haemorrhage · headache · hearing impairment · hepatic disorders · hyperbilirubinaemia · hyperhidrosis · hypersensitivity · hypotension · increased risk of infection · irritability · mucositis · multi organ failure · myalgia · nausea · neutropenia · oedema · oral disorders · pain · paraesthesia · pericardial effusion · peripheral neuropathy · psychiatric disorder · renal impairment · respiratory disorders · sepsis · sinusoidal obstruction syndrome · skin reactions · systemic inflammatory response syndrome · tachycardia · tremor · tumour lysis syndrome · vomiting · weight decreased

▸ **Frequency not known** Antibiotic associated colitis · gastrointestinal disorders · hyponatraemia · pancreatitis · severe cutaneous adverse reactions (SCARs)

- **CONCEPTION AND CONTRACEPTION** Contraceptive advice required, see *Pregnancy and reproductive function* in Cytotoxic drugs p. 575.
- **PREGNANCY** Manufacturer advises avoid (teratogenic in *animal* studies). See also *Pregnancy and reproductive function* in Cytotoxic drugs p. 575.
- **BREAST FEEDING** Discontinue breast-feeding.
- **HEPATIC IMPAIRMENT** Manufacturer advises use with caution in mild-to-moderate impairment; avoid in severe impairment—no information available.
- **RENAL IMPAIRMENT** Manufacturer advises caution in mild to moderate impairment. Avoid in severe impairment.
- **MEDICINAL FORMS** There can be variation in the licensing of different medicines containing the same drug.

Solution for infusion

ELECTROLYTES: May contain Sodium

▸ Clofarabine (Non-proprietary)

Clofarabine 1 mg per 1 ml Clofarabine 20mg/20ml concentrate for solution for infusion vials | 1 vial PoM £1,326.18 (Hospital only)

▸ Evoltra (Sanofi) ▼

Clofarabine 1 mg per 1 ml Evoltra 20mg/20ml concentrate for solution for infusion vials | 1 vial PoM £1,326.18 (Hospital only)

Cytarabine

02-Dec-2019

- **DRUG ACTION** Cytarabine acts by interfering with pyrimidine synthesis.
- **INDICATIONS AND DOSE**

Acute lymphoblastic leukaemia | Acute myeloid leukaemia | Non-Hodgkin's lymphoma

▸ BY INTRAVENOUS INJECTION, OR BY INTRAVENOUS INFUSION, OR BY SUBCUTANEOUS INJECTION

▸ Child: (consult local protocol)

Meningeal leukaemia | Meningeal neoplasms

▸ BY INTRATHECAL INJECTION

▸ Child: (consult local protocol)

- **UNLICENSED USE** *Depocyte*® intrathecal injection not licensed for use in children.

IMPORTANT SAFETY INFORMATION
Not all cytarabine preparations can be given by intrathecal injection—consult product literature.

- **INTERACTIONS** → Appendix 1: cytarabine
- **SIDE-EFFECTS**

▸ **Common or very common** Alopecia · anaemia · appetite decreased · consciousness impaired · diarrhoea · dysarthria · dysphagia · eye disorders · eye inflammation · eye stinging · fever · gastrointestinal discomfort · gastrointestinal disorders · haemorrhagic conjunctivitis (consider

prophylactic corticosteroid eye drops) · hyperuricaemia · leucopenia · nausea · oral disorders · renal impairment · skin reactions · thrombocytopenia · urinary retention · vasculitis · vision disorders · vomiting
- **Uncommon** Arthralgia · dyspnoea · headache · increased risk of infection · myalgia · nerve disorders · pain · paralysis · pericarditis · sepsis · skin ulcer · throat pain
- **Rare or very rare** Arrhythmias
- **Frequency not known** Acute respiratory distress syndrome (ARDS) · amenorrhoea · ataxia · azoospermia · bone marrow disorders · cardiomyopathy · cerebellar dysfunction · chest pain · coma · confusion · cytarabine syndrome · dizziness · drowsiness · haemorrhage · hepatic disorders · hyperbilirubinaemia · neurotoxicity · neurotoxicity rash · neutropenia · pancreatitis · personality change · pulmonary oedema · reticulocytopenia · rhabdomyolysis · seizure · tremor

- **CONCEPTION AND CONTRACEPTION** Contraceptive advice required, see *Pregnancy and reproductive function* in Cytotoxic drugs p. 575.
- **PREGNANCY** Avoid (teratogenic in *animal* studies). See also *Pregnancy and reproductive function* in Cytotoxic drugs p. 575.
- **BREAST FEEDING** Discontinue breast-feeding.
- **HEPATIC IMPAIRMENT** Manufacturer advises caution (increased risk of CNS toxicity).
  Dose adjustments Manufacturer advises dose reduction—consult product literature.
- **RENAL IMPAIRMENT** Consult local treatment protocols.
- **MONITORING REQUIREMENTS**
  - Haematological monitoring Cytarabine is a potent myelosuppressant and requires careful haematological monitoring.
- **PRESCRIBING AND DISPENSING INFORMATION** Cytarabine is available as *conventional* and *liposomal* formulations. These different formulations vary in their licensed indications, pharmacokinetics, dosage and administration, and are **not** interchangeable.

  Dose is based on weight or body-surface area, children may tolerate higher doses of cytarabine than adults.

- **MEDICINAL FORMS** There can be variation in the licensing of different medicines containing the same drug. Forms available from special-order manufacturers include: solution for injection

Solution for injection

- Cytarabine (Non-proprietary)
  Cytarabine 20 mg per 1 ml Cytarabine 500mg/25ml solution for injection vials | 1 vial PoM £19.50
  Cytarabine 100mg/5ml solution for injection vials | 5 vial PoM £30.00 (Hospital only)
  Cytarabine 500mg/25ml solution for injection Cytosafe vials | 1 vial PoM £19.50 (Hospital only)
  Cytarabine 100 mg per 1 ml Cytarabine 1g/10ml solution for injection Cytosafe vials | 1 vial PoM £39.00 (Hospital only)
  Cytarabine 1g/10ml solution for injection vials | 1 vial PoM £37.05–£52.27 (Hospital only) | 1 vial PoM £39.00
  Cytarabine 500mg/5ml solution for injection vials | 5 vial PoM £89.78–£100.00 (Hospital only)
  Cytarabine 100mg/1ml solution for injection vials | 5 vial PoM £26.93 (Hospital only)
  Cytarabine 2g/20ml solution for injection Cytosafe vials | 1 vial PoM £77.50 (Hospital only)
  Cytarabine 2g/20ml solution for injection vials | 1 vial PoM £73.63–£103.87 (Hospital only) | 1 vial PoM £77.50

Fludarabine phosphate

- **INDICATIONS AND DOSE**

Poor prognosis or relapsed acute myeloid leukaemia | Relapsed acute lymphoblastic leukaemia | Conditioning before bone marrow transplantation

- BY MOUTH, OR BY INTRAVENOUS INJECTION, OR BY INTRAVENOUS INFUSION
  - Child: (consult local protocol)

- **UNLICENSED USE** Not licensed for use in children.

IMPORTANT SAFETY INFORMATION

RISKS OF INCORRECT DOSING OF ORAL ANTI-CANCER MEDICINES

See Cytotoxic drugs p. 575.

- **CONTRA-INDICATIONS** Haemolytic anaemia
- **CAUTIONS** Increased susceptibility to skin cancer · worsening of existing skin cancer
  CAUTIONS, FURTHER INFORMATION
  - Immunosuppression Fludarabine has a potent and prolonged immunosuppresive effect. Patients treated with fludarabine are more prone to serious bacterial, opportunistic fungal, and viral infections, and prophylactic therapy is recommended in those at risk. To prevent potentially fatal transfusion-related graft-versus-host reaction, only irradiated blood products should be administered. Prescribers should consult specialist literature when using highly immunosuppressive drugs.
- **INTERACTIONS** → Appendix 1: fludarabine
- **SIDE-EFFECTS**
  GENERAL SIDE-EFFECTS
  - **Common or very common** Anaemia · appetite decreased · asthenia · bone marrow depression (may be cumulative) · chills · cough · diarrhoea · fever · increased risk of infection · malaise · mucositis · nausea · neoplasms · nerve disorders · neutropenia · oedema · stomatitis · thrombocytopenia · vision disorders · vomiting
  - **Uncommon** Autoimmune disorder · confusion · dyspnoea · haemorrhage · respiratory disorders · tumour lysis syndrome
  - **Rare or very rare** Agitation · arrhythmia · coma · heart failure · seizure · severe cutaneous adverse reactions (SCARs)

  SPECIFIC SIDE-EFFECTS
  - **Common or very common**
    - With oral use Progressive multifocal leukoencephalopathy (PML) · skin reactions · viral infection reactivation
    - With parenteral use Rash
  - **Uncommon**
    - With oral use Acquired haemophilia · crystalluria · electrolyte imbalance · haemolytic anaemia · hyperuricaemia · metabolic acidosis · renal failure
  - **Frequency not known**
    - With parenteral use Encephalopathy · intracranial haemorrhage
- **CONCEPTION AND CONTRACEPTION** Manufacturer advises effective contraception during and for at least 6 months after treatment in men or women.
- **PREGNANCY** Avoid (embryotoxic and teratogenic in *animal* studies). See also *Pregnancy and reproductive function* in Cytotoxic drugs p. 575.
- **BREAST FEEDING** Discontinue breast-feeding.
- **RENAL IMPAIRMENT** Avoid if creatinine clearance less than 30 mL/minute/1.73 m^2.
  Dose adjustments Reduce dose by up to 50% if creatinine clearance 30–70 mL/minute/1.73 m^2.
- **MONITORING REQUIREMENTS**
  - Monitor for signs of haemolysis.
  - Monitor for neurological toxicity.

- **DIRECTIONS FOR ADMINISTRATION** Concentrate for intravenous injection or infusion must be diluted before administration (consult product literature).

- **MEDICINAL FORMS** There can be variation in the licensing of different medicines containing the same drug.

Solution for injection

- Fludarabine phosphate (Non-proprietary)

Fludarabine phosphate 25 mg per 1 ml Fludarabine phosphate 50mg/2ml concentrate for solution for injection vials | 1 vial PoM £155.00–£156.00 (Hospital only)

Tablet

- Fludara (Sanofi)

Fludarabine phosphate 10 mg Fludara 10mg tablets | 15 tablet PoM £302.48 (Hospital only) | 20 tablet PoM £403.31 (Hospital only)

Powder for solution for injection

- Fludarabine phosphate (Non-proprietary)

Fludarabine phosphate 50 mg Fludarabine phosphate 50mg powder for solution for injection vials | 1 vial PoM £155.00 (Hospital only)

- Fludara (Sanofi)

Fludarabine phosphate 50 mg Fludara 50mg powder for solution for injection vials | 5 vial PoM £735.34 (Hospital only)

Mercaptopurine

02-Dec-2019

(6-Mercaptopurine)

- **INDICATIONS AND DOSE**

Severe ulcerative colitis | Severe Crohn's disease

▶ BY MOUTH

- Child 2–17 years: Initially 1–1.5 mg/kg once daily (max. per dose 50 mg), then increased if necessary up to 75 mg once daily

Acute lymphoblastic leukaemia | Lymphoblastic lymphomas

▶ BY MOUTH

- Child: (consult local protocol)

DOSE ADJUSTMENTS DUE TO INTERACTIONS

- Manufacturer advises reduce dose to one-quarter of the usual dose with concurrent use of allopurinol.

DOSE EQUIVALENCE AND CONVERSION

- Mercaptopurine tablets and *Xaluprine®* oral suspension are **not** bioequivalent, haematological monitoring is advised when switching formulations.

- **UNLICENSED USE** Not licensed for use in severe ulcerative colitis and Crohn's disease.

Not licensed for use in children for acute lymphoblastic lymphoma or T-cell non-Hodgkins lymphoma.

> IMPORTANT SAFETY INFORMATION
>
> SAFE PRACTICE
>
> Mercaptopurine has been confused with mercaptamine; care must be taken to ensure the correct drug is prescribed and dispensed.
>
> RISKS OF INCORRECT DOSING OF ORAL ANTI-CANCER MEDICINES
>
> See Cytotoxic drugs p. 575.

- **CONTRA-INDICATIONS** Absent thiopurine methyltransferase activity
- **CAUTIONS** Reduced thiopurine methyltransferase activity

CAUTIONS, FURTHER INFORMATION

- Thiopurine methyltransferase The enzyme thiopurine methyltransferase (TPMT) metabolises thiopurine drugs (azathioprine, mercaptopurine, tioguanine); the risk of myelosuppression is increased in patients with reduced activity of the enzyme, particularly for the few individuals in whom TPMT activity is undetectable. Patients with absent TPMT activity should not receive thiopurine drugs; those with reduced TPMT activity may be treated under specialist supervision.

- **INTERACTIONS** → Appendix 1: mercaptopurine
- **SIDE-EFFECTS**
- **Common or very common** Anaemia · appetite decreased · bone marrow depression · diarrhoea · hepatic disorders · hepatotoxicity (more common at high doses) · leucopenia · nausea · oral disorders · pancreatitis · thrombocytopenia · vomiting
- **Uncommon** Arthralgia · fever · increased risk of infection · neutropenia · rash
- **Rare or very rare** Alopecia · face oedema · intestinal ulcer · neoplasms · oligozoospermia
- **Frequency not known** Hypoglycaemia · photosensitivity reaction

- **CONCEPTION AND CONTRACEPTION** Contraceptive advice required, see *Pregnancy and reproductive function* in Cytotoxic drugs p. 575.
- **PREGNANCY** Avoid (teratogenic). See also *Pregnancy and reproductive function* in Cytotoxic drugs p. 575.
- **BREAST FEEDING** Discontinue breast-feeding.
- **HEPATIC IMPAIRMENT** Manufacturer advises caution (risk of increased exposure).

Dose adjustments Manufacturer advises consider dose reduction.

- **RENAL IMPAIRMENT**

Dose adjustments Manufacturer advises consider reducing dose.

- **PRE-TREATMENT SCREENING** Consider measuring thiopurine methyltransferase (TPMT) activity before starting mercaptopurine therapy.
- **MONITORING REQUIREMENTS**
- Monitor liver function—discontinue if jaundice develops.
- When used for Severe ulcerative colitis or Severe Crohn's disease Monitor for toxicity throughout treatment. Monitor full blood count weekly (more frequently with higher doses or if severe hepatic or renal impairment) for first 4 weeks (manufacturer advises weekly monitoring for 8 weeks but evidence of practical value unsatisfactory), thereafter reduce frequency of monitoring to at least every 3 months.

- **PRESCRIBING AND DISPENSING INFORMATION** Flavours of oral liquid formulations may include raspberry.

- **MEDICINAL FORMS** There can be variation in the licensing of different medicines containing the same drug. Forms available from special-order manufacturers include: tablet, capsule, oral suspension

Oral suspension

EXCIPIENTS: May contain Aspartame

- Xaluprine (Nova Laboratories Ltd)

Mercaptopurine 20 mg per 1 ml Xaluprine 20mg/ml oral suspension | 100 ml PoM £170.00 DT = £170.00

Tablet

- Mercaptopurine (Non-proprietary)

Mercaptopurine 10 mg Mercaptopurine 10mg tablets | 100 tablet PoM 🅂

Mercaptopurine 50 mg Mercaptopurine 50mg tablets | 25 tablet PoM £49.15 DT = £49.15

Hanixol 50mg tablets | 25 tablet PoM £34.39 DT = £49.15

Methotrexate

25-Jul-2019

- **DRUG ACTION** Methotrexate inhibits the enzyme dihydrofolate reductase, essential for the synthesis of purines and pyrimidines.

- **INDICATIONS AND DOSE**

Severe Crohn's disease

▶ BY SUBCUTANEOUS INJECTION, OR BY INTRAMUSCULAR INJECTION

▸ Child 7–17 years: 15 mg/m^2 once weekly (max. per dose 25 mg)

Maintenance of remission of severe Crohn's disease

▶ BY MOUTH, OR BY SUBCUTANEOUS INJECTION, OR BY INTRAMUSCULAR INJECTION

▸ Child 7–17 years: 15 mg/m^2 once weekly (max. per dose 25 mg), dose reduced according to response to lowest effective dose

Juvenile idiopathic arthritis | Juvenile dermatomyositis | Vasculitis | Uveitis | Systemic lupus erythematosus | Localised scleroderma | Sarcoidosis

▶ BY MOUTH, OR BY SUBCUTANEOUS INJECTION, OR BY INTRAMUSCULAR INJECTION

▸ Child: Initially 10–15 mg/m^2 once weekly, then increased if necessary up to 25 mg/m^2 once weekly

Maintenance and remission of acute lymphoblastic leukaemia, lymphoblastic lymphoma

▶ BY MOUTH

▸ Child: (consult local protocol)

Treatment of early stage Burkitt's lymphoma, non-Hodgkin's lymphoma, osteogenic sarcoma, some CNS tumours including infant brain tumours, acute lymphoblastic leukaemia

▶ BY INTRAVENOUS INJECTION, OR BY INTRAVENOUS INFUSION

▸ Child: (consult local protocol)

Meningeal leukaemia, treatment and prevention of CNS involvement of leukaemia

▶ BY INTRATHECAL INJECTION

▸ Child: (consult local protocol)

Severe psoriasis unresponsive to conventional therapy (specialist use only)

▶ BY MOUTH

▸ Child 2–17 years: Initially 200 micrograms/kg once weekly (max. per dose 10 mg), then increased if necessary to 400 micrograms/kg once weekly (max. per dose 25 mg), adjusted according to response, stop treatment if inadequate response after 3 months at the optimum dose

- **UNLICENSED USE** *Metoject*® is licensed for use in children over 3 years for polyarticular forms of juvenile idiopathic arthritis; other preparations not licensed for use in children for non-malignant conditions.

IMPORTANT SAFETY INFORMATION

NHS NEVER EVENT: OVERDOSE OF METHOTREXATE FOR NON-CANCER TREATMENT (JANUARY 2018)

Patients given methotrexate, by any route, for non-cancer treatment should not be given more than their intended weekly dose.

WEEKLY DOSING

Note that the dose is a **weekly** dose. To avoid error with low-dose methotrexate, it is recommended that:

- the child or their carer is carefully advised of the **dose** and **frequency** and the reason for taking methotrexate and any other prescribed medication (e.g. folic acid);
- only one strength of methotrexate tablet (usually 2.5 mg) is prescribed and dispensed;
- the prescription and the dispensing label clearly show the dose and frequency of methotrexate administration;
- the child or their carer is warned to report immediately the onset of any feature of blood disorders (e.g. sore throat, bruising, and mouth ulcers), liver toxicity (e.g. nausea, vomiting, abdominal discomfort, and dark urine), and respiratory effects (e.g. shortness of breath).

- **CONTRA-INDICATIONS** Active infection · ascites · immunodeficiency syndromes · significant pleural effusion
- **CAUTIONS** Photosensitivity—psoriasis lesions aggravated by UV radiation (skin ulceration reported) · diarrhoea · extreme caution in blood disorders (avoid if severe) · peptic ulceration · risk of accumulation in pleural effusion or ascites— drain before treatment · ulcerative colitis · ulcerative stomatitis

CAUTIONS, FURTHER INFORMATION

▸ Blood count Bone marrow suppression can occur abruptly; factors likely to increase toxicity include advanced age, renal impairment, and concomitant use with another anti-folate drug (e.g. trimethoprim). A clinically significant drop in white cell count or platelet count calls for immediate withdrawal of methotrexate and introduction of supportive therapy.

▸ Gastro-intestinal toxicity Withdraw treatment if stomatitis develops—may be first sign of gastro-intestinal toxicity.

▸ Liver toxicity Persistent 2–fold rise in liver transaminases may necessitate dose reduction or rarely discontinuation; abrupt withdrawal should be avoided as this can lead to disease flare.

▸ Pulmonary toxicity Acute pulmonary toxicity is rare in children treated for juvenile idiopathic arthritis, but children and carers should seek medical attention if dyspnoea, cough or fever develops; discontinue if pneumonitis suspected.

- **INTERACTIONS** → Appendix 1: methotrexate
- **SIDE-EFFECTS**

▶ **Common or very common**

▸ With intrathecal use Necrotising demyelinating leukoencephalopathy · neurotoxicity

▸ With oral use Anaemia · appetite decreased · diarrhoea · drowsiness · fatigue · gastrointestinal discomfort · headache · increased risk of infection · leucopenia · nausea · oral disorders · respiratory disorders · skin reactions · throat ulcer · thrombocytopenia · vomiting

▸ With parenteral use Anaemia · appetite decreased · chest pain · cough · diarrhoea · drowsiness · dyspnoea · fatigue · fever · gastrointestinal discomfort · headache · leucopenia · malaise · nausea · oral disorders · respiratory disorders · skin reactions · throat complaints · thrombocytopenia · vomiting

▶ **Uncommon**

▸ With oral use Agranulocytosis · alopecia · arthralgia · bone marrow disorders · chills · confusion · cystitis · depression · diabetes mellitus · dysuria · fever · gastrointestinal disorders · haemorrhage · healing impaired · hepatic disorders · myalgia · neoplasms · nephropathy · osteoporosis · photosensitivity reaction · rheumatoid arthritis aggravated · seizure · severe cutaneous adverse reactions (SCARs) · vasculitis · vertigo · vulvovaginal disorders

▸ With parenteral use Agranulocytosis · alopecia · arthralgia · bone marrow disorders · confusion · cystitis · depression · diabetes mellitus · drug toxicity · dysuria · gastrointestinal disorders · haemorrhage · healing impaired · hepatic disorders · increased risk of infection · lipoatrophy · local reaction · myalgia · neoplasms · osteoporosis · pain · paraesthesia · photosensitivity reaction · rheumatoid arthritis aggravated · seizure · severe cutaneous adverse reactions (SCARs) · sterile abscess · vasculitis · vertigo · vulvovaginal disorders

- **Rare or very rare**
- With oral use Azotaemia · brain oedema · cognitive impairment · conjunctivitis · cough · dyspnoea · eosinophilia · gynaecomastia · hypotension · immune deficiency · infertility · insomnia · lymphadenopathy · meningitis aseptic · menstrual disorder · mood altered · muscle weakness · nail discolouration · neutropenia · oligozoospermia · pain · pancreatitis · paresis · pericardial disorders · pericarditis · proteinuria · psychosis · radiation injuries · renal impairment · retinopathy · sensation abnormal · sepsis · sexual dysfunction · speech impairment · stress fracture · taste metallic · telangiectasia · tinnitus · visual impairment
- With parenteral use Apnoea · asthma-like conditions · azotaemia · conjunctivitis · embolism and thrombosis · eosinophilia · gynaecomastia · hypotension · immune deficiency · infertility · influenza like illness · insomnia · lymphadenopathy · meningism · meningitis aseptic · menstrual disorder · mood altered · muscle weakness · nail discolouration · necrosis · neutropenia · paralysis · pericardial disorders · pericarditis · proteinuria · reactivation of infection · renal impairment · retinopathy · sepsis · sexual dysfunction · sperm abnormalities · stress fracture · taste altered · telangiectasia · vision disorders
- **Frequency not known**
- With oral use Encephalopathy
- With parenteral use Aphasia · chills · cognitive disorder · defective oogenesis · dizziness · hemiparesis · leukoencephalopathy · metabolic change · mucositis · nephropathy · pancreatitis · pulmonary oedema · skin ulcer · sudden death · tinnitus

SIDE-EFFECTS, FURTHER INFORMATION Give folic acid to reduce side-effects. Folic acid decreases mucosal and gastrointestinal side-effects of methotrexate and may prevent hepatotoxicity; there is no evidence of a reduction in haematological side-effects.

Withdraw treatment if ulcerative stomatitis develops—may be first sign of gastro-intestinal toxicity.

Treatment with folinic acid (as calcium folinate) may be required in acute toxicity.

- **CONCEPTION AND CONTRACEPTION** Manufacturer advises effective contraception during and for at least 6 months after treatment in men and women.
- **PREGNANCY** Avoid (teratogenic; fertility may be reduced during therapy but this may be reversible).
- **BREAST FEEDING** Discontinue breast-feeding—present in milk.
- **HEPATIC IMPAIRMENT** When used for malignancy, avoid in severe hepatic impairment—consult local treatment protocol for details. Avoid with hepatic impairment in non-malignant conditions—dose-related toxicity.
- **RENAL IMPAIRMENT** Risk of nephrotoxicity at high doses. Avoid in severe impairment.

Dose adjustments Reduce dose.

- **PRE-TREATMENT SCREENING** Exclude pregnancy before treatment.

Patients should have full blood count and renal and liver function tests before starting treatment.

Check immunity to varicella-zoster and consider vaccination before initiating therapy.

- **MONITORING REQUIREMENTS** Full blood count and liver function tests repeated fortnightly for at least the first 4 weeks of treatment and at this frequency after any change in dose until therapy stabilised, thereafter monthly; renal function tests should be performed regularly during treatment.
- **PRESCRIBING AND DISPENSING INFORMATION** Folinic acid following methotrexate administration helps to prevent methotrexate-induced mucositis and myelosuppression.

The licensed routes of administration for parenteral preparations vary—further information can be found in the product literature for the individual preparations.

- **PATIENT AND CARER ADVICE** Patients and their carers should be warned to report immediately the onset of any feature of blood disorders (e.g. sore throat, bruising, and mouth ulcers), liver toxicity (e.g. nausea, vomiting, abdominal discomfort and dark urine), and respiratory effects (e.g. shortness of breath).

Children and carers should be advised to avoid self-medication with over-the-counter ibuprofen

Children and their carers should be counselled on the dose and use of NSAIDs.

Medicines for Children leaflet: Methotrexate for skin conditions www.medicinesforchildren.org.uk/methotrexate-skin-conditions

- **MEDICINAL FORMS** There can be variation in the licensing of different medicines containing the same drug. Forms available from special-order manufacturers include: oral suspension, oral solution, solution for injection

Tablet

- Methotrexate (Non-proprietary)

Methotrexate 2.5 mg Methotrexate 2.5mg tablets | 24 tablet PoM £1.29–£3.75 | 28 tablet PoM £3.82 DT = £2.34 | 100 tablet PoM £5.39–£14.10

Methotrexate 10 mg Methotrexate 10mg tablets | 100 tablet PoM £55.74 DT = £52.64

- Maxtrex (Pfizer Ltd)

Methotrexate 2.5 mg Maxtrex 2.5mg tablets | 24 tablet PoM £2.39 | 100 tablet PoM £9.96

Methotrexate 10 mg Maxtrex 10mg tablets | 100 tablet PoM £45.16 DT = £52.64

Solution for injection

- Methotrexate (Non-proprietary)

Methotrexate (as Methotrexate sodium) 2.5 mg per 1 ml Methotrexate 5mg/2ml solution for injection vials | 5 vial PoM £36.00 (Hospital only)

Methotrexate (as Methotrexate sodium) 25 mg per 1 ml Methotrexate 500mg/20ml solution for injection vials | 1 vial PoM £48.00–£726.28 (Hospital only)
Methotrexate 50mg/2ml solution for injection vials | 1 vial PoM £72.63 (Hospital only) | 5 vial PoM £35.00 (Hospital only)

Methotrexate (as Methotrexate sodium) 100 mg per 1 ml Methotrexate 1g/10ml solution for injection vials | 1 vial PoM £85.00 (Hospital only) | 1 vial PoM £80.75

- Methofill (Accord Healthcare Ltd)

Methotrexate 50 mg per 1 ml Methofill 12.5mg/0.25ml solution for injection pre-filled injector | 1 pre-filled disposable injection PoM £14.34 DT = £14.35
Methofill 22.5mg/0.45ml solution for injection pre-filled injector | 1 pre-filled disposable injection PoM £16.10 DT = £16.11
Methofill 30mg/0.6ml solution for injection pre-filled injector | 1 pre-filled disposable injection PoM £16.55 DT = £16.56
Methofill 27.5mg/0.55ml solution for injection pre-filled injector | 1 pre-filled disposable injection PoM £16.49 DT = £16.50
Methofill 7.5mg/0.15ml solution for injection pre-filled injector | 1 pre-filled disposable injection PoM £12.86 DT = £12.87
Methofill 20mg/0.4ml solution for injection pre-filled injector | 1 pre-filled disposable injection PoM £15.55 DT = £15.56
Methofill 10mg/0.2ml solution for injection pre-filled injector | 1 pre-filled disposable injection PoM £13.25 DT = £13.26
Methofill 15mg/0.3ml solution for injection pre-filled injector | 1 pre-filled disposable injection PoM £14.40 DT = £14.41
Methofill 17.5mg/0.35ml solution for injection pre-filled injector | 1 pre-filled disposable injection PoM £15.24 DT = £15.25
Methofill 25mg/0.5ml solution for injection pre-filled injector | 1 pre-filled disposable injection PoM £16.12 DT = £16.13

Methotrexate (as Methotrexate sodium) 50 mg per 1 ml Methofill 15mg/0.3ml solution for injection pre-filled syringes | 1 pre-filled disposable injection PoM £12.40
Methofill 25mg/0.5ml solution for injection pre-filled syringes | 1 pre-filled disposable injection PoM £14.24
Methofill 10mg/0.2ml solution for injection pre-filled syringes | 1 pre-filled disposable injection PoM £11.25
Methofill 7.5mg/0.15ml solution for injection pre-filled syringes | 1 pre-filled disposable injection PoM £10.86
Methofill 17.5mg/0.35ml solution for injection pre-filled syringes | 1 pre-filled disposable injection PoM £13.24

Methofill 27.5mg/0.55ml solution for injection pre-filled syringes | 1 pre-filled disposable injection PoM £14.49
Methofill 22.5mg/0.45ml solution for injection pre-filled syringes | 1 pre-filled disposable injection PoM £14.10
Methofill 12.5mg/0.25ml solution for injection pre-filled syringes | 1 pre-filled disposable injection PoM £12.34
Methofill 20mg/0.4ml solution for injection pre-filled syringes | 1 pre-filled disposable injection PoM £13.55
Methofill 30mg/0.6ml solution for injection pre-filled syringes | 1 pre-filled disposable injection PoM £14.55

▸ Metoject PEN (medac UK)
Methotrexate 50 mg per 1 ml Metoject PEN 27.5mg/0.55ml solution for injection pre-filled pens | 1 pre-filled disposable injection PoM £16.50 DT = £16.50
Metoject PEN 17.5mg/0.35ml solution for injection pre-filled pens | 1 pre-filled disposable injection PoM £15.25 DT = £15.25
Metoject PEN 30mg/0.6ml solution for injection pre-filled pens | 1 pre-filled disposable injection PoM £16.56 DT = £16.56
Metoject PEN 12.5mg/0.25ml solution for injection pre-filled pens | 1 pre-filled disposable injection PoM £14.35 DT = £14.35
Metoject PEN 10mg/0.2ml solution for injection pre-filled pens | 1 pre-filled disposable injection PoM £13.26 DT = £13.26
Metoject PEN 15mg/0.3ml solution for injection pre-filled pens | 1 pre-filled disposable injection PoM £14.41 DT = £14.41
Metoject PEN 22.5mg/0.45ml solution for injection pre-filled pens | 1 pre-filled disposable injection PoM £16.11 DT = £16.11
Metoject PEN 7.5mg/0.15ml solution for injection pre-filled pens | 1 pre-filled disposable injection PoM £12.87 DT = £12.87
Metoject PEN 25mg/0.5ml solution for injection pre-filled pens | 1 pre-filled disposable injection PoM £16.13 DT = £16.13
Metoject PEN 20mg/0.4ml solution for injection pre-filled pens | 1 pre-filled disposable injection PoM £15.56 DT = £15.56

▸ Nordimet (Nordic Pharma Ltd)
Methotrexate 25 mg per 1 ml Nordimet 15mg/0.6ml solution for injection pre-filled pens | 1 pre-filled disposable injection PoM £14.92 DT = £14.92
Nordimet 20mg/0.8ml solution for injection pre-filled pens | 1 pre-filled disposable injection PoM £16.06 DT = £16.06
Nordimet 22.5mg/0.9ml solution for injection pre-filled pens | 1 pre-filled disposable injection PoM £16.61 DT = £16.61
Nordimet 12.5mg/0.5ml solution for injection pre-filled pens | 1 pre-filled disposable injection PoM £14.85 DT = £14.85
Nordimet 10mg/0.4ml solution for injection pre-filled pens | 1 pre-filled disposable injection PoM £13.77 DT = £13.77
Nordimet 17.5mg/0.7ml solution for injection pre-filled pens | 1 pre-filled disposable injection PoM £15.75 DT = £15.75
Nordimet 25mg/1ml solution for injection pre-filled pens | 1 pre-filled disposable injection PoM £16.64 DT = £16.64
Nordimet 7.5mg/0.3ml solution for injection pre-filled pens | 1 pre-filled disposable injection PoM £13.37 DT = £13.37

▸ Zlatal (Nordic Pharma Ltd)
Methotrexate (as Methotrexate sodium) 25 mg per 1 ml Zlatal 17.5mg/0.7ml solution for injection pre-filled syringes | 1 pre-filled disposable injection PoM £15.75 DT = £15.75
Zlatal 10mg/0.4ml solution for injection pre-filled syringes | 1 pre-filled disposable injection PoM £13.77 DT = £13.77
Zlatal 25mg/1ml solution for injection pre-filled syringes | 1 pre-filled disposable injection PoM £16.64 DT = £16.64
Zlatal 20mg/0.8ml solution for injection pre-filled syringes | 1 pre-filled disposable injection PoM £16.06 DT = £16.06
Zlatal 12.5mg/0.5ml solution for injection pre-filled syringes | 1 pre-filled disposable injection PoM £14.85 DT = £14.85
Zlatal 7.5mg/0.3ml solution for injection pre-filled syringes | 1 pre-filled disposable injection PoM £13.37 DT = £13.37
Zlatal 22.5mg/0.9ml solution for injection pre-filled syringes | 1 pre-filled disposable injection PoM £16.61 DT = £16.61
Zlatal 15mg/0.6ml solution for injection pre-filled syringes | 1 pre-filled disposable injection PoM £14.92 DT = £14.92

Solution for infusion

▸ Methotrexate (Non-proprietary)
Methotrexate (as Methotrexate sodium) 100 mg per 1 ml Methotrexate 5g/50ml solution for infusion vials | 1 vial PoM £400.00 (Hospital only) | 1 vial PoM £380.00

Oral solution

▸ Methotrexate (Non-proprietary)
Methotrexate (as Methotrexate sodium) 2 mg per 1 ml Methotrexate 2mg/ml oral solution sugar free sugar-free | 35 ml PoM £114.00 DT = £95.00 sugar-free | 65 ml PoM £125.00 DT = £125.00

▸ Jylamvo (Intrapharm Laboratories Ltd)
Methotrexate (as Methotrexate sodium) 2 mg per 1 ml Jylamvo 2mg/ml oral solution sugar-free | 60 ml PoM £112.50

8 Immune system and malignant disease

Nelarabine

24-Jul-2018

● **INDICATIONS AND DOSE**

T-cell acute lymphoblastic leukaemia and T-cell lymphoblastic lymphoma in children who have relapsed or who are refractory after receiving at least two previous regimens

▸ BY INTRAVENOUS INFUSION
▸ Child: (consult local protocol)

● **CAUTIONS** Previous or concurrent craniospinal irradiation (increased risk of neurotoxicity) · previous or concurrent intrathecal chemotherapy (increased risk of neurotoxicity)

● **INTERACTIONS** → Appendix 1: nelarabine

● **SIDE-EFFECTS**

▸ **Common or very common** Anaemia · arthralgia · asthenia · ataxia · confusion · constipation · diarrhoea · drowsiness · electrolyte imbalance · fever · headache · hyperbilirubinaemia · hypoglycaemia · increased risk of infection · leucopenia · nausea · neutropenia · pain in extremity · peripheral neuropathy · seizures · sensation abnormal · sepsis · stomatitis · thrombocytopenia · tremor · vomiting

▸ **Rare or very rare** Rhabdomyolysis

SIDE-EFFECTS, FURTHER INFORMATION If neurotoxicity occurs, treatment should be discontinued.

● **CONCEPTION AND CONTRACEPTION** Manufacturer advises effective contraception during and for at least 3 months after treatment in men and women.

● **PREGNANCY** Avoid (toxicity in *animal* studies). See also *Pregnancy and reproductive function* in Cytotoxic drugs p. 575.

● **BREAST FEEDING** Discontinue breast-feeding.

● **MONITORING REQUIREMENTS**

▸ Neurotoxicity Close monitoring for neurological events is strongly recommended—discontinue if neurotoxicty occurs.

● **PATIENT AND CARER ADVICE**

Driving and skilled tasks Drowsiness may affect performance of skilled tasks (e.g. cycling or driving).

● **NATIONAL FUNDING/ACCESS DECISIONS**

Scottish Medicines Consortium (SMC) decisions

The *Scottish Medicines Consortium* has advised (April 2008) that the use of nelarabine (*Atriance*®) within NHS Scotland is restricted to bridging treatment before stem cell transplantation and restricted to use by haemato-oncology specialists.

● **MEDICINAL FORMS** There can be variation in the licensing of different medicines containing the same drug.

Solution for infusion

ELECTROLYTES: May contain Sodium

▸ Atriance (Novartis Pharmaceuticals UK Ltd) ▼
Nelarabine 5 mg per 1 ml Atriance 250mg/50ml solution for infusion vials | 6 vial PoM £1,332.00

Tioguanine
(Thioguanine)

● **INDICATIONS AND DOSE**

Infant acute lymphoblastic leukaemia

▸ BY MOUTH
▸ Child: Can be given at various stages of treatment in short-term cycles (consult local protocol)

IMPORTANT SAFETY INFORMATION

RISKS OF INCORRECT DOSING OF ORAL ANTI-CANCER MEDICINES
See Cytotoxic drugs p. 575.

- **CONTRA-INDICATIONS** Absent thiopurine methyltransferase activity
- **CAUTIONS** Thiopurine methyltransferase status

CAUTIONS, FURTHER INFORMATION

- ▸ **Thiopurine methyltransferase** The enzyme thiopurine methyltransferase (TPMT) metabolises thiopurine drugs (azathioprine, mercaptopurine, tioguanine); the risk of myelosuppression is increased in patients with reduced activity of the enzyme, particularly for the few individuals in whom TPMT activity is undetectable. Patients with absent TPMT activity should not receive thiopurine drugs; those with reduced TPMT activity may be treated under specialist supervision.
- ▸ **Long-term therapy** Long-term therapy is no longer recommended because of the high risk of liver toxicity.
- **INTERACTIONS** → Appendix 1: tioguanine
- **SIDE-EFFECTS**
- ▸ **Common or very common** Bone marrow failure · gastrointestinal disorders · hepatic disorders · hyperbilirubinaemia · hyperuricaemia · hyperuricosuria · nodular regenerative hyperplasia · oesophageal varices · sinusoidal obstruction syndrome · splenomegaly · stomatitis · thrombocytopenia · uric acid nephropathy · weight increased
- ▸ **Frequency not known** Photosensitivity reaction
- **CONCEPTION AND CONTRACEPTION** Ensure effective contraception during treatment in men or women.
- **PREGNANCY** Avoid (teratogenicity reported when men receiving tioguanine have fathered children). See also *Pregnancy and reproductive function* in Cytotoxic drugs p. 575.
- **BREAST FEEDING** Discontinue breast-feeding.
- **HEPATIC IMPAIRMENT** Manufacturer advises caution.

  Dose adjustments Manufacturer advises consider dose reduction.
- **RENAL IMPAIRMENT**

  Dose adjustments Reduce dose.
- **PRE-TREATMENT SCREENING** Consider measuring thiopurine methyltransferase (TPMT) activity before starting tioguanine therapy.
- **MONITORING REQUIREMENTS** Monitor liver function weekly—discontinue if liver toxicity develops.

- **MEDICINAL FORMS** There can be variation in the licensing of different medicines containing the same drug. Forms available from special-order manufacturers include: capsule

Tablet

▸ Tioguanine (Non-proprietary)

Tioguanine 40 mg Tioguanine 40mg tablets | 25 tablet [PoM] £109.57 DT = £109.57

ANTINEOPLASTIC DRUGS › CYTOTOXIC ANTIBIOTICS AND RELATED SUBSTANCES

Bleomycin

- **INDICATIONS AND DOSE**

Some germ cell tumours | Hodgkin's lymphoma

▸ BY INTRAVENOUS INFUSION

▸ Child: (consult local protocol)

- **UNLICENSED USE** Not licensed for use in children.
- **CONTRA-INDICATIONS** Acute pulmonary infection · significantly reduced lung function
- **CAUTIONS** Caution in handling—irritant to tissues
- **INTERACTIONS** → Appendix 1: bleomycin
- **SIDE-EFFECTS**
- ▸ **Common or very common** Alopecia · angular stomatitis · appetite decreased · chills · fever (after administration) · haemorrhage · headache · interstitial pneumonia · leucopenia · malaise · nail discolouration · nail disorder · nausea · pain · pulmonary fibrosis (dose-related) · scleroderma · skin reactions · stomatitis · vomiting · weight decreased
- ▸ **Uncommon** Diarrhoea · dizziness · hepatocellular injury · oliguria · shock · urinary disorders · vein wall hypertrophy · venous stenosis
- **CONCEPTION AND CONTRACEPTION** Contraceptive advice required, see *Pregnancy and reproductive function* in Cytotoxic drugs p. 575.
- **PREGNANCY** Avoid (teratogenic and carcinogenic in *animal* studies). See also *Pregnancy and reproductive function* in Cytotoxic drugs p. 575
- **BREAST FEEDING** Discontinue breast feeding.
- **RENAL IMPAIRMENT**

  Dose adjustments Reduce dose—consult local treatment protocol for details.
- **MONITORING REQUIREMENTS** Ensure monitoring of pulmonary function—investigate any shortness of breath before initiation.
- **PRESCRIBING AND DISPENSING INFORMATION** To conform to the European Pharmacopoeia vials previously labelled as containing '15 units' of bleomycin are now labelled as containing 15 000 units. The amount of bleomycin in the vial has not changed.

- **MEDICINAL FORMS** There can be variation in the licensing of different medicines containing the same drug.

Powder for solution for injection

▸ Bleo-Kyowa (Kyowa Kirin Ltd)

Bleomycin (as Bleomycin sulfate) 15000 unit Bleo-Kyowa 15,000unit powder for solution for injection vials | 10 vial [PoM] £190.60

Dactinomycin

(Actinomycin D)

- **INDICATIONS AND DOSE**

Wilms' tumour | Childhood rhabdomyosarcoma and other soft-tissue sarcomas | Ewing's sarcoma

▸ BY INTRAVENOUS INJECTION

▸ Child: (consult local protocol)

- **UNLICENSED USE** Not licensed for use in children under 12 years.
- **CAUTIONS** Caution in handling—irritant to tissues
- **INTERACTIONS** → Appendix 1: dactinomycin
- **SIDE-EFFECTS** Agranulocytosis · alopecia · anaemia · appetite decreased · ascites · bone marrow disorders · diarrhoea · dysphagia · fatigue · fever · gastrointestinal discomfort · gastrointestinal disorders · growth retardation · healing impaired · hepatic disorders · hypocalcaemia · increased risk of infection · lethargy · leucopenia · leukaemia secondary · malaise · myalgia · nausea · neutropenia · oedema · oral disorders · pneumonitis · renal impairment · reticulocytopenia · secondary neoplasm · sepsis · severe cutaneous adverse reactions (SCARs) · sinusoidal obstruction syndrome · skin reactions · soft tissue damage · thrombocytopenia · tumour lysis syndrome · venous thrombosis · vomiting
- **CONCEPTION AND CONTRACEPTION** Exclude pregnancy before treatment with cytotoxic drugs. Contraceptive advice should be given to men and women before cytotoxic therapy begins (and should cover the duration of contraception required after therapy has ended). Regimens that do not contain an alkylating drug or procarbazine may have less effect on fertility, but those with an alkylating drug or procarbazine carry the risk of causing permanent male sterility (there is no effect on potency). Pretreatment counselling and consideration of sperm storage may be

appropriate. Women are less severely affected, though the span of reproductive life may be shortened by the onset of a premature menopause. No increase in fetal abnormalities or abortion rate has been recorded in patients who remain fertile after cytotoxic chemotherapy.

- **PREGNANCY** Avoid (teratogenic in *animal* studies). Most cytotoxic drugs are teratogenic and should not be administered during pregnancy, especially during the first trimester. Considerable caution is necessary if a pregnant woman presents with cancer requiring chemotherapy, and specialist advice should always be sought.
- **BREAST FEEDING** Discontinue breast-feeding.
- **HEPATIC IMPAIRMENT**
Dose adjustments Consider dose reduction if raised serum bilirubin or biliary obstruction; consult local treatment protocols.

- **MEDICINAL FORMS** There can be variation in the licensing of different medicines containing the same drug.

Powder for solution for injection

▸ Cosmegen (Recordati Rare Diseases UK Ltd)
Dactinomycin 500 microgram Cosmegen Lyovac 500microgram powder for solution for injection vials | 1 vial [PoM] £52.58

ANTINEOPLASTIC DRUGS > PLATINUM COMPOUNDS

Carboplatin

08-Mar-2019

- **INDICATIONS AND DOSE**

Stage 4 neuroblastoma | Germ cell tumours | Low-grade gliomas (including astrocytomas) | Neuroectodermal tumours (including medulloblastoma) | Rhabdomyosarcoma (metastatic and non-metastatic disease) | Soft-tissue sarcomas | Retinoblastoma | High risk Wilms' tumour | Some liver tumours

▸ BY INTRAVENOUS INFUSION
▸ Child: (consult local protocol)

- **UNLICENSED USE** Not licensed for use in children.
- **INTERACTIONS** → Appendix 1: platinum compounds
- **SIDE-EFFECTS**

▸ **Common or very common** Alopecia · anaemia · asthenia · cardiovascular disorder · constipation · diarrhoea · gastrointestinal discomfort · haemorrhage · hypersensitivity · increased risk of infection · leucopenia · mucosal abnormalities · musculoskeletal disorder · nausea · neutropenia · ototoxicity · peripheral neuropathy · reflexes decreased · respiratory disorders · sensation abnormal · skin reactions · taste altered · thrombocytopenia · urogenital disorder · vision disorders · vomiting

▸ **Rare or very rare** Angioedema

▸ **Frequency not known** Appetite decreased · bone marrow failure · chills · dehydration · embolism · encephalopathy · extravasation necrosis · fever · haemolytic uraemic syndrome · heart failure · hypertension · hyponatraemia · hypotension · injection site necrosis · malaise · pancreatitis · stomatitis · stroke · treatment related secondary malignancy · tumour lysis syndrome

- **CONCEPTION AND CONTRACEPTION** Contraceptive advice required, see *Pregnancy and reproductive function* in Cytotoxic drugs p. 575.
- **PREGNANCY** Avoid (teratogenic and embryotoxic in *animal* studies). See also *Pregnancy and reproductive function* in Cytotoxic drugs p. 575.
- **BREAST FEEDING** Discontinue breast-feeding.
- **RENAL IMPAIRMENT** Avoid if creatinine clearance less than 20 mL/minute/1.73 m^2.
Dose adjustments Reduce dose.
Monitoring Monitor haematological parameters in renal impairment.
Monitor renal function in renal impairment.
- **MONITORING REQUIREMENTS**

▸ Consider therapeutic drug monitoring.

- **PRESCRIBING AND DISPENSING INFORMATION** Carboplatin can be given in an outpatient setting.
- **NATIONAL FUNDING/ACCESS DECISIONS**

NICE decisions

▸ **Bevacizumab in combination with paclitaxel and carboplatin for the first-line treatment of advanced ovarian cancer (May 2013)** NICE TA284
Bevacizumab in combination with paclitaxel and carboplatin is **not** recommended for the first-line treatment of advanced ovarian cancer (including fallopian tube and primary peritoneal cancer).
Patients whose treatment was started before this guidance was published should have the option to continue treatment until they and their clinician consider it appropriate to stop.
www.nice.org.uk/guidance/ta284

▸ **Bevacizumab in combination with gemcitabine and carboplatin for treating the first recurrence of platinum-sensitive advanced ovarian cancer (May 2013)** NICE TA285
Bevacizumab in combination with gemcitabine and carboplatin is **not** recommended within its marketing authorisation, that is, for the treatment of the first recurrence of platinum-sensitive advanced ovarian cancer (including fallopian tube and primary peritoneal cancer) that has not been previously treated with bevacizumab or other vascular endothelial growth factor (VEGF) inhibitors or VEGF receptor-targeted agents.
Patients whose treatment was started before this guidance was published should have the option to continue treatment until they and their clinician consider it appropriate to stop.
www.nice.org.uk/guidance/ta285

- **MEDICINAL FORMS** There can be variation in the licensing of different medicines containing the same drug.

Solution for infusion

▸ Carboplatin (Non-proprietary)
Carboplatin 10 mg per 1 ml Carboplatin 50mg/5ml concentrate for solution for infusion vials | 1 vial [PoM] £20.20–£21.70 (Hospital only)
Carboplatin 150mg/15ml concentrate for solution for infusion vials | 1 vial [PoM] £56.06–£60.59 (Hospital only)
Carboplatin 600mg/60ml concentrate for solution for infusion vials | 1 vial [PoM] £232.64–£264.53 (Hospital only)
Carboplatin 600mg/60ml solution for infusion vials | 1 vial [PoM] £260.00 (Hospital only) | 1 vial [PoM] £260.00
Carboplatin 450mg/45ml concentrate for solution for infusion vials | 1 vial [PoM] £166.32–£181.77 (Hospital only)
Carboplatin 450mg/45ml solution for infusion vials | 1 vial [PoM] £197.48 (Hospital only) | 1 vial [PoM] £197.48
Carboplatin 150mg/15ml solution for infusion vials | 1 vial [PoM] £65.83 (Hospital only) | 1 vial [PoM] £65.83
Carboplatin 50mg/5ml solution for infusion vials | 1 vial [PoM] £22.86 (Hospital only) | 1 vial [PoM] £22.86

Cisplatin

- **INDICATIONS AND DOSE**

Osteogenic sarcoma | Stage 4 neuroblastoma | Some liver tumours | Infant brain tumours | Intra-cranial germ-cell tumours

▸ BY INTRAVENOUS INFUSION
▸ Child: (consult local protocol)

- **UNLICENSED USE** Not licensed for use in children.
- **CAUTIONS**
Hydration Cisplatin requires intensive intravenous hydration; routine use of intravenous fluids containing

potassium or magnesium may also be required to help control hypokalaemia and hypomagnesaemia. Treatment may be complicated by severe nausea and vomiting; delayed vomiting may occur and is difficult to control.

- INTERACTIONS → Appendix 1: platinum compounds
- SIDE-EFFECTS
  - **Common or very common** Anaemia · arrhythmias · bone marrow failure · electrolyte imbalance · extravasation necrosis · fever · leucopenia · nephrotoxicity (dose-related and potentially cumulative) · sepsis · thrombocytopenia
  - **Uncommon** Anaphylactoid reaction · ototoxicity (dose-related and potentially cumulative) · spermatogenesis abnormal
  - **Rare or very rare** Acute leukaemia · cardiac arrest · encephalopathy · myocardial infarction · nerve disorders · seizure · stomatitis
  - **Frequency not known** Alopecia · appetite decreased · asthenia · autonomic dysfunction · cardiac disorder · cerebrovascular insufficiency · deafness · dehydration · diarrhoea · haemolytic anaemia · hiccups · hyperuricaemia · infection · Lhermitte's sign · malaise · muscle spasms · myelopathy · nausea · papilloedema · pulmonary embolism · rash · Raynaud's phenomenon · renal impairment · renal tubular disorder · retinal discolouration · SIADH · taste loss · tetany · thrombotic microangiopathy · tinnitus · vision disorders · vomiting
- CONCEPTION AND CONTRACEPTION Manufacturer advises effective contraception during and for at least 6 months after treatment in men or women.
- PREGNANCY Avoid (teratogenic and toxic in *animal* studies. See also *Pregnancy and reproductive function* in Cytotoxic drugs p. 575.
- BREAST FEEDING Discontinue breast-feeding.
- RENAL IMPAIRMENT Avoid if possible—nephrotoxic.
  Monitoring Baseline testing of renal function is required; for children with pre-existing renal impairment, consideration should be given to withholding treatment or using another drug.
- MONITORING REQUIREMENTS
  - Monitor full blood count.
  - Monitor audiology.
  - Monitor plasma electrolytes.
  - Baseline testing of hearing is required; for children with pre-existing hearing impairment, consideration should be given to withholding treatment or using another drug.
  - For children with pre-existing marked bone-marrow suppression, consideration should be given to withholding treatment or using another drug.
  - Monitor renal function.
- MEDICINAL FORMS There can be variation in the licensing of different medicines containing the same drug.

Solution for infusion

- Cisplatin (Non-proprietary)
  Cisplatin 1 mg per 1 ml Cisplatin 50mg/50ml concentrate for solution for infusion vials | 1 vial PoM £24.50–£28.11 DT = £19.50 (Hospital only)
  Cisplatin 100mg/100ml solution for infusion vials | 1 vial PoM £50.22 DT = £29.83 (Hospital only) | 1 vial PoM £8.12 DT = £29.83
  Cisplatin 50mg/50ml solution for infusion vials | 1 vial PoM £4.36–£28.11 DT = £19.50 | 1 vial PoM £25.37 DT = £19.50 (Hospital only)
  Cisplatin 10mg/10ml concentrate for solution for infusion vials | 1 vial PoM £5.36–£5.90 (Hospital only)
  Cisplatin 100mg/100ml concentrate for solution for infusion vials | 1 vial PoM £50.22–£55.64 DT = £29.83 (Hospital only)

ANTINEOPLASTIC DRUGS > PODOPHYLLOTOXIN DERIVATIVES

Etoposide

12-Jul-2018

- INDICATIONS AND DOSE

Stage 4 neuroblastoma | Germ-cell tumours | Intracranial germ-cell tumours | Rhabdomyosarcoma | Soft-tissue sarcomas | Neuroectodermal tumours (including medulloblastoma) | Relapsed Hodgkin's disease | Non-Hodgkin's lymphoma | Ewing tumour | Acute lymphoblastic leukaemia | Acute myeloid leukaemia

- BY MOUTH, OR BY INTRAVENOUS INFUSION
  - Child: (consult local protocol)

- UNLICENSED USE Not licensed for use in children.

> IMPORTANT SAFETY INFORMATION
> RISKS OF INCORRECT DOSING OF ORAL ANTI-CANCER MEDICINES
> See Cytotoxic drugs p. 575.

- INTERACTIONS → Appendix 1: etoposide
- SIDE-EFFECTS

GENERAL SIDE-EFFECTS
  - **Common or very common** Abdominal pain · acute leukaemia · alopecia · anaemia · appetite decreased · arrhythmia · asthenia · bone marrow depression · constipation · diarrhoea · dizziness · hepatotoxicity · hypertension · leucopenia · malaise · mucositis · myocardial infarction · nausea · neutropenia · skin reactions · thrombocytopenia · vomiting
  - **Uncommon** Nerve disorders
  - **Rare or very rare** Dysphagia · neurotoxicity · radiation recall reaction · respiratory disorders · seizure · severe cutaneous adverse reactions (SCARs) · taste altered · vision loss

SPECIFIC SIDE-EFFECTS
  - **Common or very common**
  - With intravenous use Anaphylactic reaction · hypotension · infection
  - With oral use Oesophagitis · stomatitis · transient systolic hypotension
  - **Uncommon**
  - With intravenous use Haemorrhage
  - **Rare or very rare**
  - With intravenous use Fever
  - With oral use Drowsiness
  - **Frequency not known**
  - With intravenous use Angioedema · extravasation necrosis · infertility · tumour lysis syndrome
- CONCEPTION AND CONTRACEPTION Contraceptive advice required, see *Pregnancy and reproductive function* in Cytotoxic drugs p. 575.
- PREGNANCY Avoid (teratogenic in *animal* studies). See also *Pregnancy and reproductive function* in Cytotoxic drugs p. 575.
- BREAST FEEDING Discontinue breast-feeding.
- HEPATIC IMPAIRMENT Manufacturer advises caution (increased risk of accumulation).
- RENAL IMPAIRMENT
  Dose adjustments Consider dose reduction—consult local treatment protocol for details.
- DIRECTIONS FOR ADMINISTRATION Etoposide is usually given by slow intravenous infusion. It may also be given by mouth, but it is unpredictably absorbed.

- **MEDICINAL FORMS** There can be variation in the licensing of different medicines containing the same drug.

Solution for infusion

▸ Etoposide (Non-proprietary)
Etoposide 20 mg per 1 ml Etoposide 100mg/5ml concentrate for solution for infusion vials | 1 vial [PoM] £11.50–£16.29 (Hospital only)
Etoposide 200mg/10ml concentrate for solution for infusion vials | 1 vial [PoM] [X] (Hospital only)
Etoposide 500mg/25ml concentrate for solution for infusion vials | 1 vial [PoM] £60.70–£81.42 (Hospital only)

Capsule

CAUTIONARY AND ADVISORY LABELS 23

▸ Vepesid (Cheplapharm Arzneimittel GmbH)
Etoposide 50 mg Vepesid 50mg capsules | 20 capsule [PoM] £99.82
Etoposide 100 mg Vepesid 100mg capsules | 10 capsule [PoM] £87.23

Powder for solution for injection

▸ Etopophos (Cheplapharm Arzneimittel GmbH)
Etoposide (as Etoposide phosphate) 100 mg Etopophos 100mg powder for solution for injection vials | 10 vial [PoM] £261.68

8 Immune system and malignant disease

ANTINEOPLASTIC DRUGS > VINCA ALKALOIDS

Vinblastine sulfate

03-Dec-2019

- **INDICATIONS AND DOSE**

Hodgkin's disease and other lymphomas

▸ BY INTRAVENOUS INJECTION
▸ Child: (consult local protocol)

- **UNLICENSED USE** Licensed for use in children (age range not specified by manufacturer).

IMPORTANT SAFETY INFORMATION

Vinblastine is for **intravenous administration only**. Inadvertent intrathecal administration can cause severe neurotoxicity, which is usually fatal.

The National Patient Safety Agency has advised (August 2008) that adult and teenage patients treated in an adult or adolescent unit should receive their vinca alkaloid dose in a 50 mL minibag. Teenagers and children treated in a child unit may receive their vinca alkaloid dose in a syringe.

- **CONTRA-INDICATIONS**

CONTRA-INDICATIONS, FURTHER INFORMATION
Intrathecal injection **contra-indicated.**

- **CAUTIONS** Caution in handling—irritant to tissues
- **INTERACTIONS** → Appendix 1: vinca alkaloids
- **SIDE-EFFECTS**

▸ **Rare or very rare** Hearing impairment · nerve disorders · vestibular damage
▸ **Frequency not known** Abdominal pain · acute respiratory distress syndrome (ARDS) · alopecia (reversible) · anaemia · appetite decreased · asthenia · balance impaired · cancer pain · constipation · depression · diarrhoea · dizziness · dyspnoea · haemorrhage · headache · hypertension · ileus · increased risk of infection · leucopenia (dose-limiting) · malaise · mediastinal disorder · myalgia · myocardial infarction · nausea · nystagmus · oral blistering · pain · Raynaud's phenomenon · reflexes absent · seizure · sensation abnormal · SIADH · skin reactions · stroke · thrombocytopenia · vertigo · vomiting

SIDE-EFFECTS, FURTHER INFORMATION **Constipation** Prophylactic use of laxatives may be considered.

- **CONCEPTION AND CONTRACEPTION** Contraceptive advice required, see *Pregnancy and reproductive function* in Cytotoxic drugs p. 575.
- **PREGNANCY** Avoid (limited experience suggests fetal harm; teratogenic in *animal* studies). See also *Pregnancy and reproductive function* in Cytotoxic drugs p. 575.
- **BREAST FEEDING** Discontinue breast-feeding.
- **HEPATIC IMPAIRMENT** Manufacturer advises caution in significantly impaired hepatic or biliary function.

Dose adjustments Manufacturer advises consider initial dose reduction in significantly impaired hepatic or biliary function.

- **MEDICINAL FORMS** There can be variation in the licensing of different medicines containing the same drug.

Solution for injection

▸ Vinblastine sulfate (Non-proprietary)
Vinblastine sulfate 1 mg per 1 ml Vinblastine 10mg/10ml solution for injection vials | 5 vial [PoM] £85.00 (Hospital only)

Vincristine sulfate

03-Dec-2019

- **INDICATIONS AND DOSE**

Acute leukaemias | Lymphomas | Paediatric solid tumours

▸ BY INTRAVENOUS INJECTION
▸ Child: (consult local protocol)

- **UNLICENSED USE** Licensed for use in children (age range not specified by manufacturer).

IMPORTANT SAFETY INFORMATION

Vincristine injections are for **intravenous administration only**. Inadvertent intrathecal administration can cause severe neurotoxicity, which is usually fatal.

The National Patient Safety Agency has advised (August 2008) that adult and teenage patients treated in an adult or adolescent unit should receive their vinca alkaloid dose in a 50 mL minibag. Teenagers and children treated in a child unit may receive their vinca alkaloid dose in a syringe.

- **CONTRA-INDICATIONS** Avoid injections containing benzyl alcohol in neonates

CONTRA-INDICATIONS, FURTHER INFORMATION
Intrathecal injection **contra-indicated.**

- **CAUTIONS** Caution in handling—irritant to tissues · ileus · neuromuscular disease
- **INTERACTIONS** → Appendix 1: vinca alkaloids
- **SIDE-EFFECTS**

▸ **Rare or very rare** Hypersensitivity · rash · SIADH
▸ **Frequency not known** Abdominal cramps · adrenal disorder · alopecia · anaemia · appetite decreased · azotaemia · bladder atony · bronchospasm · connective tissue disorders · constipation · coronary artery disease · dehydration · diarrhoea · dizziness · dyspnoea · eighth cranial nerve damage · eye disorders · fever · gait abnormalities · gastrointestinal disorders · haemolytic anaemia · headache · hearing impairment · hypertension · hyponatraemia · hypotension · infection · leucopenia · movement disorders · muscle atrophy · myalgia · myocardial infarction · nausea · neuromuscular effects (dose-limiting) · neutropenia · oedema · oral disorders · pain · paralysis · paresis · reflexes absent · renal disorder · secondary malignancy · seizure · sensation abnormal · sepsis · throat pain · thrombocytopenia · urinary disorders · vertigo · vestibular damage · vision loss · vomiting · weight decreased

SIDE-EFFECTS, FURTHER INFORMATION **Bronchospasm** Severe bronchospasm following administration is more common when used in combination with mitomycin-C.

Neurotoxicity Sensory and motor neuropathies are common and are cumulative. Manufacturer advises monitoring patients for symptoms of neuropathy, such as hypoesthesia, hyperesthesia, paresthesia, hyporeflexia, areflexia, neuralgia, jaw pain, decreased vibratory sense, cranial neuropathy, ileus, burning sensation, arthralgia, myalgia, muscle spasm, or weakness, both before and during treatment—requires dose reduction, treatment interruption or treatment discontinuation, depending on severity.

Motor weakness can also occur and dose reduction or discontinuation of therapy may be appropriate if motor weakness increases. Recovery from neurotoxic effects is usually slow but complete.

Constipation Prophylactic use of laxatives may be considered.

- **CONCEPTION AND CONTRACEPTION** Contraceptive advice required, see *Pregnancy and reproductive function* in Cytotoxic drugs p. 575.
- **PREGNANCY** Avoid (teratogenicity and fetal loss in *animal* studies). See also *Pregnancy and reproductive function* in Cytotoxic drugs p. 575.
- **BREAST FEEDING** Discontinue breast-feeding.
- **HEPATIC IMPAIRMENT** Manufacturer advises caution. **Dose adjustments** Manufacturer advises dose reduction.

- **MEDICINAL FORMS** There can be variation in the licensing of different medicines containing the same drug.

Solution for injection

- Vincristine sulfate (Non-proprietary)

Vincristine sulfate 1 mg per 1 ml Vincristine 1mg/1ml solution for injection vials | 1 vial PoM £13.47 (Hospital only) | 5 vial PoM £67.35 (Hospital only)
Vincristine 2mg/2ml solution for injection vials | 1 vial PoM £26.66 (Hospital only) | 5 vial PoM £133.30 (Hospital only)
Vincristine 5mg/5ml solution for injection vials | 5 vial PoM £329.50 (Hospital only)

ANTINEOPLASTIC DRUGS > OTHER

Asparaginase

11-Sep-2018

- **DRUG ACTION** Asparaginase is an enzyme which acts by breaking down L-asparagine to aspartic acid and ammonia, this disrupts protein synthesis of tumour cells.

- **INDICATIONS AND DOSE**

Acute lymphoblastic leukaemia (in combination with other antineoplastic drugs) (specialist use only)

- BY INTRAVENOUS INFUSION
  - Neonate: (consult product literature or local protocols).
  - Child 1–11 months: (consult product literature or local protocols)
  - Child 1–17 years: 5000 units/m^2 every 3 days

- **CONTRA-INDICATIONS** History of pancreatitis related to asparaginase therapy · history of serious haemorrhage related to asparaginase therapy · history of serious thrombosis related to asparaginase therapy · pancreatitis · pre-existing known coagulopathy
- **CAUTIONS** Diabetes (may raise blood glucose) · hypersensitivity reactions · hypertriglyceridaemia (severe)—increased risk of acute pancreatitis

CAUTIONS, FURTHER INFORMATION

- Hypersensitivity reactions Serious hypersensitivity reactions, including life-threatening anaphylaxis, can occur—asparaginase should only be administered when appropriately trained staff and resuscitation facilities are immediately available; in the event of a hypersensitivity reaction, treatment should be stopped immediately and appropriate management initiated. Manufacturer advises an intracutaneous or small intravenous test dose can be used but is of limited value for predicting which patients will experience an allergic reaction.

- **INTERACTIONS** → Appendix 1: asparaginase
- **SIDE-EFFECTS**
  - **Common or very common** Abdominal pain · agitation · anaemia · angioedema · appetite decreased · arthralgia · back pain · bronchospasm · confusion · depression · diarrhoea · disseminated intravascular coagulation · dizziness · drowsiness · dyspnoea · embolism and thrombosis · fatigue · flushing · haemorrhage · hallucination · hyperglycaemia · hypersensitivity · hypoalbuminaemia · hypoglycaemia · hypotension · increased risk of infection · leucopenia · nausea · neurological effects · oedema · pancreatitis · skin reactions · thrombocytopenia · vomiting · weight decreased
  - **Uncommon** Headache · hyperammonaemia · hyperuricaemia
  - **Rare or very rare** Coma · consciousness impaired · diabetic ketoacidosis · hepatic disorders · hyperparathyroidism · hypoparathyroidism · ischaemic stroke · necrotising pancreatitis · pancreatic pseudocyst · posterior reversible encephalopathy syndrome (PRES) · seizure · tremor

SIDE-EFFECTS, FURTHER INFORMATION There have been rare reports of cholestasis, icterus, hepatic cell necrosis and hepatic failure with fatal outcome; manufacturer advises interrupt treatment if these symptoms develop.

- **CONCEPTION AND CONTRACEPTION** Manufacturer advises effective contraception in men and women of child-bearing potential during treatment and for at least 3 months after last dose; asparaginase may reduce effectiveness of oral contraceptives—additional precautions (e.g. barrier method) are required, see also *Pregnancy and reproductive function* in Cytotoxic drugs p. 575.
- **PREGNANCY** Manufacturer advises avoid unless essential—toxicity in *animal* studies. See also *Pregnancy and reproductive function* in Cytotoxic drugs p. 575.
- **BREAST FEEDING** Manufacturer advises avoid—no information available.
- **HEPATIC IMPAIRMENT** Manufacturer advises avoid in severe impairment—no information available.
- **MONITORING REQUIREMENTS**
  - Manufacturer advises monitor trough serum asparaginase levels 3 days after administration; consider switching to a different asparaginase preparation if target levels not reached—seek expert advice.
  - Manufacturer advises monitor bilirubin, hepatic transaminases, and coagulation parameters before and during treatment; in addition, monitor plasma and urinary glucose, amylase, lipase, triglycerides, cholesterol and serum protein levels during treatment.
- **HANDLING AND STORAGE** Manufacturer advises store in a refrigerator (2–8°C)—consult product literature for storage conditions after reconstitution and dilution.
- **PATIENT AND CARER ADVICE**

Driving and skilled tasks Manufacturer advises asparaginase has moderate influence on driving and performance of skilled tasks—increased risk of dizziness and somnolence.

- **NATIONAL FUNDING/ACCESS DECISIONS**

Scottish Medicines Consortium (SMC) decisions

SMC No. 1319/18
The *Scottish Medicines Consortium* has advised (April 2018) that asparaginase (*Spectrila*®) is accepted for use within NHS Scotland when used as a component of antineoplastic combination therapy for the treatment of acute lymphoblastic leukaemia in paediatric patients from birth to 18 years and adults.

- **MEDICINAL FORMS** There can be variation in the licensing of different medicines containing the same drug.

Powder for solution for infusion

- Spectrila (medac UK) ▼

Asparaginase 10000 unit Spectrila 10,000unit powder for concentrate for solution for infusion vials | 1 vial PoM £450.00 (Hospital only)

Crisantaspase

16-Mar-2017

- **DRUG ACTION** Crisantaspase is the enzyme asparaginase produced by *Erwinia chrysanthemi*.

- **INDICATIONS AND DOSE**

Acute lymphoblastic leukaemia | Acute myeloid leukaemia | Non-Hodgkin's lymphoma

▸ BY INTRAVENOUS INJECTION, OR BY INTRAMUSCULAR INJECTION, OR BY SUBCUTANEOUS INJECTION

▸ Child: (consult local protocol)

- **UNLICENSED USE** Preparations of asparaginase derived from *Escherichia coli* are available but they are not licensed, they include: *Medac*® asparaginase and *Elspar*® asparaginase.
- **CONTRA-INDICATIONS** History of pancreatitis related to asparaginase therapy
- **CAUTIONS** Diabetes (may raise blood glucose)
- **INTERACTIONS** → Appendix 1: crisantaspase
- **SIDE-EFFECTS**

▸ **Common or very common** Chills · coagulation disorders · confusion · diarrhoea · dizziness · drowsiness · dyspnoea · face oedema · fever · headache · hepatic disorders · hypersensitivity · limb swelling · lip swelling · neurotoxicity · pain · pallor · pancreatitis · seizures · skin reactions · thrombosis

▸ **Uncommon** Hyperglycaemia · hyperlipidaemia · hypoxia · increased risk of infection · respiratory disorders

▸ **Rare or very rare** Arthritis reactive · coma · diabetic ketoacidosis · dysphagia · dysphasia · encephalopathy · haemorrhage · level of consciousness decreased · myalgia · myocardial infarction · necrotising pancreatitis · neutropenia · paresis · sepsis · thrombocytopenia

▸ **Frequency not known** Abdominal pain · flushing · hyperammonaemia · hypertension · hypotension · nausea · pseudocyst · vomiting

- **ALLERGY AND CROSS-SENSITIVITY** Children who are hypersensitive to asparaginase derived from one organism may tolerate asparaginase derived from another organism but cross-sensitivity occurs in about 20–30% of individuals.
- **CONCEPTION AND CONTRACEPTION** Contraceptive advice required, see *Pregnancy and reproductive function* in Cytotoxic drugs p. 575.
- **PREGNANCY** Avoid. See also, *Pregnancy and reproductive function* in Cytotoxic drugs p. 575.
- **BREAST FEEDING** Discontinue breast-feeding.
- **DIRECTIONS FOR ADMINISTRATION** Facilities for the management of anaphylaxis should be available.

- **MEDICINAL FORMS** There can be variation in the licensing of different medicines containing the same drug.

Powder for solution for injection

▸ Erwinase (Jazz Pharmaceuticals UK)

Crisantaspase 10000 unit Erwinase 10,000unit powder for solution for injection vials | 5 vial PoM £3,065.00

Hydroxycarbamide

16-Oct-2019

(Hydroxyurea)

- **INDICATIONS AND DOSE**

SIKLOS®

Sickle-cell disease [prevention of recurrent vaso-occlusive crises] (initiated by a specialist)

▸ BY MOUTH

▸ Child 2–17 years: Initially 10–15 mg/kg once daily, increased in steps of 2.5–5 mg/kg daily, dose to be increased every 12 weeks according to response; usual dose 15–30 mg/kg daily; maximum 35 mg/kg per day

XROMI®

Sickle-cell disease [prevention of vaso-occlusive complications] (specialist use only)

▸ BY MOUTH

▸ Child 2–17 years: Initially 15 mg/kg daily, increased in steps of 5 mg/kg daily, dose to be increased every 8 weeks according to response; usual maintenance 20–25 mg/kg daily; maximum 35 mg/kg per day

IMPORTANT SAFETY INFORMATION

RISKS OF INCORRECT DOSING OF ORAL ANTI-CANCER MEDICINES

See Cytotoxic drugs p. 575.

- **CAUTIONS** Leg ulcers (review treatment if cutaneous vasculitic ulcerations develop)
- **INTERACTIONS** → Appendix 1: hydroxycarbamide
- **SIDE-EFFECTS**

▸ **Common or very common** Alopecia · anaemia · appetite decreased · asthenia · bone marrow disorders · chills · constipation · cutaneous vasculitis · dermatomyositis · diarrhoea · disorientation · dizziness · drowsiness · dyspnoea · dysuria · fever · gastrointestinal discomfort · haemorrhage · hallucination · headache · hepatic disorders · leucopenia · malaise · mucositis · nail discolouration · nail disorder · nausea · neoplasms · neutropenia · oral disorders · pancreatitis · peripheral neuropathy · pulmonary oedema · red blood cell abnormalities · respiratory disorders · seizure · skin reactions · skin ulcers · sperm abnormalities · thrombocytopenia · vomiting

▸ **Rare or very rare** Cutaneous lupus erythematosus · gangrene · systemic lupus erythematosus (SLE)

▸ **Frequency not known** Amenorrhoea · gastrointestinal disorders · hypomagnesaemia · Parvovirus B19 infection · vitamin D deficiency · weight increased

- **CONCEPTION AND CONTRACEPTION** Manufacturer advises effective contraception before and during treatment.
- **PREGNANCY** Avoid (teratogenic in *animal* studies). See also *Pregnancy and reproductive function* in Cytotoxic drugs p. 575.
- **BREAST FEEDING** Discontinue breast-feeding.
- **HEPATIC IMPAIRMENT** Manufacturer advises caution in mild to moderate impairment; avoid in severe impairment (unless used for malignant conditions).
- **RENAL IMPAIRMENT** In sickle-cell disease, avoid if estimated glomerular filtration rate less than 30 mL/minute/1.73 m^2.

Dose adjustments In sickle-cell disease, reduce initial dose by 50% if estimated glomerular filtration rate less than 60 mL/minute/1.73 m^2.

- **MONITORING REQUIREMENTS**

▸ Monitor renal and hepatic function before and during treatment.

▸ Monitor full blood count before treatment, and repeatedly throughout use; in sickle-cell disease monitor every 2 weeks for the first 2 months and then every 2 to 3 months thereafter (or every 2 weeks if on maximum dose).

▸ Patients receiving long-term therapy for malignant disease should be monitored for secondary malignancies.

- **PATIENT AND CARER ADVICE** Patients receiving long-term therapy with hydroxycarbamide should be advised to protect skin from sun exposure.

Medicines for Children leaflet: Hydroxycarbamide for sickle cell disease www.medicinesforchildren.org.uk/hydroxycarbamide-sickle-cell-disease

● **MEDICINAL FORMS** There can be variation in the licensing of different medicines containing the same drug. Forms available from special-order manufacturers include: capsule, oral suspension, oral solution

Oral solution

CAUTIONARY AND ADVISORY LABELS 27

EXCIPIENTS: May contain Hydroxybenzoates (parabens)

▸ Xromi (Nova Laboratories Ltd)

Hydroxycarbamide 100 mg per 1 ml Xromi 100mg/ml oral solution sugar-free | 150 ml PoM £250.00

Tablet

▸ Siklos (Masters Pharmaceuticals Ltd)

Hydroxycarbamide 100 mg Siklos 100mg tablets | 60 tablet PoM £100.00 DT = £100.00

Hydroxycarbamide 1 gram Siklos 1000mg tablets | 30 tablet PoM £500.00 DT = £500.00

Mitotane

● **DRUG ACTION** Mitotane selectively inhibits the activity of the adrenal cortex, necessitating corticosteroid replacement therapy.

● **INDICATIONS AND DOSE**

Symptomatic treatment of advanced or inoperable adrenocortical carcinoma

▸ BY MOUTH

▸ Child: (consult local protocol)

● **UNLICENSED USE** Not licensed for use in children.

IMPORTANT SAFETY INFORMATION

RISKS OF INCORRECT DOSING OF ORAL ANTI-CANCER MEDICINES

See Cytotoxic drugs p. 575.

● **CAUTIONS** Avoid in Acute porphyrias p. 652 · risk of accumulation in overweight patients

● **INTERACTIONS** → Appendix 1: mitotane

● **SIDE-EFFECTS**

▸ **Common or very common** Adrenal insufficiency · anaemia · appetite decreased · asthenia · cognitive impairment · confusion · diarrhoea · dizziness · drowsiness · dyslipidaemia · gastrointestinal discomfort · gynaecomastia · headache · hepatic disorders · leucopenia · movement disorders · mucositis · muscle weakness · nausea · paraesthesia · polyneuropathy · rash · thrombocytopenia · vertigo · vomiting

▸ **Frequency not known** Encephalopathy · eye disorders · flushing · fungal infection · generalised pain · growth retardation · haemorrhage · hyperpyrexia · hypersalivation · hypertension · hypothyroidism · hypouricaemia · lens opacity · neuro-psychological retardation · ovarian cyst · postural hypotension · proteinuria · taste altered · thyroid disorder · vision disorders

● **CONCEPTION AND CONTRACEPTION** Contraceptive advice required, see *Pregnancy and reproductive* function in Cytotoxic drugs p. 575.

● **PREGNANCY** Manufacturer advises avoid. See also *Pregnancy and reproductive function* in Cytotoxic drugs p. 575.

● **BREAST FEEDING** Discontinue breast-feeding.

● **HEPATIC IMPAIRMENT** Manufacturer advises caution in mild to moderate impairment; avoid in severe impairment (limited information available).

Monitoring In mild to moderate hepatic impairment, monitoring of plasma-mitotane concentration is recommended.

● **RENAL IMPAIRMENT** Manufacturer advises caution in mild to moderate impairment. Avoid in severe impairment.

Monitoring In mild to moderate renal impairment, monitoring of plasma-mitotane concentration is recommended.

● **MONITORING REQUIREMENTS**

▸ Monitor plasma-mitotane concentration—consult product literature.

● **PRESCRIBING AND DISPENSING INFORMATION**

Corticosteroid replacement therapy Corticosteroid replacement therapy is necessary with treatment with mitotane. The dose of glucocorticoid should be increased in case of shock, trauma, or infection.

● **PATIENT AND CARER ADVICE** Patients should be warned to contact doctor immediately if injury, infection, or illness occurs (because of risk of acute adrenal insufficiency).

Driving and skilled tasks Central nervous system toxicity may affect performance of skilled tasks (e.g. driving).

● **MEDICINAL FORMS** There can be variation in the licensing of different medicines containing the same drug.

Tablet

CAUTIONARY AND ADVISORY LABELS 2, 10, 21

▸ Lysodren (HRA Pharma UK Ltd)

Mitotane 500 mg Lysodren 500mg tablets | 100 tablet PoM £590.97 DT = £590.97

Pegaspargase

24-Jul-2018

● **DRUG ACTION** Pegaspargase breaks down the amino acid L-asparagine, thereby interfering with the growth of malignant cells, which are unable to synthesise L-asparagine.

● **INDICATIONS AND DOSE**

Acute lymphoblastic leukaemia (in combination with other antineoplastic drugs) (specialist use only)

▸ BY INTRAMUSCULAR INJECTION, OR BY INTRAVENOUS INFUSION

▸ Neonate: 82.5 units/kg every 14 days.

▸ Child (body surface area up to 0.6 m^2): 82.5 units/kg every 14 days

▸ Child (body surface area 0.6 m^2 and above): 2500 units/m^2 every 14 days

IMPORTANT SAFETY INFORMATION

Be aware that doses are calculated either using units/kg or units/m^2, depending on the size of the child.

● **CONTRA-INDICATIONS** History of pancreatitis · history of serious haemorrhagic event with previous L-asparaginase therapy · history of serious thrombosis with previous L-asparaginase therapy

● **CAUTIONS** Concomitant use of other hepatotoxic drugs (particularly in pre-existing hepatic impairment)—monitor hepatic function · diabetes (may raise blood glucose) · hypersensitivity reactions · marked decrease of leukocyte count at start of treatment is possible—may be associated with significant rise in serum uric acid and development of uric acid nephropathy

CAUTIONS, FURTHER INFORMATION

▸ Hypersensitivity reactions Serious hypersensitivity reactions, including life-threatening anaphylaxis, can occur—pegaspargase should only be administered when appropriately trained staff and resuscitation facilities are immediately available; manufacturer advises patients should be closely monitored for signs of hypersensitivity during treatment and for an hour after administration. In the event of a hypersensitivity reaction, treatment should be stopped immediately and appropriate management initiated.

● **INTERACTIONS** → Appendix 1: pegaspargase

● **SIDE-EFFECTS**

▸ **Common or very common** Abdominal pain · anaemia · appetite decreased · ascites · bone marrow disorders · coagulation disorders · diarrhoea · dyslipidaemia ·

embolism and thrombosis · febrile neutropenia · hepatic disorders · hyperglycaemia · hypersensitivity · hypoalbuminaemia · hypokalaemia · hypoxia · increased risk of infection · nausea · pain in extremity · pancreatitis (discontinue if suspected and do not restart if confirmed) · peripheral neuropathy · seizure · sepsis · skin reactions · stomatitis · syncope · vomiting · weight decreased

- **Rare or very rare** Haemorrhage · necrotising pancreatitis · posterior reversible encephalopathy syndrome (PRES)
- **Frequency not known** Acute kidney injury · confusion · diabetic ketoacidosis · drowsiness · fever · hyperammonaemia (monitor if symptoms present) · hypoglycaemia · pancreatic pseudocyst · stroke · toxic epidermal necrolysis · tremor

SIDE-EFFECTS, FURTHER INFORMATION There have been rare reports of cholestasis, icterus, hepatic cell necrosis and hepatic failure with fatal outcome in patients receiving pegaspargase.

- **CONCEPTION AND CONTRACEPTION** Manufacturer advises effective contraception in men and women of child-bearing potential during treatment and for at least 6 months after discontinuing treatment; pegaspargase may reduce effectiveness of oral contraceptives—additional precautions (e.g. barrier method) are required, see also *Pregnancy and reproductive function* in Cytotoxic drugs p. 575.
- **PREGNANCY** Manufacturer advises avoid unless essential. See also *Pregnancy and reproductive function* in Cytotoxic drugs p. 575.
- **BREAST FEEDING** Manufacturer advises avoid—no information available.
- **HEPATIC IMPAIRMENT** Manufacturer advises avoid in severe impairment.
- **MONITORING REQUIREMENTS**
  - Manufacturer advises trough serum asparaginase activity levels may be measured before the next administration of pegaspargase; consider switching to a different asparaginase preparation if target levels not reached—seek expert advice.
  - Manufacturer advises monitor plasma and urine glucose levels during treatment; monitor coagulation profile at baseline and periodically during and after treatment (particularly with concomitant use of other drugs that inhibit coagulation); monitor serum amylase.
- **DIRECTIONS FOR ADMINISTRATION** Manufacturer advises *for intramuscular injection,* volumes over 2 mL must be divided between more than one site.
- **HANDLING AND STORAGE** Manufacturer advises store in a refrigerator between 2–8°C.
- **PATIENT AND CARER ADVICE**

Pancreatitis Manufacturer advises patients and carers should be told how to recognise signs and symptoms of pancreatitis and advised to seek medical attention if symptoms such as persistent, severe abdominal pain develop.

Driving and skilled tasks Manufacturer advises patients and carers should be counselled on the effects on driving and performance of skilled tasks—increased risk of confusion and somnolence.

- **NATIONAL FUNDING/ACCESS DECISIONS**

NICE decisions

- **Pegaspargase for treating acute lymphoblastic leukaemia (September 2016)** NICE TA408

Pegaspargase, as part of antineoplastic combination therapy, is recommended as an option for treating acute lymphoblastic leukaemia only in patients with untreated newly diagnosed disease.

Patients whose treatment was started within the NHS before this guidance was published may continue treatment until they and their clinician consider it appropriate to stop.
www.nice.org.uk/guidance/ta408

Scottish Medicines Consortium (SMC) decisions

The *Scottish Medicines Consortium* has advised (November 2016) that pegaspargase (*Oncaspar*®) is accepted for use within NHS Scotland as a component of antineoplastic combination therapy in acute lymphoblastic leukaemia.

- **MEDICINAL FORMS** There can be variation in the licensing of different medicines containing the same drug.

Solution for injection

- Oncaspar (Servier Laboratories Ltd) ▼

Pegaspargase 750 unit per 1 ml Oncaspar 3,750units/5ml solution for injection vials | 1 vial PoM £1,296.19

Powder for solution for injection

- Pegaspargase (non-proprietary) ▼

Pegaspargase 3750 unit Oncaspar 3,750unit powder for solution for injection vials | 1 vial PoM £1,296.19 (Hospital only)

Procarbazine

- **DRUG ACTION** Procarbazine is a mild monoamine-oxidase inhibitor.

- **INDICATIONS AND DOSE**

Hodgkin's lymphoma

- BY MOUTH
- Child: (consult local protocol)

IMPORTANT SAFETY INFORMATION

RISKS OF INCORRECT DOSING OF ORAL ANTI-CANCER MEDICINES

See Cytotoxic drugs p. 575.

- **CONTRA-INDICATIONS** Pre-existing severe leucopenia · pre-existing severe thrombocytopenia
- **CAUTIONS** Cardiovascular disease · cerebrovascular disease · epilepsy · phaeochromocytoma · procarbazine is a mild monoamineoxidase inhibitor (dietary restriction is rarely considered necessary)
- **INTERACTIONS** → Appendix 1: procarbazine
- **SIDE-EFFECTS**
  - **Common or very common** Appetite decreased
  - **Frequency not known** Azoospermia · hepatic disorders · infection · lethargy · leucopenia · nausea · neutropenia · ovarian failure · pneumonitis · skin reactions · thrombocytopenia · vomiting
- **CONCEPTION AND CONTRACEPTION** Contraceptive advice required, see *Pregnancy and reproductive function* in Cytotoxic drugs p. 575.
- **PREGNANCY** Avoid (teratogenic in *animal* studies and isolated reports in humans). See also *Pregnancy and reproductive function* in Cytotoxic drugs p. 575.
- **BREAST FEEDING** Discontinue breast-feeding.
- **HEPATIC IMPAIRMENT** Manufacturer advises caution in mild to moderate impairment; avoid in severe impairment.
- **RENAL IMPAIRMENT** Caution in mild to moderate impairment. Avoid in severe impairment.
- **MEDICINAL FORMS** There can be variation in the licensing of different medicines containing the same drug.

Capsule

CAUTIONARY AND ADVISORY LABELS 4

- Procarbazine (Non-proprietary)

Procarbazine (as Procarbazine hydrochloride)

50 mg Procarbazine 50mg capsules | 50 capsule PoM £411.35–£479.63 DT = £445.49

RETINOID AND RELATED DRUGS

Tretinoin

15-Jan-2020

● **INDICATIONS AND DOSE**

Induction of remission in acute promyelocytic leukaemia (used in previously untreated patients as well as in those who have relapsed after standard chemotherapy or who are refractory to it)

▶ BY MOUTH

▸ Child: (consult local protocol)

IMPORTANT SAFETY INFORMATION

MHRA/CHM ADVICE: ORAL RETINOID MEDICINES: REVISED AND SIMPLIFIED PREGNANCY PREVENTION EDUCATIONAL MATERIALS FOR HEALTHCARE PROFESSIONALS AND WOMEN (JUNE 2019)

Materials to support the Pregnancy Prevention Programme in women and girls of childbearing potential taking oral acitretin, alitretinoin, or isotretinoin have been updated. Oral tretinoin and bexarotene do not have a Pregnancy Prevention Programme in light of their oncology indication and specialist care setting. However, healthcare professionals are advised that these medicines are extremely teratogenic and product information should be consulted for contraceptive and pregnancy testing requirements when used in females of childbearing potential.

Neuropsychiatric reactions have been reported in patients taking oral retinoids. Healthcare professionals are advised to monitor patients for signs of depression or suicidal ideation and refer for appropriate treatment, if necessary; particular care is needed in those with a history of depression. Patients should be advised to speak to their doctor if they experience any changes in mood or behaviour, and encouraged to ask family and friends to look out for any change in mood.

● CAUTIONS History of depression (risk of neuropsychiatric reactions) · increased risk of thromboembolism during first month of treatment

● INTERACTIONS → Appendix 1: retinoids

● SIDE-EFFECTS

▶ **Common or very common** Abdominal pain · alopecia · anxiety · appetite decreased · arrhythmia · asthma · bone pain · cheilitis · chest pain · chills · confusion · constipation · depression · diarrhoea · dizziness · dry mouth · flushing · headache · hearing impairment · hyperhidrosis · idiopathic intracranial hypertension (children particularly susceptible - consider dose reduction if intractable headache in children) · insomnia · intracranial pressure increased · malaise · nasal dryness · nausea · pancreatitis · paraesthesia · respiratory disorders · skin reactions · visual impairment · vomiting

▶ **Frequency not known** Embolism and thrombosis · erythema nodosum · genital ulceration · hepatotoxicity · hypercalcaemia · increased leucocytes · myocardial infarction · myositis · necrotising fasciitis · QT interval prolongation · stroke · thrombocytosis · vasculitis

SIDE-EFFECTS, FURTHER INFORMATION Children are particularly susceptible to nervous system effects.

Retinoic acid syndrome Fever, dyspnoea, acute respiratory distress, pulmonary infiltrates, pleural effusion, hyperleucocytosis, hypotension, oedema, weight gain, hepatic, renal and multi-organ failure requires immediate treatment—consult product literature.

● CONCEPTION AND CONTRACEPTION Effective contraception must be used for at least 1 month before oral treatment, during treatment and for at least 1 month after stopping (oral progestogen-only contraceptives not considered effective).

● PREGNANCY Teratogenic. See *Pregnancy and reproductive function* in Cytotoxic drugs p. 575.

● BREAST FEEDING Avoid (discontinue breast-feeding).

● HEPATIC IMPAIRMENT Manufacturer advises caution.

Dose adjustments Manufacturer advises dose reduction.

● RENAL IMPAIRMENT

Dose adjustments Reduce dose—consult local treatment protocol for details.

● MONITORING REQUIREMENTS Monitor haematological and coagulation profile, liver function, serum calcium and plasma lipids before and during treatment.

● PRESCRIBING AND DISPENSING INFORMATION Tretinoin is the acid form of vitamin A.

● PATIENT AND CARER ADVICE

Risk of neuropsychiatric reactions The MHRA advises patients and carers to seek medical attention if changes in mood or behaviour occur.

● MEDICINAL FORMS There can be variation in the licensing of different medicines containing the same drug.

Capsule

CAUTIONARY AND ADVISORY LABELS 21, 25

▸ **Tretinoin (Non-proprietary)**

Tretinoin 10 mg Tretinoin 10mg capsules | 100 capsule PoM
£300.00–£315.00 DT = £300.00

2.1 Cytotoxic drug-induced side effects

DETOXIFYING DRUGS > UROPROTECTIVE DRUGS

Mesna

● **INDICATIONS AND DOSE**

Urothelial toxicity following oxazaphosphorine therapy

▶ BY INTRAVENOUS INJECTION, OR BY CONTINUOUS INTRAVENOUS INFUSION

▸ Child: (consult local protocol)

Mucolytic in cystic fibrosis

▶ BY INHALATION OF NEBULISED SOLUTION

▸ Child: 3–6 mL twice daily, use a 20% solution

● UNLICENSED USE Not licensed for use in children.

● SIDE-EFFECTS

▶ **Common or very common** Appetite decreased · arthralgia · asthenia · chest pain · chills · concentration impaired · conjunctivitis · constipation · cough · dehydration · diarrhoea · dizziness · drowsiness · dry mouth · dyspnoea · dysuria · fever · flatulence · flushing · gastrointestinal discomfort · haemorrhage · headache · hyperhidrosis · influenza like illness · laryngeal discomfort · lymphadenopathy · malaise · myalgia · nasal congestion · nausea · oral irritation · pain · palpitations · respiratory disorders · sensation abnormal · skin reactions · sleep disorders · syncope · vision disorders · vomiting

▶ **Frequency not known** Acute kidney injury · angioedema · drug reaction with eosinophilia and systemic symptoms (DRESS) · hypotension · hypoxia · oedema · tachycardia · ulcer · vulvovaginal rash

● ALLERGY AND CROSS-SENSITIVITY Contra-indicated if history of hypersensitivity to thiol-containing compounds.

● PREGNANCY Not known to be harmful. See also *Pregnancy and reproductive function* in Cytotoxic drugs p. 575.

- **MEDICINAL FORMS** There can be variation in the licensing of different medicines containing the same drug.

Solution for injection

- Mesna (Non-proprietary)
  Mesna 100 mg per 1 ml Mesna 1g/10ml solution for injection ampoules | 15 ampoule PoM £441.15–£447.15
  Mesna 400mg/4ml solution for injection ampoules | 5 ampoule PoM £17.00 | 15 ampoule PoM £201.15

VITAMINS AND TRACE ELEMENTS > FOLATES

Folinic acid

12-Apr-2019

- **INDICATIONS AND DOSE**

Reduction of methotrexate-induced toxicity

- BY MOUTH, OR BY INTRAVENOUS INFUSION, OR BY INTRAVENOUS INJECTION
- Child: (consult local protocol)

Methotrexate overdose

- BY INTRAVENOUS INFUSION, OR BY INTRAVENOUS INJECTION
- Child: (consult local protocol)

Megaloblastic anaemia due to folate deficiency

- BY MOUTH
- Child 1 month–11 years: 250 micrograms/kg once daily
- Child 12–17 years: 15 mg once daily

Metabolic disorders leading to folate deficiency

- BY MOUTH, OR BY INTRAVENOUS INFUSION
- Child: 15 mg once daily, larger doses may be required in older children

Prevention of megaloblastic anaemia associated with pyrimethamine and sulfadiazine treatment of congenital toxoplasmosis

- BY MOUTH
- Neonate: 5 mg 3 times a week; increased if necessary up to 20 mg 3 times a week, if the patient is neutropenic.
- Child 1–11 months: 10 mg 3 times a week

SODIOFOLIN®

As an antidote to methotrexate

- BY INTRAVENOUS INFUSION, OR BY INTRAVENOUS INJECTION
- Child: (consult product literature)

- **UNLICENSED USE** Consult product literature for licensing status of individual preparations.
- **CONTRA-INDICATIONS** Intrathecal injection
- **CAUTIONS** Avoid simultaneous administration of methotrexate · **not** indicated for pernicious anaemia or other megaloblastic anaemias caused by vitamin B_{12} deficiency
- **INTERACTIONS** → Appendix 1: folates
- **SIDE-EFFECTS**

GENERAL SIDE-EFFECTS

- **Common or very common** Diarrhoea
- **Uncommon** Fever
- **Rare or very rare** Agitation (with high doses) · depression (with high doses) · epilepsy exacerbated · gastrointestinal disorder (with high doses) · insomnia (with high doses)

SPECIFIC SIDE-EFFECTS

- **Common or very common**
- With intravenous use Bone marrow failure · dehydration · mucositis · nausea · oral disorders · skin reactions · vomiting
- **Rare or very rare**
- With intravenous use Sensitisation
- **Frequency not known**
- With intravenous use Hyperammonaemia
- With oral use Leucopenia · stomatitis · thrombocytopenia

- **PREGNANCY** Not known to be harmful; benefit outweighs risk.
- **BREAST FEEDING** Presence in milk unknown but benefit outweighs risk.
- **MEDICINAL FORMS** There can be variation in the licensing of different medicines containing the same drug. Forms available from special-order manufacturers include: oral suspension, oral solution

Tablet

- Folinic acid (Non-proprietary)
  Folinic acid (as Calcium folinate) 15 mg Calcium folinate 15mg tablets | 10 tablet PoM £49.00 DT = £43.26
- Refolinon (Pfizer Ltd)
  Folinic acid (as Calcium folinate) 15 mg Refolinon 15mg tablets | 30 tablet PoM £85.74

Solution for injection

- Folinic acid (Non-proprietary)
  Folinic acid (as Calcium folinate) 7.5 mg per 1 ml Calcium folinate 15mg/2ml solution for injection ampoules | 5 ampoule PoM £39.00 DT = £39.00 | 5 ampoule PoM £39.00 DT = £39.00 (Hospital only)
  Folinic acid (as Calcium folinate) 10 mg per 1 ml Calcium folinate 350mg/35ml solution for injection vials | 10 vial PoM £1,277.60 (Hospital only)
  Calcium folinate 50mg/5ml solution for injection vials | 1 vial PoM £20.00 (Hospital only)
  Calcium folinate 300mg/30ml solution for injection vials | 1 vial PoM £100.00 (Hospital only)
  Calcium folinate 100mg/10ml solution for injection vials | 1 vial PoM £37.50 (Hospital only) | 10 vial PoM £404.50 (Hospital only)
- Sodiofolin (medac UK)
  Folinic acid (as Disodium folinate) 50 mg per 1 ml Sodiofolin 400mg/8ml solution for injection vials | 1 vial PoM £126.25 (Hospital only)
  Sodiofolin 100mg/2ml solution for injection vials | 1 vial PoM £35.09 (Hospital only)

Levofolinic acid

18-May-2020

- **DRUG ACTION** Levofolinic acid is an isomer of folinic acid.

- **INDICATIONS AND DOSE**

Reduction of methotrexate-induced toxicity

- BY INTRAMUSCULAR INJECTION, OR BY INTRAVENOUS INJECTION, OR BY INTRAVENOUS INFUSION
- Child: (consult local protocol)

Methotrexate overdose

- BY INTRAMUSCULAR INJECTION, OR BY INTRAVENOUS INJECTION, OR BY INTRAVENOUS INFUSION
- Child: (consult local protocol)

- **CONTRA-INDICATIONS** Intrathecal injection
- **CAUTIONS** Avoid simultaneous administration of methotrexate · **not** indicated for pernicious anaemia or other megaloblastic anaemias caused by vitamin B_{12} deficiency
- **INTERACTIONS** → Appendix 1: folates
- **SIDE-EFFECTS**
- **Common or very common** Dehydration · diarrhoea · mucosal toxicity · nausea · vomiting
- **Uncommon** Fever
- **Rare or very rare** Agitation (with high doses) · depression (with high doses) · epilepsy exacerbated · gastrointestinal disorder · insomnia (with high doses) · urticaria
- **PREGNANCY** Not known to be harmful; benefit outweighs risk.
- **BREAST FEEDING** Presence in milk unknown but benefit outweighs risk.
- **MEDICINAL FORMS** There can be variation in the licensing of different medicines containing the same drug.

Solution for injection

- Levofolinic acid (Non-proprietary)
  Levofolinic acid (as Disodium levofolinate) 50 mg per 1 ml Levofolinic acid 50mg/1ml solution for injection vials | 1 vial PoM £24.70 (Hospital only)

Levofolinic acid 200mg/4ml solution for injection vials | 1 vial PoM £80.40 (Hospital only)

▸ Isovorin (Pfizer Ltd)
Levofolinic acid (as Calcium levofolinate) 10 mg per 1 ml Isovorin 175mg/17.5ml solution for injection vials | 1 vial PoM £81.33 (Hospital only)
Isovorin 25mg/2.5ml solution for injection vials | 1 vial PoM £11.62 (Hospital only)

2.1a Hyperuricaemia associated with cytotoxic drugs

Other drugs used for Hyperuricaemia associated with cytotoxic drugs Allopurinol, below

DETOXIFYING DRUGS > URATE OXIDASES

Rasburicase

● **INDICATIONS AND DOSE**

Prophylaxis and treatment of acute hyperuricaemia with initial chemotherapy for haematological malignancy
▸ BY INTRAVENOUS INFUSION
▸ Child: (consult local protocol)

● **UNLICENSED USE** Not licensed for use in children.
● **CONTRA-INDICATIONS** G6PD deficiency
● **CAUTIONS** Atopic allergies
● **SIDE-EFFECTS**
▸ **Common or very common** Diarrhoea · fever · headache · nausea · skin reactions · vomiting
▸ **Uncommon** Bronchospasm · haemolysis · haemolytic anaemia · hypersensitivity · hypotension · methaemoglobinaemia · seizure
▸ **Rare or very rare** Rhinitis
▸ **Frequency not known** Muscle contractions involuntary
● **PREGNANCY** Manufacturer advises avoid—no information available.
● **BREAST FEEDING** Manufacturer advises avoid—no information available.
● **MONITORING REQUIREMENTS** Monitor closely for hypersensitivity.
● **EFFECT ON LABORATORY TESTS** May interfere with test for uric acid—consult product literature.

● **MEDICINAL FORMS** There can be variation in the licensing of different medicines containing the same drug.
Powder and solvent for solution for infusion
▸ Fasturtec (Sanofi)
Rasburicase 1.5 mg Fasturtec 1.5mg powder and solvent for solution for infusion vials | 3 vial PoM £208.39 (Hospital only)
Rasburicase 7.5 mg Fasturtec 7.5mg powder and solvent for solution for infusion vials | 1 vial PoM £347.32 (Hospital only)

XANTHINE OXIDASE INHIBITORS

Allopurinol

03-Mar-2020

● **INDICATIONS AND DOSE**

Prophylaxis of hyperuricaemia associated with cancer chemotherapy | Prophylaxis of hyperuricaemic nephropathy, enzyme disorders causing increased serum urate e.g Lesch-Nyhan syndrome
▸ BY MOUTH
▸ Child 1 month–14 years: 10–20 mg/kg daily, dose to be taken preferably after food; maximum 400 mg per day
▸ Child 15–17 years: Initially 100 mg daily, taken preferably after food; dose to be increased according to response, up to 900 mg daily in divided doses (max. per dose 300 mg)

● **CAUTIONS** Ensure adequate fluid intake · for hyperuricaemia associated with cancer therapy, allopurinol treatment should be started before cancer therapy
● **INTERACTIONS** → Appendix 1: allopurinol
● **SIDE-EFFECTS**
▸ **Common or very common** Rash (discontinue therapy; if rash mild re-introduce cautiously but discontinue immediately if recurrence)
▸ **Uncommon** Hypersensitivity · nausea · vomiting
▸ **Rare or very rare** Agranulocytosis · alopecia · angina pectoris · angioedema · angioimmunoblastic T-cell lymphoma · aplastic anaemia · asthenia · ataxia · boil · bradycardia · cataract · coma · depression · diabetes mellitus · drowsiness · erectile dysfunction · fever · gastrointestinal disorders · gynaecomastia · haemorrhage · hair colour changes · headache · hepatic disorders · hyperlipidaemia · hypertension · infertility male · maculopathy · malaise · oedema · paraesthesia · paralysis · peripheral neuropathy · severe cutaneous adverse reactions (SCARs) · skin reactions · stomatitis · taste altered · thrombocytopenia · vertigo · visual impairment
● **PREGNANCY** Toxicity not reported. Manufacturer advises use only if no safer alternative and disease carries risk for mother or child.
● **BREAST FEEDING** Present in milk—not known to be harmful.
● **HEPATIC IMPAIRMENT** Manufacturer advises monitor liver function periodically during early stages of therapy.
Dose adjustments Manufacturer advises reduce dose.
● **RENAL IMPAIRMENT**
Dose adjustments Manufacturer advises reduce dose or increase dose interval in severe impairment; adjust dose to maintain plasma-oxipurinol concentration below 100 micromol/litre.
● **PATIENT AND CARER ADVICE**
Medicines for Children leaflet: Allopurinol for hyperuricaemia www.medicinesforchildren.org.uk/allopurinol-hyperuricaemia

● **MEDICINAL FORMS** There can be variation in the licensing of different medicines containing the same drug. Forms available from special-order manufacturers include: oral suspension, oral solution
Tablet
CAUTIONARY AND ADVISORY LABELS 8, 21, 27
▸ Allopurinol (Non-proprietary)
Allopurinol 100 mg Allopurinol 100mg tablets | 28 tablet PoM £8.15 DT = £1.11
Allopurinol 300 mg Allopurinol 300mg tablets | 28 tablet PoM £5.85 DT = £1.62
▸ Uricto (Ennogen Pharma Ltd)
Allopurinol 100 mg Uricto 100mg tablets | 28 tablet PoM £0.78 DT = £1.11
Allopurinol 300 mg Uricto 300mg tablets | 28 tablet PoM £1.85 DT = £1.62
▸ Zyloric (Aspen Pharma Trading Ltd)
Allopurinol 100 mg Zyloric 100mg tablets | 100 tablet PoM £10.19
Allopurinol 300 mg Zyloric 300mg tablets | 28 tablet PoM £7.31 DT = £1.62

8 Immune system and malignant disease

3 Immunotherapy responsive malignancy

IMMUNOSTIMULANTS > INTERFERONS

Interferon alfa

30-Mar-2017

- DRUG ACTION Interferon alfa has shown some antitumour effect in certain lymphomas and solid tumours.

- INDICATIONS AND DOSE

Induction of early regression of life-threatening corticosteroid resistant haemangiomata of infancy

- BY SUBCUTANEOUS INJECTION
- Child: (consult local protocol)

INTRONA ® PEN

Chronic active hepatitis B

- BY SUBCUTANEOUS INJECTION
- Child 2–17 years: 5 000 000–10 000 000 units/m^2 3 times a week

Chronic active hepatitis C (in combination with oral ribavirin)

- BY SUBCUTANEOUS INJECTION
- Child 3–17 years: 3 000 000 units/m^2 3 times a week

INTRONA ® VIALS

Chronic active hepatitis B

- BY SUBCUTANEOUS INJECTION
- Child 2–17 years: 5 000 000–10 000 000 units/m^2 3 times a week

Chronic active hepatitis C (in combination with ribavirin)

- BY SUBCUTANEOUS INJECTION
- Child 3–17 years: 3 000 000 units/m^2 3 times a week

ROFERON-A ®

Chronic active hepatitis B

- BY SUBCUTANEOUS INJECTION
- Child 2–17 years: 2 500 000–5 000 000 units/m^2 3 times a week, up to 10 000 000 units/m^2 has been used 3 times a week

- UNLICENSED USE Not licensed for use in children for chronic active hepatitis B.

ROFERON-A ® *Roferon-A* ® not licensed for use in children.

- CONTRA-INDICATIONS Avoid injections containing benzyl alcohol in neonates (in neonates) · history of severe psychiatric illness

CONTRA-INDICATIONS, FURTHER INFORMATION
For contra-indications consult product literature and local treatment protocol.

- CAUTIONS For cautions consult product literature and local treatment protocol.

Interferon alfa should always be used under the close supervision of a specialist; the decision to treat should be made only after careful assessment of the expected benefits versus the potential risks, in particular the risk of growth inhibition caused by combination therapy.

- INTERACTIONS → Appendix 1: interferons
- SIDE-EFFECTS
- **Common or very common** Alopecia · anaemia · anxiety · appetite abnormal · arthralgia · asthenia · behaviour abnormal · chest pain · chills · concentration impaired · confusion · conjunctivitis · constipation · cough · depression · diarrhoea · dizziness · drowsiness · dysphonia · dyspnoea · epistaxis · eye pain · fever · flushing · gastrointestinal discomfort · gastrointestinal disorders · growth retardation · headache · hepatic function abnormal · hyperhidrosis · hyperkinesia · hyperthyroidism · hypertriglyceridaemia (sometimes severe) · hyperuricaemia · hypothyroidism · increased risk of infection · influenza like illness · lacrimation disorder · lymphadenopathy · malaise · menstrual cycle irregularities · mood altered · musculoskeletal pain · myalgia · nail disorder · nasal complaints · nausea · neoplasms · neutropenia · oedema · oral disorders · pallor · photosensitivity reaction · sensation abnormal · skin reactions · sleep disorders · suicidal ideation · tachypnoea · testicular pain · thrombocytopenia · tremor · urinary disorders · vaginal disorder · virilism · visual impairment · vomiting

SIDE-EFFECTS, FURTHER INFORMATION Respiratory symptoms should be investigated and if pulmonary infiltrates are suspected or lung function is impaired the discontinuation of interferon alfa should be considered.

- CONCEPTION AND CONTRACEPTION Effective contraception required during treatment—consult product literature.
- PREGNANCY Avoid unless potential benefit outweighs risk (toxicity in *animal* studies).
- BREAST FEEDING Unlikely to be harmful.
- HEPATIC IMPAIRMENT Manufacturer advises caution in mild to moderate impairment; avoid in severe impairment.
Monitoring Close monitoring required in mild to moderate hepatic impairment.
- RENAL IMPAIRMENT Avoid in severe renal impairment.
Monitoring Close monitoring required in mild to moderate renal impairment.
- MONITORING REQUIREMENTS
- Monitoring of lipid concentration is recommended.
- Monitoring of hepatic function is recommended.
- DIRECTIONS FOR ADMINISTRATION

INTRONA ® VIALS *IntronA* ® injection vials for subcutaneous injection or intravenous infusion.

ROFERON-A ® *Roferon-A* ® injection for subcutaneous injection.

- MEDICINAL FORMS There can be variation in the licensing of different medicines containing the same drug.

Solution for injection

EXCIPIENTS: May contain Benzyl alcohol

- Roferon-A (Roche Products Ltd)
Interferon alfa-2a 9 mega unit per 1 ml Roferon-A 4.5million units/0.5ml solution for injection pre-filled syringes | 1 pre-filled disposable injection PoM £21.29 DT = £21.29
Interferon alfa-2a 12 mega unit per 1 ml Roferon-A 6million units/0.5ml solution for injection pre-filled syringes | 1 pre-filled disposable injection PoM £28.37 DT = £28.37

Interferon gamma-1b

(Immune interferon)

- INDICATIONS AND DOSE

To reduce the frequency of serious infection in chronic granulomatous disease

- BY SUBCUTANEOUS INJECTION
- Child 6 months–17 years (body surface area up to 0.6 m^2): 1.5 micrograms/kg 3 times a week
- Child 6 months–17 years (body surface area 0.6 m^2 and above): 50 micrograms/m^2 3 times a week

To reduce the frequency of serious infection in severe malignant osteopetrosis

- BY SUBCUTANEOUS INJECTION
- Child (body surface area up to 0.6 m^2): 1.5 micrograms/kg 3 times a week
- Child (body surface area 0.6 m^2 and above): 50 micrograms/m^2 3 times a week

- **CONTRA-INDICATIONS** Simultaneous administration of foreign proteins including immunological products (such as vaccines)—risk of exaggerated immune response
- **CAUTIONS** Arrhythmias · cardiac disease · congestive heart failure · ischaemia · seizure disorders (including seizures associated with fever)
- **SIDE-EFFECTS**
  - **Common or very common** Abdominal pain · arthralgia · back pain · chills · depression · diarrhoea · fatigue · fever · headache · nausea · rash · vomiting
  - **Frequency not known** Atrioventricular block · chest discomfort · confusion · connective tissue disorders · embolism and thrombosis · gait abnormal · gastrointestinal haemorrhage · hallucination · heart failure · hepatic failure · hypertriglyceridaemia · hypoglycaemia · hyponatraemia · hypotension · influenza like illness · myocardial infarction · neutropenia · pancreatitis · parkinsonism · proteinuria · renal failure · respiratory disorders · seizure · syncope · systemic lupus erythematosus (SLE) · tachycardia · thrombocytopenia · transient ischaemic attack
- **CONCEPTION AND CONTRACEPTION** Effective contraception required during treatment—consult product literature.
- **PREGNANCY** Manufacturers recommend avoid unless potential benefit outweighs risk (toxicity in *animal* studies).
- **BREAST FEEDING** Manufacturers advise avoid—no information available.
- **HEPATIC IMPAIRMENT** Manufacturer advises caution in severe impairment (increased risk of accumulation).
- **RENAL IMPAIRMENT** Manufacturer advises caution in severe impairment—risk of accumulation.
- **MONITORING REQUIREMENTS** Monitor before and during treatment: haematological tests (including full blood count, differential white cell count, and platelet count), blood chemistry tests (including renal and liver function tests) and urinalysis.

- **MEDICINAL FORMS** There can be variation in the licensing of different medicines containing the same drug.

Solution for injection

- Immukin (Clinigen Healthcare Ltd)
  Interferon gamma-1b (recombinant human) 200 microgram per 1 ml Immukin 100micrograms/0.5ml solution for injection vials | 6 vial PoM £450.00

IMMUNOSTIMULANTS > OTHER

Mifamurtide

- **INDICATIONS AND DOSE**

Treatment of high-grade, resectable, non-metastatic osteosarcoma after complete surgical resection (in combination with chemotherapy)

- BY INTRAVENOUS INFUSION
- Child 2–17 years: Infusion to be given over 1 hour (consult product literature or local protocols)

- **UNLICENSED USE** Not licensed for use in patients under 2 years of age at initial diagnosis.
- **CAUTIONS** Asthma—consider prophylactic bronchodilator therapy · chronic obstructive pulmonary disease—consider prophylactic bronchodilator therapy · history of autoimmune disease · history of collagen disease · history of inflammatory disease
- **INTERACTIONS** → Appendix 1: mifamurtide
- **SIDE-EFFECTS**
  - **Common or very common** Alopecia · anaemia · anxiety · appetite decreased · arthralgia · asthenia · cancer pain · chest discomfort · chills · confusion · constipation · cough · cyanosis · dehydration · depression · diarrhoea · dizziness · drowsiness · dysmenorrhoea · dyspnoea · feeling cold · fever · flushing · gastrointestinal discomfort · haemorrhage · headache · hearing loss · hepatic pain · hyperhidrosis · hypertension · hypokalaemia · hypotension · hypothermia · increased risk of infection · insomnia · laryngeal pain · leucopenia · malaise · mucositis · muscle complaints · musculoskeletal stiffness · nasal congestion · nausea · neutropenia · oedema · pain · pallor · palpitations · respiratory disorders · sensation abnormal · sepsis · skin reactions · tachycardia · thrombocytopenia · tinnitus · tremor · urinary disorders · vertigo · vision blurred · vomiting · weight decreased
- **CONCEPTION AND CONTRACEPTION** Effective contraception required.
- **PREGNANCY** Avoid.
- **BREAST FEEDING** Avoid—no information available.
- **HEPATIC IMPAIRMENT** Manufacturer advises caution in moderate impairment (risk of increased half-life and exposure); avoid in severe impairment (no information available).
- **RENAL IMPAIRMENT** Use with caution—no information available.
- **MONITORING REQUIREMENTS**
  - Monitor renal function, hepatic function and clotting parameters.
  - Monitor patients with history of venous thrombosis, vasculitis, or unstable cardiovascular disorders for persistent or worsening symptoms during administration—consult product literature.
- **NATIONAL FUNDING/ACCESS DECISIONS**

NICE decisions

- **Mifamurtide for the treatment of osteosarcoma (October 2011)** NICE TA235
  Mifamurtide (*Mepact*®) in combination with postoperative multi-agent chemotherapy is recommended (within its licensed indication), as an option for the treatment of high-grade resectable non-metastatic osteosarcoma after macroscopically complete surgical resection in children, adolescents and young adults and when mifamurtide is made available at a reduced cost to the NHS under the patient access scheme. www.nice.org.uk/guidance/ta235

- **MEDICINAL FORMS** There can be variation in the licensing of different medicines containing the same drug.

Powder for suspension for infusion

- Mepact (Takeda UK Ltd)
  Mifamurtide 4 mg Mepact 4mg powder for suspension for infusion vials | 1 vial PoM £2,375.00

4 Targeted therapy responsive malignancy

ANTINEOPLASTIC DRUGS > PROTEIN KINASE INHIBITORS

Dasatinib

05-Dec-2019

- **DRUG ACTION** Dasatinib is a tyrosine kinase inhibitor.
- **INDICATIONS AND DOSE**

Chronic phase chronic myeloid leukaemia (initiated by a specialist) | Acute lymphoblastic leukaemia [in combination with chemotherapy] (initiated by a specialist)

- BY MOUTH USING TABLETS
- Child 1–17 years (body-weight 10–19 kg): 40 mg once daily, adjust dose based on changes in body-weight every 3 months or more often if necessary; for continued →

dose escalation, or dose adjustment due to side-effects—consult product literature
- Child 1–17 years (body-weight 20–29 kg): 60 mg once daily, adjust dose based on changes in body-weight every 3 months or more often if necessary; for dose escalation, or dose adjustment due to side-effects—consult product literature
- Child 1–17 years (body-weight 30–44 kg): 70 mg once daily, adjust dose based on changes in body-weight every 3 months or more often if necessary; for dose escalation, or dose adjustment due to side-effects—consult product literature
- Child 1–17 years (body-weight 45 kg and above): 100 mg once daily, adjust dose based on changes in body-weight every 3 months or more often if necessary; for dose escalation, or dose adjustment due to side-effects—consult product literature

▶ BY MOUTH USING ORAL SUSPENSION
- Child 1–17 years (body-weight 5–9 kg): 40 mg once daily, adjust dose based on changes in body-weight every 3 months or more often if necessary; for dose escalation, or dose adjustment due to side-effects—consult product literature
- Child 1–17 years (body-weight 10–19 kg): 60 mg once daily, adjust dose based on changes in body-weight every 3 months or more often if necessary; for dose escalation, or dose adjustment due to side-effects—consult product literature
- Child 1–17 years (body-weight 20–29 kg): 90 mg once daily, adjust dose based on changes in body-weight every 3 months or more often if necessary; for dose escalation, or dose adjustment due to side-effects—consult product literature
- Child 1–17 years (body-weight 30–44 kg): 105 mg once daily, adjust dose based on changes in body-weight every 3 months or more often if necessary; for dose escalation, or dose adjustment due to side-effects—consult product literature
- Child 1–17 years (body-weight 45 kg and above): 120 mg once daily, adjust dose based on changes in body-weight every 3 months or more often if necessary; for dose escalation, or dose adjustment due to side-effects—consult product literature

DOSE EQUIVALENCE AND CONVERSION
- *Sprycel*® film-coated tablets and *Sprycel*® powder for oral suspension are **not** bioequivalent. Follow correct dosing recommendations for the dosage form when switching formulations.

IMPORTANT SAFETY INFORMATION

RISKS OF INCORRECT DOSING OF ORAL ANTI-CANCER MEDICINES
See Cytotoxic drugs p. 575.

MHRA/CHM ADVICE (MAY 2016): RISK OF HEPATITIS B VIRUS REACTIVATION WITH BCR-ABL TYROSINE KINASE INHIBITORS
An EU wide review has concluded that dasatinib can cause hepatitis B reactivation; the MHRA recommends establishing hepatitis B virus status in all patients before initiation of treatment.

- **CAUTIONS** Hepatitis B infection · risk of cardiac dysfunction (monitor closely) · susceptibility to QT-interval prolongation (correct hypokalaemia or hypomagnesaemia before starting treatment)

CAUTIONS, FURTHER INFORMATION
- Hepatitis B infection The MHRA advises that patients who are carriers of hepatitis B virus should be closely monitored for signs and symptoms of active infection throughout treatment and for several months after stopping treatment; expert advice should be sought for patients who test positive for hepatitis B virus and in those with active infection.

- **INTERACTIONS** → Appendix 1: dasatinib
- **SIDE-EFFECTS**
- **Common or very common** Alopecia · anaemia · appetite abnormal · arrhythmias · arthralgia · asthenia · bone disorders · bone marrow depression · cardiac disorder · cardiomyopathy · chest pain · chills · constipation · cough · depression · diarrhoea · dizziness · drowsiness · dry eye · dyspnoea · eye inflammation · facial swelling · fever · fluid imbalance · flushing · gastrointestinal discomfort · gastrointestinal disorders · genital abnormalities · growth retardation · haemorrhage · headache · heart failure · hypertension · hyperuricaemia · increased risk of infection · insomnia · milia · mucositis · muscle complaints · muscle weakness · musculoskeletal stiffness · myocardial dysfunction · nausea · nerve disorders · neutropenia · oedema · oral disorders · pain · palpitations · pericardial effusion · perinephric effusion · peripheral swelling · pulmonary hypertension · pulmonary oedema · respiratory disorders · sepsis · skin reactions · sweat changes · taste altered · thrombocytopenia · tinnitus · vision disorders · vomiting · weight changes
- **Uncommon** Acute coronary syndrome · anxiety · arthritis · ascites · asthma · cardiac inflammation · cardiomegaly · cerebrovascular insufficiency · cholecystitis · CNS haemorrhage · confusion · dysphagia · embolism and thrombosis · emotional lability · excessive tearing · gynaecomastia · hair disorder · hearing loss · hepatic disorders · hypercholesterolaemia · hypoalbuminaemia · hypotension · hypothyroidism · ischaemic heart disease · libido decreased · lymphadenopathy · lymphopenia · malaise · memory loss · menstrual disorder · movement disorders · myopathy · nail disorder · osteonecrosis · pancreatitis · panniculitis · penile disorders · photosensitivity reaction · proteinuria · QT interval prolongation · renal impairment · scrotal oedema · skin ulcer · syncope · tendinitis · testicular swelling · tremor · tumour lysis syndrome · urinary frequency increased · vertigo · vulvovaginal swelling
- **Rare or very rare** Cardiac arrest · dementia · diabetes mellitus · facial paralysis · gait abnormal · hypersensitivity vasculitis · hyperthyroidism · pure red cell aplasia · seizure · thyroiditis
- **Frequency not known** Hepatitis B reactivation · nephrotic syndrome · Stevens-Johnson syndrome · thrombotic microangiopathy
- **CONCEPTION AND CONTRACEPTION** Effective contraception required during treatment.
- **PREGNANCY** Manufacturer advises avoid unless potential benefit outweighs risk—toxicity in *animal* studies. See also *Pregnancy and reproductive function* in Cytotoxic drugs p. 575.
- **BREAST FEEDING** Discontinue breast-feeding.
- **HEPATIC IMPAIRMENT** Manufacturer advises caution.
- **MONITORING REQUIREMENTS**
- Manufacturer advises evaluate for signs and symptoms of underlying cardiopulmonary disease before initiation of therapy—echocardiography should be performed at treatment initiation in patients with symptoms of cardiac disease and considered for patients with risk factors for cardiac or pulmonary disease.
- Manufacturer advises monitor patients with risk factors or a history of cardiac disease for signs or symptoms of cardiac dysfunction during treatment.
- When used for Chronic phase chronic myeloid leukaemia Manufacturer advises monitor full blood count every 2 weeks for 3 months, then every 3 months or as clinically indicated thereafter.
- When used for Acute lymphoblastic leukaemia Manufacturer advises monitor full blood count prior to each treatment cycle and as clinically indicated thereafter. During

consolidation treatment, manufacturer advises monitor full blood count every 2 days until recovery.

- **NATIONAL FUNDING/ACCESS DECISIONS**

Scottish Medicines Consortium (SMC) decisions

SMC No. SMC2142

The *Scottish Medicines Consortium* has advised (April 2019) that dasatinib (*Sprycel*®) is accepted for use within NHS Scotland for the treatment of paediatric patients with newly diagnosed chronic phase Philadelphia chromosome-positive chronic myeloid leukaemia (Ph+ CML-CP) or Ph+ CML-CP resistant or intolerant to prior therapy including imatinib. This advice is contingent upon the continuing availability of the patient access scheme in NHS Scotland or a list price that is equivalent or lower.

All Wales Medicines Strategy Group (AWMSG) decisions

AWMSG No. 1514

The *All Wales Medicines Strategy Group* has advised (April 2019) that dasatinib (*Sprycel*®) is recommended as an option for use within NHS Wales for the treatment of paediatric patients weighing 10 kg and above with newly diagnosed chronic phase Philadelphia chromosome-positive chronic myeloid leukaemia (Ph+ CML-CP) or Ph+ CML-CP resistant or intolerant to prior therapy including imatinib. This recommendation applies only in circumstances where the approved Patient Access Scheme (PAS) is utilised or where the list/contract price is equivalent or lower than the PAS price.

- **MEDICINAL FORMS** There can be variation in the licensing of different medicines containing the same drug.

Oral suspension

EXCIPIENTS: May contain Benzyl alcohol, sucrose

- Sprycel (Bristol-Myers Squibb Pharmaceuticals Ltd)
  Dasatinib (as Dasatinib monohydrate) 10 mg per 1 ml Sprycel 10mg/ml oral suspension | 99 ml PoM £626.74

Tablet

CAUTIONARY AND ADVISORY LABELS 25

- **Dasatinib (Non-proprietary)**
  Dasatinib (as Dasatinib monohydrate) 20 mg Dasatinib 20mg tablets | 60 tablet PoM £650.00 DT = £1,252.48
  Dasatinib (as Dasatinib monohydrate) 50 mg Dasatinib 50mg tablets | 60 tablet PoM £1,200.00 DT = £2,504.96
  Dasatinib (as Dasatinib monohydrate) 80 mg Dasatinib 80mg tablets | 30 tablet PoM £1,200.00 DT = £2,504.96
  Dasatinib (as Dasatinib monohydrate) 100 mg Dasatinib 100mg tablets | 30 tablet PoM £1,200.00 DT = £2,504.96
  Dasatinib (as Dasatinib monohydrate) 140 mg Dasatinib 140mg tablets | 30 tablet PoM £1,200.00 DT = £2,504.96
- **Sprycel** (Bristol-Myers Squibb Pharmaceuticals Ltd)
  Dasatinib (as Dasatinib monohydrate) 20 mg Sprycel 20mg tablets | 60 tablet PoM £1,252.48 DT = £1,252.48
  Dasatinib (as Dasatinib monohydrate) 50 mg Sprycel 50mg tablets | 60 tablet PoM £2,504.96 DT = £2,504.96
  Dasatinib (as Dasatinib monohydrate) 80 mg Sprycel 80mg tablets | 30 tablet PoM £2,504.96 DT = £2,504.96
  Dasatinib (as Dasatinib monohydrate) 100 mg Sprycel 100mg tablets | 30 tablet PoM £2,504.96 DT = £2,504.96
  Dasatinib (as Dasatinib monohydrate) 140 mg Sprycel 140mg tablets | 30 tablet PoM £2,504.96 DT = £2,504.96

Everolimus

24-May-2019

- **DRUG ACTION** Everolimus is a protein kinase inhibitor.

- **INDICATIONS AND DOSE**

VOTUBIA ® DISPERSIBLE TABLETS

Subependymal giant cell astrocytoma associated with tuberous sclerosis complex

- BY MOUTH USING DISPERSIBLE TABLETS
- Child 1–17 years: (consult product literature)

Adjunctive treatment of refractory partial-onset seizures, with or without secondary generalisation, associated with tuberous sclerosis complex

- BY MOUTH USING DISPERSIBLE TABLETS
- Child 2–17 years: (consult product literature)

VOTUBIA ® TABLETS

Subependymal giant cell astrocytoma associated with tuberous sclerosis complex

- BY MOUTH USING TABLETS
- Child 1–17 years: (consult product literature)

IMPORTANT SAFETY INFORMATION

RISKS OF INCORRECT DOSING OF ORAL ANTI-CANCER MEDICINES

See Cytotoxic drugs p. 575.

- **CAUTIONS** History of bleeding disorders · peri-surgical period (impaired wound healing)
- **INTERACTIONS** → Appendix 1: everolimus
- **SIDE-EFFECTS**
  - **Common or very common** Alopecia · anaemia · appetite decreased · arthralgia · asthenia · cough · decreased leucocytes · dehydration · diabetes mellitus · diarrhoea · dry mouth · dyslipidaemia · dysphagia · dyspnoea · electrolyte imbalance · eye inflammation · fever · gastrointestinal discomfort · haemorrhage · headache · hyperglycaemia · hypertension · increased risk of infection · insomnia · menstrual cycle irregularities · mucositis · nail disorders · nausea · neutropenia · oral disorders · peripheral oedema · proteinuria · renal impairment · respiratory disorders · skin reactions · taste altered · thrombocytopenia · vomiting · weight decreased
  - **Uncommon** Congestive heart failure · embolism and thrombosis · flushing · healing impaired · hepatitis B · musculoskeletal chest pain · pancytopenia · sepsis · urinary frequency increased
  - **Rare or very rare** Pure red cell aplasia
  - **Frequency not known** Hepatitis B reactivation

  SIDE-EFFECTS, FURTHER INFORMATION Reduce dose or discontinue if severe side-effects occur—consult product literature.
- **CONCEPTION AND CONTRACEPTION** Effective contraception must be used during and for up to 8 weeks after treatment.
- **PREGNANCY** Manufacturer advises avoid (toxicity in *animal* studies). See also *Pregnancy and reproductive function* in Cytotoxic drugs p. 575.
- **BREAST FEEDING** Manufacturer advises avoid.
- **HEPATIC IMPAIRMENT** Consult product literature.
- **MONITORING REQUIREMENTS**
  - For *Votubia*® preparations: manufacturer advises everolimus blood concentration monitoring is required—consult product literature.
  - Manufacturer advises monitor blood-glucose concentration, complete blood count, serum-triglycerides and serum-cholesterol before treatment and periodically thereafter.
  - Manufacturer advises monitor renal function before treatment and periodically thereafter.
  - Manufacturer advises monitor for signs and symptoms of infection before and during treatment.
- **DIRECTIONS FOR ADMINISTRATION**

  VOTUBIA ® DISPERSIBLE TABLETS Manufacturer advises tablets must be dispersed in water before administration—consult product literature for details.

  VOTUBIA ® TABLETS Tablets may be dispersed in approximately 30 mL of water by gently stirring, immediately before drinking. After solution has been swallowed, any residue must be re-dispersed in the same volume of water and swallowed.

- **PRESCRIBING AND DISPENSING INFORMATION** *Votubia®* is available as both *tablets* and *dispersible tablets*. These formulations vary in their licensed indications and are not interchangeable—consult product literature for information on switching between formulations.
- **PATIENT AND CARER ADVICE**
Pneumonitis Non-infectious pneumonitis reported. Manufacturer advises patients and their carers should be informed to seek urgent medical advice if new or worsening respiratory symptoms occur.
Infections Manufacturer advises patients and their carers should be informed of the risk of infection.
- **NATIONAL FUNDING/ACCESS DECISIONS**
VOTUBIA® DISPERSIBLE TABLETS
Scottish Medicines Consortium (SMC) decisions
SMC No. 1331/18
The *Scottish Medicines Consortium* has advised (June 2018) that everolimus (*Votubia®* dispersible tablets) are accepted for use within NHS Scotland for the adjunctive treatment of patients aged two years and older whose refractory partial-onset seizures, with or without secondary generalisation, are associated with tuberous sclerosis complex. This advice is contingent upon the continuing availability of the patient access scheme in NHS Scotland or a list price that is equivalent or lower.

- **MEDICINAL FORMS** There can be variation in the licensing of different medicines containing the same drug.

Dispersible tablet
CAUTIONARY AND ADVISORY LABELS 13
▸ Votubia (Novartis Pharmaceuticals UK Ltd)
Everolimus 2 mg Votubia 2mg dispersible tablets sugar-free | 30 tablet PoM £960.00
Everolimus 3 mg Votubia 3mg dispersible tablets sugar-free | 30 tablet PoM £1,440.00
Everolimus 5 mg Votubia 5mg dispersible tablets sugar-free | 30 tablet PoM £2,250.00

Tablet
CAUTIONARY AND ADVISORY LABELS 25
▸ Votubia (Novartis Pharmaceuticals UK Ltd)
Everolimus 2.5 mg Votubia 2.5mg tablets | 30 tablet PoM £1,200.00
Everolimus 5 mg Votubia 5mg tablets | 30 tablet PoM £2,250.00
Everolimus 10 mg Votubia 10mg tablets | 30 tablet PoM £2,970.00

Imatinib

05-Dec-2019

- **DRUG ACTION** Imatinib is a tyrosine kinase inhibitor.

- **INDICATIONS AND DOSE**

Treatment of newly diagnosed Philadelphia-chromosome-positive chronic myeloid leukaemia when bone marrow transplantation is not considered first line treatment | Treatment of Philadelphia-chromosome-positive chronic myeloid leukaemia in chronic phase after failure of interferon alfa, or in accelerated phase, or in blast crisis | Treatment of newly diagnosed Philadelphia-chromosome-positive acute lymphoblastic leukaemia in combination with chemotherapy
▸ BY MOUTH
▸ Child: (consult local protocol)

IMPORTANT SAFETY INFORMATION
RISKS OF INCORRECT DOSING OF ORAL ANTI-CANCER MEDICINES
See Cytotoxic drugs p. 575.
MHRA/CHM ADVICE (MAY 2016): RISK OF HEPATITIS B VIRUS REACTIVATION WITH BCR-ABL TYROSINE KINASE INHIBITORS
An EU wide review has concluded that imatinib can cause hepatitis B reactivation; the MHRA recommends establishing hepatitis B virus status in all patients before initiation of treatment.

- **CAUTIONS** Cardiac disease · hepatitis B infection · history of renal failure · risk factors for heart failure
CAUTIONS, FURTHER INFORMATION
▸ Hepatitis B infection The MHRA advises that patients who are carriers of hepatitis B virus should be closely monitored for signs and symptoms of active infection throughout treatment and for several months after stopping treatment; expert advice should be sought for patients who test positive for hepatitis B virus and in those with active infection.
- **INTERACTIONS** → Appendix 1: imatinib
- **SIDE-EFFECTS**
▸ **Common or very common** Alopecia · anaemia · appetite abnormal · asthenia · bone marrow disorders · chills · constipation · cough · diarrhoea · dizziness · dry eye · dry mouth · dyspnoea · excessive tearing · eye inflammation · fever · fluid imbalance · flushing · gastrointestinal discomfort · gastrointestinal disorders · haemorrhage · headaches · insomnia · joint disorders · muscle complaints · nausea · neutropenia · oedema · pain · photosensitivity reaction · sensation abnormal · skin reactions · sweat changes · taste altered · thrombocytopenia · vision blurred · vomiting · weight changes
▸ **Uncommon** Anxiety · arrhythmias · ascites · breast abnormalities · broken nails · burping · chest pain · CNS haemorrhage · congestive heart failure · depression · drowsiness · dysphagia · electrolyte imbalance · eosinophilia · eye discomfort · gout · gynaecomastia · hearing loss · hepatic disorders · hyperbilirubinaemia · hyperglycaemia · hypertension · hyperuricaemia · hypotension · increased risk of infection · laryngeal pain · lymphadenopathy · lymphopenia · malaise · memory loss · menstrual cycle irregularities · nerve disorders · oral disorders · palpitations · pancreatitis · peripheral coldness · pulmonary oedema · Raynaud's phenomenon · renal impairment · renal pain · respiratory disorders · restless legs · scrotal oedema · sepsis · sexual dysfunction · syncope · thrombocytosis · tinnitus · tremor · urinary frequency increased · vertigo
▸ **Rare or very rare** Angina pectoris · angioedema · arthritis · cardiac arrest · cataract · confusion · glaucoma · haemolytic anaemia · haemorrhagic ovarian cyst · hepatic failure (including fatal cases) · hypersensitivity vasculitis · inflammatory bowel disease · intracranial pressure increased · muscle weakness · myocardial infarction · myopathy · nail discolouration · pericardial disorders · pulmonary hypertension · seizure · severe cutaneous adverse reactions (SCARs) · tumour lysis syndrome
▸ **Frequency not known** Embolism and thrombosis · growth retardation · hepatitis B reactivation · neoplasm complications · osteonecrosis · pericarditis
- **CONCEPTION AND CONTRACEPTION** Effective contraception required during treatment.
- **PREGNANCY** Manufacturer advises avoid unless potential benefit outweighs risk. See also *Pregnancy and reproductive function* in Cytotoxic drugs p. 575.
- **BREAST FEEDING** Discontinue breast-feeding.
- **HEPATIC IMPAIRMENT** Manufacturer advises caution.
Dose adjustments In adults, manufacturer advises dosing at minimum recommended dose and consider further dose reduction if not tolerated—consult product literature.
- **RENAL IMPAIRMENT**
Dose adjustments Start with minimum recommended dose; reduce dose further if not tolerated; consult local treatment protocol.
- **MONITORING REQUIREMENTS**
▸ Monitor for gastrointestinal haemorrhage.
▸ Monitor complete blood counts regularly.
▸ Monitor for fluid retention.
▸ Monitor liver function.

- ▸ Monitor growth in children (may cause growth retardation).
- ● **DIRECTIONS FOR ADMINISTRATION** Tablets may be dispersed in water or apple juice.
- ● **PATIENT AND CARER ADVICE** Patients or carers should be given advice on how to administer imatinib tablets.

- ● **MEDICINAL FORMS** There can be variation in the licensing of different medicines containing the same drug.

Tablet

CAUTIONARY AND ADVISORY LABELS 21, 27

▸ Imatinib (Non-proprietary)
Imatinib (as Imatinib mesilate) 100 mg Imatinib 100mg tablets | 30 tablet PoM £486.66 | 60 tablet PoM £104.49 DT = £478.08 (Hospital only) | 60 tablet PoM £973.32 DT = £478.08
Imatinib (as Imatinib mesilate) 400 mg Imatinib 400mg tablets | 30 tablet PoM £208.98 DT = £1,133.41 (Hospital only) | 30 tablet PoM £1,946.67 DT = £1,133.41 | 60 tablet PoM £3,893.34

▸ Glivec (Novartis Pharmaceuticals UK Ltd) ▼
Imatinib (as Imatinib mesilate) 100 mg Glivec 100mg tablets | 60 tablet PoM £973.32 DT = £478.08
Imatinib (as Imatinib mesilate) 400 mg Glivec 400mg tablets | 30 tablet PoM £1,946.67 DT = £1,133.41

Larotrectinib

22-Oct-2019

- ● **DRUG ACTION** Larotrectinib is a tropomyosin receptor kinase inhibitor.

● **INDICATIONS AND DOSE**

Solid tumours with neurotrophic tyrosine receptor kinase gene fusion (initiated by a specialist)

▸ BY MOUTH

▸ Child: 100 mg/m^2 twice daily (max. per dose 100 mg), for dose adjustments, treatment interruption, or discontinuation due to side-effects—consult product literature

DOSE ADJUSTMENTS DUE TO INTERACTIONS

▸ Manufacturer advises if concomitant use with potent CYP3A4 inhibitors is unavoidable, reduce dose by 50%.

IMPORTANT SAFETY INFORMATION

RISKS OF INCORRECT DOSING OF ORAL ANTI-CANCER MEDICINES

See Cytotoxic drugs p. 575.

- ● **INTERACTIONS** → Appendix 1: larotrectinib
- ● **SIDE-EFFECTS**
- ▸ **Common or very common** Anaemia · constipation · dizziness · fatigue · gait abnormal · leucopenia · muscle weakness · myalgia · nausea · neutropenia · paraesthesia · taste altered · vomiting · weight increased
- ● **CONCEPTION AND CONTRACEPTION** Manufacturer advises effective contraception in females of childbearing potential and in men with a partner of childbearing potential, during treatment and for 1 month after last treatment; additional barrier method recommended in women using hormonal contraceptives. See also *Pregnancy and reproductive function* in Cytotoxic drugs p. 575.
- ● **PREGNANCY** Manufacturer advises avoid—limited information available. See also *Pregnancy and reproductive function* in Cytotoxic drugs p. 575.
- ● **BREAST FEEDING** Manufacturer advises avoid during treatment and for 3 days after last treatment—no information available.
- ● **HEPATIC IMPAIRMENT** Manufacturer advises caution in moderate to severe impairment (increased risk of exposure).
  Dose adjustments Manufacturer advises dose reduction by 50 % in moderate to severe impairment.
- ● **MONITORING REQUIREMENTS** Manufacturer advises monitor liver function (including ALT and AST) at baseline, then monthly during the first 3 months of treatment, and periodically thereafter; more frequent monitoring should be performed in patients who develop transaminase elevations. Treatment should be withheld or permanently discontinued based on severity—consult product literature.
- ● **HANDLING AND STORAGE** For *oral solution*, manufacturer advises store in a refrigerator (2–8°C).
- ● **PATIENT AND CARER ADVICE**
  Driving and skilled tasks Manufacturer advises patients and carers should be counselled on the effects on driving and performance of skilled tasks—increased risk of dizziness and fatigue.

- ● **MEDICINAL FORMS** There can be variation in the licensing of different medicines containing the same drug.

Oral solution

EXCIPIENTS: May contain Hydroxybenzoates (parabens), potassium sorbate, propylene glycol, sorbitol, sucrose

▸ Vitrakvi (Bayer Plc) ▼
Larotrectinib (as Larotrectinib sulfate) 20 mg per 1 ml Vitrakvi 20mg/ml oral solution | 100 ml PoM £5,000.00 (Hospital only)

Nilotinib

05-Dec-2019

- ● **DRUG ACTION** Nilotinib is a tyrosine kinase inhibitor.

● **INDICATIONS AND DOSE**

Newly diagnosed chronic phase Philadelphia chromosome-positive chronic myeloid leukaemia (initiated by a specialist)

▸ BY MOUTH

▸ Child 10–17 years: (consult product literature)

Chronic phase Philadelphia chromosome-positive chronic myeloid leukaemia resistant or intolerant to previous therapy, including imatinib (initiated by a specialist)

▸ BY MOUTH

▸ Child 6–17 years: (consult product literature)

IMPORTANT SAFETY INFORMATION

RISKS OF INCORRECT DOSING OF ORAL ANTI-CANCER MEDICINES

See Cytotoxic drugs p. 575.

MHRA/CHM ADVICE (MAY 2016): RISK OF HEPATITIS B VIRUS REACTIVATION WITH TYROSINE KINASE INHIBITORS

An EU wide review has concluded that nilotinib can cause hepatitis B virus reactivation; the MHRA recommends establishing hepatitis B virus status in all patients before initiation of treatment.

- ● **CAUTIONS** Clinically significant bradycardia · congestive heart failure · hepatitis B infection · history of pancreatitis · recent myocardial infarction · susceptibility to QT-interval prolongation (including electrolyte disturbances) · unstable angina
  CAUTIONS, FURTHER INFORMATION
  ▸ Hepatitis B infection The MHRA advises that patients who are carriers of hepatitis B virus should be closely monitored for signs and symptoms of active infection throughout treatment and for several months after stopping treatment; expert advice should be sought for patients who test positive for hepatitis B virus and in those with active infection.
- ● **INTERACTIONS** → Appendix 1: nilotinib
- ● **SIDE-EFFECTS**
- ▸ **Common or very common** Alopecia · anaemia · angina pectoris · anxiety · appetite abnormal · arrhythmias · arthralgia · asthenia · bone marrow disorders · cardiac conduction disorders · chest discomfort · constipation · cough · decreased leucocytes · depression · diabetes mellitus · diarrhoea · dizziness · dry eye · dyslipidaemia · dyspnoea · electrolyte imbalance · eosinophilia ·

eye discomfort · eye disorders · eye inflammation · fever · flushing · gastrointestinal discomfort · gastrointestinal disorders · headaches · hepatic disorders · hyperbilirubinaemia · hyperglycaemia · hypertension · increased risk of infection · insomnia · muscle complaints · muscle weakness · myocardial infarction · nausea · neoplasms · neutropenia · oedema · pain · palpitations · peripheral neuropathy · QT interval prolongation · respiratory disorders · sensation abnormal · skin reactions · sweat changes · taste altered · thrombocytopenia · vertigo · vomiting · weight changes

- **Uncommon** Atherosclerosis · cerebrovascular insufficiency · chills · cyanosis · erectile dysfunction · gout · haemorrhage · heart failure · hyperaemia · malaise · oral disorders · pancreatitis · peripheral vascular disease · temperature sensation altered · vision disorders
- **Frequency not known** Breast abnormalities · chorioretinopathy · diastolic dysfunction · dry mouth · facial swelling · gynaecomastia · hepatitis B reactivation · hyperparathyroidism · hyperuricaemia · hypoglycaemia · lethargy · memory loss · menorrhagia · oesophageal pain · oropharyngeal pain · pericardial effusion · pericarditis · restless legs · sebaceous hyperplasia · syncope · tremor · urinary disorders · urine discolouration

- **CONCEPTION AND CONTRACEPTION** Manufacturer advises highly effective contraception in women of childbearing potential during treatment and for up to two weeks after stopping treatment.
- **PREGNANCY** Manufacturer advises avoid unless potential benefit outweighs risk—toxicity in *animal* studies; see also *Pregnancy and reproductive function* in Cytotoxic drugs p. 575.
- **BREAST FEEDING** Manufacturer advises avoid—present in milk in *animal* studies.
- **HEPATIC IMPAIRMENT** Manufacturer advises caution (risk of increased exposure).
- **MONITORING REQUIREMENTS**
  - Manufacturer advises monitor lipid profiles before initiating treatment, at 3 and 6 months, and then yearly thereafter; monitor blood glucose before initiating treatment and then periodically during treatment, as clinically indicated.
  - Manufacturer advises monitor full blood count every 2 weeks for the first 2 months of treatment, then monthly thereafter, or as clinically indicated.
  - Manufacturer advises perform baseline ECG before treatment and as clinically indicated thereafter; correct any electrolyte disturbances before treatment and monitor periodically during treatment.
  - Manufacturer advises monitor and actively manage cardiovascular risk factors during treatment.
  - Manufacturer advises monitor liver function (including bilirubin and hepatic transaminases) monthly or as clinically indicated.
- **DIRECTIONS FOR ADMINISTRATION** Manufacturer advises capsules should either be swallowed whole or the contents of each capsule may be dispersed in one teaspoon of apple sauce and taken immediately.
- **PRESCRIBING AND DISPENSING INFORMATION** All prescribers should be familiar with the *Summary of Key Safety Recommendations for Tasigna ® (nilotinib)* provided by the manufacturer.
- **PATIENT AND CARER ADVICE** Manufacturer advises patients and carers should seek immediate medical attention if signs or symptoms of cardiovascular events occur.

  All patients should be provided with the *Important Information About How to Take Your Medication* leaflet provided by the manufacturer.

- **MEDICINAL FORMS** There can be variation in the licensing of different medicines containing the same drug.

Capsule

CAUTIONARY AND ADVISORY LABELS 23, 25, 27

- Tasigna (Novartis Pharmaceuticals UK Ltd)
  Nilotinib (as Nilotinib hydrochloride monohydrate)
  50 mg Tasigna 50mg capsules | 120 capsule PoM £2,432.85 DT = £2,432.85
  Nilotinib (as Nilotinib hydrochloride monohydrate)
  150 mg Tasigna 150mg capsules | 112 capsule PoM £2,432.85 DT = £2,432.85
  Nilotinib (as Nilotinib hydrochloride monohydrate)
  200 mg Tasigna 200mg capsules | 112 capsule PoM £2,432.85 DT = £2,432.85

Chapter 9
Blood and nutrition

CONTENTS

9 Blood and nutrition

Blood and blood-forming organs

1 Anaemias

Anaemias

Anaemia treatment considerations

Before initiating treatment for anaemia it is essential to determine which type is present. Iron salts may be harmful and result in iron overload if given alone to patients with anaemias other than those due to iron deficiency.

Sickle-cell anaemia

Sickle-cell disease is caused by a structural abnormality of haemoglobin resulting in deformed, less flexible red blood cells. Acute complications in the more severe forms include sickle-cell crisis, where infarction of the microvasculature and blood supply to organs results in severe pain. Sickle-cell crisis requires hospitalisation, intravenous fluids, analgesia and treatment of any concurrent infection. Chronic complications include skin ulceration, renal failure, and increased susceptibility to infection. Pneumococcal vaccine, haemophilus influenzae type b vaccine, an annual influenza vaccine and prophylactic penicillin reduce the risk of infection. Hepatitis B vaccine should be considered if the patient is not immune.

In most forms of sickle-cell disease, varying degrees of haemolytic anaemia are present accompanied by increased erythropoiesis; this may increase folate requirements and folate supplementation may be necessary.

Hydroxycarbamide p. 596 can reduce the frequency of crises and the need for blood transfusions in sickle-cell disease. The beneficial effects of hydroxycarbamide may not become evident for several months.

G6PD deficiency

Glucose 6-phosphate dehydrogenase (G6PD) deficiency is highly prevalent in individuals originating from most parts of Africa, from most parts of Asia, from Oceania, and from Southern Europe; it can also occur, rarely, in any other individuals. G6PD deficiency is more common in males than it is in females.

Individuals with G6PD deficiency are susceptible to developing acute haemolytic anaemia when they take a number of common drugs. They are also susceptible to developing acute haemolytic anaemia when they eat fava beans (broad beans, *Vicia faba*); this is termed *favism* and can be more severe in children or when the fresh fava beans are eaten raw.

When prescribing drugs for patients with G6PD deficiency, the following three points should be kept in mind:

- G6PD deficiency is genetically heterogeneous; susceptibility to the haemolytic risk from drugs varies; thus, a drug found to be safe in some G6PD-deficient individuals may not be equally safe in others;
- manufacturers do not routinely test drugs for their effects in G6PD-deficient individuals;
- the risk and severity of haemolysis is almost always dose-related.

The lists below should be read with these points in mind. Ideally, information about G6PD deficiency should be available before prescribing a drug listed below. However, in the absence of this information, the possibility of haemolysis should be considered, especially if the patient belongs to a group in which G6PD deficiency is common.

A very few G6PD-deficient individuals with chronic non-spherocytic haemolytic anaemia have haemolysis even in the absence of an exogenous trigger. These patients must be regarded as being at high risk of severe exacerbation of haemolysis following administration of any of the drugs listed below.

Drugs with definite risk of haemolysis in most G6PD-deficient individuals

- Dapsone and other sulfones (higher doses for dermatitis herpetiformis more likely to cause problems)
- Fluoroquinolones (including ciprofloxacin, moxifloxacin, norfloxacin, and ofloxacin)
- Methylthioninium chloride
- Niridazole [not on UK market]
- Nitrofurantoin
- Pamaquin [not on UK market]
- Primaquine (30 mg weekly for 8 weeks has been found to be without undue harmful effects in African and Asian people)
- Quinolones (such as nalidixic acid [not on UK market])
- Rasburicase
- Sulfonamides (including co-trimoxazole; some sulfonamides, e.g. sulfadiazine, have been tested and found not to be haemolytic in many G6PD-deficient individuals)

Drugs with possible risk of haemolysis in some G6PD-deficient individuals

- Aspirin (acceptable up to a dose of at least 1 g daily in most G6PD-deficient individuals)
- Chloroquine (acceptable in acute malaria and malaria chemoprophylaxis)
- Menadione, water-soluble derivatives (e.g. menadiol sodium phosphate)
- Quinidine (acceptable in acute malaria) [not on UK market]
- Quinine (acceptable in acute malaria)
- Sulfonylureas

Naphthalene in mothballs also causes haemolysis in individuals with G6PD deficiency.

Hypoplastic, haemolytic, and renal anaemias

Anabolic steroids, pyridoxine hydrochloride p. 678, antilymphocyte immunoglobulin, rituximab [unlicensed] p. 574, and various corticosteroids are used in hypoplastic and haemolytic anaemias.

Antilymphocyte immunoglobulin given intravenously through a central line over 12–18 hours each day for 5 days produces a response in about 50% of cases of acquired *aplastic anaemia*; the response rate may be increased when ciclosporin p. 559 is given as well. Severe reactions are common in the first 2 days and profound immunosuppression can occur; antilymphocyte immunoglobulin should be given under specialist supervision with appropriate resuscitation facilities.

Alternatively, oxymetholone tablets (available from 'special order' manufacturers or specialist importing companies) can be used in aplastic anaemia for 3 to 6 months.

It is unlikely that dietary deprivation of pyridoxine hydrochloride produces clinically relevant haematological effects. However, certain forms of *sideroblastic anaemia* respond to pharmacological doses, possibly reflecting its role as a co-enzyme during haemoglobin synthesis. Pyridoxine hydrochloride is indicated in both *idiopathic acquired* and *hereditary sideroblastic anaemias*. Although complete cures have not been reported, some increase in haemoglobin can occur with high doses. *Reversible sideroblastic anaemias* respond to treatment of the underlying cause but pyridoxine hydrochloride is indicated in pregnancy, haemolytic anaemias, or during isoniazid p. 399 treatment.

Corticosteroids have an important place in the management of haematological disorders including *autoimmune haemolytic anaemia*, *idiopathic thrombocytopenias* and *neutropenias*, and *major transfusion reactions*. They are also used in chemotherapy schedules for many types of *lymphoma*, *lymphoid leukaemias*, and *paraproteinaemias*, including *multiple myeloma*.

Erythropoietins

Epoetins (recombinant human erythropoietins) are used to treat the anaemia associated with erythropoietin deficiency in chronic renal failure.

Epoetin beta p. 613 is also used for the prevention of anaemia in preterm neonates of low birth-weight; a therapeutic response may take several weeks.

There is insufficient information to support the use of erythropoietins in children with leukaemia or in those receiving cancer chemotherapy.

Darbepoetin is a glycosylated derivative of epoetin; it persists longer in the body and can be administered less frequently than epoetin.

1.1 Hypoplastic, haemolytic, and renal anaemias

Other drugs used for Hypoplastic, haemolytic, and renal anaemias Eltrombopag, p. 629

ANABOLIC STEROIDS > ANDROSTAN DERIVATIVES

Oxymetholone

● **INDICATIONS AND DOSE**

Aplastic anaemia

▶ BY MOUTH

▶ Child: 1–5 mg/kg daily for 3 to 6 months

● **INTERACTIONS** → Appendix 1: oxymetholone

● **MEDICINAL FORMS** There can be variation in the licensing of different medicines containing the same drug. Forms available from special-order manufacturers include: oral suspension

Capsule

▶ Oxymetholone (Non-proprietary)

Oxymetholone 50 mg Oxymetholone 50mg capsules | 50 capsule PoM £475.00 CD4-2

EPOETINS

Epoetins 

IMPORTANT SAFETY INFORMATION

MHRA/CHM ADVICE: RECOMBINANT HUMAN ERYTHROPOIETINS: VERY RARE RISK OF SEVERE CUTANEOUS ADVERSE REACTIONS (UPDATED JANUARY 2018)

The MHRA is aware of very rare cases of severe cutaneous adverse reactions, including Stevens-Johnson syndrome and toxic epidermal necrolysis, in patients treated with erythropoietins; some cases were fatal. More severe cases were recorded with long-acting agents (darbepoetin alfa and methoxy polyethylene glycol-epoetin beta).

Patients and their carers should be advised of the signs and symptoms of severe skin reactions when starting treatment and instructed to stop treatment and seek immediate medical attention if they develop widespread rash and blistering; these rashes often follow fever or flu-like symptoms—discontinue treatment permanently if such reactions occur.

ERYTHROPOIETINS—HAEMOGLOBIN CONCENTRATION

In chronic kidney disease, the use of erythropoietins can be considered in a child with anaemia. The aim of treatment is to relieve symptoms of anaemia and to avoid the need for blood transfusion. Manufacturer advises haemoglobin concentration should not be increased beyond that which provides adequate control of symptoms of anaemia. In *adults*, overcorrection of haemoglobin concentration with erythropoietins in those with chronic kidney disease may increase the risk of serious cardiovascular events and death; haemoglobin concentrations higher than 12 g/100 mL should be avoided in children.

- **CONTRA-INDICATIONS** Pure red cell aplasia following erythropoietin therapy · uncontrolled hypertension
- **CAUTIONS** Aluminium toxicity (can impair the response to erythropoietin) · concurrent infection (can impair the response to erythropoietin) · correct factors that contribute to the anaemia of chronic renal failure, such as iron or folate deficiency, before treatment · during dialysis (increase in unfractionated or low molecular weight heparin dose may be needed) · epilepsy · inadequately treated or poorly controlled blood pressure—interrupt treatment if blood pressure uncontrolled · ischaemic vascular disease · malignant disease · other inflammatory disease (can impair the response to erythropoietin) · sickle-cell disease (lower target haemoglobin concentration may be appropriate) · sudden stabbing migraine-like pain (warning of a hypertensive crisis) · thrombocytosis (monitor platelet count for first 8 weeks)
- **SIDE-EFFECTS**
  - **Common or very common** Arthralgia · embolism and thrombosis · headache · hypertension (dose-dependent) · influenza like illness · skin reactions · stroke
  - **Uncommon** Hypertensive crisis (in isolated patients with normal or low blood pressure) · respiratory tract congestion · seizure
  - **Rare or very rare** Thrombocytosis
  - **Frequency not known** Pure red cell aplasia (more common following subcutaneous administration in patients with chronic renal failure) · severe cutaneous adverse reactions (SCARs)

SIDE-EFFECTS, FURTHER INFORMATION

Hypertensive crisis In isolated patients with normal or low blood pressure, hypertensive crisis with encephalopathy-like symptoms and generalised tonic-clonic seizures requiring immediate medical attention has occurred with epoetin.

Pure red cell aplasia There have been very rare reports of pure red cell aplasia in patients treated with erythropoietins. In patients who develop a lack of efficacy with erythropoietin therapy and with a diagnosis of pure red cell aplasia, treatment with erythropoietins must be discontinued and testing for erythropoietin antibodies considered. Patients who develop pure red cell aplasia should not be switched to another form of erythropoietin.

- **MONITORING REQUIREMENTS**
  - Monitor closely blood pressure, reticulocyte counts, haemoglobin, and electrolytes—interrupt treatment if blood pressure uncontrolled.
  - Other factors, such as iron or folate deficiency, that contribute to the anaemia of chronic renal failure should be corrected before treatment and monitored during therapy. Supplemental iron may improve the response in resistant patients and in preterm neonates.

above

Darbepoetin alfa

30-Apr-2019

- **INDICATIONS AND DOSE**

Symptomatic anaemia associated with chronic renal failure in patients on dialysis

▶ BY SUBCUTANEOUS INJECTION, OR BY INTRAVENOUS INJECTION

▶ Child 11–17 years: Initially 450 nanograms/kg once weekly, dose to be adjusted according to response by approximately 25% at intervals of at least 4 weeks, maintenance dose to be given once weekly or once every 2 weeks, reduce dose by approximately 25% if rise in haemoglobin concentration exceeds 2 g/100 mL over 4 weeks or if haemoglobin concentration exceeds 12 g/100 mL; if haemoglobin concentration continues to rise, despite dose reduction, suspend treatment until haemoglobin concentration decreases and then restart at a dose approximately 25% lower than the previous dose, when changing route give same dose then adjust according to weekly or fortnightly haemoglobin measurements, adjust doses not more frequently than every 2 weeks during maintenance treatment

Symptomatic anaemia associated with chronic renal failure in patients not on dialysis

▶ BY SUBCUTANEOUS INJECTION

▶ Child 11–17 years: Initially 450 nanograms/kg once weekly, alternatively initially 750 nanograms/kg every 2 weeks, dose to be adjusted according to response by approximately 25% at intervals of at least 4 weeks, maintenance dose can be given once weekly, every 2 weeks, or once a month, subcutaneous route preferred in patients not on haemodialysis, reduce dose by approximately 25% if rise in haemoglobin concentration exceeds 2 g/100 mL over 4 weeks or if haemoglobin concentration exceeds 12 g/100 mL; if haemoglobin concentration continues to rise, despite dose reduction, suspend treatment until haemoglobin concentration decreases and then restart at a dose approximately 25% lower than the previous dose, when changing route give same dose then adjust according to weekly or fortnightly haemoglobin measurements, adjust doses not more frequently than every 2 weeks during maintenance treatment

Symptomatic anaemia associated with chronic renal failure in patients not on dialysis

▶ BY INTRAVENOUS INJECTION

▶ Child 11–17 years: Initially 450 nanograms/kg once weekly, dose to be adjusted according to response by approximately 25% at intervals of at least 4 weeks, maintenance dose given once weekly, subcutaneous route preferred in patients not on haemodialysis, reduce dose by approximately 25% if rise in haemoglobin concentration exceeds

continued →

2 g/100 mL over 4 weeks or if haemoglobin concentration exceeds 12 g/100 mL; if haemoglobin concentration continues to rise, despite dose reduction, suspend treatment until haemoglobin concentration decreases and then restart at a dose approximately 25% lower than the previous dose, when changing route give same dose then adjust according to weekly or fortnightly haemoglobin measurements, adjust doses not more frequently than every 2 weeks during maintenance treatment

- **INTERACTIONS** → Appendix 1: darbepoetin alfa
- **SIDE-EFFECTS**
  - ▶ **Common or very common** Hypersensitivity · oedema
- **PREGNANCY** No evidence of harm in *animal* studies—manufacturer advises caution.
- **BREAST FEEDING** Manufacturer advises avoid—no information available.
- **HEPATIC IMPAIRMENT** Manufacturer advises caution (no information available).

- **MEDICINAL FORMS** There can be variation in the licensing of different medicines containing the same drug.

Solution for injection

▶ Aranesp (Amgen Ltd)

Darbepoetin alfa 25 microgram per 1 ml Aranesp 10micrograms/0.4ml solution for injection pre-filled syringes | 4 pre-filled disposable injection PoM £58.72 DT = £58.72

Darbepoetin alfa 40 microgram per 1 ml Aranesp 20micrograms/0.5ml solution for injection pre-filled syringes | 4 pre-filled disposable injection PoM £117.45 DT = £117.45

Darbepoetin alfa 100 microgram per 1 ml Aranesp 50micrograms/0.5ml solution for injection pre-filled syringes | 4 pre-filled disposable injection PoM £293.62 DT = £293.62
Aranesp 40micrograms/0.4ml solution for injection pre-filled syringes | 4 pre-filled disposable injection PoM £234.90 DT = £234.90
Aranesp 30micrograms/0.3ml solution for injection pre-filled syringes | 4 pre-filled disposable injection PoM £176.17 DT = £176.17

Darbepoetin alfa 200 microgram per 1 ml Aranesp 130micrograms/0.65ml solution for injection pre-filled syringes | 4 pre-filled disposable injection PoM £763.42 DT = £763.42
Aranesp 100micrograms/0.5ml solution for injection pre-filled syringes | 4 pre-filled disposable injection PoM £587.24 DT = £587.24
Aranesp 60micrograms/0.3ml solution for injection pre-filled syringes | 4 pre-filled disposable injection PoM £352.35 DT = £352.35
Aranesp 80micrograms/0.4ml solution for injection pre-filled syringes | 4 pre-filled disposable injection PoM £469.79 DT = £469.79

Darbepoetin alfa 500 microgram per 1 ml Aranesp 300micrograms/0.6ml solution for injection pre-filled syringes | 1 pre-filled disposable injection PoM £440.43 DT = £440.43
Aranesp 500micrograms/1ml solution for injection pre-filled syringes | 1 pre-filled disposable injection PoM £734.05 DT = £734.05
Aranesp 150micrograms/0.3ml solution for injection pre-filled syringes | 4 pre-filled disposable injection PoM £880.86 DT = £880.86

▶ Aranesp SureClick (Amgen Ltd)

Darbepoetin alfa 40 microgram per 1 ml Aranesp SureClick 20micrograms/0.5ml solution for injection pre-filled pens | 1 pre-filled disposable injection PoM £29.36 DT = £29.36

Darbepoetin alfa 100 microgram per 1 ml Aranesp SureClick 40micrograms/0.4ml solution for injection pre-filled pens | 1 pre-filled disposable injection PoM £58.72 DT = £58.72
Aranesp SureClick 80micrograms/0.4ml solution for injection pre-filled pens | 1 pre-filled disposable injection PoM £117.45 DT = £117.45

Darbepoetin alfa 200 microgram per 1 ml Aranesp SureClick 100micrograms/0.5ml solution for injection pre-filled pens | 1 pre-filled disposable injection PoM £146.81 DT = £146.81
Aranesp SureClick 60micrograms/0.3ml solution for injection pre-filled pens | 1 pre-filled disposable injection PoM £88.09 DT = £88.09

Darbepoetin alfa 500 microgram per 1 ml Aranesp SureClick 300micrograms/0.6ml solution for injection pre-filled pens | 1 pre-filled disposable injection PoM £440.43 DT = £440.43
Aranesp SureClick 150micrograms/0.3ml solution for injection pre-filled pens | 1 pre-filled disposable injection PoM £220.22 DT = £220.22
Aranesp SureClick 500micrograms/1ml solution for injection pre-filled pens | 1 pre-filled disposable injection PoM £734.05 DT = £734.05

611

Epoetin alfa

30-Apr-2019

- **INDICATIONS AND DOSE**

EPREX® PRE-FILLED SYRINGES

Symptomatic anaemia associated with chronic renal failure in patients on haemodialysis

▶ BY INTRAVENOUS INJECTION

- ▶ Child (body-weight up to 10 kg): Initially 50 units/kg 3 times a week, adjusted in steps of 25 units/kg 3 times a week, dose adjusted according to response at intervals of at least 4 weeks; maintenance 75–150 units/kg 3 times a week, intravenous injection to be given over 1–5 minutes, reduce dose by approximately 25% if rise in haemoglobin concentration exceeds 2 g/100 mL over 4 weeks or if haemoglobin concentration exceeds 12 g/100 mL; if haemoglobin concentration continues to rise, despite dose reduction, suspend treatment until haemoglobin concentration decreases and then restart at a dose approximately 25% lower than the previous dose
- ▶ Child (body-weight 10–30 kg): Initially 50 units/kg 3 times a week, adjusted in steps of 25 units/kg 3 times a week, dose adjusted according to response at intervals of at least 4 weeks; maintenance 60–150 units/kg 3 times a week, intravenous injection to be given over 1–5 minutes, reduce dose by approximately 25% if rise in haemoglobin concentration exceeds 2 g/100 mL over 4 weeks or if haemoglobin concentration exceeds 12 g/100 mL; if haemoglobin concentration continues to rise, despite dose reduction, suspend treatment until haemoglobin concentration decreases and then restart at a dose approximately 25% lower than the previous dose
- ▶ Child (body-weight 31–60 kg): Initially 50 units/kg 3 times a week, adjusted in steps of 25 units/kg 3 times a week, dose adjusted according to response at intervals of at least 4 weeks; maintenance 30–100 units/kg 3 times a week, intravenous injection to be given over 1–5 minutes, reduce dose by approximately 25% if rise in haemoglobin concentration exceeds 2 g/100 mL over 4 weeks or if haemoglobin concentration exceeds 12 g/100 mL; if haemoglobin concentration continues to rise, despite dose reduction, suspend treatment until haemoglobin concentration decreases and then restart at a dose approximately 25% lower than the previous dose
- ▶ Child (body-weight 61 kg and above): Initially 50 units/kg 3 times a week, adjusted in steps of 25 units/kg 3 times a week, dose adjusted according to response at intervals of at least 4 weeks; maintenance 75–300 units/kg once weekly, maintenance dose can be given as a single dose or in divided doses, intravenous injection to be given over 1–5 minutes, reduce dose by approximately 25% if rise in haemoglobin concentration exceeds 2 g/100 mL over 4 weeks or if haemoglobin concentration exceeds 12 g/100 mL; if haemoglobin concentration continues to rise, despite dose reduction, suspend treatment until haemoglobin concentration decreases and then restart at a dose approximately 25% lower than the previous dose

- **INTERACTIONS** → Appendix 1: epoetin alfa
- **SIDE-EFFECTS**
  - ▶ **Common or very common** Chills · cough · diarrhoea · fever · myalgia · nausea · pain · peripheral oedema · vomiting
  - ▶ **Uncommon** Hyperkalaemia
- **PREGNANCY** No evidence of harm. Benefits probably outweigh risk of anaemia and of blood transfusion in pregnancy.

- **BREAST FEEDING** Unlikely to be present in milk. Minimal effect on infant.
- **HEPATIC IMPAIRMENT** Manufacturer advises caution in chronic hepatic failure.
- **PRESCRIBING AND DISPENSING INFORMATION** Epoetin alfa is a biological medicine. Biological medicines must be prescribed and dispensed by brand name, see *Biological medicines* and *Biosimilar medicines*, under Guidance on prescribing p. 1.

- **MEDICINAL FORMS** There can be variation in the licensing of different medicines containing the same drug.

Solution for injection

▸ Eprex (Janssen-Cilag Ltd)

Epoetin alfa 2000 unit per 1 ml Eprex 1,000units/0.5ml solution for injection pre-filled syringes | 6 pre-filled disposable injection PoM £33.18 DT = £33.18

Epoetin alfa 4000 unit per 1 ml Eprex 2,000units/0.5ml solution for injection pre-filled syringes | 6 pre-filled disposable injection PoM £66.37 DT = £66.37

Epoetin alfa 10000 unit per 1 ml Eprex 6,000units/0.6ml solution for injection pre-filled syringes | 6 pre-filled disposable injection PoM £199.11 DT = £199.11

Eprex 4,000units/0.4ml solution for injection pre-filled syringes | 6 pre-filled disposable injection PoM £132.74 DT = £132.74

Eprex 5,000units/0.5ml solution for injection pre-filled syringes | 6 pre-filled disposable injection PoM £165.92 DT = £165.92

Eprex 3,000units/0.3ml solution for injection pre-filled syringes | 6 pre-filled disposable injection PoM £99.55 DT = £99.55

Eprex 10,000units/1ml solution for injection pre-filled syringes | 6 pre-filled disposable injection PoM £331.85 DT = £331.85

Eprex 8,000units/0.8ml solution for injection pre-filled syringes | 6 pre-filled disposable injection PoM £265.48 DT = £265.48

Epoetin alfa 40000 unit per 1 ml Eprex 20,000units/0.5ml solution for injection pre-filled syringes | 1 pre-filled disposable injection PoM £110.62 DT = £110.62

Eprex 30,000units/0.75ml solution for injection pre-filled syringes | 1 pre-filled disposable injection PoM £199.11 DT = £199.11

Eprex 40,000units/1ml solution for injection pre-filled syringes | 1 pre-filled disposable injection PoM £265.48 DT = £265.48

F 611

Epoetin beta

06-Dec-2019

- **INDICATIONS AND DOSE**

Symptomatic anaemia associated with chronic renal failure

▸ BY SUBCUTANEOUS INJECTION

▸ Neonate: Initially 20 units/kg 3 times a week for 4 weeks, increased in steps of 20 units/kg 3 times a week, according to response at intervals of 4 weeks, total weekly dose may be divided into daily doses; maintenance dose, initially reduce dose by half then adjust according to response at intervals of 1–2 weeks, total weekly maintenance dose may be given as a single dose or in 3 or 7 divided doses. Subcutaneous route preferred in patients not on haemodialysis. Reduce dose by approximately 25% if rise in haemoglobin concentration exceeds 2 g/100 mL over 4 weeks or if haemoglobin concentration approaches or exceeds 12 g/100 mL; if haemoglobin concentration continues to rise, despite dose reduction, suspend treatment until haemoglobin concentration decreases and then restart at a dose approximately 25% lower than the previous dose; maximum 720 units/kg per week.

▸ Child: Initially 20 units/kg 3 times a week for 4 weeks, increased in steps of 20 units/kg 3 times a week, according to response at intervals of 4 weeks, total weekly dose may be divided into daily doses; maintenance dose, initially reduce dose by half then adjust according to response at intervals of 1–2 weeks, total weekly maintenance dose may be given as a single dose or in 3 or 7 divided doses. Subcutaneous route preferred in patients not on haemodialysis. Reduce dose by approximately 25% if rise in haemoglobin concentration exceeds 2 g/100 mL over 4 weeks or if haemoglobin concentration approaches or exceeds 12 g/100 mL; if haemoglobin concentration continues to rise, despite dose reduction, suspend treatment until haemoglobin concentration decreases and then restart at a dose approximately 25% lower than the previous dose; maximum 720 units/kg per week

▸ BY INTRAVENOUS INJECTION

▸ Neonate: Initially 40 units/kg 3 times a week for 4 weeks, then increased to 80 units/kg 3 times a week, then increased in steps of 20 units/kg 3 times a week if required, at intervals of 4 weeks; maintenance dose, initially reduce dose by half then adjust according to response at intervals of 1–2 weeks. Intravenous injection to be administered over 2 minutes. Subcutaneous route preferred in patients not on haemodialysis. Reduce dose by approximately 25% if rise in haemoglobin concentration exceeds 2 g/100 mL over 4 weeks or if haemoglobin concentration approaches or exceeds 12 g/100 mL; if haemoglobin concentration continues to rise, despite dose reduction, suspend treatment until haemoglobin concentration decreases and then restart at a dose approximately 25% lower than the previous dose; maximum 720 units/kg per week.

▸ Child: Initially 40 units/kg 3 times a week for 4 weeks, then increased to 80 units/kg 3 times a week, then increased in steps of 20 units/kg 3 times a week if required, at intervals of 4 weeks; maintenance dose, initially reduce dose by half then adjust according to response at intervals of 1–2 weeks. Intravenous injection to be administered over 2 minutes. Subcutaneous route preferred in patients not on haemodialysis. Reduce dose by approximately 25% if rise in haemoglobin concentration exceeds 2 g/100 mL over 4 weeks or if haemoglobin concentration approaches or exceeds 12 g/100 mL; if haemoglobin concentration continues to rise, despite dose reduction, suspend treatment until haemoglobin concentration decreases and then restart at a dose approximately 25% lower than the previous dose; maximum 720 units/kg per week

Prevention of anaemias of prematurity in neonates

▸ BY SUBCUTANEOUS INJECTION

▸ Neonate up to 33 weeks corrected gestational age (body-weight 0.75–1.5 kg): 250 units/kg 3 times a week preferably started within 3 days of birth and continued for 6 weeks, using single-dose unpreserved injection.

IMPORTANT SAFETY INFORMATION

MHRA/CHM ADVICE (MAY 2015) EPOETIN BETA (NEORECORMON): INCREASED RISK OF RETINOPATHY IN PRETERM INFANTS CANNOT BE EXCLUDED

There is a possible increased risk of retinopathy in premature infants, when epoetin beta is used for preventing anaemia of prematurity. When using epoetin beta in preterm infants:

- consider the benefits and risks of treatment, including the possible risk of retinopathy,
- monitor the infant for features of retinopathy, and
- advise parents or carers that their baby's eyes will be carefully monitored for any ill effects.

- **INTERACTIONS** → Appendix 1: epoetin beta
- **PREGNANCY** No evidence of harm. Benefits probably outweigh risk of anaemia and of blood transfusion in pregnancy.

9 Blood and nutrition

- **BREAST FEEDING** Unlikely to be present in milk. Minimal effect on infant.
- **HEPATIC IMPAIRMENT** Manufacturer advises caution in chronic hepatic failure.

- **MEDICINAL FORMS** There can be variation in the licensing of different medicines containing the same drug.

Solution for injection

EXCIPIENTS: May contain Phenylalanine

▸ NeoRecormon (Roche Products Ltd)

Epoetin beta 1667 unit per 1 ml NeoRecormon 500units/0.3ml solution for injection pre-filled syringes | 6 pre-filled disposable injection PoM £21.05 DT = £21.05

Epoetin beta 6667 unit per 1 ml NeoRecormon 2,000units/0.3ml solution for injection pre-filled syringes | 6 pre-filled disposable injection PoM £84.17 DT = £84.17

Epoetin beta 10000 unit per 1 ml NeoRecormon 3,000units/0.3ml solution for injection pre-filled syringes | 6 pre-filled disposable injection PoM £126.25 DT = £126.25

Epoetin beta 13333 unit per 1 ml NeoRecormon 4,000units/0.3ml solution for injection pre-filled syringes | 6 pre-filled disposable injection PoM £168.34 DT = £168.34

Epoetin beta 16667 unit per 1 ml NeoRecormon 10,000units/0.6ml solution for injection pre-filled syringes | 6 pre-filled disposable injection PoM £420.85 DT = £420.85

NeoRecormon 5,000units/0.3ml solution for injection pre-filled syringes | 6 pre-filled disposable injection PoM £210.42 DT = £210.42

Epoetin beta 20000 unit per 1 ml NeoRecormon 6,000units/0.3ml solution for injection pre-filled syringes | 6 pre-filled disposable injection PoM £252.50 DT = £252.50

Epoetin beta 33333 unit per 1 ml NeoRecormon 20,000units/0.6ml solution for injection pre-filled syringes | 6 pre-filled disposable injection PoM £841.71 DT = £841.71

Epoetin beta 50000 unit per 1 ml NeoRecormon 30,000units/0.6ml solution for injection pre-filled syringes | 4 pre-filled disposable injection PoM £841.71 DT = £841.71

F 611

Epoetin zeta

30-Apr-2019

- **INDICATIONS AND DOSE**

Symptomatic anaemia associated with chronic renal failure in patients on haemodialysis

▸ BY INTRAVENOUS INJECTION

- Child (body-weight up to 10 kg): Initially 50 units/kg 3 times a week, adjusted according to response, adjusted in steps of 25 units/kg 3 times a week, dose to be adjusted at intervals of at least 4 weeks; maintenance 75–150 units/kg 3 times a week, to be administered over 1–5 minutes, avoid increasing haemoglobin concentration at a rate exceeding 2 g/100 mL over 4 weeks
- Child (body-weight 10-30 kg): Initially 50 units/kg 3 times a week, adjusted according to response, adjusted in steps of 25 units/kg 3 times a week, dose to be adjusted at intervals of at least 4 weeks; maintenance 60–150 units/kg 3 times a week, to be administered over 1–5 minutes, avoid increasing haemoglobin concentration at a rate exceeding 2 g/100 mL over 4 weeks
- Child (body-weight 31 kg and above): Initially 50 units/kg 3 times a week, adjusted according to response, adjusted in steps of 25 units/kg 3 times a week, dose to be adjusted at intervals of at least 4 weeks; maintenance 30–100 units/kg 3 times a week, to be administered over 1–5 minutes, avoid increasing haemoglobin concentration at a rate exceeding 2 g/100 mL over 4 weeks

- **INTERACTIONS** → Appendix 1: epoetin zeta
- **SIDE-EFFECTS**
  - ▸ **Common or very common** Asthenia · dizziness
  - ▸ **Uncommon** Intracranial haemorrhage
  - ▸ **Rare or very rare** Angioedema
  - ▸ **Frequency not known** Aneurysm · cerebrovascular insufficiency · hypertensive encephalopathy · myocardial infarction · myocardial ischaemia
- **PREGNANCY** No evidence of harm. Benefits probably outweigh risk of anaemia and of blood transfusion in pregnancy.
- **BREAST FEEDING** Unlikely to be present in milk. Minimal effect on infant.
- **HEPATIC IMPAIRMENT** Manufacturer advises caution in chronic hepatic failure.
- **PRESCRIBING AND DISPENSING INFORMATION** Epoetin zeta is a biological medicine. Biological medicines must be prescribed and dispensed by brand name, see *Biological medicines* and *Biosimilar medicines*, under Guidance on prescribing p. 1.

- **MEDICINAL FORMS** There can be variation in the licensing of different medicines containing the same drug.

Solution for injection

EXCIPIENTS: May contain Phenylalanine

▸ Retacrit (Pfizer Ltd)

Epoetin zeta 3333 unit per 1 ml Retacrit 2,000units/0.6ml solution for injection pre-filled syringes | 6 pre-filled disposable injection PoM £57.70 DT = £57.70

Retacrit 3,000units/0.9ml solution for injection pre-filled syringes | 6 pre-filled disposable injection PoM £86.55 DT = £86.55

Retacrit 1,000units/0.3ml solution for injection pre-filled syringes | 6 pre-filled disposable injection PoM £28.85 DT = £28.85

Epoetin zeta 10000 unit per 1 ml Retacrit 6,000units/0.6ml solution for injection pre-filled syringes | 6 pre-filled disposable injection PoM £173.09 DT = £173.09

Retacrit 10,000units/1ml solution for injection pre-filled syringes | 6 pre-filled disposable injection PoM £288.48 DT = £288.48

Retacrit 8,000units/0.8ml solution for injection pre-filled syringes | 6 pre-filled disposable injection PoM £230.79 DT = £230.79

Retacrit 4,000units/0.4ml solution for injection pre-filled syringes | 6 pre-filled disposable injection PoM £115.40 DT = £115.40

Retacrit 5,000units/0.5ml solution for injection pre-filled syringes | 6 pre-filled disposable injection PoM £144.25 DT = £144.25

Epoetin zeta 40000 unit per 1 ml Retacrit 20,000units/0.5ml solution for injection pre-filled syringes | 1 pre-filled disposable injection PoM £96.16 DT = £96.16

Retacrit 40,000units/1ml solution for injection pre-filled syringes | 1 pre-filled disposable injection PoM £193.32 DT = £193.32

Retacrit 30,000units/0.75ml solution for injection pre-filled syringes | 1 pre-filled disposable injection PoM £144.25 DT = £144.25

1.1a Atypical haemolytic uraemic syndrome and paroxysmal nocturnal haemoglobinuria

IMMUNOSUPPRESSANTS > MONOCLONAL ANTIBODIES

Eculizumab

22-Apr-2020

- **DRUG ACTION** Eculizumab, a recombinant monoclonal antibody, inhibits terminal complement activation at the C5 protein and thereby reduces haemolysis and thrombotic microangiopathy.

- **INDICATIONS AND DOSE**

Reduce haemolysis in paroxysmal nocturnal haemoglobinuria (PNH), in those with a history of blood transfusions (under expert supervision)

▸ BY INTRAVENOUS INFUSION

- Child: Refer for specialist advice, experience very limited

Reduce thrombotic microangiopathy in atypical haemolytic uraemic syndrome (aHUS) (specialist use only)

- BY INTRAVENOUS INFUSION
- Child 2 months–17 years (body-weight 5–9 kg): Initially 300 mg once weekly for 2 weeks, followed by 300 mg every 3 weeks
- Child 2 months–17 years (body-weight 10–19 kg): Initially 600 mg once weekly for 1 week, then reduced to 300 mg once weekly for 1 week, followed by 300 mg every 2 weeks
- Child 2 months–17 years (body-weight 20–29 kg): Initially 600 mg once weekly for 3 weeks, followed by 600 mg every 2 weeks
- Child 2 months–17 years (body-weight 30–39 kg): Initially 600 mg once weekly for 2 weeks, then increased to 900 mg once weekly for 1 week, followed by 900 mg every 2 weeks
- Child 2 months–17 years (body-weight 40 kg and above): Initially 900 mg once weekly for 4 weeks, then increased to 1.2 g once weekly for 1 week, followed by 1.2 g every 2 weeks

- **UNLICENSED USE** Not licensed for use in children for paroxysmal nocturnal haemoglobinuria.
- **CONTRA-INDICATIONS** Patients unvaccinated against *Neisseria meningitidis* · unresolved *Neisseria meningitidis* infection
- **CAUTIONS** Active systemic infection

CAUTIONS, FURTHER INFORMATION

- Meningococcal infection Manufacturer advises vaccinate against *Neisseria meningitidis* at least 2 weeks before treatment (vaccines against serotypes A, C, Y, W135 and B where available, are recommended); revaccinate according to current medical guidelines. Patients receiving eculizumab less than 2 weeks after receiving meningococcal vaccine must be given prophylactic antibiotics until 2 weeks after vaccination. Advise patient to report promptly any signs of meningococcal infection. Other immunisations should also be up to date.

- **INTERACTIONS** → Appendix 1: monoclonal antibodies
- **SIDE-EFFECTS**
- **Common or very common** Alopecia · asthenia · chills · cough · decreased leucocytes · diarrhoea · dizziness · fever · gastrointestinal discomfort · headache · hypertension · increased risk of infection · influenza like illness · joint disorders · muscle complaints · nausea · oropharyngeal pain · pain · skin reactions · sleep disorders · taste altered · tremor · vomiting
- **Uncommon** Abscess · anxiety · appetite decreased · chest discomfort · constipation · cystitis · depression · dysuria · haemorrhage · hot flush · hyperhidrosis · hypersensitivity · hypotension · meningitis meningococcal · mood swings · nasal complaints · oedema · palpitations · paraesthesia · sepsis · spontaneous penile erection · throat irritation · tinnitus · vascular disorders · vertigo · vision blurred
- **Rare or very rare** Abnormal clotting factor · conjunctival irritation · feeling hot · gastrooesophageal reflux disease · gingival discomfort · Grave's disease · infusion related reaction · jaundice · malignant melanoma · menstrual disorder · syncope · urogenital tract gonococcal infection

- **CONCEPTION AND CONTRACEPTION** Manufacturer advises effective contraception during and for 5 months after treatment.
- **PREGNANCY** Manufacturer advises use only if potential benefit outweighs risk—limited information available. Eculizumab is an immunoglobulin G (IgG) monoclonal antibody; human IgG antibodies are known to cross the placenta.
- **BREAST FEEDING** Manufacturer advises use with caution—limited information available; unlikely to be present in milk.
- **MONITORING REQUIREMENTS**
- Monitor for 1 hour after infusion.
- For *paroxysmal nocturnal haemoglobinuria*, monitor for intravascular haemolysis (including serum-lactate dehydrogenase concentration) during treatment and for at least 8 weeks after discontinuation.
- For *atypical haemolytic uraemic syndrome*, monitor for thrombotic microangiopathy (measure platelet count, serum-lactate dehydrogenase concentration, and serum creatinine) during treatment and for at least 12 weeks after discontinuation.

- **DIRECTIONS FOR ADMINISTRATION** Dilute requisite dose to a concentration of 5 mg/mL with Glucose 5% or Sodium Chloride 0.9% and mix gently; give over 25–45 minutes. If infusion-related reactions occur, infusion time may be increased to 4 hours in child under 12 years or 2 hours in child over 12 years.
- **PRESCRIBING AND DISPENSING INFORMATION** Consult product literature for details of supplemental doses with concomitant plasmapheresis, plasma exchange, or plasma infusion.
- **PATIENT AND CARER ADVICE** Patients or carers should be advised to report promptly any signs of meningococcal infection. Advice about prevention of gonorrhoea should also be given.

  A patient information card and a patient safety card should be provided.
- **NATIONAL FUNDING/ACCESS DECISIONS**

NICE decisions

- **Eculizumab for treating atypical haemolytic uraemic syndrome (January 2015) NICE HST1**

Eculizumab, within its marketing authorisation, is recommended for funding for treating atypical haemolytic uraemic syndrome, only if all the following arrangements are in place:

- coordination of eculizumab use through an expert centre, **and**
- monitoring systems to record the number of people with a diagnosis of atypical haemolytic uraemic syndrome and the number who have eculizumab, and the dose and duration of treatment, **and**
- a national protocol for starting and stopping eculizumab for clinical reasons, **and**
- a research programme with robust methods to evaluate when stopping treatment or dose adjustment might occur.

The long-term budget impact of eculizumab for treating atypical haemolytic uraemic syndrome is uncertain but will be considerable. NHS England and the manufacturer should consider what opportunities might exist to reduce the cost of eculizumab to the NHS.
www.nice.org.uk/guidance/HST1

- **MEDICINAL FORMS** There can be variation in the licensing of different medicines containing the same drug.

Solution for infusion

ELECTROLYTES: May contain Sodium

- Soliris (Alexion Pharma UK Ltd)

Eculizumab 10 mg per 1 ml Soliris 300mg/30ml concentrate for solution for infusion vials | 1 vial PoM £3,150.00 (Hospital only)

9

Blood and nutrition

1.2 Iron deficiency anaemia

Anaemia, iron deficiency

Iron deficiency, treatment and prophylaxis

Treatment with an iron preparation is justified only in the presence of a demonstrable iron-deficiency state. Before starting treatment, it is important to exclude any serious underlying cause of the anaemia (e.g. gastro-intestinal bleeding). The possibility of thalassaemia should be considered in children of Mediterranean or Indian subcontinent descent.

Prophylaxis with an iron preparation may be appropriate in those with a poor diet, malabsorption, menorrhagia, pregnancy, in haemodialysis patients, and in the management of low birth-weight infants such as preterm neonates.

Oral iron

Iron salts should be given by mouth unless there are good reasons for using another route.

Ferrous salts show only marginal differences between one another in efficiency of absorption of iron. Haemoglobin regeneration rate is little affected by the type of salt used provided sufficient iron is given, and in most patients the speed of response is not critical. Choice of preparation is thus usually decided by formulation, palatability, incidence of side-effects, and cost.

Treatment of iron-deficiency anaemia

The oral dose of elemental iron to treat deficiency is 3–6 mg/kg (max. 200 mg) daily given in 2–3 divided doses. Iron supplementation may also be required to produce an optimum response to erythropoietins in iron-deficient children with chronic renal failure or in preterm neonates.

When prescribing, express the dose in terms of elemental iron and iron salt and select the most appropriate preparation; specify both the iron salt and formulation on the prescription. The iron content of artificial formula feeds should also be considered.

Iron content of different iron salts

Iron salt/amount	Content of ferrous iron
ferrous fumarate 200 mg	65 mg
ferrous gluconate 300 mg	35 mg
ferrous sulfate 300 mg	60 mg
ferrous sulfate, dried 200 mg	65 mg
sodium feredetate 190 mg	27.5 mg

Prophylaxis of iron deficiency

In neonates, haemoglobin and haematocrit concentrations change rapidly. These changes are not due to iron deficiency and cannot be corrected by iron supplementation. Similarly, neonatal anaemia resulting from repeated blood sampling does not respond to iron therapy.

All babies, including preterm neonates, are born with substantial iron stores but these stores can become depleted unless dietary intake is adequate. All babies require an iron intake of 400–700 nanograms daily to maintain body stores. Iron in breast milk is well absorbed but that in artificial feeds or in cow's milk is less so. Most artificial formula feeds are sufficiently fortified with iron to prevent deficiency and their iron content should be taken into account when considering further iron supplementation.

Prophylactic iron supplementation may be required in babies of low birth-weight who are solely breast-fed; supplementation is started 4–6 weeks after birth and continued until mixed feeding is established.

Infants with a poor diet may become anaemic in the second year of life, particularly if cow's milk, rather than fortified formula feed, is a major part of the diet.

Compound preparations

Some oral preparations contain ascorbic acid p. 680 to aid absorption of the iron, but the therapeutic advantage of such preparations is minimal and cost may be increased.

There is no justification for the inclusion of other ingredients, such as the **B group of vitamins**, except folic acid p. 620 for pregnant women.

Parenteral iron

Iron can be administered parenterally as iron dextran p. 617, iron sucrose p. 617 or ferric carboxymaltose p. 617. Parenteral iron is generally reserved for use when oral therapy is unsuccessful because the child cannot tolerate oral iron, or does not take it reliably, or if there is continuing blood loss, or in malabsorption.

Many children with chronic renal failure who are receiving haemodialysis (and some who are receiving peritoneal dialysis) also require iron by the intravenous route on a regular basis.

With the exception of children with severe renal failure receiving haemodialysis, parenteral iron does not produce a faster haemoglobin response than oral iron provided that the oral iron preparation is taken reliably and is absorbed adequately. If parenteral iron is necessary, the dose should be calculated according to the child's body-weight and total iron deficit. Depending on the preparation used, parenteral iron is given as a total dose or in divided doses. Further treatment should be guided by monitoring haemoglobin and serum iron concentrations.

MINERALS AND TRACE ELEMENTS > IRON, INJECTABLE

Iron (injectable)

IMPORTANT SAFETY INFORMATION

MHRA/CHM ADVICE: SERIOUS HYPERSENSITIVITY REACTIONS WITH INTRAVENOUS IRON (AUGUST 2013)

Serious hypersensitivity reactions, including life-threatening and fatal anaphylactic reactions, have been reported in patients receiving intravenous iron. These reactions can occur even when a previous administration has been tolerated (including a negative test dose). Test doses are no longer recommended and caution is needed with every dose of intravenous iron.

Intravenous iron products should only be administered when appropriately trained staff and resuscitation facilities are immediately available; patients should be closely monitored for signs of hypersensitivity during and for at least 30 minutes after every administration. In the event of a hypersensitivity reaction, treatment should be stopped immediately and appropriate management initiated.

The risk of hypersensitivity is increased in patients with known allergies, immune or inflammatory conditions, or those with a history of severe asthma, eczema, or other atopic allergy; in these patients, intravenous iron should only be used if the benefits outweigh the risks.

Intravenous iron should be avoided in the first trimester of pregnancy and used in the second or third trimesters only if the benefit outweighs the potential risks for both mother and fetus.

- **CONTRA-INDICATIONS** Disturbances in utilisation of iron · iron overload
- **CAUTIONS** Allergic disorders · eczema · hepatic dysfunction · immune conditions · infection (discontinue if ongoing bacteraemia) · inflammatory conditions · oral iron

should not be given until 5 days after the last injection · severe asthma

- **SIDE-EFFECTS**
  - **Common or very common** Dizziness · flushing · headache · hypertension · hypophosphataemia · hypotension · nausea · skin reactions · taste altered
  - **Uncommon** Arrhythmias · arthralgia · bronchospasm · chest pain · chills · constipation · diarrhoea · dyspnoea · fatigue · fever · gastrointestinal discomfort · hyperhidrosis · hypersensitivity · loss of consciousness · muscle complaints · pain · peripheral oedema · sensation abnormal · vision blurred · vomiting
  - **Rare or very rare** Angioedema · anxiety · circulatory collapse · influenza like illness · malaise · pallor · palpitations · psychiatric disorder · seizure · syncope · tremor
  - **Frequency not known** Kounis syndrome

  SIDE-EFFECTS, FURTHER INFORMATION Anaphylactic reactions can occur with parenteral administration of iron complexes and facilities for cardiopulmonary resuscitation must be available. If children complain of acute symptoms particularly nausea, back pain, breathlessness, or develop hypotension, the infusion should be stopped.

  Overdose For details on the management of poisoning, see Iron salts, under Emergency treatment of poisoning p. 891.

616

Ferric carboxymaltose

09-Apr-2019

- **INDICATIONS AND DOSE**

Iron-deficiency anaemia
- BY SLOW INTRAVENOUS INJECTION, OR BY INTRAVENOUS INFUSION
  - Child: Dose calculated according to body-weight and iron deficit (consult product literature)

- **UNLICENSED USE** Not licensed for use in children under 14 years.
- **INTERACTIONS** → Appendix 1: iron (injectable)
- **SIDE-EFFECTS**
  - **Rare or very rare** Face oedema · flatulence
- **PREGNANCY** Avoid in first trimester; crosses the placenta in *animal* studies. May influence skeletal development.
- **HEPATIC IMPAIRMENT** Manufacturer advises caution—monitor iron status to avoid iron overload; avoid where iron overload increases risk of impairment (particularly porphyria cutanea tarda).
- **PRESCRIBING AND DISPENSING INFORMATION** A ferric carboxymaltose complex containing 5% (50 mg/mL) of iron.

- **MEDICINAL FORMS** There can be variation in the licensing of different medicines containing the same drug.

Solution for injection

ELECTROLYTES: May contain Sodium

- Ferinject (Vifor Pharma UK Ltd) ▼
  Iron (as Ferric carboxymaltose) 50 mg per 1 ml Ferinject 1000mg/20ml solution for injection vials | 1 vial PoM £154.23
  Ferinject 100mg/2ml solution for injection vials | 5 vial PoM £95.50
  Ferinject 500mg/10ml solution for injection vials | 5 vial PoM £477.50

616

Iron dextran

09-Apr-2019

- **INDICATIONS AND DOSE**

Iron-deficiency anaemia
- BY DEEP INTRAMUSCULAR INJECTION
  - Child 14–17 years: Intramuscular injection to be administered into the gluteal muscle, doses calculated according to body-weight and iron deficit (consult product literature)
- BY SLOW INTRAVENOUS INJECTION, OR BY INTRAVENOUS INFUSION
  - Child: Doses calculated according to body-weight and iron deficit (consult product literature)

- **UNLICENSED USE** Not licensed for use in children under 14 years.
- **INTERACTIONS** → Appendix 1: iron (injectable)
- **SIDE-EFFECTS**
  - **Uncommon** Feeling hot
  - **Rare or very rare** Deafness (transient) · haemolysis
  - **Frequency not known** Injection site necrosis · rheumatoid arthritis aggravated
- **PREGNANCY** Avoid in first trimester.
- **HEPATIC IMPAIRMENT** Manufacturer advises avoid in decompensated cirrhosis and hepatitis.
- **RENAL IMPAIRMENT** Avoid in acute renal failure.
- **PRESCRIBING AND DISPENSING INFORMATION** A complex of ferric hydroxide with dextran containing 5% (50 mg/mL) of iron.

- **MEDICINAL FORMS** There can be variation in the licensing of different medicines containing the same drug.

Solution for injection

- CosmoFer (Pharmacosmos UK Ltd) ▼
  Iron (as Iron dextran) 50 mg per 1 ml CosmoFer 500mg/10ml solution for injection ampoules | 2 ampoule PoM £79.70 DT = £79.70
  CosmoFer 100mg/2ml solution for injection ampoules | 5 ampoule PoM £39.85 DT = £39.85

616

Iron sucrose

29-Nov-2019

- **INDICATIONS AND DOSE**

Iron-deficiency anaemia
- BY SLOW INTRAVENOUS INJECTION, OR BY INTRAVENOUS INFUSION
  - Child (body-weight up to 67 kg): Dose calculated according to body-weight and iron deficit, each divided dose should not exceed 3 mg/kg/dose (consult product literature)
  - Child (body-weight 67 kg and above): Dose calculated according to body-weight and iron deficit, each divided dose should not exceed max. 200 mg/dose (consult product literature)

- **UNLICENSED USE** Not licensed for use in children.
- **INTERACTIONS** → Appendix 1: iron (injectable)
- **SIDE-EFFECTS**
  - **Uncommon** Asthenia
  - **Rare or very rare** Drowsiness · urine discolouration
  - **Frequency not known** Cold sweat · confusion · level of consciousness decreased · thrombophlebitis
- **PREGNANCY** Avoid in first trimester.
- **HEPATIC IMPAIRMENT** Manufacturer advises caution—monitor iron status to avoid iron overload; avoid where iron overload is a precipitating factor (particularly porphyria cutanea tarda).
- **PRESCRIBING AND DISPENSING INFORMATION** A complex of ferric hydroxide with sucrose containing 2% (20 mg/mL) of iron.

- **MEDICINAL FORMS** There can be variation in the licensing of different medicines containing the same drug.

Solution for injection

- Venofer (Vifor Pharma UK Ltd, Imported (United States)) ▼
  Iron (as Iron sucrose) 20 mg per 1 ml Venofer 100mg/5ml solution for injection vials | 5 vial PoM £43.52
  Venofer 50mg/2.5ml solution for injection vials | 5 vial PoM

MINERALS AND TRACE ELEMENTS > IRON, ORAL

Iron (oral)

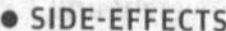

- **SIDE-EFFECTS**
- ▸ **Common or very common** Constipation · diarrhoea · gastrointestinal discomfort · nausea
- ▸ **Uncommon** Vomiting
- ▸ **Frequency not known** Appetite decreased · faeces discoloured

SIDE-EFFECTS, FURTHER INFORMATION Iron can be constipating and occasionally lead to faecal impaction. Oral iron, particularly modified-release preparations, can exacerbate diarrhoea in patients with inflammatory bowel disease; care is also needed in patients with intestinal strictures and diverticular disease.

Overdose Iron preparations are an important cause of accidental overdose in children and as little as 20 mg/kg of elemental iron can lead to symptoms of toxicity.

For details on the management of poisoning, see Iron salts, under Emergency treatment of poisoning p. 891.

- **MONITORING REQUIREMENTS**
- ▸ Therapeutic response The haemoglobin concentration should rise by about 100–200 mg/100 mL (1–2 g/litre) per day *or* 2 g/100 mL (20 g/litre) over 3–4 weeks. When the haemoglobin is in the normal range, treatment should be continued for a further 3 months to replenish the iron stores. Epithelial tissue changes such as atrophic glossitis and koilonychia are usually improved, but the response is often slow.

- **PRESCRIBING AND DISPENSING INFORMATION** Express the dose in terms of elemental iron and iron salt and select the most appropriate preparation; specify both the iron salt and formulation on the prescription.

The iron content of artificial formula feeds should also be considered.

The most common reason for lack of response in children is poor compliance; poor absorption is rare in children.

- **PATIENT AND CARER ADVICE** Although iron preparations are best absorbed on an empty stomach they can be taken after food to reduce gastro-intestinal side-effects. May discolour stools.

above

Ferrous fumarate

10-Mar-2020

- **INDICATIONS AND DOSE**

Iron-deficiency anaemia (prophylactic)

▸ BY MOUTH USING TABLETS
- ▸ Child 12–17 years: 210 mg 1–2 times a day

▸ BY MOUTH USING SYRUP
- ▸ Child 12–17 years: 140 mg twice daily

Iron-deficiency anaemia (therapeutic)

▸ BY MOUTH USING TABLETS
- ▸ Child 12–17 years: 210 mg 2–3 times a day

▸ BY MOUTH USING SYRUP
- ▸ Child 12–17 years: 280 mg twice daily

GALFER® CAPSULES

Iron-deficiency anaemia (prophylactic)

▸ BY MOUTH
- ▸ Child 12–17 years: 305 mg daily

Iron-deficiency anaemia (therapeutic)

▸ BY MOUTH
- ▸ Child 12–17 years: 305 mg twice daily

GALFER® SYRUP

Iron-deficiency anaemia (prophylaxis)

▸ BY MOUTH
- ▸ Neonate up to 36 weeks corrected gestational age (body-weight up to 3 kg): 0.5 mL daily, prophylactic iron supplementation may be required in babies of low birth-weight who are solely breast-fed; supplementation is started 4–6 weeks after birth and continued until mixed feeding is established.
- ▸ Neonate: 0.25 mL/kilogram twice daily, the total daily dose may alternatively be given in 3 divided doses, prophylactic iron supplementation may be required in babies of low birth-weight who are solely breast-fed; supplementation is started 4–6 weeks after birth and continued until mixed feeding is established.
- ▸ Child 1 month–11 years: 0.25 mL/kilogram twice daily, the total daily dose may alternatively be given in 3 divided doses, prophylactic iron supplementation may be required in babies of low birth-weight who are solely breast-fed; supplementation is started 4–6 weeks after birth and continued until mixed feeding is established; maximum 20 mL per day
- ▸ Child 12–17 years: 10 mL once daily

Iron-deficiency anaemia (therapeutic)

▸ BY MOUTH
- ▸ Neonate: 0.25 mL/kilogram twice daily, the total daily dose may alternatively be given in 3 divided doses.
- ▸ Child 1 month–11 years: 0.25 mL/kilogram twice daily, the total daily dose may alternatively be given in 3 divided doses; maximum 20 mL per day
- ▸ Child 12–17 years: 10 mL 1–2 times a day

- **INTERACTIONS** → Appendix 1: iron (oral)
- **SIDE-EFFECTS** Faecal impaction · haemosiderosis
- **PRESCRIBING AND DISPENSING INFORMATION** Non-proprietary ferrous fumarate tablets may contain 210 mg (68 mg iron), syrup may contain approx. 140 mg (45 mg iron)/5 mL; *Galfer®* capsules contain ferrous fumarate 305 mg (100 mg iron).
- **PATIENT AND CARER ADVICE**
Medicines for Children leaflet: Ferrous fumarate for iron-deficiency anaemia www.medicinesforchildren.org.uk/ferrous-fumarate-iron-deficiency-anaemia

- **MEDICINAL FORMS** There can be variation in the licensing of different medicines containing the same drug.

Oral solution

- ▸ Ferrous fumarate (Non-proprietary)
Ferrous fumarate 28 mg per 1 ml Ferrous fumarate 140mg/5ml oral solution | 200 ml [P] £3.92 DT = £3.92
- ▸ Galfer (Thornton & Ross Ltd)
Ferrous fumarate 28 mg per 1 ml Galfer 140mg/5ml syrup sugar-free | 300 ml [P] £5.33 DT = £5.33

Tablet

- ▸ Ferrous fumarate (Non-proprietary)
Ferrous fumarate 210 mg Ferrous fumarate 210mg tablets | 84 tablet [P] £3.99 DT = £3.99 | 84 tablet [NHS] DT = £3.99
Ferrous fumarate 322 mg Ferrous fumarate 322mg tablets | 28 tablet [PoM] [NHS] DT = £1.00 | 28 tablet [P] £1.00 DT = £1.00
- ▸ FerroEss (Essential-Healthcare Ltd)
Ferrous fumarate 210 mg FerroEss 210mg tablets | 84 tablet £2.47 DT = £3.99
Ferrous fumarate 322 mg FerroEss 322mg tablets | 28 tablet £0.83 DT = £1.00

Capsule

- ▸ Galfer (Thornton & Ross Ltd)
Ferrous fumarate 305 mg Galfer 305mg capsules | 100 capsule [P] £5.00 DT = £5.00 | 250 capsule [P] £12.50

618

Ferrous gluconate

10-Mar-2020

- **INDICATIONS AND DOSE**

Prophylaxis of iron-deficiency anaemia

▶ BY MOUTH USING TABLETS

- Child 6–11 years: 300–900 mg daily
- Child 12–17 years: 600 mg daily

Treatment of iron-deficiency anaemia

▶ BY MOUTH USING TABLETS

- Child 6–11 years: 300–900 mg daily
- Child 12–17 years: 1.2–1.8 g daily in divided doses

- **INTERACTIONS** → Appendix 1: iron (oral)
- **SIDE-EFFECTS** Gastrointestinal disorders
- **PRESCRIBING AND DISPENSING INFORMATION** Ferrous gluconate 300 mg contains 35 mg iron.
- **PATIENT AND CARER ADVICE** Medicines for Children leaflet: Ferrous gluconate for iron-deficiency anaemia www.medicinesforchildren.org.uk/ferrous-gluconate-iron-deficiency-anaemia

- **MEDICINAL FORMS** There can be variation in the licensing of different medicines containing the same drug.

Tablet

▸ Ferrous gluconate (Non-proprietary)
Ferrous gluconate 300 mg Ferrous gluconate 300mg tablets | 28 tablet [P] £3.35 DT = £1.09 | 1000 tablet [P] £36.07–£119.64

618

Ferrous sulfate

10-Mar-2020

- **INDICATIONS AND DOSE**

Iron-deficiency anaemia (prophylactic)

▶ BY MOUTH USING TABLETS

- Child 6–17 years: 200 mg daily

Iron-deficiency anaemia (therapeutic)

▶ BY MOUTH USING TABLETS

- Child 6–17 years: 200 mg 2–3 times a day

FEOSPAN®

Iron-deficiency anaemia

▶ BY MOUTH

- Child 1–17 years: 1 capsule daily, capsule can be opened and sprinkled on food

FERROGRAD®

Iron-deficiency anaemia (prophylactic and therapeutic)

▶ BY MOUTH

- Child 12–17 years: 1 tablet daily

IRONORM® DROPS

Iron-deficiency anaemia (prophylactic)

▶ BY MOUTH

- Child 1 month–5 years: 0.2 mL daily until mixed feeding established, higher doses up to max. 0.08 mL/kg daily may be needed, then 0.5–1.2 mL daily
- Child 6–11 years: 2.4 mL daily
- Child 12–17 years: 2.4–4.8 mL daily

Iron-deficiency anaemia (therapeutic)

▶ BY MOUTH

- Child 1 month–5 years: 0.12–0.24 mL/kilogram daily in 2–3 divided doses; maximum 8 mL per day
- Child 6–11 years: 0.12–0.24 mL/kilogram daily in 2–3 divided doses; maximum 8 mL per day
- Child 12–17 years: 4 mL 1–2 times a day

- **INTERACTIONS** → Appendix 1: iron (oral)
- **SIDE-EFFECTS** Tooth discolouration
- **PRESCRIBING AND DISPENSING INFORMATION** Iron content Ferrous sulfate 200 mg is equivalent to 65 mg iron; *Ironorm®* drops contain ferrous sulfate 125 mg (equivalent to 25 mg iron)/mL; *Feospan®* spansules contains ferrous sulfate 150 mg (47 mg iron) (spansule (= capsules m/r)); *Ferrograd®* tablets contain ferrous sulfate 325 mg (105 mg iron).
- **PATIENT AND CARER ADVICE** Medicines for Children leaflet: Ferrous sulfate for iron-deficiency anaemia www.medicinesforchildren.org.uk/ferrous-sulfate-iron-deficiency-anaemia
- **NATIONAL FUNDING/ACCESS DECISIONS** NHS restrictions *Feospan®* is not prescribable in NHS primary care.
- **LESS SUITABLE FOR PRESCRIBING** *Feospan®* is less suitable for prescribing. *Ferrograd®* is less suitable for prescribing.

- **MEDICINAL FORMS** There can be variation in the licensing of different medicines containing the same drug.

Modified-release tablet

CAUTIONARY AND ADVISORY LABELS 25

▸ Ferrograd (Teofarma)
Ferrous sulfate dried 325 mg Ferrograd 325mg modified-release tablets | 30 tablet [P] £2.58 DT = £2.58

Tablet

▸ Ferrous sulfate (Non-proprietary)
Ferrous sulfate dried 200 mg Ferrous sulfate 200mg tablets | 28 tablet [P] £8.15 DT = £1.29 | 60 tablet [P] £1.80–£3.05 | 100 tablet [P] £4.32–£5.04 | 1000 tablet [P] £43.21–£46.07

Modified-release capsule

CAUTIONARY AND ADVISORY LABELS 25

▸ Feospan Spansules (Intrapharm Laboratories Ltd)
Ferrous sulfate dried 150 mg Feospan 150mg Spansules | 30 capsule [P] £3.95

Oral drops

▸ Ironorm (Wallace Manufacturing Chemists Ltd)
Ferrous sulfate 125 mg per 1 ml Ironorm 125mg/ml oral drops sugar-free | 15 ml [P] £30.00 DT = £30.00

Ferrous sulfate with folic acid

07-May-2020

The properties listed below are those particular to the combination only. For the properties of the components please consider, ferrous sulfate above, folic acid p. 620.

- **INDICATIONS AND DOSE**

Iron-deficiency anaemia

▶ BY MOUTH USING MODIFIED-RELEASE TABLETS

- Child 12–17 years: 1 tablet daily, to be taken before food

- **INTERACTIONS** → Appendix 1: folates · iron (oral)
- **LESS SUITABLE FOR PRESCRIBING** *Ferrograd Folic®* is less suitable for prescribing.

- **MEDICINAL FORMS** There can be variation in the licensing of different medicines containing the same drug.

Modified-release tablet

CAUTIONARY AND ADVISORY LABELS 25

▸ Ferrograd Folic (Teofarma)
Folic acid 350 microgram, Ferrous sulfate dried 325 mg Ferrograd Folic 325mg/350microgram modified-release tablets | 30 tablet [P] £2.64 DT = £2.64

618

Sodium feredetate

10-Mar-2020

(Sodium ironedetate)

- **INDICATIONS AND DOSE**

Iron-deficiency anaemia (therapeutic)

▶ BY MOUTH USING ORAL SOLUTION

- Neonate: Up to 2.5 mL twice daily, smaller doses to be used initially.
- Child 1–11 months: Up to 2.5 mL twice daily, smaller doses to be used initially
- Child 1–4 years: 2.5 mL 3 times a day

continued →

- Child 5–11 years: 5 mL 3 times a day
- Child 12–17 years: 5 mL 3 times a day, increased to 10 mL 3 times a day, dose to be increased gradually

Iron-deficiency anaemia (prophylactic)

▶ BY MOUTH USING ORAL SOLUTION

- Neonate: 1 mL daily, prophylactic iron supplementation may be required in babies of low birth-weight who are solely breast-fed; supplementation is started 4–6 weeks after birth and continued until mixed feeding is established.
- Child 1–11 months: 1 mL daily, prophylactic iron supplementation may be required in babies of low birth-weight who are solely breast-fed; supplementation is started 4–6 weeks after birth and continued until mixed feeding is established

- **UNLICENSED USE** Not licensed for prophylaxis of iron deficiency.
- **INTERACTIONS** → Appendix 1: iron (oral)
- **PRESCRIBING AND DISPENSING INFORMATION** *Sytron®* contains 207.5 mg sodium feredetate trihydrate, which is equivalent to 27.5 mg of iron/5 mL.
- **PATIENT AND CARER ADVICE**
Medicines for Children leaflet: Sytron (sodium feredetate) for the prevention of anaemia www.medicinesforchildren.org.uk/sytron-prevention-anaemia
Medicines for Children leaflet: Sytron (sodium feredetate) for the treatment of anaemia www.medicinesforchildren.org.uk/sytron-treatment-anaemia

- **MEDICINAL FORMS** There can be variation in the licensing of different medicines containing the same drug.

Oral solution

- Sodium feredetate (Non-proprietary)
Iron (as Sodium feredetate) 5.5 mg per 1 ml SodiFer 190mg/5ml oral solution sugar-free | 500 ml £12.07 DT = £14.95
- Sytron (Forum Health Products Ltd)
Iron (as Sodium feredetate) 5.5 mg per 1 ml Sytron oral solution sugar-free | 500 ml Ⓟ £14.95 DT = £14.95

1.3 Megaloblastic anaemia

Anaemia, megaloblastic

Overview

Megaloblastic anaemias are rare in children; they may result from a lack of either vitamin B_{12} or folate and it is essential to establish in every case which deficiency is present and the underlying cause. In emergencies, when delay might be dangerous, it is sometimes necessary to administer both substances after the bone marrow test while plasma assay results are awaited. Normally, however, appropriate treatment should not be instituted until the results of tests are available.

Vitamin B_{12} is used in the treatment of megaloblastosis caused by *prolonged nitrous oxide anaesthesia*, which inactivates the vitamin, and in the rare disorders of *congenital transcobalamin II deficiency* and *homocystinuria*.

Vitamin B_{12} should be given prophylactically after *total ileal resection*.

Apart from dietary deficiency, all other causes of vitamin B_{12} deficiency are attributable to malabsorption. There is little place for the use of low-dose vitamin B_{12} orally and none for vitamin B_{12} intrinsic factor complexes given by mouth. Vitamin B_{12} in large oral doses [unlicensed] may be effective.

Hydroxocobalamin p. 621 has completely replaced cyanocobalamin p. 621 as the form of vitamin B_{12} of choice for therapy; it is retained in the body longer than cyanocobalamin and thus for maintenance therapy can be given at intervals of up to 3 months. Treatment is generally initiated with frequent administration of intramuscular injections to replenish the depleted body stores. Thereafter, maintenance treatment, which is usually for life, can be instituted. There is no evidence that doses larger than those recommended provide any additional benefit in vitamin B_{12} neuropathy.

Folic acid below has few indications for long-term therapy since most causes of folate deficiency are self-limiting or will yield to a short course of treatment. It should not be used in undiagnosed megaloblastic anaemia unless vitamin B_{12} is administered concurrently otherwise neuropathy may be precipitated.

In *folate-deficient megaloblastic anaemia* (e.g. because of poor nutrition, pregnancy, or antiepileptic drugs), daily folic acid supplementation for 4 months brings about haematological remission and replenishes body stores; higher doses may be necessary in malabsorption states. In pregnancy, folic acid daily is continued to term.

For prophylaxis in *chronic haemolytic states*, *malabsorption*, or *in renal dialysis*, folic acid is given daily or sometimes weekly, depending on the diet and the rate of haemolysis.

Folic acid is also used for the prevention of methotrexate-induced side-effects in juvenile idiopathic arthritis, severe Crohn's disease and severe psoriasis.

Folic acid is actively excreted in breast milk and is well absorbed by the infant. It is also present in cow's milk and artificial formula feeds but is heat labile. Serum and red cell folate concentrations fall after delivery and urinary losses are high, particularly in low birth-weight neonates. Although symptomatic deficiency is rare in the absence of malabsorption or prolonged diarrhoea, it is common for neonatal units to give supplements of folic acid to all preterm neonates from 2 weeks of age until full-term corrected age is reached, particularly if heated breast milk is used without an artificial formula fortifier.

Folinic acid p. 600 is also effective in the treatment of folate deficient megaloblastic anaemia but it is normally only used in association with cytotoxic drugs; it is given as calcium folinate.

There is **no** justification for prescribing multiple ingredient vitamin preparations containing vitamin B_{12} or folic acid.

For the use of folic acid before and during pregnancy, see Neural tube defects (prevention in pregnancy) p. 688.

VITAMINS AND TRACE ELEMENTS > FOLATES

Folic acid

10-Mar-2020

- **INDICATIONS AND DOSE**

Folate-deficient megaloblastic anaemia

▶ BY MOUTH

- Neonate: Initially 500 micrograms/kg once daily for up to 4 months.
- Child 1–11 months: Initially 500 micrograms/kg once daily (max. per dose 5 mg) for up to 4 months, doses up to 10 mg daily may be required in malabsorption states
- Child 1–17 years: 5 mg daily for 4 months (until term in pregnant women), doses up to 15 mg daily may be required in malabsorption states

Folate supplementation in neonates

▶ BY MOUTH

- Neonate: 50 micrograms once daily.

Prevention of neural tube defects (in those at a low risk of conceiving a child with a neural tube defect see Neural tube defects (prevention in pregnancy) p. 688)

- ▶ BY MOUTH
- ▸ Females of childbearing potential: 400 micrograms daily, to be taken before conception and until week 12 of pregnancy

Prevention of neural tube defects (in those in the high-risk group who wish to become pregnant or who are at risk of becoming pregnant see Neural tube defects (prevention in pregnancy) p. 688)

- ▶ BY MOUTH
- ▸ Females of childbearing potential: 5 mg daily, to be taken before conception and until week 12 of pregnancy

Prevention of neural tube defects (in those with sickle-cell disease)

- ▶ BY MOUTH
- ▸ Females of childbearing potential: 5 mg daily, patient should continue taking their normal dose of folic acid 5 mg daily (or increase the dose to 5 mg daily) before conception and continue this throughout pregnancy

Prevention of methotrexate side-effects in severe Crohn's disease | Prevention of methotrexate side-effects in severe psoriasis

- ▶ BY MOUTH
- ▸ Child: 5 mg once weekly, dose to be taken on a different day to methotrexate dose

Prophylaxis of folate deficiency in dialysis

- ▶ BY MOUTH
- ▸ Child 1 month–11 years: 250 micrograms/kg once daily (max. per dose 10 mg)
- ▸ Child 12–17 years: 5–10 mg once daily

Haemolytic anaemia | Metabolic disorders

- ▶ BY MOUTH
- ▸ Child 1 month–11 years: 2.5–5 mg once daily
- ▸ Child 12–17 years: 5–10 mg once daily

Prevention of methotrexate side-effects in juvenile idiopathic arthritis

- ▶ BY MOUTH
- ▸ Child: 1 mg daily, alternatively 5 mg once weekly, dose to be adjusted according to local guidelines, weekly dose to be taken on a different day to methotrexate dose

- **UNLICENSED USE** Unlicensed for limiting methotrexate toxicity.
- **CAUTIONS** Should never be given alone for pernicious anaemia (may precipitate subacute combined degeneration of the spinal cord)
- **INTERACTIONS** → Appendix 1: folates
- **SIDE-EFFECTS** Abdominal distension · appetite decreased · flatulence · nausea · vitamin B12 deficiency exacerbated
- **PATIENT AND CARER ADVICE**
Medicines for Children leaflet: Folic acid for megaloblastic anaemia caused by folate deficiency and haemolytic anaemia www.medicinesforchildren.org.uk/folic-acid-megaloblastic-anaemia-caused-folate-deficiency-and-haemolytic-anaemia
- **EXCEPTIONS TO LEGAL CATEGORY**
  - ▸ With oral use Can be sold to the public provided daily doses do not exceed 500 micrograms.

- **MEDICINAL FORMS** There can be variation in the licensing of different medicines containing the same drug. Forms available from special-order manufacturers include: capsule, oral suspension, oral solution

Tablet

- ▸ Folic acid (Non-proprietary)
Folic acid 400 microgram Folic acid 400microgram tablets | 90 tablet [PoM] [X] DT = £3.52
Folic acid 5 mg Folic acid 5mg tablets | 28 tablet [PoM] £2.00 DT = £0.98 | 1000 tablet [PoM] £34.29–£35.00

Oral solution

- ▸ Folic acid (Non-proprietary)
Folic acid 500 microgram per 1 ml Folic acid 2.5mg/5ml oral solution sugar-free | 150 ml [PoM] £9.16 DT = £9.16 sugar-free
Folic acid 1 mg per 1 ml Folic acid 5mg/5ml oral solution sugar free | 150 ml [PoM] £43.91–£48.27 DT = £47.20
- ▸ Lexpec (Rosemont Pharmaceuticals Ltd)
Folic acid 500 microgram per 1 ml Lexpec Folic Acid 2.5mg/5ml oral solution sugar-free | 150 ml [PoM] £9.16 DT = £9.16

VITAMINS AND TRACE ELEMENTS > VITAMIN B GROUP

Cyanocobalamin

29-Mar-2019

- **INDICATIONS AND DOSE**

Vitamin B_{12} deficiency of dietary origin

- ▶ BY MOUTH
- ▸ Child: 50–105 micrograms daily in 1–3 divided doses

- **PRESCRIBING AND DISPENSING INFORMATION** Currently available brands of the tablet may not be suitable for vegans.
- **NATIONAL FUNDING/ACCESS DECISIONS**
NHS restrictions *Cyanocobalamin* solution and *Cytamen®* injection are not prescribable in NHS primary care.
- **LESS SUITABLE FOR PRESCRIBING** Cyanocobalamin is less suitable for prescribing.

- **MEDICINAL FORMS** There can be variation in the licensing of different medicines containing the same drug. Forms available from special-order manufacturers include: tablet

Tablet

- ▸ Cyanocobalamin (Non-proprietary)
Cyanocobalamin 50 microgram Cyanocobalamin 50microgram tablets | 50 tablet [P] £12.99 DT = £11.33
- ▸ Behepan (Imported (Sweden))
Cyanocobalamin 1 mg High Potency Behepan 1mg tablets | 100 tablet [PoM] [X]

Hydroxocobalamin

20-Jul-2017

- **INDICATIONS AND DOSE**

Macrocytic anaemia without neurological involvement

- ▶ BY INTRAMUSCULAR INJECTION
- ▸ Child: Initially 0.25–1 mg once daily on alternate days for 1–2 weeks, then 0.25 mg once weekly until blood count normal, then 1 mg every 2–3 months

Macrocytic anaemia with neurological involvement

- ▶ BY INTRAMUSCULAR INJECTION
- ▸ Child: Initially 1 mg once daily on alternate days until no further improvement, then 1 mg every 2 months

Prophylaxis of macrocytic anaemias associated with vitamin B_{12} deficiency

- ▶ BY INTRAMUSCULAR INJECTION
- ▸ Child: 1 mg every 2–3 months

Leber's optic atrophy

- ▶ BY INTRAMUSCULAR INJECTION
- ▸ Child: Initially 1 mg daily for 2 weeks, then 1 mg twice weekly until no further improvement, then 1 mg every 1–3 months

Congenital transcobalamin II deficiency

- ▶ BY INTRAMUSCULAR INJECTION
- ▸ Neonate: 1 mg 3 times a week for 1 year, then reduced to 1 mg once weekly, adjusted as appropriate.
- ▸ Child: 1 mg 3 times a week for 1 year, then reduced to 1 mg once weekly, adjusted as appropriate

continued →

Methylmalonic acidaemia and homocystinuria
- ▶ BY INTRAMUSCULAR INJECTION
  - ▶ Child: Initially 1 mg daily for 5–7 days, then adjusted according to response to up to 1 mg 1–2 times a week, this is the maintenance dose

Methylmalonic acidaemia, maintenance once intramuscular response established
- ▶ BY MOUTH
  - ▶ Child: 5–10 mg 1–2 times a week, some children do not respond to oral route

CYANOKIT®

Poisoning with cyanides
- ▶ BY INTRAVENOUS INFUSION
  - ▶ Child (body-weight 5 kg and above): Initially 70 mg/kg (max. per dose 5 g), to be given over 15 minutes, then 70 mg/kg (max. per dose 5 g) if required, this second dose can be given over 15 minutes–2 hours depending on severity of poisoning and patient stability

- **UNLICENSED USE**
  - ▶ With intramuscular use or oral use Licensed for use in children (age not specified by manufacturers). Not licensed for use in inborn errors of metabolism.
- **CAUTIONS**
  - ▶ With intramuscular use or oral use Should not be given before diagnosis fully established
- **SIDE-EFFECTS**

  GENERAL SIDE-EFFECTS Diarrhoea · dizziness · headache · hot flush · nausea · skin reactions · urine discolouration

  SPECIFIC SIDE-EFFECTS
  - ▶ With intramuscular use Arrhythmia · chills · drug fever · hypokalaemia · malaise · pain · thrombocytosis · tremor · vomiting
  - ▶ With intravenous use Angioedema · dysphagia · extrasystole · gastrointestinal discomfort · memory loss · mucosal discolouration red · peripheral oedema · pleural effusion · rash pustular · red discolouration of plasma · restlessness · swelling · throat complaints
- **BREAST FEEDING** Present in milk but not known to be harmful.
- **EFFECT ON LABORATORY TESTS**
  - ▶ With intravenous use Deep red colour of hydroxocobalamin may interfere with laboratory tests.
- **DIRECTIONS FOR ADMINISTRATION**
  - ▶ With intravenous use For *intravenous infusion (Cyanokit)®*, given intermittently *in* Sodium chloride 0.9%, reconstitute 5 g vial with 200 mL Sodium Chloride 0.9%; gently invert vial for at least 1 minute to mix (do not shake).
  - ▶ With oral use For administration by *mouth*, injection solution may be given orally; it will not have prolonged effect via this route.
- **PRESCRIBING AND DISPENSING INFORMATION**
  - ▶ With intramuscular use The BP directs that when vitamin B_{12} injection is prescribed or demanded, hydroxocobalamin injection shall be dispensed or supplied.

  Poisoning by cyanides
  - ▶ With intravenous use *Cyanokit®* is the only preparation of hydroxocobalamin that is suitable for use in victims of smoke inhalation who show signs of significant cyanide poisoning.
- **NATIONAL FUNDING/ACCESS DECISIONS**

  NHS restrictions *Cobalin-H®* is not prescribable in NHS primary care.

  Neo-Cytamen® is not prescribable in NHS primary care.
- **MEDICINAL FORMS** There can be variation in the licensing of different medicines containing the same drug. Forms available from special-order manufacturers include: oral suspension, oral solution

Solution for injection
- ▶ Hydroxocobalamin (Non-proprietary)
  Hydroxocobalamin 1 mg per 1 ml Hydroxocobalamin 1mg/1ml solution for injection ampoules | 5 ampoule PoM £12.49 DT = £8.18
- ▶ Hepavit (Imported (Austria))
  Hydroxocobalamin 2.5 mg per 1 ml Hepavit 5mg/2ml solution for injection ampoules | 2 ampoule PoM ⊠
- ▶ Megamilbedoce (Imported (Spain))
  Hydroxocobalamin 5 mg per 1 ml Megamilbedoce 10mg/2ml solution for injection ampoules | 10 ampoule PoM ⊠
- ▶ Cobalin (Advanz Pharma)
  Hydroxocobalamin 1 mg per 1 ml Cobalin-H 1mg/1ml solution for injection ampoules | 5 ampoule PoM £9.50 DT = £8.18
- ▶ Neo-Cytamen (RPH Pharmaceuticals AB)
  Hydroxocobalamin 1 mg per 1 ml Neo-Cytamen 1000micrograms/1ml solution for injection ampoules | 5 ampoule PoM £12.49 DT = £8.18

Powder for solution for infusion
- ▶ Cyanokit (SERB)
  Hydroxocobalamin 5 gram Cyanokit 5g powder for solution for infusion vials | 1 vial PoM £772.00

2 Iron overload

Iron overload

Overview

Severe tissue iron overload can occur in aplastic and other refractory anaemias, mainly as the result of repeated blood transfusions. It is a particular problem in refractory anaemias with hyperplastic bone marrow, especially *thalassaemia major*, where excessive iron absorption from the gut and inappropriate iron therapy can add to the tissue siderosis.

Iron overload associated with haemochromatosis can be treated with repeated venesection. Venesection may also be used for patients who have received multiple transfusions and whose bone marrow has recovered. Where venesection is contra-indicated, and in thalassaemia, the long-term administration of the iron chelating compound desferrioxamine mesilate p. 624 is useful. Desferrioxamine mesilate (up to 2 g per unit of blood) may also be given at the time of blood transfusion, provided that the desferrioxamine mesilate is **not** added to the blood and is **not** given through the same line as the blood (but the two may be given through the same cannula).

Iron excretion induced by desferrioxamine mesilate is enhanced by ascorbic acid (vitamin C) p. 680 daily by mouth; it should be given separately from food since it also enhances iron absorption. Ascorbic acid should not be given to children with cardiac dysfunction; in children with normal cardiac function ascorbic acid should be introduced 1 month after starting desferrioxamine mesilate.

Desferrioxamine mesilate infusion can be used to treat *aluminium overload* in dialysis patients; theoretically 100 mg of desferrioxamine binds with 4.1 mg of aluminium.

ANTIDOTES AND CHELATORS > IRON CHELATORS

Deferasirox

28-Jun-2018

● **DRUG ACTION** Deferasirox is an oral iron chelator.

● **INDICATIONS AND DOSE**

Transfusion-related chronic iron overload when desferrioxamine is contra-indicated or inadequate in patients with beta thalassaemia major who receive frequent blood transfusions (7 mL/kg/month or more of packed red blood cells) (specialist use only)

▶ BY MOUTH

▸ Child 2–5 years: Initially 7–21 mg/kg once daily, dose adjusted according to serum-ferritin concentration and amount of transfused blood—consult product literature, then adjusted in steps of 3.5–7 mg/kg every 3–6 months, maintenance dose adjusted according to serum-ferritin concentration; maximum 28 mg/kg per day; Usual maximum 21 mg/kg

Transfusion-related chronic iron overload in patients with beta thalassaemia major who receive frequent blood transfusions (7 mL/kg/month or more of packed red blood cells) (specialist use only)

▶ BY MOUTH

▸ Child 6–17 years: Initially 7–21 mg/kg once daily, dose adjusted according to serum-ferritin concentration and amount of transfused blood—consult product literature, then adjusted in steps of 3.5–7 mg/kg every 3–6 months, maintenance dose adjusted according to serum-ferritin concentration; maximum 28 mg/kg per day; Usual maximum 21 mg/kg

Transfusion-related chronic iron overload when desferrioxamine is contra-indicated or inadequate in patients with beta thalassaemia major who receive infrequent blood transfusions (less than 7 mL/kg/month of packed red blood cells) (specialist use only) | Transfusion-related chronic iron overload when desferrioxamine is contra-indicated or inadequate in patients with other anaemias (specialist use only)

▶ BY MOUTH

▸ Child 2–17 years: Initially 7–21 mg/kg once daily, dose adjusted according to serum-ferritin concentration and amount of transfused blood—consult product literature, then adjusted in steps of 3.5–7 mg/kg every 3–6 months, maintenance dose adjusted according to serum-ferritin concentration; maximum 28 mg/kg per day; Usual maximum 21 mg/kg

Chronic iron overload when desferrioxamine is contra-indicated or inadequate in non-transfusion-dependent thalassaemia syndromes (specialist use only)

▶ BY MOUTH

▸ Child 10–17 years: Initially 7 mg/kg once daily, maintenance dose adjusted according to serum-ferritin concentration and liver-iron concentration (consult product literature); maximum 7 mg/kg per day

● **CAUTIONS** History of liver cirrhosis · not recommended in conditions which may reduce life expectancy (e.g. high-risk myelodysplastic syndromes) · platelet count less than 50×10^9/litre · risk of gastro-intestinal ulceration and haemorrhage · unexplained cytopenia—consider treatment interruption

● **INTERACTIONS** → Appendix 1: iron chelators

● **SIDE-EFFECTS**

▶ **Common or very common** Constipation · diarrhoea · gastrointestinal discomfort · headache · nausea · skin reactions · urine abnormalities · vomiting

▶ **Uncommon** Anxiety · cataract · cholelithiasis · dizziness · fatigue · fever · gastrointestinal disorders · gastrointestinal haemorrhage (including fatal cases) · hearing impairment · hepatic disorders · laryngeal pain · maculopathy · oedema · renal tubular disorders · sleep disorder

▶ **Rare or very rare** Optic neuritis · severe cutaneous adverse reactions (SCARs)

▶ **Frequency not known** Acute kidney injury · alopecia · anaemia aggravated · hyperammonaemic encephalopathy · hypersensitivity vasculitis · lens opacity · leucopenia · metabolic acidosis · nephritis tubulointerstitial · nephrolithiasis · neutropenia · pancreatitis acute · pancytopenia · renal tubular necrosis · thrombocytopenia

● **PREGNANCY** Manufacturer advises avoid unless essential— toxicity in *animal* studies.

● **BREAST FEEDING** Manufacturer advises avoid—present in milk in *animal* studies.

● **HEPATIC IMPAIRMENT** Manufacturer advises caution in moderate impairment; avoid in severe impairment.

Dose adjustments Manufacturer advises reduce initial dose considerably then gradually increase to max. 50% of normal dose in moderate impairment.

● **RENAL IMPAIRMENT** Manufacturer advises avoid if estimated creatinine clearance less than 60 mL/minute.

Dose adjustments Manufacturer advises reduce dose if serum-creatinine increased above age-appropriate limits or creatinine clearance less than 90 mL/minute on 2 consecutive occasions—consult product literature.

● **MONITORING REQUIREMENTS**

▶ Manufacturer advises monitoring of the following patient parameters: baseline serum creatinine twice and creatinine clearance once before initiation of treatment, weekly in the first month after treatment initiation or modification, then monthly thereafter; proteinuria before treatment initiation then monthly thereafter, and other markers of renal tubular function as needed; liver function before treatment initiation, every 2 weeks during the first month of treatment, then monthly thereafter; eye and ear examinations before treatment and annually during treatment; serum-ferritin concentration monthly.

▶ Manufacturer advises monitor liver-iron concentration every three months in children with non-transfusion-dependent thalassaemia syndromes when serum ferritin is ≤800 micrograms/litre.

▶ Manufacturer advises monitor body-weight, height, and sexual development before treatment and then annually thereafter.

● **DIRECTIONS FOR ADMINISTRATION** For *film-coated tablets*, manufacturer advises tablets may be crushed and sprinkled on to soft food (yoghurt or apple sauce), then administered immediately.

● **PATIENT AND CARER ADVICE** Patient or carers should be given advice on how to administer deferasirox tablets.

Medicines for Children leaflet: Deferasirox for removing excess iron www.medicinesforchildren.org.uk/deferasirox-removing-excess-iron-0

● **NATIONAL FUNDING/ACCESS DECISIONS**

Scottish Medicines Consortium (SMC) decisions

The *Scottish Medicines Consortium* has advised (June 2017) that deferasirox (*Exjade*®) is accepted for restricted use within NHS Scotland for the treatment of chronic iron overload associated with the treatment of rare acquired or inherited anaemias requiring recurrent blood transfusions. It is not recommended for patients with myelodysplastic syndromes.

Patients with myelodysplastic syndromes, the commonest cause of transfusion-dependent anaemia, were poorly represented in the clinical trial population and the economic case was not demonstrated in this group.

- **MEDICINAL FORMS** There can be variation in the licensing of different medicines containing the same drug.

Tablet

CAUTIONARY AND ADVISORY LABELS 25

- Exjade (Novartis Pharmaceuticals UK Ltd) ▼
  - **Deferasirox 90 mg** Exjade 90mg tablets | 30 tablet PoM £126.00 DT = £126.00
  - **Deferasirox 180 mg** Exjade 180mg tablets | 30 tablet PoM £252.00 DT = £252.00
  - **Deferasirox 360 mg** Exjade 360mg tablets | 30 tablet PoM £504.00 DT = £504.00

Deferiprone

28-Jun-2018

- **DRUG ACTION** Deferiprone is an oral iron chelator.

- **INDICATIONS AND DOSE**

Treatment of iron overload in patients with thalassaemia major in whom desferrioxamine is contra-indicated or is inadequate

▶ BY MOUTH

- Child 6–17 years: 25 mg/kg 3 times a day; maximum 100 mg/kg per day

- **CONTRA-INDICATIONS** History of agranulocytosis or recurrent neutropenia
- **INTERACTIONS** → Appendix 1: iron chelators
- **SIDE-EFFECTS**
  - **Common or very common** Abdominal pain (reducing dose and increasing gradually may improve tolerance) · agranulocytosis · appetite increased · arthralgia · diarrhoea (reducing dose and increasing gradually may improve tolerance) · fatigue · headache · nausea (reducing dose and increasing gradually may improve tolerance) · neutropenia · urine discolouration · vomiting (reducing dose and increasing gradually may improve tolerance)
  - **Frequency not known** Skin reactions · zinc deficiency
- **CONCEPTION AND CONTRACEPTION** Manufacturer advises avoid before intended conception—teratogenic and embryotoxic in *animal* studies. Contraception advised in females of child-bearing potential.
- **PREGNANCY** Manufacturer advises avoid during pregnancy—teratogenic and embryotoxic in *animal* studies.
- **BREAST FEEDING** Manufacturer advises avoid—no information available.
- **HEPATIC IMPAIRMENT** Manufacturer advises caution (no information available)—monitor hepatic function and consider interrupting treatment if persistent elevation in serum alanine aminotransferase. Manufacturer advises caution in patients with hepatitis C (ensure iron chelation is optimal)—monitor liver histology.
- **RENAL IMPAIRMENT** Manufacturer advises caution—no information available.
- **MONITORING REQUIREMENTS** Monitor neutrophil count weekly and discontinue treatment if neutropenia develops.
- **PATIENT AND CARER ADVICE**

Blood disorders Patients or their carers should be told how to recognise signs of neutropenia and advised to seek immediate medical attention if symptoms such as fever or sore throat develop.

- **MEDICINAL FORMS** There can be variation in the licensing of different medicines containing the same drug. Forms available from special-order manufacturers include: capsule, oral suspension, oral solution

Oral solution

CAUTIONARY AND ADVISORY LABELS 14

- Ferriprox (Apotex B.V.)
  - **Deferiprone 100 mg per 1 ml** Ferriprox 100mg/ml oral solution sugar-free | 500 ml PoM £152.39 DT = £152.39

Tablet

CAUTIONARY AND ADVISORY LABELS 14

- Deferiprone (Non-proprietary)
  - **Deferiprone 500 mg** Deferiprone 500mg tablets | 100 tablet PoM £130.00 DT = £152.39
- Ferriprox (Apotex B.V.)
  - **Deferiprone 500 mg** Ferriprox 500mg tablets | 100 tablet PoM £152.39 DT = £152.39
  - **Deferiprone 1 gram** Ferriprox 1000mg tablets | 50 tablet PoM £175.25 DT = £175.25

Desferrioxamine mesilate

17-Mar-2020

(Deferoxamine Mesilate)

- **INDICATIONS AND DOSE**

Iron poisoning

▶ BY CONTINUOUS INTRAVENOUS INFUSION

- Neonate: Initially up to 15 mg/kg/hour, max. 80 mg/kg in 24 hours, dose to be reduced after 4–6 hours, in severe cases, higher doses may be given on advice from the National Poisons Information Service.
- Child: Initially up to 15 mg/kg/hour, max. 80 mg/kg in 24 hours, dose to be reduced after 4–6 hours, in severe cases, higher doses may be given on advice from the National Poisons Information Service

Aluminium overload in dialysis patients

▶ BY INTRAVENOUS INFUSION

- Child: 5 mg/kg once weekly

Chronic iron overload (low iron overload)

▶ BY SUBCUTANEOUS INFUSION

- Child: Initially up to 30 mg/kg 3–7 times a week, to be given over 8–12 hours, the dose should reflect the degree of iron overload

Chronic iron overload (established overload)

▶ BY SUBCUTANEOUS INFUSION

- Child: 20–50 mg/kg daily

- **UNLICENSED USE**
  - When used for Iron poisoning Licensed for use in children (age range not specified by manufacturer).
- **CAUTIONS** Aluminium-related encephalopathy (may exacerbate neurological dysfunction)
- **INTERACTIONS** → Appendix 1: iron chelators
- **SIDE-EFFECTS**
  - **Common or very common** Arthralgia · bone disorder · fever · growth retardation · headache · muscle complaints · nausea · skin reactions
  - **Uncommon** Abdominal pain · asthma · deafness neurosensory · tinnitus · vomiting
  - **Rare or very rare** Angioedema · blood disorder · cataract · diarrhoea · dizziness · encephalopathy · eye disorders · hypersensitivity · hypotension (more common when given too rapidly by intravenous injection) · increased risk of infection · nerve disorders · nervous system disorder · paraesthesia · respiratory disorders · shock · tachycardia · thrombocytopenia · vision disorders
  - **Frequency not known** Acute kidney injury · hypocalcaemia · leucopenia · renal tubular disorder · seizure · urine red
- **PREGNANCY** Teratogenic in *animal* studies. Manufacturer advises use only if potential benefit outweighs risk.
- **BREAST FEEDING** Manufacturer advises use only if potential benefit outweighs risk—no information available.
- **RENAL IMPAIRMENT** Use with caution.
- **MONITORING REQUIREMENTS**
  - Eye and ear examinations before treatment and at 3-month intervals during treatment.
  - Monitor body-weight and height in children at 3-month intervals—risk of growth retardation with excessive doses.

- **DIRECTIONS FOR ADMINISTRATION** For full details and warnings relating to administration, consult product literature.
- When used for Chronic iron overload or Aluminium overload in dialysis patients For *intravenous* or *subcutaneous infusion*, reconstitute powder with Water for Injection to a concentration of 100 mg/mL; dilute with Glucose 5% or Sodium Chloride 0.9%. In *haemodialysis* or *haemo-filtration* administer over the last hour of dialysis (may be given via the dialysis fistula). *Intraperitoneal*: may be added to dialysis fluid. In CAPD give prior to the last exchange of the day.

- **MEDICINAL FORMS** There can be variation in the licensing of different medicines containing the same drug.

Powder for solution for injection

- Desferrioxamine mesilate (Non-proprietary)
  Desferrioxamine mesilate 500 mg Desferrioxamine 500mg powder for solution for injection vials | 10 vial PoM £46.63 DT = £46.63
  Desferrioxamine mesilate 2 gram Desferrioxamine 2g powder for solution for injection vials | 10 vial PoM £186.60
- Desferal (Novartis Pharmaceuticals UK Ltd)
  Desferrioxamine mesilate 500 mg Desferal 500mg powder for solution for injection vials | 10 vial PoM £46.63 DT = £46.63

3 Neutropenia and stem cell mobilisation

3.1 Neutropenia

Neutropenia

Management

Recombinant human granulocyte-colony stimulating factor (rhG-CSF) stimulates the production of neutrophils and may reduce the duration of chemotherapy-induced neutropenia and thereby reduce the incidence of associated sepsis; there is as yet no evidence that it improves overall survival. Filgrastim (unglycosylated rhG-CSF) below and lenograstim (glycosylated rhG-CSF) p. 626 have similar effects; both have been used in a variety of clinical settings, including cytotoxic-induced neutropenia, and neutropenia following bone marrow transplantation, but they do not have any clear-cut routine indications. In congenital neutropenia filgrastim usually increases the neutrophil count with an appropriate clinical response. Prolonged use may be associated with an increased risk of myeloid malignancy.

Treatment with granulocyte-colony stimulating factors should only be prescribed by those experienced in their use.

Neonatal neutropenia

Filgrastim has been used to treat sepsis-induced neutropenia in preterm neonates. There is no clear evidence that granulocyte–colony stimulating factors improve survival or long–term outcomes.

IMMUNOSTIMULANTS > GRANULOCYTE-COLONY STIMULATING FACTORS

Granulocyte-colony stimulating factors

- **DRUG ACTION** Recombinant human granulocyte-colony stimulating factor (rhG-CSF) stimulates the production of neutrophils.
- **CAUTIONS** Malignant myeloid conditions · pre-malignant myeloid conditions · risk of splenomegaly and rupture—spleen size should be monitored · sickle-cell disease

CAUTIONS, FURTHER INFORMATION
- Acute respiratory distress syndrome There have been reports of pulmonary infiltrates leading to acute respiratory distress syndrome—patients with a recent history of pulmonary infiltrates or pneumonia may be at higher risk.

- **SIDE-EFFECTS**
- **Common or very common** Arthralgia · cutaneous vasculitis · dyspnoea · haemoptysis · headache · hypersensitivity · leucocytosis · pain · spleen abnormalities · thrombocytopenia
- **Uncommon** Acute febrile neutrophilic dermatosis · capillary leak syndrome · hypoxia · pulmonary oedema · respiratory disorders · sickle cell anaemia with crisis

SIDE-EFFECTS, FURTHER INFORMATION Treatment should be withdrawn in patients who develop signs of pulmonary infiltration.

- **PREGNANCY** Manufacturers advise avoid—toxicity in *animal* studies.
- **BREAST FEEDING** There is no evidence for the use of granulocyte-colony stimulating factors during breast-feeding and manufacturers advise avoiding their use.
- **MONITORING REQUIREMENTS**
- Full blood counts including differential white cell and platelet counts should be monitored.
- Spleen size should be monitored during treatment—risk of splenomegaly and rupture.

F above

Filgrastim

05-Aug-2019

(Recombinant human granulocyte-colony stimulating factor; G-CSF)

- **INDICATIONS AND DOSE**

Reduction in duration of neutropenia and incidence of febrile neutropenia in cytotoxic chemotherapy for malignancy (except chronic myeloid leukaemia and myelodysplastic syndromes) (specialist use only)

- BY SUBCUTANEOUS INJECTION, OR BY INTRAVENOUS INFUSION
- Child: 5 micrograms/kg daily until neutrophil count in normal range, usually for up to 14 days (up to 38 days in acute myeloid leukaemia), to be started at least 24 hours after cytotoxic chemotherapy. Preferably given by subcutaneous injection; if given by intravenous infusion, administer over 30 minutes

Reduction in duration of neutropenia (and associated sequelae) in myeloablative therapy followed by bone-marrow transplantation (specialist use only)

- BY SUBCUTANEOUS INFUSION, OR BY INTRAVENOUS INFUSION
- Child: 10 micrograms/kg daily, to be started at least 24 hours following cytotoxic chemotherapy and within 24 hours of bone-marrow infusion, then adjusted according to neutrophil count— consult product literature, doses administered over 30 minutes or 24 hours via intravenous route and over 24 hours via subcutaneous route

Mobilisation of peripheral blood progenitor cells for autologous infusion, used alone (specialist use only)

- BY SUBCUTANEOUS INFUSION, OR BY SUBCUTANEOUS INJECTION
- Child: 10 micrograms/kg daily for 5–7 days, to be administered over 24 hours if given by subcutaneous infusion

Mobilisation of peripheral blood progenitor cells for autologous infusion, used following adjunctive myelosuppressive chemotherapy—to improve yield (specialist use only)

- BY SUBCUTANEOUS INJECTION
- Child: 5 micrograms/kg daily until neutrophil count in normal range, to be started the day after

continued →

completing chemotherapy, for timing of leucopheresis, consult product literature

Mobilisation of peripheral blood progenitor cells in normal donors for allogeneic infusion (specialist use only)

▶ BY SUBCUTANEOUS INJECTION

▸ Child 16–17 years: 10 micrograms/kg daily for 4–5 days, for timing of leucopheresis, consult product literature

Severe congenital neutropenia and history of severe or recurrent infections (distinguish carefully from other haematological disorders) (specialist use only)

▶ BY SUBCUTANEOUS INJECTION

▸ Child: Initially 12 micrograms/kg daily, adjusted according to response, can be given in single or divided doses, consult product literature and local protocol

Severe cyclic neutropenia, or idiopathic neutropenia and history of severe or recurrent infections (distinguish carefully from other haematological disorders) (specialist use only)

▶ BY SUBCUTANEOUS INJECTION

▸ Child: Initially 5 micrograms/kg daily, adjusted according to response, can be given in single or divided doses, consult product literature and local protocol

Persistent neutropenia in HIV infection (specialist use only)

▶ BY SUBCUTANEOUS INJECTION

▸ Child: Initially 1 microgram/kg daily, subsequent doses increased as necessary until neutrophil count in normal range, then adjusted to maintain neutrophil count in normal range—consult product literature; maximum 4 micrograms/kg per day

Neonatal neutropenia (specialist use only)

▶ BY SUBCUTANEOUS INJECTION

▸ Neonate: 10 micrograms/kg daily, to be discontinued if white cell count exceeds 50 x 10^9/litre.

Glycogen storage disease type 1b (specialist use only)

▶ BY SUBCUTANEOUS INJECTION

▸ Child: Initially 5 micrograms/kg daily, dose to be adjusted as necessary

● UNLICENSED USE Not licensed for treatment of glycogen storage disease or neonatal neutropenia.

● CONTRA-INDICATIONS Severe congenital neutropenia who develop leukaemia or have evidence of leukaemic evolution

● CAUTIONS Osteoporotic bone disease (monitor bone density if given for more than 6 months) · secondary acute myeloid leukaemia

● SIDE-EFFECTS

▶ **Common or very common** Anaemia · diarrhoea · dysuria · haemorrhage · hepatomegaly · hyperuricaemia · hypotension · osteoporosis · rash

▶ **Uncommon** Fluid imbalance · graft versus host disease · peripheral vascular disease · pseudogout · rheumatoid arthritis aggravated · urine abnormalities

● MONITORING REQUIREMENTS Regular morphological and cytogenetic bone-marrow examinations recommended in severe congenital neutropenia (possible risk of myelodysplastic syndromes or leukaemia).

● DIRECTIONS FOR ADMINISTRATION For *subcutaneous* or *intravenous infusion*, dilute with Glucose 5% to a concentration of not less than 15 micrograms/mL; to dilute to a concentration of 2–15 micrograms/mL, add albumin solution (human albumin solution) to produce a final albumin solution of 2 mg/mL; not compatible with Sodium Chloride solutions.

● PRESCRIBING AND DISPENSING INFORMATION Filgrastim is a biological medicine. Biological medicines must be prescribed and dispensed by brand name, see *Biological medicines* and *Biosimilar medicines*, under Guidance on prescribing p. 1.

1 million units of filgrastim solution for injection contains 10 micrograms filgrastim.

● MEDICINAL FORMS There can be variation in the licensing of different medicines containing the same drug.

Solution for injection

▸ Accofil (Accord Healthcare Ltd)

Filgrastim 60 mega unit per 1 ml Accofil 30million units/0.5ml solution for injection pre-filled syringes | 5 pre-filled disposable injection [PoM] £284.20 DT = £250.75 (Hospital only)

Filgrastim 96 mega unit per 1 ml Accofil 48million units/0.5ml solution for injection pre-filled syringes | 5 pre-filled disposable injection [PoM] £455.70 DT = £399.50 (Hospital only)

▸ Neupogen (Amgen Ltd)

Filgrastim 30 mega unit per 1 ml Neupogen 30million units/1ml solution for injection vials | 5 vial [PoM] £263.52 DT = £263.52

▸ Neupogen Singleject (Amgen Ltd)

Filgrastim 60 mega unit per 1 ml Neupogen Singleject 30million units/0.5ml solution for injection pre-filled syringes | 1 pre-filled disposable injection [PoM] £52.70

Filgrastim 96 mega unit per 1 ml Neupogen Singleject 48million units/0.5ml solution for injection pre-filled syringes | 1 pre-filled disposable injection [PoM] £84.06

▸ Nivestim (Pfizer Ltd)

Filgrastim 60 mega unit per 1 ml Nivestim 30million units/0.5ml solution for injection pre-filled syringes | 5 pre-filled disposable injection [PoM] £246.50 DT = £250.75

Nivestim 12million units/0.2ml solution for injection pre-filled syringes | 5 pre-filled disposable injection [PoM] £153.00

Filgrastim 96 mega unit per 1 ml Nivestim 48million units/0.5ml solution for injection pre-filled syringes | 5 pre-filled disposable injection [PoM] £395.25 DT = £399.50

▸ Zarzio (Sandoz Ltd)

Filgrastim 60 mega unit per 1 ml Zarzio 30million units/0.5ml solution for injection pre-filled syringes | 5 pre-filled disposable injection [PoM] £250.75 DT = £250.75

Filgrastim 96 mega unit per 1 ml Zarzio 48million units/0.5ml solution for injection pre-filled syringes | 5 pre-filled disposable injection [PoM] £399.50 DT = £399.50

F 625

Lenograstim

(Recombinant human granulocyte-colony stimulating factor; rHuG-CSF)

● INDICATIONS AND DOSE

Reduction in the duration of neutropenia and associated complications following bone-marrow transplantation for non-myeloid malignancy (specialist use only) | Reduction in the duration of neutropenia and associated complications following peripheral stem cells transplantation for non-myeloid malignancy (specialist use only)

▶ BY INTRAVENOUS INFUSION, OR BY SUBCUTANEOUS INJECTION

▸ Child 2–17 years: 150 micrograms/m^2 daily until neutrophil count stable in acceptable range (max. 28 days), to be started the day after transplantation. Intravenous infusion to be given over 30 minutes

Reduction in the duration of neutropenia and associated complications following treatment with cytotoxic chemotherapy associated with a significant incidence of febrile neutropenia (specialist use only)

▶ BY SUBCUTANEOUS INJECTION

▸ Child 2–17 years: 150 micrograms/m^2 daily until neutrophil count stable in acceptable range (max. 28 days), to be started on the day after completion of chemotherapy

Mobilisation of peripheral blood progenitor cells for harvesting and subsequent infusion, used alone (specialist use only)

▶ BY SUBCUTANEOUS INJECTION

▸ Child 2-17 years: 10 micrograms/kg daily for 4–6 days (5–6 days in healthy donors)

Mobilisation of peripheral blood progenitor cells, used following adjunctive myelosuppressive chemotherapy (to improve yield) (specialist use only)

▶ BY SUBCUTANEOUS INJECTION

▸ Child 2-17 years: 150 micrograms/m^2 daily until neutrophil count stable in acceptable range, to be started 1–5 days after completion of chemotherapy, for timing of leucopheresis, consult product literature

● UNLICENSED USE Not licensed for use in children for cytotoxic-induced neutropenia, mobilisation of peripheral blood progenitor cells (monotherapy or adjunctive therapy), or following peripheral stem cells transplantation.

● SIDE-EFFECTS

▶ **Common or very common** Abdominal pain · asthenia

▶ **Rare or very rare** Erythema nodosum · pyoderma gangrenosum · toxic epidermal necrolysis

● DIRECTIONS FOR ADMINISTRATION For *intravenous infusion*, dilute reconstituted solution to a concentration of not less than 2 micrograms/mL (*Granocyte*-13) or 2.5 micrograms/mL (*Granocyte*-34) with Sodium Chloride 0.9%.

● PRESCRIBING AND DISPENSING INFORMATION *Granocyte®* solution for injection contains 105 micrograms of lenograstim per 13.4 mega unit vial and 263 micrograms lenograstim per 33.6 mega unit vial.

● MEDICINAL FORMS There can be variation in the licensing of different medicines containing the same drug.

Powder and solvent for solution for injection

EXCIPIENTS: May contain Phenylalanine

▸ Granocyte (Chugai Pharma UK Ltd)

Lenograstim 13.4 mega unit Granocyte 13million unit powder and solvent for solution for injection pre-filled syringes | 1 pre-filled disposable injection PoM £40.11 DT = £40.11 | 5 pre-filled disposable injection PoM £200.55

Lenograstim 33.6 mega unit Granocyte 34million unit powder and solvent for solution for injection pre-filled syringes | 1 pre-filled disposable injection PoM £62.54 DT = £62.54 | 5 pre-filled disposable injection PoM £312.69

3.2 Stem cell mobilisation

IMMUNOSTIMULANTS › CHEMOKINE RECEPTOR ANTAGONISTS

Plerixafor

13-Mar-2020

● DRUG ACTION Plerixafor is a chemokine receptor antagonist.

● INDICATIONS AND DOSE

Mobilise haematopoietic stem cells to peripheral blood for collection and subsequent autologous transplantation in patients with lymphoma or solid malignant tumours (specialist use only)

▶ BY SUBCUTANEOUS INJECTION

▸ Child 1-17 years: 240 micrograms/kg daily usually for 2–4 days (and up to 7 days), to be administered 6–11 hours before initiation of apheresis, dose to be given following 4 days treatment with a granulocyte-colony stimulating factor; maximum 40 mg per day

● SIDE-EFFECTS

▶ **Common or very common** Arthralgia · constipation · diarrhoea · dizziness · dry mouth · erythema · fatigue · flatulence · gastrointestinal discomfort · headache · hyperhidrosis · malaise · musculoskeletal pain · nausea · oral hypoaesthesia · sleep disorders · vomiting

▶ **Frequency not known** Postural hypotension · splenomegaly · syncope

● CONCEPTION AND CONTRACEPTION Use effective contraception during treatment— teratogenic in *animal* studies.

● PREGNANCY Manufacturer advises avoid unless essential— teratogenic in *animal* studies.

● BREAST FEEDING Manufacturer advises avoid—no information available.

● RENAL IMPAIRMENT No information available if creatinine clearance less than 20 mL/minute.

Dose adjustments Manufacturer advises reduce dose to 160 micrograms/kg (maximum 27 mg) daily if creatinine clearance 20–50 mL/minute.

● MONITORING REQUIREMENTS Monitor platelets and white blood cell count.

● PATIENT AND CARER ADVICE

Driving and skilled tasks Manufacturer advises patients and carers should be cautioned on the effects on driving and performance of skilled tasks—increased risk of dizziness, fatigue, or vasovagal reactions.

● NATIONAL FUNDING/ACCESS DECISIONS

Scottish Medicines Consortium (SMC) decisions

SMC No. SMC2249

The *Scottish Medicines Consortium* has advised (February 2020) that plerixafor (*Mozobil®*) is accepted for use within NHS Scotland in combination with granulocyte-colony stimulating factor to enhance mobilisation of haematopoietic stem cells to the peripheral blood for collection and subsequent autologous transplantation in children aged 1 year to less than 18 years with lymphoma or solid malignant tumours.

All Wales Medicines Strategy Group (AWMSG) decisions

AWMSG No. 3297

The *All Wales Medicines Strategy Group* has advised (February 2020) that plerixafor (*Mozobil®*) is recommended for use within NHS Wales in combination with granulocyte colony stimulating factor to enhance mobilisation of haematopoietic stem cells to the peripheral blood for collection and subsequent autologous transplantation in children aged 1 year to less than 18 years with lymphoma or solid malignant tumours.

● MEDICINAL FORMS There can be variation in the licensing of different medicines containing the same drug.

Solution for injection

▸ Mozobil (Sanofi)

Plerixafor 20 mg per 1 ml Mozobil 24mg/1.2ml solution for injection vials | 1 vial PoM £4,882.77

4 Platelet disorders

4.1 Essential thrombocythaemia

Other drugs used for Essential thrombocythaemia

Hydroxycarbamide, p. 596

ANTITHROMBOTIC DRUGS > CYCLIC AMP PHOSPHODIESTERASE III INHIBITORS

Anagrelide

28-May-2018

- **INDICATIONS AND DOSE**

Essential thrombocythaemia in patients at risk of thrombo-haemorrhagic events who have not responded adequately to other drugs or who cannot tolerate other drugs (initiated under specialist supervision)

- BY MOUTH
- Child 7–17 years: Initially 500 micrograms daily, dose to be adjusted at weekly intervals according to response, increased in steps of 500 micrograms daily; usual dose 1–3 mg daily in divided doses (max. per dose 2.5 mg); maximum 10 mg per day

- **UNLICENSED USE** Not licensed for use in children.
- **CAUTIONS** Cardiovascular disease—assess cardiac function before and regularly during treatment · concomitant use of drugs that prolong QT-interval—assess cardiac function before and regularly during treatment · risk factors for QT-interval prolongation—assess cardiac function before and regularly during treatment
- **INTERACTIONS** → Appendix 1: anagrelide
- **SIDE-EFFECTS**
- **Common or very common** Anaemia · arrhythmias · asthenia · diarrhoea · dizziness · fluid retention · gastrointestinal discomfort · gastrointestinal disorders · headaches · nausea · palpitations · skin reactions · vomiting
- **Uncommon** Alopecia · appetite decreased · arthralgia · chest pain · chills · confusion · congestive heart failure · constipation · depression · dry mouth · dyspnoea · erectile dysfunction · fever · haemorrhage · hypertension · insomnia · malaise · memory loss · myalgia · nervousness · oedema · pain · pancreatitis · pancytopenia · pneumonia · pulmonary hypertension · respiratory disorders · sensation abnormal · syncope · thrombocytopenia · weight changes
- **Rare or very rare** Angina pectoris · cardiomegaly · cardiomyopathy · coordination abnormal · drowsiness · dysarthria · influenza like illness · myocardial infarction · nocturia · pericardial effusion · postural hypotension · renal failure · tinnitus · vasodilation · vision disorders
- **Frequency not known** Hepatitis · nephritis tubulointerstitial
- **CONCEPTION AND CONTRACEPTION** Effective contraception required during treatment.
- **PREGNANCY** Manufacturer advises avoid (toxicity in *animal* studies).
- **BREAST FEEDING** Manufacturer advises avoid—present in milk in *animal* studies.
- **HEPATIC IMPAIRMENT** Manufacturer advises use with caution in mild impairment; avoid in moderate-to-severe impairment or if serum transaminases exceed 5 times the upper limit of normal.
- **RENAL IMPAIRMENT** Manufacturer advises avoid if estimated glomerular filtration rate less than 50 mL/minute/1.73 m^2
- **MONITORING REQUIREMENTS**
- Monitor full blood count (monitor platelet count every 2 days for 1 week, then weekly until maintenance dose established).
- Monitor liver function.
- Monitor serum creatinine.
- Monitor urea.
- Monitor electrolytes (including potassium, magnesium and calcium) before and during treatment.
- Monitor closely for further signs of disease progression such as malignant transformation.
- **PRESCRIBING AND DISPENSING INFORMATION** Initiate only when signs of disease progression or patient suffers from thrombosis.

Consider stopping treatment after 3 months if inadequate response.
- **PATIENT AND CARER ADVICE**

Driving and skilled tasks Dizziness may affect performance of skilled tasks (e.g. cycling, driving).

- **MEDICINAL FORMS** There can be variation in the licensing of different medicines containing the same drug.

Capsule

- Anagrelide (Non-proprietary)
  Anagrelide (as Anagrelide hydrochloride)
  500 microgram Anagrelide 500microgram capsules | 100 capsule PoM £404.57 DT = £402.87
- Xagrid (Shire Pharmaceuticals Ltd)
  Anagrelide (as Anagrelide hydrochloride) 500 microgram Xagrid 500microgram capsules | 100 capsule PoM £404.57 DT = £402.87

4.2 Thrombocytopenias

4.2a Immune thrombocytopenia

Immune thrombocytopenic purpura

Overview

Acute immune (idiopathic) thrombocytopenic purpura is usually self-limiting in children. A corticosteroid, such as prednisolone p. 478, is sometimes used if immune thrombocytopenic purpura does not resolve spontaneously or if it is associated with severe cutaneous symptoms or mucous membrane bleeding; corticosteroid treatment should not be continued longer than 14 days regardless of the response.

Immunoglobulin preparations may be used in immune thrombocytopenic purpura or where a temporary rapid rise in platelets is needed, as in pregnancy or pre-operatively; they are often used in preference to a corticosteroid. Anti-D (Rh_0) immunoglobulin p. 822 is licensed for the management of immune thrombocytopenic purpura.

Other therapies that have been tried under specialist supervision in refractory immune thrombocytopenic purpura include: azathioprine p. 558, cyclophosphamide p. 579, vincristine sulfate p. 594, and ciclosporin p. 559. Rituximab [unlicensed] p. 574 is also used in specialist centres but experience of its use in children is limited. For patients with chronic severe thrombocytopenia refractory to other therapy, tranexamic acid p. 87 may be given to reduce the severity of haemorrhage.

Eltrombopag p. 629 and romiplostim p. 630 are thrombopoietin receptor agonists. They are licensed for the treatment of chronic immune thrombocytopenic purpura in children who are refractory to other treatments, such as corticosteroids or immunoglobulins. They should both be used under the supervision of a specialist.

Splenectomy is considered in chronic thrombocytopenic purpura if a satisfactory platelet count is not achieved with regular immunoglobulin infusions, if there is a relapse on withdrawing or reducing the dose of corticosteroid, and if other therapies are considered inappropriate.

ANTIHAEMORRHAGICS > THROMBOPOIETIN RECEPTOR AGONISTS

Eltrombopag

22-Jan-2020

- **DRUG ACTION** Eltrombopag is a thrombopoietin receptor agonist that binds to and activates the thrombopoietin (TPO) receptor, thereby increasing platelet production.

- **INDICATIONS AND DOSE**

Chronic immune (idiopathic) thrombocytopenic purpura in patients refractory to other treatments (such as corticosteroids or immunoglobulins) (under expert supervision)

▶ BY MOUTH

- Child 1–5 years: Initially 25 mg once daily, dose to be adjusted to achieve a platelet count of $50x10^9$/litre or more—consult product literature for dose adjustments, discontinue if inadequate response after 4 weeks treatment at maximum dose; maximum 75 mg per day
- Child 6–17 years: Initially 50 mg once daily, dose to be adjusted to achieve a platelet count of $50x10^9$/litre or more—consult product literature for dose adjustments, discontinue if inadequate response after 4 weeks treatment at maximum dose; maximum 75 mg per day
- Child 6–17 years (patients of East Asian origin): Initially 25 mg once daily, dose to be adjusted to achieve a platelet count of $50x10^9$/litre or more—consult product literature for dose adjustments, discontinue if inadequate response after 4 weeks treatment at maximum dose; maximum 75 mg per day.

IMPORTANT SAFETY INFORMATION

MHRA/CHM ADVICE: ELTROMBOPAG (*REVOLADE®*): REPORTS OF INTERFERENCE WITH BILIRUBIN AND CREATININE TEST RESULTS (JULY 2018)

See *Effect on laboratory tests*.

- **CAUTIONS** Patients of East Asian origin · risk factors for thromboembolism
- **INTERACTIONS** → Appendix 1: eltrombopag
- **SIDE-EFFECTS**

▶ **Common or very common** Alopecia · anaemia · appetite decreased · asthenia · cough · depression · diarrhoea · dry eye · dry mouth · fever · gastrointestinal discomfort · gastrointestinal disorders · haemolytic anaemia · hepatic disorders · hyperbilirubinaemia · increased risk of infection · malaise · menorrhagia · muscle complaints · nasal complaints · nausea · oral disorders · oropharyngeal complaints · pain · peripheral oedema · QT interval prolongation · sensation abnormal · skin reactions · sleep disorder · sweat changes · vertigo · vision disorders · vomiting

▶ **Uncommon** Anisocytosis · arrhythmias · balance impaired · cardiovascular disorder · cataract cortical · chest pain · cyanosis · drowsiness · ear pain · electrolyte imbalance · embolism and thrombosis · eosinophilia · excessive tearing · eye inflammation · eye pain · feeling hot · feeling jittery · food poisoning · gout · haemorrhage · headaches · hemiparesis · increased leucocytes · lens opacity · mood altered · muscle weakness · myocardial infarction · nephritis lupus · nerve disorders · nocturia · rectosigmoid cancer · renal failure · retinal pigment epitheliopathy · sinus disorder · sleep apnoea · speech disorder · sunburn · thrombocytopenia · tremor · urine abnormalities · vasodilation · wound inflammation

- **CONCEPTION AND CONTRACEPTION** Ensure effective contraception during treatment.
- **PREGNANCY** Avoid—toxicity in *animal* studies.
- **BREAST FEEDING** Manufacturer advises avoid.
- **HEPATIC IMPAIRMENT** Manufacturer advises consider avoiding.

Dose adjustments Manufacturer advises initial dose reduction to 25 mg once daily and wait at least 3 weeks before upwards titration of dose.

- **RENAL IMPAIRMENT** Use with caution.
- **MONITORING REQUIREMENTS**

▶ Manufacturer advises monitor liver function before treatment, every two weeks when adjusting the dose, and monthly thereafter.

▶ Manufacturer advises regular ophthalmological examinations for cataract formation.

▶ Manufacturer advises peripheral blood smear prior to initiation to establish baseline level of cellular morphologic abnormalities; once stabilised, full blood count with white blood cell count differential should be performed monthly.

▶ Manufacturer advises monitor full blood count including platelet count and peripheral blood smears every week during treatment until a stable platelet count is reached ($50x10^9$/litre or more for at least 4 weeks), then monthly thereafter; monitor platelet count weekly for 4 weeks following treatment discontinuation.

- **EFFECT ON LABORATORY TESTS** Eltrombopag is highly coloured and can cause serum discolouration and interference with total bilirubin and creatinine testing. If laboratory results are inconsistent with clinical observations, manufacturer advises re-testing using another method to help determine the validity of the result.
- **DIRECTIONS FOR ADMINISTRATION** Each dose should be taken at least 4 hours before or after any dairy products (or foods containing calcium), indigestion remedies, or medicines containing aluminium, calcium, iron, magnesium, zinc, or selenium to reduce possible interference with absorption.
- **PATIENT AND CARER ADVICE** Patient counselling is advised on how to administer eltrombopag tablets.
- **NATIONAL FUNDING/ACCESS DECISIONS**

Scottish Medicines Consortium (SMC) decisions

SMC No. 1206/17

The *Scottish Medicines Consortium* has advised (January 2017) that eltrombopag (*Revolade®*) is accepted for restricted use within NHS Scotland for the treatment of chronic immune (idiopathic) thrombocytopenic purpura (ITP) in patients aged 1 year to 17 years who have severe symptomatic ITP or a high risk of bleeding, **and** are refractory to other treatments (e.g. corticosteroids, immunoglobulins). This advice is contingent upon the continuing availability of the patient access scheme in NHS Scotland, or a list price that is equivalent or lower.

All Wales Medicines Strategy Group (AWMSG) decisions

AWMSG No. 2692

The *All Wales Medicines Strategy Group* has advised (October 2016) that eltrombopag (*Revolade®*) is recommended as an option for use within NHS Wales for the treatment of chronic immune (idiopathic) thrombocytopenic purpura (ITP) in patients aged 1 year to 17 years who are refractory to other treatments (e.g. corticosteroids, immunoglobulins). This recommendation applies only if the approved Wales Patient Access Scheme is used or where the list/contract price is equivalent or lower.

- **MEDICINAL FORMS** There can be variation in the licensing of different medicines containing the same drug.

Tablet

▶ Revolade (Novartis Pharmaceuticals UK Ltd)

Eltrombopag (as Eltrombopag olamine) 25 mg Revolade 25mg tablets | 28 tablet PoM £770.00 DT = £770.00

Eltrombopag (as Eltrombopag olamine) 50 mg Revolade 50mg tablets | 28 tablet PoM £1,540.00 DT = £1,540.00
Eltrombopag (as Eltrombopag olamine) 75 mg Revolade 75mg tablets | 28 tablet PoM £2,310.00 DT = £2,310.00

Romiplostim

28-Jan-2019

- **DRUG ACTION** Romiplostim is an Fc–peptide fusion protein that binds to and activates the thrombopoietin (TPO) receptor, thereby increasing platelet production.

- **INDICATIONS AND DOSE**

Chronic immune (idiopathic) thrombocytopenic purpura in patients refractory to other treatments (such as corticosteroids or immunoglobulins) (under expert supervision)

▶ BY SUBCUTANEOUS INJECTION

▸ Child 1–17 years: Initially 1 microgram/kg once weekly, adjusted in steps of 1 microgram/kg once weekly (max. per dose 10 micrograms/kg once weekly) until a stable platelet count of $50x10^9$/litre or more is reached, consult product literature for further details of dose adjustments; reassess bodyweight every 12 weeks, discontinue treatment if inadequate response after 4 weeks at maximum dose

- **CAUTIONS** Risk factors for thromboembolism
- **SIDE-EFFECTS**

▶ **Common or very common** Anaemia · angioedema · arthralgia · asthenia · bone marrow disorders · chills · constipation · cough · diarrhoea · dizziness · embolism and thrombosis · eye inflammation · fever · flushing · gastrointestinal discomfort · headaches · hypersensitivity · increased risk of infection · influenza like illness · muscle complaints · nausea · oropharyngeal pain · pain · palpitations · peripheral oedema · peripheral swelling · sensation abnormal · skin reactions · sleep disorders

▶ **Uncommon** Alopecia · appetite decreased · chest pain · clonus · dehydration · depression · dry throat · dysphagia · dyspnoea · erythromelalgia · eye disorders · eye pruritus · feeling hot · feeling jittery · gastrooesophageal reflux disease · gout · haemorrhage · hair growth abnormal · hypotension · irritability · leucocytosis · malaise · muscle weakness · myocardial infarction · nasal complaints · neoplasms · oral disorders · peripheral ischaemia · peripheral neuropathy · photosensitivity reaction · pleuritic pain · portal vein thrombosis · skin nodule · splenomegaly · taste altered · thrombocytosis · tooth discolouration · vertigo · vision disorders · vomiting · weight changes

- **PREGNANCY** Manufacturer advises avoid—toxicity in *animal* studies.
- **BREAST FEEDING** Manufacturer advises avoid—no information available.
- **HEPATIC IMPAIRMENT** Manufacturer advises caution; consider avoiding in moderate to severe impairment (risk of thromboembolic complications).
- **RENAL IMPAIRMENT** Manufacturer advises caution—no information available.
- **MONITORING REQUIREMENTS**

▶ Manufacturer advises monitor full blood count and peripheral blood smears for morphological abnormalities before and during treatment.

▶ Manufacturer advises monitor platelet count weekly until platelet count reaches $50x10^9$/litre or more for at least 4 weeks without dose adjustment, then monthly thereafter.

▶ Manufacturer advises monitor platelet count following treatment discontinuation—risk of bleeding.

- **PATIENT AND CARER ADVICE**

Driving and skilled tasks Manufacturer advises that patients and their carers should be counselled on the effects on driving and the performance of skilled tasks—increased risk of dizziness.

- **NATIONAL FUNDING/ACCESS DECISIONS**

Scottish Medicines Consortium (SMC) decisions
SMC No. SMC2126
The *Scottish Medicines Consortium* has advised (February 2019) that romiplostim (*Nplate*®) is accepted for restricted use within NHS Scotland for the treatment of chronic immune (idiopathic) thrombocytopenic purpura (ITP) in patients aged one year and older who are refractory to other treatments (e.g. corticosteroids, immunoglobulins). Romiplostim is restricted to those with severe symptomatic ITP or those with a high risk of bleeding.

All Wales Medicines Strategy Group (AWMSG) decisions
AWMSG No. 3103
The *All Wales Medicines Strategy Group* has advised (March 2019) that romiplostim (*Nplate*®) is recommended as an option for use within NHS Wales for the treatment of chronic immune (idiopathic) thrombocytopenic purpura in patients from 1 year of age up to 18 years of age who are refractory to other treatments (e.g. corticosteroids, immunoglobulins). This recommendation applies only in circumstances where the approved Patient Access Scheme (PAS) is utilised or where the list/contract price is equivalent or lower than the PAS price.

- **MEDICINAL FORMS** There can be variation in the licensing of different medicines containing the same drug.

Powder for solution for injection

▸ Nplate (Amgen Ltd)
Romiplostim 125 microgram Nplate 125microgram powder for solution for injection vials | 1 vial PoM £241.00

Nutrition and metabolic disorders

1 Acid-base imbalance

1.1 Metabolic acidosis

ALKALISING DRUGS

Trometamol

(Tris(hydroxymethyl)aminomethane, THAM)

- **INDICATIONS AND DOSE**

Metabolic acidosis

▶ BY INTRAVENOUS INFUSION

▸ Child: To be administered at an amount appropriate to the body base deficit

- **UNLICENSED USE** Unlicensed preparation.
- **CONTRA-INDICATIONS** Anuria · chronic respiratory acidosis
- **CAUTIONS** Extravasation can cause severe tissue damage
- **SIDE-EFFECTS** Hepatic necrosis (following administration via umbilical vein) (in neonates) · hyperkalaemia (in renal impairment) · hypoglycaemia · respiratory depression

SIDE-EFFECTS, FURTHER INFORMATION Respiratory support may be required because trometamol induces respiratory depression.

- **PREGNANCY** Limited information available, hypoglycaemia may harm fetus.
- **BREAST FEEDING** No information available.

● **RENAL IMPAIRMENT** Use with caution, may cause hyperkalaemia.

● **MEDICINAL FORMS** There can be variation in the licensing of different medicines containing the same drug. Forms available from special-order manufacturers include: solution for infusion

Solution for infusion

▸ Tris(Imported (Germany))

Trometamol 363.4 mg per 1 ml Tris 36.34% solution for infusion 20ml ampoules | 10 ampoule PoM

2 Fluid and electrolyte imbalances

Fluids and electrolytes

Electrolyte replacement therapy

The electrolyte concentrations (intravenous fluid) table and the electrolyte content (gastro-inestinal secretions) table may be helpful in planning replacement electrolyte therapy; faeces, vomit, or aspiration should be saved and analysed where possible if abnormal losses are suspected.

Oral preparations for fluid and electrolyte imbalance

Sodium and potassium salts, may be given by mouth to prevent deficiencies or to treat established deficiencies of mild or moderate degree.

Oral potassium

Compensation for potassium loss is especially necessary:

- in children in whom secondary hyperaldosteronism occurs, e.g. renal artery stenosis, renal tubule disorder, the nephrotic syndrome, and severe heart failure;
- in children with excessive losses of potassium in the faeces, e.g. chronic diarrhoea associated with intestinal malabsorption or laxative abuse;
- in those taking digoxin or anti-arrhythmic drugs, where potassium depletion may induce arrhythmias.

Measures to compensate for potassium loss may be required during long-term administration of drugs known to induce potassium loss (e.g. corticosteroids). Potassium supplements are **seldom required** with the small doses of diuretics given to treat hypertension; **potassium-sparing diuretics** (rather than potassium supplements) are recommended for prevention of hypokalaemia due to diuretics such as furosemide p. 148 or the thiazides when these are given to eliminate oedema.

If potassium salts are used for the *prevention of hypokalaemia*, then doses of potassium chloride p. 651 daily by mouth are suitable in patients taking a normal diet. Smaller doses must be used if there is renal insufficiency to reduce the risk of **hyperkalaemia**.

Potassium salts cause nausea and vomiting and poor compliance is a major limitation to their effectiveness (small divided doses may minimise gastric irritation); when appropriate, potassium-sparing diuretics are preferable. When there is *established potassium depletion* larger doses may be necessary, the quantity depending on the severity of any continuing potassium loss (monitoring of plasma-potassium concentration and specialist advice would be required). Potassium depletion is frequently associated with chloride depletion and with metabolic alkalosis, and these disorders require correction.

Management of hyperkalaemia

Acute severe hyperkalaemia calls for urgent treatment with intravenous infusion of **soluble insulin** (0.3–0.6 units/kg/hour in neonates and 0.05–0.2 units/kg/hour in children over 1 month) with glucose 0.5–1 g/kg/hour (5–10 mL/kg of glucose 10%; 2.5–5 mL/kg of glucose 20% via a central venous catheter may also be considered). If insulin cannot be used, salbutamol p. 164 can be given by intravenous injection, but it has a slower onset of action and may be less effective for reducing plasma-potassium concentration.

Calcium gluconate p. 642 is given by slow intravenous injection to manage cardiac excitability caused by hyperkalaemia.

The correction of causal or compounding acidosis with sodium bicarbonate p. 634 infusion should be considered (**important**: preparations of sodium bicarbonate and calcium salts should not be administered in the same line—risk of precipitation). Intravenous furosemide can also be given but is less effective in children with renal impairment. Drugs exacerbating hyperkalaemia should be reviewed and stopped as appropriate; dialysis may occasionally be required.

Ion-exchange resins may be used to remove excess potassium in *mild hyperkalaemia* or in *moderate hyperkalaemia* when there are no ECG changes. Calcium polystyrene sulfonate is preferred unless plasma-calcium concentrations are high.

Oral sodium and water

Sodium chloride p. 636 is indicated in states of sodium depletion. In preterm neonates in the first few weeks of life and in chronic conditions associated with mild or moderate degrees of sodium depletion, e.g. in salt-losing bowel or renal disease, oral supplements of sodium chloride may be sufficient. Sodium chloride solutions suitable for use by mouth in neonates are available from 'special-order' manufacturers or specialist importing companies, they should be used with care because they are hypertonic. Supplementation with sodium chloride may be required to replace losses in children with cystic fibrosis particularly in warm weather.

Oral rehydration therapy (ORT)

Diarrhoea in children is usually self-limiting, however, in children under 6 months of age, and more particularly in those under 3 months, symptoms of dehydration may be less obvious and there is a risk of rapid and severe deterioration. Intestinal absorption of sodium and water is enhanced by glucose (and other carbohydrates). Replacement of fluid and electrolytes lost through diarrhoea can therefore be achieved by giving solutions containing sodium, potassium, and glucose or another carbohydrate such as rice starch.

Oral rehydration solutions should:

- enhance the absorption of water and electrolytes;
- replace the electrolyte deficit adequately and safely;
- contain an alkalinising agent to counter acidosis;
- be slightly hypo-osmolar (about 250 mmol/litre) to prevent the possible induction of osmotic diarrhoea;
- be simple to use in hospital and at home;
- be palatable and acceptable, especially to children;
- be readily available.

It is the policy of the World Health Organization (WHO) to promote a single oral rehydration solution but to use it flexibly (e.g. by giving extra water between drinks of oral rehydration solution to moderately dehydrated infants).

The WHO oral rehydration salts formulation contains sodium chloride 2.6 g, potassium chloride 1.5 g, sodium citrate 2.9 g, anhydrous glucose 13.5 g. It is dissolved in sufficient water to produce 1 litre (providing Na^+ 75 mmol, K^+ 20 mmol, Cl^- 65 mmol, citrate 10 mmol, glucose 75 mmol/litre). This formulation is recommended by the WHO and the United Nations Children's fund, but it is not commonly used in the UK.

Oral rehydration solutions used in the UK are lower in sodium (50–60 mmol/litre) than the WHO formulation since, in general, patients suffer less severe sodium loss.

Rehydration should be rapid over 3 to 4 hours (except in hypernatraemic dehydration in which case rehydration should occur more slowly over 12 hours). The patient should be reassessed after initial rehydration and if still dehydrated rapid fluid replacement should continue.

Once rehydration is complete further dehydration is prevented by encouraging the patient to drink normal volumes of an appropriate fluid and by replacing continuing losses with an oral rehydration solution; in infants, breast-feeding or formula feeds should be offered between oral rehydration drinks.

Oral bicarbonate

Sodium bicarbonate is given by mouth for *chronic acidotic states* such as uraemic acidosis or renal tubular acidosis. The dose for correction of metabolic acidosis is not predictable and the response must be assessed. For severe *metabolic acidosis*, sodium bicarbonate can be given intravenously.

Sodium supplements may increase blood pressure or cause fluid retention and pulmonary oedema in those at risk; hypokalaemia may be exacerbated.

Sodium bicarbonate p. 634 may affect the stability or absorption of other drugs if administered at the same time. If possible, allow 1–2 hours before administering other drugs orally.

Where *hyperchloraemic acidosis* is associated with potassium deficiency, as in some renal tubular and gastrointestinal disorders it may be appropriate to give oral **potassium bicarbonate**, although acute or severe deficiency should be managed by intravenous therapy.

Parenteral preparations for fluid and electrolyte imbalance

Electrolytes and water

Solutions of electrolytes are given intravenously, to meet normal fluid and electrolyte requirements or to replenish substantial deficits or continuing losses when it is not possible or desirable to use the oral route. When intravenous administration is not possible, fluid (as sodium chloride 0.9% p. 636 or glucose 5% p. 638) can also be given subcutaneously by hypodermoclysis.

In an individual patient the nature and severity of the electrolyte imbalance must be assessed from the history and clinical and biochemical examination. Sodium, potassium, chloride, magnesium, phosphate, and water depletion can occur singly and in combination with or without disturbances of acid-base balance.

Isotonic solutions may be infused safely into a peripheral vein. Solutions more concentrated than plasma, for example 15% glucose, are best given through an indwelling catheter positioned in a large vein.

Maintenance fluid requirements in children are usually derived from the relationship that exists between body-weight and metabolic rate; the figures in the table below may be used as a guide outside the neonatal period. The glucose requirement is that needed to minimise gluconeogenesis from amino acids obtained as substrate from muscle breakdown. Maintenance fluids are intended only to provide hydration for a short period until enteral or parenteral nutrition can be established.

It is usual to meet these requirements by using a standard solution of sodium chloride with glucose p. 638. Solutions containing 20 mmol/litre of potassium chloride p. 651 meet usual potassium requirements when given in the suggested volumes; adjustments may be needed if there is an inability to excrete fluids or electrolytes, excessive renal loss or continuing extra-renal losses. The exact requirements depend upon the nature of the clinical situation and types of losses incurred.

Fluid requirements for children over 1 month:

Body-weight	24-hour fluid requirement
Under 10 kg	100 mL/kg
10–20 kg	100 mL/kg for the first 10 kg + 50 mL/kg for each 1 kg body-weight over 10 kg
Over 20 kg	100 mL/kg for the first 10 kg + 50 mL/kg for each 1 kg body-weight between 10–20 kg + 20 mL/kg for each 1 kg body-weight over 20 kg (max. 2 litres in females, 2.5 litres in males)

Important The baseline fluid requirements shown in the table should be adjusted to take account of factors that reduce water loss (e.g. increased antidiuretic hormone, renal failure, hypothermia, and high ambient humidity) or increase water loss (e.g. pyrexia or burns).

Replacement therapy: initial intravenous replacement fluid is generally required if the child is over 10% dehydrated, or if 5–10% dehydrated and oral or enteral rehydration is not tolerated or possible. Oral rehydration is adequate, if tolerated, in the majority of those less than 10% dehydrated. Subsequent fluid and electrolyte requirements are determined by clinical assessment of fluid balance.

Intravenous sodium

Intravenous sodium chloride in isotonic (0.9%) solution provides the most important extracellular ions in near physiological concentrations and is indicated in *sodium depletion*. It may be given for initial treatment of acute fluid loss and to replace ongoing gastro-intestinal losses from the upper gastro-intestinal tract. Intravenous sodium chloride is commonly given as a component of maintenance and replacement therapy, usually in combination with other electrolytes and glucose.

Chronic hyponatraemia should ideally be corrected by fluid restriction. However, if sodium chloride is required, the deficit should be corrected slowly to avoid the risk of osmotic demyelination syndrome; the rise in plasma sodium concentration should be no more than 10 mmol/litre in 24 hours.

Sodium chloride with glucose solutions are indicated when there is combined *water and sodium depletion*. A 1:1 mixture of isotonic sodium chloride and glucose 5% allows some of the water (free of sodium) to enter body cells which suffer most from dehydration while the sodium salt with a volume of water determined by the normal plasma Na^+ remains extracellular.

Combined sodium, potassium, chloride, and water depletion may occur, for example, with severe diarrhoea or persistent vomiting; replacement is carried out with sodium chloride 0.9% intravenous infusion and glucose 5% intravenous infusion with potassium as appropriate

Compound sodium lactate (Hartmann's solution) can be used instead of isotonic sodium chloride solution during or after surgery, or in the initial management of the injured or wounded.

Intravenous glucose

Glucose solutions are used mainly to replace water deficit. Water depletion (dehydration) tends to occur when losses are not matched by a comparable intake, as may occur in coma or dysphagia.

Water loss rarely exceeds electrolyte losses but this can occur in fevers, hyperthyroidism, and in uncommon water-losing renal states such as diabetes insipidus or hypercalcaemia. The volume of glucose solution needed to replace deficits varies with the severity of the disorder; the rate of infusion should be adjusted to return the plasma-sodium concentration to normal over 48 hours.

Glucose solutions are also used to correct and prevent hypoglycaemia and to provide a source of energy in those

Electrolyte concentrations—intravenous fluids

Intravenous infusion	Millimoles per litre				
	Na$^+$	K$^+$	HCO_3^-	Cl$^-$	Ca^{2+}
Normal plasma values	142	4.5	26	103	2.5
Sodium Chloride 0.9%	150	-	-	150	-
Compound Sodium Lactate (Hartmann's)	131	5	29	111	2
Sodium Chloride 0.18% and Glucose 4% (Adults only)	30	-	-	30	-
Sodium Chloride 0.45% and Glucose 5% (Children only)	75	-	-	75	-
Potassium Chloride 0.15% and Glucose 5% (Children only)	-	20	-	20	-
Potassium Chloride 0.15% and Sodium Chloride 0.9% (Children only)	150	20	-	170	-
Potassium Chloride 0.3% and Glucose 5%	-	40	-	40	-
Potassium Chloride 0.3% and Sodium Chloride 0.9%	150	40	-	190	-
To correct metabolic acidosis					
Sodium Bicarbonate 1.26%	150	-	150	-	-
Sodium Bicarbonate 8.4% for cardiac arrest	1000	-	1000	-	-
Sodium Lactate (m/6)	167	-	167	-	-

Electrolyte content—gastro-intestinal secretions

Type of fluid	Millimoles per litre				
	H$^+$	Na$^+$	K$^+$	HCO_3^-	Cl$^-$
Gastric	40-60	20-80	5-20	-	100-150
Biliary	-	120-140	5-15	30-50	80-120
Pancreatic	-	120-140	5-15	70-110	40-80
Small bowel	-	120-140	5-15	20-40	90-130

too ill to be fed adequately by mouth; glucose solutions are a key component of parenteral nutrition.

Glucose solutions are given with insulin for the emergency management of *hyperkalaemia*. They are also given, after correction of hyperglycaemia, during treatment of diabetic ketoacidosis, when they must be accompanied by continuous insulin infusion.

Intravenous potassium

Potassium chloride with sodium chloride intravenous infusion p. 636 is the initial treatment for the correction of *severe hypokalaemia* and when sufficient potassium cannot be taken by mouth.

Repeated measurements of plasma-potassium concentration are necessary to determine whether further infusions are required and to avoid the development of hyperkalaemia, which is especially likely in renal impairment.

Initial potassium replacement therapy should **not** involve glucose infusions, because glucose may cause a further decrease in the plasma-potassium concentration.

Bicarbonate and trometamol

Sodium bicarbonate is used to control severe *metabolic acidosis* (pH < 7.1) particularly that caused by loss of bicarbonate (as in renal tubular acidosis or from excessive gastro-intestinal losses). Mild metabolic acidosis associated with volume depletion should first be managed by appropriate fluid replacement because acidosis usually resolves as tissue and renal perfusion are restored. In more severe metabolic acidosis or when the acidosis remains unresponsive to correction of anoxia or hypovolaemia, sodium bicarbonate (1.26%) p. 634 can be infused over 3–4 hours with plasma-pH and electrolyte monitoring. In severe shock, for example in cardiac arrest, metabolic acidosis can develop without sodium depletion; in these circumstances sodium bicarbonate is best given intravenously as a small volume of hypertonic solution, such as 8.4%; plasma pH and electrolytes should be monitored. For *chronic acidotic states*, sodium bicarbonate can be given by mouth.

Trometamol (tris(hydroxymethyl)aminomethane, THAM) p. 630, an organic buffer, corrects metabolic acidosis by causing an increase in urinary pH and an osmotic diuresis. It is indicated when sodium bicarbonate is unsuitable as in carbon dioxide retention, hypernatraemia, or renal impairment. It is also used during cardiac bypass surgery and, very rarely, in cardiac arrest.

Plasma and plasma substitutes

Albumin solution p. 643, prepared from whole blood, contain soluble proteins and electrolytes but no clotting factors, blood group antibodies, or plasma cholinesterases; they may be given without regard to the recipient's blood group.

Albumin is usually used after the acute phase of illness to correct a plasma-volume deficit; hypoalbuminaemia itself is not an appropriate indication. The use of albumin solution in acute plasma or blood loss may be wasteful; plasma substitutes are more appropriate. Concentrated albumin solution may also be used to obtain a diuresis in hypoalbuminaemic patients (e.g. in nephrotic syndrome).

Recent evidence does not support the previous view that the use of albumin increases mortality.

Plasma substitutes

Gelatin p. 644 is a macromolecular substance that is metabolised slowly. Gelatin may be used at the outset to expand and maintain blood volume in shock arising from conditions such as burns or septicaemia; it may also be used as an immediate short-term measure to treat haemorrhage until blood is available. Gelatin is rarely needed when shock is due to sodium and water depletion because, in these circumstances, the shock responds to water and electrolyte repletion; see also the management of shock.

Plasma substitutes should **not** be used to maintain plasma volume in conditions such as burns or peritonitis where there is loss of plasma protein, water, and electrolytes over periods of several days or weeks. In these situations, plasma or plasma protein fractions containing large amounts of albumin should be given.

Large volumes of *some* plasma substitutes can increase the risk of bleeding through depletion of coagulation factors.

Parenteral preparations for fluid and electrolyte imbalance

Electrolytes and water

Neonates lose water through the skin and nose, particularly if preterm or if the skin is damaged. The basic fluid requirement for a term baby in average ambient humidity is 40–60 mL/kg/day plus urinary losses. Preterm babies have very high transepidermal losses particularly in the first few days of life; they may need more fluid replacement than full term babies and up to 180 mL/kg/day may be required. Local guidelines for fluid management in the neonatal period should be consulted.

Intravenous sodium

The sodium requirement for most healthy neonates is 3 mmol/kg daily. Preterm neonates, particularly below 30 weeks gestation, may require up to 6 mmol/kg daily. *Hyponatraemia* may be caused by excessive renal loss of sodium; it may also be dilutional and restriction of fluid intake may be appropriate. Sodium supplementation is likely to be required if the serum sodium concentration is significantly reduced.

Hypernatraemia may also occur, most often due to dehydration (e.g. breast milk insufficiency). Severe hypernatraemia and hyponatraemia can cause fits and rarely brain damage. Sodium in drug preparations, delivered via continuous infusions, or in infusions to maintain the patency of intravascular or umbilical lines, can result in significant amounts of sodium being delivered, (e.g. 1 mL/hour of 0.9% sodium chloride infused over 24 hours is equivalent to 3.6 mmol/day of sodium).

BICARBONATE

Sodium bicarbonate

29-Jul-2019

● **INDICATIONS AND DOSE**

Chronic acidotic states such as uraemic acidosis or renal tubular acidosis

▶ BY MOUTH

▶ Neonate: Initially 1–2 mmol/kg daily in divided doses, adjusted according to response.

▶ Child: Initially 1–2 mmol/kg daily in divided doses, adjusted according to response

Severe metabolic acidosis

▶ BY SLOW INTRAVENOUS INJECTION, OR BY INTRAVENOUS INFUSION

▶ Child: Administer an amount appropriate to the body base deficit, to be given by slow intravenous injection of a strong solution (up to 8.4%), or by continuous intravenous infusion of a weaker solution (usually 1.26%)

Renal hyperkalaemia

▶ BY SLOW INTRAVENOUS INJECTION

▶ Neonate: 1 mmol/kg daily.

▶ Child: 1 mmol/kg daily

Persistent cyanotic spell in a child with congenital heart disease despite optimal use of 100% oxygen and propranolol

▶ BY INTRAVENOUS INFUSION

▶ Child: 1 mmol/kg, dose given to correct acidosis (or dose calculated according to arterial blood gas results), sodium bicarbonate 4.2% intravenous infusion is appropriate for a child under 1 year and sodium bicarbonate 8.4% intravenous infusion in children over 1 year

● **CONTRA-INDICATIONS** Salt restricted diet

● **CAUTIONS** Respiratory acidosis

● **INTERACTIONS** → Appendix 1: sodium bicarbonate

● **SIDE-EFFECTS**

▶ With intravenous use Skin exfoliation · soft tissue necrosis · ulcer

▶ With oral use Abdominal cramps · burping · flatulence · hypokalaemia · metabolic alkalosis

● **HEPATIC IMPAIRMENT**

▶ With oral use Manufacturer advises caution in cirrhosis.

● **MONITORING REQUIREMENTS**

▶ With intravenous use Plasma-pH and electrolytes should be monitored.

● **DIRECTIONS FOR ADMINISTRATION**

▶ With intravenous use For *peripheral infusion* dilute 8.4% solution at least 1 in 10. For *central line infusion* dilute 1 in 5 with Glucose 5% or 10% *or* Sodium Chloride 0.9%. Extravasation can cause severe tissue damage.

▶ With oral use Sodium bicarbonate may affect the stability or absorption of other drugs if administered at the same time. If possible, allow 1–2 hours before administering other drugs orally.

● **PRESCRIBING AND DISPENSING INFORMATION**

▶ With oral use *Sodium bicarbonate* 500*mg* capsules contain approximately 6 mmol each of Na^+ and HCO_3^-; *Sodium bicarbonate* 600*mg* capsules contain approximately 7 mmol each of Na^+ and HCO_3^-. Oral solutions of sodium bicarbonate are required occasionally; these are available from 'special-order' manufacturers or specialist importing companies; the strength of sodium bicarbonate should be stated on the prescription.

▶ With intravenous use Usual strength Sodium bicarbonate 1.26% (12.6 g, 150 mmol each of Na^+ and HCO_3^-/litre), various other strengths available.

● **PATIENT AND CARER ADVICE** Patients or carers should be given advice on the administration of sodium bicarbonate oral medicines.

Medicines for Children leaflet: Sodium bicarbonate for acidosis www.medicinesforchildren.org.uk/sodium-bicarbonate-acidosis

● **MEDICINAL FORMS** There can be variation in the licensing of different medicines containing the same drug. Forms available from special-order manufacturers include: capsule, oral suspension, oral solution, solution for injection

Tablet

▶ Sodium bicarbonate (Non-proprietary)

Sodium bicarbonate 600 mg Sodium bicarbonate 600mg tablets | 100 tablet GSL £29.75 DT = £26.79 | 100 tablet £26.79–£125.50 DT = £26.79

Solution for injection

▶ Sodium bicarbonate (Non-proprietary)

Sodium bicarbonate 84 mg per 1 ml Sodium bicarbonate 8.4% (1mmol/ml) solution for injection 10ml ampoules | 10 ampoule PoM £113.59 DT = £113.59

Sodium bicarbonate 8.4% (1mmol/ml) solution for injection 250ml bottles | 10 bottle PoM £100.00 DT = £100.00

Sodium bicarbonate 8.4% (1mmol/ml) solution for injection 100ml bottles | 10 bottle PoM £100.00 DT = £100.00

Oral solution

▸ Thamicarb (Thame Laboratories Ltd)

Sodium bicarbonate 84 mg per 1 ml Thamicarb 84mg/1ml oral solution sugar-free | 100 ml PoM £39.80 DT = £39.80 sugar-free | 500 ml PoM £199.20 DT = £199.20

Capsule

▸ Sodium bicarbonate (Non-proprietary)

Sodium bicarbonate 500 mg Sodium bicarbonate 500mg capsules | 56 capsule PoM ☒ DT = £1.69 | 100 capsule £2.89

Infusion

▸ Sodium bicarbonate (Non-proprietary)

Sodium bicarbonate 12.6 mg per 1 ml Polyfusor sodium bicarbonate 1.26% solution for infusion 500ml bottles | 1 bottle PoM £11.98

Sodium bicarbonate 14 mg per 1 ml Polyfusor sodium bicarbonate 1.4% solution for infusion 500ml bottles | 1 bottle PoM £11.98

Sodium bicarbonate 27.4 mg per 1 ml Polyfusor sodium bicarbonate 2.74% solution for infusion 500ml bottles | 1 bottle PoM £11.98

Sodium bicarbonate 42 mg per 1 ml Polyfusor sodium bicarbonate 4.2% solution for infusion 500ml bottles | 1 bottle PoM £11.98

Sodium bicarbonate 84 mg per 1 ml Polyfusor sodium bicarbonate 8.4% solution for infusion 200ml bottles | 1 bottle PoM £11.98

ELECTROLYTES AND MINERALS > POTASSIUM

Potassium chloride with calcium chloride dihydrate and sodium chloride

(Ringer's solution)

The properties listed below are those particular to the combination only. For the properties of the components please consider, potassium chloride p. 651, sodium chloride p. 636.

● **INDICATIONS AND DOSE**

Electrolyte imbalance

▶ BY INTRAVENOUS INFUSION

▸ Child: Dosed according to the deficit or daily maintenance requirements (consult product literature)

● **INTERACTIONS** → Appendix 1: potassium chloride

● **PRESCRIBING AND DISPENSING INFORMATION** Ringer's solution for injection provides the following ions (in mmol/litre), Ca^{2+} 2.2, K^+ 4, Na^+ 147, Cl^- 156.

● **MEDICINAL FORMS** There can be variation in the licensing of different medicines containing the same drug.

Infusion

▸ Potassium chloride with calcium chloride dihydrate and sodium chloride (Non-proprietary)

Potassium chloride 300 microgram per 1 ml, Calcium chloride 320 microgram per 1 ml, Sodium chloride 8.6 mg per 1 ml Steriflex No.9 ringers infusion 500ml bags | 1 bag PoM £1.96 Steriflex No.9 ringers infusion 1litre bags | 1 bag PoM £2.22 Polyfusor Ringers solution for infusion 500ml bottles | 1 bottle PoM £3.58

Potassium chloride with calcium chloride, sodium chloride and sodium lactate

(Sodium Lactate Intravenous Infusion, Compound; Compound, Hartmann's Solution for Injection; Ringer-Lactate Solution for Injection)

The properties listed below are those particular to the combination only. For the properties of the components please consider, potassium chloride p. 651, sodium chloride p. 636, calcium chloride p. 642.

● **INDICATIONS AND DOSE**

For prophylaxis, and replacement therapy, requiring the use of sodium chloride and lactate, with minimal amounts of calcium and potassium

▶ BY INTRAVENOUS INFUSION

▸ Child: (consult product literature)

● **INTERACTIONS** → Appendix 1: calcium salts · potassium chloride

● **PRESCRIBING AND DISPENSING INFORMATION** Compound sodium lactate intravenous infusion contains Na^+ 131 mmol, K^+ 5 mmol, Ca^{2+} 2 mmol, HCO_3^- (as lactate) 29 mmol, Cl^- 111 mmol/litre.

● **MEDICINAL FORMS** There can be variation in the licensing of different medicines containing the same drug.

Infusion

▸ Potassium chloride with calcium chloride, sodium chloride and sodium lactate (Non-proprietary)

Calcium chloride 270 microgram per 1 ml, Potassium chloride 400 microgram per 1 ml, Sodium lactate 3.17 mg per 1 ml, Sodium chloride 6 mg per 1 ml Sodium lactate compound infusion 1litre bags | 1 bag PoM ☒

Potassium chloride with glucose

The properties listed below are those particular to the combination only. For the properties of the components please consider, potassium chloride p. 651, glucose p. 638.

● **INDICATIONS AND DOSE**

Electrolyte imbalance

▶ BY INTRAVENOUS INFUSION

▸ Child: Dosed according to the deficit or daily maintenance requirements

● **INTERACTIONS** → Appendix 1: potassium chloride

● **PRESCRIBING AND DISPENSING INFORMATION** Potassium chloride 0.3% contains 40 mmol each of K^+ and Cl^-/litre or 0.15% contains 20 mmol each of K^+ and Cl^-/litre with 5% of anhydrous glucose.

● **MEDICINAL FORMS** There can be variation in the licensing of different medicines containing the same drug. Forms available from special-order manufacturers include: infusion, solution for infusion

Infusion

▸ Potassium chloride with glucose (Non-proprietary)

Potassium chloride 3 mg per 1 ml, Glucose anhydrous 50 mg per 1 ml Potassium chloride 0.3% (potassium 20mmol/500ml) / Glucose 5% infusion 500ml bags | 1 bag PoM ☒ Potassium chloride 0.3% (potassium 40mmol/1litre) / Glucose 5% infusion 1litre bags | 1 bag PoM £1.30

Potassium chloride 2 mg per 1 ml, Glucose anhydrous 50 mg per 1 ml Steriflex No.29 potassium chloride 0.2% (potassium 27mmol/1litre) / glucose 5% infusion 1litre bags | 1 bag PoM £2.20 Steriflex No.29 potassium chloride 0.2% (potassium 13.3mmol/500ml) / glucose 5% infusion 500ml bags | 1 bag PoM £1.67

Potassium chloride 1.5 mg per 1 ml, Glucose anhydrous 50 mg per 1 ml Potassium chloride 0.15% (potassium 20mmol/1litre) / Glucose 5% infusion 1litre bags | 1 bag PoM ☒

Potassium chloride 0.15% (potassium 10mmol/500ml) / Glucose 5% infusion 500ml bags | 1 bag PoM £1.30

Potassium chloride with glucose and sodium chloride

The properties listed below are those particular to the combination only. For the properties of the components please consider, potassium chloride p. 651, glucose p. 638, sodium chloride below.

● **INDICATIONS AND DOSE**

Electrolyte imbalance

▶ BY INTRAVENOUS INFUSION

▸ Child: Dosed according to the deficit or daily maintenance requirements

● **INTERACTIONS** → Appendix 1: potassium chloride

● **PRESCRIBING AND DISPENSING INFORMATION**
Concentration of potassium chloride to be specified by the prescriber (usually K^+ 10–40 mmol/litre).

● **MEDICINAL FORMS** There can be variation in the licensing of different medicines containing the same drug. Forms available from special-order manufacturers include: infusion, solution for infusion

Infusion

▸ Potassium chloride with glucose and sodium chloride (Non-proprietary)
Sodium chloride 1.8 mg per 1 ml, Potassium chloride 3 mg per 1 ml, Glucose anhydrous 40 mg per 1 ml Potassium chloride 0.3% (potassium 20mmol/500ml) / Glucose 4% / Sodium chloride 0.18% infusion 500ml bags | 1 bag PoM
Potassium chloride 0.3% (potassium 40mmol/1litre) / Glucose 4% / Sodium chloride 0.18% infusion 1litre bags | 1 bag PoM
Potassium chloride 1.5 mg per 1 ml, Sodium chloride 1.8 mg per 1 ml, Glucose anhydrous 40 mg per 1 ml Potassium chloride 0.15% (potassium 20mmol/1litre) / Glucose 4% / Sodium chloride 0.18% infusion 1litre bags | 1 bag PoM
Potassium chloride 0.15% (potassium 10mmol/500ml) / Glucose 4% / Sodium chloride 0.18% infusion 500ml bags | 1 bag PoM
Sodium chloride 1.8 mg per 1 ml, Potassium chloride 2 mg per 1 ml, Glucose anhydrous 40 mg per 1 ml Steriflex No.30 potassium chloride 0.2% (potassium 13.3mmol/500ml) / glucose 4% / sodium chloride 0.18% infusion 500ml bags | 1 bag PoM £1.67
Steriflex No.30 potassium chloride 0.2% (potassium 27mmol/1litre) / glucose 4% / sodium chloride 0.18% infusion 1litre bags | 1 bag PoM £2.20
Potassium chloride 1.5 mg per 1 ml, Sodium chloride 4.5 mg per 1 ml, Glucose anhydrous 50 mg per 1 ml Intraven potassium chloride 0.15% (potassium 10mmol/500ml) / glucose 5% / sodium chloride 0.45% infusion 500ml bags | 1 bag PoM £3.76

Potassium chloride with potassium bicarbonate

10-Mar-2020

The properties listed below are those particular to the combination only. For the properties of the components please consider, potassium chloride p. 651.

● **INDICATIONS AND DOSE**

Potassium depletion

▶ BY MOUTH

▸ Child: Dosed according to the deficit or daily maintenance requirements (consult product literature)

● **INTERACTIONS** → Appendix 1: potassium chloride

● **PRESCRIBING AND DISPENSING INFORMATION** Each *Sando-K®* tablet contains potassium 470 mg (12 mmol of K^+) and chloride 285mg (8 mmol of Cl^-).

● **PATIENT AND CARER ADVICE**
Medicines for Children leaflet: Potassium chloride for potassium depletion www.medicinesforchildren.org.uk/potassium-chloride-potassium-depletion

● **MEDICINAL FORMS** There can be variation in the licensing of different medicines containing the same drug.

Effervescent tablet

CAUTIONARY AND ADVISORY LABELS 13, 21

▸ Sando-K (HK Pharma Ltd)
Potassium bicarbonate 400 mg, Potassium chloride 600 mg Sando-K effervescent tablets | 100 tablet P £9.95 DT = £9.95

Potassium chloride with sodium chloride

The properties listed below are those particular to the combination only. For the properties of the components please consider, potassium chloride p. 651, sodium chloride below.

● **INDICATIONS AND DOSE**

Electrolyte imbalance

▶ BY INTRAVENOUS INFUSION

▸ Child: Depending on the deficit or the daily maintenance requirements (consult product literature)

● **INTERACTIONS** → Appendix 1: potassium chloride

● **PRESCRIBING AND DISPENSING INFORMATION** Potassium chloride 0.15% with sodium chloride 0.9% contains K^+ 20 mmol, Na^+ 150 mmol, and Cl^- 170 mmol/litre or potassium chloride 0.3% with sodium chloride 0.9% contains K^+ 40 mmol, Na^+ 150 mmol, and Cl^- 190 mmol/litre.

● **MEDICINAL FORMS** There can be variation in the licensing of different medicines containing the same drug. Forms available from special-order manufacturers include: infusion, solution for infusion

Infusion

▸ Potassium chloride with sodium chloride (Non-proprietary)
Potassium chloride 3 mg per 1 ml, Sodium chloride 9 mg per 1 ml Potassium chloride 0.3% (potassium 20mmol/500ml) / Sodium chloride 0.9% infusion 500ml bags | 1 bag PoM
Potassium chloride 0.3% (potassium 40mmol/1litre) / Sodium chloride 0.9% infusion 1litre bags | 1 bag PoM
Potassium chloride 1.5 mg per 1 ml, Sodium chloride 9 mg per 1 ml Potassium chloride 0.15% (potassium 20mmol/1litre) / Sodium chloride 0.9% infusion 1litre bags | 1 bag PoM
Potassium chloride 0.15% (potassium 10mmol/500ml) / Sodium chloride 0.9% infusion 500ml bags | 1 bag PoM £1.30
Potassium chloride 2 mg per 1 ml, Sodium chloride 9 mg per 1 ml Steriflex No.28 potassium chloride 0.2% (potassium 13.3mmol/500ml) / sodium chloride 0.9% infusion 500ml bags | 1 bag PoM £1.67
Steriflex No.28 potassium chloride 0.2% (potassium 27mmol/1litre) / sodium chloride 0.9% infusion 1litre bags | 1 bag PoM £2.20

ELECTROLYTES AND MINERALS > SODIUM CHLORIDE

Sodium chloride

01-May-2020

● **INDICATIONS AND DOSE**

Chronic renal salt wasting

▶ BY MOUTH

▸ Child: 1–2 mmol/kg daily in divided doses, adjusted according to requirements

Sodium supplementation in neonates

▶ INITIALLY BY MOUTH

▸ Neonate up to 36 weeks corrected gestational age: 2 mmol, dose to be administered in 100 ml of formula feed (consult dietician), alternatively (by mouth using modified-release tablets) 3–4 mmol, dose to be administered in 100 ml of breast milk (consult dietician).

Sodium replacement
- ▶ BY MOUTH USING MODIFIED-RELEASE TABLETS
- ▸ Child: 1–2 mmol/kg daily in divided doses, adjusted according to requirements, higher doses may be needed in severe depletion

Management of diabetic ketoacidosis (to restore circulating volume if systolic blood pressure is below 90 mmHg and adjusted for age, sex, and medication as appropriate)
- ▶ BY INTRAVENOUS INFUSION
- ▸ Child: (consult local protocol)

Diluent for instillation of drugs to the bladder
- ▶ BY INTRAVESICAL INSTILLATION
- ▸ Child: (consult product literature)

Skin cleansing
- ▶ TO THE SKIN
- ▸ Child: Use for topical irrigation of wounds

● CAUTIONS
- ▸ With intravenous use Avoid excessive administration · cardiac failure · cardio-respiratory diseases · children receiving glucocorticoids · dilutional hyponatraemia · hepatic cirrhosis · hypertension · peripheral oedema · pulmonary oedema · reduced fluid loss · renal insufficiency · restrict intake in impaired renal function · toxaemia of pregnancy

CAUTIONS, FURTHER INFORMATION
- ▸ Reduced fluid loss
- ▸ With intravenous use The volume of fluid infused should take into account the possibility of reduced fluid loss owing to increased antidiuretic hormone and factors such as renal failure, hypothermia, and high humidity.
- ▸ Dilutional hyponatraemia
- ▸ With intravenous use Dilutional hyponatraemia is a rare but potentially fatal risk of parenteral hydration. It may be caused by inappropriate use of hypotonic fluids such as sodium chloride 0.18% and glucose 4% intravenous infusion, especially in the postoperative period when antidiuretic hormone secretion is increased. Dilutional hyponatraemia is characterized by a rapid fall in plasma-sodium concentration leading to cerebral oedema and seizures; any child with severe hyponatraemia or rapidly changing plasma-sodium concentration should be referred urgently to a paediatric high dependency facility.

● SIDE-EFFECTS
- ▸ With intravenous use Chills · fever · hypervolaemia · hypotension · local reaction · localised pain · paraesthesia · skin reactions · tremor · vascular irritation · venous thrombosis
- ▸ With oral use Abdominal cramps · acidosis hyperchloraemic · diarrhoea · generalised oedema · hypertension · hypotension · irritability · muscle complaints · nausea · vomiting

● MONITORING REQUIREMENTS
- ▸ With intravenous use During parenteral hydration, fluids and electrolytes should be monitored closely and any disturbance corrected by slow infusion of an appropriate solution.

● PRESCRIBING AND DISPENSING INFORMATION
- ▸ With intravenous use Sodium chloride 0.9% intravenous infusion contains Na^+ and Cl^- each 150 mmol/litre. The term 'normal saline' should not be used to describe sodium chloride intravenous infusion 0.9%; the term 'physiological saline' is acceptable but it is preferable to give the composition (i.e. sodium chloride intravenous infusion 0.9%).
- ▸ With oral use Each *Slow Sodium*® tablet contains approximately 10 mmol each of Na^+ and Cl^-; EvGr tablets can be crushed before administration ⟨E⟩.

The RCPCH and NPPG recommend that, when a liquid special of sodium chloride is required, the following strength is used: 5 mmol/mL.

● PATIENT AND CARER ADVICE
Medicines for Children leaflet: Sodium chloride for hyponatraemia
- ▸ With systemic use www.medicinesforchildren.org.uk/sodium-chloride-hyponatraemia

● MEDICINAL FORMS There can be variation in the licensing of different medicines containing the same drug. Forms available from special-order manufacturers include: capsule, solution for injection, infusion, solution for infusion

Modified-release tablet
CAUTIONARY AND ADVISORY LABELS 25
- ▸ Slow Sodium (HK Pharma Ltd)
Sodium chloride 600 mg Slow Sodium 600mg tablets | 100 tablet GSL £9.20 DT = £9.20

Solution for injection
- ▸ Sodium chloride (Non-proprietary)
Sodium chloride 9 mg per 1 ml Sodium chloride 0.9% solution for injection 50ml vials | 25 vial PoM £85.00–£85.01 DT = £85.01
Sodium chloride 0.9% solution for injection 10ml ampoules | 10 ampoule PoM £3.24–£3.70 DT = £3.24 | 20 ampoule PoM £10.21 | 50 ampoule PoM £25.50 | 100 ampoule PoM £51.00
Sodium chloride 0.9% solution for injection 20ml ampoules | 20 ampoule PoM £18.93 DT = £19.87
Sodium chloride 0.9% solution for injection 2ml ampoules | 10 ampoule PoM £2.33–£2.60 DT = £2.33
Sodium chloride 0.9% solution for injection 5ml ampoules | 10 ampoule PoM £2.50–£2.70 DT = £2.50 | 50 ampoule PoM £22.00
Sodium chloride 300 mg per 1 ml Sodium chloride 30% solution for injection 10ml ampoules | 10 ampoule PoM £77.47 DT = £77.47

Solution for infusion
- ▸ Sodium chloride (Non-proprietary)
Sodium chloride 300 mg per 1 ml Sodium chloride 30% concentrate for solution for infusion 100ml vials | 10 vial PoM £59.80 DT = £59.80
Sodium chloride 30% concentrate for solution for infusion 50ml vials | 1 vial PoM £15.36 DT = £15.36 | 10 vial PoM £83.30 DT = £83.30
Sodium chloride 30% concentrate for solution for infusion 10ml ampoules | 10 ampoule PoM £82.70

Infusion
- ▸ Sodium chloride (Non-proprietary)
Sodium chloride 1.8 mg per 1 ml Polyfusor O sodium chloride 0.18% infusion 500ml bottles | 1 bottle PoM £4.18
Sodium chloride 4.5 mg per 1 ml Sodium chloride 0.45% infusion 500ml bags | 1 bag PoM ⊠
Sodium chloride 0.45% infusion 500ml bottles | 1 bottle PoM £3.98
Sodium chloride 9 mg per 1 ml Sodium chloride 0.9% infusion 100ml bags | 1 bag PoM £0.58
Sodium chloride 0.9% infusion 250ml bags | 1 bag PoM ⊠
Sodium chloride 0.9% infusion 1litre bags | 1 bag PoM ⊠
Sodium chloride 0.9% infusion 500ml bags | 1 bag PoM ⊠
Sodium chloride 0.9% infusion 50ml bags | 1 bag PoM ⊠
Sodium chloride 0.9% infusion 100ml polyethylene bottles | 1 bottle PoM £0.55 | 20 bottle PoM £11.00
Sodium chloride 0.9% infusion 50ml bags | 1 bag PoM ⊠
Polyfusor S sodium chloride 0.9% infusion 500ml bottles | 1 bottle PoM £2.84 DT = £2.84
Polyfusor S sodium chloride 0.9% infusion 1litre bottles | 1 bottle PoM £3.77 DT = £3.77
Sodium chloride 18 mg per 1 ml Polyfusor SC sodium chloride 1.8% infusion 500ml bottles | 1 bottle PoM £4.18
Sodium chloride 27 mg per 1 ml Polyfusor SD sodium chloride 2.7% infusion 500ml bottles | 1 bottle PoM £4.18
Sodium chloride 50 mg per 1 ml Polyfusor SE sodium chloride 5% infusion 500ml bottles | 1 bottle PoM £4.18

Combinations available: ***Potassium chloride with calcium chloride dihydrate and sodium chloride,*** p. 635 · ***Potassium chloride with calcium chloride, sodium chloride and sodium lactate,*** p. 635 · ***Potassium chloride with glucose and sodium chloride,*** p. 636 · ***Potassium chloride with sodium chloride,*** p. 636

Sodium chloride with glucose

The properties listed below are those particular to the combination only. For the properties of the components please consider, sodium chloride p. 636, glucose below.

● **INDICATIONS AND DOSE**

Combined water and sodium depletion

▶ BY INTRAVENOUS INFUSION

▸ Child: (consult product literature)

● CAUTIONS Sodium chloride 0.18% and glucose 4% intravenous infusion fluid should not be used for fluid replacement in children aged 16 years or less because of the risk of hyponatraemia; availability of this infusion should be restricted to high dependency and intensive care units, and specialist wards, such as renal, liver, and cardiac units. Local guidelines on intravenous fluids should be consulted.

● MONITORING REQUIREMENTS

▸ Maintenance fluid should accurately reflect daily requirements and close monitoring is required to avoid fluid and electrolyte imbalance.

▸ During parenteral hydration, fluids and electrolytes should be monitored closely and any disturbance corrected by slow infusion of an appropriate solution.

● MEDICINAL FORMS There can be variation in the licensing of different medicines containing the same drug. Forms available from special-order manufacturers include: solution for infusion

Infusion

▸ Sodium chloride with glucose (Non-proprietary)
Sodium chloride 4.5 mg per 1 ml, Glucose anhydrous 25 mg per 1 ml Sodium chloride 0.45% / Glucose 2.5% infusion 500ml Viaflo bags | 1 bag PoM ☒
Sodium chloride 1.8 mg per 1 ml, Glucose anhydrous 40 mg per 1 ml Glucose 4% / sodium chloride 0.18% infusion 500ml bottles | 1 bottle PoM £2.40 DT = £2.40
Sodium chloride 0.18% / Glucose 4% infusion 500ml bags | 1 bag PoM ☒
Sodium chloride 0.18% / Glucose 4% infusion 1litre bags | 1 bag PoM ☒
Sodium chloride 9 mg per 1 ml, Glucose 50 mg per 1 ml Steriflex No.3 glucose 5% / sodium chloride 0.9% infusion 500ml bags | 1 bag PoM £1.47
Steriflex No.3 glucose 5% / sodium chloride 0.9% infusion 1litre bags | 1 bag PoM £2.10
Sodium chloride 4.5 mg per 1 ml, Glucose anhydrous 50 mg per 1 ml Steriflex No.45 glucose 5% / sodium chloride 0.45% infusion 500ml bags | 1 bag PoM £2.46
Sodium chloride 1.8 mg per 1 ml, Glucose anhydrous 100 mg per 1 ml Steriflex No.19 glucose 10% / sodium chloride 0.18% infusion 500ml bags | 1 bag PoM £2.46

NUTRIENTS > SUGARS

Glucose

06-Feb-2020

(Dextrose Monohydrate)

● **INDICATIONS AND DOSE**

Establish presence of gestational diabetes

▶ BY MOUTH

▸ Child: Test dose 75 g, anhydrous glucose to be given to the fasting patient and blood-glucose concentrations measured at intervals, to be given with 200–300 mL fluid

Oral glucose tolerance test

▶ BY MOUTH

▸ Child: Test dose 1.75 g/kg (max. per dose 75 g), anhydrous glucose to be given to the fasting patient and blood-glucose concentrations measured at intervals. To be given with 200–300 mL fluid

Neonatal hypoglycaemia

▶ BY INTRAVENOUS INFUSION

▸ Neonate: 500 mg/kg/hour, to be administered as Glucose 10% intravenous infusion, an initial dose of 250 mg/kg over 5 minutes may be required if hypoglycaemia is severe enough to cause loss of consciousness or seizures.

Hypoglycaemia

▶ BY INTRAVENOUS INFUSION

▸ Child: 500 mg/kg, to be administered as Glucose 10% intravenous infusion into a large vein through a large-gauge needle; care is required since this concentration is irritant

Energy source

▶ BY INTRAVENOUS INFUSION

▸ Child: (consult product literature)

Water replacement

▶ BY INTRAVENOUS INFUSION

▸ Child: The volume of glucose solution needed to replace deficits may vary (consult product literature)

Persistent cyanosis (in combination with propranolol) when blood glucose less than 3 mmol/litre (followed by morphine)

▶ BY INTRAVENOUS INFUSION

▸ Child: 200 mg/kg, to be administered as Glucose 10% intravenous infusion over 10 minutes

Management of diabetic ketoacidosis

▶ BY INTRAVENOUS INFUSION

▸ Child: Glucose 5% or 10% should be added to replacement fluid once blood-glucose concentration falls below 14 mmol/litre

DOSE EQUIVALENCE AND CONVERSION

▸ 75 g anhydrous glucose is equivalent to Glucose BP 82.5 g.

● CAUTIONS Do not give alone except when there is no significant loss of electrolytes · prolonged administration of glucose solutions without electrolytes can lead to hyponatraemia and other electrolyte disturbances

● SIDE-EFFECTS Chills · electrolyte imbalance · fever · fluid imbalance · hypersensitivity · local reaction · localised pain · polyuria · rash · venous thrombosis

● DIRECTIONS FOR ADMINISTRATION

▸ With intravenous use Injections containing more than 10% glucose can be irritant and should be given into a central venous line; however, solutions containing up to 12.5% can be administered for a short period into a peripheral line.

● PRESCRIBING AND DISPENSING INFORMATION Glucose BP is the monohydrate but Glucose Intravenous Infusion BP is a sterile solution of anhydrous glucose or glucose monohydrate, potency being expressed in terms of anhydrous glucose.

● EXCEPTIONS TO LEGAL CATEGORY

▸ With intravenous use Prescription only medicine restriction does not apply to 50% solution where administration is for saving life in emergency.

● MEDICINAL FORMS There can be variation in the licensing of different medicines containing the same drug. Forms available from special-order manufacturers include: oral solution, solution for injection, solution for infusion

Solution for infusion

▸ Glucose (Non-proprietary)
Glucose anhydrous 200 mg per 1 ml Glucose 20% solution for infusion 100ml vials | 1 vial PoM £6.00
Glucose anhydrous 500 mg per 1 ml Glucose 50% solution for infusion 20ml ampoules | 10 ampoule PoM £14.00 DT = £14.00
Glucose 50% solution for infusion 50ml vials | 25 vial PoM £59.97-£60.00 DT = £59.97

Oral solution

- Rapilose OGTT (Galen Ltd)
  Glucose 250 mg per 1 ml Rapilose OGTT solution | 300 ml £3.48

Oral gel

- Dextrogel (Neoceuticals Ltd)
  Glucose 400 mg per 1 gram Dextrogel 40% gel | 75 gram £4.30 DT = £7.16 | 80 gram £4.30
- GlucoBoost (Ennogen Healthcare Ltd)
  Glucose 400 mg per 1 gram GlucoBoost 40% gel | 75 gram £5.72 DT = £7.16 | 80 gram £6.11
- GlucoGel (BBI Healthcare Ltd)
  Glucose 400 mg per 1 gram GlucoGel 40% gel berry | 75 gram £7.16 DT = £7.16
  GlucoGel 40% gel original | 75 gram £7.16 DT = £7.16 | 80 gram £6.84
- Rapilose (Galen Ltd)
  Glucose 400 mg per 1 gram Rapilose 40% gel | 75 gram £5.49 DT = £7.16

Infusion

- Glucose (Non-proprietary)
  Glucose anhydrous 50 mg per 1 ml Glucose 5% infusion 1litre bags | 1 bag [PoM] [X]
  Glucose 5% infusion 500ml bags | 1 bag [PoM] [X]
  Glucose 5% infusion 100ml bags | 1 bag [PoM] [X]
  Glucose 5% infusion 250ml bags | 1 bag [PoM] [X]
  Glucose 5% infusion 1litre bottles | 1 bottle [PoM] £3.68
  Glucose 5% infusion 50ml bags | 1 bag [PoM] [X]
  Glucose 5% infusion 500ml bottles | 1 bottle [PoM] £2.73
  Glucose anhydrous 100 mg per 1 ml Glucose 10% infusion 1litre bags | 1 bag [PoM] [X]
  Glucose 10% infusion 500ml bags | 1 bag [PoM] [X]
  Glucose anhydrous 200 mg per 1 ml Steriflex No.31 glucose 20% infusion 500ml bags | 1 bag [PoM] £2.64
  Glucose (as Glucose monohydrate) 300 mg per 1 ml Glucose 30% infusion 500ml polyethylene bottles | 10 bottle [PoM] £40.21
  Glucose anhydrous 400 mg per 1 ml Steriflex No.33 glucose 40% infusion 500ml bags | 1 bag [PoM] £2.81
  Glucose anhydrous 500 mg per 1 ml Steriflex No.34 glucose 50% infusion 500ml bags | 1 bag [PoM] £3.11
  Glucose anhydrous 700 mg per 1 ml Glucose 70% concentrate for solution for infusion 500ml Viaflex bags | 1 bag [PoM] [X]

Combinations available: ***Potassium chloride with glucose,*** p. 635 · ***Potassium chloride with glucose and sodium chloride,*** p. 636 · ***Sodium chloride with glucose,*** p. 638

ORAL REHYDRATION SALTS

Disodium hydrogen citrate with glucose, potassium chloride and sodium chloride

(Formulated as oral rehydration salts)

● **INDICATIONS AND DOSE**

Fluid and electrolyte loss in diarrhoea

▶ BY MOUTH

- Child 1-11 months: 1–1½ times usual feed volume to be given
- Child 1-11 years: 200 mL, to be given after every loose motion
- Child 12-17 years: 200–400 mL, to be given after every loose motion, dose according to fluid loss

● **DIRECTIONS FOR ADMINISTRATION** Reconstitute 1 sachet with 200mL of water (freshly boiled and cooled for infants); 5 sachets reconstituted with 1 litre of water provide Na^{+} 60 mmol, K^{+} 20 mmol, Cl^{-} 60 mmol, citrate 10 mmol, and glucose 90 mmol.

● **PRESCRIBING AND DISPENSING INFORMATION** Flavours of oral powder formulations may include black currant, citrus, or natural.

● **PATIENT AND CARER ADVICE** After reconstitution any unused solution should be discarded no later than 1 hour after preparation unless stored in a refrigerator when it may be kept for up to 24 hours.

Medicines for Children leaflet: Oral rehydration salts www.medicinesforchildren.org.uk/oral-rehydration-salts

● **MEDICINAL FORMS** There can be variation in the licensing of different medicines containing the same drug.

Powder

- Dioralyte (Sanofi)
  Potassium chloride 300 mg, Sodium chloride 470 mg, Disodium hydrogen citrate 530 mg, Glucose 3.56 gram Dioralyte oral powder sachets citrus | 20 sachet [P] £6.72
  Dioralyte oral powder sachets plain | 20 sachet [P] £6.72
  Dioralyte oral powder sachets blackcurrant | 20 sachet [P] £6.72

Potassium chloride with rice powder, sodium chloride and sodium citrate

(Formulated as oral rehydation salts)

● **INDICATIONS AND DOSE**

Fluid and electrolyte loss in diarrhoea

▶ BY MOUTH

- Child 1-11 months: 1–1½ times usual feed volume to be given
- Child 1-11 years: 200 mL, to be given after every loose motion
- Child 12-17 years: 200–400 mL, to be given after every loose motion, dose according to fluid loss

● **UNLICENSED USE** *Dioralyte Relief®* not licensed for use in children under 3 months.

● **DIRECTIONS FOR ADMINISTRATION** Reconstitute 1 sachet with 200 mL of water (freshly boiled and cooled for infants); 5 sachets when reconstituted with 1 litre of water provide Na^{+} 60 mmol, K^{+} 20 mmol, Cl^{-} 50 mmol and citrate 10 mmol.

● **PRESCRIBING AND DISPENSING INFORMATION** Flavours of oral powder formulations may include apricot, black currant, or raspberry.

● **PATIENT AND CARER ADVICE** Patients and carers should be advised how to reconstitute *Dioralyte®* Relief oral powder. After reconstitution any unused solution should be discarded no later than 1 hour after preparation unless stored in a refrigerator when it may be kept for up to 24 hours.

Medicines for Children leaflet: Oral rehydration salts www.medicinesforchildren.org.uk/oral-rehydration-salts

● **MEDICINAL FORMS** There can be variation in the licensing of different medicines containing the same drug.

Powder

EXCIPIENTS: May contain Aspartame

- Dioralyte Relief (Sanofi)
  Potassium chloride 300 mg, Sodium chloride 350 mg, Sodium citrate 580 mg, Rice powder pre-cooked 6 gram Dioralyte Relief oral powder sachets blackcurrant sugar-free | 20 sachet [P] £7.13

2.1 Calcium imbalance

Calcium imbalance

Calcium supplements

Calcium supplements are usually only required where dietary calcium intake is deficient. This dietary requirement varies with age and is relatively greater in childhood, pregnancy, and lactation, due to an increased demand. Hypocalcaemia may be caused by vitamin D deficiency (see Vitamin D under Vitamins p. 674), impaired metabolism, a failure of secretion (hypoparathyroidism), or resistance to parathyroid hormone (pseudohypoparathyroidism).

Mild asymptomatic hypocalcaemia may be managed with oral calcium supplements. *Severe symptomatic hypocalcaemia* requires an intravenous infusion of calcium gluconate 10% p. 642 over 5 to 10 minutes, repeating the dose if symptoms persist; in exceptional cases it may be necessary to maintain a continuous calcium infusion over a day or more. Calcium chloride injection p. 642 is also available, but is more irritant; care should be taken to prevent extravasation.

See the role of calcium gluconate in temporarily reducing the toxic effects of *hyperkalaemia*.

Persistent hypocalcaemia requires oral calcium supplements and either a vitamin D analogue (alfacalcidol p. 680 or calcitriol p. 681) for hypoparathyroidism and pseudohypoparathyroidism or natural vitamin D (calciferol) if due to vitamin D deficiency. It is important to monitor plasma and urinary calcium during long-term maintenance therapy.

Severe hypercalcaemia

Severe hypercalcaemia calls for urgent treatment before detailed investigation of the cause. Dehydration should be corrected first with intravenous infusion of sodium chloride **0.9%** p. 636. Drugs (such as thiazides and vitamin D compounds) which promote hypercalcaemia, should be discontinued and dietary calcium should be restricted.

If *severe hypercalcaemia persists* drugs which inhibit mobilisation of calcium from the skeleton may be required. The **bisphosphonates** are useful and pamidronate disodium p. 506 is probably the most effective.

Corticosteroids are widely given, but may only be useful where hypercalcaemia is due to sarcoidosis or vitamin D intoxication; they often take several days to achieve the desired effect.

Calcitonin (salmon) p. 508 can be used by specialists for the treatment of hypercalcaemia associated with malignancy; it is rarely effective where bisphosphonates have failed to reduce serum calcium adequately.

After treatment of severe hypercalcaemia the underlying cause must be established. *Further treatment* is governed by the same principles as for initial therapy. Salt and water depletion and drugs promoting hypercalcaemia should be avoided; oral administration of a bisphosphonate may be useful. Parathyroidectomy may be indicated for hyperparathyroidism.

Hypercalciuria

Hypercalciuria should be investigated for an underlying cause, which should be treated. Reducing dietary calcium intake may be beneficial but severe restriction of calcium intake has not proved beneficial and may even be harmful.

Calcium supplements in neonates

Hypocalcaemia is common in the first few days of life, particularly following birth asphyxia or respiratory distress. Late onset at 4–10 days after birth may be secondary to vitamin D deficiency, hypoparathyroidism or hypomagnesaemia and may be associated with seizures.

2.1a Hypercalcaemia and hypercalciuria

CALCIUM REGULATING DRUGS › BONE RESORPTION INHIBITORS

Cinacalcet

22-Jan-2020

- **DRUG ACTION** Cinacalcet reduces parathyroid hormone which leads to a decrease in serum calcium concentrations.

- **INDICATIONS AND DOSE**

Secondary hyperparathyroidism [in patients with end-stage renal disease on dialysis] (under expert supervision)

▸ BY MOUTH

▸ Child 3–17 years: (consult product literature)

- **CONTRA-INDICATIONS** Hypocalcaemia
- **CAUTIONS** Conditions that may worsen with a decrease in serum-calcium concentrations

CAUTIONS, FURTHER INFORMATION Manufacturer advises caution with use in patients with conditions that may worsen with a decrease in serum-calcium concentrations, including predisposition to QT-interval prolongation, history of seizures, and history of impaired cardiac function—serum-calcium concentration should be closely monitored.

- **INTERACTIONS** → Appendix 1: cinacalcet
- **SIDE-EFFECTS**

▸ **Common or very common** Appetite decreased · asthenia · back pain · constipation · cough · diarrhoea · dizziness · dyspnoea · electrolyte imbalance · gastrointestinal discomfort · headache · hypersensitivity · hypotension · muscle complaints · nausea · paraesthesia · rash · seizure · upper respiratory tract infection · vomiting

▸ **Frequency not known** Heart failure aggravated · QT interval prolongation · ventricular arrhythmia

- **PREGNANCY** Manufacturer advises use only if potential benefit outweighs risk—no information available.
- **BREAST FEEDING** Manufacturer advises avoid—present in milk in *animal* studies.
- **HEPATIC IMPAIRMENT** Manufacturer advises caution in moderate to severe impairment.
- **MONITORING REQUIREMENTS** Manufacturer advises measure serum-calcium concentration before initiation of treatment and within 1 week after starting treatment or adjusting dose, then weekly thereafter. Measure parathyroid hormone concentration 1–4 weeks after starting treatment or adjusting dose.
- **DIRECTIONS FOR ADMINISTRATION** Manufacturer advises capsules containing granules should be opened and the granules sprinkled on to a small amount of soft food (apple sauce or yogurt) or liquid, then administered immediately. Capsules should not be swallowed whole. For administration advice via nasogastric or gastrostomy tube—consult product literature.
- **PATIENT AND CARER ADVICE** Manufacturer advises patients and their carers should be counselled on the symptoms of hypocalcaemia and importance of serum-calcium monitoring.

Driving and skilled tasks Manufacturer advises patients and carers should be counselled on the effects on driving and performance of skilled tasks—increased risk of dizziness and seizures.

● **MEDICINAL FORMS** There can be variation in the licensing of different medicines containing the same drug.

Granules

CAUTIONARY AND ADVISORY LABELS 21

▸ Mimpara (Amgen Ltd)

Cinacalcet (as Cinacalcet hydrochloride) 1 mg Mimpara 1mg granules in capsules for opening | 30 capsule PoM £161.16 (Hospital only)

Cinacalcet (as Cinacalcet hydrochloride) 2.5 mg Mimpara 2.5mg granules in capsules for opening | 30 capsule PoM £161.16 (Hospital only)

Cinacalcet (as Cinacalcet hydrochloride) 5 mg Mimpara 5mg granules in capsules for opening | 30 capsule PoM £161.16 (Hospital only)

Tablet

CAUTIONARY AND ADVISORY LABELS 21

▸ Cinacalcet (Non-proprietary)

Cinacalcet (as Cinacalcet hydrochloride) 30 mg Cinacalcet 30mg tablets | 28 tablet PoM £125.74–£125.75 DT = £125.75

Cinacalcet (as Cinacalcet hydrochloride) 60 mg Cinacalcet 60mg tablets | 28 tablet PoM £231.96–£231.97 DT = £231.97

Cinacalcet (as Cinacalcet hydrochloride) 90 mg Cinacalcet 90mg tablets | 28 tablet PoM £347.95–£347.96 DT = £347.96

▸ Mimpara (Amgen Ltd)

Cinacalcet (as Cinacalcet hydrochloride) 30 mg Mimpara 30mg tablets | 28 tablet PoM £125.75 DT = £125.75

Cinacalcet (as Cinacalcet hydrochloride) 60 mg Mimpara 60mg tablets | 28 tablet PoM £231.97 DT = £231.97

Cinacalcet (as Cinacalcet hydrochloride) 90 mg Mimpara 90mg tablets | 28 tablet PoM £347.96 DT = £347.96

2.1b Hypocalcaemia

ELECTROLYTES AND MINERALS › CALCIUM

Calcium salts

● **CONTRA-INDICATIONS** Conditions associated with hypercalcaemia (e.g. some forms of malignant disease) · conditions associated with hypercalciuria (e.g. some forms of malignant disease)

● **CAUTIONS** History of nephrolithiasis · sarcoidosis

● **SIDE-EFFECTS**

▸ **Uncommon** Constipation · diarrhoea · hypercalcaemia · nausea

● **RENAL IMPAIRMENT** Use with caution. Risk of hypercalcaemia and renal calculi.

above

Calcium carbonate

10-Mar-2020

● **INDICATIONS AND DOSE**

Phosphate binding in renal failure and hyperphosphataemia

▸ BY MOUTH

▸ Child 1–11 months: 120 mg 3–4 times a day, dose to be adjusted as necessary, to be taken with feeds
▸ Child 1–5 years: 300 mg 3–4 times a day, dose to be adjusted as necessary, to be taken prior to or with meals
▸ Child 6–11 years: 600 mg 3–4 times a day, dose to be adjusted as necessary, to be taken prior to or with meals
▸ Child 12–17 years: 1.25 g 3–4 times a day, dose to be adjusted as necessary, to be taken prior to or with meals

Calcium deficiency

▸ BY MOUTH

▸ Neonate: 0.25 mmol/kg 4 times a day, adjusted according to response.
▸ Child 1 month–4 years: 0.25 mmol/kg 4 times a day, adjusted according to response
▸ Child 5–11 years: 0.2 mmol/kg 4 times a day, adjusted according to response
▸ Child 12–17 years: 10 mmol 4 times a day, adjusted according to response

● **INTERACTIONS** → Appendix 1: calcium salts

● **SIDE-EFFECTS**

▸ **Uncommon** Hypercalciuria

▸ **Rare or very rare** Flatulence · gastrointestinal discomfort · milk-alkali syndrome · skin reactions

● **PRESCRIBING AND DISPENSING INFORMATION** *Adcal®* contains calcium carbonate 1.5 g (calcium 600 mg or Ca^{2+} 15 mmol); *Calcichew®* contains calcium carbonate 1.25 g (calcium 500 mg or Ca^{2+} 12.5 mmol); *Calcichew Forte®* contains calcium carbonate 2.5 g (calcium 1 g or Ca^{2+} 25 mmol); *Cacit®* contains calcium carbonate 1.25 g, providing calcium citrate when dispersed in water (calcium 500 mg or Ca^{2+} 12.5 mmol); consult product literature for details of other available products.

Flavours of chewable tablet formulations may include orange or fruit flavour.

● **PATIENT AND CARER ADVICE**

Medicines for Children leaflet: Calcium salts for kidney disease www.medicinesforchildren.org.uk/calcium-salts-kidney-disease-0

● **MEDICINAL FORMS** There can be variation in the licensing of different medicines containing the same drug. Forms available from special-order manufacturers include: tablet, capsule, oral suspension

Effervescent tablet

CAUTIONARY AND ADVISORY LABELS 13

▸ Cacit (Accord Healthcare Ltd)

Calcium carbonate 1.25 gram Cacit 500mg effervescent tablets sugar-free | 76 tablet P £11.81 DT = £11.81

Chewable tablet

CAUTIONARY AND ADVISORY LABELS 24

EXCIPIENTS: May contain Aspartame

▸ Adcal (Kyowa Kirin Ltd)

Calcium carbonate 1.5 gram Adcal 1500mg chewable tablets sugar-free | 100 tablet P £8.70 DT = £8.70

▸ Calcichew (Takeda UK Ltd)

Calcium carbonate 1.25 gram Calcichew 500mg chewable tablets sugar-free | 100 tablet P £9.33 DT = £9.33

Calcium carbonate 2.5 gram Calcichew Forte chewable tablets sugar-free | 60 tablet P £13.16 DT = £13.16

▸ Remegel (SSL International Plc)

Calcium carbonate 800 mg Remegel 800mg chewable tablets mint | 24 tablet GSL £2.58

▸ Rennie (Bayer Plc)

Calcium carbonate 500 mg Rennie Orange 500mg chewable tablets | 24 tablet GSL £1.59 | 48 tablet GSL £2.72 DT = £2.72

▸ Setlers Antacid (Thornton & Ross Ltd)

Calcium carbonate 500 mg Setlers Antacid spearmint chewable tablets | 36 tablet GSL £1.40

Setlers Antacid peppermint chewable tablets | 36 tablet GSL £1.40

Calcium carbonate with calcium lactate gluconate

The properties listed below are those particular to the combination only. For the properties of the components please consider, calcium carbonate above.

● **INDICATIONS AND DOSE**

Calcium deficiency

▸ BY MOUTH

▸ Neonate: 0.25 mmol/kg 4 times a day, adjusted according to response.

continued →

- Child 1 month–4 years: 0.25 mmol/kg 4 times a day, adjusted according to response
- Child 5–11 years: 0.2 mmol/kg 4 times a day, adjusted according to response
- Child 12–17 years: 10 mmol 4 times a day, adjusted according to response

- **INTERACTIONS** → Appendix 1: calcium salts
- **PRESCRIBING AND DISPENSING INFORMATION** Each *Sandocal®* tablet contains 1 g calcium (Ca^{2+} 25 mmol); flavours of soluble tablet formulations may include orange.

- **MEDICINAL FORMS** There can be variation in the licensing of different medicines containing the same drug.

Effervescent tablet

CAUTIONARY AND ADVISORY LABELS 13

EXCIPIENTS: May contain Aspartame

- Sandocal (GlaxoSmithKline Consumer Healthcare)
  Calcium carbonate 1.75 gram, Calcium lactate gluconate 2.263 gram Sandocal 1000 effervescent tablets sugar-free | 30 tablet [P] £12.82 DT = £12.82

641

Calcium chloride

- **INDICATIONS AND DOSE**

Acute hypocalcaemia

▶ BY INTRAVENOUS INJECTION

- Child: (consult product literature)

- **CAUTIONS** Avoid in respiratory acidosis · avoid in respiratory failure
- **INTERACTIONS** → Appendix 1: calcium salts
- **SIDE-EFFECTS** Soft tissue calcification · taste unpleasant · vasodilation
- **DIRECTIONS FOR ADMINISTRATION** Care should be taken to avoid extravasation.
- **PRESCRIBING AND DISPENSING INFORMATION** Non-proprietary *Calcium chloride dihydrate* 7.35%(calcium 20 mg or Ca^{2+} 500 micromol/mL); *Calcium chloride dihydrate* 10%(calcium 27.3 mg or Ca^{2+} 680 micromol/mL); *Calcium chloride dihydrate* 14.7%(calcium 40.1 mg or Ca^{2+} 1000 micromol/mL).

- **MEDICINAL FORMS** There can be variation in the licensing of different medicines containing the same drug. Forms available from special-order manufacturers include: solution for infusion

Solution for injection

- Calcium chloride (Non-proprietary)
  Calcium chloride dihydrate 100 mg per 1 ml Calcium chloride 10% solution for injection 10ml pre-filled syringes | 1 pre-filled disposable injection [PoM] £9.42 DT = £9.42
  Calcium chloride dihydrate 147 mg per 1 ml Calcium chloride 14.7% solution for injection 5ml ampoules | 10 ampoule [PoM] £139.73
  Calcium chloride 14.7% solution for injection 10ml ampoules | 10 ampoule [PoM] £101.96 DT = £101.96

641

Calcium gluconate

20-Nov-2019

- **INDICATIONS AND DOSE**

Calcium deficiency | Mild asymptomatic hypocalcaemia

▶ BY MOUTH

- Neonate: 0.25 mmol/kg 4 times a day, adjusted according to response.

- Child 1 month–4 years: 0.25 mmol/kg 4 times a day, adjusted according to response
- Child 5–11 years: 0.2 mmol/kg 4 times a day, adjusted according to response
- Child 12–17 years: 10 mmol 4 times a day, adjusted according to response

Acute hypocalcaemia, urgent correction | Hyperkalaemia (prevention of arrhythmias)

▶ BY SLOW INTRAVENOUS INJECTION

- Neonate: 0.11 mmol/kg for 1 dose, to be given over 5–10 minutes, some units use a dose of 0.46 mmol/kg (2 mL/kg calcium gluconate 10%) for hypocalcaemia in line with US practice.

- Child: 0.11 mmol/kg, to be given over 5–10 minutes, maximum 4.5 mmol (20 mL calcium gluconate 10%)

Acute hypocalcaemia, maintenance

▶ BY CONTINUOUS INTRAVENOUS INFUSION

- Neonate: 0.5 mmol/kg daily, adjusted according to response, dose to be given over 24 hours, use oral route as soon as possible due to risk of extravasation.

- Child 1 month–1 year: 1 mmol/kg daily, adjusted according to response, dose to be given over 24 hours, use oral route as soon as possible due to risk of extravasation; Usual maximum 8.8 mmol
- Child 2–17 years: 8.8 mmol daily, adjusted according to response, dose to be given over 24 hours, use oral route as soon as possible due to risk of extravasation

DOSE EQUIVALENCE AND CONVERSION

- 0.11 mmol/kg is equivalent to 0.5 mL/kg of calcium gluconate 10%.

IMPORTANT SAFETY INFORMATION

The MHRA has advised that repeated or prolonged administration of calcium gluconate injection packaged in 10 mL glass containers is contra-indicated in children under 18 years and in patients with renal impairment owing to the risk of aluminium accumulation; in these patients the use of calcium gluconate injection packaged in plastic containers is recommended.

- **INTERACTIONS** → Appendix 1: calcium salts
- **SIDE-EFFECTS**

GENERAL SIDE-EFFECTS Arrhythmias

SPECIFIC SIDE-EFFECTS

- With intravenous use Circulatory collapse · feeling hot · hyperhidrosis · hypotension · vasodilation · vomiting
- With oral use Gastrointestinal disorder

- **MONITORING REQUIREMENTS**

- With intravenous use Plasma-calcium and ECG monitoring required for administration by slow intravenous injection (risk of arrhythmias if given too rapidly).

- **DIRECTIONS FOR ADMINISTRATION** For intravenous infusion dilute to at least 45 micromol/mL with Glucose 5% *or* Sodium Chloride 0.9%. Maximum administration rate 45 micromol/kg/hour (or in neonates max. 22 micromol/kg/hour). May be given more concentrated via a central venous catheter. May be used undiluted (10% calcium gluconate) in emergencies. Avoid extravasation; should not be given by intramuscular injection. Incompatible with sodium bicarbonate and phosphate solutions.
- **PRESCRIBING AND DISPENSING INFORMATION** Calcium gluconate 1 g contains calcium 89 mg or Ca^{2+} 2.23 mmol.

● MEDICINAL FORMS There can be variation in the licensing of different medicines containing the same drug. Forms available from special-order manufacturers include: tablet, capsule, oral suspension, oral solution, solution for injection, solution for infusion

Solution for injection

▸ Calcium gluconate (Non-proprietary)
Calcium gluconate 100 mg per 1 ml Calcium gluconate 10% solution for injection 10ml ampoules | 10 ampoule PoM £12.00–£14.37 DT = £14.37 | 20 ampoule PoM £30.00–£31.50

Effervescent tablet

CAUTIONARY AND ADVISORY LABELS 13
ELECTROLYTES: May contain Sodium

▸ Calcium gluconate (Non-proprietary)
Calcium gluconate 1 gram Calcium gluconate 1g effervescent tablets | 28 tablet GSL £16.09 DT = £16.09

F 641

Calcium lactate

● INDICATIONS AND DOSE

Calcium deficiency

▸ BY MOUTH

▸ Neonate: 0.25 mmol/kg 4 times a day, adjusted according to response.

▸ Child 1 month–4 years: 0.25 mmol/kg 4 times a day, adjusted according to response
▸ Child 5–11 years: 0.2 mmol/kg 4 times a day, adjusted according to response
▸ Child 12–17 years: 10 mmol 4 times a day, adjusted according to response

● INTERACTIONS → Appendix 1: calcium salts

● MEDICINAL FORMS There can be variation in the licensing of different medicines containing the same drug.

Tablet

▸ Calcium lactate (Non-proprietary)
Calcium lactate 300 mg Calcium lactate 300mg tablets | 84 tablet [X] DT = £4.57 | 84 tablet GSL £4.57 DT = £4.57

F 641

Calcium phosphate

● INDICATIONS AND DOSE

Indications listed in combination monographs (available in the UK only in combination with other drugs)

▸ BY MOUTH
▸ Child: Doses listed in combination monographs

● INTERACTIONS → Appendix 1: calcium salts

● SIDE-EFFECTS Epigastric pain · gastrointestinal disorder · hypercalciuria

● MEDICINAL FORMS No licensed medicines listed.

2.2 Low blood volume

BLOOD AND RELATED PRODUCTS › PLASMA PRODUCTS

Albumin solution

30-Jan-2020

(Human Albumin Solution)

● INDICATIONS AND DOSE

Acute or sub-acute loss of plasma volume e.g. in burns, pancreatitis, trauma, and complications of surgery (with isotonic solutions) | Plasma exchange (with isotonic solutions) | Severe hypoalbuminaemia associated with low plasma volume and generalised oedema where salt and water restriction with plasma volume expansion are required (with concentrated solutions 20%) | Paracentesis of large volume ascites associated with portal hypertension (with concentrated solutions 20%)

▸ BY INTRAVENOUS INFUSION
▸ Child: (consult product literature)

Adjunct in the treatment of hyperbilirubinaemia by exchange transfusion in the newborn (with concentrated solutions 20%)

▸ BY INTRAVENOUS INFUSION
▸ Child: (consult product literature)

● CAUTIONS Correct dehydration when administering concentrated solution · history of cardiovascular disease · increased capillary permeability · risk of haemodilution (e.g. severe anaemia or haemorrhagic disorders) · risk of hypervolaemia (e.g. oesophageal varices or pulmonary oedema) · vaccination against hepatitis A and hepatitis B may be required

CAUTIONS, FURTHER INFORMATION

▸ Volume status Manufacturer advises adjust dose and rate of infusion to avoid fluid overload.

● SIDE-EFFECTS

▸ **Rare or very rare** Fever · flushing · nausea · shock · urticaria

● MONITORING REQUIREMENTS Plasma and plasma substitutes are often used in very ill patients whose condition is unstable. Therefore, close monitoring is required and fluid and electrolyte therapy should be adjusted according to the patient's condition at all times.

● PRESCRIBING AND DISPENSING INFORMATION A solution containing protein derived from plasma, serum, or normal placentas; at least 95% of the protein is albumin. The solution may be isotonic (containing 3.5–5% protein) or concentrated (containing 15–25% protein).

● MEDICINAL FORMS There can be variation in the licensing of different medicines containing the same drug.

Infusion

▸ Flexbumin (Baxalta UK Ltd)
Albumin solution human 200 gram per 1 litre Flexbumin 20% infusion 100ml bags | 1 bag PoM [X]
Flexbumin 20% infusion 50ml bags | 1 bag PoM [X]

Solution for infusion

▸ Albunorm (Octapharma Ltd)
Albumin solution human 50 mg per 1 ml Albunorm 5% solution for infusion 250ml bottles | 1 bottle PoM £33.75
Albunorm 5% solution for infusion 100ml bottles | 1 bottle PoM £13.50
Albunorm 5% solution for infusion 500ml bottles | 1 bottle PoM £67.50
Albumin solution human 200 mg per 1 ml Albunorm 20% solution for infusion 100ml bottles | 1 bottle PoM £54.00
Albunorm 20% solution for infusion 50ml bottles | 1 bottle PoM £27.00

▸ Alburex (CSL Behring UK Ltd)
Albumin solution human 50 mg per 1 ml Alburex 5% solution for infusion 500ml vials | 1 vial PoM £50.00

Albumin solution human 200 mg per 1 ml Alburex 20% solution for infusion 100ml vials | 1 vial [PoM] £40.00

- Albutein (Grifols UK Ltd)

Albumin solution human 50 mg per 1 ml Albutein 5% solution for infusion 500ml vials | 1 vial [PoM]
Albutein 5% solution for infusion 250ml vials | 1 vial [PoM]
Albumin solution human 200 mg per 1 ml Albutein 20% solution for infusion 100ml vials | 1 vial [PoM]
Albutein 20% solution for infusion 50ml vials | 1 vial [PoM]

- Biotest (Biotest (UK) Ltd)

Albumin solution human 50 mg per 1 ml Human Albumin Biotest 5% solution for infusion 250ml vials | 1 vial [PoM]
Albumin solution human 200 mg per 1 ml Human Albumin Biotest 20% solution for infusion 50ml vials | 1 vial [PoM]
Human Albumin Biotest 20% solution for infusion 100ml vials | 1 vial [PoM]

- Grifols (Grifols UK Ltd)

Albumin solution human 50 mg per 1 ml Human albumin Grifols 5% solution for infusion 500ml bottles | 1 bottle [PoM] £42.75
Human albumin Grifols 5% solution for infusion 250ml bottles | 1 bottle [PoM] £21.38
Albumin solution human 200 mg per 1 ml Human Albumin Grifols 20% solution for infusion 50ml vials | 1 vial [PoM] £23.40
Human Albumin Grifols 20% solution for infusion 100ml vials | 1 vial [PoM] £46.80

- Zenalb (Bio Products Laboratory Ltd)

Albumin solution human 45 mg per 1 ml Zenalb 4.5% solution for infusion 250ml bottles | 1 bottle [PoM] £27.51
Zenalb 4.5% solution for infusion 500ml bottles | 1 bottle [PoM] £55.02
Albumin solution human 200 mg per 1 ml Zenalb 20% solution for infusion 100ml bottles | 1 bottle [PoM] £54.00
Zenalb 20% solution for infusion 50ml bottles | 1 bottle [PoM] £27.00

- Zenbumin (Bio Products Laboratory Ltd)

Albumin solution human 200 mg per 1 ml Zenbumin 20% solution for infusion 50ml vials | 1 vial [PoM] £27.00

PLASMA SUBSTITUTES

Gelatin

- **INDICATIONS AND DOSE**

Low blood volume in hypovolaemic shock, burns and cardiopulmonary bypass

- BY INTRAVENOUS INFUSION
    - Child: Initially 10–20 mL/kilogram, use 3.5–4% solution

- **CAUTIONS** Cardiac disease · severe liver disease

CAUTIONS, FURTHER INFORMATION The use of plasma substitutes in children requires specialist supervision due to the risk of fluid overload; use is best restricted to an intensive care setting.

- **SIDE-EFFECTS**
- **Rare or very rare** Chills · dyspnoea · fever · hyperhidrosis · hypersensitivity · hypertension · hypotension · hypoxia · tachycardia · tremor · urticaria · wheezing
- **PREGNANCY** Manufacturer of *Geloplasma*® advises avoid at the end of pregnancy.
- **HEPATIC IMPAIRMENT** Manufacturers advise avoid preparations that contain lactate (risk of impaired lactate metabolism).
- **RENAL IMPAIRMENT** Use with caution in renal impairment.
- **MONITORING REQUIREMENTS**
- Urine output should be monitored. Care should be taken to avoid haematocrit concentration from falling below 25–30% and the patient should be monitored for hypersensitivity reactions.
- Plasma and plasma substitutes are often used in very ill patients whose condition is unstable. Therefore, close monitoring is required and fluid and electrolyte therapy should be adjusted according to the patient's condition at all times.
- **PRESCRIBING AND DISPENSING INFORMATION** The gelatin is partially degraded.

Gelaspan® contains succinylated gelatin (modified fluid gelatin, average molecular weight 26 500) 40 g, Na^+ 151 mmol, K^+ 4 mmol, Mg^{2+} 1 mmol, Cl^- 103 mmol, Ca^{2+} 1 mmol, acetate 24 mmol/litre; *Gelofusine*® contains succinylated gelatin (modified fluid gelatin, average molecular weight 30 000) 40 g (4%), Na^+ 154 mmol, Cl^- 124 mmol/litre; *Geloplasma*® contains partially hydrolysed and succinylated gelatin (modified liquid gelatin) (as anhydrous gelatin) 30 g (3%), Na^+ 150 mmol, K^+ 5 mmol, Mg^{2+} 1.5mmol, Cl^- 100 mmol, lactate 30 mmol/litre; *Isoplex*® contains succinylated gelatin (modified fluid gelatin, average molecular weight 30 000) 40g (4%), Na^+ 145 mmol, K^+ 4 mmol, Mg^{2+} 0.9 mmol, Cl^- 105 mmol, lactate 25mmol/litre; *Volplex*® contains succinylated gelatin (modified fluid gelatin, average molecular weight 30 000) 40 g (4%), Na^+ 154 mmol, Cl^- 125 mmol/litre.

- **MEDICINAL FORMS** There can be variation in the licensing of different medicines containing the same drug.

Infusion

- Gelaspan (B.Braun Medical Ltd)

Gelatin 40 mg per 1 ml Gelaspan 4% infusion 500ml Ecobags | 1 bag [PoM] £5.95 (Hospital only)

- Gelofusine (B.Braun Medical Ltd)

Gelatin 40 mg per 1 ml Gelofusine 4% infusion 1litre Ecobags | 1 bag [PoM] £9.31
Gelofusine 4% infusion 500ml Ecobags | 1 bag [PoM] £4.97

- Geloplasma (Fresenius Kabi Ltd)

Gelatin 30 mg per 1 ml Geloplasma 3% infusion 500ml Freeflex bags | 20 bag [PoM] (Hospital only)

- Isoplex (Kent Pharmaceuticals Ltd)

Gelatin 40 mg per 1 ml Isoplex 4% infusion 500ml bags | 10 bag [PoM] £75.00 (Hospital only)

- Volplex (Kent Pharmaceuticals Ltd)

Gelatin 40 mg per 1 ml Volplex 4% infusion 500ml bags | 10 bag [PoM] £47.00 (Hospital only)

2.3 Magnesium imbalance

Magnesium imbalance

Overview

Magnesium is an essential constituent of many enzyme systems, particularly those involved in energy generation; the largest stores are in the skeleton.

Magnesium salts are not well absorbed from the gastrointestinal tract, which explains the use of magnesium sulfate p. 646 as an osmotic laxative.

Magnesium is excreted mainly by the kidneys and is therefore retained in renal failure, but significant *hypermagnesaemia* (causing muscle weakness and arrhythmias) is rare.

Hypomagnesaemia

Since magnesium is secreted in large amounts in the gastro-intestinal fluid, excessive losses in diarrhoea, stoma or fistula are the most common causes of *hypomagnesaemia*; deficiency may also occur as a result of treatment with certain drugs. Hypomagnesaemia often causes secondary hypocalcaemia (with which it may be confused), particularly in neonates, and also hypokalaemia and hyponatraemia.

Symptomatic *hypomagnesaemia* is associated with a deficit of 0.5–1 mmol/kg. Magnesium is given initially by intravenous infusion or by intramuscular injection of magnesium sulfate; the intramuscular injection is painful. Plasma magnesium concentration should be measured to determine the rate and duration of infusion and the dose should be reduced in renal impairment. To prevent *recurrence of the deficit*, magnesium may be given by mouth in divided doses, but there is limited evidence of benefit. Magnesium aspartate p. 645 powder for oral solution is available as a licensed preparation.

9 Blood and nutrition

Arrhythmias
Magnesium sulfate injection has also been recommended for the emergency treatment of *serious arrhythmias*, especially in the presence of hypokalaemia (when hypomagnesaemia may also be present) and when salvos of rapid ventricular tachycardia show the characteristic twisting wave front known as *torsade de pointes*.

2.3a Hypomagnesaemia

ELECTROLYTES AND MINERALS > MAGNESIUM

Magnesium aspartate

● **INDICATIONS AND DOSE**

Treatment and prevention of magnesium deficiency

▶ BY MOUTH

- Child 2–3 years: 4.5 mmol daily, given as one level 5 mL spoonful of *Magnaspartate®* powder.
- Child 4–9 years: 4.5 mmol daily, given as a 5 mL level spoonful of *Magnaspartate®* powder, alternatively 10 mmol daily, given as 1 sachet of *Magnaspartate®* powder.
- Child 10–17 years: 10 mmol daily, given as 1 sachet of *Magnaspartate®* powder.

● CONTRA-INDICATIONS Disorders of cardiac conduction

● INTERACTIONS → Appendix 1: magnesium

● SIDE-EFFECTS

▶ **Uncommon** Diarrhoea · faeces soft

▶ **Rare or very rare** Fatigue · hypermagnesaemia

▶ **Frequency not known** Gastrointestinal irritation

SIDE-EFFECTS, FURTHER INFORMATION Side-effects generally occur at higher doses; if side-effects (such as diarrhoea) occur, consider interrupting treatment and restarting at a reduced dose.

Overdose Symptoms of hypermagnesaemia may include nausea, vomiting, flushing, thirst, hypotension, drowsiness, confusion, reflexes absent (due to neuromuscular blockade), respiratory depression, speech slurred, diplopia, muscle weakness, arrhythmias, coma, and cardiac arrest.

● RENAL IMPAIRMENT Avoid in severe impairment (estimated glomerular filtration rate less than 30 mL/minute/1.73^2).

● DIRECTIONS FOR ADMINISTRATION Dissolve sachet contents in 50–200 mL water, tea or orange juice and take immediately.

● PRESCRIBING AND DISPENSING INFORMATION *Magnaspartate®* contains magnesium aspartate 6.5 g (10 mmol Mg^{2+})/sachet.

● PATIENT AND CARER ADVICE Patients and carers should be given advice on how to administer magnesium aspartate powder.

● MEDICINAL FORMS There can be variation in the licensing of different medicines containing the same drug. Forms available from special-order manufacturers include: powder

Powder

EXCIPIENTS: May contain Sucrose

▶ Magnaspartate (KoRa Healthcare)
Magnesium (as Magnesium aspartate) 243 mg Magnaspartate 243mg (magnesium 10mmol) oral powder sachets | 10 sachet PoM £9.45 DT = £8.95

Magnesium glycerophosphate 24-Oct-2017

● **INDICATIONS AND DOSE**

Hypomagnesaemia

▶ BY MOUTH

- Child 1 month–11 years: Initially 0.2 mmol/kg 3 times a day, dose to be adjusted as necessary, dose expressed as Mg^{2+}
- Child 12–17 years: Initially 4–8 mmol 3 times a day, dose to be adjusted as necessary, dose expressed as Mg^{2+}

DOSE EQUIVALENCE AND CONVERSION

- Magnesium glycerophosphate 1 g is approximately equivalent to Mg^{2+} 4 mmol *or* magnesium 97 mg.

NEOMAG® CHEWABLE TABLETS

Hypomagnesaemia

▶ BY MOUTH

- Child 4–11 years: Initially 1 tablet twice daily, dose to be adjusted according to the serum total magnesium level
- Child 12–17 years: Initially 1 tablet 3 times a day, dose to be adjusted according to the serum total magnesium level

DOSE EQUIVALENCE AND CONVERSION

- Each *Neomag®* chewable tablet contains Mg^{2+} 4 mmol *or* magnesium 97 mg.

● UNLICENSED USE Preparations other than *Neomag®* are not licensed for use.

● INTERACTIONS → Appendix 1: magnesium

● SIDE-EFFECTS Diarrhoea · hypermagnesaemia

Overdose Symptoms of hypermagnesaemia may include nausea, vomiting, flushing, thirst, hypotension, drowsiness, confusion, reflexes absent (due to neuromuscular blockade), respiratory depression, speech slurred, diplopia, muscle weakness, arrhythmias, coma, and cardiac arrest.

● RENAL IMPAIRMENT Increased risk of toxicity.

Dose adjustments Avoid or reduce dose.

NEOMAG® CHEWABLE TABLETS Manufacturer advises avoid in severe impairment.

● MONITORING REQUIREMENTS Manufacturer advises to monitor serum magnesium levels every 3–6 months.

● DIRECTIONS FOR ADMINISTRATION

NEOMAG® CHEWABLE TABLETS Manufacturer advises that tablets may be broken into quarters and chewed or swallowed with water.

● NATIONAL FUNDING/ACCESS DECISIONS

NEOMAG® CHEWABLE TABLETS

Scottish Medicines Consortium (SMC) decisions

The *Scottish Medicines Consortium* has advised (September 2017) that magnesium glycerophosphate (*Neomag®*) is accepted for use within NHS Scotland as an oral magnesium supplement for the treatment of patients with chronic magnesium loss or hypomagnesaemia.

● MEDICINAL FORMS There can be variation in the licensing of different medicines containing the same drug. Forms available from special-order manufacturers include: tablet, capsule, oral suspension, oral solution, powder

Tablet

▶ Mag-4 (Ennogen Healthcare Ltd)
Magnesium (as Magnesium glycerophosphate) 97.2 mg Mag-4 (magnesium 97.2mg (4mmol)) tablets | 30 tablet £84.50

Oral solution

▶ Magnesium glycerophosphate (Non-proprietary)
Magnesium (as Magnesium glycerophosphate) 19.44 mg per 1 ml MagnEss Gly 97.2mg/5ml (4mmol/5ml) oral solution sugar-free | 200 ml £29.97
Magnesium (as Magnesium glycerophosphate) 24.25 mg per 1 ml MagnEss Gly 121.25mg/5ml (5mmol/5ml) oral solution sugar-free | 200 ml £31.97

9 Blood and nutrition

- LiquaMag GP (Fontus Health Ltd)
  Magnesium (as Magnesium glycerophosphate) 24.25 mg per 1 ml LiquaMag GP (magnesium 121.25mg/5ml (5mmol/5ml)) oral solution sugar-free | 200 ml £49.99
- MagnaPhos (TriOn Pharma Ltd)
  Magnesium (as Magnesium glycerophosphate) 19.44 mg per 1 ml MagnaPhos 97.2mg/5ml (4mmol/5ml) oral solution | 200 ml £37.87 DT = £41.97
  Magnesium (as Magnesium glycerophosphate) 24.25 mg per 1 ml MagnaPhos 121.25mg/5ml (5mmol/5ml) oral solution | 200 ml £37.87 DT = £37.87

Chewable tablet

EXCIPIENTS: May contain Aspartame

- MagnEss Gly (Essential-Healthcare Ltd)
  Magnesium (as Magnesium glycerophosphate) 97.2 mg MagnEss Gly 97.2mg (4mmol) chewable tablets sugar-free | 50 tablet £13.89 DT = £22.77
- MagnaPhate (Arjun Products Ltd)
  Magnesium (as Magnesium glycerophosphate) 97.2 mg MagnaPhate (magnesium 97.2mg (4mmol)) chewable tablets sugar-free | 50 tablet £22.64 DT = £22.77
- MagnaPhos (TriOn Pharma Ltd)
  Magnesium (as Magnesium glycerophosphate) 97.2 mg MagnaPhos 97.2mg (4mmol) chewable tablets sugar-free | 50 tablet £15.44 DT = £22.77
- Neomag (Neoceuticals Ltd)
  Magnesium (as Magnesium glycerophosphate) 97.2 mg Neomag (magnesium 97.2mg (4mmol)) chewable tablets sugar free sugar-free | 50 tablet [PoM] £22.77 DT = £22.77

Capsule

- MagnEss Gly (Essential-Healthcare Ltd)
  Magnesium (as Magnesium glycerophosphate) 39.5 mg MagnEss Gly 39.5mg (1.6mmol) capsules | 50 capsule £28.17
  Magnesium (as Magnesium glycerophosphate) 48.6 mg MagnEss Gly 48.6mg (2mmol) capsules | 50 capsule £25.97
  Magnesium (as Magnesium glycerophosphate) 97.2 mg MagnEss Gly 97.2mg (4mmol) capsules | 50 capsule £27.83
- MagnaPhos (TriOn Pharma Ltd)
  Magnesium (as Magnesium glycerophosphate) 48.6 mg MagnaPhos 48.6mg (2mmol) capsules | 50 capsule £28.86
  Magnesium (as Magnesium glycerophosphate) 97.2 mg MagnaPhos 97.2mg (4mmol) capsules | 50 capsule £31.86

Magnesium sulfate

13-Mar-2020

● INDICATIONS AND DOSE

Severe acute asthma | Continuing respiratory deterioration in anaphylaxis

- BY INTRAVENOUS INFUSION
- Child 2–17 years: 40 mg/kg (max. per dose 2 g), to be given over 20 minutes

Persistent pulmonary hypertension of the newborn

- INITIALLY BY INTRAVENOUS INFUSION
- Neonate: Initially 200 mg/kg, to be given over 20–30 minutes, then (by continuous intravenous infusion) 20–75 mg/kg/hour for up to 5 days if response occurs after initial dose (to maintain plasma magnesium concentration between 3.5–5.5 mmol/ litre).

Hypomagnesaemia

- BY INTRAVENOUS INJECTION
- Neonate: 100 mg/kg every 6–12 hours as required, to be given over at least 10 minutes.
- Child 1 month–11 years: 50 mg/kg every 12 hours as required, to be given over at least 10 minutes
- Child 12–17 years: 1 g every 12 hours as required, to be given over at least 10 minutes

Hypomagnesaemia maintenance (e.g. in intravenous nutrition)

- BY INTRAVENOUS INFUSION, OR BY INTRAMUSCULAR INJECTION
- Child: 50–100 mg/kg daily; maximum 5 g per day

Neonatal hypocalcaemia

- BY DEEP INTRAMUSCULAR INJECTION, OR BY INTRAVENOUS INFUSION
- Neonate: 100 mg/kg every 12 hours for 2–3 doses.

Torsade de pointes

- BY INTRAVENOUS INJECTION
- Child: 25–50 mg/kg (max. per dose 2 g), to be given over 10–15 minutes, dose may be repeated once if necessary (consult local protocol)

DOSE EQUIVALENCE AND CONVERSION

- Magnesium sulfate heptahydrate 1 g equivalent to Mg^{2+} approx. 4 mmol.

● **UNLICENSED USE** Unlicensed indication in severe acute asthma and continuing respiratory deterioration in anaphylaxis.

IMPORTANT SAFETY INFORMATION

MHRA/CHM ADVICE: MAGNESIUM SULFATE: RISK OF SKELETAL ADVERSE EFFECTS IN THE NEONATE FOLLOWING PROLONGED OR REPEATED USE IN PREGNANCY (MAY 2019)

Maternal administration of magnesium sulfate for longer than 5–7 days in pregnancy has been associated with hypocalcaemia, hypermagnesaemia, and skeletal side-effects in neonates. Healthcare professionals are advised to consider monitoring neonates for abnormal calcium and magnesium levels, and skeletal side-effects if maternal treatment with magnesium sulfate during pregnancy is prolonged or repeated beyond current recommendations.

● **INTERACTIONS** → Appendix 1: magnesium

● **SIDE-EFFECTS** Bone demineralisation (reported in neonates following prolonged or repeated use in pregnancy) · electrolyte imbalance · osteopenia (reported in neonates following prolonged or repeated use in pregnancy)

Overdose Symptoms of hypermagnesaemia may include nausea, vomiting, flushing, thirst, hypotension, drowsiness, confusion, reflexes absent (due to neuromuscular blockade), respiratory depression, speech slurred, diplopia, muscle weakness, arrhythmias, coma, and cardiac arrest.

● **PREGNANCY** For information on the risk of side-effects in neonates following prolonged or repeated maternal use of magnesium sulfate during pregnancy, see *Important Safety Information*.

- When used for Neonatal hypocalcaemia or Hypomagnesaemia or Torsade de pointes or Severe acute asthma or Continuing respiratory deterioration in anaphylaxis Sufficient amount may cross the placenta in mothers treated with high doses e.g. in pre-eclampsia, causing hypotonia and respiratory depression in newborns.

● **HEPATIC IMPAIRMENT** Avoid in hepatic coma if risk of renal failure.

● **RENAL IMPAIRMENT** Increased risk of toxicity.

Dose adjustments Avoid or reduce dose.

● **MONITORING REQUIREMENTS** Monitor blood pressure, respiratory rate, urinary output and for signs of overdosage (loss of patellar reflexes, weakness, nausea, sensation of warmth, flushing, drowsiness, double vision, and slurred speech).

● **DIRECTIONS FOR ADMINISTRATION**

- With intravenous use In severe hypomagnesaemia administer initially via controlled infusion device (preferably syringe pump). For *intravenous infusion*, in persistent pulmonary hypertension of the newborn, dilute to a max. concentration of 100 mg/mL (10%) (0.4 mmol/mL Mg^{2+}) magnesium sulfate heptahydrate (200 mg/mL (0.8 mmol/mL Mg^{2+}) if fluid restricted) with Glucose 5% *or*

Sodium Chloride 0.9%. For neonatal hypocalcaemia, hypomagnaesemia, and torsade de pointes, dilute to 10% (100 mg magnesium sulfate heptahydrate (0.4 mmol Mg^{2+}) in 1 mL) with Glucose 5% *or* 10%, Sodium Chloride 0.45% *or* 0.9% *or* Glucose and Sodium Chloride combinations. Up to 20% solution may be given in fluid restriction. Rate of administration should not exceed 10 mg/kg/minute (0.04 mmol/kg/minute Mg^{2+}) of magnesium sulfate heptahydrate.

- **PRESCRIBING AND DISPENSING INFORMATION** The BP directs that the label states the strength as the % w/v of magnesium sulfate heptahydrate and as the approximate concentration of magnesium ions (Mg^{2+}) in mmol/mL. Magnesium Sulfate Injection BP is a sterile solution of Magnesium Sulfate Heptahydrate.

- **MEDICINAL FORMS** There can be variation in the licensing of different medicines containing the same drug. Forms available from special-order manufacturers include: solution for injection, infusion, solution for infusion

Solution for injection

- Magnesium sulfate (Non-proprietary)
  Magnesium sulfate heptahydrate 500 mg per 1 ml Magnesium sulfate 50% (magnesium 2mmol/ml) solution for injection 10ml ampoules | 10 ampoule PoM £21.71–£55.00 DT = £21.71 | 50 ampoule PoM £21.71
  Magnesium sulfate 50% (magnesium 2mmol/ml) solution for injection 20ml vials | 10 vial PoM £61.70
  Magnesium sulfate 50% (magnesium 2mmol/ml) solution for injection 5ml ampoules | 10 ampoule PoM £45.20–£67.39
  Magnesium sulfate 50% (magnesium 2mmol/ml) solution for injection 2ml ampoules | 10 ampoule PoM £17.35–£22.00 DT = £17.35

Solution for infusion

- Magnesium sulfate (Non-proprietary)
  Magnesium sulfate heptahydrate 100 mg per 1 ml Magnesium sulfate 10% (magnesium 0.4mmol/ml) solution for injection 10ml ampoules | 10 ampoule PoM £66.26–£84.18 DT = £84.18
  Magnesium sulfate 10% (magnesium 0.4mmol/ml) solution for infusion 10ml ampoules | 10 ampoule PoM DT = £84.18 (Hospital only)
  Magnesium sulfate heptahydrate 200 mg per 1 ml Magnesium sulfate 20% (magnesium 0.8mmol/ml) solution for infusion 10ml ampoules | 10 ampoule PoM (Hospital only)
  Magnesium sulfate heptahydrate 500 mg per 1 ml Magnesium sulfate 50% (magnesium 2mmol/ml) solution for infusion 100ml vials | 10 vial PoM £81.70
  Magnesium sulfate 50% (magnesium 2mmol/ml) solution for infusion 50ml vials | 10 vial PoM £87.20

2.4 Phosphate imbalance

Phosphate imbalance

Phosphate supplements

Oral phosphate supplements p. 649 may be required in addition to vitamin D in children with hypophosphataemic vitamin D-resistant rickets, see also Vitamin D, under Vitamins p. 674.

Phosphate infusion is occasionally needed in phosphate deficiency arising from use of parenteral nutrition deficient in phosphate supplements; phosphate depletion also occurs in severe diabetic ketoacidosis. It is difficult to provide detailed guidelines for the treatment of *severe hypophosphatemia* because the extent of total body deficits and response to therapy are difficult to predict. High doses of phosphate may result in a transient serum elevation followed by redistribution into intracellular compartments or bone tissue. It is recommended that severe hypophosphataemia be treated intravenously as large doses of oral phosphate may cause diarrhoea; intestinal absorption may be unreliable and dose adjustment may be necessary.

Phosphate is not the first choice for the treatment of hypercalcaemia because of the risk of precipitation of calcium phosphate in the kidney and other tissues. If used, the child should be well hydrated and electrolytes monitored.

Phosphate-binding agents

Calcium-containing preparations are used as phosphate-binding agents in the management of hyperphosphataemia complicating renal failure. Aluminium- containing preparations are rarely used as phosphate- binding agents and can cause aluminium accumulation.

Sevelamer hydrochloride is licensed for the treatment of hyperphosphataemia in adults on haemodialysis or peritoneal dialysis. Although experience is limited in children sevelamer hydrochloride may be useful when hypercalcaemia prevents the use of calcium carbonate p. 641.

Phosphate supplements in neonates

Phosphate deficiency may occur in very low-birthweight infants and may compromise bone growth if not corrected. Parenterally fed infants may be at risk of phosphate deficiency due to the limited solubility of phosphate. Some units routinely supplement expressed breast milk with phosphate, although the effect on the osmolality of the milk should be considered.

2.4a Hyperphosphataemia

ELECTROLYTES AND MINERALS › CALCIUM

641

Calcium acetate

03-Mar-2020

- **INDICATIONS AND DOSE**

PHOSEX ® TABLETS

Phosphate binding in renal failure and hyperphosphataemia

- BY MOUTH
- Child: Dose to be adjusted according to requirements of patient, dose to be taken with meals (consult product literature)

- **INTERACTIONS** → Appendix 1: calcium salts
- **SIDE-EFFECTS**
  - **Uncommon** Vomiting
- **DIRECTIONS FOR ADMINISTRATION**
  PHOSEX ® TABLETS *Phosex*® tablets are taken with meals. Tablets can be broken to aid swallowing, but not chewed (bitter taste).
- **PRESCRIBING AND DISPENSING INFORMATION**
  PHOSEX ® TABLETS *Phosex*® tablets contain calcium acetate 1 g (equivalent to calcium 250 mg or Ca^{2+} 6.2 mmol).
- **PATIENT AND CARER ADVICE**
  Medicines for Children leaflet: Calcium salts for kidney disease www.medicinesforchildren.org.uk/calcium-salts-kidney-disease-0
  PHOSEX ® TABLETS Patients or carers should be given advice on how to administer *Phosex*® tablets.

- **MEDICINAL FORMS** There can be variation in the licensing of different medicines containing the same drug.

Tablet

CAUTIONARY AND ADVISORY LABELS 25

- Phosex (Pharmacosmos UK Ltd)
  Calcium acetate 1 gram Phosex 1g tablets | 180 tablet PoM £19.79 DT = £19.79

PHOSPHATE BINDERS

Sevelamer

28-Apr-2020

● **INDICATIONS AND DOSE**

RENAGEL ®

Hyperphosphataemia in patients on haemodialysis or peritoneal dialysis

▶ BY MOUTH

▶ Child 12–17 years: Initially 0.8–1.6 g 3 times a day, dose to be given with meals and adjusted according to serum-phosphate concentration

RENVELA ® 2.4G ORAL POWDER SACHETS

Hyperphosphataemia in chronic kidney disease

▶ BY MOUTH

▶ Child 6–17 years (body surface area 0.75–1.1 m^2): Initially 2.4 g daily in 3 divided doses, dose to be taken with meals and adjusted according to serum-phosphate concentration every 2–4 weeks—consult product literature

▶ Child 6–17 years (body surface area 1.2 m^2 and above): Initially 4.8 g daily in 3 divided doses, dose to be taken with meals and adjusted according to serum-phosphate concentration every 2–4 weeks—consult product literature

● **UNLICENSED USE**

RENAGEL ® Not licensed for use in children under 18 years.

● **CONTRA-INDICATIONS** Bowel obstruction

● **CAUTIONS** Gastro-intestinal disorders

● **SIDE-EFFECTS**

▶ **Common or very common** Constipation · diarrhoea · gastrointestinal discomfort · gastrointestinal disorders · nausea · vomiting

▶ **Frequency not known** Skin reactions

● **PREGNANCY** Manufacturer advises use only if potential benefit outweighs risk.

● **BREAST FEEDING**

RENVELA ® 2.4G ORAL POWDER SACHETS Unlikely to be present in milk (however, manufacturer advises avoid).

RENAGEL ® Manufacturer advises use only if potential benefit outweighs risk.

● **DIRECTIONS FOR ADMINISTRATION**

RENVELA ® 2.4G ORAL POWDER SACHETS Manufacturer advises each sachet should be dispersed in 60 mL water, or mixed with a small amount of cool food (100 g), prior to administration and discarded if unused after 30 minutes.

● **PATIENT AND CARER ADVICE**

Medicines for Children leaflet: Sevelamer in dialysis www.medicinesforchildren.org.uk/sevelamer-dialysis

RENVELA ® 2.4G ORAL POWDER SACHETS Patients and carers should be advised on how to administer powder for oral suspension.

● **NATIONAL FUNDING/ACCESS DECISIONS**

RENVELA ® 2.4G ORAL POWDER SACHETS

Scottish Medicines Consortium (SMC) decisions

The *Scottish Medicines Consortium* has advised (February 2018) that sevelamer carbonate (*Renvela*®) is accepted for restricted use within NHS Scotland as second-line management of hyperphosphataemia in paediatric patients (greater than 6 years of age and a Body Surface Area greater than 0.75m^2) with chronic kidney disease receiving haemodialysis.

● **MEDICINAL FORMS** There can be variation in the licensing of different medicines containing the same drug.

Powder

CAUTIONARY AND ADVISORY LABELS 13

▶ Renvela (Sanofi)

Sevelamer carbonate 2.4 gram Renvela 2.4g oral powder sachets sugar-free | 60 sachet PoM £167.04 DT = £167.04

Tablet

CAUTIONARY AND ADVISORY LABELS 25

EXCIPIENTS: May contain Propylene glycol

▶ Renagel (Sanofi)

Sevelamer 800 mg Renagel 800mg tablets | 180 tablet PoM £167.04 DT = £49.83

2.4b Hypophosphataemia

DRUGS AFFECTING BONE STRUCTURE AND MINERALISATION › MONOCLONAL ANTIBODIES

Burosumab

16-Nov-2018

● **DRUG ACTION** Burosumab is a human monoclonal antibody that inhibits the activity of fibroblast growth factor 23, thereby increasing renal tubular reabsorption of phosphate and increasing serum concentration of vitamin D.

● **INDICATIONS AND DOSE**

X-linked hypophosphataemia with radiographic evidence of bone disease in children and adolescents with growing skeletons (initiated by a specialist)

▶ BY SUBCUTANEOUS INJECTION

▶ Child 1–17 years: Initially 0.4 mg/kg, subsequent doses adjusted according to response and administered every 2 weeks. Dose may be increased in steps of 0.4 mg/kg at intervals of at least 4 weeks up to a maximum of 2 mg/kg (maximum dose 90 mg)—consult product literature; usual maintenance 0.8 mg/kg every 2 weeks (max. per dose 90 mg), to be administered into the arm, abdomen, buttock or thigh, each dose should be rounded to the nearest 10 mg

● **CONTRA-INDICATIONS** Concurrent use of oral phosphate or vitamin D analogues—discontinue 1 week before initiation of burosumab

● **SIDE-EFFECTS**

▶ **Common or very common** Dizziness · headache · myalgia · pain in extremity · rash · tooth abscess · toothache

● **PREGNANCY** Manufacturer advises avoid— toxicity in *animal* studies.

● **BREAST FEEDING** Manufacturer advises avoid—no information available.

● **RENAL IMPAIRMENT** Manufacturer advises avoid in severe impairment— no information available.

● **MONITORING REQUIREMENTS**

▶ Manufacturer advises monitor fasting serum-phosphate concentration before treatment initiation, every 2 weeks for the first month, every 4 weeks for the following 2 months, 4 weeks after dose adjustment, and as appropriate thereafter—target the lower end of the normal reference range for age to decrease the risk of ectopic mineralisation. Periodic measurement of post-prandial serum-phosphate concentration is also advised.

▶ Manufacturer advises monitor for signs and symptoms of nephrocalcinosis at treatment initiation, every 6 months for the first 12 months, and annually thereafter. Also monitor plasma alkaline phosphatases, calcium, parathyroid hormone, and creatinine every 6 months (every 3 months for children aged 1–2 years) or as indicated, and urine calcium and phosphate every 3 months.

● **DIRECTIONS FOR ADMINISTRATION** Maximum volume per injection site is 1.5 mL. If a volume over 1.5 mL is required on a given dosing day, manufacturer advises the total volume should be split and given at 2 different injection sites.

● **HANDLING AND STORAGE** Manufacturer advises store in a refrigerator (2-8°C).

● **NATIONAL FUNDING/ACCESS DECISIONS**

NICE decisions

▸ **Burosumab for treating X-linked hypophosphataemia in children and young people (October 2018)** NICE HST8
Burosumab (*Crysvita®*) is recommended, within its marketing authorisation, for treating X-linked hypophosphataemia with radiographic evidence of bone disease in children aged 1 year and over, and in young people with growing bones. It is recommended only if the manufacturer provides burosumab according to the commercial arrangement.
www.nice.org.uk/guidance/hst8

● **MEDICINAL FORMS** There can be variation in the licensing of different medicines containing the same drug.

Solution for injection

EXCIPIENTS: May contain Polysorbates, sorbitol

▸ Crysvita (Kyowa Kirin Ltd) ▼

Burosumab 10 mg per 1 ml Crysvita 10mg/1ml solution for injection vials | 1 vial PoM £2,992.00

Burosumab 20 mg per 1 ml Crysvita 20mg/1ml solution for injection vials | 1 vial PoM £5,984.00

Burosumab 30 mg per 1 ml Crysvita 30mg/1ml solution for injection vials | 1 vial PoM £8,976.00

LAXATIVES > OSMOTIC LAXATIVES

Phosphate

13-Mar-2020

● **INDICATIONS AND DOSE**

Hypophosphataemia | Hypophosphataemic rickets | Osteomalacia

▶ BY MOUTH USING EFFERVESCENT TABLETS

▸ Neonate: 1 mmol/kg daily in 1–2 divided doses, dose can be taken as a supplement in breast milk—caution advised as solubility in breast milk is limited to 1.2 mmol in 100 mL if calcium also added, contact pharmacy department for details.

▸ Child 1 month–4 years: 2–3 mmol/kg daily in 2–4 divided doses, dose to be adjusted as necessary, dose can be taken as a supplement in breast milk—caution advised as solubility in breast milk is limited to 1.2 mmol in 100 mL if calcium also added, contact pharmacy department for details; maximum 48 mmol per day

▸ Child 5-17 years: 2–3 mmol/kg daily in 2–4 divided doses, dose to be adjusted as necessary; maximum 97 mmol per day

▶ BY INTRAVENOUS INFUSION

▸ Neonate: 1 mmol/kg daily, dose to be adjusted as necessary.

▸ Child 1 month–1 year: 0.7 mmol/kg daily, dose to be adjusted as necessary

▸ Child 2-17 years: 0.4 mmol/kg daily, dose to be adjusted as necessary

> **IMPORTANT SAFETY INFORMATION**
> Some phosphate injection preparations also contain potassium. For peripheral intravenous administration the *concentration* of potassium should not usually exceed 40 mmol/litre. The infusion solution should be **thoroughly mixed**. Local policies on avoiding inadvertent use of potassium concentrate should be followed. The potassium content of some phosphate preparations may also limit the *rate* at which they may be administered.

● **CAUTIONS**

GENERAL CAUTIONS Cardiac disease · dehydration · diabetes mellitus · sodium and potassium concentrations of preparations

SPECIFIC CAUTIONS

▸ With intravenous use Avoid extravasation · severe tissue necrosis

● **SIDE-EFFECTS**

▸ With intravenous use Electrolyte imbalance

▸ With oral use Abdominal distress · diarrhoea · nausea

SIDE-EFFECTS, FURTHER INFORMATION Diarrhoea is a common side-effect and should prompt a reduction in dosage.

● **RENAL IMPAIRMENT**

Dose adjustments Reduce dose.

Monitoring Monitor closely in renal impairment.

● **MONITORING REQUIREMENTS** It is essential to monitor closely plasma concentrations of calcium, phosphate, potassium, and other electrolytes—excessive doses of phosphates may cause hypocalcaemia and metastatic calcification.

● **DIRECTIONS FOR ADMINISTRATION**

▸ With intravenous use Dilute injection with Sodium Chloride 0.9% or 0.45% or Glucose 5% or 10%. Administration rate of phosphate should not exceed 0.05 mmol/kg/hour. In emergencies in intensive care faster rates may be used—seek specialist advice.

● **PRESCRIBING AND DISPENSING INFORMATION** *Phosphate Sandoz®* contains sodium dihydrogen phosphate anhydrous (anhydrous sodium acid phosphate) 1.936 g, sodium bicarbonate 350 mg, potassium bicarbonate 315 mg, equivalent to phosphorus 500 mg (phosphate 16.1 mmol), sodium 468.8 mg (Na^+ 20.4 mmol), potassium 123 mg (K^+ 3.1 mmol); *Polyfusor NA®* contains Na^+ 162 mmol/litre, K^+ 19 mmol/litre, PO_4^{3-} 100 mmol/litre; non-proprietary *potassium dihydrogen phosphate injection* (potassium acid phosphate) 13.6% may contain 1 mmol/mL phosphate, 1 mmol/mL potassium.

● **PATIENT AND CARER ADVICE**

Medicines for Children leaflet: Phosphate supplements for low phosphate levels www.medicinesforchildren.org.uk/phosphate-supplements-low-phosphate-levels

● **MEDICINAL FORMS** There can be variation in the licensing of different medicines containing the same drug. Forms available from special-order manufacturers include: infusion, solution for infusion

Effervescent tablet

CAUTIONARY AND ADVISORY LABELS 13

▸ Phosphate Sandoz (HK Pharma Ltd)

Sodium dihydrogen phosphate anhydrous 1.936 gram Phosphate Sandoz effervescent tablets | 100 tablet PoM £19.39 DT = £19.39

Solution for infusion

▸ Phosphate (Non-proprietary)

Potassium dihydrogen phosphate 136 mg per 1 ml Potassium dihydrogen phosphate 13.6% (potassium 10mmol/10ml) solution for infusion 10ml ampoules | 10 ampoule PoM £117.77 DT = £117.77

Infusion

▸ Phosphate (Non-proprietary)

Potassium dihydrogen phosphate 1.295 gram per 1 litre, Disodium hydrogen phosphate anhydrous 5.75 gram per 1 litre Polyfusor NA phosphates infusion 500ml bottles | 1 bottle PoM £5.15

Blood and nutrition 9

2.5 Potassium imbalance

2.5a Hyperkalaemia

Other drugs used for Hyperkalaemia Calcium gluconate, p. 642 · Insulin, p. 491

ANTIDOTES AND CHELATORS › CATION EXCHANGE COMPOUNDS

Calcium polystyrene sulfonate

● **INDICATIONS AND DOSE**

Hyperkalaemia associated with anuria or severe oliguria, and in dialysis patients

▶ BY MOUTH

▸ Child: 0.5–1 g/kg daily in divided doses; maximum 60 g per day

▶ BY RECTUM

▸ Neonate: 0.5–1 g/kg daily, irrigate colon to remove resin after 8–12 hours.

▸ Child: 0.5–1 g/kg daily, irrigate colon to remove resin after 8–12 hours; maximum 30 g per day

● **CONTRA-INDICATIONS** Hyperparathyroidism · metastatic carcinoma · multiple myeloma · obstructive bowel disease · reduced gut motility (in neonates) · sarcoidosis

● **CAUTIONS** Impaction of resin with excessive dosage or inadequate dilution

● **INTERACTIONS** → Appendix 1: polystyrene sulfonate

● **SIDE-EFFECTS** Appetite decreased · constipation (discontinue—avoid magnesium-containing laxatives) · diarrhoea · electrolyte imbalance · epigastric discomfort · gastrointestinal disorders · gastrointestinal necrosis (in combination with sorbitol) · hypercalcaemia (in dialysed patients and occasionally in those with renal impairment) · increased risk of infection · nausea · vomiting

● **PREGNANCY** Manufacturers advise use only if potential benefit outweighs risk—no information available.

● **BREAST FEEDING** Manufacturers advise use only if potential benefit outweighs risk—no information available.

● **MONITORING REQUIREMENTS** Monitor for electrolyte disturbances (stop if plasma-potassium concentration below 5 mmol/litre).

● **DIRECTIONS FOR ADMINISTRATION**

▸ With rectal use Mix each 1 g of resin with 5 mL of water or 10% glucose.

● **MEDICINAL FORMS** There can be variation in the licensing of different medicines containing the same drug. Forms available from special-order manufacturers include: enema

Powder

CAUTIONARY AND ADVISORY LABELS 13, 21 (Sorbisterit® powder only)

EXCIPIENTS: May contain Sucrose

▸ Calcium Resonium (Sanofi)

Calcium polystyrene sulfonate 999.34 mg per 1 gram Calcium Resonium powder sugar-free | 300 gram Ⓟ £82.16 DT = £82.16

Sodium polystyrene sulfonate

● **INDICATIONS AND DOSE**

Hyperkalaemia associated with anuria or severe oliguria, and in dialysis patients

▶ BY MOUTH

▸ Child: 0.5–1 g/kg daily in divided doses; maximum 60 g per day

▶ BY RECTUM

▸ Neonate: 0.5–1 g/kg daily, irrigate colon to remove resin after 8–12 hours.

▸ Child: 0.5–1 g/kg daily, irrigate colon to remove resin after 8–12 hours; maximum 30 g per day

● **CONTRA-INDICATIONS** Obstructive bowel disease · reduced gut motility (in neonates)

● **CAUTIONS** Congestive heart failure · hypertension · impaction of resin with excessive dosage or inadequate dilution · oedema

● **INTERACTIONS** → Appendix 1: polystyrene sulfonate

● **SIDE-EFFECTS** Appetite decreased · bezoar · constipation (discontinue—avoid magnesium-containing laxatives) · diarrhoea · electrolyte imbalance · epigastric discomfort · gastrointestinal disorders · increased risk of infection · nausea · necrosis (in combination with sorbitol) · vomiting

● **PREGNANCY** Manufacturers advise use only if potential benefit outweighs risk—no information available.

● **BREAST FEEDING** Manufacturers advise use only if potential benefit outweighs risk—no information available.

● **RENAL IMPAIRMENT** Use with caution.

● **MONITORING REQUIREMENTS** Monitor for electrolyte disturbances (stop if plasma-potassium concentration below 5 mmol/litre).

● **DIRECTIONS FOR ADMINISTRATION**

▸ With rectal use Mix each 1 g of resin with 5 mL of water or 10% glucose.

▸ With oral use Administer dose (powder) in a small amount of water or honey—do not give with fruit juice or squash, which have a high potassium content.

● **MEDICINAL FORMS** There can be variation in the licensing of different medicines containing the same drug. Forms available from special-order manufacturers include: oral suspension

Powder

CAUTIONARY AND ADVISORY LABELS 13

▸ Resonium A (Sanofi)

Sodium polystyrene sulfonate 999.34 mg per 1 gram Resonium A powder sugar-free | 454 gram Ⓟ £81.11 DT = £81.11

2.5b Hypokalaemia

ELECTROLYTES AND MINERALS › POTASSIUM

Potassium bicarbonate with potassium acid tartrate

● **INDICATIONS AND DOSE**

Hyperchloraemic acidosis associated with potassium deficiency (as in some renal tubular and gastro-intestinal disorders)

▶ BY MOUTH

▸ Child: (consult product literature)

● **CONTRA-INDICATIONS** Hypochloraemia · plasma-potassium concentration above 5 mmol/litre

● **CAUTIONS** Cardiac disease

● **SIDE-EFFECTS** Abdominal discomfort · flatulence

- **RENAL IMPAIRMENT** Avoid in severe impairment.
  Monitoring Close monitoring required in renal impairment—high risk of hyperkalaemia.
- **DIRECTIONS FOR ADMINISTRATION** To be dissolved in water before administration.
- **PRESCRIBING AND DISPENSING INFORMATION** These tablets do not contain chloride.

- **MEDICINAL FORMS** There can be variation in the licensing of different medicines containing the same drug.

Effervescent tablet

CAUTIONARY AND ADVISORY LABELS 13, 21

▸ Potassium bicarbonate with potassium acid tartrate (Non-proprietary)

Potassium acid tartrate 300 mg, Potassium bicarbonate 500 mg Potassium (potassium 6.5mmol) effervescent tablets BPC 1968 | 56 tablet GSL £91.66–£92.15 DT = £92.15

Potassium chloride

20-Nov-2019

- **INDICATIONS AND DOSE**

Prevention of hypokalaemia (patients with normal diet)

▸ BY MOUTH

▸ Child: 1–2 mmol/kg daily; Usual maximum 50 mmol

Electrolyte imbalance

▸ BY INTRAVENOUS INFUSION

▸ Neonate: 1–2 mmol/kg daily, dose dependent on deficit or the daily maintenance requirements.

▸ Child: 1–2 mmol/kg daily, dose dependent on deficit or the daily maintenance requirements

Potassium depletion

▸ BY MOUTH

▸ Neonate: 0.5–1 mmol/kg twice daily, total daily dose may alternatively be given in 3 divided doses, dose to be adjusted according to plasma-potassium concentration.

▸ Child: 0.5–1 mmol/kg twice daily, total daily dose may alternatively be given in 3 divided doses, dose to be adjusted according to plasma-potassium concentration

> **IMPORTANT SAFETY INFORMATION**
>
> SAFE PRACTICE
>
> Potassium overdose can be fatal. Ready-mixed infusion solutions containing potassium should be used. Exceptionally, if potassium chloride concentrate is used for preparing an infusion, the infusion solution should be **thoroughly mixed**. Local policies on avoiding inadvertent use of potassium chloride concentrate should be followed.
>
> NHS NEVER EVENT: MIS-SELECTION OF A STRONG POTASSIUM SOLUTION (JANUARY 2018)
>
> Patients should not be inadvertently given a strong potassium solution (≥10% potassium w/v) intravenously, rather than the intended medication.

- **CONTRA-INDICATIONS** Plasma-potassium concentration above 5 mmol/litre
- **CAUTIONS**

▸ With intravenous use seek specialist advice in very severe potassium depletion or difficult cases

▸ With oral use Cardiac disease · hiatus hernia (*with modified-release preparations*) · history of peptic ulcer (*with modified-release preparations*) · intestinal stricture (*with modified-release preparations*)

- **INTERACTIONS** → Appendix 1: potassium chloride
- **SIDE-EFFECTS**

GENERAL SIDE-EFFECTS

Hyperkalaemia

SPECIFIC SIDE-EFFECTS

▸ With oral use Abdominal cramps · diarrhoea · gastrointestinal disorders · nausea · vomiting

- **RENAL IMPAIRMENT** Avoid in severe impairment.
  Dose adjustments Smaller doses must be used in the prevention of hypokalaemia, to reduce the risk of hyperkalaemia.
  Monitoring Close monitoring required in renal impairment—high risk of hyperkalaemia.
- **MONITORING REQUIREMENTS**

▸ Regular monitoring of plasma-potassium concentration is essential in those taking potassium supplements.

▸ With intravenous use ECG monitoring should be performed in difficult cases.

- **DIRECTIONS FOR ADMINISTRATION**

▸ With oral use in neonates Potassium chloride solutions suitable for use by mouth in neonates are available from 'special order' manufacturers or specialist importing companies; they should be used with care because they are hypertonic and can damage the gastric mucosa.

▸ With oral use Potassium salts are preferably given as a liquid (or effervescent) preparation, rather than modified-release tablets; they should be given as the chloride (the use of effervescent potassium tablets BPC 1968 should be restricted to *hyperchloraemic* states).

▸ With intravenous use Potassium chloride concentrate must be diluted with **not less** than 50 times its volume of sodium chloride intravenous infusion 0.9% or other suitable diluent and **mixed well**.

▸ With intravenous use Ready-mixed infusion solutions should be used when possible. For *peripheral intravenous infusion*, the concentration of potassium should not usually exceed 40 mmol/L. Potassium infusions should be given slowly over at least 2–3 hours and at a rate not exceeding 0.2 mmol/kg/hour with specialist advice and ECG monitoring in difficult cases. Higher concentrations of potassium chloride or faster infusion rates may be given in very severe depletion, but require specialist advice.

- **PRESCRIBING AND DISPENSING INFORMATION** Kay-Cee-L® contains 1 mmol/mL each of K^+ and Cl^-.
  Potassium Tablets Do not confuse Effervescent Potassium Tablets BPC 1968 with effervescent potassium chloride tablets. Effervescent Potassium Tablets BPC 1968 do not contain chloride ions and their use should be restricted to hyperchloraemic states.
- **PATIENT AND CARER ADVICE** Patient or carers should be given advice on how to administer potassium chloride modified-release tablets.
  Salt substitutes A number of salt substitutes which contain significant amounts of potassium chloride are readily available as health food products (e.g. *LoSalt*® and *Ruthmol*®). These should not be used by patients with renal failure as potassium intoxication may result.
- **LESS SUITABLE FOR PRESCRIBING** Modified-release tablets are less suitable for prescribing. Modified-release preparations should be avoided unless effervescent tablets or liquid preparations inappropriate.

- **MEDICINAL FORMS** There can be variation in the licensing of different medicines containing the same drug. Forms available from special-order manufacturers include: modified-release tablet, oral solution, solution for injection, infusion, solution for infusion

Modified-release tablet

CAUTIONARY AND ADVISORY LABELS 25, 27

▸ Potassium chloride (Imported)

Potassium chloride 600 mg Kaleorid LP 600mg tablets | 30 tablet PoM
Duro-K 600mg tablets | 100 tablet PoM

Solution for infusion

▸ Potassium chloride (Non-proprietary)

Potassium chloride 150 mg per 1 ml Potassium chloride 15% (potassium 20mmol/10ml) solution for infusion 10ml ampoules | 10 ampoule PoM £7.00–£10.00 | 20 ampoule PoM £6.50–£11.24
Potassium chloride 15% (potassium 20mmol/10ml) solution for infusion 10ml Mini-Plasco ampoules | 20 ampoule PoM £10.70

Potassium chloride 200 mg per 1 ml Potassium chloride 20% (potassium 13.3mmol/5ml) solution for infusion 5ml ampoules | 10 ampoule PoM £8.00

Oral solution

CAUTIONARY AND ADVISORY LABELS 21

▸ Kay-Cee-L (Geistlich Sons Ltd)

Potassium chloride 75 mg per 1 ml Kay-Cee-L syrup sugar-free | 500 ml P £8.77 DT = £8.77

Infusion

▸ Potassium chloride (Non-proprietary)

Potassium chloride 30 mg per 1 ml Potassium chloride 3% (potassium 40mmol/100ml) infusion 100ml bags | 1 bag PoM
Potassium chloride 3% (potassium 20mmol/50ml) infusion 50ml bags | 1 bag PoM

3 Metabolic disorders

Metabolic disorders

Use of medicines in metabolic disorders

Metabolic disorders should be managed under the guidance of a specialist. As many preparations are unlicensed and may be difficult to obtain, arrangements for continued prescribing and supply should be made in primary care.

General advice on the use of medicines in metabolic disorders can be obtained from:
Alder Hey Children's Hospital, Medicines Information Centre
(0151) 252 5381
and
Great Ormond Street Hospital for Children, pharmacy
(020) 7405 9200

Urea cycle disorders

Sodium benzoate p. 664 and sodium phenylbutyrate p. 665 are used in the management of urea cycle disorders. Both, either singly or in combination, are indicated as adjunctive therapy in all patients with neonatal-onset disease and in those with late-onset disease who have a history of hyperammonaemic encephalopathy. Sodium benzoate is also used in non-ketotic hyperglycinaemia.

The long-term management of urea cycle disorders includes oral maintenance treatment with sodium benzoate and sodium phenylbutyrate combined with a low protein diet and other drugs such as arginine p. 662 or citrulline p. 663, depending on the specific disorder.

Emergency management

For further information on the emergency management of urea cycle disorders consult the British Inherited Metabolic Disease Group (BIMDG) website at: www.bimdg.org.uk.

3.1 Acute porphyrias

Acute porphyrias

01-Oct-2017

Overview

The acute porphyrias (acute intermittent porphyria, variegate porphyria, hereditary coproporphyria, and 5-aminolaevulinic acid dehydratase deficiency porphyria) are hereditary disorders of haem biosynthesis; they have a prevalence of about 1 in 75 000 of the population.

Great care must be taken when prescribing for patients with acute porphyria, since certain drugs can induce acute porphyric crises. Since acute porphyrias are hereditary, relatives of affected individuals should be screened and advised about the potential danger of certain drugs.

EvGr Where there is no safe alternative, drug treatment for serious or life-threatening conditions should not be withheld from patients with acute porphyria. Where possible, the clinical situation should be discussed with a porphyria specialist for advice on how to proceed and monitor the patient. In the UK clinical advice can be obtained from the National Acute Porphyria Service or from the UK Porphyria Medicines Information Service (UKPMIS)—see details below. ⟨E⟩

Haem arginate p. 653 is administered by short intravenous infusion as haem replacement in moderate, severe, or unremitting acute porphyria crises.

In the United Kingdom the National Acute Porphyria Service (NAPS) provides clinical support and treatment with haem arginate from two centres (University Hospital of Wales and King's College Hospital). To access the service telephone (029) 2074 7747 and ask for the Acute Porphyria Service.

Drugs unsafe for use in acute porphyrias

EvGr The following list contains drugs on the UK market that have been classified as 'unsafe' in porphyria because they have been shown to be porphyrinogenic in animals or in vitro, or have been associated with acute attacks in patients. Absence of a drug from the following lists does not necessarily imply that the drug is safe. For many drugs no information about porphyria is available. ⟨E⟩

An up-to-date list of drugs considered safe in acute porphyrias is available from the UKPMIS, see *Useful resources* below.

Further information may be obtained from: porphyria.eu/ and also from:
The UK Porphyria Medicines Information Service (UKPMIS)
University Hospital of Wales
CF14 4XW
Cardiff
(029) 2074 2979/3877

Quite modest changes in chemical structure can lead to changes in porphyrinogenicity but where possible general statements have been made about groups of drugs; these should be checked first.

Unsafe Drug Groups (check first)

- Anabolic steroids
- Antidepressants, MAOIs (contact UKPMIS for advice)
- Antidepressants, Tricyclic and related (contact UKPMIS for advice)
- Barbiturates (includes primidone and thiopental)
- Contraceptives, hormonal (for detailed advice contact UKPMIS or a porphyria specialist)
- Hormone replacement therapy (for detailed advice contact UKPMIS or a porphyria specialist)
- Imidazole antifungals (applies to oral and intravenous use; topical antifungals are thought to be safe due to low systemic exposure)
- Non-nucleoside reverse transcriptase inhibitors (contact UKPMIS for advice)
- Progestogens (for detailed advice contact UKPMIS or a porphyria specialist)
- Protease inhibitors (contact UKPMIS for advice)
- Sulfonamides (includes co-trimoxazole and sulfasalazine)
- Sulfonylureas (glipizide and glimepiride are thought to be safe)
- Taxanes (contact UKPMIS for advice)
- Triazole antifungals (applies to oral and intravenous use; topical antifungals are thought to be safe due to low systemic exposure)

Unsafe Drugs (check groups above first)

- Aceclofenac
- Alcohol
- Amiodarone
- Aprepitant
- Artemether with lumefantrine
- Bexarotene
- Bosentan
- Busulfan
- Carbamazepine
- Chloral hydrate (although evidence of hazard is uncertain, manufacturer advises avoid)
- Chloramphenicol
- Chloroform (small amounts in medicines probably safe)
- Clemastine
- Clindamycin
- Cocaine
- Danazol
- Dapsone
- Diltiazem
- Disopyramide
- Disulfiram
- Ergometrine
- Ergotamine
- Erythromycin
- Etamsylate
- Ethosuximide
- Etomidate
- Flutamide
- Fosaprepitant
- Fosphenytoin
- Griseofulvin
- Hydralazine
- Ifosfamide
- Indapamide
- Isometheptene mucate
- Isoniazid (safety uncertain, contact UKPMIS for advice)
- Ketamine
- Mefenamic acid (safety uncertain, contact UKPMIS for advice)
- Meprobamate
- Methyldopa
- Metolazone
- Metyrapone
- Mifepristone
- Minoxidil (safety uncertain, contact UKPMIS for advice)
- Mitotane
- Nalidixic acid
- Nitrazepam
- Nitrofurantoin
- Orphenadrine
- Oxcarbazepine
- Oxybutynin
- Pentazocine
- Pentoxifylline
- Pergolide
- Phenoxybenzamine
- Phenytoin
- Pivmecillinam
- Pizotifen
- Porfimer
- Raloxifene
- Rifabutin (safety uncertain, contact UKPMIS for advice)
- Rifampicin
- Riluzole
- Risperidone
- Spironolactone
- Sulfinpyrazone
- Tamoxifen
- Temoporfin
- Thiotepa
- Tiagabine
- Tibolone
- Topiramate
- Toremifene
- Trimethoprim
- Valproate
- Verapamil
- Xipamide

Useful Resources

Acute porphyrias safe list. UK Porphyria Medicines Information Service. 2017.
www.wmic.wales.nhs.uk/specialist-services/drugs-in-porphyria

BLOOD AND RELATED PRODUCTS › HAEM DERIVATIVES

Haem arginate

(Human hemin)

● **INDICATIONS AND DOSE**

Acute porphyrias | Acute intermittent porphyria | Porphyria variegata | Hereditary coproporphyria

▸ BY INTRAVENOUS INFUSION

▸ Child: Initially 3 mg/kg once daily for 4 days, if response inadequate, repeat 4-day course with close biochemical monitoring; maximum 250 mg per day

● **SIDE-EFFECTS**

▸ **Common or very common** Poor venous access

▸ **Rare or very rare** Fever

▸ **Frequency not known** Headache · injection site necrosis · skin discolouration · venous thrombosis

● **PREGNANCY** Manufacturer advises avoid unless essential.

● **BREAST FEEDING** Manufacturer advises avoid unless essential—no information available.

● **DIRECTIONS FOR ADMINISTRATION** Administer over at least 30 minutes through a filter via large antebrachial or central vein; dilute requisite dose in 100 mL Sodium Chloride 0.9% in glass bottle; administer within 1 hour after dilution; max. concentration 2.5 mg/mL.

● **MEDICINAL FORMS** There can be variation in the licensing of different medicines containing the same drug.

Solution for infusion

▸ Normosang (Recordati Rare Diseases UK Ltd)
Haem arginate 25 mg per 1 ml Normosang 250mg/10ml solution for infusion ampoules | 4 ampoule PoM £1,737.00

3.2 Carnitine deficiency

AMINO ACIDS AND DERIVATIVES

Levocarnitine

29-Apr-2020

(Carnitine)

● **INDICATIONS AND DOSE**

Primary carnitine deficiency due to inborn errors of metabolism

▸ BY MOUTH

▸ Neonate: Up to 200 mg/kg daily in 2–4 divided doses.

▸ Child: Up to 200 mg/kg daily in 2–4 divided doses; maximum 3 g per day

▸ INITIALLY BY INTRAVENOUS INFUSION

▸ Neonate: Initially 100 mg/kg, to be administered over 30 minutes, followed by (by continuous intravenous infusion) 4 mg/kg/hour.

continued →

- Child: Initially 100 mg/kg, to be administered over 30 minutes, followed by (by continuous intravenous infusion) 4 mg/kg/hour
- BY SLOW INTRAVENOUS INJECTION
- Neonate: Up to 100 mg/kg daily in 2–4 divided doses, to be administered over 2–3 minutes.
- Child: Up to 100 mg/kg daily in 2–4 divided doses, to be administered over 2–3 minutes

Secondary carnitine deficiency in haemodialysis patients
- INITIALLY BY SLOW INTRAVENOUS INJECTION
- Child: 20 mg/kg, to be administered over 2–3 minutes, after each dialysis session, dosage adjusted according to plasma-carnitine concentration, then (by mouth) maintenance 1 g daily, administered if benefit is gained from first intravenous course

Organic acidaemias
- BY MOUTH
- Neonate: Up to 200 mg/kg daily in 2–4 divided doses.
- Child: Up to 200 mg/kg daily in 2–4 divided doses; maximum 3 g per day
- INITIALLY BY INTRAVENOUS INFUSION
- Neonate: Initially 100 mg/kg, to be administered over 30 minutes, followed by (by continuous intravenous infusion) 4 mg/kg/hour.
- Child: Initially 100 mg/kg, to be administered over 30 minutes, followed by (by continuous intravenous infusion) 4 mg/kg/hour
- BY SLOW INTRAVENOUS INJECTION
- Neonate: Up to 100 mg/kg daily in 2–4 divided doses, to be administered over 2–3 minutes.
- Child: Up to 100 mg/kg daily in 2–4 divided doses, to be administered over 2–3 minutes

- **UNLICENSED USE**
- With intravenous use Not licensed for use by intravenous infusion.
- With oral use Tablets, chewable tablets, and oral liquid (10%) not licensed in children under 12 years. Paediatric oral solution (30%) not licensed in children over 12 years. Not licensed for use in organic acidaemias.
- **CAUTIONS** Diabetes mellitus
- **SIDE-EFFECTS**
- **Rare or very rare** Abdominal cramps · diarrhoea · nausea · skin odour abnormal · vomiting

SIDE-EFFECTS, FURTHER INFORMATION Side-effects may be dose-related—monitor tolerance during first week and after any dose increase.

- **PREGNANCY** Appropriate to use; no evidence of teratogenicity in *animal* studies.
- **RENAL IMPAIRMENT** Accumulation of metabolites may occur with chronic oral administration in severe impairment.
- **MONITORING REQUIREMENTS**
- Monitoring of free and acyl carnitine in blood and urine recommended.
- **DIRECTIONS FOR ADMINISTRATION** For *intravenous infusion*, dilute injection with Sodium Chloride 0.9% or Glucose 5% or 10%.
- **PRESCRIBING AND DISPENSING INFORMATION**
- When used for Organic acidaemias Levocarnitine is used in the treatment of some organic acidaemias; however, use in fatty acid oxidation is controversial.
- **PATIENT AND CARER ADVICE**

Medicines for Children leaflet: Carnitine for metabolic disorders www.medicinesforchildren.org.uk/carnitine-metabolic-disorders-0

- **MEDICINAL FORMS** There can be variation in the licensing of different medicines containing the same drug. Forms available from special-order manufacturers include: capsule

Solution for injection
- Carnitor (Logixx Pharma Solutions Ltd)

L-Carnitine 200 mg per 1 ml Carnitor 1g/5ml solution for injection ampoules | 5 ampoule PoM £59.50 DT = £59.50

Oral solution
- Levocarnitine (Non-proprietary)

L-Carnitine 300 mg per 1 ml Levocarnitine 1.5g/5ml (30%) oral solution paediatric | 20 ml PoM £71.40 DT = £71.40 | 40 ml PoM £118.00
- Carnitor (Logixx Pharma Solutions Ltd)

L-Carnitine 100 mg per 1 ml Carnitor oral single dose 1g solution sugar-free | 10 unit dose PoM £35.00 DT = £35.00

Chewable tablet
- Carnitor (Logixx Pharma Solutions Ltd)

L-Carnitine 1 gram Carnitor 1g chewable tablets | 10 tablet PoM £35.00 DT = £35.00

Capsule
- Levocarnitine (Non-proprietary)

L-Carnitine 250 mg Bio-Carnitine 250mg capsules | 125 capsule £11.06

3.3 Cystinosis

3.3a Nephropathic cystinosis

AMINO ACIDS AND DERIVATIVES

Mercaptamine

29-Apr-2020

(Cysteamine)

- **INDICATIONS AND DOSE**

Nephropathic cystinosis (specialist use only)
- BY MOUTH
- Neonate: Initially one-sixth to one-quarter of the expected maintenance dose, increased gradually over 4–6 weeks to avoid intolerance, maintenance 1.3 g/m^2 daily in 4 divided doses.
- Child 1 month–11 years (body-weight up to 50 kg): Initially one-sixth to one-quarter of the expected maintenance dose, increased gradually over 4–6 weeks to avoid intolerance, maintenance 1.3 g/m^2 daily in 4 divided doses
- Child 12–17 years (body-weight up to 50 kg): Initially one-sixth to one-quarter of the expected maintenance dose, increased gradually over 4–6 weeks to avoid intolerance, maintenance 1.3 g/m^2 daily in 4 divided doses
- Child 12–17 years (body-weight 50 kg and above): Initially one-sixth to one-quarter of the expected maintenance dose, increased gradually over 4–6 weeks to avoid intolerance, maintenance 2 g daily in 4 divided doses

DOSE EQUIVALENCE AND CONVERSION
- With oral use
- 1.3 g/m^2 is approximately equivalent to 50 mg/kg.

Corneal cystine crystal deposits in patients with cystinosis (specialist use only)
- TO THE EYE
- Child 2–17 years: Apply 1 drop 4 times a day, to be applied to both eyes (minimum 4 hours between doses); dose may be reduced according to response (minimum daily dose 1 drop in each eye)

9 Blood and nutrition

> **IMPORTANT SAFETY INFORMATION**
> SAFE PRACTICE
> Mercaptamine has been confused with mercaptopurine; care must be taken to ensure the correct drug is prescribed and dispensed.

- **CAUTIONS**
- When used by eye Contact lens wearers
- With oral use Dose of phosphate supplement may need to be adjusted if transferring from phosphocysteamine to mercaptamine
- **SIDE-EFFECTS**
- **Common or very common**
- When used by eye Dry eye · eye discomfort · eye disorders · vision blurred
- With oral use Appetite decreased · asthenia · breath odour · diarrhoea · drowsiness · encephalopathy · fever · gastroenteritis · gastrointestinal discomfort · headache · nausea · skin reactions · vomiting
- **Uncommon**
- With oral use Compression fracture · gastrointestinal ulcer · hair colour changes · hallucination · joint hyperextension · leg pain · leucopenia · musculoskeletal disorders · nephrotic syndrome · nervousness · osteopenia · seizure
- **Frequency not known**
- With oral use Depression · intracranial pressure increased · papilloedema
- **ALLERGY AND CROSS-SENSITIVITY** Contra-indicated if history of hypersensitivity to penicillamine.
- **PREGNANCY**
- With oral use Manufacturer advises avoid—teratogenic and toxic in *animal* studies.
- **BREAST FEEDING**
- With oral use Manufacturer advises avoid—no information available.
- **MONITORING REQUIREMENTS**
- With oral use Leucocyte-cystine concentration and haematological monitoring required—consult product literature.
- All patients receiving mercaptamine should be registered (contact local specialist centre for details).
- **DIRECTIONS FOR ADMINISTRATION**
- With oral use For children under 6 years at risk of aspiration, capsules can be opened and contents sprinkled on food (at a temperature suitable for eating); avoid adding to acidic drinks (e.g. orange juice).
- **PRESCRIBING AND DISPENSING INFORMATION** Mercaptamine has a very unpleasant taste and smell, which can affect compliance.
- **HANDLING AND STORAGE**
- When used by eye Manufacturer advises store in a refrigerator (2–8°C)—after opening store at room temperature up to 25°C for up to 7 days; protect from light.
- **PATIENT AND CARER ADVICE**
Medicines for Children leaflet: Mercaptamine eye drops for ocular symptoms of cystinosis www.medicinesforchildren.org.uk/mercaptamine-eye-drops-ocular-symptoms-cystinosis
- **NATIONAL FUNDING/ACCESS DECISIONS**

Scottish Medicines Consortium (SMC) decisions
- With oral use The *Scottish Medicines Consortium* has advised (November 2017) that mercaptamine (*Procysbi®*) is **not** recommended for use within NHS Scotland for the treatment of proven nephropathic cystinosis.

- **MEDICINAL FORMS** There can be variation in the licensing of different medicines containing the same drug. Forms available from special-order manufacturers include: eye drops

Gastro-resistant capsule
- Procysbi (Chiesi Ltd)
Mercaptamine (as Mercaptamine bitartrate) 25 mg Procysbi 25mg gastro-resistant capsules | 60 capsule PoM £335.97
Mercaptamine (as Mercaptamine bitartrate) 75 mg Procysbi 75mg gastro-resistant capsules | 250 capsule PoM £4,199.65

Eye drops
EXCIPIENTS: May contain Benzalkonium chloride, disodium edetate
- Cystaran (Imported (United States))
Mercaptamine (as Mercaptamine hydrochloride) 4.4 mg per 1 ml Cystaran 0.44% eye drops | 15 ml PoM
- Cystadrops (Recordati Rare Diseases UK Ltd)
Mercaptamine (as Mercaptamine hydrochloride) 3.8 mg per 1 ml Cystadrops 3.8mg/ml eye drops | 5 ml PoM £865.00

Capsule
CAUTIONARY AND ADVISORY LABELS 21
- Cystagon (Recordati Rare Diseases UK Ltd)
Mercaptamine (as Mercaptamine bitartrate) 50 mg Cystagon 50mg capsules | 100 capsule PoM £70.00 DT = £70.00
Mercaptamine (as Mercaptamine bitartrate) 150 mg Cystagon 150mg capsules | 100 capsule PoM £190.00 DT = £190.00

3.4 Fabry's disease

ENZYMES

Agalsidase alfa

24-Apr-2020

- **DRUG ACTION** Agalsidase alfa, an enzyme produced by recombinant DNA technology are licensed for long-term enzyme replacement therapy in Fabry's disease (a lysosomal storage disorder caused by deficiency of alpha-galactosidase A).

- **INDICATIONS AND DOSE**

Fabry's disease (specialist use only)
- BY INTRAVENOUS INFUSION
- Child 7–17 years: 200 micrograms/kg every 2 weeks

- **INTERACTIONS** → Appendix 1: agalsidase alfa
- **SIDE-EFFECTS**
- **Common or very common** Arrhythmias · asthenia · chest discomfort · chills · cough · diarrhoea · dizziness · dyspnoea · excessive tearing · fever · flushing · gastrointestinal discomfort · headache · hoarseness · hypersomnia · hypertension · increased risk of infection · influenza like illness · joint disorders · malaise · musculoskeletal discomfort · myalgia · nausea · ototoxicity · pain · palpitations · peripheral oedema · peripheral swelling · rhinorrhoea · sensation abnormal · skin reactions · taste altered · temperature sensation altered · throat complaints · tremor · vomiting
- **Uncommon** Altered smell sensation · angioedema · hypersensitivity · sensation of pressure
- **Frequency not known** Heart failure · hyperhidrosis · hypotension · myocardial ischaemia

SIDE-EFFECTS, FURTHER INFORMATION Infusion-related reactions; manage by interrupting the infusion, or minimise by pre-treatment with an antihistamine or corticosteroid — consult product literature.
- **PREGNANCY** Use with caution.
- **BREAST FEEDING** Use with caution—no information available.
- **DIRECTIONS FOR ADMINISTRATION** Administration for *intravenous infusion*, dilute requisite dose with 100 mL Sodium Chloride 0.9% and give over 40 minutes using an in-line filter; use within 3 hours of dilution.

- **MEDICINAL FORMS** There can be variation in the licensing of different medicines containing the same drug.

Solution for infusion
- Replagal (Shire Pharmaceuticals Ltd)
Agalsidase alfa 1 mg per 1 ml Replagal 3.5mg/3.5ml solution for infusion vials | 1 vial PoM £1,049.94

Agalsidase beta

24-Apr-2020

- **DRUG ACTION** Agalsidase beta, an enzyme produced by recombinant DNA technology are licensed for long-term enzyme replacement therapy in Fabry's disease (a lysosomal storage disorder caused by deficiency of alpha-galactosidase A).

- **INDICATIONS AND DOSE**

Fabry's disease (specialist use only)

▶ BY INTRAVENOUS INFUSION

▸ Child 8–17 years: 1 mg/kg every 2 weeks

- **INTERACTIONS** → Appendix 1: agalsidase beta
- **SIDE-EFFECTS**
  - ▶ **Common or very common** Angioedema · arrhythmias · arthralgia · asthenia · chest discomfort · chills · cough · diarrhoea · dizziness · drowsiness · dyspnoea · eye disorders · fever · gastrointestinal discomfort · headache · hypertension · hyperthermia · hypotension · increased risk of infection · muscle complaints · musculoskeletal stiffness · nasal complaints · nausea · oedema · oral hypoaesthesia · pain · pallor · palpitations · respiratory disorders · sensation abnormal · skin reactions · syncope · temperature sensation altered · throat complaints · tinnitus · vasodilation · vertigo · vomiting
  - ▶ **Uncommon** Dysphagia · ear discomfort · eye pruritus · influenza like illness · malaise · peripheral coldness · tremor
  - ▶ **Frequency not known** Anaphylactoid reaction · hypersensitivity vasculitis · hypoxia

  SIDE-EFFECTS, FURTHER INFORMATION Infusion-related reactions; manage by slowing the infusion rate, or minimise by pre-treatment with an antihistamine, antipyretic, or corticosteroid — consult product literature.
- **PREGNANCY** Use with caution.
- **BREAST FEEDING** Use with caution—no information available.
- **DIRECTIONS FOR ADMINISTRATION** For *intravenous infusion*, given intermittently *in* Sodium chloride 0.9%, reconstitute initially with Water for Injections (5 mg in 1.1 mL, 35 mg in 7.2 mL) to produce a solution containing 5 mg/mL. Dilute with Sodium Chloride 0.9% (for doses less than 35 mg dilute with at least 50 mL; doses 35–70 mg dilute with at least 100 mL; doses 70–100 mg dilute with at least 250 mL; doses greater than 100 mg dilute with 500 mL) and give through an in-line low protein-binding 0.2 micron filter at an initial rate of no more than 15 mg/hour; for subsequent infusions, infusion rate may be increased gradually once tolerance has been established.

- **MEDICINAL FORMS** There can be variation in the licensing of different medicines containing the same drug.

Powder for solution for infusion

▸ Fabrazyme (Genzyme Therapeutics Ltd)

Agalsidase beta 5 mg Fabrazyme 5mg powder for solution for infusion vials | 1 vial [PoM] £315.08

Agalsidase beta 35 mg Fabrazyme 35mg powder for solution for infusion vials | 1 vial [PoM] £2,196.59

ENZYME STABILISER

Migalastat

24-Nov-2017

- **DRUG ACTION** Migalastat is a pharmacological chaperone that binds to the active sites of certain mutant forms of alpha-galactosidase A, thereby stabilising these mutant forms in the endoplasmic reticulum, and facilitating normal trafficking to lysosomes.

- **INDICATIONS AND DOSE**

Fabry's disease (specialist use only)

▶ BY MOUTH

▸ Child 16–17 years: 123 mg once daily on alternate days, take at the same time of day, at least 2 hours before or after food

- **SIDE-EFFECTS**
  - ▶ **Common or very common** Constipation · defaecation urgency · depression · diarrhoea · dizziness · dry mouth · dyspnoea · epistaxis · fatigue · gastrointestinal discomfort · headache · muscle complaints · nausea · pain · palpitations · proteinuria · sensation abnormal · skin reactions · torticollis · vertigo · weight increased
- **PREGNANCY** Manufacturer advises avoid—toxicity in *animal* studies.
- **BREAST FEEDING** Manufacturer advises avoid—present in milk in *animal* studies.
- **RENAL IMPAIRMENT** Manufacturer advises avoid if estimated glomerular filtration rate less than 30 mL/minute/1.73 m^2.
- **MONITORING REQUIREMENTS** Manufacturer advises monitor renal function, echocardiographic parameters and biochemical markers every 6 months.
- **PATIENT AND CARER ADVICE**

  Missed doses Manufacturer advises if a dose is missed entirely for the day, the missed dose should not be taken and the next dose should be taken on the normal day and at the normal time (not to be taken on 2 consecutive days).
- **NATIONAL FUNDING/ACCESS DECISIONS**

NICE decisions

▶ **Migalastat for treating Fabry disease (February 2017)**
NICE HST4

Migalastat is recommended, within its marketing authorisation, as an option for treating Fabry disease in people over 16 years of age with an amenable mutation, only if migalastat is provided with the discount agreed in the patient access scheme, and only if enzyme replacement therapy would otherwise be offered.
www.nice.org.uk/guidance/hst4

Scottish Medicines Consortium (SMC) decisions

The *Scottish Medicines Consortium* (November 2016) has advised that migalastat (*Galafold®*) is accepted for restricted use within NHS Scotland for long-term treatment of adults and adolescents aged 16 years and older with a confirmed diagnosis of Fabry disease (α-galactosidase A deficiency) and who have an amenable mutation—consult SMC advice for full details of restriction.

- **MEDICINAL FORMS** There can be variation in the licensing of different medicines containing the same drug.

Capsule

▸ Galafold (Amicus Therapeutics UK Ltd) ▼

Migalastat (as Migalastat hydrochloride) 123 mg Galafold 123mg capsules | 14 capsule [PoM] £16,153.85

3.5 Gaucher's disease

Other drugs used for Gaucher's disease Miglustat, p. 661

ENZYMES

Imiglucerase

27-Apr-2020

- DRUG ACTION Imiglucerase is an enzyme produced by recombinant DNA technology that is administered as enzyme replacement therapy for non-neurological manifestations of type I or type III Gaucher's disease, a familial disorder affecting principally the liver, spleen, bone marrow, and lymph nodes.

- INDICATIONS AND DOSE

Gaucher's disease type I (specialist use only)

▶ BY INTRAVENOUS INFUSION

- Neonate: Initially 60 units/kg every 2 weeks, adjusted according to response, doses as low as 30 units/kg once every 2 weeks may be appropriate.
- Child: Initially 60 units/kg every 2 weeks, adjusted according to response, doses as low as 30 units/kg once every 2 weeks may be appropriate

Gaucher's disease type III (specialist use only)

▶ BY INTRAVENOUS INFUSION

- Neonate: Initially 60–120 units/kg every 2 weeks, adjusted according to response.
- Child: Initially 60–120 units/kg every 2 weeks, adjusted according to response

- UNLICENSED USE Expert sources advise that imiglucerase is used in the given doses for the treatment of Gaucher's disease, but these may differ from those licensed.
- SIDE-EFFECTS
  - ▶ **Common or very common** Angioedema · cough · dyspnoea · hypersensitivity · skin reactions
  - ▶ **Uncommon** Abdominal cramps · arthralgia · back pain · chest discomfort · chills · cyanosis · diarrhoea · dizziness · fatigue · fever · flushing · headache · hypotension · nausea · paraesthesia · tachycardia · vomiting
- PREGNANCY Manufacturer advises use with caution—limited information available.
- BREAST FEEDING No information available.
- MONITORING REQUIREMENTS
  - ▶ Monitor for immunoglobulin G (IgG) antibodies to imiglucerase.
  - ▶ When stabilised, monitor all parameters and response to treatment at intervals of 6–12 months.
- DIRECTIONS FOR ADMINISTRATION For *intravenous infusion* (*Cerezyme*®), give intermittently in Sodium chloride 0.9%; initially reconstitute with water for injections (200 units in 5.1 mL, 400 units in 10.2 mL) to give 40 units/mL solution; dilute requisite dose with infusion fluid to a final volume of 100–200 mL and give initial dose at a rate not exceeding 0.5 units/kg/minute, subsequent doses to be given at a rate not exceeding 1 unit/kg/minute; administer within 3 hours after reconstitution.

- MEDICINAL FORMS There can be variation in the licensing of different medicines containing the same drug.

Powder for solution for infusion

ELECTROLYTES: May contain Sodium

▶ Cerezyme (Genzyme Therapeutics Ltd)

Imiglucerase 400 unit Cerezyme 400unit powder for solution for infusion vials | 1 vial PoM £1,071.29 (Hospital only)

Velaglucerase alfa

23-Apr-2020

- DRUG ACTION Velaglucerase alfa is an enzyme produced by recombinant DNA technology that is administered as enzyme replacement therapy for the treatment of type I Gaucher's disease.

- INDICATIONS AND DOSE

Type I Gaucher's disease (specialist use only)

▶ BY INTRAVENOUS INFUSION

- Child 4-17 years: Initially 60 units/kg every 2 weeks; adjusted according to response to 15–60 units/kg every 2 weeks

- SIDE-EFFECTS
  - ▶ **Common or very common** Arthralgia · asthenia · chest discomfort · dizziness · dyspnoea · fever · flushing · gastrointestinal discomfort · headache · hypersensitivity · hypertension · hypotension · infusion related reaction · nausea · pain · skin reactions · tachycardia

  SIDE-EFFECTS, FURTHER INFORMATION Infusion-related reactions are very common; manage by slowing the infusion rate, or interrupting the infusion, or minimise by pre-treatment with an antihistamine, antipyretic, or corticosteroid—consult product literature.
- PREGNANCY Manufacturer advises use with caution—limited information available.
- BREAST FEEDING Manufacturer advises use with caution—no information available.
- MONITORING REQUIREMENTS Monitor immunoglobulin G (IgG) antibody concentration in severe infusion-related reactions or if there is a lack or loss of effect with velaglucerase alfa.
- DIRECTIONS FOR ADMINISTRATION For *intravenous infusion*, reconstitute each 400-unit vial with 4.3 mL water for injections; dilute requisite dose in 100 mL Sodium Chloride 0.9% and give over 60 minutes through a 0.22 micron filter; start infusion within 24 hours of reconstitution.

- MEDICINAL FORMS There can be variation in the licensing of different medicines containing the same drug.

Powder for solution for infusion

ELECTROLYTES: May contain Sodium

▶ VPRIV (Shire Pharmaceuticals Ltd)

Velaglucerase alfa 400 unit VPRIV 400units powder for solution for infusion vials | 1 vial PoM £1,410.20

3.6 Homocystinuria

METHYL DONORS

Betaine

27-Apr-2019

- INDICATIONS AND DOSE

Adjunctive treatment of homocystinuria involving deficiencies or defects in cystathionine beta-synthase, 5,10-methylene-tetrahydrofolate reductase, or cobalamin cofactor metabolism (specialist use only)

▶ BY MOUTH

- Neonate: Initially 50 mg/kg twice daily (max. per dose 75 mg/kg), adjusted according to response; maximum 150 mg/kg per day.
- Child 1 month-9 years: Initially 50 mg/kg twice daily (max. per dose 75 mg/kg), adjusted according to response; maximum 150 mg/kg per day
- Child 10-17 years: 3 g twice daily (max. per dose 10 g), adjusted according to response; maximum 20 g per day

9 Blood and nutrition

- **SIDE-EFFECTS**
- ▸ **Uncommon** Abdominal discomfort · agitation · alopecia · appetite decreased · brain oedema · diarrhoea · glossitis · irritability · nausea · skin reactions · urinary incontinence · vomiting
- **PREGNANCY** Manufacturer advises avoid unless essential—limited information available.
- **BREAST FEEDING** Manufacturer advises caution—no information available.
- **MONITORING REQUIREMENTS** Monitor plasma-methionine concentration before and during treatment—interrupt treatment if symptoms of cerebral oedema occur.
- **DIRECTIONS FOR ADMINISTRATION** Powder should be mixed with water, juice, milk, formula, or food until completely dissolved and taken immediately; measuring spoons are provided to measure 1 g, 150 mg, and 100 mg of *Cystadane®* powder.
- **PRESCRIBING AND DISPENSING INFORMATION** Betaine should be used in conjunction with dietary restrictions and may be given with supplements of Vitamin B_{12}, pyridoxine, and folate under specialist advice.
- **NATIONAL FUNDING/ACCESS DECISIONS**

Scottish Medicines Consortium (SMC) decisions

SMC No. 407/07

The *Scottish Medicines Consortium* has advised (August 2010) that betaine anhydrous (*Cystadane®*) is accepted for restricted use within NHS Scotland for the adjunctive treatment of homocystinuria involving deficiencies or defects in cystathionine beta-synthase, 5,10-methylene-tetrahydrofolate reductase, or cobalamin cofactor metabolism in patients who are not responsive to pyridoxine treatment.

- **MEDICINAL FORMS** There can be variation in the licensing of different medicines containing the same drug. Forms available from special-order manufacturers include: tablet, oral solution

Powder

▸ Cystadane (Recordati Rare Diseases UK Ltd)
Betaine 1 gram per 1 gram Cystadane oral powder | 180 gram [PoM] £347.00 DT = £347.00

3.7 Hypophosphatasia

ENZYMES

Asfotase alfa

04-Dec-2017

- **DRUG ACTION** Asfotase alfa is a human recombinant tissue-nonspecific alkaline phosphatase that promotes mineralisation of the skeleton.

- **INDICATIONS AND DOSE**

Paediatric-onset hypophosphatasia (initiated by a specialist)

▸ BY SUBCUTANEOUS INJECTION

▸ Neonate: 2 mg/kg 3 times a week, alternatively 1 mg/kg 6 times a week, dosing frequency depends on body-weight—consult product literature for further information.

▸ Child: 2 mg/kg 3 times a week, alternatively 1 mg/kg 6 times a week, dosing frequency depends on body-weight—consult product literature for further information

- **CAUTIONS** Hypersensitivity reactions

CAUTIONS, FURTHER INFORMATION

▸ Hypersensitivity reactions Reactions, including signs and symptoms consistent with anaphylaxis, have occurred within minutes of administration and can occur in patients on treatment for more than one year; if these reactions occur, manufacturer advises immediate discontinuation of treatment and initiation of appropriate medical treatment. For information on re-administration, consult product literature.

- **SIDE-EFFECTS**
- ▸ **Common or very common** Bruising tendency · chills · cutis laxa · fever · headache · hypersensitivity · irritability · lipohypertrophy · myalgia · nausea · oral hypoaesthesia · pain · skin reactions · vasodilation

SIDE-EFFECTS, FURTHER INFORMATION Injection-site reactions including hypertrophy, induration, skin discolouration, and cellulitis may occur, particularly in patients receiving treatment 6 times a week. Manufacturer advises rotation of injection sites to manage these reactions; interrupt treatment if severe reactions occur and administer appropriate medical therapy.

- **PREGNANCY** Manufacturer advises avoid—no information available.
- **BREAST FEEDING** Manufacturer advises avoid—no information available.
- **MONITORING REQUIREMENTS**
- ▸ Manufacturer advises monitor serum parathyroid hormone and calcium concentrations—supplements of calcium and oral vitamin D may be required.
- ▸ Manufacturer advises periodic ophthalmological examination and renal ultrasounds.
- ▸ Manufacturer advises monitor for increased intracranial pressure (including fundoscopy for signs of papilloedema) periodically in patients below 5 years of age—prompt intervention required if increased intracranial pressure develops.
- **DIRECTIONS FOR ADMINISTRATION** Manufacturer advises max. 1 mL per injection site; administer multiple injections if more than 1 mL is required—consult product literature.
- **HANDLING AND STORAGE** Manufacturer advises store in a refrigerator (2–8 °C).
- **PATIENT AND CARER ADVICE**

Injection guides The manufacturer has produced injection guides for patients and carers to support training given by health care professionals.

- **NATIONAL FUNDING/ACCESS DECISIONS**

NICE decisions

▸ **Asfotase alfa for treating paediatric-onset hypophosphatasia (August 2017)** NICE HST6

Asfotase alfa is recommended as an option for treating paediatric-onset hypophosphatasia only:

- for people who meet the criteria for treatment within the managed access arrangement (see section 4.18 of the guidance), **and**
- for the duration of this arrangement and in line with the other conditions it specifies, **and**
- when the manufacturer provides asfotase alfa with the confidential commercial terms agreed with NHS England.

Patients whose treatment was started within the NHS before this guidance was published should have the option to continue treatment, without change to their funding arrangements, until they and their NHS clinician consider it appropriate to stop.

www.nice.org.uk/guidance/HST6

- **MEDICINAL FORMS** There can be variation in the licensing of different medicines containing the same drug.

Solution for injection

▸ Strensiq (Alexion Pharma UK Ltd) ▼
Asfotase alfa 40 mg per 1 ml Strensiq 18mg/0.45ml solution for injection vials | 12 vial [PoM] £12,700.80 (Hospital only)
Strensiq 28mg/0.7ml solution for injection vials | 12 vial [PoM] £19,756.80 (Hospital only)

Strensiq 40mg/1ml solution for injection vials | 12 vial PoM £28,224.00 (Hospital only)

Asfotase alfa 100 mg per 1 ml Strensiq 80mg/0.8ml solution for injection vials | 12 vial PoM £56,448.00 (Hospital only)

3.8 Mitochondrial disorders

VITAMINS AND TRACE ELEMENTS

Ubidecarenone

10-Mar-2020

(Ubiquinone; Co-enzyme Q10)

● **INDICATIONS AND DOSE**

Mitochondrial disorders

▸ BY MOUTH

▸ Neonate: Initially 5 mg 1–2 times a day, adjusted according to response, dose too be taken with food, increased if necessary up to 200 mg daily.

▸ Child: Initially 5 mg 1–2 times a day, adjusted according to response, dose to be taken with food, increased if necessary up to 300 mg daily

● **UNLICENSED USE** Not licensed.

● **CAUTIONS** May reduce insulin requirement in diabetes mellitus

● **SIDE-EFFECTS**

▸ **Common or very common** Diarrhoea · dyspepsia · nausea

▸ **Rare or very rare** Agitation · dizziness · headache · irritability

● **HEPATIC IMPAIRMENT**

Dose adjustments Reduce dose in moderate and severe impairment.

● **PATIENT AND CARER ADVICE**

Medicines for Children leaflet: Ubidecarenone for mitochondrial disease www.medicinesforchildren.org.uk/ubidecarenone-mitochondrial-disease

● **MEDICINAL FORMS** There can be variation in the licensing of different medicines containing the same drug. Forms available from special-order manufacturers include: oral solution, oral drops

Tablet

▸ Ubidecarenone (Non-proprietary)

Ubidecarenone 30 mg Co-enzyme Q10 30mg tablets | 30 tablet £7.23 | 90 tablet £20.16

Oral drops

▸ Ubicor (Imported (Italy))

Ubidecarenone 5 mg per 1 ml Ubicor 5mg/ml oral drops | 10 ml PoM

Chewable tablet

▸ Ubidecarenone (Non-proprietary)

Ubidecarenone 25 mg Coenzyme Q10 25mg chewable tablets sugar-free | 250 tablet PoM

Capsule

▸ BioActive Q10 Uniquinol (Pharma Nord (UK) Ltd)

Ubidecarenone 30 mg BioActive Q10 Uniquinol 30mg capsules | 60 capsule £11.06 | 150 capsule £22.11

Ubidecarenone 100 mg BioActive Q10 Uniquinol 100mg capsules | 60 capsule £29.23 | 150 capsule £53.14

▸ Super Bio-Quinone (Pharma Nord (UK) Ltd)

Ubidecarenone 30 mg Super Bio-Quinone Q10 30mg capsules | 30 capsule £4.96 | 60 capsule £9.73 | 150 capsule £17.71

3.9 Mucopolysaccharidosis

ENZYMES

Elosulfase alfa

24-Apr-2020

● **DRUG ACTION** Elosulfase alfa is an enzyme produced by recombinant DNA technology that provides replacement therapy in conditions caused by N-acetylgalactosamine-6-sulfatase (GALNS) deficiency.

● **INDICATIONS AND DOSE**

Mucopolysaccharidosis IVA (specialist use only)

▸ BY INTRAVENOUS INFUSION

▸ Neonate: 2 mg/kg once weekly.

▸ Child: 2 mg/kg once weekly

● **CAUTIONS** Infusion-related reactions

CAUTIONS, FURTHER INFORMATION Infusion-related reactions can occur; manufacturer advises these may be minimised by pre-treatment with an antihistamine and antipyretic, given 30-60 minutes before treatment. If reaction is severe, stop infusion and start appropriate treatment. Caution and close monitoring is advised during re-administration following a severe reaction.

● **SIDE-EFFECTS**

▸ **Common or very common** Chills · diarrhoea · dizziness · dyspnoea · fever · gastrointestinal discomfort · headache · hypersensitivity · myalgia · nausea · oropharyngeal pain · vomiting

▸ **Frequency not known** Infusion related reaction

● **PREGNANCY** Manufacturer advises avoid unless essential—limited information available.

● **BREAST FEEDING** Manufacturer advises use only if potential benefit outweighs risk—present in milk in *animal* studies.

● **DIRECTIONS FOR ADMINISTRATION** For *intravenous infusion* (*Vimizim*®), give intermittently *in* Sodium chloride 0.9%; body-weight under 25 kg, dilute requisite dose to final volume of 100 mL infusion fluid and mix gently, give over 4 hours through in-line filter (0.2 micron) initially at a rate of 3 mL/hour, then increase to a rate of 6 mL/hour after 15 minutes, then increase gradually if tolerated every 15 minutes by 6 mL/hour to max. 36 mL/hour; body-weight 25 kg or over, dilute requisite dose to final volume of 250 mL and mix gently, give over 4 hours through in-line filter (0.2 micron) initially at a rate of 6 mL/hour, then increase to a rate of 12 mL/hour after 15 minutes, then increase gradually if tolerated every 15 minutes by 12 mL/hour to max. 72 mL/hour.

● **HANDLING AND STORAGE** Manufacturer advises store in a refrigerator at 2–8°C. After dilution use immediately or, if necessary, store at 2-8°C for max. 24 hours, followed by up to 24 hours at 23–27°C.

● **PATIENT AND CARER ADVICE**

Driving and skilled tasks Manufacturer advises patients and carers should be counselled about the effects on driving and performance of skilled tasks—increased risk of dizziness.

● **NATIONAL FUNDING/ACCESS DECISIONS**

NICE decisions

▸ **Elosulfase alfa for treating mucopolysaccharidosis type IVa (December 2015)** NICE HST2

Elosulfase alfa, within its marketing authorisation, is recommended for funding for treating mucopolysaccharidosis type IVa (MPS IVa) according to

the conditions in the managed access agreement for elosulfase alfa.
www.nice.org.uk/guidance/HST2

- **MEDICINAL FORMS** There can be variation in the licensing of different medicines containing the same drug.

Solution for infusion

EXCIPIENTS: May contain Polysorbates, sorbitol
ELECTROLYTES: May contain Sodium

▸ Vimizim (BioMarin Europe Ltd) ▼
Elosulfase alfa 1 mg per 1 ml Vimizim 5mg/5ml concentrate for solution for infusion vials | 1 vial PoM £750.00

Galsulfase

24-Apr-2020

- **DRUG ACTION** Galsulfase is a recombinant form of human N-acetylgalactosamine-4-sulfatase.

- **INDICATIONS AND DOSE**

Mucopolysaccharidosis VI (specialist use only)

▸ BY INTRAVENOUS INFUSION
▸ Child 5–17 years: 1 mg/kg once weekly

- **CAUTIONS** Acute febrile illness (consider delaying treatment) · acute respiratory illness (consider delaying treatment) · infusion-related reactions can occur · respiratory disease
- **SIDE-EFFECTS**

▸ **Common or very common** Abdominal pain · angioedema · apnoea · arthralgia · asthma · chest pain · chills · conjunctivitis · corneal opacity · cough · dyspnoea · ear pain · fever · headache · hearing impairment · hypertension · hypotension · increased risk of infection · malaise · nasal congestion · nausea · pain · reflexes absent · respiratory disorders · skin reactions · tremor · umbilical hernia · vomiting

▸ **Frequency not known** Arrhythmias · cyanosis · hypoxia · infusion related reaction · nerve disorders · pallor · paraesthesia · shock

SIDE-EFFECTS, FURTHER INFORMATION Infusion-related reactions often occur, they can be managed by slowing the infusion rate or interrupting the infusion, and can be minimised by pre-treatment with an antihistamine and an antipyretic. Recurrent infusion-related reactions may require pre-treatment with a corticosteroid — consult product literature for details.

- **PREGNANCY** Manufacturer advises avoid unless essential.
- **BREAST FEEDING** Manufacturer advises avoid—no information available.
- **DIRECTIONS FOR ADMINISTRATION** For *intravenous infusion*, dilute requisite dose with Sodium Chloride 0.9% to a final volume of 250 mL and mix gently; infuse through a 0.2 micron in-line filter; give approx. 2.5% of the total volume over 1 hour, then infuse remaining volume over next 3 hours; if body-weight under 20 kg and at risk of fluid overload, dilute requisite dose in 100 mL Sodium Chloride 0.9% and give over at least 4 hours.

- **MEDICINAL FORMS** There can be variation in the licensing of different medicines containing the same drug.

Solution for infusion

▸ Naglazyme (BioMarin Europe Ltd) ▼
Galsulfase 1 mg per 1 ml Naglazyme 5mg/5ml solution for infusion vials | 1 vial PoM £982.00

Idursulfase

27-Apr-2020

- **DRUG ACTION** Idursulfase is an enzyme produced by recombinant DNA technology licensed for long-term replacement therapy in mucopolysaccharidosis II (Hunter syndrome), a lysosomal storage disorder caused by deficiency of iduronate-2-sulfatase.

- **INDICATIONS AND DOSE**

Mucopolysaccharidosis II (specialist use only)

▸ BY INTRAVENOUS INFUSION
▸ Child 16 months–17 years: 500 micrograms/kg once weekly

- **CAUTIONS** Acute febrile respiratory illness (consider delaying treatment) · infusion-related reactions can occur · severe respiratory disease
- **SIDE-EFFECTS**

▸ **Common or very common** Arrhythmias · arthralgia · chest pain · cough · cyanosis · diarrhoea · dizziness · dyspnoea · fever · flushing · gastrointestinal discomfort · headache · hypertension · hypotension · hypoxia · infusion related reaction · nausea · oedema · respiratory disorders · skin reactions · tongue swelling · tremor · vomiting

▸ **Frequency not known** Hypersensitivity

SIDE-EFFECTS, FURTHER INFORMATION Infusion-related reactions often occur, they can be managed by slowing the infusion rate or interrupting the infusion, and can be minimised by pre-treatment with an antihistamine and an antipyretic. Recurrent infusion-related reactions may require pre-treatment with a corticosteroid—consult product literature for details.

- **CONCEPTION AND CONTRACEPTION** Contra-indicated in women of child-bearing potential.
- **PREGNANCY** Manufacturer advises avoid.
- **BREAST FEEDING** Manufacturer advises avoid—present in milk in *animal* studies.
- **DIRECTIONS FOR ADMINISTRATION** For *intravenous infusion*, dilute requisite dose in 100 mL Sodium Chloride 0.9% and mix gently (do not shake); give over 3 hours (gradually reduced to 1 hour if no infusion-related reactions).

- **MEDICINAL FORMS** There can be variation in the licensing of different medicines containing the same drug.

Solution for infusion

▸ Elaprase (Shire Pharmaceuticals Ltd) ▼
Idursulfase 2 mg per 1 ml Elaprase 6mg/3ml concentrate for solution for infusion vials | 1 vial PoM £1,985.00

Laronidase

24-Apr-2020

- **DRUG ACTION** Laronidase is an enzyme produced by recombinant DNA technology licensed for long-term replacement therapy in the treatment of non-neurological manifestations of mucopolysaccharidosis I, a lysosomal storage disorder caused by deficiency of alpha-L-iduronidase.

- **INDICATIONS AND DOSE**

Non-neurological manifestations of mucopolysaccharidosis I (specialist use only)

▸ BY INTRAVENOUS INFUSION
▸ Child: 100 units/kg once weekly

- **CAUTIONS** Infusion-related reactions can occur
- **INTERACTIONS** → Appendix 1: laronidase
- **SIDE-EFFECTS**

▸ **Common or very common** Abdominal pain · alopecia · anaphylactic reaction · angioedema · chills · cough · diarrhoea · dizziness · dyspnoea · fatigue · fever · flushing ·

headache · hypotension · influenza like illness · joint disorders · nausea · pain · pallor · paraesthesia · peripheral coldness · respiratory disorders · restlessness · skin reactions · sweat changes · tachycardia · temperature sensation altered · vomiting
- **Frequency not known** Cyanosis · hypoxia · oedema

SIDE-EFFECTS, FURTHER INFORMATION Infusion-related reactions often occur, they can be managed by slowing the infusion rate or interrupting the infusion, and can be minimised by pre-treatment with an antihistamine and an antipyretic. Recurrent infusion-related reactions may require pre-treatment with a corticosteroid—consult product literature for details.

- **PREGNANCY** Manufacturer advises avoid unless essential—no information available.
- **BREAST FEEDING** Manufacturer advises avoid—no information available.
- **MONITORING REQUIREMENTS** Monitor immunoglobulin G (IgG) antibody concentration.
- **DIRECTIONS FOR ADMINISTRATION** For *intravenous infusion*, dilute with Sodium Chloride 0.9%; body-weight under 20 kg, dilute to 100 mL, body-weight over 20 kg dilute to 250 mL; give through in-line filter (0.22 micron) initially at a rate of 2 units/kg/hour then increase gradually every 15 minutes to max. 43 units/kg/hour.

- **MEDICINAL FORMS** There can be variation in the licensing of different medicines containing the same drug.

Solution for infusion

ELECTROLYTES: May contain Sodium

- Aldurazyme (Genzyme Therapeutics Ltd)
  Laronidase 100 unit per 1 ml Aldurazyme 500units/5ml solution for infusion vials | 1 vial PoM £444.70

3.10 Niemann-pick type C disease

ENZYME INHIBITORS > GLUCOSYLCERAMIDE SYNTHASE INHIBITORS

Miglustat

- **DRUG ACTION** Miglustat is an inhibitor of glucosylceramide synthase.

- **INDICATIONS AND DOSE**

Treatment of progressive neurological manifestations of Niemann-Pick type C disease (under expert supervision)

- BY MOUTH
- Child 4-11 years (body surface area up to 0.48 m^2): 100 mg once daily
- Child 4-11 years (body surface area 0.48–0.73 m^2): 100 mg twice daily
- Child 4-11 years (body surface area 0.74–0.88 m^2): 100 mg 3 times a day
- Child 4-11 years (body surface area 0.89-1.25 m^2): 200 mg twice daily
- Child 4-11 years (body surface area 1.26 m^2 and above): 200 mg 3 times a day
- Child 12-17 years: 200 mg 3 times a day

- **SIDE-EFFECTS**
- **Common or very common** Appetite decreased · asthenia · chills · constipation · depression · diarrhoea · dizziness · flatulence · gastrointestinal discomfort · headache · insomnia · libido decreased · malaise · muscle spasms · muscle weakness · nausea · peripheral neuropathy · sensation abnormal · thrombocytopenia · tremor · vomiting · weight decreased
- **Frequency not known** Growth retardation

- **CONCEPTION AND CONTRACEPTION** Effective contraception must be used during treatment. Men should avoid fathering a child during and for 3 months after treatment.
- **PREGNANCY** Manufacturer advises avoid—toxicity in *animal* studies.
- **BREAST FEEDING** Manufacturer advises avoid—no information available.
- **HEPATIC IMPAIRMENT** Manufacturer advises caution (no information available).
- **RENAL IMPAIRMENT** Avoid if estimated glomerular filtration less than 30 mL/minute/1.73 m^2. Child under 12 years—consult product literature.
  Dose adjustments Child 12–17 years, initially 200 mg twice daily if estimated glomerular filtration rate 50–70 mL/minute/1.73 m^2. Initially 100 mg twice daily if estimated glomerular filtration rate 30–50 mL/minute/1.73 m^2.
- **MONITORING REQUIREMENTS**
  - Monitor cognitive and neurological function.
  - Monitor growth and platelet count in Niemann-Pick type C disease.

- **MEDICINAL FORMS** There can be variation in the licensing of different medicines containing the same drug.

Capsule

- Miglustat (Non-proprietary)
  Miglustat 100 mg Miglustat 100mg capsules | 84 capsule PoM £3,934.00 (Hospital only)
- Zavesca (Actelion Pharmaceuticals UK Ltd)
  Miglustat 100 mg Zavesca 100mg capsules | 84 capsule PoM £3,934.17 (Hospital only)

3.11 Pompe disease

ENZYMES

Alglucosidase alfa

23-Apr-2020

- **DRUG ACTION** Alglucosidase alfa is an enzyme produced by recombinant DNA technology licensed for long-term replacement therapy in Pompe disease, a lysosomal storage disorder caused by deficiency of acid alpha-glucosidase.

- **INDICATIONS AND DOSE**

Pompe disease (specialist use only)

- BY INTRAVENOUS INFUSION
- Neonate: 20 mg/kg every 2 weeks.
- Child: 20 mg/kg every 2 weeks

- **CAUTIONS** Cardiac dysfunction · infusion-related reactions—consult product literature · respiratory dysfunction
- **SIDE-EFFECTS**
- **Common or very common** Anxiety · arrhythmias · chest discomfort · chills · cough · cyanosis · diarrhoea · dizziness · fatigue · feeling hot · fever · flushing · hyperhidrosis · hypersensitivity · hypertension · irritability · local swelling · muscle complaints · nausea · oedema · pallor · paraesthesia · respiratory disorders · skin reactions · throat complaints · tremor · vomiting
- **Frequency not known** Abdominal pain · angioedema · apnoea · arthralgia · cardiac arrest · dyspnoea · excessive tearing · eye inflammation · headache · hypotension · nephrotic syndrome · peripheral coldness · proteinuria · vasoconstriction

SIDE-EFFECTS, FURTHER INFORMATION Infusion-related reactions are very common, calling for use of antihistamine, antipyretic, or corticosteroid; consult product literature for details.

- **PREGNANCY** Toxicity in *animal* studies, but treatment should not be withheld.
- **BREAST FEEDING** Manufacturer advises avoid—no information available.
- **MONITORING REQUIREMENTS**
  - Monitor closely if cardiac dysfunction.
  - Monitor closely if respiratory dysfunction.
  - Monitor immunoglobulin G (IgG) antibody concentration.
- **DIRECTIONS FOR ADMINISTRATION** For *intravenous infusion*, reconstitute 50 mg with 10.3 mL water for injections to produce 5 mg/mL solution; gently rotate vial without shaking; dilute requisite dose with Sodium Chloride 0.9% to give a final concentration of 0.5–4 mg/mL; give through a low protein-binding in-line filter (0.2 micron) at an initial rate of 1 mg/kg/hour increased by 2 mg/kg/hour every 30 minutes to max. 7mg/kg/hour.

- **MEDICINAL FORMS** There can be variation in the licensing of different medicines containing the same drug.

Powder for solution for infusion

- Myozyme (Genzyme Therapeutics Ltd)
  Alglucosidase alfa 50 mg Myozyme 50mg powder for concentrate for solution for infusion vials | 1 vial PoM £356.06 (Hospital only)

3.12 Tyrosinaemia type I

ENZYME INHIBITORS › 4-HYDROXYPHENYLPYRUVATE DIOXYGENASE INHIBITORS

Nitisinone

(NTBC)

- **INDICATIONS AND DOSE**

Hereditary tyrosinaemia type I (in combination with dietary restriction of tyrosine and phenylalanine) (specialist use only)

- BY MOUTH
  - Neonate: Initially 500 micrograms/kg twice daily, adjusted according to response; maximum 2 mg/kg per day.
  - Child: Initially 500 micrograms/kg twice daily, adjusted according to response; maximum 2 mg/kg per day

- **INTERACTIONS** → Appendix 1: nitisinone
- **SIDE-EFFECTS**
  - **Common or very common** Corneal opacity · eye inflammation · eye pain · granulocytopenia · leucopenia · photophobia · thrombocytopenia
  - **Uncommon** Leucocytosis · skin reactions
- **PREGNANCY** Manufacturer advises avoid unless potential benefit outweighs risk—toxicity in *animal* studies.
- **BREAST FEEDING** Manufacturer advises avoid—adverse effects in *animal* studies.
- **PRE-TREATMENT SCREENING** Slit-lamp examination of eyes recommended before treatment.
- **MONITORING REQUIREMENTS**
  - Monitor liver function regularly.
  - Monitor platelet and white blood cell count every 6 months.
- **DIRECTIONS FOR ADMINISTRATION** Capsules can be opened and the contents suspended in a small amount of water or formula diet and taken immediately.
- **MEDICINAL FORMS** There can be variation in the licensing of different medicines containing the same drug.

Oral suspension

- Orfadin (Swedish Orphan Biovitrum Ltd)
  Nitisinone 4 mg per 1 ml Orfadin 4mg/1ml oral suspension sugar-free | 90 ml PoM £1,692.00 DT = £1,692.00

Capsule

- Nitisinone (Non-proprietary)
  Nitisinone 2 mg Nitisinone 2mg capsules | 60 capsule PoM £423.00
  Nitisinone 5 mg Nitisinone 5mg capsules | 60 capsule PoM £845.25
  Nitisinone 10 mg Nitisinone 10mg capsules | 60 capsule PoM £1,546.50
- Orfadin (Swedish Orphan Biovitrum Ltd)
  Nitisinone 2 mg Orfadin 2mg capsules | 60 capsule PoM £564.00
  Nitisinone 5 mg Orfadin 5mg capsules | 60 capsule PoM £1,127.00
  Nitisinone 10 mg Orfadin 10mg capsules | 60 capsule PoM £2,062.00
  Nitisinone 20 mg Orfadin 20mg capsules | 60 capsule PoM £4,512.00 DT = £4,512.00

3.13 Urea cycle disorders

AMINO ACIDS AND DERIVATIVES

Arginine

03-Mar-2020

- **INDICATIONS AND DOSE**

Acute hyperammonaemia in carbamylphosphate synthetase deficiency (specialist use only) | Acute hyperammonaemia in ornithine transcarbamylase deficiency (specialist use only)

- BY INTRAVENOUS INFUSION
  - Neonate: 6 mg/kg/hour.
  - Child (body-weight up to 40 kg): 6 mg/kg/hour
  - Child (body-weight 40 kg and above): 4 mg/kg/hour

Maintenance treatment of hyperammonaemia in carbamylphosphate synthetase deficiency (specialist use only) | Maintenance treatment of hyperammonaemia in ornithine transcarbamylase deficiency (specialist use only)

- BY MOUTH
  - Neonate: 100–200 mg/kg daily in 3–4 divided doses, dose to be taken with feeds.
  - Child (body-weight up to 20 kg): 100–200 mg/kg daily in 3–4 divided doses, dose to be given with feeds or meals
  - Child (body-weight 20 kg and above): 2.5–6 g/m^2 daily in 3–4 divided doses, dose to be taken with meals; maximum 6 g per day

Acute hyperammonaemia in citrullinaemia (specialist use only) | Acute hyperammonaemia in arginosuccinic aciduria (specialist use only)

- BY INTRAVENOUS INFUSION
  - Neonate: Initially 300 mg/kg, to be administered over 90 minutes, followed by 12.5 mg/kg/hour, to be administered over 24 hours (maximum 25 mg/kg/hour thereafter).
  - Child (body-weight up to 40 kg): Initially 300 mg/kg, to be administered over 90 minutes, followed by 12.5 mg/kg/hour, to be administered over 24 hours (maximum 25 mg/kg/hour thereafter)
  - Child (body-weight 40 kg and above): 21 mg/kg/hour

Maintenance treatment of hyperammonaemia in citrullinaemia (specialist use only) | Maintenance treatment of hyperammonaemia in arginosuccinic aciduria (specialist use only)

▶ BY MOUTH

- Neonate: 100–300 mg/kg daily in 3–4 divided doses, dose to be taken with feeds.
- Child (body-weight up to 20 kg): 100–300 mg/kg daily in 3–4 divided doses, dose to be taken with feed or meals
- Child (body-weight 20 kg and above): 2.5–6 g/m^2 daily in 3–4 divided doses, doses to be taken with meals; maximum 6 g per day

● **UNLICENSED USE**
- With intravenous use Injection not licensed in children.
- With oral use Tablets not licensed in children. Powder licensed for urea cycle disorders in children.

● **CONTRA-INDICATIONS** Not to be used in the treatment of arginase deficiency

● **SIDE-EFFECTS** Acidosis hyperchloraemic · flushing · headache · hypotension · nausea · numbness · vomiting

● **PREGNANCY** No information available.

● **BREAST FEEDING** No information available.

● **MONITORING REQUIREMENTS** Monitor plasma pH and chloride.

● **DIRECTIONS FOR ADMINISTRATION** For *intravenous infusion*, dilute to a max. concentration of 50 mg/mL with glucose 10%.

● **PRESCRIBING AND DISPENSING INFORMATION**
- With oral use Powder to be prescribed as a borderline substance (ACBS). For use as a supplement in urea cycle disorders other than arginase deficiency, such as hyperammonaemia types I and II, citrullinaemia, arginosuccinic aciduria, and deficiency of N-acetyl glutamate synthetase.

● **PATIENT AND CARER ADVICE**
Medicines for Children leaflet: Arginine for urea cycle disorders www.medicinesforchildren.org.uk/arginine-urea-cycle-disorders-0

● **MEDICINAL FORMS** There can be variation in the licensing of different medicines containing the same drug. Forms available from special-order manufacturers include: tablet, capsule, oral solution, solution for infusion

Tablet
- Arginine (Non-proprietary)
  L-Arginine 500 mg L-Arginine 500mg tablets | 60 tablet £5.86
  L-Arginine 1 gram Arginine 1g tablets | 90 tablet £11.59

Solution for infusion
- Arginine (Non-proprietary)
  L-Arginine monohydrochloride 210.7 mg per 1 ml L-Arginin-Hydrochlorid 21% concentrate for solution for infusion 20ml ampoules | 5 ampoule PoM ⊠

Capsule
- Arginine (Non-proprietary)
  L-Arginine 500 mg L-Arginine 500mg capsules | 60 capsule £19.99
  L-Arginine 500mg capsules | 30 capsule £4.02

Powder
- Arginine (Non-proprietary)
  L-Arginine 1 gram per 1 gram L-Arginine powder | 100 gram £47.28

Carglumic acid

● **INDICATIONS AND DOSE**

Hyperammonaemia due to N-acetylglutamate synthase deficiency (under expert supervision)

▶ BY MOUTH

- Neonate: Initially 50–125 mg/kg twice daily, to be taken immediately before feeds, dose adjusted according to plasma–ammonia concentration; maintenance 5–50 mg/kg twice daily, the total daily dose may alternatively be given in 3–4 divided doses.
- Child: Initially 50–125 mg/kg twice daily, to be taken immediately before food, dose adjusted according to plasma–ammonia concentration; maintenance 5–50 mg/kg twice daily, the total daily dose may alternatively be given in 3–4 divided doses

Hyperammonaemia due to organic acidaemia (under expert supervision)

▶ BY MOUTH

- Neonate: Initially 50–125 mg/kg twice daily, to be taken immediately before feeds, dose adjusted according to plasma-ammonia concentration, the total daily dose may alternatively be given in 3–4 divided doses.
- Child: Initially 50–125 mg/kg twice daily, to be taken immediately before food, dose adjusted according to plasma-ammonia concentration, the total daily dose may alternatively be given in 3–4 divided doses

IMPORTANT SAFETY INFORMATION

EMERGENCY MANAGEMENT OF UREA CYCLE DISORDERS

For further information on the emergency management of urea cycle disorders consult the British Inherited Metabolic Disease Group (BIMDG) website at www.bimdg.org.uk.

● **SIDE-EFFECTS**
- **Common or very common** Hyperhidrosis
- **Uncommon** Bradycardia · diarrhoea · fever · vomiting
- **Frequency not known** Rash

● **PREGNANCY** Manufacturer advises avoid unless essential—no information available.

● **BREAST FEEDING** Manufacturer advises avoid—present in milk in *animal* studies.

● **DIRECTIONS FOR ADMINISTRATION** Dispersible tablets must be dispersed in at least 5–10 mL of water and taken orally immediately, or administered via a nasogastric tube.

● **MEDICINAL FORMS** There can be variation in the licensing of different medicines containing the same drug.

Dispersible tablet

CAUTIONARY AND ADVISORY LABELS 13
- Carglumic acid (Non-proprietary)
  Carglumic acid 200 mg Carglumic acid 200mg dispersible tablets sugar free sugar-free | 5 tablet PoM £218.69 sugar-free | 15 tablet PoM £625.37 sugar-free | 60 tablet PoM £2,624.30
- Carbaglu (Recordati Rare Diseases UK Ltd)
  Carglumic acid 200 mg Carbaglu 200mg dispersible tablets sugar-free | 5 tablet PoM £299.00 sugar-free | 15 tablet PoM £897.00 sugar-free | 60 tablet PoM £3,499.00
- Ucedane (Eurocept International bv)
  Carglumic acid 200 mg Ucedane 200mg dispersible tablets sugar-free | 12 tablet PoM £660.00 sugar-free | 60 tablet PoM £3,300.00

Citrulline

● **INDICATIONS AND DOSE**

Carbamyl phosphate synthase deficiency | Ornithine carbamyl transferase deficiency

▶ BY MOUTH

- Neonate: 150 mg/kg daily in 3–4 divided doses, adjusted according to response.
- Child: 150 mg/kg daily in 3–4 divided doses, adjusted according to response

● **PREGNANCY** No information available.

● **BREAST FEEDING** No information available.

- **DIRECTIONS FOR ADMINISTRATION** Powder may be mixed with drinks or taken as a paste.

- **MEDICINAL FORMS** There can be variation in the licensing of different medicines containing the same drug. Forms available from special-order manufacturers include: tablet, oral solution, powder

Oral solution

- Citrulline (Non-proprietary)
  L-citrulline 100 mg per 1 ml Stimol oral solution 10ml sachets sugar-free | 36 sachet [PoM] [X]

Powder

- Citrulline (Non-proprietary)
  L-citrulline 1 mg per 1 mg L-Citrulline powder | 100 gram £249.99

BENZOATES

Sodium benzoate

10-Mar-2020

- **INDICATIONS AND DOSE**

Acute hyperammonaemia due to urea cycle disorder (specialist use only)

▶ BY INTRAVENOUS INFUSION

- Neonate: Initially 250 mg/kg, to be administered over 90 minutes, followed by 10 mg/kg/hour, adjusted according to response.
- Child: Initially 250 mg/kg, to be administered over 90 minutes, followed by 10 mg/kg/hour, adjusted according to response

Maintenance treatment of hyperammonaemia due to urea cycle disorders (specialist use only) | Non-ketotic hyperglycinaemia (specialist use only)

▶ BY MOUTH

- Neonate: Up to 250 mg/kg daily in 3–4 divided doses, dose to be taken with feeds.
- Child: Up to 250 mg/kg daily in 3–4 divided doses, dose to be taken with feeds or meals; maximum 12 g per day

- **UNLICENSED USE** Not licensed for use in children.
- **CAUTIONS** Conditions involving sodium retention with oedema (preparations contain significant amounts of sodium) · congestive heart failure (preparations contain significant amounts of sodium) · neonates (risk of kernicterus and increased side-effects)
- **SIDE-EFFECTS** Appetite decreased · coma · irritability · lethargy · nausea · vomiting
  SIDE-EFFECTS, FURTHER INFORMATION Gastro-intestinal side-effects may be reduced by giving smaller doses more frequently.
- **PREGNANCY** No information available.
- **BREAST FEEDING** No information available.
- **RENAL IMPAIRMENT** Caution in renal insufficiency—preparations contain significant amounts of sodium.
- **DIRECTIONS FOR ADMINISTRATION**
  - With oral use For administration *by mouth*, oral solution or powder may be administered in fruit drinks; less soluble in acidic drinks.
  - With intravenous use For *intravenous infusion*, dilute to a max. concentration of 50 mg/mL with Glucose 10%.
- **PATIENT AND CARER ADVICE**
  Medicines for Children leaflet: Sodium benzoate for urea cycle disorders www.medicinesforchildren.org.uk/sodium-benzoate-urea-cycle-disorders

- **MEDICINAL FORMS** Forms available from special-order manufacturers include: tablet, capsule, oral solution, solution for infusion

DRUGS FOR METABOLIC DISORDERS > ACETIC ACIDS

Sodium dichloroacetate

- **INDICATIONS AND DOSE**

Pyruvate dehydrogenase defects

▶ BY MOUTH

- Neonate: Initially 12.5 mg/kg 4 times a day, adjusted according to response, increased if necessary up to 200 mg/kg daily.
- Child: Initially 12.5 mg/kg 4 times a day, adjusted according to response, increased if necessary up to 200 mg/kg daily

- **SIDE-EFFECTS** Metabolic acidosis · oxalate metabolism abnormal · polyneuropathy (long term use)
- **PREGNANCY** No information available.
- **BREAST FEEDING** No information available.

- **MEDICINAL FORMS** No licensed medicines listed.

DRUGS FOR METABOLIC DISORDERS > AMMONIA LOWERING DRUGS

Glycerol phenylbutyrate

13-Sep-2018

- **DRUG ACTION** Glycerol phenylbutyrate is a nitrogen-binding agent that provides an alternative vehicle for waste nitrogen excretion.

- **INDICATIONS AND DOSE**

Urea cycle disorders (specialist use only)

▶ BY MOUTH, OR BY GASTROSTOMY TUBE, OR BY NASOGASTRIC TUBE

- Neonate (body surface area up to 1.3 m^2): Initially 9.4 g/m^2 daily in divided doses, usual maintenance 5.3–12.4 g/m^2 daily in divided doses, each dose should be rounded up to the nearest 0.1 mL and given with each feed. For dose adjustments based on individual requirements—consult product literature.
- Child 1–23 months (body surface area up to 1.3 m^2): Initially 9.4 g/m^2 daily in divided doses, usual maintenance 5.3–12.4 g/m^2 daily in divided doses, each dose should be rounded up to the nearest 0.1 mL and given with each meal or feed. For dose adjustments based on individual requirements—consult product literature
- Child 2–17 years (body surface area up to 1.3 m^2): Initially 9.4 g/m^2 daily in divided doses, usual maintenance 5.3–12.4 g/m^2 daily in divided doses, each dose should be rounded up to the nearest 0.5 mL and given with each meal. For dose adjustments based on individual requirements—consult product literature
- Child 2–17 years (body surface area 1.3 m^2 and above): Initially 8 g/m^2 daily in divided doses, usual maintenance 5.3–12.4 g/m^2 daily in divided doses, each dose should be rounded up to the nearest 0.5 mL and given with each meal. For dose adjustments based on individual requirements—consult product literature

DOSE EQUIVALENCE AND CONVERSION

- 1 mL of liquid contains 1.1 g of glycerol phenylbutyrate.
- For patients switching from sodium phenylbutyrate or sodium benzoate—consult product literature.

> **IMPORTANT SAFETY INFORMATION**
> EMERGENCY MANAGEMENT OF UREA CYCLE DISORDERS
> For further information on the emergency management of urea cycle disorders consult the British Inherited Metabolic Disease Group (BIMDG) website at www.bimdg.org.uk.

- **CONTRA-INDICATIONS** Treatment of acute hyperammonaemia
- **CAUTIONS** Intestinal malabsorption · pancreatic insufficiency
- **INTERACTIONS** → Appendix 1: glycerol phenylbutyrate
- **SIDE-EFFECTS**
  - **Common or very common** Appetite abnormal · constipation · diarrhoea · dizziness · fatigue · food aversion · gastrointestinal discomfort · gastrointestinal disorders · headache · menstrual cycle irregularities · nausea · oral disorders · peripheral oedema · skin reactions · tremor · vomiting
  - **Uncommon** Akathisia · alopecia · biliary colic · bladder pain · burping · confusion · depressed mood · drowsiness · dry mouth · dysphonia · epistaxis · fever · gastrointestinal infection viral · hot flush · hyperhidrosis · hypoalbuminaemia · hypokalaemia · hypothyroidism · joint swelling · muscle spasms · nasal congestion · oropharyngeal pain · pain · paraesthesia · plantar fasciitis · speech disorder · taste altered · throat irritation · ventricular arrhythmia · weight changes
  - **Frequency not known** Anaemia · nail ridging · thrombocytosis
- **PREGNANCY** Manufacturer advises avoid unless essential—toxicity in *animal* studies.
- **BREAST FEEDING** Manufacturer advises avoid—no information available.
- **HEPATIC IMPAIRMENT** Manufacturer advises caution (risk of increased exposure).
  Dose adjustments Manufacturer advises use lowest possible dose—consult product literature.
- **RENAL IMPAIRMENT** Manufacturer advises use with caution in severe impairment—no information available.
- **DIRECTIONS FOR ADMINISTRATION** Manufacturer advises may be added to a small amount of apple sauce, ketchup, or squash puree and used within 2 hours. For administration advice via nasogastric or gastrostomy tube—consult product literature.
- **HANDLING AND STORAGE** Manufacturer advises discard contents of bottle 14 days after opening.
- **PATIENT AND CARER ADVICE**
  Driving and skilled tasks Manufacturer advises patients and carers should be counselled on the effects on driving and performance of skilled tasks—increased risk of dizziness.
- **NATIONAL FUNDING/ACCESS DECISIONS**

Scottish Medicines Consortium (SMC) decisions
SMC No. 1342/18
The *Scottish Medicines Consortium* has advised (August 2018) that glycerol phenylbutyrate (*Ravicti*®) is accepted for use within NHS Scotland as an adjunctive therapy for chronic management of adult and paediatric patients aged 2 months and older with urea cycle disorders who cannot be managed by dietary protein restriction and/or amino acid supplementation alone. Glycerol phenylbutyrate must be used with dietary protein restriction and, in some cases, dietary supplements. This advice is contingent upon the continuing availability of the patient access scheme in NHS Scotland or a list price that is equivalent or lower.

All Wales Medicines Strategy Group (AWMSG) decisions
AWMSG No. 2127
The *All Wales Medicines Strategy Group* has advised (December 2019) that glycerol phenylbutyrate (*Ravicti*®) is recommended as an option for use within NHS Wales for use as an adjunctive therapy for chronic management of patients with urea cycle disorders who cannot be managed by dietary protein restriction and/or amino acid supplementation alone. *Ravicti*® must be used with dietary protein restriction and, in some cases, dietary supplements. This recommendation applies only in circumstances where the approved Wales Patient Access Scheme (WPAS) is utilised or where the list/contract price is equivalent or lower than the PAS/WPAS price.

- **MEDICINAL FORMS** There can be variation in the licensing of different medicines containing the same drug.

Liquid
- Ravicti (Immedica Pharma AB) ▼
  Glycerol phenylbutyrate 1.1 gram per 1 ml Ravicti 1.1g/ml oral liquid | 25 ml PoM £161.00

Sodium phenylbutyrate 29-Apr-2020

- **INDICATIONS AND DOSE**

Acute hyperammonaemia due to urea cycle disorders (specialist use only)
- BY INTRAVENOUS INFUSION
  - Neonate: Initially 250 mg/kg, to be administered over 90 minutes, followed by 10 mg/kg/hour, adjusted according to response.
  - Child: Initially 250 mg/kg, to be administered over 90 minutes, followed by 10 mg/kg/hour, adjusted according to response

Maintenance treatment of hyperammonaemia due to urea cycle disorders (specialist use only)
- BY MOUTH
  - Neonate: Up to 250 mg/kg daily in 3–4 divided doses, with feeds.
  - Child (body-weight up to 20 kg): Up to 250 mg/kg daily in 3–4 divided doses, with feeds or meals
  - Child (body-weight 20 kg and above): 5 g/m^2 daily in 3–4 divided doses, with meals; maximum 12 g per day

- **UNLICENSED USE** Injection not licensed for use in children.

> **IMPORTANT SAFETY INFORMATION**
> EMERGENCY MANAGEMENT OF UREA CYCLE DISORDERS
> For further information on the emergency management of urea cycle disorders consult the British Inherited Metabolic Disease Group (BIMDG) website at www.bimdg.org.uk.

- **CAUTIONS** Conditions involving sodium retention with oedema (preparations contain significant amounts of sodium) · congestive heart failure (preparations contain significant amounts of sodium)
- **INTERACTIONS** → Appendix 1: sodium phenylbutyrate
- **SIDE-EFFECTS**
  - **Common or very common** Abdominal pain · anaemia · appetite decreased · constipation · depression · headache · irritability · leucocytosis · leucopenia · menstrual cycle irregularities · metabolic acidosis · metabolic alkalosis · nausea · oedema · renal tubular acidosis · skin reactions · syncope · taste altered · thrombocytopenia · thrombocytosis · vomiting · weight increased
  - **Uncommon** Anorectal haemorrhage · aplastic anaemia · arrhythmia · gastrointestinal disorders · pancreatitis

9 Blood and nutrition

- **CONCEPTION AND CONTRACEPTION** Manufacturer advises adequate contraception during administration in women of child-bearing potential.
- **PREGNANCY** Avoid—toxicity in *animal* studies.
- **BREAST FEEDING** Manufacturer advises avoid—no information available.
- **HEPATIC IMPAIRMENT** Manufacturer advises caution.
- **RENAL IMPAIRMENT** Manufacturer advises use with caution (preparations contain significant amounts of sodium).
- **DIRECTIONS FOR ADMINISTRATION**
  - With oral use Oral dose may be mixed with fruit drinks, milk, or feeds. Granules should be mixed with food before taking. *Pheburane*® granules must not be administered by nasogastric or gastrostromy tubes.
  - With intravenous use For *intravenous infusion*, dilute to a maximum concentration of 50 mg/mL with Glucose 10%.
- **PATIENT AND CARER ADVICE**
  Medicines for Children leaflet: Sodium phenylbutyrate for urea cycle disorders www.medicinesforchildren.org.uk/sodium-phenylbutyrate-urea-cycle-disorders

- **MEDICINAL FORMS** There can be variation in the licensing of different medicines containing the same drug. Forms available from special-order manufacturers include: capsule, oral suspension, oral solution, solution for infusion

Granules
- Ammonaps (Immedica Pharma AB)
  Sodium phenylbutyrate 940 mg per 1 gram Ammonaps 940mg/g granules sugar-free | 266 gram PoM £860.00 DT = £860.00
- Pheburane (Eurocept International bv)
  Sodium phenylbutyrate 483 mg per 1 gram Pheburane 483mg/g granules | 174 gram PoM £331.00

Tablet
- Ammonaps (Immedica Pharma AB)
  Sodium phenylbutyrate 500 mg Ammonaps 500mg tablets | 250 tablet PoM £493.00 DT = £493.00

3.14 Wilson's disease

Other drugs used for Wilson's disease Penicillamine, below

ANTIDOTES AND CHELATORS › COPPER ABSORPTION INHIBITORS

Zinc acetate

- **DRUG ACTION** Zinc prevents the absorption of copper in Wilson's disease.

- **INDICATIONS AND DOSE**

Wilson's disease (initiated under specialist supervision)
- BY MOUTH
  - Child 1–5 years: 25 mg twice daily
  - Child 6–15 years (body-weight up to 57 kg): 25 mg 3 times a day
  - Child 6–15 years (body-weight 57 kg and above): 50 mg 3 times a day
  - Child 16–17 years: 50 mg 3 times a day

DOSE EQUIVALENCE AND CONVERSION
- Doses expressed as elemental zinc.

PHARMACOKINETICS
- Symptomatic Wilson's disease patients should be treated initially with a chelating agent because zinc has a slow onset of action. When transferring from chelating treatment to zinc maintenance therapy, chelating treatment should be co-administered for 2–3 weeks until zinc produces its maximal effect.

- **CAUTIONS** Portal hypertension (risk of hepatic decompensation when switching from chelating agent)
- **INTERACTIONS** → Appendix 1: zinc
- **SIDE-EFFECTS**
  - **Common or very common** Epigastric discomfort (usually transient)
  - **Uncommon** Leucopenia · sideroblastic anaemia
  - **Frequency not known** Condition aggravated

  SIDE-EFFECTS, FURTHER INFORMATION Transient gastric irritation may be reduced if first dose is taken mid-morning or with a little protein.
- **PREGNANCY**
  Dose adjustments Usual dose 25 mg 3 times daily adjusted according to plasma-copper concentration and urinary copper excretion.
- **BREAST FEEDING** Manufacturer advises avoid; present in milk—may cause zinc-induced copper deficiency in infant.
- **MONITORING REQUIREMENTS** Monitor full blood count and serum cholesterol.
- **DIRECTIONS FOR ADMINISTRATION** Capsules may be opened and the contents mixed with water.

- **MEDICINAL FORMS** There can be variation in the licensing of different medicines containing the same drug.

Capsule

CAUTIONARY AND ADVISORY LABELS 23
- Wilzin (Recordati Rare Diseases UK Ltd)
  Zinc (as Zinc acetate) 25 mg Wilzin 25mg capsules | 250 capsule PoM £132.00 DT = £132.00
  Zinc (as Zinc acetate) 50 mg Wilzin 50mg capsules | 250 capsule PoM £242.00 DT = £242.00

ANTIDOTES AND CHELATORS › COPPER CHELATORS

Penicillamine

- **DRUG ACTION** Penicillamine aids the elimination of copper ions in Wilson's disease (hepatolenticular degeneration).

- **INDICATIONS AND DOSE**

Wilson's disease
- BY MOUTH
  - Child 1 month–11 years: 20 mg/kg daily in 2–3 divided doses, to be taken 1 hour before food; maximum 2 g per day
  - Child 12–17 years: Initially 20 mg/kg daily in 2–3 divided doses, maintenance 0.75–1 g daily, to be taken 1 hour before food; maximum 2 g per day

Cystinuria
- BY MOUTH
  - Child: 20–30 mg/kg daily in 2–3 divided doses, lower doses may be used initially and increased gradually, doses to be adjusted to maintain 24-hour urinary cystine below 1 mmol/litre, maintain adequate fluid intake, to be taken 1 hour before food; maximum 3 g per day

- **CONTRA-INDICATIONS** Lupus erythematosus
- **CAUTIONS** Neurological involvement in Wilson's disease
- **INTERACTIONS** → Appendix 1: penicillamine
- **SIDE-EFFECTS**
  - **Common or very common** Proteinuria · thrombocytopenia
  - **Rare or very rare** Alopecia · breast enlargement (males and females) · connective tissue disorders · haematuria (discontinue immediately if cause unknown) · hypersensitivity · oral disorders · skin reactions
  - **Frequency not known** Agranulocytosis · aplastic anaemia · appetite decreased · fever · glomerulonephritis · Goodpasture's syndrome · haemolytic anaemia · increased risk of infection · jaundice cholestatic · leucopenia · lupus-

like syndrome · myasthenia gravis · nausea · nephrotic syndrome · neurological deterioration in Wilson's Disease · neutropenia · pancreatitis · polymyositis · pulmonary haemorrhage · rash (consider dose reduction) · respiratory disorders · Stevens-Johnson syndrome · taste loss (mineral supplements not recommended) · vomiting · yellow nail syndrome

- **ALLERGY AND CROSS-SENSITIVITY** Patients who are hypersensitive to penicillin may react rarely to penicillamine.
- **PREGNANCY** Fetal abnormalities reported rarely; avoid if possible.
- **BREAST FEEDING** Manufacturer advises avoid unless potential benefit outweighs risk—no information available.
- **RENAL IMPAIRMENT**
  Dose adjustments Reduce dose and monitor renal function or avoid (consult product literature).
- **MONITORING REQUIREMENTS**
  - Consider withdrawal if platelet count falls below 120 000/mm^3 or white blood cells below 2500/mm^3 or if 3 successive falls within reference range (can restart at reduced dose when counts return to within reference range but permanent withdrawal necessary if recurrence of leucopenia or thrombocytopenia).
  - Monitor urine for proteinuria.
  - Monitor blood and platelet count regularly.
- **PATIENT AND CARER ADVICE** Counselling on the symptoms of blood disorders is advised. Warn patient and carers to tell doctor immediately if sore throat, fever, infection, non-specific illness, unexplained bleeding and bruising, purpura, mouth ulcers, or rashes develop.

- **MEDICINAL FORMS** There can be variation in the licensing of different medicines containing the same drug. Forms available from special-order manufacturers include: oral solution

Tablet

CAUTIONARY AND ADVISORY LABELS 6, 22

- Penicillamine (Non-proprietary)
  Penicillamine 125 mg Penicillamine 125mg tablets | 56 tablet PoM £59.61 DT = £51.79
  Penicillamine 250 mg Penicillamine 250mg tablets | 56 tablet PoM £113.70 DT = £104.23

Trientine dihydrochloride

03-Dec-2019

- **INDICATIONS AND DOSE**

Wilson's disease in patients intolerant of penicillamine

- BY MOUTH USING CAPSULES
  - Child 2–11 years: Initially 0.6–1.5 g daily in 2–4 divided doses, adjusted according to response, to be taken before food
  - Child 12–17 years: 1.2–2.4 g daily in 2–4 divided doses, adjusted according to response, to be taken before food

DOSE EQUIVALENCE AND CONVERSION

- Doses expressed as trientine dihydrochloride.
- Capsules and tablets are not interchangeable on a milligram-for-milligram basis due to differences in bioavailability.

CUPRIOR®

Wilson's disease in patients intolerant of penicillamine

- BY MOUTH USING FILM-COATED TABLETS
  - Child 5–17 years: 225–600 mg daily in 2–4 divided doses, adjusted according to response

DOSE EQUIVALENCE AND CONVERSION

- Each tablet contains trientine tetrahydrochloride equivalent to 150 mg of trientine base; doses expressed as trientine base.
- Tablets and capsules are not interchangeable on a milligram-for-milligram basis due to differences in bioavailability.

- **INTERACTIONS** → Appendix 1: trientine
- **SIDE-EFFECTS**
  - **Common or very common** Nausea
  - **Uncommon** Skin reactions
  - **Frequency not known** Anaemia · gastrointestinal disorders · neurological deterioration in Wilson's Disease
- **PREGNANCY** Teratogenic in *animal* studies—use only if benefit outweighs risk.
  Monitoring Monitor maternal and neonatal serum-copper concentrations.
- **BREAST FEEDING** EvGr Specialist sources indicate caution—limited information available; effect on copper levels in milk conflicting and impact on infant unknown. ⟨D⟩
- **DIRECTIONS FOR ADMINISTRATION**
  CUPRIOR® Tablets can be divided into 2 equal halves.
- **PRESCRIBING AND DISPENSING INFORMATION** Trientine is **not** an alternative to penicillamine for rheumatoid arthritis or cystinuria. Penicillamine-induced systemic lupus erythematosus may not resolve on transfer to trientine.
- **HANDLING AND STORAGE** Manufacturer advises store *capsules* in a refrigerator (2–8°C)—keep in the original container with the silica gel sachet to protect from moisture.
- **NATIONAL FUNDING/ACCESS DECISIONS**

Scottish Medicines Consortium (SMC) decisions

SMC No. SMC2222

The *Scottish Medicines Consortium* has advised (November 2019) that trientine tetrahydrochloride (*Cuprior*®) is accepted for use within NHS Scotland for the treatment of Wilson's disease in adults, adolescents and children aged 5 years and older, intolerant to D-penicillamine therapy.

- **MEDICINAL FORMS** There can be variation in the licensing of different medicines containing the same drug.

Tablet

CAUTIONARY AND ADVISORY LABELS 7, 23

- Trientine dihydrochloride (Non-proprietary)
  Trientine tetrahydrochloride 150 mg Cuprior 150mg tablets | 72 tablet PoM £2,725.00

Capsule

CAUTIONARY AND ADVISORY LABELS 6, 22

- Trientine dihydrochloride (Non-proprietary)
  Trientine dihydrochloride 300 mg Trientine dihydrochloride 300mg capsules | 100 capsule PoM £3,090.00 DT = £3,090.00
- Metalite (Imported (Japan))
  Trientine dihydrochloride 250 mg Metalite 250mg capsules | 100 capsule PoM ☒

4 Mineral and trace elements deficiencies

4.1 Zinc deficiency

Zinc deficiency

Overview

Zinc supplements should not be given unless there is good evidence of deficiency (hypoproteinaemia spuriously lowers plasma-zinc concentration) or in zinc-losing conditions. Zinc deficiency can occur as a result of inadequate diet or malabsorption; excessive loss of zinc can occur in trauma, burns, and protein-losing conditions. A zinc supplement is given until clinical improvement occurs, but it may need to be continued in severe malabsorption, metabolic disease, or in zinc-losing states.

Zinc is used in the treatment of Wilson's disease and acrodermatitis enteropathica, a rare inherited abnormality of zinc absorption.

Parenteral nutrition regimens usually include trace amounts of zinc, see also Intravenous nutrition below. If necessary, further zinc can be added to intravenous feeding regimens.

ELECTROLYTES AND MINERALS > ZINC

Zinc sulfate

● **INDICATIONS AND DOSE**

Zinc deficiency or supplementation in zinc-losing conditions

▶ BY MOUTH USING EFFERVESCENT TABLETS

- Neonate: 1 mg/kg daily, dose expressed as elemental zinc, to be dissolved in water and taken after food.
- Child (body-weight up to 10 kg): 22.5 mg daily, dose to be adjusted as necessary, to be dissolved in water and taken after food, dose expressed as elemental zinc
- Child (body-weight 10-30 kg): 22.5 mg 1–3 times a day, dose to be adjusted as necessary, to be dissolved in water and taken after food, dose expressed as elemental zinc
- Child (body-weight 31 kg and above): 45 mg 1–3 times a day, dose to be adjusted as necessary, to be dissolved in water and taken after food, dose expressed as elemental zinc

Acrodermatitis enteropathica

▶ BY MOUTH USING EFFERVESCENT TABLETS

- Neonate: 0.5–1 mg/kg twice daily, dose to be adjusted as necessary, total daily dose may alternatively be given in 3 divided doses, dose expressed as elemental zinc.
- Child: 0.5–1 mg/kg twice daily, dose to be adjusted as necessary, total daily dose may alternatively be given in 3 divided doses, dose expressed as elemental zinc

● **UNLICENSED USE** *Solvazinc*® is not licensed for use in acrodermatitis enteropathica.

● **INTERACTIONS** → Appendix 1: zinc

● **SIDE-EFFECTS** Diarrhoea · gastritis · gastrointestinal discomfort · nausea · vomiting

● **PREGNANCY** Crosses placenta; risk theoretically minimal, but no information available.

● **BREAST FEEDING** Present in milk; risk theoretically minimal, but no information available.

● **RENAL IMPAIRMENT** Accumulation may occur in acute renal failure.

● **PRESCRIBING AND DISPENSING INFORMATION** Each *Solvazinc*® tablet contains zinc sulfate monohydrate 125 mg (45 mg zinc).

● **MEDICINAL FORMS** There can be variation in the licensing of different medicines containing the same drug.

Effervescent tablet

CAUTIONARY AND ADVISORY LABELS 13, 21

▶ Solvazinc (Galen Ltd)

Zinc sulfate monohydrate 125 mg Solvazinc 125mg effervescent tablets sugar-free | 90 tablet [P] £17.20 DT = £17.20

5 Nutrition (intravenous)

Intravenous nutrition

Overview

When adequate feeding through the alimentary tract is not possible, nutrients may be given by intravenous infusion. This may be in addition to oral or enteral tube feeding—**supplemental parenteral nutrition**, or may be the sole source of nutrition— **total parenteral nutrition** (TPN). Complete enteral starvation is undesirable and total parenteral nutrition is a last resort.

Indications for parenteral nutrition include prematurity; severe or prolonged disorders of the gastro-intestinal tract; preparation of undernourished patients for surgery, chemotherapy, or radiation therapy; major surgery, trauma, or burns; prolonged coma or inability to eat; and some patients with renal or hepatic failure. The composition of proprietary preparations used in children is given under Proprietary Infusion Fluids for Parenteral Feeding p. 669.

Parenteral nutrition requires the use of a solution containing amino acids, glucose, lipids, electrolytes, trace elements, and vitamins. This is now commonly provided by the pharmacy in the form of an amino-acid, glucose, electrolyte bag, and a separate lipid infusion or, in older children a single 'all-in-one' bag. If the patient is able to take small amounts by mouth, vitamins may be given orally.

The nutrition solution is infused through a central venous catheter inserted under full surgical precautions. Alternatively, infusion through a peripheral vein may be used for supplementary as well as total parenteral nutrition, depending on the availability of peripheral veins; factors prolonging cannula life and preventing thrombophlebitis include the use of soft polyurethane paediatric cannulas and use of nutritional solutions of low osmolality and neutral pH. Nutritional fluids should be given by a dedicated intravenous line; if not possible, compatibility with any drugs or fluids should be checked as precipitation of components may occur. Extravasation of parenteral nutrition solution can cause severe tissue damage and injury; the infusion site should be regularly monitored.

Before starting intravenous nutrition the patient should be clinically stable and renal function and acid-base status should be assessed. Appropriate biochemical tests should have been carried out beforehand and serious deficits corrected. Nutritional and electrolyte status must be monitored throughout treatment. The nutritional components of parenteral nutrition regimens are usually increased gradually over a number of days to prevent metabolic complications and to allow metabolic adaptation to the infused nutrients. The solutions are usually infused over 24 hours but this may be gradually reduced if long-term nutrition is required. Home parenteral nutrition is usually infused over 12 hours overnight.

Complications of long-term parenteral nutrition include gall bladder sludging, gall stones, cholestasis and abnormal liver function tests. For details of the prevention and management of parenteral nutrition complications, specialist literature should be consulted.

Protein (nitrogen) is given as mixtures of essential and non-essential synthetic L-amino acids. Ideally, all essential amino acids should be included with a wide variety of non-essential ones to provide sufficient nitrogen together with electrolytes. Solutions vary in their composition of amino acids; they often contain an energy source (usually glucose) and electrolytes. Solutions for use in neonates and children under 1 year of age are based on the amino acid profile of umbilical cord blood (*Primene*®) or breast milk (*Vaminolact*®) and contain amino acids that are essential in this age group;

Proprietary Infusion Fluids for Parenteral Feeding

Preparation	Nitrogen g/litre	1,2 Energy kJ/litre	Electrolytes K^{+}	Mg^{2+}	Na^{+}	Acet^{-}	Cl^{-}	Other components/litre
ClinOleic 20% (Baxter Healthcare Ltd) Net price 100 ml: no price available; Net price 500 ml: no price available	-	8360	-	-	-	-	-	purified olive and soya oil 200 g, glycerol 22.5 g, egg phosphatides 12 g
Intralipid 10% (Fresenius Kabi Ltd) Net price 100 ml = £4.12; Net price 500 ml = £9.01	-	4600	-	-	-	-	-	soya oil 100 g, glycerol 22 g, purified egg phospholipids 12 g, phosphate 15 mmol
Intralipid 20% (Fresenius Kabi Ltd) Net price 100 ml = £6.21; Net price 250 ml = £10.16; Net price 500 ml = £13.52	-	8400	-	-	-	-	-	soya oil 200 g, glycerol 22 g, purified egg phospholipids 12 g, phosphate 15 mmol
Lipofundin MCT/LCT 10% (B.Braun Medical Ltd) Net price 500 ml = £13.69	-	4430	-	-	-	-	-	soya oil 50 g, medium-chain triglycerides 50 g
Lipofundin MCT/LCT 20% (B.Braun Medical Ltd) Net price 100 ml = £13.28; Net price 500 ml = £20.36	-	8000	-	-	-	-	-	soya oil 100 g, medium-chain triglycerides 100 g
Primene 10% (Baxter Healthcare Ltd) Net price 100 ml: no price available; Net price 250 ml: no price available	15.0	-	-	-	-	-	19.0	
Synthamin 9 (Baxter Healthcare Ltd) Net price 500 ml: no price available	9.1	-	60.0	5.0	70.0	100.0	70.0	acid phosphate 30 mmol
Synthamin 9 EF (electrolyte-free) (Baxter Healthcare Ltd) Net price 500 ml: no price available; Net price 1 litre: no price available	9.1	-	-	-	-	44.0	22.0	
Vaminolact (Fresenius Kabi Ltd) Net price 100 ml = £3.70; Net price 500 ml = £8.50	9.3	-	-	-	-	-	-	

1 1000 kcal = 4200kJ; 1000 kJ = 238.8 kcal. All entries are Prescription-only medicines.
2 Excludes protein- or amino acid-derived energy

these amino acids may not be present in sufficient quantities in preparations designed for older children and adults.

Energy requirements must be met if amino acids are to be utilised for tissue maintenance. An appropriate energy to protein ratio is essential and requirements will vary depending on the child's age and condition. A mixture of carbohydrate and fat energy sources (usually 30–50% as fat) gives better utilisation of amino acids than glucose alone.

Glucose p. 638 is the preferred source of carbohydrate, but frequent monitoring of blood glucose is required particularly during initiation and build-up of the regimen; insulin may be necessary. Glucose above a concentration of 12.5% must be infused through a central venous catheter to avoid thrombosis; the maximum concentration of glucose that should normally be infused in fluid restricted children is 20–25%.

In parenteral nutrition regimens, it is necessary to provide adequate **phosphate** in order to allow phosphorylation of glucose and to prevent hypophosphataemia. Neonates, particularly preterm neonates, and young children also require phosphorus and calcium to ensure adequate bone mineralisation. The compatibility and solubility of calcium and phosphorus salts is complex and unpredictable; precipitation is a risk and specialist pharmacy advice should be sought.

Fat (lipid) emulsions have the advantages of a high energy to fluid volume ratio, neutral pH, and iso-osmolarity with plasma, and provide essential fatty acids. Several days of adaptation may be required to attain maximal utilisation. Reactions include occasional febrile episodes (usually only with 20% emulsions) and rare anaphylactic responses. Interference with biochemical measurements such as those for blood gases and calcium may occur if samples are taken before fat has been cleared. Regular monitoring of plasma cholesterol and triglyceride is necessary to ensure clearance from the plasma, particularly in conditions where fat metabolism may be disturbed e.g. infection. Emulsions containing 20% or 30% fat should be used in neonates as they are cleared more efficiently. **Additives should not be mixed with fat emulsions unless compatibility is known.**

Electrolytes are usually provided as the chloride salts of potassium and sodium. Acetate salts can be used to reduce the amount of chloride infused; hyperchloraemic acidosis or hypochloraemic alkalosis can occur in preterm neonates or children with renal impairment.

Adminstration

Because of the complex requirements relating to parenteral nutrition full details relating to administration have been omitted. In all cases *specialist pharmacy advice, product literature and other specialist literature should be consulted.*

NUTRIENTS > PARENTERAL NUTRITION

Parenteral nutrition supplements

27-Apr-2020

● **INDICATIONS AND DOSE**

Supplement in intravenous nutrition

▶ BY INTRAVENOUS INFUSION, OR BY SLOW INTRAVENOUS INJECTION

▶ Child: (consult product literature)

continued →

DIPEPTIVEN 20G/100ML CONCENTRATE FOR SOLUTION FOR INFUSION BOTTLES

Amino acid supplement for hypercatabolic or hypermetabolic states

- BY INTRAVENOUS INFUSION
- Child: 300–400 mg/kg daily, dose not to exceed 20% of total amino acid intake

IMPORTANT SAFETY INFORMATION

MHRA/CHM ADVICE: PARENTERAL NUTRITION PRODUCTS: LIGHT PROTECTION REQUIRED TO REDUCE THE RISK OF SERIOUS ADVERSE EFFECTS IN PREMATURE NEONATES (SEPTEMBER 2019)

- In neonates

Containers and administration sets of parenteral nutrition products containing amino acids and/or lipids should be protected from light during administration to neonates and children under 2 years of age. Studies found that light exposure caused formation of peroxides and other degradation products that may lead to adverse effects when given to premature neonates (who are considered to be at high risk of oxidative stress); this advice was extended to all neonates and children aged under 2 years as a precautionary measure.

- **CAUTIONS**

PEDITRACE SOLUTION FOR INFUSION 10ML VIALS Reduced biliary excretion · reduced biliary excretion in cholestatic liver disease · reduced biliary excretion in markedly reduced urinary excretion (careful biochemical monitoring required) · total parenteral nutrition exceeding one month

CAUTIONS, FURTHER INFORMATION

- Total parenteral nutrition exceeding one month Measure serum manganese concentration and check liver function before commencing treatment and regularly during treatment—discontinue if manganese concentration raised or if cholestasis develops.

- **DIRECTIONS FOR ADMINISTRATION** Because of the complex requirements relating to parenteral nutrition, full details relating to administration have been omitted. In all cases *specialist pharmacy advice, product literature, and other specialist literature should be consulted.* Compatibility with the infusion solution must be ascertained before adding supplementary preparations. **Additives should not be mixed with fat emulsions unless compatibility is known.**

PEDITRACE SOLUTION FOR INFUSION 10ML VIALS For addition to *Vaminolact*®, *Vamin*® 14 *Electrolyte-Free* solutions, and glucose intravenous infusions.

ADDITRACE SOLUTION FOR INFUSION 10ML AMPOULES For addition to *Vamin*® solutions and glucose intravenous infusions.

DIPEPTIVEN 20G/100ML CONCENTRATE FOR SOLUTION FOR INFUSION BOTTLES For addition to infusion solutions containing amino acids.

ADDIPHOS® VIALS For addition to *Vamin*® solutions and glucose intravenous infusions.

DECAN CONCENTRATE FOR SOLUTION FOR INFUSION 40ML BOTTLES For addition to infusion solutions.

SOLIVITO N POWDER FOR SOLUTION FOR INFUSION VIALS Dissolve in water for injections or glucose intravenous infusion for adding to glucose intravenous infusion or *Intralipid*®; dissolve in *Vitlipid N*® or *Intralipid*® for adding to *Intralipid*® only.

VITLIPID N ADULT EMULSION FOR INJECTION 10ML AMPOULES For addition to *Intralipid*®.

VITLIPID N INFANT EMULSION FOR INJECTION 10ML AMPOULES For addition to *Intralipid*®.

CERNEVIT® POWDER FOR SOLUTION FOR INJECTION VIALS Dissolve in 5 mL water for injections or Glucose 5% or Sodium Chloride 0.9% for adding to infusion solutions.

- **PRESCRIBING AND DISPENSING INFORMATION**

PEDITRACE SOLUTION FOR INFUSION 10ML VIALS For use in neonates (when kidney function established, usually second day of life), infants, and children.

Peditrace® solution contains traces of Zn^{2+}, Cu^{2+}, Mn^{2+}, Se^{4+}, F^-, I^-.

ADDITRACE SOLUTION FOR INFUSION 10ML AMPOULES For patients over 40 kg.

Additrace® solution contains traces of Fe^{3+}, Zn^{2+}, Mn^{2+}, Cu^{2+}, Cr^{3+}, Se^{4+}, Mo^{6+}, F^-, I^-.

DIPEPTIVEN 20G/100ML CONCENTRATE FOR SOLUTION FOR INFUSION BOTTLES *Dipeptiven*® solution contains N(2)-L-alanyl-L-glutamine 200 mg/mL (providing L-alanine 82 mg, L-glutamine 134.6 mg).

ADDIPHOS® VIALS *Addiphos*® sterile solution contains phosphate 40 mmol, K^+ 30 mmol, Na^+ 30 mmol/20 mL.

DECAN CONCENTRATE FOR SOLUTION FOR INFUSION 40ML BOTTLES For patients over 40 kg.

Decan® solution contains trace elements Fe^{2+}, Zn^{2+}, Cu^{2+}, Mn^{2+}, F^-, Co^{2+}, I^-, Se^{4+}, Mo^{6+}, Cr^{3+}.

SOLIVITO N POWDER FOR SOLUTION FOR INFUSION VIALS *Solivito N*® powder for reconstitution contains biotin 60 micrograms, cyanocobalamin 5 micrograms, folic acid 400 micrograms, glycine 300 mg, nicotinamide 40 mg, pyridoxine hydrochloride 4.9 mg, riboflavin sodium phosphate 4.9 mg, sodium ascorbate 113 mg, sodium pantothenate 16.5 mg, thiamine mononitrate 3.1 mg.

VITLIPID N ADULT EMULSION FOR INJECTION 10ML AMPOULES *Vitlipid N*® adult emulsion contains vitamin A 330 units, ergocalciferol 20 units, *dl*-alpha tocopherol 1 unit, phytomenadione 15 micrograms/mL.

For adults and children over 11 years.

VITLIPID N INFANT EMULSION FOR INJECTION 10ML AMPOULES *Vitlipid N*® infant emulsion contains vitamin A 230 units, ergocalciferol 40 units, *dl*-alpha tocopherol 0.7 unit, phytomenadione 20 micrograms/mL.

CERNEVIT® POWDER FOR SOLUTION FOR INJECTION VIALS *Cernevit*® powder for reconstitution contains *dl*-alpha tocopherol 10.2 mg, ascorbic acid 125 mg, biotin 69 micrograms, colecalciferol 220 units, cyanocobalamin 6 micrograms, folic acid 414 micrograms, nicotinamide 46 mg, pantothenic acid (as dexpanthenol) 17.25 mg, pyridoxine hydrochloride 5.5 mg, retinol (as palmitate) 3500 units, riboflavin (as dihydrated sodium phosphate) 4.14 mg, thiamine (as cocarboxylase tetrahydrate) 3.51 mg.

For adults and children over 11 years.

- **MEDICINAL FORMS** There can be variation in the licensing of different medicines containing the same drug. Forms available from special-order manufacturers include: solution for infusion

Solution for infusion

- Parenteral nutrition supplements (Non-proprietary)

Sodium glycerophosphate 216 mg per 1 ml Sodium glycerophosphate 4.32g/20ml concentrate for solution for infusion vials | 1 vial PoM £5.60

- Additrace (Fresenius Kabi Ltd)

Sodium molybdate 4.85 microgram per 1 ml, Chromic chloride 5.33 microgram per 1 ml, Sodium selenite 10.5 microgram per 1 ml, Potassium iodide 16.6 microgram per 1 ml, Manganese chloride 99 microgram per 1 ml, Sodium fluoride 210 microgram per 1 ml, Copper chloride 340 microgram per 1 ml, Ferric chloride 544 microgram per 1 ml, Zinc chloride 1.36 mg per 1 ml Additrace concentrate for solution for infusion 10ml ampoules | 1 ampoule PoM £1.96

- ▸ Dipeptiven (Fresenius Kabi Ltd)
  N(2)-L-alanyl-L-glutamine 200 mg per 1 ml Dipeptiven 20g/100ml concentrate for solution for infusion bottles | 1 bottle PoM £25.93
  Dipeptiven 10g/50ml concentrate for solution for infusion bottles | 1 bottle PoM £13.94
- ▸ Peditrace (Fresenius Kabi Ltd)
  Manganese (as Manganese chloride) 1 microgram per 1 ml, Iodine (as Potassium iodide) 1 microgram per 1 ml, Selenium (as Sodium selenite) 2 microgram per 1 ml, Copper (as Copper chloride) 20 microgram per 1 ml, Fluoride (as Sodium fluoride) 57 microgram per 1 ml, Zinc (as Zinc chloride) 250 microgram per 1 ml Peditrace solution for infusion 10ml vials | 1 vial PoM £3.55
- ▸ Tracutil (B.Braun Melsungen AG)
  Sodium molybdate dihydrate 2.42 microgram per 1 ml, Chromic chloride 5.3 microgram per 1 ml, Sodium selenite pentahydrate 7.89 microgram per 1 ml, Potassium iodide 16.6 microgram per 1 ml, Sodium fluoride 126 microgram per 1 ml, Manganese chloride 197.9 microgram per 1 ml, Copper chloride 204.6 microgram per 1 ml, Zinc chloride 681.5 microgram per 1 ml, Ferrous chloride 695.8 microgram per 1 ml Tracutil concentrate for solution for infusion 10ml ampoules | 5 ampoule PoM £7.96

Powder for solution for infusion

- ▸ Solivito N (Fresenius Kabi Ltd)
  Cyanocobalamin 5 microgram, Biotin 60 microgram, Folic acid 400 microgram, Thiamine nitrate 3.1 mg, Pyridoxine hydrochloride 4.9 mg, Riboflavin sodium phosphate 4.9 mg, Sodium pantothenate 16.5 mg, Nicotinamide 40 mg, Sodium ascorbate 113 mg Solivito N powder for solution for infusion vials | 1 vial PoM £1.97

Emulsion for injection

- ▸ Vitlipid N Adult (Fresenius Kabi Ltd)
  Ergocalciferol 500 nanogram per 1 ml, Phytomenadione 15 microgram per 1 ml, Retinol palmitate 99 microgram per 1 ml, Alpha tocopherol 910 microgram per 1 ml Vitlipid N Adult emulsion for infusion 10ml ampoules | 1 ampoule PoM £1.97
- ▸ Vitlipid N Infant (Fresenius Kabi Ltd)
  Ergocalciferol 1 microgram per 1 ml, Phytomenadione 20 microgram per 1 ml, Retinol palmitate 69 microgram per 1 ml, Alpha tocopherol 640 microgram per 1 ml Vitlipid N Infant emulsion for infusion 10ml ampoules | 1 ampoule PoM £1.97

Powder for solution for injection

EXCIPIENTS: May contain Glycocholic acid

- ▸ Cernevit (Baxter Healthcare Ltd)
  Cyanocobalamin 6 microgram, Biotin 69 microgram, Folic acid 414 microgram, Thiamine 3.51 mg, Riboflavin (as Riboflavin sodium phosphate) 4.14 mg, Pyridoxine (as Pyridoxine hydrochloride) 4.53 mg, Pantothenic acid (as Dexpanthenol) 17.25 mg, Nicotinamide 46 mg, Ascorbic acid 125 mg, Alpha tocopherol 11.2 unit, Colecalciferol 220 unit, Retinol 3500 unit Cernevit powder for solution for injection vials | 10 vial PoM

6 Nutrition (oral)

Enteral nutrition

Overview

Children have higher nutrient requirements per kg bodyweight, different metabolic rates, and physiological responses compared to adults. They have low nutritional stores and are particularly vulnerable to growth and nutritional problems during critical periods of development. Major illness, operations, or trauma impose increased metabolic demands and can rapidly exhaust nutritional reserves.

Every effort should be made to optimise oral food intake before beginning enteral tube feeding; this may include change of posture, special seating, feeding equipment, oral desensitisation, food texture changes, thickening of liquids, increasing energy density of food, treatment of reflux or oesophagitis, as well as using age-specific nutritional supplements.

Enteral tube feeding has a role in both short-term rehabilitation and long-term nutritional management in paediatrics. It can be used as supportive therapy, in which the enteral feed supplies a proportion of the required nutrients, or as primary therapy, in which the enteral feed delivers all the necessary nutrients. Most children receiving tube feeds should also be encouraged to take oral food and drink. Tube feeding should be considered in the following situations:

- unsafe swallowing and risk of aspiration
- inability to consume at least 60% of energy needs by mouth
- total feeding time of more than 4 hours per day
- weight loss or no weight gain for a period of 3 months (less for younger children and infants)
- weight for height (or length) less than 2nd percentile for age and sex

Most feeds for enteral use contain protein derived from cows' milk or soya. Elemental feeds containing protein hydrolysates or free amino acids can be used for children who have diminished ability to break down protein, for example in inflammatory bowel disease or pancreatic insufficiency.

Even when nutritionally complete feeds are given, water and electrolyte balance should be monitored. Haematological and biochemical parameters should also be monitored, particularly in the clinically unstable child. Extra minerals (e.g. magnesium and zinc) may be needed in patients where gastro-intestinal secretions are being lost. Additional vitamins may also be needed.

Choosing the best formula for children depends on several factors including: nutritional requirements, gastro-intestinal function, underlying disease, nutrient restrictions, age, and feed characteristics (nutritional composition, viscosity, osmolality, availability and cost). Children have specific dietary requirements and in many situations liquid feeds prepared for adults are totally unsuitable and should not be given. Expert advice from a dietician should be sought before prescribing enteral feeds for a child.

Infant formula feeds

Child 0–12 months. Term infants with normal gastro-intestinal function are given either breast milk or normal infant formula during the first year of life. The average intake is between 150 mL and 200 mL/kg/day. Infant milk formulas are based on whey- or casein-dominant protein, lactose with or without maltodextrin, amylose, vegetable oil and milk fat. The composition of all normal and soya infant formulas have to meet The Infant Formula and Follow-on Formula Regulations (England and Wales) 2007, which enact the European Community Regulations 2006/141/EC; the composition of other enteral and specialist feeds has to meet the Commission Directive (1999/21/EC) on Dietary Foods for Special Medical Purposes.

A high-energy feed, which contains 9–11% of energy derived from protein can be used for infants who fail to grow adequately. Alternatively, energy supplements may be added to normal infant formula to achieve a higher energy content (but this will reduce the protein to energy ratio) or the normal infant formula concentration may be increased slightly. Care should be taken not to present an osmotic load of more than 500 milliosmols/kg water to the normal functioning gut, otherwise osmotic diarrhoea will result. Concentrating or supplementing feeds should not be attempted without the advice of a paediatric dietician.

Enteral feeds

Child 1–6 years (body-weight 8–20 kg). Ready-to-use feeds based on caseinates, maltodextrin and vegetable oils (with or without added medium chain triglyceride (MCT) oil or fibre) are well tolerated and effective in improving nutritional status in this age group. Although originally designed for children 1–6 years (body-weight 8–20 kg),

9 Blood and nutrition

some products have ACBS approval for use in children weighing up to 30 kg (approx. 10 years of age). Enteral feeds formulated for children 1–6 years are low in sodium and potassium; electrolyte intake and biochemical status should be monitored. Older children in this age range taking small feed volumes may need to be given additional micronutrients. Fibre-enriched feeds may be helpful for children with chronic constipation or diarrhoea.

Child 7–12 years (body-weight 21–45 kg). Depending on age, weight, clinical condition and nutritional requirements, ready-to-use feeds formulated for 7–12 year olds may be given at appropriate rates.

Child over 12 years (body-weight over 45 kg). As there are no standard enteral feeds formulated for this age group, adult formulations are used. The intake of protein, electrolytes, vitamins, and trace minerals should be carefully assessed and monitored. Note: Adult feeds containing more than 6 g/100 mL protein or 2 g/100 mL fibre should be used with caution and expert advice.

Specialised formula

It is essential that any infant who is intolerant of breast milk or normal infant formula, or whose condition requires nutrient-specific adaptation, is prescribed an adequate volume of a nutritionally complete replacement formula. In the first 4 months of life, a volume of 150–200 mL/kg/day is recommended. After 6 months, should the formula still be required, a volume of 600 mL/day should be maintained, in addition to solid food.

Products for cow's milk protein intolerance or lactose intolerance. There are a number of infant formulas formulated for cow's milk protein intolerance or lactose intolerance; these feeds may contain a residual amount of lactose (less than 1 g/100 mL formula)—sometimes described as clinically lactose-free or 'lactose-free' by manufacturers. If the total daily intake of these formulas is low, it may be necessary to supplement with calcium, and a vitamin and mineral supplement.

Soya-based infant formulas have a high phytoestrogen content and this may be a long-term reproductive health risk. The Chief Medical Officer has advised that soya-based infant formulas should not be used as the first choice for the management of infants with proven cow's milk sensitivity, lactose intolerance, galactokinase deficiency and galactosaemia. Most UK paediatricians with expertise in inherited metabolic disease still advocate soya-based formulations for infants with galactosaemia as there are concerns about the residual lactose content of low lactose formulas and protein hydrolysates based on cow's milk protein.

Low lactose infant formulations, based on whole cow's milk protein, are unsuitable for children with cow's milk protein intolerance. Liquid soya milks purchased from supermarkets and health food stores are not nutritionally complete and should never be used for infants under 1 year of age.

Protein hydrolysate formulas. Non-milk, peptide-based feeds containing hydrolysates of casein, whey, meat and soya protein, are suitable for infants with disaccharide or whole protein intolerance. The total daily intake of electrolytes, vitamins and minerals should be carefully assessed and modified to meet the child's nutritional requirements; these feeds have a high osmolality when given at recommended dilution and need gradual and careful introduction.

Elemental (amino acid based formula). Specially formulated elemental feeds containing essential and nonessential amino acids are available for use in infants and children under 6 years with proven whole protein intolerance. Adult elemental formula may be used for children over 6 years; the intake of electrolytes, vitamins and minerals should be carefully assessed and modified to meet nutritional requirements. These feeds have a high osmolality when given at the recommended concentration and therefore need gradual and careful introduction.

Modular feeds. Modular feeds (see Specialised Formulas for Specific Clinical Conditions) are based on individual protein, fat, carbohydrate, vitamin and mineral components or modules which can be combined to meet the specific needs of a child. Modular feeds are used when nutritionally complete specialised formula are not tolerated, or if the fluid and nutrient requirements change e.g. in gastro-intestinal, renal or liver disease. The main advantage of modular feeds is their flexibility; disadvantages include their complexity and preparation difficulties. Modular feeds should not be used without the supervision of a paediatric dietician.

Specialised formula. Highly specialised formulas are designed to meet the specific requirements in various clinical conditions such as renal and liver diseases. When using these formulas, both the biochemical status of the child and their growth parameters need to be monitored.

Feed thickeners

Carob based thickeners may be used to thicken feeds for infants under 1 year with significant gastro-oesophageal reflux. Breast-fed infants can be given the thickener mixed to a paste with water or breast-milk prior to feeds.

Pre-thickened formula Milk-protein- or casein-dominant infant formula, which contains small quantities of pre-gelatinized starch, is recommended primarily for infants with mild gastro-oesophageal reflux. Pre-thickened formula is prepared in the same way as normal infant formula and flows through a standard teat. The feeds do not thicken on standing but thicken in the stomach when exposed to acid pH.

Starched based thickeners can be used to thicken liquids and feeds for children over 1 year of age with dysphagia.

Dietary supplements for oral use

Three types of prescribable fortified dietary supplements are available: fortified milk and non-milk tasting (juice-style) drinks, and fortified milk-based semi-solid preparations. The recommended daily quantity is age-dependent. The following is a useful guide: 1–2 years, 200 kcal (840 kJ); 3–5 years, 400 kcal (1680 kJ); 6–11 years, 600 kcal (2520 kJ); and over 12 years, 800 kcal (3360 kJ). Supplements containing 1.5 kcal/mL are high in protein and should not be used for children under 3 years of age. Many supplements are high in sugar or maltodextrin; care should be taken to prevent prolonged contact with teeth. Ideally supplements should be administered after meals or at bedtime so as not to affect appetite.

Products for metabolic diseases

There is a large range of disease-specific infant formulas and amino acid-based supplements available for use in children with metabolic diseases (see under specific metabolic diseases. Some of these formulas are nutritionally incomplete and supplementation with vitamins and other nutrients may be necessary. Many of the product names are similar; to prevent metabolic complications in children who cannot tolerate specific amino acids it is important to ensure the correct supplement is supplied.

Enteral feeding tubes

Care is required in choosing an appropriate formulation of a drug for administration through a nasogastric narrow-bore feeding tube or through a percutaneous endoscopic gastrostomy (PEG) or jejunostomy tube. Liquid preparations (or soluble tablets) are preferred; injection solutions may also be suitable for administration through an enteral tube.

If a solid formulation of a medicine needs to be given, it should be given as a suspension of particles fine enough to pass through the tube. It is possible to crush many immediate-release tablets but enteric-coated or modified-release preparations should **not** be crushed.

Enteral feeds may affect the absorption of drugs and it is therefore important to consider the timing of drug administration in relation to feeds. If more than one drug needs to be given, they should be given separately and the tube should be flushed with water after each drug has been given.

Clearing blockages

Carbonated (sugar-free) drinks may be marginally more effective than water in unblocking feeding tubes, but mildly acidic liquids (such as pineapple juice or cola-based drinks) can coagulate protein in feeds, causing further blockage. If these measures fail to clear the enteral feeding tube, an alkaline solution containing pancreatic enzymes may be introduced into the tube (followed after at least 5 minutes by water). Specific products designed to break up blockages caused by formula feeds are also available.

6.1 Special diets

Nutrition in special diets

Overview

These are preparations that have been modified to eliminate a particular constituent from a food or that are nutrient mixtures formulated as food substitutes for children who either cannot tolerate or cannot metabolise certain common constituents of food.

Coeliac disease

Coeliac disease is caused by an abnormal immune response to gluten. For management and further information, see Coeliac disease p. 30.

Phenylketonuria

Phenylketonuria (hyperphenylalaninaemia, PKU), which results from the inability to metabolise **phenylalanine**, is managed by restricting dietary intake of **phenylalanine** to a small amount sufficient for tissue building and repair.

Aspartame (used as a sweetener in some foods and medicines) contributes to the **phenylalanine** intake and may affect control of *phenylketonuria*. If alternatives are unavailable, children with phenylketonuria should not be denied access to appropriate medication; the amount of **aspartame** consumed can be taken in to account in the management of the condition. Where the presence of **aspartame** in a preparation is specified in the product literature, **aspartame** is listed as an excipient in the relevant product entry in *BNF for Children*; the child or carer should be informed of this.

Some rare forms *of phenylketonuria* are caused by a deficiency of **tetrahydrobiopterin**. Treatment involves oral supplementation of tetrahydrobiopterin p. 674; in some severe cases, the addition of the neurotransmitter precursors, levodopa and 5-hydroxytryptophan, is also necessary.

Sapropterin dihydrochloride below, a synthetic form of tetrahydrobiopterin p. 674, is licensed as an adjunct to dietary restriction of **phenylalanine** in the management of patients with *phenylketonuria* and *tetrahydrobiopterin deficiency*.

Products for metabolic diseases

There is a large range of disease-specific infant formulas and amino acid-based supplements available for use in children with metabolic diseases (see under specific metabolic diseases). Some of these formulas are nutritionally incomplete and supplementation with vitamins and other nutrients may be necessary. Many of the product names are similar; to prevent metabolic complications in children who cannot tolerate specific amino acids it is important to ensure the correct supplement is supplied.

6.1a Phenylketonuria

DRUGS FOR METABOLIC DISORDERS › TETRAHYDROBIOPTERIN AND DERIVATIVES

Sapropterin dihydrochloride 29-Apr-2020

- **INDICATIONS AND DOSE**

Phenylketonuria (adjunct to dietary restriction of phenylalanine) (specialist use only)

▶ BY MOUTH

▶ Child 4–17 years: Initially 10 mg/kg once daily, adjusted according to response; usual dose 5–20 mg/kg once daily, dose to be taken preferably in the morning

Tetrahydrobiopterin deficiency (adjunct to dietary restriction of phenylalanine) (specialist use only)

▶ BY MOUTH

▶ Neonate: Initially 2–5 mg/kg once daily, adjusted according to response, dose to be taken preferably in the morning, the total daily dose may alternatively be given in 2–3 divided doses; maximum 20 mg/kg per day.

▶ Child: Initially 2–5 mg/kg once daily, adjusted according to response, dose to be taken preferably in the morning, the total daily dose may alternatively be given in 2–3 divided doses; maximum 20 mg/kg per day

- **CAUTIONS** History of convulsions
- **INTERACTIONS** → Appendix 1: sapropterin
- **SIDE-EFFECTS**

▶ **Common or very common** Cough · diarrhoea · gastrointestinal discomfort · headache · laryngeal pain · nasal complaints · nausea · vomiting

▶ **Frequency not known** Gastrointestinal disorders · rash

- **PREGNANCY** Manufacturer advises caution—consider only if strict dietary management inadequate.
- **BREAST FEEDING** Manufacturer advises avoid—no information available.
- **HEPATIC IMPAIRMENT** Manufacturer advises caution (no information available).
- **RENAL IMPAIRMENT** Manufacturer advises caution—no information available.
- **MONITORING REQUIREMENTS**

▶ Monitor blood-phenylalanine concentration before and after first week of treatment—if unsatisfactory response increase dose at weekly intervals to max. dose and monitor blood-phenylalanine concentration weekly; discontinue treatment if unsatisfactory response after 1 month.

▶ Monitor blood-phenylalanine and tyrosine concentrations 1–2 weeks after dose adjustment and during treatment.

- **DIRECTIONS FOR ADMINISTRATION** Tablets should be dissolved in water and taken within 20 minutes.
- **PRESCRIBING AND DISPENSING INFORMATION** Sapropterin is a synthetic form of tetrahydrobiopterin.
- **PATIENT AND CARER ADVICE** Patient or carers should be given advice on how to administer sapropterin dihydrochloride dispersible tablets.
- **NATIONAL FUNDING/ACCESS DECISIONS**

Scottish Medicines Consortium (SMC) decisions

SMC No. 558/09

The *Scottish Medicines Consortium* has advised (August 2018) that sapropterin dihydrochloride (*Kuvan*®) is **not** recommended for use within NHS Scotland for the treatment of hyperphenylalaninaemia in adults and paediatric patients of all ages with phenylketonuria (who have been shown to be responsive to such treatment) as the economic case was not demonstrated.

- **MEDICINAL FORMS** There can be variation in the licensing of different medicines containing the same drug.

Soluble tablet

CAUTIONARY AND ADVISORY LABELS 13, 21

▸ Kuvan(BioMarin Europe Ltd)

Sapropterin dihydrochloride 100 mg Kuvan 100mg soluble tablets sugar-free | 30 tablet PoM £597.22

Tetrahydrobiopterin

- **INDICATIONS AND DOSE**

Monotherapy in tetrahydrobiopterin-sensitive phenylketonuria (specialist use only)

▸ BY MOUTH

▸ Child: 10 mg/kg twice daily, adjusted according to response, total daily dose may alternatively be given in 3 divided doses

In combination with neurotransmitter precursors for tetrahydrobiopterin-sensitive phenylketonuria (specialist use only)

▸ BY MOUTH

▸ Child 1 month–1 year: Initially 250–750 micrograms/kg 4 times a day, adjusted according to response, total daily dose may alternatively be given in 3 divided doses; maximum 7 mg/kg per day

▸ Child 2–17 years: Initially 250–750 micrograms/kg 4 times a day, adjusted according to response, total daily dose may alternatively be given in 3 divided doses; maximum 10 mg/kg per day

- **UNLICENSED USE** Not licensed.
- **SIDE-EFFECTS** Diarrhoea · sleep disorder · urinary frequency increased
- **PREGNANCY** Crosses the placenta; use only if benefit outweighs risk.
- **BREAST FEEDING** Present in milk, effects unknown.
- **RENAL IMPAIRMENT** Use with caution—accumulation of metabolites.

- **MEDICINAL FORMS** No licensed medicines listed.

7 Vitamin deficiency

Vitamins

Overview

Vitamins are used for the prevention and treatment of specific deficiency states or where the diet is known to be inadequate; they may be prescribed in the NHS to prevent or treat deficiency but not as dietary supplements. Except for iron-deficiency anaemia, a primary vitamin or mineral deficiency due to simple dietary inadequacy is rare in the developed world. Some children may be at risk of developing deficiencies because of an inadequate intake, impaired vitamin synthesis or malabsorption in disease states such as cystic fibrosis and Crohn's disease.

The use of vitamins as general 'pick-me-ups' is of unproven value and, the 'fad' for mega-vitamin therapy with water-soluble vitamins, such as ascorbic acid p. 680 and pyridoxine hydrochloride p. 678, is unscientific and can be harmful. Many vitamin supplements are described as 'multivitamin' but few contain the whole range of essential vitamins and many contain relatively high amounts of vitamins A and D. Care should be taken to ensure the correct dose is not exceeded.

Dietary reference values for vitamins are available in the Department of Health publication:

Dietary Reference Values for Food Energy and Nutrients for the United Kingdom: Report of the Panel on Dietary Reference Values of the Committee on Medical Aspects of Food Policy. *Report on Health and Social Subjects* 41. London: HMSO, 1991.

Dental patients

It is unjustifiable to treat stomatitis or glossitis with mixtures of vitamin preparations; this delays diagnosis and correct treatment.

Most patients who develop a nutritional deficiency despite an adequate intake of vitamins have malabsorption and if this is suspected the patient should be referred to a medical practitioner.

Vitamin A

Deficiency of vitamin A (retinol) p. 677 is associated with ocular defects (particularly xerophthalmia) and an increased susceptibility to infections, but deficiency is rare in the UK (even in disorders of fat absorption).

Vitamin A supplementation may be required in children with liver disease, particularly cholestatic liver disease, due to the malabsorption of fat soluble vitamins. In those with complete biliary obstruction an intramuscular dose once a month may be appropriate.

Preterm neonates have low plasma concentrations of vitamin A and are usually given vitamin A supplements, often as part of an oral multivitamin preparation once enteral feeding has been established.

Vitamin B group

Deficiency of the B vitamins, other than vitamin B_{12}, is rare in the UK and is usually treated by preparations containing thiamine (B_1) p. 678, and riboflavin (B_2). Other members (or substances traditionally classified as members) of the vitamin B complex such as aminobenzoic acid, biotin, choline, inositol nicotinate, and pantothenic acid or panthenol may be included in vitamin B preparations, but there is no evidence of their value as supplements; however, they can be used in the management of certain metabolic disorders. Anaphylaxis has been reported with parenteral B vitamins.

As with other vitamins of the B group, pyridoxine hydrochloride (B_6) deficiency is rare, but it may occur during isoniazid p. 399 therapy or penicillamine p. 666 treatment in Wilson's disease and is characterised by peripheral neuritis. High doses of pyridoxine hydrochloride are given in some metabolic disorders, such as hyperoxaluria, cystathioninuria and homocystinuria; folic acid p. 620 supplementation may also be beneficial in these disorders. Pyridoxine hydrochloride is also used in sideroblastic anaemia. Rarely, seizures in the neonatal period or during infancy respond to pyridoxine hydrochloride treatment; pyridoxine hydrochloride should be tried in all cases of early-onset intractable seizures and status epilepticus. Pyridoxine hydrochloride has been tried for a wide variety of other disorders, but there is little sound evidence to support the claims of efficacy.

A number of mitochondrial disorders may respond to treatment with certain B vitamins but these disorders require specialist management. Thiamine is used in the treatment of maple syrup urine disease, mitochondrial respiratory chain defects and, together with riboflavin, in the treatment of congenital lactic acidosis; riboflavin is also used in glutaric acidaemias and cytochrome oxidase deficiencies; biotin is used in carboxylase defects.

Folic acid and vitamin B_{12} are used in the treatment of megaloblastic anaemia. Folinic acid p. 600 (available as calcium folinate) is used in association with cytotoxic therapy.

Vitamin C

Vitamin C (ascorbic acid) therapy is essential in scurvy, but less florid manifestations of vitamin C deficiency have been reported. Vitamin C is used to enhance the excretion of iron one month after starting desferrioxamine mesilate p. 624 therapy; it is given separately from food as it also enhances iron absorption. Vitamin C is also used in the treatment of some inherited metabolic disorders, particularly mitochondrial disorders; specialist management of these conditions is required.

Severe scurvy causes gingival swelling and bleeding margins as well as petechiae on the skin. This is, however, exceedingly rare and a child with these signs is more likely to have leukaemia. Investigation should not be delayed by a trial period of vitamin treatment.

Claims that vitamin C ameliorates colds or promotes wound healing have not been proved.

Vitamin D

The term Vitamin D is used for a range of compounds including ergocalciferol (calciferol, vitamin D_2) p. 684, colecalciferol (vitamin D_3) p. 681, dihydrotachysterol, alfacalcidol (1α-hydroxycholecalciferol) p. 680, and calcitriol (1,25- dihydroxycholecalciferol) p. 681.

Asymptomatic vitamin D deficiency is common in the United Kingdom; symptomatic deficiency may occur in certain ethnic groups, particularly as rickets or hypocalcaemia, and rarely in association with malabsorption. The amount of vitamin D required in infancy is related to the stores built up *in-utero* and subsequent exposure to sunlight. The amount of vitamin D in breast milk varies and some breast-fed babies, particularly if preterm or born to vitamin D deficient mothers, may become deficient. Most formula milk and supplement feeds contain adequate vitamin D to prevent deficiency.

Simple, nutritional vitamin D deficiency can be prevented by oral supplementation of ergocalciferol (calciferol, vitamin D_2) or colecalciferol (vitamin D_3) daily, using multi-vitamin drops, preparations of vitamins A and D, manufactured 'special' solutions, or as calcium and ergocalciferol tablets (although the calcium and other vitamins in supplements are unnecessary); excessive supplementation may cause hypercalcaemia.

Inadequate bone mineralisation can be caused by a deficiency, or a lack of action of vitamin D or its active metabolite. In childhood this causes bowing and distortion of bones (rickets). In nutritional vitamin D deficiency rickets, initial high doses of ergocalciferol or colecalciferol should be reduced to supplemental doses after 8–12 weeks, as there is a significant risk of hypercalcaemia. However, calcium supplements are recommended if there is hypocalcaemia or evidence of a poor dietary calcium intake. A single large dose of ergocalciferol p. 684 or colecalciferol p. 681 can also be effective for the treatment of nutritional vitamin D deficiency rickets.

Poor bone mineralisation in neonates and young children may also be due to inadequate intake of phosphate or calcium particularly during long-term parenteral nutrition—supplementation with phosphate or calcium may be required.

Hypophosphataemic rickets occurs due to abnormal phosphate excretion; treatment with high doses of oral phosphate, and hydroxylated (activated) forms of vitamin D allow bone mineralisation and optimise growth.

Nutritional deficiency of vitamin D is best treated with colecalciferol or ergocalciferol. Preparations containing calcium and colecalciferol are also occasionally used in children where there is evidence of combined calcium and vitamin D deficiency. Vitamin D deficiency caused by *intestinal malabsorption* or *chronic liver disease* usually requires vitamin D in pharmacological doses; the hypocalcaemia of *hypoparathyroidism* often requires higher doses in order to achieve normocalcaemia and alfacalcidol p. 680 is generally preferred.

Vitamin D supplementation is often given in combination with calcium supplements for persistent hypocalcaemia in neonates, and in chronic renal disease

Vitamin D requires hydroxylation, by the kidney and liver, to its active form therefore the hydroxylated derivatives alfacalcidol or calcitriol p. 681 should be prescribed if patients with *severe liver or renal impairment* require vitamin D therapy. Alfacalcidol is generally preferred in children as there is more experience of its use and appropriate formulations are available. Calcitriol is unlicensed for use in children and is generally reserved for those with severe liver disease.

Paricalcitol p. 685, a synthetic vitamin D analogue, is licensed for the prevention and treatment of secondary hyperparathyroidism associated with chronic kidney disease.

Vitamin E

The daily requirement of vitamin E (tocopherol) has not been well defined. Vitamin E supplements are given to children with fat malabsorption such as in cystic fibrosis and cholestatic liver disease. In children with abetalipoproteinaemia abnormally low vitamin E concentrations may occur in association with neuromuscular problems; this usually responds to high doses of vitamin E. Some neonatal units still administer a single intramuscular dose of vitamin E at birth to preterm neonates to reduce the risk of complications; no trials of long-term outcome have been carried out. The intramuscular route should also be considered in children with severe liver disease when response to oral therapy is inadequate.

Vitamin E has been tried for various other conditions but there is little scientific evidence of its value.

Vitamin K

Vitamin K is necessary for the production of blood clotting factors and proteins necessary for the normal calcification of bone.

Because vitamin K is fat soluble, children with fat malabsorption, especially in biliary obstruction or hepatic disease, may become deficient. For oral administration to prevent vitamin K deficiency in malabsorption syndromes, a water-soluble synthetic vitamin K derivative, menadiol sodium phosphate p. 686 can be used if supplementation with phytomenadione p. 687 by mouth has been insufficient.

Oral coumarin anticoagulants act by interfering with vitamin K metabolism in the hepatic cells and their effects can be antagonised by giving vitamin K; see advice on the use of vitamin K in haemorrhage.

Vitamin K deficiency bleeding

Neonates are relatively deficient in vitamin K and those who do not receive supplements of vitamin K are at risk of serious bleeding including intracranial bleeding. The Chief Medical Officer and the Chief Nursing Officer have recommended that all newborn babies should receive vitamin K to prevent vitamin K deficiency bleeding (previously termed haemorrhagic disease of the newborn). An appropriate regimen should be selected after discussion with parents in the antenatal period.

Vitamin K (as phytomenadione) may be given by a single intramuscular injection at birth; this prevents vitamin K deficiency bleeding in virtually all babies.

Alternatively, in healthy babies who are not at particular risk of bleeding disorders, vitamin K may be given by mouth, and arrangements must be in place to ensure the appropriate regimen is followed. Two doses of a colloidal (mixed micelle) preparation of phytomenadione should be given by mouth in the first week, the first dose being given at birth and the second dose at 4–7 days. For exclusively breast-fed babies, a third dose of colloidal phytomenadione is given by mouth at 1 month of age; the third dose is omitted in formula-fed babies because formula feeds contain adequate vitamin K. An alternative regimen is to give one dose of phytomenadione by mouth at birth (using the contents of a phytomenadione capsule) to protect from the risk of vitamin K deficiency bleeding in the first week; for exclusively breast-fed babies, further doses of phytomenadione are given by mouth (using the contents of a phytomenadione capsule) at weekly intervals for 12 weeks.

Multivitamins

Multivitamin supplements are used in children with vitamin deficiencies and also in malabsorption conditions such as cystic fibrosis or liver disease. Supplementation is not required if nutrient enriched feeds are used; consult a dietician for further advice.

VITAMINS AND TRACE ELEMENTS › MULTIVITAMINS

Vitamins A and D

● **INDICATIONS AND DOSE**

Prevention of vitamin A and D deficiency

▶ BY MOUTH

▸ Child: 1 capsule daily, 1 capsule contains 4000 units vitamin A and 400 units (10 micrograms) vitamin D

● **UNLICENSED USE** Not licensed in children under 6 months of age.

● **SIDE-EFFECTS**

Overdose Prolonged excessive ingestion of vitamins A and D can lead to hypervitaminosis.

● **PRESCRIBING AND DISPENSING INFORMATION** This drug contains vitamin D; consult individual vitamin D monographs.

● **MEDICINAL FORMS** There can be variation in the licensing of different medicines containing the same drug.

Capsule

▸ Vitamins A and D (Non-proprietary)
Vitamin D 400 unit, Vitamin A 4000 unit Vitamins A and D capsules BPC 1973 | 28 capsule £2.81 | 84 capsule £8.42 DT = £8.42

Vitamins A, B group, C and D

● **INDICATIONS AND DOSE**

Prevention of deficiency

▶ BY MOUTH USING CAPSULES

▸ Child 1–11 years: 1 capsule daily

▸ Child 12–17 years: 2 capsules daily

Cystic Fibrosis: prevention of deficiency

▶ BY MOUTH USING CAPSULES

▸ Child 1–17 years: 2–3 capsules daily

ABIDEC MULTIVITAMIN DROPS®

Prevention of deficiency

▶ BY MOUTH USING ORAL DROPS

▸ Preterm neonate: 0.6 mL daily.

▸ Neonate: 0.3 mL daily.

▸ Child 1–11 months: 0.3 mL daily

▸ Child 1–17 years: 0.6 mL daily

Cystic Fibrosis: prevention of deficiency

▶ BY MOUTH USING ORAL DROPS

▸ Child 1–11 months: 0.6 mL daily

▸ Child 1–17 years: 1.2 mL daily

DALIVIT ORAL DROPS®

Prevention of deficiency

▶ BY MOUTH USING ORAL DROPS

▸ Preterm neonate: 0.3 mL daily.

▸ Neonate: 0.3 mL daily.

▸ Child 1–11 months: 0.3 mL daily

▸ Child 1–17 years: 0.6 mL daily

Cystic Fibrosis: prevention of deficiency

▶ BY MOUTH USING ORAL DROPS

▸ Child 1–11 months: 0.6 mL daily

▸ Child 1–17 years: 1 mL daily

● **UNLICENSED USE** *Dalivit®* not licensed for use in children under 6 weeks.

● **PRESCRIBING AND DISPENSING INFORMATION** This drug contains vitamin D; consult individual vitamin D monographs.

To avoid potential toxicity, the content of all vitamin preparations, particularly vitamin A, should be considered when used together with other supplements.

Vitamin A concentration of preparations varies.

ABIDEC MULTIVITAMIN DROPS® *Abidec®* contains 1333 units of vitamin A (as palmitate) per 0.6 mL dose.

DALIVIT ORAL DROPS® *Dalivit®* contains 5000 units of vitamin A (as palmitate) per 0.6 mL dose.

● **MEDICINAL FORMS** There can be variation in the licensing of different medicines containing the same drug.

Oral drops

EXCIPIENTS: May contain Arachis (peanut) oil, sucrose

▸ Abidec Multivitamin (Omega Pharma Ltd)
Nicotinamide 1333 microgram per 1 ml, Pyridoxine hydrochloride 1333 microgram per 1 ml, Riboflavin 1333 microgram per 1 ml, Thiamine hydrochloride 1.67 mg per 1 ml, Ascorbic acid 66.7 mg per 1 ml, Ergocalciferol 667 iu per 1 ml, Retinol (as Vitamin A palmitate) 2222 iu per 1 ml Abidec Multivitamin drops | 25 ml GSL £3.87

▸ Dalivit (Boston Healthcare Ltd)
Riboflavin 667 microgram per 1 ml, Pyridoxine 833 microgram per 1 ml, Thiamine 1667 microgram per 1 ml, Nicotinamide 8.3 mg per 1 ml, Ascorbic acid 83 mg per 1 ml, Ergocalciferol 667 iu per 1 ml, Vitamin A 8333 iu per 1 ml Dalivit oral drops | 25 ml GSL £6.50 | 50 ml GSL £11.36

Capsule

▸ Vitamins A, B group, C and D (Non-proprietary)
Riboflavin 500 microgram, Thiamine hydrochloride 1 mg, Nicotinamide 7.5 mg, Ascorbic acid 15 mg, Vitamin D 300 unit, Vitamin A 2500 unit Vitamins capsules | 1000 capsule £48.20 DT = £15.49

Vitamins A, C and D

05-May-2020

The properties listed below are those particular to the combination only. For the properties of the components please consider, vitamin A p. 677, ascorbic acid p. 680.

● **INDICATIONS AND DOSE**

Prevention of vitamin deficiency

▶ BY MOUTH

▸ Child 1 month–4 years: 5 drops daily, 5 drops contain vitamin A approx. 700 units, vitamin D approx. 300 units (7.5 micrograms), ascorbic acid approx. 20 mg

● **INTERACTIONS** → Appendix 1: ascorbic acid · vitamin A

● **PRESCRIBING AND DISPENSING INFORMATION** This drug contains vitamin D; consult individual vitamin D monographs.

Available free of charge to children under 4 years in families on the Healthy Start Scheme, or alternatively may be available direct to the public—further information for healthcare professionals can be accessed at www.healthystart.nhs.uk. Beneficiaries can contact their midwife or health visitor for further information on where to obtain supplies.

Healthy Start Vitamins for women (containing ascorbic acid, vitamin D, and folic acid) are also available free of charge to women on the Healthy Start Scheme during pregnancy and until their baby is one year old, or alternatively may be available direct to the public—further information for healthcare professionals can be accessed at www.healthystart.nhs.uk. Beneficiaries can contact their midwife or health visitor for further information on where to obtain supplies.

- **MEDICINAL FORMS** There can be variation in the licensing of different medicines containing the same drug.

Oral drops

- Healthy Start Children's Vitamin (Secretary of State for Health)
  Vitamin A and D3 concentrate.55 mg per 1 ml, Sodium ascorbate 18.58 mg per 1 ml, Ascorbic acid 150 mg per 1 ml, Vitamin D 2000 iu per 1 ml, Vitamin A 5000 iu per 1 ml Healthy Start Children's Vitamin drops | 10 ml [NHS]

VITAMINS AND TRACE ELEMENTS > VITAMIN A

Vitamin A

(Retinol)

- **INDICATIONS AND DOSE**

Vitamin A deficiency

▶ BY MOUTH

- Neonate: 5000 units daily, higher doses may be used initially for treatment of severe deficiency.
- Child 1–11 months: 5000 units daily, to be taken with or after food, higher doses may be used initially for treatment of severe deficiency
- Child 1–17 years: 10 000 units daily, to be taken with or after food, higher doses may be used initially for treatment of severe deficiency

Prevention of deficiency in complete biliary obstruction

▶ BY INTRAMUSCULAR INJECTION

- Neonate: 50 000 units once a month.
- Child 1–11 months: 50 000 units once a month

- **UNLICENSED USE** Preparations containing only vitamin A are not licensed.
- **INTERACTIONS** → Appendix 1: vitamin A
- **SIDE-EFFECTS**
  Overdose Massive overdose can cause rough skin, dry hair, an enlarged liver, and increases in erythrocyte sedimentation rate, serum calcium and serum alkaline phosphatase concentration.
- **PREGNANCY** Excessive doses may be teratogenic. In view of evidence suggesting that high levels of vitamin A may cause birth defects, women who are (or may become) pregnant are advised not to take vitamin A supplements (including tablets and fish liver oil drops), except on the advice of a doctor or an antenatal clinic; nor should they eat liver or products such as liver paté or liver sausage.
- **BREAST FEEDING** Theoretical risk of toxicity in infants of mothers taking large doses.
- **MONITORING REQUIREMENTS** Treatment is sometimes initiated with very high doses of vitamin A and the child should be monitored closely; very high doses are associated with acute toxicity.

- **MEDICINAL FORMS** There can be variation in the licensing of different medicines containing the same drug. Forms available from special-order manufacturers include: oral drops, solution for injection

Solution for injection

- Vitamin A (Imported)
  Retinol (as Vitamin A palmitate) 50000 unit per 1 ml Aquasol A Parenteral 100,000units/2ml solution for injection vials | 1 vial [PoM] [NHS]
  Nepalm Vitamin A 100,000units/2ml solution for injection ampoules | 6 ampoule [PoM] [NHS]

Oral drops

- Arovit (Imported (Italy))
  Vitamin A 150000 unit per 1 ml Arovit 150,000units/ml drops | 7.5 ml [PoM] [NHS]

Combinations available: ***Vitamins A, C and D***, p. 676

VITAMINS AND TRACE ELEMENTS > VITAMIN B GROUP

Biotin

03-Mar-2020

(Vitamin H)

- **INDICATIONS AND DOSE**

Isolated carboxylase defects

▶ BY MOUTH, OR BY SLOW INTRAVENOUS INJECTION

- Neonate: 5 mg once daily, adjusted according to response, maintenance 10–50 mg daily, higher doses may be required.
- Child: 10 mg once daily, adjusted according to response; maintenance 10–50 mg daily, increased if necessary up to 100 mg daily

Defects of biotin metabolism

▶ BY MOUTH, OR BY SLOW INTRAVENOUS INJECTION

- Neonate: Initially 10 mg once daily, adjusted according to response; maintenance 5–20 mg daily, higher doses may be required.
- Child: Initially 10 mg once daily, adjusted according to response; maintenance 5–20 mg daily, higher doses may be required

- **PREGNANCY** No information available.
- **BREAST FEEDING** No information available.
- **DIRECTIONS FOR ADMINISTRATION** For administration *by mouth*, tablets may be crushed and mixed with food or drink.
- **PATIENT AND CARER ADVICE**
  Medicines for Children leaflet: Biotin for metabolic disorders www.medicinesforchildren.org.uk/biotin-metabolic-disorders-0

- **MEDICINAL FORMS** There can be variation in the licensing of different medicines containing the same drug. Forms available from special-order manufacturers include: tablet, oral suspension, oral solution

Solution for injection

- Biodermatin (Imported (Italy))
  Biotin 5 mg per 1 ml Biodermatin 5mg/1ml solution for injection vials | 10 vial [PoM] [NHS]

Tablet

- Biotisan (Imported (Germany))
  Biotin 10 mg Biotisan Biotin S 10mg FORTE tablets | 30 tablet [NHS]
- BiotEss (Essential-Healthcare Ltd)
  Biotin 5 mg BiotEss 5mg tablets | 30 tablet £11.47
- OroB7 (Rhodes Pharma Ltd)
  Biotin 5 mg OroB7 5mg tablets | 30 tablet £33.99

Pyridoxine hydrochloride
(Vitamin B_6)

● **INDICATIONS AND DOSE**

Isoniazid-induced neuropathy (prophylaxis)
▶ BY MOUTH
▸ Neonate: 5 mg daily.
▸ Child 1 month–11 years: 5–10 mg daily
▸ Child 12–17 years: 10 mg daily

Isoniazid-induced neuropathy (treatment)
▶ BY MOUTH
▸ Neonate: 5–10 mg daily.
▸ Child 1 month–11 years: 10–20 mg 2–3 times a day
▸ Child 12–17 years: 30–50 mg 2–3 times a day

Prevention of penicillamine-induced neuropathy in Wilson's disease
▶ BY MOUTH
▸ Child 1–11 years: 5–10 mg daily
▸ Child 12–17 years: 10 mg daily

Metabolic diseases | Cystathioninuria | Homocystinuria
▶ BY MOUTH
▸ Neonate: 50–100 mg 1–2 times a day.
▸ Child: 50–250 mg 1–2 times a day

Pyridoxine-dependent seizures
▶ INITIALLY BY INTRAVENOUS INJECTION
▸ Neonate: Test dose 50–100 mg, repeated if necessary, if responsive, followed by an oral maintenance dose; (by mouth) maintenance 50–100 mg once daily, dose to be adjusted as necessary.
▸ Child 1 month–11 years: Test dose 50–100 mg daily, if responsive, followed by an oral maintenance dose, (by mouth) maintenance 20–50 mg 1–2 times a day, dose to be adjusted as necessary, (by mouth) increased if necessary up to 30 mg/kg daily, alternatively (by mouth) increased if necessary up to 1 g daily

● **UNLICENSED USE** Not licensed for prophylaxis of penicillamine-induced neuropathy in Wilson's disease. Not licensed for use in children.

● **CAUTIONS** Risk of cardiovascular collapse (with intravenous injection—resuscitation facilities must be available and monitor closely)

● **SIDE-EFFECTS** Peripheral neuritis

Overdose Overdosage induces toxic effects.

● **MEDICINAL FORMS** There can be variation in the licensing of different medicines containing the same drug. Forms available from special-order manufacturers include: capsule, oral suspension, oral solution, solution for injection

Tablet
▸ Pyridoxine hydrochloride (Non-proprietary)
Pyridoxine hydrochloride 10 mg Pyridoxine 10mg tablets | 28 tablet PoM £16.95–£16.98 DT = £16.98 | 500 tablet £15.99
Pyridoxine hydrochloride 20 mg Pyridoxine 20mg tablets | 500 tablet GSL ⊠
Pyridoxine hydrochloride 50 mg Pyridoxine 50mg tablets | 28 tablet PoM £31.02 DT = £18.90

Solution for injection
▸ Pyridoxine hydrochloride (Non-proprietary)
Pyridoxine hydrochloride 50 mg per 1 ml Vitamin B6 100mg/2ml solution for injection ampoules | 10 ampoule PoM ⊠
▸ Sicovit (Imported (Romania))
Pyridoxine hydrochloride 25 mg per 1 ml Sicovit B6 50mg/2ml solution for injection vials | 5 vial PoM ⊠

Oral solution
▸ PyriDose (TriOn Pharma Ltd)
Pyridoxine hydrochloride 20 mg per 1 ml PyriDose 100mg/5ml oral solution | 100 ml £29.86 DT = £25.19

Capsule
▸ Pyridoxine hydrochloride (Non-proprietary)
Pyridoxine hydrochloride 100 mg Vitamin B6 100mg capsules | 100 capsule ⊠ | 120 capsule £5.50

Riboflavin
(Riboflavine; Vitamin B_2)

● **INDICATIONS AND DOSE**

Metabolic diseases
▶ BY MOUTH
▸ Neonate: 50 mg 1–2 times a day, adjusted according to response.
▸ Child: 50–100 mg 1–2 times a day, adjusted according to response to up to 400 mg daily

● **UNLICENSED USE** Not licensed in children.

● **SIDE-EFFECTS** Urine discolouration

● **PREGNANCY** Crosses the placenta but no adverse effects reported, information at high doses limited.

● **BREAST FEEDING** Present in breast milk but no adverse effects reported, information at high doses limited.

● **MEDICINAL FORMS** There can be variation in the licensing of different medicines containing the same drug. Forms available from special-order manufacturers include: tablet, modified-release tablet, capsule, oral suspension, oral solution

Modified-release tablet
▸ Riboflavin (Non-proprietary)
Riboflavin 100 mg Vitamin B2 100mg modified-release tablets | 60 tablet £4.46

Tablet
▸ Riboflavin (Non-proprietary)
Riboflavin 100 mg Vitamin B2 100mg tablets | 100 tablet ⊠
▸ Beflavine (Imported (France))
Riboflavin 10 mg Beflavine 10mg tablets | 20 tablet ⊠

Capsule
▸ Riboflavin (Non-proprietary)
Riboflavin 50 mg RiboEss 50mg capsules | 30 capsule £41.59
Riboflavin 50mg capsules | 30 capsule £3.13
Riboflavin 100 mg RiboEss 100mg capsules | 30 capsule £47.29
▸ B-2-50 (Bio-Tech Pharmacal Inc)
Riboflavin 50 mg B-2-50 capsules | 100 capsule ⊠
▸ E-B2 (Ennogen Healthcare Ltd)
Riboflavin 100 mg E-B2 100mg capsules | 30 capsule £89.20

Thiamine
28-Nov-2019

(Vitamin B_1)

● **INDICATIONS AND DOSE**

Maple syrup urine disease
▶ BY MOUTH
▸ Neonate: 5 mg/kg daily, dose to be adjusted as necessary.
▸ Child: 5 mg/kg daily, dose to be adjusted as necessary

Metabolic disorders | Congenital lactic acidosis
▶ INITIALLY BY MOUTH, OR BY INTRAVENOUS INFUSION
▸ Neonate: 50–200 mg once daily, dose to be adjusted as necessary, the total dose may alternatively be given in 2–3 divided doses, administer intravenous infusion over 30 minutes.
▸ Child: 100–300 mg once daily, dose to be adjusted as necessary, the total dose may alternatively be given in 2–3 divided doses, administer intravenous infusion over 30 minutes, (by mouth) increased if necessary up to 2 g daily

- **UNLICENSED USE** Not licensed in children.

IMPORTANT SAFETY INFORMATION
MHRA/CHM ADVICE (SEPTEMBER 2007)
Although potentially serious allergic adverse reactions may rarely occur during, or shortly after, parenteral administration, the CHM has recommended that:
- This should not preclude the use of parenteral thiamine in patients where this route of administration is required, particularly in patients at risk of Wernicke-Korsakoff syndrome where treatment with thiamine is essential;
- Intravenous administration should be by infusion over 30 minutes;
- Facilities for treating anaphylaxis (including resuscitation facilities) should be available when parenteral thiamine is administered.

- **CAUTIONS** Anaphylaxis may occasionally follow injection
- **BREAST FEEDING** Severely thiamine-deficient mothers should avoid breast-feeding as toxic methyl-glyoxal present in milk.
- **PRESCRIBING AND DISPENSING INFORMATION**
  - With intravenous use Some preparations may contain phenol as a preservative.

- **MEDICINAL FORMS** There can be variation in the licensing of different medicines containing the same drug. Forms available from special-order manufacturers include: oral suspension, oral solution

Modified-release tablet
- Thiamine (Non-proprietary)
  Thiamine hydrochloride 100 mg Vitamin B1 100mg modified-release tablets | 90 tablet £4.46

Tablet
- Thiamine (Non-proprietary)
  Thiamine hydrochloride 25 mg Vitamin B1 25mg tablets | 100 tablet [P] [CD]
  Thiamine hydrochloride 50 mg Thiamine 50mg tablets | 28 tablet [P] £1.22–£1.80 | 100 tablet [CD] DT = £4.35 | 100 tablet [P] £6.72 DT = £4.35
  Thiamine hydrochloride 100 mg Thiamine 100mg tablets | 28 tablet [P] £1.63–£6.72 | 100 tablet [CD] DT = £5.83 | 100 tablet [P] £11.55 DT = £5.83
- Benerva (Teofarma)
  Thiamine hydrochloride 50 mg Benerva 50mg tablets | 100 tablet [P] £4.00 DT = £4.35
  Thiamine hydrochloride 100 mg Benerva 100mg tablets | 100 tablet [P] £6.29 DT = £5.83

Solution for injection
- Thiamine (Imported)
  Thiamine hydrochloride 50 mg per 1 ml Bevitine 100mg/2ml solution for injection ampoules | 5 ampoule [PoM] [CD]
  Thiamine hydrochloride 100 mg per 1 ml Vitamin B1 Streuli 100mg/1ml solution for injection ampoules | 10 ampoule [PoM] [CD]

Vitamin B complex

01-May-2020

- **INDICATIONS AND DOSE**

Treatment of deficiency
- BY MOUTH USING SYRUP
  - Child 1–11 months: 5 mL 3 times a day, this dose is for *Vigranon B®* syrup.
  - Child 1–11 years: 10 mL 3 times a day, this dose is for *Vigranon B®* syrup.
  - Child 12–17 years: 10–15 mL 3 times a day, this dose is for *Vigranon B®* syrup.

Prophylaxis of deficiency
- BY MOUTH USING SYRUP
  - Child 1–11 months: 5 mL once daily, this dose is for *Vigranon B®* syrup.
  - Child 1–11 years: 5 mL twice daily, this dose is for *Vigranon B®* syrup.
  - Child 12–17 years: 5 mL 3 times a day, this dose is for *Vigranon B®* syrup.

- **NATIONAL FUNDING/ACCESS DECISIONS**
  NHS restrictions *Vigranon B®* syrup is not prescribable in NHS primary care.
- **LESS SUITABLE FOR PRESCRIBING** Vitamin B compound tablets, vitamin B compound strong tablets, and *Vigranon B®* syrup are less suitable for prescribing.

- **MEDICINAL FORMS** There can be variation in the licensing of different medicines containing the same drug.

Oral solution
- Vigranon-B (Wallace Manufacturing Chemists Ltd)
  Pyridoxine hydrochloride 400 microgram per 1 ml, Riboflavin sodium phosphate 548 microgram per 1 ml, Dexpanthenol 600 microgram per 1 ml, Thiamine hydrochloride 1 mg per 1 ml, Nicotinamide 4 mg per 1 ml Vigranon-B syrup sugar-free | 150 ml [P] £26.00

Vitamins with minerals and trace elements

13-May-2020

- **INDICATIONS AND DOSE**

FORCEVAL® CAPSULES

Vitamin and mineral deficiency and as adjunct in synthetic diets
- BY MOUTH
  - Child 12–17 years: 1 capsule daily, one hour after a meal

KETOVITE® LIQUID

Prevention of vitamin deficiency in disorders of carbohydrate or amino-acid metabolism | Adjunct in restricted, specialised, or synthetic diets
- BY MOUTH
  - Child: 5 mL daily, use with *Ketovite® Tablets* for complete vitamin supplementation.

KETOVITE® TABLETS

Prevention of vitamin deficiency in disorders of carbohydrate or amino-acid metabolism | Adjunct in restricted, specialised, or synthetic diets
- BY MOUTH
  - Child: 1 tablet 3 times a day, use with *Ketovite® Liquid* for complete vitamin supplementation.

- **PRESCRIBING AND DISPENSING INFORMATION** To avoid potential toxicity, the content of all vitamin preparations, particularly vitamin A, should be considered when used together with other supplements.
- **PATIENT AND CARER ADVICE**
  Medicines for Children leaflet: Multivitamin preparations for vitamin deficiency www.medicinesforchildren.org.uk/multivitamin-preparations-vitamin-deficiency
  KETOVITE® LIQUID *Ketovite®* liquid may be mixed with milk, cereal, or fruit juice.
  KETOVITE® TABLETS Tablets may be crushed immediately before use.

- **MEDICINAL FORMS** There can be variation in the licensing of different medicines containing the same drug.

Oral emulsion
- Ketovite (Essential Pharmaceuticals Ltd)
  Cyanocobalamin 2.5 microgram per 1 ml, Choline chloride 30 mg per 1 ml, Ergocalciferol 80 unit per 1 ml, Vitamin A 500 unit per 1 ml Ketovite liquid sugar-free | 150 ml [P] £119.10

Tablet
- Ketovite (Essential Pharmaceuticals Ltd)
  Biotin 170 microgram, Folic acid 250 microgram, Pyridoxine hydrochloride 330 microgram, Acetomenaphthone

500 microgram, Riboflavin 1 mg, Thiamine hydrochloride 1 mg, Calcium pantothenate 1.16 mg, Nicotinamide 3.3 mg, Alpha tocopheryl acetate 5 mg, Ascorbic acid 16.6 mg, Inositol 50 mg Ketovite tablets | 100 tablet £28.77

Capsule

▸ Forceval (Forum Health Products Ltd)
Cyanocobalamin 3 microgram, Selenium 50 microgram, Biotin 100 microgram, Iodine 140 microgram, Chromium 200 microgram, Molybdenum 250 microgram, Folic acid 400 microgram, Thiamine 1.2 mg, Riboflavin 1.6 mg, Copper 2 mg, Pyridoxine 2 mg, Manganese 3 mg, Pantothenic acid 4 mg, Potassium 4 mg, Tocopheryl acetate 10 mg, Iron 12 mg, Zinc 15 mg, Nicotinamide 18 mg, Magnesium 30 mg, Ascorbic acid 60 mg, Phosphorus 77 mg, Calcium 100 mg, Ergocalciferol 400 unit, Vitamin A 2500 unit Forceval capsules | 15 **capsule** P £5.46 | 30 capsule P £9.92 | 90 capsule P £28.77

9 Blood and nutrition

VITAMINS AND TRACE ELEMENTS › VITAMIN C

Ascorbic acid

08-Jul-2019

(Vitamin C)

● **INDICATIONS AND DOSE**

Treatment of scurvy

▸ BY MOUTH

▸ Child 1 month–3 years: 125–250 mg daily in 1–2 divided doses

▸ Child 4–11 years: 250–500 mg daily in 1–2 divided doses

▸ Child 12–17 years: 0.5–1 g daily in 1–2 divided doses

Adjunct to desferrioxamine (to enhance the excretion of iron 1 month after treatment)

▸ BY MOUTH

▸ Child: 100–200 mg daily, to be taken 1 hour before food

Metabolic disorders | Tyrosinaemia type III | Transient tyrosinaemia of the newborn | Glutathione synthase deficiency | Hawkinsinuria

▸ BY MOUTH

▸ Neonate: 50–200 mg daily, dose to be adjusted as necessary.

▸ Child: 200–400 mg daily in 1–2 divided doses, dose to be adjusted as necessary, increased if necessary up to 1 g daily

● **UNLICENSED USE** Not licensed for metabolic disorders.

● **CONTRA-INDICATIONS** Hyperoxaluria

● **CAUTIONS**

Iron overload Ascorbic acid should not be given to patients with cardiac dysfunction.

In patients with normal cardiac function ascorbic acid should be introduced 1 month after starting desferrioxamine.

● **INTERACTIONS** → Appendix 1: ascorbic acid

● **SIDE-EFFECTS** Diarrhoea · gastrointestinal disorder · hyperoxaluria · oxalate nephrolithiasis · polyuria

● **PRESCRIBING AND DISPENSING INFORMATION** It is rarely necessary to prescribe more than 100 mg daily except early in the treatment of scurvy.

● **MEDICINAL FORMS** There can be variation in the licensing of different medicines containing the same drug. Forms available from special-order manufacturers include: tablet, oral suspension, oral solution

Tablet

EXCIPIENTS: May contain Aspartame

▸ **Ascorbic acid (Non-proprietary)**
Ascorbic acid 50 mg Ascorbic acid 50mg tablets | 28 tablet DT = £15.08 | 28 tablet GSL £15.08 DT = £15.08
Ascorb 50mg tablets | 28 tablet £3.29 DT = £15.08
Ascorbic acid 100 mg Ascorbic acid 100mg tablets | 28 tablet GSL £14.30 DT = £14.30 | 28 tablet DT = £14.30
Ascorb 100mg tablets | 28 tablet £3.59 DT = £14.30
Ascorbic acid 200 mg Ascorbic acid 200mg tablets | 28 tablet GSL £19.88 DT = £19.88 | 28 tablet DT = £19.88
Ascorb 200mg tablets | 28 tablet £4.37 DT = £19.88
Ascorbic acid 250 mg Ascorbic acid 250mg tablets | 1000 tablet PoM
Ascorbic acid 500 mg Ascorbic acid 500mg tablets | 28 tablet DT = £26.89 | 28 tablet GSL £26.89 DT = £26.89

Chewable tablet

CAUTIONARY AND ADVISORY LABELS 24

EXCIPIENTS: May contain Aspartame

▸ Ascur (Ennogen Healthcare Ltd)
Ascorbic acid 100 mg Ascur 100mg chewable tablets | 30 tablet £3.95
Ascorbic acid (as Sodium ascorbate) 500 mg Ascur 500mg chewable tablets sugar-free | 30 tablet £2.99

Capsule

▸ Ascorbic acid (Non-proprietary)
Ascorbic acid 500 mg BioCare Vitamin C 500mg capsules | 60 capsule £7.73 | 180 capsule £19.82

Combinations available: ***Vitamins A, C and D***, p. 676

VITAMINS AND TRACE ELEMENTS › VITAMIN D AND ANALOGUES

Vitamin D and analogues (systemic)

● **CONTRA-INDICATIONS** Hypercalcaemia · metastatic calcification

● **SIDE-EFFECTS**

▸ **Common or very common** Abdominal pain · headache · hypercalcaemia · hypercalciuria · nausea · skin reactions

▸ **Uncommon** Appetite decreased · constipation · vomiting

▸ **Frequency not known** Thirst

Overdose Symptoms of overdosage include anorexia, lassitude, nausea and vomiting, diarrhoea, constipation, weight loss, polyuria, sweating, headache, thirst, vertigo, and raised concentrations of calcium and phosphate in plasma and urine.

● **PREGNANCY** High doses teratogenic in *animals* but therapeutic doses unlikely to be harmful.

● **BREAST FEEDING** Caution with high doses; may cause hypercalcaemia in infant—monitor serum-calcium concentration.

● **MONITORING REQUIREMENTS** **Important**: all patients receiving pharmacological doses of vitamin D should have their plasma-calcium concentration checked at intervals (initially once or twice weekly) and whenever nausea or vomiting occur.

above

Alfacalcidol

(1α-Hydroxycholecalciferol)

● **INDICATIONS AND DOSE**

Hypophosphataemic rickets | Persistent hypocalcaemia due to hypoparathyroidism or pseudohypoparathyroidism

▸ BY MOUTH, OR BY INTRAVENOUS INJECTION

▸ Child 1 month–11 years: 25–50 nanograms/kg once daily, dose to be adjusted as necessary; maximum 1 microgram per day

▸ Child 12–17 years: 1 microgram once daily, dose to be adjusted as necessary

Persistent neonatal hypocalcaemia

▸ BY MOUTH, OR BY INTRAVENOUS INJECTION

▸ Neonate: 50–100 nanograms/kg once daily, dose to be adjusted as necessary, in resistant cases higher doses may be needed; increased if necessary up to 2 micrograms/kg daily.

Prevention of vitamin D deficiency in renal or cholestatic liver disease

▶ BY MOUTH, OR BY INTRAVENOUS INJECTION

- Neonate: 20 nanograms/kg once daily, dose to be adjusted as necessary.
- Child 1 month–11 years (body-weight up to 20 kg): 15–30 nanograms/kg once daily (max. per dose 500 nanograms)
- Child 1 month–11 years (body-weight 20 kg and above): 250–500 nanograms once daily, dose to be adjusted as necessary
- Child 12–17 years: 250–500 nanograms once daily, dose to be adjusted as necessary

DOSE EQUIVALENCE AND CONVERSION
- One drop of alfacalcidol 2 microgram/mL oral drops contains approximately 100 nanograms alfacalcidol.

- **CAUTIONS** Nephrolithiasis · take care to ensure correct dose in infants
- **INTERACTIONS** → Appendix 1: vitamin D substances
- **SIDE-EFFECTS**
- ▶ **Common or very common** Abdominal discomfort · hyperphosphataemia · rash pustular
- ▶ **Uncommon** Asthenia · diarrhoea · malaise · myalgia · urolithiases
- ▶ **Rare or very rare** Dizziness
- ▶ **Frequency not known** Confusion · renal impairment
- **RENAL IMPAIRMENT**
  Monitoring Monitor plasma-calcium concentration in renal impairment.
- **MONITORING REQUIREMENTS** Monitor plasma-calcium concentration in patients receiving high doses.
- **DIRECTIONS FOR ADMINISTRATION** For injection, shake ampoule for at least 5 seconds before use, and give over 30 seconds.

- **MEDICINAL FORMS** There can be variation in the licensing of different medicines containing the same drug. Forms available from special-order manufacturers include: oral suspension, oral solution

Solution for injection

EXCIPIENTS: May contain Alcohol, propylene glycol

▶ One-Alpha (LEO Pharma)
Alfacalcidol 2 microgram per 1 ml One-Alpha 2micrograms/1ml solution for injection ampoules | 10 ampoule [PoM] £41.13
One-Alpha 1micrograms/0.5ml solution for injection ampoules | 10 ampoule [PoM] £21.57

Oral drops

EXCIPIENTS: May contain Alcohol

▶ One-Alpha (LEO Pharma)
Alfacalcidol 2 microgram per 1 ml One-Alpha 2micrograms/ml oral drops sugar-free | 10 ml [PoM] £21.30 DT = £21.30

Capsule

EXCIPIENTS: May contain Sesame oil

▶ Alfacalcidol (Non-proprietary)
Alfacalcidol 250 nanogram Alfacalcidol 250nanogram capsules | 30 capsule [PoM] £5.00 DT = £4.93
AlfacalEss 0.25microgram capsules | 30 capsule £1.29 DT = £4.93
Alfacalcidol 500 nanogram Alfacalcidol 500nanogram capsules | 30 capsule [PoM] £10.00 DT = £9.90
AlfacalEss 0.5microgram capsules | 30 capsule £2.37 DT = £9.90
Alfacalcidol 1 microgram Alfacalcidol 1microgram capsules | 30 capsule [🅇] DT = £13.82 | 30 capsule [PoM] £14.00 DT = £13.82
AlfacalEss 1microgram capsules | 30 capsule £2.71 DT = £13.82

▶ One-Alpha (LEO Pharma)
Alfacalcidol 250 nanogram One-Alpha 250nanogram capsules | 30 capsule [PoM] £3.37 DT = £4.93
Alfacalcidol 500 nanogram One-Alpha 0.5microgram capsules | 30 capsule [PoM] £6.27 DT = £9.90
Alfacalcidol 1 microgram One-Alpha 1microgram capsules | 30 capsule [PoM] £8.75 DT = £13.82

680

Calcitriol

04-Mar-2020

(1,25-Dihydroxycholecalciferol)

- **INDICATIONS AND DOSE**

Vitamin D dependent rickets | Hypophosphataemic rickets | Persistent hypocalcaemia due to hypoparathyroidism | Pseudo-hypoparathyroidism (limited experience)

▶ BY MOUTH
- Child 1 month–11 years: Initially 15 nanograms/kg once daily (max. per dose 250 nanograms), increased in steps of 5 nanograms/kg daily (max. per dose 250 nanograms) if required, dose to be increased every 2–4 weeks
- Child 12–17 years: Initially 250 nanograms once daily, increased in steps of 5 nanograms/kg daily (max. per dose 250 nanograms) if required, dose to be increased every 2–4 weeks; usual dose 0.5–1 microgram daily

- **UNLICENSED USE** Not licensed for use in children.
- **CAUTIONS** Take care to ensure correct dose in infants
- **INTERACTIONS** → Appendix 1: vitamin D substances
- **SIDE-EFFECTS**
- ▶ **Common or very common** Urinary tract infection
- ▶ **Frequency not known** Abdominal pain upper · apathy · arrhythmia · dehydration · drowsiness · fever · growth retardation · muscle weakness · paralytic ileus · polydipsia · psychiatric disorder · sensory disorder · urinary disorders · weight decreased
- **RENAL IMPAIRMENT** Manufacturer advises avoid—no information available.
  Monitoring Monitor plasma-calcium concentration in renal impairment.
- **MONITORING REQUIREMENTS**
- ▶ Monitor plasma calcium, phosphate, and creatinine during dosage titration.
- ▶ Monitor plasma-calcium concentration in patients receiving high doses.
- **DIRECTIONS FOR ADMINISTRATION** Contents of capsule may be administered by oral syringe.

- **MEDICINAL FORMS** There can be variation in the licensing of different medicines containing the same drug. Forms available from special-order manufacturers include: oral suspension, oral solution

Oral solution

▶ Calcitriol (Non-proprietary)
Calcitriol 1 microgram per 1 ml Rocaltrol 1micrograms/ml oral solution sugar-free | 10 ml [PoM] [🅇]

Capsule

▶ Calcitriol (Non-proprietary)
Calcitriol 250 nanogram Calcitriol 250nanogram capsules | 30 capsule [PoM] £5.41–£18.04
Calcitriol 500 nanogram Calcitriol 500nanogram capsules | 30 capsule [PoM] £32.25

▶ Rocaltrol (Roche Products Ltd)
Calcitriol 250 nanogram Rocaltrol 250nanogram capsules | 100 capsule [PoM] £18.04 DT = £18.04
Calcitriol 500 nanogram Rocaltrol 500nanogram capsules | 100 capsule [PoM] £32.25 DT = £32.25

680

Colecalciferol

(Cholecalciferol; Vitamin D_3)

- **INDICATIONS AND DOSE**

Prevention of vitamin D deficiency

▶ BY MOUTH
- Child: 400 units daily

- **UNLICENSED USE** *Adcal-D3®*, *Calceos®*, and *Fultium-D$_3$®* 800 units and *Fultium-D$_3$®* 20000 units are not licensed for use in children under 12 years. *Cacit® D3*, *Calcichew- D$_3$® Forte*, *Calcichew- D$_3$®* 500 mg/400 unit, and *Kalcipos- D®* not licensed for use in children (age range not specified by manufacturers). *Accrete D3®*, *Calfovit D3®*, and *Natecal D3®* not licensed for use in children under 18 years.
- **CAUTIONS** Take care to ensure correct dose in infants
- **INTERACTIONS** → Appendix 1: vitamin D substances
- **SIDE-EFFECTS** Laryngeal oedema
- **RENAL IMPAIRMENT**

Monitoring Monitor plasma-calcium concentration in renal impairment.
- **MONITORING REQUIREMENTS** Monitor plasma-calcium concentration in patients receiving high doses.
- **DIRECTIONS FOR ADMINISTRATION**

INVITA D3® ORAL SOLUTION May be mixed with a small amount of milk or cold or lukewarm food immediately before administration.

9 Blood and nutrition

- **MEDICINAL FORMS** There can be variation in the licensing of different medicines containing the same drug. Forms available from special-order manufacturers include: tablet, capsule, oral suspension, oral solution, oral drops

Tablet

▸ Colecalciferol (Non-proprietary)
Colecalciferol 400 unit Colecalciferol 400unit tablets | 60 tablet £15.50
Colecalciferol 800 unit Colecalciferol 800unit tablets | 30 tablet PoM £4.59 DT = £4.59
Colecalciferol 5000 unit Vitamin D3 High Strength 5,000unit tablets | 60 tablet £5.24

▸ Aciferol D3(Rhodes Pharma Ltd)
Colecalciferol 400 unit Aciferol D3 400unit tablets | 90 tablet £9.99
Colecalciferol 2200 unit Aciferol D3 2,200unit tablets | 90 tablet £25.99
Colecalciferol 3000 unit Aciferol D3 3,000unit tablets | 60 tablet £14.99
Colecalciferol 5000 unit Aciferol D3 5,000unit tablets | 60 tablet £19.99
Colecalciferol 10000 unit Aciferol D3 10,000unit tablets | 30 tablet £13.99
Colecalciferol 20000 unit Aciferol D3 20,000unit tablets | 30 tablet £18.99

▸ Cubicole D3(Cubic Pharmaceuticals Ltd)
Colecalciferol 400 unit Cubicole D3 400unit tablets | 30 tablet £5.95

▸ Desunin(Mylan)
Colecalciferol 800 unit Desunin 800unit tablets | 30 tablet PoM £3.60 DT = £4.59 | 90 tablet PoM £10.17
Colecalciferol 4000 unit Desunin 4,000unit tablets | 70 tablet PoM £15.90 DT = £15.90

▸ E-D3(Ennogen Healthcare Ltd)
Colecalciferol 400 unit E-D3 400unit tablets | 30 tablet £78.50
Colecalciferol 1000 unit E-D3 1,000unit tablets | 30 tablet £2.95
Colecalciferol 10000 unit E-D3 10,000unit tablets | 30 tablet £95.00
Colecalciferol 20000 unit E-D3 20,000unit tablets | 30 tablet £95.90

▸ Iso D3(Nutri Advanced Ltd)
Colecalciferol 2000 unit Vitamin D3 + Isoflavones 2,000unit tablets | 90 tablet £17.54

▸ Stexerol-D3(Kyowa Kirin Ltd)
Colecalciferol 1000 unit Stexerol-D3 1,000unit tablets | 28 tablet PoM £2.95 DT = £2.95
Colecalciferol 25000 unit Stexerol-D3 25,000unit tablets | 12 tablet PoM £17.00 DT = £17.00

▸ SunVit D3(SunVit-D3 Ltd)
Colecalciferol 400 unit SunVit-D3 400unit Vegan tablets | 60 tablet £4.16
SunVit-D3 400unit tablets | 28 tablet £2.55
Colecalciferol 2000 unit SunVit-D3 2,000unit tablets | 28 tablet £3.99
Colecalciferol 3000 unit SunVit-D3 3,000unit tablets | 28 tablet £5.49
Colecalciferol 5000 unit SunVit-D3 5,000unit tablets | 28 tablet £4.99
Colecalciferol 10000 unit SunVit-D3 10,000unit tablets | 28 tablet £6.99
Colecalciferol 20000 unit SunVit-D3 20,000unit tablets | 28 tablet £4.40
Colecalciferol 50000 unit SunVit-D3 50,000unit tablets | 15 tablet £19.99

Oral drops

▸ Colecalciferol (Non-proprietary)
Colecalciferol 1000 unit per 1 ml Vitamin D3 1,000unit oral drops sugar-free | 30 ml £6.44
Colecalciferol 2000 unit per 1 ml Pro D3 2,000units/ml Vegan liquid drops sugar-free | 20 ml £11.00
Colecalciferol 20000 unit per 1 ml Vigantol 20,000units/ml oral drops | 10 ml ☒

▸ E-D3(Ennogen Healthcare Ltd)
Colecalciferol 2000 unit per 1 ml E-D3 2,000units/ml oral drops sugar-free | 20 ml ☒

▸ Fultium-D3(Internis Pharmaceuticals Ltd)
Colecalciferol 2740 unit per 1 ml Fultium-D3 2,740units/ml oral drops sugar-free | 25 ml PoM £10.70 DT = £10.70

▸ InVita D3(Consilient Health Ltd)
Colecalciferol 2400 unit per 1 ml InVita D3 2,400units/ml oral drops sugar-free | 10 ml PoM £3.60 DT = £3.60

▸ Pro D3(Synergy Biologics Ltd)
Colecalciferol 2000 unit per 1 ml Pro D3 2,000units/ml liquid drops sugar-free | 20 ml £9.80

▸ Sapvit-D3(Stirling Anglian Pharmaceuticals Ltd)
Colecalciferol 14400 unit per 1 ml Sapvit-D3 14,400units/ml oral drops sugar-free | 12.5 ml PoM £8.95 DT = £8.95

▸ SunVit D3(SunVit-D3 Ltd)
Colecalciferol 2000 unit per 1 ml SunVit-D3 2,000units/ml oral drops sugar-free | 20 ml £6.20

▸ Thorens(Galen Ltd)
Colecalciferol 10000 unit per 1 ml Thorens 10,000units/ml oral drops sugar-free | 10 ml PoM £5.85 DT = £5.85

Oral solution

CAUTIONARY AND ADVISORY LABELS 21

▸ Colecalciferol (Non-proprietary)
Colecalciferol 2000 unit per 1 ml Pro D3 2,000units/ml Vegan liquid | 50 ml £17.80
Colecalciferol 3000 unit per 1 ml Colecalciferol 3,000units/ml oral solution | 100 ml PoM £144.00 DT = £144.00
E-D3 15,000units/5ml oral solution | 50 ml ☒
Colecalciferol 10000 unit per 1 ml ZymaD 10,000units/ml oral solution | 10 ml PoM ☒

▸ Aciferol D3(Rhodes Pharma Ltd)
Colecalciferol 2000 unit per 1 ml Aciferol D3 2,000units/ml liquid | 100 ml £18.00

▸ Baby D(KoRa Healthcare)
Colecalciferol 1000 unit per 1 ml Baby D 1,000units/ml oral solution | 30 ml £4.50

▸ E-D3(Ennogen Healthcare Ltd)
Colecalciferol 1000 unit per 1 ml E-D3 1,000units/ml oral solution | 15 ml ☒

▸ InVita D3(Consilient Health Ltd)
Colecalciferol 25000 unit per 1 ml InVita D3 25,000units/1ml oral solution sugar-free | 3 ampoule PoM £4.45 DT = £4.45
Colecalciferol 50000 unit per 1 ml InVita D3 50,000units/1ml oral solution sugar-free | 3 ampoule PoM £6.25 DT = £6.25

▸ Pro D3(Synergy Biologics Ltd)
Colecalciferol 2000 unit per 1 ml Pro D3 2,000units/ml liquid | 50 ml £16.80 | 100 ml £22.50

▸ SunVit D3(SunVit-D3 Ltd)
Colecalciferol 2000 unit per 1 ml SunVit-D3 10,000units/5ml oral solution sugar-free | 50 ml £8.90
SunVit-D3 2,000units/ml oral solution sugar-free | 50 ml £8.90

▸ Thorens(Galen Ltd)
Colecalciferol 10000 unit per 1 ml Thorens 25,000units/2.5ml oral solution sugar-free | 2.5 ml PoM £1.55 DT = £1.55 sugar-free | 10 ml PoM £5.85 DT = £5.85

Chewable tablet

▸ EveryDay-D(Vega Nutritionals Ltd)
Colecalciferol 400 unit EveryDay-D 400unit chewable tablets | 100 tablet £3.22 | 500 tablet £14.60

▸ Urgent-D(Vega Nutritionals Ltd)
Colecalciferol 2000 unit Urgent-D 2,000unit chewable tablets | 60 tablet £4.31

Capsule

CAUTIONARY AND ADVISORY LABELS 25

- Colecalciferol (Non-proprietary)
  Colecalciferol 5000 unit Colecalciferol 5,000unit capsules | 40 capsule [X]
  Colecalciferol 20000 unit Colecalciferol 20,000unit capsules | 20 capsule £2.62–£22.72 | 20 capsule [PoM] £20.50 | 30 capsule £35.99 DT = £29.00
- Aciferol D3 (Rhodes Pharma Ltd)
  Colecalciferol 30000 unit Aciferol D3 30,000unit capsules | 10 capsule £19.99
- Bio-Vitamin D3(Pharma Nord (UK) Ltd)
  Colecalciferol 5000 unit Bio-Vitamin D3 5,000unit capsules | 40 capsule £5.51
- Cubicole D3 (Cubic Pharmaceuticals Ltd)
  Colecalciferol 600 unit Cubicole D3 600unit capsules | 30 capsule £6.95
  Colecalciferol 2200 unit Cubicole D3 2,200unit capsules | 30 capsule £9.95
  Colecalciferol 3000 unit Cubicole D3 3,000unit capsules | 30 capsule £11.95
  Colecalciferol 10000 unit Cubicole D3 10,000unit capsules | 30 capsule £12.95
- D-Max (Nutraconcepts Ltd)
  Colecalciferol 5000 unit D-Max 5,000unit capsules | 30 capsule £4.85
  Colecalciferol 10000 unit D-Max 10,000unit capsules | 30 capsule £6.89
- E-D3 (Ennogen Healthcare Ltd)
  Colecalciferol 600 unit E-D3 600unit capsules | 30 capsule £82.10
  Colecalciferol 2200 unit E-D3 2,200unit capsules | 30 capsule £86.20
  Colecalciferol 2500 unit E-D3 2,500unit capsules | 30 capsule £86.20
  Colecalciferol 3000 unit E-D3 3,000unit capsules | 30 capsule £88.60
  Colecalciferol 30000 unit E-D3 30,000unit capsules | 10 capsule £94.40
- Fultium-D3 (Internis Pharmaceuticals Ltd)
  Colecalciferol 800 unit Fultium-D3 800unit capsules | 30 capsule [PoM] £3.60 DT = £3.60 | 90 capsule [PoM] £8.85
  Colecalciferol 3200 unit Fultium-D3 3,200unit capsules | 30 capsule [PoM] £13.32 DT = £13.32 | 90 capsule [PoM] £39.96
  Colecalciferol 20000 unit Fultium-D3 20,000unit capsules | 15 capsule [PoM] £17.04 DT = £17.04 | 30 capsule [PoM] £29.00 DT = £29.00
- InVita D3 (Consilient Health Ltd)
  Colecalciferol 400 unit InVita D3 400unit capsules | 28 capsule [PoM] £1.85 DT = £1.85
  Colecalciferol 800 unit InVita D3 800unit capsules | 28 capsule [PoM] £2.50
  Colecalciferol 5600 unit InVita D3 5,600unit capsules | 4 capsule [PoM] £2.50 DT = £2.50
  Colecalciferol 25000 unit InVita D3 25,000unit capsules | 3 capsule [PoM] £3.95 DT = £3.95
  Colecalciferol 50000 unit InVita D3 50,000unit capsules | 3 capsule [PoM] £4.95 DT = £4.95
- Plenachol (Accord Healthcare Ltd)
  Colecalciferol 20000 unit Plenachol D3 20,000unit capsules | 10 capsule [PoM] £9.00
  Colecalciferol 40000 unit Plenachol D3 40,000unit capsules | 10 capsule [PoM] £15.00 DT = £15.00
- Pro D3 (Synergy Biologics Ltd)
  Colecalciferol 2500 unit Pro D3 2,500unit capsules | 30 capsule £9.99
  Colecalciferol 10000 unit Pro D3 10,000unit capsules | 30 capsule £14.99
  Colecalciferol 30000 unit Pro D3 30,000unit capsules | 10 capsule £24.99
- Strivit-D3 (Strides Pharma UK Ltd)
  Colecalciferol 800 unit Strivit-D3 800unit capsules | 30 capsule [PoM] £2.50 DT = £3.60
- SunVit D3 (SunVit-D3 Ltd)
  Colecalciferol 2200 unit SunVit-D3 2,200unit capsules | 28 capsule £4.99
  Colecalciferol 2500 unit SunVit-D3 2,500unit capsules | 28 capsule £5.49
  Colecalciferol 3200 unit SunVit-D3 3,200unit capsules | 28 capsule £5.99
  Colecalciferol 10000 unit SunVit-D3 10,000unit capsules | 28 capsule £6.99

Orodispersible tablet

- Colecalciferol (Non-proprietary)
  Colecalciferol 2000 unit Vitamin D3 Lemon Melts 2,000unit tablets sugar-free | 120 tablet £5.12

Colecalciferol with calcium carbonate

The properties listed below are those particular to the combination only. For the properties of the components please consider, colecalciferol p. 681, calcium carbonate p. 641.

● **INDICATIONS AND DOSE**

Prevention and treatment of vitamin D and calcium deficiency

▶ BY MOUTH

- Child: Dosed according to the deficit or daily maintenance requirements (consult product literature)

● **UNLICENSED USE** *Adcal-D3*® and *Calceos*® are not licensed for use in children under 12 years. *Cacit*® D3, *Calcichew-D*$_3$® *Forte*, *Calcichew- D*$_3$® and *Kalcipos- D*® not licensed for use in children (age range not specified by manufacturers). *Accrete D3*® and *Natecal D3*® not licensed for use in children under 18 years.

● **INTERACTIONS** → Appendix 1: calcium salts · vitamin D substances

● **PRESCRIBING AND DISPENSING INFORMATION** *Accrete D3*® contains calcium carbonate 1.5 g (calcium 600 mg or Ca^{2+} 15 mmol), colecalciferol 10 micrograms (400 units); *Adcal-D3*® tablets contain calcium carbonate 1.5 g (calcium 600 mg or Ca^{2+} 15 mmol), colecalciferol 10 micrograms (400 units); *Cacit*® *D3* contains calcium carbonate 1.25 g (calcium 500 mg or Ca^{2+} 12.5 mmol), colecalciferol 11 micrograms (440 units)/sachet; *Calceos*® contains calcium carbonate 1.25 g (calcium 500 mg or Ca^{2+} 12.5 mmol), colecalciferol 10 micrograms (400 units); *Calcichew-D3*® tablets contain calcium carbonate 1.25 g (calcium 500 mg or Ca^{2+} 12.5 mmol), colecalciferol 5 micrograms (200 units); *Calcichew-D3*® *Forte* tablets contain calcium carbonate 1.25 g (calcium 500 mg or Ca^{2+} 12.5 mmol), colecalciferol 10 micrograms (400 units); *Calcichew-D3*® 500 mg/400 unit caplets contain calcium carbonate (calcium 500 mg or Ca^{2+} 12.5 mmol), colecalciferol 10 micrograms (400 units); *Kalcipos-D*® contains calcium carbonate (calcium 500 mg or Ca^{2+} 12.5 mmol), colecalciferol 20 micrograms (800 units); *Natecal D3*® contains calcium carbonate 1.5 g (calcium 600 mg or Ca^{2+} 15 mmol), colecalciferol 10 micrograms (400 units); consult product literature for details of other available products.

Flavours of chewable and soluble forms may include orange, lemon, aniseed, peppermint, molasses, or tutti-frutti.

● **MEDICINAL FORMS** There can be variation in the licensing of different medicines containing the same drug.

Effervescent granules

CAUTIONARY AND ADVISORY LABELS 13

- Colecalciferol with calcium carbonate (Non-proprietary)
  Calcium carbonate 2.5 gram, Colecalciferol 880 unit Colecalciferol 880unit / Calcium carbonate 2.5g effervescent granules sachets | 24 sachet [PoM] [X]
- Cacit D3 (Theramex HQ UK Ltd)
  Calcium carbonate 1.25 gram, Colecalciferol 440 unit Cacit D3 effervescent granules sachets | 30 sachet [P] £4.06 DT = £4.06

Effervescent tablet

CAUTIONARY AND ADVISORY LABELS 13

- Colecalciferol with calcium carbonate (Non-proprietary)

  Calcium carbonate 1.5 gram, Colecalciferol 400 unit ColeKal-D3 Dissolve 400unit/1500mg effervescent tablets | 56 tablet £4.97 DT = £5.99

- Adcal-D3 (Kyowa Kirin Ltd)

  Calcium carbonate 1.5 gram, Colecalciferol 400 unit Adcal-D3 Dissolve 1500mg/400unit effervescent tablets | 56 tablet [P] £5.99 DT = £5.99

Tablet

EXCIPIENTS: May contain Propylene glycol

- Accrete D3 (Internis Pharmaceuticals Ltd)

  Calcium carbonate 1.5 gram, Colecalciferol 400 unit Accrete D3 tablets | 60 tablet [P] £2.95 DT = £2.95

- Adcal-D3 (Kyowa Kirin Ltd)

  Calcium carbonate 750 mg, Colecalciferol 200 unit Adcal-D3 750mg/200unit caplets | 112 tablet [P] £2.95 DT = £2.95

Chewable tablet

CAUTIONARY AND ADVISORY LABELS 24

EXCIPIENTS: May contain Aspartame

- Colecalciferol with calcium carbonate (Non-proprietary)

  Calcium carbonate 1.5 gram, Colecalciferol 400 unit SunVit-D3 400unit with Calcium 600mg chewable tablets lemon | 56 tablet £2.69 DT = £3.65

  SunVit-D3 400unit with Calcium 600mg chewable tablets tutti frutti | 56 tablet £2.69 DT = £3.65

  Colecalciferol 400unit / Calcium carbonate 1.5g chewable tablets | 56 tablet [P] £3.65 DT = £3.65 | 60 tablet [P] £5.05

- Accrete D3 One a Day (Internis Pharmaceuticals Ltd)

  Calcium carbonate 2.5 gram, Colecalciferol 880 unit Accrete D3 One a Day 1000mg/880unit chewable tablets | 30 tablet [P] £2.95 DT = £2.95

- Adcal-D3 (Kyowa Kirin Ltd)

  Calcium carbonate 1.5 gram, Colecalciferol 400 unit Adcal-D3 Lemon chewable tablets | 56 tablet [P] £3.65 DT = £3.65 | 112 tablet [P] £7.49

  Adcal-D3 chewable tablets tutti frutti | 56 tablet [P] £3.65 DT = £3.65 | 112 tablet [P] £7.49

- Calceos (Galen Ltd)

  Calcium carbonate 1.25 gram, Colecalciferol 400 unit Calceos 500mg/400unit chewable tablets | 60 tablet [P] £3.94 DT = £4.24

- Calci-D (Consilient Health Ltd)

  Calcium carbonate 2.5 gram, Colecalciferol 1000 iu Calci-D 1000mg/1,000unit chewable tablets | 28 tablet [PoM] £2.25 DT = £2.25

- Calcichew D3 (Takeda UK Ltd)

  Calcium carbonate 2.5 gram, Colecalciferol 800 iu Calcichew D3 1000mg/800unit Once Daily chewable tablets | 30 tablet [P] £6.75 DT = £6.75

  Calcium carbonate 1.25 gram, Colecalciferol 200 unit Calcichew D3 chewable tablets | 100 tablet [P] £7.68 DT = £7.68

- Calcichew D3 Forte (Takeda UK Ltd)

  Calcium carbonate 1.25 gram, Colecalciferol 400 unit Calcichew D3 Forte chewable tablets | 60 tablet [P] £4.24 DT = £4.24 | 100 tablet [P] £7.08

- Evacal D3 (Teva UK Ltd)

  Calcium carbonate 1.5 gram, Colecalciferol 400 unit Evacal D3 1500mg/400unit chewable tablets | 56 tablet [P] £2.75 DT = £3.65 | 112 tablet [P] £5.50

- Kalcipos-D (Mylan)

  Calcium carbonate 1.25 gram, Colecalciferol 800 unit Kalcipos-D 500mg/800unit chewable tablets | 30 tablet [PoM] £4.21 DT = £4.21

- Natecal (Chiesi Ltd)

  Calcium carbonate 1.5 gram, Colecalciferol 400 unit Natecal D3 600mg/400unit chewable tablets | 60 tablet [P] £3.63

- TheiCal-D3 (Stirling Anglian Pharmaceuticals Ltd)

  Calcium carbonate 2.5 gram, Colecalciferol 880 unit TheiCal-D3 1000mg/880unit chewable tablets | 30 tablet [P] £2.95 DT = £2.95

9

Blood and nutrition

Colecalciferol with calcium phosphate

The properties listed below are those particular to the combination only. For the properties of the components please consider, colecalciferol p. 681, calcium phosphate p. 643.

● **INDICATIONS AND DOSE**

Calcium and vitamin D deficiency

▶ BY MOUTH

- Child: (consult product literature)

● **INTERACTIONS** → Appendix 1: calcium salts · vitamin D substances

● **MEDICINAL FORMS** There can be variation in the licensing of different medicines containing the same drug.

Powder

CAUTIONARY AND ADVISORY LABELS 13, 21

- Calfovit D3 (A. Menarini Farmaceutica Internazionale SRL)

  Calcium phosphate 3.1 gram, Colecalciferol 800 unit Calfovit D3 oral powder sachets | 30 sachet [P] £4.32 DT = £4.32

680

Ergocalciferol

(Calciferol; Vitamin D_2)

● **INDICATIONS AND DOSE**

Nutritional vitamin-D deficiency rickets

▶ BY MOUTH

- Child 1–5 months: 3000 units daily, dose to be adjusted as necessary
- Child 6 months–11 years: 6000 units daily, dose to be adjusted as necessary
- Child 12–17 years: 10 000 units daily, dose to be adjusted as necessary

Nutritional or physiological supplement | Prevention of rickets

▶ BY MOUTH

- Neonate: 400 units daily.
- Child: 400–600 units daily

Vitamin D deficiency in intestinal malabsorption or in chronic liver disease

▶ BY MOUTH, OR BY INTRAMUSCULAR INJECTION

- Child 1–11 years: 10 000–25 000 units daily, dose to be adjusted as necessary
- Child 12–17 years: 10 000–40 000 units daily, dose to be adjusted as necessary

● **CAUTIONS** Take care to ensure correct dose in infants

● **INTERACTIONS** → Appendix 1: vitamin D substances

● **RENAL IMPAIRMENT**

Monitoring Monitor plasma-calcium concentration in renal impairment.

● **MONITORING REQUIREMENTS** Monitor plasma-calcium concentration in patients receiving high doses.

● **PRESCRIBING AND DISPENSING INFORMATION** The BP directs that when calciferol is prescribed or demanded, colecalciferol or ergocalciferol should be dispensed or supplied.

When the strength of the tablets ordered or prescribed is not clear, the intention of the prescriber with respect to the strength (expressed in micrograms or milligrams per tablet) should be ascertained.

● **MEDICINAL FORMS** There can be variation in the licensing of different medicines containing the same drug. Forms available from special-order manufacturers include: tablet, capsule, oral suspension, oral solution, solution for injection

Tablet

- Ergo-D2 (Ennogen Healthcare Ltd)
  Ergocalciferol 12.5 microgram Ergo-D2 12.5microgram tablets | 30 tablet
- Ergoral (Cubic Pharmaceuticals Ltd)
  Ergocalciferol 125 microgram Ergoral D2 5,000unit tablets | 30 tablet £14.95
  Ergocalciferol 250 microgram Ergoral D2 10,000unit tablets | 30 tablet £17.95

Solution for injection

- Ergocalciferol (Non-proprietary)
  Ergocalciferol 300000 unit per 1 ml Ergocalciferol 300,000units/1ml solution for injection ampoules | 10 ampoule PoM £93.51 DT = £93.51
  Ergocalciferol 400000 unit per 1 ml Sterogyl 15H 600,000units/1.5ml solution for injection ampoules | 1 ampoule PoM

Oral solution

- Uvesterol D (Imported (France))
  Ergocalciferol 1500 unit per 1 ml Uvesterol D 1,500units/ml oral solution sugar-free | 20 ml PoM
- Eciferol (Rhodes Pharma Ltd)
  Ergocalciferol 3000 unit per 1 ml Eciferol D2 3,000units/ml liquid | 60 ml £55.00 DT = £55.98

Capsule

- Ergo-D2 (Ennogen Healthcare Ltd)
  Ergocalciferol 1.25 mg Ergo-D2 1.25mg capsules | 30 capsule £96.80
- Eciferol (Rhodes Pharma Ltd)
  Ergocalciferol 1.25 mg Eciferol D2 50,000unit capsules | 10 capsule £29.99
- Ergoral (Cubic Pharmaceuticals Ltd)
  Ergocalciferol 1.25 mg Ergoral D2 50,000unit capsules | 10 capsule £19.95

Ergocalciferol with calcium lactate and calcium phosphate

(Calcium and vitamin D)

The properties listed below are those particular to the combination only. For the properties of the components please consider, ergocalciferol p. 684, calcium lactate p. 643.

● **INDICATIONS AND DOSE**

Prevention of calcium and vitamin D deficiency | Treatment of calcium and vitamin D deficiency

▶ BY MOUTH

- Child: (consult product literature)

● **UNLICENSED USE** Calcium and Ergocalciferol tablets not licensed for use in children under 6 years.

● **INTERACTIONS** → Appendix 1: calcium salts · vitamin D substances

● **DIRECTIONS FOR ADMINISTRATION** Tablets may be crushed before administration, or may be chewed.

● **PRESCRIBING AND DISPENSING INFORMATION** Each tablet contains calcium lactate 300 mg, calcium phosphate 150 mg (calcium 97 mg or Ca^{2+} 2.4 mmol), ergocalciferol 10 micrograms (400 units).

● **PATIENT AND CARER ADVICE** Patient or carers should be given advice on how to administer calcium and ergocalciferol tablets.

● **MEDICINAL FORMS** There can be variation in the licensing of different medicines containing the same drug.

Tablet

- Ergocalciferol with calcium lactate and calcium phosphate (Non-proprietary)
  Ergocalciferol 10 microgram, Calcium phosphate 150 mg, Calcium lactate 300 mg Calcium and Ergocalciferol tablets | 28 tablet P £40.53 DT = £21.49

F 680

Paricalcitol

24-Jul-2018

● **INDICATIONS AND DOSE**

Prevention and treatment of secondary hyperparathyroidism associated with chronic kidney disease

▶ BY MOUTH

- Child 10–17 years: (consult product literature)

● **INTERACTIONS** → Appendix 1: vitamin D substances

● **SIDE-EFFECTS**

▶ **Common or very common** Electrolyte imbalance

▶ **Uncommon** Asthenia · breast tenderness · diarrhoea · dizziness · dry mouth · gastrointestinal discomfort · gastrooesophageal reflux disease · hypoparathyroidism · malaise · muscle complaints · pain · palpitations · peripheral oedema · pneumonia · taste altered

▶ **Frequency not known** Angioedema · laryngeal oedema

● **PREGNANCY** Manufacturer advises avoid—toxicity in *animal* studies.

● **BREAST FEEDING** Manufacturer advises avoid—no information available.

● **MONITORING REQUIREMENTS**

▶ Monitor plasma calcium and phosphate during dose titration and at least monthly when stabilised.

▶ Monitor parathyroid hormone concentration.

● **MEDICINAL FORMS** There can be variation in the licensing of different medicines containing the same drug.

Capsule

EXCIPIENTS: May contain Ethanol

- Zemplar (AbbVie Ltd)
  Paricalcitol 1 microgram Zemplar 1microgram capsules | 28 capsule PoM £69.44 DT = £69.44
  Paricalcitol 2 microgram Zemplar 2microgram capsules | 28 capsule PoM £138.88 DT = £138.88

VITAMINS AND TRACE ELEMENTS > VITAMIN E

Alpha tocopherol

06-May-2020

(Tocopherol)

● **INDICATIONS AND DOSE**

Vitamin E deficiency because of malabsorption in congenital or hereditary chronic cholestasis

▶ BY MOUTH USING ORAL SOLUTION

- Neonate: 17 mg/kg daily, dose to be adjusted as necessary.
- Child: 17 mg/kg daily, dose to be adjusted as necessary

● **CONTRA-INDICATIONS** Preterm neonates (in neonates)

● **CAUTIONS** Predisposition to thrombosis

● **INTERACTIONS** → Appendix 1: vitamin E substances

● **SIDE-EFFECTS**

▶ **Common or very common** Diarrhoea

▶ **Uncommon** Alopecia · asthenia · headache · skin reactions

▶ **Frequency not known** Abdominal pain

● **PREGNANCY** Manufacturer advises caution, no evidence of harm in *animal* studies.

- **BREAST FEEDING** Manufacturer advises use only if potential benefit outweighs risk—no information available.
- **HEPATIC IMPAIRMENT** Manufacturer advises caution.
- **RENAL IMPAIRMENT** Manufacturer advises caution. Risk of renal toxicity due to polyethylene glycol content.
  Monitoring Manufacturer advises monitor closely in renal impairment.
- **PRESCRIBING AND DISPENSING INFORMATION**
  Tocofersolan is a water-soluble form of D-alpha tocopherol.

- **MEDICINAL FORMS** There can be variation in the licensing of different medicines containing the same drug.

Oral solution

- Vedrop (Recordati Rare Diseases UK Ltd) ▼
  D-alpha tocopherol (as Tocofersolan) 50 mg per 1 ml Vedrop 50mg/ml oral solution sugar-free | 20 ml PoM £54.55 DT = £54.55 sugar-free | 60 ml PoM £163.65

Alpha tocopheryl acetate
(Tocopherol)

- **INDICATIONS AND DOSE**

Vitamin E deficiency

▶ BY MOUTH
- Neonate: 10 mg/kg once daily.
- Child: 2–10 mg/kg daily, increased if necessary up to 20 mg/kg daily

Malabsorption in cystic fibrosis

▶ BY MOUTH
- Child 1-11 months: 50 mg once daily, dose to be adjusted as necessary, to be taken with food and pancreatic enzymes
- Child 1-11 years: 100 mg once daily, dose to be adjusted as necessary, to be taken with food and pancreatic enzymes
- Child 12-17 years: 100–200 mg once daily, dose to be adjusted as necessary, to be taken with food and pancreatic enzymes

Vitamin E deficiency in cholestasis and severe liver disease

▶ BY MOUTH
- Neonate: 10 mg/kg daily.
- Child 1 month-11 years: Initially 100 mg daily, adjusted according to response, increased if necessary up to 200 mg/kg daily
- Child 12-17 years: Initially 200 mg daily, adjusted according to response, increased if necessary up to 200 mg/kg daily

▶ BY INTRAMUSCULAR INJECTION
- Neonate: 10 mg/kg once a month.
- Child: 10 mg/kg once a month (max. per dose 100 mg)

Malabsorption in abetalipoproteinaemia

▶ BY MOUTH
- Neonate: 100 mg/kg once daily.
- Child: 50–100 mg/kg once daily

- **CAUTIONS** Increased risk of necrotising enterocolitis in neonate weighing less than 1.5 kg or in a preterm neonate (in neonates) · predisposition to thrombosis
- **INTERACTIONS** → Appendix 1: vitamin E substances
- **SIDE-EFFECTS** Abdominal pain (more common at high doses) · bleeding tendency · diarrhoea (more common at high doses) · increased risk of thrombosis
- **PREGNANCY** No evidence of safety of high doses.
- **BREAST FEEDING** Excreted in milk; minimal risk, although caution with large doses.
- **MONITORING REQUIREMENTS** Increased bleeding tendency in vitamin-K deficient patients or those taking anticoagulants (prothrombin time and INR should be monitored).
- **DIRECTIONS FOR ADMINISTRATION** Consider dilution of oral suspension for use in neonates due to high osmolality.

- **MEDICINAL FORMS** There can be variation in the licensing of different medicines containing the same drug. Forms available from special-order manufacturers include: chewable tablet, solution for injection

Solution for injection

- Alpha tocopheryl acetate (Non-proprietary)
  Alpha tocopheryl acetate 50 mg per 1 ml E-Vicotrat 100mg/2ml solution for injection ampoules | 10 ampoule PoM ⊠

Oral suspension

EXCIPIENTS: May contain Sucrose

- Alpha tocopheryl acetate (Non-proprietary)
  Alpha tocopheryl acetate 100 mg per 1 ml AlphaToc-E 500mg/5ml oral suspension sugar-free | 100 ml £47.19
  Alpha tocopheryl acetate 500mg/5ml oral suspension | 100 ml GSL £69.67 DT = £67.21

Chewable tablet

- E-Tabs (Ennogen Healthcare Ltd)
  Alpha tocopheryl acetate 100 mg E-Tabs 100mg chewable tablets | 30 tablet £87.30
- Ephynal (Imported (Italy))
  Alpha tocopheryl acetate 100 mg Ephynal 100mg chewable tablets | 30 tablet ⊠

Capsule

- Alpha tocopheryl acetate (Non-proprietary)
  Alpha tocopherol 75 unit Vitamin E 75unit capsules | 100 capsule £13.05
  Alpha tocopherol 200 unit Vitamin E 200unit capsules | 30 capsule £10.05
  Bio-E-Vitamin 200unit capsules | 150 capsule £9.40
  Alpha tocopherol 400 unit Vitamin E 400unit capsules | 30 capsule £15.12
- E-Caps (Ennogen Healthcare Ltd)
  Alpha tocopherol 75 unit E-Caps 75unit capsules | 100 capsule £109.50
  Alpha tocopherol 100 unit E-Caps 100unit capsules | 30 capsule £84.40
  Alpha tocopherol 200 unit E-Caps 200unit capsules | 30 capsule £89.50
  Alpha tocopherol 400 unit E-Caps 400unit capsules | 30 capsule £128.50
  Alpha tocopherol 1000 unit E-Caps 1,000unit capsules | 30 capsule £130.20
- Nutra-E (TriOn Pharma Ltd)
  Alpha tocopherol 75 unit Nutra-E 75unit capsules | 100 capsule £5.86
  Alpha tocopherol 200 unit Nutra-E 200unit capsules | 100 capsule £12.88
  Alpha tocopherol 400 unit Nutra-E 400unit capsules | 100 capsule £19.82
- Vita-E (Typharm Ltd)
  Alpha tocopherol 75 unit Vita-E 75unit capsules | 100 capsule £6.99
  Alpha tocopherol 200 unit Vita-E 200unit capsules | 30 capsule £5.35 | 100 capsule £14.99
  Alpha tocopherol 400 unit Vita-E 400unit capsules | 30 capsule £7.99 | 100 capsule £21.85

VITAMINS AND TRACE ELEMENTS > VITAMIN K

Menadiol sodium phosphate

- **INDICATIONS AND DOSE**

Supplementation in vitamin K malabsorption

▶ BY MOUTH
- Child 1-11 years: 5–10 mg daily, dose to be adjusted as necessary
- Child 12-17 years: 10–20 mg daily, dose to be adjusted as necessary

- **CONTRA-INDICATIONS** Infants · neonates
- **CAUTIONS** G6PD deficiency (risk of haemolysis) · vitamin E deficiency (risk of haemolysis)
- **PREGNANCY** Avoid in late pregnancy and labour unless benefit outweighs risk of neonatal haemolytic anaemia, hyperbilirubinaemia, and kernicterus in neonate.

- **MEDICINAL FORMS** There can be variation in the licensing of different medicines containing the same drug.

Tablet
- Menadiol sodium phosphate (Non-proprietary)
  Menadiol phosphate (as Menadiol sodium phosphate) 10 mg Menadiol 10mg tablets | 100 tablet [P] £214.71 DT = £214.71

Phytomenadione
26-Mar-2019

(Vitamin K_1)

- **INDICATIONS AND DOSE**

Neonatal prophylaxis of vitamin-K deficiency bleeding

▶ BY INTRAMUSCULAR INJECTION

- Preterm neonate: 400 micrograms/kg (max. per dose 1 mg) for 1 dose, to be given at birth, the intravenous route may be used in preterm neonates with very low birth-weight if intramuscular injection is not possible, however, it may not provide the prolonged protection of the intramuscular injection, any neonate receiving intravenous vitamin K should be given subsequent oral doses.
- Neonate: 1 mg for 1 dose, to be given at birth.

Neonatal hypoprothrombinaemia | Vitamin-K deficiency bleeding

▶ BY INTRAVENOUS INJECTION

- Neonate: 1 mg every 8 hours if required.

Neonatal biliary atresia and liver disease

▶ BY MOUTH

- Neonate: 1 mg daily.

Reversal of coumarin anticoagulation when continued anticoagulation required or if no significant bleeding—seek specialist advice

▶ BY INTRAVENOUS INJECTION

- Child: 15–30 micrograms/kg (max. per dose 1 mg) for 1 dose, dose may be repeated as necessary

Reversal of coumarin anticoagulation when anticoagulation not required or if significant bleeding—seek specialist advice | Treatment of haemorrhage associated with vitamin-K deficiency—seek specialist advice

▶ BY INTRAVENOUS INJECTION

- Child: 250–300 micrograms/kg (max. per dose 10 mg) for 1 dose

KONAKION® MM PAEDIATRIC

Neonatal prophylaxis of vitamin-K deficiency bleeding in healthy babies who are not at risk of bleeding disorders

▶ BY MOUTH

- Neonate: Initially 2 mg for 1 dose at birth, then 2 mg after 4–7 days.

Neonatal prophylaxis of vitamin-K deficiency bleeding in healthy babies who are not at risk of bleeding disorders (exclusively breast fed babies)

▶ BY MOUTH

- Neonate: Initially 2 mg for 1 dose at birth, then 2 mg after 4–7 days for a further 1 dose, then 2 mg for a further 1 dose 1 month after birth.

NEOKAY

Neonatal prophylaxis of vitamin-K deficiency bleeding in healthy babies who are not at particular risk of bleeding disorders

▶ BY MOUTH

- Neonate: 1 mg for 1 dose at birth (to protect from the risk of vitamin K deficiency bleeding in the first week).

Neonatal prophylaxis of vitamin-K deficiency bleeding in healthy babies who are not at particular risk of bleeding disorders (exclusively breast-fed babies)

▶ BY MOUTH

- Neonate: Initially 1 mg for 1 dose at birth, then 1 mg every week for 12 weeks.

- **CAUTIONS** Intravenous injections should be given very slowly—risk of vascular collapse

KONAKION® MM PAEDIATRIC
- With intravenous use Parenteral administration in premature infant or neonate of less than 2.5 kg (increased risk of kernicterus)

- **PREGNANCY** Use if potential benefit outweighs risk.
- **BREAST FEEDING** Present in milk.
- **HEPATIC IMPAIRMENT**

KONAKION® MM Manufacturer advises caution—monitor INR in patients with severe impairment (contains glycocholic acid which may displace bilirubin).

- **DIRECTIONS FOR ADMINISTRATION**

- With oral use in neonates The contents of one capsule should be administered by cutting the narrow tubular tip off and squeezing the liquid contents into the mouth; if the baby spits out the dose or is sick within three hours of administration a replacement dose should be given.

KONAKION® MM PAEDIATRIC *Konakion® MM Paediatric* may be administered *by mouth* or *by intramuscular injection* or *by intravenous injection*. For *intravenous injection*, may be diluted with Glucose 5% if necessary.

KONAKION® MM *Konakion® MM* may be administered by slow intravenous injection or by intravenous infusion in glucose 5%; **not** for intramuscular injection.

- **MEDICINAL FORMS** There can be variation in the licensing of different medicines containing the same drug. Forms available from special-order manufacturers include: capsule, oral suspension, oral solution

Solution for injection

EXCIPIENTS: May contain Glycocholic acid, lecithin
- Konakion MM (Cheplapharm Arzneimittel GmbH)
  Phytomenadione 10 mg per 1 ml Konakion MM Paediatric 2mg/0.2ml solution for injection ampoules | 5 ampoule [PoM] £4.71 DT = £4.71
  Konakion MM 10mg/1ml solution for injection ampoules | 10 ampoule [PoM] £3.78 DT = £3.78

Capsule
- K-Cap (Transdermal Ltd)
  Phytomenadione 1 mg K-Cap 1mg capsules | 30 capsule £15.80
- Neokay (Neoceuticals Ltd)
  Phytomenadione 1 mg NeoKay 1mg capsules | 12 capsule [PoM] £3.95 DT = £3.95 | 100 capsule [PoM] £34.00

7.1 Neural tube defects (prevention in pregnancy)

Neural tube defects (prevention in pregnancy) 01-Aug-2017

Description of condition

Neural tube defects represent a group of congenital defects, caused by incomplete closure of the neural tube within 28 days of conception. The most common forms are anencephaly, spina bifida and encephalocele.

The main risk factors are maternal folate deficiency, maternal vitamin B_{12} deficiency, previous history of having an infant with a neural tube defect, smoking, diabetes, obesity, and use of antiepileptic drugs. For information on smoking cessation see Smoking cessation p. 313.

Prevention in pregnancy

EvGr Pregnant women or women who wish to become pregnant should be advised to take supplementation with folic acid p. 620 before conception and until week 12 of pregnancy.

A higher daily dose (see folic acid) is recommended for women at a high risk of conceiving a child with a neural tube defect, including women who have previously had an infant with a neural tube defect, who are receiving antiepileptic medication (see Epilepsy p. 203), or who have diabetes or sickle-cell disease. ⟨A⟩

Useful Resources

Antenatal care for uncomplicated pregnancies. National Institute for Health and Care Excellence. Clinical guideline 62. March 2008 (Updated March 2016).
www.nice.org.uk/guidance/cg62

Fertility problems: assessment and treatment. National Institute for Health and Care Excellence. Clinical guideline 156. June 2015.
www.nice.org.uk/guidance/cg156

Chapter 10
Musculoskeletal system

CONTENTS

1 Arthritis

Juvenile idiopathic arthritis

Management

Rheumatic diseases require symptomatic treatment to relieve pain, swelling, and stiffness, together with treatment to control and suppress disease activity. Treatment of juvenile idiopathic arthritis may involve Non-steroidal anti-inflammatory drugs p. 703 (NSAIDs), a disease modifying anti-rheumatic drug (DMARD) such as methotrexate p. 588 or a cytokine modulator, and intra-articular, intravenous, or oral corticosteroids.

Rheumatic disease, suppressing drugs

Overview

Certain drugs, such as methotrexate p. 588, cytokine modulators, and sulfasalazine p. 36, are used to suppress the disease process in *juvenile idiopathic arthritis* (juvenile chronic arthritis); these drugs are known as disease-modifying antirheumatic drugs (DMARDs). In children, DMARDs should be used under specialist supervision.

Some children with juvenile idiopathic arthritis do not require DMARDs. Methotrexate is effective in juvenile idiopathic arthritis; sulfasalazine is an alternative but should be avoided in *systemic-onset juvenile idiopathic arthritis*. Gold and penicillamine p. 666 are no longer used. Cytokine modulators have a role in *polyarticular juvenile idiopathic arthritis*.

Unlike NSAIDs, DMARDs can affect the progression of disease but they may require 3–6 months of treatment for a full therapeutic response. Response to a DMARD may allow the dose of the NSAID to be reduced.

DMARDs can improve not only the symptoms of inflammatory joint disease but also extra-articular manifestations. They reduce the erythrocyte sedimentation rate and C-reactive protein.

Antimalarials

The antimalarial hydroxychloroquine sulfate p. 690 is rarely used to treat juvenile idiopathic arthritis. Hydroxychloroquine sulfate can also be useful for systemic or discoid lupus erythematosus, particularly involving the skin and joints, and in sarcoidosis.

Retinopathy rarely occurs provided that the recommended doses are not exceeded.

Mepacrine hydrochloride is used on rare occasions to treat discoid lupus erythematosus [unlicensed].

Drugs affecting the immune response

Methotrexate, given as a once weekly dose, is the DMARD of choice in the treatment of juvenile idiopathic arthritis and also has a role in juvenile dermatomyositis, vasculitis, uveitis, systemic lupus erythematosus, localised scleroderma, and sarcoidosis; for these indications it is given by the subcutaneous, oral, or rarely, the intramuscular route. Absorption from intramuscular or subcutaneous routes may be more predictable than from the oral route; if the oral route is ineffective subcutaneous administration is generally preferred. Folic acid may reduce mucosal or gastro-intestinal side-effects of methotrexate. The dosage regimen for folic acid p. 620 has not been established—in children over 2 years a weekly dose [unlicensed indication], may be given on a different day from the methotrexate.

Azathioprine p. 558 may be used in children for vasculitis which has failed to respond to other treatments, for the management of severe cases of *systemic lupus erythematosus* and other connective tissue disorders, in conjunction with corticosteroids for patients with severe or progressive renal disease, and in cases of *polymyositis* which are resistant to corticosteroids. Azathioprine has a corticosteroid-sparing effect in patients whose corticosteroid requirements are excessive.

Ciclosporin p. 559 is rarely used in juvenile idiopathic arthritis, connective tissue diseases, vasculitis, and uveitis; it may be considered if the condition has failed to respond to other treatments.

Cytokine modulators

Cytokine modulators should be used under specialist supervision.

Adalimumab p. 693, etanercept p. 696, and infliximab p. 38 inhibit the activity of tumour necrosis factor alpha (TNF-α). Adalimumab can be used for the management of active polyarticular juvenile idiopathic arthritis and enthesitis-related arthritis. Etanercept is licensed for the treatment of the following subtypes of juvenile idiopathic arthritis: polyarticular juvenile idiopathic arthritis in children who have had an inadequate response to methotrexate or who cannot tolerate it, oligoarthritis in children who have had an inadequate response to methotrexate or who cannot tolerate it, psoriatic arthritis in children over 12 years who have had an inadequate response to methotrexate or cannot tolerate it, and enthesitis-related arthritis in children over 12 years who have had an inadequate response to conventional therapy or cannot tolerate it. Infliximab has been used in refractory polyarticular juvenile idiopathic arthritis [unlicensed indication] when other treatments, such as etanercept, have failed.

Abatacept p. 693 prevents the full activation of T-lymphocytes; it can be used for the management of active polyarticular juvenile idiopathic arthritis. Abatacept is not recommended for use in combination with TNF inhibitors.

Canakinumab p. 565 inhibits the activity of interleukin-1 beta (IL-1β) and is licensed for the treatment of active systemic juvenile idiopathic arthritis in children over 2 years, when there has been an inadequate response to NSAIDs and systemic corticosteroids.

Tocilizumab p. 691 antagonises the actions of interleukin-6; it can be used for the management of active systemic juvenile idiopathic arthritis when there has been an inadequate response to NSAIDs and systemic corticosteroids and polyarticular juvenile idiopathic arthritis when there has been an inadequate response to methotrexate. Tocilizumab can be used in combination with methotrexate, or as monotherapy if methotrexate is not tolerated or is contra-indicated. Tocilizumab is not recommended for use with other cytokine modulators.

Sulfasalazine

Sulfasalazine has a beneficial effect in suppressing the inflammatory activity associated with some forms of juvenile idiopathic arthritis; it is generally not used in systemic-onset disease.

Other drugs used for Arthritis Cyclophosphamide, p. 579 · Diclofenac potassium, p. 704 · Diclofenac sodium, p. 704 · Etoricoxib, p. 706 · Flurbiprofen, p. 707 · Ibuprofen, p. 707 · Indometacin, p. 710 · Mefenamic acid, p. 711 · Meloxicam, p. 711 · Naproxen, p. 712 · Piroxicam, p. 713

DISEASE-MODIFYING ANTI-RHEUMATIC DRUGS

Hydroxychloroquine sulfate

11-May-2020

● **INDICATIONS AND DOSE**

Active rheumatoid arthritis (including juvenile idiopathic arthritis) (administered on expert advice) | Systemic and discoid lupus erythematosus (administered on expert advice) | Dermatological conditions caused or aggravated by sunlight (administered on expert advice)

▶ BY MOUTH

▶ Child: 5–6.5 mg/kg once daily (max. per dose 400 mg), dose given based on ideal body-weight

● **UNLICENSED USE** *Plaquenil*® not licensed for use in children for dermatological conditions caused or aggravated by sunlight.

● **CAUTIONS** Acute porphyrias p. 652 · diabetes (may lower blood glucose) · G6PD deficiency · maculopathy · may aggravate myasthenia gravis · may exacerbate psoriasis · neurological disorders (especially in those with a history of epilepsy—may lower seizure threshold) · severe gastro-intestinal disorders

CAUTIONS, FURTHER INFORMATION

▶ **Monitoring for retinopathy** A review group convened by the Royal College of Ophthalmologists has updated guidelines on monitoring for chloroquine and hydroxychloroquine retinopathy (*Hydroxychloroquine and Chloroquine Retinopathy: Recommendations on Monitoring* 2020). There are no reports of hydroxychloroquine retinopathy in patients under the age of 18 years, or evidence for monitoring paediatric patients for drug toxicity. However, the guideline recommends long-term users of hydroxychloroquine under the age of 18 years who otherwise satisfy the monitoring criteria should be referred for monitoring.

● **INTERACTIONS** → Appendix 1: hydroxychloroquine

● **SIDE-EFFECTS**

▶ **Common or very common** Abdominal pain · appetite decreased · diarrhoea · emotional lability · headache · nausea · skin reactions · vision disorders · vomiting

▶ **Uncommon** Alopecia · corneal oedema · dizziness · eye disorders · hair colour changes · nervousness · neuromuscular dysfunction · retinopathy · seizure · tinnitus · vertigo

▶ **Frequency not known** Acute hepatic failure · agranulocytosis · anaemia · angioedema · bone marrow disorders · bronchospasm · cardiac conduction disorders · cardiomyopathy · hearing loss · hypoglycaemia · leucopenia · movement disorders · muscle weakness · myopathy · photosensitivity reaction · psychosis · reflexes absent · severe cutaneous adverse reactions (SCARs) · thrombocytopenia · tremor · ventricular hypertrophy

Overdose Hydroxychloroquine is very toxic in overdosage; overdosage is extremely hazardous and difficult to treat. Urgent advice from the National Poisons Information Service is essential. Life-threatening features include arrhythmias (which can have a very rapid onset) and convulsions (which can be intractable).

● **PREGNANCY** It is not necessary to withdraw an antimalarial drug during pregnancy if the rheumatic disease is well controlled; however, the manufacturer of hydroxychloroquine advises avoiding use.

● **BREAST FEEDING** Manufacturer advises use with caution—present in milk in small amounts. Specialist sources indicate risk of accumulation in infant due to long half-life; monitor infant for symptoms of uveitis e.g. eye redness or sensitivity to light.

● **HEPATIC IMPAIRMENT** Manufacturer advises caution.

Dose adjustments Manufacturer advises consider dose adjustment in severe impairment.

● **RENAL IMPAIRMENT** Manufacturer advises caution.

Monitoring Monitor plasma-hydroxychloroquine concentration in severe renal impairment.

● **MONITORING REQUIREMENTS** Manufacturer advises regular ophthalmological examination but the evidence of practical value is unsatisfactory (see *Cautions, further information* for advice of the Royal College of Ophthalmologists).

● **PRESCRIBING AND DISPENSING INFORMATION** To avoid excessive dosage in obese patients, the dose of hydroxychloroquine should be calculated on the basis of ideal body-weight.

● **MEDICINAL FORMS** There can be variation in the licensing of different medicines containing the same drug. Forms available from special-order manufacturers include: oral suspension, oral solution

Tablet

CAUTIONARY AND ADVISORY LABELS 21

▶ **Hydroxychloroquine sulfate (Non-proprietary)**
Hydroxychloroquine sulfate 200 mg Hydroxychloroquine 200mg tablets | 60 tablet PoM £32.49 DT = £5.79

▶ **Quinoric** (Bristol Laboratories Ltd)
Hydroxychloroquine sulfate 200 mg Quinoric 200mg tablets | 60 tablet PoM £8.25 DT = £5.79

IMMUNOSUPPRESSANTS › INTERLEUKIN INHIBITORS

Anakinra

13-Nov-2018

● **INDICATIONS AND DOSE**

Cryopyrin-associated periodic syndromes (specialist use only)

▶ BY SUBCUTANEOUS INJECTION

▸ Child 8 months–17 years (body-weight 10 kg and above): 1–2 mg/kg daily, for severe cryopyrin-associated periodic syndromes, usual maintenance is 3–4 mg/kg daily, up to a maximum of 8 mg/kg daily

Still's disease (specialist use only)

▶ BY SUBCUTANEOUS INJECTION

▸ Child 8 months–17 years (body-weight 10–49 kg): 1–2 mg/kg daily, increased if necessary up to 4 mg/kg daily

▸ Child 8 months–17 years (body-weight 50 kg and above): 100 mg daily, increased if necessary up to 4 mg/kg daily

● **CONTRA-INDICATIONS** Active infection · neutropenia (absolute neutrophil count less than 1.5×10^9/litre)—do not initiate · pre-existing malignancy

● **CAUTIONS** History of asthma (increased risk of serious infection) · history of recurrent infection · predisposition to infection

● **INTERACTIONS** → Appendix 1: anakinra

● **SIDE-EFFECTS**

▶ **Common or very common** Headache · infection · neutropenia · thrombocytopenia

▶ **Uncommon** Skin reactions

▶ **Frequency not known** Hepatitis

SIDE-EFFECTS, FURTHER INFORMATION Neutropenia reported commonly—discontinue if neutropenia develops.

● **PREGNANCY** Manufacturer advises avoid.

● **BREAST FEEDING** Manufacturer advises avoid—no information available.

● **HEPATIC IMPAIRMENT** Manufacturer advises caution in severe impairment.

● **RENAL IMPAIRMENT** Manufacturer advises caution in moderate impairment.

Dose adjustments Manufacturer advises consider alternate day dosing in severe impairment.

● **PRE-TREATMENT SCREENING** Manufacturer advises patients should be screened for latent tuberculosis and viral hepatitis prior to initiation of treatment.

● **MONITORING REQUIREMENTS**

▶ Manufacturer advises monitor neutrophil count before treatment, then every month for 6 months, then every 3 months thereafter.

▸ When used for Cryopyrin-associated periodic syndromes Manufacturer advises monitor for CNS inflammation (including ear and eye tests) 3 months after starting treatment, then every 6 months until effective treatment doses have been identified, then yearly thereafter.

▸ When used for Still's disease Manufacturer advises consider routine monitoring of hepatic enzymes during the first month of treatment.

● **PRESCRIBING AND DISPENSING INFORMATION**

▸ When used for Cryopyrin-associated periodic syndromes or Still's disease The manufacturer of *Kineret®* has provided a *Guide for Healthcare Professionals*.

● **PATIENT AND CARER ADVICE**

Blood disorders Patients should be instructed to seek medical advice if symptoms suggestive of neutropenia (such as fever, sore throat, bruising or, bleeding) develop.

▸ When used for Still's disease A patient card and patient booklet should be provided.

▸ When used for Cryopyrin-associated periodic syndromes A patient booklet should be provided.

● **NATIONAL FUNDING/ACCESS DECISIONS**

Scottish Medicines Consortium (SMC) decisions

SMC No. SMC2104

The *Scottish Medicines Consortium* has advised (October 2018) that anakinra (*Kineret®*) is accepted for use within NHS Scotland for the treatment of Still's disease, as monotherapy or in combination with other anti-inflammatory drugs and disease-modifying anti-rheumatic drugs.

● **MEDICINAL FORMS** There can be variation in the licensing of different medicines containing the same drug.

Solution for injection

▸ Kineret (Swedish Orphan Biovitrum Ltd)

Anakinra 150 mg per 1 ml Kineret 100mg/0.67ml solution for injection pre-filled syringes | 7 pre-filled disposable injection [PoM] £183.61 DT = £183.61

Tocilizumab

20-Aug-2019

● **INDICATIONS AND DOSE**

Active systemic juvenile idiopathic arthritis [in combination with methotrexate or alone if methotrexate inappropriate, in children who have had an inadequate response to NSAIDs and systemic corticosteroids]

▶ BY INTRAVENOUS INFUSION

▸ Child 2–17 years (body-weight up to 30 kg): 12 mg/kg every 2 weeks, for dose adjustments in patients with liver enzyme abnormalities, or low absolute neutrophil or platelet count—consult product literature, review treatment if no improvement within 6 weeks

▸ Child 2–17 years (body-weight 30 kg and above): 8 mg/kg every 2 weeks, for dose adjustments in patients with liver enzyme abnormalities, or low absolute neutrophil or platelet count— consult product literature, review treatment if no improvement within 6 weeks

Polyarticular juvenile idiopathic arthritis [in combination with methotrexate or alone if methotrexate inappropriate, in children who have had an inadequate response to methotrexate]

▶ BY INTRAVENOUS INFUSION

▸ Child 2–17 years (body-weight up to 30 kg): 10 mg/kg every 4 weeks, for dose adjustments in patients with liver enzyme abnormalities, or low absolute neutrophil or platelet count— consult product literature, review treatment if no improvement within 12 weeks

▸ Child 2–17 years (body-weight 30 kg and above): 8 mg/kg every 4 weeks, for dose adjustments in patients with liver enzyme abnormalities, or low absolute neutrophil or platelet count—consult product literature, review treatment if no improvement within 12 weeks

ROACTEMRA® PRE-FILLED SYRINGE

Polyarticular juvenile idiopathic arthritis [in combination with methotrexate or alone if methotrexate inappropriate, in children who have had an inadequate response to methotrexate]

▶ BY SUBCUTANEOUS INJECTION

▸ Child 2–17 years (body-weight up to 30 kg): 162 mg every 3 weeks, administer to abdomen, thigh or upper arm, for dose adjustments in patients with liver enzyme abnormalities, or low absolute neutrophil or platelet count—consult product literature, review treatment if no improvement within 12 weeks

▸ Child 2–17 years (body-weight 30 kg and above): 162 mg every 2 weeks, administer to abdomen, thigh or upper arm, for dose adjustments in patients with continued →

liver enzyme abnormalities, or low absolute neutrophil or platelet count—consult product literature, review treatment if no improvement within 12 weeks

IMPORTANT SAFETY INFORMATION

MHRA/CHM ADVICE: TOCILIZUMAB (*ROACTEMRA*®): RARE RISK OF SERIOUS LIVER INJURY INCLUDING CASES REQUIRING TRANSPLANTATION (JULY 2019)

There have been reports of rare but serious cases of drug-induced liver injury, including acute liver failure and hepatitis, in patients treated with tocilizumab; some cases required liver transplantation. Serious liver injury was reported from 2 weeks to more than 5 years after initiation of tocilizumab.

Healthcare professionals are advised to initiate tocilizumab treatment with caution in patients with hepatic transaminases (ALT or AST) more than 1.5 times the upper limit of normal (ULN); initiation is not recommended in those with ALT or AST more than 5 times the ULN (see *Monitoring requirements*). Patients and their carers should be advised to seek immediate medical attention if signs and symptoms of liver injury, such as tiredness, abdominal pain, and jaundice, occur.

- **CONTRA-INDICATIONS** Do not initiate if absolute neutrophil count less than 2×10^9/litre · severe active infection
- **CAUTIONS** History of diverticulitis · history of intestinal ulceration · history of recurrent or chronic infection (interrupt treatment if serious infection occurs) · low absolute neutrophil count · low platelet count · predisposition to infection (interrupt treatment if serious infection occurs)

CAUTIONS, FURTHER INFORMATION

- Tuberculosis Patients with latent tuberculosis should be treated with standard therapy before starting tocilizumab.

- **INTERACTIONS** → Appendix 1: monoclonal antibodies
- **SIDE-EFFECTS**
- **Common or very common** Diarrhoea · headache · increased risk of infection · infusion related reaction · nausea
- **Frequency not known** Hepatic disorders

SIDE-EFFECTS, FURTHER INFORMATION **Neutrophil and platelet counts** Manufacturer advises discontinue if absolute neutrophil count less than 0.5×10^9/litre or platelet count less than 50×10^3/microlitre.

Abnormal hepatic function Manufacturer advises caution if hepatic enzymes more than 1.5 times the upper limit of normal.

Manufacturer advises discontinue if hepatic enzymes more than 5 times the upper limit of normal.

- **CONCEPTION AND CONTRACEPTION** Effective contraception required during and for 3 months after treatment.
- **PREGNANCY** Manufacturer advises avoid unless essential—toxicity in *animal* studies.
- **BREAST FEEDING** Manufacturer advises avoid—no information available.
- **HEPATIC IMPAIRMENT** Manufacturer advises caution—consult product literature.
- **RENAL IMPAIRMENT**
- With intravenous use Manufacturer advises monitor renal function closely in moderate-to-severe impairment—no information available.
- With subcutaneous use Manufacturer advises monitor renal function closely in severe impairment—no information available.
- **PRE-TREATMENT SCREENING**

Tuberculosis Patients should be evaluated for tuberculosis before treatment.

- **MONITORING REQUIREMENTS**
- Manufacturer advises monitor lipid profile 4–8 weeks after starting treatment and then as indicated.
- Manufacturer advises monitor for demyelinating disorders.
- MHRA advises monitor hepatic transaminases before starting treatment, every 4–8 weeks for first 6 months of treatment, then every 12 weeks thereafter.
- Manufacturer advises monitor neutrophil and platelet count at the time of the second administration, and then as indicated.
- **DIRECTIONS FOR ADMINISTRATION**
- With intravenous use For *intravenous infusion*, manufacturer advises for body-weight less than 30 kg, give intermittently in Sodium chloride 0.9%, dilute requisite dose to a volume of 50 mL with infusion fluid and give over 1 hour; body-weight 30 kg or greater, give intermittently in Sodium chloride 0.9%, dilute requisite dose to a volume of 100 mL with infusion fluid and give over 1 hour.
- With subcutaneous use For *subcutaneous injection*, manufacturer advises rotate injection site and avoid skin that is tender, damaged or scarred. Patients may self-administer RoActemra ®, after appropriate training in subcutaneous injection technique.
- **PRESCRIBING AND DISPENSING INFORMATION** Manufacturer advises to record the brand name and batch number after each administration.
- **HANDLING AND STORAGE** Manufacturer advises protect from light and store in a refrigerator (2–8 °C)—consult product literature for further information regarding storage conditions outside refrigerator and after preparation of the infusion.
- **PATIENT AND CARER ADVICE** Manufacturer advises patients and their carers should be advised to seek immediate medical attention if symptoms of infection occur, or if symptoms of diverticular perforation such as abdominal pain, haemorrhage, or fever accompanying change in bowel habits occur.

An alert card should be provided.

Driving and skilled tasks Manufacturer advises patients should be counselled on the effects on driving and performance of skilled tasks—increased risk of dizziness.

- **NATIONAL FUNDING/ACCESS DECISIONS**

NICE decisions

- **Tocilizumab for the treatment of systemic juvenile idiopathic arthritis (December 2011)** NICE TA238

Tocilizumab (*RoActemra*®) is recommended for the treatment of systemic juvenile idiopathic arthritis in children aged 2 years and older who have not responded adequately to NSAIDs, systemic corticosteroids and methotrexate, if the manufacturer makes tocilizumab available with the discount agreed as part of the patient access scheme.

Tocilizumab is **not** recommended for the treatment of systemic juvenile idiopathic arthritis in children whose disease continues to respond to methotrexate or who have not been treated with methotrexate.

Patients currently receiving tocilizumab for systemic juvenile idiopathic arthritis who do not meet these criteria should have the option to continue treatment until it is considered appropriate to stop.

www.nice.org.uk/guidance/ta238

- **Abatacept, adalimumab, etanercept and tocilizumab for treating juvenile idiopathic arthritis (December 2015)** NICE TA373

Tocilizumab (*RoActemra*®) is recommended as an option for treatment of polyarticular juvenile idiopathic arthritis (JIA), including polyarticular-onset, polyarticular-course and extended oligoarticular JIA in children 2 years and older whose disease has responded inadequately to previous therapy with methotrexate and if the

manufacturer provides tocilizumab with the discounts agreed in the patient access schemes.
www.nice.org.uk/guidance/ta373

- **MEDICINAL FORMS** There can be variation in the licensing of different medicines containing the same drug.

Solution for injection

- ▸ **RoActemra** (Roche Products Ltd)
  Tocilizumab 180 mg per 1 ml RoActemra 162mg/0.9ml solution for injection pre-filled syringes | 4 pre-filled disposable injection PoM £913.12 DT = £913.12 (Hospital only)
  RoActemra 162mg/0.9ml solution for injection pre-filled pens | 4 pre-filled disposable injection PoM £913.12 DT = £913.12

Solution for infusion

ELECTROLYTES: May contain Sodium

- ▸ **RoActemra** (Roche Products Ltd)
  Tocilizumab 20 mg per 1 ml RoActemra 400mg/20ml concentrate for solution for infusion vials | 1 vial PoM £512.00 (Hospital only)
  RoActemra 200mg/10ml concentrate for solution for infusion vials | 1 vial PoM £256.00 (Hospital only)
  RoActemra 80mg/4ml concentrate for solution for infusion vials | 1 vial PoM £102.40 (Hospital only)

IMMUNOSUPPRESSANTS › T-CELL ACTIVATION INHIBITORS

Abatacept

01-Dec-2017

- **INDICATIONS AND DOSE**

Moderate-to-severe active polyarticular juvenile idiopathic arthritis (specialist use only)

▸ BY INTRAVENOUS INFUSION

- ▸ Child 6–17 years (body-weight up to 75 kg): 10 mg/kg every 2 weeks for 3 doses, then 10 mg/kg every 4 weeks, review treatment if no response within 6 months
- ▸ Child 6–17 years (body-weight 75–100 kg): 750 mg every 2 weeks for 3 doses, then 750 mg every 4 weeks, review treatment if no response within 6 months
- ▸ Child 6–17 years (body-weight 101 kg and above): 1 g every 2 weeks for 3 doses, then 1 g every 4 weeks, review treatment if no response within 6 months

Moderate-to-severe active polyarticular juvenile idiopathic arthritis (specialist use only)

▸ BY SUBCUTANEOUS INJECTION

- ▸ Child 2–17 years (body-weight 10–24 kg): 50 mg once weekly, review treatment if no response within 6 months
- ▸ Child 2–17 years (body-weight 25–49 kg): 87.5 mg once weekly, review treatment if no response within 6 months
- ▸ Child 2–17 years (body-weight 50 kg and above): 125 mg once weekly, review treatment if no response within 6 months

- **CONTRA-INDICATIONS** Severe infection
- **CAUTIONS** Children should be brought up to date with current immunisation schedule before initiating therapy · do not initiate until active infections are controlled · predisposition to infection (screen for latent tuberculosis and viral hepatitis) · progressive multifocal leucoencephalopathy (discontinue treatment if neurological symptoms present)
- **INTERACTIONS** → Appendix 1: abatacept
- **SIDE-EFFECTS**

▸ **Common or very common** Asthenia · cough · diarrhoea · dizziness · gastrointestinal discomfort · headaches · hypertension · increased risk of infection · nausea · oral ulceration · skin reactions · vomiting

▸ **Uncommon** Alopecia · anxiety · arrhythmias · arthralgia · bruising tendency · conjunctivitis · depression · dry eye · dyspnoea · gastritis · hyperhidrosis · hypotension · influenza like illness · leucopenia · menstrual cycle irregularities · neoplasms · pain in extremity · palpitations · paraesthesia · respiratory disorders · sepsis · sleep disorders · throat tightness · thrombocytopenia · vasculitis · vasodilation · vertigo · visual acuity decreased · weight increased

▸ **Rare or very rare** Pelvic inflammatory disease

- **CONCEPTION AND CONTRACEPTION** Effective contraception required during treatment and for 14 weeks after last dose.
- **PREGNANCY** Manufacturer advises avoid unless essential.
- **BREAST FEEDING** Present in milk in *animal* studies—manufacturer advises avoid breast-feeding during treatment and for 14 weeks after last dose.
- **DIRECTIONS FOR ADMINISTRATION** For *intravenous infusion*, given intermittently *in* Sodium chloride 0.9%; reconstitute each vial with 10 mL water for injections using the silicone-free syringe provided; dilute requisite dose in Sodium Chloride 0.9% to 100 mL (using the same silicone-free syringe); give over 30 minutes through a low protein-binding filter (pore size 0.2–1.2 micron).
- **NATIONAL FUNDING/ACCESS DECISIONS**

NICE decisions

▸ **Abatacept, adalimumab, etanercept and tocilizumab for treating juvenile idiopathic arthritis (December 2015)** NICE TA373

Abatacept is recommended as options for treating polyarticular juvenile idiopathic arthritis (JIA), including polyarticular-onset, polyarticular-course and extended oligoarticular JIA in patients 6 years and older whose disease has responded inadequately to other disease-modifying anti-rheumatic drugs (DMARDs) including at least 1 tumour necrosis factor (TNF) inhibitor, **only** if the manufacturer provides abatacept with the discounts agreed in the patient access schemes.
www.nice.org.uk/guidance/TA373

- **MEDICINAL FORMS** There can be variation in the licensing of different medicines containing the same drug.

Solution for injection

- ▸ **Orencia** (Bristol-Myers Squibb Pharmaceuticals Ltd)
  Abatacept 125 mg per 1 ml Orencia 50mg/0.4ml solution for injection pre-filled syringes | 4 pre-filled disposable injection PoM (Hospital only)
  Orencia 87.5mg/0.7ml solution for injection pre-filled syringes | 4 pre-filled disposable injection PoM (Hospital only)
  Orencia 125mg/1ml solution for injection pre-filled syringes | 4 pre-filled disposable injection PoM £1,209.60 DT = £1,209.60 (Hospital only)
- ▸ **Orencia ClickJect** (Bristol-Myers Squibb Pharmaceuticals Ltd)
  Abatacept 125 mg per 1 ml Orencia ClickJect 125mg/1ml solution for injection pre-filled pens | 4 pre-filled disposable injection PoM £1,209.60 DT = £1,209.60

Powder for solution for infusion

ELECTROLYTES: May contain Sodium

- ▸ **Orencia** (Bristol-Myers Squibb Pharmaceuticals Ltd)
  Abatacept 250 mg Orencia 250mg powder for concentrate for solution for infusion vials | 1 vial PoM £302.40 (Hospital only)

IMMUNOSUPPRESSANTS › TUMOR NECROSIS FACTOR ALPHA (TNF-α) INHIBITORS

Adalimumab

13-Dec-2018

- **INDICATIONS AND DOSE**

Plaque psoriasis (initiated by a specialist)

▸ BY SUBCUTANEOUS INJECTION

- ▸ Child 4–17 years (body-weight 15–29 kg): Initially 20 mg once weekly for 2 doses, then 20 mg every 2 weeks, review treatment if no response within 16 weeks
- ▸ Child 4–17 years (body-weight 30 kg and above): Initially 40 mg once weekly for 2 doses, then 40 mg every 2 weeks, review treatment if no response within 16 weeks

continued →

10 Musculoskeletal system

Polyarticular juvenile idiopathic arthritis (initiated by a specialist)
- BY SUBCUTANEOUS INJECTION
- Child 2–17 years (body-weight 10–29 kg): 20 mg every 2 weeks, review treatment if no response within 12 weeks
- Child 2–17 years (body-weight 30 kg and above): 40 mg every 2 weeks, review treatment if no response within 12 weeks

Enthesitis-related arthritis (initiated by a specialist)
- BY SUBCUTANEOUS INJECTION
- Child 6–17 years (body-weight 15–29 kg): 20 mg every 2 weeks
- Child 6–17 years (body-weight 30 kg and above): 40 mg every 2 weeks

Crohn's disease (initiated by a specialist)
- BY SUBCUTANEOUS INJECTION
- Child 6–17 years (body-weight up to 40 kg): Initially 40 mg, then 20 mg after 2 weeks; maintenance 20 mg every 2 weeks, increased if necessary to 20 mg once weekly, review treatment if no response within 12 weeks
- Child 6–17 years (body-weight 40 kg and above): Initially 80 mg, then 40 mg after 2 weeks; maintenance 40 mg every 2 weeks, increased if necessary to 40 mg once weekly, alternatively 80 mg every 2 weeks, review treatment if no response within 12 weeks

Crohn's disease (accelerated regimen) (initiated by a specialist)
- BY SUBCUTANEOUS INJECTION
- Child 6–17 years (body-weight up to 40 kg): Initially 80 mg, then 40 mg after 2 weeks; maintenance 20 mg every 2 weeks, increased if necessary to 20 mg once weekly, review treatment if no response within 12 weeks
- Child 6–17 years (body-weight 40 kg and above): Initially 160 mg, dose can alternatively be given as divided injections over 2 days, then 80 mg after 2 weeks; maintenance 40 mg every 2 weeks, then increased if necessary to 40 mg once weekly, alternatively 80 mg every 2 weeks, review treatment if no response within 12 weeks

Hidradenitis suppurativa (initiated by a specialist)
- BY SUBCUTANEOUS INJECTION
- Child 12–17 years (body-weight 30 kg and above): Initially 80 mg, followed by 40 mg after 1 week, then maintenance 40 mg every 2 weeks; increased if necessary to 40 mg once weekly, alternatively 80 mg every 2 weeks, review treatment if no response within 12 weeks; if treatment interrupted—consult product literature

Uveitis (initiated by a specialist)
- BY SUBCUTANEOUS INJECTION
- Child 2–17 years (body-weight up to 30 kg): Initially 40 mg, then 20 mg after 1 week; maintenance 20 mg every 2 weeks
- Child 2–17 years (body-weight 30 kg and above): Initially 80 mg, then 40 mg after 1 week; maintenance 40 mg every 2 weeks

- **CONTRA-INDICATIONS** Moderate or severe heart failure · severe infections
- **CAUTIONS** Children should be brought up to date with current immunisation schedule before initiating therapy · demyelinating disorders (risk of exacerbation) · development of malignancy · do not initiate until active infections are controlled (discontinue if new serious infection develops) · hepatitis B virus—monitor for active infection · history of malignancy · mild heart failure (discontinue if symptoms develop or worsen) · predisposition to infection

CAUTIONS, FURTHER INFORMATION
- Tuberculosis Active tuberculosis should be treated with standard treatment for at least 2 months before starting adalimumab. Patients who have previously received adequate treatment for tuberculosis can start adalimumab but should be monitored every 3 months for possible recurrence. In patients without active tuberculosis but who were previously not treated adequately, chemoprophylaxis should ideally be completed before starting adalimumab. In patients at high risk of tuberculosis who cannot be assessed by tuberculin skin test, chemoprophylaxis can be given concurrently with adalimumab.

- **INTERACTIONS** → Appendix 1: monoclonal antibodies
- **SIDE-EFFECTS**
- **Common or very common** Agranulocytosis · alopecia · anaemia · anxiety · arrhythmias · arterial occlusion · asthma · broken nails · chest pain · coagulation disorder · connective tissue disorders · cough · dehydration · depression · dyspnoea · electrolyte imbalance · embolism and thrombosis · eye inflammation · fever · flushing · gastrointestinal discomfort · gastrointestinal disorders · haemorrhage · headaches · healing impaired · hyperglycaemia · hypersensitivity · hypertension · increased risk of infection · insomnia · leucocytosis · leucopenia · mood altered · muscle spasms · musculoskeletal pain · nausea · neoplasms · nerve disorders · neutropenia · oedema · renal impairment · seasonal allergy · sensation abnormal · sepsis · skin reactions · sweat changes · thrombocytopenia · vasculitis · vertigo · vision disorders · vomiting
- **Uncommon** Aortic aneurysm · congestive heart failure · deafness · demyelinating disorders · dysphagia · erectile dysfunction · gallbladder disorders · hepatic disorders · inflammation · lupus erythematosus · meningitis viral · myocardial infarction · nocturia · pancreatitis · respiratory disorders · rhabdomyolysis · sarcoidosis · solid organ neoplasm · stroke · tinnitus · tremor
- **Rare or very rare** Cardiac arrest · pancytopenia · Stevens-Johnson syndrome

SIDE-EFFECTS, FURTHER INFORMATION Associated with infections, sometimes severe, including tuberculosis, septicaemia, and hepatitis B reactivation.

- **CONCEPTION AND CONTRACEPTION** Manufacturer advises effective contraception required during treatment and for at least 5 months after last dose.
- **PREGNANCY** Manufacturer advises use only if potential benefit outweighs risk.
- **BREAST FEEDING** Manufacturer advises can be used—excreted in breast milk at very low concentrations (limited information available).
- **PRE-TREATMENT SCREENING**
Tuberculosis Manufacturer advises patients should be evaluated for active and latent tuberculosis before treatment.
- **MONITORING REQUIREMENTS**
- Manufacturer advises monitor for infection before, during, and for 4 months after treatment.
- Manufacturer advises monitor for non-melanoma skin cancer before and during treatment, especially in patients with a history of PUVA treatment for psoriasis or extensive immunosuppressant therapy.
- *For uveitis*, manufacturer advises patients should be assessed for pre-existing or developing central demyelinating disorders before and at regular intervals during treatment.
- **PRESCRIBING AND DISPENSING INFORMATION**
Adalimumab is a biological medicine. Biological medicines must be prescribed and dispensed by brand name, see *Biological medicines* and *Biosimilar medicines*, under Guidance on prescribing p. 1.

- **PATIENT AND CARER ADVICE** When used to treat *hidradenitis suppurativa*, patients and their carers should be advised to use a daily topical antiseptic wash on lesions during treatment with adalimumab.
Tuberculosis Patients and their carers should be advised to seek medical attention if symptoms suggestive of tuberculosis (e.g. persistent cough, weight loss, or, and fever) develop.
Blood disorders Patients and their carers should be advised to seek medical attention if symptoms suggestive of blood disorders (such as fever, sore throat, bruising, or bleeding) develop.
Alert card An alert card should be provided.
- **NATIONAL FUNDING/ACCESS DECISIONS**

NICE decisions

▸ **Abatacept, adalimumab, etanercept and tocilizumab for treating juvenile idiopathic arthritis (December 2015)** NICE TA373
Adalimumab is recommended as an option for treating polyarticular juvenile idiopathic arthritis (JIA), including polyarticular-onset, polyarticular-course and extended oligoarticular JIA in patients 2 years and older whose disease has responded inadequately to 1 or more disease-modifying antirheumatic drugs (DMARDs) and for treating enthesitis-related JIA in patients 6 years and older whose disease has responded inadequately to, or who are intolerant of, conventional therapy.
www.nice.org.uk/guidance/ta373

▸ **Adalimumab, etanercept and ustekinumab for treating plaque psoriasis in children and young people (July 2017)** NICE TA455
Adalimumab is recommended as an option for treating plaque psoriasis in children and young people aged 4 years or older, only if the disease:
- is severe, as defined by a total Psoriasis Area and Severity Index (PASI) of 10 or more and
- has not responded to standard systemic therapy, such as ciclosporin, methotrexate or phototherapy, or these options are contra-indicated or not tolerated.

Stop treatment at 16 weeks if the psoriasis has not responded adequately. An adequate response is defined as a 75% reduction in the PASI score from the start of treatment.

Patients currently receiving adalimumab who do not meet the above criteria and whose treatment was started within the NHS before this guidance was published, should have the option to continue treatment until they and their clinician consider it appropriate to stop.
www.nice.org.uk/guidance/ta455

Scottish Medicines Consortium (SMC) decisions

The *Scottish Medicines Consortium* has advised (May 2015) that adalimumab (*Humira*®) is accepted for restricted use within NHS Scotland for the treatment of active enthesitis-related arthritis in children 6 years of age and over who have had an inadequate response to, or who are intolerant of, conventional therapy, and is used within specialist rheumatology services (including those working within the network for paediatric rheumatology).

The *Scottish Medicines Consortium* has advised (June 2017) that adalimumab (*Humira*®) is accepted for use within NHS Scotland for the treatment of active moderate-to-severe hidradenitis suppurativa (HS) (acne inversa) in adolescents from 12 years of age with an inadequate response to conventional systemic HS therapy.

All Wales Medicines Strategy Group (AWMSG) decisions

The *All Wales Medicines Strategy Group* has advised (January 2017) that adalimumab (*Humira*®) is recommended as an option for use within NHS Wales for the treatment of moderately to severely active Crohn's disease in children 6 years and over, who have had an inadequate response to conventional therapy including primary nutrition therapy and a corticosteroid and/or an immunomodulator, or who are intolerant to or have contra-indications for such therapies.

The *All Wales Medicines Strategy Group* has advised (August 2017) that adalimumab (*Humira*®) is recommended as an option for use within NHS Wales for the treatment of active moderate to severe hidradenitis suppurativa (acne inversa) in adolescents from 12 years of age with an inadequate response to conventional systemic hidradenitis suppurativa therapy. This advice is contingent upon the continuing availability of the Wales Patient Access Scheme or a list price that is equivalent or lower.

The *All Wales Medicines Strategy Group* has advised (December 2017) that adalimumab (*Humira*®) is recommended as an option for use within NHS Wales for the treatment of paediatric chronic non-infectious anterior uveitis in patients from two years of age who have had an inadequate response to or are intolerant to conventional therapy, or in whom conventional therapy is inappropriate.

- **MEDICINAL FORMS** There can be variation in the licensing of different medicines containing the same drug.

Solution for injection

CAUTIONARY AND ADVISORY LABELS 10

▸ **Amgevita** (Amgen Ltd) ▼
Adalimumab 50 mg per 1 ml Amgevita 20mg/0.4ml solution for injection pre-filled syringes | 1 pre-filled disposable injection PoM £158.40
Amgevita 40mg/0.8ml solution for injection pre-filled syringes | 2 pre-filled disposable injection PoM £633.60
Amgevita 40mg/0.8ml solution for injection pre-filled pens | 2 pre-filled disposable injection PoM £633.60

▸ **Hulio** (Mylan) ▼
Adalimumab 50 mg per 1 ml Hulio 40mg/0.8ml solution for injection pre-filled pens | 2 pre-filled disposable injection PoM £616.25

▸ **Humira** (AbbVie Ltd)
Adalimumab 100 mg per 1 ml Humira 40mg/0.4ml solution for injection pre-filled pens | 2 pre-filled disposable injection PoM £704.28 DT = £704.28
Humira 40mg/0.4ml solution for injection pre-filled syringes | 2 pre-filled disposable injection PoM £704.28 DT = £704.28
Humira 20mg/0.2ml solution for injection pre-filled syringes | 2 pre-filled disposable injection PoM £352.14 DT = £352.14
Humira 80mg/0.8ml solution for injection pre-filled syringes | 1 pre-filled disposable injection PoM £704.28
Humira 80mg/0.8ml solution for injection pre-filled pens | 1 pre-filled disposable injection PoM £704.28

▸ **Hyrimoz** (Sandoz Ltd) ▼
Adalimumab 50 mg per 1 ml Hyrimoz 40mg/0.8ml solution for injection pre-filled pens | 2 pre-filled disposable injection PoM £646.18
Hyrimoz 40mg/0.8ml solution for injection pre-filled syringes | 2 pre-filled disposable injection PoM £646.18

▸ **Idacio** (Fresenius Kabi Ltd) ▼
Adalimumab 50 mg per 1 ml Idacio 40mg/0.8ml solution for injection vials | 1 vial PoM £316.93
Idacio 40mg/0.8ml solution for injection pre-filled syringes | 2 pre-filled disposable injection PoM £633.86
Idacio 40mg/0.8ml solution for injection pre-filled pens | 2 pre-filled disposable injection PoM £633.86

▸ **Imraldi** (Biogen Idec Ltd) ▼
Adalimumab 50 mg per 1 ml Imraldi 40mg/0.8ml solution for injection pre-filled pens | 2 pre-filled disposable injection PoM £633.85
Imraldi 40mg/0.8ml solution for injection pre-filled syringes | 2 pre-filled disposable injection PoM £633.85

Etanercept

02-Aug-2018

● **INDICATIONS AND DOSE**

BENEPALI ® SOLUTION FOR INJECTION

Polyarthritis in children who have had an inadequate response to methotrexate or who cannot tolerate it | Extended oligoarthritis in children who have had an inadequate response to methotrexate or who cannot tolerate it

▶ BY SUBCUTANEOUS INJECTION

▸ Child 2–17 years: 800 micrograms/kg once weekly (max. per dose 50 mg), consider discontinuation if no response after 4 months

Psoriatic arthritis in adolescents who have had an inadequate response to methotrexate or who cannot tolerate it | Enthesitis-related arthritis in adolescents who have had an inadequate response to conventional therapy or who cannot tolerate it

▶ BY SUBCUTANEOUS INJECTION

▸ Child 12–17 years: 800 micrograms/kg once weekly (max. per dose 50 mg), consider discontinuation if no response after 4 months

Chronic, severe plaque psoriasis in children who have had an inadequate response to other systemic therapies or phototherapies or who cannot tolerate them

▶ BY SUBCUTANEOUS INJECTION

▸ Child 6–17 years: 800 micrograms/kg once weekly (max. per dose 50 mg) for up to 24 weeks, discontinue if no response after 12 weeks

ENBREL ® POWDER AND SOLVENT FOR SOLUTION FOR INJECTION

Polyarthritis in children who have had an inadequate response to methotrexate or who cannot tolerate it | Extended oligoarthritis in children who have had an inadequate response to methotrexate or who cannot tolerate it

▶ BY SUBCUTANEOUS INJECTION

▸ Child 2–17 years: 400 micrograms/kg twice weekly (max. per dose 25 mg), to be given at an interval of 3—4 days between doses, alternatively 800 micrograms/kg once weekly (max. per dose 50 mg), consider discontinuation if no response after 4 months

Psoriatic arthritis in adolescents who have had an inadequate response to methotrexate or who cannot tolerate it | Enthesitis-related arthritis in adolescents who have had an inadequate response to conventional therapy or who cannot tolerate it

▶ BY SUBCUTANEOUS INJECTION

▸ Child 12–17 years: 400 micrograms/kg twice weekly (max. per dose 25 mg), to be given at an interval of 3—4 days between doses, alternatively 800 micrograms/kg once weekly (max. per dose 50 mg), consider discontinuation if no response after 4 months

Chronic, severe plaque psoriasis in children who have had an inadequate response to other systemic therapies or phototherapies or who cannot tolerate them

▶ BY SUBCUTANEOUS INJECTION

▸ Child 6–17 years: 800 micrograms/kg once weekly (max. per dose 50 mg) for up to 24 weeks, discontinue if no response after 12 weeks

ENBREL ® SOLUTION FOR INJECTION

Polyarthritis in children who have had an inadequate response to methotrexate or who cannot tolerate it | Extended oligoarthritis in children who have had an inadequate response to methotrexate or who cannot tolerate it

▶ BY SUBCUTANEOUS INJECTION

▸ Child 2–17 years: 400 micrograms/kg twice weekly (max. per dose 25 mg), to be given at an interval of 3–4 days between doses, alternatively 800 micrograms/kg once weekly (max. per dose 50 mg), consider discontinuation if no response after 4 months

Psoriatic arthritis in adolescents who have had an inadequate response to methotrexate or who cannot tolerate it | Enthesitis-related arthritis in adolescents who have had an inadequate response to conventional therapy or who cannot tolerate it

▶ BY SUBCUTANEOUS INJECTION

▸ Child 12–17 years: 400 micrograms/kg twice weekly (max. per dose 25 mg), to be given at an interval of 3–4 days between doses, alternatively 800 micrograms/kg once weekly (max. per dose 50 mg), consider discontinuation if no response after 4 months

Chronic, severe plaque psoriasis in children who have had an inadequate response to other systemic therapies or phototherapies or who cannot tolerate them

▶ BY SUBCUTANEOUS INJECTION

▸ Child 6–17 years: 800 micrograms/kg once weekly (max. per dose 50 mg) for up to 24 weeks, discontinue if no response after 12 weeks

● **CONTRA-INDICATIONS** Active infection · avoid injections containing benzyl alcohol in neonates

● **CAUTIONS** Children should be brought up to date with current immunisation schedule before initiating therapy · development of malignancy · diabetes mellitus · heart failure (risk of exacerbation) · hepatitis B virus—monitor for active infection · hepatitis C infection (monitor for worsening infection) · history of blood disorders · history of malignancy · history or increased risk of demyelinating disorders · predisposition to infection (avoid if predisposition to septicaemia) · significant exposure to herpes zoster virus—interrupt treatment and consider varicella–zoster immunoglobulin

CAUTIONS, FURTHER INFORMATION

▸ **Tuberculosis** Active tuberculosis should be treated with standard treatment for at least 2 months before starting etanercept. Patients who have previously received adequate treatment for tuberculosis can start etanercept but should be monitored every 3 months for possible recurrence. In patients without active tuberculosis but who were previously not treated adequately, chemoprophylaxis should ideally be completed before starting etanercept. In patients at high risk of tuberculosis who cannot be assessed by tuberculin skin test, chemoprophylaxis can be given concurrently with etanercept.

● **INTERACTIONS** → Appendix 1: etanercept

● **SIDE-EFFECTS**

▶ **Common or very common** Cystitis · fever · hypersensitivity · increased risk of infection · pain · skin reactions · swelling

▶ **Uncommon** Abscess · bursitis · cholecystitis · diarrhoea · endocarditis · eye inflammation · gastritis · hepatic disorders · myositis · neoplasms · respiratory disorders · sepsis · skin ulcers · thrombocytopenia · vasculitis

▶ **Rare or very rare** Anaemia · bone marrow disorders · congestive heart failure · cutaneous lupus erythematosus · demyelination · leucopenia · lupus-like syndrome · nerve disorders · neutropenia · sarcoidosis · seizure · severe cutaneous adverse reactions (SCARs) · transverse myelitis

▶ **Frequency not known** Abdominal pain · depression · dermatomyositis exacerbated · headache · hepatitis B reactivation · inflammatory bowel disease · macrophage activation syndrome · nausea · personality disorder · post procedural infection · type 1 diabetes mellitus · vomiting

SIDE-EFFECTS, FURTHER INFORMATION Associated with infections, sometimes severe, including tuberculosis, septicaemia, and hepatitis B reactivation.

- **CONCEPTION AND CONTRACEPTION** Manufacturer advises effective contraception required during treatment and for 3 weeks after last dose.
- **PREGNANCY** Avoid—limited information available.
- **BREAST FEEDING** Manufacturer advises avoid—present in milk in *animal* studies.
- **HEPATIC IMPAIRMENT** Manufacturer advises caution in moderate to severe alcoholic hepatitis.
- **PRE-TREATMENT SCREENING**
Tuberculosis Patients should be evaluated for tuberculosis before treatment.
- **MONITORING REQUIREMENTS** Monitor for skin cancer before and during treatment, particularly in those at risk (including patients with psoriasis or a history of PUVA treatment).
- **PRESCRIBING AND DISPENSING INFORMATION** Etanercept is a biological medicine. Biological medicines must be prescribed and dispensed by brand name, see *Biological medicines* and *Biosimilar medicines*, under Guidance on prescribing p. 1.
BENEPALI® SOLUTION FOR INJECTION Manufacturer advises patients requiring less than the full 50 mg dose should **not** receive *Benepali*®—if an alternate dose is required, other etanercept formulations providing this option should be used.
- **PATIENT AND CARER ADVICE**
Blood disorders Patients and their carers should be advised to seek medical attention if symptoms suggestive of blood disorders (such as fever, sore throat, bruising, or bleeding) develop.
Tuberculosis Patients and their carers should be advised to seek medical attention if symptoms suggestive of tuberculosis (e.g. persistent cough, weight loss, and fever) develop.
Alert card An alert card should be provided.
Medicines for Children leaflet: Etanercept for juvenile idiopathic arthritis www.medicinesforchildren.org.uk/etanercept-juvenile-idiopathic-arthritis
- **NATIONAL FUNDING/ACCESS DECISIONS**

NICE decisions

▸ **Abatacept, adalimumab, etanercept and tocilizumab for treating juvenile idiopathic arthritis (December 2015)** NICE TA373

Etanercept is recommended as an option for treating:
- polyarticular juvenile idiopathic arthritis (JIA), including polyarticular-onset, polyarticular-course and extended oligoarticular JIA, in patients 2 years and over whose disease has responded inadequately to, or who are intolerant of, methotrexate;
- enthesitis-related JIA in patients 12 years and over whose disease has responded inadequately to, or who are intolerant of, conventional therapy;
- psoriatic JIA in patients 12 years and over whose disease has responded inadequately to, or who are intolerant of, methotrexate.

www.nice.org.uk/guidance/ta373

▸ **Adalimumab, etanercept and ustekinumab for treating plaque psoriasis in children and young people (July 2017)**

Etanercept is recommended as an option for treating plaque psoriasis in children and young people aged 6 years and older, only if the disease:
- is severe, as defined by a total Psoriasis Area and Severity Index (PASI) of 10 or more, and
- has not responded to standard systemic therapy, such as ciclosporin, methotrexate or phototherapy, or these options are contra-indicated or not tolerated.

If the psoriasis has not responded adequately, stop treatment at 12 weeks. An adequate response is defined as a 75% reduction in PASI score from the start of treatment.

Patients currently receiving etanercept who do not meet the above criteria and whose treatment was started within the NHS before this guidance was published, should have the option to continue treatment until they and their clinician consider it appropriate to stop.
www.nice.org.uk/guidance/TA455

Scottish Medicines Consortium (SMC) decisions

The *Scottish Medicines Consortium* has advised (February 2013) that etanercept (*Enbrel*®) is accepted for restricted use within NHS Scotland for the treatment of polyarthritis (rheumatoid factor positive or negative) and extended oligoarthritis in children and adolescents from the age of 2 years who have had an inadequate response to or are intolerant of methotrexate, psoriatic arthritis in adolescents from the age of 12 years who have had an inadequate response to or are intolerant of methotrexate, and enthesitis-related arthritis in adolescents from the age of 12 years who have had an inadequate response to or are intolerant of conventional therapy. It is restricted to use within specialist rheumatology services (including those working within the network for paediatric rheumatology).

- **MEDICINAL FORMS** There can be variation in the licensing of different medicines containing the same drug.

Solution for injection

CAUTIONARY AND ADVISORY LABELS 10

▸ **Benepali** (Biogen Idec Ltd) ▼
Etanercept 50 mg per 1 ml Benepali 50mg/1ml solution for injection pre-filled pens | 4 pre-filled disposable injection PoM £656.00 DT = £715.00
Benepali 50mg/1ml solution for injection pre-filled syringes | 4 pre-filled disposable injection PoM £656.00 DT = £715.00

▸ **Enbrel** (Pfizer Ltd)
Etanercept 50 mg per 1 ml Enbrel 50mg/1ml solution for injection pre-filled syringes | 4 pre-filled disposable injection PoM £715.00 DT = £715.00 (Hospital only)
Enbrel 25mg/0.5ml solution for injection pre-filled syringes | 4 pre-filled disposable injection PoM £357.50 DT = £357.50 (Hospital only)

▸ **Enbrel MyClic** (Pfizer Ltd)
Etanercept 50 mg per 1 ml Enbrel 25mg/0.5ml solution for injection pre-filled MyClic pens | 4 pre-filled disposable injection PoM £357.50 (Hospital only)
Enbrel 50mg/1ml solution for injection pre-filled MyClic pens | 4 pre-filled disposable injection PoM £715.00 DT = £715.00 (Hospital only)

Powder and solvent for solution for injection

CAUTIONARY AND ADVISORY LABELS 10
EXCIPIENTS: May contain Benzyl alcohol

▸ **Enbrel** (Pfizer Ltd)
Etanercept 10 mg Enbrel Paediatric 10mg powder and solvent for solution for injection vials | 4 vial PoM £143.00 (Hospital only)
Etanercept 25 mg Enbrel 25mg powder and solvent for solution for injection vials | 4 vial PoM £357.50 (Hospital only)

Golimumab

03-Aug-2018

- **INDICATIONS AND DOSE**

Polyarticular juvenile idiopathic arthritis (initiated by a specialist)

▸ BY SUBCUTANEOUS INJECTION
▸ Child (body-weight 40 kg and above): 50 mg once a month, on the same date each month, review treatment if no response after 3–4 doses

- **CONTRA-INDICATIONS** Moderate or severe heart failure · severe active infection
- **CAUTIONS** Active infection (do not initiate until active infections are controlled; discontinue if new serious infection develops until infection controlled) · children should be brought up to date with current immunisation schedule before initiating therapy · demyelinating disorders (risk of exacerbation) · hepatitis B virus—monitor for active infection · history or development of malignancy · mild heart failure (discontinue if symptoms develop or worsen) · predisposition to infection · risk factors for

10 Musculoskeletal system

dysplasia or carcinoma of the colon—screen for dysplasia regularly

CAUTIONS, FURTHER INFORMATION

▸ Tuberculosis Active tuberculosis should be treated with standard treatment for at least 2 months before starting golimumab. Patients who have previously received adequate treatment for tuberculosis can start golimumab but should be monitored every 3 months for possible recurrence. In patients without active tuberculosis but who were previously not treated adequately, chemoprophylaxis should ideally be completed before starting golimumab. In patients at high risk of tuberculosis who cannot be assessed by tuberculin skin test, chemoprophylaxis can be given concurrently with golimumab. Patients who have tested negative for latent tuberculosis, and those who are receiving or who have completed treatment for latent tuberculosis, should be monitored closely for symptoms of active infection.

- **INTERACTIONS** → Appendix 1: monoclonal antibodies
- **SIDE-EFFECTS**

▸ **Common or very common** Abscess · alopecia · anaemia · asthenia · asthma · bone fracture · chest discomfort · depression · dizziness · fever · gastrointestinal discomfort · gastrointestinal disorders · gastrointestinal inflammatory disorders · headache · hypersensitivity · hypertension · increased risk of infection · insomnia · nausea · paraesthesia · respiratory disorders · skin reactions · stomatitis

▸ **Uncommon** Arrhythmia · balance impaired · bone marrow disorders · breast disorder · cholelithiasis · constipation · eye inflammation · eye irritation · flushing · goitre · hyperthyroidism · hypothyroidism · leucopenia · liver disorder · menstrual disorder · myocardial ischaemia · neoplasms · sepsis · thrombocytopenia · thrombosis · thyroid disorder · vision disorders

▸ **Rare or very rare** Bladder disorder · congestive heart failure · demyelination · healing impaired · hepatitis B reactivation · lupus-like syndrome · Raynaud's phenomenon · renal disorder · sarcoidosis · taste altered · vasculitis

SIDE-EFFECTS, FURTHER INFORMATION Associated with infections, sometimes severe, including tuberculosis, septicaemia, and hepatitis B reactivation.

- **CONCEPTION AND CONTRACEPTION** Manufacturer advises adequate contraception during treatment and for at least 6 months after last dose.
- **PREGNANCY** Use only if essential.
- **BREAST FEEDING** Manufacturer advises avoid during and for at least 6 months after treatment—present in milk in *animal* studies.
- **HEPATIC IMPAIRMENT** Manufacturer advises caution (no information available).
- **PRE-TREATMENT SCREENING**
Tuberculosis Patients should be evaluated for tuberculosis before treatment.
- **MONITORING REQUIREMENTS** Monitor for infection before, during, and for 5 months after treatment.
- **DIRECTIONS FOR ADMINISTRATION**
Missed dose If dose administered more than 2 weeks late, subsequent doses should be administered on the new monthly due date.
- **PATIENT AND CARER ADVICE**
Tuberculosis All patients and their carers should be advised to seek medical attention if symptoms suggestive of tuberculosis (e.g. persistent cough, weight loss, and fever) develop.
Blood disorders Patients and their carers should be advised to seek medical attention if symptoms suggestive of blood disorders (such as fever, sore throat, bruising, or bleeding) develop.
Alert card An alert card should be provided.

- **MEDICINAL FORMS** There can be variation in the licensing of different medicines containing the same drug.

Solution for injection

CAUTIONARY AND ADVISORY LABELS 10

▸ **Simponi** (Merck Sharp & Dohme Ltd)
Golimumab 100 mg per 1 ml Simponi 100mg/1ml solution for injection pre-filled pens | 1 pre-filled disposable injection PoM £1,525.94 DT = £1,525.94
Simponi 50mg/0.5ml solution for injection pre-filled syringes | 1 pre-filled disposable injection PoM £762.97 DT = £762.97
Simponi 50mg/0.5ml solution for injection pre-filled pens | 1 pre-filled disposable injection PoM £762.97 DT = £762.97

2 Neuromuscular disorders

Neuromuscular disorders

Drugs that enhance neuromuscular transmission

Anticholinesterases are used as first-line treatment in *ocular myasthenia gravis* and as an adjunct to immunosuppressant therapy for *generalised myasthenia gravis*.

Corticosteroids are used when anticholinesterases do not control symptoms completely. A second-line immunosuppressant such as azathioprine p. 558 is frequently used to reduce the dose of corticosteroid.

Plasmapheresis or infusion of intravenous immunoglobulin [unlicensed indication] may induce temporary remission in severe relapses, particularly where bulbar or respiratory function is compromised or before thymectomy.

Anticholinesterases

Anticholinesterase drugs enhance neuromuscular transmission in voluntary and involuntary muscle in myasthenia gravis. Excessive dosage of these drugs can impair neuromuscular transmission and precipitate cholinergic crises by causing a depolarising block. This may be difficult to distinguish from a worsening myasthenic state.

Muscarinic side-effects of anticholinesterases include increased sweating, increased salivary and gastric secretions, increased gastro-intestinal and uterine motility, and bradycardia. These parasympathomimetic effects are antagonised by atropine sulfate p. 869.

Neostigmine p. 700 produces a therapeutic effect for up to 4 hours. Its pronounced muscarinic action is a disadvantage, and simultaneous administration of an antimuscarinic drug such as atropine sulfate or propantheline bromide p. 68 may be required to prevent colic, excessive salivation, or diarrhoea. In severe disease neostigmine can be given every 2 hours. In infants, neostigmine by either subcutaneous or intramuscular injection is preferred for the short-term management of myasthenia.

Pyridostigmine bromide p. 701 is less powerful and slower in action than neostigmine but it has a longer duration of action. It is preferable to neostigmine because of its smoother action and the need for less frequent dosage. It is particularly preferred in patients whose muscles are weak on waking. It has a comparatively mild gastrointestinal effect but an antimuscarinic drug may still be required. It is inadvisable to use excessive doses because acetylcholine receptor down regulation may occur. Immunosuppressant therapy may be considered if high doses of pyridostigmine bromide are needed.

Neostigmine and pyridostigmine bromide should be given to neonates 30 minutes before feeds to improve suckling.

Neostigmine is also used to reverse the actions of the non-depolarising neuromuscular blocking drugs.

Immunosuppressant therapy
A course of **corticosteroids** is an established treatment in severe cases of myasthenia gravis and may be particularly useful when antibodies to the acetylcholine receptor are present in high titre. Short courses of high-dose ('pulsed') methylprednisolone p. 478 followed by maintenance therapy with oral corticosteroids may also be useful.

Corticosteroid treatment is usually initiated under specialist supervision. Transient but very serious worsening of symptoms can occur in the first 2–3 weeks, especially if the corticosteroid is started at a high dose. Once remission has occurred (usually after 2– 6 months), the dose of prednisolone p. 478 should be reduced slowly to the minimum effective dose.

Skeletal muscle relaxants

The drugs described are used for the relief of chronic muscle spasm or spasticity associated with neurological damage; they are not indicated for spasm associated with minor injuries. They act principally on the central nervous system with the exception of dantrolene, which has a peripheral site of action. They differ in action from the muscle relaxants used in anaesthesia, which block transmission at the neuromuscular junction.

The underlying cause of spasticity should be treated and any aggravating factors (e.g. pressure sores, infection) remedied. Skeletal muscle relaxants are effective in most forms of spasticity except the rare alpha variety. The major disadvantage of treatment with these drugs is that reduction in muscle tone can cause a loss of splinting action of the spastic leg and trunk muscles and sometimes lead to an increase in disability.

Dantrolene sodium p. 880 acts directly on skeletal muscle and produces fewer central adverse effects. It is generally used in resistant cases. The dose should be increased slowly.

Baclofen p. 701 inhibits transmission at spinal level and also depresses the central nervous system. The dose should be increased slowly to avoid the major side-effects of sedation and muscular hypotonia (other adverse events are uncommon).

Diazepam p. 236 has undoubted efficacy in some children. Sedation and occasionally extensor hypotonus are disadvantages. Other benzodiazepines also have muscle-relaxant properties.

2.1 Muscular dystrophy

DRUGS FOR NEUROMUSCULAR DISORDERS

Ataluren 08-May-2019

- **DRUG ACTION** Ataluren restores the synthesis of dystrophin by allowing ribosomes to read through premature stop codons that cause incomplete dystrophin synthesis in nonsense mutation Duchenne muscular dystrophy.

- **INDICATIONS AND DOSE**

Duchenne muscular dystrophy resulting from a nonsense mutation in the dystrophin gene, in ambulatory patients (initiated by a specialist)
▶ BY MOUTH
▶ Child 2-17 years (body-weight 12 kg and above): (consult product literature)

- **INTERACTIONS** → Appendix 1: ataluren
- **SIDE-EFFECTS**
▶ **Common or very common** Appetite decreased · constipation · cough · enuresis · fever · flatulence · gastrointestinal discomfort · haemorrhage · headache · hypertension · hypertriglyceridaemia · nausea · pain · skin reactions · vomiting · weight decreased
▶ **Frequency not known** Ear infection · malaise
- **PREGNANCY** Manufacturer advises avoid—toxicity in *animal* studies.
- **BREAST FEEDING** Manufacturer advises discontinue breastfeeding—present in milk in *animal* studies.
- **RENAL IMPAIRMENT** Manufacturer advises close monitoring—safety and efficacy not established.
- **MONITORING REQUIREMENTS** Manufacturer advises monitor renal function at least every 6–12 months, and cholesterol and triglyceride concentrations at least annually.
- **DIRECTIONS FOR ADMINISTRATION** Manufacturer advises the contents of each sachet should be mixed with at least 30 mL of liquid (water, milk, fruit juice), or 3 tablespoons of semi-solid food (yoghurt or apple sauce).
- **PATIENT AND CARER ADVICE** Manufacturer advises patients should maintain adequate hydration during treatment.
Missed doses Manufacturer advises if a morning or midday dose is more than 3 hours late, or an evening dose is more than 6 hours late, the missed dose should not be taken and the next dose should be taken at the normal time.
- **NATIONAL FUNDING/ACCESS DECISIONS**

NICE decisions
▶ **Ataluren for treating Duchenne muscular dystrophy with a nonsense mutation in the dystrophin gene (July 2016)**
NICE HST3
Ataluren, within its marketing authorisation, is recommended for treating Duchenne muscular dystrophy resulting from a nonsense mutation in the dystrophin gene in people aged 5 years and older who can walk, only when:
- the manufacturer provides ataluren with the discount agreed in the patient access scheme, **and**
- the conditions under which ataluren is made available are set out in the managed access agreement between the manufacturer and NHS England, which should include the conditions set out in sections 5.12–5.15 and 5.23 of the guidance.

Patients whose treatment was started within the NHS before this guidance was published should have the option to continue treatment, without change to their funding arrangements, until they and their NHS clinician consider it appropriate to stop.
www.nice.org.uk/guidance/HST3

Scottish Medicines Consortium (SMC) decisions
The *Scottish Medicines Consortium* has advised (April 2016) that ataluren (*Translarna*®) is **not** recommended for use within NHS Scotland for the treatment of Duchenne muscular dystrophy resulting from a nonsense mutation in the dystrophin gene, in ambulatory patients aged 5 years and older as the economic case was not demonstrated.

All Wales Medicines Strategy Group (AWMSG) decisions
AWMSG No. 940
The *All Wales Medicines Strategy Group* has advised (August 2016) that the NICE HST advice for ataluren (*Translarna*®) for the treatment of Duchenne muscular dystrophy resulting from a nonsense mutation in the dystrophin gene, in ambulatory patients aged 5 years and older should be implemented within NHS Wales.
AWMSG No. 3911
The *All Wales Medicines Strategy Group* has advised (April 2019) that ataluren (*Translarna*®) is recommended for use within NHS Wales for the treatment of Duchenne muscular dystrophy resulting from a nonsense mutation in the dystrophin gene, in ambulatory patients aged from 2 years up to 5 years. This recommendation applies only in circumstances where the approved Patient Access Scheme

(PAS) is utilised or where the list/contract price is equivalent or lower than the PAS price.

● **MEDICINAL FORMS** There can be variation in the licensing of different medicines containing the same drug.

Granules

▸ Translarna (PTC Therapeutics Ltd) ▼

Ataluren 125 mg Translarna 125mg granules for oral suspension sachets | 30 sachet PoM £2,532.00

Ataluren 250 mg Translarna 250mg granules for oral suspension sachets | 30 sachet PoM £5,064.00

Ataluren 1 gram Translarna 1,000mg granules for oral suspension sachets | 30 sachet PoM £20,256.00

Nusinersen

31-Aug-2018

● **DRUG ACTION** Nusinersen is an antisense oligonucleotide that increases the production of survival motor neurone (SMN) protein, thereby helping to compensate for the defect in the SMN1 gene found in 5q spinal muscular atrophy.

● **INDICATIONS AND DOSE**

5q spinal muscular atrophy (initiated by a specialist)

▸ BY INTRATHECAL INJECTION

▸ Neonate: Initially 12 mg for 4 doses on days 0, 14, 28 and 63, then 12 mg every 4 months, for advice on missed doses—consult product literature.

▸ Child: Initially 12 mg for 4 doses on days 0, 14, 28 and 63, then 12 mg every 4 months, for advice on missed doses—consult product literature

● **UNLICENSED USE** Licensed for use in children (age range not specified by manufacturer).

IMPORTANT SAFETY INFORMATION

MHRA/CHM ADVICE: NUSINERSEN (*SPINRAZA*®): REPORTS OF COMMUNICATING HYDROCEPHALUS NOT RELATED TO MENINGITIS OR BLEEDING (JULY 2018)

Communicating hydrocephalus not related to meningitis or bleeding has been reported in patients treated with *Spinraza*®. Patients and caregivers should be informed about the signs and symptoms of hydrocephalus before *Spinraza*® is started and should be instructed to seek medical attention in case of: persistent vomiting or headache, unexplained decrease in consciousness, and in children increase in head circumference. Patients with signs and symptoms suggestive of hydrocephalus should be further investigated by a physician with expertise in its management.

● **CAUTIONS** Risk factors for renal toxicity—monitor urine protein (preferably using a first morning urine specimen) · risk factors for thrombocytopenia and coagulation disorders—monitor platelet and coagulation profile before treatment

● **PREGNANCY** Manufacturer advises avoid—no information available.

● **BREAST FEEDING** Manufacturer advises avoid—no information available.

● **RENAL IMPAIRMENT** Manufacturer advises close monitoring—safety and efficacy not established.

● **HANDLING AND STORAGE** Manufacturer advises store in a refrigerator (2–8 °C); may be stored (in the original carton, protected from light) at or below 30 °C, for up to 14 days.

● **NATIONAL FUNDING/ACCESS DECISIONS**

NICE decisions

▸ **Nusinersen for treating spinal muscular atrophy (July 2019)** NICE TA588

Nusinersen (*Spinraza*®) is recommended as an option for treating 5q spinal muscular atrophy (SMA) only if:

- patients have pre-symptomatic SMA, or SMA types 1, 2 or 3, **and**
- the conditions in the managed access agreement are followed.

www.nice.org.uk/guidance/ta588

Scottish Medicines Consortium (SMC) decisions

SMC No. 1318/18

The *Scottish Medicines Consortium* has advised (May 2018) that nusinersen (*Spinraza*®) is accepted for restricted use within NHS Scotland for the treatment of 5q spinal muscular atrophy (SMA) in patients with symptomatic type 1 SMA (infantile onset). This advice is contingent upon the continuing availability of the patient access scheme in NHS Scotland or a list price that is equivalent or lower.

● **MEDICINAL FORMS** There can be variation in the licensing of different medicines containing the same drug.

Solution for injection

▸ Spinraza (Biogen Idec Ltd) ▼

Nusinersen (as Nusinersen sodium) 2.4 mg per 1 ml Spinraza 12mg/5ml solution for injection vials | 1 vial PoM £75,000.00

2.2 Myasthenia gravis and Lambert-Eaton myasthenic syndrome

ANTICHOLINESTERASES

Anticholinesterases

● **DRUG ACTION** They prolong the action of acetylcholine by inhibiting the action of the enzyme acetylcholinesterase.

● **CONTRA-INDICATIONS** Intestinal obstruction · urinary obstruction

● **CAUTIONS** Arrhythmias · asthma (extreme caution) · atropine or other antidote to muscarinic effects may be necessary (particularly when neostigmine is given by injection) but not given routinely because it may mask signs of overdosage · bradycardia · epilepsy · hyperthyroidism · hypotension · parkinsonism · peptic ulceration · recent myocardial infarction · vagotonia

● **SIDE-EFFECTS** Abdominal cramps · diarrhoea · excessive tearing · hypersalivation · nausea · vomiting

Overdose Signs of overdosage include bronchoconstriction, increased bronchial secretions, lacrimation, excessive sweating, involuntary defaecation, involuntary micturition, miosis, nystagmus, bradycardia, heart block, arrhythmias, hypotension, agitation, excessive dreaming, and weakness eventually leading to fasciculation and paralysis.

● **PREGNANCY** Manufacturer advises use only if potential benefit outweighs risk.

● **BREAST FEEDING** Amount probably too small to be harmful.

above

Neostigmine

(Neostigmine methylsulfate)

● **INDICATIONS AND DOSE**

Treatment of myasthenia gravis

▸ BY MOUTH

▸ Neonate: Initially 1–2 mg, then 1–5 mg every 4 hours, given 30 minutes before feeds.

- Child 1 month–5 years: Initially 7.5 mg, dose repeated at suitable intervals throughout the day, total daily dose 15–90 mg
- Child 6–11 years: Initially 15 mg, dose repeated at suitable intervals throughout the day, total daily dose 15–90 mg
- Child 12–17 years: Initially 15–30 mg, dose repeated at suitable intervals throughout the day, total daily dose 75–300 mg, the maximum that most patients can tolerate is 180 mg daily

▶ BY SUBCUTANEOUS INJECTION, OR BY INTRAMUSCULAR INJECTION

- Neonate: 150 micrograms/kg every 6–8 hours, to be given 30 minutes before feeds, then increased if necessary up to 300 micrograms/kg every 4 hours.
- Child 1 month–11 years: 200–500 micrograms, dose repeated at suitable intervals throughout the day
- Child 12–17 years: 1–2.5 mg, dose repeated at suitable intervals throughout the day

Reversal of non-depolarising (competitive) neuromuscular blockade

▶ BY INTRAVENOUS INJECTION

- Neonate: 50 micrograms/kg, to be given over 1 minute after or with glycopyrronium or atropine, followed by 25 micrograms/kg if required.
- Child 1 month–11 years: 50 micrograms/kg (max. per dose 2.5 mg), to be given over 1 minute after or with glycopyrronium or atropine, then 25 micrograms/kg if required
- Child 12–17 years: 50 micrograms/kg (max. per dose 2.5 mg), to be given over 1 minute after or with glycopyrronium or atropine, then 25 micrograms/kg (max. per dose 2.5 mg) if required

● **UNLICENSED USE**
- In neonates Dose for treatment of myasthenia gravis by subcutaneous or intramuscular injection is unlicensed.

● **CAUTIONS**
- With intravenous use glycopyrronium or atropine should also be given when reversing neuromuscular blockade

● **INTERACTIONS** → Appendix 1: neostigmine

● **SIDE-EFFECTS**
- With parenteral use Intestinal hypermotility · muscle spasms

● **RENAL IMPAIRMENT**
Dose adjustments May need dose reduction.

● **DIRECTIONS FOR ADMINISTRATION** For *intravenous injection*, give undiluted *or* dilute with Glucose 5% *or* Sodium Chloride 0.9%.

● **MEDICINAL FORMS** There can be variation in the licensing of different medicines containing the same drug. Forms available from special-order manufacturers include: oral solution

Solution for injection
- Neostigmine (Non-proprietary)
  Neostigmine metilsulfate 2.5 mg per 1 ml Neostigmine 2.5mg/1ml solution for injection ampoules | 10 ampoule PoM £7.50–£7.51 DT = £7.51

Tablet
- Neostigmine (Non-proprietary)
  Neostigmine bromide 15 mg Neostigmine 15mg tablets | 140 tablet PoM £120.52 DT = £120.52

F 700

Pyridostigmine bromide

● **DRUG ACTION** Pyridostigmine bromide has weaker muscarinic action than neostigmine.

● **INDICATIONS AND DOSE**

Myasthenia gravis

▶ INITIALLY BY MOUTH

- Neonate: Initially 1–1.5 mg/kg, dose repeated throughout the day, then (by mouth using immediate-release medicines) increased if necessary up to 10 mg, to be increased gradually and given 30–60 minutes before feeds.
- Child 1 month–11 years: Initially 1–1.5 mg/kg daily, then (by mouth using immediate-release medicines) increased to 7 mg/kg daily in 6 divided doses, to be increased gradually; (by mouth using immediate-release medicines) usual dose 30–360 mg daily in divided doses
- Child 12–17 years: 30–120 mg, dose repeated throughout the day; (by mouth using immediate-release medicines) usual dose 300–600 mg daily in divided doses, consider immunosuppressant therapy if total daily dose exceeds 360 mg, down-regulation of acetylcholine receptors possible if total daily dose exceeds 450 mg

● **INTERACTIONS** → Appendix 1: pyridostigmine

● **SIDE-EFFECTS** Gastrointestinal hypermotility · muscle cramps · rash

● **RENAL IMPAIRMENT**
Dose adjustments Reduce dose; excreted by kidney.

● **MEDICINAL FORMS** There can be variation in the licensing of different medicines containing the same drug. Forms available from special-order manufacturers include: tablet, oral suspension, oral solution

Tablet
- Pyridostigmine bromide (Non-proprietary)
  Pyridostigmine bromide 60 mg Pyridostigmine bromide 60mg tablets | 200 tablet PoM £45.48 DT = £41.75
- Mestinon (Mylan)
  Pyridostigmine bromide 60 mg Mestinon 60mg tablets | 200 tablet PoM £45.57 DT = £41.75

2.3 Spasticity

Other drugs used for Spasticity Dantrolene sodium, p. 880 · Diazepam, p. 236

MUSCLE RELAXANTS > CENTRALLY ACTING

Baclofen

08-Jan-2020

● **INDICATIONS AND DOSE**

Chronic severe spasticity of voluntary muscle

▶ BY MOUTH

- Child 1 month–7 years: Initially 300 micrograms/kg daily in 4 divided doses, increased gradually at weekly intervals until satisfactory response; maintenance 0.75–2 mg/kg daily in divided doses, review treatment if no benefit within 6 weeks of achieving maximum dose; maximum 40 mg per day
- Child 8–17 years: Initially 300 micrograms/kg daily in 4 divided doses, increased gradually at weekly intervals until satisfactory response; maintenance 0.75–2 mg/kg daily in divided doses, review treatment if no benefit within 6 weeks of achieving maximum dose; maximum 60 mg per day

continued →

Severe chronic spasticity of cerebral or spinal origin unresponsive to oral antispastic drugs (or oral therapy not tolerated) (specialist use only)

▸ BY INTRATHECAL INJECTION

▸ Child 4–17 years: Test dose 25–50 micrograms, to be given over at least 1 minute via catheter or lumbar puncture, then increased in steps of 25 micrograms (max. per dose 100 micrograms), not more often than every 24 hours to determine initial maintenance dose; maintenance 25–200 micrograms daily, adjusted according to response, dose-titration phase, most often using infusion pump (implanted into chest wall or abdominal wall tissues) to establish maintenance dose retaining some spasticity to avoid sensation of paralysis

> IMPORTANT SAFETY INFORMATION
> Consult product literature for details on test dose and titration—important to monitor patients closely in appropriately equipped and staffed environment during screening and immediately after pump implantation. Resuscitation equipment must be available for immediate use. Treatment with continuous pump-administered intrathecal baclofen should be initiated within 3 months of a satisfactory response to intrathecal baclofen testing.

● CONTRA-INDICATIONS

▸ With intrathecal use Local infection · systemic infection

▸ With oral use Active peptic ulceration

● CAUTIONS

GENERAL CAUTIONS Diabetes · epilepsy · history of peptic ulcer · hypertonic bladder sphincter · psychiatric illness · respiratory impairment

SPECIFIC CAUTIONS

▸ With intrathecal use Coagulation disorders · malnutrition (increased risk of post-surgical complications) · previous spinal fusion procedure

● INTERACTIONS → Appendix 1: baclofen

● SIDE-EFFECTS

GENERAL SIDE-EFFECTS

▸ **Common or very common** Confusion · constipation · depression · diarrhoea · dizziness · drowsiness · dry mouth · euphoric mood · hallucination · headache · hyperhidrosis · hypotension · nausea · paraesthesia · skin reactions · urinary disorders · vision disorders · vomiting

▸ **Uncommon** Bradycardia · hypothermia

▸ **Rare or very rare** Withdrawal syndrome

SPECIFIC SIDE-EFFECTS

▸ **Common or very common**

▸ With intrathecal use Anxiety · appetite decreased · asthenia · chills · dyspnoea · fever · hypersalivation · insomnia · neuromuscular dysfunction · oedema · pain · pneumonia · respiratory disorders · seizure · sexual dysfunction

▸ With oral use Fatigue · gastrointestinal disorder · muscle weakness · myalgia · respiratory depression · sleep disorders

▸ **Uncommon**

▸ With intrathecal use Alopecia · deep vein thrombosis · dehydration · flushing · hypertension · hypogeusia · ileus · memory loss · pallor · paranoia · suicidal tendencies

▸ **Rare or very rare**

▸ With oral use Abdominal pain · erectile dysfunction · hepatic function abnormal · taste altered

▸ **Frequency not known**

▸ With intrathecal use Scoliosis

● PREGNANCY Manufacturer advises use only if potential benefit outweighs risk (toxicity in *animal* studies).

● BREAST FEEDING Present in milk—amount probably too small to be harmful.

● HEPATIC IMPAIRMENT

▸ With oral use Manufacturer advises use with caution—no information available.

● RENAL IMPAIRMENT Excreted by the kidney.

Dose adjustments ▸ With oral use Risk of toxicity—use smaller oral doses and if necessary increase dosage interval; if estimated glomerular filtration rate less than 15 mL/minute/1.73 m^2 use by mouth only if potential benefit outweighs risk.

● TREATMENT CESSATION Avoid abrupt withdrawal (risk of hyperactive state, may exacerbate spasticity, and precipitate autonomic dysfunction including hyperthermia, psychiatric reactions and convulsions; to minimise risk, discontinue by gradual dose reduction over at least 1–2 weeks (longer if symptoms occur)).

● PRESCRIBING AND DISPENSING INFORMATION Flavours of oral liquid formulations may include raspberry.

● PATIENT AND CARER ADVICE

Medicines for Children leaflet: Baclofen for muscle spasm www.medicinesforchildren.org.uk/baclofen-muscle-spasm

Driving and skilled tasks Drowsiness may affect performance of skilled tasks (e.g. driving); effects of alcohol enhanced.

● MEDICINAL FORMS There can be variation in the licensing of different medicines containing the same drug. Forms available from special-order manufacturers include: oral suspension, oral solution, solution for injection

Tablet

CAUTIONARY AND ADVISORY LABELS 2, 8, 21

EXCIPIENTS: May contain Gluten

▸ **Baclofen (Non-proprietary)**

Baclofen 10 mg Baclofen 10mg tablets | 84 tablet [PoM] £9.99 DT = £1.64 | 250 tablet [PoM] £9.75

▸ **Lioresal** (Novartis Pharmaceuticals UK Ltd)

Baclofen 10 mg Lioresal 10mg tablets | 100 tablet [PoM] £14.86

Solution for injection

▸ **Baclofen (Non-proprietary)**

Baclofen 50 microgram per 1 ml Baclofen 50micrograms/1ml solution for injection ampoules | 10 ampoule [PoM] £25.00

▸ **Gablofen** (Imported (United States))

Baclofen 1 mg per 1 ml Gablofen 20mg/20ml solution for injection pre-filled syringes | 1 pre-filled disposable injection [PoM] [X]
Gablofen 20mg/20ml solution for injection vials | 1 vial [PoM] [X]

▸ **Lioresal** (Novartis Pharmaceuticals UK Ltd)

Baclofen 50 microgram per 1 ml Lioresal Intrathecal 50micrograms/1ml solution for injection ampoules | 1 ampoule [PoM] £3.16 DT = £3.16

Solution for infusion

▸ **Baclofen (Non-proprietary)**

Baclofen 500 microgram per 1 ml Baclofen 10mg/20ml solution for infusion ampoules | 1 ampoule [PoM] £50.00 DT = £70.01

Baclofen 2 mg per 1 ml Baclofen 40mg/20ml solution for infusion ampoules | 1 ampoule [PoM] £250.00
Baclofen 10mg/5ml solution for infusion ampoules | 10 ampoule [PoM] £500.00

▸ **Lioresal** (Novartis Pharmaceuticals UK Ltd)

Baclofen 500 microgram per 1 ml Lioresal Intrathecal 10mg/20ml solution for infusion ampoules | 1 ampoule [PoM] £70.01 DT = £70.01

Baclofen 2 mg per 1 ml Lioresal Intrathecal 10mg/5ml solution for infusion ampoules | 1 ampoule [PoM] £70.01 DT = £70.01

Oral solution

CAUTIONARY AND ADVISORY LABELS 2, 8, 21

▸ **Baclofen (Non-proprietary)**

Baclofen 1 mg per 1 ml Baclofen 5mg/5ml oral solution sugar free sugar-free | 300 ml [PoM] £24.78 DT = £4.72

▸ **Lioresal** (Novartis Pharmaceuticals UK Ltd)

Baclofen 1 mg per 1 ml Lioresal 5mg/5ml liquid sugar-free | 300 ml [PoM] £10.31 DT = £4.72

▸ **Lyflex** (Chemidex Pharma Ltd)

Baclofen 1 mg per 1 ml Lyflex 5mg/5ml oral solution sugar-free | 300 ml [PoM] £7.95 DT = £4.72

3 Pain and inflammation in musculoskeletal disorders

Non-steroidal anti-inflammatory drugs

Therapeutic effects

In *single doses* non-steroidal anti-inflammatory drugs (NSAIDs) have analgesic activity comparable to that of paracetamol p. 288 but paracetamol is preferred.

In regular *full dosage* NSAIDs have both a lasting analgesic and an anti-inflammatory effect which makes them particularly useful for the treatment of continuous or regular pain associated with inflammation.

Choice

Differences in anti-inflammatory activity between NSAIDs are small, but there is considerable variation in individual response and tolerance of these drugs. A large proportion of children will respond to any NSAID; of the others, those who do not respond to one may well respond to another. Pain relief starts soon after taking the first dose and a full analgesic effect should normally be obtained within a week, whereas an anti-inflammatory effect may not be achieved (or may not be clinically assessable) for up to 3 weeks. However, in juvenile idiopathic arthritis NSAIDs may take 4–12 weeks to be effective. If appropriate responses are not obtained within these times, another NSAID should be tried. The availability of appropriate formulations needs to be considered when prescribing NSAIDs for children.

NSAIDs reduce the production of prostaglandins by inhibiting the enzyme cyclo-oxygenase. They vary in their selectivity for inhibiting different types of cyclo-oxygenase; selective inhibition of cyclo-oxygenase-2 is associated with less gastro-intestinal intolerance. However, in children gastro-intestinal symptoms are rare in those taking NSAIDs for short periods. The role of selective inhibitors of cyclo-oxygenase-2 is undetermined in children.

Ibuprofen p. 707 and naproxen p. 712 are propionic acid derivatives used in children.

Ibuprofen combines anti-inflammatory, analgesic, and antipyretic properties. It has fewer side-effects than other NSAIDs but its anti-inflammatory properties are weaker.

Naproxen combines good efficacy with a low incidence of side-effects.

Diclofenac sodium p. 704, diclofenac potassium p. 704, indometacin p. 710, mefenamic acid p. 711, and piroxicam p. 713 have properties similar to those of propionic acid derivatives:

Diclofenac sodium and diclofenac potassium are similar in efficacy to naproxen.

Indometacin has an action equal to or superior to that of naproxen, but with a high incidence of side-effects including headache, dizziness, and gastro-intestinal disturbances. It is rarely used in children and should be reserved for when other NSAIDs have been unsuccessful.

Mefenamic acid has minor anti-inflammatory properties. It has occasionally been associated with diarrhoea and haemolytic anaemia which require discontinuation of treatment.

Piroxicam is as effective as naproxen and has a long duration of action which permits once-daily administration. However, it has more gastro-intestinal side-effects than most other NSAIDs, and is associated with more frequent serious skin reactions.

Meloxicam p. 711 is a selective inhibitor of cyclo-oxygenase-2. Its use may be considered in adolescents intolerant to other NSAIDs.

Ketorolac trometamol p. 876 can be used for the short-term management of postoperative pain.

Etoricoxib p. 706, a selective inhibitor of cyclo-oxygenase-2, is licensed for the relief of pain in osteoarthritis, rheumatoid arthritis, ankylosing spondylitis, and acute gout in children aged 16 years and over.

Dental and orofacial pain

Most mild to moderate dental pain and inflammation is effectively relieved by ibuprofen, diclofenac potassium or diclofenac sodium.

NSAIDs and cardiovascular events

The risk of cardiovascular events secondary to NSAID use is undetermined in children. In adults, all NSAID use (including cyclo-oxygenase-2 selective inhibitors) can, to varying degrees, be associated with a small increased risk of thrombotic events (e.g. myocardial infarction and stroke) independent of baseline cardiovascular risk factors or duration of NSAID use; however, the greatest risk may be in those patients receiving high doses long term. A small increased thrombotic risk cannot be excluded in children.

In adults, cyclo-oxygenase-2 selective inhibitors, diclofenac (150 mg daily) and ibuprofen (2.4 g daily) are associated with an increased risk of thrombotic events. The increased risk for diclofenac is similar to that of etoricoxib. Naproxen (in adults, 1 g daily) is associated with a lower thrombotic risk, and lower doses of ibuprofen (in adults, 1.2 g daily or less) have not been associated with an increased risk of myocardial infarction.

The lowest effective dose of NSAID should be prescribed for the shortest period of time to control symptoms, and the need for long-term treatment should be reviewed periodically.

NSAIDs and gastro-intestinal events

All NSAIDs are associated with gastro-intestinal toxicity. In adults, evidence on the relative safety of NSAIDs indicates differences in the risks of serious upper gastro-intestinal side-effects—piroxicam and ketorolac trometamol are associated with the highest risk; indometacin, diclofenac, and naproxen are associated with intermediate risk, and ibuprofen with the lowest risk (although high doses of ibuprofen have been associated with intermediate risk). Selective inhibitors of cyclo-oxygenase-2 are associated with a *lower risk* of serious upper gastro-intestinal side-effects than non-selective NSAIDs.

Children appear to tolerate NSAIDs better than adults and gastro-intestinal side-effects are less common although they do still occur and can be significant; use of gastro-protective drugs may be necessary.

Asthma

All NSAIDs have the potential to worsen asthma, either acutely or as a gradual worsening of symptoms; consider both prescribed NSAIDs and those that are purchased over the counter.

Advanced Pharmacy Services

Children taking NSAIDs may be eligible for the Medicines Use Review service provided by a community pharmacist. For further information, see *Advanced Pharmacy Services* in Medicines optimisation p. 25.

ANALGESICS > NON-STEROIDAL ANTI-INFLAMMATORY DRUGS

Diclofenac potassium

16-Apr-2020

● **INDICATIONS AND DOSE**

Pain and inflammation in rheumatic disease and other musculoskeletal disorders

▶ BY MOUTH

▸ Child 14–17 years: 75–100 mg daily in 2–3 divided doses

Postoperative pain

▶ BY MOUTH

▸ Child 9–13 years (body-weight 35 kg and above): Up to 2 mg/kg daily in 3 divided doses; maximum 100 mg per day

▸ Child 14–17 years: 75–100 mg daily in 2–3 divided doses

Fever in ear, nose, or throat infection

▶ BY MOUTH

▸ Child 9–17 years (body-weight 35 kg and above): Up to 2 mg/kg daily in 3 divided doses; maximum 100 mg per day

● UNLICENSED USE *Voltarol® Rapid* not licensed for use in children under 14 years or in fever.

● CONTRA-INDICATIONS Active gastro-intestinal bleeding · active gastro-intestinal ulceration · cerebrovascular disease · history of gastro-intestinal bleeding related to previous NSAID therapy · history of gastro-intestinal perforation related to previous NSAID therapy · history of recurrent gastro-intestinal haemorrhage (two or more distinct episodes) · history of recurrent gastro-intestinal ulceration (two or more distinct episodes) · ischaemic heart disease · mild to severe heart failure · peripheral arterial disease

● CAUTIONS Allergic disorders · cardiac impairment (NSAIDs may impair renal function) · coagulation defects · connective-tissue disorders · dehydration (risk of renal impairment) · history of cardiac failure · history of gastro-intestinal disorders (e.g. ulcerative colitis, Crohn's disease) · hypertension · oedema · risk factors for cardiovascular events

● INTERACTIONS → Appendix 1: NSAIDs

● SIDE-EFFECTS

▶ **Common or very common** Appetite decreased · diarrhoea · dizziness · gastrointestinal discomfort · gastrointestinal disorders · headache · nausea · skin reactions · vertigo · vomiting

▶ **Uncommon** Chest pain · heart failure · myocardial infarction · palpitations

▶ **Rare or very rare** Acute kidney injury · agranulocytosis · alopecia · anaemia · angioedema · anxiety · aplastic anaemia · asthma · confusion · constipation · depression · drowsiness · dyspnoea · erectile dysfunction · fatigue · haemolytic anaemia · haemorrhage · hearing impairment · hepatic disorders · hypersensitivity · hypertension · hypotension · inflammatory bowel disease · irritability · leucopenia · memory loss · meningitis aseptic (patients with connective-tissue disorders such as systemic lupus erythematosus may be especially susceptible) · nephritis tubulointerstitial · nephrotic syndrome · oedema · oesophageal disorder · oral disorders · pancreatitis · photosensitivity reaction · pneumonitis · proteinuria · psychotic disorder · renal papillary necrosis · seizure · sensation abnormal · severe cutaneous adverse reactions (SCARs) · shock · sleep disorders · stroke · taste altered · thrombocytopenia · tinnitus · tremor · vasculitis · vision disorders

▶ **Frequency not known** Hallucination · malaise · optic neuritis

SIDE-EFFECTS, FURTHER INFORMATION For information about cardiovascular and gastrointestinal side-effects, and a possible exacerbation of symptoms in asthma, see Non-steroidal anti-inflammatory drugs.

● ALLERGY AND CROSS-SENSITIVITY Contra-indicated in patients with a history of hypersensitivity to aspirin or any other NSAID—which includes those in whom attacks of asthma, angioedema, urticaria or rhinitis have been precipitated by aspirin or any other NSAID.

● PREGNANCY Avoid unless the potential benefit outweighs the risk. Avoid during the third trimester (risk of closure of fetal ductus arteriosus *in utero* and possibly persistent pulmonary hypertension of the newborn); onset of labour may be delayed and duration may be increased.

● BREAST FEEDING Use with caution during breast-feeding. Amount in milk too small to be harmful.

● HEPATIC IMPAIRMENT Manufacturer advises caution in mild to moderate impairment; avoid in severe impairment.

● RENAL IMPAIRMENT Avoid if possible or use with caution. Avoid in severe impairment.

Dose adjustments The lowest effective dose should be used for the shortest possible duration.

Monitoring In renal impairment monitor renal function; sodium and water retention may occur and renal function may deteriorate, possibly leading to renal failure.

● PATIENT AND CARER ADVICE

Medicines for Children leaflet: Diclofenac for pain and inflammation www.medicinesforchildren.org.uk/diclofenac-pain-and-inflammation

● MEDICINAL FORMS There can be variation in the licensing of different medicines containing the same drug.

Tablet

CAUTIONARY AND ADVISORY LABELS 21

▸ Diclofenac potassium (Non-proprietary)

Diclofenac potassium 25 mg Diclofenac potassium 25mg tablets | 28 tablet [PoM] £3.86 DT = £3.86

Diclofenac potassium 50 mg Diclofenac potassium 50mg tablets | 28 tablet [PoM] £7.41 DT = £7.41

▸ Voltarol Rapid (Novartis Pharmaceuticals UK Ltd)

Diclofenac potassium 50 mg Voltarol Rapid 50mg tablets | 30 tablet [PoM] £7.94

Diclofenac sodium

28-Apr-2020

● **INDICATIONS AND DOSE**

Pain and inflammation in rheumatic disease including juvenile idiopathic arthritis

▶ BY MOUTH USING IMMEDIATE-RELEASE MEDICINES

▸ Child 6 months–17 years: 1.5–2.5 mg/kg twice daily, total daily dose may alternatively be given in 3 divided doses; maximum 150 mg per day

Postoperative pain

▶ BY RECTUM

▸ Child 6 months–17 years (body-weight 8–11 kg): 12.5 mg twice daily for maximum 4 days

▸ Child 6 months–17 years (body-weight 12 kg and above): 1 mg/kg 3 times a day (max. per dose 50 mg) for maximum 4 days

Inflammation | Mild to moderate pain

▶ BY MOUTH USING IMMEDIATE-RELEASE MEDICINES, OR BY RECTUM

▸ Child 6 months–17 years: 0.3–1 mg/kg 3 times a day (max. per dose 50 mg)

DICLOMAX RETARD®

Pain and inflammation

▶ BY MOUTH

▸ Child 12–17 years: 1 capsule once daily

DICLOMAX SR®

Pain and inflammation

▶ BY MOUTH

▸ Child 12-17 years: 1 capsule 1–2 times a day

MOTIFENE®

Pain and inflammation

▶ BY MOUTH

▸ Child 12-17 years: 1 capsule 1–2 times a day

VOLTAROL® 75MG SR TABLETS

Pain and inflammation

▶ BY MOUTH

▸ Child 12-17 years: 1 tablet 1–2 times a day

VOLTAROL® RETARD

Pain and inflammation

▶ BY MOUTH

▸ Child 12-17 years: 1 tablet once daily

VOLTAROL® SOLUTION FOR INJECTION

Postoperative pain

▶ BY INTRAVENOUS INFUSION, OR BY DEEP INTRAMUSCULAR INJECTION

▸ Child 2-17 years: 0.3–1 mg/kg 1–2 times a day for maximum 2 days, for intramuscular injection, to be injected into the gluteal muscle; maximum 150 mg per day

● UNLICENSED USE Not licensed for use in children under 1 year. *Suppositories* not licensed for use in children under 6 years except for use in children over 1 year for juvenile idiopathic arthritis. Solid dose forms containing more than 25 mg not licensed for use in children. *Injection* not licensed for use in children.

● CONTRA-INDICATIONS Active gastro-intestinal bleeding · active gastro-intestinal ulceration · avoid suppositories in proctitis · cerebrovascular disease · history of gastro-intestinal bleeding related to previous NSAID therapy · history of gastro-intestinal perforation related to previous NSAID therapy · history of recurrent gastro-intestinal haemorrhage (two or more distinct episodes) · history of recurrent gastro-intestinal ulceration (two or more distinct episodes) · ischaemic heart disease · mild to severe heart failure · peripheral arterial disease

▸ With intravenous use avoid injections containing benzyl alcohol in neonates · dehydration · history of asthma · history of confirmed or suspected cerebrovascular bleeding · history of haemorrhagic diathesis · hypovolaemia · operations with high risk of haemorrhage

● CAUTIONS Allergic disorders · cardiac impairment (NSAIDs may impair renal function) · coagulation defects · connective-tissue disorders · dehydration (risk of renal impairment) · history of cardiac failure · history of gastro-intestinal disorders (e.g. ulcerative colitis, Crohn's disease) · hypertension · oedema · risk factors for cardiovascular events

● INTERACTIONS → Appendix 1: NSAIDs

● SIDE-EFFECTS

GENERAL SIDE-EFFECTS

▶ **Common or very common** Appetite decreased · diarrhoea · dizziness · gastrointestinal discomfort · gastrointestinal disorders · headache · nausea · rash (discontinue) · vertigo · vomiting

▶ **Uncommon** Chest pain · heart failure · myocardial infarction · palpitations

▶ **Rare or very rare** Acute kidney injury · agranulocytosis · alopecia · anaemia · angioedema · anxiety · aplastic anaemia · asthma · confusion · constipation · depression · drowsiness · dyspnoea · erectile dysfunction · fatigue · haemolytic anaemia · haemorrhage · hearing impairment · hepatic disorders · hypersensitivity · hypertension · hypotension · irritability · leucopenia · memory loss · meningitis aseptic (patients with connective-tissue disorders such as systemic lupus erythematosus may be especially susceptible) · nephritis tubulointerstitial · nephrotic syndrome · oedema · oesophageal disorder · oral disorders · pancreatitis · photosensitivity reaction · pneumonitis · proteinuria · psychotic disorder · renal papillary necrosis · seizure · sensation abnormal · severe cutaneous adverse reactions (SCARs) · skin reactions · shock · sleep disorders · stroke · taste altered · thrombocytopenia · tinnitus · tremor · vasculitis · vision disorders

▶ **Frequency not known** Fertility decreased female · fluid retention · hallucination · malaise · optic neuritis · platelet aggregation inhibition

SPECIFIC SIDE-EFFECTS

▶ **Rare or very rare**

▸ With rectal use Ulcerative colitis aggravated

▸ With parenteral use Injection site necrosis

SIDE-EFFECTS, FURTHER INFORMATION For information about cardiovascular and gastrointestinal side-effects, and a possible exacerbation of symptoms in asthma, see Non-steroidal anti-inflammatory drugs p. 703

● ALLERGY AND CROSS-SENSITIVITY Contra-indicated in patients with a history of hypersensitivity to aspirin or any other NSAID—which includes those in whom attacks of asthma, angioedema, urticaria or rhinitis have been precipitated by aspirin or any other NSAID.

● PREGNANCY Avoid unless the potential benefit outweighs the risk. Avoid during the third trimester (risk of closure of fetal ductus arteriosus *in utero* and possibly persistent pulmonary hypertension of the newborn); onset of labour may be delayed and duration may be increased.

● BREAST FEEDING Use with caution during breast-feeding. Amount in milk too small to be harmful.

● HEPATIC IMPAIRMENT Manufacturer advises caution in mild to moderate impairment; avoid in severe impairment.

● RENAL IMPAIRMENT Avoid if possible or use with caution. Avoid in severe impairment.

▸ With intravenous use Contra-indicated in moderate or severe renal impairment.

Dose adjustments The lowest effective dose should be used for the shortest possible duration.

Monitoring In renal impairment monitor renal function; sodium and water retention may occur and renal function may deteriorate, possibly leading to renal failure.

● DIRECTIONS FOR ADMINISTRATION For *intravenous infusion*, dilute 75 mg with 100–500 mL Glucose 5% *or* Sodium Chloride 0.9% (previously buffered with 0.5 mL Sodium Bicarbonate 8.4% solution *or* with 1 mL Sodium Bicarbonate 4.2% solution); give over 30–120 minutes.

● PATIENT AND CARER ADVICE

Medicines for Children leaflet: Diclofenac for pain and inflammation www.medicinesforchildren.org.uk/diclofenac-pain-and-inflammation

---

● MEDICINAL FORMS There can be variation in the licensing of different medicines containing the same drug. Forms available from special-order manufacturers include: dispersible tablet, oral suspension, oral solution

Gastro-resistant tablet

CAUTIONARY AND ADVISORY LABELS 5, 25

▸ Diclofenac sodium (Non-proprietary)

Diclofenac sodium 25 mg Diclofenac sodium 25mg gastro-resistant tablets | 28 tablet PoM £8.99 DT = £1.69 | 84 tablet PoM £1.50-£26.97

Diclofenac sodium 50 mg Diclofenac sodium 50mg gastro-resistant tablets | 28 tablet PoM £4.97 DT = £1.63 | 84 tablet PoM £2.48-£15.00

▸ Fenactol (Dexcel-Pharma Ltd)

Diclofenac sodium 50 mg Fenactol 50mg gastro-resistant tablets | 100 tablet PoM £3.70

Suppository
- Econac (Advanz Pharma)
  Diclofenac sodium 100 mg Econac 100mg suppositories | 10 suppository PoM £3.04 DT = £3.64
- Voltarol (Novartis Pharmaceuticals UK Ltd)
  Diclofenac sodium 12.5 mg Voltarol 12.5mg suppositories | 10 suppository PoM £0.70 DT = £0.70
  Diclofenac sodium 25 mg Voltarol 25mg suppositories | 10 suppository PoM £1.24 DT = £1.24
  Diclofenac sodium 50 mg Voltarol 50mg suppositories | 10 suppository PoM £2.04 DT = £2.04
  Diclofenac sodium 100 mg Voltarol 100mg suppositories | 10 suppository PoM £3.64 DT = £3.64

Solution for injection
EXCIPIENTS: May contain Benzyl alcohol, propylene glycol
- Voltarol (Novartis Pharmaceuticals UK Ltd)
  Diclofenac sodium 25 mg per 1 ml Voltarol 75mg/3ml solution for injection ampoules | 10 ampoule PoM £9.91 DT = £9.91

Modified-release capsule
CAUTIONARY AND ADVISORY LABELS 21 (does not apply to Motifene® 75 mg), 25
EXCIPIENTS: May contain Propylene glycol
- Diclomax Retard (Galen Ltd)
  Diclofenac sodium 100 mg Diclomax Retard 100mg capsules | 28 capsule PoM £8.20 DT = £8.20
- Diclomax SR (Galen Ltd)
  Diclofenac sodium 75 mg Diclomax SR 75mg capsules | 56 capsule PoM £11.40 DT = £11.40
- Motifene (Daiichi Sankyo UK Ltd)
  Diclofenac sodium 75 mg Motifene 75mg modified-release capsules | 56 capsule PoM £8.00 DT = £8.00

Etoricoxib

15-Apr-2020

● **INDICATIONS AND DOSE**

Pain and inflammation in osteoarthritis
▶ BY MOUTH
- Child 16–17 years: 30 mg once daily, increased if necessary to 60 mg once daily

Pain and inflammation in rheumatoid arthritis | Ankylosing spondylitis
▶ BY MOUTH
- Child 16–17 years: 60 mg once daily, increased if necessary to 90 mg once daily

Acute gout
▶ BY MOUTH
- Child 16–17 years: 120 mg once daily for maximum 8 days

● **CONTRA-INDICATIONS** Active gastro-intestinal bleeding · active gastro-intestinal ulceration · cerebrovascular disease · inflammatory bowel disease · ischaemic heart disease · mild to severe heart failure · peripheral arterial disease · uncontrolled hypertension (persistently above 140/90 mmHg)

● **CAUTIONS** Allergic disorders · cardiac impairment (NSAIDs may impair renal function) · coagulation defects · connective-tissue disorders · dehydration (risk of renal impairment) · history of cardiac failure · history of gastro-intestinal disorders · hypertension · left ventricular dysfunction · oedema · risk factors for cardiovascular events

● **INTERACTIONS** → Appendix 1: NSAIDs

● **SIDE-EFFECTS**
- **Common or very common** Arrhythmias · asthenia · bronchospasm · constipation · diarrhoea · dizziness · fluid retention · gastrointestinal discomfort · gastrointestinal disorders · headache · hypertension · increased risk of infection · influenza like illness · nausea · oedema · oral ulceration · palpitations · skin reactions · vomiting
- **Uncommon** Alertness decreased · anaemia · angina pectoris · anxiety · appetite abnormal · cerebrovascular insufficiency · chest pain · congestive heart failure · conjunctivitis · cough · depression · drowsiness · dry mouth · dyspnoea · flushing · haemorrhage · hallucination · hyperkalaemia · hypersensitivity · insomnia · irritable bowel syndrome · leucopenia · myocardial infarction · pancreatitis · proteinuria · renal failure (more common in patients with pre-existing renal impairment) · sensation abnormal · taste altered · thrombocytopenia · tinnitus · vasculitis · vertigo · vision blurred · weight increased
- **Rare or very rare** Angioedema · confusion · hepatic disorders · muscle complaints · severe cutaneous adverse reactions (SCARs) · shock
- **Frequency not known** Nephritis tubulointerstitial · nephropathy

SIDE-EFFECTS, FURTHER INFORMATION For information about cardiovascular and gastrointestinal side-effects, and a possible exacerbation of symptoms in asthma, see Non-steroidal anti-inflammatory drugs.

● **ALLERGY AND CROSS-SENSITIVITY** Contra-indicated in patients with a history of hypersensitivity to aspirin or any other NSAID—which includes those in whom attacks of asthma, angioedema, urticaria or rhinitis have been precipitated by aspirin or any other NSAID.

● **CONCEPTION AND CONTRACEPTION** Caution—long-term use of some NSAIDs is associated with reduced female fertility, which is reversible on stopping treatment.

● **PREGNANCY** Manufacturer advises avoid (teratogenic in *animal* studies). Avoid during the third trimester (risk of closure of fetal ductus arteriosus *in utero* and possibly persistent pulmonary hypertension of the newborn); onset of labour may be delayed and duration may be increased.

● **BREAST FEEDING** Use with caution during breast-feeding. Manufacturer advises avoid—present in milk in *animal* studies.

● **HEPATIC IMPAIRMENT** Manufacturer advises caution in mild to moderate impairment; avoid in severe impairment (no information available).
Dose adjustments Manufacturer advises max. 60 mg once daily in mild impairment; max. 30 mg once daily in moderate impairment.

● **RENAL IMPAIRMENT** Avoid if possible or use with caution. Avoid if estimated glomerular filtration rate less than 30 mL/minute/1.73 m^2.
Dose adjustments The lowest effective dose should be used for the shortest possible duration.
Monitoring In renal impairment monitor renal function; sodium and water retention may occur and renal function may deteriorate, possibly leading to renal failure.

● **MONITORING REQUIREMENTS** Monitor blood pressure before treatment, 2 weeks after initiation and periodically during treatment.

● **MEDICINAL FORMS** There can be variation in the licensing of different medicines containing the same drug.

Tablet
- Etoricoxib (Non-proprietary)
  Etoricoxib 30 mg Etoricoxib 30mg tablets | 28 tablet PoM £13.99 DT = £8.18
  Etoricoxib 60 mg Etoricoxib 60mg tablets | 28 tablet PoM £20.11 DT = £2.79
  Etoricoxib 90 mg Etoricoxib 90mg tablets | 28 tablet PoM £22.96 DT = £2.89
  Etoricoxib 120 mg Etoricoxib 120mg tablets | 7 tablet PoM £1.90-£5.73 | 28 tablet PoM £24.11 DT = £13.71
- Arcoxia (Merck Sharp & Dohme Ltd)
  Etoricoxib 30 mg Arcoxia 30mg tablets | 28 tablet PoM £13.99 DT = £8.18
  Etoricoxib 60 mg Arcoxia 60mg tablets | 28 tablet PoM £20.11 DT = £2.79
  Etoricoxib 90 mg Arcoxia 90mg tablets | 28 tablet PoM £22.96 DT = £2.89
  Etoricoxib 120 mg Arcoxia 120mg tablets | 7 tablet PoM £6.03 | 28 tablet PoM £24.11 DT = £13.71

Flurbiprofen

27-Apr-2020

● **INDICATIONS AND DOSE**

Pain and inflammation in rheumatic disease and other musculoskeletal disorders | Migraine | Postoperative analgesia | Mild to moderate pain

▶ BY MOUTH

▸ Child 12–17 years: 150–200 mg daily in 2–4 divided doses, then increased to 300 mg daily, dose to be increased only in acute conditions

Dysmenorrhoea

▶ BY MOUTH

▸ Child 12–17 years: Initially 100 mg, then 50–100 mg every 4–6 hours; maximum 300 mg per day

● **CONTRA-INDICATIONS** Active gastro-intestinal bleeding · active gastro-intestinal ulceration · Crohn's disease (may be exacerbated) · history of gastro-intestinal bleeding related to previous NSAID therapy · history of gastro-intestinal perforation related to previous NSAID therapy · history of recurrent gastro-intestinal haemorrhage (two or more distinct episodes) · history of recurrent gastro-intestinal ulceration (two or more distinct episodes) · severe heart failure · ulcerative colitis (may be exacerbated)

● **CAUTIONS** Allergic disorders · cardiac impairment (NSAIDs may impair renal function) · cerebrovascular disease · coagulation defects · connective-tissue disorders · dehydration (risk of renal impairment) · heart failure · history of gastro-intestinal disorders · ischaemic heart disease · peripheral arterial disease · risk factors for cardiovascular events · uncontrolled hypertension

● **INTERACTIONS** → Appendix 1: NSAIDs

● **SIDE-EFFECTS** Agranulocytosis · angioedema · aplastic anaemia · asthma · bronchospasm · confusion · constipation · Crohn's disease · depression · diarrhoea · dizziness · drowsiness · dyspnoea · fatigue · fertility decreased female · gastrointestinal discomfort · gastrointestinal disorders · haemolytic anaemia · haemorrhage · hallucination · headache · heart failure · hepatic disorders · hypersensitivity · hypertension · malaise · meningitis aseptic (patients with connective-tissue disorders such as systemic lupus erythematosus may be especially susceptible) · nausea · nephritis tubulointerstitial · nephropathy · neutropenia · oedema · optic neuritis · oral ulceration · pancreatitis · paraesthesia · photosensitivity reaction · platelet aggregation inhibition · renal failure (more common in patients with pre-existing renal impairment) · respiratory tract reaction · severe cutaneous adverse reactions (SCARs) · skin reactions · stroke · thrombocytopenia · tinnitus · vertigo · visual impairment · vomiting

SIDE-EFFECTS, FURTHER INFORMATION For information about cardiovascular and gastrointestinal side-effects, and a possible exacerbation of symptoms in asthma, see Non-steroidal anti-inflammatory drugs. p. 703

● **ALLERGY AND CROSS-SENSITIVITY** Contra-indicated in patients with a history of hypersensitivity to aspirin or any other NSAID—which includes those in whom attacks of asthma, angioedema, urticaria or rhinitis have been precipitated by aspirin or any other NSAID.

● **PREGNANCY** Avoid unless the potential benefit outweighs the risk. Avoid during the third trimester (risk of closure of fetal ductus arteriosus *in utero* and possibly persistent pulmonary hypertension of the newborn); onset of labour may be delayed and duration may be increased.

● **BREAST FEEDING** Use with caution during breast-feeding. Small amount present in milk—manufacturer advises avoid.

● **HEPATIC IMPAIRMENT** Manufacturer advises caution in mild to moderate impairment; avoid in severe impairment.

● **RENAL IMPAIRMENT** Avoid if possible or use with caution. Avoid in severe impairment.

Dose adjustments The lowest effective dose should be used for the shortest possible duration.

Monitoring In renal impairment monitor renal function; sodium and water retention may occur and renal function may deteriorate, possibly leading to renal failure.

● **MEDICINAL FORMS** There can be variation in the licensing of different medicines containing the same drug.

Tablet

CAUTIONARY AND ADVISORY LABELS 21

▸ **Flurbiprofen (Non-proprietary)**

Flurbiprofen 50 mg Flurbiprofen 50mg tablets | 100 tablet PoM £21.30–£51.81 DT = £47.49

Flurbiprofen 100 mg Flurbiprofen 100mg tablets | 100 tablet PoM £38.10–£92.64 DT = £84.92

Ibuprofen

14-Apr-2020

● **INDICATIONS AND DOSE**

Closure of ductus arteriosus

▶ BY SLOW INTRAVENOUS INJECTION

▸ Neonate: Initially 10 mg/kg for 1 dose, followed by 5 mg/kg every 24 hours for 2 doses, the course may be repeated after 48 hours if necessary.

Mild to moderate pain | Pain and inflammation of soft-tissue injuries | Pyrexia with discomfort

▶ BY MOUTH USING IMMEDIATE-RELEASE MEDICINES

▸ Child 1–2 months: 5 mg/kg 3–4 times a day

▸ Child 3–5 months: 50 mg 3 times a day, maximum daily dose to be given in 3–4 divided doses; maximum 30 mg/kg per day

▸ Child 6–11 months: 50 mg 3–4 times a day, maximum daily dose to be given in 3–4 divided doses; maximum 30 mg/kg per day

▸ Child 1–3 years: 100 mg 3 times a day, maximum daily dose to be given in 3–4 divided doses; maximum 30 mg/kg per day

▸ Child 4–6 years: 150 mg 3 times a day, maximum daily dose to be given in 3–4 divided doses; maximum 30 mg/kg per day

▸ Child 7–9 years: 200 mg 3 times a day, maximum daily dose to be given in 3–4 divided doses; maximum 30 mg/kg per day; maximum 2.4 g per day

▸ Child 10–11 years: 300 mg 3 times a day, maximum daily dose to be given in 3–4 divided doses; maximum 30 mg/kg per day; maximum 2.4 g per day

▸ Child 12–17 years: Initially 300–400 mg 3–4 times a day; increased if necessary up to 600 mg 4 times a day; maintenance 200–400 mg 3 times a day, may be adequate

Pain and inflammation

▶ BY MOUTH USING MODIFIED-RELEASE MEDICINES

▸ Child 12–17 years: 1.6 g once daily, dose preferably taken in the early evening, increased to 2.4 g daily in 2 divided doses, dose to be increased only in severe cases

Pain and inflammation in rheumatic disease including juvenile idiopathic arthritis

▶ BY MOUTH USING IMMEDIATE-RELEASE MEDICINES

▸ Child 3 months–17 years: 30–40 mg/kg daily in 3–4 divided doses; maximum 2.4 g per day continued →

Pain and inflammation in systemic juvenile idiopathic arthritis
- ▶ BY MOUTH USING IMMEDIATE-RELEASE MEDICINES
- ▶ Child 3 months–17 years: Up to 60 mg/kg daily in 4–6 divided doses; maximum 2.4 g per day

Post-immunisation pyrexia in infants (on doctor's advice only)
- ▶ BY MOUTH USING IMMEDIATE-RELEASE MEDICINES
- ▶ Child 2–3 months: 50 mg for 1 dose, followed by 50 mg after 6 hours if required

Pain and inflammation in rheumatic disease and other musculoskeletal disorders (dose approved for use by community practitioner nurse prescribers) | Mild to moderate pain including dysmenorrhoea (dose approved for use by community practitioner nurse prescribers) | Migraine (dose approved for use by community practitioner nurse prescribers) | Dental pain (dose approved for use by community practitioner nurse prescribers) | Headache (dose approved for use by community practitioner nurse prescribers) | Fever (dose approved for use by community practitioner nurse prescribers) | Symptoms of colds and influenza (dose approved for use by community practitioner nurse prescribers) | Neuralgia (dose approved for use by community practitioner nurse prescribers)
- ▶ BY MOUTH USING IMMEDIATE-RELEASE MEDICINES
- ▶ Child 12–17 years: 200–400 mg 3 times a day, if symptoms worsen or persist for more than 3 days refer to doctor

Mild to moderate pain (dose approved for use by community practitioner nurse prescribers) | Pain and inflammation of soft-tissue injuries (dose approved for use by community practitioner nurse prescribers) | Pyrexia with discomfort (dose approved for use by community practitioner nurse prescribers)
- ▶ BY MOUTH USING IMMEDIATE-RELEASE MEDICINES
- ▶ Child 3–5 months (body-weight 5 kg and above): 20–30 mg/kg daily in divided doses, alternatively 50 mg 3 times a day for maximum of 24 hours, refer to doctor if symptoms persist for more than 24 hours
- ▶ Child 6–11 months: 50 mg 3–4 times a day, refer to doctor if symptoms persist for more than 3 days
- ▶ Child 1–3 years: 100 mg 3 times a day, refer to doctor if symptoms persist for more than 3 days
- ▶ Child 4–6 years: 150 mg 3 times a day, refer to doctor if symptoms persist for more than 3 days
- ▶ Child 7–9 years: 200 mg 3 times a day, refer to doctor if symptoms persist for more than 3 days
- ▶ Child 10–11 years: 300 mg 3 times a day, refer to doctor if symptoms persist for more than 3 days

Post-immunisation pyrexia in infants (dose approved for use by community practitioner nurse prescribers) (on doctor's advice only)
- ▶ BY MOUTH USING IMMEDIATE-RELEASE MEDICINES
- ▶ Child 3 months: 50 mg for 1 dose, followed by 50 mg after 6 hours if required, if pyrexia persists refer to doctor

● **UNLICENSED USE**
- ▶ With intravenous use Orphan licence for the injection for closure of ductus arteriosus in premature neonates less than 34 weeks corrected gestational age.
- ▶ With oral use Not licensed for use in children under 3 months or body-weight under 5 kg. Maximum dose for systemic juvenile idiopathic arthritis is unlicensed.

● **CONTRA-INDICATIONS** Active gastro-intestinal bleeding · active gastro-intestinal ulceration · history of gastro-intestinal bleeding related to previous NSAID therapy · history of gastro-intestinal perforation related to previous NSAID therapy · history of recurrent gastro-intestinal haemorrhage (two or more distinct episodes) · history of recurrent gastro-intestinal ulceration (two or more distinct episodes) · severe heart failure · varicella infection
- ▶ With intravenous use Active bleeding (especially intracranial or gastro-intestinal) · coagulation defects · ductal-dependent congential heart disease · known or suspected necrotising enterocolitis · life-threatening infection · marked unconjugated hyperbilirubinaemia · pulmonary hypertension · thrombocytopenia

● **CAUTIONS** Allergic disorders · cardiac impairment (NSAIDs may impair renal function) · cerebrovascular disease · coagulation defects · connective-tissue disorders · dehydration (risk of renal impairment) · heart failure · history of gastro-intestinal disorders (e.g. ulcerative colitis, Crohn's disease) · ischaemic heart disease · peripheral arterial disease · risk factors for cardiovascular events · uncontrolled hypertension
- ▶ With intravenous use May mask symptoms of infection (in neonates)

CAUTIONS, FURTHER INFORMATION
- ▶ High-dose ibuprofen A small increase in cardiovascular risk, similar to the risk associated with cyclo-oxygenase-2 inhibitors and diclofenac, has been reported with high-dose ibuprofen ($\geq$ 2.4 g daily); use should be avoided in patients with established ischaemic heart disease, peripheral arterial disease, cerebrovascular disease, congestive heart failure (New York Heart Association classification II–III), and uncontrolled hypertension.

● **INTERACTIONS** → Appendix 1: NSAIDs

● **SIDE-EFFECTS**

GENERAL SIDE-EFFECTS
- ▶ **Rare or very rare** Gastrointestinal disorders (very common in neonates) · haemorrhage (very common in neonates) · thrombocytopenia (very common in neonates)
- ▶ **Frequency not known** Fluid retention (very common in neonates)

SPECIFIC SIDE-EFFECTS
- ▶ **Common or very common**
- ▶ With intravenous use Intraventricular haemorrhage ; neutropenia ; periventricular leukomalacia ; renal impairment
- ▶ **Uncommon**
- ▶ With oral use Gastrointestinal discomfort · headache · hypersensitivity · nausea · rash (discontinue) · skin reactions
- ▶ **Rare or very rare**
- ▶ With oral use Acute kidney injury · agranulocytosis · anaemia · angioedema · constipation · diarrhoea · dyspnoea · leucopenia · liver disorder · meningitis aseptic (patients with connective-tissue disorders such as systemic lupus erythematosus may be especially susceptible) · oedema · oral ulceration · pancytopenia · renal papillary necrosis · severe cutaneous adverse reactions (SCARs) · shock · vomiting
- ▶ **Frequency not known**
- ▶ With oral use Asthma · Crohn's disease · fertility decreased female · heart failure · hypertension · increased risk of arterial thromboembolism · renal failure (more common in patients with pre-existing renal impairment) · respiratory disorders · respiratory tract reaction

SIDE-EFFECTS, FURTHER INFORMATION For information about cardiovascular and gastrointestinal side-effects, and a possible exacerbation of symptoms in asthma, see Non-steroidal anti-inflammatory drugs. p. 703

Overdose Overdosage with ibuprofen may cause nausea, vomiting, epigastric pain, and tinnitus, but more serious toxicity is very uncommon. Charcoal, activated followed by symptomatic measures are indicated if more than 100 mg/kg has been ingested within the preceding hour.

For details on the management of poisoning, see Emergency treatment of poisoning p. 891.

- **ALLERGY AND CROSS-SENSITIVITY** Contra-indicated in patients with a history of hypersensitivity to aspirin or any other NSAID—which includes those in whom attacks of asthma, angioedema, urticaria or rhinitis have been precipitated by aspirin or any other NSAID.
- **PREGNANCY** Avoid unless the potential benefit outweighs the risk. Avoid during the third trimester (risk of closure of fetal ductus arteriosus *in utero* and possibly persistent pulmonary hypertension of the newborn); onset of labour may be delayed and duration may be increased.
- **BREAST FEEDING**
  - With oral use Use with caution during breast-feeding. Amount too small to be harmful but some manufacturers advise avoid.
- **HEPATIC IMPAIRMENT**
  - With oral use Manufacturer advises caution in mild to moderate impairment; avoid in severe impairment.
- **RENAL IMPAIRMENT**
  - With intravenous use Avoid if possible in severe impairment.
  - With oral use Avoid if possible or use with caution. Avoid in severe impairment.

  Dose adjustments ▶ With intravenous use Use lowest effective dose.

  ▶ With oral use The lowest effective dose should be used for the shortest possible duration.

  Monitoring In renal impairment monitor renal function; sodium and water retention may occur and renal function may deteriorate, possibly leading to renal failure.
- **MONITORING REQUIREMENTS**
  - With intravenous use Monitor for bleeding. Monitor gastro-intestinal function.
- **DIRECTIONS FOR ADMINISTRATION**
  - With intravenous use For *slow intravenous injection*, give over 15 minutes, preferably undiluted. May be diluted with Glucose 5% *or* Sodium Chloride 0.9%.
- **PRESCRIBING AND DISPENSING INFORMATION**
  - With oral use Flavours of syrup may include orange.
- **PATIENT AND CARER ADVICE**
  Medicines for Children leaflet: Ibuprofen for pain and inflammation www.medicinesforchildren.org.uk/ibuprofen-pain-and-inflammation
- **PROFESSION SPECIFIC INFORMATION**
  Dental practitioners' formulary
  Ibuprofen Oral Suspension Sugar-free may be prescribed. Ibuprofen Tablets may be prescribed.
- **EXCEPTIONS TO LEGAL CATEGORY** Oral preparations can be sold to the public in certain circumstances.

- **MEDICINAL FORMS** There can be variation in the licensing of different medicines containing the same drug. Forms available from special-order manufacturers include: oral suspension

Effervescent granules

CAUTIONARY AND ADVISORY LABELS 13, 21

ELECTROLYTES: May contain Sodium

▶ **Brufen** (Mylan)

Ibuprofen 600 mg Brufen 600mg effervescent granules sachets | 20 sachet [PoM] £6.80 DT = £6.80

Modified-release tablet

CAUTIONARY AND ADVISORY LABELS 25, 27

▶ **Brufen Retard** (Mylan)

Ibuprofen 800 mg Brufen Retard 800mg tablets | 56 tablet [PoM] £7.74 DT = £7.74

Tablet

CAUTIONARY AND ADVISORY LABELS 21

▶ **Ibuprofen (Non-proprietary)**

Ibuprofen 200 mg Ibuprofen 200mg tablets | 16 tablet [P] £0.25 | 24 tablet [P] £0.99 DT = £0.99 | 48 tablet [P] £0.80–£1.98 | 84 tablet [P] £3.82 DT = £3.47 | 96 tablet [P] £1.69

Ibuprofen 200mg caplets | 16 tablet [P] £0.25 | 24 tablet [P] [X] DT = £0.99

Ibuprofen 400 mg Ibuprofen 400mg tablets film coated | 24 tablet [P] [X] DT = £1.11

Ibuprofen 400mg caplets | 24 tablet [P] [X] DT = £1.11

Ibuprofen 400mg tablets | 250 tablet [PoM] £13.04

Ibuprofen 600 mg Ibuprofen 600mg tablets | 84 tablet [PoM] £4.08 DT = £4.08

Ibuprofen 600mg tablets film coated | 84 tablet [PoM] £4.08 DT = £4.08

▶ **Brufen** (Mylan)

Ibuprofen 400 mg Brufen 400mg tablets | 60 tablet [PoM] £4.90

Ibuprofen 600 mg Brufen 600mg tablets | 60 tablet [PoM] £7.34

▶ **Feminax Express** (Bayer Plc)

Ibuprofen (as Ibuprofen lysine) 200 mg Feminax Express 342mg tablets | 8 tablet [GSL] £1.76 DT = £1.76 | 16 tablet [GSL] £2.67 DT = £2.67

▶ **Nurofen Express** (Reckitt Benckiser Healthcare (UK) Ltd)

Ibuprofen (as Ibuprofen lysine) 400 mg Nurofen Express 684mg caplets | 24 tablet [P] £6.40 DT = £6.40

▶ **Nurofen Joint & Back Pain Relief** (Reckitt Benckiser Healthcare (UK) Ltd)

Ibuprofen (as Ibuprofen sodium dihydrate) 200 mg Nurofen Joint & Back Pain Relief 256mg caplets | 16 tablet [GSL] £2.44

Nurofen Joint & Back Pain Relief 256mg tablets | 16 tablet [GSL] £2.30

Ibuprofen (as Ibuprofen sodium dihydrate) 400 mg Nurofen Max Strength Joint & Back Pain Relief 512mg tablets | 24 tablet [P] £6.46

▶ **Nurofen Migraine Pain** (Reckitt Benckiser Healthcare (UK) Ltd)

Ibuprofen (as Ibuprofen lysine) 200 mg Nurofen Migraine Pain 342mg tablets | 12 tablet [GSL] £2.09

Oral suspension

CAUTIONARY AND ADVISORY LABELS 21

▶ **Ibuprofen (Non-proprietary)**

Ibuprofen 20 mg per 1 ml Ibuprofen 100mg/5ml oral suspension sugar-free | 500 ml [PoM] £7.85

Ibuprofen 40 mg per 1 ml Ibuprofen Twelve Plus Pain Relief 200mg/5ml oral suspension sugar-free | 100 ml [P] £3.49 DT = £3.49

Ibuprofen Seven Plus Pain Relief 200mg/5ml oral suspension sugar-free | 100 ml [P] £3.49 DT = £3.49

▶ **Brufen** (Mylan)

Ibuprofen 20 mg per 1 ml Brufen 100mg/5ml syrup | 500 ml [PoM] £8.88 DT = £8.88

Modified-release capsule

▶ **Nurofen Back Pain SR** (Reckitt Benckiser Healthcare (UK) Ltd)

Ibuprofen 300 mg Nurofen Back Pain SR 300mg capsules | 24 capsule [P] £4.85 DT = £4.85

Solution for infusion

▶ **Ibuprofen (Non-proprietary)**

Ibuprofen (as Ibuprofen lysine) 10 mg per 1 ml NeoProfen 20mg/2ml solution for infusion vials | 3 vial [PoM] [X]

▶ **Pedea** (Recordati Rare Diseases UK Ltd)

Ibuprofen 5 mg per 1 ml Pedea 10mg/2ml solution for infusion ampoules | 4 ampoule [PoM] £288.00 (Hospital only)

Chewable capsule

▶ **Nurofen** (Reckitt Benckiser Healthcare (UK) Ltd)

Ibuprofen 100 mg Nurofen for Children 100mg chewable capsules | 12 capsule [P] £3.23

Capsule

▶ **Ibuprofen (Non-proprietary)**

Ibuprofen 200 mg Ibuprofen 200mg capsules | 30 capsule [P] [X] DT = £4.85

▶ **Flarin** (infirst Healthcare Ltd)

Ibuprofen 200 mg Flarin 200mg capsules | 12 capsule [P] £4.13 | 30 capsule [P] £6.22 DT = £4.85

▶ **Nurofen Express** (Reckitt Benckiser Healthcare (UK) Ltd)

Ibuprofen 200 mg Nurofen Express 200mg liquid capsules | 30 capsule [P] £4.85 DT = £4.85

Ibuprofen 400 mg Nurofen Express 400mg liquid capsules | 10 capsule [P] £3.88 | 20 capsule [P] £6.47 DT = £6.47

Orodispersible tablet

▶ **Nurofen Meltlets** (Reckitt Benckiser Healthcare (UK) Ltd)

Ibuprofen 200 mg Nurofen Meltlets 200mg tablets sugar-free | 12 tablet [GSL] £2.58 DT = £2.58

Indometacin

20-Apr-2020

(Indomethacin)

● **INDICATIONS AND DOSE**

Symptomatic ductus arteriosus

▸ BY INTRAVENOUS INFUSION

▸ Neonate: Initially 100–200 micrograms/kg for 1 dose, followed by 100 micrograms/kg after 24 hours for 2 doses, at 24-hour intervals, doses to be given over 20–30 minutes, if residual patency present, 100 micrograms/kg to be given for a further 3 doses at 24-hour intervals.

Relief of pain and inflammation in rheumatic diseases including juvenile idiopathic arthritis

▸ BY MOUTH USING IMMEDIATE-RELEASE MEDICINES

▸ Child: 0.5–1 mg/kg twice daily, higher doses may be used under specialist supervision

● **UNLICENSED USE**

▸ With oral use Not licensed for use in children.

● **CONTRA-INDICATIONS**

▸ With intravenous use Bleeding (especially with active intracranial haemorrhage or gastro-intestinal bleeding) ; coagulation defects · necrotising enterocolitis · thrombocytopenia · untreated infection

▸ With oral use Active gastro-intestinal bleeding · active gastro-intestinal ulceration · history of gastro-intestinal bleeding related to previous NSAID therapy · history of gastro-intestinal perforation related to previous NSAID therapy · history of recurrent gastro-intestinal haemorrhage (two or more distinct episodes) · history of recurrent gastro-intestinal ulceration (two or more distinct episodes) · severe heart failure

● **CAUTIONS**

GENERAL CAUTIONS Heart failure

SPECIFIC CAUTIONS

▸ With intravenous use Inhibition of platelet aggregation (monitor for bleeding) ; may induce hyponatraemia · may mask symptoms of infection · may reduce urine output by 50% or more and precipitate renal impairment especially if extracellular volume depleted ; sepsis

▸ With oral use Allergic disorders · cardiac impairment (NSAIDs may impair renal function) · cerebrovascular disease · coagulation defects · connective-tissue disorders · dehydration (risk of renal impairment) · epilepsy · history of gastro-intestinal disorders (e.g. ulcerative colitis, Crohn's disease) · ischaemic heart disease · peripheral arterial disease · psychiatric disturbances · risk factors for cardiovascular events · uncontrolled hypertension

● **INTERACTIONS** → Appendix 1: NSAIDs

● **SIDE-EFFECTS** Agranulocytosis · alopecia · anaphylactic reaction · angioedema · anxiety · appetite decreased · arrhythmias · asthma · blood disorder · bone marrow disorders · breast abnormalities · chest pain · coma · confusion · congestive heart failure · constipation · corneal deposits · depression · diarrhoea · disseminated intravascular coagulation · dizziness · drowsiness · dysarthria · dyspnoea · erythema nodosum · eye disorder · eye pain · fatigue · fluid retention · flushing · gastrointestinal discomfort · gastrointestinal disorders · gynaecomastia · haemolytic anaemia · haemorrhage · hallucination · headache · hearing impairment · hepatic disorders · hyperglycaemia · hyperhidrosis · hyperkalaemia · hypotension · inflammatory bowel disease · insomnia · leucopenia · malaise · movement disorders · muscle weakness · nausea · nephritis tubulointerstitial · nephrotic syndrome · oedema · oral disorders · palpitations · pancreatitis · paraesthesia · peripheral neuropathy · photosensitivity reaction · platelet aggregation inhibition · psychiatric disorders · pulmonary oedema · renal failure (more common in patients with pre-existing renal impairment) · respiratory disorders · seizures · severe cutaneous adverse reactions (SCARs) · sigmoid lesion perforation · skin reactions · syncope · thrombocytopenia · tinnitus · urine abnormalities · vasculitis · vertigo · vision disorders · vomiting

SIDE-EFFECTS, FURTHER INFORMATION For information about cardiovascular and gastrointestinal side-effects, and a possible exacerbation of symptoms in asthma, see Non-steroidal anti-inflammatory drugs. p. 703

● **ALLERGY AND CROSS-SENSITIVITY** Contra-indicated in patients with a history of hypersensitivity to aspirin or any other NSAID—which includes those in whom attacks of asthma, angioedema, urticaria or rhinitis have been precipitated by aspirin or any other NSAID.

● **PREGNANCY**

▸ With oral use Avoid unless the potential benefit outweighs the risk. Avoid during the third trimester (risk of closure of fetal ductus arteriosus *in utero* and possibly persistent pulmonary hypertension of the newborn); onset of labour may be delayed and duration may be increased.

● **BREAST FEEDING**

▸ With oral use Amount probably too small to be harmful—manufacturers advise avoid. Use with caution during breast-feeding.

● **HEPATIC IMPAIRMENT**

▸ With intravenous use in neonates Increased risk of gastro-intestinal bleeding and fluid retention. Avoid in severe impairment.

▸ With oral use Use with caution; there is an increased risk of gastro-intestinal bleeding and fluid retention. Avoid in severe liver disease.

● **RENAL IMPAIRMENT**

▸ With intravenous use in neonates Avoid if possible in severe impairment.

Anuria or oliguria

▸ With intravenous use in neonates If anuria or marked oliguria (urinary output less than 0.6 mL/kg/hour), delay further doses until renal function returns to normal.

▸ With oral use Avoid if possible or use with caution. Avoid in severe impairment.

Dose adjustments ▸ With intravenous use in neonates Use lowest effective dose.

▸ With oral use The lowest effective dose should be used for the shortest possible duration.

Monitoring In renal impairment monitor renal function; sodium and water retention may occur and renal function may deteriorate, possibly leading to renal failure.

● **MONITORING REQUIREMENTS**

▸ With oral use During prolonged therapy ophthalmic and blood examinations particularly advisable.

● **DIRECTIONS FOR ADMINISTRATION** For *intravenous infusion*, dilute each vial with 1–2 mL Sodium Chloride 0.9% *or* Water for Injections.

● **PATIENT AND CARER ADVICE**

Driving and skilled tasks Dizziness may affect performance of skilled tasks (e.g. driving).

● **MEDICINAL FORMS** There can be variation in the licensing of different medicines containing the same drug. Forms available from special-order manufacturers include: oral suspension, oral solution

Capsule

CAUTIONARY AND ADVISORY LABELS 21

▸ **Indometacin (Non-proprietary)**

Indometacin 25 mg Indometacin 25mg capsules | 28 capsule PoM £1.32 DT = £1.29

Indometacin 50 mg Indometacin 50mg capsules | 28 capsule PoM £1.93 DT = £1.59

Mefenamic acid

17-Apr-2020

- **INDICATIONS AND DOSE**

Acute pain including dysmenorrhoea | Menorrhagia

▶ BY MOUTH

▸ Child 12–17 years: 500 mg 3 times a day

- **CONTRA-INDICATIONS** Active gastro-intestinal bleeding · active gastro-intestinal ulceration · following coronary artery bypass graft (CABG) surgery · history of gastro-intestinal bleeding related to previous NSAID therapy · history of gastro-intestinal perforation related to previous NSAID therapy · history of recurrent gastro-intestinal haemorrhage (two or more distinct episodes) · history of recurrent gastro-intestinal ulceration (two or more distinct episodes) · inflammatory bowel disease · severe heart failure
- **CAUTIONS** Acute porphyrias p. 652 · allergic disorders · cardiac impairment (NSAIDs may impair renal function) · cerebrovascular disease · coagulation defects · connective-tissue disorders · dehydration (risk of renal impairment) · epilepsy · heart failure · history of gastro-intestinal disorders (e.g. ulcerative colitis, Crohn's disease) · ischaemic heart disease · peripheral arterial disease · risk factors for cardiovascular events · uncontrolled hypertension
- **INTERACTIONS** → Appendix 1: NSAIDs
- **SIDE-EFFECTS** Agranulocytosis · anaemia · angioedema · appetite decreased · asthma · bone marrow disorders · confusion · constipation · Crohn's disease · depression · diarrhoea (discontinue) · disseminated intravascular coagulation · dizziness · drowsiness · dyspnoea · dysuria · ear pain · eosinophilia · eye irritation · fatigue · fertility decreased female · gastrointestinal discomfort · gastrointestinal disorders · glomerulonephritis · glucose tolerance impaired · haemolytic anaemia · haemorrhage · hallucination · headache · heart failure · hepatic disorders · hyperhidrosis · hypersensitivity · hypertension · hyponatraemia · hypotension · insomnia · leucopenia · malaise · meningitis aseptic (patients with connective-tissue disorders such as systemic lupus erythematosus may be especially susceptible) · multi organ failure · nausea · nephritis acute interstitial · nephrotic syndrome · nervousness · neutropenia · oedema · optic neuritis · oral ulceration · palpitations · pancreatitis · paraesthesia · photosensitivity reaction · proteinuria · rash (discontinue) · renal failure (more common in patients with pre-existing renal impairment) · renal failure non-oliguric · renal papillary necrosis · respiratory disorders · seizure · sepsis · severe cutaneous adverse reactions (SCARs) · skin reactions · thrombocytopenia · tinnitus · vertigo · vision disorders · vomiting

  SIDE-EFFECTS, FURTHER INFORMATION For information about cardiovascular and gastrointestinal side-effects, and a possible exacerbation of symptoms in asthma, see Non-steroidal anti-inflammatory drugs. p. 703

  Overdose Mefenamic acid has important consequences in overdosage because it can cause convulsions, which if prolonged or recurrent, require treatment.

  For details on the management of poisoning, see Emergency treatment of poisoning p. 891, in particular, Convulsions.
- **ALLERGY AND CROSS-SENSITIVITY** Contra-indicated in patients with a history of hypersensitivity to aspirin or any other NSAID—which includes those in whom attacks of asthma, angioedema, urticaria or rhinitis have been precipitated by aspirin or any other NSAID.
- **PREGNANCY** Avoid unless the potential benefit outweighs the risk. Avoid during the third trimester (risk of closure of fetal ductus arteriosus *in utero* and possibly persistent pulmonary hypertension of the newborn); onset of labour may be delayed and duration may be increased.
- **BREAST FEEDING** Use with caution during breast-feeding. Amount too small to be harmful but manufacturer advises avoid.
- **HEPATIC IMPAIRMENT** Manufacturer advises caution in mild to moderate impairment; avoid in severe impairment.
- **RENAL IMPAIRMENT** Avoid if possible or use with caution. Avoid in severe impairment.

  Dose adjustments The lowest effective dose should be used for the shortest possible duration.

  Monitoring In renal impairment monitor renal function; sodium and water retention may occur and renal function may deteriorate, possibly leading to renal failure.

- **MEDICINAL FORMS** There can be variation in the licensing of different medicines containing the same drug. Forms available from special-order manufacturers include: oral suspension

Oral suspension

CAUTIONARY AND ADVISORY LABELS 21

EXCIPIENTS: May contain Ethanol

▸ **Mefenamic acid (Non-proprietary)**

Mefenamic acid 10 mg per 1 ml Mefenamic acid 50mg/5ml oral suspension | 125 ml [PoM] £179.00 DT = £179.00

Tablet

CAUTIONARY AND ADVISORY LABELS 21

▸ **Mefenamic acid (Non-proprietary)**

Mefenamic acid 500 mg Mefenamic acid 500mg tablets | 28 tablet [PoM] £60.00 DT = £25.82 | 84 tablet [PoM] £77.00–£170.00

▸ **Ponstan** (Chemidex Pharma Ltd)

Mefenamic acid 500 mg Ponstan Forte 500mg tablets | 100 tablet [PoM] £15.72

Capsule

CAUTIONARY AND ADVISORY LABELS 21

▸ **Mefenamic acid (Non-proprietary)**

Mefenamic acid 250 mg Mefenamic acid 250mg capsules | 100 capsule [PoM] £60.10 DT = £22.64

▸ **Ponstan** (Chemidex Pharma Ltd)

Mefenamic acid 250 mg Ponstan 250mg capsules | 100 capsule [PoM] £8.17 DT = £22.64

Meloxicam

17-Apr-2020

- **INDICATIONS AND DOSE**

Exacerbation of osteoarthritis (short-term)

▶ BY MOUTH

▸ Child 16–17 years: 7.5 mg once daily, then increased if necessary up to 15 mg once daily

Pain and inflammation in rheumatic disease | Ankylosing spondylitis

▶ BY MOUTH

▸ Child 16–17 years: 15 mg once daily, then reduced to 7.5 mg once daily if required

Relief of pain and inflammation in juvenile idiopathic arthritis and other musculoskeletal disorders in children intolerant to other NSAIDs

▶ BY MOUTH

▸ Child 12–17 years (body-weight up to 50 kg): 7.5 mg once daily

▸ Child 12–17 years (body-weight 50 kg and above): 15 mg once daily

- **UNLICENSED USE** Not licensed for use in children under 16 years.
- **CONTRA-INDICATIONS** Active gastro-intestinal bleeding · active gastro-intestinal ulceration · following coronary artery bypass graft surgery · history of gastro-intestinal bleeding related to previous NSAID therapy · history of gastro-intestinal perforation related to previous NSAID therapy · history of recurrent gastro-intestinal haemorrhage (two or more distinct episodes) · history of

recurrent gastro-intestinal ulceration (two or more distinct episodes) · severe heart failure

- **CAUTIONS** Allergic disorders · cardiac impairment (NSAIDs may impair renal function) · cerebrovascular disease · coagulation defects · connective-tissue disorders · dehydration (risk of renal impairment) · heart failure · history of gastro-intestinal disorders (e.g. ulcerative colitis, Crohn's disease) · ischaemic heart disease · peripheral arterial disease · risk factors for cardiovascular events · uncontrolled hypertension
- **INTERACTIONS** → Appendix 1: NSAIDs
- **SIDE-EFFECTS**
  - **Common or very common** Constipation · diarrhoea · gastrointestinal discomfort · gastrointestinal disorders · headache · nausea · vomiting
  - **Uncommon** Anaemia · angioedema · burping · dizziness · drowsiness · electrolyte imbalance · fluid retention · flushing · haemorrhage · hepatic disorders · hypersensitivity · oedema · skin reactions · stomatitis · vertigo
  - **Rare or very rare** Acute kidney injury · asthma · conjunctivitis · leucopenia · mood altered · nightmare · palpitations · severe cutaneous adverse reactions (SCARs) · thrombocytopenia · tinnitus · vision disorders
  - **Frequency not known** Agranulocytosis · confusion · fertility decreased female · heart failure · increased risk of arterial thromboembolism · nephritis tubulointerstitial · nephrotic syndrome · photosensitivity reaction · renal necrosis

  SIDE-EFFECTS, FURTHER INFORMATION For information about cardiovascular and gastrointestinal side-effects, and a possible exacerbation of symptoms in asthma, see Non-steroidal anti-inflammatory drugs. p. 703
- **ALLERGY AND CROSS-SENSITIVITY** Contra-indicated in patients with a history of hypersensitivity to aspirin or any other NSAID—which includes those in whom attacks of asthma, angioedema, urticaria or rhinitis have been precipitated by aspirin or any other NSAID.
- **PREGNANCY** Avoid unless the potential benefit outweighs the risk. Avoid during the third trimester (risk of closure of fetal ductus arteriosus *in utero* and possibly persistent pulmonary hypertension of the newborn); onset of labour may be delayed and duration may be increased.
- **BREAST FEEDING** Use with caution during breast-feeding. Present in milk in *animal* studies—manufacturer advises avoid.
- **HEPATIC IMPAIRMENT** Manufacturer advises caution in mild to moderate impairment; avoid in severe impairment.
- **RENAL IMPAIRMENT** Avoid if possible or use with caution. Avoid if estimated glomerular filtration rate less than 25 mL/minute/1.73 m^2.

  Dose adjustments The lowest effective dose should be used for the shortest possible duration.

  Monitoring In renal impairment monitor renal function; sodium and water retention may occur and renal function may deteriorate, possibly leading to renal failure.

- **MEDICINAL FORMS** There can be variation in the licensing of different medicines containing the same drug. Forms available from special-order manufacturers include: oral suspension

Orodispersible tablet

- Meloxicam (Non-proprietary)

  Meloxicam 7.5 mg Meloxicam 7.5mg orodispersible tablets sugar-free | 30 tablet [PoM] £25.50 DT = £25.50

  Meloxicam 15 mg Meloxicam 15mg orodispersible tablets sugar-free | 30 tablet [PoM] £25.50 DT = £25.50

Tablet

CAUTIONARY AND ADVISORY LABELS 21

- Meloxicam (Non-proprietary)

  Meloxicam 7.5 mg Meloxicam 7.5mg tablets | 30 tablet [PoM] £3.60 DT = £2.92

  Meloxicam 15 mg Meloxicam 15mg tablets | 30 tablet [PoM] £7.35 DT = £5.26

10 Musculoskeletal system

Naproxen

19-Apr-2020

- **INDICATIONS AND DOSE**

Pain and inflammation in musculoskeletal disorders | Dysmenorrhoea

- BY MOUTH
  - Child: 5 mg/kg twice daily; maximum 1 g per day

Pain and inflammation in juvenile idiopathic arthritis

- BY MOUTH
  - Child 2-17 years: 5–7.5 mg/kg twice daily; maximum 1 g per day

- **UNLICENSED USE** Not licensed for use in children under 5 years for juvenile idiopathic arthritis. Not licensed for use in children under 16 years for musculoskeletal disorders or dysmenorrhoea.
- **CONTRA-INDICATIONS** Active gastro-intestinal bleeding · active gastro-intestinal ulceration · history of gastro-intestinal bleeding related to previous NSAID therapy · history of gastro-intestinal perforation related to previous NSAID therapy · history of recurrent gastro-intestinal haemorrhage (two or more distinct episodes) · history of recurrent gastro-intestinal ulceration (two or more distinct episodes) · severe heart failure
- **CAUTIONS** Allergic disorders · cardiac impairment (NSAIDs may impair renal function) · cerebrovascular disease · coagulation defects · connective-tissue disorders · dehydration (risk of renal impairment) · heart failure · history of gastro-intestinal disorders (e.g. ulcerative colitis, Crohn's disease) · ischaemic heart disease · peripheral arterial disease · risk factors for cardiovascular events · uncontrolled hypertension
- **INTERACTIONS** → Appendix 1: NSAIDs
- **SIDE-EFFECTS** Agranulocytosis · alopecia · angioedema · aplastic anaemia · asthma · cognitive impairment · concentration impaired · confusion · constipation · corneal opacity · depression · diarrhoea · dizziness · drowsiness · dyspnoea · erythema nodosum · fatigue · gastrointestinal discomfort · gastrointestinal disorders · glomerulonephritis · haemolytic anaemia · haemorrhage · hallucination · headache · hearing impairment · heart failure · hepatic disorders · hyperhidrosis · hyperkalaemia · hypersensitivity · hypertension · increased risk of arterial thromboembolism · infertility female · inflammatory bowel disease · malaise · meningitis aseptic (patients with connective-tissue disorders such as systemic lupus erythematosus may be especially susceptible) · muscle weakness · myalgia · nausea · nephritis tubulointerstitial · nephropathy · neutropenia · oedema · optic neuritis · oral disorders · palpitations · pancreatitis · papillitis · papilloedema · paraesthesia · photosensitivity reaction · platelet aggregation inhibition · pulmonary oedema · rash pustular · renal failure (more common in patients with pre-existing renal impairment) · renal papillary necrosis · respiratory disorders · seizure · severe cutaneous adverse reactions (SCARs) · skin reactions · sleep disorders · thirst · thrombocytopenia · tinnitus · vasculitis · vertigo · visual impairment · vomiting

  SIDE-EFFECTS, FURTHER INFORMATION For information about cardiovascular and gastrointestinal side-effects, and a possible exacerbation of symptoms in asthma, see Non-steroidal anti-inflammatory drugs. p. 703
- **ALLERGY AND CROSS-SENSITIVITY** Contra-indicated in patients with a history of hypersensitivity to aspirin or any other NSAID—which includes those in whom attacks of asthma, angioedema, urticaria or rhinitis have been precipitated by aspirin or any other NSAID.
- **PREGNANCY** Avoid unless the potential benefit outweighs the risk. Avoid during the third trimester (risk of closure of fetal ductus arteriosus *in utero* and possibly persistent

pulmonary hypertension of the newborn); onset of labour may be delayed and duration may be increased.

- **BREAST FEEDING** Use with caution during breast-feeding. Amount too small to be harmful but manufacturer advises avoid.
- **HEPATIC IMPAIRMENT** Manufacturer advises caution in mild to moderate impairment; avoid in severe impairment. **Dose adjustments** Manufacturer advises consider dose reduction in mild to moderate impairment.
- **RENAL IMPAIRMENT** Avoid if possible or use with caution. Avoid if estimated glomerular filtration rate less than 30 mL/minute/1.73 m^2.
Dose adjustments The lowest effective dose should be used for the shortest possible duration.
Monitoring In renal impairment monitor renal function; sodium and water retention may occur and renal function may deteriorate, possibly leading to renal failure.
- **EXCEPTIONS TO LEGAL CATEGORY** Can be sold to the public for the treatment of primary dysmenorrhoea in women aged 15–50 years subject to max. single dose of 500 mg, max. daily dose of 750 mg for max. 3 days, and a max. pack size of 9 × 250 mg tablets.

- **MEDICINAL FORMS** There can be variation in the licensing of different medicines containing the same drug. Forms available from special-order manufacturers include: oral suspension

Gastro-resistant tablet

CAUTIONARY AND ADVISORY LABELS 5, 25

- Naproxen (Non-proprietary)
  Naproxen 250 mg Naproxen 250mg gastro-resistant tablets | 56 tablet PoM £11.69 DT = £9.73
  Naproxen 375 mg Naproxen 375mg gastro-resistant tablets | 56 tablet PoM £27.78 DT = £27.77
  Naproxen 500 mg Naproxen 500mg gastro-resistant tablets | 56 tablet PoM £23.79 DT = £19.54
- Naprosyn EC (Atnahs Pharma UK Ltd)
  Naproxen 250 mg Naprosyn EC 250mg tablets | 56 tablet PoM £4.29 DT = £9.73
  Naproxen 375 mg Naprosyn EC 375mg tablets | 56 tablet PoM £6.42 DT = £27.77
  Naproxen 500 mg Naprosyn EC 500mg tablets | 56 tablet PoM £8.56 DT = £19.54
- Nexocin EC (Noumed Life Sciences Ltd)
  Naproxen 250 mg Nexocin EC 250mg gastro-resistant tablets | 56 tablet PoM ⊠ DT = £9.73
  Naproxen 375 mg Nexocin EC 375mg gastro-resistant tablets | 56 tablet PoM ⊠ DT = £27.77
  Naproxen 500 mg Nexocin EC 500mg gastro-resistant tablets | 56 tablet PoM ⊠ DT = £19.54

Tablet

CAUTIONARY AND ADVISORY LABELS 21

- Naproxen (Non-proprietary)
  Naproxen 250 mg Naproxen 250mg tablets | 28 tablet PoM £5.35 DT = £2.91 | 56 tablet PoM £10.70
  Naproxen 500 mg Naproxen 500mg tablets | 28 tablet PoM £8.14 DT = £2.47 | 56 tablet PoM £14.30
- Naprosyn (Atnahs Pharma UK Ltd)
  Naproxen 250 mg Naprosyn 250mg tablets | 56 tablet PoM £4.29
  Naproxen 500 mg Naprosyn 500mg tablets | 56 tablet PoM £8.56

Oral suspension

- Naproxen (Non-proprietary)
  Naproxen 25 mg per 1 ml Naproxen 25mg/ml oral suspension sugar-free | 100 ml PoM £110.00 DT = £119.00
  Naproxen 125mg/5ml oral suspension sugar-free | 100 ml PoM £110.00–£128.00 DT = £119.00
  Naproxen 50 mg per 1 ml Naproxen 50mg/ml oral suspension | 100 ml PoM £45.01 DT = £45.01

Effervescent tablet

- Stirlescent (Stirling Anglian Pharmaceuticals Ltd)
  Naproxen 250 mg Stirlescent 250mg effervescent tablets sugar-free | 20 tablet PoM £52.72 DT = £52.72

Piroxicam

20-Apr-2020

- **INDICATIONS AND DOSE**

Relief of pain and inflammation in juvenile idiopathic arthritis

▶ BY MOUTH
- Child 6–17 years (body-weight up to 15 kg): 5 mg daily
- Child 6–17 years (body-weight 15–25 kg): 10 mg daily
- Child 6–17 years (body-weight 26–45 kg): 15 mg daily
- Child 6–17 years (body-weight 46 kg and above): 20 mg daily

- **UNLICENSED USE** Not licensed for use in children.

IMPORTANT SAFETY INFORMATION

CHMP ADVICE—PIROXICAM (JUNE 2007)

The CHMP has recommended restrictions on the use of piroxicam because of the increased risk of gastro-intestinal side effects and serious skin reactions. The CHMP has advised that:
- piroxicam should be initiated only by physicians experienced in treating inflammatory or degenerative rheumatic diseases
- piroxicam should not be used as first-line treatment
- in adults, use of piroxicam should be limited to the symptomatic relief of osteoarthritis, rheumatoid arthritis, and ankylosing spondylitis
- piroxicam dose should not exceed 20 mg daily
- piroxicam should no longer be used for the treatment of acute painful and inflammatory conditions
- treatment should be reviewed 2 weeks after initiating piroxicam, and periodically thereafter
- concomitant administration of a gastro-protective agent should be considered.

Topical preparations containing piroxicam are not affected by these restrictions.

- **CONTRA-INDICATIONS** Active gastro-intestinal bleeding · active gastro-intestinal ulceration · history of gastro-intestinal bleeding · history of gastro-intestinal perforation · history of gastro-intestinal ulceration · inflammatory bowel disease · severe heart failure
- **CAUTIONS** Allergic disorders · cardiac impairment (NSAIDs may impair renal function) · cerebrovascular disease · coagulation defects · connective-tissue disorders · dehydration (risk of renal impairment) · heart failure · history of gastro-intestinal disorders · ischaemic heart disease · peripheral arterial disease · risk factors for cardiovascular events · uncontrolled hypertension
- **INTERACTIONS** → Appendix 1: NSAIDs
- **SIDE-EFFECTS**
  - **Common or very common** Anaemia · appetite decreased · constipation · diarrhoea · dizziness · drowsiness · eosinophilia · gastrointestinal discomfort · gastrointestinal disorders · headache · hyperglycaemia · leucopenia · nausea · oedema · rash (discontinue) · skin reactions · thrombocytopenia · tinnitus · vertigo · vomiting · weight changes
  - **Uncommon** Hypoglycaemia · palpitations · stomatitis · vision blurred
  - **Rare or very rare** Nephritis tubulointerstitial · nephrotic syndrome · renal failure · renal papillary necrosis · severe cutaneous adverse reactions (SCARs)
  - **Frequency not known** Alopecia · angioedema · aplastic anaemia · bronchospasm · confusion · depression · dyspnoea · embolism and thrombosis · eye irritation · eye swelling · fertility decreased female · fluid retention · haemolytic anaemia · haemorrhage · hallucination · hearing impairment · heart failure · hepatic disorders · hypersensitivity · hypertension · malaise · mood altered · nervousness · onycholysis · pancreatitis · paraesthesia · photosensitivity reaction · sleep disorders · vasculitis

SIDE-EFFECTS, FURTHER INFORMATION For information about cardiovascular and gastrointestinal side-effects, and a possible exacerbation of symptoms in asthma, see Non-steroidal anti-inflammatory drugs. p. 703

- **ALLERGY AND CROSS-SENSITIVITY** Contra-indicated in patients with a history of hypersensitivity to aspirin or any other NSAID—which includes those in whom attacks of asthma, angioedema, urticaria or rhinitis have been precipitated by aspirin or any other NSAID.
- **PREGNANCY** Avoid unless the potential benefit outweighs the risk. Avoid during the third trimester (risk of closure of fetal ductus arteriosus *in utero* and possibly persistent pulmonary hypertension of the newborn); onset of labour may be delayed and duration may be increased.
- **BREAST FEEDING** Use with caution during breast-feeding. Amount too small to be harmful.
- **HEPATIC IMPAIRMENT** Manufacturer advises caution.
- **RENAL IMPAIRMENT** Avoid if possible or use with caution.

Dose adjustments The lowest effective dose should be used for the shortest possible duration.

Monitoring In renal impairment monitor renal function; sodium and water retention may occur and renal function may deteriorate, possibly leading to renal failure.

- **DIRECTIONS FOR ADMINISTRATION** Piroxicam orodispersible tablets can be taken by placing on the tongue and allowing to dissolve or by swallowing.

Piroxicam orodispersible tablets may be halved to give 10 mg dose [unlicensed].

- **LESS SUITABLE FOR PRESCRIBING**

▸ With oral use Piroxicam is less suitable for prescribing.

- **MEDICINAL FORMS** There can be variation in the licensing of different medicines containing the same drug.

Orodispersible tablet

CAUTIONARY AND ADVISORY LABELS 10, 21

EXCIPIENTS: May contain Aspartame

▸ **Feldene Melt** (Pfizer Ltd)

Piroxicam 20 mg Feldene Melt 20mg tablets sugar-free | 30 tablet PoM £10.53 DT = £10.53

Capsule

CAUTIONARY AND ADVISORY LABELS 21

▸ **Piroxicam (Non-proprietary)**

Piroxicam 10 mg Piroxicam 10mg capsules | 56 capsule PoM £5.77 DT = £4.90

Piroxicam 20 mg Piroxicam 20mg capsules | 28 capsule PoM £5.76 DT = £4.48

▸ **Feldene** (Pfizer Ltd)

Piroxicam 10 mg Feldene 10mg capsules | 30 capsule PoM £3.86

Piroxicam 20 mg Feldene 20 capsules | 30 capsule PoM £7.71

4 Soft tissue and joint disorders

4.1 Local inflammation of joints and soft tissue

Other drugs used for Local inflammation of joints and soft tissue Dexamethasone, p. 475 · Prednisolone, p. 478

CORTICOSTEROIDS

Corticosteroids, inflammatory disorders

Systemic corticosteroids

In children with rheumatic diseases corticosteroids should be reserved for specific indications (e.g. when other therapies are unsuccessful or while waiting for DMARDs to take effect) and should be used only under the supervision of a specialist.

Systemic corticosteroids may be considered for the management of juvenile idiopathic arthritis in systemic disease or when several joints are affected. Systemic corticosteroids may also be considered in severe, possibly life-threatening conditions such as systemic lupus erythematosus, systemic vasculitis, juvenile dermatomyositis, Behçet's disease, and polyarticular joint disease.

In severe conditions, short courses ('pulses') of high dose intravenous methylprednisolone p. 478 or a pulsed oral corticosteroid may be particularly effective for providing rapid relief, and has fewer long-term adverse effects than continuous treatment.

Corticosteroid doses should be reduced with care because of the possibility of relapse if the reduction is too rapid. If complete discontinuation of corticosteroids is not possible, consideration should be given to alternate-day (or alternate high-dose, low-dose) administration; on days when no corticosteroid is given, or a lower dose is given, an additional dose of a NSAID may be helpful. In some conditions, alternative treatment using an antimalarial or concomitant use of an immunosuppressant drug, such as azathioprine p. 558, methotrexate p. 588 or cyclophosphamide p. 579 may prove useful; in less severe conditions treatment with a NSAID alone may be adequate.

Administration of corticosteroids may result in suppression of growth and may affect the development of puberty. The risk of corticosteroid-induced osteoporosis should be considered for those on long-term corticosteroid treatment; corticosteroids may also increase the risk of osteopenia in those unable to exercise. See the disadvantages of corticosteroid treatment.

Local corticosteroid injections

Corticosteroids are injected locally for an anti-inflammatory effect. In inflammatory conditions of the joints, including juvenile idiopathic arthritis, they are given by intra-articular injection as monotherapy, or as an adjunct to long-term therapy to reduce swelling and deformity in one or a few joints. Aseptic precautions (e.g. a no-touch technique) are essential, as is a clinician skilled in the technique; infected areas should be avoided and general anaesthesia, or local anaesthesia, or conscious sedation should be used. Occasionally an acute inflammatory reaction develops after an intra-articular or soft-tissue injection of a corticosteroid. This may be a reaction to the microcrystalline suspension of the corticosteroid used, but must be distinguished from sepsis introduced into the injection site.

Triamcinolone hexacetonide p. 715 [unlicensed] is preferred for intra-articular injection because it is almost insoluble and has a long-acting (depot) effect. Triamcinolone acetonide p. 715 and methylprednisolone may also be considered for intra-articular injection into larger joints, whilst hydrocortisone acetate p. 715 should be reserved for smaller joints or for soft-tissue injections. Intra-articular corticosteroid injections can cause flushing and, in adults, may affect the hyaline cartilage. Each joint should usually be treated no more than 3–4 times in one year.

A smaller amount of corticosteroid may also be injected directly into soft tissues for the relief of inflammation in conditions such as *tennis* or *golfer's elbow* or *compression neuropathies*, which occur rarely in children. In *tendinitis*, injections should be made into the tendon sheath and not directly into the tendon (due to the absence of a true tendon sheath and a high risk of rupture, the Achilles tendon should not be injected).

Corticosteroid injections are also injected into soft tissues for the treatment of skin lesions.

472

Hydrocortisone
17-Dec-2019

● **INDICATIONS AND DOSE**

HYDROCORTISTAB ®

Local inflammation of joints and soft-tissues

▶ BY INTRA-ARTICULAR INJECTION

▸ Child 1 month–11 years: 5–30 mg, select dose according to size of child and joint; where appropriate dose may be repeated at intervals of 21 days. Not more than 3 joints should be treated on any one day, for details consult product literature

▸ Child 12–17 years: 5–50 mg, select dose according to size of patient and joint; where appropriate dose may be repeated at intervals of 21 days. Not more than 3 joints should be treated on any one day, for details consult product literature

● **INTERACTIONS** → Appendix 1: corticosteroids

● **SIDE-EFFECTS** Myocardial rupture (following recent myocardial infarction)

● **MEDICINAL FORMS** There can be variation in the licensing of different medicines containing the same drug.

Suspension for injection

▸ Hydrocortistab (Advanz Pharma)

Hydrocortisone acetate 25 mg per 1 ml Hydrocortistab 25mg/1ml suspension for injection ampoules | 10 ampoule PoM £68.72 DT = £68.72

472

Methylprednisolone
11-Oct-2019

● **INDICATIONS AND DOSE**

DEPO-MEDRONE ®

Local inflammation of joints and soft tissues

▶ BY INTRA-ARTICULAR INJECTION

▸ Child: (consult product literature)

● **INTERACTIONS** → Appendix 1: corticosteroids

● **SIDE-EFFECTS** Angioedema · cataract · confusion · delusions · depressed mood · diarrhoea · dizziness · drug dependence · dyslipidaemia · embolism and thrombosis · epidural lipomatosis · gastrointestinal disorders · glucose tolerance impaired · hallucination · hepatitis · hiccups · hypopituitarism · increased insulin requirement · intracranial pressure increased · memory loss · metabolic acidosis · muscle weakness · myalgia · neuropathic arthropathy · peripheral oedema · psychiatric disorder · schizophrenia exacerbated · sterile abscess · suicidal ideation · vision loss · withdrawal syndrome

● **PATIENT AND CARER ADVICE** Patient counselling is advised for methylprednisolone tablets and injections (steroid card).

● **MEDICINAL FORMS** There can be variation in the licensing of different medicines containing the same drug.

Suspension for injection

CAUTIONARY AND ADVISORY LABELS 10

▸ Depo-Medrone (Pfizer Ltd)

Methylprednisolone acetate 40 mg per 1 ml Depo-Medrone 40mg/1ml suspension for injection vials | 1 vial PoM £3.44 DT = £3.44 | 10 vial PoM £34.04

Depo-Medrone 80mg/2ml suspension for injection vials | 1 vial PoM £6.18 DT = £6.18 | 10 vial PoM £61.39

Depo-Medrone 120mg/3ml suspension for injection vials | 1 vial PoM £8.96 DT = £8.96 | 10 vial PoM £88.81

472

Triamcinolone acetonide
26-Nov-2019

● **INDICATIONS AND DOSE**

ADCORTYL ® INTRA-ARTICULAR/INTRADERMAL

Local inflammation of joints and soft tissues

▶ BY INTRA-ARTICULAR INJECTION

▸ Child 1–17 years: 2 mg/kg (max. per dose 15 mg), for details consult product literature, dose applies for larger joints. For doses above 15 mg use *Kenalog® Intra-articular/Intramuscular*. If appropriate repeat treatment for relapse.

KENALOG ® VIALS

Local inflammation of joints and soft tissues

▶ BY INTRA-ARTICULAR INJECTION

▸ Child 1–17 years: 2 mg/kg, for details consult product literature, if appropriate repeat treatment for relapse, higher doses than usual maximum have been used; Usual maximum 40 mg

● **UNLICENSED USE** Not licensed for use in children under 6 years.

● **INTERACTIONS** → Appendix 1: corticosteroids

● **PATIENT AND CARER ADVICE** Patient counselling is advised for triamcinolone acetonide injection (steroid card).

● **MEDICINAL FORMS** There can be variation in the licensing of different medicines containing the same drug.

Suspension for injection

CAUTIONARY AND ADVISORY LABELS 10

EXCIPIENTS: May contain Benzyl alcohol

▸ Adcortyl Intra-articular / Intradermal (Bristol-Myers Squibb Pharmaceuticals Ltd)

Triamcinolone acetonide 10 mg per 1 ml Adcortyl Intra-articular / Intradermal 50mg/5ml suspension for injection vials | 1 vial PoM £3.63 DT = £3.63

Adcortyl Intra-articular / Intradermal 10mg/1ml suspension for injection ampoules | 5 ampoule PoM £4.47 DT = £4.47

▸ Kenalog (Bristol-Myers Squibb Pharmaceuticals Ltd)

Triamcinolone acetonide 40 mg per 1 ml Kenalog Intra-articular / Intramuscular 40mg/1ml suspension for injection vials | 5 vial PoM £7.45 DT = £7.45

472

Triamcinolone hexacetonide
28-Nov-2019

● **INDICATIONS AND DOSE**

Symptomatic treatment of subacute and chronic inflammatory joint diseases (for details, consult product literature)

▶ BY INTRA-ARTICULAR INJECTION

▸ Child 12–17 years: 2–20 mg, according to size of the joint; if appropriate repeat treatment at intervals of 3–4 weeks, no more than 2 joints should be treated on any one day

▶ BY PERI-ARTICULAR INJECTION

▸ Child 12–17 years: 10–20 mg, according to size of the joint, no more than 2 joints should be treated on any one day

Juvenile idiopathic arthritis

▶ BY INTRA-ARTICULAR INJECTION

▸ Child 3–11 years: (consult product literature)

● **CONTRA-INDICATIONS** Avoid injections containing benzyl alcohol in neonates ; consult product literature

● **CAUTIONS** Consult product literature

● **INTERACTIONS** → Appendix 1: corticosteroids

● **SIDE-EFFECTS** Protein catabolism

● **PRESCRIBING AND DISPENSING INFORMATION** Various strengths available from 'special order' manufacturers or specialist importing companies.

● **NATIONAL FUNDING/ACCESS DECISIONS**

All Wales Medicines Strategy Group (AWMSG) decisions
The *All Wales Medicines Strategy Group* has advised (August 2017) that triamcinolone hexacetonide 20 mg/mL suspension for injection is recommended as an option for use within NHS Wales for the treatment of juvenile idiopathic arthritis.

● **MEDICINAL FORMS** There can be variation in the licensing of different medicines containing the same drug.

Suspension for injection
EXCIPIENTS: May contain Benzyl alcohol
▸ Triamcinolone hexacetonide (Non-proprietary)
Triamcinolone hexacetonide 20 mg per 1 ml Triamcinolone hexacetonide 20mg/1ml suspension for injection ampoules | 10 ampoule PoM £120.00 DT = £120.00

4.2 Soft tissue disorders

Soft-tissue disorders

Soft-tissue and musculoskeletal disorders

The management of children with soft-tissue injuries and strains, and musculoskeletal disorders, may include temporary rest together with the local application of heat or cold, local massage and physiotherapy. For pain relief, paracetamol p. 288 is often adequate and should be used first. Alternatively, the lowest effective dose of a **NSAID** (e.g. ibuprofen p. 707) can be used. If pain relief with either drug is inadequate, both paracetamol (in a full dose appropriate for the child) and a low dose of a NSAID may be required.

Extravasation

Local guidelines for the management of extravasation should be followed where they exist or specialist advice sought.

Extravasation injury follows leakage of drugs or intravenous fluids from the veins or inadvertent administration into the subcutaneous or subdermal tissue. It must be dealt with **promptly** to prevent tissue necrosis.

Acidic or alkaline preparations and those with an osmolarity greater than that of plasma can cause extravasation injury; excipients including alcohol and polyethylene glycol have also been implicated. Cytotoxic drugs commonly cause extravasation injury. Very young children are at increased risk. Those receiving anticoagulants are more likely to lose blood into surrounding tissues if extravasation occurs, while those receiving sedatives or analgesics may not notice the early signs or symptoms of extravasation.

Extravasation prevention

Precautions should be taken to avoid extravasation; ideally, drugs likely to cause extravasation injury should be given through a central line and children receiving repeated doses of hazardous drugs peripherally should have the cannula resited at regular intervals. Attention should be paid to the manufacturers' recommendations for administration. Placing a glyceryl trinitrate p. 142 patch or using glyceryl trinitrate ointment distal to the cannula may improve the patency of the vessel in children with small veins or in those whose veins are prone to collapse. Children or their carers should be asked to report any pain or burning at the site of injection immediately.

Extravasation management

If extravasation is suspected the infusion should be stopped immediately but the cannula should not be removed until after an attempt has been made to aspirate the area (through the cannula) in order to remove as much of the drug as possible. Aspiration is sometimes possible if the extravasation presents with a raised bleb or blister at the injection site and is surrounded by hardened tissue, but it is often unsuccessful if the tissue is soft or soggy. **Corticosteroids** are usually given to treat inflammation, although there is little evidence to support their use in extravasation. Hydrocortisone p. 476 or dexamethasone p. 475 can be given either locally by subcutaneous injection or intravenously at a site distant from the injury. Antihistamines and analgesics may be required for symptom relief.

The management of extravasation beyond these measures is not well standardised and calls for specialist advice. Treatment depends on the nature of the offending substance; one approach is to localise and neutralise the substance whereas another is to spread and dilute it. The first method may be appropriate following extravasation of vesicant drugs and involves administration of an antidote (if available) and the application of cold compresses 3–4 times a day (consult specialist literature for details of specific antidotes). Spreading and diluting the offending substance involves infiltrating the area with physiological saline, applying warm compresses, elevating the affected limb, and administering hyaluronidase below. A saline flush-out technique (involving flushing the subcutaneous tissue with physiological saline) may be effective but requires specialist advice. Hyaluronidase should **not** be administered following extravasation of vesicant drugs (unless it is either specifically indicated or used in the saline flush-out technique).

Enzymes used in soft-tissue disorders

Hyaluronidase is used for the management of extravasation.

ENZYMES

Hyaluronidase

24-Feb-2020

● **INDICATIONS AND DOSE**

Extravasation
▶ BY LOCAL INFILTRATION
▸ Child: (consult product literature)

● **UNLICENSED USE** Licensed for use in children, but age range not specified by the manufacturer.

● **CONTRA-INDICATIONS** Avoid sites where infection is present · avoid sites where malignancy is present · do not apply direct to cornea · not for anaesthesia in unexplained premature labour · not for intravenous administration · not to be used to enhance the absorption and dispersion of dopamine and/or alpha-adrenoceptor agonists · not to be used to reduce swelling of bites · not to be used to reduce swelling of stings

● **SIDE-EFFECTS** Oedema · periorbital oedema

● **MEDICINAL FORMS** There can be variation in the licensing of different medicines containing the same drug.

Powder for solution for injection
▸ Hyaluronidase (Non-proprietary)
Hyaluronidase 1500 unit Hyaluronidase 1,500unit powder for solution for injection ampoules | 10 ampoule PoM £136.55

Chapter 11
Eye

CONTENTS

Eye

Eye treatment: drug administration

Drugs are most commonly administered to the eye by topical application as eye drops or eye ointments. When a higher drug concentration is required within the eye, a local injection may be necessary.

Eye-drop dispenser devices are available to aid the instillation of eye drops from plastic bottles and some are prescribable on the NHS (consult Drug Tariff—see Appliances and Reagents). Product-specific devices may be supplied by manufacturers—contact individual manufacturers for further information. They are particularly useful for children in whom normal application is difficult, for the visually impaired, or otherwise physically limited patients.

Eye drops and eye ointments

Eye drops are generally instilled into the pocket formed by gently pulling down the lower eyelid and keeping the eye closed for as long as possible after application; in neonates and infants it may be more appropriate to administer the drop in the inner angle of the open eye. One drop is all that is needed; instillation of more than one drop at a time should be discouraged because it may increase systemic side-effects. A small amount of eye ointment is applied similarly; the ointment melts rapidly and blinking helps to spread it.

When two different eye-drop preparations are used at the same time of day, dilution and overflow can occur when one immediately follows the other. The carer or child should therefore leave an interval of at least 5 minutes between the two; the interval should be extended when eye drops with a prolonged contact time, such as gels and suspensions, are used. Eye ointment should be applied after drops. Both drops and ointment can cause transient blurred vision; children should be warned, where appropriate, not to perform skilled tasks (e.g. cycling or driving) until vision is clear.

Systemic effects may arise from absorption of drugs into the general circulation from conjunctival vessels or from the nasal mucosa after the excess preparation has drained down through the tear ducts. The extent of systemic absorption following ocular administration is highly variable; nasal drainage of drugs is associated with eye drops much more often than with eye ointments. Pressure on the lacrimal punctum for at least a minute after applying eye drops reduces nasolacrimal drainage and therefore decreases systemic absorption from the nasal mucosa.

Also see warnings relating to eye drops and contact lenses.

Eye lotions

These are solutions for the irrigation of the conjunctival sac. They act mechanically to flush out irritants or foreign bodies as a first-aid treatment. Sterile sodium chloride 0.9% solution p. 726 is usually used. Clean water will suffice in an emergency.

Other preparations administered to the eye

Subconjunctival injection may be used to administer anti-infective drugs, mydriatics, or corticosteroids for conditions not responding to topical therapy; intracameral and intravitreal routes can also be used to administer certain drugs, for example antibacterials. These injections should only be used under specialist supervision.

Drugs such as antimicrobials and corticosteroids may be administered systemically to treat susceptible eye conditions.

Ophthalmic Specials

The Royal College of Ophthalmologists and the UK Ophthalmic Pharmacy Group have produced the Ophthalmic Specials Guidance to help prescribers and pharmacists manage and restrict the use of unlicensed eye preparations. 'Specials' should only be prescribed in situations where a licensed product will not be suitable for a child's needs. The Ophthalmic Specials Guidance can be accessed on the Royal College of Ophthalmologists website (www.rcophth.ac.uk). The guidance will be reviewed every six months to ensure the most accurate and up-to-date information is available.

Preservatives and sensitisers

Information on preservatives and substances identified as skin sensitisers is provided under Excipients statements in preparation entries. Very rarely, cases of corneal calcification have been reported with the use of phosphate-containing eye drops in patients with significantly damaged corneas—consult product literature for further information.

Eye preparations: control of microbial contamination

Preparations for the eye should be sterile when issued. Care should be taken to avoid contamination of the contents during use.

Eye drops in multiple-application containers for *domiciliary use* should not be used for more than 4 weeks after first opening (unless otherwise stated by the manufacturer).

Multiple application eye drops for use in *hospital wards* are normally discarded 1 week after first opening—local practice may vary. Individual containers should be provided for each patient. A separate container should be supplied for each eye only if there are special concerns about contamination. Containers used before an eye operation should be discarded at the time of the operation and fresh containers supplied postoperatively. A fresh supply should also be provided upon discharge from hospital; in specialist ophthalmology units, it may be acceptable to issue containers that have been dispensed to the patient on the day of discharge.

In *out-patient departments* single-application containers should be used; if multiple-application containers are used, they should be discarded after single patient use within one clinical session.

In *eye surgery* single-application containers should be used if possible; if a multiple-application container is used, it should be discarded after single use. Preparations used during intra-ocular procedures and others that may penetrate into the anterior chamber must be isotonic and without preservatives and buffered if necessary to a neutral pH. Specially formulated fluids should be used for intra-ocular surgery; intravenous infusion preparations are not usually suitable for this purpose (Hartmann's solution may be used in some ocular surgery). For all surgical procedures, a previously unopened container is used for each patient.

Contact lenses

For cosmetic reasons many people prefer to wear contact lenses rather than spectacles; contact lenses are also sometimes required for medical indications. Visual defects are corrected by either rigid ('hard' or gas permeable) lenses or soft (hydrogel or silicone hydrogel—in adults only) lenses; soft lenses are the most popular type, because they are initially the most comfortable, but they may not give the best vision. Lenses should usually be worn for a specified number of hours each day and removed for sleeping. The risk of infectious and non-infectious keratitis is increased by extended continuous contact lens wear, which is not recommended, except when medically indicated.

Contact lenses require meticulous care. Poor compliance with directions for use, and with daily cleaning and disinfection, can result in complications including ulcerative keratitis or conjunctivitis. One-day disposable lenses, which are worn only once and therefore require no disinfection or cleaning, are becoming increasingly popular.

Acanthamoeba keratitis, a painful and sight-threatening condition, is associated with ineffective lens cleaning and disinfection, the use of contaminated lens cases, or tap water coming into contact with the lenses. The condition is especially associated with the use of soft lenses (including frequently replaced lenses) and should be treated by specialists.

Contact lenses and drug treatment

Special care is required in prescribing eye preparations for contact lens users. Some drugs and preservatives in eye preparations can accumulate in hydrogel lenses and may induce toxic and adverse reactions. Therefore, unless medically indicated, the lenses should be removed before instillation of the eye preparation and not worn during the period of treatment. Alternatively, unpreserved drops can be used. Eye drops may, however, be instilled while patients are wearing rigid corneal contact lenses. Ointment preparations should never be used in conjunction with contact lens wear; oily eye drops should also be avoided.

Many drugs given systemically can also have adverse effects on contact lens wear. These include oral contraceptives (particularly those with a higher oestrogen content), drugs which reduce blink rate (e.g. anxiolytics, hypnotics, antihistamines, and muscle relaxants), drugs which reduce lacrimation (e.g. antihistamines, antimuscarinics, phenothiazines and related drugs, some beta-blockers, diuretics, and tricyclic antidepressants), and drugs which increase lacrimation (including ephedrine hydrochloride p. 130 and hydralazine hydrochloride p. 123). Other drugs that may affect contact lens wear are isotretinoin p. 809 (can cause conjunctival inflammation), aspirin p. 98 (salicylic acid appears in tears and can be absorbed by contact lenses—leading to irritation), and rifampicin p. 396 and sulfasalazine p. 36 (can discolour lenses).

1 Allergic and inflammatory eye conditions

Eye, allergy and inflammation

Corticosteroids

Corticosteroids administered locally to the eye or given by mouth are effective for treating anterior segment inflammation, including that which results from surgery.

Topical corticosteroids should normally only be used under expert supervision; three main dangers are associated with their use:

- a 'red eye', when the diagnosis is unconfirmed, may be due to herpes simplex virus, and a corticosteroid may aggravate the condition, leading to corneal ulceration, with possible damage to vision and even loss of the eye. Bacterial, fungal, and amoebic infections pose a similar hazard;
- 'steroid glaucoma' can follow the use of corticosteroid eye preparations in susceptible individuals;
- a 'steroid cataract' can follow prolonged use.

Products combining a corticosteroid with an antimicrobial are used after ocular surgery to reduce inflammation and prevent infection: use of combination products is otherwise rarely justified.

Systemic corticosteroids may be useful for ocular conditions. The risk of producing a 'steroid cataract' increases with the dose and duration of corticosteroid use.

Eye care, other anti-inflammatory preparations

Eye drops containing **antihistamines**, such as antazoline with xylometazoline below as *Otrivine-Antistin®*), azelastine hydrochloride p. 719, epinastine hydrochloride p. 719, ketotifen p. 719, and olopatadine p. 719, can be used for allergic conjunctivitis.

Sodium cromoglicate p. 720 and nedocromil sodium eye drops p. 720 may be useful for vernal keratoconjunctivitis and other allergic forms of conjunctivitis.

Lodoxamide eye drops p. 719 are used for allergic conjunctival conditions including seasonal allergic conjunctivitis.

1.1 Allergic conjunctivitis

ANTIHISTAMINES

Antazoline with xylometazoline 06-Apr-2020

- **INDICATIONS AND DOSE**

Allergic conjunctivitis

▶ TO THE EYE

▸ Child 12–17 years: Apply 2–3 times a day for maximum 7 days

- **CAUTIONS** Angle-closure glaucoma · cardiovascular disease · diabetes mellitus · hypertension · hyperthyroidism · phaeochromocytoma · urinary retention
- **INTERACTIONS** → Appendix 1: antihistamines, sedating · sympathomimetics, vasoconstrictor

- **SIDE-EFFECTS** Drowsiness · eye irritation · headache · hyperhidrosis · hypertension · mydriasis · nausea · palpitations · vascular disorders · vision blurred

  SIDE-EFFECTS, FURTHER INFORMATION Absorption of antazoline and xylometazoline may result in systemic side-effects.

- **MEDICINAL FORMS** There can be variation in the licensing of different medicines containing the same drug.

Eye drops

EXCIPIENTS: May contain Benzalkonium chloride, disodium edetate

- Otrivine Antistin (Thea Pharmaceuticals Ltd)

  Xylometazoline hydrochloride 500 microgram per 1 ml, Antazoline sulfate 5 mg per 1 ml Otrivine Antistin 0.5%/0.05% eye drops | 10 ml P £3.35 DT = £3.35

Azelastine hydrochloride 11-May-2020

- **INDICATIONS AND DOSE**

Seasonal allergic conjunctivitis

▶ TO THE EYE

- Child 4–17 years: Apply twice daily, increased if necessary to 4 times a day

Perennial conjunctivitis

▶ TO THE EYE

- Child 12–17 years: Apply twice daily; increased if necessary to 4 times a day, maximum duration of treatment 6 weeks

- **INTERACTIONS** → Appendix 1: antihistamines, non-sedating
- **SIDE-EFFECTS**
  - **Common or very common** Eye irritation · taste bitter (if applied incorrectly)
- **MEDICINAL FORMS** There can be variation in the licensing of different medicines containing the same drug.

Eye drops

EXCIPIENTS: May contain Benzalkonium chloride, disodium edetate

- Optilast (Mylan)

  Azelastine hydrochloride 500 microgram per 1 ml Optilast 0.05% eye drops | 8 ml PoM £6.40 DT = £6.40

Epinastine hydrochloride 26-Mar-2020

- **INDICATIONS AND DOSE**

Seasonal allergic conjunctivitis

▶ TO THE EYE

- Child 12–17 years: Apply twice daily for maximum 8 weeks

- **SIDE-EFFECTS**
  - **Common or very common** Eye discomfort
  - **Uncommon** Dry eye · eye disorders · headache · nasal irritation · rhinitis · taste altered · visual impairment
- **MEDICINAL FORMS** There can be variation in the licensing of different medicines containing the same drug.

Eye drops

EXCIPIENTS: May contain Benzalkonium chloride, disodium edetate

- Relestat (Allergan Ltd)

  Epinastine hydrochloride 500 microgram per 1 ml Relestat 500micrograms/ml eye drops | 5 ml PoM £9.90 DT = £9.90

Ketotifen 13-May-2020

- **INDICATIONS AND DOSE**

Seasonal allergic conjunctivitis

▶ TO THE EYE

- Child 3–17 years: Apply twice daily

- **INTERACTIONS** → Appendix 1: antihistamines, sedating
- **SIDE-EFFECTS**
  - **Common or very common** Eye discomfort · eye disorders · eye inflammation
  - **Uncommon** Conjunctival haemorrhage · drowsiness · dry eye · dry mouth · headache · skin reactions · vision disorders
  - **Frequency not known** Asthma exacerbated · facial swelling · oedema
- **MEDICINAL FORMS** There can be variation in the licensing of different medicines containing the same drug.

Eye drops

EXCIPIENTS: May contain Benzalkonium chloride

- Ketofall (Scope Ophthalmics Ltd)

  Ketotifen (as Ketotifen hydrogen fumarate) 250 microgram per 1 ml Ketofall 0.25mg/ml eye drops 0.4ml unit dose | 30 unit dose PoM £6.95 DT = £6.95

- Zaditen (Thea Pharmaceuticals Ltd)

  Ketotifen (as Ketotifen fumarate) 250 microgram per 1 ml Zaditen 250micrograms/ml eye drops | 5 ml PoM £7.80 DT = £7.80

Olopatadine 25-Mar-2020

- **INDICATIONS AND DOSE**

Seasonal allergic conjunctivitis

▶ TO THE EYE

- Child 3–17 years: Apply twice daily for maximum 4 months

- **SIDE-EFFECTS**
  - **Common or very common** Asthenia · dry eye · eye discomfort · headache · nasal dryness · taste altered
  - **Uncommon** Dizziness · eye disorders · eye inflammation · increased risk of infection · numbness · skin reactions · vision disorders
  - **Frequency not known** Drowsiness · dyspnoea · malaise · nausea · vomiting
- **MEDICINAL FORMS** There can be variation in the licensing of different medicines containing the same drug.

Eye drops

EXCIPIENTS: May contain Benzalkonium chloride

- Olopatadine (Non-proprietary)

  Olopatadine (as Olopatadine hydrochloride) 1 mg per 1 ml Olopatadine 1mg/ml eye drops | 5 ml PoM £6.14 DT = £4.68

- Opatanol (Novartis Pharmaceuticals UK Ltd)

  Olopatadine (as Olopatadine hydrochloride) 1 mg per 1 ml Opatanol 1mg/ml eye drops | 5 ml PoM £4.68 DT = £4.68

MAST-CELL STABILISERS

Lodoxamide 06-Apr-2020

- **INDICATIONS AND DOSE**

Allergic conjunctivitis

▶ TO THE EYE

- Child 4–17 years: Apply 4 times a day, improvement of symptoms may sometimes require treatment for up to 4 weeks

- **SIDE-EFFECTS**
  - **Common or very common** Dry eye · eye discomfort · eye disorders · vision disorders
  - **Uncommon** Corneal deposits · dizziness · eye inflammation · headache · nausea
  - **Rare or very rare** Nasal complaints · rash · taste altered
- **EXCEPTIONS TO LEGAL CATEGORY** Lodoxamide 0.1% eye drops can be sold to the public for treatment of allergic conjunctivitis in adults and children over 4 years.

- **MEDICINAL FORMS** There can be variation in the licensing of different medicines containing the same drug.

Eye drops

EXCIPIENTS: May contain Benzalkonium chloride, disodium edetate

- Alomide (Novartis Pharmaceuticals UK Ltd)
  Lodoxamide (as Lodoxamide trometamol) 1 mg per 1 ml Alomide 0.1% eye drops | 10 ml PoM £5.21 DT = £5.21

Nedocromil sodium

25-Jul-2018

- **INDICATIONS AND DOSE**

Seasonal and perennial conjunctivitis

- TO THE EYE
- Child 6–17 years: Apply twice daily, increased if necessary to 4 times a day, max.12 weeks duration of treatment for seasonal allergic conjunctivitis

Seasonal keratoconjunctivitis

- TO THE EYE
- Child 6–17 years: Apply 4 times a day

- **SIDE-EFFECTS**
- **Common or very common** Eye discomfort · eye strain · taste altered

- **MEDICINAL FORMS** No licensed medicines listed.

Sodium cromoglicate

21-May-2020

(Sodium cromoglycate)

- **INDICATIONS AND DOSE**

Allergic conjunctivitis | Seasonal keratoconjunctivitis

- TO THE EYE
- Child: Apply 4 times a day

- **SIDE-EFFECTS** Eye stinging
- **EXCEPTIONS TO LEGAL CATEGORY** Sodium cromoglicate 2% eye drops can be sold to the public (in max. pack size of 10 mL) for treatment of acute seasonal and perennial allergic conjunctivitis.

- **MEDICINAL FORMS** There can be variation in the licensing of different medicines containing the same drug. Forms available from special-order manufacturers include: eye drops

Eye drops

- Sodium cromoglicate (Non-proprietary)
  Sodium cromoglicate 20 mg per 1 ml Sodium cromoglicate 2% eye drops | 13.5 ml PoM £13.13 DT = £11.46
- Opticrom (Sanofi)
  Sodium cromoglicate 20 mg per 1 ml Opticrom Aqueous 2% eye drops | 13.5 ml PoM £8.03 DT = £11.46

1.2 Inflammatory eye conditions

Other drugs used for Inflammatory eye conditions

Adalimumab, p. 693 · Fluocinolone acetonide, p. 789 · Hydrocortisone, p. 476

CORTICOSTEROIDS

Betamethasone

F 472

28-Nov-2019

- **DRUG ACTION** Betamethasone has very high glucocorticoid activity and insignificant mineralocorticoid activity.

- **INDICATIONS AND DOSE**

Local treatment of inflammation (short-term)

- TO THE EYE USING EYE DROP
- Child: Apply every 1–2 hours until controlled then reduce frequency
- TO THE EYE USING EYE OINTMENT
- Child: Apply 2–4 times a day, alternatively apply at night when used in combination with eye drops

- **INTERACTIONS** → Appendix 1: corticosteroids
- **SIDE-EFFECTS** Vision disorders

- **MEDICINAL FORMS** There can be variation in the licensing of different medicines containing the same drug.

Ear/eye/nose drops solution

EXCIPIENTS: May contain Benzalkonium chloride, disodium edetate

- Betnesol (RPH Pharmaceuticals AB)
  Betamethasone sodium phosphate 1 mg per 1 ml Betnesol 0.1% eye/ear/nose drops | 10 ml PoM £2.32 DT = £2.32
- Vistamethasone (Martindale Pharmaceuticals Ltd)
  Betamethasone sodium phosphate 1 mg per 1 ml Vistamethasone 0.1% ear/eye/nose drops | 5 ml PoM £1.02 | 10 ml PoM £1.16 DT = £2.32

Combinations available: *Betamethasone with neomycin*, p. 721

Dexamethasone

F 472

10-Mar-2020

- **DRUG ACTION** Dexamethasone has very high glucocorticoid activity and insignificant mineralocorticoid activity.

- **INDICATIONS AND DOSE**

Local treatment of inflammation (short-term)

- TO THE EYE USING EYE DROP
- Child: Apply 4–6 times a day

Short term local treatment of inflammation (severe conditions)

- TO THE EYE USING EYE DROP
- Child: Apply every 30–60 minutes until controlled, reduce frequency when control achieved

- **UNLICENSED USE** *Maxidex*® not licensed for use in children under 2 years. *Dropodex*® not licensed for use in children.
- **INTERACTIONS** → Appendix 1: corticosteroids
- **SIDE-EFFECTS**
- **Common or very common** Eye discomfort
- **Uncommon** Photophobia · taste altered
- **PREGNANCY** Dexamethasone readily crosses the placenta.
- **PRESCRIBING AND DISPENSING INFORMATION** Although multi-dose dexamethasone eye drops commonly contain preservatives, preservative-free unit dose vials may be available.

- **MEDICINAL FORMS** There can be variation in the licensing of different medicines containing the same drug. Forms available from special-order manufacturers include:eye drops

Eye drops

EXCIPIENTS: May contain Benzalkonium chloride, disodium edetate, polysorbates

- Dexamethasone (Bausch & Lomb UK Ltd)
  Dexamethasone sodium phosphate 1 mg per 1 ml Minims dexamethasone 0.1% eye drops 0.5ml unit dose | 20 unit dose PoM £11.46 DT = £11.46

▸ Dexafree (Thea Pharmaceuticals Ltd)
Dexamethasone sodium phosphate 1 mg per 1 ml Dexafree 1mg/1ml eye drops 0.4ml unit dose | 30 unit dose PoM £9.70

▸ Dropodex (Rayner Pharmaceuticals Ltd)
Dexamethasone sodium phosphate 1 mg per 1 ml Dropodex 0.1% eye drops 0.4ml unit dose | 20 unit dose PoM £10.48 DT = £10.48

▸ Eythalm (Aspire Pharma Ltd)
Dexamethasone 1 mg per 1 ml Eythalm 1mg/ml eye drops | 6 ml PoM £9.75 DT = £9.75

▸ Maxidex (Novartis Pharmaceuticals UK Ltd)
Dexamethasone 1 mg per 1 ml Maxidex 0.1% eye drops | 5 ml PoM £1.42 DT = £1.42 | 10 ml PoM £2.80 DT = £2.80

Combinations available: *Dexamethasone with framycetin sulfate and gramicidin,* below · ***Dexamethasone with hypromellose, neomycin and polymyxin B sulfate,*** p. 722

Fluorometholone

21-Dec-2017

● **INDICATIONS AND DOSE**

Local treatment of inflammation (short term)

▸ TO THE EYE

▸ Child 2–17 years: Apply every 1 hour for 24–48 hours, then reduced to 2–4 times a day

IMPORTANT SAFETY INFORMATION

MHRA/CHM ADVICE: CORTICOSTEROIDS: RARE RISK OF CENTRAL SEROUS CHORIORETINOPATHY WITH LOCAL AS WELL AS SYSTEMIC ADMINISTRATION (AUGUST 2017)

See Corticosteroids, general use p. 470.

● **SIDE-EFFECTS** Cataract · eye discomfort · eye disorders · eye infection · eye inflammation · rash · taste altered · vision disorders

● **MEDICINAL FORMS** There can be variation in the licensing of different medicines containing the same drug.

Eye drops

EXCIPIENTS: May contain Benzalkonium chloride, disodium edetate, polysorbates

▸ FML Liquifilm (Allergan Ltd)
Fluorometholone 1 mg per 1 ml FML Liquifilm 0.1% ophthalmic suspension | 5 ml PoM £1.71 DT = £1.71 | 10 ml PoM £2.95 DT = £2.95

F 472

Prednisolone

29-Nov-2019

● **DRUG ACTION** Prednisolone exerts predominantly glucocorticoid effects with minimal mineralocorticoid effects.

● **INDICATIONS AND DOSE**

Local treatment of inflammation (short-term)

▸ TO THE EYE

▸ Child: Apply every 1–2 hours until controlled then reduce frequency

● **UNLICENSED USE** *Pred Forte®* not licensed for use in children (age range not specified by manufacturer).

● **INTERACTIONS** → Appendix 1: corticosteroids

● **SIDE-EFFECTS** Eye discomfort · taste altered · visual impairment

● **PRESCRIBING AND DISPENSING INFORMATION** Although multi-dose prednisolone eye drops commonly contain preservatives, preservative-free unit dose vials may be available.

● **MEDICINAL FORMS** There can be variation in the licensing of different medicines containing the same drug. Forms available from special-order manufacturers include: eye drops

Eye drops

EXCIPIENTS: May contain Benzalkonium chloride, disodium edetate, polysorbates

▸ Prednisolone (Bausch & Lomb UK Ltd)
Prednisolone sodium phosphate 5 mg per 1 ml Minims prednisolone sodium phosphate 0.5% eye drops 0.5ml unit dose | 20 unit dose PoM £12.25 DT = £12.25

▸ Pred Forte (Allergan Ltd)
Prednisolone acetate 10 mg per 1 ml Pred Forte 1% eye drops | 5 ml PoM £1.82 DT = £1.82 | 10 ml PoM £3.66 DT = £3.66

Ear/eye drops solution

EXCIPIENTS: May contain Benzalkonium chloride, disodium edetate

▸ Prednisolone (Non-proprietary)
Prednisolone sodium phosphate 5 mg per 1 ml Prednisolone sodium phosphate 0.5% ear/eye drops | 10 ml PoM £2.57 DT = £2.57

CORTICOSTEROIDS > CORTICOSTEROID COMBINATIONS WITH ANTI-INFECTIVES

Betamethasone with neomycin

The properties listed below are those particular to the combination only. For the properties of the components please consider, betamethasone p. 720, neomycin sulfate p. 774.

● **INDICATIONS AND DOSE**

Local treatment of eye inflammation and bacterial infection (short-term)

▸ TO THE EYE USING EYE DROP

▸ Child: (consult product literature)

● **INTERACTIONS** → Appendix 1: corticosteroids · neomycin

● **LESS SUITABLE FOR PRESCRIBING** Betamethasone with neomycin eye-drops are less suitable for prescribing.

● **MEDICINAL FORMS** There can be variation in the licensing of different medicines containing the same drug.

Ear/eye/nose drops solution

EXCIPIENTS: May contain Benzalkonium chloride, disodium edetate

▸ Betnesol-N (RPH Pharmaceuticals AB)
Betamethasone (as Betamethasone sodium phosphate) 1 mg per 1 ml, Neomycin sulfate 5 mg per 1 ml Betnesol-N ear/eye/nose drops | 10 ml PoM £2.39 DT = £2.39

Dexamethasone with framycetin sulfate and gramicidin

21-Dec-2017

The properties listed below are those particular to the combination only. For the properties of the components please consider, dexamethasone p. 720, framycetin sulfate p. 742.

● **INDICATIONS AND DOSE**

Local treatment of inflammation (short-term)

▸ TO THE EYE

▸ Child: Apply 4–6 times a day, may be administered every 30–60 minutes in severe conditions until controlled, then reduce frequency

● **CAUTIONS** Avoid prolonged use

● **INTERACTIONS** → Appendix 1: corticosteroids

● **LESS SUITABLE FOR PRESCRIBING** *Sofradex®* is less suitable for prescribing.

● **MEDICINAL FORMS** There can be variation in the licensing of different medicines containing the same drug.

Ear/eye drops solution

EXCIPIENTS: May contain Polysorbates

▸ Sofradex (Sanofi)
Gramicidin 50 microgram per 1 ml, Dexamethasone (as Dexamethasone sodium metasulfobenzoate) 500 microgram per 1 ml, Framycetin sulfate 5 mg per 1 ml Sofradex ear/eye drops | 8 ml PoM £7.50

Dexamethasone with hypromellose, neomycin and polymyxin B sulfate

The properties listed below are those particular to the combination only. For the properties of the components please consider, dexamethasone p. 720, neomycin sulfate p. 774.

- **INDICATIONS AND DOSE**

Local treatment of inflammation (short-term)

▶ TO THE EYE USING EYE DROP
- Child: Apply every 30–60 minutes until controlled, then reduced to 4–6 times a day

Local treatment of inflammation (short-term)

▶ TO THE EYE USING EYE OINTMENT
- Child: Apply 3–4 times a day, alternatively, apply at night when used with eye drops

- **INTERACTIONS** → Appendix 1: corticosteroids · neomycin
- **LESS SUITABLE FOR PRESCRIBING** Dexamethasone with neomycin and polymixin B sulfate is less suitable for prescribing.

- **MEDICINAL FORMS** There can be variation in the licensing of different medicines containing the same drug.

Eye ointment

EXCIPIENTS: May contain Hydroxybenzoates (parabens), woolfat and related substances (including lanolin)

▶ Maxitrol (Novartis Pharmaceuticals UK Ltd)
Dexamethasone 1 mg per 1 gram, Neomycin (as Neomycin sulfate) 3500 unit per 1 gram, Polymyxin B sulfate 6000 unit per 1 gram Maxitrol eye ointment | 3.5 gram [PoM] £1.44

Eye drops

EXCIPIENTS: May contain Benzalkonium chloride, polysorbates

▶ Maxitrol (Novartis Pharmaceuticals UK Ltd)
Dexamethasone 1 mg per 1 ml, Hypromellose 5 mg per 1 ml, Neomycin (as Neomycin sulfate) 3500 unit per 1 ml, Polymyxin B sulfate 6000 unit per 1 ml Maxitrol eye drops | 5 ml [PoM] £1.68

IMMUNOSUPPRESSANTS › CALCINEURIN INHIBITORS AND RELATED DRUGS

Ciclosporin

26-Nov-2019

(Cyclosporin)

- **DRUG ACTION** Ciclosporin inhibits production and release of lymphokines, thereby suppressing cell-mediated immune response.

- **INDICATIONS AND DOSE**

VERKAZIA ®

Severe vernal keratoconjunctivitis (initiated by a specialist)

▶ TO THE EYE
- Child 4-17 years: Apply 1 drop 4 times a day, to be applied to the affected eye(s) during the vernal keratoconjunctivitis season, if signs and symptoms persist after the end of the season, treatment may be continued at the recommended dose or decreased to 1 drop twice daily once adequate control is achieved. Once resolved, treatment should be discontinued, and re-initiated upon recurrence

- **CONTRA-INDICATIONS** Active or suspected ocular or peri-ocular infection · Ocular or peri-ocular malignancies or premalignant conditions
- **CAUTIONS** History of ocular herpes—no information available
- **INTERACTIONS** → Appendix 1: ciclosporin
- **SIDE-EFFECTS**
  ▶ **Common or very common** Cough · eye discomfort · eye disorders · eye inflammation · headache · increased risk of infection · vision blurred
- **PREGNANCY** Manufacturer advises avoid unless potential benefit outweighs risk—no information available.
- **BREAST FEEDING** Manufacturer advises avoid—limited information.
- **MONITORING REQUIREMENTS** Manufacturer advises regular eye examinations when used for more than 12 months (efficacy and safety have not been studied beyond 12 months).
- **DIRECTIONS FOR ADMINISTRATION** Manufacturer advises keep eyes closed for 2 minutes after using eye drops to increase local drug action and reduce systemic absorption.
- **PATIENT AND CARER ADVICE**

Driving and skilled tasks Manufacturer advises patients and carers should be counselled on the effects on driving and performance of skilled tasks—increased risk of blurred vision.

- **NATIONAL FUNDING/ACCESS DECISIONS**

Scottish Medicines Consortium (SMC) decisions

SMC No. SMC2111

The *Scottish Medicines Consortium* has advised (December 2018) that ciclosporin 1 mg/mL (0.1%) eye drops emulsion (*Verkazia*®) is accepted for use within NHS Scotland for the treatment of severe vernal keratoconjunctivitis in patients from 4 to 17 years of age.

All Wales Medicines Strategy Group (AWMSG) decisions

AWMSG No. 2908

The *All Wales Medicines Strategy Group* has advised (March 2019) that ciclosporin (*Verkazia*®) is recommended as an option for use within NHS Wales for the treatment of severe vernal keratoconjunctivitis in patients from 4 years of age up to 18 years of age.

- **MEDICINAL FORMS** There can be variation in the licensing of different medicines containing the same drug.

Eye drops

▶ Verkazia (Santen UK Ltd)
Ciclosporin 1 mg per 1 ml Verkazia 0.1% eye drops 0.3ml unit dose | 120 unit dose [PoM] £288.00

1.2a Anterior uveitis

ANTIMUSCARINICS

Antimuscarinics (eye)

- **CAUTIONS** Children under 3 months owing to the possible association between cycloplegia and the development of amblyopia · darkly pigmented iris is more resistant to pupillary dilatation and caution should be exercised to avoid overdosage · mydriasis can precipitate acute angle-closure glaucoma (usually in those who are predisposed to the condition because of a shallow anterior chamber) · neonates at increased risk of systemic toxicity
- **SIDE-EFFECTS** Dizziness · photophobia · skin reactions · tachycardia
- **PATIENT AND CARER ADVICE** Patients may not be able to undertake skilled tasks until vision clears after mydriasis.

722

Atropine sulfate

05-Dec-2019

● **INDICATIONS AND DOSE**

Cycloplegia

▶ TO THE EYE USING EYE DROP

▸ Child 3 months–17 years: Apply twice daily for 3 days, before procedure

Anterior uveitis

▶ TO THE EYE USING EYE DROP

▸ Child 2–17 years: Apply 1 drop up to 4 times a day

● **UNLICENSED USE** Not licensed for use in children for uveitis.

● **INTERACTIONS** → Appendix 1: atropine

● **SIDE-EFFECTS**

SIDE-EFFECTS, FURTHER INFORMATION Systemic side-effects can occur.

● **PRESCRIBING AND DISPENSING INFORMATION** Although multi-dose atropine sulphate eye drops commonly contain preservatives, preservative-free unit dose vials may be available.

● **MEDICINAL FORMS** There can be variation in the licensing of different medicines containing the same drug. Forms available from special-order manufacturers include: eye drops, eye ointment

Eye drops

▸ Atropine sulfate (Non-proprietary)

Atropine sulfate 10 mg per 1 ml Atropine 1% eye drops | 10 ml PoM £131.89 DT = £131.89

▸ Atropine sulfate (Bausch & Lomb UK Ltd)

Atropine sulfate 10 mg per 1 ml Minims atropine sulfate 1% eye drops 0.5ml unit dose | 20 unit dose PoM £15.10 DT = £15.10

722

Cyclopentolate hydrochloride

● **INDICATIONS AND DOSE**

Cycloplegia

▶ TO THE EYE

▸ Child 3 months–11 years: Apply 1 drop, 30–60 minutes before examination, using 1% eye drops

▸ Child 12–17 years: Apply 1 drop, 30–60 minutes before examination, using 0.5% eye drops

Uveitis

▶ TO THE EYE

▸ Child 3 months–17 years: Apply 1 drop 2–4 times a day, using 0.5% eye drops (1% for deeply pigmented eyes)

● **INTERACTIONS** → Appendix 1: cyclopentolate

● **SIDE-EFFECTS** Abdominal distension · arrhythmias · behaviour abnormal · cardio-respiratory distress · conjunctivitis (on prolonged administration) · constipation · dry mouth · eye oedema (on prolonged administration) · flushing · gastrointestinal disorders · hyperaemia (on prolonged administration) · mydriasis · palpitations · psychotic disorder · staggering · urinary disorders · vomiting

SIDE-EFFECTS, FURTHER INFORMATION Systemic side-effects can occur.

● **PRESCRIBING AND DISPENSING INFORMATION** Although multi-dose cyclopentolate eye drops commonly contain preservatives, preservative-free unit dose vials may be available.

● **MEDICINAL FORMS** There can be variation in the licensing of different medicines containing the same drug.

Eye drops

EXCIPIENTS: May contain Benzalkonium chloride

▸ Cyclopentolate hydrochloride (Bausch & Lomb UK Ltd)

Cyclopentolate hydrochloride 5 mg per 1 ml Minims cyclopentolate hydrochloride 0.5% eye drops 0.5ml unit dose | 20 unit dose PoM £11.41 DT = £11.41

Cyclopentolate hydrochloride 10 mg per 1 ml Minims cyclopentolate hydrochloride 1% eye drops 0.5ml unit dose | 20 unit dose PoM £11.68 DT = £11.68

▸ Mydrilate (Intrapharm Laboratories Ltd)

Cyclopentolate hydrochloride 5 mg per 1 ml Mydrilate 0.5% solution | 5 ml PoM £8.08 DT = £8.08

Cyclopentolate hydrochloride 10 mg per 1 ml Mydrilate 1% solution | 5 ml PoM £8.08 DT = £8.08

722

Homatropine hydrobromide

● **INDICATIONS AND DOSE**

Anterior uveitis

▶ TO THE EYE

▸ Child 3 months–1 year: Apply 1 drop daily, alternatively apply 1 drop once daily on alternate days, adjusted according to response, only 0.5% eye drops to be used

▸ Child 2–17 years: Apply 1 drop twice daily, adjusted according to response

● **INTERACTIONS** → Appendix 1: homatropine

● **MEDICINAL FORMS** Forms available from special-order manufacturers include: eye drops

2 Dry eye conditions

Dry eye

08-Feb-2020

Description of condition

Dry eye presents as chronic soreness and inflammation of ocular surface associated with reduced or abnormal tear secretion (e.g. in Sjögren's syndrome). It often responds to tear replacement therapy in the form of eye drops (preferably preservative-free), eye ointment (used at night), or gels. Choice of preparation is based on the type of dry eye (e.g. aqueous-deficient or evaporative), symptoms, and patient preference.

Drug treatment

EvGr Young children presenting with symptoms of dry eye should be referred to an optometrist for specialist assessment. Urgent referral to an ophthalmologist is required for children with any corneal change (e.g. staining or vascularisation).

Hypromellose p. 725 is the most frequently used treatment for tear deficiency in patients with mild dry eye. Ⓐ Initially, it may need to be instilled frequently (e.g. hourly) for adequate symptom relief, then at a reduced frequency. EvGr Carbomers p. 724 and polyvinyl alcohol p. 725 are suitable alternatives. Ⓐ The ability of carbomers p. 724 and polyvinyl alcohol to cling to the eye surface and their higher viscosity may help reduce frequency of application to 4 times daily. Carbomers p. 724 can be less tolerated than hypromellose due to their impact on vision. EvGr Preservative-free tear replacement is preferred in cases of frequent and chronic application.

Ocular lubricants containing sodium hyaluronate p. 726, hydroxypropyl guar, or carmellose sodium p. 724 can be used for moderate to severe dry eye following a suitable trial (6–8 weeks) of treatment options for mild dry eye.

Eye ointments containing a paraffin (e.g. liquid paraffin with white soft paraffin and wool alcohols p. 725) can be used in addition to other options to lubricate the eye surface, especially in cases of recurrent corneal epithelial erosion. They may cause temporary visual disturbance and are best suited for application before sleep. Ointments should not be used during contact lens wear. (A)

OCULAR LUBRICANTS

Acetylcysteine

07-Feb-2017

● **INDICATIONS AND DOSE**

Tear deficiency | Impaired or abnormal mucus production

▶ TO THE EYE

▸ Child: Apply 3–4 times a day

● **SIDE-EFFECTS** Eye discomfort · eye redness

● **MEDICINAL FORMS** There can be variation in the licensing of different medicines containing the same drug. Forms available from special-order manufacturers include: eye drops

Eye drops

EXCIPIENTS: May contain Benzalkonium chloride, disodium edetate

▸ **Ilube** (Rayner Pharmaceuticals Ltd)
Acetylcysteine 50 mg per 1 ml Ilube 5% eye drops | 10 ml [PoM] £33.46 DT = £33.46

Carbomers

27-Mar-2020

(Polyacrylic acid)

● **INDICATIONS AND DOSE**

Dry eyes including keratoconjunctivitis sicca, unstable tear film

▶ TO THE EYE

▸ Child: Apply 3–4 times a day or when required

● **PRESCRIBING AND DISPENSING INFORMATION** Synthetic high molecular weight polymers of acrylic acid cross-linked with either allyl ethers of sucrose or allyl ethers of pentaerithrityl.

● **MEDICINAL FORMS** There can be variation in the licensing of different medicines containing the same drug.

Eye gel

EXCIPIENTS: May contain Benzalkonium chloride, cetrimide, disodium edetate

▸ **Blephagel** (Thea Pharmaceuticals Ltd)
Carbomer 3.6 mg per 1 gram Blephagel 0.36% eye gel preservative free | 30 gram £7.53

▸ **Liquivisc** (Thea Pharmaceuticals Ltd)
Carbomer 974P 2.5 mg per 1 gram Liquivisc 0.25% eye gel | 10 gram [P] £4.50 DT = £4.50

Eye drops

▸ **GelTears** (Bausch & Lomb UK Ltd)
Carbomer 980 2 mg per 1 gram GelTears 0.2% gel | 10 gram [P] £2.80 DT = £2.80

▸ **Viscotears** (Bausch & Lomb UK Ltd)
Carbomer 980 2 mg per 1 gram Viscotears 2mg/g liquid gel | 10 gram [P] £1.59 DT = £2.80
Viscotears 2mg/g eye gel 0.6ml unit dose | 30 unit dose [P] £5.42 DT = £5.42

Carmellose sodium

23-Mar-2020

● **INDICATIONS AND DOSE**

Dry eye conditions

▶ TO THE EYE

▸ Child: Apply as required

● **PRESCRIBING AND DISPENSING INFORMATION** Some preparations are contained units which are resealable and may be used for up to 12 hours.

● **MEDICINAL FORMS** There can be variation in the licensing of different medicines containing the same drug.

Eye drops

▸ **Carmellose sodium (Non-proprietary)**
Carmellose 0.5% eye drops | 10 ml £7.49
Carmellose 1% eye drops 0.4ml unit dose preservative free | 30 unit dose £3.00 DT = £3.00

▸ **Carmellose** (Aspire Pharma Ltd, Medicom Healthcare Ltd)
PF Drops Carmellose 0.5% eye drops preservative free | 10 ml £7.49
PF Drops Carmellose 1% eye drops preservative free | 10 ml £7.49

▸ **Carmize** (Aspire Pharma Ltd)
Carmize 1% eye drops | 10 ml £8.49
Carmize 0.5% eye drops | 10 ml £7.49

▸ **Cellusan** (Farmigea S.p.A.)
Cellusan 1% eye drops preservative free | 10 ml £4.80
Cellusan Light 0.5% eye drops preservative free | 10 ml £4.80

▸ **Celluvisc** (Allergan Ltd)
Celluvisc 1% eye drops 0.4ml unit dose | 30 unit dose [P] £3.00 DT = £3.00 | 60 unit dose [P] £10.99
Celluvisc 0.5% eye drops 0.4ml unit dose | 30 unit dose [P] £4.80 DT = £4.80 | 90 unit dose [P] £15.53

▸ **Ocu-Lube Carmellose** (Sai-Meds Ltd)
Ocu-Lube Carmellose 0.5% eye drops preservative free | 10 ml £7.49
Ocu-Lube Carmellose 1% eye drops preservative free | 10 ml £7.49

▸ **Optho-Lique** (Essential-Healthcare Ltd)
Optho-Lique 0.5% eye drops | 10 ml £3.73
Optho-Lique Forte 1% eye drops | 10 ml £3.97

▸ **Optive** (Allergan Ltd)
Optive 0.5% eye drops | 10 ml £7.49

▸ **Optive Plus** (Allergan Ltd)
Optive Plus 0.5% eye drops | 10 ml £7.49

▸ **Tearvis** (Sai-Meds Ltd)
Tearvis 1% eye drops | 10 ml £8.49
Tearvis 0.5% eye drops | 10 ml £7.49

Hydroxyethylcellulose

23-Mar-2020

● **INDICATIONS AND DOSE**

Tear deficiency

▶ TO THE EYE

▸ Child: Apply as required

● **PRESCRIBING AND DISPENSING INFORMATION** Although multi-dose hydroxyethylcellulose eye drops commonly contain preservatives, preservative-free unit dose vials may be available.

● **MEDICINAL FORMS** There can be variation in the licensing of different medicines containing the same drug.

Eye drops

▸ **Artificial tears** (Bausch & Lomb UK Ltd)
Hydroxyethylcellulose 4.4 mg per 1 ml Minims artificial tears 0.44% eye drops 0.5ml unit dose | 20 unit dose [P] £9.33 DT = £9.33

Hydroxypropyl guar with polyethylene glycol and propylene glycol

(Formulated as an ocular lubricant)

● **INDICATIONS AND DOSE**

Dry eye conditions

▶ TO THE EYE

▸ Child: Apply as required

● **MEDICINAL FORMS** No licensed medicines listed.

Hypromellose 23-Mar-2020

● **INDICATIONS AND DOSE**

Tear deficiency

▶ TO THE EYE

▸ Child: Apply as required

● **PRESCRIBING AND DISPENSING INFORMATION** Although multi-dose hypromellose eye drops commonly contain preservatives, preservative-free unit dose vials may be available.

● **MEDICINAL FORMS** There can be variation in the licensing of different medicines containing the same drug. Forms available from special-order manufacturers include: eye drops

Eye drops

EXCIPIENTS: May contain Benzalkonium chloride, cetrimide, disodium edetate

▸ Hypromellose (Non-proprietary)
Hypromellose 3 mg per 1 ml Hypromellose 0.3% eye drops | 10 ml £0.99 DT = £0.90 | 10 ml [P] £1.31 DT = £0.90

▸ Artelac (Bausch & Lomb UK Ltd)
Hypromellose 3.2 mg per 1 ml Artelac Single Dose Unit 0.32% eye drops 0.5ml unit dose | 30 unit dose [P] £16.95 DT = £16.95
Artelac 0.32% eye drops | 10 ml [P] £4.99 DT = £4.99

▸ Hydromoor (Rayner Pharmaceuticals Ltd)
Hydromoor 0.3% eye drops 0.4ml unit dose preservative free | 30 unit dose £5.75

▸ Isopto Plain (Alcon Eye Care Ltd)
Hypromellose 5 mg per 1 ml Isopto Plain 0.5% eye drops | 10 ml [P] £0.81 DT = £0.81

▸ Tear-Lac (Scope Ophthalmics Ltd)
Hypromellose 3 mg per 1 ml Tear-Lac Hypromellose 0.3% eye drops preservative free | 10 ml £5.80

Hypromellose with dextran 70 07-Apr-2020

The properties listed below are those particular to the combination only. For the properties of the components please consider, hypromellose above.

● **INDICATIONS AND DOSE**

Tear deficiency

▶ TO THE EYE

▸ Child: Apply as required

● **MEDICINAL FORMS** There can be variation in the licensing of different medicines containing the same drug.

Eye drops

EXCIPIENTS: May contain Benzalkonium chloride, disodium edetate

▸ Tears Naturale (Alcon Eye Care Ltd)
Dextran 70 1 mg per 1 ml, Hypromellose 3 mg per 1 ml Tears Naturale eye drops | 15 ml [P] £1.89 DT = £1.89
Tears Naturale eye drops 0.4ml unit dose | 28 unit dose [P] £13.26 DT = £13.26

Liquid paraffin with white soft paraffin and wool alcohols 18-May-2020

● **INDICATIONS AND DOSE**

Dry eye conditions

▶ TO THE EYE

▸ Child: Apply as required, best suited for application before sleep

● **PATIENT AND CARER ADVICE** May cause temporary visual disturbance. Should not be used during contact lens wear.

● **MEDICINAL FORMS** There can be variation in the licensing of different medicines containing the same drug.

Eye ointment

▸ Liquid paraffin with white soft paraffin and wool alcohols (Non-proprietary)
Xailin Night eye ointment preservative free | 5 gram £2.56

▸ Lacri-Lube (Allergan Ltd)
Wool alcohols 2 mg per 1 gram, Liquid paraffin 425 mg per 1 gram, White soft paraffin 573 mg per 1 gram Lacri-lube eye ointment | 3.5 gram [P] £3.01 | 5 gram [P] £3.98

Paraffin, yellow, soft 16-Apr-2020

● **INDICATIONS AND DOSE**

Eye surface lubrication

▶ TO THE EYE

▸ Child: Apply as required

● **PATIENT AND CARER ADVICE** Ophthalmic preparations may cause temporary visual disturbance. Should not be used during contact lens wear.

● **MEDICINAL FORMS** There can be variation in the licensing of different medicines containing the same drug.

Eye ointment

▸ Paraffin, yellow, soft (Non-proprietary)
Liquid paraffin 100 mg per 1 gram, Wool fat 100 mg per 1 gram, Yellow soft paraffin 800 mg per 1 gram Simple eye ointment | 4 gram [P] £41.49 DT = £37.62

Polyvinyl alcohol 17-Apr-2020

● **INDICATIONS AND DOSE**

Tear deficiency

▶ TO THE EYE

▸ Child: Apply as required

● **PRESCRIBING AND DISPENSING INFORMATION** Although multi-dose polyvinyl alcohol eye drops commonly contain preservatives, preservative-free unit dose vials may be available.

● **MEDICINAL FORMS** There can be variation in the licensing of different medicines containing the same drug. Forms available from special-order manufacturers include: eye drops

Eye drops

EXCIPIENTS: May contain Benzalkonium chloride, disodium edetate

▸ Liquifilm Tears (Allergan Ltd)
Polyvinyl alcohol 14 mg per 1 ml Liquifilm Tears 1.4% eye drops | 15 ml £1.93
Liquifilm Tears 1.4% eye drops 0.4ml unit dose preservative free | 30 unit dose £5.35

▸ Refresh Ophthalmic (Allergan Ltd)
Polyvinyl alcohol 14 mg per 1 ml Refresh Ophthalmic 1.4% eye drops 0.4ml unit dose | 30 unit dose £2.25

▸ Sno Tears (Bausch & Lomb UK Ltd)
Polyvinyl alcohol 14 mg per 1 ml Sno Tears 1.4% eye drops | 10 ml £1.06

Retinol palmitate with white soft paraffin, light liquid paraffin, liquid paraffin and wool fat

(Formulated as an ocular lubricant)

● **INDICATIONS AND DOSE**

Dry eye conditions

▶ TO THE EYE

▸ Child: Apply as required

- **MEDICINAL FORMS** There can be variation in the licensing of different medicines containing the same drug.

Eye ointment

- Hylo Night (Scope Ophthalmics Ltd)
  Hylo Night eye ointment preservative free | 5 gram £2.75

Sodium chloride

01-May-2020

- **INDICATIONS AND DOSE**

Tear deficiency | Ocular lubricants and astringents | Irrigation, including first-aid removal of harmful substances | Intra-ocular or topical irrigation during surgical procedures

▶ TO THE EYE
- Child: Apply as required, use 0.9% eye preparations

- **PRESCRIBING AND DISPENSING INFORMATION** Although multi-dose sodium chloride eye drops commonly contain preservatives, preservative-free unit dose vials may be available.

- **MEDICINAL FORMS** There can be variation in the licensing of different medicines containing the same drug. Forms available from special-order manufacturers include: eye drops, eye ointment, irrigation

Eye drops

- Saline (Bausch & Lomb UK Ltd)
  Sodium chloride 9 mg per 1 ml Minims saline 0.9% eye drops 0.5ml unit dose | 20 unit dose [P] £7.43 DT = £7.43

Sodium hyaluronate

23-Mar-2020

- **INDICATIONS AND DOSE**

Dry eye conditions

▶ TO THE EYE
- Child: Apply as required

- **PRESCRIBING AND DISPENSING INFORMATION** Some preparations are contained in units which are resealable and may be used for up to 12 hours.
  Although multi-dose sodium hyaluronate eye drops commonly contain preservatives, preservative-free unit dose vials may be available.

- **MEDICINAL FORMS** There can be variation in the licensing of different medicines containing the same drug.

Eye drops

- Artelac Rebalance (Bausch & Lomb UK Ltd)
  Artelac Rebalance 0.15% eye drops | 10 ml £4.00
- Artelac Splash (Bausch & Lomb UK Ltd)
  Artelac Splash 0.2% eye drops 0.5ml unit dose | 30 unit dose £7.00 | 60 unit dose £11.20
- Blink Intensive (AMO UK Ltd)
  Blink Intensive Tears 0.2% eye drops 0.4ml unit dose | 20 unit dose £2.97
  Blink Intensive Tears 0.2% eye drops | 10 ml £2.97
- Clinitas (Altacor Ltd)
  Clinitas Multi 0.4% eye drops preservative free | 10 ml £6.99
  Clinitas 0.4% eye drops 0.5ml unit dose | 30 unit dose £5.70
- Evolve HA (Medicom Healthcare Ltd)
  Evolve HA 0.2% eye drops preservative free | 10 ml £5.99
- Hy-Opti (Alissa Healthcare Research Ltd)
  Hy-Opti 0.1% eye drops preservative free | 10 ml £8.50
  Hy-Opti 0.2% eye drops preservative free | 10 ml £9.50
- Hyabak (Thea Pharmaceuticals Ltd)
  Hyabak 0.15% eye drops preservative free | 10 ml £7.99
- Hycosan (Scope Ophthalmics Ltd)
  Hycosan Extra 0.2% eye drops | 7.5 ml [X]
  Hycosan 0.1% eye drops | 7.5 ml [X]
- HydraMed (Farmigea S.p.A.)
  HydraMed 0.2% eye drops preservative free | 10 ml £5.60
  HydraMed 0.2% eye drops 0.5ml unit dose preservative free | 30 unit dose £5.60
- Hylo-Comod (Scope Ophthalmics Ltd)
  Hylo-Tear 0.1% eye drops preservative free | 10 ml £8.50
  Hylo-Forte 0.2% eye drops preservative free | 10 ml £9.50
- Hylo-fresh (Scope Ophthalmics Ltd)
  Hylo-Fresh 0.03% eye drops preservative free | 10 ml £4.95
- Lubristil (Rayner Pharmaceuticals Ltd)
  Lubristil 0.15% eye drops 0.3ml unit dose preservative free | 20 unit dose £4.99
- Ocu-Lube HA (Sai-Meds Ltd)
  Ocu-Lube HA 0.1% eye drops preservative free | 10 ml £8.00
- Ocusan (Agepha Pharma s.r.o.)
  Ocusan 0.2% eye drops 0.5ml unit dose | 20 unit dose £5.47
- Optive Fusion (Allergan Ltd)
  Optive Fusion 0.1% eye drops | 10 ml £7.49
- Oxyal (Bausch & Lomb UK Ltd)
  Oxyal 0.15% eye drops | 10 ml £4.15
- Vismed (TRB Chemidica (UK) Ltd)
  Vismed Gel Multi 0.3% eye drops preservative free | 10 ml £8.01
  Vismed Multi 0.18% eye drops preservative free | 10 ml £6.87
  Vismed 0.18% eye drops 0.3ml unit dose preservative free | 20 unit dose £5.14
- Xailin HA (Visufarma UK Ltd)
  Xailin HA 0.2% eye drops | 10 ml £7.34

Eye gel

- Lubristil (Rayner Pharmaceuticals Ltd)
  Lubristil 0.15% eye gel 0.4ml unit dose preservative free | 20 unit dose £6.49
- Vismed (TRB Chemidica (UK) Ltd)
  Vismed Gel 0.3% eye gel 0.45ml unit dose preservative free | 20 unit dose £6.03

Sodium hyaluronate with trehalose

21-Nov-2017

- **INDICATIONS AND DOSE**

Dry eye conditions

▶ TO THE EYE
- Child: Apply 1 drop 4–6 times a day

- **PRESCRIBING AND DISPENSING INFORMATION** Sodium hyaluronate and trehalose preparations do not contain preservatives; multi-dose preparation can be used for up to 3 months.

- **MEDICINAL FORMS** There can be variation in the licensing of different medicines containing the same drug.

Eye drops

- Thealoz Duo (Thea Pharmaceuticals Ltd)
  Thealoz Duo eye drops preservative free | 10 ml £8.99
  Thealoz Duo UD eye drops 0.4ml unit dose preservative free | 30 unit dose £7.07

Soybean oil

- **INDICATIONS AND DOSE**

Dry eye conditions

▶ TO THE EYE
- Child: Apply up to 4 times a day

- **MEDICINAL FORMS** There can be variation in the licensing of different medicines containing the same drug.

Eye drops

- Emustil (Rayner Pharmaceuticals Ltd)
  Emustil eye drops 0.3ml unit dose preservative free | 20 unit dose £6.22

3 Eye infections

Eye, infections

Eye infections

Most acute superficial eye infections can be treated topically. Blepharitis and conjunctivitis are often caused by staphylococci; keratitis and endophthalmitis may be bacterial, viral, or fungal.

Bacterial *blepharitis* is treated by lid hygiene and application of antibacterial eye drops to the conjunctival sac or to the lid margins. Systemic treatment may be required and may be necessary for 3 months or longer.

Most cases of acute bacterial conjunctivitis are self-limiting; where treatment is appropriate, antibacterial eye drops or an eye ointment are used. A poor response might indicate viral or allergic conjunctivitis or antibiotic resistance.

Corneal *ulcer* and *keratitis* require specialist treatment, usually under inpatient care, and may call for intensive topical, subconjunctival, or systemic administration of antimicrobials.

Endophthalmitis is a medical emergency which also calls for specialist management and requires intravitreal administration of antimicrobials; concomitant systemic treatment is required in some cases. Surgical intervention, such as vitrectomy, is sometimes indicated.

See reference to the treatment of *crab lice of the eyelashes*.

Antibacterials for eye infections

Bacterial eye infections are generally treated topically with eye drops and eye ointments. Systemic administration is sometimes appropriate in blepharitis.

Chloramphenicol p. 729 has a broad spectrum of activity and is the drug of choice for *superficial eye infections*. Chloramphenicol eye drops are well tolerated and the recommendation that chloramphenicol eye drops should be avoided because of an increased risk of aplastic anaemia is not well founded.

Other antibacterials with a broad spectrum of activity include the quinolones, ciprofloxacin p. 728, levofloxacin p. 728, moxifloxacin p. 729, and ofloxacin p. 729; the aminoglycosides, gentamicin below and tobramycin p. 728 are also active against a wide variety of bacteria. Gentamicin, tobramycin, quinolones (except moxifloxacin), and **polymyxin B** are effective for infections caused by *Pseudomonas aeruginosa*.

Ciprofloxacin eye drops are licensed for corneal ulcers; intensive application (especially in the first 2 days) is required throughout the day and night.

Azithromycin eye drops p. 728 are licensed for trachomatous conjunctivitis caused by *Chlamydia trachomatis* and for purulent bacterial conjunctivitis. *Trachoma* which results from chronic infection with *Chlamydia trachomatis* can be treated with azithromycin by mouth [unlicensed indication].

Fusidic acid is useful for staphylococcal infections.

Propamidine isetionate p. 729 is of little value in bacterial infections but is used by specialists to treat the rare, but potentially sight-threatening, condition of *acanthamoeba keratitis* [unlicensed indication].

Other antibacterial eye drops may be prepared aseptically in a specialist manufacturing unit from material supplied for injection.

With corticosteroids

Many antibacterial preparations also incorporate a corticosteroid but such mixtures should **not** be used unless a patient is under close specialist supervision. In particular they should not be prescribed for undiagnosed 'red eye' which is sometimes caused by the herpes simplex virus and may be difficult to diagnose.

Administration

Frequency of application depends on the severity of the infection and the potential for irreversible ocular damage; antibacterial eye preparations are usually administered as follows:

- *Eye drops*, apply 1 drop at least every 2 hours in severe infection then reduce frequency as infection is controlled and continue for 48 hours after healing. For less severe infection 3–4 times daily is generally sufficient.
- *Eye ointment*, apply *either* at night (if eye drops used during the day) *or* 3–4 times daily (if eye ointment used alone).

Antifungals for eye infections

Fungal infections of the cornea are rare. Orbital mycosis is rarer, and when it occurs it is usually because of direct spread of infection from the paranasal sinuses. Debility or immunosuppression can encourage fungal proliferation. The spread of infection through blood occasionally produces metastatic endophthalmitis.

Many different fungi are capable of producing ocular infection; they can be identified by appropriate laboratory procedures.

Antifungal preparations for the eye are not generally available. Treatment will normally be carried out at specialist centres, but requests for information about supplies of preparations not available commercially should be addressed to the Strategic Health Authority (or equivalent in Scotland or Northern Ireland), or to the nearest hospital ophthalmology unit, or to Moorfields Eye Hospital, 162 City Road, London EC1V 2PD (tel. (020) 7253 3411) or www.moorfields.nhs.uk.

Antivirals for eye infections

Herpes simplex infections producing, for example, dendritic corneal ulcers can be treated with aciclovir p. 730. Aciclovir eye ointment is used in combination with systemic treatment for ophthalmic zoster.

Also see systemic treatment of CMV retinitis.

Antibacterials for eye infections in neonates

Antibacterial eye drops are used to treat acute bacterial conjunctivitis in neonates (ophthalmia neonatorum); where possible the causative microorganism should be identified. Chloramphenicol eye drops are used to treat mild conjunctivitis; more serious infections also require a systemic antibacterial. Failure to respond to initial treatment requires further investigation; chlamydial infection is one of the most frequent causes of neonatal conjunctivitis and should be considered.

Azithromycin eye drops are licensed to treat trachomatous conjunctivitis caused by *Chlamydia trachomatis* and purulent bacterial conjunctivitis in neonates. However, as there is a risk of simultaneous infection at other sites in neonates and children under 3 months presenting with conjunctivitis caused by *Chlamydia trachomatis*, systemic treatment with oral erythromycin p. 355 is required.

Gonococcal eye infections are treated with a single-dose of parenteral cefotaxime p. 342 or ceftriaxone p. 343. Gentamicin eye drops together with appropriate systemic antibacterials are used in the treatment of *pseudomonal eye infections*; high-strength gentamicin eye drops (1.5%) [unlicensed] are available for severe infections.

3.1 Bacterial eye infection

ANTIBACTERIALS > AMINOGLYCOSIDES

F 332

Gentamicin

19-Mar-2020

● INDICATIONS AND DOSE

Bacterial eye infections

▶ TO THE EYE

▸ Child: Apply 1 drop at least every 2 hours in severe infection, reduce frequency as infection is controlled and continue for 48 hours after healing,

continued →

11 Eye

frequency of eye drops depends on the severity of the infection and the potential for irreversible ocular damage; for less severe infection 3–4 times daily is generally sufficient

- **UNLICENSED USE** Gentamicin doses in BNF publications may differ from those in product literature.
- **INTERACTIONS** → Appendix 1: aminoglycosides
- **PRESCRIBING AND DISPENSING INFORMATION** Eye drops may be sourced as a manufactured special or from specialist importing companies.

- **MEDICINAL FORMS** There can be variation in the licensing of different medicines containing the same drug. Forms available from special-order manufacturers include: eye drops

Ear/eye drops solution

EXCIPIENTS: May contain Benzalkonium chloride

▸ Gentamicin (Non-proprietary)

Gentamicin (as Gentamicin sulfate) 3 mg per 1 ml Gentamicin 0.3% ear/eye drops | 10 ml PoM £2.85 DT = £2.86

332

Tobramycin

16-Mar-2020

- **INDICATIONS AND DOSE**

Local treatment of infections

▸ TO THE EYE

▸ Child 1–17 years: Apply twice daily for 6–8 days

Local treatment of infections (severe infection)

▸ TO THE EYE

▸ Child 1–17 years: Apply 4 times a day for first day, then apply twice daily for 5–7 days

- **INTERACTIONS** → Appendix 1: aminoglycosides

- **MEDICINAL FORMS** No licensed medicines listed

ANTIBACTERIALS › MACROLIDES

352

Azithromycin

03-Mar-2020

- **INDICATIONS AND DOSE**

Trachomatous conjunctivitis caused by *Chlamydia trachomatis* | Purulent bacterial conjunctivitis

▸ TO THE EYE

▸ Child: Apply twice daily for 3 days, review if no improvement after 3 days of treatment

- **INTERACTIONS** → Appendix 1: macrolides
- **SIDE-EFFECTS**

▸ **Common or very common** Eye discomfort

▸ **Uncommon** Eye allergy

- **MEDICINAL FORMS** There can be variation in the licensing of different medicines containing the same drug.

Eye drops

▸ Azyter (Thea Pharmaceuticals Ltd)

Azithromycin dihydrate 15 mg per 1 gram Azyter 15mg/g eye drops 0.25g unit dose | 6 unit dose PoM £6.99 DT = £6.99

ANTIBACTERIALS › QUINOLONES

376

Ciprofloxacin

17-Apr-2020

- **INDICATIONS AND DOSE**

Superficial bacterial eye infection

▸ TO THE EYE USING EYE DROP

▸ Child: Apply 4 times a day for maximum duration of treatment 21 days

▸ TO THE EYE USING EYE OINTMENT

▸ Child 1–17 years: Apply 1.25 centimetres 3 times a day for 2 days, then apply 1.25 centimetres twice daily for 5 days

Superficial bacterial eye infection (severe infection)

▸ TO THE EYE USING EYE DROP

▸ Child: Apply every 2 hours during waking hours for 2 days, then apply 4 times a day for maximum duration of treatment 21 days

Corneal ulcer

▸ TO THE EYE USING EYE DROP

▸ Child: Apply every 15 minutes for 6 hours, then apply every 30 minutes for the remainder of day 1, then apply every 1 hour on day 2, then apply every 4 hours on days 3–14, maximum duration of treatment 21 days, to be administered throughout the day and night

▸ TO THE EYE USING EYE OINTMENT

▸ Child 1–17 years: Apply 1.25 centimetres every 1–2 hours for 2 days, then apply 1.25 centimetres every 4 hours for the next 12 days, to be administered throughout the day and night

- **INTERACTIONS** → Appendix 1: quinolones
- **SIDE-EFFECTS**

▸ **Rare or very rare** Ear pain · hordeolum · paranasal sinus hypersecretion

- **PREGNANCY** Manufacturer advises use only if potential benefit outweighs risk.
- **BREAST FEEDING** Manufacturer advises caution.
- **PRESCRIBING AND DISPENSING INFORMATION** For choice of antibacterial therapy, see Eye, infections p. 726.

- **MEDICINAL FORMS** There can be variation in the licensing of different medicines containing the same drug. Forms available from special-order manufacturers include: eye drops, eye ointment

Eye drops

EXCIPIENTS: May contain Benzalkonium chloride

▸ Ciloxan (Novartis Pharmaceuticals UK Ltd)

Ciprofloxacin (as Ciprofloxacin hydrochloride) 3 mg per 1 ml Ciloxan 0.3% eye drops | 5 ml PoM £4.70 DT = £4.70

376

Levofloxacin

17-Apr-2020

- **INDICATIONS AND DOSE**

Local treatment of eye infections

▸ TO THE EYE

▸ Child 1–17 years: Apply every 2 hours for first 2 days, to be applied maximum 8 times a day, then apply 4 times a day for 3 days

- **INTERACTIONS** → Appendix 1: quinolones
- **PREGNANCY** Manufacturer advises use only if potential benefit outweighs risk.
- **BREAST FEEDING** Manufacturer advises use only if potential benefit outweighs risk.
- **PRESCRIBING AND DISPENSING INFORMATION** Although multi-dose levofloxacin eye drops commonly contain preservatives, preservative-free unit dose vials may be available.

- **MEDICINAL FORMS** There can be variation in the licensing of different medicines containing the same drug.

Eye drops

EXCIPIENTS: May contain Benzalkonium chloride

▸ Levofloxacin (Non-proprietary)

Levofloxacin (as Levofloxacin hemihydrate) 5 mg per 1 ml Levofloxacin 5mg/ml eye drops | 5 ml PoM £6.95 DT = £7.71 (Hospital only) | 5 ml PoM £8.10 DT = £7.71

▸ Oftaquix (Santen UK Ltd)

Levofloxacin (as Levofloxacin hemihydrate) 5 mg per 1 ml Oftaquix 5mg/ml eye drops 0.3ml unit dose | 30 unit dose PoM £17.95 DT = £17.95

Oftaquix 5mg/ml eye drops | 5 ml PoM £6.95 DT = £7.71

F 376

Moxifloxacin
17-Apr-2020

● **INDICATIONS AND DOSE**

Local treatment of infections

▶ TO THE EYE

▸ Child: Apply 3 times a day continue treatment for 2–3 days after infection improves; review if no improvement within 5 days

● **CAUTIONS** Not recommended for neonates

● **INTERACTIONS** → Appendix 1: quinolones

● **SIDE-EFFECTS**

▶ **Uncommon** Conjunctival haemorrhage

▶ **Rare or very rare** Laryngeal pain · nasal discomfort

● **MEDICINAL FORMS** There can be variation in the licensing of different medicines containing the same drug.

Eye drops

▸ Moxivig (Novartis Pharmaceuticals UK Ltd)
Moxifloxacin (as Moxifloxacin hydrochloride) 5 mg per 1 ml Moxivig 0.5% eye drops | 5 ml PoM £9.80 DT = £9.80

F 376

Ofloxacin
17-Apr-2020

● **INDICATIONS AND DOSE**

Local treatment of infections

▶ TO THE EYE

▸ Child 1–17 years: Apply every 2–4 hours for the first 2 days, then reduced to 4 times a day for maximum 10 days treatment

● **CAUTIONS** Corneal ulcer (risk of corneal perforation) · epithelial defect (risk of corneal perforation)

● **INTERACTIONS** → Appendix 1: quinolones

● **SIDE-EFFECTS** Oropharyngeal swelling · tongue swelling

● **PREGNANCY** Manufacturer advises use only if benefit outweighs risk (systemic quinolones have caused arthropathy in *animal* studies).

● **BREAST FEEDING** Manufacturer advises avoid.

● **MEDICINAL FORMS** There can be variation in the licensing of different medicines containing the same drug.

Eye drops

EXCIPIENTS: May contain Benzalkonium chloride

▸ Exocin (Allergan Ltd)
Ofloxacin 3 mg per 1 ml Exocin 0.3% eye drops | 5 ml PoM £2.17 DT = £2.17

ANTIBACTERIALS > OTHER

Chloramphenicol
13-May-2020

● **DRUG ACTION** Chloramphenicol is a potent broad-spectrum antibiotic.

● **INDICATIONS AND DOSE**

Superficial eye infections

▶ TO THE EYE USING EYE DROP

▸ Child: Apply 1 drop every 2 hours then reduce frequency as infection is controlled and continue for 48 hours after healing, frequency dependent on the severity of the infection. For less severe infection 3–4 times daily is generally sufficient

▶ TO THE EYE USING EYE OINTMENT

▸ Child: Apply daily, to be applied at night (if eye drops used during the day), alternatively apply 3–4 times a day, if ointment used alone

● **INTERACTIONS** → Appendix 1: chloramphenicol

● **SIDE-EFFECTS** Angioedema · bone marrow disorders · eye stinging · fever · paraesthesia · skin reactions

● **PREGNANCY** Avoid unless essential—no information on *topical* use but risk of 'neonatal grey-baby syndrome' with *oral* use in third trimester.

● **BREAST FEEDING** Avoid unless essential— *theoretical* risk of bone-marrow toxicity.

● **PRESCRIBING AND DISPENSING INFORMATION** Although multi-dose chloramphenicol eye drops commonly contain preservatives, preservative-free unit dose vials may be available.

● **PATIENT AND CARER ADVICE**
Medicines for Children leaflet: Chloramphenicol for eye infections www.medicinesforchildren.org.uk/chloramphenicol-eye-infections-0

● **EXCEPTIONS TO LEGAL CATEGORY** Chloramphenicol 0.5% eye drops (in max. pack size 10 mL) and 1% eye ointment (in max. pack size 4 g) can be sold to the public for treatment of acute bacterial conjunctivitis in adults and children over 2 years; max. duration of treatment 5 days.

● **MEDICINAL FORMS** There can be variation in the licensing of different medicines containing the same drug.

Eye drops

EXCIPIENTS: May contain Phenylmercuric acetate

▸ Chloramphenicol (Bausch & Lomb UK Ltd)
Chloramphenicol 5 mg per 1 ml Minims chloramphenicol 0.5% eye drops 0.5ml unit dose | 20 unit dose PoM £11.43 DT = £11.43
Chloramphenicol 0.5% eye drops | 10 ml PoM £5.65 DT = £4.13

▸ Eykappo (Aspire Pharma Ltd)
Chloramphenicol 5 mg per 1 ml Eykappo 5mg/ml eye drops | 10 ml PoM £10.12 DT = £10.12

Eye ointment

▸ Chloramphenicol (Non-proprietary)
Chloramphenicol 10 mg per 1 gram Chloramphenicol 1% eye ointment | 4 gram PoM £2.03 DT = £1.75

Fusidic acid
30-Apr-2020

● **DRUG ACTION** Fusidic acid and its salts are narrow-spectrum antibiotics used for staphylococcal infections.

● **INDICATIONS AND DOSE**

Staphylococcal eye infections

▶ TO THE EYE

▸ Child: Apply twice daily

● **INTERACTIONS** → Appendix 1: fusidate

● **SIDE-EFFECTS**

▶ **Common or very common** Dry eye · eye discomfort · vision blurred

▶ **Uncommon** Crying on application · skin reactions · watering eye

▶ **Frequency not known** Angioedema · eye inflammation

● **MEDICINAL FORMS** There can be variation in the licensing of different medicines containing the same drug.

Modified-release drops

EXCIPIENTS: May contain Benzalkonium chloride, disodium edetate

▸ Fusidic acid (Non-proprietary)
Fusidic acid 10 mg per 1 gram Fusidic acid 1% modified-release eye drops | 5 gram PoM £35.00 DT = £35.00

ANTIPROTOZOALS

Propamidine isetionate

● **INDICATIONS AND DOSE**

***Acanthamoeba keratitis* infections (specialist use only) | Local treatment of eye infections**

▶ TO THE EYE USING EYE OINTMENT

▸ Child: Apply 1–2 times a day

▶ TO THE EYE USING EYE DROP

▸ Child: Apply up to 4 times a day

- **UNLICENSED USE** Not licensed for *acanthamoeba keratitis* infections.
- **SIDE-EFFECTS** Eye discomfort · vision blurred
- **PREGNANCY** Manufacturer advises avoid unless essential—no information available.
- **BREAST FEEDING** Manufacturer advises avoid unless essential—no information available.

- **MEDICINAL FORMS** There can be variation in the licensing of different medicines containing the same drug.

Eye ointment

▸ Golden Eye (dibrompropamidine) (Cambridge Healthcare Supplies Ltd)
Dibrompropamidine isetionate 1.5 mg per 1 gram Golden Eye 0.15% ointment | 5 gram [P] £4.15 DT = £4.15

Eye drops

EXCIPIENTS: May contain Benzalkonium chloride

▸ Brolene (Propamidine) (Sanofi)
Propamidine isetionate 1 mg per 1 ml Brolene 0.1% eye drops | 10 ml [P] £2.80 DT = £2.80

▸ Golden Eye (propamidine) (Cambridge Healthcare Supplies Ltd)
Propamidine isetionate 1 mg per 1 ml Golden Eye 0.1% drops | 10 ml [P] £3.95 DT = £2.80

3.2 Viral eye infection

3.2a Ophthalmic herpes simplex

ANTIVIRALS › NUCLEOSIDE ANALOGUES

Aciclovir
10-Mar-2020

(Acyclovir)

- **INDICATIONS AND DOSE**

Herpes simplex infection (local treatment)

▸ TO THE EYE USING EYE OINTMENT

▸ Child: Apply 1 centimetre 5 times a day continue for at least 3 days after complete healing

- **INTERACTIONS** → Appendix 1: aciclovir
- **SIDE-EFFECTS**

▸ **Common or very common** Eye inflammation · eye pain

- **PATIENT AND CARER ADVICE**
Medicines for Children leaflet: Aciclovir eye ointment for herpes simplex infections
www.medicinesforchildren.org.uk/aciclovir-eye-ointment-herpes-simplex-infection-0

- **MEDICINAL FORMS** There can be variation in the licensing of different medicines containing the same drug.

Eye ointment

▸ Aciclovir (Non-proprietary)
Aciclovir 30 mg per 1 gram Aciclovir 3% eye ointment | 4.5 gram [PoM] £45.00 DT = £45.00

4 Eye procedures

Mydriatics and cycloplegics
25-Apr-2020

Overview

Antimuscarinics dilate the pupil and paralyse the ciliary muscle; they vary in potency and duration of action.

Short-acting, relatively weak mydriatics, such as tropicamide below (action lasts for up to 6 hours), facilitate the examination of the fundus of the eye. Cyclopentolate hydrochloride p. 723 (complete recovery can take up to 24 hours) or atropine sulfate p. 723 (action up to 7 days) are also licensed for producing cycloplegia for refraction in young children. Expert sources advise tropicamide may be preferred in neonates.

Phenylephrine hydrochloride p. 731 is licensed for mydriasis in diagnostic or therapeutic procedures; mydriasis occurs within 60–90 minutes and lasts up to 5–7 hours.

[EvGr] Mydriatics and cycloplegics are used in the treatment of anterior uveitis, usually as an adjunct to corticosteroids. Atropine sulfate or cyclopentolate hydrochloride can prevent posterior synechiae and relieve ciliary spasm when used for anterior uveitis. ⟨A⟩

ANTIMUSCARINICS

722

Tropicamide

- **INDICATIONS AND DOSE**

Funduscopy

▸ TO THE EYE

▸ Neonate: 0.5% eye drops to be applied 20 minutes before examination.

▸ Child: 0.5% eye drops to be applied 20 minutes before examination

- **INTERACTIONS** → Appendix 1: tropicamide
- **SIDE-EFFECTS** Eye erythema · eye irritation (on prolonged administration) · eye pain · headache · hypotension · nausea · syncope · vision blurred
- **PRESCRIBING AND DISPENSING INFORMATION** Although multi-dose tropicamide eye drops commonly contain preservatives, preservative-free unit dose vials may be available.

- **MEDICINAL FORMS** There can be variation in the licensing of different medicines containing the same drug.

Eye drops

EXCIPIENTS: May contain Benzalkonium chloride, edetic acid (edta)

▸ Mydriacyl (Alcon Eye Care Ltd)
Tropicamide 10 mg per 1 ml Mydriacyl 1% eye drops | 5 ml [PoM] £1.60

▸ Tropicamide (Bausch & Lomb UK Ltd)
Tropicamide 5 mg per 1 ml Minims tropicamide 0.5% eye drops 0.5ml unit dose | 20 unit dose [PoM] £11.18 DT = £11.18
Tropicamide 10 mg per 1 ml Minims tropicamide 1% eye drops 0.5ml unit dose | 20 unit dose [PoM] £11.31 DT = £11.31

ANTISEPTICS AND DISINFECTANTS › IODINE PRODUCTS

Povidone-iodine

- **INDICATIONS AND DOSE**

Cutaneous peri-ocular and conjunctival antisepsis before ocular surgery

▸ TO THE EYE

▸ Neonate: Apply, leave for 2 minutes, then irrigate thoroughly with sodium chloride 0.9%.

▸ Child: Apply, leave for 2 minutes, then irrigate thoroughly with sodium chloride 0.9%

- **CONTRA-INDICATIONS** Concomitant use of ocular antimicrobial drugs · concomitant use of ocular formulations containing mercury-based preservatives · preterm neonates
- **SIDE-EFFECTS**

▸ **Rare or very rare** Eye erythema · punctate keratitis

▸ **Frequency not known** Cytotoxicity · eye discolouration · hypothyroidism

- **BREAST FEEDING** Avoid regular or excessive use.
- **PRESCRIBING AND DISPENSING INFORMATION** Although multi-dose povidone iodine eye drops commonly contain

preservatives, preservative-free unit dose vials may be available.

- **MEDICINAL FORMS** There can be variation in the licensing of different medicines containing the same drug. Forms available from special-order manufacturers include: eye drops, eye lotion

Eye drops

- Povidone iodine (Bausch & Lomb UK Ltd)
  Povidone-Iodine 50 mg per 1 ml Minims povidone iodine 5% eye drops 0.4ml unit dose | 20 unit dose [PoM] £16.00

DIAGNOSTIC AGENTS > DYES

Fluorescein sodium

- **INDICATIONS AND DOSE**

Detection of lesions and foreign bodies

- TO THE EYE
- Child: Use sufficient amount to stain damaged areas

- **PRESCRIBING AND DISPENSING INFORMATION** Although multi-dose fluorescein eye drops commonly contain preservatives, preservative-free unit dose vials may be available.

- **MEDICINAL FORMS** There can be variation in the licensing of different medicines containing the same drug.

Eye drops

- Fluorescein sodium (Bausch & Lomb UK Ltd)
  Fluorescein sodium 10 mg per 1 ml Minims fluorescein sodium 1% eye drops 0.5ml unit dose | 20 unit dose [P] £9.25
  Fluorescein sodium 20 mg per 1 ml Minims fluorescein sodium 2% eye drops 0.5ml unit dose | 20 unit dose [P] £9.25

MIOTICS > PARASYMPATHOMIMETICS

Acetylcholine chloride

- **INDICATIONS AND DOSE**

Cataract surgery | Penetrating keratoplasty | Iridectomy | Anterior segment surgery requiring rapid complete miosis

- TO THE EYE
- Child: (consult product literature)

- **UNLICENSED USE** Not licensed for use in children.
- **CAUTIONS** Asthma · gastro-intestinal spasm · heart failure · hyperthyroidism · peptic ulcer · urinary-tract obstruction
- **SIDE-EFFECTS** Bradycardia · corneal decompensation · corneal oedema · dyspnoea · flushing · hyperhidrosis · hypotension
- **PREGNANCY** Avoid unless potential benefit outweighs risk—no information available.
- **BREAST FEEDING** Avoid unless potential benefit outweighs risk—no information available.

- **MEDICINAL FORMS** There can be variation in the licensing of different medicines containing the same drug.

Irrigation

- Miochol-E (Bausch & Lomb UK Ltd)
  Acetylcholine chloride 20 mg Miochol-E 20mg powder and solvent for solution for intraocular irrigation vials | 1 vial [PoM] £7.28
- Miphtel (Farmigea S.p.A.)
  Acetylcholine chloride 20 mg Miphtel 20mg powder and solvent for solution for intraocular irrigation ampoules | 6 ampoule [PoM] £43.68 (Hospital only)

SYMPATHOMIMETICS > VASOCONSTRICTOR

Phenylephrine hydrochloride

- **INDICATIONS AND DOSE**

Mydriasis

- TO THE EYE
- Child: Apply 1 drop, to be administered before procedure, a drop of proxymetacaine topical anaesthetic may be applied to the eye a few minutes before using phenylephrine to prevent stinging

- **CONTRA-INDICATIONS** 10% strength eye drops in children · 10% strength eye drops in neonates · aneurysms · cardiovascular disease · hypertension · thyrotoxicosis
- **CAUTIONS** Asthma · corneal epithelial damage · darkly pigmented iris is more resistant to pupillary dilatation and caution should be exercised to avoid overdosage · diabetes (avoid eye drops in long standing diabetes) · mydriasis can precipitate acute angle-closure glaucoma in the very few children who are predisposed to the condition because of a shallow anterior chamber · neonates are at an increased risk of systemic toxicity · ocular hyperaemia · susceptibility to angle-closure glaucoma
- **INTERACTIONS** → Appendix 1: sympathomimetics, vasoconstrictor
- **SIDE-EFFECTS** Arrhythmias · conjunctivitis allergic · eye discomfort · hypertension · myocardial infarction (usually after use of 10% strength in patients with pre-existing cardiovascular disease) · palpitations · periorbital pallor · vision disorders
- **PREGNANCY** Use only if potential benefit outweighs risk.
- **BREAST FEEDING** Use only if potential benefit outweighs risk—no information available.
- **PRESCRIBING AND DISPENSING INFORMATION** Although multi-dose phenylephrine eye drops commonly contain preservatives, preservative-free unit dose vials may be available.
- **PATIENT AND CARER ADVICE**
  Driving and skilled tasks Patients should be warned not to undertake skilled tasks (e.g. driving) until vision clears after mydriasis.

- **MEDICINAL FORMS** There can be variation in the licensing of different medicines containing the same drug. Forms available from special-order manufacturers include: eye drops

Eye drops

EXCIPIENTS: May contain Disodium edetate, sodium metabisulfite

- Phenylephrine hydrochloride (Bausch & Lomb UK Ltd)
  Phenylephrine hydrochloride 25 mg per 1 ml Minims phenylephrine hydrochloride 2.5% eye drops 0.5ml unit dose | 20 unit dose [P] £11.87 DT = £11.87

4.1 Post-operative pain and inflammation

Eye, surgical and peri-operative drug use

Ocular peri-operative drugs

Drugs used to prepare the eye for surgery and drugs that are injected into the anterior chamber at the time of surgery are included here.

Sodium hyaluronate p. 726 is used during surgical procedures on the eye.

Apraclonidine p. 739, an alpha$_2$-adrenoceptor agonist, reduces intra-ocular pressure possibly by reducing the production of aqueous humour. It is used for short-term treatment only.

Balanced Salt Solution is used routinely in intra-ocular surgery.

Povidone-iodine p. 730 is used for peri-ocular and conjunctival antisepsis before ocular surgery to support postoperative infection control.

Ocular local anaesthetics

Oxybuprocaine hydrochloride below and tetracaine below are widely used topical local anaesthetics. Proxymetacaine hydrochloride below causes less initial stinging and is useful for children. Oxybuprocaine hydrochloride or a combined preparation of lidocaine hydrochloride p. 884 and fluorescein sodium p. 731 is used for tonometry. Tetracaine produces a more profound anaesthesia and is suitable for use before minor surgical procedures, such as the removal of corneal sutures. It has a temporary disruptive effect on the corneal epithelium. Lidocaine hydrochloride, with or without adrenaline/epinephrine p. 143, is injected into the eyelids for minor surgery. Local anaesthetics should never be used for the management of ocular symptoms.

Local anaesthetic eye drops should be avoided in preterm neonates because of the immaturity of the metabolising enzyme system.

ANAESTHETICS, LOCAL

Fluorescein with lidocaine

● **INDICATIONS AND DOSE**

Local anaesthesia

▶ TO THE EYE
▸ Child: Apply as required

● **CONTRA-INDICATIONS** Avoid in pre-term neonate (immature metabolising enzyme system)

● **PRESCRIBING AND DISPENSING INFORMATION** Although multi-dose lidocaine and fluorescein eye drops commonly contain preservatives, preservative-free unit dose vials may be available.

● **MEDICINAL FORMS** There can be variation in the licensing of different medicines containing the same drug.

Eye drops

▸ Lidocaine and Fluorescein (Bausch & Lomb UK Ltd)
Fluorescein sodium 2.5 mg per 1 ml, Lidocaine hydrochloride 40 mg per 1 ml Minims lidocaine and fluorescein eye drops 0.5ml unit dose | 20 unit dose PoM £11.69

Oxybuprocaine hydrochloride

(Benoxinate hydrochloride)

● **INDICATIONS AND DOSE**

Local anaesthetic

▶ TO THE EYE
▸ Child: Apply as required

● **CONTRA-INDICATIONS** Avoid in preterm neonates

● **INTERACTIONS** → Appendix 1: anaesthetics, local

● **PRESCRIBING AND DISPENSING INFORMATION** Although multi-dose oxybuprocaine eye drops commonly contain preservatives, preservative-free unit dose vials may be available.

● **MEDICINAL FORMS** There can be variation in the licensing of different medicines containing the same drug.

Eye drops

▸ Oxybuprocaine hydrochloride (Bausch & Lomb UK Ltd)
Oxybuprocaine hydrochloride 4 mg per 1 ml Minims oxybuprocaine hydrochloride 0.4% eye drops 0.5ml unit dose | 20 unit dose PoM £10.56

Proxymetacaine hydrochloride

● **INDICATIONS AND DOSE**

Local anaesthetic

▶ TO THE EYE
▸ Child: Apply as required

● **CONTRA-INDICATIONS** Avoid in preterm neonates

● **INTERACTIONS** → Appendix 1: anaesthetics, local

● **PRESCRIBING AND DISPENSING INFORMATION** Although multi-dose proxymetacaine eye drops commonly contain preservatives, preservative-free unit dose vials may be available.

● **MEDICINAL FORMS** There can be variation in the licensing of different medicines containing the same drug.

Eye drops

▸ Proxymetacaine (Bausch & Lomb UK Ltd)
Proxymetacaine hydrochloride 5 mg per 1 ml Minims proxymetacaine 0.5% eye drops 0.5ml unit dose | 20 unit dose PoM £12.12

Tetracaine

10-Mar-2020

(Amethocaine)

● **INDICATIONS AND DOSE**

Local anaesthetic

▶ TO THE EYE
▸ Child: Apply as required

● **UNLICENSED USE** Not licensed for use in neonates.

● **CONTRA-INDICATIONS** Avoid in preterm neonates

● **INTERACTIONS** → Appendix 1: anaesthetics, local

● **SIDE-EFFECTS** Dermatitis · eye disorders · eye inflammation · paraesthesia

● **PRESCRIBING AND DISPENSING INFORMATION** Although multi-dose tetracaine eye drops commonly contain preservatives, preservative-free unit dose vials may be available.

● **MEDICINAL FORMS** There can be variation in the licensing of different medicines containing the same drug.

Eye drops

▸ Tetracaine (Bausch & Lomb UK Ltd)
Tetracaine hydrochloride 5 mg per 1 ml Minims tetracaine hydrochloride 0.5% eye drops 0.5ml unit dose | 20 unit dose PoM £10.57 DT = £10.57
Tetracaine hydrochloride 10 mg per 1 ml Minims tetracaine hydrochloride 1% eye drops 0.5ml unit dose | 20 unit dose PoM £10.57 DT = £10.57

ANALGESICS > NON-STEROIDAL ANTI-INFLAMMATORY DRUGS

Diclofenac sodium

28-Apr-2020

- **INDICATIONS AND DOSE**

Inhibition of intra-operative miosis during cataract surgery (but does not possess intrinsic mydriatic properties) | Postoperative inflammation in cataract surgery, strabismus surgery, argon laser trabeculoplasty

▶ TO THE EYE
▶ Child: (consult product literature)

- **UNLICENSED USE** Not licensed for use in children.
- **INTERACTIONS** → Appendix 1: NSAIDs
- **SIDE-EFFECTS**
▶ **Rare or very rare** Asthma exacerbated · dyspnoea · eye disorders · eye inflammation · hypersensitivity · oedema · skin reactions
▶ **Frequency not known** Eye discomfort · rhinitis · vision blurred
- **ALLERGY AND CROSS-SENSITIVITY** Contra-indicated in patients with a history of hypersensitivity to aspirin or any other NSAID—which includes those in whom attacks of asthma, angioedema, urticaria or rhinitis have been precipitated by aspirin or any other NSAID.
- **PRESCRIBING AND DISPENSING INFORMATION** Although multi-dose diclofenac sodium eye drops commonly contain preservatives, preservative-free unit dose vials may be available.

- **MEDICINAL FORMS** There can be variation in the licensing of different medicines containing the same drug.

Eye drops

EXCIPIENTS: May contain Benzalkonium chloride, disodium edetate, propylene glycol

▶ **Voltarol Ophtha** (Thea Pharmaceuticals Ltd)
Diclofenac sodium 1 mg per 1 ml Voltarol Ophtha 0.1% eye drops 0.3ml unit dose | 5 unit dose [PoM] £4.00 DT = £4.00 | 40 unit dose [PoM] £32.00 DT = £32.00
▶ **Voltarol Ophtha Multidose** (Thea Pharmaceuticals Ltd)
Diclofenac sodium 1 mg per 1 ml Voltarol Ophtha Multidose 0.1% eye drops | 5 ml [PoM] £6.68 DT = £6.68

Flurbiprofen

27-Apr-2020

- **INDICATIONS AND DOSE**

Inhibition of intra-operative miosis (but does not possess intrinsic mydriatic properties) | Control of anterior segment inflammation following postoperative and post-laser trabeculoplasty when corticosteroids contra-indicated

▶ TO THE EYE
▶ Child: (consult product literature)

- **UNLICENSED USE** Not licensed for use in children.
- **INTERACTIONS** → Appendix 1: NSAIDs
- **SIDE-EFFECTS**
▶ **Common or very common** Eye discomfort · haemorrhage
▶ **Frequency not known** Eye disorders
- **ALLERGY AND CROSS-SENSITIVITY** Contra-indicated in patients with a history of hypersensitivity to aspirin or any other NSAID—which includes those in whom attacks of asthma, angioedema, urticaria or rhinitis have been precipitated by aspirin or any other NSAID.

- **MEDICINAL FORMS** There can be variation in the licensing of different medicines containing the same drug.

Eye drops

▶ **Ocufen** (Allergan Ltd)
Flurbiprofen sodium 300 microgram per 1 ml Ocufen 0.03% eye drops 0.4ml unit dose | 40 unit dose [PoM] £37.15 DT = £37.15

Ketorolac trometamol

17-Apr-2020

- **INDICATIONS AND DOSE**

Prophylaxis and reduction of inflammation and associated symptoms following ocular surgery

▶ TO THE EYE
▶ Child: (consult product literature)

- **UNLICENSED USE** Not licensed for use in children.
- **INTERACTIONS** → Appendix 1: NSAIDs
- **SIDE-EFFECTS**
▶ **Common or very common** Eye discomfort · eye disorders · eye infection · eye inflammation · headache · hypersensitivity · keratic deposits · paraesthesia · retinal haemorrhage · vision disorders
▶ **Uncommon** Dry eye
▶ **Frequency not known** Asthma exacerbated · bronchospasm
- **ALLERGY AND CROSS-SENSITIVITY** Contra-indicated in patients with a history of hypersensitivity to aspirin or any other NSAID—which includes those in whom attacks of asthma, angioedema, urticaria or rhinitis have been precipitated by aspirin or any other NSAID.

- **MEDICINAL FORMS** There can be variation in the licensing of different medicines containing the same drug.

Eye drops

EXCIPIENTS: May contain Benzalkonium chloride, disodium edetate

▶ **Ketorolac trometamol (Non-proprietary)**
Ketorolac trometamol 5 mg per 1 ml Ketorolac 0.5% eye drops | 5 ml [PoM] £3.99 DT = £3.99
▶ **Acular** (Allergan Ltd)
Ketorolac trometamol 5 mg per 1 ml Acular 0.5% eye drops | 5 ml [PoM] £3.00 DT = £3.99

5 Glaucoma and ocular hypertension

Glaucoma

Overview

Glaucoma describes a group of disorders characterised by a loss of visual field associated with cupping of the optic disc and optic nerve damage and is generally associated with raised intra-ocular pressure.

Glaucoma is rare in children and should always be managed by a specialist. *Primary congenital glaucoma* is the most common form of glaucoma in children, followed by *secondary glaucomas*, such as following hereditary anterior segment malformations; *juvenile open-angle glaucoma* is less common and usually occurs in older children.

Treatment of glaucoma is determined by the pathophysiology and usually involves controlling raised intra-ocular pressure with surgery. Drug therapy is generally supportive, and can be used temporarily, pre- or post-operatively, or both, to reduce intra-ocular pressure. In secondary glaucomas, drug therapy is often used first-line, and long-term treatment may be required. Drugs that reduce intra-ocular pressure by different mechanisms are available for managing glaucoma. A topical beta-blocker or a prostaglandin analogue can be used. It may be necessary to combine these drugs or add others, such as carbonic anhydrase inhibitors, or miotics to control intra-ocular pressure.

Children with an acute form of glaucoma (usually presenting with pain in older children, a cloudy cornea, and may be associated with a previous history of controlled glaucoma or recent intra-ocular surgery) need immediate referral for specialist ophthalmology assessment and treatment.

Beta-blockers for glaucoma

Topical application of a beta-blocker to the eye reduces intra-ocular pressure effectively in primary and secondary glaucomas, probably by reducing the rate of production of aqueous humour.

Prostaglandin analogues for glaucoma

The prostaglandin analogues latanoprost p. 738, and travoprost, and the synthetic prostamide, bimatoprost, increase uveoscleral outflow and subsequently reduce intra-ocular pressure. They are used to reduce intra-ocular pressure. Only latanoprost (*Xalatan*® and certain non-proprietary preparations of latanoprost) is licensed for use in children. Children receiving prostaglandin analogues should be managed by a specialist.

Sympathomimetics for glaucoma

Apraclonidine p. 739 is an alpha$_2$-adrenoceptor agonist that lowers intra-ocular pressure by reducing aqueous humour formation. Eye drops containing apraclonidine 0.5% are used for a short period to delay laser treatment or surgery for glaucoma in patients not adequately controlled by another drug; eye drops containing 1% are used for control of intra-ocular pressure after anterior segment laser surgery.

Brimonidine tartrate, an alpha$_2$-adrenoceptor agonist, is thought to lower intra-ocular pressure by reducing aqueous humour formation and increasing uveoscleral outflow.

Carbonic anhydrase inhibitors and systemic drugs for glaucoma

The **carbonic anhydrase inhibitors**, acetazolamide p. 735, brinzolamide p. 736, and dorzolamide p. 737, reduce intra-ocular pressure by reducing aqueous humour production. Systemic use of acetazolamide also produces weak diuresis.

Acetazolamide is given by mouth or, rarely in children, by intravenous injection (intramuscular injections are painful because of the alkaline pH of the solution). It is used as an adjunct to other treatment for reducing intra-ocular pressure. Acetazolamide is not generally recommended for long-term use.

Dorzolamide and brinzolamide are topical carbonic anhydrase inhibitors. They are unlicensed in children but are used in those resistant to beta-blockers or those in whom beta-blockers are contra-indicated. They are used alone or as an adjunct to a topical beta-blocker. Brinzolamide can also be used as an adjunct to a prostaglandin analogue. Systemic absorption can rarely cause sulfonamide-like side-effects and may require discontinuation if severe.

Metabolic acidosis can occur in children using topical carbonic anhydrase inhibitors; symptoms may include poor feeding and lack of weight gain.

Miotics for glaucoma

Miotics act by opening up the inefficient drainage channels in the trabecular meshwork. Pilocarpine p. 737 is a miotic used pre- and post-operatively in goniotomy and trabeculotomy; it is used occasionally for aphakic glaucoma.

BETA-ADRENOCEPTOR BLOCKERS

Betaxolol

03-Apr-2020

● **INDICATIONS AND DOSE**

Primary and secondary glaucomas

▶ TO THE EYE

▸ Child: Apply twice daily

● **UNLICENSED USE** Not licensed for use in children.

● **CONTRA-INDICATIONS** Also consider contra-indications listed for systemically administered beta blockers · bradycardia · heart block

● **CAUTIONS** Patients with corneal disease

CAUTIONS, FURTHER INFORMATION Systemic absorption can follow topical application to the eyes; consider cautions listed for systemically administered beta blockers.

● **INTERACTIONS** → Appendix 1: beta blockers, selective

● **SIDE-EFFECTS**

▸ **Common or very common** Eye discomfort · eye disorders · vision disorders

▸ **Uncommon** Dry eye · eye inflammation · rhinitis

▸ **Rare or very rare** Cataract · rhinorrhoea · skin reactions

▸ **Frequency not known** Angioedema · hypersensitivity

SIDE-EFFECTS, FURTHER INFORMATION Systemic absorption can follow topical application to the eyes; consider side effects listed for systemically administered beta blockers.

● **PRESCRIBING AND DISPENSING INFORMATION** Although multi-dose bextaxolol eye drops commonly contain preservatives, preservative-free unit dose vials may be available.

● **MEDICINAL FORMS** There can be variation in the licensing of different medicines containing the same drug.

Eye drops

EXCIPIENTS: May contain Benzalkonium chloride, disodium edetate

▸ Betaxolol (Non-proprietary)

Betaxolol (as Betaxolol hydrochloride) 5 mg per 1 ml Betaxolol 0.5% eye drops | 5 ml [PoM] [NHS] DT = £1.90

▸ Betoptic (Novartis Pharmaceuticals UK Ltd)

Betaxolol (as Betaxolol hydrochloride) 2.5 mg per 1 ml Betoptic 0.25% suspension eye drops | 5 ml [PoM] £2.66 DT = £2.66

Betoptic 0.25% eye drops suspension 0.25ml unit dose | 50 unit dose [PoM] £13.77 DT = £13.77

Betaxolol (as Betaxolol hydrochloride) 5 mg per 1 ml Betoptic 0.5% eye drops | 5 ml [PoM] £1.90 DT = £1.90

Levobunolol hydrochloride

03-Apr-2020

● **INDICATIONS AND DOSE**

Primary and secondary glaucomas

▶ TO THE EYE

▸ Child: Apply 1–2 times a day

● **UNLICENSED USE** Not licensed for use in children.

● **CONTRA-INDICATIONS** Also consider contra-indications listed for systemically administered beta blockers · bradycardia · heart block

● **CAUTIONS** Patients with corneal disease

CAUTIONS, FURTHER INFORMATION Systemic absorption can follow topical application to the eyes; consider cautions listed for systemically administered beta blockers.

● **INTERACTIONS** → Appendix 1: beta blockers, non-selective

● **SIDE-EFFECTS**

▸ **Common or very common** Eye discomfort · eye inflammation

▸ **Frequency not known** Dry eye · eye disorders · vision blurred

Dorzolamide

20-Jan-2020

● **INDICATIONS AND DOSE**

Raised intra-ocular pressure in primary and secondary glaucoma used alone in patients unresponsive to beta-blockers or if beta-blockers contra-indicated

▶ TO THE EYE

▸ Child: Apply 3 times a day

Raised intra-ocular pressure in primary and secondary glaucoma as adjunct to a beta-blocker

▶ TO THE EYE

▸ Child: Apply twice daily

● **UNLICENSED USE** Not licensed for use in children.

● **CONTRA-INDICATIONS** Hyperchloraemic acidosis

● **CAUTIONS** Chronic corneal defects · history of intra-ocular surgery · history of renal calculi · immature renal tubules (neonates and infants)—risk of metabolic acidosis · low endothelial cell count · systemic absorption follows topical application

● **INTERACTIONS** → Appendix 1: dorzolamide

● **SIDE-EFFECTS**

▶ **Common or very common** Asthenia · eye discomfort · eye disorders · eye inflammation · headache · nausea · paraesthesia · taste bitter · vision disorders

▶ **Rare or very rare** Angioedema · bronchospasm · dizziness · dry mouth · dyspnoea · epistaxis · local reaction · pain · severe cutaneous adverse reactions (SCARs) · skin reactions · throat irritation · urolithiasis

SIDE-EFFECTS, FURTHER INFORMATION Systemic absorption can cause sulfonamide-like side-effects and may require discontinuation if severe.

● **ALLERGY AND CROSS-SENSITIVITY** Contra-indicated if history of sulfonamide hypersensitivity.

● **PREGNANCY** Manufacturer advises avoid—toxicity in *animal* studies.

● **BREAST FEEDING** Manufacturer advises avoid—no information available.

● **HEPATIC IMPAIRMENT** Manufacturer advises caution—no information available.

● **RENAL IMPAIRMENT** Avoid if estimated glomerular filtration rate less than 30 mL/minute/1.73 m^2.

● **PRESCRIBING AND DISPENSING INFORMATION** Although multi-dose dorzolamide eye drops commonly contain preservatives, preservative-free unit dose vials may be available.

● **MEDICINAL FORMS** There can be variation in the licensing of different medicines containing the same drug.

Eye drops

EXCIPIENTS: May contain Benzalkonium chloride

▸ **Dorzolamide (Non-proprietary)**

Dorzolamide (as Dorzolamide hydrochloride) 20 mg per 1 ml Dorzolamide 20mg/ml eye drops | 5 ml PoM £5.69 DT = £2.46

▸ **Eydelto** (Aspire Pharma Ltd)

Dorzolamide (as Dorzolamide hydrochloride) 20 mg per 1 ml Eydelto 20mg/ml eye drops | 5 ml PoM £12.09 DT = £12.09

▸ **Trusopt** (Santen UK Ltd)

Dorzolamide (as Dorzolamide hydrochloride) 20 mg per 1 ml Trusopt 20mg/ml eye drops 0.2ml unit dose preservative free | 60 unit dose PoM £24.18 DT = £24.18
Trusopt 20mg/ml eye drops | 5 ml PoM £6.33 DT = £2.46

Dorzolamide with timolol

The properties listed below are those particular to the combination only. For the properties of the components please consider, dorzolamide above, timolol maleate p. 735.

● **INDICATIONS AND DOSE**

Raised intra-ocular pressure in open-angle glaucoma when beta-blockers alone not adequate | Raised intra-ocular pressure in pseudo-exfoliative glaucoma when beta-blockers alone not adequate

▶ TO THE EYE

▸ Child: Apply twice daily

● **INTERACTIONS** → Appendix 1: beta blockers, non-selective · dorzolamide

● **PRESCRIBING AND DISPENSING INFORMATION** Although multi-dose dorzolamide with timolol eye drops commonly contain preservatives, preservative-free unit dose vials may be available.

● **MEDICINAL FORMS** There can be variation in the licensing of different medicines containing the same drug.

Eye drops

EXCIPIENTS: May contain Benzalkonium chloride

▸ **Dorzolamide with timolol (Non-proprietary)**

Timolol (as Timolol maleate) 5 mg per 1 ml, Dorzolamide (as Dorzolamide hydrochloride) 20 mg per 1 ml Dorzolamide 20mg/ml / Timolol 5mg/ml eye drops 0.2ml unit dose preservative free | 60 unit dose PoM £31.99 DT = £28.59
Dorzolamide 20mg/ml / Timolol 5mg/ml eye drops | 5 ml PoM £27.16 DT = £2.33

▸ **Cosopt** (Santen UK Ltd)

Timolol (as Timolol maleate) 5 mg per 1 ml, Dorzolamide (as Dorzolamide hydrochloride) 20 mg per 1 ml Cosopt 20mg/ml / 5mg/ml eye drops 0.2ml unit dose preservative free | 60 unit dose PoM £28.59 DT = £28.59
Cosopt 20mg/ml / 5mg/ml eye drops | 5 ml PoM £10.05 DT = £2.33

▸ **Cosopt iMulti** (Santen UK Ltd)

Timolol (as Timolol maleate) 5 mg per 1 ml, Dorzolamide (as Dorzolamide hydrochloride) 20 mg per 1 ml Cosopt iMulti 20mg/ml / 5mg/ml eye drops preservative free | 10 ml PoM £28.00

▸ **Eylamdo** (Aspire Pharma Ltd)

Timolol (as Timolol maleate) 5 mg per 1 ml, Dorzolamide (as Dorzolamide hydrochloride) 20 mg per 1 ml Eylamdo 20mg/ml / 5mg/ml eye drops | 5 ml PoM £13.99 DT = £14.29

MIOTICS > PARASYMPATHOMIMETICS

Pilocarpine

31-Oct-2019

● **DRUG ACTION** Pilocarpine acts by opening the inefficient drainage channels in the trabecular meshwork.

● **INDICATIONS AND DOSE**

Raised intra-ocular pressure

▶ TO THE EYE

▸ Child 1 month–1 year: Apply 1 drop 3 times a day, doses are for 0.5% or 1% solution

▸ Child 2–17 years: Apply 1 drop 4 times a day

Pre- and postoperatively in goniotomy and trabeculotomy

▶ TO THE EYE

▸ Child: Apply once daily, 1% or 2% solution to be applied

● **UNLICENSED USE** Not licensed for use in children.

● **CONTRA-INDICATIONS** Acute iritis · anterior uveitis · conditions where pupillary constriction is undesirable · some forms of secondary glaucoma (where pupillary constriction is undesirable)

- **CAUTIONS** A darkly pigmented iris may require a higher concentration of the miotic or more frequent administration and care should be taken to avoid overdosage · asthma · cardiac disease · care in conjunctival damage · care in corneal damage · epilepsy · gastro-intestinal spasm · hypertension · hyperthyroidism · hypotension · peptic ulceration · retinal detachment has occurred in susceptible individuals and those with retinal disease · urinary-tract obstruction
- **INTERACTIONS** → Appendix 1: pilocarpine
- **SIDE-EFFECTS**
  - **Common or very common** Diarrhoea · headache · hyperhidrosis · hypersalivation · nausea · skin reactions · vision disorders · vomiting
  - **Frequency not known** Bradycardia · bronchospasm · conjunctival vascular congestion · eye disorder (long term use) · eye disorders · hypotension · lens changes (long term use) · pain · paraesthesia · pulmonary oedema · sensitisation · vitreous haemorrhage
- **PREGNANCY** Avoid unless the potential benefit outweighs risk—limited information available.
- **BREAST FEEDING** Avoid unless the potential benefit outweighs risk—no information available.
- **PRE-TREATMENT SCREENING** Fundus examination is advised before starting treatment with a miotic (retinal detachment has occurred).
- **MONITORING REQUIREMENTS** Intra-ocular pressure and visual fields should be monitored in those with chronic simple glaucoma and those receiving long-term treatment with a miotic.
- **PRESCRIBING AND DISPENSING INFORMATION** Although multi-dose pilocarpine eye drops commonly contain preservatives, preservative-free unit dose vials may be available.
- **PATIENT AND CARER ADVICE**

Driving and skilled tasks Blurred vision may affect performance of skilled tasks (e.g. driving) particularly at night or in reduced lighting.

- **MEDICINAL FORMS** There can be variation in the licensing of different medicines containing the same drug. Forms available from special-order manufacturers include: eye drops

Eye drops

EXCIPIENTS: May contain Benzalkonium chloride

- Pilocarpine (Non-proprietary)
  - **Pilocarpine hydrochloride 10 mg per 1 ml** Pilocarpine hydrochloride 1% eye drops | 10 ml [PoM] £22.20 DT = £22.20
  - **Pilocarpine hydrochloride 20 mg per 1 ml** Pilocarpine hydrochloride 2% eye drops | 10 ml [PoM] £22.79 DT = £22.79
  - **Pilocarpine hydrochloride 40 mg per 1 ml** Pilocarpine hydrochloride 4% eye drops | 10 ml [PoM] £28.40 DT = £28.40
- Pilocarpine nitrate (Bausch & Lomb UK Ltd)
  - **Pilocarpine nitrate 20 mg per 1 ml** Minims pilocarpine nitrate 2% eye drops 0.5ml unit dose | 20 unit dose [PoM] £12.47 DT = £12.47

PROSTAGLANDINS AND ANALOGUES

Latanoprost

20-Apr-2020

- **INDICATIONS AND DOSE**

Reduction of intra-ocular pressure in raised intra-ocular pressure and glaucoma

- TO THE EYE
  - Child: Apply once daily, to be administered preferably in the evening

IMPORTANT SAFETY INFORMATION

MHRA/CHM ADVICE: LATANOPROST (*XALATAN*®): INCREASED REPORTING OF EYE IRRITATION SINCE REFORMULATION (JULY 2015)

Following reformulation of *Xalatan*®, to allow for long-term storage at room temperature, there has been an increase in the number of reports of eye irritation from across the EU. Patients should be advised to tell their health professional promptly (within a week) if they experience eye irritation (e.g. excessive watering) severe enough to make them consider stopping treatment. Review treatment and prescribe a different formulation if necessary.

- **CONTRA-INDICATIONS** Active herpes simplex keratitis · history of recurrent herpetic keratitis associated with prostaglandin analogues
- **CAUTIONS** Aphakia · asthma · children less than 1 year—limited information available · contact lens wearers · do not use within 5 minutes of thiomersal-containing preparations · history of significant ocular viral infections · peri-operative period of cataract surgery · preterm neonates less than 36 weeks gestational age—no information available · pseudophakia with torn posterior lens capsule or anterior chamber lenses · risk factors for cystoid macular oedema · risk factors for iritis · risk factors for uveitis
- **SIDE-EFFECTS**
  - **Common or very common** Eye discolouration · eye discomfort · eye disorders · eye inflammation · vision disorders
  - **Uncommon** Dry eye · rash
  - **Rare or very rare** Asthma · chest pain · dyspnoea · unstable angina
  - **Frequency not known** Arthralgia · dizziness · headache · myalgia · ophthalmic herpes simplex · palpitations
- **PREGNANCY** Manufacturer advises avoid.
- **BREAST FEEDING** May be present in milk—manufacturer advises avoid.
- **MONITORING REQUIREMENTS** Monitor for changes to eye coloration.
- **PRESCRIBING AND DISPENSING INFORMATION** Although multi-dose latanoprost eye drops commonly contain preservatives, preservative-free unit dose vials may be available.
- **PATIENT AND CARER ADVICE**

Changes in eye colour Before initiating treatment, patients should be warned of a possible change in eye colour as an increase in the brown pigment in the iris can occur, which may be permanent; particular care is required in those with mixed coloured irides and those receiving treatment to one eye only. Changes in eyelashes and vellus hair can also occur, and patients should also be advised to avoid repeated contact of the eye drop solution with skin as this can lead to hair growth or skin pigmentation.

- **NATIONAL FUNDING/ACCESS DECISIONS**

MONOPOST® **Scottish Medicines Consortium (SMC) decisions**

The *Scottish Medicines Consortium* has advised (July 2013) that *Monopost*® is accepted for restricted use within NHS Scotland for the reduction of elevated intra-ocular pressure in patients with open-angle glaucoma and ocular hypertension who have proven sensitivity to benzalkonium chloride.

- **MEDICINAL FORMS** There can be variation in the licensing of different medicines containing the same drug.

Eye drops

EXCIPIENTS: May contain Benzalkonium chloride

- Latanoprost (Non-proprietary)
  - **Latanoprost 50 microgram per 1 ml** Latanoprost 50micrograms/ml eye drops | 2.5 ml [PoM] £12.48 DT = £4.05
- Medizol (Medicom Healthcare Ltd)
  - **Latanoprost 50 microgram per 1 ml** Medizol 0.005% eye drops | 2.5 ml [PoM] [X] DT = £4.05

- Monopost (Thea Pharmaceuticals Ltd)
  Latanoprost 50 microgram per 1 ml Monopost 50micrograms/ml eye drops 0.2ml unit dose | 30 unit dose PoM £8.49 DT = £8.49 | 90 unit dose PoM £25.47 DT = £25.47
- Xalatan (Upjohn UK Ltd)
  Latanoprost 50 microgram per 1 ml Xalatan 50micrograms/ml eye drops | 2.5 ml PoM £12.48 DT = £4.05

SYMPATHOMIMETICS › ALPHA$_2$-ADRENOCEPTOR AGONISTS

Apraclonidine

03-Apr-2020

- **DRUG ACTION** Apraclonidine is an alpha$_2$-adrenoceptor agonist that lowers intra-ocular pressure by reducing aqueous humour formation. It is a derivative of clonidine.

- **INDICATIONS AND DOSE**

Control or prevention of postoperative elevation of intra-ocular pressure after anterior segment laser surgery

▸ TO THE EYE

- Child: Apply 1 drop, 1 hour before laser procedure, then 1 drop, immediately after completion of procedure, 1% eye drops to be administered

Short-term adjunctive treatment of chronic glaucoma in patients not adequately controlled by another drug

▸ TO THE EYE

- Child 12–17 years: Apply 1 drop 3 times a day usually for maximum 1 month, 0.5% eye drops to be administered, may not provide additional benefit if patient already using two drugs that suppress the production of aqueous humour

- **UNLICENSED USE** 1% drops are not licensed for use in children.
- **CONTRA-INDICATIONS** History of severe or unstable and uncontrolled cardiovascular disease
- **CAUTIONS** Cerebrovascular disease · depression · heart failure · history of angina · hypertension · loss of effect may occur over time · Raynaud's syndrome · recent myocardial infarction · reduction in vision in end-stage glaucoma (suspend treatment) · severe coronary insufficiency · thromboangiitis obliterans · vasovagal attack
- **INTERACTIONS** → Appendix 1: apraclonidine
- **SIDE-EFFECTS**

▸ **Common or very common** Eye disorders

▸ **Uncommon** Bradycardia · conjunctival haemorrhage · diarrhoea · dry eye · eye discomfort · eye inflammation · gastrointestinal discomfort · irritability · libido decreased · nasal dryness · palpitations · postural hypotension · sensation abnormal · sleep disorders · syncope · vision disorders · vomiting

▸ **Rare or very rare** Chest pain · dry mouth · fatigue · headache · hyperhidrosis · pain in extremity · pruritus · taste altered · temperature sensation altered

SIDE-EFFECTS, FURTHER INFORMATION Since absorption may follow topical application, systemic effects may occur– see clonidine hydrochloride p. 108.

Ocular intolerance Manufacturer advises withdrawal if eye pruritus, ocular hyperaemia, increased lacrimation, or oedema of the eyelids and conjunctiva occur.

- **PREGNANCY** Manufacturer advises avoid—no information available.
- **BREAST FEEDING** Manufacturer advises avoid—no information available.
- **HEPATIC IMPAIRMENT** Manufacturer advises use with caution and monitor, including close monitoring of cardiovascular parameters—no information available.
- **RENAL IMPAIRMENT** Use with caution in chronic renal failure.
- **MONITORING REQUIREMENTS**

▸ Monitor intra-ocular pressure and visual fields.

▸ Monitor for excessive reduction in intra-ocular pressure following peri-operative use.

- **PATIENT AND CARER ADVICE**

Driving and skilled tasks Drowsiness may affect performance of skilled tasks (e.g. driving).

- **MEDICINAL FORMS** There can be variation in the licensing of different medicines containing the same drug.

Eye drops

EXCIPIENTS: May contain Benzalkonium chloride

- Iopidine (Novartis Pharmaceuticals UK Ltd)
  Apraclonidine (as Apraclonidine hydrochloride) 5 mg per 1 ml Iopidine 5mg/ml eye drops | 5 ml PoM £10.88 DT = £10.88
  Apraclonidine (as Apraclonidine hydrochloride) 10 mg per 1 ml Iopidine 1% eye drops 0.25ml unit dose | 24 unit dose PoM £77.85 DT = £77.85

6 Retinal disorders

6.1 Optic neuropathy

DRUGS FOR METABOLIC DISORDERS › ANTIOXIDANTS

Idebenone

10-Mar-2020

- **DRUG ACTION** Idebenone is a nootropic and antioxidant that is thought to act by restoring cellular ATP generation, thereby reactivating retinal ganglion cells.

- **INDICATIONS AND DOSE**

Leber's Hereditary Optic Neuropathy (initiated by a specialist)

▸ BY MOUTH

- Child 12–17 years: 300 mg 3 times a day

- **SIDE-EFFECTS**

▸ **Common or very common** Cough · diarrhoea · increased risk of infection · pain

▸ **Frequency not known** Agranulocytosis · anaemia · anxiety · appetite decreased · azotaemia · delirium · dizziness · dyspepsia · hallucination · headache · hepatitis · leucopenia · malaise · movement disorders · nausea · neutropenia · poriomania · seizure · skin reactions · stupor · thrombocytopenia · urine discolouration · vomiting

SIDE-EFFECTS, FURTHER INFORMATION The metabolites of idebenone may cause red-brown discolouration of the urine. This effect is harmless, but the manufacturer advises caution as this may mask colour changes due to other causes (e.g. renal or blood disorders).

- **PREGNANCY** Manufacturer advises avoid unless potential benefit outweighs risk—no information available.
- **BREAST FEEDING** Manufacturer advises avoid—present in milk in *animal* studies.
- **HEPATIC IMPAIRMENT** Manufacturer advises caution (no information available).
- **RENAL IMPAIRMENT** Manufacturer advises use with caution—no information available.
- **PATIENT AND CARER ADVICE**

Medicines for Children leaflet: Idebenone for Friedreich's ataxia www.medicinesforchildren.org.uk/idebenone-friedreich's-ataxia

● **NATIONAL FUNDING/ACCESS DECISIONS**

Scottish Medicines Consortium (SMC) decisions

The *Scottish Medicines Consortium* has advised (May 2017) that idebenone (*Raxone*®) is accepted for restricted use within NHS Scotland for the treatment of visual impairment in patients with Leber's Hereditary Optic Neuropathy (LHON) who are not yet blind i.e. they do not meet the UK criteria to be registered as severely sight impaired. This advice is contingent upon the continuing availability of the Patient Access Scheme in NHS Scotland or a list price that is equivalent or lower.

● **MEDICINAL FORMS** There can be variation in the licensing of different medicines containing the same drug. Forms available from special-order manufacturers include: tablet

Tablet

CAUTIONARY AND ADVISORY LABELS 14, 21

▸ **Raxone** (Chiesi Ltd) ▼

Idebenone 150 mg Raxone 150mg tablets | 180 tablet PoM
£6,364.00 DT = £6,364.00

Chapter 12
Ear, nose and oropharynx

CONTENTS

Ear

Ear

03-Sep-2018

Otitis externa

Otitis externa is an inflammatory reaction of the lining of the ear canal usually associated with an underlying seborrhoeic dermatitis or eczema; it is important to exclude an underlying chronic otitis media before treatment is commenced. Many cases recover after thorough cleansing of the external ear canal by suction or dry mopping.

A frequent problem in resistant cases is the difficulty in applying lotions and ointments satisfactorily to the relatively inaccessible affected skin. The most effective method is to introduce a ribbon gauze dressing or sponge wick soaked with **corticosteroid** ear drops or with an astringent such as aluminium acetate solution p. 746. When this is not practical, the ear should be gently cleansed with a probe covered in cotton wool and the patient encouraged to lie with the affected ear uppermost for ten minutes after the canal has been filled with a liberal quantity of the appropriate solution.

Secondary infection in otitis externa may be of bacterial, fungal, or viral origin. If infection is present, a topical anti-infective which is not used systemically (such as neomycin sulfate p. 743 or **clioquinol**) may be used, but for only about a week because excessive use may result in fungal infections that are difficult to treat. Sensitivity to the anti-infective or solvent may occur and resistance to antibacterials is a possibility with prolonged use. Aluminium acetate ear drops are also effective against bacterial infection and inflammation of the ear. Chloramphenicol p. 744 may be used, but the ear drops contain propylene glycol and cause hypersensitivity reactions in about 10% of patients. Solutions containing an anti-infective and a corticosteroid are used for treating children when infection is present with inflammation and eczema. Clotrimazole 1% solution p. 744 is used topically to treat fungal infection in otitis externa.

In view of reports of ototoxicity, manufacturers contra-indicate treatment with topical **aminoglycosides** or **polymyxins** in children with a perforated tympanic membrane (eardrum) or patent grommet. However, some specialists do use these drops cautiously in the presence of a perforation or patent grommet in children with chronic suppurative otitis media and when other measures have failed for otitis externa; treatment should be considered only **by specialists** in the following circumstances:

- drops should only be used in the presence of obvious infection;
- treatment should be for no longer than 2 weeks;
- the carer and child should be counselled on the risk of ototoxicity and given justification for the use of these topical antibiotics;
- baseline audiometry should be performed, if possible, before treatment is commenced.

Clinical expertise and judgement should be used to assess the risk of treatment versus the benefit to the patient in such circumstances.

A solution of **acetic acid** 2% acts as an antifungal and antibacterial in the external ear canal. It may be used to treat mild otitis externa but in severe cases an anti-inflammatory preparation with or without an anti-infective drug is required. A proprietary preparation containing acetic acid 2% (*EarCalm*® spray) is on sale to the public for children over 12 years.

For severe pain associated with otitis externa, a simple analgesic, such as paracetamol p. 288 or ibuprofen p. 707, can be used. A systemic antibacterial can be used if there is spreading cellulitis or if the patient is systemically unwell. When a resistant staphylococcal infection (a boil) is present in the external auditory meatus, flucloxacillin p. 373 is the drug of choice; oral ciprofloxacin p. 377 or a systemic aminoglycoside may be needed for pseudomonal infections, particularly in children with diabetes or compromised immunity.

The skin of the pinna adjacent to the ear canal is often affected by eczema. Topical corticosteroid creams and ointments are then required, but prolonged use should be avoided.

Otitis media

Acute otitis media

Acute otitis media is a self-limiting condition that mainly affects children. It is characterised by inflammation in the middle ear associated with effusion and accompanied by the rapid onset of signs and symptoms of an ear infection. The infection can be caused by viruses or bacteria; often both are present simultaneously.

Children with acute otitis media usually present with symptoms such as ear pain, rubbing of the ear, fever, irritability, crying, poor feeding, restlessness at night, cough, or rhinorrhoea. Symptoms usually improve within 3 to 7 days without antibacterial drugs. The use of antibacterials generally does not prevent common complications of acute otitis media such as short-term hearing loss, perforated eardrum, or recurrent infection. Acute complications such as mastoiditis, meningitis, intracranial abscess, sinus thrombosis, and facial nerve paralysis, are rare.

EvGr Children and their carers should be given advice about the usual duration of acute otitis media, self-care of symptoms such as pain and fever with paracetamol or ibuprofen p. 707, and when to seek medical help. In children aged 3 years and over who do not have a perforated eardrum, pain can be relieved with anaesthetic ear drops in addition to oral analgesics [unlicensed use]. Children and their carers should be reassured that antibacterial drugs are usually not required.

An immediate antibacterial drug should be given if the child is systemically very unwell, has signs or symptoms of a more serious illness, or is at high risk of complications such as significant heart, lung, renal, liver or neuromuscular disease, immunosuppression, cystic fibrosis, and young children who were born prematurely. An immediate antibacterial drug can also be considered if otorrhoea is present, or in children under 2 years of age with bilateral otitis media. See *Antibacterial therapy for otitis media* in Ear infections, antibacterial therapy p. 324.

Children with acute otitis media associated with a severe systemic infection or acute complications should be referred to hospital. (A)

Otitis media with effusion

Otitis media with effusion (glue ear) occurs in about 10% of children and in 90% of children with cleft palates. Antimicrobials, corticosteroids, decongestants, and antihistamines have little place in the routine management of otitis media with effusion. If glue ear persists for more than a month or two, the child should be referred for assessment and follow up because of the risk of long-term hearing impairment which can delay language development. Untreated or resistant glue ear may be responsible for some types of *chronic otitis media*.

Chronic otitis media

Opportunistic organisms are often present in the debris, keratin, and necrotic bone of the middle ear and mastoid in children with chronic otitis media. The mainstay of treatment is thorough cleansing with aural microsuction, which may completely resolve long-standing infection. Cleansing may be followed by topical treatment as for otitis externa; this is particularly beneficial for discharging ears or infections of the mastoid cavity. Acute exacerbations of chronic infection may require treatment with an oral antibacterial; a swab should be taken to identify infecting organisms and antibacterial sensitivity.

In view of reports of ototoxicity, manufacturers contraindicate topical treatment with ototoxic antibacterials in the presence of a tympanic perforation or patent grommet. Ciprofloxacin p. 743 or ofloxacin eye drops p. 729 used in the ear [unlicensed use] or ear drops [both unlicensed; available from 'special-order' manufacturers or specialist importing companies] are an effective alternative to such ototoxic ear drops for chronic otitis media in patients with perforation of the tympanic membrane.

However, some specialists do use ear drops containing **aminoglycosides** or **polymyxins** [unlicensed indications] cautiously in children with chronic suppurative otitis media and perforation of the tympanic membrane, if the otitis media has failed to settle with systemic antibacterials; treatment should be considered only **by specialists** in the following circumstances:

- drops should only be used in the presence of obvious infection;
- treatment should be for no longer than 2 weeks;
- the carer and child should be counselled on the risk of ototoxicity and given justification for the use of these topical antibiotics;
- baseline audiometry should be performed, if possible, before treatment is commenced.

Clinical expertise and judgement should be used to assess the risk of treatment versus the benefit to the patient in such circumstances. It is considered that the pus in the middle ear associated with otitis media also carries a risk of ototoxicity.

Removal of ear wax

Ear wax (cerumen) is a normal bodily secretion which provides a protective film on the meatal skin and need only be removed if it causes hearing loss or interferes with a proper view of the ear drum.

Ear wax causing discomfort or impaired hearing may be softened using simple remedies such as **olive oil** ear drops or **almond oil** ear drops; sodium bicarbonate ear drops p. 746 are also effective, but may cause dryness of the ear canal. If the wax is hard and impacted, the drops can be used twice daily for several days and this may reduce the need for mechanical removal of the wax. The child should lie with the affected ear uppermost for 5 to 10 minutes after a generous amount of the softening remedy has been introduced into the ear. Proprietary preparations containing organic solvents can irritate the meatal skin, and in most cases the simple remedies indicated above are just as effective and less likely to cause irritation. Docusate sodium p. 747 or urea hydrogen peroxide p. 747 are ingredients in a number of proprietary preparations for softening ear wax.

If necessary, wax may be removed by irrigation with water (warmed to body temperature). Ear irrigation is generally best avoided in young children, in children unable to co-operate with the procedure, in children who have had otitis media in the last six weeks, in otitis externa, in children with cleft palate, a history of ear drum perforation, or previous ear surgery. A child who has hearing in one ear only should not have that ear irrigated because even a very slight risk of damage is unacceptable in this situation.

Administration

To administer ear drops, lay the child down with the head turned to one side; for an infant pull the earlobe back and down, for an older child pull the earlobe back and up.

1 Otitis externa

ANTIBACTERIALS > AMINOGLYCOSIDES

Framycetin sulfate

- **INDICATIONS AND DOSE**

Bacterial infection in otitis externa

▶ TO THE EAR

▸ Child: (consult product literature)

- **CONTRA-INDICATIONS** Perforated tympanic membrane
- **CAUTIONS** Avoid prolonged use
- **MEDICINAL FORMS** No licensed medicines listed.

Combinations available: *Dexamethasone with framycetin sulfate and gramicidin*, p. 746

332

Gentamicin

19-Mar-2020

● **INDICATIONS AND DOSE**

Bacterial infection in otitis externa

▶ TO THE EAR

▸ Child: Apply 2–3 drops 4–5 times a day, (including a dose at bedtime)

● **UNLICENSED USE** Gentamicin doses in BNF publications may differ from those in product literature.

● **CONTRA-INDICATIONS** Patent grommet (although may be used by specialists, see Ear p. 741) · perforated tympanic membrane (although may be used by specialists, see Ear p. 741)

● **CAUTIONS** Avoid prolonged use

● **INTERACTIONS** → Appendix 1: aminoglycosides

● **MEDICINAL FORMS** There can be variation in the licensing of different medicines containing the same drug. Forms available from special-order manufacturers include: eye drops

Ear/eye drops solution

EXCIPIENTS: May contain Benzalkonium chloride

▸ **Gentamicin (Non-proprietary)**
Gentamicin (as Gentamicin sulfate) 3 mg per 1 ml Gentamicin 0.3% ear/eye drops | 10 ml PoM £2.85 DT = £2.86

Gentamicin with hydrocortisone

13-Mar-2020

● **INDICATIONS AND DOSE**

Eczematous inflammation in otitis externa

▶ TO THE EAR

▸ Child: Apply 2–4 drops 4–5 times a day, (including a dose at bedtime)

IMPORTANT SAFETY INFORMATION

MHRA/CHM ADVICE: CORTICOSTEROIDS: RARE RISK OF CENTRAL SEROUS CHORIORETINOPATHY WITH LOCAL AS WELL AS SYSTEMIC ADMINISTRATION (AUGUST 2017)

See Corticosteroids, general use p. 470.

● **CONTRA-INDICATIONS** Patent grommet (although may be used by specialists, see Ear p. 741) · perforated tympanic membrane (although may be used by specialists, see Ear p. 741)

● **CAUTIONS** Avoid prolonged use

● **SIDE-EFFECTS** Local reaction

● **PATIENT AND CARER ADVICE**
Medicines for Children leaflet: Gentamicin and hydrocortisone ear drops for inflammatory ear infections
www.medicinesforchildren.org.uk/gentamicin-and-hydrocortisone-ear-drops-inflammatory-ear-infections

● **MEDICINAL FORMS** There can be variation in the licensing of different medicines containing the same drug.

Ear drops

EXCIPIENTS: May contain Benzalkonium chloride, disodium edetate

▸ **Gentamicin with hydrocortisone (Non-proprietary)**
Gentamicin (as Gentamicin sulfate) 3 mg per 1 ml, Hydrocortisone acetate 10 mg per 1 ml Gentamicin 0.3% / Hydrocortisone acetate 1% ear drops | 10 ml PoM £33.26 DT = £33.26

Neomycin sulfate

● **INDICATIONS AND DOSE**

Bacterial infection in otitis externa

▶ TO THE EAR

▸ Child: (consult product literature)

● **CONTRA-INDICATIONS** Patent grommet (although may be used by specialists, see Ear p. 741) · perforated tympanic membrane (although may be used by specialists, see Ear p. 741)

● **CAUTIONS** Avoid prolonged use

● **INTERACTIONS** → Appendix 1: neomycin

● **SIDE-EFFECTS** Local reaction

● **MEDICINAL FORMS** No licensed medicines listed.

Combinations available: ***Betamethasone with neomycin,*** p. 745 · ***Dexamethasone with glacial acetic acid and neomycin sulfate,*** p. 746 · ***Hydrocortisone with neomycin and polymyxin B sulfate,*** p. 746

ANTIBACTERIALS › QUINOLONES

376

Ciprofloxacin

17-Apr-2020

● **INDICATIONS AND DOSE**

Acute otitis externa

▶ TO THE EAR

▸ Child 1–17 years: Apply 0.25 mL twice daily for 7 days, each 0.25 mL dose contains 0.5 mg ciprofloxacin

● **CAUTIONS** Known (or at risk of) perforated tympanic membrane

● **INTERACTIONS** → Appendix 1: quinolones

● **SIDE-EFFECTS**

▶ **Uncommon** Ear pruritus

● **PRESCRIBING AND DISPENSING INFORMATION** For choice of antibacterial therapy, see Ear infections, antibacterial therapy p. 324.

● **HANDLING AND STORAGE** Manufacturer advises discard any ampoules remaining 8 days after opening the pouch.

● **PATIENT AND CARER ADVICE**
Medicines for Children leaflet: Ciprofloxacin drops for infection
www.medicinesforchildren.org.uk/ciprofloxacin-drops-infection

● **NATIONAL FUNDING/ACCESS DECISIONS**

Scottish Medicines Consortium (SMC) decisions

SMC No. 1320/18

The *Scottish Medicines Consortium* has advised (April 2018) that ciprofloxacin ear drops (*Cetraxal*®) are recommended for use within NHS Scotland for treatment of acute otitis externa in adults and children over 1 year with an intact tympanic membrane, caused by ciprofloxacin susceptible microorganisms when off-label or unlicensed ciprofloxacin formulations would otherwise be used.

All Wales Medicines Strategy Group (AWMSG) decisions

AWMSG No. 1343

The *All Wales Medicines Strategy Group* has advised (July 2018) that ciprofloxacin (*Cetraxal*®) is recommended as an option for use within NHS Wales for the treatment of acute otitis externa in adults and children older than 1 year with an intact tympanic membrane, caused by ciprofloxacin susceptible microorganisms.

● **MEDICINAL FORMS** There can be variation in the licensing of different medicines containing the same drug. Forms available from special-order manufacturers include: ear drops

Ear drops

▸ **Cetraxal** (Aspire Pharma Ltd)
Ciprofloxacin (as Ciprofloxacin hydrochloride) 2 mg per 1 ml Cetraxal 2mg/ml ear drops 0.25ml unit dose | 15 unit dose PoM £6.01 DT = £6.01

Combinations available: ***Ciprofloxacin with dexamethasone,*** p. 745 · ***Ciprofloxacin with fluocinolone acetonide,*** p. 745

ANTIBACTERIALS > OTHER

Chloramphenicol

13-May-2020

- **DRUG ACTION** Chloramphenicol is a potent broad-spectrum antibiotic.

- **INDICATIONS AND DOSE**

Bacterial infection in otitis externa

▶ TO THE EAR

▸ Child: Apply 2–3 drops 2–3 times a day

- **CAUTIONS** Avoid prolonged use
- **INTERACTIONS** → Appendix 1: chloramphenicol
- **SIDE-EFFECTS** Blood disorder · bone marrow depression
- **PATIENT AND CARER ADVICE** Medicines for Children leaflet: Chloramphenicol ear drops for ear infections (otitis externa) www.medicinesforchildren.org.uk/chloramphenicol-ear-drops-ear-infections-otitis-externa-0
- **LESS SUITABLE FOR PRESCRIBING** Chloramphenicol ear drops are less suitable for prescribing.

- **MEDICINAL FORMS** There can be variation in the licensing of different medicines containing the same drug.

Ear drops

EXCIPIENTS: May contain Propylene glycol

▸ Chloramphenicol (Non-proprietary)
Chloramphenicol 50 mg per 1 ml Chloramphenicol 5% ear drops | 10 ml PoM £97.69 DT = £97.69
Chloramphenicol 100 mg per 1 ml Chloramphenicol 10% ear drops | 10 ml PoM £94.26 DT = £90.03

ANTIFUNGALS > IMIDAZOLE ANTIFUNGALS

Clotrimazole

10-Mar-2020

- **INDICATIONS AND DOSE**

Fungal infection in otitis externa

▶ TO THE EAR

▸ Child: Apply 2–3 times a day continue for at least 14 days after disappearance of infection

- **INTERACTIONS** → Appendix 1: antifungals, azoles
- **SIDE-EFFECTS** Hypersensitivity · oedema · pain · paraesthesia · skin reactions
- **PATIENT AND CARER ADVICE** Medicines for Children leaflet: Clotrimazole for fungal infections www.medicinesforchildren.org.uk/clotrimazole-fungal-infections

- **MEDICINAL FORMS** There can be variation in the licensing of different medicines containing the same drug.

Liquid

▸ Canesten (clotrimazole) (Bayer Plc)
Clotrimazole 10 mg per 1 ml Canesten 1% solution | 20 ml P £2.53 DT = £2.53

CORTICOSTEROIDS

F 472

Betamethasone

28-Nov-2019

- **INDICATIONS AND DOSE**

BETNESOL®

Eczematous inflammation in otitis externa

▶ TO THE EAR

▸ Child: Apply 2–3 drops every 2–3 hours, reduce frequency when relief obtained

VISTAMETHASONE®

Eczematous inflammation in otitis externa

▶ TO THE EAR

▸ Child: Apply 2–3 drops every 3–4 hours, reduce frequency when relief obtained

- **CONTRA-INDICATIONS** Avoid alone in the presence of untreated infection (combine with suitable anti-infective)
- **CAUTIONS** Avoid prolonged use
- **INTERACTIONS** → Appendix 1: corticosteroids

- **MEDICINAL FORMS** There can be variation in the licensing of different medicines containing the same drug.

Ear/eye/nose drops solution

EXCIPIENTS: May contain Benzalkonium chloride, disodium edetate

▸ Betnesol (RPH Pharmaceuticals AB)
Betamethasone sodium phosphate 1 mg per 1 ml Betnesol 0.1% eye/ear/nose drops | 10 ml PoM £2.32 DT = £2.32

▸ Vistamethasone (Martindale Pharmaceuticals Ltd)
Betamethasone sodium phosphate 1 mg per 1 ml Vistamethasone 0.1% ear/eye/nose drops | 5 ml PoM £1.02 | 10 ml PoM £1.16 DT = £2.32

Combinations available: *Betamethasone with neomycin*, p. 745

Flumetasone pivalate with clioquinol

21-Dec-2017

- **INDICATIONS AND DOSE**

Eczematous inflammation in otitis externa | Mild bacterial or fungal infections in otitis externa

▶ TO THE EAR

▸ Child 2-17 years: 2–3 drops twice daily for 7–10 days, to be instilled into the ear

IMPORTANT SAFETY INFORMATION

MHRA/CHM ADVICE: CORTICOSTEROIDS: RARE RISK OF CENTRAL SEROUS CHORIORETINOPATHY WITH LOCAL AS WELL AS SYSTEMIC ADMINISTRATION (AUGUST 2017)

See Corticosteroids, general use p. 470.

- **CONTRA-INDICATIONS** Iodine sensitivity
- **CAUTIONS** Avoid prolonged use · manufacturer advises avoid in perforated tympanic membrane (but used by specialists for short periods)
- **SIDE-EFFECTS** Paraesthesia · skin reactions
- **PATIENT AND CARER ADVICE** Clioquinol stains skin and clothing

- **MEDICINAL FORMS** There can be variation in the licensing of different medicines containing the same drug.

Ear drops

▸ Flumetasone pivalate with clioquinol (Non-proprietary)
Flumetasone pivalate 200 microgram per 1 ml, Clioquinol 10 mg per 1 ml Flumetasone 0.02% / Clioquinol 1% ear drops | 7.5 ml PoM £11.34 DT = £11.34 | 10 ml PoM £15.13 DT = £15.13

F 472

Prednisolone

29-Nov-2019

- **INDICATIONS AND DOSE**

Eczematous inflammation in otitis externa

▶ TO THE EAR

▸ Child: Apply 2–3 drops every 2–3 hours, frequency to be reduced when relief obtained

- **CONTRA-INDICATIONS** Avoid alone in the presence of untreated infection (combine with suitable anti-infective)
- **CAUTIONS** Avoid prolonged use
- **INTERACTIONS** → Appendix 1: corticosteroids
- **SIDE-EFFECTS** Local reaction

- **MEDICINAL FORMS** There can be variation in the licensing of different medicines containing the same drug. Forms available from special-order manufacturers include: ear drops

Ear/eye drops solution

EXCIPIENTS: May contain Benzalkonium chloride, disodium edetate

- Prednisolone (Non-proprietary)
  Prednisolone sodium phosphate 5 mg per 1 ml Prednisolone sodium phosphate 0.5% ear/eye drops | 10 ml PoM £2.57 DT = £2.57

CORTICOSTEROIDS > CORTICOSTEROID COMBINATIONS WITH ANTI-INFECTIVES

Betamethasone with neomycin

The properties listed below are those particular to the combination only. For the properties of the components please consider, betamethasone p. 744, neomycin sulfate p. 743.

- **INDICATIONS AND DOSE**

Eczematous inflammation in otitis externa

- TO THE EAR USING EAR DROPS
- Child: Apply 2–3 drops 3–4 times a day

- **CONTRA-INDICATIONS** Patent grommet (although may be used by specialists, see Ear p. 741) · perforated tympanic membrane (although may be used by specialists, see Ear p. 741)
- **CAUTIONS** Avoid prolonged use
- **INTERACTIONS** → Appendix 1: corticosteroids · neomycin

- **MEDICINAL FORMS** There can be variation in the licensing of different medicines containing the same drug.

Ear/eye/nose drops solution

EXCIPIENTS: May contain Benzalkonium chloride, disodium edetate

- Betnesol-N (RPH Pharmaceuticals AB)
  Betamethasone (as Betamethasone sodium phosphate) 1 mg per 1 ml, Neomycin sulfate 5 mg per 1 ml Betnesol-N ear/eye/nose drops | 10 ml PoM £2.39 DT = £2.39

Ciprofloxacin with dexamethasone

21-Dec-2017

The properties listed below are those particular to the combination only. For the properties of the components please consider, dexamethasone p. 475, ciprofloxacin p. 743.

- **INDICATIONS AND DOSE**

Acute otitis media in patients with tympanostomy tubes

- TO THE EAR
- Child 6 months–17 years: Apply 4 drops twice daily for 7 days

Acute otitis externa

- TO THE EAR
- Child 1–17 years: Apply 4 drops twice daily for 7 days

- **CONTRA-INDICATIONS** Fungal ear infections · viral ear infections
- **CAUTIONS** Avoid prolonged use
- **INTERACTIONS** → Appendix 1: corticosteroids · quinolones
- **SIDE-EFFECTS**
- **Common or very common** Ear discomfort
- **Uncommon** Ear infection fungal · flushing · irritability · malaise · otorrhoea · paraesthesia · skin reactions · taste altered · vomiting
- **Rare or very rare** Dizziness · headache · hearing loss · tinnitus

SIDE-EFFECTS, FURTHER INFORMATION Manufacturer advises further evaluation of underlying conditions if otorrhoea persists after a full course, or if at least two episodes of otorrhoea occur within 6 months.

- **PREGNANCY** Manufacturer advises use only if potential benefit outweighs risk—no information available.
- **BREAST FEEDING** Manufacturer advises caution—no information available.
- **PATIENT AND CARER ADVICE** Manufacturer advises counselling on administration.
- **NATIONAL FUNDING/ACCESS DECISIONS**

Scottish Medicines Consortium (SMC) decisions

The *Scottish Medicines Consortium* has advised (July 2017) that dexamethasone with ciprofloxacin (*Cilodex*®) is accepted for restricted use within NHS Scotland for the treatment of acute otitis media in patients with tympanostomy tubes (AOMT).

- **MEDICINAL FORMS** There can be variation in the licensing of different medicines containing the same drug.

Ear drops

EXCIPIENTS: May contain Benzalkonium chloride, disodium edetate

- Cilodex (Consilient Health Ltd)
  Dexamethasone 1 mg per 1 ml, Ciprofloxacin (as Ciprofloxacin hydrochloride) 3 mg per 1 ml Cilodex ear drops | 5 ml PoM £6.12 DT = £6.12

Ciprofloxacin with fluocinolone acetonide

08-Dec-2018

The properties listed below are those particular to the combination only. For the properties of the components please consider, ciprofloxacin p. 743.

- **INDICATIONS AND DOSE**

Acute otitis externa | Acute otitis media in patients with tympanostomy tubes

- TO THE EAR
- Child 6 months–17 years: Apply 0.25 mL twice daily for 7 days

DOSE EQUIVALENCE AND CONVERSION

- Each 0.25 mL dose contains 0.75 mg ciprofloxacin and 0.0625 mg of fluocinolone acetonide.

> **IMPORTANT SAFETY INFORMATION**
>
> MHRA/CHM ADVICE: CORTICOSTEROIDS: RARE RISK OF CENTRAL SEROUS CHORIORETINOPATHY WITH LOCAL AS WELL AS SYSTEMIC ADMINISTRATION (AUGUST 2017)
>
> See Corticosteroids, general use p. 470.

- **CONTRA-INDICATIONS** Fungal ear infections · viral ear infections
- **INTERACTIONS** → Appendix 1: fluocinolone · quinolones
- **SIDE-EFFECTS**
- **Common or very common** Ear discomfort · taste altered
- **Uncommon** Crying · dizziness · fatigue · flushing · headache · hearing impairment · increased risk of infection · irritability · otorrhoea · paraesthesia · skin reactions · tinnitus · tympanic membrane disorder · vomiting

SIDE-EFFECTS, FURTHER INFORMATION Manufacturer advises further evaluation of underlying conditions if otorrhoea persists after a full course, or if at least two episodes of otorrhoea occur within 6 months.

- **PREGNANCY** Manufacturer advises use only if potential benefit outweighs risk—limited information available.
- **BREAST FEEDING** Manufacturer advises caution.
- **PATIENT AND CARER ADVICE** Manufacturer advises counselling on administration.

● MEDICINAL FORMS There can be variation in the licensing of different medicines containing the same drug.

Ear drops

EXCIPIENTS: May contain Polysorbates

▸ Cetraxal Plus (Aspire Pharma Ltd)

Fluocinolone acetonide.25 mg per 1 ml, Ciprofloxacin (as Ciprofloxacin hydrochloride) 3 mg per 1 ml Cetraxal Plus 3mg/ml + 0.25mg/ml ear drops 0.25ml unit dose | 15 unit dose PoM £6.01 DT = £6.01

Dexamethasone with framycetin sulfate and gramicidin

21-Dec-2017

The properties listed below are those particular to the combination only. For the properties of the components please consider, dexamethasone p. 475, framycetin sulfate p. 742.

● **INDICATIONS AND DOSE**

Eczematous inflammation in otitis externa

▸ TO THE EAR

▸ Child: 2–3 drops 3–4 times a day

● CAUTIONS Avoid prolonged use

● INTERACTIONS → Appendix 1: corticosteroids

● LESS SUITABLE FOR PRESCRIBING *Sofradex®* is less suitable for prescribing.

● MEDICINAL FORMS

▸ Sofradex (Sanofi)

Dexamethasone (as Dexamethasone sodium metasulfobenzoate) 500 microgram per 1 ml, Framycetin sulfate 5 mg per 1 ml, Gramicidin 50 microgram per 1 ml Sofradex ear/eye drops | 8ml PoM £7.50

Dexamethasone with glacial acetic acid and neomycin sulfate

21-Dec-2017

The properties listed below are those particular to the combination only. For the properties of the components please consider, dexamethasone p. 475, neomycin sulfate p. 743.

● **INDICATIONS AND DOSE**

Eczematous inflammation in otitis externa

▸ TO THE EAR

▸ Child 2-17 years: Apply 1 spray 3 times a day

● CONTRA-INDICATIONS Patent grommet (although may be used by specialists, see Ear p. 741) · perforated tympanic membrane (although may be used by specialists, see Ear p. 741)

● CAUTIONS Avoid prolonged use

● INTERACTIONS → Appendix 1: corticosteroids · neomycin

● SIDE-EFFECTS Paraesthesia · skin reactions · vision blurred

● MEDICINAL FORMS There can be variation in the licensing of different medicines containing the same drug.

Spray

EXCIPIENTS: May contain Hydroxybenzoates (parabens)

▸ Otomize (Teva UK Ltd)

Dexamethasone 1 mg per 1 gram, Neomycin sulfate 5 mg per 1 gram, Acetic acid glacial 20 mg per 1 gram Otomize ear spray | 5 ml PoM £3.27

Hydrocortisone with neomycin and polymyxin B sulfate

21-Dec-2017

The properties listed below are those particular to the combination only. For the properties of the components please consider, hydrocortisone p. 476, neomycin sulfate p. 743.

● **INDICATIONS AND DOSE**

Bacterial infection in otitis externa

▸ TO THE EAR

▸ Child 3-17 years: Apply 3 drops 3–4 times a day for 7 days (review treatment if there is no clinical improvement)

● INTERACTIONS → Appendix 1: corticosteroids · neomycin · polymyxin b

● RENAL IMPAIRMENT Manufacturer advises avoid prolonged, unsupervised use.

Dose adjustments Manufacturer advises reduce dose.

● MEDICINAL FORMS There can be variation in the licensing of different medicines containing the same drug.

Ear drops

EXCIPIENTS: May contain Cetostearyl alcohol (including cetyl and stearyl alcohol), hydroxybenzoates (parabens), polysorbates

▸ Otosporin (Phoenix Labs Ltd)

Hydrocortisone 10 mg per 1 ml, Neomycin sulfate 3400 unit per 1 ml, Polymyxin B sulfate 10000 unit per 1 ml Otosporin ear drops | 10 ml PoM £7.45

DERMATOLOGICAL DRUGS › ASTRINGENTS

Aluminium acetate

● **INDICATIONS AND DOSE**

Inflammation in otitis externa

▸ TO THE EAR

▸ Child: To be inserted into meatus or apply on a ribbon gauze dressing or sponge wick which should be kept saturated with the ear drops

● UNLICENSED USE Not licensed for use in children.

● DIRECTIONS FOR ADMINISTRATION For ear drops 8%—dilute 8 parts aluminium acetate ear drops (13%) with 5 parts purified water. Must be freshly prepared.

● MEDICINAL FORMS Forms available from special-order manufacturers include: ear drops

2 Removal of earwax

BICARBONATE

Sodium bicarbonate

29-Jul-2019

● **INDICATIONS AND DOSE**

Removal of earwax (with 5% ear drop solution)

▸ TO THE EAR

▸ Child: (consult product literature)

● INTERACTIONS → Appendix 1: sodium bicarbonate

● SIDE-EFFECTS Dry ear

● MEDICINAL FORMS There can be variation in the licensing of different medicines containing the same drug.

Ear drops

▸ Sodium bicarbonate (Non-proprietary)

Sodium bicarbonate 50 mg per 1 ml Sodium bicarbonate 5% ear drops | 10 ml £1.23–£1.25

- ▸ KliarVax Sodium Bicarbonate (Essential-Healthcare Ltd)
  Sodium bicarbonate 50 mg per 1 ml KliarVax Sodium Bicarbonate ear drops | 10 ml £0.97

SOFTENING DRUGS

Almond oil

● **INDICATIONS AND DOSE**

Removal of earwax

▶ TO THE EAR

▸ Child: Allow drops to warm to room temperature before use (consult product literature)

● **DIRECTIONS FOR ADMINISTRATION** The patient should lie with the affected ear uppermost for 5 to 10 minutes after a generous amount of the softening remedy has been introduced into the ear.

● **MEDICINAL FORMS** There can be variation in the licensing of different medicines containing the same drug.

Liquid

- ▸ Almond oil (Non-proprietary)
  Almond oil 1 ml per 1 ml Almond oil liquid | 50 ml £0.95 DT = £0.95 | 70 ml £0.85 | 200 ml £2.68

Docusate sodium

16-Mar-2020

(Dioctyl sodium sulphosuccinate)

● **INDICATIONS AND DOSE**

Removal of ear wax

▶ TO THE EAR

▸ Child 1–17 years: (consult product literature)

● **INTERACTIONS** → Appendix 1: docusate sodium

● **SIDE-EFFECTS** Skin reactions

● **LESS SUITABLE FOR PRESCRIBING** Ear drops less suitable for prescribing.

● **MEDICINAL FORMS** There can be variation in the licensing of different medicines containing the same drug.

Ear drops

EXCIPIENTS: May contain Propylene glycol

- ▸ Molcer (Wallace Manufacturing Chemists Ltd)
  Docusate sodium 50 mg per 1 ml Molcer ear drops | 15 ml [P] £5.60
- ▸ Waxsol (Mylan)
  Docusate sodium 5 mg per 1 ml Waxsol ear drops | 10 ml [P] £1.95 DT = £1.95

Olive oil

● **INDICATIONS AND DOSE**

Removal of earwax

▶ TO THE EAR

▸ Child: Apply twice daily for several days (if wax is hard and impacted)

Removal of earwax (dose approved for use by community practitioner nurse prescribers)

▶ TO THE EAR

▸ Child: (consult product literature)

● **DIRECTIONS FOR ADMINISTRATION** The patient should lie with the affected ear uppermost for 5 to 10 minutes after a generous amount of the softening remedy has been introduced into the ear. Allow ear drops to warm to room temperature before use.

● **MEDICINAL FORMS** There can be variation in the licensing of different medicines containing the same drug.

Spray

- ▸ Earol (HL Healthcare Ltd)
  Earol olive oil ear spray | 10 ml [X]

Ear drops

- ▸ Olive oil (Non-proprietary)
  Olive oil ear drops | 10 ml £1.35–£1.42
- ▸ Arjun (Arjun Products Ltd)
  Arjun ear drops | 10 ml £1.26
- ▸ Cerumol (olive oil) (Thornton & Ross Ltd)
  Cerumol olive oil ear drops | 10 ml [X]
- ▸ KliarVax (Essential-Healthcare Ltd)
  KliarVax Olive Oil ear drops | 10 ml £0.97

Urea hydrogen peroxide

07-Feb-2020

● **INDICATIONS AND DOSE**

Softening and removal of earwax

▶ TO THE EAR

▸ Child: (consult product literature)

● **PATIENT AND CARER ADVICE** The patient should lie with the affected ear uppermost for 5 to 10 minutes after a generous amount of the softening remedy has been introduced into the ear.

● **LESS SUITABLE FOR PRESCRIBING** Urea-hydrogen peroxide ear drops are less suitable for prescribing.

● **MEDICINAL FORMS** There can be variation in the licensing of different medicines containing the same drug.

Ear drops

- ▸ Exterol (Dermal Laboratories Ltd)
  Urea hydrogen peroxide 50 mg per 1 gram Exterol 5% ear drops | 8 ml [P] £1.75 DT = £2.89
- ▸ Otex (Dendron Ltd)
  Urea hydrogen peroxide 50 mg per 1 gram Otex 5% ear drops | 8 ml [P] £2.89 DT = £2.89

Nose

Nose

30-Mar-2020

Rhinitis

Rhinitis may be acute or chronic, allergic or non-allergic. Nasal spray and drop preparations often carry indications for the management of allergic rhinitis and perennial rhinitis. Many nasal preparations contain sympathomimetic drugs which may irritate the nasal mucosa.

Drugs used in nasal allergy

[EvGr] Sodium chloride 0.9% solution p. 636 may be used as nasal irrigation in allergic rhinitis for modest symptom reduction, and to reduce the need for other drug treatment.

Mild allergic rhinitis is controlled by **antihistamines** (see under Antihistamines, allergen immunotherapy and allergic emergencies p. 180) or topical **nasal corticosteroids**. Topical antihistamines (e.g. azelastine hydrochloride p. 751) are faster acting than oral antihistamines and therefore useful for controlling breakthrough symptoms in allergic rhinitis; they are less effective than topical nasal corticosteroids. Topical nasal decongestants can be used for a short period to provide quick relief from congestion and allow penetration of a topical nasal corticosteroid. Systemic nasal decongestants are weakly effective in reducing nasal obstruction but have considerable potential for side-effects, and therefore are not recommended. Sodium cromoglicate is a weakly effective alternative in children with mild symptoms, sporadic seasonal problems, or limited allergen exposure.

Moderate to severe allergic rhinitis can be relieved by topical **nasal corticosteroids** during periods of allergen exposure. Severe allergic rhinitis causing very disabling symptoms despite conventional treatment may justify the use of **oral corticosteroids** for short periods. In severe cases, oral corticosteroids may also be used in combination with nasal corticosteroids during treatment initiation to relieve severe mucosal oedema and allow the spray to penetrate the nasal cavity.

Nasal ipratropium bromide p. 751 may be added to allergic rhinitis treatment when watery rhinorrhoea persists despite treatment with topical nasal steroids and antihistamines; it has no effect on other nasal symptoms.

In seasonal allergic rhinitis (e.g. hay fever), treatment should begin 2 to 3 weeks before the season commences and/or exposure to the allergen.

Montelukast p. 174 is less effective than topical nasal corticosteroids but can be used in children with seasonal allergic rhinitis and concomitant asthma. (A)

Corticosteroids

EvGr Topical nasal corticosteroid preparations should be avoided in the presence of untreated nasal infections, after nasal surgery (until healing has occurred), and in pulmonary tuberculosis. Systemic absorption may follow nasal administration particularly if high doses are used or if treatment is prolonged. The extent of absorption varies between steroids; mometasone furoate p. 753 and fluticasone p. 753 have negligible systemic absorption, others have modest absorption, whilst betamethasone p. 752 has high systemic absorption and should only be used short-term. The growth of children receiving treatment with corticosteroids should be monitored; especially in those receiving corticosteroids via multiple routes. (A)

Nasal polyps

EvGr All children presenting with nasal polyps must be screened for cystic fibrosis and referred to an ear, nose and throat specialist for initial review. Nasal polyps may be treated with topical nasal corticosteroids (drops or spray). There may be a higher risk of side-effects with use of nasal drops compared to nasal spray due to greater systemic absorption and incorrect administration of drops. To reduce the risk, the drops must be administered with the child in the 'head down' position. A short course of a systemic corticosteroid can provide symptomatic relief but effects may be temporary and its use is rare due to concerns of systemic side-effects. If systemic corticosteroids are given, they should be used in combination with topical nasal corticosteroids. (A)

Pregnancy

EvGr If a pregnant female cannot tolerate the symptoms of allergic rhinitis, treatment may be given. (A) Although the safety of nasal corticosteroids in pregnancy has not been established through clinical trials, only minimal amounts of nasal corticosteroids are systemically absorbed. Beclometasone dipropionate p. 752, budesonide p. 752, and fluticasone are widely used in asthmatic pregnant females; fluticasone has the lowest systemic absorption when used intra-nasally. EvGr Decongestants are not recommended however, some antihistamines and sodium cromoglicate may be used. (A)

Topical nasal decongestants

The nasal mucosa is sensitive to changes in atmospheric temperature and humidity and these alone may cause slight nasal congestion. EvGr Sodium chloride 0.9% given as nasal drops, spray, or irrigation may relieve nasal congestion.

Symptoms of nasal congestion associated with allergic rhinitis, the common cold, and sinusitis may be relieved by the short-term use (usually not longer than 7 days) of decongestant nasal drops and sprays. (A) These all contain sympathomimetic drugs which exert their effect by vasoconstriction of the mucosal blood vessels which in turn reduces oedema of the nasal mucosa. Their use, especially with longer durations, can give rise to rebound congestion (rhinitis medicamentosa) on withdrawal, due to a secondary vasodilatation with a subsequent temporary increase in nasal congestion. This in turn tempts the further use of the decongestant, leading to a vicious cycle of events; tolerance with reduced effect may also be seen with excessive use.

EvGr Non-allergic watery rhinorrhoea often responds to treatment with nasal antimuscarinic ipratropium bromide. (A)

Nasal preparations for infection

Nasal staphylococci

EvGr Elimination of organisms such as staphylococci from the nasal vestibule can be achieved by the use of antimicrobial preparations such as chlorhexidine with neomycin cream (*Naseptin*®) p. 750. A nasal ointment containing mupirocin p. 750 is available if *Naseptin*® is unsuitable or ineffective.

In hospitals or in care establishments, mupirocin nasal ointment can be used for eradication of nasal carriage of meticillin-resistant *Staphylococcus aureus* (MRSA). (A)

For information on eradication of MRSA, consult local infection control policy. See also management of MRSA p. 392.

1 Nasal congestion

SYMPATHOMIMETICS › VASOCONSTRICTOR

Ephedrine hydrochloride

04-Dec-2019

● **INDICATIONS AND DOSE**

Nasal congestion | Sinusitis affecting the maxillary antrum

▶ BY INTRANASAL ADMINISTRATION

▶ Child 12–17 years: Apply 1–2 drops up to 4 times a day as required for a maximum of 7 days, to be instilled into each nostril, administer ephedrine 0.5% nasal drops

IMPORTANT SAFETY INFORMATION

CHM/MHRA ADVICE

The CHM/MHRA has stated that non-prescription cough and cold medicines containing ephedrine can be considered for up to 5 days' treatment in children aged 6–12 years after basic principles of best care have been tried; these medicines should not be used in children under 6 years of age.

● **CAUTIONS** Avoid excessive or prolonged use · cardiovascular disease · diabetes mellitus · hypertension · hyperthyroidism

● **INTERACTIONS** → Appendix 1: sympathomimetics, vasoconstrictor

● **SIDE-EFFECTS**

▶ **Common or very common** Anxiety · headache · insomnia · nausea

▶ **Frequency not known** Appetite decreased · arrhythmia · circulation impaired · dermatitis · dizziness · drug dependence · dry mouth · dyspnoea · hallucination · hyperglycaemia · hyperhidrosis · hypersalivation · hypertension · hypokalaemia · hypotension · irritability · muscle weakness · mydriasis · pain · palpitations · paranoia · piloerection · rebound congestion · syncope · thirst · tremor · urinary disorders · vasoconstriction · vasodilation · vomiting

● **PREGNANCY** Manufacturer advises avoid.

● **BREAST FEEDING** Present in milk; manufacturer advises avoid—irritability and disturbed sleep reported.

- **PRESCRIBING AND DISPENSING INFORMATION** For nasal drops, the BP directs that if no strength is specified 0.5% drops should be supplied.
- **PROFESSION SPECIFIC INFORMATION**

Dental practitioners' formulary

Ephedrine nasal drops may be prescribed.

- **EXCEPTIONS TO LEGAL CATEGORY** Ephedrine nasal drops can be sold to the public provided no more than 180 mg of ephedrine base (or salts) are supplied at one time, and pseudoephedrine salts are not supplied at the same time; for conditions that apply to supplies made at the request of a patient, see *Medicines, Ethics and Practice*, London, Pharmaceutical Press (always consult latest edition).

- **MEDICINAL FORMS** There can be variation in the licensing of different medicines containing the same drug. Forms available from special-order manufacturers include: nasal drops

Nasal drops

- ▸ **Ephedrine hydrochloride (Non-proprietary)**
  Ephedrine hydrochloride 5 mg per 1 ml Ephedrine 0.5% nasal drops | 10 ml [P] £1.90 DT = £1.90
  Ephedrine hydrochloride 10 mg per 1 ml Ephedrine 1% nasal drops | 10 ml [P] £1.94 DT = £1.94

Pseudoephedrine hydrochloride

06-Apr-2020

- **INDICATIONS AND DOSE**

Congestion of mucous membranes of upper respiratory tract

▸ BY MOUTH

- ▸ Child 6–11 years: 30 mg 3–4 times a day
- ▸ Child 12–17 years: 60 mg 3–4 times a day

> **IMPORTANT SAFETY INFORMATION**
> MHRA/CHM ADVICE: OVER-THE-COUNTER COUGH AND COLD MEDICINES FOR CHILDREN (APRIL 2009)
> Children under 6 years should not be given over-the-counter cough and cold medicines containing pseudoephedrine.

- **CAUTIONS** Diabetes · heart disease · hypertension · hyperthyroidism · raised intra-ocular pressure
- **INTERACTIONS** → Appendix 1: sympathomimetics, vasoconstrictor
- **SIDE-EFFECTS** Angle closure glaucoma · anxiety · arrhythmias · circulation impaired · dry mouth · hallucination · headache · hypertension · irritability · nausea · palpitations · psychotic disorder · skin reactions · sleep disorders · tremor · urinary retention · vomiting
- **PREGNANCY** Defective closure of the abdominal wall (gastroschisis) reported very rarely in newborns after first trimester exposure.
- **BREAST FEEDING** May suppress lactation; avoid if lactation not well established or if milk production insufficient.
- **HEPATIC IMPAIRMENT** Manufacturer advises caution in severe impairment.
- **RENAL IMPAIRMENT** Use with caution in mild to moderate renal impairment. Manufacturer advises avoid in severe renal impairment.
- **LESS SUITABLE FOR PRESCRIBING** Pseudoephedrine hydrochloride is less suitable for prescribing.
- **EXCEPTIONS TO LEGAL CATEGORY** *Galpseud®* and *Sudafed®* can be sold to the public provided no more than 720 mg of pseudoephedrine salts are supplied, and ephedrine base (or salts) are not supplied at the same time; for details see *Medicines, Ethics and Practice*, London, Pharmaceutical Press (always consult latest edition).
- **MEDICINAL FORMS** There can be variation in the licensing of different medicines containing the same drug.

Oral solution

EXCIPIENTS: May contain Alcohol

- ▸ **Galpseud** (Thornton & Ross Ltd)
  Pseudoephedrine hydrochloride 6 mg per 1 ml Galpseud 30mg/5ml linctus sugar-free | 2000 ml [PoM] £14.00
- ▸ **Sudafed Non-Drowsy Decongestant (pseudoephedrine)** (McNeil Products Ltd)
  Pseudoephedrine hydrochloride 6 mg per 1 ml Sudafed Decongestant 30mg/5ml liquid | 100 ml [P] £2.22 DT = £2.22

Tablet

- ▸ **Galpseud** (Thornton & Ross Ltd)
  Pseudoephedrine hydrochloride 60 mg Galpseud 60mg tablets | 24 tablet [PoM] £2.25
- ▸ **Sudafed Non-Drowsy Decongestant (pseudoephedrine)** (McNeil Products Ltd)
  Pseudoephedrine hydrochloride 60 mg Sudafed Decongestant 60mg tablets | 12 tablet [P] £2.43

Xylometazoline hydrochloride

13-Feb-2020

- **DRUG ACTION** Xylometazoline is a sympathomimetic.
- **INDICATIONS AND DOSE**

Nasal congestion

▸ BY INTRANASAL ADMINISTRATION USING NASAL DROPS

- ▸ Child 6–11 years: 1–2 drops 1–2 times a day as required for maximum duration of 5 days, 0.05% solution to be administered into each nostril
- ▸ Child 12–17 years: 2–3 drops 2–3 times a day as required for maximum duration of 7 days, 0.1% solution to be administered into each nostril

▸ BY INTRANASAL ADMINISTRATION USING NASAL SPRAY

- ▸ Child 12–17 years: 1 spray 1–3 times a day as required for maximum duration of 7 days, to be administered into each nostril

> **IMPORTANT SAFETY INFORMATION**
> The CHM/MHRA has stated that non-prescription cough and cold medicines containing oxymetazoline or xylometazoline can be considered for up to 5 days' treatment in children aged 6–12 years after basic principles of best care have been tried; these medicines should not be used in children under 6 years of age.

- **CAUTIONS** Angle-closure glaucoma · avoid excessive or prolonged use · cardiovascular disease · diabetes mellitus · hypertension · hyperthyroidism · rebound congestion

CAUTIONS, FURTHER INFORMATION

- ▸ Rebound congestion Sympathomimetic drugs are of limited value in the treatment of nasal congestion because they can, following prolonged use (more than 7 days), give rise to a rebound congestion (rhinitis medicamentosa) on withdrawal, due to a secondary vasodilatation with a subsequent temporary increase in nasal congestion. This in turn tempts the further use of the decongestant, leading to a vicious cycle of events.

- **INTERACTIONS** → Appendix 1: sympathomimetics, vasoconstrictor
- **SIDE-EFFECTS** Cardiovascular effects · headache · hypersensitivity · nasal dryness · nausea · paraesthesia · visual impairment

SIDE-EFFECTS, FURTHER INFORMATION Use of decongestants in infants and children under 6 years has been associated with agitated psychosis, ataxia, hallucinations, and even death—avoid.

- **PREGNANCY** Manufacturer advises avoid.
- **BREAST FEEDING** Manufacturer advises caution—no information available.

- **MEDICINAL FORMS** There can be variation in the licensing of different medicines containing the same drug.

Spray

- Otrivine (GlaxoSmithKline Consumer Healthcare)
  Xylometazoline hydrochloride 1 mg per 1 ml Otrivine Congestion Relief 0.1% nasal spray | 10 ml GSL £3.05 DT = £2.18
  Otrivine Adult Measured Dose Sinusitis spray | 10 ml GSL £2.62 DT = £2.18
  Otrivine Allergy Relief 0.1% nasal spray | 10 ml GSL £2.62 DT = £2.18
  Otrivine Adult nasal spray | 10 ml GSL £2.18 DT = £2.18
  Otrivine Adult Metered Dose 0.1% nasal spray | 10 ml GSL £2.62 DT = £2.18
- Sudafed Congestion Relief (McNeil Products Ltd)
  Xylometazoline hydrochloride 1 mg per 1 ml Sudafed Congestion Relief 0.1% nasal spray | 10 ml GSL £3.46 DT = £2.18
- Sudafed Non-Drowsy Decongestant (xylometazoline) (McNeil Products Ltd)
  Xylometazoline hydrochloride 1 mg per 1 ml Sudafed Blocked Nose 0.1% spray | 15 ml GSL £2.76
- Sudafed Sinus-Ease (McNeil Products Ltd)
  Xylometazoline hydrochloride 1 mg per 1 ml Sudafed Sinus-Ease 0.1% nasal spray | 15 ml GSL £2.80

Nasal drops

- Otrivine (GlaxoSmithKline Consumer Healthcare)
  Xylometazoline hydrochloride 500 microgram per 1 ml Otrivine Child nasal drops | 10 ml P £1.91 DT = £1.91
  Xylometazoline hydrochloride 1 mg per 1 ml Otrivine Adult 0.1% nasal drops | 10 ml GSL £2.18 DT = £2.18

12

Ear, nose and oropharynx

2 Nasal infection

Sinusitis (acute)

31-Oct-2017

Description of condition

Sinusitis is an inflammation of the mucosal lining of the paranasal sinuses. Acute sinusitis (rhinosinusitis) is a self-limiting condition usually triggered by a viral upper-respiratory tract infection such as the 'common cold'. Occasionally, acute sinusitis may become complicated by a bacterial infection (*see Antibacterial therapy for acute sinusitis* in Nose infections, antibacterial therapy p. 326).

Children with acute sinusitis, particularly young children, often present with non-specific symptoms in the upper respiratory tract, including nasal blockage or congestion, discoloured nasal discharge, or cough during the day or night.

Symptoms usually improve within 2 to 3 weeks without requiring treatment.

Rarely, acute sinusitis may lead to orbital, intracranial or skeletal complications (e.g. periorbital cellulitis, symptoms or signs of meningitis).

Aims of treatment

Treatment is aimed at managing symptoms including pain, fever, and nasal congestion as well as treatment of bacterial infection if present.

Treatment

EvGr Children presenting with symptoms for around 10 *days or less*, should be given advice about the usual duration of acute sinusitis, self-care of pain or fever with paracetamol p. 288 or ibuprofen p. 707, and when to seek medical help. Children and their carers should be reassured that antibiotics are usually not required.

Children (over the age of 12) presenting with symptoms for around 10 *days or more* with no improvement could be considered for treatment with a high-dose nasal corticosteroid, such as mometasone furoate p. 753 [unlicensed use] or fluticasone p. 753 [unlicensed use] for 14 days.

If the child is systemically very unwell, has signs and symptoms of a more serious illness or condition, or is at high-risk of complications, an immediate antibiotic could be offered if deemed appropriate. (A) *(see Antibacterial therapy for acute sinusitis* in Nose infections, antibacterial therapy p. 326).

EvGr Children presenting with symptoms of acute sinusitis associated with a severe systemic infection or with orbital or intracranial complications should be referred to hospital. (A)

Useful Resources

Sinusitis (acute): antimicrobial prescribing. National Institute for Health and Care Excellence. NICE guideline 79. October 2017.
www.nice.org.uk/guidance/ng79

ANTIBACTERIALS > AMINOGLYCOSIDES

Chlorhexidine with neomycin

- **INDICATIONS AND DOSE**

Eradication of nasal carriage of staphylococci
- BY INTRANASAL ADMINISTRATION
- Child: Apply 4 times a day for 10 days

Preventing nasal carriage of staphylococci
- BY INTRANASAL ADMINISTRATION
- Child: Apply twice daily

- **MEDICINAL FORMS** There can be variation in the licensing of different medicines containing the same drug.

Cream

EXCIPIENTS: May contain Arachis (peanut) oil, cetostearyl alcohol (including cetyl and stearyl alcohol)

- Naseptin (Alliance Pharmaceuticals Ltd)
  Chlorhexidine hydrochloride 1 mg per 1 gram, Neomycin sulfate 5 mg per 1 gram Naseptin nasal cream | 15 gram PoM £1.99 DT = £1.99

ANTIBACTERIALS > OTHER

Mupirocin

18-May-2020

- **INDICATIONS AND DOSE**

BACTROBAN NASAL ®

For eradication of nasal carriage of staphylococci, including meticillin-resistant *Staphylococcus aureus* (MRSA)
- BY INTRANASAL ADMINISTRATION
- Child: Apply 2–3 times a day for 5 days; a sample should be taken 2 days after treatment to confirm eradication. Course may be repeated once if sample positive (and throat not colonised), dose to be applied to the inner surface of each nostril

- **SIDE-EFFECTS**
  - **Common or very common** Skin reactions
  - **Uncommon** Nasal mucosal disorder
- **PREGNANCY** Manufacturer advises avoid unless potential benefit outweighs risk—no information available.
- **BREAST FEEDING** No information available.
- **RENAL IMPAIRMENT** Manufacturer advises caution when mupirocin ointment used in moderate or severe impairment because it contains macrogols (polyethylene glycol).

- **MEDICINAL FORMS** There can be variation in the licensing of different medicines containing the same drug.

Nasal ointment

- Bactroban (GlaxoSmithKline UK Ltd)
  Mupirocin (as Mupirocin calcium) 20 mg per 1 gram Bactroban 2% nasal ointment | 3 gram PoM £4.24 DT = £4.24

CORTICOSTEROIDS > CORTICOSTEROID COMBINATIONS WITH ANTI-INFECTIVES

Betamethasone with neomycin

The properties listed below are those particular to the combination only. For the properties of the components please consider, betamethasone p. 752, neomycin sulfate p. 774.

- **INDICATIONS AND DOSE**

Nasal infection

- BY INTRANASAL ADMINISTRATION USING NASAL DROPS
- Child: Apply 2–3 drops 2–3 times a day, to be applied into each nostril

- **INTERACTIONS** → Appendix 1: corticosteroids · neomycin
- **LESS SUITABLE FOR PRESCRIBING** Betamethasone with neomycin nasal-drops are less suitable for prescribing; there is no evidence that topical anti-infective nasal preparations have any therapeutic value in rhinitis or sinusitis.

- **MEDICINAL FORMS** There can be variation in the licensing of different medicines containing the same drug.

Ear/eye/nose drops solution

EXCIPIENTS: May contain Benzalkonium chloride, disodium edetate

- Betnesol-N (RPH Pharmaceuticals AB)
  Betamethasone (as Betamethasone sodium phosphate) 1 mg per 1 ml, Neomycin sulfate 5 mg per 1 ml Betnesol-N ear/eye/nose drops | 10 ml PoM £2.39 DT = £2.39

3 Nasal inflammation, nasal polyps and rhinitis

Other drugs used for Nasal inflammation, nasal polyps and rhinitis Desloratadine, p. 183 · Fexofenadine hydrochloride, p. 184 · Ketotifen, p. 188 · Rupatadine, p. 185 · Sodium cromoglicate, p. 176

ANTIHISTAMINES

Azelastine hydrochloride

11-May-2020

- **INDICATIONS AND DOSE**

Allergic rhinitis

- BY INTRANASAL ADMINISTRATION
- Child 6–17 years: 1 spray twice daily, to be administered into each nostril

DOSE EQUIVALENCE AND CONVERSION

- 1 spray equivalent to 140 micrograms.

- **INTERACTIONS** → Appendix 1: antihistamines, non-sedating
- **SIDE-EFFECTS**
  - **Common or very common** Taste bitter (if applied incorrectly)
  - **Uncommon** Epistaxis · nasal complaints

- **MEDICINAL FORMS** There can be variation in the licensing of different medicines containing the same drug.

Spray

- Rhinolast (Mylan)
  Azelastine hydrochloride 140 microgram per 1 actuation Rhinolast 140micrograms/dose nasal spray | 22 ml PoM £10.50 DT = £10.50

Combinations available: *Fluticasone with azelastine*, p. 753

ANTIMUSCARINICS

F 161

Ipratropium bromide

25-Jul-2018

- **INDICATIONS AND DOSE**

Rhinorrhoea associated with allergic and non-allergic rhinitis

- BY INTRANASAL ADMINISTRATION
- Child 12–17 years: 2 sprays 2–3 times a day, dose to be sprayed into each nostril

DOSE EQUIVALENCE AND CONVERSION

- 1 metered spray of nasal spray = 21 micrograms.

- **CAUTIONS** Avoid spraying near eyes · bladder outflow obstruction · cystic fibrosis · susceptibility to angle-closure glaucoma
- **INTERACTIONS** → Appendix 1: ipratropium
- **SIDE-EFFECTS**
  - **Common or very common** Epistaxis · gastrointestinal motility disorder · headache · nasal complaints · throat complaints
  - **Uncommon** Corneal oedema · eye disorders · eye pain · nausea · respiratory disorders · stomatitis · vision disorders
  - **Rare or very rare** Palpitations
- **ALLERGY AND CROSS-SENSITIVITY** Contra-indicated in patients with hypersensitivity to atropine or its derivatives.
- **PREGNANCY** Manufacturer advises only use if potential benefit outweighs the risk.
- **BREAST FEEDING** No information available—manufacturer advises only use if potential benefit outweighs risk.
- **PATIENT AND CARER ADVICE** Patients or carers should be counselled on appropriate administration technique and warned against accidental contact with the eye (due to risk of ocular complications).
  Driving and skilled tasks Manufacturer advises patients and carers should be counselled on the effects on driving and performance of skilled tasks—increased risk of dizziness and vision disorders.

- **MEDICINAL FORMS** There can be variation in the licensing of different medicines containing the same drug.

Spray

EXCIPIENTS: May contain Benzalkonium chloride, disodium edetate

- Rinatec (Sanofi)
  Ipratropium bromide 21 microgram per 1 dose Rinatec 21micrograms/dose nasal spray | 180 dose PoM £6.54 DT = £6.54

CORTICOSTEROIDS

Corticosteroids (intranasal)

IMPORTANT SAFETY INFORMATION

MHRA/CHM ADVICE: CORTICOSTEROIDS: RARE RISK OF CENTRAL SEROUS CHORIORETINOPATHY WITH LOCAL AS WELL AS SYSTEMIC ADMINISTRATION (AUGUST 2017)

Central serous chorioretinopathy is a retinal disorder that has been linked to the systemic use of corticosteroids. Recently, it has also been reported after local administration of corticosteroids via inhaled and intranasal, epidural, intra-articular, topical dermal, and periocular routes. The MHRA recommends that patients should be advised to report any blurred vision or other visual disturbances with corticosteroid treatment given by any route; consider referral to an ophthalmologist for evaluation of possible causes if a patient presents with vision problems.

- **CAUTIONS** Avoid after nasal surgery (until healing has occurred) · avoid in pulmonary tuberculosis · avoid in the presence of untreated nasal infections · patients transferred from systemic corticosteroids may experience exacerbation of some symptoms

  CAUTIONS, FURTHER INFORMATION
  - Systemic absorption Systemic absorption may follow nasal administration particularly if high doses are used or if treatment is prolonged; therefore also consider the cautions and side-effects of systemic corticosteroids. The risk of systemic effects may be greater with nasal drops than with nasal sprays; drops are administered incorrectly more often than sprays.

- **SIDE-EFFECTS**
  - **Common or very common** Altered smell sensation · epistaxis · headache · nasal complaints · taste altered · throat irritation
  - **Rare or very rare** Glaucoma · nasal septum perforation (more common following nasal surgery) · vision blurred

  SIDE-EFFECTS, FURTHER INFORMATION Systemic absorption may follow nasal administration particularly if high doses are used or if treatment is prolonged. Therefore also consider the side-effects of systemic corticosteroids.
- **MONITORING REQUIREMENTS** The height of children receiving prolonged treatment with nasal corticosteroids should be monitored; if growth is slowed, referral to a paediatrician should be considered.

751

Beclometasone dipropionate

15-May-2020

(Beclomethasone dipropionate)

- **INDICATIONS AND DOSE**

Prophylaxis and treatment of allergic and vasomotor rhinitis

- BY INTRANASAL ADMINISTRATION
  - Child 6–17 years: 100 micrograms twice daily, dose to be administered into each nostril, reduced to 50 micrograms twice daily, dose to be administered into each nostril, dose to be reduced when symptoms controlled; maximum 400 micrograms per day

- **INTERACTIONS** → Appendix 1: corticosteroids
- **MEDICINAL FORMS** There can be variation in the licensing of different medicines containing the same drug.

Spray

EXCIPIENTS: May contain Benzalkonium chloride, polysorbates

- Beclometasone dipropionate (Non-proprietary)
  Beclometasone dipropionate 50 microgram per 1 dose Beclometasone 50micrograms/dose nasal spray | 200 dose [PoM] [X] DT = £2.63
- Beconase (GlaxoSmithKline UK Ltd, Omega Pharma Ltd)
  Beclometasone dipropionate 50 microgram per 1 dose Beconase Aqueous 50micrograms/dose nasal spray | 200 dose [PoM] £2.63 DT = £2.63
- Nasobec (Teva UK Ltd)
  Beclometasone dipropionate 50 microgram per 1 dose Nasobec Aqueous 50micrograms/dose nasal spray | 200 dose [PoM] £3.06 DT = £2.63

751

Betamethasone

28-Nov-2019

- **INDICATIONS AND DOSE**

BETNESOL®

Non-infected inflammatory conditions of nose

- BY INTRANASAL ADMINISTRATION
  - Child: Apply 2–3 drops 2–3 times a day, dose to be applied into each nostril

VISTAMETHASONE®

Non-infected inflammatory conditions of nose

- BY INTRANASAL ADMINISTRATION
  - Child: Apply 2–3 drops twice daily, dose to be applied into each nostril

- **INTERACTIONS** → Appendix 1: corticosteroids
- **MEDICINAL FORMS** There can be variation in the licensing of different medicines containing the same drug.

Ear/eye/nose drops solution

EXCIPIENTS: May contain Benzalkonium chloride, disodium edetate

- Betnesol (RPH Pharmaceuticals AB)
  Betamethasone sodium phosphate 1 mg per 1 ml Betnesol 0.1% eye/ear/nose drops | 10 ml [PoM] £2.32 DT = £2.32
- Vistamethasone (Martindale Pharmaceuticals Ltd)
  Betamethasone sodium phosphate 1 mg per 1 ml Vistamethasone 0.1% ear/eye/nose drops | 5 ml [PoM] £1.02 | 10 ml [PoM] £1.16 DT = £2.32

751

Budesonide

21-Dec-2017

- **INDICATIONS AND DOSE**

Allergic rhinitis | Nasal polyps

- BY INTRANASAL ADMINISTRATION
  - Child 6–17 years: 128 micrograms once daily, dose to be administered into each nostril in the morning, alternatively 64 micrograms twice daily, dose to be administered to each nostril, reduce dose when control achieved

Prophylaxis and treatment of allergic and vasomotor rhinitis

- BY INTRANASAL ADMINISTRATION
  - Child 12–17 years: Initially 200 micrograms once daily, dose to be administered into each nostril in the morning, alternatively initially 100 micrograms twice daily, dose to be administered to each nostril; reduced to 100 micrograms once daily, dose to be administered into each nostril, dose can be reduced when control achieved

Nasal polyps

- BY INTRANASAL ADMINISTRATION
  - Child 12–17 years: 100 micrograms twice daily for up to 3 months, dose to be administered into each nostril

RHINOCORT AQUA®

Rhinitis

- BY INTRANASAL ADMINISTRATION
  - Child 12–17 years: 128 micrograms once daily, dose to be administered into each nostril in the morning, alternatively 64 micrograms twice daily, dose to be administered into each nostril; reduced to 64 micrograms once daily when control achieved. Use for maximum 3 months, doses to be administered into each nostril

Nasal polyps

- BY INTRANASAL ADMINISTRATION
  - Child 12–17 years: 64 micrograms twice daily for up to 3 months, dose to be administered into each nostril

- **UNLICENSED USE** *Rhinocort Aqua®* is not licensed for use in children.

- **INTERACTIONS** → Appendix 1: corticosteroids
- **SIDE-EFFECTS**
  - ▸ **Rare or very rare** Adrenal suppression

- **MEDICINAL FORMS** There can be variation in the licensing of different medicines containing the same drug.

Spray

EXCIPIENTS: May contain Disodium edetate, polysorbates, potassium sorbate

▸ Aircort (Imported (Italy))
Budesonide 100 microgram per 1 dose Aircort 100micrograms/dose nasal spray | 200 dose PoM

▸ Budeflam Aquanase (Imported (South Africa))
Budesonide 100 microgram per 1 dose Budeflam Aquanase 100micrograms/dose nasal spray | 150 dose PoM

▸ Rhinocort (Johnson & Johnson Ltd)
Budesonide 64 microgram per 1 dose Rhinocort Aqua 64 nasal spray | 120 dose PoM £3.77 DT = £5.25

751

Fluticasone

21-Dec-2017

- **INDICATIONS AND DOSE**

Prophylaxis and treatment of allergic rhinitis and perennial rhinitis

▸ BY INTRANASAL ADMINISTRATION USING NASAL SPRAY

- ▸ Child 4–11 years: 50 micrograms once daily, to be administered into each nostril preferably in the morning, increased if necessary to 50 micrograms twice daily
- ▸ Child 12–17 years: 100 micrograms once daily, to be administered into each nostril preferably in the morning, increased if necessary to 100 micrograms twice daily; reduced to 50 micrograms once daily, dose to be administered into each nostril, dose to be reduced when control achieved

Nasal polyps

▸ BY INTRANASAL ADMINISTRATION USING NASAL DROPS

- ▸ Child 16–17 years: 200 micrograms 1–2 times a day, to be administered into each nostril, alternative treatment should be considered if no improvement after 4–6 weeks, (200 micrograms is equivalent to approximately 6 drops)

AVAMYS ® SPRAY

Prophylaxis and treatment of allergic rhinitis

▸ BY INTRANASAL ADMINISTRATION

- ▸ Child 6–11 years: 27.5 micrograms once daily, dose to be sprayed into each nostril, then increased if necessary to 55 micrograms once daily, dose to be sprayed into each nostril, reduced to 27.5 micrograms once daily, to be sprayed into each nostril, dose to be reduced once control achieved; use minimum effective dose
- ▸ Child 12–17 years: 55 micrograms once daily, dose to be sprayed into each nostril, reduced to 27.5 micrograms once daily, to be sprayed into each nostril, dose to be reduced once control achieved; use minimum effective dose

DOSE EQUIVALENCE AND CONVERSION

- ▸ For *Avamys ® spray*: 1 spray equivalent to 27.5 micrograms.

- **INTERACTIONS** → Appendix 1: corticosteroids
- **SIDE-EFFECTS** Adrenal suppression

SIDE-EFFECTS, FURTHER INFORMATION Nasal ulceration occurs commonly with nasal preparations containing fluticasone furoate.

- **MEDICINAL FORMS** There can be variation in the licensing of different medicines containing the same drug.

Spray

EXCIPIENTS: May contain Benzalkonium chloride, disodium edetate, polysorbates

▸ Avamys (GlaxoSmithKline UK Ltd)
Fluticasone furoate 27.5 microgram per 1 dose Avamys 27.5micrograms/dose nasal spray | 120 dose PoM £6.44 DT = £6.44

▸ Flixonase (GlaxoSmithKline Consumer Healthcare, GlaxoSmithKline UK Ltd)
Fluticasone propionate 50 microgram per 1 dose Flixonase 50micrograms/dose aqueous nasal spray | 150 dose PoM £11.01 DT = £6.87

▸ Nasofan (Teva UK Ltd)
Fluticasone propionate 50 microgram per 1 dose Nasofan 50micrograms/dose aqueous nasal spray | 150 dose PoM £8.04 DT = £6.87

Nasal drops

EXCIPIENTS: May contain Polysorbates

▸ Flixonase (GlaxoSmithKline UK Ltd)
Fluticasone propionate 400 microgram Flixonase Nasule 400microgram/unit dose nasal drops | 28 unit dose PoM £12.99 DT = £12.99

Fluticasone with azelastine

The properties listed below are those particular to the combination only. For the properties of the components please consider, fluticasone p. 753, azelastine hydrochloride p. 719.

- **INDICATIONS AND DOSE**

Moderate to severe seasonal and perennial allergic rhinitis, if monotherapy with antihistamine or corticosteroid is inadequate

▸ BY INTRANASAL ADMINISTRATION

- ▸ Child 12–17 years: 1 spray twice daily, dose to be administered into each nostril

- **INTERACTIONS** → Appendix 1: antihistamines, non-sedating · corticosteroids

- **MEDICINAL FORMS** There can be variation in the licensing of different medicines containing the same drug.

Spray

EXCIPIENTS: May contain Benzalkonium chloride, polysorbates

▸ Dymista (Mylan)
Fluticasone propionate 50 microgram per 1 actuation, Azelastine hydrochloride 137 microgram per 1 actuation Dymista 137micrograms/dose / 50micrograms/dose nasal spray | 120 dose PoM £14.80 DT = £14.80

751

Mometasone furoate

21-Dec-2017

- **INDICATIONS AND DOSE**

Prophylaxis and treatment of seasonal allergic or perennial rhinitis

▸ BY INTRANASAL ADMINISTRATION

- ▸ Child 3–11 years: 50 micrograms daily, dose to be sprayed into each nostril
- ▸ Child 12–17 years: 100 micrograms daily, increased if necessary up to 200 micrograms daily, dose to be sprayed into each nostril; reduced to 50 micrograms daily, dose to be reduced when control achieved, dose to be sprayed into each nostril

- **INTERACTIONS** → Appendix 1: corticosteroids
- **SIDE-EFFECTS**

SIDE-EFFECTS, FURTHER INFORMATION Nasal ulceration occurs commonly with preparations containing mometasone furoate.

- **MEDICINAL FORMS** There can be variation in the licensing of different medicines containing the same drug.

Spray

EXCIPIENTS: May contain Benzalkonium chloride, polysorbates

▸ Mometasone furoate (Non-proprietary)
Mometasone furoate 50 microgram per 1 dose Mometasone 50micrograms/dose nasal spray | 140 dose PoM £6.50 DT = £4.61

- Nasonex (Merck Sharp & Dohme Ltd)
  Mometasone furoate 50 microgram per 1 dose Nasonex 50micrograms/dose nasal spray | 140 dose PoM £7.68 DT = £4.61

F 751

Triamcinolone acetonide

26-Nov-2019

- **INDICATIONS AND DOSE**

Prophylaxis and treatment of allergic rhinitis

▸ BY INTRANASAL ADMINISTRATION

- Child 2–5 years: 55 micrograms once daily for maximum 3 months, dose to be sprayed into each nostril
- Child 6–11 years: 55 micrograms once daily, dose to be sprayed into each nostril, increased if necessary to 110 micrograms once daily, dose to be sprayed into each nostril; reduced to 55 micrograms once daily, dose to be sprayed into each nostril, reduce dose when control achieved; maximum duration of treatment 3 months
- Child 12–17 years: 110 micrograms once daily, dose to be sprayed into each nostril, reduced to 55 micrograms once daily, dose to be sprayed into each nostril, reduce dose when control achieved

- **UNLICENSED USE** Not licensed for use in children under 6 years.
- **INTERACTIONS** → Appendix 1: corticosteroids
- **MEDICINAL FORMS** There can be variation in the licensing of different medicines containing the same drug.

Spray

EXCIPIENTS: May contain Benzalkonium chloride, disodium edetate, polysorbates

- Nasacort (Sanofi)
  Triamcinolone acetonide 55 microgram per 1 dose Nasacort 55micrograms/dose nasal spray | 120 dose PoM £7.39 DT = £7.39

Oropharynx

1 Dry mouth

Treatment of dry mouth

Overview

Dry mouth (xerostomia) may be caused by drugs with antimuscarinic (anticholinergic) side-effects (e.g. antispasmodics and sedating antihistamines), by irradiation of the head and neck region or by damage to or disease of the salivary glands. Children with a persistently dry mouth may develop a burning or scalded sensation and have poor oral hygiene; they may develop dental caries, periodontal disease, and oral infections (particularly candidiasis). Dry mouth may be relieved in many patients by simple measures such as frequent sips of cool drinks or sucking pieces of ice or sugar-free fruit pastilles. Sugar-free chewing gum stimulates salivation in patients with residual salivary function.

Artificial saliva can provide useful relief of dry mouth. A properly balanced artificial saliva should be of a neutral pH and contain electrolytes (including fluoride) to correspond approximately to the composition of saliva. The acidic pH of some artificial saliva products may be inappropriate.

Artificial saliva products

- **ARTIFICIAL SALIVA PRODUCTS**

AS SALIVA ORTHANA® LOZENGES

Mucin 65 mg, xylitol 59 mg, in a sorbitol basis, pH neutral

- **INDICATIONS AND DOSE**

Dry mouth as a result of having (or having undergone) radiotherapy (ACBS) | Dry mouth as a result of sicca syndrome (ACBS)

▸ BY MOUTH

- Child: 1 lozenge as required, allow to dissolve slowly in the mouth

- **PRESCRIBING AND DISPENSING INFORMATION** *AS Saliva Orthana®* lozenges do not contain fluoride.

AS Saliva Orthana lozenges (CCMed Ltd)
30 lozenge(ACBS) • NHS indicative price = £3.04 • Drug Tariff (Part VIIIA Category C) price = £3.50

AS SALIVA ORTHANA® SPRAY

Gastric mucin (porcine) 3.5%, xylitol 2%, sodium fluoride 4.2 mg/litre, with preservatives and flavouring agents, pH neutral.

- **INDICATIONS AND DOSE**

Symptomatic treatment of dry mouth

▸ BY MOUTH

- Child: Apply 2–3 sprays as required, spray onto oral and pharyngeal mucosa

- **PROFESSION SPECIFIC INFORMATION**

Dental practitioners' formulary

AS Saliva Orthana® Oral Spray may be prescribed.

AS Saliva Orthana spray (CCMed Ltd)
50 ml • NHS indicative price = £4.92 • Drug Tariff (Part IXa)

BIOXTRA® GEL

Lactoperoxidase, lactoferrin, lysozyme, whey colostrum, xylitol and other ingredients.

- **INDICATIONS AND DOSE**

Dry mouth as a result of having (or having undergone) radiotherapy | Dry mouth as a result of sicca syndrome

▸ BY MOUTH

- Child: Apply as required, apply to oral mucosa

- **PROFESSION SPECIFIC INFORMATION**

Dental practitioners' formulary

BioXtra® Gel may be prescribed.

BioXtra Dry Mouth oral gel (R.I.S. Products Ltd)
40 ml • NHS indicative price = £3.98 • Drug Tariff (Part IXa)

BIOTENE ORALBALANCE®

Lactoperoxidase, lactoferrin, lysozyme, glucose oxidase, xylitol in a gel basis

- **INDICATIONS AND DOSE**

Symptomatic treatment of dry mouth

▸ BY MOUTH

- Child: Apply as required, apply to gums and tongue

- **PATIENT AND CARER ADVICE** Avoid use with toothpastes containing detergents (including foaming agents).
- **PROFESSION SPECIFIC INFORMATION**

Dental practitioners' formulary

Biotene Oralbalance® Saliva Replacement Gel may be prescribed as Artificial Saliva Gel.

Biotene Oralbalance dry mouth saliva replacement gel (GlaxoSmithKline Consumer Healthcare) **Glucose oxidase 12000 unit, Lactoferrin 12 mg, Lactoperoxidase 12000 unit, Muramidase 12 mg** 50 gram • NHS indicative price = £4.46 • Drug Tariff (Part IXa)

GLANDOSANE®

Carmellose sodium 500 mg, sorbitol 1.5 g, potassium chloride 60 mg, sodium chloride 42.2 mg, magnesium chloride 2.6 mg, calcium chloride 7.3 mg, and dipotassium hydrogen phosphate 17.1 mg/50 g, pH 5.75.

● **INDICATIONS AND DOSE**

Dry mouth as a result of having (or having undergone) radiotherapy (ACBS) | Dry mouth as a result of sicca syndrome (ACBS)

▶ BY MOUTH

▸ Child: Apply as required, spray onto oral and pharyngeal mucosa

● **PROFESSION SPECIFIC INFORMATION**

Dental practitioners' formulary
Glandosane® Aerosol Spray may be prescribed.

Glandosane synthetic saliva spray lemon (Fresenius Kabi Ltd)
50 ml • NHS indicative price = £5.68 • Drug Tariff (Part IXa)

Glandosane synthetic saliva spray natural (Fresenius Kabi Ltd)
50 ml • NHS indicative price = £5.68 • Drug Tariff (Part IXa)

Glandosane synthetic saliva spray peppermint (Fresenius Kabi Ltd)
50 ml • NHS indicative price = £5.68 • Drug Tariff (Part IXa)

ORALIEVE MOISTURISING MOUTH SPRAY
Aqua, glycerin, xylitol, poloxamer 407, sodium benzoate, monosodium phosphate, xanthan gum, aroma, disodium phosphate, benzoic acid, whey protein, lactoferrin, lactoperoxidase, potassium thiocyanate, glucose oxidase, SLS free, alcohol free, pH 5.8

Oralieve moisturising mouth spray (Oralieve UK)
50 ml • NHS indicative price = £4.95 • Drug Tariff (Part IXa)

ORALIEVE GEL

● **INDICATIONS AND DOSE**

Symptomatic treatment of dry mouth

▶ BY MOUTH

▸ Child: Apply as required, particularly at night, to oral mucosa

● **PRESCRIBING AND DISPENSING INFORMATION** Contains traces of milk protein and egg white protein.

Oralieve moisturising mouth gel (Oralieve UK)
50 ml • NHS indicative price = £2.96 • Drug Tariff (Part IXa)

SST®
Sugar-free, citric acid, malic acid and other ingredients in a sorbitol base.

● **INDICATIONS AND DOSE**

Symptomatic treatment of dry mouth in patients with impaired salivary gland function and patent salivary ducts

▶ BY MOUTH

▸ Child: 1 tablet as required, allow tablet to dissolve slowly in the mouth

● **PROFESSION SPECIFIC INFORMATION**

Dental practitioners' formulary
May be prescribed as Saliva Stimulating Tablets.

SST saliva stimulating tablets (Sinclair IS Pharma Plc)
100 tablet • NHS indicative price = £4.86 • Drug Tariff (Part IXa)

SALIVEZE®
Carmellose sodium (sodium carboxymethylcellulose), calcium chloride, magnesium chloride, potassium chloride, sodium chloride, and dibasic sodium phosphate, pH neutral

● **INDICATIONS AND DOSE**

Dry mouth as a result of having (or having undergone) radiotherapy (ACBS) | Dry mouth as a result of sicca syndrome (ACBS)

▶ BY MOUTH

▸ Child: Apply 1 spray as required, spray onto oral mucosa

● **PROFESSION SPECIFIC INFORMATION**

Dental practitioners' formulary
Saliveze® Oral Spray may be prescribed.

Saliveze mouth spray (Wyvern Medical Ltd)
50 ml • NHS indicative price = £3.50 • Drug Tariff (Part IXa)

SALIVIX®
Sugar-free, reddish-amber, acacia, malic acid and other ingredients.

● **INDICATIONS AND DOSE**

Symptomatic treatment of dry mouth

▶ BY MOUTH USING PASTILLES

▸ Child: 1 unit as required, suck pastille

● **PROFESSION SPECIFIC INFORMATION**

Dental practitioners' formulary
Salivix® Pastilles may be prescribed as Artificial Saliva Pastilles.

Salivix pastilles (Galen Ltd)
50 pastille • NHS indicative price = £3.59 • Drug Tariff (Part IXa)

XEROTIN®
Sugar-free, water, sorbitol, carmellose (carboxymethylcellulose), potassium chloride, sodium chloride, potassium phosphate, magnesium chloride, calcium chloride and other ingredients, pH neutral.

● **INDICATIONS AND DOSE**

Symptomatic treatment of dry mouth

▶ BY MOUTH

▸ Child: 1 spray as required

● **PROFESSION SPECIFIC INFORMATION**

Dental practitioners' formulary
Xerotin® Oral Spray may be prescribed as Artificial Saliva Oral Spray.

Xerotin spray (SpePharm UK Ltd)
100 ml • NHS indicative price = £6.86 • Drug Tariff (Part IXa)

2 Oral hygiene

Mouthwashes and other preparations for oropharyngeal use

Lozenges and sprays

There is no convincing evidence that antiseptic lozenges and sprays have a beneficial action and they sometimes irritate and cause sore tongue and sore lips. Some of these preparations also contain local anaesthetics which relieve pain but may cause sensitisation.

Mouthwashes and gargles

Superficial infections of the mouth are often helped by warm mouthwashes which have a mechanical cleansing effect and cause some local hyperaemia. However, to be effective, they must be used frequently and vigorously. Mouthwashes may not be suitable for children under 7 years (risk of the solution being swallowed); the mouthwash or dental gel may be applied using a cotton bud.

A warm saline mouthwash is ideal and can be prepared either by dissolving half a teaspoonful of salt in a glassful of warm water or by diluting compound sodium chloride mouthwash p. 757 with an equal volume of warm water.

Mouthwashes containing an oxidising agent, such as hydrogen peroxide p. 757, may be useful in the treatment of acute ulcerative gingivitis (Vincent's infection) since the organisms involved are anaerobes. It also has a mechanical cleansing effect arising from frothing when in contact with oral debris. Concentrations greater than 1.5% in children may cause ulceration and tissue damage.

Chlorhexidine below is an effective antiseptic which has the advantage of inhibiting plaque formation on the teeth. It does not, however, completely control plaque deposition and is not a substitute for effective toothbrushing. Moreover, chlorhexidine preparations do not penetrate significantly into stagnation areas and are therefore of little value in the control of dental caries or of periodontal disease once pocketing has developed. Chlorhexidine preparations are of little value in the control of acute necrotising ulcerative gingivitis. With prolonged use, chlorhexidine causes reversible brown staining of teeth and tongue. Chlorhexidine may be incompatible with some ingredients in toothpaste, causing an unpleasant taste in the mouth; rinse the mouth thoroughly with water between using toothpaste and chlorhexidine-containing products.

Chlorhexidine can be used as a mouthwash, spray or gel for secondary infection in mucosal ulceration and for controlling gingivitis, as an adjunct to other oral hygiene measures. These preparations may also be used instead of toothbrushing where there is a painful periodontal condition (e.g. primary herpetic stomatitis) or if the patient has a haemorrhagic disorder, or is disabled. Chlorhexidine mouthwash is used in the prevention of oral candidiasis in immunocompromised patients. Chlorhexidine mouthwash reduces the incidence of alveolar osteitis following tooth extraction. Chlorhexidine mouthwash should not be used for the prevention of endocarditis in children undergoing dental procedures.

ANTISEPTICS AND DISINFECTANTS

Chlorhexidine

21-Nov-2019

● **INDICATIONS AND DOSE**

Oral hygiene and plaque inhibition | Oral candidiasis | Gingivitis | Management of aphthous ulcers

▸ BY MOUTH USING MOUTHWASH

▸ Child: Rinse or gargle 10 mL twice daily (rinse or gargle for about 1 minute)

Oral hygiene and plaque inhibition and gingivitis

▸ BY MOUTH USING DENTAL GEL

▸ Child: Apply 1–2 times a day, to be brushed on the teeth

Oral candidiasis | Management of aphthous ulcers

▸ BY MOUTH USING DENTAL GEL

▸ Child: Apply 1–2 times a day, to affected areas

Oral hygiene and plaque inhibition | Oral candidiasis | Gingivitis | Management of aphthous ulcers

▸ BY MOUTH USING OROMUCOSAL SPRAY

▸ Child: Apply up to 12 sprays twice daily as required, to be applied tooth, gingival, or ulcer surfaces

Bladder irrigation and catheter patency solutions

▸ BY INTRAVESICAL INSTILLATION

▸ Child: (consult product literature)

● **UNLICENSED USE**

▸ With oral (topical) use *Corsodyl®* not licensed for use in children under 12 years (unless on the advice of a healthcare professional).

● **SIDE-EFFECTS**

▸ **Common or very common**

▸ With oromucosal use Dry mouth · hypersensitivity · oral disorders · taste altered · tongue discolouration · tooth discolouration

SIDE-EFFECTS, FURTHER INFORMATION If desquamation occurs with mucosal irritation, discontinue treatment.

● **PATIENT AND CARER ADVICE**

▸ With oral (topical) use Chlorhexidine gluconate may be incompatible with some ingredients in toothpaste; rinse the mouth thoroughly with water between using toothpaste and chlorhexidine-containing product.

● **PROFESSION SPECIFIC INFORMATION**

Dental practitioners' formulary

▸ With oral (topical) use *Corsodyl®* dental gel may be prescribed as Chlorhexidine Gluconate Gel; *Corsodyl®* mouthwash may be prescribed as Chlorhexidine Mouthwash; *Corsodyl®* oral spray may be prescribed as Chlorhexidine Oral Spray.

● **MEDICINAL FORMS** There can be variation in the licensing of different medicines containing the same drug. Forms available from special-order manufacturers include: liquid, irrigation solution

Dental gel

▸ Corsodyl (GlaxoSmithKline Consumer Healthcare)
Chlorhexidine gluconate 10 mg per 1 gram Corsodyl 1% dental gel sugar-free | 50 gram [P] £2.23 DT = £2.23

Irrigation

▸ Chlorhexidine (Non-proprietary)
Chlorhexidine acetate 200 microgram per 1 ml Chlorhexidine acetate 0.02% catheter maintenance solution | 100 ml [P] [X] DT = £2.70

▸ Uro-Tainer (chlorhexidine) (B.Braun Medical Ltd)
Chlorhexidine acetate 200 microgram per 1 ml Uro-Tainer chlorhexidine 1:5000 catheter maintenance solution | 100 ml [P] £2.70 DT = £2.70

Mouthwash

▸ Chlorhexidine (Non-proprietary)
Chlorhexidine gluconate 2 mg per 1 ml Chlorhexidine gluconate 0.2% mouthwash aniseed | 300 ml [GSL] £2.09 DT = £3.19
Chlorhexidine gluconate 0.2% mouthwash natural | 300 ml [GSL] £4.18 DT = £3.19
Chlorhexidine gluconate 0.2% mouthwash plain | 300 ml [GSL] £3.19 DT = £3.19
Chlorhexidine gluconate 0.2% mouthwash peppermint | 300 ml [GSL] £4.19 DT = £3.19
Chlorhexidine gluconate 0.2% mouthwash original | 300 ml [GSL] £4.18 DT = £3.19

▸ Corsodyl (GlaxoSmithKline Consumer Healthcare)
Chlorhexidine gluconate 2 mg per 1 ml Corsodyl Mint 0.2% mouthwash | 300 ml [GSL] £2.99 DT = £3.19 | 600 ml [GSL] £4.50
Corsodyl 0.2% mouthwash aniseed | 300 ml [GSL] £2.99 DT = £3.19
Corsodyl 0.2% mouthwash alcohol free | 300 ml [GSL] £3.57 DT = £3.19

▸ Curasept (Curaprox (UK) Ltd)
Chlorhexidine gluconate 2 mg per 1 ml Curasept 0.2% oral rinse | 200 ml [X]

Irrigation solution

▸ Chlorhexidine (Non-proprietary)
Chlorhexidine acetate 200 microgram per 1 ml Chlorhexidine acetate 0.02% irrigation solution 1litre bottles | 1 bottle [P] [X]
Chlorhexidine acetate 500 microgram per 1 ml Chlorhexidine acetate 0.05% irrigation solution 1litre bottles | 1 bottle [P] [X]

Hexetidine

06-Aug-2018

● **INDICATIONS AND DOSE**

Oral hygiene

▸ BY MOUTH USING MOUTHWASH

▸ Child 12–17 years: Rinse or gargle 15 mL 2–3 times a day, to be used undiluted

● **SIDE-EFFECTS**

▸ **Rare or very rare** Anaesthesia · taste altered

▸ **Frequency not known** Cough · dry mouth · dysphagia · dyspnoea · nausea · salivary gland enlargement · vomiting

● **MEDICINAL FORMS** There can be variation in the licensing of different medicines containing the same drug.

Mouthwash

▸ Oraldene (McNeil Products Ltd)
Hexetidine 1 mg per 1 ml Oraldene 0.1% mouthwash peppermint sugar-free | 200 ml [GSL] £2.92 DT = £2.92

Hydrogen peroxide

03-Mar-2020

● **DRUG ACTION** Hydrogen peroxide is an oxidising agent.

● **INDICATIONS AND DOSE**

Oral hygiene (with hydrogen peroxide 6%)

▶ BY MOUTH USING MOUTHWASH

▸ Child: Rinse or gargle 15 mL 2–3 times a day for 2–3 minutes, to be diluted in half a tumblerful of warm water

PEROXYL ®

Oral hygiene

▶ BY MOUTH USING MOUTHWASH

▸ Child 6-17 years: Rinse or gargle 10 mL 3 times a day for about 1 minute, for maximum 7 days, to be used after meals and at bedtime

● **PRESCRIBING AND DISPENSING INFORMATION** When prepared extemporaneously, the BP states Hydrogen Peroxide Mouthwash, BP consists of hydrogen peroxide 6% solution (= approx. 20 volume) BP.

● **HANDLING AND STORAGE** Hydrogen peroxide bleaches fabric.

● **PROFESSION SPECIFIC INFORMATION**

Dental practitioners' formulary
Hydrogen Peroxide Mouthwash may be prescribed.

● **MEDICINAL FORMS** There can be variation in the licensing of different medicines containing the same drug. Forms available from special-order manufacturers include: liquid

Mouthwash

▸ Peroxyl (Colgate-Palmolive (UK) Ltd)
Hydrogen peroxide 15 mg per 1 ml Peroxyl 1.5% mouthwash sugar-free | 300 ml GSL £2.94 DT = £2.94

Sodium bicarbonate with sodium chloride

● **INDICATIONS AND DOSE**

Oral hygiene

▶ BY MOUTH USING MOUTHWASH

▸ Child: (consult product literature)

● **DIRECTIONS FOR ADMINISTRATION** For mouthwash, extemporaneous preparations should be prepared according to the following formula: sodium chloride 1.5 g, sodium bicarbonate 1 g, concentrated peppermint emulsion 2.5 mL, double-strength chloroform water 50 mL, water to 100 mL. To be diluted with an equal volume of warm water prior to administration.

● **PRESCRIBING AND DISPENSING INFORMATION** Flavours of mouthwash may include peppermint.

● **PROFESSION SPECIFIC INFORMATION**

Dental practitioners' formulary
Compound sodium chloride mouthwash may be prescribed.

● **MEDICINAL FORMS** Forms available from special-order manufacturers include: oral solution, mouthwash

Sodium chloride

01-May-2020

● **INDICATIONS AND DOSE**

Oral hygiene

▶ BY MOUTH USING MOUTHWASH

▸ Child: Rinse or gargle as required

● **DIRECTIONS FOR ADMINISTRATION** Extemporaneous mouthwash preparations should be prepared according to the following formula: sodium chloride 1.5 g, sodium bicarbonate 1 g, concentrated peppermint emulsion 2.5 mL, double-strength chloroform water 50 mL, water to 100 mL. To be diluted with an equal volume of warm water.

● **PRESCRIBING AND DISPENSING INFORMATION** No mouthwash preparations available—when prepared extemporaneously, the BP states Sodium Chloride Mouthwash, Compound, BP consists of sodium bicarbonate 1%, sodium chloride 1.5% in a suitable vehicle with peppermint flavour.

● **PROFESSION SPECIFIC INFORMATION**

Dental practitioners' formulary Compound Sodium Chloride Mouthwash may be prescribed.

● **MEDICINAL FORMS** No licensed medicines listed.

2.1 Dental caries

Fluoride imbalance

Overview

Availability of adequate fluoride confers significant resistance to dental caries. It is now considered that the topical action of fluoride on enamel and plaque is more important than the systemic effect.

When the fluoride content of drinking water is less than 700 micrograms per litre (0.7 parts per million), daily administration of fluoride tablets or drops provides suitable supplementation. Systemic fluoride supplements should not be prescribed without reference to the fluoride content of the local water supply. Infants need not receive fluoride supplements until the age of 6 months.

Dentifrices which incorporate sodium fluoride or monofluorophosphate are also a convenient source of fluoride.

Individuals who are either particularly caries prone or medically compromised may be given additional protection by use of fluoride rinses or by application of fluoride gels. Rinses may be used daily or weekly; daily use of a less concentrated rinse is more effective than weekly use of a more concentrated one. High-strength gels must be applied regularly under professional supervision; extreme caution is necessary to prevent children from swallowing any excess. Less concentrated gels are available for home use. Varnishes are also available and are particularly valuable for young or disabled children since they adhere to the teeth and set in the presence of moisture.

VITAMINS AND TRACE ELEMENTS

Sodium fluoride

28-Feb-2020

● **INDICATIONS AND DOSE**

Prophylaxis of dental caries for water content less than 300micrograms/litre (0.3 parts per million) of fluoride ion

▶ BY MOUTH USING TABLETS

▸ Child 6 months-2 years: 250 micrograms daily, doses expressed as fluoride ion (F^-)

▸ Child 3-5 years: 500 micrograms daily, doses expressed as fluoride ion (F^-)

▸ Child 6-17 years: 1 mg daily, doses expressed as fluoride ion (F^-)

Prophylaxis of dental caries for water content between 300 and 700micrograms/litre (0.3–0.7 parts per million) of fluoride ion

▶ BY MOUTH USING TABLETS

▸ Child 3-5 years: 250 micrograms daily, doses expressed as fluoride ion (F^-)

continued →

12 Ear, nose and oropharynx

- Child 6–17 years: 500 micrograms daily, doses expressed as fluoride ion (F^-)

Prophylaxis of dental caries

▶ BY MOUTH USING MOUTHWASH

- Child 6–17 years: Rinse or gargle 5–10 mL daily

DOSE EQUIVALENCE AND CONVERSION

- Sodium fluoride 2.2 mg provides approx. 1 mg fluoride ion.

COLGATE DURAPHAT® 2800PPM FLUORIDE TOOTHPASTE

Prophylaxis of dental caries

▶ BY MOUTH USING PASTE

- Child 10–17 years: Apply 1 centimetre twice daily, to be applied using a toothbrush

COLGATE DURAPHAT® 5000PPM FLUORIDE TOOTHPASTE

Prophylaxis of dental caries

▶ BY MOUTH USING PASTE

- Child 16–17 years: Apply 2 centimetres 3 times a day, to be applied after meals using a toothbrush

EN-DE-KAY® FLUORINSE

Prophylaxis of dental caries

▶ BY MOUTH USING MOUTHWASH

- Child 8–17 years: 5 drops daily, dilute 5 drops to 10 mL of water, alternatively 20 drops once weekly, dilute 20 drops to 10 mL

12 Ear, nose and oropharynx

- **SIDE-EFFECTS** Dental fluorosis
- **DIRECTIONS FOR ADMINISTRATION** Tablets should be sucked or dissolved in the mouth and taken preferably in the evening.
For mouthwash, rinse mouth for 1 minute and then spit out.
COLGATE DURAPHAT® 5000PPM FLUORIDE TOOTHPASTE Brush teeth for 3 minutes before spitting out.
COLGATE DURAPHAT® 2800PPM FLUORIDE TOOTHPASTE Brush teeth for 1 minute before spitting out.
- **PRESCRIBING AND DISPENSING INFORMATION** Flavours of oral tablet formulations may include orange.
- **PATIENT AND CARER ADVICE**
Mouthwash Avoid eating, drinking, or rinsing mouth for 15 minutes after use.
COLGATE DURAPHAT® 5000PPM FLUORIDE TOOTHPASTE Patients or carers should be given advice on how to administer Sodium fluoride toothpaste.
COLGATE DURAPHAT® 2800PPM FLUORIDE TOOTHPASTE Patients or carers should be given advice on how to administer sodium fluoride toothpaste.
Avoid drinking or rinsing mouth for 30 minutes after use.
- **PROFESSION SPECIFIC INFORMATION**

Dental practitioners' formulary

Tablets may be prescribed as Sodium Fluoride Tablets.

Oral drops may be prescribed as Sodium Fluoride Oral Drops.

Mouthwashes may be prescribed as Sodium Fluoride Mouthwash 0.05% or Sodium Fluoride Mouthwash 2%.

COLGATE DURAPHAT® 5000PPM FLUORIDE TOOTHPASTE May be prescribed as Sodium Fluoride Toothpaste 1.1%.

COLGATE DURAPHAT® 2800PPM FLUORIDE TOOTHPASTE May be prescribed as Sodium Fluoride Toothpaste 0.619%.

Dental information

Fluoride mouthwash, oral drops, tablets and toothpaste are prescribable on form FP10D (GP14 in Scotland, WP10D in Wales).

There are also arrangements for health authorities to supply fluoride tablets in the course of pre-school dental schemes, and they may also be supplied in school dental schemes.

Fluoride gels are not prescribable on form FP10D (GP14 in Scotland, WP10D in Wales).

- **MEDICINAL FORMS** There can be variation in the licensing of different medicines containing the same drug. Forms available from special-order manufacturers include: oral solution

Tablet

- **Endekay** (Manx Healthcare Ltd)
Sodium fluoride 1.1 mg Endekay Fluotabs 3-6 Years 1.1mg tablets | 200 tablet [P] £2.38 DT = £2.38
Sodium fluoride 2.2 mg Endekay Fluotabs 6+ Years 2.2mg tablets | 200 tablet [P] £2.38 DT = £2.38

Paste

- **Sodium fluoride (Non-proprietary)**
Fluoride (as Sodium fluoride) 2.8 mg per 1 gram Sodium fluoride 0.619% dental paste sugar free sugar-free | 75 ml [PoM] £4.17 DT = £3.81
Fluoride (as Sodium fluoride) 5 mg per 1 gram Sodium fluoride 1.1% dental paste sugar free sugar-free | 51 gram [PoM] £7.88 DT = £6.88
- **Colgate Duraphat** (Colgate-Palmolive (UK) Ltd)
Fluoride (as Sodium fluoride) 2.8 mg per 1 gram Colgate Duraphat 2800ppm fluoride toothpaste sugar-free | 75 ml [PoM] £3.26 DT = £3.81
Fluoride (as Sodium fluoride) 5 mg per 1 gram Colgate Duraphat 5000ppm fluoride toothpaste sugar-free | 51 gram [PoM] £6.50 DT = £6.88

Mouthwash

- **Sodium fluoride (Non-proprietary)**
Sodium fluoride 500 microgram per 1 ml Sodium fluoride 0.05% mouthwash sugar free sugar-free | 250 ml [GSL] [X] DT = £1.51
- **Colgate FluoriGard** (Colgate-Palmolive (UK) Ltd)
Sodium fluoride 500 microgram per 1 ml Colgate FluoriGard 0.05% daily dental rinse alcohol free sugar-free | 400 ml £2.99
Colgate FluoriGard 0.05% daily dental rinse sugar-free | 400 ml [GSL] £2.99
- **Endekay** (Manx Healthcare Ltd)
Sodium fluoride 500 microgram per 1 ml Endekay 0.05% daily fluoride mouthrinse sugar-free | 250 ml [GSL] £1.51 DT = £1.51
sugar-free | 500 ml [GSL] £2.45

3 Oral ulceration and inflammation

Oral ulceration and inflammation

Ulceration and inflammation

Ulceration of the oral mucosa may be caused by trauma (physical or chemical), recurrent aphthae, infections, carcinoma, dermatological disorders, nutritional deficiencies, gastro-intestinal disease, haematopoietic disorders, and drug therapy. It is important to establish the diagnosis in each case as the majority of these lesions require specific management in addition to local treatment. Local treatment aims to protect the ulcerated area, to relieve pain, to reduce inflammation, or to control secondary infection. Children with an unexplained mouth ulcer of more than 3 weeks' duration require urgent referral to hospital to exclude oral cancer in adults or secondary causes such as leukaemia.

Simple mouthwashes

A **saline** mouthwash may relieve the pain of traumatic ulceration. The mouthwash is made up with warm water and used at frequent intervals until the discomfort and swelling subsides.

Antiseptic mouthwashes

Secondary bacterial infection may be a feature of any mucosal ulceration; it can increase discomfort and delay healing. Use of chlorhexidine mouthwash p. 756 is often beneficial and may accelerate healing of recurrent aphthae.

Corticosteroids

Topical corticosteroid therapy may be used for some forms of oral ulceration. In the case of aphthous ulcers it is most effective if applied in the 'prodromal' phase. Thrush or other types of candidiasis are recognised complications of corticosteroid treatment.

Hydrocortisone oromucosal tablets p. 760 are allowed to dissolve next to an ulcer and are useful in recurrent aphthae and erosive lichenoid lesions.

Beclometasone dipropionate inhaler p. 167 sprayed on the oral mucosa is used to manage oral ulceration [unlicensed indication]. Alternatively, betamethasone soluble tablets p. 760 dissolved in water can be used as a mouthwash to treat oral ulceration [unlicensed indication].

Systemic corticosteroid therapy (see under Corticosteroids, inflammatory disorders p. 714) is reserved for severe conditions such as pemphigus vulgaris.

Local analgesics

Local analgesics have a limited role in the management of oral ulceration. When applied topically their action is of a relatively short duration so that analgesia cannot be maintained continuously throughout the day. When local anaesthetics are used in the mouth, care must be taken not to produce anaesthesia of the pharynx before meals as this might lead to choking.

Benzydamine hydrochloride below and flurbiprofen p. 707 are non-steroidal anti-inflammatory drugs (NSAIDs). Benzydamine hydrochloride mouthwash or spray may be useful in reducing the discomfort associated with a variety of ulcerative conditions. It has also been found to be effective in reducing the discomfort of tonsillectomy and post-irradiation mucositis. Some patients find the full-strength mouthwash causes some stinging and, for them, it should be diluted with an equal volume of water. Flurbiprofen lozenges are licensed for the relief of sore throat in adolescents.

Choline salicylate p. 761 is a derivative of salicylic acid and has some analgesic action. The dental gel may provide relief for recurrent aphthae, but excessive application or confinement under a denture irritates the mucosa and can itself cause ulceration in adults and children over 16 years of age.

Other preparations

Doxycycline p. 761 rinsed in the mouth may be of value for recurrent aphthous ulceration.

Periodontitis

Low-dose doxycycline (*Periostat®*) is licensed as an adjunct to scaling and root planing for the treatment of periodontitis; a low dose of doxycycline reduces collagenase activity without inhibiting bacteria associated with periodontitis.

For anti-infectives used in the treatment of destructive (refractory) forms of periodontal disease, see under Oropharyngeal infections, antibacterial therapy p. 761. See also Mouthwashes and other preparations for oropharyngeal use p. 755 for mouthwashes used for oral hygiene and plaque inhibition.

ANAESTHETICS, LOCAL

Lidocaine hydrochloride 11-Dec-2019

(Lignocaine hydrochloride)

● **INDICATIONS AND DOSE**

Dental practice

▶ BY BUCCAL ADMINISTRATION USING OINTMENT

▸ Child: Rub gently into dry gum

XYLOCAINE®

Bronchoscopy | Laryngoscopy | Oesophagoscopy | Endotracheal intubation

▶ TO MUCOUS MEMBRANES

▸ Child: Up to 3 mg/kg

● **CAUTIONS** Can damage plastic cuffs of endotracheal tubes

● **INTERACTIONS** → Appendix 1: antiarrhythmics

● **ALLERGY AND CROSS-SENSITIVITY**

▸ Hypersensitivity and cross-sensitivity Hypersensitivity reactions occur mainly with the ester-type local anaesthetics, such as tetracaine; reactions are less frequent with the amide types, such as articaine, bupivacaine, levobupivacaine, lidocaine, mepivacaine, prilocaine, and ropivacaine. Cross-sensitivity reactions may be avoided by using the alternative chemical type.

● **PREGNANCY** Crosses the placenta but not known to be harmful in *animal* studies—use if benefit outweighs risk. When used as a local anaesthetic, large doses can cause fetal bradycardia; if given during delivery can also cause neonatal respiratory depression, hypotonia, or bradycardia after paracervical or epidural block.

● **BREAST FEEDING** Present in milk but amount too small to be harmful.

● **HEPATIC IMPAIRMENT** Manufacturer advises caution (risk of increased exposure).

● **RENAL IMPAIRMENT** Possible accumulation of lidocaine and active metabolite; caution in severe impairment.

● **PROFESSION SPECIFIC INFORMATION**

Dental practitioners' formulary

Lidocaine ointment 5% may be prescribed. Spray may be prescribed as Lidocaine Spray 10%

XYLOCAINE® May be prescribed as lidocaine spray 10%.

● **MEDICINAL FORMS** There can be variation in the licensing of different medicines containing the same drug. Forms available from special-order manufacturers include: liquid, ointment

Spray

▸ Xylocaine (Aspen Pharma Trading Ltd)

Lidocaine 10 mg per 1 actuation Xylocaine 10mg/dose spray sugar-free | 50 ml Ⓟ £6.29 DT = £6.29

Ointment

▸ Lidocaine hydrochloride (Non-proprietary)

Lidocaine hydrochloride 50 mg per 1 gram Lidocaine 5% ointment | 15 gram Ⓟ £9.00 DT = £8.28

ANALGESICS > NON-STEROIDAL ANTI-INFLAMMATORY DRUGS

Benzydamine hydrochloride 18-Feb-2020

● **INDICATIONS AND DOSE**

Painful inflammatory conditions of oropharynx

▶ TO THE LESION USING MOUTHWASH

▸ Child 13–17 years: Rinse or gargle 15 mL every 1.5–3 hours as required usually for not more than 7 days, dilute with an equal volume of water if stinging occurs

▶ TO THE LESION USING OROMUCOSAL SPRAY

▸ Child 1 month–5 years (body-weight 4–7 kg): 1 spray every 1.5–3 hours, to be administered onto the affected area

▸ Child 1 month–5 years (body-weight 8–11 kg): 2 sprays every 1.5–3 hours, to be administered onto the affected area

▸ Child 1 month–5 years (body-weight 12–15 kg): 3 sprays every 1.5–3 hours, to be administered onto the affected area

▸ Child 1 month–5 years (body-weight 16 kg and above): 4 sprays every 1.5–3 hours, to be administered onto the affected area

continued →

- Child 6–11 years: 4 sprays every 1.5–3 hours, to be administered onto affected area
- Child 12–17 years: 4–8 sprays every 1.5–3 hours, to be administered onto affected area

- **INTERACTIONS** → Appendix 1: NSAIDs
- **SIDE-EFFECTS**
  - **Uncommon** Oral disorders
  - **Rare or very rare** Photosensitivity reaction · respiratory disorders · skin reactions
  - **Frequency not known** Angioedema
- **PROFESSION SPECIFIC INFORMATION**

Dental practitioners' formulary
Benzydamine Oromucosal Spray 0.15% may be prescribed.
Benzydamine mouthwash may be prescribed as Benzydamine Mouthwash 0.15%.

- **MEDICINAL FORMS** There can be variation in the licensing of different medicines containing the same drug.

Spray
- Benzydamine hydrochloride (Non-proprietary)
  Benzydamine hydrochloride 1.5 mg per 1 ml Benzydamine 0.15% oromucosal spray sugar free sugar-free | 30 ml Ⓟ £4.24 DT = £2.91
- Difflam (Mylan)
  Benzydamine hydrochloride 1.5 mg per 1 ml Difflam 0.15% spray sugar-free | 30 ml Ⓟ £4.24 DT = £2.91

Mouthwash
- Benzydamine hydrochloride (Non-proprietary)
  Benzydamine hydrochloride 1.5 mg per 1 ml Benzydamine 0.15% mouthwash sugar free sugar-free | 300 ml Ⓟ £9.75 DT = £7.79
- Difflam (Mylan)
  Benzydamine hydrochloride 1.5 mg per 1 ml Difflam Oral Rinse 0.15% solution sugar-free | 300 ml Ⓟ £6.50 DT = £7.79
  Difflam 0.15% Sore Throat Rinse sugar-free | 200 ml Ⓟ £4.64

Flurbiprofen

27-Apr-2020

- **INDICATIONS AND DOSE**

Relief of sore throat
- BY MOUTH USING LOZENGES
  - Child 12–17 years: 1 lozenge every 3–6 hours for maximum 3 days, allow lozenge to dissolve slowly in the mouth; maximum 5 lozenges per day

- **INTERACTIONS** → Appendix 1: NSAIDs
- **SIDE-EFFECTS** Oral ulceration (move lozenge around mouth) · taste altered
- **ALLERGY AND CROSS-SENSITIVITY** Contra-indicated in patients with a history of hypersensitivity to aspirin or any other NSAID—which includes those in whom attacks of asthma, angioedema, urticaria or rhinitis have been precipitated by aspirin or any other NSAID.

- **MEDICINAL FORMS** There can be variation in the licensing of different medicines containing the same drug.

Lozenge
- Strefen (Reckitt Benckiser Healthcare (UK) Ltd)
  Flurbiprofen 8.75 mg Strefen Honey and Lemon 8.75mg lozenges | 16 lozenge Ⓟ £3.42 DT = £3.42

CORTICOSTEROIDS

F 472

Betamethasone

28-Nov-2019

- **INDICATIONS AND DOSE**

Oral ulceration
- TO THE LESION USING SOLUBLE TABLETS
  - Child 12–17 years: 500 micrograms 4 times a day, to be dissolved in 20 mL water and rinsed around the mouth; not to be swallowed

- **UNLICENSED USE** Betamethasone soluble tablets not licensed for use as mouthwash or in oral ulceration.
- **CONTRA-INDICATIONS** Untreated local infection
- **INTERACTIONS** → Appendix 1: corticosteroids
- **PATIENT AND CARER ADVICE** Patient counselling is advised for betamethasone soluble tablets (administration).
- **PROFESSION SPECIFIC INFORMATION**

Dental practitioners' formulary Betamethasone Soluble Tablets 500 micrograms may be prescribed.

- **MEDICINAL FORMS** There can be variation in the licensing of different medicines containing the same drug.

Soluble tablet

CAUTIONARY AND ADVISORY LABELS 10, 13, 21 (not for use as mouthwash for oral ulceration)
- Betamethasone (Non-proprietary)
  Betamethasone (as Betamethasone sodium phosphate)
  500 microgram Betamethasone 500microgram soluble tablets sugar free sugar-free | 100 tablet [PoM] £58.15 DT = £58.15

F 472

Hydrocortisone

17-Dec-2019

- **INDICATIONS AND DOSE**

Oral and perioral lesions
- TO THE LESION USING BUCCAL TABLET
  - Child 1 month–11 years: Only on medical advice
  - Child 12–17 years: 1 lozenge 4 times a day, allowed to dissolve slowly in the mouth in contact with the ulcer

- **UNLICENSED USE** *Hydrocortisone mucoadhesive buccal tablets* licensed for use in children (under 12 years—on medical advice only).

IMPORTANT SAFETY INFORMATION

MHRA/CHM ADVICE: HYDROCORTISONE MUCO-ADHESIVE BUCCAL TABLETS: SHOULD NOT BE USED OFF-LABEL FOR ADRENAL INSUFFICIENCY IN CHILDREN DUE TO SERIOUS RISKS (DECEMBER 2018)

The MHRA has received reports of off-label use of hydrocortisone muco-adhesive buccal tablets for adrenal insufficiency in children.

Healthcare professionals are advised that:
- hydrocortisone muco-adhesive buccal tablets are indicated only for local use in the mouth for aphthous ulceration and should not be used to treat adrenal insufficiency;
- substitution of licensed oral hydrocortisone formulations with muco-adhesive buccal tablets can result in insufficient cortisol absorption and, in stress situations, life-threatening adrenal crisis;
- only hydrocortisone products licensed for adrenal replacement therapy should be used.

- **CONTRA-INDICATIONS** Untreated local infection
- **INTERACTIONS** → Appendix 1: corticosteroids
- **PROFESSION SPECIFIC INFORMATION**

Dental practitioners' formulary Mucoadhesive buccal tablets may be prescribed as Hydrocortisone Oromucosal Tablets.

- **MEDICINAL FORMS** There can be variation in the licensing of different medicines containing the same drug.

Muco-adhesive buccal tablet
- Hydrocortisone (Non-proprietary)
  Hydrocortisone (as Hydrocortisone sodium succinate)
  2.5 mg Hydrocortisone 2.5mg muco-adhesive buccal tablets sugar free sugar-free | 20 tablet Ⓟ £8.96 DT = £8.96

SALICYLIC ACID AND DERIVATIVES

Choline salicylate

14-Feb-2020

● **INDICATIONS AND DOSE**

Mild oral and perioral lesions

▸ TO THE LESION

▸ Child 16–17 years: Apply 0.5 inch, apply with gentle massage, not more often than every 3 hours

● **CONTRA-INDICATIONS** Children under 16 years

CONTRA-INDICATIONS, FURTHER INFORMATION

▸ Reye's syndrome The CHM has advised that topical oral pain relief products containing salicylate salts should not be used in children under 16 years, as a cautionary measure due to the theoretical risk of Reye's syndrome.

● **CAUTIONS** Frequent application, especially in children, may give rise to salicylate poisoning

● **INTERACTIONS** → Appendix 1: choline salicylate

● **SIDE-EFFECTS** Bronchospasm

● **PRESCRIBING AND DISPENSING INFORMATION** When prepared extemporaneously, the BP states Choline Salicylate Dental Gel, BP consists of choline salicylate 8.7% in a flavoured gel basis.

● **PROFESSION SPECIFIC INFORMATION**

Dental practitioners' formulary

Choline Salicylate Dental Gel may be prescribed.

● **MEDICINAL FORMS** There can be variation in the licensing of different medicines containing the same drug.

Oromucosal gel

▸ Bonjela (Reckitt Benckiser Healthcare (UK) Ltd)

Choline salicylate 87 mg per 1 gram Bonjela Cool Mint gel sugar-free | 15 gram GSL £3.55 DT = £2.91

Bonjela Original gel sugar-free | 15 gram GSL £2.91 DT = £2.91

Salicylic acid with rhubarb extract

18-Feb-2020

● **INDICATIONS AND DOSE**

Mild oral and perioral lesions

▸ TO THE LESION

▸ Child 16–17 years: Apply 3–4 times a day maximum duration 7 days

● **CONTRA-INDICATIONS** Children under 16 years

CONTRA-INDICATIONS, FURTHER INFORMATION

▸ Reye's syndrome The CHM has advised that topical oral pain relief products containing salicylate salts should not be used in children under 16 years, as a cautionary measure due to the theoretical risk of Reye's syndrome.

● **CAUTIONS** Frequent application, especially in children, may give rise to salicylate poisoning

● **SIDE-EFFECTS**

▸ **Common or very common** Oral discolouration · tooth discolouration

● **PATIENT AND CARER ADVICE** May cause temporary discolouration of teeth and oral mucosa.

● **MEDICINAL FORMS** There can be variation in the licensing of different medicines containing the same drug.

Paint

EXCIPIENTS: May contain Ethanol

▸ Pyralvex (Mylan)

Salicylic acid 10 mg per 1 ml, Rhubarb extract 50 mg per 1 ml Pyralvex solution | 10 ml P £3.25

4 Oropharyngeal bacterial infections

Oropharyngeal infections, antibacterial therapy

Pericoronitis

Antibacterial required only in presence of systemic features of infection, or of trismus, or persistent swelling despite local treatment.

● Metronidazole p. 358, or *alternatively*, amoxicillin p. 366

▸ *Suggested duration of treatment* 3 days or until symptoms resolve.

Gingivitis (acute necrotising ulcerative)

Antibacterial required only if systemic features of infection.

● Metronidazole, or *alternatively*, amoxicillin

▸ *Suggested duration of treatment* 3 days or until symptoms resolve.

Abscess (periapical or periodontal)

Antibacterial required only in severe disease with cellulitis or if systemic features of infection.

● Amoxicillin, or *alternatively*, metronidazole

▸ *Suggested duration of treatment* 5 days.

Periodontitis

Antibacterial used as an adjunct to debridement in severe disease or disease unresponsive to local treatment alone.

● Metronidazole, or *alternatively in adults and children over 12 years*, doxycycline p. 381

Sore throat (acute)

Acute sore throat is usually triggered by a viral infection and is self-limiting. Symptoms can last for around 1 week, and most people will improve within this time without treatment with antibiotics, regardless of the cause.

EvGr Antibacterial therapy is required only in patients with severe systemic symptoms, signs and symptoms of a more serious illness or condition, or those at high risk of complications. Patients with severe systemic infection or severe suppurative complications such as peri-tonsillar abscess (quinsy), acute otitis media, acute sinusitis or cellulitis should be referred to hospital. Ⓐ

● Phenoxymethylpenicillin p. 365

▸ *Suggested duration of treatment* 5 to 10 days.

● *If penicillin-allergic*, clarithromycin p. 353 (*or* erythromycin p. 355)

▸ *Suggested duration of treatment* 5 days.

ANTIBACTERIALS › TETRACYCLINES AND RELATED DRUGS

F 380

Doxycycline

18-May-2020

● **INDICATIONS AND DOSE**

Treatment of recurrent aphthous ulceration

▸ BY MOUTH USING SOLUBLE TABLETS

▸ Child 12–17 years: 100 mg 4 times a day usually for 3 days, dispersible tablet can be stirred into a small amount of water then rinsed around the mouth for 2–3 minutes, it should preferably not be swallowed

● **UNLICENSED USE** Doxycycline may be used as detailed below, although these situations are considered outside the scope of its licence:
- recurrent aphthous ulceration.

● **CAUTIONS** Alcohol dependence

- **INTERACTIONS** → Appendix 1: tetracyclines
- **SIDE-EFFECTS**
  - ▸ **Common or very common** Dyspnoea · hypotension · peripheral oedema · tachycardia
  - ▸ **Uncommon** Gastrointestinal discomfort
  - ▸ **Rare or very rare** Antibiotic associated colitis · anxiety · arthralgia · flushing · intracranial pressure increased with papilloedema · Jarisch-Herxheimer reaction · myalgia · photoonycholysis · severe cutaneous adverse reactions (SCARs) · skin hyperpigmentation (long term use) · tinnitus · vision disorders
- **RENAL IMPAIRMENT** Use with caution (avoid excessive doses).
- **PATIENT AND CARER ADVICE** Counselling on administration advised.
  Photosensitivity Patients should be advised to avoid exposure to sunlight or sun lamps.
- **PROFESSION SPECIFIC INFORMATION**
  Dental practitioners' formulary
  Dispersible tablets may be prescribed as Dispersible Doxycycline Tablets.

- **MEDICINAL FORMS** There can be variation in the licensing of different medicines containing the same drug.
  Dispersible tablet
  CAUTIONARY AND ADVISORY LABELS 6, 9, 11, 13
  - ▸ Vibramycin-D (Pfizer Ltd)
    Doxycycline (as Doxycycline monohydrate) 100 mg Vibramycin-D 100mg dispersible tablets sugar-free | 8 tablet PoM £4.91 DT = £4.91

5 Oropharyngeal fungal infections

Oropharyngeal fungal infections

Overview

Fungal infections of the mouth are usually caused by *Candida* spp. (candidiasis or candidosis). Different types of oropharyngeal candidiasis are managed as follows:

Thrush

Acute pseudomembranous candidiasis (thrush), is usually an acute infection but it may persist for months in patients receiving inhaled corticosteroids, cytotoxics, or broad-spectrum antibacterials. Thrush also occurs in patients with serious systemic disease associated with reduced immunity such as leukaemia, other malignancies, and HIV infection. Any predisposing condition should be managed appropriately. When thrush is associated with corticosteroid inhalers, rinsing the mouth with water (or cleaning a child's teeth) immediately after using the inhaler may avoid the problem. Treatment with nystatin p. 763 or miconazole below may be needed. Fluconazole p. 407 is effective for unresponsive infections or if a topical antifungal drug cannot be used. Topical therapy may not be adequate in immunocompromised children and an oral triazole antifungal is preferred.

Acute erythematous candidiasis

Acute erythematous (atrophic) candidiasis is a relatively uncommon condition associated with corticosteroid and broad-spectrum antibacterial use and with HIV disease. It is usually treated with fluconazole.

Angular cheilitis

Angular cheilitis (angular stomatitis) is characterised by soreness, erythema and fissuring at the angles of the mouth. It may represent a nutritional deficiency or it may be related to orofacial granulomatosis or HIV infection. Both yeasts (*Candida* spp.) and bacteria (*Staphylococcus aureus* and beta-haemolytic streptococci) are commonly involved as interacting, infective factors. While the underlying cause is being identified and treated, it is often helpful to apply miconazole cream or fusidic acid ointment p. 387; if the angular cheilitis is unresponsive to treatment, hydrocortisone with miconazole cream or ointment p. 795 can be used.

Immunocompromised patients

See advice on prevention of fungal infections under *Immunocompromised children* in Antifungals, systemic use p. 403.

Antiseptic mouthwashes can have a role in the prevention of oral candidiasis in immunocompromised children.

Drugs used in oropharyngeal candidiasis

Nystatin is not absorbed from the gastro-intestinal tract and is applied locally (as a suspension) to the mouth for treating local fungal infections. Miconazole is used by local application (as an oral gel) in the mouth but it is also absorbed to the extent that potential interactions need to be considered. Miconazole also has some activity against Gram-positive bacteria including streptococci and staphylococci. In neonates, nystatin oral suspension or miconazole oral gel is used for the treatment of oropharyngeal candidiasis; to prevent re-infection it is important to ensure that the mother's breast nipples and the teats of feeding bottles are cleaned adequately.

Fluconazole given by mouth is reliably absorbed; it is used for infections that do not respond to topical therapy or when topical therapy cannot be used. Itraconazole p. 409 can be used for fluconazole-resistant infections.

If candidal infection fails to respond after 1 to 2 weeks of treatment with antifungal drugs the child should be sent for investigation to eliminate the possibility of underlying disease. Persistent infection may also be caused by re-infection from the genito-urinary or gastro-intestinal tract.

ANTIFUNGALS > IMIDAZOLE ANTIFUNGALS

Miconazole

20-Jan-2020

- **INDICATIONS AND DOSE**

Oral candidiasis

▸ BY MOUTH USING ORAL GEL

- ▸ Neonate: 1 mL 2–4 times a day treatment should be continued for at least 7 days after lesions have healed or symptoms have cleared, to be smeared around the inside of the mouth after feeds.
- ▸ Child 1–23 months: 1.25 mL 4 times a day treatment should be continued for at least 7 days after lesions have healed or symptoms have cleared, to be smeared around the inside of the mouth after feeds
- ▸ Child 2–17 years: 2.5 mL 4 times a day treatment should be continued for at least 7 days after lesions have healed or symptoms have cleared, to be administered after meals, retain near oral lesions before swallowing (dental prostheses and orthodontic appliances should be removed at night and brushed with gel)

Intestinal candidiasis

▸ BY MOUTH USING ORAL GEL

- ▸ Child 4 months–17 years: 5 mg/kg 4 times a day (max. per dose 250 mg) treatment should be continued for at least 7 days after lesions have healed or symptoms have cleared

Prevention and treatment of oral candidiasis (dose approved for use by community practitioner nurse prescribers)

▸ BY MOUTH USING ORAL GEL

- ▸ Child 4–23 months: 1.25 mL 4 times a day treatment should be continued for at least 7 days after lesions

have healed or symptoms have cleared, to be smeared around the inside of the mouth after feeds
- Child 2-17 years: 2.5 mL 4 times a day treatment should be continued for at least 7 days after lesions have healed or symptoms have cleared, to be administered after meals, retain near oral lesions before swallowing (dental prostheses and orthodontic appliances should be removed at night and brushed with gel)

- **UNLICENSED USE** Not licensed for use in children under 4 months of age or during first 5–6 months of life of an infant born pre-term.
- **CONTRA-INDICATIONS** Infants with impaired swallowing reflex
- **CAUTIONS** Avoid in Acute porphyrias p. 652
- **INTERACTIONS** → Appendix 1: antifungals, azoles
- **SIDE-EFFECTS**
  - **Uncommon** Skin reactions
  - **Frequency not known** Angioedema
- **PREGNANCY** Manufacturer advises avoid if possible—toxicity at high doses in *animal* studies.
- **BREAST FEEDING** Manufacturer advises caution—no information available.
- **HEPATIC IMPAIRMENT** Manufacturer advises avoid.
- **DIRECTIONS FOR ADMINISTRATION** Oral gel should be held in mouth, after food.
- **PRESCRIBING AND DISPENSING INFORMATION** Flavours of oral gel may include orange.
- **PATIENT AND CARER ADVICE** Patients or carers should be given advice on how to administer miconazole oromucosal gel.
- **PROFESSION SPECIFIC INFORMATION**
  Dental practitioners' formulary Miconazole Oromucosal Gel may be prescribed.
- **EXCEPTIONS TO LEGAL CATEGORY** 15-g tube of oral gel can be sold to the public.

- **MEDICINAL FORMS** There can be variation in the licensing of different medicines containing the same drug.

Oromucosal gel

CAUTIONARY AND ADVISORY LABELS 9
- Daktarin (Johnson & Johnson Ltd, Janssen-Cilag Ltd)
  Miconazole 20 mg per 1 gram Daktarin 20mg/g oromucosal gel sugar-free | 15 gram [P] £4.01 DT = £4.01 sugar-free | 80 gram [PoM] £4.38 DT = £4.38

ANTIFUNGALS > POLYENE ANTIFUNGALS

Nystatin

05-May-2020

- **INDICATIONS AND DOSE**

Oral candidiasis
- BY MOUTH
  - Neonate: 100 000 units 4 times a day usually for 7 days, and continued for 48 hours after lesions have resolved, to be given after feeds.
  - Child: 100 000 units 4 times a day usually for 7 days, and continued for 48 hours after lesions have resolved

Oral and perioral fungal infections (dose approved for use by community practitioner nurse prescribers)
- BY MOUTH
  - Neonate: 100 000 units 4 times a day usually for 7 days, and continued for 48 hours after lesions have resolved, to be given after feeds.
  - Child: 100 000 units 4 times a day usually for 7 days, and continued for 48 hours after lesions have resolved

- **UNLICENSED USE** [EvGr] Nystatin may be used in neonates, ⟨E⟩ but it is not licensed for use in this patient group.
  Suspension not licensed for use in neonates for the treatment of candidiasis but the Department of Health has advised that a Community Practitioner Nurse Prescriber may prescribe nystatin oral suspension for a neonate, in the doses provided in the BNFC, provided that there is a clear diagnosis of oral thrush. The nurse prescriber must only prescribe within their own competence and must accept clinical and medicolegal responsibility for prescribing.
- **SIDE-EFFECTS** Abdominal distress · angioedema · diarrhoea · face oedema · nausea · sensitisation · skin reactions · Stevens-Johnson syndrome · vomiting
- **PATIENT AND CARER ADVICE** Counselling advised with oral suspension (use of pipette, hold in mouth, after food).
  Medicines for Children leaflet: Nystatin for Candida infection www.medicinesforchildren.org.uk/nystatin-candida-infection
- **PROFESSION SPECIFIC INFORMATION**
  Dental practitioners' formulary
  Nystatin Oral Suspension may be prescribed.

- **MEDICINAL FORMS** There can be variation in the licensing of different medicines containing the same drug. Forms available from special-order manufacturers include: tablet, capsule, oral suspension

Oral suspension

CAUTIONARY AND ADVISORY LABELS 9

EXCIPIENTS: May contain Ethanol
- Nystatin (Non-proprietary)
  Nystatin 100000 unit per 1 ml Nystatin 100,000units/ml oral suspension | 30 ml [PoM] £2.74 DT = £2.69

6 Oropharyngeal viral infections

Oropharyngeal viral infections

Management

Viral infections are the most common cause of a sore throat. It is usually a self-limiting condition which does not benefit from anti-infective treatment. Adequate analgesia may be all that is required.

Children with varicella–zoster infection often develop painful lesions in the mouth and throat. Benzydamine hydrochloride p. 759 may be used to provide local analgesia. Chlorhexidine mouthwash or gel p. 756 will control plaque accumulation if toothbrushing is painful and will also help to control secondary infection in general.

In severe herpetic stomatitis systemic aciclovir p. 440 or valaciclovir p. 442 may be used for oral lesions associated with herpes zoster. Aciclovir and valaciclovir are also used to prevent frequently recurring herpes simplex lesions of the mouth particularly when associated with the initiation of erythema multiforme. See the treatment of labial herpes simplex infections.

Chapter 13 Skin

CONTENTS

Skin conditions, management

Topical preparations

When prescribing topical preparations for the treatment of skin conditions in children, the site of application, the condition being treated, and the child's (and carer's) preference for a particular vehicle all need to be taken into consideration.

Vehicles

The British Association of Dermatologists list of preferred unlicensed dermatological preparations (specials) is available at www.bad.org.uk.

The vehicle in topical preparations for the skin affects the degree of hydration, has a mild anti-inflammatory effect, and aids the penetration of the active drug. Therefore, the vehicle, as well as the active drug, should be chosen on the basis of their suitability for the child's skin condition.

Applications are usually viscous solutions, emulsions, or suspensions for application to the skin (including the scalp) or nails.

Collodions are painted on the skin and allowed to dry to leave a flexible film over the site of application.

Creams are emulsions of oil and water and are generally well absorbed into the skin. They may contain an antimicrobial preservative unless the active ingredient or basis is intrinsically bactericidal and fungicidal. Generally, creams are cosmetically more acceptable than ointments because they are less greasy and easier to apply.

Gels consist of active ingredients in suitable hydrophilic or hydrophobic bases; they generally have a high water content. Gels are particularly suitable for application to the face and scalp.

Lotions have a cooling effect and may be preferred to ointments or creams for application over a hairy area. Lotions in alcoholic basis can sting if used on broken skin. *Shake lotions* (such as calamine lotion) contain insoluble powders which leave a deposit on the skin surface.

Ointments are greasy preparations which are normally anhydrous and insoluble in water, and are more occlusive than creams. They are particularly suitable for chronic, dry lesions. The most commonly used ointment bases consist of soft paraffin or a combination of soft, liquid, and hard paraffin. Some ointment bases have both *hydrophilic and lipophilic* properties; they may have occlusive properties on the skin surface, encourage hydration, and also be miscible with water; they often have a mild anti-inflammatory effect. *Water-soluble ointments* contain macrogols which are freely soluble in water and are therefore readily washed off; they have a limited but useful role where ready removal is desirable.

Pastes are stiff preparations containing a high proportion of finely powdered solids such as zinc oxide and starch suspended in an ointment. They are used for circumscribed lesions such as those which occur in lichen simplex, chronic eczema, or psoriasis. They are less occlusive than ointments and can be used to protect inflamed, lichenified, or excoriated skin.

Dusting powders are used only rarely. They reduce friction between opposing skin surfaces. Dusting powders should not be applied to moist areas because they can cake and abrade the skin. Talc is a lubricant but it does not absorb moisture; it can cause respiratory irritation. Starch is less lubricant but absorbs water.

Dilution

The BP directs that creams and ointments should **not** normally be diluted but that should dilution be necessary care should be taken, in particular, to prevent microbial contamination. The appropriate diluent should be used and heating should be avoided during mixing; excessive dilution may affect the stability of some creams. Diluted creams should normally be used within 2 weeks of preparation.

Suitable quantities for prescribing

Suitable quantities of dermatological preparations to be prescribed for specific areas of the body

Area of body	Creams and Ointments	Lotions
Face	15–30 g	100 ml
Both hands	25–50 g	200 ml
Scalp	50–100 g	200 ml
Both arms or both legs	100–200 g	200 ml
Trunk	400 g	500 ml
Groins and genitalia	15–25 g	100 ml

These amounts are usually suitable for children 12-18 years for twice daily application for 1 week; smaller quantities will be required for children under 12 years. These recommendations **do not apply** to corticosteroid preparations.

Excipients and sensitisation

Excipients in topical products rarely cause problems. If a patch test indicates allergy to an excipient, products containing the substance should be avoided (see also Anaphylaxis). The following excipients in topical preparations are associated, rarely, with sensitisation; the presence of these excipients is indicated in the entries for topical products. See also Excipients, under General Guidance.

- Beeswax
- Benzyl alcohol
- Butylated hydroxyanisole
- Butylated hydroxytoluene
- Cetostearyl alcohol (including cetyl and stearyl alcohol)
- Chlorocresol
- Edetic acid (EDTA)
- Ethylenediamine
- Fragrances
- Hydroxybenzoates (parabens)
- Imidurea
- Isopropyl palmitate
- N-(3-Chloroallyl)hexaminium chloride (quaternium 15)
- Polysorbates
- Propylene glycol
- Sodium metabisulfite
- Sorbic acid
- Wool fat and related substances including lanolin (purified versions of wool fat have reduced the problem)

Neonates

Caution is required when prescribing topical preparations for neonates—their large body surface area in relation to body mass increases susceptibility to toxicity from systemic absorption of substances applied to the skin. Topical preparations containing potentially sensitising substances such as corticosteroids, aminoglycosides, iodine, and parasiticidal drugs should be avoided. Preparations containing alcohol should be avoided because they can dehydrate the skin, cause pain if applied to raw areas, and the alcohol can cause necrosis. In *preterm neonates*, the skin is more fragile and offers a poor barrier, especially in the first fortnight after birth. Preterm infants, especially if below 32 weeks corrected gestational age, may also require special measures to maintain skin hydration.

1 Dry and scaling skin disorders

Emollient and barrier preparations

28-Jan-2019

Borderline substances

The preparations marked 'ACBS' are regarded as drugs when prescribed in accordance with the advice of the Advisory Committee on Borderline Substances for the clinical conditions listed. Prescriptions issued in accordance with this advice and endorsed 'ACBS' will normally not be investigated.

Emollients

Emollients hydrate the skin, soften the skin, act as barrier to water and external irritants, and are indicated for all dry or scaling disorders. Their effects are short-lived and they should be applied frequently even after improvement occurs. They are useful in dry and eczematous disorders, and to a lesser extent in psoriasis; they should be applied immediately after washing or bathing to maximise the effect of skin hydration. The choice of an appropriate emollient will depend on the severity of the condition, the child's (or carer's) preference, and the site of application. Ointments may exacerbate acne and folliculitis. Some ingredients rarely cause sensitisation and this should be suspected if an eczematous reaction occurs. The use of aqueous cream as a leave-on emollient may increase the risk of skin reactions, particularly in eczema.

Preparations such as **aqueous cream** and **emulsifying ointment** can be used as soap substitutes for handwashing and in the bath; the preparation is rubbed on the skin before rinsing off completely. The addition of a bath oil may also be helpful.

Urea is occasionally used with other topical agents such as corticosteroids to enhance penetration of the skin.

Emollient bath and shower preparations

In dry skin conditions soap should be avoided.

The quantities of bath additives recommended for older children are suitable for an adult-size bath. Proportionately less should be used for a child-size bath or a washbasin; recommended bath additive quantities for younger children reflect this.

MHRA/CHM advice (updated December 2018): Emollients: new information about risk of severe and fatal burns with paraffin-containing and paraffin-free emollients

Emollients are an important and effective treatment for chronic dry skin disorders and people should continue to use these products. However, healthcare professionals must ensure that patients and their carers understand the fire risk associated with the build-up of residue on clothing and bedding and can take action to minimise the risk. There is a fire risk with all paraffin-containing emollients, regardless of paraffin concentration, and it cannot be excluded with paraffin-free emollients. A similar risk may apply to products that are applied to the skin over large body areas, or in large volumes for repeated use for more than a few days.

Healthcare professionals should advise patients not to smoke or go near naked flames because clothing, bedding, dressings, and other fabrics that have been in contact with an emollient or emollient-treated skin can rapidly ignite. Washing these materials at high temperature may reduce emollient build-up but not totally remove it.

Barrier preparations

Barrier preparations often contain water-repellent substances such as dimeticone (see barrier creams and ointments p. 766), natural oils, and paraffins, to help protect the skin from abrasion and irritation; they are used to protect intact skin around stomas and pressure sores, and as a barrier against nappy rash. In neonates, barrier preparations which do not contain potentially sensitising excipients are preferred. Where the skin has broken down, barrier preparations have a limited role in protecting adjacent skin. Barrier preparations with zinc oxide or titanium salts are used to aid healing of uninfected, excoriated skin.

Nappy rash (Dermatitis)

The first line of treatment is to ensure that nappies are changed frequently and that tightly fitting water-proof pants are avoided. The rash may clear when left exposed to the air and a barrier preparation, applied with each nappy change, can be helpful. A mild corticosteroid such as hydrocortisone 0.5% or 1% p. 790 can be used if inflammation is causing discomfort, but it should be avoided in neonates. The barrier preparation should be applied after the corticosteroid preparation to prevent further damage. Preparations containing hydrocortisone should be applied for no more than a week; the hydrocortisone should be discontinued as soon as the inflammation subsides. The occlusive effect of nappies and waterproof pants may increase absorption of corticosteroids (see cautions). If the rash is associated with candidal infection, a topical antifungal such as clotrimazole cream p. 776 can be used. Topical antibacterial preparations can be used if bacterial infection is present; treatment with an oral antibacterial may occasionally be required in severe or recurrent infection. Hydrocortisone may be used in combination with antimicrobial preparations if there is considerable inflammation, erosion, and infection.

Emollients for neonates

In the *neonate*, a preservative-free paraffin-based emollient hydrates the skin without affecting the normal skin flora; substances such as olive oil are also used. The development of blisters (epidermolysis bullosa) or ichthyosis may be alleviated by applying liquid and white soft paraffin ointment while awaiting dermatological investigation.

DERMATOLOGICAL DRUGS > BARRIER PREPARATIONS

13 Skin

Barrier creams and ointments

13-Feb-2020

● **INDICATIONS AND DOSE**

For use as a barrier preparation

▶ TO THE SKIN
▶ Child: (consult product literature)

● **MEDICINAL FORMS** There can be variation in the licensing of different medicines containing the same drug.

Ointment

EXCIPIENTS: May contain Woolfat and related substances (including lanolin)

▶ Barrier creams and ointments (Non-proprietary)
Cetostearyl alcohol 20 mg per 1 gram, Zinc oxide 75 mg per 1 gram, Beeswax white 100 mg per 1 gram, Arachis oil 305 mg per 1 gram, Castor oil 500 mg per 1 gram Zinc and Castor oil ointment | 500 gram GSL £5.14–£5.46 DT = £5.46
Zinc and Castor oil cream | 100 gram GSL £1.46

▶ Metanium (Thornton & Ross Ltd)
Titanium salicylate 30 mg per 1 gram, Titanium peroxide 50 mg per 1 gram, Titanium dioxide 200 mg per 1 gram Metanium Nappy Rash ointment | 30 gram GSL £2.24 DT = £2.24

Spray

CAUTIONARY AND ADVISORY LABELS 15
EXCIPIENTS: May contain Cetostearyl alcohol (including cetyl and stearyl alcohol), hydroxybenzoates (parabens), woolfat and related substances (including lanolin)

▶ Sprilon (J M Loveridge Ltd)
Dimeticone 10.4 mg per 1 gram, Zinc oxide 125 mg per 1 gram Sprilon aerosol spray | 115 gram GSL £8.90 DT = £8.90

Cream

EXCIPIENTS: May contain Beeswax, butylated hydroxyanisole, butylated hydroxytoluene, cetostearyl alcohol (including cetyl and stearyl alcohol), chlorocresol, fragrances, hydroxybenzoates (parabens), propylene glycol, woolfat and related substances (including lanolin)

▶ Conotrane (Karo Pharma)
Benzalkonium chloride 1 mg per 1 gram, Dimeticone 220 mg per 1 gram Conotrane cream | 100 gram GSL £0.88 DT = £0.88 | 500 gram GSL £3.51

▶ Drapolene (Supra Enterprises Ltd)
Benzalkonium chloride 100 microgram per 1 gram, Cetrimide 2 mg per 1 gram Drapolene cream | 100 gram GSL £2.81 DT = £2.81 | 200 gram GSL £3.74 DT = £3.74 | 350 gram GSL £4.99 DT = £4.99

▶ Siopel (Derma UK Ltd)
Cetrimide 3 mg per 1 gram, Dimeticone 1000 100 mg per 1 gram Siopel cream | 50 gram GSL £4.65 DT = £4.65

▶ Sudocrem (Teva UK Ltd)
Benzyl cinnamate 1.5 mg per 1 gram, Benzyl alcohol 3.9 mg per 1 gram, Benzyl benzoate 10.1 mg per 1 gram, Wool fat hydrous 40 mg per 1 gram, Zinc oxide 152.5 mg per 1 gram Sudocrem antiseptic healing cream | 60 gram GSL £1.45 | 125 gram GSL £2.15 | 250 gram GSL £3.67 | 400 gram GSL £5.25

DERMATOLOGICAL DRUGS > EMOLLIENTS

Emollient bath and shower products, antimicrobial-containing

31-Aug-2016

● **INDICATIONS AND DOSE**

DERMOL ® 200 SHOWER EMOLLIENT

Dry and pruritic skin conditions including eczema and dermatitis

▶ TO THE SKIN
▶ Child: To be applied to the skin or used as a soap substitute

DERMOL ® 600 BATH EMOLLIENT

Dry and pruritic skin conditions including eczema and dermatitis

▶ TO THE SKIN
▶ Child 1–23 months: 5–15 mL/bath, not to be used undiluted
▶ Child 2–17 years: 15–30 mL/bath, not to be used undiluted

DERMOL ® WASH EMULSION

Dry and pruritic skin conditions including eczema and dermatitis

▶ TO THE SKIN
▶ Child: To be applied to the skin or used as a soap substitute

EMULSIDERM ®

Dry skin conditions including eczema and ichthyosis

▶ TO THE SKIN
▶ Child 1–23 months: 5–10 mL/bath, alternatively, to be rubbed into dry skin until absorbed
▶ Child 2–17 years: 7–30 mL/bath, alternatively, to be rubbed into dry skin until absorbed

OILATUM ® PLUS

Topical treatment of eczema, including eczema at risk from infection

▶ TO THE SKIN
▶ Child 6–11 months: 1 mL/bath, not to be used undiluted
▶ Child 1–17 years: 1–2 capfuls/bath, not to be used undiluted

IMPORTANT SAFETY INFORMATION

These preparations make skin and surfaces slippery—particular care is needed when bathing.

MHRA/CHM ADVICE (UPDATED DECEMBER 2018): EMOLLIENTS: NEW INFORMATION ABOUT RISK OF SEVERE AND FATAL BURNS WITH PARAFFIN-CONTAINING AND PARAFFIN-FREE EMOLLIENTS

See Emollient and barrier preparations p. 765.

● **DIRECTIONS FOR ADMINISTRATION** Emollient bath additives should be added to bath water; hydration can be improved by soaking in the bath for 10–20 minutes. Some bath emollients can be applied to wet skin undiluted and rinsed off. Emollient preparations contained in tubs should be removed with a clean spoon or spatula to reduce bacterial contamination of the emollient. Emollients should be applied in the direction of hair growth to reduce the risk of folliculitis.

● **PRESCRIBING AND DISPENSING INFORMATION** Preparations containing an antibacterial should be avoided unless infection is present or is a frequent complication.

● **MEDICINAL FORMS** There can be variation in the licensing of different medicines containing the same drug.

Bath additive

CAUTIONARY AND ADVISORY LABELS 15
EXCIPIENTS: May contain Acetylated lanolin alcohols, isopropyl palmitate, polysorbates

- Dermol 600 (Dermal Laboratories Ltd)
  Benzalkonium chloride 5 mg per 1 gram, Isopropyl myristate 250 mg per 1 gram, Liquid paraffin 250 mg per 1 gram Dermol 600 bath emollient | 600 ml [P] £7.55
- Emulsiderm (Dermal Laboratories Ltd)
  Benzalkonium chloride 5 mg per 1 gram, Isopropyl myristate 250 mg per 1 gram, Liquid paraffin 250 mg per 1 gram Emulsiderm emollient | 300 ml [P] £3.85 | 1000 ml [P] £12.00
- Oilatum Plus (Thornton & Ross Ltd)
  Triclosan 20 mg per 1 gram, Benzalkonium chloride 60 mg per 1 gram, Liquid paraffin light 525 mg per 1 gram Oilatum Plus bath additive | 500 ml [GSL] £7.94

Liquid

CAUTIONARY AND ADVISORY LABELS 15

EXCIPIENTS: May contain Cetostearyl alcohol (including cetyl and stearyl alcohol)

- Dermol 200 (Dermal Laboratories Ltd)
  Benzalkonium chloride 1 mg per 1 gram, Chlorhexidine hydrochloride 1 mg per 1 gram, Isopropyl myristate 25 mg per 1 gram, Liquid paraffin 25 mg per 1 gram Dermol 200 shower emollient | 200 ml [P] £3.55
- Dermol Wash (Dermal Laboratories Ltd)
  Benzalkonium chloride 1 mg per 1 gram, Chlorhexidine hydrochloride 1 mg per 1 gram, Isopropyl myristate 25 mg per 1 gram, Liquid paraffin 25 mg per 1 gram Dermol Wash cutaneous emulsion | 200 ml [P] £3.55

Emollient bath and shower products, paraffin-containing

08-May-2020

● **INDICATIONS AND DOSE**

Dry skin conditions (using Aqueous Cream BP)

▶ TO THE SKIN

- Child: To be used as a soap substitute

AQUAMAX ® WASH

Dry skin conditions

▶ TO THE SKIN

- Child: To be applied to wet or dry skin and rinse

CETRABEN ® BATH

Dry skin conditions, including eczema

▶ TO THE SKIN

- Neonate: 0.5 capful/bath, alternatively, to be applied to wet skin and rinse.
- Child 1 month–11 years: 0.5–1 capful/bath, alternatively, to be applied to wet skin and rinse
- Child 12–17 years: 1–2 capfuls/bath, alternatively, to be applied to wet skin and rinse

DERMALO ®

Dermatitis | Dry skin conditions, including ichthyosis

▶ TO THE SKIN

- Neonate: 5 mL/bath, alternatively, to be applied to wet skin and rinse.
- Child 1 month–11 years: 5–10 mL/bath, alternatively, to be applied to wet skin and rinse
- Child 12–17 years: 15–20 mL/bath, alternatively, to be applied to wet skin and rinse

DOUBLEBASE ® EMOLLIENT BATH ADDITIVE

Dry skin conditions including dermatitis and ichthyosis

▶ TO THE SKIN

- Neonate: 5–10 mL/bath.
- Child 1 month–11 years: 5–10 mL/bath
- Child 12–17 years: 15–20 mL/bath

DOUBLEBASE ® EMOLLIENT SHOWER GEL

Dry, chapped, or itchy skin conditions

▶ TO THE SKIN

- Child: To be applied to wet or dry skin and rinse, or apply to dry skin after showering

DOUBLEBASE ® EMOLLIENT WASH GEL

Dry, chapped, or itchy skin conditions

▶ TO THE SKIN

- Child: To be used as a soap substitute

E45 ® BATH OIL

Endogenous and exogenous eczema, xeroderma, and ichthyosis

▶ TO THE SKIN

- Neonate: 5 mL/bath, alternatively, to be applied to wet skin and rinse.
- Child 1 month–11 years: 5–10 mL/bath, alternatively, to be applied to wet skin and rinse
- Child 12–17 years: 15 mL/bath, alternatively, to be applied to wet skin and rinse

E45 ® WASH CREAM

Endogenous and exogenous eczema, xeroderma, and ichthyosis

▶ TO THE SKIN

- Child: To be used as a soap substitute

HYDROMOL ® BATH AND SHOWER EMOLLIENT

Dry skin conditions | Eczema | Ichthyosis

▶ TO THE SKIN

- Neonate: 0.5 capful/bath, alternatively apply to wet skin and rinse.
- Child 1 month–11 years: 0.5–2 capfuls/bath, alternatively apply to wet skin and rinse
- Child 12–17 years: 1–3 capfuls/bath, alternatively apply to wet skin and rinse

LPL 63.4 ®

Dry skin conditions

▶ TO THE SKIN

- Neonate: 0.5 capful/bath, alternatively, to be applied to wet skin and rinse.
- Child 1 month–11 years: 0.5–2 capfuls/bath, alternatively, to be applied to wet skin and rinse
- Child 12–17 years: 1–3 capfuls/bath, alternatively, to be applied to wet skin and rinse

OILATUM ® EMOLLIENT BATH ADDITIVE

Dry skin conditions including dermatitis and ichthyosis

▶ TO THE SKIN

- Neonate: 0.5 capful/bath, alternatively, to be applied to wet skin and rinse.
- Child 1 month–11 years: Apply 0.5–2 capfuls/bath, alternatively, to be applied to wet skin and rinse
- Child 12–17 years: 1–3 capfuls/bath, alternatively, to be applied to wet skin and rinse

OILATUM ® JUNIOR BATH ADDITIVE

Dry skin conditions including dermatitis and ichthyosis

▶ TO THE SKIN

- Neonate: 0.5 capful/bath, alternatively, apply to wet skin and rinse.
- Child 1 month–11 years: 0.5–2 capfuls/bath, alternatively, apply to wet skin and rinse
- Child 12–17 years: 1–3 capfuls/bath, alternatively, apply to wet skin and rinse

continued →

QV ® BATH OIL

Dry skin conditions including eczema, psoriasis, ichthyosis, and pruritus

▸ TO THE SKIN

- Neonate: 5 mL/bath, alternatively, to be applied to wet skin and rinse.
- Child 1–11 months: 5 mL/bath, alternatively, to be applied to wet skin and rinse
- Child 1–17 years: 10 mL/bath, alternatively, to be applied to wet skin and rinse

QV ® GENTLE WASH

Dry skin conditions including eczema, psoriasis, ichthyosis, and pruritus

▸ TO THE SKIN

- Child: To be used as a soap substitute

ZEROLATUM ®

Dry skin conditions | Dermatitis | Ichthyosis

▸ TO THE SKIN

- Child 1 month–11 years: 5–10 mL/bath
- Child 12–17 years: 15–20 mL/bath

IMPORTANT SAFETY INFORMATION

These preparations make the skin and surfaces slippery—particular care is needed when bathing.

MHRA/CHM ADVICE (UPDATED DECEMBER 2018): EMOLLIENTS: NEW INFORMATION ABOUT RISK OF SEVERE AND FATAL BURNS WITH PARAFFIN-CONTAINING AND PARAFFIN-FREE EMOLLIENTS

See Emollient and barrier preparations p. 765.

● **DIRECTIONS FOR ADMINISTRATION** Emollient bath additives should be added to bath water; hydration can be improved by soaking in the bath for 10–20 minutes. Some bath emollients can be applied to wet skin undiluted and rinsed off. Emollient preparations contained in tubs should be removed with a clean spoon or spatula to reduce bacterial contamination of the emollient. Emollients should be applied in the direction of hair growth to reduce the risk of folliculitis.

● **MEDICINAL FORMS** There can be variation in the licensing of different medicines containing the same drug.

Bath additive

CAUTIONARY AND ADVISORY LABELS 15

EXCIPIENTS: May contain Acetylated lanolin alcohols, cetostearyl alcohol (including cetyl and stearyl alcohol), fragrances, isopropyl palmitate

- **Cetraben** (Genus Pharmaceuticals Ltd)
  Liquid paraffin light 828 mg per 1 gram Cetraben emollient 82.8% bath additive | 500 ml [GSL] £5.75 DT = £5.75
- **Dermalo** (Dermal Laboratories Ltd)
  Acetylated wool alcohols 50 mg per 1 gram, Liquid paraffin 650 mg per 1 gram Dermalo bath emollient | 500 ml [GSL] £3.44
- **Doublebase** (Dermal Laboratories Ltd)
  Liquid paraffin 650 mg per 1 gram Doublebase emollient bath additive | 500 ml [GSL] £5.45 DT = £5.45
- **E45 emollient bath** (Forum Health Products Ltd)
  E45 emollient bath oil | 500 ml £5.29
- **Hydromol** (Alliance Pharmaceuticals Ltd)
  Isopropyl myristate 130 mg per 1 ml, Liquid paraffin light 378 mg per 1 ml Hydromol Bath & Shower emollient | 350 ml £3.91 | 500 ml £4.46 | 1000 ml £8.87
- **LPL** (Huxley Europe Ltd)
  Liquid paraffin light 634 mg per 1 ml LPL 63.4 bath additive and emollient | 500 ml £3.13 DT = £5.80
- **Oilatum** (Thornton & Ross Ltd)
  Liquid paraffin light 634 mg per 1 ml Oilatum Bath Formula | 150 ml [GSL] £2.95 DT = £2.95 | 300 ml [GSL] £5.02 DT = £5.02
  Oilatum Emollient | 500 ml [GSL] £5.80 DT = £5.80
- **Oilatum junior** (Thornton & Ross Ltd)
  Liquid paraffin light 634 mg per 1 ml Oilatum Junior bath additive | 150 ml [GSL] £2.95 DT = £2.95 | 300 ml [GSL] £5.02 DT = £5.02 | 600 ml [GSL] £7.34 DT = £7.34
- **QV** (Crawford Healthcare Ltd)
  Liquid paraffin light 850.9 mg per 1 gram QV 85.09% bath oil | 250 ml £2.93 | 500 ml £4.79
- **Zerolatum** (Thornton & Ross Ltd)
  Acetylated wool alcohols 50 mg per 1 gram, Liquid paraffin 650 mg per 1 gram Zerolatum Emollient bath additive | 500 ml £4.79

Gel

CAUTIONARY AND ADVISORY LABELS 15

EXCIPIENTS: May contain Cetostearyl alcohol (including cetyl and stearyl alcohol)

- **Doublebase** (Dermal Laboratories Ltd)
  Isopropyl myristate 150 mg per 1 gram, Liquid paraffin 150 mg per 1 gram Doublebase Dayleve gel | 100 gram [P] £2.65 DT = £2.65 | 500 gram [P] £6.29 DT = £5.83
  Doublebase gel | 100 gram [P] £2.65 DT = £2.65 | 500 gram [P] £5.83 DT = £5.83 | 1000 gram [P] £10.98
  Doublebase emollient wash gel | 200 gram [P] £5.21
  Doublebase emollient shower gel | 200 gram [P] £5.21

Cream

CAUTIONARY AND ADVISORY LABELS 15

EXCIPIENTS: May contain Cetostearyl alcohol (including cetyl and stearyl alcohol)

- **Emollient bath and shower products, paraffin-containing (Non-proprietary)**
  Phenoxyethanol 10 mg per 1 gram, Liquid paraffin 60 mg per 1 gram, Emulsifying wax 90 mg per 1 gram, White soft paraffin 150 mg per 1 gram, Purified water 690 mg per 1 gram Aqueous cream | 100 gram [GSL] £1.41 DT = £0.94 | 500 gram [GSL] £6.35 DT = £4.70

Wash

CAUTIONARY AND ADVISORY LABELS 15

EXCIPIENTS: May contain Cetostearyl alcohol (including cetyl and stearyl alcohol), hydroxybenzoates (parabens), polysorbates

- **Aquamax** (Intrapharm Laboratories Ltd)
  Aquamax wash | 250 gram £2.99
- **E45 emollient wash** (Forum Health Products Ltd)
  E45 emollient wash cream | 250 ml £3.30
- **QV Gentle** (Crawford Healthcare Ltd)
  QV Gentle wash | 250 ml £3.19 | 500 ml £5.32

Emollient bath and shower products, soya-bean oil-containing

● **INDICATIONS AND DOSE**

BALNEUM ® BATH OIL

Dry skin conditions including those associated with dermatitis and eczema

▸ TO THE SKIN

- Neonate: 5–15 mL/bath, not to be used undiluted.
- Child 1–23 months: 5–15 mL/bath, not to be used undiluted
- Child 2–17 years: 20–60 mL/bath, not to be used undiluted

BALNEUM ® PLUS BATH OIL

Dry skin conditions including those associated with dermatitis and eczema where pruritus also experienced

▸ TO THE SKIN

- Neonate: 5 mL/bath, alternatively, to be applied to wet skin and rinse.
- Child 1–23 months: 5 mL/bath, alternatively, to be applied to wet skin and rinse
- Child 2–17 years: 10–20 mL/bath, alternatively, to be applied to wet skin and rinse

ZERONEUM ®

Dry skin conditions, including eczema

▸ TO THE SKIN

- Child 1 month–11 years: 5 mL/bath
- Child 12–17 years: 20 mL/bath

IMPORTANT SAFETY INFORMATION

These preparations make skin and surfaces slippery—particular care is needed when bathing.

MHRA/CHM ADVICE (UPDATED DECEMBER 2018): EMOLLIENTS: NEW INFORMATION ABOUT RISK OF SEVERE AND FATAL BURNS WITH PARAFFIN-CONTAINING AND PARAFFIN-FREE EMOLLIENTS

See Emollient and barrier preparations p. 765.

- **DIRECTIONS FOR ADMINISTRATION** Emollient bath additives should be added to bath water; hydration can be improved by soaking in the bath for 10–20 minutes. Some bath emollients can be applied to wet skin undiluted and rinsed off. Emollient preparations contained in tubs should be removed with a clean spoon or spatula to reduce bacterial contamination of the emollient. Emollients should be applied in the direction of hair growth to reduce the risk of folliculitis.

- **MEDICINAL FORMS** There can be variation in the licensing of different medicines containing the same drug.

Bath additive

CAUTIONARY AND ADVISORY LABELS 15
EXCIPIENTS: May contain Butylated hydroxytoluene, fragrances, propylene glycol

- Balneum (Almirall Ltd)
  Lauromacrogols 150 mg per 1 gram, Soya oil 829.5 mg per 1 gram Balneum Plus bath oil | 500 ml GSL £6.66 DT = £6.66
  Soya oil 847.5 mg per 1 gram Balneum 84.75% bath oil | 500 ml GSL £5.38 DT = £5.38 | 1000 ml GSL £10.39 DT = £10.39
- Zeroneum (Thornton & Ross Ltd)
  Soya oil 833.5 mg per 1 gram Zeroneum 83.35% bath additive | 500 ml £4.48

Emollient bath and shower products, tar-containing

17-Aug-2016

- **INDICATIONS AND DOSE**

POLYTAR EMOLLIENT®

Psoriasis, eczema, atopic and pruritic dermatoses

- TO THE SKIN
- Child: 2–4 capfuls/bath, add 15–30 mL to an adult-size bath and proportionally less for a child's bath; soak for 20 minutes

PSORIDERM® EMULSION

Psoriasis

- TO THE SKIN
- Child: Up to 30 mL/bath, use 30mL in adult-size bath, and proportionally less for a child's bath, soak for 5 minutes

IMPORTANT SAFETY INFORMATION

These preparations make skin and surfaces slippery—particular care is needed when bathing.

MHRA/CHM ADVICE (UPDATED DECEMBER 2018): EMOLLIENTS: NEW INFORMATION ABOUT RISK OF SEVERE AND FATAL BURNS WITH PARAFFIN-CONTAINING AND PARAFFIN-FREE EMOLLIENTS

See Emollient and barrier preparations p. 765.

- **DIRECTIONS FOR ADMINISTRATION** Emollient bath additives should be added to bath water; hydration can be improved by soaking in the bath for 10–20 minutes. Some bath emollients can be applied to wet skin undiluted and rinsed off. Emollient preparations contained in tubs should be removed with a clean spoon or spatula to reduce bacterial contamination of the emollient. Emollients should be applied in the direction of hair growth to reduce the risk of folliculitis.

- **MEDICINAL FORMS** There can be variation in the licensing of different medicines containing the same drug.

Bath additive

CAUTIONARY AND ADVISORY LABELS 15
EXCIPIENTS: May contain Isopropyl palmitate, polysorbates

- Psoriderm (Dermal Laboratories Ltd)
  Coal tar distilled 400 mg per 1 ml Psoriderm Emulsion 40% bath additive | 200 ml P £2.74 DT = £2.74

Emollient creams and ointments, antimicrobial-containing

14-Feb-2020

- **INDICATIONS AND DOSE**

Dry and pruritic skin conditions including eczema and dermatitis

- TO THE SKIN
- Child: To be applied to the skin or used as a soap substitute

IMPORTANT SAFETY INFORMATION

These preparations make skin and surfaces slippery—particular care is needed when bathing.

MHRA/CHM ADVICE (UPDATED DECEMBER 2018): EMOLLIENTS: NEW INFORMATION ABOUT RISK OF SEVERE AND FATAL BURNS WITH PARAFFIN-CONTAINING AND PARAFFIN-FREE EMOLLIENTS

See Emollient and barrier preparations p. 765.

- **DIRECTIONS FOR ADMINISTRATION** Emollients should be applied immediately after washing or bathing to maximise the effect of skin hydration. Emollient preparations contained in tubs should be removed with a clean spoon or spatula to reduce bacterial contamination of the emollient. Emollients should be applied in the direction of hair growth to reduce the risk of folliculitis.
- **PRESCRIBING AND DISPENSING INFORMATION** Preparations containing an antibacterial should be avoided unless infection is present or is a frequent complication.

- **MEDICINAL FORMS** There can be variation in the licensing of different medicines containing the same drug.

Cream

CAUTIONARY AND ADVISORY LABELS 15
EXCIPIENTS: May contain Cetostearyl alcohol (including cetyl and stearyl alcohol)

- Dermol (Dermal Laboratories Ltd)
  Benzalkonium chloride 1 mg per 1 gram, Chlorhexidine hydrochloride 1 mg per 1 gram, Isopropyl myristate 100 mg per 1 gram, Liquid paraffin 100 mg per 1 gram Dermol cream | 100 gram P £2.86 | 500 gram P £6.63

Liquid

CAUTIONARY AND ADVISORY LABELS 15
EXCIPIENTS: May contain Cetostearyl alcohol (including cetyl and stearyl alcohol)

- Dermol 500 (Dermal Laboratories Ltd)
  Benzalkonium chloride 1 mg per 1 gram, Chlorhexidine hydrochloride 1 mg per 1 gram, Isopropyl myristate 25 mg per 1 gram, Liquid paraffin 25 mg per 1 gram Dermol 500 lotion | 500 ml P £6.04

Emollient creams and ointments, colloidal oatmeal-containing

15-Jan-2019

● **INDICATIONS AND DOSE**

Endogenous and exogenous eczema | Xeroderma | Ichthyosis

▶ TO THE SKIN

▸ Child: (consult product literature)

IMPORTANT SAFETY INFORMATION

MHRA/CHM ADVICE (UPDATED DECEMBER 2018): EMOLLIENTS: NEW INFORMATION ABOUT RISK OF SEVERE AND FATAL BURNS WITH PARAFFIN-CONTAINING AND PARAFFIN-FREE EMOLLIENTS

See Emollient and barrier preparations p. 765.

● **DIRECTIONS FOR ADMINISTRATION** Emollients should be applied immediately after washing or bathing to maximise the effect of skin hydration. Emollient preparations contained in tubs should be removed with a clean spoon or spatula to reduce bacterial contamination of the emollient. Emollients should be applied in the direction of hair growth to reduce the risk of folliculitis.

● **MEDICINAL FORMS** There can be variation in the licensing of different medicines containing the same drug.

Cream and lotion

CAUTIONARY AND ADVISORY LABELS 15

EXCIPIENTS: May contain Benzyl alcohol, cetostearyl alcohol (including cetyl and stearyl alcohol), isopropyl palmitate

▸ **Aveeno** (Johnson & Johnson Ltd)
Aveeno lotion | 500 ml(ACBS) £6.66
Aveeno cream | 100 ml(ACBS) £3.97 | 300 ml(ACBS) £6.80 | 500 ml (ACBS) £6.47

Emollient creams and ointments, paraffin-containing

14-Feb-2020

● **INDICATIONS AND DOSE**

Dry skin conditions | Eczema | Psoriasis | Ichthyosis | Pruritus

▶ TO THE SKIN

▸ Child: (consult product literature)

IMPORTANT SAFETY INFORMATION

MHRA/CHM ADVICE (UPDATED DECEMBER 2018): EMOLLIENTS: NEW INFORMATION ABOUT RISK OF SEVERE AND FATAL BURNS WITH PARAFFIN-CONTAINING AND PARAFFIN-FREE EMOLLIENTS

See Emollient and barrier preparations p. 765.

● **DIRECTIONS FOR ADMINISTRATION** Emollients should be applied immediately after washing or bathing to maximise the effect of skin hydration. Emollient preparations contained in tubs should be removed with a clean spoon or spatula to reduce bacterial contamination of the emollient. Emollients should be applied in the direction of hair growth to reduce the risk of folliculitis.

● **MEDICINAL FORMS** There can be variation in the licensing of different medicines containing the same drug.

Spray

CAUTIONARY AND ADVISORY LABELS 15

▸ **Dermamist** (Alliance Pharmaceuticals Ltd)
White soft paraffin 100 mg per 1 gram Dermamist 10% spray | 250 ml [P] £5.97 DT = £5.97

▸ **Emollin** (C D Medical Ltd)
Emollin aerosol spray | 150 ml £4.00 | 240 ml £6.39

Gel

CAUTIONARY AND ADVISORY LABELS 15

▸ **Emollient creams and ointments, paraffin-containing (Non-proprietary)**
Isopropyl myristate 150 mg per 1 gram, Liquid paraffin 150 mg per 1 gram MyriBase emollient shower gel | 200 ml £4.17

▸ **AproDerm (isopropyl myristate / liquid paraffin)** (Fontus Health Ltd)
Isopropyl myristate 150 mg per 1 gram, Liquid paraffin 150 mg per 1 gram AproDerm gel | 100 gram £1.99 DT = £2.65 | 500 gram £3.99 DT = £5.83

▸ **Doublebase** (Dermal Laboratories Ltd)
Isopropyl myristate 150 mg per 1 gram, Liquid paraffin 150 mg per 1 gram Doublebase Dayleve gel | 100 gram [P] £2.65 DT = £2.65 | 500 gram [P] £6.29 DT = £5.83
Doublebase gel | 100 gram [P] £2.65 DT = £2.65 | 500 gram [P] £5.83 DT = £5.83 | 1000 gram [P] £10.98
Doublebase emollient wash gel | 200 gram [P] £5.21
Doublebase emollient shower gel | 200 gram [P] £5.21

▸ **Exmabase** (Ascot Laboratories Ltd)
Isopropyl myristate 150 mg per 1 gram, Liquid paraffin 150 mg per 1 gram Exmabase gel | 500 gram £2.85 DT = £5.83

▸ **HypoBase** (Galen Ltd)
Isopropyl myristate 150 mg per 1 gram, Liquid paraffin 150 mg per 1 gram HypoBase gel | 500 gram £5.83 DT = £5.83

▸ **MyriBase** (Galen Ltd)
Isopropyl myristate 150 mg per 1 gram, Liquid paraffin 150 mg per 1 gram MyriBase gel | 100 gram £2.12 DT = £2.65 | 500 ml £4.66

▸ **Zerodouble** (Thornton & Ross Ltd)
Isopropyl myristate 150 mg per 1 gram, Liquid paraffin 150 mg per 1 gram Zerodouble gel | 100 gram £2.25 DT = £2.65 | 500 gram £4.90 DT = £5.83

▸ **Isomol** (Aspire Pharma Ltd)
Isopropyl myristate 150 mg per 1 gram, Liquid paraffin 150 mg per 1 gram Epimax isomol gel | 100 gram £1.99 DT = £2.65 | 500 gram £2.92 DT = £5.83

Cream

CAUTIONARY AND ADVISORY LABELS 15

EXCIPIENTS: May contain Benzyl alcohol, cetostearyl alcohol (including cetyl and stearyl alcohol), chlorocresol, disodium edetate, fragrances, hydroxybenzoates (parabens), polysorbates, propylene glycol, sorbic acid, lanolin

▸ **Aquamol** (Thornton & Ross Ltd)
Aquamol cream | 50 gram £1.22 | 500 gram £6.40

▸ **Cetraben** (Thornton & Ross Ltd)
Liquid paraffin light 105 mg per 1 gram, White soft paraffin 132 mg per 1 gram Cetraben cream | 50 gram £1.40 | 150 gram £3.98 | 500 gram £5.99 | 1050 gram £11.62

▸ **Diprobase** (Bayer Plc)
Diprobase cream | 50 gram £1.28 | 500 gram £6.32

▸ **E45** (Forum Health Products Ltd)
Wool fat 10 mg per 1 gram, Liquid paraffin light 126 mg per 1 gram, White soft paraffin 145 mg per 1 gram E45 cream | 50 gram [GSL] £1.93 | 125 gram [GSL] £3.22 | 350 gram [GSL] £5.81 | 500 gram [GSL] £5.99

▸ **Enopen** (Ennogen Healthcare Ltd)
Liquid paraffin light 105 mg per 1 gram, White soft paraffin 132 mg per 1 gram Enopen cream | 50 gram £1.40 | 150 gram £3.98 | 500 gram £5.99 | 1050 gram £11.62

▸ **Epaderm** (Molnlycke Health Care Ltd)
Epaderm cream | 50 gram £1.71 | 150 gram £3.58 | 500 gram £7.01

▸ **Epimax original cream** (Aspire Pharma Ltd)
Epimax original cream | 100 gram £0.75 | 500 gram £2.49

▸ **ExCetra** (Aspire Pharma Ltd)
Liquid paraffin light 105 mg per 1 gram, White soft paraffin 132 mg per 1 gram Epimax excetra cream | 100 gram £1.75 | 500 gram £2.95

▸ **ExmaQS** (Ascot Laboratories Ltd)
Liquid paraffin light 60 mg per 1 gram, White soft paraffin 150 mg per 1 gram ExmaQS cream | 500 gram £2.95

▸ **Exmaben** (Ascot Laboratories Ltd)
Liquid paraffin light 105 mg per 1 gram, White soft paraffin 132 mg per 1 gram Exmaben cream | 500 gram £4.25

▸ **Exmalatum** (Ascot Laboratories Ltd)
Liquid paraffin light 60 mg per 1 gram, White soft paraffin 150 mg per 1 gram Exmalatum cream | 500 gram £4.45

▸ **Hydromol** (Alliance Pharmaceuticals Ltd)
Sodium lactate 10 mg per 1 gram, Sodium pidolate 25 mg per 1 gram, Isopropyl myristate 50 mg per 1 gram, Liquid paraffin

100 mg per 1 gram Hydromol 2.5% cream | 50 gram £2.25 | 100 gram £4.20 | 500 gram £12.25

- **Lipobase** (Karo Pharma)
  Lipobase cream | 50 gram [P] £1.46
- **Oilatum** (Thornton & Ross Ltd)
  Liquid paraffin light 60 mg per 1 gram, White soft paraffin 150 mg per 1 gram Oilatum cream | 150 gram [GSL] £3.06 DT = £3.06 | 500 ml [GSL] £5.28 DT = £5.28
- **Oilatum junior** (Thornton & Ross Ltd)
  Liquid paraffin light 60 mg per 1 gram, White soft paraffin 150 mg per 1 gram Oilatum Junior cream | 150 gram [GSL] £3.06 DT = £3.06 | 350 ml [GSL] £4.65 DT = £4.65 | 500 ml [GSL] £5.28 DT = £5.28
- **Soffen** (Vitame Ltd)
  Liquid paraffin light 105 mg per 1 gram, White soft paraffin 132 mg per 1 gram Soffen cream | 500 gram £4.79
- **Ultrabase** (Derma UK Ltd)
  Ultrabase cream | 500 gram [GSL] £8.67
- **Unguentum M** (Almirall Ltd)
  Unguentum M cream | 100 gram [GSL] £2.78 | 500 gram [GSL] £8.48
- **ZeroAQS** (Thornton & Ross Ltd)
  ZeroAQS emollient cream | 500 gram £3.29
- **Zerobase** (Thornton & Ross Ltd)
  Liquid paraffin 110 mg per 1 gram Zerobase 11% cream | 50 gram £1.04 | 500 gram £5.26
- **Zerocream** (Thornton & Ross Ltd)
  Liquid paraffin 126 mg per 1 gram, White soft paraffin 145 mg per 1 gram Zerocream | 50 gram £1.17 | 500 gram £4.08
- **Zeroguent** (Thornton & Ross Ltd)
  White soft paraffin 40 mg per 1 gram, Soya oil 50 mg per 1 gram, Liquid paraffin light 80 mg per 1 gram Zeroguent cream | 100 gram £2.33 | 500 gram £6.99

Ointment

CAUTIONARY AND ADVISORY LABELS 15

EXCIPIENTS: May contain Cetostearyl alcohol (including cetyl and stearyl alcohol), polysorbates

- **Emollient creams and ointments, paraffin-containing (Non-proprietary)**
  Liquid paraffin 200 mg per 1 gram, Emulsifying wax 300 mg per 1 gram, White soft paraffin 500 mg per 1 gram Emulsifying ointment | 500 gram [GSL] £4.82
  Liquid paraffin 500 mg per 1 gram, White soft paraffin 500 mg per 1 gram White soft paraffin 50% / Liquid paraffin 50% ointment | 250 gram £1.92–£2.03 | 500 gram £4.32 DT = £4.57 | 500 gram [P] £4.57 DT = £4.57
  Magnesium sulfate dried 5 mg per 1 gram, Phenoxyethanol 10 mg per 1 gram, Wool alcohols ointment 500 mg per 1 gram AquaDerm Hydrous ointment | 500 gram £4.15
  Hydrous ointment | 500 gram [GSL] [X]
  White soft paraffin 1 mg per 1 mg White soft paraffin solid | 500 gram [GSL] £5.18 DT = £4.03 | 4500 gram [GSL] £22.72
  Yellow soft paraffin 1 mg per 1 mg Yellow soft paraffin solid | 15 gram [GSL] £1.21 | 500 gram [GSL] £4.26 DT = £4.18 | 4500 gram [GSL] £21.99
- **Diprobase** (Bayer Plc)
  Liquid paraffin 50 mg per 1 gram, White soft paraffin 950 mg per 1 gram Diprobase ointment | 50 gram [GSL] £1.28 DT = £1.28 | 500 gram [GSL] £5.99 DT = £5.99
- **Emelpin** (Vitame Ltd)
  Emulsifying wax 300 mg per 1 gram, Yellow soft paraffin 300 mg per 1 gram Emelpin ointment | 125 gram £3.08 | 500 gram £3.97
- **Epaderm** (Molnlycke Health Care Ltd)
  Emulsifying wax 300 mg per 1 gram, Yellow soft paraffin 300 mg per 1 gram Epaderm ointment | 125 gram £3.88 | 500 gram £6.58 | 1000 gram £12.25
- **Epaderm Junior** (Molnlycke Health Care Ltd)
  Emulsifying wax 300 mg per 1 gram, Yellow soft paraffin 300 mg per 1 gram Epaderm Junior ointment | 125 gram £3.85
- **Fifty:50** (Ennogen Healthcare Ltd)
  Liquid paraffin 500 mg per 1 gram, White soft paraffin 500 mg per 1 gram Fifty:50 ointment | 250 gram £1.83 | 500 gram £3.66 DT = £4.57
- **Hydromol** (Alliance Pharmaceuticals Ltd)
  Emulsifying wax 300 mg per 1 gram, Yellow soft paraffin 300 mg per 1 gram Hydromol ointment | 100 gram £3.20 | 125 gram £2.92 | 500 gram £4.96 | 1000 gram £8.20
- **KreaMoint** (Essential-Healthcare Ltd)
  Liquid paraffin 500 mg per 1 gram, White soft paraffin 500 mg per 1 gram KreaMoint 50:50 ointment | 500 gram £3.17 DT = £4.57
- **Thirty:30** (Ennogen Healthcare Ltd)
  Emulsifying wax 300 mg per 1 gram, Yellow soft paraffin 300 mg per 1 gram Thirty:30 ointment | 125 gram £3.81 | 250 gram £4.29 | 500 gram £6.47
- **Vaseline** (Unilever UK Home & Personal Care)
  White soft paraffin 1 mg per 1 mg Vaseline Pure Petroleum jelly | 50 ml [GSL] [X]

Liquid

CAUTIONARY AND ADVISORY LABELS 15

EXCIPIENTS: May contain Benzyl alcohol, cetostearyl alcohol (including cetyl and stearyl alcohol), hydroxybenzoates (parabens), isopropyl palmitate

- **E45** (Forum Health Products Ltd)
  E45 lotion | 200 ml £2.45 | 500 ml £4.59
- **QV** (Crawford Healthcare Ltd)
  White soft paraffin 50 mg per 1 gram QV 5% skin lotion | 250 ml £3.19 | 500 ml £5.32

Emollients, urea-containing

15-Jan-2019

● **DRUG ACTION** Urea is a keratin softener and hydrating agent used in the treatment of dry, scaling conditions (including ichthyosis) and may be useful in elderly patients.

● **INDICATIONS AND DOSE**

AQUADRATE ®

Dry, scaling, and itching skin

▶ TO THE SKIN
- Child: Apply twice daily, to be applied thinly

BALNEUM ® CREAM

Dry skin conditions

▶ TO THE SKIN
- Child: Apply twice daily

BALNEUM ® PLUS CREAM

Dry, scaling, and itching skin

▶ TO THE SKIN
- Child: Apply twice daily

CALMURID ®

Dry, scaling, and itching skin

▶ TO THE SKIN
- Child: Apply twice daily, apply a thick layer for 3–5 minutes, massage into area, and remove excess. Can be diluted with aqueous cream (life of diluted cream is 14 days). Half-strength cream can be used for 1 week if stinging occurs

DERMATONICS ONCE HEEL BALM ®

Dry skin on soles of feet

▶ TO THE SKIN
- Child 12–17 years: Apply once daily

E45 ® ITCH RELIEF CREAM

Dry, scaling, and itching skin

▶ TO THE SKIN
- Child: Apply twice daily

EUCERIN ® INTENSIVE CREAM

Dry skin conditions including eczema, ichthyosis, xeroderma, and hyperkeratosis

▶ TO THE SKIN
- Child: Apply twice daily, to be applied thinly and rubbed into area

EUCERIN ® INTENSIVE LOTION

Dry skin conditions including eczema, ichthyosis, xeroderma, and hyperkeratosis

▶ TO THE SKIN
- Child: Apply twice daily, to be applied sparingly and rubbed into area

continued →

FLEXITOL ®

Dry skin on soles of feet and heels

▸ TO THE SKIN

▸ Child 12-17 years: Apply 1–2 times a day

HYDROMOL ® INTENSIVE

Dry, scaling, and itching skin

▸ TO THE SKIN

▸ Child: Apply twice daily, to be applied thinly

IMUDERM ® EMOLLIENT

Dry skin conditions including eczema, psoriasis or dermatitis

▸ TO THE SKIN

▸ Child: Apply to skin or use as a soap substitute

NUTRAPLUS ®

Dry, scaling, and itching skin

▸ TO THE SKIN

▸ Child: Apply 2–3 times a day

IMPORTANT SAFETY INFORMATION

MHRA/CHM ADVICE (UPDATED DECEMBER 2018): EMOLLIENTS: NEW INFORMATION ABOUT RISK OF SEVERE AND FATAL BURNS WITH PARAFFIN-CONTAINING AND PARAFFIN-FREE EMOLLIENTS

See Emollient and barrier preparations p. 765.

● DIRECTIONS FOR ADMINISTRATION Emollients should be applied immediately after washing or bathing to maximise the effect of skin hydration. Emollient preparations contained in tubs should be removed with a clean spoon or spatula to reduce bacterial contamination of the emollient. Emollients should be applied in the direction of hair growth to reduce the risk of folliculitis.

● MEDICINAL FORMS There can be variation in the licensing of different medicines containing the same drug.

Cream

CAUTIONARY AND ADVISORY LABELS 15

EXCIPIENTS: May contain Benzyl alcohol, cetostearyl alcohol (including cetyl and stearyl alcohol), hydroxybenzoates (parabens), isopropyl palmitate, polysorbates, propylene glycol, woolfat and related substances (including lanolin)

▸ **Aquadrate** (Alliance Pharmaceuticals Ltd)
Urea 100 mg per 1 gram Aquadrate 10% cream | 30 gram £1.64 | 100 gram £4.45

▸ **Balneum** (Almirall Ltd)
Balneum cream | 50 gram £2.85 | 500 gram £9.97

▸ **Balneum Plus** (Almirall Ltd)
Lauromacrogols 30 mg per 1 gram, Urea 50 mg per 1 gram Balneum Plus cream | 100 gram GSL £3.29 DT = £4.28 | 500 gram GSL £14.99 DT = £14.99

▸ **E45 Itch Relief** (Forum Health Products Ltd)
Lauromacrogols 30 mg per 1 gram, Urea 50 mg per 1 gram E45 Itch Relief cream | 50 gram GSL £2.81 DT = £2.81 | 100 gram GSL £4.28 DT = £4.28 | 500 gram GSL £14.99 DT = £14.99

▸ **Eucerin Intensive** (Beiersdorf UK Ltd)
Urea 100 mg per 1 gram Eucerin Intensive 10% cream | 100 ml GSL £7.59

▸ **Hydromol Intensive** (Alliance Pharmaceuticals Ltd)
Urea 100 mg per 1 gram Hydromol Intensive 10% cream | 30 gram £1.67 | 100 gram £4.45

▸ **imuDERM emollient** (CliniSupplies Ltd)
imuDERM emollient | 500 gram £6.62

▸ **Nutraplus** (Galderma (UK) Ltd)
Urea 100 mg per 1 gram Nutraplus 10% cream | 100 gram P £4.37

Liquid

CAUTIONARY AND ADVISORY LABELS 15

EXCIPIENTS: May contain Benzyl alcohol, isopropyl palmitate

▸ **Eucerin Intensive** (Beiersdorf UK Ltd)
Urea 100 mg per 1 gram Eucerin Intensive 10% lotion | 250 ml GSL £7.93 DT = £7.93

Balm

CAUTIONARY AND ADVISORY LABELS 15

EXCIPIENTS: May contain Beeswax, benzyl alcohol, cetostearyl alcohol (including cetyl and stearyl alcohol), fragrances, lanolin

▸ **Dermatonics Once** (Dermatonics Ltd)
Dermatonics Once Heel Balm | 75 ml £3.60 | 200 ml £8.50

▸ **Flexitol** (Thornton & Ross Ltd)
Flexitol 25% Urea Heel Balm | 40 gram £2.75 | 75 gram £3.80 | 200 gram £9.40 | 500 gram £14.75

2 Infections of the skin

Skin infections

22-Mar-2020

Antibacterial preparations for the skin

Topical antibacterial preparations are used to treat localised bacterial skin infections caused by Gram-positive organisms (particularly by staphylococci or streptococci). Systemic antibacterial treatment is more appropriate for deep-seated skin infections.

Problems associated with the use of topical antibacterials include bacterial resistance, contact sensitisation, and superinfection. In order to minimise the development of resistance, antibacterials used systemically (e.g. fusidic acid p. 387) should not generally be chosen for topical use. *Resistant organisms* are more common in hospitals, and whenever possible swabs should be taken for bacteriological examination before beginning treatment.

Neomycin sulfate p. 774 applied topically may cause sensitisation and cross-sensitivity with other aminoglycoside antibacterials such as gentamicin p. 333 may occur. Topical antibacterials applied over large areas can cause systemic toxicity; ototoxicity with neomycin sulfate is a particular risk for neonates and children with renal impairment.

Superficial bacterial infection of the skin may be treated with a topical antiseptic such as povidone-iodine p. 813 which also softens crusts, or hydrogen peroxide 1% cream p. 814.

Bacterial infections such as *folliculitis* can be treated with a short course of topical fusidic acid; mupirocin p. 776 should be used only to treat meticillin-resistant *Staphylococcus aureus*.

Impetigo requires topical antiseptic/antibacterial or systemic antibacterial treatment, see Skin infections, antibacterial therapy p. 329.

Cellulitis and *erysipelas* require systemic antibacterial treatment, see Skin infections, antibacterial therapy p. 329.

Staphylococcal scalded-skin syndrome requires urgent treatment with a systemic antibacterial, such as flucloxacillin p. 373.

Mupirocin is not related to any other antibacterial in use; it is effective for skin infections, particularly those due to Gram-positive organisms but it is not indicated for pseudomonal infection. Although *Staphylococcus aureus* strains with low-level resistance to mupirocin are emerging, it is generally useful in infections resistant to other antibacterials. To avoid the development of resistance, mupirocin or fusidic acid should not be used for longer than 10 days and local microbiology advice should be sought before using it in hospital. In the presence of mupirocin-resistant MRSA infection, a topical antiseptic, such as povidone-iodine, chlorhexidine p. 813, or alcohol, can be used; their use should be discussed with the local microbiologist.

Mupirocin ointment contains macrogols; extensive absorption of macrogols through the mucous membranes or through application to thin or damaged skin may result in renal toxicity, especially in neonates. Mupirocin nasal ointment is formulated in a paraffin base and may be more suitable for the treatment of MRSA-infected open wound in neonates.

Metronidazole p. 775 gel is used topically in children to reduce the odour associated with anaerobic infections and for the treatment of periorificial rosacea; oral metronidazole is used to treat wounds infected with anaerobic bacteria.

Silver sulfadiazine p. 775 is licensed for the prevention and treatment of infection in burns but the use of appropriate dressings may be more effective. Systemic effects may occur following extensive application of silver sulfadiazine; its use is not recommended in neonates.

Antibacterial preparations also used systemically
Fusidic acid is a narrow-spectrum antibacterial used for staphylococcal infections.

An ointment containing fusidic acid is used in the fissures of angular cheilitis when associated with staphylococcal infection. See Oropharyngeal fungal infections p. 762 for further information on angular cheilitis.

Metronidazole is used topically to treat rosacea and to reduce the odour associated with anaerobic infections; oral metronidazole is used to treat wounds infected with anaerobic bacteria.

Antifungal preparations for the skin

Most localised fungal infections are treated with topical preparations. To prevent relapse, local antifungal treatment should be continued for 1–2 weeks after the disappearance of all signs of infection. Systemic therapy is necessary for scalp infection or if the skin infection is widespread, disseminated or intractable; although topical therapy may be used to treat some nail infections, systemic therapy is more effective. Specimens of scale, nail or hair should be sent for mycological examination before starting treatment, unless the diagnosis is certain.

Dermatophytoses
Ringworm infection can affect the scalp (tinea capitis), body (tinea corporis), groin (tinea cruris), hand (tinea manuum), foot (tinea pedis, athlete's foot), or nail (tinea unguium, onychomycosis). Tinea capitis is a common childhood infection that requires systemic treatment with an oral antifungal; additional application of a topical antifungal, during the early stages of treatment, may reduce the risk of transmission. A topical antifungal can also be used to treat asymptomatic carriers of scalp ringworm.

Tinea corporis and tinea pedis infections in children respond to treatment with a topical **imidazole** (clotrimazole p. 776, econazole nitrate p. 776, or miconazole p. 777) or terbinafine cream p. 778. Nystatin p. 763 is less effective against tinea.

Compound benzoic acid ointment (Whitfield's ointment) has been used for ringworm infections but it is cosmetically less acceptable than proprietary preparations. Antifungal dusting powders are of little therapeutic value in the treatment of fungal skin infections and may cause skin irritation; they may have some role in preventing re-infection.

Antifungal treatment may not be necessary in asymptomatic children with tinea infection of the nails. If treatment is necessary, a systemic antifungal is more effective than topical therapy. However, topical application of tioconazole p. 777 may be useful for treating early onychomycosis when involvement is limited to mild distal disease, or for superficial white onychomycosis, or where there are contra-indications to systemic therapy. Chronic paronychia on the fingers (usually due to a candidal infection) should be treated with topical clotrimazole or nystatin, but these preparations should be used with caution in children who suck their fingers. Chronic paronychia of the toes (usually due to dermatophyte infection) can be treated with topical terbinafine.

Pityriasis versicolor
Pityriasis (tinea) versicolor can be treated with ketoconazole shampoo p. 777 or **selenium sulfide** shampoo. Topical imidazole antifungals such as clotrimazole, econazole nitrate and miconazole or topical terbinafine are alternatives, but large quantities may be required.

If topical therapy fails, or if the infection is widespread, pityriasis versicolor is treated systemically with an azole antifungal. Relapse is common, especially in the immunocompromised.

Candidiasis
Candidal skin infections can be treated with topical imidazole antifungals clotrimazole, econazole nitrate, or miconazole; topical terbinafine is an alternative. Topical application of nystatin is also effective for candidiasis but it is ineffective against dermatophytosis. Refractory candidiasis requires systemic treatment generally with a triazole such as fluconazole p. 407; systemic treatment with griseofulvin p. 412 or terbinafine is **not appropriate** for refractory candidiasis. See the treatment of oral candiasis and for the management of nappy rash.

Angular cheilitis
Miconazole cream is used in the fissures of angular cheilitis when associated with *Candida*.

Compound topical preparations
Combination of an imidazole and a mild corticosteroid (such as hydrocortisone 1% p. 790) may be of value in the treatment of eczematous intertrigo and, in the first few days only, of a severely inflamed patch of ringworm. Combination of a mild corticosteroid with either an imidazole or nystatin p. 763 may be of use in the treatment of *intertriginous eczema* associated with candida.

Antiviral preparations for the skin

Aciclovir cream p. 781 is used for the treatment of initial and recurrent labial, cutaneous, and genital *herpes simplex infections* in children; treatment should begin as early as possible. Systemic treatment is necessary for buccal or vaginal infections or if cold sores recur frequently.

Herpes labialis
Aciclovir cream can be used for the treatment of initial and recurrent labial herpes simplex infections (cold sores). It is best applied at the earliest possible stage, usually when prodromal changes of sensation are felt in the lip and before vesicles appear.

Penciclovir cream is also licensed for the treatment of herpes labialis; it needs to be applied more frequently than aciclovir cream.

Parasiticidal preparations for the skin

Suitable quantities of parasiticidal preparations

Area of body	Skin creams	Lotions	Cream rinses
Scalp (head lice)		50-100 mL	50-100 mL
Body (scabies)	30-60 g	100 mL	
Body (crab lice)	30-60 g	100 mL	

These amounts are usually suitable for a child 12-17 years for single application.

Scabies
Permethrin p. 780 is used for the treatment of *scabies* (*Sarcoptes scabiei*); malathion p. 780 can be used if permethrin is inappropriate.

Benzyl benzoate is an irritant and should be avoided in children; it is less effective than malathion and permethrin.

Ivermectin p. 416 (available from 'special-order' manufacturers or specialist importing companies) by mouth has been used, in combination with topical drugs, for the treatment of hyperkeratotic (crusted or 'Norwegian') scabies that does not respond to topical treatment alone.

Application
Although acaricides have traditionally been applied after a hot bath, this is **not** necessary and there is even evidence that a hot bath may increase absorption into the blood, removing them from their site of action on the skin.

All members of the affected household should be treated simultaneously. Treatment should be applied to the whole body including the scalp, neck, face, and ears. Particular attention should be paid to the webs of the fingers and toes and lotion brushed under the ends of nails. It is now recommended that malathion and permethrin should be applied twice, one week apart; in the case of benzyl benzoate in adults, up to 3 applications on consecutive days may be needed. It is important to warn users to reapply treatment to the hands if they are washed. Patients with hyperkeratotic scabies may require 2 or 3 applications of acaricide on consecutive days to ensure that enough penetrates the skin crusts to kill all the mites.

Itching
The *itch* and *eczema* of scabies persists for some weeks after the infestation has been eliminated and treatment for pruritus and eczema may be required. Application of crotamiton p. 804 can be used to control itching after treatment with more effective acaricides. A topical corticosteroid may help to reduce itch and inflammation after scabies has been treated successfully; however, persistent symptoms suggest that scabies eradication was not successful. Oral administration of a **sedating antihistamine** at night may also be useful.

Head lice
Dimeticone p. 780 is effective against head lice (*Pediculus humanus capitis*) and acts on the surface of the organism. Malathion, an organophosphorus insecticide, is an alternative, but resistance has been reported. Benzyl benzoate is licensed for the treatment of head lice but it is not recommended for use in children.

Head lice infestation (pediculosis) should be treated using lotion or liquid formulations only if live lice are present. Shampoos are diluted too much in use to be effective. A contact time of 8–12 hours or overnight treatment is recommended for lotions and liquids; a 2-hour treatment is not sufficient to kill eggs.

In general, a course of treatment for head lice should be 2 applications of product 7 days apart to kill lice emerging from any eggs that survive the first application. All affected household members should be treated at the same time.

MHRA/CHM advice: Head lice eradication products: risk of serious burns if treated hair is exposed to open flames or other sources of ignition (March 2018)
Some products for the eradication of head lice infestations are combustible/flammable when on the hair and can ignite and cause serious harm in the presence of an open flame or other source of ignition such as when lighting cigarettes.

Patients and carers should be advised on the safe and correct use of head lice eradication treatments and if appropriate, should be advised that they should not smoke around treated hair and that it should be kept away from open flames or other sources of ignition, including in the morning after overnight application until hair is washed.

Wet combing methods
Head lice can be mechanically removed by combing wet hair meticulously with a plastic detection comb (probably for at least 30 minutes each time) over the whole scalp at 4-day intervals for a minimum of 2 weeks, and continued until no lice are found on 3 consecutive sessions; hair conditioner or vegetable oil can be used to facilitate the process.

Several devices for the removal of head lice such as combs and topical solutions, are available and some are prescribable on the NHS.

The Drug Tariffs can be accessed online at:

- National Health Service Drug Tariff for England and Wales: www.ppa.org.uk/ppa/edt_intro.htm
- Health and Personal Social Services for Northern Ireland Drug Tariff: www.hscbusiness.hscni.net/services/2034.htm
- Scottish Drug Tariff: www.isdscotland.org/Health-topics/Prescribing-and-Medicines/Scottish-Drug-Tariff/

Crab lice
Permethrin and malathion are used to eliminate *crab lice* (*Pthirus pubis*); permethrin is not licensed for treatment of crab lice in children under 18 years. An aqueous preparation should be applied, allowed to dry naturally and washed off after 12 hours; a second treatment is needed after 7 days to kill lice emerging from surviving eggs. All surfaces of the body should be treated, including the scalp, neck, and face (paying particular attention to the eyebrows and other facial hair). A different insecticide should be used if a course of treatment fails.

Parasiticidal preparations
Dimeticone coats head lice and interferes with water balance in lice by preventing the excretion of water; it is less active against eggs and treatment should be repeated after 7 days.

Malathion is recommended for *scabies*, *head lice* and *crab lice*. The risk of systemic effects associated with 1–2 applications of malathion p. 780 is considered to be very low; however, except in the treatment of hyperkeratofic scabies in children, applications of malathion liquid repeated at intervals of less than 1 week or application for more than 3 consecutive weeks should be **avoided** since the likelihood of eradication of lice is not increased.

Permethrin p. 780 is effective for *scabies*. It is also active against *head lice* but the formulation and licensed methods of application of the current products make them unsuitable for the treatment of head lice. Permethrin is also effective against *crab lice* but it is not licensed for this purpose in children under 18 years.

2.1 Bacterial skin infections

ANTIBACTERIALS > AMINOGLYCOSIDES

Neomycin sulfate

- **INDICATIONS AND DOSE**

Bacterial skin infections
▸ TO THE SKIN
▸ Child: Apply up to 3 times a day, for short-term use only

- **UNLICENSED USE** *Neomycin Cream BPC*—no information available.
- **CONTRA-INDICATIONS** Neonates
- **CAUTIONS**
Large areas If large areas of skin are being treated ototoxicity may be a hazard in children, particularly in those with renal impairment.
- **INTERACTIONS** → Appendix 1: neomycin
- **SIDE-EFFECTS** Sensitisation (cross sensitivity with other aminoglycosides may occur)
- **RENAL IMPAIRMENT** Ototoxicity may be a hazard if large areas of skin are treated.
- **LESS SUITABLE FOR PRESCRIBING** Neomycin sulfate cream is less suitable for prescribing.

- **MEDICINAL FORMS** Forms available from special-order manufacturers include: cream

ANTIBACTERIALS > NITROIMIDAZOLE DERIVATIVES

Metronidazole

18-May-2020

● **DRUG ACTION** Metronidazole is an antimicrobial drug with high activity against anaerobic bacteria and protozoa.

● **INDICATIONS AND DOSE**

ACEA®

Acute inflammatory exacerbation of rosacea

▶ TO THE SKIN

▸ Child 1–17 years: Apply twice daily, to be applied thinly

ANABACT®

Malodorous fungating tumours and malodorous gravitational and decubitus ulcers

▶ TO THE SKIN

▸ Child: Apply 1–2 times a day, to be applied to clean wound and covered with non-adherent dressing

METROGEL®

Acute inflammatory exacerbation of rosacea

▶ TO THE SKIN

▸ Child 1–17 years: Apply twice daily, to be applied thinly

Malodorous fungating tumours

▶ TO THE SKIN

▸ Child: Apply 1–2 times a day, to be applied to clean wound and covered with non-adherent dressing

METROSA®

Acute exacerbation of rosacea

▶ TO THE SKIN

▸ Child 1–17 years: Apply twice daily, to be applied thinly

ROSICED®

Inflammatory papules and pustules of rosacea

▶ TO THE SKIN

▸ Child 1–17 years: Apply twice daily for 6 weeks (longer if necessary)

ROZEX® CREAM

Inflammatory papules, pustules and erythema of rosacea

▶ TO THE SKIN

▸ Child 1–17 years: Apply twice daily

ROZEX® GEL

Inflammatory papules, pustules and erythema of rosacea

▶ TO THE SKIN

▸ Child 1–17 years: Apply twice daily

ZYOMET®

Acute inflammatory exacerbation of rosacea

▶ TO THE SKIN

▸ Child 1–17 years: Apply twice daily, to be applied thinly

● **UNLICENSED USE**
METROGEL®, METROSA®, ROSICED®, ROZEX® CREAM, ROZEX® GEL, ZYOMET® Not licensed for use in children.
ACEA®, ANABACT® Not licensed for use in children under 12 years.

● **CAUTIONS** Avoid exposure to strong sunlight or UV light

● **INTERACTIONS** → Appendix 1: metronidazole

● **SIDE-EFFECTS**

▶ **Common or very common** Skin reactions

● **PRESCRIBING AND DISPENSING INFORMATION** For choice of antibacterial therapy, see Skin infections, antibacterial therapy p. 329.

● **PATIENT AND CARER ADVICE**
Medicines for Children leaflet: Metronidazole for bacterial infections www.medicinesforchildren.org.uk/metronidazole-bacterial-infections

● **MEDICINAL FORMS** There can be variation in the licensing of different medicines containing the same drug.

Gel

EXCIPIENTS: May contain Benzyl alcohol, disodium edetate, hydroxybenzoates (parabens), propylene glycol

▸ Acea (Ferndale Pharmaceuticals Ltd)
Metronidazole 7.5 mg per 1 gram Acea 0.75% gel | 40 gram PoM £9.95 DT = £22.63

▸ Anabact (Cambridge Healthcare Supplies Ltd)
Metronidazole 7.5 mg per 1 gram Anabact 0.75% gel | 15 gram PoM £5.64 DT = £5.64 | 30 gram PoM £7.89 | 40 gram PoM £15.89 DT = £22.63

▸ Metrogel (Galderma (UK) Ltd)
Metronidazole 7.5 mg per 1 gram Metrogel 0.75% gel | 40 gram PoM £22.63 DT = £22.63

▸ Metrosa (M & A Pharmachem Ltd)
Metronidazole 7.5 mg per 1 gram Metrosa 0.75% gel | 30 gram PoM £12.00 | 40 gram PoM £19.90 DT = £22.63

▸ Rozex (Galderma (UK) Ltd)
Metronidazole 7.5 mg per 1 gram Rozex 0.75% gel | 30 gram PoM £6.60 | 40 gram PoM £9.88 DT = £22.63

▸ Zyomet (Advanz Pharma)
Metronidazole 7.5 mg per 1 gram Zyomet 0.75% gel | 30 gram PoM £12.00

Cream

EXCIPIENTS: May contain Benzyl alcohol, isopropyl palmitate, propylene glycol

▸ Rosiced (Pierre Fabre Dermo-Cosmetique)
Metronidazole 7.5 mg per 1 gram Rosiced 0.75% cream | 30 gram PoM £6.60 DT = £6.60

▸ Rozex (Galderma (UK) Ltd)
Metronidazole 7.5 mg per 1 gram Rozex 0.75% cream | 30 gram PoM £6.60 DT = £6.60 | 40 gram PoM £9.88 DT = £9.88

ANTIBACTERIALS > SULFONAMIDES

Silver sulfadiazine

20-May-2020

● **INDICATIONS AND DOSE**

Prophylaxis and treatment of infection in burn wounds

▶ TO THE SKIN

▸ Child: Apply daily, may be applied more frequently if very exudative

For conservative management of finger-tip injuries

▶ TO THE SKIN

▸ Child: Apply every 2–3 days, consult product literature for details

Adjunct to prophylaxis of infection in skin graft donor sites and extensive abrasions

▶ TO THE SKIN

▸ Child: (consult product literature)

Adjunct to short-term treatment of infection in pressure sores

▶ TO THE SKIN

▸ Child: (consult product literature)

● **UNLICENSED USE** No age range specified by manufacturer.

● **CONTRA-INDICATIONS** Not recommended for neonates

● **CAUTIONS** G6PD deficiency

CAUTIONS, FURTHER INFORMATION

▸ Large areas Plasma-sulfadiazine concentrations may approach therapeutic levels with *side-effects* and *interactions* as for sulfonamides if large areas of skin are treated.

● **INTERACTIONS** → Appendix 1: silver sulfadiazine

● **SIDE-EFFECTS**

▶ **Common or very common** Leucopenia · skin reactions

▶ **Rare or very rare** Argyria (following treatment of large areas of skin or long term use) · renal failure

SIDE-EFFECTS, FURTHER INFORMATION Leucopenia developing 2–3 days after starting treatment of burns patients is reported usually to be self-limiting and silver sulfadiazine need not usually be discontinued provided

13 Skin

blood counts are monitored carefully to ensure return to normality within a few days.

- **ALLERGY AND CROSS-SENSITIVITY** Contra-indicated in patients with sensitivity to sulfonamides.
- **PREGNANCY** Risk of neonatal haemolysis and methaemoglobinaemia in third trimester.
- **BREAST FEEDING** Small risk of kernicterus in jaundiced infants and of haemolysis in G6PD-deficient infants.
- **HEPATIC IMPAIRMENT** Manufacturer advises caution in significant hepatic impairment.
- **RENAL IMPAIRMENT** Manufacturer advises caution if significant impairment.
- **MONITORING REQUIREMENTS** Monitor for leucopenia.
- **DIRECTIONS FOR ADMINISTRATION** Apply with sterile applicator.

- **MEDICINAL FORMS** There can be variation in the licensing of different medicines containing the same drug.

Cream

EXCIPIENTS: May contain Cetostearyl alcohol (including cetyl and stearyl alcohol), polysorbates, propylene glycol

- Flamazine (Smith & Nephew Healthcare Ltd)
  Sulfadiazine silver 10 mg per 1 gram Flamazine 1% cream | 20 gram PoM £2.91 | 50 gram PoM £3.85 DT = £3.85 | 250 gram PoM £10.32 DT = £10.32 | 500 gram PoM £18.27 DT = £18.27

ANTIBACTERIALS > OTHER

Mupirocin

18-May-2020

- **INDICATIONS AND DOSE**

Bacterial skin infections, particularly those caused by Gram-positive organisms (except pseudomonal infection)

- TO THE SKIN
- Child: Apply up to 3 times a day for up to 10 days

Non-bullous impetigo [in patients who are not systemically unwell or at high risk of complications]

- TO THE SKIN
- Child: Apply 3 times a day for 5–7 days

- **UNLICENSED USE** Mupirocin ointment licensed for use in children (age range not specified by manufacturer). *Bactroban*® cream not recommended for use in children under 1 year.
- **SIDE-EFFECTS**
- **Common or very common** Skin reactions
- **PREGNANCY** Manufacturer advises avoid unless potential benefit outweighs risk—no information available.
- **BREAST FEEDING** No information available.
- **RENAL IMPAIRMENT** Manufacturer advises caution when mupirocin ointment used in moderate or severe impairment because it contains macrogols (polyethylene glycol).
- **PRESCRIBING AND DISPENSING INFORMATION** For choice of antibacterial therapy, see Skin infections, antibacterial therapy p. 329.

- **MEDICINAL FORMS** There can be variation in the licensing of different medicines containing the same drug.

Ointment

- Mupirocin (Non-proprietary)
  Mupirocin 20 mg per 1 gram Mupirocin 2% ointment | 15 gram PoM £12.50 DT = £5.26
- Bactroban (GlaxoSmithKline UK Ltd)
  Mupirocin 20 mg per 1 gram Bactroban 2% ointment | 15 gram PoM £5.26 DT = £5.26

Cream

EXCIPIENTS: May contain Benzyl alcohol, cetostearyl alcohol (including cetyl and stearyl alcohol)

- Bactroban (GlaxoSmithKline UK Ltd)
  Mupirocin (as Mupirocin calcium) 20 mg per 1 gram Bactroban 2% cream | 15 gram PoM £5.26 DT = £5.26

2.2 Fungal skin infections

Other drugs used for Fungal skin infections Griseofulvin, p. 412 · Hydrocortisone with clotrimazole, p. 794

ANTIFUNGALS > IMIDAZOLE ANTIFUNGALS

Clotrimazole

10-Mar-2020

- **INDICATIONS AND DOSE**

Fungal skin infections

- TO THE SKIN
- Child: Apply 2–3 times a day

- **CAUTIONS** Contact with eyes and mucous membranes should be avoided
- **INTERACTIONS** → Appendix 1: antifungals, azoles
- **SIDE-EFFECTS** Oedema · pain · paraesthesia · skin reactions
- **PREGNANCY** Minimal absorption from skin; not known to be harmful.
- **PRESCRIBING AND DISPENSING INFORMATION** Spray may be useful for application of clotrimazole to large or hairy areas of the skin.
- **PATIENT AND CARER ADVICE**
  Medicines for Children leaflet: Clotrimazole for fungal infections www.medicinesforchildren.org.uk/clotrimazole-fungal-infections

- **MEDICINAL FORMS** There can be variation in the licensing of different medicines containing the same drug. Forms available from special-order manufacturers include: powder

Cream

EXCIPIENTS: May contain Benzyl alcohol, cetostearyl alcohol (including cetyl and stearyl alcohol), polysorbates

- Clotrimazole (Non-proprietary)
  Clotrimazole 10 mg per 1 gram Clotrimazole 1% cream | 20 gram P £2.06 DT = £1.29 | 50 gram P £5.45 DT = £3.23
- Canesten (clotrimazole) (Bayer Plc)
  Clotrimazole 10 mg per 1 gram Canesten 1% cream | 20 gram P £2.20 DT = £1.29 | 50 gram P £3.64 DT = £3.23
  Canesten Antifungal 1% cream | 20 gram P £1.85 DT = £1.29
  Clotrimazole 20 mg per 1 gram Canesten 2% thrush cream | 20 gram P £4.76 DT = £4.76

Liquid

- Canesten (clotrimazole) (Bayer Plc)
  Clotrimazole 10 mg per 1 ml Canesten 1% solution | 20 ml P £2.53 DT = £2.53

Combinations available: ***Hydrocortisone with clotrimazole***, p. 794

Econazole nitrate

08-May-2020

- **INDICATIONS AND DOSE**

Fungal skin infections

- TO THE SKIN
- Child: Apply twice daily

Fungal nail infections

- BY TRANSUNGUAL APPLICATION
- Child: Apply once daily, applied under occlusive dressing

- **CAUTIONS** Avoid contact with eyes and mucous membranes
- **SIDE-EFFECTS**
- **Common or very common** Pain · skin reactions

▶ **Uncommon** Swelling
▶ **Frequency not known** Angioedema

SIDE-EFFECTS, FURTHER INFORMATION Treatment should be discontinued if side-effects are severe.

● PREGNANCY Minimal absorption from skin; not known to be harmful.

● PRESCRIBING AND DISPENSING INFORMATION *Pevaryl®* 1% cream should be used.

● MEDICINAL FORMS There can be variation in the licensing of different medicines containing the same drug.

Cream

EXCIPIENTS: May contain Butylated hydroxyanisole, fragrances

▸ Pevaryl (Janssen-Cilag Ltd)
Econazole nitrate 10 mg per 1 gram Pevaryl 1% cream | 30 gram [P] £3.71 DT = £3.78

Ketoconazole

04-Feb-2020

● INDICATIONS AND DOSE

Treatment of seborrhoeic dermatitis and dandruff

▶ TO THE SKIN USING SHAMPOO

▸ Child 12-17 years: Apply twice weekly for 2–4 weeks, leave preparation on for 3–5 minutes before rinsing

Prophylaxis of seborrhoeic dermatitis and dandruff

▶ TO THE SKIN USING SHAMPOO

▸ Child 12-17 years: Apply every 1–2 weeks, leave preparation on for 3–5 minutes before rinsing

Treatment of pityriasis versicolor

▶ TO THE SKIN USING SHAMPOO

▸ Child 12-17 years: Apply once daily for maximum 5 days, leave preparation on for 3–5 minutes before rinsing

Prophylaxis of pityriasis versicolor

▶ TO THE SKIN USING SHAMPOO

▸ Child 12-17 years: Apply once daily for up to 3 days before sun exposure, leave preparation on for 3–5 minutes before rinsing

● CONTRA-INDICATIONS Acute porphyrias p. 652

● CAUTIONS Avoid contact with eyes · avoid contact with mucous membranes

● INTERACTIONS → Appendix 1: antifungals, azoles

● SIDE-EFFECTS

▶ **Common or very common** Skin reactions
▶ **Uncommon** Alopecia · angioedema · excessive tearing · folliculitis · hair changes
▶ **Rare or very rare** Eye irritation · taste altered

● EXCEPTIONS TO LEGAL CATEGORY

▸ For Seborrhoeic dermatitis and dandruff Can be sold to the public for the prevention and treatment of dandruff and seborrhoeic dermatitis of the scalp as a shampoo formulation containing ketoconazole maximum 2%, in a pack containing maximum 120 mL and labelled to show a maximum frequency of application of once every 3 days.

● MEDICINAL FORMS There can be variation in the licensing of different medicines containing the same drug.

Shampoo

EXCIPIENTS: May contain Imidurea

▸ Ketoconazole (Non-proprietary)
Ketoconazole 20 mg per 1 gram Ketoconazole 2% shampoo | 120 ml [PoM] £4.81 DT = £4.53

▸ Dandrazol (Transdermal Ltd)
Ketoconazole 20 mg per 1 gram Dandrazol 2% shampoo | 120 ml [PoM] £3.39 DT = £4.53

▸ Nizoral (Thornton & Ross Ltd)
Ketoconazole 20 mg per 1 gram Nizoral 2% shampoo | 120 ml [PoM] £3.59 DT = £4.53

Miconazole

20-Jan-2020

● INDICATIONS AND DOSE

Fungal skin infections

▶ TO THE SKIN

▸ Neonate: Apply twice daily continuing for 10 days after lesions have healed.

▸ Child: Apply twice daily continuing for 10 days after lesions have healed

Fungal nail infections

▶ TO THE SKIN

▸ Child: Apply 1–2 times a day

● UNLICENSED USE Licensed for use in children (age range not specified by manufacturer).

● CAUTIONS Avoid in Acute porphyrias p. 652 · contact with eyes and mucous membranes should be avoided

● INTERACTIONS → Appendix 1: antifungals, azoles

● SIDE-EFFECTS

▶ **Uncommon** Skin reactions
▶ **Frequency not known** Angioedema

● PREGNANCY Absorbed from the skin in small amounts; manufacturer advises caution.

● BREAST FEEDING Manufacturer advises caution—no information available.

● PROFESSION SPECIFIC INFORMATION

Dental practitioners' formulary

Miconazole cream may be prescribed.

● NATIONAL FUNDING/ACCESS DECISIONS

NHS restrictions *Daktarin®* powder and *Daktarin®* cream 15 g is not prescribable in NHS primary care.

● MEDICINAL FORMS There can be variation in the licensing of different medicines containing the same drug.

Cream

EXCIPIENTS: May contain Butylated hydroxyanisole

▸ Daktarin (McNeil Products Ltd, Janssen-Cilag Ltd, Johnson & Johnson Ltd)
Miconazole nitrate 20 mg per 1 gram Daktarin 2% cream | 15 gram [P] £2.66 | 30 gram [P] £1.82 DT = £1.82

Powder

▸ Daktarin (McNeil Products Ltd)
Miconazole nitrate 20 mg per 1 gram Daktarin 2% powder | 20 gram [P] £3.13 DT = £3.13

Tioconazole

03-Feb-2020

● INDICATIONS AND DOSE

Fungal nail infection

▶ BY TRANSUNGUAL APPLICATION

▸ Child: Apply twice daily usually for up to 6 months (may be extended to 12 months), apply to nails and surrounding skin

● UNLICENSED USE Licensed for use in children (age range not specified by manufacturer).

● CAUTIONS Contact with eyes and mucous membranes should be avoided · use with caution if child likely to suck affected digits

● SIDE-EFFECTS

▶ **Common or very common** Peripheral oedema
▶ **Uncommon** Skin reactions
▶ **Frequency not known** Nail disorder · pain · paraesthesia · periorbital oedema

● PREGNANCY Manufacturer advises avoid.

- **MEDICINAL FORMS** There can be variation in the licensing of different medicines containing the same drug.

Paint

- Tioconazole (Non-proprietary)
  Tioconazole 283 mg per 1 ml Tioconazole 283mg/ml medicated nail lacquer | 12 ml [PoM] £28.74 DT = £28.74
- Trosyl (Pfizer Ltd)
  Tioconazole 283 mg per 1 ml Trosyl 283mg/ml nail solution | 12 ml [PoM] £27.38 DT = £28.74

ANTIFUNGALS › OTHER

Amorolfine

20-Jan-2020

- **INDICATIONS AND DOSE**

Fungal nail infections

▶ BY TRANSUNGUAL APPLICATION

- Child 1 month–11 years: Apply 1–2 times a week for 6 months to treat finger nails and for toe nails 9–12 months (review at intervals of 3 months), apply to infected nails after filing and cleansing, allow to dry for approximately 3 minutes
- Child 12–17 years: Apply 1–2 times a week for 6 months to treat finger nails and for toe nails 9–12 months (review at intervals of 3 months), apply to infected nails after filing and cleansing, allow to dry for approximately 3 minutes

- **UNLICENSED USE** Not licensed for use in children under 12 years.
- **CAUTIONS** Avoid contact with ears · avoid contact with eyes and mucous membranes · use with caution in child likely to suck affected digits
- **SIDE-EFFECTS**
  ▶ **Rare or very rare** Nail discolouration · skin reactions
- **PATIENT AND CARER ADVICE** Avoid nail varnish or artificial nails during treatment.

- **MEDICINAL FORMS** There can be variation in the licensing of different medicines containing the same drug.

Medicated nail lacquer

CAUTIONARY AND ADVISORY LABELS 10

- Amorolfine (Non-proprietary)
  Amorolfine (as Amorolfine hydrochloride) 50 mg per 1 ml Amorolfine 5% medicated nail lacquer | 5 ml [PoM] £16.21 DT = £8.36
- Loceryl (Galderma (UK) Ltd)
  Amorolfine (as Amorolfine hydrochloride) 50 mg per 1 ml Loceryl 5% medicated nail lacquer | 5 ml [PoM] £9.08 DT = £8.36
- Omicur (Morningside Healthcare Ltd)
  Amorolfine (as Amorolfine hydrochloride) 50 mg per 1 ml Omicur 5% medicated nail lacquer | 2.5 ml [PoM] £9.09 | 5 ml [PoM] £9.09 DT = £8.36

Terbinafine

12-May-2020

- **INDICATIONS AND DOSE**

Tinea pedis

▶ TO THE SKIN USING CREAM

- Child: Apply 1–2 times a day for up to 1 week, to be applied thinly

▶ BY MOUTH USING TABLETS

- Child 1–17 years (body-weight 10–19 kg): 62.5 mg once daily for 2–6 weeks
- Child 1–17 years (body-weight 20–39 kg): 125 mg once daily for 2–6 weeks
- Child 1–17 years (body-weight 40 kg and above): 250 mg once daily for 2–6 weeks

Tinea corporis

▶ TO THE SKIN USING CREAM

- Child: Apply 1–2 times a day for up to 1–2 weeks, to be applied thinly, review treatment after 2 weeks

▶ BY MOUTH USING TABLETS

- Child 1–17 years (body-weight 10–19 kg): 62.5 mg once daily for 4 weeks
- Child 1–17 years (body-weight 20–39 kg): 125 mg once daily for 4 weeks
- Child 1–17 years (body-weight 40 kg and above): 250 mg once daily for 4 weeks

Tinea cruris

▶ TO THE SKIN USING CREAM

- Child: Apply 1–2 times a day for up to 1–2 weeks, to be applied thinly, review treatment after 2 weeks

▶ BY MOUTH USING TABLETS

- Child 1–17 years (body-weight 10–19 kg): 62.5 mg once daily for 2–4 weeks
- Child 1–17 years (body-weight 20–39 kg): 125 mg once daily for 2–4 weeks
- Child 1–17 years (body-weight 40 kg and above): 250 mg once daily for 2–4 weeks

Tinea capitis

▶ BY MOUTH USING TABLETS

- Child 1–17 years (body-weight 10–19 kg): 62.5 mg once daily for 4 weeks
- Child 1–17 years (body-weight 20–39 kg): 125 mg once daily for 4 weeks
- Child 1–17 years (body-weight 40 kg and above): 250 mg once daily for 4 weeks

Dermatophyte infections of the nails

▶ BY MOUTH USING TABLETS

- Child 1–17 years (body-weight 10–19 kg): 62.5 mg once daily for 6 weeks–3 months (occasionally longer in toenail infections)
- Child 1–17 years (body-weight 20–39 kg): 125 mg once daily for 6 weeks–3 months (occasionally longer in toenail infections)
- Child 1–17 years (body-weight 40 kg and above): 250 mg once daily for 6 weeks–3 months (occasionally longer in toenail infections)

Cutaneous candidiasis | Pityriasis versicolor

▶ TO THE SKIN USING CREAM

- Child: Apply 1–2 times a day for 2 weeks, to be applied thinly, review treatment after 2 weeks

- **UNLICENSED USE** Not licensed for use in children.
- **CAUTIONS**
  - With oral use Psoriasis (risk of exacerbation) · risk of lupus erythematosus
  - With topical use contact with eyes and mucous membranes should be avoided
- **INTERACTIONS** → Appendix 1: terbinafine
- **SIDE-EFFECTS**

GENERAL SIDE-EFFECTS

▶ **Common or very common** Skin reactions

SPECIFIC SIDE-EFFECTS

▶ **Common or very common**
- With oral use Appetite decreased · arthralgia · diarrhoea · gastrointestinal discomfort · gastrointestinal disorder · headache · myalgia · nausea

▶ **Uncommon**
- With oral use Taste altered
- With topical use Pain

▶ **Rare or very rare**
- With oral use Agranulocytosis · alopecia · cutaneous lupus erythematosus · dizziness · hepatic disorders · malaise · neutropenia · photosensitivity reaction · sensation abnormal · severe cutaneous adverse reactions (SCARs) ·

systemic lupus erythematosus (SLE) · thrombocytopenia · vertigo

- **Frequency not known**
- With oral use Anaemia · anxiety · depressive symptom · fatigue · fever · hearing impairment · influenza like illness · pancreatitis · pancytopenia · rhabdomyolysis · serum sickness-like reaction · smell altered · tinnitus · vasculitis · vision disorders
- With topical use Hypersensitivity

SIDE-EFFECTS, FURTHER INFORMATION

Liver toxicity With oral use; discontinue treatment if liver toxicity develops (including jaundice, cholestasis and hepatitis).

Serious skin reactions With oral use; discontinue treatment in progressive skin rash (including Stevens-Johnson syndrome and toxic epidermal necrolysis).

- **PREGNANCY**
  - With topical use Manufacturer advises use only if potential benefit outweighs risk— *animal* studies suggest no adverse effects.
  - With oral use Manufacturer advises use only if potential benefit outweighs risk—no information available.
- **BREAST FEEDING**
  - With topical use Manufacturer advises avoid—present in milk. Less than 5% of the dose is absorbed after topical application of terbinafine; avoid application to mother's chest.
  - With oral use Avoid—present in milk.
- **HEPATIC IMPAIRMENT**
  - With oral use Manufacturer advises avoid (risk of increased exposure).
- **RENAL IMPAIRMENT**

Dose adjustments ▸ With oral use Use half normal dose if estimated glomerular filtration rate less than 50 mL/minute/1.73 m^2 and no suitable alternative available.

- **MONITORING REQUIREMENTS**
  - With oral use Monitor hepatic function before treatment and then periodically after 4–6 weeks of treatment—discontinue if abnormalities in liver function tests.
- **PATIENT AND CARER ADVICE**
  - With oral use Manufacturer advises that patients should immediately report any signs or symptoms suggestive of liver dysfunction such as pruritus, unexplained persistent nausea, decreased appetite, anorexia, jaundice, vomiting, fatigue, right upper abdominal pain, dark urine, or pale stools. Patients with these symptoms should discontinue taking terbinafine and the patient's liver function should be immediately evaluated.
- **EXCEPTIONS TO LEGAL CATEGORY**
  - With topical use Preparations of terbinafine hydrochloride (maximum 1%) can be sold to the public for use in those over 16 years for external use for the treatment of tinea pedis as a cream in a pack containing maximum 15 g, or for the treatment of tinea pedis and cruris as a cream in a pack containing maximum 15 g, or for the treatment of tinea pedis, cruris, and corporis as a spray in a pack containing maximum 30 mL spray or as a gel in a pack containing maximum 30 g gel.

- **MEDICINAL FORMS** There can be variation in the licensing of different medicines containing the same drug.

Tablet

CAUTIONARY AND ADVISORY LABELS 9

- Terbinafine (Non-proprietary)

Terbinafine (as Terbinafine hydrochloride) 250 mg Terbinafine 250mg tablets | 14 tablet [PoM] £18.11 DT = £1.80 | 28 tablet [PoM] £3.56–£34.93

- Lamisil (Novartis Pharmaceuticals UK Ltd)

Terbinafine (as Terbinafine hydrochloride) 250 mg Lamisil 250mg tablets | 14 tablet [PoM] £21.30 DT = £1.80 | 28 tablet [PoM] £41.09

Cream

EXCIPIENTS: May contain Benzyl alcohol, cetostearyl alcohol (including cetyl and stearyl alcohol), polysorbates

- Terbinafine (Non-proprietary)

Terbinafine hydrochloride 10 mg per 1 gram Terbinafine 1% cream | 15 gram [PoM] £3.17 DT = £1.54 | 30 gram [PoM] £6.33 DT = £3.08

- Lamisil (GlaxoSmithKline Consumer Healthcare)

Terbinafine hydrochloride 10 mg per 1 gram Lamisil 1% cream | 30 gram [PoM] £8.76 DT = £3.08

ANTISEPTICS AND DISINFECTANTS › UNDECENOATES

Undecenoic acid with zinc undecenoate

- **INDICATIONS AND DOSE**

Treatment of athletes foot

- TO THE SKIN
  - Child: Apply twice daily, continue use for 7 days after lesions have healed

Prevention of athletes foot

- TO THE SKIN
  - Child: Apply once daily

- **UNLICENSED USE** *Mycota*® licensed for use in children (age range not specified by manufacturer).
- **CAUTIONS** Avoid broken skin · contact with eyes should be avoided · contact with mucous membranes should be avoided
- **SIDE-EFFECTS**
  - **Rare or very rare** Skin irritation

SIDE-EFFECTS, FURTHER INFORMATION Treatment should be discontinued if irritation is severe.

- **MEDICINAL FORMS** There can be variation in the licensing of different medicines containing the same drug.

Cream

EXCIPIENTS: May contain Cetostearyl alcohol (including cetyl and stearyl alcohol), fragrances

- Mycota (zinc undecenoate / undecenoic acid) (Thornton & Ross Ltd)

Undecenoic acid 50 mg per 1 gram, Zinc undecenoate 200 mg per 1 gram Mycota cream | 25 gram [GSL] £2.01

Powder

EXCIPIENTS: May contain Fragrances

- Mycota (zinc undecenoate / undecenoic acid) (Thornton & Ross Ltd)

Undecenoic acid 20 mg per 1 gram, Zinc undecenoate 200 mg per 1 gram Mycota powder | 70 gram [GSL] £3.04

ANTISEPTICS AND DISINFECTANTS › OTHER

Chlorhexidine with nystatin

- **INDICATIONS AND DOSE**

Skin infections due to Candida spp.

- TO THE SKIN
  - Child: Apply 2–3 times a day, continuing for 7 days after lesions have healed

- **UNLICENSED USE** Licensed for use in children (age range not specified by manufacturer).
- **CAUTIONS** Avoid contact with eyes and mucous membranes
- **SIDE-EFFECTS** Hypersensitivity · skin reactions

- **MEDICINAL FORMS** There can be variation in the licensing of different medicines containing the same drug.

Cream

EXCIPIENTS: May contain Benzyl alcohol, cetostearyl alcohol (including cetyl and stearyl alcohol), polysorbates

- Chlorhexidine with nystatin (Non-proprietary)
  Chlorhexidine hydrochloride 10 mg per 1 gram, Nystatin 100000 unit per 1 gram Nystatin 100,000units/g / Chlorhexidine hydrochloride 1% cream | 30 gram PoM £4.99 DT = £4.99

BENZOATES

Benzoic acid with salicylic acid

● **INDICATIONS AND DOSE**

Ringworm (tinea)

▶ TO THE SKIN

- Child: Apply twice daily

● **UNLICENSED USE** Licensed for use in children (age range not specified by manufacturer).

● **CAUTIONS** Avoid broken or inflamed skin · avoid contact with eyes · avoid contact with mucous membranes

CAUTIONS, FURTHER INFORMATION

- Salicylate toxicity Salicylate toxicity may occur particularly if applied on large areas of skin.

● **SIDE-EFFECTS** Drug toxicity · eye irritation · mucosal irritation · skin reactions

● **PRESCRIBING AND DISPENSING INFORMATION** Benzoic Acid Ointment, Compound, BP has also been referred to as Whitfield's ointment.

● **MEDICINAL FORMS** Forms available from special-order manufacturers include: cream, ointment

13 Skin

2.3 Parasitic skin infections

PARASITICIDES

Dimeticone

04-Feb-2020

● **INDICATIONS AND DOSE**

Head lice

▶ TO THE SKIN

- Child: Apply once weekly for 2 doses, rub into dry hair and scalp, allow to dry naturally, shampoo after minimum 8 hours (or overnight)

● **UNLICENSED USE** Not licensed for use in children under 6 months except under medical supervision.

IMPORTANT SAFETY INFORMATION

MHRA/CHM ADVICE: HEAD LICE ERADICATION PRODUCTS: RISK OF SERIOUS BURNS IF TREATED HAIR IS EXPOSED TO OPEN FLAMES OR OTHER SOURCES OF IGNITION (MARCH 2018)

See Skin infections p. 772.

● **CAUTIONS** Avoid contact with eyes · children under 6 months, medical supervision required

● **SIDE-EFFECTS** Alopecia · dyspnoea · eye irritation · hypersensitivity · scalp changes · skin reactions

● **MEDICINAL FORMS** There can be variation in the licensing of different medicines containing the same drug.

Liquid

- Hedrin (Thornton & Ross Ltd)
  Dimeticone 40 mg per 1 gram Hedrin 4% lotion | 50 ml P £3.28 DT = £3.28 | 150 ml P £7.62 DT = £7.62
- Lyclear (dimeticone) (Omega Pharma Ltd)
  Dimeticone 40 mg per 1 gram Lyclear lotion | 100 ml [NHS]

Cutaneous spray solution

- Hedrin (Thornton & Ross Ltd)
  Dimeticone 40 mg per 1 gram Hedrin 4% spray | 120 ml P £7.85 DT = £7.85

Malathion

04-Feb-2020

● **INDICATIONS AND DOSE**

Head lice

▶ TO THE SKIN

- Child: Apply once weekly for 2 doses, rub preparation into dry hair and scalp, allow to dry naturally, remove by washing after 12 hours

Crab lice

▶ TO THE SKIN

- Child: Apply once weekly for 2 doses, apply preparation over whole body, allow to dry naturally, wash off after 12 hours or overnight

Scabies

▶ TO THE SKIN

- Child: Apply once weekly for 2 doses, apply preparation over whole body, and wash off after 24 hours, if hands are washed with soap within 24 hours, they should be retreated

● **UNLICENSED USE** Not licensed for use in children under 6 months except under medical supervision.

IMPORTANT SAFETY INFORMATION

MHRA/CHM ADVICE: HEAD LICE ERADICATION PRODUCTS: RISK OF SERIOUS BURNS IF TREATED HAIR IS EXPOSED TO OPEN FLAMES OR OTHER SOURCES OF IGNITION (MARCH 2018)

See Skin infections p. 772.

● **CAUTIONS** Alcoholic lotions **not** recommended for head lice in children with severe eczema or asthma, or for scabies or crab lice · avoid contact with eyes · children under 6 months, medical supervision required · do not use lotion more than once a week for 3 consecutive weeks · do not use on broken or secondarily infected skin

● **SIDE-EFFECTS** Angioedema · eye swelling · hypersensitivity · skin reactions

● **PRESCRIBING AND DISPENSING INFORMATION** For scabies, manufacturer recommends application to the body but not necessarily to the head and neck. However, application should be extended to the scalp, neck, face, and ears.

● **MEDICINAL FORMS** There can be variation in the licensing of different medicines containing the same drug.

Liquid

EXCIPIENTS: May contain Cetostearyl alcohol (including cetyl and stearyl alcohol), fragrances, hydroxybenzoates (parabens)

- Derbac-M (G.R. Lane Health Products Ltd)
  Malathion 5 mg per 1 gram Derbac-M 0.5% liquid | 50 ml P £4.26 DT = £4.26 | 200 ml P £9.91 DT = £9.91

Permethrin

04-Feb-2020

● **INDICATIONS AND DOSE**

Scabies

▶ TO THE SKIN

- Child: Apply once weekly for 2 doses, apply 5% preparation over whole body including face, neck, scalp and ears then wash off after 8–12 hours. If hands are washed with soap within 8 hours of application, they should be treated again with cream

● **UNLICENSED USE** *Dermal Cream* (scabies), not licensed for use in children under 2 months; not licensed for treatment of crab lice in children under 18 years. *Creme Rinse* (head lice) not licensed for use in children under 6 months except under medical supervision.

IMPORTANT SAFETY INFORMATION

MHRA/CHM ADVICE: HEAD LICE ERADICATION PRODUCTS: RISK OF SERIOUS BURNS IF TREATED HAIR IS EXPOSED TO OPEN FLAMES OR OTHER SOURCES OF IGNITION (MARCH 2018)

See Skin infections p. 772.

- **CAUTIONS** Avoid contact with eyes · children aged 2 months–2 years, medical supervision required for dermal cream (scabies) · children under 6 months, medical supervision required for cream rinse (head lice) · do not use on broken or secondarily infected skin
- **SIDE-EFFECTS** Scalp irritation · skin reactions
- **PRESCRIBING AND DISPENSING INFORMATION** Manufacturer recommends application to the body but to exclude head and neck. However, application should be extended to the scalp, neck, face, and ears.
  Larger patients may require up to two 30-g packs for adequate treatment.
- **LESS SUITABLE FOR PRESCRIBING** Lyclear® Creme Rinse is less suitable for prescribing.
- **MEDICINAL FORMS** There can be variation in the licensing of different medicines containing the same drug.

Cream

CAUTIONARY AND ADVISORY LABELS 10 (Dermal cream only)

EXCIPIENTS: May contain Butylated hydroxytoluene, woolfat and related substances (including lanolin)

- Permethrin (Non-proprietary)
  Permethrin 50 mg per 1 gram Permethrin 5% cream | 30 gram [P] £7.46 DT = £7.46
- Lyclear (Omega Pharma Ltd)
  Permethrin 50 mg per 1 gram Lyclear 5% dermal cream | 30 gram [P] £5.71 DT = £7.46

Liquid

EXCIPIENTS: May contain Cetostearyl alcohol (including cetyl and stearyl alcohol)

- Lyclear (Omega Pharma Ltd)
  Permethrin 10 mg per 1 gram Lyclear 1% creme rinse | 59 ml [P] £4.20 DT = £4.20 | 118 ml [P] £7.11 DT = £7.11

2.4 Viral skin infections

ANTIVIRALS › NUCLEOSIDE ANALOGUES

Aciclovir

10-Mar-2020

(Acyclovir)

- **INDICATIONS AND DOSE**

Herpes simplex infection (local treatment)

- TO THE SKIN
- Child: Apply 5 times a day for 5–10 days, to be applied to lesions approximately every 4 hours, starting at first sign of attack

- **UNLICENSED USE** Cream licensed for use in children (age range not specified by manufacturer).
- **CAUTIONS** Avoid cream coming in to contact with eyes and mucous membranes
- **INTERACTIONS** → Appendix 1: aciclovir
- **SIDE-EFFECTS**
  - **Uncommon** Skin reactions
- **PREGNANCY** Limited absorption from topical aciclovir preparations.
- **PATIENT AND CARER ADVICE**
  Medicines for Children leaflet: Aciclovir cream for herpes www.medicinesforchildren.org.uk/aciclovir-cream-herpes-0
- **PROFESSION SPECIFIC INFORMATION**
  Dental practitioners' formulary
  Aciclovir Cream may be prescribed.
- **EXCEPTIONS TO LEGAL CATEGORY** A 2-g tube and a pump pack are on sale to the public for the treatment of cold sores.
- **MEDICINAL FORMS** There can be variation in the licensing of different medicines containing the same drug.

Cream

EXCIPIENTS: May contain Cetostearyl alcohol (including cetyl and stearyl alcohol), propylene glycol

- Aciclovir (Non-proprietary)
  Aciclovir 50 mg per 1 gram Aciclovir 5% cream | 2 gram [PoM] £1.26 DT = £1.26 | 10 gram [PoM] £6.38 DT = £6.31
- Zovirax (GlaxoSmithKline Consumer Healthcare, GlaxoSmithKline UK Ltd)
  Aciclovir 50 mg per 1 gram Zovirax 5% cream | 2 gram [PoM] £4.63 DT = £1.26 | 10 gram [PoM] £13.96 DT = £6.31

3 Inflammatory skin conditions

3.1 Eczema and psoriasis

Eczema

Types and management

The main types of eczema (dermatitis) in children are atopic, irritant and allergic contact; different types may co-exist. *Atopic eczema* is the most common type and it usually involves dry skin as well as infection and lichenification caused by scratching and rubbing. *Seborrhoeic dermatitis* is also common in infants.

Management of eczema involves the removal or treatment of contributory factors; known or suspected irritants and contact allergens should be avoided. Rarely, ingredients in topical medicinal products may sensitise the skin; *BNF for Children* lists active ingredients together with excipients that have been associated with skin sensitisation.

Skin dryness and the consequent irritant eczema requires **emollients** applied regularly (at least twice daily) and liberally to the affected area; this can be supplemented with bath or shower emollients. The use of emollients should continue even if the eczema improves or if other treatment is being used.

Topical corticosteroids are also required in the management of eczema; the potency of the corticosteroid should be appropriate to the severity and site of the condition, and the age of the child. Mild corticosteroids are generally used on the face and on flexures; the more potent corticosteroids are generally required for use on lichenified areas of eczema or for severe eczema on the scalp, limbs, and trunk. Treatment should be reviewed regularly, especially if a potent corticosteroid is required. In children with frequent flares (2–3 per month), a topical corticosteroid can be applied on 2 consecutive days each week to prevent further flares.

Bandages (including those containing ichthammol with zinc oxide p. 795) are sometimes applied over topical corticosteroids or emollients to treat eczema of the limbs. Dry-wrap dressings can be used to provide a physical barrier to help prevent scratching and improve retention of emollients. Wet elasticated viscose stockinette is used for 'wet-wrap' bandaging over topical corticosteroids or emollients to cool the skin and relieve itching, but there is an increased risk of infection and excessive absorption of the corticosteroid; 'wet-wrap' bandaging should be used under specialist supervision.

See *Wound management products and elasticated garments* for details of elasticated viscose stockinette tubular bandages and garments, and silk clothing.

See Eczema and psoriasis, drugs affecting the immune response p. 783 for the role of topical pimecrolimus p. 797 and tacrolimus p. 798 in atopic eczema.

Infection

Bacterial infection (commonly with *Staphylococcus aureus* and occasionally with *Streptococcus pyogenes*) can exacerbate eczema. A topical antibacterial may be used for small areas of mild infection; treatment should be limited to a short course (typically 1 week) to reduce the risk of drug resistance or skin sensitisation. Associated eczema is treated simultaneously with a topical corticosteroid which can be combined with a topical antimicrobial.

Eczema involving moderate to severe, widespread, or recurrent infection requires the use of a systemic antibacterial that is active against the infecting organism. Preparations that combine an antiseptic with an emollient application and with a bath emollient can also be used; antiseptic shampoos can be used on the scalp.

Intertriginous eczema commonly involves candida and bacteria; it is best treated with a mild or moderately potent topical corticosteroid combined with a suitable antimicrobial drug.

Widespread *herpes simplex infection* may complicate atopic eczema (eczema herpeticum) and treatment under specialist supervision with a systemic antiviral drug is indicated. Secondary bacterial infection often exacerbates eczema herpeticum.

Management of other features of eczema

Lichenification, which results from repeated scratching, is treated initially with a potent corticosteroid. Bandages containing ichthammol p. 795 (to reduce pruritus) and other substances such as **zinc oxide** can be applied over the corticosteroid or emollient. **Coal tar** and ichthammol can be useful in some cases of *chronic eczema*. *Discoid eczema*, with thickened plaques in chronic atopic eczema, is usually treated with a topical antiseptic preparation, a potent topical corticosteroid, and paste bandages containing ichthammol with zinc oxide.

A *non-sedating* antihistamine may be of some value in relieving severe itching or urticaria associated with eczema. A *sedating* antihistamine can be used at night if itching causes sleep disturbance, but a large dose may be needed and drowsiness may persist on the following day.

Exudative ('weeping') eczema requires a potent corticosteroid initially; infection may also be present and require specific treatment. Potassium permanganate solution (1 in 10,000) p. 812 can be used as a soak in exudating eczema for its antiseptic and astringent effects; treatment should be stopped when exudation stops.

Severe refractory eczema is best managed under specialist supervision; it may require phototherapy or drugs that act on the immune system.

Seborrhoeic dermatitis

Seborrhoeic dermatitis (seborrhoeic eczema) is associated with species of the yeast *Malassezia*. *Infantile seborrhoeic dermatitis* affects particularly the body folds, nappy area and scalp; it is treated with emollients and mild topical corticosteroids with suitable antimicrobials. Infantile seborrhoeic dermatitis affecting the scalp (*cradle cap*) is treated by hydrating the scalp using natural oils and the use of mild shampoo.

In older children, seborrhoeic dermatitis affects the scalp, paranasal areas, and eyebrows. Shampoos active against the yeast (including those containing ketoconazole p. 777 and coal tar) and combinations of mild topical corticosteroids with suitable antimicrobials are used to treat older children.

Medicated bandages

Zinc paste bandages (see *Wound management products and elasticated garments*) are used with **coal tar** or ichthammol in chronic lichenified skin conditions such as chronic eczema (ichthammol often being preferred since its action is considered to be milder). They are also used with calamine in milder eczematous skin conditions.

Psoriasis

Management

Psoriasis is characterised by epidermal thickening and scaling. It commonly affects extensor surfaces and the scalp. For mild psoriasis, reassurance and treatment with an emollient may be all that is necessary. *Guttate psoriasis* is a distinctive form of psoriasis that characteristically occurs in children and young adults, often following a streptococcal throat infection or tonsillitis.

Occasionally psoriasis is provoked or exacerbated by drugs such as lithium, chloroquine and hydroxychloroquine, beta-blockers, non-steroidal anti-inflammatory drugs, and ACE inhibitors. Psoriasis may not occur until the drug has been taken for weeks or months.

Emollients, in addition to their effects on dryness, scaling and cracking, may have an antiproliferative effect in psoriasis. They are particularly useful in *inflammatory psoriasis* and in *chronic stable plaque psoriasis*.

For *chronic stable plaque psoriasis* on extensor surfaces of trunk and limbs preparations containing **coal tar** are moderately effective, but the smell is unacceptable to some children. **Vitamin D** and its analogues are effective and cosmetically acceptable alternatives to preparations containing coal tar or dithranol p. 795. Dithranol is an effective topical antipsoriatic agent but it irritates and stains the skin and it should be used only under specialist supervision. Adverse effects of dithranol are minimised by using a 'short-contact technique' and by starting with low concentration preparations. Tazarotene, a topical retinoid for the treatment of mild to moderate plaque psoriasis, is not recommended for use in children under 18 years. These medications can irritate the skin particularly in the flexures and they are not suitable for the more inflammatory forms of psoriasis; their use should be suspended during an inflammatory phase of psoriasis. The efficacy and the irritancy of each substance varies between patients. If a substance irritates significantly, it should be stopped or the concentration reduced; if it is tolerated, its effects should be assessed after 4 to 6 weeks and treatment continued if it is effective.

Widespread *unstable psoriasis* of erythrodermic or generalised pustular type requires urgent specialist assessment. Initial topical treatment should be limited to using emollients frequently and generously. More localised acute or subacute *inflammatory psoriasis* with hot, spreading or itchy lesions, should be treated topically with emollients or with a corticosteroid of moderate potency.

Scalp psoriasis is usually scaly, and the scale may be thick and adherent. This requires softening with an emollient ointment, cream, or oil and usually combined with salicylic acid p. 820 as a keratolytic.

Some preparations for psoriasis affecting the scalp combine salicylic acid with coal tar or **sulfur**. The preparation should be applied generously and left on for at least an hour, often more conveniently overnight, before washing it off. If a corticosteroid lotion or gel is required (e.g. for itch), it can be used in the morning.

Flexural psoriasis can be managed with short-term use of a mild potency topical corticosteroid. Calcitriol p. 802 or tacalcitol p. 802 can be used in the longer term; calcipotriol p. 802 is more likely to cause irritation in flexures and should be avoided. Low-strength tar preparations can also be used.

Facial psoriasis can be treated with short-term use of a mild topical corticosteroid; if this is ineffective, calcitriol, tacalcitol, or a low-strength tar preparation can be used.

Calcipotriol and tacalcitol are analogues of vitamin D that affect cell division and differentiation. Calcitriol is an active form of vitamin D. Vitamin D and its analogues are used as first-line treatment for plaque psoriasis; they do not smell or stain and they may be more acceptable than tar or dithranol products. Of the vitamin D analogues, tacalcitol and calcitriol are less likely to irritate.

Coal tar p. 796 has anti-inflammatory properties that are useful in chronic plaque psoriasis; it also has antiscaling properties. Contact of coal tar products with normal skin is not normally harmful and preparations containing coal tar can be used for widespread small lesions; however, irritation, contact allergy, and sterile folliculitis can occur. Leave-on preparations that remain in contact with the skin, such as creams or ointments, containing up to 6% coal tar may be used on children 1 month to 2 years; leave-on preparations containing coal tar 10% may be used on children over 2 years with more severe psoriasis. Tar baths and tar shampoos may also be helpful.

Dithranol is effective for chronic plaque psoriasis. Its major disadvantages are irritation (for which individual susceptibility varies) and staining of skin and of clothing. Dithranol is not generally suitable for widespread small lesions nor should it be used in the flexures or on the face. Proprietary preparations are more suitable for home use; they are usually washed off after 20–30 minutes ('short contact' technique). Specialist nurses may apply intensive treatment with dithranol paste which is covered by stockinette dressings and usually retained overnight. Dithranol should be discontinued if even a low concentration causes acute inflammation; continued use can result in the psoriasis becoming unstable.

A topical **corticosteroid** is not generally suitable for long-term use or as the sole treatment of extensive chronic plaque psoriasis; any early improvement is not usually maintained and there is a risk of the condition deteriorating or of precipitating an unstable form of psoriasis e.g. erythrodermic psoriasis or generalised pustular psoriasis on withdrawal. Topical use of potent corticosteroids on widespread psoriasis can also lead to systemic as well as local side-effects. However, topical corticosteroids used short-term may be appropriate to treat psoriasis in specific sites such as the face or flexures with a mild corticosteroid, and psoriasis of the scalp, palms, and soles with a potent corticosteroid. Very potent topical corticosteroids should only be used under specialist supervision.

Combining the use of a corticosteroid with another specific topical treatment may be beneficial in chronic plaque psoriasis; the drugs may be used separately at different times of the day or used together in a single formulation. *Eczema* co-existing with psoriasis may be treated with a corticosteroid, or coal tar, or both.

Phototherapy

Phototherapy is available in specialist centres under the supervision of a dermatologist. Narrow band ultraviolet B (UVB) radiation is usually effective for *chronic stable psoriasis* and for *guttate psoriasis*. It can be considered for children with moderately severe psoriasis in whom topical treatment has failed, but it may irritate inflammatory psoriasis. The use of phototherapy and photochemotherapy in children is limited by concerns over carcinogenicity and premature ageing.

Photochemotherapy combining long-wave ultraviolet A radiation with a psoralen (PUVA) is available in specialist centres under the supervision of a dermatologist. The psoralen, which enhances the effect of irradiation, is administered either by mouth or topically. PUVA is effective in most forms of psoriasis, including the *localised palmoplantar pustular psoriasis*. Early adverse effects include phototoxicity and pruritus. Higher cumulative doses exaggerate skin ageing, increase the risk of dysplastic and neoplastic skin lesions especially squamous cancer, and pose a theoretical risk of cataracts.

Phototherapy combined with coal tar, dithranol, topical vitamin D or vitamin D analogues, or oral acitretin, allows reduction of the cumulative dose of phototherapy required to treat psoriasis.

Systemic treatment

Systemic treatment is required for severe, resistant, unstable or complicated forms of psoriasis, and it should be initiated only under specialist supervision. Systemic drugs for psoriasis include acitretin and drugs that affect the immune response (see Eczema and psoriasis, drugs affecting the immune response below).

Acitretin p. 800, a metabolite of etretinate, is a retinoid (vitamin A derivative); it is prescribed by specialists. The main indication of acitretin is severe psoriasis resistant to other forms of therapy. It is also used in disorders of keratinisation such as severe *Darier's disease* (keratosis follicularis), and some forms of *ichthyosis*. Although a minority of cases of psoriasis respond well to acitretin alone, it is only moderately effective in many cases; adverse effects are a limiting factor. A therapeutic effect occurs after 2 to 4 weeks and the maximum benefit after 4 months. Consideration should be given to stopping acitretin if the response is inadequate after 4 months at the optimum dose. Continuous treatment for longer than 6 months is not usually necessary in psoriasis. However, some patients, particularly those with severe ichthyosis, may benefit from longer treatment, provided that the lowest effective dose is used, patients are monitored carefully for adverse effects, and the need for treatment is reviewed regularly. Topical preparations containing keratolytics should normally be stopped before administration of acitretin. Liberal use of emollients should be encouraged and topical corticosteroids can be continued if necessary.

Acitretin is teratogenic; in females of child-bearing age, the possibility of pregnancy must be excluded before treatment and effective contraception must be used during treatment and for at least 3 years afterwards (oral progestogen-only contraceptives not considered effective).

Topical treatment

The vitamin D and analogues, calcipotriol p. 802, calcitriol p. 802, and tacalcitol p. 802 are used for the management of plaque psoriasis. They should be avoided by those with calcium metabolism disorders, and used with caution in generalised pustular or erythrodermic exfoliative psoriasis (enhanced risk of hypercalcaemia).

Eczema and psoriasis, drugs affecting the immune response

Overview

Drugs affecting the immune response are used for eczema or psoriasis. Pimecrolimus p. 797 by topical application is licensed for *mild to moderate atopic eczema*. Tacrolimus p. 798 is licensed for topical use in *moderate to severe atopic eczema*. Both are drugs whose long-term safety is still being evaluated and they should not usually be considered first-line treatment unless there is a specific reason to avoid or reduce the use of topical corticosteroids. Treatment with topical pimecrolimus or topical tacrolimus should be initiated only by prescribers experienced in treating atopic eczema.

Topical corticosteroids have a role in eczema and a limited role in psoriasis. A systemic corticosteroid such as prednisolone p. 478 may be used in severe refractory eczema.

Systemic drugs acting on the immune system are generally used by **specialists** in a hospital setting.

Ciclosporin p. 559 by mouth can be used for *severe psoriasis* and for *severe eczema*. Azathioprine p. 558 or mycophenolate mofetil p. 566 are also used for severe refractory eczema in children.

Methotrexate p. 588 can be used for *severe resistant* psoriasis; the dose is given **once weekly** and adjusted according to severity of the condition and haematological and biochemical measurements. Folic acid p. 620 should be given to reduce the possibility of methotrexate toxicity [unlicensed indication]. Folic acid can be given once weekly on a different day to the methotrexate; alternative regimens may be used in some settings.

Etanercept p. 696 (a cytokine modulator) is licensed in children over 6 years of age for the treatment of *severe plaque psoriasis* that is inadequately controlled by other systemic treatments and photochemotherapy, or when these other treatments cannot be used because of intolerance or contra-indications.

Adalimumab p. 693 (a cytokine modulator) is licensed in children over 4 years for the treatment of *severe chronic plaque psoriasis* that is inadequately controlled by other topical treatments and phototherapies, or when these treatments are inappropriate.

CORTICOSTEROIDS

Topical corticosteroids

Overview

Topical corticosteroids are used for the treatment of inflammatory conditions of the skin (other than those arising from an infection), particularly eczema, contact dermatitis, insect stings, and eczema of scabies. Corticosteroids suppress the inflammatory reaction during use; they are not curative and on discontinuation a rebound exacerbation of the condition may occur. They are generally used to relieve symptoms and suppress signs of the disorder when other measures such as emollients are ineffective.

Children, especially infants, are particularly susceptible to side-effects. However, concern about the safety of topical corticosteroids in children should not result in the child being undertreated. The aim is to control the condition as well as possible; inadequate treatment will perpetuate the condition. Carers of young children should be advised that treatment should **not** necessarily be reserved to 'treat only the worst areas' and they may need to be advised that patient information leaflets may contain inappropriate advice for the child's condition.

In an acute flare-up of atopic eczema, it may be appropriate to use more potent formulations of topical corticosteroids for a short period to regain control of the condition.

Topical corticosteroids are not recommended in the routine treatment of urticaria; treatment should only be initiated and supervised by a specialist. Topical corticosteroids may worsen ulcerated or secondarily infected lesions. They should not be used indiscriminately in pruritus (where they will only benefit if inflammation is causing the itch) and are **not** recommended for acne vulgaris.

Systemic or very potent topical corticosteroids should be avoided or given only under specialist supervision in psoriasis because, although they may suppress the psoriasis in the short term, relapse or vigorous rebound occurs on withdrawal (sometimes precipitating severe pustular psoriasis). Topical use of potent corticosteroids on widespread psoriasis can lead to systemic as well as to local side-effects. It is reasonable, however, to prescribe a mild topical corticosteroid for a short period (2–4 weeks) for *flexural* and *facial psoriasis*, and to use a more potent corticosteroid such as betamethasone p. 786 or fluocinonide p. 789 for *psoriasis* of the *scalp, palms*, or *soles*.

In general, the most potent topical corticosteroids should be reserved for recalcitrant dermatoses such as *chronic discoid lupus erythematosus, lichen simplex chronicus, hypertrophic lichen planus*, and *palmoplantar pustulosis*. Potent corticosteroids should generally be avoided on the face and skin flexures, but specialists occasionally prescribe them for use on these areas in certain circumstances.

When topical treatment has failed, intralesional corticosteroid injections may be used. These are more effective than the very potent topical corticosteroid preparations and should be reserved for severe cases where there are localised lesions such as *keloid scars, hypertrophic lichen planus*, or *localised alopecia areata*.

Perioral lesions

Hydrocortisone 1% cream p. 790 can be used for up to 7 days to treat uninfected inflammatory lesions on the lips. Hydrocortisone with miconazole cream or ointment p. 795 is useful where infection by susceptible organisms and inflammation co-exist, particularly for initial treatment (up to 7 days) e.g. in angular cheilitis. Organisms susceptible to miconazole include *Candida* spp. and many Gram-positive bacteria including streptococci and staphylococci.

Choice

Water-miscible corticosteroid creams are suitable for moist or weeping lesions whereas ointments are generally chosen for dry, lichenified or scaly lesions or where a more occlusive effect is required. Lotions may be useful when minimal application to a large or hair-bearing area is required or for the treatment of exudative lesions. *Occlusive polythene* or *hydrocolloid dressings* increase absorption, but also increase the risk of side-effects; they are therefore used only under supervision on a short-term basis for areas of very thick skin (such as the palms and soles). Disposable nappies and tight fitting pants also increase the risk of side-effects by increasing absorption of the corticosteroid. The inclusion of urea or salicylic acid p. 820 also increases the penetration of the corticosteroid.

In the *BNF for Children*, topical corticosteroids for the skin are categorised as 'mild', 'moderately potent', 'potent' or 'very potent'; the least potent preparation which is effective should be chosen but dilution should be avoided whenever possible.

Topical hydrocortisone is usually used in children under 1 year of age. Moderately potent and potent topical corticosteroids should be used with great care in children and for short periods (1–2 weeks) only. A very potent corticosteroid should be initiated under the supervision of a specialist.

Appropriate topical corticosteroids for specific conditions are:

- *insect bites and stings*—mild corticosteroid such as hydrocortisone 1% cream;
- *inflamed nappy rash causing discomfort* in infant over 1 month—mild corticosteroid such as hydrocortisone 0.5% or 1% for up to 7 days (combined with antimicrobial if infected);
- *mild to moderate eczema, flexural and facial eczema or psoriasis*—mild corticosteroid such as hydrocortisone 1%;
- *severe eczema of the face and neck*—moderately potent corticosteroid for 3–5 days only, if not controlled by a mild corticosteroid;
- *severe eczema on the trunk and limbs*—moderately potent or potent corticosteroid for 1–2 weeks only, switching to a less potent preparation as the condition improves;
- *eczema affecting area with thickened skin (e.g. soles of feet)*—potent topical corticosteroid in combination with urea or salicylic acid (to increase penetration of corticosteroid).

Absorption through the skin

Mild and *moderately potent* topical corticosteroids are associated with few side-effects but particular care is required when treating neonates and infants, and in the use of *potent* and *very potent* corticosteroids. Absorption through the skin can rarely cause adrenal suppression and even Cushing's syndrome, depending on the area of the body being treated and the duration of treatment. Absorption of corticosteroid is greatest from severely inflamed skin, thin skin (especially on the face or genital area), from flexural sites (e.g. axillae, groin), and in infants where skin surface area is higher in relation to body-weight; absorption is increased by occlusion.

Compound preparations

The advantages of including other substances (such as antibacterials or antifungals) with corticosteroids in topical preparations are uncertain, but such combinations may have a place where inflammatory skin conditions are associated with bacterial or fungal infection, such as infected eczema. In these cases the antimicrobial drug should be chosen according to the sensitivity of the infecting organism and used regularly for a short period (typically twice daily for 1 week). Longer use increases the likelihood of resistance and of sensitisation.

The keratolytic effect of salicylic acid p. 820 facilitates the absorption of topical corticosteroids; however, excessive and prolonged use of topical preparations containing salicylic acid may cause salicylism.

Topical corticosteroid preparation potencies

Potency of a topical corticosteroid preparation is a result of the formulation as well as the corticosteroid. Therefore, proprietary names are shown.

Mild
- Hydrocortisone 0.1–2.5%
- Dioderm
- Mildison
- Synalar 1 in 10 dilution

Mild with antimicrobials
- Canesten HC
- Daktacort
- Econacort
- Fucidin H
- Hydrocortisone with chlorhexidine hydrochloride and nystatin
- Terra-Cortril
- Timodine

Moderate
- Betnovate-RD
- Eumovate
- Haelan
- Modrasone
- Synalar 1 in 4 Dilution
- Ultralanum Plain

Moderate with antimicrobials
- Trimovate

Moderate with urea:
- Alphaderm

Potent
- Beclometasone dipropionate 0.025%
- Betamethasone valerate 0.1%
- Betacap
- Betesil
- Bettamousse
- Betnovate
- Cutivate
- Diprosone
- Elocon
- Hydrocortisone butyrate
- Locoid
- Locoid Crelo
- Metosyn
- Mometasone furoate 0.1%
- Nerisone
- Synalar

Potent with antimicrobials
- Aureocort
- Betamethasone and clioquinol
- Betamethasone and neomycin
- Fucibet
- Lotriderm
- Synalar C
- Synalar N

Potent with salicylic acid
- Diprosalic

Very potent
- Dermovate
- Nerisone Forte

Very potent with antimicrobials
- Clobetasol propionate 0.05% with neomycin and nystatin

Corticosteroids (topical) 

IMPORTANT SAFETY INFORMATION

MHRA/CHM ADVICE: CORTICOSTEROIDS: RARE RISK OF CENTRAL SEROUS CHORIORETINOPATHY WITH LOCAL AS WELL AS SYSTEMIC ADMINISTRATION (AUGUST 2017)

Central serous chorioretinopathy is a retinal disorder that has been linked to the systemic use of corticosteroids. Recently, it has also been reported after local administration of corticosteroids via inhaled and intranasal, epidural, intra-articular, topical dermal, and periocular routes. The MHRA recommends that patients should be advised to report any blurred vision or other visual disturbances with corticosteroid treatment given by any route; consider referral to an ophthalmologist for evaluation of possible causes if a patient presents with vision problems.

- **CONTRA-INDICATIONS** Acne · perioral dermatitis · potent corticosteroids in widespread plaque psoriasis · rosacea · untreated bacterial, fungal or viral skin lesions
- **CAUTIONS** Avoid prolonged use (particularly on the face) · cautions applicable to systemic corticosteroids may also apply if absorption occurs following topical and local use · dermatoses of infancy, including nappy rash (extreme caution required—treatment should be limited to 5–7 days) · infection · keep away from eyes · use potent or very potent topical corticosteroids under specialist supervision
- **SIDE-EFFECTS**
  - **Common or very common** Skin reactions · telangiectasia
  - **Rare or very rare** Adrenal suppression · hypertrichosis · skin depigmentation (may be reversible)
  - **Frequency not known** Local reaction · vasodilation

  SIDE-EFFECTS, FURTHER INFORMATION Side-effects applicable to systemic corticosteroids may also apply if absorption occurs following topical and local use. In order to minimise the side-effects of a topical corticosteroid, it is important to apply it thinly to affected areas only, no more frequently than twice daily, and to use the least potent formulation which is fully effective.
- **DIRECTIONS FOR ADMINISTRATION** Topical corticosteroid preparations should be applied no more frequently than twice daily; once daily is often sufficient. Topical corticosteroids should be spread thinly on the skin but in sufficient quantity to cover the affected areas. The length of cream or ointment expelled from a tube may be used to

specify the quantity to be applied to a given area of skin. This length can be measured in terms of a *fingertip unit* (the distance from the tip of the adult index finger to the first crease). One fingertip unit (approximately 500 mg from a tube with a standard 5 mm diameter nozzle) is sufficient to cover an area that is twice that of the flat adult handprint (palm and fingers). Mixing topical preparations on the skin should be avoided where possible; several minutes should elapse between application of different preparations.

'Wet-wrap bandaging' increases absorption into the skin, but should be initiated only by a dermatologist and application supervised by a healthcare professional trained in the technique.

- **PRESCRIBING AND DISPENSING INFORMATION** The potency of each topical corticosteroid should be included on the label with the directions for use. The label should be attached to the container (for example, the tube) rather than the outer packaging.
- **PATIENT AND CARER ADVICE** Patients or carers should be given advice on how to administer corticosteroid creams and ointments. If a patient is using topical corticosteroids of different potencies, the patient should be told when to use each corticosteroid. Patients and their carers should be reassured that side effects such as skin thinning and systemic effects rarely occur when topical corticosteroids are used appropriately.

785

Alclometasone dipropionate

21-Dec-2017

- **INDICATIONS AND DOSE**

Inflammatory skin disorders such as eczemas

▶ TO THE SKIN
▸ Child: Apply 1–2 times a day, to be applied thinly

POTENCY
▸ Alclometasone dipropionate cream 0.05%: moderate

- **UNLICENSED USE** Licensed for use in children (age range not specified by manufacturer).
- **PATIENT AND CARER ADVICE** Patients or carers should be counselled on the application of alclometasone dipropionate cream.
- **MEDICINAL FORMS** There can be variation in the licensing of different medicines containing the same drug.

Cream

CAUTIONARY AND ADVISORY LABELS 28
EXCIPIENTS: May contain Cetostearyl alcohol (including cetyl and stearyl alcohol), chlorocresol, propylene glycol

▸ Alclometasone dipropionate (Non-proprietary)
Alclometasone dipropionate 500 microgram per 1 gram Boots Derma Care Eczema & Dermatitis Flare-Up 0.05% cream | 15 gram P ☒

785

Beclometasone dipropionate

15-May-2020

(Beclomethasone dipropionate)

- **INDICATIONS AND DOSE**

Severe inflammatory skin disorders such as eczemas unresponsive to less potent corticosteroids | Psoriasis

▶ TO THE SKIN
▸ Child: Apply 1–2 times a day, to be applied thinly

POTENCY
▸ Beclometasone dipropionate cream and ointment 0.025%: potent.

- **UNLICENSED USE** Not licensed for use in children under 1 year.
- **INTERACTIONS** → Appendix 1: corticosteroids
- **SIDE-EFFECTS** Vision blurred
- **MEDICINAL FORMS** There can be variation in the licensing of different medicines containing the same drug. Forms available from special-order manufacturers include: cream, ointment

Cream

CAUTIONARY AND ADVISORY LABELS 28

▸ Beclometasone dipropionate (Non-proprietary)
Beclometasone dipropionate 250 microgram per 1 gram Beclometasone 0.025% cream | 30 gram PoM £68.00 DT = £68.00

Ointment

CAUTIONARY AND ADVISORY LABELS 28

▸ Beclometasone dipropionate (Non-proprietary)
Beclometasone dipropionate 250 microgram per 1 gram Beclometasone 0.025% ointment | 30 gram PoM £68.00 DT = £68.00

785

Betamethasone

28-Nov-2019

- **DRUG ACTION** Betamethasone has very high glucocorticoid activity and insignificant mineralocorticoid activity.
- **INDICATIONS AND DOSE**

Severe inflammatory skin disorders such as eczemas unresponsive to less potent corticosteroids | Psoriasis

▶ TO THE SKIN
▸ Child: Apply 1–2 times a day, to be applied thinly

POTENCY
▸ Betamethasone valerate 0.025% cream and ointment: moderate. Betamethasone valerate 0.1% cream, lotion, ointment, and scalp application: potent. Betamethasone valerate 0.12% foam: potent. Betamethasone dipropionate 0.05% cream, lotion, and ointment: potent.

- **UNLICENSED USE** *Betacap*®, *Betnovate*® and *Betnovate-RD*® are not licensed for use in children under 1 year. *Bettamousse*® is not licensed for use in children under 6 years.
- **CAUTIONS** Use of more than 100 g per week of 0.1% preparation likely to cause adrenal suppression
- **INTERACTIONS** → Appendix 1: corticosteroids
- **PATIENT AND CARER ADVICE** Patient counselling is advised for betamethasone cream, ointment, scalp application and foam (application).
- **MEDICINAL FORMS** There can be variation in the licensing of different medicines containing the same drug. Forms available from special-order manufacturers include: cream, ointment

Foam

CAUTIONARY AND ADVISORY LABELS 15, 28
EXCIPIENTS: May contain Cetostearyl alcohol (including cetyl and stearyl alcohol), polysorbates, propylene glycol

▸ Bettamousse (RPH Pharmaceuticals AB)
Betamethasone (as Betamethasone valerate) 1 mg per 1 gram Bettamousse 0.1% cutaneous foam | 100 gram PoM £9.75 DT = £9.75

Cream

CAUTIONARY AND ADVISORY LABELS 28
EXCIPIENTS: May contain Cetostearyl alcohol (including cetyl and stearyl alcohol), chlorocresol

▸ Betamethasone (Non-proprietary)
Betamethasone (as Betamethasone valerate) 1 mg per 1 gram Betamethasone valerate 0.1% cream | 15 gram PoM £3.00 | 30 gram PoM £3.01 DT = £2.30 | 100 gram PoM £7.64 DT = £7.64

▸ Audavate (Accord Healthcare Ltd)
Betamethasone (as Betamethasone valerate) 250 microgram per 1 gram Audavate RD 0.025% cream | 100 gram PoM £2.99 DT = £3.15

Betamethasone (as Betamethasone valerate) 1 mg per 1 gram Audavate 0.1% cream | 30 gram PoM £1.14 DT = £2.30 | 100 gram PoM £3.24 DT = £7.64

▸ Betnovate (GlaxoSmithKline UK Ltd)
Betamethasone (as Betamethasone valerate) 250 microgram per 1 gram Betnovate RD 0.025% cream | 100 gram PoM £3.15 DT = £3.15

Betamethasone (as Betamethasone valerate) 1 mg per 1 gram Betnovate 0.1% cream | 30 gram PoM £1.43 DT = £2.30 | 100 gram PoM £4.05 DT = £7.64

▸ Diprosone (Merck Sharp & Dohme Ltd)
Betamethasone (as Betamethasone dipropionate) 500 microgram per 1 gram Diprosone 0.05% cream | 30 gram PoM £2.16 DT = £2.16 | 100 gram PoM £6.12 DT = £6.12

Ointment

CAUTIONARY AND ADVISORY LABELS 28

▸ Betamethasone (Non-proprietary)
Betamethasone (as Betamethasone valerate) 1 mg per 1 gram Betamethasone valerate 0.1% ointment | 30 gram PoM £1.97 DT = £1.97 | 100 gram PoM £6.57 DT = £6.57

▸ Audavate (Accord Healthcare Ltd, Auden McKenzie (Pharma Division) Ltd)
Betamethasone (as Betamethasone valerate) 250 microgram per 1 gram Audavate RD 0.025% ointment | 100 gram PoM £2.99 DT = £3.15
Betamethasone (as Betamethasone valerate) 1 mg per 1 gram Audavate 0.1% ointment | 30 gram PoM £1.36 DT = £1.97 | 100 gram PoM £3.85 DT = £6.57

▸ Betnovate (GlaxoSmithKline UK Ltd)
Betamethasone (as Betamethasone valerate) 250 microgram per 1 gram Betnovate RD 0.025% ointment | 100 gram PoM £3.15 DT = £3.15
Betamethasone (as Betamethasone valerate) 1 mg per 1 gram Betnovate 0.1% ointment | 30 gram PoM £1.43 DT = £1.97 | 100 gram PoM £4.05 DT = £6.57

▸ Diprosone (Merck Sharp & Dohme Ltd)
Betamethasone (as Betamethasone dipropionate) 500 microgram per 1 gram Diprosone 0.05% ointment | 30 gram PoM £2.16 DT = £2.16 | 100 gram PoM £6.12 DT = £6.12

Liquid

CAUTIONARY AND ADVISORY LABELS 15(scalp lotion only), 28
EXCIPIENTS: May contain Cetostearyl alcohol (including cetyl and stearyl alcohol), hydroxybenzoates (parabens)

▸ Betacap (Dermal Laboratories Ltd)
Betamethasone (as Betamethasone valerate) 1 mg per 1 gram Betacap 0.1% scalp application | 100 ml PoM £3.75 DT = £3.75

▸ Betnovate (GlaxoSmithKline UK Ltd)
Betamethasone (as Betamethasone valerate) 1 mg per 1 gram Betnovate 0.1% scalp application | 100 ml PoM £4.99 DT = £3.75
Betnovate 0.1% lotion | 100 ml PoM £4.58 DT = £4.58

▸ Diprosone (Merck Sharp & Dohme Ltd)
Betamethasone (as Betamethasone dipropionate) 500 microgram per 1 ml Diprosone 0.05% lotion | 100 ml PoM £7.80 DT = £7.80

Combinations available: ***Betamethasone with clioquinol,*** p. 791 · ***Betamethasone with clotrimazole,*** p. 791 · ***Betamethasone with fusidic acid,*** p. 792 · ***Betamethasone with neomycin,*** p. 792 · ***Betamethasone with salicylic acid,*** p. 792

Calcipotriol with betamethasone

30-May-2017

The properties listed below are those particular to the combination only. For the properties of the components please consider, calcipotriol p. 802, betamethasone p. 786.

● **INDICATIONS AND DOSE**

DOVOBET ® GEL

Scalp psoriasis

▶ TO THE SKIN
▸ Child 12–17 years (specialist use only): Apply 1–4 g once daily usual duration of therapy 4 weeks; if necessary, treatment may be continued beyond 4 weeks or repeated, on the advice of a specialist, shampoo off after leaving on scalp overnight or during day, when different preparations containing calcipotriol used together, maximum total calcipiotriol 3.75 mg in any one week

Mild to moderate plaque psoriasis

▶ TO THE SKIN
▸ Child 12–17 years (specialist use only): Apply once daily usual duration for up to 4 weeks; if necessary treatment should be continued beyond 4 weeks, or repeated, only on the advice of a specialist, apply to maximum 30% of body surface, when different preparations containing calcipotriol used together, max. total calcipotriol 3.75 mg in any one week; maximum 75 g per week

DOVOBET ® OINTMENT

Stable plaque psoriasis

▶ TO THE SKIN
▸ Child 12–17 years (specialist use only): Apply once daily for up to 4 weeks; if necessary, treatment may be continued beyond 4 weeks or repeated, on the advice of a specialist, apply to a maximum 30% of body surface, when different preparations containing calcipotriol used together, max. total calcipotriol 3.75 mg in any one week; maximum 75 g per week

● **UNLICENSED USE** *Dovobet*® not licensed for use in children.

● **CONTRA-INDICATIONS** Erythrodermic psoriasis · pustular psoriasis

● **INTERACTIONS** → Appendix 1: corticosteroids · vitamin D substances

● **MEDICINAL FORMS** There can be variation in the licensing of different medicines containing the same drug.

Ointment

CAUTIONARY AND ADVISORY LABELS 28
EXCIPIENTS: May contain Butylated hydroxytoluene

▸ Dovobet (LEO Pharma)
Calcipotriol (as Calcipotriol hydrate) 50 microgram per 1 gram, Betamethasone (as Betamethasone dipropionate) 500 microgram per 1 gram Dovobet ointment | 30 gram PoM £19.84 DT = £19.84 | 60 gram PoM £39.68 | 120 gram PoM £73.86

Gel

CAUTIONARY AND ADVISORY LABELS 28
EXCIPIENTS: May contain Butylated hydroxytoluene

▸ Dovobet (LEO Pharma)
Calcipotriol (as Calcipotriol monohydrate) 50 microgram per 1 gram, Betamethasone (as Betamethasone dipropionate) 500 microgram per 1 gram Dovobet gel | 60 gram PoM £37.21 DT = £37.21 | 120 gram PoM £69.11

F 785

Clobetasol propionate

21-Dec-2017

● **INDICATIONS AND DOSE**

Short-term treatment only of severe resistant inflammatory skin disorders such as recalcitrant eczemas unresponsive to less potent corticosteroids | Psoriasis

▶ TO THE SKIN
▸ Child 1–17 years: Apply 1–2 times a day for up to 4 weeks, to be applied thinly

POTENCY
▸ Clobetasol propionate 0.05% cream, foam, ointment, scalp application, and shampoo: very potent.

● **UNLICENSED USE** *Dermovate*® not licensed for use in children under 1 year.

● **PATIENT AND CARER ADVICE** Patients or carers should be given advice on how to administer clobetasol propionate foam, liquid (scalp application), cream, ointment and shampoo.
Scalp application Patients or carers should be advised to apply foam directly to scalp lesions (foam begins to subside immediately on contact with skin).

● **MEDICINAL FORMS** There can be variation in the licensing of different medicines containing the same drug. Forms available from special-order manufacturers include: cream, ointment, paste

Cream

CAUTIONARY AND ADVISORY LABELS 28

EXCIPIENTS: May contain Beeswax, cetostearyl alcohol (including cetyl and stearyl alcohol), chlorocresol, propylene glycol

▸ ClobaDerm (Accord Healthcare Ltd)
Clobetasol propionate 500 microgram per 1 gram ClobaDerm 0.05% cream | 30 gram PoM £2.56 DT = £2.69 | 100 gram PoM £7.51 DT = £7.90

▸ Dermovate (GlaxoSmithKline UK Ltd)
Clobetasol propionate 500 microgram per 1 gram Dermovate 0.05% cream | 30 gram PoM £2.69 DT = £2.69 | 100 gram PoM £7.90 DT = £7.90

Ointment

CAUTIONARY AND ADVISORY LABELS 28

EXCIPIENTS: May contain Propylene glycol

▸ ClobaDerm (Accord Healthcare Ltd)
Clobetasol propionate 500 microgram per 1 gram ClobaDerm 0.05% ointment | 30 gram PoM £2.56 DT = £2.69 | 100 gram PoM £7.51 DT = £7.90

▸ Dermovate (GlaxoSmithKline UK Ltd)
Clobetasol propionate 500 microgram per 1 gram Dermovate 0.05% ointment | 30 gram PoM £2.69 DT = £2.69 | 100 gram PoM £7.90 DT = £7.90

Liquid

CAUTIONARY AND ADVISORY LABELS 15, 28

▸ Dermovate (GlaxoSmithKline UK Ltd)
Clobetasol propionate 500 microgram per 1 gram Dermovate 0.05% scalp application | 30 ml PoM £3.07 DT = £3.07 | 100 ml PoM £10.42 DT = £10.42

Combinations available: ***Clobetasol propionate with neomycin sulfate and nystatin,*** p. 793

785

Clobetasone butyrate

21-Dec-2017

● **INDICATIONS AND DOSE**

Eczemas and dermatitis of all types | Maintenance between courses of more potent corticosteroids

▸ TO THE SKIN

▸ Child: Apply 1–2 times a day, to be applied thinly

POTENCY

▸ Clobetasone butyrate 0.05% cream and ointment: moderate.

● **UNLICENSED USE** Licensed for use in children (age range not specified by manufacturer).

● **PATIENT AND CARER ADVICE** Patients or carers should be advised on the application of clobetasone butyrate containing preparations.

● **EXCEPTIONS TO LEGAL CATEGORY** Cream can be sold to the public for short-term symptomatic treatment and control of patches of eczema and dermatitis (but not seborrhoeic dermatitis) in adults and children over 12 years provided pack does not contain more than 15 g.

● **MEDICINAL FORMS** There can be variation in the licensing of different medicines containing the same drug. Forms available from special-order manufacturers include: cream, ointment

Ointment

CAUTIONARY AND ADVISORY LABELS 28

▸ Clobavate (Teva UK Ltd)
Clobetasone butyrate 500 microgram per 1 gram Clobavate 0.05% ointment | 30 gram PoM £1.49 DT = £1.86 | 100 gram PoM £4.35 DT = £5.44

▸ Eumovate (GlaxoSmithKline UK Ltd)
Clobetasone butyrate 500 microgram per 1 gram Eumovate 0.05% ointment | 30 gram PoM £1.86 DT = £1.86 | 100 gram PoM £5.44 DT = £5.44

Cream

CAUTIONARY AND ADVISORY LABELS 28

EXCIPIENTS: May contain Cetostearyl alcohol (including cetyl and stearyl alcohol), chlorocresol

▸ Eumovate (GlaxoSmithKline Consumer Healthcare, GlaxoSmithKline UK Ltd)
Clobetasone butyrate 500 microgram per 1 gram Eumovate 0.05% cream | 30 gram PoM £1.86 DT = £1.86 | 100 gram PoM £5.44 DT = £5.44

Combinations available: ***Clobetasone butyrate with nystatin and oxytetracycline,*** p. 793

785

Diflucortolone valerate

21-Dec-2017

● **INDICATIONS AND DOSE**

Severe inflammatory skin disorders such as eczemas unresponsive to less potent corticosteroids (using 0.3% diflucortolone valerate) | Short-term treatment of severe exacerbations (using 0.3% diflucortolone valerate) | Psoriasis (using 0.3% diflucortolone valerate)

▸ TO THE SKIN

▸ Child 1 month–3 years: Apply 1–2 times a day for up to 2 weeks, reducing strength as condition responds, to be applied thinly

▸ Child 4–17 years: Apply 1–2 times a day for up to 2 weeks, reducing strength as condition responds, to be applied thinly; maximum 60 g per week

Severe inflammatory skin disorders such as eczemas unresponsive to less potent corticosteroids (using 0.1% diflucortolone valerate) | Psoriasis (using 0.1% diflucortolone valerate)

▸ TO THE SKIN

▸ Child: Apply 1–2 times a day for up to 4 weeks, to be applied thinly

POTENCY

▸ Diflucortolone valerate 0.1% cream and ointment: potent.

▸ Diflucortolone valerate 0.3% cream and ointment: very potent.

● **UNLICENSED USE** *Nerisone®* licensed for use in children (age range not specified by manufacturer); *Nerisone Forte®* not licensed for use in children under 4 years.

● **PRESCRIBING AND DISPENSING INFORMATION** Patients or carers should be advised on application of diflucortolone valerate containing preparations.

● **MEDICINAL FORMS** There can be variation in the licensing of different medicines containing the same drug.

Ointment

CAUTIONARY AND ADVISORY LABELS 28

▸ Nerisone (Meadow Laboratories Ltd)
Diflucortolone valerate 1 mg per 1 gram Nerisone 0.1% ointment | 30 gram PoM £3.98 DT = £3.98
Diflucortolone valerate 3 mg per 1 gram Nerisone Forte 0.3% ointment | 15 gram PoM £4.70 DT = £4.70

Cream

CAUTIONARY AND ADVISORY LABELS 28

EXCIPIENTS: May contain Beeswax, cetostearyl alcohol (including cetyl and stearyl alcohol), disodium edetate, hydroxybenzoates (parabens)

▸ Nerisone (Meadow Laboratories Ltd)
Diflucortolone valerate 1 mg per 1 gram Nerisone 0.1% cream | 30 gram PoM £3.98 DT = £3.98
Nerisone 0.1% oily cream | 30 gram PoM £4.95 DT = £4.95
Diflucortolone valerate 3 mg per 1 gram Nerisone Forte 0.3% oily cream | 15 gram PoM £4.70 DT = £4.70

785

Fludroxycortide (Flurandrenolone)

21-Dec-2017

● **INDICATIONS AND DOSE**

Inflammatory skin disorders such as eczemas

▸ TO THE SKIN

▸ Child: Apply 1–2 times a day, to be applied thinly

POTENCY
- Fludroxycortide 0.0125% cream and ointment: moderate

HAELAN® TAPE

Chronic localised recalcitrant dermatoses (but not acute or weeping)
- TO THE SKIN
- Child: Cut tape to fit lesion, apply to clean, dry skin shorn of hair, usually for 12 hours daily

- **UNLICENSED USE** Licensed for use in children (age range not specified by manufacturer).
- **SIDE-EFFECTS** Cushing's syndrome · increased risk of infection
- **PATIENT AND CARER ADVICE** Patients or carers should be counselled on application of fludroxycortide cream and ointment.

- **MEDICINAL FORMS** There can be variation in the licensing of different medicines containing the same drug.

Ointment
CAUTIONARY AND ADVISORY LABELS 28
EXCIPIENTS: May contain Beeswax, cetostearyl alcohol (including cetyl and stearyl alcohol), polysorbates
- Fludroxycortide (Non-proprietary)
  Fludroxycortide 125 microgram per 1 gram Fludroxycortide 0.0125% ointment | 60 gram [PoM] £5.99

Cream
CAUTIONARY AND ADVISORY LABELS 28
EXCIPIENTS: May contain Cetostearyl alcohol (including cetyl and stearyl alcohol), propylene glycol
- Fludroxycortide (Non-proprietary)
  Fludroxycortide 125 microgram per 1 gram Fludroxycortide 0.0125% cream | 60 gram [PoM] £5.99 DT = £5.99

Impregnated dressing
- Fludroxycortide (Non-proprietary)
  Fludroxycortide 4 microgram per 1 square cm Fludroxycortide 4micrograms/square cm tape 7.5cm | 20 cm [PoM] £12.49–£13.67 DT = £13.67 | 50 cm [PoM] £18.75

F 785

Fluocinolone acetonide

28-Nov-2019

- **INDICATIONS AND DOSE**

Severe inflammatory skin disorders such as eczemas | Psoriasis
- TO THE SKIN
- Child 1–17 years: Apply 1–2 times a day, to be applied thinly, reduce strength as condition responds

POTENCY
- Fluocinolone acetonide 0.025% cream, gel, and ointment: potent.
- Fluocinolone acetonide 0.00625% cream and ointment: moderate.
- Fluocinolone acetonide 0.0025% cream: mild.

- **UNLICENSED USE** Not licensed for use in children under 1 year.
- **INTERACTIONS** → Appendix 1: fluocinolone
- **PRESCRIBING AND DISPENSING INFORMATION** Gel is useful for application to the scalp and other hairy areas.
- **PATIENT AND CARER ADVICE** Patient counselling is advised for fluocinolone acetonide cream, gel and ointment (application).

- **MEDICINAL FORMS** There can be variation in the licensing of different medicines containing the same drug.

Ointment
CAUTIONARY AND ADVISORY LABELS 28
EXCIPIENTS: May contain Propylene glycol, woolfat and related substances (including lanolin)
- Synalar (Reig Jofre UK Ltd)
  Fluocinolone acetonide 62.5 microgram per 1 gram Synalar 1 in 4 Dilution 0.00625% ointment | 50 gram [PoM] £4.84 DT = £4.84
  Fluocinolone acetonide 250 microgram per 1 gram Synalar 0.025% ointment | 30 gram [PoM] £4.14 DT = £4.14 | 100 gram [PoM] £11.75 DT = £11.75

Cream
CAUTIONARY AND ADVISORY LABELS 28
EXCIPIENTS: May contain Benzyl alcohol, cetostearyl alcohol (including cetyl and stearyl alcohol), polysorbates, propylene glycol
- Synalar (Reig Jofre UK Ltd)
  Fluocinolone acetonide 62.5 microgram per 1 gram Synalar 1 in 4 Dilution 0.00625% cream | 50 gram [PoM] £4.84 DT = £4.84
  Fluocinolone acetonide 250 microgram per 1 gram Synalar 0.025% cream | 30 gram [PoM] £4.14 DT = £4.14 | 100 gram [PoM] £11.75 DT = £11.75

Gel
CAUTIONARY AND ADVISORY LABELS 28
EXCIPIENTS: May contain Hydroxybenzoates (parabens), propylene glycol
- Synalar (Reig Jofre UK Ltd)
  Fluocinolone acetonide 250 microgram per 1 gram Synalar 0.025% gel | 30 gram [PoM] £5.56 DT = £5.56 | 60 gram [PoM] £10.02 DT = £10.02

Combinations available: *Fluocinolone acetonide with clioquinol*, p. 793 · ***Fluocinolone acetonide with neomycin*,** p. 793

F 785

Fluocinonide

21-Dec-2017

- **INDICATIONS AND DOSE**

Severe inflammatory skin disorders such as eczemas unresponsive to less potent corticosteroids | Psoriasis
- TO THE SKIN
- Child: Apply 1–2 times a day, to be applied thinly

POTENCY
- Fluocinonide 0.05% cream and ointment: potent.

- **UNLICENSED USE** Not licensed for use in children under 1 year.
- **PATIENT AND CARER ADVICE** Patients or carers should be advised on the application of fluocinonide preparations.

- **MEDICINAL FORMS** There can be variation in the licensing of different medicines containing the same drug. Forms available from special-order manufacturers include: ointment

Ointment
CAUTIONARY AND ADVISORY LABELS 28
EXCIPIENTS: May contain Propylene glycol, woolfat and related substances (including lanolin)
- Metosyn (Reig Jofre UK Ltd)
  Fluocinonide 500 microgram per 1 gram Metosyn 0.05% ointment | 25 gram [PoM] £3.50 DT = £3.50 | 100 gram [PoM] £13.15 DT = £13.15

Cream
CAUTIONARY AND ADVISORY LABELS 28
EXCIPIENTS: May contain Propylene glycol
- Metosyn FAPG (Reig Jofre UK Ltd)
  Fluocinonide 500 microgram per 1 gram Metosyn FAPG 0.05% cream | 25 gram [PoM] £3.96 DT = £3.96 | 100 gram [PoM] £13.34 DT = £13.34

F 785

Fluticasone

21-Dec-2017

- **INDICATIONS AND DOSE**

Severe inflammatory skin disorders such as dermatitis and eczemas unresponsive to less potent corticosteroids | Psoriasis
- TO THE SKIN
- Child 1–2 months: Apply 1–2 times a day, to be applied thinly
- Child 3 months–17 years: Apply 1–2 times a day, to be applied thinly

POTENCY
- Fluticasone cream 0.05%: potent.
- Fluticasone ointment 0.005%: potent.

- **UNLICENSED USE** Not licensed for use in children under 3 months.
- **INTERACTIONS** → Appendix 1: corticosteroids
- **PATIENT AND CARER ADVICE** Patients or carers should be given advice on application of fluticasone creams and ointments.

- **MEDICINAL FORMS** There can be variation in the licensing of different medicines containing the same drug.

Cream
CAUTIONARY AND ADVISORY LABELS 28
EXCIPIENTS: May contain Cetostearyl alcohol (including cetyl and stearyl alcohol), imidurea, propylene glycol
- ▸ Fluticasone (Non-proprietary)
  Fluticasone propionate 500 microgram per 1 gram Fluticasone 0.05% cream | 30 gram PoM £5.08 DT = £4.24
- ▸ Cutivate (GlaxoSmithKline UK Ltd)
  Fluticasone propionate 500 microgram per 1 gram Cutivate 0.05% cream | 15 gram PoM £2.27 DT = £2.27 | 30 gram PoM £4.24 DT = £4.24

Ointment
CAUTIONARY AND ADVISORY LABELS 28
EXCIPIENTS: May contain Propylene glycol
- ▸ Cutivate (GlaxoSmithKline UK Ltd)
  Fluticasone propionate 50 microgram per 1 gram Cutivate 0.005% ointment | 15 gram PoM £2.27 DT = £2.27 | 30 gram PoM £4.24 DT = £4.24

785

Hydrocortisone

17-Dec-2019

- **DRUG ACTION** Hydrocortisone has equal glucocorticoid and mineralocorticoid activity.

- **INDICATIONS AND DOSE**

Mild inflammatory skin disorders such as eczemas
▸ TO THE SKIN
▸ Child: Apply 1–2 times a day, to be applied thinly

Nappy rash
▸ TO THE SKIN
▸ Child: Apply 1–2 times a day for no longer than 1 week, discontinued as soon as the inflammation subsides

POTENCY
▸ Hydrocortisone cream and ointment 0.5 to 2.5%: mild

- **INTERACTIONS** → Appendix 1: corticosteroids
- **PRESCRIBING AND DISPENSING INFORMATION** When hydrocortisone cream or ointment is prescribed and no strength is stated, the 1% strength should be supplied. Although *Dioderm*® contains only 0.1% hydrocortisone, the formulation is designed to provide a clinical activity comparable to that of Hydrocortisone Cream 1% BP.
- **PATIENT AND CARER ADVICE** Patient counselling is advised for hydrocortisone cream and ointment (application).
- **PROFESSION SPECIFIC INFORMATION**
  Dental practitioners' formulary
  Hydrocortisone Cream 1% 15 g may be prescribed.
- **EXCEPTIONS TO LEGAL CATEGORY** Skin creams and ointments containing hydrocortisone (alone or with other ingredients) can be sold to the public for the treatment of allergic contact dermatitis, irritant dermatitis, insect bite reactions and mild to moderate eczema in patients over 10 years, to be applied sparingly over the affected area 1–2 times daily for max. 1 week. Over-the-counter hydrocortisone preparations should not be sold without medical advice for children under 10 years or for pregnant women; they should **not** be sold for application to the face, anogenital region, broken or infected skin (including cold sores, acne, and athlete's foot).

- **MEDICINAL FORMS** There can be variation in the licensing of different medicines containing the same drug. Forms available from special-order manufacturers include: cream, ointment

Cream
CAUTIONARY AND ADVISORY LABELS 28
EXCIPIENTS: May contain Benzyl alcohol, cetostearyl alcohol (including cetyl and stearyl alcohol), hydroxybenzoates (parabens), propylene glycol
- ▸ Hydrocortisone (Non-proprietary)
  Hydrocortisone 5 mg per 1 gram Hydrocortisone 0.5% cream | 15 gram PoM £44.00 DT = £1.22 | 30 gram PoM £2.44–£88.00
  Hydrocortisone 10 mg per 1 gram Hydrocortisone 1% cream | 15 gram PoM £18.88 DT = £1.06 | 30 gram PoM £29.32 DT = £2.12 | 50 gram PoM £44.12 DT = £3.53
  Hydrocortisone 25 mg per 1 gram Hydrocortisone 2.5% cream | 15 gram PoM £44.00 DT = £4.99 | 30 gram PoM £9.98–£88.00
- ▸ Dioderm (Dermal Laboratories Ltd)
  Hydrocortisone 1 mg per 1 gram Dioderm 0.1% cream | 30 gram PoM £2.39 DT = £2.39
- ▸ Mildison Lipocream (Karo Pharma)
  Hydrocortisone 10 mg per 1 gram Mildison Lipocream 1% cream | 30 gram PoM £1.71 DT = £2.12

Ointment
CAUTIONARY AND ADVISORY LABELS 28
- ▸ Hydrocortisone (Non-proprietary)
  Hydrocortisone 5 mg per 1 gram Hydrocortisone 0.5% ointment | 15 gram PoM £44.00 DT = £44.00 | 30 gram PoM £88.00
  Hydrocortisone 10 mg per 1 gram Hydrocortisone 1% ointment | 15 gram PoM £16.55 DT = £1.30 | 30 gram PoM £24.96 DT = £2.60 | 50 gram PoM £39.41 DT = £4.33
  Hydrocortisone 25 mg per 1 gram Hydrocortisone 2.5% ointment | 15 gram PoM £44.00 DT = £24.48 | 30 gram PoM £48.96–£88.00

Combinations available: *Hydrocortisone with benzalkonium chloride, dimeticone and nystatin,* p. 794 · ***Hydrocortisone with chlorhexidine hydrochloride and nystatin,*** p. 794 · ***Hydrocortisone with clotrimazole,*** p. 794 · ***Hydrocortisone with fusidic acid,*** p. 794 · ***Hydrocortisone with miconazole,*** p. 795 · ***Hydrocortisone with oxytetracycline,*** p. 795

785

Hydrocortisone butyrate

21-Dec-2017

- **INDICATIONS AND DOSE**

Severe inflammatory skin disorders such as eczemas unresponsive to less potent corticosteroids | Psoriasis
▸ TO THE SKIN
▸ Child 1–17 years: Apply 1–2 times a day, to be applied thinly

POTENCY
▸ Hydrocortisone butyrate 0.1% cream, liquid, and ointment: potent

- **PATIENT AND CARER ADVICE** Patients or carers should be given advice on how to administer hydrocortisone butyrate lotion, cream, ointment and scalp lotion.
  Medicines for Children leaflet: Hydrocortisone (topical) for eczema www.medicinesforchildren.org.uk/hydrocortisone-topical-eczema

- **MEDICINAL FORMS** There can be variation in the licensing of different medicines containing the same drug. Forms available from special-order manufacturers include: ointment

Ointment
CAUTIONARY AND ADVISORY LABELS 28
- ▸ Locoid (LEO Pharma)
  Hydrocortisone butyrate 1 mg per 1 gram Locoid 0.1% ointment | 30 gram PoM £1.60 DT = £1.60 | 100 gram PoM £4.93 DT = £4.93

Cream
CAUTIONARY AND ADVISORY LABELS 28
EXCIPIENTS: May contain Benzyl alcohol, cetostearyl alcohol (including cetyl and stearyl alcohol), hydroxybenzoates (parabens)
- ▸ Locoid (LEO Pharma)
  Hydrocortisone butyrate 1 mg per 1 gram Locoid 0.1% cream | 30 gram PoM £1.60 DT = £1.60 | 100 gram PoM £4.93 DT = £4.93
- ▸ Locoid Lipocream (LEO Pharma)
  Hydrocortisone butyrate 1 mg per 1 gram Locoid 0.1% Lipocream | 30 gram PoM £1.69 DT = £1.60 | 100 gram PoM £5.17 DT = £4.93

Liquid
CAUTIONARY AND ADVISORY LABELS 15(excluding Locoid Crelo topical emulsion), 28
EXCIPIENTS: May contain Butylated hydroxytoluene, cetostearyl alcohol (including cetyl and stearyl alcohol), hydroxybenzoates (parabens), propylene glycol
- Locoid (LEO Pharma)
  Hydrocortisone butyrate 1 mg per 1 ml Locoid 0.1% scalp lotion | 100 ml PoM £6.83 DT = £6.83
- Locoid Crelo (LEO Pharma)
  Hydrocortisone butyrate 1 mg per 1 gram Locoid Crelo 0.1% topical emulsion | 100 gram PoM £5.91 DT = £5.91

F 785

Mometasone furoate 21-Dec-2017

● **INDICATIONS AND DOSE**

Severe inflammatory skin disorders such as eczemas unresponsive to less potent corticosteroids | Psoriasis
- TO THE SKIN
- Child 1 month–1 year: Apply once daily, to be applied thinly (to scalp in case of lotion)
- Child 2–17 years: Apply once daily, to be applied thinly (to scalp in case of lotion)

POTENCY
- Mometasone furoate 0.1% cream, ointment, and scalp lotion: potent.

● **UNLICENSED USE** Not licensed for use in children under 2 years.
● **INTERACTIONS** → Appendix 1: corticosteroids

● **MEDICINAL FORMS** There can be variation in the licensing of different medicines containing the same drug. Forms available from special-order manufacturers include: ointment

Cream
CAUTIONARY AND ADVISORY LABELS 28
EXCIPIENTS: May contain Beeswax
- Mometasone furoate (Non-proprietary)
  Mometasone furoate 1 mg per 1 gram Mometasone 0.1% cream | 30 gram PoM £4.39 DT = £2.85 | 100 gram PoM £12.58 DT = £9.50
- Elocon (Merck Sharp & Dohme Ltd)
  Mometasone furoate 1 mg per 1 gram Elocon 0.1% cream | 30 gram PoM £4.80 DT = £2.85 | 100 gram PoM £15.10 DT = £9.50

Ointment
CAUTIONARY AND ADVISORY LABELS 28
EXCIPIENTS: May contain Beeswax, propylene glycol
- Mometasone furoate (Non-proprietary)
  Mometasone furoate 1 mg per 1 gram Mometasone 0.1% ointment | 15 gram PoM £4.32 | 30 gram PoM £4.45 DT = £2.98 | 50 gram PoM £12.44 | 100 gram PoM £12.82 DT = £9.93
- Elocon (Merck Sharp & Dohme Ltd)
  Mometasone furoate 1 mg per 1 gram Elocon 0.1% ointment | 30 gram PoM £4.32 DT = £2.98 | 100 gram PoM £12.44 DT = £9.93

Liquid
CAUTIONARY AND ADVISORY LABELS 28
EXCIPIENTS: May contain Propylene glycol
- Elocon (Merck Sharp & Dohme Ltd)
  Mometasone furoate 1 mg per 1 gram Elocon 0.1% scalp lotion | 30 ml PoM £4.36 DT = £4.36

CORTICOSTEROIDS > CORTICOSTEROID COMBINATIONS WITH ANTI-INFECTIVES

Betamethasone with clioquinol 20-Mar-2020

The properties listed below are those particular to the combination only. For the properties of the components please consider, betamethasone p. 786.

● **INDICATIONS AND DOSE**

Severe inflammatory skin disorders such as eczemas associated with infection and unresponsive to less potent corticosteroids | Psoriasis (excluding widespread plaque psoriasis)
- TO THE SKIN
- Child 1-17 years: (consult product literature)

POTENCY
- Betamethasone (as valerate) 0.1% with clioquinol cream and ointment: potent.

● **INTERACTIONS** → Appendix 1: corticosteroids
● **PATIENT AND CARER ADVICE** Stains clothing. Patients or carers should be counselled on application of betamethasone with clioquinol preparations.

● **MEDICINAL FORMS** There can be variation in the licensing of different medicines containing the same drug.

Ointment
CAUTIONARY AND ADVISORY LABELS 28
- Betamethasone with clioquinol (Non-proprietary)
  Betamethasone (as Betamethasone valerate) 1 mg per 1 gram, Clioquinol 30 mg per 1 gram Betamethasone valerate 0.1% / Clioquinol 3% ointment | 30 gram PoM £38.88 DT = £38.88

Cream
CAUTIONARY AND ADVISORY LABELS 28
EXCIPIENTS: May contain Cetostearyl alcohol (including cetyl and stearyl alcohol), chlorocresol
- Betamethasone with clioquinol (Non-proprietary)
  Betamethasone (as Betamethasone valerate) 1 mg per 1 gram, Clioquinol 30 mg per 1 gram Betamethasone valerate 0.1% / Clioquinol 3% cream | 30 gram PoM £38.88 DT = £38.88

Betamethasone with clotrimazole

06-Nov-2019

The properties listed below are those particular to the combination only. For the properties of the components please consider, betamethasone p. 786, clotrimazole p. 776.

● **INDICATIONS AND DOSE**

Short-term treatment of tinea infections and candidiasis
- TO THE SKIN
- Child 12-17 years: Apply twice daily for 2 weeks for tinea cruris, tinea corporis or candidiasis, or for 4 weeks for tinea pedis

POTENCY
- Betamethasone dipropionate 0.064% (=betamethasone 0.05%) with clotrimazole cream: potent.

● **INTERACTIONS** → Appendix 1: antifungals, azoles · corticosteroids
● **PATIENT AND CARER ADVICE** Patients or carers should be given advice on how to administer betamethasone with clotrimazole cream.

● **MEDICINAL FORMS** There can be variation in the licensing of different medicines containing the same drug.

Cream
CAUTIONARY AND ADVISORY LABELS 28
EXCIPIENTS: May contain Benzyl alcohol, cetostearyl alcohol (including cetyl and stearyl alcohol), propylene glycol
- Lotriderm (Merck Sharp & Dohme Ltd)
  Betamethasone dipropionate 640 microgram per 1 gram, Clotrimazole 10 mg per 1 gram Lotriderm cream | 30 gram PoM £6.34 DT = £6.34

Betamethasone with fusidic acid

20-Mar-2020

The properties listed below are those particular to the combination only. For the properties of the components please consider, betamethasone p. 786, fusidic acid p. 387.

- **INDICATIONS AND DOSE**

Severe inflammatory skin disorders such as eczemas associated with infection and unresponsive to less potent corticosteroids

▶ TO THE SKIN

▸ Child: (consult product literature)

POTENCY

▸ Betamethasone (as valerate) 0.1% with fusidic acid cream: potent.

- **UNLICENSED USE** *Fucibet® Lipid Cream* is not licensed for use in children under 6 years.
- **INTERACTIONS** → Appendix 1: corticosteroids · fusidate
- **PATIENT AND CARER ADVICE** Patients or carers should be counselled on application of betamethasone with fusidic acid preparations.

- **MEDICINAL FORMS** There can be variation in the licensing of different medicines containing the same drug.

Cream

CAUTIONARY AND ADVISORY LABELS 28

EXCIPIENTS: May contain Cetostearyl alcohol (including cetyl and stearyl alcohol), chlorocresol, hydroxybenzoates (parabens)

▸ Fucibet (LEO Pharma)
Betamethasone (as Betamethasone valerate) 1 mg per 1 gram, Fusidic acid 20 mg per 1 gram Fucibet cream | 30 gram PoM £6.38 DT = £6.38 | 60 gram PoM £12.76 DT = £12.76
Fucibet Lipid cream | 30 gram PoM £6.74 DT = £6.38

▸ Xemacort (Mylan)
Betamethasone (as Betamethasone valerate) 1 mg per 1 gram, Fusidic acid 20 mg per 1 gram Xemacort 20mg/g / 1mg/g cream | 30 gram PoM £6.05 DT = £6.38 | 60 gram PoM £12.45 DT = £12.76

Betamethasone with neomycin

The properties listed below are those particular to the combination only. For the properties of the components please consider, betamethasone p. 786, neomycin sulfate p. 774.

- **INDICATIONS AND DOSE**

Severe inflammatory skin disorders such as eczemas unresponsive to less potent corticosteroids | Psoriasis

▶ TO THE SKIN USING OINTMENT, OR TO THE SKIN USING CREAM

▸ Child 1-23 months: Apply 1–2 times a day, to be applied thinly

▸ Child 2-17 years: Apply 1–2 times a day, to be applied thinly

POTENCY

▸ Betamethasone (as valerate) 0.1% with neomycin cream and ointment: potent.

- **UNLICENSED USE** Betamethasone and neomycin preparations not licensed for use in children under 2 years.
- **INTERACTIONS** → Appendix 1: corticosteroids · neomycin
- **PATIENT AND CARER ADVICE** Patient counselling is advised for betamethasone with neomycin cream and ointment (application).

- **MEDICINAL FORMS** There can be variation in the licensing of different medicines containing the same drug.

Ointment

CAUTIONARY AND ADVISORY LABELS 28

▸ Betamethasone with neomycin (Non-proprietary)
Betamethasone (as Betamethasone valerate) 1 mg per 1 gram, Neomycin sulfate 5 mg per 1 gram Betamethasone valerate 0.1% / Neomycin 0.5% ointment | 30 gram PoM £38.88 DT = £31.36 | 100 gram PoM £97.00 DT = £104.52

Cream

CAUTIONARY AND ADVISORY LABELS 28

EXCIPIENTS: May contain Cetostearyl alcohol (including cetyl and stearyl alcohol), chlorocresol

▸ Betamethasone with neomycin (Non-proprietary)
Betamethasone (as Betamethasone valerate) 1 mg per 1 gram, Neomycin sulfate 5 mg per 1 gram Betamethasone valerate 0.1% / Neomycin 0.5% cream | 30 gram PoM £38.88 DT = £31.36 | 100 gram PoM £97.00 DT = £104.52

Betamethasone with salicylic acid

11-Mar-2020

The properties listed below are those particular to the combination only. For the properties of the components please consider, betamethasone p. 786, salicylic acid p. 820.

- **INDICATIONS AND DOSE**

DIPROSALIC® OINTMENT

Severe inflammatory skin disorders such as eczemas unresponsive to less potent corticosteroids | Psoriasis

▶ TO THE SKIN

▸ Child: Apply 1–2 times a day, max. 60 g per week

POTENCY

▸ Betamethasone (as dipropionate) 0.05% with salicylic acid 3%: potent.

DIPROSALIC® SCALP APPLICATION

Severe inflammatory skin disorders such as eczemas unresponsive to less potent corticosteroids | Psoriasis

▶ TO THE SKIN

▸ Child: Apply 1–2 times a day, apply a few drops

POTENCY

▸ Betamethasone (as dipropionate) 0.05% with salicylic acid 2%: potent.

- **INTERACTIONS** → Appendix 1: corticosteroids
- **PATIENT AND CARER ADVICE**

DIPROSALIC® OINTMENT Patients or carers should be counselled on application of betamethasone and salicylic acid preparations.

DIPROSALIC® SCALP APPLICATION Patients or carers should be counselled on application of betamethasone and salicylic acid scalp application.

- **MEDICINAL FORMS** There can be variation in the licensing of different medicines containing the same drug.

Ointment

CAUTIONARY AND ADVISORY LABELS 28

▸ Diprosalic (Merck Sharp & Dohme Ltd)
Betamethasone (as Betamethasone dipropionate) 500 microgram per 1 gram, Salicylic acid 30 mg per 1 gram Diprosalic 0.05%/3% ointment | 30 gram PoM £3.18 DT = £3.18 | 100 gram PoM £9.14 DT = £9.14

Liquid

CAUTIONARY AND ADVISORY LABELS 28

EXCIPIENTS: May contain Disodium edetate

▸ Diprosalic (Merck Sharp & Dohme Ltd)
Betamethasone (as Betamethasone dipropionate) 500 microgram per 1 ml, Salicylic acid 20 mg per 1 ml Diprosalic 0.05%/2% scalp application | 100 ml PoM £10.10 DT = £10.10

Clobetasol propionate with neomycin sulfate and nystatin

The properties listed below are those particular to the combination only. For the properties of the components please consider, clobetasol propionate p. 787, neomycin sulfate p. 774.

- **INDICATIONS AND DOSE**

Short-term treatment only of severe resistant inflammatory skin disorders such as recalcitrant eczemas associated with infection and unresponsive to less potent corticosteroids | Psoriasis associated with infection

▶ TO THE SKIN

▸ Child: (consult product literature)

POTENCY

▸ Clobetasol propionate 0.05% with neomycin sulfate and nystatin cream and ointment: very potent.

- **UNLICENSED USE** Clobetasol with neomycin and nystatin preparations not licensed for use in children under 2 years.
- **INTERACTIONS** → Appendix 1: neomycin
- **PATIENT AND CARER ADVICE** Patients or carers should be advised on application of clobetasol propionate, neomycin sulfate and nystatin containing preparations.

- **MEDICINAL FORMS** There can be variation in the licensing of different medicines containing the same drug.

Ointment

CAUTIONARY AND ADVISORY LABELS 28

▸ Clobetasol propionate with neomycin sulfate and nystatin (Non-proprietary)
Clobetasol propionate 500 microgram per 1 gram, Neomycin sulfate 5 mg per 1 gram, Nystatin 100000 unit per 1 gram Clobetasol 500microgram / Neomycin 5mg / Nystatin 100,000units/g ointment | 30 gram PoM £87.00 DT = £87.00

Cream

CAUTIONARY AND ADVISORY LABELS 28

▸ Clobetasol propionate with neomycin sulfate and nystatin (Non-proprietary)
Clobetasol propionate 500 microgram per 1 gram, Neomycin sulfate 5 mg per 1 gram, Nystatin 100000 unit per 1 gram Clobetasol 500microgram / Neomycin 5mg / Nystatin 100,000units/g cream | 30 gram PoM £87.00 DT = £87.00

Clobetasone butyrate with nystatin and oxytetracycline

06-Mar-2020

The properties listed below are those particular to the combination only. For the properties of the components please consider, clobetasone butyrate p. 788, oxytetracycline p. 383.

- **INDICATIONS AND DOSE**

Steroid-responsive dermatoses where candidal or bacterial infection is present

▶ TO THE SKIN

▸ Child: (consult product literature)

POTENCY

▸ Clobetasone butyrate 0.05% with nystatin and oxytetracyline cream: moderate.

- **INTERACTIONS** → Appendix 1: tetracyclines
- **PATIENT AND CARER ADVICE** Stains clothing.

- **MEDICINAL FORMS** There can be variation in the licensing of different medicines containing the same drug.

Cream

CAUTIONARY AND ADVISORY LABELS 28

EXCIPIENTS: May contain Cetostearyl alcohol (including cetyl and stearyl alcohol), chlorocresol, sodium metabisulfite

▸ Trimovate (Ennogen Healthcare Ltd)
Clobetasone butyrate 500 microgram per 1 gram, Oxytetracycline (as Oxytetracycline calcium) 30 mg per 1 gram, Nystatin 100000 unit per 1 gram Trimovate cream | 30 gram PoM £12.45 DT = £12.45

Fluocinolone acetonide with clioquinol

20-Mar-2020

The properties listed below are those particular to the combination only. For the properties of the components please consider, fluocinolone acetonide p. 789.

- **INDICATIONS AND DOSE**

Inflammatory skin disorders such as eczemas associated with infection

▶ TO THE SKIN

▸ Child 1–17 years: Apply 2–3 times a day, to be applied thinly

POTENCY

▸ Clioquinol 3% with fluocinolone acetonide 0.025% cream and ointment: potent

- **INTERACTIONS** → Appendix 1: fluocinolone
- **PATIENT AND CARER ADVICE** Patient counselling is advised for clioquinol with fluocinolone acetonide cream and ointment (application). Ointment stains clothing.

- **MEDICINAL FORMS** There can be variation in the licensing of different medicines containing the same drug.

Ointment

CAUTIONARY AND ADVISORY LABELS 28

EXCIPIENTS: May contain Propylene glycol, woolfat and related substances (including lanolin)

▸ Synalar C (Reig Jofre UK Ltd)
Fluocinolone acetonide 250 microgram per 1 gram, Clioquinol 30 mg per 1 gram Synalar C ointment | 15 gram PoM £2.66 DT = £2.66

Cream

CAUTIONARY AND ADVISORY LABELS 28

EXCIPIENTS: May contain Cetostearyl alcohol (including cetyl and stearyl alcohol), disodium edetate, hydroxybenzoates (parabens), polysorbates, propylene glycol

▸ Synalar C (Reig Jofre UK Ltd)
Fluocinolone acetonide 250 microgram per 1 gram, Clioquinol 30 mg per 1 gram Synalar C cream | 15 gram PoM £2.66 DT = £2.66

Fluocinolone acetonide with neomycin

The properties listed below are those particular to the combination only. For the properties of the components please consider, fluocinolone acetonide p. 789, neomycin sulfate p. 774.

- **INDICATIONS AND DOSE**

Inflammatory skin disorders such as eczemas associated with infection | Psoriasis associated with infection

▶ TO THE SKIN

▸ Child 1–11 months: Apply 1–2 times a day, to be applied thinly, reducing strength as condition responds

▸ Child 1–17 years: Apply 1–2 times a day, to be applied thinly, reducing strength as condition responds

POTENCY

▸ Fluocinolone acetonide 0.025% with neomycin 0.5% cream and ointment: potent.

- **INTERACTIONS** → Appendix 1: fluocinolone · neomycin
- **PATIENT AND CARER ADVICE** Patients or carers should be counselled on the application of fluocinolone acetonide with neomycin preparations.

- **MEDICINAL FORMS** No licensed medicines listed.

Hydrocortisone with benzalkonium chloride, dimeticone and nystatin

06-Mar-2020

The properties listed below are those particular to the combination only. For the properties of the components please consider, hydrocortisone p. 790, dimeticone p. 780.

- **INDICATIONS AND DOSE**

Mild inflammatory skin disorders such as eczemas associated with infection

▸ TO THE SKIN

▸ Child: Apply 3 times a day until lesion has healed, to be applied thinly

POTENCY

▸ Benzalkonium with dimeticone, hydrocortisone acetate 0.5%, and nystatin cream: mild.

- **INTERACTIONS** → Appendix 1: corticosteroids
- **PATIENT AND CARER ADVICE** Patients or carers should be advised on application of benzalkonium with dimeticone and hydrocortisone and nystatin preparations.

- **MEDICINAL FORMS** There can be variation in the licensing of different medicines containing the same drug.

Cream

CAUTIONARY AND ADVISORY LABELS 28

EXCIPIENTS: May contain Butylated hydroxyanisole, cetostearyl alcohol (including cetyl and stearyl alcohol), hydroxybenzoates (parabens), sodium metabisulfite, sorbic acid

▸ **Timodine** (Alliance Pharmaceuticals Ltd)
Benzalkonium chloride 1 mg per 1 gram, Hydrocortisone 5 mg per 1 gram, Dimeticone 350 100 mg per 1 gram, Nystatin 100000 unit per 1 gram Timodine cream | 30 gram PoM £3.37

Hydrocortisone with chlorhexidine hydrochloride and nystatin

10-Mar-2020

The properties listed below are those particular to the combination only. For the properties of the components please consider, hydrocortisone p. 790, chlorhexidine p. 813.

- **INDICATIONS AND DOSE**

Mild inflammatory skin disorders such as eczemas associated with infection

▸ TO THE SKIN

▸ Child: (consult product literature)

POTENCY

▸ Hydrocortisone 0.5% with chlorhexidine hydrochloride 1% and nystatin cream: mild

▸ Hydrocortisone 1% with chlorhexidine hydrochloride 1% and nystatin ointment: mild

- **INTERACTIONS** → Appendix 1: corticosteroids
- **PATIENT AND CARER ADVICE** Patients or carers should be given advice on application of chlorhexidine hydrochloride with hydrocortisone and nystatin preparations.

- **MEDICINAL FORMS** There can be variation in the licensing of different medicines containing the same drug.

Ointment

CAUTIONARY AND ADVISORY LABELS 28

▸ **Hydrocortisone with chlorhexidine hydrochloride and nystatin (Non-proprietary)**
Chlorhexidine acetate 10 mg per 1 gram, Hydrocortisone 10 mg per 1 gram, Nystatin 100000 unit per 1 gram Nystatin 100,000units/g / Chlorhexidine acetate 1% / Hydrocortisone 1% ointment | 30 gram PoM £5.29 DT = £5.29

Cream

CAUTIONARY AND ADVISORY LABELS 28

EXCIPIENTS: May contain Benzyl alcohol, cetostearyl alcohol (including cetyl and stearyl alcohol), polysorbates

▸ **Hydrocortisone with chlorhexidine hydrochloride and nystatin (Non-proprietary)**
Hydrocortisone 5 mg per 1 gram, Chlorhexidine hydrochloride 10 mg per 1 gram, Nystatin 100000 unit per 1 gram Nystatin 100,000units/g / Chlorhexidine hydrochloride 1% / Hydrocortisone 0.5% cream | 30 gram PoM £5.29 DT = £5.29

Hydrocortisone with clotrimazole

17-Mar-2020

The properties listed below are those particular to the combination only. For the properties of the components please consider, hydrocortisone p. 790, clotrimazole p. 776.

- **INDICATIONS AND DOSE**

Mild inflammatory skin disorders such as eczemas (associated with fungal infection)

▸ TO THE SKIN

▸ Child: (consult product literature)

POTENCY

▸ Clotrimazole with hydrocortisone 1% cream: mild

- **INTERACTIONS** → Appendix 1: antifungals, azoles · corticosteroids
- **PATIENT AND CARER ADVICE** Patients or carers should be given advice on how to administer clotrimazole with hydrocortisone cream.
- **EXCEPTIONS TO LEGAL CATEGORY** A 15-g tube is on sale to the public for the treatment of athlete's foot and fungal infection of skin folds with associated inflammation in patients 10 years and over.

- **MEDICINAL FORMS** There can be variation in the licensing of different medicines containing the same drug.

Cream

CAUTIONARY AND ADVISORY LABELS 28

EXCIPIENTS: May contain Benzyl alcohol, cetostearyl alcohol (including cetyl and stearyl alcohol)

▸ **Canesten HC** (Bayer Plc)
Clotrimazole 10 mg per 1 gram, Hydrocortisone 10 mg per 1 gram Canesten HC cream | 30 gram PoM £2.42 DT = £2.42

Hydrocortisone with fusidic acid

13-Mar-2020

The properties listed below are those particular to the combination only. For the properties of the components please consider, hydrocortisone p. 790, fusidic acid p. 387.

- **INDICATIONS AND DOSE**

Mild inflammatory skin disorders such as eczemas associated with infection

▸ TO THE SKIN

▸ Child: (consult product literature)

POTENCY

▸ Hydrocortisone with fusidic acid cream: mild

- **INTERACTIONS** → Appendix 1: corticosteroids · fusidate
- **PATIENT AND CARER ADVICE** Patients or carers should be advised on application of hydrocortisone with fusidic acid preparations.

- **MEDICINAL FORMS** There can be variation in the licensing of different medicines containing the same drug.

Cream

CAUTIONARY AND ADVISORY LABELS 28

EXCIPIENTS: May contain Butylated hydroxyanisole, cetostearyl alcohol (including cetyl and stearyl alcohol), polysorbates, potassium sorbate

▸ **Fucidin H (Fusidic acid / Hydrocortisone)** (LEO Pharma)
Hydrocortisone acetate 10 mg per 1 gram, Fusidic acid 20 mg per 1 gram Fucidin H cream | 30 gram PoM £6.02 DT = £6.02 | 60 gram PoM £12.05 DT = £12.05

Hydrocortisone with miconazole

17-Mar-2020

The properties listed below are those particular to the combination only. For the properties of the components please consider, hydrocortisone p. 790, miconazole p. 777.

- **INDICATIONS AND DOSE**

Mild inflammatory skin disorders such as eczemas associated with infections

▶ TO THE SKIN

▸ Child: (consult product literature)

POTENCY

▸ Hydrocortisone 1% with miconazole cream and ointment: mild

- **INTERACTIONS** → Appendix 1: antifungals, azoles · corticosteroids
- **PATIENT AND CARER ADVICE** Patients or carers should be advised on application of hydrocortisone with miconazole preparations.
- **PROFESSION SPECIFIC INFORMATION**

Dental practitioners' formulary

May be prescribed as Miconazole and Hydrocortisone Cream or Ointment for max. 7 days.

- **EXCEPTIONS TO LEGAL CATEGORY** A 15-g tube of hydrocortisone with miconazole cream is on sale to the public for the treatment of athlete's foot and candidal intertrigo in children over 10 years.
- **MEDICINAL FORMS** There can be variation in the licensing of different medicines containing the same drug.

Ointment

CAUTIONARY AND ADVISORY LABELS 28

▸ Daktacort (Janssen-Cilag Ltd)

Hydrocortisone 10 mg per 1 gram, Miconazole nitrate 20 mg per 1 gram Daktacort ointment | 30 gram PoM £2.50 DT = £2.50

Cream

CAUTIONARY AND ADVISORY LABELS 28

EXCIPIENTS: May contain Butylated hydroxyanisole, disodium edetate

▸ Daktacort (McNeil Products Ltd, Janssen-Cilag Ltd)

Hydrocortisone 10 mg per 1 gram, Miconazole nitrate 20 mg per 1 gram Daktacort Hydrocortisone cream | 15 gram P £3.63 DT = £3.63

Daktacort 2%/1% cream | 30 gram PoM £2.49 DT = £2.49

Hydrocortisone with oxytetracycline

The properties listed below are those particular to the combination only. For the properties of the components please consider, hydrocortisone p. 790, oxytetracycline p. 383.

- **INDICATIONS AND DOSE**

Mild inflammatory skin disorders such as eczemas

▶ TO THE SKIN

▸ Child 12–17 years: (consult product literature)

POTENCY

▸ Hydrocortisone 1% with oxytetracycline ointment: mild.

- **CONTRA-INDICATIONS** Children under 12 years
- **INTERACTIONS** → Appendix 1: corticosteroids · tetracyclines
- **PREGNANCY** Tetracyclines should not be given to pregnant women. Effects on skeletal development have been documented when tetracyclines have been used in the first trimester in animal studies. Administration during the second or third trimester may cause discoloration of the child's teeth.
- **BREAST FEEDING** Tetracyclines should not be given to women who are breast-feeding (although absorption and therefore discoloration of teeth in the infant is probably usually prevented by chelation with calcium in milk).
- **PATIENT AND CARER ADVICE** Patients should be given advice on the application of hydrocortisone with oxytetracycline ointment.
- **MEDICINAL FORMS** There can be variation in the licensing of different medicines containing the same drug.

Ointment

CAUTIONARY AND ADVISORY LABELS 28

▸ Terra-Cortril (Intrapharm Laboratories Ltd)

Hydrocortisone 10 mg per 1 gram, Oxytetracycline (as Oxytetracycline hydrochloride) 30 mg per 1 gram Terra-Cortril ointment | 30 gram PoM £5.01 DT = £5.01

DERMATOLOGICAL DRUGS › ANTI-INFECTIVES

Ichthammol

- **INDICATIONS AND DOSE**

Chronic lichenified eczema

▶ TO THE SKIN

▸ Child 1–17 years: Apply 1–3 times a day

- **UNLICENSED USE** No information available.
- **SIDE-EFFECTS** Skin irritation
- **MEDICINAL FORMS** There can be variation in the licensing of different medicines containing the same drug. Forms available from special-order manufacturers include: ointment, paste

Form unstated

▸ Ichthammol (Non-proprietary)

Ichthammol 1 mg per 1 mg Ichthammol liquid | 100 gram GSL £12.99 DT = £12.86 | 500 gram GSL £41.88

Ichthammol with zinc oxide

The properties listed below are those particular to the combination only. For the properties of the components please consider, ichthammol above.

- **INDICATIONS AND DOSE**

Chronic lichenified eczema

▶ TO THE SKIN

▸ Child: (consult product literature)

- **MEDICINAL FORMS** There can be variation in the licensing of different medicines containing the same drug. Forms available from special-order manufacturers include: cream, ointment

Impregnated dressing

▸ Ichthopaste (Evolan Pharma AB)

Ichthopaste bandage 7.5cm × 6m | 1 bandage £3.82

DERMATOLOGICAL DRUGS › ANTRACEN DERIVATIVES

Dithranol

(Anthralin)

- **INDICATIONS AND DOSE**

Subacute and chronic psoriasis

▶ TO THE SKIN

▸ Child: (consult product literature)

DITHROCREAM®

Subacute and chronic psoriasis

▶ TO THE SKIN

▸ Child: For application to skin or scalp, 0.1–0.5% cream suitable for overnight treatment, 1–2% cream for maximum 1 hour (consult product literature)

continued →

MICANOL®
Subacute and chronic psoriasis
▶ TO THE SKIN
▸ Child: Apply once daily, for application to skin or scalp, to be applied for up to 30 minutes, apply 1% cream, if necessary 3% cream can be used under medical supervision

- **UNLICENSED USE**
MICANOL® *Micanol*® licensed for use in children, but not recommended for infants or young children (age range not specified by manufacturer).
DITHROCREAM® *Dithrocream*® is licensed for use in children (age range not specified by manufacturer).
- **CONTRA-INDICATIONS** Acute and pustular psoriasis · hypersensitivity
- **CAUTIONS** Avoid sensitive areas of skin · avoid use near eyes
- **SIDE-EFFECTS** Skin reactions
- **PREGNANCY** No adverse effects reported.
- **BREAST FEEDING** No adverse effects reported.
- **DIRECTIONS FOR ADMINISTRATION** When applying dithranol, hands should be protected by gloves or they should be washed thoroughly afterwards. Dithranol should be applied to chronic extensor plaques only, carefully avoiding normal skin.
MICANOL® At the end of contact time, use plenty of lukewarm (not hot) water to rinse off cream; soap may be used after the cream has been rinsed off; use shampoo before applying cream to scalp and if necessary after cream has been rinsed off.
- **PRESCRIBING AND DISPENSING INFORMATION** Treatment should be started with a low concentration such as dithranol 0.1%, and the strength increased gradually every few days up to 3%, according to tolerance.
- **PATIENT AND CARER ADVICE** Dithranol can stain the skin, hair and fabrics.
- **EXCEPTIONS TO LEGAL CATEGORY** Prescription only medicine if dithranol content more than 1%, otherwise may be sold to the public.

- **MEDICINAL FORMS** There can be variation in the licensing of different medicines containing the same drug. Forms available from special-order manufacturers include: ointment

Cream
CAUTIONARY AND ADVISORY LABELS 28
EXCIPIENTS: May contain Cetostearyl alcohol (including cetyl and stearyl alcohol), chlorocresol
▸ Dithrocream (Dermal Laboratories Ltd)
Dithranol 1 mg per 1 gram Dithrocream 0.1% cream | 50 gram [P] £3.77 DT = £3.77
Dithranol 2.5 mg per 1 gram Dithrocream 0.25% cream | 50 gram [P] £4.04 DT = £4.04
Dithranol 5 mg per 1 gram Dithrocream 0.5% cream | 50 gram [P] £4.66 DT = £4.66
Dithranol 10 mg per 1 gram Dithrocream 1% cream | 50 gram [P] £5.42 DT = £5.42
Dithranol 20 mg per 1 gram Dithrocream 2% cream | 50 gram [PoM] £6.79 DT = £6.79

Combinations available: *Coal tar with dithranol and salicylic acid*, p. 797

Dithranol with salicylic acid and zinc oxide

The properties listed below are those particular to the combination only. For the properties of the components please consider, dithranol p. 795, salicylic acid p. 820.

- **INDICATIONS AND DOSE**
Subacute and chronic psoriasis
▶ TO THE SKIN
▸ Child: (consult local protocol)

- **MEDICINAL FORMS** Forms available from special-order manufacturers include: ointment, paste

DERMATOLOGICAL DRUGS › TARS

Coal tar

07-Apr-2020

- **INDICATIONS AND DOSE**
Psoriasis | Scaly scalp disorders such as psoriasis, eczema, seborrhoeic dermatitis and dandruff
▶ TO THE SKIN
▸ Child: (consult product literature)

- **CONTRA-INDICATIONS** Avoid broken or inflamed skin · avoid eye area · avoid genital area · avoid mucosal areas · avoid rectal area · infection · sore, acute, or pustular psoriasis
- **CAUTIONS**
GENERAL CAUTIONS Application to face
SPECIFIC CAUTIONS
▸ When used for scaly scalp disorders, using shampoo children under 12 years (consult product literature)
- **SIDE-EFFECTS** Photosensitivity reaction · skin reactions
- **PRESCRIBING AND DISPENSING INFORMATION** Coal Tar Solution BP contains coal tar 20%, Strong Coal Tar Solution BP contains coal tar 40%.
- **HANDLING AND STORAGE** Use suitable chemical protection gloves for extemporaneous preparation. May stain skin, hair and fabric.
- **PATIENT AND CARER ADVICE** May stain skin, hair and fabric.

- **MEDICINAL FORMS** There can be variation in the licensing of different medicines containing the same drug. Forms available from special-order manufacturers include: cream, ointment, paste

Cutaneous emulsion
EXCIPIENTS: May contain Hydroxybenzoates (parabens)
▸ Exorex (Teva UK Ltd)
Coal tar solution 50 mg per 1 gram Exorex lotion | 100 ml [GSL] £8.11 DT = £8.11 | 250 ml [GSL] £16.24 DT = £16.24

Shampoo
EXCIPIENTS: May contain Fragrances, hydroxybenzoates (parabens)
▸ Alphosyl 2 in 1 (Omega Pharma Ltd)
Coal tar extract alcoholic 50 mg per 1 gram Alphosyl 2 in 1 shampoo | 250 ml [GSL] £5.81 DT = £5.81
▸ Neutrogena T/Gel Therapeutic (Johnson & Johnson Ltd)
Coal tar extract 20 mg per 1 gram Neutrogena T/Gel Therapeutic shampoo | 125 ml [GSL] £3.90 DT = £3.90 | 250 ml [GSL] £5.86 DT = £5.86
▸ Polytar Scalp (Thornton & Ross Ltd)
Coal tar solution 40 mg per 1 ml Polytar Scalp shampoo | 150 ml [GSL] £3.46 DT = £3.46
▸ Psoriderm (Dermal Laboratories Ltd)
Coal tar distilled 25 mg per 1 ml Psoriderm scalp lotion | 250 ml [P] £4.74 DT = £4.74

Cream
EXCIPIENTS: May contain Isopropyl palmitate, lecithin, propylene glycol
▸ Psoriderm (Dermal Laboratories Ltd)
Coal tar distilled 60 mg per 1 gram Psoriderm cream | 225 ml [P] £9.42 DT = £9.42

13 Skin

Coal tar with coconut oil and salicylic acid

19-Mar-2020

The properties listed below are those particular to the combination only. For the properties of the components please consider, coal tar p. 796, salicylic acid p. 820.

- **INDICATIONS AND DOSE**

Scaly scalp disorders | Psoriasis | Seborrhoeic dermatitis | Dandruff | Cradle cap

▶ TO THE SKIN USING SHAMPOO

▸ Child: Apply daily as required

- **MEDICINAL FORMS** There can be variation in the licensing of different medicines containing the same drug.

Shampoo

▸ Capasal (Dermal Laboratories Ltd)
Salicylic acid 5 mg per 1 gram, Coal tar distilled 10 mg per 1 gram, Coconut oil 10 mg per 1 gram Capasal Therapeutic shampoo | 250 ml [P] £4.69

Coal tar with dithranol and salicylic acid

The properties listed below are those particular to the combination only. For the properties of the components please consider, coal tar p. 796, dithranol p. 795, salicylic acid p. 820.

- **INDICATIONS AND DOSE**

Subacute and chronic psoriasis

▶ TO THE SKIN

▸ Child: Apply up to twice daily

- **UNLICENSED USE** *Psorin*® is licensed for use in children (age range not specified by manufacturer).
- **MEDICINAL FORMS** Forms available from special-order manufacturers include: ointment

Coal tar with salicylic acid and precipitated sulfur

20-Mar-2020

The properties listed below are those particular to the combination only. For the properties of the components please consider, coal tar p. 796, salicylic acid p. 820.

- **INDICATIONS AND DOSE**

COCOIS® OINTMENT

Scaly scalp disorders including psoriasis, eczema, seborrhoeic dermatitis and dandruff

▶ TO THE SKIN USING SCALP OINTMENT

▸ Child 6-11 years: Medical supervision required

▸ Child 12-17 years: Apply once weekly as required, alternatively apply daily for the first 3–7 days (if severe), shampoo off after 1 hour

SEBCO® OINTMENT

Scaly scalp disorders including psoriasis, eczema, seborrhoeic dermatitis and dandruff

▶ TO THE SKIN USING SCALP OINTMENT

▸ Child 6-11 years: Medical supervision required

▸ Child 12-17 years: Apply as required, alternatively apply daily for the first 3–7 days (if severe), shampoo off after 1 hour

- **MEDICINAL FORMS** There can be variation in the licensing of different medicines containing the same drug.

Ointment

EXCIPIENTS: May contain Cetostearyl alcohol (including cetyl and stearyl alcohol)

▸ Cocois (RPH Pharmaceuticals AB)
Salicylic acid 20 mg per 1 gram, Sulfur precipitated 40 mg per 1 gram, Coal tar solution 120 mg per 1 gram Cocois ointment | 40 gram [GSL] £6.22 | 100 gram [GSL] £11.69

▸ Sebco (Derma UK Ltd)
Salicylic acid 20 mg per 1 gram, Sulfur precipitated 40 mg per 1 gram, Coal tar solution 120 mg per 1 gram Sebco ointment | 40 gram [GSL] £7.91 | 100 gram [GSL] £13.38

Coal tar with zinc oxide

16-Jan-2019

The properties listed below are those particular to the combination only. For the properties of the components please consider, coal tar p. 796.

- **INDICATIONS AND DOSE**

Psoriasis | Chronic atopic eczema

▶ TO THE SKIN

▸ Child: Apply 1–2 times a day

IMPORTANT SAFETY INFORMATION

MHRA/CHM ADVICE (UPDATED DECEMBER 2018): EMOLLIENTS: NEW INFORMATION ABOUT RISK OF SEVERE AND FATAL BURNS WITH PARAFFIN-CONTAINING AND PARAFFIN-FREE EMOLLIENTS

See Emollient and barrier preparations p. 765.

- **PRESCRIBING AND DISPENSING INFORMATION** No preparations available—when prepared extemporaneously, the BP states Zinc and Coal Tar Paste, BP consists of zinc oxide 6%, coal tar 6%, emulsifying wax 5%, starch 38%, yellow soft paraffin 45%.
- **MEDICINAL FORMS** Forms available from special-order manufacturers include: ointment, paste

IMMUNOSUPPRESSANTS > CALCINEURIN INHIBITORS AND RELATED DRUGS

Pimecrolimus

- **INDICATIONS AND DOSE**

Short-term treatment of mild to moderate atopic eczema (including flares) when topical corticosteroids cannot be used (initiated by a specialist)

▶ TO THE SKIN

▸ Child 2-17 years: Apply twice daily until symptoms resolve (stop treatment if eczema worsens or no response after 6 weeks)

- **CONTRA-INDICATIONS** Application to malignant or potentially malignant skin lesions · application under occlusion · congenital epidermal barrier defects · contact with eyes · contact with mucous membranes · generalised erythroderma · immunodeficiency · infection at treatment site
- **CAUTIONS** Alcohol consumption (risk of facial flushing and skin irritation) · avoid other topical treatments except emollients at treatment site · UV light (avoid excessive exposure to sunlight and sunlamps)
- **INTERACTIONS** → Appendix 1: pimecrolimus
- **SIDE-EFFECTS**

▸ **Common or very common** Increased risk of infection

▸ **Rare or very rare** Skin discolouration

▸ **Frequency not known** Skin papilloma

- **PREGNANCY** Manufacturer advises avoid; toxicity in *animal* studies following systemic administration.
- **BREAST FEEDING** Manufacturer advises caution; ensure infant does not come in contact with treated areas.

● NATIONAL FUNDING/ACCESS DECISIONS

NICE decisions

▸ **Tacrolimus and pimecrolimus for atopic eczema (August 2004)** NICE TA82

Topical pimecrolimus is an option for atopic eczema not controlled by maximal topical corticosteroid treatment or if there is a risk of important corticosteroid side-effects (particularly skin atrophy).

Topical pimecrolimus is recommended for moderate atopic eczema on the face and neck of children aged 2–16 years. Pimecrolimus should be used within its licensed indications.
www.nice.org.uk/TA82

● MEDICINAL FORMS There can be variation in the licensing of different medicines containing the same drug.

Cream

CAUTIONARY AND ADVISORY LABELS 4, 11, 28
EXCIPIENTS: May contain Benzyl alcohol, cetostearyl alcohol (including cetyl and stearyl alcohol), propylene glycol

▸ Elidel (Mylan)
Pimecrolimus 10 mg per 1 gram Elidel 1% cream | 30 gram PoM £19.69 DT = £19.69 | 60 gram PoM £37.41 DT = £37.41 | 100 gram PoM £59.07 DT = £59.07

13 Skin

Tacrolimus

19-Nov-2019

● DRUG ACTION Tacrolimus is a calcineurin inhibitor.

● INDICATIONS AND DOSE

Short-term treatment of moderate to severe atopic eczema (including flares) in patients unresponsive to, or intolerant of conventional therapy (initiated by a specialist)

▸ TO THE SKIN
- Child 2–15 years: Apply twice daily for up to 3 weeks (consider other treatment if eczema worsens or if no improvement after 2 weeks), 0.03% ointment to be applied thinly, then reduced to once daily until lesion clears
- Child 16–17 years: Apply twice daily until lesion clears (consider other treatment if eczema worsens or no improvement after 2 weeks), initially 0.1% ointment to be applied thinly, reduce frequency to once daily or strength of ointment to 0.03% if condition allows

Prevention of flares in patients with moderate to severe atopic eczema and 4 or more flares a year who have responded to initial treatment with topical tacrolimus (initiated by a specialist)

▸ TO THE SKIN
- Child 2–15 years: Apply twice weekly, 0.03% ointment to be applied thinly, with an interval of 2–3 days between applications, use short-term treatment regimen during an acute flare; review need for preventative therapy after 1 year
- Child 16–17 years: Apply twice weekly, 0.1% ointment to be applied thinly, with an interval of 2–3 days between applications, use short-term treatment regimen during an acute flare; review need for preventative therapy after 1 year

● CONTRA-INDICATIONS Application to malignant or potentially malignant skin lesions · application under occlusion · avoid contact with eyes · avoid contact with mucous membranes · congenital epidermal barrier defects · generalised erythroderma · immunodeficiency · infection at treatment site

● CAUTIONS UV light (avoid excessive exposure to sunlight and sunlamps)

● INTERACTIONS → Appendix 1: tacrolimus

● SIDE-EFFECTS

▸ **Common or very common** Alcohol intolerance · increased risk of infection · sensation abnormal · skin reactions

▸ **Uncommon** Lymphadenopathy

▸ **Frequency not known** Malignancy · neoplasms

● ALLERGY AND CROSS-SENSITIVITY Contra-indicated if history of hypersensitivity to macrolides.

● PREGNANCY Manufacturer advises avoid unless essential; toxicity in *animal* studies following systemic administration.

● BREAST FEEDING Avoid—present in breast milk (following systemic administration).

● HEPATIC IMPAIRMENT Manufacturer advises caution in hepatic failure.

● PATIENT AND CARER ADVICE Avoid excessive exposure to UV light including sunlight.

● NATIONAL FUNDING/ACCESS DECISIONS

NICE decisions

▸ **Tacrolimus and pimecrolimus for atopic eczema (August 2004)** NICE TA82

Topical tacrolimus is an option for atopic eczema not controlled by maximal topical corticosteroid treatment or if there is a risk of important corticosteroid side-effects (particularly skin atrophy).

Topical tacrolimus is recommended as an option for the second-line treatment for moderate to severe atopic eczema in adults and children over 2 years.Tacrolimus should be used within its licensed indications.
www.nice.org.uk/guidance/TA82

Scottish Medicines Consortium (SMC) decisions

The *Scottish Medicines Consortium* has advised (March 2010) that tacrolimus 0.03 % ointment (*Protopic*®) is accepted for restricted use within NHS Scotland for the prevention of flares in children aged 2 to 15 years with moderate-to-severe atopic eczema in accordance with the licensed indications; initiation of treatment is restricted to doctors (including general practitioners) with a specialist interest and experience in treating atopic eczema with immunomodulatory therapy.

The *Scottish Medicines Consortium* has advised (April 2010) that tacrolimus 0.1 % ointment (*Protopic*®) is accepted for restricted use within NHS Scotland for the prevention of flares in patients aged 16 years and over with moderate-to-severe atopic eczema in accordance with the licensed indications; initiation of treatment is restricted to doctors (including general practitioners) with a specialist interest and experience in treating atopic eczema with immunomodulatory therapy.

● MEDICINAL FORMS There can be variation in the licensing of different medicines containing the same drug.

Ointment

CAUTIONARY AND ADVISORY LABELS 4, 11, 28
EXCIPIENTS: May contain Beeswax

▸ Tacrolimus (Non-proprietary)
Tacrolimus (as Tacrolimus monohydrate) 1 mg per 1 gram Tacrolimus 0.1% ointment | 30 gram PoM £25.96 DT = £18.88 | 60 gram PoM £51.91 DT = £37.76

▸ Protopic (LEO Pharma)
Tacrolimus (as Tacrolimus monohydrate) 300 microgram per 1 gram Protopic 0.03% ointment | 30 gram PoM £23.33 DT = £23.33 | 60 gram PoM £42.55 DT = £42.55
Tacrolimus (as Tacrolimus monohydrate) 1 mg per 1 gram Protopic 0.1% ointment | 30 gram PoM £25.92 DT = £18.88 | 60 gram PoM £47.28 DT = £37.76

IMMUNOSUPPRESSANTS › INTERLEUKIN INHIBITORS

Dupilumab

21-Oct-2019

- **DRUG ACTION** Dupilumab is a recombinant human monoclonal antibody that inhibits interleukin-4 and interleukin-13 signaling.

- **INDICATIONS AND DOSE**

Moderate-to-severe atopic eczema (initiated by a specialist)

▶ BY SUBCUTANEOUS INJECTION

▶ Child 12–17 years (body-weight up to 59 kg): Initially 400 mg, followed by 200 mg every 2 weeks, the initial dose should be administered as two consecutive 200 mg injections at different injection sites, review treatment if no response after 16 weeks

▶ Child 12–17 years (body-weight 60 kg and above): Initially 600 mg, followed by 300 mg every 2 weeks, the initial dose should be administered as two consecutive 300 mg injections at different injection sites, review treatment if no response after 16 weeks

Severe asthma with type 2 inflammation [add-on maintenance therapy] (initiated by a specialist)

▶ BY SUBCUTANEOUS INJECTION

▶ Child 12–17 years: Initially 400 mg, followed by 200 mg every 2 weeks, the initial dose should be administered as two consecutive 200 mg injections at different injection sites, review need for treatment yearly

Severe asthma with type 2 inflammation [add-on maintenance therapy for patients currently treated with oral corticosteroids or patients with co-morbid moderate-to-severe atopic dermatitis] (initiated by a specialist)

▶ BY SUBCUTANEOUS INJECTION

▶ Child 12–17 years: Initially 600 mg, followed by 300 mg every 2 weeks, the initial dose should be administered as two consecutive 300 mg injections at different injection sites, review need for treatment yearly

- **CAUTIONS** Helminth infection

CAUTIONS, FURTHER INFORMATION

▶ Risk of infection Dupilumab may influence the immune response to helminth infections. Resolve pre-existing infection before initiating treatment; suspend treatment if resistant infection develops during therapy.

Manufacturer advises patients should be brought up-to-date with live and live attenuated vaccines before initiating treatment.

- **INTERACTIONS** → Appendix 1: monoclonal antibodies
- **SIDE-EFFECTS**

▶ **Common or very common** Eosinophilia · eye inflammation · eye pruritus · headache · oral herpes

▶ **Rare or very rare** Hypersensitivity

▶ **Frequency not known** Pneumonia eosinophilic · vasculitis

SIDE-EFFECTS, FURTHER INFORMATION **Eosinophilic granulomatosis with polyangiitis (Churg-Strauss syndrome)** Churg-Strauss syndrome has occurred in patients given dupilumab; the reaction may be associated with the reduction of oral corticosteroid therapy. Churg-Strauss syndrome can present as vasculitic rash, cardiac complications, worsening pulmonary symptoms, or peripheral neuropathy in patients with eosinophilia.

- **PREGNANCY** Manufacturer advises use only if potential benefit outweighs risk—limited information available.
- **BREAST FEEDING** Manufacturer advises avoid—no information available.
- **DIRECTIONS FOR ADMINISTRATION** Manufacturer advises to inject into the thigh or abdomen (except for the 5 cm around the navel), or upper arm (if not self-administered); rotate injection site and avoid skin that is tender, damaged or scarred. Patients may self-administer *Dupixent®* after appropriate training in preparation and administration.
- **PRESCRIBING AND DISPENSING INFORMATION** Dupilumab is a biological medicine. Biological medicines must be prescribed and dispensed by brand name, see *Biological medicines* and *Biosimilar medicines*, under Guidance on prescribing p. 1; manufacturer advises to record the brand name and batch number after each administration.
- **HANDLING AND STORAGE** Manufacturer advises store in a refrigerator (2–8°C) and protect from light; pre-filled syringes may be kept at room temperature (max. 25°C) for max. 14 days.
- **NATIONAL FUNDING/ACCESS DECISIONS**

Scottish Medicines Consortium (SMC) decisions

SMC No. SMC2232

The *Scottish Medicines Consortium* has advised (January 2020) that dupilumab (*Dupixent®*) is accepted for restricted use within NHS Scotland for the treatment of moderate-to-severe atopic dermatitis in patients aged 12 years up to 18 years, who have had an inadequate response to existing systemic immunosuppressants such as ciclosporin, or in whom such treatment is considered unsuitable. This advice is contingent upon the continuing availability of the patient access scheme in NHS Scotland or a list price that is equivalent or lower.

All Wales Medicines Strategy Group (AWMSG) decisions

AWMSG No. 4089

The *All Wales Medicines Strategy Group* has advised (November 2019) that dupilumab (*Dupixent®*) is recommended as an option for restricted use within NHS Wales for the treatment of moderate-to-severe atopic dermatitis in patients aged 12 years or older, who are candidates for systemic therapy, only if the disease has not responded to at least one other systemic therapy, or these are contra-indicated or not tolerated. It is not recommended for use within NHS Wales outside of this subpopulation. This recommendation only applies in circumstances where the approved Patient Access Scheme (PAS) is utilised or where the list/contract price is equivalent or lower than the PAS price.

- **MEDICINAL FORMS** There can be variation in the licensing of different medicines containing the same drug.

Solution for injection

EXCIPIENTS: May contain Polysorbates

▶ Dupixent (Sanofi) ▼

Dupilumab 150 mg per 1 ml Dupixent 300mg/2ml solution for injection pre-filled syringes | 2 pre-filled disposable injection PoM £1,264.89

Dupixent 300mg/2ml solution for injection pre-filled pens | 2 pre-filled disposable injection PoM £1,264.89

Dupilumab 175 mg per 1 ml Dupixent 200mg/1.14ml solution for injection pre-filled syringes | 2 pre-filled disposable injection PoM £1,264.89

Dupixent 200mg/1.14ml solution for injection pre-filled pens | 2 pre-filled disposable injection PoM £1,264.89

Ustekinumab

11-Dec-2019

- **INDICATIONS AND DOSE**

Plaque psoriasis (specialist use only)

▶ BY SUBCUTANEOUS INJECTION

▶ Child 12–17 years (body-weight up to 60 kg): Initially 750 micrograms/kg, then 750 micrograms/kg after 4 weeks, then 750 micrograms/kg every 12 weeks, consider discontinuation if no response within 28 weeks, consult product literature for advice on calculating volume of injection to be given

▶ Child 12–17 years (body-weight 60–100 kg): Initially 45 mg, then 45 mg after 4 weeks, then continued →

45 mg every 12 weeks, consider discontinuation if no response within 28 weeks
- Child 12–17 years (body-weight 100 kg and above): Initially 90 mg, then 90 mg after 4 weeks, then 90 mg every 12 weeks, consider discontinuation if no response within 28 weeks

- **CONTRA-INDICATIONS** Active infection
- **CAUTIONS** Development of malignancy · history of malignancy · predisposition to infection · start appropriate treatment if widespread erythema and skin exfoliation develop, and stop ustekinumab treatment if exfoliative dermatitis suspected

CAUTIONS, FURTHER INFORMATION
- Tuberculosis Active tuberculosis should be treated with standard treatment for at least 2 months before starting ustekinumab. Patients who have previously received adequate treatment for tuberculosis can start ustekinumab but should be monitored every 3 months for possible recurrence. In patients without active tuberculosis but who were previously not treated adequately, chemoprophylaxis should ideally be completed before starting ustekinumab. In patients at high risk of tuberculosis who cannot be assessed by tuberculin skin test, chemoprophylaxis can be given concurrently with ustekinumab.

- **INTERACTIONS** → Appendix 1: monoclonal antibodies
- **SIDE-EFFECTS**
  - **Common or very common** Arthralgia · asthenia · back pain · diarrhoea · dizziness · headache · increased risk of infection · myalgia · nausea · oropharyngeal pain · skin reactions · vomiting
  - **Uncommon** Depression · facial paralysis · hypersensitivity (may be delayed) · nasal congestion
  - **Rare or very rare** Respiratory disorders
  - **Frequency not known** Increased risk of cancer
- **CONCEPTION AND CONTRACEPTION** Manufacturer advises effective contraception during treatment and for 15 weeks after stopping treatment.
- **PREGNANCY** Avoid.
- **BREAST FEEDING** Manufacturer advises avoid—present in milk in *animal* studies.
- **PRE-TREATMENT SCREENING**
Tuberculosis Patients should be evaluated for tuberculosis before treatment.
- **MONITORING REQUIREMENTS**
  - Monitor for non-melanoma skin cancer, especially in patients with a history of PUVA treatment or prolonged immunosuppressant therapy, or those over 60 years of age.
  - Monitor for signs and symptoms of exfoliative dermatitis or erythrodermic psoriasis.
- **PATIENT AND CARER ADVICE**
Exfoliative dermatitis Patients should be advised to seek prompt medical attention if symptoms suggestive of exfoliative dermatitis or erythrodermic psoriasis (such as increased redness and shedding of skin over a larger area of the body) develop.
Tuberculosis Patients should be advised to seek medical attention if symptoms suggestive of tuberculosis (e.g. persistent cough, weight loss, and fever) develop.
- **NATIONAL FUNDING/ACCESS DECISIONS**

NICE decisions
- **Adalimumab, etanercept and ustekinumab for treating plaque psoriasis in children and young people (July 2017)** NICE TA455
Ustekinumab is recommended as an option for treating plaque psoriasis in children and young people aged 12 years or older, only if the disease:
  - is severe, as defined by a total PASI of 10 or more, **and**
  - has not responded to standard systemic therapy, such as ciclosporin, methotrexate or phototherapy, or these options are contra-indicated or not tolerated.

If the psoriasis has not responded adequately, stop treatment at 16 weeks. An adequate response is defined as a 75% reduction in PASI score from the start of treatment.
Patients currently receiving ustekinumab who do not meet the above criteria and whose treatment was started within the NHS before this guidance was published, should have the option to continue treatment until they and their clinician consider it appropriate to stop.
www.nice.org.uk/guidance/ta455

- **MEDICINAL FORMS** There can be variation in the licensing of different medicines containing the same drug.

Solution for injection
CAUTIONARY AND ADVISORY LABELS 10
- Stelara (Janssen-Cilag Ltd)
Ustekinumab 90 mg per 1 ml Stelara 90mg/1ml solution for injection pre-filled syringes | 1 pre-filled disposable injection PoM £2,147.00 (Hospital only)
Stelara 45mg/0.5ml solution for injection vials | 1 vial PoM £2,147.00 (Hospital only)
Stelara 45mg/0.5ml solution for injection pre-filled syringes | 1 pre-filled disposable injection PoM £2,147.00 (Hospital only)

RETINOID AND RELATED DRUGS

Acitretin

28-Jan-2020

- **DRUG ACTION** Acitretin is a metabolite of etretinate.

- **INDICATIONS AND DOSE**

Severe extensive psoriasis resistant to other forms of therapy (under expert supervision) | Palmoplantar pustular psoriasis (under expert supervision) | Severe congenital ichthyosis (under expert supervision)
- BY MOUTH
  - Child 1 month–11 years: 0.5 mg/kg once daily; increased if necessary to 1 mg/kg once daily, to be taken with food or milk, careful monitoring of musculoskeletal development required; maximum 35 mg per day
  - Child 12–17 years: Initially 25–30 mg daily for 2–4 weeks, then adjusted according to response to 25–50 mg daily, increased to up to 75 mg daily, dose only increased to 75 mg daily for short periods in psoriasis

Severe Darier's disease (keratosis follicularis) (under expert supervision)
- BY MOUTH
  - Child 1 month–11 years: 0.5 mg/kg once daily; increased if necessary to 1 mg/kg once daily, to be taken with food or milk, careful monitoring of musculoskeletal development required; maximum 35 mg per day
  - Child 12–17 years: Initially 10 mg daily for 2–4 weeks, then adjusted according to response to 25–50 mg daily

Harlequin ichthyosis (under expert supervision)
- BY MOUTH
  - Neonate: 0.5 mg/kg once daily; increased if necessary to 1 mg/kg once daily, to be taken with food or milk, careful monitoring of musculoskeletal development required.

IMPORTANT SAFETY INFORMATION
MHRA/CHM ADVICE: ORAL RETINOID MEDICINES: REVISED AND SIMPLIFIED PREGNANCY PREVENTION EDUCATIONAL MATERIALS FOR HEALTHCARE PROFESSIONALS AND WOMEN (JUNE 2019)
New prescriber checklists, patient reminder cards, and pharmacy checklists are available to support the Pregnancy Prevention Programme in women and girls of childbearing potential taking oral acitretin, alitretinoin, or isotretinoin. Healthcare professionals are reminded

that the use of oral retinoids is contra-indicated in pregnancy due to a high risk of serious congenital malformations, and any use in females must be within the conditions of the Pregnancy Prevention Programme (see *Conception and contraception* and *Prescribing and dispensing information*).

Neuropsychiatric reactions have been reported in patients taking oral retinoids. Healthcare professionals are advised to monitor patients for signs of depression or suicidal ideation and refer for appropriate treatment, if necessary; particular care is needed in those with a history of depression. Patients should be advised to speak to their doctor if they experience any changes in mood or behaviour, and encouraged to ask family and friends to look out for any change in mood.

- **CONTRA-INDICATIONS** Hyperlipidaemia
- **CAUTIONS** Avoid excessive exposure to sunlight and unsupervised use of sunlamps · diabetes (can alter glucose tolerance—initial frequent blood glucose checks) · do not donate blood during and for 3 years after stopping therapy (teratogenic risk) · history of depression (risk of neuropsychiatric reactions) · in children use only in exceptional circumstances and monitor growth parameters and bone development (premature epiphyseal closure reported) · investigate atypical musculoskeletal symptoms
- **INTERACTIONS** → Appendix 1: retinoids
- **SIDE-EFFECTS**
  - **Common or very common** Abdominal pain · arthralgia · brittle nails · conjunctivitis · diarrhoea · dry mouth · gastrointestinal disorder · haemorrhage · hair texture abnormal · headache · increased risk of infection · mucosal abnormalities · myalgia · nausea · oral disorders · peripheral oedema · skin reactions · thirst · vomiting · xerophthalmia
  - **Uncommon** Dizziness · hepatic disorders · photosensitivity reaction · vision disorders
  - **Rare or very rare** Bone pain · exostosis · idiopathic intracranial hypertension · peripheral neuropathy
  - **Frequency not known** Angioedema · capillary leak syndrome · drowsiness · dysphonia · flushing · glucose tolerance impaired · granuloma · hearing impairment · hyperhidrosis · malaise · pyogenic granuloma · retinoic acid syndrome · taste altered · tinnitus

SIDE-EFFECTS, FURTHER INFORMATION **Exostosis** Skeletal hyperostosis and extra-osseous calcification reported following long-term treatment with etretinate (of which acitretin is a metabolite) and premature epiphyseal closure in children.

Benign intracranial hypertension Discontinue if severe headache, nausea, vomiting, or visual disturbances occur.

- **CONCEPTION AND CONTRACEPTION** The MHRA advises that women and girls of childbearing potential being treated with the oral retinoids acitretin, alitretinoin, or isotretinoin must be supported on a Pregnancy Prevention Programme with regular follow-up and pregnancy testing.

Pregnancy prevention Effective contraception must be used.

In females of childbearing potential (including those with a history of infertility), exclude pregnancy up to 3 days before treatment, every month during treatment, and every 1–3 months for 3 years after stopping treatment. Treatment should be started on day 2 or 3 of menstrual cycle. Females of childbearing age must practise effective contraception for at least 1 month before starting treatment, during treatment, and for at least 3 years after stopping treatment. Females should be advised to use at least 1 method of contraception, but ideally they should use 2 methods of contraception. Oral progestogen-only contraceptives are not considered effective. Barrier methods should not be used alone but can be used in conjunction with other contraceptive methods. Females should be advised to seek medical attention immediately if they become pregnant during treatment or within 3 years of stopping treatment. They should also be advised to avoid alcohol during treatment and for 2 months after stopping treatment.

- **PREGNANCY** Manufacturer advises avoid—teratogenic.
- **BREAST FEEDING** Avoid.
- **HEPATIC IMPAIRMENT** Manufacturer advises avoid in severe impairment.
- **RENAL IMPAIRMENT** Avoid in severe impairment; increased risk of toxicity.
- **MONITORING REQUIREMENTS**
  - Monitor serum-triglyceride and serum-cholesterol concentrations before treatment, 1 month after starting, then every 3 months.
  - Check liver function at start, at least every 4 weeks for first 2 months and then every 3 months.
- **PRESCRIBING AND DISPENSING INFORMATION**

Prescribing for females of childbearing potential The Pregnancy Prevention Programme is supported by the following materials provided by the manufacturer: *Checklists for prescribers and pharmacists*, and *Patient reminder cards*.

Each prescription for oral acitretin should be limited to a supply of up to 30 days' treatment. Pregnancy testing should ideally be carried out on the same day as prescription issuing and dispensing.

- **PATIENT AND CARER ADVICE**

Risk of neuropsychiatric reactions The MHRA advises patients and carers to seek medical attention if changes in mood or behaviour occur.

Pregnancy Prevention Programme Pharmacists must ensure that female patients have a patient card—see also *Important safety information*.

- **MEDICINAL FORMS** There can be variation in the licensing of different medicines containing the same drug. Forms available from special-order manufacturers include: oral suspension, oral solution

Capsule

CAUTIONARY AND ADVISORY LABELS 10, 11, 21

- Acitretin (Non-proprietary)
  - **Acitretin 10 mg** Acitretin 10mg capsules | 60 capsule PoM £26.98 DT = £26.98
  - **Acitretin 25 mg** Acitretin 25mg capsules | 60 capsule PoM £55.24 DT = £43.75
- Neotigason (Teva UK Ltd)
  - **Acitretin 10 mg** Neotigason 10mg capsules | 60 capsule PoM £17.30 DT = £26.98
  - **Acitretin 25 mg** Neotigason 25mg capsules | 60 capsule PoM £43.00 DT = £43.75

SALICYLIC ACID AND DERIVATIVES

Salicylic acid with zinc oxide

- **INDICATIONS AND DOSE**

Hyperkeratotic skin disorders

- TO THE SKIN
  - Child: Apply twice daily

- **CAUTIONS** Avoid broken skin · avoid inflamed skin

CAUTIONS, FURTHER INFORMATION

- Salicylate toxicity Salicylate toxicity may occur particularly if applied on large areas of skin or neonatal skin.

- **SIDE-EFFECTS** Skin irritation
- **PRESCRIBING AND DISPENSING INFORMATION** Zinc and Salicylic Acid Paste BP is also referred to as Lassar's Paste. When prepared extemporaneously, the BP states Zinc and Salicylic Acid Paste, BP (Lassar's Paste) consists of zinc oxide 24%, salicylic acid 2%, starch 24%, white soft paraffin 50%.

- **MEDICINAL FORMS** Forms available from special-order manufacturers include: paste

VITAMINS AND TRACE ELEMENTS › VITAMIN D AND ANALOGUES

Calcipotriol

- **INDICATIONS AND DOSE**

Plaque psoriasis

▶ TO THE SKIN USING OINTMENT

▸ Child 6–11 years: Apply twice daily, when preparations used together maximum total calcipotriol 2.5 mg in any one week (e.g. scalp solution 20 mL with ointment 30 g); maximum 50 g per week

▸ Child 12–17 years: Apply twice daily, when preparations used together maximum total calcipotriol 3.75 mg in any one week (e.g. scalp solution 30 mL with ointment 45 g); maximum 75 g per week

Scalp psoriasis

▶ TO THE SKIN USING SCALP LOTION

▸ Child 6–11 years (specialist use only): Apply twice daily, when preparations used together max. total calcipotriol 2.5 mg in any one week (e.g. scalp solution 20 mL with ointment 30 g); maximum 30 mL per week

▸ Child 12–17 years (specialist use only): Apply twice daily, when preparations used together maximum total calcipotriol 3.75 mg in any one week (e.g. scalp solution 30 mL with ointment 45 g); maximum 45 mL per week

- **UNLICENSED USE** Calcipotriol ointment and scalp solution not licensed for use in children.
- **CONTRA-INDICATIONS** Calcium metabolism disorders
- **CAUTIONS** Avoid excessive exposure to sunlight and sunlamps · avoid use on face · erythrodermic exfoliative psoriasis (enhanced risk of hypercalcaemia) · generalised pustular psoriasis (enhanced risk of hypercalcaemia)
- **INTERACTIONS** → Appendix 1: vitamin D substances
- **SIDE-EFFECTS**

▶ **Common or very common** Skin reactions

▶ **Uncommon** Increased risk of infection

▶ **Rare or very rare** Hypercalcaemia · hypercalciuria · photosensitivity reaction

- **PREGNANCY** Manufacturers advise avoid unless essential.
- **BREAST FEEDING** No information available.
- **HEPATIC IMPAIRMENT** Manufacturers advise avoid in severe impairment (no information available).
- **RENAL IMPAIRMENT** Manufacturers advise avoid in severe impairment.
- **PATIENT AND CARER ADVICE**

Advice on application Patient information leaflet for *Dovonex*® ointment advises liberal application. However, patients should be advised of maximum recommended weekly dose.

Hands should be washed thoroughly after application to avoid inadvertent transfer to other body areas.

- **MEDICINAL FORMS** There can be variation in the licensing of different medicines containing the same drug. Forms available from special-order manufacturers include: ointment

Ointment

EXCIPIENTS: May contain Disodium edetate, propylene glycol

▸ Calcipotriol (Non-proprietary)

Calcipotriol 50 microgram per 1 gram Calcipotriol 50micrograms/g ointment | 30 gram PoM £7.43 DT = £7.42 | 60 gram PoM £11.56–£14.86 | 120 gram PoM £23.10–£29.72

▸ Dovonex (LEO Pharma)

Calcipotriol 50 microgram per 1 gram Dovonex 50micrograms/g ointment | 30 gram PoM £5.78 DT = £7.42 | 60 gram PoM £11.56

Liquid

▸ Calcipotriol (Non-proprietary)

Calcipotriol (as Calcipotriol hydrate) 50 microgram per 1 ml Calcipotriol 50micrograms/ml scalp solution | 60 ml PoM £56.94 DT = £56.94 | 120 ml PoM £113.88 DT = £113.88

Combinations available: *Calcipotriol with betamethasone*, p. 787

F 680

Calcitriol

04-Mar-2020

(1,25-Dihydroxycholecalciferol)

- **INDICATIONS AND DOSE**

Mild to moderate plaque psoriasis

▶ TO THE SKIN

▸ Child 12–17 years: Apply twice daily, not more than 35% of body surface to be treated daily; maximum 30 g per day

- **CONTRA-INDICATIONS** Do not apply under occlusion · patients with calcium metabolism disorders
- **CAUTIONS** Erythrodermic exfoliative psoriasis (enhanced risk of hypercalcaemia) · generalised pustular psoriasis (enhanced risk of hypercalcaemia)
- **INTERACTIONS** → Appendix 1: vitamin D substances
- **PREGNANCY** Manufacturer advises use in restricted amounts only if clearly necessary.

Monitoring Monitor urine- and serum-calcium concentration in pregnancy.

- **BREAST FEEDING** Manufacturer advises avoid.
- **HEPATIC IMPAIRMENT** Manufacturer advises avoid.
- **RENAL IMPAIRMENT** Manufacturer advises avoid—no information available.
- **HANDLING AND STORAGE** Hands should be washed thoroughly after application to avoid inadvertent transfer to other body areas.

- **MEDICINAL FORMS** There can be variation in the licensing of different medicines containing the same drug.

Ointment

▸ Silkis (Galderma (UK) Ltd)

Calcitriol 3 microgram per 1 gram Silkis ointment | 100 gram PoM £18.06 DT = £18.06

Tacalcitol

18-Feb-2020

- **INDICATIONS AND DOSE**

Plaque psoriasis

▶ TO THE SKIN

▸ Child 12–17 years: Apply once daily, preferably at bedtime, maximum 10 g ointment or 10 mL lotion daily, when lotion and ointment used together, maximum total tacalcitol 280 micrograms in any one week (e.g. lotion 30 mL with ointment 40 g)

- **UNLICENSED USE** Expert sources advise that tacalcitol may be used in children from the age of 12 years, but it is not licensed for this age group.
- **CONTRA-INDICATIONS** Calcium metabolism disorders
- **CAUTIONS** Avoid eyes · erythrodermic exfoliative psoriasis (enhanced risk of hypercalcaemia) · generalised pustular psoriasis (enhanced risk of hypercalcaemia) · if used in conjunction with UV treatment

CAUTIONS, FURTHER INFORMATION

▸ UV treatment If tacalcitol is used in conjunction with UV treatment, UV radiation should be given in the morning and tacalcitol applied at bedtime.

- **INTERACTIONS** → Appendix 1: vitamin D substances

- **SIDE-EFFECTS**
  - ▸ **Uncommon** Skin reactions
  - ▸ **Frequency not known** Hypercalcaemia
- **PREGNANCY** Manufacturer advises avoid unless no safer alternative—no information available.
- **BREAST FEEDING** Manufacturer advises avoid application to breast area; no information available on presence in milk.
- **RENAL IMPAIRMENT**
  Monitoring Monitor serum calcium concentration.
- **MONITORING REQUIREMENTS** Monitor serum calcium if risk of hypercalcaemia.
- **PATIENT AND CARER ADVICE** Hands should be washed thoroughly after application to avoid inadvertent transfer to other body areas.

- **MEDICINAL FORMS** There can be variation in the licensing of different medicines containing the same drug.

Ointment

▸ Curatoderm (Almirall Ltd)
Tacalcitol (as Tacalcitol monohydrate) 4 microgram per 1 gram Curatoderm 4micrograms/g ointment | 30 gram [PoM] £13.40 DT = £13.40 | 100 gram [PoM] £30.86 DT = £30.86

Liquid

EXCIPIENTS: May contain Disodium edetate, propylene glycol

▸ Curatoderm (Almirall Ltd)
Tacalcitol (as Tacalcitol monohydrate) 4 microgram per 1 gram Curatoderm 4micrograms/g lotion | 30 ml [PoM] £12.73 DT = £12.73

4 Perspiration

4.1 Hyperhidrosis

Hyperhidrosis

Overview

Aluminium chloride hexahydrate below is a potent antiperspirant used in the treatment of axillary, palmar, and plantar hyperhidrosis. Aluminium salts are also incorporated in preparations used for minor fungal skin infections associated with hyperhidrosis.

In more severe cases specialists use tap water or glycopyrronium bromide below (as a 0.05% solution) in the iontophoretic treatment of hyperhidrosis of palms and soles.

Botox® contains botulinum toxin type A complex p. 275 and is available for use intradermally for severe hyperhidrosis of the axillae unresponsive to topical antiperspirant or other antihidrotic treatment; intradermal treatment is unlikely to be tolerated by most children and should be administered under hospital specialist supervision.

ANTIMUSCARINICS 527

Glycopyrronium bromide

19-Dec-2019

(Glycopyrrolate)

- **INDICATIONS AND DOSE**

Iontophoretic treatment of hyperhidrosis

▸ TO THE SKIN
▸ Child: Only 1 site to be treated at a time, maximum 2 sites treated in any 24 hours, treatment not to be repeated within 7 days (consult product literature)

- **UNLICENSED USE** Licensed for use in children (age range not specified by manufacturer).
- **CONTRA-INDICATIONS** Infections affecting the treatment site

  CONTRA-INDICATIONS, FURTHER INFORMATION Contra-indications applicable to systemic use should be considered; however, glycopyrronium is poorly absorbed and systemic effects unlikely with topical use.
- **CAUTIONS**

  CAUTIONS, FURTHER INFORMATION Cautions applicable to systemic use should be considered; however, glycopyrronium is poorly absorbed and systemic effects unlikely with topical use.
- **INTERACTIONS** → Appendix 1: glycopyrronium
- **SIDE-EFFECTS** Abdominal discomfort · eating disorder · pain · paraesthesia

  SIDE-EFFECTS, FURTHER INFORMATION The possibility of systemic side-effects should be considered; however, glycopyrronium is poorly absorbed and systemic effects are unlikely with topical use.

- **MEDICINAL FORMS** There can be variation in the licensing of different medicines containing the same drug.

Powder for solution for iontophoresis

▸ Glycopyrronium bromide (Non-proprietary)
Glycopyrronium bromide 1 mg per 1 mg Glycopyrronium bromide powder for solution for iontophoresis | 3 gram [PoM] £327.00 DT = £327.00

DERMATOLOGICAL DRUGS › ASTRINGENTS

Aluminium chloride hexahydrate

- **INDICATIONS AND DOSE**

Hyperhidrosis affecting axillae, hands or feet

▸ TO THE SKIN
▸ Child: Apply once daily, apply liquid formulation at night to dry skin, wash off the following morning, reduce frequency as condition improves—do not bathe immediately before use

Hyperhidrosis | Bromidrosis | Intertrigo | Prevention of tinea pedis and related conditions

▸ TO THE SKIN
▸ Child: Apply powder to dry skin

- **UNLICENSED USE** Licensed for use in children (age range not specified by manufacturer).
- **CAUTIONS** Avoid contact with eyes · avoid contact with mucous membranes · avoid use on broken or irritated skin · do not shave axillae or use depilatories within 12 hours of application
- **SIDE-EFFECTS** Skin reactions
- **PATIENT AND CARER ADVICE** Avoid contact with clothing.
- **EXCEPTIONS TO LEGAL CATEGORY** A 30 mL pack of aluminium chloride hexahydrate 20% is on sale to the public.

- **MEDICINAL FORMS** There can be variation in the licensing of different medicines containing the same drug.

Liquid

CAUTIONARY AND ADVISORY LABELS 15

▸ Anhydrol (Dermal Laboratories Ltd)
Aluminium chloride 200 mg per 1 ml Anhydrol Forte 20% solution | 60 ml [P] £2.51 DT = £2.51

▸ Driclor (GlaxoSmithKline Consumer Healthcare)
Aluminium chloride 200 mg per 1 ml Driclor 20% solution | 60 ml [P] £5.41 DT = £2.51

5 Pruritus

Topical local antipruritics

Overview

Pruritus may be caused by systemic disease (such as obstructive jaundice, endocrine disease, chronic renal disease, iron deficiency, and certain malignant diseases), skin disease (such as eczema, psoriasis, urticaria, and scabies), drug hypersensitivity, or as a side-effect of opioid analgesics. Where possible, the underlying cause should be treated. Local antipruritics have a role in the treatment of pruritus in palliative care. Pruritus caused by cholestasis generally requires a bile acid sequestrant.

An **emollient** may be of value where the pruritus is associated with dry skin. Preparations containing calamine or crotamiton below are sometimes used but are of uncertain value.

A topical preparation containing doxepin 5% below is licensed for the relief of pruritus in eczema in children over 12 years; it can cause drowsiness and there may be a risk of sensitisation.

Topical antihistamines and local anaesthetics are only marginally effective and occasionally cause sensitisation. For *insect stings* and *insect bites*, a short course of a topical corticosteroid is appropriate. Short-term treatment with a **sedating antihistamine** may help in insect stings and in intractable pruritus where sedation is desirable. Calamine preparations are of little value for the treatment of insect stings or bites.

In *pruritus ani*, the underlying cause such as faecal soiling, eczema, psoriasis, or helminth infection should be treated.

Other drugs used for Pruritus Alimemazine tartrate, p. 186 · Cetirizine hydrochloride, p. 183 · Chlorphenamine maleate, p. 186 · Hydroxyzine hydrochloride, p. 187 · Levocetirizine hydrochloride, p. 184

ANTIPRURITICS

Calamine with zinc oxide

11-Mar-2020

● **INDICATIONS AND DOSE**

Minor skin conditions

▶ TO THE SKIN

▸ Child: (consult product literature)

IMPORTANT SAFETY INFORMATION

MHRA/CHM ADVICE (UPDATED DECEMBER 2018): EMOLLIENTS: NEW INFORMATION ABOUT RISK OF SEVERE AND FATAL BURNS WITH PARAFFIN-CONTAINING AND PARAFFIN-FREE EMOLLIENTS

See Emollient and barrier preparations p. 765.

● **CONTRA-INDICATIONS** Avoid application of preparations containing zinc oxide prior to x-ray (zinc oxide may affect outcome of x-ray)

● **LESS SUITABLE FOR PRESCRIBING** Less suitable for prescribing.

● **MEDICINAL FORMS** There can be variation in the licensing of different medicines containing the same drug.

Cream

CAUTIONARY AND ADVISORY LABELS 15

▸ Calamine with zinc oxide (Non-proprietary)
Phenoxyethanol 5 mg per 1 gram, Zinc oxide 30 mg per 1 gram, Calamine 40 mg per 1 gram, Cetomacrogol emulsifying wax 50 mg per 1 gram, Self-emulsifying glyceryl monostearate 50 mg per 1 gram, Liquid paraffin 200 mg per 1 gram Aqueous calamine cream | 100 gram GSL £1.43 DT = £1.43

▸ Cala Soothe (Ennogen Healthcare Ltd)
Phenoxyethanol 5 mg per 1 gram, Zinc oxide 30 mg per 1 gram, Calamine 40 mg per 1 gram, Cetomacrogol emulsifying wax 50 mg per 1 gram, Self-emulsifying glyceryl monostearate 50 mg per 1 gram, Liquid paraffin 200 mg per 1 gram Cala Soothe cream | 100 ml £18.80

Liquid

▸ Calamine with zinc oxide (Non-proprietary)
Phenol liquefied 5 mg per 1 ml, Sodium citrate 5 mg per 1 ml, Bentonite 30 mg per 1 ml, Glycerol 50 mg per 1 ml, Zinc oxide 50 mg per 1 ml, Calamine 150 mg per 1 ml Calamine lotion | 200 ml GSL £0.94–£1.09 DT = £1.09

▸ Cala Soothe (Ennogen Healthcare Ltd)
Phenol liquefied 5 mg per 1 ml, Sodium citrate 5 mg per 1 ml, Bentonite 30 mg per 1 ml, Glycerol 50 mg per 1 ml, Zinc oxide 50 mg per 1 ml, Calamine 150 mg per 1 ml Cala Soothe lotion | 200 ml £19.50 DT = £1.09

Crotamiton

29-Apr-2020

● **INDICATIONS AND DOSE**

Pruritus (including pruritus after scabies)

▶ TO THE SKIN

▸ Child 1 month–2 years (on doctor's advice only): Apply once daily

▸ Child 3–17 years: Apply 2–3 times a day

● **CONTRA-INDICATIONS** Acute exudative dermatoses

● **CAUTIONS** Avoid use in buccal mucosa · avoid use near eyes · avoid use on broken skin · avoid use on very inflamed skin · use on doctor's advice for children under 3 years

● **PREGNANCY** Manufacturer advises avoid, especially during the first trimester—no information available.

● **BREAST FEEDING** No information available; avoid application to nipple area.

● **MEDICINAL FORMS** There can be variation in the licensing of different medicines containing the same drug.

Cream

EXCIPIENTS: May contain Beeswax, cetostearyl alcohol (including cetyl and stearyl alcohol), fragrances, hydroxybenzoates (parabens)

▸ Eurax (Thornton & Ross Ltd)
Crotamiton 100 mg per 1 gram Eurax 10% cream | 30 gram GSL £2.50 DT = £2.50 | 100 gram GSL £4.35 DT = £4.35

Doxepin

05-Jul-2019

● **INDICATIONS AND DOSE**

Pruritus in eczema

▶ TO THE SKIN

▸ Child 12–17 years: Apply up to 3 g 3–4 times a day, apply thinly; coverage should be less than 10% of body surface area; maximum 12 g per day

● **CAUTIONS** Arrhythmias · avoid application to large areas · mania · severe heart disease · susceptibility to angle-closure glaucoma · urinary retention

● **INTERACTIONS** → Appendix 1: tricyclic antidepressants

● **SIDE-EFFECTS** Constipation · diarrhoea · dizziness · drowsiness · dry eye · dry mouth · dyspepsia · fever · headache · nausea · paraesthesia · skin reactions · suicidal tendencies · taste altered · urinary retention · vision blurred · vomiting

● **PREGNANCY** Manufacturer advises use only if potential benefit outweighs risk.

● **BREAST FEEDING** Manufacturer advises use only if potential benefit outweighs risk.

● **HEPATIC IMPAIRMENT** Manufacturer advises caution in severe impairment.

● **PATIENT AND CARER ADVICE** A patient information leaflet should be provided.

Driving and skilled tasks Drowsiness may affect performance of skilled tasks (e.g. driving).
Effects of alcohol enhanced.

● MEDICINAL FORMS There can be variation in the licensing of different medicines containing the same drug.

Cream
CAUTIONARY AND ADVISORY LABELS 2, 10
EXCIPIENTS: May contain Benzyl alcohol
▸ Xepin (Cambridge Healthcare Supplies Ltd)
Doxepin hydrochloride 50 mg per 1 gram Xepin 5% cream | 30 gram [PoM] £13.66 DT = £13.66

6 Rosacea and acne

Rosacea and Acne

Acne vulgaris in children

Acne vulgaris commonly affects children around puberty and occasionally affects infants. Treatment of acne should be commenced early to prevent scarring; lesions may worsen before improving. The choice of treatment depends on age, severity, and whether the acne is predominantly inflammatory or comedonal.

Mild to moderate acne is generally treated with topical preparations, such as benzoyl peroxide p. 807, azelaic acid p. 808, and retinoids.

For *moderate to severe inflammatory acne* or where topical preparations are not tolerated or are ineffective or where application to the site is difficult, systemic treatment with oral antibacterials may be effective. Co-cyprindiol p. 806 (cyproterone acetate with ethinylestradiol) has anti-androgenic properties and may be useful in young women with acne refractory to other treatments.

Severe acne, acne unresponsive to prolonged courses of oral antibacterials, acne with scarring, or acne associated with psychological problems calls for early referral to a consultant dermatologist who may prescribe oral isotretinoin p. 809.

Acne in neonates and infants

Inflammatory papules, pustules, and occasionally comedones may develop at birth or within the first month; most neonates with acne do not require treatment. Acne developing at 3–6 months of age may be more severe and persistent; lesions are usually confined to the face. Topical preparations containing benzoyl peroxide (at the lowest strength possible to avoid irritation), adapalene p. 808, or tretinoin (available from 'special-order' manufacturers) may be used if treatment for infantile acne is necessary. In infants with inflammatory acne, oral erythromycin p. 355 is used because topical preparations for acne are not well tolerated. In cases of erythromycin-resistant acne, oral isotretinoin can be given on the advice of a consultant dermatologist.

Acne: topical preparations

In mild to moderate acne, comedones and inflamed lesions respond well to benzoyl peroxide or topical retinoids. Alternatively, topical application of an antibacterial such as erythromycin or clindamycin p. 807 may be effective for inflammatory acne. However, topical antibacterials are probably no more effective than benzoyl peroxide and may promote the emergence of resistant organisms. If topical preparations prove inadequate, oral preparations may be needed. The choice of product and formulation (gel, solution, lotion, or cream) is largely determined by skin type, patient preference, and previous usage of acne products.

Benzoyl peroxide and azelaic acid

Benzoyl peroxide is effective in mild to moderate acne. Both comedones and inflamed lesions respond well to benzoyl peroxide. The lower concentrations seem to be as effective as higher concentrations in reducing inflammation. It is usual to start with a lower strength and to increase the concentration of benzoyl peroxide gradually. The usefulness of benzoyl peroxide washes is limited by the short time the products are in contact with the skin. Adverse effects include local skin irritation, particularly when therapy is initiated, but the scaling and redness often subside with a reduction in benzoyl peroxide concentration, frequency, and area of application. If the acne does not respond after 2 months then use of a topical antibacterial should be considered.

Azelaic acid has antimicrobial and anticomedonal properties. It may be used as an alternative to benzoyl peroxide or to a topical retinoid for treating mild to moderate comedonal acne, particularly of the face; azelaic acid is less likely to cause local irritation than benzoyl peroxide.

Topical antibacterials for acne

In the treatment of mild to moderate inflammatory acne, topical antibacterials may be no more effective than topical benzoyl peroxide or tretinoin. Topical antibacterials are probably best reserved for children who wish to avoid oral antibacterials or who cannot tolerate them.

Topical preparations of erythromycin and clindamycin may be used to treat *inflamed lesions* in mild to moderate acne when topical benzoyl peroxide or tretinoin is ineffective or poorly tolerated. Topical benzoyl peroxide, azelaic acid, or retinoids used in combination with an antibacterial (topical or systemic) may be more effective than an antibacterial used alone. Topical antibacterials can produce mild irritation of the skin, and on rare occasions cause sensitisation; gastro-intestinal disturbances have been reported with topical clindamycin.

Antibacterial resistance of *Propionibacterium acnes* is increasing; there is cross-resistance between erythromycin and clindamycin. To avoid development of resistance:

- when possible use non-antibiotic antimicrobials (such as benzoyl peroxide or azelaic acid);
- avoid concomitant treatment with different oral and topical antibacterials;
- if a particular antibacterial is effective, use it for repeat courses if needed (short intervening courses of benzoyl peroxide or azelaic acid may eliminate any resistant propionibacteria);
- do not continue treatment for longer than necessary (but treatment with a topical preparation should be continued for at least 6 months).

Topical retinoids and related preparations for acne

Topical tretinoin (available from 'special-order' manufacturers), its isomer isotretinoin, and adapalene (a retinoid-like drug), are useful for treating comedones and inflammatory lesions in mild to moderate acne. Patients should be warned that some redness and skin peeling can occur initially but settles with time. If undue irritation occurs, the frequency of application should be reduced or treatment suspended until the reaction subsides; if irritation persists, discontinue treatment. Several months of treatment may be needed to achieve an optimal response and the treatment should be continued until no new lesions develop.

Tretinoin can be used under specialist supervision to treat infantile acne; adapalene can also be used.

Other topical preparations for acne

A topical preparation of nicotinamide p. 811 is available for inflammatory acne.

Acne: oral preparations

Oral antibacterials for acne

Oral antibacterials may be used in *moderate to severe inflammatory acne* when topical treatment is not adequately effective or is inappropriate. Concomitant anticomedonal

13 Skin

treatment with topical benzoyl peroxide or azelaic acid may also be required.

Tetracyclines should not be given to children under 12 years. In children over 12 years, either oxytetracycline p. 383 or tetracycline p. 384 is usually given for acne. If there is no improvement after the first 3 months another oral antibacterial should be used. Maximum improvement usually occurs after 4 to 6 months but in more severe cases treatment may need to be continued for 2 years or longer. Doxycycline p. 381 and lymecycline p. 383 are alternatives to tetracycline in children over 12 years.

Although minocycline p. 383 is as effective as other tetracyclines for acne, it is associated with a greater risk of lupus erythematosus-like syndrome. Minocycline sometimes causes irreversible pigmentation.

Erythromycin is an alternative for the management of moderate to severe acne with inflamed lesions, but propionibacteria strains resistant to erythromycin are becoming widespread and this may explain poor response. In cases of erythromycin-resistant *P. acnes* in infants, oral isotretinoin may be used on the advice of a consultant dermatologist.

Concomitant use of different topical and systemic antibacterials is undesirable owing to the increased likelihood of the development of bacterial resistance.

Hormone treatment for acne

Co-cyprindiol below (cyproterone acetate with ethinylestradiol) contains an anti-androgen. It is no more effective than an oral broad-spectrum antibacterial but is useful in females of childbearing age who also wish to receive oral contraception.

Improvement of acne with co-cyprindiol probably occurs because of decreased sebum secretion which is under androgen control. Some females with moderately severe hirsutism may also benefit because hair growth is also androgen-dependent.

Oral retinoid for acne

The retinoid isotretinoin p. 809 reduces sebum secretion. It is used for the systemic treatment of nodulo-cystic and conglobate acne, severe acne, acne with scarring, or for acne which has not responded to an adequate course of a systemic antibacterial. Isotretinoin is used for the treatment of severe infantile acne resistant to erythromycin p. 355.

Isotretinoin is a toxic drug that should be prescribed **only** by, or under the supervision of, a consultant dermatologist. It is given for at least 16 weeks; repeat courses are not normally required. The drug is **teratogenic** and must **not** be given to females of child-bearing age unless they practise effective contraception (oral progestogen-only contraceptives not considered effective) and then only after detailed assessment and explanation by the physician. They must also be registered with a pregnancy prevention programme.

Although a causal link between isotretinoin use and psychiatric changes (including suicidal ideation) has not been established, the possibility should be considered before initiating treatment; if psychiatric changes occur during treatment, isotretinoin should be stopped, the prescriber informed, and specialist psychiatric advice should be sought.

Rosacea

The adult form of rosacea rarely occurs in children. Persistent or repeated use of potent topical corticosteroids may cause periorificial rosacea (steroid acne). The pustules and papules of rosacea may be treated for at least 6 weeks with a topical metronidazole p. 775 preparation, or a systemic antibacterial such as erythromycin, or for a child over 12 years, oxytetracycline p. 383. Tetracyclines are **contra-indicated** in children under 12 years of age.

6.1 Acne

ANTI-ANDROGENS

Co-cyprindiol

02-Mar-2017

● **INDICATIONS AND DOSE**

Moderate to severe acne in females of child-bearing age refractory to topical therapy or oral antibacterials | Moderately severe hirsutism

▸ BY MOUTH

▸ Females of childbearing potential: 1 tablet daily for 21 days, to be started on day 1 of menstrual cycle; subsequent courses repeated after a 7-day interval (during which withdrawal bleeding occurs), time to symptom remission, at least 3 months; review need for treatment regularly

● **CONTRA-INDICATIONS** Acute porphyrias p. 652 · gallstones · heart disease associated with pulmonary hypertension or risk of embolus · history during pregnancy of cholestatic jaundice · history during pregnancy of chorea · history during pregnancy of pemphigoid gestationis · history during pregnancy of pruritus · history of breast cancer but can be used after 5 years if no evidence of disease and non-hormonal methods unacceptable · history of haemolytic uraemic syndrome · migraine with aura · personal history of venous or arterial thrombosis · presence or history of liver tumours · sclerosing treatment for varicose veins · severe or multiple risk factors for arterial disease or for venous thromboembolism · systemic lupus erythematosus with (or unknown) antiphospholipid antibodies · transient cerebral ischaemic attacks without headaches · undiagnosed vaginal bleeding

● **CAUTIONS** Active trophoblastic disease (until return to normal of urine- and plasma-gonadotrophin concentration)—seek specialist advice · arterial disease · gene mutations associated with breast cancer (e.g. BRCA 1) · history of severe depression especially if induced by hormonal contraceptive · hyperprolactinaemia—seek specialist advice · inflammatory bowel disease including Crohn's disease · migraine · personal or family history of hypertriglyceridaemia (increased risk of pancreatitis) · risk factors for venous thromboembolism · sickle-cell disease · undiagnosed breast mass

CAUTIONS, FURTHER INFORMATION

▸ **Venous thromboembolism** There is an increased risk of venous thromboembolism in women taking co-cyprindiol, particularly during the first year of use. The incidence of venous thromboembolism is 1.5–2 times higher in women using co-cyprindiol than in women using combined oral contraceptives containing levonorgestrel, but the risk may be similar to that associated with use of combined oral contraceptives containing third generation progestogens (desogestrel and gestodene) or drospirenone. Women requiring co-cyprindiol may have an inherently increased risk of cardiovascular disease.

● **INTERACTIONS** → Appendix 1: combined hormonal contraceptives

● **SIDE-EFFECTS**

▸ **Common or very common** Abdominal pain · breast abnormalities · depression · headaches · mood altered · nausea · weight changes

▸ **Uncommon** Diarrhoea · fluid retention · sexual dysfunction · skin reactions · vomiting

▸ **Rare or very rare** Contact lens intolerance · erythema nodosum · thromboembolism · vaginal discharge

▸ **Frequency not known** Amenorrhoea (on discontinuation) · angioedema aggravated · chorea exacerbated · hepatic function abnormal · hepatic neoplasm · hypertension ·

hypertriglyceridaemia · inflammatory bowel disease · menstrual cycle irregularities · suicidal tendencies

- **PREGNANCY** Avoid—risk of feminisation of male fetus with cyproterone.
- **BREAST FEEDING** Manufacturer advises avoid; possibility of anti-androgen effects in neonate with cyproterone.
- **HEPATIC IMPAIRMENT** Manufacturer advises caution; avoid in severe or active disease
- **PRESCRIBING AND DISPENSING INFORMATION** A mixture of cyproterone acetate and ethinylestradiol in the mass proportions 2000 parts to 35 parts, respectively.

- **MEDICINAL FORMS** There can be variation in the licensing of different medicines containing the same drug.

Tablet

- Co-cyprindiol (Non-proprietary)
  Ethinylestradiol 35 microgram, Cyproterone acetate 2 mg Co-cyprindiol 2000microgram/35microgram tablets | 63 tablet PoM £16.65 DT = £10.78
- Clairette (Stragen UK Ltd)
  Ethinylestradiol 35 microgram, Cyproterone acetate 2 mg Clairette 2000/35 tablets | 63 tablet PoM £5.90 DT = £10.78
- Dianette (Bayer Plc)
  Ethinylestradiol 35 microgram, Cyproterone acetate 2 mg Dianette tablets | 63 tablet PoM £7.71 DT = £10.78
- Teragezza (Morningside Healthcare Ltd)
  Ethinylestradiol 35 microgram, Cyproterone acetate 2 mg Teragezza 2000microgram/35microgram tablets | 63 tablet PoM £11.10 DT = £10.78

ANTIBACTERIALS > LINCOSAMIDES

Clindamycin 18-May-2020

- **INDICATIONS AND DOSE**

DALACIN T® LOTION

Acne vulgaris

- TO THE SKIN
  - Child: Apply twice daily, to be applied thinly

DALACIN T® SOLUTION

Acne vulgaris

- TO THE SKIN
  - Child: Apply twice daily, to be applied thinly

ZINDACLIN® GEL

Acne vulgaris

- TO THE SKIN
  - Child 12-17 years: Apply once daily, to be applied thinly

- **INTERACTIONS** → Appendix 1: clindamycin
- **SIDE-EFFECTS**
  - **Common or very common** Skin reactions
  - **Frequency not known** Abdominal pain · antibiotic associated colitis · folliculitis gram-negative · gastrointestinal disorder
- **PATIENT AND CARER ADVICE** Patients and their carers should be advised to discontinue and contact a doctor immediately if severe, prolonged or bloody diarrhoea develops.

- **MEDICINAL FORMS** There can be variation in the licensing of different medicines containing the same drug.

Gel

EXCIPIENTS: May contain Propylene glycol

- Zindaclin (Crawford Healthcare Ltd)
  Clindamycin (as Clindamycin phosphate) 10 mg per 1 gram Zindaclin 1% gel | 30 gram PoM £8.66 DT = £8.66

Liquid

EXCIPIENTS: May contain Cetostearyl alcohol (including cetyl and stearyl alcohol), hydroxybenzoates (parabens), propylene glycol

- Dalacin T (Pfizer Ltd)
  Clindamycin (as Clindamycin phosphate) 10 mg per 1 ml Dalacin T 1% topical lotion | 30 ml PoM £5.08 DT = £5.08 | 60 ml PoM £10.16
  Dalacin T 1% topical solution | 30 ml PoM £4.34 DT = £4.34 | 50 ml PoM £7.23

Combinations available: ***Benzoyl peroxide with clindamycin,*** p. 808 · ***Tretinoin with clindamycin,*** p. 810

ANTIBACTERIALS > MACROLIDES

Erythromycin with zinc acetate 20-Apr-2020

The properties listed below are those particular to the combination only. For the properties of the components please consider, erythromycin p. 355.

- **INDICATIONS AND DOSE**

Acne vulgaris

- TO THE SKIN
  - Child: Apply twice daily

- **INTERACTIONS** → Appendix 1: macrolides

- **MEDICINAL FORMS** There can be variation in the licensing of different medicines containing the same drug.

Liquid

- Zineryt (LEO Pharma)
  Zinc acetate 12 mg per 1 ml, Erythromycin 40 mg per 1 ml Zineryt lotion | 30 ml PoM £9.25 DT = £9.25 | 90 ml PoM £20.02 DT = £20.02

ANTISEPTICS AND DISINFECTANTS > PEROXIDES

Benzoyl peroxide

- **INDICATIONS AND DOSE**

Acne vulgaris

- TO THE SKIN
  - Child 12-17 years: Apply 1–2 times a day, preferably apply after washing with soap and water, start treatment with lower-strength preparations

Infantile acne

- TO THE SKIN
  - Child 1 month-1 year: Apply 1–2 times a day, start treatment with lower-strength preparations

- **UNLICENSED USE** Not licensed for use in treatment of infantile acne.
- **CAUTIONS** Avoid contact with broken skin · avoid contact with eyes · avoid contact with mouth · avoid contact with mucous membranes · avoid excessive exposure to sunlight
- **SIDE-EFFECTS**
  - **Common or very common** Skin reactions
  - **Frequency not known** Facial swelling

  SIDE-EFFECTS, FURTHER INFORMATION Reduce frequency or suspend use until skin irritation subsides and re-introduce at reduced frequency.
- **PATIENT AND CARER ADVICE** May bleach fabrics and hair.

- **MEDICINAL FORMS** There can be variation in the licensing of different medicines containing the same drug.

Gel

EXCIPIENTS: May contain Fragrances, propylene glycol

- Acnecide (Galderma (UK) Ltd)
  Benzoyl peroxide 50 mg per 1 gram Acnecide 5% gel | 30 gram P £5.44 DT = £5.44 | 60 gram P £10.68 DT = £10.68
  Acnecide Wash 5% gel | 50 gram P £5.44 DT = £5.44

Combinations available: ***Adapalene with benzoyl peroxide,*** p. 808

13 Skin

Benzoyl peroxide with clindamycin

09-Mar-2020

The properties listed below are those particular to the combination only. For the properties of the components please consider, benzoyl peroxide p. 807, clindamycin p. 807.

- **INDICATIONS AND DOSE**

Acne vulgaris

▶ TO THE SKIN

▸ Child 12–17 years: Apply once daily, dose to be applied in the evening

- **INTERACTIONS** → Appendix 1: clindamycin

- **MEDICINAL FORMS** There can be variation in the licensing of different medicines containing the same drug.

Gel

EXCIPIENTS: May contain Disodium edetate

▸ Duac (Stiefel Laboratories (UK) Ltd)

Clindamycin (as Clindamycin phosphate) 10 mg per 1 gram, Benzoyl peroxide 30 mg per 1 gram Duac Once Daily gel (3% and 1%) | 30 gram [PoM] £13.14 DT = £13.14 | 60 gram [PoM] £26.28

Clindamycin (as Clindamycin phosphate) 10 mg per 1 gram, Benzoyl peroxide 50 mg per 1 gram Duac Once Daily gel (5% and 1%) | 30 gram [PoM] £13.14 DT = £13.14 | 60 gram [PoM] £26.28 DT = £26.28

DERMATOLOGICAL DRUGS › ANTICOMEDONALS

Azelaic acid

10-Mar-2020

- **INDICATIONS AND DOSE**

FINACEA®

Facial acne vulgaris

▶ TO THE SKIN

▸ Child 12–17 years: Apply twice daily, discontinue if no improvement after 1 month

SKINOREN®

Acne vulgaris

▶ TO THE SKIN

▸ Child 12–17 years: Apply twice daily

Acne vulgaris in patients with sensitive skin

▶ TO THE SKIN

▸ Child 12–17 years: Apply once daily for 1 week, then apply twice daily

- **CAUTIONS** Avoid contact with eyes · avoid contact with mouth · avoid contact with mucous membranes
- **SIDE-EFFECTS**
  - ▶ **Uncommon** Skin reactions
  - ▶ **Rare or very rare** Asthma exacerbated · cheilitis
  - ▶ **Frequency not known** Angioedema · eye swelling

- **MEDICINAL FORMS** There can be variation in the licensing of different medicines containing the same drug.

Cream

EXCIPIENTS: May contain Propylene glycol

▸ Skinoren (LEO Pharma)

Azelaic acid 200 mg per 1 gram Skinoren 20% cream | 30 gram [PoM] £4.49 DT = £4.49

Gel

EXCIPIENTS: May contain Disodium edetate, polysorbates, propylene glycol

▸ Finacea (LEO Pharma)

Azelaic acid 150 mg per 1 gram Finacea 15% gel | 30 gram [PoM] £7.48 DT = £7.48

RETINOID AND RELATED DRUGS

Adapalene

16-Jan-2020

- **INDICATIONS AND DOSE**

Mild to moderate acne vulgaris

▶ TO THE SKIN

▸ Child 12–17 years: Apply once daily, apply thinly in the evening

Infantile acne

▶ TO THE SKIN

▸ Child 1 month–1 year: Apply once daily, apply thinly in the evening

- **UNLICENSED USE** Not licensed for use in infantile acne.
- **CAUTIONS** Avoid accumulation in angles of the nose · avoid contact with eyes, nostrils, mouth and mucous membranes, eczematous, broken or sunburned skin · avoid exposure to UV light (including sunlight, solariums) · avoid in severe acne involving large areas · caution in sensitive areas such as the neck
- **INTERACTIONS** → Appendix 1: retinoids
- **CONCEPTION AND CONTRACEPTION** Females of child-bearing age must use effective contraception (oral progestogen-only contraceptives not considered effective).
- **PREGNANCY** Avoid.
- **BREAST FEEDING** Amount of drug in milk probably too small to be harmful; ensure infant does not come in contact with treated areas.
- **PATIENT AND CARER ADVICE** If sun exposure is unavoidable, an appropriate sunscreen or protective clothing should be used.

- **MEDICINAL FORMS** There can be variation in the licensing of different medicines containing the same drug.

Cream

CAUTIONARY AND ADVISORY LABELS 11

EXCIPIENTS: May contain Disodium edetate, hydroxybenzoates (parabens)

▸ Differin (Galderma (UK) Ltd)

Adapalene 1 mg per 1 gram Differin 0.1% cream | 45 gram [PoM] £16.43 DT = £16.43

Gel

CAUTIONARY AND ADVISORY LABELS 11

EXCIPIENTS: May contain Disodium edetate, hydroxybenzoates (parabens), propylene glycol

▸ Differin (Galderma (UK) Ltd)

Adapalene 1 mg per 1 gram Differin 0.1% gel | 45 gram [PoM] £16.43 DT = £16.43

Adapalene with benzoyl peroxide

09-Mar-2020

The properties listed below are those particular to the combination only. For the properties of the components please consider, adapalene above, benzoyl peroxide p. 807.

- **INDICATIONS AND DOSE**

Acne vulgaris

▶ TO THE SKIN

▸ Child 9–17 years: Apply once daily, to be applied thinly in the evening

- **INTERACTIONS** → Appendix 1: retinoids
- **CONCEPTION AND CONTRACEPTION** Females of child-bearing age must use effective contraception (oral progestogen-only contraceptives not considered effective).
- **PATIENT AND CARER ADVICE** Gel may bleach clothing and hair.

- **NATIONAL FUNDING/ACCESS DECISIONS**

Scottish Medicines Consortium (SMC) decisions

The *Scottish Medicines Consortium* has advised (April 2014) that *Epiduo*® should be restricted for use in mild to moderate facial acne when monotherapy with benzoyl peroxide or adapalene is inappropriate.

- **MEDICINAL FORMS** There can be variation in the licensing of different medicines containing the same drug.

Gel

CAUTIONARY AND ADVISORY LABELS 11

EXCIPIENTS: May contain Disodium edetate, polysorbates, propylene glycol

▸ Adapalene with benzoyl peroxide (Non-proprietary)
Adapalene 3 mg per 1 gram, Benzoyl peroxide 25 mg per 1 gram Epiduo 0.3%/2.5% gel | 45 gram PoM £19.53

▸ Epiduo (Galderma (UK) Ltd)
Adapalene 1 mg per 1 gram, Benzoyl peroxide 25 mg per 1 gram Epiduo 0.1%/2.5% gel | 45 gram PoM £19.53 DT = £19.53

Isotretinoin

12-May-2020

- **INDICATIONS AND DOSE**

Severe acne (under expert supervision) | Acne which is associated with psychological problems (under expert supervision) | Acne which has not responded to an adequate course of a systemic antibacterial (under expert supervision) | Acne with scarring (under expert supervision) | Systemic treatment of nodulo-cystic and conglobate acne (under expert supervision)

▸ BY MOUTH

▸ Child 12–17 years: Initially 500 micrograms/kg daily in 1–2 divided doses, increased if necessary to 1 mg/kg daily for 16–24 weeks, repeat treatment course after a period of at least 8 weeks if relapse after first course; maximum 150 mg/kg per course

Severe infantile acne (under expert supervision)

▸ BY MOUTH

▸ Child 1 month–1 year: Initially 200 micrograms/kg daily in 1–2 divided doses, increased if necessary to 1 mg/kg daily for 16–24 weeks; maximum 150 mg/kg per course

- **UNLICENSED USE** Not licensed for use in infantile acne.

IMPORTANT SAFETY INFORMATION

MHRA/CHM ADVICE: ISOTRETINOIN (*ROACCUTANE*®): RARE REPORTS OF ERECTILE DYSFUNCTION AND DECREASED LIBIDO (OCTOBER 2017)

An EU-wide review has concluded that on rare occasions, oral isotretinoin, indicated for severe acne, may cause sexual side-effects, including erectile dysfunction and decreased libido.

MHRA/CHM ADVICE: ORAL RETINOID MEDICINES: REVISED AND SIMPLIFIED PREGNANCY PREVENTION EDUCATIONAL MATERIALS FOR HEALTHCARE PROFESSIONALS AND WOMEN (JUNE 2019)

New prescriber checklists, patient reminder cards, and pharmacy checklists are available to support the Pregnancy Prevention Programme in women and girls of childbearing potential taking oral acitretin, alitretinoin, or isotretinoin. Healthcare professionals are reminded that the use of oral retinoids is contra-indicated in pregnancy due to a high risk of serious congenital malformations, and any use in females must be within the conditions of the Pregnancy Prevention Programme (see *Conception and contraception* and *Prescribing and dispensing information*).

Neuropsychiatric reactions have been reported in patients taking oral retinoids. Healthcare professionals are advised to monitor patients for signs of depression or suicidal ideation and refer for appropriate treatment, if necessary; particular care is needed in those with a history of depression. Patients should be advised to speak to their doctor if they experience any changes in mood or behaviour, and encouraged to ask family and friends to look out for any change in mood.

- **CONTRA-INDICATIONS** Hyperlipidaemia · hypervitaminosis A
- **CAUTIONS** Avoid blood donation during treatment and for at least 1 month after treatment · diabetes · dry eye syndrome (associated with risk of keratitis) · history of depression (risk of neuropsychiatric reactions)
- **INTERACTIONS** → Appendix 1: retinoids
- **SIDE-EFFECTS**

▸ **Common or very common** Alopecia · anaemia · arthralgia · back pain · cheilitis · dry eye · eye discomfort · eye inflammation · haemorrhage · headache · increased risk of infection · myalgia · nasal dryness · neutropenia · proteinuria · skin fragility (trauma may cause blistering) · skin reactions · thrombocytopenia · thrombocytosis

▸ **Rare or very rare** Anxiety · arthritis · behaviour abnormal · bone disorders · bronchospasm · cataract · corneal opacity · depression · diabetes mellitus · dizziness · drowsiness · dry throat · gastrointestinal disorders · glomerulonephritis · hair changes · hearing impairment · hepatitis · hoarseness · hyperhidrosis · hyperuricaemia · idiopathic intracranial hypertension · inflammatory bowel disease · lymphadenopathy · malaise · mood altered · nail dystrophy · nausea · pancreatitis · photosensitivity reaction · psychotic disorder · pyogenic granuloma · seizure · suicidal tendencies · tendinitis · vasculitis · vision disorders

▸ **Frequency not known** Rhabdomyolysis · severe cutaneous adverse reactions (SCARs)

SIDE-EFFECTS, FURTHER INFORMATION Risk of pancreatitis if triglycerides above 9 mmol/litre—discontinue if uncontrolled hypertriglyceridaemia or pancreatitis.

Discontinue treatment if skin peeling severe or haemorrhagic diarrhoea develops.

Visual disturbances require expert referral and possible withdrawal.

Psychiatric side-effects could require expert referral.

- **CONCEPTION AND CONTRACEPTION** The MHRA advises that women and girls of childbearing potential being treated with the oral retinoids acitretin, alitretinoin, or isotretinoin must be supported on a Pregnancy Prevention Programme with regular follow-up and pregnancy testing.

Pregnancy prevention Effective contraception must be used.

In females of childbearing potential, exclude pregnancy a few days before treatment, every month during treatment (unless there are compelling reasons to indicate that there is no risk of pregnancy), and 4 weeks after stopping treatment. Females must practise effective contraception for at least 1 month before starting treatment, during treatment, and for at least 1 month after stopping treatment. They should be advised to use at least 1 method of contraception, but ideally they should use 2 methods of contraception. Oral progestogen-only contraceptives are not considered effective. Barrier methods should not be used alone, but can be used in conjunction with other contraceptive methods. Females should be advised to discontinue treatment and to seek prompt medical attention if they become pregnant during treatment or within 1 month of stopping treatment.

- **PREGNANCY** Manufacturer advises avoid—teratogenic.
- **BREAST FEEDING** Avoid.
- **HEPATIC IMPAIRMENT** Manufacturer advises avoid—limited information available.
- **RENAL IMPAIRMENT**

Dose adjustments In severe impairment, reduce initial dose and increase gradually, if necessary, up to 1 mg/kg daily as tolerated.

- **MONITORING REQUIREMENTS** Measure hepatic function and serum lipids before treatment, 1 month after starting and then every 3 months (reduce dose or discontinue if transaminase or serum lipids persistently raised).
- **PRESCRIBING AND DISPENSING INFORMATION** Isotretinoin is an isomer of tretinoin.
Prescribing for females of childbearing potential The Pregnancy Prevention Programme is supported by the following materials provided by the manufacturer: *Checklists for prescribers and pharmacists*, and *Patient reminder cards*.
Each prescription for oral isotretinoin should be limited to a supply of up to 30 days' treatment. Pregnancy testing should ideally be carried out on the same day as prescription issuing and dispensing.
- **PATIENT AND CARER ADVICE** Warn patient to avoid wax epilation (risk of epidermal stripping), dermabrasion, and laser skin treatments (risk of scarring) during treatment and for at least 6 months after stopping; patient should avoid exposure to UV light (including sunlight) and use sunscreen and emollient (including lip balm) preparations from the start of treatment.
Risk of neuropsychiatric reactions The MHRA advises patients and carers to seek medical attention if changes in mood or behaviour occur.
Pregnancy Prevention Programme Pharmacists must ensure that female patients have a patient card—see also *Important safety information*.

13 Skin

- **MEDICINAL FORMS** There can be variation in the licensing of different medicines containing the same drug.

Capsule

CAUTIONARY AND ADVISORY LABELS 10, 11, 21

- ▸ **Isotretinoin (Non-proprietary)**
Isotretinoin 5 mg Isotretinoin 5mg capsules | 30 capsule PoM £10.10–£10.15 | 56 capsule PoM £14.78–£14.79 DT = £14.79
Isotretinoin 10 mg Isotretinoin 10mg capsules | 30 capsule PoM £14.54 DT = £14.53
Isotretinoin 20 mg Isotretinoin 20mg capsules | 30 capsule PoM £20.00 DT = £16.66 | 56 capsule PoM £31.10–£37.85
Isotretinoin 40 mg Isotretinoin 40mg capsules | 30 capsule PoM £38.98 DT = £38.98
- ▸ **Roaccutane** (Roche Products Ltd)
Isotretinoin 10 mg Roaccutane 10mg capsules | 30 capsule PoM £14.54 DT = £14.53
Isotretinoin 20 mg Roaccutane 20mg capsules | 30 capsule PoM £20.02 DT = £16.66

Tretinoin with clindamycin

10-Mar-2020

The properties listed below are those particular to the combination only. For the properties of the components please consider, tretinoin p. 599, clindamycin p. 807.

- **INDICATIONS AND DOSE**

Facial acne

▸ TO THE SKIN

▸ Child 12–17 years: Apply daily, (to be applied thinly at bedtime)

- **CONTRA-INDICATIONS** Perioral dermatitis · personal or familial history of skin cancer · rosacea
- **CAUTIONS** Allow peeling (resulting from other irritant treatments) to subside before using a topical retinoid · avoid accumulation in angles of the nose · avoid contact with eyes, nostrils, mouth and mucous membranes, eczematous, broken or sunburned skin · avoid exposure to UV light (including sunlight, solariums) · avoid use of topical retinoids with keratolytic agents, abrasive cleaners, comedogenic or astringent cosmetics · caution in sensitive areas such as the neck · severe acne
- **INTERACTIONS** → Appendix 1: clindamycin · retinoids
- **SIDE-EFFECTS** Dry skin (discontinue if severe) · eye irritation · oedema · photosensitivity reaction · skin pigmentation change (transient) · skin reactions
- **CONCEPTION AND CONTRACEPTION** Females of child-bearing age must use effective contraception (oral progestogen-only contraceptives not considered effective).
- **PREGNANCY** Contra-indicated in pregnancy.
- **BREAST FEEDING** Amount of drug in milk after topical application probably too small to be harmful; ensure infant does not come in contact with treated areas.
- **PATIENT AND CARER ADVICE** If sun exposure is unavoidable, an appropriate sunscreen or protective clothing should be used.
Patients and carers should be warned that some redness and skin peeling can occur initially but settles with time. If undue irritation occurs, the frequency of application should be reduced or treatment suspended until the reaction subsides; if irritation persists, discontinue treatment. Several months of treatment may be needed to achieve an optimal response and the treatment should be continued until no new lesions develop.

- **MEDICINAL FORMS** There can be variation in the licensing of different medicines containing the same drug.

Gel

CAUTIONARY AND ADVISORY LABELS 11

EXCIPIENTS: May contain Butylated hydroxytoluene, hydroxybenzoates (parabens), polysorbates

- ▸ **Treclin** (Mylan)
Tretinoin 250 microgram per 1 gram, Clindamycin (as Clindamycin phosphate) 10 mg per 1 gram Treclin 1%/0.025% gel | 30 gram PoM £11.94 DT = £11.94

Tretinoin with erythromycin

03-Apr-2020

The properties listed below are those particular to the combination only. For the properties of the components please consider, tretinoin p. 599, erythromycin p. 355.

- **INDICATIONS AND DOSE**

Acne

▸ TO THE SKIN

▸ Child: Apply 1–2 times a day, apply thinly

- **CONTRA-INDICATIONS** Perioral dermatitis · personal or familial history of skin cancer · rosacea
- **CAUTIONS** Allow peeling (resulting from other irritant treatments) to subside before using a topical retinoid · avoid accumulation in angles of the nose · avoid contact with eyes, nostrils, mouth and mucous membranes, eczematous, broken or sunburned skin · avoid exposure to UV light (including sunlight, solariums) · avoid use of topical retinoids with keratolytic agents, abrasive cleaners, comedogenic or astringent cosmetics · caution in sensitive areas such as the neck · severe acne
- **INTERACTIONS** → Appendix 1: macrolides · retinoids
- **SIDE-EFFECTS** Dry skin (discontinue if severe) · eye irritation · oedema · photosensitivity reaction · skin eruption · skin pigmentation change (transient)
- **CONCEPTION AND CONTRACEPTION** Females of child-bearing age must use effective contraception (oral progestogen-only contraceptives not considered effective).
- **PREGNANCY** Contra-indicated in pregnancy.
- **BREAST FEEDING** Amount of drug in milk after topical application probably too small to be harmful; ensure infant does not come in contact with treated areas.
- **PATIENT AND CARER ADVICE** Patients and carers should be warned that some redness and skin peeling can occur initially but settles with time. If undue irritation occurs,

the frequency of application should be reduced or treatment suspended until the reaction subsides; if irritation persists, discontinue treatment. Several months of treatment may be needed to achieve an optimal response and the treatment should be continued until no new lesions develop. If sun exposure is unavoidable, an appropriate sunscreen or protective clothing should be used.

- **MEDICINAL FORMS** There can be variation in the licensing of different medicines containing the same drug.

Liquid

CAUTIONARY AND ADVISORY LABELS 11

- Aknemycin Plus (Almirall Ltd)
  Tretinoin 250 microgram per 1 gram, Erythromycin 40 mg per 1 gram Aknemycin Plus solution | 25 ml PoM £7.05 DT = £7.05

VITAMINS AND TRACE ELEMENTS > VITAMIN B GROUP

Nicotinamide

06-May-2020

- **INDICATIONS AND DOSE**

Inflammatory acne vulgaris

- TO THE SKIN
- Child: Apply twice daily, reduced to once daily or on alternate days, dose reduced if irritation occurs

- **CAUTIONS** Avoid contact with eyes · avoid contact with mucous membranes (including nose and mouth) · reduce frequency of application if excessive dryness, irritation or peeling
- **SIDE-EFFECTS** Paraesthesia · skin reactions

- **MEDICINAL FORMS** There can be variation in the licensing of different medicines containing the same drug.

Gel

- Freederm (Dendron Ltd)
  Nicotinamide 40 mg per 1 gram Freederm Treatment 4% gel | 25 gram P £5.56 DT = £5.56
- Nicam (Dermal Laboratories Ltd)
  Nicotinamide 40 mg per 1 gram Nicam 4% gel | 60 gram P £7.10 DT = £7.10

7 Scalp and hair conditions

Scalp and hair conditions

Overview

The detergent action of shampoo removes grease (sebum) from hair. Prepubertal children produce very little grease and require shampoo less frequently than adults. Shampoos can be used as vehicles for medicinal products, but their usefulness is limited by the short time the product is in contact with the scalp and by their irritant nature.

Oils and ointments are very useful for scaly, dry scalp conditions; if a greasy appearance is cosmetically unacceptable, the preparation may be applied at night and washed out in the morning. Alcohol-based lotions are rarely used in children; alcohol causes painful stinging on broken skin and the fumes may exacerbate asthma.

Itchy, inflammatory, eczematous scalp conditions may be relieved by a simple emollient oil such as **olive oil** or **coconut oil** (arachis oil (ground nut oil, peanut oil) is best avoided in children under 5 years). In more severe cases a topical **corticosteroid** may be required. Preparations containing **coal tar** are used for the common scaly scalp conditions of childhood including seborrhoeic dermatitis, dandruff (a mild form of seborrhoeic dermatitis), and psoriasis; salicylic acid p. 820 is used as a keratolytic in some scalp preparations.

Shampoos containing antimicrobials such as selenium below or ketoconazole p. 777 are used for seborrhoeic dermatitis and dandruff in which yeast infection has been implicated, and for tinea capitis (ringworm of the scalp). Bacterial infection affecting the scalp (usually secondary to eczema, head lice, or ringworm) may be treated with shampoos containing antimicrobials such as **pyrithione zinc**, cetrimide, or povidone-iodine p. 813

In neonates and infants, *cradle cap* (which is also a form of seborrhoeic eczema) can be treated by massaging **coconut oil** or **olive oil** into the scalp; a bland emollient such as **emulsifying ointment** can be rubbed onto the affected area once or twice daily before bathing and a mild shampoo used.

Other drugs used for Scalp and hair conditions Coal tar, p. 796 · Coal tar with salicylic acid and precipitated sulfur, p. 797

ANTISEPTICS AND DISINFECTANTS > UNDECENOATES

Cetrimide with undecenoic acid

- **INDICATIONS AND DOSE**

Scalp psoriasis | Seborrhoeic dermatitis | Dandruff

- TO THE SKIN
- Child: Apply 3 times a week for 1 week, then apply twice weekly

- **MEDICINAL FORMS** There can be variation in the licensing of different medicines containing the same drug.

Shampoo

- Ceanel (Alliance Pharmaceuticals Ltd)
  Undecenoic acid 10 mg per 1 ml, Phenylethyl alcohol 75 mg per 1 ml, Cetrimide 100 mg per 1 ml Ceanel Concentrate shampoo | 150 ml P £3.40 | 500 ml P £9.80

ANTISEPTICS AND DISINFECTANTS > OTHER

Benzalkonium chloride

26-Mar-2020

- **INDICATIONS AND DOSE**

Seborrhoeic scalp conditions associated with dandruff and scaling

- TO THE SKIN
- Child: Apply as required

- **MEDICINAL FORMS** There can be variation in the licensing of different medicines containing the same drug.

Shampoo

- Dermax (Dermal Laboratories Ltd)
  Benzalkonium chloride 5 mg per 1 ml Dermax Therapeutic 0.5% shampoo | 250 ml P £5.69 DT = £5.69

VITAMINS AND TRACE ELEMENTS

Selenium

- **INDICATIONS AND DOSE**

Seborrhoeic dermatitis | Dandruff

- TO THE SKIN USING SHAMPOO
- Child 5–17 years: Apply twice weekly for 2 weeks, then apply once weekly for 2 weeks, then apply as required

Pityriasis versicolor

- TO THE SKIN USING SHAMPOO
- Child 5–17 years: Apply once daily for 7 days, apply to the affected area and leave on for 10 minutes before rinsing off. The course may be repeated if continued →

necessary. Diluting with a small amount of water prior to application can reduce irritation

- **UNLICENSED USE** The use of selenium sulfide shampoo as a lotion for the treatment of pityriasis (tinea) versicolor is an unlicensed indication.
- **INTERACTIONS** → Appendix 1: selenium
- **PATIENT AND CARER ADVICE** Avoid using 48 hours before or after applying hair colouring, straightening or waving preparations.

- **MEDICINAL FORMS** There can be variation in the licensing of different medicines containing the same drug.

Shampoo

EXCIPIENTS: May contain Fragrances

- Selsun (Chattem (U.K.) Ltd)

  Selenium sulfide 25 mg per 1 ml Selsun 2.5% shampoo | 50 ml [P] £1.61 DT = £1.61 | 100 ml [P] £2.15 DT = £2.15 | 150 ml [P] £3.06 DT = £3.06

8 Skin cleansers, antiseptics and desloughing agents

Skin cleansers, antiseptics and desloughing agents

Skin cleansers and antiseptics

Soap or detergent is used with water to cleanse intact skin but they can irritate infantile skin; emollient preparations such as aqueous cream or emulsifying ointment can be used in place of soap or detergent for cleansing dry or irritated skin.

An antiseptic is used for skin that is infected or that is susceptible to recurrent infection. Detergent preparations containing chlorhexidine p. 813 or povidone-iodine p. 813, which should be thoroughly rinsed off, are used. Emollients may also contain antiseptics.

Antiseptics such as chlorhexidine or povidone-iodine are used on intact skin before surgical procedures; their antiseptic effect is enhanced by an alcoholic solvent. Antiseptic solutions containing cetrimide can be used if a detergent effect is also required.

Preparations containing alcohol, and regular use of povidone-iodine, should be avoided on neonatal skin.

Hydrogen peroxide p. 814, an oxidising agent, is available as a cream and can be used for superficial bacterial skin infections.

For irrigating ulcers or wounds, lukewarm sterile sodium chloride 0.9% solution p. 636 is used but tap water is often appropriate.

Potassium permanganate 1 in 10 000 solution below, a mild antiseptic with astringent properties, can be used as a soak for exudative eczematous areas; treatment should be stopped when the skin becomes dry.

Desloughing agents

Alginate, hydrogel, and hydrocolloid dressings are effective in wound debridement. Sterile larvae (maggots) (available from BioMonde) are also used for managing sloughing wounds and are prescribable on the NHS.

Desloughing solutions and creams are of little clinical value. Substances applied to an open area are easily absorbed and perilesional skin is easily sensitised.

ANTISEPTICS AND DISINFECTANTS

Potassium permanganate

26-Jun-2019

- **INDICATIONS AND DOSE**

Cleansing and deodorising suppurating eczematous reactions and wounds

- TO THE SKIN
- Child: For wet dressings or baths, use approximately 0.01% (1 in 10 000) solution

IMPORTANT SAFETY INFORMATION

NHS IMPROVEMENT PATIENT SAFETY ALERT: RISK OF DEATH OR SERIOUS HARM FROM ACCIDENTAL INGESTION OF POTASSIUM PERMANGANATE PREPARATIONS (DECEMBER 2014)

Potassium permanganate is for external use only. Oral ingestion can cause fatality due to local inflammatory reactions that block the airways or cause perforations of the gastrointestinal tract, or through toxicity and organ failure. Following a number of reports of ingestion, NHS England advises that healthcare professionals should consider whether action needs to be taken locally to reduce the risk of accidental ingestion occurring.

Potassium permanganate is subject to the requirements of Control of Substances Hazardous to Health including: separate storage, additional hazard labelling, and issue only to staff and patients who have been educated to understand its safe use. Accidental ingestion should be treated as a medical emergency.

- **CAUTIONS** Irritant to mucous membranes
- **DIRECTIONS FOR ADMINISTRATION** Potassium permanganate 0.1% solution to be diluted 1 in 10 to provide a 0.01% (1 in 10 000) solution. With potassium permanganate tablets for solution, 1 tablet dissolved in 4 litres of water provides a 0.01% (1 in 10 000) solution.
- **PATIENT AND CARER ADVICE** Can stain clothing, skin and nails (especially with prolonged use).

- **MEDICINAL FORMS** There can be variation in the licensing of different medicines containing the same drug. Forms available from special-order manufacturers include: liquid

Tablet for cutaneous solution

- EN-Potab (Ennogen Healthcare Ltd)

  Potassium permanganate 400 mg EN-Potab 400mg tablets for cutaneous solution | 30 tablet [S] DT = £19.92
- Permitabs (Alliance Pharmaceuticals Ltd)

  Potassium permanganate 400 mg Permitabs 400mg tablets for cutaneous solution | 30 tablet £19.92 DT = £19.92

ANTISEPTICS AND DISINFECTANTS > ALCOHOL DISINFECTANTS

Alcohol

(Industrial methylated spirit)

- **INDICATIONS AND DOSE**

Skin preparation before injection

- TO THE SKIN
- Child: Apply as required

- **CONTRA-INDICATIONS** Neonates
- **CAUTIONS** Avoid broken skin · flammable · patients have suffered severe burns when diathermy has been preceded by application of alcoholic skin disinfectants
- **PRESCRIBING AND DISPENSING INFORMATION** Industrial methylated spirits defined by the BP as a mixture of 19 volumes of ethyl alcohol of an appropriate strength with 1 volume of approved wood naphtha.

- **MEDICINAL FORMS** There can be variation in the licensing of different medicines containing the same drug.

Liquid

- Alcohol (Non-proprietary)
  Industrial methylated spirit 70% | 600 ml £6.56–£7.01

ANTISEPTICS AND DISINFECTANTS > IODINE PRODUCTS

Povidone-iodine

- **INDICATIONS AND DOSE**

Skin disinfection

- TO THE SKIN
- Child: (consult product literature)

BETADINE® DRY POWDER SPRAY

Skin disinfection, particularly minor wounds and infections

- TO THE SKIN
- Child 2–17 years: Not for use in serous cavities (consult product literature)

VIDENE® SOLUTION

Skin disinfection

- TO THE SKIN
- Child: Apply undiluted in pre-operative skin disinfection and general antisepsis

VIDENE® SURGICAL SCRUB®

Skin disinfection

- TO THE SKIN
- Child: Use as a pre-operative scrub for hand and skin disinfection

VIDENE® TINCTURE

Skin disinfection

- TO THE SKIN
- Child: Apply undiluted in pre-operative skin disinfection

- **CONTRA-INDICATIONS** Concomitant use of lithium · corrected gestational age under 32 weeks · infants body-weight under 1.5 kg · regular use in neonates
  VIDENE® TINCTURE Neonates
- **CAUTIONS** Broken skin · large open wounds
  CAUTIONS, FURTHER INFORMATION
  - Large open wounds The application of povidone–iodine to large wounds or severe burns may produce systemic adverse effects such as metabolic acidosis, hypernatraemia and impairment of renal function.
  VIDENE® TINCTURE Procedures involving hot wire cautery and diathermy
- **SIDE-EFFECTS** Acute kidney injury · goitre · hyperthyroidism · hypothyroidism · metabolic acidosis · skin burning sensation
- **PREGNANCY** Sufficient iodine may be absorbed to affect the fetal thyroid in the second and third trimester.
- **BREAST FEEDING** Avoid regular or excessive use.
- **RENAL IMPAIRMENT** Avoid regular application to inflamed or broken skin or mucosa.
- **EFFECT ON LABORATORY TESTS** May interfere with thyroid function tests.

- **MEDICINAL FORMS** There can be variation in the licensing of different medicines containing the same drug. Forms available from special-order manufacturers include: eye drops, eye lotion, liquid

Spray

- Betadine (Aspire Pharma Ltd)
  Povidone-Iodine 25 mg per 1 gram Betadine 2.5% dry powder spray | 100 ml GSL £9.95 DT = £9.95

Liquid

CAUTIONARY AND ADVISORY LABELS 15 (Only for use with alcoholic solutions)

- Videne (Ecolab Healthcare Division)
  Povidone-Iodine 75 mg per 1 ml Videne 7.5% surgical scrub solution | 500 ml P £7.97 DT = £7.97
  Povidone-Iodine 100 mg per 1 ml Videne 10% antiseptic solution | 500 ml P £7.97 DT = £7.97
  Videne 10% alcoholic tincture | 500 ml P £7.97 DT = £7.97

ANTISEPTICS AND DISINFECTANTS > OTHER

Chlorhexidine

21-Nov-2019

- **INDICATIONS AND DOSE**

CEPTON® LOTION

For skin disinfection in acne

- TO THE SKIN
- Child: (consult product literature)

CEPTON® SKIN WASH

For use as skin wash in acne

- TO THE SKIN
- Child: (consult product literature)

HIBITANE® PLUS 5% CONCENTRATE SOLUTION

General and pre-operative skin disinfection

- TO THE SKIN
- Child: (consult product literature)

HIBISCRUB®

Pre-operative hand and skin disinfection | General hand and skin disinfection

- TO THE SKIN
- Child: Use as alternative to soap (consult product literature)

HIBITANE OBSTETRIC®

For use in obstetrics and gynaecology as an antiseptic and lubricant

- TO THE SKIN
- Child: To be applied to skin around vulva and perineum and to hands of midwife or doctor

HIBI® LIQUID HAND RUB+

Hand and skin disinfection

- TO THE SKIN
- Child: To be used undiluted (consult product literature)

HYDREX® SOLUTION

For pre-operative skin disinfection

- TO THE SKIN
- Child: (consult product literature)

HYDREX® SURGICAL SCRUB

For pre-operative hand and skin disinfection | General hand disinfection

- TO THE SKIN
- Child: (consult product literature)

UNISEPT®

For cleansing and disinfecting wounds and burns and swabbing in obstetrics

- TO THE SKIN
- Child: (consult product literature)

IMPORTANT SAFETY INFORMATION

MHRA/CHM ADVICE: CHLORHEXIDINE SOLUTIONS: REMINDER OF THE RISK OF CHEMICAL BURNS IN PREMATURE INFANTS (NOVEMBER 2014)

In premature infants, use sparingly, monitor for skin reactions, and do not allow solution to pool—risk of severe chemical burns.

- **CONTRA-INDICATIONS** Alcoholic solutions not suitable for use on neonatal skin · not for use in body cavities

13 Skin

- **CAUTIONS** Avoid contact with brain · avoid contact with eyes · avoid contact with meninges · avoid contact with middle ear · use prior to diathermy (alcohol containing skin disinfectants)
- **SIDE-EFFECTS** Skin reactions
- **DIRECTIONS FOR ADMINISTRATION**

HIBITANE® PLUS 5% CONCENTRATE SOLUTION For pre-operative skin preparation, dilute 1 in 10 (0.5%) with alcohol 70%. For general skin disinfection, dilute 1 in 100 (0.05%) with water. Alcoholic solutions not suitable for use before diathermy or on neonatal skin.

- **MEDICINAL FORMS** There can be variation in the licensing of different medicines containing the same drug.

Cream

- Hibitane Obstetric (Derma UK Ltd)
  Chlorhexidine gluconate 10 mg per 1 gram Hibitane Obstetric 1% cream | 250 ml GSL £19.23 DT = £19.23

Liquid

CAUTIONARY AND ADVISORY LABELS 15 (For ethanolic solutions (e.g. ChloraPrep® and Hydrex® only)
EXCIPIENTS: May contain Fragrances

- Cepton (Boston Healthcare Ltd)
  Chlorhexidine gluconate 10 mg per 1 ml Cepton 1% medicated skin wash | 150 ml GSL £34.75 DT = £34.75
- HiBiTane Plus (Molnlycke Health Care Ltd)
  Chlorhexidine gluconate 50 mg per 1 ml HiBiTane Plus 5% concentrate solution | 5000 ml GSL £14.50 DT = £14.50
- Hibi (Molnlycke Health Care Ltd)
  Chlorhexidine gluconate 5 mg per 1 ml HiBi Liquid Hand Rub+ 0.5% solution | 500 ml GSL £5.25 DT = £5.25
- Hibiscrub (Molnlycke Health Care Ltd)
  Chlorhexidine gluconate 40 mg per 1 ml HiBiScrub 4% solution | 125 ml GSL £1.50 | 250 ml GSL £4.25 DT = £4.25 | 500 ml GSL £5.25 DT = £5.25 | 5000 ml GSL £24.00 DT = £24.00
- Hydrex (Ecolab Healthcare Division)
  Chlorhexidine gluconate 5 mg per 1 ml Hydrex pink chlorhexidine gluconate 0.5% solution | 600 ml GSL £4.91 DT = £4.91
  Hydrex clear chlorhexidine gluconate 0.5% solution | 600 ml GSL £4.91 DT = £4.91
  Chlorhexidine gluconate 40 mg per 1 ml Hydrex 4% Surgical Scrub | 250 ml GSL £4.47 DT = £4.25 | 500 ml GSL £4.96 DT = £5.25
- Sterets Unisept (Molnlycke Health Care Ltd)
  Chlorhexidine gluconate 500 microgram per 1 ml Sterets Unisept 0.05% solution 25ml sachets | 25 sachet P £5.54 DT = £5.54
  Sterets Unisept 0.05% solution 100ml sachets | 10 sachet P £6.83 DT = £6.83

Chlorhexidine gluconate with isopropyl alcohol

The properties listed below are those particular to the combination only. For the properties of the components please consider, chlorhexidine p. 813.

- **INDICATIONS AND DOSE**

Skin disinfection before invasive procedures

▶ TO THE SKIN
- Child 2 months–17 years: (consult product literature)

- **MEDICINAL FORMS** There can be variation in the licensing of different medicines containing the same drug. Forms available from special-order manufacturers include: liquid

Liquid

CAUTIONARY AND ADVISORY LABELS 15

- ChloraPrep (CareFusion U.K. Ltd)
  Chlorhexidine gluconate 20 mg per 1 ml, Isopropyl alcohol 700 ml per 1 litre ChloraPrep with Tint solution 10.5ml applicators | 25 applicator GSL £76.65 DT = £73.00
  ChloraPrep with Tint solution 26ml applicators | 25 applicator GSL £170.75 DT = £162.50
  ChloraPrep solution 3ml applicators | 25 applicator GSL £21.25 DT = £21.25
  ChloraPrep solution 1.5ml applicators | 20 applicator GSL £11.00 DT = £11.00
  ChloraPrep with Tint solution 3ml applicators | 25 applicator GSL £22.31 DT = £21.25
  ChloraPrep solution 0.67ml applicators | 200 applicator GSL £60.00 DT = £60.00
  ChloraPrep solution 10.5ml applicators | 25 applicator GSL £73.00 DT = £73.00
  ChloraPrep solution 26ml applicators | 25 applicator GSL £162.50 DT = £162.50

Chlorhexidine with cetrimide

The properties listed below are those particular to the combination only. For the properties of the components please consider, chlorhexidine p. 813.

- **INDICATIONS AND DOSE**

Skin disinfection such as wound cleansing and obstetrics

▶ TO THE SKIN
- Child: To be used undiluted

- **MEDICINAL FORMS** There can be variation in the licensing of different medicines containing the same drug.

Cream

- Savlon (Thornton & Ross Ltd)
  Chlorhexidine gluconate 1 mg per 1 gram, Cetrimide 5 mg per 1 gram Savlon antiseptic cream | 15 gram GSL £0.90 DT = £0.90 | 30 gram GSL £1.19 DT = £1.19 | 60 gram GSL £1.91 DT = £1.91 | 100 gram GSL £2.78 DT = £2.78

Irrigation solution

- Chlorhexidine with cetrimide (Non-proprietary)
  Chlorhexidine acetate 150 microgram per 1 ml, Cetrimide 1.5 mg per 1 ml Chlorhexidine acetate 0.015% / Cetrimide 0.15% irrigation solution 1litre bottles | 1 bottle P

Liquid

- Sterets Tisept (Molnlycke Health Care Ltd)
  Chlorhexidine gluconate 150 microgram per 1 ml, Cetrimide 1.5 mg per 1 ml Sterets Tisept solution 25ml sachets | 25 sachet P £5.33 DT = £5.33
  Sterets Tisept solution 100ml sachets | 10 sachet P £6.85 DT = £6.85

Diethyl phthalate with methyl salicylate

- **INDICATIONS AND DOSE**

Skin preparation before injection

▶ TO THE SKIN
- Child: Apply to the area to be disinfected

- **MEDICINAL FORMS** There can be variation in the licensing of different medicines containing the same drug.

Liquid

CAUTIONARY AND ADVISORY LABELS 15

- Diethyl phthalate with methyl salicylate (Non-proprietary)
  Methyl salicylate 5 ml per 1 litre, Diethyl phthalate 20 ml per 1 litre, Castor oil 25 ml per 1 litre, Industrial methylated spirit 950 ml per 1 litre Surgical spirit | 200 ml GSL £1.17 DT = £1.17 | 1000 ml GSL £4.03

Hydrogen peroxide

29-Apr-2020

- **DRUG ACTION** Hydrogen peroxide is an oxidising agent.

- **INDICATIONS AND DOSE**

CRYSTACIDE®

Superficial bacterial skin infection

▶ TO THE SKIN
- Child: Apply 2–3 times a day for up to 3 weeks

Localised non-bullous impetigo [in patients who are not systemically unwell or at high risk of complications]

▶ TO THE SKIN
- Child: Apply 2–3 times a day for 5–7 days

- **UNLICENSED USE** Licensed for use in children (age range not specified by manufacturer).
- **CONTRA-INDICATIONS** Deep wounds · large wounds
- **CAUTIONS** Avoid on eyes · avoid on healthy skin · incompatible with products containing iodine or potassium permanganate
- **PRESCRIBING AND DISPENSING INFORMATION** The BP directs that when hydrogen peroxide is prescribed, hydrogen peroxide solution 6% (20 vols) should be dispensed.

  Strong solutions of hydrogen peroxide which contain 27% (90 vols) and 30% (100 vols) are only for the preparation of weaker solutions.

  CRYSTACIDE ® For choice of therapy, see Skin infections, antibacterial therapy p. 329.
- **HANDLING AND STORAGE** Hydrogen peroxide bleaches fabric.

- **MEDICINAL FORMS** There can be variation in the licensing of different medicines containing the same drug. Forms available from special-order manufacturers include: liquid

Cream

EXCIPIENTS: May contain Edetic acid (edta), propylene glycol

▸ Crystacide (Reig Jofre UK Ltd)
Hydrogen peroxide 10 mg per 1 gram Crystacide 1% cream | 25 gram Ⓟ £8.07 DT = £8.07 | 40 gram Ⓟ £11.62

Proflavine

- **INDICATIONS AND DOSE**

Infected wounds | Infected burns

▸ TO THE SKIN
▸ Child: (consult product literature)

- **PATIENT AND CARER ADVICE** Stains clothing.

- **MEDICINAL FORMS** Forms available from special-order manufacturers include: liquid

Irrigation solutions

- **IRRIGATION SOLUTIONS**

Flowfusor sodium chloride 0.9% irrigation solution 120ml bottles (Fresenius Kabi Ltd) **Sodium chloride 9 mg per 1 ml** 1 bottle · NHS indicative price = £1.71 · Drug Tariff (Part IXa)

Irriclens sodium chloride 0.9% irrigation solution aerosol spray (ConvaTec Ltd) **Sodium chloride 9 mg per 1 ml** 240 ml · NHS indicative price = £3.64 · Drug Tariff (Part IXa)

Normasol sodium chloride 0.9% irrigation solution 100ml sachets (Molnlycke Health Care Ltd) **Sodium chloride 9 mg per 1 ml** 10 unit dose · NHS indicative price = £8.06 · Drug Tariff (Part IXa)

Normasol sodium chloride 0.9% irrigation solution 25ml sachets (Molnlycke Health Care Ltd) **Sodium chloride 9 mg per 1 ml** 25 unit dose · NHS indicative price = £6.53 · Drug Tariff (Part IXa)

Sodium chloride 0.9% irrigation solution 20ml Clinipod unit dose (Mayors Healthcare Ltd) **Sodium chloride 9 mg per 1 ml** 25 unit dose · NHS indicative price = £4.80 · Drug Tariff (Part IXa)

Sodium chloride 0.9% irrigation solution 20ml ISO-POD unit dose (St Georges Medical Ltd) **Sodium chloride 9 mg per 1 ml** 25 unit dose · NHS indicative price = £4.95 · Drug Tariff (Part IXa)

Sodium chloride 0.9% irrigation solution 20ml Irripod unit dose (C D Medical Ltd) **Sodium chloride 9 mg per 1 ml** 25 unit dose · NHS indicative price = £5.90 · Drug Tariff (Part IXa)

Sodium chloride 0.9% irrigation solution 20ml Sal-e Pods unit dose (Ennogen Healthcare Ltd) **Sodium chloride 9 mg per 1 ml** 25 unit dose · NHS indicative price = £4.80 · Drug Tariff (Part IXa)

Sodium chloride 0.9% irrigation solution 20ml Salipod unit dose (Sai-Meds Ltd) **Sodium chloride 9 mg per 1 ml** 25 unit dose · NHS indicative price = £4.99 · Drug Tariff (Part IXa)

Sodium chloride 0.9% irrigation solution 20ml Steripod unit dose (Molnlycke Health Care Ltd) **Sodium chloride 9 mg per 1 ml** 25 unit dose · NHS indicative price = £5.00 · Drug Tariff (Part IXa)

Sodium chloride 0.9% irrigation solution 20ml Sterowash unit dose (Steroplast Healthcare Ltd) **Sodium chloride 9 mg per 1 ml** 25 unit dose · NHS indicative price = £5.40 · Drug Tariff (Part IXa)

Sodium chloride 0.9% irrigation solution 20ml unit dose (Alissa Healthcare Research Ltd) **Sodium chloride 9 mg per 1 ml** 25 unit dose · NHS indicative price = £7.36 · Drug Tariff (Part IXa)

Sodium chloride 0.9% irrigation solution 20ml unit dose (Bell, Sons & Co (Druggists) Ltd) **Sodium chloride 9 mg per 1 ml** 25 unit dose · NHS indicative price = £6.76 · Drug Tariff (Part IXa)

Sodium chloride 0.9% irrigation solution 20ml unit dose (Crest Medical Ltd) **Sodium chloride 9 mg per 1 ml** 25 unit dose · NHS indicative price = £4.99 · Drug Tariff (Part IXa)

Sodium chloride 0.9% irrigation solution 20ml unit dose (Mylan) **Sodium chloride 9 mg per 1 ml** 25 unit dose · NHS indicative price = £5.50 · Drug Tariff (Part IXa)

Stericlens sodium chloride 0.9% irrigation solution aerosol spray (C D Medical Ltd) **Sodium chloride 9 mg per 1 ml** 100 ml · NHS indicative price = £2.07 · Drug Tariff (Part IXa)240 ml · NHS indicative price = £3.15 · Drug Tariff (Part IXa)

8.1 Minor cuts and abrasions

Minor cuts and abrasions

Management

Many preparations traditionally used to manage minor burns, and abrasions have fallen out of favour. Preparations containing camphor and sulfonamides should be avoided. Preparations such as magnesium sulfate paste are now rarely used to treat carbuncles and boils as these are best treated with antibiotics.

Cetrimide is used to treat minor cuts and abrasions and proflavine above may be used to treat infected wounds or burns, but its use has now been largely superseded by other antispetics or suitable antibacterials. The effervescent effect of hydrogen peroxide p. 814 is used to clean minor cuts and abrasions.

Flexible collodion (see castor oil with collodion and colophony below) may be used to seal minor cuts and wounds that have partially healed; skin tissue adhesives are used similarly, and also for additional suture support.

DERMATOLOGICAL DRUGS › COLLODIONS

Castor oil with collodion and colophony

- **INDICATIONS AND DOSE**

Used to seal minor cuts and wounds that have partially healed

▸ TO THE SKIN
▸ Child: (consult product literature)

- **ALLERGY AND CROSS-SENSITIVITY** Contra-indicated if patient has an allergy to colophony in elastic adhesive plasters and tape.

- **MEDICINAL FORMS** There can be variation in the licensing of different medicines containing the same drug.

Flexible collodion

▸ Castor oil with collodion and colophony (Non-proprietary)
Castor oil 25 mg per 1 ml, Colophony 25 mg per 1 ml, Collodion methylated 950 microlitre per 1 ml Flexible collodion methylated | 100 ml £13.81–£14.37 | 500 ml £29.91

Skin adhesives

- **SKIN ADHESIVES**

Derma+Flex skin adhesive (Chemence Ltd)
0.5 ml • NHS indicative price = £5.36 • Drug Tariff (Part IXa)

Dermabond ProPen skin adhesive (Ethicon Ltd)
0.5 ml • NHS indicative price = £19.46 • Drug Tariff (Part IXa)

Histoacryl L skin adhesive (B.Braun Medical Ltd)
0.5 ml • NHS indicative price = £6.72 • Drug Tariff (Part IXa)

Histoacryl skin adhesive (B.Braun Medical Ltd)
0.5 ml • NHS indicative price = £6.50 • Drug Tariff (Part IXa)

Indermil skin adhesive (Covidien (UK) Commercial Ltd)
0.5 gram • NHS indicative price = £6.50 • Drug Tariff (Part IXa)

LiquiBand flow control tissue adhesive (Advanced Medical Solutions Ltd)
0.5 gram • NHS indicative price = £5.50 • Drug Tariff (Part IXa)

LiquiBand tissue adhesive (Advanced Medical Solutions Ltd)
0.5 gram • NHS indicative price = £5.50 • Drug Tariff (Part IXa)

9 Skin disfigurement

Camouflagers

Overview

Disfigurement of the skin can be very distressing to patients and may have a marked psychological effect. In skilled hands, or with experience, camouflage cosmetics can be very effective in concealing scars and birthmarks. The depigmented patches in vitiligo are also very disfiguring and camouflage creams are of great cosmetic value.

Opaque cover foundation or cream is used to mask skin pigment abnormalities; careful application using a combination of dark- and light-coloured cover creams set with powder helps to minimise the appearance of skin deformities.

Borderline substances

The preparations marked 'ACBS' can be prescribed on the NHS for postoperative scars and other deformities and as adjunctive therapy in the relief of emotional disturbances due to disfiguring skin disease, such as vitiligo.

Camouflages

- **CAMOUFLAGES**

Covermark classic foundation (Derma UK Ltd)
15 ml(ACBS) • NHS indicative price = £11.86

Covermark finishing powder (Derma UK Ltd)
25 gram(ACBS) • NHS indicative price = £11.86

Covermark removing cream (Derma UK Ltd)
200 ml • No NHS indicative price available

Dermablend Dermasmooth Corrective Foundation (Vichy)
30 ml • No NHS indicative price available

Dermacolor Creme Effectiv (Kryolan UK Ltd)
50 ml • NHS indicative price = £5.73

Dermacolor body camouflage (Kryolan UK Ltd)
50 ml • NHS indicative price = £8.94

Dermacolor camouflage creme (Kryolan UK Ltd)
30 gram • NHS indicative price = £11.00

Dermacolor cleansing cream (Kryolan UK Ltd)
75 gram • No NHS indicative price available

Dermacolor fixing powder (Kryolan UK Ltd)
60 gram(ACBS) • NHS indicative price = £9.85

Keromask finishing powder (Bellava Ltd)
20 gram(ACBS) • NHS indicative price = £6.46

Keromask masking cream (Bellava Ltd)
15 ml(ACBS) • NHS indicative price = £6.46

Veil cover cream (Thomas Blake Cosmetic Creams Ltd)
19 gram(ACBS) • NHS indicative price = £22.4244 gram(ACBS) • NHS indicative price = £33.3570 gram(ACBS) • NHS indicative price = £42.10

Veil finishing powder(Thomas Blake Cosmetic Creams Ltd)
35 gram(ACBS) • NHS indicative price = £24.58

10 Sun protection and photodamage

Sunscreen

05-Feb-2020

Sunscreen preparations

Solar ultraviolet irradiation can be harmful to the skin. It is responsible for disorders such as *polymorphic light eruption, solar urticaria,* and it provokes the various *cutaneous porphyrias*. It also provokes (or at least aggravates) skin lesions of *lupus erythematosus* and may aggravate some other *dermatoses*. Certain drugs, such as demeclocycline, phenothiazines, or amiodarone, can cause photosensitivity. All these conditions (as well as *sunburn*) may occur after relatively short periods of exposure to the sun. Solar ultraviolet irradiation may provoke attacks of recurrent herpes labialis (but it is not known whether the effect of sunlight exposure is local or systemic).

The effects of exposure over longer periods include *ageing changes* and more importantly the initiation of *skin cancer*.

Solar ultraviolet radiation is approximately 200–400 m in wavelength. The medium wavelengths (290–320 nm, known as UVB) cause sunburn. The long wavelengths (320–400 nm, known as UVA) are responsible for many *photosensitivity reactions* and *photodermatoses*. Both UVA and UVB contribute to long-term *photodamage* and to the changes responsible for *skin cancer* and ageing.

Sunscreen preparations contain substances that protect the skin against UVA and UVB radiation, but they are no substitute for covering the skin and avoiding sunlight. Protective clothing and sun avoidance (rather than the use of sunscreen preparations) are recommended for children under 6 months of age.

The sun protection factor (SPF, usually indicated in the preparation title) provides guidance on the degree of protection offered against UVB; it indicates the multiples of protection provided against burning, compared with unprotected skin; for example, an SPF of 8 should enable a child to remain 8 times longer in the sun without burning. However, in practice users do not apply sufficient sunscreen product and the protection is lower than that found in experimental studies. Some manufacturers use a star rating system to indicate the protection against UVA relative to protection against UVB for sunscreen products. However, the usefulness of the star rating system remains controversial. The EU Commission (September 2006) has recommended that the UVA protection factor for a sunscreen should be at least one-third of the sun protection factor (SPF); products that achieve this requirement will be labelled with a UVA logo alongside the SPF classification. Preparations that also contain reflective substances, such as titanium dioxide, provide the most effective protection against UVA.

Sunscreen preparations may rarely cause allergic reactions.

For optimum photoprotection, sunscreen preparations should be applied **thickly** and **frequently** (approximately 2 hourly). In photodermatoses, they should be used from spring to autumn. As maximum protection from sunlight is desirable, preparations with the highest SPF should be prescribed.

Ingredient nomenclature in sunscreen preparations

rINN	INCI
amiloxate	isoamyl *p*-methoxycinnamate
avobenzone	butyl methoxydibenzoylmethane
bemotrizinol	bis-ethylhexyloxyphenol methoxyphenyl triazine
bisoctrizole	methylene bis-benzotriazolyl tetramethylbutylphenol
ecamsule	terephthalylidene dicamphor sulfonic acid
ensulizole	phenylbenzimidazole sulfonic acid
enzacamene	4-methylbenzylidene camphor
octinoxate	octyl (*or* ethylhexyl) methoxycinnamate
octocrilene	octocrylene
oxybenzone	benzophenone-3

The European Commission Cosmetic Products Regulation (EC) 1223/2009 requires the use of INCI (International Nomenclature of Cosmetic Ingredients) for cosmetics and sunscreens. This table includes the rINN and the INCI synonym for the active ingredients of sunscreen preparations in the BNFC

Borderline substances

LA Roche-Posay Anthelios® XL SPF 50+ Cream; *Sunsense*® Ultra (Ego) SPF 50+; *Uvistat*® Lipscreen SPF 50; and *Uvistat*® Suncream SPF 30 and 50 (see *About Borderline Substances*) are regarded as drugs when prescribed for skin protection against ultraviolet radiation and/or visible light in abnormal cutaneous photosensitivity causing severe cutaneous reactions in genetic disorders (including xeroderma pigmentosum and porphyrias), severe photodermatoses (both idiopathic and acquired) and in those with increased risk of ultraviolet radiation causing adverse effects due to chronic disease (such as haematological malignancies), medical therapies and/or procedures.

Photodamage

Overview

Actinic (solar) keratoses occur very rarely in healthy children; actinic cheilitis may occur on the lips of adolescents following excessive sun exposure.

Diclofenac gel (Solaraze®) and topical preparations of fluorouracil are licensed for the treatment of actinic keratoses but they are not licensed for use in children.

In children with photosensitivity disorders, such as erythropoietic protoporphyria, specialists may use betacarotene below, mepacrine, chloroquine or hydroxychloroquine to reduce skin reactions.

VITAMINS AND TRACE ELEMENTS › VITAMIN A

Betacarotene

- **DRUG ACTION** Betacarotene is a precursor to vitamin A.

- **INDICATIONS AND DOSE**

Management of photosensitivity reactions in erythropoietic protoporphyria (specialist use only)

▶ BY MOUTH

- Child 1–4 years: 60–90 mg daily, to be given as a single dose or in divided doses
- Child 5–8 years: 90–120 mg daily, to be given as a single dose or in divided doses
- Child 9–11 years: 120–150 mg daily, to be given as a single dose or in divided doses
- Child 12–15 years: 150–180 mg daily, to be given as a single dose or in divided doses
- Child 16–17 years: 180–300 mg daily, to be given as a single dose or in divided doses

- **UNLICENSED USE** Not licensed.
- **CAUTIONS** Monitor vitamin A intake

CAUTIONS, FURTHER INFORMATION Protection not total—avoid strong sunlight and use sunscreen preparations; generally 2–6 weeks of treatment (resulting in yellow coloration of palms and soles) necessary before increasing exposure to sunlight; dose should be adjusted according to level of exposure to sunlight.

- **SIDE-EFFECTS**

▶ **Rare or very rare** Arthralgia · skin reactions

▶ **Frequency not known** Diarrhoea

- **PREGNANCY** Partially converted to vitamin A, but does not give rise to abnormally high serum concentration; manufacturer advises use only if potential benefit outweighs risk.
- **BREAST FEEDING** Use with caution—present in milk.
- **HEPATIC IMPAIRMENT** Avoid.
- **RENAL IMPAIRMENT** Use with caution.

- **MEDICINAL FORMS** There can be variation in the licensing of different medicines containing the same drug. Forms available from special-order manufacturers include: tablet, capsule

Capsule

CAUTIONARY AND ADVISORY LABELS 21

▶ **Bio-Carotene** (Pharma Nord (UK) Ltd)
Betacarotene 9 mg Bio-Carotene 9mg capsules | 150 capsule £5.51

▶ **Carotaben** (Imported (Germany))
Betacarotene 25 mg Carotaben 25mg capsules | 100 capsule [P] [X]

▶ **Lumitene** (Imported (United States))
Betacarotene 30 mg Lumitene 30mg capsules | 100 capsule [PoM] [X]

▶ **Super Betavit** (Health+Plus Ltd)
Betacarotene 15 mg Super Betavit 15mg capsules | 30 capsule £3.59

11 Superficial soft-tissue injuries and superficial thrombophlebitis

Topical circulatory preparations

Overview

These preparations are used to improve circulation in conditions such as bruising and superficial thrombophlebitis but are of little value. First aid measures such as rest, ice, compression, and elevation should be used. Chilblains are best managed by avoidance of exposure to cold; neither systemic nor topical vasodilator therapy is established as being effective.

HEPARINOIDS

Heparinoid

- **INDICATIONS AND DOSE**

Superficial thrombophlebitis | Bruising | Haematoma

▶ TO THE SKIN

- Child 5–17 years: Apply up to 4 times a day

- **CONTRA-INDICATIONS** Should not be used on large areas of skin, broken or sensitive skin, or mucous membranes

- **LESS SUITABLE FOR PRESCRIBING** Hirudoid® is less suitable for prescribing.

- **MEDICINAL FORMS** There can be variation in the licensing of different medicines containing the same drug.

Cream

EXCIPIENTS: May contain Cetostearyl alcohol (including cetyl and stearyl alcohol), hydroxybenzoates (parabens)

- Hirudoid (Genus Pharmaceuticals Ltd)
  Heparinoid 3 mg per 1 gram Hirudoid 0.3% cream | 50 gram [P] £3.99 DT = £3.99

Gel

EXCIPIENTS: May contain Fragrances, propylene glycol

- Hirudoid (Genus Pharmaceuticals Ltd)
  Heparinoid 3 mg per 1 gram Hirudoid 0.3% gel | 50 gram [P] £3.99 DT = £3.99

12 Warts and calluses

Warts and calluses

Overview

Warts (verruca vulgaris) are common, benign, self-limiting, and usually asymptomatic. They are caused by a human papillomavirus, which most frequently affects the hands, feet (plantar warts), and the anogenital region; treatment usually relies on local tissue destruction and is required only if the warts are painful, unsightly, persistent, or cause distress. In immunocompromised children, warts may be more difficult to eradicate.

Preparations of salicylic acid p. 820, formaldehyde below, glutaraldehyde p. 819 or silver nitrate p. 819 are used for the removal of warts on hands and feet. Salicylic acid is a useful keratolytic which may be considered first-line in the treatment of warts; it is also suitable for the removal of *corns and calluses*. Preparations of salicylic acid in a collodion basis are available but some patients may develop an allergy to colophony in the formulation; collodion should be avoided in children allergic to elastic adhesive plaster. Cryotherapy causes pain, swelling, and blistering, and may be no more effective than topical salicylic acid in the treatment of warts.

Anogenital warts

Anogenital warts (condylomata acuminata) in children are often asymptomatic and require only a simple barrier preparation. If treatment is required it should be supervised by a hospital specialist. Persistent warts on genital skin may require treatment with cryotherapy or other forms of physical ablation under general anaesthesia.

Podophyllotoxin below (the major active ingredient of podophyllum), or imiquimod p. 819 are used to treat external anogenital warts; these preparations can cause considerable irritation of the treated area and are therefore suitable only for children who are able to co-operate with the treatment.

ANTINEOPLASTIC DRUGS › PLANT ALKALOIDS

Podophyllotoxin

- **INDICATIONS AND DOSE**

CONDYLINE®

Condylomata acuminata affecting the penis or the female external genitalia

▶ TO THE LESION

- Child 2–17 years (initiated under specialist supervision): Apply twice daily for 3 consecutive days, treatment may be repeated at weekly intervals if necessary for a total of five 3-day treatment courses, direct medical supervision for lesions in the female and for lesions greater than 4 cm^2 in the male, maximum 50 single applications ('loops') per session (consult product literature)

WARTICON® CREAM

Condylomata acuminata affecting the penis or the female external genitalia

▶ TO THE LESION

- Child 2–17 years (initiated under specialist supervision): Apply twice daily for 3 consecutive days, treatment may be repeated at weekly intervals if necessary for a total of four 3-day treatment courses, direct medical supervision for lesions greater than 4 cm^2

WARTICON® LIQUID

Condylomata acuminata affecting the penis or the female external genitalia

▶ TO THE LESION

- Child 2–17 years (initiated under specialist supervision): Apply twice daily for 3 consecutive days, treatment may be repeated at weekly intervals if necessary for a total of four 3-day treatment courses, direct medical supervision for lesions greater than 4 cm^2, maximum 50 single applications ('loops') per session (consult product literature)

- **UNLICENSED USE** Not licensed for use in children.
- **CAUTIONS** Avoid normal skin · avoid open wounds · keep away from face · very irritant to eyes
- **SIDE-EFFECTS** Balanoposthitis · skin irritation
- **PREGNANCY** Avoid.
- **BREAST FEEDING** Avoid.

- **MEDICINAL FORMS** There can be variation in the licensing of different medicines containing the same drug.

Cream

EXCIPIENTS: May contain Butylated hydroxyanisole, cetostearyl alcohol (including cetyl and stearyl alcohol), hydroxybenzoates (parabens), sorbic acid

- Warticon (Phoenix Labs Ltd)
  Podophyllotoxin 1.5 mg per 1 gram Warticon 0.15% cream | 5 gram [PoM] £17.83 DT = £17.83

Liquid

CAUTIONARY AND ADVISORY LABELS 15

- Condyline (Takeda UK Ltd)
  Podophyllotoxin 5 mg per 1 ml Condyline 0.5% solution | 3.5 ml [PoM] £14.49 DT = £14.49
- Warticon (Phoenix Labs Ltd)
  Podophyllotoxin 5 mg per 1 ml Warticon 0.5% solution | 3 ml [PoM] £14.86 DT = £14.86

ANTISEPTICS AND DISINFECTANTS › ALDEHYDES AND DERIVATIVES

Formaldehyde

- **INDICATIONS AND DOSE**

Warts, particularly plantar warts

▶ TO THE LESION

- Child: Apply twice daily

- **UNLICENSED USE** Licensed for use in children (age range not specified by manufacturer).
- **CAUTIONS** Impaired peripheral circulation · not suitable for application to anogenital region · not suitable for application to face · not suitable for application to large areas · patients with diabetes at risk of neuropathic ulcers · protect surrounding skin and avoid broken skin · significant peripheral neuropathy
- **SIDE-EFFECTS** Asthma · cough · dysphagia · eye irritation · increased risk of infection · laryngospasm · skin reactions

● **MEDICINAL FORMS** There can be variation in the licensing of different medicines containing the same drug. Forms available from special-order manufacturers include: liquid

Form unstated
- Formaldehyde (Non-proprietary)
  Formaldehyde 350 mg per 1 gram Formaldehyde solution | 500 ml £7.31 DT = £7.24 | 2000 ml £18.72

Liquid
- Formaldehyde (Non-proprietary)
  Formaldehyde 40 mg per 1 ml Formaldehyde (Buffered) 4% solution | 1000 ml £3.90 DT = £3.90

Glutaraldehyde

● **INDICATIONS AND DOSE**

Warts, particularly plantar warts
- TO THE LESION
- Child: Apply twice daily

● **UNLICENSED USE** Licensed for use in children (age range not specified by manufacturer).

● **CAUTIONS** Not for application to anogenital areas · not for application to face · not for application to mucosa · protect surrounding skin

● **SIDE-EFFECTS**
- **Rare or very rare** Severe cutaneous adverse reactions (SCARs)
- **Frequency not known** Rash · skin irritation (discontinue if severe)

● **MEDICINAL FORMS** There can be variation in the licensing of different medicines containing the same drug.

Paint
- Glutarol (Dermal Laboratories Ltd)
  Glutaraldehyde 100 mg per 1 ml Glutarol 10% cutaneous solution | 10 ml [P] £2.07 DT = £2.07

ANTISEPTICS AND DISINFECTANTS > OTHER

Silver nitrate

● **INDICATIONS AND DOSE**

Common warts
- TO THE LESION
- Child: Apply every 24 hours for up to 3 applications, apply moistened caustic pencil tip for 1–2 minutes. Instructions in proprietary packs generally incorporate advice to remove dead skin before use by gentle filing and to cover with adhesive dressing after application

Verrucas
- TO THE LESION
- Child: Apply every 24 hours for up to 6 applications, apply moistened caustic pencil tip for 1–2 minutes. Instructions in proprietary packs generally incorporate advice to remove dead skin before use by gentle filing and to cover with adhesive dressing after application

Umbilical granulomas
- TO THE SKIN
- Child: Apply moistened caustic pencil tip (usually containing silver nitrate 40%) for 1–2 minutes, protect surrounding skin with soft paraffin

● **UNLICENSED USE** No age range specified by manufacturer.

● **CAUTIONS** Avoid broken skin · not suitable for application to ano-genital region · not suitable for application to face · not suitable for application to large areas · protect surrounding skin

● **SIDE-EFFECTS**
- **Rare or very rare** Argyria · methaemoglobinaemia

● **PATIENT AND CARER ADVICE** Patients should be advised that silver nitrate may stain fabric.

● **MEDICINAL FORMS** There can be variation in the licensing of different medicines containing the same drug.

Stick
- Avoca (Bray Group Ltd)
  Silver nitrate 400 mg per 1 gram Avoca 40% silver nitrate pencils | 1 applicator [P] £1.16 DT = £1.16
  Silver nitrate 750 mg per 1 gram Avoca 75% silver nitrate applicators | 100 applicator [P] £49.16 DT = £49.16
  Avoca 75% silver nitrate applicators with thick handles | 50 applicator [P] £48.51
  Silver nitrate 950 mg per 1 gram Avoca 95% silver nitrate applicators | 100 applicator [P] £52.60 DT = £52.60
  Avoca 95% silver nitrate pencils | 1 applicator [P] £2.63 DT = £3.08
  Avoca wart and verruca treatment set | 1 applicator [P] £3.08 DT = £3.08

ANTIVIRALS > IMMUNE RESPONSE MODIFIERS

Imiquimod

20-May-2020

● **INDICATIONS AND DOSE**

ALDARA ®

Warts (external genital and perianal)
- TO THE LESION
- Child (initiated under specialist supervision): Apply 3 times a week until lesions resolve (maximum 16 weeks), to be applied thinly at night

● **UNLICENSED USE**

ALDARA ® Not licensed for use in children.

● **CAUTIONS** Autoimmune disease · avoid broken skin · avoid normal skin · avoid open wounds · immunosuppressed patients · not suitable for internal genital warts · uncircumcised males (risk of phimosis or stricture of foreskin)

● **SIDE-EFFECTS**
- **Common or very common** Appetite decreased · arthralgia · asthenia · headaches · increased risk of infection · lymphadenopathy · myalgia · nausea · pain
- **Uncommon** Anorectal disorder · chills · conjunctival irritation · depression · diarrhoea · dizziness · drowsiness · dry mouth · dysuria · erectile dysfunction · eyelid oedema · face oedema · fever · flushing · gastrointestinal discomfort · genital pain · hyperhidrosis · inflammation · influenza like illness · insomnia · irritability · laryngeal pain · malaise · nasal congestion · painful sexual intercourse · paraesthesia · penis disorder · skin reactions · skin ulcer · tinnitus · uterovaginal prolapse · vomiting · vulvovaginal disorders
- **Rare or very rare** Autoimmune disorder exacerbated
- **Frequency not known** Alopecia · cutaneous lupus erythematosus · severe cutaneous adverse reactions (SCARs)

● **CONCEPTION AND CONTRACEPTION** May damage latex condoms and diaphragms.

● **PREGNANCY** No evidence of teratogenicity or toxicity in *animal* studies; manufacturer advises caution.

● **BREAST FEEDING** No information available.

● **DIRECTIONS FOR ADMINISTRATION**

ALDARA ® ▸ **Important** Should be rubbed in and allowed to stay on the treated area for 6–10 hours then washed off with mild soap and water (uncircumcised males treating warts under foreskin should wash the area daily). The cream should be washed off before sexual contact.

● **PATIENT AND CARER ADVICE** A patient information leaflet should be provided.

● **MEDICINAL FORMS** There can be variation in the licensing of different medicines containing the same drug.

Cream

CAUTIONARY AND ADVISORY LABELS 10

EXCIPIENTS: May contain Benzyl alcohol, cetostearyl alcohol (including cetyl and stearyl alcohol), hydroxybenzoates (parabens), polysorbates

▸ Aldara (Mylan)
Imiquimod 50 mg per 1 gram Aldara 5% cream 250mg sachets | 12 sachet [PoM] £48.60 DT = £48.60

SALICYLIC ACID AND DERIVATIVES

Salicylic acid

● **INDICATIONS AND DOSE**

OCCLUSAL ®

Common and plantar warts

▸ TO THE LESION

▸ Child: Apply daily, treatment may need to be continued for up to 3 months

VERRUGON ®

For plantar warts

▸ TO THE LESION

▸ Child: Apply daily, treatment may need to be continued for up to 3 months

● **UNLICENSED USE** Not licensed for use in children under 2 years.

● **CAUTIONS** Avoid broken skin · impaired peripheral circulation · not suitable for application to anogenital region · not suitable for application to face · not suitable for application to large areas · patients with diabetes at risk of neuropathic ulcers · significant peripheral neuropathy

● **SIDE-EFFECTS** Skin irritation

● **PATIENT AND CARER ADVICE** Advise patient to apply carefully to wart and to protect surrounding skin (e.g. with soft paraffin or specially designed plaster); rub wart surface gently with file or pumice stone once weekly.

● **MEDICINAL FORMS** There can be variation in the licensing of different medicines containing the same drug.

Ointment

▸ Verrugon (Optima Consumer Health Ltd)
Salicylic acid 500 mg per 1 gram Verrugon complete 50% ointment | 6 gram [P] £4.44 DT = £4.44

Liquid

CAUTIONARY AND ADVISORY LABELS 15

▸ Occlusal (Alliance Pharmaceuticals Ltd)
Salicylic acid 260 mg per 1 ml Occlusal 26% solution | 10 ml [P] £3.56 DT = £3.56

Salicylic acid with lactic acid

The properties listed below are those particular to the combination only. For the properties of the components please consider, salicylic acid above.

● **INDICATIONS AND DOSE**

DUOFILM ®

Plantar and mosaic warts

▸ TO THE LESION

▸ Child: Apply daily, treatment may need to be continued for up to 3 months

SALACTOL ®

Warts, particularly plantar warts | Verrucas | Corns | Calluses

▸ TO THE LESION

▸ Child: Apply daily, treatment may need to be continued for up to 3 months

SALATAC ®

Warts | Verrucas | Corns | Calluses

▸ TO THE LESION

▸ Child: Apply daily, treatment may need to be continued for up to 3 months

● **PRESCRIBING AND DISPENSING INFORMATION** Preparation of salicylic acid in a collodion basis (*Salactol*®) is available but some patients may develop an allergy to colophony in the formulation.

● **MEDICINAL FORMS** There can be variation in the licensing of different medicines containing the same drug.

Paint

CAUTIONARY AND ADVISORY LABELS 15

▸ Duofilm (GlaxoSmithKline Consumer Healthcare)
Lactic acid 150 mg per 1 gram, Salicylic acid 167 mg per 1 gram Duofilm paint | 15 ml [P] £2.78 DT = £2.78

▸ Salactol (Dermal Laboratories Ltd)
Lactic acid 167 mg per 1 gram, Salicylic acid 167 mg per 1 gram Salactol paint | 10 ml [P] £1.71 DT = £1.71

Gel

CAUTIONARY AND ADVISORY LABELS 15

▸ Salatac (Dermal Laboratories Ltd)
Lactic acid 40 mg per 1 gram, Salicylic acid 120 mg per 1 gram Salatac gel | 8 gram [P] £2.98 DT = £2.98

Chapter 14 Vaccines

CONTENTS

1 Immunoglobulin therapy

IMMUNE SERA AND IMMUNOGLOBULINS › IMMUNOGLOBULINS

Immunoglobulins

04-Oct-2017

Passive immunity

Immunity with immediate protection against certain infective organisms can be obtained by injecting preparations made from the plasma of immune individuals with adequate levels of antibody to the disease for which protection is sought. The duration of this passive immunity varies according to the dose and the type of immunoglobulin. Passive immunity may last only a few weeks; when necessary, passive immunisation can be repeated. Antibodies of human origin are usually termed immunoglobulins. The term antiserum is applied to material prepared in animals. Because of serum sickness and other allergic-type reactions that may follow injections of antisera, this therapy has been replaced wherever possible by the use of immunoglobulins. Reactions are theoretically possible after injection of human immunoglobulins but reports of such reactions are very rare.

Two types of human immunoglobulin preparation are available, normal immunoglobulin p. 825 and **disease-specific immunoglobulins.**

Human immunoglobulin is a sterile preparation of concentrated antibodies (immune globulins) recovered from pooled human plasma or serum obtained from outside the UK, tested and found non-reactive for hepatitis B surface antigen and for antibodies against hepatitis C virus and human immunodeficiency virus (types 1 and 2). A global shortage of human immunoglobulin and the rapidly increasing range of clinical indications for treatment with immunoglobulins has resulted in the need for a Demand Management programme in the UK, for further information consult www.ivig.nhs.uk and *Clinical Guidelines for Immunoglobulin Use*, www.gov.uk/dh.

Further information on the use of immunoglobulins is included in Public Health England's *Immunoglobulin Handbook*, www.gov.uk/phe, and in the Department of Health's publication, *Immunisation against Infectious Disease*, www.gov.uk/dh.

Availability

Normal immunoglobulin for intramuscular administration is available from some regional Public Health laboratories for protection of contacts and the control of outbreaks of hepatitis A, measles, and rubella only. For other indications, subcutaneous or intravenous normal immunoglobulin should be purchased from the manufacturer.

Disease-specific immunoglobulins are available from some regional Public Health laboratories, with the exception of tetanus immunoglobulin p. 826 which is available from BPL, hospital pharmacies, or blood transfusion departments. Rabies immunoglobulin p. 826 is available from the Specialist and Reference Microbiology Division, Public Health England, Colindale. Hepatitis B immunoglobulin p. 824 required by transplant centres should be obtained commercially.

In Scotland all immunoglobulins are available from the *Scottish National Blood Transfusion Service* (SNBTS).

In Wales all immunoglobulins are available from the *Welsh Blood Service* (WBS).

In Northern Ireland all immunoglobulins are available from the *Northern Ireland Blood Transfusion Service* (NIBTS).

Normal immunoglobulin

Human normal immunoglobulin ('HNIG') is prepared from pools of at least 1000 donations of human plasma; it contains immunoglobulin G (IgG) and antibodies to hepatitis A, measles, mumps, rubella, varicella, and other viruses that are currently prevalent in the general population.

Uses

Normal immunoglobulin (containing 10–18% protein) is administered by *intramuscular injection* for the protection of susceptible contacts against **hepatitis A** virus (infectious hepatitis), **measles** and, to a lesser extent, **rubella**. Injection of immunoglobulin produces immediate protection lasting for several weeks.

Normal immunoglobulin (containing 3–12% protein) for *intravenous administration* is used as *replacement therapy* for children with congenital agammaglobulinaemia and hypogammaglobulinaemia, and for the short-term treatment of idiopathic thrombocytopenic purpura and Kawasaki disease; it is also used for the prophylaxis of infection following bone-marrow transplantation and in children with symptomatic HIV infection who have recurrent bacterial infections. Normal immunoglobulin for replacement therapy may also be given intramuscularly or subcutaneously, but intravenous formulations are normally preferred. Intravenous immunoglobulin is also used in the treatment of Guillain-Barré syndrome as an alternative to plasma exchange.

The dose of normal immunoglobulin used as replacement therapy in patients with immunodeficiencies is **not the same** as the dose required for treatment of acute conditions. For Kawasaki disease a single dose by intravenous infusion should be given with concomitant aspirin p. 98 within 10 days of onset of symptoms (but children with a delayed diagnosis may also benefit).

For guidance on the use of intravenous normal immunoglobulin and alternative therapies for other conditions, consult *Clinical Guidelines for Immunoglobulin Use* (www.gov.uk/dh).

Hepatitis A

Hepatitis A vaccine p. 852 is recommended for individuals at risk of infection including those visiting areas where the disease is highly endemic (all countries excluding Northern and Western Europe, North America, Japan, Australia, and

New Zealand). In unimmunised individuals, transmission of hepatitis A is reduced by good hygiene. Intramuscular normal immunoglobulin is no longer recommended for prophylaxis in travellers.

Public Health England recommends the use of normal immunoglobulin in addition to hepatitis A vaccine for prevention of infection in close contacts (of confirmed cases of hepatitis A) who have chronic liver disease (including chronic hepatitis B or C infection), or HIV infection (with a CD4 count < 200 cells per microlitre), or who are immunosuppressed; normal immunoglobulin should be given as soon as possible, preferably within 14 days of exposure to the primary case. However, normal immunoglobulin can still be given to contacts with chronic liver disease up to 28 days after exposure to the primary case. Hepatitis A vaccine can be given at the same time, but it should be given at a separate injection site.

Measles

Intravenous or subcutaneous normal immunoglobulin may be given to prevent or attenuate an attack of measles in individuals who do not have adequate immunity. Children with compromised immunity who have come into contact with measles should receive intravenous or subcutaneous normal immunoglobulin as soon as possible after exposure. It is most effective if given within 72 hours but can be effective if given within 6 days.

Subcutaneous or intramuscular normal immunoglobulin should also be considered for the following individuals if they have been in contact with a confirmed case of measles or with a person associated with a local outbreak:

- non-immune pregnant women
- infants under 9 months

Further advice should be sought from the Centre for Infections, Public Health England (tel. (020) 8200 6868).

Individuals with normal immunity who are not in the above categories and who have not been fully immunised against measles, can be given measles, mumps and rubella vaccine, live p. 857 for prophylaxis following exposure to measles.

Rubella

Intramuscular immunoglobulin after exposure to rubella does **not** prevent infection in non-immune contacts and is **not** recommended for protection of pregnant women exposed to rubella. It may, however, reduce the likelihood of a clinical attack which may possibly reduce the risk to the fetus. Risk of intra-uterine transmission is greatest in the first 11 weeks of pregnancy, between 16 and 20 weeks there is minimal risk of deafness only, after 20 weeks there is no increased risk. Intramuscular normal immunoglobulin p. 825 should be used only if termination of pregnancy would be unacceptable to the pregnant woman—it should be given as soon as possible after exposure. Serological follow-up of recipients is essential to determine if the woman has become infected despite receiving immunoglobulin.

For routine prophylaxis against Rubella, see measles, mumps and rubella vaccine, live p. 857.

Disease-specific immunoglobulins

Specific immunoglobulins are prepared by pooling the plasma of selected human donors with high levels of the specific antibody required. For further information, see *Immunoglobulin Handbook* (www.gov.uk/phe).

There are no specific immunoglobulins for hepatitis A, measles, or rubella—normal immunoglobulin is used in certain circumstances. There is no specific immunoglobulin for mumps; neither normal immunoglobulin nor measles, mumps and rubella vaccine, live is effective as postexposure prophylaxis.

Hepatitis B immunoglobulin

Disease-specific hepatitis B immunoglobulin p. 824 ('HBIG') is available for use in association with hepatitis B vaccine p. 853 for the prevention of infection in infants born to mothers who have become infected with this virus in pregnancy or who are high-risk carriers (see hepatitis B vaccine). Hepatitis B immunoglobulin will not inhibit the antibody response when given at the same time as hepatitis B vaccine but should be given at different sites.

An intravenous and preparation of hepatitis B immunoglobulin is licensed for the prevention of hepatitis B recurrence in HBV-DNA negative patients who have undergone liver transplantation for liver failure caused by the virus.

Rabies immunoglobulin

Following exposure of an unimmunised individual to an animal in or from a country where the risk of rabies is high the site of the bite should be washed with soapy water and specific rabies immunoglobulin p. 826 of human origin administered. All of the dose should be injected around the site of the wound; if this is difficult or the wound has completely healed it can be given in the anterolateral thigh (remote from the site used for vaccination).

Rabies vaccine p. 858 should also be given intramuscularly at a different site (for details see rabies vaccine). If there is delay in giving the rabies immunoglobulin, it should be given within 7 days of starting the course of rabies vaccine.

Tetanus immunoglobulin

For the management of tetanus-prone wounds, tetanus immunoglobulin p. 826 should be used in addition to wound cleansing and, where appropriate, antibacterial prophylaxis and a tetanus-containing vaccine. Tetanus immunoglobulin, together with metronidazole p. 358 and wound cleansing, should also be used for the treatment of established cases of tetanus.

Varicella–zoster immunoglobulin

Varicella-zoster immunoglobulin (VZIG) p. 827 is recommended for individuals who are at increased risk of severe varicella (neonates, pregnant women, and immunosuppressed individuals with varicella-zoster virus immunoglobulin G antibody less than 150 mIU/mL) *and* who have no antibodies to varicella-zoster virus *and* who have significant exposure to chickenpox (varicella) or shingles (herpes zoster) during the infectious period.

Immunosuppressed children receiving regular intravenous immunoglobulin replacement therapy only require varicella-zoster immunoglobulin if the most recent dose was administered more than 3 weeks before exposure.

Immunosuppressed children on long term aciclovir p. 440 or valaciclovir prophylaxis p. 442 will require a temporary increase in their dose following exposure; for children within 12 months of a stem cell transplant, varicella-zoster immunoglobulin should also be considered.

Important: for full details consult *Guidance for issuing varicella-zoster immunoglobulin (VZIG)* and *Immunisation against infectious disease* from Public Health England (www.gov.uk).

Anti-D (Rh_0) immunoglobulin

03-Mar-2020

- **INDICATIONS AND DOSE**

To rhesus-negative woman for prevention of Rh_0(D) sensitisation, following birth of rhesus-positive infant

▸ BY DEEP INTRAMUSCULAR INJECTION

▸ Females of childbearing potential: 500 units, dose to be administered immediately or within 72 hours; for transplacental bleed of over 4 mL fetal red cells, extra 100–125 units per mL fetal red cells, subcutaneous route used for patients with bleeding disorders

To rhesus-negative woman for prevention of Rh_0(D) sensitisation, following any potentially sensitising episode (e.g. stillbirth, abortion, amniocentesis) up to 20 weeks' gestation
- BY DEEP INTRAMUSCULAR INJECTION
- Females of childbearing potential: 250 units per episode, dose to be administered immediately or within 72 hours, subcutaneous route used for patients with bleeding disorders

To rhesus-negative woman for prevention of Rh_0(D) sensitisation, following any potentially sensitising episode (e.g. stillbirth, abortion, amniocentesis) after 20 weeks' gestation
- BY DEEP INTRAMUSCULAR INJECTION
- Females of childbearing potential: 500 units per episode, dose to be administered immediately or within 72 hours, subcutaneous route used for patients with bleeding disorders

To rhesus-negative woman for prevention of Rh_0(D) sensitisation, antenatal prophylaxis
- BY DEEP INTRAMUSCULAR INJECTION
- Females of childbearing potential: 500 units, dose to be given at weeks 28 and 34 of pregnancy, if infant rhesus-positive, a further dose is still needed immediately or within 72 hours of delivery, subcutaneous route used for patients with bleeding disorders

To rhesus-negative woman for prevention of Rh_0(D) sensitisation, antenatal prophylaxis (alternative NICE recommendation)
- BY DEEP INTRAMUSCULAR INJECTION
- Females of childbearing potential: 1000–1650 units, dose to be given at weeks 28 and 34 of pregnancy, alternatively 1500 units for 1 dose, dose to be given between 28 and 30 weeks gestation

To rhesus-negative woman for prevention of Rh_0(D) sensitisation, following Rh_0(D) incompatible blood transfusion
- BY DEEP INTRAMUSCULAR INJECTION
- Females of childbearing potential: 100–125 units per mL of transfused rhesus-positive red cells, subcutaneous route used for patients with bleeding disorders

RHOPHYLAC®

To rhesus-negative woman for prevention of Rh_0(D) sensitisation, following birth of rhesus-positive infant
- BY INTRAMUSCULAR INJECTION, OR BY INTRAVENOUS INJECTION
- Females of childbearing potential: 1000–1500 units, dose to administered immediately or within 72 hours; for large transplacental bleed, extra 100 units per mL fetal red cells (preferably by intravenous injection), intravenous route recommended for patients with bleeding disorders

To rhesus-negative woman for prevention of Rh_0(D) sensitisation, following any potentially sensitising episode (e.g. abortion, amniocentesis, chorionic villous sampling) up to 12 weeks' gestation
- BY INTRAMUSCULAR INJECTION, OR BY INTRAVENOUS INJECTION
- Females of childbearing potential: 1000 units per episode, dose to be administered immediately or within 72 hours, intravenous route recommended for patients with bleeding disorders, higher doses may be required after 12 weeks gestation

To rhesus-negative woman for prevention of Rh_0(D) sensitisation, antenatal prophylaxis
- BY INTRAMUSCULAR INJECTION, OR BY INTRAVENOUS INJECTION
- Females of childbearing potential: 1500 units, dose to be given between weeks 28–30 of pregnancy; if infant rhesus-positive, a further dose is still needed immediately or within 72 hours of delivery, intravenous route recommended for patients with bleeding disorders

To rhesus-negative woman for prevention of Rh_0(D) sensitisation, following Rh_0(D) incompatible blood transfusion
- BY INTRAVENOUS INJECTION
- Females of childbearing potential: 50 units per mL of transfused rhesus-positive blood, alternatively 100 units per of mL of erythrocyte concentrate, intravenous route recommended for patients with bleeding disorders

- **CAUTIONS** Immunoglobulin A deficiency · possible interference with live virus vaccines

CAUTIONS, FURTHER INFORMATION
- MMR vaccine MMR vaccine may be given in the postpartum period with anti-D (Rh_0) immunoglobulin injection provided that separate syringes are used and the products are administered into different limbs. If blood is transfused, the antibody response to the vaccine may be inhibited—measure rubella antibodies after 6–8 weeks and revaccinate if necessary.

- **INTERACTIONS** → Appendix 1: immunoglobulins
- **SIDE-EFFECTS**
- **Uncommon** Chills · fever · headache · malaise · skin reactions
- **Rare or very rare** Arthralgia · dyspnoea · hypersensitivity · hypotension · nausea · tachycardia · vomiting
- **Frequency not known** Intravascular haemolysis
- **HANDLING AND STORAGE** Care must be taken to store all immunological products under the conditions recommended in the product literature, otherwise the preparation may become ineffective. **Refrigerated storage** is usually necessary; many immunoglobulins need to be stored at 2–8°C and not allowed to freeze. Immunoglobulins should be protected from light. Opened multidose vials must be used within the period recommended in the product literature.
- **NATIONAL FUNDING/ACCESS DECISIONS**

NICE decisions
- **Routine antenatal anti-D prophylaxis for rhesus-negative women (August 2008) NICE TA156**
  Routine antenatal anti-D prophylaxis should be offered to all non-sensitised pregnant women who are rhesus negative.
  www.nice.org.uk/guidance/ta156

- **MEDICINAL FORMS** There can be variation in the licensing of different medicines containing the same drug.

Solution for injection
- D-Gam (Bio Products Laboratory Ltd)
  Anti-D (RHO) immunoglobulin 500 unit D-Gam Anti-D immunoglobulin 500unit solution for injection vials | 1 vial PoM £38.25
  Anti-D (RHO) immunoglobulin 1500 unit D-Gam Anti-D immunoglobulin 1,500unit solution for injection vials | 1 vial PoM £58.00
- Rhophylac (CSL Behring UK Ltd)
  Anti-D (RHO) immunoglobulin 750 unit per 1 ml Rhophylac 1,500units/2ml solution for injection pre-filled syringes | 1 pre-filled disposable injection PoM £46.50

Cytomegalovirus immunoglobulin

16-Apr-2020

- **INDICATIONS AND DOSE**

Prophylaxis of cytomegalovirus infection in patients taking immunosuppressants, particularly transplant recipients (specialist use only)

▶ BY INTRAVENOUS INFUSION

- Child: (consult product literature)

- **CONTRA-INDICATIONS** Selective IgA deficiency with IgA antibodies
- **CAUTIONS** Interference with live virus vaccines

CAUTIONS, FURTHER INFORMATION

- Interference with live virus vaccines Cytomegalovirus immunoglobulin may impair the immune response to live virus vaccines; such vaccines should only be given 3 months after CMV immunoglobulin treatment. Patients receiving measles vaccines should have their antibody status checked as impairment of immune response may persist for up to 1 year.

14

Vaccines

- **INTERACTIONS** → Appendix 1: immunoglobulins
- **SIDE-EFFECTS** Arthralgia · back pain · chills · cutaneous lupus erythematosus · dizziness · embolism and thrombosis · fatigue · fever · haemolysis · haemolytic anaemia · headache · hypotension · infusion related reaction · meningitis aseptic · myocardial infarction · nausea · neutropenia · renal impairment · skin reactions · stroke · transfusion-related acute lung injury · vomiting
- **MONITORING REQUIREMENTS**

▶ Manufacturer advises monitor for signs of infusion-related reactions during and for at least one hour after each infusion in patients receiving cytomegalovirus immunoglobulin for the first time, or following a prolonged period between treatments, or when a different human immunoglobulin has been used previously; monitor all other patients for at least 20 minutes after each infusion—in case of reaction, reduce rate or stop infusion as clinically appropriate.

▶ Manufacturer advises monitor urine output and serum creatinine.

- **HANDLING AND STORAGE** Care must be taken to store all immunological products under the conditions recommended in the product literature, otherwise the preparation may become ineffective. **Refrigerated storage** is usually necessary; many immunoglobulins need to be stored at 2–8°C and not allowed to freeze. Immunoglobulins should be protected from light. Opened multidose vials must be used within the period recommended in the product literature.

- **MEDICINAL FORMS** There can be variation in the licensing of different medicines containing the same drug.

Solution for infusion

- Cytotect CP Biotest (Biotest (UK) Ltd)'

Cytomegalovirus immunoglobulin human 100 unit per 1 ml Cytotect CP Biotest 5,000units/50ml solution for infusion vials | 1 vial PoM £917.70

Cytotect CP Biotest 1,000units/10ml solution for infusion vials | 1 vial PoM £183.54

Hepatitis B immunoglobulin

06-Mar-2020

- **INDICATIONS AND DOSE**

Prophylaxis against hepatitis B infection

▶ BY INTRAMUSCULAR INJECTION

- Neonate: 200 units, dose to be administered as soon as possible after exposure; ideally within 12–48 hours, but no later than 7 days after exposure.
- Child 1 month–4 years: 200 units, dose to be administered as soon as possible after exposure; ideally within 12–48 hours, but no later than 7 days after exposure
- Child 5–9 years: 300 units, dose to be administered as soon as possible after exposure; ideally within 12–48 hours, but no later than 7 days after exposure
- Child 10–17 years: 500 units, dose to be administered as soon as possible after exposure; ideally within 12–48 hours, but no later than 7 days after exposure

Prevention of transmitted infection at birth

▶ BY INTRAMUSCULAR INJECTION

- Neonate: 200 units, dose to be administered as soon as possible after birth; for full details consult Immunisation against Infectious Disease (www.dh.gov.uk).

▶ BY INTRAVENOUS INFUSION

- Neonate: (consult product literature).

Prophylaxis against hepatitis B infection, after exposure to hepatitis B virus-contaminated material

▶ BY INTRAVENOUS INFUSION

- Child: Dose to be administered as soon as possible after exposure, but no later than 72 hours (consult product literature)

Prophylaxis against re-infection of transplanted liver

▶ BY INTRAVENOUS INFUSION

- Child: (consult product literature)

- **CAUTIONS** IgA deficiency · interference with live virus vaccines
- **INTERACTIONS** → Appendix 1: immunoglobulins
- **SIDE-EFFECTS**

▶ **Uncommon** Abdominal pain upper · headache

▶ **Rare or very rare** Cardiac discomfort · fatigue · hypersensitivity · hypertension · hypotension · muscle spasms · nasopharyngitis · oropharyngeal pain · palpitations · skin reactions

- **PRESCRIBING AND DISPENSING INFORMATION** Vials containing 200 units or 500 units (for intramuscular injection), available from selected Public Health England and NHS laboratories (except for Transplant Centres), also available from BPL.
- **HANDLING AND STORAGE** Care must be taken to store all immunological products under the conditions recommended in the product literature, otherwise the preparation may become ineffective. **Refrigerated storage** is usually necessary; many immunoglobulins need to be stored at 2–8°C and not allowed to freeze. Immunoglobulins should be protected from light. Opened multidose vials must be used within the period recommended in the product literature.

- **MEDICINAL FORMS** There can be variation in the licensing of different medicines containing the same drug.

Solution for injection

- Hepatitis B immunoglobulin (Non-proprietary)

Hepatitis B immunoglobulin human 200 unit Hepatitis B immunoglobulin human 200unit solution for injection vials | 1 vial PoM £200.00

Hepatitis B immunoglobulin human 500 unit Hepatitis B immunoglobulin human 500unit solution for injection vials | 1 vial PoM £400.00

- Zutectra (Biotest (UK) Ltd)

Zutectra 500units/1ml solution for injection pre-filled syringes | 5 syringe PoM £1,500.00

Solution for infusion

- Hepatect CP (Biotest (UK) Ltd)

Hepatitis B immunoglobulin human 50 unit per 1 ml Hepatect CP 100units/2ml solution for infusion vials | 1 vial PoM £55.00

Hepatect CP 2000units/40ml solution for infusion vials | 1 vial PoM £1,100.00

Hepatect CP 500units/10ml solution for infusion vials | 1 vial PoM £275.00
Hepatect CP 5000units/100ml solution for infusion vials | 1 vial PoM £2,750.00

- **Omri-Hep-B** (Imported (Israel))
  Hepatitis B immunoglobulin human 50 unit per 1 ml Omri-Hep-B 5000units/100ml solution for infusion vials | 1 vial PoM

Normal immunoglobulin

17-Mar-2020

● **INDICATIONS AND DOSE**

To control outbreaks of hepatitis A

▶ BY DEEP INTRAMUSCULAR INJECTION
- Child 1 month–9 years: 250 mg
- Child 10–17 years: 500 mg

Rubella in pregnancy, prevention of clinical attack

▶ BY DEEP INTRAMUSCULAR INJECTION
- Females of childbearing potential: 750 mg

Antibody deficiency syndromes

▶ BY SUBCUTANEOUS INFUSION
- Child: (consult product literature)

Kawasaki disease (with concomitant aspirin)

▶ BY INTRAVENOUS INFUSION
- Child: 2 g/kg daily for 1 dose, treatment should be given within 10 days of onset of symptom (but children with a delayed diagnosis may also benefit)

SUBGAM®

Hepatitis A prophylaxis in outbreaks

▶ BY INTRAMUSCULAR INJECTION
- Child 1 month–9 years: 500 mg
- Child 10–17 years: 750 mg

● **UNLICENSED USE**
SUBGAM® *Subgam®* is not licensed for prophylactic use, but due to difficulty in obtaining suitable immunoglobulin products, Public Health England recommends intramuscular use for prophylaxis against Hepatitis A or rubella.

● **CONTRA-INDICATIONS** Patients with selective IgA deficiency who have known antibody against IgA

PRIVIGEN® Hyperprolinaemia (contains L-proline)

FLEBOGAMMA® DIF Hereditary fructose intolerance (contains sorbitol)

HIZENTRA® Hyperprolinaemia (contains L-proline)

GAMMAPLEX® Hereditary fructose intolerance (contains sorbitol)

● **CAUTIONS**
GENERAL CAUTIONS Agammaglobulinaemia with or without IgA deficiency · hypogammaglobulinaemia with or without IgA deficiency · interference with live virus vaccines

SPECIFIC CAUTIONS
- With intravenous use Ensure adequate hydration · obesity · renal insufficiency · risk factors for arterial or venous thromboembolic events · thrombophilic disorders

CAUTIONS, FURTHER INFORMATION
- Interference with live virus vaccines Normal immunoglobulin may **interfere with the immune response to live virus vaccines** which should therefore only be given **at least 3 weeks before or 3 months after** an injection of normal immunoglobulin (this does not apply to yellow fever vaccine since normal immunoglobulin does not contain antibody to this virus).

OCTAGAM® Falsely elevated results with blood glucose testing systems (contains maltose)

● **INTERACTIONS** → Appendix 1: immunoglobulins

● **SIDE-EFFECTS**

▶ **Common or very common**
- With intramuscular use Chills
- With subcutaneous use Diarrhoea · dizziness · drowsiness · fatigue · gastrointestinal discomfort · headaches · hypotension · local reaction · myalgia · nausea · pain · skin reactions

▶ **Uncommon**
- With intramuscular use Dizziness · fatigue · feeling hot · headache · nausea · pain · skin reactions
- With subcutaneous use Paraesthesia

▶ **Rare or very rare**
- With intramuscular use Abdominal pain · arthralgia · musculoskeletal stiffness · myalgia · peripheral coldness · tremor

▶ **Frequency not known**
- With intramuscular use Chest discomfort · dyspnoea · facial swelling · fever · flushing · hyperhidrosis · hypertension · hypotension · malaise · oral paraesthesia · pallor · paraesthesia · tachycardia · vomiting
- With intravenous use Embolism and thrombosis · gastrointestinal discomfort · haemolytic anaemia · myocardial infarction · stroke

SIDE-EFFECTS, FURTHER INFORMATION Adverse reactions are more likely to occur in patients receiving normal immunoglobulin for the first time, or following a prolonged period between treatments, or when a different brand of normal immunoglobulin is administered.

● **MONITORING REQUIREMENTS** Monitor for acute renal failure; consider discontinuation if renal function deteriorates. Intravenous preparations with added sucrose have been associated with cases of renal dysfunction and acute renal failure.

● **DIRECTIONS FOR ADMINISTRATION**
Preparations for subcutaneous use May be administered by intramuscular injection if subcutaneous route not possible; intramuscular route **not** for patients with thrombocytopenia or other bleeding disorders.

GAMUNEX® Use Glucose 5% intravenous infusion if dilution prior to infusion is required.

KIOVIG® Use Glucose 5% intravenous infusion if dilution prior to infusion is required.

● **PRESCRIBING AND DISPENSING INFORMATION** Antibody titres can vary widely between normal immunoglobulin preparations from different manufacturers—formulations are **not interchangeable**; patients should be maintained on the same formulation throughout long-term treatment to avoid adverse effects.
- With intramuscular use Available from the Centre for Infections and other regional Public Health England offices (for contacts and control of outbreaks only).

● **HANDLING AND STORAGE** Care must be taken to store all immunological products under the conditions recommended in the product literature, otherwise the preparation may become ineffective. **Refrigerated storage** is usually necessary; many immunoglobulins need to be stored at 2–8°C and not allowed to freeze. Immunoglobulins should be protected from light. Opened multidose vials must be used within the period recommended in the product literature.

● **MEDICINAL FORMS** There can be variation in the licensing of different medicines containing the same drug.

Solution for injection

ELECTROLYTES: May contain Sodium

- **Hizentra** (CSL Behring UK Ltd)
  Normal immunoglobulin human 200 mg per 1 ml Hizentra 2g/10ml solution for injection pre-filled syringes | 1 pre-filled disposable injection PoM £108.00
- **Subgam** (Bio Products Laboratory Ltd)
  Normal immunoglobulin human 160 mg per 1 ml Subgam 1.5g/9.375ml solution for injection vials | 1 vial PoM £75.00

Subgam 4g/25ml solution for injection vials | 1 vial PoM £200.00
Subgam 2g/12.5ml solution for injection vials | 1 vial PoM £100.00
Subgam 1g/6.25ml solution for injection vials | 1 vial PoM £50.00
Subgam 750mg/4.6875ml solution for injection vials | 1 vial PoM £37.50

Solution for infusion

EXCIPIENTS: May contain Glucose, maltose, sorbitol, sucrose

▸ Normal immunoglobulin (Non-proprietary)
Normal immunoglobulin human 100 mg per 1 ml Normal immunoglobulin human 5g/50ml solution for infusion vials | 1 vial PoM
Normal immunoglobulin human 2.5g/25ml solution for infusion vials | 1 vial PoM
Normal immunoglobulin human 20g/200ml solution for infusion vials | 1 vial PoM
Normal immunoglobulin human 10g/100ml solution for infusion vials | 1 vial PoM
Normal immunoglobulin human 30g/300ml solution for infusion vials | 1 vial PoM

▸ Flebogammadif (Grifols UK Ltd)
Normal immunoglobulin human 50 mg per 1 ml Flebogamma DIF 2.5g/50ml solution for infusion vials | 1 vial PoM £127.50
Flebogamma DIF 10g/200ml solution for infusion vials | 1 vial PoM £510.00
Flebogamma DIF 5g/100ml solution for infusion vials | 1 vial PoM £255.00
Flebogamma DIF 20g/400ml solution for infusion vials | 1 vial PoM £1,020.00

▸ Gammaplex (Bio Products Laboratory Ltd)
Normal immunoglobulin human 50 mg per 1 ml Gammaplex 10g/200ml solution for infusion vials | 1 vial PoM £418.00 (Hospital only)
Gammaplex 5g/100ml solution for infusion vials | 1 vial PoM £209.00 (Hospital only)
Gammaplex 20g/400ml solution for infusion vials | 1 vial PoM £836.00 (Hospital only)
Normal immunoglobulin human 100 mg per 1 ml Gammaplex 5g/50ml solution for infusion vials | 1 vial PoM £325.00 (Hospital only)
Gammaplex 10g/100ml solution for infusion vials | 1 vial PoM £650.00 (Hospital only)
Gammaplex 20g/200ml solution for infusion vials | 1 vial PoM £1,300.00 (Hospital only)

▸ Gamunex (Grifols UK Ltd)
Normal immunoglobulin human 100 mg per 1 ml Gamunex 10% 1g/10ml solution for infusion vials | 1 vial PoM £42.50
Gamunex 10% 10g/100ml solution for infusion vials | 1 vial PoM £425.00
Gamunex 10% 20g/200ml solution for infusion vials | 1 vial PoM £850.00
Gamunex 10% 5g/50ml solution for infusion vials | 1 vial PoM £212.50

▸ Hizentra (CSL Behring UK Ltd)
Normal immunoglobulin human 200 mg per 1 ml Hizentra 2g/10ml solution for infusion vials | 1 vial PoM £108.00
Hizentra 1g/5ml solution for infusion vials | 1 vial PoM £54.00
Hizentra 4g/20ml solution for infusion vials | 1 vial PoM £216.00

▸ Kiovig (Baxalta UK Ltd)
Normal immunoglobulin human 100 mg per 1 ml Kiovig 5g/50ml solution for infusion vials | 1 vial PoM £245.00
Kiovig 20g/200ml solution for infusion vials | 1 vial PoM £980.00
Kiovig 10g/100ml solution for infusion vials | 1 vial PoM £490.00
Kiovig 30g/300ml solution for infusion vials | 1 vial PoM £1,470.00
Kiovig 2.5g/25ml solution for infusion vials | 1 vial PoM £122.50
Kiovig 1g/10ml solution for infusion vials | 1 vial PoM £49.00

▸ Octagam (Octapharma Ltd)
Normal immunoglobulin human 50 mg per 1 ml Octagam 5% 10g/200ml solution for infusion bottles | 1 bottle PoM £480.00 (Hospital only)
Octagam 5% 5g/100ml solution for infusion bottles | 1 bottle PoM £240.00 (Hospital only)
Normal immunoglobulin human 100 mg per 1 ml Octagam 10% 10g/100ml solution for infusion bottles | 1 bottle PoM £690.00 (Hospital only)
Octagam 10% 20g/200ml solution for infusion bottles | 1 bottle PoM £1,380.00 (Hospital only)
Octagam 10% 5g/50ml solution for infusion bottles | 1 bottle PoM £345.00 (Hospital only)
Octagam 10% 2g/20ml solution for infusion vials | 1 vial PoM £138.00 (Hospital only)

▸ Panzyga (Octapharma Ltd) ▼
Normal immunoglobulin human 100 mg per 1 ml Panzyga 10g/100ml solution for infusion bottles | 1 bottle PoM £586.50 (Hospital only)
Panzyga 20g/200ml solution for infusion bottles | 1 bottle PoM £1,173.00 (Hospital only)
Panzyga 5g/50ml solution for infusion bottles | 1 bottle PoM £293.25 (Hospital only)

▸ Privigen (CSL Behring UK Ltd)
Normal immunoglobulin human 100 mg per 1 ml Privigen 5g/50ml solution for infusion vials | 1 vial PoM £270.00
Privigen 20g/200ml solution for infusion vials | 1 vial PoM £1,080.00
Privigen 10g/100ml solution for infusion vials | 1 vial PoM £540.00
Privigen 2.5g/25ml solution for infusion vials | 1 vial PoM £135.00

Rabies immunoglobulin

16-Mar-2020

● **INDICATIONS AND DOSE**

Post-exposure prophylaxis against rabies infection

▶ BY LOCAL INFILTRATION, OR BY INTRAMUSCULAR INJECTION

▸ Child: 20 units/kg, dose administered by infiltration in and around the cleansed wound; if the wound not visible or healed or if infiltration of whole volume not possible, give remainder by intramuscular injection into anterolateral thigh (remote from vaccination site)

● **CAUTIONS** IgA deficiency · interference with live virus vaccines

● **INTERACTIONS** → Appendix 1: immunoglobulins

● **SIDE-EFFECTS**

▶ **Rare or very rare** Arthralgia · chills · fatigue · fever · headache · hypersensitivity · hypotension · influenza like illness · malaise · nausea · skin reactions · tachycardia · vomiting

● **PRESCRIBING AND DISPENSING INFORMATION** The potency of individual batches of rabies immunoglobulin from the manufacturer may vary; potency may also be described differently by different manufacturers. It is therefore critical to know the potency of the batch to be used and the weight of the patient in order to calculate the specific volume required to provide the necessary dose.

Available from Specialist and Reference Microbiology Division, Public Health England (also from BPL).

● **HANDLING AND STORAGE** Care must be taken to store all immunological products under the conditions recommended in the product literature, otherwise the preparation may become ineffective. **Refrigerated storage** is usually necessary; many immunoglobulins need to be stored at 2–8°C and not allowed to freeze. Immunoglobulins should be protected from light. Opened multidose vials must be used within the period recommended in the product literature.

● **MEDICINAL FORMS** There can be variation in the licensing of different medicines containing the same drug.

Solution for injection

▸ Rabies immunoglobulin (Non-proprietary)
Rabies immunoglobulin human 500 unit Rabies immunoglobulin human 500unit solution for injection vials | 1 vial PoM £800.00

Tetanus immunoglobulin

16-Mar-2020

● **INDICATIONS AND DOSE**

Post-exposure prophylaxis

▶ BY INTRAMUSCULAR INJECTION

▸ Child: Initially 250 units, then increased to 500 units, dose is only increased if more than 24 hours have elapsed or there is risk of heavy contamination or following burns

Treatment of tetanus infection
- ▶ BY INTRAMUSCULAR INJECTION
 - ▶ Child: 150 units/kg, dose may be given over multiple sites

- **CAUTIONS** IgA deficiency · interference with live virus vaccines
- **INTERACTIONS** → Appendix 1: immunoglobulins
- **SIDE-EFFECTS**
 - ▶ **Rare or very rare** Anaphylactic reaction · hypotension
 - ▶ **Frequency not known** Arthralgia · chest pain · dizziness · dyspnoea · face oedema · oral disorders · tremor
- **HANDLING AND STORAGE** Care must be taken to store all immunological products under the conditions recommended in the product literature, otherwise the preparation may become ineffective. **Refrigerated storage** is usually necessary; many immunoglobulins need to be stored at 2–8°C and not allowed to freeze. Immunoglobulins should be protected from light. Opened multidose vials must be used within the period recommended in the product literature.

- **MEDICINAL FORMS** There can be variation in the licensing of different medicines containing the same drug.

Solution for injection
- ▶ Tetanus immunoglobulin (Non-proprietary)
 Tetanus immunoglobulin human 250 unit Tetanus immunoglobulin human 250unit solution for injection vials | 1 vial PoM £170.00 DT = £170.00

Varicella-zoster immunoglobulin

16-Mar-2020

(Antivaricella-zoster Immunoglobulin)

- **INDICATIONS AND DOSE**

Prophylaxis against varicella infection
- ▶ BY DEEP INTRAMUSCULAR INJECTION
 - ▶ Neonate: 250 mg, to be administered as soon as possible—not later than 10 days after exposure, second dose to be given if further exposure occurs more than 3 weeks after first dose, no evidence that effective in severe disease.
 - ▶ Child 1 month–5 years: 250 mg, to be administered as soon as possible—not later than 10 days after exposure, second dose to be given if further exposure occurs more than 3 weeks after first dose, no evidence that effective in severe disease
 - ▶ Child 6–10 years: 500 mg, to be administered as soon as possible—not later than 10 days after exposure, second dose to be given if further exposure occurs more than 3 weeks after first dose, no evidence that effective in severe disease
 - ▶ Child 11–14 years: 750 mg, to be administered as soon as possible—not later than 10 days after exposure, second dose to be given if further exposure occurs more than 3 weeks after first dose, no evidence that effective in severe disease
 - ▶ Child 15–17 years: 1 g, to be administered as soon as possible—not later than 10 days after exposure, second dose to be given if further exposure occurs more than 3 weeks after first dose, no evidence that effective in severe disease

- **CAUTIONS** IgA deficiency · interference with live virus vaccines
- **INTERACTIONS** → Appendix 1: immunoglobulins
- **SIDE-EFFECTS** Arthralgia · chills · fever · headache · hypersensitivity · hypotension · malaise · nausea · skin reactions · tachycardia · vomiting
- **DIRECTIONS FOR ADMINISTRATION** Normal immunoglobulin for intravenous use may be used in those unable to receive intramuscular injections.
- **PRESCRIBING AND DISPENSING INFORMATION** Available from selected Public Health England and NHS laboratories (also from BPL).
- **HANDLING AND STORAGE** Care must be taken to store all immunological products under the conditions recommended in the product literature, otherwise the preparation may become ineffective. **Refrigerated storage** is usually necessary; many immunoglobulins need to be stored at 2–8°C and not allowed to freeze. Immunoglobulins should be protected from light. Opened multidose vials must be used within the period recommended in the product literature.

- **MEDICINAL FORMS** There can be variation in the licensing of different medicines containing the same drug.

Solution for injection
- ▶ Varicella-Zoster (Bio Products Laboratory Ltd)
 Varicella-Zoster immunoglobulin human 250 mg Varicella-Zoster immunoglobulin human 250mg solution for injection vials | 1 vial PoM £600.00 DT = £600.00

2 Post-exposure prophylaxis

IMMUNE SERA AND IMMUNOGLOBULINS ›
ANTITOXINS

Botulism antitoxin

- **DRUG ACTION** A preparation containing the specific antitoxic globulins that have the power of neutralising the toxins formed by types A, B, and E of *Clostridium botulinum*.

- **INDICATIONS AND DOSE**

Post exposure prophylaxis of botulism
- ▶ BY INTRAMUSCULAR INJECTION
 - ▶ Child: (consult product literature)

- **SIDE-EFFECTS** Hypersensitivity

 SIDE-EFFECTS, FURTHER INFORMATION It is essential to read the contra-indications, warnings, and details of sensitivity tests on the package insert. Prior to treatment checks should be made regarding previous administration of any antitoxin and history of any allergic condition, e.g. asthma, hay fever, etc.
- **PRE-TREATMENT SCREENING** All patients should be tested for sensitivity (diluting the antitoxin if history of allergy).
- **PRESCRIBING AND DISPENSING INFORMATION** Available from local designated centres, for details see TOXBASE (requires registration) www.toxbase.org. For supplies outside working hours apply to other designated centres or to the Public Health England Colindale duty doctor (Tel (020) 8200 6868). For major incidents, obtain supplies from the local blood bank.

 The BP title Botulinum Antitoxin is not used because the preparation currently in use may have a different specification.

- **MEDICINAL FORMS** No licensed medicines listed.

Diphtheria antitoxin

(Dip/Ser)

● **INDICATIONS AND DOSE**

Passive immunisation in suspected cases of diphtheria

▸ BY INTRAVENOUS INFUSION

▸ Child: Dose should be given without waiting for bacteriological confirmation (consult product literature)

● **CAUTIONS**

CAUTIONS, FURTHER INFORMATION

▸ Hypersensitivity Hypersensitivity is common after administration; resuscitation facilities should be available.

Diphtheria antitoxin is no longer used for prophylaxis because of the risk of hypersensitivity; unimmunised contacts should be promptly investigated and given antibacterial prophylaxis and vaccine.

● **SIDE-EFFECTS**

▸ **Common or very common** Hypersensitivity

● **PRE-TREATMENT SCREENING** Diphtheria antitoxin is derived from horse serum and reactions are common; tests for hypersensitivity should be carried out before use.

● **PRESCRIBING AND DISPENSING INFORMATION** Available from Centre for Infections (Tel (020) 8200 6868) or in Northern Ireland from Public Health Laboratory, Belfast City Hospital (Tel (028) 9032 9241).

● **MEDICINAL FORMS** There can be variation in the licensing of different medicines containing the same drug.

Solution for injection

▸ Diphtheria antitoxin (Non-proprietary)
Diphtheria antitoxin 1000 unit per 1 ml Antidiphtheria serum 10,000units/10ml solution for injection ampoules | 1 ampoule PoM

3 Tuberculosis diagnostic test

DIAGNOSTIC AGENTS

Tuberculin purified protein derivative

(Tuberculin PPD)

● **INDICATIONS AND DOSE**

Mantoux test

▸ BY INTRADERMAL INJECTION

▸ Child: 2 units for one dose

Mantoux test (if first test is negative and a further test is considered appropriate)

▸ BY INTRADERMAL INJECTION

▸ Child: 10 units for 1 dose

DOSE EQUIVALENCE AND CONVERSION

▸ 2 units is equivalent to 0.1 mL of 20 units/mL strength.

▸ 10 units is equivalent to 0.1 mL of 100 units/mL strength.

● **CAUTIONS**

CAUTIONS, FURTHER INFORMATION

▸ Mantoux test Response to tuberculin may be suppressed by viral infection, sarcoidosis, corticosteroid therapy, or immunosuppression due to disease or treatment and the MMR vaccine. If a tuberculin skin test has already been initiated, then the MMR should be delayed until the skin test has been read unless protection against measles is required urgently. If a child has had a recent MMR, and requires a tuberculin test, then a 4 week interval should be observed. Apart from tuberculin and MMR, all other live vaccines can be administered at any time before or after tuberculin.

● **PRESCRIBING AND DISPENSING INFORMATION** Available from ImmForm (SSI brand).

The strength of tuberculin PPD in currently available products may be different to the strengths of products used previously for the Mantoux test; care is required to select the correct strength.

● **MEDICINAL FORMS** There can be variation in the licensing of different medicines containing the same drug. Forms available from special-order manufacturers include: solution for injection

Solution for injection

▸ Tuberculin purified protein derivative (Non-proprietary)
Tuberculin purified protein derivative 20 tuberculin unit per 1 ml Tuberculin PPD RT 23 SSI 20 tuberculin units/ml solution for injection 1.5ml vials | 1 vial
Tuberculin purified protein derivative 100 tuberculin unit per 1 ml Tuberculin PPD RT 23 SSI 100 tuberculin units/ml solution for injection 1.5ml vials | 1 vial

4 Vaccination

Vaccination, general principles

06-Feb-2020

Active immunity

Active immunity can be acquired by natural disease or by vaccination. **Vaccines** stimulate production of antibodies and other components of the immune mechanism; they consist of either:

1. a *live attenuated* form of a virus (e.g. measles, mumps and rubella vaccine) or bacteria (e.g. BCG vaccine), or
2. *inactivated* preparations of the virus (e.g. influenza vaccine) or bacteria, or
3. *detoxified exotoxins* produced by a micro-organism (e.g. tetanus vaccine), or
4. *extracts of* a micro-organism, which may be derived from the organism (e.g. pneumococcal vaccine) or produced by recombinant DNA technology (e.g. hepatitis B vaccine).

Live attenuated vaccines usually produce a durable immunity, but not always as long-lasting as that resulting from natural infection.

Inactivated vaccines may require a primary series of injections of vaccine to produce an adequate antibody response, and in most cases booster (reinforcing) injections are required; the duration of immunity varies from months to many years. Some inactivated vaccines are adsorbed onto an adjuvant (such as aluminium hydroxide) to enhance the antibody response.

Passive immunity

Immunity with immediate protection against certain infective organisms can be obtained by injecting preparations made from the plasma of immune individuals with adequate levels of antibody to the disease for which protection is sought (see under *Immunoglobulins*). The duration of this passive immunity varies according to the dose and the type of immunoglobulin. Passive immunity may last only a few weeks; when necessary, passive immunisation can be repeated.

Antibodies of human origin are usually termed *immunoglobulins*. The term *antiserum* is applied to material prepared in animals. Because of serum sickness and other allergic-type reactions that may follow injections of antisera, this therapy has been replaced whenever possible by the use of immunoglobulins.

Routine immunisation schedule

When to immunise	Vaccine given and dose schedule (for details of dose, see under individual vaccines)
Neonates at risk only	▸ Bacillus Calmette-Guérin vaccine p. 847 (at birth, see Bacillus Calmette-Guérin vaccine p. 831). ▸ Hepatitis B vaccine p. 853 (at birth, 4 weeks, and 1 year, see Hepatitis B vaccine p. 834).
8 weeks	▸ Diphtheria with tetanus, pertussis, hepatitis B, poliomyelitis and haemophilus influenzae type b vaccine p. 846 (*Infanrix hexa*®). First dose. ▸ Meningococcal group B vaccine (rDNA, component, adsorbed) p. 849 (*Bexsero*®). First dose. ▸ Changes have been made to the immunisation schedule for children born on or after 1st January 2020, see *12 weeks*. **For children born on or before 31st December** 2019, give pneumococcal polysaccharide conjugate vaccine (adsorbed) p. 850 (*Prevenar 13*®). First dose. ▸ Rotavirus vaccine p. 859 (*Rotarix*®). First dose.
12 weeks	▸ Diphtheria with tetanus, pertussis, hepatitis B, poliomyelitis and haemophilus influenzae type b vaccine (*Infanrix hexa*®). Second dose. ▸ **For children born on or after 1st January** 2020, give pneumococcal polysaccharide conjugate vaccine (adsorbed) (*Prevenar 13*®). Single dose. ▸ Rotavirus vaccine (*Rotarix*®). Second dose.
16 weeks	▸ Diphtheria with tetanus, pertussis, hepatitis B, poliomyelitis and haemophilus influenzae type b vaccine (*Infanrix hexa*®). Third dose. ▸ Meningococcal group B vaccine (rDNA, component, adsorbed) (*Bexsero*®). Second dose. ▸ **For children born on or before 31st December** 2019, give pneumococcal polysaccharide conjugate vaccine (adsorbed) (*Prevenar 13*®). Second dose.
1 year (on or after first birthday)	▸ Measles, mumps and rubella vaccine, live p. 857 (*MMR VaxPRO*® or *Priorix*®). First dose. ▸ Meningococcal group B vaccine (rDNA, component, adsorbed) (*Bexsero*®). Single booster dose. ▸ Pneumococcal polysaccharide conjugate vaccine (adsorbed) (*Prevenar 13*®). **Single booster dose regardless of birth date.** ▸ Haemophilus influenzae type b with meningococcal group C vaccine p. 848 (*Menitorix*®). Single booster dose.
2-10 years on 31st August 2019 (including children in reception class and school years 1, 2, 3, 4, 5, and 6).	▸ Influenza vaccine p. 856. Each year from September. **Note:** live attenuated influenza nasal spray is recommended (*Fluenz Tetra*®). If contra-indicated and child is in a clinical risk group, use inactivated influenza vaccine (see Influenza vaccine p. 835).
3 years and 4 months, or soon after	▸ Diphtheria with tetanus, pertussis and poliomyelitis vaccine p. 846 (*Boostrix-IPV*® or *Repevax*®). Single booster dose. ▸ Measles, mumps and rubella vaccine, live (*MMR VaxPRO*® or *Priorix*®). Second dose.
11-14 years. First dose of HPV vaccine will be offered to individuals aged 12-13 years in England, Wales, and Northern Ireland, and those aged 11-13 years in Scotland. For individuals aged 15 years and over, see Human papillomavirus vaccine p. 834.	▸ Human papillomavirus vaccines p. 855 (*Gardasil*®). 2 dose schedule; second dose 6-24 months after first dose. Only *Gardasil*® is offered as part of the national immunisation programme. For individuals who started the schedule with *Cervarix*®, but did not complete the vaccination course, the course can be completed with *Gardasil*®. Ideally one vaccine should be used for the entire course.
13-15 years	▸ Meningococcal groups A with C and W135 and Y vaccine p. 849 (*Nimenrix*® or *Menveo*®). Single booster dose.
13-18 years	▸ Diphtheria with tetanus and poliomyelitis vaccine p. 846 (*Revaxis*®). Single booster dose. **Note:** Can be given at the same time as the dose of meningococcal groups A with C and W135 and Y vaccine at 13-15 years of age.
Females of child-bearing age susceptible to rubella	▸ Measles, mumps and rubella vaccine, live. Females of child-bearing age who have not received 2 doses of a rubella-containing vaccine or who do not have a positive antibody test for rubella should be offered rubella immunisation (using the MMR vaccine)—exclude pregnancy before immunisation, and avoid pregnancy for one month after vaccination.
Pregnant females	▸ Acellular pertussis-containing vaccine administered as diphtheria with tetanus, pertussis and poliomyelitis vaccine (*Boostrix-IPV*® or *Repevax*®). 1 dose from the 16th week of pregnancy, preferably after the fetal anomaly scan (weeks 18-20). ▸ Influenza vaccine (inactivated). Single dose administered from September, regardless of the stage of pregnancy (see Influenza vaccine p. 835).

Reactions are theoretically possible after injection of human immunoglobulins, but reports of such reactions are very rare.

Vaccines and HIV infection

HIV-positive children with or without symptoms can receive the following live vaccines:

- MMR (but avoid if immunity significantly impaired), varicella-zoster vaccine against chickenpox (but avoid if immunity significantly impaired—consult product literature; use of normal immunoglobulin should be considered after exposure to measles and varicella–zoster immunoglobulin considered after exposure to chickenpox or herpes zoster), rotavirus;

and the following inactivated vaccines:

- anthrax, cholera (oral), diphtheria, haemophilus influenzae type b, hepatitis A, hepatitis B, human papillomavirus, influenza (injection), meningococcal, pertussis, pneumococcal, poliomyelitis (inactivated poliomyelitis vaccine is now used instead of oral poliomyelitis vaccine for routine immunisation of children), rabies, tetanus, tick-borne encephalitis, typhoid (injection).

HIV-positive children should **not** receive:

- BCG, influenza nasal spray (unless stable HIV infection and receiving antiretroviral therapy), typhoid (oral), yellow fever (if yellow fever risk is unavoidable, specialist advice should be sought).

The above advice differs from that for other immunocompromised patients; *Immunisation of HIV infected Children* issued by *Children's HIV Association* (CHIVA) are available at www.chiva.org.uk.

Vaccines and asplenia, splenic dysfunction, or complement disorders

The following vaccines are recommended for individuals with asplenia, splenic dysfunction, or complement disorders (including those taking complement inhibitors) depending on the age at which their condition is diagnosed:

- Influenza vaccine p. 856;
- Meningococcal groups A with C and W135 and Y vaccine p. 849 and meningococcal group B vaccine (rDNA, component, adsorbed) p. 849;
- 13-valent pneumococcal polysaccharide conjugate vaccine (adsorbed) p. 850 and/or 23-valent pneumococcal polysaccharide vaccine p. 851. Patients on complement inhibitor therapy with eculizumab p. 614 are not at increased risk of pneumococcal disease and do not require 23-valent pneumococcal polysaccharide vaccine p. 851 or additional doses of 13-valent pneumococcal polysaccharide conjugate vaccine (adsorbed) p. 850.

Additional booster doses of other vaccines should be considered depending on the individual's underlying condition—specialist advice may be required. For information on specific indications for immunisation of vulnerable groups, see Chapter 7, Immunisation of individuals with underlying medical conditions, in *Immunisation against infectious disease*- 'The Green Book'.

Children first diagnosed or presenting aged under *1* ***year*** should be immunised according to the Immunisation schedule p. 831. During their first year they should also be given 2 doses of meningococcal groups A with C and W135 and Y vaccine at least 4 weeks apart, and a dose of 13-valent pneumococcal polysaccharide conjugate vaccine (adsorbed) p. 850 (in order to have received a total of 2 doses of 13-valent *pneumococcal polysaccharide conjugate vaccine (adsorbed)* with an 8 week interval). 8 weeks following their routine 1 year booster vaccines, they should receive a booster dose of meningococcal groups A with C and W135 and Y vaccine. An additional dose of 13-valent pneumococcal polysaccharide conjugate vaccine (adsorbed) p. 850 should be given at least 8 weeks after the routine 13-valent pneumococcal polysaccharide conjugate vaccine (adsorbed) booster p. 850 scheduled at 1 year. After their second birthday, a dose of 23-valent pneumococcal polysaccharide vaccine p. 851 should be given at least 8 weeks after the last dose of 13-valent pneumococcal polysaccharide conjugate vaccine (adsorbed) p. 850. The influenza vaccine should be given annually in children aged 6 months or older.

Children first diagnosed or presenting aged *1* ***year to under*** *2* ***years*** should be immunised according to the Immunisation schedule p. 831, including any routine vaccines due at 1 year of age if not yet administered. 8 weeks following the routine 1 year booster vaccines a dose of meningococcal groups A with C and W135 and Y vaccine should be given. An additional dose of 13-valent pneumococcal polysaccharide conjugate vaccine (adsorbed) p. 850 should be given at least 8 weeks after the 1 year 13-valent pneumococcal polysaccharide conjugate vaccine (adsorbed) booster dose p. 850. After their second birthday, a dose of 23-valent pneumococcal polysaccharide vaccine p. 851 should be given at least 8 weeks after the last dose of 13-valent pneumococcal polysaccharide conjugate vaccine (adsorbed) p. 850. The influenza vaccine should be given annually.

Children first diagnosed or presenting aged *2* ***years to under*** *10* ***years*** should be immunised according to the Immunisation schedule p. 831. Additionally, they should be given a dose of meningococcal groups A with C and W135 and Y vaccine and 23-valent pneumococcal polysaccharide vaccine p. 851. For children who have not received the full routine immunisation for meningococcal group B vaccine (rDNA, component, adsorbed), ensure that 2 doses, 8 weeks apart have been given since their first birthday. For children who have not received any 13-valent pneumococcal polysaccharide conjugate vaccine (adsorbed) p. 850 previously, a single dose should be given, followed by a dose of 23-valent pneumococcal polysaccharide vaccine p. 851 at least 8 weeks later. The influenza vaccine should be given annually.

Individuals first diagnosed aged *10* ***years and over*** regardless of previous immunisations, should be given a dose of 23-valent pneumococcal polysaccharide vaccine p. 851, meningococcal group B vaccine (rDNA, component, adsorbed) and meningococcal groups A with C and W135 and Y vaccine. After 4 weeks, an additional dose of meningococcal group B vaccine (rDNA, component, adsorbed) should be given. The influenza vaccine should be given annually.

Vaccines and antisera availability

Anthrax vaccine and yellow fever vaccine, live p. 860, botulism antitoxin p. 827, diphtheria antitoxin p. 828, and snake and spider venom antitoxins are available from local designated holding centres.

For antivenom, see Emergency Treatment of Poisoning.

Enquiries for vaccines not available commercially can also be made to:

Vaccines and Countermeasures Response Department
Public Health England
Wellington House
133–155 Waterloo Road
London
SE1 8UG
Email: vaccinesupply@phe.gov.uk

In Scotland information about availability of vaccines can be obtained from a Specialist in Pharmaceutical Public Health.

In Wales enquiries for vaccines not available commercially should be directed to:

Welsh Medicines Information Centre
University Hospital of Wales
Cardiff
CF14 4XW
(029) 2074 2979

In Northern Ireland:

Pharmacy and Medicines Management Centre
Northern Health and Social Care Trust
Beech House
Antrim Hospital Site
Bush Road
Antrim
BT41 2RL
Email: rphps.admin@northerntrust.hscni.net

For further details of availability, see under individual vaccines.

Useful Resources

Recommendations reflect advice from *Immunisation against Infectious Disease*- 'The Green Book'. Public Health England, (2013). Chapters from the handbook (including updates since 2013) are available at:

www.gov.uk/government/collections/immunisation-against-infectious-disease-the-green-book

Immunisation schedule

21-Apr-2020

Routine immunisations, sources of information

The Joint Committee on Vaccination and Immunisation have issued a statement on immunisation prioritisation during the COVID-19 pandemic, available at: www.gov.uk/government/publications/jcvi-statement-on-immunisation-prioritisation/statement-from-jcvi-on-immunisation-prioritisation

The following recommendations reflect advice produced by Public Health England. Recommendations specific to each vaccine can be found in *Immunisation against infectious disease*– 'The Green Book'. Public Health England at: www.gov.uk/government/collections/immunisation-against-infectious-disease-the-green-book

The immunisation schedule reflects advice from 'The complete routine immunisation schedule' produced by Public Health England (2019). For the most up to date immunisation schedule, see: www.gov.uk/government/publications/the-complete-routine-immunisation-schedule

The Influenza immunisation recommendations reflect advice from the 'National flu immunisation programme plan 2019/2020' produced by Public Health England, Department of Health and Social Care, and NHS England. For the most up-to-date letter, see: www.gov.uk/government/publications/national-flu-immunisation-programme-plan

Vaccines for the immunisation schedule should be obtained from ImmForm at: www.immform.dh.gov.uk

Preterm birth

Babies born preterm should receive all routine immunisations based on their actual date of birth. The risk of apnoea following vaccination is increased in preterm babies, particularly in those born at or before 28 weeks gestational age. If babies at risk of apnoea are in hospital at the time of their first immunisation, they should be monitored for respiratory complications for 48–72 hours after immunisation. If a baby develops apnoea, bradycardia, or desaturation after the first immunisation, the second immunisation should also be given in hospital with similar monitoring.

Individuals with unknown or incomplete immunisation history

For children born in the UK who present with an inadequate or unknown immunisation history, investigation into immunisations received should be carried out. Outstanding doses should be administered where the routine childhood immunisation schedule has not been completed.

For advice on dosing schedules for missed vaccinations, and the immunisation of individuals coming to the UK, consult Chapter 11, The UK immunisation schedule, in *Immunisation against infectious disease*– 'The Green Book'. Public Health England, available at: www.gov.uk/government/publications/immunisation-schedule-the-green-book-chapter-11

Anthrax vaccine

31-Oct-2018

Overview

Anthrax vaccine is rarely required for children.

Useful Resources

Recommendations reflect Chapter 13, Anthrax, in *Immunisation against infectious disease*– 'The 'Green Book'. Public Health England. February 2017.
www.gov.uk/government/publications/anthrax-the-green-book-chapter-13

Bacillus Calmette-Guérin vaccine

24-Oct-2019

Overview

The Bacillus Calmette-Guérin vaccine p. 847 (BCG vaccine) contains a live attenuated strain derived from *Mycobacterium bovis* which is indicated for the prevention of Tuberculosis p. 392.

BCG vaccine is recommended for the following children if immunisation has not previously been carried out and they are tuberculin-negative:

- all neonates and infants (aged 0–12 months) living in areas of the UK where the annual incidence of tuberculosis is 40 cases per 100 000 or greater;
- all neonates and infants (aged 0–12 months) with a parent or grandparent born in a country where the annual incidence of tuberculosis is 40 cases per 100 000 or greater;
- previously unvaccinated children (aged 1–5 years) with a parent or grandparent born in a country where the annual incidence of tuberculosis is 40 cases per 100 000 or greater (tuberculin testing is not usually required);
- previously unvaccinated children (aged 6–15 years) with a parent or grandparent born in a country where the annual incidence of tuberculosis is 40 cases per 100 000 or greater;
- previously unvaccinated children (aged under 16 years) with close contact to cases of sputum smear-positive pulmonary or laryngeal tuberculosis;
- previously unvaccinated children (aged under 16 years) who were born in, or lived for at least 3 months in a country where the annual incidence of tuberculosis is 40 cases per 100 000 or greater.

Although protection provided by BCG vaccine may decrease with time, there is no evidence that repeat vaccination offers significant additional protection and therefore repeat BCG vaccination is not recommended.

The Bacillus Calmette-Guérin vaccine is contra-indicated in all HIV-infected children. For advice on BCG vaccination in immunosuppressed children, consult Chapter 32: Tuberculosis - 'The Green Book', Public Health England (see useful resources).

For advice on drug treatment, see Tuberculosis p. 392; for treatment of infection following vaccination, seek expert advice.

Travel

The risk of a child acquiring tuberculosis infection while travelling depends on several factors including the incidence of tuberculosis in that country, the duration of travel, the degree of contact with the local population, the reason for travel and the susceptibility and age of the child.

BCG vaccine is recommended for previously unvaccinated, tuberculin-negative children aged under 16 years who intend to travel for 3 months or more in a country where the annual incidence of tuberculosis is 40 cases per 100 000 or greater, or where the risk of multi-drug resistant tuberculosis is high. The risk of children acquiring tuberculosis infection while travelling is low and BCG vaccine is not required if no other factors are present.

A list of countries where the annual incidence of tuberculosis is 40 cases per 100 000 or greater, is available at www.gov.uk/government/publications/tuberculosis-tb-by-country-rates-per-100000-people.

Tuberculin skin testing

The tuberculin skin test (*Mantoux test*) is used to assess a child's sensitivity to tuberculin protein when BCG vaccination is being considered or as an aid to diagnosis of tuberculosis. A tuberculin skin test involves administration of tuberculin purified protein derivative by intradermal injection p. 828. It is necessary before BCG vaccination for:

- children aged 6 years and over;

- children aged under 6 years living in a country for more than 3 months with an annual tuberculosis incidence of 40 cases per 100 000 or greater;
- those who have had close contact with a person with known tuberculosis;
- those who have a family history of tuberculosis within the last 5 years.

BCG vaccination can be given up to three months following a negative tuberculin test.

The BCG vaccine should not be administered to an individual with a positive tuberculin test—it is unnecessary and may cause a more severe local reaction. Those with a *Mantoux test* induration of 5 mm and greater should be referred to a tuberculosis clinic for assessment of the need for further investigation and treatment.

All suspected cases of tuberculosis must be notified to the local health protection unit. Where there is a community level outbreak, specialist advice should be sought from Public Health England (tel. 020 8200 4400) or, in Scotland, Health Protection Scotland (tel. 0140 300 1191).

Useful Resources

Recommendations reflect Chapter 32, Tuberculosis, in *Immunisation against infectious disease*– 'The Green Book'. Public Health England, August 2018.
www.gov.uk/government/publications/tuberculosis-the-green-book-chapter-32

Botulism antitoxin

Overview

A polyvalent botulism antitoxin p. 827 is available for the post-exposure prophylaxis of botulism and for the treatment of persons thought to be suffering from botulism. It specifically neutralises the toxins produced by *Clostridium botulinum* types A, B, and E. It is not effective against infantile botulism as the toxin (type A) is seldom, if ever, found in the blood in this type of infection.

Hypersensitivity reactions are a problem. It is essential to read the contra-indications, warnings, and details of sensitivity tests on the package insert. Prior to treatment checks should be made regarding previous administration of any antitoxin and history of any allergic condition, e.g. asthma, hay fever, etc. All patients should be tested for sensitivity (diluting the antitoxin if history of allergy).

Useful Resources

Advice reflects that in the handbook Immunisation against Infectious Disease (2013), which in turn reflects the guidance of the Joint Committee on Vaccination and Immunisation (JCVI). The advice also incorporates changes announced by the Chief Medical Officer and Health Department Updates. Chapters from the handbook (including updates since 2013) are available at:
www.gov.uk/government/collections/immunisation-against-infectious-disease-the-green-book

Cholera vaccine

07-Nov-2018

Overview

Oral cholera vaccine p. 848 contains inactivated Inaba (including El-Tor biotype) and Ogawa strains of *Vibrio cholerae*, serotype O1 together with recombinant B-subunit of the cholera toxin produced in Inaba strains of *V. cholerae*, serotype O1.

Oral cholera vaccine is licensed for children from 2 years of age who are travelling to endemic or epidemic areas on the basis of current recommendations. Immunisation should be completed at least one week before potential exposure. However, there is no requirement for cholera vaccination for international travel. After a full risk assessment, immunisation can be considered for the following children:

- children travelling with remote itineraries in areas where cholera epidemics are occurring and there is limited access to medical care;
- children travelling to potential cholera risk areas, for whom vaccination is considered potentially beneficial.

For dosing schedule, see cholera vaccine.

Immunisation with cholera vaccine does not provide complete protection and all travellers to a country where cholera exists should be warned that scrupulous attention to food, water, and personal hygiene is essential.

All suspected cases of cholera must be notified to the local health protection unit. Where there is a community level outbreak, specialist advice should be sought from Public Health England (tel. 020 8200 4400) or, in Scotland, Health Protection Scotland (tel. 0140 300 1191).

Contacts

Contacts of children with cholera should maintain high standards of personal hygiene to avoid becoming infected. Cholera vaccine should not be used in the management of contacts of cases or in controlling the spread of infection.

Useful Resources

Recommendations reflect Chapter 14, Cholera, in *Immunisation against infectious disease*– 'The Green Book'. Public Health England, December 2013.
www.gov.uk/government/publications/cholera-the-green-book-chapter-14

Diphtheria vaccine

Overview

Diphtheria vaccines are prepared from the toxin of *Corynebacterium diphtheriae* and adsorption on aluminium hydroxide or aluminium phosphate improves antigenicity. The vaccine stimulates the production of the protective antitoxin. The quantity of diphtheria toxoid in a preparation determines whether the vaccine is defined as 'high dose' or 'low dose'. Vaccines containing the higher dose of diphtheria toxoid are used for primary immunisation of children under 10 years of age. Vaccines containing the lower dose of diphtheria toxoid are used for primary immunisation in adults and children over 10 years. Single-antigen diphtheria vaccine is not available and adsorbed diphtheria vaccine is given as a combination product containing other vaccines.

For primary immunisation *of children aged between 2 months and* 10 *years* vaccination is recommended usually in the form of 3 doses (separated by 1-month intervals) of diphtheria with tetanus, pertussis, hepatitis B, poliomyelitis and haemophilus influenzae type b vaccine p. 846 (*Infanrix hexa*®) (see Immunisation schedule). In unimmunised individuals aged *over* 10 *years* the primary course comprises of 3 doses of **adsorbed diphtheria** [low dose], **tetanus and poliomyelitis (inactivated) vaccine.**

A booster dose should be given 3 years after the primary course (this interval can be reduced to a minimum of 1 year if the primary course was delayed). Children *under* 10 *years* should receive *either* **adsorbed diphtheria, tetanus, pertussis (acellular, component) and poliomyelitis (inactivated) vaccine** *or***adsorbed diphtheria** [low dose], **tetanus, pertussis (acellular, component) and poliomyelitis (inactivated) vaccine** . Individuals aged *over* 10 *years* should receive **adsorbed diphtheria** [low dose], **tetanus, and poliomyelitis (inactivated) vaccine**.

A second booster dose, of adsorbed diphtheria [low dose], tetanus and poliomyelitis (inactivated) vaccine, should be given 10 years after the previous booster dose (this interval can be reduced to a minimum of 5 years if previous doses were delayed). For children who have been vaccinated following a tetanus-prone wound, see tetanus vaccines.

Travel
Those intending to travel to areas with a risk of diphtheria infection should be fully immunised according to the UK schedule. If more than 10 years have lapsed since completion of the UK schedule, a dose of **adsorbed diphtheria** [low dose], **tetanus and poliomyelitis (inactivated) vaccine** should be administered.

Contacts
Advice on the management of cases of diphtheria, carriers, contacts and outbreaks must be sought from health protection units. The immunisation history of infected children and their contacts should be determined; those who have been incompletely immunised should complete their immunisation and fully immunised individuals should receive a reinforcing dose. Also see advice on antibacterial treatment to prevent a secondary case of diphtheria in a non-immune child.

Useful Resources
Advice reflects that in the handbook Immunisation against Infectious Disease (2013), which in turn reflects the guidance of the Joint Committee on Vaccination and Immunisation (JCVI). The advice also incorporates changes announced by the Chief Medical Officer and Health Department Updates. Chapters from the handbook (including updates since 2013) are available at:
www.gov.uk/government/collections/immunisation-against-infectious-disease-the-green-book

Haemophilus influenzae type B conjugate vaccine

Overview
Haemophilus influenzae type b (Hib) vaccine is made from capsular polysaccharide; it is conjugated with a protein such as tetanus toxoid to increase immunogenicity, especially in young children. *Haemophilus influenzae type b vaccine* immunisation is given in combination with diphtheria, tetanus, pertussis, hepatitis B and poliomyelitis vaccine (*Infanrix hexa*®), as a component of the primary course of childhood immunisation (see Immunisation schedule). For infants under 1 year, the course consists of 3 doses of a vaccine containing *Haemophilus influenzae* type b component with an interval of 1 month between doses. A booster dose of Haemophilus influenzae type b vaccine (combined with meningococcal group C conjugate vaccine) should be given at 1 year of age, on or after the child's first birthday.

Children 1–10 years who have not been immunised against *Haemophilus influenzae* type b need to receive only 1 dose of *Haemophilus influenzae* type b vaccine (combined with meningococcal group C conjugate vaccine). However, if a primary course of immunisation has not been completed, children born before August 2017 should be given 3 doses of the combined vaccine they were started on. The risk of infection falls sharply in older children and the vaccine is not normally required for children over 10 years.

Haemophilus influenzae type b vaccine may be given to those over 10 years who are considered to be at increased risk of invasive *H. influenzae* type b disease (such as those with sickle-cell disease or complement deficiency, or those receiving treatment for malignancy).

Invasive *Haemophilus influenzae* type b disease
After recovery from infection, unimmunised and partially immunised index cases under 10 years of age should complete their age-specific course of immunisation. Previously vaccinated cases under 10 years of age should be given an additional dose of haemophilus influenzae type b vaccine (combined with meningococcal group C conjugate vaccine) if Hib antibody concentrations are low or if it is not possible to measure antibody concentrations. Index cases of any age with asplenia or splenic dysfunction should complete their immunisation according to the recommendations below; fully vaccinated cases with asplenia or splenic dysfunction should be given an additional dose of haemophilus influenzae type b vaccine (combined with meningococcal group C conjugate vaccine) if they received their previous dose over 1 year ago.

Also see use of rifampicin p. 396 in the prevention of secondary cases of *Haemophilus influenzae* type b disease.

Useful Resources
Advice reflects that in the handbook Immunisation against Infectious Disease (2013), which in turn reflects the guidance of the Joint Committee on Vaccination and Immunisation (JCVI). The advice also incorporates changes announced by the Chief Medical Officer and Health Department Updates. Chapters from the handbook (including updates since 2013) are available at:
www.gov.uk/government/collections/immunisation-against-infectious-disease-the-green-book

Hepatitis A vaccine

Overview
Hepatitis A vaccine p. 852 is prepared from formaldehyde-inactivated hepatitis A virus grown in human diploid cells.

Immunisation is recommended for:

- residents of homes for those with severe learning difficulties;
- children with haemophilia or other conditions treated with plasma-derived clotting factors;
- children with severe liver disease;
- children travelling to high-risk areas;
- adolescents who are at risk due to their sexual behaviour;
- parenteral drug abusers.

Immunisation should be considered for:

- children with chronic liver disease including chronic hepatitis B or chronic hepatitis C;
- prevention of secondary cases in close contacts of confirmed cases of hepatitis A, within 14 days of exposure to the primary case (within 8 weeks of exposure to the primary case where there is more than 1 contact in the household).

A booster dose of hepatitis A vaccine is usually given 6–12 months after the initial dose. A second booster dose can be given 20 years after the previous booster dose to those who continue to be at risk. Specialist advice should be sought on re-immunisation of immunocompromised individuals.

In children under 16 years, a single dose of the combined vaccine *Ambirix*® can be used to provide rapid protection against hepatitis A. Public Health England recommends the use of intramuscular normal immunoglobulin p. 825 in addition to hepatitis A vaccine for prevention of infection in close contacts (of confirmed cases of hepatitis A) who have chronic liver disease or HIV infection, or who are immunosuppressed. For further guidance, see Immunoglobulins p. 821.

Post-exposure prophylaxis is not required for healthy children under 1 year of age, so long as all those involved in nappy changing are vaccinated against hepatitis A. However, children 2–12 months of age can be given a dose of hepatitis A vaccine if it is not possible to vaccinate their carers, or if the child becomes a source of infection to others [unlicensed use]; in these cases, if the child goes on to require long-term protection against hepatitis A after the first birthday, the full course of 2 doses should be given.

Useful Resources

Advice reflects that in the handbook Immunisation against Infectious Disease (2013), which in turn reflects the guidance of the Joint Committee on Vaccination and Immunisation (JCVI). The advice also incorporates changes announced by the Chief Medical Officer and Health Department Updates. Chapters from the handbook (including updates since 2013) are available at:
www.gov.uk/government/collections/immunisation-against-infectious-disease-the-green-book

Hepatitis B vaccine

Overview

Hepatitis B vaccine p. 853 contains inactivated hepatitis B virus surface antigen (HBsAg) adsorbed onto an adjuvant. It is made biosynthetically using recombinant DNA technology.

From August 2017, vaccination against hepatitis B is recommended as part of the **routine immunisation schedule**. Primary immunisation (see *Routine immunisation schedule*) requires 3 doses, given at intervals of 1 month from the age of 2 months, to be given as part of the combined diphtheria with tetanus, pertussis, hepatitis B, poliomyelitis and haemophilus influenzae type b vaccine p. 846 (*Infanrix hexa*®).

As part of the **selective neonatal immunisation programme**, vaccination is recommended for neonates whose mothers have had acute hepatitis B during pregnancy *or* are positive for hepatitis B surface antigen (regardless of e-antigen markers). Hepatitis B vaccination is started immediately after birth with a dose of the monovalent hepatitis B vaccine (no later than 24 hours after delivery), followed by a second dose at 4 weeks; the routine immunisation combination vaccine (*Infanrix hexa*®) at weeks 8, 12 and 16; and a further dose of the monovalent hepatitis B vaccine at one year of age.

Neonates born to highly infectious mothers should also receive hepatitis B immunoglobulin p. 824 at the same time as the first dose of monovalent hepatitis B vaccine, but administered at a different site—more detailed guidance is given in the handbook *Immunisation against Infectious Disease* www.gov.uk/government/publications/hepatitis-b-the-green-book-chapter-18

Following **significant exposure to hepatitis B** (e.g. through needle-stick injury or unprotected sex) and for **pre-exposure prophylaxis in high-risk groups**, 'an accelerated schedule' using the single, monovalent hepatitis B vaccine is recommended immediately, with the second dose given 1 month after the initial dose, and the third dose given 2 months after the initial dose. For those at continued high risk following exposure, a fourth dose should be given 12 months after the first dose. More detailed guidance is given in the handbook *Immunisation against Infectious Disease*.

Specific hepatitis B immunoglobulin can also be indicated for use with the vaccine in those accidentally inoculated and in neonates at special risk of infection. If hepatitis B immunoglobulin is indicated, it should be given as soon as possible, ideally at the same time or within 24 hours of the first dose of vaccine, but not after seven days have elapsed since exposure. See also *hepatitis B immunoglobulin* in Immunoglobulins p. 821.

In the UK, groups at high-risk of hepatitis B include:

- parenteral drug misusers, their sexual partners, and household contacts; other drug misusers who are likely to 'progress' to injecting;
- adolescents who are at risk from their sexual behaviour;
- close family contacts of an individual with chronic hepatitis B infection;
- children with haemophilia, those receiving regular blood transfusions or blood products, and carers responsible for the administration of such products;
- children with chronic renal failure including those on haemodialysis. Children receiving haemodialysis should be monitored for antibodies annually and re-immunised if necessary. Home carers (of dialysis patients) should be vaccinated;
- children with chronic liver disease
- patients of day-care or residential accommodation for those with severe learning difficulties;
- children in custodial institutions;
- children travelling to areas of high or intermediate prevalence who are at increased risk or who plan to remain there for lengthy periods;
- families adopting children from countries with a high or intermediate prevalence of hepatitis B;
- foster carers and their families.

Following a primary course of immunisation, most children do not require a reinforcing dose of a hepatitis B-containing vaccine. A single booster dose should be offered to healthcare workers around five years after primary immunisation, to patients on renal dialysis with anti-HBs levels below 10mIU/mL, and at the time of a subsequent significant exposure.

Immunisation does not eliminate the need for commonsense precautions for avoiding the risk of infection from known carriers by the routes of infection which have been clearly established, consult *Guidance for Clinical Health Care Workers: Protection against Infection with Blood-borne Viruses* (available at www.dh.gov.uk).
Accidental inoculation of hepatitis B virus-infected blood into a wound, incision, needle-prick, or abrasion may lead to infection, whereas it is unlikely that indirect exposure to a carrier will do so.

A combined hepatitis A and B vaccine p. 852 is also available.

Useful Resources

Advice reflects that in the handbook Immunisation against Infectious Disease (2013), which in turn reflects the guidance of the Joint Committee on Vaccination and Immunisation (JCVI). The advice also incorporates changes announced by the Chief Medical Officer and Health Department Updates. Chapters from the handbook (including updates since 2013) are available at:
www.gov.uk/government/collections/immunisation-against-infectious-disease-the-green-book

Human papillomavirus vaccine

15-Jan-2019

Overview

The human papillomavirus vaccines p. 855 consist of virus-like particles prepared from the major protein of the viral coat or capsid and mimic the structure of the native virus, but do not contain any viral DNA. The vaccines are available as a bivalent vaccine (*Cervarix*®, containing human papillomavirus (HPV) types 16 and 18), a quadrivalent vaccine (*Gardasil*®, containing HPV types 6, 11, 16 and 18), and a nine-valent vaccine (*Gardasil 9*®, containing HPV types 6, 11, 16, 18, 31, 33, 45, 52 and 58). All are adjuvanted and used for the prevention of cervical and anal cancers, and pre-cancerous genital (cervical, vulvar, and vaginal) and anal lesions associated with HPV types 16 and 18. *Gardasil*® and *Gardasil 9*® are also effective at preventing genital warts. The vaccines may also provide some cross-protection against infection caused by other high-risk HPV types.

Although there is emerging evidence on interchangeability of the HPV vaccines, the same vaccine product should be used for an entire course. Only *Gardasil®* is offered as part of the national HPV programme and is recommended for eligible children aged 11 years and over, and for males who have sex with males aged 15 years and over.

As the vaccines do not protect against all strains of HPV, safe sex precautions should always be practiced; and for all females, routine cervical screening should continue at the scheduled age.

Children aged 9 to 14 years

The human papillomavirus vaccines are licensed for individuals from 9 years of age, however, vaccination in children aged 9 to 10 years is not offered as part of the national programme. A 2 dose schedule is recommended for children who receive the first dose before the age of 15 years. The first dose is usually given to children from 11 years, with the second dose given 6–24 months after the first dose. See Immunisation schedule p. 831 for guidance on immunisation in different countries within the UK.

2 doses given less than 6 months apart should not be considered adequate to provide long term protection. A third dose should be given according to human papillomavirus vaccines dosing schedule.

Children aged 15 years and over

Under the national programme in England, individuals remain eligible to receive the HPV vaccine up to the age of 25 years if they did not receive the vaccine when scheduled. A 3 dose schedule is recommended, with the second and third dose given 1 month and 4–6 months after the first dose respectively. All 3 doses should be given within a 12-month period (see human papillomavirus vaccines).

In cases where the second dose is given late and there is a high likelihood that the individual will not return, or it is not practical for the third dose to be given after three months, then the third dose can be given at least one month after the second dose.

Where appropriate, immunisation with the HPV vaccine should be offered to children coming into the UK, as they may not have been offered protection in their country of origin.

Vaccination of males who have sex with males and other at risk individuals

Males aged 15 years and over, who have sex with other males and attend Specialist Sexual Health Services or HIV clinics are eligible for vaccination if they have not previously been vaccinated. Immunisation should still be offered to eligible males who have sex with males, regardless of CD4 cell count, antiretroviral therapy use, viral load, or if known to be immunocompromised at the time of immunisation. A 3 dose schedule of *Gardasil®* should be given, with administration of doses aligned with clinic appointments. All 3 doses should be given within a 24 month period.

There may be considerable benefit in offering the HPV vaccination to individuals who attend Specialist Sexual Health Services or HIV clinics, who are not eligible under the national immunisation programme and are deemed to have a similar risk profile to that seen in males who have sex with males. This includes some transgender individuals, sex workers, and males and females living with HIV infection. For these individuals a 3 dose schedule of *Gardasil®* is recommended.

Booster doses

Protection from human papillomavirus vaccines is maintained for at least 10 years, although protection is expected to last longer. There is no recommendation for the need for booster doses.

Useful Resources

Recommendations reflect Chapter 18a, Human papillomavirus, in *Immunisation against infectious disease-* 'The Green Book'. Public Health England, July 2019.
www.gov.uk/government/publications/human-papillomavirus-hpv-the-green-book-chapter-18a

HPV vaccination programme for men who have sex with men (MSM) - Clinical and operational guidance. Public Health England, April 2018.
www.gov.uk/government/collections/hpv-vaccination-for-men-who-have-sex-with-men-msm-programme

Influenza vaccine

23-Apr-2019

Overview

While most viruses are antigenically stable, the influenza viruses A and B (especially A) are constantly altering their antigenic structure, as indicated by changes in the haemagglutinins (H) and neuraminidases (N) on the surface of the viruses. It is essential that influenza vaccine p. 856 in use contain the H and N components of the prevalent strain or strains recommended each year by the World Health Organization.

The influenza vaccines recommended for immunisation in children are the standard egg-grown quadrivalent influenza vaccine (inactivated), and the live attenuated influenza vaccine. The choice of vaccine is dependent on the child's age and contra-indications.

The ideal time for immunisation is between September and early November.

Immunisation is recommended *for children at high risk* from influenza, and to reduce transmission of infection. Annual immunisation is strongly recommended for children (including infants that were preterm or low birth-weight) aged 6 months and over with the following conditions:

- chronic respiratory disease;
- chronic heart disease;
- chronic liver disease;
- chronic renal disease at stage 3, 4 or 5;
- chronic neurological disease;
- complement disorders;
- diabetes mellitus;
- immunosuppression because of disease (including asplenia or splenic dysfunction) or treatment (including prolonged systemic corticosteroid treatment [for over 1 month at dose equivalents of prednisolone p. 478: *child under* 20 *kg*, 1 mg/kg or more daily; *child over* 20 *kg*, 20 mg or more daily], and chemotherapy);
- HIV infection (regardless of immune status);
- morbid obesity (BMI of 40 kg/m^2 and above).

Annual influenza vaccine is also recommended for:

- children of specific ages see Immunisation schedule p. 831;
- all pregnant females (including those who become pregnant during the flu season);
- children living in long-stay facilities;
- carers of children whose welfare may be at risk if the carer falls ill;
- household contacts of immunocompromised individuals.

Children aged 6 months to less than 2 years of age in clinical risk groups should be offered the standard egg-grown quadrivalent inactivated influenza vaccine.

Children aged 2–17 years of age (including those in clinical risk groups) should be offered the live attenuated influenza vaccine administered as a nasal spray (*Fluenz tetra®*). The live attenuated vaccine is thought to provide broader protection than inactivated vaccines. If the child is in a clinical risk group and the live attenuated vaccine is contra-indicated or otherwise unsuitable, offer standard egg-grown quadrivalent inactivated influenza vaccine.

Children aged 6 months to less than 9 years of age in clinical risk groups who have not had the influenza vaccine previously should be offered two doses of the appropriate influenza vaccine, four weeks apart.

In the 2019/2020 national influenza immunisation programme, annual influenza vaccine will be offered to all children aged 2–10 years on 31st August 2019 (including those in reception class and school years 1, 2, 3, 4, 5, and 6).

For the management of influenza, see Influenza p. 463.

Further information on pandemic influenza, avian influenza, swine influenza, and annual flu programme may be found at www.gov.uk/government/collections/pandemic-flu-public-health-response and at www.gov.uk/government/collections/annual-flu-programme.

Useful Resources

Recommendations reflect Chapter 19, Influenza, in *Immunisation against infectious disease*– 'The Green Book'. Public Health England. April 2019.
www.gov.uk/government/publications/influenza-the-green-book-chapter-19

'National flu immunisation programme plan 2019/2020' Public Health England, Department of Health and Social Care, and NHS England. March 2019.
www.gov.uk/government/publications/national-flu-immunisation-programme-plan

Japanese encephalitis vaccine 14-Nov-2018

Overview

Japanese encephalitis is a mosquito-borne viral encephalitis caused by a *Flavivirus*.

Japanese encephalitis vaccine p. 857 (*IXIARO*) ® is an inactivated vaccine adsorbed onto an adjuvant. It is recommended for children who are going to reside in an area where Japanese encephalitis is endemic or epidemic. Children travelling to South and South-East Asia and the Far East should be immunised if staying for a month or longer in endemic areas during the transmission season. Other children travelling with shorter exposure periods should also be immunised if the risk is considered sufficient.

The primary immunisation course of 2 doses should be completed at least one week before potential exposure to Japanese encephalitis virus.

Children (aged 2 months and over) at ongoing risk (such as long-term travellers), should receive a single booster dose 12 months after the primary immunisation course. For other children travelling, a single booster dose should be given within 12–24 months after primary immunisation, before potential re-exposure to the Japanese encephalitis virus.

Cases of Japanese encephalitis should be managed with supportive treatment.

Up-to-date information on the risk of Japanese encephalitis in specific countries can be obtained from the National Travel Health Network and Centre.

Useful Resources

Recommendations reflect Chapter 20, Japanese encephalitis, in *Immunisation against infectious disease*– 'The 'Green book'. Public Health England, June 2018.
www.gov.uk/government/publications/japanese-encephalitis-the-green-book-chapter-20

National Travel Health Network and Centre
nathnac.net

Measles, Mumps and Rubella vaccine

Overview

Measles vaccine has been replaced by a combined measles, mumps and rubella vaccine, live p. 857 (MMR vaccine).

A combined measles, mumps and rubella vaccine, live (MMR vaccine) aims to eliminate measles, mumps, and rubella (German measles) and congenital rubella syndrome. Every child should receive two doses of measles, mumps and rubella vaccine, live by entry to primary school, unless there is a valid contra-indication. Measles, mumps and rubella vaccine, live should be given irrespective of previous measles, mumps, or rubella infection or vaccination.

The first dose of measles, mumps and rubella vaccine, live is given to children at 1 year of age, on or after their first birthday. A second dose is given before starting school at 3 years and 4 months of age, or soon after (see Immunisation Schedule).

Children presenting for pre-school booster who have not received the first dose of measles, mumps and rubella vaccine, live should be given a dose of measles, mumps and rubella vaccine, live followed 3 months later by a second dose.

At school-leaving age or at entry into further education, MMR immunisation should be offered to individuals of both sexes who have not received 2 doses during childhood. In those who have received only a single dose of MMR in childhood, a second dose is recommended to achieve full protection. If 2 doses of measles, mumps and rubella vaccine, live are required, the second dose should be given one month after the initial dose.

Measles, mumps and rubella vaccine, live should be used to protect against rubella in *seronegative women of child-bearing age* (see Immunisation Schedule); unimmunised healthcare workers who might put pregnant women and other vulnerable groups at risk of rubella or measles should be vaccinated. Measles, mumps and rubella vaccine, live may also be offered to previously *unimmunised and seronegative post-partum women* (see measles, mumps and rubella vaccine, live)—vaccination a few days after delivery is important because about 60% of congenital abnormalities from rubella infection occur in babies of women who have borne more than one child. Immigrants arriving after the age of school immunisation are particularly likely to require immunisation.

Contacts

Measles, mumps and rubella vaccine, live may also be used in the control of outbreaks of measles and should be offered to susceptible children aged over 6 months who are contacts of a case, within 3 days of exposure to infection. Children immunised before 12 months of age should still receive two doses of measles, mumps and rubella vaccine, live at the recommended ages. If one dose of measles, mumps and rubella vaccine, live has already been given to a child, then the second dose may be brought forward to at least one month after the first, to ensure complete protection. If the child is under 18 months of age and the second dose is given within 3 months of the first, then the routine dose before starting school at 3 years and 4 months of age (or soon after) should still be given. Children aged under 9 months for whom avoidance of measles infection is particularly important (such as those with history of recent severe illness) can be given normal immunoglobulin p. 825 after exposure to measles; routine MMR immunisation should then be given after at least 3 months at the appropriate age.

Measles, mumps and rubella vaccine, live is **not suitable** for prophylaxis following exposure to mumps or rubella since the antibody response to the mumps and rubella components is too slow for effective prophylaxis.

Children with impaired immune response should not receive live vaccines (for advice on HIV). If they have been exposed to measles infection they should be given normal immunoglobulin.

Travel

Unimmunised travellers, including children over 6 months, to areas where measles is endemic or epidemic should receive measles, mumps and rubella vaccine, live. Children immunised before 12 months of age should still receive two doses of measles, mumps and rubella vaccine, live at the recommended ages. If one dose of measles, mumps and rubella vaccine, live has already been given to a child, then the second dose should be brought forward to at least one month after the first, to ensure complete protection. If the child is under 18 months of age and the second dose is given within 3 months of the first, then the routine dose before starting school at 3 years and 4 months of age (or soon after) should still be given.

Useful Resources

Advice reflects that in the handbook Immunisation against Infectious Disease (2013), which in turn reflects the guidance of the Joint Committee on Vaccination and Immunisation (JCVI). The advice also incorporates changes announced by the Chief Medical Officer and Health Department Updates. Chapters from the handbook (including updates since 2013) are available at:
www.gov.uk/government/collections/immunisation-against-infectious-disease-the-green-book

Meningococcal vaccine

Overview

Almost all childhood meningococcal disease in the UK is caused by *Neisseria meningitidis* serogroups B and C. **Meningococcal group C conjugate vaccine** protects only against infection by serogroup C and **meningococcal group B vaccine** protects only against infection by serogroup B. The risk of meningococcal disease declines with age—immunisation is not generally recommended after the age of 25 years.

Tetravalent meningococcal vaccines that cover serogroups A, C, W135, and Y are available. Although the duration of protection has not been established, the **meningococcal groups A, C, W135, and Y conjugate vaccine** is likely to provide longer-lasting protection than the unconjugated meningococcal polysaccharide vaccine. The antibody response to serogroup C in unconjugated meningococcal polysaccharide vaccines in young children may be suboptimal [not currently available in the UK].

Meningococcal group B vaccines, *Bexsero®* and *Trumenba®*, are licensed in the UK against infection caused by *Neisseria meningitidis* serogroup B. The use of *Bexsero®* is recommended in the Immunisation Schedule. *Bexsero®* contains 3 recombinant *Neisseria meningitidis* serogroup B proteins and the outer membrane vesicles from the NZ 98/254 strain, in order to achieve broad protection against *Neisseria meningitidis* serogroup B. *Trumenba®* contains 2 recombinant *Neisseria meningitidis* serogroup B proteins. The proteins are adsorbed onto an aluminium compound to stimulate an enhanced immune response.

Childhood immunisation

Meningococcal group C conjugate vaccine provides long-term protection against infection by serogroup C of *Neisseria meningitidis*. Immunisation consists of 1 dose given at 12 months of age (as the haemophilus influenzae type b with meningococcal group C vaccine p. 848) and a second dose given at 13–15 years of age (as the meningococcal groups A with C and W135 and Y vaccine p. 849) (see Immunisation Schedule).

Meningococcal group B vaccine provides protection against infection by serogroup B of *Neisseria meningitidis*. Immunisation consists of 1 dose given at 2 months of age, a second dose at 4 months of age, and a booster dose at 12 months of age (see *Immunisation Schedule* above).

Unimmunised children aged under 12 months should be given 1 dose of meningococcal group B vaccine (rDNA, component, adsorbed) p. 849 followed by a second dose two months later. They should then be vaccinated according to the Immunisation Schedule (ensuring at least a two month interval between doses of meningococcal group B vaccines). Unimmunised children aged 12–23 months should be given 2 doses of meningococcal group B vaccine (rDNA, component, adsorbed) separated by an interval of two months if they have received less than 2 doses in the first year of life. Unimmunised children aged 2–9 years should be given a single dose of meningococcal group C vaccine (as the haemophilus influenzae type b with meningococcal group C vaccine), followed by a booster dose of meningococcal groups A with C and W135 and Y vaccine at 13–15 years of age.

From 2015, unimmunised individuals aged 10–25 years, including those aged under 25 years who are attending university for the first time, should be given a single dose of meningococcal groups A with C and W135 and Y vaccine; a booster dose is not required.

Children with confirmed serogroup C disease, who have previously been immunised with meningococcal group C vaccine, should be offered meningococcal group C conjugate vaccine before discharge from hospital.

Travel

Individuals travelling to countries of risk should be immunised with meningococcal groups A, C, W135, and Y conjugate vaccine, even if they have previously received meningococcal group C conjugate vaccine. If an individual has recently received meningococcal group C conjugate vaccine, an interval of at least 4 weeks should be allowed before administration of the tetravalent (meningococcal groups A, C, W135, and Y) vaccine.

Vaccination is particularly important for those living or working with local people or visiting an area of risk during outbreaks.

Immunisation recommendations and requirements for visa entry for individual countries should be checked before travelling, particularly to countries in Sub-Saharan Africa, Asia, and the Indian sub-continent where epidemics of meningococcal outbreaks and infection are reported. Country-by-country information is available from the National Travel Health Network and Centre (www.nathnac.org/).

Proof of vaccination with the tetravalent (meningococcal groups A, C, W135, and Y) vaccine is required for those travelling to Saudi Arabia during the Hajj and Umrah pilgrimages (where outbreaks of the W135 strain have occurred).

Contacts

For advice on the immunisation of *laboratory workers and close contacts* of cases of meningococcal disease in the UK and on the role of the vaccine in the control of *local outbreaks*, consult Guidelines for Public Health Management of Meningococcal Disease in the UK at www.gov.uk/phe. Also see antibacterial prophylaxis for prevention of secondary cases of meningococcal meningitis.

Useful Resources

Advice reflects that in the handbook Immunisation against Infectious Disease (2013), which in turn reflects the guidance of the Joint Committee on Vaccination and Immunisation (JCVI). The advice also incorporates changes announced by the Chief Medical Officer and Health Department Updates. Chapters from the handbook (including updates since 2013) are available at:
www.gov.uk/government/collections/immunisation-against-infectious-disease-the-green-book

Pertussis vaccine

Overview

Pertussis vaccine is given as a combination preparation containing other vaccines. Acellular vaccines are derived from highly purified components of *Bordetella pertussis*. Primary immunisation against pertussis (whooping cough) requires 3 doses of an acellular pertussis-containing vaccine (see Immunisation schedule), given at intervals of 1 month from the age of 2 months.

All children up to the age of 10 years should receive primary immunisation with a combination vaccine of diphtheria with tetanus, pertussis, hepatitis B, poliomyelitis and haemophilus influenzae type b vaccine p. 846 (*Infanrix hexa*®).

A booster dose of an acellular pertussis-containing vaccine should ideally be given 3 years after the primary course, although, the interval can be reduced to 1 year if the primary course was delayed.

Children aged 1–10 years who have not received a *pertussis-containing* vaccine as part of their primary immunisation should be offered 1 dose of a suitable pertussis-containing vaccine; after an interval of at least 1 year, a booster dose of a suitable pertussis-containing vaccine should be given. Immunisation against pertussis is not routinely recommended in individuals over 10 years of age.

Vaccination of pregnant women against pertussis

In response to the pertussis outbreak, the UK health departments introduced a temporary programme (October 2012) to vaccinate pregnant women against pertussis, and this programme will continue until further notice. The aim of the programme is to boost the levels of pertussis–specific antibodies that are transferred, through the placenta, from the mother to the fetus, so that the newborn is protected before routine immunisation begins at 2 months of age.

Pregnant women should be offered a single dose of acellular pertussis-containing vaccine (as adsorbed diphtheria [low dose], tetanus, pertussis (acellular, component) and poliomyelitis (inactivated) vaccine; *Boostrix-IPV*®) between 16 and 32 weeks of pregnancy. Public Health England has advised (2016) that the vaccine is probably best offered on or after the fetal anomaly scan at around 18–20 weeks. Pregnant women should be offered a single dose of acellular pertussis-containing vaccine up to the onset of labour if they missed the opportunity for vaccination at 16–32 weeks of pregnancy. A single dose of acellular pertussis-containing vaccine may also be offered to new mothers, who have never previously been vaccinated against pertussis, until the child receives the first vaccination.

While this programme is in place, women who become pregnant again should be offered vaccination during each pregnancy to maximise transplacental transfer of antibody.

Contacts

Vaccination against pertussis should be considered for close contacts of cases with pertussis who have been offered antibacterial prophylaxis. Unimmunised or partially immunised contacts under 10 years of age should complete their vaccination against pertussis. A booster dose of an acellular pertussis-containing vaccine is recommended for contacts aged over 10 years who have not received a pertussis-containing vaccine in the last 5 years and who have not received adsorbed diphtheria [low dose], tetanus, and poliomyelitis (inactivated) vaccine in the last month.

Side-effects

Local reactions do not contra-indicate further doses.

The vaccine should not be withheld from children with a history to a preceding dose of:

- fever, irrespective of severity;
- persistent crying or screaming for more than 3 hours;
- severe local reaction, irrespective of extent.

Useful Resources

Advice reflects that in the handbook Immunisation against Infectious Disease (2013), which in turn reflects the guidance of the Joint Committee on Vaccination and Immunisation (JCVI). The advice also incorporates changes announced by the Chief Medical Officer and Health Department Updates. Chapters from the handbook (including updates since 2013) are available at:
www.gov.uk/government/collections/immunisation-against-infectious-disease-the-green-book

Pneumococcal vaccine

07-Jan-2020

Overview

The pneumococcal polysaccharide conjugate vaccine (adsorbed) p. 850 and the pneumococcal polysaccharide vaccine p. 851 protect against infection with *Streptococcus pneumoniae* (pneumococcus). Both vaccines contain polysaccharide from capsular pneumococci. The pneumococcal polysaccharide vaccine contains purified polysaccharide from **23 capsular types** of pneumococcus, whereas the pneumococcal polysaccharide conjugate vaccine (adsorbed) contains polysaccharide from either **10 capsular types** (*Synflorix*®) or **13 capsular types** (*Prevenar* 13®). Both vaccines are inactivated.

Prevenar 13® is the 13-valent pneumococcal polysaccharide conjugate vaccine (adsorbed) used in childhood immunisation. For children born on or before December 31st 2019, the schedule consists of 3 doses given at separate intervals. For children born on or after January 1st 2020, the schedule consists of 2 doses given at separate intervals. For more information, see Immunisation schedule p. 831. Children who present late for vaccination should be immunised according to *Children with unknown or incomplete vaccination histories*.

The 23-valent pneumococcal polysaccharide vaccine is recommended for children aged 2 years and over in the following at-risk groups:

- asplenia or splenic dysfunction (including homozygous sickle cell disease and coeliac syndrome which could lead to splenic dysfunction);
- chronic respiratory disease (including severe asthma treated with continuous or frequent use of a systemic corticosteroid);
- chronic heart disease;
- chronic renal disease;
- chronic liver disease;
- diabetes mellitus requiring insulin or anti-diabetic medication;
- immunosuppression because of disease (e.g. HIV infection, and genetic disorders affecting the immune system) or treatment (including prolonged systemic corticosteroid treatment for over 1 month at dose equivalents of prednisolone: *child under* 20 *kg*, 1 mg/kg or more daily; *child over* 20 *kg*, 20 mg or more daily, and chemotherapy);
- presence of cochlear implant;
- conditions where leakage of cerebrospinal fluid may occur.

Where possible, the vaccine should be given at least 2 weeks (ideally 4–6 weeks) before splenectomy, chemotherapy or radiotherapy; children and their parents, or carers should be given advice about the increased risk of pneumococcal infection. If it is not possible to vaccinate at least 2 weeks before splenectomy, chemotherapy or radiotherapy, the vaccine should be given at least 2 weeks after the splenectomy, and at least 3 months after completion of chemotherapy or radiotherapy. Vaccination advice for children with leukaemia or those who have had a bone marrow transplant, and information on patient cards and leaflets for children with apslenia, are available in Chapter 25, Pneumococcal, in *Immunisation against infectious disease*- 'The Green Book'.

Vaccination regimens may differ depending on the child's age, risk of pneumococcal disease, vaccination history, and immune status. Children in at-risk groups may require additional protection.

For information on revaccination with 23-valent pneumococcal polysaccharide vaccine for children in whom the antibody concentration is likely to decline rapidly, see *Revaccination*.

Children with unknown or incomplete vaccination histories

Individuals born on or before December 31st 2019

Unimmunised or partially immunised children who present late for vaccination and before the age of 1 year should receive 2 doses of the 13-valent pneumococcal polysaccharide conjugate vaccine (adsorbed) 2 months apart, and a booster dose on or after their first birthday, at least 2 months after the previous dose (intervals can be reduced to 1 month to allow the immunisation schedule to be completed promptly).

Children aged 1 year to under 2 years who are unimmunised or partially immunised should receive a single dose of the 13-valent pneumococcal polysaccharide conjugate vaccine (adsorbed).

Individuals born on or after January 1st 2020

Unimmunised or partially immunised children who present late for vaccination and before the age of 1 year should receive a single dose of the 13-valent pneumococcal polysaccharide conjugate vaccine (adsorbed), and a booster dose on or after their first birthday, at least 4 weeks after the previous dose.

Children aged 1 year to under 2 years who are unimmunised or partially immunised should receive a single dose of the 13-valent pneumococcal polysaccharide conjugate vaccine (adsorbed).

For the management of children who received one or more doses of 10-valent pneumococcal polysaccharide conjugate vaccine (adsorbed) in another country, refer to Chapter 25 (for infants born on or after 1 January 2020), Pneumococcal, in *Immunisation against infectious disease*- 'The Green Book'.

Individuals with an at-risk condition born on or before December 31st 2019

Children diagnosed with at-risk conditions aged under 2 years

Children diagnosed with an at-risk condition aged under 1 year should receive the 13-valent pneumococcal polysaccharide conjugate vaccine (adsorbed) according to the Immunisation schedule p. 831. Those who present late for vaccination should be immunised according to *Children with unknown or incomplete vaccination histories*. A single dose of the 23-valent pneumococcal polysaccharide vaccine should then be given at 2 years of age, at least 2 months after the last dose of 13-valent pneumococcal polysaccharide conjugate vaccine (adsorbed).

Children aged under 2 years who are severely immunocompromised, or those with asplenia, splenic dysfunction or complement disorders, should have an additional dose of the 13-valent pneumococcal polysaccharide conjugate vaccine (adsorbed), given at least 2 months after the booster dose due on or after their first birthday (the interval can be reduced to 1 month to allow the immunisation schedule to be completed promptly). A single dose of the 23-valent pneumococcal polysaccharide vaccine should then be given at 2 years of age, at least 2 months after the last dose of 13-valent pneumococcal polysaccharide conjugate vaccine (adsorbed).

For further information on vaccination in individuals with asplenia, splenic dysfunction, or complement disorders, see Vaccination, general principles p. 828.

Children diagnosed with at-risk conditions aged 2 years to under 10 years

Children diagnosed or first presenting with an at-risk condition who have completed their routine immunisation schedule should receive a single dose of 23-valent pneumococcal polysaccharide vaccine, at least 2 months after the last dose of 13-valent pneumococcal polysaccharide conjugate vaccine (adsorbed).

Children previously unvaccinated or partially vaccinated with the 13-valent pneumococcal polysaccharide conjugate vaccine (adsorbed) should receive a single dose of the 13-valent pneumococcal polysaccharide conjugate vaccine (adsorbed), followed by a single dose of the 23-valent pneumococcal polysaccharide vaccine at least 2 months later.

For further information on vaccination in individuals with asplenia, splenic dysfunction, or complement disorders, see Vaccination, general principles p. 828.

Severely immunocompromised children may have a sub-optimal immunological response to the vaccine and should be given an additional dose of the 13-valent pneumococcal polysaccharide conjugate vaccine (adsorbed), even if they are fully vaccinated. This should be followed by a single dose of the 23-valent pneumococcal polysaccharide vaccine, at least 2 months after the last dose of 13-valent pneumococcal polysaccharide conjugate vaccine (adsorbed). If the 23-valent pneumococcal polysaccharide vaccine has already been given, the 13-valent pneumococcal polysaccharide conjugate vaccine (adsorbed) should be given at least 6 months after.

Individuals diagnosed with at-risk conditions aged 10 years and over

Individuals diagnosed or first presenting with an at-risk condition should be given a single dose of the 23-valent pneumococcal polysaccharide vaccine p. 851; no additional 23-valent pneumococcal polysaccharide vaccine is required at 65 years of age.

For further information on vaccination in individuals with asplenia, splenic dysfunction, or complement disorders, see Vaccination, general principles p. 828.

Severely immunocompromised individuals should be given a single dose of the 13-valent pneumococcal polysaccharide conjugate vaccine (adsorbed) p. 850 followed by the 23-valent pneumococcal polysaccharide vaccine at least 2 months after, irrespective of their previous pneumococcal vaccinations. If the 23-valent pneumococcal polysaccharide vaccine has already been given, the 13-valent pneumococcal polysaccharide conjugate vaccine (adsorbed) should be given at least 6 months after.

Individuals with an at-risk condition born on or after January 1st 2020

Children diagnosed with at-risk conditions aged under 1 year

Children in an at-risk group (excluding those with asplenia, splenic dysfunction or complement disorder, or who are severely immunocompromised) should receive the 13-valent pneumococcal polysaccharide conjugate vaccine (adsorbed) according to the Immunisation schedule p. 831. Those who present late for vaccination should be immunised according to *Children with unknown or incomplete vaccination histories*. A single dose of the 23-valent pneumococcal polysaccharide vaccine should then be given at 2 years of age, at least 8 weeks after the last dose of 13-valent pneumococcal polysaccharide conjugate vaccine (adsorbed).

Children who are severely immunocompromised, or those with asplenia, splenic dysfunction or complement disorders, should receive 2 doses of the 13-valent pneumococcal polysaccharide conjugate vaccine (adsorbed) at least 8 weeks apart (commencing no earlier than 6 weeks of age), followed by a single booster dose given on or after their first birthday. An additional dose of 13-valent pneumococcal polysaccharide conjugate vaccine (adsorbed) should be given at least 8 weeks after the booster dose. A single dose of the 23-valent pneumococcal polysaccharide vaccine should then be given at 2 years of age, at least 8 weeks after the last dose of 13-valent pneumococcal polysaccharide conjugate vaccine (adsorbed).

For further information on vaccination in individuals with asplenia, splenic dysfunction, or complement disorders, see Vaccination, general principles p. 828.

Children diagnosed with at-risk conditions aged 1 year to under 2 years

Children in an at-risk group (excluding those with asplenia, splenic dysfunction or complement disorder, or who are severely immunocompromised) should receive their 13-valent pneumococcal polysaccharide conjugate vaccine (adsorbed) booster dose according to the Immunisation schedule p. 831. Those who present late for vaccination should be immunised according to *Children with unknown or incomplete vaccination histories*. A single dose of the 23-valent pneumococcal polysaccharide vaccine should then be given at 2 years of age, at least 8 weeks after the last dose of 13-valent pneumococcal polysaccharide conjugate vaccine (adsorbed).

Children who are severely immunocompromised, or those with asplenia, splenic dysfunction or complement disorders, should receive their 13-valent pneumococcal polysaccharide conjugate vaccine (adsorbed) booster dose according to the Immunisation schedule p. 831. Those who present late for vaccination should be immunised according to *Children with unknown or incomplete vaccination histories*. An additional dose of the 13-valent pneumococcal polysaccharide conjugate vaccine (adsorbed) should be given at least 8 weeks after the booster dose. A single dose of the 23-valent pneumococcal polysaccharide vaccine should then be given at 2 years of age, at least 8 weeks after the last dose of 13-valent pneumococcal polysaccharide conjugate vaccine (adsorbed).

For further information on vaccination in individuals with asplenia, splenic dysfunction, or complement disorders, see Vaccination, general principles p. 828.

Children diagnosed with at-risk conditions aged 2 years to under 10 years

Children diagnosed or first presenting with an at-risk condition (excluding those severely immunocompromised) who have completed their routine immunisation schedule should receive a single dose of 23-valent pneumococcal polysaccharide vaccine, at least 8 weeks after the last dose of 13-valent pneumococcal polysaccharide conjugate vaccine (adsorbed).

Children diagnosed or first presenting with an at-risk condition (excluding those severely immunocompromised) who are previously unimmunised or partially immunised with the 13-valent pneumococcal polysaccharide conjugate vaccine (adsorbed), should receive a single dose of the 13-valent pneumococcal polysaccharide conjugate vaccine (adsorbed), followed by a single dose of the 23-valent pneumococcal polysaccharide vaccine at least 8 weeks later.

For further information on vaccination in individuals with asplenia, splenic dysfunction, or complement disorders, see Vaccination, general principles p. 828.

Severely immunocompromised children should be given a single dose of the 13-valent pneumococcal polysaccharide conjugate vaccine (adsorbed), regardless of immunisation status. This should be followed by a single dose of the 23-valent pneumococcal polysaccharide vaccine, at least 8 weeks after the last dose of 13-valent pneumococcal polysaccharide conjugate vaccine (adsorbed).

Individuals diagnosed with at-risk conditions aged 10 years and over

Individuals diagnosed or first presenting with an at-risk condition (excluding those who are severely immunocompromised) should be given a single dose of the 23-valent pneumococcal polysaccharide vaccine. The 23-valent pneumococcal polysaccharide vaccine is not required for individuals with asplenia, splenic dysfunction or complement disorders if they have already received a dose within the previous 2 years (due to a theoretical risk of pneumococcal serotype-specific hypo-responsiveness with revaccination).

For further information on vaccination in individuals with asplenia, splenic dysfunction, or complement disorders, see Vaccination, general principles p. 828.

Severely immunocompromised individuals should be given a single dose of the 13-valent pneumococcal polysaccharide conjugate vaccine (adsorbed), followed by a single dose of the 23-valent pneumococcal polysaccharide vaccine at least 8 weeks after. The 13-valent pneumococcal polysaccharide conjugate vaccine (adsorbed) or additional 23-valent pneumococcal polysaccharide vaccine are not required if a 23-valent pneumococcal polysaccharide vaccine has already been received within the previous 2 years, due to a theoretical risk of pneumococcal serotype-specific hypo-responsiveness with re-vaccination.

Revaccination

Revaccination is not recommended for any clinical risk groups or age groups, except for individuals in whom the antibody concentration is likely to decline rapidly (e.g. asplenia, splenic dysfunction, or chronic renal disease), where revaccination is recommended every 5 years.

Management of cases

For the management of cases, contacts and outbreaks, refer to Chapter 25, Pneumococcal, in *Immunisation against infectious disease*- 'The Green Book' (see *Useful resources*).

Useful Resources

Recommendations reflect Chapter 25 (for infants born up to and including 31 December 2019), Pneumococcal, in *Immunisation against infectious disease*- 'The Green Book'. Public Health England, January 2018.
www.gov.uk/government/publications/pneumococcal-the-green-book-chapter-25

Recommendations reflect Chapter 25 (for infants born on or after 1 January 2020), Pneumococcal, in *Immunisation against infectious disease*- 'The Green Book'. Public Health England, January 2020.
www.gov.uk/government/publications/pneumococcal-the-green-book-chapter-25

Poliomyelitis vaccine

Overview

Two types of poliomyelitis vaccines (containing strains of poliovirus types 1, 2, and 3) are available, inactivated poliomyelitis vaccines (for injection) and live (oral) poliomyelitis vaccines. **Inactivated** poliomyelitis vaccines, only available in combined preparation, is recommended for routine immunisation; it is given by injection and contains inactivated strains of human poliovirus types 1, 2 and 3.

A course of primary immunisation consists of 3 doses of a combined preparation containing inactivated poliomyelitis vaccines starting at 2 months of age with intervals of 1 month between doses (see Immunisation schedule). A course of 3 doses should also be given to all unimmunised children; no child should remain unimmunised against poliomyelitis.

Two booster doses of a preparation containing inactivated poliomyelitis vaccines are recommended, the first before school entry and the second before leaving school (see Immunisation schedule). Further booster doses should be given every 10 years only to individuals at special risk.

Live (oral) poliomyelitis vaccines is no longer available for routine use; its use may be considered during large outbreaks, but advice should be sought from Public Health England. The live (oral) vaccine poses a very rare risk of vaccine-associated paralytic polio because the attenuated strain of the virus can revert to a virulent form. For this reason the live (oral) vaccine must **not** be used for immunosuppressed individuals or their household contacts. The use of inactivated poliomyelitis vaccines removes the risk of vaccine-associated paralytic polio altogether.

Travel

Unimmunised travellers to areas with a high incidence of poliomyelitis should receive a full 3-dose course of a preparation containing inactivated poliomyelitis vaccines. Those who have not been vaccinated in the last 10 years should receive a booster dose of **adsorbed diphtheria [low dose], tetanus and poliomyelitis (inactivated) vaccine**. Information about countries with a high incidence of poliomyelitis can be obtained from www.travax.nhs.uk/ or from the National Travel Health Network and Centre, (www.nathnac.org/).

Useful Resources

Advice reflects that in the handbook Immunisation against Infectious Disease (2013), which in turn reflects the guidance of the Joint Committee on Vaccination and Immunisation (JCVI). The advice also incorporates changes announced by the Chief Medical Officer and Health Department Updates. Chapters from the handbook (including updates since 2013) are available at:
www.gov.uk/government/collections/immunisation-against-infectious-disease-the-green-book

Rabies vaccine

Overview

Rabies vaccine p. 858 contains inactivated rabies virus cultivated in either human diploid cells or purified chick embryo cells; vaccines are used for pre- and postexposure prophylaxis.

Pre-exposure prophylaxis

Immunisation should be offered to children at high risk of exposure to rabies—where there is limited access to prompt medical care for those living in areas where rabies is enzootic, for those travelling to such areas for longer than 1 month, and for those on shorter visits who may be exposed to unusual risk. Transmission of rabies by humans has not been recorded but it is advised that those caring for children with the disease should be vaccinated.

Up-to-date country-by-country information on the incidence of rabies can be obtained from the National Travel Health Network and Centre (www.nathnac.org/) and, in Scotland, from Health Protection Scotland (www.hps.scot.nhs.uk/).

Immunisation against rabies requires 3 doses of rabies vaccine, with further booster doses for those who remain at frequent risk.

Post-exposure management

Following potential exposure to rabies, the wound or site of exposure (e.g. mucous membrane) should be cleansed under running water and washed for several minutes with soapy water as soon as possible after exposure. Disinfectant and a simple dressing can be applied, but suturing should be delayed because it may increase the risk of introducing rabies virus into the nerves.

Post-exposure prophylaxis against rabies depends on the level of risk in the country, the nature of exposure, and the individual's immunity. In each case, expert risk assessment and advice on appropriate management should be obtained from the local Public Health England Centre or Public Health England's Virus Reference Department, Colindale (tel. (020) 8200 4400) or the PHE Colindale Duty Doctor (tel. (020) 8200 6868), in Wales from the Public Health Wales local Health Protection Team or Public Health Wales Virus Reference Laboratory (tel. (029) 2074 7747), in Scotland from the local on-call infectious diseases consultant, and in Northern Ireland from the Public Health Agency Duty Room (tel (028) 9055 3997/(028) 9063 2662) or the Regional Virology Service (tel. (028) 9024 0503).

There are no specific contra-indications to the use of rabies vaccine for post-exposure prophylaxis and its use should be considered whenever a child has been attacked by an animal in a country where rabies is enzootic, even if there is no direct evidence of rabies in the attacking animal. Because of the potential consequences of untreated rabies exposure and because rabies vaccination has not been associated with fetal abnormalities, pregnancy is not considered a contra-indication to post-exposure prophylaxis.

For post-exposure prophylaxis of *fully immunised* individuals (who have previously received pre-exposure or post-exposure prophylaxis with cell-derived rabies vaccine), 2 doses of cell-derived vaccine are likely to be sufficient; the first dose is given on day 0 and the second dose is given between day 3–7. Rabies immunoglobulin p. 826 is not necessary in such cases.

Post-exposure treatment for *unimmunised individuals* (or those whose prophylaxis is possibly incomplete) comprises 5 doses of rabies vaccine given over 1 month (on days 0, 3, 7, 14, and the fifth dose is given between day 28–30); also, depending on the level of risk (determined by factors such as the nature of the bite and the country where it was sustained), rabies immunoglobulin is given to unimmunised individuals on day 0 or within 7 days of starting the course of rabies vaccine. The immunisation course can be discontinued if it is proved that the child was not at risk.

Useful Resources

Advice reflects that in the handbook Immunisation against Infectious Disease (2013), which in turn reflects the guidance of the Joint Committee on Vaccination and Immunisation (JCVI). The advice also incorporates changes announced by the Chief Medical Officer and Health Department Updates. Chapters from the handbook (including updates since 2013) are available at:
www.gov.uk/government/collections/immunisation-against-infectious-disease-the-green-book

Rotavirus vaccine

02-Aug-2019

Overview

Rotavirus vaccine p. 859 is a live, oral vaccine that protects young children against gastro-enteritis caused by rotavirus infection. The recommended schedule consists of 2 doses, the first at 8 weeks of age, and the second at 12 weeks of age (see Immunisation schedule p. 831). The first dose of rotavirus vaccine must be given between 6 weeks and under 15 weeks of age and the second dose should be given after an interval of at least 4 weeks; the vaccine should not be started in children 15 weeks of age or older. Ideally, the full course should be completed before 16 weeks of age to provide protection before the main burden of disease, and to avoid a temporal association between vaccination and intussusception; the course must be completed before 24 weeks of age.

Children who inadvertently receive the first dose of rotavirus vaccine at 15 weeks of age or older should still receive a second dose after at least 4 weeks, providing that they will still be under 24 weeks of age at the time.

The rotavirus vaccine virus is excreted in the stool and may be transmitted to close contacts; however, vaccination of children with *immunosuppressed* close contacts may protect the contacts from wild-type rotavirus disease and outweigh any risk from transmission of vaccine virus. Carers of a recently vaccinated child should be advised of the need to wash their hands after changing the child's nappies.

Useful Resources

Recommendations reflect Chapter 27b, Rotavirus, in *Immunisation against infectious disease*– 'The Green book'. Public Health England, August 2015.
www.gov.uk/government/publications/rotavirus-the-green-book-chapter-27b

Smallpox vaccine

Overview

Limited supplies of **smallpox vaccine** are held at the Specialist and Reference Microbiology Division, Public Health England Colindale (Tel. (020) 8200 4400) for the exclusive use of workers in laboratories where pox viruses (such as vaccinia) are handled.

If a wider use of the vaccine is being considered, *Guidelines for smallpox response and management in the post-eradication era* should be consulted at www.gov.uk/phe.

Useful Resources

Advice reflects that in the handbook Immunisation against Infectious Disease (2013), which in turn reflects the guidance of the Joint Committee on Vaccination and Immunisation (JCVI). The advice also incorporates changes announced by the Chief Medical Officer and Health Department Updates. Chapters from the handbook (including updates since 2013) are available at:
www.gov.uk/government/collections/immunisation-against-infectious-disease-the-green-book

Tetanus vaccine

Overview

Tetanus vaccine contains a cell-free purified toxin of *Clostridium tetani* adsorbed on aluminium hydroxide or aluminium phosphate to improve antigenicity.

Primary immunisation for children under 10 years consists of 3 doses of a combined preparation containing adsorbed tetanus vaccine, with an interval of 1 month between doses. Following routine childhood vaccination, 2 booster doses of a preparation containing adsorbed tetanus vaccine are recommended, the first before school entry and the second before leaving school (see Immunisation schedule).

The recommended schedule of tetanus vaccination not only gives protection against tetanus in childhood but also gives the basic immunity for subsequent booster doses. In most circumstances, a total of 5 doses of tetanus vaccine is considered sufficient for long term protection.

For primary immunisation of adults and children over 10 years previously unimmunised against tetanus, 3 doses of **adsorbed diphtheria [low dose], tetanus and poliomyelitis (inactivated) vaccine** are given with an interval of 1 month between doses.

When an individual presents for a booster dose but has been vaccinated following a tetanus-prone wound, the vaccine preparation administered at the time of injury should be determined. If this is not possible, the booster should still be given to ensure adequate protection against all antigens in the booster vaccine.

Very rarely, tetanus has developed after abdominal surgery; patients awaiting elective surgery should be asked about tetanus immunisation and immunised if necessary.

Parenteral drug abuse is also associated with tetanus; those abusing drugs by injection should be vaccinated if unimmunised—booster doses should be given if there is any doubt about their immunisation status.

All laboratory staff should be offered a primary course if unimmunised.

Wounds

Wounds are considered to be tetanus-prone if they are sustained more than 6 hours before surgical treatment or at any interval after injury and are puncture-type (particularly if contaminated with soil or manure) *or* show much devitalised tissue *or* are septic *or* are compound fractures *or* contain foreign bodies. All wounds should receive thorough cleansing.

- For *clean wounds*: fully immunised individuals (those who have received a total of 5 doses of a tetanus-containing vaccine at appropriate intervals) and those whose primary immunisation is complete (with boosters up to date), do not require tetanus vaccine; individuals whose primary immunisation is incomplete or whose boosters are not up to date require a reinforcing dose of a tetanus-containing vaccine (followed by further doses as required to complete the schedule); non-immunised individuals (or those whose immunisation status is not known or who have been fully immunised but are now immunocompromised) should be given a dose of the appropriate tetanus-containing vaccine immediately (followed by completion of the full course of the vaccine if records confirm the need)
- For *tetanus-prone wounds*: management is as for clean wounds with the addition of a dose of tetanus immunoglobulin given at a different site; in fully immunised individuals and those whose primary immunisation is complete (with boosters up to date) the immunoglobulin is needed only if the risk of infection is especially high (e.g. contamination with manure). Antibacterial prophylaxis (with benzylpenicillin, co-amoxiclav, or metronidazole) may also be required for tetanus-prone wounds.

Useful Resources

Advice reflects that in the handbook Immunisation against Infectious Disease (2013), which in turn reflects the guidance of the Joint Committee on Vaccination and Immunisation (JCVI). The advice also incorporates changes announced by the Chief Medical Officer and Health Department Updates. Chapters from the handbook (including updates since 2013) are available at:
www.gov.uk/government/collections/immunisation-against-infectious-disease-the-green-book

Tick-borne encephalitis vaccine

Overview

Tick-borne encephalitis vaccine, inactivated p. 859 contains inactivated tick-borne encephalitis virus cultivated in chick embryo cells. It is recommended for immunisation of those working in, or visiting, high-risk areas (see International Travel). Those working, walking or camping in warm forested areas of Central and Eastern Europe, Scandinavia, Northern and Eastern China, and some parts of Japan, particularly from April to November when ticks are most prevalent, are at greatest risk of tick-borne encephalitis. For full protection, 3 doses of the vaccine are required; booster doses are required every 3–5 years for those still at risk. Ideally, immunisation should be completed at least one month before travel.

Useful Resources

Advice reflects that in the handbook Immunisation against Infectious Disease (2013), which in turn reflects the guidance of the Joint Committee on Vaccination and Immunisation (JCVI). The advice also incorporates changes announced by the Chief Medical Officer and Health Department Updates. Chapters from the handbook (including updates since 2013) are available at:
www.gov.uk/government/collections/immunisation-against-infectious-disease-the-green-book

Typhoid vaccine

29-Jul-2019

Overview

Typhoid vaccine p. 851 is available as Vi capsular polysaccharide (from *Salmonella typhi*) vaccine for injection and as live, attenuated *Salmonella typhi* vaccine for oral use.

Typhoid immunisation is advised for children travelling to:

- areas where typhoid is endemic and whose planned activities put them at higher risk (country-by-country information is available from the National Travel Health Network and Centre);
- endemic areas where frequent or prolonged exposure to poor sanitation and poor food hygiene is likely.

Capsular polysaccharide typhoid vaccine is given as a single dose, usually by intramuscular injection. Children under 2 years [unlicensed] may respond suboptimally to the vaccine, but children aged between 1–2 years should be immunised if the risk of typhoid fever is considered high (immunisation is not recommended for infants under 12 months). A single booster dose should be given at 3-year intervals in children over 2 years of age who remain at risk from typhoid fever.

Oral typhoid vaccine is a live, attenuated vaccine contained in an enteric-coated capsule recommended in children aged 5 years and over. One capsule taken on alternate days for a total of 3 doses provides protection 7–10 days after the last dose. If travelling from a non-endemic area to an area where typhoid is endemic, a booster consisting of 3 doses is recommended every 3 years. The oral typhoid vaccine should be avoided in immunosuppressed and HIV-infected children.

Prevention of typhoid primarily depends on improving sanitation and water supplies in endemic areas and on scrupulous personal, food and water hygiene.

All suspected cases of typhoid fever must be notified to the local health protection unit. Where there is a community level outbreak, specialist advice should be sought from Public Health England (tel. 020 8200 4400) or, in Scotland, Health Protection Scotland (tel. 0140 300 1191).

Useful Resources

Recommendations reflect Chapter 33, Typhoid, in *Immunisation against infectious disease*– 'The Green Book'. Public Health England, May 2019.
www.gov.uk/government/publications/typhoid-the-green-book-chapter-33

National Travel Health Network and Centre
nathnac.net

Varicella-zoster vaccine

Overview

Varicella-zoster vaccine p. 860 (live) is licensed for immunisation against varicella (chickenpox) in seronegative individuals. It is not recommended for routine use in children but can be given to seronegative healthy children over 1 year who come into close contact with individuals at high risk of severe varicella infections.

Rarely, the varicella-zoster vaccine virus has been transmitted from the vaccinated individual to close contacts. Therefore, contact with the following should be avoided if a vaccine-related cutaneous rash develops within 4–6 weeks of the first or second dose:

- varicella-susceptible pregnant females;
- individuals at high risk of severe varicella, including those with immunodeficiency or those receiving immunosuppressive therapy.

Varicella-zoster immunoglobulin p. 827 is used to protect susceptible children at increased risk of severe varicella infection (*see* Immunoglobulins p. 821).

Useful Resources

Advice reflects that in the handbook Immunisation against Infectious Disease (2013), which in turn reflects the guidance of the Joint Committee on Vaccination and Immunisation (JCVI). The advice also incorporates changes announced by the Chief Medical Officer and Health Department Updates. Chapters from the handbook (including updates since 2013) are available at:
www.gov.uk/government/collections/immunisation-against-infectious-disease-the-green-book

Yellow fever vaccine

23-Jan-2020

MHRA/CHM advice: stronger precautions in people with weakened immunity

The MHRA and CHM have released important safety information regarding the use of the live yellow fever vaccine in those with weakened immunity. For further information, see *Important safety information* for yellow fever vaccine, live p. 860.

Overview

Yellow fever vaccine, live is an attenuated preparation of yellow fever virus grown in chick eggs. Yellow fever vaccine, live is recommended for:

- children aged 9 months or older who are travelling to, or living in areas or countries with a risk of yellow fever transmission;
- children aged 9 months or older who are travelling to, or living in countries that require an International Certificate of Vaccination or Prophylaxis (ICVP) for entry (information about countries at risk of yellow fever is available from the National Health Network and Centre).

Children aged under 9 months are at higher risk of vaccine-associated encephalitis, with the risk being inversely proportional to age. Children aged under 6 months should **not** be vaccinated. Children aged 6–9 months should only be vaccinated following a detailed risk assessment, and vaccination is generally only recommended if the risk of yellow fever transmission is high (such as during epidemics/outbreaks). If travel is unavoidable, seek expert advice on whether to vaccinate.

Yellow fever vaccine, live should be avoided in children with primary or acquired immunodeficiency due to a congenital condition or disease process, and in children who are immunosuppressed as a result of treatment.

If the yellow fever risk is unavoidable in HIV-infected children, consult the Children's HIV Association of UK and Ireland (www.chiva.org.uk/guidelines/immunisation) or other specialist advice.

For additional guidance on the suitability of immunisation against yellow fever, standardised checklists are available from: National Travel Health Network and Centre (see *Useful resources*) or Health Protection Scotland (www.Travax.nhs.uk).

A single-dose of yellow fever vaccine, live confers life-long immunity against yellow fever disease. Immunisation should be performed at least 10 days before travelling to an endemic area to allow protective immunity to develop and for the ICVP (if required) to become valid.

Reinforcing immunisation is not needed, except for a small subset of children at continued risk who may not have developed long-term protection from their initial yellow fever vaccine, live vaccination–seek expert advice.

All suspected cases of yellow fever must be notified to the local health protection unit. Where there is a community level outbreak, specialist advice should be sought from Public Health England (tel. 020 8200 4400) or, in Scotland, Health Protection Scotland (tel. 0140 300 1191).

Useful Resources

Recommendations reflect Chapter 35, Yellow fever, in *Immunisation against infectious disease*- 'The Green Book'. Public Health England, January 2020.
www.gov.uk/government/publications/yellow-fever-the-green-book-chapter-35

National Travel Health Network and Centre
travelhealthpro.org.uk

Vaccines for travel

Immunisation for travel

See advice on Malaria, treatment p. 426.

No special immunisation is required for travellers to the United States, Europe, Australia, or New Zealand, although all travellers should have immunity to tetanus and poliomyelitis (and childhood immunisations should be up to date); Tick-borne encephalitis vaccine is recommended for immunisation of those working in, or visiting, high-risk areas. Certain special precautions are required in non-European areas surrounding the Mediterranean, in Africa, the Middle East, Asia, and South America.

Travellers to areas that have a high incidence of **poliomyelitis** or **tuberculosis** should be immunised with the appropriate vaccine; in the case of poliomyelitis previously immunised travellers may be given a booster dose of a preparation containing inactivated poliomyelitis vaccine. For guidance on immunisation against tuberculosis, see *Travel* in Bacillus Calmette-Guérin vaccine p. 831.

For guidance on immunisation against **yellow fever**, see Yellow fever vaccine p. 843.

Immunisation against **meningococcal meningitis** is recommended for a number of areas of the world.

Protection against **hepatitis A** is recommended for travellers to high-risk areas outside Northern and Western Europe, North America, Japan, Australia and New Zealand. Hepatitis A vaccine is recommended and it is likely to be effective even if given shortly before departure; Public Health England recommends travellers can be vaccinated with hepatitis A vaccine up to the day of travel, and no longer recommends the use of normal immunoglobulin for travel prophylaxis. Special care must also be taken with food hygiene.

Hepatitis B vaccine is recommended for those travelling to areas of high or intermediate prevalence who intend to seek employment as healthcare workers or who plan to remain there for lengthy periods and who may therefore be at increased risk of acquiring infection as the result of medical or dental procedures carried out in those countries. Short-term tourists or business travellers are not generally at increased risk of infection but may put themselves at risk by their sexual behaviour when abroad.

Prophylactic immunisation against **rabies** is recommended for travellers to enzootic areas on long journeys or to areas out of reach of immediate medical attention.

Travellers who have not had a **tetanus** booster in the last 10 years and are visiting areas where medical attention may not be accessible should receive a booster dose of adsorbed diphtheria [low dose], tetanus and poliomyelitis (inactivated) vaccine, even if they have received 5 doses of a tetanus-containing vaccine previously.

Typhoid vaccine is indicated for travellers to countries where typhoid is endemic, but the vaccine is no substitute for personal precautions.

There is no requirement for cholera vaccination as a condition for entry into any country, but **oral cholera vaccine** should be considered for backpackers and those travelling to situations where the risk is greatest (e.g. refugee camps). Regardless of vaccination, travellers to areas where cholera is endemic should take special care with food hygiene.

Advice on **diphtheria**, on **Japanese encephalitis**, and on **tick-borne encephalitis** is included in *Health Information for Overseas Travel*.

Food hygiene

In areas where sanitation is poor, good food hygiene is important to help prevent hepatitis A, typhoid, cholera, and other diarrhoeal diseases (including travellers' diarrhoea). Food should be freshly prepared and hot, and uncooked vegetables (including green salads) should be avoided; only fruits which can be peeled should be eaten. Only suitable bottled water, or tap water that has been boiled or treated with sterilising tablets, should be used for drinking.

Information on health advice for travellers

Health professionals and travellers can find the latest information on immunisation requirements and precautions for avoiding disease while travelling from: nathnac.net.

The handbook, *Health Information for Overseas Travel* (2010), which draws together essential information *for healthcare professionals* regarding health advice for travellers, can also be obtained from this website.

Immunisation requirements change from time to time, and information on the current requirements for any particular country may be obtained from the embassy or legation of the appropriate country or from:

National Travel Health Network and Centre
UCLH NHS Foundation Trust
3rd Floor Central,
250 Euston Road,
London, NW1 2PG
Tel: 0845 602 6712
(Monday and Friday: 9–11 a.m. and 1–2 p.m. Tuesday to Thursday: 9–11 a.m. and 1–3:30 p.m. For healthcare professionals only) www.travelhealthpro.org.uk/

Travel Medicine Team
Health Protection Scotland
Meridian Court,
5 Cadogan Street,
Glasgow, G2 6QE
Tel: (0141) 300 1130
(2–4 p.m. Monday to Wednesday, 9:30–11:30 a.m. Friday; for registered TRAVAX users only) www.travax.nhs.uk

(TRAVAX is free for NHS Scotland users (registration required); subscription fee may be payable for users outside NHS Scotland)

Welsh Assembly Government
Tel (029) 2082 5397
(9 a.m.–5:30 p.m. weekdays)
Department of Health, Social Services and Public Safety
Castle Buildings,
Stormont,
Belfast, BT4 3SQ
Tel: (028) 9052 2118
(9 a.m.–5 p.m. weekdays) www.health-ni.gov.uk/contact

VACCINES

Vaccines

IMPORTANT SAFETY INFORMATION

MHRA/CHM ADVICE (UPDATED NOVEMBER 2017)
Following reports of death in neonates who received a live attenuated vaccine after exposure to a tumor necrosis factor alpha (TNF-a) inhibitor in utero, the MHRA has issued the following advice:
- any infant who has been exposed to immunosuppressive treatment from the mother either in utero during pregnancy or via breastfeeding should have any live attenuated vaccination deferred for as long as a postnatal influence on the immune status of the infant remains possible;
- in the case of infants who have been exposed to TNF-a inhibitors and other immunosuppressive biological medicines in utero, PHE advise that any live attenuated vaccination (e.g. BCG vaccine) should be deferred until the infant is age 6 months;
- PHE advise if there is any doubt as to whether an infant due to receive a live attenuated vaccine may be immunosuppressed due to the mother's therapy, including exposure through breast-feeding, specialist advice should be sought.

- **CONTRA-INDICATIONS**

CONTRA-INDICATIONS, FURTHER INFORMATION
- **Impaired immune response** Public Health England advises severely immunosuppressed patients should not be given live vaccines (including those with severe primary immunodeficiency).

- **CAUTIONS** Acute illness · minor illnesses

CAUTIONS, FURTHER INFORMATION Vaccination may be postponed if the individual is suffering from an acute illness; however, it is not necessary to postpone immunisation in patients with minor illnesses without fever or systemic upset.
- **Impaired immune response and drugs affecting immune response** Immune response to vaccines may be reduced in immunosuppressed patients and there is also a risk of generalised infection with live vaccines.

Specialist advice should be sought for those being treated with high doses of corticosteroids (dose equivalents of prednisolone: **adults**, at least 40 mg daily for more than 1 week; **children**, 2 mg/kg (or more than 40 mg) daily for at least 1 week or 1 mg/kg daily for 1 month), or other immunosuppressive drugs, and those being treated for malignant conditions with chemotherapy or generalised radiotherapy. Live vaccines should be postponed until at least 3 months after stopping high-dose systemic corticosteroids and at least 6 months after stopping other immunosuppressive drugs or generalised radiotherapy (at least 12 months after discontinuing immunosuppressants following bone-marrow transplantation).

The Royal College of Paediatrics and Child Health has produced a statement, *Immunisation of the Immunocompromised Child (*2002) (available at www.rcpch.ac.uk).

- **Predisposition to neurological problems** When there is a personal or family history of *febrile* convulsions, there is an increased risk of these occurring during fever from any cause including immunisation, but this is not a contra-indication to immunisation. In children who have had a seizure associated with fever without neurological deterioration, immunisation is *recommended*; advice on the *management of fever* (see Post-immunisation Pyrexia in Infants) should be given before immunisation. When a child has had a convulsion not associated with fever, and the neurological condition is not deteriorating, immunisation is *recommended.*

Children with stable neurological disorders (e.g. spina bifida, congenital brain abnormality, and peri-natal hypoxic-ischaemic encephalopathy) should be immunised according to the recommended schedule.

When there is a *still evolving neurological problem*, including poorly controlled epilepsy, immunisation should be deferred and the child referred to a specialist. Immunisation is recommended if a cause for the neurological disorder is identified. If a cause is not identified, immunisation should be deferred until the condition is stable.

- **SIDE-EFFECTS**
- **Common or very common** Appetite decreased · arthralgia · diarrhoea · dizziness · fatigue · fever · headache · irritability · lymphadenopathy · malaise · myalgia · nausea · skin reactions · vomiting
- **Uncommon** Hypersensitivity
- **ALLERGY AND CROSS-SENSITIVITY** Contra-indicated in patients with a confirmed anaphylactic reaction to a preceding dose of a vaccine containing the same antigens or vaccine component (such as antibacterials in viral vaccines).
- **PREGNANCY** Live vaccines should not be administered routinely to pregnant women because of the theoretical risk of fetal infection but where there is a significant risk of exposure to disease, the need for vaccination usually outweighs any possible risk to the fetus. Termination of pregnancy following inadvertent immunisation is not recommended. There is no evidence of risk from vaccinating pregnant women with inactivated viral or bacterial vaccines or toxoids.
- **BREAST FEEDING** Although there is a theoretical risk of live vaccine being present in breast milk, vaccination is not contra-indicated for women who are breast-feeding when there is significant risk of exposure to disease. There is no evidence of risk from vaccinating women who are breast-feeding, with inactivated viral or bacterial vaccines or toxoids.
- **DIRECTIONS FOR ADMINISTRATION** If alcohol or disinfectant is used for cleansing the skin it should be allowed to evaporate before vaccination to prevent possible inactivation of live vaccines.

When 2 or more live vaccines are required (and are not available as a combined preparation), they can be administered at any time before or after each other at different sites, preferably in a different limb; if more than one injection is to be given in the same limb, they should be administered at least 2.5 cm apart. See also Bacillus Calmette-Guérin vaccine p. 847, and Cautions, further information in measles, mumps and rubella vaccine, live p. 857.

Vaccines should not be given intravenously. Most vaccines are given by the intramuscular route, although some are given by either the intradermal, deep subcutaneous, or oral route. The intramuscular route should not be used in patients with **bleeding disorders** such as haemophilia or thrombocytopenia, vaccines usually given by the intramuscular route should be given by deep subcutaneous injection instead.

The Department of Health has advised *against the use of jet guns* for vaccination owing to the risk of transmitting blood borne infections, such as HIV.

Particular attention must be paid to instructions on the use of diluents. Vaccines which are liquid suspensions or are reconstituted before use should be adequately mixed to ensure uniformity of the material to be injected.

- HANDLING AND STORAGE Care must be taken to store all vaccines under the conditions recommended in the product literature, otherwise the preparation may become ineffective. **Refrigerated storage** is usually necessary; many vaccines need to be stored at 2–8°C and not allowed to freeze. Vaccines should be protected from light. Reconstituted vaccines and opened multidose vials must be used within the period recommended in the product literature. Unused vaccines should be disposed of by incineration at a registered disposal contractor.

VACCINES > BACTERIAL AND VIRAL VACCINES, COMBINED

845

Diphtheria with tetanus and poliomyelitis vaccine

- **INDICATIONS AND DOSE**

Primary immunisation

▶ BY INTRAMUSCULAR INJECTION

- Child 10–17 years: 0.5 mL every month for 3 doses

Booster doses

▶ BY INTRAMUSCULAR INJECTION

- Child 10–17 years: 0.5 mL for 1 dose, first booster dose—should be given 3 years after primary course (this interval can be reduced to a minimum of 1 year if the primary course was delayed), then 0.5 mL for 1 dose, second booster dose—should be given 10 years after first booster dose (this interval can be reduced to a minimum of 5 years if previous doses were delayed), second booster dose may also be used as first booster dose in those over 10 years who have received only 3 previous doses of a diphtheria-containing vaccine

- SIDE-EFFECTS

▶ **Common or very common** Vertigo

▶ **Frequency not known** Abdominal pain · asthenia · chills · face oedema · influenza like illness · nerve disorders · pallor · seizure · shock · syncope · vaccination reactions

- PRESCRIBING AND DISPENSING INFORMATION Available as part of childhood schedule from health organisations or ImmForm.

- MEDICINAL FORMS There can be variation in the licensing of different medicines containing the same drug.

Suspension for injection

EXCIPIENTS: May contain Neomycin, polymyxin b, streptomycin

- Revaxis (Sanofi Pasteur)
  Revaxis vaccine suspension for injection 0.5ml pre-filled syringes | 1 pre-filled disposable injection PoM £7.80 DT = £7.80

845

Diphtheria with tetanus, pertussis and poliomyelitis vaccine

- **INDICATIONS AND DOSE**

First booster dose

▶ BY INTRAMUSCULAR INJECTION

- Child 3–9 years: 0.5 mL, to be given 3 years after primary immunisation

Vaccination of pregnant women against pertussis (using low dose vaccines)

▶ BY INTRAMUSCULAR INJECTION

- Females of childbearing potential: 0.5 mL for 1 dose

- SIDE-EFFECTS

▶ **Common or very common** Abdominal pain · drowsiness · extensive swelling of vaccinated limb

▶ **Uncommon** Apathy · asthma · chills · dry throat · oral herpes · pain · paraesthesia · sleep disorder

▶ **Frequency not known** Angioedema · asthenia · hypotonic-hyporesponsiveness episode · seizure

SIDE-EFFECTS, FURTHER INFORMATION The incidence of local and systemic reactions is lower with acellular pertussis vaccines than with whole-cell pertussis vaccines used previously.

Compared with primary vaccination, injection site reactions are more common with booster doses of vaccines containing acellular pertussis.

Public Health England has advised (2016) that the vaccine should not be withheld from children with a history to a preceding dose of: fever, irrespective of severity; hypotonic-hyporesonsive episodes; persistent crying or screaming for more than 3 hours; severe local reaction, irrespective of extent.

- PREGNANCY Contra-indicated in pregnant women with a history of encephalopathy of unknown origin within 7 days of previous immunisation with a pertussis-containing vaccine. Contra-indicated in pregnant women with a history of transient thrombocytopenia or neurological complications following previous immunisation against diphtheria or tetanus.

- PRESCRIBING AND DISPENSING INFORMATION Pregnant women should be vaccinated using low dose vaccines (brands may include *Boostrix-IPV*® or *Repevax*®).

Available as part of childhood immunisation schedule from health organisations or ImmForm.

Available for vaccination of pregnant women from ImmForm.

- MEDICINAL FORMS There can be variation in the licensing of different medicines containing the same drug.

Suspension for injection

EXCIPIENTS: May contain Neomycin, polymyxin b, streptomycin

- Boostrix-IPV (GlaxoSmithKline UK Ltd)
  Boostrix-IPV suspension for injection 0.5ml pre-filled syringes | 1 pre-filled disposable injection PoM £22.74 DT = £20.00
- Repevax (Sanofi Pasteur)
  Repevax vaccine suspension for injection 0.5ml pre-filled syringes | 1 pre-filled disposable injection PoM £20.00 DT = £20.00

845

Diphtheria with tetanus, pertussis, hepatitis B, poliomyelitis and haemophilus influenzae type b vaccine

12-Oct-2017

- **INDICATIONS AND DOSE**

Primary immunisation (first dose)

▶ BY DEEP INTRAMUSCULAR INJECTION

- Child 2 months: 0.5 mL for 1 dose

Primary immunisation (second dose)

▶ BY DEEP INTRAMUSCULAR INJECTION

- Child 3 months: 0.5 mL for 1 dose, preferably administer at a different injection site to that of first dose

Primary immunisation (third dose)

▶ BY DEEP INTRAMUSCULAR INJECTION

- Child 4 months: 0.5 mL for 1 dose, preferably administer at a different injection site to that of second dose

- **SIDE-EFFECTS**
- ▶ **Common or very common** Anxiety · crying abnormal
- ▶ **Uncommon** Cough · drowsiness · extensive swelling of vaccinated limb · increased risk of infection
- ▶ **Rare or very rare** Angioedema · apnoea · hypotonic-hyporesponsiveness episode · seizure · swelling · thrombocytopenia
- **PRESCRIBING AND DISPENSING INFORMATION** Available as part of childhood schedule from health organisations or ImmForm.

- **MEDICINAL FORMS** There can be variation in the licensing of different medicines containing the same drug.

Powder and suspension for suspension for injection

EXCIPIENTS: May contain Neomycin, polymyxin b

- ▶ Infanrix Hexa (GlaxoSmithKline UK Ltd)
  Infanrix Hexa vaccine powder and suspension for suspension for injection 0.5ml pre-filled syringes | 1 pre-filled disposable injection [PoM] [X]

F 845

Diphtheria with tetanus, pertussis, poliomyelitis and haemophilus influenzae type b vaccine

- **INDICATIONS AND DOSE**

Primary immunisation

▶ BY INTRAMUSCULAR INJECTION

- ▶ Child 2 months–9 years: 0.5 mL every month for 3 doses

- **UNLICENSED USE** *Infanrix-IPV+ Hib®* not licensed for use in children over 36 months; *Pediacel®* not licensed in children over 4 years. However, the Department of Health recommends that these be used for children up to 10 years.
- **SIDE-EFFECTS**
- ▶ **Common or very common** Crying abnormal · drowsiness · restlessness
- ▶ **Uncommon** Cough · extensive swelling of vaccinated limb · increased risk of infection · rhinorrhoea
- ▶ **Frequency not known** Angioedema · apnoea · hypotonic-hyporesponsiveness episode · seizure

SIDE-EFFECTS, FURTHER INFORMATION The incidence of local and systemic reactions is lower with acellular pertussis vaccines than with whole-cell pertussis vaccines used previously.

Compared with primary vaccination, injection site reactions are more common with booster doses of vaccines containing acellular pertussis.

Public Health England has advised (2016) that the vaccine should not be withheld from children with a history to a preceding dose of: fever, irrespective of severity; hypotonic-hyporesonsive episodes; persistent crying or screaming for more than 3 hours; severe local reaction, irrespective of extent.

- **PRESCRIBING AND DISPENSING INFORMATION** Available as part of childhood schedule from health organisations or ImmForm.

- **MEDICINAL FORMS** There can be variation in the licensing of different medicines containing the same drug.

Powder and suspension for suspension for injection

- ▶ Infanrix-IPV + Hib (GlaxoSmithKline UK Ltd)
  Infanrix-IPV + Hib vaccine powder and suspension for suspension for injection 0.5ml pre-filled syringes | 1 pre-filled disposable injection [PoM] £27.86

VACCINES > BACTERIAL VACCINES

F 845

Bacillus Calmette-Guérin vaccine

12-Nov-2019

(BCG Vaccine)

- **DRUG ACTION** BCG (Bacillus Calmette-Guérin) is a live attenuated strain derived from *Mycobacterium bovis* which stimulates the development of immunity to *M. tuberculosis*.

- **INDICATIONS AND DOSE**

Immunisation against tuberculosis

▶ BY INTRADERMAL INJECTION

- ▶ Neonate: 0.05 mL, to be injected at insertion of deltoid muscle onto humerus (keloid formation more likely with sites higher on arm); tip of shoulder should be **avoided.**
- ▶ Child 1–11 months: 0.05 mL, to be injected at insertion of deltoid muscle onto humerus (keloid formation more likely with sites higher on arm); tip of shoulder should be **avoided**
- ▶ Child 1–17 years: 0.1 mL, to be injected at insertion of deltoid muscle onto humerus (keloid formation more likely with sites higher on arm); tip of shoulder should be **avoided**

- **CONTRA-INDICATIONS** Children less than 2 years of age in household contact with known or suspected case of active tuberculosis · generalised septic skin conditions

CONTRA-INDICATIONS, FURTHER INFORMATION Manufacturer advises using a lesion-free site to administer BCG vaccine to patients with eczema.

- **CAUTIONS**

CAUTIONS, FURTHER INFORMATION When BCG is given to infants, there is no need to delay routine primary immunisations. No further vaccination should be given in the arm used for BCG vaccination for at least 3 months because of the risk of regional lymphadenitis.

- **INTERACTIONS** → Appendix 1: live vaccines
- **SIDE-EFFECTS**
- ▶ **Uncommon** Lymphadenitis suppurative
- ▶ **Rare or very rare** Osteitis · osteomyelitis
- ▶ **Frequency not known** Seizure · syncope
- **PRE-TREATMENT SCREENING** Apart from children under 6 years, any person being considered for BCG immunisation must first be given a skin test for hypersensitivity to tuberculoprotein (see tuberculin purified protein derivative p. 828). A skin test is not necessary for a child under 6 years provided that the child has not stayed for longer than 3 months in a country with an incidence of tuberculosis greater than 40 per 100 000, the child has not had contact with a person with tuberculosis, and there is no family history of tuberculosis within the last 5 years.
- **DIRECTIONS FOR ADMINISTRATION**

Intradermal injection technique Skin is stretched between thumb and forefinger and needle (size 25G or 26G) inserted (bevel upwards) for about 3 mm into superficial layers of dermis (almost parallel with surface). Needle should be short with short bevel (can usually be seen through epidermis during insertion). Tense raised blanched bleb showing tips of hair follicles is sign of correct injection; 7 mm bleb ≡ 0.1 mL injection, 3 mm bleb ≡ 0.05 mL injection; if considerable resistance not felt, needle too deep and should be removed and reinserted before giving more vaccine.

- **PRESCRIBING AND DISPENSING INFORMATION** Available from health organisations or direct from ImmForm

14 Vaccines

www.immform.dh.gov.uk (SSI brand, multidose vial with diluent).

- **MEDICINAL FORMS** There can be variation in the licensing of different medicines containing the same drug.

Powder for injection

- BCG Vaccine AJV (AJ Vaccines)
  BCG Vaccine AJV powder for suspension for injection 1ml vials | 10 vial PoM

Powder and solvent for suspension for injection

- InterVax BCG vaccine (InterVax Ltd)
  InterVax BCG vaccine powder and solvent for suspension for injection ampoules | 20 ampoule PoM

F 845

Cholera vaccine

- **INDICATIONS AND DOSE**

Immunisation against cholera (for travellers to endemic or epidemic areas on the basis of current recommendations)

- BY MOUTH
- Child 2–5 years: 1 dose every 1–6 weeks for 3 doses, if more than 6 weeks have elapsed between doses, the primary course should be restarted, immunisation should be completed at least one week before potential exposure
- Child 6–17 years: 1 dose every 1–6 weeks for 2 doses, if more than 6 weeks have elapsed between doses, the primary course should be restarted, immunisation should be completed at least one week before potential exposure

Booster

- BY MOUTH
- Child 2–5 years: A single booster dose can be given within 6 months after primary course, if more than 6 months have elapsed since the last vaccination, the primary course should be repeated
- Child 6–17 years: A single booster dose can be given within 2 years after primary course, if more than 2 years have elapsed since the last vaccination, the primary course should be repeated

- **CONTRA-INDICATIONS** Acute gastro-intestinal illness
- **INTERACTIONS** → Appendix 1: cholera vaccine
- **SIDE-EFFECTS**
- **Uncommon** Gastrointestinal discomfort · gastrointestinal disorders
- **Rare or very rare** Chills · cough · dehydration · drowsiness · hyperhidrosis · increased risk of infection · insomnia · pulmonary reaction · syncope · taste altered · throat pain
- **Frequency not known** Angioedema · asthenia · dyspnoea · hypertension · influenza like illness · lymphadenitis · pain · paraesthesia · sputum increased
- **DIRECTIONS FOR ADMINISTRATION** Dissolve effervescent sodium bicarbonate granules in a glassful of water *or* chlorinated water (approximately 150 mL). For children over 6 years, add vaccine suspension to make one dose. For child 2–5 years, discard half (approximately 75 mL) of the solution, then add vaccine suspension to make one dose. Drink within 2 hours. Food, drink, and other oral medicines should be avoided for 1 hour before and after vaccination.
- **PATIENT AND CARER ADVICE** Counselling on administration advised. Immunisation with cholera vaccine does not provide complete protection and all travellers to a country where cholera exists should be warned that scrupulous attention to food, water, and personal hygiene is **essential**.
- **MEDICINAL FORMS** There can be variation in the licensing of different medicines containing the same drug.

Oral suspension

- Dukoral (Valneva UK Ltd)
  Dukoral cholera vaccine oral suspension | 2 dose PoM £26.35 DT = £26.35

F 845

Haemophilus influenzae type b with meningococcal group C vaccine

- **INDICATIONS AND DOSE**

Booster dose (for infants who have received primary immunisation with a vaccine containing *Haemophilus influenzae* type b component) and primary immunisation against *Neisseria meningitidis*

- BY INTRAMUSCULAR INJECTION
- Child 12–13 months: 0.5 mL for 1 dose

Immunisation against *Neisseria meningitidis* in an unimmunised patient

- BY INTRAMUSCULAR INJECTION
- Child 1–9 years: 0.5 mL for 1 dose

Booster dose (for children who have not been immunised against *Haemophilus influenza* type b) | Booster dose after recovery from *Haemophilus influenzae* type b disease (for index cases previously vaccinated, with low Hib antibody concentration or if it is not possible to measure antibody concentration)

- BY INTRAMUSCULAR INJECTION
- Child 1–9 years: 0.5 mL for 1 dose

Booster dose after recovery from *Haemophilus influenzae* type b disease (for fully vaccinated index cases with asplenia or splenic dysfunction, if previous dose received over 1 year ago)

- BY INTRAMUSCULAR INJECTION
- Child 1–17 years: 0.5 mL for 1 dose

Booster dose (for patients diagnosed with asplenia, splenic dysfunction or complement deficiency at under 2 years of age)

- BY INTRAMUSCULAR INJECTION
- Child 2–17 years: 0.5 mL for 1 dose, this booster dose should be given after the second birthday, this is the second dose of haemophilus influenzae type B vaccine combined with meningococcal group C conjugate vaccine (the first dose is given during the routine immunisation schedule)

Booster dose (for patients diagnosed with asplenia, splenic dysfunction or complement deficiency at over 2 years of age)

- BY INTRAMUSCULAR INJECTION
- Child 2–17 years: 0.5 mL for 1 dose, this booster dose should be followed 2 months later by one dose of meningococcal A, C, W135, and Y conjugate vaccine (in patients from 11 years of age, this interval can be reduced to one month)

- **UNLICENSED USE** Not licensed for use in patients over 2 years.
- **SIDE-EFFECTS**
- **Common or very common** Drowsiness
- **Uncommon** Crying
- **Rare or very rare** Abdominal pain · insomnia
- **Frequency not known** Apnoea (in neonates) · febrile seizure · meningism (but no evidence that vaccine causes meningococcal C meningitis) · muscle tone decreased
- **PRESCRIBING AND DISPENSING INFORMATION** Available as part of the childhood immunisation schedule from ImmForm.

● **MEDICINAL FORMS** There can be variation in the licensing of different medicines containing the same drug.

Powder and solvent for solution for injection

▸ Menitorix (GlaxoSmithKline UK Ltd)
Menitorix vaccine powder and solvent for solution for injection 0.5ml vials | 1 vial PoM £37.76 DT = £37.76

⚑ 845

Meningococcal group B vaccine (rDNA, component, adsorbed)

19-Oct-2017

● **INDICATIONS AND DOSE**

BEXSERO®

Immunisation against *Neisseria meningitidis*, primary immunisation

▸ BY DEEP INTRAMUSCULAR INJECTION

▸ Child 2 months: 0.5 mL for 1 dose, injected preferably into deltoid region (or anterolateral thigh in infants), for information about the use of paracetamol for prophylaxis of post-immunisation pyrexia, see paracetamol p. 288.

▸ Child 4 months: 0.5 mL for 1 dose, injected preferably into deltoid region (or anterolateral thigh in infants), for information about the use of paracetamol for prophylaxis of post-immunisation pyrexia, see paracetamol p. 288.

Immunisation against *Neisseria meningitidis*, primary immunisation booster dose

▸ BY DEEP INTRAMUSCULAR INJECTION

▸ Child 12-23 months: 0.5 mL for 1 dose, injected preferably into deltoid region (or anterolateral thigh in infants)

Immunisation against *Neisseria meningitidis*, primary immunisation (in unimmunised patients)

▸ BY DEEP INTRAMUSCULAR INJECTION

▸ Child 6-11 months: 0.5 mL for 2 doses, separated by an interval of at least 2 months; booster dose of 0.5 mL given between 1–2 years of age and at least 2 months after completion of primary immunisation, injected preferably into deltoid region (or anterolateral thigh in infants)

▸ Child 12-23 months: 0.5 mL for 2 doses, separated by an interval of at least 2 months; booster dose of 0.5 mL given 12–24 months after completion of primary immunisation, injected preferably into deltoid region (or anterolateral thigh in infants)

▸ Child 2-10 years: 0.5 mL for 2 doses, separated by an interval of at least 2 months. Injected preferably into deltoid region (or anterolateral thigh in infants)

▸ Child 11-17 years: 0.5 mL for 2 doses, separated by an interval of at least 1 month. Injected preferably into deltoid region

TRUMENBA®

Immunisation against *Neisseria meningitidis*, primary immunisation

▸ BY INTRAMUSCULAR INJECTION

▸ Child 10-17 years: 0.5 mL for 2 doses, separated by an interval of 6 months, alternatively 0.5 mL for 2 doses, separated by an interval of at least 1 month, followed by 0.5 mL as a third dose, given at least 4 months after the second dose, injected preferably into deltoid region, a booster dose should be considered for individuals at continued risk—consult product literature

● **SIDE-EFFECTS**

▸ **Common or very common** Crying abnormal · drowsiness · eating disorder

▸ **Uncommon** Seizures · vascular disorders

▸ **Frequency not known** Extensive swelling of vaccinated limb · hypotonic-hyporesponsiveness episode

● **MEDICINAL FORMS** There can be variation in the licensing of different medicines containing the same drug.

Suspension for injection

EXCIPIENTS: May contain Kanamycin

▸ Bexsero (GlaxoSmithKline UK Ltd)
Bexsero vaccine suspension for injection 0.5ml pre-filled syringes | 1 pre-filled disposable injection PoM £75.00

▸ Trumenba (Pfizer Ltd) ▼
Trumenba vaccine suspension for injection 0.5ml pre-filled syringes | 1 pre-filled disposable injection PoM £75.00

⚑ 845

Meningococcal group C vaccine

● **INDICATIONS AND DOSE**

Patients with confirmed serogroup C disease (who have previously been immunised)

▸ BY INTRAMUSCULAR INJECTION

▸ Child 1-17 years: 0.5 mL for 1 dose, dose to be given before discharge from hospital

● **SIDE-EFFECTS**

▸ **Common or very common** Anxiety · cough · crying · drowsiness · gastrointestinal discomfort · hyperhidrosis · increased risk of infection · pain · sleep disorders

▸ **Uncommon** Asthenia · chills · eyelid oedema · flushing · joint stiffness · musculoskeletal stiffness · nasal congestion · oedema · respiratory disorders · seizures · sensation abnormal · syncope

▸ **Rare or very rare** Circulatory collapse · influenza like illness

▸ **Frequency not known** Angioedema · apnoea · dyspnoea · hypotonic-hyporesponsiveness episode · immune thrombocytopenic purpura · meningism (but no evidence that vaccine causes meningococcal C meningitis) · Stevens-Johnson syndrome

● **PRESCRIBING AND DISPENSING INFORMATION** Available as part of childhood immunisation schedule from www.immform.dh.gov.uk.

● **MEDICINAL FORMS** There can be variation in the licensing of different medicines containing the same drug.

Suspension for injection

▸ NeisVac-C (Pfizer Ltd)
NeisVac-C vaccine suspension for injection 0.5ml pre-filled syringes | 10 pre-filled disposable injection PoM £187.50

⚑ 845

Meningococcal groups A with C and W135 and Y vaccine

● **INDICATIONS AND DOSE**

MENVEO®

Primary immunisation against *Neisseria meningitidis*

▸ BY INTRAMUSCULAR INJECTION

▸ Child 13-15 years: 0.5 mL for 1 dose, dose preferably injected into deltoid region

Immunisation against *Neisseria meningitidis* in an unimmunised patient

▸ BY INTRAMUSCULAR INJECTION

▸ Child 10-17 years: 0.5 mL for 1 dose, booster dose is not required

Immunisation against *Neisseria meningitidis* in those at risk of exposure to prevent invasive disease

▸ BY INTRAMUSCULAR INJECTION

▸ Child 3-11 months: 0.5 mL every month for 2 doses, dose preferably injected into deltoid region

▸ Child 1-17 years: 0.5 mL for 1 dose, dose preferably injected into deltoid region

continued →

Patients attending university for the first time (who have not received the routine meningococcal groups A with C and W135 and Y conjugate vaccine over the age of 10 years)
- ▶ BY INTRAMUSCULAR INJECTION
- ▸ Child 16–17 years: 0.5 mL for 1 dose

NIMENRIX ®

Primary immunisation against *Neisseria meningitidis*
- ▶ BY INTRAMUSCULAR INJECTION
- ▸ Child 13–15 years: 0.5 mL for 1 dose, to be injected preferably into deltoid region

Immunisation against *Neisseria meningitidis* in an unimmunised patient
- ▶ BY INTRAMUSCULAR INJECTION
- ▸ Child 10–17 years: 0.5 mL for 1 dose, booster dose is not required

Immunisation against *Neisseria meningitidis* in those at risk of exposure
- ▶ BY INTRAMUSCULAR INJECTION
- ▸ Child 1–17 years: 0.5 mL for 1 dose, to be injected preferably into deltoid region (or anterolateral thigh in child 12–23 months), then 0.5 mL after 1 year if required for 1 dose, second dose should be considered in those who continue to be at risk of *Neisseria meningitidis* serogroup A infection

Patients attending university for the first time (who have not received the routine meningococcal groups A with C and W135 and Y conjugate vaccine over the age of 10 years)
- ▶ BY INTRAMUSCULAR INJECTION
- ▸ Child 16–17 years: 0.5 mL for 1 dose

● **UNLICENSED USE**

MENVEO ® *Menveo*® is not licensed for use in children under 2 years.

● **SIDE-EFFECTS**
- ▶ **Common or very common** Drowsiness
- ▶ **Uncommon** Crying · insomnia · numbness · pain in extremity
- ▶ **Frequency not known** Extensive swelling of vaccinated limb

● **MEDICINAL FORMS** There can be variation in the licensing of different medicines containing the same drug.

Powder and solvent for solution for injection
- ▸ Menveo (GlaxoSmithKline UK Ltd)
  Menveo vaccine powder and solvent for solution for injection 0.5ml vials | 1 vial PoM £30.00 DT = £30.00
- ▸ Nimenrix (Pfizer Ltd)
  Nimenrix vaccine powder and solvent for solution for injection 0.5ml pre-filled syringes | 1 pre-filled disposable injection PoM £30.00 DT = £30.00

F 845

Pneumococcal polysaccharide conjugate vaccine (adsorbed)

12-Nov-2019

● **INDICATIONS AND DOSE**

PREVENAR 13 ®

Primary immunisation against pneumococcal infection—first dose [infants born on or after 1 January 2020]
- ▶ BY INTRAMUSCULAR INJECTION
- ▸ Child 12 weeks: 0.5 mL for 1 dose, anterolateral thigh is preferred site of injection in infants under 1 year

Primary immunisation against pneumococcal infection—booster dose [infants born on or after 1 January 2020]
- ▶ BY INTRAMUSCULAR INJECTION
- ▸ Child 1 year: 0.5 mL for 1 dose, anterolateral thigh is preferred site of injection in infants under 1 year; deltoid muscle is preferred in older children

Primary immunisation against pneumococcal infection—in those with asplenia, splenic dysfunction, complement disorder or severe immunocompromise [infants born on or after 1 January 2020]
- ▶ BY INTRAMUSCULAR INJECTION
- ▸ Child 6 weeks–11 months: 0.5 mL for 4 doses, the first two doses to be given at least 8 weeks apart, the third dose to be given on or after their first birthday, and the fourth dose to be given at least 8 weeks later. Anterolateral thigh is preferred site of injection in infants under 1 year; deltoid muscle is preferred in children
- ▸ Child 1–2 years: 0.5 mL for 2 doses, the first dose to be given on or after their first birthday and the second dose to be given at least 8 weeks later. Deltoid muscle is preferred site of injection in children

Immunisation against pneumococcal infection—unimmunised or partially immunised patients [infants born on or after 1 January 2020]
- ▶ BY INTRAMUSCULAR INJECTION
- ▸ Child 3–11 months: 0.5 mL for 1 dose, followed by 0.5 mL for 1 dose on or after their first birthday, given at least 4 weeks after the first dose. Anterolateral thigh is preferred site of injection in infants under 1 year
- ▸ Child 12–23 months: 0.5 mL for 1 dose, deltoid muscle is preferred site of injection in children

Immunisation against pneumococcal infection—unimmunised or partially immunised patients at increased risk [born on or after 1 January 2020]
- ▶ BY INTRAMUSCULAR INJECTION
- ▸ Child 2–9 years: 0.5 mL for 1 dose, deltoid muscle is preferred site of injection in children

Immunisation against pneumococcal infection—immunised patients with severe immunocompromise [born on or after 1 January 2020]
- ▶ BY INTRAMUSCULAR INJECTION
- ▸ Child 2–17 years: 0.5 mL for 1 dose, deltoid muscle is preferred site of injection in children

Primary immunisation against pneumococcal infection—first dose [infants born on or before 31 December 2019]
- ▶ BY INTRAMUSCULAR INJECTION
- ▸ Child 8 weeks: 0.5 mL for 1 dose, anterolateral thigh is preferred site of injection in infants under 1 year

Primary immunisation against pneumococcal infection—second dose [infants born on or before 31 December 2019]
- ▶ BY INTRAMUSCULAR INJECTION
- ▸ Child 16 weeks: 0.5 mL for 1 dose, anterolateral thigh is preferred site of injection in infants under 1 year

Primary immunisation against pneumococcal infection—booster dose [infants born on or before 31 December 2019]
- ▶ BY INTRAMUSCULAR INJECTION
- ▸ Child 1 year: 0.5 mL for 1 dose, anterolateral thigh is preferred site of injection in infants under 1 year; deltoid muscle is preferred in older children

Immunisation against pneumococcal infection—unimmunised or partially immunised patients [infants born on or before 31 December 2019]
- ▶ BY INTRAMUSCULAR INJECTION
- ▸ Child 3–11 months: 0.5 mL for 2 doses, given 2 months apart (interval may be reduced to 1 month to ensure immunisation schedule is completed), followed by 0.5 mL for 1 dose on their first birthday, given at least 2 months after the last dose. Anterolateral thigh is preferred site of injection in infants under 1 year
- ▸ Child 12–23 months: 0.5 mL for 1 dose, deltoid muscle is preferred site of injection in children

Immunisation against pneumococcal infection—immunised patients at increased risk [born on or before 31 December 2019]
- ▶ BY INTRAMUSCULAR INJECTION
  - Child 14 months–17 years: 0.5 mL for 1 dose, given at least 2 months after primary immunisation booster dose, deltoid muscle is preferred site of injection in children

Immunisation against pneumococcal infection—unimmunised or partially immunised patients at increased risk [born on or before 31 December 2019]
- ▶ BY INTRAMUSCULAR INJECTION
  - Child 3–11 months: 0.5 mL for 2 doses, given 2 months apart (interval may be reduced to 1 month to ensure immunisation schedule is completed), followed by 0.5 mL for 1 dose on their first birthday, given at least 2 months after the last dose, followed by 0.5 mL for 1 dose, given at least 2 months after the last dose. Anterolateral thigh is preferred site of injection in infants under 1 year
  - Child 1–9 years: 0.5 mL for 1 dose, an additional dose is recommended (at least 2 months later) in those who are severely immunocompromised. Deltoid muscle is preferred site of injection in children
  - Child 10–17 years: 0.5 mL for 1 dose, deltoid muscle is preferred site of injection in children

SYNFLORIX ®

Immunisation against pneumococcal infection
- ▶ BY INTRAMUSCULAR INJECTION
  - Child 6 weeks–4 years: Deltoid muscle is preferred site of injection in young children; anterolateral thigh is preferred site in infants (consult product literature)

- **UNLICENSED USE**

PREVENAR 13 ® The dose in BNF publications may differ from that in product literature.

- **SIDE-EFFECTS**
- ▶ **Common or very common** Drowsiness
- ▶ **Uncommon** Apnoea · crying abnormal · extensive swelling of vaccinated limb
- ▶ **Rare or very rare** Angioedema · hypotonic-hyporesponsiveness episode · Kawasaki disease · seizure

- **PRESCRIBING AND DISPENSING INFORMATION**

PREVENAR 13 ® Available as part of childhood immunisation schedule from ImmForm www.immform.dh.gov.uk.

- **MEDICINAL FORMS** There can be variation in the licensing of different medicines containing the same drug.

Suspension for injection
- Prevenar (Pfizer Ltd)
  Prevenar 13 vaccine suspension for injection 0.5ml pre-filled syringes | 1 pre-filled disposable injection PoM £49.10 DT = £49.10 | 10 pre-filled disposable injection PoM £491.00

F 845

Pneumococcal polysaccharide vaccine

01-May-2019

- **INDICATIONS AND DOSE**

Immunisation against pneumococcal infection [in patients at increased risk]
- ▶ BY INTRAMUSCULAR INJECTION
  - Child 2–17 years: 0.5 mL for 1 dose, dose should be administered at least 2 months after the last dose of the 13-valent pneumococcal polysaccharide conjugate vaccine (adsorbed), deltoid muscle is preferred site of injection in children and adults

Immunisation against pneumococcal infection [revaccination; booster dose in patients with no spleen, splenic dysfunction or chronic kidney disease]
- ▶ BY INTRAMUSCULAR INJECTION
  - Child 7–17 years: 0.5 mL every 5 years, deltoid muscle is preferred site of injection in children and adults

- **SIDE-EFFECTS** Angioedema · arthritis · asthenia · chills · febrile seizure · haemolytic anaemia · injected limb mobility decreased · leucocytosis · lymphadenitis · nerve disorders · paraesthesia · peripheral oedema · thrombocytopenia

- **MEDICINAL FORMS** There can be variation in the licensing of different medicines containing the same drug.

Solution for injection
- Pneumococcal polysaccharide vaccine (Non-proprietary)
  Pneumococcal polysaccharide vaccine solution for injection 0.5ml vials | 1 vial PoM £8.32 DT = £8.32
- Pneumovax 23 (Merck Sharp & Dohme Ltd)
  Pneumovax 23 solution for injection 0.5ml pre-filled syringes | 1 pre-filled disposable injection PoM £16.80 DT = £16.80

F 845

Typhoid vaccine

17-Mar-2020

- **DRUG ACTION** Typhoid vaccine protects against typhoid fever caused by *Salmonella typhi* infection; it is available as an oral live attenuated vaccine and an injectable polysaccharide vaccine.

- **INDICATIONS AND DOSE**

Immunisation against typhoid fever [in children at high risk of typhoid fever]
- ▶ BY INTRAMUSCULAR INJECTION
  - Child 12–23 months: 0.5 mL for 1 dose, dose should be given at least 2 weeks before potential exposure to typhoid infection, response may be suboptimal

Immunisation against typhoid fever
- ▶ BY INTRAMUSCULAR INJECTION
  - Child 2–17 years: 0.5 mL for 1 dose, dose should be given at least 2 weeks before potential exposure to typhoid infection
- ▶ BY MOUTH
  - Child 5–17 years: 1 capsule every 2 days for 3 doses (on days 1, 3, and 5), course should be completed at least 1 week before potential exposure to typhoid infection

Booster
- ▶ BY INTRAMUSCULAR INJECTION
  - Child 2–17 years: 0.5 mL for 1 dose every 3 years
- ▶ BY MOUTH
  - Child 5–17 years: 1 capsule every 2 days for 3 doses (on days 1, 3, and 5) every 3 years

- **UNLICENSED USE**
- ▶ With intramuscular use Not licensed for use in children under 2 years.
- **CONTRA-INDICATIONS**
- ▶ With oral use Acute gastro-intestinal illness
- **INTERACTIONS** → Appendix 1: live vaccines
- **SIDE-EFFECTS**

GENERAL SIDE-EFFECTS
Shock

SPECIFIC SIDE-EFFECTS
- ▶ **Common or very common**
  - With oral use Gastrointestinal discomfort
- ▶ **Frequency not known**
  - With oral use Asthenia · back pain · chills · flatulence · influenza like illness · paraesthesia
  - With parenteral use Abdominal pain · asthma · syncope

14 Vaccines

- **DIRECTIONS FOR ADMINISTRATION** Capsule should be taken one hour before a meal. Swallow as soon as possible after placing in mouth with a cold or lukewarm drink.
- **HANDLING AND STORAGE**
  - With oral use It is important to store capsules in a refrigerator.
- **PATIENT AND CARER ADVICE**
  - With oral use Patients or carers should be given advice on how to administer and store typhoid vaccine capsules.
- **MEDICINAL FORMS** There can be variation in the licensing of different medicines containing the same drug.

Solution for injection

- Typhim Vi (Sanofi Pasteur)
  Salmonella typhi Vi capsular polysaccharide 50 microgram per 1 ml Typhim Vi 25micrograms/0.5ml vaccine solution for injection pre-filled syringes | 1 pre-filled disposable injection PoM £11.16 DT = £11.16 | 10 pre-filled disposable injection PoM £111.60 DT = £111.60

Gastro-resistant capsule

CAUTIONARY AND ADVISORY LABELS 25

- Vivotif (Emergent BioSolutions UK)
  Vivotif vaccine gastro-resistant capsules | 3 capsule PoM £14.77 DT = £14.77

Combinations available: ***Hepatitis A with typhoid vaccine,*** p. 853.

14 Vaccines

VACCINES > VIRAL VACCINES

Hepatitis A and B vaccine

03-Dec-2019

The properties listed below are those particular to the combination only. For the properties of the components please consider, hepatitis A vaccine below, hepatitis B vaccine p. 853.

- **INDICATIONS AND DOSE**

AMBIRIX®

Immunisation against hepatitis A and hepatitis B infection (primary course)

- BY INTRAMUSCULAR INJECTION
  - Child 1–15 years: Initially 1 mL for 1 dose, then 1 mL after 6–12 months for 1 dose, the deltoid region is the preferred site of injection in older children; anterolateral thigh is the preferred site in infants; not to be injected into the buttock (vaccine efficacy reduced), subcutaneous route used for patients with bleeding disorders (but immune response may be reduced)

TWINRIX® ADULT

Immunisation against hepatitis A and hepatitis B infection (primary course)

- BY INTRAMUSCULAR INJECTION
  - Child 16–17 years: Initially 1 mL every month for 2 doses, then 1 mL after 5 months for 1 dose, the deltoid region is the preferred site of injection; not to be injected into the buttock (vaccine efficacy reduced), subcutaneous route used for patients with bleeding disorders (but immune response may be reduced)

Immunisation against hepatitis A and hepatitis B infection—accelerated schedule for travellers departing within 1 month

- BY INTRAMUSCULAR INJECTION
  - Child 16–17 years: Initially 1 mL for 1 dose, then 1 mL after 7 days for 1 dose, then 1 mL after 14 days for 1 dose, then 1 mL for 1 dose given 12 months after the first dose, the deltoid region is the preferred site of injection; not to be injected into the buttock (vaccine efficacy reduced), subcutaneous route used for patients with bleeding disorders (but immune response may be reduced)

TWINRIX® PAEDIATRIC

Immunisation against hepatitis A and hepatitis B infection (primary course)

- BY INTRAMUSCULAR INJECTION
  - Child 1–15 years: Initially 0.5 mL every month for 2 doses, then 0.5 mL after 5 months for 1 dose, the deltoid region is the preferred site of injection in older children; anterolateral thigh is the preferred site in infants; not to be injected into the buttock (vaccine efficacy reduced), subcutaneous route used for patients with bleeding disorders (but immune response may be reduced)

IMPORTANT SAFETY INFORMATION

Ambirix® and *Twinrix®* are not recommended for post-exposure prophylaxis following percutaneous (needle-stick), ocular, or mucous membrane exposure to hepatitis B virus.

- **PRESCRIBING AND DISPENSING INFORMATION**

TWINRIX® PAEDIATRIC Primary course should be completed with *Twinrix®* (single component vaccines given at appropriate intervals may be used for booster dose).

TWINRIX® ADULT Primary course should be completed with *Twinrix®* (single component vaccines given at appropriate intervals may be used for booster dose).

AMBIRIX® Primary course should be completed with *Ambirix®* (single component vaccines given at appropriate intervals may be used for booster dose).

- **MEDICINAL FORMS** There can be variation in the licensing of different medicines containing the same drug.

Suspension for injection

EXCIPIENTS: May contain Neomycin

- Ambirix (GlaxoSmithKline UK Ltd)
  Ambirix vaccine suspension for injection 1ml pre-filled syringes | 1 pre-filled disposable injection PoM £31.18 DT = £31.18
- Twinrix (GlaxoSmithKline UK Ltd)
  Twinrix Paediatric vaccine suspension for injection 0.5ml pre-filled syringes | 1 pre-filled disposable injection PoM £20.79 DT = £20.79
  Twinrix Adult vaccine suspension for injection 1ml pre-filled syringes | 1 pre-filled disposable injection PoM £33.31 DT = £31.18 | 10 pre-filled disposable injection PoM £333.13

845

Hepatitis A vaccine

- **INDICATIONS AND DOSE**

AVAXIM®

Immunisation against hepatitis A infection

- BY INTRAMUSCULAR INJECTION
  - Child 16–17 years: Initially 0.5 mL for 1 dose, then 0.5 mL after 6–12 months, dose given as booster; booster dose may be delayed by up to 3 years if not given after recommended interval following primary dose, the deltoid region is the preferred site of injection. The subcutaneous route may be used for patients with bleeding disorders; not to be injected into the buttock (vaccine efficacy reduced)

HAVRIX MONODOSE®

Immunisation against hepatitis A infection

- BY INTRAMUSCULAR INJECTION
  - Child 1–15 years: Initially 0.5 mL for 1 dose, then 0.5 mL after 6–12 months, dose given as booster; booster dose may be delayed by up to 3 years if not given after recommended interval following primary dose, the deltoid region is the preferred site of injection. The subcutaneous route may be used for patients with bleeding disorders

- Child 16–17 years: Initially 1 mL for 1 dose, then 1 mL after 6–12 months, dose given as booster; booster dose may be delayed by up to 3 years if not given after recommended interval following primary dose, the deltoid region is the preferred site of injection. The subcutaneous route may be used for patients with bleeding disorders

VAQTA® PAEDIATRIC

Immunisation against hepatitis A infection

- BY INTRAMUSCULAR INJECTION
- Child 1–17 years: Initially 0.5 mL for 1 dose, then 0.5 mL after 6–18 months, dose given as booster, the deltoid region is the preferred site of injection. The subcutaneous route may be used for patients with bleeding disorders (but immune response may be reduced)

● **SIDE-EFFECTS**

- **Uncommon** Anxiety · asthenia · cough · crying · drowsiness · gastrointestinal discomfort · nasal complaints · pain · sleep disorders
- **Rare or very rare** Allergic rhinitis · asthma · ataxia · burping · chest pain · constipation · dehydration · ear pain · eyelid crusting · feeling hot · flushing · gait abnormal · gastrointestinal disorders · infantile spitting up · influenza like illness · musculoskeletal stiffness · oropharyngeal pain · paraesthesia · respiratory tract congestion · screaming · sensation of tightness · sweat changes · synovitis
- **Frequency not known** Guillain-Barre syndrome · thrombocytopenia

● **MEDICINAL FORMS** There can be variation in the licensing of different medicines containing the same drug.

Suspension for injection

EXCIPIENTS: May contain Neomycin

- **Avaxim** (Sanofi Pasteur)
  Avaxim vaccine suspension for injection 0.5ml pre-filled syringes | 1 pre-filled disposable injection [PoM] £21.72 | 10 pre-filled disposable injection [PoM] £217.20
- **Havrix** (GlaxoSmithKline UK Ltd)
  Havrix Monodose vaccine suspension for injection 1ml pre-filled syringes | 1 pre-filled disposable injection [PoM] £22.14 DT = £22.14 | 10 pre-filled disposable injection [PoM] £221.43
  Havrix Junior Monodose vaccine suspension for injection 0.5ml pre-filled syringes | 1 pre-filled disposable injection [PoM] £16.77 | 10 pre-filled disposable injection [PoM] £167.68
- **VAQTA** (Merck Sharp & Dohme Ltd)
  VAQTA Paediatric vaccine suspension for injection 0.5ml pre-filled syringes | 1 pre-filled disposable injection [PoM] £14.74

Hepatitis A with typhoid vaccine

The properties listed below are those particular to the combination only. For the properties of the components please consider, hepatitis A vaccine p. 852, typhoid vaccine p. 851.

● **INDICATIONS AND DOSE**

HEPATYRIX®

Immunisation against hepatitis A and typhoid infection (primary course)

- BY INTRAMUSCULAR INJECTION
- Child 15–17 years: 1 mL for 1 dose, the deltoid region is the preferred site of injection; not to be injected into the buttock (vaccine efficacy reduced). The subcutaneous route may be used for patients with bleeding disorders, booster dose given using single component vaccines

VIATIM®

Immunisation against hepatitis A and typhoid infection (primary course)

- BY INTRAMUSCULAR INJECTION
- Child 16–17 years: 1 mL for 1 dose, the deltoid region is the preferred site of injection; not to be injected into the buttock (vaccine efficacy reduced). The subcutaneous route may be used for patients with bleeding disorders, booster dose given using single component vaccines

● **MEDICINAL FORMS** There can be variation in the licensing of different medicines containing the same drug.

Suspension for injection

EXCIPIENTS: May contain Neomycin

- **ViATIM** (Sanofi Pasteur)
  ViATIM vaccine suspension for injection 1ml pre-filled syringes | 1 pre-filled disposable injection [PoM] £35.76 DT = £35.76

F 845

Hepatitis B vaccine

● **INDICATIONS AND DOSE**

ENGERIX B®

Immunisation against hepatitis B infection

- BY INTRAMUSCULAR INJECTION
- Neonate: 10 micrograms for 1 dose, then 10 micrograms after 1 month for 1 dose, followed by 10 micrograms after 5 months for 1 dose, anterolateral thigh is preferred site in neonates; not to be injected into the buttock (vaccine efficacy reduced), this dose should not be given to neonates born to hepatitis B surface antigen positive mother.
- Child 1 month–15 years: 10 micrograms for 1 dose, then 10 micrograms after 1 month for 1 dose, followed by 10 micrograms after 5 months for 1 dose, deltoid muscle is preferred site of injection in older children; anterolateral thigh is preferred site in infants and young children; not to be injected into the buttock (vaccine efficacy reduced)
- Child 16–17 years: 20 micrograms for 1 dose, then 20 micrograms after 1 month for 1 dose, followed by 20 micrograms after 5 months for 1 dose, deltoid muscle is preferred site of injection; not to be injected into the buttock (vaccine efficacy reduced)

Immunisation against hepatitis B infection (accelerated schedule)

- BY INTRAMUSCULAR INJECTION
- Neonate: 10 micrograms every month for 3 doses, followed by 10 micrograms after 10 months for 1 dose, anterolateral thigh is preferred site in neonates; not to be injected into the buttock (vaccine efficacy reduced), this dose should not be given to neonates born to hepatitis B surface antigen positive mother.
- Child 1 month–15 years: 10 micrograms every month for 3 doses, followed by 10 micrograms after 10 months for 1 dose, deltoid muscle is preferred site of injection in older children; anterolateral thigh is preferred site in infants and young children; not to be injected into the buttock (vaccine efficacy reduced)
- Child 16–17 years: 20 micrograms every month for 3 doses, followed by 20 micrograms after 10 months for 1 dose, deltoid muscle is preferred site of injection; not to be injected into the buttock (vaccine efficacy reduced)

continued →

Immunisation against hepatitis B infection, alternative accelerated schedule

▶ BY INTRAMUSCULAR INJECTION

- Child 11–15 years: 20 micrograms for 1 dose, followed by 20 micrograms after 6 months, this schedule is not suitable if high risk of infection between doses or if compliance with second dose uncertain, deltoid muscle is preferred site of injection; not to be injected into the buttock (vaccine efficacy reduced)

Immunisation against hepatitis B infection (for neonates born to hepatitis B surface antigen positive mother)

▶ BY INTRAMUSCULAR INJECTION

- Neonate: 10 micrograms once a month for 3 doses, first dose to be given at birth with hepatitis B immunoglobulin injection (separate site), followed by 10 micrograms after 10 months for 1 dose, anterolateral thigh is preferred site in neonates; not to be injected into the buttock (vaccine efficacy reduced).

Immunisation against hepatitis B infection (in renal insufficiency, including haemodialysis patients)

▶ BY INTRAMUSCULAR INJECTION

- Neonate: 10 micrograms every month for 2 doses, followed by 10 micrograms after 5 months for 1 dose, immunisation schedule and booster doses may need to be adjusted in those with low antibody concentration, anterolateral thigh is preferred site in neonates; not to be injected into the buttock (vaccine efficacy reduced), this dose should not be given to neonates born to hepatitis B surface antigen positive mother.
- Child 1 month–15 years: 10 micrograms every month for 2 doses, followed by 10 micrograms after 5 months for 1 dose, immunisation schedule and booster doses may need to be adjusted in those with low antibody concentration, deltoid muscle is preferred site of injection in older children; anterolateral thigh is preferred site in infants and young children; not to be injected into the buttock (vaccine efficacy reduced)
- Child 16–17 years: 40 micrograms every month for 3 doses, followed by 40 micrograms after 4 months for 1 dose, immunisation schedule and booster doses may need to be adjusted in those with low antibody concentration, deltoid muscle is preferred site of injection; not to be injected into the buttock (vaccine efficacy reduced)

Immunisation against hepatitis B infection (in renal insufficiency, including haemodialysis patients (accelerated schedule))

▶ BY INTRAMUSCULAR INJECTION

- Neonate: 10 micrograms every month for 3 doses, followed by 10 micrograms after 10 months for 1 dose, immunisation schedule and booster doses may need to be adjusted in those with low antibody concentration, anterolateral thigh is preferred site in neonates; not to be injected into the buttock (vaccine efficacy reduced), this dose should not be given to neonates born to hepatitis B surface antigen positive mother.
- Child 1 month–15 years: 10 micrograms every month for 3 doses, followed by 10 micrograms after 10 months for 1 dose, immunisation schedule and booster doses may need to be adjusted in those with low antibody concentration, deltoid muscle is preferred site of injection in older children; anterolateral thigh is preferred site in infants and young children; not to be injected into the buttock (vaccine efficacy reduced)

FENDRIX®

Immunisation against hepatitis B infection in renal insufficiency (including pre-haemodialysis and haemodialysis patients)

▶ BY INTRAMUSCULAR INJECTION

- Child 15–17 years: 20 micrograms every month for 3 doses, followed by 20 micrograms after 4 months for 1 dose, immunisation schedule and booster doses may need to be adjusted in those with low antibody concentration, deltoid muscle is preferred site of injection; not to be injected into the buttock (vaccine efficacy reduced)

HBVAXPRO®

Immunisation against hepatitis B infection

▶ BY INTRAMUSCULAR INJECTION

- Neonate: 5 micrograms for 1 dose, followed by 5 micrograms after 1 month for 1 dose, then 5 micrograms after 5 months for 1 dose, booster doses may be required in immunocompromised patients with low antibody concentration, anterolateral thigh is preferred site in neonates; not to be injected into the buttock (vaccine efficacy reduced), dose not to be used for neonate born to hepatitis B surface antigen positive mother.
- Child 1 month–15 years: 5 micrograms for 1 dose, followed by 5 micrograms after 1 month for 1 dose, then 5 micrograms after 5 months for 1 dose, booster doses may be required in immunocompromised patients with low antibody concentration, deltoid muscle is preferred site of injection in adults and older children; anterolateral thigh is preferred site in infants; not to be injected into the buttock (vaccine efficacy reduced)
- Child 16–17 years: 10 micrograms for 1 dose, followed by 10 micrograms after 1 month for 1 dose, followed by 10 micrograms after 5 months for 1 dose, booster doses may be required in immunocompromised patients with low antibody concentration, deltoid muscle is preferred site of injection in adults and older children; not to be injected into the buttock (vaccine efficacy reduced)

Immunisation against hepatitis B infection (accelerated schedule)

▶ BY INTRAMUSCULAR INJECTION

- Neonate: 5 micrograms every month for 3 doses, followed by 5 micrograms after 10 months for 1 dose, booster doses may be required in immunocompromised patients with low antibody concentration, anterolateral thigh is preferred site in neonates; not to be injected into the buttock (vaccine efficacy reduced), dose not to be used for neonate born to hepatitis B surface antigen positive mother.
- Child 1 month–15 years: 5 micrograms every month for 3 doses, followed by 5 micrograms after 10 months for 1 dose, booster doses may be required in immunocompromised patients with low antibody concentration, deltoid muscle is preferred site of injection in older children; anterolateral thigh is preferred site in infants; not to be injected into the buttock (vaccine efficacy reduced)
- Child 16–17 years: 10 micrograms every month for 3 doses, followed by 10 micrograms after 10 months for 1 dose, booster doses may be required in immunocompromised patients with low antibody concentration, deltoid muscle is preferred site of injection in older children; not to be injected into the buttock (vaccine efficacy reduced)

Neonate born to hepatitis B surface antigen-positive mother

▶ BY INTRAMUSCULAR INJECTION

▸ Neonate: 5 micrograms every month for 3 doses, first dose given at birth with hepatitis B immunoglobulin injection (separate site), followed by 5 micrograms after 10 months for 1 dose, anterolateral thigh is preferred site in neonates; not to be injected into the buttock (vaccine efficacy reduced).

Chronic haemodialysis patients

▶ BY INTRAMUSCULAR INJECTION

▸ Child 16–17 years: 40 micrograms every month for 2 doses, followed by 40 micrograms after 5 months for 1 dose, booster doses may be required in those with low antibody concentration, deltoid muscle is preferred site of injection in older children; not to be injected into the buttock (vaccine efficacy reduced)

● **SIDE-EFFECTS**

▶ **Common or very common** Drowsiness · gastrointestinal disorder

▶ **Uncommon** Influenza like illness

▶ **Rare or very rare** Sensation abnormal

▶ **Frequency not known** Angioedema · apnoea · arthritis · encephalitis · encephalopathy · hypotension · meningitis · multiple sclerosis · muscle weakness · nerve disorders · paralysis · seizure · thrombocytopenia · vasculitis

● **MEDICINAL FORMS** There can be variation in the licensing of different medicines containing the same drug.

Suspension for injection

EXCIPIENTS: May contain Thiomersal

▸ **Engerix B** (GlaxoSmithKline UK Ltd)

Hepatitis B virus surface antigen 20 microgram per 1 ml Engerix B 10micrograms/0.5ml vaccine suspension for injection pre-filled syringes | 1 pre-filled disposable injection PoM £9.67 DT = £9.67
Engerix B 20micrograms/1ml vaccine suspension for injection pre-filled syringes | 1 pre-filled disposable injection PoM £12.99 DT = £12.99 | 10 pre-filled disposable injection PoM £129.92

▸ **Fendrix** (GlaxoSmithKline UK Ltd)

Hepatitis B virus surface antigen 40 microgram per 1 ml Fendrix 20micrograms/0.5ml vaccine suspension for injection pre-filled syringes | 1 pre-filled disposable injection PoM £38.10 DT = £38.10

▸ **HBVAXPRO** (Merck Sharp & Dohme Ltd)

Hepatitis B virus surface antigen 10 microgram per 1 ml HBVAXPRO 10micrograms/1ml vaccine suspension for injection pre-filled syringes | 1 pre-filled disposable injection PoM £12.20
HBVAXPRO 5micrograms/0.5ml vaccine suspension for injection pre-filled syringes | 1 pre-filled disposable injection PoM £8.95 DT = £8.95

Hepatitis B virus surface antigen 40 microgram per 1 ml HBvaxPRO 40micrograms/1ml vaccine suspension for injection vials | 1 vial PoM £27.60 DT = £27.60

F 845

Human papillomavirus vaccines

29-Oct-2019

● **INDICATIONS AND DOSE**

CERVARIX®

Immunisation against HPV-related premalignant lesions and cancer (cervical, vulvar, vaginal, and anal) [2 dose schedule]

▶ BY INTRAMUSCULAR INJECTION

▸ Child 9–14 years: 0.5 mL for 1 dose, followed by 0.5 mL after 5–24 months for 1 dose, if second dose administered earlier than 5 months after the first, a third dose should be administered, to be administered into deltoid region, if the 2 dose schedule is interrupted, it should be resumed (using the same vaccine) but not repeated, even if more than 24 months have elapsed since the first dose or if the patient is now older than 14 years

Immunisation against HPV-related premalignant lesions and cancer (cervical, vulvar, vaginal, and anal) [3 dose schedule]

▶ BY INTRAMUSCULAR INJECTION

▸ Child 15–17 years: 0.5 mL for 1 dose, followed by 0.5 mL after 1–2.5 months for 1 dose, then 0.5 mL after 5–12 months from the first dose for 1 dose, to be administered into deltoid region, if the 3 dose schedule is interrupted, it should be resumed (using the same vaccine) but not repeated, allowing the appropriate interval between the remaining doses

GARDASIL 9®

Immunisation against HPV-related premalignant lesions and cancer (cervical, vulvar, vaginal, and anal) and genital warts [2 dose schedule]

▶ BY INTRAMUSCULAR INJECTION

▸ Child 9–14 years: 0.5 mL for 1 dose, followed by 0.5 mL after 5–24 months for 1 dose, to be administered preferably into deltoid region or higher anterolateral thigh, if the 2 dose schedule is interrupted, it should be resumed (using the same vaccine) but not repeated, even if more than 24 months have elapsed since the first dose or if the patient is now older than 14 years

Immunisation against HPV-related premalignant lesions and cancer (cervical, vulvar, vaginal, and anal) and genital warts [3 dose schedule]

▶ BY INTRAMUSCULAR INJECTION

▸ Child 9–17 years: 0.5 mL for 1 dose, followed by 0.5 mL for 1 dose, second dose to be given at least 1 month after the first dose, then 0.5 mL for 1 dose, third dose to be given at least 3 months after the second dose, to be administered preferably into deltoid region or higher anterolateral thigh, the 3 dose schedule should be completed within 12 months of the first dose. If the schedule is interrupted, it should be resumed (using the same vaccine) but not repeated, allowing the appropriate interval between the remaining doses

GARDASIL®

Immunisation against HPV-related premalignant lesions and cancer (cervical, vulvar, vaginal, and anal) and genital warts [2 dose schedule]

▶ BY INTRAMUSCULAR INJECTION

▸ Child 9–14 years: 0.5 mL for 1 dose, followed by 0.5 mL after 6–24 months for 1 dose, to be administered preferably into deltoid region or higher anterolateral thigh, if the 2 dose schedule is interrupted, it should be resumed (using the same vaccine) but not repeated, even if more than 24 months have elapsed since the first dose or if the patient is now older than 14 years

Immunisation against HPV-related premalignant lesions and cancer (cervical, vulvar, vaginal, and anal) and genital warts [3 dose schedule]

▶ BY INTRAMUSCULAR INJECTION

▸ Child 9–17 years: 0.5 mL for 1 dose, followed by 0.5 mL for 1 dose, second dose to be given at least 1 month after the first dose, then 0.5 mL for 1 dose, third dose to be given at least 3 months after the second dose, to be administered preferably into deltoid region or higher anterolateral thigh, the 3 dose schedule should be completed within 12 months of the first dose, if the schedule is interrupted, it should be resumed (using the same vaccine) but not repeated, allowing the appropriate interval between the remaining doses

● **UNLICENSED USE** EvGr Human papillomavirus vaccines are used in a 2 dose immunisation schedule, (A) but the interval between doses may differ from licensing.

GARDASIL® EvGr The 2 dose schedule is not licensed for use in children aged 14 years. (A)

● SIDE-EFFECTS
▸ **Common or very common** Abdominal pain · gastrointestinal disorder · pain in extremity
▸ **Uncommon** Upper respiratory tract infection
▸ **Frequency not known** Acute disseminated encephalomyelitis · angioedema · asthenia · bronchospasm · chills · Guillain-Barre syndrome · immune thrombocytopenic purpura · syncope
● PREGNANCY Not known to be harmful, but vaccination should be postponed until completion of pregnancy.
● PRESCRIBING AND DISPENSING INFORMATION To avoid confusion, prescribers should specify the brand to be dispensed.

● MEDICINAL FORMS There can be variation in the licensing of different medicines containing the same drug.
Suspension for injection
▸ Cervarix (GlaxoSmithKline UK Ltd)
Cervarix vaccine suspension for injection 0.5ml pre-filled syringes | 1 pre-filled disposable injection PoM £80.50
▸ Gardasil (Merck Sharp & Dohme Ltd)
Gardasil vaccine suspension for injection 0.5ml pre-filled syringes | 1 pre-filled disposable injection PoM £86.50 DT = £86.50
▸ Gardasil 9 (Merck Sharp & Dohme Ltd)
Gardasil 9 vaccine suspension for injection 0.5ml pre-filled syringes | 1 pre-filled disposable injection PoM £105.00 DT = £105.00

845

Influenza vaccine

12-Nov-2019

● DRUG ACTION Influenza vaccines protect people at high risk from influenza and reduce transmission of infection; the nasal spray contains live attenuated strains, all other vaccines are inactivated.

● INDICATIONS AND DOSE
Annual immunisation against seasonal influenza
▸ BY INTRAMUSCULAR INJECTION
▸ Child 6 months–17 years: 0.5 mL for 1 dose
▸ BY INTRANASAL ADMINISTRATION
▸ Child 2–17 years: 0.1 mL for 1 dose, dose to be administered into each nostril

Annual immunisation against seasonal influenza (for children in clinical risk groups who have not received seasonal influenza vaccine previously)
▸ BY INTRAMUSCULAR INJECTION
▸ Child 6 months–8 years: 0.5 mL for 1 dose, followed by 0.5 mL for 1 dose, after at least 4 weeks
▸ BY INTRANASAL ADMINISTRATION
▸ Child 2–8 years: 0.1 mL for 1 dose, followed by 0.1 mL for 1 dose, after at least 4 weeks. 0.1 mL dose to be administered to each nostril

● UNLICENSED USE The Joint Committee on Vaccination and Immunisation advises offering a second dose of vaccine for annual immunisation against seasonal influenza to children in clinical risk groups only.
● CONTRA-INDICATIONS Preparations marketed by Pfizer, or CSL Biotherapies in child under 5 years—increased risk of febrile convulsions
FLUENZ TETRA ® Active wheezing · concomitant use with antiviral therapy for influenza · concomitant use with salicylates · severe asthma
CONTRA-INDICATIONS, FURTHER INFORMATION
▸ Concomitant use with antiviral therapy for influenza Public Health England advises avoid immunisation for at least 48 hours after stopping the influenza antiviral agent. Administration of influenza antiviral agents within two weeks of Fluenz Tetra® administration may reduce the effectiveness of the vaccine.
● CAUTIONS Increased risk of fever in child 5–9 years with preparations marketed by Pfizer or CSL Biotherapies—use alternative influenza vaccine if available
● INTERACTIONS → Appendix 1: live vaccines
● SIDE-EFFECTS
▸ **Common or very common**
▸ With intramuscular use Chills · hyperhidrosis · induration · local reactions · pain
▸ With intranasal use Nasal complaints
▸ **Uncommon**
▸ With intranasal use Epistaxis · face oedema
▸ **Frequency not known**
▸ With intramuscular use Angioedema · encephalomyelitis · extensive swelling of vaccinated limb · febrile seizure · nerve disorders · nervous system disorder · paraesthesia · shock · syncope · thrombocytopenia · vasculitis
▸ With intranasal use Guillain-Barre syndrome
● ALLERGY AND CROSS-SENSITIVITY Individuals with a history of egg allergy can be immunised with either an egg free influenza vaccine, if available, or an influenza vaccine with an ovalbumin content less than 120 nanograms/mL (facilities should be available to treat anaphylaxis). Vaccines with an ovalbumin content more than 120 nanograms/mL or where content is not stated should not be used in individuals with egg allergy. If an influenza vaccine containing ovalbumin is being considered in those with a history of anaphylaxis to egg or egg allergy with uncontrolled asthma, these individuals should be referred to a specialist in hospital.
● PREGNANCY Inactivated vaccines not known to be harmful.
FLUENZ TETRA ® Avoid in pregnancy.
● BREAST FEEDING Inactivated vaccines not known to be harmful.
FLUENZ TETRA ® Avoid in breast-feeding.
● PRESCRIBING AND DISPENSING INFORMATION The available preparations are not licensed for use in all age-groups—further information can be found in the product literature for the individual vaccines.
FLUARIX TETRA ® Ovalbumin content less than 100 nanograms/mL.
● PATIENT AND CARER ADVICE
FLUENZ TETRA ® Avoid close contact with severely immunocompromised patients for 1–2 weeks after vaccination.

● MEDICINAL FORMS There can be variation in the licensing of different medicines containing the same drug.
Spray
EXCIPIENTS: May contain Gelatin, gentamicin
▸ Fluenz Tetra (AstraZeneca UK Ltd)
Fluenz Tetra vaccine nasal suspension 0.2ml unit dose | 10 unit dose PoM £180.00

Suspension for injection
EXCIPIENTS: May contain Gentamicin, kanamycin, neomycin, polymyxin b
▸ Influenza vaccine (non-proprietary) ▼
Influenza vaccine (split virion, inactivated) suspension for injection 0.5ml pre-filled syringes | 10 pre-filled disposable injection PoM £65.90
Quadrivalent influenza vaccine (split virion, inactivated) suspension for injection 0.5ml pre-filled syringes | 1 pre-filled disposable injection PoM £8.00 | 10 pre-filled disposable injection PoM £80.00
Influenza Tetra MYL vaccine suspension for injection 0.5ml pre-filled syringes | 1 pre-filled disposable injection PoM £8.00 | 10 pre-filled disposable injection PoM £80.00
Fluad vaccine suspension for injection 0.5ml pre-filled syringes | 1 pre-filled disposable injection PoM £9.79 | 10 pre-filled disposable injection PoM £97.90
Adjuvanted trivalent influenza vaccine (surface antigen, inactivated) suspension for injection 0.5ml pre-filled syringes | 1 pre-filled disposable injection PoM £9.79 | 10 pre-filled disposable injection PoM £97.90
▸ Fluarix Tetra (GlaxoSmithKline UK Ltd)
Fluarix Tetra vaccine suspension for injection 0.5ml pre-filled syringes | 1 pre-filled disposable injection PoM £9.94 | 10 pre-filled disposable injection PoM £99.40

- ▸ **Flucelvax Tetra** (Seqirus Vaccines Ltd) ▼
  Flucelvax Tetra vaccine suspension for injection 0.5ml pre-filled syringes | 1 pre-filled disposable injection PoM £9.94 | 10 pre-filled disposable injection PoM £99.40
- ▸ **Imuvac** (Mylan)
  Imuvac vaccine suspension for injection 0.5ml pre-filled syringes | 1 pre-filled disposable injection PoM £6.59 | 10 pre-filled disposable injection PoM £65.90
- ▸ **Influvac Sub-unit** (Mylan) ▼
  Influvac sub-unit Tetra vaccine suspension for injection 0.5ml pre-filled syringes | 1 pre-filled disposable injection PoM £9.94 | 10 pre-filled disposable injection PoM £99.40

F 845

Japanese encephalitis vaccine

22-Feb-2019

● **INDICATIONS AND DOSE**

Immunisation against Japanese encephalitis

▸ BY INTRAMUSCULAR INJECTION

- ▸ Child 2–35 months: 0.25 mL every 28 days for 2 doses, alternatively 0.25 mL every 7 days for 2 doses, anterolateral thigh may be used as the injection site in infants; deltoid muscle is preferred site in older children, immunisation should be completed at least 1 week before potential exposure
- ▸ Child 3–17 years: 0.5 mL every 28 days for 2 doses, alternatively 0.5 mL every 7 days for 2 doses, deltoid muscle is preferred site in older children, immunisation should be completed at least 1 week before potential exposure

First booster

▸ BY INTRAMUSCULAR INJECTION

- ▸ Child 14–35 months: 0.25 mL after 1–2 years, anterolateral thigh may be used as the injection site in infants; deltoid muscle is preferred site in older children, for those at continued risk, the booster dose should be given 1 year after completing the primary course
- ▸ Child 3–17 years: 0.5 mL after 1–2 years, deltoid muscle is preferred site in older children, for those at continued risk, the booster dose should be given 1 year after completing the primary course

● **UNLICENSED USE**

▸ When used for Immunisation against Japanese encephalitis The rapid schedule administered at days 0 and 7 is not licensed in children or the elderly.

● **SIDE-EFFECTS** Abdominal pain · cough · influenza like illness

● **PREGNANCY** Although manufacturer advises avoid because of limited information, miscarriage has been associated with Japanese encephalitis virus infection acquired during the first 2 trimesters of pregnancy.

● **MEDICINAL FORMS** There can be variation in the licensing of different medicines containing the same drug.

Solution for injection

- ▸ **Japanese encephalitis vaccine (Non-proprietary)**
  Japanese encephalitis GCVC vaccine solution for injection 1ml vials | 1 vial ℞
  Japanese encephalitis GCVC vaccine solution for injection 20ml vials | 1 vial ℞
  Japanese encephalitis GCVC vaccine solution for injection 10ml vials | 1 vial ℞

Suspension for injection

- ▸ **Ixiaro** (Valneva UK Ltd)
  Ixiaro vaccine suspension for injection 0.5ml pre-filled syringes | 1 pre-filled disposable injection PoM £59.50 DT = £59.50

F 845

Measles, mumps and rubella vaccine, live

● **INDICATIONS AND DOSE**

Primary immunisation against measles, mumps, and rubella (first dose)

▸ BY INTRAMUSCULAR INJECTION, OR BY DEEP SUBCUTANEOUS INJECTION

- ▸ Child 12–13 months: 0.5 mL for 1 dose

Primary immunisation against measles, mumps, and rubella (second dose)

▸ BY INTRAMUSCULAR INJECTION, OR BY DEEP SUBCUTANEOUS INJECTION

- ▸ Child 40 months–5 years: 0.5 mL for 1 dose

Rubella immunisation (in seronegative women, susceptible to rubella and in unimmunised, seronegative women, post-partum)

▸ BY INTRAMUSCULAR INJECTION, OR BY DEEP SUBCUTANEOUS INJECTION

- ▸ Females of childbearing potential: (consult product literature or local protocols)

Children presenting for pre-school booster, who have not received the primary immunisation (first dose) | Immunisation for patients at school-leaving age or at entry into further education, who have not completed the primary immunisation course | Control of measles outbreak | Immunisation for patients travelling to areas where measles is endemic or epidemic, who have not completed the primary immunisation

▸ BY INTRAMUSCULAR INJECTION, OR BY DEEP SUBCUTANEOUS INJECTION

- ▸ Child 6 months–17 years: (consult product literature or local protocols)

● **UNLICENSED USE** Not licensed for use in children under 9 months.

> **IMPORTANT SAFETY INFORMATION**
>
> MMR VACCINATION AND BOWEL DISEASE OR AUTISM
>
> Reviews undertaken on behalf of the CSM, the Medical Research Council, and the Cochrane Collaboration, have not found any evidence of a link between MMR vaccination and bowel disease or autism. The Chief Medical Officers have advised that the MMR vaccine is the safest and best way to protect children against measles, mumps, and rubella. Information (including fact sheets and a list of references) may be obtained from www.dh.gov.uk/immunisation.

● **CAUTIONS** Antibody response to measles component may be reduced after immunoglobulin administration or blood transfusion—leave an interval of at least 3 months before MMR immunisation

CAUTIONS, FURTHER INFORMATION

▸ Administration with other vaccines MMR vaccine should not be administered on the same day as yellow fever vaccine; there should be a 4-week minimum interval between the vaccines. When protection is rapidly required, the vaccines can be given at any interval and an additional dose of MMR may be considered.

MMR and varicella-zoster vaccine can be given on the same day or separated by a 4-week minimum interval. When protection is rapidly required, the vaccines can be given at any interval and an additional dose of the vaccine given second may be considered.

● **INTERACTIONS** → Appendix 1: live vaccines

● **SIDE-EFFECTS**

▸ **Uncommon** Increased risk of infection · rhinorrhoea

▸ **Frequency not known** Angioedema · arthritis · ataxia · cough · encephalopathy · eye inflammation · meningitis aseptic · nerve deafness · nerve disorders · oculomotor nerve paralysis · oedema · panniculitis · papillitis · paraesthesia · regional lymphadenopathy · respiratory disorders · seizures · Stevens-Johnson syndrome · subacute sclerosing panencephalitis · syncope · throat pain · thrombocytopenia · vasculitis

SIDE-EFFECTS, FURTHER INFORMATION Malaise, fever, or a rash can occur after the first dose of MMR vaccine–most commonly about a week after vaccination and lasting about 2 to 3 days.

Febrile seizures occur rarely 6 to 11 days after MMR vaccination (the incidence is lower than that following measles infection).

Idiopathic thrombocytopenic purpura Idiopathic thrombocytopenic purpura has occurred rarely following MMR vaccination, usually within 6 weeks of the first dose. The risk of idiopathic thrombocytopenic purpura after MMR vaccine is much less than the risk after infection with wild measles or rubella virus. Children who develop idiopathic thrombocytopenic purpura within 6 weeks of the first dose of MMR should undergo serological testing before the second dose is due; if the results suggest incomplete immunity against measles, mumps or rubella then a second dose of MMR is recommended. Samples should be sent to the Virus Reference Laboratory of the Health Protection Agency.

Frequency of side effects Adverse reactions are considerably less frequent after the second dose of MMR vaccine than after the first.

- **ALLERGY AND CROSS-SENSITIVITY** MMR vaccine can be given safely even when the child has had an anaphylactic reaction to food containing egg. Dislike of eggs, refusal to eat egg, or confirmed anaphylactic reactions to egg-containing food is not a contra-indication to MMR vaccination. Children with a confirmed anaphylactic reaction to the MMR vaccine should be assessed by a specialist.
- **CONCEPTION AND CONTRACEPTION** Exclude pregnancy before immunisation. Avoid pregnancy for at least 1 month after vaccination.
- **PRESCRIBING AND DISPENSING INFORMATION** Available as part of childhood immunisation schedule from health organisations or ImmForm www.immform.dh.gov.uk.

- **MEDICINAL FORMS** There can be variation in the licensing of different medicines containing the same drug.

Powder and solvent for suspension for injection

EXCIPIENTS: May contain Gelatin, neomycin

▸ **M-M-RVAXPRO** (Merck Sharp & Dohme Ltd)
M-M-RVAXPRO vaccine powder and solvent for suspension for injection 0.5ml pre-filled syringes | 1 pre-filled disposable injection PoM £11.00 DT = £11.00

Powder and solvent for solution for injection

EXCIPIENTS: May contain Neomycin

▸ **Priorix** (GlaxoSmithKline UK Ltd)
Priorix vaccine powder and solvent for solution for injection 0.5ml pre-filled syringes | 1 pre-filled disposable injection PoM £7.64 DT = £7.64

F 845

Rabies vaccine

- **INDICATIONS AND DOSE**

Pre-exposure prophylaxis

▸ BY INTRAMUSCULAR INJECTION

▸ Child: 1 mL for 2 doses (on days 0 and 7), followed by 1 mL for 1 dose (on day 28), to be administered in deltoid region or anterolateral thigh in infants, for those at continuous risk, measure plasma-concentration of antirabies antibodies every 6 months and give a booster dose if the titre is less than 0.5 units/mL, final dose may be given from day 21, if insufficient time before travel

Pre-exposure prophylaxis booster dose (for patients at frequent risk of exposure)

▸ BY INTRAMUSCULAR INJECTION

▸ Child: 1 mL after 1 year for 1 dose, to be given 1 year after primary course is completed, then 1 mL every 3–5 years, to be administered in deltoid region or anterolateral thigh in infants, the frequency of booster doses may alternatively be determined according to plasma-concentration of antirabies antibodies

Pre-exposure prophylaxis booster dose (for patients at infrequent risk of exposure)

▸ BY INTRAMUSCULAR INJECTION

▸ Child: 1 mL for 1 dose, to be given 10 years after primary course is completed, administered in deltoid region or anterolateral thigh in infants

Post-exposure prophylaxis of fully immunised individuals (who have previously received pre-exposure or post-exposure prophylaxis with cell-derived rabies vaccine)

▸ BY INTRAMUSCULAR INJECTION

▸ Child (administered on expert advice): 1 mL for 1 dose, followed by 1 mL after 3–7 days for 1 dose, to be administered in deltoid region or anterolateral thigh in infants, rabies immunoglobulin is not necessary

Post-exposure treatment for unimmunised individuals (or those whose prophylaxis is possibly incomplete)

▸ BY INTRAMUSCULAR INJECTION

▸ Child (administered on expert advice): 1 mL 5 times a month for 1 month, doses should be given on days 0, 3, 7, 14, and the fifth dose is given between day 28–30, to be administered in deltoid region or anterolateral thigh in infants, depending on the level of risk (determined by factors such as the nature of the bite and the country where it was sustained), rabies immunoglobulin is given to unimmunised individuals on day 0 or within 7 days of starting the course of rabies vaccine, the immunisation course can be discontinued if it is proved that the individual was not at risk

- **INTERACTIONS** → Appendix 1: rabies vaccine
- **SIDE-EFFECTS**

▸ **Common or very common** Asthenia · gastrointestinal discomfort

▸ **Rare or very rare** Angioedema · chills · encephalitis · Guillain-Barre syndrome · hyperhidrosis · paraesthesia · syncope · vertigo

- **PREGNANCY** Because of the potential consequences of untreated rabies exposure and because rabies vaccination has not been associated with fetal abnormalities, pregnancy is not considered a contra-indication to post-exposure prophylaxis. Immunisation against rabies is indicated during pregnancy if there is substantial risk of exposure to rabies and rapid access to post-exposure prophylaxis is likely to be limited.

- **MEDICINAL FORMS** There can be variation in the licensing of different medicines containing the same drug.

Powder and solvent for suspension for injection

EXCIPIENTS: May contain Neomycin

▸ **Rabies vaccine (Non-proprietary)**
Rabies vaccine powder and solvent for suspension for injection 1ml vials | 1 vial PoM £40.84

▸ **Verorab** (Imported (France))
Verorab powder and solvent for suspension for injection 0.5ml vials | 1 vial PoM

Powder and solvent for solution for injection

EXCIPIENTS: May contain Neomycin

▸ **Rabipur** (GlaxoSmithKline UK Ltd)
Rabipur vaccine powder and solvent for solution for injection 1ml pre-filled syringes | 1 pre-filled disposable injection PoM £34.56

845

Rotavirus vaccine

12-Nov-2019

- **DRUG ACTION** Rotavirus vaccine is a live, oral vaccine that protects young children against gastro-enteritis caused by rotavirus infection.

- **INDICATIONS AND DOSE**

Immunisation against gastro-enteritis caused by rotavirus

▶ BY MOUTH

- Child 6–23 weeks: 1.5 mL for 2 doses separated by an interval of at least 4 weeks, first dose must be given between 6–14 weeks of age; course should be completed before 24 weeks of age (preferably before 16 weeks)

IMPORTANT SAFETY INFORMATION

PUBLIC HEALTH ENGLAND: UPDATE TO GREEN BOOK (OCTOBER 2017)

Public Health England advises that immunisation with live vaccines should be delayed until 6 months of age in children born to mothers who received immunosuppressive biological therapy during pregnancy. In practice, this means that children born to mothers who were on immunosuppressive biological therapy during pregnancy will not be eligible to receive rotavirus vaccine.

- **CONTRA-INDICATIONS** History of intussusception · predisposition to intussusception · severe combined immunodeficiency disorder

CONTRA-INDICATIONS, FURTHER INFORMATION

- Immunosuppression With the exception of severe combined immunodeficiency disorder (and children born to mothers who received immunosuppressive biological therapy during pregnancy, see *Important safety information*), rotavirus vaccine is not contra-indicated in immunosuppressed patients—benefit from vaccination is likely to outweigh the risk, if there is any doubt, Public Health England recommends seek specialist advice.

- **CAUTIONS** Diarrhoea (postpone vaccination) · immunosuppressed close contacts · vomiting (postpone vaccination)

CAUTIONS, FURTHER INFORMATION The rotavirus vaccine virus is excreted in the stool and may be transmitted to close contacts; however, vaccination of those with immunosuppressed close contacts may protect the contacts from wild-type rotavirus disease and outweigh any risk from transmission of vaccine virus.

- **INTERACTIONS** → Appendix 1: live vaccines
- **SIDE-EFFECTS**
  - **Uncommon** Abdominal pain · gastrointestinal disorders
  - **Frequency not known** Apnoea · haematochezia
- **PATIENT AND CARER ADVICE** The rotavirus vaccine virus is excreted in the stool and may be transmitted to close contacts; carers of a recently vaccinated baby should be advised of the need to wash their hands after changing the baby's nappies.

- **MEDICINAL FORMS** There can be variation in the licensing of different medicines containing the same drug.

Oral suspension

- Rotarix (GlaxoSmithKline UK Ltd)
  Rotarix vaccine live oral suspension 1.5ml tube | 1 tube PoM £34.76 DT = £34.76

845

Tick-borne encephalitis vaccine, inactivated

- **INDICATIONS AND DOSE**

Initial immunisation against tick-borne encephalitis

▶ BY INTRAMUSCULAR INJECTION

- Child 1–15 years: 0.25 mL for 1 dose, followed by 0.25 mL after 1–3 months for 1 dose, then 0.25 mL after further 5–12 months for 1 dose, to achieve more rapid protection, second dose may be given 14 days after first dose, dose to be administered in deltoid region or anterolateral thigh in infants, in immunocompromised patients (including those receiving immunosuppressants), antibody concentration may be measured 4 weeks after second dose and dose repeated if protective levels not achieved
- Child 16–17 years: 0.5 mL for 1 dose, followed by 0.5 mL after 1–3 months for 1 dose, then 0.5 mL after further 5–12 months for 1 dose, to achieve more rapid protection, second dose may be given 14 days after first dose, dose to be administered in deltoid region, in immunocompromised patients (including those receiving immunosuppressants), antibody concentration may be measured 4 weeks after second dose and dose repeated if protective levels not achieved

Immunisation against tick-borne encephalitis, booster doses

▶ BY INTRAMUSCULAR INJECTION

- Child 1–17 years: First dose to be given within 3 years after initial course completed and then every 3–5 years, dose to be administered in deltoid region or anterolateral thigh in infants (consult product literature)

- **SIDE-EFFECTS**
  - **Common or very common** Restlessness · sleep disorder
  - **Uncommon** Chills · gastrointestinal discomfort
  - **Rare or very rare** Asthenia · dyspnoea · encephalitis · eye pain · gait abnormal · hyperhidrosis · influenza like illness · meningism · motor dysfunction · musculoskeletal stiffness · nerve disorders · oedema · pain · seizures · sensory disorder · tinnitus · vertigo · vision disorders
- **ALLERGY AND CROSS-SENSITIVITY** Individuals with evidence of previous anaphylactic reaction to egg should not be given tick-borne encephalitis vaccine.

- **MEDICINAL FORMS** There can be variation in the licensing of different medicines containing the same drug.

Suspension for injection

EXCIPIENTS: May contain Gentamicin, neomycin

- TicoVac (Pfizer Ltd)
  TicoVac Junior vaccine suspension for injection 0.25ml pre-filled syringes | 1 pre-filled disposable injection PoM £28.00
  TicoVac vaccine suspension for injection 0.5ml pre-filled syringes | 1 pre-filled disposable injection PoM £32.00

845

Varicella-zoster vaccine

21-Oct-2019

● **DRUG ACTION** *Varilrix*® and *Varivax*® are live attenuated vaccines that protect against varicella (chickenpox) caused by varicella-zoster virus infection. *Zostavax*® is a live attenuated vaccine that protects against herpes zoster (shingles) caused by varicella-zoster virus infection.

● **INDICATIONS AND DOSE**

VARILRIX®

Prevention of varicella infection (chickenpox)

▶ BY SUBCUTANEOUS INJECTION

▸ Child 1–17 years: 0.5 mL every 4–6 weeks for 2 doses, to be administered into the deltoid region or anterolateral thigh

VARIVAX®

Prevention of varicella infection (chickenpox)

▶ BY SUBCUTANEOUS INJECTION, OR BY INTRAMUSCULAR INJECTION

▸ Child 1–12 years: 0.5 mL for 2 doses, interval of at least 4 weeks between each dose, to be administered into the deltoid region (or higher anterolateral thigh in young children)

▸ Child 13–17 years: 0.5 mL for 2 doses, interval of 4–8 weeks between each dose, to be administered preferably into the deltoid region

Prevention of varicella infection (chickenpox) in children with asymptomatic HIV infection

▶ BY SUBCUTANEOUS INJECTION, OR BY INTRAMUSCULAR INJECTION

▸ Child 1–12 years: 0.5 mL for 2 doses, interval of 12 weeks between each dose, to be administered into the deltoid region (or higher anterolateral thigh in young children)

● **CAUTIONS** Post-vaccination close contact with susceptible individuals

CAUTIONS, FURTHER INFORMATION Rarely, the varicella–zoster vaccine virus has been transmitted from the vaccinated individual to close contacts. Therefore, contact with the following should be avoided if a vaccine-related cutaneous rash develops within 4–6 weeks of the first or second dose:

- varicella-susceptible pregnant women;
- individuals at high risk of severe varicella, including those with immunodeficiency or those receiving immunosuppressive therapy.

Healthcare workers who develop a generalised papular or vesicular rash on vaccination should avoid contact with patients until the lesions have crusted. Those who develop a localised rash after vaccination should cover the lesions and be allowed to continue working unless in contact with patients at high risk of severe varicella.

▸ Administration with MMR vaccine Varicella–zoster and MMR vaccines can be given on the same day or separated by a 4-week minimum interval. When protection is rapidly required, the vaccines can be given at any interval and an additional dose of the vaccine given second may be considered.

● **INTERACTIONS** → Appendix 1: live vaccines

● **SIDE-EFFECTS**

▶ **Uncommon** Cough · drowsiness · increased risk of infection

▶ **Rare or very rare** Abdominal pain · conjunctivitis · Kawasaki disease · seizure · stroke · thrombocytopenia · vasculitis

● **CONCEPTION AND CONTRACEPTION** Avoid pregnancy for 3 months after vaccination.

● **MEDICINAL FORMS** There can be variation in the licensing of different medicines containing the same drug.

Powder and solvent for suspension for injection

EXCIPIENTS: May contain Gelatin, neomycin

▸ **Varivax** (Merck Sharp & Dohme Ltd)
Varivax vaccine powder and solvent for suspension for injection 0.5ml vials | 1 vial PoM £30.28 DT = £30.28

Powder and solvent for solution for injection

EXCIPIENTS: May contain Neomycin

▸ **Varilrix** (GlaxoSmithKline UK Ltd)
Varilrix vaccine powder and solvent for solution for injection 0.5ml vials | 1 vial PoM £27.31 DT = £27.31

845

Yellow fever vaccine, live

22-May-2019

● **INDICATIONS AND DOSE**

Immunisation against yellow fever

▶ BY DEEP SUBCUTANEOUS INJECTION

▸ Child 6–8 months (administered on expert advice): Infants under 9 months should be vaccinated only if the risk of yellow fever is high and unavoidable (consult product literature or local protocols)

▸ Child 9 months–17 years: 0.5 mL for 1 dose

IMPORTANT SAFETY INFORMATION

MHRA/CHM ADVICE (UPDATED NOVEMBER 2019): YELLOW FEVER VACCINE: STRONGER PRECAUTIONS IN PEOPLE WITH WEAKENED IMMUNITY

The yellow fever vaccine (*Stamaril*®) has been associated with the very rare, life-threatening reactions viscerotropic disease (YEL-AVD) and neurotropic disease (YEL-AND), which both resemble yellow fever infection. It must not be given to patients who have had a thymectomy, who are taking immunosuppressive or immunomodulating biological drugs, or who have a first-degree family history of YEL-AVD or YEL-AND following vaccination that was unrelated to a known medical risk factor. It must only be administered by healthcare professionals specifically trained in the benefit-risk evaluation of yellow fever vaccine. Healthcare professionals must inform patients and carers about the early signs and symptoms of YEL-AVD and YEL-AND, and advise them to seek urgent medical attention if they occur; the manufacturer's patient information leaflet should also be provided.

Healthcare professionals administering vaccines should consult information in the YF Vaccine Centre code of practice and strengthen protocols and checklists to avoid inappropriate administration.

● **CONTRA-INDICATIONS** Children under 6 months · history of thymus dysfunction

● **CAUTIONS**

CAUTIONS, FURTHER INFORMATION

▸ Administration with MMR vaccine Yellow fever and MMR vaccines should not be administered on the same day; there should be a 4-week minimum interval between the vaccines. When protection is rapidly required, the vaccines can be given at any interval and an additional dose of MMR may be considered.

● **INTERACTIONS** → Appendix 1: live vaccines

● **SIDE-EFFECTS**

▶ **Common or very common** Asthenia · crying · drowsiness

▶ **Uncommon** Abdominal pain

▶ **Rare or very rare** Rhinitis · yellow fever vaccine-associated neurotropic disease · yellow fever vaccine-associated viscerotropic disease

▶ **Frequency not known** Angioedema · influenza like illness · paraesthesia

SIDE-EFFECTS, FURTHER INFORMATION Very rare vaccine-associated adverse effects may occur, such as viscerotropic disease (yellow-fever vaccine-associated viscerotropic disease, YEL-AVD), a syndrome which may include metabolic acidosis, muscle and liver cirrhosis, and multi-organ failure. Neurological disorders (yellow fever vaccine-associated neurotropic disease, YEL-AND) such as encephalitis have also been reported. These very rare adverse effects usually occur after the first dose of yellow fever vaccine in those with no previous immunity. Increased risk of fatal reactions reported in patients aged 60 years and older and those who are immunosuppressed.

- **ALLERGY AND CROSS-SENSITIVITY** Yellow fever vaccine should only be considered under the guidance of a specialist in individuals with evidence of previous anaphylactic reaction to egg.
- **PREGNANCY** Live yellow fever vaccine should not be given during pregnancy because there is a theoretical risk of fetal infection. Pregnant women should be advised not to travel to areas at high risk of yellow fever. If exposure cannot be avoided during pregnancy, then the vaccine should be given if the risk from disease in the mother outweighs the risk to the fetus from vaccination.
- **BREAST FEEDING** Avoid; seek specialist advice if exposure to virus cannot be avoided.

- **MEDICINAL FORMS** There can be variation in the licensing of different medicines containing the same drug.

Powder and solvent for suspension for injection

▸ Stamaril (Sanofi Pasteur)
Stamaril vaccine powder and solvent for suspension for injection 0.5ml vials | 1 vial [PoM] £39.72 DT = £39.72

Chapter 15 Anaesthesia

CONTENTS

General anaesthesia

Anaesthesia (general)

Overview

Several different types of drug are given together during general anaesthesia. Anaesthesia is induced with either a volatile drug given by inhalation or with an intravenously administered drug; anaesthesia is maintained with an intravenous or inhalational anaesthetic. Analgesics, usually short-acting opioids, are also used. The use of neuromuscular blocking drugs necessitates intermittent positive-pressure ventilation. Following surgery, anticholinesterases can be given to reverse the effects of neuromuscular blocking drugs; specific antagonists can be used to reverse central and respiratory depression caused by some drugs used in surgery. A local topical anaesthetic can be used to reduce pain at the injection site.

Individual requirements vary considerably and the recommended doses are only a guide. Smaller doses are indicated in ill, shocked, or debilitated children and in significant hepatic impairment, while robust individuals may require larger doses. The required dose of induction agent may be less if the patient has been premedicated with a sedative agent or if an opioid analgesic has been used.

Intravenous anaesthetics

Intravenous anaesthetics may be used either to induce anaesthesia or for maintenance of anaesthesia throughout surgery. Intravenous anaesthetics nearly all produce their effect in one arm-brain circulation time. Extreme care is required in surgery of the mouth, pharynx, or larynx where the airway may be difficult to maintain (e.g. in the presence of a tumour in the pharynx or larynx).

To facilitate tracheal intubation, induction is usually followed by a neuromuscular blocking drug or a short-acting opioid.

The doses of all intravenous anaesthetic drugs should be titrated to effect (except when using 'rapid sequence induction').

Total intravenous anaesthesia

This is a technique in which major surgery is carried out with all drugs given intravenously. Respiration can be spontaneous, or controlled with oxygen-enriched air. Neuromuscular blocking drugs can be used to provide relaxation and prevent reflex muscle movements. The main problem to be overcome is the assessment of depth of anaesthesia. Target Controlled Infusion (TCI) systems can be used to titrate intravenous anaesthetic infusions to predicted plasma-drug concentrations; specific models with paediatric pharmacokinetic data should be used for children.

Drugs used for intravenous anaesthesia

Propofol p. 864, the most widely used intravenous anaesthetic, can be used for induction or maintenance of anaesthesia in children, but it is not commonly used in neonates. Propofol is associated with rapid recovery and less hangover effect than other intravenous anaesthetics. Propofol can also be used for sedation during diagnostic procedures.

Thiopental sodium p. 237 is a barbiturate that is used for induction of anaesthesia, but has no analgesic properties. Induction is generally smooth and rapid, but dose-related cardiovascular and respiratory depression can occur. Awakening from a moderate dose of thiopental sodium is rapid because the drug redistributes into other tissues, particularly fat. However, metabolism is slow and sedative effects can persist for 24 hours. Repeated doses have a cumulative effect particularly in neonates and recovery is much slower.

Etomidate p. 863 is an intravenous agent associated with rapid recovery without a hangover effect. Etomidate causes less hypotension than thiopental sodium and propofol during induction. It produces a high incidence of extraneous muscle movements, which can be minimised by an opioid analgesic or a short-acting benzodiazepine given just before induction.

Ketamine p. 879 causes less hypotension than thiopental sodium and propofol during induction. It is sometimes used in children requiring repeat anaesthesia (such as for serial burns dressings), however recovery is relatively slow and there is a high incidence of extraneous muscle movements. Ketamine can cause hallucinations, nightmares, and other transient psychotic effects; these can be reduced by a benzodiazepine such as diazepam p. 236 or midazolam p. 239.

Inhalational anaesthetics

Inhalational anaesthetics include gases and volatile liquids. *Gaseous anaesthetics* require suitable equipment for storage and administration. *Volatile liquid anaesthetics* are administered using calibrated vaporisers, using air, oxygen, or nitrous oxide-oxygen mixtures as the carrier gas. To prevent hypoxia, the inspired gas mixture should contain a minimum of 25% oxygen at all times. Higher concentrations of oxygen (greater than 30%) are usually required during inhalational anaesthesia when nitrous oxide p. 867 is being administered.

Volatile liquid anaesthetics

Volatile liquid anaesthetics can be used for induction and maintenance of anaesthesia, and following induction with an intravenous anaesthetic.

Isoflurane p. 866 is a volatile liquid anaesthetic. Heart rhythm is generally stable during isoflurane anaesthesia, but heart-rate can rise. Systemic arterial pressure and cardiac output can fall, owing to a decrease in systemic vascular resistance. Muscle relaxation occurs and the effects of muscle relaxant drugs are potentiated. Isoflurane is not recommended for induction of anaesthesia in infants and children of all ages because of the occurrence of cough, breath-holding, desaturation, increased secretions, and laryngospasm. Isoflurane is the preferred inhalational anaesthetic for use in obstetrics.

Desflurane p. 866 is a rapid acting volatile liquid anaesthetic; it is reported to have about one-fifth the potency of isoflurane. Emergence and recovery from anaesthesia are particularly rapid because of its low solubility. Desflurane is not recommended for induction of anaesthesia as it is irritant to the upper respiratory tract.

Sevoflurane p. 867 is a rapid acting volatile liquid anaesthetic and is more potent than desflurane. Emergence and recovery are particularly rapid, but slower than desflurane. Sevoflurane is non-irritant and is therefore often used for inhalational induction of anaesthesia.

Nitrous oxide

Nitrous oxide is used for maintenance of anaesthesia and, in sub-anaesthetic concentrations, for analgesia. For *anaesthesia*, it is commonly used in a concentration of 50 to 66% in oxygen as part of a balanced technique in association with other inhalational or intravenous agents. Nitrous oxide is unsatisfactory as a sole anaesthetic owing to lack of potency, but is useful as part of a combination of drugs since it allows a significant reduction in dosage.

For analgesia (without loss of consciousness), a mixture of nitrous oxide and oxygen containing 50% of each gas (*Entonox*®, *Equanox*®) is used. Self-administration using a demand valve may be used in children who are able to self-regulate their intake (usually over 5 years of age) for painful dressing changes, as an aid to postoperative physiotherapy, for wound debridement and in emergency ambulances.

Nitrous oxide may have a deleterious effect if used in children with an air-containing closed space since nitrous oxide diffuses into such a space with a resulting increase in pressure. This effect may be dangerous in conditions such as pneumothorax, which may enlarge to compromise respiration, or in the presence of intracranial air after head injury, entrapped air following recent underwater dive, or recent intra-ocular gas injection.

Malignant hyperthermia

Malignant hyperthermia is a rare but potentially lethal complication of anaesthesia. It is characterised by a rapid rise in temperature, increased muscle rigidity, tachycardia, and acidosis. The most common triggers of malignant hyperthermia are the volatile anaesthetics. Suxamethonium chloride p. 872 has also been implicated, but malignant hyperthermia is more likely if it is given following a volatile anaesthetic. Volatile anaesthetics and suxamethonium chloride should be avoided during anaesthesia in children at high risk of malignant hyperthermia.

Dantrolene sodium p. 880 is used in the treatment of malignant hyperthermia.

Sedation, anaesthesia, and resuscitation in dental practice

Overview

Sedation for dental procedures should be limited to conscious sedation whenever possible. Nitrous oxide p. 867 alone and midazolam p. 239 are effective for many children.

For details of anaesthesia, sedation, and resuscitation in dental practice see *A Conscious Decision*: *A review of the use of general anaesthesia and conscious sedation in primary dental care* ; report by a group chaired by the Chief Medical Officer and Chief Dental Officer, July 2000 and associated documents. Further details can also be found in *Standards for Conscious Sedation in the Provision of Dental Care*; report of an Intercollegiate Advisory Committee for Sedation in Dentistry, 2015 www.rcseng.ac.uk/-/media/files/rcs/library-and-publications/non-journal-publications/dental-sedation-report.pdf.

Surgery and long-term medication

Overview

The risk of losing disease control on stopping long-term medication before surgery is often greater than the risk posed by continuing it during surgery. It is vital that the anaesthetist knows about **all** drugs that a patient is (or has been) taking.

Patients with adrenal atrophy resulting from long-term corticosteroid use may suffer a precipitous fall in blood pressure unless corticosteroid cover is provided during anaesthesia and in the immediate postoperative period. Anaesthetists must therefore know whether a patient is, or has been, receiving corticosteroids (including high-dose inhaled corticosteroids).

Other drugs that should normally not be stopped before surgery include drugs for epilepsy, asthma, immunosuppression, and metabolic, endocrine and cardiovascular disorders (but see potassium sparing diuretics). Expert advice is required for children receiving antivirals for HIV infection. See general advice on surgery in children with diabetes in Diabetes, surgery and medical illness p. 486.

Children taking antiplatelet medication or an oral anticoagulant present an increased risk for surgery. In these circumstances, the anaesthetist and surgeon should assess the relative risks and decide jointly whether the antiplatelet or the anticoagulant drug should be stopped or replaced with heparin (unfractionated) p. 101 or low molecular weight heparin therapy.

Drugs that should be stopped before surgery include combined oral contraceptives, see Contraceptives, hormonal p. 532. If antidepressants need to be stopped, they should be withdrawn gradually to avoid withdrawal symptoms. Tricyclic antidepressants need not be stopped, but there may be an increased risk of arrhythmias and hypotension (and dangerous interactions with vasopressor drugs); therefore, the anaesthetist should be informed if they are not stopped. Lithium should be stopped 24 hours before major surgery but the normal dose can be continued for minor surgery (with careful monitoring of fluids and electrolytes). Potassium-sparing diuretics may need to be withheld on the morning of surgery because hyperkalaemia may develop if renal perfusion is impaired or if there is tissue damage. Herbal medicines may be associated with adverse effects when given with anaesthetic drugs and consideration should be given to stopping them before surgery.

ANAESTHETICS, GENERAL > INTRAVENOUS

Etomidate

04-Dec-2019

● INDICATIONS AND DOSE

Induction of anaesthesia

▸ BY SLOW INTRAVENOUS INJECTION

▸ Child 1 month–14 years: 150–300 micrograms/kg (max. per dose 60 mg), to be administered over 30–60 seconds (60 seconds for children in whom hypotension might be hazardous), increased if necessary to 400 micrograms/kg

▸ Child 15–17 years: 150–300 micrograms/kg (max. per dose 60 mg), to be administered over 30–60 seconds (60 seconds for children in whom hypotension might be hazardous)

- **UNLICENSED USE** *Hypnomidate*® licensed for use in children (age range not specified by manufacturer). *Etomidate-Lipuro*® not licensed for children under 6 months except for imperative indications during inpatient treatment. Doses in *BNF for Children* may differ from those in the product literature.

> **IMPORTANT SAFETY INFORMATION**
> Etomidate should only be administered by, or under the direct supervision of, personnel experienced in its use, with adequate training in anaesthesia and airway management, and when resuscitation equipment is available.

- **CAUTIONS** Acute circulatory failure (shock) · adrenal insufficiency · Avoid in Acute porphyrias p. 652 · cardiovascular disease · fixed cardiac output · hypovolaemia

  CAUTIONS, FURTHER INFORMATION
  - Adrenal insufficiency Etomidate suppresses adrenocortical function, particularly during continuous administration, and it should not be used for maintenance of anaesthesia. It should be used with caution in patients with underlying adrenal insufficiency, for example, those with sepsis.
- **INTERACTIONS** → Appendix 1: etomidate
- **SIDE-EFFECTS**
  - **Common or very common** Apnoea · hypotension · movement disorders · nausea · respiratory disorders · skin reactions · vascular pain · vomiting
  - **Uncommon** Arrhythmias · cough · hiccups · hypersalivation · hypertension · muscle rigidity · neuromuscular dysfunction · nystagmus · procedural complications
  - **Frequency not known** Adrenal insufficiency · atrioventricular block · cardiac arrest · embolism and thrombosis · seizures · shock · Stevens-Johnson syndrome · trismus

  SIDE-EFFECTS, FURTHER INFORMATION **Pain on injection** Can be reduced by injecting into a larger vein or by giving an opioid analgesic just before induction.

  Extraneous muscle movements Extraneous muscle movements can be minimised by an opioid analgesic or a short-acting benzodiazepine given just before induction.
- **PREGNANCY** May depress neonatal respiration if used during delivery.
- **BREAST FEEDING** Breast-feeding can be resumed as soon as mother has recovered sufficiently from anaesthesia.
- **HEPATIC IMPAIRMENT**
  Dose adjustments Manufacturer advises reduce dose in liver cirrhosis.
- **DIRECTIONS FOR ADMINISTRATION** To be administered over 30–60 seconds (60 seconds in patients in whom hypotension might be hazardous).
- **PATIENT AND CARER ADVICE**
  Driving and skilled tasks Patients given sedatives and analgesics during minor outpatient procedures should be very carefully warned about the risk of driving or undertaking skilled tasks afterwards. For a short general anaesthetic the risk extends to **at least 24 hours** after administration. Responsible persons should be available to take patients home. The dangers of taking **alcohol** should also be emphasised.

- **MEDICINAL FORMS** There can be variation in the licensing of different medicines containing the same drug.

Solution for injection

EXCIPIENTS: May contain Propylene glycol

- Hypnomidate (Piramal Critical Care Ltd)
  Etomidate 2 mg per 1 ml Hypnomidate 20mg/10ml solution for injection ampoules | 5 ampoule PoM £6.90

Emulsion for injection

- Etomidate-Lipuro (B.Braun Medical Ltd)
  Etomidate 2 mg per 1 ml Etomidate-Lipuro 20mg/10ml emulsion for injection ampoules | 10 ampoule PoM £16.09

Propofol

04-Dec-2019

- **INDICATIONS AND DOSE**

Induction of anaesthesia using 0.5% or 1% injection
- BY SLOW INTRAVENOUS INJECTION, OR BY INTRAVENOUS INFUSION
  - Child 1 month–16 years: Usual dose 2.5–4 mg/kg, dose adjusted according to age, body-weight and response
  - Child 17 years: Usual dose 1.5–2.5 mg/kg, to be administered at a rate of 20–40 mg every 10 seconds until response

Induction of anaesthesia using 2% injection
- BY INTRAVENOUS INFUSION
  - Child 3–16 years: Usual dose 2.5–4 mg/kg, dose adjusted according to age, body-weight and response
  - Child 17 years: Usual dose 1.5–2.5 mg/kg, to be administered at a rate of 20–40 mg every 10 seconds until response

Maintenance of anaesthesia using 1% injection
- BY CONTINUOUS INTRAVENOUS INFUSION
  - Child 1 month–16 years: Usual dose 9–15 mg/kg/hour, dose adjusted according to age, body-weight and response
  - Child 17 years: Usual dose 4–12 mg/kg/hour, adjusted according to response

Maintenance of anaesthesia using 2% injection
- BY CONTINUOUS INTRAVENOUS INFUSION
  - Child 3–16 years: Usual dose 9–15 mg/kg/hour, dose adjusted according to age, body-weight and response
  - Child 17 years: Usual dose 4–12 mg/kg/hour, adjusted according to response

Sedation of ventilated patients in intensive care using 1% or 2% injection
- BY CONTINUOUS INTRAVENOUS INFUSION
  - Child 16–17 years: Usual dose 0.3–4 mg/kg/hour, adjusted according to response

Induction of sedation for surgical and diagnostic procedures using 0.5% or 1% injection
- BY SLOW INTRAVENOUS INJECTION
  - Child 1 month–16 years: Initially 1–2 mg/kg, dose and rate of administration adjusted according to desired level of sedation and response
  - Child 17 years: Initially 0.5–1 mg/kg, to be administered over 1–5 minutes, dose and rate of administration adjusted according to desired level of sedation and response

Maintenance of sedation for surgical and diagnostic procedures using 0.5% injection
- INITIALLY BY INTRAVENOUS INFUSION
  - Child 17 years: Initially 1.5–4.5 mg/kg/hour, dose and rate of administration adjusted according to desired level of sedation and response, followed by (by slow intravenous injection) 10–20 mg, (if rapid increase in sedation required)

Maintenance of sedation for surgical and diagnostic procedures using 1% injection
- INITIALLY BY INTRAVENOUS INFUSION
  - Child 1 month–16 years: Usual dose 1.5–9 mg/kg/hour, dose and rate of administration adjusted according to desired level of sedation and response, followed by (by slow intravenous injection) up to 1 mg/kg, (if rapid increase in sedation required)
  - Child 17 years: Initially 1.5–4.5 mg/kg/hour, dose and rate of administration adjusted according to desired level of sedation and response, followed by (by slow

intravenous injection) 10–20 mg, (if rapid increase in sedation required)

Maintenance of sedation for surgical and diagnostic procedures using 2% injection
- INITIALLY BY INTRAVENOUS INFUSION
- Child 3–16 years: Usual dose 1.5–9 mg/kg/hour, dose and rate of administration adjusted according to desired level of sedation and response
- Child 17 years: Initially 1.5–4.5 mg/kg/hour, dose and rate of administration adjusted according to desired level of sedation and response, followed by (by slow intravenous injection) 10–20 mg, using 0.5% or 1% injection (if rapid increase in sedation required)

IMPORTANT SAFETY INFORMATION
Propofol should only be administered by, or under the direct supervision of, personnel experienced in its use, with adequate training in anaesthesia and airway management, and when resuscitation equipment is available.

- **CONTRA-INDICATIONS** Children under 16 years receiving intensive care

CONTRA-INDICATIONS, FURTHER INFORMATION
Use in intensive care associated with a risk of propofol infusion syndrome (potentially fatal effects, including metabolic acidosis, arrhythmias, cardiac failure, rhabdomyolysis, hyperlipidaemia, hyperkalaemia, hepatomegaly, and renal failure).

- **CAUTIONS** Acute circulatory failure (shock) · cardiac impairment · cardiovascular disease · epilepsy · fixed cardiac output · hypotension · hypovolaemia · raised intracranial pressure · respiratory impairment
- **INTERACTIONS** → Appendix 1: propofol
- **SIDE-EFFECTS**
- **Common or very common** Apnoea · arrhythmias · headache · hypotension · localised pain · nausea · vomiting
- **Uncommon** Thrombosis
- **Rare or very rare** Epileptiform seizure (may be delayed) · pancreatitis · post procedural complications · pulmonary oedema · sexual disinhibition · soft tissue necrosis · urine discolouration
- **Frequency not known** Drug use disorders · dyskinesia · euphoric mood · heart failure · hepatomegaly · hyperkalaemia · hyperlipidaemia · metabolic acidosis · renal failure · respiratory depression · rhabdomyolysis

SIDE-EFFECTS, FURTHER INFORMATION **Bradycardia** Bradycardia may be profound and may be treated with intravenous administration of an antimuscarinic drug.

Pain on injection Pain on injection can be reduced by intravenous lidocaine.

Propofol infusion syndrome Prolonged infusion of propofol doses exceeding 4mg/kg/hour may result in potentially fatal effects, including metabolic acidosis, arrhythmias, cardiac failure, rhabdomyolysis, hyperlipidaemia, hyperkalaemia, hepatomegaly, and renal failure.

- **PREGNANCY** May depress neonatal respiration if used during delivery.

Dose adjustments Max. dose for maintenance of anaesthesia 6 mg/kg/hour.

- **BREAST FEEDING** Breast-feeding can be resumed as soon as mother has recovered sufficiently from anaesthesia.
- **HEPATIC IMPAIRMENT** Manufacturer advises caution.
- **RENAL IMPAIRMENT** Use with caution.
- **MONITORING REQUIREMENTS** Monitor blood-lipid concentration if risk of fat overload or if sedation longer than 3 days.
- **DIRECTIONS FOR ADMINISTRATION** Shake before use; microbiological filter not recommended; may be administered via a Y-piece close to injection site co-administered with Glucose 5% *or* Sodium chloride 0.9%. 0.5% **emulsion** for injection or intermittent infusion; may be administered undiluted, or diluted with Glucose 5% *or* Sodium chloride 0.9%; dilute to a concentration not less than 1 mg/mL. 1% **emulsion** for injection or infusion; may be administered undiluted, or diluted with Glucose 5% (*Diprivan*®) or (*Propofol-Lipuro*®) *or* Sodium chloride 0.9% (*Propofol-Lipuro*® only); dilute to a concentration not less than 2 mg/mL; use within 6 hours of preparation. 2% **emulsion** for infusion; do not dilute.
- **PATIENT AND CARER ADVICE**

Driving and skilled tasks Patients given sedatives and analgesics during minor outpatient procedures should be very carefully warned about the risk of driving or undertaking skilled tasks afterwards. For a short general anaesthetic the risk extends to **at least 24 hours** after administration. Responsible persons should be available to take patients home. The dangers of taking **alcohol** should also be emphasised.

- **MEDICINAL FORMS** There can be variation in the licensing of different medicines containing the same drug.

Emulsion for infusion
- Propofol (Non-proprietary)

Propofol 10 mg per 1 ml Propofol 500mg/50ml emulsion for infusion vials | 1 vial PoM £15.00 (Hospital only)
Propofol-Lipuro 1% emulsion for infusion 50ml vials | 10 vial PoM £97.56 (Hospital only)
Propofol 1g/100ml emulsion for infusion vials | 1 vial PoM £15.00 (Hospital only)
Propofol-Lipuro 1% emulsion for infusion 100ml vials | 10 vial PoM £186.66 (Hospital only)

Propofol 20 mg per 1 ml Propofol 1g/50ml emulsion for infusion vials | 1 vial PoM £15.00 (Hospital only)
Propofol-Lipuro 2% emulsion for infusion 50ml vials | 10 vial PoM £186.64 (Hospital only)

- Diprivan (Aspen Pharma Trading Ltd)

Propofol 10 mg per 1 ml Diprivan 1% emulsion for infusion 50ml pre-filled syringes | 1 pre-filled disposable injection PoM £10.68

Propofol 20 mg per 1 ml Diprivan 2% emulsion for infusion 50ml pre-filled syringes | 1 pre-filled disposable injection PoM £15.16

- Propoven (Fresenius Kabi Ltd)

Propofol 10 mg per 1 ml Propoven 1% emulsion for infusion 50ml vials | 10 vial PoM £120.60 (Hospital only)
Propoven 1% emulsion for infusion 100ml vials | 10 vial PoM £241.50 (Hospital only)

Propofol 20 mg per 1 ml Propoven 2% emulsion for infusion 50ml vials | 10 vial PoM £241.50 (Hospital only)

Emulsion for injection
- Propofol (Non-proprietary)

Propofol 10 mg per 1 ml Propofol 200mg/20ml emulsion for injection vials | 5 vial PoM £20.00 (Hospital only)
Propofol-Lipuro 1% emulsion for injection 20ml ampoules | 5 ampoule PoM £20.16 (Hospital only)

- Diprivan (Aspen Pharma Trading Ltd)

Propofol 10 mg per 1 ml Diprivan 1% emulsion for injection 20ml ampoules | 5 ampoule PoM £15.36 (Hospital only)

- Propofol-Lipuro (B.Braun Melsungen AG)

Propofol 5 mg per 1 ml Propofol-Lipuro 0.5% emulsion for injection 20ml ampoules | 5 ampoule PoM £15.15

- Propoven (Fresenius Kabi Ltd)

Propofol 10 mg per 1 ml Propoven 1% emulsion for injection 20ml ampoules | 5 ampoule PoM £23.90 (Hospital only)

ANAESTHETICS, GENERAL > VOLATILE LIQUID

Volatile halogenated anaesthetics

IMPORTANT SAFETY INFORMATION
Should only be administered by, or under the direct supervision of, personnel experienced in their use, with

adequate training in anaesthesia and airway management, and when resuscitation equipment is available.

- **CONTRA-INDICATIONS** Susceptibility to malignant hyperthermia
- **CAUTIONS** Can trigger malignant hyperthermia · neuromuscular disease (inhalational anaesthetics are very rarely associated with hyperkalaemia, resulting in cardiac arrhythmias and death) · raised intracranial pressure (can increase cerebrospinal pressure)
- **SIDE-EFFECTS**
  - **Common or very common** Agitation · apnoea · arrhythmias · chills · cough · dizziness · headache · hypersalivation · hypertension · hypotension · nausea · respiratory disorders · vomiting
  - **Uncommon** Hypoxia
  - **Frequency not known** Breath holding · cardiac arrest · haemorrhage · hepatic disorders · hyperkalaemia · malignant hyperthermia · QT interval prolongation · rhabdomyolysis · seizure
- **ALLERGY AND CROSS-SENSITIVITY** Can cause hepatotoxicity in those sensitised to halogenated anaesthetics.
- **DIRECTIONS FOR ADMINISTRATION** Volatile liquid anaesthetics are administered using calibrated vaporisers, using air, oxygen, or nitrous oxide-oxygen mixtures as the carrier gas. To prevent hypoxia, the inspired gas mixture should contain a minimum of 25% oxygen at all times.
- **PATIENT AND CARER ADVICE**

Driving and skilled tasks Patients given sedatives and analgesics during minor outpatient procedures should be very carefully warned about the risks of driving or undertaking skilled tasks afterwards. For a short general anaesthetic, the risk extends **to at least 24 hours** after administration. Responsible persons should be available to take patients home. The dangers of taking **alcohol** should also be emphasised.

F 865

Desflurane

- **INDICATIONS AND DOSE**

Induction of anaesthesia (but not recommended)

▶ BY INHALATION

- Child 12–17 years: 4–11 %, to be inhaled through specifically calibrated vaporiser

Maintenance of anaesthesia (in nitrous oxide–oxygen)

▶ BY INHALATION

- Neonate: 2–6 %, to be inhaled through a specifically calibrated vaporiser.
- Child: 2–6 %, to be inhaled through a specifically calibrated vaporiser

Maintenance of anaesthesia (in oxygen or oxygen-enriched air)

▶ BY INHALATION

- Neonate: 2.5–8.5 %, to be inhaled through a specifically calibrated vaporiser.
- Child: 2.5–8.5 %, to be inhaled through a specifically calibrated vaporiser

- **INTERACTIONS** → Appendix 1: volatile halogenated anaesthetics
- **SIDE-EFFECTS**
  - **Common or very common** Coagulation disorder · conjunctivitis
  - **Uncommon** Myalgia · myocardial infarction · myocardial ischaemia · vasodilation
  - **Frequency not known** Abdominal pain · asthenia · heart failure · hypokalaemia · malaise · metabolic acidosis · pancreatitis acute · shock · skin reactions · ventricular dysfunction · visual acuity decreased
- **PREGNANCY** May depress neonatal respiration if used during delivery.
- **BREAST FEEDING** Breast-feeding can be resumed as soon as mother has recovered sufficiently from anaesthesia.
- **MEDICINAL FORMS** There can be variation in the licensing of different medicines containing the same drug.

Inhalation vapour

▶ Desflurane (Non-proprietary)

Desflurane 1 ml per 1 ml Desflurane volatile liquid | 240 ml PoM 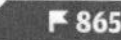 (Hospital only)

F 865

Isoflurane

12-Dec-2019

- **INDICATIONS AND DOSE**

Induction of anaesthesia (in oxygen or nitrous oxide-oxygen) (but indication not recommended in infants and children of all ages)

▶ BY INHALATION

- Neonate: Initially 0.5 %, increased to 3 %, adjusted according to response, administered using specifically calibrated vaporiser.
- Child: Initially 0.5 %, increased to 3 %, adjusted according to response, administered using specifically calibrated vaporiser

Maintenance of anaesthesia (in nitrous oxide–oxygen)

▶ BY INHALATION

- Neonate: 1–2.5 %, to be administered using specifically calibrated vaporiser; an additional 0.5–1% may be required when given with oxygen alone.
- Child: 1–2.5 %, to be administered using specifically calibrated vaporiser; an additional 0.5–1% may be required when given with oxygen alone

Maintenance of anaesthesia in caesarean section (in nitrous oxide–oxygen)

▶ BY INHALATION

- Child: 0.5–0.75 %, to be administered using specifically calibrated vaporiser

IMPORTANT SAFETY INFORMATION

Isoflurane is not recommended for induction of anaesthesia in infants and children of all ages because of the occurrence of cough, breath-holding, desaturation, increased secretions, and laryngospasm.

- **CAUTIONS** Children under 2 years—limited experience
- **INTERACTIONS** → Appendix 1: volatile halogenated anaesthetics
- **SIDE-EFFECTS** Carboxyhaemoglobinaemia · chest discomfort · cognitive impairment · delirium · dyspnoea · ileus · mood altered (that can last several days) · myoglobinuria · skin reactions
- **PREGNANCY** May depress neonatal respiration if used during delivery.
- **BREAST FEEDING** Breast-feeding can be resumed as soon as mother has recovered sufficiently from anaesthesia.
- **MEDICINAL FORMS** There can be variation in the licensing of different medicines containing the same drug.

Inhalation vapour

▶ Isoflurane (Non-proprietary)

Isoflurane 1 ml per 1 ml Isoflurane inhalation vapour | 250 ml PoM £35.29 (Hospital only)

15 Anaesthesia

▸ AErrane (Baxter Healthcare Ltd)
Isoflurane 1 ml per 1 ml AErrane volatile liquid | 250 ml PoM ⊠ (Hospital only)

Nitrous oxide

10-Mar-2020

● **INDICATIONS AND DOSE**

Maintenance of anaesthesia in conjunction with other anaesthetic agents

▸ BY INHALATION

▸ Neonate: 50–66 %, to be administered using suitable anaesthetic apparatus in oxygen.

▸ Child: 50–66 %, to be administered using suitable anaesthetic apparatus in oxygen

Analgesia

▸ BY INHALATION

▸ Neonate: Up to 50 %, to be administered using suitable anaesthetic apparatus in oxygen, adjusted according to the patient's needs.

▸ Child: Up to 50 %, to be administered using suitable anaesthetic apparatus in oxygen, adjusted according to the patient's needs

IMPORTANT SAFETY INFORMATION
Nitrous oxide should only be administered by, or under the direct supervision of, personnel experienced in its use, with adequate training in anaesthesia and airway management, and when resuscitation equipment is available.

● **CAUTIONS** Entrapped air following recent underwater dive · pneumothorax · presence of intracranial air after head injury · recent intra-ocular gas injection

CAUTIONS, FURTHER INFORMATION Nitrous oxide may have a deleterious effect if used in patients with an air-containing closed space since nitrous oxide diffuses into such a space with a resulting increase in pressure. This effect may be dangerous in conditions such as pneumothorax, which may enlarge to compromise respiration, or in the presence of intracranial air after head injury, entrapped air following recent underwater dive, or recent intra-ocular gas injection.

● **INTERACTIONS** → Appendix 1: nitrous oxide

● **SIDE-EFFECTS** Abdominal distension · addiction · agranulocytosis · disorientation · dizziness · euphoric mood · megaloblastic anaemia · middle ear damage · myeloneuropathy · nausea · paraesthesia · sedation · subacute combined cord degeneration · tympanic membrane perforation · vomiting

SIDE-EFFECTS, FURTHER INFORMATION Exposure of patients to nitrous oxide for prolonged periods, either by continuous or by intermittent administration, may result in megaloblastic anaemia owing to interference with the action of vitamin B_{12}; neurological toxic effects can occur without preceding overt haematological changes. Depression of white cell formation may also occur.

● **PREGNANCY** May depress neonatal respiration if used during delivery.

● **BREAST FEEDING** Breast-feeding can be resumed as soon as mother has recovered sufficiently from anaesthesia.

● **MONITORING REQUIREMENTS**

▸ Assessment of plasma-vitamin B_{12} concentration should be considered in those at risk of deficiency, including the elderly, those who have a poor, vegetarian, or vegan diet, and those with a history of anaemia.

▸ Nitrous oxide should **not** be given continuously for longer than 24 hours or more frequently than every 4 days without close supervision and haematological monitoring.

● **DIRECTIONS FOR ADMINISTRATION** For analgesia (without loss of consciousness), a mixture of nitrous oxide and oxygen containing 50% of each gas (*Entonox®*, *Equanox®*) is used.

● **HANDLING AND STORAGE** Exposure of theatre staff to nitrous oxide should be minimised (risk of serious side-effects).

● **PATIENT AND CARER ADVICE**
Medicines for Children leaflet: Nitrous oxide for pain
www.medicinesforchildren.org.uk/nitrous-oxide-pain

● **MEDICINAL FORMS** There can be variation in the licensing of different medicines containing the same drug.

Inhalation gas

▸ Nitrous oxide (Non-proprietary)
Nitrous oxide 1 ml per 1 ml Nitrous oxide cylinders size E | 1800 litre P ⊠
Medical Nitrous Oxide cylinders size D | 900 litre P ⊠
Medical Nitrous Oxide cylinders size G | 9000 litre P ⊠
Nitrous oxide cylinders size F | 3600 litre P ⊠
Nitrous oxide cylinders size J | 18000 litre P ⊠
Nitrous oxide cylinders size G | 9000 litre P ⊠
Medical Nitrous Oxide cylinders size F | 3600 litre P ⊠
Nitrous oxide cylinders size D | 900 litre P ⊠
Medical Nitrous Oxide cylinders size E | 1800 litre P ⊠

F 865

Sevoflurane

● **INDICATIONS AND DOSE**

Induction of anaesthesia (in oxygen or nitrous oxide-oxygen)

▸ BY INHALATION

▸ Neonate: Up to 4 %, adjusted according to response, to be administered using specifically calibrated vaporiser.

▸ Child: Initially 0.5–1 %, then increased to up to 8 %, increased gradually, according to response, to be administered using specifically calibrated vaporiser

Maintenance of anaesthesia (in oxygen or nitrous oxide-oxygen)

▸ BY INHALATION

▸ Neonate: 0.5–2 %, adjusted according to response, to be administered using specifically calibrated vaporiser.

▸ Child: 0.5–3 %, adjusted according to response, to be administered using specifically calibrated vaporiser

● **CAUTIONS** Susceptibility to QT-interval prolongation

● **INTERACTIONS** → Appendix 1: volatile halogenated anaesthetics

● **SIDE-EFFECTS**

▸ **Common or very common** Drowsiness · fever · hypothermia

▸ **Uncommon** Asthma · atrioventricular block · confusion

▸ **Frequency not known** Dystonia · intracranial pressure increased · muscle rigidity · nephritis tubulointerstitial · oedema · pancreatitis

● **PREGNANCY** May depress neonatal respiration if used during delivery.

● **BREAST FEEDING** Breast-feeding can be resumed as soon as mother has recovered sufficiently from anaesthesia.

● **RENAL IMPAIRMENT** Use with caution.

● **MEDICINAL FORMS** There can be variation in the licensing of different medicines containing the same drug.

Inhalation vapour

▸ Sevoflurane (Non-proprietary)
Sevoflurane 1 ml per 1 ml Sevoflurane volatile liquid | 250 ml PoM £123.00 (Hospital only)

15 Anaesthesia

1 Anaesthesia adjuvants

Pre-medication and peri-operative drugs

Drugs that affect gastric pH

Regurgitation and aspiration of gastric contents (Mendelson's syndrome) can be a complication of general anaesthesia, particularly in obstetrics and in gastro-oesophageal reflux disease; prophylaxis against acid aspiration is not routinely used in children but may be required in high-risk cases.

An **H_2-receptor antagonist** can be used before surgery to increase the pH and reduce the volume of gastric fluid. It does not affect the pH of fluid already in the stomach and this limits its value in emergency procedures; an oral H_2-receptor antagonist can be given 1–2 hours before the procedure.

Antimuscarinic drugs

Antimuscarinic drugs are used (less commonly nowadays) as premedicants to dry bronchial and salivary secretions which are increased by intubation, upper airway surgery, or some inhalational anaesthetics. They are also used before or with neostigmine p. 700 to prevent bradycardia, excessive salivation, and other muscarinic actions of neostigmine. They also prevent bradycardia and hypotension associated with drugs such as propofol p. 864 and suxamethonium chloride p. 872.

Atropine sulfate p. 869 is now rarely used for premedication but still has an emergency role in the treatment of vagotonic side-effects. Atropine sulfate may have a role in cardiopulmonary resuscitation.

Hyoscine hydrobromide p. 283 reduces secretions and also provides a degree of amnesia, sedation, and anti-emesis. Unlike atropine sulfate it may produce bradycardia rather than tachycardia.

Glycopyrronium bromide p. 870 reduces salivary secretions. When given intravenously it produces less tachycardia than atropine sulfate. It is widely used with neostigmine for reversal of non-depolarising muscle relaxants.

Glycopyrronium bromide or hyoscine hydrobromide are also used to control excessive secretions in upper airways or hypersalivation in palliative care and in children unable to control posture or with abnormal swallowing reflex; effective dose varies and tolerance may develop. The intramuscular route should be avoided if possible. Hyoscine hydrobromide transdermal patches may also be used.

Sedative drugs

Premedication

Fear and anxiety before a procedure (including the night before) can be minimised by using a sedative drug, usually a **benzodiazepine**. Premedication may also augment the action of anaesthetics and provide some degree of pre-operative amnesia. The choice of drug depends on the individual, the nature of the procedure, the anaesthetic to be used, and other prevailing circumstances such as outpatients, obstetrics, and availability of recovery facilities. The choice also varies between elective and emergency procedures. Oral administration is preferred if possible; the rectal route should only be used in exceptional circumstances.

Premedicants can be given the night before major surgery; a further, smaller dose may be required before surgery. Alternatively, the first dose may be given on the day of the procedure.

Oral midazolam p. 239 is the most common premedicant for children; temazepam p. 879 may be used in older children. The antihistamine alimemazine tartrate p. 186 is occasionally used orally, but when given alone it may cause postoperative restlessness in the presence of pain.

Benzodiazepines

Benzodiazepines possess useful properties for premedication including relief of anxiety, sedation, and amnesia; short-acting benzodiazepines taken by mouth are the most common premedicants. Benzodiazepines are also used for sedation prior to clinical procedures and for sedation in intensive care.

Benzodiazepines may occasionally cause marked respiratory depression and facilities for its treatment are essential; flumazenil p. 899 is used to antagonise the effects of benzodiazepines.

Midazolam, a water-soluble benzodiazepine, is the preferred benzodiazepine for premedication and for sedation for clinical procedures in children. It has a fast onset of action, and recovery is faster than for other benzodiazepines. Recovery may be longer in children with a low cardiac output, or after repeated dosing.

Midazolam can be given by mouth [unlicensed], but its bitter acidic taste may need to be disguised. It can also be given buccally [unlicensed indication] or intranasally [unlicensed]. Midazolam is associated with profound sedation when high doses are given or when it is used with certain other drugs. It can cause severe disinhibition and restlessness in some children. Midazolam is not recommended for prolonged sedation in neonates; drug accumulation is likely to occur.

Temazepam is given by mouth for premedication in older children and has a short duration of action. Anxiolytic and sedative effects last about 90 minutes, although there may be residual drowsiness. Temazepam is rarely used for dental procedures in children.

Lorazepam p. 238 produces more prolonged sedation than temazepam and it has marked amnesic effects.

Peri-operative use of diazepam p. 236 is not recommended in children; onset and magnitude of response are unreliable, and paradoxical effects may occur. Diazepam is not used for dental procedures in children.

Antagonists for central and respiratory depression

Respiratory depression is a major concern with opioid analgesics and it may be treated by artificial ventilation or be reversed by an opioid antagonist. Naloxone hydrochloride p. 901 given intravenously immediately reverses opioid-induced respiratory depression but the dose may have to be repeated because of its **short duration of action**. Intramuscular injection of naloxone hydrochloride produces a more gradual and prolonged effect but absorption may be erratic. Care is required in children requiring pain relief because naloxone hydrochloride also antagonises the analgesic effect of opioids.

Flumazenil is a benzodiazepine antagonist for the reversal of the central sedative effects of benzodiazepines after anaesthetic and similar procedures. Flumazenil has a shorter half-life and duration of action than diazepam or midazolam so patients may become resedated.

Neonates

Naloxone hydrochloride is used in newborn infants to reverse respiratory depression and sedation resulting from the use of opioids by the mother, usually for pain during labour. In neonates the effects of opioids may persist for up to 48 hours and in such cases naloxone hydrochloride is often given by intramuscular injection for its prolonged effect. In severe respiratory depression after birth, breathing should first be established (using artificial means if necessary) and naloxone hydrochloride administered only if use of opioids by the mother is thought to cause the respiratory depression; the infant should be monitored closely and further doses of naloxone hydrochloride administered as necessary.

ANTIMUSCARINICS

F 527

Atropine sulfate

05-Dec-2019

● **INDICATIONS AND DOSE**

Bradycardia due to acute massive overdosage of beta-blockers

▶ BY INTRAVENOUS INJECTION

▸ Child: 40 micrograms/kg (max. per dose 3 mg)

Treatment of poisoning by organophosphorus insecticide or nerve agent (in combination with pralidoxime chloride)

▶ BY INTRAVENOUS INJECTION

▸ Child: 20 micrograms/kg every 5–10 minutes (max. per dose 2 mg) until the skin becomes flushed and dry, the pupils dilate, and bradycardia is abolished, frequency of administration dependent on the severity of poisoning

Premedication

▶ BY INTRAVENOUS INJECTION

▸ Neonate: 10 micrograms/kg, to be administered immediately before induction of anaesthesia.

▸ Child 1 month–11 years: 20 micrograms/kg, to be administered immediately before induction of anaesthesia (minimum 100 micrograms, max. 600 micrograms)

▸ Child 12–17 years: 300–600 micrograms, to be administered immediately before induction of anaesthesia

▶ BY SUBCUTANEOUS INJECTION, OR BY INTRAMUSCULAR INJECTION

▸ Neonate: 10 micrograms/kg, to be administered 30–60 minutes before induction of anaesthesia.

▸ Child 1 month–11 years: 10–30 micrograms/kg, to be administered 30–60 minutes before induction of anaesthesia (minimum 100 micrograms, max. 600 micrograms)

▸ Child 12–17 years: 300–600 micrograms, to be administered 30–60 minutes before induction of anaesthesia

▶ BY MOUTH

▸ Neonate: 20–40 micrograms/kg, to be administered 1–2 hours before induction of anaesthesia.

▸ Child: 20–40 micrograms/kg (max. per dose 900 micrograms), to be administered 1–2 hours before induction of anaesthesia

Intra-operative bradycardia

▶ BY INTRAVENOUS INJECTION

▸ Neonate: 10–20 micrograms/kg.

▸ Child 1 month–11 years: 10–20 micrograms/kg

▸ Child 12–17 years: 300–600 micrograms, larger doses may be used in emergencies

Control of muscarinic side-effects of neostigmine in reversal of competitive neuromuscular block

▶ BY INTRAVENOUS INJECTION

▸ Neonate: 20 micrograms/kg.

▸ Child 1 month–11 years: 20 micrograms/kg (max. per dose 1.2 mg)

▸ Child 12–17 years: 0.6–1.2 mg

● **UNLICENSED USE** Not licensed for use in children under 12 years for intra-operative bradycardia or by intravenous route for premedication. Not licensed for use by oral route.

IMPORTANT SAFETY INFORMATION

▸ With systemic use for Premedication

Antimuscarinic drugs used for premedication to general anaesthesia should only be administered by, or under the direct supervision of, personnel experienced in their use.

● **INTERACTIONS** → Appendix 1: atropine

● **SIDE-EFFECTS**

▶ **Common or very common**

▸ With intravenous use Abdominal distension · anhidrosis · anxiety · arrhythmias · bronchial secretion decreased · dysphagia · gastrointestinal disorders · hallucination · hyperthermia · movement disorders · mydriasis · speech disorder · taste loss · thirst

▶ **Uncommon**

▸ With intravenous use Psychotic disorder

▶ **Rare or very rare**

▸ With intravenous use Angina pectoris · hypertensive crisis · seizure

▶ **Frequency not known**

▸ With intravenous use Insomnia

▸ With oral use Angle closure glaucoma · arrhythmias · bronchial secretion altered · chest pain · dysphagia · fever · gastrointestinal disorders · mydriasis · staggering · thirst

● **PREGNANCY** Not known to be harmful; manufacturer advises caution.

● **BREAST FEEDING** May suppress lactation; small amount present in milk—manufacturer advises caution.

● **MONITORING REQUIREMENTS**

▸ Control of muscarinic side-effects of neostigmine in reversal of competitive neuromuscular block Since atropine has a shorter duration of action than neostigmine, late unopposed bradycardia may result; close monitoring of the patient is necessary.

● **DIRECTIONS FOR ADMINISTRATION** For administration *by mouth*, injection solution may be given orally.

● **EXCEPTIONS TO LEGAL CATEGORY**

▸ With intramuscular use or intravenous use or subcutaneous use Prescription only medicine restriction does not apply where administration is for saving life in emergency.

● **MEDICINAL FORMS** There can be variation in the licensing of different medicines containing the same drug. Forms available from special-order manufacturers include: oral suspension, oral solution, solution for injection, solution for infusion, eye drops, eye ointment

Tablet

▸ Atropine sulfate (Non-proprietary)

Atropine sulfate 600 microgram Atropine 600microgram tablets | 28 tablet PoM £52.92 DT = £52.92

Solution for injection

▸ Atropine sulfate (Non-proprietary)

Atropine sulfate 100 microgram per 1 ml Atropine 500micrograms/5ml solution for injection pre-filled syringes | 1 pre-filled disposable injection PoM £13.00 | 10 pre-filled disposable injection PoM £130.00

Atropine sulfate 200 microgram per 1 ml Atropine 1mg/5ml solution for injection pre-filled syringes | 1 pre-filled disposable injection PoM £13.00 | 10 pre-filled disposable injection PoM £130.00

Atropine sulfate 300 microgram per 1 ml Atropine 3mg/10ml solution for injection pre-filled syringes | 1 pre-filled disposable injection PoM £7.29–£13.00 DT = £7.29 | 10 pre-filled disposable injection PoM £130.00

Atropine sulfate 600 microgram per 1 ml Atropine 600micrograms/1ml solution for injection ampoules | 10 ampoule PoM £11.71 DT = £11.71

Atropine sulfate 1 mg per 1 ml Atropine 1mg/1ml solution for injection ampoules | 10 ampoule PoM £109.35 DT = £109.35

527

Glycopyrronium bromide (Glycopyrrolate)

19-Dec-2019

● **INDICATIONS AND DOSE**

Premedication at induction

▶ BY INTRAMUSCULAR INJECTION, OR BY INTRAVENOUS INJECTION

▸ Neonate: 5 micrograms/kg.

▸ Child 1 month–11 years: 4–8 micrograms/kg (max. per dose 200 micrograms)
▸ Child 12–17 years: 200–400 micrograms, alternatively 4–5 micrograms/kg (max. per dose 400 micrograms)

Intra-operative bradycardia

▶ BY INTRAVENOUS INJECTION

▸ Neonate: 10 micrograms/kg, repeated if necessary.

▸ Child: 4–8 micrograms/kg (max. per dose 200 micrograms), repeated if necessary

Control of muscarinic side-effects of neostigmine in reversal of non-depolarising neuromuscular block

▶ BY INTRAVENOUS INJECTION

▸ Neonate: 10 micrograms/kg.

▸ Child 1 month–11 years: 10 micrograms/kg (max. per dose 500 micrograms)
▸ Child 12–17 years: 10–15 micrograms/kg, alternatively, 200 micrograms per 1 mg of neostigmine to be administered

Control of upper airways secretion | Hypersalivation

▶ BY MOUTH
▸ Child: 40–100 micrograms/kg 3–4 times a day (max. per dose 2 mg), adjusted according to response, dose to be administered using tablets or injection solution, see *Directions for administration*

▶ BY SUBCUTANEOUS INFUSION
▸ Child 1 month–11 years: 12–40 micrograms/kg (max. per dose 1.2 mg) over 24 hours
▸ Child 12–17 years: 0.6–1.2 mg/24 hours

▶ BY SUBCUTANEOUS INJECTION, OR BY INTRAMUSCULAR INJECTION, OR BY INTRAVENOUS INJECTION
▸ Child 1 month–11 years: 4–10 micrograms/kg 4 times a day (max. per dose 200 micrograms) as required
▸ Child 12–17 years: 200 micrograms every 4 hours as required

SIALANAR® ORAL SOLUTION

Severe sialorrhoea (chronic pathological drooling)

▶ BY MOUTH
▸ Child 3–17 years: (consult product literature)

● **UNLICENSED USE** Not licensed for use in control of upper airways secretion and hypersalivation.

> **IMPORTANT SAFETY INFORMATION**
> Antimuscarinic drugs used for premedication to general anaesthesia should only be administered by, or under the direct supervision of, personnel experienced in their use.

● **CAUTIONS**

SIALANAR® ORAL SOLUTION Compromised blood-brain barrier—monitor for behavioural changes

● **INTERACTIONS** → Appendix 1: glycopyrronium

● **SIDE-EFFECTS**

▶ **Common or very common**
▸ With oral use Akathisia · anxiety · behaviour abnormal · bronchial secretion decreased · concentration impaired · crying · depressed mood · diarrhoea · fever · increased risk of infection · mood altered · nasal congestion

▶ **Uncommon**
▸ With oral use Breath odour · dehydration · eye disorders · gastrointestinal disorders · insomnia · seizure · thirst

▶ **Frequency not known**
▸ With oral use Anhidrosis · dry eye · dysphagia · epistaxis · speech disorder
▸ With parenteral use Anhidrosis · bronchial secretion decreased · mydriasis

● **PREGNANCY**

SIALANAR® ORAL SOLUTION Manufacturer advises avoid—no information available.

● **BREAST FEEDING**

SIALANAR® ORAL SOLUTION Manufacturer advises avoid—no information available.

● **RENAL IMPAIRMENT**

SIALANAR® ORAL SOLUTION Manufacturer advises avoid if estimated glomerular filtration rate is less than 30 mL/minute/1.73 m^2.

Dose adjustments Manufacturer advises reduce dose by 30% if estimated glomerular filtration rate is 30–89 mL/minute/1.73 m^2—consult product literature.

● **DIRECTIONS FOR ADMINISTRATION**

▸ With oral use for Control of upper airways secretion or Hypersalivation For administration *by mouth*, injection solution may be given or crushed tablets suspended in water.

SIALANAR® ORAL SOLUTION Doses should be given at least 1 hour before or 2 hours after food, or at consistent times with respect to food if co-administration with food is required—high-fat food should be avoided; for administration by a nasogastric or feeding tube, flush with 10 mL of water immediately after dosing.

● **PRESCRIBING AND DISPENSING INFORMATION**

▸ With oral use Tablets may be available on a named-patient basis from specialist importing companies.

● **PATIENT AND CARER ADVICE**

SIALANAR® ORAL SOLUTION Manufacturer advises patients and their carers should be informed to stop treatment and seek medical advice if constipation, urinary retention, pneumonia, allergic reaction, pyrexia, or changes in behaviour occur; treatment should also be stopped and medical advice sought in very hot weather.

● **NATIONAL FUNDING/ACCESS DECISIONS**

Scottish Medicines Consortium (SMC) decisions

The *Scottish Medicines Consortium* has advised (July 2017) that glycopyrronium bromide (*Sialanar®*) is accepted for use within NHS Scotland for the symptomatic treatment of severe sialorrhoea (chronic pathological drooling) in children and adolescents aged 3 years and older with chronic neurological disorders.

● **MEDICINAL FORMS** There can be variation in the licensing of different medicines containing the same drug. Forms available from special-order manufacturers include: oral solution

Tablet

▸ Glycopyrronium bromide (Non-proprietary)
Glycopyrronium bromide 1 mg Glycopyrronium bromide 1mg tablets | 30 tablet [PoM] £230.72 DT = £230.71
Glycopyrronium bromide 2 mg Glycopyrronium bromide 2mg tablets | 30 tablet [PoM] £254.24 DT = £254.23

Solution for injection

▸ Glycopyrronium bromide (Non-proprietary)
Glycopyrronium bromide 200 microgram per 1 ml Glycopyrronium bromide 200micrograms/1ml solution for injection ampoules | 10 ampoule [PoM] £14.00 DT = £9.95 | 10 ampoule [PoM] £5.72 DT = £9.95 (Hospital only)
Glycopyrronium bromide 600micrograms/3ml solution for injection ampoules | 3 ampoule [PoM] £8.00 | 10 ampoule [PoM] £9.61 DT = £14.99 (Hospital only) | 10 ampoule [PoM] £14.99 DT = £14.99

Oral solution

- **Glycopyrronium bromide (Non-proprietary)**
  Glycopyrronium bromide 200 microgram per 1 ml Glycopyrronium bromide 1mg/5ml oral solution sugar free sugar-free | 150 ml [PoM] £91.00 DT = £91.00
- **Sialanar** (Proveca Ltd)
  Glycopyrronium bromide 400 microgram per 1 ml Sialanar 320micrograms/ml oral solution sugar-free | 60 ml [PoM] £76.80 DT = £76.80 sugar-free | 250 ml [PoM] £320.00 DT = £320.00

1.1 Neuromuscular blockade

Neuromuscular blockade

Neuromuscular blocking drugs

Neuromuscular blocking drugs used in anaesthesia are also known as **muscle relaxants**. By specific blockade of the neuromuscular junction they enable light anaesthesia to be used with adequate relaxation of the muscles of the abdomen and diaphragm. They also relax the vocal cords and allow the passage of a tracheal tube. Their action differs from the muscle relaxants used in musculoskeletal disorders that act on the spinal cord or brain.

Children who have received a neuromuscular blocking drug should **always** have their respiration assisted or controlled until the drug has been inactivated or antagonised. They should also receive sufficient concomitant inhalational or intravenous anaesthetic or sedative drugs to prevent awareness.

Non-depolarising neuromuscular blocking drugs

Non-depolarising neuromuscular blocking drugs (also known as competitive muscle relaxants) compete with acetylcholine for receptor sites at the neuromuscular junction and their action can be reversed with anticholinesterases such as neostigmine p. 700. Non-depolarising neuromuscular blocking drugs can be divided into the **aminosteroid** group, comprising pancuronium bromide p. 874, rocuronium bromide p. 874, and vecuronium bromide p. 875, and the **benzylisoquinolinium** group, comprising atracurium besilate p. 872, cisatracurium p. 873, and mivacurium p. 873.

Non-depolarising neuromuscular blocking drugs have a slower onset of action than suxamethonium chloride p. 872. These drugs can be classified by their duration of action as short-acting (15–30 minutes), intermediate-acting (30–40 minutes), and long-acting (60–120 minutes), although duration of action is dose-dependent. Drugs with a shorter or intermediate duration of action, such as atracurium besilate and vecuronium bromide p. 875, are more widely used than those with a longer duration of action, such as pancuronium bromide.

Non-depolarising neuromuscular blocking drugs have no sedative or analgesic effects and are not considered to trigger malignant hyperthermia.

For patients receiving intensive care and who require tracheal intubation and mechanical ventilation, a non-depolarising neuromuscular blocking drug is chosen according to its onset of effect, duration of action, and side-effects. Rocuronium bromide, with a rapid onset of effect, may facilitate intubation. Atracurium besilate or cisatracurium may be suitable for long-term neuromuscular blockade since their duration of action is not dependent on elimination by the liver or the kidneys.

Atracurium besilate, a mixture of 10 isomers, is a benzylisoquinolinium neuromuscular blocking drug with an intermediate duration of action. It undergoes non-enzymatic metabolism which is independent of liver and kidney function, thus allowing its use in children with hepatic or renal impairment. Cardiovascular effects are associated with significant histamine release; histamine release can be minimised by administering slowly or in divided doses over at least 1 minute. Neonates may be more sensitive to the effects of atracurium besilate and lower doses may be required.

Cisatracurium is a single isomer of atracurium besilate. It is more potent and has a slightly longer duration of action than atracurium besilate and provides greater cardiovascular stability because cisatracurium lacks histamine-releasing effects. In children aged 1 month to 12 years, cisatracurium has a shorter duration of action and produces faster spontaneous recovery.

Mivacurium, a benzylisoquinolinium neuromuscular blocking drug, has a short duration of action. It is metabolised by plasma cholinesterase and muscle paralysis is prolonged in individuals deficient in this enzyme. It is not associated with vagolytic activity or ganglionic blockade although histamine release can occur, particularly with rapid injection. In children under 12 years mivacurium has a faster onset, shorter duration of action, and produces more rapid spontaneous recovery.

Pancuronium bromide, an aminosteroid neuromuscular blocking drug, has a long duration of action and is often used in children receiving long-term mechanical ventilation in intensive care units. It lacks a histamine-releasing effect, but vagolytic and sympathomimetic effects can cause tachycardia and hypertension. The half-life of pancuronium bromide is prolonged in neonates; neonates should receive postoperative intermittent positive pressure ventilation.

Rocuronium bromide exerts an effect within 2 minutes and has the most rapid onset of any of the non-depolarising neuromuscular blocking drugs. It is an aminosteroid neuromuscular blocking drug with an intermediate duration of action. It is reported to have minimal cardiovascular effects; high doses produce mild vagolytic activity. In most children, the duration of action of rocuronium bromide may be shorter than in adults; however, in neonates and children under 2 years, usual doses may produce a more prolonged action.

Vecuronium bromide p. 875, an aminosteroid neuromuscular blocking drug, has an intermediate duration of action. It does not generally produce histamine release and lacks cardiovascular effects. In most children, the duration of action of vecuronium bromide may be shorter than in adults; however, in neonates and children under 2 years, usual doses may produce a more prolonged action.

Depolarising neuromuscular blocking drugs

Suxamethonium chloride has the most rapid onset of action of any of the neuromuscular blocking drugs and is ideal if fast onset and brief duration of action are required e.g. with tracheal intubation. Neonates and young children are less sensitive to suxamethonium chloride and a higher dose may be required. Unlike the non-depolarising neuromuscular blocking drugs, its action cannot be reversed and recovery is spontaneous; anticholinesterases such as neostigmine potentiate the neuromuscular block.

Suxamethonium chloride should be given after anaesthetic induction because paralysis is usually preceded by painful muscle fasciculations. Bradycardia may occur; premedication with atropine sulfate p. 869 reduces bradycardia as well as the excessive salivation associated with suxamethonium chloride use.

Prolonged paralysis may occur in dual block, which occurs with high or repeated doses of suxamethonium chloride and is caused by the development of a non-depolarising block following the initial depolarising block. Children with myasthenia gravis are resistant to suxamethonium chloride but can develop dual block resulting in delayed recovery. Prolonged paralysis may also occur in those with low or atypical plasma cholinesterase. Assisted ventilation should be continued until muscle function is restored.

NEUROMUSCULAR BLOCKING DRUGS › DEPOLARISING

Suxamethonium chloride

26-Nov-2019

(Succinylcholine chloride)

- **DRUG ACTION** Suxamethonium acts by mimicking acetylcholine at the neuromuscular junction but hydrolysis is much slower than for acetylcholine; depolarisation is therefore prolonged, resulting in neuromuscular blockade.

- **INDICATIONS AND DOSE**

Neuromuscular blockade (short duration) during surgery

▶ BY INTRAVENOUS INJECTION

- Neonate: 2 mg/kg, produces 5–10 minutes neuromuscular blockade.
- Child 1–11 months: 2 mg/kg
- Child 1–17 years: 1 mg/kg

▶ BY INTRAMUSCULAR INJECTION

- Neonate: Up to 4 mg/kg, produces 10–30 minutes neuromuscular blockade.
- Child 1–11 months: Up to 5 mg/kg
- Child 1–11 years: Up to 4 mg/kg (max. per dose 150 mg)

PHARMACOKINETICS

- Intramuscular injection has a duration of onset of 2–3 minutes.

> **IMPORTANT SAFETY INFORMATION**
> Should only be administered by, or under the direct supervision of, personnel experienced in its use.

- **CONTRA-INDICATIONS** Hyperkalaemia · low plasma-cholinesterase activity (including severe liver disease) · major trauma · neurological disease involving acute wasting of major muscle · personal or family history of congenital myotonic disease · personal or family history of malignant hyperthermia · prolonged immobilisation (risk of hyperkalaemia) · severe burns · skeletal muscle myopathies (e.g. Duchenne muscular dystrophy)
- **CAUTIONS** Cardiac disease · neuromuscular disease · raised intra-ocular pressure (avoid in penetrating eye injury) · respiratory disease · severe sepsis (risk of hyperkalaemia)
- **INTERACTIONS** → Appendix 1: suxamethonium
- **SIDE-EFFECTS**
  - **Common or very common** Arrhythmias · flushing · muscle contractions involuntary · myoglobinaemia · myoglobinuria · post procedural muscle pain · rash
  - **Rare or very rare** Apnoea · cardiac arrest · hypersensitivity · malignant hyperthermia · respiratory disorders · trismus

  SIDE-EFFECTS, FURTHER INFORMATION Premedication with atropine reduces bradycardia associated with suxamethonium use.
- **ALLERGY AND CROSS-SENSITIVITY** Allergic cross-reactivity between neuromuscular blocking drugs has been reported; caution is advised in cases of hypersensitivity to these drugs.
- **PREGNANCY** Mildly prolonged maternal neuromuscular blockade may occur.
- **BREAST FEEDING** Unlikely to be present in breast milk in significant amounts (ionised at physiological pH). Breast-feeding may be resumed once the mother recovered from neuromuscular block.
- **HEPATIC IMPAIRMENT** Manufacturer advises caution, particularly in end stage hepatic failure (increased risk of prolonged apnoea due to reduced hepatic synthesis of plasma cholinesterase).
- **DIRECTIONS FOR ADMINISTRATION** For *intravenous injection*, give undiluted or dilute with Glucose 5% or Sodium Chloride 0.9%.
- **MEDICINAL FORMS** There can be variation in the licensing of different medicines containing the same drug. Forms available from special-order manufacturers include: solution for injection

Solution for injection

- Suxamethonium chloride (Non-proprietary)
  Suxamethonium chloride 50 mg per 1 ml Suxamethonium chloride 100mg/2ml solution for injection ampoules | 10 ampoule PoM £28.80–£50.00
- Anectine (Aspen Pharma Trading Ltd)
  Suxamethonium chloride 50 mg per 1 ml Anectine 100mg/2ml solution for injection ampoules | 5 ampoule PoM £3.57 (Hospital only)

NEUROMUSCULAR BLOCKING DRUGS › NON-DEPOLARISING

Non-depolarising neuromuscular blocking drugs

> **IMPORTANT SAFETY INFORMATION**
> Non-depolarising neuromuscular blocking drugs should only be administered by, or under direct supervision of, personnel experienced in their use, with adequate training in anaesthesia and airway management.

- **CAUTIONS** Burns (resistance can develop, increased doses may be required) · cardiovascular disease (reduce rate of administration) · electrolyte disturbances (response unpredictable) · fluid disturbances (response unpredictable) · hypothermia (activity prolonged, lower doses required) · myasthenia gravis (activity prolonged, lower doses required) · neuromuscular disorders (response unpredictable)
- **SIDE-EFFECTS**
  - **Common or very common** Flushing · hypotension
  - **Uncommon** Bronchospasm · hypersensitivity · skin reactions · tachycardia
  - **Rare or very rare** Circulatory collapse · muscle weakness (after prolonged use in intensive care) · myopathy (after prolonged use in intensive care) · shock
- **ALLERGY AND CROSS-SENSITIVITY** Allergic cross-reactivity between neuromuscular blocking drugs has been reported; caution is advised in cases of hypersensitivity to these drugs.
- **PREGNANCY** Non-depolarising neuromuscular blocking drugs are highly ionised at physiological pH and are therefore unlikely to cross the placenta in significant amounts.
- **BREAST FEEDING** Non-depolarising neuromuscular blocking drugs are ionised at physiological pH and are unlikely to be present in milk in significant amounts. Breast-feeding may be resumed once the mother has recovered from neuromuscular block.

above

Atracurium besilate

(Atracurium besylate)

- **INDICATIONS AND DOSE**

Neuromuscular blockade (short to intermediate duration) for surgery

▶ INITIALLY BY INTRAVENOUS INJECTION

- Neonate: Initially 300–500 micrograms/kg, followed by (by intravenous injection) 100–200 micrograms/kg, repeated if necessary, alternatively (by intravenous infusion) 300–400 micrograms/kg/hour, adjusted according to response.

- Child: Initially 300–600 micrograms/kg, then (by intravenous injection) 100–200 micrograms/kg, repeated if necessary, alternatively (by intravenous injection) initially 300–600 micrograms/kg, followed by (by intravenous infusion) 300–600 micrograms/kg/hour, adjusted according to response

Neuromuscular blockade during intensive care

- INITIALLY BY INTRAVENOUS INJECTION
- Neonate: Initially 300–500 micrograms/kg, followed by (by intravenous injection) 100–200 micrograms/kg, repeated if necessary, alternatively (by intravenous infusion) 300–400 micrograms/kg/hour, adjusted according to response, higher doses may be necessary.
- Child: Initially 300–600 micrograms/kg, initial dose is optional, then (by intravenous infusion) 270–1770 micrograms/kg/hour; (by intravenous infusion) usual dose 650–780 micrograms/kg/hour

DOSES AT EXTREMES OF BODY-WEIGHT

- To avoid excessive dosage in obese patients, dose should be calculated on the basis of ideal body-weight.

- **UNLICENSED USE** Not licensed for use in neonates.
- **INTERACTIONS** → Appendix 1: neuromuscular blocking drugs, non-depolarising
- **SIDE-EFFECTS**
  - **Rare or very rare** Cardiac arrest
  - **Frequency not known** Seizure

SIDE-EFFECTS, FURTHER INFORMATION Hypotension, skin flushing, and bronchospasm is associated with histamine release. Manufacturer advises minimising effects of histamine release by administering over 1 minute in patients with cardiovascular disease or sensitivity to hypotension. Neonates may be more sensitive to the effects of atracurium and lower doses may be required.

- **DIRECTIONS FOR ADMINISTRATION** For *continuous intravenous infusion*, dilute to a concentration of 0.5–5 mg/mL with Glucose 5% or Sodium Chloride 0.9%; stability varies with diluent.
  - In neonates *Neonatal intensive care*, dilute 60 mg/kg body-weight to a final volume of 50 mL with Glucose 5% or Sodium Chloride 0.9%; minimum concentration of 500 micrograms/mL, maximum concentration of 5 mg/mL; an intravenous infusion rate of 0.1 mL/hour provides a dose of 120 micrograms/kg/hour.

- **MEDICINAL FORMS** There can be variation in the licensing of different medicines containing the same drug. Forms available from special-order manufacturers include: solution for injection

Solution for injection

- Atracurium besilate (Non-proprietary)
  Atracurium besilate 10 mg per 1 ml Atracurium besilate 250mg/25ml solution for injection vials | 1 vial PoM £16.50 (Hospital only)
  Atracurium besilate 25mg/2.5ml solution for injection ampoules | 5 ampoule PoM £9.25 (Hospital only) | 5 ampoule PoM £11.50 | 10 ampoule PoM £18.50 | 10 ampoule PoM £16.56 (Hospital only)
  Atracurium besilate 50mg/5ml solution for injection ampoules | 5 ampoule PoM £17.50 (Hospital only) | 5 ampoule PoM £17.50 | 10 ampoule PoM £35.00 | 10 ampoule PoM £30.04 (Hospital only)
- Tracrium (Aspen Pharma Trading Ltd)
  Atracurium besilate 10 mg per 1 ml Tracrium 250mg/25ml solution for injection vials | 2 vial PoM £25.81 (Hospital only)
  Tracrium 25mg/2.5ml solution for injection ampoules | 5 ampoule PoM £8.28 (Hospital only)
  Tracrium 50mg/5ml solution for injection ampoules | 5 ampoule PoM £15.02 (Hospital only)

F 872

Cisatracurium

- **INDICATIONS AND DOSE**

Neuromuscular blockade (intermediate duration) during surgery

- INITIALLY BY INTRAVENOUS INJECTION
- Child 1 month–1 year: Initially 150 micrograms/kg, then (by intravenous injection) 30 micrograms/kg every 20 minutes as required
- Child 2–11 years: Initially 150 micrograms/kg, 80–100 micrograms/kg if not for intubation, then (by intravenous injection) 20 micrograms/kg every 10 minutes as required, alternatively (by intravenous injection) initially 150 micrograms/kg, followed by (by intravenous infusion) 180 micrograms/kg/hour, (by intravenous infusion) reduced to 60–120 micrograms/kg/hour, adjusted according to response
- Child 12–17 years: Initially 150 micrograms/kg, then (by intravenous injection) 30 micrograms/kg every 20 minutes as required, alternatively (by intravenous injection) initially 150 micrograms/kg, followed by (by intravenous infusion) 180 micrograms/kg/hour, (by intravenous infusion) reduced to 60–120 micrograms/kg/hour, adjusted according to response

DOSES AT EXTREMES OF BODY-WEIGHT

- To avoid excessive dosage in obese patients, dose should be calculated on the basis of ideal body-weight.

- **INTERACTIONS** → Appendix 1: neuromuscular blocking drugs, non-depolarising
- **SIDE-EFFECTS**
  - **Common or very common** Bradycardia
- **DIRECTIONS FOR ADMINISTRATION** For *continuous intravenous infusion*, dilute to a concentration of 0.1–2 mg/mL with Glucose 5% or Sodium Chloride 0.9%; solutions of 2 mg/mL and 5 mg/mL may be infused undiluted.

- **MEDICINAL FORMS** There can be variation in the licensing of different medicines containing the same drug.

Solution for injection

- Cisatracurium (Non-proprietary)
  Cisatracurium (as Cisatracurium besilate) 2 mg per 1 ml Cisatracurium besilate 10mg/5ml solution for injection ampoules | 5 ampoule PoM 🅇 (Hospital only)
  Cisatracurium besilate 20mg/10ml solution for injection ampoules | 5 ampoule PoM £37.75 (Hospital only) | 5 ampoule PoM £32.09-£37.75 | 10 ampoule PoM £75.50
  Cisatracurium besilate 20mg/10ml solution for injection vials | 5 vial PoM £37.75 (Hospital only)
  Cisatracurium (as Cisatracurium besilate) 5 mg per 1 ml Cisatracurium besilate 150mg/30ml solution for injection vials | 1 vial PoM £45.00 (Hospital only) | 1 vial PoM £26.43
- Nimbex (Aspen Pharma Trading Ltd)
  Cisatracurium (as Cisatracurium besilate) 2 mg per 1 ml Nimbex 20mg/10ml solution for injection ampoules | 5 ampoule PoM £37.75
  Cisatracurium (as Cisatracurium besilate) 5 mg per 1 ml Nimbex Forte 150mg/30ml solution for injection vials | 1 vial PoM £31.09

F 872

Mivacurium

- **INDICATIONS AND DOSE**

Neuromuscular blockade (short duration) during surgery

- INITIALLY BY INTRAVENOUS INJECTION
- Child 2–5 months: Initially 150 micrograms/kg, then (by intravenous injection) 100 micrograms/kg every 6–9 minutes as required, alternatively (by intravenous infusion) 8–10 micrograms/kg/minute, (by intravenous infusion) adjusted in steps of continued →

1 microgram/kg/minute every 3 minutes if required; (by intravenous infusion) usual dose 11–14 micrograms/kg/minute
- Child 6 months–11 years: Initially 200 micrograms/kg, then (by intravenous injection) 100 micrograms/kg every 6–9 minutes as required, alternatively (by intravenous infusion) 8–10 micrograms/kg/minute, (by intravenous infusion) adjusted in steps of 1 microgram/kg/minute every 3 minutes if required; (by intravenous infusion) usual dose 11–14 micrograms/kg/minute
- Child 12–17 years: Initially 70–250 micrograms/kg, then (by intravenous injection) 100 micrograms/kg every 15 minutes as required, alternatively (by intravenous infusion) 8–10 micrograms/kg/minute, (by intravenous infusion) adjusted in steps of 1 microgram/kg/minute every 3 minutes if required; (by intravenous infusion) usual dose 6–7 micrograms/kg/minute

DOSES AT EXTREMES OF BODY-WEIGHT
- To avoid excessive dosage in obese patients, dose should be calculated on the basis of ideal body-weight.

- **CAUTIONS** Burns (low plasma cholinesterase activity; dose titration required)
- **INTERACTIONS** → Appendix 1: neuromuscular blocking drugs, non-depolarising
- **HEPATIC IMPAIRMENT** Manufacturer advises caution in hepatic failure (increased duration of action).
  Dose adjustments Manufacturer advises dose reduction in hepatic failure.
- **RENAL IMPAIRMENT**
  Dose adjustments Clinical effect prolonged in renal failure—reduce dose according to response.
- **DIRECTIONS FOR ADMINISTRATION** For *intravenous injection*, give undiluted or dilute in Glucose 5% or Sodium Chloride 0.9%. Doses up to 150 micrograms/kg may be given over 5–15 seconds, higher doses should be given over 30 seconds. In asthma, cardiovascular disease or in those sensitive to reduced arterial blood pressure, give over 60 seconds.

- **MEDICINAL FORMS** There can be variation in the licensing of different medicines containing the same drug.

Solution for injection
- Mivacron (Aspen Pharma Trading Ltd)
  Mivacurium (as Mivacurium chloride) 2 mg per 1 ml Mivacron 10mg/5ml solution for injection ampoules | 5 ampoule [PoM] £13.95 (Hospital only)
  Mivacron 20mg/10ml solution for injection ampoules | 5 ampoule [PoM] £22.57 (Hospital only)

F 872

Pancuronium bromide

- **INDICATIONS AND DOSE**

Neuromuscular blockade (long duration) during surgery
- BY INTRAVENOUS INJECTION
- Neonate: Initially 100 micrograms/kg, then 50 micrograms/kg, repeated if necessary.
- Child: Initially 100 micrograms/kg, then 20 micrograms/kg, repeated if necessary

DOSES AT EXTREMES OF BODY-WEIGHT
- To avoid excessive dosage in obese patients, dose should be calculated on the basis of ideal body-weight.

- **INTERACTIONS** → Appendix 1: neuromuscular blocking drugs, non-depolarising
- **SIDE-EFFECTS** Apnoea · arrhythmia · hypersalivation · increased cardiac output · miosis
  SIDE-EFFECTS, FURTHER INFORMATION Pancuronium lacks histamine-releasing effect, but vagolytic and sympathomimetic effects can cause tachycardia.
- **HEPATIC IMPAIRMENT** Manufacturer advises caution (possibly slower onset and higher dose requirements due to resistance to neuromuscular blocking action which may lead to a prolonged recovery time).
- **RENAL IMPAIRMENT** Use with caution; prolonged duration of block.
- **DIRECTIONS FOR ADMINISTRATION** For *intravenous injection*, give undiluted or dilute in Glucose 5% or Sodium Chloride 0.9%.

- **MEDICINAL FORMS** There can be variation in the licensing of different medicines containing the same drug.

Solution for injection
- Pancuronium bromide (Non-proprietary)
  Pancuronium bromide 2 mg per 1 ml Pancuronium bromide 4mg/2ml solution for injection ampoules | 10 ampoule [PoM] £50.00 (Hospital only)

F 872

Rocuronium bromide

- **INDICATIONS AND DOSE**

Neuromuscular blockade (intermediate duration) during surgery
- INITIALLY BY INTRAVENOUS INJECTION
- Neonate: Initially 600 micrograms/kg, then (by intravenous injection) 150 micrograms/kg, repeated if necessary, alternatively (by intravenous infusion) 300–600 micrograms/kg/hour, adjusted according to response.
- Child: Initially 600 micrograms/kg, then (by intravenous injection) 150 micrograms/kg, repeated if necessary, alternatively (by intravenous infusion) 300–600 micrograms/kg/hour, adjusted according to response

Assisted ventilation in intensive care
- INITIALLY BY INTRAVENOUS INJECTION
- Child: Initially 600 micrograms/kg, initial dose is optional, then (by intravenous infusion) 300–600 micrograms/kg/hour for first hour, then (by intravenous infusion), adjusted according to response

DOSES AT EXTREMES OF BODY-WEIGHT
- To avoid excessive dosage in obese patients, dose should be calculated on the basis of ideal body-weight.

- **UNLICENSED USE** Not licensed for use in children for assisted ventilation in intensive care.
- **INTERACTIONS** → Appendix 1: neuromuscular blocking drugs, non-depolarising
- **SIDE-EFFECTS**
  - **Uncommon** Procedural complications
  - **Rare or very rare** Angioedema · face oedema · malignant hyperthermia · paralysis
- **HEPATIC IMPAIRMENT** Manufacturer advises caution (may prolong duration of action).
  Dose adjustments Manufacturer advises consider dose reduction—consult product literature.
- **RENAL IMPAIRMENT**
  Dose adjustments Reduce maintenance dose; prolonged paralysis.
- **DIRECTIONS FOR ADMINISTRATION** For *continuous intravenous infusion* or via drip tubing, may be diluted with Glucose 5% or Sodium Chloride 0.9%.

- **MEDICINAL FORMS** There can be variation in the licensing of different medicines containing the same drug.

Solution for injection
- Rocuronium bromide (Non-proprietary)
  Rocuronium bromide 10 mg per 1 ml Rocuronium bromide 50mg/5ml solution for injection ampoules | 10 ampoule [PoM] £24.00–£28.00

Rocuronium bromide 50mg/5ml solution for injection vials | 10 vial PoM £28.00–£38.30 | 10 vial PoM £28.00 (Hospital only)
Rocuronium bromide 100mg/10ml solution for injection vials | 10 vial PoM £57.00–£76.70 | 10 vial PoM £57.00 (Hospital only)
Rocuronium bromide 100mg/10ml solution for injection ampoules | 10 ampoule PoM £57.00

- Esmeron (Merck Sharp & Dohme Ltd)
  Rocuronium bromide 10 mg per 1 ml Esmeron 50mg/5ml solution for injection vials | 10 vial PoM £28.92 (Hospital only)

F 872

Vecuronium bromide

22-May-2019

- **INDICATIONS AND DOSE**

Neuromuscular blockade (intermediate duration) during surgery

- BY INTRAVENOUS INJECTION
- Neonate: (consult product literature).
- Child: (consult product literature)

DOSES AT EXTREMES OF BODY-WEIGHT

- To avoid excessive dosage in obese patients, dose should be calculated on the basis of ideal body-weight.

- **INTERACTIONS** → Appendix 1: neuromuscular blocking drugs, non-depolarising
- **SIDE-EFFECTS**
- **Uncommon** Procedural complications
- **Rare or very rare** Angioedema · face oedema · paralysis
- **HEPATIC IMPAIRMENT** Manufacturer advises caution in significant impairment.
- **RENAL IMPAIRMENT** Use with caution.
- **MEDICINAL FORMS** There can be variation in the licensing of different medicines containing the same drug.

Powder for solution for injection

- Vecuronium bromide (Non-proprietary)
  Vecuronium bromide 10 mg Vecuronium bromide 10mg powder for solution for injection vials | 10 vial PoM £57.85 (Hospital only)

1.2 Neuromuscular blockade reversal

Neuromuscular blockade reversal

Neuromuscular blockade reversal

Anticholinesterases

Anticholinesterases reverse the effects of the non-depolarising (competitive) neuromuscular blocking drugs such as pancuronium bromide p. 874 but they prolong the action of the depolarising neuromuscular blocking drug suxamethonium chloride p. 872.

Neostigmine p. 700 is used specifically for reversal of non-depolarising (competitive) blockade. It acts within one minute of intravenous injection and its effects last for 20 to 30 minutes; a second dose may then be necessary. Glycopyrronium bromide p. 870 or alternatively atropine sulfate p. 869, given before or with neostigmine, prevent bradycardia, excessive salivation, and other muscarinic effects of neostigmine.

Other drugs for reversal of neuromuscular blockade

Sugammadex below is a modified gamma cyclodextrin that can be used in children for the routine reversal of neuromuscular blockade induced by rocuronium bromide p. 874.

ANTICHOLINESTERASES

Neostigmine with glycopyrronium bromide

The properties listed below are those particular to the combination only. For the properties of the components please consider, neostigmine p. 700, glycopyrronium bromide p. 870.

- **INDICATIONS AND DOSE**

Reversal of non-depolarising neuromuscular blockade

- BY INTRAVENOUS INJECTION
- Child: 0.02 mL/kilogram, repeated if necessary, alternatively dilute to 1 in 10 solution and give 0.2 mL/kg; maximum 2 mL per course

- **INTERACTIONS** → Appendix 1: glycopyrronium · neostigmine
- **DIRECTIONS FOR ADMINISTRATION** For *intravenous injection,* may be diluted with Sodium Chloride 0.9%, give over 10–30 seconds
- **MEDICINAL FORMS** There can be variation in the licensing of different medicines containing the same drug.

Solution for injection

- Neostigmine with glycopyrronium bromide (Non-proprietary)
  Glycopyrronium bromide 500 microgram per 1 ml, Neostigmine metilsulfate 2.5 mg per 1 ml Neostigmine 2.5mg/1ml / Glycopyrronium bromide 500micrograms/1ml solution for injection ampoules | 10 ampoule PoM £11.50

ANTIDOTES AND CHELATORS

Sugammadex

18-Nov-2019

- **INDICATIONS AND DOSE**

Routine reversal of neuromuscular blockade induced by rocuronium

- BY INTRAVENOUS INJECTION
- Child 2–17 years: 2 mg/kg (consult product literature)

> IMPORTANT SAFETY INFORMATION
> Should only be administered by, or under the direct supervision of, personnel experienced in its use.

- **CAUTIONS** Cardiovascular disease (recovery may be delayed) · pre-existing coagulation disorders · recurrence of neuromuscular blockade— monitor respiratory function until fully recovered · use of anticoagulants (unrelated to surgery) · wait 24 hours before re-administering rocuronium
- **INTERACTIONS** → Appendix 1: sugammadex
- **SIDE-EFFECTS**
- **Common or very common** Abdominal pain · arrhythmias · cough · dizziness · headache · nausea · procedural complications · skin reactions · taste altered · vomiting
- **Uncommon** Hypersensitivity
- **Frequency not known** Bronchospasm
- **PREGNANCY** Use with caution—no information available.
- **RENAL IMPAIRMENT** Avoid if estimated glomerular filtration rate less than 30 mL/minute/1.73 m^2.
- **DIRECTIONS FOR ADMINISTRATION** For *intravenous injection* dose may be diluted to a concentration of 10 mg/mL with Sodium Chloride 0.9%.
- **NATIONAL FUNDING/ACCESS DECISIONS**

Scottish Medicines Consortium (SMC) decisions

The *Scottish Medicines Consortium*, has advised (February 2013) that sugammadex (*Bridion*®) is accepted for restricted use within NHS Scotland for the routine reversal of neuromuscular blockade in high-risk patients only, or where prompt reversal of neuromuscular block is required.

- **MEDICINAL FORMS** There can be variation in the licensing of different medicines containing the same drug.

Solution for injection

ELECTROLYTES: May contain Sodium

- ▸ **Bridion** (Merck Sharp & Dohme Ltd)

Sugammadex (as Sugammadex sodium) 100 mg per 1 ml Bridion 500mg/5ml solution for injection vials | 10 vial PoM £1,491.00 (Hospital only)

Bridion 200mg/2ml solution for injection vials | 10 vial PoM £596.40 (Hospital only)

1.3 Peri-operative analgesia

Peri-operative analgesia

Non-opioid analgesics

Since non-steroidal anti-inflammatory drugs (NSAIDs) do not depress respiration, do not impair gastro-intestinal motility, and do not cause dependence, they may be useful alternatives or adjuncts to opioids for the relief of postoperative pain. NSAIDs may be inadequate for the relief of severe pain.

Diclofenac sodium p. 704, diclofenac potassium p. 704, ibuprofen p. 707, paracetamol p. 288, and ketorolac trometamol below are used to relieve postoperative pain in children; diclofenac sodium and paracetamol can be given parenterally and rectally as well as by mouth. Ketorolac trometamol is given by intravenous injection.

Opioid analgesics

Opioid analgesics are now rarely used as premedicants; they are more likely to be administered at induction. Pre-operative use of opioid analgesics is generally limited to children who require control of existing pain. The main side-effects of opioid analgesics are respiratory depression, cardiovascular depression, nausea, and vomiting; see general notes on opioid analgesics and their use in postoperative pain.

See the management of opioid-induced respiratory depression in Pre-medication and peri-operative drugs p. 868.

Intra-operative analgesia

Opioid analgesics given in small doses before or with induction reduce the dose requirement of some drugs used during anaesthesia.

Alfentanil p. 877, fentanyl p. 296, and remifentanil p. 878 are particularly useful because they act within 1–2 minutes and have short durations of action. The initial doses of alfentanil or fentanyl are followed either by successive intravenous injections or by an intravenous infusion; prolonged infusions increase the duration of effect.

In contrast to other opioids which are metabolised in the liver, remifentanil undergoes rapid metabolism by nonspecific blood and tissue esterases; its short duration of action allows prolonged administration at high dosage, without accumulation, and with little risk of residual postoperative respiratory depression. Remifentanil should not be given by intravenous injection intraoperatively, but it is well suited to continuous infusion; a supplementary analgesic is given before stopping the infusion of remifentanil.

ANALGESICS > NON-STEROIDAL ANTI-INFLAMMATORY DRUGS

Ketorolac trometamol

17-Apr-2020

- **INDICATIONS AND DOSE**

Short-term management of moderate to severe acute postoperative pain only

▸ BY INTRAMUSCULAR INJECTION, OR BY INTRAVENOUS INJECTION

- ▸ Child 16–17 years (body-weight up to 50 kg): Initially 10 mg, then 10–30 mg every 4–6 hours as required for maximum duration of treatment 2 days, frequency may be increased to up to every 2 hours during initial postoperative period; maximum 60 mg per day
- ▸ Child 16–17 years (body-weight 50 kg and above): Initially 10 mg, then 10–30 mg every 4–6 hours as required for maximum duration of treatment 2 days, frequency may be increased to up to every 2 hours during initial postoperative period; maximum 90 mg per day

▸ BY INTRAVENOUS INJECTION

- ▸ Child 6 months–15 years: Initially 0.5–1 mg/kg (max. per dose 15 mg), then 500 micrograms/kg every 6 hours (max. per dose 15 mg) as required for maximum duration of treatment 2 days; maximum 60 mg per day

- **UNLICENSED USE** Not licensed for use in children under 16 years.
- **CONTRA-INDICATIONS** Active or history of gastro-intestinal bleeding · active or history of gastro-intestinal ulceration · coagulation disorders · complete or partial syndrome of nasal polyps · confirmed or suspected cerebrovascular bleeding · dehydration · following operations with high risk of haemorrhage or incomplete haemostasis · haemorrhagic diatheses · history of gastro-intestinal bleeding related to previous NSAID therapy · history of gastro-intestinal perforation related to previous NSAID therapy · hypovolaemia · severe heart failure
- **CAUTIONS** Allergic disorders · cardiac impairment (NSAIDs may impair renal function) · cerebrovascular disease · connective-tissue disorders · heart failure · history of gastro-intestinal disorders (e.g. ulcerative colitis, Crohn's disease) · ischaemic heart disease · peripheral arterial disease · risk factors for cardiovascular events · uncontrolled hypertension
- **INTERACTIONS** → Appendix 1: NSAIDs
- **SIDE-EFFECTS**

▸ **Common or very common** Headache · hypersensitivity · paraesthesia

▸ **Frequency not known** Agranulocytosis · angioedema · anxiety · aplastic anaemia · appetite decreased · asthenia · asthma · azotaemia · bradycardia · burping · chest pain · concentration impaired · confusion · constipation · Crohn's disease aggravated · depression · diarrhoea · dizziness · drowsiness · dry mouth · dyspnoea · electrolyte imbalance · embolism and thrombosis · euphoric mood · fever · flank pain · fluid retention · flushing · gastrointestinal discomfort · gastrointestinal disorders · haemolytic anaemia · haemorrhage · hallucination · hearing loss · heart failure · hepatic disorders · hyperhidrosis · hyperkinesia · hypertension · hypotension · infertility female · malaise · meningitis aseptic (patients with connective-tissue disorders such as systemic lupus erythematosus may be especially susceptible) · musculoskeletal disorder · myalgia · myocardial infarction · nausea · nephritis tubulointerstitial · nephropathy · neutropenia · oedema · optic neuritis · oral disorders · pallor · palpitations · pancreatitis · perforation · photosensitivity reaction · platelet aggregation inhibition · psychotic disorder · pulmonary oedema · renal impairment · respiratory disorders · seizure · severe cutaneous adverse reactions

(SCARs) · skin reactions · sleep disorders · stroke · taste altered · thinking abnormal · thirst · thrombocytopenia · tinnitus · ulcer · urinary disorders · vertigo · visual impairment · vomiting · weight increased · wound haemorrhage

SIDE-EFFECTS, FURTHER INFORMATION For information about cardiovascular and gastrointestinal side-effects, and a possible exacerbation of symptoms in asthma, see Non-steroidal anti-inflammatory drugs. p. 703

- **ALLERGY AND CROSS-SENSITIVITY** Contra-indicated in patients with a history of hypersensitivity to aspirin or any other NSAID—which includes those in whom attacks of asthma, angioedema, urticaria or rhinitis have been precipitated by aspirin or any other NSAID.
- **PREGNANCY** Avoid unless the potential benefit outweighs the risk. Avoid during the third trimester (risk of closure of fetal ductus arteriosus *in utero* and possibly persistent pulmonary hypertension of the newborn); onset of labour may be delayed and duration may be increased.
- **BREAST FEEDING** Amount too small to be harmful.
- **HEPATIC IMPAIRMENT** Manufacturer advises caution—may increase risk of renal impairment; avoid in hepatic failure.
- **RENAL IMPAIRMENT** Avoid if possible or use with caution. Avoid if serum creatinine greater than 160 micromol/litre.
  Dose adjustments The lowest effective dose should be used for the shortest possible duration. Max. 60 mg daily by intramuscular injection or intravenous injection.
  Monitoring In renal impairment monitor renal function; sodium and water retention may occur and renal function may deteriorate, possibly leading to renal failure.
- **DIRECTIONS FOR ADMINISTRATION** For *intravenous injection*, give over at least 15 seconds.

- **MEDICINAL FORMS** There can be variation in the licensing of different medicines containing the same drug.

Solution for injection

- Ketorolac trometamol (Non-proprietary)
  Ketorolac trometamol 30 mg per 1 ml Ketorolac 30mg/1ml solution for injection ampoules | 5 ampoule PoM £20.00-£30.00 DT = £5.36 (Hospital only)
- Toradol (Atnahs Pharma UK Ltd)
  Ketorolac trometamol 30 mg per 1 ml Toradol 30mg/1ml solution for injection ampoules | 5 ampoule PoM £5.36 DT = £5.36 (Hospital only)

ANALGESICS > OPIOIDS

F 290

Alfentanil

- **INDICATIONS AND DOSE**

Assisted ventilation: analgesia and enhancement of anaesthesia for short procedures

▶ BY INTRAVENOUS INJECTION

- Neonate: Initially 5–20 micrograms/kg, dose to be administered over 30 seconds; supplemental doses up to 10 micrograms/kg.
- Child: Initially 10–20 micrograms/kg, dose to be administered over 30 seconds; supplemental doses up to 10 micrograms/kg

Assisted ventilation: analgesia and enhancement of anaesthesia during maintenance of anaesthesia for longer procedures

▶ BY INTRAVENOUS INFUSION

- Neonate: Initially 10–50 micrograms/kg, dose to be administered over 10 minutes, followed by 30–60 micrograms/kg/hour.
- Child: Initially 50–100 micrograms/kg, dose to be administered over 10 minutes, followed by 30–120 micrograms/kg/hour, usual dose with intravenous anaesthetic, 60 micrograms/kg/hour

DOSES AT EXTREMES OF BODY-WEIGHT

- To avoid excessive dosage in obese patients, dose should be calculated on the basis of ideal body-weight.

PHARMACOKINETICS

- Half-life is prolonged in neonates and accumulation is likely with prolonged use. Clearance may be increased in children 1 month–12 years and higher infusion doses might be needed.

- **CAUTIONS**

CAUTIONS, FURTHER INFORMATION

- Repeated intra-operative doses Repeated intra-operative doses of alfentanil should be given with care since the resulting respiratory depression can persist postoperatively and occasionally it may become apparent for the first time postoperatively when monitoring of the patient might be less intensive.

- **INTERACTIONS** → Appendix 1: opioids
- **SIDE-EFFECTS**
  - **Common or very common** Apnoea · chills · fatigue · hypertension · movement disorders · muscle rigidity · procedural complications
  - **Uncommon** Coma · hiccups · hypercapnia · pain · post procedural complications · respiratory disorders
  - **Rare or very rare** Agitation · crying · epistaxis · vascular pain
  - **Frequency not known** Cardiac arrest · cough · fever · loss of consciousness · seizure

  SIDE-EFFECTS, FURTHER INFORMATION Alfentanil can cause muscle rigidity, particularly of the chest wall or jaw; this can be managed by the use of neuromuscular blocking drugs.
- **BREAST FEEDING** Present in milk—withhold breast-feeding for 24 hours.
- **HEPATIC IMPAIRMENT** Manufacturer advises caution.
  Dose adjustments Manufacturer advises dose reduction and cautious titration.
- **RENAL IMPAIRMENT** Avoid use or reduce dose; opioid effects increased and prolonged and increased cerebral sensitivity occurs.
- **DIRECTIONS FOR ADMINISTRATION** 5 mg/mL injection to be diluted before use. For *continuous or intermittent intravenous infusion* dilute in Glucose 5% *or* Sodium Chloride 0.9%.

- **MEDICINAL FORMS** There can be variation in the licensing of different medicines containing the same drug. Forms available from special-order manufacturers include: solution for injection

Solution for injection

- Alfentanil (Non-proprietary)
  Alfentanil (as Alfentanil hydrochloride) 500 microgram per 1 ml Alfentanil 1mg/2ml solution for injection ampoules | 10 ampoule PoM £5.95 DT = £6.34 CD2
  Alfentanil 25mg/50ml solution for injection vials | 1 vial PoM £14.90 CD2
  Alfentanil 5mg/10ml solution for injection ampoules | 10 ampoule PoM £27.80 DT = £27.80 CD2
  Alfentanil (as Alfentanil hydrochloride) 5 mg per 1 ml Alfentanil 5mg/1ml solution for injection ampoules | 10 ampoule PoM £21.95 DT = £23.19 CD2
- Rapifen (Piramal Critical Care Ltd)
  Alfentanil (as Alfentanil hydrochloride) 500 microgram per 1 ml Rapifen 5mg/10ml solution for injection ampoules | 5 ampoule PoM £16.00 DT = £14.50 CD2
  Rapifen 1mg/2ml solution for injection ampoules | 10 ampoule PoM £6.34 DT = £6.34 CD2
  Alfentanil (as Alfentanil hydrochloride) 5 mg per 1 ml Rapifen Intensive Care 5mg/1ml solution for injection ampoules | 10 ampoule PoM £23.19 DT = £23.19 (Hospital only) CD2

15 Anaesthesia

F 290

Remifentanil

● **INDICATIONS AND DOSE**

Analgesia and enhancement of anaesthesia at induction (initial bolus injection)

▶ BY INTRAVENOUS INJECTION

▶ Child 12–17 years: Initially 0.25–1 microgram/kg, dose to be administered over at least 30 seconds, if child is to be intubated more than 8 minutes after start of intravenous infusion, initial bolus intravenous injection dose is not necessary

Analgesia and enhancement of anaesthesia at induction with or without initial bolus dose

▶ BY INTRAVENOUS INFUSION

▶ Child 12–17 years: 30–60 micrograms/kg/hour, if child is to be intubated more than 8 minutes after start of intravenous infusion, initial bolus intravenous injection dose is not necessary

Assisted ventilation: analgesia and enhancement of anaesthesia during maintenance of anaesthesia (initial bolus injection)

▶ BY INTRAVENOUS INJECTION

▶ Child 1 month–11 years: Initially 0.1–1 microgram/kg, dose to be administered over at least 30 seconds (omitted if not required)

▶ Child 12–17 years: Initially 0.1–1 microgram/kg, dose to be administered over at least 30 seconds (omitted if not required)

Assisted ventilation: analgesia and enhancement of anaesthesia during maintenance of anaesthesia with or without initial bolus dose

▶ BY INTRAVENOUS INFUSION

▶ Neonate: 24–60 micrograms/kg/hour, additional doses of 1 microgram/kg can be given *by intravenous injection* during the intravenous infusion.

▶ Child 1 month–11 years: 3–78 micrograms/kg/hour, dose to be administered according to anaesthetic technique and adjusted according to response, additional doses can be given *by intravenous injection* during the intravenous infusion

▶ Child 12–17 years: 3–120 micrograms/kg/hour, dose to be administered according to anaesthetic technique and adjusted according to response, additional doses can be given *by intravenous injection* during the intravenous infusion

Spontaneous respiration: analgesia and enhancement of anaesthesia during maintenance of anaesthesia

▶ BY INTRAVENOUS INFUSION

▶ Child 12–17 years: Initially 2.4 micrograms/kg/hour, adjusted according to response; usual dose 1.5–6 micrograms/kg/hour

DOSES AT EXTREMES OF BODY-WEIGHT

▶ To avoid excessive dosage in obese patients, dose should be calculated on the basis of ideal body-weight.

● **UNLICENSED USE** Not licensed for use in children under 1 year.

● **CONTRA-INDICATIONS** Analgesia in conscious patients

● **INTERACTIONS** → Appendix 1: opioids

● **SIDE-EFFECTS**

▶ **Common or very common** Apnoea · muscle rigidity · post procedural complications

▶ **Uncommon** Hypoxia

▶ **Rare or very rare** Cardiac arrest

▶ **Frequency not known** Agitation · atrioventricular block · hypertension · seizure

SIDE-EFFECTS, FURTHER INFORMATION In contrast to other opioids which are metabolised in the liver, remifentanil undergoes rapid metabolism by plasma esterases; it has short duration of action which is independent of dose and duration of infusion.

Muscle rigidity Remifentanil can cause muscle rigidity that can be managed by the use of neuromuscular blocking drugs.

● **PREGNANCY** No information available.

● **BREAST FEEDING** Avoid breast-feeding for 24 hours after administration—present in milk in *animal* studies.

● **HEPATIC IMPAIRMENT** Manufacturer advises caution in severe impairment (limited information available).

● **RENAL IMPAIRMENT**

Dose adjustments No dose adjustment necessary in renal impairment.

● **DIRECTIONS FOR ADMINISTRATION** For *intravenous injection*, reconstitute to a concentration of 1 mg/mL; for *continuous intravenous infusion*, dilute further with Glucose 5% or Sodium Chloride 0.9% to a concentration of 20–25 micrograms/mL for child 1–12 years or 20–250 micrograms/mL (usually 50 micrograms/mL) for child 12–18 years.

● **PRESCRIBING AND DISPENSING INFORMATION** Remifentanil should not be given by intravenous injection intra-operatively, but it is well suited to continuous infusion; a supplementary analgesic is given before stopping the infusion of remifentanil.

● **MEDICINAL FORMS** There can be variation in the licensing of different medicines containing the same drug.

Powder for solution for injection

▶ Remifentanil (Non-proprietary)

Remifentanil (as Remifentanyl hydrochloride) 1 mg Remifentanil 1mg powder for concentrate for solution for injection vials | 5 vial PoM £25.60 (Hospital only) CD2

Remifentanil (as Remifentanyl hydrochloride) 2 mg Remifentanil 2mg powder for concentrate for solution for injection vials | 5 vial PoM £51.13 (Hospital only) CD2

Remifentanil (as Remifentanyl hydrochloride) 5 mg Remifentanil 5mg powder for concentrate for solution for injection vials | 5 vial PoM £127.90–£131.74 (Hospital only) CD2

▶ **Ultiva** (Aspen Pharma Trading Ltd)

Remifentanil (as Remifentanyl hydrochloride) 1 mg Ultiva 1mg powder for solution for injection vials | 5 vial PoM £25.58 (Hospital only) CD2

Remifentanil (as Remifentanyl hydrochloride) 2 mg Ultiva 2mg powder for solution for injection vials | 5 vial PoM £51.15 (Hospital only) CD2

Remifentanil (as Remifentanyl hydrochloride) 5 mg Ultiva 5mg powder for solution for injection vials | 5 vial PoM £127.88 (Hospital only) CD2

1.4 Peri-operative sedation

Conscious sedation for clinical procedures

Overview

Sedation of children during diagnostic and therapeutic procedures is used to reduce fear and anxiety, to control pain, and to minimise excessive movement. The choice of sedative drug will depend upon the intended procedure and whether the child is cooperative; some procedures are safer and more successful under anaesthesia.

Midazolam p. 239 and chloral hydrate p. 311 are suitable for sedating children for painless procedures, such as imaging. For painful procedures, alternative choices include nitrous oxide p. 867, local anaesthesia, ketamine p. 879, or concomitant use of sedation with **opioid** or **non-opioid analgesia**.

ANAESTHETICS, GENERAL › NMDA RECEPTOR ANTAGONISTS

Ketamine

04-Dec-2019

● **INDICATIONS AND DOSE**

Induction and maintenance of anaesthesia for short procedures

▶ BY INTRAMUSCULAR INJECTION

▶ Neonate: 4 mg/kg, adjusted according to response, a dose of 4 mg/kg usually produces 15 minutes of surgical anaesthesia.

▶ Child: 4–13 mg/kg, adjusted according to response, a dose of 4 mg/kg sufficient for some diagnostic procedures, a dose of 10 mg/kg usually produces 12–25 minutes of surgical anaesthesia

▶ BY INTRAVENOUS INJECTION

▶ Neonate: 1–2 mg/kg, adjusted according to response, to be given over at least 60 seconds, a dose of 1–2 mg/kg produces 5–10 minutes of surgical anaesthesia.

▶ Child 1 month–11 years: 1–2 mg/kg, adjusted according to response, to be given over at least 60 seconds, a dose of 1–2 mg/kg produces 5–10 minutes of surgical anaesthesia

▶ Child 12–17 years: 1–4.5 mg/kg, adjusted according to response, to be given over at least 60 seconds, a dose of 2 mg/kg usually produces 5–10 minutes of surgical anaesthesia

Induction and maintenance of anaesthesia for long procedures

▶ INITIALLY BY INTRAVENOUS INJECTION

▶ Neonate: Initially 0.5–2 mg/kg, followed by (by continuous intravenous infusion) 8 micrograms/kg/minute, adjusted according to response, doses up to 30 micrograms/kg/minute may be used to produce deep anaesthesia.

▶ Child: Initially 0.5–2 mg/kg, followed by (by continuous intravenous infusion) 10–45 micrograms/kg/minute, adjusted according to response

Sedation prior to invasive or painful procedures

▶ BY INTRAVENOUS INJECTION

▶ Child: 1–2 mg/kg for 1 dose

IMPORTANT SAFETY INFORMATION

Ketamine should only be administered by, or under the direct supervision of, personnel experienced in its use, with adequate training in anaesthesia and airway management, and when resuscitation equipment is available.

● **CONTRA-INDICATIONS** Acute porphyrias p. 652 · eclampsia · head trauma · hypertension · pre-eclampsia · raised intracranial pressure · severe cardiac disease · stroke

● **CAUTIONS** Acute circulatory failure (shock) · cardiovascular disease · dehydration · fixed cardiac output · hallucinations · head injury · hypertension · hypovolaemia · increased cerebrospinal fluid pressure · intracranial mass lesions · nightmares · predisposition to seizures · psychotic disorders · raised intra-ocular pressure · respiratory tract infection · thyroid dysfunction

● **INTERACTIONS** → Appendix 1: ketamine

● **SIDE-EFFECTS**

▶ **Common or very common** Anxiety · behaviour abnormal · confusion · diplopia · hallucination · muscle tone increased · nausea · nystagmus · skin reactions · sleep disorders · tonic clonic movements · vomiting

▶ **Uncommon** Appetite decreased · arrhythmias · hypotension · respiratory disorders

▶ **Rare or very rare** Apnoea · cystitis · cystitis haemorrhagic · delirium · dysphoria · flashback · hypersalivation

▶ **Frequency not known** Drug-induced liver injury

SIDE-EFFECTS, FURTHER INFORMATION Incidence of hallucinations can be reduced by premedicaton with a benzodiazepine (such as midazolam).

● **PREGNANCY** May depress neonatal respiration if used during delivery.

● **BREAST FEEDING** Avoid for at least 12 hours after last dose.

● **HEPATIC IMPAIRMENT** Manufacturer advises caution (risk of prolonged duration of action).

Dose adjustments Manufacturer advises consider dose reduction.

● **DIRECTIONS FOR ADMINISTRATION** For *intravenous injection*, dilute 100 mg/mL strength to a concentration of not more than 50 mg/mL with Glucose 5% *or* Sodium Chloride 0.9%. For *continuous intravenous infusion*, dilute to a concentration of 1 mg/mL with Glucose 5% *or* Sodium Chloride 0.9%; use microdrip infusion for maintenance of anaesthesia.

● **PATIENT AND CARER ADVICE**

Driving and skilled tasks Patients given sedatives and analgesics during minor outpatient procedures should be very carefully warned about the risk of driving or undertaking skilled tasks afterwards. For a short general anaesthetic the risk extends to **at least 24 hours** after administration. Responsible persons should be available to take patients home. The dangers of taking **alcohol** should also be emphasised.

For information on 2015 legislation regarding driving whilst taking certain controlled drugs, including ketamine, see *Drugs and skilled tasks* under Guidance on prescribing p. 1.

● **MEDICINAL FORMS** There can be variation in the licensing of different medicines containing the same drug. Forms available from special-order manufacturers include:solution for injection

Solution for injection

▶ Ketamine (Non-proprietary)

Ketamine (as Ketamine hydrochloride) 10 mg per 1 ml Ketamin 10 Curamed 50mg/5ml solution for injection ampoules | 10 ampoule PoM CD2

Ketamine (as Ketamine hydrochloride) 50 mg per 1 ml Ketamine 500mg/10ml solution for injection vials | 10 vial PoM £70.00 CD2 | 10 vial PoM £70.00 (Hospital only) CD2

Ketamin 100mg/2ml solution for injection ampoules | 10 ampoule PoM CD2

Ketamine 500mg/10ml solution for injection ampoules | 10 ampoule PoM £70.00 CD2

▶ Ketalar (Pfizer Ltd)

Ketamine (as Ketamine hydrochloride) 10 mg per 1 ml Ketalar 200mg/20ml solution for injection vials | 1 vial PoM £5.06 DT = £5.06 CD2

Ketamine (as Ketamine hydrochloride) 50 mg per 1 ml Ketalar 500mg/10ml solution for injection vials | 1 vial PoM £8.77 DT = £8.77 CD2

HYPNOTICS, SEDATIVES AND ANXIOLYTICS › BENZODIAZEPINES

233

Temazepam

21-Oct-2019

● **INDICATIONS AND DOSE**

Premedication before surgery or investigatory procedures

▶ BY MOUTH

▶ Child 12–17 years: 10–20 mg, to be taken 1 hour before procedure

● **UNLICENSED USE** Tablets not licensed for use in children.

● **CONTRA-INDICATIONS** Chronic psychosis · CNS depression · compromised airway · respiratory depression

15 Anaesthesia

- **CAUTIONS** Hypoalbuminaemia · muscle weakness · organic brain changes

CAUTIONS, FURTHER INFORMATION

- ▸ Paradoxical effects A paradoxical increase in hostility and aggression may be reported by patients taking benzodiazepines. The effects range from talkativeness and excitement to aggressive and antisocial acts. Adjustment of the dose (up or down) sometimes attenuates the impulses. Increased anxiety and perceptual disorders are other paradoxical effects.
- **INTERACTIONS** → Appendix 1: temazepam
- **SIDE-EFFECTS** Drug abuse · dry mouth · hypersalivation · speech slurred
- **BREAST FEEDING** Benzodiazepines are present in milk, and should be avoided if possible during breast-feeding.
- **RENAL IMPAIRMENT**

Dose adjustments Start with small doses in severe impairment.

- **PATIENT AND CARER ADVICE**

Driving and skilled tasks Patients given sedatives and analgesics during minor outpatient procedures should be very carefully warned about the risks of undertaking skilled tasks (e.g. driving) afterwards. Responsible persons should be available to take patients home afterwards. The dangers of taking **alcohol** should be emphasised.

- **PROFESSION SPECIFIC INFORMATION**

Dental practitioners' formulary
Temazepam tablets and oral Solution may be prescribed.

- **MEDICINAL FORMS** There can be variation in the licensing of different medicines containing the same drug. Forms available from special-order manufacturers include: oral suspension, oral solution

Oral solution

CAUTIONARY AND ADVISORY LABELS 19

▸ Temazepam (Non-proprietary)
Temazepam 2 mg per 1 ml Temazepam 10mg/5ml oral solution sugar free sugar-free | 300 ml PoM £183.28 DT = £183.28 CD3

Tablet

CAUTIONARY AND ADVISORY LABELS 19

▸ Temazepam (Non-proprietary)
Temazepam 10 mg Temazepam 10mg tablets | 28 tablet PoM £35.00 DT = £1.62 CD3 | 500 tablet PoM £26.07–£624.82 CD3
Temazepam 20 mg Temazepam 20mg tablets | 28 tablet PoM £35.00 DT = £1.56 CD3 | 250 tablet PoM £13.93–£307.94 CD3

2 Malignant hyperthermia

MUSCLE RELAXANTS › DIRECTLY ACTING

Dantrolene sodium

29-Nov-2019

- **DRUG ACTION** Acts on skeletal muscle cells by interfering with calcium efflux, thereby stopping the contractile process.

- **INDICATIONS AND DOSE**

Malignant hyperthermia

▸ BY RAPID INTRAVENOUS INJECTION

- ▸ Child: Initially 2–3 mg/kg, then 1 mg/kg, repeated if necessary; maximum 10 mg/kg per course

Chronic severe spasticity of voluntary muscle

▸ BY MOUTH

- ▸ Child 5–11 years: Initially 500 micrograms/kg once daily for 7 days, then increased to 500 micrograms/kg/dose 3 times a day, then increased in steps of 500 micrograms/kg/dose every 7 days (max. per dose 2 mg/kg 3–4 times a day) until satisfactory response; maximum 400 mg per day
- ▸ Child 12–17 years: Initially 25 mg once daily for 7 days, then increased to 25 mg 3 times a day, then increased in steps of 500 micrograms/kg/dose every 7 days (max. per dose 2 mg/kg 3–4 times a day) until satisfactory response; maximum 400 mg per day

- **UNLICENSED USE** Not licensed for use in children.

IMPORTANT SAFETY INFORMATION
Should only be administered by, or under the direct supervision of, personnel experienced in the use of dantrolene when used for malignant hyperthermia.

- **CONTRA-INDICATIONS**
  - ▸ With oral use Acute muscle spasm · avoid when spasticity is useful, for example, locomotion
- **CAUTIONS**
  - ▸ With intravenous use Avoid extravasation (risk of tissue necrosis)
  - ▸ With oral use Females (hepatotoxicity) · history of liver disorders (hepatotoxicity) · if doses greater than 400 mg daily (hepatotoxicity) · impaired cardiac function · impaired pulmonary function · therapeutic effect may take a few weeks to develop— discontinue if no response within 6–8 weeks
- **INTERACTIONS** → Appendix 1: dantrolene
- **SIDE-EFFECTS**

GENERAL SIDE-EFFECTS

- ▸ **Common or very common** Abdominal pain · hepatic disorders · nausea · respiratory disorders · skin reactions · speech disorder · vomiting
- ▸ **Uncommon** Crystalluria · hyperhidrosis
- ▸ **Frequency not known** Arrhythmias · dizziness · drowsiness

SPECIFIC SIDE-EFFECTS

- ▸ **Common or very common**
  - ▸ With oral use Appetite decreased · chills · confusion · depression · eosinophilia · fever · headache · insomnia · nervousness · pericarditis · visual impairment
- ▸ **Uncommon**
  - ▸ With oral use Constipation · dysphagia · haemorrhage · heart failure aggravated · urinary disorders
- ▸ **Frequency not known**
  - ▸ With intravenous use Gastrointestinal haemorrhage · heart failure · localised pain · pulmonary oedema · seizure · thrombophlebitis
  - ▸ With oral use Asthenia · diarrhoea · dyspnoea · hypertension · malaise

- **PREGNANCY**
  - ▸ With intravenous use Use only if potential benefit outweighs risk.
  - ▸ With oral use Although teratological studies in *animals* have proved satisfactory, dantrolene sodium does cross the placenta, therefore manufacturer advises avoid.
- **BREAST FEEDING**
  - ▸ With intravenous use Present in milk—use only if potential benefit outweighs risk.
  - ▸ With oral use Present in milk—manufacturer advises avoid.
- **HEPATIC IMPAIRMENT**
  - ▸ With oral use Manufacturer advises avoid in hepatic impairment.
- **MONITORING REQUIREMENTS**
  - ▸ With oral use Test liver function before and at intervals during therapy.
- **PATIENT AND CARER ADVICE**

Hepatotoxicity ▸ With oral use Patients should be told how to recognise signs of liver disorder and advised to seek prompt medical attention if symptoms such as anorexia, nausea, vomiting, fatigue, abdominal pain, dark urine, or pruritus develop.

Driving and skilled tasks ▸ With oral use Drowsiness may affect performance of skilled tasks (e.g. driving); effects of alcohol enhanced.

- **MEDICINAL FORMS** There can be variation in the licensing of different medicines containing the same drug. Forms available from special-order manufacturers include: oral suspension, oral solution

Powder for solution for injection

▸ Dantrium (Forum Health Products Ltd)
Dantrolene sodium 20 mg Dantrium Intravenous 20mg powder for solution for injection vials | 12 vial PoM £612.00 (Hospital only) | 36 vial PoM £1,836.00 (Hospital only)

Capsule

CAUTIONARY AND ADVISORY LABELS 2

▸ Dantrium (Forum Health Products Ltd)
Dantrolene sodium 25 mg Dantrium 25mg capsules | 100 capsule PoM £16.87 DT = £16.87
Dantrolene sodium 100 mg Dantrium 100mg capsules | 100 capsule PoM £43.07 DT = £43.07

Local anaesthesia

Anaesthesia (local)

Local anaesthetic drugs

The use of local anaesthetics by injection or by application to mucous membranes to produce local analgesia is discussed in this section.

Local anaesthetic drugs act by causing a reversible block to conduction along nerve fibres. They vary widely in their potency, toxicity, duration of action, stability, solubility in water, and ability to penetrate mucous membranes. These factors determine their application, e.g. topical (surface), infiltration, peripheral nerve block, intravenous regional anaesthesia (Bier's block), plexus, epidural (extradural), or spinal (intrathecal or subarachnoid) block. Local anaesthetics may also be used for postoperative pain relief, thereby reducing the need for analgesics such as opioids.

Bupivacaine hydrochloride p. 883 has a longer duration of action than other local anaesthetics. It has a slow onset of action, taking up to 30 minutes for full effect. It is often used in lumbar epidural blockade and is particularly suitable for continuous epidural analgesia in labour, or for postoperative pain relief. It is the principal drug used for spinal anaesthesia. Hyperbaric solutions containing glucose may be used for spinal block.

Levobupivacaine p. 884, an isomer of bupivacaine hydrochloride, has anaesthetic and analgesic properties similar to bupivacaine hydrochloride, but is thought to have fewer adverse effects.

Lidocaine hydrochloride p. 884 is effectively absorbed from mucous membranes and is a useful surface anaesthetic in concentrations up to 10%. Except for surface anaesthesia and dental anaesthesia, solutions should **not** usually exceed 1% in strength. The duration of the block (with adrenaline/epinephrine p. 143) is about 90 minutes.

Application of a mixture of lidocaine and prilocaine (*EMLA*®) under an occlusive dressing provides surface anaesthesia for 1–2 hours. *EMLA*® does not appear to be effective in providing local anaesthesia for heel lancing in neonates.

Prilocaine hydrochloride p. 888 is a local anaesthetic of low toxicity which is similar to lidocaine hydrochloride.

Ropivacaine hydrochloride p. 889 is an amide-type local anaesthetic agent similar to bupivacaine hydrochloride. It is less cardiotoxic than bupivacaine hydrochloride, but also less potent.

Tetracaine p. 890, a para-aminobenzoic acid ester, is an effective local anaesthetic for topical application; a 4% gel is indicated for anaesthesia before venepuncture or venous cannulation. Tetracaine is effective for 4–6 hours after a single application in most children. It is not recommended prior to neonatal heel lancing.

Tetracaine is rapidly absorbed from mucous membranes and should never be applied to inflamed, traumatised, or highly vascular surfaces. It should never be used to provide anaesthesia for bronchoscopy or cystoscopy because lidocaine hydrochloride is a safer alternative.

Administration by injection

The dose of local anaesthetic depends on the injection site and the procedure used. In determining the safe dosage, it is important to take account of the rate of absorption and excretion, and of the potency. The child's age, weight, physique, and clinical condition, and the vascularity of the administration site and the duration of administration, must also be considered.

Uptake of local anaesthetics into the systemic circulation determines their duration of action and produces toxicity.

NHS Improvement has advised (September 2016) that, prior to administration, all injectable medicines must be drawn directly from their original ampoule or container into a syringe and should **never** be decanted into gallipots or open containers. This is to avoid the risk of medicines being confused with other substances, e.g. skin disinfectants, and to reduce the risk of contamination.

Great care must be taken to avoid accidental intravascular injection; local anaesthetic injections should be given slowly in order to detect inadvertent intravascular administration. When prolonged analgesia is required, a long-acting local anaesthetic is preferred to minimise the likelihood of cumulative systemic toxicity. Local anaesthesia around the oral cavity may impair swallowing and therefore increases the risk of aspiration.

Epidural anaesthesia is combined with general anaesthesia for certain surgical procedures in children.

Vasoconstrictors in combination with local anaesthetics

Local anaesthetics cause dilatation of blood vessels. The addition of a vasoconstrictor such as adrenaline/epinephrine to the local anaesthetic preparation diminishes local blood flow, slowing the rate of absorption and thereby prolonging the anaesthetic effect. Great care should be taken to avoid inadvertent intravenous administration of a preparation containing adrenaline/epinephrine, and it is not advisable to give adrenaline/epinephrine with a local anaesthetic injection in digits or appendages because of the risk of ischaemic necrosis.

Adrenaline/epinephrine must be used in a low concentration when administered with a local anaesthetic. Care must also be taken to calculate a safe maximum dose of local anaesthetic when using combination products.

In children with severe hypertension or unstable cardiac rhythm, the use of adrenaline/epinephrine with a local anaesthetic may be hazardous. For these children an anaesthetic without adrenaline/epinephrine should be used.

Dental anaesthesia

Lidocaine hydrochloride is widely used in dental procedures; it is most often used in combination with adrenaline/epinephrine. Lidocaine hydrochloride 2% combined with adrenaline/epinephrine 1 in 80 000 (12.5 micrograms/mL) is a safe and effective preparation; there is no justification for using higher concentrations of adrenaline/epinephrine. The amide-type local anaesthetics articaine and mepivacaine hydrochloride p. 887 are also used in dentistry; they are available in cartridges suitable for dental use. Mepivacaine hydrochloride is available with or without adrenaline/epinephrine, and articaine is available with adrenaline/epinephrine. In children with severe hypertension or unstable cardiac rhythm, mepivacaine hydrochloride without adrenaline/epinephrine may be used.

Alternatively, prilocaine hydrochloride with or without felypressin can be used but there is no evidence that it is any safer. Felypressin can cause coronary vasoconstriction when used at high doses; limit dose in children with coronary artery disease.

Toxicity induced by local anaesthesia

For management of toxicity see Severe local anaesthetic-induced cardiovascular toxicity below.

Severe local anaesthetic-induced cardiovascular toxicity

Overview

After injection of a bolus of local anaesthetic, toxicity may develop at any time in the following hour. In the event of signs of toxicity during injection, the administration of the local anaesthetic must be stopped immediately.

Cardiovascular status must be assessed and cardiopulmonary resuscitation procedures must be followed.

In the event of local anaesthetic-induced cardiac arrest, standard cardiopulmonary resuscitation should be initiated immediately. Lidocaine must not be used as anti-arrhythmic therapy.

If the patient does not respond rapidly to standard procedures, 20% lipid emulsion such as *Intralipid*® [unlicensed indication] should be given intravenously at an initial bolus dose of 1.5 mL/kg over 1 minute, followed by an infusion of 15 mL/kg/hour. After 5 minutes, if cardiovascular stability has not been restored or circulation deteriorates, give a maximum of two further bolus doses of 1.5 mL/kg over 1 minute, 5 minutes apart, and increase the infusion rate to 30 mL/kg/hour. Continue infusion until cardiovascular stability and adequate circulation are restored or maximum cumulative dose of 12 mL/kg is given.

Standard cardiopulmonary resuscitation must be maintained throughout lipid emulsion treatment.

Propofol is not a suitable alternative to lipid emulsion.

Further advice on ongoing treatment should be obtained from the National Poisons Information Service.

Detailed treatment algorithms and accompanying notes are available at www.toxbase.org *or* can be found in the Association of Anaesthetists of Great Britain and Ireland safety guideline, Management of Severe Local Anaesthetic Toxicity and Management of Severe Local Anaesthetic Toxicity - Accompanying notes.

ANAESTHETICS, LOCAL

Adrenaline with articaine hydrochloride

19-Dec-2019

(Carticaine hydrochloride with epinephrine)

- **INDICATIONS AND DOSE**

Infiltration anaesthesia in dentistry

▸ BY REGIONAL ADMINISTRATION

▸ Child 4–17 years: Consult expert dental sources

DOSES AT EXTREMES OF BODY-WEIGHT

▸ To avoid excessive dosage in obese patients, dose should be calculated on the basis of ideal body-weight.

> IMPORTANT SAFETY INFORMATION
> Should only be administered by, or under the direct supervision of, personnel experienced in their use, with adequate training in anaesthesia and airway management, and should not be administered parenterally unless adequate resuscitation equipment is available.

- **CONTRA-INDICATIONS** Injection into infected tissues · injection into inflamed tissues · preparations containing preservatives should not be used for caudal, epidural, or spinal block

CONTRA-INDICATIONS, FURTHER INFORMATION

▸ Injection site Manufacturer advises the local anaesthetic effect may be reduced when injected into an inflamed or infected area, due to altered local pH. Increased absorption into the blood also increases the possibility of systemic side-effects.

- **CAUTIONS** Arrhythmias · cardiovascular disease · cerebrovascular disease · children (consider dose reduction) · cor pulmonale · debilitated patients (consider dose reduction) · diabetes mellitus · epilepsy · hypercalcaemia · hyperreflexia · hypertension · hyperthyroidism · hypokalaemia · hypovolaemia · impaired cardiac conduction · impaired respiratory function · ischaemic heart disease · myasthenia gravis · obstructive cardiomyopathy · occlusive vascular disease · organic brain damage · phaeochromocytoma · prostate disorders · psychoneurosis · severe angina · shock · susceptibility to angle-closure glaucoma

CAUTIONS, FURTHER INFORMATION

▸ Use of vasoconstrictors In patients with severe hypertension or unstable cardiac rhythm, the use of adrenaline with a local anaesthetic may be hazardous. For these patients an anaesthetic without adrenaline should be used.

- **INTERACTIONS** → Appendix 1: articaine · sympathomimetics, vasoconstrictor
- **SIDE-EFFECTS** Face oedema · gingivitis · headache · nausea · sensation abnormal

SIDE-EFFECTS, FURTHER INFORMATION Toxic effects after administration of local anaesthetics are a result of excessively high plasma concentrations; severe toxicity usually results from inadvertent intravascular injection. The toxicity mainly involves the central nervous and cardiovascular systems. The onset of toxicity can be unpredictable and delayed. Monitor as per local protocol for at least 30 minutes after administration.

- **ALLERGY AND CROSS-SENSITIVITY**

▸ Hypersensitivity and cross-sensitivity Hypersensitivity reactions occur mainly with the ester-type local anaesthetics, such as tetracaine; reactions are less frequent with the amide types, such as articaine, bupivacaine, levobupivacaine, lidocaine, mepivacaine, prilocaine, and ropivacaine. Cross-sensitivity reactions may be avoided by using the alternative chemical type.

- **PREGNANCY** Use only if potential benefit outweighs risk—no information available.
- **BREAST FEEDING** Avoid breast-feeding for 48 hours after administration.
- **HEPATIC IMPAIRMENT** Manufacturer advises caution (increased risk of toxicity in severe impairment).
- **RENAL IMPAIRMENT** Manufacturers advise use with caution in severe impairment.
- **MONITORING REQUIREMENTS** Consider monitoring blood pressure and ECG (advised with systemic adrenaline/epinephrine).

- **MEDICINAL FORMS** There can be variation in the licensing of different medicines containing the same drug.

Solution for injection

EXCIPIENTS: May contain Sulfites

▸ Septanest (Septodont Ltd)

Adrenaline (as Adrenaline acid tartrate) 10 microgram per 1 ml, Articaine hydrochloride 40 mg per 1 ml Septanest 1 in 100,000 solution for injection cartridges | 50 cartridge PoM £24.95

Adrenaline (as Adrenaline acid tartrate) 5 microgram per 1 ml, Articaine hydrochloride 40 mg per 1 ml Septanest 1 in 200,000 solution for injection cartridges | 50 cartridge PoM £24.95

Bupivacaine hydrochloride
09-Dec-2019

● **INDICATIONS AND DOSE**

Surgical anaesthesia | Acute pain

▶ BY REGIONAL ADMINISTRATION

▸ Child: Doses adjusted according to child's physical status and nature of procedure, seek expert advice (consult product literature or local protocols)

DOSES AT EXTREMES OF BODY-WEIGHT

▸ To avoid excessive dosage in obese patients, dose should be calculated on the basis of ideal body-weight.

IMPORTANT SAFETY INFORMATION

The licensed doses stated may not be appropriate in some settings and expert advice should be sought.

Should only be administered by, or under the direct supervision of, personnel experienced in their use, with adequate training in anaesthesia and airway management, and should not be administered parenterally unless adequate resuscitation equipment is available.

● **CONTRA-INDICATIONS** Avoid injection into infected tissues · avoid injection into inflamed tissues · intravenous regional anaesthesia (Bier's block) · preparations containing preservatives should not be used for caudal, epidural, or spinal block

CONTRA-INDICATIONS, FURTHER INFORMATION

▸ Injection site Manufacturer advises local anaesthetics should not be injected into inflamed or infected tissues. Increased absorption into the blood increases the possibility of systemic side-effects, and the local anaesthetic effect may also be reduced by altered local pH.

● **CAUTIONS** Cardiovascular disease · cerebral atheroma · children (consider dose reduction) · complete heart block · debilitated patients (consider dose reduction) · epilepsy · hypertension · hypotension · hypovolaemia · impaired cardiac conduction · impaired respiratory function · myasthenia gravis · myocardial depression may be more severe and more resistant to treatment · shock

● **INTERACTIONS** → Appendix 1: anaesthetics, local

● **SIDE-EFFECTS**

▶ **Common or very common** Arrhythmias · dizziness · hypertension · hypotension · nausea · paraesthesia · urinary retention · vomiting

▶ **Uncommon** Neurotoxicity

▶ **Rare or very rare** Arachnoiditis · cardiac arrest · diplopia · nerve disorders · paraplegia · paresis · respiratory depression

SIDE-EFFECTS, FURTHER INFORMATION Toxic effects after administration of local anaesthetics are a result of excessively high plasma concentrations; severe toxicity usually results from inadvertent intravascular injection. The systemic toxicity of local anaesthetics mainly involves the central nervous and cardiovascular systems. The onset of toxicity can be unpredictable and delayed. Monitor as per local protocol for at least 30 minutes after administration.

● **ALLERGY AND CROSS-SENSITIVITY**

▸ Hypersensitivity and cross-sensitivity Hypersensitivity reactions occur mainly with the ester-type local anaesthetics, such as tetracaine; reactions are less frequent with the amide types, such as articaine, bupivacaine, levobupivacaine, lidocaine, mepivacaine, prilocaine, and ropivacaine. Cross-sensitivity reactions may be avoided by using the alternative chemical type.

● **PREGNANCY** Large doses during delivery can cause neonatal respiratory depression, hypotonia, and bradycardia after epidural block.

Dose adjustments Use lower doses for intrathecal use during late pregnancy.

● **BREAST FEEDING** Amount too small to be harmful.

● **HEPATIC IMPAIRMENT** Manufacturer advises use with caution in advanced liver dysfunction.

● **RENAL IMPAIRMENT** Use with caution in severe impairment.

● **MEDICINAL FORMS** There can be variation in the licensing of different medicines containing the same drug. Forms available from special-order manufacturers include: solution for injection, infusion, solution for infusion

Solution for injection

▸ Bupivacaine hydrochloride (Non-proprietary)

Bupivacaine hydrochloride 2.5 mg per 1 ml Bupivacaine 25mg/10ml (0.25%) solution for injection vials | 10 vial PoM ☒
Bupivacaine 0.25% solution for injection 10ml Sure-Amp ampoules | 20 ampoule PoM £17.50 DT = £17.50

Bupivacaine hydrochloride 5 mg per 1 ml Bupivacaine 0.5% solution for injection 10ml Sure-Amp ampoules | 20 ampoule PoM £18.30 DT = £18.30
Bupivacaine 100mg/20ml (0.5%) solution for injection vials | 10 vial PoM ☒
Bupivacaine 50mg/10ml (0.5%) solution for injection ampoules | 10 ampoule PoM £7.56 DT = £7.56 | 10 ampoule PoM £17.58 DT = £7.56 (Hospital only)

Bupivacaine hydrochloride anhydrous 40 mg per 1 ml Bupivacain Sintetica 40mg/ml (4%) solution for injection ampoules | 10 ampoule PoM ☒

▸ Marcain (Aspen Pharma Trading Ltd)

Bupivacaine hydrochloride 2.5 mg per 1 ml Marcain 0.25% solution for injection 10ml Polyamp Steripack ampoules | 5 ampoule PoM £7.92 DT = £7.92 (Hospital only)

Bupivacaine hydrochloride 5 mg per 1 ml Marcain 0.5% solution for injection 10ml Polyamp Steripack ampoules | 5 ampoule PoM £9.25 DT = £9.25 (Hospital only)

Infusion

▸ Bupivacaine hydrochloride (Non-proprietary)

Bupivacaine hydrochloride 1 mg per 1 ml Bupivacaine 100mg/100ml (0.1%) infusion bags | 20 bag PoM ☒
Bupivacaine 250mg/250ml (0.1%) infusion bags | 5 bag PoM £60.87 | 20 bag PoM £243.48

Bupivacaine hydrochloride 1.25 mg per 1 ml Bupivacaine 312.5mg/250ml (0.125%) infusion bags | 5 bag PoM £62.12 | 20 bag PoM £248.47

Bupivacaine with adrenaline
19-Dec-2019

The properties listed below are those particular to the combination only. For the properties of the components please consider, bupivacaine hydrochloride above, adrenaline/epinephrine p. 143.

● **INDICATIONS AND DOSE**

Surgical anaesthesia

▶ BY LUMBAR EPIDURAL, OR BY LOCAL INFILTRATION, OR BY CAUDAL EPIDURAL

▸ Child 12–17 years: (consult product literature)

Acute pain management

▶ BY LUMBAR EPIDURAL, OR BY LOCAL INFILTRATION

▸ Child 1–17 years: (consult product literature)

● **CAUTIONS**

CAUTIONS, FURTHER INFORMATION In patients with severe hypertension or unstable cardiac rhythm, the use of adrenaline with a local anaesthetic may be hazardous. For these patients an anaesthetic without adrenaline should be used.

● **INTERACTIONS** → Appendix 1: anaesthetics, local · sympathomimetics, vasoconstrictor

- **MEDICINAL FORMS** There can be variation in the licensing of different medicines containing the same drug.

Solution for injection

- Bupivacaine with adrenaline (Non-proprietary)
  Adrenaline (as Adrenaline acid tartrate) 5 microgram per 1 ml, Bupivacaine hydrochloride 2.5 mg per 1 ml Bupivacaine 25mg/10ml (0.25%) / Adrenaline (base) 50micrograms/10ml (1 in 200,000) solution for injection ampoules | 10 ampoule PoM £46.00 DT = £46.00
  Adrenaline (as Adrenaline acid tartrate) 5 microgram per 1 ml, Bupivacaine hydrochloride 5 mg per 1 ml Bupivacaine 50mg/10ml (0.5%) / Adrenaline (base) 50micrograms/10ml (1 in 200,000) solution for injection ampoules | 10 ampoule PoM £51.75 DT = £51.75

Levobupivacaine

09-Dec-2019

- **INDICATIONS AND DOSE**

Surgical anaesthesia | Acute pain

▶ BY REGIONAL ADMINISTRATION

- Child: Doses adjusted according to child's physical status and nature of procedure, seek expert advice (consult product literature or local protocols)

DOSES AT EXTREMES OF BODY-WEIGHT

- To avoid excessive dosage in obese patients, dose should be calculated on the basis of ideal body-weight.

- **UNLICENSED USE** Not licensed for use in children except for analgesia by ilioinguinal or iliohypogastric block.

IMPORTANT SAFETY INFORMATION

The licensed doses stated may not be appropriate in some settings and expert advice should be sought.

Should only be administered by, or under the direct supervision of, personnel experienced in their use, with adequate training in anaesthesia and airway management, and should not be administered parenterally unless adequate resuscitation equipment is available.

- **CONTRA-INDICATIONS** Avoid injection into infected tissues · avoid injection into inflamed tissues · intravenous regional anaesthesia (Bier's block) · preparations containing preservatives should not be used for caudal, epidural, or spinal block

CONTRA-INDICATIONS, FURTHER INFORMATION

- Injection site Manufacturer advises local anaesthetics should not be injected into inflamed or infected tissues. Increased absorption into the blood increases the possibility of systemic side-effects, and the local anaesthetic effect may also be reduced by altered local pH.

- **CAUTIONS** Cardiovascular disease · children (consider dose reduction) · complete heart block · debilitated patients (consider dose reduction) · epilepsy · hypovolaemia · impaired cardiac conduction · impaired respiratory function · myasthenia gravis · shock
- **INTERACTIONS** → Appendix 1: anaesthetics, local
- **SIDE-EFFECTS**

▶ **Common or very common** Anaemia · back pain · dizziness · fever · headache · hypotension · nausea · procedural pain · vomiting

▶ **Frequency not known** Angioedema · apnoea · arrhythmias · asthenia · atrioventricular block · bladder disorder · cardiac arrest · drowsiness · eye disorders · faecal incontinence · flushing · loss of consciousness · muscle twitching · muscle weakness · nerve disorders · neurological injury · oral hypoaesthesia · paralysis · priapism · respiratory disorders · seizure · sensation abnormal · skin reactions · sneezing · sweat changes · syncope · vision blurred

SIDE-EFFECTS, FURTHER INFORMATION The systemic toxicity of local anaesthetics mainly involves the central nervous and cardiovascular systems. Systemic toxicity can occur due to inadvertent intravascular injection. The onset of toxicity can be unpredictable and delayed. Monitor as per local protocol for at least 30 minutes after administration.

- **ALLERGY AND CROSS-SENSITIVITY**

- Hypersensitivity and cross-sensitivity Hypersensitivity reactions occur mainly with the ester-type local anaesthetics, such as tetracaine; reactions are less frequent with the amide types, such as articaine, bupivacaine, levobupivacaine, lidocaine, mepivacaine, prilocaine, and ropivacaine. Cross-sensitivity reactions may be avoided by using the alternative chemical type.

- **PREGNANCY** Large doses during delivery can cause neonatal respiratory depression, hypotonia, and bradycardia after epidural block. Avoid if possible in the first trimester—toxicity in *animal* studies. May cause fetal distress syndrome. Do not use for paracervical block in obstetrics. Do not use 7.5 mg/mL strength in obstetrics.
- **BREAST FEEDING** Amount too small to be harmful.
- **HEPATIC IMPAIRMENT** Manufacturer advises caution in impairment or patients with reduced hepatic blood flow (no information available).
- **DIRECTIONS FOR ADMINISTRATION** For 1.25 mg/mL concentration dilute standard solutions with sodium chloride 0.9%.
- **PRESCRIBING AND DISPENSING INFORMATION** Levobupivacaine is an isomer of bupivacaine.

- **MEDICINAL FORMS** There can be variation in the licensing of different medicines containing the same drug.

Solution for injection

- Levobupivacaine (Non-proprietary)
  Levobupivacaine (as Levobupivacaine hydrochloride) 2.5 mg per 1 ml Levobupivacaine 25mg/10ml solution for injection ampoules | 5 ampoule PoM £9.45 (Hospital only)
  Levobupivacaine (as Levobupivacaine hydrochloride) 5 mg per 1 ml Levobupivacaine 50mg/10ml solution for injection ampoules | 5 ampoule PoM £10.85 (Hospital only)
  Levobupivacaine (as Levobupivacaine hydrochloride) 7.5 mg per 1 ml Levobupivacaine 75mg/10ml solution for injection ampoules | 5 ampoule PoM £16.20 (Hospital only)
- Chirocaine (AbbVie Ltd)
  Levobupivacaine (as Levobupivacaine hydrochloride) 2.5 mg per 1 ml Chirocaine 25mg/10ml solution for injection ampoules | 10 ampoule PoM £14.11 (Hospital only)
  Levobupivacaine (as Levobupivacaine hydrochloride) 5 mg per 1 ml Chirocaine 50mg/10ml solution for injection ampoules | 10 ampoule PoM £16.15 (Hospital only)
  Levobupivacaine (as Levobupivacaine hydrochloride) 7.5 mg per 1 ml Chirocaine 75mg/10ml solution for injection ampoules | 10 ampoule PoM £24.23 (Hospital only)

Infusion

- Levobupivacaine (Non-proprietary)
  Levobupivacaine (as Levobupivacaine hydrochloride).625 mg per 1 ml Levobupivacaine 62.5mg/100ml infusion bags | 5 bag PoM
  Levobupivacaine 125mg/200ml infusion bags | 5 bag PoM
  Levobupivacaine (as Levobupivacaine hydrochloride) 1.25 mg per 1 ml Levobupivacaine 125mg/100ml infusion bags | 5 bag PoM
- Chirocaine (AbbVie Ltd)
  Levobupivacaine (as Levobupivacaine hydrochloride) 1.25 mg per 1 ml Chirocaine 125mg/100ml infusion bags | 24 bag PoM £174.22
  Chirocaine 250mg/200ml infusion bags | 12 bag PoM £124.44

Lidocaine hydrochloride

11-Dec-2019

(Lignocaine hydrochloride)

- **INDICATIONS AND DOSE**

Infiltration anaesthesia

▶ BY LOCAL INFILTRATION

- Neonate: Up to 3 mg/kg, dose to be given according to patient's weight and nature of procedure, dose may be repeated not more often than every 4 hours, 3 mg/kg equivalent to 0.3 mL/kg of 1% solution.

- Child 1 month–11 years: Up to 3 mg/kg, dose to be given according to patient's weight and nature of procedure, dose may be repeated not more often than every 4 hours, 3 mg/kg equivalent to 0.3 mL/kg of 1% solution
- Child 12–17 years: (max. per dose 200 mg), dose to be given according to child's weight and nature of procedure, dose may be repeated not more often than every 4 hours

DOSES AT EXTREMES OF BODY-WEIGHT

- When used by local infiltration To avoid excessive dosage in obese patients, weight-based doses for non-emergency indications may need to be calculated on the basis of ideal body-weight.

Intravenous regional anaesthesia and nerve block

- BY REGIONAL ADMINISTRATION
- Child: Seek expert advice

Dental anaesthesia

- BY REGIONAL ADMINISTRATION
- Child: Seek expert advice

Pain relief (in anal fissures, haemorrhoids, pruritus ani, pruritus vulvae, herpes zoster, or herpes labialis) | Lubricant in cystoscopy | Lubricant in proctoscopy

- TO THE SKIN USING OINTMENT
- Child: Apply 1–2 mL as required, avoid long-term use

LMX 4®

Anaesthesia before venous cannulation or venepuncture

- TO THE SKIN
- Child 1–2 months: Apply up to 1 g, apply thick layer to small area (2.5 cm × 2.5 cm) of non-irritated skin at least 30 minutes before procedure; may be applied under an occlusive dressing; max. application time 60 minutes, remove cream with gauze and perform procedure after approximately 5 minutes
- Child 3–11 months: Apply up to 1 g, apply thick layer to small area (2.5 cm × 2.5 cm) of non-irritated skin at least 30 minutes before procedure; may be applied under an occlusive dressing; max. application time 4 hours, remove cream with gauze and perform procedure after approximately 5 minutes
- Child 1–17 years: Apply 1–2.5 g, apply thick layer to small area (2.5 cm × 2.5 cm) of non-irritated skin at least 30 minutes before procedure; may be applied under an occlusive dressing; max. application time 5 hours, remove cream with gauze and perform procedure after approximately 5 minutes

IMPORTANT SAFETY INFORMATION

- When used by local infiltration

The licensed doses stated may not be appropriate in some settings and expert advice should be sought. Should only be administered by, or under the direct supervision of, personnel experienced in their use, with adequate training in anaesthesia and airway management, and should not be administered parenterally unless adequate resuscitation equipment is available.

- **CONTRA-INDICATIONS**
- When used by regional administration Avoid injection into infected tissues · avoid injection into inflamed tissues · complete heart block · preparations containing preservatives should not be used for caudal, epidural, or spinal block, or for intravenous regional anaesthesia (Bier's block)
- With topical use Application to the middle ear (can cause ototoxicity) · should not be applied to damaged skin

CONTRA-INDICATIONS, FURTHER INFORMATION

- Administration site
- With topical use or when used by regional administration Manufacturer advises local anaesthetics should not be injected into inflamed or infected tissues nor should they be applied to damaged skin. Increased absorption into the blood increases the possibility of systemic side-effects, and the local anaesthetic effect may also be reduced by altered local pH.

- **CAUTIONS**
- When used by regional administration Acute porphyrias p. 652 (consider infusion with glucose for its anti-porphyrinogenic effects) · children (consider dose reduction) · congestive cardiac failure (consider lower dose) · debilitated patients (consider dose reduction) · epilepsy · hypovolaemia · impaired cardiac conduction · impaired respiratory function · myasthenia gravis · ; post cardiac surgery (consider lower dose) · shock

- **INTERACTIONS** → Appendix 1: antiarrhythmics
- **SIDE-EFFECTS**
- With parenteral use Anxiety · arrhythmias · atrioventricular block · cardiac arrest · circulatory collapse · confusion · dizziness · drowsiness · euphoric mood · headache · hypotension (may lead to cardiac arrest) · loss of consciousness · methaemoglobinaemia · muscle twitching · myocardial contractility decreased · nausea · neurological effects · nystagmus · pain · psychosis · respiratory disorders · seizure · sensation abnormal · temperature sensation altered · tinnitus · tremor · vision blurred · vomiting

SIDE-EFFECTS, FURTHER INFORMATION **Toxic effects** The systemic toxicity of local anaesthetics mainly involves the central nervous and cardiovascular systems.

Methaemoglobinaemia Methylthioninium chloride can be used for the acute symptomatic treatment of drug-induced methaemoglobinaemia.

- **ALLERGY AND CROSS-SENSITIVITY**
- Hypersensitivity and cross-sensitivity Hypersensitivity reactions occur mainly with the ester-type local anaesthetics, such as tetracaine; reactions are less frequent with the amide types, such as articaine, bupivacaine, levobupivacaine, lidocaine, mepivacaine, prilocaine, and ropivacaine. Cross-sensitivity reactions may be avoided by using the alternative chemical type.

- **PREGNANCY** Crosses the placenta but not known to be harmful in *animal* studies—use if benefit outweighs risk. When used as a local anaesthetic, large doses can cause fetal bradycardia; if given during delivery can also cause neonatal respiratory depression, hypotonia, or bradycardia after paracervical or epidural block.
- **BREAST FEEDING** Present in milk but amount too small to be harmful.
- **HEPATIC IMPAIRMENT** Manufacturer advises caution (risk of increased exposure).
- **RENAL IMPAIRMENT** Possible accumulation of lidocaine and active metabolite; caution in severe impairment.
- **MONITORING REQUIREMENTS**
- With systemic use Monitor ECG and have resuscitation facilities available.

- **MEDICINAL FORMS** There can be variation in the licensing of different medicines containing the same drug. Forms available from special-order manufacturers include: solution for injection, ointment

Solution for injection

- Lidocaine hydrochloride (Non-proprietary)

Lidocaine hydrochloride 5 mg per 1 ml Lidocaine 50mg/10ml (0.5%) solution for injection ampoules | 10 ampoule PoM £7.00

Lidocaine hydrochloride 10 mg per 1 ml Lidocaine 100mg/10ml (1%) solution for injection Mini-Plasco ampoules | 20 ampoule PoM £1.15–£11.21

Lidocaine 100mg/10ml (1%) solution for injection ampoules | 10 ampoule PoM £5.00 DT = £5.00

15 Anaesthesia

Lidocaine 200mg/20ml (1%) solution for injection vials | 10 vial PoM £22.00 DT = £22.00
Lidocaine 200mg/20ml (1%) solution for injection ampoules | 10 ampoule PoM £10.00-£11.00 DT = £11.00
Lidocaine 50mg/5ml (1%) solution for injection ampoules | 10 ampoule PoM £3.00-£12.00 DT = £3.00
Lidocaine 200mg/20ml (1%) solution for injection Mini-Plasco ampoules | 20 ampoule PoM
Lidocaine 20mg/2ml (1%) solution for injection ampoules | 10 ampoule PoM £12.00 DT = £2.50
Lidocaine 50mg/5ml (1%) solution for injection Mini-Plasco ampoules | 20 ampoule PoM £6.50
Lidocaine 50mg/5ml (1%) solution for injection Sure-Amp ampoules | 20 ampoule PoM £6.00
Lidocaine hydrochloride 20 mg per 1 ml Lidocaine 100mg/5ml (2%) solution for injection ampoules | 10 ampoule PoM £3.20-£12.00 DT = £3.20
Lidocaine 400mg/20ml (2%) solution for injection vials | 10 vial PoM £23.00 DT = £23.00
Lidocaine 200mg/10ml (2%) solution for injection Mini-Plasco ampoules | 20 ampoule PoM £14.95 DT = £14.95
Lidocaine 400mg/20ml (2%) solution for injection Mini-Plasco ampoules | 20 ampoule PoM
Lidocaine 40mg/2ml (2%) solution for injection ampoules | 10 ampoule PoM £12.00 DT = £2.70
Lidocaine 100mg/5ml (2%) solution for injection Mini-Plasco ampoules | 20 ampoule PoM £7.50
Lidocaine 400mg/20ml (2%) solution for injection ampoules | 10 ampoule PoM £11.00-£11.40 DT = £11.40

Cream

EXCIPIENTS: May contain Benzyl alcohol, propylene glycol

- LMX 4 (Ferndale Pharmaceuticals Ltd)
  Lidocaine 40 mg per 1 gram LMX 4 cream | 5 gram P £2.98 DT = £2.98 | 30 gram P £14.90 DT = £14.90
- Vagisil medicated (Combe International Ltd)
  Lidocaine 20 mg per 1 gram Vagisil 2% medicated cream | 30 gram GSL £2.99 DT = £2.99

Ointment

- Lidocaine hydrochloride (Non-proprietary)
  Lidocaine hydrochloride 50 mg per 1 gram Lidocaine 5% ointment | 15 gram P £9.00 DT = £8.28

Lidocaine with adrenaline

19-Dec-2019

The properties listed below are those particular to the combination only. For the properties of the components please consider, lidocaine hydrochloride p. 884, adrenaline/epinephrine p. 143.

- **INDICATIONS AND DOSE**

Local anaesthesia

- BY LOCAL INFILTRATION
- Child 12-17 years: Dosed according to the type of nerve block required (consult product literature)

- **INTERACTIONS** → Appendix 1: antiarrhythmics · sympathomimetics, vasoconstrictor
- **PROFESSION SPECIFIC INFORMATION**

Dental information A variety of lidocaine injections with adrenaline is available in dental cartridges.

Consult expert dental sources for specific advice in relation to dose of lidocaine for dental anaesthesia.

- **MEDICINAL FORMS** There can be variation in the licensing of different medicines containing the same drug. Forms available from special-order manufacturers include: solution for injection

Solution for injection

EXCIPIENTS: May contain Sulfites

- Lignospan Special (Septodont Ltd)
  Adrenaline (as Adrenaline acid tartrate) 12.5 microgram per 1 ml, Lidocaine hydrochloride 20 mg per 1 ml Lignospan Special 20mg/ml / 12.5micrograms/ml solution for injection 2.2ml cartridges | 50 cartridge PoM £21.95 DT = £21.95
  Lignospan Special 20mg/ml / 12.5micrograms/ml solution for injection 1.8ml cartridges | 50 cartridge PoM £21.95
- Rexocaine (Henry Schein Ltd)
  Adrenaline (as Adrenaline acid tartrate) 12.5 microgram per 1 ml, Lidocaine hydrochloride 20 mg per 1 ml Rexocaine 2% injection 2.2ml cartridges | 50 cartridge PoM £23.29 DT = £21.95
- Xylocaine with Adrenaline (Aspen Pharma Trading Ltd)
  Adrenaline (as Adrenaline acid tartrate) 5 microgram per 1 ml, Lidocaine hydrochloride 10 mg per 1 ml Xylocaine 1% with Adrenaline 100micrograms/20ml (1 in 200,000) solution for injection vials | 5 vial PoM £9.66 DT = £9.66 (Hospital only)
  Adrenaline (as Adrenaline acid tartrate) 5 microgram per 1 ml, Lidocaine hydrochloride 20 mg per 1 ml Xylocaine 2% with Adrenaline 100micrograms/20ml (1 in 200,000) solution for injection vials | 5 vial PoM £8.85 DT = £8.85 (Hospital only)

Lidocaine with cetrimide

27-Apr-2018

The properties listed below are those particular to the combination only. For the properties of the components please consider, lidocaine hydrochloride p. 884.

- **INDICATIONS AND DOSE**

Anaesthesia and disinfection in dental practice

- TO MUCOUS MEMBRANES USING OROMUCOSAL SPRAY
- Child 4-17 years: 10–20 mg, no more than 30 mg should be applied to the same quadrant of the buccal cavity—consult product literature, dose expressed as lidocaine

Anaesthesia in dental practice

- TO MUCOUS MEMBRANES USING DENTAL GEL
- Child 4-17 years: Apply 100–500 mg, use cotton pellet for application to dried mucosa, dose expressed as weight of gel

DOSE EQUIVALENCE AND CONVERSION

- 1 metered dose of *Xylonor®* spray is equivalent to 10 mg of lidocaine.
- 2 millimetres of *Xylonor®* gel is approximately equivalent to 100 mg of gel (approximately equivalent to 5 mg of lidocaine).

- **CAUTIONS** Sepsis (risk of rapid systemic absorption) · traumatised mucosa (risk of rapid systemic absorption)
- **INTERACTIONS** → Appendix 1: antiarrhythmics
- **MEDICINAL FORMS** There can be variation in the licensing of different medicines containing the same drug.

Oromucosal gel

- Xylonor (Septodont Ltd)
  Cetrimide 1.5 mg per 1 gram, Lidocaine 50 mg per 1 gram Xylonor 50mg/g / 1.5mg/g gel sugar-free | 15 gram PoM £4.00

Spray

- Xylonor (Septodont Ltd)
  Cetrimide 100 microgram per 1 gram, Lidocaine 10 mg per 1 gram Xylonor 150mg/g / 1.5mg/g oromucosal spray sugar-free | 36 gram PoM £20.15

Lidocaine with phenylephrine

The properties listed below are those particular to the combination only. For the properties of the components please consider, lidocaine hydrochloride p. 884, phenylephrine hydrochloride p. 132.

- **INDICATIONS AND DOSE**

Anaesthesia before nasal surgery, endoscopy, laryngoscopy, or removal of foreign bodies from the nose

- BY INTRANASAL ADMINISTRATION
- Child 12-17 years: Up to 8 sprays

- **INTERACTIONS** → Appendix 1: antiarrhythmics · sympathomimetics, vasoconstrictor

- **MEDICINAL FORMS** There can be variation in the licensing of different medicines containing the same drug.

Spray

- Lidocaine with phenylephrine (Non-proprietary)
Phenylephrine hydrochloride 5 mg per 1 ml, Lidocaine hydrochloride 50 mg per 1 ml Lidocaine 5% / Phenylephrine 0.5% nasal spray | 2.5 ml PoM £14.19 DT = £14.19

Lidocaine with prilocaine

10-Mar-2020

The properties listed below are those particular to the combination only. For the properties of the components please consider, lidocaine hydrochloride p. 884, prilocaine hydrochloride p. 888.

- **INDICATIONS AND DOSE**

Anaesthesia before minor skin procedures including venepuncture

- TO THE SKIN
- Neonate: Apply up to 1 g for maximum 1 hour before procedure, to be applied under occlusive dressing, shorter application time of 15–30 minutes is recommended for children with atopic dermatitis (30 minutes before removal of mollusca); maximum 1 dose per day.
- Child 1–2 months: Apply up to 1 g for maximum 1 hour before procedure, to be applied under occlusive dressing, shorter application time of 15–30 minutes is recommended for children with atopic dermatitis (30 minutes before removal of mollusca); maximum 1 dose per day
- Child 3–11 months: Apply up to 2 g for maximum 1 hour before procedure, to be applied under occlusive dressing, shorter application time of 15–30 minutes is recommended for children with atopic dermatitis (30 minutes before removal of mollusca); maximum 2 doses per day
- Child 1–11 years: Apply 1–5 hours before procedure, a thick layer should be applied under occlusive dressing, shorter application time of 15–30 minutes is recommended for children with atopic dermatitis (30 minutes before removal of mollusca); maximum 2 doses per day
- Child 12–17 years: Apply 1–5 hours before procedure (2–5 hours before procedures on large areas e.g. split skin grafting), a thick layer should be applied under occlusive dressing, shorter application time of 15–30 minutes is recommended for children with atopic dermatitis (30 minutes before removal of mollusca)

Anaesthesia on genital skin before injection of local anaesthetics

- TO THE SKIN
- Child 12–17 years: Apply under occlusive dressing for 15 minutes (males) or 60 minutes (females) before procedure

Anaesthesia before surgical treatment of lesions on genital mucosa

- TO THE SKIN
- Child 12–17 years: Apply up to 10 g, to be applied 5–10 minutes before procedure, maximum dose should be proportionally reduced in adolescents with body-weight less than 20 kg

Anaesthesia before cervical curettage

- TO THE SKIN
- Child 12–17 years: Apply 10 g in lateral vaginal fornices for 10 minutes

- **CONTRA-INDICATIONS** Use in child less than 37 weeks corrected gestational age
- **INTERACTIONS** → Appendix 1: anaesthetics, local · antiarrhythmics
- **SIDE-EFFECTS**
- **Rare or very rare** Methaemoglobinaemia · skin reactions
- **PATIENT AND CARER ADVICE**
Medicines for Children leaflet: EMLA cream for local anaesthesia www.medicinesforchildren.org.uk/emla-cream-local-anaesthesia

- **MEDICINAL FORMS** There can be variation in the licensing of different medicines containing the same drug.

Cream

- Denela (Teva UK Ltd)
Lidocaine 25 mg per 1 gram, Prilocaine 25 mg per 1 gram Denela 5% cream | 5 gram P £3.29 | 25 gram P £12.99 | 30 gram P £14.75 DT = £12.30
- Emla (Aspen Pharma Trading Ltd)
Lidocaine 25 mg per 1 gram, Prilocaine 25 mg per 1 gram Emla 5% cream | 5 gram P £2.25–£2.99 | 25 gram P £11.70 | 30 gram P £12.30 DT = £12.30
- Nulbia (Glenmark Pharmaceuticals Europe Ltd)
Lidocaine 25 mg per 1 gram, Prilocaine 25 mg per 1 gram Nulbia 5% cream | 5 gram P £1.58 | 25 gram P £7.88 | 30 gram P £8.61 DT = £12.30

Mepivacaine hydrochloride

04-Dec-2019

- **INDICATIONS AND DOSE**

Infiltration anaesthesia and nerve block in dentistry

- Child 3–17 years: Consult expert dental sources

DOSES AT EXTREMES OF BODY-WEIGHT

- To avoid excessive dosage in obese patients, dose should be calculated on the basis of ideal body-weight.

IMPORTANT SAFETY INFORMATION
Should only be administered by, or under the direct supervision of, personnel experienced in their use, with adequate training in anaesthesia and airway management, and should not be administered parenterally unless adequate resuscitation equipment is available.

- **CONTRA-INDICATIONS** Avoid injection into infected tissues · avoid injection into inflamed tissues · intravenous regional anaesthesia (Bier's block) · preparations containing preservatives should not be used for caudal, epidural, or spinal block · severe atrio-ventricular conduction disorders not controlled by a pacemaker

CONTRA-INDICATIONS, FURTHER INFORMATION

- Injection site Manufacturer advises the local anaesthetic effect may be reduced when injected into an inflamed or infected area, due to altered local pH. Increased absorption into the blood also increases the possibility of systemic side-effects.

- **CAUTIONS** Cardiovascular disease · children (consider dose reduction) · debilitated patients (consider dose reduction) · epilepsy · hypovolaemia · impaired cardiac conduction · impaired respiratory function · myasthenia gravis · shock
- **INTERACTIONS** → Appendix 1: anaesthetics, local
- **SIDE-EFFECTS**
- **Common or very common** Arrhythmias · dizziness · hypertension · hypotension · nausea · paraesthesia · vomiting
- **Uncommon** Neurotoxicity
- **Rare or very rare** Arachnoiditis · cardiac arrest · diplopia · nerve disorders · respiratory depression

SIDE-EFFECTS, FURTHER INFORMATION Toxic effects after administration of local anaesthetics are a result of excessively high plasma concentrations; severe toxicity usually results from inadvertent intravascular injection or too rapid injection. The systemic toxicity of local anaesthetics mainly involves the central nervous and cardiovascular systems. The onset of toxicity can be unpredictable and delayed. Monitor as per local protocol for at least 30 minutes after administration.

- **ALLERGY AND CROSS-SENSITIVITY**
- ▶ Hypersensitivity and cross-sensitivity Hypersensitivity reactions occur mainly with the ester-type local anaesthetics, such as tetracaine; reactions are less frequent with the amide types, such as articaine, bupivacaine, levobupivacaine, lidocaine, mepivacaine, prilocaine, and ropivacaine. Cross-sensitivity reactions may be avoided by using the alternative chemical type.
- **PREGNANCY** Use with caution in early pregnancy.
- **BREAST FEEDING** Use with caution.
- **HEPATIC IMPAIRMENT** Manufacturer advises caution; increased risk of toxic plasma concentrations in severe impairment.
- **RENAL IMPAIRMENT** Use with caution; increased risk of side-effects.

- **MEDICINAL FORMS** There can be variation in the licensing of different medicines containing the same drug.

Solution for injection

▶ Scandonest plain (Septodont Ltd)
Mepivacaine hydrochloride 30 mg per 1 ml Scandonest plain 3% solution for injection 2.2ml cartridges | 50 cartridge PoM £21.95

Mepivacaine with adrenaline 19-Dec-2019

The properties listed below are those particular to the combination only. For the properties of the components please consider, mepivacaine hydrochloride p. 887, adrenaline/epinephrine p. 143.

- **INDICATIONS AND DOSE**

Infiltration anaesthesia and nerve block in dentistry

▶ BY LOCAL INFILTRATION
▶ Child: (consult product literature)

- **INTERACTIONS** → Appendix 1: anaesthetics, local · sympathomimetics, vasoconstrictor

- **MEDICINAL FORMS** There can be variation in the licensing of different medicines containing the same drug.

Solution for injection

EXCIPIENTS: May contain Sulfites

▶ Scandonest special (Septodont Ltd)
Adrenaline 10 microgram per 1 ml, Mepivacaine hydrochloride 20 mg per 1 ml Scandonest special 2% solution for injection 2.2ml cartridges | 50 cartridge PoM £21.95

Prilocaine hydrochloride 09-Dec-2019

- **INDICATIONS AND DOSE**

DOSES AT EXTREMES OF BODY-WEIGHT
To avoid excessive dosage in obese patients, dose should be calculated on the basis of ideal body-weight.

CITANEST 1%®

Infiltration anaesthesia | Nerve block

▶ BY REGIONAL ADMINISTRATION
▶ Child 6 months–11 years: Up to 5 mg/kg, dose adjusted according to site of administration and response; maximum 400 mg per course
▶ Child 12–17 years: 100–200 mg/minute, alternatively, may be given in incremental doses; dose adjusted according to site of administration and response; maximum 400 mg per course

IMPORTANT SAFETY INFORMATION
Should only be administered by, or under the direct supervision of, personnel experienced in their use, with adequate training in anaesthesia and airway management, and should not be administered parenterally unless adequate resuscitation equipment is available.

- **CONTRA-INDICATIONS** Acquired methaemoglobinaemia · anaemia · avoid injection into infected tissues · avoid injection into inflamed tissues · congenital methaemoglobinaemia · preparations containing preservatives should not be used for caudal, epidural, or spinal block

CONTRA-INDICATIONS, FURTHER INFORMATION
▶ Injection site Manufacturer advises local anaesthetics should not be injected into inflamed or infected tissues. Increased absorption into the blood increases the possibility of systemic side-effects, and the local anaesthetic effect may also be reduced by altered local pH.

- **CAUTIONS** Cardiovascular disease · children (consider dose reduction) · debilitated patients (consider dose reduction) · epilepsy · hypovolaemia · impaired cardiac conduction · impaired respiratory function · myasthenia gravis · neonates and infants under 6 months are particularly susceptible to methaemoglobinaemia · severe or untreated hypertension · shock
- **INTERACTIONS** → Appendix 1: anaesthetics, local
- **SIDE-EFFECTS**

▶ **Common or very common** Arrhythmias · dizziness · hypertension · hypotension · nausea · paraesthesia · vomiting
▶ **Uncommon** Neurotoxicity
▶ **Rare or very rare** Cardiac arrest · methaemoglobinaemia · nerve disorders
▶ **Frequency not known** Diplopia · respiratory depression

SIDE-EFFECTS, FURTHER INFORMATION **Toxic effects** Toxic effects after administration of local anaesthetics are a result of excessively high plasma concentrations; severe toxicity usually results from inadvertent intravascular injection or too rapid injection. The systemic toxicity of local anaesthetics mainly involves the central nervous and cardiovascular systems. The onset of toxicity can be unpredictable and delayed. Monitor as per local protocol for at least 30 minutes after administration.

Methaemoglobinaemia Methaemoglobinaemia can be treated with an intravenous injection of methylthioninium chloride.

- **ALLERGY AND CROSS-SENSITIVITY**
- ▶ Hypersensitivity and cross-sensitivity Hypersensitivity reactions occur mainly with the ester-type local anaesthetics, such as tetracaine; reactions are less frequent with the amide types, such as articaine, bupivacaine, levobupivacaine, lidocaine, mepivacaine, prilocaine, and ropivacaine. Cross-sensitivity reactions may be avoided by using the alternative chemical type.
- **PREGNANCY** Large doses during delivery can cause neonatal respiratory depression, hypotonia, and bradycardia after epidural block. Avoid paracervical or pudendal block in obstetrics (neonatal methaemoglobinaemia reported).
Dose adjustments Use lower doses for intrathecal use during late pregnancy.
- **BREAST FEEDING** Present in milk but not known to be harmful.
- **HEPATIC IMPAIRMENT** Manufacturer advises caution.
- **RENAL IMPAIRMENT** Use with caution.
Dose adjustments Lower doses may be required for intrathecal anaesthesia.

● **MEDICINAL FORMS** There can be variation in the licensing of different medicines containing the same drug.

Solution for injection

▸ Citanest (Aspen Pharma Trading Ltd)
Prilocaine hydrochloride 10 mg per 1 ml Citanest 1% solution for injection 50ml vials | 1 vial PoM £5.06

Prilocaine with felypressin

The properties listed below are those particular to the combination only. For the properties of the components please consider, prilocaine hydrochloride p. 888.

● **INDICATIONS AND DOSE**

Dental anaesthesia

▸ BY REGIONAL ADMINISTRATION

▸ Child: Consult expert dental sources for specific advice

● **INTERACTIONS** → Appendix 1: anaesthetics, local

● **SIDE-EFFECTS** Bradycardia · cardiac arrest · dizziness · drowsiness · hypotension · loss of consciousness · methaemoglobinaemia · myocardial contractility decreased · nervousness · respiratory arrest · seizure · tremor · vision blurred

● **MEDICINAL FORMS** There can be variation in the licensing of different medicines containing the same drug.

Solution for injection

▸ Citanest with Octapressin (Dentsply Ltd)
Prilocaine hydrochloride 30 mg per 1 ml, Felypressin.03 unit per 1 ml Citanest 3% with Octapressin Dental 0.066units/2.2ml solution for injection self aspirating cartridges | 50 cartridge PoM

Ropivacaine hydrochloride

09-Dec-2019

● **INDICATIONS AND DOSE**

Acute pain | Surgical anaesthesia

▸ BY REGIONAL ADMINISTRATION

▸ Child: Adjust according to child's physical status and nature of procedure, seek expert advice

DOSES AT EXTREMES OF BODY-WEIGHT

▸ To avoid excessive dosage in obese patients, dose may need to be calculated on the basis of ideal bodyweight.

● **UNLICENSED USE** 2 mg/mL strength not licensed for use in children under 12 years except for acute pain management by caudal epidural block and continuous epidural infusion. 7.5 mg/mL and 10 mg/mL strengths not licensed for use in children under 12 years.

IMPORTANT SAFETY INFORMATION

Should only be administered by, or under the direct supervision of, personnel experienced in their use, with adequate training in anaesthesia and airway management, and should not be administered parenterally unless adequate resuscitation equipment is available.

● **CONTRA-INDICATIONS** Avoid injection into infected tissues · avoid injection into inflamed tissues · intravenous regional anaesthesia (Bier's block) · preparations containing preservatives should not be used for caudal, epidural, or spinal block

CONTRA-INDICATIONS, FURTHER INFORMATION

▸ Injection site Manufacturer advises local anaesthetics should not be injected into inflamed or infected tissues. Increased absorption into the blood increases the possibility of systemic side-effects, and the local anaesthetic effect may also be reduced by altered local pH.

● **CAUTIONS** Acute porphyrias p. 652 · cardiovascular disease · children (consider dose reduction) · complete heart block · debilitated patients (consider dose reduction) · epilepsy · hypovolaemia · impaired cardiac conduction · impaired respiratory function · myasthenia gravis · shock

● **INTERACTIONS** → Appendix 1: anaesthetics, local

● **SIDE-EFFECTS**

▸ **Common or very common** Arrhythmias · back pain · chills · dizziness · headache · hypertension · hypotension · nausea · sensation abnormal · urinary retention · vomiting

▸ **Uncommon** Anxiety · dyspnoea · hypothermia · neurotoxicity · syncope

▸ **Rare or very rare** Cardiac arrest

▸ **Frequency not known** Dyskinesia

SIDE-EFFECTS, FURTHER INFORMATION Toxic effects after administration of local anaesthetics are a result of excessively high plasma concentrations; severe toxicity usually results from inadvertent intravascular injection. The systemic toxicity of local anaesthetics mainly involves the central nervous and cardiovascular systems. The onset of toxicity can be unpredictable and delayed. Monitor as per local protocol for at least 30 minutes after administration.

● **ALLERGY AND CROSS-SENSITIVITY**

▸ Hypersensitivity and cross-sensitivity Hypersensitivity reactions occur mainly with the ester-type local anaesthetics, such as tetracaine; reactions are less frequent with the amide types, such as articaine, bupivacaine, levobupivacaine, lidocaine, mepivacaine, prilocaine, and ropivacaine. Cross-sensitivity reactions may be avoided by using the alternative chemical type.

● **PREGNANCY** Not known to be harmful. Do not use for paracervical block in obstetrics.

● **BREAST FEEDING** Not known to be harmful.

● **HEPATIC IMPAIRMENT** Manufacturer advises caution in severe impairment.

Dose adjustments Manufacturer advises consider dose reduction for repeat doses in severe impairment.

● **RENAL IMPAIRMENT** Caution in severe impairment. Increased risk of systemic toxicity in chronic renal failure.

● **MEDICINAL FORMS** There can be variation in the licensing of different medicines containing the same drug.

Solution for injection

ELECTROLYTES: May contain Sodium

▸ Ropivacaine hydrochloride (Non-proprietary)
Ropivacaine hydrochloride 2 mg per 1 ml Ropivacaine 20mg/10ml solution for injection ampoules | 10 ampoule PoM £16.50–£27.84 (Hospital only)
Ropivacaine hydrochloride 7.5 mg per 1 ml Ropivacaine 75mg/10ml solution for injection ampoules | 10 ampoule PoM £25.00–£28.40 (Hospital only)
Ropivacaine hydrochloride 10 mg per 1 ml Ropivacaine 100mg/10ml solution for injection ampoules | 10 ampoule PoM £30.00–£31.74 (Hospital only)

▸ Naropin (Aspen Pharma Trading Ltd)
Ropivacaine hydrochloride 2 mg per 1 ml Naropin 20mg/10ml solution for injection ampoules | 5 ampoule PoM £12.79
Ropivacaine hydrochloride 7.5 mg per 1 ml Naropin 75mg/10ml solution for injection ampoules | 5 ampoule PoM £15.90 (Hospital only)
Ropivacaine hydrochloride 10 mg per 1 ml Naropin 100mg/10ml solution for injection ampoules | 5 ampoule PoM £19.22 (Hospital only)

Infusion

ELECTROLYTES: May contain Sodium

▸ Ropivacaine hydrochloride (Non-proprietary)
Ropivacaine hydrochloride 2 mg per 1 ml Ropivacaine 400mg/200ml infusion bags | 5 bag PoM £79.35–£82.05 (Hospital only) | 10 bag PoM £137.00 (Hospital only)

▸ Naropin (Aspen Pharma Trading Ltd)
Ropivacaine hydrochloride 2 mg per 1 ml Naropin 400mg/200ml infusion Polybags | 5 bag PoM £86.70 (Hospital only)

Tetracaine

10-Mar-2020

(Amethocaine)

● **INDICATIONS AND DOSE**

Anaesthesia before venepuncture or venous cannulation

▸ TO THE SKIN

▸ Neonate: Apply contents of tube (or appropriate proportion) to site of venepuncture or venous cannulation and cover with occlusive dressing; remove gel and dressing after 30 minutes for venepuncture and after 45 minutes for venous cannulation.

▸ Child 1 month–4 years: Apply contents of up to 1 tube (applied at separate sites at a single time or appropriate proportion) to site of venepuncture or venous cannulation and cover with occlusive dressing; remove gel and dressing after 30 minutes for venepuncture and after 45 minutes for venous cannulation

▸ Child 5–17 years: Apply contents of up to 5 tubes (applied at separate sites at a single time or appropriate proportion) to site of venepuncture or venous cannulation and cover with occlusive dressing; remove gel and dressing after 30 minutes for venepuncture and after 45 minutes for venous cannulation

● **UNLICENSED USE** Not licensed for use in neonates.

● **CONTRA-INDICATIONS** Should not be applied to damaged skin

● **INTERACTIONS** → Appendix 1: anaesthetics, local

● **SIDE-EFFECTS** Oedema · skin reactions

SIDE-EFFECTS, FURTHER INFORMATION The systemic toxicity of local anaesthetics mainly involves the central nervous system; systemic side effects unlikely as minimal absorption following topical application.

● **ALLERGY AND CROSS-SENSITIVITY**

▸ Hypersensitivity and cross-sensitivity Hypersensitivity reactions occur mainly with the ester-type local anaesthetics, such as tetracaine; reactions are less frequent with the amide types, such as articaine, bupivacaine, levobupivacaine, lidocaine, mepivacaine, prilocaine, and ropivacaine. Cross-sensitivity reactions may be avoided by using the alternative chemical type.

● **BREAST FEEDING** Not known to be harmful.

● **PATIENT AND CARER ADVICE**

Medicines for Children leaflet: Tetracaine gel for local anaesthesia www.medicinesforchildren.org.uk/tetracaine-gel-local-anaesthesia

● **MEDICINAL FORMS** There can be variation in the licensing of different medicines containing the same drug.

Gel

EXCIPIENTS: May contain Hydroxybenzoates (parabens)

▸ Ametop (Forum Health Products Ltd)

Tetracaine 40 mg per 1 gram Ametop 4% gel | 1.5 gram [P] £1.08 DT = £1.08

15 Anaesthesia

Chapter 16
Emergency treatment of poisoning

CONTENTS

Poisoning, emergency treatment

28-Apr-2020

Overview

These notes provide only an overview of the treatment of poisoning, and it is strongly recommended that either **TOXBASE** or the **UK National Poisons Information Service** be consulted when there is doubt about the degree of risk or about management.

Most childhood poisoning is accidental. Other causes include intentional overdose, drug abuse, iatrogenic and deliberate poisoning. The drugs most commonly involved in childhood poisoning are paracetamol p. 288, ibuprofen p. 707, orally ingested creams, aspirin p. 98, iron preparations, cough medicines, and the contraceptive pill.

Hospital admission

Children who have features of poisoning should generally be admitted to hospital. Children who have taken poisons with delayed actions should also be admitted, even if they appear well. Delayed-action poisons include aspirin, iron, paracetamol, tricyclic antidepressants, and co-phenotrope (diphenoxylate with atropine, *Lomotil*®) p. 53; the effects of modified-release preparations are also delayed. A note of all relevant information, including what treatment has been given, should accompany the patient to hospital.

Further information

TOXBASE, the primary clinical toxicology database of the National Poisons Information Service, is available on the internet to registered users at www.toxbase.org (a backup site is available at www.toxbasebackup.org if the main site cannot be accessed). It provides information about routine diagnosis, treatment, and management of patients exposed to drugs, household products, and industrial and agricultural chemicals.

Specialist information and advice on the treatment of poisoning is available day and night from the **UK National Poisons Information Service** on the following number: Tel: 0344 892 0111.

Advice on laboratory analytical services can be obtained from TOXBASE or from the National Poisons Information Service. Help with identifying capsules or tablets may be available from a regional medicines information centre or from the National Poisons Information Service (out of hours).

General care

It is often impossible to establish with certainty the identity of the poison and the size of the dose. This is not usually important because only a few poisons (such as opioids, paracetamol, and iron) have specific antidotes; few patients require active removal of the poison. In most patients, treatment is directed at managing symptoms as they arise. Nevertheless, knowledge of the type and timing of poisoning can help in anticipating the course of events. All relevant information should be sought from the poisoned individual and from carers or parents. However, such information should be interpreted with care because it may not be complete or entirely reliable. Sometimes symptoms arise from other illnesses and patients should be assessed carefully. Accidents may involve domestic and industrial products (the contents of which are not generally known). The **National Poisons Information Service** should be consulted when there is doubt about any aspect of suspected poisoning.

Respiration

Respiration is often impaired in unconscious patients. An obstructed airway requires immediate attention. In the absence of trauma, the airway should be opened with simple measures such as chin lift or jaw thrust. An oropharyngeal or nasopharyngeal airway may be useful in patients with reduced consciousness to prevent obstruction, provided ventilation is adequate. Intubation and ventilation should be considered in patients whose airway cannot be protected or who have respiratory acidosis because of inadequate ventilation; such patients should be monitored in a critical care area.

Most poisons that impair consciousness also depress respiration. Assisted ventilation (either mouth-to-mouth or using a bag-valve-mask device) may be needed. Oxygen is not a substitute for adequate ventilation, although it should be given in the highest concentration possible in poisoning with carbon monoxide and irritant gases.

The potential for pulmonary aspiration of gastric contents should be considered.

Blood pressure

Hypotension is common in severe poisoning with central nervous system depressants; if severe, this may lead to irreversible brain damage or renal tubular necrosis. Hypotension should be corrected initially by raising the foot of the bed and administration of an infusion of either sodium chloride p. 636 or a colloid. Vasoconstrictor sympathomimetics are rarely required and their use may be discussed with the National Poisons Information Service or a paediatric intensive care unit.

Fluid depletion without hypotension is common after prolonged coma and after aspirin poisoning due to vomiting, sweating, and hyperpnoea.

Hypertension, often transient, occurs less frequently than hypotension in poisoning; it may be associated with sympathomimetic drugs such as amfetamines, phencyclidine, and cocaine.

Heart

Cardiac conduction defects and arrhythmias can occur in acute poisoning, notably with tricyclic antidepressants, some antipsychotics, and some antihistamines. Arrhythmias often respond to correction of underlying hypoxia, acidosis, or other biochemical abnormalities, but ventricular arrhythmias that cause serious hypotension require treatment. If the QT interval is prolonged, specialist advice should be sought because the use of some anti-arrhythmic drugs may be inappropriate. Supraventricular arrhythmias are seldom life-threatening and drug treatment is best withheld until the patient reaches hospital.

Body temperature

Hypothermia may develop in patients of any age who have been deeply unconscious for some hours, particularly following overdose with barbiturates or phenothiazines. It may be missed unless core temperature is measured using a low-reading rectal thermometer or by some other means. Hypothermia should be managed by prevention of further heat loss and appropriate rewarming as clinically indicated.

Hyperthermia can develop in patients taking CNS stimulants; children and the elderly are also at risk when taking therapeutic doses of drugs with antimuscarinic properties. Hyperthermia is initially managed by removing all unnecessary clothing and using a fan. Sponging with **tepid** water will promote evaporation. Advice should be sought from the National Poisons Information Service on the management of severe hyperthermia resulting from conditions such as the serotonin syndrome.

Both hypothermia and hyperthermia require **urgent** hospitalisation for assessment and supportive treatment.

Convulsions during poisoning

Single short-lived convulsions (lasting less than 5 minutes) do not require treatment. If convulsions are protracted or recur frequently, lorazepam p. 238 or diazepam p. 236 (preferably as emulsion) should be given by slow intravenous injection into a large vein. Benzodiazepines should not be given by the intramuscular route for convulsions. If the intravenous route is not readily available, midazolam oromucosal solution p. 239 can be given by the buccal route or diazepam can be administered as a rectal solution.

Methaemoglobinaemia

Drug- or chemical-induced methaemoglobinaemia should be treated with **methylthioninium chloride p. 903** if the methaemoglobin concentration is 30% or higher, *or* if symptoms of tissue hypoxia are present despite oxygen therapy. Methylthioninium chloride p. 903 reduces the ferric iron of methaemoglobin back to the ferrous iron of haemoglobin; in high doses, methylthioninium chloride can itself cause methaemoglobinaemia.

Poison removal and elimination

Prevention of absorption

Given by mouth, **charcoal, activated p. 898** can adsorb many poisons in the gastro-intestinal system, thereby reducing their absorption. The **sooner** it is given the **more effective** it is, but it may still be effective up to 1 hour after ingestion of the poison—longer in the case of modified-release preparations or of drugs with antimuscarinic (anticholinergic) properties. It is particularly useful for the prevention of absorption of poisons that are toxic in small amounts, such as antidepressants.

A second dose may occasionally be required when blood-drug concentration continues to rise suggesting delayed drug release or delayed gastric emptying.

Active elimination techniques

Repeated doses of **charcoal, activated** by mouth may *enhance the elimination* of some drugs after they have been absorbed; repeated doses are given after overdosage with:

- Carbamazepine
- Dapsone
- Phenobarbital
- Quinine
- Theophylline

If vomiting occurs after dosing, it should be treated (e.g. with an antiemetic drug) since it may reduce the efficacy of charcoal treatment. In cases of intolerance, the dose may be reduced and the frequency increased but this may compromise efficacy.

Charcoal, activated should **not** be used for poisoning with petroleum distillates, corrosive substances, alcohols, malathion, cyanides and metal salts including iron and lithium salts.

Other techniques intended to enhance the elimination of poisons after absorption are only practicable in hospital and are only suitable for a small number of severely poisoned patients. Moreover, they only apply to a limited number of poisons. Examples include:

- haemodialysis for ethylene glycol, lithium, methanol, phenobarbital, salicylates, and sodium valproate;
- alkalinisation of the urine for salicylates.

Removal from the gastro-intestinal tract

Gastric lavage is rarely required as benefit rarely outweighs risk; advice should be sought from the National Poisons Information Service if a significant quantity of iron or lithium has been ingested within the previous hour.

Whole bowel irrigation (by means of a bowel cleansing preparation) has been used in poisoning with certain modified-release or enteric-coated formulations, in severe poisoning with lithium salts, and if illicit drugs are carried in the gastro-intestinal tract ('body-packing'). However, it is not clear that the procedure improves outcome and advice should be sought from the National Poisons Information Service.

The administration of **laxatives** alone has no role in the management of the poisoned child and is not a recommended method of gut decontamination. The routine use of a laxative in combination with charcoal, activated has mostly been abandoned. Laxatives should not be administered to young children because of the likelihood of fluid and electrolyte imbalance.

Alcohol, acute intoxication

Acute intoxication with **alcohol** (ethanol) is common in adults but also occurs in children. The features include ataxia, dysarthria, nystagmus, and drowsiness, which may progress to coma, with hypotension and acidosis. Aspiration of vomit is a special hazard and hypoglycaemia may occur. Patients are managed supportively, with particular attention to maintaining a clear airway and measures to reduce the risk of aspiration of gastric contents. The blood glucose is measured and glucose given if indicated.

Aspirin poisoning

The main features of salicylate poisoning are hyperventilation, tinnitus, deafness, vasodilatation, and sweating. Coma is uncommon but indicates very severe poisoning. The associated acid-base disturbances are complex.

Treatment must be in hospital, where plasma salicylate, pH, and electrolytes can be measured; absorption of aspirin may be slow and the plasma-salicylate concentration may continue to rise for several hours, requiring repeated measurement. Plasma-salicylate concentration may not correlate with clinical severity in the young, and clinical and biochemical assessment is necessary. Generally, the clinical severity of poisoning is less below a plasma-salicylate concentration of 500 mg/litre (3.6 mmol/litre), unless there is evidence of metabolic acidosis. Activated charcoal can be given within 1 hour of ingesting more than 125 mg/kg of aspirin. Fluid losses should be replaced and intravenous sodium bicarbonate may be given (ensuring plasma-potassium concentration is within the reference range) to enhance urinary salicylate excretion (optimum urinary pH 7.5–8.5).

Plasma-potassium concentration should be corrected before giving sodium bicarbonate as hypokalaemia may complicate alkalinisation of the urine.

Haemodialysis is the treatment of choice for severe salicylate poisoning and should be considered when the plasma-salicylate concentration exceeds 700 mg/litre (5.1 mmol/litre) or in the presence of severe metabolic acidosis, convulsions, respiratory failure, pulmonary oedema or persistently high plasma-salicylate concentrations unresponsive to urinary alkalinisation.

Opioid poisoning

Opioids (narcotic analgesics) cause varying degrees of coma, respiratory depression, and pinpoint pupils. The specific antidote naloxone hydrochloride p. 901 is indicated if there is coma or bradypnoea. Since naloxone has a shorter duration of action than many opioids, close monitoring and repeated injections are necessary according to the respiratory rate and depth of coma. When repeated administration of naloxone is required, it can be given by continuous intravenous infusion instead and the rate of infusion adjusted according to vital signs. All children should be observed for at least 6 hours after the last dose of naloxone. The effects of some opioids, such as buprenorphine, are only partially reversed by naloxone. Dextropropoxyphene and methadone have very long durations of action; patients may need to be monitored for long periods following large overdoses.

Naloxone reverses the opioid effects of dextropropoxyphene. The long duration of action of dextropropoxyphene calls for prolonged monitoring and further doses of naloxone may be required. Norpropoxyphene, a metabolite of dextropropoxyphene, also has cardiotoxic effects which may require treatment with sodium bicarbonate p. 634 or magnesium sulfate p. 646, or both. Arrhythmias may occur for up to 12 hours.

Paracetamol poisoning

In all cases of **intravenous paracetamol poisoning** clinicians are encouraged to contact the National Poisons Information Service for advice on risk assessment and management.

Toxic doses of paracetamol may cause severe hepatocellular necrosis and, much less frequently, renal tubular necrosis. Nausea and vomiting, the only early features of poisoning, usually settle within 24 hours. Persistence beyond this time, often associated with the onset of right subcostal pain and tenderness, usually indicates development of hepatic necrosis. Liver damage is maximal 3–4 days after paracetamol overdose and may lead to hepatic failure, encephalopathy, coma, and death.

The following guidance provides only an overview of the management of paracetamol overdosage from the *National Poisons Information Service TOXBASE* database.

To avoid underestimating the potentially toxic paracetamol dose ingested by obese children who weigh more than 110 kg, use a body-weight of 110 kg (rather than their actual body-weight) when calculating the total dose of paracetamol ingested (in mg/kg).

Acetylcysteine p. 902 prevents or reduces the severity of liver damage if given up to, and possibly beyond (in those at risk of severe liver disease) 24 hours of ingesting paracetamol. It is most effective if given within 8 hours of paracetamol ingestion, after which effectiveness declines. Very rarely, giving acetylcysteine by mouth [unlicensed route] is an alternative if intravenous access is not possible.

Neonates less than 45 weeks corrected gestational age may be more susceptible to paracetamol-induced liver toxicity, therefore, treatment with acetylcysteine should be considered in all paracetamol overdoses, and if uncertain advice should be sought from the National Poisons Information Service.

Acute overdose

Acute overdose involves ingestion of a potentially toxic dose of paracetamol in 1 hour or less. Serious toxicity is unlikely to occur from a single ingestion of less than 75 mg/kg. All children should be referred to hospital for medical assessment if they have ingested paracetamol in the context of self-harm, are symptomatic, have ingested 75 mg/kg or more of paracetamol in 1 hour or less, or where the time of ingestion is uncertain but the dose ingested is 75 mg/kg or more. Although the benefit of gastric decontamination is uncertain, charcoal, activated p. 898 should be considered if the child presents within 1 hour of ingesting paracetamol in excess of 150 mg/kg.

Children at risk of liver damage and therefore requiring acetylcysteine, can be identified from a single measurement of the plasma-paracetamol concentration related to the time from ingestion, provided this time interval is not less than 4 hours; earlier samples cannot be interpreted. The concentration is plotted on a paracetamol treatment graph, with a reference line ('treatment line') joining plots of 100 mg/litre (0.66 mmol/litre) at 4 hours and 3.13 mg/litre (0.02 mmol/litre) at 24 hours, see *Paracetamol overdose treatment graph*.

Acetylcysteine treatment should commence in children:

- whose plasma-paracetamol concentration falls on or above the *treatment line* on the paracetamol treatment graph;
- who present within 8 hours of ingestion of more than 150 mg/kg of paracetamol, if there is going to be a delay of 8 hours or more in obtaining the paracetamol concentration after the overdose;
- who present 8–24 hours of ingestion of an acute overdose of more than 150 mg/kg of paracetamol, even if the plasma-paracetamol concentration is not yet available;
- who present more than 24 hours of ingestion of an overdose, if they are clearly jaundiced or have hepatic tenderness, their ALT is above the upper limit of normal (patients with chronically elevated ALT should be discussed with the National Poisons Information Service), their INR is greater than 1.3 (in the absence of another cause), or the paracetamol concentration is detectable.

Consider acetylcysteine treatment in children who present within 24 hours of an overdose if biochemical tests suggest acute liver injury, even if the plasma paracetamol concentration is below the treatment line on the paracetamol treatment graph.

If the child is not at risk of liver toxicity (i.e. the paracetamol concentration is below the treatment line or undetectable; the INR and ALT are normal; and the patient is asymptomatic) no treatment with an antidote is indicated; acetylcysteine may be discontinued if it has been started.

Where the time of ingestion is unknown, patients should be managed as a *staggered overdose*.

Staggered overdose or therapeutic excess

Children who have ingested more than 150 mg/kg of paracetamol in any 24-hour period are at risk of serious toxicity. Toxicity rarely occurs with paracetamol doses between 75–150 mg/kg in any 24-hour period. Doses consistently less than 75 mg/kg in any 24-hour period are

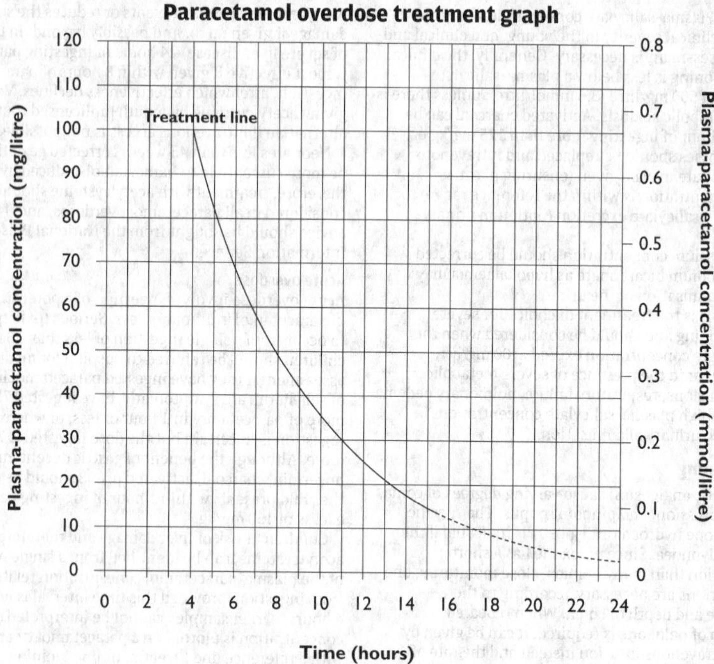

Patients whose plasma-paracetamol concentrations are on or above the **treatment line** should be treated with acetylcysteine by intravenous infusion.

The prognostic accuracy after 15 hours is uncertain, but a plasma-paracetamol concentration on or above the treatment line should be regarded as carrying a serious risk of liver damage.

Graph reproduced courtesy of Medicines and Healthcare products Regulatory Agency

very unlikely to be toxic; however risk may be increased if this dose is repeatedly ingested over 2 or more days. Ingestion of a licensed dose of paracetamol is not considered an overdose.

A **staggered overdose** involves ingestion of a potentially toxic dose of paracetamol over more than 1 hour, with the possible intention of causing self-harm. All children who have taken a staggered overdose should be referred to hospital for medical assessment. The MHRA advises that all children who have ingested a staggered overdose should be treated with acetylcysteine without delay.

Therapeutic excess is the ingestion of a potentially toxic dose of paracetamol with intent to treat pain or fever and without self-harm intent during its clinical use. All children should be referred to hospital for medical assessment if they are symptomatic, have ingested more than a licensed dose and more than or equal to 75 mg/kg in any 24-hour period, or have ingested more than the licensed dose but less than 75 mg/kg/24 hours on each of the preceding 2 or more days. Children with clinical features of hepatic injury such as jaundice or hepatic tenderness should be treated urgently with acetylcysteine. For other children, management is determined by the maximum dose of paracetamol ingested in any 24-hour period.

When there is uncertainty about whether the presentation was due to therapeutic excess, the patient should be managed as a *staggered overdose*.

Clinically significant toxicity is unlikely and the child is not considered to be at risk if, there has been at least 4 hours or more since the last paracetamol ingestion, the child has no symptoms suggesting liver damage, the paracetamol concentration is less than 10 mg/L, their ALT is within the normal range, and INR is 1.3 or less. Acetylcysteine can be discontinued in children not considered to be at risk of clinically significant liver damage. If there is uncertainty about a child's risk of toxicity after paracetamol overdose, advice should be sought from the National Poisons Information Service.

Acetylcysteine dose and administration

For paracetamol overdosage, acetylcysteine is given in a total dose that is divided into 3 consecutive intravenous infusions over a total of 21 hours. For further information on dosing/administration, see **Acetylcysteine Doses—Children** (for children who weigh less than 40 kg) and **Acetylcysteine Doses—Adults** (for children who weigh 40 kg or more), available from TOXBASE.

Antidepressant poisoning

Tricyclic and related antidepressants

Tricyclic and related antidepressants cause dry mouth, coma of varying degree, hypotension, hypothermia, hyperreflexia, extensor plantar responses, convulsions, respiratory failure, cardiac conduction defects, and arrhythmias. Dilated pupils and urinary retention also occur. Metabolic acidosis may complicate severe poisoning; delirium with confusion, agitation, and visual and auditory hallucinations are common during recovery.

Assessment in hospital is strongly advised in case of poisoning by tricyclic and related antidepressants but symptomatic treatment can be given before transfer. Supportive measures to ensure a clear airway and adequate ventilation during transfer are mandatory. Intravenous lorazepam or intravenous diazepam (preferably in emulsion form) may be required to treat convulsions. Activated charcoal given within 1 hour of the overdose reduces absorption of the drug. Although arrhythmias are worrying, some will respond to correction of hypoxia and acidosis. The use of anti-arrhythmic drugs is best avoided, but intravenous infusion of sodium bicarbonate can arrest arrhythmias or prevent them in those with an extended QRS duration. Diazepam p. 236 given by mouth is usually adequate to sedate delirious patients but large doses may be required.

Selective serotonin re-uptake inhibitors (SSRIs)

Symptoms of poisoning by selective serotonin re-uptake inhibitors include nausea, vomiting, agitation, tremor, nystagmus, drowsiness, and sinus tachycardia; convulsions may occur. Rarely, severe poisoning results in the serotonin syndrome, with marked neuropsychiatric effects, neuromuscular hyperactivity, and autonomic instability; hyperthermia, rhabdomyolysis, renal failure, and coagulopathies may develop.

Management of SSRI poisoning is supportive. Activated charcoal given within 1 hour of the overdose reduces absorption of the drug. Convulsions can be treated with lorazepam p. 238, diazepam, or buccal midazolam p. 239 (see *Convulsions*). Contact the National Poisons Information Service for the management of hyperthermia or the serotonin syndrome.

Antimalarial poisoning

Overdosage with quinine, chloroquine, or hydroxychloroquine is extremely hazardous and difficult to treat. Urgent advice from the National Poisons Information Service is essential. Life-threatening features include arrhythmias (which can have a very rapid onset) and convulsions (which can be intractable).

Antipsychotic poisoning

Phenothiazines and related drugs

Phenothiazines cause less depression of consciousness and respiration than other sedatives. Hypotension, hypothermia, sinus tachycardia, and arrhythmias may complicate poisoning. Dystonic reactions can occur with therapeutic doses (particularly with prochlorperazine and trifluoperazine), and convulsions may occur in severe cases. Arrhythmias may respond to correction of hypoxia, acidosis, and other biochemical abnormalities, but specialist advice should be sought if arrhythmias result from a prolonged QT interval; the use of some anti-arrhythmic drugs can worsen such arrhythmias. Dystonic reactions are rapidly abolished by injection of drugs such as procyclidine hydrochloride p. 273 or diazepam (emulsion preferred).

Second-generation antipsychotic drugs

Features of poisoning by second-generation antipsychotic drugs include drowsiness, convulsions, extrapyramidal symptoms, hypotension, and ECG abnormalities (including prolongation of the QT interval). Management is supportive. Charcoal, activated p. 898 can be given within 1 hour of ingesting a significant quantity of a second-generation antipsychotic drug.

Benzodiazepine poisoning

Benzodiazepines taken alone cause drowsiness, ataxia, dysarthria, nystagmus, and occasionally respiratory depression, and coma. Charcoal, activated can be given within 1 hour of ingesting a significant quantity of benzodiazepine, provided the patient is awake and the airway is protected. Benzodiazepines potentiate the effects of other central nervous system depressants taken concomitantly. Use of the benzodiazepine antagonist flumazenil p. 899 [unlicensed indication] can be hazardous, particularly in mixed overdoses involving tricyclic antidepressants or in benzodiazepine-dependent patients. Flumazenil may prevent the need for ventilation, particularly in patients with severe respiratory disorders; it should be used on expert advice only and not as a diagnostic test in children with a reduced level of consciousness.

Beta blockers poisoning

Overdosages with beta-blockers may cause cardiac effects such as bradycardia, hypotension, syncope, conduction abnormalities, and heart failure. Bradycardia is the most common arrhythmia, but some beta-blockers may induce ventricular tachyarrhythmias secondary to prolongation of QT interval (e.g. sotalol) or QRS duration (e.g. propranolol). Although the predominant effects of beta-blocker overdose are on the heart, other features may also occur, such as central nervous system effects (including drowsiness, confusion, convulsions, hallucinations, and in severe cases coma), respiratory depression, and bronchospasm. The effects of overdosage can vary from one beta-blocker to another; propranolol overdosage in particular may cause coma and convulsions.

The following guidance provides only an overview of the management of beta-blocker overdosage from the *National Poisons Information Service TOXBASE database*.

All children who have been exposed to beta-blockers as a result of self-harm should be referred for assessment. Medical assessment is recommended for all children who are symptomatic or have ingested more than a toxic dose; and in those who are treatment naive or have taken more than their therapeutic dose, and have a significant cardiac history or asthma. All children who have exceeded their prescribed daily dose of 2 or more cardiotoxic agents should also be referred for medical assessment irrespective of the dose ingested. Hospital clinicians are encouraged to discuss all serious cases with the UK National Poisons Information Service.

For children presenting with overdose, maintain a clear airway and adequate ventilation. Although the benefit of gastric decontamination is uncertain, charcoal, activated can be considered if the child presents within 1 hour of ingestion of more than a potentially toxic dose.

For the management of hypotension, ensure adequate fluid resuscitation; in an emergency, vasopressors and inotropes can be initiated under the advice of an experienced physician. Intravenous glucagon [unlicensed] p. 502 is a treatment option for severe hypotension, heart failure, or cardiogenic shock. In severe cases, an insulin and glucose infusion can improve myocardial contractility and systemic perfusion, especially in the presence of acidosis. Consider intravenous sodium bicarbonate p. 634 for correction of metabolic acidosis that persists despite correction of hypoxia and adequate fluid resuscitation—rapid correction is particularly important if QRS duration is prolonged. For symptomatic bradycardia give intravenous atropine sulfate p. 869; dobutamine [unlicensed] p. 129 or isoprenaline [unlicensed] (available from 'special-order' manufacturers or specialist importing companies) may be considered if bradycardia is associated with hypotension. A temporary cardiac pacemaker can be used to increase the heart rate.

Treat bronchospasm with nebulised bronchodilators and corticosteroids.

If convulsions occur give oxygen, and correct acid-base and metabolic disturbances as required. Prolonged or frequent convulsions should be controlled with intravenous diazepam, lorazepam, or midazolam. If convulsions are unresponsive to treatment, the child should be referred urgently to critical care.

Calcium-channel blockers poisoning

Features of calcium-channel blocker poisoning include nausea, vomiting, dizziness, agitation, confusion, and coma in severe poisoning. Metabolic acidosis and hyperglycaemia may occur. Verapamil and diltiazem have a profound cardiac depressant effect causing hypotension and arrhythmias, including complete heart block and asystole. The dihydropyridine calcium-channel blockers cause severe hypotension secondary to profound peripheral vasodilatation.

Charcoal, activated p. 898 should be considered if the patient presents within 1 hour of overdosage with a calcium-channel blocker; repeated doses of activated charcoal are considered if a modified-release preparation is involved. In patients with significant features of poisoning, calcium chloride p. 642 or calcium gluconate p. 642 is given by injection; atropine sulfate p. 869 is given to correct symptomatic bradycardia. In severe cases, an insulin and glucose infusion may be required in the management of hypotension and myocardial failure. For the management of hypotension, the choice of inotropic sympathomimetic depends on whether hypotension is secondary to vasodilatation or to myocardial depression—advice should be sought from the National Poisons Information Service.

Iron salts poisoning

Iron poisoning in childhood is usually accidental. The symptoms are nausea, vomiting, abdominal pain, diarrhoea, haematemesis, and rectal bleeding. Hypotension and hepatocellular necrosis can occur later. Coma, shock, and metabolic acidosis indicate severe poisoning.

Advice should be sought from the National Poisons Information Service if a significant quantity of iron has been ingested within the previous hour.

Mortality is reduced by intensive and specific therapy with desferrioxamine mesilate p. 624, which chelates iron. The serum-iron concentration is measured as an emergency and intravenous desferrioxamine mesilate given to chelate absorbed iron in excess of the expected iron binding capacity. In severe toxicity intravenous desferrioxamine mesilate should be given immediately without waiting for the result of the serum-iron measurement.

Lithium poisoning

Most cases of lithium intoxication occur as a complication of long-term therapy and are caused by reduced excretion of the drug because of a variety of factors including dehydration, deterioration of renal function, infections, and co-administration of diuretics or NSAIDs (or other drugs that interact). Acute deliberate overdoses may also occur with delayed onset of symptoms (12 hours or more) owing to slow entry of lithium into the tissues and continuing absorption from modified-release formulations.

The early clinical features are non-specific and may include apathy and restlessness which could be confused with mental changes arising from the child's depressive illness. Vomiting, diarrhoea, ataxia, weakness, dysarthria, muscle twitching, and tremor may follow. Severe poisoning is associated with convulsions, coma, renal failure, electrolyte imbalance, dehydration, and hypotension.

Therapeutic serum-lithium concentrations are within the range of 0.4–1 mmol/litre; concentrations in excess of 2 mmol/litre are usually associated with serious toxicity and such cases may need treatment with haemodialysis if neurological symptoms or renal failure are present. In acute overdosage much higher serum-lithium concentrations may be present without features of toxicity and all that is usually necessary is to take measures to increase urine output (e.g. by increasing fluid intake but avoiding diuretics). Otherwise, treatment is supportive with special regard to electrolyte balance, renal function, and control of convulsions. Whole-bowel irrigation should be considered for significant ingestion, but advice should be sought from the National Poisons Information Service.

Stimulant-drug poisoning

Amfetamines

Amfetamines cause wakefulness, excessive activity, paranoia, hallucinations, and hypertension followed by exhaustion, convulsions, hyperthermia, and coma. The early stages can be controlled by diazepam p. 236 or lorazepam p. 238; advice should be sought from the National Poisons Information Service on the management of hypertension. Later, tepid sponging, anticonvulsants, and artificial respiration may be needed.

Cocaine

Cocaine stimulates the central nervous system, causing agitation, dilated pupils, tachycardia, hypertension, hallucinations, hyperthermia, hypertonia, and hyperreflexia; cardiac effects include chest pain, myocardial infarction, and arrhythmias.

Initial treatment of cocaine poisoning involves cooling measures for hyperthermia (see Body temperature); agitation, hypertension and cardiac effects require specific treatment and expert advice should be sought.

Ecstasy

Ecstasy (methylenedioxymethamfetamine, MDMA) may cause severe reactions, even at doses that were previously tolerated. The most serious effects are delirium, coma, convulsions, ventricular arrhythmias, hyperthermia, rhabdomyolysis, acute renal failure, acute hepatitis, disseminated intravascular coagulation, adult respiratory distress syndrome, hyperreflexia, hypotension and intracerebral haemorrhage; hyponatraemia has also been associated with ecstasy use and syndrome of inappropriate antidiuretic hormone secretion (SIADH) can occur.

Treatment of methylenedioxymethamfetamine poisoning is supportive, with diazepam to control persistent convulsions and close monitoring including ECG. For the management of agitation, seek specialist advice. Self-induced water intoxication should be considered in patients with ecstasy poisoning.

'Liquid ecstasy' is a term used for sodium oxybate (gamma-hydroxybutyrate, GHB), which is a sedative.

Theophylline poisoning

Theophylline and related drugs are often prescribed as modified-release formulations and toxicity can therefore be delayed. They cause vomiting (which may be severe and intractable), agitation, restlessness, dilated pupils, sinus tachycardia, and hyperglycaemia. More serious effects are haematemesis, convulsions, and supraventricular and ventricular arrhythmias. Severe hypokalaemia may develop rapidly.

Repeated doses of charcoal, activated can be used to eliminate theophylline even if more than 1 hour has elapsed after ingestion and especially if a modified-release preparation has been taken (see also under Active Elimination Techniques). Ondansetron p. 281 may be effective for severe vomiting that is resistant to other antiemetics. Hypokalaemia is corrected by intravenous infusion of potassium chloride p. 651 and may be so severe as to require high doses under ECG monitoring. Convulsions should be controlled by intravenous administration of lorazepam or diazepam (see Convulsions). For the management of agitation associated with theophylline overdosage, seek specialist advice.

Provided the child does **not** suffer from asthma, a short-acting beta-blocker can be administered intravenously to reverse severe tachycardia, hypokalaemia, and hyperglycaemia.

Cyanide poisoning

Oxygen should be administered to children with cyanide poisoning. The choice of antidote depends on the severity of poisoning, certainty of diagnosis, and the cause. Dicobalt edetate p. 898 is the antidote of choice when there is a strong clinical suspicion of severe cyanide poisoning, but it should **not** be used as a precautionary measure. Dicobalt edetate itself is toxic, associated with anaphylactoid reactions, and is potentially fatal if administered in the absence of cyanide poisoning. A regimen of sodium nitrite p. 899 followed by sodium thiosulfate p. 899 is an alternative if dicobalt edetate is not available.

Hydroxocobalamin (*Cyanokit*®—no other preparation of hydroxocobalamin is suitable) p. 621 can be considered for use in victims of smoke inhalation who show signs of significant cyanide poisoning.

Ethylene glycol and methanol poisoning

Fomepizole (available from 'special-order' manufacturers or specialist importing companies) is the treatment of choice for ethylene glycol and methanol (methyl alcohol) poisoning. If necessary, **ethanol** (by mouth or by intravenous infusion) can be used, but with caution. Advice on the treatment of ethylene glycol and methanol poisoning should be obtained from the National Poisons Information Service. It is important to start antidote treatment promptly in cases of suspected poisoning with these agents.

Heavy metal poisoning

Heavy metal antidotes include succimer (DMSA) [unlicensed], unithiol (DMPS) [unlicensed], sodium calcium edetate [unlicensed], and dimercaprol. Dimercaprol in the management of heavy metal poisoning has been superseded by other chelating agents. In all cases of heavy metal poisoning, the advice of the National Poisons Information Service should be sought.

Noxious gases poisoning

Carbon monoxide

Carbon monoxide poisoning is usually due to inhalation of smoke, car exhaust, or fumes caused by blocked flues or incomplete combustion of fuel gases in confined spaces.

Immediate treatment of carbon monoxide poisoning is essential. The patient should be moved to fresh air, the airway cleared, and high-flow **oxygen** 100% administered as soon as available. Artificial respiration should be given as necessary and continued until adequate spontaneous breathing starts, or stopped only after persistent and efficient treatment of cardiac arrest has failed. The child should be admitted to hospital because complications may arise after a delay of hours or days. Cerebral oedema may occur in severe poisoning and is treated with an intravenous infusion of mannitol p. 149. Referral for hyperbaric oxygen treatment should be discussed with the National Poisons Information Service if the patient is pregnant or in cases of severe poisoning such as if the patient is or has been unconscious, or has psychiatric or neurological features other than a headache or has myocardial ischaemia or an arrhythmia, or has a blood carboxyhaemoglobin concentration of more than 20%.

Sulfur dioxide, chlorine, phosgene, and ammonia

All of these gases can cause upper respiratory tract and conjunctival irritation. Pulmonary oedema, with severe breathlessness and cyanosis may develop suddenly up to 36 hours after exposure. Death may occur. Patients are kept under observation and those who develop pulmonary oedema are given oxygen. Assisted ventilation may be necessary in the most serious cases.

CS spray poisoning

CS spray, which is used for riot control, irritates the eyes (hence 'tear gas') and the respiratory tract; symptoms normally settle spontaneously within 15 minutes. If symptoms persist, the patient should be removed to a well-ventilated area, and the exposed skin washed with soap and water after removal of contaminated clothing. Contact lenses should be removed and rigid ones washed (soft ones should be discarded). Eye symptoms should be treated by irrigating the eyes with physiological saline (or water if saline is not available) and advice sought from an ophthalmologist. Patients with features of severe poisoning, particularly respiratory complications, should be admitted to hospital for symptomatic treatment.

Nerve agents poisoning

Treatment of nerve agent poisoning is similar to organophosphorus insecticide poisoning, but advice must be sought from the National Poisons Information Service. The risk of cross-contamination is significant; adequate decontamination and protective clothing for healthcare personnel are essential. In emergencies involving the release of **nerve agents**, kits ('NAAS pods') containing **pralidoxime chloride p. 899** can be obtained through the Ambulance Service from the National Blood Service (or the Welsh Blood Service in South Wales or designated hospital pharmacies in Northern Ireland and Scotland—see TOXBASE for list of designated centres).

Pesticide poisoning

Organophosphorus insecticides

Organophosphorus insecticides are usually supplied as powders or dissolved in organic solvents. All are absorbed through the bronchi and intact skin as well as through the gut and inhibit cholinesterase activity, thereby prolonging and intensifying the effects of acetylcholine. Toxicity between different compounds varies considerably, and onset may be delayed after skin exposure.

Anxiety, restlessness, dizziness, headache, miosis, nausea, hypersalivation, vomiting, abdominal colic, diarrhoea, bradycardia, and sweating are common features of organophosphorus poisoning. Muscle weakness and fasciculation may develop and progress to generalised flaccid paralysis, including the ocular and respiratory muscles. Convulsions, coma, pulmonary oedema with copious bronchial secretions, hypoxia, and arrhythmias occur in severe cases. Hyperglycaemia and glycosuria without ketonuria may also be present.

Further absorption of the organophosphorus insecticide should be prevented by moving the child to fresh air, removing soiled clothing, and washing contaminated skin. In severe poisoning it is vital to ensure a clear airway, frequent removal of bronchial secretions, and adequate ventilation and oxygenation; gastric lavage may be considered provided that the airway is protected. Atropine sulfate p. 869 will reverse the muscarinic effects of acetylcholine and is given by intravenous injection until the skin becomes flushed and dry, the pupils dilate, and bradycardia is abolished.

Pralidoxime chloride, a cholinesterase reactivator, is used as an adjunct to atropine sulfate in moderate or severe poisoning. It improves muscle tone within 30 minutes of administration. Pralidoxime chloride is continued until the patient has not required atropine sulfate for 12 hours. Pralidoxime chloride can be obtained from designated centres, the names of which are held by the National Poisons Information Service.

Snake bites and animal stings

Snake bites

Envenoming from snake bite is uncommon in the UK. Many exotic snakes are kept, some illegally, but the only indigenous venomous snake is the adder (*Vipera berus*). The bite may cause local and systemic effects. Local effects include pain, swelling, bruising, and tender enlargement of regional lymph nodes. Systemic effects include early anaphylactic symptoms (transient hypotension with syncope, angioedema, urticaria, abdominal colic, diarrhoea, and vomiting), with later persistent or recurrent hypotension, ECG abnormalities, spontaneous systemic bleeding, coagulopathy, adult respiratory distress syndrome, and acute renal failure. Fatal envenoming is rare but the potential for severe envenoming must not be underestimated.

Early anaphylactic symptoms should be treated with adrenaline/epinephrine p. 143. Indications for european viper snake venom antiserum p. 904 treatment include *systemic envenoming*, especially hypotension, ECG abnormalities, vomiting, haemostatic abnormalities, and marked local envenoming such that after bites on the hand or foot, swelling extends beyond the wrist or ankle within 4 hours of the bite. For those children who present with clinical features of *severe envenoming* (e.g. shock, ECG abnormalities, or local swelling that has advanced from the foot to above the knee or from the hand to above the elbow within 2 hours of the bite), a higher initial dose of the european viper snake venom antiserum is recommended; if symptoms of *systemic envenoming* persist contact the National Poisons Information Service.
Adrenaline/epinephrine injection must be immediately to hand for treatment of anaphylactic reactions to the european viper snake venom antiserum.

Antivenom is available for bites by certain foreign snakes and spiders, stings by scorpions and fish. For information on identification, management, and for supply in an emergency, telephone the National Poisons Information Service. Whenever possible the TOXBASE entry should be read, and relevant information collected, before telephoning the National Poisons Information Service.

16

Emergency treatment of poisoning

Insect stings

Stings from ants, wasps, hornets, and bees cause local pain and swelling but seldom cause severe direct toxicity unless many stings are inflicted at the same time. If the sting is in the mouth or on the tongue local swelling may threaten the upper airway. The stings from these insects are usually treated by cleaning the area with a topical antiseptic. Bee stings should be removed as quickly as possible.
Anaphylactic reactions require immediate treatment with intramuscular **adrenaline/epinephrine** **p. 143**; self-administered (or administered by a carer) intramuscular adrenaline/epinephrine (e.g. *EpiPen®*) is the best first-aid treatment for patients with severe hypersensitivity. An inhaled bronchodilator should be used for asthmatic reactions, see also the management of anaphylaxis. A short course of an **oral antihistamine** or a **topical corticosteroid** may help to reduce inflammation and relieve itching. A vaccine containing extracts of bee and wasp venom can be used to reduce the risk of anaphylaxis and systemic reactions in patients with systemic hypersensitivity to bee or wasp stings.

Marine stings

The severe pain of weeverfish (*Trachinus vipera*) and Portuguese man-o'-war stings can be relieved by immersing the stung area immediately in uncomfortably hot, but not scalding, water (not more than 45° C). People stung by jellyfish and Portuguese man-o'-war around the UK coast should be removed from the sea as soon as possible. Adherent tentacles should be lifted off carefully (wearing gloves or using tweezers) or washed off with seawater. Alcoholic solutions, including suntan lotions, should **not** be applied because they can cause further discharge of stinging hairs. Ice packs can be used to reduce pain.

Other poisons

Consult either the National Poisons Information Service day and night or TOXBASE.

The **National Poisons Information Service** (Tel: 0344 892 0111) will provide specialist advice on all aspects of poisoning day and night.

1 Active elimination from the gastro-intestinal tract

ANTIDOTES AND CHELATORS › INTESTINAL ADSORBENTS

Charcoal, activated

● **INDICATIONS AND DOSE**

Reduction of absorption of poisons in the gastro-intestinal system

▶ BY MOUTH

- Neonate: 1 g/kg.
- Child 1 month–11 years: 1 g/kg (max. per dose 50 g)
- Child 12–17 years: 50 g

Active elimination of poisons

▶ BY MOUTH

- Neonate: 1 g/kg every 4 hours, dose may be reduced and the frequency increased if not tolerated, reduced dose may compromise efficacy.
- Child 1 month–11 years: 1 g/kg every 4 hours (max. per dose 50 g), dose may be reduced and the frequency increased if not tolerated, reduced dose may compromise efficacy
- Child 12–17 years: Initially 50 g, then 50 g every 4 hours, reduced if not tolerated to 25 g every 2 hours, alternatively 12.5 g every 1 hour, reduced dose may compromise efficacy

● **CAUTIONS** Comatose patient (risk of aspiration—ensure airway is protected) · drowsy patient (risk of aspiration—ensure airway protected) · reduced gastrointestinal motility (risk of obstruction)

● **SIDE-EFFECTS** Bezoar · constipation · diarrhoea · gastrointestinal disorders

● **DIRECTIONS FOR ADMINISTRATION** Suspension or reconstituted powder may be mixed with soft drinks (e.g. caffeine-free diet cola) or fruit juices to mask the taste.

● **MEDICINAL FORMS** There can be variation in the licensing of different medicines containing the same drug.

Oral suspension

▸ Charcodote (Teva UK Ltd)
Activated charcoal 200 mg per 1 ml Charcodote 200mg/ml oral suspension sugar-free | 250 ml Ⓟ £11.88

Granules

▸ Carbomix (Kent Pharmaceuticals Ltd)
Activated charcoal 813 mg per 1 gram Carbomix 81.3% granules sugar-free | 50 gram Ⓟ £11.90

2 Chemical toxicity

2.1 Cyanide toxicity

ANTIDOTES AND CHELATORS

Dicobalt edetate

● **INDICATIONS AND DOSE**

Severe poisoning with cyanides

▶ BY INTRAVENOUS INJECTION

- Child: Consult the National Poisons Information Service

- **CAUTIONS** Owing to toxicity to be used only for definite cyanide poisoning when patient tending to lose, or has lost, consciousness
- **SIDE-EFFECTS** Reflex tachycardia · vomiting
- **EXCEPTIONS TO LEGAL CATEGORY** Prescription only medicine restriction does not apply where administration is for saving life in emergency.

- **MEDICINAL FORMS** No licensed medicines listed.

Sodium nitrite

16-Mar-2018

- **INDICATIONS AND DOSE**

Poisoning with cyanides (used in conjunction with sodium thiosulfate)

▶ BY INTRAVENOUS INJECTION

▸ Child: Consult the National Poisons Information Service

- **SIDE-EFFECTS** Arrhythmias · dizziness · headache · hypotension · palpitations
- **EXCEPTIONS TO LEGAL CATEGORY** Prescription only medicine restriction does not apply where administration is for saving life in emergency.

- **MEDICINAL FORMS** There can be variation in the licensing of different medicines containing the same drug.

Solution for injection

▸ Sodium nitrite (Non-proprietary)
Sodium nitrite 30 mg per 1 ml Sodium nitrite 300mg/10ml solution for injection vials | 1 vial PoM ☒ (Hospital only)

Sodium thiosulfate

16-Mar-2018

- **INDICATIONS AND DOSE**

Poisoning with cyanides

▶ BY INTRAVENOUS INJECTION

▸ Child: Consult the National Poisons Information Service

DOSE EQUIVALENCE AND CONVERSION

▸ 12.5 g equates to 50 mL of a 25% solution *or* 25 mL of a 50% solution.

- **EXCEPTIONS TO LEGAL CATEGORY** Prescription only medicine restriction does not apply where administration is for saving life in emergency.

- **MEDICINAL FORMS** There can be variation in the licensing of different medicines containing the same drug. Forms available from special-order manufacturers include: solution for injection

Solution for injection

▸ Sodium thiosulfate (Non-proprietary)
Sodium thiosulfate 250 mg per 1 ml Sodium thiosulfate 12.5g/50ml solution for injection vials | 1 vial PoM ☒ (Hospital only)

2.2 Organophosphorus toxicity

Other drugs used for Organophosphorus toxicity Atropine sulfate, p. 869

ANTIDOTES AND CHELATORS

Pralidoxime chloride

- **INDICATIONS AND DOSE**

Adjunct to atropine in the treatment of poisoning by organophosphorus insecticide or nerve agent

▶ BY INTRAVENOUS INFUSION

▸ Child: Initially 30 mg/kg, to be given over 20 minutes, followed by 8 mg/kg/hour; maximum 12 g per day

- **UNLICENSED USE** Pralidoxime chloride doses may differ from those in product literature.
  Licensed for use in children (age range not specified by manufacturer).
- **CONTRA-INDICATIONS** Poisoning with carbamates · poisoning with organophosphorus compounds without anticholinesterase activity
- **CAUTIONS** Myasthenia gravis
- **SIDE-EFFECTS** Dizziness · drowsiness · headache · hyperventilation · muscle weakness · nausea · tachycardia · vision disorders
- **RENAL IMPAIRMENT** Use with caution.
- **DIRECTIONS FOR ADMINISTRATION** The loading dose may be administered by intravenous injection (diluted to a concentration of 50 mg/mL with water for injections) over at least 5 minutes if pulmonary oedema is present or if it is not practical to administer an intravenous infusion.
  For *intravenous infusion*, reconstitute each vial with 20 mL Water for Injections, then dilute to a concentration of 10–20 mg/mL with Sodium Chloride 0.9%.
- **PRESCRIBING AND DISPENSING INFORMATION** Available from designated centres for organophosphorus insecticide poisoning or from the National Blood Service (or Welsh Ambulance Services for Mid West and South East Wales)—see TOXBASE for list of designated centres).
- **EXCEPTIONS TO LEGAL CATEGORY** Prescription only medicine restriction does not apply where administration is for saving life in emergency.

- **MEDICINAL FORMS** There can be variation in the licensing of different medicines containing the same drug.

Powder for solution for injection

▸ Protopam Chloride (Imported (United States))
Pralidoxime chloride 1 gram Protopam Chloride 1g powder for solution for injection vials | 6 vial PoM ☒

3 Drug toxicity

3.1 Benzodiazepine toxicity

ANTIDOTES AND CHELATORS › BENZODIAZEPINE ANTAGONISTS

Flumazenil

19-Nov-2019

- **INDICATIONS AND DOSE**

Reversal of sedative effects of benzodiazepines

▶ BY INTRAVENOUS INJECTION

▸ Neonate: 10 micrograms/kg every 1 minute if required, dose to be administered over 15 seconds.

▸ Child: 10 micrograms/kg every 1 minute (max. per dose 200 micrograms) if required, dose to be administered over 15 seconds; maximum 1 mg per course; maximum 50 micrograms/kg per course

continued →

Reversal of sedative effects of benzodiazepines (if drowsiness recurs after injection)

▶ BY INTRAVENOUS INFUSION

▸ Neonate: 2–10 micrograms/kg/hour, adjusted according to response.

▸ Child: 2–10 micrograms/kg/hour (max. per dose 400 micrograms/hour), adjusted according to response

Reversal of sedative effects of benzodiazepines in intensive care

▶ BY INTRAVENOUS INJECTION

▸ Child: 10 micrograms/kg every 1 minute (max. per dose 200 micrograms) if required, dose to be administered over 15 seconds; maximum 2 mg per course; maximum 50 micrograms/kg per course

- **UNLICENSED USE** Not licensed for use in children under 1 year. Not licensed for use by intravenous infusion in children. Not licensed for use in children in intensive care.

IMPORTANT SAFETY INFORMATION
Flumazenil should only be administered by, or under the direct supervision of, personnel experienced in its use.

- **CONTRA-INDICATIONS** Life-threatening condition (e.g. raised intracranial pressure, status epilepticus) controlled by benzodiazepines
- **CAUTIONS** Avoid rapid injection following major surgery · avoid rapid injection in high-risk or anxious patients · benzodiazepine dependence (may precipitate withdrawal symptoms) · children · ensure neuromuscular blockade cleared before giving · head injury (rapid reversal of benzodiazepine sedation may cause convulsions) · history of panic disorders (risk of recurrence) · prolonged benzodiazepine therapy for epilepsy (risk of convulsions) · short-acting (repeat doses may be necessary—benzodiazepine effects may persist for at least 24 hours)
- **SIDE-EFFECTS**

▶ **Common or very common** Anxiety · diplopia · dry mouth · eye disorders · flushing · headache · hiccups · hyperhidrosis · hyperventilation · hypotension · insomnia · nausea · palpitations · paraesthesia · speech disorder · tremor · vertigo · vomiting

▶ **Uncommon** Abnormal hearing · arrhythmias · chest pain · chills · cough · dyspnoea · nasal congestion · seizure (more common in patients with epilepsy)

▶ **Frequency not known** Withdrawal syndrome

- **PREGNANCY** Not known to be harmful.
- **BREAST FEEDING** Avoid breast-feeding for 24 hours.
- **HEPATIC IMPAIRMENT** Manufacturer advises caution (risk of increased half-life).
  Dose adjustments Manufacturer advises cautious dose titration.
- **DIRECTIONS FOR ADMINISTRATION** For *continuous intravenous infusion*, dilute with Glucose 5% or Sodium Chloride 0.9%.

- **MEDICINAL FORMS** There can be variation in the licensing of different medicines containing the same drug.

Solution for injection

▸ Flumazenil (Non-proprietary)
Flumazenil 100 microgram per 1 ml Flumazenil 500micrograms/5ml solution for injection ampoules | 5 ampoule [PoM] £72.46 (Hospital only) | 5 ampoule [PoM] £65.50-£70.00 | 10 ampoule [PoM] £140.00

3.2 Digoxin toxicity

ANTIDOTES AND CHELATORS > ANTIBODIES

Digoxin-specific antibody

- **INDICATIONS AND DOSE**

Treatment of known or strongly suspected life-threatening digoxin toxicity associated with ventricular arrhythmias or bradyarrhythmias unresponsive to atropine and when measures beyond the withdrawal of digoxin and correction of any electrolyte abnormalities are considered necessary

▶ BY INTRAVENOUS INFUSION

▸ Child: Serious cases of digoxin toxicity should be discussed with the National Poisons Information Service (consult product literature)

- **MEDICINAL FORMS** There can be variation in the licensing of different medicines containing the same drug.

Powder for solution for infusion

▸ DigiFab (BTG International Ltd)
Digoxin-specific antibody fragments 40 mg DigiFab 40mg powder for solution for infusion vials | 1 vial [PoM] £750.00 (Hospital only)

3.3 Heparin toxicity

ANTIDOTES AND CHELATORS

Protamine sulfate

- **INDICATIONS AND DOSE**

Overdosage with intravenous injection or intravenous infusion of unfractionated heparin (less than 30 minutes lapsed since overdose)

▶ BY INTRAVENOUS INJECTION

▸ Child: 1 mg (max. per dose 50 mg), to be administered at a rate not exceeding 5 mg/minute, to neutralise each 100 units of unfractionated heparin

Overdosage with intravenous injection or intravenous infusion of unfractionated heparin (if 30–60 minutes lapsed since overdose)

▶ BY INTRAVENOUS INJECTION

▸ Child: 500–750 micrograms (max. per dose 50 mg), to be administered at a rate not exceeding 5 mg/minute, to neutralise each 100 units of unfractionated heparin

Overdosage with intravenous injection or intravenous infusion of unfractionated heparin (if 60–120 minutes lapsed since overdose)

▶ BY INTRAVENOUS INJECTION

▸ Child: 375–500 micrograms (max. per dose 50 mg), to be administered at a rate not exceeding 5 mg/minute, to neutralise each 100 units of unfractionated heparin

Overdosage with intravenous injection or intravenous infusion of unfractionated heparin (if over 120 minutes lapsed since overdose)

▶ BY INTRAVENOUS INJECTION

▸ Child: 250–375 micrograms (max. per dose 50 mg), to be administered at a rate not exceeding 5 mg/minute, to neutralise each 100 units of unfractionated heparin

Overdosage with subcutaneous injection of unfractionated heparin

▶ BY INTRAVENOUS INJECTION, OR BY INTRAVENOUS INFUSION

▸ Child: (max. per dose 50 mg), 50–100% of the total dose to be given by intravenous injection (rate not exceeding 5 mg/minute), then give any remainder of dose by intravenous infusion over 8–16 hours, 1 mg neutralises approx. 100 units of unfractionated heparin

Overdosage with subcutaneous injection of low molecular weight heparin

▶ BY INTRAVENOUS INJECTION, OR BY CONTINUOUS INTRAVENOUS INFUSION

▸ Child: (max. per dose 50 mg), to be administered by intermittent intravenous injection at a rate not exceeding 5 mg/minute or by continuous intravenous infusion, 1 mg neutralises approx. 100 units of low molecular weight heparin, consult product literature of low molecular weight heparin for details

● **CAUTIONS** Excessive doses can have an anticoagulant effect

● **SIDE-EFFECTS**

▶ **Rare or very rare** Hypertension · pulmonary oedema non-cardiogenic

▶ **Frequency not known** Acute pulmonary vasoconstriction · back pain · bradycardia · circulatory collapse · dyspnoea · fatigue · feeling hot · flushing · nausea · pulmonary hypertension · vomiting

● **ALLERGY AND CROSS-SENSITIVITY** Caution if increased risk of allergic reaction to protamine (includes previous treatment with protamine or protamine insulin, allergy to fish, men who are infertile or who have had a vasectomy and who may have antibodies to protamine).

● **MONITORING REQUIREMENTS** Monitor activated partial thromboplastin time or other appropriate blood clotting parameters.

● **DIRECTIONS FOR ADMINISTRATION** May be diluted if necessary with Sodium Chloride 0.9%.

● **PRESCRIBING AND DISPENSING INFORMATION** The long half-life of low molecular weight heparins should be taken into consideration when determining the dose of protamine sulfate; the effects of low molecular weight heparins can persist for up to 24 hours after administration.

● **MEDICINAL FORMS** There can be variation in the licensing of different medicines containing the same drug.

Solution for injection

▸ Protamine sulfate (Non-proprietary)

Protamine sulfate 10 mg per 1 ml Protamine sulfate 100mg/10ml solution for injection ampoules | 5 ampoule [PoM] [S]
Protamine sulfate 50mg/5ml solution for injection ampoules | 10 ampoule [PoM] £49.55

3.4 Opioid toxicity

OPIOID RECEPTOR ANTAGONISTS

Naloxone hydrochloride

08-Jan-2020

● **INDICATIONS AND DOSE**

Overdosage with opioids

▶ BY INTRAVENOUS INJECTION

▸ Neonate: Initially 100 micrograms/kg, if no response, repeat at intervals of 1 minute to a max. of 2 mg, then review diagnosis; further doses may be required if respiratory function deteriorates, doses can be given by subcutaneous or intramuscular routes but only if intravenous route is not feasible; intravenous administration has more rapid onset of action.

▸ Child 1 month–11 years: Initially 100 micrograms/kg (max. per dose 2 mg), if no response, repeat at intervals of 1 minute to a max. of 2 mg, then review diagnosis; further doses may be required if respiratory function deteriorates, doses can be given by subcutaneous or intramuscular routes but only if intravenous route is not feasible; intravenous administration has more rapid onset of action

▸ Child 12–17 years: Initially 400 micrograms, then 800 micrograms for up to 2 doses at 1 minute intervals if no response to preceding dose, then increased to 2 mg for 1 dose if still no response (4 mg dose may be required in seriously poisoned patients), then review diagnosis; further doses may be required if respiratory function deteriorates, doses can be given by subcutaneous or intramuscular routes but only if intravenous route is not feasible; intravenous administration has more rapid onset of action

▶ BY CONTINUOUS INTRAVENOUS INFUSION

▸ Neonate: Using an infusion pump, adjust rate according to response (initially, rate may be set at 60% of the initial resuscitative intravenous injection dose per hour). The initial resuscitative *intravenous injection* dose is that which maintained satisfactory ventilation for at least 15 minutes.

▸ Child: Using an infusion pump, adjust rate according to response (initially, rate may be set at 60% of the initial resuscitative intravenous injection dose per hour). The initial resuscitative *intravenous injection* dose is that which maintained satisfactory ventilation for at least 15 minutes

▶ BY INTRANASAL ADMINISTRATION

▸ Child 14–17 years: 1.8 mg, administered into one nostril, if no response, give a second dose after 2–3 minutes. If the patient responds to the first dose then relapses into respiratory depression, give the second dose immediately. Further doses should be administered into alternate nostrils

Overdosage with opioids in a non-medical setting

▶ BY INTRANASAL ADMINISTRATION

▸ Child 14–17 years: 1.8 mg, administered into one nostril, if no response, give a second dose after 2–3 minutes. If the patient responds to the first dose then relapses into respiratory depression, give the second dose immediately. Further doses should be administered into alternate nostrils

Reversal of postoperative respiratory depression

▶ INITIALLY BY INTRAVENOUS INJECTION

▸ Neonate: 1 microgram/kg, repeated every 2–3 minutes if required.

▸ Child 1 month–11 years: 1 microgram/kg, repeated every 2–3 minutes if required

▸ Child 12–17 years: Initially 100–200 micrograms, alternatively (by intravenous injection) initially 1.5–3 micrograms/kg, if response inadequate, give subsequent doses, (by intravenous injection) 100 micrograms every 2 minutes, alternatively (by intramuscular injection) 100 micrograms every 1–2 hours

Reversal of respiratory and CNS depression resulting from opioid administration to mother during labour

▶ BY INTRAMUSCULAR INJECTION

▸ Neonate: 200 micrograms, alternatively 60 micrograms/kg, to be given as a single dose at birth.

▶ BY INTRAVENOUS INJECTION, OR BY SUBCUTANEOUS INJECTION

▸ Neonate: 10 micrograms/kg, repeated every 2–3 minutes if required.

DOSE EQUIVALENCE AND CONVERSION

▸ With intranasal use

▸ 1 spray equivalent to 1.8 mg.

continued →

PHARMACOKINETICS
- Naloxone has a short duration of action; repeated doses or infusion may be necessary to reverse effects of opioids with longer duration of action.

- **UNLICENSED USE** Naloxone doses in BNF may differ from those in product literature.

IMPORTANT SAFETY INFORMATION

SAFE PRACTICE

Doses used in acute opioid overdosage may not be appropriate for the management of opioid-induced respiratory depression and sedation in those receiving palliative care and in chronic opioid use.

- **CAUTIONS** Cardiovascular disease or those receiving cardiotoxic drugs (serious adverse cardiovascular effects reported) · maternal physical dependence on opioids (may precipitate withdrawal in newborn) · pain · physical dependence on opioids (precipitates withdrawal)

CAUTIONS, FURTHER INFORMATION
- Titration of dose In postoperative use, the dose should be titrated for each patient in order to obtain sufficient respiratory response; however, naloxone antagonises analgesia.
- **SIDE-EFFECTS**

GENERAL SIDE-EFFECTS
- **Common or very common** Arrhythmias · dizziness · headache · hypertension · hypotension · nausea · vomiting
- **Uncommon** Diarrhoea · dry mouth · hyperhidrosis · hyperventilation · tremor
- **Rare or very rare** Cardiac arrest · erythema multiforme · pulmonary oedema

SPECIFIC SIDE-EFFECTS
- **Uncommon**
- With parenteral use Inflammation localised · pain · vascular irritation
- **Rare or very rare**
- With parenteral use Anxiety · seizure
- **Frequency not known**
- With parenteral use Analgesia reversed · asthenia · chills · death · dyspnoea · fever · irritability · nasal complaints · piloerection · yawning
- **PREGNANCY** Use only if potential benefit outweighs risk.
- **BREAST FEEDING** Not orally bioavailable.
- **DIRECTIONS FOR ADMINISTRATION**
- With intravenous use For *continuous intravenous infusion*, dilute to a concentration of up to 200 micrograms/mL with Glucose 5% or Sodium Chloride 0.9%.
- **PRESCRIBING AND DISPENSING INFORMATION**
- With intranasal use The manufacturer has provided a *Healthcare Professional Guidance Document*.
- **PATIENT AND CARER ADVICE** Patients and carers should be given advice on how to administer naloxone nasal spray.
- With intranasal use Patient training and information cards should be provided.

- **MEDICINAL FORMS** There can be variation in the licensing of different medicines containing the same drug.

Solution for injection
- Naloxone hydrochloride (Non-proprietary)
  Naloxone hydrochloride 20 microgram per 1 ml Naloxone 40micrograms/2ml solution for injection ampoules | 10 ampoule PoM £55.00
  Naloxone hydrochloride (as Naloxone hydrochloride dihydrate) 400 microgram per 1 ml Naloxone 400micrograms/1ml solution for injection ampoules | 10 ampoule PoM £36.00–£53.70 DT = £40.51
  Naloxone hydrochloride 1 mg per 1 ml Naloxone 2mg/2ml solution for injection pre-filled syringes | 1 pre-filled disposable injection PoM £16.80

Spray
- Nyxoid (Napp Pharmaceuticals Ltd)
  Naloxone (as Naloxone hydrochloride dihydrate) 18 mg per 1 ml Nyxoid 1.8mg/0.1ml nasal spray 0.1ml unit dose | 2 unit dose PoM £27.50

3.5 Paracetamol toxicity

ANTIDOTES AND CHELATORS

Acetylcysteine

03-Apr-2018

- **INDICATIONS AND DOSE**

Paracetamol overdosage

▶ BY INTRAVENOUS INFUSION
- Neonate: Initially 150 mg/kg over 1 hour, dose to be administered in 3 mL/kg glucose 5%, followed by 50 mg/kg over 4 hours, dose to be administered in 7 mL/kg glucose 5%, then 100 mg/kg over 16 hours, dose to be administered in 14 mL/kg glucose 5%.
- Child (body-weight up to 20 kg): Initially 150 mg/kg over 1 hour, dose to be administered in 3 mL/kg glucose 5%, followed by 50 mg/kg over 4 hours, dose to be administered in 7 mL/kg glucose 5%, then 100 mg/kg over 16 hours, dose to be administered in 14 mL/kg glucose 5%
- Child (body-weight 20-39 kg): Initially 150 mg/kg over 1 hour, dose to be administered in 100 mL glucose 5%, followed by 50 mg/kg over 4 hours, dose to be administered in 250 mL glucose 5%, then 100 mg/kg over 16 hours, dose to be administered in 500 mL glucose 5%
- Child (body-weight 40 kg and above): 150 mg/kg over 1 hour, dose to be administered in 200 mL Glucose Intravenous Infusion 5%, then 50 mg/kg over 4 hours, to be started immediately after completion of first infusion, dose to be administered in 500 mL Glucose Intravenous Infusion 5%, then 100 mg/kg over 16 hours, to be started immediately after completion of second infusion, dose to be administered in 1 litre Glucose Intravenous Infusion 5%

Meconium ileus

▶ BY MOUTH
- Neonate: 200–400 mg up to 3 times a day if required.

Treatment of distal intestinal obstructive syndrome

▶ BY MOUTH
- Child 1 month–1 year: 0.4–3 g as a single dose
- Child 2-6 years: 2–3 g as a single dose
- Child 7-17 years: 4–6 g as a single dose

Prevention of distal intestinal obstruction syndrome

▶ BY MOUTH
- Child 1 month–1 year: 100–200 mg 3 times a day
- Child 2-11 years: 200 mg 3 times a day
- Child 12-17 years: 200–400 mg 3 times a day

DOSES AT EXTREMES OF BODY-WEIGHT
- To avoid excessive dosage in obese patients, a ceiling weight of 110 kg should be used when calculating the dose for paracetamol overdosage.

● **UNLICENSED USE**

▸ With oral use Not licensed for use in meconium ileus or for distal intestinal obstructive syndrome in children with cystic fibrosis.

IMPORTANT SAFETY INFORMATION

MHRA/CHM ADVICE: INTRAVENOUS ACETYLCYSTEINE FOR PARACETAMOL OVERDOSE: REMINDER OF AUTHORISED DOSE REGIMEN; POSSIBLE NEED FOR CONTINUED TREATMENT (JANUARY 2017)

The authorised dose regimen for acetylcysteine in paracetamol overdose is 3 consecutive intravenous infusions given over a total of 21 hours.

Continued treatment (given at the dose and rate as used in the third infusion) may be necessary depending on the clinical evaluation of the individual patient.

● **CAUTIONS**

▸ With intravenous use asthma (see Side-effects for management of asthma but do not delay acetylcysteine treatment) · atopy · may slightly increase INR · may slightly increase prothrombin time

▸ With oral use Asthma · history of peptic ulceration

● **SIDE-EFFECTS**

▸ With parenteral use Acidosis · anaphylactoid reaction · angioedema · anxiety · arrhythmias · cardiac arrest · chest discomfort · cough · cyanosis · eye pain · eye swelling · generalised seizure · hyperhidrosis · hypertension · hypotension · joint disorders · malaise · nausea · pain facial · respiratory disorders · skin reactions · syncope · thrombocytopenia · vasodilation · vision blurred · vomiting

SIDE-EFFECTS, FURTHER INFORMATION Anaphylactoid reactions (with intravenous use) can be managed by suspending treatment and initiating appropriate management. Treatment may then be restarted at lower rate.

● **DIRECTIONS FOR ADMINISTRATION**

▸ With oral use For *oral* administration, use oral granules, *or* dilute injection solution (200 mg/mL) to a concentration of 50 mg/mL; orange or blackcurrant juice or cola drink may be used as a diluent to mask the bitter taste.

▸ With intravenous use Glucose 5% is preferred fluid; Sodium Chloride 0.9% is an alternative if Glucose 5% unsuitable.

● **MEDICINAL FORMS** There can be variation in the licensing of different medicines containing the same drug. Forms available from special-order manufacturers include: effervescent tablet, granules, solution for infusion

Granules

CAUTIONARY AND ADVISORY LABELS 13

▸ Fluimucil N (Imported (Germany))

Acetylcysteine 100 mg Fluimucil N 100mg granules sachets | 20 sachet PoM

Acetylcysteine 200 mg Fluimucil N 200mg granules sachets | 20 sachet PoM

▸ A-CYS (Ennogen Healthcare Ltd)

Acetylcysteine 200 mg A-CYS 200mg granules sachets | 20 sachet £75.00

Solution for infusion

ELECTROLYTES: May contain Sodium

▸ Acetylcysteine (Non-proprietary)

Acetylcysteine 200 mg per 1 ml Acetylcysteine 2g/10ml solution for infusion ampoules | 10 ampoule PoM £21.26 DT = £21.26

▸ Parvolex (Phoenix Labs Ltd)

Acetylcysteine 200 mg per 1 ml Parvolex 2g/10ml concentrate for solution for infusion ampoules | 10 ampoule PoM £22.50 DT = £21.26

4 Methaemoglobinaemia

ANTIDOTES AND CHELATORS

Methylthioninium chloride

(Methylene blue)

● **INDICATIONS AND DOSE**

Drug- or chemical-induced methaemoglobinaemia

▸ BY SLOW INTRAVENOUS INJECTION

▸ Neonate: Seek advice from National Poisons Information Service.

▸ Child 1-2 months: Seek advice from National Poisons Information Service

▸ Child 3 months–17 years: Initially 1–2 mg/kg, then 1–2 mg/kg after 30–60 minutes if required, to be given over 5 minutes, seek advice from National Poisons Information Service if further repeat doses are required; maximum 7 mg/kg per course

Aniline- or dapsone-induced methaemoglobinaemia

▸ BY SLOW INTRAVENOUS INJECTION

▸ Child 3 months–17 years: Initially 1–2 mg/kg, then 1–2 mg/kg after 30–60 minutes if required, to be given over 5 minutes, seek advice from National Poisons Information Service if further repeat doses are required; maximum 4 mg/kg per course

● **CAUTIONS** Children under 3 months (more susceptible to methaemoglobinaemia from high doses of methylthioninium) · chlorate poisoning (reduces efficacy of methylthioninium) · G6PD deficiency (seek advice from National Poisons Information Service) · methaemoglobinaemia due to treatment of cyanide poisoning with sodium nitrite (seek advice from National Poisons Information Service) · pulse oximetry may give false estimation of oxygen saturation

● **INTERACTIONS** → Appendix 1: methylthioninium chloride

● **SIDE-EFFECTS**

▸ **Common or very common** Abdominal pain · anxiety · chest pain · dizziness · headache · hyperhidrosis · nausea · pain in extremity · paraesthesia · skin reactions · taste altered · urine discolouration · vomiting

▸ **Frequency not known** Aphasia · arrhythmias · confusion · faeces discoloured · fever · haemolytic anaemia · hyperbilirubinaemia (in infants) · hypertension · hypotension · injection site necrosis · mydriasis · tremor

● **PREGNANCY** No information available, but risk to fetus of untreated methaemoglobinaemia likely to be significantly higher than risk of treatment.

● **BREAST FEEDING** Manufacturer advises avoid breastfeeding for up to 6 days after administration—no information available.

● **RENAL IMPAIRMENT**

Dose adjustments Use with caution in severe impairment; dose reduction may be required.

● **DIRECTIONS FOR ADMINISTRATION** For *intravenous injection*, may be diluted with Glucose 5% to minimise injection-site pain; not compatible with Sodium Chloride 0.9%.

● **MEDICINAL FORMS** There can be variation in the licensing of different medicines containing the same drug. Forms available from special-order manufacturers include: solution for injection

Solution for injection

▸ Methylthioninium chloride (Non-proprietary)

Methylthioninium chloride 5 mg per 1 ml Methylthioninium chloride Proveblue 50mg/10ml solution for injection ampoules | 5 ampoule PoM £196.89

Methylthioninium chloride 10 mg per 1 ml Methylthioninium chloride 50mg/5ml concentrate for solution for injection vials | 5 vial PoM £150.00 (Hospital only)

5 Snake bites

IMMUNE SERA AND IMMUNOGLOBULINS › ANTITOXINS

European viper snake venom antiserum

● **INDICATIONS AND DOSE**

Systemic envenoming from snake bites | Marked local envenoming

▶ BY INTRAVENOUS INJECTION, OR BY INTRAVENOUS INFUSION

▶ Child: Initially 10 mL for 1 dose, then 10 mL after 1–2 hours if required, the second dose should only be given if symptoms of systemic envenoming persist after the first dose, if symptoms of systemic envenoming persist contact the National Poisons Information Service

Severe systemic envenoming from snake bites in patients presenting with clinical features

▶ BY INTRAVENOUS INJECTION, OR BY INTRAVENOUS INFUSION

▶ Child: Initially 20 mL for 1 dose, if symptoms of systemic envenoming persist contact the National Poisons Information Service

● **DIRECTIONS FOR ADMINISTRATION** By *intravenous injection* given over 10–15 minutes or by *intravenous infusion* over 30 minutes after diluting in sodium chloride 0.9% (use 5 mL diluent/kg body-weight).

● **PRESCRIBING AND DISPENSING INFORMATION** To order, email immform@dh.gsi.gov.uk.

● **MEDICINAL FORMS** There can be variation in the licensing of different medicines containing the same drug.

Solution for injection

▶ European viper snake venom antiserum (Non-proprietary)
European viper snake venom antiserum 100 mg per 1 ml Viper venom antiserum, European (equine) 1g/10ml solution for injection vials | 1 vial PoM ☒

Appendix 1 Interactions

Changes have been made to the interactions content in BNF publications. For more information, see www.bnf.org/new-bnf-interactions/.

Two or more drugs given at the same time can exert their effects independently or they can interact. Interactions may be beneficial and exploited therapeutically; this type of interaction is not within the scope of this appendix. Many interactions are harmless, and even those that are potentially harmful can often be managed, allowing the drugs to be used safely together. Nevertheless, adverse drug interactions should be reported to the Medicines and Healthcare products Regulatory Agency (MHRA), through the Yellow Card Scheme (see Adverse reactions to drugs p. 13), as for other adverse drug reactions.

Potentially harmful drug interactions may occur in only a small number of patients, but the true incidence is often hard to establish. Furthermore the severity of a harmful interaction is likely to vary from one patient to another. Patients at increased risk from drug interactions include the elderly and those with impaired renal or hepatic function.

Interactions can result in the potentiation or antagonism of one drug by another, or result in another effect, such as renal impairment. Drug interactions may develop either through pharmacokinetic or pharmacodynamic mechanisms.

Pharmacodynamic interactions

These are interactions between drugs which have similar or antagonistic pharmacological effects or side-effects. They might be due to competition at receptor sites, or occur between drugs acting on the same physiological system. They are usually predictable from a knowledge of the pharmacology of the interacting drugs; in general, those demonstrated with one drug are likely to occur with related drugs.

Pharmacokinetic interactions

These occur when one drug alters the absorption, distribution, metabolism, or excretion of another, thus increasing or decreasing the amount of drug available to produce its pharmacological effects. Pharmacokinetic interactions occurring with one drug do not necessarily occur uniformly across a group of related drugs.

Affecting absorption The rate of absorption and the total amount absorbed can both be altered by drug interactions. Delayed absorption is rarely of clinical importance unless a rapid effect is required (e.g. when giving an analgesic). Reduction in the total amount absorbed, however, can result in ineffective therapy.

Affecting distribution *Due to changes in protein binding*: To a variable extent most drugs are loosely bound to plasma proteins. Protein-binding sites are non-specific and one drug can displace another thereby increasing the proportion free to diffuse from plasma to its site of action. This only produces a detectable increase in effect if it is an extensively bound drug (more than 90%) that is not widely distributed throughout the body. Even so displacement rarely produces more than transient potentiation because this increased concentration of free drug will usually be eliminated.

Displacement from protein binding plays a part in the potentiation of warfarin by sulfonamides but these interactions become clinically relevant mainly because warfarin metabolism is also inhibited.

Induction or inhibition of drug transporter proteins: Drug transporter proteins, such as P-glycoprotein, actively transport drugs across biological membranes. Transporters can be induced or inhibited, resulting in changes in the concentrations of drugs that are substrates for the transporter. For example, rifampicin induces P-glycoprotein, particularly in the gut wall, resulting in decreased plasma concentrations of digoxin, a P-glycoprotein substrate.

Affecting metabolism Many drugs are metabolised in the liver. Drugs are either metabolised by phase I reactions (oxidation, reduction, or hydrolysis) or by phase II reactions (e.g. glucoronidation).

Phase I reactions are mainly carried out by the cytochrome P450 family of isoenzymes, of which CYP3A4 is the most important isoenzyme involved in the metabolism of drugs. Induction of cytochrome P450 isoenzymes by one drug can increase the rate of metabolism of another, resulting in lower plasma concentrations and a reduced effect. On withdrawal of the inducing drug, plasma concentrations increase and toxicity can occur.

Conversely when one drug inhibits cytochrome P450 isoenzymes, it can decrease the metabolism of another, leading to higher plasma concentrations, resulting in an increased effect with a risk of toxicity.

Isoenzymes of the hepatic cytochrome P450 system interact with a wide range of drugs. With knowledge of which isoenzymes are involved in a drug's metabolism, it is possible to predict whether certain pharmacokinetic interactions will occur. For example, carbamazepine is a potent inducer of CYP3A4, ketoconazole is potent inhibitor of CYP3A4, and midazolam is a substrate of CYP3A4. Carbamazepine reduces midazolam concentrations, and it is therefore likely that other drugs that are potent inducers of CYP3A4 will interact similarly with midazolam. Ketoconazole, however, increases midazolam concentrations, and it can be predicted that other drugs that are potent inhibitors of CYP3A4 will interact similarly.

Less is known about the enzymes involved in phase II reactions. These include UDP-glucuronyltransferases which, for example, might be induced by rifampicin, resulting in decreased metabolism of mycophenolate (a substrate for this enzyme) to its active form, mycophenolic acid.

Affecting renal excretion Drugs are eliminated through the kidney both by glomerular filtration and by active tubular secretion. Competition occurs between those which share active transport mechanisms in the proximal tubule. For example, salicylates and some other NSAIDs delay the excretion of methotrexate; serious methotrexate toxicity is possible. Changes in urinary pH can also affect the reabsorption of a small number of drugs, including methenamine.

Relative importance of interactions

Levels of severity: Most interactions have been assigned a severity; this describes the likely effect of an unmanaged interaction on the patient.

Severe—the result may be a life-threatening event or have a permanent detrimental effect.

Moderate—the result could cause considerable distress or partially incapacitate a patient; they are unlikely to be life-threatening or result in long-term effects.

Mild—the result is unlikely to cause concern or incapacitate the majority of patients.

Unknown—used for those interactions that are predicted, but there is insufficient evidence to hazard a guess at the outcome.

Levels of evidence: Most interactions have been assigned a rating to indicate the weight of evidence behind the interaction.

Study—for interactions where the information is based on formal study including those for other drugs with same mechanism (e.g. known inducers, inhibitors, or substrates of cytochrome P450 isoenzymes or P-glycoprotein).

Anecdotal—interactions based on either a single case report or a limited number of case reports.

Theoretical—interactions that are predicted based on sound theoretical considerations. The information may have been derived from *in vitro* studies or based on the way other members in the same class act.

Action messages: Each interaction describes the effect that occurs, and the action to be taken, either based on manufacturer's advice from the relevant Summary of Product Characteristics or advice from a relevant authority (e.g. MHRA). An action message is only included where the combination is to be avoided, where a dose adjustment is required, or where specific administration requirements (e.g timing of doses) are recommended. **Pharmacodynamic interactions**, with the exception of interactions with drugs that may prolong the QT interval, do not have an action message included as these will depend on individual patient circumstances.

Appendix 1 structure

A1 Interactions | Appendix 1

❶ Drugs

Drugs are listed alphabetically. If a drug is a member of a drug class, all interactions for that drug will be listed under the drug class entry; in this case the drug entry provides direction to the relevant drug class where its interactions can be found.

Within a drug or drug class entry, interactions are listed alphabetically by the interacting drug or drug class. The interactions describe the effect that occurs, and the action to be taken, either based on manufacturer's advice from the relevant Summary of Product Characteristics or advice from a relevant authority (e.g. MHRA). An action message is only included where the combination is to be avoided, where a dose adjustment is required, or where specific administration requirements (e.g. timing of doses) are recommended. If two drugs have a pharmacodynamic effect in addition to a pharmacokinetic interaction, a cross-reference to the relevant pharmacodynamic effect table is included at the end of the pharmacokinetic message.

❷ Drug classes

The drugs that are members of a drug class are listed underneath the drug class entry in a blue box. Interactions for the class are then listed alphabetically by the interacting drug or drug class. If the interaction only applies to certain drugs in the class, these drugs will be shown in brackets after the drug class name.

❸ Supplementary information

If a drug has additional important information to be considered, this is shown in a blue box underneath the drug or drug class entry. This information might be food and lifestyle advice (including smoking), relate to the pharmacology of the drug or applicability of interactions to certain routes of administration, or it might be advice about separating administration times.

❶ **Drug entry**

- Details of interaction between **drug entry** and another drug or drug class. Action statement. [Severity] Evidence
- Details of interaction between **drug entry** and another drug or drug class. Action statement. [Severity] Evidence
  → Also see **TABLE 1**

Drug entry → see Drug class entry

❷ **Drug class entry**

Drug A • Drug B • Drug C • Drug D

- Details of interaction between **drug class entry** and another drug or drug class. Action statement. [Severity] Evidence

❸ **Drug entry or Drug class entry**

Supplementary information

❹ **Drug entry or Drug class entry** → see **TABLE 1**

TABLE 1

Name of pharmacodynamic effect

Explanation of the effect

Drug	Drug	Drug
Drug	Drug	Drug

❹ Pharmacodynamic effects

Tables at the beginning of Appendix 1 cover pharmacodynamic effects. If a drug is included in one or more of these tables, this will be indicated at the top of the list of interactions for the drug or drug class. In addition to the list of interactions for a drug or drug class, these tables should always be consulted.

Each table describes the relevant pharmacodynamic effect and lists those drugs that are commonly associated with the effect. Concurrent use of two or more drugs from the same table is expected to increase the risk of the pharmacodynamic effect occurring. Please note these tables are not exhaustive.

TABLE 1

Drugs that cause hepatotoxicity

The following is a list of some drugs that cause hepatotoxicity (note that this list is not exhaustive). Concurrent use of two or more drugs from the list might increase this risk.

alcohol (beverage)
alectinib
asparaginase
atorvastatin
bedaquiline
carbamazepine
clavulanate
crisantaspase
dactinomycin
dantrolene
demeclocycline
doxycycline
flucloxacillin
fluconazole
fluvastatin
isoniazid
itraconazole
leflunomide
lenalidomide
lomitapide
lymecycline
mercaptopurine
methotrexate
micafungin
minocycline
neratinib
oxytetracycline
paracetamol
pegaspargase
pravastatin
rosuvastatin
simvastatin
streptozocin
sulfasalazine
teriflunomide
tetracycline
tigecycline
trabectedin
valproate
vincristine

TABLE 2

Drugs that cause nephrotoxicity

The following is a list of some drugs that cause nephrotoxicity (note that this list is not exhaustive). Concurrent use of two or more drugs from the list might increase this risk.

aceclofenac
aciclovir
adefovir
amikacin
amphotericin
bacitracin
capreomycin
carboplatin
cefaclor
cefadroxil
cefalexin
cefepime
cefixime
cefotaxime
cefoxitin
cefradine
ceftaroline
ceftazidime
ceftobiprole
ceftolozane
ceftriaxone
cefuroxime
celecoxib
ciclosporin
cidofovir
cisplatin
colistimethate (particularly intravenous)
dexibuprofen
dexketoprofen
diclofenac
etodolac
etoricoxib
flurbiprofen
foscarnet
ganciclovir
gentamicin
ibuprofen
ifosfamide
indometacin
ketoprofen
ketorolac
mefenamic acid
meloxicam
methotrexate
nabumetone
naproxen
neomycin
oxaliplatin
parecoxib
pemetrexed
penicillamine
pentamidine
piroxicam
polymyxin b
streptomycin
streptozocin
sulindac
tacrolimus
telavancin
tenofovir disoproxil
tenoxicam
tiaprofenic acid
tobramycin
tolfenamic acid
trimethoprim
valaciclovir
valganciclovir
vancomycin
zidovudine
zoledronate

TABLE 3

Drugs with anticoagulant effects

The following is a list of drugs that have anticoagulant effects. Concurrent use of two or more drugs from this list might increase the risk of bleeding; concurrent use of drugs with antiplatelet effects (see table of drugs with antiplatelet effects) might also increase this risk.

acenocoumarol
alteplase
apixaban
argatroban
bivalirudin
dabigatran
dalteparin
danaparoid
edoxaban
enoxaparin
fondaparinux
heparin (unfractionated)
nicotinic acid
omega-3-acid ethyl esters
phenindione
rivaroxaban
streptokinase
tenecteplase
tinzaparin
urokinase
warfarin

TABLE 4

Drugs with antiplatelet effects

The following is a list of drugs that have antiplatelet effects (note that this list is not exhaustive). Concurrent use of two or more drugs from this list might increase the risk of bleeding; concurrent use of drugs with anticoagulant effects (see table of drugs with anticoagulant effects) might also increase this risk.

aceclofenac
anagrelide
aspirin
bevacizumab
cangrelor
celecoxib
cilostazol
citalopram
clopidogrel
dapoxetine
dasatinib
dexibuprofen
dexketoprofen
diclofenac
dipyridamole
duloxetine
epoprostenol
eptifibatide
escitalopram
etodolac
etoricoxib
fluoxetine
flurbiprofen
fluvoxamine
ibrutinib
ibuprofen
iloprost
indometacin
inotersen
ketoprofen
ketorolac
mefenamic acid
meloxicam
nabumetone
naproxen
parecoxib
paroxetine
piroxicam
prasugrel
regorafenib
sertraline
sulindac
tenoxicam
tiaprofenic acid
ticagrelor
tirofiban
tolfenamic acid
trastuzumab emtansine
venlafaxine
vortioxetine

TABLE 5

Drugs that cause thromboembolism

The following is a list of some drugs that cause thromboembolism (note that this list is not exhaustive). Concurrent use of two or more drugs from the list might increase this risk.

bleomycin
cyclophosphamide
darbepoetin alfa
doxorubicin
epoetin alfa
epoetin beta
epoetin zeta
fluorouracil
fulvestrant
lenalidomide
methotrexate
mitomycin
pentostatin
pomalidomide
raloxifene
strontium
tamoxifen
thalidomide
tibolone
toremifene
tranexamic acid
tretinoin
vinblastine
vincristine
vindesine
vinflunine
vinorelbine

TABLE 6

Drugs that cause bradycardia

The following is a list of drugs that cause bradycardia (note that this list is not exhaustive). Concurrent use of two or more drugs from the list might increase this risk.

acebutolol
alectinib
alfentanil
amiodarone
apraclonidine
atenolol
betaxolol
bisoprolol
brimonidine
carvedilol
celiprolol
cisatracurium
clonidine
crizotinib
digoxin
diltiazem
donepezil
esmolol
fentanyl
fingolimod
flecainide
galantamine
ivabradine
labetalol
levobunolol
methadone
metoprolol
nadolol
nebivolol
neostigmine
pasireotide
pindolol
propranolol
pyridostigmine
remifentanil
rivastigmine
selegiline
siponimod
sotalol
thalidomide
timolol
tizanidine
verapamil

TABLE 7

Drugs that cause first dose hypotension

The following is a list of some drugs that can cause first-dose hypotension (note that this list is not exhaustive). Concurrent use of two or more drugs from the list might increase this risk.

alfuzosin
azilsartan
candesartan
captopril
doxazosin
enalapril
eprosartan
fosinopril
glyceryl trinitrate
imidapril
indoramin
irbesartan
isosorbide dinitrate
isosorbide mononitrate
lisinopril
losartan
olmesartan
perindopril
prazosin
quinapril
ramipril
tamsulosin
telmisartan
terazosin
trandolapril
valsartan

TABLE 8

Drugs that cause hypotension

The following is a list of some drugs that cause hypotension (note that this list is not exhaustive). Concurrent use of two or more drugs from the list might increase this risk.

acebutolol
alcohol (beverage)
alfuzosin
aliskiren
alprostadil
amantadine
amitriptyline
amlodipine
apomorphine
apraclonidine
aripiprazole
asenapine
atenolol
avanafil
azilsartan
baclofen
bendroflumethiazide
benperidol
betaxolol
bisoprolol
bortezomib
brimonidine
bromocriptine
bumetanide
cabergoline
canagliflozin
candesartan
captopril
cariprazine
carvedilol
celiprolol
chlorothiazide
chlorpromazine
chlortalidone
clomipramine
clonidine
clozapine
dapagliflozin
desflurane
diazoxide
diltiazem
dipyridamole
dosulepin
doxazosin
doxepin
droperidol
empagliflozin
enalapril
eplerenone
epoprostenol
eprosartan
ertugliflozin
esketamine
esmolol
etomidate
felodipine
flupentixol
fluphenazine
fosinopril
furosemide
glyceryl trinitrate
guanfacine
haloperidol
hydralazine
hydrochlorothiazide
hydroflumethiazide
iloprost
imidapril
imipramine
indapamide
indoramin
irbesartan
isocarboxazid
isoflurane
isosorbide dinitrate
isosorbide mononitrate
ketamine
labetalol
lacidipine
lercanidipine
levobunolol
levodopa
levomepromazine
lisinopril
lofepramine
lofexidine
losartan
loxapine
lurasidone
methoxyflurane
methyldopa
metolazone
metoprolol
minoxidil
moxisylyte
moxonidine
nadolol
nebivolol
nicardipine
nicorandil
nifedipine
nimodipine
nitroprusside
nitrous oxide
nortriptyline
olanzapine
olmesartan
paliperidone
pergolide
pericyazine
perindopril
phenelzine
pimozide
pindolol
pramipexole
prazosin
prochlorperazine
promazine
propofol
propranolol
quetiapine
quinagolide
quinapril
ramipril
riociguat
risperidone
ropinirole
rotigotine
sacubitril
sapropterin
selegiline
sevoflurane
sildenafil
sodium oxybate
sotalol
spironolactone
sulpiride
tadalafil
tamsulosin
telmisartan
terazosin
thiopental
timolol
tizanidine
torasemide
trandolapril
tranylcypromine
trifluoperazine
trimipramine
valsartan
vardenafil
verapamil
vernakalant
xipamide
zuclopenthixol

TABLE 9
Drugs that prolong the QT interval

The following is a list of some drugs that prolong the QT-interval (note that this list is not exhaustive). In general, manufacturers advise that the use of two or more drugs that are associated with QT prolongation should be avoided. Increasing age, female sex, cardiac disease, and some metabolic disturbances (notably hypokalaemia) predispose to QT prolongation—concurrent use of drugs that reduce serum potassium might further increase this risk (see table of drugs that reduce serum potassium).

Drugs that are not known to prolong the QT interval but are predicted (by the manufacturer) to increase the risk of QT prolongation include: domperidone, fingolimod, granisetron, ivabradine, mefloquine, mizolastine, palonosetron, intravenous pentamidine, and siponimod. Most manufacturers advise avoiding concurrent use with drugs that prolong the QT interval.

amifampridine
amiodarone
amisulpride
anagrelide
apalutamide
apomorphine
arsenic trioxide
artemether
artenimol
bedaquiline
bosutinib
cabozantinib
ceritinib
chlorpromazine
citalopram
clarithromycin
clomipramine
crizotinib
dasatinib
delamanid
disopyramide
dronedarone
droperidol
efavirenz
encorafenib
eribulin
erythromycin
escitalopram
flecainide
fluconazole
haloperidol
hydroxyzine
inotuzumab ozogamicin
lapatinib
lenvatinib
levomepromazine
lithium
lofexidine
methadone
moxifloxacin
nilotinib
ondansetron
osimertinib
paliperidone
panobinostat
pasireotide
pazopanib
pimozide
quinine
ranolazine
ribociclib
risperidone
saquinavir
sildenafil
sorafenib
sotalol
sulpiride
sunitinib
telavancin
tetrabenazine
tizanidine
tolterodine
toremifene
vandetanib
vardenafil
vemurafenib
venlafaxine
vernakalant
vinflunine
voriconazole
zuclopenthixol

TABLE 10
Drugs with antimuscarinic effects

The following is a list of some drugs that have antimuscarinic effects (note that this list is not exhaustive). Concurrent use of two or more drugs from this list might increase the risk of these effects occurring.

aclidinium
amantadine
amitriptyline
atropine
baclofen
chlorphenamine
chlorpromazine
clemastine
clomipramine
clozapine
cyclizine
cyclopentolate
cyproheptadine
darifenacin
dicycloverine
dimenhydrinate
disopyramide
dosulepin
doxepin
fesoterodine
flavoxate
glycopyrronium
haloperidol
homatropine
hydroxyzine
hyoscine
imipramine
ipratropium
levomepromazine
lofepramine
loxapine
nefopam
nortriptyline
orphenadrine
oxybutynin
pimozide
prochlorperazine
procyclidine
promethazine
propafenone
propantheline
propiverine
solifenacin
tiotropium
tolterodine
trifluoperazine
trihexyphenidyl
trimipramine
tropicamide
trospium
umeclidinium

TABLE 11
Drugs with CNS depressant effects

The following is a list of some drugs with CNS depressant effects (note that this list is not exhaustive). Concurrent use of two or more drugs from this list might increase the risk of CNS depressant effects, such as drowsiness, which might affect the ability to perform skilled tasks (see 'Drugs and skilled tasks' in Guidance on Prescribing p. 1).

agomelatine
alcohol (beverage)
alfentanil
alimemazine
alprazolam
amisulpride
amitriptyline
apraclonidine
aripiprazole
articaine
asenapine
baclofen
benperidol
brimonidine
buclizine
bupivacaine
buprenorphine
cannabidiol
cariprazine
chloral hydrate
chlordiazepoxide
chloroprocaine
chlorphenamine
chlorpromazine
cinnarizine
clemastine
clobazam
clomethiazole
clomipramine
clonazepam
clonidine
clozapine
codeine
cyclizine
cyproheptadine
desflurane
dexmedetomidine
diamorphine
diazepam
dihydrocodeine
dipipanone
dosulepin
doxepin
dronabinol
droperidol
esketamine
etomidate
fentanyl
flupentixol
fluphenazine
flurazepam
gabapentin
guanfacine
haloperidol
hydromorphone
hydroxyzine
imipramine
isoflurane
ketamine
ketotifen
lamotrigine
levetiracetam
levomepromazine
lidocaine
lofepramine
lofexidine
loprazolam
lorazepam
lormetazepam
loxapine
lurasidone
melatonin
mepivacaine
meprobamate
meptazinol
methadone
methocarbamol
methoxyflurane
mianserin
midazolam
mirtazapine
morphine
moxonidine
nabilone
nitrazepam
nitrous oxide
nortriptyline
olanzapine
oxazepam
oxycodone
paliperidone
pentazocine
perampanel
pericyazine
pethidine
phenobarbital
pimozide
pizotifen
pregabalin
prilocaine
primidone
prochlorperazine
promazine
promethazine
propofol
quetiapine
remifentanil
risperidone
ropivacaine
sevoflurane
sodium oxybate
sulpiride
tapentadol
temazepam
tetrabenazine
tetracaine
thalidomide
thiopental
tizanidine
tramadol
trazodone
trifluoperazine
trimipramine
venlafaxine
zolpidem
zopiclone
zuclopenthixol

TABLE 12

Drugs that cause peripheral neuropathy

The following is a list of some drugs that cause peripheral neuropathy (note that this list is not exhaustive). Concurrent use of two or more drugs from the list might increase this risk.

amiodarone
bortezomib
brentuximab vedotin
cabazitaxel
cisplatin
disulfiram
docetaxel
eribulin
fosphenytoin
isoniazid
lamivudine
metronidazole
nitrofurantoin
paclitaxel
phenytoin
stavudine
thalidomide
vinblastine
vincristine
vindesine
vinflunine
vinorelbine

TABLE 13

Drugs that cause serotonin syndrome

The following is a list of some drugs that cause serotonin syndrome (note that this list is not exhaustive). See 'Serotonin Syndrome' and 'Monoamine-Oxidase Inhibitors' under Antidepressant drugs in BNF for more information and for specific advice on avoiding monoamine-oxidase inhibitors during and after administration of other serotonergic drugs.

almotriptan
bupropion
buspirone
citalopram
clomipramine
dapoxetine
dexamfetamine
duloxetine
eletriptan
escitalopram
fentanyl
fluoxetine
fluvoxamine
frovatriptan
granisetron
imipramine
isocarboxazid
linezolid
lisdexamfetamine
lithium
methadone
methylthioninium chloride
mirtazapine
moclobemide
naratriptan
ondansetron
palonosetron
paroxetine
pentazocine
pethidine
phenelzine
procarbazine
rasagiline
rizatriptan
safinamide
selegiline
sertraline
St John's Wort
sumatriptan
tramadol
tranylcypromine
trazodone
tryptophan
venlafaxine
vortioxetine
zolmitriptan

TABLE 14

Antidiabetic drugs

The following is a list of antidiabetic drugs (note that this list is not exhaustive). Concurrent use of two or more drugs from the list might increase the risk of hypoglycaemia.

acarbose
alogliptin
canagliflozin
dapagliflozin
dulaglutide
empagliflozin
ertugliflozin
exenatide
glibenclamide
gliclazide
glimepiride
glipizide
insulins
linagliptin
liraglutide
lixisenatide
metformin
nateglinide
pioglitazone
repaglinide
saxagliptin
semaglutide
sitagliptin
tolbutamide
vildagliptin

TABLE 15

Drugs that cause myelosuppression

The following is a list of some drugs that cause myelosuppression (note that this list is not exhaustive). Concurrent use of two or more drugs from the list might increase this risk.

afatinib
aflibercept
alemtuzumab
amsacrine
anakinra
arsenic trioxide
asparaginase
axitinib
azacitidine
azathioprine
balsalazide
belimumab
bendamustine
bevacizumab
bleomycin
blinatumomab
bortezomib
bosutinib
brentuximab vedotin
busulfan
cabazitaxel
cabozantinib
canakinumab
capecitabine
carbimazole
carboplatin
carfilzomib
carmustine
ceritinib
cetuximab
chlorambucil
chlormethine
cisplatin
cladribine
clofarabine
clozapine
crisantaspase
crizotinib
cyclophosphamide
cytarabine
dabrafenib
dacarbazine
dactinomycin
dasatinib
daunorubicin
decitabine
deferiprone
docetaxel
doxorubicin
epirubicin
eribulin
estramustine
ethosuximide
etoposide
everolimus
fludarabine
fluorouracil
ganciclovir
gefitinib
gemcitabine
hydroxycarbamide
ibrutinib
idarubicin
idelalisib
ifosfamide
imatinib
interferon alfa
interferon beta
irinotecan
leflunomide
lenalidomide
linezolid
lomustine
melphalan
mercaptopurine
methotrexate
mitomycin
mitotane
mitoxantrone
mycophenolate
nelarabine
nilotinib
nivolumab
obinutuzumab
olanzapine
olaparib
olsalazine
oxaliplatin
paclitaxel
panitumumab
panobinostat
pazopanib
pegaspargase
peginterferon alfa
peginterferon beta
pemetrexed
pentamidine
pentostatin
pixantrone
pomalidomide
primaquine
procarbazine
propylthiouracil
pyrimethamine
raltitrexed
ramucirumab
regorafenib
rituximab
ruxolitinib
siltuximab
sorafenib
sulfadiazine
sulfamethoxazole
sulfasalazine
sunitinib
temozolomide
temsirolimus
thalidomide
thiotepa
tioguanine
topotecan
trabectedin
trastuzumab emtansine
treosulfan
trimethoprim
valganciclovir
vinblastine
vincristine
vindesine
vinflunine
vinorelbine
vismodegib
zidovudine

TABLE 16
Drugs that increase serum potassium

The following is a list of some drugs that increase serum potassium concentrations (note that this list is not exhaustive). Concurrent use of two or more drugs from this list might increase the risk of hyperkalaemia (hyperkalaemia is particularly notable when ACE inhibitors or angiotensin-II receptor antagonists are given with spironolactone or eplerenone).

aceclofenac
aliskiren
amiloride
azilsartan
candesartan
captopril
celecoxib
ciclosporin
dalteparin
darbepoetin alfa
dexibuprofen
dexketoprofen
diclofenac
drospirenone
enalapril
enoxaparin
eplerenone
epoetin alfa
epoetin beta
epoetin zeta
eprosartan
etodolac
etoricoxib
flurbiprofen
heparin (unfractionated)
ibuprofen
imidapril
indometacin
irbesartan
ketoprofen
ketorolac
lisinopril
losartan
mefenamic acid
meloxicam
nabumetone
naproxen
olmesartan
parecoxib
perindopril
piroxicam
potassium aminobenzoate
potassium canrenoate
potassium chloride
quinapril
ramipril
spironolactone
sulindac
tacrolimus
telmisartan
tenoxicam
tiaprofenic acid
tinzaparin
tolfenamic acid
tolvaptan
trandolapril
triamterene
trimethoprim
valsartan

TABLE 17
Drugs that reduce serum potassium

The following is a list of some drugs that reduce serum potassium concentrations (note that this list is not exhaustive and that other drugs can cause hypokalaemia in overdose). Concurrent use of two or more drugs from this list might increase the risk of hypokalaemia. Hypokalaemia can increase the risk of torsade de pointes, which might be additive with the effects of drugs that prolong the QT interval (see table of drugs that prolong the QT interval).

aminophylline
amphotericin
bambuterol
beclometasone
bendroflumethiazide
betamethasone
budesonide
bumetanide
chlorothiazide
chlortalidone
deflazacort
dexamethasone
fludrocortisone
formoterol
furosemide
hydrochlorothiazide
hydrocortisone
hydroflumethiazide
indacaterol
indapamide
methylprednisolone
metolazone
olodaterol
prednisolone
salbutamol
salmeterol
terbutaline
theophylline
torasemide
triamcinolone
vilanterol
xipamide

TABLE 18
Drugs that cause hyponatraemia

The following is a list of some drugs that reduce sodium concentrations (note that this list is not exhaustive). Concurrent use of two or more drugs from this list might increase the risk of hyponatraemia.

aceclofenac
amiloride
amitriptyline
bendroflumethiazide
bumetanide
carbamazepine
celecoxib
chlorothiazide
chlortalidone
citalopram
clomipramine
dapoxetine
desmopressin
dexibuprofen
dexketoprofen
diclofenac
dosulepin
doxepin
duloxetine
eplerenone
escitalopram
etodolac
etoricoxib
fluoxetine
flurbiprofen
fluvoxamine
furosemide
gabapentin
hydrochlorothiazide
hydroflumethiazide
ibuprofen
imipramine
indapamide
indometacin
ketoprofen
ketorolac
mefenamic acid
meloxicam
metolazone
nabumetone
naproxen
nortriptyline
parecoxib
paroxetine
piroxicam
sertraline
sodium picosulfate
spironolactone
sulindac
tenoxicam
tiaprofenic acid
tolfenamic acid
torasemide
triamterene
trimethoprim
trimipramine
xipamide

TABLE 19
Drugs that cause ototoxicity

The following is a list of some drugs that cause ototoxicity (note that this list is not exhaustive). Concurrent use of two or more drugs from the list might increase this risk.

amikacin
bumetanide
capreomycin
carboplatin
cisplatin
furosemide
gentamicin
neomycin
oxaliplatin
streptomycin
telavancin
tobramycin
torasemide
vancomycin
vinblastine
vincristine
vindesine
vinflunine
vinorelbine

TABLE 20
Drugs with neuromuscular blocking effects

The following is a list of some drugs with neuromuscular blocking effects (note that this list is not exhaustive). Concurrent use of two or more drugs from the list might increase this risk.

amikacin
atracurium
botulinum toxin type A
botulinum toxin type B
cisatracurium
colistimethate
gentamicin
mivacurium
neomycin
pancuronium
polymyxin b
rocuronium
streptomycin
suxamethonium
tobramycin

List of drug interactions

The following is an alphabetical list of drugs and their interactions; to avoid excessive cross-referencing each drug or group is listed twice: in the alphabetical list and also against the drug or group with which it interacts.

Abacavir
- Antiepileptics **(carbamazepine, fosphenytoin, phenobarbital, phenytoin, primidone)** are predicted to decrease the exposure to **abacavir**. Moderate Theoretical
- HIV-protease inhibitors **(tipranavir)** slightly decrease the exposure to **abacavir**. Avoid. Severe Study

Abatacept
- **Live vaccines** are predicted to increase the risk of generalised infection (possibly life-threatening) when given with **abatacept**. Public Health England advises avoid (refer to Green Book). Severe Theoretical
- **Abatacept** is predicted to increase the risk of generalised infection (possibly life-threatening) when given with monoclonal antibodies **(golimumab)**. Avoid. Severe Theoretical

Abemaciclib
- Antiarrhythmics **(dronedarone)** are predicted to increase the exposure to **abemaciclib**. Moderate Study
- Antiepileptics **(carbamazepine, fosphenytoin, phenobarbital, phenytoin, primidone)** are predicted to markedly decrease the exposure to **abemaciclib**. Avoid. Severe Study
- Antifungals, azoles **(fluconazole, isavuconazole, posaconazole)** are predicted to increase the exposure to **abemaciclib**. Moderate Study
- Antifungals, azoles **(itraconazole, ketoconazole, voriconazole)** are predicted to increase the exposure to **abemaciclib**. Avoid or adjust **abemaciclib** dose. Severe Study
- **Apalutamide** is predicted to markedly decrease the exposure to **abemaciclib**. Avoid. Severe Study
- **Aprepitant** is predicted to increase the exposure to **abemaciclib**. Moderate Study
- Calcium channel blockers **(diltiazem, verapamil)** are predicted to increase the exposure to **abemaciclib**. Moderate Study
- **Cobicistat** is predicted to increase the exposure to **abemaciclib**. Avoid or adjust **abemaciclib** dose. Severe Study
- **Crizotinib** is predicted to increase the exposure to **abemaciclib**. Moderate Study
- **Enzalutamide** is predicted to markedly decrease the exposure to **abemaciclib**. Avoid. Severe Study
- **Grapefruit juice** is predicted to increase the exposure to **abemaciclib**. Avoid. Moderate Theoretical
- **HIV-protease inhibitors** are predicted to increase the exposure to **abemaciclib**. Avoid or adjust **abemaciclib** dose. Severe Study
- **Idelalisib** is predicted to increase the exposure to **abemaciclib**. Avoid or adjust **abemaciclib** dose. Severe Study
- **Imatinib** is predicted to increase the exposure to **abemaciclib**. Moderate Study
- Macrolides **(clarithromycin)** are predicted to increase the exposure to **abemaciclib**. Avoid or adjust **abemaciclib** dose. Severe Study
- Macrolides **(erythromycin)** are predicted to increase the exposure to **abemaciclib**. Moderate Study
- **Mitotane** is predicted to markedly decrease the exposure to **abemaciclib**. Avoid. Severe Study
- **Netupitant** is predicted to increase the exposure to **abemaciclib**. Moderate Study
- **Nilotinib** is predicted to increase the exposure to **abemaciclib**. Moderate Study
- **Rifampicin** is predicted to markedly decrease the exposure to **abemaciclib**. Avoid. Severe Study
- **St John's Wort** is predicted to decrease the exposure to **abemaciclib**. Avoid. Severe Study

Abiraterone

GENERAL INFORMATION Caution with concurrent chemotherapy—safety and efficacy not established.

- Aldosterone antagonists **(spironolactone)** are predicted to oppose the effects of **abiraterone**. Avoid. Severe Theoretical
- Antiepileptics **(carbamazepine, fosphenytoin, phenobarbital, phenytoin, primidone)** are predicted to decrease the exposure to **abiraterone**. Avoid. Severe Study
- **Apalutamide** is predicted to decrease the exposure to **abiraterone**. Avoid. Severe Study
- **Abiraterone** is predicted to increase the exposure to beta blockers, selective **(metoprolol)**. Moderate Study
- **Abiraterone** is predicted to increase the exposure to **eliglustat**. Avoid or adjust dose—consult product literature. Severe Study
- **Enzalutamide** is predicted to decrease the exposure to **abiraterone**. Avoid. Severe Study
- **Mitotane** is predicted to decrease the exposure to **abiraterone**. Avoid. Severe Study
- **Rifampicin** is predicted to decrease the exposure to **abiraterone**. Avoid. Severe Study

Acarbose → see TABLE 14 p. 910 (antidiabetic drugs)
- **Acarbose** decreases the concentration of **digoxin**. Moderate Study
- **Pancreatin** is predicted to decrease the effects of **acarbose**. Avoid. Moderate Theoretical

ACE inhibitors → see TABLE 7 p. 908 (first-dose hypotension), TABLE 8 p. 908 (hypotension), TABLE 16 p. 911 (increased serum potassium)

captopril · enalapril · fosinopril · imidapril · lisinopril · perindopril · quinapril · ramipril · trandolapril

- **ACE inhibitors** increase the risk of renal impairment when given with aliskiren. Use with caution or avoid **aliskiren** in selected patients. Severe Study → Also see TABLE 8 p. 908 → Also see TABLE 16 p. 911
- **ACE inhibitors** are predicted to increase the risk of hypersensitivity and haematological reactions when given with **allopurinol**. Severe Anecdotal
- **ACE inhibitors** are predicted to increase the risk of anaemia and/or leucopenia when given with **azathioprine**. Severe Anecdotal
- **Everolimus** potentially increases the risk of angioedema when given with **ACE inhibitors**. Severe Anecdotal
- **ACE inhibitors** are predicted to decrease the efficacy of **icatibant** and **icatibant** is predicted to decrease the efficacy of **ACE inhibitors**. Avoid. Moderate Theoretical
- **ACE inhibitors** are predicted to increase the concentration of **lithium**. Monitor and adjust dose. Severe Anecdotal
- **ACE inhibitors** are predicted to increase the risk of hypersensitivity when given with **sodium aurothiomalate**. Severe Anecdotal
- **ACE inhibitors** are predicted to increase the risk of angioedema when given with **temsirolimus**. Moderate Theoretical
- **Quinapril** (tablet) decreases the absorption of oral tetracyclines **(tetracycline)**. Avoid. Moderate Study

Acebutolol → see beta blockers, selective

Aceclofenac → see NSAIDs

Acenocoumarol → see coumarins

Acetazolamide
- **Acetazolamide** potentially increases the risk of toxicity when given with antiepileptics **(valproate)**. Severe Study
- **Acetazolamide** potentially increases the risk of overheating and dehydration when given with antiepileptics **(zonisamide)**. Avoid in children. Severe Theoretical
- **Acetazolamide** increases the risk of severe toxic reaction when given with **aspirin (high-dose)**. Severe Study
- **Acetazolamide** alters the concentration of **lithium**. Severe Anecdotal
- **Acetazolamide** is predicted to decrease the efficacy of **methenamine**. Avoid. Moderate Theoretical
- **Acetazolamide** increases the urinary excretion of **methotrexate**. Moderate Study

Aciclovir → see TABLE 2 p. 907 (nephrotoxicity)

ROUTE-SPECIFIC INFORMATION Since systemic absorption can follow topical application, the possibility of interactions should be borne in mind.

- **Aciclovir** increases the exposure to **aminophylline**. Monitor and adjust dose. Severe Anecdotal
- **Mycophenolate** is predicted to increase the risk of haematological toxicity when given with **aciclovir**. Moderate Theoretical

- **Aciclovir** is predicted to increase the exposure to **theophylline**. Monitor and adjust dose. [Severe] Theoretical

Acitretin → see retinoids
Aclidinium → see TABLE 10 p. 909 (antimuscarinics)
Acrivastine → see antihistamines, non-sedating
Adalimumab → see monoclonal antibodies
Adapalene → see retinoids
Adefovir → see TABLE 2 p. 907 (nephrotoxicity)

- **Leflunomide** is predicted to increase the exposure to **adefovir**. [Moderate] Theoretical
- **Nitisinone** is predicted to increase the exposure to **adefovir**. [Moderate] Study
- **Teriflunomide** is predicted to increase the exposure to **adefovir**. [Moderate] Study

Adenosine → see antiarrhythmics
Adrenaline/epinephrine → see sympathomimetics, vasoconstrictor
Afatinib → see TABLE 15 p. 910 (myelosuppression)

- Antiarrhythmics **(amiodarone, dronedarone)** are predicted to increase the exposure to **afatinib**. Separate administration by 12 hours. [Moderate] Study
- Antiepileptics **(carbamazepine)** are predicted to decrease the exposure to **afatinib**. [Moderate] Study
- Antifungals, azoles **(itraconazole, ketoconazole)** are predicted to increase the exposure to **afatinib**. Separate administration by 12 hours. [Moderate] Study
- Calcium channel blockers **(verapamil)** are predicted to increase the exposure to **afatinib**. Separate administration by 12 hours. [Moderate] Study
- **Ciclosporin** is predicted to increase the exposure to **afatinib**. Separate administration by 12 hours. [Moderate] Study
- HIV-protease inhibitors **(lopinavir, ritonavir, saquinavir)** are predicted to increase the exposure to **afatinib**. Separate administration by 12 hours. [Moderate] Study
- **Lapatinib** is predicted to increase the exposure to **afatinib**. Separate administration by 12 hours. [Moderate] Study
- **Macrolides** are predicted to increase the exposure to **afatinib**. Separate administration by 12 hours. [Moderate] Study
- **Ranolazine** is predicted to increase the exposure to **afatinib**. Separate administration by 12 hours. [Moderate] Study
- **Rifampicin** is predicted to decrease the exposure to **afatinib**. [Moderate] Study
- **St John's Wort** is predicted to decrease the exposure to **afatinib**. [Moderate] Study
- **Vemurafenib** is predicted to increase the exposure to **afatinib**. Separate administration by 12 hours. [Moderate] Study

Aflibercept → see TABLE 15 p. 910 (myelosuppression)

ROUTE-SPECIFIC INFORMATION Interactions do not generally apply to topical use unless specified.

Agalsidase alfa

- **Aminoglycosides** are predicted to decrease the effects of **agalsidase alfa**. Avoid. [Moderate] Theoretical
- Antiarrhythmics **(amiodarone)** are predicted to decrease the effects of **agalsidase alfa**. Avoid. [Moderate] Theoretical
- Antimalarials **(chloroquine)** are predicted to decrease the effects of **agalsidase alfa**. Avoid. [Moderate] Theoretical
- **Hydroxychloroquine** is predicted to decrease the effects of **agalsidase alfa**. [Moderate] Theoretical

Agalsidase beta

- **Aminoglycosides** are predicted to decrease the effects of **agalsidase beta**. Avoid. [Moderate] Theoretical
- Antiarrhythmics **(amiodarone)** are predicted to decrease the effects of **agalsidase beta**. Avoid. [Moderate] Theoretical
- Antimalarials **(chloroquine)** are predicted to decrease the effects of **agalsidase beta**. Avoid. [Moderate] Theoretical
- **Hydroxychloroquine** is predicted to decrease the exposure to **agalsidase beta**. [Moderate] Theoretical

Agomelatine → see TABLE 11 p. 909 (CNS depressant effects)

- Dose adjustment might be necessary if smoking started or stopped during treatment.
- Caution with concomitant use of drugs associated with hepatic injury.

- Antiepileptics **(fosphenytoin, phenytoin)** are predicted to decrease the exposure to **agomelatine**. [Moderate] Theoretical
- **Combined hormonal contraceptives** are predicted to increase the exposure to **agomelatine**. [Moderate] Study
- HIV-protease inhibitors **(ritonavir)** are predicted to decrease the exposure to **agomelatine**. [Moderate] Theoretical
- **Leflunomide** is predicted to decrease the exposure to **agomelatine**. [Moderate] Theoretical
- **Mexiletine** is predicted to increase the exposure to **agomelatine**. [Moderate] Study
- Quinolones **(ciprofloxacin)** are predicted to increase the exposure to **agomelatine**. [Moderate] Study
- **Rifampicin** is predicted to decrease the exposure to **agomelatine**. [Moderate] Theoretical
- SSRIs **(fluvoxamine)** very markedly increase the exposure to **agomelatine**. Avoid. [Severe] Study
- **Teriflunomide** is predicted to decrease the exposure to **agomelatine**. [Moderate] Theoretical

Albendazole

- Antiepileptics **(carbamazepine, fosphenytoin, phenobarbital, phenytoin, primidone)** decrease the concentration of **albendazole**. [Moderate] Study
- H_2 receptor antagonists **(cimetidine)** decrease the clearance of **albendazole**. [Moderate] Study
- HIV-protease inhibitors **(ritonavir)** decrease the exposure to **albendazole**. [Moderate] Study
- **Albendazole** slightly decreases the exposure to **levamisole** and **levamisole** moderately decreases the exposure to **albendazole**. [Moderate] Study

Alcohol (beverage) → see TABLE 1 p. 907 (hepatotoxicity), TABLE 8 p. 908 (hypotension), TABLE 11 p. 909 (CNS depressant effects)

- **Alcohol (beverage)** potentially increases the risk of visual disturbances when given with antiepileptics **(retigabine)**. [Moderate] Study
- **Alcohol (beverage)** potentially causes a disulfiram-like reaction when given with antifungals, azoles **(ketoconazole)**. Avoid. [Moderate] Anecdotal
- **Alcohol (beverage)** causes serious, potentially fatal, CNS depression when given with **clomethiazole**. Avoid. [Severe] Study → Also see TABLE 11 p. 909
- **Alcohol (beverage)** (in those who drink heavily) potentially decreases the anticoagulant effect of **coumarins**. [Severe] Study
- **Alcohol (beverage)** (excessive consumption) potentially increases the risk of gastrointestinal side-effects when given with **dimethyl fumarate**. Avoid. [Moderate] Theoretical
- **Alcohol (beverage)** causes an extremely unpleasant systemic reaction when given with **disulfiram**. Avoid for at least 24 hours before and up to 14 days after stopping treatment. [Severe] Study
- **Alcohol (beverage)** potentially causes a disulfiram-like reaction when given with **griseofulvin**. [Moderate] Anecdotal
- **Alcohol (beverage)** potentially causes a disulfiram-like reaction when given with **levamisole**. [Moderate] Study
- **Alcohol (beverage)** (excessive consumption) potentially increases the risk of lactic acidosis when given with **metformin**. Avoid excessive alcohol consumption. [Moderate] Theoretical
- **Alcohol (beverage)** potentially causes a disulfiram-like reaction when given with **metronidazole**. Avoid for at least 48 hours stopping treatment. [Moderate] Study
- **Alcohol (beverage)** causes rapid release of opioids **(hydromorphone, morphine)** (from extended-release preparations). Avoid. [Severe] Study → Also see TABLE 11 p. 909
- **Alcohol (beverage)** (in those who drink heavily) causes severe liver damage when given with **paracetamol**. [Severe] Study → Also see TABLE 1 p. 907
- **Alcohol (beverage)** increases the risk of facial flushing and skin irritation when given with topical **pimecrolimus**. [Moderate] Study
- **Alcohol (beverage)** potentially causes a disulfiram-like reaction when given with **procarbazine**. [Moderate] Anecdotal
- **Alcohol (beverage)** potentially increases the concentration of retinoids **(acitretin)**. Avoid and for 2 months after stopping **acitretin**. [Moderate] Study
- **Alcohol (beverage)** increases the risk of facial flushing and skin irritation when given with topical **tacrolimus**. [Moderate] Study

Alcohol (beverage) (continued)
- **Alcohol (beverage)** potentially causes a disulfiram-like reaction when given with tinidazole. Avoid for 72 hours stopping treatment. [Moderate] Theoretical

Aldosterone antagonists → see TABLE 18 p. 911 (hyponatraemia), TABLE 8 p. 908 (hypotension), TABLE 16 p. 911 (increased serum potassium)

eplerenone · spironolactone

- **Spironolactone** is predicted to oppose the effects of abiraterone. Avoid. [Severe] Theoretical
- Antiarrhythmics (**amiodarone**) are predicted to increase the exposure to **eplerenone**. Adjust **eplerenone** dose. [Severe] Theoretical
- Antiarrhythmics (**dronedarone**) are predicted to increase the exposure to **eplerenone**. Adjust **eplerenone** dose. [Severe] Study
- Antiepileptics (**carbamazepine, fosphenytoin, phenobarbital, phenytoin, primidone**) are predicted to decrease the exposure to **eplerenone**. Avoid. [Moderate] Theoretical → Also see TABLE 18 p. 911
- Antifungals, azoles (**fluconazole, isavuconazole, posaconazole**) are predicted to increase the exposure to **eplerenone**. Adjust **eplerenone** dose. [Severe] Study
- Antifungals, azoles (**itraconazole, ketoconazole, voriconazole**) are predicted to markedly increase the exposure to **eplerenone**. Avoid. [Severe] Study
- **Apalutamide** is predicted to decrease the exposure to **eplerenone**. Avoid. [Moderate] Theoretical
- **Aprepitant** is predicted to increase the exposure to **eplerenone**. Adjust **eplerenone** dose. [Severe] Study
- Calcium channel blockers (**diltiazem, verapamil**) are predicted to increase the exposure to **eplerenone**. Adjust **eplerenone** dose. [Severe] Study → Also see TABLE 8 p. 908
- **Cobicistat** is predicted to markedly increase the exposure to **eplerenone**. Avoid. [Severe] Study
- **Crizotinib** is predicted to increase the exposure to **eplerenone**. Adjust **eplerenone** dose. [Severe] Study
- **Eplerenone** very slightly increases the exposure to digoxin. [Mild] Study
- **Spironolactone** increases the concentration of digoxin. Monitor and adjust dose. [Moderate] Study
- **Enzalutamide** is predicted to decrease the exposure to **eplerenone**. Avoid. [Moderate] Theoretical
- **HIV-protease inhibitors** are predicted to markedly increase the exposure to **eplerenone**. Avoid. [Severe] Study
- **Idelalisib** is predicted to markedly increase the exposure to **eplerenone**. Avoid. [Severe] Study
- **Imatinib** is predicted to increase the exposure to **eplerenone**. Adjust **eplerenone** dose. [Severe] Study
- **Eplerenone** potentially increases the concentration of lithium. Avoid. [Moderate] Theoretical
- **Spironolactone** potentially increases the concentration of lithium. [Moderate] Study
- Macrolides (**clarithromycin**) are predicted to markedly increase the exposure to **eplerenone**. Avoid. [Severe] Study
- Macrolides (**erythromycin**) are predicted to increase the exposure to **eplerenone**. Adjust **eplerenone** dose. [Severe] Study
- **Mitotane** is predicted to decrease the exposure to **eplerenone**. Avoid. [Moderate] Theoretical
- **Spironolactone** is predicted to decrease the effects of **mitotane**. Avoid. [Severe] Anecdotal
- **Netupitant** is predicted to increase the exposure to **eplerenone**. Adjust **eplerenone** dose. [Severe] Study
- **Nilotinib** is predicted to increase the exposure to **eplerenone**. Adjust **eplerenone** dose. [Severe] Study
- **Rifampicin** is predicted to decrease the exposure to **eplerenone**. Avoid. [Moderate] Theoretical
- **St John's Wort** is predicted to slightly decrease the exposure to **eplerenone**. Avoid. [Moderate] Study

Alectinib → see TABLE 6 p. 908 (bradycardia), TABLE 1 p. 907 (hepatotoxicity)
Alemtuzumab → see monoclonal antibodies
Alendronate → see bisphosphonates
Alfacalcidol → see vitamin D substances
Alfentanil → see opioids
Alfuzosin → see alpha blockers
Alimemazine → see antihistamines, sedating
Aliskiren → see TABLE 8 p. 908 (hypotension), TABLE 16 p. 911 (increased serum potassium)

FOOD AND LIFESTYLE Avoid apple juice and orange juice as they greatly decrease aliskiren concentrations and plasma renin activity.

- **ACE inhibitors** increase the risk of renal impairment when given with **aliskiren**. Use with caution or avoid **aliskiren** in selected patients. [Severe] Study → Also see TABLE 8 p. 908 → Also see TABLE 16 p. 911
- **Angiotensin-II receptor antagonists** increase the risk of renal impairment when given with **aliskiren**. Use with caution or avoid **aliskiren** in selected patients. [Severe] Study → Also see TABLE 8 p. 908 → Also see TABLE 16 p. 911
- Antiarrhythmics (**amiodarone, dronedarone**) are predicted to increase the exposure to **aliskiren**. [Severe] Study
- Antiepileptics (**carbamazepine**) decrease the exposure to **aliskiren**. [Moderate] Study
- Antifungals, azoles (**itraconazole**) markedly increase the exposure to **aliskiren**. Avoid. [Severe] Study
- Antifungals, azoles (**ketoconazole**) moderately increase the exposure to **aliskiren**. [Moderate] Study
- Calcium channel blockers (**verapamil**) moderately increase the exposure to **aliskiren**. [Moderate] Study → Also see TABLE 8 p. 908
- **Ceritinib** is predicted to increase the exposure to **aliskiren**. [Moderate] Theoretical
- **Ciclosporin** markedly increases the exposure to **aliskiren**. Avoid. [Severe] Study → Also see TABLE 16 p. 911
- **Eliglustat** is predicted to increase the exposure to **aliskiren**. Adjust dose. [Moderate] Study
- **Grapefruit juice** moderately decreases the exposure to **aliskiren**. Avoid. [Severe] Study
- HIV-protease inhibitors (**ritonavir, saquinavir**) are predicted to increase the exposure to **aliskiren**. [Moderate] Theoretical
- **Lapatinib** is predicted to increase the exposure to **aliskiren**. [Moderate] Theoretical
- **Aliskiren** slightly decreases the exposure to loop diuretics (**furosemide**). [Moderate] Study → Also see TABLE 8 p. 908
- Macrolides (**azithromycin**) are predicted to increase the exposure to **aliskiren**. [Moderate] Theoretical
- Macrolides (**clarithromycin, erythromycin**) are predicted to increase the exposure to **aliskiren**. [Moderate] Study
- **Mirabegron** is predicted to increase the exposure to **aliskiren**. [Mild] Theoretical
- **Paritaprevir** (with ritonavir and ombitasvir) is predicted to increase the exposure to **aliskiren**. [Moderate] Study
- **Pibrentasvir** (with glecaprevir) is predicted to increase the exposure to **aliskiren**. [Moderate] Study
- **Pitolisant** is predicted to decrease the exposure to **aliskiren**. [Mild] Theoretical
- **Ranolazine** is predicted to increase the exposure to **aliskiren**. [Moderate] Theoretical
- **Rifampicin** decreases the exposure to **aliskiren**. [Moderate] Study
- **St John's Wort** decreases the exposure to **aliskiren**. [Moderate] Study
- Statins (**atorvastatin**) slightly to moderately increase the exposure to **aliskiren**. [Moderate] Study
- **Velpatasvir** is predicted to increase the exposure to **aliskiren**. [Severe] Theoretical
- **Vemurafenib** is predicted to increase the exposure to **aliskiren**. Use with caution and adjust dose. [Moderate] Theoretical

Alitretinoin → see retinoids
Alkylating agents → see TABLE 15 p. 910 (myelosuppression), TABLE 2 p. 907 (nephrotoxicity), TABLE 5 p. 907 (thromboembolism)

bendamustine · busulfan · carmustine · chlorambucil · cyclophosphamide · dacarbazine · estramustine · ifosfamide · lomustine · melphalan · temozolomide · thiotepa · treosulfan

- **Antacids** are predicted to decrease the absorption of **estramustine**. Avoid. [Moderate] Study
- Antifungals, azoles (**isavuconazole**) are predicted to increase the exposure to **cyclophosphamide**. [Moderate] Study
- Antifungals, azoles (**itraconazole**) increase the risk of busulfan toxicity when given with **busulfan**. Monitor and adjust dose. [Moderate] Study

- Antifungals, azoles **(miconazole)** are predicted to increase the concentration of **busulfan**. Use with caution and adjust dose. [Moderate] Theoretical
- **Aprepitant** is predicted to increase the exposure to **ifosfamide**. [Severe] Theoretical
- Oral **calcium salts** decrease the absorption of **estramustine**. [Severe] Study
- **Fosaprepitant** is predicted to increase the exposure to **ifosfamide**. [Severe] Theoretical
- **Live vaccines** are predicted to increase the risk of generalised infection (possibly life-threatening) when given with **alkylating agents**. Public Health England advises avoid (refer to Green Book). [Severe] Theoretical
- **Metronidazole** increases the risk of toxicity when given with **busulfan**. [Severe] Study
- **Netupitant** very slightly increases the exposure to **cyclophosphamide**. [Moderate] Study
- **Netupitant** is predicted to increase the exposure to **ifosfamide**. [Moderate] Study
- **Paracetamol** is predicted to decrease the clearance of **busulfan**. [Moderate] Theoretical
- **Cyclophosphamide** (high-dose) increases the risk of toxicity when given with **pentostatin**. Avoid. [Severe] Anecdotal → Also see TABLE 15 p. 910 → Also see TABLE 5 p. 907
- **Rolapitant** is predicted to increase the exposure to **bendamustine**. Avoid or monitor. [Moderate] Study
- **Cyclophosphamide** increases the risk of prolonged neuromuscular blockade when given with **suxamethonium**. [Moderate] Study

Allopurinol

- **ACE inhibitors** are predicted to increase the risk of hypersensitivity and haematological reactions when given with **allopurinol**. [Severe] Anecdotal
- **Allopurinol** potentially increases the risk of haematological toxicity when given with **azathioprine**. Adjust **azathioprine** dose, p. 558. [Severe] Study
- **Allopurinol** is predicted to decrease the effects of **capecitabine**. Avoid. [Severe] Study
- **Allopurinol** potentially increases the risk of haematological toxicity when given with **mercaptopurine**. Adjust **mercaptopurine** dose, p. 587. [Severe] Study
- **Allopurinol** increases the risk of skin rash when given with penicillins **(amoxicillin, ampicillin)**. [Moderate] Study
- **Allopurinol** is predicted to increase the risk of hyperuricaemia when given with **pyrazinamide**. [Moderate] Theoretical
- **Thiazide diuretics** are predicted to increase the risk of hypersensitivity reactions when given with **allopurinol**. [Severe] Theoretical

Almotriptan → see TABLE 13 p. 910 (serotonin syndrome)

- Antifungals, azoles **(itraconazole, ketoconazole, voriconazole)** increase the exposure to **almotriptan**. [Mild] Study
- **Cobicistat** increases the exposure to **almotriptan**. [Mild] Study
- **Almotriptan** is predicted to increase the risk of vasoconstriction when given with **ergotamine**. **Ergotamine** should be taken at least 24 hours before or 6 hours after **almotriptan**. [Severe] Theoretical
- **HIV-protease inhibitors** increase the exposure to **almotriptan**. [Mild] Study
- **Idelalisib** increases the exposure to **almotriptan**. [Mild] Study
- Macrolides **(clarithromycin)** increase the exposure to **almotriptan**. [Mild] Study

Alogliptin → see TABLE 14 p. 910 (antidiabetic drugs)

Alpha blockers → see TABLE 7 p. 908 (first-dose hypotension), TABLE 8 p. 908 (hypotension)

alfuzosin · doxazosin · indoramin · prazosin · tamsulosin · terazosin

- Antiarrhythmics **(dronedarone)** are predicted to increase the exposure to **tamsulosin**. [Moderate] Theoretical
- Antifungals, azoles **(fluconazole, isavuconazole, posaconazole)** are predicted to increase the exposure to **tamsulosin**. [Moderate] Theoretical
- Antifungals, azoles **(itraconazole, ketoconazole, voriconazole)** are predicted to increase the exposure to **doxazosin**. [Moderate] Study
- Antifungals, azoles **(itraconazole, ketoconazole, voriconazole)** are predicted to moderately increase the exposure to alpha blockers **(alfuzosin, tamsulosin)**. Use with caution or avoid. [Moderate] Study
- **Aprepitant** is predicted to increase the exposure to **tamsulosin**. [Moderate] Theoretical
- Calcium channel blockers **(diltiazem, verapamil)** are predicted to increase the exposure to **tamsulosin**. [Moderate] Theoretical → Also see TABLE 8 p. 908
- **Cobicistat** is predicted to moderately increase the exposure to alpha blockers **(alfuzosin, tamsulosin)**. Use with caution or avoid. [Moderate] Study
- **Cobicistat** is predicted to increase the exposure to **doxazosin**. [Moderate] Study
- **Crizotinib** is predicted to increase the exposure to **tamsulosin**. [Moderate] Theoretical
- **HIV-protease inhibitors** are predicted to moderately increase the exposure to alpha blockers **(alfuzosin, tamsulosin)**. Use with caution or avoid. [Moderate] Study
- **HIV-protease inhibitors** are predicted to increase the exposure to **doxazosin**. [Moderate] Study
- **Idelalisib** is predicted to moderately increase the exposure to alpha blockers **(alfuzosin, tamsulosin)**. Use with caution or avoid. [Moderate] Study
- **Idelalisib** is predicted to increase the exposure to **doxazosin**. [Moderate] Study
- **Imatinib** is predicted to increase the exposure to **tamsulosin**. [Moderate] Theoretical
- Macrolides **(clarithromycin)** are predicted to increase the exposure to **doxazosin**. [Moderate] Study
- Macrolides **(erythromycin)** are predicted to increase the exposure to **tamsulosin**. [Moderate] Theoretical
- Macrolides **(clarithromycin)** are predicted to moderately increase the exposure to alpha blockers **(alfuzosin, tamsulosin)**. Use with caution or avoid. [Moderate] Study
- **MAOIs, irreversible** are predicted to increase the effects of **indoramin**. Avoid. [Severe] Theoretical → Also see TABLE 8 p. 908
- **Netupitant** is predicted to increase the exposure to **tamsulosin**. [Moderate] Theoretical
- **Nilotinib** is predicted to increase the exposure to **tamsulosin**. [Moderate] Theoretical
- **Alpha blockers** cause significant hypotensive effects when given with **phosphodiesterase type-5 inhibitors**. Patient should be stabilised on first drug then second drug should be added at the lowest recommended dose. [Severe] Study → Also see TABLE 8 p. 908
- **Ribociclib** (high-dose) is predicted to increase the exposure to **alfuzosin**. Avoid. [Moderate] Theoretical

Alpha tocopherol → see vitamin E substances

Alpha tocopheryl acetate → see vitamin E substances

Alprazolam → see TABLE 11 p. 909 (CNS depressant effects)

- Antiarrhythmics **(dronedarone)** are predicted to increase the exposure to **alprazolam**. [Severe] Study
- Antiepileptics **(carbamazepine, fosphenytoin, phenobarbital, phenytoin, primidone)** are predicted to decrease the exposure to **alprazolam**. Adjust dose. [Moderate] Theoretical → Also see TABLE 11 p. 909
- Antifungals, azoles **(fluconazole, isavuconazole, posaconazole)** are predicted to increase the exposure to **alprazolam**. [Severe] Study
- Antifungals, azoles **(itraconazole, ketoconazole, voriconazole)** moderately increase the exposure to **alprazolam**. Avoid. [Moderate] Study
- Antifungals, azoles **(miconazole)** are predicted to increase the exposure to **alprazolam**. Use with caution and adjust dose. [Moderate] Theoretical
- **Apalutamide** is predicted to decrease the exposure to **alprazolam**. Adjust dose. [Moderate] Theoretical
- **Aprepitant** is predicted to increase the exposure to **alprazolam**. [Severe] Study
- Calcium channel blockers **(diltiazem, verapamil)** are predicted to increase the exposure to **alprazolam**. [Severe] Study
- **Cobicistat** moderately increases the exposure to **alprazolam**. Avoid. [Moderate] Study
- **Crizotinib** is predicted to increase the exposure to **alprazolam**. [Severe] Study

Alprazolam (continued)
- **Enzalutamide** is predicted to decrease the exposure to **alprazolam**. Adjust dose. [Moderate] Theoretical
- **Fosaprepitant** is predicted to increase the exposure to **alprazolam**. [Moderate] Study
- **HIV-protease inhibitors** moderately increase the exposure to **alprazolam**. Avoid. [Moderate] Study
- **Idelalisib** moderately increases the exposure to **alprazolam**. Avoid. [Moderate] Study
- **Imatinib** is predicted to increase the exposure to **alprazolam**. [Severe] Study
- **Alprazolam** is predicted to increase the exposure to **lomitapide**. Separate administration by 12 hours. [Moderate] Theoretical
- Macrolides **(clarithromycin)** moderately increase the exposure to **alprazolam**. Avoid. [Moderate] Study
- Macrolides **(erythromycin)** are predicted to increase the exposure to **alprazolam**. [Severe] Study
- **Mitotane** is predicted to decrease the exposure to **alprazolam**. Adjust dose. [Moderate] Theoretical
- Monoclonal antibodies **(tocilizumab)** are predicted to decrease the exposure to **alprazolam**. Monitor and adjust dose. [Moderate] Theoretical
- **Netupitant** is predicted to increase the exposure to **alprazolam**. [Severe] Study
- **Nilotinib** is predicted to increase the exposure to **alprazolam**. [Severe] Study
- **Rifampicin** is predicted to decrease the exposure to **alprazolam**. Adjust dose. [Moderate] Theoretical
- SSRIs **(fluvoxamine)** moderately increase the exposure to **alprazolam**. Adjust dose. [Moderate] Study
- **St John's Wort** moderately decreases the exposure to **alprazolam**. [Moderate] Study

Alprostadil → see **TABLE 8** p. 908 (hypotension)
Alteplase → see **TABLE 3** p. 907 (anticoagulant effects)
Aluminium hydroxide → see antacids
Amantadine → see dopamine receptor agonists
Ambrisentan
- **Ciclosporin** moderately increases the exposure to **ambrisentan**. Adjust **ambrisentan** dose. [Moderate] Study
- **Rifampicin** transiently increases the exposure to **ambrisentan**. [Moderate] Study

Amfetamines → see **TABLE 13** p. 910 (serotonin syndrome)

dexamfetamine · lisdexamfetamine

- **Amfetamines** are predicted to decrease the effects of **apraclonidine**. Avoid. [Severe] Theoretical
- **Amfetamines** are predicted to increase the risk of side-effects when given with **atomoxetine**. [Severe] Theoretical
- HIV-protease inhibitors **(ritonavir, tipranavir)** are predicted to increase the exposure to **amfetamines**. [Severe] Theoretical
- MAO-B inhibitors **(rasagiline, selegiline)** are predicted to increase the risk of severe hypertension when given with **amfetamines**. Avoid. [Severe] Theoretical → Also see **TABLE 13** p. 910
- MAO-B inhibitors **(safinamide)** are predicted to increase the risk of severe hypertension when given with **amfetamines**. [Severe] Theoretical → Also see **TABLE 13** p. 910
- **MAOIs, irreversible** are predicted to increase the risk of a hypertensive crisis when given with **amfetamines**. Avoid and for 14 days after stopping the MAOI. [Severe] Anecdotal → Also see **TABLE 13** p. 910
- **Moclobemide** is predicted to increase the risk of a hypertensive crisis when given with **amfetamines**. Avoid. [Severe] Theoretical → Also see **TABLE 13** p. 910
- **Nabilone** is predicted to increase the risk of cardiovascular side-effects when given with **amfetamines**. [Severe] Theoretical
- **Phenothiazines** are predicted to decrease the effects of **amfetamines** and **amfetamines** are predicted to decrease the effects of **phenothiazines**. [Moderate] Study
- SSRIs **(fluoxetine, paroxetine)** are predicted to increase the exposure to **amfetamines**. [Severe] Theoretical → Also see **TABLE 13** p. 910

Amifampridine → see **TABLE 9** p. 909 (QT-interval prolongation)
Amikacin → see aminoglycosides
Amiloride → see potassium-sparing diuretics
Aminoglycosides → see **TABLE 2** p. 907 (nephrotoxicity), **TABLE 19** p. 911 (ototoxicity), **TABLE 20** p. 911 (neuromuscular blocking effects)

amikacin · gentamicin · streptomycin · tobramycin

ROUTE-SPECIFIC INFORMATION Since systemic absorption can follow topical application, the possibility of interactions with topical **gentamicin** and topical **tobramycin** should be borne in mind.

- **Aminoglycosides** are predicted to decrease the effects of **agalsidase alfa**. Avoid. [Moderate] Theoretical
- **Aminoglycosides** are predicted to decrease the effects of **agalsidase beta**. Avoid. [Moderate] Theoretical
- Antifungals, azoles **(miconazole)** potentially decrease the exposure to **tobramycin**. [Moderate] Anecdotal
- **Ataluren** is predicted to increase the risk of nephrotoxicity when given with intravenous **aminoglycosides**. Avoid. [Severe] Study
- **Aminoglycosides** increase the risk of hypocalcaemia when given with **bisphosphonates**. [Moderate] Anecdotal → Also see **TABLE 2** p. 907
- **Aminoglycosides** potentially increase the concentration of **digoxin**. Monitor and adjust dose. [Mild] Study
- **Loop diuretics** increase the risk of nephrotoxicity when given with **aminoglycosides**. Avoid. [Moderate] Study → Also see **TABLE 19** p. 911
- **Aminoglycosides** are predicted to decrease the effects of **neostigmine**. [Moderate] Theoretical
- **Aminoglycosides** are predicted to decrease the effects of **pyridostigmine**. [Moderate] Theoretical

Aminophylline → see **TABLE 17** p. 911 (reduced serum potassium)

FOOD AND LIFESTYLE Smoking can increase aminophylline clearance and increased doses of aminophylline are therefore required; dose adjustments are likely to be necessary if smoking started or stopped during treatment.

- **Aciclovir** increases the exposure to **aminophylline**. Monitor and adjust dose. [Severe] Anecdotal
- **Aminophylline** is predicted to decrease the efficacy of antiarrhythmics **(adenosine)**. Separate administration by 24 hours. [Mild] Theoretical
- Antiepileptics **(fosphenytoin)** are predicted to decrease the exposure to **aminophylline**. Adjust dose. [Moderate] Study
- Antiepileptics **(phenobarbital)** are predicted to decrease the exposure to **aminophylline**. Adjust dose. [Moderate] Theoretical
- Antiepileptics **(phenytoin)** decrease the exposure to **aminophylline**. Adjust dose. [Moderate] Study
- Antiepileptics **(primidone)** are predicted to increase the clearance of **aminophylline**. Adjust dose. [Moderate] Theoretical
- Antiepileptics **(stiripentol)** are predicted to increase the exposure to **aminophylline**. Avoid. [Moderate] Theoretical
- **Beta blockers, non-selective** are predicted to increase the risk of bronchospasm when given with **aminophylline**. Avoid. [Severe] Theoretical
- **Beta blockers, selective** are predicted to increase the risk of bronchospasm when given with **aminophylline**. Avoid. [Severe] Theoretical
- **Combined hormonal contraceptives** are predicted to increase the exposure to **aminophylline**. Adjust dose. [Moderate] Theoretical
- **Aminophylline** increases the risk of agitation when given with **doxapram**. [Moderate] Study
- **Esketamine** is predicted to increase the risk of seizures when given with **aminophylline**. Avoid. [Severe] Theoretical
- H_2 receptor antagonists **(cimetidine)** increase the concentration of **aminophylline**. Adjust dose. [Severe] Study
- HIV-protease inhibitors **(ritonavir)** decrease the exposure to **aminophylline**. Adjust dose. [Moderate] Study
- **Interferons** are predicted to slightly increase the exposure to **aminophylline**. Adjust dose. [Moderate] Theoretical
- Iron chelators **(deferasirox)** are predicted to increase the exposure to **aminophylline**. Avoid. [Moderate] Theoretical
- **Isoniazid** is predicted to affect the clearance of **aminophylline**. [Severe] Theoretical
- **Leflunomide** decreases the exposure to **aminophylline**. Adjust dose. [Moderate] Study
- **Aminophylline** is predicted to decrease the concentration of **lithium**. [Moderate] Theoretical

- Macrolides **(azithromycin)** are predicted to increase the exposure to **aminophylline**. Moderate Theoretical
- Macrolides **(clarithromycin)** are predicted to increase the exposure to **aminophylline**. Adjust dose. Moderate Theoretical
- **Aminophylline** is predicted to decrease the exposure to macrolides **(erythromycin)**. Adjust dose. Severe Study
- **Methotrexate** is predicted to decrease the clearance of **aminophylline**. Moderate Theoretical
- **Mexiletine** is predicted to increase the exposure to **aminophylline**. Adjust dose. Moderate Theoretical
- Monoclonal antibodies **(blinatumomab)** are predicted to transiently increase the exposure to **aminophylline**. Monitor and adjust dose. Moderate Theoretical
- Monoclonal antibodies **(sarilumab)** potentially affect the exposure to **aminophylline**. Monitor and adjust dose. Moderate Theoretical
- Monoclonal antibodies **(tocilizumab)** are predicted to decrease the exposure to **aminophylline**. Monitor and adjust dose. Moderate Theoretical
- **Pentoxifylline** is predicted to increase the concentration of **aminophylline**. Use with caution or avoid. Severe Theoretical
- Quinolones **(ciprofloxacin)** are predicted to increase the exposure to **aminophylline**. Adjust dose. Moderate Theoretical
- **Rifampicin** decreases the exposure to **aminophylline**. Adjust dose. Moderate Study
- **Aminophylline** is predicted to slightly increase the exposure to **roflumilast**. Avoid. Moderate Theoretical
- **Rucaparib** is predicted to increase the exposure to **aminophylline**. Monitor and adjust dose. Moderate Study
- SSRIs **(fluvoxamine)** moderately to markedly increase the exposure to **aminophylline**. Avoid. Severe Study
- **St John's Wort** is predicted to decrease the concentration of **aminophylline**. Severe Theoretical
- Sympathomimetics, vasoconstrictor **(ephedrine)** increase the risk of side-effects when given with **aminophylline**. Avoid in children. Moderate Study
- **Teriflunomide** decreases the exposure to **aminophylline**. Adjust dose. Moderate Study
- **Valaciclovir** is predicted to increase the exposure to **aminophylline**. Severe Anecdotal

Aminosalicylic acid
- **Aminosalicylic acid** is predicted to increase the risk of methaemoglobinaemia when given with topical anaesthetics, local **(prilocaine)**. Use with caution or avoid. Severe Theoretical
- **Aminosalicylic acid** is predicted to increase the risk of methaemoglobinaemia when given with **dapsone**. Severe Theoretical

Amiodarone → see antiarrhythmics

Amisulpride → see **TABLE 9** p. 909 (QT-interval prolongation), **TABLE 11** p. 909 (CNS depressant effects)
- **Amisulpride** is predicted to decrease the effects of **dopamine receptor agonists**. Avoid. Moderate Theoretical → Also see **TABLE 9** p. 909
- **Amisulpride** is predicted to decrease the effects of **levodopa**. Avoid. Severe Theoretical

Amitriptyline → see tricyclic antidepressants

Amlodipine → see calcium channel blockers

Amoxicillin → see penicillins

Amphotericin → see **TABLE 2** p. 907 (nephrotoxicity), **TABLE 17** p. 911 (reduced serum potassium)
- **Amphotericin** increases the risk of toxicity when given with **flucytosine**. Severe Study
- **Micafungin** slightly increases the exposure to **amphotericin**. Avoid or monitor toxicity. Moderate Study
- **Sodium stibogluconate** increases the risk of cardiovascular side-effects when given with **amphotericin**. Separate administration by 14 days. Severe Study

Ampicillin → see penicillins

Amsacrine → see **TABLE 15** p. 910 (myelosuppression)
- **Live vaccines** are predicted to increase the risk of generalised infection (possibly life-threatening) when given with **amsacrine**. Public Health England advises avoid (refer to Green Book). Severe Theoretical

Anaesthetics, local → see **TABLE 11** p. 909 (CNS depressant effects)

bupivacaine · levobupivacaine · mepivacaine · oxybuprocaine · prilocaine · proxymetacaine · ropivacaine · tetracaine

ROUTE-SPECIFIC INFORMATION Since systemic absorption can follow topical application, the possibility of interactions should be borne in mind.

- **Aminosalicylic acid** is predicted to increase the risk of methaemoglobinaemia when given with topical **prilocaine**. Use with caution or avoid. Severe Theoretical
- **Anaesthetics, local** are predicted to increase the risk of cardiodepression when given with **antiarrhythmics**. Severe Theoretical → Also see **TABLE 11** p. 909
- Antiepileptics **(fosphenytoin, phenobarbital, phenytoin, primidone)** are predicted to increase the risk of methaemoglobinaemia when given with topical **prilocaine**. Use with caution or avoid. Severe Theoretical → Also see **TABLE 11** p. 909
- Antiepileptics **(phenytoin)** are predicted to decrease the exposure to **ropivacaine**. Moderate Theoretical
- Antimalarials **(chloroquine, primaquine)** are predicted to increase the risk of methaemoglobinaemia when given with topical **prilocaine**. Use with caution or avoid. Severe Theoretical
- **Dapsone** is predicted to increase the risk of methaemoglobinaemia when given with topical **prilocaine**. Use with caution or avoid. Severe Theoretical
- HIV-protease inhibitors **(ritonavir)** are predicted to decrease the exposure to **ropivacaine**. Moderate Theoretical
- **Leflunomide** is predicted to decrease the exposure to **ropivacaine**. Moderate Theoretical
- **Metoclopramide** is predicted to increase the risk of methaemoglobinaemia when given with topical **prilocaine**. Avoid. Severe Theoretical
- **Nitrates** are predicted to increase the risk of methaemoglobinaemia when given with topical **prilocaine**. Avoid. Severe Theoretical
- **Nitrofurantoin** is predicted to increase the risk of methaemoglobinaemia when given with topical **prilocaine**. Use with caution or avoid. Severe Theoretical
- **Nitroprusside** is predicted to increase the risk of methaemoglobinaemia when given with **prilocaine**. Severe Theoretical
- **Paracetamol** is predicted to increase the risk of methaemoglobinaemia when given with topical **prilocaine**. Use with caution or avoid. Severe Theoretical
- **Rifampicin** is predicted to decrease the exposure to **ropivacaine**. Moderate Theoretical
- SSRIs **(fluvoxamine)** decrease the clearance of **ropivacaine**. Avoid prolonged use. Moderate Study
- **Sulfonamides** potentially increase the risk of methaemoglobinaemia when given with topical **prilocaine**. Use with caution or avoid. Severe Anecdotal
- **Teriflunomide** is predicted to decrease the exposure to **ropivacaine**. Moderate Theoretical

Anagrelide → see **TABLE 9** p. 909 (QT-interval prolongation), **TABLE 4** p. 907 (antiplatelet effects)
- **Combined hormonal contraceptives** are predicted to increase the exposure to **anagrelide**. Moderate Theoretical
- **Mexiletine** is predicted to increase the exposure to **anagrelide**. Moderate Theoretical
- Quinolones **(ciprofloxacin)** are predicted to increase the exposure to **anagrelide**. Moderate Theoretical
- SSRIs **(fluvoxamine)** are predicted to increase the exposure to **anagrelide**. Moderate Theoretical → Also see **TABLE 4** p. 907

Anakinra → see **TABLE 15** p. 910 (myelosuppression)
- **Anakinra** is predicted to increase the risk of generalised infection (possibly life-threatening) when given with **etanercept**. Avoid. Severe Theoretical
- **Live vaccines** are predicted to increase the risk of generalised infection (possibly life-threatening) when given with **anakinra**. Public Health England advises avoid (refer to Green Book). Severe Theoretical
- **Anakinra** is predicted to increase the risk of generalised infection (possibly life-threatening) when given with monoclonal antibodies **(golimumab)**. Avoid. Severe Theoretical

Angiotensin-II receptor antagonists → see TABLE 7 p. 908 (first-dose hypotension), TABLE 8 p. 908 (hypotension), TABLE 16 p. 911 (increased serum potassium)

azilsartan · candesartan · eprosartan · irbesartan · losartan · olmesartan · telmisartan · valsartan

- **Angiotensin-II receptor antagonists** increase the risk of renal impairment when given with aliskiren. Use with caution or avoid **aliskiren** in selected patients. [Severe] Study → Also see TABLE 8 p. 908 → Also see TABLE 16 p. 911
- **Angiotensin-II receptor antagonists** potentially increase the concentration of lithium. Monitor concentration and adjust dose. [Severe] Anecdotal

Antacids

aluminium hydroxide · magnesium carbonate · magnesium trisilicate

SEPARATION OF ADMINISTRATION Antacids should preferably not be taken at the same time as other drugs since they might impair absorption. Antacids might damage enteric coatings designed to prevent dissolution in the stomach.

- **Antacids** are predicted to decrease the absorption of alkylating agents **(estramustine)**. Avoid. [Moderate] Study
- **Antacids** decrease the absorption of antiepileptics **(gabapentin)**. **Gabapentin** should be taken 2 hours after antacids. [Moderate] Study
- **Antacids** decrease the absorption of antifungals, azoles (itraconazole) (capsule). **Itraconazole** should be taken 2 hours before or 1 hour after antacids. [Moderate] Study
- **Antacids** decrease the absorption of antifungals, azoles **(ketoconazole)**. Separate administration by at least 2 hours. [Moderate] Study
- **Antacids** decrease the absorption of antihistamines, non-sedating **(fexofenadine)**. Separate administration by 2 hours. [Mild] Study
- **Antacids** decrease the absorption of antimalarials **(chloroquine)**. Separate administration by at least 4 hours. [Moderate] Study
- **Antacids** are predicted to decrease the absorption of antimalarials **(proguanil)**. Separate administration by at least 2 hours. [Moderate] Study
- **Antacids** decrease the absorption of **aspirin** (high-dose). [Moderate] Study
- **Antacids** decrease the exposure to **bictegravir**. Separate administration by at least 2 hours. [Moderate] Study
- **Antacids** decrease the absorption of bisphosphonates **(alendronate)**. **Alendronate** should be taken at least 30 minutes before antacids. [Moderate] Study
- **Antacids** decrease the absorption of bisphosphonates **(clodronate)**. Avoid antacids for 2 hours before or 1 hour after **clodronate**. [Moderate] Study
- **Antacids** are predicted to decrease the absorption of bisphosphonates **(ibandronate)**. Avoid antacids for at least 6 hours before or 1 hour after **ibandronate**. [Moderate] Theoretical
- **Antacids** decrease the absorption of bisphosphonates **(risedronate)**. Separate administration by at least 2 hours. [Moderate] Study
- **Antacids** are predicted to decrease the absorption of **bosutinib**. **Bosutinib** should be taken at least 12 hours before antacids. [Moderate] Theoretical
- **Antacids** are predicted to decrease the absorption of **ceritinib**. Separate administration by 2 hours. [Moderate] Theoretical
- Oral **aluminium hydroxide** decreases the absorption of **chenodeoxycholic acid**. [Moderate] Study
- **Antacids** are predicted to decrease the absorption of **cholic** acid. Separate administration by 5 hours. [Mild] Theoretical
- **Antacids** are predicted to decrease the absorption of corticosteroids **(deflazacort)**. Separate administration by 2 hours. [Moderate] Theoretical
- **Antacids** decrease the absorption of corticosteroids **(dexamethasone)**. [Moderate] Study
- **Antacids** decrease the absorption of **dasatinib**. Separate administration by at least 2 hours. [Moderate] Study
- **Antacids** decrease the absorption of **digoxin**. Separate administration by 2 hours. [Mild] Study
- **Antacids** are predicted to decrease the absorption of **dipyridamole** (immediate release tablets). [Moderate] Theoretical
- **Antacids** moderately decrease the exposure to **dolutegravir**. **Dolutegravir** should be taken 2 hours before or 6 hours after antacids. [Moderate] Study
- **Antacids** decrease the absorption of **eltrombopag**. **Eltrombopag** should be taken 2 hours before or 4 hours after antacids. [Severe] Study
- **Antacids** moderately decrease the exposure to **elvitegravir**. Separate administration by at least 4 hours. [Moderate] Study
- **Aluminium hydroxide** increases the risk of blocked enteral or nasogastric tubes when given with **enteral feeds**. [Moderate] Study
- **Antacids** are predicted to decrease the absorption of **erlotinib**. **Erlotinib** should be taken 2 hours before or 4 hours after antacids. [Moderate] Theoretical
- **Antacids** slightly to moderately decrease the exposure to fibrates **(gemfibrozil)**. [Moderate] Study
- **Antacids** are predicted to slightly decrease the exposure to **gefitinib**. [Moderate] Theoretical
- **Antacids** are predicted to decrease the absorption of HIV-protease inhibitors **(atazanavir)**. **Atazanavir** should be taken 2 hours before or 1 hour after antacids. [Severe] Theoretical
- **Antacids** are predicted to decrease the absorption of HIV-protease inhibitors **(tipranavir)**. Separate administration by 2 hours. [Moderate] Study
- **Antacids** decrease the absorption of **hydroxychloroquine**. Separate administration by at least 4 hours. [Moderate] Study
- **Antacids** decrease the absorption of **iron (oral)**. **Iron (oral)** should be taken 1 hour before or 2 hours after antacids. [Moderate] Study
- **Aluminium hydroxide** is predicted to decrease the exposure to iron chelators **(deferasirox)**. Avoid. [Moderate] Theoretical
- **Aluminium hydroxide** is predicted to decrease the absorption of iron chelators **(deferiprone)**. Avoid. [Moderate] Theoretical
- **Antacids** are predicted to decrease the absorption of **lapatinib**. Avoid. [Moderate] Theoretical
- **Antacids** are predicted to decrease the exposure to **ledipasvir**. Separate administration by 4 hours. [Moderate] Theoretical
- **Antacids** decrease the exposure to **mycophenolate**. [Moderate] Study
- Oral **antacids** are predicted to decrease the exposure to oral **neratinib**. Separate administration by at least 3 hours. [Mild] Theoretical
- **Antacids** are predicted to decrease the absorption of **nilotinib**. Separate administration by at least 2 hours. [Moderate] Theoretical
- **Magnesium trisilicate** decreases the absorption of **nitrofurantoin**. [Moderate] Study
- **Antacids** are predicted to decrease the absorption of **pazopanib**. **Pazopanib** should be taken 1 hour before or 2 hours after antacids. [Moderate] Theoretical
- **Antacids** decrease the absorption of **penicillamine**. Separate administration by 2 hours. [Mild] Study
- **Antacids** decrease the absorption of **phenothiazines**. [Moderate] Anecdotal
- **Antacids** increase the risk of metabolic alkalosis when given with **polystyrene sulfonate**. [Severe] Anecdotal
- **Antacids** decrease the absorption of **quinolones**. **Quinolones** should be taken 2 hours before or 4 hours after antacids. [Moderate] Study
- **Antacids** slightly decrease the exposure to **raltegravir**. Avoid. [Moderate] Study
- **Antacids** decrease the absorption of **rifampicin**. **Rifampicin** should be taken 1 hour before antacids. [Moderate] Study
- **Antacids** are predicted to decrease the exposure to **rilpivirine**. **Rilpivirine** should be taken 4 hours before or 2 hours after antacids. [Severe] Theoretical
- **Antacids** slightly decrease the exposure to **riociguat**. **Riociguat** should be taken 1 hour before or 2 hours after antacids. [Mild] Study
- **Antacids** moderately decrease the absorption of statins **(rosuvastatin)**. Separate administration by 2 hours. [Moderate] Study
- **Antacids** decrease the absorption of **strontium**. Separate administration by 2 hours. [Moderate] Study

▸ **Antacids** decrease the absorption of **sulpiride**. Separate administration by 2 hours. [Moderate] Study
▸ **Antacids** decrease the absorption of **tetracyclines**. Separate administration by 2 to 3 hours. [Moderate] Study
▸ **Antacids** are predicted to decrease the absorption of thyroid hormones **(levothyroxine)**. Separate administration by at least 4 hours. [Moderate] Anecdotal
▸ **Antacids** are predicted to decrease the absorption of **ursodeoxycholic acid**. Separate administration by 2 hours. [Moderate] Theoretical
▸ **Antacids** are predicted to decrease the concentration of **velpatasvir**. Separate administration by 4 hours. [Moderate] Theoretical

Antazoline → see antihistamines, sedating

Anthracyclines → see **TABLE 15** p. 910 (myelosuppression), **TABLE 5** p. 907 (thromboembolism)

daunorubicin · doxorubicin · epirubicin · idarubicin · mitoxantrone · pixantrone

GENERAL INFORMATION Caution is necessary with concurrent use of cardiotoxic drugs, or drugs that reduce cardiac contractility.

▸ Calcium channel blockers **(verapamil)** moderately increase the exposure to **doxorubicin**. [Moderate] Study
▸ **Ciclosporin** increases the concentration of anthracyclines **(daunorubicin, doxorubicin, epirubicin, idarubicin, mitoxantrone)**. [Severe] Study
▸ H_2 receptor antagonists **(cimetidine)** slightly increase the exposure to **epirubicin**. Avoid. [Moderate] Study
▸ **Leflunomide** is predicted to increase the exposure to anthracyclines **(daunorubicin, doxorubicin, mitoxantrone)**. [Moderate] Theoretical → Also see **TABLE 15** p. 910
▸ **Live vaccines** are predicted to increase the risk of generalised infection (possibly life-threatening) when given with **anthracyclines**. Public Health England advises avoid (refer to Green Book). [Severe] Theoretical
▸ **Anthracyclines** are predicted to increase the risk of cardiotoxicity when given with monoclonal antibodies **(trastuzumab, trastuzumab emtansine)**. Avoid. [Severe] Theoretical → Also see **TABLE 15** p. 910
▸ **Rolapitant** is predicted to increase the exposure to anthracyclines **(doxorubicin, mitoxantrone)**. Avoid or monitor. [Moderate] Study
▸ **Teriflunomide** is predicted to increase the exposure to anthracyclines **(daunorubicin, doxorubicin, mitoxantrone)**. [Moderate] Theoretical

Anti-D (Rh_0) immunoglobulin → see immunoglobulins

Antiarrhythmics → see **TABLE 6** p. 908 (bradycardia), **TABLE 8** p. 908 (hypotension), **TABLE 12** p. 910 (peripheral neuropathy), **TABLE 9** p. 909 (QT-interval prolongation), **TABLE 11** p. 909 (CNS depressant effects), **TABLE 10** p. 909 (antimuscarinics)

adenosine · amiodarone · disopyramide · dronedarone · flecainide · lidocaine · propafenone · vernakalant

▸ **Amiodarone** has a long half-life; there is potential for drug interactions to occur for several weeks (or even months) after treatment with it has been stopped.
▸ Since systemic absorption can follow topical application of **lidocaine**, the possibility of interactions should be borne in mind.
▸ Avoid intravenous class I and class III antiarrhythmics for 4 hours before and after **vernakalant**.

▸ **Dronedarone** is predicted to increase the exposure to **abemaciclib**. [Moderate] Study
▸ Antiarrhythmics **(amiodarone, dronedarone)** are predicted to increase the exposure to **afatinib**. Separate administration by 12 hours. [Moderate] Study
▸ **Amiodarone** is predicted to decrease the effects of **agalsidase alfa**. Avoid. [Moderate] Theoretical
▸ **Amiodarone** is predicted to decrease the effects of **agalsidase beta**. Avoid. [Moderate] Theoretical
▸ **Amiodarone** is predicted to increase the exposure to aldosterone antagonists **(eplerenone)**. Adjust **eplerenone** dose. [Severe] Theoretical
▸ **Dronedarone** is predicted to increase the exposure to aldosterone antagonists **(eplerenone)**. Adjust **eplerenone** dose. [Severe] Study
▸ Antiarrhythmics **(amiodarone, dronedarone)** are predicted to increase the exposure to **aliskiren**. [Severe] Study
▸ **Dronedarone** is predicted to increase the exposure to alpha blockers **(tamsulosin)**. [Moderate] Theoretical
▸ **Dronedarone** is predicted to increase the exposure to **alprazolam**. [Severe] Study
▸ **Aminophylline** is predicted to decrease the efficacy of **adenosine**. Separate administration by 24 hours. [Mild] Theoretical
▸ **Anaesthetics, local** are predicted to increase the risk of cardiodepression when given with **antiarrhythmics**. [Severe] Theoretical → Also see **TABLE 11** p. 909
▸ Antiarrhythmics **(propafenone)** are predicted to increase the risk of cardiodepression when given with antiarrhythmics **(amiodarone)**. Monitor and adjust dose. [Severe] Theoretical
▸ Antiarrhythmics **(amiodarone)** increase the concentration of antiarrhythmics **(flecainide)**. Adjust **flecainide** dose and monitor side effects. [Severe] Study → Also see **TABLE 6** p. 908 → Also see **TABLE 9** p. 909
▸ Antiarrhythmics **(propafenone)** are predicted to increase the risk of cardiodepression when given with antiarrhythmics **(lidocaine)**. [Moderate] Study
▸ Antiarrhythmics **(dronedarone)** are predicted to increase the exposure to antiarrhythmics **(propafenone)**. Monitor and adjust dose. [Moderate] Study
▸ Antiepileptics **(carbamazepine, fosphenytoin, phenobarbital, phenytoin, primidone)** are predicted to decrease the efficacy of **propafenone**. [Moderate] Study
▸ Antiepileptics **(fosphenytoin, phenytoin)** are predicted to decrease the exposure to **lidocaine**. [Severe] Anecdotal
▸ Antiepileptics **(carbamazepine, fosphenytoin, phenobarbital, phenytoin, primidone)** are predicted to decrease the exposure to antiarrhythmics **(disopyramide, dronedarone)**. Avoid. [Severe] Study
▸ **Amiodarone** is predicted to slightly increase the concentration of antiepileptics **(fosphenytoin, phenytoin)**. Monitor and adjust dose. [Severe] Study → Also see **TABLE 12** p. 910
▸ Antifungals, azoles **(fluconazole)** are predicted to increase the exposure to **dronedarone**. [Severe] Theoretical → Also see **TABLE 9** p. 909
▸ Antifungals, azoles **(fluconazole, isavuconazole, posaconazole)** are predicted to increase the exposure to **propafenone**. Monitor and adjust dose. [Moderate] Study
▸ Antifungals, azoles **(itraconazole, ketoconazole, voriconazole)** are predicted to increase the exposure to **disopyramide**. Avoid. [Severe] Theoretical → Also see **TABLE 9** p. 909
▸ Antifungals, azoles **(itraconazole, ketoconazole, voriconazole)** very markedly increase the exposure to **dronedarone**. Avoid. [Severe] Study → Also see **TABLE 9** p. 909
▸ Antifungals, azoles **(itraconazole, ketoconazole, voriconazole)** are predicted to increase the exposure to **propafenone**. Monitor and adjust dose. [Severe] Study
▸ Antifungals, azoles **(miconazole)** are predicted to increase the exposure to **disopyramide**. Use with caution and adjust dose. [Severe] Theoretical
▸ Antifungals, azoles **(posaconazole)** are predicted to increase the exposure to antiarrhythmics **(disopyramide, dronedarone)**. Avoid. [Severe] Theoretical
▸ **Dronedarone** is predicted to increase the exposure to antihistamines, non-sedating **(fexofenadine, mizolastine)**. [Severe] Theoretical
▸ **Dronedarone** is predicted to increase the exposure to antihistamines, non-sedating **(rupatadine)**. Avoid. [Moderate] Study
▸ **Dronedarone** is predicted to increase the concentration of antimalarials **(piperaquine)**. [Severe] Theoretical
▸ **Apalutamide** is predicted to decrease the exposure to antiarrhythmics **(disopyramide, dronedarone)**. Avoid. [Severe] Study → Also see **TABLE 9** p. 909
▸ **Apalutamide** is predicted to decrease the efficacy of **propafenone**. [Moderate] Study
▸ **Dronedarone** is predicted to increase the exposure to **apixaban**. [Moderate] Theoretical

Antiarrhythmics (continued)

- **Aprepitant** increases the exposure to **dronedarone.** [Severe] Theoretical
- **Aprepitant** is predicted to increase the exposure to **propafenone**. Monitor and adjust dose. [Moderate] Study
- **Dronedarone** is predicted to increase the exposure to **axitinib**. [Moderate] Theoretical
- **Dronedarone** is predicted to increase the exposure to **bedaquiline**. Avoid prolonged use. [Mild] Theoretical → Also see **TABLE 9** p. 909
- Antiarrhythmics **(amiodarone, disopyramide, dronedarone, flecainide, lidocaine)** are predicted to increase the risk of cardiovascular side-effects when given with **beta blockers, non-selective**. Use with caution or avoid. [Severe] Study → Also see **TABLE 6** p. 908 → Also see **TABLE 9** p. 909
- **Propafenone** is predicted to increase the risk of cardiovascular side-effects when given with beta blockers, non-selective **(labetalol, levobunolol, nadolol, pindolol, sotalol)**. Use with caution or avoid. [Severe] Study
- **Propafenone** increases the risk of cardiovascular side-effects when given with beta blockers, non-selective **(propranolol)**. Use with caution or avoid. [Severe] Study
- **Propafenone** is predicted to increase the exposure to beta blockers, non-selective **(timolol)** and beta blockers, non-selective **(timolol)** are predicted to increase the risk of cardiodepression when given with **propafenone.** [Severe] Anecdotal
- Antiarrhythmics **(amiodarone, disopyramide, dronedarone, flecainide, lidocaine)** are predicted to increase the risk of cardiovascular side-effects when given with **beta blockers, selective**. Use with caution or avoid. [Severe] Study → Also see **TABLE 6** p. 908
- **Propafenone** is predicted to increase the risk of cardiovascular side-effects when given with beta blockers, selective **(acebutolol, atenolol, betaxolol, bisoprolol, celiprolol, esmolol)**. Use with caution or avoid. [Severe] Study
- **Propafenone** is predicted to increase the exposure to beta blockers, selective **(metoprolol)**. [Moderate] Study
- **Propafenone** is predicted to increase the exposure to beta blockers, selective **(nebivolol)** and beta blockers, selective **(nebivolol)** are predicted to increase the risk of cardiodepression when given with **propafenone.** Avoid. [Severe] Theoretical
- Antiarrhythmics **(amiodarone, dronedarone)** are predicted to increase the exposure to **bictegravir**. Use with caution or avoid. [Moderate] Theoretical
- **Bosentan** is predicted to decrease the exposure to **dronedarone.** [Severe] Theoretical
- **Dronedarone** is predicted to increase the exposure to **bosutinib**. Avoid or adjust dose. [Severe] Theoretical → Also see **TABLE 9** p. 909
- **Dronedarone** is predicted to increase the exposure to **buspirone**. Use with caution and adjust dose. [Moderate] Study
- **Dronedarone** is predicted to increase the exposure to **cabozantinib**. [Moderate] Theoretical → Also see **TABLE 9** p. 909
- **Caffeine citrate** decreases the efficacy of **adenosine**. Separate administration by 24 hours. [Mild] Study
- Calcium channel blockers **(diltiazem, verapamil)** increase the exposure to **dronedarone** and **dronedarone** increases the exposure to calcium channel blockers **(diltiazem, verapamil)**. [Moderate] Study
- Calcium channel blockers **(diltiazem, verapamil)** are predicted to increase the exposure to **propafenone**. Monitor and adjust dose. [Moderate] Study
- Calcium channel blockers **(verapamil)** increase the risk of cardiodepression when given with **flecainide.** [Severe] Anecdotal → Also see **TABLE 6** p. 908
- **Dronedarone** is predicted to increase the exposure to calcium channel blockers **(amlodipine, felodipine, lacidipine, lercanidipine, nicardipine, nifedipine, nimodipine)**. Monitor and adjust dose. [Moderate] Study
- **Amiodarone** is predicted to increase the risk of cardiodepression when given with calcium channel blockers **(diltiazem, verapamil)**. Avoid. [Severe] Theoretical → Also see **TABLE 6** p. 908
- **Disopyramide** is predicted to increase the risk of cardiodepression when given with calcium channel blockers **(verapamil)**. [Severe] Theoretical
- **Dronedarone** is predicted to increase the exposure to **cariprazine**. Avoid. [Severe] Study
- **Amiodarone** is predicted to increase the exposure to **ceritinib**. [Moderate] Theoretical → Also see **TABLE 9** p. 909
- **Chloroprocaine** is predicted to increase the risk of cardiovascular side-effects when given with antiarrhythmics **(amiodarone, dronedarone, vernakalant)**. [Severe] Theoretical
- **Amiodarone** increases the concentration of **ciclosporin**. Monitor concentration and adjust dose. [Severe] Study
- **Dronedarone** is predicted to increase the concentration of **ciclosporin**. [Severe] Study
- **Cobicistat** potentially increases the concentration of antiarrhythmics **(amiodarone, disopyramide, flecainide, lidocaine)**. [Severe] Theoretical
- **Cobicistat** very markedly increases the exposure to **dronedarone**. Avoid. [Severe] Study
- **Cobicistat** is predicted to increase the exposure to **propafenone.** Monitor and adjust dose. [Severe] Study
- **Dronedarone** is predicted to increase the exposure to **cobimetinib**. [Severe] Theoretical
- **Amiodarone** is predicted to increase the exposure to **colchicine**. Avoid P-glycoprotein inhibitors or adjust **colchicine** dose. [Severe] Theoretical
- **Dronedarone** is predicted to increase the exposure to colchicine. Adjust **colchicine** dose with moderate inhibitors of CYP3A4. [Severe] Study
- **Dronedarone** is predicted to increase the exposure to corticosteroids **(methylprednisolone)**. Monitor and adjust dose. [Moderate] Study
- **Amiodarone** increases the anticoagulant effect of **coumarins**. [Severe] Study
- **Propafenone** increases the anticoagulant effect of **coumarins**. Monitor INR and adjust dose. [Moderate] Study
- **Crizotinib** is predicted to increase the exposure to **propafenone**. Monitor and adjust dose. [Moderate] Study
- **Amiodarone** increases the exposure to **dabigatran**. Adjust **dabigatran** dose. [Moderate] Study
- **Dronedarone** slightly increases the exposure to **dabigatran**. Avoid. [Severe] Study
- **Dronedarone** is predicted to slightly increase the exposure to **darifenacin**. [Moderate] Study
- **Darifenacin** is predicted to increase the concentration of **flecainide**. [Moderate] Theoretical
- **Dronedarone** is predicted to increase the exposure to **dasatinib**. [Severe] Study → Also see **TABLE 9** p. 909
- **Dronedarone** is predicted to slightly increase the exposure to **dienogest**. [Moderate] Study
- Antiarrhythmics **(amiodarone, dronedarone)** are predicted to moderately increase the exposure to **digoxin**. Monitor and adjust **digoxin** dose, p. 86. [Severe] Study → Also see **TABLE 6** p. 908
- **Propafenone** increases the concentration of **digoxin**. Monitor and adjust dose. [Severe] Study
- **Dipyridamole** increases the exposure to **adenosine**. Avoid or adjust dose. [Severe] Study
- **Dronedarone** increases the risk of QT-prolongation when given with **domperidone**. Avoid. [Severe] Study
- **Dronedarone** is predicted to increase the exposure to dopamine receptor agonists **(bromocriptine)**. [Severe] Theoretical
- **Dronedarone** is predicted to increase the concentration of dopamine receptor agonists **(cabergoline)**. [Severe] Anecdotal
- **Dronedarone** is predicted to moderately increase the exposure to **dutasteride**. [Mild] Study
- **Dronedarone** slightly increases the exposure to **edoxaban**. Adjust **edoxaban** dose. [Severe] Study
- **Efavirenz** is predicted to decrease the exposure to **dronedarone**. [Severe] Theoretical → Also see **TABLE 9** p. 909
- Antiarrhythmics **(dronedarone, propafenone)** are predicted to increase the exposure to **eliglustat**. Avoid or adjust dose—consult product literature. [Severe] Study
- **Dronedarone** is predicted to moderately increase the exposure to **encorafenib**. [Moderate] Study → Also see **TABLE 9** p. 909

- **Enzalutamide** is predicted to decrease the exposure to antiarrhythmics **(disopyramide, dronedarone)**. Avoid. Severe Study
- **Enzalutamide** is predicted to decrease the efficacy of **propafenone**. Moderate Study
- **Dronedarone** is predicted to increase the risk of ergotism when given with **ergometrine**. Severe Theoretical
- **Dronedarone** is predicted to increase the risk of ergotism when given with **ergotamine**. Severe Theoretical
- Antiarrhythmics **(amiodarone, dronedarone)** are predicted to increase the exposure to **erlotinib**. Moderate Theoretical
- **Dronedarone** is predicted to increase the concentration of **everolimus**. Avoid or adjust dose. Moderate Study
- **Dronedarone** is predicted to increase the exposure to **fesoterodine**. Adjust **fesoterodine** dose with moderate inhibitors of CYP3A4 in hepatic and renal impairment. Mild Study
- Antiarrhythmics **(amiodarone, dronedarone)** are predicted to increase the exposure to **fidaxomicin**. Avoid. Moderate Study
- **Dronedarone** is predicted to increase the exposure to **gefitinib**. Moderate Theoretical
- **Dronedarone** potentially increases the exposure to **glecaprevir**. Moderate Theoretical
- **Grapefruit juice** increases the exposure to **amiodarone**. Avoid. Moderate Study
- **Grapefruit juice** moderately increases the exposure to **dronedarone**. Avoid. Severe Study
- **Grapefruit juice** increases the exposure to **propafenone**. Monitor and adjust dose. Moderate Study
- **Dronedarone** is predicted to increase the concentration of **guanfacine**. Adjust **guanfacine** dose, p. 247. Moderate Theoretical
- H_2 receptor antagonists **(cimetidine)** increase the exposure to **amiodarone**. Moderate Study
- H_2 receptor antagonists **(cimetidine)** slightly increase the exposure to **flecainide**. Monitor and adjust dose. Mild Study
- H_2 receptor antagonists **(cimetidine)** increase the exposure to **lidocaine**. Monitor and adjust dose. Moderate Study
- H_2 receptor antagonists **(cimetidine)** are predicted to increase the exposure to **propafenone**. Monitor and adjust dose. Moderate Theoretical
- **HIV-protease inhibitors** are predicted to increase the exposure to **amiodarone**. Avoid. Severe Theoretical → Also see **TABLE 9** p. 909
- **HIV-protease inhibitors** are predicted to increase the exposure to **disopyramide**. Severe Theoretical → Also see **TABLE 9** p. 909
- **HIV-protease inhibitors** very markedly increase the exposure to **dronedarone**. Avoid. Severe Study → Also see **TABLE 9** p. 909
- HIV-protease inhibitors **(ritonavir)** are predicted to increase the exposure to **flecainide**. Avoid or monitor side effects. Severe Theoretical
- **HIV-protease inhibitors** are predicted to increase the exposure to **lidocaine**. Avoid. Severe Study
- **HIV-protease inhibitors** are predicted to increase the exposure to **propafenone**. Monitor and adjust dose. Severe Study
- **Amiodarone** is predicted to increase the exposure to **ibrutinib**. Adjust **ibrutinib** dose. Severe Theoretical
- **Dronedarone** is predicted to increase the exposure to **ibrutinib**. Adjust **ibrutinib** dose with moderate inhibitors of CYP3A4. Severe Study
- **Idelalisib** is predicted to increase the exposure to **amiodarone**. Avoid. Moderate Theoretical
- **Idelalisib** very markedly increases the exposure to **dronedarone**. Avoid. Severe Study
- **Idelalisib** is predicted to increase the exposure to **propafenone**. Monitor and adjust dose. Severe Study
- **Imatinib** is predicted to increase the exposure to **dronedarone**. Severe Theoretical
- **Imatinib** is predicted to increase the exposure to **propafenone**. Monitor and adjust dose. Moderate Study
- **Dronedarone** is predicted to increase the exposure to **ivabradine**. Adjust **ivabradine** dose. Severe Theoretical
- **Dronedarone** is predicted to increase the exposure to **ivacaftor**. Adjust ivacaftor p. 196 or tezacaftor with ivacaftor p. 198 dose with moderate inhibitors of CYP3A4. Severe Study
- **Dronedarone** is predicted to increase the exposure to **lapatinib**. Moderate Study → Also see **TABLE 9** p. 909
- Antiarrhythmics **(amiodarone, dronedarone)** are predicted to increase the exposure to **larotrectinib**. Mild Theoretical
- **Ledipasvir** increases the risk of severe bradycardia or heart block when given with **amiodarone**. Refer to specialist literature. Severe Anecdotal
- **Letermovir** is predicted to increase the concentration of **amiodarone**. Moderate Theoretical
- **Amiodarone** is predicted to increase the exposure to **lomitapide**. Separate administration by 12 hours. Moderate Theoretical
- **Dronedarone** is predicted to increase the exposure to **lomitapide**. Avoid. Moderate Theoretical
- **Dronedarone** is predicted to increase the exposure to **loperamide**. Severe Theoretical
- **Dronedarone** is predicted to increase the exposure to **lurasidone**. Adjust **lurasidone** dose. Moderate Study
- Macrolides **(clarithromycin)** very markedly increase the exposure to **dronedarone**. Avoid. Severe Study → Also see **TABLE 9** p. 909
- Macrolides **(clarithromycin)** are predicted to increase the exposure to **propafenone**. Monitor and adjust dose. Severe Study
- Macrolides **(clarithromycin, erythromycin)** are predicted to increase the exposure to **lidocaine**. Moderate Theoretical
- Macrolides **(erythromycin)** are predicted to moderately increase the exposure to **dronedarone**. Avoid. Severe Theoretical → Also see **TABLE 9** p. 909
- Macrolides **(erythromycin)** are predicted to increase the exposure to **propafenone**. Monitor and adjust dose. Moderate Study
- **Mexiletine** increases the risk of torsade de pointes when given with **antiarrhythmics**. Avoid. Severe Theoretical
- **Dronedarone** is predicted to increase the exposure to **midazolam**. Monitor side effects and adjust dose. Severe Study
- **Dronedarone** is predicted to increase the exposure to **midostaurin**. Moderate Theoretical
- **Mitotane** is predicted to decrease the exposure to antiarrhythmics **(disopyramide, dronedarone)**. Avoid. Severe Study
- **Mitotane** is predicted to decrease the efficacy of **propafenone**. Moderate Study
- **Dronedarone** increases the risk of neutropenia when given with monoclonal antibodies **(brentuximab vedotin)**. Monitor and adjust dose. Severe Theoretical
- Antiarrhythmics **(amiodarone, dronedarone)** are predicted to increase the exposure to **naldemedine**. Moderate Study
- **Dronedarone** is predicted to increase the exposure to **naloxegol**. Adjust **naloxegol** dose and monitor side effects. Moderate Study
- **Dronedarone** is predicted to increase the exposure to **neratinib**. Avoid. Severe Study
- **Netupitant** is predicted to increase the exposure to **propafenone**. Monitor and adjust dose. Moderate Study
- **Nevirapine** is predicted to decrease the exposure to **dronedarone**. Severe Theoretical
- **Nilotinib** is predicted to increase the exposure to **propafenone**. Monitor and adjust dose. Moderate Study
- Antiarrhythmics **(amiodarone, dronedarone)** are predicted to increase the exposure to **nintedanib**. Moderate Study
- NSAIDs **(celecoxib)** are predicted to increase the exposure to antiarrhythmics **(flecainide, propafenone)**. Monitor and adjust dose. Moderate Theoretical
- **Dronedarone** is predicted to increase the exposure to **olaparib**. Avoid moderate inhibitors of CYP3A4 or adjust **olaparib** dose. Moderate Theoretical
- **Dronedarone** is predicted to increase the exposure to opioids **(alfentanil, buprenorphine, fentanyl, oxycodone)**. Monitor and adjust dose. Moderate Study
- **Amiodarone** is predicted to increase the concentration of opioids **(fentanyl)**. Moderate Theoretical → Also see **TABLE 6** p. 908
- **Dronedarone** is predicted to increase the exposure to opioids **(methadone)**. Moderate Theoretical → Also see **TABLE 9** p. 909
- **Dronedarone** is predicted to increase the exposure to **oxybutynin**. Mild Theoretical

Antiarrhythmics (continued)

- Antiarrhythmics **(amiodarone, dronedarone)** are predicted to increase the exposure to **panobinostat**. Adjust dose. Moderate Theoretical → Also see **TABLE 9** p. 909
- **Dronedarone** is predicted to increase the exposure to **pazopanib**. Moderate Theoretical → Also see **TABLE 9** p. 909
- **Propafenone** is predicted to increase the anticoagulant effect of **phenindione**. Monitor and adjust dose. Moderate Theoretical
- **Dronedarone** is predicted to increase the exposure to phosphodiesterase type-5 inhibitors **(avanafil)**. Adjust **avanafil** dose. Moderate Theoretical
- **Dronedarone** is predicted to increase the exposure to phosphodiesterase type-5 inhibitors **(sildenafil)**. Monitor or adjust **sildenafil** dose with moderate inhibitors of CYP3A4, p. 125. Moderate Study → Also see **TABLE 9** p. 909
- **Dronedarone** is predicted to increase the exposure to phosphodiesterase type-5 inhibitors **(tadalafil)**. Severe Theoretical
- **Dronedarone** is predicted to increase the exposure to phosphodiesterase type-5 inhibitors **(vardenafil)**. Adjust dose. Severe Theoretical → Also see **TABLE 9** p. 909
- **Amiodarone** is predicted to increase the exposure to **pibrentasvir**. Moderate Theoretical
- **Dronedarone** potentially increases the exposure to **pibrentasvir**. Moderate Theoretical
- **Dronedarone** is predicted to increase the exposure to **pimozide**. Avoid. Severe Theoretical → Also see **TABLE 9** p. 909
- **Dronedarone** is predicted to increase the exposure to **quetiapine**. Avoid. Moderate Study
- Quinolones **(ciprofloxacin)** slightly increase the exposure to **lidocaine**. Mild Study
- **Dronedarone** is predicted to increase the exposure to **ranolazine**. Severe Study → Also see **TABLE 9** p. 909
- **Amiodarone** is predicted to increase the exposure to retinoids **(alitretinoin)**. Adjust **alitretinoin** dose. Moderate Theoretical
- **Ribociclib** (high-dose) is predicted to increase the exposure to **amiodarone**. Avoid. Moderate Theoretical → Also see **TABLE 9** p. 909
- **Dronedarone** is predicted to increase the exposure to **ribociclib**. Moderate Study → Also see **TABLE 9** p. 909
- **Rifampicin** is predicted to decrease the exposure to antiarrhythmics **(disopyramide, dronedarone)**. Avoid. Severe Study
- **Rifampicin** is predicted to decrease the efficacy of **propafenone**. Moderate Study
- **Dronedarone** is predicted to increase the exposure to **rivaroxaban**. Avoid. Moderate Theoretical
- **Rolapitant** is predicted to increase the exposure to **propafenone**. Severe Study
- **Dronedarone** is predicted to increase the exposure to **ruxolitinib**. Moderate Theoretical
- **Dronedarone** is predicted to increase the exposure to **saxagliptin**. Mild Study
- **Amiodarone** is predicted to increase the exposure to **siponimod**. Avoid depending on other drugs taken—consult product literature. Severe Study → Also see **TABLE 6** p. 908
- **Amiodarone** is predicted to increase the concentration of **sirolimus**. Severe Anecdotal
- **Dronedarone** increases the concentration of **sirolimus**. Monitor and adjust dose. Moderate Study
- **Sofosbuvir** is predicted to increase the risk of severe bradycardia or heart block when given with **amiodarone**. Refer to specialist literature. Severe Anecdotal
- SSRIs **(fluvoxamine)** are predicted to increase the exposure to **propafenone**. Monitor and adjust dose. Moderate Study
- **Dronedarone** is predicted to increase the exposure to SSRIs **(citalopram, escitalopram, fluoxetine, fluvoxamine, paroxetine, sertraline)**. Severe Theoretical → Also see **TABLE 9** p. 909
- **Dronedarone** is predicted to increase the exposure to SSRIs (dapoxetine). Adjust **dapoxetine** dose with moderate inhibitors of CYP3A4. Moderate Theoretical
- **St John's Wort** is predicted to decrease the exposure to **dronedarone**. Avoid. Severe Theoretical
- **Amiodarone** is predicted to increase the risk of rhabdomyolysis when given with statins **(atorvastatin)**. Monitor and adjust dose. Moderate Theoretical
- **Dronedarone** slightly increases the exposure to statins **(atorvastatin)**. Monitor and adjust dose. Severe Study
- **Amiodarone** is predicted to increase the exposure to statins **(fluvastatin)**. Severe Theoretical
- **Dronedarone** slightly increases the exposure to statins **(rosuvastatin)**. Adjust dose. Severe Study
- **Amiodarone** increases the risk of rhabdomyolysis when given with statins **(simvastatin)**. Adjust **simvastatin** dose, p. 141. Severe Study
- **Dronedarone** moderately increases the exposure to statins **(simvastatin)**. Monitor and adjust dose. Severe Study
- **Amiodarone** is predicted to increase the exposure to **sulfonylureas**. Use with caution and adjust dose. Moderate Study
- **Dronedarone** is predicted to increase the exposure to **sunitinib**. Moderate Theoretical → Also see **TABLE 9** p. 909
- **Lidocaine** is predicted to increase the effects of **suxamethonium**. Moderate Study
- **Amiodarone** is predicted to increase the concentration of **tacrolimus**. Severe Anecdotal
- **Dronedarone** is predicted to increase the concentration of **tacrolimus**. Severe Study
- Antiarrhythmics **(amiodarone, dronedarone)** are predicted to slightly increase the exposure to **talazoparib**. Avoid or adjust **talazoparib** dose. Severe Study
- **Dronedarone** is predicted to increase the exposure to taxanes **(cabazitaxel)**. Moderate Theoretical
- **Dronedarone** is predicted to increase the exposure to taxanes **(paclitaxel)**. Severe Theoretical
- **Dronedarone** is predicted to increase the concentration of **temsirolimus**. Use with caution or avoid. Moderate Theoretical
- **Dronedarone** is predicted to increase the exposure to **tezacaftor**. Adjust tezacaftor with ivacaftor p. 198 dose with moderate inhibitors of CYP3A4. Severe Study
- **Theophylline** decreases the efficacy of **adenosine**. Separate administration by 24 hours. Mild Study
- **Amiodarone** is predicted to increase the risk of thyroid dysfunction when given with **thyroid hormones**. Avoid. Moderate Study
- **Amiodarone** is predicted to increase the exposure to **ticagrelor**. Use with caution or avoid. Severe Study
- **Dronedarone** given with a potent CYP2C19 inhibitor is predicted to increase the exposure to **tofacitinib**. Adjust **tofacitinib** dose. Moderate Study
- **Dronedarone** is predicted to increase the exposure to **tolterodine**. Mild Theoretical → Also see **TABLE 9** p. 909
- **Dronedarone** is predicted to increase the exposure to **tolvaptan**. Manufacturer advises caution or adjust **tolvaptan** dose with moderate inhibitors of CYP3A4. Moderate Study
- Antiarrhythmics **(amiodarone, dronedarone)** are predicted to increase the exposure to **topotecan**. Severe Study
- Antiarrhythmics **(amiodarone, dronedarone)** are predicted to increase the concentration of **trametinib**. Moderate Theoretical
- **Dronedarone** is predicted to increase the exposure to **trazodone**. Moderate Theoretical
- **Dronedarone** is predicted to increase the exposure to **tricyclic antidepressants**. Avoid. Severe Theoretical → Also see **TABLE 9** p. 909
- **Propafenone** is predicted to increase the concentration of **tricyclic antidepressants**. Moderate Theoretical → Also see **TABLE 10** p. 909
- **Dronedarone** is predicted to increase the exposure to **ulipristal**. Avoid if used for uterine fibroids. Moderate Study
- **Amiodarone** is predicted to increase the concentration of **velpatasvir**. Avoid or monitor. Moderate Theoretical
- **Amiodarone** is predicted to increase the exposure to **venetoclax**. Avoid or monitor for toxicity. Severe Theoretical
- **Dronedarone** is predicted to increase the exposure to **venetoclax**. Avoid or adjust dose—consult product literature. Severe Study
- **Dronedarone** is predicted to increase the exposure to **vinca alkaloids**. Severe Theoretical → Also see **TABLE 9** p. 909
- **Dronedarone** is predicted to increase the exposure to **zopiclone**. Adjust dose. Moderate Study

Anticholinesterases, centrally acting → see TABLE 6 p. 908 (bradycardia)

donepezil · galantamine · rivastigmine

- Antiepileptics **(carbamazepine, fosphenytoin, phenobarbital, phenytoin, primidone)** are predicted to decrease the exposure to **donepezil**. Mild Study
- Antifungals, azoles **(itraconazole, ketoconazole, voriconazole)** are predicted to increase the exposure to **galantamine**. Monitor and adjust dose. Moderate Study
- **Apalutamide** is predicted to decrease the exposure to **donepezil**. Mild Study
- **Bupropion** is predicted to increase the exposure to **galantamine**. Monitor and adjust dose. Moderate Study
- **Cinacalcet** is predicted to increase the exposure to **galantamine**. Monitor and adjust dose. Moderate Study
- **Cobicistat** is predicted to increase the exposure to **galantamine**. Monitor and adjust dose. Moderate Study
- **Enzalutamide** is predicted to decrease the exposure to **donepezil**. Mild Study
- **HIV-protease inhibitors** are predicted to increase the exposure to **galantamine**. Monitor and adjust dose. Moderate Study
- **Idelalisib** is predicted to increase the exposure to **galantamine**. Monitor and adjust dose. Moderate Study
- Macrolides **(clarithromycin)** are predicted to increase the exposure to **galantamine**. Monitor and adjust dose. Moderate Study
- **Mitotane** is predicted to decrease the exposure to **donepezil**. Mild Study
- **Anticholinesterases, centrally acting** are predicted to decrease the effects of **neuromuscular blocking drugs, non-depolarising**. Moderate Theoretical → Also see TABLE 6 p. 908
- **Rifampicin** is predicted to decrease the exposure to **donepezil**. Mild Study
- SSRIs **(fluoxetine, paroxetine)** are predicted to increase the exposure to **galantamine**. Monitor and adjust dose. Moderate Study
- **Anticholinesterases, centrally acting** increase the effects of **suxamethonium**. Moderate Theoretical
- **Terbinafine** is predicted to increase the exposure to **galantamine**. Monitor and adjust dose. Moderate Study

Antiepileptics → see TABLE 1 p. 907 (hepatotoxicity), TABLE 18 p. 911 (hyponatraemia), TABLE 15 p. 910 (myelosuppression), TABLE 12 p. 910 (peripheral neuropathy), TABLE 11 p. 909 (CNS depressant effects)

brivaracetam · carbamazepine · eslicarbazepine · ethosuximide · fosphenytoin · gabapentin · lacosamide · lamotrigine · levetiracetam · oxcarbazepine · paraldehyde · perampanel · phenobarbital · phenytoin · pregabalin · primidone · retigabine · rufinamide · stiripentol · tiagabine · topiramate · valproate · vigabatrin · zonisamide

FOOD AND LIFESTYLE Avoid taking milk, dairy products, carbonated drinks, fruit juices, or caffeine-containing food and drinks at the same time as **stiripentol**.

- Antiepileptics **(carbamazepine, fosphenytoin, phenobarbital, phenytoin, primidone)** are predicted to decrease the exposure to **abacavir**. Moderate Theoretical
- Antiepileptics **(carbamazepine, fosphenytoin, phenobarbital, phenytoin, primidone)** are predicted to markedly decrease the exposure to **abemaciclib**. Avoid. Severe Study
- Antiepileptics **(carbamazepine, fosphenytoin, phenobarbital, phenytoin, primidone)** are predicted to decrease the exposure to **abiraterone**. Avoid. Severe Study
- **Acetazolamide** potentially increases the risk of toxicity when given with **valproate**. Severe Study
- **Acetazolamide** potentially increases the risk of overheating and dehydration when given with **zonisamide**. Avoid in children. Severe Theoretical
- **Carbamazepine** is predicted to decrease the exposure to **afatinib**. Moderate Study
- Antiepileptics **(fosphenytoin, phenytoin)** are predicted to decrease the exposure to **agomelatine**. Moderate Theoretical
- Antiepileptics **(carbamazepine, fosphenytoin, phenobarbital, phenytoin, primidone)** decrease the concentration of **albendazole**. Moderate Study
- **Alcohol (beverage)** potentially increases the risk of visual disturbances when given with **retigabine**. Moderate Study
- Antiepileptics **(carbamazepine, fosphenytoin, phenobarbital, phenytoin, primidone)** are predicted to decrease the exposure to aldosterone antagonists **(eplerenone)**. Avoid. Moderate Theoretical → Also see TABLE 18 p. 911
- **Carbamazepine** decreases the exposure to **aliskiren**. Moderate Study
- Antiepileptics **(carbamazepine, fosphenytoin, phenobarbital, phenytoin, primidone)** are predicted to decrease the exposure to **alprazolam**. Adjust dose. Moderate Theoretical → Also see TABLE 11 p. 909
- **Fosphenytoin** is predicted to decrease the exposure to **aminophylline**. Adjust dose. Moderate Study
- **Phenobarbital** is predicted to decrease the exposure to **aminophylline**. Adjust dose. Moderate Theoretical
- **Phenytoin** decreases the exposure to **aminophylline**. Adjust dose. Moderate Study
- **Primidone** is predicted to increase the clearance of **aminophylline**. Adjust dose. Moderate Theoretical
- **Stiripentol** is predicted to increase the exposure to **aminophylline**. Avoid. Moderate Theoretical
- Antiepileptics **(fosphenytoin, phenobarbital, phenytoin, primidone)** are predicted to increase the risk of methaemoglobinaemia when given with topical anaesthetics, local **(prilocaine)**. Use with caution or avoid. Severe Theoretical → Also see TABLE 11 p. 909
- **Phenytoin** is predicted to decrease the exposure to anaesthetics, local **(ropivacaine)**. Moderate Theoretical
- **Antacids** decrease the absorption of **gabapentin**. **Gabapentin** should be taken 2 hours after antacids. Moderate Study
- Antiepileptics **(carbamazepine, fosphenytoin, phenobarbital, phenytoin, primidone)** are predicted to decrease the exposure to antiarrhythmics **(disopyramide, dronedarone)**. Avoid. Severe Study
- Antiarrhythmics **(amiodarone)** are predicted to slightly increase the concentration of antiepileptics **(fosphenytoin, phenytoin)**. Monitor and adjust dose. Severe Study → Also see TABLE 12 p. 910
- Antiepileptics **(fosphenytoin, phenytoin)** are predicted to decrease the exposure to antiarrhythmics **(lidocaine)**. Severe Anecdotal
- Antiepileptics **(carbamazepine, fosphenytoin, phenobarbital, phenytoin, primidone)** are predicted to decrease the efficacy of antiarrhythmics **(propafenone)**. Moderate Study
- Antiepileptics **(carbamazepine, fosphenytoin, phenobarbital, phenytoin, primidone)** are predicted to decrease the exposure to anticholinesterases, centrally acting **(donepezil)**. Mild Study
- Antiepileptics **(carbamazepine)** decrease the concentration of antiepileptics **(brivaracetam)**. Moderate Study
- Antiepileptics **(fosphenytoin, phenytoin)** decrease the concentration of antiepileptics **(brivaracetam)**. Moderate Study
- Antiepileptics **(lamotrigine)** potentially increase the concentration of antiepileptics **(carbamazepine)** and antiepileptics **(carbamazepine)** decrease the concentration of antiepileptics **(lamotrigine)**. Adjust **lamotrigine** dose and monitor **carbamazepine** concentration, p. 216, p. 209. Moderate Study
- Antiepileptics **(phenobarbital)** affect the concentration of antiepileptics **(carbamazepine)** and antiepileptics **(carbamazepine)** increase the concentration of antiepileptics **(phenobarbital)**. Adjust dose. Moderate Study
- Antiepileptics **(topiramate)** increase the risk of carbamazepine toxicity when given with antiepileptics **(carbamazepine)**. Moderate Study
- Antiepileptics **(stiripentol)** increase the concentration of antiepileptics **(carbamazepine, phenobarbital)**. Avoid in Dravet syndrome. Severe Study
- Antiepileptics **(carbamazepine)** slightly decrease the exposure to antiepileptics **(eslicarbazepine, oxcarbazepine)**. Monitor and adjust dose. Moderate Study
- Antiepileptics **(oxcarbazepine)** are predicted to increase the concentration of antiepileptics **(fosphenytoin)**. Monitor concentration and adjust dose. Moderate Study
- Antiepileptics **(stiripentol)** are predicted to increase the concentration of antiepileptics **(fosphenytoin)**. Severe Study

Antiepileptics (continued)

- Antiepileptics **(carbamazepine)** affect the concentration of antiepileptics **(fosphenytoin, phenytoin)** and antiepileptics **(fosphenytoin, phenytoin)** decrease the concentration of antiepileptics **(carbamazepine)**. Monitor and adjust dose. [Severe] Study
- Antiepileptics **(eslicarbazepine)** increase the exposure to antiepileptics **(fosphenytoin, phenytoin)** and antiepileptics **(fosphenytoin, phenytoin)** decrease the exposure to antiepileptics **(eslicarbazepine)**. Monitor and adjust dose. [Moderate] Study
- Antiepileptics **(valproate)** affect the concentration of antiepileptics **(fosphenytoin, phenytoin)** and antiepileptics **(fosphenytoin, phenytoin)** decrease the concentration of antiepileptics **(valproate)**. [Severe] Study
- Antiepileptics **(vigabatrin)** decrease the concentration of antiepileptics **(fosphenytoin, phenytoin)**. [Mild] Study
- Antiepileptics **(fosphenytoin)** decrease the concentration of antiepileptics **(lamotrigine)**. Monitor and adjust **lamotrigine** dose, p. 216. [Moderate] Study
- Antiepileptics **(phenobarbital, phenytoin, primidone)** decrease the concentration of antiepileptics **(lamotrigine)**. Monitor and adjust **lamotrigine** dose, p. 216. [Moderate] Study → Also see **TABLE 11** p. 909
- Antiepileptics **(valproate)** increase the exposure to antiepileptics **(lamotrigine)**. Adjust **lamotrigine** dose and monitor rash, p. 216. [Severe] Study
- Antiepileptics **(lamotrigine)** are predicted to increase the concentration of antiepileptics **(oxcarbazepine)** and antiepileptics **(oxcarbazepine)** are predicted to decrease the concentration of antiepileptics **(lamotrigine)**. Monitor side effects and adjust dose. [Moderate] Study
- Antiepileptics **(carbamazepine, fosphenytoin)** are predicted to decrease the exposure to antiepileptics **(perampanel)**. Monitor and adjust dose. [Moderate] Study
- Antiepileptics **(oxcarbazepine)** decrease the concentration of antiepileptics **(perampanel)** and antiepileptics **(perampanel)** increase the concentration of antiepileptics **(oxcarbazepine)**. Monitor and adjust dose. [Moderate] Study
- Antiepileptics **(phenobarbital, phenytoin, primidone)** are predicted to decrease the exposure to antiepileptics **(perampanel)**. Monitor and adjust dose. [Moderate] Study → Also see **TABLE 11** p. 909
- Antiepileptics **(phenytoin)** increase the concentration of antiepileptics **(phenobarbital)** and antiepileptics **(phenobarbital)** affect the concentration of antiepileptics **(phenytoin)**. [Moderate] Study
- Antiepileptics **(fosphenytoin)** increase the concentration of antiepileptics **(phenobarbital, primidone)** and antiepileptics **(phenobarbital, primidone)** affect the concentration of antiepileptics **(fosphenytoin)**. [Moderate] Study
- Antiepileptics **(oxcarbazepine)** are predicted to increase the concentration of antiepileptics **(phenytoin)**. Monitor concentration and adjust dose. [Moderate] Study
- Antiepileptics **(stiripentol)** are predicted to increase the concentration of antiepileptics **(phenytoin)**. Avoid in Dravet syndrome. [Severe] Study
- Antiepileptics **(carbamazepine)** potentially decrease the concentration of antiepileptics **(primidone)** and antiepileptics **(primidone)** potentially decrease the concentration of antiepileptics **(carbamazepine)**. Adjust dose. [Moderate] Anecdotal
- Antiepileptics **(phenytoin)** increase the concentration of antiepileptics **(primidone)** and antiepileptics **(primidone)** affect the concentration of antiepileptics **(phenytoin)**. [Moderate] Study
- Antiepileptics **(stiripentol)** are predicted to increase the concentration of antiepileptics **(primidone)**. [Severe] Theoretical
- Antiepileptics **(valproate)** affect the concentration of antiepileptics **(primidone)**. Monitor and adjust dose. [Severe] Study
- Antiepileptics **(carbamazepine)** slightly increase the clearance of antiepileptics **(retigabine)**. [Moderate] Study
- Antiepileptics **(fosphenytoin, phenytoin)** are predicted to slightly increase the clearance of antiepileptics **(retigabine)**. [Moderate] Study
- Antiepileptics **(valproate)** increase the exposure to antiepileptics **(rufinamide)**. Adjust **rufinamide** dose, p. 222. [Moderate] Study
- Antiepileptics **(carbamazepine, fosphenytoin, phenobarbital, phenytoin, primidone)** decrease the exposure to antiepileptics **(tiagabine)**. Monitor and adjust **tiagabine** dose, p. 227. [Moderate] Study
- Antiepileptics **(fosphenytoin, phenytoin)** decrease the concentration of antiepileptics **(topiramate)** and antiepileptics **(topiramate)** increase the concentration of antiepileptics **(fosphenytoin, phenytoin)**. Monitor and adjust dose. [Moderate] Study
- Antiepileptics **(phenobarbital, primidone)** are predicted to decrease the concentration of antiepileptics **(topiramate)**. [Mild] Study
- Antiepileptics **(phenobarbital)** decrease the concentration of antiepileptics **(valproate)** and antiepileptics **(valproate)** increase the concentration of antiepileptics **(phenobarbital)**. Monitor and adjust dose. [Moderate] Study
- Antiepileptics **(topiramate)** increase the risk of toxicity when given with antiepileptics **(valproate)**. [Severe] Study
- Antiepileptics **(carbamazepine)** slightly to moderately decrease the concentration of antiepileptics **(zonisamide)** and antiepileptics **(zonisamide)** affect the concentration of antiepileptics **(carbamazepine)**. Monitor and adjust dose. [Moderate] Study
- Antiepileptics **(fosphenytoin, phenytoin)** slightly to moderately decrease the concentration of antiepileptics **(zonisamide)**. Monitor and adjust dose. [Moderate] Study
- Antiepileptics **(phenobarbital, primidone)** are predicted to decrease the concentration of antiepileptics **(zonisamide)**. Monitor and adjust dose. [Moderate] Study
- Antiepileptics **(topiramate)** potentially increase the risk of overheating and dehydration when given with antiepileptics **(zonisamide)**. Avoid in children. [Severe] Theoretical
- Antifungals, azoles **(itraconazole, ketoconazole, voriconazole)** are predicted to very slightly increase the exposure to **perampanel**. [Mild] Study
- Antifungals, azoles **(miconazole)** increase the risk of carbamazepine toxicity when given with **carbamazepine**. Monitor and adjust dose. [Severe] Anecdotal
- Antifungals, azoles **(miconazole)** increase the risk of phenytoin toxicity when given with **fosphenytoin**. Monitor and adjust dose. [Severe] Anecdotal
- Antifungals, azoles **(miconazole)** increase the risk of phenytoin toxicity when given with **phenytoin**. Monitor and adjust dose. [Severe] Anecdotal
- **Carbamazepine** is predicted to decrease the efficacy of antifungals, azoles **(fluconazole)** and antifungals, azoles **(fluconazole)** increase the concentration of **carbamazepine**. Avoid or monitor **carbamazepine** concentration and adjust dose accordingly, p. 209. [Severe] Theoretical → Also see **TABLE 1** p. 907
- Antifungals, azoles **(fluconazole)** increase the concentration of antiepileptics **(fosphenytoin, phenytoin)**. Monitor concentration and adjust dose. [Moderate] Study
- Antiepileptics **(carbamazepine, fosphenytoin, phenobarbital, phenytoin, primidone)** are predicted to decrease the exposure to antifungals, azoles **(isavuconazole)**. Avoid. [Severe] Study
- **Fosphenytoin** very markedly decreases the exposure to antifungals, azoles **(itraconazole)**. Avoid and for 14 days after stopping **fosphenytoin**. [Moderate] Study
- **Phenobarbital** decreases the concentration of antifungals, azoles **(itraconazole)**. Avoid and for 14 days after stopping **phenobarbital**. [Moderate] Study
- **Phenytoin** very markedly decreases the exposure to antifungals, azoles **(itraconazole)**. Avoid and for 14 days after stopping **phenytoin**. [Moderate] Study
- **Primidone** is predicted to decrease the concentration of antifungals, azoles **(itraconazole)**. [Moderate] Theoretical
- **Carbamazepine** is predicted to decrease the efficacy of antifungals, azoles **(itraconazole, voriconazole)** and antifungals, azoles **(itraconazole, voriconazole)** increase the concentration of **carbamazepine**. Avoid or adjust dose. [Moderate] Theoretical → Also see **TABLE 1** p. 907

- **Carbamazepine** is predicted to decrease the efficacy of antifungals, azoles **(ketoconazole)** and antifungals, azoles **(ketoconazole)** slightly increase the concentration of **carbamazepine**. Avoid or monitor **carbamazepine** concentration and adjust dose accordingly, p. 209. Moderate Study
- **Phenobarbital** is predicted to decrease the concentration of antifungals, azoles **(ketoconazole)**. Avoid. Moderate Study
- Antiepileptics **(fosphenytoin, phenytoin)** decrease the exposure to antifungals, azoles **(ketoconazole)**. Avoid. Moderate Study
- **Primidone** is predicted to decrease the concentration of antifungals, azoles **(ketoconazole, posaconazole)**. Avoid. Moderate Study
- **Carbamazepine** is predicted to decrease the efficacy of antifungals, azoles **(posaconazole)** and antifungals, azoles **(posaconazole)** increase the concentration of **carbamazepine**. Avoid. Moderate Theoretical
- **Phenobarbital** is predicted to decrease the concentration of antifungals, azoles **(posaconazole)**. Avoid. Moderate Study
- Antiepileptics **(fosphenytoin, phenytoin)** are predicted to decrease the exposure to antifungals, azoles **(posaconazole)**. Avoid. Moderate Study
- **Fosphenytoin** decreases the exposure to antifungals, azoles **(voriconazole)** and antifungals, azoles **(voriconazole)** increase the exposure to **fosphenytoin**. Avoid or adjust **voriconazole** dose and monitor phenytoin concentration, p. 410. Moderate Study
- **Phenytoin** decreases the exposure to antifungals, azoles **(voriconazole)** and antifungals, azoles **(voriconazole)** increase the exposure to **phenytoin**. Avoid or adjust **voriconazole** dose and monitor **phenytoin** concentration, p. 410, p. 220. Moderate Study
- Antiepileptics **(phenobarbital, primidone)** are predicted to decrease the concentration of antifungals, azoles **(voriconazole)**. Avoid. Moderate Theoretical
- Antihistamines, sedating **(hydroxyzine)** potentially increase the risk of overheating and dehydration when given with **zonisamide**. Avoid in children. Severe Theoretical
- Antiepileptics **(carbamazepine, fosphenytoin, phenobarbital, phenytoin, primidone)** are predicted to decrease the exposure to antimalarials **(artemether)** (with lumefantrine). Avoid. Severe Study
- Antimalarials **(pyrimethamine)** increase the risk of haematological toxicity when given with antiepileptics **(fosphenytoin, phenytoin)**. Severe Study
- Antimalarials **(pyrimethamine)** are predicted to increase the risk of haematological toxicity when given with antiepileptics **(phenobarbital, primidone)**. Severe Theoretical
- Antiepileptics **(carbamazepine, fosphenytoin, phenobarbital, phenytoin, primidone)** are predicted to decrease the concentration of antimalarials **(piperaquine)**. Avoid. Moderate Theoretical
- Antiepileptics **(carbamazepine, phenobarbital, primidone)** potentially increase the risk of toxicity when given with antimalarials **(quinine)**. Unknown Study
- **Apalutamide** is predicted to decrease the exposure to **perampanel**. Monitor and adjust dose. Moderate Study
- **Apalutamide** potentially decreases the exposure to **valproate**. Mild Theoretical
- Antiepileptics **(carbamazepine, fosphenytoin, phenobarbital, phenytoin, primidone)** are predicted to moderately decrease the exposure to **apixaban**. Use with caution or avoid. Severe Study
- Antiepileptics **(carbamazepine, fosphenytoin, phenobarbital, phenytoin, primidone)** moderately decrease the exposure to **apremilast**. Avoid. Severe Study
- Antiepileptics **(carbamazepine, fosphenytoin, phenobarbital, phenytoin, primidone)** are predicted to markedly decrease the exposure to **aprepitant**. Avoid. Moderate Study
- Antiepileptics **(carbamazepine, fosphenytoin, phenobarbital, phenytoin, primidone)** are predicted to moderately decrease the exposure to **aripiprazole**. Adjust **aripiprazole** dose, p. 265. Moderate Study → Also see **TABLE 11** p. 909
- Antiepileptics **(carbamazepine, fosphenytoin, phenobarbital, phenytoin, primidone)** are predicted to decrease the exposure to **axitinib**. Avoid or adjust dose. Moderate Study
- Antiepileptics **(carbamazepine, fosphenytoin, phenobarbital, phenytoin, primidone)** are predicted to decrease the exposure to **bazedoxifene**. Moderate Theoretical
- Antiepileptics **(carbamazepine, fosphenytoin, phenobarbital, phenytoin, primidone)** decrease the exposure to **bedaquiline**. Avoid. Severe Study → Also see **TABLE 1** p. 907
- Antiepileptics **(phenobarbital, primidone)** are predicted to decrease the exposure to beta blockers, non-selective **(carvedilol, labetalol)**. Moderate Theoretical
- Antiepileptics **(phenobarbital, primidone)** are predicted to decrease the exposure to beta blockers, non-selective **(propranolol)**. Moderate Study
- Antiepileptics **(phenobarbital, primidone)** are predicted to decrease the exposure to beta blockers, selective **(acebutolol, bisoprolol, metoprolol, nebivolol)**. Moderate Study
- Antiepileptics **(carbamazepine, fosphenytoin, phenobarbital, phenytoin, primidone)** are predicted to decrease the exposure to **bictegravir**. Avoid. Moderate Study
- **Oxcarbazepine** is predicted to decrease the exposure to **bictegravir**. Avoid. Moderate Theoretical
- Antiepileptics **(carbamazepine, fosphenytoin, phenobarbital, phenytoin, primidone)** slightly decrease the exposure to **bortezomib**. Avoid. Severe Study → Also see **TABLE 12** p. 910
- Antiepileptics **(carbamazepine, fosphenytoin, phenobarbital, phenytoin, primidone)** affect the exposure to **bosentan**. Avoid. Severe Study
- Antiepileptics **(carbamazepine, fosphenytoin, phenobarbital, phenytoin, primidone)** are predicted to very markedly decrease the exposure to **bosutinib**. Avoid. Severe Study
- Antiepileptics **(carbamazepine, fosphenytoin, phenobarbital, phenytoin, primidone)** are predicted to decrease the exposure to **brigatinib**. Avoid. Severe Study
- Antiepileptics **(carbamazepine, fosphenytoin, phenobarbital, phenytoin, primidone)** are predicted to markedly decrease the exposure to **bupropion**. Severe Study
- **Valproate** increases the exposure to **bupropion**. Severe Study
- Antiepileptics **(carbamazepine, fosphenytoin, phenobarbital, phenytoin, primidone)** are predicted to decrease the exposure to **buspirone**. Use with caution and adjust dose. Severe Study
- Antiepileptics **(carbamazepine, fosphenytoin, phenobarbital, phenytoin, primidone)** moderately decrease the exposure to **cabozantinib**. Avoid. Moderate Study
- Antiepileptics **(fosphenytoin, phenytoin)** are predicted to moderately increase the clearance of **caffeine citrate**. Monitor and adjust dose. Moderate Study
- Calcium channel blockers **(diltiazem)** increase the concentration of **carbamazepine** and **carbamazepine** is predicted to decrease the exposure to calcium channel blockers **(diltiazem)**. Monitor concentration and adjust dose. Severe Anecdotal
- Calcium channel blockers **(verapamil)** increase the concentration of **carbamazepine** and **carbamazepine** is predicted to decrease the exposure to calcium channel blockers **(verapamil)**. Severe Anecdotal
- Antiepileptics **(carbamazepine, fosphenytoin, phenobarbital, phenytoin, primidone)** are predicted to decrease the exposure to calcium channel blockers **(amlodipine, felodipine, lacidipine, lercanidipine, nicardipine, nifedipine, nimodipine)**. Monitor and adjust dose. Moderate Study
- Antiepileptics **(phenobarbital, primidone)** are predicted to decrease the exposure to calcium channel blockers **(diltiazem, verapamil)**. Severe Study
- Calcium channel blockers **(diltiazem, verapamil)** potentially increase the concentration of antiepileptics **(fosphenytoin, phenytoin)** and antiepileptics **(fosphenytoin, phenytoin)** are predicted to decrease the exposure to calcium channel blockers **(diltiazem, verapamil)**. Severe Study
- **Valproate** increases the exposure to calcium channel blockers **(nimodipine)**. Adjust dose. Moderate Study
- Antiepileptics **(carbamazepine, fosphenytoin, phenobarbital, phenytoin, primidone)** are predicted to decrease the exposure to **cannabidiol**. Adjust dose. Moderate Study → Also see **TABLE 11** p. 909

Antiepileptics (continued)

- Cannabidiol increases the risk of increased ALT concentrations when given with **valproate**. Avoid or adjust dose. Severe Study
- Capecitabine increases the concentration of antiepileptics **(fosphenytoin, phenytoin)**. Severe Anecdotal
- Carbapenems decrease the concentration of **valproate**. Avoid. Severe Anecdotal
- Antiepileptics **(carbamazepine, fosphenytoin, phenobarbital, phenytoin, primidone)** are predicted to decrease the exposure to cariprazine. Avoid. Severe Theoretical → Also see **TABLE 11** p. 909
- Antiepileptics **(carbamazepine, fosphenytoin, phenytoin)** are predicted to decrease the concentration of caspofungin. Adjust **caspofungin** dose, p. 405. Moderate Theoretical
- Antiepileptics **(carbamazepine, fosphenytoin, phenobarbital, phenytoin, primidone)** are predicted to decrease the exposure to ceritinib. Avoid. Severe Study
- Antiepileptics **(phenobarbital, primidone)** are predicted to affect the efficacy of chenodeoxycholic acid. Monitor and adjust dose. Moderate Theoretical
- Antiepileptics **(phenobarbital, primidone)** decrease the concentration of chloramphenicol. Moderate Study
- Intravenous chloramphenicol increases the concentration of antiepileptics **(fosphenytoin, phenytoin)** and antiepileptics **(fosphenytoin, phenytoin)** affect the concentration of intravenous chloramphenicol. Monitor concentration and adjust dose. Severe Study
- Chlordiazepoxide affects the concentration of antiepileptics **(fosphenytoin, phenytoin)**. Severe Study
- **Phenobarbital** decreases the effects of cholic acid. Avoid. Moderate Study
- Antiepileptics **(carbamazepine, fosphenytoin, phenobarbital, phenytoin, primidone)** decrease the concentration of ciclosporin. Severe Study
- **Oxcarbazepine** decreases the concentration of ciclosporin. Severe Anecdotal
- Antiepileptics **(carbamazepine, fosphenytoin, phenobarbital, phenytoin, primidone)** are predicted to alter the effects of cilostazol. Moderate Theoretical
- Antiepileptics **(carbamazepine, fosphenytoin, phenobarbital, phenytoin, primidone)** are predicted to decrease the exposure to cinacalcet. Monitor and adjust dose. Moderate Study
- **Carbamazepine** is predicted to increase the risk of haematological toxicity when given with oral cladribine. Moderate Theoretical
- Clobazam potentially affects the concentration of antiepileptics **(fosphenytoin, phenytoin)**. Severe Anecdotal
- **Stiripentol** increases the concentration of clobazam. Severe Study
- Antiepileptics **(carbamazepine, fosphenytoin, phenobarbital, phenytoin, primidone)** decrease the exposure to clomethiazole. Monitor and adjust dose. Moderate Study → Also see **TABLE 11** p. 909
- Clonazepam potentially affects the concentration of antiepileptics **(fosphenytoin, phenytoin)**. Severe Anecdotal
- Antiepileptics **(fosphenytoin, phenobarbital, phenytoin, primidone)** are predicted to decrease the exposure to clozapine. Moderate Anecdotal → Also see **TABLE 11** p. 909
- **Carbamazepine** is predicted to increase the risk of myelosuppression when given with clozapine. Avoid. Severe Anecdotal
- Antiepileptics **(carbamazepine, fosphenytoin, phenobarbital, phenytoin, primidone)** are predicted to decrease the exposure to cobicistat. Avoid. Severe Theoretical
- **Oxcarbazepine** is predicted to decrease the concentration of cobicistat. Severe Theoretical
- Cobicistat is predicted to very slightly increase the exposure to **perampanel**. Mild Study
- Antiepileptics **(carbamazepine, fosphenytoin, phenobarbital, phenytoin, primidone)** are predicted to decrease the exposure to cobimetinib. Avoid. Severe Theoretical
- Antiepileptics **(carbamazepine, eslicarbazepine, fosphenytoin, oxcarbazepine, perampanel, phenobarbital, phenytoin, primidone, rufinamide, topiramate)** are predicted to decrease the efficacy of combined hormonal contraceptives. For FSRH guidance, see Contraceptives, interactions p. 536. Severe Study
- Combined hormonal contraceptives alter the exposure to **lamotrigine**. Adjust dose. Moderate Study
- Antiepileptics **(carbamazepine, fosphenytoin, phenobarbital, phenytoin, primidone)** are predicted to decrease the exposure to corticosteroids **(budesonide, deflazacort, dexamethasone, fludrocortisone, hydrocortisone, methylprednisolone, prednisolone, triamcinolone)**. Monitor and adjust dose. Moderate Study
- Antiepileptics **(carbamazepine, fosphenytoin, phenobarbital, phenytoin, primidone)** are predicted to decrease the exposure to corticosteroids **(fluticasone)**. Unknown Theoretical
- Antiepileptics **(fosphenytoin, phenytoin)** are predicted to alter the anticoagulant effect of coumarins. Moderate Anecdotal
- Antiepileptics **(phenobarbital, primidone)** decrease the anticoagulant effect of coumarins. Monitor INR and adjust dose. Moderate Study
- **Carbamazepine** decreases the effects of coumarins. Monitor and adjust dose. Severe Study
- Antiepileptics **(carbamazepine, fosphenytoin, phenobarbital, phenytoin, primidone)** are predicted to markedly decrease the exposure to crizotinib. Avoid. Severe Study
- **Carbamazepine** is predicted to decrease the exposure to dabigatran. Avoid. Severe Study
- **Phenytoin** is predicted to decrease the exposure to **dabigatran**. Avoid. Severe Theoretical
- Antiepileptics **(carbamazepine, fosphenytoin, phenobarbital, phenytoin, primidone)** are predicted to decrease the exposure to dabrafenib. Avoid. Moderate Theoretical
- Danazol moderately increases the concentration of **carbamazepine**. Monitor and adjust dose. Severe Study
- Antiepileptics **(fosphenytoin, phenobarbital, phenytoin, primidone)** are predicted to increase the risk of methaemoglobinaemia when given with dapsone. Severe Theoretical
- Antiepileptics **(carbamazepine, fosphenytoin, phenobarbital, phenytoin, primidone)** are predicted to decrease the exposure to darifenacin. Moderate Theoretical
- Antiepileptics **(carbamazepine, fosphenytoin, phenobarbital, phenytoin, primidone)** are predicted to decrease the exposure to dasabuvir. Avoid. Severe Theoretical
- Antiepileptics **(carbamazepine, fosphenytoin, phenobarbital, phenytoin, primidone)** are predicted to markedly decrease the exposure to dasatinib. Avoid. Severe Study
- Antiepileptics **(carbamazepine, fosphenytoin, phenobarbital, phenytoin, primidone)** are predicted to slightly decrease the exposure to delamanid. Avoid. Moderate Study
- **Lamotrigine** is predicted to increase the risk of hyponatraemia when given with desmopressin. Severe Theoretical
- Antiepileptics **(carbamazepine, eslicarbazepine, fosphenytoin, oxcarbazepine, perampanel, phenobarbital, phenytoin, primidone, rufinamide, topiramate)** are predicted to decrease the efficacy of desogestrel. For FSRH guidance, see Contraceptives, interactions p. 536. Severe Theoretical
- Desogestrel is predicted to increase the exposure to **lamotrigine**. Moderate Study
- Diazepam potentially affects the concentration of antiepileptics **(fosphenytoin, phenytoin)**. Monitor concentration and adjust dose. Severe Study
- Diazoxide decreases the concentration of antiepileptics **(fosphenytoin, phenytoin)** and antiepileptics **(fosphenytoin, phenytoin)** are predicted to decrease the effects of diazoxide. Monitor concentration and adjust dose. Moderate Anecdotal
- Antiepileptics **(carbamazepine, fosphenytoin, phenobarbital, phenytoin, primidone)** are predicted to markedly decrease the exposure to dienogest. Severe Study
- Antiepileptics **(fosphenytoin, phenytoin)** are predicted to decrease the concentration of digoxin. Moderate Anecdotal
- Disulfiram increases the concentration of antiepileptics **(fosphenytoin, phenytoin)**. Monitor concentration and adjust dose. Severe Study → Also see **TABLE 12** p. 910
- Antiepileptics **(carbamazepine, fosphenytoin, phenobarbital, phenytoin, primidone)** decrease the exposure to dolutegravir. Adjust dose. Severe Study
- **Oxcarbazepine** is predicted to decrease the exposure to dolutegravir. Adjust dose. Severe Theoretical

- Antiepileptics **(carbamazepine, fosphenytoin, phenobarbital, phenytoin, primidone)** are predicted to decrease the exposure to doravirine. Avoid. [Severe] Study
- **Oxcarbazepine** is predicted to decrease the exposure to doravirine. Avoid. [Severe] Theoretical
- Antiepileptics **(carbamazepine, fosphenytoin, phenobarbital, phenytoin, primidone)** are predicted to decrease the exposure to dronabinol. Avoid or adjust dose. [Mild] Study → Also see TABLE 11 p. 909
- **Phenytoin** is predicted to decrease the exposure to **duloxetine**. [Moderate] Theoretical
- **Carbamazepine** is predicted to decrease the exposure to edoxaban. [Moderate] Study
- **Phenytoin** is predicted to decrease the exposure to **edoxaban**. [Moderate] Theoretical
- Antiepileptics **(fosphenytoin, phenytoin)** slightly decrease the exposure to efavirenz and efavirenz affects the concentration of antiepileptics **(fosphenytoin, phenytoin)**. [Severe] Theoretical
- **Carbamazepine** slightly decreases the exposure to efavirenz and efavirenz slightly decreases the exposure to **carbamazepine**. [Severe] Study
- **Phenobarbital** is predicted to decrease the exposure to efavirenz and efavirenz affects the concentration of **phenobarbital**. [Severe] Theoretical
- Efavirenz is predicted to affect the efficacy of **primidone** and **primidone** is predicted to slightly decrease the exposure to efavirenz. [Severe] Theoretical
- Antiepileptics **(carbamazepine, fosphenytoin, phenobarbital, phenytoin, primidone)** are predicted to decrease the exposure to elbasvir. Avoid. [Severe] Study
- Antiepileptics **(carbamazepine, fosphenytoin, phenobarbital, phenytoin, primidone)** are predicted to decrease the exposure to eliglustat. Avoid. [Severe] Study
- Antiepileptics **(carbamazepine, fosphenytoin, phenobarbital, phenytoin, primidone)** are predicted to decrease the concentration of elvitegravir. Avoid. [Severe] Theoretical
- Antiepileptics **(carbamazepine, fosphenytoin, phenobarbital, phenytoin, primidone)** are predicted to decrease the exposure to encorafenib. [Severe] Theoretical
- Enteral feeds decrease the absorption of **phenytoin**. [Severe] Study
- Enzalutamide is predicted to slightly decrease the exposure to **brivaracetam**. [Moderate] Theoretical
- Enzalutamide is predicted to decrease the exposure to **perampanel**. Monitor and adjust dose. [Moderate] Study
- Antiepileptics **(carbamazepine, fosphenytoin, phenobarbital, phenytoin, primidone)** are predicted to decrease the effects of ergotamine. [Moderate] Theoretical
- Antiepileptics **(carbamazepine, fosphenytoin, phenobarbital, phenytoin, primidone)** are predicted to decrease the exposure to erlotinib. Avoid or adjust **erlotinib** dose. [Severe] Study
- Antiepileptics **(carbamazepine, fosphenytoin, phenobarbital, phenytoin, primidone)** are predicted to decrease the exposure to esketamine. Adjust dose. [Moderate] Theoretical → Also see TABLE 11 p. 909
- Antiepileptics **(carbamazepine, eslicarbazepine, fosphenytoin, oxcarbazepine, perampanel, phenobarbital, phenytoin, primidone, rufinamide, topiramate)** are predicted to decrease the efficacy of etonogestrel. For FSRH guidance, see Contraceptives, interactions p. 536. [Severe] Theoretical
- Antiepileptics **(carbamazepine, fosphenytoin, phenobarbital, phenytoin, primidone)** are predicted to decrease the efficacy of etoposide. [Moderate] Study
- Antiepileptics **(carbamazepine, fosphenytoin, phenobarbital, phenytoin, primidone)** are predicted to decrease the exposure to etravirine. Avoid. [Severe] Theoretical
- Antiepileptics **(carbamazepine, fosphenytoin, phenobarbital, phenytoin, primidone)** are predicted to decrease the concentration of everolimus. Avoid or adjust dose. [Severe] Study
- Antiepileptics **(carbamazepine, fosphenytoin, phenobarbital, phenytoin, primidone)** moderately decrease the exposure to exemestane. [Moderate] Study
- Antiepileptics **(carbamazepine, fosphenytoin, phenobarbital, phenytoin, primidone)** are predicted to decrease the exposure to fesoterodine. Avoid. [Moderate] Study
- Antiepileptics **(carbamazepine, fosphenytoin, phenobarbital, phenytoin, primidone)** are predicted to decrease the exposure to fingolimod. [Moderate] Study
- Fluorouracil increases the concentration of antiepileptics **(fosphenytoin, phenytoin)**. Monitor concentration and adjust dose. [Severe] Anecdotal
- Folates are predicted to decrease the concentration of antiepileptics **(fosphenytoin, phenobarbital, phenytoin, primidone)**. Monitor concentration and adjust dose. [Severe] Study
- Antiepileptics **(carbamazepine, fosphenytoin, phenobarbital, phenytoin, primidone)** are predicted to decrease the exposure to fosaprepitant. Avoid. [Moderate] Theoretical
- Antiepileptics **(carbamazepine, fosphenytoin, phenobarbital, phenytoin, primidone)** are predicted to decrease the exposure to gefitinib. Avoid. [Severe] Study
- Antiepileptics **(carbamazepine, fosphenytoin, phenytoin)** are predicted to decrease the exposure to gilteritinib. Avoid. [Severe] Study
- Antiepileptics **(carbamazepine, fosphenytoin, phenobarbital, phenytoin, primidone)** are predicted to moderately decrease the exposure to glecaprevir. Avoid. [Severe] Study
- Antiepileptics **(eslicarbazepine, oxcarbazepine)** potentially decrease the exposure to glecaprevir. Avoid. [Severe] Theoretical
- **Valproate** potentially opposes the effects of glycerol phenylbutyrate. [Moderate] Theoretical
- Grapefruit juice slightly increases the exposure to **carbamazepine**. Monitor and adjust dose. [Moderate] Study
- Antiepileptics **(carbamazepine, fosphenytoin, phenobarbital, phenytoin, primidone)** are predicted to decrease the exposure to grazoprevir. Avoid. [Severe] Study
- Antiepileptics **(phenobarbital, primidone)** decrease the effects of griseofulvin. [Moderate] Study
- Antiepileptics **(carbamazepine, fosphenytoin, phenobarbital, phenytoin, primidone)** are predicted to decrease the concentration of guanfacine. Adjust **guanfacine** dose, p. 247. [Moderate] Study → Also see TABLE 11 p. 909
- **Oxcarbazepine** is predicted to decrease the concentration of guanfacine. Monitor and adjust **guanfacine** dose, p. 247. [Moderate] Theoretical
- Guanfacine increases the concentration of **valproate**. Monitor and adjust dose. [Moderate] Study
- H_2 receptor antagonists **(cimetidine)** transiently increase the concentration of **carbamazepine**. Monitor concentration and adjust dose. [Moderate] Study
- H_2 receptor antagonists **(cimetidine)** increase the concentration of antiepileptics **(fosphenytoin, phenytoin)**. Monitor concentration and adjust dose. [Severe] Study
- Antiepileptics **(carbamazepine, fosphenytoin, phenobarbital, phenytoin, primidone)** decrease the concentration of haloperidol. Adjust dose. [Moderate] Study → Also see TABLE 11 p. 909
- Haloperidol potentially increases the risk of overheating and dehydration when given with **zonisamide**. Avoid in children. [Severe] Theoretical
- HIV-protease inhibitors are predicted to affect the exposure to antiepileptics **(fosphenytoin, phenytoin)** and antiepileptics **(fosphenytoin, phenytoin)** decrease the concentration of HIV-protease inhibitors. [Severe] Theoretical
- HIV-protease inhibitors are predicted to affect the concentration of antiepileptics **(phenobarbital, primidone)** and antiepileptics **(phenobarbital, primidone)** are predicted to decrease the concentration of HIV-protease inhibitors. [Severe] Theoretical
- HIV-protease inhibitors are predicted to increase the exposure to **carbamazepine** and **carbamazepine** is predicted to decrease the exposure to HIV-protease inhibitors. Monitor and adjust dose. [Severe] Theoretical
- HIV-protease inhibitors **(ritonavir)** slightly decrease the exposure to **lamotrigine**. [Severe] Study
- HIV-protease inhibitors are predicted to very slightly increase the exposure to **perampanel**. [Mild] Study
- HIV-protease inhibitors **(ritonavir)** are predicted to decrease the concentration of **valproate**. [Severe] Anecdotal

Antiepileptics (continued)

- Antiepileptics **(carbamazepine, eslicarbazepine, fosphenytoin, oxcarbazepine, perampanel, phenobarbital, phenytoin, primidone, rufinamide, topiramate)** are predicted to decrease the effects of **hormone replacement therapy**. [Moderate] Anecdotal
- **Hormone replacement therapy** is predicted to alter the exposure to **lamotrigine**. [Moderate] Theoretical
- Antiepileptics **(carbamazepine, fosphenytoin, phenobarbital, phenytoin, primidone)** are predicted to decrease the exposure to **ibrutinib**. Avoid or adjust **ibrutinib** dose. [Severe] Study
- Antiepileptics **(carbamazepine, fosphenytoin, phenobarbital, phenytoin, primidone)** are predicted to decrease the exposure to **idelalisib**. Avoid. [Severe] Study
- **Idelalisib** is predicted to very slightly increase the exposure to **perampanel**. [Mild] Study
- Antiepileptics **(carbamazepine, fosphenytoin, phenobarbital, phenytoin, primidone)** are predicted to decrease the exposure to **imatinib**. Avoid. [Moderate] Study
- **Oxcarbazepine** decreases the exposure to **imatinib**. Avoid. [Moderate] Study
- Antiepileptics **(carbamazepine, fosphenytoin, phenobarbital, phenytoin, primidone)** are predicted to decrease the exposure to **irinotecan**. Avoid. [Severe] Study
- Antiepileptics **(carbamazepine, fosphenytoin, phenobarbital, phenytoin, primidone)** are predicted to decrease the exposure to iron chelators **(deferasirox)**. Monitor serum ferritin and adjust dose. [Moderate] Theoretical
- **Isoniazid** increases the concentration of antiepileptics **(fosphenytoin, phenytoin)**. [Moderate] Study → Also see TABLE 12 p. 910
- **Isoniazid** markedly increases the concentration of **carbamazepine** and **carbamazepine** increases the risk of hepatotoxicity when given with **isoniazid**. Monitor concentration and adjust dose. [Severe] Study → Also see TABLE 1 p. 907
- Antiepileptics **(carbamazepine, fosphenytoin, phenobarbital, phenytoin, primidone)** are predicted to decrease the exposure to **ivabradine**. Adjust dose. [Moderate] Theoretical
- Antiepileptics **(carbamazepine, fosphenytoin, phenobarbital, phenytoin, primidone)** are predicted to moderately to markedly decrease the exposure to **ivacaftor**. Avoid. [Severe] Study
- Antiepileptics **(carbamazepine, fosphenytoin, phenobarbital, phenytoin, primidone)** are predicted to decrease the exposure to **ixazomib**. Avoid. [Severe] Study
- Antiepileptics **(carbamazepine, fosphenytoin, phenobarbital, phenytoin, primidone)** are predicted to decrease the exposure to **lapatinib**. Avoid. [Severe] Study
- Antiepileptics **(carbamazepine, fosphenytoin, phenobarbital, phenytoin, primidone)** are predicted to moderately decrease the exposure to **larotrectinib**. Avoid. [Moderate] Study
- Antiepileptics **(fosphenytoin, oxcarbazepine, phenobarbital, phenytoin, primidone)** are predicted to decrease the exposure to **ledipasvir**. Avoid. [Severe] Theoretical
- **Carbamazepine** is predicted to decrease the exposure to **ledipasvir**. Avoid. [Severe] Study
- Antiepileptics **(carbamazepine, phenobarbital, primidone)** are predicted to decrease the concentration of **letermovir**. [Moderate] Theoretical
- **Letermovir** is predicted to decrease the concentration of antiepileptics **(fosphenytoin, phenytoin)** and antiepileptics **(fosphenytoin, phenytoin)** are predicted to decrease the concentration of **letermovir**. [Moderate] Theoretical
- Antiepileptics **(fosphenytoin, phenytoin)** decrease the effects of **levodopa**. [Moderate] Study
- Antiepileptics **(carbamazepine, eslicarbazepine, fosphenytoin, oxcarbazepine, perampanel, phenobarbital, phenytoin, primidone, rufinamide, topiramate)** are predicted to decrease the efficacy of **levonorgestrel**. For FSRH guidance, see Contraceptives, interactions p. 536. [Severe] Theoretical
- Antiepileptics **(carbamazepine, fosphenytoin, phenobarbital, phenytoin, primidone)** are predicted to decrease the exposure to **linagliptin**. [Moderate] Study
- Antiepileptics **(carbamazepine, oxcarbazepine)** are predicted to increase the risk of neurotoxicity when given with **lithium**. [Severe] Anecdotal
- Antiepileptics **(carbamazepine, fosphenytoin, phenobarbital, phenytoin, primidone)** are predicted to decrease the exposure to **lomitapide**. Monitor and adjust dose. [Moderate] Theoretical → Also see TABLE 1 p. 907
- Antiepileptics **(fosphenytoin, phenytoin)** decrease the effects of loop diuretics **(furosemide)**. [Moderate] Study
- Antiepileptics **(carbamazepine, fosphenytoin, phenobarbital, phenytoin, primidone)** are predicted to decrease the exposure to **lorlatinib**. Avoid. [Severe] Study
- **Lumacaftor** is predicted to decrease the exposure to antiepileptics **(carbamazepine, fosphenytoin, phenobarbital, phenytoin, primidone)**. Avoid. [Severe] Theoretical
- Antiepileptics **(carbamazepine, fosphenytoin, phenobarbital, phenytoin, primidone)** are predicted to decrease the exposure to **lurasidone**. Avoid. [Moderate] Study → Also see TABLE 11 p. 909
- Antiepileptics **(carbamazepine, fosphenytoin, phenobarbital, phenytoin, primidone)** are predicted to decrease the exposure to **macitentan**. Avoid. [Severe] Study
- Macrolides **(clarithromycin)** slightly increase the concentration of **carbamazepine**. Monitor concentration and adjust dose. [Severe] Study
- Macrolides **(clarithromycin)** are predicted to very slightly increase the exposure to **perampanel**. [Mild] Study
- Macrolides **(erythromycin)** markedly increase the concentration of **carbamazepine**. Monitor concentration and adjust dose. [Severe] Study
- Antiepileptics **(phenobarbital, primidone)** are predicted to increase the effects of **MAOIs, irreversible**. [Severe] Theoretical
- **Carbamazepine** is predicted to increase the risk of severe toxic reaction when given with **MAOIs, irreversible**. Avoid and for 14 days after stopping the MAOI. [Severe] Theoretical
- Antiepileptics **(carbamazepine, fosphenytoin, phenobarbital, phenytoin, primidone)** are predicted to decrease the exposure to **maraviroc**. Adjust dose. [Severe] Study
- **Phenytoin** is predicted to decrease the exposure to **melatonin**. [Moderate] Theoretical
- **Levetiracetam** decreases the clearance of **methotrexate**. [Severe] Anecdotal
- Antiepileptics **(phenobarbital, primidone)** are predicted to decrease the exposure to **metronidazole**. [Moderate] Study
- Antiepileptics **(fosphenytoin, phenobarbital, phenytoin, primidone)** are predicted to decrease the effects of **metyrapone**. Avoid. [Moderate] Study
- **Phenytoin** is predicted to increase the clearance of **mexiletine**. Monitor and adjust dose. [Moderate] Study
- Antiepileptics **(phenobarbital, primidone)** are predicted to decrease the exposure to **mianserin**. [Moderate] Study → Also see TABLE 11 p. 909
- **Carbamazepine** markedly decreases the exposure to **mianserin**. Adjust dose. [Moderate] Study
- Antiepileptics **(carbamazepine, fosphenytoin, phenobarbital, phenytoin, primidone)** are predicted to decrease the exposure to **midazolam**. Monitor and adjust dose. [Moderate] Study → Also see TABLE 11 p. 909
- Antiepileptics **(carbamazepine, fosphenytoin, phenobarbital, phenytoin, primidone)** are predicted to decrease the exposure to **midostaurin**. Avoid. [Severe] Study
- Antiepileptics **(carbamazepine, fosphenytoin, phenobarbital, phenytoin, primidone)** are predicted to decrease the exposure to **mirtazapine**. Adjust dose. [Moderate] Study → Also see TABLE 11 p. 909
- **Mitotane** is predicted to decrease the exposure to **perampanel**. Monitor and adjust dose. [Moderate] Study
- Antiepileptics **(carbamazepine, phenobarbital, primidone)** are predicted to decrease the exposure to **modafinil**. [Mild] Theoretical
- Antiepileptics **(fosphenytoin, phenytoin)** are predicted to decrease the exposure to **modafinil** and **modafinil** is predicted to increase the concentration of antiepileptics **(fosphenytoin, phenytoin)**. Monitor concentration and adjust dose. [Moderate] Theoretical
- **Carbamazepine** is predicted to decrease the effects of monoclonal antibodies **(brentuximab vedotin)**. [Severe] Theoretical

- Monoclonal antibodies **(tocilizumab)** are predicted to decrease the exposure to antiepileptics **(fosphenytoin, phenytoin)**. Monitor and adjust dose. Moderate Theoretical
- Antiepileptics **(carbamazepine, fosphenytoin, phenobarbital, phenytoin, primidone)** are predicted to decrease the exposure to monoclonal antibodies **(polatuzumab vedotin)**. Moderate Theoretical
- Antiepileptics **(carbamazepine, fosphenytoin, phenobarbital, phenytoin, primidone)** are predicted to decrease the exposure to **montelukast**. Mild Study
- Antiepileptics **(carbamazepine, fosphenytoin, phenobarbital, phenytoin, primidone)** are predicted to markedly decrease the exposure to **naldemedine**. Avoid. Severe Study
- Antiepileptics **(carbamazepine, fosphenytoin, phenobarbital, phenytoin, primidone)** are predicted to markedly decrease the exposure to **naloxegol**. Avoid. Moderate Study
- Antiepileptics **(carbamazepine, fosphenytoin, phenobarbital, phenytoin, primidone)** are predicted to slightly decrease the exposure to **nateglinide**. Mild Study
- Antiepileptics **(carbamazepine, fosphenytoin, phenobarbital, phenytoin, primidone)** are predicted to decrease the exposure to **neratinib**. Avoid. Severe Study → Also see TABLE 1 p. 907
- Antiepileptics **(carbamazepine, fosphenytoin, phenobarbital, phenytoin, primidone)** are predicted to decrease the exposure to **netupitant**. Avoid. Severe Study
- **Carbamazepine** is predicted to decrease the effects of (but acute use increases the effects of) neuromuscular blocking drugs, non-depolarising **(atracurium, cisatracurium, pancuronium, rocuronium, vecuronium)**. Monitor and adjust dose. Moderate Study
- Antiepileptics **(fosphenytoin, phenytoin)** decrease the effects of (but acute use increases the effects of) neuromuscular blocking drugs, non-depolarising **(atracurium, cisatracurium, pancuronium, rocuronium, vecuronium)**. Moderate Study
- **Nevirapine** is predicted to decrease the concentration of antiepileptics **(carbamazepine, fosphenytoin, phenobarbital, phenytoin, primidone)** and antiepileptics **(carbamazepine, fosphenytoin, phenobarbital, phenytoin, primidone)** are predicted to decrease the concentration of **nevirapine**. Severe Study
- Antiepileptics **(carbamazepine, fosphenytoin, phenobarbital, phenytoin, primidone)** are predicted to moderately decrease the exposure to **nilotinib**. Avoid. Severe Study
- **Carbamazepine** is predicted to decrease the exposure to **nintedanib**. Moderate Study
- Antiepileptics **(carbamazepine, fosphenytoin, phenobarbital, phenytoin, primidone)** are predicted to decrease the exposure to **nitisinone**. Adjust dose. Moderate Theoretical
- Antiepileptics **(carbamazepine, eslicarbazepine, fosphenytoin, oxcarbazepine, perampanel, phenobarbital, phenytoin, primidone, rufinamide, topiramate)** are predicted to decrease the efficacy of **norethisterone**. For FSRH guidance, see Contraceptives, interactions p. 536. Severe Anecdotal
- **Carbamazepine** potentially decreases the exposure to **olanzapine**. Monitor and adjust dose. Moderate Study
- **Phenytoin** is predicted to decrease the exposure to **olanzapine**. Monitor and adjust dose. Moderate Study
- Antiepileptics **(carbamazepine, fosphenytoin, phenobarbital, phenytoin, primidone)** are predicted to decrease the exposure to **olaparib**. Avoid. Moderate Theoretical
- Antiepileptics **(carbamazepine, fosphenytoin, phenobarbital, phenytoin)** are predicted to decrease the exposure to **ombitasvir**. Avoid. Severe Theoretical
- Antiepileptics **(carbamazepine, fosphenytoin, phenobarbital, phenytoin, primidone)** are predicted to decrease the exposure to **ondansetron**. Moderate Study
- Antiepileptics **(carbamazepine, fosphenytoin, phenobarbital, phenytoin, primidone)** are predicted to decrease the exposure to opioids **(alfentanil, fentanyl)**. Moderate Study → Also see TABLE 11 p. 909
- Antiepileptics **(carbamazepine, fosphenytoin, phenobarbital, phenytoin, primidone)** are predicted to decrease the exposure to opioids **(buprenorphine)**. Monitor and adjust dose. Moderate Theoretical → Also see TABLE 11 p. 909
- Antiepileptics **(carbamazepine, fosphenytoin, phenobarbital, phenytoin, primidone)** decrease the exposure to opioids (methadone). Monitor and adjust dose. Severe Study → Also see TABLE 11 p. 909
- Antiepileptics **(carbamazepine, fosphenytoin, phenobarbital, phenytoin, primidone)** are predicted to decrease the exposure to opioids **(oxycodone)**. Monitor and adjust dose. Moderate Study → Also see TABLE 11 p. 909
- **Carbamazepine** decreases the concentration of opioids (tramadol). Adjust dose. Severe Study
- Antiepileptics **(carbamazepine, fosphenytoin, phenobarbital, phenytoin, primidone)** are predicted to moderately decrease the exposure to osimertinib. Avoid. Moderate Study
- Antiepileptics **(carbamazepine, fosphenytoin, phenobarbital, phenytoin, primidone)** are predicted to moderately decrease the exposure to **ospemifene**. Moderate Study
- Oxybutynin potentially increases the risk of overheating and dehydration when given with **zonisamide**. Avoid in children. Severe Theoretical
- Antiepileptics **(carbamazepine, fosphenytoin, phenobarbital, phenytoin, primidone)** are predicted to decrease the exposure to **palbociclib**. Avoid. Severe Study
- Antiepileptics **(carbamazepine, fosphenytoin, phenobarbital, phenytoin, primidone)** are predicted to decrease the exposure to **paliperidone**. Monitor and adjust dose. Severe Study → Also see TABLE 11 p. 909
- **Valproate** slightly increases the exposure to **paliperidone**. Adjust dose. Moderate Study
- Antiepileptics **(carbamazepine, fosphenytoin, phenobarbital, phenytoin, primidone)** are predicted to decrease the exposure to **panobinostat**. Avoid. Moderate Theoretical
- Antiepileptics **(carbamazepine, fosphenytoin, phenobarbital, phenytoin, primidone)** decrease the exposure to **paracetamol**. Moderate Study → Also see TABLE 1 p. 907
- Antiepileptics **(carbamazepine, fosphenytoin, phenobarbital, phenytoin, primidone)** are predicted to decrease the exposure to paritaprevir (with ritonavir and ombitasvir). Avoid. Severe Study
- Antiepileptics **(carbamazepine, fosphenytoin, phenobarbital, phenytoin, primidone)** are predicted to decrease the exposure to **pazopanib**. Avoid. Severe Theoretical
- **Valproate** increases the risk of side-effects when given with penicillins **(pivmecillinam)**. Avoid. Severe Anecdotal
- Phenothiazines **(chlorpromazine)** decrease the concentration of antiepileptics **(phenobarbital, primidone)** and antiepileptics **(phenobarbital, primidone)** decrease the concentration of phenothiazines **(chlorpromazine)**. Moderate Study → Also see TABLE 11 p. 909
- Antiepileptics **(carbamazepine, fosphenytoin, phenobarbital, phenytoin, primidone)** are predicted to decrease the exposure to phosphodiesterase type-5 inhibitors **(avanafil, tadalafil)**. Avoid. Severe Study
- Antiepileptics **(carbamazepine, fosphenytoin, phenobarbital, phenytoin, primidone)** are predicted to decrease the exposure to phosphodiesterase type-5 inhibitors **(sildenafil, vardenafil)**. Moderate Theoretical
- Antiepileptics **(carbamazepine, fosphenytoin, phenobarbital, phenytoin, primidone)** are predicted to moderately to markedly decrease the exposure to **pibrentasvir**. Avoid. Severe Study
- Antiepileptics **(eslicarbazepine, oxcarbazepine)** potentially decrease the exposure to **pibrentasvir**. Avoid. Severe Theoretical
- Antiepileptics **(fosphenytoin, phenytoin)** are predicted to decrease the exposure to **pirfenidone**. Moderate Theoretical
- Antiepileptics **(carbamazepine, fosphenytoin, phenobarbital, phenytoin, primidone)** are predicted to moderately decrease the exposure to **pitolisant**. Moderate Study
- Antiepileptics **(carbamazepine, fosphenytoin, phenobarbital, phenytoin, primidone)** are predicted to decrease the exposure to **ponatinib**. Avoid. Moderate Theoretical
- Antiepileptics **(carbamazepine, fosphenytoin, phenobarbital, phenytoin, primidone)** are predicted to markedly decrease the exposure to **praziquantel**. Avoid. Moderate Study
- Antiepileptics **(carbamazepine, phenobarbital, phenytoin, primidone)** are predicted to increase the risk of

Antiepileptics (continued)
hypersensitivity reactions when given with **procarbazine.** Severe Anecdotal

- **Fosphenytoin** is predicted to increase the risk of hypersensitivity when given with **procarbazine.** Severe Anecdotal
- **Valproate** potentially increases the concentration of **propofol.** Adjust dose. Severe Theoretical
- Antiepileptics **(carbamazepine, fosphenytoin, phenobarbital, phenytoin, primidone)** are predicted to decrease the exposure to **quetiapine.** Moderate Study → Also see **TABLE 11** p. 909
- **Valproate** potentially increases the risk of neutropenia when given with **quetiapine.** Moderate Study
- Quinolones **(ciprofloxacin)** affect the concentration of antiepileptics **(fosphenytoin, phenytoin).** Monitor concentration and adjust dose. Severe Study
- Antiepileptics **(fosphenytoin, phenobarbital, phenytoin, primidone)** are predicted to affect the exposure to **raltegravir.** Use with caution or avoid. Moderate Theoretical
- **Carbamazepine** is predicted to affect the exposure to **raltegravir.** Moderate Theoretical
- Antiepileptics **(carbamazepine, fosphenytoin, phenobarbital, phenytoin, primidone)** are predicted to decrease the exposure to **ranolazine.** Avoid. Severe Study
- Antiepileptics **(carbamazepine, fosphenytoin, phenobarbital, phenytoin, primidone)** are predicted to decrease the exposure to **reboxetine.** Moderate Anecdotal
- Antiepileptics **(carbamazepine, fosphenytoin, phenobarbital, phenytoin, primidone)** are predicted to decrease the exposure to **regorafenib.** Avoid. Moderate Study
- Antiepileptics **(carbamazepine, fosphenytoin, phenobarbital, phenytoin, primidone)** are predicted to decrease the exposure to **repaglinide.** Monitor blood glucose and adjust dose. Moderate Study
- Antiepileptics **(carbamazepine, fosphenytoin, phenobarbital, phenytoin, primidone)** are predicted to markedly decrease the exposure to **ribociclib.** Avoid. Severe Study
- Antiepileptics **(phenobarbital, primidone)** are predicted to decrease the exposure to **rifampicin** and **rifampicin** is predicted to decrease the exposure to antiepileptics **(phenobarbital, primidone).** Use with caution and adjust dose. Moderate Study
- **Rifampicin** decreases the concentration of antiepileptics **(fosphenytoin, phenytoin).** Use with caution and adjust dose. Moderate Study
- **Rifampicin** slightly decreases the exposure to **brivaracetam.** Adjust dose. Moderate Study
- **Rifampicin** markedly increases the clearance of **lamotrigine.** Adjust **lamotrigine** dose, p. 216. Moderate Study
- **Rifampicin** is predicted to decrease the exposure to **perampanel.** Monitor and adjust dose. Moderate Study
- Antiepileptics **(carbamazepine, fosphenytoin, phenobarbital, phenytoin, primidone)** markedly decrease the exposure to **rilpivirine.** Avoid. Severe Study
- **Oxcarbazepine** is predicted to decrease the concentration of **rilpivirine.** Avoid. Severe Theoretical
- Antiepileptics **(carbamazepine, fosphenytoin, phenobarbital, phenytoin, primidone)** are predicted to decrease the exposure to **risperidone.** Adjust dose. Moderate Study → Also see **TABLE 11** p. 909
- Antiepileptics **(carbamazepine, fosphenytoin, phenobarbital, phenytoin, primidone)** are predicted to moderately decrease the exposure to **rivaroxaban.** Avoid unless patient can be monitored for signs of thrombosis. Severe Study
- Antiepileptics **(carbamazepine, fosphenytoin, phenobarbital, phenytoin, primidone)** are predicted to decrease the exposure to **roflumilast.** Avoid. Moderate Study
- Antiepileptics **(carbamazepine, fosphenytoin, phenobarbital, phenytoin, primidone)** are predicted to markedly decrease the exposure to **rolapitant.** Avoid. Severe Study
- **Rucaparib** is predicted to increase the exposure to **phenytoin.** Monitor and adjust dose. Moderate Study
- Antiepileptics **(carbamazepine, fosphenytoin, phenobarbital, phenytoin, primidone)** are predicted to decrease the exposure to **ruxolitinib.** Monitor and adjust dose. Moderate Study
- Antiepileptics **(carbamazepine, fosphenytoin, phenobarbital, phenytoin, primidone)** are predicted to moderately decrease the exposure to **saxagliptin.** Moderate Study
- Antiepileptics **(carbamazepine, fosphenytoin, phenytoin)** are predicted to decrease the exposure to the active metabolite of **selexipag.** Adjust dose. Moderate Study
- **Valproate** is predicted to increase the exposure to **selexipag.** Unknown Theoretical
- Antiepileptics **(carbamazepine, fosphenytoin, phenobarbital, phenytoin, primidone)** are predicted to decrease the exposure to **siponimod.** Severe Study
- Antiepileptics **(carbamazepine, fosphenytoin, phenobarbital, phenytoin, primidone)** are predicted to decrease the concentration of **sirolimus.** Avoid. Severe Study
- **Valproate** increases the exposure to **sodium oxybate.** Adjust **sodium oxybate** dose. Moderate Study
- **Valproate** potentially decreases the effects of **sodium phenylbutyrate.** Moderate Anecdotal
- Antiepileptics **(fosphenytoin, oxcarbazepine, phenobarbital, phenytoin, primidone)** are predicted to decrease the exposure to **sofosbuvir.** Avoid. Severe Theoretical
- **Carbamazepine** is predicted to decrease the exposure to **sofosbuvir.** Avoid. Severe Study
- Antiepileptics **(carbamazepine, fosphenytoin, phenobarbital, phenytoin, primidone)** are predicted to decrease the exposure to **solifenacin.** Moderate Theoretical
- Antiepileptics **(carbamazepine, fosphenytoin, phenobarbital, phenytoin, primidone)** are predicted to decrease the exposure to **sorafenib.** Moderate Theoretical
- SSRIs **(fluoxetine, fluvoxamine)** are predicted to increase the concentration of antiepileptics **(fosphenytoin, phenytoin).** Monitor and adjust dose. Severe Anecdotal
- SSRIs **(sertraline)** potentially increase the risk of toxicity when given with antiepileptics **(fosphenytoin, phenytoin).** Monitor concentration and adjust dose. Severe Anecdotal
- Antiepileptics **(fosphenytoin, phenytoin)** decrease the concentration of SSRIs **(paroxetine).** Moderate Study
- **St John's Wort** is predicted to decrease the concentration of antiepileptics **(fosphenytoin, phenobarbital, phenytoin, primidone).** Avoid. Severe Theoretical
- **St John's Wort** is predicted to decrease the exposure to **brivaracetam.** Moderate Theoretical
- **St John's Wort** is predicted to decrease the concentration of **carbamazepine.** Monitor and adjust dose. Moderate Theoretical
- **St John's Wort** is predicted to decrease the exposure to **perampanel.** Monitor and adjust dose. Moderate Theoretical
- **St John's Wort** is predicted to decrease the exposure to **tiagabine.** Avoid. Mild Theoretical
- Antiepileptics **(carbamazepine, eslicarbazepine)** are predicted to decrease the exposure to statins **(atorvastatin).** Monitor and adjust dose. Moderate Theoretical → Also see **TABLE 1** p. 907
- Antiepileptics **(fosphenytoin, phenytoin)** potentially decrease the exposure to statins **(atorvastatin, simvastatin).** Moderate Anecdotal
- **Carbamazepine** moderately decreases the exposure to statins **(simvastatin).** Monitor and adjust dose. Severe Study → Also see **TABLE 1** p. 907
- **Eslicarbazepine** moderately decreases the exposure to statins **(simvastatin).** Monitor and adjust dose. Moderate Study
- Sulfonamides **(sulfadiazine)** are predicted to increase the concentration of **fosphenytoin.** Monitor and adjust dose. Moderate Study
- Sulfonamides **(sulfadiazine)** increase the concentration of **phenytoin.** Monitor and adjust dose. Moderate Study
- Antiepileptics **(carbamazepine, fosphenytoin, phenobarbital, phenytoin, primidone)** are predicted to decrease the exposure to **sunitinib.** Avoid or adjust **sunitinib** dose. Moderate Study
- Antiepileptics **(fosphenytoin, phenytoin)** increase the effects of **suxamethonium.** Moderate Study
- **Carbamazepine** increases the risk of prolonged neuromuscular blockade when given with **suxamethonium.** Moderate Study
- Antiepileptics **(carbamazepine, fosphenytoin, phenobarbital, phenytoin, primidone)** decrease the concentration of **tacrolimus.** Monitor and adjust dose. Severe Study

- Antiepileptics **(carbamazepine, fosphenytoin, phenobarbital, phenytoin, primidone)** are predicted to decrease the exposure to taxanes (cabazitaxel, paclitaxel). Avoid. Severe Study → Also see **TABLE 12** p. 910
- Antiepileptics **(carbamazepine, fosphenytoin, phenobarbital, phenytoin, primidone)** are predicted to decrease the exposure to taxanes (docetaxel). Severe Theoretical → Also see **TABLE 12** p. 910
- **Tegafur** potentially increases the concentration of antiepileptics **(fosphenytoin, phenytoin)**. Monitor concentration and adjust dose. Severe Anecdotal
- Antiepileptics **(carbamazepine, fosphenytoin, phenobarbital, phenytoin, primidone)** are predicted to decrease the concentration of **temsirolimus**. Avoid. Severe Study
- Antiepileptics **(carbamazepine, fosphenytoin, oxcarbazepine, phenobarbital, phenytoin, primidone)** are predicted to decrease the exposure to **tenofovir alafenamide**. Avoid. Moderate Theoretical
- Antiepileptics **(carbamazepine, fosphenytoin, phenobarbital, phenytoin, primidone)** decrease the exposure to tetracyclines (doxycycline). Monitor and adjust dose. Moderate Study → Also see **TABLE 1** p. 907
- Antiepileptics **(carbamazepine, fosphenytoin, phenobarbital, phenytoin, primidone)** are predicted to decrease the exposure to **tezacaftor**. Avoid. Severe Theoretical
- Antiepileptics **(fosphenytoin, phenytoin)** are predicted to decrease the exposure to **theophylline**. Adjust dose. Moderate Study
- Antiepileptics **(phenobarbital, primidone)** are predicted to increase the clearance of **theophylline**. Adjust dose. Moderate Theoretical
- **Carbamazepine** potentially increases the clearance of **theophylline** and **theophylline** decreases the exposure to **carbamazepine**. Adjust dose. Moderate Anecdotal
- **Stiripentol** is predicted to increase the exposure to **theophylline**. Avoid. Moderate Theoretical
- Antiepileptics **(carbamazepine, fosphenytoin, phenytoin)** are predicted to increase the risk of hypothyroidism when given with **thyroid hormones**. Moderate Study
- Antiepileptics **(phenobarbital, primidone)** are predicted to decrease the effects of **thyroid hormones**. Moderate Theoretical
- Antiepileptics **(carbamazepine, fosphenytoin, phenobarbital, phenytoin, primidone)** are predicted to markedly decrease the exposure to **ticagrelor**. Avoid. Severe Study
- Antiepileptics **(carbamazepine, fosphenytoin, phenobarbital, phenytoin, primidone)** are predicted to decrease the exposure to **tivozanib**. Severe Study
- Antiepileptics **(fosphenytoin, phenytoin)** moderately decrease the exposure to **tizanidine**. Mild Study
- Antiepileptics **(carbamazepine, fosphenytoin, phenobarbital, phenytoin, primidone)** are predicted to decrease the exposure to **tofacitinib**. Avoid. Severe Study
- Antiepileptics **(carbamazepine, fosphenytoin, phenobarbital, phenytoin, primidone)** are predicted to decrease the exposure to **tolvaptan**. Use with caution or avoid depending on indication. Severe Study
- Antiepileptics **(fosphenytoin, phenytoin)** increase the clearance of **topotecan**. Moderate Study
- Antiepileptics **(carbamazepine, fosphenytoin, phenobarbital, phenytoin, primidone)** are predicted to decrease the exposure to **toremifene**. Adjust dose. Moderate Study
- Antiepileptics **(carbamazepine, fosphenytoin, phenobarbital, phenytoin, primidone)** are predicted to decrease the exposure to **trabectedin**. Avoid. Severe Theoretical → Also see **TABLE 1** p. 907
- **Carbamazepine** decreases the concentration of **trazodone**. Adjust dose. Moderate Anecdotal
- Antiepileptics **(phenobarbital, primidone)** are predicted to decrease the exposure to **tricyclic antidepressants**. Moderate Study → Also see **TABLE 11** p. 909
- **Carbamazepine** decreases the exposure to **tricyclic antidepressants**. Adjust dose. Moderate Study → Also see **TABLE 18** p. 911
- Tricyclic antidepressants **(clomipramine, imipramine)** potentially increase the risk of overheating and dehydration when given with **zonisamide**. Avoid in children. Severe Theoretical
- **Trimethoprim** increases the concentration of antiepileptics **(fosphenytoin, phenytoin)**. Moderate Study
- Antiepileptics **(carbamazepine, eslicarbazepine, fosphenytoin, oxcarbazepine, perampanel, phenobarbital, phenytoin, primidone, rufinamide, topiramate)** decrease the efficacy of **ulipristal**. For FSRH guidance, see Contraceptives, interactions p. 536. Severe Anecdotal
- Antiepileptics **(carbamazepine, fosphenytoin, phenobarbital, phenytoin, primidone)** are predicted to decrease the exposure to **upadacitinib**. Moderate Study
- Antiepileptics **(carbamazepine, fosphenytoin, phenobarbital, phenytoin, primidone)** are predicted to decrease the exposure to **vandetanib**. Avoid. Moderate Study
- Antiepileptics **(carbamazepine, fosphenytoin, phenobarbital, phenytoin, primidone)** are predicted to moderately decrease the exposure to **velpatasvir**. Avoid. Severe Study
- **Oxcarbazepine** is predicted to decrease the exposure to **velpatasvir**. Avoid. Severe Theoretical
- Antiepileptics **(carbamazepine, fosphenytoin, phenobarbital, phenytoin, primidone)** are predicted to decrease the exposure to **vemurafenib**. Avoid. Severe Theoretical
- Antiepileptics **(carbamazepine, fosphenytoin, phenobarbital, phenytoin, primidone)** are predicted to decrease the exposure to **venetoclax**. Avoid. Severe Study
- Antiepileptics **(carbamazepine, fosphenytoin, phenobarbital, phenytoin, primidone)** are predicted to decrease the exposure to vinca alkaloids **(vinblastine, vincristine, vindesine)**. Severe Theoretical → Also see **TABLE 1** p. 907 → Also see **TABLE 12** p. 910
- Antiepileptics **(carbamazepine, fosphenytoin, phenobarbital, phenytoin, primidone)** are predicted to decrease the exposure to vinca alkaloids **(vinflunine)**. Avoid. Severe Theoretical → Also see **TABLE 12** p. 910
- Antiepileptics **(carbamazepine, fosphenytoin, phenobarbital, phenytoin, primidone)** are predicted to decrease the exposure to vinca alkaloids **(vinorelbine)**. Use with caution or avoid. Severe Theoretical → Also see **TABLE 12** p. 910
- Antiepileptics **(carbamazepine, fosphenytoin, phenobarbital, phenytoin, primidone)** are predicted to decrease the exposure to **vismodegib**. Avoid. Moderate Theoretical
- Antiepileptics **(fosphenytoin, phenytoin)** decrease the effects of **vitamin D substances**. Moderate Study
- Antiepileptics **(phenobarbital, primidone)** are predicted to decrease the effects of **vitamin D substances**. Moderate Theoretical
- **Carbamazepine** is predicted to decrease the effects of **vitamin D substances**. Moderate Study
- Antiepileptics **(phenobarbital, primidone)** potentially increase the risk of nephrotoxicity when given with volatile halogenated anaesthetics **(methoxyflurane)**. Avoid. Severe Theoretical → Also see **TABLE 11** p. 909
- Antiepileptics **(carbamazepine, fosphenytoin, phenobarbital, phenytoin, primidone)** are predicted to decrease the exposure to **vortioxetine**. Monitor and adjust dose. Moderate Study
- Antiepileptics **(carbamazepine, fosphenytoin, phenobarbital, phenytoin, primidone)** are predicted to decrease the concentration of **voxilaprevir**. Avoid. Severe Study
- **Oxcarbazepine** is predicted to decrease the concentration of **voxilaprevir**. Avoid. Severe Theoretical
- **Valproate** slightly increases the exposure to **zidovudine**. Moderate Study
- **Carbamazepine** moderately decreases the exposure to **zolpidem**. Moderate Study
- Antiepileptics **(carbamazepine, fosphenytoin, phenobarbital, phenytoin, primidone)** are predicted to decrease the exposure to **zopiclone**. Adjust dose. Moderate Study → Also see **TABLE 11** p. 909

Antifungals, azoles → see **TABLE 1** p. 907 (hepatotoxicity), **TABLE 9** p. 909 (QT-interval prolongation)

clotrimazole · fluconazole · isavuconazole · itraconazole · ketoconazole · miconazole · posaconazole · voriconazole

- Since systemic absorption can follow topical application, the possibility of interactions with topical **clotrimazole** and topical **ketoconazole** should be borne in mind.

Antifungals, azoles (continued)

- In general, **fluconazole** interactions relate to multiple-dose treatment.
- The use of carbonated drinks, such as cola, improves **itraconazole**, **ketoconazole**, and **posaconazole** bioavailability.
- Interactions of **miconazole** apply to the oral gel formulation, as a sufficient quantity can be absorbed to cause systemic effects. Systemic absorption from intravaginal and topical formulations might also occur.

- Antifungals, azoles **(fluconazole, isavuconazole, posaconazole)** are predicted to increase the exposure to **abemaciclib**. Moderate Study
- Antifungals, azoles **(itraconazole, ketoconazole, voriconazole)** are predicted to increase the exposure to **abemaciclib**. Avoid or adjust **abemaciclib** dose. Severe Study
- Antifungals, azoles **(itraconazole, ketoconazole)** are predicted to increase the exposure to **afatinib**. Separate administration by 12 hours. Moderate Study
- **Alcohol (beverage)** potentially causes a disulfiram-like reaction when given with **ketoconazole**. Avoid. Moderate Anecdotal
- Antifungals, azoles **(fluconazole, isavuconazole, posaconazole)** are predicted to increase the exposure to aldosterone antagonists **(eplerenone)**. Adjust **eplerenone** dose. Severe Study
- Antifungals, azoles **(itraconazole, ketoconazole, voriconazole)** are predicted to markedly increase the exposure to aldosterone antagonists **(eplerenone)**. Avoid. Severe Study
- **Itraconazole** markedly increases the exposure to **aliskiren**. Avoid. Severe Study
- **Ketoconazole** moderately increases the exposure to **aliskiren**. Moderate Study
- **Itraconazole** increases the risk of busulfan toxicity when given with alkylating agents **(busulfan)**. Monitor and adjust dose. Moderate Study
- **Miconazole** is predicted to increase the concentration of alkylating agents **(busulfan)**. Use with caution and adjust dose. Moderate Theoretical
- **Isavuconazole** is predicted to increase the exposure to alkylating agents **(cyclophosphamide)**. Moderate Study
- Antifungals, azoles **(itraconazole, ketoconazole, voriconazole)** increase the exposure to **almotriptan**. Mild Study
- Antifungals, azoles **(itraconazole, ketoconazole, voriconazole)** are predicted to moderately increase the exposure to alpha blockers **(alfuzosin, tamsulosin)**. Use with caution or avoid. Moderate Study
- Antifungals, azoles **(itraconazole, ketoconazole, voriconazole)** are predicted to increase the exposure to alpha blockers **(doxazosin)**. Moderate Study
- Antifungals, azoles **(fluconazole, isavuconazole, posaconazole)** are predicted to increase the exposure to alpha blockers **(tamsulosin)**. Moderate Theoretical
- Antifungals, azoles **(fluconazole, isavuconazole, posaconazole)** are predicted to increase the exposure to **alprazolam**. Severe Study
- Antifungals, azoles **(itraconazole, ketoconazole, voriconazole)** moderately increase the exposure to **alprazolam**. Avoid. Moderate Study
- **Miconazole** is predicted to increase the exposure to **alprazolam**. Use with caution and adjust dose. Moderate Theoretical
- **Miconazole** potentially decreases the exposure to aminoglycosides **(tobramycin)**. Moderate Anecdotal
- **Antacids** decrease the absorption of **itraconazole** (capsule). **Itraconazole** should be taken 2 hours before or 1 hour after antacids. Moderate Study
- **Antacids** decrease the absorption of **ketoconazole**. Separate administration by at least 2 hours. Moderate Study
- **Miconazole** is predicted to increase the exposure to antiarrhythmics **(disopyramide)**. Use with caution and adjust dose. Severe Theoretical
- Antifungals, azoles **(itraconazole, ketoconazole, voriconazole)** are predicted to increase the exposure to antiarrhythmics **(disopyramide)**. Avoid. Severe Theoretical → Also see **TABLE 9** p. 909
- **Posaconazole** is predicted to increase the exposure to antiarrhythmics **(disopyramide, dronedarone)**. Avoid. Severe Theoretical
- **Fluconazole** is predicted to increase the exposure to antiarrhythmics **(dronedarone)**. Severe Theoretical → Also see **TABLE 9** p. 909
- Antifungals, azoles **(itraconazole, ketoconazole, voriconazole)** very markedly increase the exposure to antiarrhythmics **(dronedarone)**. Avoid. Severe Study → Also see **TABLE 9** p. 909
- Antifungals, azoles **(fluconazole, isavuconazole, posaconazole)** are predicted to increase the exposure to antiarrhythmics **(propafenone)**. Monitor and adjust dose. Moderate Study
- Antifungals, azoles **(itraconazole, ketoconazole, voriconazole)** are predicted to increase the exposure to antiarrhythmics **(propafenone)**. Monitor and adjust dose. Severe Study
- Antifungals, azoles **(itraconazole, ketoconazole, voriconazole)** are predicted to increase the exposure to anticholinesterases, centrally acting **(galantamine)**. Monitor and adjust dose. Moderate Study
- Antiepileptics **(carbamazepine)** are predicted to decrease the efficacy of **fluconazole** and **fluconazole** increases the concentration of antiepileptics **(carbamazepine)**. Avoid or monitor **carbamazepine** concentration and adjust dose accordingly, p. 209. Severe Theoretical → Also see **TABLE 1** p. 907
- Antiepileptics **(carbamazepine)** are predicted to decrease the efficacy of **ketoconazole** and **ketoconazole** slightly increases the concentration of antiepileptics **(carbamazepine)**. Avoid or monitor **carbamazepine** concentration and adjust dose accordingly, p. 209. Moderate Study
- Antiepileptics **(carbamazepine)** are predicted to decrease the efficacy of **posaconazole** and **posaconazole** increases the concentration of antiepileptics **(carbamazepine)**. Avoid. Moderate Theoretical
- Antiepileptics **(carbamazepine, fosphenytoin, phenobarbital, phenytoin, primidone)** are predicted to decrease the exposure to **isavuconazole**. Avoid. Severe Study
- Antiepileptics **(fosphenytoin)** very markedly decrease the exposure to **itraconazole**. Avoid and for 14 days after stopping **fosphenytoin**. Moderate Study
- Antiepileptics **(fosphenytoin)** decrease the exposure to **voriconazole** and **voriconazole** increases the exposure to antiepileptics **(fosphenytoin)**. Avoid or adjust **voriconazole** dose and monitor phenytoin concentration, p. 410. Moderate Study
- Antiepileptics **(fosphenytoin, phenytoin)** decrease the exposure to **ketoconazole**. Avoid. Moderate Study
- Antiepileptics **(fosphenytoin, phenytoin)** are predicted to decrease the exposure to **posaconazole**. Avoid. Moderate Study
- Antiepileptics **(phenobarbital)** decrease the concentration of **itraconazole**. Avoid and for 14 days after stopping **phenobarbital**. Moderate Study
- Antiepileptics **(phenobarbital)** are predicted to decrease the concentration of **ketoconazole**. Avoid. Moderate Study
- Antiepileptics **(phenobarbital)** are predicted to decrease the concentration of **posaconazole**. Avoid. Moderate Study
- Antiepileptics **(phenobarbital, primidone)** are predicted to decrease the concentration of **voriconazole**. Avoid. Moderate Theoretical
- Antiepileptics **(phenytoin)** very markedly decrease the exposure to **itraconazole**. Avoid and for 14 days after stopping **phenytoin**. Moderate Study
- Antiepileptics **(phenytoin)** decrease the exposure to **voriconazole** and **voriconazole** increases the exposure to antiepileptics **(phenytoin)**. Avoid or adjust **voriconazole** dose and monitor **phenytoin** concentration, p. 410, p. 220. Moderate Study
- Antiepileptics **(primidone)** are predicted to decrease the concentration of **itraconazole**. Moderate Theoretical
- **Miconazole** increases the risk of carbamazepine toxicity when given with antiepileptics **(carbamazepine)**. Monitor and adjust dose. Severe Anecdotal
- **Miconazole** increases the risk of phenytoin toxicity when given with antiepileptics **(fosphenytoin)**. Monitor and adjust dose. Severe Anecdotal

- **Fluconazole** increases the concentration of antiepileptics **(fosphenytoin, phenytoin)**. Monitor concentration and adjust dose. Moderate Study
- Antiepileptics **(carbamazepine)** are predicted to decrease the efficacy of antifungals, azoles **(itraconazole, voriconazole)** and antifungals, azoles **(itraconazole, voriconazole)** increase the concentration of antiepileptics **(carbamazepine)**. Avoid or adjust dose. Moderate Theoretical → Also see **TABLE 1** p. 907
- Antiepileptics **(primidone)** are predicted to decrease the concentration of antifungals, azoles **(ketoconazole, posaconazole)**. Avoid. Moderate Study
- Antifungals, azoles **(itraconazole, ketoconazole, voriconazole)** are predicted to very slightly increase the exposure to antiepileptics **(perampanel)**. Mild Study
- **Miconazole** increases the risk of phenytoin toxicity when given with antiepileptics **(phenytoin)**. Monitor and adjust dose. Severe Anecdotal
- Antifungals, azoles **(fluconazole)** are predicted to increase the exposure to antifungals, azoles **(isavuconazole)**. Severe Theoretical
- Antifungals, azoles **(itraconazole, ketoconazole, voriconazole)** are predicted to increase the exposure to antifungals, azoles **(isavuconazole)**. Avoid or monitor side effects. Severe Study
- Antifungals, azoles **(posaconazole)** are predicted to increase the exposure to antifungals, azoles **(isavuconazole)**. Moderate Theoretical
- **Miconazole** is predicted to increase the exposure to antihistamines, non-sedating **(mizolastine)**. Avoid. Moderate Theoretical
- Antifungals, azoles **(fluconazole, isavuconazole, posaconazole)** are predicted to increase the exposure to antihistamines, non-sedating **(mizolastine)**. Severe Theoretical
- Antifungals, azoles **(itraconazole, ketoconazole, voriconazole)** are predicted to increase the exposure to antihistamines, non-sedating **(mizolastine)**. Avoid. Severe Study
- Antifungals, azoles **(fluconazole, isavuconazole, itraconazole, ketoconazole, posaconazole, voriconazole)** are predicted to increase the exposure to antihistamines, non-sedating (rupatadine). Avoid. Moderate Study
- **Ketoconazole** increases the exposure to antimalarials **(mefloquine)**. Moderate Study
- Antifungals, azoles **(fluconazole, itraconazole, posaconazole, voriconazole)** are predicted to increase the exposure to antimalarials **(mefloquine)**. Moderate Theoretical
- Antifungals, azoles **(fluconazole, isavuconazole, itraconazole, ketoconazole, posaconazole, voriconazole)** are predicted to increase the concentration of antimalarials **(piperaquine)**. Severe Theoretical
- Antifungals, azoles **(itraconazole, ketoconazole, voriconazole)** are predicted to increase the exposure to **apalutamide**. Mild Study → Also see **TABLE 9** p. 909
- **Apalutamide** is predicted to decrease the exposure to **isavuconazole**. Avoid. Severe Study
- **Itraconazole** is predicted to increase the exposure to **apixaban**. Avoid. Severe Theoretical
- **Ketoconazole** slightly to moderately increases the exposure to apixaban. Avoid. Severe Study
- **Voriconazole** is predicted to increase the exposure to **apixaban**. Avoid. Moderate Theoretical
- Antifungals, azoles **(itraconazole, ketoconazole, voriconazole)** are predicted to markedly increase the exposure to **aprepitant**. Moderate Study
- **Fluconazole** is predicted to increase the exposure to aprepitant. Moderate Theoretical
- Aprepitant is predicted to increase the exposure to **isavuconazole**. Moderate Theoretical
- **Posaconazole** is predicted to increase the exposure to **aprepitant**. Moderate Study
- Antifungals, azoles **(itraconazole, ketoconazole, voriconazole)** are predicted to slightly increase the exposure to **aripiprazole**. Adjust **aripiprazole** dose, p. 265. Moderate Study
- Antifungals, azoles **(fluconazole, isavuconazole, posaconazole)** are predicted to increase the exposure to **axitinib**. Moderate Theoretical
- Antifungals, azoles **(itraconazole, ketoconazole, voriconazole)** are predicted to increase the exposure to **axitinib**. Avoid or adjust dose. Moderate Study
- Antifungals, azoles **(fluconazole, isavuconazole, posaconazole)** are predicted to increase the exposure to **bedaquiline**. Avoid prolonged use. Mild Theoretical → Also see **TABLE 1** p. 907 → Also see **TABLE 9** p. 909
- Antifungals, azoles **(itraconazole, ketoconazole, voriconazole)** are predicted to increase the exposure to **bedaquiline**. Avoid prolonged use. Mild Study → Also see **TABLE 1** p. 907 → Also see **TABLE 9** p. 909
- Antifungals, azoles **(itraconazole, ketoconazole)** are predicted to increase the exposure to beta blockers, non-selective **(nadolol)**. Moderate Study
- Antifungals, azoles **(itraconazole, ketoconazole, voriconazole)** are predicted to increase the exposure to $beta_2$ agonists **(salmeterol)**. Avoid. Severe Study
- Antifungals, azoles **(itraconazole, ketoconazole)** are predicted to increase the exposure to **bictegravir**. Use with caution or avoid. Moderate Theoretical
- **Posaconazole** is predicted to increase the exposure to **bictegravir**. Moderate Theoretical
- Antifungals, azoles **(itraconazole, ketoconazole, voriconazole)** slightly increase the exposure to **bortezomib**. Moderate Study
- **Fluconazole** is predicted to increase the exposure to **bosentan**. Avoid. Severe Study
- **Bosentan** is predicted to decrease the exposure to **isavuconazole**. Avoid. Severe Theoretical
- **Itraconazole** is predicted to increase the exposure to **bosentan**. Moderate Theoretical
- **Ketoconazole** moderately increases the exposure to **bosentan**. Moderate Study
- **Voriconazole** is predicted to increase the exposure to **bosentan**. Avoid. Severe Theoretical
- Antifungals, azoles **(fluconazole, isavuconazole, posaconazole)** are predicted to increase the exposure to **bosutinib**. Avoid or adjust dose. Severe Theoretical → Also see **TABLE 9** p. 909
- Antifungals, azoles **(itraconazole, ketoconazole, voriconazole)** are predicted to markedly increase the exposure to **bosutinib**. Avoid or adjust dose. Severe Study → Also see **TABLE 9** p. 909
- Antifungals, azoles **(itraconazole, ketoconazole, voriconazole)** are predicted to increase the exposure to **brigatinib**. Adjust **brigatinib** dose. Severe Study
- **Isavuconazole** slightly increases the exposure to **bupropion**. Adjust dose. Moderate Study
- Antifungals, azoles **(fluconazole, isavuconazole, posaconazole)** are predicted to increase the exposure to **buspirone**. Use with caution and adjust dose. Moderate Study
- Antifungals, azoles **(itraconazole, ketoconazole, voriconazole)** are predicted to increase the exposure to **buspirone**. Adjust **buspirone** dose. Severe Study
- **Miconazole** is predicted to increase the concentration of buspirone. Use with caution and adjust dose. Moderate Theoretical
- Antifungals, azoles **(fluconazole, isavuconazole, posaconazole)** are predicted to increase the exposure to **cabozantinib**. Moderate Theoretical → Also see **TABLE 9** p. 909
- Antifungals, azoles **(itraconazole, ketoconazole, voriconazole)** slightly increase the exposure to **cabozantinib**. Moderate Study → Also see **TABLE 9** p. 909
- Calcium channel blockers **(diltiazem, verapamil)** are predicted to increase the exposure to **isavuconazole**. Moderate Theoretical
- Antifungals, azoles **(fluconazole, isavuconazole, posaconazole)** are predicted to increase the exposure to calcium channel blockers **(amlodipine, felodipine, lacidipine, lercanidipine, nicardipine, nifedipine, nimodipine)**. Monitor and adjust dose. Moderate Study
- **Miconazole** is predicted to increase the exposure to calcium channel blockers **(amlodipine, felodipine, lacidipine, lercanidipine, nicardipine, nifedipine, nimodipine, verapamil)**. Use with caution and adjust dose. Moderate Theoretical
- Antifungals, azoles **(itraconazole, ketoconazole, voriconazole)** are predicted to increase the exposure to calcium channel blockers **(amlodipine, felodipine, lacidipine, nicardipine, nifedipine, nimodipine)**. Monitor and adjust dose. Moderate Study

Antifungals, azoles (continued)
- **Miconazole** is predicted to increase the exposure to calcium channel blockers **(diltiazem).** Moderate Theoretical
- **Fluconazole** (high-dose) is predicted to increase the exposure to calcium channel blockers **(diltiazem, verapamil).** Moderate Theoretical
- **Posaconazole** is predicted to increase the exposure to calcium channel blockers **(diltiazem, verapamil).** Moderate Theoretical
- Antifungals, azoles **(itraconazole, ketoconazole, voriconazole)** are predicted to increase the exposure to calcium channel blockers (diltiazem, verapamil). Severe Study
- Antifungals, azoles **(itraconazole, ketoconazole, voriconazole)** are predicted to markedly increase the exposure to calcium channel blockers (lercanidipine). Avoid. Severe Study
- Antifungals, azoles **(itraconazole, ketoconazole, voriconazole)** are predicted to increase the exposure to cannabidiol. Avoid or adjust dose. Mild Study
- **Fluconazole** is predicted to increase the exposure to cannabidiol. Moderate Theoretical
- Antifungals, azoles **(fluconazole, isavuconazole, posaconazole)** are predicted to increase the exposure to cariprazine. Avoid. Severe Study
- Antifungals, azoles **(itraconazole, ketoconazole, voriconazole)** are predicted to moderately increase the exposure to cariprazine. Avoid. Severe Study
- Antifungals, azoles **(itraconazole, ketoconazole, voriconazole)** are predicted to increase the exposure to ceritinib. Avoid or adjust **ceritinib** dose. Severe Study → Also see TABLE 9 p. 909
- Antifungals, azoles **(fluconazole, isavuconazole, posaconazole)** are predicted to increase the concentration of ciclosporin. Severe Study
- Antifungals, azoles **(itraconazole, ketoconazole, voriconazole)** increase the concentration of ciclosporin. Severe Study
- **Miconazole** increases the concentration of ciclosporin. Monitor and adjust dose. Severe Anecdotal
- Antifungals, azoles **(itraconazole, ketoconazole, voriconazole)** are predicted to moderately increase the exposure to cilostazol. Adjust **cilostazol** dose. Moderate Study
- **Fluconazole** is predicted to increase the exposure to cilostazol. Adjust **cilostazol** dose. Moderate Theoretical
- **Miconazole** is predicted to increase the exposure to cilostazol. Use with caution and adjust dose. Moderate Theoretical
- Antifungals, azoles **(itraconazole, ketoconazole, voriconazole)** are predicted to moderately increase the exposure to cinacalcet. Adjust dose. Moderate Study
- Antifungals, azoles **(fluconazole, voriconazole)** potentially increase the exposure to clobazam. Adjust dose. Moderate Theoretical
- **Fluconazole** is predicted to decrease the efficacy of clopidogrel. Avoid. Severe Theoretical
- **Voriconazole** is predicted to decrease the efficacy of clopidogrel. Avoid. Moderate Study
- Cobicistat is predicted to increase the exposure to antifungals, azoles **(fluconazole, posaconazole).** Moderate Theoretical
- Cobicistat is predicted to increase the exposure to antifungals, azoles **(itraconazole, ketoconazole).** Adjust dose. Moderate Theoretical
- Cobicistat is predicted to increase the exposure to **isavuconazole.** Avoid or monitor side effects. Severe Study
- Cobicistat is predicted to affect the exposure to **voriconazole.** Avoid. Moderate Theoretical
- Antifungals, azoles **(fluconazole, isavuconazole, miconazole, posaconazole)** are predicted to increase the exposure to cobimetinib. Severe Theoretical
- Antifungals, azoles **(itraconazole, ketoconazole, voriconazole)** are predicted to markedly increase the exposure to cobimetinib. Avoid or monitor for toxicity. Severe Study
- Antifungals, azoles **(fluconazole, isavuconazole, posaconazole)** are predicted to increase the exposure to colchicine. Adjust **colchicine** dose with moderate inhibitors of CYP3A4. Severe Study
- Antifungals, azoles **(itraconazole, ketoconazole, voriconazole)** are predicted to increase the exposure to colchicine. Avoid potent inhibitors of CYP3A4 or adjust **colchicine** dose. Severe Study
- Antifungals, azoles **(itraconazole, ketoconazole, voriconazole)** are predicted to increase the exposure to corticosteroids **(beclometasone)** (risk with beclometasone is likely to be lower than with other corticosteroids). Moderate Theoretical
- Antifungals, azoles **(itraconazole, ketoconazole, voriconazole)** are predicted to increase the exposure to corticosteroids **(betamethasone, budesonide, ciclesonide, deflazacort, dexamethasone, fludrocortisone, fluticasone, hydrocortisone, methylprednisolone, mometasone, prednisolone, triamcinolone).** Avoid or monitor side effects. Severe Study
- **Miconazole** is predicted to increase the concentration of corticosteroids **(methylprednisolone).** Monitor and adjust dose. Moderate Theoretical
- Antifungals, azoles **(fluconazole, isavuconazole, posaconazole)** are predicted to increase the exposure to corticosteroids **(methylprednisolone).** Monitor and adjust dose. Moderate Study
- **Fluconazole** increases the anticoagulant effect of **coumarins.** Monitor INR and adjust dose. Severe Study
- **Itraconazole** potentially increases the anticoagulant effect of **coumarins.** Severe Anecdotal
- **Ketoconazole** potentially increases the anticoagulant effect of coumarins **(warfarin).** Monitor INR and adjust dose. Severe Anecdotal
- **Miconazole** greatly increases the anticoagulant effect of **coumarins.** MHRA advises avoid unless INR can be monitored closely; monitor for signs of bleeding. Severe Study
- **Voriconazole** increases the anticoagulant effect of **coumarins.** Monitor INR and adjust dose. Moderate Study
- Antifungals, azoles **(itraconazole, ketoconazole, voriconazole)** are predicted to moderately increase the exposure to **crizotinib.** Avoid. Moderate Study → Also see TABLE 9 p. 909
- Antifungals, azoles **(itraconazole, ketoconazole)** are predicted to increase the exposure to dabigatran. Avoid. Severe Study
- **Isavuconazole** is predicted to increase the exposure to dabigatran. Monitor and adjust dose. Moderate Study
- Antifungals, azoles **(itraconazole, ketoconazole, voriconazole)** are predicted to increase the exposure to dabrafenib. Use with caution or avoid. Moderate Study
- Antifungals, azoles **(fluconazole, isavuconazole, posaconazole)** are predicted to slightly increase the exposure to **darifenacin.** Moderate Study
- Antifungals, azoles **(itraconazole, ketoconazole, voriconazole)** are predicted to markedly to very markedly increase the exposure to **darifenacin.** Avoid. Severe Study
- Antifungals, azoles **(fluconazole, isavuconazole, posaconazole)** are predicted to increase the exposure to dasatinib. Severe Study → Also see TABLE 9 p. 909
- Antifungals, azoles **(itraconazole, ketoconazole, voriconazole)** are predicted to markedly increase the exposure to **dasatinib.** Avoid or adjust dose—consult product literature. Severe Study → Also see TABLE 9 p. 909
- Antifungals, azoles **(itraconazole, ketoconazole, voriconazole)** very slightly increase the exposure to delamanid. Severe Study → Also see TABLE 9 p. 909
- Antifungals, azoles **(fluconazole, voriconazole)** moderately increase the exposure to diazepam. Monitor and adjust dose. Moderate Study
- Antifungals, azoles **(fluconazole, isavuconazole, posaconazole)** are predicted to slightly increase the exposure to **dienogest.** Moderate Study
- Antifungals, azoles **(itraconazole, ketoconazole, voriconazole)** are predicted to moderately increase the exposure to **dienogest.** Moderate Study
- **Isavuconazole** slightly increases the exposure to digoxin. Monitor and adjust dose. Moderate Study
- **Itraconazole** is predicted to markedly increase the concentration of digoxin. Monitor and adjust dose. Severe Study
- **Ketoconazole** is predicted to markedly increase the concentration of **digoxin.** Severe Study
- **Posaconazole** is predicted to increase the concentration of **digoxin.** Severe Study
- Antifungals, azoles **(fluconazole, isavuconazole, itraconazole, ketoconazole, posaconazole, voriconazole)** increase the risk of

QT-prolongation when given with **domperidone**. Avoid. Severe Study

- Antifungals, azoles **(fluconazole, isavuconazole, posaconazole)** are predicted to increase the exposure to dopamine receptor agonists **(bromocriptine)**. Severe Theoretical
- Antifungals, azoles **(itraconazole, ketoconazole, voriconazole)** increase the exposure to dopamine receptor agonists **(bromocriptine)**. Severe Study
- Antifungals, azoles **(fluconazole, isavuconazole, itraconazole, ketoconazole, posaconazole, voriconazole)** are predicted to increase the concentration of dopamine receptor agonists **(cabergoline)**. Moderate Anecdotal
- **Isavuconazole** is predicted to increase the exposure to dopamine receptor agonists **(pramipexole)**. Adjust dose. Moderate Study
- Antifungals, azoles **(itraconazole, ketoconazole, voriconazole)** are predicted to increase the exposure to **doravirine**. Mild Study
- Antifungals, azoles **(itraconazole, ketoconazole, voriconazole)** are predicted to increase the exposure to **dronabinol**. Adjust dose. Mild Study
- **Ketoconazole** moderately increases the exposure to **drospirenone**. Severe Study
- Antifungals, azoles **(fluconazole, isavuconazole, posaconazole)** are predicted to moderately increase the exposure to **dutasteride**. Mild Study
- Antifungals, azoles **(itraconazole, ketoconazole, voriconazole)** are predicted to increase the exposure to **dutasteride**. Monitor side effects and adjust dose. Moderate Theoretical
- **Itraconazole** is predicted to slightly increase the exposure to **edoxaban**. Severe Theoretical
- **Ketoconazole** slightly increases the exposure to **edoxaban**. Adjust **edoxaban** dose. Severe Study
- **Efavirenz** is predicted to decrease the exposure to **isavuconazole**. Avoid. Severe Theoretical
- **Efavirenz** slightly decreases the exposure to **itraconazole**. Avoid and for 14 days after stopping **efavirenz**. Moderate Study
- **Efavirenz** moderately decreases the exposure to **ketoconazole**. Severe Study
- **Efavirenz** slightly decreases the exposure to **posaconazole**. Avoid. Moderate Study
- **Efavirenz** moderately decreases the exposure to **voriconazole** and **voriconazole** slightly increases the exposure to **efavirenz**. Adjust dose. Severe Study → Also see TABLE 9 p. 909
- Antifungals, azoles **(itraconazole, ketoconazole, voriconazole)** are predicted to markedly increase the exposure to **eletriptan**. Avoid. Severe Study
- Antifungals, azoles **(fluconazole, isavuconazole, itraconazole, ketoconazole, posaconazole, voriconazole)** are predicted to increase the exposure to **eliglustat**. Avoid or adjust dose—consult product literature. Severe Study
- Antifungals, azoles **(fluconazole, isavuconazole, posaconazole)** are predicted to moderately increase the exposure to **encorafenib**. Moderate Study → Also see TABLE 9 p. 909
- Antifungals, azoles **(itraconazole, ketoconazole, voriconazole)** are predicted to increase the exposure to **encorafenib**. Avoid or monitor. Severe Study → Also see TABLE 9 p. 909
- **Enzalutamide** is predicted to decrease the exposure to **isavuconazole**. Avoid. Severe Study
- Antifungals, azoles **(fluconazole, isavuconazole, posaconazole)** are predicted to increase the risk of ergotism when given with **ergometrine**. Severe Theoretical
- Antifungals, azoles **(itraconazole, ketoconazole, voriconazole)** are predicted to increase the risk of ergotism when given with **ergometrine**. Avoid. Severe Theoretical
- **Miconazole** is predicted to increase the exposure to **ergometrine**. Avoid. Moderate Theoretical
- Antifungals, azoles **(fluconazole, isavuconazole, posaconazole)** are predicted to increase the risk of ergotism when given with **ergotamine**. Severe Theoretical
- Antifungals, azoles **(itraconazole, ketoconazole, voriconazole)** are predicted to increase the risk of ergotism when given with **ergotamine**. Avoid. Severe Theoretical
- **Miconazole** is predicted to increase the exposure to **ergotamine**. Avoid. Moderate Theoretical
- Antifungals, azoles **(fluconazole, isavuconazole, posaconazole)** are predicted to increase the exposure to **erlotinib**. Moderate Theoretical
- Antifungals, azoles **(itraconazole, ketoconazole, voriconazole)** are predicted to slightly increase the exposure to **erlotinib**. Use with caution and adjust dose. Moderate Study
- Antifungals, azoles **(itraconazole, ketoconazole, voriconazole)** are predicted to increase the exposure to **esketamine**. Adjust dose. Moderate Study
- Antifungals, azoles **(fluconazole, isavuconazole, posaconazole)** are predicted to increase the concentration of **everolimus**. Avoid or adjust dose. Moderate Study
- Antifungals, azoles **(itraconazole, ketoconazole, voriconazole)** are predicted to increase the concentration of **everolimus**. Avoid. Severe Study
- Antifungals, azoles **(fluconazole, isavuconazole, posaconazole)** are predicted to increase the exposure to **fesoterodine**. Adjust **fesoterodine** dose with moderate inhibitors of CYP3A4 in hepatic and renal impairment. Mild Study
- Antifungals, azoles **(itraconazole, ketoconazole, voriconazole)** are predicted to moderately increase the exposure to **fesoterodine**. Adjust **fesoterodine** dose with potent inhibitors of CYP3A4; avoid in hepatic and renal impairment. Severe Study
- Antifungals, azoles **(itraconazole, ketoconazole)** are predicted to increase the exposure to **fidaxomicin**. Avoid. Moderate Study
- Antifungals, azoles **(itraconazole, ketoconazole, voriconazole)** are predicted to increase the exposure to **fosaprepitant**. Moderate Theoretical
- **Posaconazole** is predicted to increase the exposure to **fosaprepitant**. Moderate Study
- Antifungals, azoles **(fluconazole, isavuconazole, posaconazole)** are predicted to increase the exposure to **gefitinib**. Moderate Theoretical
- Antifungals, azoles **(itraconazole, ketoconazole, voriconazole)** are predicted to increase the exposure to **gefitinib**. Moderate Study
- Antifungals, azoles **(itraconazole, ketoconazole, voriconazole)** are predicted to increase the exposure to **gilteritinib**. Moderate Study
- Antifungals, azoles **(itraconazole, ketoconazole)** potentially increase the exposure to **glecaprevir**. Moderate Theoretical
- Antifungals, azoles **(itraconazole, ketoconazole, voriconazole)** are predicted to moderately to markedly increase the exposure to **grazoprevir**. Avoid. Severe Study
- Antifungals, azoles **(fluconazole, isavuconazole, posaconazole)** are predicted to increase the concentration of **guanfacine**. Adjust **guanfacine** dose, p. 247. Moderate Theoretical
- Antifungals, azoles **(itraconazole, ketoconazole, voriconazole)** are predicted to increase the exposure to **guanfacine**. Adjust **guanfacine** dose, p. 247. Moderate Study
- **H_2 receptor antagonists** are predicted to decrease the absorption of **itraconazole**. Administer **itraconazole** capsules with an acidic beverage, p. 409. Moderate Study
- **H_2 receptor antagonists** are predicted to decrease the absorption of **ketoconazole**. Administer **ketoconazole** with an acidic beverage, p. 480. Moderate Study
- **H_2 receptor antagonists** are predicted to decrease the exposure to **posaconazole**. Avoid use of posaconazole oral suspension. Moderate Study
- **Itraconazole** increases the concentration of **haloperidol**. Moderate Study
- **Fluconazole** slightly increases the exposure to HIV-protease inhibitors **(tipranavir)**. Avoid or adjust dose. Moderate Study
- **HIV-protease inhibitors** are predicted to increase the exposure to **isavuconazole**. Avoid or monitor side effects. Severe Study
- **HIV-protease inhibitors** are predicted to increase the exposure to **itraconazole**. Use with caution and adjust dose. Severe Study
- **HIV-protease inhibitors** are predicted to increase the exposure to **ketoconazole**. Use with caution and adjust dose. Moderate Study
- **Miconazole** is predicted to increase the concentration of **HIV-protease inhibitors**. Use with caution and adjust dose. Moderate Theoretical
- **Posaconazole** is predicted to increase the exposure to **HIV-protease inhibitors**. Moderate Study

Antifungals, azoles (continued)

- ▸ **HIV-protease inhibitors** are predicted to affect the exposure to **voriconazole** and **voriconazole** potentially affects the exposure to **HIV-protease inhibitors**. [Severe] Study → Also see TABLE 9 p. 909
- ▸ Antifungals, azoles **(fluconazole, isavuconazole, posaconazole)** are predicted to increase the exposure to **ibrutinib**. Adjust **ibrutinib** dose with moderate inhibitors of CYP3A4. [Severe] Study
- ▸ Antifungals, azoles **(itraconazole, ketoconazole, voriconazole)** are predicted to very markedly increase the exposure to **ibrutinib**. Avoid potent inhibitors of CYP3A4 or adjust **ibrutinib** dose. [Severe] Study
- ▸ **Idelalisib** is predicted to increase the exposure to **isavuconazole**. Avoid or monitor side effects. [Severe] Study
- ▸ Antifungals, azoles **(fluconazole, posaconazole)** are predicted to increase the exposure to **imatinib**. [Moderate] Theoretical
- ▸ Antifungals, azoles **(itraconazole, ketoconazole, voriconazole)** are predicted to increase the exposure to **imatinib**. [Moderate] Study
- ▸ **Imatinib** is predicted to increase the exposure to **isavuconazole**. [Moderate] Theoretical
- ▸ Antifungals, azoles **(itraconazole, ketoconazole, voriconazole)** are predicted to increase the risk of toxicity when given with **irinotecan**. Avoid. [Moderate] Study
- ▸ Antifungals, azoles **(fluconazole, isavuconazole, posaconazole)** are predicted to increase the exposure to **ivabradine**. Adjust **ivabradine** dose. [Severe] Theoretical
- ▸ Antifungals, azoles **(itraconazole, ketoconazole, voriconazole)** are predicted to increase the exposure to **ivabradine**. Avoid. [Severe] Study
- ▸ Antifungals, azoles **(fluconazole, isavuconazole, posaconazole)** are predicted to increase the exposure to **ivacaftor**. Adjust **ivacaftor** p. 196 or **tezacaftor with ivacaftor** p. 198 dose with moderate inhibitors of CYP3A4. [Severe] Study
- ▸ Antifungals, azoles **(itraconazole, ketoconazole, voriconazole)** are predicted to increase the exposure to **ivacaftor**. Adjust **ivacaftor** p. 196 or **lumacaftor with ivacaftor** p. 197 or **tezacaftor with ivacaftor** p. 198 dose with potent inhibitors of CYP3A4. [Severe] Study
- ▸ **Lanthanum** is predicted to decrease the absorption of **ketoconazole**. Separate administration by at least 2 hours. [Moderate] Theoretical
- ▸ Antifungals, azoles **(fluconazole, isavuconazole, posaconazole)** are predicted to increase the exposure to **lapatinib**. [Moderate] Study → Also see TABLE 9 p. 909
- ▸ Antifungals, azoles **(itraconazole, ketoconazole, voriconazole)** are predicted to increase the exposure to **lapatinib**. Avoid. [Moderate] Study → Also see TABLE 9 p. 909
- ▸ Antifungals, azoles **(itraconazole, ketoconazole, voriconazole)** are predicted to moderately increase the exposure to **larotrectinib**. Avoid or adjust **larotrectinib** dose, p. 607. [Moderate] Study
- ▸ **Letermovir** slightly decreases the exposure to **voriconazole**. [Moderate] Study
- ▸ Antifungals, azoles **(fluconazole, isavuconazole, posaconazole)** are predicted to increase the exposure to **lomitapide**. Avoid. [Moderate] Theoretical → Also see TABLE 1 p. 907
- ▸ Antifungals, azoles **(itraconazole, ketoconazole, voriconazole)** are predicted to markedly increase the exposure to **lomitapide**. Avoid. [Severe] Study → Also see TABLE 1 p. 907
- ▸ **Clotrimazole** is predicted to increase the exposure to **lomitapide**. Separate administration by 12 hours. [Moderate] Theoretical
- ▸ Antifungals, azoles **(itraconazole, ketoconazole, voriconazole)** are predicted to increase the exposure to **lorlatinib**. Avoid or adjust **lorlatinib** dose. [Severe] Study
- ▸ **Lumacaftor** is predicted to decrease the exposure to antifungals, azoles **(itraconazole, ketoconazole, posaconazole, voriconazole)**. Avoid or monitor efficacy. [Moderate] Theoretical
- ▸ **Lumacaftor** is predicted to decrease the exposure to **fluconazole**. Adjust dose. [Mild] Theoretical
- ▸ Antifungals, azoles **(fluconazole, isavuconazole)** are predicted to increase the exposure to **lurasidone**. Adjust **lurasidone** dose. [Moderate] Study
- ▸ Antifungals, azoles **(itraconazole, ketoconazole, voriconazole)** are predicted to increase the exposure to **lurasidone**. Avoid. [Severe] Study
- ▸ **Posaconazole** moderately increases the exposure to **lurasidone**. Avoid. [Severe] Study
- ▸ Antifungals, azoles **(itraconazole, ketoconazole, voriconazole)** are predicted to increase the exposure to **macitentan**. [Moderate] Study
- ▸ **Macrolides (clarithromycin)** are predicted to increase the exposure to **isavuconazole**. Avoid or monitor side effects. [Severe] Study
- ▸ **Macrolides (erythromycin)** are predicted to increase the exposure to **isavuconazole**. [Moderate] Theoretical
- ▸ Antifungals, azoles **(itraconazole, ketoconazole, voriconazole)** are predicted to markedly increase the exposure to **maraviroc**. Adjust dose. [Severe] Study
- ▸ **Metoclopramide** potentially decreases the absorption of **posaconazole** (oral suspension). [Moderate] Study
- ▸ Antifungals, azoles **(fluconazole, isavuconazole, posaconazole)** are predicted to increase the exposure to **midazolam**. Monitor side effects and adjust dose. [Severe] Study
- ▸ Antifungals, azoles **(itraconazole, ketoconazole, voriconazole)** are predicted to markedly to very markedly increase the exposure to **midazolam**. Avoid or adjust dose. [Severe] Study
- ▸ **Miconazole** is predicted to increase the exposure to intravenous **midazolam**. Use with caution and adjust dose. [Moderate] Theoretical
- ▸ **Miconazole** is predicted to increase the exposure to oral **midazolam**. Avoid. [Moderate] Theoretical
- ▸ Antifungals, azoles **(fluconazole, isavuconazole, posaconazole)** are predicted to increase the exposure to **midostaurin**. [Moderate] Theoretical
- ▸ Antifungals, azoles **(itraconazole, ketoconazole, voriconazole)** are predicted to very markedly increase the exposure to **midostaurin**. Avoid or monitor for toxicity. [Severe] Study
- ▸ Antifungals, azoles **(itraconazole, ketoconazole, voriconazole)** are predicted to increase the exposure to **mirabegron**. Adjust **mirabegron** dose in hepatic and renal impairment. [Moderate] Study
- ▸ Antifungals, azoles **(itraconazole, ketoconazole, voriconazole)** are predicted to increase the exposure to **mirtazapine**. [Moderate] Study
- ▸ **Mitotane** is predicted to decrease the exposure to **isavuconazole**. Avoid. [Severe] Study
- ▸ Antifungals, azoles **(itraconazole, ketoconazole, voriconazole)** are predicted to increase the exposure to **modafinil**. [Mild] Theoretical
- ▸ Antifungals, azoles **(itraconazole, ketoconazole)** increase the risk of neutropenia when given with monoclonal antibodies **(brentuximab vedotin)**. Monitor and adjust dose. [Severe] Study
- ▸ Antifungals, azoles **(itraconazole, ketoconazole, voriconazole)** are predicted to increase the exposure to monoclonal antibodies **(polatuzumab vedotin)**. [Moderate] Theoretical
- ▸ Antifungals, azoles **(itraconazole, ketoconazole, voriconazole)** are predicted to increase the exposure to monoclonal antibodies **(trastuzumab emtansine)**. Avoid. [Severe] Theoretical
- ▸ **Isavuconazole** increases the exposure to **mycophenolate**. [Moderate] Study
- ▸ Antifungals, azoles **(fluconazole, isavuconazole, posaconazole)** are predicted to increase the exposure to **naldemedine**. [Moderate] Study
- ▸ Antifungals, azoles **(itraconazole, ketoconazole, voriconazole)** are predicted to increase the exposure to **naldemedine**. Avoid or monitor. [Moderate] Study
- ▸ Antifungals, azoles **(fluconazole, isavuconazole, posaconazole)** are predicted to increase the exposure to **naloxegol**. Adjust **naloxegol** dose and monitor side effects. [Moderate] Study
- ▸ Antifungals, azoles **(itraconazole, ketoconazole, voriconazole)** are predicted to markedly increase the exposure to **naloxegol**. Avoid. [Severe] Study
- ▸ Antifungals, azoles **(fluconazole, isavuconazole, posaconazole)** are predicted to increase the exposure to **neratinib**. Avoid. [Severe] Study → Also see TABLE 1 p. 907
- ▸ Antifungals, azoles **(itraconazole, ketoconazole, voriconazole)** are predicted to increase the exposure to **neratinib**. Avoid or adjust **neratinib** dose. [Severe] Study → Also see TABLE 1 p. 907
- ▸ Antifungals, azoles **(itraconazole, ketoconazole, voriconazole)** are predicted to increase the exposure to **netupitant**. [Moderate] Study

- Netupitant is predicted to decrease the exposure to **isavuconazole**. Moderate Theoretical
- **Fluconazole** slightly to moderately increases the exposure to **nevirapine**. Moderate Study
- **Nevirapine** is predicted to decrease the exposure to **isavuconazole**. Avoid. Severe Theoretical
- **Nevirapine** moderately decreases the exposure to **itraconazole**. Avoid and for 14 days after stopping **nevirapine**. Moderate Study
- **Nevirapine** moderately decreases the exposure to **ketoconazole**. Avoid. Severe Study
- **Nevirapine** is predicted to decrease the exposure to **voriconazole** and **voriconazole** increases the exposure to **nevirapine**. Monitor and adjust dose. Severe Theoretical
- Antifungals, azoles **(fluconazole, posaconazole)** are predicted to increase the exposure to **nilotinib**. Moderate Theoretical → Also see **TABLE 9** p. 909
- Antifungals, azoles **(itraconazole, ketoconazole, voriconazole)** are predicted to moderately increase the exposure to **nilotinib**. Avoid. Severe Study → Also see **TABLE 9** p. 909
- Antifungals, azoles **(itraconazole, ketoconazole)** are predicted to increase the exposure to **nintedanib**. Moderate Study
- Antifungals, azoles **(itraconazole, ketoconazole, voriconazole)** are predicted to increase the exposure to **nitisinone**. Adjust dose. Moderate Theoretical
- **Fluconazole** moderately increases the exposure to NSAIDs **(celecoxib)**. Adjust **celecoxib** dose. Moderate Study
- **Voriconazole** slightly increases the exposure to NSAIDs **(diclofenac)**. Monitor and adjust dose. Moderate Study
- **Voriconazole** moderately increases the exposure to NSAIDs **(ibuprofen)**. Adjust dose. Moderate Study
- **Fluconazole** increases the exposure to NSAIDs **(parecoxib)**. Monitor and adjust dose. Moderate Study
- Antifungals, azoles **(fluconazole, isavuconazole, posaconazole)** are predicted to increase the exposure to **olaparib**. Avoid moderate inhibitors of CYP3A4 or adjust **olaparib** dose. Moderate Theoretical
- Antifungals, azoles **(itraconazole, ketoconazole, voriconazole)** are predicted to increase the exposure to **olaparib**. Avoid potent inhibitors of CYP3A4 or adjust **olaparib** dose. Moderate Study
- **Miconazole** is predicted to increase the exposure to opioids **(alfentanil)**. Use with caution and adjust dose. Moderate Theoretical
- Antifungals, azoles **(fluconazole, isavuconazole, posaconazole)** are predicted to increase the exposure to opioids **(alfentanil, buprenorphine, fentanyl, oxycodone)**. Monitor and adjust dose. Moderate Study
- Antifungals, azoles **(itraconazole, ketoconazole, voriconazole)** are predicted to increase the exposure to opioids **(alfentanil, buprenorphine, fentanyl, oxycodone)**. Monitor and adjust dose. Severe Study
- Antifungals, azoles **(fluconazole, isavuconazole, posaconazole)** are predicted to increase the exposure to opioids **(methadone)**. Moderate Theoretical → Also see **TABLE 9** p. 909
- Antifungals, azoles **(itraconazole, ketoconazole, voriconazole)** are predicted to increase the exposure to opioids **(methadone)**. Adjust dose. Severe Theoretical → Also see **TABLE 9** p. 909
- Antifungals, azoles **(itraconazole, ketoconazole, voriconazole)** are predicted to increase the exposure to **ospemifene**. Avoid in poor CYP2C9 metabolisers. Moderate Study
- **Fluconazole** increases the exposure to ospemifene. Use with caution or avoid. Moderate Study
- Antifungals, azoles **(fluconazole, isavuconazole, posaconazole)** are predicted to increase the exposure to **oxybutynin**. Mild Theoretical
- Antifungals, azoles **(itraconazole, ketoconazole, voriconazole)** are predicted to increase the exposure to **oxybutynin**. Mild Study
- Antifungals, azoles **(itraconazole, ketoconazole, voriconazole)** are predicted to increase the exposure to palbociclib. Avoid or adjust **palbociclib** dose. Severe Study
- Antifungals, azoles **(itraconazole, ketoconazole, voriconazole)** are predicted to increase the exposure to panobinostat. Adjust **panobinostat** dose; in hepatic impairment avoid. Moderate Study → Also see **TABLE 9** p. 909
- **Posaconazole** is predicted to increase the exposure to panobinostat. Adjust dose. Moderate Theoretical
- Antifungals, azoles **(itraconazole, ketoconazole, voriconazole)** are predicted to increase the exposure to **paritaprevir**. Avoid. Severe Study
- **Posaconazole** is predicted to increase the exposure to paritaprevir (with ritonavir and ombitasvir) and paritaprevir (with ritonavir and ombitasvir) is predicted to increase the exposure to **posaconazole**. Avoid. Severe Study
- Antifungals, azoles **(fluconazole, isavuconazole, posaconazole)** are predicted to increase the exposure to **pazopanib**. Moderate Theoretical → Also see **TABLE 9** p. 909
- Antifungals, azoles **(itraconazole, ketoconazole, voriconazole)** are predicted to increase the exposure to pazopanib. Avoid or adjust **pazopanib** dose. Moderate Study → Also see **TABLE 9** p. 909
- **Miconazole** greatly increases the anticoagulant effect of **phenindione**. Severe Theoretical
- Antifungals, azoles **(fluconazole, isavuconazole, posaconazole)** are predicted to increase the exposure to phosphodiesterase type-5 inhibitors **(avanafil)**. Adjust **avanafil** dose. Moderate Theoretical
- Antifungals, azoles **(itraconazole, ketoconazole, voriconazole)** are predicted to increase the exposure to phosphodiesterase type-5 inhibitors **(avanafil, vardenafil)**. Avoid. Severe Study → Also see **TABLE 9** p. 909
- **Miconazole** is predicted to increase the exposure to phosphodiesterase type-5 inhibitors **(sildenafil)**. Use with caution and adjust dose. Severe Theoretical
- Antifungals, azoles **(fluconazole, isavuconazole, posaconazole)** are predicted to increase the exposure to phosphodiesterase type-5 inhibitors **(sildenafil)**. Monitor or adjust **sildenafil** dose with moderate inhibitors of CYP3A4, p. 125. Moderate Study → Also see **TABLE 9** p. 909
- Antifungals, azoles **(itraconazole, ketoconazole, voriconazole)** are predicted to increase the exposure to phosphodiesterase type-5 inhibitors **(sildenafil)**. Avoid potent inhibitors of CYP3A4 or adjust **sildenafil** dose, p. 125. Severe Study → Also see **TABLE 9** p. 909
- Antifungals, azoles **(fluconazole, isavuconazole, posaconazole)** are predicted to increase the exposure to phosphodiesterase type-5 inhibitors **(tadalafil)**. Severe Theoretical
- Antifungals, azoles **(itraconazole, ketoconazole, voriconazole)** are predicted to increase the exposure to phosphodiesterase type-5 inhibitors **(tadalafil)**. Use with caution or avoid. Severe Study
- Antifungals, azoles **(fluconazole, isavuconazole, posaconazole)** are predicted to increase the exposure to phosphodiesterase type-5 inhibitors **(vardenafil)**. Adjust dose. Severe Theoretical → Also see **TABLE 9** p. 909
- Antifungals, azoles **(itraconazole, ketoconazole)** are predicted to increase the exposure to **pibrentasvir**. Moderate Theoretical
- Antifungals, azoles **(fluconazole, isavuconazole, posaconazole)** are predicted to increase the exposure to **pimozide**. Avoid. Severe Theoretical → Also see **TABLE 9** p. 909
- Antifungals, azoles **(itraconazole, ketoconazole, voriconazole)** are predicted to increase the exposure to pimozide. Avoid. Severe Study → Also see **TABLE 9** p. 909
- **Miconazole** is predicted to increase the exposure to **pimozide**. Avoid. Moderate Theoretical
- **Pioglitazone** potentially decreases the exposure to **isavuconazole**. Use with caution or avoid. Moderate Theoretical
- Antifungals, azoles **(itraconazole, ketoconazole, voriconazole)** are predicted to slightly increase the exposure to **ponatinib**. Monitor and adjust **ponatinib** dose. Moderate Study
- Antifungals, azoles **(itraconazole, ketoconazole, voriconazole)** are predicted to moderately increase the exposure to **praziquantel**. Mild Study
- Antifungals, azoles **(itraconazole, ketoconazole, voriconazole)** given with carbimazole are predicted to increase the exposure to propiverine. Adjust starting dose. Moderate Theoretical
- **Proton pump inhibitors** decrease the absorption of **itraconazole**. Administer itraconazole capsules with an acidic beverage. Moderate Study
- **Proton pump inhibitors** decrease the absorption of **ketoconazole**. Administer ketoconazole with an acidic beverage. Moderate Study
- **Proton pump inhibitors** decrease the absorption of **posaconazole** (oral suspension). Avoid. Moderate Study

A1 Interactions | **Appendix 1**

Antifungals, azoles (continued)

- **Voriconazole** increases the exposure to proton pump inhibitors **(esomeprazole, omeprazole)**. Adjust dose. Moderate Study
- Antifungals, azoles **(fluconazole, isavuconazole, posaconazole)** are predicted to increase the exposure to **quetiapine**. Avoid. Moderate Study
- Antifungals, azoles **(itraconazole, ketoconazole, voriconazole)** are predicted to increase the exposure to **quetiapine**. Avoid. Severe Study
- Antifungals, azoles **(fluconazole, isavuconazole, posaconazole)** are predicted to increase the exposure to **ranolazine**. Severe Study → Also see TABLE 9 p. 909
- Antifungals, azoles **(itraconazole, ketoconazole, voriconazole)** are predicted to increase the exposure to **ranolazine**. Avoid. Severe Study → Also see TABLE 9 p. 909
- Antifungals, azoles **(itraconazole, ketoconazole, voriconazole)** are predicted to increase the exposure to **reboxetine**. Avoid. Moderate Study
- **Miconazole** is predicted to increase the concentration of **reboxetine**. Use with caution and adjust dose. Moderate Theoretical
- Antifungals, azoles **(itraconazole, ketoconazole, voriconazole)** are predicted to increase the exposure to **regorafenib**. Avoid. Moderate Study
- Antifungals, azoles **(itraconazole, ketoconazole, voriconazole)** are predicted to increase the exposure to **repaglinide**. Moderate Study
- Antifungals, azoles **(fluconazole, itraconazole, ketoconazole, miconazole, voriconazole)** are predicted to increase the exposure to retinoids **(alitretinoin)**. Adjust **alitretinoin** dose. Moderate Theoretical
- Antifungals, azoles **(fluconazole, ketoconazole, voriconazole)** are predicted to increase the risk of tretinoin toxicity when given with retinoids **(tretinoin)**. Moderate Study
- Antifungals, azoles **(fluconazole, isavuconazole, posaconazole)** are predicted to increase the exposure to **ribociclib**. Moderate Study → Also see TABLE 9 p. 909
- Antifungals, azoles **(itraconazole, ketoconazole, voriconazole)** are predicted to increase the exposure to **ribociclib**. Avoid or adjust **ribociclib** dose. Moderate Study → Also see TABLE 9 p. 909
- Antifungals, azoles **(itraconazole, posaconazole)** increase the concentration of **rifabutin** and **rifabutin** decreases the concentration of antifungals, azoles **(itraconazole, posaconazole)**. Avoid. Severe Study
- **Fluconazole** increases the risk of uveitis when given with **rifabutin**. Adjust dose. Severe Study
- **Rifabutin** is predicted to decrease the exposure to **isavuconazole**. Avoid. Severe Theoretical
- **Ketoconazole** is predicted to increase the concentration of **rifabutin** and **rifabutin** is predicted to decrease the concentration of **ketoconazole**. Avoid. Severe Theoretical
- **Miconazole** is predicted to increase the concentration of **rifabutin**. Use with caution and adjust dose. Moderate Theoretical
- **Rifabutin** decreases the concentration of **voriconazole** and **voriconazole** increases the concentration of **rifabutin**. Avoid or adjust **voriconazole** dose, p. 410. Severe Study
- **Rifampicin** slightly decreases the exposure to **fluconazole**. Adjust dose. Moderate Study
- **Rifampicin** is predicted to decrease the exposure to **isavuconazole**. Avoid. Severe Study
- **Rifampicin** markedly decreases the exposure to **itraconazole**. Avoid and for 14 days after stopping **rifampicin** Moderate Study
- **Rifampicin** markedly decreases the exposure to **ketoconazole** and **ketoconazole** potentially decreases the exposure to **rifampicin**. Avoid. Moderate Study
- **Rifampicin** is predicted to decrease the exposure to **posaconazole**. Avoid. Moderate Anecdotal
- **Rifampicin** very markedly decreases the exposure to **voriconazole**. Avoid. Moderate Study
- Antifungals, azoles **(itraconazole, posaconazole)** are predicted to increase the exposure to **riociguat**. Adjust **riociguat** dose and monitor blood pressure. Moderate Theoretical
- **Ketoconazole** moderately increases the exposure to **riociguat**. Adjust **riociguat** dose and monitor blood pressure. Moderate Study
- Antifungals, azoles **(itraconazole, ketoconazole, voriconazole)** are predicted to increase the exposure to **risperidone**. Adjust dose. Moderate Study → Also see TABLE 9 p. 909
- Antifungals, azoles **(itraconazole, ketoconazole)** are predicted to moderately increase the exposure to **rivaroxaban**. Avoid. Severe Study
- Antifungals, azoles **(fluconazole, isavuconazole, posaconazole)** are predicted to increase the exposure to **ruxolitinib**. Moderate Theoretical
- Antifungals, azoles **(itraconazole, ketoconazole, voriconazole)** are predicted to increase the exposure to **ruxolitinib**. Adjust dose and monitor side effects. Moderate Study
- Antifungals, azoles **(fluconazole, isavuconazole, posaconazole)** are predicted to increase the exposure to **saxagliptin**. Mild Study
- Antifungals, azoles **(itraconazole, ketoconazole, voriconazole)** are predicted to increase the exposure to **saxagliptin**. Moderate Study
- **Fluconazole** is predicted to increase the exposure to **selexipag**. Unknown Theoretical
- Antifungals, azoles **(itraconazole, ketoconazole, voriconazole)** are predicted to increase the exposure to **siponimod**. Avoid depending on other drugs taken—consult product literature. Severe Theoretical
- **Miconazole** is predicted to increase the exposure to **siponimod**. Avoid depending on other drugs taken—consult product literature. Severe Study
- Antifungals, azoles **(fluconazole, isavuconazole, posaconazole)** increase the concentration of **sirolimus**. Monitor and adjust dose. Moderate Study
- Antifungals, azoles **(itraconazole, ketoconazole, voriconazole)** are predicted to increase the concentration of **sirolimus**. Avoid. Severe Study
- **Miconazole** is predicted to increase the concentration of **sirolimus**. Monitor and adjust dose. Moderate Study
- Oral **sodium bicarbonate** decreases the absorption of **ketoconazole**. Moderate Study
- **Sodium zirconium cyclosilicate** is predicted to decrease the exposure to **antifungals, azoles**. Separate administration by at least 2 hours. Moderate Theoretical
- Antifungals, azoles **(itraconazole, ketoconazole, voriconazole)** are predicted to increase the exposure to **solifenacin**. Adjust solifenacin or tamsulosin with solifenacin dose; avoid in hepatic and renal impairment. Severe Study
- **Voriconazole** is predicted to increase the exposure to SSRIs **(citalopram)**. Severe Theoretical → Also see TABLE 9 p. 909
- Antifungals, azoles **(fluconazole, isavuconazole, posaconazole)** are predicted to increase the exposure to SSRIs **(dapoxetine)**. Adjust **dapoxetine** dose with moderate inhibitors of CYP3A4. Moderate Theoretical
- Antifungals, azoles **(itraconazole, ketoconazole, voriconazole)** are predicted to moderately increase the exposure to SSRIs **(dapoxetine)**. Avoid potent inhibitors of CYP3A4 or adjust **dapoxetine** dose. Severe Study
- **St John's Wort** is predicted to decrease the exposure to **isavuconazole**. Avoid. Severe Theoretical
- **St John's Wort** moderately decreases the exposure to **voriconazole**. Avoid. Moderate Study
- **Fluconazole** potentially increases the risk of rhabdomyolysis when given with statins **(atorvastatin)**. Monitor and adjust dose. Severe Anecdotal → Also see TABLE 1 p. 907
- **Isavuconazole** slightly increases the exposure to statins **(atorvastatin)**. Moderate Study
- **Miconazole** potentially increases the exposure to statins **(atorvastatin)**. Severe Anecdotal
- **Posaconazole** is predicted to increase the exposure to statins **(atorvastatin)**. Avoid. Severe Anecdotal
- Antifungals, azoles **(itraconazole, ketoconazole, voriconazole)** are predicted to increase the exposure to statins **(atorvastatin)**. Avoid or adjust dose and monitor rhabdomyolysis. Severe Study → Also see TABLE 1 p. 907

- Antifungals, azoles **(fluconazole, miconazole)** are predicted to increase the exposure to statins (fluvastatin). [Severe] Theoretical → Also see **TABLE 1** p. 907
- **Isavuconazole** is predicted to increase the exposure to statins (fluvastatin, rosuvastatin). [Moderate] Theoretical
- **Fluconazole** is predicted to increase the exposure to statins (simvastatin). Monitor and adjust dose. [Severe] Anecdotal → Also see **TABLE 1** p. 907
- **Isavuconazole** is predicted to increase the exposure to statins (simvastatin). Monitor and adjust dose. [Severe] Theoretical
- **Miconazole** is predicted to increase the exposure to statins (simvastatin). Avoid. [Severe] Theoretical
- **Posaconazole** markedly to very markedly increases the exposure to statins (simvastatin). Avoid. [Severe] Study
- Antifungals, azoles **(itraconazole, ketoconazole, voriconazole)** are predicted to increase the exposure to statins (simvastatin). Avoid. [Severe] Study → Also see **TABLE 1** p. 907
- **Isavuconazole** is predicted to increase the exposure to sulfasalazine. [Moderate] Theoretical
- Antifungals, azoles **(fluconazole, miconazole)** are predicted to increase the exposure to sulfonylureas. Use with caution and adjust dose. [Moderate] Study
- **Voriconazole** is predicted to increase the concentration of sulfonylureas. Use with caution and adjust dose. [Moderate] Study
- Antifungals, azoles **(fluconazole, isavuconazole, posaconazole)** are predicted to increase the exposure to sunitinib. [Moderate] Theoretical → Also see **TABLE 9** p. 909
- Antifungals, azoles **(itraconazole, ketoconazole, voriconazole)** are predicted to slightly increase the exposure to sunitinib. Avoid or adjust **sunitinib** dose. [Moderate] Study → Also see **TABLE 9** p. 909
- Antifungals, azoles **(fluconazole, isavuconazole, posaconazole)** are predicted to increase the concentration of tacrolimus. [Severe] Study
- Antifungals, azoles **(itraconazole, ketoconazole, voriconazole)** are predicted to increase the concentration of tacrolimus. Monitor and adjust dose. [Severe] Study
- **Miconazole** is predicted to increase the concentration of tacrolimus. Monitor and adjust dose. [Severe] Theoretical
- Antifungals, azoles **(itraconazole, ketoconazole)** are predicted to slightly increase the exposure to talazoparib. Avoid or adjust **talazoparib** dose. [Severe] Study
- Antifungals, azoles **(fluconazole, isavuconazole, posaconazole)** are predicted to increase the exposure to taxanes (cabazitaxel). [Moderate] Theoretical
- Antifungals, azoles **(itraconazole, ketoconazole, voriconazole)** are predicted to increase the exposure to taxanes (cabazitaxel). Avoid. [Severe] Study
- **Miconazole** is predicted to increase the concentration of taxanes (docetaxel). Use with caution and adjust dose. [Moderate] Theoretical
- Antifungals, azoles **(itraconazole, ketoconazole, voriconazole)** are predicted to moderately increase the exposure to taxanes (docetaxel). Avoid or adjust dose. [Severe] Study
- Antifungals, azoles **(itraconazole, ketoconazole, voriconazole)** are predicted to increase the exposure to taxanes (paclitaxel). [Severe] Theoretical
- Antifungals, azoles **(fluconazole, isavuconazole, posaconazole)** are predicted to increase the concentration of temsirolimus. Use with caution or avoid. [Moderate] Theoretical
- Antifungals, azoles **(itraconazole, ketoconazole, voriconazole)** are predicted to increase the concentration of temsirolimus. Avoid. [Severe] Theoretical
- Antifungals, azoles **(fluconazole, isavuconazole, posaconazole)** are predicted to increase the exposure to tezacaftor. Adjust tezacaftor with ivacaftor p. 198 dose with moderate inhibitors of CYP3A4. [Severe] Study
- Antifungals, azoles **(itraconazole, ketoconazole, voriconazole)** are predicted to increase the exposure to tezacaftor. Adjust tezacaftor with ivacaftor p. 198 dose with potent inhibitors of CYP3A4. [Severe] Study
- Antifungals, azoles **(itraconazole, ketoconazole, voriconazole)** are predicted to markedly increase the exposure to ticagrelor. Avoid. [Severe] Study
- Antifungals, azoles **(itraconazole, ketoconazole, voriconazole)** are predicted to increase the exposure to tofacitinib. Adjust **tofacitinib** dose. [Moderate] Study
- **Fluconazole** increases the exposure to tofacitinib. Adjust **tofacitinib** dose. [Moderate] Study
- **Isavuconazole** given with a potent CYP2C19 inhibitor is predicted to increase the exposure to tofacitinib. Adjust **tofacitinib** dose. [Moderate] Study
- **Posaconazole** given with a potent CYP2C19 inhibitor is predicted to increase the exposure to tofacitinib. Adjust **tofacitinib** dose. [Moderate] Theoretical
- Antifungals, azoles **(fluconazole, isavuconazole, posaconazole)** are predicted to increase the exposure to tolterodine. [Mild] Theoretical → Also see **TABLE 9** p. 909
- Antifungals, azoles **(itraconazole, ketoconazole, voriconazole)** are predicted to increase the exposure to tolterodine. Avoid. [Severe] Study → Also see **TABLE 9** p. 909
- Antifungals, azoles **(fluconazole, isavuconazole, posaconazole)** are predicted to increase the exposure to tolvaptan. Manufacturer advises caution or adjust **tolvaptan** dose with moderate inhibitors of CYP3A4. [Moderate] Study
- Antifungals, azoles **(itraconazole, ketoconazole, voriconazole)** are predicted to increase the exposure to tolvaptan. Manufacturer advises caution or adjust **tolvaptan** dose with potent inhibitors of CYP3A4. [Severe] Study
- Antifungals, azoles **(itraconazole, ketoconazole)** are predicted to increase the exposure to topotecan. [Severe] Study
- **Isavuconazole** is predicted to increase the exposure to topotecan. [Moderate] Theoretical
- Antifungals, azoles **(itraconazole, ketoconazole, voriconazole)** are predicted to increase the exposure to toremifene. [Moderate] Theoretical → Also see **TABLE 9** p. 909
- Antifungals, azoles **(itraconazole, ketoconazole, voriconazole)** are predicted to increase the exposure to trabectedin. Avoid or adjust dose. [Severe] Theoretical → Also see **TABLE 1** p. 907
- Antifungals, azoles **(itraconazole, ketoconazole)** are predicted to increase the concentration of trametinib. [Moderate] Theoretical
- Antifungals, azoles **(fluconazole, isavuconazole, posaconazole)** are predicted to increase the exposure to trazodone. [Moderate] Theoretical
- Antifungals, azoles **(itraconazole, ketoconazole, voriconazole)** are predicted to moderately increase the exposure to trazodone. Avoid or adjust dose. [Moderate] Study
- Antifungals, azoles **(fluconazole, isavuconazole, posaconazole)** are predicted to increase the exposure to ulipristal. Avoid if used for uterine fibroids. [Moderate] Study
- Antifungals, azoles **(itraconazole, ketoconazole, voriconazole)** are predicted to increase the exposure to ulipristal. Avoid if used for uterine fibroids. [Severe] Study
- Antifungals, azoles **(itraconazole, ketoconazole, voriconazole)** are predicted to increase the exposure to upadacitinib. Use with caution or avoid. [Severe] Study
- **Posaconazole** is predicted to increase the exposure to upadacitinib. Use with caution or avoid. [Moderate] Study
- Antifungals, azoles **(itraconazole, ketoconazole, voriconazole)** are predicted to increase the exposure to vemurafenib. [Severe] Theoretical → Also see **TABLE 9** p. 909
- Antifungals, azoles **(fluconazole, isavuconazole, itraconazole, ketoconazole, posaconazole, voriconazole)** are predicted to increase the exposure to venetoclax. Avoid or adjust dose—consult product literature. [Severe] Study
- Antifungals, azoles **(itraconazole, ketoconazole, voriconazole)** are predicted to increase the exposure to venlafaxine. [Moderate] Study → Also see **TABLE 9** p. 909
- Antifungals, azoles **(fluconazole, isavuconazole, itraconazole, ketoconazole, posaconazole, voriconazole)** are predicted to increase the exposure to vinca alkaloids. [Severe] Theoretical → Also see **TABLE 1** p. 907 → Also see **TABLE 9** p. 909
- **Miconazole** is predicted to increase the concentration of vinca alkaloids. Use with caution and adjust dose. [Moderate] Theoretical
- Antifungals, azoles **(clotrimazole, ketoconazole)** are predicted to decrease the exposure to vitamin D substances **(colecalciferol)**. [Moderate] Theoretical

Antifungals, azoles (continued)

- Antifungals, azoles **(itraconazole, ketoconazole, voriconazole)** are predicted to increase the exposure to vitamin D substances **(paricalcitol).** Moderate Study
- **Fluconazole** slightly increases the exposure to **zidovudine.** Moderate Study
- Antifungals, azoles **(fluconazole, isavuconazole, posaconazole)** are predicted to increase the exposure to **zopiclone**. Adjust dose. Moderate Study
- Antifungals, azoles **(itraconazole, ketoconazole, voriconazole)** are predicted to increase the exposure to **zopiclone**. Adjust dose. Moderate Theoretical

Antihistamines, non-sedating → see TABLE 9 p. 909 (QT-interval prolongation)

acrivastine · azelastine · bilastine · cetirizine · desloratadine · fexofenadine · levocetirizine · loratadine · mizolastine · rupatadine

- Since systemic absorption can follow topical application, the possibility of interactions with topical **azelastine** should be borne in mind.
- Apple juice and orange juice decrease the exposure to **fexofenadine**.

- **Antacids** decrease the absorption of **fexofenadine**. Separate administration by 2 hours. Mild Study
- Antiarrhythmics **(dronedarone)** are predicted to increase the exposure to **rupatadine.** Avoid. Moderate Study
- Antiarrhythmics **(dronedarone)** are predicted to increase the exposure to antihistamines, non-sedating **(fexofenadine, mizolastine).** Severe Theoretical
- Antifungals, azoles **(fluconazole, isavuconazole, itraconazole, ketoconazole, posaconazole, voriconazole)** are predicted to increase the exposure to **rupatadine**. Avoid. Moderate Study
- Antifungals, azoles **(fluconazole, isavuconazole, posaconazole)** are predicted to increase the exposure to **mizolastine**. Severe Theoretical
- Antifungals, azoles **(itraconazole, ketoconazole, voriconazole)** are predicted to increase the exposure to **mizolastine**. Avoid. Severe Study
- Antifungals, azoles **(miconazole)** are predicted to increase the exposure to **mizolastine**. Avoid. Moderate Theoretical
- **Apalutamide** slightly decreases the exposure to **fexofenadine**. Mild Study
- **Aprepitant** is predicted to increase the exposure to **mizolastine**. Severe Theoretical
- **Aprepitant** is predicted to increase the exposure to **rupatadine**. Avoid. Moderate Study
- **Antihistamines, non-sedating** are predicted to decrease the effects of betahistine. Moderate Theoretical
- Calcium channel blockers **(diltiazem, verapamil)** are predicted to increase the exposure to **mizolastine.** Severe Theoretical
- Calcium channel blockers **(diltiazem, verapamil)** are predicted to increase the exposure to **rupatadine**. Avoid. Moderate Study
- **Ceritinib** is predicted to increase the exposure to **fexofenadine**. Moderate Theoretical
- **Cobicistat** is predicted to increase the exposure to **mizolastine**. Avoid. Severe Study
- **Cobicistat** is predicted to increase the exposure to **rupatadine**. Avoid. Moderate Study
- **Crizotinib** is predicted to increase the exposure to **mizolastine**. Severe Theoretical
- **Crizotinib** is predicted to increase the exposure to **rupatadine**. Avoid. Moderate Study
- **Eliglustat** is predicted to increase the exposure to **fexofenadine**. Adjust dose. Moderate Study
- **Grapefruit juice** slightly decreases the exposure to **bilastine**. **Bilastine** should be taken 1 hour before or 2 hours after **grapefruit juice.** Moderate Study
- **Grapefruit juice** increases the exposure to **rupatadine**. Avoid. Moderate Study
- **HIV-protease inhibitors** are predicted to increase the exposure to **mizolastine**. Avoid. Severe Study
- **HIV-protease inhibitors** are predicted to increase the exposure to **rupatadine**. Avoid. Moderate Study
- **Idelalisib** is predicted to increase the exposure to **mizolastine**. Avoid. Severe Study
- **Idelalisib** is predicted to increase the exposure to **rupatadine.** Avoid. Moderate Study
- **Imatinib** is predicted to increase the exposure to **mizolastine.** Severe Theoretical
- **Imatinib** is predicted to increase the exposure to **rupatadine.** Avoid. Moderate Study
- **Lapatinib** is predicted to increase the exposure to **fexofenadine.** Moderate Theoretical
- **Leflunomide** is predicted to increase the exposure to **fexofenadine.** Moderate Study
- **Letermovir** is predicted to increase the concentration of **fexofenadine.** Moderate Theoretical
- Macrolides **(clarithromycin)** are predicted to increase the exposure to **mizolastine.** Avoid. Severe Study
- Macrolides **(clarithromycin, erythromycin)** are predicted to increase the exposure to **rupatadine.** Avoid. Moderate Study
- Macrolides **(erythromycin)** are predicted to increase the exposure to **mizolastine.** Severe Theoretical
- **MAOIs, irreversible** are predicted to increase the risk of antimuscarinic side-effects when given with **antihistamines, non-sedating.** Avoid. Severe Theoretical
- **Mirabegron** is predicted to increase the exposure to **fexofenadine.** Mild Theoretical
- **Neratinib** is predicted to increase the exposure to **fexofenadine.** Moderate Study
- **Netupitant** is predicted to increase the exposure to **mizolastine.** Severe Theoretical
- **Netupitant** is predicted to increase the exposure to **rupatadine.** Avoid. Moderate Study
- **Nilotinib** is predicted to increase the exposure to **mizolastine.** Severe Theoretical
- **Nilotinib** is predicted to increase the exposure to **rupatadine.** Avoid. Moderate Study
- **Pibrentasvir (with glecaprevir)** is predicted to increase the exposure to **fexofenadine.** Moderate Study
- **Pitolisant** is predicted to decrease the exposure to **fexofenadine.** Mild Theoretical
- **Rifampicin** is predicted to decrease the exposure to **bilastine.** Moderate Theoretical
- **Rifampicin** increases the clearance of **fexofenadine.** Moderate Study
- **Teriflunomide** is predicted to increase the exposure to **fexofenadine.** Moderate Study
- **Velpatasvir** is predicted to increase the exposure to **fexofenadine.** Severe Theoretical
- **Venetoclax** is predicted to increase the exposure to **fexofenadine.** Moderate Theoretical

Antihistamines, sedating → see TABLE 9 p. 909 (QT-interval prolongation), TABLE 11 p. 909 (CNS depressant effects), TABLE 10 p. 909 (antimuscarinics)

alimemazine · antazoline · buclizine · chlorphenamine · cinnarizine · clemastine · cyclizine · cyproheptadine · doxylamine · hydroxyzine · ketotifen · pizotifen · promethazine

ROUTE-SPECIFIC INFORMATION Since systemic absorption can follow topical application of **ketotifen**, the possibility of interactions should be borne in mind.

- **Hydroxyzine** potentially increases the risk of overheating and dehydration when given with antiepileptics **(zonisamide).** Avoid in children. Severe Theoretical
- **Antihistamines, sedating** are predicted to decrease the effects of betahistine. Moderate Theoretical
- **MAOIs, irreversible** are predicted to increase the risk of antimuscarinic side-effects when given with **antihistamines, sedating.** Avoid. Severe Theoretical
- **Cyproheptadine** decreases the effects of **metyrapone.** Avoid. Moderate Study
- **Antihistamines, sedating** are predicted to decrease the efficacy of **pitolisant.** Moderate Theoretical
- **Cyproheptadine** potentially decreases the effects of **SSRIs.** Moderate Anecdotal

Antimalarials → see TABLE 15 p. 910 (myelosuppression), TABLE 9 p. 909 (QT-interval prolongation) artemether · artenimol · atovaquone · chloroquine · lumefantrine · mefloquine · piperaquine · primaquine · proguanil · pyrimethamine · quinine

PHARMACOLOGY **Piperaquine** has a long half-life; there is a potential for drug interactions to occur for up to 3 months after treatment has been stopped.

- **Chloroquine** is predicted to decrease the effects of agalsidase alfa. Avoid. Moderate Theoretical
- **Chloroquine** is predicted to decrease the effects of agalsidase beta. Avoid. Moderate Theoretical
- Antimalarials **(chloroquine, primaquine)** are predicted to increase the risk of methaemoglobinaemia when given with topical anaesthetics, local **(prilocaine)**. Use with caution or avoid. Severe Theoretical
- Antacids decrease the absorption of **chloroquine**. Separate administration by at least 4 hours. Moderate Study
- Antacids are predicted to decrease the absorption of **proguanil**. Separate administration by at least 2 hours. Moderate Study
- Antiarrhythmics **(dronedarone)** are predicted to increase the concentration of **piperaquine**. Severe Theoretical
- Antiepileptics **(carbamazepine, fosphenytoin, phenobarbital, phenytoin, primidone)** are predicted to decrease the exposure to **artemether** (with lumefantrine). Avoid. Severe Study
- Antiepileptics **(carbamazepine, fosphenytoin, phenobarbital, phenytoin, primidone)** are predicted to decrease the concentration of **piperaquine**. Avoid. Moderate Theoretical
- Antiepileptics **(carbamazepine, phenobarbital, primidone)** potentially increase the risk of toxicity when given with **quinine**. Unknown Study
- **Pyrimethamine** increases the risk of haematological toxicity when given with antiepileptics **(fosphenytoin, phenytoin)**. Severe Study
- **Pyrimethamine** is predicted to increase the risk of haematological toxicity when given with antiepileptics **(phenobarbital, primidone)**. Severe Theoretical
- Antifungals, azoles **(fluconazole, isavuconazole, itraconazole, ketoconazole, posaconazole, voriconazole)** are predicted to increase the concentration of **piperaquine**. Severe Theoretical
- Antifungals, azoles **(fluconazole, itraconazole, posaconazole, voriconazole)** are predicted to increase the exposure to **mefloquine**. Moderate Theoretical
- Antifungals, azoles **(ketoconazole)** increase the exposure to **mefloquine**. Moderate Study
- Antimalarials **(proguanil)** are predicted to increase the risk of side-effects when given with antimalarials **(pyrimethamine)**. Severe Theoretical
- **Apalutamide** is predicted to decrease the exposure to **artemether** (with lumefantrine). Avoid. Severe Study → Also see TABLE 9 p. 909
- **Apalutamide** is predicted to decrease the concentration of **piperaquine**. Avoid. Moderate Theoretical
- **Aprepitant** is predicted to increase the concentration of **piperaquine**. Severe Theoretical
- **Mefloquine** is predicted to increase the risk of bradycardia when given with **beta blockers, non-selective**. Severe Theoretical
- **Mefloquine** is predicted to increase the risk of bradycardia when given with **beta blockers, selective**. Severe Theoretical
- **Mefloquine** is predicted to increase the risk of bradycardia when given with **calcium channel blockers**. Severe Theoretical
- Calcium channel blockers **(diltiazem, verapamil)** are predicted to increase the concentration of **piperaquine**. Severe Theoretical
- Calcium salts **(calcium carbonate)** decrease the absorption of **chloroquine**. Separate administration by at least 4 hours. Moderate Study
- Calcium salts **(calcium carbonate)** are predicted to decrease the absorption of **proguanil**. Separate administration by at least 2 hours. Moderate Study
- **Chloroquine** decreases the efficacy of oral **cholera vaccine**. Moderate Study
- **Cobicistat** is predicted to increase the concentration of **piperaquine**. Severe Theoretical
- **Crizotinib** is predicted to increase the concentration of **piperaquine**. Severe Theoretical
- Antimalarials **(chloroquine, primaquine)** are predicted to increase the risk of methaemoglobinaemia when given with dapsone. Severe Theoretical
- **Mefloquine** is predicted to increase the risk of bradycardia when given with digoxin. Severe Theoretical
- **Quinine** increases the concentration of digoxin. Monitor and adjust **digoxin** dose, p. 86. Severe Anecdotal
- **Efavirenz** decreases the concentration of **artemether**. Severe Study → Also see TABLE 9 p. 909
- **Efavirenz** moderately decreases the exposure to **atovaquone**. Avoid. Moderate Study
- **Efavirenz** affects the exposure to **proguanil**. Avoid. Moderate Study
- **Enzalutamide** is predicted to decrease the exposure to **artemether** (with lumefantrine). Avoid. Severe Study
- **Enzalutamide** is predicted to decrease the concentration of **piperaquine**. Avoid. Moderate Theoretical
- **Etravirine** decreases the exposure to **artemether**. Moderate Study
- **Grapefruit juice** increases the exposure to **artemether**. Unknown Study
- **Grapefruit juice** is predicted to increase the concentration of **piperaquine**. Avoid. Severe Theoretical
- H_2 receptor antagonists **(cimetidine)** decrease the clearance of **chloroquine**. Moderate Study
- H_2 receptor antagonists **(cimetidine)** slightly increase the exposure to **quinine**. Moderate Study
- **HIV-protease inhibitors** decrease the exposure to **atovaquone**. Avoid if boosted with ritonavir. Moderate Study
- **HIV-protease inhibitors** are predicted to increase the concentration of **piperaquine**. Severe Theoretical
- **HIV-protease inhibitors** are predicted to decrease the exposure to **proguanil**. Avoid. Moderate Study
- **HIV-protease inhibitors** are predicted to affect the exposure to **quinine**. Severe Study → Also see TABLE 9 p. 909
- **Idelalisib** is predicted to increase the concentration of **piperaquine**. Severe Theoretical
- **Imatinib** is predicted to increase the concentration of **piperaquine**. Severe Theoretical
- **Lanthanum** is predicted to decrease the absorption of **chloroquine**. Separate administration by at least 2 hours. Moderate Theoretical
- **Chloroquine** is predicted to decrease the exposure to laronidase. Avoid simultaneous administration. Severe Theoretical
- Macrolides **(clarithromycin, erythromycin)** are predicted to increase the concentration of **piperaquine**. Severe Theoretical
- **Mepacrine** is predicted to increase the concentration of **primaquine**. Avoid. Moderate Theoretical
- **Pyrimethamine** is predicted to increase the risk of side-effects when given with **methotrexate**. Severe Theoretical → Also see TABLE 15 p. 910
- **Metoclopramide** decreases the concentration of **atovaquone**. Avoid. Moderate Study
- **Mitotane** is predicted to decrease the exposure to **artemether** (with lumefantrine). Avoid. Severe Study
- **Mitotane** is predicted to decrease the concentration of **piperaquine**. Avoid. Moderate Theoretical
- **Netupitant** is predicted to increase the concentration of **piperaquine**. Severe Theoretical
- **Nilotinib** is predicted to increase the concentration of **piperaquine**. Severe Theoretical
- **Pyrimethamine** is predicted to increase the risk of side-effects when given with **pemetrexed**. Severe Theoretical → Also see TABLE 15 p. 910
- **Chloroquine** is predicted to increase the risk of haematological toxicity when given with **penicillamine**. Avoid. Severe Theoretical
- **Chloroquine** moderately decreases the exposure to **praziquantel**. Use with caution and adjust dose. Moderate Study
- **Chloroquine** decreases the efficacy of **rabies vaccine** (intradermal). Avoid. Moderate Study
- **Rifabutin** slightly decreases the exposure to **atovaquone**. Avoid. Moderate Study

Antimalarials (continued)
- **Rifampicin** is predicted to decrease the exposure to **artemether** (with lumefantrine). Avoid. Severe Study
- **Rifampicin** moderately decreases the exposure to **atovaquone** and **atovaquone** slightly increases the exposure to **rifampicin**. Avoid. Moderate Study
- **Rifampicin** moderately decreases the exposure to **mefloquine**. Severe Study
- **Rifampicin** is predicted to decrease the concentration of **piperaquine**. Avoid. Moderate Theoretical
- **Rifampicin** decreases the exposure to **quinine**. Severe Study
- **St John's Wort** is predicted to decrease the concentration of **piperaquine**. Avoid. Moderate Theoretical
- **Pyrimethamine** increases the risk of side-effects when given with **sulfonamides**. Severe Study → Also see TABLE 15 p. 910
- Tetracyclines **(tetracycline)** decrease the concentration of **atovaquone**. Moderate Study
- **Pyrimethamine** increases the risk of side-effects when given with **trimethoprim**. Severe Study → Also see TABLE 15 p. 910
- **Pyrimethamine** is predicted to increase the risk of side-effects when given with **zidovudine**. Severe Theoretical → Also see TABLE 15 p. 910

Antithymocyte immunoglobulin (rabbit) → see immunoglobulins

Apalutamide → see TABLE 9 p. 909 (QT-interval prolongation)
- **Apalutamide** is predicted to markedly decrease the exposure to **abemaciclib**. Avoid. Severe Study
- **Apalutamide** is predicted to decrease the exposure to **abiraterone**. Avoid. Severe Study
- **Apalutamide** is predicted to decrease the exposure to aldosterone antagonists **(eplerenone)**. Avoid. Moderate Theoretical
- **Apalutamide** is predicted to decrease the exposure to **alprazolam**. Adjust dose. Moderate Theoretical
- **Apalutamide** is predicted to decrease the exposure to antiarrhythmics **(disopyramide, dronedarone)**. Avoid. Severe Study → Also see TABLE 9 p. 909
- **Apalutamide** is predicted to decrease the efficacy of antiarrhythmics **(propafenone)**. Moderate Study
- **Apalutamide** is predicted to decrease the exposure to anticholinesterases, centrally acting **(donepezil)**. Mild Study
- **Apalutamide** is predicted to decrease the exposure to antiepileptics **(perampanel)**. Monitor and adjust dose. Moderate Study
- **Apalutamide** potentially decreases the exposure to antiepileptics **(valproate)**. Mild Theoretical
- Antifungals, azoles **(itraconazole, ketoconazole, voriconazole)** are predicted to increase the exposure to **apalutamide**. Mild Study → Also see TABLE 9 p. 909
- **Apalutamide** is predicted to decrease the exposure to antifungals, azoles **(isavuconazole)**. Avoid. Severe Study
- **Apalutamide** slightly decreases the exposure to antihistamines, non-sedating **(fexofenadine)**. Mild Study
- **Apalutamide** is predicted to decrease the exposure to antimalarials **(artemether)** (with lumefantrine). Avoid. Severe Study → Also see TABLE 9 p. 909
- **Apalutamide** is predicted to decrease the concentration of antimalarials **(piperaquine)**. Avoid. Moderate Theoretical
- **Apalutamide** is predicted to moderately decrease the exposure to **apixaban**. Use with caution or avoid. Severe Study
- **Apalutamide** moderately decreases the exposure to **apremilast**. Avoid. Severe Study
- **Apalutamide** is predicted to markedly decrease the exposure to **aprepitant**. Avoid. Moderate Study
- **Apalutamide** is predicted to moderately decrease the exposure to **aripiprazole**. Adjust **aripiprazole** dose, p. 265. Moderate Study
- **Apalutamide** is predicted to decrease the exposure to **axitinib**. Avoid or adjust dose. Moderate Study
- **Apalutamide** decreases the exposure to **bedaquiline**. Avoid. Severe Study → Also see TABLE 9 p. 909
- **Apalutamide** is predicted to decrease the exposure to beta$_2$ agonists **(salmeterol)**. Avoid or monitor. Moderate Study
- **Apalutamide** is predicted to decrease the exposure to **bictegravir**. Avoid. Moderate Study
- **Apalutamide** slightly decreases the exposure to **bortezomib**. Avoid. Severe Study
- **Apalutamide** affects the exposure to **bosentan**. Avoid. Severe Study
- **Apalutamide** is predicted to very markedly decrease the exposure to **bosutinib**. Avoid. Severe Study → Also see TABLE 9 p. 909
- **Apalutamide** is predicted to decrease the exposure to **brigatinib**. Avoid. Severe Study
- **Apalutamide** is predicted to decrease the exposure to **buspirone**. Use with caution and adjust dose. Severe Study
- **Apalutamide** moderately decreases the exposure to **cabozantinib**. Avoid. Moderate Study → Also see TABLE 9 p. 909
- **Apalutamide** is predicted to decrease the exposure to calcium channel blockers **(amlodipine, felodipine, lacidipine, lercanidipine, nicardipine, nimodipine)**. Monitor and adjust dose. Moderate Study
- **Apalutamide** is predicted to decrease the exposure to **cannabidiol**. Adjust dose. Moderate Study
- **Apalutamide** is predicted to decrease the exposure to **cariprazine**. Avoid. Severe Theoretical
- **Apalutamide** is predicted to decrease the exposure to **ceritinib**. Avoid. Severe Study → Also see TABLE 9 p. 909
- **Apalutamide** decreases the concentration of **ciclosporin**. Severe Study
- **Apalutamide** is predicted to alter the effects of **cilostazol**. Moderate Theoretical
- **Apalutamide** is predicted to decrease the exposure to **cinacalcet**. Monitor and adjust dose. Moderate Study
- **Apalutamide** decreases the exposure to **clomethiazole**. Monitor and adjust dose. Moderate Study
- **Clopidogrel** is predicted to increase the exposure to **apalutamide**. Mild Study
- **Apalutamide** is predicted to decrease the exposure to **cobicistat**. Avoid. Severe Theoretical
- **Cobicistat** is predicted to increase the exposure to **apalutamide**. Mild Study
- **Apalutamide** is predicted to decrease the exposure to **cobimetinib**. Avoid. Severe Theoretical
- **Apalutamide** is predicted to decrease the exposure to **colchicine**. Mild Study
- **Apalutamide** is predicted to decrease the exposure to corticosteroids **(budesonide, deflazacort, dexamethasone, fludrocortisone, hydrocortisone, methylprednisolone, prednisolone, triamcinolone)**. Monitor and adjust dose. Moderate Study
- **Apalutamide** is predicted to decrease the exposure to corticosteroids **(fluticasone)**. Unknown Theoretical
- **Apalutamide** is predicted to decrease the exposure to **coumarins**. Avoid or monitor. Mild Study
- **Apalutamide** is predicted to markedly decrease the exposure to **crizotinib**. Avoid. Severe Study → Also see TABLE 9 p. 909
- **Apalutamide** is predicted to decrease the exposure to **dabigatran**. Mild Study
- **Apalutamide** is predicted to decrease the exposure to **dabrafenib**. Avoid. Moderate Theoretical
- **Apalutamide** is predicted to decrease the exposure to **darifenacin**. Moderate Theoretical
- **Apalutamide** is predicted to markedly decrease the exposure to **dasatinib**. Avoid. Severe Study → Also see TABLE 9 p. 909
- **Apalutamide** is predicted to slightly decrease the exposure to **delamanid**. Avoid. Moderate Study → Also see TABLE 9 p. 909
- **Apalutamide** is predicted to decrease the exposure to **diazepam**. Avoid or monitor. Mild Study
- **Apalutamide** is predicted to markedly decrease the exposure to **dienogest**. Severe Study
- **Apalutamide** is predicted to decrease the exposure to **digoxin**. Mild Study
- **Apalutamide** decreases the exposure to **dolutegravir**. Adjust dose. Severe Study
- **Apalutamide** is predicted to decrease the exposure to **doravirine**. Avoid. Severe Study
- **Apalutamide** is predicted to decrease the exposure to **dronabinol**. Avoid or adjust dose. Mild Study
- **Apalutamide** is predicted to decrease the exposure to **elbasvir**. Avoid. Severe Study

A1 Interactions | Appendix 1

- **Apalutamide** is predicted to decrease the exposure to eliglustat. Avoid. [Severe] Study
- **Apalutamide** is predicted to decrease the concentration of elvitegravir. Avoid. [Severe] Theoretical
- **Apalutamide** is predicted to decrease the exposure to encorafenib. [Severe] Theoretical → Also see **TABLE 9** p. 909
- **Apalutamide** is predicted to decrease the effects of ergotamine. [Moderate] Theoretical
- **Apalutamide** is predicted to decrease the exposure to **erlotinib**. Avoid or adjust **erlotinib** dose. [Severe] Study
- **Apalutamide** is predicted to decrease the exposure to esketamine. Adjust dose. [Moderate] Theoretical
- **Apalutamide** is predicted to decrease the exposure to etravirine. Avoid. [Severe] Theoretical
- **Apalutamide** is predicted to decrease the concentration of everolimus. Avoid or adjust dose. [Severe] Study
- **Apalutamide** moderately decreases the exposure to exemestane. [Moderate] Study
- **Apalutamide** is predicted to decrease the exposure to fesoterodine. Avoid. [Moderate] Study
- Fibrates **(gemfibrozil)** are predicted to increase the exposure to **apalutamide**. [Mild] Study
- **Apalutamide** is predicted to decrease the exposure to fingolimod. [Moderate] Study
- **Apalutamide** is predicted to decrease the exposure to fosaprepitant. Avoid. [Moderate] Theoretical
- **Apalutamide** is predicted to decrease the exposure to **gefitinib**. Avoid. [Severe] Study
- **Apalutamide** is predicted to decrease the exposure to grazoprevir. Avoid. [Severe] Study
- **Apalutamide** is predicted to decrease the concentration of guanfacine. Adjust **guanfacine** dose, p. 247. [Moderate] Study
- **Apalutamide** decreases the concentration of **haloperidol**. Adjust dose. [Moderate] Study → Also see **TABLE 9** p. 909
- **HIV-protease inhibitors** are predicted to increase the exposure to **apalutamide**. [Mild] Study → Also see **TABLE 9** p. 909
- **Apalutamide** is predicted to decrease the exposure to **ibrutinib**. Avoid or adjust **ibrutinib** dose. [Severe] Study
- **Apalutamide** is predicted to decrease the exposure to **idelalisib**. Avoid. [Severe] Study
- **Idelalisib** is predicted to increase the exposure to **apalutamide**. [Mild] Study
- **Apalutamide** is predicted to decrease the exposure to **imatinib**. Avoid. [Moderate] Study
- **Apalutamide** is predicted to decrease the exposure to irinotecan. Avoid. [Severe] Study
- **Apalutamide** is predicted to decrease the exposure to ivabradine. Adjust dose. [Moderate] Theoretical
- **Apalutamide** is predicted to moderately to markedly decrease the exposure to **ivacaftor**. Avoid. [Severe] Study
- **Apalutamide** is predicted to decrease the exposure to **ixazomib**. Avoid. [Severe] Study
- **Apalutamide** is predicted to decrease the exposure to **lapatinib**. Avoid. [Severe] Study → Also see **TABLE 9** p. 909
- **Apalutamide** is predicted to moderately decrease the exposure to larotrectinib. Avoid. [Moderate] Study
- **Apalutamide** is predicted to decrease the exposure to linagliptin. [Moderate] Study
- **Apalutamide** is predicted to decrease the exposure to lomitapide. Monitor and adjust dose. [Moderate] Theoretical
- **Apalutamide** is predicted to decrease the exposure to lorlatinib. Avoid. [Severe] Study
- **Apalutamide** is predicted to decrease the exposure to lurasidone. Avoid. [Moderate] Study
- **Apalutamide** is predicted to decrease the exposure to macitentan. Avoid. [Severe] Study
- Macrolides **(clarithromycin)** are predicted to increase the exposure to **apalutamide**. [Mild] Study → Also see **TABLE 9** p. 909
- **Apalutamide** is predicted to decrease the exposure to maraviroc. Adjust dose. [Severe] Study
- **Apalutamide** is predicted to decrease the exposure to methotrexate. [Mild] Study
- **Apalutamide** is predicted to decrease the exposure to midazolam. Monitor and adjust dose. [Moderate] Study
- **Apalutamide** is predicted to decrease the exposure to midostaurin. Avoid. [Severe] Study
- **Apalutamide** is predicted to decrease the exposure to mirtazapine. Adjust dose. [Moderate] Study
- **Apalutamide** is predicted to decrease the exposure to moclobemide. Avoid or monitor. [Mild] Study
- **Apalutamide** is predicted to decrease the exposure to monoclonal antibodies **(polatuzumab vedotin)**. [Moderate] Theoretical
- **Apalutamide** is predicted to decrease the exposure to montelukast. [Mild] Study
- **Apalutamide** is predicted to markedly decrease the exposure to naldemedine. Avoid. [Severe] Study
- **Apalutamide** is predicted to markedly decrease the exposure to naloxegol. Avoid. [Moderate] Study
- **Apalutamide** is predicted to slightly decrease the exposure to nateglinide. [Mild] Study
- **Apalutamide** is predicted to decrease the exposure to neratinib. Avoid. [Severe] Study
- **Apalutamide** is predicted to decrease the exposure to netupitant. Avoid. [Severe] Study
- **Apalutamide** is predicted to moderately decrease the exposure to **nilotinib**. Avoid. [Severe] Study → Also see **TABLE 9** p. 909
- **Apalutamide** is predicted to decrease the exposure to nitisinone. Adjust dose. [Moderate] Theoretical
- **Apalutamide** is predicted to decrease the exposure to **olaparib**. Avoid. [Moderate] Theoretical
- **Apalutamide** is predicted to decrease the exposure to ondansetron. [Moderate] Study → Also see **TABLE 9** p. 909
- **Apalutamide** is predicted to decrease the exposure to opioids **(alfentanil, fentanyl)**. [Moderate] Study
- **Apalutamide** is predicted to decrease the exposure to opioids (buprenorphine). Monitor and adjust dose. [Moderate] Theoretical
- **Apalutamide** decreases the exposure to opioids **(methadone)**. Monitor and adjust dose. [Severe] Study → Also see **TABLE 9** p. 909
- **Apalutamide** is predicted to decrease the exposure to opioids (oxycodone). Monitor and adjust dose. [Moderate] Study
- **Apalutamide** is predicted to moderately decrease the exposure to **osimertinib**. Avoid. [Moderate] Study → Also see **TABLE 9** p. 909
- **Apalutamide** is predicted to moderately decrease the exposure to **ospemifene**. [Moderate] Study
- **Apalutamide** is predicted to decrease the exposure to palbociclib. Avoid. [Severe] Study
- **Apalutamide** is predicted to decrease the exposure to paliperidone. Monitor and adjust dose. [Severe] Study → Also see **TABLE 9** p. 909
- **Apalutamide** is predicted to decrease the exposure to panobinostat. Avoid. [Moderate] Theoretical → Also see **TABLE 9** p. 909
- **Apalutamide** is predicted to decrease the exposure to paritaprevir (with ritonavir and ombitasvir). Avoid. [Severe] Study
- **Apalutamide** is predicted to decrease the exposure to pazopanib. Avoid. [Severe] Theoretical → Also see **TABLE 9** p. 909
- **Apalutamide** is predicted to decrease the exposure to phosphodiesterase type-5 inhibitors **(avanafil, tadalafil)**. Avoid. [Severe] Study
- **Apalutamide** is predicted to decrease the exposure to phosphodiesterase type-5 inhibitors **(sildenafil, vardenafil)**. [Moderate] Theoretical → Also see **TABLE 9** p. 909
- **Apalutamide** is predicted to moderately to markedly decrease the exposure to **pibrentasvir**. Avoid. [Severe] Study
- **Apalutamide** is predicted to moderately decrease the exposure to **pitolisant**. [Moderate] Study
- **Apalutamide** is predicted to decrease the exposure to ponatinib. Avoid. [Moderate] Theoretical
- **Apalutamide** is predicted to markedly decrease the exposure to praziquantel. Avoid. [Moderate] Study
- **Apalutamide** is predicted to decrease the exposure to proton pump inhibitors **(lansoprazole, rabeprazole)**. Avoid or monitor. [Mild] Study
- **Apalutamide** markedly decreases the exposure to proton pump inhibitors **(omeprazole)**. Avoid or monitor. [Moderate] Study
- **Apalutamide** is predicted to decrease the exposure to quetiapine. [Moderate] Study

Apalutamide (continued)
- **Apalutamide** is predicted to decrease the exposure to ranolazine. Avoid. [Severe] Study → Also see **TABLE 9** p. 909
- **Apalutamide** is predicted to decrease the exposure to reboxetine. [Moderate] Anecdotal
- **Apalutamide** is predicted to decrease the exposure to regorafenib. Avoid. [Moderate] Study
- **Apalutamide** is predicted to decrease the exposure to repaglinide. Monitor blood glucose and adjust dose. [Moderate] Study
- **Apalutamide** is predicted to markedly decrease the exposure to ribociclib. Avoid. [Severe] Study → Also see **TABLE 9** p. 909
- **Apalutamide** markedly decreases the exposure to **rilpivirine**. Avoid. [Severe] Study
- **Apalutamide** is predicted to decrease the exposure to risperidone. Adjust dose. [Moderate] Study → Also see **TABLE 9** p. 909
- **Apalutamide** is predicted to moderately decrease the exposure to rivaroxaban. Avoid unless patient can be monitored for signs of thrombosis. [Severe] Study
- **Apalutamide** is predicted to decrease the exposure to roflumilast. Avoid. [Moderate] Study
- **Apalutamide** is predicted to markedly decrease the exposure to rolapitant. Avoid. [Severe] Study
- **Apalutamide** is predicted to decrease the exposure to ruxolitinib. Monitor and adjust dose. [Moderate] Study
- **Apalutamide** is predicted to moderately decrease the exposure to saxagliptin. [Moderate] Study
- **Apalutamide** is predicted to decrease the exposure to siponimod. [Severe] Study
- **Apalutamide** is predicted to decrease the concentration of sirolimus. Avoid. [Severe] Study
- **Apalutamide** is predicted to decrease the exposure to solifenacin. [Moderate] Theoretical
- **Apalutamide** is predicted to decrease the exposure to sorafenib. [Moderate] Theoretical → Also see **TABLE 9** p. 909
- **Apalutamide** is predicted to decrease the exposure to SSRIs (citalopram). Avoid or monitor. [Mild] Study → Also see **TABLE 9** p. 909
- **Apalutamide** slightly decreases the exposure to statins (rosuvastatin). [Mild] Study
- **Apalutamide** is predicted to decrease the exposure to statins (simvastatin). Avoid or monitor. [Moderate] Study
- **Apalutamide** is predicted to decrease the exposure to **sunitinib**. Avoid or adjust **sunitinib** dose. [Moderate] Study → Also see **TABLE 9** p. 909
- **Apalutamide** decreases the concentration of **tacrolimus**. Monitor and adjust dose. [Severe] Study
- **Apalutamide** is predicted to decrease the exposure to taxanes (cabazitaxel, paclitaxel). Avoid. [Severe] Study
- **Apalutamide** is predicted to decrease the exposure to taxanes (docetaxel). [Severe] Theoretical
- **Apalutamide** is predicted to decrease the concentration of temsirolimus. Avoid. [Severe] Study
- **Apalutamide** decreases the exposure to tetracyclines (doxycycline). Monitor and adjust dose. [Moderate] Study
- **Apalutamide** is predicted to decrease the exposure to tezacaftor. Avoid. [Severe] Theoretical
- **Apalutamide** potentially decreases the exposure to thyroid hormones (levothyroxine). [Mild] Theoretical
- **Apalutamide** is predicted to markedly decrease the exposure to ticagrelor. Avoid. [Severe] Study
- **Apalutamide** is predicted to decrease the exposure to tivozanib. [Severe] Study
- **Apalutamide** is predicted to decrease the exposure to tofacitinib. Avoid. [Severe] Study
- **Apalutamide** is predicted to decrease the exposure to tolvaptan. Use with caution or avoid depending on indication. [Severe] Study
- **Apalutamide** is predicted to decrease the exposure to toremifene. Adjust dose. [Moderate] Study → Also see **TABLE 9** p. 909
- **Apalutamide** is predicted to decrease the exposure to trabectedin. Avoid. [Severe] Theoretical
- **Apalutamide** is predicted to decrease the exposure to upadacitinib. [Moderate] Study
- **Apalutamide** is predicted to decrease the exposure to vandetanib. Avoid. [Moderate] Study → Also see **TABLE 9** p. 909
- **Apalutamide** is predicted to moderately decrease the exposure to velpatasvir. Avoid. [Severe] Study
- **Apalutamide** is predicted to decrease the exposure to vemurafenib. Avoid. [Severe] Theoretical → Also see **TABLE 9** p. 909
- **Apalutamide** is predicted to decrease the exposure to venetoclax. Avoid. [Severe] Study
- **Apalutamide** is predicted to decrease the exposure to vinca alkaloids (vinblastine, vincristine, vindesine). [Severe] Theoretical
- **Apalutamide** is predicted to decrease the exposure to vinca alkaloids (vinflunine). Avoid. [Severe] Theoretical → Also see **TABLE 9** p. 909
- **Apalutamide** is predicted to decrease the exposure to vinca alkaloids (vinorelbine). Use with caution or avoid. [Severe] Theoretical
- **Apalutamide** is predicted to decrease the exposure to vismodegib. Avoid. [Moderate] Theoretical
- **Apalutamide** is predicted to decrease the exposure to vortioxetine. Monitor and adjust dose. [Moderate] Study
- **Apalutamide** is predicted to decrease the concentration of voxilaprevir. Avoid. [Severe] Study
- **Apalutamide** is predicted to decrease the exposure to zopiclone. Adjust dose. [Moderate] Study

Apixaban → see **TABLE 3** p. 907 (anticoagulant effects)
- Antiarrhythmics (dronedarone) are predicted to increase the exposure to **apixaban**. [Moderate] Theoretical
- Antiepileptics (carbamazepine, fosphenytoin, phenobarbital, phenytoin, primidone) are predicted to moderately decrease the exposure to **apixaban**. Use with caution or avoid. [Severe] Study
- Antifungals, azoles (itraconazole) are predicted to increase the exposure to **apixaban**. Avoid. [Severe] Theoretical
- Antifungals, azoles (ketoconazole) slightly to moderately increase the exposure to **apixaban**. Avoid. [Severe] Study
- Antifungals, azoles (voriconazole) are predicted to increase the exposure to **apixaban**. Avoid. [Moderate] Theoretical
- Apalutamide is predicted to moderately decrease the exposure to **apixaban**. Use with caution or avoid. [Severe] Study
- Calcium channel blockers (verapamil) are predicted to increase the exposure to **apixaban**. [Moderate] Theoretical
- Cobicistat is predicted to increase the exposure to **apixaban**. Avoid. [Severe] Theoretical
- Enzalutamide is predicted to moderately decrease the exposure to **apixaban**. Use with caution or avoid. [Severe] Study
- HIV-protease inhibitors (ritonavir) are predicted to increase the exposure to **apixaban**. Avoid. [Severe] Theoretical
- Macrolides (erythromycin) are predicted to increase the exposure to **apixaban**. [Moderate] Theoretical
- Mitotane is predicted to moderately decrease the exposure to **apixaban**. Use with caution or avoid. [Severe] Study
- Rifampicin is predicted to moderately decrease the exposure to **apixaban**. Use with caution or avoid. [Severe] Study
- St John's Wort is predicted to decrease the exposure to **apixaban**. Use with caution or avoid. [Moderate] Theoretical

Apomorphine → see dopamine receptor agonists

Apraclonidine → see **TABLE 6** p. 908 (bradycardia), **TABLE 8** p. 908 (hypotension), **TABLE 11** p. 909 (CNS depressant effects)
- Amfetamines are predicted to decrease the effects of **apraclonidine**. Avoid. [Severe] Theoretical
- Methylphenidate is predicted to decrease the effects of **apraclonidine**. Avoid. [Severe] Theoretical
- Sympathomimetics, inotropic are predicted to decrease the effects of **apraclonidine**. Avoid. [Severe] Theoretical
- Sympathomimetics, vasoconstrictor are predicted to decrease the effects of **apraclonidine**. Avoid. [Severe] Theoretical

Apremilast
- Antiepileptics (carbamazepine, fosphenytoin, phenobarbital, phenytoin, primidone) moderately decrease the exposure to **apremilast**. Avoid. [Severe] Study
- Apalutamide moderately decreases the exposure to **apremilast**. Avoid. [Severe] Study
- Enzalutamide moderately decreases the exposure to **apremilast**. Avoid. [Severe] Study

- Mitotane moderately decreases the exposure to **apremilast**. Avoid. Severe Study
- Rifampicin moderately decreases the exposure to **apremilast**. Avoid. Severe Study
- St John's Wort is predicted to decrease the exposure to **apremilast**. Avoid. Severe Theoretical

Aprepitant

- **Aprepitant** is predicted to increase the exposure to **abemaciclib**. Moderate Study
- **Aprepitant** is predicted to increase the exposure to aldosterone antagonists **(eplerenone)**. Adjust **eplerenone** dose. Severe Study
- **Aprepitant** is predicted to increase the exposure to alkylating agents **(ifosfamide)**. Severe Theoretical
- **Aprepitant** is predicted to increase the exposure to alpha blockers **(tamsulosin)**. Moderate Theoretical
- **Aprepitant** is predicted to increase the exposure to **alprazolam**. Severe Study
- **Aprepitant** increases the exposure to antiarrhythmics **(dronedarone)**. Severe Theoretical
- **Aprepitant** is predicted to increase the exposure to antiarrhythmics **(propafenone)**. Monitor and adjust dose. Moderate Study
- Antiepileptics **(carbamazepine, fosphenytoin, phenobarbital, phenytoin, primidone)** are predicted to markedly decrease the exposure to **aprepitant**. Avoid. Moderate Study
- Antifungals, azoles **(fluconazole)** are predicted to increase the exposure to **aprepitant**. Moderate Theoretical
- Antifungals, azoles **(itraconazole, ketoconazole, voriconazole)** are predicted to markedly increase the exposure to **aprepitant**. Moderate Study
- Antifungals, azoles **(posaconazole)** are predicted to increase the exposure to **aprepitant**. Moderate Study
- **Aprepitant** is predicted to increase the exposure to antifungals, azoles **(isavuconazole)**. Moderate Theoretical
- **Aprepitant** is predicted to increase the exposure to antihistamines, non-sedating **(mizolastine)**. Severe Theoretical
- **Aprepitant** is predicted to increase the exposure to antihistamines, non-sedating **(rupatadine)**. Avoid. Moderate Study
- **Aprepitant** is predicted to increase the concentration of antimalarials **(piperaquine)**. Severe Theoretical
- **Apalutamide** is predicted to markedly decrease the exposure to **aprepitant**. Avoid. Moderate Study
- **Aprepitant** is predicted to increase the exposure to **axitinib**. Moderate Theoretical
- **Aprepitant** is predicted to increase the exposure to **bedaquiline**. Avoid prolonged use. Mild Theoretical
- **Aprepitant** is predicted to increase the exposure to beta$_2$ agonists **(salmeterol)**. Moderate Study
- **Bosentan** is predicted to decrease the exposure to **aprepitant**. Moderate Study
- **Aprepitant** is predicted to increase the exposure to **bosutinib**. Avoid or adjust dose. Severe Theoretical
- **Aprepitant** is predicted to increase the exposure to **buspirone**. Use with caution and adjust dose. Moderate Study
- **Aprepitant** is predicted to increase the exposure to **cabozantinib**. Moderate Theoretical
- Calcium channel blockers **(diltiazem, verapamil)** are predicted to increase the exposure to **aprepitant** and **aprepitant** is predicted to increase the exposure to calcium channel blockers **(diltiazem, verapamil)**. Moderate Study
- **Aprepitant** is predicted to increase the exposure to calcium channel blockers **(amlodipine, felodipine, lacidipine, lercanidipine, nicardipine, nifedipine, nimodipine)**. Monitor and adjust dose. Moderate Study
- **Aprepitant** is predicted to increase the exposure to **cariprazine**. Avoid. Severe Study
- **Aprepitant** is predicted to increase the concentration of **ciclosporin**. Severe Study
- **Cobicistat** is predicted to markedly increase the exposure to **aprepitant**. Moderate Study
- **Aprepitant** is predicted to increase the exposure to **cobimetinib**. Severe Theoretical
- **Aprepitant** is predicted to increase the exposure to **colchicine**. Adjust **colchicine** dose with moderate inhibitors of CYP3A4. Severe Study
- **Aprepitant** is predicted to decrease the efficacy of **combined hormonal contraceptives**. For FSRH guidance, see Contraceptives, interactions p. 536. Severe Study
- **Aprepitant** is predicted to increase the exposure to oral corticosteroids **(budesonide)**. Moderate Study
- **Aprepitant** moderately increases the exposure to corticosteroids (dexamethasone). Monitor and adjust dose. Moderate Study
- **Aprepitant** is predicted to increase the exposure to corticosteroids **(fluticasone)**. Moderate Study
- **Aprepitant** is predicted to increase the exposure to corticosteroids **(methylprednisolone)**. Monitor and adjust dose. Moderate Study
- **Aprepitant** decreases the anticoagulant effect of **coumarins**. Moderate Study
- **Aprepitant** is predicted to slightly increase the exposure to **darifenacin**. Moderate Study
- **Aprepitant** is predicted to increase the exposure to **dasatinib**. Severe Study
- **Aprepitant** is predicted to decrease the efficacy of **desogestrel**. For FSRH guidance, see Contraceptives, interactions p. 536. Severe Theoretical
- **Aprepitant** is predicted to slightly increase the exposure to **dienogest**. Moderate Study
- **Aprepitant** increases the risk of QT-prolongation when given with **domperidone**. Avoid. Severe Study
- **Aprepitant** is predicted to increase the exposure to dopamine receptor agonists **(bromocriptine)**. Severe Theoretical
- **Aprepitant** is predicted to increase the concentration of dopamine receptor agonists **(cabergoline)**. Moderate Anecdotal
- **Aprepitant** is predicted to moderately increase the exposure to **dutasteride**. Mild Study
- **Efavirenz** is predicted to decrease the exposure to **aprepitant**. Moderate Study
- **Aprepitant** is predicted to increase the exposure to **eletriptan**. Moderate Study
- **Aprepitant** is predicted to increase the exposure to **eliglustat**. Avoid or adjust dose—consult product literature. Severe Study
- **Aprepitant** is predicted to moderately increase the exposure to **encorafenib**. Moderate Study
- **Enzalutamide** is predicted to markedly decrease the exposure to **aprepitant**. Avoid. Moderate Study
- **Aprepitant** is predicted to increase the risk of ergotism when given with **ergometrine**. Severe Theoretical
- **Aprepitant** is predicted to increase the risk of ergotism when given with **ergotamine**. Severe Theoretical
- **Aprepitant** is predicted to increase the exposure to **erlotinib**. Moderate Theoretical
- **Aprepitant** is predicted to decrease the efficacy of **etonogestrel**. For FSRH guidance, see Contraceptives, interactions p. 536. Severe Theoretical
- **Aprepitant** is predicted to increase the concentration of **everolimus**. Avoid or adjust dose. Moderate Study
- **Aprepitant** is predicted to increase the exposure to **fesoterodine**. Adjust **fesoterodine** dose with moderate inhibitors of CYP3A4 in hepatic and renal impairment. Mild Study
- **Aprepitant** is predicted to increase the exposure to **gefitinib**. Moderate Theoretical
- **Aprepitant** is predicted to increase the concentration of **guanfacine**. Adjust **guanfacine** dose, p. 247. Moderate Theoretical
- **HIV-protease inhibitors** are predicted to markedly increase the exposure to **aprepitant**. Moderate Study
- **Aprepitant** is predicted to decrease the effects of **hormone replacement therapy**. Moderate Anecdotal
- **Aprepitant** is predicted to increase the exposure to **ibrutinib**. Adjust **ibrutinib** dose with moderate inhibitors of CYP3A4. Severe Study
- **Idelalisib** is predicted to markedly increase the exposure to **aprepitant**. Moderate Study
- **Aprepitant** is predicted to increase the exposure to **imatinib**. Moderate Theoretical
- **Aprepitant** is predicted to increase the exposure to intravenous **irinotecan**. Severe Theoretical
- **Aprepitant** is predicted to increase the exposure to **ivabradine**. Adjust **ivabradine** dose. Severe Theoretical

Aprepitant (continued)
- **Aprepitant** is predicted to increase the exposure to **ivacaftor.** Adjust ivacaftor p. 196 or tezacaftor with ivacaftor p. 198 dose with moderate inhibitors of CYP3A4. Severe Study
- **Aprepitant** is predicted to increase the exposure to **lapatinib.** Moderate Study
- **Aprepitant** is predicted to decrease the efficacy of levonorgestrel. For FSRH guidance, see Contraceptives, interactions p. 536. Severe Theoretical
- **Aprepitant** is predicted to increase the exposure to **lomitapide.** Avoid. Moderate Theoretical
- **Aprepitant** is predicted to increase the exposure to **lurasidone.** Adjust **lurasidone** dose. Moderate Study
- Macrolides **(clarithromycin)** are predicted to markedly increase the exposure to **aprepitant.** Moderate Study
- Macrolides **(erythromycin)** are predicted to increase the exposure to **aprepitant**. Moderate Study
- **Aprepitant** is predicted to increase the exposure to **maraviroc.** Moderate Study
- **Aprepitant** is predicted to increase the exposure to **midazolam.** Monitor side effects and adjust dose. Severe Study
- **Aprepitant** is predicted to increase the exposure to **midostaurin.** Moderate Theoretical
- **Mitotane** is predicted to markedly decrease the exposure to **aprepitant**. Avoid. Moderate Study
- **Aprepitant** is predicted to increase the exposure to **naldemedine.** Moderate Study
- **Aprepitant** is predicted to increase the exposure to **naloxegol.** Adjust **naloxegol** dose and monitor side effects. Moderate Study
- **Aprepitant** is predicted to increase the exposure to **neratinib.** Avoid. Severe Study
- **Nevirapine** is predicted to decrease the exposure to **aprepitant.** Moderate Study
- **Aprepitant** is predicted to increase the exposure to **nilotinib.** Moderate Theoretical
- **Aprepitant** is predicted to decrease the efficacy of **norethisterone.** For FSRH guidance, see Contraceptives, interactions p. 536. Severe Anecdotal
- **Aprepitant** is predicted to increase the exposure to **olaparib.** Avoid moderate inhibitors of CYP3A4 or adjust **olaparib** dose. Moderate Theoretical
- **Aprepitant** is predicted to increase the exposure to opioids **(alfentanil, buprenorphine, fentanyl, oxycodone).** Monitor and adjust dose. Moderate Study
- **Aprepitant** is predicted to increase the exposure to opioids **(methadone).** Moderate Theoretical
- **Aprepitant** is predicted to increase the exposure to **oxybutynin.** Mild Theoretical
- **Aprepitant** is predicted to increase the exposure to **pazopanib.** Moderate Theoretical
- **Aprepitant** is predicted to increase the exposure to phosphodiesterase type-5 inhibitors **(avanafil).** Adjust **avanafil** dose. Moderate Theoretical
- **Aprepitant** is predicted to increase the exposure to phosphodiesterase type-5 inhibitors **(sildenafil).** Monitor or adjust **sildenafil** dose with moderate inhibitors of CYP3A4, p. 125. Moderate Study
- **Aprepitant** is predicted to increase the exposure to phosphodiesterase type-5 inhibitors **(tadalafil).** Severe Theoretical
- **Aprepitant** is predicted to increase the exposure to phosphodiesterase type-5 inhibitors **(vardenafil).** Adjust dose. Severe Theoretical
- **Aprepitant** is predicted to increase the exposure to **pimozide.** Avoid. Severe Theoretical
- **Aprepitant** is predicted to increase the exposure to **quetiapine.** Avoid. Moderate Study
- **Aprepitant** is predicted to increase the exposure to **ranolazine.** Severe Study
- **Aprepitant** is predicted to increase the exposure to **ribociclib.** Moderate Study
- **Rifampicin** is predicted to markedly decrease the exposure to **aprepitant.** Avoid. Moderate Study
- **Aprepitant** is predicted to increase the exposure to **ruxolitinib.** Moderate Theoretical
- **Aprepitant** is predicted to increase the exposure to **saxagliptin.** Mild Study
- **Aprepitant** increases the concentration of **sirolimus.** Monitor and adjust dose. Moderate Study
- **Aprepitant** is predicted to increase the exposure to SSRIs **(dapoxetine).** Adjust **dapoxetine** dose with moderate inhibitors of CYP3A4. Moderate Theoretical
- **St John's Wort** is predicted to decrease the exposure to **aprepitant**. Avoid. Moderate Theoretical
- **Aprepitant** is predicted to increase the exposure to statins **(atorvastatin, simvastatin).** Monitor and adjust dose. Severe Theoretical
- **Aprepitant** is predicted to increase the exposure to **sunitinib.** Moderate Theoretical
- **Aprepitant** is predicted to increase the concentration of **tacrolimus.** Severe Study
- **Aprepitant** is predicted to increase the exposure to taxanes **(cabazitaxel).** Moderate Theoretical
- **Aprepitant** is predicted to increase the concentration of **temsirolimus.** Use with caution or avoid. Moderate Theoretical
- **Aprepitant** is predicted to increase the exposure to **tezacaftor.** Adjust tezacaftor with ivacaftor p. 198 dose with moderate inhibitors of CYP3A4. Severe Study
- **Aprepitant** given with a potent CYP2C19 inhibitor is predicted to increase the exposure to **tofacitinib.** Adjust **tofacitinib** dose. Moderate Study
- **Aprepitant** is predicted to increase the exposure to **tolterodine.** Mild Theoretical
- **Aprepitant** is predicted to increase the exposure to **tolvaptan.** Manufacturer advises caution or adjust **tolvaptan** dose with moderate inhibitors of CYP3A4. Moderate Study
- **Aprepitant** is predicted to increase the exposure to **trazodone.** Moderate Theoretical
- **Aprepitant** decreases the efficacy of **ulipristal.** For FSRH guidance, see Contraceptives, interactions p. 536. Severe Anecdotal
- **Aprepitant** is predicted to increase the exposure to **venetoclax.** Avoid or adjust dose—consult product literature. Severe Study
- **Aprepitant** is predicted to increase the exposure to **vinca alkaloids.** Severe Theoretical
- **Aprepitant** is predicted to increase the exposure to **zopiclone.** Adjust dose. Moderate Study

Argatroban → see TABLE 3 p. 907 (anticoagulant effects)
- **Ranibizumab** is predicted to increase the risk of bleeding events when given with **argatroban.** Severe Theoretical

Aripiprazole → see TABLE 8 p. 908 (hypotension), TABLE 11 p. 909 (CNS depressant effects)
- Antiepileptics **(carbamazepine, fosphenytoin, phenobarbital, phenytoin, primidone)** are predicted to moderately decrease the exposure to **aripiprazole.** Adjust **aripiprazole** dose, p. 265. Moderate Study → Also see TABLE 11 p. 909
- Antifungals, azoles **(itraconazole, ketoconazole, voriconazole)** are predicted to slightly increase the exposure to **aripiprazole.** Adjust **aripiprazole** dose, p. 265. Moderate Study
- **Apalutamide** is predicted to moderately decrease the exposure to **aripiprazole**. Adjust **aripiprazole** dose, p. 265. Moderate Study
- **Bupropion** is predicted to moderately increase the exposure to **aripiprazole.** Adjust **aripiprazole** dose, p. 265. Moderate Study
- **Cinacalcet** is predicted to moderately increase the exposure to **aripiprazole.** Adjust **aripiprazole** dose, p. 265. Moderate Study
- **Cobicistat** is predicted to slightly increase the exposure to **aripiprazole.** Adjust **aripiprazole** dose, p. 265. Moderate Study
- **Aripiprazole** is predicted to decrease the effects of **dopamine receptor agonists.** Moderate Theoretical → Also see TABLE 8 p. 908
- **Enzalutamide** is predicted to moderately decrease the exposure to **aripiprazole**. Adjust **aripiprazole** dose, p. 265. Moderate Study
- **HIV-protease inhibitors** are predicted to slightly increase the exposure to **aripiprazole**. Adjust **aripiprazole** dose, p. 265. Moderate Study
- **Idelalisib** is predicted to slightly increase the exposure to **aripiprazole.** Adjust **aripiprazole** dose, p. 265. Moderate Study
- **Aripiprazole** is predicted to decrease the effects of **levodopa.** Severe Theoretical → Also see TABLE 8 p. 908

- Macrolides **(clarithromycin)** are predicted to slightly increase the exposure to **aripiprazole**. Adjust **aripiprazole** dose, p. 265. Moderate Study
- **Mitotane** is predicted to moderately decrease the exposure to **aripiprazole**. Adjust **aripiprazole** dose, p. 265. Moderate Study
- **Rifampicin** is predicted to moderately decrease the exposure to **aripiprazole**. Adjust **aripiprazole** dose, p. 265. Moderate Study
- SSRIs **(fluoxetine, paroxetine)** are predicted to moderately increase the exposure to **aripiprazole**. Adjust **aripiprazole** dose, p. 265. Moderate Study
- **Terbinafine** is predicted to moderately increase the exposure to **aripiprazole**. Adjust **aripiprazole** dose, p. 265. Moderate Study

Arsenic trioxide → see **TABLE 15** p. 910 (myelosuppression), **TABLE 9** p. 909 (QT-interval prolongation)

Artemether → see antimalarials

Artenimol → see antimalarials

Articaine → see **TABLE 11** p. 909 (CNS depressant effects)

Ascorbic acid

- **Ascorbic acid** is predicted to increase the risk of cardiovascular side-effects when given with iron chelators **(deferiprone, desferrioxamine)**. Severe Theoretical

Asenapine → see **TABLE 8** p. 908 (hypotension), **TABLE 11** p. 909 (CNS depressant effects)

- **Asenapine** is predicted to decrease the effects of **dopamine receptor agonists**. Adjust dose. Moderate Theoretical → Also see **TABLE 8** p. 908
- **Asenapine** is predicted to decrease the effects of **levodopa**. Adjust dose. Severe Theoretical → Also see **TABLE 8** p. 908
- SSRIs **(fluvoxamine)** increase the exposure to **asenapine**. Moderate Study
- SSRIs **(paroxetine)** moderately increase the exposure to **asenapine**. Moderate Study

Asparaginase → see **TABLE 1** p. 907 (hepatotoxicity), **TABLE 15** p. 910 (myelosuppression)

- **Asparaginase** is predicted to increase the risk of hepatotoxicity when given with **imatinib**. Severe Theoretical → Also see **TABLE 15** p. 910
- **Asparaginase** affects the efficacy of **methotrexate**. Severe Anecdotal → Also see **TABLE 1** p. 907 → Also see **TABLE 15** p. 910
- **Asparaginase** potentially increases the risk of neurotoxicity when given with vinca alkaloids **(vincristine)**. **Vincristine** should be taken 3 to 24 hours before **asparaginase**. Severe Anecdotal → Also see **TABLE 1** p. 907 → Also see **TABLE 15** p. 910

Aspirin → see **TABLE 4** p. 907 (antiplatelet effects)

- **Acetazolamide** increases the risk of severe toxic reaction when given with **aspirin** (high-dose). Severe Study
- **Antacids** decrease the absorption of **aspirin** (high-dose). Moderate Study
- **Bismuth subsalicylate** is predicted to increase the risk of side-effects when given with **aspirin**. Avoid. Moderate Theoretical
- **Aspirin** (high-dose) is predicted to increase the risk of gastrointestinal irritation when given with bisphosphonates **(alendronate, ibandronate)**. Moderate Study
- **Aspirin** (high-dose) is predicted to increase the risk of renal impairment when given with bisphosphonates **(clodronate)**. Severe Theoretical
- **Corticosteroids** are predicted to decrease the concentration of **aspirin** (high-dose) and **aspirin** (high-dose) increases the risk of gastrointestinal bleeding when given with **corticosteroids**. Moderate Study
- **Aspirin** (high-dose) increases the risk of renal impairment when given with **daptomycin**. Moderate Theoretical
- **Erlotinib** is predicted to increase the risk of gastrointestinal perforation when given with **aspirin** (high-dose). Severe Theoretical
- **Aspirin** (high-dose) is predicted to increase the risk of gastrointestinal bleeds when given with iron chelators **(deferasirox)**. Severe Theoretical
- **Aspirin** (high-dose) is predicted to increase the risk of toxicity when given with **methotrexate**. Severe Study
- **Aspirin** is predicted to increase the risk of gastrointestinal perforation when given with **nicorandil**. Severe Theoretical
- **Aspirin** (high-dose) potentially increases the exposure to **pemetrexed**. Use with caution or avoid. Severe Theoretical
- **Aspirin** (high-dose) increases the risk of acute renal failure when given with **thiazide diuretics**. Severe Theoretical
- **Zidovudine** increases the risk of haematological toxicity when given with **aspirin** (high-dose). Severe Study

Ataluren

- **Ataluren** is predicted to increase the risk of nephrotoxicity when given with intravenous **aminoglycosides**. Avoid. Severe Study
- **Rifampicin** decreases the exposure to **ataluren**. Moderate Study

Atazanavir → see HIV-protease inhibitors

Atenolol → see beta blockers, selective

Atezolizumab → see monoclonal antibodies

Atomoxetine

- **Amfetamines** are predicted to increase the risk of side-effects when given with **atomoxetine**. Severe Theoretical
- **Atomoxetine** is predicted to increase the risk of cardiovascular side-effects when given with **beta$_2$ agonists** (high-dose). Moderate Study
- **Bupropion** is predicted to markedly increase the exposure to **atomoxetine**. Adjust dose. Severe Study
- **Cinacalcet** is predicted to markedly increase the exposure to **atomoxetine**. Adjust dose. Severe Study
- **Dacomitinib** is predicted to markedly increase the exposure to **atomoxetine**. Avoid or adjust dose. Severe Study
- **Eliglustat** is predicted to increase the exposure to **atomoxetine**. Adjust dose. Moderate Theoretical
- **MAOIs, irreversible** are predicted to increase the risk of side-effects when given with **atomoxetine**. Avoid and for 2 weeks after stopping the MAOI. Severe Theoretical
- **Panobinostat** is predicted to increase the exposure to **atomoxetine**. Monitor and adjust dose. Severe Theoretical
- SSRIs **(fluoxetine, paroxetine)** are predicted to markedly increase the exposure to **atomoxetine**. Adjust dose. Severe Study
- **Terbinafine** is predicted to markedly increase the exposure to **atomoxetine**. Adjust dose. Severe Study

Atorvastatin → see statins

Atovaquone → see antimalarials

Atracurium → see neuromuscular blocking drugs, non-depolarising

Atropine → see **TABLE 10** p. 909 (antimuscarinics)

ROUTE-SPECIFIC INFORMATION Since systemic absorption can follow topical application, the possibility of interactions should be borne in mind.

- **Atropine** increases the risk of severe hypertension when given with sympathomimetics, vasoconstrictor **(phenylephrine)**. Severe Study

Avanafil → see phosphodiesterase type-5 inhibitors

Avelumab → see monoclonal antibodies

Axitinib → see **TABLE 15** p. 910 (myelosuppression)

- Antiarrhythmics **(dronedarone)** are predicted to increase the exposure to **axitinib**. Moderate Theoretical
- Antiepileptics **(carbamazepine, fosphenytoin, phenobarbital, phenytoin, primidone)** are predicted to decrease the exposure to **axitinib**. Avoid or adjust dose. Moderate Study
- Antifungals, azoles **(fluconazole, isavuconazole, posaconazole)** are predicted to increase the exposure to **axitinib**. Moderate Theoretical
- Antifungals, azoles **(itraconazole, ketoconazole, voriconazole)** are predicted to increase the exposure to **axitinib**. Avoid or adjust dose. Moderate Study
- **Apalutamide** is predicted to decrease the exposure to **axitinib**. Avoid or adjust dose. Moderate Study
- **Aprepitant** is predicted to increase the exposure to **axitinib**. Moderate Theoretical
- **Bosentan** is predicted to decrease the exposure to **axitinib**. Moderate Theoretical
- Calcium channel blockers **(diltiazem, verapamil)** are predicted to increase the exposure to **axitinib**. Moderate Theoretical
- **Cobicistat** is predicted to increase the exposure to **axitinib**. Avoid or adjust dose. Moderate Study
- **Axitinib** is predicted to increase the risk of bleeding events when given with **coumarins**. Severe Theoretical
- **Crizotinib** is predicted to increase the exposure to **axitinib**. Moderate Theoretical → Also see **TABLE 15** p. 910

Axitinib (continued)
- Efavirenz is predicted to decrease the exposure to **axitinib.** [Moderate] Theoretical
- Enzalutamide is predicted to decrease the exposure to **axitinib.** Avoid or adjust dose. [Moderate] Study
- Grapefruit juice is predicted to increase the exposure to **axitinib.** [Moderate] Theoretical
- HIV-protease inhibitors are predicted to increase the exposure to **axitinib.** Avoid or adjust dose. [Moderate] Study
- Idelalisib is predicted to increase the exposure to **axitinib.** Avoid or adjust dose. [Moderate] Study → Also see **TABLE 15** p. 910
- Imatinib is predicted to increase the exposure to **axitinib.** [Moderate] Theoretical → Also see **TABLE 15** p. 910
- Macrolides **(clarithromycin)** are predicted to increase the exposure to **axitinib.** Avoid or adjust dose. [Moderate] Study
- Macrolides **(erythromycin)** are predicted to increase the exposure to **axitinib.** [Moderate] Theoretical
- Mitotane is predicted to decrease the exposure to **axitinib.** Avoid or adjust dose. [Moderate] Study → Also see **TABLE 15** p. 910
- Netupitant is predicted to increase the exposure to **axitinib.** [Moderate] Theoretical
- Nevirapine is predicted to decrease the exposure to **axitinib.** [Moderate] Theoretical
- Nilotinib is predicted to increase the exposure to **axitinib.** [Moderate] Theoretical → Also see **TABLE 15** p. 910
- **Axitinib** is predicted to increase the risk of bleeding events when given with phenindione. [Severe] Theoretical
- Rifampicin is predicted to decrease the exposure to **axitinib.** Avoid or adjust dose. [Moderate] Study
- St John's Wort is predicted to decrease the exposure to **axitinib.** [Moderate] Theoretical

Azacitidine → see **TABLE 15** p. 910 (myelosuppression)

Azathioprine → see **TABLE 15** p. 910 (myelosuppression)
- ACE inhibitors are predicted to increase the risk of anaemia and/or leucopenia when given with **azathioprine.** [Severe] Anecdotal
- Allopurinol potentially increases the risk of haematological toxicity when given with **azathioprine**. Adjust **azathioprine** dose, p. 558. [Severe] Study
- **Azathioprine** decreases the anticoagulant effect of coumarins. [Moderate] Study
- Febuxostat is predicted to increase the exposure to **azathioprine.** Avoid. [Severe] Theoretical
- Live vaccines are predicted to increase the risk of generalised infection (possibly life-threatening) when given with **azathioprine** (high-dose). Public Health England advises avoid (refer to Green Book). [Severe] Theoretical

Azelastine → see antihistamines, non-sedating

Azilsartan → see angiotensin-II receptor antagonists

Azithromycin → see macrolides

Bacillus Calmette-Guérin vaccine → see live vaccines

Bacitracin → see **TABLE 2** p. 907 (nephrotoxicity)

Baclofen → see **TABLE 8** p. 908 (hypotension), **TABLE 11** p. 909 (CNS depressant effects), **TABLE 10** p. 909 (antimuscarinics)
- **Baclofen** is predicted to increase the risk of side-effects when given with levodopa. [Severe] Anecdotal → Also see **TABLE 8** p. 908

Balsalazide → see **TABLE 15** p. 910 (myelosuppression)
- **Balsalazide** is predicted to decrease the concentration of digoxin. [Moderate] Theoretical

Bambuterol → see beta$_2$ agonists

Baricitinib
- Leflunomide potentially increases the exposure to **baricitinib.** [Moderate] Theoretical
- Live vaccines are predicted to increase the risk of generalised infection (possibly life-threatening) when given with **baricitinib.** Avoid. [Severe] Theoretical
- Teriflunomide potentially increases the exposure to **baricitinib.** [Moderate] Theoretical

Basiliximab → see monoclonal antibodies

Bazedoxifene
- Antiepileptics **(carbamazepine, fosphenytoin, phenobarbital, phenytoin, primidone)** are predicted to decrease the exposure to **bazedoxifene.** [Moderate] Theoretical
- Rifampicin is predicted to decrease the exposure to **bazedoxifene.** [Moderate] Theoretical

Beclometasone → see corticosteroids

Bedaquiline → see **TABLE 1** p. 907 (hepatotoxicity), **TABLE 9** p. 909 (QT-interval prolongation)
- Antiarrhythmics **(dronedarone)** are predicted to increase the exposure to **bedaquiline.** Avoid prolonged use. [Mild] Theoretical → Also see **TABLE 9** p. 909
- Antiepileptics **(carbamazepine, fosphenytoin, phenobarbital, phenytoin, primidone)** decrease the exposure to **bedaquiline.** Avoid. [Severe] Study → Also see **TABLE 1** p. 907
- Antifungals, azoles **(fluconazole, isavuconazole, posaconazole)** are predicted to increase the exposure to **bedaquiline.** Avoid prolonged use. [Mild] Theoretical → Also see **TABLE 1** p. 907 → Also see **TABLE 9** p. 909
- Antifungals, azoles **(itraconazole, ketoconazole, voriconazole)** are predicted to increase the exposure to **bedaquiline.** Avoid prolonged use. [Mild] Study → Also see **TABLE 1** p. 907 → Also see **TABLE 9** p. 909
- Apalutamide decreases the exposure to **bedaquiline.** Avoid. [Severe] Study → Also see **TABLE 9** p. 909
- Aprepitant is predicted to increase the exposure to **bedaquiline.** Avoid prolonged use. [Mild] Theoretical
- Bosentan is predicted to decrease the exposure to **bedaquiline.** Avoid. [Severe] Study
- Calcium channel blockers **(diltiazem, verapamil)** are predicted to increase the exposure to **bedaquiline.** Avoid prolonged use. [Mild] Theoretical
- Clofazimine potentially increases the risk of QT-prolongation when given with **bedaquiline.** [Severe] Study
- Cobicistat is predicted to increase the exposure to **bedaquiline.** Avoid prolonged use. [Mild] Study
- Crizotinib is predicted to increase the exposure to **bedaquiline.** Avoid prolonged use. [Mild] Theoretical → Also see **TABLE 9** p. 909
- Efavirenz is predicted to decrease the exposure to **bedaquiline.** Avoid. [Severe] Study → Also see **TABLE 9** p. 909
- Enzalutamide decreases the exposure to **bedaquiline.** Avoid. [Severe] Study
- Etravirine is predicted to decrease the exposure to **bedaquiline.** Avoid. [Severe] Theoretical
- HIV-protease inhibitors are predicted to increase the exposure to **bedaquiline.** Avoid prolonged use. [Mild] Study → Also see **TABLE 9** p. 909
- Idelalisib is predicted to increase the exposure to **bedaquiline.** Avoid prolonged use. [Mild] Study
- Imatinib is predicted to increase the exposure to **bedaquiline.** Avoid prolonged use. [Mild] Theoretical
- Macrolides **(clarithromycin)** are predicted to increase the exposure to **bedaquiline.** Avoid prolonged use. [Mild] Study → Also see **TABLE 9** p. 909
- Macrolides **(erythromycin)** are predicted to increase the exposure to **bedaquiline.** Avoid prolonged use. [Mild] Theoretical → Also see **TABLE 9** p. 909
- Mitotane decreases the exposure to **bedaquiline.** Avoid. [Severe] Study
- Netupitant is predicted to increase the exposure to **bedaquiline.** Avoid prolonged use. [Mild] Theoretical
- Nevirapine is predicted to decrease the exposure to **bedaquiline.** Avoid. [Severe] Study
- Nilotinib is predicted to increase the exposure to **bedaquiline.** Avoid prolonged use. [Mild] Theoretical → Also see **TABLE 9** p. 909
- Rifampicin decreases the exposure to **bedaquiline.** Avoid. [Severe] Study
- St John's Wort is predicted to decrease the exposure to **bedaquiline.** Avoid. [Severe] Study

Bee venom extract

GENERAL INFORMATION Desensitising vaccines should be avoided in patients taking beta-blockers (adrenaline might be ineffective in case of a hypersensitivity reaction) or ACE inhibitors (risk of severe anaphylactoid reactions).

Belatacept
- Live vaccines are predicted to increase the risk of generalised infection (possibly life-threatening) when given with **belatacept.** Public Health England advises avoid (refer to Green Book). [Severe] Theoretical

Belimumab → see monoclonal antibodies

Bendamustine → see alkylating agents

Bendroflumethiazide → see thiazide diuretics

Benperidol → see TABLE 8 p. 908 (hypotension), TABLE 11 p. 909 (CNS depressant effects)

- **Benperidol** is predicted to decrease the effects of **dopamine** receptor agonists. Avoid. Moderate Theoretical → Also see TABLE 8 p. 908
- **Benperidol** is predicted to decrease the effects of levodopa. Severe Study → Also see TABLE 8 p. 908

Benzathine benzylpenicillin → see penicillins

Benzydamine → see NSAIDs

Benzylpenicillin → see penicillins

Beta blockers, non-selective → see TABLE 6 p. 908 (bradycardia), TABLE 8 p. 908 (hypotension), TABLE 9 p. 909 (QT-interval prolongation)

carvedilol · labetalol · levobunolol · nadolol · pindolol · propranolol · sotalol · timolol

ROUTE-SPECIFIC INFORMATION Since systemic absorption can follow topical application of **levobunolol** and **timolol**, the possibility of interactions should be borne in mind.

- **Beta blockers, non-selective** are predicted to increase the risk of bronchospasm when given with **aminophylline**. Avoid. Severe Theoretical
- Antiarrhythmics **(amiodarone, disopyramide, dronedarone, flecainide, lidocaine)** are predicted to increase the risk of cardiovascular side-effects when given with **beta blockers, non-selective**. Use with caution or avoid. Severe Study → Also see TABLE 6 p. 908 → Also see TABLE 9 p. 909
- Antiarrhythmics **(propafenone)** increase the risk of cardiovascular side-effects when given with **propranolol**. Use with caution or avoid. Severe Study
- Antiarrhythmics **(propafenone)** are predicted to increase the exposure to **timolol** and **timolol** is predicted to increase the risk of cardiodepression when given with antiarrhythmics **(propafenone)**. Severe Anecdotal
- Antiarrhythmics **(propafenone)** are predicted to increase the risk of cardiovascular side-effects when given with beta blockers, non-selective **(labetalol, levobunolol, nadolol, pindolol, sotalol)**. Use with caution or avoid. Severe Study
- Antiepileptics **(phenobarbital, primidone)** are predicted to decrease the exposure to **propranolol**. Moderate Study
- Antiepileptics **(phenobarbital, primidone)** are predicted to decrease the exposure to beta blockers, non-selective **(carvedilol, labetalol)**. Moderate Theoretical
- Antifungals, azoles **(itraconazole, ketoconazole)** are predicted to increase the exposure to **nadolol**. Moderate Study
- Antimalarials **(mefloquine)** are predicted to increase the risk of bradycardia when given with **beta blockers, non-selective**. Severe Theoretical
- Calcium channel blockers **(diltiazem)** are predicted to increase the risk of cardiodepression when given with **beta blockers, non-selective**. Severe Study → Also see TABLE 6 p. 908 → Also see TABLE 8 p. 908
- **Intravenous** calcium channel blockers **(verapamil)** increase the risk of cardiovascular side-effects when given with **beta blockers, non-selective**. Avoid. Severe Study → Also see TABLE 6 p. 908 → Also see TABLE 8 p. 908
- **Oral** calcium channel blockers **(verapamil)** increase the risk of cardiovascular side-effects when given with **beta blockers, non-selective**. Severe Study → Also see TABLE 6 p. 908 → Also see TABLE 8 p. 908
- **Chloroprocaine** is predicted to increase the risk of cardiovascular side-effects when given with **sotalol**. Severe Theoretical
- **Ciclosporin** is predicted to increase the exposure to **nadolol**. Moderate Study
- **Dacomitinib** is predicted to markedly increase the exposure to **propranolol**. Avoid. Severe Study
- **Eliglustat** is predicted to increase the exposure to **propranolol**. Adjust dose. Moderate Study
- **Beta blockers, non-selective** are predicted to increase the risk of peripheral vasoconstriction when given with **ergometrine**. Severe Study
- **Beta blockers, non-selective** are predicted to increase the risk of peripheral vasoconstriction when given with **ergotamine**. Severe Study
- HIV-protease inhibitors **(lopinavir, ritonavir, saquinavir)** are predicted to increase the exposure to **nadolol**. Moderate Study
- **Beta blockers, non-selective** are predicted to increase the risk of bradycardia when given with **lanreotide**. Moderate Theoretical
- **Lapatinib** is predicted to increase the exposure to **nadolol**. Moderate Study
- **Macrolides** are predicted to increase the exposure to **nadolol**. Moderate Study
- **Mexiletine** potentially increases the risk of cardiovascular side-effects when given with **beta blockers, non-selective**. Avoid or monitor. Severe Theoretical
- **Ranolazine** is predicted to increase the exposure to **nadolol**. Moderate Study
- **Rifampicin** moderately decreases the exposure to **carvedilol**. Moderate Study
- **Rifampicin** decreases the exposure to **propranolol**. Monitor and adjust dose. Moderate Study
- **Propranolol** slightly to moderately increases the exposure to rizatriptan. Adjust **rizatriptan** dose and separate administration by at least 2 hours. Moderate Study
- SSRIs **(fluvoxamine)** moderately increase the concentration of **propranolol**. Moderate Study
- **Beta blockers, non-selective** increase the risk of hypertension and bradycardia when given with sympathomimetics, inotropic **(dobutamine)**. Severe Theoretical
- **Beta blockers, non-selective** are predicted to increase the risk of hypertension and bradycardia when given with sympathomimetics, vasoconstrictor **(adrenaline/epinephrine, noradrenaline/norepinephrine)**. Severe Study
- **Beta blockers, non-selective** are predicted to increase the risk of bronchospasm when given with **theophylline**. Avoid. Severe Theoretical
- **Vemurafenib** is predicted to increase the exposure to **nadolol**. Moderate Study

Beta blockers, selective → see TABLE 6 p. 908 (bradycardia), TABLE 8 p. 908 (hypotension)

acebutolol · atenolol · betaxolol · bisoprolol · celiprolol · esmolol · metoprolol · nebivolol

- Since systemic absorption can follow topical application of **betaxolol**, the possibility of interactions should be borne in mind.
- Orange juice greatly decreases the exposure to **celiprolol**.

- **Abiraterone** is predicted to increase the exposure to **metoprolol**. Moderate Study
- **Beta blockers, selective** are predicted to increase the risk of bronchospasm when given with **aminophylline**. Avoid. Severe Theoretical
- Antiarrhythmics **(amiodarone, disopyramide, dronedarone, flecainide, lidocaine)** are predicted to increase the risk of cardiovascular side-effects when given with **beta blockers, selective**. Use with caution or avoid. Severe Study → Also see TABLE 6 p. 908
- Antiarrhythmics **(propafenone)** are predicted to increase the exposure to **metoprolol**. Moderate Study
- Antiarrhythmics **(propafenone)** are predicted to increase the exposure to **nebivolol** and **nebivolol** is predicted to increase the risk of cardiodepression when given with antiarrhythmics **(propafenone)**. Avoid. Severe Theoretical
- Antiarrhythmics **(propafenone)** are predicted to increase the risk of cardiovascular side-effects when given with beta blockers, selective **(acebutolol, atenolol, betaxolol, bisoprolol, celiprolol, esmolol)**. Use with caution or avoid. Severe Study
- Antiepileptics **(phenobarbital, primidone)** are predicted to decrease the exposure to beta blockers, selective **(acebutolol, bisoprolol, metoprolol, nebivolol)**. Moderate Study
- Antimalarials **(mefloquine)** are predicted to increase the risk of bradycardia when given with **beta blockers, selective**. Severe Theoretical
- **Bupropion** is predicted to increase the exposure to beta blockers, selective **(metoprolol, nebivolol)**. Moderate Study
- Calcium channel blockers **(diltiazem)** are predicted to increase the risk of cardiodepression when given with **beta blockers, selective**. Severe Study → Also see TABLE 6 p. 908 → Also see TABLE 8 p. 908

Beta blockers, selective (continued)

- Intravenous calcium channel blockers **(verapamil)** increase the risk of cardiovascular side-effects when given with **beta blockers, selective**. Avoid. Severe Study → Also see TABLE 6 p. 908 → Also see TABLE 8 p. 908
- Oral calcium channel blockers **(verapamil)** increase the risk of cardiovascular side-effects when given with **beta blockers, selective**. Severe Study → Also see TABLE 6 p. 908 → Also see TABLE 8 p. 908
- Cinacalcet is predicted to increase the exposure to beta blockers, selective **(metoprolol, nebivolol)**. Moderate Study
- Dacomitinib is predicted to markedly increase the exposure to beta blockers, selective **(metoprolol, nebivolol)**. Avoid. Severe Study
- Duloxetine is predicted to increase the exposure to **metoprolol**. Moderate Study
- Eliglustat is predicted to increase the exposure to **metoprolol**. Adjust dose. Moderate Study
- **Beta blockers, selective** are predicted to increase the risk of peripheral vasoconstriction when given with ergometrine. Severe Study
- **Beta blockers, selective** are predicted to increase the risk of peripheral vasoconstriction when given with ergotamine. Severe Study
- Grapefruit juice greatly decreases the exposure to **celiprolol**. Moderate Study
- HIV-protease inhibitors **(ritonavir)** are predicted to increase the exposure to **metoprolol**. Moderate Study
- **Beta blockers, selective** are predicted to increase the risk of bradycardia when given with lanreotide. Moderate Theoretical
- Mexiletine potentially increases the risk of cardiovascular side-effects when given with **beta blockers, selective**. Avoid or monitor. Severe Theoretical
- Mirabegron is predicted to increase the exposure to **metoprolol**. Moderate Study
- Panobinostat is predicted to increase the exposure to **metoprolol**. Monitor and adjust dose. Moderate Theoretical
- Panobinostat is predicted to increase the exposure to **nebivolol**. Monitor and adjust dose. Mild Theoretical
- Rifampicin slightly decreases the exposure to beta blockers, selective **(bisoprolol, metoprolol)**. Mild Study
- Rifampicin moderately decreases the exposure to **celiprolol**. Moderate Study
- Rolapitant is predicted to moderately increase the exposure to **metoprolol**. Severe Study
- SSRIs **(fluoxetine, paroxetine)** are predicted to increase the exposure to beta blockers, selective **(metoprolol, nebivolol)**. Moderate Study
- **Beta blockers, selective** increase the risk of hypertension and bradycardia when given with sympathomimetics, inotropic **(dobutamine)**. Moderate Theoretical
- **Beta blockers, selective** are predicted to increase the risk of hypertension and bradycardia when given with sympathomimetics, vasoconstrictor **(adrenaline/epinephrine, noradrenaline/norepinephrine)**. Severe Study
- Terbinafine is predicted to increase the exposure to beta blockers, selective **(metoprolol, nebivolol)**. Moderate Study
- **Beta blockers, selective** are predicted to increase the risk of bronchospasm when given with theophylline. Avoid. Severe Theoretical
- Vaborbactam is predicted to increase the concentration of **metoprolol**. Unknown Theoretical

Beta$_2$ agonists → see TABLE 17 p. 911 (reduced serum potassium)

bambuterol · formoterol · indacaterol · olodaterol · salbutamol · salmeterol · terbutaline · vilanterol

- Antifungals, azoles **(itraconazole, ketoconazole, voriconazole)** are predicted to increase the exposure to **salmeterol**. Avoid. Severe Study
- Apalutamide is predicted to decrease the exposure to **salmeterol**. Avoid or monitor. Moderate Study
- Aprepitant is predicted to increase the exposure to **salmeterol**. Moderate Study
- Atomoxetine is predicted to increase the risk of cardiovascular side-effects when given with **beta$_2$ agonists** (high-dose). Moderate Study
- Cobicistat is predicted to increase the exposure to **salmeterol**. Avoid. Severe Study
- HIV-protease inhibitors are predicted to increase the exposure to **salmeterol**. Avoid. Severe Study
- Idelalisib is predicted to increase the exposure to **salmeterol**. Avoid. Severe Study
- **Beta$_2$ agonists** are predicted to increase the risk of glaucoma when given with ipratropium. Moderate Anecdotal
- **Beta$_2$ agonists** are predicted to increase the risk of elevated blood pressure when given with linezolid. Avoid. Severe Theoretical
- Macrolides **(clarithromycin)** are predicted to increase the exposure to **salmeterol**. Avoid. Severe Study
- MAO-B inhibitors **(rasagiline, selegiline)** are predicted to increase the risk of severe hypertension when given with **beta$_2$ agonists**. Avoid. Severe Theoretical
- MAO-B inhibitors **(safinamide)** are predicted to increase the risk of severe hypertension when given with **beta$_2$ agonists**. Severe Theoretical
- MAOIs, irreversible are predicted to increase the risk of cardiovascular side-effects when given with **beta$_2$ agonists**. Moderate Anecdotal
- Netupitant is predicted to increase the exposure to **salmeterol**. Moderate Study

Betahistine

- Antihistamines, non-sedating are predicted to decrease the effects of **betahistine**. Moderate Theoretical
- Antihistamines, sedating are predicted to decrease the effects of **betahistine**. Moderate Theoretical

Betamethasone → see corticosteroids
Betaxolol → see beta blockers, selective
Bevacizumab → see monoclonal antibodies
Bexarotene → see retinoids
Bezafibrate → see fibrates

Bicalutamide

- Bicalutamide is predicted to increase the exposure to lomitapide. Separate administration by 12 hours. Moderate Theoretical

Bictegravir

- Antacids decrease the exposure to **bictegravir**. Separate administration by at least 2 hours. Moderate Study
- Antiarrhythmics **(amiodarone, dronedarone)** are predicted to increase the exposure to **bictegravir**. Use with caution or avoid. Moderate Theoretical
- Antiepileptics **(carbamazepine, fosphenytoin, phenobarbital, phenytoin, primidone)** are predicted to decrease the exposure to **bictegravir**. Avoid. Moderate Study
- Antiepileptics **(oxcarbazepine)** are predicted to decrease the exposure to **bictegravir**. Avoid. Moderate Theoretical
- Antifungals, azoles **(itraconazole, ketoconazole)** are predicted to increase the exposure to **bictegravir**. Use with caution or avoid. Moderate Theoretical
- Antifungals, azoles **(posaconazole)** are predicted to increase the exposure to **bictegravir**. Moderate Theoretical
- Apalutamide is predicted to decrease the exposure to **bictegravir**. Avoid. Moderate Study
- Calcium channel blockers **(verapamil)** are predicted to increase the exposure to **bictegravir**. Use with caution or avoid. Moderate Theoretical
- Ciclosporin is predicted to increase the exposure to **bictegravir**. Use with caution or avoid. Moderate Theoretical
- Enzalutamide is predicted to decrease the exposure to **bictegravir**. Avoid. Moderate Study
- HIV-protease inhibitors **(atazanavir)** moderately increase the exposure to **bictegravir**. Avoid. Severe Study
- HIV-protease inhibitors **(lopinavir, ritonavir, saquinavir)** are predicted to increase the exposure to **bictegravir**. Use with caution or avoid. Moderate Theoretical
- Iron (oral) decreases the exposure to **bictegravir**. Manufacturer advises take 2 hours before **iron (oral)**. Moderate Study
- Lapatinib is predicted to increase the exposure to **bictegravir**. Use with caution or avoid. Moderate Theoretical
- Macrolides are predicted to increase the exposure to **bictegravir**. Use with caution or avoid. Moderate Theoretical

- ▸ **Bictegravir** slightly increases the exposure to **metformin**. Moderate Study
- ▸ **Mitotane** is predicted to decrease the exposure to **bictegravir**. Avoid. Moderate Study
- ▸ **Bictegravir** is predicted to increase the exposure to opioids (methadone). Moderate Theoretical
- ▸ **Ranolazine** is predicted to increase the exposure to **bictegravir**. Use with caution or avoid. Moderate Theoretical
- ▸ **Rifabutin** slightly decreases the exposure to **bictegravir**. Avoid. Moderate Study
- ▸ **Rifampicin** is predicted to decrease the exposure to **bictegravir**. Avoid. Moderate Study
- ▸ **St John's Wort** is predicted to decrease the exposure to **bictegravir**. Avoid. Moderate Theoretical
- ▸ **Sucralfate** is predicted to decrease the exposure to **bictegravir**. Avoid. Moderate Theoretical
- ▸ **Vemurafenib** is predicted to increase the exposure to **bictegravir**. Use with caution or avoid. Moderate Theoretical

Bilastine → see antihistamines, non-sedating

Bismuth

- ▸ **Bismuth** subsalicylate is predicted to increase the risk of side-effects when given with aspirin. Avoid. Moderate Theoretical
- ▸ **Bismuth** subsalicylate is predicted to increase the risk of bleeding events when given with drugs with anticoagulant effects. Moderate Theoretical
- ▸ **Bismuth** greatly decreases the efficacy of tetracyclines. Separate administration by 2 hours. Moderate Study

Bisoprolol → see beta blockers, selective

Bisphosphonates → see TABLE 2 p. 907 (nephrotoxicity)

alendronate · clodronate · ibandronate · pamidronate · risedronate · zoledronate

- ▸ **Aminoglycosides** increase the risk of hypocalcaemia when given with **bisphosphonates**. Moderate Anecdotal → Also see TABLE 2 p. 907
- ▸ **Antacids** decrease the absorption of **alendronate**. **Alendronate** should be taken at least 30 minutes before antacids. Moderate Study
- ▸ **Antacids** decrease the absorption of **clodronate**. Avoid antacids for 2 hours before or 1 hour after **clodronate**. Moderate Study
- ▸ **Antacids** are predicted to decrease the absorption of **ibandronate**. Avoid antacids for at least 6 hours before or 1 hour after **ibandronate**. Moderate Theoretical
- ▸ **Antacids** decrease the absorption of **risedronate**. Separate administration by at least 2 hours. Moderate Study
- ▸ **Aspirin** (high-dose) is predicted to increase the risk of gastrointestinal irritation when given with bisphosphonates **(alendronate, ibandronate)**. Moderate Study
- ▸ **Aspirin** (high-dose) is predicted to increase the risk of renal impairment when given with **clodronate**. Severe Theoretical
- ▸ Oral **calcium salts** decrease the absorption of **alendronate**. **Alendronate** should be taken at least 30 minutes before **calcium salts** Moderate Study
- ▸ Oral **calcium salts** decrease the absorption of **clodronate**. Avoid **calcium salts** for 2 hours before or 1 hour after **clodronate**. Moderate Study
- ▸ Oral **calcium salts** are predicted to decrease the absorption of oral **ibandronate**. Avoid **calcium salts** for at least 6 hours before or 1 hour after **ibandronate**. Moderate Theoretical
- ▸ Oral **calcium salts** decrease the absorption of **risedronate**. Separate administration by at least 2 hours. Moderate Study
- ▸ **Iron (oral)** decreases the absorption of **clodronate**. Avoid **iron (oral)** for 2 hours before or 1 hour after **clodronate**. Moderate Study
- ▸ **Iron (oral)** is predicted to decrease the absorption of oral **ibandronate**. Avoid **iron (oral)** for at least 6 hours before or 1 hour after **ibandronate**. Moderate Theoretical
- ▸ **Iron (oral)** decreases the absorption of **risedronate**. Separate administration by at least 2 hours. Moderate Study
- ▸ **Bisphosphonates** are predicted to increase the risk of gastrointestinal bleeding when given with iron chelators (deferasirox). Severe Theoretical
- ▸ Oral **magnesium** decreases the absorption of **alendronate**. **Alendronate** should be taken at least 30 minutes before **magnesium**. Moderate Study
- ▸ Oral **magnesium** decreases the absorption of **clodronate**. Avoid **magnesium** for 2 hours before or 1 hour after **clodronate**. Moderate Study
- ▸ Oral **magnesium** is predicted to decrease the absorption of oral **ibandronate**. Avoid for at least 6 hours before or 1 hour after **ibandronate**. Moderate Theoretical
- ▸ Oral **magnesium** decreases the absorption of **risedronate**. Separate administration by at least 2 hours. Moderate Study
- ▸ **NSAIDs** are predicted to increase the risk of gastrointestinal irritation when given with bisphosphonates **(alendronate, ibandronate)**. Moderate Study
- ▸ **NSAIDs** are predicted to increase the risk of renal impairment when given with **clodronate**. Moderate Study
- ▸ **Bisphosphonates** are predicted to decrease the effects of parathyroid hormone. Avoid. Moderate Study
- ▸ Oral **zinc** decreases the absorption of oral **alendronate**. **Alendronate** should be taken at least 30 minutes before **zinc**. Moderate Study
- ▸ Oral **zinc** decreases the absorption of oral **clodronate**. Avoid **zinc** for 2 hours before or 1 hour after **clodronate**. Moderate Study
- ▸ Oral **zinc** is predicted to decrease the absorption of oral **ibandronate**. Avoid **zinc** for at least 6 hours before or 1 hour after **ibandronate**. Moderate Theoretical
- ▸ Oral **zinc** decreases the absorption of oral **risedronate**. Separate administration by at least 2 hours. Moderate Study

Bivalirudin → see TABLE 3 p. 907 (anticoagulant effects)

- ▸ **Ranibizumab** is predicted to increase the risk of bleeding events when given with **bivalirudin**. Moderate Theoretical

Bleomycin → see TABLE 15 p. 910 (myelosuppression), TABLE 5 p. 907 (thromboembolism)

- ▸ **Live vaccines** are predicted to increase the risk of generalised infection (possibly life-threatening) when given with **bleomycin**. Public Health England advises avoid (refer to Green Book). Severe Theoretical
- ▸ Monoclonal antibodies **(brentuximab vedotin)** increase the risk of pulmonary toxicity when given with **bleomycin**. Avoid. Severe Study → Also see TABLE 15 p. 910
- ▸ Platinum compounds **(cisplatin)** increase the risk of pulmonary toxicity when given with **bleomycin**. Severe Study → Also see TABLE 15 p. 910

Blinatumomab → see monoclonal antibodies

Bortezomib → see TABLE 8 p. 908 (hypotension), TABLE 15 p. 910 (myelosuppression), TABLE 12 p. 910 (peripheral neuropathy)

- ▸ Antiepileptics **(carbamazepine, fosphenytoin, phenobarbital, phenytoin, primidone)** slightly decrease the exposure to **bortezomib**. Avoid. Severe Study → Also see TABLE 12 p. 910
- ▸ Antifungals, azoles **(itraconazole, ketoconazole, voriconazole)** slightly increase the exposure to **bortezomib**. Moderate Study
- ▸ **Apalutamide** slightly decreases the exposure to **bortezomib**. Avoid. Severe Study
- ▸ **Cobicistat** slightly increases the exposure to **bortezomib**. Moderate Study
- ▸ **Enzalutamide** slightly decreases the exposure to **bortezomib**. Avoid. Severe Study
- ▸ **HIV-protease inhibitors** slightly increase the exposure to **bortezomib**. Moderate Study
- ▸ **Idelalisib** slightly increases the exposure to **bortezomib**. Moderate Study → Also see TABLE 15 p. 910
- ▸ Macrolides **(clarithromycin)** slightly increase the exposure to **bortezomib**. Moderate Study
- ▸ **Mitotane** slightly decreases the exposure to **bortezomib**. Avoid. Severe Study → Also see TABLE 15 p. 910
- ▸ **Rifampicin** slightly decreases the exposure to **bortezomib**. Avoid. Severe Study

Bosentan

- ▸ **Bosentan** is predicted to decrease the exposure to antiarrhythmics **(dronedarone)**. Severe Theoretical
- ▸ Antiepileptics **(carbamazepine, fosphenytoin, phenobarbital, phenytoin, primidone)** affect the exposure to **bosentan**. Avoid. Severe Study
- ▸ Antifungals, azoles **(fluconazole)** are predicted to increase the exposure to **bosentan**. Avoid. Severe Study
- ▸ Antifungals, azoles **(itraconazole)** are predicted to increase the exposure to **bosentan**. Moderate Theoretical

Bosentan (continued)
- Antifungals, azoles (**ketoconazole**) moderately increase the exposure to **bosentan**. Moderate Study
- Antifungals, azoles (**voriconazole**) are predicted to increase the exposure to **bosentan**. Avoid. Severe Theoretical
- **Bosentan** is predicted to decrease the exposure to antifungals, azoles (**isavuconazole**). Avoid. Severe Theoretical
- **Apalutamide** affects the exposure to **bosentan**. Avoid. Severe Study
- **Bosentan** is predicted to decrease the exposure to **aprepitant**. Moderate Study
- **Bosentan** is predicted to decrease the exposure to **axitinib**. Moderate Theoretical
- **Bosentan** is predicted to decrease the exposure to **bedaquiline**. Avoid. Severe Study
- **Bosentan** is predicted to decrease the exposure to **bosutinib**. Avoid. Severe Theoretical
- **Bosentan** is predicted to decrease the exposure to **brigatinib**. Avoid. Severe Study
- **Bosentan** is predicted to decrease the exposure to **cabozantinib**. Moderate Theoretical
- **Bosentan** is predicted to decrease the exposure to calcium channel blockers (**amlodipine, felodipine, lacidipine, lercanidipine, nicardipine, nifedipine, nimodipine**). Monitor and adjust dose. Moderate Theoretical
- **Bosentan** is predicted to decrease the exposure to calcium channel blockers (**diltiazem, verapamil**). Moderate Theoretical
- **Bosentan** is predicted to decrease the exposure to **cariprazine**. Avoid. Severe Theoretical
- Cephalosporins (**ceftobiprole**) are predicted to increase the exposure to **bosentan**. Moderate Theoretical
- **Bosentan** moderately decreases the exposure to **ciclosporin** and **ciclosporin** moderately increases the exposure to **bosentan**. Avoid. Severe Study
- **Bosentan** is predicted to decrease the exposure to **cobicistat**. Avoid. Severe Theoretical
- **Bosentan** is predicted to decrease the exposure to **cobimetinib**. Avoid. Severe Theoretical
- **Bosentan** is predicted to decrease the efficacy of **combined hormonal contraceptives**. For FSRH guidance, see Contraceptives, interactions p. 536. Severe Study
- **Bosentan** decreases the anticoagulant effect of **coumarins**. Moderate Study
- **Bosentan** is predicted to decrease the exposure to **crizotinib**. Avoid. Severe Theoretical
- **Bosentan** is predicted to decrease the exposure to **dasatinib**. Severe Study
- **Bosentan** is predicted to decrease the efficacy of **desogestrel**. For FSRH guidance, see Contraceptives, interactions p. 536. Severe Theoretical
- **Bosentan** decreases the exposure to **dolutegravir**. Adjust dose. Severe Study
- **Bosentan** is predicted to decrease the exposure to **doravirine**. Avoid or adjust doravirine or lamivudine with tenofovir disoproxil and doravirine dose. Severe Theoretical
- **Bosentan** is predicted to moderately decrease the exposure to **elbasvir**. Avoid. Severe Study
- **Bosentan** is predicted to decrease the exposure to **eliglustat**. Moderate Theoretical
- **Bosentan** is predicted to decrease the concentration of **elvitegravir**. Avoid. Severe Theoretical
- **Enzalutamide** affects the exposure to **bosentan**. Avoid. Severe Study
- **Bosentan** is predicted to decrease the effects of **ergotamine**. Moderate Theoretical
- **Bosentan** is predicted to decrease the exposure to **erlotinib**. Severe Theoretical
- **Bosentan** is predicted to decrease the efficacy of **etonogestrel**. For FSRH guidance, see Contraceptives, interactions p. 536. Severe Theoretical
- **Bosentan** is predicted to decrease the exposure to **etravirine**. Avoid. Severe Study
- **Bosentan** is predicted to decrease the concentration of **everolimus**. Avoid or adjust dose. Severe Study
- **Bosentan** is predicted to decrease the exposure to **fosaprepitant**. Moderate Theoretical
- **Bosentan** is predicted to decrease the exposure to **gefitinib**. Avoid. Severe Theoretical
- **Bosentan** is predicted to decrease the exposure to **glecaprevir**. Avoid. Severe Study
- **Bosentan** is predicted to markedly decrease the exposure to **grazoprevir**. Avoid. Severe Study
- **Bosentan** is predicted to decrease the concentration of **guanfacine**. Adjust dose. Moderate Theoretical
- **HIV-protease inhibitors** are predicted to increase the exposure to **bosentan**. Severe Study
- **Bosentan** is predicted to decrease the effects of **hormone replacement therapy**. Moderate Anecdotal
- **Bosentan** is predicted to decrease the exposure to **idelalisib**. Avoid. Moderate Theoretical
- **Bosentan** is predicted to decrease the exposure to **imatinib**. Moderate Study
- **Bosentan** is predicted to decrease the exposure to **ivacaftor**. Moderate Study
- **Bosentan** is predicted to decrease the exposure to **lapatinib**. Avoid. Severe Study
- **Bosentan** is predicted to decrease the exposure to **larotrectinib**. Avoid. Moderate Study
- **Leflunomide** is predicted to increase the exposure to **bosentan**. Moderate Study
- **Letermovir** is predicted to increase the concentration of **bosentan**. Moderate Theoretical
- **Bosentan** is predicted to decrease the efficacy of **levonorgestrel**. For FSRH guidance, see Contraceptives, interactions p. 536. Severe Theoretical
- **Bosentan** is predicted to decrease the exposure to **lorlatinib**. Avoid. Severe Theoretical
- **Bosentan** is predicted to decrease the exposure to **lurasidone**. Monitor and adjust dose. Moderate Theoretical
- Macrolides (**clarithromycin**) are predicted to increase the exposure to **bosentan**. Moderate Theoretical
- **Bosentan** is predicted to decrease the exposure to **maraviroc**. Avoid. Moderate Theoretical
- **Bosentan** is predicted to decrease the concentration of **midazolam**. Monitor and adjust dose. Moderate Theoretical
- **Mitotane** affects the exposure to **bosentan**. Avoid. Severe Study
- **Bosentan** is predicted to decrease the exposure to **neratinib**. Severe Study
- **Bosentan** is predicted to decrease the exposure to **netupitant**. Moderate Theoretical
- **Bosentan** is predicted to decrease the exposure to **nevirapine**. Severe Theoretical
- **Bosentan** is predicted to decrease the exposure to **nilotinib**. Avoid. Severe Theoretical
- **Bosentan** is predicted to decrease the efficacy of **norethisterone**. For FSRH guidance, see Contraceptives, interactions p. 536. Severe Anecdotal
- **Bosentan** is predicted to decrease the exposure to **olaparib**. Avoid. Moderate Theoretical
- **Bosentan** decreases the exposure to opioids (**methadone**). Monitor and adjust dose. Severe Study
- **Bosentan** is predicted to decrease the exposure to **osimertinib**. Moderate Theoretical
- **Bosentan** is predicted to decrease the exposure to **ospemifene**. Moderate Study
- **Bosentan** is predicted to decrease the exposure to **paritaprevir** (with ritonavir and ombitasvir). Avoid. Severe Study
- **Bosentan** decreases the exposure to **phosphodiesterase type-5 inhibitors**. Moderate Study
- **Bosentan** is predicted to decrease the exposure to **pibrentasvir**. Avoid. Severe Study
- **Bosentan** is predicted to decrease the exposure to **quetiapine**. Moderate Study
- **Bosentan** is predicted to decrease the exposure to **ribociclib**. Moderate Study
- **Rifampicin** affects the exposure to **bosentan**. Avoid. Severe Study
- **Bosentan** is predicted to decrease the exposure to **rilpivirine**. Avoid. Severe Theoretical

- **Bosentan** is predicted to decrease the exposure to **rolapitant**. Avoid. [Severe] Study
- **Bosentan** is predicted to decrease the exposure to **ruxolitinib**. Monitor and adjust dose. [Moderate] Theoretical
- **Bosentan** is predicted to decrease the exposure to **siponimod**. Manufacturer advises caution depending on genotype—consult product literature. [Severe] Theoretical
- **Bosentan** is predicted to decrease the concentration of sirolimus and sirolimus potentially increases the concentration of **bosentan**. Avoid. [Severe] Theoretical
- St John's Wort is predicted to decrease the exposure to **bosentan**. Avoid. [Moderate] Theoretical
- **Bosentan** slightly decreases the exposure to statins (atorvastatin). [Mild] Study
- **Bosentan** moderately decreases the exposure to statins (simvastatin). [Moderate] Study
- **Bosentan** increases the risk of hepatotoxicity when given with sulfonylureas (glibenclamide). Avoid. [Severe] Study
- **Bosentan** is predicted to decrease the concentration of tacrolimus and tacrolimus potentially increases the concentration of **bosentan**. Avoid. [Severe] Theoretical
- **Bosentan** is predicted to decrease the exposure to taxanes (cabazitaxel). Avoid. [Severe] Study
- **Bosentan** is predicted to decrease the concentration of temsirolimus. Avoid. [Severe] Theoretical
- Teriflunomide is predicted to increase the exposure to **bosentan**. [Moderate] Study
- **Bosentan** is predicted to decrease the exposure to **ticagrelor**. [Moderate] Theoretical
- **Bosentan** is predicted to decrease the exposure to tofacitinib. [Moderate] Study
- **Bosentan** decreases the efficacy of ulipristal. For FSRH guidance, see Contraceptives, interactions p. 536. [Severe] Anecdotal
- **Bosentan** is predicted to decrease the exposure to velpatasvir. Avoid. [Moderate] Theoretical
- **Bosentan** is predicted to decrease the exposure to venetoclax. Avoid. [Severe] Study
- Venetoclax is predicted to increase the exposure to **bosentan**. [Moderate] Theoretical
- **Bosentan** is predicted to decrease the concentration of voxilaprevir. Avoid. [Severe] Theoretical

Bosutinib → see TABLE 15 p. 910 (myelosuppression), TABLE 9 p. 909 (QT-interval prolongation)

- Antacids are predicted to decrease the absorption of **bosutinib**. **Bosutinib** should be taken at least 12 hours before antacids. [Moderate] Theoretical
- Antiarrhythmics (dronedarone) are predicted to increase the exposure to **bosutinib**. Avoid or adjust dose. [Severe] Theoretical → Also see TABLE 9 p. 909
- Antiepileptics (carbamazepine, fosphenytoin, phenobarbital, phenytoin, primidone) are predicted to very markedly decrease the exposure to **bosutinib**. Avoid. [Severe] Study
- Antifungals, azoles (fluconazole, isavuconazole, posaconazole) are predicted to increase the exposure to **bosutinib**. Avoid or adjust dose. [Severe] Theoretical → Also see TABLE 9 p. 909
- Antifungals, azoles (itraconazole, ketoconazole, voriconazole) are predicted to markedly increase the exposure to **bosutinib**. Avoid or adjust dose. [Severe] Study → Also see TABLE 9 p. 909
- Apalutamide is predicted to very markedly decrease the exposure to **bosutinib**. Avoid. [Severe] Study → Also see TABLE 9 p. 909
- Aprepitant is predicted to increase the exposure to **bosutinib**. Avoid or adjust dose. [Severe] Theoretical
- Bosentan is predicted to decrease the exposure to **bosutinib**. Avoid. [Severe] Theoretical
- Calcium channel blockers (diltiazem, verapamil) are predicted to increase the exposure to **bosutinib**. Avoid or adjust dose. [Severe] Theoretical
- Cobicistat is predicted to markedly increase the exposure to **bosutinib**. Avoid or adjust dose. [Severe] Study
- **Bosutinib** is predicted to increase the risk of bleeding events when given with coumarins. [Severe] Theoretical
- Crizotinib is predicted to increase the exposure to **bosutinib**. Avoid or adjust dose. [Severe] Theoretical → Also see TABLE 15 p. 910 → Also see TABLE 9 p. 909
- Efavirenz is predicted to decrease the exposure to **bosutinib**. Avoid. [Severe] Theoretical → Also see TABLE 9 p. 909
- Enzalutamide is predicted to very markedly decrease the exposure to **bosutinib**. Avoid. [Severe] Study
- Etravirine is predicted to decrease the exposure to **bosutinib**. Avoid. [Severe] Theoretical
- Fosaprepitant is predicted to increase the exposure to **bosutinib**. [Severe] Theoretical
- Grapefruit juice is predicted to increase the exposure to **bosutinib**. Avoid. [Moderate] Theoretical
- H_2 receptor antagonists are predicted to decrease the absorption of **bosutinib**. [Moderate] Theoretical
- HIV-protease inhibitors are predicted to markedly increase the exposure to **bosutinib**. Avoid or adjust dose. [Severe] Study → Also see TABLE 9 p. 909
- Idelalisib is predicted to markedly increase the exposure to **bosutinib**. Avoid or adjust dose. [Severe] Study → Also see TABLE 15 p. 910
- Imatinib is predicted to increase the exposure to **bosutinib**. Avoid or adjust dose. [Severe] Theoretical → Also see TABLE 15 p. 910
- Macrolides (clarithromycin) are predicted to markedly increase the exposure to **bosutinib**. Avoid or adjust dose. [Severe] Study → Also see TABLE 9 p. 909
- Macrolides (erythromycin) are predicted to increase the exposure to **bosutinib**. Avoid or adjust dose. [Severe] Theoretical → Also see TABLE 9 p. 909
- Mitotane is predicted to very markedly decrease the exposure to **bosutinib**. Avoid. [Severe] Study → Also see TABLE 15 p. 910
- Modafinil is predicted to decrease the exposure to **bosutinib**. Avoid. [Severe] Theoretical
- Netupitant is predicted to increase the exposure to **bosutinib**. Avoid or adjust dose. [Severe] Theoretical
- Nevirapine is predicted to decrease the exposure to **bosutinib**. Avoid. [Severe] Theoretical
- Nilotinib is predicted to increase the exposure to **bosutinib**. Avoid or adjust dose. [Severe] Theoretical → Also see TABLE 15 p. 910 → Also see TABLE 9 p. 909
- **Bosutinib** is predicted to increase the risk of bleeding events when given with phenindione. [Severe] Theoretical
- Pitolisant is predicted to decrease the exposure to **bosutinib**. Avoid. [Severe] Theoretical
- Proton pump inhibitors are predicted to decrease the absorption of **bosutinib**. [Moderate] Study
- Rifampicin is predicted to very markedly decrease the exposure to **bosutinib**. Avoid. [Severe] Study
- St John's Wort is predicted to decrease the exposure to **bosutinib**. Avoid. [Severe] Theoretical

Botulinum toxin type A → see botulinum toxins

Botulinum toxin type B → see botulinum toxins

Botulinum toxins → see TABLE 20 p. 911 (neuromuscular blocking effects)

botulinum toxin type A · botulinum toxin type B

Bowel cleansing preparations

SEPARATION OF ADMINISTRATION Other oral drugs should not be taken 1 hour before, or after, administration of bowel cleansing preparations because absorption may be impaired. Consider withholding ACE inhibitors, angiotensin-II receptor antagonists, and NSAIDs on the day that bowel cleansing preparations are given and for up to 72 hours after the procedure. Also consider withholding diuretics on the day that bowel cleansing preparations are given.

Brentuximab vedotin → see monoclonal antibodies

Brigatinib

- Antiepileptics (carbamazepine, fosphenytoin, phenobarbital, phenytoin, primidone) are predicted to decrease the exposure to **brigatinib**. Avoid. [Severe] Study
- Antifungals, azoles (itraconazole, ketoconazole, voriconazole) are predicted to increase the exposure to **brigatinib**. Adjust **brigatinib** dose. [Severe] Study
- Apalutamide is predicted to decrease the exposure to **brigatinib**. Avoid. [Severe] Study

Brigatinib (continued)
- **Bosentan** is predicted to decrease the exposure to **brigatinib**. Avoid. [Severe] Study
- **Cobicistat** is predicted to increase the exposure to **brigatinib**. Adjust **brigatinib** dose. [Severe] Study
- **Brigatinib** decreases the exposure to **combined hormonal contraceptives**. Use additional contraceptive precautions. [Severe] Theoretical
- **Brigatinib** potentially increases the concentration of dabigatran. [Moderate] Theoretical
- **Brigatinib** potentially increases the concentration of digoxin. [Moderate] Theoretical
- **Efavirenz** is predicted to decrease the exposure to **brigatinib**. Avoid. [Severe] Study
- **Enzalutamide** is predicted to decrease the exposure to **brigatinib**. Avoid. [Severe] Study
- **Etravirine** is predicted to decrease the exposure to **brigatinib**. Avoid. [Moderate] Theoretical
- **Grapefruit juice** is predicted to increase the concentration of **brigatinib**. Avoid. [Severe] Study
- **HIV-protease inhibitors** are predicted to increase the exposure to **brigatinib**. Adjust **brigatinib** dose. [Severe] Study
- **Idelalisib** is predicted to increase the exposure to **brigatinib**. Adjust **brigatinib** dose. [Severe] Study
- Macrolides **(clarithromycin)** are predicted to increase the exposure to **brigatinib**. Adjust **brigatinib** dose. [Severe] Study
- **Brigatinib** potentially increases the concentration of methotrexate. [Moderate] Theoretical
- **Mitotane** is predicted to decrease the exposure to **brigatinib**. Avoid. [Severe] Study
- **Nevirapine** is predicted to decrease the exposure to **brigatinib**. Avoid. [Severe] Study
- **Brigatinib** potentially decreases the concentration of opioids **(alfentanil, fentanyl)**. Avoid. [Moderate] Theoretical
- **Rifabutin** is predicted to decrease the exposure to **brigatinib**. Avoid. [Moderate] Theoretical
- **Rifampicin** is predicted to decrease the exposure to **brigatinib**. Avoid. [Severe] Study
- **Brigatinib** potentially decreases the concentration of sirolimus. Avoid. [Moderate] Theoretical
- **St John's Wort** is predicted to decrease the exposure to **brigatinib**. Avoid. [Severe] Study
- **Brigatinib** potentially decreases the concentration of tacrolimus. Avoid. [Moderate] Theoretical

Brimonidine → see **TABLE 6** p. 908 (bradycardia), **TABLE 8** p. 908 (hypotension), **TABLE 11** p. 909 (CNS depressant effects)

Brinzolamide

ROUTE-SPECIFIC INFORMATION Since systemic absorption can follow topical application, the possibility of interactions should be borne in mind.

Brivaracetam → see antiepileptics
Brodalumab → see monoclonal antibodies
Bromfenac → see NSAIDs
Bromocriptine → see dopamine receptor agonists
Buclizine → see antihistamines, sedating
Budesonide → see corticosteroids
Bumetanide → see loop diuretics
Bupivacaine → see anaesthetics, local
Buprenorphine → see opioids
Bupropion → see **TABLE 13** p. 910 (serotonin syndrome)
- **Bupropion** is predicted to increase the exposure to anticholinesterases, centrally acting **(galantamine)**. Monitor and adjust dose. [Moderate] Study
- Antiepileptics **(carbamazepine, fosphenytoin, phenobarbital, phenytoin, primidone)** are predicted to markedly decrease the exposure to **bupropion**. [Severe] Study
- Antiepileptics **(valproate)** increase the exposure to **bupropion**. [Severe] Study
- Antifungals, azoles **(isavuconazole)** slightly increase the exposure to **bupropion**. Adjust dose. [Moderate] Study
- **Bupropion** is predicted to moderately increase the exposure to aripiprazole. Adjust **aripiprazole** dose, p. 265. [Moderate] Study
- **Bupropion** is predicted to markedly increase the exposure to atomoxetine. Adjust dose. [Severe] Study
- **Bupropion** is predicted to increase the exposure to beta blockers, selective **(metoprolol, nebivolol)**. [Moderate] Study
- **Bupropion** is predicted to slightly increase the exposure to darifenacin. [Mild] Study
- **Bupropion** increases the risk of side-effects when given with dopamine receptor agonists **(amantadine)**. [Moderate] Study
- **Efavirenz** is predicted to decrease the exposure to **bupropion**. [Moderate] Study
- **Bupropion** is predicted to increase the exposure to eliglustat. Avoid or adjust dose—consult product literature. [Severe] Study
- HIV-protease inhibitors **(ritonavir)** are predicted to decrease the exposure to **bupropion**. [Moderate] Study
- **Bupropion** increases the risk of side-effects when given with levodopa. [Moderate] Study
- **Bupropion** is predicted to increase the risk of intraoperative hypertension when given with linezolid. [Severe] Anecdotal → Also see **TABLE 13** p. 910
- **MAO-B inhibitors** are predicted to increase the risk of severe hypertension when given with **bupropion**. Avoid. [Moderate] Theoretical → Also see **TABLE 13** p. 910
- **MAOIs, irreversible** are predicted to increase the risk of severe hypertension when given with **bupropion**. Avoid and for 14 days after stopping the MAOI. [Severe] Theoretical → Also see **TABLE 13** p. 910
- **Methylthioninium chloride** is predicted to increase the risk of severe hypertension when given with **bupropion**. Avoid. [Severe] Theoretical → Also see **TABLE 13** p. 910
- **Bupropion** is predicted to increase the exposure to mexiletine. [Moderate] Study
- **Moclobemide** is predicted to increase the risk of severe hypertension when given with **bupropion**. Avoid. [Severe] Theoretical → Also see **TABLE 13** p. 910
- **Bupropion** is predicted to decrease the efficacy of opioids (codeine). [Moderate] Theoretical
- **Bupropion** is predicted to decrease the efficacy of opioids (tramadol). [Severe] Study → Also see **TABLE 13** p. 910
- **Bupropion** is predicted to moderately increase the exposure to pitolisant. Use with caution and adjust dose. [Moderate] Study
- **Rifampicin** is predicted to decrease the exposure to **bupropion**. [Moderate] Study
- **Bupropion** is predicted to increase the exposure to risperidone. Adjust dose. [Moderate] Study
- **Bupropion** is predicted to increase the exposure to SSRIs (dapoxetine). [Moderate] Theoretical → Also see **TABLE 13** p. 910
- **Bupropion** is predicted to decrease the efficacy of tamoxifen. Avoid. [Severe] Study
- **Bupropion** is predicted to increase the exposure to the active metabolite of tetrabenazine. [Moderate] Study
- **Bupropion** is predicted to increase the exposure to tricyclic antidepressants. Monitor for toxicity and adjust dose. [Severe] Study → Also see **TABLE 13** p. 910
- **Bupropion** is predicted to increase the exposure to vortioxetine. Monitor and adjust dose. [Moderate] Study → Also see **TABLE 13** p. 910

Buspirone → see **TABLE 13** p. 910 (serotonin syndrome)
- Antiarrhythmics **(dronedarone)** are predicted to increase the exposure to **buspirone**. Use with caution and adjust dose. [Moderate] Study
- Antiepileptics **(carbamazepine, fosphenytoin, phenobarbital, phenytoin, primidone)** are predicted to decrease the exposure to **buspirone**. Use with caution and adjust dose. [Severe] Study
- Antifungals, azoles **(fluconazole, isavuconazole, posaconazole)** are predicted to increase the exposure to **buspirone**. Use with caution and adjust dose. [Moderate] Study
- Antifungals, azoles **(itraconazole, ketoconazole, voriconazole)** are predicted to increase the exposure to **buspirone**. Adjust **buspirone** dose. [Severe] Study
- Antifungals, azoles **(miconazole)** are predicted to increase the concentration of **buspirone**. Use with caution and adjust dose. [Moderate] Theoretical
- **Apalutamide** is predicted to decrease the exposure to **buspirone**. Use with caution and adjust dose. [Severe] Study
- **Aprepitant** is predicted to increase the exposure to **buspirone**. Use with caution and adjust dose. [Moderate] Study

- Calcium channel blockers **(diltiazem, verapamil)** are predicted to increase the exposure to **buspirone**. Use with caution and adjust dose. Moderate Study
- Cobicistat is predicted to increase the exposure to **buspirone**. Adjust **buspirone** dose. Severe Study
- Crizotinib is predicted to increase the exposure to **buspirone**. Use with caution and adjust dose. Moderate Study
- Enzalutamide is predicted to decrease the exposure to **buspirone**. Use with caution and adjust dose. Severe Study
- Grapefruit juice increases the exposure to **buspirone**. Avoid. Mild Study
- HIV-protease inhibitors are predicted to increase the exposure to **buspirone**. Adjust **buspirone** dose. Severe Study
- Idelalisib is predicted to increase the exposure to **buspirone**. Adjust **buspirone** dose. Severe Study
- Imatinib is predicted to increase the exposure to **buspirone**. Use with caution and adjust dose. Moderate Study
- **Buspirone** is predicted to increase the risk of elevated blood pressure when given with linezolid. Avoid. Severe Theoretical → Also see TABLE 13 p. 910
- Macrolides **(clarithromycin)** are predicted to increase the exposure to **buspirone**. Adjust **buspirone** dose. Severe Study
- Macrolides **(erythromycin)** are predicted to increase the exposure to **buspirone**. Use with caution and adjust dose. Moderate Study
- **Buspirone** is predicted to increase the risk of elevated blood pressure when given with **MAOIs, irreversible**. Avoid. Severe Anecdotal → Also see TABLE 13 p. 910
- Mitotane is predicted to decrease the exposure to **buspirone**. Use with caution and adjust dose. Severe Study
- Netupitant is predicted to increase the exposure to **buspirone**. Use with caution and adjust dose. Moderate Study
- Nilotinib is predicted to increase the exposure to **buspirone**. Use with caution and adjust dose. Moderate Study
- Rifampicin is predicted to decrease the exposure to **buspirone**. Use with caution and adjust dose. Severe Study

Busulfan → see alkylating agents

Cabazitaxel → see taxanes

Cabergoline → see dopamine receptor agonists

Cabozantinib → see TABLE 15 p. 910 (myelosuppression), TABLE 9 p. 909 (QT-interval prolongation)

- Antiarrhythmics **(dronedarone)** are predicted to increase the exposure to **cabozantinib**. Moderate Theoretical → Also see TABLE 9 p. 909
- Antiepileptics **(carbamazepine, fosphenytoin, phenobarbital, phenytoin, primidone)** moderately decrease the exposure to **cabozantinib**. Avoid. Moderate Study
- Antifungals, azoles **(fluconazole, isavuconazole, posaconazole)** are predicted to increase the exposure to **cabozantinib**. Moderate Theoretical → Also see TABLE 9 p. 909
- Antifungals, azoles **(itraconazole, ketoconazole, voriconazole)** slightly increase the exposure to **cabozantinib**. Moderate Study → Also see TABLE 9 p. 909
- Apalutamide moderately decreases the exposure to **cabozantinib**. Avoid. Moderate Study → Also see TABLE 9 p. 909
- Aprepitant is predicted to increase the exposure to **cabozantinib**. Moderate Theoretical
- Bosentan is predicted to decrease the exposure to **cabozantinib**. Moderate Theoretical
- Calcium channel blockers **(diltiazem, verapamil)** are predicted to increase the exposure to **cabozantinib**. Moderate Theoretical
- Cobicistat slightly increases the exposure to **cabozantinib**. Moderate Study
- **Cabozantinib** is predicted to increase the risk of bleeding events when given with **coumarins**. Severe Theoretical
- Crizotinib is predicted to increase the exposure to **cabozantinib**. Moderate Theoretical → Also see TABLE 15 p. 910 → Also see TABLE 9 p. 909
- Efavirenz is predicted to decrease the exposure to **cabozantinib**. Moderate Theoretical → Also see TABLE 9 p. 909
- Enzalutamide moderately decreases the exposure to **cabozantinib**. Avoid. Moderate Study
- Grapefruit juice is predicted to increase the exposure to **cabozantinib**. Moderate Theoretical
- HIV-protease inhibitors slightly increase the exposure to **cabozantinib**. Moderate Study → Also see TABLE 9 p. 909
- Idelalisib slightly increases the exposure to **cabozantinib**. Moderate Study → Also see TABLE 15 p. 910
- Imatinib is predicted to increase the exposure to **cabozantinib**. Moderate Theoretical → Also see TABLE 15 p. 910
- Macrolides **(clarithromycin)** slightly increase the exposure to **cabozantinib**. Moderate Study → Also see TABLE 9 p. 909
- Macrolides **(erythromycin)** are predicted to increase the exposure to **cabozantinib**. Moderate Theoretical → Also see TABLE 9 p. 909
- Mitotane moderately decreases the exposure to **cabozantinib**. Avoid. Moderate Study → Also see TABLE 15 p. 910
- Netupitant is predicted to increase the exposure to **cabozantinib**. Moderate Theoretical
- Nevirapine is predicted to decrease the exposure to **cabozantinib**. Moderate Theoretical
- Nilotinib is predicted to increase the exposure to **cabozantinib**. Moderate Theoretical → Also see TABLE 15 p. 910 → Also see TABLE 9 p. 909
- **Cabozantinib** is predicted to increase the risk of bleeding events when given with phenindione. Severe Theoretical
- Rifampicin moderately decreases the exposure to **cabozantinib**. Avoid. Moderate Study
- St John's Wort is predicted to decrease the exposure to **cabozantinib**. Moderate Theoretical

Caffeine citrate

- **Caffeine citrate** decreases the efficacy of antiarrhythmics (adenosine). Separate administration by 24 hours. Mild Study
- Antiepileptics **(fosphenytoin, phenytoin)** are predicted to moderately increase the clearance of **caffeine citrate**. Monitor and adjust dose. Moderate Study
- HIV-protease inhibitors **(ritonavir)** are predicted to moderately increase the clearance of **caffeine citrate**. Monitor and adjust dose. Moderate Study
- Leflunomide is predicted to moderately increase the clearance of **caffeine citrate**. Monitor and adjust dose. Moderate Study
- Rifampicin is predicted to moderately increase the clearance of **caffeine citrate**. Monitor and adjust dose. Moderate Study
- SSRIs **(fluvoxamine)** markedly decrease the clearance of **caffeine citrate**. Monitor and adjust dose. Severe Study
- Teriflunomide is predicted to moderately increase the clearance of **caffeine citrate**. Monitor and adjust dose. Moderate Study
- **Caffeine citrate** decreases the clearance of **theophylline**. Moderate Study

Calcipotriol → see vitamin D substances

Calcitonins

- **Calcitonins** decrease the concentration of lithium. Adjust dose. Moderate Study

Calcitriol → see vitamin D substances

Calcium acetate → see calcium salts

Calcium carbonate → see calcium salts

Calcium channel blockers → see TABLE 6 p. 908 (bradycardia), TABLE 8 p. 908 (hypotension)

amlodipine · diltiazem · felodipine · lacidipine · lercanidipine · nicardipine · nifedipine · nimodipine · verapamil

- Calcium channel blockers **(diltiazem, verapamil)** are predicted to increase the exposure to abemaciclib. Moderate Study
- **Verapamil** is predicted to increase the exposure to **afatinib**. Separate administration by 12 hours. Moderate Study
- Calcium channel blockers **(diltiazem, verapamil)** are predicted to increase the exposure to aldosterone antagonists **(eplerenone)**. Adjust **eplerenone** dose. Severe Study → Also see TABLE 8 p. 908
- **Verapamil** moderately increases the exposure to **aliskiren**. Moderate Study → Also see TABLE 8 p. 908
- Calcium channel blockers **(diltiazem, verapamil)** are predicted to increase the exposure to alpha blockers **(tamsulosin)**. Moderate Theoretical → Also see TABLE 8 p. 908
- Calcium channel blockers **(diltiazem, verapamil)** are predicted to increase the exposure to **alprazolam**. Severe Study
- **Verapamil** moderately increases the exposure to anthracyclines **(doxorubicin)**. Moderate Study

Calcium channel blockers (continued)

- Antiarrhythmics **(disopyramide)** are predicted to increase the risk of cardiodepression when given with **verapamil**. Severe Theoretical
- Antiarrhythmics **(dronedarone)** are predicted to increase the exposure to calcium channel blockers **(amlodipine, felodipine, lacidipine, lercanidipine, nicardipine, nifedipine, nimodipine)**. Monitor and adjust dose. Moderate Study
- Antiarrhythmics **(amiodarone)** are predicted to increase the risk of cardiodepression when given with calcium channel blockers **(diltiazem, verapamil)**. Avoid. Severe Theoretical → Also see TABLE 6 p. 908
- Calcium channel blockers **(diltiazem, verapamil)** increase the exposure to antiarrhythmics **(dronedarone)** and antiarrhythmics **(dronedarone)** increase the exposure to calcium channel blockers **(diltiazem, verapamil)**. Moderate Study
- **Verapamil** increases the risk of cardiodepression when given with antiarrhythmics **(flecainide)**. Severe Anecdotal → Also see TABLE 6 p. 908
- Calcium channel blockers **(diltiazem, verapamil)** are predicted to increase the exposure to antiarrhythmics **(propafenone)**. Monitor and adjust dose. Moderate Study
- Antiepileptics **(valproate)** increase the exposure to **nimodipine**. Adjust dose. Moderate Study
- Antiepileptics **(carbamazepine, fosphenytoin, phenobarbital, phenytoin, primidone)** are predicted to decrease the exposure to calcium channel blockers **(amlodipine, felodipine, lacidipine, lercanidipine, nicardipine, nifedipine, nimodipine)**. Monitor and adjust dose. Moderate Study
- **Diltiazem** increases the concentration of antiepileptics **(carbamazepine)** and antiepileptics **(carbamazepine)** are predicted to decrease the exposure to **diltiazem**. Monitor concentration and adjust dose. Severe Anecdotal
- **Verapamil** increases the concentration of antiepileptics **(carbamazepine)** and antiepileptics **(carbamazepine)** are predicted to decrease the exposure to **verapamil**. Severe Anecdotal
- Antiepileptics **(phenobarbital, primidone)** are predicted to decrease the exposure to calcium channel blockers **(diltiazem, verapamil)**. Severe Study
- Calcium channel blockers **(diltiazem, verapamil)** potentially increase the concentration of antiepileptics **(fosphenytoin, phenytoin)** and antiepileptics **(fosphenytoin, phenytoin)** are predicted to decrease the exposure to calcium channel blockers **(diltiazem, verapamil)**. Severe Study
- Antifungals, azoles **(itraconazole, ketoconazole, voriconazole)** are predicted to markedly increase the exposure to **lercanidipine**. Avoid. Severe Study
- Antifungals, azoles **(miconazole)** are predicted to increase the exposure to **diltiazem**. Moderate Theoretical
- Antifungals, azoles **(fluconazole, isavuconazole, posaconazole)** are predicted to increase the exposure to calcium channel blockers **(amlodipine, felodipine, lacidipine, lercanidipine, nicardipine, nifedipine, nimodipine)**. Monitor and adjust dose. Moderate Study
- Antifungals, azoles **(miconazole)** are predicted to increase the exposure to calcium channel blockers **(amlodipine, felodipine, lacidipine, lercanidipine, nicardipine, nifedipine, nimodipine, verapamil)**. Use with caution and adjust dose. Moderate Theoretical
- Antifungals, azoles **(itraconazole, ketoconazole, voriconazole)** are predicted to increase the exposure to calcium channel blockers **(amlodipine, felodipine, lacidipine, nicardipine, nifedipine, nimodipine)**. Monitor and adjust dose. Moderate Study
- Antifungals, azoles **(fluconazole)** (high-dose) are predicted to increase the exposure to calcium channel blockers **(diltiazem, verapamil)**. Moderate Theoretical
- Antifungals, azoles **(itraconazole, ketoconazole, voriconazole)** are predicted to increase the exposure to calcium channel blockers **(diltiazem, verapamil)**. Severe Study
- Antifungals, azoles **(posaconazole)** are predicted to increase the exposure to calcium channel blockers **(diltiazem, verapamil)**. Moderate Theoretical
- Calcium channel blockers **(diltiazem, verapamil)** are predicted to increase the exposure to antifungals, azoles **(isavuconazole)**. Moderate Theoretical
- Calcium channel blockers **(diltiazem, verapamil)** are predicted to increase the exposure to antihistamines, non-sedating **(mizolastine)**. Severe Theoretical
- Calcium channel blockers **(diltiazem, verapamil)** are predicted to increase the exposure to antihistamines, non-sedating **(rupatadine)**. Avoid. Moderate Study
- Antimalarials **(mefloquine)** are predicted to increase the risk of bradycardia when given with **calcium channel blockers**. Severe Theoretical
- Calcium channel blockers **(diltiazem, verapamil)** are predicted to increase the concentration of antimalarials **(piperaquine)**. Severe Theoretical
- **Apalutamide** is predicted to decrease the exposure to calcium channel blockers **(amlodipine, felodipine, lacidipine, lercanidipine, nicardipine, nimodipine)**. Monitor and adjust dose. Moderate Study
- **Verapamil** is predicted to increase the exposure to **apixaban**. Moderate Theoretical
- Calcium channel blockers **(diltiazem, verapamil)** are predicted to increase the exposure to **aprepitant** and **aprepitant** is predicted to increase the exposure to calcium channel blockers **(diltiazem, verapamil)**. Moderate Study
- **Aprepitant** is predicted to increase the exposure to calcium channel blockers **(amlodipine, felodipine, lacidipine, lercanidipine, nicardipine, nifedipine, nimodipine)**. Monitor and adjust dose. Moderate Study
- Calcium channel blockers **(diltiazem, verapamil)** are predicted to increase the exposure to **axitinib**. Moderate Theoretical
- Calcium channel blockers **(diltiazem, verapamil)** are predicted to increase the exposure to **bedaquiline**. Avoid prolonged use. Mild Theoretical
- **Diltiazem** is predicted to increase the risk of cardiodepression when given with **beta blockers, non-selective**. Severe Study → Also see TABLE 6 p. 908 → Also see TABLE 8 p. 908
- Intravenous **verapamil** increases the risk of cardiovascular side-effects when given with **beta blockers, non-selective**. Avoid. Severe Study → Also see TABLE 6 p. 908 → Also see TABLE 8 p. 908
- Oral **verapamil** increases the risk of cardiovascular side-effects when given with **beta blockers, non-selective**. Severe Study → Also see TABLE 6 p. 908 → Also see TABLE 8 p. 908
- **Diltiazem** is predicted to increase the risk of cardiodepression when given with **beta blockers, selective**. Severe Study → Also see TABLE 6 p. 908 → Also see TABLE 8 p. 908
- Intravenous **verapamil** increases the risk of cardiovascular side-effects when given with **beta blockers, selective**. Avoid. Severe Study → Also see TABLE 6 p. 908 → Also see TABLE 8 p. 908
- Oral **verapamil** increases the risk of cardiovascular side-effects when given with **beta blockers, selective**. Severe Study → Also see TABLE 6 p. 908 → Also see TABLE 8 p. 908
- **Verapamil** is predicted to increase the exposure to **bictegravir**. Use with caution or avoid. Moderate Theoretical
- **Bosentan** is predicted to decrease the exposure to calcium channel blockers **(amlodipine, felodipine, lacidipine, lercanidipine, nicardipine, nifedipine, nimodipine)**. Monitor and adjust dose. Moderate Theoretical
- **Bosentan** is predicted to decrease the exposure to calcium channel blockers **(diltiazem, verapamil)**. Moderate Theoretical
- Calcium channel blockers **(diltiazem, verapamil)** are predicted to increase the exposure to **bosutinib**. Avoid or adjust dose. Severe Theoretical
- Calcium channel blockers **(diltiazem, verapamil)** are predicted to increase the exposure to **buspirone**. Use with caution and adjust dose. Moderate Study
- Calcium channel blockers **(diltiazem, verapamil)** are predicted to increase the exposure to **cabozantinib**. Moderate Theoretical
- Calcium channel blockers **(diltiazem)** are predicted to increase the exposure to calcium channel blockers **(amlodipine)**. Monitor and adjust dose. Moderate Study → Also see TABLE 8 p. 908
- Calcium channel blockers **(verapamil)** are predicted to increase the exposure to calcium channel blockers **(amlodipine, felodipine, lacidipine, lercanidipine, nicardipine, nifedipine,**

nimodipine). Monitor and adjust dose. [Moderate] Study → Also see **TABLE 8** p. 908
- Calcium channel blockers **(diltiazem)** are predicted to increase the exposure to calcium channel blockers **(felodipine, lacidipine, lercanidipine, nicardipine, nifedipine, nimodipine)**. Monitor and adjust dose. [Moderate] Study → Also see **TABLE 8** p. 908
- Calcium channel blockers **(diltiazem, verapamil)** are predicted to increase the exposure to **cariprazine**. Avoid. [Severe] Study → Also see **TABLE 8** p. 908
- Calcium channel blockers **(diltiazem, verapamil)** are predicted to increase the concentration of **ciclosporin**. [Severe] Study
- **Ciclosporin** moderately increases the exposure to **lercanidipine**. Use with caution or avoid. [Severe] Study
- **Nicardipine** increases the concentration of **ciclosporin**. [Severe] Study
- **Cobicistat** is predicted to increase the exposure to calcium channel blockers **(amlodipine, felodipine, lacidipine, nicardipine, nifedipine, nimodipine)**. Monitor and adjust dose. [Moderate] Study
- **Cobicistat** is predicted to increase the exposure to calcium channel blockers **(diltiazem, verapamil)**. [Severe] Study
- **Cobicistat** is predicted to markedly increase the exposure to **lercanidipine**. Avoid. [Severe] Study
- Calcium channel blockers **(diltiazem, verapamil)** are predicted to increase the exposure to **cobimetinib**. [Severe] Theoretical
- Calcium channel blockers **(diltiazem, verapamil)** are predicted to increase the exposure to **colchicine**. Adjust **colchicine** dose with moderate inhibitors of CYP3A4. [Severe] Study
- Calcium channel blockers **(diltiazem, verapamil)** are predicted to increase the exposure to corticosteroids **(methylprednisolone)**. Monitor and adjust dose. [Moderate] Study
- **Crizotinib** is predicted to increase the exposure to calcium channel blockers **(amlodipine, felodipine, lacidipine, lercanidipine, nicardipine, nifedipine, nimodipine)**. Monitor and adjust dose. [Moderate] Study
- **Verapamil** increases the exposure to **dabigatran**. Adjust **dabigatran** dose. [Severe] Study
- Intravenous **dantrolene** potentially increases the risk of acute hyperkalaemia and cardiovascular collapse when given with calcium channel blockers **(diltiazem, verapamil)**. Avoid. [Severe] Anecdotal
- Calcium channel blockers **(diltiazem, verapamil)** are predicted to slightly increase the exposure to **darifenacin**. [Moderate] Study
- Calcium channel blockers **(diltiazem, verapamil)** are predicted to increase the exposure to **dasatinib**. [Severe] Study
- Calcium channel blockers **(diltiazem, verapamil)** are predicted to slightly increase the exposure to **dienogest**. [Moderate] Study
- Calcium channel blockers **(diltiazem, verapamil)** increase the concentration of **digoxin**. Monitor and adjust dose. [Severe] Study → Also see **TABLE 6** p. 908
- Calcium channel blockers **(diltiazem, verapamil)** increase the risk of QT-prolongation when given with **domperidone**. Avoid. [Severe] Study
- Calcium channel blockers **(diltiazem, verapamil)** are predicted to increase the exposure to dopamine receptor agonists **(bromocriptine)**. [Severe] Theoretical → Also see **TABLE 8** p. 908
- Calcium channel blockers **(diltiazem, verapamil)** are predicted to increase the concentration of dopamine receptor agonists **(cabergoline)**. [Moderate] Anecdotal → Also see **TABLE 8** p. 908
- Calcium channel blockers **(diltiazem, verapamil)** are predicted to moderately increase the exposure to **dutasteride**. [Mild] Study
- **Efavirenz** is predicted to decrease the exposure to calcium channel blockers **(amlodipine, felodipine, lacidipine, lercanidipine, nicardipine, nifedipine, nimodipine)**. Monitor and adjust dose. [Moderate] Theoretical
- **Efavirenz** is predicted to decrease the exposure to calcium channel blockers **(diltiazem, verapamil)**. [Moderate] Theoretical
- Calcium channel blockers **(diltiazem, verapamil)** are predicted to increase the exposure to **eliglustat**. Avoid or adjust dose—consult product literature. [Severe] Study
- Calcium channel blockers **(diltiazem, verapamil)** are predicted to moderately increase the exposure to **encorafenib**. [Moderate] Study
- **Enzalutamide** is predicted to decrease the exposure to calcium channel blockers **(amlodipine, felodipine, lacidipine, lercanidipine, nicardipine, nifedipine, nimodipine)**. Monitor and adjust dose. [Moderate] Study
- **Enzalutamide** is predicted to decrease the exposure to calcium channel blockers **(diltiazem, verapamil)**. [Severe] Study
- Calcium channel blockers **(diltiazem, verapamil)** are predicted to increase the risk of ergotism when given with **ergometrine**. [Severe] Theoretical
- Calcium channel blockers **(diltiazem, verapamil)** are predicted to increase the risk of ergotism when given with **ergotamine**. [Severe] Theoretical
- Calcium channel blockers **(diltiazem, verapamil)** are predicted to increase the exposure to **erlotinib**. [Moderate] Theoretical
- Calcium channel blockers **(diltiazem, verapamil)** are predicted to increase the concentration of **everolimus**. Avoid or adjust dose. [Moderate] Study
- Calcium channel blockers **(diltiazem, verapamil)** are predicted to increase the exposure to **fesoterodine**. Adjust **fesoterodine** dose with moderate inhibitors of CYP3A4 in hepatic and renal impairment. [Mild] Study
- **Verapamil** is predicted to increase the exposure to **fidaxomicin**. Avoid. [Moderate] Study
- Calcium channel blockers **(diltiazem, verapamil)** are predicted to increase the exposure to **fingolimod**. Avoid. [Moderate] Theoretical → Also see **TABLE 6** p. 908
- Calcium channel blockers **(diltiazem, verapamil)** are predicted to increase the exposure to **gefitinib**. [Moderate] Theoretical
- **Grapefruit juice** very slightly increases the exposure to **amlodipine**. Avoid. [Mild] Study
- **Grapefruit juice** increases the exposure to calcium channel blockers **(nifedipine, verapamil)**. Avoid. [Mild] Study
- **Grapefruit juice** increases the exposure to **felodipine**. Avoid. [Moderate] Study
- **Grapefruit juice** is predicted to increase the exposure to **lercanidipine**. Avoid. [Moderate] Theoretical
- **Grapefruit juice** increases the exposure to **nicardipine**. [Mild] Study
- **Grazoprevir** is predicted to increase the concentration of **calcium channel blockers**. [Moderate] Theoretical
- Calcium channel blockers **(diltiazem, verapamil)** are predicted to increase the concentration of **guanfacine**. Adjust **guanfacine** dose, p. 247. [Moderate] Theoretical → Also see **TABLE 8** p. 908
- H_2 receptor antagonists **(cimetidine)** (high-dose) are predicted to increase the exposure to **lercanidipine**. [Moderate] Theoretical
- H_2 receptor antagonists **(cimetidine)** moderately increase the exposure to **nifedipine**. Monitor and adjust dose. [Severe] Study
- H_2 receptor antagonists **(cimetidine)** increase the exposure to **verapamil**. [Moderate] Study
- H_2 receptor antagonists **(cimetidine)** slightly increase the exposure to calcium channel blockers **(diltiazem, nimodipine)**. Monitor and adjust dose. [Moderate] Study
- **HIV-protease inhibitors** are predicted to increase the exposure to calcium channel blockers **(amlodipine, felodipine, lacidipine, nicardipine, nifedipine, nimodipine)**. Monitor and adjust dose. [Moderate] Study
- **HIV-protease inhibitors** are predicted to increase the exposure to calcium channel blockers **(diltiazem, verapamil)**. [Severe] Study
- **HIV-protease inhibitors** are predicted to markedly increase the exposure to **lercanidipine**. Avoid. [Severe] Study
- Calcium channel blockers **(diltiazem, verapamil)** are predicted to increase the exposure to **ibrutinib**. Adjust **ibrutinib** dose with moderate inhibitors of CYP3A4. [Severe] Study
- **Idelalisib** is predicted to increase the exposure to calcium channel blockers **(amlodipine, felodipine, lacidipine, nicardipine, nifedipine, nimodipine)**. Monitor and adjust dose. [Moderate] Study
- **Idelalisib** is predicted to increase the exposure to calcium channel blockers **(diltiazem, verapamil)**. [Severe] Study
- **Idelalisib** is predicted to markedly increase the exposure to **lercanidipine**. Avoid. [Severe] Study
- Calcium channel blockers **(diltiazem, verapamil)** are predicted to increase the exposure to **imatinib**. [Moderate] Theoretical
- **Imatinib** is predicted to increase the exposure to calcium channel blockers **(amlodipine, felodipine, lacidipine, lercanidipine, nicardipine, nifedipine, nimodipine)**. Monitor and adjust dose. [Moderate] Study

Calcium channel blockers (continued)

- Calcium channel blockers **(diltiazem, verapamil)** are predicted to increase the exposure to ivabradine. Avoid. Moderate Study → Also see TABLE 6 p. 908
- Calcium channel blockers **(diltiazem, verapamil)** are predicted to increase the exposure to ivacaftor. Adjust ivacaftor p. 196 or tezacaftor with ivacaftor p. 198 dose with moderate inhibitors of CYP3A4. Severe Study
- Calcium channel blockers **(diltiazem, verapamil)** are predicted to increase the exposure to lapatinib. Moderate Study
- **Verapamil** is predicted to increase the exposure to larotrectinib. Mild Theoretical
- Calcium channel blockers **(diltiazem, verapamil)** are predicted to increase the risk of neurotoxicity when given with lithium. Severe Anecdotal
- Calcium channel blockers **(amlodipine, lacidipine)** are predicted to increase the exposure to lomitapide. Separate administration by 12 hours. Moderate Theoretical
- Calcium channel blockers **(diltiazem, verapamil)** are predicted to increase the exposure to lomitapide. Avoid. Moderate Theoretical
- Calcium channel blockers **(diltiazem, verapamil)** are predicted to increase the exposure to lurasidone. Adjust **lurasidone** dose. Moderate Study → Also see TABLE 8 p. 908
- Macrolides **(clarithromycin)** are predicted to markedly increase the exposure to **lercanidipine**. Avoid. Severe Study
- Macrolides **(erythromycin)** are predicted to increase the exposure to **diltiazem**. Severe Theoretical
- Macrolides **(erythromycin)** are predicted to increase the exposure to **verapamil**. Severe Study
- Macrolides **(erythromycin)** are predicted to increase the exposure to calcium channel blockers **(amlodipine, felodipine, lacidipine, lercanidipine, nicardipine, nifedipine, nimodipine)**. Monitor and adjust dose. Moderate Study
- Macrolides **(clarithromycin)** are predicted to increase the exposure to calcium channel blockers **(amlodipine, felodipine, lacidipine, nicardipine, nifedipine, nimodipine)**. Monitor and adjust dose. Moderate Study
- Macrolides **(clarithromycin)** are predicted to increase the exposure to calcium channel blockers **(diltiazem, verapamil)**. Severe Study
- Intravenous **magnesium** potentially increases the risk of hypotension when given with calcium channel blockers **(amlodipine, felodipine, lacidipine, lercanidipine, nicardipine, nifedipine, nimodipine, verapamil)** in pregnant women. Severe Anecdotal
- **Mexiletine** increases the risk of cardiovascular side-effects when given with **diltiazem**. Avoid or monitor. Severe Theoretical
- **Mexiletine** potentially increases the risk of cardiovascular side-effects when given with **verapamil**. Avoid or monitor. Severe Theoretical
- Calcium channel blockers **(diltiazem, verapamil)** are predicted to increase the exposure to midazolam. Monitor side effects and adjust dose. Severe Study
- Calcium channel blockers **(diltiazem, verapamil)** are predicted to increase the exposure to midostaurin. Moderate Theoretical
- **Mitotane** is predicted to decrease the exposure to calcium channel blockers **(amlodipine, felodipine, lacidipine, lercanidipine, nicardipine, nifedipine, nimodipine)**. Monitor and adjust dose. Moderate Study
- **Mitotane** is predicted to decrease the exposure to **diltiazem**. Severe Study
- Monoclonal antibodies **(tocilizumab)** are predicted to decrease the exposure to **calcium channel blockers**. Monitor and adjust dose. Moderate Theoretical
- Calcium channel blockers **(diltiazem, verapamil)** are predicted to increase the exposure to naldemedine. Moderate Study
- Calcium channel blockers **(diltiazem, verapamil)** are predicted to increase the exposure to naloxegol. Adjust **naloxegol** dose and monitor side effects. Moderate Study
- Calcium channel blockers **(diltiazem, verapamil)** are predicted to increase the exposure to neratinib. Avoid. Severe Study
- **Netupitant** is predicted to increase the exposure to calcium channel blockers **(amlodipine, felodipine, lacidipine, lercanidipine, nicardipine, nifedipine, nimodipine)**. Monitor and adjust dose. Moderate Study
- **Nevirapine** is predicted to decrease the exposure to calcium channel blockers **(amlodipine, felodipine, lacidipine, lercanidipine, nicardipine, nifedipine, nimodipine)**. Monitor and adjust dose. Moderate Theoretical
- **Nevirapine** is predicted to decrease the exposure to calcium channel blockers **(diltiazem, verapamil)**. Moderate Theoretical
- Calcium channel blockers **(diltiazem, verapamil)** are predicted to increase the exposure to nilotinib. Moderate Theoretical
- **Nilotinib** is predicted to increase the exposure to calcium channel blockers **(amlodipine, felodipine, lacidipine, lercanidipine, nicardipine, nifedipine, nimodipine)**. Monitor and adjust dose. Moderate Study
- **Verapamil** is predicted to increase the exposure to **nintedanib**. Moderate Study
- Calcium channel blockers **(diltiazem, verapamil)** are predicted to increase the exposure to olaparib. Avoid moderate inhibitors of CYP3A4 or adjust **olaparib** dose. Moderate Theoretical
- Calcium channel blockers **(diltiazem, verapamil)** are predicted to increase the exposure to opioids **(alfentanil, buprenorphine, fentanyl, oxycodone)**. Monitor and adjust dose. Moderate Study → Also see TABLE 6 p. 908
- Calcium channel blockers **(diltiazem, verapamil)** are predicted to increase the exposure to opioids **(methadone)**. Moderate Theoretical → Also see TABLE 6 p. 908
- Calcium channel blockers **(diltiazem, verapamil)** are predicted to increase the exposure to **oxybutynin**. Mild Theoretical
- **Verapamil** is predicted to increase the exposure to panobinostat. Adjust dose. Moderate Theoretical
- Calcium channel blockers **(diltiazem, verapamil)** are predicted to increase the exposure to **pazopanib**. Moderate Theoretical
- Calcium channel blockers **(diltiazem, verapamil)** are predicted to increase the exposure to phosphodiesterase type-5 inhibitors (avanafil). Adjust **avanafil** dose. Moderate Theoretical → Also see TABLE 8 p. 908
- Calcium channel blockers **(diltiazem, verapamil)** are predicted to increase the exposure to phosphodiesterase type-5 inhibitors (sildenafil). Monitor or adjust **sildenafil** dose with moderate inhibitors of CYP3A4, p. 125. Moderate Study → Also see TABLE 8 p. 908
- Calcium channel blockers **(diltiazem, verapamil)** are predicted to increase the exposure to phosphodiesterase type-5 inhibitors (tadalafil). Severe Theoretical → Also see TABLE 8 p. 908
- Calcium channel blockers **(diltiazem, verapamil)** are predicted to increase the exposure to phosphodiesterase type-5 inhibitors (vardenafil). Adjust dose. Severe Theoretical → Also see TABLE 8 p. 908
- **Verapamil** is predicted to increase the exposure to pibrentasvir. Moderate Theoretical
- Calcium channel blockers **(diltiazem, verapamil)** are predicted to increase the exposure to pimozide. Avoid. Severe Theoretical → Also see TABLE 8 p. 908
- Calcium channel blockers **(diltiazem, verapamil)** are predicted to increase the exposure to quetiapine. Avoid. Moderate Study → Also see TABLE 8 p. 908
- Calcium channel blockers **(diltiazem, verapamil)** are predicted to increase the exposure to ranolazine. Severe Study
- Calcium channel blockers **(diltiazem, verapamil)** are predicted to increase the exposure to ribociclib. Moderate Study
- **Rifampicin** is predicted to decrease the exposure to calcium channel blockers **(amlodipine, felodipine, lacidipine, lercanidipine, nicardipine, nimodipine)**. Monitor and adjust dose. Moderate Study
- **Rifampicin** greatly decreases the exposure to calcium channel blockers **(diltiazem, verapamil)**. Severe Study
- **Rifampicin** moderately decreases the exposure to **nifedipine**. Avoid. Severe Study
- Calcium channel blockers **(diltiazem, verapamil)** are predicted to increase the exposure to ruxolitinib. Moderate Theoretical
- Calcium channel blockers **(diltiazem, verapamil)** are predicted to increase the exposure to saxagliptin. Mild Study
- Calcium channel blockers **(diltiazem, verapamil)** increase the concentration of sirolimus. Monitor and adjust dose. Moderate Study

- Calcium channel blockers **(diltiazem, verapamil)** are predicted to increase the exposure to SSRIs (dapoxetine). Adjust **dapoxetine** dose with moderate inhibitors of CYP3A4. Moderate Theoretical
- **St John's Wort** is predicted to decrease the exposure to calcium channel blockers **(amlodipine, felodipine, lacidipine, lercanidipine, nicardipine, nifedipine, nimodipine)**. Monitor and adjust dose. Moderate Theoretical
- **St John's Wort** is predicted to decrease the exposure to calcium channel blockers **(diltiazem, verapamil)**. Moderate Theoretical
- **Diltiazem** slightly to moderately increases the exposure to statins **(atorvastatin)**. Monitor and adjust dose. Severe Anecdotal
- **Verapamil** is predicted to slightly to moderately increase the exposure to statins **(atorvastatin)**. Monitor and adjust dose. Severe Theoretical
- **Amlodipine** slightly increases the exposure to statins **(simvastatin)**. Adjust **simvastatin** dose, p. 141. Mild Study
- Calcium channel blockers **(diltiazem, verapamil)** moderately increase the exposure to statins **(simvastatin)**. Monitor and adjust dose. Severe Study
- Calcium channel blockers **(diltiazem, verapamil)** are predicted to increase the exposure to **sunitinib**. Moderate Theoretical
- Calcium channel blockers **(diltiazem, verapamil)** are predicted to increase the concentration of **tacrolimus**. Severe Study
- **Nicardipine** potentially increases the concentration of **tacrolimus**. Monitor concentration and adjust dose. Severe Anecdotal
- **Verapamil** is predicted to slightly increase the exposure to talazoparib. Avoid or adjust **talazoparib** dose. Severe Study
- Calcium channel blockers **(diltiazem, verapamil)** are predicted to increase the exposure to taxanes **(cabazitaxel)**. Moderate Theoretical
- Calcium channel blockers **(diltiazem, verapamil)** are predicted to increase the concentration of and the risk of angioedema when given with **temsirolimus**. Use with caution or avoid. Moderate Theoretical
- **Temsirolimus** is predicted to increase the risk of angioedema when given with calcium channel blockers **(amlodipine, felodipine, lacidipine, lercanidipine, nicardipine, nifedipine, nimodipine)**. Moderate Theoretical
- Calcium channel blockers **(diltiazem, verapamil)** are predicted to increase the exposure to **tezacaftor**. Adjust tezacaftor with ivacaftor p. 198 dose with moderate inhibitors of CYP3A4. Severe Study
- Calcium channel blockers **(diltiazem, verapamil)** given with a potent CYP2C19 inhibitor are predicted to increase the exposure to **tofacitinib**. Adjust **tofacitinib** dose. Moderate Study
- Calcium channel blockers **(diltiazem, verapamil)** are predicted to increase the exposure to **tolterodine**. Mild Theoretical
- Calcium channel blockers **(diltiazem, verapamil)** are predicted to increase the exposure to **tolvaptan**. Manufacturer advises caution or adjust **tolvaptan** dose with moderate inhibitors of CYP3A4. Moderate Study
- **Verapamil** is predicted to increase the exposure to **topotecan**. Severe Study
- **Verapamil** is predicted to increase the concentration of **trametinib**. Moderate Theoretical
- Calcium channel blockers **(diltiazem, verapamil)** are predicted to increase the exposure to **trazodone**. Moderate Theoretical
- Calcium channel blockers **(diltiazem, verapamil)** are predicted to increase the exposure to **ulipristal**. Avoid if used for uterine fibroids. Moderate Study
- Calcium channel blockers **(diltiazem, verapamil)** are predicted to increase the exposure to **venetoclax**. Avoid or adjust dose—consult product literature. Severe Study
- Calcium channel blockers **(diltiazem, verapamil)** are predicted to increase the exposure to **vinca alkaloids**. Severe Theoretical
- Calcium channel blockers **(diltiazem, verapamil)** are predicted to increase the exposure to **zopiclone**. Adjust dose. Moderate Study

Calcium chloride → see calcium salts
Calcium gluconate → see calcium salts
Calcium lactate → see calcium salts
Calcium phosphate → see calcium salts

Calcium salts

calcium acetate · calcium carbonate · calcium chloride · calcium gluconate · calcium lactate · calcium phosphate

SEPARATION OF ADMINISTRATION **Calcium carbonate-containing antacids** should preferably not be taken at the same time as other drugs since they might impair absorption. **Antacids** might damage enteric coatings designed to prevent dissolution in the stomach.

- Oral **calcium salts** decrease the absorption of alkylating agents **(estramustine)**. Severe Study
- **Calcium carbonate** decreases the absorption of antimalarials **(chloroquine)**. Separate administration by at least 4 hours. Moderate Study
- **Calcium carbonate** is predicted to decrease the absorption of antimalarials **(proguanil)**. Separate administration by at least 2 hours. Moderate Study
- Oral **calcium salts** decrease the absorption of bisphosphonates **(alendronate)**. **Alendronate** should be taken at least 30 minutes before **calcium salts**. Moderate Study
- Oral **calcium salts** decrease the absorption of bisphosphonates **(clodronate)**. Avoid **calcium salts** for 2 hours before or 1 hour after **clodronate**. Moderate Study
- Oral **calcium salts** are predicted to decrease the absorption of oral bisphosphonates **(ibandronate)**. Avoid **calcium salts** for at least 6 hours before or 1 hour after **ibandronate**. Moderate Theoretical
- Oral **calcium salts** decrease the absorption of bisphosphonates **(risedronate)**. Separate administration by at least 2 hours. Moderate Study
- Cephalosporins **(ceftriaxone)** increase the risk of cardio-respiratory arrest when given with **calcium chloride**. Avoid. Severe Anecdotal
- Cephalosporins **(ceftriaxone)** increase the risk of cardio-respiratory arrest when given with intravenous **calcium gluconate**. Avoid. Severe Anecdotal
- Intravenous **calcium salts** increase the effects of **digoxin**. Avoid. Moderate Anecdotal
- Oral **calcium salts** decrease the absorption of **dolutegravir**. **Dolutegravir** should be taken 2 hours before or 6 hours after **calcium salts**. Moderate Study
- Oral **calcium salts** decrease the absorption of **eltrombopag**. **Eltrombopag** should be taken 2 hours before or 4 hours after **calcium salts**. Severe Study
- **Calcium carbonate** decreases the absorption of hydroxychloroquine. Separate administration by at least 4 hours. Moderate Study
- **Calcium carbonate** decreases the absorption of **iron (oral)**. **Calcium carbonate** should be taken 1 hour before or 2 hours after **iron (oral)**. Moderate Study
- **Calcium carbonate** is predicted to decrease the exposure to ledipasvir. Separate administration by 4 hours. Moderate Theoretical
- Oral **calcium carbonate** is predicted to decrease the exposure to oral neratinib. Separate administration by at least 3 hours. Mild Theoretical
- **Calcium carbonate** decreases the absorption of quinolones **(ciprofloxacin)**. Separate administration by 2 hours. Moderate Study
- **Calcium carbonate** greatly decreases the exposure to raltegravir (high-dose). Avoid. Severe Study
- **Calcium carbonate** is predicted to slightly decrease the exposure to **rilpivirine**. **Calcium carbonate** should be taken 2 hours before or 4 hours after **rilpivirine**. Severe Theoretical
- Oral **calcium salts** decrease the exposure to **strontium**. Separate administration by 2 hours. Moderate Study
- **Calcium carbonate** is predicted to decrease the absorption of tetracyclines. Separate administration by 2 to 3 hours. Moderate Theoretical
- **Thiazide diuretics** increase the risk of hypercalcaemia when given with **calcium salts**. Severe Anecdotal
- Oral **calcium salts** are predicted to decrease the absorption of thyroid hormones **(levothyroxine)**. Separate administration by at least 4 hours. Moderate Anecdotal

Calcium salts (continued)

- **Calcium carbonate** is predicted to decrease the concentration of velpatasvir. Separate administration by 4 hours. [Moderate] Anecdotal
- Oral **calcium salts** decrease the absorption of zinc. [Moderate] Study

Canagliflozin → see TABLE 14 p. 910 (antidiabetic drugs), TABLE 8 p. 908 (hypotension)

- Rifampicin moderately decreases the exposure to **canagliflozin**. Adjust **canagliflozin** dose. [Moderate] Study

Canakinumab → see monoclonal antibodies

Candesartan → see angiotensin-II receptor antagonists

Cangrelor → see TABLE 4 p. 907 (antiplatelet effects)

Cannabidiol → see TABLE 11 p. 909 (CNS depressant effects)

- Antiepileptics (carbamazepine, fosphenytoin, phenobarbital, phenytoin, primidone) are predicted to decrease the exposure to **cannabidiol**. Adjust dose. [Moderate] Study → Also see TABLE 11 p. 909
- **Cannabidiol** increases the risk of increased ALT concentrations when given with antiepileptics (valproate). Avoid or adjust dose. [Severe] Study
- Antifungals, azoles (fluconazole) are predicted to increase the exposure to **cannabidiol**. [Moderate] Theoretical
- Antifungals, azoles (itraconazole, ketoconazole, voriconazole) are predicted to increase the exposure to **cannabidiol**. Avoid or adjust dose. [Mild] Study
- Apalutamide is predicted to decrease the exposure to **cannabidiol**. Adjust dose. [Moderate] Study
- **Cannabidiol** increases the exposure to the active metabolite of clobazam and clobazam increases the exposure to the active metabolite of **cannabidiol**. Adjust dose. [Moderate] Study → Also see TABLE 11 p. 909
- Cobicistat is predicted to increase the exposure to **cannabidiol**. Avoid or adjust dose. [Mild] Study
- Enzalutamide is predicted to decrease the exposure to **cannabidiol**. Adjust dose. [Moderate] Study
- HIV-protease inhibitors are predicted to increase the exposure to **cannabidiol**. Avoid or adjust dose. [Mild] Study
- Idelalisib is predicted to increase the exposure to **cannabidiol**. Avoid or adjust dose. [Mild] Study
- Macrolides (clarithromycin) are predicted to increase the exposure to **cannabidiol**. Avoid or adjust dose. [Mild] Study
- Mitotane is predicted to decrease the exposure to **cannabidiol**. Adjust dose. [Moderate] Study
- Moclobemide is predicted to increase the exposure to **cannabidiol**. [Moderate] Theoretical
- Proton pump inhibitors (esomeprazole) are predicted to increase the exposure to **cannabidiol**. [Moderate] Theoretical
- Rifampicin is predicted to decrease the exposure to **cannabidiol**. Adjust dose. [Moderate] Study
- SSRIs (fluoxetine, fluvoxamine) are predicted to increase the exposure to **cannabidiol**. [Moderate] Theoretical
- St John's Wort is predicted to decrease the exposure to **cannabidiol**. Adjust dose. [Mild] Study

Capecitabine → see TABLE 15 p. 910 (myelosuppression)

- Allopurinol is predicted to decrease the effects of **capecitabine**. Avoid. [Severe] Study
- **Capecitabine** increases the concentration of antiepileptics (fosphenytoin, phenytoin). [Severe] Anecdotal
- **Capecitabine** increases the effects of coumarins. Monitor INR and adjust dose. [Moderate] Anecdotal
- Folates are predicted to increase the risk of toxicity when given with **capecitabine**. [Severe] Anecdotal
- H_2 receptor antagonists (cimetidine) are predicted to slightly increase the exposure to **capecitabine**. [Severe] Theoretical
- Live vaccines are predicted to increase the risk of generalised infection (possibly life-threatening) when given with **capecitabine**. Public Health England advises avoid (refer to Green Book). [Severe] Theoretical
- Metronidazole is predicted to increase the risk of capecitabine toxicity when given with **capecitabine**. [Severe] Theoretical

Caplacizumab

- **Caplacizumab** is predicted to increase the risk of bleeding events when given with drugs with anticoagulant effects (see TABLE 3 p. 907). [Severe] Theoretical
- **Caplacizumab** is predicted to increase the risk of bleeding events when given with drugs with antiplatelet effects (see TABLE 4 p. 907). [Severe] Theoretical

Capreomycin → see TABLE 2 p. 907 (nephrotoxicity), TABLE 19 p. 911 (ototoxicity)

Captopril → see ACE inhibitors

Carbamazepine → see antiepileptics

Carbapenems

ertapenem · imipenem · meropenem

- **Carbapenems** decrease the concentration of antiepileptics (valproate). Avoid. [Severe] Anecdotal
- Ganciclovir is predicted to increase the risk of seizures when given with **imipenem**. Avoid. [Severe] Anecdotal
- Valganciclovir is predicted to increase the risk of seizures when given with **imipenem**. Avoid. [Severe] Anecdotal

Carbidopa

- Iron (oral) is predicted to decrease the exposure to **carbidopa**. [Moderate] Theoretical

Carbimazole → see TABLE 15 p. 910 (myelosuppression)

- **Carbimazole** affects the concentration of digoxin. Monitor and adjust dose. [Moderate] Theoretical
- **Carbimazole** decreases the effects of metyrapone. Avoid. [Moderate] Theoretical
- **Carbimazole** given with a potent CYP3A4 inhibitor is predicted to increase the exposure to propiverine. Adjust starting dose. [Moderate] Theoretical

Carboplatin → see platinum compounds

Carfilzomib → see TABLE 15 p. 910 (myelosuppression)

- **Carfilzomib** potentially decreases the efficacy of combined hormonal contraceptives. Use additional contraceptive precautions. [Severe] Theoretical

Cariprazine → see TABLE 8 p. 908 (hypotension), TABLE 11 p. 909 (CNS depressant effects)

- Antiarrhythmics (dronedarone) are predicted to increase the exposure to **cariprazine**. Avoid. [Severe] Study
- Antiepileptics (carbamazepine, fosphenytoin, phenobarbital, phenytoin, primidone) are predicted to decrease the exposure to **cariprazine**. Avoid. [Severe] Theoretical → Also see TABLE 11 p. 909
- Antifungals, azoles (fluconazole, isavuconazole, posaconazole) are predicted to increase the exposure to **cariprazine**. Avoid. [Severe] Study
- Antifungals, azoles (itraconazole, ketoconazole, voriconazole) are predicted to moderately increase the exposure to **cariprazine**. Avoid. [Severe] Study
- Apalutamide is predicted to decrease the exposure to **cariprazine**. Avoid. [Severe] Theoretical
- Aprepitant is predicted to increase the exposure to **cariprazine**. Avoid. [Severe] Study
- Bosentan is predicted to decrease the exposure to **cariprazine**. Avoid. [Severe] Theoretical
- Calcium channel blockers (diltiazem, verapamil) are predicted to increase the exposure to **cariprazine**. Avoid. [Severe] Study → Also see TABLE 8 p. 908
- Cobicistat is predicted to moderately increase the exposure to **cariprazine**. Avoid. [Severe] Study
- Crizotinib is predicted to increase the exposure to **cariprazine**. Avoid. [Severe] Study
- Efavirenz is predicted to decrease the exposure to **cariprazine**. Avoid. [Severe] Theoretical
- Enzalutamide is predicted to decrease the exposure to **cariprazine**. Avoid. [Severe] Theoretical
- Grapefruit juice is predicted to increase the exposure to **cariprazine**. Avoid. [Moderate] Study
- HIV-protease inhibitors are predicted to moderately increase the exposure to **cariprazine**. Avoid. [Severe] Study
- Idelalisib is predicted to moderately increase the exposure to **cariprazine**. Avoid. [Severe] Study
- Imatinib is predicted to increase the exposure to **cariprazine**. Avoid. [Severe] Study
- Macrolides (clarithromycin) are predicted to moderately increase the exposure to **cariprazine**. Avoid. [Severe] Study
- Macrolides (erythromycin) are predicted to increase the exposure to **cariprazine**. Avoid. [Severe] Study
- Mitotane is predicted to decrease the exposure to **cariprazine**. Avoid. [Severe] Theoretical

- Netupitant is predicted to increase the exposure to **cariprazine.** Avoid. Severe Study
- Nevirapine is predicted to decrease the exposure to **cariprazine.** Avoid. Severe Theoretical
- Nilotinib is predicted to increase the exposure to **cariprazine.** Avoid. Severe Study
- Rifampicin is predicted to decrease the exposure to **cariprazine.** Avoid. Severe Theoretical
- St John's Wort is predicted to decrease the exposure to **cariprazine.** Avoid. Severe Theoretical

Carmustine → see alkylating agents
Carvedilol → see beta blockers, non-selective
Caspofungin

- Antiepileptics (carbamazepine, fosphenytoin, phenytoin) are predicted to decrease the concentration of **caspofungin**. Adjust **caspofungin** dose, p. 405. Moderate Theoretical
- Ciclosporin slightly increases the exposure to **caspofungin.** Severe Study
- Corticosteroids (dexamethasone) are predicted to decrease the concentration of **caspofungin**. Adjust **caspofungin** dose, p. 405. Moderate Theoretical
- Efavirenz is predicted to decrease the concentration of **caspofungin**. Adjust dose. Moderate Study
- Nevirapine is predicted to decrease the concentration of **caspofungin**. Adjust dose. Moderate Theoretical
- Rifampicin decreases the concentration of **caspofungin**. Adjust **caspofungin** dose, p. 405. Moderate Study

Cefaclor → see cephalosporins
Cefadroxil → see cephalosporins
Cefalexin → see cephalosporins
Cefepime → see cephalosporins
Cefixime → see cephalosporins
Cefotaxime → see cephalosporins
Cefoxitin → see cephalosporins
Cefradine → see cephalosporins
Ceftaroline → see cephalosporins
Ceftazidime → see cephalosporins
Ceftobiprole → see cephalosporins
Ceftolozane → see cephalosporins
Ceftriaxone → see cephalosporins
Cefuroxime → see cephalosporins
Celecoxib → see NSAIDs
Celiprolol → see beta blockers, selective
Cemiplimab → see monoclonal antibodies
Cephalosporins → see TABLE 2 p. 907 (nephrotoxicity)

cefaclor · cefadroxil · cefalexin · cefepime · cefixime · cefotaxime · cefoxitin · cefradine · ceftaroline · ceftazidime · ceftobiprole · ceftolozane · ceftriaxone · cefuroxime

ROUTE-SPECIFIC INFORMATION Interactions do not generally apply to topical use of **cefuroxime** unless specified.

- **Ceftobiprole** is predicted to increase the exposure to bosentan. Moderate Theoretical
- **Ceftriaxone** increases the risk of cardio-respiratory arrest when given with calcium salts (calcium chloride). Avoid. Severe Anecdotal
- **Ceftriaxone** increases the risk of cardio-respiratory arrest when given with intravenous calcium salts (calcium gluconate). Avoid. Severe Anecdotal
- **Ceftriaxone** potentially increases the risk of bleeding events when given with coumarins. Severe Anecdotal
- Leflunomide is predicted to increase the exposure to **cefaclor.** Moderate Theoretical
- Nitisinone is predicted to increase the exposure to **cefaclor.** Moderate Study
- **Ceftriaxone** potentially increases the risk of bleeding events when given with phenindione. Severe Anecdotal
- **Ceftobiprole** is predicted to increase the concentration of statins. Moderate Theoretical
- **Ceftobiprole** is predicted to increase the concentration of sulfonylureas (glibenclamide). Moderate Theoretical
- Teriflunomide is predicted to increase the exposure to **cefaclor.** Moderate Study

Ceritinib → see TABLE 15 p. 910 (myelosuppression), TABLE 9 p. 909 (QT-interval prolongation)

- **Ceritinib** is predicted to increase the exposure to aliskiren. Moderate Theoretical
- Antacids are predicted to decrease the absorption of **ceritinib.** Separate administration by 2 hours. Moderate Theoretical
- Antiarrhythmics (amiodarone) are predicted to increase the exposure to **ceritinib.** Moderate Theoretical → Also see TABLE 9 p. 909
- Antiepileptics (carbamazepine, fosphenytoin, phenobarbital, phenytoin, primidone) are predicted to decrease the exposure to **ceritinib.** Avoid. Severe Study
- Antifungals, azoles (itraconazole, ketoconazole, voriconazole) are predicted to increase the exposure to **ceritinib.** Avoid or adjust **ceritinib** dose. Severe Study → Also see TABLE 9 p. 909
- **Ceritinib** is predicted to increase the exposure to antihistamines, non-sedating (fexofenadine). Moderate Theoretical
- Apalutamide is predicted to decrease the exposure to **ceritinib.** Avoid. Severe Study → Also see TABLE 9 p. 909
- **Ceritinib** is predicted to increase the exposure to ciclosporin. Avoid. Severe Theoretical
- Cobicistat is predicted to increase the exposure to **ceritinib.** Avoid or adjust **ceritinib** dose. Severe Study
- **Ceritinib** is predicted to increase the exposure to colchicine. Moderate Theoretical
- **Ceritinib** is predicted to increase the exposure to coumarins (warfarin). Avoid. Severe Theoretical
- **Ceritinib** is predicted to increase the exposure to dabigatran. Moderate Theoretical
- **Ceritinib** is predicted to increase the risk of bradycardia when given with digoxin. Avoid. Severe Theoretical
- **Ceritinib** is predicted to increase the exposure to edoxaban. Moderate Theoretical
- Enzalutamide is predicted to decrease the exposure to **ceritinib.** Avoid. Severe Study
- **Ceritinib** is predicted to increase the exposure to ergotamine. Avoid. Severe Theoretical
- **Ceritinib** is predicted to increase the exposure to everolimus. Moderate Theoretical → Also see TABLE 15 p. 910
- Grapefruit juice is predicted to increase the exposure to **ceritinib.** Avoid. Severe Theoretical
- H_2 receptor antagonists are predicted to decrease the absorption of **ceritinib.** Moderate Theoretical
- HIV-protease inhibitors are predicted to increase the exposure to **ceritinib.** Avoid or adjust **ceritinib** dose. Severe Study → Also see TABLE 9 p. 909
- Idelalisib is predicted to increase the exposure to **ceritinib.** Avoid or adjust **ceritinib** dose. Severe Study → Also see TABLE 15 p. 910
- Lapatinib is predicted to increase the exposure to **ceritinib.** Moderate Theoretical → Also see TABLE 9 p. 909
- **Ceritinib** is predicted to increase the exposure to loperamide. Moderate Theoretical
- Macrolides (azithromycin) are predicted to increase the exposure to **ceritinib.** Moderate Theoretical
- Macrolides (clarithromycin) are predicted to increase the exposure to **ceritinib.** Avoid or adjust **ceritinib** dose. Severe Study → Also see TABLE 9 p. 909
- Mitotane is predicted to decrease the exposure to **ceritinib.** Avoid. Severe Study → Also see TABLE 15 p. 910
- **Ceritinib** is predicted to increase the exposure to NSAIDs (celecoxib, diclofenac). Adjust dose. Moderate Theoretical
- **Ceritinib** is predicted to increase the exposure to opioids (alfentanil, fentanyl). Avoid. Severe Theoretical
- **Ceritinib** is predicted to increase the exposure to pimozide. Avoid. Severe Theoretical → Also see TABLE 9 p. 909
- Proton pump inhibitors are predicted to decrease the absorption of **ceritinib.** Moderate Theoretical
- Ranolazine is predicted to increase the exposure to **ceritinib.** Moderate Theoretical → Also see TABLE 9 p. 909
- Rifampicin is predicted to decrease the exposure to **ceritinib.** Avoid. Severe Study
- **Ceritinib** is predicted to increase the exposure to sirolimus. Avoid. Severe Theoretical
- St John's Wort is predicted to decrease the exposure to **ceritinib.** Avoid. Severe Theoretical

Ceritinib (continued)
- **Ceritinib** is predicted to increase the exposure to sulfonylureas **(glimepiride)**. Adjust dose. Moderate Theoretical
- **Ceritinib** is predicted to increase the exposure to **tacrolimus**. Avoid. Severe Theoretical
- **Ceritinib** is predicted to increase the exposure to taxanes **(paclitaxel)**. Moderate Theoretical → Also see **TABLE 15** p. 910
- **Ceritinib** is predicted to increase the exposure to **topotecan**. Moderate Theoretical → Also see **TABLE 15** p. 910

Certolizumab pegol → see monoclonal antibodies

Cetirizine → see antihistamines, non-sedating

Cetuximab → see monoclonal antibodies

Chenodeoxycholic acid
- Oral antacids **(aluminium hydroxide)** decrease the absorption of **chenodeoxycholic acid**. Moderate Study
- Antiepileptics **(phenobarbital, primidone)** are predicted to affect the efficacy of **chenodeoxycholic acid**. Monitor and adjust dose. Moderate Theoretical
- **Ciclosporin** is predicted to affect the efficacy of **chenodeoxycholic acid**. Monitor and adjust dose. Moderate Theoretical
- **Oral combined hormonal contraceptives** potentially decrease the efficacy of **chenodeoxycholic acid**. Avoid. Moderate Theoretical
- **Sirolimus** is predicted to affect the efficacy of **chenodeoxycholic acid**. Monitor and adjust dose. Moderate Theoretical

Chloral hydrate → see **TABLE 11** p. 909 (CNS depressant effects)
- Intravenous loop diuretics **(furosemide)** potentially increase the risk of sweating, variable blood pressure, and tachycardia when given after **chloral hydrate**. Moderate Anecdotal

Chlorambucil → see alkylating agents

Chloramphenicol

ROUTE-SPECIFIC INFORMATION Since systemic absorption can follow topical application, the possibility of interactions should be borne in mind.

- Antiepileptics **(phenobarbital, primidone)** decrease the concentration of **chloramphenicol**. Moderate Study
- Intravenous **chloramphenicol** increases the concentration of antiepileptics **(fosphenytoin, phenytoin)** and antiepileptics **(fosphenytoin, phenytoin)** affect the concentration of intravenous **chloramphenicol**. Monitor concentration and adjust dose. Severe Study
- **Chloramphenicol** potentially increases the anticoagulant effect of **coumarins**. Moderate Anecdotal
- **Chloramphenicol** is predicted to increase the exposure to **guanfacine**. Adjust **guanfacine** dose, p. 247. Moderate Theoretical
- **Chloramphenicol** decreases the efficacy of intravenous **iron (injectable)**. Moderate Anecdotal
- **Chloramphenicol** decreases the efficacy of oral **iron (oral)**. Moderate Theoretical
- **Rifampicin** decreases the concentration of **chloramphenicol**. Moderate Study
- **Chloramphenicol** is predicted to increase the exposure to **sulfonylureas**. Severe Study
- **Chloramphenicol** increases the concentration of **tacrolimus**. Severe Study

Chlordiazepoxide → see **TABLE 11** p. 909 (CNS depressant effects)
- **Chlordiazepoxide** affects the concentration of antiepileptics **(fosphenytoin, phenytoin)**. Severe Study
- **Rifampicin** is predicted to decrease the exposure to **chlordiazepoxide**. Moderate Theoretical

Chlormethine → see **TABLE 15** p. 910 (myelosuppression)

ROUTE-SPECIFIC INFORMATION Since systemic absorption can follow topical application, the possibility of interactions should be borne in mind.

Chloroprocaine → see **TABLE 11** p. 909 (CNS depressant effects)
- **Chloroprocaine** is predicted to increase the risk of cardiovascular side-effects when given with antiarrhythmics **(amiodarone, dronedarone, vernakalant)**. Severe Theoretical
- **Chloroprocaine** is predicted to increase the risk of cardiovascular side-effects when given with beta blockers, non-selective **(sotalol)**. Severe Theoretical
- **Chloroprocaine** is predicted to decrease the effects of **sulfonamides**. Avoid. Severe Theoretical

Chloroquine → see antimalarials

Chlorothiazide → see thiazide diuretics

Chlorphenamine → see antihistamines, sedating

Chlorpromazine → see phenothiazines

Chlortalidone → see thiazide diuretics

Cholera vaccine
- Antimalarials **(chloroquine)** decrease the efficacy of oral **cholera vaccine**. Moderate Study
- **Hydroxychloroquine** is predicted to decrease the efficacy of oral **cholera vaccine**. Moderate Theoretical

Cholic acid
- **Antacids** are predicted to decrease the absorption of **cholic acid**. Separate administration by 5 hours. Mild Theoretical
- Antiepileptics **(phenobarbital)** decrease the effects of **cholic acid**. Avoid. Moderate Study
- **Ciclosporin** affects the concentration of **cholic acid**. Avoid. Moderate Study

Choline salicylate
- **Corticosteroids** are predicted to decrease the concentration of **choline salicylate**. Moderate Study

Ciclesonide → see corticosteroids

Ciclosporin → see **TABLE 2** p. 907 (nephrotoxicity), **TABLE 16** p. 911 (increased serum potassium)

- Pomelo juice is predicted to increase ciclosporin exposure, and purple grape juice is predicted to decrease ciclosporin exposure.
- Since systemic absorption can follow topical application, the possibility of interactions should be borne in mind.

- **Ciclosporin** is predicted to increase the exposure to **afatinib**. Separate administration by 12 hours. Moderate Study
- **Ciclosporin** markedly increases the exposure to **aliskiren**. Avoid. Severe Study → Also see **TABLE 16** p. 911
- **Ciclosporin** moderately increases the exposure to **ambrisentan**. Adjust **ambrisentan** dose. Moderate Study
- **Ciclosporin** increases the concentration of anthracyclines **(daunorubicin, doxorubicin, epirubicin, idarubicin, mitoxantrone)**. Severe Study
- Antiarrhythmics **(amiodarone)** increase the concentration of **ciclosporin**. Monitor concentration and adjust dose. Severe Study
- Antiarrhythmics **(dronedarone)** are predicted to increase the concentration of **ciclosporin**. Severe Study
- Antiepileptics **(carbamazepine, fosphenytoin, phenobarbital, phenytoin, primidone)** decrease the concentration of **ciclosporin**. Severe Study
- Antiepileptics **(oxcarbazepine)** decrease the concentration of **ciclosporin**. Severe Anecdotal
- Antifungals, azoles **(fluconazole, isavuconazole, posaconazole)** are predicted to increase the concentration of **ciclosporin**. Severe Study
- Antifungals, azoles **(itraconazole, ketoconazole, voriconazole)** increase the concentration of **ciclosporin**. Severe Study
- Antifungals, azoles **(miconazole)** increase the concentration of **ciclosporin**. Monitor and adjust dose. Severe Anecdotal
- **Apalutamide** decreases the concentration of **ciclosporin**. Severe Study
- **Aprepitant** is predicted to increase the concentration of **ciclosporin**. Severe Study
- **Ciclosporin** is predicted to increase the exposure to beta blockers, non-selective **(nadolol)**. Moderate Study
- **Ciclosporin** is predicted to increase the exposure to **bictegravir**. Use with caution or avoid. Moderate Theoretical
- **Bosentan** moderately decreases the exposure to **ciclosporin** and **ciclosporin** moderately increases the exposure to **bosentan**. Avoid. Severe Study
- Calcium channel blockers **(diltiazem, verapamil)** are predicted to increase the concentration of **ciclosporin**. Severe Study
- Calcium channel blockers **(nicardipine)** increase the concentration of **ciclosporin**. Severe Study
- **Ciclosporin** moderately increases the exposure to calcium channel blockers **(lercanidipine)**. Use with caution or avoid. Severe Study
- **Ciclosporin** slightly increases the exposure to **caspofungin**. Severe Study

- Ceritinib is predicted to increase the exposure to **ciclosporin.** Avoid. [Severe] Theoretical
- **Ciclosporin** is predicted to affect the efficacy of **chenodeoxycholic acid.** Monitor and adjust dose. [Moderate] Theoretical
- **Ciclosporin** affects the concentration of **cholic acid.** Avoid. [Moderate] Study
- Cobicistat increases the concentration of **ciclosporin.** [Severe] Study
- **Ciclosporin** increases the exposure to **colchicine.** Avoid P-glycoprotein inhibitors or adjust **colchicine** dose. [Severe] Study
- **Crizotinib** is predicted to increase the concentration of **ciclosporin.** [Severe] Study
- **Ciclosporin** is predicted to increase the exposure to **dabigatran.** Avoid. [Severe] Theoretical
- **Danazol** increases the concentration of **ciclosporin.** [Severe] Study
- **Ciclosporin** is predicted to increase the risk of rhabdomyolysis when given with **daptomycin.** [Severe] Theoretical
- **Ciclosporin** is predicted to increase the exposure to **darifenacin.** Avoid. [Moderate] Theoretical
- **Ciclosporin** increases the concentration of **digoxin.** Monitor and adjust dose. [Severe] Theoretical
- **Ciclosporin** slightly increases the exposure to **edoxaban.** Adjust **edoxaban** dose. [Severe] Study
- **Efavirenz** decreases the concentration of **ciclosporin.** Monitor concentration and adjust dose. [Moderate] Study
- **Ciclosporin** decreases the exposure to **eltrombopag.** Monitor and adjust dose. [Moderate] Study
- **Enzalutamide** decreases the concentration of **ciclosporin.** [Severe] Study
- **Ciclosporin** is predicted to increase the exposure to **erlotinib.** [Moderate] Theoretical
- **Ciclosporin** increases the exposure to **etoposide.** Monitor and adjust dose. [Severe] Study
- **Ciclosporin** moderately increases the exposure to **everolimus.** Avoid or adjust dose. [Severe] Study
- **Ciclosporin** moderately increases the exposure to **ezetimibe** and **ezetimibe** slightly increases the exposure to **ciclosporin.** [Moderate] Study
- Fibrates **(bezafibrate)** are predicted to increase the risk of nephrotoxicity when given with **ciclosporin.** [Severe] Theoretical
- Fibrates **(fenofibrate)** increase the risk of nephrotoxicity when given with **ciclosporin.** [Severe] Study
- **Ciclosporin** is predicted to increase the exposure to **fidaxomicin.** Avoid. [Moderate] Study
- **Ciclosporin** increases the exposure to **glecaprevir.** Avoid or monitor. [Severe] Study
- **Grapefruit juice** increases the concentration of **ciclosporin.** Avoid. [Severe] Study
- **Ciclosporin** greatly increases the exposure to **grazoprevir.** Avoid. [Severe] Study
- H_2 receptor antagonists **(cimetidine)** increase the concentration of **ciclosporin.** [Mild] Study
- **HIV-protease inhibitors** increase the concentration of **ciclosporin.** [Severe] Study
- **Idelalisib** increases the concentration of **ciclosporin.** [Severe] Study
- **Imatinib** is predicted to increase the concentration of **ciclosporin.** [Severe] Study
- **Lanreotide** is predicted to decrease the absorption of oral **ciclosporin.** Adjust dose. [Severe] Theoretical
- **Ciclosporin** is predicted to increase the exposure to **larotrectinib.** [Mild] Study
- **Letermovir** increases the exposure to **ciclosporin** and **ciclosporin** increases the exposure to **letermovir.** Monitor and adjust **letermovir** dose. [Severe] Study
- **Live vaccines** are predicted to increase the risk of generalised infection (possibly life-threatening) when given with **ciclosporin.** Public Health England advises avoid (refer to Green Book). [Severe] Theoretical
- **Ciclosporin** is predicted to increase the exposure to **lomitapide.** Separate administration by 12 hours. [Moderate] Theoretical
- **Lorlatinib** is predicted to decrease the exposure to **ciclosporin.** Avoid. [Moderate] Theoretical
- **Lumacaftor** is predicted to decrease the exposure to **ciclosporin.** Avoid. [Severe] Theoretical
- Macrolides **(clarithromycin)** increase the concentration of **ciclosporin.** [Severe] Study
- Macrolides **(erythromycin)** are predicted to increase the concentration of **ciclosporin.** [Severe] Study
- **Ciclosporin** is predicted to decrease the efficacy of **mifamurtide.** Avoid. [Severe] Theoretical
- **Mitotane** decreases the concentration of **ciclosporin.** [Severe] Study
- Monoclonal antibodies **(blinatumomab)** are predicted to transiently increase the exposure to **ciclosporin.** Monitor and adjust dose. [Moderate] Theoretical
- Monoclonal antibodies **(sarilumab)** potentially affect the exposure to **ciclosporin.** Monitor and adjust dose. [Moderate] Theoretical
- Monoclonal antibodies **(tocilizumab)** are predicted to decrease the exposure to **ciclosporin.** Monitor and adjust dose. [Moderate] Theoretical
- **Ciclosporin** is predicted to increase the exposure to **naldemedine.** [Moderate] Study
- **Netupitant** is predicted to increase the concentration of **ciclosporin.** [Severe] Study
- **Nevirapine** is predicted to decrease the concentration of **ciclosporin.** [Moderate] Study
- **Nilotinib** is predicted to increase the concentration of **ciclosporin.** [Severe] Study
- **Ciclosporin** is predicted to increase the exposure to **nintedanib.** [Moderate] Study
- **Ciclosporin** increases the concentration of NSAIDs **(diclofenac).** [Severe] Study → Also see TABLE 2 p. 907 → Also see TABLE 16 p. 911
- **Octreotide** decreases the absorption of oral **ciclosporin.** Adjust **ciclosporin** dose, p. 559. [Severe] Anecdotal
- **Palbociclib** is predicted to increase the exposure to **ciclosporin.** Adjust dose. [Moderate] Theoretical
- **Ciclosporin** is predicted to increase the exposure to **panobinostat.** Adjust dose. [Moderate] Theoretical
- **Pasireotide** is predicted to decrease the absorption of oral **ciclosporin.** Adjust dose. [Severe] Theoretical
- **Pitolisant** is predicted to decrease the exposure to **ciclosporin.** Avoid. [Severe] Theoretical
- **Ciclosporin** is predicted to increase the concentration of **ranolazine** and **ranolazine** is predicted to increase the concentration of **ciclosporin.** [Moderate] Theoretical
- **Ciclosporin** moderately increases the exposure to **repaglinide.** [Moderate] Study
- **Ribociclib** is predicted to increase the exposure to **ciclosporin.** Use with caution and adjust dose. [Moderate] Theoretical
- **Rifampicin** decreases the concentration of **ciclosporin.** [Severe] Study
- **Ciclosporin** very markedly increases the exposure to **rifaximin.** [Severe] Study
- **Ciclosporin** is predicted to increase the exposure to **riociguat.** [Moderate] Theoretical
- **Rucaparib** is predicted to increase the exposure to **ciclosporin.** Monitor and adjust dose. [Moderate] Study
- **Ciclosporin** moderately increases the exposure to **sirolimus.** Separate administration by 4 hours. [Severe] Study
- **St John's Wort** decreases the concentration of **ciclosporin.** Avoid. [Moderate] Study
- **Ciclosporin** very markedly increases the exposure to statins **(atorvastatin).** Avoid or adjust **atorvastatin** dose, p. 139. [Severe] Study
- **Ciclosporin** moderately increases the exposure to statins **(fluvastatin).** [Severe] Study
- **Ciclosporin** markedly to very markedly increases the exposure to statins **(pravastatin).** Adjust dose. [Severe] Study
- **Ciclosporin** markedly increases the exposure to statins **(rosuvastatin, simvastatin).** Avoid. [Severe] Study
- **Ciclosporin** increases the concentration of **tacrolimus.** Avoid. [Severe] Study → Also see TABLE 2 p. 907 → Also see TABLE 16 p. 911
- **Ciclosporin** is predicted to slightly increase the exposure to **talazoparib.** Avoid or adjust **talazoparib** dose. [Severe] Study
- **Ciclosporin** is predicted to increase the exposure to **tenofovir alafenamide.** [Moderate] Theoretical

Ciclosporin (continued)
- **Ciclosporin** is predicted to increase the exposure to **tenofovir disoproxil**. Moderate Theoretical → Also see TABLE 2 p. 907
- **Ciclosporin** is predicted to increase the exposure to **ticagrelor**. Use with caution or avoid. Severe Study
- **Ciclosporin** increases the exposure to **tofacitinib**. Avoid. Severe Study
- **Ciclosporin** is predicted to increase the exposure to **topotecan**. Severe Study
- **Ciclosporin** is predicted to increase the concentration of **trametinib**. Moderate Theoretical
- **Ursodeoxycholic acid** affects the concentration of **ciclosporin**. Use with caution and adjust dose. Severe Anecdotal
- **Ciclosporin** is predicted to increase the exposure to **venetoclax**. Avoid or monitor for toxicity. Severe Theoretical
- **Vitamin E substances** affect the exposure to **ciclosporin**. Moderate Study
- **Ciclosporin** increases the concentration of **voxilaprevir**. Avoid. Severe Study

Cidofovir → see TABLE 2 p. 907 (nephrotoxicity)

Cilostazol → see TABLE 4 p. 907 (antiplatelet effects)

GENERAL INFORMATION Concurrent use with 2 or more antiplatelets or anticoagulants is contra-indicated.

- Antiepileptics (**carbamazepine, fosphenytoin, phenobarbital, phenytoin, primidone**) are predicted to alter the effects of **cilostazol**. Moderate Theoretical
- Antifungals, azoles (**fluconazole**) are predicted to increase the exposure to **cilostazol**. Adjust **cilostazol** dose. Moderate Theoretical
- Antifungals, azoles (**itraconazole, ketoconazole, voriconazole**) are predicted to moderately increase the exposure to **cilostazol**. Adjust **cilostazol** dose. Moderate Study
- Antifungals, azoles (**miconazole**) are predicted to increase the exposure to **cilostazol**. Use with caution and adjust dose. Moderate Theoretical
- **Apalutamide** is predicted to alter the effects of **cilostazol**. Moderate Theoretical
- **Cobicistat** is predicted to moderately increase the exposure to **cilostazol**. Adjust **cilostazol** dose. Moderate Study
- **Enzalutamide** is predicted to alter the effects of **cilostazol**. Moderate Theoretical
- **HIV-protease inhibitors** are predicted to moderately increase the exposure to **cilostazol**. Adjust **cilostazol** dose. Moderate Study
- **Idelalisib** is predicted to moderately increase the exposure to **cilostazol**. Adjust **cilostazol** dose. Moderate Study
- **Cilostazol** is predicted to increase the exposure to **lomitapide**. Separate administration by 12 hours. Moderate Theoretical
- Macrolides (**clarithromycin**) are predicted to moderately increase the exposure to **cilostazol**. Adjust **cilostazol** dose. Moderate Study
- Macrolides (**erythromycin**) slightly increase the exposure to **cilostazol**. Adjust **cilostazol** dose. Moderate Study
- **Mitotane** is predicted to alter the effects of **cilostazol**. Moderate Theoretical
- **Moclobemide** is predicted to increase the exposure to **cilostazol**. Moderate Theoretical
- Proton pump inhibitors (**esomeprazole**) are predicted to increase the exposure to **cilostazol**. Moderate Theoretical
- Proton pump inhibitors (**omeprazole**) are predicted to increase the exposure to **cilostazol**. Adjust **cilostazol** dose. Moderate Study
- **Rifampicin** is predicted to alter the effects of **cilostazol**. Moderate Theoretical
- SSRIs (**fluoxetine, fluvoxamine**) are predicted to increase the exposure to **cilostazol**. Adjust **cilostazol** dose. Moderate Theoretical → Also see TABLE 4 p. 907
- **St John's Wort** is predicted to alter the effects of **cilostazol**. Moderate Theoretical

Cimetidine → see H_2 receptor antagonists

Cinacalcet

FOOD AND LIFESTYLE Dose adjustment might be necessary if smoking started or stopped during treatment.

- **Cinacalcet** is predicted to increase the exposure to anticholinesterases, centrally acting (**galantamine**). Monitor and adjust dose. Moderate Study
- Antiepileptics (**carbamazepine, fosphenytoin, phenobarbital, phenytoin, primidone**) are predicted to decrease the exposure to **cinacalcet**. Monitor and adjust dose. Moderate Study
- Antifungals, azoles (**itraconazole, ketoconazole, voriconazole**) are predicted to moderately increase the exposure to **cinacalcet**. Adjust dose. Moderate Study
- **Apalutamide** is predicted to decrease the exposure to **cinacalcet**. Monitor and adjust dose. Moderate Study
- **Cinacalcet** is predicted to moderately increase the exposure to aripiprazole. Adjust **aripiprazole** dose, p. 265. Moderate Study
- **Cinacalcet** is predicted to markedly increase the exposure to atomoxetine. Adjust dose. Severe Study
- **Cinacalcet** is predicted to increase the exposure to beta blockers, selective (**metoprolol, nebivolol**). Moderate Study
- **Cobicistat** is predicted to moderately increase the exposure to **cinacalcet**. Adjust dose. Moderate Study
- **Cinacalcet** is predicted to slightly increase the exposure to darifenacin. Mild Study
- **Cinacalcet** is predicted to increase the exposure to **eliglustat**. Avoid or adjust dose—consult product literature. Severe Study
- **Enzalutamide** is predicted to decrease the exposure to **cinacalcet**. Monitor and adjust dose. Moderate Study
- **Cinacalcet** increases the risk of hypocalcaemia when given with etelcalcetide. Avoid. Severe Theoretical
- **HIV-protease inhibitors** are predicted to moderately increase the exposure to **cinacalcet**. Adjust dose. Moderate Study
- **Idelalisib** is predicted to moderately increase the exposure to **cinacalcet**. Adjust dose. Moderate Study
- Macrolides (**clarithromycin**) are predicted to moderately increase the exposure to **cinacalcet**. Adjust dose. Moderate Study
- **Cinacalcet** is predicted to increase the exposure to **mexiletine**. Moderate Study
- **Mitotane** is predicted to decrease the exposure to **cinacalcet**. Monitor and adjust dose. Moderate Study
- **Cinacalcet** is predicted to decrease the efficacy of opioids (**codeine**). Moderate Theoretical
- **Cinacalcet** is predicted to decrease the efficacy of opioids (**tramadol**). Severe Study
- **Cinacalcet** is predicted to moderately increase the exposure to pitolisant. Use with caution and adjust dose. Moderate Study
- **Rifampicin** is predicted to decrease the exposure to **cinacalcet**. Monitor and adjust dose. Moderate Study
- **Cinacalcet** is predicted to increase the exposure to **risperidone**. Adjust dose. Moderate Study
- SSRIs (**fluvoxamine**) are predicted to increase the exposure to **cinacalcet**. Adjust dose. Moderate Theoretical
- **Cinacalcet** is predicted to increase the exposure to SSRIs (**dapoxetine**). Moderate Theoretical
- **Cinacalcet** is predicted to decrease the efficacy of **tamoxifen**. Avoid. Severe Study
- **Cinacalcet** is predicted to increase the exposure to the active metabolite of tetrabenazine. Moderate Study
- **Cinacalcet** is predicted to increase the exposure to **tricyclic antidepressants**. Monitor for toxicity and adjust dose. Severe Study
- **Cinacalcet** is predicted to increase the exposure to **vortioxetine**. Monitor and adjust dose. Moderate Study

Cinnarizine → see antihistamines, sedating

Ciprofibrate → see fibrates

Ciprofloxacin → see quinolones

Cisatracurium → see neuromuscular blocking drugs, non-depolarising

Cisplatin → see platinum compounds

Citalopram → see SSRIs

Cladribine → see TABLE 15 p. 910 (myelosuppression)

SEPARATION OF ADMINISTRATION Oral cladribine might affect the absorption of concurrently administered drugs—consider separating administration by at least 3 hours.

- Antiepileptics (**carbamazepine**) are predicted to increase the risk of haematological toxicity when given with oral **cladribine**. Moderate Theoretical

- Live vaccines are predicted to increase the risk of generalised infection (possibly life-threatening) when given with **cladribine**. Public Health England advises avoid (refer to Green Book). [Severe] Theoretical

Clarithromycin → see macrolides
Clavulanate → see TABLE 1 p. 907 (hepatotoxicity)
Clemastine → see antihistamines, sedating
Clindamycin

ROUTE-SPECIFIC INFORMATION Since systemic absorption can follow topical application, the possibility of interactions should be borne in mind.

- **Clindamycin** increases the effects of **neuromuscular blocking drugs, non-depolarising**. [Severe] Anecdotal
- **Clindamycin** increases the effects of **suxamethonium**. [Severe] Anecdotal

Clobazam → see TABLE 11 p. 909 (CNS depressant effects)
- Antiepileptics (**stiripentol**) increase the concentration of **clobazam**. [Severe] Study
- **Clobazam** potentially affects the concentration of antiepileptics (**fosphenytoin, phenytoin**). [Severe] Anecdotal
- Antifungals, azoles (**fluconazole, voriconazole**) potentially increase the exposure to **clobazam**. Adjust dose. [Moderate] Theoretical
- **Cannabidiol** increases the exposure to the active metabolite of **clobazam** and **clobazam** increases the exposure to the active metabolite of **cannabidiol**. Adjust dose. [Moderate] Study → Also see TABLE 11 p. 909
- **Moclobemide** potentially increases the exposure to **clobazam**. Adjust dose. [Moderate] Theoretical
- Proton pump inhibitors (**esomeprazole, omeprazole**) potentially increase the exposure to **clobazam**. Adjust dose. [Moderate] Theoretical
- SSRIs (**fluoxetine, fluvoxamine**) potentially increase the exposure to **clobazam**. Adjust dose. [Moderate] Theoretical

Clodronate → see bisphosphonates
Clofarabine → see TABLE 15 p. 910 (myelosuppression)
- Live vaccines are predicted to increase the risk of generalised infection (possibly life-threatening) when given with **clofarabine**. Public Health England advises avoid (refer to Green Book). [Severe] Theoretical

Clofazimine
- **Clofazimine** potentially increases the risk of QT-prolongation when given with **bedaquiline**. [Severe] Study

Clomethiazole → see TABLE 11 p. 909 (CNS depressant effects)
- **Alcohol (beverage)** causes serious, potentially fatal, CNS depression when given with **clomethiazole**. Avoid. [Severe] Study → Also see TABLE 11 p. 909
- Antiepileptics (**carbamazepine, fosphenytoin, phenobarbital, phenytoin, primidone**) decrease the exposure to **clomethiazole**. Monitor and adjust dose. [Moderate] Study → Also see TABLE 11 p. 909
- **Apalutamide** decreases the exposure to **clomethiazole**. Monitor and adjust dose. [Moderate] Study
- **Enzalutamide** decreases the exposure to **clomethiazole**. Monitor and adjust dose. [Moderate] Study
- **Mitotane** decreases the exposure to **clomethiazole**. Monitor and adjust dose. [Moderate] Study
- **Rifampicin** decreases the exposure to **clomethiazole**. Monitor and adjust dose. [Moderate] Study

Clomipramine → see tricyclic antidepressants
Clonazepam → see TABLE 11 p. 909 (CNS depressant effects)
- **Clonazepam** potentially affects the concentration of antiepileptics (**fosphenytoin, phenytoin**). [Severe] Anecdotal

Clonidine → see TABLE 6 p. 908 (bradycardia), TABLE 8 p. 908 (hypotension), TABLE 11 p. 909 (CNS depressant effects)
- **Tricyclic antidepressants** decrease the antihypertensive effects of **clonidine**. Monitor and adjust dose. [Moderate] Anecdotal → Also see TABLE 8 p. 908 → Also see TABLE 11 p. 909

Clopidogrel → see TABLE 4 p. 907 (antiplatelet effects)
- Antifungals, azoles (**fluconazole**) are predicted to decrease the efficacy of **clopidogrel**. Avoid. [Severe] Theoretical
- Antifungals, azoles (**voriconazole**) are predicted to decrease the efficacy of **clopidogrel**. Avoid. [Moderate] Study
- **Clopidogrel** is predicted to increase the exposure to **apalutamide**. [Mild] Study
- **Clopidogrel** is predicted to increase the exposure to **dabrafenib**. [Moderate] Theoretical
- **Clopidogrel** is predicted to very markedly increase the exposure to **dasabuvir**. Avoid. [Severe] Study
- **Clopidogrel** moderately increases the exposure to **enzalutamide**. Avoid or adjust **enzalutamide** dose. [Severe] Study
- **Grapefruit juice** markedly decreases the exposure to **clopidogrel**. [Severe] Study
- **Moclobemide** is predicted to decrease the efficacy of **clopidogrel**. Avoid. [Moderate] Study
- **Clopidogrel** is predicted to moderately increase the exposure to **montelukast**. [Moderate] Study
- **Clopidogrel** increases the exposure to **pioglitazone**. Monitor blood glucose and adjust dose. [Severe] Study
- Proton pump inhibitors (**esomeprazole, omeprazole**) are predicted to decrease the efficacy of **clopidogrel**. Avoid. [Moderate] Study
- **Clopidogrel** increases the exposure to **repaglinide**. Avoid. [Severe] Study
- **Clopidogrel** is predicted to increase the exposure to retinoids (**alitretinoin**). Adjust **alitretinoin** dose. [Moderate] Theoretical
- **Clopidogrel** is predicted to increase the exposure to **selexipag**. Adjust **selexipag** dose. [Moderate] Study
- SSRIs (**fluoxetine, fluvoxamine**) are predicted to decrease the efficacy of **clopidogrel**. Avoid. [Severe] Theoretical → Also see TABLE 4 p. 907
- **Clopidogrel** increases the exposure to statins (**rosuvastatin**). Adjust **rosuvastatin** dose, p. 140. [Moderate] Study
- **Clopidogrel** is predicted to increase the concentration of taxanes (**paclitaxel**). [Severe] Anecdotal

Clotrimazole → see antifungals, azoles
Clozapine → see TABLE 8 p. 908 (hypotension), TABLE 15 p. 910 (myelosuppression), TABLE 11 p. 909 (CNS depressant effects), TABLE 10 p. 909 (antimuscarinics)

- Dose adjustment might be necessary if smoking started or stopped during treatment.
- Avoid concomitant use of clozapine with drugs that have a substantial potential for causing agranulocytosis.

- Antiepileptics (**carbamazepine**) are predicted to increase the risk of myelosuppression when given with **clozapine**. Avoid. [Severe] Anecdotal
- Antiepileptics (**fosphenytoin, phenobarbital, phenytoin, primidone**) are predicted to decrease the exposure to **clozapine**. [Moderate] Anecdotal → Also see TABLE 11 p. 909
- **Combined hormonal contraceptives** increase the concentration of **clozapine**. Monitor side effects and adjust dose. [Severe] Study
- **Clozapine** is predicted to decrease the effects of **dopamine receptor agonists**. [Moderate] Theoretical → Also see TABLE 8 p. 908 → Also see TABLE 10 p. 909
- **Enzalutamide** is predicted to decrease the exposure to **clozapine**. [Moderate] Theoretical
- HIV-protease inhibitors (**ritonavir**) are predicted to affect the exposure to **clozapine**. Avoid. [Severe] Theoretical
- Iron chelators (**deferasirox**) are predicted to increase the exposure to **clozapine**. Avoid. [Moderate] Theoretical
- **Leflunomide** is predicted to decrease the exposure to **clozapine**. [Moderate] Theoretical → Also see TABLE 15 p. 910
- **Clozapine** is predicted to decrease the effects of **levodopa**. [Severe] Theoretical → Also see TABLE 8 p. 908
- Macrolides (**erythromycin**) potentially increase the risk of toxicity when given with **clozapine**. [Severe] Anecdotal
- **Mexiletine** increases the concentration of **clozapine**. Monitor side effects and adjust dose. [Severe] Study
- Quinolones (**ciprofloxacin**) increase the concentration of **clozapine**. Monitor side effects and adjust dose. [Severe] Study
- **Rifampicin** decreases the exposure to **clozapine**. [Severe] Anecdotal
- SSRIs (**fluvoxamine**) increase the concentration of **clozapine**. Monitor side effects and adjust dose. [Severe] Study
- **Teriflunomide** is predicted to decrease the exposure to **clozapine**. [Moderate] Theoretical

Cobicistat
- **Cobicistat** is predicted to increase the exposure to **abemaciclib**. Avoid or adjust **abemaciclib** dose. [Severe] Study

Cobicistat (continued)

- **Cobicistat** is predicted to markedly increase the exposure to aldosterone antagonists **(eplerenone)**. Avoid. Severe Study
- **Cobicistat** increases the exposure to **almotriptan**. Mild Study
- **Cobicistat** is predicted to moderately increase the exposure to alpha blockers **(alfuzosin, tamsulosin)**. Use with caution or avoid. Moderate Study
- **Cobicistat** is predicted to increase the exposure to alpha blockers **(doxazosin)**. Moderate Study
- **Cobicistat** moderately increases the exposure to **alprazolam**. Avoid. Moderate Study
- **Cobicistat** potentially increases the concentration of antiarrhythmics **(amiodarone, disopyramide, flecainide, lidocaine)**. Severe Theoretical
- **Cobicistat** very markedly increases the exposure to antiarrhythmics **(dronedarone)**. Avoid. Severe Study
- **Cobicistat** is predicted to increase the exposure to antiarrhythmics **(propafenone)**. Monitor and adjust dose. Severe Study
- **Cobicistat** is predicted to increase the exposure to anticholinesterases, centrally acting **(galantamine)**. Monitor and adjust dose. Moderate Study
- Antiepileptics **(carbamazepine, fosphenytoin, phenobarbital, phenytoin, primidone)** are predicted to decrease the exposure to **cobicistat**. Avoid. Severe Theoretical
- Antiepileptics **(oxcarbazepine)** are predicted to decrease the concentration of **cobicistat**. Severe Theoretical
- **Cobicistat** is predicted to very slightly increase the exposure to antiepileptics **(perampanel)**. Mild Study
- **Cobicistat** is predicted to increase the exposure to antifungals, azoles **(fluconazole, posaconazole)**. Moderate Theoretical
- **Cobicistat** is predicted to increase the exposure to antifungals, azoles **(isavuconazole)**. Avoid or monitor side effects. Severe Study
- **Cobicistat** is predicted to increase the exposure to antifungals, azoles **(itraconazole, ketoconazole)**. Adjust dose. Moderate Theoretical
- **Cobicistat** is predicted to affect the exposure to antifungals, azoles **(voriconazole)**. Avoid. Moderate Theoretical
- **Cobicistat** is predicted to increase the exposure to antihistamines, non-sedating **(mizolastine)**. Avoid. Severe Study
- **Cobicistat** is predicted to increase the exposure to antihistamines, non-sedating **(rupatadine)**. Avoid. Moderate Study
- **Cobicistat** is predicted to increase the concentration of antimalarials **(piperaquine)**. Severe Theoretical
- **Apalutamide** is predicted to decrease the exposure to **cobicistat**. Avoid. Severe Theoretical
- **Cobicistat** is predicted to increase the exposure to **apalutamide**. Mild Study
- **Cobicistat** is predicted to increase the exposure to **apixaban**. Avoid. Severe Theoretical
- **Cobicistat** is predicted to markedly increase the exposure to **aprepitant**. Moderate Study
- **Cobicistat** is predicted to slightly increase the exposure to aripiprazole. Adjust **aripiprazole** dose, p. 265. Moderate Study
- **Cobicistat** is predicted to increase the exposure to **axitinib**. Avoid or adjust dose. Moderate Study
- **Cobicistat** is predicted to increase the exposure to **bedaquiline**. Avoid prolonged use. Mild Study
- **Cobicistat** is predicted to increase the exposure to beta$_2$ agonists **(salmeterol)**. Avoid. Severe Study
- **Cobicistat** slightly increases the exposure to **bortezomib**. Moderate Study
- **Bosentan** is predicted to decrease the exposure to **cobicistat**. Avoid. Severe Theoretical
- **Cobicistat** is predicted to markedly increase the exposure to bosutinib. Avoid or adjust dose. Severe Study
- **Cobicistat** is predicted to increase the exposure to **brigatinib**. Adjust **brigatinib** dose. Severe Study
- **Cobicistat** is predicted to increase the exposure to **buspirone**. Adjust **buspirone** dose. Severe Study
- **Cobicistat** slightly increases the exposure to **cabozantinib**. Moderate Study
- **Cobicistat** is predicted to increase the exposure to calcium channel blockers **(amlodipine, felodipine, lacidipine, nicardipine, nifedipine, nimodipine)**. Monitor and adjust dose. Moderate Study
- **Cobicistat** is predicted to increase the exposure to calcium channel blockers **(diltiazem, verapamil)**. Severe Study
- **Cobicistat** is predicted to markedly increase the exposure to calcium channel blockers **(lercanidipine)**. Avoid. Severe Study
- **Cobicistat** is predicted to increase the exposure to **cannabidiol**. Avoid or adjust dose. Mild Study
- **Cobicistat** is predicted to moderately increase the exposure to cariprazine. Avoid. Severe Study
- **Cobicistat** is predicted to increase the exposure to **ceritinib**. Avoid or adjust **ceritinib** dose. Severe Study
- **Cobicistat** increases the concentration of **ciclosporin**. Severe Study
- **Cobicistat** is predicted to moderately increase the exposure to cilostazol. Adjust **cilostazol** dose. Moderate Study
- **Cobicistat** is predicted to moderately increase the exposure to cinacalcet. Adjust dose. Moderate Study
- **Cobicistat** is predicted to markedly increase the exposure to cobimetinib. Avoid or monitor for toxicity. Severe Study
- **Cobicistat** is predicted to increase the exposure to **colchicine**. Avoid potent inhibitors of CYP3A4 or adjust **colchicine** dose. Severe Study
- **Cobicistat** is predicted to decrease the efficacy of **combined hormonal contraceptives**. Avoid. Severe Study
- **Cobicistat** is predicted to increase the exposure to corticosteroids **(beclometasone)** (risk with beclometasone is likely to be lower than with other corticosteroids). Moderate Theoretical
- **Cobicistat** is predicted to increase the exposure to corticosteroids **(betamethasone, budesonide, ciclesonide, deflazacort, dexamethasone, fludrocortisone, fluticasone, hydrocortisone, methylprednisolone, mometasone, prednisolone, triamcinolone)**. Avoid or monitor side effects. Severe Study
- **Cobicistat** is predicted to moderately increase the exposure to **crizotinib**. Avoid. Moderate Study
- **Cobicistat** is predicted to increase the exposure to **dabigatran**. Avoid. Severe Theoretical
- **Cobicistat** is predicted to increase the exposure to **dabrafenib**. Use with caution or avoid. Moderate Study
- **Cobicistat** is predicted to markedly to very markedly increase the exposure to **darifenacin**. Avoid. Severe Study
- **Cobicistat** is predicted to markedly increase the exposure to **dasatinib**. Avoid or adjust dose—consult product literature. Severe Study
- **Cobicistat** very slightly increases the exposure to **delamanid**. Severe Study
- **Cobicistat** is predicted to moderately increase the exposure to **dienogest**. Moderate Study
- **Cobicistat** increases the risk of QT-prolongation when given with **domperidone**. Avoid. Severe Study
- **Cobicistat** increases the exposure to dopamine receptor agonists **(bromocriptine)**. Severe Study
- **Cobicistat** is predicted to increase the concentration of dopamine receptor agonists **(cabergoline)**. Moderate Anecdotal
- **Cobicistat** is predicted to increase the exposure to **doravirine**. Mild Study
- **Cobicistat** is predicted to increase the exposure to **dronabinol**. Adjust dose. Mild Study
- **Cobicistat** is predicted to increase the exposure to **dutasteride**. Monitor side effects and adjust dose. Moderate Theoretical
- **Cobicistat** is predicted to increase the exposure to **edoxaban**. Avoid. Severe Theoretical
- **Efavirenz** is predicted to decrease the exposure to **cobicistat**. Avoid. Severe Theoretical
- **Cobicistat** is predicted to markedly increase the exposure to eletriptan. Avoid. Severe Study
- **Cobicistat** is predicted to increase the exposure to **eliglustat**. Avoid or adjust dose—consult product literature. Severe Study
- **Cobicistat** is predicted to increase the exposure to **encorafenib**. Avoid or monitor. Severe Study
- **Enzalutamide** is predicted to decrease the exposure to **cobicistat**. Avoid. Severe Theoretical

- **Cobicistat** is predicted to increase the risk of ergotism when given with ergometrine. Avoid. Severe Theoretical
- **Cobicistat** is predicted to increase the risk of ergotism when given with ergotamine. Avoid. Severe Theoretical
- **Cobicistat** is predicted to slightly increase the exposure to erlotinib. Use with caution and adjust dose. Moderate Study
- **Cobicistat** is predicted to increase the exposure to esketamine. Adjust dose. Moderate Study
- **Cobicistat** is predicted to increase the concentration of everolimus. Avoid. Severe Study
- **Cobicistat** is predicted to moderately increase the exposure to fesoterodine. Adjust **fesoterodine** dose with potent inhibitors of CYP3A4; avoid in hepatic and renal impairment. Severe Study
- **Cobicistat** is predicted to increase the exposure to fosaprepitant. Moderate Theoretical
- **Cobicistat** is predicted to increase the exposure to gefitinib. Moderate Study
- **Cobicistat** is predicted to increase the exposure to gilteritinib. Moderate Study
- **Cobicistat** potentially increases the exposure to glecaprevir. Moderate Theoretical
- **Cobicistat** is predicted to moderately to markedly increase the exposure to grazoprevir. Avoid. Severe Study
- **Cobicistat** is predicted to increase the exposure to guanfacine. Adjust **guanfacine** dose, p. 247. Moderate Study
- **Cobicistat** is predicted to very markedly increase the exposure to ibrutinib. Avoid potent inhibitors of CYP3A4 or adjust **ibrutinib** dose. Severe Study
- **Cobicistat** is predicted to increase the exposure to imatinib. Moderate Study
- **Cobicistat** is predicted to increase the risk of toxicity when given with irinotecan. Avoid. Moderate Study
- **Cobicistat** is predicted to increase the exposure to ivabradine. Avoid. Severe Study
- **Cobicistat** is predicted to increase the exposure to ivacaftor. Adjust ivacaftor p. 196 or lumacaftor with ivacaftor p. 197 or tezacaftor with ivacaftor p. 198 dose with potent inhibitors of CYP3A4. Severe Study
- **Cobicistat** is predicted to increase the exposure to lapatinib. Avoid. Moderate Study
- **Cobicistat** is predicted to moderately increase the exposure to larotrectinib. Avoid or adjust **larotrectinib** dose, p. 607. Moderate Study
- **Cobicistat** is predicted to markedly increase the exposure to lomitapide. Avoid. Severe Study
- **Cobicistat** is predicted to increase the exposure to lorlatinib. Avoid or adjust **lorlatinib** dose. Severe Study
- **Cobicistat** is predicted to increase the exposure to lurasidone. Avoid. Severe Study
- **Cobicistat** is predicted to increase the exposure to macitentan. Moderate Study
- **Cobicistat** markedly increases the exposure to maraviroc. Refer to specialist literature. Severe Study
- **Cobicistat** potentially increases the exposure to mexiletine. Severe Theoretical
- **Cobicistat** is predicted to markedly to very markedly increase the exposure to midazolam. Avoid or adjust dose. Severe Study
- **Cobicistat** is predicted to very markedly increase the exposure to midostaurin. Avoid or monitor for toxicity. Severe Study
- **Cobicistat** is predicted to increase the exposure to mirabegron. Adjust **mirabegron** dose in hepatic and renal impairment. Moderate Study
- **Cobicistat** is predicted to increase the exposure to mirtazapine. Moderate Study
- **Mitotane** is predicted to decrease the exposure to **cobicistat**. Avoid. Severe Theoretical
- **Cobicistat** is predicted to increase the exposure to modafinil. Mild Theoretical
- **Cobicistat** is predicted to increase the exposure to monoclonal antibodies (**polatuzumab vedotin**). Moderate Theoretical
- **Cobicistat** is predicted to increase the exposure to monoclonal antibodies (**trastuzumab emtansine**). Avoid. Severe Theoretical
- **Cobicistat** is predicted to increase the exposure to naldemedine. Avoid or monitor. Moderate Study
- **Cobicistat** is predicted to markedly increase the exposure to naloxegol. Avoid. Severe Study
- **Cobicistat** is predicted to increase the exposure to neratinib. Avoid or adjust **neratinib** dose. Severe Study
- **Cobicistat** is predicted to increase the exposure to netupitant. Moderate Study
- **Nevirapine** is predicted to decrease the exposure to **cobicistat**. Avoid. Severe Theoretical
- **Cobicistat** is predicted to moderately increase the exposure to nilotinib. Avoid. Severe Study
- **Cobicistat** is predicted to increase the exposure to nitisinone. Adjust dose. Moderate Theoretical
- **Cobicistat** is predicted to increase the exposure to olaparib. Avoid potent inhibitors of CYP3A4 or adjust **olaparib** dose. Moderate Study
- **Cobicistat** is predicted to increase the exposure to opioids (**alfentanil, buprenorphine, fentanyl, oxycodone**). Monitor and adjust dose. Severe Study
- **Cobicistat** is predicted to increase the exposure to ospemifene. Avoid in poor CYP2C9 metabolisers. Moderate Study
- **Cobicistat** is predicted to increase the exposure to oxybutynin. Mild Study
- **Cobicistat** is predicted to increase the exposure to palbociclib. Avoid or adjust **palbociclib** dose. Severe Study
- **Cobicistat** is predicted to increase the exposure to panobinostat. Adjust **panobinostat** dose; in hepatic impairment avoid. Moderate Study
- **Cobicistat** is predicted to increase the exposure to paritaprevir. Avoid. Severe Study
- **Cobicistat** is predicted to increase the exposure to pazopanib. Avoid or adjust **pazopanib** dose. Moderate Study
- **Cobicistat** is predicted to increase the exposure to phosphodiesterase type-5 inhibitors (**avanafil, vardenafil**). Avoid. Severe Study
- **Cobicistat** is predicted to increase the exposure to phosphodiesterase type-5 inhibitors (**sildenafil**). Avoid potent inhibitors of CYP3A4 or adjust **sildenafil** dose, p. 125. Severe Study
- **Cobicistat** is predicted to increase the exposure to phosphodiesterase type-5 inhibitors (**tadalafil**). Use with caution or avoid. Severe Study
- **Cobicistat** is predicted to increase the exposure to pimozide. Avoid. Severe Study
- **Cobicistat** is predicted to slightly increase the exposure to ponatinib. Monitor and adjust **ponatinib** dose. Moderate Study
- **Cobicistat** is predicted to moderately increase the exposure to praziquantel. Mild Study
- **Cobicistat** given with carbimazole is predicted to increase the exposure to propiverine. Adjust starting dose. Moderate Theoretical
- **Cobicistat** is predicted to increase the exposure to quetiapine. Avoid. Severe Study
- **Cobicistat** is predicted to increase the exposure to ranolazine. Avoid. Severe Study
- **Cobicistat** is predicted to increase the exposure to reboxetine. Avoid. Moderate Study
- **Cobicistat** is predicted to increase the exposure to regorafenib. Avoid. Moderate Study
- **Cobicistat** is predicted to increase the exposure to repaglinide. Moderate Study
- **Cobicistat** is predicted to increase the exposure to retinoids (**alitretinoin**). Adjust **alitretinoin** dose. Moderate Theoretical
- **Cobicistat** is predicted to increase the exposure to ribociclib. Avoid or adjust **ribociclib** dose. Moderate Study
- **Rifabutin** decreases the concentration of **cobicistat** and **cobicistat** increases the exposure to rifabutin. Avoid or adjust dose. Severe Study
- **Rifampicin** is predicted to decrease the exposure to **cobicistat**. Avoid. Severe Theoretical
- **Cobicistat** is predicted to increase the exposure to risperidone. Adjust dose. Moderate Study
- **Cobicistat** is predicted to increase the exposure to rivaroxaban. Avoid. Severe Theoretical
- **Cobicistat** is predicted to increase the exposure to ruxolitinib. Adjust dose and monitor side effects. Moderate Study

Cobicistat (continued)
- **Cobicistat** is predicted to increase the exposure to **saxagliptin**. Moderate Study
- **Cobicistat** is predicted to increase the exposure to **siponimod**. Avoid depending on other drugs taken—consult product literature. Severe Theoretical
- **Cobicistat** is predicted to increase the concentration of **sirolimus**. Avoid. Severe Study
- **Cobicistat** is predicted to increase the exposure to **solifenacin**. Adjust solifenacin or tamsulosin with solifenacin dose; avoid in hepatic and renal impairment. Severe Study
- **Cobicistat** is predicted to moderately increase the exposure to SSRIs **(dapoxetine)**. Avoid potent inhibitors of CYP3A4 or adjust **dapoxetine** dose. Severe Study
- **St John's Wort** is predicted to decrease the exposure to **cobicistat**. Avoid. Severe Theoretical
- **Cobicistat** is predicted to increase the exposure to statins **(atorvastatin)**. Avoid or adjust dose and monitor rhabdomyolysis. Severe Study
- **Cobicistat** is predicted to increase the exposure to statins **(simvastatin)**. Avoid. Severe Study
- **Cobicistat** is predicted to slightly increase the exposure to **sunitinib**. Avoid or adjust **sunitinib** dose. Moderate Study
- **Cobicistat** is predicted to increase the concentration of **tacrolimus**. Monitor and adjust dose. Severe Study
- **Cobicistat** is predicted to increase the exposure to taxanes **(cabazitaxel)**. Avoid. Severe Study
- **Cobicistat** is predicted to moderately increase the exposure to taxanes **(docetaxel)**. Avoid or adjust dose. Severe Study
- **Cobicistat** is predicted to increase the exposure to taxanes **(paclitaxel)**. Severe Theoretical
- **Cobicistat** is predicted to increase the concentration of **temsirolimus**. Avoid. Severe Theoretical
- **Cobicistat** is predicted to increase the exposure to **tezacaftor**. Adjust tezacaftor with ivacaftor p. 198 dose with potent inhibitors of CYP3A4. Severe Study
- **Cobicistat** is predicted to markedly increase the exposure to **ticagrelor**. Avoid. Severe Study
- **Cobicistat** is predicted to increase the exposure to **tofacitinib**. Adjust **tofacitinib** dose. Moderate Study
- **Cobicistat** is predicted to increase the exposure to **tolterodine**. Avoid. Severe Study
- **Cobicistat** is predicted to increase the exposure to **tolvaptan**. Manufacturer advises caution or adjust **tolvaptan** dose with potent inhibitors of CYP3A4. Severe Study
- **Cobicistat** is predicted to increase the exposure to **toremifene**. Moderate Theoretical
- **Cobicistat** is predicted to increase the exposure to **trabectedin**. Avoid or adjust dose. Severe Theoretical
- **Cobicistat** is predicted to moderately increase the exposure to **trazodone**. Avoid or adjust dose. Moderate Study
- **Cobicistat** is predicted to slightly increase the exposure to **tricyclic antidepressants**. Mild Study
- **Cobicistat** is predicted to increase the exposure to **ulipristal**. Avoid if used for uterine fibroids. Severe Study
- **Cobicistat** is predicted to increase the exposure to **upadacitinib**. Use with caution or avoid. Severe Study
- **Cobicistat** is predicted to increase the exposure to **vemurafenib**. Severe Theoretical
- **Cobicistat** is predicted to increase the exposure to **venetoclax**. Avoid or adjust dose—consult product literature. Severe Study
- **Cobicistat** is predicted to increase the exposure to **venlafaxine**. Moderate Study
- **Cobicistat** is predicted to increase the exposure to **vinca alkaloids**. Severe Theoretical
- **Cobicistat** is predicted to increase the exposure to vitamin D substances **(paricalcitol)**. Moderate Study
- **Cobicistat** is predicted to increase the exposure to **zopiclone**. Adjust dose. Moderate Theoretical

Cobimetinib
- Antiarrhythmics **(dronedarone)** are predicted to increase the exposure to **cobimetinib**. Severe Theoretical
- Antiepileptics **(carbamazepine, fosphenytoin, phenobarbital, phenytoin, primidone)** are predicted to decrease the exposure to **cobimetinib**. Avoid. Severe Theoretical
- Antifungals, azoles **(fluconazole, isavuconazole, miconazole, posaconazole)** are predicted to increase the exposure to **cobimetinib**. Severe Theoretical
- Antifungals, azoles **(itraconazole, ketoconazole, voriconazole)** are predicted to markedly increase the exposure to **cobimetinib**. Avoid or monitor for toxicity. Severe Study
- **Apalutamide** is predicted to decrease the exposure to **cobimetinib**. Avoid. Severe Theoretical
- **Aprepitant** is predicted to increase the exposure to **cobimetinib**. Severe Theoretical
- **Bosentan** is predicted to decrease the exposure to **cobimetinib**. Avoid. Severe Theoretical
- Calcium channel blockers **(diltiazem, verapamil)** are predicted to increase the exposure to **cobimetinib**. Severe Theoretical
- **Cobicistat** is predicted to markedly increase the exposure to **cobimetinib**. Avoid or monitor for toxicity. Severe Study
- **Crizotinib** is predicted to increase the exposure to **cobimetinib**. Severe Theoretical
- **Efavirenz** is predicted to decrease the exposure to **cobimetinib**. Avoid. Severe Theoretical
- **Enzalutamide** is predicted to decrease the exposure to **cobimetinib**. Avoid. Severe Theoretical
- **Grapefruit juice** is predicted to increase the exposure to **cobimetinib**. Avoid. Severe Theoretical
- **HIV-protease inhibitors** are predicted to markedly increase the exposure to **cobimetinib**. Avoid or monitor for toxicity. Severe Study
- **Idelalisib** is predicted to markedly increase the exposure to **cobimetinib**. Avoid or monitor for toxicity. Severe Study
- **Imatinib** is predicted to increase the exposure to **cobimetinib**. Severe Theoretical
- Macrolides **(clarithromycin)** are predicted to markedly increase the exposure to **cobimetinib**. Avoid or monitor for toxicity. Severe Study
- Macrolides **(erythromycin)** are predicted to increase the exposure to **cobimetinib**. Severe Theoretical
- **Mitotane** is predicted to decrease the exposure to **cobimetinib**. Avoid. Severe Theoretical
- **Netupitant** is predicted to increase the exposure to **cobimetinib**. Severe Theoretical
- **Nevirapine** is predicted to decrease the exposure to **cobimetinib**. Avoid. Severe Theoretical
- **Nilotinib** is predicted to increase the exposure to **cobimetinib**. Severe Theoretical
- **Rifampicin** is predicted to decrease the exposure to **cobimetinib**. Avoid. Severe Theoretical
- **St John's Wort** is predicted to decrease the exposure to **cobimetinib**. Avoid. Severe Theoretical

Codeine → see opioids

Colchicine
- Antiarrhythmics **(amiodarone)** are predicted to increase the exposure to **colchicine**. Avoid P-glycoprotein inhibitors or adjust **colchicine** dose. Severe Theoretical
- Antiarrhythmics **(dronedarone)** are predicted to increase the exposure to **colchicine**. Adjust **colchicine** dose with moderate inhibitors of CYP3A4. Severe Study
- Antifungals, azoles **(fluconazole, isavuconazole, posaconazole)** are predicted to increase the exposure to **colchicine**. Adjust **colchicine** dose with moderate inhibitors of CYP3A4. Severe Study
- Antifungals, azoles **(itraconazole, ketoconazole, voriconazole)** are predicted to increase the exposure to **colchicine**. Avoid potent inhibitors of CYP3A4 or adjust **colchicine** dose. Severe Study
- **Apalutamide** is predicted to decrease the exposure to **colchicine**. Mild Study
- **Aprepitant** is predicted to increase the exposure to **colchicine**. Adjust **colchicine** dose with moderate inhibitors of CYP3A4. Severe Study
- Calcium channel blockers **(diltiazem, verapamil)** are predicted to increase the exposure to **colchicine**. Adjust **colchicine** dose with moderate inhibitors of CYP3A4. Severe Study
- **Ceritinib** is predicted to increase the exposure to **colchicine**. Moderate Theoretical
- **Ciclosporin** increases the exposure to **colchicine**. Avoid P-glycoprotein inhibitors or adjust **colchicine** dose. Severe Study

- Cobicistat is predicted to increase the exposure to **colchicine**. Avoid potent inhibitors of CYP3A4 or adjust **colchicine** dose. Severe Study
- Crizotinib is predicted to increase the exposure to **colchicine**. Adjust **colchicine** dose with moderate inhibitors of CYP3A4. Severe Study
- Eliglustat is predicted to increase the exposure to **colchicine**. Avoid or adjust **colchicine** dose. Severe Theoretical
- **Colchicine** increases the risk of rhabdomyolysis when given with fibrates. Severe Anecdotal
- HIV-protease inhibitors are predicted to increase the exposure to **colchicine**. Avoid potent inhibitors of CYP3A4 or adjust **colchicine** dose. Severe Study
- Idelalisib is predicted to increase the exposure to **colchicine**. Avoid potent inhibitors of CYP3A4 or adjust **colchicine** dose. Severe Study
- Imatinib is predicted to increase the exposure to **colchicine**. Adjust **colchicine** dose with moderate inhibitors of CYP3A4. Severe Study
- Lapatinib is predicted to increase the exposure to **colchicine**. Avoid P-glycoprotein inhibitors or adjust **colchicine** dose. Moderate Theoretical
- Macrolides (azithromycin) are predicted to increase the exposure to **colchicine**. Avoid P-glycoprotein inhibitors or adjust **colchicine** dose. Severe Theoretical
- Macrolides (clarithromycin) are predicted to increase the exposure to **colchicine**. Avoid potent inhibitors of CYP3A4 or adjust **colchicine** dose. Severe Study
- Macrolides (erythromycin) are predicted to increase the exposure to **colchicine**. Adjust **colchicine** dose with moderate inhibitors of CYP3A4. Severe Study
- Mirabegron is predicted to increase the exposure to **colchicine**. Mild Theoretical
- Netupitant is predicted to increase the exposure to **colchicine**. Adjust **colchicine** dose with moderate inhibitors of CYP3A4. Severe Study
- Nilotinib is predicted to increase the exposure to **colchicine**. Adjust **colchicine** dose with moderate inhibitors of CYP3A4. Severe Study
- Pibrentasvir (with glecaprevir) is predicted to increase the exposure to **colchicine**. Moderate Study
- Pitolisant is predicted to decrease the exposure to **colchicine**. Mild Theoretical
- Ranolazine is predicted to increase the exposure to **colchicine**. Avoid P-glycoprotein inhibitors or adjust **colchicine** dose. Severe Theoretical
- Rolapitant is predicted to increase the exposure to **colchicine**. Moderate Study
- **Colchicine** increases the risk of rhabdomyolysis when given with statins. Severe Anecdotal
- Velpatasvir is predicted to increase the exposure to **colchicine**. Severe Theoretical
- Vemurafenib is predicted to increase the exposure to **colchicine**. Avoid P-glycoprotein inhibitors or adjust **colchicine** dose. Severe Theoretical

Colecalciferol → see vitamin D substances

Colesevelam

SEPARATION OF ADMINISTRATION Manufacturer advises take 4 hours before, or after, other drugs.

Colestipol

SEPARATION OF ADMINISTRATION Manufacturer advises take other drugs at least 1 hour before, or 4 hours after, colestipol.

Colestyramine

SEPARATION OF ADMINISTRATION Manufacturer advises take other drugs at least 1 hour before, or 4–6 hours after, colestyramine.

Colistimethate → see TABLE 2 p. 907 (nephrotoxicity), TABLE 20 p. 911 (neuromuscular blocking effects)

Combined hormonal contraceptives

- **Combined hormonal contraceptives** are predicted to increase the exposure to agomelatine. Moderate Study
- **Combined hormonal contraceptives** are predicted to increase the exposure to aminophylline. Adjust dose. Moderate Theoretical
- **Combined hormonal contraceptives** are predicted to increase the exposure to anagrelide. Moderate Theoretical
- Antiepileptics (carbamazepine, eslicarbazepine, fosphenytoin, oxcarbazepine, perampanel, phenobarbital, phenytoin, primidone, rufinamide, topiramate) are predicted to decrease the efficacy of **combined hormonal contraceptives**. For FSRH guidance, see Contraceptives, interactions p. 536. Severe Study
- **Combined hormonal contraceptives** alter the exposure to antiepileptics (lamotrigine). Adjust dose. Moderate Study
- Aprepitant is predicted to decrease the efficacy of **combined hormonal contraceptives**. For FSRH guidance, see Contraceptives, interactions p. 536. Severe Study
- Bosentan is predicted to decrease the efficacy of **combined hormonal contraceptives**. For FSRH guidance, see Contraceptives, interactions p. 536. Severe Study
- Brigatinib decreases the exposure to **combined hormonal contraceptives**. Use additional contraceptive precautions. Severe Theoretical
- Carfilzomib potentially decreases the efficacy of **combined hormonal contraceptives**. Use additional contraceptive precautions. Severe Theoretical
- Oral **combined hormonal contraceptives** potentially decrease the efficacy of chenodeoxycholic acid. Avoid. Moderate Theoretical
- **Combined hormonal contraceptives** increase the concentration of clozapine. Monitor side effects and adjust dose. Severe Study
- Cobicistat is predicted to decrease the efficacy of **combined hormonal contraceptives**. Avoid. Severe Study
- **Combined hormonal contraceptives** (containing ethinylestradiol) increase the risk of increased ALT concentrations when given with dasabuvir. Avoid. Severe Study
- **Combined hormonal contraceptives** are predicted to increase the exposure to dopamine receptor agonists (ropinirole). Adjust dose. Moderate Study
- Efavirenz is predicted to decrease the efficacy of **combined hormonal contraceptives**. For FSRH guidance, see Contraceptives, interactions p. 536. Severe Study
- Encorafenib is predicted to affect the exposure to **combined hormonal contraceptives**. Severe Theoretical
- **Combined hormonal contraceptives** slightly increase the exposure to erlotinib. Monitor side effects and adjust dose. Moderate Study
- Fosaprepitant is predicted to decrease the efficacy of **combined hormonal contraceptives**. For FSRH guidance, see Contraceptives, interactions p. 536. Severe Study
- **Combined hormonal contraceptives** (containing ethinylestradiol) are predicted to increase the risk of increased ALT concentrations when given with glecaprevir. Avoid. Severe Study
- Griseofulvin potentially decreases the efficacy of **combined hormonal contraceptives**. For FSRH guidance, see Contraceptives, interactions p. 536. Severe Anecdotal
- HIV-protease inhibitors (atazanavir) (unboosted) increase the exposure to **combined hormonal contraceptives**. Adjust dose. Severe Study
- HIV-protease inhibitors (ritonavir) are predicted to decrease the efficacy of **combined hormonal contraceptives**. For FSRH guidance, see Contraceptives, interactions p. 536. Severe Study
- Larotrectinib potentially decreases the efficacy of **combined hormonal contraceptives**. Use additional contraceptive precautions. Severe Theoretical
- **Combined hormonal contraceptives** are predicted to increase the risk of venous thromboembolism when given with lenalidomide. Avoid. Severe Theoretical
- Oral **combined hormonal contraceptives** slightly increase the exposure to lomitapide. Separate administration by 12 hours. Moderate Theoretical
- Lorlatinib is predicted to decrease the exposure to **combined hormonal contraceptives**. Avoid. Moderate Theoretical
- **Combined hormonal contraceptives** are predicted to increase the exposure to loxapine. Avoid. Unknown Theoretical

Combined hormonal contraceptives (continued)

- **Lumacaftor** is predicted to decrease the efficacy of **combined hormonal contraceptives.** Use additional contraceptive precautions. [Severe] Theoretical
- **Combined hormonal contraceptives** slightly increase the exposure to MAO-B inhibitors **(rasagiline).** [Moderate] Study
- **Combined hormonal contraceptives** increase the exposure to MAO-B inhibitors **(selegiline).** Avoid. [Severe] Study
- **Combined hormonal contraceptives** are predicted to increase the exposure to **melatonin.** [Moderate] Theoretical
- **Combined hormonal contraceptives** decrease the effects of **metyrapone.** Avoid. [Moderate] Theoretical
- **Modafinil** is predicted to decrease the efficacy of **combined hormonal contraceptives.** For FSRH guidance, see Contraceptives, interactions p. 536. [Severe] Study
- Monoclonal antibodies **(sarilumab)** potentially decrease the exposure to **combined hormonal contraceptives.** [Severe] Theoretical
- **Nevirapine** is predicted to decrease the efficacy of **combined hormonal contraceptives.** For FSRH guidance, see Contraceptives, interactions p. 536. [Severe] Study
- NSAIDs **(etoricoxib)** slightly increase the exposure to **combined hormonal contraceptives.** [Moderate] Study
- **Olaparib** potentially affects the efficacy of **combined hormonal contraceptives.** Use additional contraceptive precautions. [Moderate] Theoretical
- **Combined hormonal contraceptives** potentially oppose the effects of **ospemifene.** Avoid. [Severe] Theoretical
- **Combined hormonal contraceptives** (containing ethinylestradiol) are predicted to increase the risk of increased ALT concentrations when given with **paritaprevir** (with ritonavir and ombitasvir). Avoid. [Severe] Study
- **Combined hormonal contraceptives** (containing ethinylestradiol) are predicted to increase the risk of increased ALT concentrations when given with **pibrentasvir.** Avoid. [Severe] Study
- **Combined hormonal contraceptives** are predicted to increase the exposure to **pirfenidone.** Use with caution and adjust dose. [Moderate] Study
- **Pitolisant** is predicted to decrease the efficacy of **combined hormonal contraceptives.** Avoid. [Severe] Theoretical
- **Combined hormonal contraceptives** are predicted to increase the risk of venous thromboembolism when given with **pomalidomide.** Avoid. [Severe] Theoretical
- **Combined hormonal contraceptives** potentially oppose the effects of **raloxifene.** Avoid. [Severe] Theoretical
- **Rifabutin** is predicted to decrease the efficacy of **combined hormonal contraceptives.** For FSRH guidance, see Contraceptives, interactions p. 536. [Severe] Study
- **Rifampicin** is predicted to decrease the efficacy of **combined hormonal contraceptives.** For FSRH guidance, see Contraceptives, interactions p. 536. [Severe] Study
- **Combined hormonal contraceptives** are predicted to increase the exposure to **roflumilast.** [Moderate] Theoretical
- **St John's Wort** decreases the efficacy of **combined hormonal contraceptives.** MHRA advises avoid. For FSRH guidance, see Contraceptives, interactions p. 536. [Severe] Anecdotal
- **Sugammadex** is predicted to decrease the exposure to oral **combined hormonal contraceptives.** Refer to patient information leaflet for missed pill advice. [Severe] Theoretical
- **Combined hormonal contraceptives** are predicted to increase the risk of venous thromboembolism when given with **thalidomide.** Avoid. [Severe] Study
- **Combined hormonal contraceptives** are predicted to increase the exposure to **theophylline.** Monitor and adjust dose. [Moderate] Theoretical
- **Combined hormonal contraceptives** increase the exposure to **tizanidine.** Avoid. [Moderate] Study
- **Ulipristal** is predicted to decrease the efficacy of **combined hormonal contraceptives.** Avoid. [Severe] Theoretical
- **Combined hormonal contraceptives** (containing ethinylestradiol) are predicted to increase the risk of increased ALT concentrations when given with **voxilaprevir** (with sofosbuvir and velpatasvir). Avoid. [Severe] Study
- **Combined hormonal contraceptives** are predicted to increase the exposure to **zolmitriptan.** Adjust **zolmitriptan** dose, p. 310. [Moderate] Theoretical

Corticosteroids → see **TABLE 17** p. 911 (reduced serum potassium)

beclometasone · betamethasone · budesonide · ciclesonide · deflazacort · dexamethasone · fludrocortisone · fluticasone · hydrocortisone · methylprednisolone · mometasone · prednisolone · triamcinolone

- With intravitreal use of **dexamethasone** in adults: caution with concurrent administration of anticoagulant or antiplatelet drugs—increased risk of haemorrhagic events.
- Interactions do not generally apply to corticosteroids used for topical action (including inhalation, except **budesonide** and **fluticasone**) unless specified. However, as systemic absorption might occur with **hydrocortisone** *eye drops*, the possibility of interactions should be borne in mind.

- **Antacids** are predicted to decrease the absorption of **deflazacort.** Separate administration by 2 hours. [Moderate] Theoretical
- **Antacids** decrease the absorption of **dexamethasone.** [Moderate] Study
- Antiarrhythmics **(dronedarone)** are predicted to increase the exposure to **methylprednisolone.** Monitor and adjust dose. [Moderate] Study
- Antiepileptics **(carbamazepine, fosphenytoin, phenobarbital, phenytoin, primidone)** are predicted to decrease the exposure to **fluticasone.** [Unknown] Theoretical
- Antiepileptics **(carbamazepine, fosphenytoin, phenobarbital, phenytoin, primidone)** are predicted to decrease the exposure to corticosteroids **(budesonide, deflazacort, dexamethasone, fludrocortisone, hydrocortisone, methylprednisolone, prednisolone, triamcinolone).** Monitor and adjust dose. [Moderate] Study
- Antifungals, azoles **(fluconazole, isavuconazole, posaconazole)** are predicted to increase the exposure to **methylprednisolone.** Monitor and adjust dose. [Moderate] Study
- Antifungals, azoles **(itraconazole, ketoconazole, voriconazole)** are predicted to increase the exposure to **beclometasone** (risk with beclometasone is likely to be lower than with other corticosteroids). [Moderate] Theoretical
- Antifungals, azoles **(miconazole)** are predicted to increase the concentration of **methylprednisolone.** Monitor and adjust dose. [Moderate] Theoretical
- Antifungals, azoles **(itraconazole, ketoconazole, voriconazole)** are predicted to increase the exposure to corticosteroids **(betamethasone, budesonide, ciclesonide, deflazacort, dexamethasone, fludrocortisone, fluticasone, hydrocortisone, methylprednisolone, mometasone, prednisolone, triamcinolone).** Avoid or monitor side effects. [Severe] Study
- **Apalutamide** is predicted to decrease the exposure to corticosteroids **(budesonide, deflazacort, dexamethasone, fludrocortisone, hydrocortisone, methylprednisolone, prednisolone, triamcinolone).** Monitor and adjust dose. [Moderate] Study
- **Apalutamide** is predicted to decrease the exposure to **fluticasone.** [Unknown] Theoretical
- **Aprepitant** is predicted to increase the exposure to oral **budesonide.** [Moderate] Study
- **Aprepitant** moderately increases the exposure to **dexamethasone.** Monitor and adjust dose. [Moderate] Study
- **Aprepitant** is predicted to increase the exposure to **fluticasone.** [Moderate] Study
- **Aprepitant** is predicted to increase the exposure to **methylprednisolone.** Monitor and adjust dose. [Moderate] Study
- **Corticosteroids** are predicted to decrease the concentration of **aspirin** (high-dose) and **aspirin** (high-dose) increases the risk of gastrointestinal bleeding when given with **corticosteroids.** [Moderate] Study
- Calcium channel blockers **(diltiazem, verapamil)** are predicted to increase the exposure to **methylprednisolone.** Monitor and adjust dose. [Moderate] Study
- **Dexamethasone** is predicted to decrease the concentration of caspofungin. Adjust **caspofungin** dose, p. 405. [Moderate] Theoretical

- **Corticosteroids** are predicted to decrease the concentration of choline salicylate. Moderate Study
- Cobicistat is predicted to increase the exposure to **beclometasone** (risk with beclometasone is likely to be lower than with other corticosteroids). Moderate Theoretical
- Cobicistat is predicted to increase the exposure to corticosteroids **(betamethasone, budesonide, ciclesonide, deflazacort, dexamethasone, fludrocortisone, fluticasone, hydrocortisone, methylprednisolone, mometasone, prednisolone, triamcinolone)**. Avoid or monitor side effects. Severe Study
- **Corticosteroids** are predicted to increase the effects of **coumarins**. Moderate Study
- Crizotinib is predicted to increase the exposure to **methylprednisolone**. Monitor and adjust dose. Moderate Study
- Enzalutamide is predicted to decrease the exposure to corticosteroids **(budesonide, deflazacort, dexamethasone, fludrocortisone, hydrocortisone, methylprednisolone, prednisolone, triamcinolone)**. Monitor and adjust dose. Moderate Study
- Enzalutamide is predicted to decrease the exposure to **fluticasone**. Unknown Theoretical
- **Corticosteroids** increase the risk of gastrointestinal perforation when given with **erlotinib**. Severe Theoretical
- **Corticosteroids** potentially oppose the effects of **glycerol** phenylbutyrate. Moderate Theoretical
- Grapefruit juice moderately increases the exposure to oral **budesonide**. Avoid. Moderate Study
- HIV-protease inhibitors are predicted to increase the exposure to **beclometasone** (risk with beclometasone is likely to be lower than with other corticosteroids). Moderate Theoretical
- HIV-protease inhibitors are predicted to increase the exposure to corticosteroids **(betamethasone, budesonide, ciclesonide, deflazacort, dexamethasone, fludrocortisone, fluticasone, hydrocortisone, methylprednisolone, mometasone, prednisolone, triamcinolone)**. Avoid or monitor side effects. Severe Study
- Idelalisib is predicted to increase the exposure to **beclometasone** (risk with beclometasone is likely to be lower than with other corticosteroids). Moderate Theoretical
- Idelalisib is predicted to increase the exposure to corticosteroids **(betamethasone, budesonide, ciclesonide, deflazacort, dexamethasone, fludrocortisone, fluticasone, hydrocortisone, methylprednisolone, mometasone, prednisolone, triamcinolone)**. Avoid or monitor side effects. Severe Study
- Imatinib is predicted to increase the exposure to **methylprednisolone**. Monitor and adjust dose. Moderate Study
- **Corticosteroids** are predicted to increase the risk of gastrointestinal bleeding when given with iron chelators (deferasirox). Severe Theoretical
- Live vaccines are predicted to increase the risk of generalised infection (possibly life-threatening) when given with **corticosteroids** (high-dose). Public Health England advises avoid (refer to Green Book). Severe Theoretical
- Lumacaftor is predicted to decrease the exposure to **methylprednisolone**. Adjust dose. Severe Theoretical
- Macrolides (clarithromycin) are predicted to increase the exposure to **beclometasone** (risk with beclometasone is likely to be lower than with other corticosteroids). Moderate Theoretical
- Macrolides (erythromycin) are predicted to increase the exposure to **methylprednisolone**. Monitor and adjust dose. Moderate Study
- Macrolides (clarithromycin) are predicted to increase the exposure to corticosteroids **(betamethasone, budesonide, ciclesonide, deflazacort, dexamethasone, fludrocortisone, fluticasone, hydrocortisone, methylprednisolone, mometasone, prednisolone, triamcinolone)**. Avoid or monitor side effects. Severe Study
- **Corticosteroids** are predicted to decrease the efficacy of **mifamurtide**. Avoid. Severe Theoretical
- **Mifepristone** is predicted to decrease the efficacy of **corticosteroids**. Use with caution and adjust dose. Moderate Theoretical
- **Mitotane** is predicted to decrease the exposure to corticosteroids **(budesonide, deflazacort, dexamethasone, fludrocortisone, hydrocortisone, methylprednisolone, prednisolone, triamcinolone)**. Monitor and adjust dose. Moderate Study
- **Mitotane** is predicted to decrease the exposure to **fluticasone**. Unknown Theoretical
- Corticosteroids **(betamethasone, deflazacort, dexamethasone, hydrocortisone, methylprednisolone, prednisolone)** are predicted to decrease the efficacy of monoclonal antibodies **(atezolizumab, ipilimumab, nivolumab, pembrolizumab)**. Use with caution or avoid. Severe Theoretical
- Monoclonal antibodies **(tocilizumab)** are predicted to decrease the exposure to corticosteroids **(dexamethasone, methylprednisolone)**. Monitor and adjust dose. Moderate Theoretical
- **Corticosteroids** are predicted to increase the risk of immunosuppression when given with monoclonal antibodies **(dinutuximab)**. Avoid except in life-threatening situations. Severe Theoretical
- **Netupitant** is predicted to increase the exposure to oral **budesonide**. Moderate Study
- **Netupitant** is predicted to increase the exposure to **dexamethasone**. Adjust dose. Moderate Study
- **Netupitant** is predicted to increase the exposure to **fluticasone**. Moderate Study
- **Netupitant** is predicted to increase the exposure to **methylprednisolone**. Monitor and adjust dose. Moderate Study
- **Corticosteroids** are predicted to decrease the effects of **neuromuscular blocking drugs, non-depolarising**. Severe Anecdotal
- **Corticosteroids** increase the risk of gastrointestinal perforation when given with **nicorandil**. Severe Anecdotal
- **Nilotinib** is predicted to increase the exposure to **methylprednisolone**. Monitor and adjust dose. Moderate Study
- **NSAIDs** increase the risk of gastrointestinal bleeding when given with **corticosteroids**. Severe Study
- **Corticosteroids** are predicted to increase the effects of **phenindione**. Moderate Anecdotal
- **Dexamethasone** decreases the exposure to **praziquantel**. Moderate Study
- **Rifampicin** is predicted to decrease the exposure to corticosteroids **(budesonide, deflazacort, dexamethasone, fludrocortisone, hydrocortisone, methylprednisolone, prednisolone, triamcinolone)**. Monitor and adjust dose. Moderate Study
- **Rifampicin** is predicted to decrease the exposure to **fluticasone**. Unknown Theoretical
- **Dexamethasone** is predicted to decrease the concentration of **rilpivirine**. Avoid multiple-dose dexamethasone. Severe Theoretical
- **Corticosteroids** potentially decrease the effects of **sodium phenylbutyrate**. Moderate Anecdotal
- **Corticosteroids** are predicted to decrease the effects of **somatropin**. Moderate Theoretical
- **Corticosteroids** are predicted to decrease the effects of **suxamethonium**. Severe Anecdotal

Coumarins → see TABLE 3 p. 907 (anticoagulant effects)

acenocoumarol · warfarin

FOOD AND LIFESTYLE The effects of coumarins can be reduced or abolished by vitamin K, including that found in health foods, food supplements, enteral feeds, or large amounts of some green vegetables or green tea. Major changes in diet (especially involving salads and vegetables) and in alcohol consumption can affect anticoagulant control. Pomegranate juice is predicted to increase the INR in response to **acenocoumarol** and **warfarin**.

- **Alcohol** (beverage)(in those who drink heavily) potentially decreases the anticoagulant effect of **coumarins**. Severe Study
- Antiarrhythmics **(amiodarone)** increase the anticoagulant effect of **coumarins**. Severe Study
- Antiarrhythmics **(propafenone)** increase the anticoagulant effect of **coumarins**. Monitor INR and adjust dose. Moderate Study

Coumarins (continued)

- Antiepileptics **(carbamazepine)** decrease the effects of **coumarins.** Monitor and adjust dose. Severe Study
- Antiepileptics **(fosphenytoin, phenytoin)** are predicted to alter the anticoagulant effect of **coumarins.** Moderate Anecdotal
- Antiepileptics **(phenobarbital, primidone)** decrease the anticoagulant effect of **coumarins.** Monitor INR and adjust dose. Moderate Study
- Antifungals, azoles **(fluconazole)** increase the anticoagulant effect of **coumarins.** Monitor INR and adjust dose. Severe Study
- Antifungals, azoles **(itraconazole)** potentially increase the anticoagulant effect of **coumarins.** Severe Anecdotal
- Antifungals, azoles **(ketoconazole)** potentially increase the anticoagulant effect of **warfarin.** Monitor INR and adjust dose. Severe Anecdotal
- Antifungals, azoles **(miconazole)** greatly increase the anticoagulant effect of **coumarins.** MHRA advises avoid unless INR can be monitored closely; monitor for signs of bleeding. Severe Study
- Antifungals, azoles **(voriconazole)** increase the anticoagulant effect of **coumarins.** Monitor INR and adjust dose. Moderate Study
- **Apalutamide** is predicted to decrease the exposure to **coumarins.** Avoid or monitor. Mild Study
- **Aprepitant** decreases the anticoagulant effect of **coumarins.** Moderate Study
- **Axitinib** is predicted to increase the risk of bleeding events when given with **coumarins.** Severe Theoretical
- **Azathioprine** decreases the anticoagulant effect of **coumarins.** Moderate Study
- **Bosentan** decreases the anticoagulant effect of **coumarins.** Moderate Study
- **Bosutinib** is predicted to increase the risk of bleeding events when given with **coumarins.** Severe Theoretical
- **Cabozantinib** is predicted to increase the risk of bleeding events when given with **coumarins.** Severe Theoretical
- **Capecitabine** increases the effects of **coumarins.** Monitor INR and adjust dose. Moderate Anecdotal
- Cephalosporins **(ceftriaxone)** potentially increase the risk of bleeding events when given with **coumarins.** Severe Anecdotal
- **Ceritinib** is predicted to increase the exposure to **warfarin.** Avoid. Severe Theoretical
- **Chloramphenicol** potentially increases the anticoagulant effect of **coumarins.** Moderate Anecdotal
- **Corticosteroids** are predicted to increase the effects of **coumarins.** Moderate Study
- **Cranberry juice** potentially increases the anticoagulant effect of **warfarin.** Avoid. Severe Anecdotal
- **Crizotinib** is predicted to increase the risk of bleeding events when given with **coumarins.** Severe Theoretical
- **Dabrafenib** is predicted to decrease the anticoagulant effect of **coumarins.** Severe Theoretical
- **Danazol** potentially increases the anticoagulant effect of **coumarins.** Severe Anecdotal
- **Dasatinib** is predicted to increase the risk of bleeding events when given with **coumarins.** Severe Theoretical
- **Disulfiram** increases the anticoagulant effect of **coumarins.** Monitor and adjust dose. Severe Study
- **Efavirenz** is predicted to affect the concentration of **coumarins.** Adjust dose. Moderate Theoretical
- **Elvitegravir** is predicted to decrease the anticoagulant effect of **coumarins.** Moderate Theoretical
- **Enteral feeds** (vitamin-K containing) potentially decrease the anticoagulant effect of **coumarins.** Severe Anecdotal
- **Enzalutamide** potentially decreases the exposure to **coumarins.** Avoid or adjust dose and monitor INR. Severe Study
- **Erlotinib** increases the anticoagulant effect of **coumarins.** Severe Anecdotal
- **Etravirine** increases the anticoagulant effect of **coumarins.** Moderate Theoretical
- **Fibrates** are predicted to increase the anticoagulant effect of **coumarins.** Monitor INR and adjust dose. Severe Study
- **Fluorouracil** increases the anticoagulant effect of **coumarins.** Severe Anecdotal
- **Fosaprepitant** is predicted to decrease the anticoagulant effect of **coumarins.** Moderate Theoretical
- **Gefitinib** is predicted to increase the anticoagulant effect of **coumarins.** Severe Anecdotal
- **Glucagon** increases the anticoagulant effect of **warfarin.** Severe Study
- **Glucosamine** potentially decreases the anticoagulant effect of **acenocoumarol.** Moderate Anecdotal
- **Glucosamine** potentially increases the anticoagulant effect of **warfarin.** Avoid. Moderate Anecdotal
- **Griseofulvin** potentially decreases the anticoagulant effect of **coumarins.** Moderate Anecdotal
- H_2 receptor antagonists **(cimetidine)** increase the anticoagulant effect of **coumarins.** Severe Study
- **HIV-protease inhibitors** are predicted to affect the anticoagulant effect of **coumarins.** Moderate Study
- **Imatinib** is predicted to increase the risk of bleeding events when given with **coumarins.** Severe Theoretical
- **Ivacaftor** is predicted to increase the anticoagulant effect of **warfarin.** Severe Theoretical
- **Ivermectin** potentially increases the anticoagulant effect of **coumarins.** Severe Anecdotal
- **Lapatinib** is predicted to increase the risk of bleeding events when given with **coumarins.** Severe Theoretical
- **Leflunomide** increases the anticoagulant effect of **coumarins.** Severe Anecdotal
- **Letermovir** is predicted to decrease the concentration of **warfarin.** Monitor and adjust dose. Moderate Theoretical
- **Lomitapide** increases the exposure to **warfarin.** Monitor INR and adjust dose. Severe Study
- Macrolides **(clarithromycin, erythromycin)** increase the anticoagulant effect of **coumarins.** Monitor INR and adjust dose. Severe Anecdotal
- **Mercaptopurine** decreases the anticoagulant effect of **coumarins.** Moderate Anecdotal
- **Metronidazole** increases the anticoagulant effect of **coumarins.** Monitor INR and adjust dose. Severe Study
- **Mexiletine** potentially affects the exposure to **warfarin.** Avoid. Unknown Theoretical
- Monoclonal antibodies **(blinatumomab)** are predicted to transiently increase the exposure to **warfarin.** Monitor and adjust dose. Moderate Theoretical
- Monoclonal antibodies **(sarilumab)** potentially affect the exposure to **warfarin.** Monitor and adjust dose. Severe Theoretical
- Monoclonal antibodies **(tocilizumab)** are predicted to decrease the exposure to **warfarin.** Monitor and adjust dose. Moderate Theoretical
- **Nandrolone** is predicted to increase the anticoagulant effect of **coumarins.** Monitor and adjust dose. Severe Theoretical
- **Nevirapine** potentially alters the anticoagulant effect of **coumarins.** Severe Anecdotal
- **Nilotinib** is predicted to increase the risk of bleeding events when given with **coumarins.** Severe Theoretical
- **Nitisinone** is predicted to increase the exposure to **warfarin.** Moderate Study
- **Obeticholic acid** decreases the anticoagulant effect of **warfarin.** Severe Study
- **Oxymetholone** increases the anticoagulant effect of **coumarins.** Severe Anecdotal
- **Paracetamol** increases the anticoagulant effect of **coumarins.** Moderate Study
- **Paritaprevir** (in fixed-dose combination with dasabuvir) decreases the anticoagulant effect of **acenocoumarol.** Monitor INR and adjust dose. Severe Anecdotal
- **Paritaprevir** (in fixed-dose combination) decreases the anticoagulant effect of **warfarin.** Monitor INR and adjust dose. Severe Anecdotal
- **Pazopanib** is predicted to increase the risk of bleeding events when given with **coumarins.** Severe Theoretical
- **Penicillins** potentially alter the anticoagulant effect of **coumarins.** Monitor INR and adjust dose. Severe Anecdotal
- **Pitolisant** is predicted to decrease the exposure to **warfarin.** Mild Theoretical

- **Ponatinib** is predicted to increase the risk of bleeding events when given with **coumarins.** Severe Theoretical
- **Quinolones** increase the anticoagulant effect of **coumarins.** Severe Anecdotal
- **Ranibizumab** increases the risk of bleeding events when given with **coumarins.** Severe Theoretical
- **Regorafenib** is predicted to increase the risk of bleeding events when given with **coumarins.** Severe Study
- **Rifampicin** decreases the anticoagulant effect of **coumarins.** Severe Study
- **Rucaparib** slightly increases the exposure to **warfarin.** Monitor and adjust dose. Severe Study
- **Ruxolitinib** is predicted to increase the risk of bleeding events when given with **coumarins.** Severe Theoretical
- **Sorafenib** increases the anticoagulant effect of **coumarins.** Severe Anecdotal
- **St John's Wort** decreases the anticoagulant effect of **coumarins.** Avoid. Severe Anecdotal
- Statins **(fluvastatin, rosuvastatin)** increase the anticoagulant effect of **coumarins.** Monitor INR and adjust dose. Severe Study
- **Sucralfate** potentially decreases the effects of **warfarin.** Separate administration by 2 hours. Moderate Anecdotal
- Sulfonamides **(sulfadiazine)** are predicted to increase the anticoagulant effect of **coumarins.** Severe Theoretical
- Sulfonamides **(sulfamethoxazole)** increase the anticoagulant effect of **coumarins.** Severe Study
- **Sunitinib** is predicted to increase the risk of bleeding events when given with **coumarins.** Severe Theoretical
- **Tamoxifen** increases the anticoagulant effect of **coumarins.** Severe Study
- **Tegafur** increases the anticoagulant effect of **coumarins.** Moderate Theoretical
- **Teriflunomide** affects the anticoagulant effect of **coumarins.** Severe Study
- **Tetracyclines** increase the risk of bleeding events when given with **coumarins.** Moderate Anecdotal
- **Tigecycline** increases the risk of bleeding events when given with **coumarins.** Moderate Anecdotal
- **Tinidazole** is predicted to increase the anticoagulant effect of **coumarins.** Monitor INR and adjust dose. Severe Theoretical
- **Toremifene** is predicted to increase the anticoagulant effect of **coumarins.** Severe Theoretical
- **Trimethoprim** is predicted to increase the anticoagulant effect of **coumarins.** Severe Study
- **Vandetanib** is predicted to increase the risk of bleeding events when given with **coumarins.** Severe Theoretical
- **Venetoclax** slightly increases the exposure to **warfarin.** Moderate Study

Cranberry juice

- **Cranberry juice** potentially increases the anticoagulant effect of coumarins **(warfarin).** Avoid. Severe Anecdotal

Crisantaspase → see **TABLE 1** p. 907 (hepatotoxicity), **TABLE 15** p. 910 (myelosuppression)

- **Crisantaspase** is predicted to increase the risk of hepatotoxicity when given with **imatinib.** Severe Theoretical → Also see **TABLE 15** p. 910
- **Crisantaspase** affects the efficacy of **methotrexate.** Severe Anecdotal → Also see **TABLE 1** p. 907 → Also see **TABLE 15** p. 910
- **Crisantaspase** potentially increases the risk of neurotoxicity when given with vinca alkaloids **(vincristine). Vincristine** should be taken 3 to 24 hours before **crisantaspase.** Severe Anecdotal → Also see **TABLE 1** p. 907 → Also see **TABLE 15** p. 910

Crizotinib → see **TABLE 6** p. 908 (bradycardia), **TABLE 15** p. 910 (myelosuppression), **TABLE 9** p. 909 (QT-interval prolongation)

GENERAL INFORMATION Caution with concurrent use of drugs that cause gastrointestinal perforation—discontinue treatment if gastrointestinal perforation occurs.

- **Crizotinib** is predicted to increase the exposure to **abemaciclib.** Moderate Study
- **Crizotinib** is predicted to increase the exposure to aldosterone antagonists **(eplerenone).** Adjust **eplerenone** dose. Severe Study
- **Crizotinib** is predicted to increase the exposure to alpha blockers **(tamsulosin).** Moderate Theoretical
- **Crizotinib** is predicted to increase the exposure to **alprazolam.** Severe Study
- **Crizotinib** is predicted to increase the exposure to antiarrhythmics **(propafenone).** Monitor and adjust dose. Moderate Study
- Antiepileptics **(carbamazepine, fosphenytoin, phenobarbital, phenytoin, primidone)** are predicted to markedly decrease the exposure to **crizotinib.** Avoid. Severe Study
- Antifungals, azoles **(itraconazole, ketoconazole, voriconazole)** are predicted to moderately increase the exposure to **crizotinib.** Avoid. Moderate Study → Also see **TABLE 9** p. 909
- **Crizotinib** is predicted to increase the exposure to antihistamines, non-sedating **(mizolastine).** Severe Theoretical
- **Crizotinib** is predicted to increase the exposure to antihistamines, non-sedating **(rupatadine).** Avoid. Moderate Study
- **Crizotinib** is predicted to increase the concentration of antimalarials **(piperaquine).** Severe Theoretical
- **Apalutamide** is predicted to markedly decrease the exposure to **crizotinib.** Avoid. Severe Study → Also see **TABLE 9** p. 909
- **Crizotinib** is predicted to increase the exposure to **axitinib.** Moderate Theoretical → Also see **TABLE 15** p. 910
- **Crizotinib** is predicted to increase the exposure to **bedaquiline.** Avoid prolonged use. Mild Theoretical → Also see **TABLE 9** p. 909
- **Bosentan** is predicted to decrease the exposure to **crizotinib.** Avoid. Severe Theoretical
- **Crizotinib** is predicted to increase the exposure to **bosutinib.** Avoid or adjust dose. Severe Theoretical → Also see **TABLE 15** p. 910 → Also see **TABLE 9** p. 909
- **Crizotinib** is predicted to increase the exposure to **buspirone.** Use with caution and adjust dose. Moderate Study
- **Crizotinib** is predicted to increase the exposure to **cabozantinib.** Moderate Theoretical → Also see **TABLE 15** p. 910 → Also see **TABLE 9** p. 909
- **Crizotinib** is predicted to increase the exposure to calcium channel blockers **(amlodipine, felodipine, lacidipine, lercanidipine, nicardipine, nifedipine, nimodipine).** Monitor and adjust dose. Moderate Study
- **Crizotinib** is predicted to increase the exposure to **cariprazine.** Avoid. Severe Study
- **Crizotinib** is predicted to increase the concentration of **ciclosporin.** Severe Study
- **Cobicistat** is predicted to moderately increase the exposure to **crizotinib.** Avoid. Moderate Study
- **Crizotinib** is predicted to increase the exposure to **cobimetinib.** Severe Theoretical
- **Crizotinib** is predicted to increase the exposure to **colchicine.** Adjust **colchicine** dose with moderate inhibitors of CYP3A4. Severe Study
- **Crizotinib** is predicted to increase the exposure to corticosteroids **(methylprednisolone).** Monitor and adjust dose. Moderate Study
- **Crizotinib** is predicted to increase the risk of bleeding events when given with **coumarins.** Severe Theoretical
- **Crizotinib** is predicted to slightly increase the exposure to **darifenacin.** Moderate Study
- **Crizotinib** is predicted to increase the exposure to **dasatinib.** Severe Study → Also see **TABLE 15** p. 910 → Also see **TABLE 9** p. 909
- **Crizotinib** is predicted to slightly increase the exposure to **dienogest.** Moderate Study
- **Crizotinib** increases the risk of QT-prolongation when given with **domperidone.** Avoid. Severe Study
- **Crizotinib** is predicted to increase the exposure to dopamine receptor agonists **(bromocriptine).** Severe Theoretical
- **Crizotinib** is predicted to increase the concentration of dopamine receptor agonists **(cabergoline).** Moderate Anecdotal
- **Crizotinib** is predicted to moderately increase the exposure to **dutasteride.** Mild Study
- **Efavirenz** is predicted to decrease the exposure to **crizotinib.** Avoid. Severe Theoretical → Also see **TABLE 9** p. 909
- **Crizotinib** is predicted to increase the exposure to **eliglustat.** Avoid or adjust dose—consult product literature. Severe Study
- **Crizotinib** is predicted to moderately increase the exposure to **encorafenib.** Moderate Study → Also see **TABLE 9** p. 909
- **Enzalutamide** is predicted to markedly decrease the exposure to **crizotinib.** Avoid. Severe Study
- **Crizotinib** is predicted to increase the risk of ergotism when given with **ergometrine.** Severe Theoretical

Crizotinib (continued)
- **Crizotinib** is predicted to increase the risk of ergotism when given with ergotamine. Severe Theoretical
- **Crizotinib** is predicted to increase the exposure to **erlotinib**. Moderate Theoretical
- **Crizotinib** is predicted to increase the concentration of everolimus. Avoid or adjust dose. Moderate Study → Also see **TABLE 15** p. 910
- **Crizotinib** is predicted to increase the exposure to fesoterodine. Adjust **fesoterodine** dose with moderate inhibitors of CYP3A4 in hepatic and renal impairment. Mild Study
- **Crizotinib** is predicted to increase the exposure to **gefitinib**. Moderate Theoretical → Also see **TABLE 15** p. 910
- **Crizotinib** potentially decreases the exposure to **glecaprevir**. Avoid. Severe Theoretical
- **Grapefruit juice** is predicted to increase the exposure to **crizotinib**. Avoid. Moderate Theoretical
- **Crizotinib** is predicted to increase the concentration of guanfacine. Adjust **guanfacine** dose, p. 247. Moderate Theoretical
- **HIV-protease inhibitors** are predicted to moderately increase the exposure to **crizotinib**. Avoid. Moderate Study → Also see **TABLE 9** p. 909
- **Crizotinib** is predicted to increase the exposure to **ibrutinib**. Adjust **ibrutinib** dose with moderate inhibitors of CYP3A4. Severe Study → Also see **TABLE 15** p. 910
- **Idelalisib** is predicted to moderately increase the exposure to **crizotinib**. Avoid. Moderate Study → Also see **TABLE 15** p. 910
- **Crizotinib** is predicted to increase the exposure to **ivabradine**. Adjust **ivabradine** dose. Severe Theoretical → Also see **TABLE 6** p. 908
- **Crizotinib** is predicted to increase the exposure to **ivacaftor**. Adjust ivacaftor p. 196 or **tezacaftor with ivacaftor** p. 198 dose with moderate inhibitors of CYP3A4. Severe Study
- **Crizotinib** is predicted to increase the exposure to **lapatinib**. Moderate Study → Also see **TABLE 9** p. 909
- **Crizotinib** is predicted to increase the exposure to **lomitapide**. Avoid. Moderate Theoretical
- **Crizotinib** is predicted to increase the exposure to **lurasidone**. Adjust **lurasidone** dose. Moderate Study
- Macrolides (clarithromycin) are predicted to moderately increase the exposure to **crizotinib**. Avoid. Moderate Study → Also see **TABLE 9** p. 909
- **Crizotinib** is predicted to increase the exposure to **midazolam**. Monitor side effects and adjust dose. Severe Study
- **Crizotinib** is predicted to increase the exposure to **midostaurin**. Moderate Theoretical
- **Mitotane** is predicted to markedly decrease the exposure to **crizotinib**. Avoid. Severe Study → Also see **TABLE 15** p. 910
- **Crizotinib** is predicted to increase the exposure to naldemedine. Moderate Study
- **Crizotinib** is predicted to increase the exposure to **naloxegol**. Adjust **naloxegol** dose and monitor side effects. Moderate Study
- **Crizotinib** is predicted to increase the exposure to **neratinib**. Avoid. Severe Study
- **Nevirapine** is predicted to decrease the exposure to **crizotinib**. Avoid. Severe Theoretical
- **Crizotinib** is predicted to increase the exposure to **olaparib**. Avoid moderate inhibitors of CYP3A4 or adjust **olaparib** dose. Moderate Theoretical → Also see **TABLE 15** p. 910
- **Crizotinib** is predicted to increase the exposure to opioids (alfentanil, buprenorphine, fentanyl, oxycodone). Monitor and adjust dose. Moderate Study → Also see **TABLE 6** p. 908
- **Crizotinib** is predicted to increase the exposure to opioids (methadone). Moderate Theoretical → Also see **TABLE 6** p. 908 → Also see **TABLE 9** p. 909
- **Crizotinib** is predicted to increase the exposure to **oxybutynin**. Mild Theoretical
- **Crizotinib** is predicted to increase the exposure to **pazopanib**. Moderate Theoretical → Also see **TABLE 15** p. 910 → Also see **TABLE 9** p. 909
- **Crizotinib** is predicted to increase the risk of bleeding events when given with **phenindione**. Severe Theoretical
- **Crizotinib** is predicted to increase the exposure to phosphodiesterase type-5 inhibitors **(avanafil)**. Adjust **avanafil** dose. Moderate Theoretical
- **Crizotinib** is predicted to increase the exposure to phosphodiesterase type-5 inhibitors **(sildenafil)**. Monitor or adjust **sildenafil** dose with moderate inhibitors of CYP3A4, p. 125. Moderate Study → Also see **TABLE 9** p. 909
- **Crizotinib** is predicted to increase the exposure to phosphodiesterase type-5 inhibitors **(tadalafil)**. Severe Theoretical
- **Crizotinib** is predicted to increase the exposure to phosphodiesterase type-5 inhibitors **(vardenafil)**. Adjust dose. Severe Theoretical → Also see **TABLE 9** p. 909
- **Crizotinib** potentially decreases the exposure to **pibrentasvir**. Avoid. Severe Theoretical
- **Crizotinib** is predicted to increase the exposure to **pimozide**. Avoid. Severe Theoretical → Also see **TABLE 9** p. 909
- **Pitolisant** is predicted to decrease the exposure to **crizotinib**. Avoid. Severe Theoretical
- **Crizotinib** is predicted to increase the exposure to **quetiapine**. Avoid. Moderate Study
- **Crizotinib** is predicted to increase the exposure to **ranolazine**. Severe Study → Also see **TABLE 9** p. 909
- **Crizotinib** is predicted to increase the exposure to **ribociclib**. Moderate Study → Also see **TABLE 9** p. 909
- **Rifampicin** is predicted to markedly decrease the exposure to **crizotinib**. Avoid. Severe Study
- **Crizotinib** is predicted to increase the exposure to **ruxolitinib**. Moderate Theoretical → Also see **TABLE 15** p. 910
- **Crizotinib** is predicted to increase the exposure to **saxagliptin**. Mild Study
- **Crizotinib** increases the concentration of **sirolimus**. Monitor and adjust dose. Moderate Study
- **Crizotinib** is predicted to increase the exposure to SSRIs (dapoxetine). Adjust **dapoxetine** dose with moderate inhibitors of CYP3A4. Moderate Theoretical
- **St John's Wort** is predicted to decrease the exposure to **crizotinib**. Avoid. Severe Theoretical
- **Crizotinib** is predicted to increase the exposure to statins (atorvastatin, simvastatin). Monitor and adjust dose. Severe Theoretical
- **Crizotinib** is predicted to increase the exposure to **sunitinib**. Moderate Theoretical → Also see **TABLE 15** p. 910 → Also see **TABLE 9** p. 909
- **Crizotinib** is predicted to increase the concentration of **tacrolimus**. Severe Study
- **Crizotinib** is predicted to increase the exposure to taxanes (cabazitaxel). Moderate Theoretical → Also see **TABLE 15** p. 910
- **Crizotinib** is predicted to increase the concentration of **temsirolimus**. Use with caution or avoid. Moderate Theoretical → Also see **TABLE 15** p. 910
- **Crizotinib** is predicted to increase the exposure to **tezacaftor**. Adjust tezacaftor with ivacaftor p. 198 dose with moderate inhibitors of CYP3A4. Severe Study
- **Crizotinib** given with a potent CYP2C19 inhibitor is predicted to increase the exposure to tofacitinib. Adjust **tofacitinib** dose. Moderate Study
- **Crizotinib** is predicted to increase the exposure to **tolterodine**. Mild Theoretical → Also see **TABLE 9** p. 909
- **Crizotinib** is predicted to increase the exposure to **tolvaptan**. Manufacturer advises caution or adjust **tolvaptan** dose with moderate inhibitors of CYP3A4. Moderate Study
- **Crizotinib** is predicted to increase the exposure to **trazodone**. Moderate Theoretical
- **Crizotinib** is predicted to increase the exposure to **ulipristal**. Avoid if used for uterine fibroids. Moderate Study
- **Crizotinib** is predicted to increase the exposure to **venetoclax**. Avoid or adjust dose—consult product literature. Severe Study
- **Crizotinib** is predicted to increase the exposure to vinca alkaloids. Severe Theoretical → Also see **TABLE 15** p. 910 → Also see **TABLE 9** p. 909
- **Crizotinib** is predicted to increase the exposure to **zopiclone**. Adjust dose. Moderate Study

Cyclizine → see antihistamines, sedating
Cyclopentolate → see **TABLE 10** p. 909 (antimuscarinics)
Cyclophosphamide → see alkylating agents

A1 Interactions | Appendix 1

Cycloserine
- Cycloserine increases the risk of CNS toxicity when given with isoniazid. Monitor and adjust dose. [Moderate] Study

Cyproheptadine → see antihistamines, sedating

Cytarabine → see TABLE 15 p. 910 (myelosuppression)
- Cytarabine decreases the concentration of flucytosine. Avoid. [Severe] Study
- Live vaccines are predicted to increase the risk of generalised infection (possibly life-threatening) when given with **cytarabine**. Public Health England advises avoid (refer to Green Book). [Severe] Theoretical

Cytomegalovirus immunoglobulin → see immunoglobulins

Dabigatran → see TABLE 3 p. 907 (anticoagulant effects)
- Antiarrhythmics (**amiodarone**) increase the exposure to **dabigatran**. Adjust **dabigatran** dose. [Moderate] Study
- Antiarrhythmics (**dronedarone**) slightly increase the exposure to **dabigatran**. Avoid. [Severe] Study
- Antiepileptics (**carbamazepine**) are predicted to decrease the exposure to **dabigatran**. Avoid. [Severe] Study
- Antiepileptics (**phenytoin**) are predicted to decrease the exposure to **dabigatran**. Avoid. [Severe] Theoretical
- Antifungals, azoles (**isavuconazole**) are predicted to increase the exposure to **dabigatran**. Monitor and adjust dose. [Moderate] Study
- Antifungals, azoles (**itraconazole, ketoconazole**) are predicted to increase the exposure to **dabigatran**. Avoid. [Severe] Study
- **Apalutamide** is predicted to decrease the exposure to **dabigatran**. [Mild] Study
- **Brigatinib** potentially increases the concentration of **dabigatran**. [Moderate] Theoretical
- Calcium channel blockers (**verapamil**) increase the exposure to **dabigatran**. Adjust **dabigatran** dose. [Severe] Study
- **Ceritinib** is predicted to increase the exposure to **dabigatran**. [Moderate] Theoretical
- **Ciclosporin** is predicted to increase the exposure to **dabigatran**. Avoid. [Severe] Theoretical
- **Cobicistat** is predicted to increase the exposure to **dabigatran**. Avoid. [Severe] Theoretical
- **Elbasvir** is predicted to increase the concentration of **dabigatran**. [Moderate] Theoretical
- **Eliglustat** is predicted to increase the exposure to **dabigatran**. Adjust dose. [Moderate] Study
- **Glecaprevir** (with pibrentasvir) increases the exposure to **dabigatran**. Avoid. [Moderate] Study
- HIV-protease inhibitors (**lopinavir, ritonavir, saquinavir**) are predicted to increase the exposure to **dabigatran**. Avoid. [Severe] Theoretical
- **Lapatinib** is predicted to increase the exposure to **dabigatran**. [Severe] Theoretical
- **Ledipasvir** is predicted to increase the exposure to **dabigatran**. [Moderate] Theoretical
- **Letermovir** is predicted to decrease the concentration of **dabigatran**. Avoid. [Severe] Theoretical
- **Macrolides** are predicted to increase the exposure to **dabigatran**. [Moderate] Theoretical
- **Mirabegron** is predicted to increase the exposure to **dabigatran**. [Severe] Theoretical
- **Neratinib** is predicted to increase the exposure to **dabigatran**. [Moderate] Study
- **Paritaprevir** (with ritonavir and ombitasvir) is predicted to increase the exposure to **dabigatran**. [Severe] Study
- **Pibrentasvir** (with glecaprevir) increases the exposure to **dabigatran**. Avoid. [Moderate] Study
- **Pitolisant** is predicted to decrease the exposure to **dabigatran**. [Mild] Theoretical
- **Ranolazine** is predicted to increase the exposure to **dabigatran**. [Severe] Theoretical
- **Rifampicin** is predicted to decrease the exposure to **dabigatran**. Avoid. [Severe] Study
- **Rolapitant** is predicted to increase the exposure to **dabigatran**. [Moderate] Study
- **St John's Wort** is predicted to decrease the exposure to **dabigatran**. Avoid. [Severe] Study
- **Tacrolimus** is predicted to increase the exposure to **dabigatran**. Avoid. [Severe] Theoretical
- **Velpatasvir** increases the exposure to **dabigatran**. Avoid. [Severe] Study
- **Vemurafenib** increases the exposure to **dabigatran**. Use with caution and adjust dose. [Severe] Theoretical
- **Venetoclax** is predicted to increase the exposure to **dabigatran**. Avoid or adjust dose. [Severe] Study
- **Voxilaprevir** (with sofosbuvir and velpatasvir) increases the concentration of **dabigatran**. Avoid. [Severe] Study

Dabrafenib → see TABLE 15 p. 910 (myelosuppression)
- Antiepileptics (**carbamazepine, fosphenytoin, phenobarbital, phenytoin, primidone**) are predicted to decrease the exposure to **dabrafenib**. Avoid. [Moderate] Theoretical
- Antifungals, azoles (**itraconazole, ketoconazole, voriconazole**) are predicted to increase the exposure to **dabrafenib**. Use with caution or avoid. [Moderate] Study
- **Apalutamide** is predicted to decrease the exposure to **dabrafenib**. Avoid. [Moderate] Theoretical
- **Clopidogrel** is predicted to increase the exposure to **dabrafenib**. [Moderate] Theoretical
- **Cobicistat** is predicted to increase the exposure to **dabrafenib**. Use with caution or avoid. [Moderate] Study
- **Dabrafenib** is predicted to decrease the anticoagulant effect of **coumarins**. [Severe] Theoretical
- **Dabrafenib** is predicted to decrease the exposure to **doravirine**. Avoid or adjust doravirine or lamivudine with tenofovir disoproxil and doravirine dose. [Severe] Theoretical
- **Enzalutamide** is predicted to decrease the exposure to **dabrafenib**. Avoid. [Moderate] Theoretical
- Fibrates (**gemfibrozil**) are predicted to increase the exposure to **dabrafenib**. [Moderate] Theoretical
- **HIV-protease inhibitors** are predicted to increase the exposure to **dabrafenib**. Use with caution or avoid. [Moderate] Study
- **Idelalisib** is predicted to increase the exposure to **dabrafenib**. Use with caution or avoid. [Moderate] Study → Also see TABLE 15 p. 910
- Macrolides (**clarithromycin**) are predicted to increase the exposure to **dabrafenib**. Use with caution or avoid. [Moderate] Study
- **Dabrafenib** decreases the exposure to **midazolam**. Monitor and adjust dose. [Moderate] Study
- **Mitotane** is predicted to decrease the exposure to **dabrafenib**. Avoid. [Moderate] Theoretical → Also see TABLE 15 p. 910
- **Rifampicin** is predicted to decrease the exposure to **dabrafenib**. Avoid. [Moderate] Theoretical

Dacarbazine → see alkylating agents

Dacomitinib
- **Dacomitinib** is predicted to markedly increase the exposure to atomoxetine. Avoid or adjust dose. [Severe] Study
- **Dacomitinib** is predicted to markedly increase the exposure to beta blockers, non-selective (**propranolol**). Avoid. [Severe] Study
- **Dacomitinib** is predicted to markedly increase the exposure to beta blockers, selective (**metoprolol, nebivolol**). Avoid. [Severe] Study
- **Dacomitinib** is predicted to markedly increase the exposure to eliglustat. Avoid or adjust dose—consult product literature. [Severe] Study
- H_2 **receptor antagonists** are predicted to decrease the concentration of **dacomitinib. Dacomitinib** should be taken 2 hours before or 10 hours after H_2 **receptor antagonists.** [Mild] Study
- **Proton pump inhibitors** are predicted to decrease the exposure to **dacomitinib**. Avoid. [Moderate] Study
- **Dacomitinib** is predicted to markedly increase the exposure to tolterodine. Avoid. [Severe] Study
- **Dacomitinib** is predicted to markedly increase the exposure to tricyclic antidepressants (**imipramine, nortriptyline**). Avoid. [Severe] Study

Dactinomycin → see TABLE 1 p. 907 (hepatotoxicity), TABLE 15 p. 910 (myelosuppression)
- **Live vaccines** are predicted to increase the risk of generalised infection (possibly life-threatening) when given with **dactinomycin**. Public Health England advises avoid (refer to Green Book). [Severe] Theoretical

Dairy products
- **Dairy products** are predicted to decrease the absorption of eltrombopag. **Eltrombopag** should be taken 2 hours before or 4 hours after **dairy products.** Severe Theoretical
- **Dairy products** decrease the exposure to tetracyclines **(demeclocycline, oxytetracycline, tetracycline)**. Avoid. Moderate Study

Dalteparin → see low molecular-weight heparins

Danaparoid → see TABLE 3 p. 907 (anticoagulant effects)
- Ranibizumab is predicted to increase the risk of bleeding events when given with **danaparoid**. Severe Theoretical

Danazol
- **Danazol** moderately increases the concentration of antiepileptics **(carbamazepine)**. Monitor and adjust dose. Severe Study
- **Danazol** increases the concentration of ciclosporin. Severe Study
- **Danazol** potentially increases the anticoagulant effect of coumarins. Severe Anecdotal
- **Danazol** is predicted to increase the risk of rhabdomyolysis when given with statins **(atorvastatin)**. Severe Theoretical
- **Danazol** increases the risk of rhabdomyolysis when given with statins **(simvastatin)**. Avoid. Severe Anecdotal
- **Danazol** potentially increases the concentration of tacrolimus. Severe Anecdotal

Dantrolene → see TABLE 1 p. 907 (hepatotoxicity)
- Intravenous **dantrolene** potentially increases the risk of acute hyperkalaemia and cardiovascular collapse when given with calcium channel blockers **(diltiazem, verapamil)**. Avoid. Severe Anecdotal

Dapagliflozin → see TABLE 14 p. 910 (antidiabetic drugs), TABLE 8 p. 908 (hypotension)

Dapoxetine → see SSRIs

Dapsone
- Aminosalicylic acid is predicted to increase the risk of methaemoglobinaemia when given with **dapsone**. Severe Theoretical
- **Dapsone** is predicted to increase the risk of methaemoglobinaemia when given with topical anaesthetics, local **(prilocaine)**. Use with caution or avoid. Severe Theoretical
- Antiepileptics **(fosphenytoin, phenobarbital, phenytoin, primidone)** are predicted to increase the risk of methaemoglobinaemia when given with **dapsone**. Severe Theoretical
- Antimalarials **(chloroquine, primaquine)** are predicted to increase the risk of methaemoglobinaemia when given with **dapsone**. Severe Theoretical
- Nitrates are predicted to increase the risk of methaemoglobinaemia when given with **dapsone**. Severe Theoretical
- Nitrofurantoin is predicted to increase the risk of methaemoglobinaemia when given with **dapsone**. Severe Theoretical
- Nitroprusside is predicted to increase the risk of methaemoglobinaemia when given with **dapsone**. Severe Theoretical
- Paracetamol is predicted to increase the risk of methaemoglobinaemia when given with **dapsone**. Severe Theoretical
- Rifabutin decreases the exposure to **dapsone**. Moderate Study
- Rifampicin decreases the exposure to **dapsone**. Moderate Study
- Sulfonamides are predicted to increase the risk of methaemoglobinaemia when given with **dapsone**. Severe Theoretical
- **Dapsone** increases the exposure to trimethoprim and trimethoprim increases the exposure to **dapsone**. Severe Study

Daptomycin
- Aspirin (high-dose) increases the risk of renal impairment when given with **daptomycin**. Moderate Theoretical
- Ciclosporin is predicted to increase the risk of rhabdomyolysis when given with **daptomycin**. Severe Theoretical
- Fibrates are predicted to increase the risk of rhabdomyolysis when given with **daptomycin**. Severe Theoretical
- **NSAIDs** increase the risk of renal impairment when given with **daptomycin**. Moderate Theoretical
- Statins are predicted to increase the risk of rhabdomyolysis when given with **daptomycin**. Severe Theoretical

Daratumumab → see monoclonal antibodies

Darbepoetin alfa → see TABLE 5 p. 907 (thromboembolism), TABLE 16 p. 911 (increased serum potassium)

Darifenacin → see TABLE 10 p. 909 (antimuscarinics)
- Antiarrhythmics **(dronedarone)** are predicted to slightly increase the exposure to **darifenacin**. Moderate Study
- **Darifenacin** is predicted to increase the concentration of antiarrhythmics **(flecainide)**. Moderate Theoretical
- Antiepileptics **(carbamazepine, fosphenytoin, phenobarbital, phenytoin, primidone)** are predicted to decrease the exposure to **darifenacin**. Moderate Theoretical
- Antifungals, azoles **(fluconazole, isavuconazole, posaconazole)** are predicted to slightly increase the exposure to **darifenacin**. Moderate Study
- Antifungals, azoles **(itraconazole, ketoconazole, voriconazole)** are predicted to markedly to very markedly increase the exposure to **darifenacin**. Avoid. Severe Study
- Apalutamide is predicted to decrease the exposure to **darifenacin**. Moderate Theoretical
- Aprepitant is predicted to slightly increase the exposure to **darifenacin**. Moderate Study
- Bupropion is predicted to slightly increase the exposure to **darifenacin**. Mild Study
- Calcium channel blockers **(diltiazem, verapamil)** are predicted to slightly increase the exposure to **darifenacin**. Moderate Study
- Ciclosporin is predicted to increase the exposure to **darifenacin**. Avoid. Moderate Theoretical
- Cinacalcet is predicted to slightly increase the exposure to **darifenacin**. Mild Study
- Cobicistat is predicted to markedly to very markedly increase the exposure to **darifenacin**. Avoid. Severe Study
- Crizotinib is predicted to slightly increase the exposure to **darifenacin**. Moderate Study
- Enzalutamide is predicted to decrease the exposure to **darifenacin**. Moderate Theoretical
- Grapefruit juice is predicted to increase the exposure to **darifenacin**. Moderate Study
- HIV-protease inhibitors are predicted to markedly to very markedly increase the exposure to **darifenacin**. Avoid. Severe Study
- Idelalisib is predicted to markedly to very markedly increase the exposure to **darifenacin**. Avoid. Severe Study
- Imatinib is predicted to slightly increase the exposure to **darifenacin**. Moderate Study
- Macrolides **(clarithromycin)** are predicted to markedly to very markedly increase the exposure to **darifenacin**. Avoid. Severe Study
- Macrolides **(erythromycin)** are predicted to slightly increase the exposure to **darifenacin**. Moderate Study
- Mitotane is predicted to decrease the exposure to **darifenacin**. Moderate Theoretical
- Netupitant is predicted to slightly increase the exposure to **darifenacin**. Moderate Study
- Nilotinib is predicted to slightly increase the exposure to **darifenacin**. Moderate Study
- Rifampicin is predicted to decrease the exposure to **darifenacin**. Moderate Theoretical
- SSRIs **(fluoxetine, paroxetine)** are predicted to slightly increase the exposure to **darifenacin**. Mild Study
- St John's Wort is predicted to decrease the exposure to **darifenacin**. Moderate Theoretical
- Terbinafine is predicted to slightly increase the exposure to **darifenacin**. Mild Study
- **Darifenacin** is predicted to increase the exposure to tricyclic antidepressants. Moderate Theoretical → Also see TABLE 10 p. 909

Darunavir → see HIV-protease inhibitors

Dasabuvir
- Antiepileptics **(carbamazepine, fosphenytoin, phenobarbital, phenytoin, primidone)** are predicted to decrease the exposure to **dasabuvir**. Avoid. Severe Theoretical
- Clopidogrel is predicted to very markedly increase the exposure to **dasabuvir**. Avoid. Severe Study

- Combined hormonal contraceptives (containing ethinylestradiol) increase the risk of increased ALT concentrations when given with **dasabuvir**. Avoid. Severe Study
- Efavirenz increases the risk of increased ALT concentrations when given with **dasabuvir**. Avoid. Severe Study
- Enzalutamide is predicted to decrease the exposure to **dasabuvir**. Avoid. Severe Theoretical
- Etravirine is predicted to decrease the exposure to **dasabuvir**. Avoid. Severe Theoretical
- Fibrates **(gemfibrozil)** are predicted to very markedly increase the exposure to **dasabuvir**. Avoid. Severe Study
- **Dasabuvir** (with ombitasvir, paritaprevir, and ritonavir) decreases the concentration of HIV-protease inhibitors **(darunavir)**. Avoid or adjust dose. Moderate Study
- **Dasabuvir** (with ombitasvir, paritaprevir, and ritonavir) increases the concentration of loop diuretics **(furosemide)**. Adjust dose. Moderate Study
- Mitotane is predicted to decrease the exposure to **dasabuvir**. Avoid. Severe Theoretical
- Nevirapine is predicted to decrease the exposure to **dasabuvir**. Avoid. Severe Theoretical
- Rifampicin is predicted to decrease the exposure to **dasabuvir**. Avoid. Severe Theoretical
- St John's Wort is predicted to decrease the exposure to **dasabuvir**. Avoid. Severe Theoretical
- **Dasabuvir** increases the exposure to statins **(rosuvastatin)**. Adjust **rosuvastatin** dose, p. 140. Moderate Study

Dasatinib → see TABLE 15 p. 910 (myelosuppression), TABLE 9 p. 909 (QT-interval prolongation), TABLE 4 p. 907 (antiplatelet effects)

- Antacids decrease the absorption of **dasatinib**. Separate administration by at least 2 hours. Moderate Study
- Antiarrhythmics **(dronedarone)** are predicted to increase the exposure to **dasatinib**. Severe Study → Also see TABLE 9 p. 909
- Antiepileptics **(carbamazepine, fosphenytoin, phenobarbital, phenytoin, primidone)** are predicted to markedly decrease the exposure to **dasatinib**. Avoid. Severe Study
- Antifungals, azoles **(fluconazole, isavuconazole, posaconazole)** are predicted to increase the exposure to **dasatinib**. Severe Study → Also see TABLE 9 p. 909
- Antifungals, azoles **(itraconazole, ketoconazole, voriconazole)** are predicted to markedly increase the exposure to **dasatinib**. Avoid or adjust dose—consult product literature. Severe Study → Also see TABLE 9 p. 909
- Apalutamide is predicted to markedly decrease the exposure to **dasatinib**. Avoid. Severe Study → Also see TABLE 9 p. 909
- Aprepitant is predicted to increase the exposure to **dasatinib**. Severe Study
- Bosentan is predicted to decrease the exposure to **dasatinib**. Severe Study
- Calcium channel blockers **(diltiazem, verapamil)** are predicted to increase the exposure to **dasatinib**. Severe Study
- Cobicistat is predicted to markedly increase the exposure to **dasatinib**. Avoid or adjust dose—consult product literature. Severe Study
- **Dasatinib** is predicted to increase the risk of bleeding events when given with **coumarins**. Severe Theoretical
- Crizotinib is predicted to increase the exposure to **dasatinib**. Severe Study → Also see TABLE 15 p. 910 → Also see TABLE 9 p. 909
- Efavirenz is predicted to decrease the exposure to **dasatinib**. Severe Study → Also see TABLE 9 p. 909
- Enzalutamide is predicted to markedly decrease the exposure to **dasatinib**. Avoid. Severe Study
- Grapefruit juice is predicted to increase the exposure to **dasatinib**. Avoid. Moderate Theoretical
- H_2 receptor antagonists are predicted to decrease the exposure to **dasatinib**. Avoid. Moderate Study
- HIV-protease inhibitors are predicted to markedly increase the exposure to **dasatinib**. Avoid or adjust dose—consult product literature. Severe Study → Also see TABLE 9 p. 909
- Idelalisib is predicted to markedly increase the exposure to **dasatinib**. Avoid or adjust dose—consult product literature. Severe Study → Also see TABLE 15 p. 910
- Imatinib is predicted to increase the exposure to **dasatinib**. Severe Study → Also see TABLE 15 p. 910
- Macrolides **(clarithromycin)** are predicted to markedly increase the exposure to **dasatinib**. Avoid or adjust dose—consult product literature. Severe Study → Also see TABLE 9 p. 909
- Macrolides **(erythromycin)** are predicted to increase the exposure to **dasatinib**. Severe Study → Also see TABLE 9 p. 909
- Mitotane is predicted to markedly decrease the exposure to **dasatinib**. Avoid. Severe Study → Also see TABLE 15 p. 910
- Netupitant is predicted to increase the exposure to **dasatinib**. Severe Study
- Nevirapine is predicted to decrease the exposure to **dasatinib**. Severe Study
- Nilotinib is predicted to increase the exposure to **dasatinib**. Severe Study → Also see TABLE 15 p. 910 → Also see TABLE 9 p. 909
- **Dasatinib** is predicted to increase the risk of bleeding events when given with **phenindione**. Severe Theoretical
- Pitolisant is predicted to decrease the exposure to **dasatinib**. Avoid. Severe Theoretical
- Proton pump inhibitors are predicted to slightly to moderately decrease the exposure to **dasatinib**. Avoid. Severe Study
- Rifampicin is predicted to markedly decrease the exposure to **dasatinib**. Avoid. Severe Study
- Sodium zirconium cyclosilicate is predicted to decrease the exposure to **dasatinib**. Separate administration by at least 2 hours. Moderate Theoretical
- St John's Wort is predicted to decrease the exposure to **dasatinib**. Severe Study
- **Dasatinib** is predicted to increase the exposure to statins **(simvastatin)**. Moderate Theoretical

Daunorubicin → see anthracyclines
Decitabine → see TABLE 15 p. 910 (myelosuppression)
Deferasirox → see iron chelators
Deferiprone → see iron chelators
Deflazacort → see corticosteroids
Delamanid → see TABLE 9 p. 909 (QT-interval prolongation)

- Antiepileptics **(carbamazepine, fosphenytoin, phenobarbital, phenytoin, primidone)** are predicted to slightly decrease the exposure to **delamanid**. Avoid. Moderate Study
- Antifungals, azoles **(itraconazole, ketoconazole, voriconazole)** very slightly increase the exposure to **delamanid**. Severe Study → Also see TABLE 9 p. 909
- Apalutamide is predicted to slightly decrease the exposure to **delamanid**. Avoid. Moderate Study → Also see TABLE 9 p. 909
- Cobicistat very slightly increases the exposure to **delamanid**. Severe Study
- Enzalutamide is predicted to slightly decrease the exposure to **delamanid**. Avoid. Moderate Study
- HIV-protease inhibitors very slightly increase the exposure to **delamanid**. Severe Study → Also see TABLE 9 p. 909
- Idelalisib very slightly increases the exposure to **delamanid**. Severe Study
- Macrolides **(clarithromycin)** very slightly increase the exposure to **delamanid**. Severe Study → Also see TABLE 9 p. 909
- Mitotane is predicted to slightly decrease the exposure to **delamanid**. Avoid. Moderate Study
- Rifampicin is predicted to slightly decrease the exposure to **delamanid**. Avoid. Moderate Study

Demeclocycline → see tetracyclines
Desferrioxamine → see iron chelators
Desflurane → see volatile halogenated anaesthetics
Desloratadine → see antihistamines, non-sedating
Desmopressin → see TABLE 18 p. 911 (hyponatraemia)

- Antiepileptics **(lamotrigine)** are predicted to increase the risk of hyponatraemia when given with **desmopressin**. Severe Theoretical
- Loperamide greatly increases the absorption of oral **desmopressin** (and possibly sublingual). Moderate Study
- Phenothiazines **(chlorpromazine)** are predicted to increase the risk of hyponatraemia when given with **desmopressin**. Severe Theoretical

Desogestrel

- Antiepileptics **(carbamazepine, eslicarbazepine, fosphenytoin, oxcarbazepine, perampanel, phenobarbital, phenytoin, primidone, rufinamide, topiramate)** are predicted to decrease the efficacy of **desogestrel**. For FSRH guidance, see Contraceptives, interactions p. 536. Severe Theoretical

Desogestrel (continued)

- **Desogestrel** is predicted to increase the exposure to antiepileptics **(lamotrigine).** Moderate Study
- **Aprepitant** is predicted to decrease the efficacy of **desogestrel.** For FSRH guidance, see Contraceptives, interactions p. 536. Severe Theoretical
- **Bosentan** is predicted to decrease the efficacy of **desogestrel.** For FSRH guidance, see Contraceptives, interactions p. 536. Severe Theoretical
- **Efavirenz** is predicted to decrease the efficacy of **desogestrel.** For FSRH guidance, see Contraceptives, interactions p. 536. Severe Theoretical
- **Fosaprepitant** is predicted to decrease the efficacy of **desogestrel.** For FSRH guidance, see Contraceptives, interactions p. 536. Severe Theoretical
- **Griseofulvin** potentially decreases the efficacy of **desogestrel.** For FSRH guidance, see Contraceptives, interactions p. 536. Severe Anecdotal
- HIV-protease inhibitors **(ritonavir)** are predicted to decrease the efficacy of **desogestrel.** For FSRH guidance, see Contraceptives, interactions p. 536. Severe Theoretical
- **Modafinil** is predicted to decrease the efficacy of **desogestrel.** For FSRH guidance, see Contraceptives, interactions p. 536. Severe Theoretical
- **Nevirapine** is predicted to decrease the efficacy of **desogestrel.** For FSRH guidance, see Contraceptives, interactions p. 536. Severe Theoretical
- **Rifabutin** is predicted to decrease the efficacy of **desogestrel.** For FSRH guidance, see Contraceptives, interactions p. 536. Severe Theoretical
- **Rifampicin** is predicted to decrease the efficacy of **desogestrel.** For FSRH guidance, see Contraceptives, interactions p. 536. Severe Theoretical
- **St John's Wort** is predicted to decrease the efficacy of **desogestrel.** MHRA advises avoid. For FSRH guidance, see Contraceptives, interactions p. 536. Severe Theoretical
- **Sugammadex** is predicted to decrease the exposure to **desogestrel.** Refer to patient information leaflet for missed pill advice. Severe Theoretical
- **Ulipristal** is predicted to decrease the efficacy of **desogestrel.** Avoid. Severe Theoretical

Dexamethasone → see corticosteroids

Dexamfetamine → see amfetamines

Dexibuprofen → see NSAIDs

Dexketoprofen → see NSAIDs

Dexmedetomidine → see TABLE 11 p. 909 (CNS depressant effects)

Dexrazoxane → see iron chelators

Diamorphine → see opioids

Diazepam → see TABLE 11 p. 909 (CNS depressant effects)

- **Diazepam** potentially affects the concentration of antiepileptics **(fosphenytoin, phenytoin).** Monitor concentration and adjust dose. Severe Study
- Antifungals, azoles **(fluconazole, voriconazole)** moderately increase the exposure to **diazepam.** Monitor and adjust dose. Moderate Study
- **Apalutamide** is predicted to decrease the exposure to **diazepam.** Avoid or monitor. Mild Study
- HIV-protease inhibitors **(ritonavir)** are predicted to increase the exposure to **diazepam.** Avoid. Moderate Theoretical
- Monoclonal antibodies **(tocilizumab)** are predicted to decrease the exposure to **diazepam.** Monitor and adjust dose. Moderate Theoretical
- **Rifampicin** moderately decreases the exposure to **diazepam.** Avoid. Moderate Study
- SSRIs **(fluvoxamine)** moderately increase the exposure to **diazepam.** Moderate Study

Diazoxide → see TABLE 8 p. 908 (hypotension)

- **Diazoxide** decreases the concentration of antiepileptics **(fosphenytoin, phenytoin)** and antiepileptics **(fosphenytoin, phenytoin)** are predicted to decrease the effects of **diazoxide.** Monitor concentration and adjust dose. Moderate Anecdotal
- **Diazoxide** increases the risk of severe hypotension when given with **hydralazine.** Severe Study → Also see TABLE 8 p. 908

Diclofenac → see NSAIDs

Dicycloverine → see TABLE 10 p. 909 (antimuscarinics)

Dienogest

- Antiarrhythmics **(dronedarone)** are predicted to slightly increase the exposure to **dienogest.** Moderate Study
- Antiepileptics **(carbamazepine, fosphenytoin, phenobarbital, phenytoin, primidone)** are predicted to markedly decrease the exposure to **dienogest.** Severe Study
- Antifungals, azoles **(fluconazole, isavuconazole, posaconazole)** are predicted to slightly increase the exposure to **dienogest.** Moderate Study
- Antifungals, azoles **(itraconazole, ketoconazole, voriconazole)** are predicted to moderately increase the exposure to **dienogest.** Moderate Study
- **Apalutamide** is predicted to markedly decrease the exposure to **dienogest.** Severe Study
- **Aprepitant** is predicted to slightly increase the exposure to **dienogest.** Moderate Study
- Calcium channel blockers **(diltiazem, verapamil)** are predicted to slightly increase the exposure to **dienogest.** Moderate Study
- **Cobicistat** is predicted to moderately increase the exposure to **dienogest.** Moderate Study
- **Crizotinib** is predicted to slightly increase the exposure to **dienogest.** Moderate Study
- **Enzalutamide** is predicted to markedly decrease the exposure to **dienogest.** Severe Study
- **HIV-protease inhibitors** are predicted to moderately increase the exposure to **dienogest.** Moderate Study
- **Idelalisib** is predicted to moderately increase the exposure to **dienogest.** Moderate Study
- **Imatinib** is predicted to slightly increase the exposure to **dienogest.** Moderate Study
- Macrolides **(clarithromycin)** are predicted to moderately increase the exposure to **dienogest.** Moderate Study
- Macrolides **(erythromycin)** are predicted to slightly increase the exposure to **dienogest.** Moderate Study
- **Mitotane** is predicted to markedly decrease the exposure to **dienogest.** Severe Study
- **Netupitant** is predicted to slightly increase the exposure to **dienogest.** Moderate Study
- **Nilotinib** is predicted to slightly increase the exposure to **dienogest.** Moderate Study
- **Rifampicin** is predicted to markedly decrease the exposure to **dienogest.** Severe Study

Digoxin → see TABLE 6 p. 908 (bradycardia)

- **Acarbose** decreases the concentration of **digoxin.** Moderate Study
- Aldosterone antagonists **(eplerenone)** very slightly increase the exposure to **digoxin.** Mild Study
- Aldosterone antagonists **(spironolactone)** increase the concentration of **digoxin.** Monitor and adjust dose. Moderate Study
- **Aminoglycosides** potentially increase the concentration of **digoxin.** Monitor and adjust dose. Mild Study
- **Antacids** decrease the absorption of **digoxin.** Separate administration by 2 hours. Mild Study
- Antiarrhythmics **(amiodarone, dronedarone)** are predicted to moderately increase the exposure to **digoxin.** Monitor and adjust **digoxin** dose, p. 86. Severe Study → Also see TABLE 6 p. 908
- Antiarrhythmics **(propafenone)** increase the concentration of **digoxin.** Monitor and adjust dose. Severe Study
- Antiepileptics **(fosphenytoin, phenytoin)** are predicted to decrease the concentration of **digoxin.** Moderate Anecdotal
- Antifungals, azoles **(isavuconazole)** slightly increase the exposure to **digoxin.** Monitor and adjust dose. Moderate Study
- Antifungals, azoles **(itraconazole)** are predicted to markedly increase the concentration of **digoxin.** Monitor and adjust dose. Severe Study
- Antifungals, azoles **(ketoconazole)** are predicted to markedly increase the concentration of **digoxin.** Severe Study
- Antifungals, azoles **(posaconazole)** are predicted to increase the concentration of **digoxin.** Severe Study
- Antimalarials **(mefloquine)** are predicted to increase the risk of bradycardia when given with **digoxin.** Severe Theoretical
- Antimalarials **(quinine)** increase the concentration of **digoxin.** Monitor and adjust **digoxin** dose, p. 86. Severe Anecdotal

- Apalutamide is predicted to decrease the exposure to **digoxin**. Mild Study
- Balsalazide is predicted to decrease the concentration of **digoxin**. Moderate Theoretical
- Brigatinib potentially increases the concentration of **digoxin**. Moderate Theoretical
- Calcium channel blockers **(diltiazem, verapamil)** increase the concentration of **digoxin**. Monitor and adjust dose. Severe Study → Also see **TABLE 6** p. 908
- Intravenous **calcium salts** increase the effects of **digoxin**. Avoid. Moderate Anecdotal
- Carbimazole affects the concentration of **digoxin**. Monitor and adjust dose. Moderate Theoretical
- Ceritinib is predicted to increase the risk of bradycardia when given with **digoxin**. Avoid. Severe Theoretical
- Ciclosporin increases the concentration of **digoxin**. Monitor and adjust dose. Severe Theoretical
- Drugs that reduce serum potassium (see **TABLE 17** p. 911) are predicted to increase the risk of digoxin toxicity when given with **digoxin**. Severe Study
- Eliglustat increases the exposure to **digoxin**. Adjust dose. Moderate Study
- Glecaprevir (with pibrentasvir) increases the exposure to **digoxin**. Moderate Study
- HIV-protease inhibitors **(ritonavir)** increase the concentration of **digoxin**. Adjust dose and monitor concentration. Severe Study
- Ivacaftor slightly increases the exposure to **digoxin**. Moderate Study
- Lapatinib is predicted to increase the exposure to **digoxin**. Moderate Theoretical
- Ledipasvir is predicted to increase the exposure to **digoxin**. Monitor and adjust dose. Moderate Theoretical
- Macrolides increase the concentration of **digoxin**. Severe Anecdotal
- Mirabegron slightly increases the exposure to **digoxin**. Monitor concentration and adjust dose. Severe Study
- Neomycin decreases the absorption of **digoxin**. Moderate Study
- Neratinib is predicted to slightly increase the exposure to **digoxin**. Moderate Study
- Neuromuscular blocking drugs, non-depolarising **(pancuronium)** are predicted to increase the risk of cardiovascular side-effects when given with **digoxin**. Severe Anecdotal
- NSAIDs **(indometacin)** increase the concentration of **digoxin**. Severe Study
- Paritaprevir (with ritonavir and ombitasvir) increases the exposure to **digoxin**. Monitor and adjust **digoxin** dose, p. 86. Moderate Study
- Penicillamine potentially decreases the concentration of **digoxin**. Separate administration by 2 hours. Severe Anecdotal
- Pibrentasvir (with glecaprevir) increases the exposure to **digoxin**. Moderate Study
- Pitolisant is predicted to decrease the exposure to **digoxin**. Mild Theoretical
- Ranolazine increases the concentration of **digoxin**. Moderate Study
- Ribociclib is predicted to increase the exposure to **digoxin**. Moderate Theoretical
- Rifampicin decreases the concentration of **digoxin**. Moderate Study
- Rolapitant slightly increases the exposure to **digoxin**. Moderate Study
- St John's Wort decreases the concentration of **digoxin**. Avoid. Severe Anecdotal
- Sucralfate decreases the absorption of **digoxin**. Separate administration by 2 hours. Severe Anecdotal
- Sulfasalazine decreases the concentration of **digoxin**. Moderate Study
- Suxamethonium is predicted to increase the risk of cardiovascular side-effects when given with **digoxin**. Severe Anecdotal
- Thyroid hormones are predicted to affect the concentration of **digoxin**. Monitor and adjust dose. Moderate Theoretical
- Ticagrelor increases the concentration of **digoxin**. Moderate Study
- Tolvaptan increases the concentration of **digoxin**. Mild Study
- Trimethoprim increases the concentration of **digoxin**. Moderate Study
- Vandetanib slightly increases the exposure to **digoxin**. Monitor ECG and adjust dose. Moderate Study
- Velpatasvir is predicted to increase the exposure to **digoxin**. Severe Study
- Venetoclax increases the exposure to **digoxin**. Avoid or adjust dose. Severe Study
- Vitamin D substances are predicted to increase the risk of toxicity when given with **digoxin**. Severe Theoretical
- Voxilaprevir (with sofosbuvir and velpatasvir) is predicted to increase the exposure to **digoxin**. Monitor and adjust dose. Severe Theoretical

Dihydrocodeine → see opioids

Dihydrotachysterol → see vitamin D substances

Diltiazem → see calcium channel blockers

Dimenhydrinate → see **TABLE 10** p. 909 (antimuscarinics)

Dimethyl fumarate

- Alcohol (beverage)(excessive consumption) potentially increases the risk of gastrointestinal side-effects when given with **dimethyl fumarate**. Avoid. Moderate Theoretical
- Live vaccines are predicted to increase the risk of generalised infection (possibly life-threatening) when given with **dimethyl fumarate**. Public Health England advises avoid (refer to Green Book). Severe Theoretical

Dinutuximab → see monoclonal antibodies

Diphenoxylate → see opioids

Dipipanone → see opioids

Dipyridamole → see **TABLE 8** p. 908 (hypotension), **TABLE 4** p. 907 (antiplatelet effects)

- Antacids are predicted to decrease the absorption of **dipyridamole** (immediate release tablets). Moderate Theoretical
- **Dipyridamole** increases the exposure to antiarrhythmics (adenosine). Avoid or adjust dose. Severe Study
- H_2 receptor antagonists are predicted to decrease the absorption of **dipyridamole** (immediate release tablets). Moderate Theoretical
- Proton pump inhibitors are predicted to decrease the absorption of **dipyridamole** (immediate release tablets). Moderate Theoretical

Disopyramide → see antiarrhythmics

Disulfiram → see **TABLE 12** p. 910 (peripheral neuropathy)

- Alcohol (beverage) causes an extremely unpleasant systemic reaction when given with **disulfiram**. Avoid for at least 24 hours before and up to 14 days after stopping treatment. Severe Study
- **Disulfiram** increases the concentration of antiepileptics **(fosphenytoin, phenytoin)**. Monitor concentration and adjust dose. Severe Study → Also see **TABLE 12** p. 910
- **Disulfiram** increases the anticoagulant effect of **coumarins**. Monitor and adjust dose. Severe Study
- **Disulfiram** increases the risk of acute psychoses when given with **metronidazole**. Severe Study → Also see **TABLE 12** p. 910
- **Disulfiram** is predicted to increase the anticoagulant effect of phenindione. Severe Theoretical

Dobutamine → see sympathomimetics, inotropic

Docetaxel → see taxanes

Docusate sodium

ROUTE-SPECIFIC INFORMATION Interactions do not generally apply to topical use of **docusate** unless specified.

Dolutegravir

- Antacids moderately decrease the exposure to **dolutegravir**. **Dolutegravir** should be taken 2 hours before or 6 hours after antacids. Moderate Study
- Antiepileptics **(carbamazepine, fosphenytoin, phenobarbital, phenytoin, primidone)** decrease the exposure to **dolutegravir**. Adjust dose. Severe Study
- Antiepileptics **(oxcarbazepine)** are predicted to decrease the exposure to **dolutegravir**. Adjust dose. Severe Theoretical
- Apalutamide decreases the exposure to **dolutegravir**. Adjust dose. Severe Study
- Bosentan decreases the exposure to **dolutegravir**. Adjust dose. Severe Study

Dolutegravir (continued)

- Oral calcium salts decrease the absorption of **dolutegravir. Dolutegravir** should be taken 2 hours before or 6 hours after **calcium salts.** Moderate Study
- **Dolutegravir** is predicted to increase the exposure to dopamine receptor agonists **(pramipexole)**. Adjust dose. Moderate Study
- **Efavirenz** decreases the exposure to **dolutegravir**. Adjust dose. Severe Study
- **Encorafenib** is predicted to increase the exposure to **dolutegravir.** Moderate Theoretical
- **Enzalutamide** decreases the exposure to **dolutegravir**. Adjust dose. Severe Study
- **Etravirine** moderately decreases the exposure to **dolutegravir**. Avoid unless given with atazanavir, darunavir, or lopinavir (all boosted with ritonavir). Severe Study
- HIV-protease inhibitors **(fosamprenavir)** boosted with ritonavir slightly decrease the exposure to **dolutegravir**. Avoid if resistant to HIV-integrase inhibitors. Severe Study
- HIV-protease inhibitors **(tipranavir)** moderately decrease the exposure to **dolutegravir**. Refer to specialist literature. Severe Study
- **Iron (oral)** decreases the absorption of **dolutegravir**. **Dolutegravir** should be taken 2 hours before or 6 hours after **iron (oral).** Moderate Study
- **Dolutegravir** increases the exposure to **metformin**. Use with caution and adjust dose. Severe Study
- **Mitotane** decreases the exposure to **dolutegravir**. Adjust dose. Severe Study
- **Nevirapine** decreases the exposure to **dolutegravir**. Adjust dose. Severe Study
- **Rifampicin** decreases the exposure to **dolutegravir**. Adjust dose. Severe Study
- **St John's Wort** decreases the exposure to **dolutegravir**. Adjust dose. Severe Study
- **Sucralfate** decreases the absorption of **dolutegravir**. Moderate Study

Domperidone → see **TABLE 9** p. 909 (QT-interval prolongation)

- Antiarrhythmics **(dronedarone)** increase the risk of QT-prolongation when given with **domperidone**. Avoid. Severe Study
- Antifungals, azoles **(fluconazole, isavuconazole, itraconazole, ketoconazole, posaconazole, voriconazole)** increase the risk of QT-prolongation when given with **domperidone**. Avoid. Severe Study
- **Aprepitant** increases the risk of QT-prolongation when given with **domperidone**. Avoid. Severe Study
- Calcium channel blockers **(diltiazem, verapamil)** increase the risk of QT-prolongation when given with **domperidone**. Avoid. Severe Study
- **Cobicistat** increases the risk of QT-prolongation when given with **domperidone**. Avoid. Severe Study
- **Crizotinib** increases the risk of QT-prolongation when given with **domperidone**. Avoid. Severe Study
- **Domperidone** is predicted to decrease the prolactin-lowering effect of dopamine receptor agonists **(bromocriptine, cabergoline)**. Moderate Theoretical
- **HIV-protease inhibitors** increase the risk of QT-prolongation when given with **domperidone**. Avoid. Severe Study
- **Idelalisib** increases the risk of QT-prolongation when given with **domperidone**. Avoid. Severe Study
- **Imatinib** increases the risk of QT-prolongation when given with **domperidone**. Avoid. Severe Study
- Macrolides **(clarithromycin, erythromycin)** increase the risk of QT-prolongation when given with **domperidone**. Avoid. Severe Study
- **Netupitant** increases the risk of QT-prolongation when given with **domperidone**. Avoid. Severe Study
- **Nilotinib** increases the risk of QT-prolongation when given with **domperidone**. Avoid. Severe Study

Donepezil → see anticholinesterases, centrally acting

Dopamine → see sympathomimetics, inotropic

Dopamine receptor agonists → see **TABLE 8** p. 908 (hypotension), **TABLE 9** p. 909 (QT-interval prolongation), **TABLE 10** p. 909 (antimuscarinics)

amantadine · apomorphine · bromocriptine · cabergoline · pergolide · pramipexole · quinagolide · ropinirole · rotigotine

FOOD AND LIFESTYLE Dose adjustment might be necessary if smoking started or stopped during treatment with **ropinirole.**

- **Amisulpride** is predicted to decrease the effects of **dopamine receptor agonists.** Avoid. Moderate Theoretical → Also see **TABLE 9** p. 909
- Antiarrhythmics **(dronedarone)** are predicted to increase the exposure to **bromocriptine.** Severe Theoretical
- Antiarrhythmics **(dronedarone)** are predicted to increase the concentration of **cabergoline.** Severe Anecdotal
- Antifungals, azoles **(fluconazole, isavuconazole, itraconazole, ketoconazole, posaconazole, voriconazole)** are predicted to increase the concentration of **cabergoline.** Moderate Anecdotal
- Antifungals, azoles **(fluconazole, isavuconazole, posaconazole)** are predicted to increase the exposure to **bromocriptine.** Severe Theoretical
- Antifungals, azoles **(isavuconazole)** are predicted to increase the exposure to **pramipexole**. Adjust dose. Moderate Study
- Antifungals, azoles **(itraconazole, ketoconazole, voriconazole)** increase the exposure to **bromocriptine.** Severe Study
- **Aprepitant** is predicted to increase the exposure to **bromocriptine.** Severe Theoretical
- **Aprepitant** is predicted to increase the concentration of **cabergoline.** Moderate Anecdotal
- **Aripiprazole** is predicted to decrease the effects of **dopamine receptor agonists.** Moderate Theoretical → Also see **TABLE 8** p. 908
- **Asenapine** is predicted to decrease the effects of **dopamine receptor agonists.** Adjust dose. Moderate Theoretical → Also see **TABLE 8** p. 908
- **Benperidol** is predicted to decrease the effects of **dopamine receptor agonists.** Avoid. Moderate Theoretical → Also see **TABLE 8** p. 908
- **Bupropion** increases the risk of side-effects when given with **amantadine.** Moderate Study
- Calcium channel blockers **(diltiazem, verapamil)** are predicted to increase the exposure to **bromocriptine.** Severe Theoretical → Also see **TABLE 8** p. 908
- Calcium channel blockers **(diltiazem, verapamil)** are predicted to increase the concentration of **cabergoline.** Moderate Anecdotal → Also see **TABLE 8** p. 908
- **Clozapine** is predicted to decrease the effects of **dopamine receptor agonists.** Moderate Theoretical → Also see **TABLE 8** p. 908 → Also see **TABLE 10** p. 909
- **Cobicistat** increases the exposure to **bromocriptine.** Severe Study
- **Cobicistat** is predicted to increase the concentration of **cabergoline.** Moderate Anecdotal
- **Combined hormonal contraceptives** are predicted to increase the exposure to **ropinirole.** Adjust dose. Moderate Study
- **Crizotinib** is predicted to increase the exposure to **bromocriptine.** Severe Theoretical
- **Crizotinib** is predicted to increase the concentration of **cabergoline.** Moderate Anecdotal
- **Dolutegravir** is predicted to increase the exposure to **pramipexole.** Adjust dose. Moderate Study
- **Domperidone** is predicted to decrease the prolactin-lowering effect of dopamine receptor agonists **(bromocriptine, cabergoline).** Moderate Theoretical
- Dopamine receptor agonists **(cabergoline)** are predicted to increase the risk of ergotism when given with dopamine receptor agonists **(bromocriptine)**. Avoid. Moderate Theoretical → Also see **TABLE 8** p. 908
- Dopamine receptor agonists **(bromocriptine, cabergoline)** are predicted to increase the risk of ergotism when given with dopamine receptor agonists **(pergolide)**. Avoid. Moderate Theoretical → Also see **TABLE 8** p. 908
- Dopamine receptor agonists **(amantadine)** are predicted to increase the exposure to dopamine receptor agonists **(pramipexole)**. Adjust dose. Moderate Theoretical → Also see **TABLE 8** p. 908
- **Droperidol** is predicted to decrease the effects of **dopamine receptor agonists.** Avoid. Moderate Theoretical → Also see **TABLE 8** p. 908 → Also see **TABLE 9** p. 909

- ▶ **Ergometrine** is predicted to increase the risk of ergotism when given with dopamine receptor agonists **(cabergoline, pergolide)**. Avoid. [Moderate] Theoretical
- ▶ **Ergotamine** is predicted to increase the risk of ergotism when given with dopamine receptor agonists **(bromocriptine, cabergoline)**. Avoid. [Moderate] Theoretical
- ▶ **Ergotamine** is predicted to increase the risk of ergotism when given with **pergolide**. [Moderate] Theoretical
- ▶ **Flupentixol** is predicted to decrease the effects of **dopamine receptor agonists**. Avoid. [Moderate] Theoretical → Also see **TABLE 8** p. 908
- ▶ **Apomorphine** is predicted to increase the risk of severe hypotension when given with **granisetron**. [Severe] Theoretical
- ▶ H$_2$ receptor antagonists **(cimetidine)** are predicted to increase the exposure to **pramipexole**. Adjust dose. [Moderate] Study
- ▶ **Haloperidol** is predicted to decrease the effects of **dopamine receptor agonists**. Avoid. [Moderate] Theoretical → Also see **TABLE 8** p. 908 → Also see **TABLE 9** p. 909 → Also see **TABLE 10** p. 909
- ▶ **HIV-protease inhibitors** increase the exposure to **bromocriptine**. [Severe] Study
- ▶ **HIV-protease inhibitors** are predicted to increase the concentration of **cabergoline**. [Moderate] Anecdotal
- ▶ **Hormone replacement therapy** decreases the clearance of **ropinirole**. Monitor and adjust dose. [Moderate] Study
- ▶ **Idelalisib** increases the exposure to **bromocriptine**. [Severe] Study
- ▶ **Idelalisib** is predicted to increase the concentration of **cabergoline**. [Moderate] Anecdotal
- ▶ **Imatinib** is predicted to increase the exposure to **bromocriptine**. [Severe] Theoretical
- ▶ **Imatinib** is predicted to increase the concentration of **cabergoline**. [Moderate] Anecdotal
- ▶ **Loxapine** is predicted to decrease the effects of **dopamine receptor agonists**. [Moderate] Theoretical → Also see **TABLE 8** p. 908 → Also see **TABLE 10** p. 909
- ▶ Macrolides **(clarithromycin)** increase the exposure to **bromocriptine**. [Severe] Study
- ▶ Macrolides **(clarithromycin, erythromycin)** are predicted to increase the concentration of **cabergoline**. Avoid. [Severe] Study
- ▶ Macrolides **(erythromycin)** are predicted to increase the exposure to **bromocriptine**. [Severe] Theoretical
- ▶ **Amantadine** increases the risk of CNS toxicity when given with **memantine**. Use with caution or avoid. [Severe] Theoretical
- ▶ **Memantine** is predicted to increase the effects of dopamine receptor agonists **(apomorphine, bromocriptine, cabergoline, pergolide, pramipexole, quinagolide, ropinirole, rotigotine)**. [Moderate] Theoretical
- ▶ **Metoclopramide** is predicted to decrease the effects of dopamine receptor agonists **(apomorphine, bromocriptine, cabergoline, pergolide, pramipexole, quinagolide, ropinirole, rotigotine)**. Avoid. [Moderate] Study
- ▶ **Mexiletine** is predicted to increase the exposure to **ropinirole**. Adjust dose. [Moderate] Study
- ▶ **Netupitant** is predicted to increase the exposure to **bromocriptine**. [Severe] Theoretical
- ▶ **Netupitant** is predicted to increase the concentration of **cabergoline**. [Moderate] Anecdotal
- ▶ **Nilotinib** is predicted to increase the exposure to **bromocriptine**. [Severe] Theoretical
- ▶ **Nilotinib** is predicted to increase the concentration of **cabergoline**. [Moderate] Anecdotal
- ▶ **Olanzapine** is predicted to decrease the effects of **dopamine receptor agonists**. Avoid. [Moderate] Theoretical → Also see **TABLE 8** p. 908
- ▶ **Apomorphine** increases the risk of severe hypotension when given with **ondansetron**. Avoid. [Severe] Study → Also see **TABLE 9** p. 909
- ▶ **Paliperidone** is predicted to decrease the effects of **dopamine receptor agonists**. Avoid. [Moderate] Theoretical → Also see **TABLE 8** p. 908 → Also see **TABLE 9** p. 909
- ▶ **Apomorphine** is predicted to increase the risk of severe hypotension when given with **palonosetron**. [Severe] Theoretical
- ▶ **Phenothiazines** are predicted to decrease the effects of **dopamine receptor agonists**. Avoid. [Moderate] Theoretical → Also see **TABLE 8** p. 908 → Also see **TABLE 9** p. 909 → Also see **TABLE 10** p. 909
- ▶ **Pimozide** is predicted to decrease the effects of **dopamine receptor agonists**. Avoid. [Moderate] Theoretical → Also see **TABLE 8** p. 908 → Also see **TABLE 9** p. 909 → Also see **TABLE 10** p. 909
- ▶ **Quetiapine** is predicted to decrease the effects of **dopamine receptor agonists**. Avoid. [Moderate] Theoretical → Also see **TABLE 8** p. 908
- ▶ Quinolones **(ciprofloxacin)** are predicted to increase the exposure to **ropinirole**. Adjust dose. [Moderate] Study
- ▶ **Ranolazine** is predicted to increase the exposure to **pramipexole**. Adjust dose. [Moderate] Study
- ▶ **Risperidone** is predicted to decrease the effects of **dopamine receptor agonists**. Avoid. [Moderate] Theoretical → Also see **TABLE 8** p. 908 → Also see **TABLE 9** p. 909
- ▶ **SSRIs (fluvoxamine)** are predicted to increase the exposure to **ropinirole**. Adjust dose. [Moderate] Study
- ▶ **Sulpiride** is predicted to decrease the effects of **dopamine receptor agonists**. Avoid. [Moderate] Theoretical → Also see **TABLE 8** p. 908 → Also see **TABLE 9** p. 909
- ▶ Sympathomimetics, vasoconstrictor **(isometheptene)** potentially increase the risk of side-effects when given with **bromocriptine**. Avoid. [Severe] Anecdotal
- ▶ **Trimethoprim** is predicted to increase the exposure to **pramipexole**. Adjust dose. [Moderate] Study
- ▶ **Vandetanib** is predicted to increase the exposure to **pramipexole**. Adjust dose. [Moderate] Study
- ▶ **Zuclopenthixol** is predicted to decrease the effects of **dopamine receptor agonists**. Avoid. [Moderate] Theoretical → Also see **TABLE 8** p. 908 → Also see **TABLE 9** p. 909

Doravirine

- ▶ Antiepileptics **(carbamazepine, fosphenytoin, phenobarbital, phenytoin, primidone)** are predicted to decrease the exposure to **doravirine**. Avoid. [Severe] Study
- ▶ Antiepileptics **(oxcarbazepine)** are predicted to decrease the exposure to **doravirine**. Avoid. [Severe] Theoretical
- ▶ Antifungals, azoles **(itraconazole, ketoconazole, voriconazole)** are predicted to increase the exposure to **doravirine**. [Mild] Study
- ▶ **Apalutamide** is predicted to decrease the exposure to **doravirine**. Avoid. [Severe] Study
- ▶ **Bosentan** is predicted to decrease the exposure to **doravirine**. Avoid or adjust doravirine or lamivudine with tenofovir disoproxil and doravirine dose. [Severe] Theoretical
- ▶ **Cobicistat** is predicted to increase the exposure to **doravirine**. [Mild] Study
- ▶ **Dabrafenib** is predicted to decrease the exposure to **doravirine**. Avoid or adjust doravirine or lamivudine with tenofovir disoproxil and doravirine dose. [Severe] Theoretical
- ▶ **Efavirenz** is predicted to decrease the exposure to **doravirine**. Avoid or adjust doravirine or lamivudine with tenofovir disoproxil and doravirine dose. [Severe] Theoretical
- ▶ **Enzalutamide** is predicted to decrease the exposure to **doravirine**. Avoid. [Severe] Study
- ▶ **HIV-protease inhibitors** are predicted to increase the exposure to **doravirine**. [Mild] Study
- ▶ **Idelalisib** is predicted to increase the exposure to **doravirine**. [Mild] Study
- ▶ **Lumacaftor** is predicted to decrease the exposure to **doravirine**. Avoid. [Severe] Theoretical
- ▶ Macrolides **(clarithromycin)** are predicted to increase the exposure to **doravirine**. [Mild] Study
- ▶ **Mitotane** is predicted to decrease the exposure to **doravirine**. Avoid. [Severe] Study
- ▶ **Modafinil** is predicted to decrease the exposure to **doravirine**. Avoid or adjust doravirine or lamivudine with tenofovir disoproxil and doravirine dose. [Severe] Theoretical
- ▶ **Nevirapine** is predicted to decrease the exposure to **doravirine**. Avoid or adjust doravirine or lamivudine with tenofovir disoproxil and doravirine dose. [Severe] Theoretical
- ▶ **Rifabutin** moderately decreases the exposure to **doravirine**. Adjust doravirine or lamivudine with tenofovir disoproxil and doravirine dose. [Moderate] Study
- ▶ **Rifampicin** is predicted to decrease the exposure to **doravirine**. Avoid. [Severe] Study
- ▶ **Doravirine** is predicted to decrease the exposure to **sirolimus**. Monitor **sirolimus** concentration and adjust dose, p. 561. [Moderate] Theoretical

Doravirine (continued)
- **St John's Wort** is predicted to decrease the exposure to **doravirine**. Avoid. Severe Theoretical
- **Doravirine** is predicted to decrease the exposure to **tacrolimus**. Monitor **tacrolimus** concentration and adjust dose, p. 562. Moderate Theoretical
- **Telotristat ethyl** is predicted to decrease the exposure to **doravirine**. Avoid or adjust doravirine or lamivudine with tenofovir disoproxil and doravirine dose. Severe Theoretical

Dorzolamide

ROUTE-SPECIFIC INFORMATION Since systemic absorption can follow topical application, the possibility of interactions should be borne in mind.

Dosulepin → see tricyclic antidepressants

Doxapram
- **Aminophylline** increases the risk of agitation when given with **doxapram**. Moderate Study
- **MAOIs, irreversible** are predicted to increase the effects of **doxapram**. Moderate Theoretical
- **Theophylline** increases the risk of agitation when given with **doxapram**. Moderate Study

Doxazosin → see alpha blockers

Doxepin → see tricyclic antidepressants

Doxorubicin → see anthracyclines

Doxycycline → see tetracyclines

Doxylamine → see antihistamines, sedating

Dronabinol → see TABLE 11 p. 909 (CNS depressant effects)
- Antiepileptics **(carbamazepine, fosphenytoin, phenobarbital, phenytoin, primidone)** are predicted to decrease the exposure to **dronabinol**. Avoid or adjust dose. Mild Study → Also see TABLE 11 p. 909
- Antifungals, azoles **(itraconazole, ketoconazole, voriconazole)** are predicted to increase the exposure to **dronabinol**. Adjust dose. Mild Study
- **Apalutamide** is predicted to decrease the exposure to **dronabinol**. Avoid or adjust dose. Mild Study
- **Cobicistat** is predicted to increase the exposure to **dronabinol**. Adjust dose. Mild Study
- **Enzalutamide** is predicted to decrease the exposure to **dronabinol**. Avoid or adjust dose. Mild Study
- **HIV-protease inhibitors** are predicted to increase the exposure to **dronabinol**. Adjust dose. Mild Study
- **Idelalisib** is predicted to increase the exposure to **dronabinol**. Adjust dose. Mild Study
- Macrolides **(clarithromycin)** are predicted to increase the exposure to **dronabinol**. Adjust dose. Mild Study
- **Mitotane** is predicted to decrease the exposure to **dronabinol**. Avoid or adjust dose. Mild Study
- **Rifampicin** is predicted to decrease the exposure to **dronabinol**. Avoid or adjust dose. Mild Study
- **St John's Wort** is predicted to decrease the exposure to **dronabinol**. Avoid or adjust dose. Mild Study

Dronedarone → see antiarrhythmics

Droperidol → see TABLE 8 p. 908 (hypotension), TABLE 9 p. 909 (QT-interval prolongation), TABLE 11 p. 909 (CNS depressant effects)
- **Droperidol** is predicted to decrease the effects of **dopamine receptor agonists**. Avoid. Moderate Theoretical → Also see TABLE 8 p. 908 → Also see TABLE 9 p. 909
- **Droperidol** decreases the effects of **levodopa**. Severe Study → Also see TABLE 8 p. 908

Drospirenone → see TABLE 16 p. 911 (increased serum potassium)
- Antifungals, azoles **(ketoconazole)** moderately increase the exposure to **drospirenone**. Severe Study

Drugs that reduce serum potassium
- **Drugs that reduce serum potassium** (see TABLE 17 p. 911) are predicted to increase the risk of digoxin toxicity when given with **digoxin**. Severe Study

Drugs with anticoagulant effects
- **Bismuth** subsalicylate is predicted to increase the risk of bleeding events when given with **drugs with anticoagulant effects** (see TABLE 3 p. 907). Moderate Theoretical
- **Caplacizumab** is predicted to increase the risk of bleeding events when given with **drugs with anticoagulant effects** (see TABLE 3 p. 907). Severe Theoretical
- **Volanesorsen** potentially increases the risk of bleeding events when given with **drugs with anticoagulant effects** (see TABLE 3 p. 907). Avoid depending on platelet count—consult product literature. Severe Theoretical

Drugs with antimuscarinic effects
- **Drugs with antimuscarinic effects** (see TABLE 10 p. 909) decrease the absorption of **levodopa**. Moderate Theoretical

Drugs with antiplatelet effects
- **Caplacizumab** is predicted to increase the risk of bleeding events when given with **drugs with antiplatelet effects** (see TABLE 4 p. 907). Severe Theoretical
- **Volanesorsen** potentially increases the risk of bleeding events when given with **drugs with antiplatelet effects** (see TABLE 4 p. 907). Avoid depending on platelet count—consult product literature. Severe Theoretical

Dulaglutide → see TABLE 14 p. 910 (antidiabetic drugs)

Duloxetine → see TABLE 18 p. 911 (hyponatraemia), TABLE 13 p. 910 (serotonin syndrome), TABLE 4 p. 907 (antiplatelet effects)
- Antiepileptics **(phenytoin)** are predicted to decrease the exposure to **duloxetine**. Moderate Theoretical
- **Duloxetine** is predicted to increase the exposure to beta blockers, selective **(metoprolol)**. Moderate Study
- **Duloxetine** is predicted to increase the exposure to **eliglustat**. Avoid or adjust dose—consult product literature. Severe Study
- HIV-protease inhibitors **(ritonavir)** are predicted to decrease the exposure to **duloxetine**. Moderate Theoretical
- **Leflunomide** is predicted to decrease the exposure to **duloxetine**. Moderate Theoretical
- **Duloxetine** is predicted to increase the exposure to **pitolisant**. Use with caution and adjust dose. Moderate Study
- Quinolones **(ciprofloxacin)** are predicted to increase the exposure to **duloxetine**. Avoid. Moderate Theoretical
- **Rifampicin** is predicted to decrease the exposure to **duloxetine**. Moderate Theoretical
- SSRIs **(fluvoxamine)** markedly increase the exposure to **duloxetine**. Avoid. Severe Study → Also see TABLE 18 p. 911 → Also see TABLE 13 p. 910 → Also see TABLE 4 p. 907
- **Teriflunomide** is predicted to decrease the exposure to **duloxetine**. Moderate Theoretical

Dupilumab → see monoclonal antibodies

Durvalumab → see monoclonal antibodies

Dutasteride
- Antiarrhythmics **(dronedarone)** are predicted to moderately increase the exposure to **dutasteride**. Mild Study
- Antifungals, azoles **(fluconazole, isavuconazole, posaconazole)** are predicted to moderately increase the exposure to **dutasteride**. Mild Study
- Antifungals, azoles **(itraconazole, ketoconazole, voriconazole)** are predicted to increase the exposure to **dutasteride**. Monitor side effects and adjust dose. Moderate Theoretical
- **Aprepitant** is predicted to moderately increase the exposure to **dutasteride**. Mild Study
- Calcium channel blockers **(diltiazem, verapamil)** are predicted to moderately increase the exposure to **dutasteride**. Mild Study
- **Cobicistat** is predicted to increase the exposure to **dutasteride**. Monitor side effects and adjust dose. Moderate Theoretical
- **Crizotinib** is predicted to moderately increase the exposure to **dutasteride**. Mild Study
- **HIV-protease inhibitors** are predicted to increase the exposure to **dutasteride**. Monitor side effects and adjust dose. Moderate Theoretical
- **Idelalisib** is predicted to increase the exposure to **dutasteride**. Monitor side effects and adjust dose. Moderate Theoretical
- **Imatinib** is predicted to moderately increase the exposure to **dutasteride**. Mild Study
- Macrolides **(clarithromycin)** are predicted to increase the exposure to **dutasteride**. Monitor side effects and adjust dose. Moderate Theoretical
- Macrolides **(erythromycin)** are predicted to moderately increase the exposure to **dutasteride**. Mild Study
- **Netupitant** is predicted to moderately increase the exposure to **dutasteride**. Mild Study
- **Nilotinib** is predicted to moderately increase the exposure to **dutasteride**. Mild Study

Eculizumab → see monoclonal antibodies

A1 Interactions | Appendix 1

Edoxaban → see TABLE 3 p. 907 (anticoagulant effects)
- Antiarrhythmics **(dronedarone)** slightly increase the exposure to **edoxaban**. Adjust **edoxaban** dose. [Severe] Study
- Antiepileptics **(carbamazepine)** are predicted to decrease the exposure to **edoxaban**. [Moderate] Study
- Antiepileptics **(phenytoin)** are predicted to decrease the exposure to **edoxaban**. [Moderate] Theoretical
- Antifungals, azoles **(itraconazole)** are predicted to slightly increase the exposure to **edoxaban**. [Severe] Theoretical
- Antifungals, azoles **(ketoconazole)** slightly increase the exposure to **edoxaban**. Adjust **edoxaban** dose. [Severe] Study
- **Ceritinib** is predicted to increase the exposure to **edoxaban**. [Moderate] Theoretical
- **Ciclosporin** slightly increases the exposure to **edoxaban**. Adjust **edoxaban** dose. [Severe] Study
- **Cobicistat** is predicted to increase the exposure to **edoxaban**. Avoid. [Severe] Theoretical
- **Eliglustat** is predicted to increase the exposure to **edoxaban**. Adjust dose. [Moderate] Study
- HIV-protease inhibitors **(lopinavir, ritonavir, saquinavir)** are predicted to slightly increase the exposure to **edoxaban**. [Severe] Theoretical
- **Lapatinib** is predicted to slightly increase the exposure to **edoxaban**. [Severe] Theoretical
- Macrolides **(azithromycin, clarithromycin)** are predicted to slightly increase the exposure to **edoxaban**. [Severe] Theoretical
- Macrolides **(erythromycin)** slightly increase the exposure to **edoxaban**. Adjust **edoxaban** dose. [Severe] Study
- **Mirabegron** is predicted to increase the exposure to **edoxaban**. [Mild] Theoretical
- **Neratinib** is predicted to increase the exposure to **edoxaban**. [Moderate] Study
- **Paritaprevir** (with ritonavir and ombitasvir) is predicted to increase the exposure to **edoxaban**. [Severe] Study
- **Pibrentasvir** (with glecaprevir) is predicted to increase the exposure to **edoxaban**. [Moderate] Study
- **Pitolisant** is predicted to decrease the exposure to **edoxaban**. [Mild] Theoretical
- **Ranolazine** is predicted to slightly increase the exposure to **edoxaban**. [Severe] Theoretical
- **Rifampicin** is predicted to decrease the exposure to **edoxaban**. [Moderate] Study
- **St John's Wort** is predicted to decrease the exposure to **edoxaban**. [Moderate] Study
- **Velpatasvir** is predicted to increase the exposure to **edoxaban**. [Severe] Theoretical
- **Vemurafenib** is predicted to slightly increase the exposure to **edoxaban**. [Severe] Theoretical
- **Voxilaprevir** (with sofosbuvir and velpatasvir) is predicted to increase the concentration of **edoxaban**. Avoid. [Severe] Theoretical

Efavirenz → see TABLE 9 p. 909 (QT-interval prolongation)
- **Efavirenz** is predicted to decrease the exposure to antiarrhythmics **(dronedarone)**. [Severe] Theoretical → Also see TABLE 9 p. 909
- Antiepileptics **(carbamazepine)** slightly decrease the exposure to **efavirenz** and **efavirenz** slightly decreases the exposure to antiepileptics **(carbamazepine)**. [Severe] Study
- Antiepileptics **(fosphenytoin, phenytoin)** slightly decrease the exposure to **efavirenz** and **efavirenz** affects the concentration of antiepileptics **(fosphenytoin, phenytoin)**. [Severe] Theoretical
- Antiepileptics **(phenobarbital)** are predicted to decrease the exposure to **efavirenz** and **efavirenz** affects the concentration of antiepileptics **(phenobarbital)**. [Severe] Theoretical
- **Efavirenz** is predicted to affect the efficacy of antiepileptics **(primidone)** and antiepileptics **(primidone)** are predicted to slightly decrease the exposure to **efavirenz**. [Severe] Theoretical
- **Efavirenz** is predicted to decrease the exposure to antifungals, azoles **(isavuconazole)**. Avoid. [Severe] Theoretical
- **Efavirenz** slightly decreases the exposure to antifungals, azoles **(itraconazole)**. Avoid and for 14 days after stopping **efavirenz**. [Moderate] Study
- **Efavirenz** moderately decreases the exposure to antifungals, azoles **(ketoconazole)**. [Severe] Study
- **Efavirenz** slightly decreases the exposure to antifungals, azoles **(posaconazole)**. Avoid. [Moderate] Study
- **Efavirenz** moderately decreases the exposure to antifungals, azoles **(voriconazole)** and antifungals, azoles **(voriconazole)** slightly increase the exposure to **efavirenz**. Adjust dose. [Severe] Study → Also see TABLE 9 p. 909
- **Efavirenz** decreases the concentration of antimalarials **(artemether)**. [Severe] Study → Also see TABLE 9 p. 909
- **Efavirenz** moderately decreases the exposure to antimalarials **(atovaquone)**. Avoid. [Moderate] Study
- **Efavirenz** affects the exposure to antimalarials **(proguanil)**. Avoid. [Moderate] Study
- **Efavirenz** is predicted to decrease the exposure to **aprepitant**. [Moderate] Study
- **Efavirenz** is predicted to decrease the exposure to **axitinib**. [Moderate] Theoretical
- **Efavirenz** is predicted to decrease the exposure to **bedaquiline**. Avoid. [Severe] Study → Also see TABLE 9 p. 909
- **Efavirenz** is predicted to decrease the exposure to **bosutinib**. Avoid. [Severe] Theoretical → Also see TABLE 9 p. 909
- **Efavirenz** is predicted to decrease the exposure to **brigatinib**. Avoid. [Severe] Study
- **Efavirenz** is predicted to decrease the exposure to **bupropion**. [Moderate] Study
- **Efavirenz** is predicted to decrease the exposure to **cabozantinib**. [Moderate] Theoretical → Also see TABLE 9 p. 909
- **Efavirenz** is predicted to decrease the exposure to calcium channel blockers **(amlodipine, felodipine, lacidipine, lercanidipine, nicardipine, nifedipine, nimodipine)**. Monitor and adjust dose. [Moderate] Theoretical
- **Efavirenz** is predicted to decrease the exposure to calcium channel blockers **(diltiazem, verapamil)**. [Moderate] Theoretical
- **Efavirenz** is predicted to decrease the exposure to **cariprazine**. Avoid. [Severe] Theoretical
- **Efavirenz** is predicted to decrease the concentration of **caspofungin**. Adjust dose. [Moderate] Study
- **Efavirenz** decreases the concentration of **ciclosporin**. Monitor concentration and adjust dose. [Moderate] Study
- **Efavirenz** is predicted to decrease the exposure to **cobicistat**. Avoid. [Severe] Theoretical
- **Efavirenz** is predicted to decrease the exposure to **cobimetinib**. Avoid. [Severe] Theoretical
- **Efavirenz** is predicted to decrease the efficacy of **combined hormonal contraceptives**. For FSRH guidance, see Contraceptives, interactions p. 536. [Severe] Study
- **Efavirenz** is predicted to affect the concentration of **coumarins**. Adjust dose. [Moderate] Theoretical
- **Efavirenz** is predicted to decrease the exposure to **crizotinib**. Avoid. [Severe] Theoretical → Also see TABLE 9 p. 909
- **Efavirenz** increases the risk of increased ALT concentrations when given with **dasabuvir**. Avoid. [Severe] Study
- **Efavirenz** is predicted to decrease the exposure to **dasatinib**. [Severe] Study → Also see TABLE 9 p. 909
- **Efavirenz** is predicted to decrease the efficacy of **desogestrel**. For FSRH guidance, see Contraceptives, interactions p. 536. [Severe] Theoretical
- **Efavirenz** decreases the exposure to **dolutegravir**. Adjust dose. [Severe] Study
- **Efavirenz** is predicted to decrease the exposure to **doravirine**. Avoid or adjust doravirine or lamivudine with tenofovir disoproxil and doravirine dose. [Severe] Theoretical
- **Efavirenz** is predicted to moderately decrease the exposure to **elbasvir**. Avoid. [Severe] Study
- **Efavirenz** is predicted to decrease the exposure to **eliglustat**. [Moderate] Theoretical
- **Efavirenz** is predicted to decrease the concentration of **elvitegravir**. Avoid. [Severe] Theoretical
- **Efavirenz** is predicted to decrease the effects of **ergotamine**. [Moderate] Theoretical
- **Efavirenz** is predicted to decrease the exposure to **erlotinib**. [Severe] Theoretical
- **Efavirenz** is predicted to decrease the efficacy of **etonogestrel**. For FSRH guidance, see Contraceptives, interactions p. 536. [Severe] Theoretical

Efavirenz (continued)
- ▶ **Efavirenz** is predicted to decrease the exposure to **etravirine**. Avoid. Severe Study
- ▶ **Efavirenz** is predicted to decrease the concentration of **everolimus**. Avoid or adjust dose. Severe Study
- ▶ **Efavirenz** is predicted to decrease the exposure to **fosaprepitant**. Moderate Theoretical
- ▶ **Efavirenz** is predicted to decrease the exposure to **gefitinib**. Avoid. Severe Theoretical
- ▶ **Efavirenz** is predicted to decrease the exposure to **glecaprevir**. Avoid. Severe Study
- ▶ **Efavirenz** is predicted to markedly decrease the exposure to **grazoprevir**. Avoid. Severe Study
- ▶ **Efavirenz** is predicted to decrease the concentration of **guanfacine**. Adjust dose. Moderate Theoretical
- ▶ **Efavirenz** decreases the exposure to **HIV-protease inhibitors**. Refer to specialist literature. Severe Study → Also see **TABLE 9** p. 909
- ▶ **Efavirenz** is predicted to decrease the effects of **hormone replacement therapy**. Moderate Anecdotal
- ▶ **Efavirenz** is predicted to decrease the exposure to **idelalisib**. Avoid. Moderate Theoretical
- ▶ **Efavirenz** is predicted to decrease the exposure to **imatinib**. Moderate Study
- ▶ **Efavirenz** is predicted to decrease the exposure to **ivacaftor**. Moderate Study
- ▶ **Efavirenz** is predicted to decrease the exposure to **lapatinib**. Avoid. Severe Study → Also see **TABLE 9** p. 909
- ▶ **Efavirenz** is predicted to decrease the exposure to **larotrectinib**. Avoid. Moderate Study
- ▶ **Efavirenz** is predicted to decrease the concentration of **letermovir**. Moderate Theoretical
- ▶ **Efavirenz** is predicted to decrease the efficacy of **levonorgestrel**. For FSRH guidance, see Contraceptives, interactions p. 536. Severe Theoretical
- ▶ **Efavirenz** is predicted to decrease the exposure to **lorlatinib**. Avoid. Severe Theoretical
- ▶ **Efavirenz** is predicted to decrease the exposure to **lurasidone**. Monitor and adjust dose. Moderate Theoretical
- ▶ **Efavirenz** decreases the exposure to macrolides (**clarithromycin**). Moderate Study → Also see **TABLE 9** p. 909
- ▶ **Efavirenz** decreases the exposure to **maraviroc**. Refer to specialist literature. Severe Theoretical
- ▶ **Efavirenz** is predicted to alter the effects of **midazolam**. Avoid. Moderate Theoretical
- ▶ **Efavirenz** is predicted to decrease the exposure to **neratinib**. Severe Study
- ▶ **Efavirenz** is predicted to decrease the exposure to **netupitant**. Moderate Theoretical
- ▶ **Nevirapine** decreases the concentration of **efavirenz**. Avoid. Severe Study
- ▶ **Efavirenz** is predicted to decrease the exposure to **nilotinib**. Avoid. Severe Theoretical → Also see **TABLE 9** p. 909
- ▶ **Efavirenz** is predicted to decrease the efficacy of **norethisterone**. For FSRH guidance, see Contraceptives, interactions p. 536. Severe Anecdotal
- ▶ **Efavirenz** is predicted to decrease the exposure to **olaparib**. Avoid. Moderate Theoretical
- ▶ **Efavirenz** is predicted to decrease the exposure to **ombitasvir**. Avoid. Severe Theoretical
- ▶ **Efavirenz** decreases the exposure to opioids (**methadone**). Monitor and adjust dose. Severe Study → Also see **TABLE 9** p. 909
- ▶ **Efavirenz** is predicted to decrease the exposure to **osimertinib**. Moderate Theoretical → Also see **TABLE 9** p. 909
- ▶ **Efavirenz** is predicted to decrease the exposure to **ospemifene**. Moderate Study
- ▶ **Efavirenz** is predicted to decrease the exposure to **paritaprevir** (with **ritonavir** and **ombitasvir**). Avoid. Severe Study
- ▶ **Efavirenz** is predicted to decrease the exposure to **phosphodiesterase type-5 inhibitors**. Moderate Theoretical → Also see **TABLE 9** p. 909
- ▶ **Efavirenz** is predicted to decrease the exposure to **pibrentasvir**. Avoid. Severe Study
- ▶ **Pitolisant** is predicted to decrease the exposure to **efavirenz**. Mild Theoretical
- ▶ **Efavirenz** is predicted to decrease the exposure to **quetiapine**. Moderate Study
- ▶ **Efavirenz** is predicted to decrease the exposure to **ribociclib**. Moderate Study → Also see **TABLE 9** p. 909
- ▶ **Efavirenz** slightly decreases the exposure to **rifabutin**. Adjust dose. Severe Study
- ▶ **Rifampicin** slightly decreases the exposure to **efavirenz**. Adjust dose. Severe Study
- ▶ **Efavirenz** is predicted to decrease the exposure to **rilpivirine**. Avoid. Severe Theoretical
- ▶ **Efavirenz** is predicted to decrease the exposure to **rolapitant**. Avoid. Severe Study
- ▶ **Efavirenz** is predicted to decrease the exposure to **ruxolitinib**. Monitor and adjust dose. Moderate Theoretical
- ▶ **Efavirenz** is predicted to decrease the exposure to **siponimod**. Manufacturer advises caution depending on genotype—consult product literature. Severe Theoretical
- ▶ **Efavirenz** is predicted to decrease the concentration of **sirolimus**. Monitor and adjust dose. Moderate Theoretical
- ▶ **St John's Wort** is predicted to decrease the concentration of **efavirenz**. Avoid. Severe Theoretical
- ▶ **Efavirenz** slightly decreases the exposure to statins (**atorvastatin**). Mild Study
- ▶ **Efavirenz** moderately decreases the exposure to statins (**simvastatin**). Moderate Study
- ▶ **Efavirenz** is predicted to decrease the concentration of **tacrolimus**. Monitor and adjust dose. Moderate Theoretical
- ▶ **Efavirenz** is predicted to decrease the exposure to taxanes (**cabazitaxel**). Avoid. Severe Study
- ▶ **Efavirenz** is predicted to decrease the concentration of **temsirolimus**. Avoid. Severe Theoretical
- ▶ **Efavirenz** is predicted to decrease the exposure to **ticagrelor**. Moderate Theoretical
- ▶ **Efavirenz** is predicted to decrease the exposure to **tofacitinib**. Moderate Study
- ▶ **Efavirenz** decreases the efficacy of **ulipristal**. For FSRH guidance, see Contraceptives, interactions p. 536. Severe Anecdotal
- ▶ **Efavirenz** is predicted to decrease the exposure to **velpatasvir**. Avoid. Moderate Theoretical
- ▶ **Efavirenz** is predicted to decrease the exposure to **venetoclax**. Avoid. Severe Study
- ▶ **Efavirenz** is predicted to decrease the concentration of **voxilaprevir**. Avoid. Severe Theoretical

Elbasvir
- ▶ Antiepileptics (**carbamazepine, fosphenytoin, phenobarbital, phenytoin, primidone**) are predicted to decrease the exposure to **elbasvir**. Avoid. Severe Study
- ▶ **Apalutamide** is predicted to decrease the exposure to **elbasvir**. Avoid. Severe Study
- ▶ **Bosentan** is predicted to moderately decrease the exposure to **elbasvir**. Avoid. Severe Study
- ▶ **Elbasvir** is predicted to increase the concentration of **dabigatran**. Moderate Theoretical
- ▶ **Efavirenz** is predicted to moderately decrease the exposure to **elbasvir**. Avoid. Severe Study
- ▶ **Enzalutamide** is predicted to decrease the exposure to **elbasvir**. Avoid. Severe Study
- ▶ **Etravirine** is predicted to decrease the exposure to **elbasvir**. Avoid. Unknown Theoretical
- ▶ **Mitotane** is predicted to decrease the exposure to **elbasvir**. Avoid. Severe Study
- ▶ **Modafinil** is predicted to decrease the exposure to **elbasvir**. Avoid. Unknown Theoretical
- ▶ **Nevirapine** is predicted to moderately decrease the exposure to **elbasvir**. Avoid. Severe Study
- ▶ **Rifampicin** is predicted to decrease the exposure to **elbasvir**. Avoid. Severe Study
- ▶ **St John's Wort** is predicted to moderately decrease the exposure to **elbasvir**. Avoid. Severe Study
- ▶ **Elbasvir** increases the exposure to statins (**atorvastatin**). Adjust **atorvastatin** dose, p. 139. Moderate Study
- ▶ **Elbasvir** is predicted to increase the exposure to statins (**fluvastatin**). Adjust **fluvastatin** dose, p. 139. Unknown Theoretical

- **Elbasvir** increases the exposure to statins (**rosuvastatin**). Adjust **rosuvastatin** dose, p. 140. Moderate Study
- **Elbasvir** is predicted to increase the exposure to statins (**simvastatin**). Adjust **simvastatin** dose, p. 141. Unknown Theoretical
- **Elbasvir** is predicted to increase the concentration of **sunitinib**. Use with caution and adjust dose. Moderate Theoretical

Eletriptan → see TABLE 13 p. 910 (serotonin syndrome)

- Antifungals, azoles (**itraconazole, ketoconazole, voriconazole**) are predicted to markedly increase the exposure to **eletriptan**. Avoid. Severe Study
- **Aprepitant** is predicted to increase the exposure to **eletriptan**. Moderate Study
- **Cobicistat** is predicted to markedly increase the exposure to **eletriptan**. Avoid. Severe Study
- **Eletriptan** increases the risk of vasoconstriction when given with **ergotamine**. Separate administration by 24 hours. Severe Study
- **HIV-protease inhibitors** are predicted to markedly increase the exposure to **eletriptan**. Avoid. Severe Study
- **Idelalisib** is predicted to markedly increase the exposure to **eletriptan**. Avoid. Severe Study
- Macrolides (**clarithromycin**) are predicted to markedly increase the exposure to **eletriptan**. Avoid. Severe Study
- Macrolides (**erythromycin**) moderately increase the exposure to **eletriptan**. Avoid. Moderate Study
- **Netupitant** is predicted to increase the exposure to **eletriptan**. Moderate Study

Eliglustat

- **Abiraterone** is predicted to increase the exposure to **eliglustat**. Avoid or adjust dose—consult product literature. Severe Study
- **Eliglustat** is predicted to increase the exposure to **aliskiren**. Adjust dose. Moderate Study
- Antiarrhythmics (**dronedarone, propafenone**) are predicted to increase the exposure to **eliglustat**. Avoid or adjust dose—consult product literature. Severe Study
- Antiepileptics (**carbamazepine, fosphenytoin, phenobarbital, phenytoin, primidone**) are predicted to decrease the exposure to **eliglustat**. Avoid. Severe Study
- Antifungals, azoles (**fluconazole, isavuconazole, itraconazole, ketoconazole, posaconazole, voriconazole**) are predicted to increase the exposure to **eliglustat**. Avoid or adjust dose—consult product literature. Severe Study
- **Eliglustat** is predicted to increase the exposure to antihistamines, non-sedating (**fexofenadine**). Adjust dose. Moderate Study
- **Apalutamide** is predicted to decrease the exposure to **eliglustat**. Avoid. Severe Study
- **Aprepitant** is predicted to increase the exposure to **eliglustat**. Avoid or adjust dose—consult product literature. Severe Study
- **Eliglustat** is predicted to increase the exposure to **atomoxetine**. Adjust dose. Moderate Theoretical
- **Eliglustat** is predicted to increase the exposure to beta blockers, non-selective (**propranolol**). Adjust dose. Moderate Study
- **Eliglustat** is predicted to increase the exposure to beta blockers, selective (**metoprolol**). Adjust dose. Moderate Study
- **Bosentan** is predicted to decrease the exposure to **eliglustat**. Moderate Theoretical
- **Bupropion** is predicted to increase the exposure to **eliglustat**. Avoid or adjust dose—consult product literature. Severe Study
- Calcium channel blockers (**diltiazem, verapamil**) are predicted to increase the exposure to **eliglustat**. Avoid or adjust dose—consult product literature. Severe Study
- **Cinacalcet** is predicted to increase the exposure to **eliglustat**. Avoid or adjust dose—consult product literature. Severe Study
- **Cobicistat** is predicted to increase the exposure to **eliglustat**. Avoid or adjust dose—consult product literature. Severe Study
- **Eliglustat** is predicted to increase the exposure to **colchicine**. Avoid or adjust **colchicine** dose. Severe Theoretical
- **Crizotinib** is predicted to increase the exposure to **eliglustat**. Avoid or adjust dose—consult product literature. Severe Study
- **Eliglustat** is predicted to increase the exposure to **dabigatran**. Adjust dose. Moderate Study
- **Dacomitinib** is predicted to markedly increase the exposure to **eliglustat**. Avoid or adjust dose—consult product literature. Severe Study
- **Eliglustat** increases the exposure to **digoxin**. Adjust dose. Moderate Study
- **Duloxetine** is predicted to increase the exposure to **eliglustat**. Avoid or adjust dose—consult product literature. Severe Study
- **Eliglustat** is predicted to increase the exposure to **edoxaban**. Adjust dose. Moderate Study
- **Efavirenz** is predicted to decrease the exposure to **eliglustat**. Moderate Theoretical
- **Enzalutamide** is predicted to decrease the exposure to **eliglustat**. Avoid. Severe Study
- **Eliglustat** is predicted to increase the exposure to **everolimus**. Adjust dose. Moderate Study
- **Grapefruit juice** is predicted to increase the exposure to **eliglustat**. Avoid. Severe Theoretical
- **HIV-protease inhibitors** are predicted to increase the exposure to **eliglustat**. Avoid or adjust dose—consult product literature. Severe Study
- **Idelalisib** is predicted to increase the exposure to **eliglustat**. Avoid or adjust dose—consult product literature. Severe Study
- **Imatinib** is predicted to increase the exposure to **eliglustat**. Avoid or adjust dose—consult product literature. Severe Study
- **Eliglustat** is predicted to increase the exposure to **loperamide**. Adjust dose. Moderate Study
- Macrolides (**clarithromycin, erythromycin**) are predicted to increase the exposure to **eliglustat**. Avoid or adjust dose—consult product literature. Severe Study
- **Mirabegron** is predicted to increase the exposure to **eliglustat**. Avoid or adjust dose—consult product literature. Severe Study
- **Mitotane** is predicted to decrease the exposure to **eliglustat**. Avoid. Severe Study
- **Moclobemide** is predicted to increase the exposure to **eliglustat**. Avoid or adjust dose—consult product literature. Severe Theoretical
- **Netupitant** is predicted to increase the exposure to **eliglustat**. Avoid or adjust dose—consult product literature. Severe Study
- **Nevirapine** is predicted to decrease the exposure to **eliglustat**. Moderate Theoretical
- **Nilotinib** is predicted to increase the exposure to **eliglustat**. Avoid or adjust dose—consult product literature. Severe Study
- Quinolones (**ciprofloxacin**) are predicted to increase the exposure to **eliglustat**. Avoid or adjust dose—consult product literature. Severe Theoretical
- **Rifampicin** is predicted to decrease the exposure to **eliglustat**. Avoid. Severe Study
- **Eliglustat** is predicted to increase the exposure to **sirolimus**. Adjust dose. Moderate Study
- SSRIs (**fluoxetine, paroxetine**) are predicted to increase the exposure to **eliglustat**. Avoid or adjust dose—consult product literature. Severe Study
- **St John's Wort** is predicted to increase the exposure to **eliglustat**. Avoid. Severe Study
- **Eliglustat** is predicted to increase the exposure to taxanes (**paclitaxel**). Adjust dose. Moderate Study
- **Terbinafine** is predicted to increase the exposure to **eliglustat**. Avoid or adjust dose—consult product literature. Severe Study
- **Eliglustat** is predicted to increase the exposure to **tolterodine**. Adjust dose. Moderate Theoretical
- **Eliglustat** is predicted to increase the exposure to **topotecan**. Adjust dose. Moderate Study
- **Eliglustat** is predicted to increase the exposure to tricyclic antidepressants (**nortriptyline**). Adjust dose. Moderate Theoretical

Elotuzumab → see monoclonal antibodies

Eltrombopag

- **Antacids** decrease the absorption of **eltrombopag**. **Eltrombopag** should be taken 2 hours before or 4 hours after antacids. Severe Study
- **Oral calcium salts** decrease the absorption of **eltrombopag**. **Eltrombopag** should be taken 2 hours before or 4 hours after **calcium salts**. Severe Study
- **Ciclosporin** decreases the exposure to **eltrombopag**. Monitor and adjust dose. Moderate Study

Interactions | **Appendix 1** A1

Eltrombopag (continued)
- **Dairy products** are predicted to decrease the absorption of **eltrombopag. Eltrombopag** should be taken 2 hours before or 4 hours after **dairy products.** Severe Theoretical
- **Iron (oral)** is predicted to decrease the absorption of **eltrombopag. Eltrombopag** should be taken 2 hours before or 4 hours after **iron (oral).** Severe Theoretical
- **Eltrombopag** is predicted to increase the exposure to **larotrectinib.** Mild Study
- **Eltrombopag** is predicted to increase the concentration of **letermovir.** Moderate Study
- **Eltrombopag** is predicted to increase the concentration of **methotrexate.** Moderate Theoretical
- **Rifampicin** is predicted to decrease the exposure to **eltrombopag** and **eltrombopag** is predicted to increase the concentration of **rifampicin.** Moderate Theoretical
- Oral **selenium** is predicted to decrease the absorption of **eltrombopag. Eltrombopag** should be taken 2 hours before or 4 hours after **selenium.** Severe Theoretical
- SSRIs **(fluvoxamine)** are predicted to increase the exposure to **eltrombopag.** Moderate Theoretical
- **Eltrombopag** is predicted to increase the exposure to **statins.** Monitor and adjust dose. Moderate Study
- **Eltrombopag** potentially increases the exposure to **talazoparib.** Avoid or monitor. Moderate Theoretical
- **Eltrombopag** is predicted to increase the exposure to **tenofovir alafenamide.** Moderate Theoretical
- **Eltrombopag** is predicted to increase the exposure to **tenofovir disoproxil.** Moderate Theoretical
- Oral **zinc** is predicted to decrease the absorption of **eltrombopag. Eltrombopag** should be taken 2 hours before or 4 hours after **zinc.** Severe Theoretical

Elvitegravir
- **Antacids** moderately decrease the exposure to **elvitegravir.** Separate administration by at least 4 hours. Moderate Study
- Antiepileptics **(carbamazepine, fosphenytoin, phenobarbital, phenytoin, primidone)** are predicted to decrease the concentration of **elvitegravir.** Avoid. Severe Theoretical
- **Apalutamide** is predicted to decrease the concentration of **elvitegravir.** Avoid. Severe Theoretical
- **Bosentan** is predicted to decrease the concentration of **elvitegravir.** Avoid. Severe Theoretical
- **Elvitegravir** is predicted to decrease the anticoagulant effect of **coumarins.** Moderate Theoretical
- **Efavirenz** is predicted to decrease the concentration of **elvitegravir.** Avoid. Severe Theoretical
- **Enzalutamide** is predicted to decrease the concentration of **elvitegravir.** Avoid. Severe Theoretical
- **Elvitegravir** markedly increases the exposure to **grazoprevir.** Avoid. Severe Study
- HIV-protease inhibitors **(atazanavir, lopinavir)** boosted with ritonavir increase the concentration of **elvitegravir.** Refer to specialist literature. Moderate Study
- **Mitotane** is predicted to decrease the concentration of **elvitegravir.** Avoid. Severe Theoretical
- **Nevirapine** is predicted to decrease the concentration of **elvitegravir.** Avoid. Severe Theoretical
- **Rifampicin** is predicted to decrease the concentration of **elvitegravir.** Avoid. Severe Theoretical
- **St John's Wort** is predicted to decrease the concentration of **elvitegravir.** Avoid. Severe Theoretical

Empagliflozin → see TABLE 14 p. 910 (antidiabetic drugs), TABLE 8 p. 908 (hypotension)

Enalapril → see ACE inhibitors

Encorafenib → see TABLE 9 p. 909 (QT-interval prolongation)
- Antiarrhythmics **(dronedarone)** are predicted to moderately increase the exposure to **encorafenib.** Moderate Study → Also see TABLE 9 p. 909
- Antiepileptics **(carbamazepine, fosphenytoin, phenobarbital, phenytoin, primidone)** are predicted to decrease the exposure to **encorafenib.** Severe Theoretical
- Antifungals, azoles **(fluconazole, isavuconazole, posaconazole)** are predicted to moderately increase the exposure to **encorafenib.** Moderate Study → Also see TABLE 9 p. 909
- Antifungals, azoles **(itraconazole, ketoconazole, voriconazole)** are predicted to increase the exposure to **encorafenib.** Avoid or monitor. Severe Study → Also see TABLE 9 p. 909
- **Apalutamide** is predicted to decrease the exposure to **encorafenib.** Severe Theoretical → Also see TABLE 9 p. 909
- **Aprepitant** is predicted to moderately increase the exposure to **encorafenib.** Moderate Study
- Calcium channel blockers **(diltiazem, verapamil)** are predicted to moderately increase the exposure to **encorafenib.** Moderate Study
- **Cobicistat** is predicted to increase the exposure to **encorafenib.** Avoid or monitor. Severe Study
- **Encorafenib** is predicted to affect the exposure to **combined hormonal contraceptives.** Severe Theoretical
- **Crizotinib** is predicted to moderately increase the exposure to **encorafenib.** Moderate Study → Also see TABLE 9 p. 909
- **Encorafenib** is predicted to increase the exposure to **dolutegravir.** Moderate Theoretical
- **Enzalutamide** is predicted to decrease the exposure to **encorafenib.** Severe Theoretical
- **Grapefruit juice** is predicted to increase the exposure to **encorafenib.** Avoid. Moderate Study
- **HIV-protease inhibitors** are predicted to increase the exposure to **encorafenib.** Avoid or monitor. Severe Study → Also see TABLE 9 p. 909
- **Idelalisib** is predicted to increase the exposure to **encorafenib.** Avoid or monitor. Severe Study
- **Imatinib** is predicted to moderately increase the exposure to **encorafenib.** Moderate Study
- Macrolides **(clarithromycin)** are predicted to increase the exposure to **encorafenib.** Avoid or monitor. Severe Study → Also see TABLE 9 p. 909
- Macrolides **(erythromycin)** are predicted to moderately increase the exposure to **encorafenib.** Moderate Study → Also see TABLE 9 p. 909
- **Mitotane** is predicted to decrease the exposure to **encorafenib.** Severe Theoretical
- **Netupitant** is predicted to moderately increase the exposure to **encorafenib.** Moderate Study
- **Nilotinib** is predicted to moderately increase the exposure to **encorafenib.** Moderate Study → Also see TABLE 9 p. 909
- **Encorafenib** is predicted to increase the exposure to **raltegravir.** Moderate Theoretical
- **Rifampicin** is predicted to decrease the exposure to **encorafenib.** Severe Theoretical
- **St John's Wort** is predicted to decrease the exposure to **encorafenib.** Severe Theoretical

Enoxaparin → see low molecular-weight heparins

Entacapone
- **Iron (oral)** is predicted to decrease the absorption of **entacapone.** Separate administration by at least 2 hours. Moderate Theoretical
- **Entacapone** increases the exposure to **levodopa.** Monitor side effects and adjust dose. Moderate Study
- **Entacapone** is predicted to increase the risk of elevated blood pressure when given with **MAOIs, irreversible.** Avoid. Severe Theoretical
- **Entacapone** is predicted to increase the exposure to **methyldopa.** Moderate Theoretical
- **Entacapone** is predicted to increase the risk of cardiovascular side-effects when given with **sympathomimetics, inotropic.** Moderate Theoretical
- **Entacapone** is predicted to increase the risk of cardiovascular side-effects when given with sympathomimetics, vasoconstrictor **(adrenaline/epinephrine, noradrenaline/norepinephrine).** Moderate Study

Enteral feeds
- Antacids **(aluminium hydroxide)** increase the risk of blocked enteral or nasogastric tubes when given with **enteral feeds.** Moderate Study
- **Enteral feeds** decrease the absorption of antiepileptics **(phenytoin).** Severe Study
- **Enteral feeds** (vitamin-K containing) potentially decrease the anticoagulant effect of **coumarins.** Severe Anecdotal

- **Enteral feeds** (vitamin-K containing) potentially decrease the effects of phenindione. Severe Theoretical
- **Enteral feeds** decrease the exposure to quinolones (ciprofloxacin). Moderate Study
- Sucralfate increases the risk of blocked enteral or nasogastric tubes when given with **enteral feeds**. Separate administration by 1 hour. Moderate Study
- **Enteral feeds** decrease the exposure to **theophylline**. Moderate Study

Enzalutamide

GENERAL INFORMATION Caution with concurrent chemotherapy—safety and efficacy not established.

- **Enzalutamide** is predicted to markedly decrease the exposure to abemaciclib. Avoid. Severe Study
- **Enzalutamide** is predicted to decrease the exposure to abiraterone. Avoid. Severe Study
- **Enzalutamide** is predicted to decrease the exposure to aldosterone antagonists (**eplerenone**). Avoid. Moderate Theoretical
- **Enzalutamide** is predicted to decrease the exposure to alprazolam. Adjust dose. Moderate Theoretical
- **Enzalutamide** is predicted to decrease the exposure to antiarrhythmics (**disopyramide, dronedarone**). Avoid. Severe Study
- **Enzalutamide** is predicted to decrease the efficacy of antiarrhythmics (**propafenone**). Moderate Study
- **Enzalutamide** is predicted to decrease the exposure to anticholinesterases, centrally acting (**donepezil**). Mild Study
- **Enzalutamide** is predicted to slightly decrease the exposure to antiepileptics (**brivaracetam**). Moderate Theoretical
- **Enzalutamide** is predicted to decrease the exposure to antiepileptics (**perampanel**). Monitor and adjust dose. Moderate Study
- **Enzalutamide** is predicted to decrease the exposure to antifungals, azoles (**isavuconazole**). Avoid. Severe Study
- **Enzalutamide** is predicted to decrease the exposure to antimalarials (**artemether**) (with lumefantrine). Avoid. Severe Study
- **Enzalutamide** is predicted to decrease the concentration of antimalarials (**piperaquine**). Avoid. Moderate Theoretical
- **Enzalutamide** is predicted to moderately decrease the exposure to **apixaban**. Use with caution or avoid. Severe Study
- **Enzalutamide** moderately decreases the exposure to **apremilast**. Avoid. Severe Study
- **Enzalutamide** is predicted to markedly decrease the exposure to **aprepitant**. Avoid. Moderate Study
- **Enzalutamide** is predicted to moderately decrease the exposure to **aripiprazole**. Adjust **aripiprazole** dose, p. 265. Moderate Study
- **Enzalutamide** is predicted to decrease the exposure to **axitinib**. Avoid or adjust dose. Moderate Study
- **Enzalutamide** decreases the exposure to **bedaquiline**. Avoid. Severe Study
- **Enzalutamide** is predicted to decrease the exposure to **bictegravir**. Avoid. Moderate Study
- **Enzalutamide** slightly decreases the exposure to **bortezomib**. Avoid. Severe Study
- **Enzalutamide** affects the exposure to **bosentan**. Avoid. Severe Study
- **Enzalutamide** is predicted to very markedly decrease the exposure to **bosutinib**. Avoid. Severe Study
- **Enzalutamide** is predicted to decrease the exposure to **brigatinib**. Avoid. Severe Study
- **Enzalutamide** is predicted to decrease the exposure to **buspirone**. Use with caution and adjust dose. Severe Study
- **Enzalutamide** moderately decreases the exposure to **cabozantinib**. Avoid. Moderate Study
- **Enzalutamide** is predicted to decrease the exposure to calcium channel blockers (**amlodipine, felodipine, lacidipine, lercanidipine, nicardipine, nifedipine, nimodipine**). Monitor and adjust dose. Moderate Study
- **Enzalutamide** is predicted to decrease the exposure to calcium channel blockers (**diltiazem, verapamil**). Severe Study
- **Enzalutamide** is predicted to decrease the exposure to **cannabidiol**. Adjust dose. Moderate Study
- **Enzalutamide** is predicted to decrease the exposure to **cariprazine**. Avoid. Severe Theoretical
- **Enzalutamide** is predicted to decrease the exposure to **ceritinib**. Avoid. Severe Study
- **Enzalutamide** decreases the concentration of **ciclosporin**. Severe Study
- **Enzalutamide** is predicted to alter the effects of **cilostazol**. Moderate Theoretical
- **Enzalutamide** is predicted to decrease the exposure to **cinacalcet**. Monitor and adjust dose. Moderate Study
- **Enzalutamide** decreases the exposure to **clomethiazole**. Monitor and adjust dose. Moderate Study
- Clopidogrel moderately increases the exposure to **enzalutamide**. Avoid or adjust **enzalutamide** dose. Severe Study
- **Enzalutamide** is predicted to decrease the exposure to **clozapine**. Moderate Theoretical
- **Enzalutamide** is predicted to decrease the exposure to **cobicistat**. Avoid. Severe Theoretical
- **Enzalutamide** is predicted to decrease the exposure to **cobimetinib**. Avoid. Severe Theoretical
- **Enzalutamide** is predicted to decrease the exposure to corticosteroids (**budesonide, deflazacort, dexamethasone, fludrocortisone, hydrocortisone, methylprednisolone, prednisolone, triamcinolone**). Monitor and adjust dose. Moderate Study
- **Enzalutamide** is predicted to decrease the exposure to corticosteroids (**fluticasone**). Unknown Theoretical
- **Enzalutamide** potentially decreases the exposure to **coumarins**. Avoid or adjust dose and monitor INR. Severe Study
- **Enzalutamide** is predicted to markedly decrease the exposure to **crizotinib**. Avoid. Severe Study
- **Enzalutamide** is predicted to decrease the exposure to **dabrafenib**. Avoid. Moderate Theoretical
- **Enzalutamide** is predicted to decrease the exposure to **darifenacin**. Moderate Theoretical
- **Enzalutamide** is predicted to decrease the exposure to **dasabuvir**. Avoid. Severe Theoretical
- **Enzalutamide** is predicted to markedly decrease the exposure to **dasatinib**. Avoid. Severe Study
- **Enzalutamide** is predicted to slightly decrease the exposure to **delamanid**. Avoid. Moderate Study
- **Enzalutamide** is predicted to markedly decrease the exposure to **dienogest**. Severe Study
- **Enzalutamide** decreases the exposure to **dolutegravir**. Adjust dose. Severe Study
- **Enzalutamide** is predicted to decrease the exposure to **doravirine**. Avoid. Severe Study
- **Enzalutamide** is predicted to decrease the exposure to **dronabinol**. Avoid or adjust dose. Mild Study
- **Enzalutamide** is predicted to decrease the exposure to **elbasvir**. Avoid. Severe Study
- **Enzalutamide** is predicted to decrease the exposure to **eliglustat**. Avoid. Severe Study
- **Enzalutamide** is predicted to decrease the concentration of **elvitegravir**. Avoid. Severe Theoretical
- **Enzalutamide** is predicted to decrease the exposure to **encorafenib**. Severe Theoretical
- **Enzalutamide** is predicted to decrease the effects of **ergotamine**. Moderate Theoretical
- **Enzalutamide** is predicted to decrease the exposure to **erlotinib**. Avoid or adjust **erlotinib** dose. Severe Study
- **Enzalutamide** is predicted to decrease the exposure to **esketamine**. Adjust dose. Moderate Theoretical
- **Enzalutamide** is predicted to decrease the exposure to **etravirine**. Avoid. Severe Theoretical
- **Enzalutamide** is predicted to decrease the concentration of **everolimus**. Avoid or adjust dose. Severe Study
- **Enzalutamide** moderately decreases the exposure to **exemestane**. Moderate Study
- **Enzalutamide** is predicted to decrease the exposure to **fesoterodine**. Avoid. Moderate Study
- Fibrates (**gemfibrozil**) moderately increase the exposure to **enzalutamide**. Avoid or adjust **enzalutamide** dose. Severe Study
- **Enzalutamide** is predicted to decrease the exposure to **fingolimod**. Moderate Study

Enzalutamide (continued)

- **Enzalutamide** is predicted to decrease the exposure to fosaprepitant. Avoid. Moderate Theoretical
- **Enzalutamide** is predicted to decrease the exposure to gefitinib. Avoid. Severe Study
- **Enzalutamide** is predicted to greatly decrease the concentration of **glecaprevir**. Avoid. Severe Study
- **Enzalutamide** is predicted to decrease the exposure to grazoprevir. Avoid. Severe Study
- **Enzalutamide** is predicted to decrease the concentration of guanfacine. Adjust **guanfacine** dose, p. 247. Moderate Study
- **Enzalutamide** decreases the concentration of **haloperidol**. Adjust dose. Moderate Study
- **Enzalutamide** is predicted to decrease the exposure to ibrutinib. Avoid or adjust **ibrutinib** dose. Severe Study
- **Enzalutamide** is predicted to decrease the exposure to idelalisib. Avoid. Severe Study
- **Enzalutamide** is predicted to decrease the exposure to imatinib. Avoid. Moderate Study
- **Enzalutamide** is predicted to decrease the exposure to irinotecan. Avoid. Severe Study
- **Enzalutamide** is predicted to decrease the exposure to ivabradine. Adjust dose. Moderate Theoretical
- **Enzalutamide** is predicted to moderately to markedly decrease the exposure to **ivacaftor**. Avoid. Severe Study
- **Enzalutamide** is predicted to decrease the exposure to ixazomib. Avoid. Severe Study
- **Enzalutamide** is predicted to decrease the exposure to lapatinib. Avoid. Severe Study
- **Enzalutamide** is predicted to moderately decrease the exposure to larotrectinib. Avoid. Moderate Study
- **Enzalutamide** is predicted to decrease the exposure to linagliptin. Moderate Study
- **Enzalutamide** is predicted to decrease the exposure to lomitapide. Monitor and adjust dose. Moderate Theoretical
- **Enzalutamide** is predicted to decrease the exposure to lorlatinib. Avoid. Severe Study
- **Enzalutamide** is predicted to decrease the exposure to lurasidone. Avoid. Moderate Study
- **Enzalutamide** is predicted to decrease the exposure to macitentan. Avoid. Severe Study
- **Enzalutamide** is predicted to decrease the exposure to maraviroc. Adjust dose. Severe Study
- **Enzalutamide** is predicted to decrease the exposure to midazolam. Monitor and adjust dose. Moderate Study
- **Enzalutamide** is predicted to decrease the exposure to midostaurin. Avoid. Severe Study
- **Enzalutamide** is predicted to decrease the exposure to mirtazapine. Adjust dose. Moderate Study
- **Enzalutamide** is predicted to decrease the exposure to monoclonal antibodies **(polatuzumab vedotin)**. Moderate Theoretical
- **Enzalutamide** is predicted to decrease the exposure to montelukast. Mild Study
- **Enzalutamide** is predicted to markedly decrease the exposure to naldemedine. Avoid. Severe Study
- **Enzalutamide** is predicted to markedly decrease the exposure to naloxegol. Avoid. Moderate Study
- **Enzalutamide** is predicted to slightly decrease the exposure to nateglinide. Mild Study
- **Enzalutamide** is predicted to decrease the exposure to neratinib. Avoid. Severe Study
- **Enzalutamide** is predicted to decrease the exposure to netupitant. Avoid. Severe Study
- **Enzalutamide** is predicted to decrease the exposure to nevirapine. Severe Theoretical
- **Enzalutamide** is predicted to moderately decrease the exposure to nilotinib. Avoid. Severe Study
- **Enzalutamide** is predicted to decrease the exposure to nitisinone. Adjust dose. Moderate Theoretical
- **Enzalutamide** is predicted to decrease the exposure to olaparib. Avoid. Moderate Theoretical
- **Enzalutamide** is predicted to decrease the exposure to ombitasvir. Avoid. Severe Theoretical
- **Enzalutamide** is predicted to decrease the exposure to ondansetron. Moderate Study
- **Enzalutamide** is predicted to decrease the exposure to opioids **(alfentanil, fentanyl)**. Moderate Study
- **Enzalutamide** is predicted to decrease the exposure to opioids **(buprenorphine)**. Monitor and adjust dose. Moderate Theoretical
- **Enzalutamide** decreases the exposure to opioids **(methadone)**. Monitor and adjust dose. Severe Study
- **Enzalutamide** is predicted to decrease the exposure to opioids (oxycodone). Monitor and adjust dose. Moderate Study
- **Enzalutamide** is predicted to moderately decrease the exposure to **osimertinib**. Avoid. Moderate Study
- **Enzalutamide** is predicted to moderately decrease the exposure to **ospemifene**. Moderate Study
- **Enzalutamide** is predicted to decrease the exposure to palbociclib. Avoid. Severe Study
- **Enzalutamide** is predicted to decrease the exposure to paliperidone. Monitor and adjust dose. Severe Study
- **Enzalutamide** is predicted to decrease the exposure to panobinostat. Avoid. Moderate Theoretical
- **Enzalutamide** is predicted to decrease the exposure to paritaprevir (with ritonavir and ombitasvir). Avoid. Severe Study
- **Enzalutamide** is predicted to decrease the exposure to pazopanib. Avoid. Severe Theoretical
- **Enzalutamide** is predicted to decrease the exposure to phosphodiesterase type-5 inhibitors **(avanafil, tadalafil)**. Avoid. Severe Study
- **Enzalutamide** is predicted to decrease the exposure to phosphodiesterase type-5 inhibitors **(sildenafil, vardenafil)**. Moderate Theoretical
- **Enzalutamide** is predicted to moderately to markedly decrease the exposure to **pibrentasvir**. Avoid. Severe Study
- **Enzalutamide** is predicted to moderately decrease the exposure to **pitolisant**. Moderate Study
- **Enzalutamide** is predicted to decrease the exposure to ponatinib. Avoid. Moderate Theoretical
- **Enzalutamide** is predicted to markedly decrease the exposure to praziquantel. Avoid. Moderate Study
- **Enzalutamide** is predicted to decrease the exposure to quetiapine. Moderate Study
- **Enzalutamide** is predicted to decrease the exposure to ranolazine. Avoid. Severe Study
- **Enzalutamide** is predicted to decrease the exposure to reboxetine. Moderate Anecdotal
- **Enzalutamide** is predicted to decrease the exposure to regorafenib. Avoid. Moderate Study
- **Enzalutamide** is predicted to decrease the exposure to repaglinide. Monitor blood glucose and adjust dose. Moderate Study
- **Enzalutamide** is predicted to markedly decrease the exposure to ribociclib. Avoid. Severe Study
- **Enzalutamide** markedly decreases the exposure to **rilpivirine**. Avoid. Severe Study
- **Enzalutamide** is predicted to decrease the exposure to risperidone. Adjust dose. Moderate Study
- **Enzalutamide** is predicted to moderately decrease the exposure to **rivaroxaban**. Avoid unless patient can be monitored for signs of thrombosis. Severe Study
- **Enzalutamide** is predicted to decrease the exposure to roflumilast. Avoid. Moderate Study
- **Enzalutamide** is predicted to markedly decrease the exposure to rolapitant. Avoid. Severe Study
- **Enzalutamide** is predicted to decrease the exposure to ruxolitinib. Monitor and adjust dose. Moderate Study
- **Enzalutamide** is predicted to moderately decrease the exposure to **saxagliptin**. Moderate Study
- **Enzalutamide** is predicted to decrease the exposure to siponimod. Severe Study
- **Enzalutamide** is predicted to decrease the concentration of sirolimus. Avoid. Severe Study
- **Enzalutamide** is predicted to decrease the exposure to solifenacin. Moderate Theoretical
- **Enzalutamide** is predicted to decrease the exposure to sorafenib. Moderate Theoretical

- **Enzalutamide** is predicted to decrease the exposure to statins (simvastatin). Severe Study
- **Enzalutamide** is predicted to decrease the exposure to sunitinib. Avoid or adjust **sunitinib** dose. Moderate Study
- **Enzalutamide** decreases the concentration of **tacrolimus.** Monitor and adjust dose. Severe Study
- **Enzalutamide** is predicted to decrease the exposure to taxanes **(cabazitaxel, paclitaxel).** Avoid. Severe Study
- **Enzalutamide** is predicted to decrease the exposure to taxanes **(docetaxel).** Severe Theoretical
- **Enzalutamide** is predicted to decrease the concentration of temsirolimus. Avoid. Severe Study
- **Enzalutamide** decreases the exposure to tetracyclines (doxycycline). Monitor and adjust dose. Moderate Study
- **Enzalutamide** is predicted to decrease the exposure to tezacaftor. Avoid. Severe Theoretical
- **Enzalutamide** is predicted to markedly decrease the exposure to ticagrelor. Avoid. Severe Study
- **Enzalutamide** is predicted to decrease the exposure to tivozanib. Severe Study
- **Enzalutamide** is predicted to decrease the exposure to tofacitinib. Avoid. Severe Study
- **Enzalutamide** is predicted to decrease the exposure to tolvaptan. Use with caution or avoid depending on indication. Severe Study
- **Enzalutamide** is predicted to decrease the exposure to toremifene. Adjust dose. Moderate Study
- **Enzalutamide** is predicted to decrease the exposure to trabectedin. Avoid. Severe Theoretical
- **Enzalutamide** is predicted to markedly decrease the exposure to ulipristal. Avoid and for 4 weeks after stopping **ulipristal.** Severe Theoretical
- **Enzalutamide** is predicted to decrease the exposure to upadacitinib. Moderate Study
- **Enzalutamide** is predicted to decrease the exposure to vandetanib. Avoid. Moderate Study
- **Enzalutamide** is predicted to moderately decrease the exposure to velpatasvir. Avoid. Severe Study
- **Enzalutamide** is predicted to decrease the exposure to vemurafenib. Avoid. Severe Theoretical
- **Enzalutamide** is predicted to decrease the exposure to venetoclax. Avoid. Severe Study
- **Enzalutamide** is predicted to decrease the exposure to vinca alkaloids **(vinblastine, vincristine, vindesine).** Severe Theoretical
- **Enzalutamide** is predicted to decrease the exposure to vinca alkaloids **(vinflunine).** Avoid. Severe Theoretical
- **Enzalutamide** is predicted to decrease the exposure to vinca alkaloids **(vinorelbine).** Use with caution or avoid. Severe Theoretical
- **Enzalutamide** is predicted to decrease the exposure to vismodegib. Avoid. Moderate Theoretical
- **Enzalutamide** is predicted to decrease the exposure to vortioxetine. Monitor and adjust dose. Moderate Study
- **Enzalutamide** is predicted to decrease the concentration of voxilaprevir. Avoid. Severe Study
- **Enzalutamide** is predicted to decrease the exposure to zopiclone. Adjust dose. Moderate Study

Ephedrine → see sympathomimetics, vasoconstrictor

Epirubicin → see anthracyclines

Eplerenone → see aldosterone antagonists

Epoetin alfa → see TABLE 5 p. 907 (thromboembolism), TABLE 16 p. 911 (increased serum potassium)

Epoetin beta → see TABLE 5 p. 907 (thromboembolism), TABLE 16 p. 911 (increased serum potassium)

Epoetin zeta → see TABLE 5 p. 907 (thromboembolism), TABLE 16 p. 911 (increased serum potassium)

Epoprostenol → see TABLE 8 p. 908 (hypotension), TABLE 4 p. 907 (antiplatelet effects)

Eprosartan → see angiotensin-II receptor antagonists

Eptifibatide → see TABLE 4 p. 907 (antiplatelet effects)

Ergocalciferol → see vitamin D substances

Ergometrine

- Antiarrhythmics **(dronedarone)** are predicted to increase the risk of ergotism when given with **ergometrine.** Severe Theoretical
- Antifungals, azoles **(fluconazole, isavuconazole, posaconazole)** are predicted to increase the risk of ergotism when given with **ergometrine.** Severe Theoretical
- Antifungals, azoles **(itraconazole, ketoconazole, voriconazole)** are predicted to increase the risk of ergotism when given with **ergometrine.** Avoid. Severe Theoretical
- Antifungals, azoles **(miconazole)** are predicted to increase the exposure to **ergometrine.** Avoid. Moderate Theoretical
- **Aprepitant** is predicted to increase the risk of ergotism when given with **ergometrine.** Severe Theoretical
- **Beta blockers, non-selective** are predicted to increase the risk of peripheral vasoconstriction when given with **ergometrine.** Severe Study
- **Beta blockers, selective** are predicted to increase the risk of peripheral vasoconstriction when given with **ergometrine.** Severe Study
- Calcium channel blockers **(diltiazem, verapamil)** are predicted to increase the risk of ergotism when given with **ergometrine.** Severe Theoretical
- **Cobicistat** is predicted to increase the risk of ergotism when given with **ergometrine.** Avoid. Severe Theoretical
- **Crizotinib** is predicted to increase the risk of ergotism when given with **ergometrine.** Severe Theoretical
- **Ergometrine** is predicted to increase the risk of ergotism when given with dopamine receptor agonists **(cabergoline, pergolide).** Avoid. Moderate Theoretical
- **Esketamine** is predicted to increase the risk of elevated blood pressure when given with **ergometrine.** Avoid. Severe Theoretical
- **Grapefruit juice** is predicted to increase the exposure to **ergometrine.** Severe Theoretical
- **HIV-protease inhibitors** are predicted to increase the risk of ergotism when given with **ergometrine.** Avoid. Severe Theoretical
- **Idelalisib** is predicted to increase the risk of ergotism when given with **ergometrine.** Avoid. Severe Theoretical
- **Imatinib** is predicted to increase the risk of ergotism when given with **ergometrine.** Severe Theoretical
- **Ketamine** is predicted to increase the risk of elevated blood pressure when given with **ergometrine.** Severe Theoretical
- **Letermovir** is predicted to increase the concentration of **ergometrine.** Avoid. Severe Theoretical
- Macrolides **(clarithromycin)** are predicted to increase the risk of ergotism when given with **ergometrine.** Avoid. Severe Theoretical
- Macrolides **(erythromycin)** are predicted to increase the risk of ergotism when given with **ergometrine.** Severe Theoretical
- **Netupitant** is predicted to increase the risk of ergotism when given with **ergometrine.** Severe Theoretical
- **Nilotinib** is predicted to increase the risk of ergotism when given with **ergometrine.** Severe Theoretical
- **Ergometrine** potentially increases the risk of peripheral vasoconstriction when given with sympathomimetics, inotropic **(dopamine).** Avoid. Severe Anecdotal
- **Ergometrine** is predicted to increase the risk of peripheral vasoconstriction when given with sympathomimetics, vasoconstrictor **(noradrenaline/norepinephrine).** Severe Anecdotal

Ergotamine

- **Almotriptan** is predicted to increase the risk of vasoconstriction when given with **ergotamine. Ergotamine** should be taken at least 24 hours before or 6 hours after **almotriptan.** Severe Theoretical
- Antiarrhythmics **(dronedarone)** are predicted to increase the risk of ergotism when given with **ergotamine.** Severe Theoretical
- Antiepileptics **(carbamazepine, fosphenytoin, phenobarbital, phenytoin, primidone)** are predicted to decrease the effects of **ergotamine.** Moderate Theoretical
- Antifungals, azoles **(fluconazole, isavuconazole, posaconazole)** are predicted to increase the risk of ergotism when given with **ergotamine.** Severe Theoretical
- Antifungals, azoles **(itraconazole, ketoconazole, voriconazole)** are predicted to increase the risk of ergotism when given with **ergotamine.** Avoid. Severe Theoretical
- Antifungals, azoles **(miconazole)** are predicted to increase the exposure to **ergotamine.** Avoid. Moderate Theoretical

Ergotamine (continued)
- Apalutamide is predicted to decrease the effects of **ergotamine.** Moderate Theoretical
- Aprepitant is predicted to increase the risk of ergotism when given with **ergotamine.** Severe Theoretical
- Beta blockers, non-selective are predicted to increase the risk of peripheral vasoconstriction when given with **ergotamine.** Severe Study
- Beta blockers, selective are predicted to increase the risk of peripheral vasoconstriction when given with **ergotamine.** Severe Study
- Bosentan is predicted to decrease the effects of **ergotamine.** Moderate Theoretical
- Calcium channel blockers **(diltiazem, verapamil)** are predicted to increase the risk of ergotism when given with **ergotamine.** Severe Theoretical
- Ceritinib is predicted to increase the exposure to **ergotamine.** Avoid. Severe Theoretical
- Cobicistat is predicted to increase the risk of ergotism when given with **ergotamine.** Avoid. Severe Theoretical
- Crizotinib is predicted to increase the risk of ergotism when given with **ergotamine.** Severe Theoretical
- **Ergotamine** is predicted to increase the risk of ergotism when given with dopamine receptor agonists **(bromocriptine, cabergoline).** Avoid. Moderate Theoretical
- **Ergotamine** is predicted to increase the risk of ergotism when given with dopamine receptor agonists **(pergolide).** Moderate Theoretical
- Efavirenz is predicted to decrease the effects of **ergotamine.** Moderate Theoretical
- Eletriptan increases the risk of vasoconstriction when given with **ergotamine.** Separate administration by 24 hours. Severe Study
- Enzalutamide is predicted to decrease the effects of **ergotamine.** Moderate Theoretical
- Frovatriptan is predicted to increase the risk of vasoconstriction when given with **ergotamine.** Separate administration by 24 hours. Severe Theoretical
- Grapefruit juice is predicted to increase the exposure to **ergotamine.** Severe Theoretical
- HIV-protease inhibitors are predicted to increase the risk of ergotism when given with **ergotamine.** Avoid. Severe Theoretical
- Idelalisib is predicted to increase the risk of ergotism when given with **ergotamine.** Avoid. Severe Theoretical
- Imatinib is predicted to increase the risk of ergotism when given with **ergotamine.** Severe Theoretical
- Larotrectinib is predicted to increase the exposure to **ergotamine.** Use with caution and adjust dose. Mild Theoretical
- Letermovir is predicted to increase the concentration of **ergotamine.** Avoid. Severe Theoretical
- Lorlatinib is predicted to decrease the exposure to **ergotamine.** Avoid. Moderate Theoretical
- Macrolides **(clarithromycin)** are predicted to increase the risk of ergotism when given with **ergotamine.** Avoid. Severe Theoretical
- Macrolides **(erythromycin)** are predicted to increase the risk of ergotism when given with **ergotamine.** Severe Theoretical
- Mitotane is predicted to decrease the effects of **ergotamine.** Moderate Theoretical
- Naratriptan is predicted to increase the risk of vasoconstriction when given with **ergotamine.** Separate administration by 24 hours. Severe Theoretical
- Netupitant is predicted to increase the risk of ergotism when given with **ergotamine.** Severe Theoretical
- Nevirapine is predicted to decrease the effects of **ergotamine.** Moderate Theoretical
- Nilotinib is predicted to increase the risk of ergotism when given with **ergotamine.** Severe Theoretical
- Palbociclib is predicted to increase the exposure to **ergotamine.** Adjust dose. Moderate Theoretical
- Ribociclib (high-dose) is predicted to increase the exposure to **ergotamine.** Avoid. Moderate Theoretical
- Rifampicin is predicted to decrease the effects of **ergotamine.** Moderate Theoretical
- Rizatriptan is predicted to increase the risk of vasoconstriction when given with **ergotamine. Ergotamine** should be taken at least 24 hours before or 6 hours after **rizatriptan.** Severe Theoretical
- Rucaparib is predicted to increase the exposure to **ergotamine.** Monitor and adjust dose. Moderate Study
- St John's Wort is predicted to decrease the effects of **ergotamine.** Moderate Theoretical
- Sumatriptan increases the risk of vasoconstriction when given with **ergotamine. Ergotamine** should be taken at least 24 hours before or 6 hours after **sumatriptan.** Severe Study
- Ticagrelor is predicted to increase the exposure to **ergotamine.** Avoid. Severe Theoretical
- Zolmitriptan is predicted to increase the risk of vasoconstriction when given with **ergotamine. Ergotamine** should be taken at least 24 hours before or 6 hours after **zolmitriptan.** Severe Theoretical

Eribulin → see TABLE 15 p. 910 (myelosuppression), TABLE 12 p. 910 (peripheral neuropathy), TABLE 9 p. 909 (QT-interval prolongation)

Erlotinib

FOOD AND LIFESTYLE Dose adjustment may be necessary if smoking started or stopped during treatment.

- Antacids are predicted to decrease the absorption of **erlotinib. Erlotinib** should be taken 2 hours before or 4 hours after antacids. Moderate Theoretical
- Antiarrhythmics **(amiodarone, dronedarone)** are predicted to increase the exposure to **erlotinib.** Moderate Theoretical
- Antiepileptics **(carbamazepine, fosphenytoin, phenobarbital, phenytoin, primidone)** are predicted to decrease the exposure to **erlotinib.** Avoid or adjust **erlotinib** dose. Severe Study
- Antifungals, azoles **(fluconazole, isavuconazole, posaconazole)** are predicted to increase the exposure to **erlotinib.** Moderate Theoretical
- Antifungals, azoles **(itraconazole, ketoconazole, voriconazole)** are predicted to slightly increase the exposure to **erlotinib.** Use with caution and adjust dose. Moderate Study
- Apalutamide is predicted to decrease the exposure to **erlotinib.** Avoid or adjust **erlotinib** dose. Severe Study
- Aprepitant is predicted to increase the exposure to **erlotinib.** Moderate Theoretical
- **Erlotinib** is predicted to increase the risk of gastrointestinal perforation when given with **aspirin** (high-dose). Severe Theoretical
- Bosentan is predicted to decrease the exposure to **erlotinib.** Severe Theoretical
- Calcium channel blockers **(diltiazem, verapamil)** are predicted to increase the exposure to **erlotinib.** Moderate Theoretical
- Ciclosporin is predicted to increase the exposure to **erlotinib.** Moderate Theoretical
- Cobicistat is predicted to slightly increase the exposure to **erlotinib.** Use with caution and adjust dose. Moderate Study
- Combined hormonal contraceptives slightly increase the exposure to **erlotinib.** Monitor side effects and adjust dose. Moderate Study
- Corticosteroids increase the risk of gastrointestinal perforation when given with **erlotinib.** Severe Theoretical
- **Erlotinib** increases the anticoagulant effect of **coumarins.** Severe Anecdotal
- Crizotinib is predicted to increase the exposure to **erlotinib.** Moderate Theoretical
- Efavirenz is predicted to decrease the exposure to **erlotinib.** Severe Theoretical
- Enzalutamide is predicted to decrease the exposure to **erlotinib.** Avoid or adjust **erlotinib** dose. Severe Study
- Grapefruit juice is predicted to increase the exposure to **erlotinib.** Moderate Theoretical
- H_2 receptor antagonists are predicted to decrease the exposure to **erlotinib. Erlotinib** should be taken 2 hours before or 10 hours after **H_2 receptor antagonists.** Moderate Study
- HIV-protease inhibitors are predicted to slightly increase the exposure to **erlotinib.** Use with caution and adjust dose. Moderate Study
- Idelalisib is predicted to slightly increase the exposure to **erlotinib.** Use with caution and adjust dose. Moderate Study
- Imatinib is predicted to increase the exposure to **erlotinib.** Moderate Theoretical

- Lapatinib is predicted to increase the exposure to **erlotinib**. Moderate Theoretical
- Macrolides (**azithromycin, erythromycin**) are predicted to increase the exposure to **erlotinib**. Moderate Theoretical
- Macrolides (**clarithromycin**) are predicted to slightly increase the exposure to **erlotinib**. Use with caution and adjust dose. Moderate Study
- **Mexiletine** slightly increases the exposure to **erlotinib**. Monitor side effects and adjust dose. Moderate Study
- **Mitotane** is predicted to decrease the exposure to **erlotinib**. Avoid or adjust **erlotinib** dose. Severe Study
- **Netupitant** is predicted to increase the exposure to **erlotinib**. Moderate Theoretical
- **Nevirapine** is predicted to decrease the exposure to **erlotinib**. Severe Theoretical
- **Nilotinib** is predicted to increase the exposure to **erlotinib**. Moderate Theoretical
- **Erlotinib** is predicted to increase the risk of gastrointestinal perforation when given with **NSAIDs**. Severe Theoretical
- **Erlotinib** is predicted to increase the risk of bleeding events when given with **phenindione**. Severe Theoretical
- **Proton pump inhibitors** are predicted to slightly decrease the exposure to **erlotinib**. Avoid. Moderate Study
- Quinolones (**ciprofloxacin**) slightly increase the exposure to **erlotinib**. Monitor side effects and adjust dose. Moderate Study
- **Ranolazine** is predicted to increase the exposure to **erlotinib**. Moderate Theoretical
- **Rifampicin** is predicted to decrease the exposure to **erlotinib**. Avoid or adjust **erlotinib** dose. Severe Study
- **Sodium zirconium cyclosilicate** is predicted to decrease the exposure to **erlotinib**. Separate administration by at least 2 hours. Moderate Theoretical
- SSRIs (**fluvoxamine**) are predicted to increase the exposure to **erlotinib**. Monitor side effects and adjust dose. Moderate Theoretical
- **St John's Wort** is predicted to decrease the exposure to **erlotinib**. Severe Theoretical
- **Vemurafenib** is predicted to increase the exposure to **erlotinib**. Moderate Theoretical

Ertapenem → see carbapenems

Ertugliflozin → see TABLE 14 p. 910 (antidiabetic drugs), TABLE 8 p. 908 (hypotension)

Erythromycin → see macrolides

Escitalopram → see SSRIs

Esketamine → see TABLE 8 p. 908 (hypotension), TABLE 11 p. 909 (CNS depressant effects)

- **Esketamine** is predicted to increase the risk of seizures when given with **aminophylline**. Avoid. Severe Theoretical
- Antiepileptics (**carbamazepine, fosphenytoin, phenobarbital, phenytoin, primidone**) are predicted to decrease the exposure to **esketamine**. Adjust dose. Moderate Theoretical → Also see TABLE 11 p. 909
- Antifungals, azoles (**itraconazole, ketoconazole, voriconazole**) are predicted to increase the exposure to **esketamine**. Adjust dose. Moderate Study
- **Apalutamide** is predicted to decrease the exposure to **esketamine**. Adjust dose. Moderate Theoretical
- **Cobicistat** is predicted to increase the exposure to **esketamine**. Adjust dose. Moderate Study
- **Enzalutamide** is predicted to decrease the exposure to **esketamine**. Adjust dose. Moderate Theoretical
- **Esketamine** is predicted to increase the risk of elevated blood pressure when given with **ergometrine**. Avoid. Severe Theoretical
- **HIV-protease inhibitors** are predicted to increase the exposure to **esketamine**. Adjust dose. Moderate Study
- **Idelalisib** is predicted to increase the exposure to **esketamine**. Adjust dose. Moderate Study
- Macrolides (**clarithromycin**) are predicted to increase the exposure to **esketamine**. Adjust dose. Moderate Study
- **Mitotane** is predicted to decrease the exposure to **esketamine**. Adjust dose. Moderate Theoretical
- **Rifampicin** is predicted to decrease the exposure to **esketamine**. Adjust dose. Moderate Theoretical
- **Esketamine** is predicted to increase the risk of seizures when given with **theophylline**. Avoid. Severe Theoretical

Eslicarbazepine → see antiepileptics

Esmolol → see beta blockers, selective

Esomeprazole → see proton pump inhibitors

Estramustine → see alkylating agents

Etanercept

- **Anakinra** is predicted to increase the risk of generalised infection (possibly life-threatening) when given with **etanercept**. Avoid. Severe Theoretical
- **Live vaccines** are predicted to increase the risk of generalised infection (possibly life-threatening) when given with **etanercept**. Public Health England advises avoid (refer to Green Book). Severe Theoretical

Etelcalcetide

- **Cinacalcet** increases the risk of hypocalcaemia when given with **etelcalcetide**. Avoid. Severe Theoretical

Ethambutol

- **Isoniazid** increases the risk of optic neuropathy when given with **ethambutol**. Severe Anecdotal

Ethosuximide → see antiepileptics

Etodolac → see NSAIDs

Etomidate → see TABLE 8 p. 908 (hypotension), TABLE 11 p. 909 (CNS depressant effects)

Etonogestrel

- Antiepileptics (**carbamazepine, eslicarbazepine, fosphenytoin, oxcarbazepine, perampanel, phenobarbital, phenytoin, primidone, rufinamide, topiramate**) are predicted to decrease the efficacy of **etonogestrel**. For FSRH guidance, see Contraceptives, interactions p. 536. Severe Theoretical
- **Aprepitant** is predicted to decrease the efficacy of **etonogestrel**. For FSRH guidance, see Contraceptives, interactions p. 536. Severe Theoretical
- **Bosentan** is predicted to decrease the efficacy of **etonogestrel**. For FSRH guidance, see Contraceptives, interactions p. 536. Severe Theoretical
- **Efavirenz** is predicted to decrease the efficacy of **etonogestrel**. For FSRH guidance, see Contraceptives, interactions p. 536. Severe Theoretical
- **Fosaprepitant** is predicted to decrease the efficacy of **etonogestrel**. For FSRH guidance, see Contraceptives, interactions p. 536. Severe Theoretical
- **Griseofulvin** decreases the efficacy of **etonogestrel**. For FSRH guidance, see Contraceptives, interactions p. 536. Severe Anecdotal
- HIV-protease inhibitors (**ritonavir**) are predicted to decrease the efficacy of **etonogestrel**. For FSRH guidance, see Contraceptives, interactions p. 536. Severe Theoretical
- **Modafinil** is predicted to decrease the efficacy of **etonogestrel**. For FSRH guidance, see Contraceptives, interactions p. 536. Severe Theoretical
- **Nevirapine** is predicted to decrease the efficacy of **etonogestrel**. For FSRH guidance, see Contraceptives, interactions p. 536. Severe Theoretical
- **Rifabutin** is predicted to decrease the efficacy of **etonogestrel**. For FSRH guidance, see Contraceptives, interactions p. 536. Severe Theoretical
- **Rifampicin** is predicted to decrease the efficacy of **etonogestrel**. For FSRH guidance, see Contraceptives, interactions p. 536. Severe Theoretical
- **St John's Wort** is predicted to decrease the efficacy of **etonogestrel**. MHRA advises avoid. For FSRH guidance, see Contraceptives, interactions p. 536. Severe Theoretical
- **Sugammadex** is predicted to decrease the efficacy of **etonogestrel**. Use additional contraceptive precautions. Severe Theoretical
- **Ulipristal** is predicted to decrease the efficacy of **etonogestrel**. Avoid. Severe Theoretical

Etoposide → see TABLE 15 p. 910 (myelosuppression)

- Antiepileptics (**carbamazepine, fosphenytoin, phenobarbital, phenytoin, primidone**) are predicted to decrease the efficacy of **etoposide**. Moderate Study
- **Ciclosporin** increases the exposure to **etoposide**. Monitor and adjust dose. Severe Study

Etoposide (continued)

- ▶ **Live vaccines** are predicted to increase the risk of generalised infection (possibly life-threatening) when given with **etoposide**. Public Health England advises avoid (refer to Green Book). Severe Theoretical
- ▶ **Netupitant** slightly increases the exposure to **etoposide**. Moderate Study

Etoricoxib → see NSAIDs

Etravirine

- ▶ Antiepileptics (**carbamazepine, fosphenytoin, phenobarbital, phenytoin, primidone**) are predicted to decrease the exposure to **etravirine**. Avoid. Severe Theoretical
- ▶ **Etravirine** decreases the exposure to antimalarials (**artemether**). Moderate Study
- ▶ **Apalutamide** is predicted to decrease the exposure to **etravirine**. Avoid. Severe Theoretical
- ▶ **Etravirine** is predicted to decrease the exposure to **bedaquiline**. Avoid. Severe Theoretical
- ▶ **Bosentan** is predicted to decrease the exposure to **etravirine**. Avoid. Severe Study
- ▶ **Etravirine** is predicted to decrease the exposure to **bosutinib**. Avoid. Severe Theoretical
- ▶ **Etravirine** is predicted to decrease the exposure to **brigatinib**. Avoid. Moderate Theoretical
- ▶ **Etravirine** increases the anticoagulant effect of **coumarins**. Moderate Theoretical
- ▶ **Etravirine** is predicted to decrease the exposure to **dasabuvir**. Avoid. Severe Theoretical
- ▶ **Etravirine** moderately decreases the exposure to **dolutegravir**. Avoid unless given with atazanavir, darunavir, or lopinavir (all boosted with ritonavir). Severe Study
- ▶ **Efavirenz** is predicted to decrease the exposure to **etravirine**. Avoid. Severe Study
- ▶ **Etravirine** is predicted to decrease the exposure to **elbasvir**. Avoid. Unknown Theoretical
- ▶ **Enzalutamide** is predicted to decrease the exposure to **etravirine**. Avoid. Severe Theoretical
- ▶ **Etravirine** is predicted to decrease the exposure to **grazoprevir**. Avoid. Mild Theoretical
- ▶ HIV-protease inhibitors (**tipranavir**) decrease the exposure to **etravirine**. Avoid. Severe Study
- ▶ **Etravirine** increases the exposure to HIV-protease inhibitors (**fosamprenavir**) boosted with ritonavir. Refer to specialist literature. Moderate Study
- ▶ **Etravirine** is predicted to decrease the exposure to **letermovir**. Moderate Theoretical
- ▶ **Etravirine** decreases the exposure to macrolides (**clarithromycin**) and macrolides (**clarithromycin**) slightly increase the exposure to **etravirine**. Severe Study
- ▶ **Etravirine** (with a boosted protease inhibitor) increases the exposure to **maraviroc**. Avoid or adjust dose. Moderate Study
- ▶ **Mitotane** is predicted to decrease the exposure to **etravirine**. Avoid. Severe Theoretical
- ▶ **Nevirapine** is predicted to decrease the exposure to **etravirine**. Avoid. Severe Study
- ▶ **Etravirine** is predicted to decrease the exposure to **ombitasvir**. Avoid. Severe Theoretical
- ▶ **Etravirine** is predicted to decrease the exposure to **paritaprevir**. Avoid. Severe Theoretical
- ▶ **Etravirine** moderately decreases the exposure to **phosphodiesterase type-5 inhibitors**. Adjust dose. Moderate Study
- ▶ **Rifabutin** decreases the exposure to **etravirine**. Moderate Study
- ▶ **Rifampicin** is predicted to decrease the exposure to **etravirine**. Avoid. Severe Theoretical
- ▶ **Etravirine** is predicted to decrease the exposure to **rilpivirine**. Avoid. Severe Theoretical
- ▶ **St John's Wort** is predicted to decrease the exposure to **etravirine**. Avoid. Severe Study

Everolimus → see TABLE 15 p. 910 (myelosuppression)

- ▶ **Everolimus** potentially increases the risk of angioedema when given with **ACE inhibitors**. Severe Anecdotal
- ▶ Antiarrhythmics (**dronedarone**) are predicted to increase the concentration of **everolimus**. Avoid or adjust dose. Moderate Study
- ▶ Antiepileptics (**carbamazepine, fosphenytoin, phenobarbital, phenytoin, primidone**) are predicted to decrease the concentration of **everolimus**. Avoid or adjust dose. Severe Study
- ▶ Antifungals, azoles (**fluconazole, isavuconazole, posaconazole**) are predicted to increase the concentration of **everolimus**. Avoid or adjust dose. Moderate Study
- ▶ Antifungals, azoles (**itraconazole, ketoconazole, voriconazole**) are predicted to increase the concentration of **everolimus**. Avoid. Severe Study
- ▶ **Apalutamide** is predicted to decrease the concentration of **everolimus**. Avoid or adjust dose. Severe Study
- ▶ **Aprepitant** is predicted to increase the concentration of **everolimus**. Avoid or adjust dose. Moderate Study
- ▶ **Bosentan** is predicted to decrease the concentration of **everolimus**. Avoid or adjust dose. Severe Study
- ▶ Calcium channel blockers (**diltiazem, verapamil**) are predicted to increase the concentration of **everolimus**. Avoid or adjust dose. Moderate Study
- ▶ **Ceritinib** is predicted to increase the exposure to **everolimus**. Moderate Theoretical → Also see TABLE 15 p. 910
- ▶ **Ciclosporin** moderately increases the exposure to **everolimus**. Avoid or adjust dose. Severe Study
- ▶ **Cobicistat** is predicted to increase the concentration of **everolimus**. Avoid. Severe Study
- ▶ **Crizotinib** is predicted to increase the concentration of **everolimus**. Avoid or adjust dose. Moderate Study → Also see TABLE 15 p. 910
- ▶ **Efavirenz** is predicted to decrease the concentration of **everolimus**. Avoid or adjust dose. Severe Study
- ▶ **Eliglustat** is predicted to increase the exposure to **everolimus**. Adjust dose. Moderate Study
- ▶ **Enzalutamide** is predicted to decrease the concentration of **everolimus**. Avoid or adjust dose. Severe Study
- ▶ **Grapefruit juice** is predicted to increase the exposure to **everolimus**. Avoid. Severe Theoretical
- ▶ **HIV-protease inhibitors** are predicted to increase the concentration of **everolimus**. Avoid. Severe Study
- ▶ **Idelalisib** is predicted to increase the concentration of **everolimus**. Avoid. Severe Study → Also see TABLE 15 p. 910
- ▶ **Imatinib** is predicted to increase the concentration of **everolimus**. Avoid or adjust dose. Moderate Study → Also see TABLE 15 p. 910
- ▶ **Lapatinib** is predicted to increase the exposure to **everolimus**. Moderate Theoretical
- ▶ **Letermovir** is predicted to increase the concentration of **everolimus**. Monitor and adjust dose. Severe Study
- ▶ **Live vaccines** are predicted to increase the risk of generalised infection (possibly life-threatening) when given with **everolimus**. Public Health England advises avoid (refer to Green Book). Severe Theoretical
- ▶ **Everolimus** is predicted to increase the exposure to **lomitapide**. Separate administration by 12 hours. Moderate Theoretical
- ▶ **Lumacaftor** is predicted to decrease the exposure to **everolimus**. Avoid. Severe Theoretical
- ▶ Macrolides (**clarithromycin**) are predicted to increase the concentration of **everolimus**. Avoid. Severe Study
- ▶ Macrolides (**erythromycin**) are predicted to increase the concentration of **everolimus**. Avoid or adjust dose. Moderate Study
- ▶ **Mirabegron** is predicted to increase the exposure to **everolimus**. Mild Theoretical
- ▶ **Mitotane** is predicted to decrease the concentration of **everolimus**. Avoid or adjust dose. Severe Study → Also see TABLE 15 p. 910
- ▶ **Neratinib** is predicted to increase the exposure to **everolimus**. Moderate Study
- ▶ **Netupitant** is predicted to increase the concentration of **everolimus**. Avoid or adjust dose. Moderate Study
- ▶ **Nevirapine** is predicted to decrease the concentration of **everolimus**. Avoid or adjust dose. Severe Study
- ▶ **Nilotinib** is predicted to increase the concentration of **everolimus**. Avoid or adjust dose. Moderate Study → Also see TABLE 15 p. 910
- ▶ **Palbociclib** is predicted to increase the exposure to **everolimus**. Adjust dose. Moderate Theoretical

- Pibrentasvir (with glecaprevir) is predicted to increase the exposure to **everolimus**. Moderate Study
- Pitolisant is predicted to decrease the exposure to **everolimus**. Avoid. Severe Theoretical
- Ribociclib is predicted to increase the exposure to **everolimus**. Use with caution and adjust dose. Moderate Theoretical
- Rifampicin is predicted to decrease the concentration of **everolimus**. Avoid or adjust dose. Severe Study
- St John's Wort is predicted to decrease the concentration of **everolimus**. Avoid or adjust dose. Severe Study
- Velpatasvir is predicted to increase the exposure to **everolimus**. Severe Theoretical
- Venetoclax is predicted to increase the exposure to **everolimus**. Avoid or adjust dose. Severe Study

Exemestane
- Antiepileptics (carbamazepine, fosphenytoin, phenobarbital, phenytoin, primidone) moderately decrease the exposure to **exemestane**. Moderate Study
- Apalutamide moderately decreases the exposure to **exemestane**. Moderate Study
- Enzalutamide moderately decreases the exposure to **exemestane**. Moderate Study
- Mitotane moderately decreases the exposure to **exemestane**. Moderate Study
- Rifampicin moderately decreases the exposure to **exemestane**. Moderate Study
- St John's Wort is predicted to decrease the exposure to **exemestane**. Moderate Theoretical

Exenatide → see TABLE 14 p. 910 (antidiabetic drugs)

SEPARATION OF ADMINISTRATION With standard-release exenatide: some orally administered drugs should be taken at least 1 hour before, or 4 hours after, exenatide injection.

Ezetimibe
- Ciclosporin moderately increases the exposure to **ezetimibe** and **ezetimibe** slightly increases the exposure to ciclosporin. Moderate Study
- Fibrates are predicted to increase the risk of gallstones when given with **ezetimibe**. Severe Theoretical
- **Ezetimibe** potentially increases the risk of rhabdomyolysis when given with statins. Severe Anecdotal

Famotidine → see H_2 receptor antagonists

Fampridine
- H_2 receptor antagonists (cimetidine) increase the concentration of **fampridine**. Avoid. Severe Theoretical

Febuxostat
- **Febuxostat** is predicted to increase the exposure to azathioprine. Avoid. Severe Theoretical
- **Febuxostat** is predicted to increase the exposure to mercaptopurine. Avoid. Severe Theoretical

Felbinac → see NSAIDs
Felodipine → see calcium channel blockers
Fenofibrate → see fibrates
Fentanyl → see opioids
Ferric carboxymaltose → see iron (injectable)
Ferric maltol → see iron (oral)
Ferrous fumarate → see iron (oral)
Ferrous gluconate → see iron (oral)
Ferrous sulfate → see iron (oral)
Fesoterodine → see TABLE 10 p. 909 (antimuscarinics)
- Antiarrhythmics (dronedarone) are predicted to increase the exposure to **fesoterodine**. Adjust **fesoterodine** dose with moderate inhibitors of CYP3A4 in hepatic and renal impairment. Mild Study
- Antiepileptics (carbamazepine, fosphenytoin, phenobarbital, phenytoin, primidone) are predicted to decrease the exposure to **fesoterodine**. Avoid. Moderate Study
- Antifungals, azoles (fluconazole, isavuconazole, posaconazole) are predicted to increase the exposure to **fesoterodine**. Adjust **fesoterodine** dose with moderate inhibitors of CYP3A4 in hepatic and renal impairment. Mild Study
- Antifungals, azoles (itraconazole, ketoconazole, voriconazole) are predicted to moderately increase the exposure to **fesoterodine**. Adjust **fesoterodine** dose with potent inhibitors of CYP3A4; avoid in hepatic and renal impairment. Severe Study
- Apalutamide is predicted to decrease the exposure to **fesoterodine**. Avoid. Moderate Study
- Aprepitant is predicted to increase the exposure to **fesoterodine**. Adjust **fesoterodine** dose with moderate inhibitors of CYP3A4 in hepatic and renal impairment. Mild Study
- Calcium channel blockers (diltiazem, verapamil) are predicted to increase the exposure to **fesoterodine**. Adjust **fesoterodine** dose with moderate inhibitors of CYP3A4 in hepatic and renal impairment. Mild Study
- Cobicistat is predicted to moderately increase the exposure to **fesoterodine**. Adjust **fesoterodine** dose with potent inhibitors of CYP3A4; avoid in hepatic and renal impairment. Severe Study
- Crizotinib is predicted to increase the exposure to **fesoterodine**. Adjust **fesoterodine** dose with moderate inhibitors of CYP3A4 in hepatic and renal impairment. Mild Study
- Enzalutamide is predicted to decrease the exposure to **fesoterodine**. Avoid. Moderate Study
- HIV-protease inhibitors are predicted to moderately increase the exposure to **fesoterodine**. Adjust **fesoterodine** dose with potent inhibitors of CYP3A4; avoid in hepatic and renal impairment. Severe Study
- Idelalisib is predicted to moderately increase the exposure to **fesoterodine**. Adjust **fesoterodine** dose with potent inhibitors of CYP3A4; avoid in hepatic and renal impairment. Severe Study
- Imatinib is predicted to increase the exposure to **fesoterodine**. Adjust **fesoterodine** dose with moderate inhibitors of CYP3A4 in hepatic and renal impairment. Mild Study
- Macrolides (clarithromycin) are predicted to moderately increase the exposure to **fesoterodine**. Adjust **fesoterodine** dose with potent inhibitors of CYP3A4; avoid in hepatic and renal impairment. Severe Study
- Macrolides (erythromycin) are predicted to increase the exposure to **fesoterodine**. Adjust **fesoterodine** dose with moderate inhibitors of CYP3A4 in hepatic and renal impairment. Mild Study
- Mitotane is predicted to decrease the exposure to **fesoterodine**. Avoid. Moderate Study
- Netupitant is predicted to increase the exposure to **fesoterodine**. Adjust **fesoterodine** dose with moderate inhibitors of CYP3A4 in hepatic and renal impairment. Mild Study
- Nilotinib is predicted to increase the exposure to **fesoterodine**. Adjust **fesoterodine** dose with moderate inhibitors of CYP3A4 in hepatic and renal impairment. Mild Study
- Rifampicin is predicted to decrease the exposure to **fesoterodine**. Avoid. Moderate Study
- St John's Wort is predicted to decrease the exposure to **fesoterodine**. Avoid. Severe Theoretical

Fexofenadine → see antihistamines, non-sedating

Fibrates

bezafibrate · ciprofibrate · fenofibrate · gemfibrozil

- Antacids slightly to moderately decrease the exposure to **gemfibrozil**. Moderate Study
- **Gemfibrozil** is predicted to increase the exposure to apalutamide. Mild Study
- **Bezafibrate** is predicted to increase the risk of nephrotoxicity when given with ciclosporin. Severe Theoretical
- **Fenofibrate** increases the risk of nephrotoxicity when given with ciclosporin. Severe Study
- Colchicine increases the risk of rhabdomyolysis when given with **fibrates**. Severe Anecdotal
- **Fibrates** are predicted to increase the anticoagulant effect of coumarins. Monitor INR and adjust dose. Severe Study
- **Gemfibrozil** is predicted to increase the exposure to dabrafenib. Moderate Theoretical
- **Fibrates** are predicted to increase the risk of rhabdomyolysis when given with daptomycin. Severe Theoretical
- **Gemfibrozil** is predicted to very markedly increase the exposure to dasabuvir. Avoid. Severe Study
- **Gemfibrozil** moderately increases the exposure to enzalutamide. Avoid or adjust **enzalutamide** dose. Severe Study

Fibrates (continued)

- **Fibrates** are predicted to increase the risk of gallstones when given with **ezetimibe**. Severe Theoretical
- **Fibrates** are predicted to increase the risk of hypoglycaemia when given with **insulins**. Moderate Theoretical
- **Gemfibrozil** is predicted to increase the exposure to **irinotecan**. Avoid. Moderate Theoretical
- **Gemfibrozil** is predicted to increase the concentration of **letermovir**. Moderate Study
- **Gemfibrozil** is predicted to moderately increase the exposure to **montelukast**. Moderate Study
- **Fibrates** are predicted to increase the anticoagulant effect of **phenindione**. Monitor INR and adjust dose. Severe Study
- **Gemfibrozil** increases the exposure to **pioglitazone**. Monitor blood glucose and adjust dose. Severe Study
- **Gemfibrozil** increases the exposure to **repaglinide**. Avoid. Severe Study
- **Gemfibrozil** is predicted to increase the exposure to retinoids **(alitretinoin)**. Adjust **alitretinoin** dose. Moderate Theoretical
- **Gemfibrozil** increases the concentration of retinoids **(bexarotene)**. Avoid. Severe Study
- **Gemfibrozil** increases the exposure to **selexipag**. Avoid. Severe Study
- **Ciprofibrate** increases the risk of rhabdomyolysis when given with statins **(atorvastatin)**. Avoid or adjust dose. Severe Study
- **Bezafibrate** increases the risk of rhabdomyolysis when given with statins **(atorvastatin, fluvastatin)**. Severe Study
- **Fenofibrate** increases the risk of rhabdomyolysis when given with statins **(atorvastatin, simvastatin)**. Adjust **fenofibrate** dose, p. 138. Severe Anecdotal
- **Ciprofibrate** increases the risk of rhabdomyolysis when given with statins **(fluvastatin)**. Severe Study
- **Fenofibrate** is predicted to increase the risk of rhabdomyolysis when given with statins **(fluvastatin)**. Adjust **fenofibrate** dose, p. 138. Severe Theoretical
- **Fenofibrate** is predicted to increase the risk of rhabdomyolysis when given with statins **(pravastatin)**. Avoid. Severe Theoretical
- Fibrates **(bezafibrate, ciprofibrate)** increase the risk of rhabdomyolysis when given with statins **(pravastatin)**. Avoid. Severe Study
- **Fenofibrate** increases the risk of rhabdomyolysis when given with statins **(rosuvastatin)**. Adjust **fenofibrate** and **rosuvastatin** doses, p. 138, p. 140. Severe Anecdotal
- Fibrates **(bezafibrate, ciprofibrate)** increase the risk of rhabdomyolysis when given with statins **(rosuvastatin)**. Adjust **rosuvastatin** dose, p. 140. Severe Study
- Fibrates **(bezafibrate, ciprofibrate)** increase the risk of rhabdomyolysis when given with statins **(simvastatin)**. Adjust **simvastatin** dose, p. 141. Severe Study
- **Gemfibrozil** increases the risk of rhabdomyolysis when given with **statins**. Avoid. Severe Anecdotal
- **Fibrates** are predicted to increase the risk of hypoglycaemia when given with **sulfonylureas**. Moderate Theoretical
- **Gemfibrozil** is predicted to increase the concentration of taxanes **(paclitaxel)**. Severe Anecdotal
- **Fibrates** are predicted to decrease the efficacy of **ursodeoxycholic acid**. Avoid. Severe Theoretical

Fidaxomicin

- Antiarrhythmics **(amiodarone, dronedarone)** are predicted to increase the exposure to **fidaxomicin**. Avoid. Moderate Study
- Antifungals, azoles **(itraconazole, ketoconazole)** are predicted to increase the exposure to **fidaxomicin**. Avoid. Moderate Study
- Calcium channel blockers **(verapamil)** are predicted to increase the exposure to **fidaxomicin**. Avoid. Moderate Study
- **Ciclosporin** is predicted to increase the exposure to **fidaxomicin**. Avoid. Moderate Study
- HIV-protease inhibitors **(lopinavir, ritonavir, saquinavir)** are predicted to increase the exposure to **fidaxomicin**. Avoid. Moderate Study
- **Lapatinib** is predicted to increase the exposure to **fidaxomicin**. Avoid. Moderate Study
- **Macrolides** are predicted to increase the exposure to **fidaxomicin**. Avoid. Moderate Study
- **Ranolazine** is predicted to increase the exposure to **fidaxomicin**. Avoid. Moderate Study
- **Vemurafenib** is predicted to increase the exposure to **fidaxomicin**. Avoid. Moderate Study

Fingolimod → see TABLE 6 p. 908 (bradycardia), TABLE 9 p. 909 (QT-interval prolongation)

- Antiepileptics **(carbamazepine, fosphenytoin, phenobarbital, phenytoin, primidone)** are predicted to decrease the exposure to **fingolimod**. Moderate Study
- **Apalutamide** is predicted to decrease the exposure to **fingolimod**. Moderate Study
- Calcium channel blockers **(diltiazem, verapamil)** are predicted to increase the exposure to **fingolimod**. Avoid. Moderate Theoretical → Also see TABLE 6 p. 908
- **Enzalutamide** is predicted to decrease the exposure to **fingolimod**. Moderate Study
- **Live vaccines** are predicted to increase the risk of generalised infection (possibly life-threatening) when given with **fingolimod**. Public Health England advises avoid (refer to Green Book). Severe Theoretical
- **Mitotane** is predicted to decrease the exposure to **fingolimod**. Moderate Study
- **Rifampicin** is predicted to decrease the exposure to **fingolimod**. Moderate Study
- **St John's Wort** is predicted to decrease the exposure to **fingolimod**. Avoid. Moderate Theoretical

Flavoxate → see TABLE 10 p. 909 (antimuscarinics)

Flecainide → see antiarrhythmics

Flucloxacillin → see penicillins

Fluconazole → see antifungals, azoles

Flucytosine

- **Amphotericin** increases the risk of toxicity when given with **flucytosine**. Severe Study
- **Cytarabine** decreases the concentration of **flucytosine**. Avoid. Severe Study
- **Zidovudine** increases the risk of haematological toxicity when given with **flucytosine**. Monitor and adjust dose. Severe Theoretical

Fludarabine → see TABLE 15 p. 910 (myelosuppression)

- **Live vaccines** are predicted to increase the risk of generalised infection (possibly life-threatening) when given with **fludarabine**. Public Health England advises avoid (refer to Green Book). Severe Theoretical
- **Fludarabine** increases the risk of pulmonary toxicity when given with **pentostatin**. Avoid. Severe Study → Also see TABLE 15 p. 910

Fludrocortisone → see corticosteroids

Fluocinolone

- With intravitreal use in adults: caution with concurrent administration of anticoagulant or antiplatelet drugs (higher incidence of conjunctival haemorrhage).
- Interactions do not generally apply to corticosteroids used for topical action unless specified.

Fluorouracil → see TABLE 15 p. 910 (myelosuppression), TABLE 5 p. 907 (thromboembolism)

ROUTE-SPECIFIC INFORMATION Since systemic absorption can follow topical application, the possibility of interactions should be borne in mind.

- **Fluorouracil** increases the concentration of antiepileptics **(fosphenytoin, phenytoin)**. Monitor concentration and adjust dose. Severe Anecdotal
- **Fluorouracil** increases the anticoagulant effect of **coumarins**. Severe Anecdotal
- Folates **(folic acid)** are predicted to increase the risk of toxicity when given with **fluorouracil**. Avoid. Severe Theoretical
- Folates **(folinic acid)** are predicted to increase the risk of toxicity when given with **fluorouracil**. Monitor and adjust dose. Severe Theoretical
- H_2 receptor antagonists **(cimetidine)** slightly increase the exposure to **fluorouracil**. Severe Study
- **Live vaccines** are predicted to increase the risk of generalised infection (possibly life-threatening) when given with **fluorouracil**. Public Health England advises avoid (refer to Green Book). Severe Theoretical

A1 Interactions | Appendix 1

▸ Methotrexate potentially increases the risk of severe skin reaction when given with topical **fluorouracil**. [Severe] Anecdotal → Also see **TABLE 15** p. 910 → Also see **TABLE 5** p. 907
▸ Metronidazole increases the risk of toxicity when given with **fluorouracil**. [Severe] Study

Fluoxetine → see SSRIs

Flupentixol → see **TABLE 8** p. 908 (hypotension), **TABLE 11** p. 909 (CNS depressant effects)
▸ **Flupentixol** is predicted to decrease the effects of **dopamine receptor agonists**. Avoid. [Moderate] Theoretical → Also see **TABLE 8** p. 908
▸ **Flupentixol** decreases the effects of levodopa. Avoid or monitor worsening parkinsonian symptoms. [Severe] Theoretical → Also see **TABLE 8** p. 908

Fluphenazine → see phenothiazines

Flurazepam → see **TABLE 11** p. 909 (CNS depressant effects)
▸ HIV-protease inhibitors (**ritonavir**) are predicted to increase the exposure to **flurazepam**. Avoid. [Moderate] Theoretical

Flurbiprofen → see NSAIDs

Fluticasone → see corticosteroids

Fluvastatin → see statins

Fluvoxamine → see SSRIs

Folates

folic acid · folinic acid · levofolinic acid

▸ **Folates** are predicted to decrease the concentration of antiepileptics (**fosphenytoin, phenobarbital, phenytoin, primidone**). Monitor concentration and adjust dose. [Severe] Study
▸ **Folates** are predicted to increase the risk of toxicity when given with **capecitabine**. [Severe] Anecdotal
▸ **Folic acid** is predicted to increase the risk of toxicity when given with **fluorouracil**. Avoid. [Severe] Theoretical
▸ **Folinic acid** is predicted to increase the risk of toxicity when given with **fluorouracil**. Monitor and adjust dose. [Severe] Theoretical
▸ **Folates** are predicted to alter the effects of **raltitrexed**. Avoid. [Moderate] Study
▸ Sulfasalazine is predicted to decrease the absorption of **folates**. [Moderate] Study
▸ **Folates** are predicted to increase the risk of toxicity when given with **tegafur**. [Severe] Theoretical

Folic acid → see folates

Folinic acid → see folates

Fondaparinux → see **TABLE 3** p. 907 (anticoagulant effects)

Formoterol → see $beta_2$ agonists

Fosamprenavir → see HIV-protease inhibitors

Fosaprepitant
▸ **Fosaprepitant** is predicted to increase the exposure to alkylating agents (**ifosfamide**). [Severe] Theoretical
▸ **Fosaprepitant** is predicted to increase the exposure to **alprazolam**. [Moderate] Study
▸ Antiepileptics (**carbamazepine, fosphenytoin, phenobarbital, phenytoin, primidone**) are predicted to decrease the exposure to **fosaprepitant**. Avoid. [Moderate] Theoretical
▸ Antifungals, azoles (**itraconazole, ketoconazole, voriconazole**) are predicted to increase the exposure to **fosaprepitant**. [Moderate] Theoretical
▸ Antifungals, azoles (**posaconazole**) are predicted to increase the exposure to **fosaprepitant**. [Moderate] Study
▸ Apalutamide is predicted to decrease the exposure to **fosaprepitant**. Avoid. [Moderate] Theoretical
▸ Bosentan is predicted to decrease the exposure to **fosaprepitant**. [Moderate] Theoretical
▸ **Fosaprepitant** is predicted to increase the exposure to **bosutinib**. [Severe] Theoretical
▸ Cobicistat is predicted to increase the exposure to **fosaprepitant**. [Moderate] Theoretical
▸ **Fosaprepitant** is predicted to decrease the efficacy of **combined hormonal contraceptives**. For FSRH guidance, see Contraceptives, interactions p. 536. [Severe] Study
▸ **Fosaprepitant** is predicted to decrease the anticoagulant effect of **coumarins**. [Moderate] Theoretical
▸ **Fosaprepitant** is predicted to decrease the efficacy of **desogestrel**. For FSRH guidance, see Contraceptives, interactions p. 536. [Severe] Theoretical
▸ Efavirenz is predicted to decrease the exposure to **fosaprepitant**. [Moderate] Theoretical
▸ Enzalutamide is predicted to decrease the exposure to **fosaprepitant**. Avoid. [Moderate] Theoretical
▸ **Fosaprepitant** is predicted to decrease the efficacy of **etonogestrel**. For FSRH guidance, see Contraceptives, interactions p. 536. [Severe] Theoretical
▸ **Fosaprepitant** is predicted to increase the concentration of **guanfacine**. [Moderate] Theoretical
▸ HIV-protease inhibitors are predicted to increase the exposure to **fosaprepitant**. [Moderate] Theoretical
▸ **Fosaprepitant** is predicted to decrease the effects of **hormone replacement therapy**. [Moderate] Anecdotal
▸ **Fosaprepitant** is predicted to slightly increase the exposure to **ibrutinib**. [Moderate] Theoretical
▸ Idelalisib is predicted to increase the exposure to **fosaprepitant**. [Moderate] Theoretical
▸ **Fosaprepitant** is predicted to increase the exposure to intravenous **irinotecan**. [Severe] Theoretical
▸ **Fosaprepitant** is predicted to decrease the efficacy of **levonorgestrel**. For FSRH guidance, see Contraceptives, interactions p. 536. [Severe] Theoretical
▸ **Fosaprepitant** is predicted to increase the exposure to **lomitapide**. Separate administration by 12 hours. [Moderate] Theoretical
▸ Macrolides (**clarithromycin**) are predicted to increase the exposure to **fosaprepitant**. [Moderate] Theoretical
▸ **Fosaprepitant** slightly increases the exposure to **midazolam**. [Moderate] Study
▸ Mitotane is predicted to decrease the exposure to **fosaprepitant**. Avoid. [Moderate] Theoretical
▸ Nevirapine is predicted to decrease the exposure to **fosaprepitant**. [Moderate] Theoretical
▸ **Fosaprepitant** is predicted to decrease the efficacy of **norethisterone**. For FSRH guidance, see Contraceptives, interactions p. 536. [Severe] Anecdotal
▸ **Fosaprepitant** is predicted to increase the exposure to **pimozide**. Avoid. [Severe] Theoretical
▸ Rifampicin is predicted to decrease the exposure to **fosaprepitant**. Avoid. [Moderate] Theoretical
▸ St John's Wort is predicted to decrease the exposure to **fosaprepitant**. Avoid. [Moderate] Theoretical
▸ **Fosaprepitant** decreases the efficacy of **ulipristal**. For FSRH guidance, see Contraceptives, interactions p. 536. [Severe] Anecdotal
▸ **Fosaprepitant** is predicted to increase the exposure to **vinca alkaloids**. [Severe] Theoretical

Foscarnet → see **TABLE 2** p. 907 (nephrotoxicity)
▸ **Foscarnet** increases the risk of hypocalcaemia when given with **pentamidine**. [Severe] Anecdotal → Also see **TABLE 2** p. 907

Fosinopril → see ACE inhibitors

Fosphenytoin → see antiepileptics

Frovatriptan → see **TABLE 13** p. 910 (serotonin syndrome)
▸ **Frovatriptan** is predicted to increase the risk of vasoconstriction when given with **ergotamine**. Separate administration by 24 hours. [Severe] Theoretical
▸ SSRIs (**fluvoxamine**) increase the concentration of **frovatriptan**. [Severe] Study → Also see **TABLE 13** p. 910

Fulvestrant → see **TABLE 5** p. 907 (thromboembolism)

Furosemide → see loop diuretics

Fusidate
▸ **Fusidate** increases the risk of rhabdomyolysis when given with **statins**. Avoid. [Severe] Anecdotal

Gabapentin → see antiepileptics

Galantamine → see anticholinesterases, centrally acting

Ganciclovir → see **TABLE 15** p. 910 (myelosuppression), **TABLE 2** p. 907 (nephrotoxicity)

ROUTE-SPECIFIC INFORMATION Since systemic absorption can follow topical application, the possibility of interactions should be borne in mind.

▸ **Ganciclovir** is predicted to increase the risk of seizures when given with carbapenems (**imipenem**). Avoid. [Severe] Anecdotal
▸ Leflunomide is predicted to increase the exposure to **ganciclovir**. [Moderate] Theoretical → Also see **TABLE 15** p. 910

Ganciclovir (continued)
- **Mycophenolate** is predicted to increase the risk of haematological toxicity when given with **ganciclovir**. Moderate Theoretical → Also see **TABLE 15** p. 910
- **Nitisinone** is predicted to increase the exposure to **ganciclovir**. Moderate Study
- **Teriflunomide** is predicted to increase the exposure to **ganciclovir**. Moderate Study

Gefitinib → see **TABLE 15** p. 910 (myelosuppression)
- **Antacids** are predicted to slightly decrease the exposure to **gefitinib**. Moderate Theoretical
- Antiarrhythmics **(dronedarone)** are predicted to increase the exposure to **gefitinib**. Moderate Theoretical
- Antiepileptics **(carbamazepine, fosphenytoin, phenobarbital, phenytoin, primidone)** are predicted to decrease the exposure to **gefitinib**. Avoid. Severe Study
- Antifungals, azoles **(fluconazole, isavuconazole, posaconazole)** are predicted to increase the exposure to **gefitinib**. Moderate Theoretical
- Antifungals, azoles **(itraconazole, ketoconazole, voriconazole)** are predicted to increase the exposure to **gefitinib**. Moderate Study
- **Apalutamide** is predicted to decrease the exposure to **gefitinib**. Avoid. Severe Study
- **Aprepitant** is predicted to increase the exposure to **gefitinib**. Moderate Theoretical
- **Bosentan** is predicted to decrease the exposure to **gefitinib**. Avoid. Severe Theoretical
- Calcium channel blockers **(diltiazem, verapamil)** are predicted to increase the exposure to **gefitinib**. Moderate Theoretical
- **Cobicistat** is predicted to increase the exposure to **gefitinib**. Moderate Study
- **Gefitinib** is predicted to increase the anticoagulant effect of **coumarins**. Severe Anecdotal
- **Crizotinib** is predicted to increase the exposure to **gefitinib**. Moderate Theoretical → Also see **TABLE 15** p. 910
- **Efavirenz** is predicted to decrease the exposure to **gefitinib**. Avoid. Severe Theoretical
- **Enzalutamide** is predicted to decrease the exposure to **gefitinib**. Avoid. Severe Study
- H_2 **receptor antagonists** are predicted to slightly to moderately decrease the exposure to **gefitinib**. Moderate Study
- **HIV-protease inhibitors** are predicted to increase the exposure to **gefitinib**. Moderate Study
- **Idelalisib** is predicted to increase the exposure to **gefitinib**. Moderate Study → Also see **TABLE 15** p. 910
- **Imatinib** is predicted to increase the exposure to **gefitinib**. Moderate Theoretical → Also see **TABLE 15** p. 910
- Macrolides **(clarithromycin)** are predicted to increase the exposure to **gefitinib**. Moderate Study
- Macrolides **(erythromycin)** are predicted to increase the exposure to **gefitinib**. Moderate Theoretical
- **Mitotane** is predicted to decrease the exposure to **gefitinib**. Avoid. Severe Study → Also see **TABLE 15** p. 910
- **Netupitant** is predicted to increase the exposure to **gefitinib**. Moderate Theoretical
- **Nevirapine** is predicted to decrease the exposure to **gefitinib**. Avoid. Severe Theoretical
- **Nilotinib** is predicted to increase the exposure to **gefitinib**. Moderate Theoretical → Also see **TABLE 15** p. 910
- **Gefitinib** is predicted to increase the risk of bleeding events when given with **phenindione**. Severe Theoretical
- **Proton pump inhibitors** are predicted to decrease the exposure to **gefitinib**. Severe Theoretical
- **Rifampicin** is predicted to decrease the exposure to **gefitinib**. Avoid. Severe Study
- **St John's Wort** is predicted to decrease the exposure to **gefitinib**. Avoid. Severe Theoretical

Gemcitabine → see **TABLE 15** p. 910 (myelosuppression)
- **Live vaccines** are predicted to increase the risk of generalised infection (possibly life-threatening) when given with **gemcitabine**. Public Health England advises avoid (refer to Green Book). Severe Theoretical

Gemfibrozil → see fibrates

Gentamicin → see aminoglycosides

Gilteritinib
- Antiepileptics **(carbamazepine, fosphenytoin, phenytoin)** are predicted to decrease the exposure to **gilteritinib**. Avoid. Severe Study
- Antifungals, azoles **(itraconazole, ketoconazole, voriconazole)** are predicted to increase the exposure to **gilteritinib**. Moderate Study
- **Cobicistat** is predicted to increase the exposure to **gilteritinib**. Moderate Study
- **HIV-protease inhibitors** are predicted to increase the exposure to **gilteritinib**. Moderate Study
- **Idelalisib** is predicted to increase the exposure to **gilteritinib**. Moderate Study
- Macrolides **(azithromycin, erythromycin)** are predicted to increase the exposure to **gilteritinib**. Moderate Theoretical
- Macrolides **(clarithromycin)** are predicted to increase the exposure to **gilteritinib**. Moderate Study
- **Rifampicin** moderately decreases the exposure to **gilteritinib**. Avoid. Severe Study
- **Gilteritinib** is predicted to decrease the efficacy of SSRIs **(escitalopram, fluoxetine, sertraline)**. Avoid. Moderate Theoretical
- **St John's Wort** is predicted to decrease the exposure to **gilteritinib**. Avoid. Severe Study

Glecaprevir
- Antiarrhythmics **(dronedarone)** potentially increase the exposure to **glecaprevir**. Moderate Theoretical
- Antiepileptics **(carbamazepine, fosphenytoin, phenobarbital, phenytoin, primidone)** are predicted to moderately decrease the exposure to **glecaprevir**. Avoid. Severe Study
- Antiepileptics **(eslicarbazepine, oxcarbazepine)** potentially decrease the exposure to **glecaprevir**. Avoid. Severe Theoretical
- Antifungals, azoles **(itraconazole, ketoconazole)** potentially increase the exposure to **glecaprevir**. Moderate Theoretical
- **Bosentan** is predicted to decrease the exposure to **glecaprevir**. Avoid. Severe Study
- **Ciclosporin** increases the exposure to **glecaprevir**. Avoid or monitor. Severe Study
- **Cobicistat** potentially increases the exposure to **glecaprevir**. Moderate Theoretical
- **Combined hormonal contraceptives** (containing ethinylestradiol) are predicted to increase the risk of increased ALT concentrations when given with **glecaprevir**. Avoid. Severe Study
- **Crizotinib** potentially decreases the exposure to **glecaprevir**. Avoid. Severe Theoretical
- **Glecaprevir** (with pibrentasvir) increases the exposure to dabigatran. Avoid. Moderate Study
- **Glecaprevir** (with pibrentasvir) increases the exposure to digoxin. Moderate Study
- **Efavirenz** is predicted to decrease the exposure to **glecaprevir**. Avoid. Severe Study
- **Enzalutamide** is predicted to greatly decrease the concentration of **glecaprevir**. Avoid. Severe Study
- HIV-protease inhibitors **(atazanavir, darunavir, lopinavir)** boosted with ritonavir increase the exposure to **glecaprevir**. Avoid. Severe Study
- HIV-protease inhibitors **(ritonavir)** increase the exposure to **glecaprevir**. Avoid. Severe Study
- **Lumacaftor** potentially decreases the exposure to **glecaprevir**. Avoid. Severe Theoretical
- **Mitotane** is predicted to greatly decrease the concentration of **glecaprevir**. Avoid. Severe Study
- **Nevirapine** is predicted to decrease the exposure to **glecaprevir**. Avoid. Severe Study
- **Rifampicin** markedly affects the exposure to **glecaprevir**. Avoid. Severe Study
- **St John's Wort** is predicted to decrease the exposure to **glecaprevir**. Avoid. Severe Study
- **Glecaprevir** (with pibrentasvir) markedly increases the exposure to statins **(atorvastatin)**. Avoid. Severe Study
- **Glecaprevir** (with pibrentasvir) is predicted to increase the exposure to statins **(fluvastatin)**. Moderate Theoretical

- **Glecaprevir** (with pibrentasvir) increases the exposure to statins (**pravastatin**). Use with caution and adjust **pravastatin** dose. [Moderate] Study
- **Glecaprevir** (with pibrentasvir) increases the exposure to statins (**rosuvastatin**). Use with caution and adjust **rosuvastatin** dose, p. 140. [Moderate] Study
- **Glecaprevir** (with pibrentasvir) increases the exposure to statins (**simvastatin**). Avoid. [Moderate] Study
- **Glecaprevir** (with pibrentasvir) slightly increases the exposure to tacrolimus. Monitor and adjust dose. [Mild] Study

Glibenclamide → see sulfonylureas
Gliclazide → see sulfonylureas
Glimepiride → see sulfonylureas
Glipizide → see sulfonylureas
Glucagon

- **Glucagon** increases the anticoagulant effect of coumarins (**warfarin**). [Severe] Study

Glucosamine

- **Glucosamine** potentially decreases the anticoagulant effect of coumarins (**acenocoumarol**). [Moderate] Anecdotal
- **Glucosamine** potentially increases the anticoagulant effect of coumarins (**warfarin**). Avoid. [Moderate] Anecdotal

Glycerol phenylbutyrate

- Antiepileptics (**valproate**) potentially oppose the effects of **glycerol phenylbutyrate**. [Moderate] Theoretical
- Corticosteroids potentially oppose the effects of **glycerol phenylbutyrate**. [Moderate] Theoretical
- Haloperidol potentially opposes the effects of **glycerol phenylbutyrate**. [Moderate] Theoretical

Glyceryl trinitrate → see nitrates
Glycopyrronium → see TABLE 10 p. 909 (antimuscarinics)

ROUTE-SPECIFIC INFORMATION Since systemic absorption can follow topical application, the possibility of interactions should be borne in mind.

Golimumab → see monoclonal antibodies
Granisetron → see TABLE 13 p. 910 (serotonin syndrome), TABLE 9 p. 909 (QT-interval prolongation)

- Dopamine receptor agonists (**apomorphine**) are predicted to increase the risk of severe hypotension when given with **granisetron**. [Severe] Theoretical

Grapefruit juice

- **Grapefruit juice** is predicted to increase the exposure to abemaciclib. Avoid. [Moderate] Theoretical
- **Grapefruit juice** moderately decreases the exposure to aliskiren. Avoid. [Severe] Study
- **Grapefruit juice** increases the exposure to antiarrhythmics (**amiodarone**). Avoid. [Moderate] Study
- **Grapefruit juice** moderately increases the exposure to antiarrhythmics (**dronedarone**). Avoid. [Severe] Study
- **Grapefruit juice** increases the exposure to antiarrhythmics (**propafenone**). Monitor and adjust dose. [Moderate] Study
- **Grapefruit juice** slightly increases the exposure to antiepileptics (**carbamazepine**). Monitor and adjust dose. [Moderate] Study
- **Grapefruit juice** slightly decreases the exposure to antihistamines, non-sedating (**bilastine**). **Bilastine** should be taken 1 hour before or 2 hours after **grapefruit juice**. [Moderate] Study
- **Grapefruit juice** increases the exposure to antihistamines, non-sedating (**rupatadine**). Avoid. [Moderate] Study
- **Grapefruit juice** increases the exposure to antimalarials (**artemether**). [Unknown] Study
- **Grapefruit juice** is predicted to increase the concentration of antimalarials (**piperaquine**). Avoid. [Severe] Theoretical
- **Grapefruit juice** is predicted to increase the exposure to axitinib. [Moderate] Theoretical
- **Grapefruit juice** greatly decreases the exposure to beta blockers, selective (**celiprolol**). [Moderate] Study
- **Grapefruit juice** is predicted to increase the exposure to bosutinib. Avoid. [Moderate] Theoretical
- **Grapefruit juice** is predicted to increase the concentration of brigatinib. Avoid. [Severe] Study
- **Grapefruit juice** increases the exposure to **buspirone**. Avoid. [Mild] Study
- **Grapefruit juice** is predicted to increase the exposure to cabozantinib. [Moderate] Theoretical
- **Grapefruit juice** very slightly increases the exposure to calcium channel blockers (**amlodipine**). Avoid. [Mild] Study
- **Grapefruit juice** increases the exposure to calcium channel blockers (**felodipine**). Avoid. [Moderate] Study
- **Grapefruit juice** is predicted to increase the exposure to calcium channel blockers (**lercanidipine**). Avoid. [Moderate] Theoretical
- **Grapefruit juice** increases the exposure to calcium channel blockers (**nicardipine**). [Mild] Study
- **Grapefruit juice** increases the exposure to calcium channel blockers (**nifedipine, verapamil**). Avoid. [Mild] Study
- **Grapefruit juice** is predicted to increase the exposure to cariprazine. Avoid. [Moderate] Study
- **Grapefruit juice** is predicted to increase the exposure to ceritinib. Avoid. [Severe] Theoretical
- **Grapefruit juice** increases the concentration of **ciclosporin**. Avoid. [Severe] Study
- **Grapefruit juice** markedly decreases the exposure to clopidogrel. [Severe] Study
- **Grapefruit juice** is predicted to increase the exposure to cobimetinib. Avoid. [Severe] Theoretical
- **Grapefruit juice** moderately increases the exposure to oral corticosteroids (**budesonide**). Avoid. [Moderate] Study
- **Grapefruit juice** is predicted to increase the exposure to crizotinib. Avoid. [Moderate] Theoretical
- **Grapefruit juice** is predicted to increase the exposure to darifenacin. [Moderate] Study
- **Grapefruit juice** is predicted to increase the exposure to dasatinib. Avoid. [Moderate] Theoretical
- **Grapefruit juice** is predicted to increase the exposure to eliglustat. Avoid. [Severe] Theoretical
- **Grapefruit juice** is predicted to increase the exposure to encorafenib. Avoid. [Moderate] Study
- **Grapefruit juice** is predicted to increase the exposure to ergometrine. [Severe] Theoretical
- **Grapefruit juice** is predicted to increase the exposure to ergotamine. [Severe] Theoretical
- **Grapefruit juice** is predicted to increase the exposure to erlotinib. [Moderate] Theoretical
- **Grapefruit juice** is predicted to increase the exposure to everolimus. Avoid. [Severe] Theoretical
- **Grapefruit juice** is predicted to increase the exposure to guanfacine. Avoid. [Moderate] Theoretical
- **Grapefruit juice** is predicted to increase the exposure to ibrutinib. Avoid. [Moderate] Theoretical
- **Grapefruit juice** is predicted to increase the exposure to imatinib. [Moderate] Theoretical
- **Grapefruit juice** is predicted to increase the exposure to ivabradine. Avoid. [Moderate] Study
- **Grapefruit juice** is predicted to increase the exposure to ivacaftor. Avoid. [Moderate] Theoretical
- **Grapefruit juice** is predicted to increase the exposure to lapatinib. Avoid. [Moderate] Theoretical
- **Grapefruit juice** is predicted to increase the exposure to larotrectinib. Avoid. [Moderate] Theoretical
- **Grapefruit juice** is predicted to increase the exposure to lomitapide. Separate administration by 12 hours. [Moderate] Theoretical
- **Grapefruit juice** is predicted to increase the concentration of lorlatinib. Avoid. [Moderate] Theoretical
- **Grapefruit juice** is predicted to increase the exposure to lurasidone. Avoid. [Severe] Theoretical
- **Grapefruit juice** is predicted to increase the exposure to naldemedine. Avoid or monitor. [Moderate] Theoretical
- **Grapefruit juice** is predicted to increase the exposure to naloxegol. Avoid. [Moderate] Theoretical
- **Grapefruit juice** is predicted to increase the exposure to neratinib. Avoid. [Severe] Theoretical
- **Grapefruit juice** is predicted to increase the exposure to nilotinib. Avoid. [Severe] Theoretical
- **Grapefruit juice** is predicted to increase the exposure to olaparib. Avoid. [Moderate] Theoretical
- **Grapefruit juice** is predicted to increase the exposure to palbociclib. Avoid. [Severe] Theoretical
- **Grapefruit juice** is predicted to increase the exposure to pazopanib. Avoid. [Severe] Theoretical

Grapefruit juice (continued)
- **Grapefruit juice** is predicted to increase the exposure to **phosphodiesterase type-5 inhibitors**. Use with caution or avoid. Moderate Study
- **Grapefruit juice** increases the exposure to **pimozide**. Avoid. Severe Theoretical
- **Grapefruit juice** is predicted to increase the exposure to **ponatinib**. Moderate Theoretical
- **Grapefruit juice** is predicted to increase the exposure to **praziquantel**. Moderate Study
- **Grapefruit juice** is predicted to increase the exposure to **quetiapine**. Avoid. Severe Theoretical
- **Grapefruit juice** is predicted to increase the concentration of **ranolazine**. Avoid. Severe Theoretical
- **Grapefruit juice** is predicted to increase the exposure to **regorafenib**. Avoid. Moderate Theoretical
- **Grapefruit juice** is predicted to increase the exposure to **ribociclib**. Avoid. Moderate Theoretical
- **Grapefruit juice** is predicted to increase the exposure to **ruxolitinib**. Severe Theoretical
- **Grapefruit juice** is predicted to increase the exposure to **saxagliptin**. Mild Theoretical
- **Grapefruit juice** increases the concentration of **sirolimus**. Avoid. Moderate Study
- **Grapefruit juice** moderately increases the exposure to SSRIs **(sertraline)**. Avoid. Moderate Study
- **Grapefruit juice** increases the exposure to statins **(atorvastatin)**. Mild Study
- **Grapefruit juice** increases the exposure to statins **(simvastatin)**. Avoid. Severe Study
- **Grapefruit juice** is predicted to increase the exposure to **sunitinib**. Avoid. Moderate Theoretical
- **Grapefruit juice** greatly increases the concentration of **tacrolimus**. Avoid. Severe Study
- **Grapefruit juice** is predicted to increase the concentration of **temsirolimus**. Use with caution or avoid. Moderate Theoretical
- **Grapefruit juice** is predicted to increase the exposure to **tezacaftor**. Avoid. Severe Study
- **Grapefruit juice** moderately increases the exposure to **ticagrelor**. Moderate Study
- **Grapefruit juice** increases the exposure to **tolvaptan**. Avoid. Moderate Study
- **Grapefruit juice** is predicted to increase the exposure to **ulipristal**. Avoid if used for uterine fibroids. Moderate Theoretical
- **Grapefruit juice** is predicted to increase the exposure to **venetoclax**. Avoid. Severe Theoretical

Grass pollen extract

GENERAL INFORMATION Desensitising vaccines should be avoided in patients taking beta-blockers (adrenaline might be ineffective in case of a hypersensitivity reaction) or ACE inhibitors (risk of severe anaphylactoid reactions).

Grazoprevir
- Antiepileptics **(carbamazepine, fosphenytoin, phenobarbital, phenytoin, primidone)** are predicted to decrease the exposure to **grazoprevir**. Avoid. Severe Study
- Antifungals, azoles **(itraconazole, ketoconazole, voriconazole)** are predicted to moderately to markedly increase the exposure to **grazoprevir**. Avoid. Severe Study
- **Apalutamide** is predicted to decrease the exposure to **grazoprevir**. Avoid. Severe Study
- **Bosentan** is predicted to markedly decrease the exposure to **grazoprevir**. Avoid. Severe Study
- **Grazoprevir** is predicted to increase the concentration of **calcium channel blockers**. Moderate Theoretical
- **Ciclosporin** greatly increases the exposure to **grazoprevir**. Avoid. Severe Study
- **Cobicistat** is predicted to moderately to markedly increase the exposure to **grazoprevir**. Avoid. Severe Study
- **Efavirenz** is predicted to markedly decrease the exposure to **grazoprevir**. Avoid. Severe Study
- **Elvitegravir** markedly increases the exposure to **grazoprevir**. Avoid. Severe Study
- **Enzalutamide** is predicted to decrease the exposure to **grazoprevir**. Avoid. Severe Study
- **Etravirine** is predicted to decrease the exposure to **grazoprevir**. Avoid. Mild Theoretical
- **HIV-protease inhibitors** are predicted to moderately to markedly increase the exposure to **grazoprevir**. Avoid. Severe Study
- **Idelalisib** is predicted to moderately to markedly increase the exposure to **grazoprevir**. Avoid. Severe Study
- Macrolides **(clarithromycin)** are predicted to moderately to markedly increase the exposure to **grazoprevir**. Avoid. Severe Study
- **Mitotane** is predicted to decrease the exposure to **grazoprevir**. Avoid. Severe Study
- **Modafinil** is predicted to decrease the exposure to **grazoprevir**. Avoid. Severe Theoretical
- **Nevirapine** is predicted to markedly decrease the exposure to **grazoprevir**. Avoid. Severe Study
- **Rifampicin** is predicted to decrease the exposure to **grazoprevir**. Avoid. Severe Study
- **St John's Wort** is predicted to markedly decrease the exposure to **grazoprevir**. Avoid. Severe Study
- **Grazoprevir** increases the exposure to statins **(atorvastatin)**. Adjust **atorvastatin** dose, p. 139. Moderate Study
- **Grazoprevir** is predicted to increase the exposure to statins **(fluvastatin)**. Adjust **fluvastatin** dose, p. 139. Unknown Theoretical
- **Grazoprevir** increases the exposure to statins **(rosuvastatin)**. Adjust **rosuvastatin** dose, p. 140. Moderate Study
- **Grazoprevir** is predicted to increase the exposure to statins **(simvastatin)**. Adjust **simvastatin** dose, p. 141. Unknown Theoretical
- **Grazoprevir** is predicted to increase the concentration of **sunitinib**. Use with caution and adjust dose. Moderate Theoretical
- **Grazoprevir** increases the exposure to **tacrolimus**. Moderate Study

Griseofulvin

ROUTE-SPECIFIC INFORMATION Interactions do not generally apply to topical use unless specified.

- **Alcohol (beverage)** potentially causes a disulfiram-like reaction when given with **griseofulvin**. Moderate Anecdotal
- Antiepileptics **(phenobarbital, primidone)** decrease the effects of **griseofulvin**. Moderate Study
- **Griseofulvin** potentially decreases the efficacy of **combined hormonal contraceptives**. For FSRH guidance, see Contraceptives, interactions p. 536. Severe Anecdotal
- **Griseofulvin** potentially decreases the anticoagulant effect of **coumarins**. Moderate Anecdotal
- **Griseofulvin** potentially decreases the efficacy of **desogestrel**. For FSRH guidance, see Contraceptives, interactions p. 536. Severe Anecdotal
- **Griseofulvin** decreases the efficacy of **etonogestrel**. For FSRH guidance, see Contraceptives, interactions p. 536. Severe Anecdotal
- **Griseofulvin** potentially decreases the efficacy of oral **levonorgestrel**. For FSRH guidance, see Contraceptives, interactions p. 536. Severe Anecdotal
- **Griseofulvin** potentially decreases the efficacy of **norethisterone**. For FSRH guidance, see Contraceptives, interactions p. 536. Severe Anecdotal
- **Griseofulvin** potentially decreases the efficacy of **ulipristal**. For FSRH guidance, see Contraceptives, interactions p. 536. Severe Anecdotal

Guanfacine → see TABLE 8 p. 908 (hypotension), TABLE 11 p. 909 (CNS depressant effects)
- Antiarrhythmics **(dronedarone)** are predicted to increase the concentration of **guanfacine**. Adjust **guanfacine** dose, p. 247. Moderate Theoretical
- Antiepileptics **(carbamazepine, fosphenytoin, phenobarbital, phenytoin, primidone)** are predicted to decrease the concentration of **guanfacine**. Adjust **guanfacine** dose, p. 247. Moderate Study → Also see TABLE 11 p. 909
- Antiepileptics **(oxcarbazepine)** are predicted to decrease the concentration of **guanfacine**. Monitor and adjust **guanfacine** dose, p. 247. Moderate Theoretical
- **Guanfacine** increases the concentration of antiepileptics **(valproate)**. Monitor and adjust dose. Moderate Study

- Antifungals, azoles **(fluconazole, isavuconazole, posaconazole)** are predicted to increase the concentration of **guanfacine**. Adjust **guanfacine** dose, p. 247. Moderate Theoretical
- Antifungals, azoles **(itraconazole, ketoconazole, voriconazole)** are predicted to increase the exposure to **guanfacine**. Adjust **guanfacine** dose, p. 247. Moderate Study
- **Apalutamide** is predicted to decrease the concentration of **guanfacine**. Adjust **guanfacine** dose, p. 247. Moderate Study
- **Aprepitant** is predicted to increase the concentration of **guanfacine**. Adjust **guanfacine** dose, p. 247. Moderate Theoretical
- **Bosentan** is predicted to decrease the concentration of **guanfacine**. Adjust dose. Moderate Theoretical
- Calcium channel blockers **(diltiazem, verapamil)** are predicted to increase the concentration of **guanfacine**. Adjust **guanfacine** dose, p. 247. Moderate Theoretical → Also see TABLE 8 p. 908
- **Chloramphenicol** is predicted to increase the exposure to **guanfacine**. Adjust **guanfacine** dose, p. 247. Moderate Theoretical
- **Cobicistat** is predicted to increase the exposure to **guanfacine**. Adjust **guanfacine** dose, p. 247. Moderate Study
- **Crizotinib** is predicted to increase the concentration of **guanfacine**. Adjust **guanfacine** dose, p. 247. Moderate Theoretical
- **Efavirenz** is predicted to decrease the concentration of **guanfacine**. Adjust dose. Moderate Theoretical
- **Enzalutamide** is predicted to decrease the concentration of **guanfacine**. Adjust **guanfacine** dose, p. 247. Moderate Study
- **Fosaprepitant** is predicted to increase the concentration of **guanfacine**. Moderate Theoretical
- **Grapefruit juice** is predicted to increase the exposure to **guanfacine**. Avoid. Moderate Theoretical
- **HIV-protease inhibitors** are predicted to increase the exposure to **guanfacine**. Adjust **guanfacine** dose, p. 247. Moderate Study
- **Idelalisib** is predicted to increase the exposure to **guanfacine**. Adjust **guanfacine** dose, p. 247. Moderate Study
- **Imatinib** is predicted to increase the concentration of **guanfacine**. Adjust **guanfacine** dose, p. 247. Moderate Theoretical
- Macrolides **(clarithromycin)** are predicted to increase the exposure to **guanfacine**. Adjust **guanfacine** dose, p. 247. Moderate Study
- Macrolides **(erythromycin)** are predicted to increase the concentration of **guanfacine**. Adjust **guanfacine** dose, p. 247. Moderate Theoretical
- **Guanfacine** is predicted to increase the concentration of **metformin**. Moderate Theoretical
- **Mitotane** is predicted to decrease the concentration of **guanfacine**. Adjust **guanfacine** dose, p. 247. Moderate Study
- **Netupitant** is predicted to increase the concentration of **guanfacine**. Adjust **guanfacine** dose, p. 247. Moderate Theoretical
- **Nevirapine** is predicted to decrease the concentration of **guanfacine**. Adjust dose. Moderate Theoretical
- **Nilotinib** is predicted to increase the concentration of **guanfacine**. Adjust **guanfacine** dose, p. 247. Moderate Theoretical
- **Rifampicin** is predicted to decrease the concentration of **guanfacine**. Adjust **guanfacine** dose, p. 247. Moderate Study
- **St John's Wort** is predicted to decrease the concentration of **guanfacine**. Adjust dose. Moderate Theoretical

Guselkumab → see monoclonal antibodies

H_2 receptor antagonists

cimetidine · famotidine · nizatidine · ranitidine

- **Cimetidine** decreases the clearance of **albendazole**. Moderate Study
- **Cimetidine** increases the concentration of **aminophylline**. Adjust dose. Severe Study
- **Cimetidine** slightly increases the exposure to anthracyclines **(epirubicin)**. Avoid. Moderate Study
- **Cimetidine** increases the exposure to antiarrhythmics **(amiodarone)**. Moderate Study
- **Cimetidine** slightly increases the exposure to antiarrhythmics **(flecainide)**. Monitor and adjust dose. Mild Study
- **Cimetidine** increases the exposure to antiarrhythmics **(lidocaine)**. Monitor and adjust dose. Moderate Study
- **Cimetidine** is predicted to increase the exposure to antiarrhythmics **(propafenone)**. Monitor and adjust dose. Moderate Theoretical
- **Cimetidine** transiently increases the concentration of antiepileptics **(carbamazepine)**. Monitor concentration and adjust dose. Moderate Study
- **Cimetidine** increases the concentration of antiepileptics **(fosphenytoin, phenytoin)**. Monitor concentration and adjust dose. Severe Study
- **H_2 receptor antagonists** are predicted to decrease the absorption of antifungals, azoles **(itraconazole)**. Administer **itraconazole** capsules with an acidic beverage, p. 409. Moderate Study
- **H_2 receptor antagonists** are predicted to decrease the absorption of antifungals, azoles **(ketoconazole)**. Administer **ketoconazole** with an acidic beverage, p. 480. Moderate Study
- **H_2 receptor antagonists** are predicted to decrease the exposure to antifungals, azoles **(posaconazole)**. Avoid use of posaconazole oral suspension. Moderate Study
- **Cimetidine** decreases the clearance of antimalarials **(chloroquine)**. Moderate Study
- **Cimetidine** slightly increases the exposure to antimalarials **(quinine)**. Moderate Study
- **H_2 receptor antagonists** are predicted to decrease the absorption of **bosutinib**. Moderate Theoretical
- **Cimetidine** slightly increases the exposure to calcium channel blockers **(diltiazem, nimodipine)**. Monitor and adjust dose. Moderate Study
- **Cimetidine** (high-dose) is predicted to increase the exposure to calcium channel blockers **(lercanidipine)**. Moderate Theoretical
- **Cimetidine** moderately increases the exposure to calcium channel blockers **(nifedipine)**. Monitor and adjust dose. Severe Study
- **Cimetidine** increases the exposure to calcium channel blockers **(verapamil)**. Moderate Study
- **Cimetidine** is predicted to slightly increase the exposure to **capecitabine**. Severe Theoretical
- **H_2 receptor antagonists** are predicted to decrease the absorption of **ceritinib**. Moderate Theoretical
- **Cimetidine** increases the concentration of **ciclosporin**. Mild Study
- **Cimetidine** increases the anticoagulant effect of **coumarins**. Severe Study
- **H_2 receptor antagonists** are predicted to decrease the concentration of **dacomitinib**. **Dacomitinib** should be taken 2 hours before or 10 hours after **H_2 receptor antagonists**. Mild Study
- **H_2 receptor antagonists** are predicted to decrease the exposure to **dasatinib**. Avoid. Moderate Study
- **H_2 receptor antagonists** are predicted to decrease the absorption of **dipyridamole** (immediate release tablets). Moderate Theoretical
- **Cimetidine** is predicted to increase the exposure to dopamine receptor agonists **(pramipexole)**. Adjust dose. Moderate Study
- **H_2 receptor antagonists** are predicted to decrease the exposure to **erlotinib**. **Erlotinib** should be taken 2 hours before or 10 hours after **H_2 receptor antagonists**. Moderate Study
- **Cimetidine** increases the concentration of **fampridine**. Avoid. Severe Theoretical
- **Cimetidine** slightly increases the exposure to **fluorouracil**. Severe Study
- **H_2 receptor antagonists** are predicted to slightly to moderately decrease the exposure to **gefitinib**. Moderate Study
- **H_2 receptor antagonists** decrease the exposure to HIV-protease inhibitors **(atazanavir)**. Monitor and adjust dose. Moderate Study
- **Cimetidine** is predicted to decrease the clearance of **hydroxychloroquine**. Moderate Theoretical
- **H_2 receptor antagonists** are predicted to decrease the absorption of **lapatinib**. Avoid. Moderate Theoretical
- **H_2 receptor antagonists** are predicted to decrease the exposure to **ledipasvir**. Adjust dose, see ledipasvir with sofosbuvir p. 436. Moderate Study
- **Leflunomide** is predicted to increase the exposure to H_2 receptor antagonists **(cimetidine, famotidine)**. Moderate Theoretical
- H_2 receptor antagonists **(cimetidine, ranitidine)** are predicted to increase the exposure to **lomitapide**. Separate administration by 12 hours. Moderate Theoretical

H_2 receptor antagonists (continued)
- **Cimetidine** slightly increases the exposure to macrolides (erythromycin). Moderate Study
- **Cimetidine** increases the concentration of **mebendazole.** Moderate Study
- **Cimetidine** increases the exposure to **metformin.** Monitor and adjust dose. Moderate Study
- **Cimetidine** slightly increases the exposure to **mirtazapine.** Use with caution and adjust dose. Moderate Theoretical
- **Cimetidine** increases the exposure to **moclobemide.** Adjust **moclobemide** dose. Mild Study
- **H_2 receptor antagonists** are predicted to decrease the exposure to **neratinib.** Avoid. Severe Theoretical
- **H_2 receptor antagonists** are predicted to decrease the absorption of **nilotinib. H_2 receptor antagonists** should be taken 10 hours before or 2 hours after **nilotinib.** Mild Theoretical
- Nitisinone is predicted to increase the exposure to H_2 receptor antagonists **(cimetidine, famotidine).** Moderate Study
- **Cimetidine** increases the concentration of opioids **(alfentanil).** Use with caution and adjust dose. Severe Study
- **Cimetidine** increases the exposure to opioids **(fentanyl).** Moderate Study
- **H_2 receptor antagonists** are predicted to decrease the exposure to **pazopanib. H_2 receptor antagonists** should be taken 10 hours before or 2 hours after **pazopanib.** Moderate Theoretical
- **Cimetidine** increases the exposure to **phenindione.** Severe Anecdotal
- **Cimetidine** moderately increases the exposure to **praziquantel.** Moderate Study
- **H_2 receptor antagonists** are predicted to decrease the exposure to **rilpivirine. H_2 receptor antagonists** should be taken 12 hours before or 4 hours after **rilpivirine.** Severe Study
- **Cimetidine** slightly increases the exposure to **roflumilast.** Moderate Study
- **H_2 receptor antagonists** potentially decrease the exposure to **sofosbuvir.** Adjust dose, see ledipasvir with sofosbuvir p. 436 sofosbuvir with velpatasvir, and sofosbuvir with velpatasvir and voxilaprevir. Moderate Study
- **Cimetidine** slightly increases the exposure to SSRIs **(citalopram, escitalopram).** Adjust dose. Moderate Study
- **Cimetidine** slightly increases the exposure to SSRIs **(paroxetine, sertraline).** Moderate Study
- **Cimetidine** is predicted to increase the risk of toxicity when given with **tegafur.** Severe Theoretical
- Teriflunomide is predicted to increase the exposure to H_2 receptor antagonists **(cimetidine, famotidine).** Moderate Study
- **Cimetidine** increases the concentration of **theophylline.** Adjust dose. Severe Study
- **Cimetidine** increases the exposure to **tricyclic antidepressants.** Moderate Study
- **H_2 receptor antagonists** are predicted to decrease the concentration of **velpatasvir.** Adjust dose, see sofosbuvir with velpatasvir. Moderate Study
- **Cimetidine** slightly increases the exposure to **venlafaxine.** Mild Study
- **Cimetidine** slightly increases the exposure to **zolmitriptan.** Adjust **zolmitriptan** dose, p. 310. Mild Study

Haloperidol → see **TABLE 8** p. 908 (hypotension), **TABLE 9** p. 909 (QT-interval prolongation), **TABLE 11** p. 909 (CNS depressant effects), **TABLE 10** p. 909 (antimuscarinics)

FOOD AND LIFESTYLE Dose adjustment might be necessary if smoking started or stopped during treatment.

- Antiepileptics **(carbamazepine, fosphenytoin, phenobarbital, phenytoin, primidone)** decrease the concentration of **haloperidol.** Adjust dose. Moderate Study → Also see **TABLE 11** p. 909
- **Haloperidol** potentially increases the risk of overheating and dehydration when given with antiepileptics **(zonisamide).** Avoid in children. Severe Theoretical
- Antifungals, azoles **(itraconazole)** increase the concentration of **haloperidol.** Moderate Study
- **Apalutamide** decreases the concentration of **haloperidol.** Adjust dose. Moderate Study → Also see **TABLE 9** p. 909
- **Haloperidol** is predicted to decrease the effects of **dopamine receptor agonists.** Avoid. Moderate Theoretical → Also see **TABLE 8** p. 908 → Also see **TABLE 9** p. 909 → Also see **TABLE 10** p. 909
- **Enzalutamide** decreases the concentration of **haloperidol.** Adjust dose. Moderate Study
- **Haloperidol** potentially opposes the effects of **glycerol phenylbutyrate.** Moderate Theoretical
- HIV-protease inhibitors **(ritonavir)** are predicted to increase the exposure to **haloperidol.** Severe Theoretical
- **Haloperidol** decreases the effects of **levodopa.** Severe Study → Also see **TABLE 8** p. 908
- **Mitotane** decreases the concentration of **haloperidol.** Adjust dose. Moderate Study
- **Rifampicin** decreases the concentration of **haloperidol.** Adjust dose. Moderate Study
- **Haloperidol** potentially decreases the effects of **sodium phenylbutyrate.** Moderate Anecdotal
- SSRIs **(fluoxetine)** increase the concentration of **haloperidol.** Adjust dose. Moderate Anecdotal
- SSRIs **(fluvoxamine)** increase the concentration of **haloperidol.** Adjust dose. Moderate Study
- **Venlafaxine** slightly increases the exposure to **haloperidol.** Severe Study → Also see **TABLE 9** p. 909 → Also see **TABLE 11** p. 909

Heparin (unfractionated) → see **TABLE 16** p. 911 (increased serum potassium), **TABLE 3** p. 907 (anticoagulant effects)
- **Ranibizumab** increases the risk of bleeding events when given with **heparin (unfractionated).** Severe Theoretical

Hepatitis B immunoglobulin → see immunoglobulins

HIV-protease inhibitors → see **TABLE 9** p. 909 (QT-interval prolongation)

atazanavir · darunavir · fosamprenavir · lopinavir · ritonavir · saquinavir · tipranavir

- Caution on concurrent use of **atazanavir, lopinavir with ritonavir**, and **ritonavir** with drugs that prolong the PR interval
- Concurrent use of **saquinavir** with drugs that prolong the PR interval is contra-indicated.
- Caution with concurrent use of **tipranavir** with drugs that increase risk of bleeding.

- **Tipranavir** slightly decreases the exposure to **abacavir.** Avoid. Severe Study
- **HIV-protease inhibitors** are predicted to increase the exposure to **abemaciclib.** Avoid or adjust **abemaciclib** dose. Severe Study
- HIV-protease inhibitors **(lopinavir, ritonavir, saquinavir)** are predicted to increase the exposure to **afatinib.** Separate administration by 12 hours. Moderate Study
- **Ritonavir** is predicted to decrease the exposure to **agomelatine.** Moderate Theoretical
- **Ritonavir** decreases the exposure to **albendazole.** Moderate Study
- **HIV-protease inhibitors** are predicted to markedly increase the exposure to aldosterone antagonists **(eplerenone).** Avoid. Severe Study
- HIV-protease inhibitors **(ritonavir, saquinavir)** are predicted to increase the exposure to **aliskiren.** Moderate Theoretical
- **HIV-protease inhibitors** increase the exposure to **almotriptan.** Mild Study
- **HIV-protease inhibitors** are predicted to moderately increase the exposure to alpha blockers **(alfuzosin, tamsulosin).** Use with caution or avoid. Moderate Study
- **HIV-protease inhibitors** are predicted to increase the exposure to alpha blockers **(doxazosin).** Moderate Study
- **HIV-protease inhibitors** moderately increase the exposure to **alprazolam.** Avoid. Moderate Study
- HIV-protease inhibitors **(ritonavir, tipranavir)** are predicted to increase the exposure to **amfetamines.** Severe Theoretical
- **Ritonavir** decreases the exposure to **aminophylline.** Adjust dose. Moderate Study
- **Ritonavir** is predicted to decrease the exposure to anaesthetics, local **(ropivacaine).** Moderate Theoretical
- **Antacids** are predicted to decrease the absorption of **atazanavir. Atazanavir** should be taken 2 hours before or 1 hour after antacids. Severe Theoretical

- Antacids are predicted to decrease the absorption of **tipranavir**. Separate administration by 2 hours. Moderate Study
- **HIV-protease inhibitors** are predicted to increase the exposure to antiarrhythmics **(amiodarone)**. Avoid. Severe Theoretical → Also see **TABLE 9** p. 909
- **HIV-protease inhibitors** are predicted to increase the exposure to antiarrhythmics **(disopyramide)**. Severe Theoretical → Also see **TABLE 9** p. 909
- **HIV-protease inhibitors** very markedly increase the exposure to antiarrhythmics **(dronedarone)**. Avoid. Severe Study → Also see **TABLE 9** p. 909
- **Ritonavir** is predicted to increase the exposure to antiarrhythmics **(flecainide)**. Avoid or monitor side effects. Severe Theoretical
- **HIV-protease inhibitors** are predicted to increase the exposure to antiarrhythmics **(lidocaine)**. Avoid. Severe Study
- **HIV-protease inhibitors** are predicted to increase the exposure to antiarrhythmics **(propafenone)**. Monitor and adjust dose. Severe Study
- **HIV-protease inhibitors** are predicted to increase the exposure to anticholinesterases, centrally acting **(galantamine)**. Monitor and adjust dose. Moderate Study
- **HIV-protease inhibitors** are predicted to increase the exposure to antiepileptics **(carbamazepine)** and antiepileptics **(carbamazepine)** are predicted to decrease the exposure to **HIV-protease inhibitors**. Monitor and adjust dose. Severe Theoretical
- **HIV-protease inhibitors** are predicted to affect the exposure to antiepileptics **(fosphenytoin, phenytoin)** and antiepileptics **(fosphenytoin, phenytoin)** decrease the concentration of **HIV-protease inhibitors**. Severe Theoretical
- **Ritonavir** slightly decreases the exposure to antiepileptics **(lamotrigine)**. Severe Study
- **HIV-protease inhibitors** are predicted to very slightly increase the exposure to antiepileptics **(perampanel)**. Mild Study
- **HIV-protease inhibitors** are predicted to affect the concentration of antiepileptics **(phenobarbital, primidone)** and antiepileptics **(phenobarbital, primidone)** are predicted to decrease the concentration of **HIV-protease inhibitors**. Severe Theoretical
- **Ritonavir** is predicted to decrease the concentration of antiepileptics **(valproate)**. Severe Anecdotal
- Antifungals, azoles **(fluconazole)** slightly increase the exposure to **tipranavir**. Avoid or adjust dose. Moderate Study
- Antifungals, azoles **(miconazole)** are predicted to increase the concentration of **HIV-protease inhibitors**. Use with caution and adjust dose. Moderate Theoretical
- Antifungals, azoles **(posaconazole)** are predicted to increase the exposure to **HIV-protease inhibitors**. Moderate Study
- **HIV-protease inhibitors** are predicted to increase the exposure to antifungals, azoles **(isavuconazole)**. Avoid or monitor side effects. Severe Study
- **HIV-protease inhibitors** are predicted to increase the exposure to antifungals, azoles **(itraconazole)**. Use with caution and adjust dose. Severe Study
- **HIV-protease inhibitors** are predicted to increase the exposure to antifungals, azoles **(ketoconazole)**. Use with caution and adjust dose. Moderate Study
- **HIV-protease inhibitors** are predicted to affect the exposure to antifungals, azoles **(voriconazole)** and antifungals, azoles **(voriconazole)** potentially affect the exposure to **HIV-protease inhibitors**. Severe Study → Also see **TABLE 9** p. 909
- **HIV-protease inhibitors** are predicted to increase the exposure to antihistamines, non-sedating **(mizolastine)**. Avoid. Severe Study
- **HIV-protease inhibitors** are predicted to increase the exposure to antihistamines, non-sedating **(rupatadine)**. Avoid. Moderate Study
- **HIV-protease inhibitors** decrease the exposure to antimalarials **(atovaquone)**. Avoid if boosted with ritonavir. Moderate Study
- **HIV-protease inhibitors** are predicted to increase the concentration of antimalarials **(piperaquine)**. Severe Theoretical
- **HIV-protease inhibitors** are predicted to decrease the exposure to antimalarials **(proguanil)**. Avoid. Moderate Study
- **HIV-protease inhibitors** are predicted to affect the exposure to antimalarials **(quinine)**. Severe Study → Also see **TABLE 9** p. 909
- **HIV-protease inhibitors** are predicted to increase the exposure to **apalutamide**. Mild Study → Also see **TABLE 9** p. 909
- **Ritonavir** is predicted to increase the exposure to **apixaban**. Avoid. Severe Theoretical
- **HIV-protease inhibitors** are predicted to markedly increase the exposure to **aprepitant**. Moderate Study
- **HIV-protease inhibitors** are predicted to slightly increase the exposure to **aripiprazole**. Adjust **aripiprazole** dose, p. 265. Moderate Study
- **HIV-protease inhibitors** are predicted to increase the exposure to **axitinib**. Avoid or adjust dose. Moderate Study
- **HIV-protease inhibitors** are predicted to increase the exposure to **bedaquiline**. Avoid prolonged use. Mild Study → Also see **TABLE 9** p. 909
- HIV-protease inhibitors **(lopinavir, ritonavir, saquinavir)** are predicted to increase the exposure to beta blockers, non-selective **(nadolol)**. Moderate Study
- **Ritonavir** is predicted to increase the exposure to beta blockers, selective **(metoprolol)**. Moderate Study
- **HIV-protease inhibitors** are predicted to increase the exposure to beta$_2$ agonists **(salmeterol)**. Avoid. Severe Study
- **Atazanavir** moderately increases the exposure to **bictegravir**. Avoid. Severe Study
- HIV-protease inhibitors **(lopinavir, ritonavir, saquinavir)** are predicted to increase the exposure to **bictegravir**. Use with caution or avoid. Moderate Theoretical
- **HIV-protease inhibitors** slightly increase the exposure to **bortezomib**. Moderate Study
- **HIV-protease inhibitors** are predicted to increase the exposure to **bosentan**. Severe Study
- **HIV-protease inhibitors** are predicted to markedly increase the exposure to **bosutinib**. Avoid or adjust dose. Severe Study → Also see **TABLE 9** p. 909
- **HIV-protease inhibitors** are predicted to increase the exposure to **brigatinib**. Adjust **brigatinib** dose. Severe Study
- **Ritonavir** is predicted to decrease the exposure to **bupropion**. Moderate Study
- **HIV-protease inhibitors** are predicted to increase the exposure to **buspirone**. Adjust **buspirone** dose. Severe Study
- **HIV-protease inhibitors** slightly increase the exposure to **cabozantinib**. Moderate Study → Also see **TABLE 9** p. 909
- **Ritonavir** is predicted to moderately increase the clearance of **caffeine citrate**. Monitor and adjust dose. Moderate Study
- **HIV-protease inhibitors** are predicted to increase the exposure to calcium channel blockers **(amlodipine, felodipine, lacidipine, nicardipine, nifedipine, nimodipine)**. Monitor and adjust dose. Moderate Study
- **HIV-protease inhibitors** are predicted to increase the exposure to calcium channel blockers **(diltiazem, verapamil)**. Severe Study
- **HIV-protease inhibitors** are predicted to markedly increase the exposure to calcium channel blockers **(lercanidipine)**. Avoid. Severe Study
- **HIV-protease inhibitors** are predicted to increase the exposure to **cannabidiol**. Avoid or adjust dose. Mild Study
- **HIV-protease inhibitors** are predicted to moderately increase the exposure to **cariprazine**. Avoid. Severe Study
- **HIV-protease inhibitors** are predicted to increase the exposure to **ceritinib**. Avoid or adjust **ceritinib** dose. Severe Study → Also see **TABLE 9** p. 909
- **HIV-protease inhibitors** increase the concentration of **ciclosporin**. Severe Study
- **HIV-protease inhibitors** are predicted to moderately increase the exposure to **cilostazol**. Adjust **cilostazol** dose. Moderate Study
- **HIV-protease inhibitors** are predicted to moderately increase the exposure to **cinacalcet**. Adjust dose. Moderate Study
- **Ritonavir** is predicted to affect the exposure to **clozapine**. Avoid. Severe Theoretical
- **HIV-protease inhibitors** are predicted to markedly increase the exposure to **cobimetinib**. Avoid or monitor for toxicity. Severe Study
- **HIV-protease inhibitors** are predicted to increase the exposure to **colchicine**. Avoid potent inhibitors of CYP3A4 or adjust **colchicine** dose. Severe Study

HIV-protease inhibitors (continued)
- **Atazanavir** (unboosted) increases the exposure to **combined hormonal contraceptives**. Adjust dose. [Severe] Study
- **Ritonavir** is predicted to decrease the efficacy of **combined hormonal contraceptives**. For FSRH guidance, see Contraceptives, interactions p. 536. [Severe] Study
- **HIV-protease inhibitors** are predicted to increase the exposure to corticosteroids **(beclometasone)** (risk with beclometasone is likely to be lower than with other corticosteroids). [Moderate] Theoretical
- **HIV-protease inhibitors** are predicted to increase the exposure to corticosteroids **(betamethasone, budesonide, ciclesonide, deflazacort, dexamethasone, fludrocortisone, fluticasone, hydrocortisone, methylprednisolone, mometasone, prednisolone, triamcinolone)**. Avoid or monitor side effects. [Severe] Study
- **HIV-protease inhibitors** are predicted to affect the anticoagulant effect of **coumarins**. [Moderate] Study
- **HIV-protease inhibitors** are predicted to moderately increase the exposure to **crizotinib**. Avoid. [Moderate] Study → Also see TABLE 9 p. 909
- HIV-protease inhibitors **(lopinavir, ritonavir, saquinavir)** are predicted to increase the exposure to **dabigatran**. Avoid. [Severe] Theoretical
- **HIV-protease inhibitors** are predicted to increase the exposure to **dabrafenib**. Use with caution or avoid. [Moderate] Study
- **HIV-protease inhibitors** are predicted to markedly to very markedly increase the exposure to **darifenacin**. Avoid. [Severe] Study
- **Dasabuvir** (with ombitasvir, paritaprevir, and ritonavir) decreases the concentration of **darunavir**. Avoid or adjust dose. [Moderate] Study
- **HIV-protease inhibitors** are predicted to markedly increase the exposure to **dasatinib**. Avoid or adjust dose—consult product literature. [Severe] Study → Also see TABLE 9 p. 909
- **HIV-protease inhibitors** very slightly increase the exposure to **delamanid**. [Severe] Study → Also see TABLE 9 p. 909
- **Ritonavir** is predicted to decrease the efficacy of **desogestrel**. For FSRH guidance, see Contraceptives, interactions p. 536. [Severe] Theoretical
- **Ritonavir** is predicted to increase the exposure to **diazepam**. Avoid. [Moderate] Theoretical
- **HIV-protease inhibitors** are predicted to moderately increase the exposure to **dienogest**. [Moderate] Study
- **Ritonavir** increases the concentration of **digoxin**. Adjust dose and monitor concentration. [Severe] Study
- **Fosamprenavir** boosted with ritonavir slightly decreases the exposure to **dolutegravir**. Avoid if resistant to HIV-integrase inhibitors. [Severe] Study
- **Tipranavir** moderately decreases the exposure to **dolutegravir**. Refer to specialist literature. [Severe] Study
- **HIV-protease inhibitors** increase the risk of QT-prolongation when given with **domperidone**. Avoid. [Severe] Study
- **HIV-protease inhibitors** increase the exposure to dopamine receptor agonists **(bromocriptine)**. [Severe] Study
- **HIV-protease inhibitors** are predicted to increase the concentration of dopamine receptor agonists **(cabergoline)**. [Moderate] Anecdotal
- **HIV-protease inhibitors** are predicted to increase the exposure to **doravirine**. [Mild] Study
- **HIV-protease inhibitors** are predicted to increase the exposure to **dronabinol**. Adjust dose. [Mild] Study
- **Ritonavir** is predicted to decrease the exposure to **duloxetine**. [Moderate] Theoretical
- **HIV-protease inhibitors** are predicted to increase the exposure to **dutasteride**. Monitor side effects and adjust dose. [Moderate] Theoretical
- HIV-protease inhibitors **(lopinavir, ritonavir, saquinavir)** are predicted to slightly increase the exposure to **edoxaban**. [Severe] Theoretical
- **Efavirenz** decreases the exposure to **HIV-protease inhibitors**. Refer to specialist literature. [Severe] Study → Also see TABLE 9 p. 909
- **HIV-protease inhibitors** are predicted to markedly increase the exposure to **eletriptan**. Avoid. [Severe] Study
- **HIV-protease inhibitors** are predicted to increase the exposure to **eliglustat**. Avoid or adjust dose—consult product literature. [Severe] Study
- HIV-protease inhibitors **(atazanavir, lopinavir)** boosted with ritonavir increase the concentration of **elvitegravir**. Refer to specialist literature. [Moderate] Study
- **HIV-protease inhibitors** are predicted to increase the exposure to **encorafenib**. Avoid or monitor. [Severe] Study → Also see TABLE 9 p. 909
- **HIV-protease inhibitors** are predicted to increase the risk of ergotism when given with **ergometrine**. Avoid. [Severe] Theoretical
- **HIV-protease inhibitors** are predicted to increase the risk of ergotism when given with **ergotamine**. Avoid. [Severe] Theoretical
- **HIV-protease inhibitors** are predicted to slightly increase the exposure to **erlotinib**. Use with caution and adjust dose. [Moderate] Study
- **HIV-protease inhibitors** are predicted to increase the exposure to **esketamine**. Adjust dose. [Moderate] Study
- **Ritonavir** is predicted to decrease the efficacy of **etonogestrel**. For FSRH guidance, see Contraceptives, interactions p. 536. [Severe] Theoretical
- **Etravirine** increases the exposure to **fosamprenavir** boosted with ritonavir. Refer to specialist literature. [Moderate] Study
- **Tipranavir** decreases the exposure to **etravirine**. Avoid. [Severe] Study
- **HIV-protease inhibitors** are predicted to increase the concentration of **everolimus**. Avoid. [Severe] Study
- **HIV-protease inhibitors** are predicted to moderately increase the exposure to **fesoterodine**. Adjust **fesoterodine** dose with potent inhibitors of CYP3A4; avoid in hepatic and renal impairment. [Severe] Study
- HIV-protease inhibitors **(lopinavir, ritonavir, saquinavir)** are predicted to increase the exposure to **fidaxomicin**. Avoid. [Moderate] Study
- **Ritonavir** is predicted to increase the exposure to **flurazepam**. Avoid. [Moderate] Theoretical
- **HIV-protease inhibitors** are predicted to increase the exposure to **fosaprepitant**. [Moderate] Theoretical
- **HIV-protease inhibitors** are predicted to increase the exposure to **gefitinib**. [Moderate] Study
- **HIV-protease inhibitors** are predicted to increase the exposure to **gilteritinib**. [Moderate] Study
- HIV-protease inhibitors **(atazanavir, darunavir, lopinavir)** boosted with ritonavir increase the exposure to **glecaprevir**. Avoid. [Severe] Study
- **Ritonavir** increases the exposure to **glecaprevir**. Avoid. [Severe] Study
- **HIV-protease inhibitors** are predicted to moderately to markedly increase the exposure to **grazoprevir**. Avoid. [Severe] Study
- **HIV-protease inhibitors** are predicted to increase the exposure to **guanfacine**. Adjust **guanfacine** dose, p. 247. [Moderate] Study
- **H_2 receptor antagonists** decrease the exposure to **atazanavir**. Monitor and adjust dose. [Moderate] Study
- **Ritonavir** is predicted to increase the exposure to **haloperidol**. [Severe] Theoretical
- **Ritonavir** is predicted to decrease the effects of **hormone replacement therapy**. [Moderate] Anecdotal
- **HIV-protease inhibitors** are predicted to very markedly increase the exposure to **ibrutinib**. Avoid potent inhibitors of CYP3A4 or adjust **ibrutinib** dose. [Severe] Study
- **HIV-protease inhibitors** are predicted to increase the exposure to **imatinib**. [Moderate] Study
- **HIV-protease inhibitors** are predicted to increase the risk of toxicity when given with **irinotecan**. Avoid. [Moderate] Study
- **Ritonavir** is predicted to decrease the exposure to iron chelators **(deferasirox)**. Monitor serum ferritin and adjust dose. [Moderate] Theoretical
- **HIV-protease inhibitors** are predicted to increase the exposure to **ivabradine**. Avoid. [Severe] Study
- **HIV-protease inhibitors** are predicted to increase the exposure to **ivacaftor**. Adjust ivacaftor p. 196 or lumacaftor with ivacaftor p. 197 or tezacaftor with ivacaftor p. 198 dose with potent inhibitors of CYP3A4. [Severe] Study

- **HIV-protease inhibitors** are predicted to increase the exposure to lapatinib. Avoid. [Moderate] Study → Also see **TABLE 9** p. 909
- **HIV-protease inhibitors** are predicted to moderately increase the exposure to larotrectinib. Avoid or adjust **larotrectinib** dose, p. 607. [Moderate] Study
- **Tipranavir** boosted with ritonavir is predicted to decrease the exposure to ledipasvir. Avoid. [Severe] Theoretical
- HIV-protease inhibitors **(atazanavir, lopinavir)** boosted with ritonavir are predicted to increase the concentration of letermovir. [Moderate] Study
- **Ritonavir** is predicted to decrease the concentration of letermovir. [Moderate] Theoretical
- **Ritonavir** is predicted to decrease the efficacy of levonorgestrel. For FSRH guidance, see Contraceptives, interactions p. 536. [Severe] Theoretical
- **HIV-protease inhibitors** are predicted to markedly increase the exposure to lomitapide. Avoid. [Severe] Study
- **HIV-protease inhibitors** are predicted to increase the exposure to lorlatinib. Avoid or adjust **lorlatinib** dose. [Severe] Study
- **HIV-protease inhibitors** are predicted to increase the exposure to lurasidone. Avoid. [Severe] Study
- **HIV-protease inhibitors** are predicted to increase the exposure to macitentan. [Moderate] Study
- Macrolides **(clarithromycin)** increase the exposure to **saquinavir** and **saquinavir** increases the exposure to macrolides (clarithromycin). Avoid. [Severe] Study → Also see **TABLE 9** p. 909
- Macrolides **(erythromycin)** are predicted to increase the exposure to **saquinavir**. Avoid. [Severe] Theoretical → Also see **TABLE 9** p. 909
- **Atazanavir** is predicted to increase the exposure to macrolides (clarithromycin). Adjust dose in renal impairment. [Severe] Study
- **Ritonavir** increases the exposure to macrolides **(clarithromycin)**. Adjust dose in renal impairment. [Severe] Study
- **Tipranavir** boosted with ritonavir increases the exposure to macrolides **(clarithromycin)** and macrolides **(clarithromycin)** increase the exposure to **tipranavir** boosted with ritonavir. Monitor; adjust dose in renal impairment. [Severe] Study
- HIV-protease inhibitors **(darunavir, fosamprenavir, lopinavir)** boosted with ritonavir are predicted to increase the exposure to macrolides **(clarithromycin)**. Adjust dose in renal impairment. [Severe] Study
- HIV-protease inhibitors **(atazanavir, darunavir, fosamprenavir, lopinavir, ritonavir, tipranavir)** are predicted to increase the exposure to macrolides **(erythromycin)**. [Severe] Theoretical
- **Darunavir** boosted with ritonavir markedly increases the exposure to maraviroc. Refer to specialist literature. [Severe] Study
- **Maraviroc** potentially decreases the exposure to **fosamprenavir** and **fosamprenavir** potentially decreases the exposure to maraviroc. Avoid. [Severe] Study
- HIV-protease inhibitors **(atazanavir, saquinavir)** moderately to markedly increase the exposure to maraviroc. Refer to specialist literature. [Severe] Study
- **Lopinavir** boosted with ritonavir moderately increases the exposure to maraviroc. Refer to specialist literature. [Severe] Study
- **Ritonavir** markedly increases the exposure to maraviroc. Refer to specialist literature. [Severe] Study
- **Ritonavir** is predicted to decrease the exposure to melatonin. [Moderate] Theoretical
- **Ritonavir** is predicted to increase the clearance of mexiletine. Monitor and adjust dose. [Moderate] Study
- **HIV-protease inhibitors** are predicted to markedly to very markedly increase the exposure to midazolam. Avoid or adjust dose. [Severe] Study
- **HIV-protease inhibitors** are predicted to very markedly increase the exposure to midostaurin. Avoid or monitor for toxicity. [Severe] Study
- **HIV-protease inhibitors** are predicted to increase the exposure to mirabegron. Adjust **mirabegron** dose in hepatic and renal impairment. [Moderate] Study
- **HIV-protease inhibitors** are predicted to increase the exposure to mirtazapine. [Moderate] Study
- **HIV-protease inhibitors** are predicted to increase the exposure to modafinil. [Mild] Theoretical
- HIV-protease inhibitors **(lopinavir, ritonavir, saquinavir)** are predicted to increase the risk of neutropenia when given with monoclonal antibodies **(brentuximab vedotin)**. Monitor and adjust dose. [Severe] Study
- **HIV-protease inhibitors** are predicted to increase the exposure to monoclonal antibodies **(polatuzumab vedotin)**. [Moderate] Theoretical
- **HIV-protease inhibitors** are predicted to increase the exposure to monoclonal antibodies **(trastuzumab emtansine)**. Avoid. [Severe] Theoretical
- **HIV-protease inhibitors** are predicted to increase the exposure to naldemedine. Avoid or monitor. [Moderate] Study
- **HIV-protease inhibitors** are predicted to markedly increase the exposure to naloxegol. Avoid. [Severe] Study
- **HIV-protease inhibitors** are predicted to increase the exposure to neratinib. Avoid or adjust **neratinib** dose. [Severe] Study
- **HIV-protease inhibitors** are predicted to increase the exposure to netupitant. [Moderate] Study
- **Nevirapine** decreases the exposure to **HIV-protease inhibitors**. Refer to specialist literature. [Moderate] Study
- **HIV-protease inhibitors** are predicted to moderately increase the exposure to nilotinib. Avoid. [Severe] Study → Also see **TABLE 9** p. 909
- HIV-protease inhibitors **(lopinavir, ritonavir, saquinavir)** are predicted to increase the exposure to **nintedanib**. [Moderate] Study
- **HIV-protease inhibitors** are predicted to increase the exposure to nitisinone. Adjust dose. [Moderate] Theoretical
- **Ritonavir** is predicted to decrease the efficacy of norethisterone. For FSRH guidance, see Contraceptives, interactions p. 536. [Severe] Anecdotal
- **Ritonavir** is predicted to decrease the exposure to olanzapine. Monitor and adjust dose. [Moderate] Study
- **HIV-protease inhibitors** are predicted to increase the exposure to olaparib. Avoid potent inhibitors of CYP3A4 or adjust **olaparib** dose. [Moderate] Study
- **Ombitasvir** (in fixed-dose combination with dasabuvir) decreases the concentration of **darunavir**. Avoid or adjust dose. [Moderate] Study
- **HIV-protease inhibitors** are predicted to increase the exposure to opioids **(alfentanil, buprenorphine, fentanyl, oxycodone)**. Monitor and adjust dose. [Severe] Study
- **HIV-protease inhibitors** boosted with ritonavir are predicted to decrease the exposure to opioids **(methadone)**. [Moderate] Study → Also see **TABLE 9** p. 909
- **Ritonavir** is predicted to decrease the concentration of opioids **(morphine)**. [Moderate] Theoretical
- **Ritonavir** increases the risk of CNS toxicity when given with opioids **(pethidine)**. Avoid. [Severe] Study
- **HIV-protease inhibitors** are predicted to increase the exposure to ospemifene. Avoid in poor CYP2C9 metabolisers. [Moderate] Study
- **HIV-protease inhibitors** are predicted to increase the exposure to oxybutynin. [Mild] Study
- **HIV-protease inhibitors** are predicted to increase the exposure to palbociclib. Avoid or adjust **palbociclib** dose. [Severe] Study
- **HIV-protease inhibitors** are predicted to increase the exposure to panobinostat. Adjust **panobinostat** dose; in hepatic impairment avoid. [Moderate] Study → Also see **TABLE 9** p. 909
- **Atazanavir** boosted with ritonavir markedly increases the exposure to paritaprevir. Avoid or give unboosted. [Moderate] Study
- **Darunavir** boosted with ritonavir slightly decreases the exposure to paritaprevir. Avoid or give unboosted. [Moderate] Study
- HIV-protease inhibitors **(fosamprenavir, tipranavir)** boosted with ritonavir are predicted to increase the exposure to paritaprevir. Avoid. [Severe] Study
- **Lopinavir** boosted with ritonavir moderately to markedly increases the exposure to paritaprevir. Avoid. [Severe] Study
- **Saquinavir** is predicted to increase the exposure to **paritaprevir** (in fixed-dose combination). Avoid. [Severe] Study
- **HIV-protease inhibitors** are predicted to increase the exposure to pazopanib. Avoid or adjust **pazopanib** dose. [Moderate] Study → Also see **TABLE 9** p. 909

HIV-protease inhibitors (continued)

- **HIV-protease inhibitors** are predicted to increase the exposure to phosphodiesterase type-5 inhibitors **(avanafil, vardenafil)**. Avoid. Severe Study → Also see **TABLE 9** p. 909
- **HIV-protease inhibitors** are predicted to increase the exposure to phosphodiesterase type-5 inhibitors **(sildenafil)**. Avoid potent inhibitors of CYP3A4 or adjust **sildenafil** dose, p. 125. Severe Study → Also see **TABLE 9** p. 909
- **HIV-protease inhibitors** are predicted to increase the exposure to phosphodiesterase type-5 inhibitors **(tadalafil)**. Use with caution or avoid. Severe Study
- HIV-protease inhibitors **(atazanavir, lopinavir)** boosted with ritonavir increase the exposure to **pibrentasvir**. Avoid. Severe Study
- **Ritonavir** potentially increases the exposure to **pibrentasvir**. Severe Theoretical
- **Saquinavir** is predicted to increase the exposure to **pibrentasvir**. Moderate Theoretical
- **HIV-protease inhibitors** are predicted to increase the exposure to **pimozide**. Avoid. Severe Study → Also see **TABLE 9** p. 909
- **Ritonavir** is predicted to decrease the exposure to **pirfenidone**. Moderate Theoretical
- **HIV-protease inhibitors** are predicted to slightly increase the exposure to **ponatinib**. Monitor and adjust **ponatinib** dose. Moderate Study
- **HIV-protease inhibitors** are predicted to moderately increase the exposure to **praziquantel**. Mild Study
- **HIV-protease inhibitors** given with carbimazole are predicted to increase the exposure to **propiverine**. Adjust starting dose. Moderate Theoretical
- **Proton pump inhibitors** decrease the exposure to **atazanavir**. Avoid or adjust dose. Severe Study
- **Proton pump inhibitors** increase the exposure to **saquinavir**. Avoid. Severe Study
- **Tipranavir** decreases the exposure to **proton pump inhibitors**. Avoid. Severe Study
- **HIV-protease inhibitors** are predicted to increase the exposure to **quetiapine**. Avoid. Severe Study
- **Atazanavir** increases the exposure to **raltegravir** (high-dose). Avoid. Moderate Study
- **Darunavir** increases the risk of rash when given with **raltegravir**. Moderate Study
- **Fosamprenavir** boosted with ritonavir decreases the exposure to **raltegravir** and **raltegravir** decreases the exposure to **fosamprenavir** boosted with ritonavir. Avoid. Severe Study
- **Tipranavir** boosted with ritonavir is predicted to decrease the exposure to **raltegravir** (high-dose). Avoid. Moderate Study
- **HIV-protease inhibitors** are predicted to increase the exposure to **ranolazine**. Avoid. Severe Study → Also see **TABLE 9** p. 909
- **HIV-protease inhibitors** are predicted to increase the exposure to **reboxetine**. Avoid. Moderate Study
- **HIV-protease inhibitors** are predicted to increase the exposure to **regorafenib**. Avoid. Moderate Study
- **HIV-protease inhibitors** are predicted to increase the exposure to **repaglinide**. Moderate Study
- **HIV-protease inhibitors** are predicted to increase the exposure to retinoids **(alitretinoin)**. Adjust **alitretinoin** dose. Moderate Theoretical
- **HIV-protease inhibitors** are predicted to increase the exposure to **ribociclib**. Avoid or adjust **ribociclib** dose. Moderate Study → Also see **TABLE 9** p. 909
- HIV-protease inhibitors **(atazanavir, darunavir, fosamprenavir, lopinavir, saquinavir, tipranavir)** boosted with ritonavir increase the exposure to **rifabutin**. Monitor and adjust dose. Severe Study
- **Ritonavir** markedly increases the exposure to **rifabutin**. Avoid or adjust dose. Severe Study
- **Rifampicin** is predicted to moderately to markedly decrease the exposure to HIV-protease inhibitors **(atazanavir, darunavir, fosamprenavir, lopinavir, saquinavir)**. Avoid. Severe Study
- **Rifampicin** slightly decreases the exposure to **ritonavir**. Severe Study
- **Rifampicin** is predicted to decrease the exposure to **tipranavir**. Avoid. Severe Study
- **Ritonavir** is predicted to increase the exposure to **riociguat**. Adjust dose and monitor blood pressure. Moderate Theoretical
- **HIV-protease inhibitors** are predicted to increase the exposure to **risperidone**. Adjust dose. Moderate Study → Also see **TABLE 9** p. 909
- **Ritonavir** moderately increases the exposure to **rivaroxaban**. Avoid. Severe Study
- **HIV-protease inhibitors** are predicted to increase the exposure to **ruxolitinib**. Adjust dose and monitor side effects. Moderate Study
- **HIV-protease inhibitors** are predicted to increase the exposure to **saxagliptin**. Moderate Study
- **HIV-protease inhibitors** are predicted to increase the exposure to **siponimod**. Avoid depending on other drugs taken—consult product literature. Severe Theoretical
- **HIV-protease inhibitors** are predicted to increase the concentration of **sirolimus**. Avoid. Severe Study
- **Sodium zirconium cyclosilicate** is predicted to decrease the exposure to **HIV-protease inhibitors**. Separate administration by at least 2 hours. Moderate Theoretical
- **Tipranavir** is predicted to decrease the exposure to **sofosbuvir**. Avoid. Severe Theoretical
- **HIV-protease inhibitors** are predicted to increase the exposure to **solifenacin**. Adjust solifenacin or tamsulosin with solifenacin dose; avoid in hepatic and renal impairment. Severe Study
- **HIV-protease inhibitors** are predicted to moderately increase the exposure to SSRIs **(dapoxetine)**. Avoid potent inhibitors of CYP3A4 or adjust **dapoxetine** dose. Severe Study
- **St John's Wort** is predicted to decrease the exposure to **HIV-protease inhibitors**. Avoid. Severe Study
- **HIV-protease inhibitors** are predicted to increase the exposure to statins **(atorvastatin)**. Avoid or adjust dose and monitor rhabdomyolysis. Severe Study
- **HIV-protease inhibitors** slightly to moderately increase the exposure to statins **(rosuvastatin)**. Avoid or adjust dose. Severe Study
- **HIV-protease inhibitors** are predicted to increase the exposure to statins **(simvastatin)**. Avoid. Severe Study
- **HIV-protease inhibitors** are predicted to slightly increase the exposure to **sunitinib**. Avoid or adjust **sunitinib** dose. Moderate Study → Also see **TABLE 9** p. 909
- **HIV-protease inhibitors** are predicted to increase the concentration of **tacrolimus**. Monitor and adjust dose. Severe Study
- HIV-protease inhibitors **(lopinavir, ritonavir, saquinavir)** are predicted to slightly increase the exposure to **talazoparib**. Avoid or adjust **talazoparib** dose. Severe Study
- **HIV-protease inhibitors** are predicted to increase the exposure to taxanes **(cabazitaxel)**. Avoid. Severe Study
- **HIV-protease inhibitors** are predicted to moderately increase the exposure to taxanes **(docetaxel)**. Avoid or adjust dose. Severe Study
- **HIV-protease inhibitors** are predicted to increase the exposure to taxanes **(paclitaxel)**. Severe Theoretical
- **HIV-protease inhibitors** are predicted to increase the concentration of **temsirolimus**. Avoid. Severe Theoretical
- HIV-protease inhibitors **(atazanavir, darunavir, lopinavir)** increase the exposure to **tenofovir alafenamide**. Avoid or adjust dose. Moderate Study
- **Tipranavir** is predicted to decrease the exposure to **tenofovir alafenamide**. Avoid. Moderate Theoretical
- HIV-protease inhibitors **(atazanavir, darunavir, lopinavir)** are predicted to increase the risk of renal impairment when given with **tenofovir disoproxil**. Severe Anecdotal
- **HIV-protease inhibitors** are predicted to increase the exposure to **tezacaftor**. Adjust tezacaftor with ivacaftor p. 198 dose with potent inhibitors of CYP3A4. Severe Study
- **Ritonavir** is predicted to decrease the exposure to **theophylline**. Adjust dose. Moderate Study
- **Ritonavir** decreases the concentration of thyroid hormones **(levothyroxine)**. MHRA advises monitor TSH for at least one month after starting or stopping ritonavir. Moderate Anecdotal
- **HIV-protease inhibitors** are predicted to markedly increase the exposure to **ticagrelor**. Avoid. Severe Study

- **Ritonavir** moderately decreases the exposure to **tizanidine.** Mild Study
- **HIV-protease inhibitors** are predicted to increase the exposure to tofacitinib. Adjust **tofacitinib** dose. Moderate Study
- **HIV-protease inhibitors** are predicted to increase the exposure to tolterodine. Avoid. Severe Study → Also see **TABLE 9** p. 909
- **HIV-protease inhibitors** are predicted to increase the exposure to tolvaptan. Manufacturer advises caution or adjust **tolvaptan** dose with potent inhibitors of CYP3A4. Severe Study
- HIV-protease inhibitors **(lopinavir, ritonavir, saquinavir)** are predicted to increase the exposure to **topotecan.** Severe Study
- **HIV-protease inhibitors** are predicted to increase the exposure to **toremifene.** Moderate Theoretical → Also see **TABLE 9** p. 909
- **HIV-protease inhibitors** are predicted to increase the exposure to trabectedin. Avoid or adjust dose. Severe Theoretical
- HIV-protease inhibitors **(lopinavir, ritonavir, saquinavir)** are predicted to increase the concentration of **trametinib.** Moderate Theoretical
- **HIV-protease inhibitors** are predicted to moderately increase the exposure to **trazodone.** Avoid or adjust dose. Moderate Study
- HIV-protease inhibitors **(ritonavir, tipranavir)** are predicted to increase the exposure to **tricyclic antidepressants.** Moderate Theoretical
- HIV-protease inhibitors **(atazanavir, darunavir, fosamprenavir, lopinavir, saquinavir, tipranavir)** are predicted to increase the exposure to **ulipristal.** Avoid if used for uterine fibroids. Severe Study
- **Ritonavir** decreases the efficacy of **ulipristal.** For FSRH guidance, see Contraceptives, interactions p. 536. Severe Anecdotal
- **HIV-protease inhibitors** are predicted to increase the exposure to **upadacitinib.** Use with caution or avoid. Severe Study
- **Tipranavir** is predicted to increase the exposure to **velpatasvir.** Severe Theoretical
- **HIV-protease inhibitors** are predicted to increase the exposure to **vemurafenib.** Severe Theoretical → Also see **TABLE 9** p. 909
- **HIV-protease inhibitors** are predicted to increase the exposure to **venetoclax.** Avoid or adjust dose—consult product literature. Severe Study
- **HIV-protease inhibitors** are predicted to increase the exposure to **venlafaxine.** Moderate Study → Also see **TABLE 9** p. 909
- **HIV-protease inhibitors** are predicted to increase the exposure to **vinca alkaloids.** Severe Theoretical → Also see **TABLE 9** p. 909
- **HIV-protease inhibitors** are predicted to increase the exposure to vitamin D substances **(paricalcitol).** Moderate Study
- **Atazanavir** boosted with ritonavir increases the concentration of **voxilaprevir.** Avoid. Severe Study
- **Lopinavir** boosted with ritonavir is predicted to increase the concentration of **voxilaprevir.** Avoid. Severe Theoretical
- **Tipranavir** boosted with ritonavir is predicted to increase the concentration of **voxilaprevir.** Severe Theoretical
- **Tipranavir** slightly decreases the exposure to **zidovudine.** Avoid. Moderate Study
- **HIV-protease inhibitors** are predicted to increase the exposure to **zopiclone.** Adjust dose. Moderate Theoretical

Homatropine → see **TABLE 10** p. 909 (antimuscarinics)

Hormone replacement therapy

- Antiepileptics **(carbamazepine, eslicarbazepine, fosphenytoin, oxcarbazepine, perampanel, phenobarbital, phenytoin, primidone, rufinamide, topiramate)** are predicted to decrease the effects of **hormone replacement therapy.** Moderate Anecdotal
- **Hormone replacement therapy** is predicted to alter the exposure to antiepileptics **(lamotrigine).** Moderate Theoretical
- **Aprepitant** is predicted to decrease the effects of **hormone replacement therapy.** Moderate Anecdotal
- **Bosentan** is predicted to decrease the effects of **hormone replacement therapy.** Moderate Anecdotal
- **Hormone replacement therapy** decreases the clearance of dopamine receptor agonists **(ropinirole).** Monitor and adjust dose. Moderate Study
- **Efavirenz** is predicted to decrease the effects of **hormone replacement therapy.** Moderate Anecdotal
- **Fosaprepitant** is predicted to decrease the effects of **hormone replacement therapy.** Moderate Anecdotal
- HIV-protease inhibitors **(ritonavir)** are predicted to decrease the effects of **hormone replacement therapy.** Moderate Anecdotal
- **Hormone replacement therapy** is predicted to increase the risk of venous thromboembolism when given with **lenalidomide.** Severe Theoretical
- **Hormone replacement therapy** is predicted to increase the exposure to MAO-B inhibitors **(selegiline).** Avoid. Moderate Study
- **Modafinil** is predicted to decrease the effects of **hormone replacement therapy.** Moderate Anecdotal
- **Nevirapine** is predicted to decrease the effects of **hormone replacement therapy.** Moderate Anecdotal
- NSAIDs **(etoricoxib)** slightly increase the exposure to **hormone replacement therapy.** Moderate Study
- **Hormone replacement therapy** potentially opposes the effects of **ospemifene.** Avoid. Severe Theoretical
- **Hormone replacement therapy** is predicted to increase the risk of venous thromboembolism when given with **pomalidomide.** Severe Theoretical
- **Hormone replacement therapy** potentially opposes the effects of **raloxifene.** Avoid. Severe Theoretical
- **Rifabutin** is predicted to decrease the effects of **hormone replacement therapy.** Moderate Anecdotal
- **Rifampicin** is predicted to decrease the effects of **hormone replacement therapy.** Moderate Anecdotal
- **St John's Wort** is predicted to decrease the efficacy of **hormone replacement therapy.** Moderate Theoretical
- **Hormone replacement therapy** is predicted to increase the risk of venous thromboembolism when given with **thalidomide.** Severe Theoretical
- Oral **hormone replacement therapy** is predicted to decrease the effects of **thyroid hormones.** Moderate Theoretical

Hydralazine → see **TABLE 8** p. 908 (hypotension)

- **Diazoxide** increases the risk of severe hypotension when given with **hydralazine.** Severe Study → Also see **TABLE 8** p. 908

Hydrochlorothiazide → see thiazide diuretics

Hydrocortisone → see corticosteroids

Hydroflumethiazide → see thiazide diuretics

Hydromorphone → see opioids

Hydroxycarbamide → see **TABLE 15** p. 910 (myelosuppression)

- **Live vaccines** are predicted to increase the risk of generalised infection (possibly life-threatening) when given with **hydroxycarbamide.** Public Health England advises avoid (refer to Green Book). Severe Theoretical
- **Hydroxycarbamide** increases the risk of toxicity when given with **stavudine.** Avoid. Severe Study

Hydroxychloroquine

- **Hydroxychloroquine** is predicted to decrease the effects of **agalsidase alfa.** Moderate Theoretical
- **Hydroxychloroquine** is predicted to decrease the exposure to **agalsidase beta.** Moderate Theoretical
- **Antacids** decrease the absorption of **hydroxychloroquine.** Separate administration by at least 4 hours. Moderate Study
- Calcium salts **(calcium carbonate)** decrease the absorption of **hydroxychloroquine.** Separate administration by at least 4 hours. Moderate Study
- **Hydroxychloroquine** is predicted to decrease the efficacy of **oral cholera vaccine.** Moderate Theoretical
- H_2 receptor antagonists **(cimetidine)** are predicted to decrease the clearance of **hydroxychloroquine.** Moderate Theoretical
- **Lanthanum** is predicted to decrease the absorption of **hydroxychloroquine.** Separate administration by at least 2 hours. Moderate Theoretical
- **Hydroxychloroquine** is predicted to decrease the exposure to **laronidase.** Avoid simultaneous administration. Severe Theoretical
- **Hydroxychloroquine** is predicted to increase the risk of haematological toxicity when given with **penicillamine.** Avoid. Severe Theoretical
- **Hydroxychloroquine** is predicted to decrease efficacy **rabies vaccine.** Moderate Theoretical

Hydroxyzine → see antihistamines, sedating

Hyoscine → see **TABLE 10** p. 909 (antimuscarinics)

Ibandronate → see bisphosphonates

Ibrutinib → see **TABLE 15** p. 910 (myelosuppression), **TABLE 4** p. 907 (antiplatelet effects)

Ibrutinib (continued)

FOOD AND LIFESTYLE Avoid food or drink containing bitter (Seville) oranges as they are predicted to increase the exposure to ibrutinib.

- Antiarrhythmics **(amiodarone)** are predicted to increase the exposure to **ibrutinib**. Adjust **ibrutinib** dose. Severe Theoretical
- Antiarrhythmics **(dronedarone)** are predicted to increase the exposure to **ibrutinib**. Adjust **ibrutinib** dose with moderate inhibitors of CYP3A4. Severe Study
- Antiepileptics **(carbamazepine, fosphenytoin, phenobarbital, phenytoin, primidone)** are predicted to decrease the exposure to **ibrutinib**. Avoid or adjust **ibrutinib** dose. Severe Study
- Antifungals, azoles **(fluconazole, isavuconazole, posaconazole)** are predicted to increase the exposure to **ibrutinib**. Adjust **ibrutinib** dose with moderate inhibitors of CYP3A4. Severe Study
- Antifungals, azoles **(itraconazole, ketoconazole, voriconazole)** are predicted to very markedly increase the exposure to **ibrutinib**. Avoid potent inhibitors of CYP3A4 or adjust **ibrutinib** dose. Severe Study
- **Apalutamide** is predicted to decrease the exposure to **ibrutinib**. Avoid or adjust **ibrutinib** dose. Severe Study
- **Aprepitant** is predicted to increase the exposure to **ibrutinib**. Adjust **ibrutinib** dose with moderate inhibitors of CYP3A4. Severe Study
- Calcium channel blockers **(diltiazem, verapamil)** are predicted to increase the exposure to **ibrutinib**. Adjust **ibrutinib** dose with moderate inhibitors of CYP3A4. Severe Study
- **Cobicistat** is predicted to very markedly increase the exposure to **ibrutinib**. Avoid potent inhibitors of CYP3A4 or adjust **ibrutinib** dose. Severe Study
- **Crizotinib** is predicted to increase the exposure to **ibrutinib**. Adjust **ibrutinib** dose with moderate inhibitors of CYP3A4. Severe Study → Also see TABLE 15 p. 910
- **Enzalutamide** is predicted to decrease the exposure to **ibrutinib**. Avoid or adjust **ibrutinib** dose. Severe Study
- **Fosaprepitant** is predicted to slightly increase the exposure to **ibrutinib**. Moderate Theoretical
- **Grapefruit juice** is predicted to increase the exposure to **ibrutinib**. Avoid. Moderate Theoretical
- **HIV-protease inhibitors** are predicted to very markedly increase the exposure to **ibrutinib**. Avoid potent inhibitors of CYP3A4 or adjust **ibrutinib** dose. Severe Study
- **Idelalisib** is predicted to very markedly increase the exposure to **ibrutinib**. Avoid potent inhibitors of CYP3A4 or adjust **ibrutinib** dose. Severe Study → Also see TABLE 15 p. 910
- **Imatinib** is predicted to increase the exposure to **ibrutinib**. Adjust **ibrutinib** dose with moderate inhibitors of CYP3A4. Severe Study → Also see TABLE 15 p. 910
- Macrolides **(clarithromycin)** are predicted to very markedly increase the exposure to **ibrutinib**. Avoid potent inhibitors of CYP3A4 or adjust **ibrutinib** dose. Severe Study
- Macrolides **(erythromycin)** are predicted to increase the exposure to **ibrutinib**. Adjust **ibrutinib** dose with moderate inhibitors of CYP3A4. Severe Study
- **Mitotane** is predicted to decrease the exposure to **ibrutinib**. Avoid or adjust **ibrutinib** dose. Severe Study → Also see TABLE 15 p. 910
- **Netupitant** is predicted to increase the exposure to **ibrutinib**. Adjust **ibrutinib** dose with moderate inhibitors of CYP3A4. Severe Study
- **Nilotinib** is predicted to increase the exposure to **ibrutinib**. Adjust **ibrutinib** dose with moderate inhibitors of CYP3A4. Severe Study → Also see TABLE 15 p. 910
- Quinolones **(ciprofloxacin)** are predicted to increase the exposure to **ibrutinib**. Adjust **ibrutinib** dose. Severe Theoretical
- **Rifampicin** is predicted to decrease the exposure to **ibrutinib**. Avoid or adjust **ibrutinib** dose. Severe Study
- **St John's Wort** is predicted to decrease the exposure to **ibrutinib**. Avoid. Severe Theoretical

Ibuprofen → see NSAIDs

Icatibant

- **ACE inhibitors** are predicted to decrease the efficacy of **icatibant** and **icatibant** is predicted to decrease the efficacy of **ACE inhibitors**. Avoid. Moderate Theoretical

Idarubicin → see anthracyclines

Idelalisib → see TABLE 15 p. 910 (myelosuppression)

- **Idelalisib** is predicted to increase the exposure to **abemaciclib**. Avoid or adjust **abemaciclib** dose. Severe Study
- **Idelalisib** is predicted to markedly increase the exposure to aldosterone antagonists **(eplerenone)**. Avoid. Severe Study
- **Idelalisib** increases the exposure to **almotriptan**. Mild Study
- **Idelalisib** is predicted to moderately increase the exposure to alpha blockers **(alfuzosin, tamsulosin)**. Use with caution or avoid. Moderate Study
- **Idelalisib** is predicted to increase the exposure to alpha blockers **(doxazosin)**. Moderate Study
- **Idelalisib** moderately increases the exposure to **alprazolam**. Avoid. Moderate Study
- **Idelalisib** is predicted to increase the exposure to antiarrhythmics **(amiodarone)**. Avoid. Moderate Theoretical
- **Idelalisib** very markedly increases the exposure to antiarrhythmics **(dronedarone)**. Avoid. Severe Study
- **Idelalisib** is predicted to increase the exposure to antiarrhythmics **(propafenone)**. Monitor and adjust dose. Severe Study
- **Idelalisib** is predicted to increase the exposure to anticholinesterases, centrally acting **(galantamine)**. Monitor and adjust dose. Moderate Study
- Antiepileptics **(carbamazepine, fosphenytoin, phenobarbital, phenytoin, primidone)** are predicted to decrease the exposure to **idelalisib**. Avoid. Severe Study
- **Idelalisib** is predicted to very slightly increase the exposure to antiepileptics **(perampanel)**. Mild Study
- **Idelalisib** is predicted to increase the exposure to antifungals, azoles **(isavuconazole)**. Avoid or monitor side effects. Severe Study
- **Idelalisib** is predicted to increase the exposure to antihistamines, non-sedating **(mizolastine)**. Avoid. Severe Study
- **Idelalisib** is predicted to increase the exposure to antihistamines, non-sedating **(rupatadine)**. Avoid. Moderate Study
- **Idelalisib** is predicted to increase the concentration of antimalarials **(piperaquine)**. Severe Theoretical
- **Apalutamide** is predicted to decrease the exposure to **idelalisib**. Avoid. Severe Study
- **Idelalisib** is predicted to increase the exposure to **apalutamide**. Mild Study
- **Idelalisib** is predicted to markedly increase the exposure to **aprepitant**. Moderate Study
- **Idelalisib** is predicted to slightly increase the exposure to **aripiprazole**. Adjust **aripiprazole** dose, p. 265. Moderate Study
- **Idelalisib** is predicted to increase the exposure to **axitinib**. Avoid or adjust dose. Moderate Study → Also see TABLE 15 p. 910
- **Idelalisib** is predicted to increase the exposure to **bedaquiline**. Avoid prolonged use. Mild Study
- **Idelalisib** is predicted to increase the exposure to beta$_2$ agonists **(salmeterol)**. Avoid. Severe Study
- **Idelalisib** slightly increases the exposure to **bortezomib**. Moderate Study → Also see TABLE 15 p. 910
- **Bosentan** is predicted to decrease the exposure to **idelalisib**. Avoid. Moderate Theoretical
- **Idelalisib** is predicted to markedly increase the exposure to **bosutinib**. Avoid or adjust dose. Severe Study → Also see TABLE 15 p. 910
- **Idelalisib** is predicted to increase the exposure to **brigatinib**. Adjust **brigatinib** dose. Severe Study
- **Idelalisib** is predicted to increase the exposure to **buspirone**. Adjust **buspirone** dose. Severe Study
- **Idelalisib** slightly increases the exposure to **cabozantinib**. Moderate Study → Also see TABLE 15 p. 910
- **Idelalisib** is predicted to increase the exposure to calcium channel blockers **(amlodipine, felodipine, lacidipine, nicardipine, nifedipine, nimodipine)**. Monitor and adjust dose. Moderate Study
- **Idelalisib** is predicted to increase the exposure to calcium channel blockers **(diltiazem, verapamil)**. Severe Study
- **Idelalisib** is predicted to markedly increase the exposure to calcium channel blockers **(lercanidipine)**. Avoid. Severe Study
- **Idelalisib** is predicted to increase the exposure to **cannabidiol**. Avoid or adjust dose. Mild Study

A1 Interactions | Appendix 1

- **Idelalisib** is predicted to moderately increase the exposure to cariprazine. Avoid. Severe Study
- **Idelalisib** is predicted to increase the exposure to **ceritinib**. Avoid or adjust **ceritinib** dose. Severe Study → Also see **TABLE 15** p. 910
- **Idelalisib** increases the concentration of ciclosporin. Severe Study
- **Idelalisib** is predicted to moderately increase the exposure to cilostazol. Adjust **cilostazol** dose. Moderate Study
- **Idelalisib** is predicted to moderately increase the exposure to cinacalcet. Adjust dose. Moderate Study
- **Idelalisib** is predicted to markedly increase the exposure to cobimetinib. Avoid or monitor for toxicity. Severe Study
- **Idelalisib** is predicted to increase the exposure to colchicine. Avoid potent inhibitors of CYP3A4 or adjust **colchicine** dose. Severe Study
- **Idelalisib** is predicted to increase the exposure to corticosteroids **(beclometasone)** (risk with beclometasone is likely to be lower than with other corticosteroids). Moderate Theoretical
- **Idelalisib** is predicted to increase the exposure to corticosteroids **(betamethasone, budesonide, ciclesonide, deflazacort, dexamethasone, fludrocortisone, fluticasone, hydrocortisone, methylprednisolone, mometasone, prednisolone, triamcinolone)**. Avoid or monitor side effects. Severe Study
- **Idelalisib** is predicted to moderately increase the exposure to crizotinib. Avoid. Moderate Study → Also see **TABLE 15** p. 910
- **Idelalisib** is predicted to increase the exposure to dabrafenib. Use with caution or avoid. Moderate Study → Also see **TABLE 15** p. 910
- **Idelalisib** is predicted to markedly to very markedly increase the exposure to darifenacin. Avoid. Severe Study
- **Idelalisib** is predicted to markedly increase the exposure to dasatinib. Avoid or adjust dose—consult product literature. Severe Study → Also see **TABLE 15** p. 910
- **Idelalisib** very slightly increases the exposure to **delamanid**. Severe Study
- **Idelalisib** is predicted to moderately increase the exposure to dienogest. Moderate Study
- **Idelalisib** increases the risk of QT-prolongation when given with domperidone. Avoid. Severe Study
- **Idelalisib** increases the exposure to dopamine receptor agonists **(bromocriptine)**. Severe Study
- **Idelalisib** is predicted to increase the concentration of dopamine receptor agonists **(cabergoline)**. Moderate Anecdotal
- **Idelalisib** is predicted to increase the exposure to doravirine. Mild Study
- **Idelalisib** is predicted to increase the exposure to dronabinol. Adjust dose. Mild Study
- **Idelalisib** is predicted to increase the exposure to dutasteride. Monitor side effects and adjust dose. Moderate Theoretical
- Efavirenz is predicted to decrease the exposure to **idelalisib**. Avoid. Moderate Theoretical
- **Idelalisib** is predicted to markedly increase the exposure to eletriptan. Avoid. Severe Study
- **Idelalisib** is predicted to increase the exposure to eliglustat. Avoid or adjust dose—consult product literature. Severe Study
- **Idelalisib** is predicted to increase the exposure to encorafenib. Avoid or monitor. Severe Study
- Enzalutamide is predicted to decrease the exposure to **idelalisib**. Avoid. Severe Study
- **Idelalisib** is predicted to increase the risk of ergotism when given with ergometrine. Avoid. Severe Theoretical
- **Idelalisib** is predicted to increase the risk of ergotism when given with ergotamine. Avoid. Severe Theoretical
- **Idelalisib** is predicted to slightly increase the exposure to erlotinib. Use with caution and adjust dose. Moderate Study
- **Idelalisib** is predicted to increase the exposure to esketamine. Adjust dose. Moderate Study
- **Idelalisib** is predicted to increase the concentration of everolimus. Avoid. Severe Study → Also see **TABLE 15** p. 910
- **Idelalisib** is predicted to moderately increase the exposure to fesoterodine. Adjust **fesoterodine** dose with potent inhibitors of CYP3A4; avoid in hepatic and renal impairment. Severe Study
- **Idelalisib** is predicted to increase the exposure to fosaprepitant. Moderate Theoretical
- **Idelalisib** is predicted to increase the exposure to gefitinib. Moderate Study → Also see **TABLE 15** p. 910
- **Idelalisib** is predicted to increase the exposure to gilteritinib. Moderate Study
- **Idelalisib** is predicted to moderately to markedly increase the exposure to grazoprevir. Avoid. Severe Study
- **Idelalisib** is predicted to increase the exposure to guanfacine. Adjust **guanfacine** dose, p. 247. Moderate Study
- **Idelalisib** is predicted to very markedly increase the exposure to ibrutinib. Avoid potent inhibitors of CYP3A4 or adjust **ibrutinib** dose. Severe Study → Also see **TABLE 15** p. 910
- **Idelalisib** is predicted to increase the exposure to imatinib. Moderate Study → Also see **TABLE 15** p. 910
- **Idelalisib** is predicted to increase the risk of toxicity when given with irinotecan. Avoid. Moderate Study → Also see **TABLE 15** p. 910
- **Idelalisib** is predicted to increase the exposure to ivabradine. Avoid. Severe Study
- **Idelalisib** is predicted to increase the exposure to **ivacaftor**. Adjust ivacaftor p. 196 or lumacaftor with ivacaftor p. 197 or tezacaftor with ivacaftor p. 198 dose with potent inhibitors of CYP3A4. Severe Study
- **Idelalisib** is predicted to increase the exposure to lapatinib. Avoid. Moderate Study
- **Idelalisib** is predicted to moderately increase the exposure to larotrectinib. Avoid or adjust **larotrectinib** dose, p. 607. Moderate Study
- **Idelalisib** is predicted to markedly increase the exposure to lomitapide. Avoid. Severe Study
- **Idelalisib** is predicted to increase the exposure to lorlatinib. Avoid or adjust **lorlatinib** dose. Severe Study
- **Idelalisib** is predicted to increase the exposure to lurasidone. Avoid. Severe Study
- **Idelalisib** is predicted to increase the exposure to macitentan. Moderate Study
- **Idelalisib** markedly increases the exposure to maraviroc. Adjust dose. Severe Theoretical
- **Idelalisib** is predicted to markedly to very markedly increase the exposure to **midazolam**. Avoid or adjust dose. Severe Study
- **Idelalisib** is predicted to very markedly increase the exposure to **midostaurin**. Avoid or monitor for toxicity. Severe Study
- **Idelalisib** is predicted to increase the exposure to mirabegron. Adjust **mirabegron** dose in hepatic and renal impairment. Moderate Study
- **Idelalisib** is predicted to increase the exposure to mirtazapine. Moderate Study
- Mitotane is predicted to decrease the exposure to **idelalisib**. Avoid. Severe Study → Also see **TABLE 15** p. 910
- **Idelalisib** is predicted to increase the exposure to modafinil. Mild Theoretical
- **Idelalisib** is predicted to increase the exposure to monoclonal antibodies **(polatuzumab vedotin)**. Moderate Theoretical
- **Idelalisib** is predicted to increase the exposure to monoclonal antibodies **(trastuzumab emtansine)**. Avoid. Severe Theoretical → Also see **TABLE 15** p. 910
- **Idelalisib** is predicted to increase the exposure to naldemedine. Avoid or monitor. Moderate Study
- **Idelalisib** is predicted to markedly increase the exposure to naloxegol. Avoid. Severe Study
- **Idelalisib** is predicted to increase the exposure to neratinib. Avoid or adjust **neratinib** dose. Severe Study
- **Idelalisib** is predicted to increase the exposure to netupitant. Moderate Study
- Nevirapine is predicted to decrease the exposure to **idelalisib**. Avoid. Moderate Theoretical
- **Idelalisib** is predicted to moderately increase the exposure to nilotinib. Avoid. Severe Study → Also see **TABLE 15** p. 910
- **Idelalisib** is predicted to increase the exposure to nitisinone. Adjust dose. Moderate Theoretical

Idelalisib (continued)
- **Idelalisib** is predicted to increase the exposure to **olaparib**. Avoid potent inhibitors of CYP3A4 or adjust **olaparib** dose. [Moderate] Study → Also see **TABLE 15** p. 910
- **Idelalisib** is predicted to increase the exposure to opioids (alfentanil, buprenorphine, fentanyl, oxycodone). Monitor and adjust dose. [Severe] Study
- **Idelalisib** is predicted to increase the exposure to opioids (methadone). [Severe] Theoretical
- **Idelalisib** is predicted to increase the exposure to **ospemifene**. Avoid in poor CYP2C9 metabolisers. [Moderate] Study
- **Idelalisib** is predicted to increase the exposure to **oxybutynin**. [Mild] Study
- **Idelalisib** is predicted to increase the exposure to **palbociclib**. Avoid or adjust **palbociclib** dose. [Severe] Study
- **Idelalisib** is predicted to increase the exposure to panobinostat. Adjust **panobinostat** dose; in hepatic impairment avoid. [Moderate] Study → Also see **TABLE 15** p. 910
- Paritaprevir is predicted to increase the exposure to **idelalisib**. Avoid. [Severe] Study
- **Idelalisib** is predicted to increase the exposure to **pazopanib**. Avoid or adjust **pazopanib** dose. [Moderate] Study → Also see **TABLE 15** p. 910
- **Idelalisib** is predicted to increase the exposure to phosphodiesterase type-5 inhibitors **(avanafil, vardenafil)**. Avoid. [Severe] Study
- **Idelalisib** is predicted to increase the exposure to phosphodiesterase type-5 inhibitors **(sildenafil)**. Avoid potent inhibitors of CYP3A4 or adjust **sildenafil** dose, p. 125. [Severe] Study
- **Idelalisib** is predicted to increase the exposure to phosphodiesterase type-5 inhibitors **(tadalafil)**. Use with caution or avoid. [Severe] Study
- **Idelalisib** is predicted to increase the exposure to **pimozide**. Avoid. [Severe] Study
- **Idelalisib** is predicted to slightly increase the exposure to ponatinib. Monitor and adjust **ponatinib** dose. [Moderate] Study
- **Idelalisib** is predicted to moderately increase the exposure to praziquantel. [Mild] Study
- **Idelalisib** given with carbimazole is predicted to increase the exposure to propiverine. Adjust starting dose. [Moderate] Theoretical
- **Idelalisib** is predicted to increase the exposure to **quetiapine**. Avoid. [Severe] Study
- **Idelalisib** is predicted to increase the exposure to **ranolazine**. Avoid. [Severe] Study
- **Idelalisib** is predicted to increase the exposure to **reboxetine**. Avoid. [Moderate] Study
- **Idelalisib** is predicted to increase the exposure to **regorafenib**. Avoid. [Moderate] Study → Also see **TABLE 15** p. 910
- **Idelalisib** is predicted to increase the exposure to **repaglinide**. [Moderate] Study
- **Idelalisib** is predicted to increase the exposure to retinoids (alitretinoin). Adjust **alitretinoin** dose. [Moderate] Theoretical
- **Idelalisib** is predicted to increase the exposure to **ribociclib**. Avoid or adjust **ribociclib** dose. [Moderate] Study
- Rifampicin is predicted to decrease the exposure to **idelalisib**. Avoid. [Severe] Study
- **Idelalisib** is predicted to increase the exposure to **risperidone**. Adjust dose. [Moderate] Study
- **Idelalisib** is predicted to increase the exposure to **ruxolitinib**. Adjust dose and monitor side effects. [Moderate] Study → Also see **TABLE 15** p. 910
- **Idelalisib** is predicted to increase the exposure to **saxagliptin**. [Moderate] Study
- **Idelalisib** is predicted to increase the exposure to **siponimod**. Avoid depending on other drugs taken—consult product literature. [Severe] Theoretical
- **Idelalisib** is predicted to increase the concentration of sirolimus. Avoid. [Severe] Study
- **Idelalisib** is predicted to increase the exposure to **solifenacin**. Adjust solifenacin or tamsulosin with solifenacin dose; avoid in hepatic and renal impairment. [Severe] Study
- **Idelalisib** is predicted to moderately increase the exposure to SSRIs (dapoxetine). Avoid potent inhibitors of CYP3A4 or adjust **dapoxetine** dose. [Severe] Study
- **St John's Wort** is predicted to decrease the exposure to **idelalisib**. Avoid. [Moderate] Theoretical
- **Idelalisib** is predicted to increase the exposure to statins (atorvastatin). Avoid or adjust dose and monitor rhabdomyolysis. [Severe] Study
- **Idelalisib** is predicted to increase the exposure to statins (simvastatin). Avoid. [Severe] Study
- **Idelalisib** is predicted to slightly increase the exposure to sunitinib. Avoid or adjust **sunitinib** dose. [Moderate] Study → Also see **TABLE 15** p. 910
- **Idelalisib** is predicted to increase the concentration of tacrolimus. Monitor and adjust dose. [Severe] Study
- **Idelalisib** is predicted to increase the exposure to taxanes (cabazitaxel). Avoid. [Severe] Study → Also see **TABLE 15** p. 910
- **Idelalisib** is predicted to moderately increase the exposure to taxanes **(docetaxel)**. Avoid or adjust dose. [Severe] Study → Also see **TABLE 15** p. 910
- **Idelalisib** is predicted to increase the exposure to taxanes (paclitaxel). [Severe] Theoretical → Also see **TABLE 15** p. 910
- **Idelalisib** is predicted to increase the concentration of temsirolimus. Avoid. [Severe] Theoretical → Also see **TABLE 15** p. 910
- **Idelalisib** is predicted to increase the exposure to **tezacaftor**. Adjust tezacaftor with ivacaftor p. 198 dose with potent inhibitors of CYP3A4. [Severe] Study
- **Idelalisib** is predicted to markedly increase the exposure to ticagrelor. Avoid. [Severe] Study
- **Idelalisib** is predicted to increase the exposure to **tofacitinib**. Adjust **tofacitinib** dose. [Moderate] Study
- **Idelalisib** is predicted to increase the exposure to **tolterodine**. Avoid. [Severe] Study
- **Idelalisib** is predicted to increase the exposure to **tolvaptan**. Manufacturer advises caution or adjust **tolvaptan** dose with potent inhibitors of CYP3A4. [Severe] Study
- **Idelalisib** is predicted to increase the exposure to **toremifene**. [Moderate] Theoretical
- **Idelalisib** is predicted to increase the exposure to **trabectedin**. Avoid or adjust dose. [Severe] Theoretical → Also see **TABLE 15** p. 910
- **Idelalisib** is predicted to moderately increase the exposure to trazodone. Avoid or adjust dose. [Moderate] Study
- **Idelalisib** is predicted to increase the exposure to **ulipristal**. Avoid if used for uterine fibroids. [Severe] Study
- **Idelalisib** is predicted to increase the exposure to **upadacitinib**. Use with caution or avoid. [Severe] Study
- **Idelalisib** is predicted to increase the exposure to **vemurafenib**. [Severe] Theoretical
- **Idelalisib** is predicted to increase the exposure to **venetoclax**. Avoid or adjust dose—consult product literature. [Severe] Study
- **Idelalisib** is predicted to increase the exposure to **venlafaxine**. [Moderate] Study
- **Idelalisib** is predicted to increase the exposure to **vinca** alkaloids. [Severe] Theoretical → Also see **TABLE 15** p. 910
- **Idelalisib** is predicted to increase the exposure to vitamin D substances **(paricalcitol)**. [Moderate] Study
- **Idelalisib** is predicted to increase the exposure to **zopiclone**. Adjust dose. [Moderate] Theoretical

Ifosfamide → see alkylating agents

Iloprost → see **TABLE 8** p. 908 (hypotension), **TABLE 4** p. 907 (antiplatelet effects)

Imatinib → see **TABLE 15** p. 910 (myelosuppression)
- **Imatinib** is predicted to increase the exposure to **abemaciclib**. [Moderate] Study
- **Imatinib** is predicted to increase the exposure to aldosterone antagonists **(eplerenone)**. Adjust **eplerenone** dose. [Severe] Study
- **Imatinib** is predicted to increase the exposure to alpha blockers **(tamsulosin)**. [Moderate] Theoretical
- **Imatinib** is predicted to increase the exposure to **alprazolam**. [Severe] Study
- **Imatinib** is predicted to increase the exposure to antiarrhythmics **(dronedarone)**. [Severe] Theoretical
- **Imatinib** is predicted to increase the exposure to antiarrhythmics (propafenone). Monitor and adjust dose. [Moderate] Study

- Antiepileptics **(carbamazepine, fosphenytoin, phenobarbital, phenytoin, primidone)** are predicted to decrease the exposure to **imatinib**. Avoid. Moderate Study
- Antiepileptics **(oxcarbazepine)** decrease the exposure to **imatinib**. Avoid. Moderate Study
- Antifungals, azoles **(fluconazole, posaconazole)** are predicted to increase the exposure to **imatinib**. Moderate Theoretical
- Antifungals, azoles **(itraconazole, ketoconazole, voriconazole)** are predicted to increase the exposure to **imatinib**. Moderate Study
- **Imatinib** is predicted to increase the exposure to antifungals, azoles **(isavuconazole)**. Moderate Theoretical
- **Imatinib** is predicted to increase the exposure to antihistamines, non-sedating **(mizolastine)**. Severe Theoretical
- **Imatinib** is predicted to increase the exposure to antihistamines, non-sedating **(rupatadine)**. Avoid. Moderate Study
- **Imatinib** is predicted to increase the concentration of antimalarials **(piperaquine)**. Severe Theoretical
- **Apalutamide** is predicted to decrease the exposure to **imatinib**. Avoid. Moderate Study
- **Aprepitant** is predicted to increase the exposure to **imatinib**. Moderate Theoretical
- **Asparaginase** is predicted to increase the risk of hepatotoxicity when given with **imatinib**. Severe Theoretical → Also see TABLE 15 p. 910
- **Imatinib** is predicted to increase the exposure to **axitinib**. Moderate Theoretical → Also see TABLE 15 p. 910
- **Imatinib** is predicted to increase the exposure to **bedaquiline**. Avoid prolonged use. Mild Theoretical
- **Bosentan** is predicted to decrease the exposure to **imatinib**. Moderate Study
- **Imatinib** is predicted to increase the exposure to **bosutinib**. Avoid or adjust dose. Severe Theoretical → Also see TABLE 15 p. 910
- **Imatinib** is predicted to increase the exposure to **buspirone**. Use with caution and adjust dose. Moderate Study
- **Imatinib** is predicted to increase the exposure to **cabozantinib**. Moderate Theoretical → Also see TABLE 15 p. 910
- Calcium channel blockers **(diltiazem, verapamil)** are predicted to increase the exposure to **imatinib**. Moderate Theoretical
- **Imatinib** is predicted to increase the exposure to calcium channel blockers **(amlodipine, felodipine, lacidipine, lercanidipine, nicardipine, nifedipine, nimodipine)**. Monitor and adjust dose. Moderate Study
- **Imatinib** is predicted to increase the exposure to **cariprazine**. Avoid. Severe Study
- **Imatinib** is predicted to increase the concentration of **ciclosporin**. Severe Study
- **Cobicistat** is predicted to increase the exposure to **imatinib**. Moderate Study
- **Imatinib** is predicted to increase the exposure to **cobimetinib**. Severe Theoretical
- **Imatinib** is predicted to increase the exposure to **colchicine**. Adjust **colchicine** dose with moderate inhibitors of CYP3A4. Severe Study
- **Imatinib** is predicted to increase the exposure to corticosteroids **(methylprednisolone)**. Monitor and adjust dose. Moderate Study
- **Imatinib** is predicted to increase the risk of bleeding events when given with **coumarins**. Severe Theoretical
- **Crisantaspase** is predicted to increase the risk of hepatotoxicity when given with **imatinib**. Severe Theoretical → Also see TABLE 15 p. 910
- **Imatinib** is predicted to slightly increase the exposure to **darifenacin**. Moderate Study
- **Imatinib** is predicted to increase the exposure to **dasatinib**. Severe Study → Also see TABLE 15 p. 910
- **Imatinib** is predicted to slightly increase the exposure to **dienogest**. Moderate Study
- **Imatinib** increases the risk of QT-prolongation when given with **domperidone**. Avoid. Severe Study
- **Imatinib** is predicted to increase the exposure to dopamine receptor agonists **(bromocriptine)**. Severe Theoretical
- **Imatinib** is predicted to increase the concentration of dopamine receptor agonists **(cabergoline)**. Moderate Anecdotal
- **Imatinib** is predicted to moderately increase the exposure to **dutasteride**. Mild Study
- **Efavirenz** is predicted to decrease the exposure to **imatinib**. Moderate Study
- **Imatinib** is predicted to increase the exposure to **eliglustat**. Avoid or adjust dose—consult product literature. Severe Study
- **Imatinib** is predicted to moderately increase the exposure to **encorafenib**. Moderate Study
- **Enzalutamide** is predicted to decrease the exposure to **imatinib**. Avoid. Moderate Study
- **Imatinib** is predicted to increase the risk of ergotism when given with **ergometrine**. Severe Theoretical
- **Imatinib** is predicted to increase the risk of ergotism when given with **ergotamine**. Severe Theoretical
- **Imatinib** is predicted to increase the exposure to **erlotinib**. Moderate Theoretical
- **Imatinib** is predicted to increase the concentration of **everolimus**. Avoid or adjust dose. Moderate Study → Also see TABLE 15 p. 910
- **Imatinib** is predicted to increase the exposure to **fesoterodine**. Adjust **fesoterodine** dose with moderate inhibitors of CYP3A4 in hepatic and renal impairment. Mild Study
- **Imatinib** is predicted to increase the exposure to **gefitinib**. Moderate Theoretical → Also see TABLE 15 p. 910
- **Grapefruit juice** is predicted to increase the exposure to **imatinib**. Moderate Theoretical
- **Imatinib** is predicted to increase the concentration of **guanfacine**. Adjust **guanfacine** dose, p. 247. Moderate Theoretical
- **HIV-protease inhibitors** are predicted to increase the exposure to **imatinib**. Moderate Study
- **Imatinib** is predicted to increase the exposure to **ibrutinib**. Adjust **ibrutinib** dose with moderate inhibitors of CYP3A4. Severe Study → Also see TABLE 15 p. 910
- **Idelalisib** is predicted to increase the exposure to **imatinib**. Moderate Study → Also see TABLE 15 p. 910
- **Imatinib** is predicted to increase the exposure to **ivabradine**. Adjust **ivabradine** dose. Severe Theoretical
- **Imatinib** is predicted to increase the exposure to **ivacaftor**. Adjust ivacaftor p. 196 or tezacaftor with ivacaftor p. 198 dose with moderate inhibitors of CYP3A4. Severe Study
- **Imatinib** is predicted to increase the exposure to **lapatinib**. Moderate Study
- **Imatinib** is predicted to increase the exposure to **lomitapide**. Avoid. Moderate Theoretical
- **Imatinib** is predicted to increase the exposure to **lurasidone**. Adjust **lurasidone** dose. Moderate Study
- Macrolides **(clarithromycin)** are predicted to increase the exposure to **imatinib**. Moderate Study
- Macrolides **(erythromycin)** are predicted to increase the exposure to **imatinib**. Moderate Theoretical
- **Imatinib** is predicted to increase the exposure to **midazolam**. Monitor side effects and adjust dose. Severe Study
- **Imatinib** is predicted to increase the exposure to **midostaurin**. Moderate Theoretical
- **Mitotane** is predicted to decrease the exposure to **imatinib**. Avoid. Moderate Study → Also see TABLE 15 p. 910
- **Imatinib** is predicted to increase the exposure to **naldemedine**. Moderate Study
- **Imatinib** is predicted to increase the exposure to **naloxegol**. Adjust **naloxegol** dose and monitor side effects. Moderate Study
- **Imatinib** is predicted to increase the exposure to **neratinib**. Avoid. Severe Study
- **Netupitant** is predicted to increase the exposure to **imatinib**. Moderate Theoretical
- **Nevirapine** is predicted to decrease the exposure to **imatinib**. Moderate Study
- **Imatinib** is predicted to increase the exposure to **olaparib**. Avoid moderate inhibitors of CYP3A4 or adjust **olaparib** dose. Moderate Theoretical → Also see TABLE 15 p. 910
- **Imatinib** is predicted to increase the exposure to opioids **(alfentanil, buprenorphine, fentanyl, oxycodone)**. Monitor and adjust dose. Moderate Study
- **Imatinib** is predicted to increase the exposure to opioids **(methadone)**. Moderate Theoretical
- **Imatinib** is predicted to increase the exposure to **oxybutynin**. Mild Theoretical

Imatinib (continued)

- ▶ **Imatinib** increases the risk of hepatotoxicity when given with paracetamol. Severe Anecdotal
- ▶ **Imatinib** is predicted to increase the exposure to **pazopanib**. Moderate Theoretical → Also see **TABLE 15** p. 910
- ▶ **Pegaspargase** is predicted to increase the risk of hepatotoxicity when given with **imatinib**. Severe Theoretical → Also see **TABLE 15** p. 910
- ▶ **Imatinib** is predicted to increase the risk of bleeding events when given with **phenindione**. Severe Theoretical
- ▶ **Imatinib** is predicted to increase the exposure to phosphodiesterase type-5 inhibitors **(avanafil)**. Adjust **avanafil** dose. Moderate Theoretical
- ▶ **Imatinib** is predicted to increase the exposure to phosphodiesterase type-5 inhibitors **(sildenafil)**. Monitor or adjust **sildenafil** dose with moderate inhibitors of CYP3A4, p. 125. Moderate Study
- ▶ **Imatinib** is predicted to increase the exposure to phosphodiesterase type-5 inhibitors **(tadalafil)**. Severe Theoretical
- ▶ **Imatinib** is predicted to increase the exposure to phosphodiesterase type-5 inhibitors **(vardenafil)**. Adjust dose. Severe Theoretical
- ▶ **Imatinib** is predicted to increase the exposure to **pimozide**. Avoid. Severe Theoretical
- ▶ **Imatinib** is predicted to increase the exposure to **quetiapine**. Avoid. Moderate Study
- ▶ **Imatinib** is predicted to increase the exposure to **ranolazine**. Severe Study
- ▶ **Imatinib** is predicted to increase the exposure to **ribociclib**. Moderate Study
- ▶ **Rifampicin** is predicted to decrease the exposure to **imatinib**. Avoid. Moderate Study
- ▶ **Imatinib** is predicted to increase the exposure to **ruxolitinib**. Moderate Theoretical → Also see **TABLE 15** p. 910
- ▶ **Imatinib** is predicted to increase the exposure to **saxagliptin**. Mild Study
- ▶ **Imatinib** increases the concentration of **sirolimus**. Monitor and adjust dose. Moderate Study
- ▶ **Imatinib** is predicted to increase the exposure to SSRIs **(dapoxetine)**. Adjust **dapoxetine** dose with moderate inhibitors of CYP3A4. Moderate Theoretical
- ▶ **St John's Wort** is predicted to decrease the exposure to **imatinib**. Moderate Study
- ▶ **Imatinib** is predicted to increase the exposure to statins **(atorvastatin)**. Monitor and adjust dose. Severe Theoretical
- ▶ **Imatinib** moderately increases the exposure to statins **(simvastatin)**. Monitor and adjust dose. Severe Study
- ▶ **Imatinib** is predicted to increase the exposure to **sunitinib**. Moderate Theoretical → Also see **TABLE 15** p. 910
- ▶ **Imatinib** is predicted to increase the concentration of **tacrolimus**. Severe Study
- ▶ **Imatinib** is predicted to increase the exposure to taxanes **(cabazitaxel)**. Moderate Theoretical → Also see **TABLE 15** p. 910
- ▶ **Tedizolid** is predicted to increase the exposure to **imatinib**. Avoid. Moderate Theoretical
- ▶ **Imatinib** is predicted to increase the concentration of **temsirolimus**. Use with caution or avoid. Moderate Theoretical → Also see **TABLE 15** p. 910
- ▶ **Imatinib** is predicted to increase the exposure to **tezacaftor**. Adjust **tezacaftor** with **ivacaftor** p. 198 dose with moderate inhibitors of CYP3A4. Severe Study
- ▶ **Imatinib** given with a potent CYP2C19 inhibitor is predicted to increase the exposure to **tofacitinib**. Adjust **tofacitinib** dose. Moderate Study
- ▶ **Imatinib** is predicted to increase the exposure to **tolterodine**. Mild Theoretical
- ▶ **Imatinib** is predicted to increase the exposure to **tolvaptan**. Manufacturer advises caution or adjust **tolvaptan** dose with moderate inhibitors of CYP3A4. Moderate Study
- ▶ **Imatinib** is predicted to increase the exposure to **trazodone**. Moderate Theoretical
- ▶ **Imatinib** is predicted to increase the exposure to **ulipristal**. Avoid if used for uterine fibroids. Moderate Study
- ▶ **Imatinib** is predicted to increase the exposure to **venetoclax**. Avoid or adjust dose—consult product literature. Severe Study
- ▶ **Imatinib** is predicted to increase the exposure to **vinca alkaloids**. Severe Theoretical → Also see **TABLE 15** p. 910
- ▶ **Imatinib** is predicted to increase the exposure to **zopiclone**. Adjust dose. Moderate Study

Imidapril → see ACE inhibitors

Imipenem → see carbapenems

Imipramine → see tricyclic antidepressants

Immunoglobulins

Anti-D (Rh_0) immunoglobulin · antithymocyte immunoglobulin (rabbit) · cytomegalovirus immunoglobulin · hepatitis B immunoglobulin · normal immunoglobulin · rabies immunoglobulin · tetanus immunoglobulin · varicella-zoster immunoglobulin

- ▶ **Cytomegalovirus immunoglobulin** is predicted to decrease the efficacy of **live vaccines**. Avoid. Severe Theoretical
- ▶ **Cytomegalovirus immunoglobulin** is predicted to increase the risk of side-effects when given with **loop diuretics**. Avoid. Moderate Theoretical
- ▶ **Immunoglobulins** are predicted to alter the effects of monoclonal antibodies **(dinutuximab)**. Avoid. Severe Theoretical

Indacaterol → see beta₂ agonists

Indapamide → see thiazide diuretics

Indometacin → see NSAIDs

Indoramin → see alpha blockers

Infliximab → see monoclonal antibodies

Influenza vaccine (live) → see live vaccines

Inotersen → see **TABLE 4** p. 907 (antiplatelet effects)

Inotuzumab ozogamicin → see monoclonal antibodies

Insulins → see **TABLE 14** p. 910 (antidiabetic drugs)

- ▶ **Fibrates** are predicted to increase the risk of hypoglycaemia when given with **insulins**. Moderate Theoretical

Interferon alfa → see interferons

Interferon beta → see interferons

Interferons → see **TABLE 15** p. 910 (myelosuppression)

interferon alfa · interferon beta · peginterferon alfa

- ▶ **Interferons** are predicted to slightly increase the exposure to **aminophylline**. Adjust dose. Moderate Theoretical
- ▶ **Interferon alfa** is predicted to increase the risk of peripheral neuropathy when given with **telbivudine**. Avoid. Severe Theoretical
- ▶ **Peginterferon alfa** increases the risk of peripheral neuropathy when given with **telbivudine**. Avoid. Severe Study
- ▶ **Interferons** slightly increase the exposure to **theophylline**. Adjust dose. Moderate Study

Ipilimumab → see monoclonal antibodies

Ipratropium → see **TABLE 10** p. 909 (antimuscarinics)

- ▶ **Beta₂ agonists** are predicted to increase the risk of glaucoma when given with **ipratropium**. Moderate Anecdotal

Irbesartan → see angiotensin-II receptor antagonists

Irinotecan → see **TABLE 15** p. 910 (myelosuppression)

- ▶ Antiepileptics **(carbamazepine, fosphenytoin, phenobarbital, phenytoin, primidone)** are predicted to decrease the exposure to **irinotecan**. Avoid. Severe Study
- ▶ Antifungals, azoles **(itraconazole, ketoconazole, voriconazole)** are predicted to increase the risk of toxicity when given with **irinotecan**. Avoid. Moderate Study
- ▶ **Apalutamide** is predicted to decrease the exposure to **irinotecan**. Avoid. Severe Study
- ▶ **Aprepitant** is predicted to increase the exposure to intravenous **irinotecan**. Severe Theoretical
- ▶ **Cobicistat** is predicted to increase the risk of toxicity when given with **irinotecan**. Avoid. Moderate Study
- ▶ **Enzalutamide** is predicted to decrease the exposure to **irinotecan**. Avoid. Severe Study
- ▶ Fibrates **(gemfibrozil)** are predicted to increase the exposure to **irinotecan**. Avoid. Moderate Theoretical
- ▶ **Fosaprepitant** is predicted to increase the exposure to intravenous **irinotecan**. Severe Theoretical
- ▶ **HIV-protease inhibitors** are predicted to increase the risk of toxicity when given with **irinotecan**. Avoid. Moderate Study
- ▶ **Idelalisib** is predicted to increase the risk of toxicity when given with **irinotecan**. Avoid. Moderate Study → Also see **TABLE 15** p. 910
- ▶ **Live vaccines** are predicted to increase the risk of generalised infection (possibly life-threatening) when given with

irinotecan. Public Health England advises avoid (refer to Green Book). Severe Theoretical
- Macrolides (clarithromycin) are predicted to increase the risk of toxicity when given with irinotecan. Avoid. Moderate Study
- Mitotane is predicted to decrease the exposure to irinotecan. Avoid. Severe Study → Also see TABLE 15 p. 910
- Netupitant is predicted to increase the exposure to irinotecan. Moderate Study
- Irinotecan is predicted to decrease the effects of neuromuscular blocking drugs, non-depolarising. Moderate Theoretical
- Pitolisant is predicted to decrease the exposure to irinotecan. Mild Theoretical
- Rifampicin is predicted to decrease the exposure to irinotecan. Avoid. Severe Study
- Rolapitant is predicted to increase the exposure to irinotecan. Avoid or monitor. Moderate Study
- St John's Wort slightly decreases the exposure to irinotecan. Avoid. Severe Study
- Irinotecan is predicted to increase the risk of prolonged neuromuscular blockade when given with suxamethonium. Moderate Theoretical

Iron (injectable)

ferric carboxymaltose · iron dextran · iron isomaltoside 1000 · iron sucrose

- Chloramphenicol decreases the efficacy of intravenous iron (injectable). Moderate Anecdotal

Iron (oral)

ferric maltol · ferrous fumarate · ferrous gluconate · ferrous sulfate · sodium feredetate

- Antacids decrease the absorption of iron (oral). Iron (oral) should be taken 1 hour before or 2 hours after antacids. Moderate Study
- Iron (oral) decreases the exposure to bictegravir. Manufacturer advises take 2 hours before iron (oral). Moderate Study
- Iron (oral) decreases the absorption of bisphosphonates (clodronate). Avoid iron (oral) for 2 hours before or 1 hour after clodronate. Moderate Study
- Iron (oral) is predicted to decrease the absorption of oral bisphosphonates (ibandronate). Avoid iron (oral) for at least 6 hours before or 1 hour after ibandronate. Moderate Theoretical
- Iron (oral) decreases the absorption of bisphosphonates (risedronate). Separate administration by at least 2 hours. Moderate Study
- Calcium salts (calcium carbonate) decrease the absorption of iron (oral). Calcium carbonate should be taken 1 hour before or 2 hours after iron (oral). Moderate Study
- Iron (oral) is predicted to decrease the exposure to carbidopa. Moderate Theoretical
- Chloramphenicol decreases the efficacy of oral iron (oral). Moderate Theoretical
- Iron (oral) decreases the absorption of dolutegravir. Dolutegravir should be taken 2 hours before or 6 hours after iron (oral). Moderate Study
- Iron (oral) is predicted to decrease the absorption of eltrombopag. Eltrombopag should be taken 2 hours before or 4 hours after iron (oral). Severe Theoretical
- Iron (oral) is predicted to decrease the absorption of entacapone. Separate administration by at least 2 hours. Moderate Theoretical
- Iron (oral) are predicted to decrease the absorption of iron chelators (deferiprone). Moderate Theoretical
- Iron (oral) decreases the absorption of levodopa. Moderate Study
- Iron (oral) decreases the effects of methyldopa. Moderate Study
- Iron (oral) is predicted to decrease the absorption of penicillamine. Separate administration by at least 2 hours. Mild Study
- Iron (oral) decreases the exposure to quinolones. Separate administration by at least 2 hours. Moderate Study
- Iron (oral) decreases the absorption of tetracyclines. Tetracyclines should be taken 2 to 3 hours after iron (oral). Moderate Study
- Iron (oral) decreases the absorption of thyroid hormones (levothyroxine). Separate administration by at least 4 hours. Moderate Study
- Trientine potentially decreases the absorption of iron (oral). Moderate Theoretical
- Zinc is predicted to decrease the efficacy of iron (oral) and iron (oral) is predicted to decrease the efficacy of zinc. Moderate Study

Iron chelators → see TABLE 15 p. 910 (myelosuppression)

deferasirox · deferiprone · desferrioxamine · dexrazoxane

- Deferasirox is predicted to increase the exposure to aminophylline. Avoid. Moderate Theoretical
- Antacids (aluminium hydroxide) are predicted to decrease the exposure to deferasirox. Avoid. Moderate Theoretical
- Antacids (aluminium hydroxide) are predicted to decrease the absorption of deferiprone. Avoid. Moderate Theoretical
- Antiepileptics (carbamazepine, fosphenytoin, phenobarbital, phenytoin, primidone) are predicted to decrease the exposure to deferasirox. Monitor serum ferritin and adjust dose. Moderate Theoretical
- Ascorbic acid is predicted to increase the risk of cardiovascular side-effects when given with iron chelators (deferiprone, desferrioxamine). Severe Theoretical
- Aspirin (high-dose) is predicted to increase the risk of gastrointestinal bleeds when given with deferasirox. Severe Theoretical
- Bisphosphonates are predicted to increase the risk of gastrointestinal bleeding when given with deferasirox. Severe Theoretical
- Deferasirox is predicted to increase the exposure to clozapine. Avoid. Moderate Theoretical
- Corticosteroids are predicted to increase the risk of gastrointestinal bleeding when given with deferasirox. Severe Theoretical
- HIV-protease inhibitors (ritonavir) are predicted to decrease the exposure to deferasirox. Monitor serum ferritin and adjust dose. Moderate Theoretical
- Iron (oral) are predicted to decrease the absorption of deferiprone. Moderate Theoretical
- Live vaccines are predicted to increase the risk of generalised infection (possibly life-threatening) when given with dexrazoxane. Avoid. Severe Theoretical
- Deferasirox is predicted to increase the exposure to montelukast. Moderate Theoretical
- NSAIDs are predicted to increase the risk of gastrointestinal bleeding when given with deferasirox. Severe Theoretical
- NSAIDs (diclofenac) are predicted to increase the exposure to deferiprone. Moderate Theoretical
- Deferasirox is predicted to increase the exposure to pioglitazone. Moderate Study
- Deferasirox moderately increases the exposure to repaglinide. Avoid. Moderate Study
- Rifampicin is predicted to decrease the exposure to deferasirox. Monitor serum ferritin and adjust dose. Moderate Study
- Deferasirox is predicted to increase the exposure to selexipag. Adjust selexipag dose. Moderate Study
- Deferasirox is predicted to increase the concentration of taxanes (paclitaxel). Severe Anecdotal
- Deferasirox increases the exposure to theophylline. Avoid. Moderate Study
- Deferasirox is predicted to increase the exposure to tizanidine. Avoid. Moderate Theoretical
- Oral zinc is predicted to decrease the absorption of oral deferiprone. Moderate Theoretical

Iron dextran → see iron (injectable)
Iron isomaltoside 1000 → see iron (injectable)
Iron sucrose → see iron (injectable)
Isavuconazole → see antifungals, azoles
Isocarboxazid → see MAOIs, irreversible
Isoflurane → see volatile halogenated anaesthetics
Isometheptene → see sympathomimetics, vasoconstrictor
Isoniazid → see TABLE 1 p. 907 (hepatotoxicity), TABLE 12 p. 910 (peripheral neuropathy)

Isoniazid (continued)

FOOD AND LIFESTYLE Avoid tyramine-rich foods (such as mature cheeses, salami, pickled herring, *Bovril*®, *Oxo*®, *Marmite*® or any similar meat or yeast extract or fermented soya bean extract, and some beers, lagers or wines) or histamine-rich foods (such as very mature cheese or fish from the scromboid family (e.g. tuna, mackerel, salmon)), as tachycardia, palpitation, hypotension, flushing, headache, dizziness, and sweating reported.

- **Isoniazid** is predicted to affect the clearance of **aminophylline**. Severe Theoretical
- **Isoniazid** markedly increases the concentration of antiepileptics **(carbamazepine)** and antiepileptics **(carbamazepine)** increase the risk of hepatotoxicity when given with **isoniazid**. Monitor concentration and adjust dose. Severe Study → Also see **TABLE 1** p. 907
- **Isoniazid** increases the concentration of antiepileptics **(fosphenytoin, phenytoin)**. Moderate Study → Also see **TABLE 12** p. 910
- **Cycloserine** increases the risk of CNS toxicity when given with **isoniazid**. Monitor and adjust dose. Moderate Study
- **Isoniazid** increases the risk of optic neuropathy when given with **ethambutol**. Severe Anecdotal
- **Isoniazid** decreases the effects of **levodopa**. Moderate Study
- **Isoniazid** is predicted to increase the exposure to **lomitapide**. Separate administration by 12 hours. Unknown Theoretical → Also see **TABLE 1** p. 907
- **Isoniazid** is predicted to increase the risk of peripheral neuropathy when given with **stavudine**. Severe Theoretical → Also see **TABLE 12** p. 910
- **Isoniazid** is predicted to affect the clearance of **theophylline**. Severe Anecdotal
- **Isoniazid** potentially increases the risk of nephrotoxicity when given with volatile halogenated anaesthetics **(methoxyflurane)**. Avoid. Severe Theoretical

Isosorbide dinitrate → see nitrates
Isosorbide mononitrate → see nitrates
Isotretinoin → see retinoids
Itraconazole → see antifungals, azoles
Ivabradine → see **TABLE 6** p. 908 (bradycardia)

- Antiarrhythmics **(dronedarone)** are predicted to increase the exposure to **ivabradine**. Adjust **ivabradine** dose. Severe Theoretical
- Antiepileptics **(carbamazepine, fosphenytoin, phenobarbital, phenytoin, primidone)** are predicted to decrease the exposure to **ivabradine**. Adjust dose. Moderate Theoretical
- Antifungals, azoles **(fluconazole, isavuconazole, posaconazole)** are predicted to increase the exposure to **ivabradine**. Adjust **ivabradine** dose. Severe Theoretical
- Antifungals, azoles **(itraconazole, ketoconazole, voriconazole)** are predicted to increase the exposure to **ivabradine**. Avoid. Severe Study
- **Apalutamide** is predicted to decrease the exposure to **ivabradine**. Adjust dose. Moderate Theoretical
- **Aprepitant** is predicted to increase the exposure to **ivabradine**. Adjust **ivabradine** dose. Severe Theoretical
- Calcium channel blockers **(diltiazem, verapamil)** are predicted to increase the exposure to **ivabradine**. Avoid. Moderate Study → Also see **TABLE 6** p. 908
- **Cobicistat** is predicted to increase the exposure to **ivabradine**. Avoid. Severe Study
- **Crizotinib** is predicted to increase the exposure to **ivabradine**. Adjust **ivabradine** dose. Severe Theoretical → Also see **TABLE 6** p. 908
- **Enzalutamide** is predicted to decrease the exposure to **ivabradine**. Adjust dose. Moderate Theoretical
- **Grapefruit juice** is predicted to increase the exposure to **ivabradine**. Avoid. Moderate Study
- **HIV-protease inhibitors** are predicted to increase the exposure to **ivabradine**. Avoid. Severe Study
- **Idelalisib** is predicted to increase the exposure to **ivabradine**. Avoid. Severe Study
- **Imatinib** is predicted to increase the exposure to **ivabradine**. Adjust **ivabradine** dose. Severe Theoretical
- Macrolides **(clarithromycin)** are predicted to increase the exposure to **ivabradine**. Avoid. Severe Study
- Macrolides **(erythromycin)** are predicted to increase the exposure to **ivabradine**. Avoid. Severe Theoretical
- **Mitotane** is predicted to decrease the exposure to **ivabradine**. Adjust dose. Moderate Theoretical
- **Netupitant** is predicted to increase the exposure to **ivabradine**. Adjust **ivabradine** dose. Severe Theoretical
- **Nilotinib** is predicted to increase the exposure to **ivabradine**. Adjust **ivabradine** dose. Severe Theoretical
- **Rifampicin** is predicted to decrease the exposure to **ivabradine**. Adjust dose. Moderate Theoretical
- **St John's Wort** decreases the exposure to **ivabradine**. Avoid. Moderate Study

Ivacaftor

FOOD AND LIFESTYLE Avoid bitter (Seville) oranges as they are predicted to increase the exposure to ivacaftor.

- Antiarrhythmics **(dronedarone)** are predicted to increase the exposure to **ivacaftor**. Adjust ivacaftor p. 196 or tezacaftor with ivacaftor p. 198 dose with moderate inhibitors of CYP3A4. Severe Study
- Antiepileptics **(carbamazepine, fosphenytoin, phenobarbital, phenytoin, primidone)** are predicted to moderately to markedly decrease the exposure to **ivacaftor**. Avoid. Severe Study
- Antifungals, azoles **(fluconazole, isavuconazole, posaconazole)** are predicted to increase the exposure to **ivacaftor**. Adjust ivacaftor p. 196 or tezacaftor with ivacaftor p. 198 dose with moderate inhibitors of CYP3A4. Severe Study
- Antifungals, azoles **(itraconazole, ketoconazole, voriconazole)** are predicted to increase the exposure to **ivacaftor**. Adjust ivacaftor p. 196 or lumacaftor with ivacaftor p. 197 or tezacaftor with ivacaftor p. 198 dose with potent inhibitors of CYP3A4. Severe Study
- **Apalutamide** is predicted to moderately to markedly decrease the exposure to **ivacaftor**. Avoid. Severe Study
- **Aprepitant** is predicted to increase the exposure to **ivacaftor**. Adjust ivacaftor p. 196 or tezacaftor with ivacaftor p. 198 dose with moderate inhibitors of CYP3A4. Severe Study
- **Bosentan** is predicted to decrease the exposure to **ivacaftor**. Moderate Study
- Calcium channel blockers **(diltiazem, verapamil)** are predicted to increase the exposure to **ivacaftor**. Adjust ivacaftor p. 196 or tezacaftor with ivacaftor p. 198 dose with moderate inhibitors of CYP3A4. Severe Study
- **Cobicistat** is predicted to increase the exposure to **ivacaftor**. Adjust ivacaftor p. 196 or lumacaftor with ivacaftor p. 197 or tezacaftor with ivacaftor p. 198 dose with potent inhibitors of CYP3A4. Severe Study
- **Ivacaftor** is predicted to increase the anticoagulant effect of coumarins **(warfarin)**. Severe Theoretical
- **Crizotinib** is predicted to increase the exposure to **ivacaftor**. Adjust ivacaftor p. 196 or tezacaftor with ivacaftor p. 198 dose with moderate inhibitors of CYP3A4. Severe Study
- **Ivacaftor** slightly increases the exposure to **digoxin**. Moderate Study
- **Efavirenz** is predicted to decrease the exposure to **ivacaftor**. Moderate Study
- **Enzalutamide** is predicted to moderately to markedly decrease the exposure to **ivacaftor**. Avoid. Severe Study
- **Grapefruit juice** is predicted to increase the exposure to **ivacaftor**. Avoid. Moderate Theoretical
- **HIV-protease inhibitors** are predicted to increase the exposure to **ivacaftor**. Adjust ivacaftor p. 196 or lumacaftor with ivacaftor p. 197 or tezacaftor with ivacaftor p. 198 dose with potent inhibitors of CYP3A4. Severe Study
- **Idelalisib** is predicted to increase the exposure to **ivacaftor**. Adjust ivacaftor p. 196 or lumacaftor with ivacaftor p. 197 or tezacaftor with ivacaftor p. 198 dose with potent inhibitors of CYP3A4. Severe Study
- **Imatinib** is predicted to increase the exposure to **ivacaftor**. Adjust ivacaftor p. 196 or tezacaftor with ivacaftor p. 198 dose with moderate inhibitors of CYP3A4. Severe Study
- **Ivacaftor** is predicted to increase the exposure to **lomitapide**. Separate administration by 12 hours. Moderate Theoretical

- Macrolides **(clarithromycin)** are predicted to increase the exposure to **ivacaftor**. Adjust ivacaftor p. 196 or lumacaftor with ivacaftor p. 197 or tezacaftor with ivacaftor p. 198 dose with potent inhibitors of CYP3A4. [Severe] Study
- Macrolides **(erythromycin)** are predicted to increase the exposure to **ivacaftor**. Adjust ivacaftor p. 196 or tezacaftor with ivacaftor p. 198 dose with moderate inhibitors of CYP3A4. [Severe] Study
- **Mitotane** is predicted to moderately to markedly decrease the exposure to **ivacaftor**. Avoid. [Severe] Study
- **Netupitant** is predicted to increase the exposure to **ivacaftor**. Adjust ivacaftor p. 196 or tezacaftor with ivacaftor p. 198 dose with moderate inhibitors of CYP3A4. [Severe] Study
- **Nevirapine** is predicted to decrease the exposure to **ivacaftor**. [Moderate] Study
- **Nilotinib** is predicted to increase the exposure to **ivacaftor**. Adjust ivacaftor p. 196 or tezacaftor with ivacaftor p. 198 dose with moderate inhibitors of CYP3A4. [Severe] Study
- **Rifampicin** is predicted to moderately to markedly decrease the exposure to **ivacaftor**. Avoid. [Severe] Study
- **St John's Wort** is predicted to decrease the exposure to **ivacaftor**. Avoid. [Severe] Study

Ivermectin

ROUTE-SPECIFIC INFORMATION Since systemic absorption can follow topical application, the possibility of interactions should be borne in mind.

- **Ivermectin** potentially increases the anticoagulant effect of **coumarins**. [Severe] Anecdotal
- **Levamisole** increases the exposure to **ivermectin**. [Moderate] Study

Ixazomib

- Antiepileptics **(carbamazepine, fosphenytoin, phenobarbital, phenytoin, primidone)** are predicted to decrease the exposure to **ixazomib**. Avoid. [Severe] Study
- **Apalutamide** is predicted to decrease the exposure to **ixazomib**. Avoid. [Severe] Study
- **Enzalutamide** is predicted to decrease the exposure to **ixazomib**. Avoid. [Severe] Study
- **Mitotane** is predicted to decrease the exposure to **ixazomib**. Avoid. [Severe] Study
- **Rifampicin** is predicted to decrease the exposure to **ixazomib**. Avoid. [Severe] Study
- **St John's Wort** is predicted to decrease the exposure to **ixazomib**. Avoid. [Severe] Theoretical

Ixekizumab → see monoclonal antibodies

Kaolin

- **Kaolin** is predicted to decrease the absorption of **tetracyclines**. [Moderate] Theoretical

Ketamine → see TABLE 8 p. 908 (hypotension), TABLE 11 p. 909 (CNS depressant effects)

- **Ketamine** is predicted to increase the risk of elevated blood pressure when given with **ergometrine**. [Severe] Theoretical
- **Memantine** is predicted to increase the risk of CNS side-effects when given with **ketamine**. Avoid. [Severe] Theoretical

Ketoconazole → see antifungals, azoles

Ketoprofen → see NSAIDs

Ketorolac → see NSAIDs

Ketotifen → see antihistamines, sedating

Labetalol → see beta blockers, non-selective

Lacidipine → see calcium channel blockers

Lacosamide → see antiepileptics

Lamivudine → see TABLE 12 p. 910 (peripheral neuropathy)

- **Trimethoprim** slightly increases the exposure to **lamivudine**. [Moderate] Study
- **Zidovudine** increases the risk of toxicity when given with **lamivudine**. [Severe] Anecdotal

Lamotrigine → see antiepileptics

Lanreotide

- **Beta blockers, non-selective** are predicted to increase the risk of bradycardia when given with **lanreotide**. [Moderate] Theoretical
- **Beta blockers, selective** are predicted to increase the risk of bradycardia when given with **lanreotide**. [Moderate] Theoretical
- **Lanreotide** is predicted to decrease the absorption of oral **ciclosporin**. Adjust dose. [Severe] Theoretical

Lansoprazole → see proton pump inhibitors

Lanthanum

- **Lanthanum** is predicted to decrease the absorption of antifungals, azoles **(ketoconazole)**. Separate administration by at least 2 hours. [Moderate] Theoretical
- **Lanthanum** is predicted to decrease the absorption of antimalarials **(chloroquine)**. Separate administration by at least 2 hours. [Moderate] Theoretical
- **Lanthanum** is predicted to decrease the absorption of **hydroxychloroquine**. Separate administration by at least 2 hours. [Moderate] Theoretical
- **Lanthanum** moderately decreases the exposure to **quinolones**. **Quinolones** should be taken 2 hours before or 4 hours after **lanthanum**. [Moderate] Study
- **Lanthanum** is predicted to decrease the absorption of **tetracyclines**. Separate administration by 2 hours. [Moderate] Theoretical
- **Lanthanum** decreases the absorption of **thyroid hormones**. Separate administration by 2 hours. [Moderate] Study

Lapatinib → see TABLE 9 p. 909 (QT-interval prolongation)

- **Lapatinib** is predicted to increase the exposure to **afatinib**. Separate administration by 12 hours. [Moderate] Study
- **Lapatinib** is predicted to increase the exposure to **aliskiren**. [Moderate] Theoretical
- **Antacids** are predicted to decrease the absorption of **lapatinib**. Avoid. [Moderate] Theoretical
- Antiarrhythmics **(dronedarone)** are predicted to increase the exposure to **lapatinib**. [Moderate] Study → Also see TABLE 9 p. 909
- Antiepileptics **(carbamazepine, fosphenytoin, phenobarbital, phenytoin, primidone)** are predicted to decrease the exposure to **lapatinib**. Avoid. [Severe] Study
- Antifungals, azoles **(fluconazole, isavuconazole, posaconazole)** are predicted to increase the exposure to **lapatinib**. [Moderate] Study → Also see TABLE 9 p. 909
- Antifungals, azoles **(itraconazole, ketoconazole, voriconazole)** are predicted to increase the exposure to **lapatinib**. Avoid. [Moderate] Study → Also see TABLE 9 p. 909
- **Lapatinib** is predicted to increase the exposure to antihistamines, non-sedating **(fexofenadine)**. [Moderate] Theoretical
- **Apalutamide** is predicted to decrease the exposure to **lapatinib**. Avoid. [Severe] Study → Also see TABLE 9 p. 909
- **Aprepitant** is predicted to increase the exposure to **lapatinib**. [Moderate] Study
- **Lapatinib** is predicted to increase the exposure to beta blockers, non-selective **(nadolol)**. [Moderate] Study
- **Lapatinib** is predicted to increase the exposure to **bictegravir**. Use with caution or avoid. [Moderate] Theoretical
- **Bosentan** is predicted to decrease the exposure to **lapatinib**. Avoid. [Severe] Study
- Calcium channel blockers **(diltiazem, verapamil)** are predicted to increase the exposure to **lapatinib**. [Moderate] Study
- **Lapatinib** is predicted to increase the exposure to **ceritinib**. [Moderate] Theoretical → Also see TABLE 9 p. 909
- **Cobicistat** is predicted to increase the exposure to **lapatinib**. Avoid. [Moderate] Study
- **Lapatinib** is predicted to increase the exposure to **colchicine**. Avoid P-glycoprotein inhibitors or adjust **colchicine** dose. [Moderate] Theoretical
- **Lapatinib** is predicted to increase the risk of bleeding events when given with **coumarins**. [Severe] Theoretical
- **Crizotinib** is predicted to increase the exposure to **lapatinib**. [Moderate] Study → Also see TABLE 9 p. 909
- **Lapatinib** is predicted to increase the exposure to **dabigatran**. [Severe] Theoretical
- **Lapatinib** is predicted to increase the exposure to **digoxin**. [Moderate] Theoretical
- **Lapatinib** is predicted to slightly increase the exposure to **edoxaban**. [Severe] Theoretical
- **Efavirenz** is predicted to decrease the exposure to **lapatinib**. Avoid. [Severe] Study → Also see TABLE 9 p. 909
- **Enzalutamide** is predicted to decrease the exposure to **lapatinib**. Avoid. [Severe] Study
- **Lapatinib** is predicted to increase the exposure to **erlotinib**. [Moderate] Theoretical
- **Lapatinib** is predicted to increase the exposure to **everolimus**. [Moderate] Theoretical

Lapatinib (continued)

- **Lapatinib** is predicted to increase the exposure to **fidaxomicin**. Avoid. Moderate Study
- **Grapefruit juice** is predicted to increase the exposure to **lapatinib**. Avoid. Moderate Theoretical
- **H_2 receptor antagonists** are predicted to decrease the absorption of **lapatinib**. Avoid. Moderate Theoretical
- **HIV-protease inhibitors** are predicted to increase the exposure to **lapatinib**. Avoid. Moderate Study → Also see TABLE 9 p. 909
- **Idelalisib** is predicted to increase the exposure to **lapatinib**. Avoid. Moderate Study
- **Imatinib** is predicted to increase the exposure to **lapatinib**. Moderate Study
- **Lapatinib** is predicted to increase the exposure to **larotrectinib**. Mild Theoretical
- **Lapatinib** is predicted to increase the exposure to **lomitapide**. Separate administration by 12 hours. Moderate Theoretical
- **Lapatinib** is predicted to increase the exposure to **loperamide**. Moderate Theoretical
- Macrolides **(clarithromycin)** are predicted to increase the exposure to **lapatinib**. Avoid. Moderate Study → Also see TABLE 9 p. 909
- Macrolides **(erythromycin)** are predicted to increase the exposure to **lapatinib**. Moderate Study → Also see TABLE 9 p. 909
- **Mitotane** is predicted to decrease the exposure to **lapatinib**. Avoid. Severe Study
- **Netupitant** is predicted to increase the exposure to **lapatinib**. Moderate Study
- **Nevirapine** is predicted to decrease the exposure to **lapatinib**. Avoid. Severe Study
- **Nilotinib** is predicted to increase the exposure to **lapatinib**. Moderate Study → Also see TABLE 9 p. 909
- **Lapatinib** is predicted to increase the exposure to **nintedanib**. Moderate Study
- **Lapatinib** is predicted to increase the exposure to **panobinostat**. Adjust dose. Moderate Theoretical → Also see TABLE 9 p. 909
- **Lapatinib** is predicted to increase the risk of bleeding events when given with **phenindione**. Severe Theoretical
- **Lapatinib** is predicted to increase the exposure to **pibrentasvir**. Moderate Theoretical
- **Pitolisant** is predicted to decrease the exposure to **lapatinib**. Avoid. Severe Theoretical
- **Rifampicin** is predicted to decrease the exposure to **lapatinib**. Avoid. Severe Study
- **Lapatinib** is predicted to increase the exposure to **sirolimus**. Moderate Theoretical
- **St John's Wort** is predicted to decrease the exposure to **lapatinib**. Avoid. Severe Study
- **Lapatinib** is predicted to slightly increase the exposure to **talazoparib**. Avoid or adjust **talazoparib** dose. Severe Study
- **Lapatinib** slightly increases the exposure to taxanes **(paclitaxel)**. Severe Study
- **Tedizolid** is predicted to increase the exposure to **lapatinib**. Avoid. Moderate Theoretical
- **Lapatinib** is predicted to increase the exposure to **topotecan**. Severe Study
- **Lapatinib** is predicted to increase the concentration of **trametinib**. Moderate Theoretical
- **Lapatinib** is predicted to increase the exposure to **venetoclax**. Avoid or monitor for toxicity. Severe Theoretical

Laronidase

- Antimalarials **(chloroquine)** are predicted to decrease the exposure to **laronidase**. Avoid simultaneous administration. Severe Theoretical
- **Hydroxychloroquine** is predicted to decrease the exposure to **laronidase**. Avoid simultaneous administration. Severe Theoretical

Larotrectinib

- Antiarrhythmics **(amiodarone, dronedarone)** are predicted to increase the exposure to **larotrectinib**. Mild Theoretical
- Antiepileptics **(carbamazepine, fosphenytoin, phenobarbital, phenytoin, primidone)** are predicted to moderately decrease the exposure to **larotrectinib**. Avoid. Moderate Study
- Antifungals, azoles **(itraconazole, ketoconazole, voriconazole)** are predicted to moderately increase the exposure to **larotrectinib**. Avoid or adjust **larotrectinib** dose, p. 607. Moderate Study
- **Apalutamide** is predicted to moderately decrease the exposure to **larotrectinib**. Avoid. Moderate Study
- **Bosentan** is predicted to decrease the exposure to **larotrectinib**. Avoid. Moderate Study
- Calcium channel blockers **(verapamil)** are predicted to increase the exposure to **larotrectinib**. Mild Theoretical
- **Ciclosporin** is predicted to increase the exposure to **larotrectinib**. Mild Study
- **Cobicistat** is predicted to moderately increase the exposure to **larotrectinib**. Avoid or adjust **larotrectinib** dose, p. 607. Moderate Study
- **Larotrectinib** potentially decreases the efficacy of **combined hormonal contraceptives**. Use additional contraceptive precautions. Severe Theoretical
- **Efavirenz** is predicted to decrease the exposure to **larotrectinib**. Avoid. Moderate Study
- **Eltrombopag** is predicted to increase the exposure to **larotrectinib**. Mild Study
- **Enzalutamide** is predicted to moderately decrease the exposure to **larotrectinib**. Avoid. Moderate Study
- **Larotrectinib** is predicted to increase the exposure to **ergotamine**. Use with caution and adjust dose. Mild Theoretical
- **Grapefruit juice** is predicted to increase the exposure to **larotrectinib**. Avoid. Moderate Theoretical
- **HIV-protease inhibitors** are predicted to moderately increase the exposure to **larotrectinib**. Avoid or adjust **larotrectinib** dose, p. 607. Moderate Study
- **Idelalisib** is predicted to moderately increase the exposure to **larotrectinib**. Avoid or adjust **larotrectinib** dose, p. 607. Moderate Study
- **Lapatinib** is predicted to increase the exposure to **larotrectinib**. Mild Theoretical
- **Leflunomide** is predicted to increase the exposure to **larotrectinib**. Mild Study
- Macrolides **(azithromycin, erythromycin)** are predicted to increase the exposure to **larotrectinib**. Mild Theoretical
- Macrolides **(clarithromycin)** are predicted to moderately increase the exposure to **larotrectinib**. Avoid or adjust **larotrectinib** dose, p. 607. Moderate Study
- **Larotrectinib** slightly increases the exposure to **midazolam**. Use with caution and adjust dose. Mild Study
- **Mitotane** is predicted to moderately decrease the exposure to **larotrectinib**. Avoid. Moderate Study
- **Nevirapine** is predicted to decrease the exposure to **larotrectinib**. Avoid. Moderate Study
- **Larotrectinib** is predicted to increase the exposure to opioids **(alfentanil, fentanyl)**. Use with caution and adjust dose. Mild Theoretical
- **Larotrectinib** is predicted to increase the exposure to **pimozide**. Use with caution and adjust dose. Mild Theoretical
- **Ranolazine** is predicted to increase the exposure to **larotrectinib**. Mild Theoretical
- **Rifampicin** is predicted to moderately decrease the exposure to **larotrectinib**. Avoid. Moderate Study
- **Larotrectinib** is predicted to increase the exposure to **sirolimus**. Use with caution and adjust dose. Mild Theoretical
- **St John's Wort** is predicted to decrease the exposure to **larotrectinib**. Avoid. Moderate Study
- **Larotrectinib** is predicted to increase the exposure to **tacrolimus**. Use with caution and adjust dose. Mild Theoretical
- **Teriflunomide** is predicted to increase the exposure to **larotrectinib**. Mild Study
- **Vemurafenib** is predicted to increase the exposure to **larotrectinib**. Mild Theoretical

Ledipasvir

- **Antacids** are predicted to decrease the exposure to **ledipasvir**. Separate administration by 4 hours. Moderate Theoretical
- **Ledipasvir** increases the risk of severe bradycardia or heart block when given with antiarrhythmics **(amiodarone)**. Refer to specialist literature. Severe Anecdotal
- Antiepileptics **(carbamazepine)** are predicted to decrease the exposure to **ledipasvir**. Avoid. Severe Study

- Antiepileptics (**fosphenytoin, oxcarbazepine, phenobarbital, phenytoin, primidone**) are predicted to decrease the exposure to **ledipasvir**. Avoid. Severe Theoretical
- Calcium salts (**calcium carbonate**) are predicted to decrease the exposure to **ledipasvir**. Separate administration by 4 hours. Moderate Theoretical
- **Ledipasvir** is predicted to increase the exposure to dabigatran. Moderate Theoretical
- **Ledipasvir** is predicted to increase the exposure to digoxin. Monitor and adjust dose. Moderate Theoretical
- H_2 receptor antagonists are predicted to decrease the exposure to **ledipasvir**. Adjust dose, see ledipasvir with sofosbuvir p. 436. Moderate Study
- HIV-protease inhibitors (**tipranavir**) boosted with ritonavir are predicted to decrease the exposure to **ledipasvir**. Avoid. Severe Theoretical
- Proton pump inhibitors are predicted to decrease the exposure to **ledipasvir**. Adjust dose, see ledipasvir with sofosbuvir p. 436. Moderate Theoretical
- Rifabutin is predicted to decrease the exposure to **ledipasvir**. Avoid. Severe Theoretical
- Rifampicin is predicted to decrease the exposure to **ledipasvir**. Avoid. Severe Study
- Sodium zirconium cyclosilicate is predicted to decrease the exposure to **ledipasvir**. Separate administration by at least 2 hours. Moderate Theoretical
- St John's Wort is predicted to decrease the exposure to **ledipasvir**. Avoid. Severe Study
- **Ledipasvir** is predicted to increase the exposure to statins (**atorvastatin, fluvastatin, pravastatin, simvastatin**). Monitor and adjust dose. Moderate Theoretical
- **Ledipasvir** is predicted to increase the exposure to statins (**rosuvastatin**). Avoid. Severe Theoretical
- **Ledipasvir** (with sofosbuvir) slightly increases the exposure to tenofovir disoproxil. Moderate Study

Leflunomide → see **TABLE 1** p. 907 (hepatotoxicity), **TABLE 15** p. 910 (myelosuppression)

PHARMACOLOGY Leflunomide has a long half-life; washout procedure recommended before switching to other DMARDs (consult product literature).

- **Leflunomide** is predicted to increase the exposure to adefovir. Moderate Theoretical
- **Leflunomide** is predicted to decrease the exposure to agomelatine. Moderate Theoretical
- **Leflunomide** decreases the exposure to aminophylline. Adjust dose. Moderate Study
- **Leflunomide** is predicted to decrease the exposure to anaesthetics, local (**ropivacaine**). Moderate Theoretical
- **Leflunomide** is predicted to increase the exposure to anthracyclines (**daunorubicin, doxorubicin, mitoxantrone**). Moderate Theoretical → Also see **TABLE 15** p. 910
- **Leflunomide** is predicted to increase the exposure to antihistamines, non-sedating (**fexofenadine**). Moderate Study
- **Leflunomide** potentially increases the exposure to baricitinib. Moderate Theoretical
- **Leflunomide** is predicted to increase the exposure to bosentan. Moderate Study
- **Leflunomide** is predicted to moderately increase the clearance of caffeine citrate. Monitor and adjust dose. Moderate Study
- **Leflunomide** is predicted to increase the exposure to cephalosporins (**cefaclor**). Moderate Theoretical
- **Leflunomide** is predicted to decrease the exposure to clozapine. Moderate Theoretical → Also see **TABLE 15** p. 910
- **Leflunomide** increases the anticoagulant effect of coumarins. Severe Anecdotal
- **Leflunomide** is predicted to decrease the exposure to duloxetine. Moderate Theoretical
- **Leflunomide** is predicted to increase the exposure to ganciclovir. Moderate Theoretical → Also see **TABLE 15** p. 910
- **Leflunomide** is predicted to increase the exposure to H_2 receptor antagonists (**cimetidine, famotidine**). Moderate Theoretical
- **Leflunomide** is predicted to increase the exposure to larotrectinib. Mild Study
- **Leflunomide** is predicted to increase the concentration of letermovir. Moderate Study
- Live vaccines are predicted to increase the risk of generalised infection (possibly life-threatening) when given with **leflunomide**. Public Health England advises avoid (refer to Green Book). Severe Theoretical
- **Leflunomide** is predicted to increase the exposure to loop diuretics (**furosemide**). Moderate Theoretical
- **Leflunomide** is predicted to decrease the exposure to melatonin. Moderate Theoretical
- **Leflunomide** is predicted to increase the exposure to methotrexate. Moderate Theoretical → Also see **TABLE 1** p. 907 → Also see **TABLE 15** p. 910
- **Leflunomide** is predicted to increase the clearance of mexiletine. Monitor and adjust dose. Moderate Study
- **Leflunomide** is predicted to increase the exposure to montelukast. Moderate Theoretical
- **Leflunomide** is predicted to increase the exposure to nateglinide. Moderate Theoretical
- **Leflunomide** is predicted to increase the exposure to NSAIDs (**indometacin, ketoprofen**). Moderate Theoretical
- **Leflunomide** is predicted to decrease the exposure to olanzapine. Monitor and adjust dose. Moderate Study → Also see **TABLE 15** p. 910
- **Leflunomide** is predicted to increase the exposure to oseltamivir. Moderate Theoretical
- **Leflunomide** is predicted to increase the exposure to penicillins (**benzylpenicillin**). Moderate Theoretical
- **Leflunomide** is predicted to increase the exposure to pioglitazone. Moderate Study
- **Leflunomide** is predicted to decrease the exposure to pirfenidone. Moderate Theoretical
- **Leflunomide** is predicted to increase the exposure to quinolones (**ciprofloxacin**). Moderate Theoretical
- **Leflunomide** is predicted to increase the exposure to repaglinide. Moderate Study
- **Leflunomide** is predicted to increase the exposure to rifampicin. Moderate Theoretical
- **Leflunomide** is predicted to increase the exposure to **selexipag**. Adjust **selexipag** dose. Moderate Study
- **Leflunomide** is predicted to increase the exposure to statins (**atorvastatin, fluvastatin, pravastatin, simvastatin**). Moderate Study → Also see **TABLE 1** p. 907
- **Leflunomide** is predicted to increase the exposure to statins (**rosuvastatin**). Adjust dose. Moderate Study → Also see **TABLE 1** p. 907
- **Leflunomide** is predicted to increase the exposure to sulfasalazine. Moderate Study → Also see **TABLE 1** p. 907 → Also see **TABLE 15** p. 910
- **Leflunomide** is predicted to increase the exposure to sulfonylureas (**glibenclamide**). Moderate Study
- **Leflunomide** potentially increases the exposure to **talazoparib**. Avoid or monitor. Moderate Theoretical
- **Leflunomide** is predicted to increase the concentration of taxanes (**paclitaxel**). Severe Anecdotal → Also see **TABLE 15** p. 910
- **Leflunomide** is predicted to increase the exposure to **tenofovir alafenamide**. Moderate Theoretical
- **Leflunomide** is predicted to increase the exposure to **tenofovir disoproxil**. Moderate Theoretical
- **Leflunomide** is predicted to decrease the exposure to theophylline. Adjust dose. Moderate Study
- **Leflunomide** moderately decreases the exposure to **tizanidine**. Mild Study
- **Leflunomide** is predicted to increase the exposure to topotecan. Moderate Study → Also see **TABLE 15** p. 910
- **Leflunomide** is predicted to increase the exposure to zidovudine. Moderate Theoretical → Also see **TABLE 15** p. 910

Lenalidomide → see **TABLE 1** p. 907 (hepatotoxicity), **TABLE 15** p. 910 (myelosuppression), **TABLE 5** p. 907 (thromboembolism)

- Combined hormonal contraceptives are predicted to increase the risk of venous thromboembolism when given with **lenalidomide**. Avoid. Severe Theoretical
- Hormone replacement therapy is predicted to increase the risk of venous thromboembolism when given with **lenalidomide**. Severe Theoretical

Lenvatinib → see TABLE 9 p. 909 (QT-interval prolongation)
Lercanidipine → see calcium channel blockers
Letermovir
- **Letermovir** is predicted to increase the concentration of antiarrhythmics **(amiodarone)**. Moderate Theoretical
- Antiepileptics **(carbamazepine, phenobarbital, primidone)** are predicted to decrease the concentration of **letermovir**. Moderate Theoretical
- **Letermovir** is predicted to decrease the concentration of antiepileptics **(fosphenytoin, phenytoin)** and antiepileptics **(fosphenytoin, phenytoin)** are predicted to decrease the concentration of **letermovir**. Moderate Theoretical
- **Letermovir** slightly decreases the exposure to antifungals, azoles **(voriconazole)**. Moderate Study
- **Letermovir** is predicted to increase the concentration of antihistamines, non-sedating **(fexofenadine)**. Moderate Theoretical
- **Letermovir** is predicted to increase the concentration of **bosentan**. Moderate Theoretical
- **Letermovir** increases the exposure to **ciclosporin** and **ciclosporin** increases the exposure to **letermovir**. Monitor and adjust **letermovir** dose. Severe Study
- **Letermovir** is predicted to decrease the concentration of coumarins **(warfarin)**. Monitor and adjust dose. Moderate Theoretical
- **Letermovir** is predicted to decrease the concentration of **dabigatran**. Avoid. Severe Theoretical
- **Efavirenz** is predicted to decrease the concentration of **letermovir**. Moderate Theoretical
- **Eltrombopag** is predicted to increase the concentration of **letermovir**. Moderate Study
- **Letermovir** is predicted to increase the concentration of **ergometrine**. Avoid. Severe Theoretical
- **Letermovir** is predicted to increase the concentration of **ergotamine**. Avoid. Severe Theoretical
- **Etravirine** is predicted to decrease the exposure to **letermovir**. Moderate Theoretical
- **Letermovir** is predicted to increase the concentration of **everolimus**. Monitor and adjust dose. Severe Study
- Fibrates **(gemfibrozil)** are predicted to increase the concentration of **letermovir**. Moderate Study
- HIV-protease inhibitors **(atazanavir, lopinavir)** boosted with ritonavir are predicted to increase the concentration of **letermovir**. Moderate Study
- HIV-protease inhibitors **(ritonavir)** are predicted to decrease the concentration of **letermovir**. Moderate Theoretical
- **Leflunomide** is predicted to increase the concentration of **letermovir**. Moderate Study
- Macrolides **(clarithromycin, erythromycin)** are predicted to increase the concentration of **letermovir**. Moderate Study
- **Letermovir** slightly to moderately increases the exposure to **midazolam**. Monitor and adjust dose. Moderate Study
- **Modafinil** is predicted to decrease the concentration of **letermovir**. Moderate Theoretical
- **Letermovir** is predicted to increase the exposure to opioids **(alfentanil, fentanyl)**. Monitor and adjust dose. Moderate Study
- **Letermovir** is predicted to increase the concentration of **pimozide**. Avoid. Severe Theoretical
- **Letermovir** is predicted to increase the concentration of **repaglinide**. Avoid. Moderate Theoretical
- **Rifabutin** is predicted to decrease the concentration of **letermovir**. Moderate Theoretical
- **Rifampicin** is predicted to affect the concentration of **letermovir**. Severe Theoretical
- **Letermovir** moderately increases the exposure to **sirolimus**. Monitor and adjust dose. Severe Study
- **St John's Wort** is predicted to decrease the concentration of **letermovir**. Moderate Theoretical
- **Letermovir** moderately increases the exposure to statins **(atorvastatin)**. Avoid or adjust **atorvastatin** dose, p. 139. Severe Study
- **Letermovir** is predicted to increase the exposure to statins **(fluvastatin)**. Monitor and adjust dose. Moderate Theoretical
- **Letermovir** is predicted to increase the exposure to statins **(pravastatin)**. Avoid or adjust dose. Moderate Theoretical
- **Letermovir** is predicted to increase the exposure to statins **(rosuvastatin, simvastatin)**. Avoid. Severe Study
- **Letermovir** is predicted to increase the concentration of sulfonylureas **(glibenclamide)**. Moderate Theoretical
- **Letermovir** moderately increases the exposure to **tacrolimus**. Monitor and adjust dose. Severe Study
- **Teriflunomide** is predicted to increase the concentration of **letermovir**. Moderate Study

Levamisole
- **Albendazole** slightly decreases the exposure to **levamisole** and **levamisole** moderately decreases the exposure to **albendazole**. Moderate Study
- **Alcohol (beverage)** potentially causes a disulfiram-like reaction when given with **levamisole**. Moderate Study
- **Levamisole** increases the exposure to **ivermectin**. Moderate Study

Levetiracetam → see antiepileptics
Levobunolol → see beta blockers, non-selective
Levobupivacaine → see anaesthetics, local
Levocetirizine → see antihistamines, non-sedating
Levodopa → see TABLE 8 p. 908 (hypotension)
- **Amisulpride** is predicted to decrease the effects of **levodopa**. Avoid. Severe Theoretical
- Antiepileptics **(fosphenytoin, phenytoin)** decrease the effects of **levodopa**. Moderate Study
- **Aripiprazole** is predicted to decrease the effects of **levodopa**. Severe Theoretical → Also see TABLE 8 p. 908
- **Asenapine** is predicted to decrease the effects of **levodopa**. Adjust dose. Severe Theoretical → Also see TABLE 8 p. 908
- **Baclofen** is predicted to increase the risk of side-effects when given with **levodopa**. Severe Anecdotal → Also see TABLE 8 p. 908
- **Benperidol** is predicted to decrease the effects of **levodopa**. Severe Study → Also see TABLE 8 p. 908
- **Bupropion** increases the risk of side-effects when given with **levodopa**. Moderate Study
- **Clozapine** is predicted to decrease the effects of **levodopa**. Severe Theoretical → Also see TABLE 8 p. 908
- **Droperidol** decreases the effects of **levodopa**. Severe Study → Also see TABLE 8 p. 908
- **Drugs with antimuscarinic effects** (see TABLE 10 p. 909) decrease the absorption of **levodopa**. Moderate Theoretical
- **Entacapone** increases the exposure to **levodopa**. Monitor side effects and adjust dose. Moderate Study
- **Flupentixol** decreases the effects of **levodopa**. Avoid or monitor worsening parkinsonian symptoms. Severe Theoretical → Also see TABLE 8 p. 908
- **Haloperidol** decreases the effects of **levodopa**. Severe Study → Also see TABLE 8 p. 908
- **Iron (oral)** decreases the absorption of **levodopa**. Moderate Study
- **Isoniazid** decreases the effects of **levodopa**. Moderate Study
- **Levodopa** is predicted to increase the risk of elevated blood pressure when given with **linezolid**. Avoid. Severe Theoretical
- **Loxapine** is predicted to decrease the effects of **levodopa**. Severe Theoretical → Also see TABLE 8 p. 908
- **Lurasidone** is predicted to decrease the effects of **levodopa**. Severe Theoretical → Also see TABLE 8 p. 908
- **MAO-B inhibitors** are predicted to increase the effects of **levodopa**. Adjust dose. Mild Study → Also see TABLE 8 p. 908
- **Levodopa** increases the risk of a hypertensive crisis when given with **MAOIs, irreversible**. Avoid and for 14 days after stopping the MAOI. Severe Study → Also see TABLE 8 p. 908
- **Memantine** is predicted to increase the effects of **levodopa**. Moderate Theoretical
- **Metoclopramide** decreases the effects of **levodopa**. Avoid. Moderate Study
- **Levodopa** increases the risk of side-effects when given with **moclobemide**. Moderate Study
- **Olanzapine** decreases the effects of **levodopa**. Avoid or monitor worsening parkinsonian symptoms. Severe Anecdotal → Also see TABLE 8 p. 908
- **Opicapone** increases the exposure to **levodopa**. Adjust dose. Moderate Study
- **Paliperidone** is predicted to decrease the effects of **levodopa**. Severe Theoretical → Also see TABLE 8 p. 908

- **Phenothiazines** decrease the effects of **levodopa**. Avoid or monitor worsening parkinsonian symptoms. Severe Study → Also see **TABLE 8** p. 908
- **Pimozide** decreases the effects of **levodopa**. Severe Theoretical → Also see **TABLE 8** p. 908
- **Quetiapine** decreases the effects of **levodopa**. Severe Anecdotal → Also see **TABLE 8** p. 908
- **Risperidone** is predicted to decrease the effects of **levodopa**. Avoid or adjust dose. Severe Anecdotal → Also see **TABLE 8** p. 908
- **Sulpiride** is predicted to decrease the effects of **levodopa**. Avoid. Severe Theoretical → Also see **TABLE 8** p. 908
- **Tetrabenazine** is predicted to decrease the effects of **levodopa**. Use with caution or avoid. Moderate Theoretical
- **Tolcapone** increases the exposure to **levodopa**. Monitor and adjust dose. Moderate Study
- **Tryptophan** greatly decreases the concentration of **levodopa**. Moderate Study
- **Zuclopenthixol** is predicted to decrease the effects of **levodopa**. Avoid or monitor worsening parkinsonian symptoms. Severe Theoretical → Also see **TABLE 8** p. 908

Levofloxacin → see quinolones

Levofolinic acid → see folates

Levomepromazine → see phenothiazines

Levonorgestrel

- Antiepileptics **(carbamazepine, eslicarbazepine, fosphenytoin, oxcarbazepine, perampanel, phenobarbital, phenytoin, primidone, rufinamide, topiramate)** are predicted to decrease the efficacy of **levonorgestrel**. For FSRH guidance, see Contraceptives, interactions p. 536. Severe Theoretical
- **Aprepitant** is predicted to decrease the efficacy of **levonorgestrel**. For FSRH guidance, see Contraceptives, interactions p. 536. Severe Theoretical
- **Bosentan** is predicted to decrease the efficacy of **levonorgestrel**. For FSRH guidance, see Contraceptives, interactions p. 536. Severe Theoretical
- **Efavirenz** is predicted to decrease the efficacy of **levonorgestrel**. For FSRH guidance, see Contraceptives, interactions p. 536. Severe Theoretical
- **Fosaprepitant** is predicted to decrease the efficacy of **levonorgestrel**. For FSRH guidance, see Contraceptives, interactions p. 536. Severe Theoretical
- **Griseofulvin** potentially decreases the efficacy of oral **levonorgestrel**. For FSRH guidance, see Contraceptives, interactions p. 536. Severe Anecdotal
- HIV-protease inhibitors **(ritonavir)** are predicted to decrease the efficacy of **levonorgestrel**. For FSRH guidance, see Contraceptives, interactions p. 536. Severe Theoretical
- **Lumacaftor** is predicted to decrease the efficacy of **levonorgestrel**. Use additional contraceptive precautions. Severe Theoretical
- **Modafinil** is predicted to decrease the efficacy of **levonorgestrel**. For FSRH guidance, see Contraceptives, interactions p. 536. Severe Theoretical
- **Nevirapine** is predicted to decrease the efficacy of **levonorgestrel**. For FSRH guidance, see Contraceptives, interactions p. 536. Severe Theoretical
- **Rifabutin** is predicted to decrease the efficacy of **levonorgestrel**. For FSRH guidance, see Contraceptives, interactions p. 536. Severe Theoretical
- **Rifampicin** is predicted to decrease the efficacy of **levonorgestrel**. For FSRH guidance, see Contraceptives, interactions p. 536. Severe Theoretical
- **St John's Wort** is predicted to decrease the efficacy of **levonorgestrel**. MHRA advises avoid. For FSRH guidance, see Contraceptives, interactions p. 536. Severe Theoretical
- **Sugammadex** is predicted to decrease the exposure to **levonorgestrel**. Use additional contraceptive precautions. Severe Theoretical
- **Ulipristal** is predicted to decrease the efficacy of **levonorgestrel**. Avoid. Severe Theoretical

Levothyroxine → see thyroid hormones

Lidocaine → see antiarrhythmics

Linagliptin → see **TABLE 14** p. 910 (antidiabetic drugs)

- Antiepileptics **(carbamazepine, fosphenytoin, phenobarbital, phenytoin, primidone)** are predicted to decrease the exposure to **linagliptin**. Moderate Study
- **Apalutamide** is predicted to decrease the exposure to **linagliptin**. Moderate Study
- **Enzalutamide** is predicted to decrease the exposure to **linagliptin**. Moderate Study
- **Linagliptin** is predicted to increase the exposure to **lomitapide**. Separate administration by 12 hours. Moderate Theoretical
- **Mitotane** is predicted to decrease the exposure to **linagliptin**. Moderate Study
- **Rifampicin** is predicted to decrease the exposure to **linagliptin**. Moderate Study

Linezolid → see **TABLE 15** p. 910 (myelosuppression), **TABLE 13** p. 910 (serotonin syndrome)

FOOD AND LIFESTYLE Patients taking linezolid should avoid consuming large amounts of tyramine-rich foods (such as mature cheese, salami, pickled herring, *Bovril®*, *Oxo®*, *Marmite®* or any similar meat or yeast extract or fermented soya bean extract, and some beers, lagers or wines).

- **Beta$_2$ agonists** are predicted to increase the risk of elevated blood pressure when given with **linezolid**. Avoid. Severe Theoretical
- **Bupropion** is predicted to increase the risk of intraoperative hypertension when given with **linezolid**. Severe Anecdotal → Also see **TABLE 13** p. 910
- **Buspirone** is predicted to increase the risk of elevated blood pressure when given with **linezolid**. Avoid. Severe Theoretical → Also see **TABLE 13** p. 910
- **Levodopa** is predicted to increase the risk of elevated blood pressure when given with **linezolid**. Avoid. Severe Theoretical
- Macrolides **(clarithromycin)** increase the exposure to **linezolid**. Moderate Anecdotal
- MAO-B inhibitors **(rasagiline, selegiline)** are predicted to increase the risk of side-effects when given with **linezolid**. Avoid and for 14 days after stopping the MAOI. Severe Theoretical → Also see **TABLE 13** p. 910
- MAO-B inhibitors **(safinamide)** are predicted to increase the risk of side-effects when given with **linezolid**. Avoid and for 1 week after stopping **safinamide**. Severe Theoretical → Also see **TABLE 13** p. 910
- **MAOIs, irreversible** are predicted to increase the risk of side-effects when given with **linezolid**. Avoid and for 14 days after stopping the MAOI. Severe Theoretical → Also see **TABLE 13** p. 910
- **Methylphenidate** is predicted to increase the risk of elevated blood pressure when given with **linezolid**. Avoid. Severe Theoretical
- **Moclobemide** is predicted to increase the risk of side-effects when given with **linezolid**. Avoid and for 14 days after stopping **moclobemide**. Severe Theoretical → Also see **TABLE 13** p. 910
- **Reboxetine** is predicted to increase the risk of a hypertensive crisis when given with **linezolid**. Avoid. Severe Theoretical
- **Rifampicin** slightly decreases the exposure to **linezolid**. Moderate Study
- **Sympathomimetics, inotropic** are predicted to increase the risk of elevated blood pressure when given with **linezolid**. Avoid. Severe Theoretical
- Sympathomimetics, vasoconstrictor **(adrenaline/epinephrine, ephedrine, isometheptene, noradrenaline/norepinephrine, phenylephrine)** are predicted to increase the risk of elevated blood pressure when given with **linezolid**. Avoid. Severe Theoretical
- Sympathomimetics, vasoconstrictor **(pseudoephedrine)** increase the risk of elevated blood pressure when given with **linezolid**. Avoid. Severe Study

Liothyronine → see thyroid hormones

Liraglutide → see **TABLE 14** p. 910 (antidiabetic drugs)

Lisdexamfetamine → see amfetamines

Lisinopril → see ACE inhibitors

Lithium → see **TABLE 13** p. 910 (serotonin syndrome), **TABLE 9** p. 909 (QT-interval prolongation)

- **ACE inhibitors** are predicted to increase the concentration of **lithium**. Monitor and adjust dose. Severe Anecdotal

Lithium (continued)
- **Acetazolamide** alters the concentration of **lithium**. Severe Anecdotal
- Aldosterone antagonists **(eplerenone)** potentially increase the concentration of **lithium**. Avoid. Moderate Theoretical
- Aldosterone antagonists **(spironolactone)** potentially increase the concentration of **lithium**. Moderate Study
- **Aminophylline** is predicted to decrease the concentration of **lithium**. Moderate Theoretical
- **Angiotensin-II receptor antagonists** potentially increase the concentration of **lithium**. Monitor concentration and adjust dose. Severe Anecdotal
- Antiepileptics **(carbamazepine, oxcarbazepine)** are predicted to increase the risk of neurotoxicity when given with **lithium**. Severe Anecdotal
- **Calcitonins** decrease the concentration of **lithium**. Adjust dose. Moderate Study
- Calcium channel blockers **(diltiazem, verapamil)** are predicted to increase the risk of neurotoxicity when given with **lithium**. Severe Anecdotal
- **Loop diuretics** increase the concentration of **lithium**. Monitor and adjust dose. Severe Study
- **Methyldopa** increases the risk of neurotoxicity when given with **lithium**. Severe Anecdotal
- **Metronidazole** is predicted to increase the concentration of **lithium**. Avoid or adjust dose. Severe Anecdotal
- **Mexiletine** potentially affects the exposure to **lithium**. Avoid. Unknown Theoretical
- **NSAIDs** increase the concentration of **lithium**. Monitor and adjust dose. Severe Study
- **Phenothiazines** potentially increase the risk of neurotoxicity when given with **lithium**. Severe Anecdotal → Also see TABLE 9 p. 909
- Potassium-sparing diuretics **(triamterene)** potentially increase the clearance of **lithium**. Moderate Study
- **Quetiapine** potentially increases the risk of neurotoxicity when given with **lithium**. Severe Anecdotal
- **Risperidone** potentially increases the risk of neurotoxicity when given with **lithium**. Severe Anecdotal → Also see TABLE 9 p. 909
- **Sodium bicarbonate** decreases the concentration of **lithium**. Severe Anecdotal
- **Sulpiride** potentially increases the risk of neurotoxicity when given with **lithium**. Severe Anecdotal → Also see TABLE 9 p. 909
- **Tetracyclines** are predicted to increase the risk of lithium toxicity when given with **lithium**. Avoid or adjust dose. Severe Anecdotal
- **Theophylline** is predicted to decrease the concentration of **lithium**. Monitor concentration and adjust dose. Moderate Anecdotal
- **Thiazide diuretics** increase the concentration of **lithium**. Avoid or adjust dose and monitor concentration. Severe Study
- **Tricyclic antidepressants** potentially increase the risk of neurotoxicity when given with **lithium**. Severe Anecdotal → Also see TABLE 13 p. 910 → Also see TABLE 9 p. 909
- **Zuclopenthixol** potentially increases the risk of neurotoxicity when given with **lithium**. Severe Anecdotal → Also see TABLE 9 p. 909

Live vaccines

Bacillus Calmette-Guérin vaccine · influenza vaccine (live) · measles, mumps and rubella vaccine, live · rotavirus vaccine · typhoid vaccine, oral · varicella-zoster vaccine · yellow fever vaccine, live

GENERAL INFORMATION **Oral typhoid vaccine** is inactivated by concurrent administration of antibacterials or antimalarials: antibacterials should be avoided for 3 days before and after oral typhoid vaccination; *mefloquine* should be avoided for at least 12 hours before or after oral typhoid vaccination; for other antimalarials oral typhoid vaccine vaccination should be completed at least 3 days before the first dose of the antimalarial (except proguanil hydrochloride with atovaquone, which can be given concurrently).

- **Live vaccines** are predicted to increase the risk of generalised infection (possibly life-threatening) when given with abatacept. Public Health England advises avoid (refer to Green Book). Severe Theoretical
- **Live vaccines** are predicted to increase the risk of generalised infection (possibly life-threatening) when given with alkylating agents. Public Health England advises avoid (refer to Green Book). Severe Theoretical
- **Live vaccines** are predicted to increase the risk of generalised infection (possibly life-threatening) when given with amsacrine. Public Health England advises avoid (refer to Green Book). Severe Theoretical
- **Live vaccines** are predicted to increase the risk of generalised infection (possibly life-threatening) when given with anakinra. Public Health England advises avoid (refer to Green Book). Severe Theoretical
- **Live vaccines** are predicted to increase the risk of generalised infection (possibly life-threatening) when given with anthracyclines. Public Health England advises avoid (refer to Green Book). Severe Theoretical
- **Live vaccines** are predicted to increase the risk of generalised infection (possibly life-threatening) when given with azathioprine (high-dose). Public Health England advises avoid (refer to Green Book). Severe Theoretical
- **Live vaccines** are predicted to increase the risk of generalised infection (possibly life-threatening) when given with baricitinib. Avoid. Severe Theoretical
- **Live vaccines** are predicted to increase the risk of generalised infection (possibly life-threatening) when given with belatacept. Public Health England advises avoid (refer to Green Book). Severe Theoretical
- **Live vaccines** are predicted to increase the risk of generalised infection (possibly life-threatening) when given with bleomycin. Public Health England advises avoid (refer to Green Book). Severe Theoretical
- **Live vaccines** are predicted to increase the risk of generalised infection (possibly life-threatening) when given with capecitabine. Public Health England advises avoid (refer to Green Book). Severe Theoretical
- **Live vaccines** are predicted to increase the risk of generalised infection (possibly life-threatening) when given with ciclosporin. Public Health England advises avoid (refer to Green Book). Severe Theoretical
- **Live vaccines** are predicted to increase the risk of generalised infection (possibly life-threatening) when given with cladribine. Public Health England advises avoid (refer to Green Book). Severe Theoretical
- **Live vaccines** are predicted to increase the risk of generalised infection (possibly life-threatening) when given with clofarabine. Public Health England advises avoid (refer to Green Book). Severe Theoretical
- **Live vaccines** are predicted to increase the risk of generalised infection (possibly life-threatening) when given with corticosteroids (high-dose). Public Health England advises avoid (refer to Green Book). Severe Theoretical
- **Live vaccines** are predicted to increase the risk of generalised infection (possibly life-threatening) when given with cytarabine. Public Health England advises avoid (refer to Green Book). Severe Theoretical
- **Live vaccines** are predicted to increase the risk of generalised infection (possibly life-threatening) when given with dactinomycin. Public Health England advises avoid (refer to Green Book). Severe Theoretical
- **Live vaccines** are predicted to increase the risk of generalised infection (possibly life-threatening) when given with dimethyl fumarate. Public Health England advises avoid (refer to Green Book). Severe Theoretical
- **Live vaccines** are predicted to increase the risk of generalised infection (possibly life-threatening) when given with etanercept. Public Health England advises avoid (refer to Green Book). Severe Theoretical
- **Live vaccines** are predicted to increase the risk of generalised infection (possibly life-threatening) when given with etoposide. Public Health England advises avoid (refer to Green Book). Severe Theoretical
- **Live vaccines** are predicted to increase the risk of generalised infection (possibly life-threatening) when given with

everolimus. Public Health England advises avoid (refer to Green Book). Severe Theoretical
- **Live vaccines** are predicted to increase the risk of generalised infection (possibly life-threatening) when given with **fingolimod**. Public Health England advises avoid (refer to Green Book). Severe Theoretical
- **Live vaccines** are predicted to increase the risk of generalised infection (possibly life-threatening) when given with **fludarabine**. Public Health England advises avoid (refer to Green Book). Severe Theoretical
- **Live vaccines** are predicted to increase the risk of generalised infection (possibly life-threatening) when given with **fluorouracil**. Public Health England advises avoid (refer to Green Book). Severe Theoretical
- **Live vaccines** are predicted to increase the risk of generalised infection (possibly life-threatening) when given with **gemcitabine**. Public Health England advises avoid (refer to Green Book). Severe Theoretical
- **Live vaccines** are predicted to increase the risk of generalised infection (possibly life-threatening) when given with **hydroxycarbamide**. Public Health England advises avoid (refer to Green Book). Severe Theoretical
- Immunoglobulins **(cytomegalovirus immunoglobulin)** are predicted to decrease the efficacy of **live vaccines**. Avoid. Severe Theoretical
- **Live vaccines** are predicted to increase the risk of generalised infection (possibly life-threatening) when given with **irinotecan**. Public Health England advises avoid (refer to Green Book). Severe Theoretical
- **Live vaccines** are predicted to increase the risk of generalised infection (possibly life-threatening) when given with iron chelators **(dexrazoxane)**. Avoid. Severe Theoretical
- **Live vaccines** are predicted to increase the risk of generalised infection (possibly life-threatening) when given with **leflunomide**. Public Health England advises avoid (refer to Green Book). Severe Theoretical
- **Live vaccines** are predicted to increase the risk of generalised infection (possibly life-threatening) when given with **mercaptopurine** (high-dose). Public Health England advises avoid (refer to Green Book). Severe Theoretical
- **Live vaccines** are predicted to increase the risk of generalised infection (possibly life-threatening) when given with **methotrexate** (high-dose). Public Health England advises avoid (refer to Green Book). Severe Theoretical
- **Live vaccines** are predicted to increase the risk of generalised infection (possibly life-threatening) when given with **mitomycin**. Public Health England advises avoid (refer to Green Book). Severe Theoretical
- **Live vaccines** are predicted to increase the risk of generalised infection (possibly life-threatening) when given with **monoclonal antibodies**. Public Health England advises avoid (refer to Green Book). Severe Theoretical
- **Live vaccines** are predicted to increase the risk of generalised infection (possibly life-threatening) when given with **mycophenolate**. Public Health England advises avoid (refer to Green Book). Severe Theoretical
- **Live vaccines** are predicted to increase the risk of generalised infection (possibly life-threatening) when given with **pemetrexed**. Public Health England advises avoid (refer to Green Book). Severe Theoretical
- **Live vaccines** are predicted to increase the risk of generalised infection (possibly life-threatening) when given with **platinum compounds**. Public Health England advises avoid (refer to Green Book). Severe Theoretical
- **Live vaccines** are predicted to increase the risk of generalised infection (possibly life-threatening) when given with **procarbazine**. Public Health England advises avoid (refer to Green Book). Severe Theoretical
- **Live vaccines** are predicted to increase the risk of generalised infection (possibly life-threatening) when given with **raltitrexed**. Public Health England advises avoid (refer to Green Book). Severe Theoretical
- **Live vaccines** are predicted to increase the risk of generalised infection (possibly life-threatening) when given with siponimod. Avoid and for 4 weeks after stopping **siponimod**. Severe Theoretical
- **Live vaccines** are predicted to increase the risk of generalised infection (possibly life-threatening) when given with **sirolimus**. Public Health England advises avoid (refer to Green Book). Severe Theoretical
- **Live vaccines** are predicted to increase the risk of generalised infection (possibly life-threatening) when given with **streptozocin**. Public Health England advises avoid (refer to Green Book). Severe Theoretical
- **Live vaccines** are predicted to increase the risk of generalised infection (possibly life-threatening) when given with **tacrolimus**. Public Health England advises avoid (refer to Green Book). Severe Theoretical
- **Live vaccines** are predicted to increase the risk of generalised infection (possibly life-threatening) when given with taxanes **(docetaxel, paclitaxel)**. Public Health England advises avoid (refer to Green Book). Severe Theoretical
- **Live vaccines** are predicted to increase the risk of generalised infection (possibly life-threatening) when given with **tegafur**. Public Health England advises avoid (refer to Green Book). Severe Theoretical
- **Live vaccines** are predicted to increase the risk of generalised infection (possibly life-threatening) when given with **temsirolimus**. Public Health England advises avoid (refer to Green Book). Severe Theoretical
- **Live vaccines** are predicted to increase the risk of generalised infection (possibly life-threatening) when given with **teriflunomide**. Public Health England advises avoid (refer to Green Book). Severe Theoretical
- **Live vaccines** are predicted to increase the risk of generalised infection (possibly life-threatening) when given with **tioguanine**. Public Health England advises avoid (refer to Green Book). Severe Theoretical
- **Live vaccines** potentially increase the risk of generalised infection (possibly life-threatening) when given with **tofacitinib**. Avoid. Severe Theoretical
- **Live vaccines** are predicted to increase the risk of generalised infection (possibly life-threatening) when given with **topotecan**. Public Health England advises avoid (refer to Green Book). Severe Theoretical
- **Live vaccines** are predicted to increase the risk of generalised infection (possibly life-threatening) when given with **trabectedin**. Public Health England advises avoid (refer to Green Book). Severe Theoretical
- **Live vaccines** are predicted to increase the risk of generalised infection (possibly life-threatening) when given with **upadacitinib**. Avoid. Severe Theoretical
- **Venetoclax** potentially decreases the efficacy of **live vaccines**. Avoid. Severe Theoretical
- **Live vaccines** are predicted to increase the risk of generalised infection (possibly life-threatening) when given with **vinca alkaloids**. Public Health England advises avoid (refer to Green Book). Severe Theoretical

Lixisenatide → see TABLE 14 p. 910 (antidiabetic drugs)

SEPARATION OF ADMINISTRATION Some orally administered drugs should be taken at least 1 hour before, or 4 hours after, lixisenatide injection.

Lofepramine → see tricyclic antidepressants

Lofexidine → see TABLE 8 p. 908 (hypotension), TABLE 9 p. 909 (QT-interval prolongation), TABLE 11 p. 909 (CNS depressant effects)

Lomitapide → see TABLE 1 p. 907 (hepatotoxicity)

FOOD AND LIFESTYLE Bitter (Seville) orange is predicted to increase the exposure to lomitapide; separate administration by 12 hours.

- Alprazolam is predicted to increase the exposure to **lomitapide**. Separate administration by 12 hours. Moderate Theoretical
- Antiarrhythmics **(amiodarone)** are predicted to increase the exposure to **lomitapide**. Separate administration by 12 hours. Moderate Theoretical
- Antiarrhythmics **(dronedarone)** are predicted to increase the exposure to **lomitapide**. Avoid. Moderate Theoretical
- Antiepileptics **(carbamazepine, fosphenytoin, phenobarbital, phenytoin, primidone)** are predicted to decrease the exposure

Lomitapide (continued)
to **lomitapide**. Monitor and adjust dose. Moderate Theoretical → Also see TABLE 1 p. 907
- Antifungals, azoles **(clotrimazole)** are predicted to increase the exposure to **lomitapide**. Separate administration by 12 hours. Moderate Theoretical
- Antifungals, azoles **(fluconazole, isavuconazole, posaconazole)** are predicted to increase the exposure to **lomitapide**. Avoid. Moderate Theoretical → Also see TABLE 1 p. 907
- Antifungals, azoles **(itraconazole, ketoconazole, voriconazole)** are predicted to markedly increase the exposure to **lomitapide**. Avoid. Severe Study → Also see TABLE 1 p. 907
- **Apalutamide** is predicted to decrease the exposure to **lomitapide**. Monitor and adjust dose. Moderate Theoretical
- **Aprepitant** is predicted to increase the exposure to **lomitapide**. Avoid. Moderate Theoretical
- **Bicalutamide** is predicted to increase the exposure to **lomitapide**. Separate administration by 12 hours. Moderate Theoretical
- Calcium channel blockers **(amlodipine, lacidipine)** are predicted to increase the exposure to **lomitapide**. Separate administration by 12 hours. Moderate Theoretical
- Calcium channel blockers **(diltiazem, verapamil)** are predicted to increase the exposure to **lomitapide**. Avoid. Moderate Theoretical
- **Ciclosporin** is predicted to increase the exposure to **lomitapide**. Separate administration by 12 hours. Moderate Theoretical
- **Cilostazol** is predicted to increase the exposure to **lomitapide**. Separate administration by 12 hours. Moderate Theoretical
- **Cobicistat** is predicted to markedly increase the exposure to **lomitapide**. Avoid. Severe Study
- Oral **combined hormonal contraceptives** slightly increase the exposure to **lomitapide**. Separate administration by 12 hours. Moderate Theoretical
- **Lomitapide** increases the exposure to coumarins **(warfarin)**. Monitor INR and adjust dose. Severe Study
- **Crizotinib** is predicted to increase the exposure to **lomitapide**. Avoid. Moderate Theoretical
- **Enzalutamide** is predicted to decrease the exposure to **lomitapide**. Monitor and adjust dose. Moderate Theoretical
- **Everolimus** is predicted to increase the exposure to **lomitapide**. Separate administration by 12 hours. Moderate Theoretical
- **Fosaprepitant** is predicted to increase the exposure to **lomitapide**. Separate administration by 12 hours. Moderate Theoretical
- **Grapefruit juice** is predicted to increase the exposure to **lomitapide**. Separate administration by 12 hours. Moderate Theoretical
- H_2 receptor antagonists **(cimetidine, ranitidine)** are predicted to increase the exposure to **lomitapide**. Separate administration by 12 hours. Moderate Theoretical
- **HIV-protease inhibitors** are predicted to markedly increase the exposure to **lomitapide**. Avoid. Severe Study
- **Idelalisib** is predicted to markedly increase the exposure to **lomitapide**. Avoid. Severe Study
- **Imatinib** is predicted to increase the exposure to **lomitapide**. Avoid. Moderate Theoretical
- **Isoniazid** is predicted to increase the exposure to **lomitapide**. Separate administration by 12 hours. Unknown Theoretical → Also see TABLE 1 p. 907
- **Ivacaftor** is predicted to increase the exposure to **lomitapide**. Separate administration by 12 hours. Moderate Theoretical
- **Lapatinib** is predicted to increase the exposure to **lomitapide**. Separate administration by 12 hours. Moderate Theoretical
- **Linagliptin** is predicted to increase the exposure to **lomitapide**. Separate administration by 12 hours. Moderate Theoretical
- Macrolides **(azithromycin)** are predicted to increase the exposure to **lomitapide**. Separate administration by 12 hours. Moderate Theoretical
- Macrolides **(clarithromycin)** are predicted to markedly increase the exposure to **lomitapide**. Avoid. Severe Study
- Macrolides **(erythromycin)** are predicted to increase the exposure to **lomitapide**. Avoid. Moderate Theoretical
- **Mitotane** is predicted to decrease the exposure to **lomitapide**. Monitor and adjust dose. Moderate Theoretical
- **Netupitant** is predicted to increase the exposure to **lomitapide**. Avoid. Moderate Theoretical
- **Nilotinib** is predicted to increase the exposure to **lomitapide**. Avoid. Moderate Theoretical
- **Pazopanib** is predicted to increase the exposure to **lomitapide**. Separate administration by 12 hours. Moderate Theoretical
- **Peppermint** oil is predicted to increase the exposure to **lomitapide**. Separate administration by 12 hours. Moderate Theoretical
- **Propiverine** is predicted to increase the exposure to **lomitapide**. Separate administration by 12 hours. Moderate Theoretical
- **Ranolazine** is predicted to increase the exposure to **lomitapide**. Separate administration by 12 hours. Moderate Theoretical
- **Rifampicin** is predicted to decrease the exposure to **lomitapide**. Monitor and adjust dose. Moderate Theoretical
- SSRIs **(fluoxetine)** are predicted to increase the exposure to **lomitapide**. Separate administration by 12 hours. Unknown Theoretical
- SSRIs **(fluvoxamine)** are predicted to increase the exposure to **lomitapide**. Separate administration by 12 hours. Moderate Theoretical
- **Lomitapide** increases the exposure to statins **(atorvastatin)**. Adjust **lomitapide** dose or separate administration by 12 hours. Mild Study → Also see TABLE 1 p. 907
- **Lomitapide** increases the exposure to statins **(simvastatin)**. Monitor and adjust **simvastatin** dose, p. 141. Moderate Study → Also see TABLE 1 p. 907
- **Tacrolimus** is predicted to increase the exposure to **lomitapide**. Separate administration by 12 hours. Moderate Theoretical
- **Ticagrelor** is predicted to increase the exposure to **lomitapide**. Separate administration by 12 hours. Moderate Theoretical
- **Tolvaptan** is predicted to increase the exposure to **lomitapide**. Separate administration by 12 hours. Moderate Theoretical

Lomustine → see alkylating agents

Loop diuretics → see TABLE 18 p. 911 (hyponatraemia), TABLE 8 p. 908 (hypotension), TABLE 19 p. 911 (ototoxicity), TABLE 17 p. 911 (reduced serum potassium)

bumetanide · furosemide · torasemide

- **Aliskiren** slightly decreases the exposure to **furosemide**. Moderate Study → Also see TABLE 8 p. 908
- **Loop diuretics** increase the risk of nephrotoxicity when given with **aminoglycosides**. Avoid. Moderate Study → Also see TABLE 19 p. 911
- Antiepileptics **(fosphenytoin, phenytoin)** decrease the effects of **furosemide**. Moderate Study
- Intravenous **furosemide** potentially increases the risk of sweating, variable blood pressure, and tachycardia when given after **chloral hydrate**. Moderate Anecdotal
- **Dasabuvir** (with ombitasvir, paritaprevir, and ritonavir) increases the concentration of **furosemide**. Adjust dose. Moderate Study
- Immunoglobulins **(cytomegalovirus immunoglobulin)** are predicted to increase the risk of side-effects when given with **loop diuretics**. Avoid. Moderate Theoretical
- **Leflunomide** is predicted to increase the exposure to **furosemide**. Moderate Theoretical
- **Loop diuretics** increase the concentration of **lithium**. Monitor and adjust dose. Severe Study
- **Nitisinone** is predicted to increase the exposure to **furosemide**. Moderate Study
- **Paritaprevir** (with ritonavir and ombitasvir) is predicted to increase the exposure to **furosemide**. Adjust dose. Moderate Theoretical
- **Reboxetine** is predicted to increase the risk of hypokalaemia when given with **loop diuretics**. Moderate Theoretical
- **Teriflunomide** is predicted to increase the exposure to **furosemide**. Moderate Study

Loperamide
- Antiarrhythmics **(dronedarone)** are predicted to increase the exposure to **loperamide**. Severe Theoretical
- **Ceritinib** is predicted to increase the exposure to **loperamide**. Moderate Theoretical
- **Loperamide** greatly increases the absorption of oral **desmopressin** (and possibly sublingual). Moderate Study

- Eliglustat is predicted to increase the exposure to **loperamide**. Adjust dose. [Moderate] Study
- Lapatinib is predicted to increase the exposure to **loperamide**. [Moderate] Theoretical
- Mirabegron is predicted to increase the exposure to **loperamide**. [Mild] Theoretical
- Opicapone is predicted to increase the exposure to **loperamide**. Avoid. [Moderate] Study
- Paritaprevir (with ritonavir and ombitasvir) is predicted to increase the exposure to **loperamide**. [Moderate] Study
- Pibrentasvir (with glecaprevir) is predicted to increase the exposure to **loperamide**. [Moderate] Study
- Pitolisant is predicted to decrease the exposure to **loperamide**. [Mild] Theoretical
- Velpatasvir is predicted to increase the exposure to **loperamide**. [Severe] Theoretical

Lopinavir → see HIV-protease inhibitors

Loprazolam → see TABLE 11 p. 909 (CNS depressant effects)

Loratadine → see antihistamines, non-sedating

Lorazepam → see TABLE 11 p. 909 (CNS depressant effects)

- Rifampicin increases the clearance of **lorazepam**. [Moderate] Study

Lorlatinib

- Antiepileptics **(carbamazepine, fosphenytoin, phenobarbital, phenytoin, primidone)** are predicted to decrease the exposure to **lorlatinib**. Avoid. [Severe] Study
- Antifungals, azoles **(itraconazole, ketoconazole, voriconazole)** are predicted to increase the exposure to **lorlatinib**. Avoid or adjust **lorlatinib** dose. [Severe] Study
- Apalutamide is predicted to decrease the exposure to **lorlatinib**. Avoid. [Severe] Study
- Bosentan is predicted to decrease the exposure to **lorlatinib**. Avoid. [Severe] Theoretical
- **Lorlatinib** is predicted to decrease the exposure to **ciclosporin**. Avoid. [Moderate] Theoretical
- Cobicistat is predicted to increase the exposure to **lorlatinib**. Avoid or adjust **lorlatinib** dose. [Severe] Study
- **Lorlatinib** is predicted to decrease the exposure to **combined hormonal contraceptives**. Avoid. [Moderate] Theoretical
- Efavirenz is predicted to decrease the exposure to **lorlatinib**. Avoid. [Severe] Theoretical
- Enzalutamide is predicted to decrease the exposure to **lorlatinib**. Avoid. [Severe] Study
- **Lorlatinib** is predicted to decrease the exposure to **ergotamine**. Avoid. [Moderate] Theoretical
- Grapefruit juice is predicted to increase the concentration of **lorlatinib**. Avoid. [Moderate] Theoretical
- **HIV-protease inhibitors** are predicted to increase the exposure to **lorlatinib**. Avoid or adjust **lorlatinib** dose. [Severe] Study
- Idelalisib is predicted to increase the exposure to **lorlatinib**. Avoid or adjust **lorlatinib** dose. [Severe] Study
- Macrolides **(clarithromycin)** are predicted to increase the exposure to **lorlatinib**. Avoid or adjust **lorlatinib** dose. [Severe] Study
- **Lorlatinib** moderately decreases the exposure to **midazolam**. Avoid. [Moderate] Study
- Mitotane is predicted to decrease the exposure to **lorlatinib**. Avoid. [Severe] Study
- Nevirapine is predicted to decrease the exposure to **lorlatinib**. Avoid. [Severe] Theoretical
- **Lorlatinib** is predicted to decrease the exposure to opioids **(alfentanil, fentanyl)**. Avoid. [Moderate] Theoretical
- **Lorlatinib** is predicted to decrease the exposure to **pimozide**. Avoid. [Moderate] Theoretical
- Rifampicin is predicted to decrease the exposure to **lorlatinib**. Avoid. [Severe] Study
- **Lorlatinib** is predicted to decrease the exposure to **sirolimus**. Avoid. [Moderate] Theoretical
- St John's Wort is predicted to decrease the exposure to **lorlatinib**. Avoid. [Severe] Theoretical
- **Lorlatinib** is predicted to decrease the exposure to **tacrolimus**. Avoid. [Moderate] Theoretical

Lormetazepam → see TABLE 11 p. 909 (CNS depressant effects)

Losartan → see angiotensin-II receptor antagonists

Low molecular-weight heparins → see TABLE 16 p. 911 (increased serum potassium), TABLE 3 p. 907 (anticoagulant effects)

dalteparin · enoxaparin · tinzaparin

- Ranibizumab increases the risk of bleeding events when given with **low molecular-weight heparins**. [Severe] Theoretical

Loxapine → see TABLE 8 p. 908 (hypotension), TABLE 11 p. 909 (CNS depressant effects), TABLE 10 p. 909 (antimuscarinics)

- **Combined hormonal contraceptives** are predicted to increase the exposure to **loxapine**. Avoid. [Unknown] Theoretical
- **Loxapine** is predicted to decrease the effects of **dopamine receptor agonists**. [Moderate] Theoretical → Also see TABLE 8 p. 908 → Also see TABLE 10 p. 909
- **Loxapine** is predicted to decrease the effects of **levodopa**. [Severe] Theoretical → Also see TABLE 8 p. 908
- Mexiletine is predicted to increase the exposure to **loxapine**. Avoid. [Unknown] Theoretical
- Quinolones **(ciprofloxacin)** are predicted to increase the exposure to **loxapine**. Avoid. [Unknown] Theoretical
- SSRIs **(fluvoxamine)** are predicted to increase the exposure to **loxapine**. Avoid. [Unknown] Theoretical

Lumacaftor

- **Lumacaftor** is predicted to decrease the exposure to antiepileptics **(carbamazepine, fosphenytoin, phenobarbital, phenytoin, primidone)**. Avoid. [Severe] Theoretical
- **Lumacaftor** is predicted to decrease the exposure to antifungals, azoles **(fluconazole)**. Adjust dose. [Mild] Theoretical
- **Lumacaftor** is predicted to decrease the exposure to antifungals, azoles **(itraconazole, ketoconazole, posaconazole, voriconazole)**. Avoid or monitor efficacy. [Moderate] Theoretical
- **Lumacaftor** is predicted to decrease the exposure to **ciclosporin**. Avoid. [Severe] Theoretical
- **Lumacaftor** is predicted to decrease the efficacy of **combined hormonal contraceptives**. Use additional contraceptive precautions. [Severe] Theoretical
- **Lumacaftor** is predicted to decrease the exposure to corticosteroids **(methylprednisolone)**. Adjust dose. [Severe] Theoretical
- **Lumacaftor** is predicted to decrease the exposure to **doravirine**. Avoid. [Severe] Theoretical
- **Lumacaftor** is predicted to decrease the exposure to **everolimus**. Avoid. [Severe] Theoretical
- **Lumacaftor** potentially decreases the exposure to **glecaprevir**. Avoid. [Severe] Theoretical
- **Lumacaftor** is predicted to decrease the efficacy of **levonorgestrel**. Use additional contraceptive precautions. [Severe] Theoretical
- **Lumacaftor** is predicted to decrease the exposure to macrolides **(clarithromycin, erythromycin)**. [Moderate] Theoretical
- **Lumacaftor** is predicted to decrease the exposure to **midazolam**. Avoid. [Severe] Theoretical
- **Lumacaftor** potentially decreases the exposure to **pibrentasvir**. Avoid. [Severe] Theoretical
- **Lumacaftor** is predicted to decrease the exposure to **rifabutin**. Adjust dose. [Moderate] Theoretical
- **Lumacaftor** is predicted to decrease the exposure to **sirolimus**. Avoid. [Severe] Theoretical
- **Lumacaftor** is predicted to decrease the exposure to **tacrolimus**. Avoid. [Severe] Theoretical
- **Lumacaftor** is predicted to decrease the exposure to **temsirolimus**. Avoid. [Severe] Theoretical
- **Lumacaftor** is predicted to decrease the efficacy of **ulipristal**. Use additional contraceptive precautions. [Severe] Theoretical

Lumefantrine → see antimalarials

Lurasidone → see TABLE 8 p. 908 (hypotension), TABLE 11 p. 909 (CNS depressant effects)

- Antiarrhythmics **(dronedarone)** are predicted to increase the exposure to **lurasidone**. Adjust **lurasidone** dose. [Moderate] Study
- Antiepileptics **(carbamazepine, fosphenytoin, phenobarbital, phenytoin, primidone)** are predicted to decrease the exposure to **lurasidone**. Avoid. [Moderate] Study → Also see TABLE 11 p. 909
- Antifungals, azoles **(fluconazole, isavuconazole)** are predicted to increase the exposure to **lurasidone**. Adjust **lurasidone** dose. [Moderate] Study

Lurasidone (continued)
- Antifungals, azoles **(itraconazole, ketoconazole, voriconazole)** are predicted to increase the exposure to **lurasidone**. Avoid. [Severe] Study
- Antifungals, azoles **(posaconazole)** moderately increase the exposure to **lurasidone**. Avoid. [Severe] Study
- **Apalutamide** is predicted to decrease the exposure to **lurasidone**. Avoid. [Moderate] Study
- **Aprepitant** is predicted to increase the exposure to **lurasidone**. Adjust **lurasidone** dose. [Moderate] Study
- **Bosentan** is predicted to decrease the exposure to **lurasidone**. Monitor and adjust dose. [Moderate] Theoretical
- Calcium channel blockers **(diltiazem, verapamil)** are predicted to increase the exposure to **lurasidone**. Adjust **lurasidone** dose. [Moderate] Study → Also see TABLE 8 p. 908
- **Cobicistat** is predicted to increase the exposure to **lurasidone**. Avoid. [Severe] Study
- **Crizotinib** is predicted to increase the exposure to **lurasidone**. Adjust **lurasidone** dose. [Moderate] Study
- **Efavirenz** is predicted to decrease the exposure to **lurasidone**. Monitor and adjust dose. [Moderate] Theoretical
- **Enzalutamide** is predicted to decrease the exposure to **lurasidone**. Avoid. [Moderate] Study
- **Grapefruit juice** is predicted to increase the exposure to **lurasidone**. Avoid. [Severe] Theoretical
- **HIV-protease inhibitors** are predicted to increase the exposure to **lurasidone**. Avoid. [Severe] Study
- **Idelalisib** is predicted to increase the exposure to **lurasidone**. Avoid. [Severe] Study
- **Imatinib** is predicted to increase the exposure to **lurasidone**. Adjust **lurasidone** dose. [Moderate] Study
- **Lurasidone** is predicted to decrease the effects of **levodopa**. [Severe] Theoretical → Also see TABLE 8 p. 908
- Macrolides **(clarithromycin)** are predicted to increase the exposure to **lurasidone**. Avoid. [Severe] Study
- Macrolides **(erythromycin)** are predicted to increase the exposure to **lurasidone**. Adjust **lurasidone** dose. [Moderate] Study
- **Mitotane** is predicted to decrease the exposure to **lurasidone**. Avoid. [Moderate] Study
- **Netupitant** is predicted to increase the exposure to **lurasidone**. Adjust **lurasidone** dose. [Moderate] Study
- **Nevirapine** is predicted to decrease the exposure to **lurasidone**. Monitor and adjust dose. [Moderate] Theoretical
- **Nilotinib** is predicted to increase the exposure to **lurasidone**. Adjust **lurasidone** dose. [Moderate] Study
- **Rifampicin** is predicted to decrease the exposure to **lurasidone**. Avoid. [Moderate] Study
- **St John's Wort** is predicted to decrease the exposure to **lurasidone**. Monitor and adjust dose. [Moderate] Theoretical

Lymecycline → see tetracyclines

Macitentan
- Antiepileptics **(carbamazepine, fosphenytoin, phenobarbital, phenytoin, primidone)** are predicted to decrease the exposure to **macitentan**. Avoid. [Severe] Study
- Antifungals, azoles **(itraconazole, ketoconazole, voriconazole)** are predicted to increase the exposure to **macitentan**. [Moderate] Study
- **Apalutamide** is predicted to decrease the exposure to **macitentan**. Avoid. [Severe] Study
- **Cobicistat** is predicted to increase the exposure to **macitentan**. [Moderate] Study
- **Enzalutamide** is predicted to decrease the exposure to **macitentan**. Avoid. [Severe] Study
- **HIV-protease inhibitors** are predicted to increase the exposure to **macitentan**. [Moderate] Study
- **Idelalisib** is predicted to increase the exposure to **macitentan**. [Moderate] Study
- Macrolides **(clarithromycin)** are predicted to increase the exposure to **macitentan**. [Moderate] Study
- **Mitotane** is predicted to decrease the exposure to **macitentan**. Avoid. [Severe] Study
- **Rifampicin** is predicted to decrease the exposure to **macitentan**. Avoid. [Severe] Study
- **St John's Wort** is predicted to decrease the exposure to **macitentan**. Avoid. [Severe] Theoretical

Macrolides → see TABLE 9 p. 909 (QT-interval prolongation)

azithromycin · clarithromycin · erythromycin

- Interactions do not generally apply to topical use of **azithromycin** unless specified.
- Since systemic absorption can follow topical application of **erythromycin**, the possibility of interactions should be borne in mind.

- **Clarithromycin** is predicted to increase the exposure to abemaciclib. Avoid or adjust **abemaciclib** dose. [Severe] Study
- **Erythromycin** is predicted to increase the exposure to abemaciclib. [Moderate] Study
- **Macrolides** are predicted to increase the exposure to **afatinib**. Separate administration by 12 hours. [Moderate] Study
- **Clarithromycin** is predicted to markedly increase the exposure to aldosterone antagonists **(eplerenone)**. Avoid. [Severe] Study
- **Erythromycin** is predicted to increase the exposure to aldosterone antagonists **(eplerenone)**. Adjust **eplerenone** dose. [Severe] Study
- **Azithromycin** is predicted to increase the exposure to **aliskiren**. [Moderate] Theoretical
- Macrolides **(clarithromycin, erythromycin)** are predicted to increase the exposure to aliskiren. [Moderate] Study
- **Clarithromycin** increases the exposure to almotriptan. [Mild] Study
- **Clarithromycin** is predicted to moderately increase the exposure to alpha blockers **(alfuzosin, tamsulosin)**. Use with caution or avoid. [Moderate] Study
- **Clarithromycin** is predicted to increase the exposure to alpha blockers **(doxazosin)**. [Moderate] Study
- **Erythromycin** is predicted to increase the exposure to alpha blockers **(tamsulosin)**. [Moderate] Theoretical
- **Clarithromycin** moderately increases the exposure to alprazolam. Avoid. [Moderate] Study
- **Erythromycin** is predicted to increase the exposure to alprazolam. [Severe] Study
- **Azithromycin** is predicted to increase the exposure to **aminophylline**. [Moderate] Theoretical
- **Clarithromycin** is predicted to increase the exposure to aminophylline. Adjust dose. [Moderate] Theoretical
- **Aminophylline** is predicted to decrease the exposure to **erythromycin**. Adjust dose. [Severe] Study
- **Clarithromycin** very markedly increases the exposure to antiarrhythmics **(dronedarone)**. Avoid. [Severe] Study → Also see TABLE 9 p. 909
- **Erythromycin** is predicted to moderately increase the exposure to antiarrhythmics **(dronedarone)**. Avoid. [Severe] Theoretical → Also see TABLE 9 p. 909
- Macrolides **(clarithromycin, erythromycin)** are predicted to increase the exposure to antiarrhythmics **(lidocaine)**. [Moderate] Theoretical
- **Clarithromycin** is predicted to increase the exposure to antiarrhythmics **(propafenone)**. Monitor and adjust dose. [Severe] Study
- **Erythromycin** is predicted to increase the exposure to antiarrhythmics **(propafenone)**. Monitor and adjust dose. [Moderate] Study
- **Clarithromycin** is predicted to increase the exposure to anticholinesterases, centrally acting **(galantamine)**. Monitor and adjust dose. [Moderate] Study
- **Clarithromycin** slightly increases the concentration of antiepileptics **(carbamazepine)**. Monitor concentration and adjust dose. [Severe] Study
- **Erythromycin** markedly increases the concentration of antiepileptics **(carbamazepine)**. Monitor concentration and adjust dose. [Severe] Study
- **Clarithromycin** is predicted to very slightly increase the exposure to antiepileptics **(perampanel)**. [Mild] Study
- **Clarithromycin** is predicted to increase the exposure to antifungals, azoles **(isavuconazole)**. Avoid or monitor side effects. [Severe] Study
- **Erythromycin** is predicted to increase the exposure to antifungals, azoles **(isavuconazole)**. [Moderate] Theoretical
- **Clarithromycin** is predicted to increase the exposure to antihistamines, non-sedating **(mizolastine)**. Avoid. [Severe] Study

- **Erythromycin** is predicted to increase the exposure to antihistamines, non-sedating **(mizolastine)**. Severe Theoretical
- Macrolides **(clarithromycin, erythromycin)** are predicted to increase the exposure to antihistamines, non-sedating (rupatadine). Avoid. Moderate Study
- Macrolides **(clarithromycin, erythromycin)** are predicted to increase the concentration of antimalarials **(piperaquine)**. Severe Theoretical
- **Clarithromycin** is predicted to increase the exposure to apalutamide. Mild Study → Also see **TABLE 9** p. 909
- **Erythromycin** is predicted to increase the exposure to apixaban. Moderate Theoretical
- **Clarithromycin** is predicted to markedly increase the exposure to aprepitant. Moderate Study
- **Erythromycin** is predicted to increase the exposure to aprepitant. Moderate Study
- **Clarithromycin** is predicted to slightly increase the exposure to aripiprazole. Adjust **aripiprazole** dose, p. 265. Moderate Study
- **Clarithromycin** is predicted to increase the exposure to axitinib. Avoid or adjust dose. Moderate Study
- **Erythromycin** is predicted to increase the exposure to **axitinib**. Moderate Theoretical
- **Clarithromycin** is predicted to increase the exposure to bedaquiline. Avoid prolonged use. Mild Study → Also see **TABLE 9** p. 909
- **Erythromycin** is predicted to increase the exposure to bedaquiline. Avoid prolonged use. Mild Theoretical → Also see **TABLE 9** p. 909
- **Macrolides** are predicted to increase the exposure to beta blockers, non-selective **(nadolol)**. Moderate Study
- **Clarithromycin** is predicted to increase the exposure to $beta_2$ agonists **(salmeterol)**. Avoid. Severe Study
- **Macrolides** are predicted to increase the exposure to bictegravir. Use with caution or avoid. Moderate Theoretical
- **Clarithromycin** slightly increases the exposure to **bortezomib**. Moderate Study
- **Clarithromycin** is predicted to increase the exposure to bosentan. Moderate Theoretical
- **Clarithromycin** is predicted to markedly increase the exposure to bosutinib. Avoid or adjust dose. Severe Study → Also see **TABLE 9** p. 909
- **Erythromycin** is predicted to increase the exposure to bosutinib. Avoid or adjust dose. Severe Theoretical → Also see **TABLE 9** p. 909
- **Clarithromycin** is predicted to increase the exposure to brigatinib. Adjust **brigatinib** dose. Severe Study
- **Clarithromycin** is predicted to increase the exposure to buspirone. Adjust **buspirone** dose. Severe Study
- **Erythromycin** is predicted to increase the exposure to buspirone. Use with caution and adjust dose. Moderate Study
- **Clarithromycin** slightly increases the exposure to **cabozantinib**. Moderate Study → Also see **TABLE 9** p. 909
- **Erythromycin** is predicted to increase the exposure to cabozantinib. Moderate Theoretical → Also see **TABLE 9** p. 909
- **Erythromycin** is predicted to increase the exposure to calcium channel blockers **(amlodipine, felodipine, lacidipine, lercanidipine, nicardipine, nifedipine, nimodipine)**. Monitor and adjust dose. Moderate Study
- **Clarithromycin** is predicted to increase the exposure to calcium channel blockers **(amlodipine, felodipine, lacidipine, nicardipine, nifedipine, nimodipine)**. Monitor and adjust dose. Moderate Study
- **Erythromycin** is predicted to increase the exposure to calcium channel blockers **(diltiazem)**. Severe Theoretical
- **Clarithromycin** is predicted to increase the exposure to calcium channel blockers **(diltiazem, verapamil)**. Severe Study
- **Clarithromycin** is predicted to markedly increase the exposure to calcium channel blockers **(lercanidipine)**. Avoid. Severe Study
- **Erythromycin** is predicted to increase the exposure to calcium channel blockers **(verapamil)**. Severe Study
- **Clarithromycin** is predicted to increase the exposure to cannabidiol. Avoid or adjust dose. Mild Study
- **Clarithromycin** is predicted to moderately increase the exposure to cariprazine. Avoid. Severe Study
- **Erythromycin** is predicted to increase the exposure to cariprazine. Avoid. Severe Study
- **Azithromycin** is predicted to increase the exposure to **ceritinib**. Moderate Theoretical
- **Clarithromycin** is predicted to increase the exposure to ceritinib. Avoid or adjust **ceritinib** dose. Severe Study → Also see **TABLE 9** p. 909
- **Clarithromycin** increases the concentration of **ciclosporin**. Severe Study
- **Erythromycin** is predicted to increase the concentration of ciclosporin. Severe Study
- **Clarithromycin** is predicted to moderately increase the exposure to cilostazol. Adjust **cilostazol** dose. Moderate Study
- **Erythromycin** slightly increases the exposure to **cilostazol**. Adjust **cilostazol** dose. Moderate Study
- **Clarithromycin** is predicted to moderately increase the exposure to cinacalcet. Adjust dose. Moderate Study
- **Erythromycin** potentially increases the risk of toxicity when given with clozapine. Severe Anecdotal
- **Clarithromycin** is predicted to markedly increase the exposure to cobimetinib. Avoid or monitor for toxicity. Severe Study
- **Erythromycin** is predicted to increase the exposure to cobimetinib. Severe Theoretical
- **Azithromycin** is predicted to increase the exposure to colchicine. Avoid P-glycoprotein inhibitors or adjust **colchicine** dose. Severe Theoretical
- **Clarithromycin** is predicted to increase the exposure to colchicine. Avoid potent inhibitors of CYP3A4 or adjust **colchicine** dose. Severe Study
- **Erythromycin** is predicted to increase the exposure to colchicine. Adjust **colchicine** dose with moderate inhibitors of CYP3A4. Severe Study
- **Clarithromycin** is predicted to increase the exposure to corticosteroids **(beclometasone)** (risk with beclometasone is likely to be lower than with other corticosteroids). Moderate Theoretical
- **Clarithromycin** is predicted to increase the exposure to corticosteroids **(betamethasone, budesonide, ciclesonide, deflazacort, dexamethasone, fludrocortisone, fluticasone, hydrocortisone, methylprednisolone, mometasone, prednisolone, triamcinolone)**. Avoid or monitor side effects. Severe Study
- **Erythromycin** is predicted to increase the exposure to corticosteroids **(methylprednisolone)**. Monitor and adjust dose. Moderate Study
- Macrolides **(clarithromycin, erythromycin)** increase the anticoagulant effect of coumarins. Monitor INR and adjust dose. Severe Anecdotal
- **Clarithromycin** is predicted to moderately increase the exposure to **crizotinib**. Avoid. Moderate Study → Also see **TABLE 9** p. 909
- **Macrolides** are predicted to increase the exposure to dabigatran. Moderate Theoretical
- **Clarithromycin** is predicted to increase the exposure to dabrafenib. Use with caution or avoid. Moderate Study
- **Clarithromycin** is predicted to markedly to very markedly increase the exposure to darifenacin. Avoid. Severe Study
- **Erythromycin** is predicted to slightly increase the exposure to darifenacin. Moderate Study
- **Clarithromycin** is predicted to markedly increase the exposure to dasatinib. Avoid or adjust dose—consult product literature. Severe Study → Also see **TABLE 9** p. 909
- **Erythromycin** is predicted to increase the exposure to dasatinib. Severe Study → Also see **TABLE 9** p. 909
- **Clarithromycin** very slightly increases the exposure to delamanid. Severe Study → Also see **TABLE 9** p. 909
- **Clarithromycin** is predicted to moderately increase the exposure to **dienogest**. Moderate Study
- **Erythromycin** is predicted to slightly increase the exposure to dienogest. Moderate Study
- **Macrolides** increase the concentration of **digoxin**. Severe Anecdotal
- Macrolides **(clarithromycin, erythromycin)** increase the risk of QT-prolongation when given with **domperidone**. Avoid. Severe Study

Macrolides (continued)

- **Clarithromycin** increases the exposure to dopamine receptor agonists **(bromocriptine)**. Severe Study
- **Erythromycin** is predicted to increase the exposure to dopamine receptor agonists **(bromocriptine)**. Severe Theoretical
- Macrolides **(clarithromycin, erythromycin)** are predicted to increase the concentration of dopamine receptor agonists **(cabergoline)**. Avoid. Severe Study
- **Clarithromycin** is predicted to increase the exposure to **doravirine**. Mild Study
- **Clarithromycin** is predicted to increase the exposure to **dronabinol**. Adjust dose. Mild Study
- **Clarithromycin** is predicted to increase the exposure to **dutasteride**. Monitor side effects and adjust dose. Moderate Theoretical
- **Erythromycin** is predicted to moderately increase the exposure to **dutasteride**. Mild Study
- **Erythromycin** slightly increases the exposure to **edoxaban**. Adjust **edoxaban** dose. Severe Study
- Macrolides **(azithromycin, clarithromycin)** are predicted to slightly increase the exposure to **edoxaban**. Severe Theoretical
- Efavirenz decreases the exposure to **clarithromycin**. Moderate Study → Also see **TABLE 9** p. 909
- **Clarithromycin** is predicted to markedly increase the exposure to **eletriptan**. Avoid. Severe Study
- **Erythromycin** moderately increases the exposure to **eletriptan**. Avoid. Moderate Study
- Macrolides **(clarithromycin, erythromycin)** are predicted to increase the exposure to **eliglustat**. Avoid or adjust dose—consult product literature. Severe Study
- **Clarithromycin** is predicted to increase the exposure to **encorafenib**. Avoid or monitor. Severe Study → Also see **TABLE 9** p. 909
- **Erythromycin** is predicted to moderately increase the exposure to **encorafenib**. Moderate Study → Also see **TABLE 9** p. 909
- **Clarithromycin** is predicted to increase the risk of ergotism when given with **ergometrine**. Avoid. Severe Theoretical
- **Erythromycin** is predicted to increase the risk of ergotism when given with **ergometrine**. Severe Theoretical
- **Clarithromycin** is predicted to increase the risk of ergotism when given with **ergotamine**. Avoid. Severe Theoretical
- **Erythromycin** is predicted to increase the risk of ergotism when given with **ergotamine**. Severe Theoretical
- **Clarithromycin** is predicted to slightly increase the exposure to **erlotinib**. Use with caution and adjust dose. Moderate Study
- Macrolides **(azithromycin, erythromycin)** are predicted to increase the exposure to **erlotinib**. Moderate Theoretical
- **Clarithromycin** is predicted to increase the exposure to **esketamine**. Adjust dose. Moderate Study
- Etravirine decreases the exposure to **clarithromycin** and **clarithromycin** slightly increases the exposure to **etravirine**. Severe Study
- **Clarithromycin** is predicted to increase the concentration of **everolimus**. Avoid. Severe Study
- **Erythromycin** is predicted to increase the concentration of **everolimus**. Avoid or adjust dose. Moderate Study
- **Clarithromycin** is predicted to moderately increase the exposure to **fesoterodine**. Adjust **fesoterodine** dose with potent inhibitors of CYP3A4; avoid in hepatic and renal impairment. Severe Study
- **Erythromycin** is predicted to increase the exposure to **fesoterodine**. Adjust **fesoterodine** dose with moderate inhibitors of CYP3A4 in hepatic and renal impairment. Mild Study
- **Macrolides** are predicted to increase the exposure to **fidaxomicin**. Avoid. Moderate Study
- **Clarithromycin** is predicted to increase the exposure to **fosaprepitant**. Moderate Theoretical
- **Clarithromycin** is predicted to increase the exposure to **gefitinib**. Moderate Study
- **Erythromycin** is predicted to increase the exposure to **gefitinib**. Moderate Theoretical
- **Clarithromycin** is predicted to increase the exposure to **gilteritinib**. Moderate Study
- Macrolides **(azithromycin, erythromycin)** are predicted to increase the exposure to **gilteritinib**. Moderate Theoretical
- **Clarithromycin** is predicted to moderately to markedly increase the exposure to **grazoprevir**. Avoid. Severe Study
- **Clarithromycin** is predicted to increase the exposure to **guanfacine**. Adjust **guanfacine** dose, p. 247. Moderate Study
- **Erythromycin** is predicted to increase the concentration of **guanfacine**. Adjust **guanfacine** dose, p. 247. Moderate Theoretical
- H_2 receptor antagonists **(cimetidine)** slightly increase the exposure to **erythromycin**. Moderate Study
- HIV-protease inhibitors **(atazanavir)** are predicted to increase the exposure to **clarithromycin**. Adjust dose in renal impairment. Severe Study
- HIV-protease inhibitors **(atazanavir, darunavir, fosamprenavir, lopinavir, ritonavir, tipranavir)** are predicted to increase the exposure to **erythromycin**. Severe Theoretical
- HIV-protease inhibitors **(darunavir, fosamprenavir, lopinavir)** boosted with ritonavir are predicted to increase the exposure to **clarithromycin**. Adjust dose in renal impairment. Severe Study
- HIV-protease inhibitors **(ritonavir)** increase the exposure to **clarithromycin**. Adjust dose in renal impairment. Severe Study
- HIV-protease inhibitors **(tipranavir)** boosted with ritonavir increase the exposure to **clarithromycin** and **clarithromycin** increases the exposure to HIV-protease inhibitors **(tipranavir)** boosted with ritonavir. Monitor; adjust dose in renal impairment. Severe Study
- **Clarithromycin** increases the exposure to HIV-protease inhibitors **(saquinavir)** and HIV-protease inhibitors **(saquinavir)** increase the exposure to **clarithromycin**. Avoid. Severe Study → Also see **TABLE 9** p. 909
- **Erythromycin** is predicted to increase the exposure to HIV-protease inhibitors **(saquinavir)**. Avoid. Severe Theoretical → Also see **TABLE 9** p. 909
- **Clarithromycin** is predicted to very markedly increase the exposure to **ibrutinib**. Avoid potent inhibitors of CYP3A4 or adjust **ibrutinib** dose. Severe Study
- **Erythromycin** is predicted to increase the exposure to **ibrutinib**. Adjust **ibrutinib** dose with moderate inhibitors of CYP3A4. Severe Study
- **Clarithromycin** is predicted to increase the exposure to **imatinib**. Moderate Study
- **Erythromycin** is predicted to increase the exposure to **imatinib**. Moderate Theoretical
- **Clarithromycin** is predicted to increase the risk of toxicity when given with **irinotecan**. Avoid. Moderate Study
- **Clarithromycin** is predicted to increase the exposure to **ivabradine**. Avoid. Severe Study
- **Erythromycin** is predicted to increase the exposure to **ivabradine**. Avoid. Severe Theoretical
- **Clarithromycin** is predicted to increase the exposure to **ivacaftor**. Adjust ivacaftor p. 196 or lumacaftor with ivacaftor p. 197 or **tezacaftor with ivacaftor** p. 198 dose with potent inhibitors of CYP3A4. Severe Study
- **Erythromycin** is predicted to increase the exposure to **ivacaftor**. Adjust ivacaftor p. 196 or tezacaftor with ivacaftor p. 198 dose with moderate inhibitors of CYP3A4. Severe Study
- **Clarithromycin** is predicted to increase the exposure to **lapatinib**. Avoid. Moderate Study → Also see **TABLE 9** p. 909
- **Erythromycin** is predicted to increase the exposure to **lapatinib**. Moderate Study → Also see **TABLE 9** p. 909
- **Clarithromycin** is predicted to moderately increase the exposure to **larotrectinib**. Avoid or adjust **larotrectinib** dose, p. 607. Moderate Study
- Macrolides **(azithromycin, erythromycin)** are predicted to increase the exposure to **larotrectinib**. Mild Theoretical
- Macrolides **(clarithromycin, erythromycin)** are predicted to increase the concentration of **letermovir**. Moderate Study
- **Clarithromycin** increases the exposure to **linezolid**. Moderate Anecdotal
- **Azithromycin** is predicted to increase the exposure to **lomitapide**. Separate administration by 12 hours. Moderate Theoretical
- **Clarithromycin** is predicted to markedly increase the exposure to **lomitapide**. Avoid. Severe Study

- ▸ **Erythromycin** is predicted to increase the exposure to lomitapide. Avoid. Moderate Theoretical
- ▸ **Clarithromycin** is predicted to increase the exposure to lorlatinib. Avoid or adjust **lorlatinib** dose. Severe Study
- ▸ Lumacaftor is predicted to decrease the exposure to macrolides **(clarithromycin, erythromycin)**. Moderate Theoretical
- ▸ **Clarithromycin** is predicted to increase the exposure to lurasidone. Avoid. Severe Study
- ▸ **Erythromycin** is predicted to increase the exposure to lurasidone. Adjust **lurasidone** dose. Moderate Study
- ▸ **Clarithromycin** is predicted to increase the exposure to macitentan. Moderate Study
- ▸ **Clarithromycin** is predicted to markedly increase the exposure to maraviroc. Adjust dose. Severe Study
- ▸ **Clarithromycin** is predicted to markedly to very markedly increase the exposure to midazolam. Avoid or adjust dose. Severe Study
- ▸ **Erythromycin** is predicted to increase the exposure to midazolam. Monitor side effects and adjust dose. Severe Study
- ▸ **Clarithromycin** is predicted to very markedly increase the exposure to midostaurin. Avoid or monitor for toxicity. Severe Study
- ▸ **Erythromycin** is predicted to increase the exposure to midostaurin. Moderate Theoretical
- ▸ **Clarithromycin** is predicted to increase the exposure to mirabegron. Adjust **mirabegron** dose in hepatic and renal impairment. Moderate Study
- ▸ **Clarithromycin** is predicted to increase the exposure to mirtazapine. Moderate Study
- ▸ **Clarithromycin** is predicted to increase the exposure to modafinil. Mild Theoretical
- ▸ **Clarithromycin** increases the risk of neutropenia when given with monoclonal antibodies **(brentuximab vedotin)**. Monitor and adjust dose. Severe Theoretical
- ▸ **Clarithromycin** is predicted to increase the exposure to monoclonal antibodies **(polatuzumab vedotin)**. Moderate Theoretical
- ▸ **Clarithromycin** is predicted to increase the exposure to monoclonal antibodies **(trastuzumab emtansine)**. Avoid. Severe Theoretical
- ▸ **Clarithromycin** is predicted to increase the exposure to naldemedine. Avoid or monitor. Moderate Study
- ▸ Macrolides **(azithromycin, erythromycin)** are predicted to increase the exposure to naldemedine. Moderate Study
- ▸ **Clarithromycin** is predicted to markedly increase the exposure to naloxegol. Avoid. Severe Study
- ▸ **Erythromycin** is predicted to increase the exposure to naloxegol. Adjust **naloxegol** dose and monitor side effects. Moderate Study
- ▸ **Clarithromycin** is predicted to increase the exposure to neratinib. Avoid or adjust **neratinib** dose. Severe Study
- ▸ **Erythromycin** is predicted to increase the exposure to neratinib. Avoid. Severe Study
- ▸ **Clarithromycin** is predicted to increase the exposure to netupitant. Moderate Study
- ▸ **Nevirapine** decreases the exposure to **clarithromycin**. Moderate Study
- ▸ **Clarithromycin** is predicted to moderately increase the exposure to nilotinib. Avoid. Severe Study → Also see **TABLE 9** p. 909
- ▸ **Erythromycin** is predicted to increase the exposure to nilotinib. Moderate Theoretical → Also see **TABLE 9** p. 909
- ▸ **Macrolides** are predicted to increase the exposure to nintedanib. Moderate Study
- ▸ **Clarithromycin** is predicted to increase the exposure to nitisinone. Adjust dose. Moderate Theoretical
- ▸ **Clarithromycin** is predicted to increase the exposure to olaparib. Avoid potent inhibitors of CYP3A4 or adjust **olaparib** dose. Moderate Study
- ▸ **Erythromycin** is predicted to increase the exposure to olaparib. Avoid moderate inhibitors of CYP3A4 or adjust **olaparib** dose. Moderate Theoretical
- ▸ **Clarithromycin** is predicted to increase the exposure to opioids (alfentanil, buprenorphine, fentanyl, oxycodone). Monitor and adjust dose. Severe Study
- ▸ **Erythromycin** is predicted to increase the exposure to opioids **(alfentanil, buprenorphine, fentanyl, oxycodone)**. Monitor and adjust dose. Moderate Study
- ▸ **Clarithromycin** is predicted to increase the concentration of opioids **(methadone)**. Severe Theoretical → Also see **TABLE 9** p. 909
- ▸ **Erythromycin** is predicted to increase the exposure to opioids **(methadone)**. Moderate Theoretical → Also see **TABLE 9** p. 909
- ▸ **Clarithromycin** is predicted to increase the exposure to ospemifene. Avoid in poor CYP2C9 metabolisers. Moderate Study
- ▸ **Clarithromycin** is predicted to increase the exposure to oxybutynin. Mild Study
- ▸ **Erythromycin** is predicted to increase the exposure to oxybutynin. Mild Theoretical
- ▸ **Clarithromycin** is predicted to increase the exposure to palbociclib. Avoid or adjust **palbociclib** dose. Severe Study
- ▸ **Clarithromycin** is predicted to increase the exposure to panobinostat. Adjust **panobinostat** dose; in hepatic impairment avoid. Moderate Study → Also see **TABLE 9** p. 909
- ▸ Macrolides **(azithromycin, erythromycin)** are predicted to increase the exposure to panobinostat. Adjust dose. Moderate Theoretical → Also see **TABLE 9** p. 909
- ▸ **Clarithromycin** is predicted to increase the exposure to paritaprevir. Avoid. Severe Study
- ▸ **Erythromycin** is predicted to increase the exposure to paritaprevir. Moderate Theoretical
- ▸ **Clarithromycin** is predicted to increase the exposure to pazopanib. Avoid or adjust **pazopanib** dose. Moderate Study → Also see **TABLE 9** p. 909
- ▸ **Erythromycin** is predicted to increase the exposure to pazopanib. Moderate Theoretical → Also see **TABLE 9** p. 909
- ▸ **Erythromycin** is predicted to increase the exposure to phosphodiesterase type-5 inhibitors **(avanafil)**. Adjust **avanafil** dose. Moderate Theoretical
- ▸ **Clarithromycin** is predicted to increase the exposure to phosphodiesterase type-5 inhibitors **(avanafil, vardenafil)**. Avoid. Severe Study → Also see **TABLE 9** p. 909
- ▸ **Clarithromycin** is predicted to increase the exposure to phosphodiesterase type-5 inhibitors **(sildenafil)**. Avoid potent inhibitors of CYP3A4 or adjust **sildenafil** dose, p. 125. Severe Study → Also see **TABLE 9** p. 909
- ▸ **Erythromycin** is predicted to increase the exposure to phosphodiesterase type-5 inhibitors **(sildenafil)**. Monitor or adjust **sildenafil** dose with moderate inhibitors of CYP3A4, p. 125. Moderate Study → Also see **TABLE 9** p. 909
- ▸ **Clarithromycin** is predicted to increase the exposure to phosphodiesterase type-5 inhibitors **(tadalafil)**. Use with caution or avoid. Severe Study
- ▸ **Erythromycin** is predicted to increase the exposure to phosphodiesterase type-5 inhibitors **(tadalafil)**. Severe Theoretical
- ▸ **Erythromycin** is predicted to increase the exposure to phosphodiesterase type-5 inhibitors **(vardenafil)**. Adjust dose. Severe Theoretical → Also see **TABLE 9** p. 909
- ▸ **Macrolides** are predicted to increase the exposure to pibrentasvir. Moderate Theoretical
- ▸ **Clarithromycin** is predicted to increase the exposure to pimozide. Avoid. Severe Study → Also see **TABLE 9** p. 909
- ▸ **Erythromycin** is predicted to increase the exposure to pimozide. Avoid. Severe Theoretical → Also see **TABLE 9** p. 909
- ▸ **Clarithromycin** is predicted to slightly increase the exposure to ponatinib. Monitor and adjust **ponatinib** dose. Moderate Study
- ▸ **Clarithromycin** is predicted to moderately increase the exposure to praziquantel. Mild Study
- ▸ **Clarithromycin** given with carbimazole is predicted to increase the exposure to propiverine. Adjust starting dose. Moderate Theoretical
- ▸ **Clarithromycin** is predicted to increase the exposure to quetiapine. Avoid. Severe Study
- ▸ **Erythromycin** is predicted to increase the exposure to quetiapine. Avoid. Moderate Study
- ▸ **Clarithromycin** is predicted to increase the exposure to ranolazine. Avoid. Severe Study → Also see **TABLE 9** p. 909
- ▸ **Erythromycin** is predicted to increase the exposure to ranolazine. Severe Study → Also see **TABLE 9** p. 909

Macrolides (continued)
- **Clarithromycin** is predicted to increase the exposure to reboxetine. Avoid. Moderate Study
- **Clarithromycin** is predicted to increase the exposure to regorafenib. Avoid. Moderate Study
- **Clarithromycin** is predicted to increase the exposure to repaglinide. Moderate Study
- **Clarithromycin** is predicted to increase the exposure to retinoids **(alitretinoin)**. Adjust **alitretinoin** dose. Moderate Theoretical
- **Clarithromycin** is predicted to increase the exposure to ribociclib. Avoid or adjust **ribociclib** dose. Moderate Study → Also see TABLE 9 p. 909
- **Erythromycin** is predicted to increase the exposure to ribociclib. Moderate Study → Also see TABLE 9 p. 909
- **Azithromycin** increases the risk of neutropenia when given with rifabutin. Severe Study
- **Clarithromycin** increases the risk of uveitis when given with rifabutin. Adjust dose. Severe Study
- **Erythromycin** is predicted to increase the risk of uveitis when given with rifabutin. Adjust dose. Severe Theoretical
- Rifampicin decreases the concentration of **clarithromycin.** Severe Study
- **Clarithromycin** is predicted to increase the exposure to risperidone. Adjust dose. Moderate Study → Also see TABLE 9 p. 909
- **Clarithromycin** is predicted to increase the exposure to ruxolitinib. Adjust dose and monitor side effects. Moderate Study
- **Erythromycin** is predicted to increase the exposure to ruxolitinib. Moderate Theoretical
- **Clarithromycin** is predicted to increase the exposure to saxagliptin. Moderate Study
- **Erythromycin** is predicted to increase the exposure to saxagliptin. Mild Study
- **Clarithromycin** is predicted to increase the exposure to siponimod. Avoid depending on other drugs taken—consult product literature. Severe Theoretical
- **Clarithromycin** is predicted to increase the concentration of sirolimus. Avoid. Severe Study
- **Erythromycin** increases the concentration of sirolimus. Monitor and adjust dose. Moderate Study
- **Clarithromycin** is predicted to increase the exposure to solifenacin. Adjust solifenacin or tamsulosin with solifenacin dose; avoid in hepatic and renal impairment. Severe Study
- **Clarithromycin** is predicted to moderately increase the exposure to SSRIs **(dapoxetine)**. Avoid potent inhibitors of CYP3A4 or adjust **dapoxetine** dose. Severe Study
- **Erythromycin** is predicted to increase the exposure to SSRIs (dapoxetine). Adjust **dapoxetine** dose with moderate inhibitors of CYP3A4. Moderate Theoretical
- **Clarithromycin** is predicted to increase the exposure to statins (atorvastatin). Avoid or adjust dose and monitor rhabdomyolysis. Severe Study
- **Erythromycin** slightly increases the exposure to statins (atorvastatin). Monitor and adjust dose. Severe Anecdotal
- **Clarithromycin** moderately increases the exposure to statins (pravastatin). Severe Study
- **Erythromycin** is predicted to increase the exposure to statins (pravastatin). Severe Study
- **Clarithromycin** is predicted to increase the exposure to statins (simvastatin). Avoid. Severe Study
- **Erythromycin** markedly increases the exposure to statins (simvastatin). Avoid. Severe Study
- **Clarithromycin** is predicted to slightly increase the exposure to sulfonylureas. Moderate Theoretical
- **Clarithromycin** is predicted to slightly increase the exposure to sunitinib. Avoid or adjust **sunitinib** dose. Moderate Study → Also see TABLE 9 p. 909
- **Erythromycin** is predicted to increase the exposure to sunitinib. Moderate Theoretical → Also see TABLE 9 p. 909
- **Clarithromycin** is predicted to increase the concentration of tacrolimus. Monitor and adjust dose. Severe Study
- **Erythromycin** is predicted to increase the concentration of tacrolimus. Severe Study
- **Macrolides** are predicted to slightly increase the exposure to talazoparib. Avoid or adjust **talazoparib** dose. Severe Study
- **Clarithromycin** is predicted to increase the exposure to taxanes (cabazitaxel). Avoid. Severe Study
- **Erythromycin** is predicted to increase the exposure to taxanes (cabazitaxel). Moderate Theoretical
- **Clarithromycin** is predicted to moderately increase the exposure to taxanes **(docetaxel)**. Avoid or adjust dose. Severe Study
- **Clarithromycin** is predicted to increase the exposure to taxanes (paclitaxel). Severe Theoretical
- **Clarithromycin** is predicted to increase the concentration of temsirolimus. Avoid. Severe Theoretical
- **Erythromycin** is predicted to increase the concentration of temsirolimus. Use with caution or avoid. Moderate Theoretical
- **Clarithromycin** is predicted to increase the exposure to tezacaftor. Adjust tezacaftor with ivacaftor p. 198 dose with potent inhibitors of CYP3A4. Severe Study
- **Erythromycin** is predicted to increase the exposure to tezacaftor. Adjust tezacaftor with ivacaftor p. 198 dose with moderate inhibitors of CYP3A4. Severe Study
- **Erythromycin** decreases the clearance of theophylline and theophylline potentially decreases the clearance of **erythromycin.** Adjust dose. Severe Study
- Macrolides **(azithromycin, clarithromycin)** are predicted to increase the exposure to theophylline. Adjust dose. Moderate Anecdotal
- **Azithromycin** is predicted to increase the exposure to ticagrelor. Use with caution or avoid. Severe Study
- **Clarithromycin** is predicted to markedly increase the exposure to ticagrelor. Avoid. Severe Study
- **Clarithromycin** is predicted to increase the exposure to tofacitinib. Adjust **tofacitinib** dose. Moderate Study
- **Erythromycin** given with a potent CYP2C19 inhibitor is predicted to increase the exposure to tofacitinib. Adjust **tofacitinib** dose. Moderate Study
- **Clarithromycin** is predicted to increase the exposure to tolterodine. Avoid. Severe Study → Also see TABLE 9 p. 909
- **Erythromycin** is predicted to increase the exposure to tolterodine. Mild Theoretical → Also see TABLE 9 p. 909
- **Clarithromycin** is predicted to increase the exposure to tolvaptan. Manufacturer advises caution or adjust **tolvaptan** dose with potent inhibitors of CYP3A4. Severe Study
- **Erythromycin** is predicted to increase the exposure to tolvaptan. Manufacturer advises caution or adjust **tolvaptan** dose with moderate inhibitors of CYP3A4. Moderate Study
- **Macrolides** are predicted to increase the exposure to topotecan. Severe Study
- **Clarithromycin** is predicted to increase the exposure to toremifene. Moderate Theoretical → Also see TABLE 9 p. 909
- **Clarithromycin** is predicted to increase the exposure to trabectedin. Avoid or adjust dose. Severe Theoretical
- **Macrolides** are predicted to increase the concentration of trametinib. Moderate Theoretical
- **Clarithromycin** is predicted to moderately increase the exposure to trazodone. Avoid or adjust dose. Moderate Study
- **Erythromycin** is predicted to increase the exposure to trazodone. Moderate Theoretical
- **Clarithromycin** is predicted to increase the exposure to ulipristal. Avoid if used for uterine fibroids. Severe Study
- **Erythromycin** is predicted to increase the exposure to ulipristal. Avoid if used for uterine fibroids. Moderate Study
- **Clarithromycin** is predicted to increase the exposure to upadacitinib. Use with caution or avoid. Severe Study
- **Clarithromycin** is predicted to increase the exposure to vemurafenib. Severe Theoretical → Also see TABLE 9 p. 909
- Macrolides **(clarithromycin, erythromycin)** are predicted to increase the exposure to venetoclax. Avoid or adjust dose—consult product literature. Severe Study
- **Clarithromycin** is predicted to increase the exposure to venlafaxine. Moderate Study → Also see TABLE 9 p. 909
- Macrolides **(clarithromycin, erythromycin)** are predicted to increase the exposure to vinca alkaloids. Severe Theoretical → Also see TABLE 9 p. 909

- **Clarithromycin** is predicted to increase the exposure to vitamin D substances **(paricalcitol).** Moderate Study
- **Clarithromycin** decreases the absorption of **zidovudine.** Separate administration by at least 2 hours. Moderate Study
- **Clarithromycin** is predicted to increase the exposure to **zopiclone.** Adjust dose. Moderate Theoretical
- **Erythromycin** is predicted to increase the exposure to **zopiclone.** Adjust dose. Moderate Study

Magnesium

- Oral **magnesium** decreases the absorption of bisphosphonates **(alendronate). Alendronate** should be taken at least 30 minutes before **magnesium** . Moderate Study
- Oral **magnesium** decreases the absorption of bisphosphonates **(clodronate).** Avoid **magnesium** for 2 hours before or 1 hour after **clodronate.** Moderate Study
- Oral **magnesium** is predicted to decrease the absorption of oral bisphosphonates **(ibandronate).** Avoid for at least 6 hours before or 1 hour after **ibandronate.** Moderate Theoretical
- Oral **magnesium** decreases the absorption of bisphosphonates **(risedronate).** Separate administration by at least 2 hours. Moderate Study
- Intravenous **magnesium** potentially increases the risk of hypotension when given with calcium channel blockers **(amlodipine, felodipine, lacidipine, lercanidipine, nicardipine, nifedipine, nimodipine, verapamil)** in pregnant women. Severe Anecdotal
- Intravenous **magnesium** increases the effects of **neuromuscular blocking drugs, non-depolarising.** Moderate Study
- Intravenous **magnesium** is predicted to increase the effects of **suxamethonium.** Moderate Study

Magnesium carbonate → see antacids

Magnesium trisilicate → see antacids

MAO-B inhibitors → see **TABLE 6** p. 908 (bradycardia), **TABLE 8** p. 908 (hypotension), **TABLE 13** p. 910 (serotonin syndrome)

rasagiline · safinamide · selegiline

FOOD AND LIFESTYLE Hypertension is predicted to occur when high-dose **selegiline** is taken with tyramine-rich foods (such as mature cheese, salami, pickled herring, *Bovril®*, *Oxo®*, *Marmite®* or any similar meat or yeast extract or fermented soya bean extract, and some beers, lagers or wines).

- MAO-B inhibitors **(rasagiline, selegiline)** are predicted to increase the risk of severe hypertension when given with **amfetamines.** Avoid. Severe Theoretical → Also see **TABLE 13** p. 910
- **Safinamide** is predicted to increase the risk of severe hypertension when given with **amfetamines.** Severe Theoretical → Also see **TABLE 13** p. 910
- MAO-B inhibitors **(rasagiline, selegiline)** are predicted to increase the risk of severe hypertension when given with **beta$_2$ agonists.** Avoid. Severe Theoretical
- **Safinamide** is predicted to increase the risk of severe hypertension when given with **beta$_2$ agonists.** Severe Theoretical
- **MAO-B inhibitors** are predicted to increase the risk of severe hypertension when given with **bupropion.** Avoid. Moderate Theoretical → Also see **TABLE 13** p. 910
- **Combined hormonal contraceptives** slightly increase the exposure to **rasagiline.** Moderate Study
- **Combined hormonal contraceptives** increase the exposure to **selegiline.** Avoid. Severe Study
- **Hormone replacement therapy** is predicted to increase the exposure to **selegiline.** Avoid. Moderate Study
- **MAO-B inhibitors** are predicted to increase the effects of **levodopa.** Adjust dose. Mild Study → Also see **TABLE 8** p. 908
- MAO-B inhibitors **(rasagiline, selegiline)** are predicted to increase the risk of side-effects when given with **linezolid.** Avoid and for 14 days after stopping the MAOI. Severe Theoretical → Also see **TABLE 13** p. 910
- **Safinamide** is predicted to increase the risk of side-effects when given with **linezolid.** Avoid and for 1 week after stopping **safinamide.** Severe Theoretical → Also see **TABLE 13** p. 910
- MAO-B inhibitors **(rasagiline, selegiline)** are predicted to increase the risk of side-effects when given with **MAOIs, irreversible.** Avoid and for 14 days after stopping the MAOI. Severe Theoretical → Also see **TABLE 8** p. 908 → Also see **TABLE 13** p. 910
- **Safinamide** is predicted to increase the risk of side-effects when given with **MAOIs, irreversible.** Avoid and for 1 week after stopping **safinamide.** Severe Theoretical → Also see **TABLE 13** p. 910
- MAO-B inhibitors **(rasagiline, selegiline)** are predicted to increase the risk of a hypertensive crisis when given with **methylphenidate.** Avoid. Severe Theoretical
- **Mexiletine** slightly increases the exposure to **rasagiline.** Moderate Study
- **Moclobemide** is predicted to increase the effects of MAO-B inhibitors **(rasagiline, selegiline).** Avoid. Severe Theoretical → Also see **TABLE 13** p. 910
- **Moclobemide** is predicted to increase the risk of side-effects when given with **safinamide.** Avoid and for 1 week after stopping **safinamide.** Severe Theoretical → Also see **TABLE 13** p. 910
- **Rasagiline** is predicted to increase the risk of side-effects when given with opioids **(pethidine).** Avoid and for 14 days after stopping **rasagiline.** Severe Theoretical → Also see **TABLE 13** p. 910
- **Safinamide** is predicted to increase the risk of side-effects when given with opioids **(pethidine).** Avoid and for 1 week after stopping **safinamide.** Severe Theoretical → Also see **TABLE 13** p. 910
- **Selegiline** increases the risk of side-effects when given with opioids **(pethidine).** Avoid. Severe Anecdotal → Also see **TABLE 13** p. 910
- Quinolones **(ciprofloxacin)** slightly increase the exposure to **rasagiline.** Moderate Study
- **Reboxetine** is predicted to increase the risk of a hypertensive crisis when given with MAO-B inhibitors **(rasagiline, selegiline).** Avoid. Severe Theoretical
- **MAO-B inhibitors** are predicted to increase the risk of a hypertensive crisis when given with **sympathomimetics, inotropic.** Avoid. Severe Anecdotal
- **MAO-B inhibitors** are predicted to increase the risk of a hypertensive crisis when given with **sympathomimetics, vasoconstrictor.** Avoid. Severe Anecdotal
- **Tetrabenazine** potentially increases the risk of CNS excitation and hypertension when given with **MAO-B inhibitors.** Severe Theoretical

MAOIs, irreversible → see **TABLE 8** p. 908 (hypotension), **TABLE 13** p. 910 (serotonin syndrome)

isocarboxazid · phenelzine · tranylcypromine

FOOD AND LIFESTYLE Potentially life-threatening hypertensive crisis can develop in those taking MAOIs who eat tyramine-rich food (such as mature cheese, salami, pickled herring, *Bovril®*, *Oxo®*, *Marmite®* or any similar meat or yeast extract or fermented soya bean extract, and some beers, lagers or wines) or foods containing dopa (such as broad bean pods). Avoid tyramine-rich or dopa-rich food or drinks with, or for 2 to 3 weeks after stopping, the MAOI.

- **MAOIs, irreversible** are predicted to increase the effects of alpha blockers **(indoramin).** Avoid. Severe Theoretical → Also see **TABLE 8** p. 908
- **MAOIs, irreversible** are predicted to increase the risk of a hypertensive crisis when given with **amfetamines.** Avoid and for 14 days after stopping the MAOI. Severe Anecdotal → Also see **TABLE 13** p. 910
- Antiepileptics **(carbamazepine)** are predicted to increase the risk of severe toxic reaction when given with **MAOIs, irreversible.** Avoid and for 14 days after stopping the MAOI. Severe Theoretical
- Antiepileptics **(phenobarbital, primidone)** are predicted to increase the effects of **MAOIs, irreversible.** Severe Theoretical
- **MAOIs, irreversible** are predicted to increase the risk of antimuscarinic side-effects when given with **antihistamines, non-sedating.** Avoid. Severe Theoretical
- **MAOIs, irreversible** are predicted to increase the risk of antimuscarinic side-effects when given with **antihistamines, sedating.** Avoid. Severe Theoretical
- **MAOIs, irreversible** are predicted to increase the risk of side-effects when given with **atomoxetine.** Avoid and for 2 weeks after stopping the MAOI. Severe Theoretical
- **MAOIs, irreversible** are predicted to increase the risk of cardiovascular side-effects when given with **beta$_2$ agonists.** Moderate Anecdotal

Interactions | **Appendix 1** A1

MAOIs, irreversible (continued)
- **MAOIs, irreversible** are predicted to increase the risk of severe hypertension when given with bupropion. Avoid and for 14 days after stopping the MAOI. [Severe] Theoretical → Also see **TABLE 13** p. 910
- **Buspirone** is predicted to increase the risk of elevated blood pressure when given with **MAOIs, irreversible**. Avoid. [Severe] Anecdotal → Also see **TABLE 13** p. 910
- **MAOIs, irreversible** are predicted to increase the effects of doxapram. [Moderate] Theoretical
- **Entacapone** is predicted to increase the risk of elevated blood pressure when given with **MAOIs, irreversible**. Avoid. [Severe] Theoretical
- **Levodopa** increases the risk of a hypertensive crisis when given with **MAOIs, irreversible**. Avoid and for 14 days after stopping the MAOI. [Severe] Study → Also see **TABLE 8** p. 908
- **MAOIs, irreversible** are predicted to increase the risk of side-effects when given with linezolid. Avoid and for 14 days after stopping the MAOI. [Severe] Theoretical → Also see **TABLE 13** p. 910
- MAO-B inhibitors **(rasagiline, selegiline)** are predicted to increase the risk of side-effects when given with **MAOIs, irreversible**. Avoid and for 14 days after stopping the MAOI. [Severe] Theoretical → Also see **TABLE 8** p. 908 → Also see **TABLE 13** p. 910
- MAO-B inhibitors **(safinamide)** are predicted to increase the risk of side-effects when given with **MAOIs, irreversible**. Avoid and for 1 week after stopping **safinamide**. [Severe] Theoretical → Also see **TABLE 13** p. 910
- **MAOIs, irreversible** are predicted to alter the antihypertensive effects of methyldopa. Avoid. [Severe] Theoretical → Also see **TABLE 8** p. 908
- **Methylphenidate** is predicted to increase the risk of a hypertensive crisis when given with **MAOIs, irreversible**. Avoid and for 14 days after stopping the MAOI. [Severe] Theoretical
- **Mianserin** is predicted to increase the risk of toxicity when given with **MAOIs, irreversible**. Avoid and for 14 days after stopping the MAOI. [Severe] Theoretical
- **Nefopam** is predicted to increase the risk of serious elevations in blood pressure when given with **MAOIs, irreversible**. Avoid. [Severe] Theoretical
- **Opicapone** is predicted to increase the risk of elevated blood pressure when given with **MAOIs, irreversible**. Avoid. [Severe] Theoretical
- **Opioids** are predicted to increase the risk of CNS excitation or depression when given with **MAOIs, irreversible**. Avoid. [Severe] Study → Also see **TABLE 13** p. 910
- **MAOIs, irreversible** are predicted to increase the risk of neuroleptic malignant syndrome when given with phenothiazines. [Severe] Theoretical → Also see **TABLE 8** p. 908
- **Pholcodine** is predicted to increase the risk of CNS excitation or depression when given with **MAOIs, irreversible**. Avoid and for 14 days after stopping the MAOI. [Severe] Theoretical
- **Reboxetine** is predicted to increase the risk of a hypertensive crisis when given with **MAOIs, irreversible**. Avoid. [Severe] Theoretical
- **MAOIs, irreversible** are predicted to increase the exposure to rizatriptan. Avoid and for 14 days after stopping the MAOI. [Severe] Theoretical → Also see **TABLE 13** p. 910
- **MAOIs, irreversible** are predicted to increase the exposure to sumatriptan. Avoid and for 14 days after stopping the MAOI. [Severe] Theoretical → Also see **TABLE 13** p. 910
- **MAOIs, irreversible** are predicted to increase the risk of a hypertensive crisis when given with sympathomimetics, inotropic. Avoid and for 14 days after stopping the MAOI. [Severe] Theoretical
- **MAOIs, irreversible** are predicted to increase the risk of a hypertensive crisis when given with sympathomimetics, vasoconstrictor. Avoid and for 14 days after stopping the MAOI. [Severe] Study
- **Tetrabenazine** potentially increases the risk of CNS excitation and hypertension when given with **MAOIs, irreversible**. Avoid and for 14 days after stopping the MAOI. [Severe] Theoretical
- **Tolcapone** is predicted to increase the effects of **MAOIs, irreversible**. Avoid. [Severe] Theoretical
- **Tricyclic antidepressants** are predicted to increase the risk of severe toxic reaction when given with **MAOIs, irreversible**. Avoid and for 14 days after stopping the MAOI. [Severe] Theoretical → Also see **TABLE 8** p. 908 → Also see **TABLE 13** p. 910
- **Tryptophan** increases the risk of side-effects when given with **MAOIs, irreversible**. [Severe] Anecdotal → Also see **TABLE 13** p. 910
- **MAOIs, irreversible** are predicted to increase the exposure to zolmitriptan. [Severe] Theoretical → Also see **TABLE 13** p. 910

Maraviroc
- Antiepileptics **(carbamazepine, fosphenytoin, phenobarbital, phenytoin, primidone)** are predicted to decrease the exposure to **maraviroc**. Adjust dose. [Severe] Study
- Antifungals, azoles **(itraconazole, ketoconazole, voriconazole)** are predicted to markedly increase the exposure to **maraviroc**. Adjust dose. [Severe] Study
- **Apalutamide** is predicted to decrease the exposure to **maraviroc**. Adjust dose. [Severe] Study
- **Aprepitant** is predicted to increase the exposure to **maraviroc**. [Moderate] Study
- **Bosentan** is predicted to decrease the exposure to **maraviroc**. Avoid. [Moderate] Theoretical
- **Cobicistat** markedly increases the exposure to **maraviroc**. Refer to specialist literature. [Severe] Study
- **Efavirenz** decreases the exposure to **maraviroc**. Refer to specialist literature. [Severe] Theoretical
- **Enzalutamide** is predicted to decrease the exposure to **maraviroc**. Adjust dose. [Severe] Study
- **Etravirine** (with a boosted protease inhibitor) increases the exposure to **maraviroc**. Avoid or adjust dose. [Moderate] Study
- HIV-protease inhibitors **(atazanavir, saquinavir)** moderately to markedly increase the exposure to **maraviroc**. Refer to specialist literature. [Severe] Study
- HIV-protease inhibitors **(darunavir)** boosted with ritonavir markedly increase the exposure to **maraviroc**. Refer to specialist literature. [Severe] Study
- HIV-protease inhibitors **(lopinavir)** boosted with ritonavir moderately increase the exposure to **maraviroc**. Refer to specialist literature. [Severe] Study
- HIV-protease inhibitors **(ritonavir)** markedly increase the exposure to **maraviroc**. Refer to specialist literature. [Severe] Study
- **Maraviroc** potentially decreases the exposure to HIV-protease inhibitors **(fosamprenavir)** and HIV-protease inhibitors **(fosamprenavir)** potentially decrease the exposure to **maraviroc**. Avoid. [Severe] Study
- **Idelalisib** markedly increases the exposure to **maraviroc**. Adjust dose. [Severe] Theoretical
- Macrolides **(clarithromycin)** are predicted to markedly increase the exposure to **maraviroc**. Adjust dose. [Severe] Study
- **Mitotane** is predicted to decrease the exposure to **maraviroc**. Adjust dose. [Severe] Study
- **Netupitant** is predicted to increase the exposure to **maraviroc**. [Moderate] Study
- **Rifampicin** is predicted to decrease the exposure to **maraviroc**. Adjust dose. [Severe] Study
- **St John's Wort** is predicted to decrease the exposure to **maraviroc**. Avoid. [Severe] Theoretical

Measles, mumps and rubella vaccine, live → see live vaccines

Mebendazole
- H_2 receptor antagonists **(cimetidine)** increase the concentration of **mebendazole**. [Moderate] Study

Medroxyprogesterone
- **Sugammadex** is predicted to decrease the exposure to **medroxyprogesterone**. Use additional contraceptive precautions. [Severe] Theoretical

Mefenamic acid → see NSAIDs

Mefloquine → see antimalarials

Melatonin → see **TABLE 11** p. 909 (CNS depressant effects)
- Antiepileptics **(phenytoin)** are predicted to decrease the exposure to **melatonin**. [Moderate] Theoretical
- **Combined hormonal contraceptives** are predicted to increase the exposure to **melatonin**. [Moderate] Theoretical
- HIV-protease inhibitors **(ritonavir)** are predicted to decrease the exposure to **melatonin**. [Moderate] Theoretical
- **Leflunomide** is predicted to decrease the exposure to **melatonin**. [Moderate] Theoretical

- Mexiletine is predicted to increase the exposure to **melatonin.** [Moderate] Theoretical
- Quinolones **(ciprofloxacin)** are predicted to increase the exposure to **melatonin.** [Moderate] Theoretical
- Rifampicin is predicted to decrease the exposure to **melatonin.** [Moderate] Theoretical
- SSRIs **(fluvoxamine)** very markedly increase the exposure to **melatonin.** Avoid. [Severe] Study
- Teriflunomide is predicted to decrease the exposure to **melatonin.** [Moderate] Theoretical

Meloxicam → see NSAIDs

Melphalan → see alkylating agents

Memantine

- Dopamine receptor agonists **(amantadine)** increase the risk of CNS toxicity when given with **memantine.** Use with caution or avoid. [Severe] Theoretical
- **Memantine** is predicted to increase the effects of dopamine receptor agonists **(apomorphine, bromocriptine, cabergoline, pergolide, pramipexole, quinagolide, ropinirole, rotigotine).** [Moderate] Theoretical
- **Memantine** is predicted to increase the risk of CNS side-effects when given with **ketamine.** Avoid. [Severe] Theoretical
- **Memantine** is predicted to increase the effects of **levodopa.** [Moderate] Theoretical

Mepacrine

- **Mepacrine** is predicted to increase the concentration of antimalarials **(primaquine).** Avoid. [Moderate] Theoretical

Mepivacaine → see anaesthetics, local

Meprobamate → see TABLE 11 p. 909 (CNS depressant effects)

Meptazinol → see opioids

Mercaptopurine → see TABLE 1 p. 907 (hepatotoxicity), TABLE 15 p. 910 (myelosuppression)

- Allopurinol potentially increases the risk of haematological toxicity when given with **mercaptopurine.** Adjust **mercaptopurine** dose, p. 587. [Severe] Study
- **Mercaptopurine** decreases the anticoagulant effect of **coumarins.** [Moderate] Anecdotal
- Febuxostat is predicted to increase the exposure to **mercaptopurine.** Avoid. [Severe] Theoretical
- Live vaccines are predicted to increase the risk of generalised infection (possibly life-threatening) when given with **mercaptopurine** (high-dose). Public Health England advises avoid (refer to Green Book). [Severe] Theoretical

Meropenem → see carbapenems

Mesalazine

ROUTE-SPECIFIC INFORMATION The manufacturers of some mesalazine gastro-resistant and modified-release medicines (*Asacol MR* tablets, *Ipocol*, *Salofalk* granules) suggest that preparations that lower stool pH (e.g. lactulose) might prevent the release of mesalazine.

Metaraminol → see sympathomimetics, vasoconstrictor

Metformin → see TABLE 14 p. 910 (antidiabetic drugs)

- Alcohol (beverage)(excessive consumption) potentially increases the risk of lactic acidosis when given with **metformin.** Avoid excessive alcohol consumption. [Moderate] Theoretical
- Bictegravir slightly increases the exposure to **metformin.** [Moderate] Study
- Dolutegravir increases the exposure to **metformin.** Use with caution and adjust dose. [Severe] Study
- Guanfacine is predicted to increase the concentration of **metformin.** [Moderate] Theoretical
- H_2 receptor antagonists **(cimetidine)** increase the exposure to **metformin.** Monitor and adjust dose. [Moderate] Study
- Mexiletine is predicted to affect the exposure to **metformin.** [Unknown] Theoretical
- Pitolisant is predicted to increase the exposure to **metformin.** [Mild] Theoretical
- Ribociclib is predicted to increase the exposure to **metformin.** [Moderate] Theoretical
- Vandetanib increases the exposure to **metformin.** Monitor and adjust dose. [Moderate] Study

Methadone → see opioids

Methenamine

- Acetazolamide is predicted to decrease the efficacy of **methenamine.** Avoid. [Moderate] Theoretical
- Potassium citrate is predicted to decrease the efficacy of **methenamine.** Avoid. [Moderate] Theoretical
- Sodium bicarbonate is predicted to decrease the efficacy of **methenamine.** Avoid. [Moderate] Theoretical
- Sodium citrate is predicted to decrease the efficacy of **methenamine.** Avoid. [Moderate] Theoretical

Methocarbamol → see TABLE 11 p. 909 (CNS depressant effects)

Methotrexate → see TABLE 1 p. 907 (hepatotoxicity), TABLE 15 p. 910 (myelosuppression), TABLE 2 p. 907 (nephrotoxicity), TABLE 5 p. 907 (thromboembolism)

- Acetazolamide increases the urinary excretion of **methotrexate.** [Moderate] Study
- **Methotrexate** is predicted to decrease the clearance of **aminophylline.** [Moderate] Theoretical
- Antiepileptics **(levetiracetam)** decrease the clearance of **methotrexate.** [Severe] Anecdotal
- Antimalarials **(pyrimethamine)** are predicted to increase the risk of side-effects when given with **methotrexate.** [Severe] Theoretical → Also see TABLE 15 p. 910
- Apalutamide is predicted to decrease the exposure to **methotrexate.** [Mild] Study
- Asparaginase affects the efficacy of **methotrexate.** [Severe] Anecdotal → Also see TABLE 1 p. 907 → Also see TABLE 15 p. 910
- Aspirin (high-dose) is predicted to increase the risk of toxicity when given with **methotrexate.** [Severe] Study
- Brigatinib potentially increases the concentration of **methotrexate.** [Moderate] Theoretical
- Crisantaspase affects the efficacy of **methotrexate.** [Severe] Anecdotal → Also see TABLE 1 p. 907 → Also see TABLE 15 p. 910
- Eltrombopag is predicted to increase the concentration of **methotrexate.** [Moderate] Theoretical
- **Methotrexate** potentially increases the risk of severe skin reaction when given with topical **fluorouracil.** [Severe] Anecdotal → Also see TABLE 15 p. 910 → Also see TABLE 5 p. 907
- Leflunomide is predicted to increase the exposure to **methotrexate.** [Moderate] Theoretical → Also see TABLE 1 p. 907 → Also see TABLE 15 p. 910
- Live vaccines are predicted to increase the risk of generalised infection (possibly life-threatening) when given with **methotrexate** (high-dose). Public Health England advises avoid (refer to Green Book). [Severe] Theoretical
- Nitisinone is predicted to increase the exposure to **methotrexate.** [Moderate] Study
- Nitrous oxide potentially increases the risk of methotrexate toxicity when given with **methotrexate.** Avoid. [Severe] Study
- NSAIDs are predicted to increase the risk of toxicity when given with **methotrexate.** [Severe] Study → Also see TABLE 2 p. 907
- Pegaspargase affects the efficacy of **methotrexate.** [Severe] Anecdotal → Also see TABLE 1 p. 907 → Also see TABLE 15 p. 910
- Penicillins are predicted to increase the risk of toxicity when given with **methotrexate.** [Severe] Anecdotal → Also see TABLE 1 p. 907
- Potassium aminobenzoate increases the concentration of **methotrexate.** [Moderate] Theoretical
- Proton pump inhibitors decrease the clearance of **methotrexate** (high-dose). Use with caution or avoid. [Severe] Study
- Quinolones **(ciprofloxacin)** potentially increase the risk of toxicity when given with **methotrexate.** [Severe] Anecdotal
- Regorafenib is predicted to increase the exposure to **methotrexate.** [Moderate] Theoretical → Also see TABLE 15 p. 910
- Retinoids **(acitretin)** are predicted to increase the concentration of **methotrexate.** Avoid. [Moderate] Anecdotal
- Rolapitant is predicted to increase the exposure to **methotrexate.** Avoid or monitor. [Moderate] Study
- **Methotrexate** is predicted to decrease the efficacy of **sapropterin.** [Moderate] Theoretical
- Sulfonamides are predicted to increase the exposure to **methotrexate.** Use with caution or avoid. [Severe] Theoretical → Also see TABLE 15 p. 910
- Tedizolid is predicted to increase the exposure to **methotrexate.** Avoid. [Moderate] Theoretical

Methotrexate (continued)
- **Methotrexate** is predicted to increase the risk of toxicity when given with tegafur. Severe Theoretical
- **Teriflunomide** is predicted to increase the exposure to **methotrexate**. Moderate Study → Also see TABLE 1 p. 907
- **Methotrexate** decreases the clearance of **theophylline**. Moderate Study
- **Trimethoprim** increases the risk of side-effects when given with **methotrexate**. Avoid. Severe Anecdotal → Also see TABLE 15 p. 910 → Also see TABLE 2 p. 907

Methoxyflurane → see volatile halogenated anaesthetics

Methyldopa → see TABLE 8 p. 908 (hypotension)
- **Entacapone** is predicted to increase the exposure to **methyldopa**. Moderate Theoretical
- **Iron (oral)** decreases the effects of **methyldopa**. Moderate Study
- **Methyldopa** increases the risk of neurotoxicity when given with lithium. Severe Anecdotal
- **MAOIs, irreversible** are predicted to alter the antihypertensive effects of **methyldopa**. Avoid. Severe Theoretical → Also see TABLE 8 p. 908

Methylphenidate
- **Methylphenidate** is predicted to decrease the effects of apraclonidine. Avoid. Severe Theoretical
- **Methylphenidate** is predicted to increase the risk of elevated blood pressure when given with **linezolid**. Avoid. Severe Theoretical
- MAO-B inhibitors **(rasagiline, selegiline)** are predicted to increase the risk of a hypertensive crisis when given with **methylphenidate**. Avoid. Severe Theoretical
- **Methylphenidate** is predicted to increase the risk of a hypertensive crisis when given with **MAOIs, irreversible**. Avoid and for 14 days after stopping the MAOI. Severe Theoretical
- **Methylphenidate** is predicted to increase the risk of a hypertensive crisis when given with **moclobemide**. Severe Theoretical
- **Methylphenidate** increases the risk of dyskinesias when given with **paliperidone**. Severe Theoretical
- **Risperidone** increases the risk of dyskinesias when given with **methylphenidate**. Severe Anecdotal

Methylprednisolone → see corticosteroids

Methylthioninium chloride → see TABLE 13 p. 910 (serotonin syndrome)
- **Methylthioninium chloride** is predicted to increase the risk of severe hypertension when given with **bupropion**. Avoid. Severe Theoretical → Also see TABLE 13 p. 910

Metoclopramide
- **Metoclopramide** is predicted to increase the risk of methaemoglobinaemia when given with topical anaesthetics, local **(prilocaine)**. Avoid. Severe Theoretical
- **Metoclopramide** potentially decreases the absorption of antifungals, azoles **(posaconazole)** (oral suspension). Moderate Study
- **Metoclopramide** decreases the concentration of antimalarials **(atovaquone)**. Avoid. Moderate Study
- **Metoclopramide** is predicted to decrease the effects of dopamine receptor agonists **(apomorphine, bromocriptine, cabergoline, pergolide, pramipexole, quinagolide, ropinirole, rotigotine)**. Avoid. Moderate Study
- **Metoclopramide** decreases the effects of **levodopa**. Avoid. Moderate Study
- **Metoclopramide** is predicted to increase the effects of **neuromuscular blocking drugs, non-depolarising**. Moderate Theoretical
- **Metoclopramide** increases the effects of **suxamethonium**. Moderate Study

Metolazone → see thiazide diuretics

Metoprolol → see beta blockers, selective

Metronidazole → see TABLE 12 p. 910 (peripheral neuropathy)

ROUTE-SPECIFIC INFORMATION Since systemic absorption can follow topical application, the possibility of interactions should be borne in mind.

- **Alcohol (beverage)** potentially causes a disulfiram-like reaction when given with **metronidazole**. Avoid for at least 48 hours stopping treatment. Moderate Study
- **Metronidazole** increases the risk of toxicity when given with alkylating agents **(busulfan)**. Severe Study
- Antiepileptics **(phenobarbital, primidone)** are predicted to decrease the exposure to **metronidazole**. Moderate Study
- **Metronidazole** is predicted to increase the risk of capecitabine toxicity when given with **capecitabine**. Severe Theoretical
- **Metronidazole** increases the anticoagulant effect of **coumarins**. Monitor INR and adjust dose. Severe Study
- **Disulfiram** increases the risk of acute psychoses when given with **metronidazole**. Severe Study → Also see TABLE 12 p. 910
- **Metronidazole** increases the risk of toxicity when given with **fluorouracil**. Severe Study
- **Metronidazole** is predicted to increase the concentration of **lithium**. Avoid or adjust dose. Severe Anecdotal

Metyrapone
- Antiepileptics **(fosphenytoin, phenobarbital, phenytoin, primidone)** are predicted to decrease the effects of **metyrapone**. Avoid. Moderate Study
- Antihistamines, sedating **(cyproheptadine)** decrease the effects of **metyrapone**. Avoid. Moderate Study
- **Carbimazole** decreases the effects of **metyrapone**. Avoid. Moderate Theoretical
- **Combined hormonal contraceptives** decrease the effects of **metyrapone**. Avoid. Moderate Theoretical
- Phenothiazines **(chlorpromazine)** decrease the effects of **metyrapone**. Avoid. Moderate Theoretical
- **Propylthiouracil** is predicted to decrease the effects of **metyrapone**. Avoid. Moderate Theoretical
- Tricyclic antidepressants **(amitriptyline)** decrease the effects of **metyrapone**. Avoid. Moderate Theoretical

Mexiletine

FOOD AND LIFESTYLE Dose adjustment might be necessary if smoking started or stopped during treatment.

- **Mexiletine** is predicted to increase the exposure to **agomelatine**. Moderate Study
- **Mexiletine** is predicted to increase the exposure to **aminophylline**. Adjust dose. Moderate Theoretical
- **Mexiletine** is predicted to increase the exposure to **anagrelide**. Moderate Theoretical
- **Mexiletine** increases the risk of torsade de pointes when given with **antiarrhythmics**. Avoid. Severe Theoretical
- Antiepileptics **(phenytoin)** are predicted to increase the clearance of **mexiletine**. Monitor and adjust dose. Moderate Study
- **Mexiletine** potentially increases the risk of cardiovascular side-effects when given with **beta blockers, non-selective**. Avoid or monitor. Severe Theoretical
- **Mexiletine** potentially increases the risk of cardiovascular side-effects when given with **beta blockers, selective**. Avoid or monitor. Severe Theoretical
- **Bupropion** is predicted to increase the exposure to **mexiletine**. Moderate Study
- **Mexiletine** increases the risk of cardiovascular side-effects when given with calcium channel blockers **(diltiazem)**. Avoid or monitor. Severe Theoretical
- **Mexiletine** potentially increases the risk of cardiovascular side-effects when given with calcium channel blockers **(verapamil)**. Avoid or monitor. Severe Theoretical
- **Cinacalcet** is predicted to increase the exposure to **mexiletine**. Moderate Study
- **Mexiletine** increases the concentration of **clozapine**. Monitor side effects and adjust dose. Severe Study
- **Cobicistat** potentially increases the exposure to **mexiletine**. Severe Theoretical
- **Mexiletine** potentially affects the exposure to coumarins **(warfarin)**. Avoid. Unknown Theoretical
- **Mexiletine** is predicted to increase the exposure to dopamine receptor agonists **(ropinirole)**. Adjust dose. Moderate Study
- **Mexiletine** slightly increases the exposure to **erlotinib**. Monitor side effects and adjust dose. Moderate Study
- HIV-protease inhibitors **(ritonavir)** are predicted to increase the clearance of **mexiletine**. Monitor and adjust dose. Moderate Study
- **Leflunomide** is predicted to increase the clearance of **mexiletine**. Monitor and adjust dose. Moderate Study

- **Mexiletine** potentially affects the exposure to **lithium**. Avoid. Unknown Theoretical
- **Mexiletine** is predicted to increase the exposure to **loxapine**. Avoid. Unknown Theoretical
- **Mexiletine** slightly increases the exposure to MAO-B inhibitors **(rasagiline)**. Moderate Study
- **Mexiletine** is predicted to increase the exposure to **melatonin**. Moderate Theoretical
- **Mexiletine** is predicted to affect the exposure to **metformin**. Unknown Theoretical
- **Mexiletine** is predicted to increase the exposure to **olanzapine**. Adjust dose. Moderate Anecdotal
- **Opioids** potentially decrease the absorption of oral **mexiletine**. Moderate Study
- **Mexiletine** is predicted to increase the exposure to phenothiazines **(chlorpromazine)**. Moderate Theoretical
- **Mexiletine** is predicted to increase the exposure to **pirfenidone**. Use with caution and adjust dose. Moderate Study
- **Rifampicin** is predicted to increase the clearance of **mexiletine**. Monitor and adjust dose. Moderate Study
- **Mexiletine** is predicted to increase the exposure to **riluzole**. Moderate Theoretical
- **Mexiletine** is predicted to increase the exposure to **roflumilast**. Moderate Theoretical
- SSRIs **(fluoxetine, fluvoxamine, paroxetine)** are predicted to increase the exposure to **mexiletine**. Moderate Study
- **Terbinafine** is predicted to increase the exposure to **mexiletine**. Moderate Study
- **Teriflunomide** is predicted to increase the clearance of **mexiletine**. Monitor and adjust dose. Moderate Study
- **Mexiletine** is predicted to increase the exposure to **theophylline**. Monitor and adjust dose. Moderate Theoretical
- **Mexiletine** increases the exposure to **tizanidine**. Avoid. Moderate Study
- **Mexiletine** is predicted to increase the exposure to **zolmitriptan**. Adjust **zolmitriptan** dose, p. 310. Moderate Theoretical

Mianserin → see TABLE 11 p. 909 (CNS depressant effects)

- Antiepileptics **(carbamazepine)** markedly decrease the exposure to **mianserin**. Adjust dose. Moderate Study
- Antiepileptics **(phenobarbital, primidone)** are predicted to decrease the exposure to **mianserin**. Moderate Study → Also see TABLE 11 p. 909
- **Mianserin** is predicted to increase the risk of toxicity when given with **MAOIs, irreversible**. Avoid and for 14 days after stopping the MAOI. Severe Theoretical
- **Mianserin** is predicted to increase the risk of toxicity when given with **moclobemide**. Avoid and for 1 week after stopping **mianserin**. Severe Theoretical
- **Mianserin** is predicted to decrease the efficacy of **pitolisant**. Moderate Theoretical
- **Mianserin** decreases the effects of sympathomimetics, vasoconstrictor **(ephedrine)**. Severe Anecdotal

Micafungin → see TABLE 1 p. 907 (hepatotoxicity)

- **Micafungin** slightly increases the exposure to **amphotericin**. Avoid or monitor toxicity. Moderate Study

Miconazole → see antifungals, azoles

Midazolam → see TABLE 11 p. 909 (CNS depressant effects)

- Antiarrhythmics **(dronedarone)** are predicted to increase the exposure to **midazolam**. Monitor side effects and adjust dose. Severe Study
- Antiepileptics **(carbamazepine, fosphenytoin, phenobarbital, phenytoin, primidone)** are predicted to decrease the exposure to **midazolam**. Monitor and adjust dose. Moderate Study → Also see TABLE 11 p. 909
- Antifungals, azoles **(fluconazole, isavuconazole, posaconazole)** are predicted to increase the exposure to **midazolam**. Monitor side effects and adjust dose. Severe Study
- Antifungals, azoles **(itraconazole, ketoconazole, voriconazole)** are predicted to markedly to very markedly increase the exposure to **midazolam**. Avoid or adjust dose. Severe Study
- Antifungals, azoles **(miconazole)** are predicted to increase the exposure to intravenous **midazolam**. Use with caution and adjust dose. Moderate Theoretical
- Antifungals, azoles **(miconazole)** are predicted to increase the exposure to oral **midazolam**. Avoid. Moderate Theoretical
- **Apalutamide** is predicted to decrease the exposure to **midazolam**. Monitor and adjust dose. Moderate Study
- **Aprepitant** is predicted to increase the exposure to **midazolam**. Monitor side effects and adjust dose. Severe Study
- **Bosentan** is predicted to decrease the concentration of **midazolam**. Monitor and adjust dose. Moderate Theoretical
- Calcium channel blockers **(diltiazem, verapamil)** are predicted to increase the exposure to **midazolam**. Monitor side effects and adjust dose. Severe Study
- **Cobicistat** is predicted to markedly to very markedly increase the exposure to **midazolam**. Avoid or adjust dose. Severe Study
- **Crizotinib** is predicted to increase the exposure to **midazolam**. Monitor side effects and adjust dose. Severe Study
- **Dabrafenib** decreases the exposure to **midazolam**. Monitor and adjust dose. Moderate Study
- **Efavirenz** is predicted to alter the effects of **midazolam**. Avoid. Moderate Theoretical
- **Enzalutamide** is predicted to decrease the exposure to **midazolam**. Monitor and adjust dose. Moderate Study
- **Fosaprepitant** slightly increases the exposure to **midazolam**. Moderate Study
- **HIV-protease inhibitors** are predicted to markedly to very markedly increase the exposure to **midazolam**. Avoid or adjust dose. Severe Study
- **Idelalisib** is predicted to markedly to very markedly increase the exposure to **midazolam**. Avoid or adjust dose. Severe Study
- **Imatinib** is predicted to increase the exposure to **midazolam**. Monitor side effects and adjust dose. Severe Study
- **Larotrectinib** slightly increases the exposure to **midazolam**. Use with caution and adjust dose. Mild Study
- **Letermovir** slightly to moderately increases the exposure to **midazolam**. Monitor and adjust dose. Moderate Study
- **Lorlatinib** moderately decreases the exposure to **midazolam**. Avoid. Moderate Study
- **Lumacaftor** is predicted to decrease the exposure to **midazolam**. Avoid. Severe Theoretical
- Macrolides **(clarithromycin)** are predicted to markedly to very markedly increase the exposure to **midazolam**. Avoid or adjust dose. Severe Study
- Macrolides **(erythromycin)** are predicted to increase the exposure to **midazolam**. Monitor side effects and adjust dose. Severe Study
- **Mitotane** is predicted to decrease the exposure to **midazolam**. Monitor and adjust dose. Moderate Study
- Monoclonal antibodies **(tocilizumab)** are predicted to decrease the exposure to **midazolam**. Monitor and adjust dose. Moderate Theoretical
- **Netupitant** is predicted to increase the exposure to **midazolam**. Monitor side effects and adjust dose. Severe Study
- **Nevirapine** decreases the concentration of **midazolam**. Monitor and adjust dose. Moderate Study
- **Nilotinib** is predicted to increase the exposure to **midazolam**. Monitor side effects and adjust dose. Severe Study
- **Palbociclib** increases the exposure to **midazolam**. Moderate Study
- **Ribociclib** moderately increases the exposure to **midazolam**. Avoid. Moderate Study
- **Rifampicin** is predicted to decrease the exposure to **midazolam**. Monitor and adjust dose. Moderate Study
- **Rucaparib** slightly increases the exposure to **midazolam**. Monitor and adjust dose. Severe Study
- **St John's Wort** moderately decreases the exposure to **midazolam**. Monitor and adjust dose. Moderate Study
- **Telotristat ethyl** decreases the exposure to **midazolam**. Moderate Study

Midodrine → see sympathomimetics, vasoconstrictor

Midostaurin

- Antiarrhythmics **(dronedarone)** are predicted to increase the exposure to **midostaurin**. Moderate Theoretical
- Antiepileptics **(carbamazepine, fosphenytoin, phenobarbital, phenytoin, primidone)** are predicted to decrease the exposure to **midostaurin**. Avoid. Severe Study

Midostaurin (continued)
- Antifungals, azoles **(fluconazole, isavuconazole, posaconazole)** are predicted to increase the exposure to **midostaurin**. Moderate Theoretical
- Antifungals, azoles **(itraconazole, ketoconazole, voriconazole)** are predicted to very markedly increase the exposure to **midostaurin**. Avoid or monitor for toxicity. Severe Study
- **Apalutamide** is predicted to decrease the exposure to **midostaurin**. Avoid. Severe Study
- **Aprepitant** is predicted to increase the exposure to **midostaurin**. Moderate Theoretical
- Calcium channel blockers **(diltiazem, verapamil)** are predicted to increase the exposure to **midostaurin**. Moderate Theoretical
- **Cobicistat** is predicted to very markedly increase the exposure to **midostaurin**. Avoid or monitor for toxicity. Severe Study
- **Crizotinib** is predicted to increase the exposure to **midostaurin**. Moderate Theoretical
- **Enzalutamide** is predicted to decrease the exposure to **midostaurin**. Avoid. Severe Study
- **HIV-protease inhibitors** are predicted to very markedly increase the exposure to **midostaurin**. Avoid or monitor for toxicity. Severe Study
- **Idelalisib** is predicted to very markedly increase the exposure to **midostaurin**. Avoid or monitor for toxicity. Severe Study
- **Imatinib** is predicted to increase the exposure to **midostaurin**. Moderate Theoretical
- Macrolides **(clarithromycin)** are predicted to very markedly increase the exposure to **midostaurin**. Avoid or monitor for toxicity. Severe Study
- Macrolides **(erythromycin)** are predicted to increase the exposure to **midostaurin**. Moderate Theoretical
- **Mitotane** is predicted to decrease the exposure to **midostaurin**. Avoid. Severe Study
- **Netupitant** is predicted to increase the exposure to **midostaurin**. Moderate Theoretical
- **Nilotinib** is predicted to increase the exposure to **midostaurin**. Moderate Theoretical
- **Rifampicin** is predicted to decrease the exposure to **midostaurin**. Avoid. Severe Study
- **St John's Wort** is predicted to decrease the exposure to **midostaurin**. Avoid. Severe Theoretical

Mifamurtide
- **Ciclosporin** is predicted to decrease the efficacy of **mifamurtide**. Avoid. Severe Theoretical
- **Corticosteroids** are predicted to decrease the efficacy of **mifamurtide**. Avoid. Severe Theoretical
- **NSAIDs** (high-dose) are predicted to decrease the efficacy of **mifamurtide**. Avoid. Severe Theoretical
- **Pimecrolimus** is predicted to decrease the efficacy of **mifamurtide**. Avoid. Severe Theoretical
- **Sirolimus** is predicted to decrease the efficacy of **mifamurtide**. Avoid. Severe Theoretical
- **Tacrolimus** is predicted to affect the efficacy of **mifamurtide**. Avoid. Severe Theoretical

Mifepristone
- **Mifepristone** is predicted to decrease the efficacy of **corticosteroids**. Use with caution and adjust dose. Moderate Theoretical

Minocycline → see tetracyclines

Minoxidil → see TABLE 8 p. 908 (hypotension)

ROUTE-SPECIFIC INFORMATION Since systemic absorption can follow topical application, the possibility of interactions should be borne in mind.

Mirabegron
- **Mirabegron** is predicted to increase the exposure to **aliskiren**. Mild Theoretical
- Antifungals, azoles **(itraconazole, ketoconazole, voriconazole)** are predicted to increase the exposure to **mirabegron**. Adjust **mirabegron** dose in hepatic and renal impairment. Moderate Study
- **Mirabegron** is predicted to increase the exposure to antihistamines, non-sedating **(fexofenadine)**. Mild Theoretical
- **Mirabegron** is predicted to increase the exposure to beta blockers, selective **(metoprolol)**. Moderate Study
- **Cobicistat** is predicted to increase the exposure to **mirabegron**. Adjust **mirabegron** dose in hepatic and renal impairment. Moderate Study
- **Mirabegron** is predicted to increase the exposure to **colchicine**. Mild Theoretical
- **Mirabegron** is predicted to increase the exposure to **dabigatran**. Severe Theoretical
- **Mirabegron** slightly increases the exposure to **digoxin**. Monitor concentration and adjust dose. Severe Study
- **Mirabegron** is predicted to increase the exposure to **edoxaban**. Mild Theoretical
- **Mirabegron** is predicted to increase the exposure to **eliglustat**. Avoid or adjust dose—consult product literature. Severe Study
- **Mirabegron** is predicted to increase the exposure to **everolimus**. Mild Theoretical
- **HIV-protease inhibitors** are predicted to increase the exposure to **mirabegron**. Adjust **mirabegron** dose in hepatic and renal impairment. Moderate Study
- **Idelalisib** is predicted to increase the exposure to **mirabegron**. Adjust **mirabegron** dose in hepatic and renal impairment. Moderate Study
- **Mirabegron** is predicted to increase the exposure to **loperamide**. Mild Theoretical
- Macrolides **(clarithromycin)** are predicted to increase the exposure to **mirabegron**. Adjust **mirabegron** dose in hepatic and renal impairment. Moderate Study
- **Mirabegron** is predicted to increase the exposure to **sirolimus**. Mild Theoretical
- **Mirabegron** is predicted to increase the exposure to taxanes **(paclitaxel)**. Mild Theoretical
- **Mirabegron** is predicted to increase the exposure to **topotecan**. Mild Theoretical

Mirtazapine → see TABLE 13 p. 910 (serotonin syndrome), TABLE 11 p. 909 (CNS depressant effects)
- Antiepileptics **(carbamazepine, fosphenytoin, phenobarbital, phenytoin, primidone)** are predicted to decrease the exposure to **mirtazapine**. Adjust dose. Moderate Study → Also see TABLE 11 p. 909
- Antifungals, azoles **(itraconazole, ketoconazole, voriconazole)** are predicted to increase the exposure to **mirtazapine**. Moderate Study
- **Apalutamide** is predicted to decrease the exposure to **mirtazapine**. Adjust dose. Moderate Study
- **Cobicistat** is predicted to increase the exposure to **mirtazapine**. Moderate Study
- **Enzalutamide** is predicted to decrease the exposure to **mirtazapine**. Adjust dose. Moderate Study
- H_2 receptor antagonists **(cimetidine)** slightly increase the exposure to **mirtazapine**. Use with caution and adjust dose. Moderate Theoretical
- **HIV-protease inhibitors** are predicted to increase the exposure to **mirtazapine**. Moderate Study
- **Idelalisib** is predicted to increase the exposure to **mirtazapine**. Moderate Study
- Macrolides **(clarithromycin)** are predicted to increase the exposure to **mirtazapine**. Moderate Study
- **Mitotane** is predicted to decrease the exposure to **mirtazapine**. Adjust dose. Moderate Study
- **Mirtazapine** is predicted to decrease the efficacy of **pitolisant**. Moderate Theoretical
- **Rifampicin** is predicted to decrease the exposure to **mirtazapine**. Adjust dose. Moderate Study

Mitomycin → see TABLE 15 p. 910 (myelosuppression), TABLE 5 p. 907 (thromboembolism)
- **Live vaccines** are predicted to increase the risk of generalised infection (possibly life-threatening) when given with **mitomycin**. Public Health England advises avoid (refer to Green Book). Severe Theoretical

Mitotane → see TABLE 15 p. 910 (myelosuppression)
- **Mitotane** is predicted to markedly decrease the exposure to **abemaciclib**. Avoid. Severe Study
- **Mitotane** is predicted to decrease the exposure to **abiraterone**. Avoid. Severe Study
- Aldosterone antagonists **(spironolactone)** are predicted to decrease the effects of **mitotane**. Avoid. Severe Anecdotal

- **Mitotane** is predicted to decrease the exposure to aldosterone antagonists **(eplerenone)**. Avoid. [Moderate] Theoretical
- **Mitotane** is predicted to decrease the exposure to **alprazolam**. Adjust dose. [Moderate] Theoretical
- **Mitotane** is predicted to decrease the exposure to antiarrhythmics **(disopyramide, dronedarone)**. Avoid. [Severe] Study
- **Mitotane** is predicted to decrease the efficacy of antiarrhythmics **(propafenone)**. [Moderate] Study
- **Mitotane** is predicted to decrease the exposure to anticholinesterases, centrally acting **(donepezil)**. [Mild] Study
- **Mitotane** is predicted to decrease the exposure to antiepileptics **(perampanel)**. Monitor and adjust dose. [Moderate] Study
- **Mitotane** is predicted to decrease the exposure to antifungals, azoles **(isavuconazole)**. Avoid. [Severe] Study
- **Mitotane** is predicted to decrease the exposure to antimalarials **(artemether)** (with lumefantrine). Avoid. [Severe] Study
- **Mitotane** is predicted to decrease the concentration of antimalarials **(piperaquine)**. Avoid. [Moderate] Theoretical
- **Mitotane** is predicted to moderately decrease the exposure to **apixaban**. Use with caution or avoid. [Severe] Study
- **Mitotane** moderately decreases the exposure to **apremilast**. Avoid. [Severe] Study
- **Mitotane** is predicted to markedly decrease the exposure to **aprepitant**. Avoid. [Moderate] Study
- **Mitotane** is predicted to moderately decrease the exposure to **aripiprazole**. Adjust **aripiprazole** dose, p. 265. [Moderate] Study
- **Mitotane** is predicted to decrease the exposure to **axitinib**. Avoid or adjust dose. [Moderate] Study → Also see **TABLE 15** p. 910
- **Mitotane** decreases the exposure to **bedaquiline**. Avoid. [Severe] Study
- **Mitotane** is predicted to decrease the exposure to **bictegravir**. Avoid. [Moderate] Study
- **Mitotane** slightly decreases the exposure to **bortezomib**. Avoid. [Severe] Study → Also see **TABLE 15** p. 910
- **Mitotane** affects the exposure to **bosentan**. Avoid. [Severe] Study
- **Mitotane** is predicted to very markedly decrease the exposure to **bosutinib**. Avoid. [Severe] Study → Also see **TABLE 15** p. 910
- **Mitotane** is predicted to decrease the exposure to **brigatinib**. Avoid. [Severe] Study
- **Mitotane** is predicted to decrease the exposure to **buspirone**. Use with caution and adjust dose. [Severe] Study
- **Mitotane** moderately decreases the exposure to **cabozantinib**. Avoid. [Moderate] Study → Also see **TABLE 15** p. 910
- **Mitotane** is predicted to decrease the exposure to calcium channel blockers **(amlodipine, felodipine, lacidipine, lercanidipine, nicardipine, nifedipine, nimodipine)**. Monitor and adjust dose. [Moderate] Study
- **Mitotane** is predicted to decrease the exposure to calcium channel blockers **(diltiazem)**. [Severe] Study
- **Mitotane** is predicted to decrease the exposure to **cannabidiol**. Adjust dose. [Moderate] Study
- **Mitotane** is predicted to decrease the exposure to **cariprazine**. Avoid. [Severe] Theoretical
- **Mitotane** is predicted to decrease the exposure to **ceritinib**. Avoid. [Severe] Study → Also see **TABLE 15** p. 910
- **Mitotane** decreases the concentration of **ciclosporin**. [Severe] Study
- **Mitotane** is predicted to alter the effects of **cilostazol**. [Moderate] Theoretical
- **Mitotane** is predicted to decrease the exposure to **cinacalcet**. Monitor and adjust dose. [Moderate] Study
- **Mitotane** decreases the exposure to **clomethiazole**. Monitor and adjust dose. [Moderate] Study
- **Mitotane** is predicted to decrease the exposure to **cobicistat**. Avoid. [Severe] Theoretical
- **Mitotane** is predicted to decrease the exposure to **cobimetinib**. Avoid. [Severe] Theoretical
- **Mitotane** is predicted to decrease the exposure to corticosteroids **(budesonide, deflazacort, dexamethasone, fludrocortisone, hydrocortisone, methylprednisolone, prednisolone, triamcinolone)**. Monitor and adjust dose. [Moderate] Study
- **Mitotane** is predicted to decrease the exposure to corticosteroids **(fluticasone)**. [Unknown] Theoretical
- **Mitotane** is predicted to markedly decrease the exposure to **crizotinib**. Avoid. [Severe] Study → Also see **TABLE 15** p. 910
- **Mitotane** is predicted to decrease the exposure to **dabrafenib**. Avoid. [Moderate] Theoretical → Also see **TABLE 15** p. 910
- **Mitotane** is predicted to decrease the exposure to **darifenacin**. [Moderate] Theoretical
- **Mitotane** is predicted to decrease the exposure to **dasabuvir**. Avoid. [Severe] Theoretical
- **Mitotane** is predicted to markedly decrease the exposure to **dasatinib**. Avoid. [Severe] Study → Also see **TABLE 15** p. 910
- **Mitotane** is predicted to slightly decrease the exposure to **delamanid**. Avoid. [Moderate] Study
- **Mitotane** is predicted to markedly decrease the exposure to **dienogest**. [Severe] Study
- **Mitotane** decreases the exposure to **dolutegravir**. Adjust dose. [Severe] Study
- **Mitotane** is predicted to decrease the exposure to **doravirine**. Avoid. [Severe] Study
- **Mitotane** is predicted to decrease the exposure to **dronabinol**. Avoid or adjust dose. [Mild] Study
- **Mitotane** is predicted to decrease the exposure to **elbasvir**. Avoid. [Severe] Study
- **Mitotane** is predicted to decrease the exposure to **eliglustat**. Avoid. [Severe] Study
- **Mitotane** is predicted to decrease the concentration of **elvitegravir**. Avoid. [Severe] Theoretical
- **Mitotane** is predicted to decrease the exposure to **encorafenib**. [Severe] Theoretical
- **Mitotane** is predicted to decrease the effects of **ergotamine**. [Moderate] Theoretical
- **Mitotane** is predicted to decrease the exposure to **erlotinib**. Avoid or adjust **erlotinib** dose. [Severe] Study
- **Mitotane** is predicted to decrease the exposure to **esketamine**. Adjust dose. [Moderate] Theoretical
- **Mitotane** is predicted to decrease the exposure to **etravirine**. Avoid. [Severe] Theoretical
- **Mitotane** is predicted to decrease the concentration of **everolimus**. Avoid or adjust dose. [Severe] Study → Also see **TABLE 15** p. 910
- **Mitotane** moderately decreases the exposure to **exemestane**. [Moderate] Study
- **Mitotane** is predicted to decrease the exposure to **fesoterodine**. Avoid. [Moderate] Study
- **Mitotane** is predicted to decrease the exposure to **fingolimod**. [Moderate] Study
- **Mitotane** is predicted to decrease the exposure to **fosaprepitant**. Avoid. [Moderate] Theoretical
- **Mitotane** is predicted to decrease the exposure to **gefitinib**. Avoid. [Severe] Study → Also see **TABLE 15** p. 910
- **Mitotane** is predicted to greatly decrease the concentration of **glecaprevir**. Avoid. [Severe] Study
- **Mitotane** is predicted to decrease the exposure to **grazoprevir**. Avoid. [Severe] Study
- **Mitotane** is predicted to decrease the concentration of **guanfacine**. Adjust **guanfacine** dose, p. 247. [Moderate] Study
- **Mitotane** decreases the concentration of **haloperidol**. Adjust dose. [Moderate] Study
- **Mitotane** is predicted to decrease the exposure to **ibrutinib**. Avoid or adjust **ibrutinib** dose. [Severe] Study → Also see **TABLE 15** p. 910
- **Mitotane** is predicted to decrease the exposure to **idelalisib**. Avoid. [Severe] Study → Also see **TABLE 15** p. 910
- **Mitotane** is predicted to decrease the exposure to **imatinib**. Avoid. [Moderate] Study → Also see **TABLE 15** p. 910
- **Mitotane** is predicted to decrease the exposure to **irinotecan**. Avoid. [Severe] Study → Also see **TABLE 15** p. 910
- **Mitotane** is predicted to decrease the exposure to **ivabradine**. Adjust dose. [Moderate] Theoretical
- **Mitotane** is predicted to moderately to markedly decrease the exposure to **ivacaftor**. Avoid. [Severe] Study
- **Mitotane** is predicted to decrease the exposure to **ixazomib**. Avoid. [Severe] Study
- **Mitotane** is predicted to decrease the exposure to **lapatinib**. Avoid. [Severe] Study

Mitotane (continued)
- **Mitotane** is predicted to moderately decrease the exposure to **larotrectinib**. Avoid. Moderate Study
- **Mitotane** is predicted to decrease the exposure to **linagliptin**. Moderate Study
- **Mitotane** is predicted to decrease the exposure to **lomitapide**. Monitor and adjust dose. Moderate Theoretical
- **Mitotane** is predicted to decrease the exposure to **lorlatinib**. Avoid. Severe Study
- **Mitotane** is predicted to decrease the exposure to **lurasidone**. Avoid. Moderate Study
- **Mitotane** is predicted to decrease the exposure to **macitentan**. Avoid. Severe Study
- **Mitotane** is predicted to decrease the exposure to **maraviroc**. Adjust dose. Severe Study
- **Mitotane** is predicted to decrease the exposure to **midazolam**. Monitor and adjust dose. Moderate Study
- **Mitotane** is predicted to decrease the exposure to **midostaurin**. Avoid. Severe Study
- **Mitotane** is predicted to decrease the exposure to **mirtazapine**. Adjust dose. Moderate Study
- **Mitotane** is predicted to decrease the exposure to monoclonal antibodies **(polatuzumab vedotin)**. Moderate Theoretical
- **Mitotane** is predicted to decrease the exposure to **montelukast**. Mild Study
- **Mitotane** is predicted to markedly decrease the exposure to **naldemedine**. Avoid. Severe Study
- **Mitotane** is predicted to markedly decrease the exposure to **naloxegol**. Avoid. Moderate Study
- **Mitotane** is predicted to slightly decrease the exposure to **nateglinide**. Mild Study
- **Mitotane** is predicted to decrease the exposure to **neratinib**. Avoid. Severe Study
- **Mitotane** is predicted to decrease the exposure to **netupitant**. Avoid. Severe Study
- **Mitotane** is predicted to decrease the exposure to **nevirapine**. Severe Theoretical
- **Mitotane** is predicted to moderately decrease the exposure to **nilotinib**. Avoid. Severe Study → Also see **TABLE 15** p. 910
- **Mitotane** is predicted to decrease the exposure to **nitisinone**. Adjust dose. Moderate Theoretical
- **Mitotane** is predicted to decrease the exposure to **olaparib**. Avoid. Moderate Theoretical → Also see **TABLE 15** p. 910
- **Mitotane** is predicted to decrease the exposure to **ombitasvir**. Avoid. Severe Theoretical
- **Mitotane** is predicted to decrease the exposure to **ondansetron**. Moderate Study
- **Mitotane** is predicted to decrease the exposure to opioids **(alfentanil, fentanyl)**. Moderate Study
- **Mitotane** is predicted to decrease the exposure to opioids **(buprenorphine)**. Monitor and adjust dose. Moderate Theoretical
- **Mitotane** decreases the exposure to opioids **(methadone)**. Monitor and adjust dose. Severe Study
- **Mitotane** is predicted to decrease the exposure to opioids **(oxycodone)**. Monitor and adjust dose. Moderate Study
- **Mitotane** is predicted to moderately decrease the exposure to **osimertinib**. Avoid. Moderate Study
- **Mitotane** is predicted to moderately decrease the exposure to **ospemifene**. Moderate Study
- **Mitotane** is predicted to decrease the exposure to **palbociclib**. Avoid. Severe Study
- **Mitotane** is predicted to decrease the exposure to **paliperidone**. Monitor and adjust dose. Severe Study
- **Mitotane** is predicted to decrease the exposure to **panobinostat**. Avoid. Moderate Theoretical → Also see **TABLE 15** p. 910
- **Mitotane** is predicted to decrease the exposure to **paritaprevir** (with ritonavir and ombitasvir). Avoid. Severe Study
- **Mitotane** is predicted to decrease the exposure to **pazopanib**. Avoid. Severe Theoretical → Also see **TABLE 15** p. 910
- **Mitotane** is predicted to decrease the exposure to phosphodiesterase type-5 inhibitors **(avanafil, tadalafil)**. Avoid. Severe Study
- **Mitotane** is predicted to decrease the exposure to phosphodiesterase type-5 inhibitors **(sildenafil, vardenafil)**. Moderate Theoretical
- **Mitotane** is predicted to moderately to markedly decrease the exposure to **pibrentasvir**. Avoid. Severe Study
- **Mitotane** is predicted to moderately decrease the exposure to **pitolisant**. Moderate Study
- **Mitotane** is predicted to decrease the exposure to **ponatinib**. Avoid. Moderate Theoretical
- **Mitotane** is predicted to markedly decrease the exposure to **praziquantel**. Avoid. Moderate Study
- **Mitotane** is predicted to decrease the exposure to **quetiapine**. Moderate Study
- **Mitotane** is predicted to decrease the exposure to **ranolazine**. Avoid. Severe Study
- **Mitotane** is predicted to decrease the exposure to **reboxetine**. Moderate Anecdotal
- **Mitotane** is predicted to decrease the exposure to **regorafenib**. Avoid. Moderate Study → Also see **TABLE 15** p. 910
- **Mitotane** is predicted to decrease the exposure to **repaglinide**. Monitor blood glucose and adjust dose. Moderate Study
- **Mitotane** is predicted to markedly decrease the exposure to **ribociclib**. Avoid. Severe Study
- **Mitotane** markedly decreases the exposure to **rilpivirine**. Avoid. Severe Study
- **Mitotane** is predicted to decrease the exposure to **risperidone**. Adjust dose. Moderate Study
- **Mitotane** is predicted to moderately decrease the exposure to **rivaroxaban**. Avoid unless patient can be monitored for signs of thrombosis. Severe Study
- **Mitotane** is predicted to decrease the exposure to **roflumilast**. Avoid. Moderate Study
- **Mitotane** is predicted to markedly decrease the exposure to **rolapitant**. Avoid. Severe Study
- **Mitotane** is predicted to decrease the exposure to **ruxolitinib**. Monitor and adjust dose. Moderate Study → Also see **TABLE 15** p. 910
- **Mitotane** is predicted to moderately decrease the exposure to **saxagliptin**. Moderate Study
- **Mitotane** is predicted to decrease the exposure to **siponimod**. Severe Study
- **Mitotane** is predicted to decrease the concentration of **sirolimus**. Avoid. Severe Study
- **Mitotane** is predicted to decrease the exposure to **solifenacin**. Moderate Theoretical
- **Mitotane** is predicted to decrease the exposure to **sorafenib**. Moderate Theoretical → Also see **TABLE 15** p. 910
- **Mitotane** is predicted to decrease the exposure to statins **(simvastatin)**. Severe Study
- **Mitotane** is predicted to decrease the exposure to **sunitinib**. Avoid or adjust **sunitinib** dose. Moderate Study → Also see **TABLE 15** p. 910
- **Mitotane** decreases the concentration of **tacrolimus**. Monitor and adjust dose. Severe Study
- **Mitotane** is predicted to decrease the exposure to taxanes **(cabazitaxel, paclitaxel)**. Avoid. Severe Study → Also see **TABLE 15** p. 910
- **Mitotane** is predicted to decrease the exposure to taxanes **(docetaxel)**. Severe Theoretical → Also see **TABLE 15** p. 910
- **Mitotane** is predicted to decrease the concentration of **temsirolimus**. Avoid. Severe Study → Also see **TABLE 15** p. 910
- **Mitotane** decreases the exposure to tetracyclines **(doxycycline)**. Monitor and adjust dose. Moderate Study
- **Mitotane** is predicted to decrease the exposure to **tezacaftor**. Avoid. Severe Theoretical
- **Mitotane** is predicted to markedly decrease the exposure to **ticagrelor**. Avoid. Severe Study
- **Mitotane** is predicted to decrease the exposure to **tivozanib**. Severe Study
- **Mitotane** is predicted to decrease the exposure to **tofacitinib**. Avoid. Severe Study
- **Mitotane** is predicted to decrease the exposure to **tolvaptan**. Use with caution or avoid depending on indication. Severe Study

- **Mitotane** is predicted to decrease the exposure to **toremifene**. Adjust dose. [Moderate] Study
- **Mitotane** is predicted to decrease the exposure to **trabectedin**. Avoid. [Severe] Theoretical → Also see **TABLE 15** p. 910
- **Mitotane** is predicted to decrease the exposure to **upadacitinib**. [Moderate] Study
- **Mitotane** is predicted to decrease the exposure to **vandetanib**. Avoid. [Moderate] Study
- **Mitotane** is predicted to moderately decrease the exposure to velpatasvir. Avoid. [Severe] Study
- **Mitotane** is predicted to decrease the exposure to **vemurafenib**. Avoid. [Severe] Theoretical
- **Mitotane** is predicted to decrease the exposure to **venetoclax**. Avoid. [Severe] Study
- **Mitotane** is predicted to decrease the exposure to vinca alkaloids **(vinblastine, vincristine, vindesine)**. [Severe] Theoretical → Also see **TABLE 15** p. 910
- **Mitotane** is predicted to decrease the exposure to vinca alkaloids **(vinflunine)**. Avoid. [Severe] Theoretical → Also see **TABLE 15** p. 910
- **Mitotane** is predicted to decrease the exposure to vinca alkaloids **(vinorelbine)**. Use with caution or avoid. [Severe] Theoretical → Also see **TABLE 15** p. 910
- **Mitotane** is predicted to decrease the exposure to **vismodegib**. Avoid. [Moderate] Theoretical → Also see **TABLE 15** p. 910
- **Mitotane** is predicted to decrease the exposure to **vortioxetine**. Monitor and adjust dose. [Moderate] Study
- **Mitotane** is predicted to decrease the concentration of voxilaprevir. Avoid. [Severe] Study
- **Mitotane** is predicted to decrease the exposure to **zopiclone**. Adjust dose. [Moderate] Study

Mitoxantrone → see anthracyclines

Mivacurium → see neuromuscular blocking drugs, non-depolarising

Mizolastine → see antihistamines, non-sedating

Moclobemide → see **TABLE 13** p. 910 (serotonin syndrome)

FOOD AND LIFESTYLE Moclobemide is claimed to cause less potentiation of the pressor effect of tyramine than the traditional (irreversible) MAOIs, but patients should avoid consuming large amounts of tyramine-rich foods (such as mature cheese, salami, pickled herring, *Bovril*®, *Oxo*®, *Marmite*® or any similar meat or yeast extract or fermented soya bean extract, and some beers, lagers or wines).

- **Moclobemide** is predicted to increase the risk of a hypertensive crisis when given with **amfetamines**. Avoid. [Severe] Theoretical → Also see **TABLE 13** p. 910
- **Apalutamide** is predicted to decrease the exposure to **moclobemide**. Avoid or monitor. [Mild] Study
- **Moclobemide** is predicted to increase the risk of severe hypertension when given with **bupropion**. Avoid. [Severe] Theoretical → Also see **TABLE 13** p. 910
- **Moclobemide** is predicted to increase the exposure to **cannabidiol**. [Moderate] Theoretical
- **Moclobemide** is predicted to increase the exposure to **cilostazol**. [Moderate] Theoretical
- **Moclobemide** potentially increases the exposure to **clobazam**. Adjust dose. [Moderate] Theoretical
- **Moclobemide** is predicted to decrease the efficacy of **clopidogrel**. Avoid. [Moderate] Study
- **Moclobemide** is predicted to increase the exposure to **eliglustat**. Avoid or adjust dose—consult product literature. [Severe] Theoretical
- H_2 receptor antagonists **(cimetidine)** increase the exposure to **moclobemide**. Adjust **moclobemide** dose. [Mild] Study
- **Levodopa** increases the risk of side-effects when given with **moclobemide**. [Moderate] Study
- **Moclobemide** is predicted to increase the risk of side-effects when given with **linezolid**. Avoid and for 14 days after stopping **moclobemide**. [Severe] Theoretical → Also see **TABLE 13** p. 910
- **Moclobemide** is predicted to increase the effects of MAO-B inhibitors **(rasagiline, selegiline)**. Avoid. [Severe] Theoretical → Also see **TABLE 13** p. 910
- **Moclobemide** is predicted to increase the risk of side-effects when given with MAO-B inhibitors **(safinamide)**. Avoid and for 1 week after stopping **safinamide**. [Severe] Theoretical → Also see **TABLE 13** p. 910
- **Methylphenidate** is predicted to increase the risk of a hypertensive crisis when given with **moclobemide**. [Severe] Theoretical
- **Mianserin** is predicted to increase the risk of toxicity when given with **moclobemide**. Avoid and for 1 week after stopping **mianserin**. [Severe] Theoretical
- **Opicapone** is predicted to increase the risk of elevated blood pressure when given with **moclobemide**. Avoid. [Severe] Theoretical
- **Moclobemide** increases the risk of side-effects when given with phenothiazines **(levomepromazine)**. [Moderate] Study
- **Reboxetine** is predicted to increase the risk of a hypertensive crisis when given with **moclobemide**. Avoid. [Severe] Theoretical
- **Moclobemide** moderately increases the exposure to **rizatriptan**. Avoid. [Moderate] Study → Also see **TABLE 13** p. 910
- **Moclobemide** moderately increases the exposure to **sumatriptan**. Avoid. [Moderate] Study → Also see **TABLE 13** p. 910
- **Moclobemide** is predicted to increase the risk of a hypertensive crisis when given with sympathomimetics, vasoconstrictor **(ephedrine, isometheptene, phenylephrine, pseudoephedrine)**. Avoid. [Severe] Study
- **Tetrabenazine** potentially increases the risk of CNS excitation and hypertension when given with **moclobemide**. [Severe] Theoretical
- **Tricyclic antidepressants** are predicted to increase the risk of severe toxic reaction when given with **moclobemide**. Avoid. [Severe] Theoretical → Also see **TABLE 13** p. 910
- **Moclobemide** slightly increases the exposure to **zolmitriptan**. Adjust **zolmitriptan** dose, p. 310. [Moderate] Study → Also see **TABLE 13** p. 910

Modafinil

- Antiepileptics **(carbamazepine, phenobarbital, primidone)** are predicted to decrease the exposure to **modafinil**. [Mild] Theoretical
- Antiepileptics **(fosphenytoin, phenytoin)** are predicted to decrease the exposure to **modafinil** and **modafinil** is predicted to increase the concentration of antiepileptics **(fosphenytoin, phenytoin)**. Monitor concentration and adjust dose. [Moderate] Theoretical
- Antifungals, azoles **(itraconazole, ketoconazole, voriconazole)** are predicted to increase the exposure to **modafinil**. [Mild] Theoretical
- **Modafinil** is predicted to decrease the exposure to **bosutinib**. Avoid. [Severe] Theoretical
- **Cobicistat** is predicted to increase the exposure to **modafinil**. [Mild] Theoretical
- **Modafinil** is predicted to decrease the efficacy of **combined hormonal contraceptives**. For FSRH guidance, see Contraceptives, interactions p. 536. [Severe] Study
- **Modafinil** is predicted to decrease the efficacy of **desogestrel**. For FSRH guidance, see Contraceptives, interactions p. 536. [Severe] Theoretical
- **Modafinil** is predicted to decrease the exposure to **doravirine**. Avoid or adjust doravirine or lamivudine with tenofovir disoproxil and doravirine dose. [Severe] Theoretical
- **Modafinil** is predicted to decrease the exposure to **elbasvir**. Avoid. [Unknown] Theoretical
- **Modafinil** is predicted to decrease the efficacy of **etonogestrel**. For FSRH guidance, see Contraceptives, interactions p. 536. [Severe] Theoretical
- **Modafinil** is predicted to decrease the exposure to **grazoprevir**. Avoid. [Severe] Theoretical
- **HIV-protease inhibitors** are predicted to increase the exposure to **modafinil**. [Mild] Theoretical
- **Modafinil** is predicted to decrease the effects of **hormone replacement therapy**. [Moderate] Anecdotal
- **Idelalisib** is predicted to increase the exposure to **modafinil**. [Mild] Theoretical
- **Modafinil** is predicted to decrease the concentration of **letermovir**. [Moderate] Theoretical
- **Modafinil** is predicted to decrease the efficacy of **levonorgestrel**. For FSRH guidance, see Contraceptives, interactions p. 536. [Severe] Theoretical

Modafinil (continued)

- Macrolides **(clarithromycin)** are predicted to increase the exposure to **modafinil**. [Mild] Theoretical
- **Modafinil** is predicted to decrease the efficacy of norethisterone. For FSRH guidance, see Contraceptives, interactions p. 536. [Severe] Anecdotal
- **Rifampicin** is predicted to decrease the exposure to **modafinil**. [Moderate] Theoretical
- **Modafinil** is predicted to decrease the exposure to **sofosbuvir**. Avoid. [Severe] Theoretical
- **Modafinil** decreases the efficacy of **ulipristal**. For FSRH guidance, see Contraceptives, interactions p. 536. [Severe] Anecdotal
- **Modafinil** is predicted to decrease the exposure to **velpatasvir**. Avoid. [Severe] Theoretical
- **Modafinil** is predicted to decrease the concentration of voxilaprevir. Avoid. [Severe] Theoretical

Mogamulizumab → see monoclonal antibodies

Mometasone → see corticosteroids

Monoclonal antibodies → see TABLE 15 p. 910 (myelosuppression), TABLE 12 p. 910 (peripheral neuropathy), TABLE 9 p. 909 (QT-interval prolongation), TABLE 4 p. 907 (antiplatelet effects)

adalimumab · alemtuzumab · atezolizumab · avelumab · basiliximab · belimumab · bevacizumab · blinatumomab · brentuximab vedotin · brodalumab · canakinumab · cemiplimab · certolizumab pegol · cetuximab · daratumumab · dinutuximab · dupilumab · durvalumab · eculizumab · elotuzumab · golimumab · guselkumab · infliximab · inotuzumab ozogamicin · ipilimumab · ixekizumab · mogamulizumab · natalizumab · necitumumab · nivolumab · obinutuzumab · ocrelizumab · panitumumab · pembrolizumab · pertuzumab · polatuzumab vedotin · ramucirumab · risankizumab · rituximab · sarilumab · secukinumab · siltuximab · tildrakizumab · tocilizumab · trastuzumab · trastuzumab emtansine · ustekinumab · vedolizumab

- **Abatacept** is predicted to increase the risk of generalised infection (possibly life-threatening) when given with **golimumab**. Avoid. [Severe] Theoretical
- **Tocilizumab** is predicted to decrease the exposure to alprazolam. Monitor and adjust dose. [Moderate] Theoretical
- **Blinatumomab** is predicted to transiently increase the exposure to **aminophylline**. Monitor and adjust dose. [Moderate] Theoretical
- **Sarilumab** potentially affects the exposure to **aminophylline**. Monitor and adjust dose. [Moderate] Theoretical
- **Tocilizumab** is predicted to decrease the exposure to **aminophylline**. Monitor and adjust dose. [Moderate] Theoretical
- **Anakinra** is predicted to increase the risk of generalised infection (possibly life-threatening) when given with **golimumab**. Avoid. [Severe] Theoretical
- **Anthracyclines** are predicted to increase the risk of cardiotoxicity when given with monoclonal antibodies **(trastuzumab, trastuzumab emtansine)**. Avoid. [Severe] Theoretical → Also see TABLE 15 p. 910
- Antiarrhythmics **(dronedarone)** increase the risk of neutropenia when given with **brentuximab vedotin**. Monitor and adjust dose. [Severe] Theoretical
- Antiepileptics **(carbamazepine)** are predicted to decrease the effects of **brentuximab vedotin**. [Severe] Theoretical
- Antiepileptics **(carbamazepine, fosphenytoin, phenobarbital, phenytoin, primidone)** are predicted to decrease the exposure to **polatuzumab vedotin**. [Moderate] Theoretical
- **Tocilizumab** is predicted to decrease the exposure to antiepileptics **(fosphenytoin, phenytoin)**. Monitor and adjust dose. [Moderate] Theoretical
- Antifungals, azoles **(itraconazole, ketoconazole)** increase the risk of neutropenia when given with **brentuximab vedotin**. Monitor and adjust dose. [Severe] Study
- Antifungals, azoles **(itraconazole, ketoconazole, voriconazole)** are predicted to increase the exposure to **polatuzumab vedotin**. [Moderate] Theoretical
- Antifungals, azoles **(itraconazole, ketoconazole, voriconazole)** are predicted to increase the exposure to **trastuzumab emtansine**. Avoid. [Severe] Theoretical
- **Apalutamide** is predicted to decrease the exposure to **polatuzumab vedotin**. [Moderate] Theoretical
- **Brentuximab vedotin** increases the risk of pulmonary toxicity when given with **bleomycin**. Avoid. [Severe] Study → Also see TABLE 15 p. 910
- **Tocilizumab** is predicted to decrease the exposure to **calcium channel blockers**. Monitor and adjust dose. [Moderate] Theoretical
- **Blinatumomab** is predicted to transiently increase the exposure to **ciclosporin**. Monitor and adjust dose. [Moderate] Theoretical
- **Sarilumab** potentially affects the exposure to **ciclosporin**. Monitor and adjust dose. [Moderate] Theoretical
- **Tocilizumab** is predicted to decrease the exposure to ciclosporin. Monitor and adjust dose. [Moderate] Theoretical
- **Cobicistat** is predicted to increase the exposure to **polatuzumab vedotin**. [Moderate] Theoretical
- **Cobicistat** is predicted to increase the exposure to **trastuzumab emtansine**. Avoid. [Severe] Theoretical
- **Sarilumab** potentially decreases the exposure to **combined hormonal contraceptives**. [Severe] Theoretical
- **Corticosteroids** are predicted to increase the risk of immunosuppression when given with **dinutuximab**. Avoid except in life-threatening situations. [Severe] Theoretical
- Corticosteroids **(betamethasone, deflazacort, dexamethasone, hydrocortisone, methylprednisolone, prednisolone)** are predicted to decrease the efficacy of monoclonal antibodies **(atezolizumab, ipilimumab, nivolumab, pembrolizumab)**. Use with caution or avoid. [Severe] Theoretical
- **Tocilizumab** is predicted to decrease the exposure to corticosteroids **(dexamethasone, methylprednisolone)**. Monitor and adjust dose. [Moderate] Theoretical
- **Blinatumomab** is predicted to transiently increase the exposure to coumarins **(warfarin)**. Monitor and adjust dose. [Moderate] Theoretical
- **Sarilumab** potentially affects the exposure to coumarins **(warfarin)**. Monitor and adjust dose. [Severe] Theoretical
- **Tocilizumab** is predicted to decrease the exposure to coumarins **(warfarin)**. Monitor and adjust dose. [Moderate] Theoretical
- **Tocilizumab** is predicted to decrease the exposure to **diazepam**. Monitor and adjust dose. [Moderate] Theoretical
- **Enzalutamide** is predicted to decrease the exposure to **polatuzumab vedotin**. [Moderate] Theoretical
- HIV-protease inhibitors **(lopinavir, ritonavir, saquinavir)** are predicted to increase the risk of neutropenia when given with **brentuximab vedotin**. Monitor and adjust dose. [Severe] Study
- **HIV-protease inhibitors** are predicted to increase the exposure to **polatuzumab vedotin**. [Moderate] Theoretical
- **HIV-protease inhibitors** are predicted to increase the exposure to **trastuzumab emtansine**. Avoid. [Severe] Theoretical
- **Idelalisib** is predicted to increase the exposure to **polatuzumab vedotin**. [Moderate] Theoretical
- **Idelalisib** is predicted to increase the exposure to **trastuzumab emtansine**. Avoid. [Severe] Theoretical → Also see TABLE 15 p. 910
- **Immunoglobulins** are predicted to alter the effects of **dinutuximab**. Avoid. [Severe] Theoretical
- **Live vaccines** are predicted to increase the risk of generalised infection (possibly life-threatening) when given with **monoclonal antibodies**. Public Health England advises avoid (refer to Green Book). [Severe] Theoretical
- Macrolides **(clarithromycin)** increase the risk of neutropenia when given with **brentuximab vedotin**. Monitor and adjust dose. [Severe] Theoretical
- Macrolides **(clarithromycin)** are predicted to increase the exposure to **polatuzumab vedotin**. [Moderate] Theoretical
- Macrolides **(clarithromycin)** are predicted to increase the exposure to **trastuzumab emtansine**. Avoid. [Severe] Theoretical
- **Tocilizumab** is predicted to decrease the exposure to midazolam. Monitor and adjust dose. [Moderate] Theoretical
- **Mitotane** is predicted to decrease the exposure to **polatuzumab vedotin**. [Moderate] Theoretical
- **Rifampicin** decreases the effects of **brentuximab vedotin**. [Severe] Study
- **Rifampicin** is predicted to decrease the exposure to **polatuzumab vedotin**. [Moderate] Theoretical
- **Siponimod** potentially increases the risk of immunosuppression when given with **alemtuzumab**. Avoid. [Severe] Theoretical

- **Sarilumab** potentially affects the exposure to **sirolimus**. Monitor and adjust dose. Moderate Theoretical
- **Sarilumab** is predicted to decrease the exposure to statins **(atorvastatin, simvastatin)**. Moderate Study
- **Tocilizumab** is predicted to decrease the exposure to statins **(atorvastatin, simvastatin)**. Monitor and adjust dose. Moderate Study
- **Sarilumab** potentially affects the exposure to **tacrolimus**. Monitor and adjust dose. Moderate Theoretical
- **Blinatumomab** is predicted to transiently increase the exposure to **theophylline**. Monitor and adjust dose. Moderate Theoretical
- **Sarilumab** potentially affects the exposure to **theophylline**. Monitor and adjust dose. Moderate Theoretical
- **Tocilizumab** is predicted to decrease the exposure to **theophylline**. Monitor and adjust dose. Moderate Theoretical

Montelukast
- Antiepileptics **(carbamazepine, fosphenytoin, phenobarbital, phenytoin, primidone)** are predicted to decrease the exposure to **montelukast**. Mild Study
- **Apalutamide** is predicted to decrease the exposure to **montelukast**. Mild Study
- **Clopidogrel** is predicted to moderately increase the exposure to **montelukast**. Moderate Study
- **Enzalutamide** is predicted to decrease the exposure to **montelukast**. Mild Study
- Fibrates **(gemfibrozil)** are predicted to moderately increase the exposure to **montelukast**. Moderate Study
- Iron chelators **(deferasirox)** are predicted to increase the exposure to **montelukast**. Moderate Theoretical
- **Leflunomide** is predicted to increase the exposure to **montelukast**. Moderate Theoretical
- **Mitotane** is predicted to decrease the exposure to **montelukast**. Mild Study
- **Opicapone** is predicted to increase the exposure to **montelukast**. Avoid. Moderate Study
- **Rifampicin** is predicted to decrease the exposure to **montelukast**. Mild Study
- **Teriflunomide** is predicted to increase the exposure to **montelukast**. Moderate Theoretical

Morphine → see opioids

Moxifloxacin → see quinolones

Moxisylyte → see TABLE 8 p. 908 (hypotension)

Moxonidine → see TABLE 8 p. 908 (hypotension), TABLE 11 p. 909 (CNS depressant effects)
- **Tricyclic antidepressants** are predicted to decrease the effects of **moxonidine**. Avoid. Moderate Theoretical → Also see TABLE 8 p. 908 → Also see TABLE 11 p. 909

Mycophenolate → see TABLE 15 p. 910 (myelosuppression)
- **Mycophenolate** is predicted to increase the risk of haematological toxicity when given with **aciclovir**. Moderate Theoretical
- **Antacids** decrease the exposure to **mycophenolate**. Moderate Study
- Antifungals, azoles **(isavuconazole)** increase the exposure to **mycophenolate**. Moderate Study
- **Mycophenolate** is predicted to increase the risk of haematological toxicity when given with **ganciclovir**. Moderate Theoretical → Also see TABLE 15 p. 910
- **Live vaccines** are predicted to increase the risk of generalised infection (possibly life-threatening) when given with **mycophenolate**. Public Health England advises avoid (refer to Green Book). Severe Theoretical
- **Rifampicin** decreases the concentration of **mycophenolate**. Monitor and adjust dose. Severe Study
- **Mycophenolate** is predicted to increase the risk of haematological toxicity when given with **valaciclovir**. Moderate Theoretical
- **Mycophenolate** is predicted to increase the risk of haematological toxicity when given with **valganciclovir**. Moderate Theoretical → Also see TABLE 15 p. 910

Nabilone → see TABLE 11 p. 909 (CNS depressant effects)
- **Nabilone** is predicted to increase the risk of cardiovascular side-effects when given with **amfetamines**. Severe Theoretical

Nabumetone → see NSAIDs

Nadolol → see beta blockers, non-selective

Naldemedine
- Antiarrhythmics **(amiodarone, dronedarone)** are predicted to increase the exposure to **naldemedine**. Moderate Study
- Antiepileptics **(carbamazepine, fosphenytoin, phenobarbital, phenytoin, primidone)** are predicted to markedly decrease the exposure to **naldemedine**. Avoid. Severe Study
- Antifungals, azoles **(fluconazole, isavuconazole, posaconazole)** are predicted to increase the exposure to **naldemedine**. Moderate Study
- Antifungals, azoles **(itraconazole, ketoconazole, voriconazole)** are predicted to increase the exposure to **naldemedine**. Avoid or monitor. Moderate Study
- **Apalutamide** is predicted to markedly decrease the exposure to **naldemedine**. Avoid. Severe Study
- **Aprepitant** is predicted to increase the exposure to **naldemedine**. Moderate Study
- Calcium channel blockers **(diltiazem, verapamil)** are predicted to increase the exposure to **naldemedine**. Moderate Study
- **Ciclosporin** is predicted to increase the exposure to **naldemedine**. Moderate Study
- **Cobicistat** is predicted to increase the exposure to **naldemedine**. Avoid or monitor. Moderate Study
- **Crizotinib** is predicted to increase the exposure to **naldemedine**. Moderate Study
- **Enzalutamide** is predicted to markedly decrease the exposure to **naldemedine**. Avoid. Severe Study
- **Grapefruit juice** is predicted to increase the exposure to **naldemedine**. Avoid or monitor. Moderate Theoretical
- **HIV-protease inhibitors** are predicted to increase the exposure to **naldemedine**. Avoid or monitor. Moderate Study
- **Idelalisib** is predicted to increase the exposure to **naldemedine**. Avoid or monitor. Moderate Study
- **Imatinib** is predicted to increase the exposure to **naldemedine**. Moderate Study
- Macrolides **(azithromycin, erythromycin)** are predicted to increase the exposure to **naldemedine**. Moderate Study
- Macrolides **(clarithromycin)** are predicted to increase the exposure to **naldemedine**. Avoid or monitor. Moderate Study
- **Mitotane** is predicted to markedly decrease the exposure to **naldemedine**. Avoid. Severe Study
- **Netupitant** is predicted to increase the exposure to **naldemedine**. Moderate Study
- **Nilotinib** is predicted to increase the exposure to **naldemedine**. Moderate Study
- **Ranolazine** is predicted to increase the exposure to **naldemedine**. Moderate Study
- **Rifampicin** is predicted to markedly decrease the exposure to **naldemedine**. Avoid. Severe Study
- **St John's Wort** is predicted to decrease the exposure to **naldemedine**. Avoid. Severe Study
- **Vemurafenib** is predicted to increase the exposure to **naldemedine**. Moderate Study

Nalmefene

GENERAL INFORMATION Discontinue treatment 1 week before anticipated use of opioids; if emergency analgesia is required during treatment, an increased dose of opioid analgesic might be necessary (monitor for opioid intoxication).

- **Nalmefene** is predicted to decrease the efficacy of **opioids**. Avoid. Severe Theoretical

Naloxegol
- Antiarrhythmics **(dronedarone)** are predicted to increase the exposure to **naloxegol**. Adjust **naloxegol** dose and monitor side effects. Moderate Study
- Antiepileptics **(carbamazepine, fosphenytoin, phenobarbital, phenytoin, primidone)** are predicted to markedly decrease the exposure to **naloxegol**. Avoid. Moderate Study
- Antifungals, azoles **(fluconazole, isavuconazole, posaconazole)** are predicted to increase the exposure to **naloxegol**. Adjust **naloxegol** dose and monitor side effects. Moderate Study
- Antifungals, azoles **(itraconazole, ketoconazole, voriconazole)** are predicted to markedly increase the exposure to **naloxegol**. Avoid. Severe Study
- **Apalutamide** is predicted to markedly decrease the exposure to **naloxegol**. Avoid. Moderate Study

Naloxegol (continued)
- Aprepitant is predicted to increase the exposure to **naloxegol**. Adjust **naloxegol** dose and monitor side effects. [Moderate] Study
- Calcium channel blockers **(diltiazem, verapamil)** are predicted to increase the exposure to **naloxegol**. Adjust **naloxegol** dose and monitor side effects. [Moderate] Study
- Cobicistat is predicted to markedly increase the exposure to **naloxegol**. Avoid. [Severe] Study
- Crizotinib is predicted to increase the exposure to **naloxegol**. Adjust **naloxegol** dose and monitor side effects. [Moderate] Study
- Enzalutamide is predicted to markedly decrease the exposure to **naloxegol**. Avoid. [Moderate] Study
- Grapefruit juice is predicted to increase the exposure to **naloxegol**. Avoid. [Moderate] Theoretical
- HIV-protease inhibitors are predicted to markedly increase the exposure to **naloxegol**. Avoid. [Severe] Study
- Idelalisib is predicted to markedly increase the exposure to **naloxegol**. Avoid. [Severe] Study
- Imatinib is predicted to increase the exposure to **naloxegol**. Adjust **naloxegol** dose and monitor side effects. [Moderate] Study
- Macrolides **(clarithromycin)** are predicted to markedly increase the exposure to **naloxegol**. Avoid. [Severe] Study
- Macrolides **(erythromycin)** are predicted to increase the exposure to **naloxegol**. Adjust **naloxegol** dose and monitor side effects. [Moderate] Study
- Mitotane is predicted to markedly decrease the exposure to **naloxegol**. Avoid. [Moderate] Study
- Netupitant is predicted to increase the exposure to **naloxegol**. Adjust **naloxegol** dose and monitor side effects. [Moderate] Study
- Nilotinib is predicted to increase the exposure to **naloxegol**. Adjust **naloxegol** dose and monitor side effects. [Moderate] Study
- Rifampicin is predicted to markedly decrease the exposure to **naloxegol**. Avoid. [Moderate] Study
- St John's Wort is predicted to decrease the exposure to **naloxegol**. Avoid. [Moderate] Theoretical

Naltrexone

GENERAL INFORMATION Avoid concurrent use of opioids.

Nandrolone
- **Nandrolone** is predicted to increase the anticoagulant effect of coumarins. Monitor and adjust dose. [Severe] Theoretical
- **Nandrolone** is predicted to increase the anticoagulant effect of phenindione. Monitor and adjust dose. [Severe] Theoretical

Naproxen → see NSAIDs

Naratriptan → see TABLE 13 p. 910 (serotonin syndrome)
- **Naratriptan** is predicted to increase the risk of vasoconstriction when given with **ergotamine**. Separate administration by 24 hours. [Severe] Theoretical

Natalizumab → see monoclonal antibodies

Nateglinide → see TABLE 14 p. 910 (antidiabetic drugs)
- Antiepileptics **(carbamazepine, fosphenytoin, phenobarbital, phenytoin, primidone)** are predicted to slightly decrease the exposure to **nateglinide**. [Mild] Study
- Apalutamide is predicted to slightly decrease the exposure to **nateglinide**. [Mild] Study
- Enzalutamide is predicted to slightly decrease the exposure to **nateglinide**. [Mild] Study
- Leflunomide is predicted to increase the exposure to **nateglinide**. [Moderate] Theoretical
- Mitotane is predicted to slightly decrease the exposure to **nateglinide**. [Mild] Study
- Rifampicin is predicted to slightly decrease the exposure to **nateglinide**. [Mild] Study
- Teriflunomide is predicted to increase the exposure to **nateglinide**. [Moderate] Theoretical

Nebivolol → see beta blockers, selective

Necitumumab → see monoclonal antibodies

Nefopam → see TABLE 10 p. 909 (antimuscarinics)
- **Nefopam** is predicted to increase the risk of serious elevations in blood pressure when given with **MAOIs**, irreversible. Avoid. [Severe] Theoretical

Nelarabine → see TABLE 15 p. 910 (myelosuppression)

Neomycin → see TABLE 2 p. 907 (nephrotoxicity), TABLE 19 p. 911 (ototoxicity), TABLE 20 p. 911 (neuromuscular blocking effects)

ROUTE-SPECIFIC INFORMATION Since systemic absorption can follow topical application, the possibility of interactions should be borne in mind.

- **Neomycin** decreases the absorption of digoxin. [Moderate] Study
- **Neomycin** moderately decreases the exposure to **sorafenib**. [Moderate] Study

Neostigmine → see TABLE 6 p. 908 (bradycardia)
- Aminoglycosides are predicted to decrease the effects of **neostigmine**. [Moderate] Theoretical

Nepafenac → see NSAIDs

Neratinib → see TABLE 1 p. 907 (hepatotoxicity)
- Oral antacids are predicted to decrease the exposure to oral **neratinib**. Separate administration by at least 3 hours. [Mild] Theoretical
- Antiarrhythmics **(dronedarone)** are predicted to increase the exposure to **neratinib**. Avoid. [Severe] Study
- Antiepileptics **(carbamazepine, fosphenytoin, phenobarbital, phenytoin, primidone)** are predicted to decrease the exposure to **neratinib**. Avoid. [Severe] Study → Also see TABLE 1 p. 907
- Antifungals, azoles **(fluconazole, isavuconazole, posaconazole)** are predicted to increase the exposure to **neratinib**. Avoid. [Severe] Study → Also see TABLE 1 p. 907
- Antifungals, azoles **(itraconazole, ketoconazole, voriconazole)** are predicted to increase the exposure to **neratinib**. Avoid or adjust **neratinib** dose. [Severe] Study → Also see TABLE 1 p. 907
- **Neratinib** is predicted to increase the exposure to antihistamines, non-sedating **(fexofenadine)**. [Moderate] Study
- Apalutamide is predicted to decrease the exposure to **neratinib**. Avoid. [Severe] Study
- Aprepitant is predicted to increase the exposure to **neratinib**. Avoid. [Severe] Study
- Bosentan is predicted to decrease the exposure to **neratinib**. [Severe] Study
- Calcium channel blockers **(diltiazem, verapamil)** are predicted to increase the exposure to **neratinib**. Avoid. [Severe] Study
- Oral calcium salts **(calcium carbonate)** are predicted to decrease the exposure to oral **neratinib**. Separate administration by at least 3 hours. [Mild] Theoretical
- Cobicistat is predicted to increase the exposure to **neratinib**. Avoid or adjust **neratinib** dose. [Severe] Study
- Crizotinib is predicted to increase the exposure to **neratinib**. Avoid. [Severe] Study
- **Neratinib** is predicted to increase the exposure to **dabigatran**. [Moderate] Study
- **Neratinib** is predicted to slightly increase the exposure to digoxin. [Moderate] Study
- **Neratinib** is predicted to increase the exposure to **edoxaban**. [Moderate] Study
- Efavirenz is predicted to decrease the exposure to **neratinib**. [Severe] Study
- Enzalutamide is predicted to decrease the exposure to **neratinib**. Avoid. [Severe] Study
- **Neratinib** is predicted to increase the exposure to **everolimus**. [Moderate] Study
- Grapefruit juice is predicted to increase the exposure to **neratinib**. Avoid. [Severe] Theoretical
- **H_2 receptor antagonists** are predicted to decrease the exposure to **neratinib**. Avoid. [Severe] Theoretical
- HIV-protease inhibitors are predicted to increase the exposure to **neratinib**. Avoid or adjust **neratinib** dose. [Severe] Study
- Idelalisib is predicted to increase the exposure to **neratinib**. Avoid or adjust **neratinib** dose. [Severe] Study
- Imatinib is predicted to increase the exposure to **neratinib**. Avoid. [Severe] Study
- Macrolides **(clarithromycin)** are predicted to increase the exposure to **neratinib**. Avoid or adjust **neratinib** dose. [Severe] Study
- Macrolides **(erythromycin)** are predicted to increase the exposure to **neratinib**. Avoid. [Severe] Study
- Mitotane is predicted to decrease the exposure to **neratinib**. Avoid. [Severe] Study
- Netupitant is predicted to increase the exposure to **neratinib**. Avoid. [Severe] Study
- Nevirapine is predicted to decrease the exposure to **neratinib**. [Severe] Study

- **Nilotinib** is predicted to increase the exposure to **neratinib**. Avoid. Severe Study
- **Proton pump inhibitors** are predicted to decrease the exposure to **neratinib**. Avoid. Severe Study
- **Rifampicin** is predicted to decrease the exposure to **neratinib**. Avoid. Severe Study
- **Neratinib** is predicted to increase the exposure to **sirolimus**. Moderate Study
- **St John's Wort** is predicted to decrease the exposure to **neratinib**. Avoid. Severe Theoretical

Netupitant

- **Netupitant** is predicted to increase the exposure to **abemaciclib**. Moderate Study
- **Netupitant** is predicted to increase the exposure to aldosterone antagonists **(eplerenone)**. Adjust **eplerenone** dose. Severe Study
- **Netupitant** very slightly increases the exposure to alkylating agents **(cyclophosphamide)**. Moderate Study
- **Netupitant** is predicted to increase the exposure to alkylating agents **(ifosfamide)**. Moderate Study
- **Netupitant** is predicted to increase the exposure to alpha blockers **(tamsulosin)**. Moderate Theoretical
- **Netupitant** is predicted to increase the exposure to **alprazolam**. Severe Study
- **Netupitant** is predicted to increase the exposure to antiarrhythmics **(propafenone)**. Monitor and adjust dose. Moderate Study
- Antiepileptics **(carbamazepine, fosphenytoin, phenobarbital, phenytoin, primidone)** are predicted to decrease the exposure to **netupitant**. Avoid. Severe Study
- Antifungals, azoles **(itraconazole, ketoconazole, voriconazole)** are predicted to increase the exposure to **netupitant**. Moderate Study
- **Netupitant** is predicted to decrease the exposure to antifungals, azoles **(isavuconazole)**. Moderate Theoretical
- **Netupitant** is predicted to increase the exposure to antihistamines, non-sedating **(mizolastine)**. Severe Theoretical
- **Netupitant** is predicted to increase the exposure to antihistamines, non-sedating **(rupatadine)**. Avoid. Moderate Study
- **Netupitant** is predicted to increase the concentration of antimalarials **(piperaquine)**. Severe Theoretical
- **Apalutamide** is predicted to decrease the exposure to **netupitant**. Avoid. Severe Study
- **Netupitant** is predicted to increase the exposure to **axitinib**. Moderate Theoretical
- **Netupitant** is predicted to increase the exposure to **bedaquiline**. Avoid prolonged use. Mild Theoretical
- **Netupitant** is predicted to increase the exposure to beta$_2$ agonists **(salmeterol)**. Moderate Study
- **Bosentan** is predicted to decrease the exposure to **netupitant**. Moderate Theoretical
- **Netupitant** is predicted to increase the exposure to **bosutinib**. Avoid or adjust dose. Severe Theoretical
- **Netupitant** is predicted to increase the exposure to **buspirone**. Use with caution and adjust dose. Moderate Study
- **Netupitant** is predicted to increase the exposure to **cabozantinib**. Moderate Theoretical
- **Netupitant** is predicted to increase the exposure to calcium channel blockers **(amlodipine, felodipine, lacidipine, lercanidipine, nicardipine, nifedipine, nimodipine)**. Monitor and adjust dose. Moderate Study
- **Netupitant** is predicted to increase the exposure to **cariprazine**. Avoid. Severe Study
- **Netupitant** is predicted to increase the concentration of **ciclosporin**. Severe Study
- **Cobicistat** is predicted to increase the exposure to **netupitant**. Moderate Study
- **Netupitant** is predicted to increase the exposure to **cobimetinib**. Severe Theoretical
- **Netupitant** is predicted to increase the exposure to **colchicine**. Adjust **colchicine** dose with moderate inhibitors of CYP3A4. Severe Study
- **Netupitant** is predicted to increase the exposure to oral corticosteroids **(budesonide)**. Moderate Study
- **Netupitant** is predicted to increase the exposure to corticosteroids **(dexamethasone)**. Adjust dose. Moderate Study
- **Netupitant** is predicted to increase the exposure to corticosteroids **(fluticasone)**. Moderate Study
- **Netupitant** is predicted to increase the exposure to corticosteroids **(methylprednisolone)**. Monitor and adjust dose. Moderate Study
- **Netupitant** is predicted to slightly increase the exposure to **darifenacin**. Moderate Study
- **Netupitant** is predicted to increase the exposure to **dasatinib**. Severe Study
- **Netupitant** is predicted to slightly increase the exposure to **dienogest**. Moderate Study
- **Netupitant** increases the risk of QT-prolongation when given with **domperidone**. Avoid. Severe Study
- **Netupitant** is predicted to increase the exposure to dopamine receptor agonists **(bromocriptine)**. Severe Theoretical
- **Netupitant** is predicted to increase the concentration of dopamine receptor agonists **(cabergoline)**. Moderate Anecdotal
- **Netupitant** is predicted to moderately increase the exposure to **dutasteride**. Mild Study
- **Efavirenz** is predicted to decrease the exposure to **netupitant**. Moderate Theoretical
- **Netupitant** is predicted to increase the exposure to **eletriptan**. Moderate Study
- **Netupitant** is predicted to increase the exposure to **eliglustat**. Avoid or adjust dose—consult product literature. Severe Study
- **Netupitant** is predicted to moderately increase the exposure to **encorafenib**. Moderate Study
- **Enzalutamide** is predicted to decrease the exposure to **netupitant**. Avoid. Severe Study
- **Netupitant** is predicted to increase the risk of ergotism when given with **ergometrine**. Severe Theoretical
- **Netupitant** is predicted to increase the risk of ergotism when given with **ergotamine**. Severe Theoretical
- **Netupitant** is predicted to increase the exposure to **erlotinib**. Moderate Theoretical
- **Netupitant** slightly increases the exposure to **etoposide**. Moderate Study
- **Netupitant** is predicted to increase the concentration of **everolimus**. Avoid or adjust dose. Moderate Study
- **Netupitant** is predicted to increase the exposure to **fesoterodine**. Adjust **fesoterodine** dose with moderate inhibitors of CYP3A4 in hepatic and renal impairment. Mild Study
- **Netupitant** is predicted to increase the exposure to **gefitinib**. Moderate Theoretical
- **Netupitant** is predicted to increase the concentration of **guanfacine**. Adjust **guanfacine** dose, p. 247. Moderate Theoretical
- **HIV-protease inhibitors** are predicted to increase the exposure to **netupitant**. Moderate Study
- **Netupitant** is predicted to increase the exposure to **ibrutinib**. Adjust **ibrutinib** dose with moderate inhibitors of CYP3A4. Severe Study
- **Idelalisib** is predicted to increase the exposure to **netupitant**. Moderate Study
- **Netupitant** is predicted to increase the exposure to **imatinib**. Moderate Theoretical
- **Netupitant** is predicted to increase the exposure to **irinotecan**. Moderate Study
- **Netupitant** is predicted to increase the exposure to **ivabradine**. Adjust **ivabradine** dose. Severe Theoretical
- **Netupitant** is predicted to increase the exposure to **ivacaftor**. Adjust ivacaftor p. 196 or tezacaftor with ivacaftor p. 198. Severe Study
- **Netupitant** is predicted to increase the exposure to **lapatinib**. Moderate Study
- **Netupitant** is predicted to increase the exposure to **lomitapide**. Avoid. Moderate Theoretical
- **Netupitant** is predicted to increase the exposure to **lurasidone**. Adjust **lurasidone** dose. Moderate Study
- Macrolides **(clarithromycin)** are predicted to increase the exposure to **netupitant**. Moderate Study
- **Netupitant** is predicted to increase the exposure to **maraviroc**. Moderate Study
- **Netupitant** is predicted to increase the exposure to **midazolam**. Monitor side effects and adjust dose. Severe Study

Netupitant (continued)

- **Netupitant** is predicted to increase the exposure to **midostaurin.** Moderate Theoretical
- **Mitotane** is predicted to decrease the exposure to **netupitant.** Avoid. Severe Study
- **Netupitant** is predicted to increase the exposure to **naldemedine.** Moderate Study
- **Netupitant** is predicted to increase the exposure to **naloxegol.** Adjust **naloxegol** dose and monitor side effects. Moderate Study
- **Netupitant** is predicted to increase the exposure to **neratinib.** Avoid. Severe Study
- **Nevirapine** is predicted to decrease the exposure to **netupitant.** Moderate Theoretical
- **Netupitant** is predicted to increase the exposure to **nilotinib.** Moderate Theoretical
- **Netupitant** is predicted to increase the exposure to **olaparib.** Avoid moderate inhibitors of CYP3A4 or adjust **olaparib** dose. Moderate Theoretical
- **Netupitant** is predicted to increase the exposure to opioids **(alfentanil, buprenorphine, fentanyl, oxycodone).** Monitor and adjust dose. Moderate Study
- **Netupitant** is predicted to increase the exposure to opioids **(methadone).** Moderate Theoretical
- **Netupitant** is predicted to increase the exposure to **oxybutynin.** Mild Theoretical
- **Netupitant** is predicted to increase the exposure to **pazopanib.** Moderate Theoretical
- **Netupitant** is predicted to increase the exposure to phosphodiesterase type-5 inhibitors **(avanafil).** Adjust **avanafil** dose. Moderate Theoretical
- **Netupitant** is predicted to increase the exposure to phosphodiesterase type-5 inhibitors **(sildenafil).** Monitor or adjust **sildenafil** dose with moderate inhibitors of CYP3A4, p. 125. Moderate Study
- **Netupitant** is predicted to increase the exposure to phosphodiesterase type-5 inhibitors **(tadalafil).** Severe Theoretical
- **Netupitant** is predicted to increase the exposure to phosphodiesterase type-5 inhibitors **(vardenafil).** Adjust dose. Severe Theoretical
- **Netupitant** is predicted to increase the exposure to **pimozide.** Avoid. Severe Theoretical
- **Netupitant** is predicted to increase the exposure to **quetiapine.** Avoid. Moderate Study
- **Netupitant** is predicted to increase the exposure to **ranolazine.** Severe Study
- **Netupitant** is predicted to increase the exposure to **ribociclib.** Moderate Study
- **Rifampicin** is predicted to decrease the exposure to **netupitant.** Avoid. Severe Study
- **Netupitant** is predicted to increase the exposure to **ruxolitinib.** Moderate Theoretical
- **Netupitant** is predicted to increase the exposure to **saxagliptin.** Mild Study
- **Netupitant** increases the concentration of **sirolimus.** Monitor and adjust dose. Moderate Study
- **Netupitant** is predicted to increase the exposure to SSRIs **(dapoxetine).** Adjust **dapoxetine** dose with moderate inhibitors of CYP3A4. Moderate Theoretical
- **St John's Wort** is predicted to decrease the exposure to **netupitant.** Moderate Theoretical
- **Netupitant** is predicted to increase the exposure to statins **(atorvastatin, simvastatin).** Monitor and adjust dose. Severe Theoretical
- **Netupitant** is predicted to increase the exposure to **sunitinib.** Moderate Theoretical
- **Netupitant** is predicted to increase the concentration of **tacrolimus.** Severe Study
- **Netupitant** is predicted to increase the exposure to taxanes **(cabazitaxel).** Moderate Theoretical
- **Netupitant** slightly increases the exposure to taxanes **(docetaxel).** Moderate Study
- **Netupitant** is predicted to increase the exposure to taxanes **(paclitaxel).** Moderate Study
- **Netupitant** is predicted to increase the concentration of **temsirolimus.** Use with caution or avoid. Moderate Theoretical
- **Netupitant** is predicted to increase the exposure to **tezacaftor.** Adjust tezacaftor with ivacaftor p. 198 dose with moderate inhibitors of CYP3A4. Severe Study
- **Netupitant** given with a potent CYP2C19 inhibitor is predicted to increase the exposure to **tofacitinib.** Adjust **tofacitinib** dose. Moderate Study
- **Netupitant** is predicted to increase the exposure to **tolterodine.** Mild Theoretical
- **Netupitant** is predicted to increase the exposure to **tolvaptan.** Manufacturer advises caution or adjust **tolvaptan** dose with moderate inhibitors of CYP3A4. Moderate Study
- **Netupitant** is predicted to increase the exposure to **trazodone.** Moderate Theoretical
- **Netupitant** is predicted to increase the exposure to **ulipristal.** Avoid if used for uterine fibroids. Moderate Study
- **Netupitant** is predicted to increase the exposure to **venetoclax.** Avoid or adjust dose—consult product literature. Severe Study
- **Netupitant** is predicted to increase the exposure to **vinca alkaloids.** Severe Theoretical
- **Netupitant** is predicted to increase the exposure to **zopiclone.** Adjust dose. Moderate Study

Neuromuscular blocking drugs, non-depolarising → see TABLE 6 p. 908 (bradycardia), TABLE 20 p. 911 (neuromuscular blocking effects)

atracurium · cisatracurium · mivacurium · pancuronium · rocuronium · vecuronium

- **Anticholinesterases, centrally acting** are predicted to decrease the effects of **neuromuscular blocking drugs, non-depolarising.** Moderate Theoretical → Also see TABLE 6 p. 908
- Antiepileptics **(carbamazepine)** are predicted to decrease the effects of (but acute use increases the effects of) neuromuscular blocking drugs, non-depolarising **(atracurium, cisatracurium, pancuronium, rocuronium, vecuronium).** Monitor and adjust dose. Moderate Study
- Antiepileptics **(fosphenytoin, phenytoin)** decrease the effects of (but acute use increases the effects of) neuromuscular blocking drugs, non-depolarising **(atracurium, cisatracurium, pancuronium, rocuronium, vecuronium).** Moderate Study
- **Clindamycin** increases the effects of **neuromuscular blocking drugs, non-depolarising.** Severe Anecdotal
- **Corticosteroids** are predicted to decrease the effects of **neuromuscular blocking drugs, non-depolarising.** Severe Anecdotal
- **Pancuronium** is predicted to increase the risk of cardiovascular side-effects when given with **digoxin.** Severe Anecdotal
- **Irinotecan** is predicted to decrease the effects of **neuromuscular blocking drugs, non-depolarising.** Moderate Theoretical
- Intravenous **magnesium** increases the effects of **neuromuscular blocking drugs, non-depolarising.** Moderate Study
- **Metoclopramide** is predicted to increase the effects of **neuromuscular blocking drugs, non-depolarising.** Moderate Theoretical
- Penicillins **(piperacillin)** increase the effects of **neuromuscular blocking drugs, non-depolarising.** Moderate Study
- **SSRIs** potentially increase the risk of prolonged neuromuscular blockade when given with **mivacurium.** Unknown Theoretical

Nevirapine

- **Nevirapine** is predicted to decrease the exposure to antiarrhythmics **(dronedarone).** Severe Theoretical
- **Nevirapine** is predicted to decrease the concentration of antiepileptics **(carbamazepine, fosphenytoin, phenobarbital, phenytoin, primidone)** and antiepileptics **(carbamazepine, fosphenytoin, phenobarbital, phenytoin, primidone)** are predicted to decrease the concentration of **nevirapine.** Severe Study
- Antifungals, azoles **(fluconazole)** slightly to moderately increase the exposure to **nevirapine.** Moderate Study
- **Nevirapine** is predicted to decrease the exposure to antifungals, azoles **(isavuconazole).** Avoid. Severe Theoretical
- **Nevirapine** moderately decreases the exposure to antifungals, azoles **(itraconazole).** Avoid and for 14 days after stopping **nevirapine.** Moderate Study
- **Nevirapine** moderately decreases the exposure to antifungals, azoles **(ketoconazole).** Avoid. Severe Study

- ▸ **Nevirapine** is predicted to decrease the exposure to antifungals, azoles **(voriconazole)** and antifungals, azoles **(voriconazole)** increase the exposure to **nevirapine**. Monitor and adjust dose. Severe Theoretical
- ▸ **Nevirapine** is predicted to decrease the exposure to **aprepitant**. Moderate Study
- ▸ **Nevirapine** is predicted to decrease the exposure to **axitinib**. Moderate Theoretical
- ▸ **Nevirapine** is predicted to decrease the exposure to **bedaquiline**. Avoid. Severe Study
- ▸ **Bosentan** is predicted to decrease the exposure to **nevirapine**. Severe Theoretical
- ▸ **Nevirapine** is predicted to decrease the exposure to **bosutinib**. Avoid. Severe Theoretical
- ▸ **Nevirapine** is predicted to decrease the exposure to **brigatinib**. Avoid. Severe Study
- ▸ **Nevirapine** is predicted to decrease the exposure to **cabozantinib**. Moderate Theoretical
- ▸ **Nevirapine** is predicted to decrease the exposure to calcium channel blockers **(amlodipine, felodipine, lacidipine, lercanidipine, nicardipine, nifedipine, nimodipine)**. Monitor and adjust dose. Moderate Theoretical
- ▸ **Nevirapine** is predicted to decrease the exposure to calcium channel blockers **(diltiazem, verapamil)**. Moderate Theoretical
- ▸ **Nevirapine** is predicted to decrease the exposure to **cariprazine**. Avoid. Severe Theoretical
- ▸ **Nevirapine** is predicted to decrease the concentration of **caspofungin**. Adjust dose. Moderate Theoretical
- ▸ **Nevirapine** is predicted to decrease the concentration of **ciclosporin**. Moderate Study
- ▸ **Nevirapine** is predicted to decrease the exposure to **cobicistat**. Avoid. Severe Theoretical
- ▸ **Nevirapine** is predicted to decrease the exposure to **cobimetinib**. Avoid. Severe Theoretical
- ▸ **Nevirapine** is predicted to decrease the efficacy of **combined hormonal contraceptives**. For FSRH guidance, see Contraceptives, interactions p. 536. Severe Study
- ▸ **Nevirapine** potentially alters the anticoagulant effect of **coumarins**. Severe Anecdotal
- ▸ **Nevirapine** is predicted to decrease the exposure to **crizotinib**. Avoid. Severe Theoretical
- ▸ **Nevirapine** is predicted to decrease the exposure to **dasabuvir**. Avoid. Severe Theoretical
- ▸ **Nevirapine** is predicted to decrease the exposure to **dasatinib**. Severe Study
- ▸ **Nevirapine** is predicted to decrease the efficacy of **desogestrel**. For FSRH guidance, see Contraceptives, interactions p. 536. Severe Theoretical
- ▸ **Nevirapine** decreases the exposure to **dolutegravir**. Adjust dose. Severe Study
- ▸ **Nevirapine** is predicted to decrease the exposure to **doravirine**. Avoid or adjust doravirine or lamivudine with tenofovir disoproxil and doravirine dose. Severe Theoretical
- ▸ **Nevirapine** decreases the concentration of **efavirenz**. Avoid. Severe Study
- ▸ **Nevirapine** is predicted to moderately decrease the exposure to **elbasvir**. Avoid. Severe Study
- ▸ **Nevirapine** is predicted to decrease the exposure to **eliglustat**. Moderate Theoretical
- ▸ **Nevirapine** is predicted to decrease the concentration of **elvitegravir**. Avoid. Severe Theoretical
- ▸ **Enzalutamide** is predicted to decrease the exposure to **nevirapine**. Severe Theoretical
- ▸ **Nevirapine** is predicted to decrease the effects of **ergotamine**. Moderate Theoretical
- ▸ **Nevirapine** is predicted to decrease the exposure to **erlotinib**. Severe Theoretical
- ▸ **Nevirapine** is predicted to decrease the efficacy of **etonogestrel**. For FSRH guidance, see Contraceptives, interactions p. 536. Severe Theoretical
- ▸ **Nevirapine** is predicted to decrease the exposure to **etravirine**. Avoid. Severe Study
- ▸ **Nevirapine** is predicted to decrease the concentration of **everolimus**. Avoid or adjust dose. Severe Study
- ▸ **Nevirapine** is predicted to decrease the exposure to **fosaprepitant**. Moderate Theoretical
- ▸ **Nevirapine** is predicted to decrease the exposure to **gefitinib**. Avoid. Severe Theoretical
- ▸ **Nevirapine** is predicted to decrease the exposure to **glecaprevir**. Avoid. Severe Study
- ▸ **Nevirapine** is predicted to markedly decrease the exposure to **grazoprevir**. Avoid. Severe Study
- ▸ **Nevirapine** is predicted to decrease the concentration of **guanfacine**. Adjust dose. Moderate Theoretical
- ▸ **Nevirapine** decreases the exposure to **HIV-protease inhibitors**. Refer to specialist literature. Moderate Study
- ▸ **Nevirapine** is predicted to decrease the effects of **hormone replacement therapy**. Moderate Anecdotal
- ▸ **Nevirapine** is predicted to decrease the exposure to **idelalisib**. Avoid. Moderate Theoretical
- ▸ **Nevirapine** is predicted to decrease the exposure to **imatinib**. Moderate Study
- ▸ **Nevirapine** is predicted to decrease the exposure to **ivacaftor**. Moderate Study
- ▸ **Nevirapine** is predicted to decrease the exposure to **lapatinib**. Avoid. Severe Study
- ▸ **Nevirapine** is predicted to decrease the exposure to **larotrectinib**. Avoid. Moderate Study
- ▸ **Nevirapine** is predicted to decrease the efficacy of **levonorgestrel**. For FSRH guidance, see Contraceptives, interactions p. 536. Severe Theoretical
- ▸ **Nevirapine** is predicted to decrease the exposure to **lorlatinib**. Avoid. Severe Theoretical
- ▸ **Nevirapine** is predicted to decrease the exposure to **lurasidone**. Monitor and adjust dose. Moderate Theoretical
- ▸ **Nevirapine** decreases the exposure to macrolides **(clarithromycin)**. Moderate Study
- ▸ **Nevirapine** decreases the concentration of **midazolam**. Monitor and adjust dose. Moderate Study
- ▸ **Mitotane** is predicted to decrease the exposure to **nevirapine**. Severe Theoretical
- ▸ **Nevirapine** is predicted to decrease the exposure to **neratinib**. Severe Study
- ▸ **Nevirapine** is predicted to decrease the exposure to **netupitant**. Moderate Theoretical
- ▸ **Nevirapine** is predicted to decrease the exposure to **nilotinib**. Avoid. Severe Theoretical
- ▸ **Nevirapine** is predicted to decrease the efficacy of **norethisterone**. For FSRH guidance, see Contraceptives, interactions p. 536. Severe Anecdotal
- ▸ **Nevirapine** is predicted to decrease the exposure to **olaparib**. Avoid. Moderate Theoretical
- ▸ **Nevirapine** is predicted to decrease the exposure to **ombitasvir**. Avoid. Severe Theoretical
- ▸ **Nevirapine** decreases the exposure to opioids **(methadone)**. Monitor and adjust dose. Severe Study
- ▸ **Nevirapine** is predicted to decrease the exposure to **osimertinib**. Severe Theoretical
- ▸ **Nevirapine** is predicted to decrease the exposure to **ospemifene**. Moderate Study
- ▸ **Nevirapine** is predicted to decrease the exposure to paritaprevir (with ritonavir and ombitasvir). Avoid. Severe Study
- ▸ **Nevirapine** is predicted to decrease the exposure to **phosphodiesterase type-5 inhibitors**. Moderate Theoretical
- ▸ **Nevirapine** is predicted to decrease the exposure to **pibrentasvir**. Avoid. Severe Study
- ▸ **Nevirapine** is predicted to decrease the exposure to **quetiapine**. Moderate Study
- ▸ **Nevirapine** is predicted to decrease the exposure to **ribociclib**. Moderate Study
- ▸ **Rifampicin** decreases the concentration of **nevirapine**. Avoid. Severe Study
- ▸ **Nevirapine** is predicted to decrease the exposure to **rilpivirine**. Avoid. Severe Theoretical
- ▸ **Nevirapine** is predicted to decrease the exposure to **rolapitant**. Avoid. Severe Study
- ▸ **Nevirapine** is predicted to decrease the exposure to **ruxolitinib**. Monitor and adjust dose. Moderate Theoretical

Nevirapine (continued)

- **Nevirapine** is predicted to decrease the exposure to **siponimod**. Manufacturer advises caution depending on genotype—consult product literature. Severe Theoretical
- **Nevirapine** is predicted to decrease the concentration of **sirolimus**. Monitor and adjust dose. Moderate Theoretical
- **St John's Wort** is predicted to decrease the concentration of **nevirapine**. Avoid. Severe Theoretical
- **Nevirapine** slightly decreases the exposure to statins **(atorvastatin)**. Mild Study
- **Nevirapine** moderately decreases the exposure to statins **(simvastatin)**. Moderate Study
- **Nevirapine** is predicted to decrease the concentration of **tacrolimus**. Monitor and adjust dose. Moderate Theoretical
- **Nevirapine** is predicted to decrease the exposure to taxanes **(cabazitaxel)**. Avoid. Severe Study
- **Nevirapine** is predicted to decrease the concentration of **temsirolimus**. Avoid. Severe Theoretical
- **Nevirapine** is predicted to decrease the exposure to **ticagrelor**. Moderate Theoretical
- **Nevirapine** is predicted to decrease the exposure to **tofacitinib**. Moderate Study
- **Nevirapine** decreases the efficacy of **ulipristal**. For FSRH guidance, see Contraceptives, interactions p. 536. Severe Anecdotal
- **Nevirapine** is predicted to decrease the exposure to **velpatasvir**. Avoid. Moderate Theoretical
- **Nevirapine** is predicted to decrease the exposure to **venetoclax**. Avoid. Severe Study
- **Nevirapine** is predicted to decrease the concentration of **voxilaprevir**. Avoid. Severe Theoretical
- **Nevirapine** is predicted to decrease the concentration of **zidovudine**. Refer to specialist literature. Severe Theoretical

Nicardipine → see calcium channel blockers

Nicorandil → see **TABLE 8** p. 908 (hypotension)

- **Aspirin** is predicted to increase the risk of gastrointestinal perforation when given with **nicorandil**. Severe Theoretical
- **Corticosteroids** increase the risk of gastrointestinal perforation when given with **nicorandil**. Severe Anecdotal
- **Nicorandil** is predicted to increase the risk of gastrointestinal perforation when given with **NSAIDs**. Severe Theoretical
- **Nicorandil** is predicted to increase the risk of hypotension when given with **phosphodiesterase type-5 inhibitors**. Avoid. Severe Theoretical → Also see **TABLE 8** p. 908

Nicotinic acid → see **TABLE 3** p. 907 (anticoagulant effects)

- **Nicotinic acid** is predicted to increase the risk of rhabdomyolysis when given with **statins**. Severe Theoretical

Nifedipine → see calcium channel blockers

Nilotinib → see **TABLE 15** p. 910 (myelosuppression), **TABLE 9** p. 909 (QT-interval prolongation)

- **Nilotinib** is predicted to increase the exposure to **abemaciclib**. Moderate Study
- **Nilotinib** is predicted to increase the exposure to aldosterone antagonists **(eplerenone)**. Adjust **eplerenone** dose. Severe Study
- **Nilotinib** is predicted to increase the exposure to alpha blockers **(tamsulosin)**. Moderate Theoretical
- **Nilotinib** is predicted to increase the exposure to **alprazolam**. Severe Study
- **Antacids** are predicted to decrease the absorption of **nilotinib**. Separate administration by at least 2 hours. Moderate Theoretical
- **Nilotinib** is predicted to increase the exposure to antiarrhythmics **(propafenone)**. Monitor and adjust dose. Moderate Study
- Antiepileptics **(carbamazepine, fosphenytoin, phenobarbital, phenytoin, primidone)** are predicted to moderately decrease the exposure to **nilotinib**. Avoid. Severe Study
- Antifungals, azoles **(fluconazole, posaconazole)** are predicted to increase the exposure to **nilotinib**. Moderate Theoretical → Also see **TABLE 9** p. 909
- Antifungals, azoles **(itraconazole, ketoconazole, voriconazole)** are predicted to moderately increase the exposure to **nilotinib**. Avoid. Severe Study → Also see **TABLE 9** p. 909
- **Nilotinib** is predicted to increase the exposure to antihistamines, non-sedating **(mizolastine)**. Severe Theoretical
- **Nilotinib** is predicted to increase the exposure to antihistamines, non-sedating **(rupatadine)**. Avoid. Moderate Study
- **Nilotinib** is predicted to increase the concentration of antimalarials **(piperaquine)**. Severe Theoretical
- **Apalutamide** is predicted to moderately decrease the exposure to **nilotinib**. Avoid. Severe Study → Also see **TABLE 9** p. 909
- **Aprepitant** is predicted to increase the exposure to **nilotinib**. Moderate Theoretical
- **Nilotinib** is predicted to increase the exposure to **axitinib**. Moderate Theoretical → Also see **TABLE 15** p. 910
- **Nilotinib** is predicted to increase the exposure to **bedaquiline**. Avoid prolonged use. Mild Theoretical → Also see **TABLE 9** p. 909
- **Bosentan** is predicted to decrease the exposure to **nilotinib**. Avoid. Severe Theoretical
- **Nilotinib** is predicted to increase the exposure to **bosutinib**. Avoid or adjust dose. Severe Theoretical → Also see **TABLE 15** p. 910 → Also see **TABLE 9** p. 909
- **Nilotinib** is predicted to increase the exposure to **buspirone**. Use with caution and adjust dose. Moderate Study
- **Nilotinib** is predicted to increase the exposure to **cabozantinib**. Moderate Theoretical → Also see **TABLE 15** p. 910 → Also see **TABLE 9** p. 909
- Calcium channel blockers **(diltiazem, verapamil)** are predicted to increase the exposure to **nilotinib**. Moderate Theoretical
- **Nilotinib** is predicted to increase the exposure to calcium channel blockers **(amlodipine, felodipine, lacidipine, lercanidipine, nicardipine, nifedipine, nimodipine)**. Monitor and adjust dose. Moderate Study
- **Nilotinib** is predicted to increase the exposure to **cariprazine**. Avoid. Severe Study
- **Nilotinib** is predicted to increase the concentration of **ciclosporin**. Severe Study
- **Cobicistat** is predicted to moderately increase the exposure to **nilotinib**. Avoid. Severe Study
- **Nilotinib** is predicted to increase the exposure to **cobimetinib**. Severe Theoretical
- **Nilotinib** is predicted to increase the exposure to **colchicine**. Adjust **colchicine** dose with moderate inhibitors of CYP3A4. Severe Study
- **Nilotinib** is predicted to increase the exposure to corticosteroids **(methylprednisolone)**. Monitor and adjust dose. Moderate Study
- **Nilotinib** is predicted to increase the risk of bleeding events when given with **coumarins**. Severe Theoretical
- **Nilotinib** is predicted to slightly increase the exposure to **darifenacin**. Moderate Study
- **Nilotinib** is predicted to increase the exposure to **dasatinib**. Severe Study → Also see **TABLE 15** p. 910 → Also see **TABLE 9** p. 909
- **Nilotinib** is predicted to slightly increase the exposure to **dienogest**. Moderate Study
- **Nilotinib** increases the risk of QT-prolongation when given with **domperidone**. Avoid. Severe Study
- **Nilotinib** is predicted to increase the exposure to dopamine receptor agonists **(bromocriptine)**. Severe Theoretical
- **Nilotinib** is predicted to increase the concentration of dopamine receptor agonists **(cabergoline)**. Moderate Anecdotal
- **Nilotinib** is predicted to moderately increase the exposure to **dutasteride**. Mild Study
- **Efavirenz** is predicted to decrease the exposure to **nilotinib**. Avoid. Severe Theoretical → Also see **TABLE 9** p. 909
- **Nilotinib** is predicted to increase the exposure to **eliglustat**. Avoid or adjust dose—consult product literature. Severe Study
- **Nilotinib** is predicted to moderately increase the exposure to **encorafenib**. Moderate Study → Also see **TABLE 9** p. 909
- **Enzalutamide** is predicted to moderately decrease the exposure to **nilotinib**. Avoid. Severe Study
- **Nilotinib** is predicted to increase the risk of ergotism when given with **ergometrine**. Severe Theoretical
- **Nilotinib** is predicted to increase the risk of ergotism when given with **ergotamine**. Severe Theoretical
- **Nilotinib** is predicted to increase the exposure to **erlotinib**. Moderate Theoretical
- **Nilotinib** is predicted to increase the concentration of **everolimus**. Avoid or adjust dose. Moderate Study → Also see **TABLE 15** p. 910

A1 Interactions | Appendix 1

- ▸ **Nilotinib** is predicted to increase the exposure to **fesoterodine.** Adjust **fesoterodine** dose with moderate inhibitors of CYP3A4 in hepatic and renal impairment. [Mild] Study
- ▸ **Nilotinib** is predicted to increase the exposure to **gefitinib.** [Moderate] Theoretical → Also see **TABLE 15** p. 910
- ▸ **Grapefruit juice** is predicted to increase the exposure to **nilotinib.** Avoid. [Severe] Theoretical
- ▸ **Nilotinib** is predicted to increase the concentration of **guanfacine.** Adjust **guanfacine** dose, p. 247. [Moderate] Theoretical
- ▸ **H_2 receptor antagonists** are predicted to decrease the absorption of **nilotinib. H_2 receptor antagonists** should be taken 10 hours before or 2 hours after **nilotinib.** [Mild] Theoretical
- ▸ **HIV-protease inhibitors** are predicted to moderately increase the exposure to **nilotinib.** Avoid. [Severe] Study → Also see **TABLE 9** p. 909
- ▸ **Nilotinib** is predicted to increase the exposure to **ibrutinib.** Adjust **ibrutinib** dose with moderate inhibitors of CYP3A4. [Severe] Study → Also see **TABLE 15** p. 910
- ▸ **Idelalisib** is predicted to moderately increase the exposure to **nilotinib.** Avoid. [Severe] Study → Also see **TABLE 15** p. 910
- ▸ **Nilotinib** is predicted to increase the exposure to **ivabradine.** Adjust **ivabradine** dose. [Severe] Theoretical
- ▸ **Nilotinib** is predicted to increase the exposure to **ivacaftor.** Adjust ivacaftor p. 196 or tezacaftor with ivacaftor p. 198 dose with moderate inhibitors of CYP3A4. [Severe] Study
- ▸ **Nilotinib** is predicted to increase the exposure to **lapatinib.** [Moderate] Study → Also see **TABLE 9** p. 909
- ▸ **Nilotinib** is predicted to increase the exposure to **lomitapide.** Avoid. [Moderate] Theoretical
- ▸ **Nilotinib** is predicted to increase the exposure to **lurasidone.** Adjust **lurasidone** dose. [Moderate] Study
- ▸ Macrolides **(clarithromycin)** are predicted to moderately increase the exposure to **nilotinib.** Avoid. [Severe] Study → Also see **TABLE 9** p. 909
- ▸ Macrolides **(erythromycin)** are predicted to increase the exposure to **nilotinib.** [Moderate] Theoretical → Also see **TABLE 9** p. 909
- ▸ **Nilotinib** is predicted to increase the exposure to **midazolam.** Monitor side effects and adjust dose. [Severe] Study
- ▸ **Nilotinib** is predicted to increase the exposure to **midostaurin.** [Moderate] Theoretical
- ▸ **Mitotane** is predicted to moderately decrease the exposure to **nilotinib.** Avoid. [Severe] Study → Also see **TABLE 15** p. 910
- ▸ **Nilotinib** is predicted to increase the exposure to **naldemedine.** [Moderate] Study
- ▸ **Nilotinib** is predicted to increase the exposure to **naloxegol.** Adjust **naloxegol** dose and monitor side effects. [Moderate] Study
- ▸ **Nilotinib** is predicted to increase the exposure to **neratinib.** Avoid. [Severe] Study
- ▸ **Netupitant** is predicted to increase the exposure to **nilotinib.** [Moderate] Theoretical
- ▸ **Nevirapine** is predicted to decrease the exposure to **nilotinib.** Avoid. [Severe] Theoretical
- ▸ **Nilotinib** is predicted to increase the exposure to **olaparib.** Avoid moderate inhibitors of CYP3A4 or adjust **olaparib** dose. [Moderate] Theoretical → Also see **TABLE 15** p. 910
- ▸ **Nilotinib** is predicted to increase the exposure to opioids **(alfentanil, buprenorphine, fentanyl, oxycodone).** Monitor and adjust dose. [Moderate] Study
- ▸ **Nilotinib** is predicted to increase the exposure to opioids **(methadone).** [Moderate] Theoretical → Also see **TABLE 9** p. 909
- ▸ **Nilotinib** is predicted to increase the exposure to **oxybutynin.** [Mild] Theoretical
- ▸ **Nilotinib** is predicted to increase the exposure to **pazopanib.** [Moderate] Theoretical → Also see **TABLE 15** p. 910 → Also see **TABLE 9** p. 909
- ▸ **Nilotinib** is predicted to increase the risk of bleeding events when given with **phenindione.** [Severe] Theoretical
- ▸ **Nilotinib** is predicted to increase the exposure to phosphodiesterase type-5 inhibitors **(avanafil).** Adjust **avanafil** dose. [Moderate] Theoretical
- ▸ **Nilotinib** is predicted to increase the exposure to phosphodiesterase type-5 inhibitors **(sildenafil).** Monitor or adjust **sildenafil** dose with moderate inhibitors of CYP3A4, p. 125. [Moderate] Study → Also see **TABLE 9** p. 909
- ▸ **Nilotinib** is predicted to increase the exposure to phosphodiesterase type-5 inhibitors **(tadalafil).** [Severe] Theoretical
- ▸ **Nilotinib** is predicted to increase the exposure to phosphodiesterase type-5 inhibitors **(vardenafil).** Adjust dose. [Severe] Theoretical → Also see **TABLE 9** p. 909
- ▸ **Nilotinib** is predicted to increase the exposure to **pimozide.** Avoid. [Severe] Theoretical → Also see **TABLE 9** p. 909
- ▸ **Pitolisant** is predicted to decrease the exposure to **nilotinib.** Avoid. [Severe] Theoretical
- ▸ **Nilotinib** is predicted to increase the exposure to **quetiapine.** Avoid. [Moderate] Study
- ▸ **Nilotinib** is predicted to increase the exposure to **ranolazine.** [Severe] Study → Also see **TABLE 9** p. 909
- ▸ **Nilotinib** is predicted to increase the exposure to **ribociclib.** [Moderate] Study → Also see **TABLE 9** p. 909
- ▸ **Rifampicin** is predicted to moderately decrease the exposure to **nilotinib.** Avoid. [Severe] Study
- ▸ **Nilotinib** is predicted to increase the exposure to **ruxolitinib.** [Moderate] Theoretical → Also see **TABLE 15** p. 910
- ▸ **Nilotinib** is predicted to increase the exposure to **saxagliptin.** [Mild] Study
- ▸ **Nilotinib** increases the concentration of **sirolimus.** Monitor and adjust dose. [Moderate] Study
- ▸ **Sodium zirconium cyclosilicate** is predicted to decrease the exposure to **nilotinib.** Separate administration by at least 2 hours. [Moderate] Theoretical
- ▸ **Nilotinib** is predicted to increase the exposure to SSRIs **(dapoxetine).** Adjust **dapoxetine** dose with moderate inhibitors of CYP3A4. [Moderate] Theoretical
- ▸ **St John's Wort** is predicted to decrease the exposure to **nilotinib.** Avoid. [Severe] Theoretical
- ▸ **Nilotinib** is predicted to slightly increase the exposure to statins **(atorvastatin).** Monitor and adjust dose. [Severe] Theoretical
- ▸ **Nilotinib** is predicted to increase the exposure to statins **(simvastatin).** Monitor and adjust dose. [Severe] Theoretical
- ▸ **Nilotinib** is predicted to increase the exposure to **sunitinib.** [Moderate] Theoretical → Also see **TABLE 15** p. 910 → Also see **TABLE 9** p. 909
- ▸ **Nilotinib** is predicted to increase the concentration of **tacrolimus.** [Severe] Study
- ▸ **Nilotinib** is predicted to increase the exposure to taxanes **(cabazitaxel).** [Moderate] Theoretical → Also see **TABLE 15** p. 910
- ▸ **Nilotinib** is predicted to increase the concentration of **temsirolimus.** Use with caution or avoid. [Moderate] Theoretical → Also see **TABLE 15** p. 910
- ▸ **Nilotinib** is predicted to increase the exposure to **tezacaftor.** Adjust tezacaftor with ivacaftor p. 198 dose with moderate inhibitors of CYP3A4. [Severe] Study
- ▸ **Nilotinib** given with a potent CYP2C19 inhibitor is predicted to increase the exposure to **tofacitinib.** Adjust **tofacitinib** dose. [Moderate] Study
- ▸ **Nilotinib** is predicted to increase the exposure to **tolterodine.** [Mild] Theoretical → Also see **TABLE 9** p. 909
- ▸ **Nilotinib** is predicted to increase the exposure to **tolvaptan.** Manufacturer advises caution or adjust **tolvaptan** dose with moderate inhibitors of CYP3A4. [Moderate] Study
- ▸ **Nilotinib** is predicted to increase the exposure to **trazodone.** [Moderate] Theoretical
- ▸ **Nilotinib** is predicted to increase the exposure to **ulipristal.** Avoid if used for uterine fibroids. [Moderate] Study
- ▸ **Nilotinib** is predicted to increase the exposure to **venetoclax.** Avoid or adjust dose—consult product literature. [Severe] Study
- ▸ **Nilotinib** is predicted to increase the exposure to **vinca alkaloids.** [Severe] Theoretical → Also see **TABLE 15** p. 910 → Also see **TABLE 9** p. 909
- ▸ **Nilotinib** is predicted to increase the exposure to **zopiclone.** Adjust dose. [Moderate] Study

Nimodipine → see calcium channel blockers

Nintedanib

- ▸ Antiarrhythmics **(amiodarone, dronedarone)** are predicted to increase the exposure to **nintedanib.** [Moderate] Study
- ▸ Antiepileptics **(carbamazepine)** are predicted to decrease the exposure to **nintedanib.** [Moderate] Study

Nintedanib (continued)

- Antifungals, azoles **(itraconazole, ketoconazole)** are predicted to increase the exposure to **nintedanib.** Moderate Study
- Calcium channel blockers **(verapamil)** are predicted to increase the exposure to **nintedanib.** Moderate Study
- **Ciclosporin** is predicted to increase the exposure to **nintedanib.** Moderate Study
- HIV-protease inhibitors **(lopinavir, ritonavir, saquinavir)** are predicted to increase the exposure to **nintedanib.** Moderate Study
- **Lapatinib** is predicted to increase the exposure to **nintedanib.** Moderate Study
- **Macrolides** are predicted to increase the exposure to **nintedanib.** Moderate Study
- **Ranolazine** is predicted to increase the exposure to **nintedanib.** Moderate Study
- **Rifampicin** is predicted to decrease the exposure to **nintedanib.** Moderate Study
- **St John's Wort** is predicted to decrease the exposure to **nintedanib.** Moderate Study
- **Vemurafenib** is predicted to increase the exposure to **nintedanib.** Moderate Study

Nitisinone

- **Nitisinone** is predicted to increase the exposure to **adefovir.** Moderate Study
- Antiepileptics **(carbamazepine, fosphenytoin, phenobarbital, phenytoin, primidone)** are predicted to decrease the exposure to **nitisinone.** Adjust dose. Moderate Theoretical
- Antifungals, azoles **(itraconazole, ketoconazole, voriconazole)** are predicted to increase the exposure to **nitisinone.** Adjust dose. Moderate Theoretical
- **Apalutamide** is predicted to decrease the exposure to **nitisinone.** Adjust dose. Moderate Theoretical
- **Nitisinone** is predicted to increase the exposure to cephalosporins **(cefaclor).** Moderate Study
- **Cobicistat** is predicted to increase the exposure to **nitisinone.** Adjust dose. Moderate Theoretical
- **Nitisinone** is predicted to increase the exposure to coumarins **(warfarin).** Moderate Study
- **Enzalutamide** is predicted to decrease the exposure to **nitisinone.** Adjust dose. Moderate Theoretical
- **Nitisinone** is predicted to increase the exposure to **ganciclovir.** Moderate Study
- **Nitisinone** is predicted to increase the exposure to H_2 receptor antagonists **(cimetidine, famotidine).** Moderate Study
- **HIV-protease inhibitors** are predicted to increase the exposure to **nitisinone.** Adjust dose. Moderate Theoretical
- **Idelalisib** is predicted to increase the exposure to **nitisinone.** Adjust dose. Moderate Theoretical
- **Nitisinone** is predicted to increase the exposure to loop diuretics **(furosemide).** Moderate Study
- Macrolides **(clarithromycin)** are predicted to increase the exposure to **nitisinone.** Adjust dose. Moderate Theoretical
- **Nitisinone** is predicted to increase the exposure to **methotrexate.** Moderate Study
- **Mitotane** is predicted to decrease the exposure to **nitisinone.** Adjust dose. Moderate Theoretical
- **Nitisinone** is predicted to increase the exposure to NSAIDs **(celecoxib).** Moderate Study
- **Nitisinone** is predicted to increase the exposure to **oseltamivir.** Moderate Study
- **Nitisinone** is predicted to increase the exposure to penicillins **(benzylpenicillin).** Moderate Study
- **Rifampicin** is predicted to decrease the exposure to **nitisinone.** Adjust dose. Moderate Theoretical
- **Nitisinone** is predicted to increase the exposure to sulfonylureas **(glimepiride, tolbutamide).** Moderate Study

Nitrates → see TABLE 7 p. 908 (first-dose hypotension), TABLE 8 p. 908 (hypotension)

glyceryl trinitrate · isosorbide dinitrate · isosorbide mononitrate

PHARMACOLOGY Drugs with antimuscarinic effects can cause dry mouth, which can reduce the effectiveness of sublingual glyceryl trinitrate tablets.

- **Nitrates** are predicted to increase the risk of methaemoglobinaemia when given with topical anaesthetics, local **(prilocaine).** Avoid. Severe Theoretical
- **Nitrates** are predicted to increase the risk of methaemoglobinaemia when given with **dapsone.** Severe Theoretical
- **Nitrates** potentially increase the risk of hypotension when given with **phosphodiesterase type-5 inhibitors.** Avoid. Severe Study → Also see TABLE 8 p. 908

Nitrazepam → see TABLE 11 p. 909 (CNS depressant effects)

- **Rifampicin** increases the clearance of **nitrazepam.** Moderate Study

Nitrofurantoin → see TABLE 12 p. 910 (peripheral neuropathy)

- **Nitrofurantoin** is predicted to increase the risk of methaemoglobinaemia when given with topical anaesthetics, local **(prilocaine).** Use with caution or avoid. Severe Theoretical
- Antacids **(magnesium trisilicate)** decrease the absorption of **nitrofurantoin.** Moderate Study
- **Nitrofurantoin** is predicted to increase the risk of methaemoglobinaemia when given with **dapsone.** Severe Theoretical

Nitroprusside → see TABLE 8 p. 908 (hypotension)

- **Nitroprusside** is predicted to increase the risk of methaemoglobinaemia when given with anaesthetics, local **(prilocaine).** Severe Theoretical
- **Nitroprusside** is predicted to increase the risk of methaemoglobinaemia when given with **dapsone.** Severe Theoretical

Nitrous oxide → see TABLE 8 p. 908 (hypotension), TABLE 11 p. 909 (CNS depressant effects)

- **Nitrous oxide** potentially increases the risk of methotrexate toxicity when given with **methotrexate.** Avoid. Severe Study

Nivolumab → see monoclonal antibodies

Nizatidine → see H_2 receptor antagonists

Noradrenaline/norepinephrine → see sympathomimetics, vasoconstrictor

Norethisterone

- Antiepileptics **(carbamazepine, eslicarbazepine, fosphenytoin, oxcarbazepine, perampanel, phenobarbital, phenytoin, primidone, rufinamide, topiramate)** are predicted to decrease the efficacy of **norethisterone.** For FSRH guidance, see Contraceptives, interactions p. 536. Severe Anecdotal
- **Aprepitant** is predicted to decrease the efficacy of **norethisterone.** For FSRH guidance, see Contraceptives, interactions p. 536. Severe Anecdotal
- **Bosentan** is predicted to decrease the efficacy of **norethisterone.** For FSRH guidance, see Contraceptives, interactions p. 536. Severe Anecdotal
- **Efavirenz** is predicted to decrease the efficacy of **norethisterone.** For FSRH guidance, see Contraceptives, interactions p. 536. Severe Anecdotal
- **Fosaprepitant** is predicted to decrease the efficacy of **norethisterone.** For FSRH guidance, see Contraceptives, interactions p. 536. Severe Anecdotal
- **Griseofulvin** potentially decreases the efficacy of **norethisterone.** For FSRH guidance, see Contraceptives, interactions p. 536. Severe Anecdotal
- HIV-protease inhibitors **(ritonavir)** are predicted to decrease the efficacy of **norethisterone.** For FSRH guidance, see Contraceptives, interactions p. 536. Severe Anecdotal
- **Modafinil** is predicted to decrease the efficacy of **norethisterone.** For FSRH guidance, see Contraceptives, interactions p. 536. Severe Anecdotal
- **Nevirapine** is predicted to decrease the efficacy of **norethisterone.** For FSRH guidance, see Contraceptives, interactions p. 536. Severe Anecdotal
- **Rifabutin** is predicted to decrease the efficacy of **norethisterone.** For FSRH guidance, see Contraceptives, interactions p. 536. Severe Anecdotal
- **Rifampicin** is predicted to decrease the efficacy of **norethisterone.** For FSRH guidance, see Contraceptives, interactions p. 536. Severe Anecdotal
- **St John's Wort** is predicted to decrease the efficacy of **norethisterone.** MHRA advises avoid. For FSRH guidance, see Contraceptives, interactions p. 536. Severe Anecdotal

- ▸ Sugammadex is predicted to decrease the exposure to **norethisterone**. Use additional contraceptive precautions. [Severe] Theoretical
- ▸ Ulipristal is predicted to decrease the efficacy of **norethisterone**. Avoid. [Severe] Theoretical

Normal immunoglobulin → see immunoglobulins

Nortriptyline → see tricyclic antidepressants

NSAIDs → see TABLE 18 p. 911 (hyponatraemia), TABLE 2 p. 907 (nephrotoxicity), TABLE 16 p. 911 (increased serum potassium), TABLE 4 p. 907 (antiplatelet effects)

aceclofenac · benzydamine · bromfenac · celecoxib · dexibuprofen · dexketoprofen · diclofenac · etodolac · etoricoxib · felbinac · flurbiprofen · ibuprofen · indometacin · ketoprofen · ketorolac · mefenamic acid · meloxicam · nabumetone · naproxen · nepafenac · parecoxib · piroxicam · sulindac · tenoxicam · tiaprofenic acid · tolfenamic acid

ROUTE-SPECIFIC INFORMATION Since systemic absorption can follow topical application, the possibility of interactions should be borne in mind.

- ▸ **Celecoxib** is predicted to increase the exposure to antiarrhythmics **(flecainide, propafenone)**. Monitor and adjust dose. [Moderate] Theoretical
- ▸ Antifungals, azoles **(fluconazole)** moderately increase the exposure to **celecoxib**. Adjust **celecoxib** dose. [Moderate] Study
- ▸ Antifungals, azoles **(fluconazole)** increase the exposure to **parecoxib**. Monitor and adjust dose. [Moderate] Study
- ▸ Antifungals, azoles **(voriconazole)** slightly increase the exposure to **diclofenac**. Monitor and adjust dose. [Moderate] Study
- ▸ Antifungals, azoles **(voriconazole)** moderately increase the exposure to **ibuprofen**. Adjust dose. [Moderate] Study
- ▸ **NSAIDs** are predicted to increase the risk of gastrointestinal irritation when given with bisphosphonates **(alendronate, ibandronate)**. [Moderate] Study
- ▸ **NSAIDs** are predicted to increase the risk of renal impairment when given with bisphosphonates **(clodronate)**. [Moderate] Study
- ▸ Ceritinib is predicted to increase the exposure to NSAIDs **(celecoxib, diclofenac)**. Adjust dose. [Moderate] Theoretical
- ▸ Ciclosporin increases the concentration of **diclofenac**. [Severe] Study → Also see TABLE 2 p. 907 → Also see TABLE 16 p. 911
- ▸ **Etoricoxib** slightly increases the exposure to combined hormonal contraceptives. [Moderate] Study
- ▸ **NSAIDs** increase the risk of gastrointestinal bleeding when given with corticosteroids. [Severe] Study
- ▸ **NSAIDs** increase the risk of renal impairment when given with daptomycin. [Moderate] Theoretical
- ▸ **Indometacin** increases the concentration of digoxin. [Severe] Study
- ▸ Erlotinib is predicted to increase the risk of gastrointestinal perforation when given with **NSAIDs**. [Severe] Theoretical
- ▸ **Etoricoxib** slightly increases the exposure to hormone replacement therapy. [Moderate] Study
- ▸ **NSAIDs** are predicted to increase the risk of gastrointestinal bleeding when given with iron chelators **(deferasirox)**. [Severe] Theoretical
- ▸ **Diclofenac** is predicted to increase the exposure to iron chelators **(deferiprone)**. [Moderate] Theoretical
- ▸ Leflunomide is predicted to increase the exposure to NSAIDs **(indometacin, ketoprofen)**. [Moderate] Theoretical
- ▸ **NSAIDs** increase the concentration of lithium. Monitor and adjust dose. [Severe] Study
- ▸ **NSAIDs** are predicted to increase the risk of toxicity when given with methotrexate. [Severe] Study → Also see TABLE 2 p. 907
- ▸ **NSAIDs** (high-dose) are predicted to decrease the efficacy of mifamurtide. Avoid. [Severe] Theoretical
- ▸ Nicorandil is predicted to increase the risk of gastrointestinal perforation when given with **NSAIDs**. [Severe] Theoretical
- ▸ Nitisinone is predicted to increase the exposure to **celecoxib**. [Moderate] Study
- ▸ **NSAIDs** are predicted to increase the exposure to pemetrexed. Use with caution or avoid. [Severe] Theoretical → Also see TABLE 2 p. 907
- ▸ **NSAIDs** potentially increase the risk of seizures when given with quinolones. [Severe] Theoretical
- ▸ Regorafenib is predicted to increase the exposure to **mefenamic acid**. Avoid. [Moderate] Theoretical → Also see TABLE 4 p. 907
- ▸ Rifampicin moderately decreases the exposure to NSAIDs **(celecoxib, diclofenac, etoricoxib)**. [Moderate] Study
- ▸ Teriflunomide is predicted to increase the exposure to NSAIDs **(indometacin, ketoprofen)**. [Moderate] Theoretical
- ▸ **NSAIDs** increase the risk of acute renal failure when given with thiazide diuretics. [Severe] Theoretical → Also see TABLE 18 p. 911
- ▸ Zidovudine increases the risk of haematological toxicity when given with **NSAIDs**. [Severe] Study → Also see TABLE 2 p. 907

Obeticholic acid

- ▸ **Obeticholic acid** decreases the anticoagulant effect of coumarins **(warfarin)**. [Severe] Study
- ▸ **Obeticholic acid** is predicted to increase the exposure to theophylline. [Severe] Theoretical
- ▸ **Obeticholic acid** is predicted to increase the exposure to tizanidine. [Severe] Theoretical

Obinutuzumab → see monoclonal antibodies

Ocrelizumab → see monoclonal antibodies

Octreotide

- ▸ **Octreotide** decreases the absorption of oral ciclosporin. Adjust ciclosporin dose, p. 559. [Severe] Anecdotal
- ▸ **Octreotide** (short-acting) decreases the exposure to telotristat ethyl. **Telotristat ethyl** should be taken at least 30 minutes before **octreotide**. [Moderate] Study

Ofloxacin → see quinolones

Olanzapine → see TABLE 8 p. 908 (hypotension), TABLE 15 p. 910 (myelosuppression), TABLE 11 p. 909 (CNS depressant effects)

FOOD AND LIFESTYLE Dose adjustment might be necessary if smoking started or stopped during treatment.

- ▸ Antiepileptics **(carbamazepine)** potentially decrease the exposure to **olanzapine**. Monitor and adjust dose. [Moderate] Study
- ▸ Antiepileptics **(phenytoin)** are predicted to decrease the exposure to **olanzapine**. Monitor and adjust dose. [Moderate] Study
- ▸ **Olanzapine** is predicted to decrease the effects of dopamine receptor agonists. Avoid. [Moderate] Theoretical → Also see TABLE 8 p. 908
- ▸ HIV-protease inhibitors **(ritonavir)** are predicted to decrease the exposure to **olanzapine**. Monitor and adjust dose. [Moderate] Study
- ▸ **Leflunomide** is predicted to decrease the exposure to **olanzapine**. Monitor and adjust dose. [Moderate] Study → Also see TABLE 15 p. 910
- ▸ **Olanzapine** decreases the effects of levodopa. Avoid or monitor worsening parkinsonian symptoms. [Severe] Anecdotal → Also see TABLE 8 p. 908
- ▸ Mexiletine is predicted to increase the exposure to **olanzapine**. Adjust dose. [Moderate] Anecdotal
- ▸ Quinolones **(ciprofloxacin)** are predicted to increase the exposure to **olanzapine**. Adjust dose. [Moderate] Anecdotal
- ▸ Rifampicin is predicted to decrease the exposure to **olanzapine**. Monitor and adjust dose. [Moderate] Study
- ▸ SSRIs **(fluvoxamine)** moderately increase the exposure to **olanzapine**. Adjust dose. [Severe] Anecdotal
- ▸ Teriflunomide is predicted to decrease the exposure to **olanzapine**. Monitor and adjust dose. [Moderate] Study

Olaparib → see TABLE 15 p. 910 (myelosuppression)

FOOD AND LIFESTYLE Bitter (Seville) orange is predicted to increase the exposure to olaparib.

- ▸ Antiarrhythmics **(dronedarone)** are predicted to increase the exposure to **olaparib**. Avoid moderate inhibitors of CYP3A4 or adjust **olaparib** dose. [Moderate] Theoretical
- ▸ Antiepileptics **(carbamazepine, fosphenytoin, phenobarbital, phenytoin, primidone)** are predicted to decrease the exposure to **olaparib**. Avoid. [Moderate] Theoretical
- ▸ Antifungals, azoles **(fluconazole, isavuconazole, posaconazole)** are predicted to increase the exposure to **olaparib**. Avoid moderate inhibitors of CYP3A4 or adjust **olaparib** dose. [Moderate] Theoretical

Olaparib (continued)
- Antifungals, azoles (**itraconazole, ketoconazole, voriconazole**) are predicted to increase the exposure to **olaparib**. Avoid potent inhibitors of CYP3A4 or adjust **olaparib** dose. Moderate Study
- Apalutamide is predicted to decrease the exposure to **olaparib**. Avoid. Moderate Theoretical
- Aprepitant is predicted to increase the exposure to **olaparib**. Avoid moderate inhibitors of CYP3A4 or adjust **olaparib** dose. Moderate Theoretical
- Bosentan is predicted to decrease the exposure to **olaparib**. Avoid. Moderate Theoretical
- Calcium channel blockers (**diltiazem, verapamil**) are predicted to increase the exposure to **olaparib**. Avoid moderate inhibitors of CYP3A4 or adjust **olaparib** dose. Moderate Theoretical
- Cobicistat is predicted to increase the exposure to **olaparib**. Avoid potent inhibitors of CYP3A4 or adjust **olaparib** dose. Moderate Study
- **Olaparib** potentially affects the efficacy of combined hormonal contraceptives. Use additional contraceptive precautions. Moderate Theoretical
- Crizotinib is predicted to increase the exposure to **olaparib**. Avoid moderate inhibitors of CYP3A4 or adjust **olaparib** dose. Moderate Theoretical → Also see **TABLE 15** p. 910
- Efavirenz is predicted to decrease the exposure to **olaparib**. Avoid. Moderate Theoretical
- Enzalutamide is predicted to decrease the exposure to **olaparib**. Avoid. Moderate Theoretical
- Grapefruit juice is predicted to increase the exposure to **olaparib**. Avoid. Moderate Theoretical
- HIV-protease inhibitors are predicted to increase the exposure to **olaparib**. Avoid potent inhibitors of CYP3A4 or adjust **olaparib** dose. Moderate Study
- Idelalisib is predicted to increase the exposure to **olaparib**. Avoid potent inhibitors of CYP3A4 or adjust **olaparib** dose. Moderate Study → Also see **TABLE 15** p. 910
- Imatinib is predicted to increase the exposure to **olaparib**. Avoid moderate inhibitors of CYP3A4 or adjust **olaparib** dose. Moderate Theoretical → Also see **TABLE 15** p. 910
- Macrolides (**clarithromycin**) are predicted to increase the exposure to **olaparib**. Avoid potent inhibitors of CYP3A4 or adjust **olaparib** dose. Moderate Study
- Macrolides (**erythromycin**) are predicted to increase the exposure to **olaparib**. Avoid moderate inhibitors of CYP3A4 or adjust **olaparib** dose. Moderate Theoretical
- Mitotane is predicted to decrease the exposure to **olaparib**. Avoid. Moderate Theoretical → Also see **TABLE 15** p. 910
- Netupitant is predicted to increase the exposure to **olaparib**. Avoid moderate inhibitors of CYP3A4 or adjust **olaparib** dose. Moderate Theoretical
- Nevirapine is predicted to decrease the exposure to **olaparib**. Avoid. Moderate Theoretical
- Nilotinib is predicted to increase the exposure to **olaparib**. Avoid moderate inhibitors of CYP3A4 or adjust **olaparib** dose. Moderate Theoretical → Also see **TABLE 15** p. 910
- Rifampicin is predicted to decrease the exposure to **olaparib**. Avoid. Moderate Theoretical
- St John's Wort is predicted to decrease the exposure to **olaparib**. Avoid. Moderate Theoretical

Olmesartan → see angiotensin-II receptor antagonists

Olodaterol → see beta$_2$ agonists

Olsalazine → see **TABLE 15** p. 910 (myelosuppression)

Ombitasvir
- Antiepileptics (**carbamazepine, fosphenytoin, phenobarbital, phenytoin**) are predicted to decrease the exposure to **ombitasvir**. Avoid. Severe Theoretical
- Efavirenz is predicted to decrease the exposure to **ombitasvir**. Avoid. Severe Theoretical
- Enzalutamide is predicted to decrease the exposure to **ombitasvir**. Avoid. Severe Theoretical
- Etravirine is predicted to decrease the exposure to **ombitasvir**. Avoid. Severe Theoretical
- **Ombitasvir** (in fixed-dose combination with dasabuvir) decreases the concentration of HIV-protease inhibitors (**darunavir**). Avoid or adjust dose. Moderate Study
- Mitotane is predicted to decrease the exposure to **ombitasvir**. Avoid. Severe Theoretical
- Nevirapine is predicted to decrease the exposure to **ombitasvir**. Avoid. Severe Theoretical
- Rifampicin is predicted to decrease the exposure to **ombitasvir**. Avoid. Severe Theoretical
- St John's Wort is predicted to decrease the exposure to **ombitasvir**. Avoid. Severe Theoretical

Omega-3-acid ethyl esters → see **TABLE 3** p. 907 (anticoagulant effects)

Omeprazole → see proton pump inhibitors

Ondansetron → see **TABLE 13** p. 910 (serotonin syndrome), **TABLE 9** p. 909 (QT-interval prolongation)
- Antiepileptics (**carbamazepine, fosphenytoin, phenobarbital, phenytoin, primidone**) are predicted to decrease the exposure to **ondansetron**. Moderate Study
- Apalutamide is predicted to decrease the exposure to **ondansetron**. Moderate Study → Also see **TABLE 9** p. 909
- Dopamine receptor agonists (**apomorphine**) increase the risk of severe hypotension when given with **ondansetron**. Avoid. Severe Study → Also see **TABLE 9** p. 909
- Enzalutamide is predicted to decrease the exposure to **ondansetron**. Moderate Study
- Mitotane is predicted to decrease the exposure to **ondansetron**. Moderate Study
- Rifampicin is predicted to decrease the exposure to **ondansetron**. Moderate Study

Opicapone
- **Opicapone** increases the exposure to **levodopa**. Adjust dose. Moderate Study
- **Opicapone** is predicted to increase the exposure to **loperamide**. Avoid. Moderate Study
- **Opicapone** is predicted to increase the risk of elevated blood pressure when given with **MAOIs**, irreversible. Avoid. Severe Theoretical
- **Opicapone** is predicted to increase the risk of elevated blood pressure when given with **moclobemide**. Avoid. Severe Theoretical
- **Opicapone** is predicted to increase the exposure to **montelukast**. Avoid. Moderate Study
- **Opicapone** is predicted to increase the exposure to **pioglitazone**. Avoid. Moderate Study
- **Opicapone** is predicted to increase the exposure to **repaglinide**. Avoid. Moderate Study
- **Opicapone** is predicted to increase the risk of cardiovascular side-effects when given with **sympathomimetics, inotropic**. Severe Theoretical
- **Opicapone** is predicted to increase the risk of cardiovascular side-effects when given with sympathomimetics, vasoconstrictor (**adrenaline/epinephrine, noradrenaline/norepinephrine**). Severe Theoretical

Opioids → see **TABLE 6** p. 908 (bradycardia), **TABLE 13** p. 910 (serotonin syndrome), **TABLE 9** p. 909 (QT-interval prolongation), **TABLE 11** p. 909 (CNS depressant effects)

alfentanil · buprenorphine · codeine · diamorphine · dihydrocodeine · diphenoxylate · dipipanone · fentanyl · hydromorphone · meptazinol · methadone · morphine · oxycodone · pentazocine · pethidine · remifentanil · tapentadol · tramadol

- Alcohol (beverage) causes rapid release of opioids (**hydromorphone, morphine**) (from extended-release preparations). Avoid. Severe Study → Also see **TABLE 11** p. 909
- Antiarrhythmics (**amiodarone**) are predicted to increase the concentration of **fentanyl**. Moderate Theoretical → Also see **TABLE 6** p. 908
- Antiarrhythmics (**dronedarone**) are predicted to increase the exposure to **methadone**. Moderate Theoretical → Also see **TABLE 9** p. 909
- Antiarrhythmics (**dronedarone**) are predicted to increase the exposure to opioids (**alfentanil, buprenorphine, fentanyl, oxycodone**). Monitor and adjust dose. Moderate Study
- Antiepileptics (**carbamazepine**) decrease the concentration of **tramadol**. Adjust dose. Severe Study
- Antiepileptics (**carbamazepine, fosphenytoin, phenobarbital, phenytoin, primidone**) are predicted to decrease the exposure

to **buprenorphine**. Monitor and adjust dose. Moderate Theoretical → Also see **TABLE 11** p. 909
- Antiepileptics **(carbamazepine, fosphenytoin, phenobarbital, phenytoin, primidone)** decrease the exposure to **methadone**. Monitor and adjust dose. Severe Study → Also see **TABLE 11** p. 909
- Antiepileptics **(carbamazepine, fosphenytoin, phenobarbital, phenytoin, primidone)** are predicted to decrease the exposure to **oxycodone**. Monitor and adjust dose. Moderate Study → Also see **TABLE 11** p. 909
- Antiepileptics **(carbamazepine, fosphenytoin, phenobarbital, phenytoin, primidone)** are predicted to decrease the exposure to opioids **(alfentanil, fentanyl)**. Moderate Study → Also see **TABLE 11** p. 909
- Antifungals, azoles **(fluconazole, isavuconazole, posaconazole)** are predicted to increase the exposure to **methadone**. Moderate Theoretical → Also see **TABLE 9** p. 909
- Antifungals, azoles **(itraconazole, ketoconazole, voriconazole)** are predicted to increase the exposure to **methadone**. Adjust dose. Severe Theoretical → Also see **TABLE 9** p. 909
- Antifungals, azoles **(miconazole)** are predicted to increase the exposure to **alfentanil**. Use with caution and adjust dose. Moderate Theoretical
- Antifungals, azoles **(fluconazole, isavuconazole, posaconazole)** are predicted to increase the exposure to opioids **(alfentanil, buprenorphine, fentanyl, oxycodone)**. Monitor and adjust dose. Moderate Study
- Antifungals, azoles **(itraconazole, ketoconazole, voriconazole)** are predicted to increase the exposure to opioids **(alfentanil, buprenorphine, fentanyl, oxycodone)**. Monitor and adjust dose. Severe Study
- **Apalutamide** is predicted to decrease the exposure to **buprenorphine**. Monitor and adjust dose. Moderate Theoretical
- **Apalutamide** decreases the exposure to **methadone**. Monitor and adjust dose. Severe Study → Also see **TABLE 9** p. 909
- **Apalutamide** is predicted to decrease the exposure to opioids **(alfentanil, fentanyl)**. Moderate Study
- **Apalutamide** is predicted to decrease the exposure to **oxycodone**. Monitor and adjust dose. Moderate Study
- **Aprepitant** is predicted to increase the exposure to **methadone**. Moderate Theoretical
- **Aprepitant** is predicted to increase the exposure to opioids **(alfentanil, buprenorphine, fentanyl, oxycodone)**. Monitor and adjust dose. Moderate Study
- **Bictegravir** is predicted to increase the exposure to **methadone**. Moderate Theoretical
- **Bosentan** decreases the exposure to **methadone**. Monitor and adjust dose. Severe Study
- **Brigatinib** potentially decreases the concentration of opioids **(alfentanil, fentanyl)**. Avoid. Moderate Theoretical
- **Bupropion** is predicted to decrease the efficacy of **codeine**. Moderate Theoretical
- **Bupropion** is predicted to decrease the efficacy of **tramadol**. Severe Study → Also see **TABLE 13** p. 910
- Calcium channel blockers **(diltiazem, verapamil)** are predicted to increase the exposure to **methadone**. Moderate Theoretical → Also see **TABLE 6** p. 908
- Calcium channel blockers **(diltiazem, verapamil)** are predicted to increase the exposure to opioids **(alfentanil, buprenorphine, fentanyl, oxycodone)**. Monitor and adjust dose. Moderate Study → Also see **TABLE 6** p. 908
- **Ceritinib** is predicted to increase the exposure to opioids **(alfentanil, fentanyl)**. Avoid. Severe Theoretical
- **Cinacalcet** is predicted to decrease the efficacy of **codeine**. Moderate Theoretical
- **Cinacalcet** is predicted to decrease the efficacy of **tramadol**. Severe Study
- **Cobicistat** is predicted to increase the exposure to opioids **(alfentanil, buprenorphine, fentanyl, oxycodone)**. Monitor and adjust dose. Severe Study
- **Crizotinib** is predicted to increase the exposure to **methadone**. Moderate Theoretical → Also see **TABLE 6** p. 908 → Also see **TABLE 9** p. 909
- **Crizotinib** is predicted to increase the exposure to opioids **(alfentanil, buprenorphine, fentanyl, oxycodone)**. Monitor and adjust dose. Moderate Study → Also see **TABLE 6** p. 908
- **Efavirenz** decreases the exposure to **methadone**. Monitor and adjust dose. Severe Study → Also see **TABLE 9** p. 909
- **Enzalutamide** is predicted to decrease the exposure to **buprenorphine**. Monitor and adjust dose. Moderate Theoretical
- **Enzalutamide** decreases the exposure to **methadone**. Monitor and adjust dose. Severe Study
- **Enzalutamide** is predicted to decrease the exposure to opioids **(alfentanil, fentanyl)**. Moderate Study
- **Enzalutamide** is predicted to decrease the exposure to **oxycodone**. Monitor and adjust dose. Moderate Study
- H_2 receptor antagonists **(cimetidine)** increase the concentration of **alfentanil**. Use with caution and adjust dose. Severe Study
- H_2 receptor antagonists **(cimetidine)** increase the exposure to **fentanyl**. Moderate Study
- **HIV-protease inhibitors** boosted with ritonavir are predicted to decrease the exposure to **methadone**. Moderate Study → Also see **TABLE 9** p. 909
- HIV-protease inhibitors **(ritonavir)** are predicted to decrease the concentration of **morphine**. Moderate Theoretical
- HIV-protease inhibitors **(ritonavir)** increase the risk of CNS toxicity when given with **pethidine**. Avoid. Severe Study
- **HIV-protease inhibitors** are predicted to increase the exposure to opioids **(alfentanil, buprenorphine, fentanyl, oxycodone)**. Monitor and adjust dose. Severe Study
- **Idelalisib** is predicted to increase the exposure to **methadone**. Severe Theoretical
- **Idelalisib** is predicted to increase the exposure to opioids **(alfentanil, buprenorphine, fentanyl, oxycodone)**. Monitor and adjust dose. Severe Study
- **Imatinib** is predicted to increase the exposure to **methadone**. Moderate Theoretical
- **Imatinib** is predicted to increase the exposure to opioids **(alfentanil, buprenorphine, fentanyl, oxycodone)**. Monitor and adjust dose. Moderate Study
- **Larotrectinib** is predicted to increase the exposure to opioids **(alfentanil, fentanyl)**. Use with caution and adjust dose. Mild Theoretical
- **Letermovir** is predicted to increase the exposure to opioids **(alfentanil, fentanyl)**. Monitor and adjust dose. Moderate Study
- **Lorlatinib** is predicted to decrease the exposure to opioids **(alfentanil, fentanyl)**. Avoid. Moderate Theoretical
- Macrolides **(clarithromycin)** are predicted to increase the concentration of **methadone**. Severe Theoretical → Also see **TABLE 9** p. 909
- Macrolides **(erythromycin)** are predicted to increase the exposure to **methadone**. Moderate Theoretical → Also see **TABLE 9** p. 909
- Macrolides **(clarithromycin)** are predicted to increase the exposure to opioids **(alfentanil, buprenorphine, fentanyl, oxycodone)**. Monitor and adjust dose. Severe Study
- Macrolides **(erythromycin)** are predicted to increase the exposure to opioids **(alfentanil, buprenorphine, fentanyl, oxycodone)**. Monitor and adjust dose. Moderate Study
- MAO-B inhibitors **(rasagiline)** are predicted to increase the risk of side-effects when given with **pethidine**. Avoid and for 14 days after stopping **rasagiline**. Severe Theoretical → Also see **TABLE 13** p. 910
- MAO-B inhibitors **(safinamide)** are predicted to increase the risk of side-effects when given with **pethidine**. Avoid and for 1 week after stopping **safinamide**. Severe Theoretical → Also see **TABLE 13** p. 910
- MAO-B inhibitors **(selegiline)** increase the risk of side-effects when given with **pethidine**. Avoid. Severe Anecdotal → Also see **TABLE 13** p. 910
- **Opioids** are predicted to increase the risk of CNS excitation or depression when given with **MAOIs, irreversible**. Avoid. Severe Study → Also see **TABLE 13** p. 910
- **Opioids** potentially decrease the absorption of oral mexiletine. Moderate Study
- **Mitotane** is predicted to decrease the exposure to **buprenorphine**. Monitor and adjust dose. Moderate Theoretical
- **Mitotane** decreases the exposure to **methadone**. Monitor and adjust dose. Severe Study
- **Mitotane** is predicted to decrease the exposure to opioids **(alfentanil, fentanyl)**. Moderate Study

A1

Interactions | **Appendix 1**

Opioids (continued)

- ▸ **Mitotane** is predicted to decrease the exposure to **oxycodone**. Monitor and adjust dose. Moderate Study
- ▸ **Nalmefene** is predicted to decrease the efficacy of **opioids**. Avoid. Severe Theoretical
- ▸ **Netupitant** is predicted to increase the exposure to **methadone**. Moderate Theoretical
- ▸ **Netupitant** is predicted to increase the exposure to opioids **(alfentanil, buprenorphine, fentanyl, oxycodone)**. Monitor and adjust dose. Moderate Study
- ▸ **Nevirapine** decreases the exposure to **methadone**. Monitor and adjust dose. Severe Study
- ▸ **Nilotinib** is predicted to increase the exposure to **methadone**. Moderate Theoretical → Also see TABLE 9 p. 909
- ▸ **Nilotinib** is predicted to increase the exposure to opioids **(alfentanil, buprenorphine, fentanyl, oxycodone)**. Monitor and adjust dose. Moderate Study
- ▸ Opioids **(buprenorphine)** are predicted to increase the risk of opiate withdrawal when given with opioids **(alfentanil)**. Severe Theoretical → Also see TABLE 11 p. 909
- ▸ Opioids **(pentazocine)** are predicted to increase the risk of opiate withdrawal when given with opioids **(alfentanil, codeine, diamorphine, dihydrocodeine, dipipanone, fentanyl, hydromorphone, meptazinol, methadone, morphine, oxycodone)**. Severe Theoretical → Also see TABLE 13 p. 910 → Also see TABLE 11 p. 909
- ▸ Opioids **(buprenorphine)** are predicted to increase the risk of opiate withdrawal when given with opioids **(codeine, diamorphine, dihydrocodeine, dipipanone, fentanyl, hydromorphone, meptazinol, methadone, morphine, oxycodone, pentazocine, pethidine, remifentanil, tapentadol, tramadol)**. Severe Theoretical → Also see TABLE 11 p. 909
- ▸ Opioids **(pentazocine)** are predicted to increase the risk of opiate withdrawal when given with opioids **(pethidine, remifentanil, tapentadol, tramadol)**. Severe Theoretical → Also see TABLE 13 p. 910 → Also see TABLE 11 p. 909
- ▸ **Palbociclib** is predicted to increase the exposure to opioids **(alfentanil, fentanyl)**. Adjust dose. Moderate Theoretical
- ▸ **Pitolisant** is predicted to decrease the exposure to **morphine**. Mild Theoretical
- ▸ **Ribociclib** is predicted to increase the exposure to opioids **(alfentanil, fentanyl)**. Use with caution and adjust dose. Moderate Theoretical
- ▸ **Rifampicin** is predicted to decrease the exposure to **buprenorphine**. Monitor and adjust dose. Moderate Theoretical
- ▸ **Rifampicin** decreases the exposure to **methadone**. Monitor and adjust dose. Severe Study
- ▸ **Rifampicin** is predicted to decrease the exposure to opioids **(alfentanil, fentanyl)**. Moderate Study
- ▸ **Rifampicin** decreases the exposure to opioids **(codeine, morphine)**. Moderate Study
- ▸ **Rifampicin** is predicted to decrease the exposure to **oxycodone**. Monitor and adjust dose. Moderate Study
- ▸ **Rucaparib** is predicted to increase the exposure to opioids **(alfentanil, fentanyl)**. Monitor and adjust dose. Moderate Study
- ▸ SSRIs **(fluoxetine, paroxetine)** are predicted to decrease the efficacy of **codeine**. Moderate Theoretical
- ▸ SSRIs **(fluoxetine, paroxetine)** are predicted to decrease the efficacy of **tramadol**. Severe Study → Also see TABLE 13 p. 910
- ▸ **St John's Wort** decreases the exposure to **methadone**. Monitor and adjust dose. Severe Study → Also see TABLE 13 p. 910
- ▸ **St John's Wort** moderately decreases the exposure to **oxycodone**. Adjust dose. Moderate Study
- ▸ **Terbinafine** is predicted to decrease the efficacy of **codeine**. Moderate Theoretical
- ▸ **Terbinafine** is predicted to decrease the efficacy of **tramadol**. Severe Study

Orlistat

SEPARATION OF ADMINISTRATION Orlistat might affect the absorption of concurrently administered drugs—consider separating administration. Particular care should be taken with antiepileptics, antiretrovirals, and drugs that have a narrow therapeutic index.

Orphenadrine → see TABLE 10 p. 909 (antimuscarinics)

Oseltamivir

- ▸ **Leflunomide** is predicted to increase the exposure to **oseltamivir**. Moderate Theoretical
- ▸ **Nitisinone** is predicted to increase the exposure to **oseltamivir**. Moderate Study
- ▸ **Teriflunomide** is predicted to increase the exposure to **oseltamivir**. Moderate Study

Osimertinib → see TABLE 9 p. 909 (QT-interval prolongation)

- ▸ Antiepileptics **(carbamazepine, fosphenytoin, phenobarbital, phenytoin, primidone)** are predicted to moderately decrease the exposure to **osimertinib**. Avoid. Moderate Study
- ▸ **Apalutamide** is predicted to moderately decrease the exposure to **osimertinib**. Avoid. Moderate Study → Also see TABLE 9 p. 909
- ▸ **Bosentan** is predicted to decrease the exposure to **osimertinib**. Moderate Theoretical
- ▸ **Efavirenz** is predicted to decrease the exposure to **osimertinib**. Moderate Theoretical → Also see TABLE 9 p. 909
- ▸ **Enzalutamide** is predicted to moderately decrease the exposure to **osimertinib**. Avoid. Moderate Study
- ▸ **Mitotane** is predicted to moderately decrease the exposure to **osimertinib**. Avoid. Moderate Study
- ▸ **Nevirapine** is predicted to decrease the exposure to **osimertinib**. Severe Theoretical
- ▸ **Rifampicin** is predicted to moderately decrease the exposure to **osimertinib**. Avoid. Moderate Study
- ▸ **St John's Wort** is predicted to decrease the exposure to **osimertinib**. Avoid. Moderate Theoretical
- ▸ **Osimertinib** slightly increases the exposure to statins **(rosuvastatin)**. Moderate Study

Ospemifene

- ▸ Antiepileptics **(carbamazepine, fosphenytoin, phenobarbital, phenytoin, primidone)** are predicted to moderately decrease the exposure to **ospemifene**. Moderate Study
- ▸ Antifungals, azoles **(fluconazole)** increase the exposure to **ospemifene**. Use with caution or avoid. Moderate Study
- ▸ Antifungals, azoles **(itraconazole, ketoconazole, voriconazole)** are predicted to increase the exposure to **ospemifene**. Avoid in poor CYP2C9 metabolisers. Moderate Study
- ▸ **Apalutamide** is predicted to moderately decrease the exposure to **ospemifene**. Moderate Study
- ▸ **Bosentan** is predicted to decrease the exposure to **ospemifene**. Moderate Study
- ▸ **Cobicistat** is predicted to increase the exposure to **ospemifene**. Avoid in poor CYP2C9 metabolisers. Moderate Study
- ▸ **Combined hormonal contraceptives** potentially oppose the effects of **ospemifene**. Avoid. Severe Theoretical
- ▸ **Efavirenz** is predicted to decrease the exposure to **ospemifene**. Moderate Study
- ▸ **Enzalutamide** is predicted to moderately decrease the exposure to **ospemifene**. Moderate Study
- ▸ **HIV-protease inhibitors** are predicted to increase the exposure to **ospemifene**. Avoid in poor CYP2C9 metabolisers. Moderate Study
- ▸ **Hormone replacement therapy** potentially opposes the effects of **ospemifene**. Avoid. Severe Theoretical
- ▸ **Idelalisib** is predicted to increase the exposure to **ospemifene**. Avoid in poor CYP2C9 metabolisers. Moderate Study
- ▸ Macrolides **(clarithromycin)** are predicted to increase the exposure to **ospemifene**. Avoid in poor CYP2C9 metabolisers. Moderate Study
- ▸ **Mitotane** is predicted to moderately decrease the exposure to **ospemifene**. Moderate Study
- ▸ **Nevirapine** is predicted to decrease the exposure to **ospemifene**. Moderate Study
- ▸ **Rifampicin** is predicted to moderately decrease the exposure to **ospemifene**. Moderate Study
- ▸ **St John's Wort** is predicted to decrease the exposure to **ospemifene**. Moderate Study

Oxaliplatin → see platinum compounds

Oxazepam → see TABLE 11 p. 909 (CNS depressant effects)

Oxcarbazepine → see antiepileptics

Oxybuprocaine → see anaesthetics, local

Oxybutynin → see TABLE 10 p. 909 (antimuscarinics)

- ▸ Antiarrhythmics **(dronedarone)** are predicted to increase the exposure to **oxybutynin**. Mild Theoretical

- **Oxybutynin** potentially increases the risk of overheating and dehydration when given with antiepileptics **(zonisamide)**. Avoid in children. Severe Theoretical
- Antifungals, azoles **(fluconazole, isavuconazole, posaconazole)** are predicted to increase the exposure to **oxybutynin**. Mild Theoretical
- Antifungals, azoles **(itraconazole, ketoconazole, voriconazole)** are predicted to increase the exposure to **oxybutynin**. Mild Study
- **Aprepitant** is predicted to increase the exposure to **oxybutynin**. Mild Theoretical
- Calcium channel blockers **(diltiazem, verapamil)** are predicted to increase the exposure to **oxybutynin**. Mild Theoretical
- **Cobicistat** is predicted to increase the exposure to **oxybutynin**. Mild Study
- **Crizotinib** is predicted to increase the exposure to **oxybutynin**. Mild Theoretical
- **HIV-protease inhibitors** are predicted to increase the exposure to **oxybutynin**. Mild Study
- **Idelalisib** is predicted to increase the exposure to **oxybutynin**. Mild Study
- **Imatinib** is predicted to increase the exposure to **oxybutynin**. Mild Theoretical
- Macrolides **(clarithromycin)** are predicted to increase the exposure to **oxybutynin**. Mild Study
- Macrolides **(erythromycin)** are predicted to increase the exposure to **oxybutynin**. Mild Theoretical
- **Netupitant** is predicted to increase the exposure to **oxybutynin**. Mild Theoretical
- **Nilotinib** is predicted to increase the exposure to **oxybutynin**. Mild Theoretical

Oxycodone → see opioids

Oxymetholone

- **Oxymetholone** increases the anticoagulant effect of **coumarins**. Severe Anecdotal
- **Oxymetholone** increases the anticoagulant effect of **phenindione**. Severe Anecdotal

Oxytetracycline → see tetracyclines

Paclitaxel → see taxanes

Palbociclib

- Antiepileptics **(carbamazepine, fosphenytoin, phenobarbital, phenytoin, primidone)** are predicted to decrease the exposure to **palbociclib**. Avoid. Severe Study
- Antifungals, azoles **(itraconazole, ketoconazole, voriconazole)** are predicted to increase the exposure to **palbociclib**. Avoid or adjust **palbociclib** dose. Severe Study
- **Apalutamide** is predicted to decrease the exposure to **palbociclib**. Avoid. Severe Study
- **Palbociclib** is predicted to increase the exposure to **ciclosporin**. Adjust dose. Moderate Theoretical
- **Cobicistat** is predicted to increase the exposure to **palbociclib**. Avoid or adjust **palbociclib** dose. Severe Study
- **Enzalutamide** is predicted to decrease the exposure to **palbociclib**. Avoid. Severe Study
- **Palbociclib** is predicted to increase the exposure to **ergotamine**. Adjust dose. Moderate Theoretical
- **Palbociclib** is predicted to increase the exposure to **everolimus**. Adjust dose. Moderate Theoretical
- **Grapefruit juice** is predicted to increase the exposure to **palbociclib**. Avoid. Severe Theoretical
- **HIV-protease inhibitors** are predicted to increase the exposure to **palbociclib**. Avoid or adjust **palbociclib** dose. Severe Study
- **Idelalisib** is predicted to increase the exposure to **palbociclib**. Avoid or adjust **palbociclib** dose. Severe Study
- Macrolides **(clarithromycin)** are predicted to increase the exposure to **palbociclib**. Avoid or adjust **palbociclib** dose. Severe Study
- **Palbociclib** increases the exposure to **midazolam**. Moderate Study
- **Mitotane** is predicted to decrease the exposure to **palbociclib**. Avoid. Severe Study
- **Palbociclib** is predicted to increase the exposure to opioids **(alfentanil, fentanyl)**. Adjust dose. Moderate Theoretical
- **Palbociclib** is predicted to increase the exposure to **pimozide**. Adjust dose. Moderate Theoretical
- **Rifampicin** is predicted to decrease the exposure to **palbociclib**. Avoid. Severe Study
- **Palbociclib** is predicted to increase the exposure to **sirolimus**. Adjust dose. Moderate Theoretical
- **St John's Wort** is predicted to decrease the exposure to **palbociclib**. Avoid. Severe Theoretical
- **Palbociclib** is predicted to increase the exposure to **tacrolimus**. Adjust dose. Moderate Theoretical

Paliperidone → see TABLE 8 p. 908 (hypotension), TABLE 9 p. 909 (QT-interval prolongation), TABLE 11 p. 909 (CNS depressant effects)

- Antiepileptics **(carbamazepine, fosphenytoin, phenobarbital, phenytoin, primidone)** are predicted to decrease the exposure to **paliperidone**. Monitor and adjust dose. Severe Study → Also see TABLE 11 p. 909
- Antiepileptics **(valproate)** slightly increase the exposure to **paliperidone**. Adjust dose. Moderate Study
- **Apalutamide** is predicted to decrease the exposure to **paliperidone**. Monitor and adjust dose. Severe Study → Also see TABLE 9 p. 909
- **Paliperidone** is predicted to decrease the effects of **dopamine receptor agonists**. Avoid. Moderate Theoretical → Also see TABLE 8 p. 908 → Also see TABLE 9 p. 909
- **Enzalutamide** is predicted to decrease the exposure to **paliperidone**. Monitor and adjust dose. Severe Study
- **Paliperidone** is predicted to decrease the effects of **levodopa**. Severe Theoretical → Also see TABLE 8 p. 908
- **Methylphenidate** increases the risk of dyskinesias when given with **paliperidone**. Severe Theoretical
- **Mitotane** is predicted to decrease the exposure to **paliperidone**. Monitor and adjust dose. Severe Study
- **Rifampicin** is predicted to decrease the exposure to **paliperidone**. Monitor and adjust dose. Severe Study
- **St John's Wort** is predicted to decrease the exposure to **paliperidone**. Severe Theoretical

Palonosetron → see TABLE 9 p. 909 (QT-interval prolongation), TABLE 13 p. 910 (serotonin syndrome)

- Dopamine receptor agonists **(apomorphine)** are predicted to increase the risk of severe hypotension when given with **palonosetron**. Severe Theoretical

Pamidronate → see bisphosphonates

Pancreatin

- **Pancreatin** is predicted to decrease the effects of **acarbose**. Avoid. Moderate Theoretical

Pancuronium → see neuromuscular blocking drugs, non-depolarising

Panitumumab → see monoclonal antibodies

Panobinostat → see TABLE 15 p. 910 (myelosuppression), TABLE 9 p. 909 (QT-interval prolongation)

FOOD AND LIFESTYLE Avoid pomegranate, pomegranate juice, and star fruit as they are predicted to increase panobinostat exposure.

- Antiarrhythmics **(amiodarone, dronedarone)** are predicted to increase the exposure to **panobinostat**. Adjust dose. Moderate Theoretical → Also see TABLE 9 p. 909
- Antiepileptics **(carbamazepine, fosphenytoin, phenobarbital, phenytoin, primidone)** are predicted to decrease the exposure to **panobinostat**. Avoid. Moderate Theoretical
- Antifungals, azoles **(itraconazole, ketoconazole, voriconazole)** are predicted to increase the exposure to **panobinostat**. Adjust **panobinostat** dose; in hepatic impairment avoid. Moderate Study → Also see TABLE 9 p. 909
- Antifungals, azoles **(posaconazole)** are predicted to increase the exposure to **panobinostat**. Adjust dose. Moderate Theoretical
- **Apalutamide** is predicted to decrease the exposure to **panobinostat**. Avoid. Moderate Theoretical → Also see TABLE 9 p. 909
- **Panobinostat** is predicted to increase the exposure to **atomoxetine**. Monitor and adjust dose. Severe Theoretical
- **Panobinostat** is predicted to increase the exposure to beta blockers, selective **(metoprolol)**. Monitor and adjust dose. Moderate Theoretical
- **Panobinostat** is predicted to increase the exposure to beta blockers, selective **(nebivolol)**. Monitor and adjust dose. Mild Theoretical
- Calcium channel blockers **(verapamil)** are predicted to increase the exposure to **panobinostat**. Adjust dose. Moderate Theoretical

Panobinostat (continued)
- **Ciclosporin** is predicted to increase the exposure to **panobinostat**. Adjust dose. Moderate Theoretical
- **Cobicistat** is predicted to increase the exposure to **panobinostat**. Adjust **panobinostat** dose; in hepatic impairment avoid. Moderate Study
- **Enzalutamide** is predicted to decrease the exposure to **panobinostat**. Avoid. Moderate Theoretical
- **HIV-protease inhibitors** are predicted to increase the exposure to **panobinostat**. Adjust **panobinostat** dose; in hepatic impairment avoid. Moderate Study → Also see TABLE 9 p. 909
- **Idelalisib** is predicted to increase the exposure to **panobinostat**. Adjust **panobinostat** dose; in hepatic impairment avoid. Moderate Study → Also see TABLE 15 p. 910
- **Lapatinib** is predicted to increase the exposure to **panobinostat**. Adjust dose. Moderate Theoretical → Also see TABLE 9 p. 909
- Macrolides **(azithromycin, erythromycin)** are predicted to increase the exposure to **panobinostat**. Adjust dose. Moderate Theoretical → Also see TABLE 9 p. 909
- Macrolides **(clarithromycin)** are predicted to increase the exposure to **panobinostat**. Adjust **panobinostat** dose; in hepatic impairment avoid. Moderate Study → Also see TABLE 9 p. 909
- **Mitotane** is predicted to decrease the exposure to **panobinostat**. Avoid. Moderate Theoretical → Also see TABLE 15 p. 910
- **Panobinostat** is predicted to increase the exposure to **pimozide**. Avoid. Severe Theoretical → Also see TABLE 9 p. 909
- **Ranolazine** is predicted to increase the exposure to **panobinostat**. Adjust dose. Moderate Theoretical → Also see TABLE 9 p. 909
- **Rifampicin** is predicted to decrease the exposure to **panobinostat**. Avoid. Moderate Theoretical
- **St John's Wort** is predicted to decrease the exposure to **panobinostat**. Avoid. Moderate Theoretical
- **Vemurafenib** is predicted to increase the exposure to **panobinostat**. Adjust dose. Moderate Theoretical → Also see TABLE 9 p. 909

Pantoprazole → see proton pump inhibitors

Paracetamol → see TABLE 1 p. 907 (hepatotoxicity)
- **Alcohol (beverage)**(in those who drink heavily) causes severe liver damage when given with **paracetamol**. Severe Study → Also see TABLE 1 p. 907
- **Paracetamol** is predicted to decrease the clearance of alkylating agents **(busulfan)**. Moderate Theoretical
- **Paracetamol** is predicted to increase the risk of methaemoglobinaemia when given with topical anaesthetics, local **(prilocaine)**. Use with caution or avoid. Severe Theoretical
- Antiepileptics **(carbamazepine, fosphenytoin, phenobarbital, phenytoin, primidone)** decrease the exposure to **paracetamol**. Moderate Study → Also see TABLE 1 p. 907
- **Paracetamol** increases the anticoagulant effect of **coumarins**. Moderate Study
- **Paracetamol** is predicted to increase the risk of methaemoglobinaemia when given with **dapsone**. Severe Theoretical
- **Imatinib** increases the risk of hepatotoxicity when given with **paracetamol**. Severe Anecdotal
- **Paracetamol** potentially increases the risk of high anion gap metabolic acidosis when given with penicillins **(flucloxacillin)**. Severe Theoretical → Also see TABLE 1 p. 907
- **Paracetamol** is predicted to increase the anticoagulant effect of **phenindione**. Severe Theoretical
- **Pitolisant** is predicted to decrease the exposure to **paracetamol**. Mild Theoretical
- **Rifampicin** decreases the exposure to **paracetamol**. Moderate Study

Paraldehyde → see antiepileptics

Parathyroid hormone
- **Bisphosphonates** are predicted to decrease the effects of **parathyroid hormone**. Avoid. Moderate Study

Parecoxib → see NSAIDs

Paricalcitol → see vitamin D substances

Paritaprevir
- **Paritaprevir** (with ritonavir and ombitasvir) is predicted to increase the exposure to **aliskiren**. Moderate Study
- Antiepileptics **(carbamazepine, fosphenytoin, phenobarbital, phenytoin, primidone)** are predicted to decrease the exposure to **paritaprevir** (with ritonavir and ombitasvir). Avoid. Severe Study
- Antifungals, azoles **(itraconazole, ketoconazole, voriconazole)** are predicted to increase the exposure to **paritaprevir**. Avoid. Severe Study
- Antifungals, azoles **(posaconazole)** are predicted to increase the exposure to **paritaprevir** (with ritonavir and ombitasvir) and **paritaprevir** (with ritonavir and ombitasvir) is predicted to increase the exposure to antifungals, azoles **(posaconazole)**. Avoid. Severe Study
- **Apalutamide** is predicted to decrease the exposure to **paritaprevir** (with ritonavir and ombitasvir). Avoid. Severe Study
- **Bosentan** is predicted to decrease the exposure to **paritaprevir** (with ritonavir and ombitasvir). Avoid. Severe Study
- **Cobicistat** is predicted to increase the exposure to **paritaprevir**. Avoid. Severe Study
- **Combined hormonal contraceptives** (containing ethinylestradiol) are predicted to increase the risk of increased ALT concentrations when given with **paritaprevir** (with ritonavir and ombitasvir). Avoid. Severe Study
- **Paritaprevir** (in fixed-dose combination with dasabuvir) decreases the anticoagulant effect of coumarins **(acenocoumarol)**. Monitor INR and adjust dose. Severe Anecdotal
- **Paritaprevir** (in fixed-dose combination) decreases the anticoagulant effect of coumarins **(warfarin)**. Monitor INR and adjust dose. Severe Anecdotal
- **Paritaprevir** (with ritonavir and ombitasvir) is predicted to increase the exposure to **dabigatran**. Severe Study
- **Paritaprevir** (with ritonavir and ombitasvir) increases the exposure to digoxin. Monitor and adjust **digoxin** dose, p. 86. Moderate Study
- **Paritaprevir** (with ritonavir and ombitasvir) is predicted to increase the exposure to **edoxaban**. Severe Study
- **Efavirenz** is predicted to decrease the exposure to **paritaprevir** (with ritonavir and ombitasvir). Avoid. Severe Study
- **Enzalutamide** is predicted to decrease the exposure to **paritaprevir** (with ritonavir and ombitasvir). Avoid. Severe Study
- **Etravirine** is predicted to decrease the exposure to **paritaprevir**. Avoid. Severe Theoretical
- HIV-protease inhibitors **(atazanavir)** boosted with ritonavir markedly increase the exposure to **paritaprevir**. Avoid or give unboosted. Moderate Study
- HIV-protease inhibitors **(darunavir)** boosted with ritonavir slightly decrease the exposure to **paritaprevir**. Avoid or give unboosted. Moderate Study
- HIV-protease inhibitors **(fosamprenavir, tipranavir)** boosted with ritonavir are predicted to increase the exposure to **paritaprevir**. Avoid. Severe Study
- HIV-protease inhibitors **(lopinavir)** boosted with ritonavir moderately to markedly increase the exposure to **paritaprevir**. Avoid. Severe Study
- HIV-protease inhibitors **(saquinavir)** are predicted to increase the exposure to **paritaprevir** (in fixed-dose combination). Avoid. Severe Study
- **Paritaprevir** is predicted to increase the exposure to **idelalisib**. Avoid. Severe Study
- **Paritaprevir** (with ritonavir and ombitasvir) is predicted to increase the exposure to loop diuretics **(furosemide)**. Adjust dose. Moderate Theoretical
- **Paritaprevir** (with ritonavir and ombitasvir) is predicted to increase the exposure to **loperamide**. Moderate Study
- Macrolides **(clarithromycin)** are predicted to increase the exposure to **paritaprevir**. Avoid. Severe Study
- Macrolides **(erythromycin)** are predicted to increase the exposure to **paritaprevir**. Moderate Theoretical
- **Mitotane** is predicted to decrease the exposure to **paritaprevir** (with ritonavir and ombitasvir). Avoid. Severe Study

A1 Interactions | **Appendix 1**

- Nevirapine is predicted to decrease the exposure to **paritaprevir** (with ritonavir and ombitasvir). Avoid. Severe Study
- Rifampicin is predicted to decrease the exposure to **paritaprevir** (with ritonavir and ombitasvir). Avoid. Severe Study
- St John's Wort is predicted to decrease the exposure to **paritaprevir** (with ritonavir and ombitasvir). Avoid. Severe Study
- **Paritaprevir** (in fixed-dose combination) is predicted to increase the risk of rhabdomyolysis when given with statins (atorvastatin). Avoid. Severe Theoretical
- **Paritaprevir** (with ritonavir and ombitasvir) is predicted to increase the exposure to statins (fluvastatin). Avoid. Moderate Theoretical
- **Paritaprevir** (with ritonavir and ombitasvir) increases the exposure to statins (pravastatin). Adjust **pravastatin** dose. Moderate Study
- **Paritaprevir** (with ritonavir and ombitasvir) slightly to moderately increases the exposure to statins (rosuvastatin). Adjust **rosuvastatin** dose, p. 140. Moderate Study
- **Paritaprevir** (in fixed-dose combination) is predicted to increase the risk of rhabdomyolysis when given with statins (simvastatin). Avoid. Severe Theoretical
- **Paritaprevir** (with ritonavir and ombitasvir) is predicted to increase the exposure to taxanes (paclitaxel). Moderate Study
- **Paritaprevir** (with ritonavir and ombitasvir) is predicted to increase the exposure to thyroid hormones (levothyroxine). Monitor and adjust dose. Moderate Theoretical
- **Paritaprevir** (with ritonavir and ombitasvir) is predicted to increase the exposure to topotecan. Moderate Study

Paroxetine → see SSRIs

Pasireotide → see TABLE 6 p. 908 (bradycardia), TABLE 9 p. 909 (QT-interval prolongation)

- **Pasireotide** is predicted to decrease the absorption of oral ciclosporin. Adjust dose. Severe Theoretical

Patiromer

SEPARATION OF ADMINISTRATION Manufacturer advises take 3 hours before, or after, other drugs.

Pazopanib → see TABLE 15 p. 910 (myelosuppression), TABLE 9 p. 909 (QT-interval prolongation)

- Antacids are predicted to decrease the absorption of **pazopanib**. **Pazopanib** should be taken 1 hour before or 2 hours after antacids. Moderate Theoretical
- Antiarrhythmics (dronedarone) are predicted to increase the exposure to **pazopanib**. Moderate Theoretical → Also see TABLE 9 p. 909
- Antiepileptics (carbamazepine, fosphenytoin, phenobarbital, phenytoin, primidone) are predicted to decrease the exposure to **pazopanib**. Avoid. Severe Theoretical
- Antifungals, azoles (fluconazole, isavuconazole, posaconazole) are predicted to increase the exposure to **pazopanib**. Moderate Theoretical → Also see TABLE 9 p. 909
- Antifungals, azoles (itraconazole, ketoconazole, voriconazole) are predicted to increase the exposure to **pazopanib**. Avoid or adjust **pazopanib** dose. Moderate Study → Also see TABLE 9 p. 909
- Apalutamide is predicted to decrease the exposure to **pazopanib**. Avoid. Severe Theoretical → Also see TABLE 9 p. 909
- Aprepitant is predicted to increase the exposure to **pazopanib**. Moderate Theoretical
- Calcium channel blockers (diltiazem, verapamil) are predicted to increase the exposure to **pazopanib**. Moderate Theoretical
- Cobicistat is predicted to increase the exposure to **pazopanib**. Avoid or adjust **pazopanib** dose. Moderate Study
- **Pazopanib** is predicted to increase the risk of bleeding events when given with coumarins. Severe Theoretical
- Crizotinib is predicted to increase the exposure to **pazopanib**. Moderate Theoretical → Also see TABLE 15 p. 910 → Also see TABLE 9 p. 909
- Enzalutamide is predicted to decrease the exposure to **pazopanib**. Avoid. Severe Theoretical
- Grapefruit juice is predicted to increase the exposure to **pazopanib**. Avoid. Severe Theoretical
- H_2 receptor antagonists are predicted to decrease the exposure to **pazopanib**. **H_2 receptor antagonists** should be taken 10 hours before or 2 hours after **pazopanib**. Moderate Theoretical
- HIV-protease inhibitors are predicted to increase the exposure to **pazopanib**. Avoid or adjust **pazopanib** dose. Moderate Study → Also see TABLE 9 p. 909
- Idelalisib is predicted to increase the exposure to **pazopanib**. Avoid or adjust **pazopanib** dose. Moderate Study → Also see TABLE 15 p. 910
- Imatinib is predicted to increase the exposure to **pazopanib**. Moderate Theoretical → Also see TABLE 15 p. 910
- **Pazopanib** is predicted to increase the exposure to **lomitapide**. Separate administration by 12 hours. Moderate Theoretical
- Macrolides (clarithromycin) are predicted to increase the exposure to **pazopanib**. Avoid or adjust **pazopanib** dose. Moderate Study → Also see TABLE 9 p. 909
- Macrolides (erythromycin) are predicted to increase the exposure to **pazopanib**. Moderate Theoretical → Also see TABLE 9 p. 909
- Mitotane is predicted to decrease the exposure to **pazopanib**. Avoid. Severe Theoretical → Also see TABLE 15 p. 910
- Netupitant is predicted to increase the exposure to **pazopanib**. Moderate Theoretical
- Nilotinib is predicted to increase the exposure to **pazopanib**. Moderate Theoretical → Also see TABLE 15 p. 910 → Also see TABLE 9 p. 909
- **Pazopanib** is predicted to increase the risk of bleeding events when given with phenindione. Severe Theoretical
- Proton pump inhibitors are predicted to decrease the exposure to **pazopanib**. Avoid or administer concurrently without food. Moderate Study
- Rifampicin is predicted to decrease the exposure to **pazopanib**. Avoid. Severe Theoretical
- **Pazopanib** is predicted to affect the exposure to statins (atorvastatin). Moderate Anecdotal
- **Pazopanib** is predicted to affect the exposure to statins (pravastatin, rosuvastatin, simvastatin). Moderate Theoretical

Pegaspargase → see TABLE 1 p. 907 (hepatotoxicity), TABLE 15 p. 910 (myelosuppression)

- **Pegaspargase** is predicted to increase the risk of hepatotoxicity when given with **imatinib**. Severe Theoretical → Also see TABLE 15 p. 910
- **Pegaspargase** affects the efficacy of **methotrexate**. Severe Anecdotal → Also see TABLE 1 p. 907 → Also see TABLE 15 p. 910
- **Pegaspargase** potentially increases the risk of neurotoxicity when given with vinca alkaloids (vincristine). **Vincristine** should be taken 3 to 24 hours before **pegaspargase**. Severe Anecdotal → Also see TABLE 1 p. 907 → Also see TABLE 15 p. 910

Peginterferon alfa → see interferons

Peginterferon beta → see TABLE 15 p. 910 (myelosuppression)

Pembrolizumab → see monoclonal antibodies

Pemetrexed → see TABLE 15 p. 910 (myelosuppression), TABLE 2 p. 907 (nephrotoxicity)

- Antimalarials (pyrimethamine) are predicted to increase the risk of side-effects when given with **pemetrexed**. Severe Theoretical → Also see TABLE 15 p. 910
- Aspirin (high-dose) potentially increases the exposure to **pemetrexed**. Use with caution or avoid. Severe Theoretical
- Live vaccines are predicted to increase the risk of generalised infection (possibly life-threatening) when given with **pemetrexed**. Public Health England advises avoid (refer to Green Book). Severe Theoretical
- NSAIDs are predicted to increase the exposure to **pemetrexed**. Use with caution or avoid. Severe Theoretical → Also see TABLE 2 p. 907

Penicillamine → see TABLE 2 p. 907 (nephrotoxicity)

- Antacids decrease the absorption of **penicillamine**. Separate administration by 2 hours. Mild Study
- Antimalarials (chloroquine) are predicted to increase the risk of haematological toxicity when given with **penicillamine**. Avoid. Severe Theoretical
- **Penicillamine** potentially decreases the concentration of digoxin. Separate administration by 2 hours. Severe Anecdotal

Interactions | **Appendix 1** A1

Penicillamine (continued)
- **Hydroxychloroquine** is predicted to increase the risk of haematological toxicity when given with **penicillamine**. Avoid. [Severe] Theoretical
- **Iron (oral)** is predicted to decrease the absorption of **penicillamine**. Separate administration by at least 2 hours. [Mild] Study
- **Sodium aurothiomalate** potentially increases the risk of side-effects when given with **penicillamine** (in those who have had previous adverse reactions to gold). Avoid. [Severe] Study
- **Zinc** is predicted to decrease the absorption of **penicillamine**. [Mild] Theoretical

Penicillins → see TABLE 1 p. 907 (hepatotoxicity)

amoxicillin · ampicillin · benzathine benzylpenicillin · benzylpenicillin · flucloxacillin · phenoxymethylpenicillin · piperacillin · pivmecillinam · temocillin · ticarcillin

- **Allopurinol** increases the risk of skin rash when given with penicillins **(amoxicillin, ampicillin)**. [Moderate] Study
- Antiepileptics **(valproate)** increase the risk of side-effects when given with **pivmecillinam**. Avoid. [Severe] Anecdotal
- **Penicillins** potentially alter the anticoagulant effect of coumarins. Monitor INR and adjust dose. [Severe] Anecdotal
- **Leflunomide** is predicted to increase the exposure to **benzylpenicillin**. [Moderate] Theoretical
- **Penicillins** are predicted to increase the risk of toxicity when given with methotrexate. [Severe] Anecdotal → Also see TABLE 1 p. 907
- **Piperacillin** increases the effects of neuromuscular blocking drugs, non-depolarising. [Moderate] Study
- **Nitisinone** is predicted to increase the exposure to **benzylpenicillin**. [Moderate] Study
- **Paracetamol** potentially increases the risk of high anion gap metabolic acidosis when given with **flucloxacillin**. [Severe] Theoretical → Also see TABLE 1 p. 907
- **Penicillins** are predicted to increase the risk of bleeding events when given with phenindione. [Severe] Theoretical
- **Piperacillin** increases the effects of suxamethonium. [Moderate] Study
- **Teriflunomide** is predicted to increase the exposure to **benzylpenicillin**. [Moderate] Study

Pentamidine → see TABLE 9 p. 909 (QT-interval prolongation), TABLE 15 p. 910 (myelosuppression), TABLE 2 p. 907 (nephrotoxicity)
- **Foscarnet** increases the risk of hypocalcaemia when given with **pentamidine**. [Severe] Anecdotal → Also see TABLE 2 p. 907

Pentazocine → see opioids

Pentostatin → see TABLE 15 p. 910 (myelosuppression), TABLE 5 p. 907 (thromboembolism)
- Alkylating agents **(cyclophosphamide)** (high-dose) increase the risk of toxicity when given with **pentostatin**. Avoid. [Severe] Anecdotal → Also see TABLE 15 p. 910 → Also see TABLE 5 p. 907
- **Fludarabine** increases the risk of pulmonary toxicity when given with **pentostatin**. Avoid. [Severe] Study → Also see TABLE 15 p. 910

Pentoxifylline
- **Pentoxifylline** is predicted to increase the concentration of aminophylline. Use with caution or avoid. [Severe] Theoretical
- Quinolones **(ciprofloxacin)** very slightly increase the exposure to **pentoxifylline**. [Moderate] Study
- SSRIs **(fluvoxamine)** are predicted to increase the exposure to **pentoxifylline**. [Moderate] Theoretical
- **Pentoxifylline** increases the concentration of **theophylline**. Monitor and adjust dose. [Severe] Study

Peppermint
- **Peppermint** oil is predicted to increase the exposure to lomitapide. Separate administration by 12 hours. [Moderate] Theoretical

Perampanel → see antiepileptics

Pergolide → see dopamine receptor agonists

Pericyazine → see phenothiazines

Perindopril → see ACE inhibitors

Pertuzumab → see monoclonal antibodies

Pethidine → see opioids

Phenelzine → see MAOIs, irreversible

Phenindione → see TABLE 3 p. 907 (anticoagulant effects)

FOOD AND LIFESTYLE The effects of phenindione can be reduced or abolished by vitamin K, including that found in health foods, food supplements, enteral feeds, or large amounts of some green vegetables or green tea. Major changes in diet (especially involving salads and vegetables) and in alcohol consumption can affect anticoagulant control.

- Antiarrhythmics **(propafenone)** are predicted to increase the anticoagulant effect of **phenindione**. Monitor and adjust dose. [Moderate] Theoretical
- Antifungals, azoles **(miconazole)** greatly increase the anticoagulant effect of **phenindione**. [Severe] Theoretical
- **Axitinib** is predicted to increase the risk of bleeding events when given with **phenindione**. [Severe] Theoretical
- **Bosutinib** is predicted to increase the risk of bleeding events when given with **phenindione**. [Severe] Theoretical
- **Cabozantinib** is predicted to increase the risk of bleeding events when given with **phenindione**. [Severe] Theoretical
- Cephalosporins **(ceftriaxone)** potentially increase the risk of bleeding events when given with **phenindione**. [Severe] Anecdotal
- **Corticosteroids** are predicted to increase the effects of **phenindione**. [Moderate] Anecdotal
- **Crizotinib** is predicted to increase the risk of bleeding events when given with **phenindione**. [Severe] Theoretical
- **Dasatinib** is predicted to increase the risk of bleeding events when given with **phenindione**. [Severe] Theoretical
- **Disulfiram** is predicted to increase the anticoagulant effect of **phenindione**. [Severe] Theoretical
- **Enteral feeds (vitamin-K containing)** potentially decrease the effects of **phenindione**. [Severe] Theoretical
- **Erlotinib** is predicted to increase the risk of bleeding events when given with **phenindione**. [Severe] Theoretical
- **Fibrates** are predicted to increase the anticoagulant effect of **phenindione**. Monitor INR and adjust dose. [Severe] Study
- **Gefitinib** is predicted to increase the risk of bleeding events when given with **phenindione**. [Severe] Theoretical
- H_2 receptor antagonists **(cimetidine)** increase the exposure to **phenindione**. [Severe] Anecdotal
- **Imatinib** is predicted to increase the risk of bleeding events when given with **phenindione**. [Severe] Theoretical
- **Lapatinib** is predicted to increase the risk of bleeding events when given with **phenindione**. [Severe] Theoretical
- **Nandrolone** is predicted to increase the anticoagulant effect of **phenindione**. Monitor and adjust dose. [Severe] Theoretical
- **Nilotinib** is predicted to increase the risk of bleeding events when given with **phenindione**. [Severe] Theoretical
- **Oxymetholone** increases the anticoagulant effect of **phenindione**. [Severe] Anecdotal
- **Paracetamol** is predicted to increase the anticoagulant effect of **phenindione**. [Severe] Theoretical
- **Pazopanib** is predicted to increase the risk of bleeding events when given with **phenindione**. [Severe] Theoretical
- **Penicillins** are predicted to increase the risk of bleeding events when given with **phenindione**. [Severe] Theoretical
- **Ponatinib** is predicted to increase the risk of bleeding events when given with **phenindione**. [Severe] Theoretical
- **Ranibizumab** is predicted to increase the risk of bleeding events when given with **phenindione**. [Severe] Theoretical
- **Regorafenib** is predicted to increase the risk of bleeding events when given with **phenindione**. [Severe] Theoretical
- **Ruxolitinib** is predicted to increase the risk of bleeding events when given with **phenindione**. [Severe] Theoretical
- **Sorafenib** is predicted to increase the risk of bleeding events when given with **phenindione**. [Severe] Theoretical
- Statins **(rosuvastatin)** are predicted to increase the anticoagulant effect of **phenindione**. Monitor INR and adjust dose. [Severe] Theoretical
- **Sunitinib** is predicted to increase the risk of bleeding events when given with **phenindione**. [Severe] Theoretical
- **Vandetanib** is predicted to increase the risk of bleeding events when given with **phenindione**. [Severe] Theoretical

Phenobarbital → see antiepileptics

Phenothiazines → see TABLE 8 p. 908 (hypotension), TABLE 9 p. 909 (QT-interval prolongation), TABLE 11 p. 909 (CNS depressant effects), TABLE 10 p. 909 (antimuscarinics) chlorpromazine · fluphenazine · levomepromazine · pericyazine · prochlorperazine · promazine · trifluoperazine

FOOD AND LIFESTYLE **Chlorpromazine** and **fluphenazine** dose adjustment might be necessary if smoking started or stopped during treatment.

- **Phenothiazines** are predicted to decrease the effects of **amfetamines** and **amfetamines** are predicted to decrease the effects of **phenothiazines.** Moderate Study
- **Antacids** decrease the absorption of **phenothiazines.** Moderate Anecdotal
- **Chlorpromazine** decreases the concentration of antiepileptics **(phenobarbital, primidone)** and antiepileptics **(phenobarbital, primidone)** decrease the concentration of **chlorpromazine.** Moderate Study → Also see **TABLE 11** p. 909
- **Chlorpromazine** is predicted to increase the risk of hyponatraemia when given with **desmopressin.** Severe Theoretical
- **Phenothiazines** are predicted to decrease the effects of **dopamine receptor agonists.** Avoid. Moderate Theoretical → Also see **TABLE 8** p. 908 → Also see **TABLE 9** p. 909 → Also see **TABLE 10** p. 909
- **Phenothiazines** decrease the effects of **levodopa.** Avoid or monitor worsening parkinsonian symptoms. Severe Study → Also see **TABLE 8** p. 908
- **Phenothiazines** potentially increase the risk of neurotoxicity when given with **lithium.** Severe Anecdotal → Also see **TABLE 9** p. 909
- **MAOIs, irreversible** are predicted to increase the risk of neuroleptic malignant syndrome when given with **phenothiazines.** Severe Theoretical → Also see **TABLE 8** p. 908
- **Chlorpromazine** decreases the effects of **metyrapone.** Avoid. Moderate Theoretical
- **Mexiletine** is predicted to increase the exposure to **chlorpromazine.** Moderate Theoretical
- **Moclobemide** increases the risk of side-effects when given with **levomepromazine.** Moderate Study
- Quinolones **(ciprofloxacin)** are predicted to increase the exposure to **chlorpromazine.** Moderate Theoretical
- SSRIs **(fluvoxamine)** are predicted to increase the exposure to **chlorpromazine.** Moderate Theoretical

Phenoxymethylpenicillin → see penicillins

Phenylephrine → see sympathomimetics, vasoconstrictor

Phenytoin → see antiepileptics

Pholcodine

- **Pholcodine** is predicted to increase the risk of CNS excitation or depression when given with **MAOIs, irreversible.** Avoid and for 14 days after stopping the MAOI. Severe Theoretical

Phosphodiesterase type-5 inhibitors → see **TABLE 8** p. 908 (hypotension), **TABLE 9** p. 909 (QT-interval prolongation)

avanafil · sildenafil · tadalafil · vardenafil

- **Alpha blockers** cause significant hypotensive effects when given with **phosphodiesterase type-5 inhibitors.** Patient should be stabilised on first drug then second drug should be added at the lowest recommended dose. Severe Study → Also see **TABLE 8** p. 908
- Antiarrhythmics **(dronedarone)** are predicted to increase the exposure to **avanafil.** Adjust **avanafil** dose. Moderate Theoretical
- Antiarrhythmics **(dronedarone)** are predicted to increase the exposure to **sildenafil.** Monitor or adjust **sildenafil** dose with moderate inhibitors of CYP3A4, p. 125. Moderate Study → Also see **TABLE 9** p. 909
- Antiarrhythmics **(dronedarone)** are predicted to increase the exposure to **tadalafil.** Severe Theoretical
- Antiarrhythmics **(dronedarone)** are predicted to increase the exposure to **vardenafil.** Adjust dose. Severe Theoretical → Also see **TABLE 9** p. 909
- Antiepileptics **(carbamazepine, fosphenytoin, phenobarbital, phenytoin, primidone)** are predicted to decrease the exposure to phosphodiesterase type-5 inhibitors **(avanafil, tadalafil).** Avoid. Severe Study
- Antiepileptics **(carbamazepine, fosphenytoin, phenobarbital, phenytoin, primidone)** are predicted to decrease the exposure to phosphodiesterase type-5 inhibitors **(sildenafil, vardenafil).** Moderate Theoretical
- Antifungals, azoles **(fluconazole, isavuconazole, posaconazole)** are predicted to increase the exposure to **avanafil.** Adjust **avanafil** dose. Moderate Theoretical
- Antifungals, azoles **(fluconazole, isavuconazole, posaconazole)** are predicted to increase the exposure to **sildenafil.** Monitor or adjust **sildenafil** dose with moderate inhibitors of CYP3A4, p. 125. Moderate Study → Also see **TABLE 9** p. 909
- Antifungals, azoles **(fluconazole, isavuconazole, posaconazole)** are predicted to increase the exposure to **tadalafil.** Severe Theoretical
- Antifungals, azoles **(fluconazole, isavuconazole, posaconazole)** are predicted to increase the exposure to **vardenafil.** Adjust dose. Severe Theoretical → Also see **TABLE 9** p. 909
- Antifungals, azoles **(itraconazole, ketoconazole, voriconazole)** are predicted to increase the exposure to **sildenafil.** Avoid potent inhibitors of CYP3A4 or adjust **sildenafil** dose, p. 125. Severe Study → Also see **TABLE 9** p. 909
- Antifungals, azoles **(itraconazole, ketoconazole, voriconazole)** are predicted to increase the exposure to **tadalafil.** Use with caution or avoid. Severe Study
- Antifungals, azoles **(miconazole)** are predicted to increase the exposure to **sildenafil.** Use with caution and adjust dose. Severe Theoretical
- Antifungals, azoles **(itraconazole, ketoconazole, voriconazole)** are predicted to increase the exposure to phosphodiesterase type-5 inhibitors **(avanafil, vardenafil).** Avoid. Severe Study → Also see **TABLE 9** p. 909
- **Apalutamide** is predicted to decrease the exposure to phosphodiesterase type-5 inhibitors **(avanafil, tadalafil).** Avoid. Severe Study
- **Apalutamide** is predicted to decrease the exposure to phosphodiesterase type-5 inhibitors **(sildenafil, vardenafil).** Moderate Theoretical → Also see **TABLE 9** p. 909
- **Aprepitant** is predicted to increase the exposure to **avanafil.** Adjust **avanafil** dose. Moderate Theoretical
- **Aprepitant** is predicted to increase the exposure to **sildenafil.** Monitor or adjust **sildenafil** dose with moderate inhibitors of CYP3A4, p. 125. Moderate Study
- **Aprepitant** is predicted to increase the exposure to **tadalafil.** Severe Theoretical
- **Aprepitant** is predicted to increase the exposure to **vardenafil.** Adjust dose. Severe Theoretical
- **Bosentan** decreases the exposure to **phosphodiesterase type-5 inhibitors.** Moderate Study
- Calcium channel blockers **(diltiazem, verapamil)** are predicted to increase the exposure to **avanafil.** Adjust **avanafil** dose. Moderate Theoretical → Also see **TABLE 8** p. 908
- Calcium channel blockers **(diltiazem, verapamil)** are predicted to increase the exposure to **sildenafil.** Monitor or adjust **sildenafil** dose with moderate inhibitors of CYP3A4, p. 125. Moderate Study → Also see **TABLE 8** p. 908
- Calcium channel blockers **(diltiazem, verapamil)** are predicted to increase the exposure to **tadalafil.** Severe Theoretical → Also see **TABLE 8** p. 908
- Calcium channel blockers **(diltiazem, verapamil)** are predicted to increase the exposure to **vardenafil.** Adjust dose. Severe Theoretical → Also see **TABLE 8** p. 908
- **Cobicistat** is predicted to increase the exposure to phosphodiesterase type-5 inhibitors **(avanafil, vardenafil).** Avoid. Severe Study
- **Cobicistat** is predicted to increase the exposure to **sildenafil.** Avoid potent inhibitors of CYP3A4 or adjust **sildenafil** dose, p. 125. Severe Study
- **Cobicistat** is predicted to increase the exposure to **tadalafil.** Use with caution or avoid. Severe Study
- **Crizotinib** is predicted to increase the exposure to **avanafil.** Adjust **avanafil** dose. Moderate Theoretical
- **Crizotinib** is predicted to increase the exposure to **sildenafil.** Monitor or adjust **sildenafil** dose with moderate inhibitors of CYP3A4, p. 125. Moderate Study → Also see **TABLE 9** p. 909
- **Crizotinib** is predicted to increase the exposure to **tadalafil.** Severe Theoretical

Phosphodiesterase type-5 inhibitors (continued)

- **Crizotinib** is predicted to increase the exposure to **vardenafil**. Adjust dose. Severe Theoretical → Also see **TABLE 9** p. 909
- **Efavirenz** is predicted to decrease the exposure to **phosphodiesterase type-5 inhibitors**. Moderate Theoretical → Also see **TABLE 9** p. 909
- **Enzalutamide** is predicted to decrease the exposure to phosphodiesterase type-5 inhibitors **(avanafil, tadalafil)**. Avoid. Severe Study
- **Enzalutamide** is predicted to decrease the exposure to phosphodiesterase type-5 inhibitors **(sildenafil, vardenafil)**. Moderate Theoretical
- **Etravirine** moderately decreases the exposure to **phosphodiesterase type-5 inhibitors**. Adjust dose. Moderate Study
- **Grapefruit juice** is predicted to increase the exposure to **phosphodiesterase type-5 inhibitors**. Use with caution or avoid. Moderate Study
- **HIV-protease inhibitors** are predicted to increase the exposure to phosphodiesterase type-5 inhibitors **(avanafil, vardenafil)**. Avoid. Severe Study → Also see **TABLE 9** p. 909
- **HIV-protease inhibitors** are predicted to increase the exposure to **sildenafil**. Avoid potent inhibitors of CYP3A4 or adjust **sildenafil** dose, p. 125. Severe Study → Also see **TABLE 9** p. 909
- **HIV-protease inhibitors** are predicted to increase the exposure to **tadalafil**. Use with caution or avoid. Severe Study
- **Idelalisib** is predicted to increase the exposure to phosphodiesterase type-5 inhibitors **(avanafil, vardenafil)**. Avoid. Severe Study
- **Idelalisib** is predicted to increase the exposure to **sildenafil**. Avoid potent inhibitors of CYP3A4 or adjust **sildenafil** dose, p. 125. Severe Study
- **Idelalisib** is predicted to increase the exposure to **tadalafil**. Use with caution or avoid. Severe Study
- **Imatinib** is predicted to increase the exposure to **avanafil**. Adjust **avanafil** dose. Moderate Theoretical
- **Imatinib** is predicted to increase the exposure to **sildenafil**. Monitor or adjust **sildenafil** dose with moderate inhibitors of CYP3A4, p. 125. Moderate Study
- **Imatinib** is predicted to increase the exposure to **tadalafil**. Severe Theoretical
- **Imatinib** is predicted to increase the exposure to **vardenafil**. Adjust dose. Severe Theoretical
- Macrolides **(clarithromycin)** are predicted to increase the exposure to **sildenafil**. Avoid potent inhibitors of CYP3A4 or adjust **sildenafil** dose, p. 125. Severe Study → Also see **TABLE 9** p. 909
- Macrolides **(clarithromycin)** are predicted to increase the exposure to **tadalafil**. Use with caution or avoid. Severe Study
- Macrolides **(erythromycin)** are predicted to increase the exposure to **avanafil**. Adjust **avanafil** dose. Moderate Theoretical
- Macrolides **(erythromycin)** are predicted to increase the exposure to **sildenafil**. Monitor or adjust **sildenafil** dose with moderate inhibitors of CYP3A4, p. 125. Moderate Study → Also see **TABLE 9** p. 909
- Macrolides **(erythromycin)** are predicted to increase the exposure to **tadalafil**. Severe Theoretical
- Macrolides **(erythromycin)** are predicted to increase the exposure to **vardenafil**. Adjust dose. Severe Theoretical → Also see **TABLE 9** p. 909
- Macrolides **(clarithromycin)** are predicted to increase the exposure to phosphodiesterase type-5 inhibitors **(avanafil, vardenafil)**. Avoid. Severe Study → Also see **TABLE 9** p. 909
- **Mitotane** is predicted to decrease the exposure to phosphodiesterase type-5 inhibitors **(avanafil, tadalafil)**. Avoid. Severe Study
- **Mitotane** is predicted to decrease the exposure to phosphodiesterase type-5 inhibitors **(sildenafil, vardenafil)**. Moderate Theoretical
- **Netupitant** is predicted to increase the exposure to **avanafil**. Adjust **avanafil** dose. Moderate Theoretical
- **Netupitant** is predicted to increase the exposure to **sildenafil**. Monitor or adjust **sildenafil** dose with moderate inhibitors of CYP3A4, p. 125. Moderate Study
- **Netupitant** is predicted to increase the exposure to **tadalafil**. Severe Theoretical
- **Netupitant** is predicted to increase the exposure to **vardenafil**. Adjust dose. Severe Theoretical
- **Nevirapine** is predicted to decrease the exposure to **phosphodiesterase type-5 inhibitors**. Moderate Theoretical
- **Nicorandil** is predicted to increase the risk of hypotension when given with **phosphodiesterase type-5 inhibitors**. Avoid. Severe Theoretical → Also see **TABLE 8** p. 908
- **Nilotinib** is predicted to increase the exposure to **avanafil**. Adjust **avanafil** dose. Moderate Theoretical
- **Nilotinib** is predicted to increase the exposure to **sildenafil**. Monitor or adjust **sildenafil** dose with moderate inhibitors of CYP3A4, p. 125. Moderate Study → Also see **TABLE 9** p. 909
- **Nilotinib** is predicted to increase the exposure to **tadalafil**. Severe Theoretical
- **Nilotinib** is predicted to increase the exposure to **vardenafil**. Adjust dose. Severe Theoretical → Also see **TABLE 9** p. 909
- **Nitrates** potentially increase the risk of hypotension when given with **phosphodiesterase type-5 inhibitors**. Avoid. Severe Study → Also see **TABLE 8** p. 908
- **Ribociclib** is predicted to increase the exposure to **sildenafil**. Avoid. Moderate Theoretical → Also see **TABLE 9** p. 909
- **Rifampicin** is predicted to decrease the exposure to phosphodiesterase type-5 inhibitors **(avanafil, tadalafil)**. Avoid. Severe Study
- **Rifampicin** is predicted to decrease the exposure to phosphodiesterase type-5 inhibitors **(sildenafil, vardenafil)**. Moderate Theoretical
- **Riociguat** is predicted to increase the risk of hypotension when given with **phosphodiesterase type-5 inhibitors**. Avoid. Severe Theoretical → Also see **TABLE 8** p. 908
- **Phosphodiesterase type-5 inhibitors** are predicted to increase the risk of hypotension when given with **sapropterin**. Moderate Theoretical → Also see **TABLE 8** p. 908
- **St John's Wort** is predicted to decrease the exposure to **phosphodiesterase type-5 inhibitors**. Moderate Theoretical

Pibrentasvir

- **Pibrentasvir** (with glecaprevir) is predicted to increase the exposure to **aliskiren**. Moderate Study
- Antiarrhythmics **(amiodarone)** are predicted to increase the exposure to **pibrentasvir**. Moderate Theoretical
- Antiarrhythmics **(dronedarone)** potentially increase the exposure to **pibrentasvir**. Moderate Theoretical
- Antiepileptics **(carbamazepine, fosphenytoin, phenobarbital, phenytoin, primidone)** are predicted to moderately to markedly decrease the exposure to **pibrentasvir**. Avoid. Severe Study
- Antiepileptics **(eslicarbazepine, oxcarbazepine)** potentially decrease the exposure to **pibrentasvir**. Avoid. Severe Theoretical
- Antifungals, azoles **(itraconazole, ketoconazole)** are predicted to increase the exposure to **pibrentasvir**. Moderate Theoretical
- **Pibrentasvir** (with glecaprevir) is predicted to increase the exposure to antihistamines, non-sedating **(fexofenadine)**. Moderate Study
- **Apalutamide** is predicted to moderately to markedly decrease the exposure to **pibrentasvir**. Avoid. Severe Study
- **Bosentan** is predicted to decrease the exposure to **pibrentasvir**. Avoid. Severe Study
- Calcium channel blockers **(verapamil)** are predicted to increase the exposure to **pibrentasvir**. Moderate Theoretical
- **Pibrentasvir** (with glecaprevir) is predicted to increase the exposure to **colchicine**. Moderate Study
- **Combined hormonal contraceptives** (containing ethinylestradiol) are predicted to increase the risk of increased ALT concentrations when given with **pibrentasvir**. Avoid. Severe Study
- **Crizotinib** potentially decreases the exposure to **pibrentasvir**. Avoid. Severe Theoretical
- **Pibrentasvir** (with glecaprevir) increases the exposure to **dabigatran**. Avoid. Moderate Study
- **Pibrentasvir** (with glecaprevir) increases the exposure to **digoxin**. Moderate Study
- **Pibrentasvir** (with glecaprevir) is predicted to increase the exposure to **edoxaban**. Moderate Study

- Efavirenz is predicted to decrease the exposure to **pibrentasvir**. Avoid. Severe Study
- Enzalutamide is predicted to moderately to markedly decrease the exposure to **pibrentasvir**. Avoid. Severe Study
- **Pibrentasvir** (with glecaprevir) is predicted to increase the exposure to everolimus. Moderate Study
- HIV-protease inhibitors **(atazanavir, lopinavir)** boosted with ritonavir increase the exposure to **pibrentasvir**. Avoid. Severe Study
- HIV-protease inhibitors **(ritonavir)** potentially increase the exposure to **pibrentasvir**. Severe Theoretical
- HIV-protease inhibitors **(saquinavir)** are predicted to increase the exposure to **pibrentasvir**. Moderate Theoretical
- Lapatinib is predicted to increase the exposure to **pibrentasvir**. Moderate Theoretical
- **Pibrentasvir** (with glecaprevir) is predicted to increase the exposure to loperamide. Moderate Study
- Lumacaftor potentially decreases the exposure to **pibrentasvir**. Avoid. Severe Theoretical
- Macrolides are predicted to increase the exposure to **pibrentasvir**. Moderate Theoretical
- Mitotane is predicted to moderately to markedly decrease the exposure to **pibrentasvir**. Avoid. Severe Study
- Nevirapine is predicted to decrease the exposure to **pibrentasvir**. Avoid. Severe Study
- Ranolazine is predicted to increase the exposure to **pibrentasvir**. Moderate Theoretical
- Rifampicin is predicted to moderately to markedly decrease the exposure to **pibrentasvir**. Avoid. Severe Study
- **Pibrentasvir** (with glecaprevir) is predicted to increase the exposure to sirolimus. Moderate Study
- St John's Wort is predicted to decrease the exposure to **pibrentasvir**. Avoid. Severe Study
- **Pibrentasvir** (with glecaprevir) markedly increases the exposure to statins **(atorvastatin)**. Avoid. Severe Study
- **Pibrentasvir** (with glecaprevir) is predicted to increase the exposure to statins **(fluvastatin)**. Moderate Theoretical
- **Pibrentasvir** (with glecaprevir) increases the exposure to statins **(pravastatin)**. Use with caution and adjust **pravastatin** dose. Moderate Study
- **Pibrentasvir** (with glecaprevir) increases the exposure to statins **(rosuvastatin)**. Use with caution and adjust **rosuvastatin** dose, p. 140. Moderate Study
- **Pibrentasvir** (with glecaprevir) increases the exposure to statins **(simvastatin)**. Avoid. Moderate Study
- **Pibrentasvir** (with glecaprevir) slightly increases the exposure to tacrolimus. Monitor and adjust dose. Mild Study
- **Pibrentasvir** (with glecaprevir) is predicted to increase the exposure to taxanes **(paclitaxel)**. Moderate Study
- **Pibrentasvir** (with glecaprevir) is predicted to increase the exposure to topotecan. Moderate Study
- Vemurafenib is predicted to increase the exposure to **pibrentasvir**. Moderate Theoretical

Pilocarpine

ROUTE-SPECIFIC INFORMATION Since systemic absorption can follow topical application, the possibility of interactions should be borne in mind.

Pimecrolimus

- Alcohol (beverage) increases the risk of facial flushing and skin irritation when given with topical **pimecrolimus**. Moderate Study
- **Pimecrolimus** is predicted to decrease the efficacy of mifamurtide. Avoid. Severe Theoretical

Pimozide → see TABLE 8 p. 908 (hypotension), TABLE 9 p. 909 (QT-interval prolongation), TABLE 11 p. 909 (CNS depressant effects), TABLE 10 p. 909 (antimuscarinics)

- Antiarrhythmics **(dronedarone)** are predicted to increase the exposure to **pimozide**. Avoid. Severe Theoretical → Also see TABLE 9 p. 909
- Antifungals, azoles **(fluconazole, isavuconazole, posaconazole)** are predicted to increase the exposure to **pimozide**. Avoid. Severe Theoretical → Also see TABLE 9 p. 909
- Antifungals, azoles **(itraconazole, ketoconazole, voriconazole)** are predicted to increase the exposure to **pimozide**. Avoid. Severe Study → Also see TABLE 9 p. 909
- Antifungals, azoles **(miconazole)** are predicted to increase the exposure to **pimozide**. Avoid. Moderate Theoretical
- Aprepitant is predicted to increase the exposure to **pimozide**. Avoid. Severe Theoretical
- Calcium channel blockers **(diltiazem, verapamil)** are predicted to increase the exposure to **pimozide**. Avoid. Severe Theoretical → Also see TABLE 8 p. 908
- Ceritinib is predicted to increase the exposure to **pimozide**. Avoid. Severe Theoretical → Also see TABLE 9 p. 909
- Cobicistat is predicted to increase the exposure to **pimozide**. Avoid. Severe Study
- Crizotinib is predicted to increase the exposure to **pimozide**. Avoid. Severe Theoretical → Also see TABLE 9 p. 909
- **Pimozide** is predicted to decrease the effects of **dopamine receptor agonists**. Avoid. Moderate Theoretical → Also see TABLE 8 p. 908 → Also see TABLE 9 p. 909 → Also see TABLE 10 p. 909
- Fosaprepitant is predicted to increase the exposure to **pimozide**. Avoid. Severe Theoretical
- Grapefruit juice increases the exposure to **pimozide**. Avoid. Severe Theoretical
- HIV-protease inhibitors are predicted to increase the exposure to **pimozide**. Avoid. Severe Study → Also see TABLE 9 p. 909
- Idelalisib is predicted to increase the exposure to **pimozide**. Avoid. Severe Study
- Imatinib is predicted to increase the exposure to **pimozide**. Avoid. Severe Theoretical
- Larotrectinib is predicted to increase the exposure to **pimozide**. Use with caution and adjust dose. Mild Theoretical
- Letermovir is predicted to increase the concentration of **pimozide**. Avoid. Severe Theoretical
- **Pimozide** decreases the effects of **levodopa**. Severe Theoretical → Also see TABLE 8 p. 908
- Lorlatinib is predicted to decrease the exposure to **pimozide**. Avoid. Moderate Theoretical
- Macrolides **(clarithromycin)** are predicted to increase the exposure to **pimozide**. Avoid. Severe Study → Also see TABLE 9 p. 909
- Macrolides **(erythromycin)** are predicted to increase the exposure to **pimozide**. Avoid. Severe Theoretical → Also see TABLE 9 p. 909
- Netupitant is predicted to increase the exposure to **pimozide**. Avoid. Severe Theoretical
- Nilotinib is predicted to increase the exposure to **pimozide**. Avoid. Severe Theoretical → Also see TABLE 9 p. 909
- Palbociclib is predicted to increase the exposure to **pimozide**. Adjust dose. Moderate Theoretical
- Panobinostat is predicted to increase the exposure to **pimozide**. Avoid. Severe Theoretical → Also see TABLE 9 p. 909
- Pitolisant is predicted to decrease the exposure to **pimozide**. Avoid. Severe Theoretical
- Ribociclib (high-dose) is predicted to increase the exposure to **pimozide**. Avoid. Moderate Theoretical → Also see TABLE 9 p. 909
- Rolapitant is predicted to increase the exposure to **pimozide**. Severe Study
- Rucaparib is predicted to increase the exposure to **pimozide**. Monitor and adjust dose. Moderate Study

Pindolol → see beta blockers, non-selective

Pioglitazone → see TABLE 14 p. 910 (antidiabetic drugs)

- **Pioglitazone** potentially decreases the exposure to antifungals, azoles **(isavuconazole)**. Use with caution or avoid. Moderate Theoretical
- Clopidogrel increases the exposure to **pioglitazone**. Monitor blood glucose and adjust dose. Severe Study
- Fibrates **(gemfibrozil)** increase the exposure to **pioglitazone**. Monitor blood glucose and adjust dose. Severe Study
- Iron chelators **(deferasirox)** are predicted to increase the exposure to **pioglitazone**. Moderate Study
- Leflunomide is predicted to increase the exposure to **pioglitazone**. Moderate Study
- Opicapone is predicted to increase the exposure to **pioglitazone**. Avoid. Moderate Study
- Rifampicin moderately decreases the exposure to **pioglitazone**. Monitor and adjust dose. Moderate Study
- St John's Wort slightly decreases the exposure to **pioglitazone**. Mild Study

Pioglitazone (continued)

- **Teriflunomide** is predicted to increase the exposure to **pioglitazone**. [Moderate] Study

Piperacillin → see penicillins

Piperaquine → see antimalarials

Pirfenidone

FOOD AND LIFESTYLE Smoking increases pirfenidone clearance; patients should be encouraged to stop smoking before and during treatment with pirfenidone.

- Antiepileptics **(fosphenytoin, phenytoin)** are predicted to decrease the exposure to **pirfenidone**. [Moderate] Theoretical
- **Combined hormonal contraceptives** are predicted to increase the exposure to **pirfenidone**. Use with caution and adjust dose. [Moderate] Study
- HIV-protease inhibitors **(ritonavir)** are predicted to decrease the exposure to **pirfenidone**. [Moderate] Theoretical
- **Leflunomide** is predicted to decrease the exposure to **pirfenidone**. [Moderate] Theoretical
- **Mexiletine** is predicted to increase the exposure to **pirfenidone**. Use with caution and adjust dose. [Moderate] Study
- Quinolones **(ciprofloxacin)** are predicted to increase the exposure to **pirfenidone**. Use with caution and adjust dose. [Moderate] Study
- **Rifampicin** is predicted to decrease the exposure to **pirfenidone**. Avoid. [Moderate] Theoretical
- SSRIs **(fluvoxamine)** are predicted to moderately increase the exposure to **pirfenidone**. Avoid. [Moderate] Study
- **Teriflunomide** is predicted to decrease the exposure to **pirfenidone**. [Moderate] Theoretical

Piroxicam → see NSAIDs

Pitolisant

- **Pitolisant** is predicted to decrease the exposure to **aliskiren**. [Mild] Theoretical
- Antiepileptics **(carbamazepine, fosphenytoin, phenobarbital, phenytoin, primidone)** are predicted to moderately decrease the exposure to **pitolisant**. [Moderate] Study
- **Pitolisant** is predicted to decrease the exposure to antihistamines, non-sedating **(fexofenadine)**. [Mild] Theoretical
- **Antihistamines, sedating** are predicted to decrease the efficacy of **pitolisant**. [Moderate] Theoretical
- **Apalutamide** is predicted to moderately decrease the exposure to **pitolisant**. [Moderate] Study
- **Pitolisant** is predicted to decrease the exposure to **bosutinib**. Avoid. [Severe] Theoretical
- **Bupropion** is predicted to moderately increase the exposure to **pitolisant**. Use with caution and adjust dose. [Moderate] Study
- **Pitolisant** is predicted to decrease the exposure to **ciclosporin**. Avoid. [Severe] Theoretical
- **Cinacalcet** is predicted to moderately increase the exposure to **pitolisant**. Use with caution and adjust dose. [Moderate] Study
- **Pitolisant** is predicted to decrease the exposure to **colchicine**. [Mild] Theoretical
- **Pitolisant** is predicted to decrease the efficacy of **combined hormonal contraceptives**. Avoid. [Severe] Theoretical
- **Pitolisant** is predicted to decrease the exposure to coumarins **(warfarin)**. [Mild] Theoretical
- **Pitolisant** is predicted to decrease the exposure to **crizotinib**. Avoid. [Severe] Theoretical
- **Pitolisant** is predicted to decrease the exposure to **dabigatran**. [Mild] Theoretical
- **Pitolisant** is predicted to decrease the exposure to **dasatinib**. Avoid. [Severe] Theoretical
- **Pitolisant** is predicted to decrease the exposure to **digoxin**. [Mild] Theoretical
- **Duloxetine** is predicted to increase the exposure to **pitolisant**. Use with caution and adjust dose. [Moderate] Study
- **Pitolisant** is predicted to decrease the exposure to **edoxaban**. [Mild] Theoretical
- **Pitolisant** is predicted to decrease the exposure to **efavirenz**. [Mild] Theoretical
- **Enzalutamide** is predicted to moderately decrease the exposure to **pitolisant**. [Moderate] Study
- **Pitolisant** is predicted to decrease the exposure to **everolimus**. Avoid. [Severe] Theoretical
- **Pitolisant** is predicted to decrease the exposure to **irinotecan**. [Mild] Theoretical
- **Pitolisant** is predicted to decrease the exposure to **lapatinib**. Avoid. [Severe] Theoretical
- **Pitolisant** is predicted to decrease the exposure to **loperamide**. [Mild] Theoretical
- **Pitolisant** is predicted to increase the exposure to **metformin**. [Mild] Theoretical
- **Mianserin** is predicted to decrease the efficacy of **pitolisant**. [Moderate] Theoretical
- **Mirtazapine** is predicted to decrease the efficacy of **pitolisant**. [Moderate] Theoretical
- **Mitotane** is predicted to moderately decrease the exposure to **pitolisant**. [Moderate] Study
- **Pitolisant** is predicted to decrease the exposure to **nilotinib**. Avoid. [Severe] Theoretical
- **Pitolisant** is predicted to decrease the exposure to opioids **(morphine)**. [Mild] Theoretical
- **Pitolisant** is predicted to decrease the exposure to **paracetamol**. [Mild] Theoretical
- **Pitolisant** is predicted to decrease the exposure to **pimozide**. Avoid. [Severe] Theoretical
- **Pitolisant** is predicted to decrease the exposure to **repaglinide**. [Mild] Theoretical
- **Rifampicin** is predicted to moderately decrease the exposure to **pitolisant**. [Moderate] Study
- **Pitolisant** is predicted to decrease the exposure to **sirolimus**. Avoid. [Severe] Theoretical
- SSRIs **(fluoxetine, paroxetine)** are predicted to moderately increase the exposure to **pitolisant**. Use with caution and adjust dose. [Moderate] Study
- **St John's Wort** is predicted to decrease the exposure to **pitolisant**. Monitor and adjust dose. [Moderate] Theoretical
- **Pitolisant** is predicted to decrease the exposure to **tacrolimus**. Avoid. [Severe] Theoretical
- **Pitolisant** is predicted to decrease the exposure to taxanes **(docetaxel)**. Avoid. [Severe] Theoretical
- **Pitolisant** is predicted to decrease the exposure to taxanes **(paclitaxel)**. [Mild] Theoretical
- **Pitolisant** is predicted to decrease the exposure to **temsirolimus**. Avoid. [Severe] Theoretical
- **Terbinafine** is predicted to moderately increase the exposure to **pitolisant**. Use with caution and adjust dose. [Moderate] Study
- **Pitolisant** is predicted to decrease the exposure to **topotecan**. [Mild] Theoretical
- **Tricyclic antidepressants** are predicted to decrease the efficacy of **pitolisant**. [Mild] Theoretical
- **Venlafaxine** is predicted to increase the exposure to **pitolisant**. Use with caution and adjust dose. [Mild] Theoretical

Pivmecillinam → see penicillins

Pixantrone → see anthracyclines

Pizotifen → see antihistamines, sedating

Platinum compounds → see TABLE 15 p. 910 (myelosuppression), TABLE 2 p. 907 (nephrotoxicity), TABLE 19 p. 911 (ototoxicity), TABLE 12 p. 910 (peripheral neuropathy)

carboplatin · cisplatin · oxaliplatin

- **Cisplatin** increases the risk of pulmonary toxicity when given with **bleomycin**. [Severe] Study → Also see TABLE 15 p. 910
- **Live vaccines** are predicted to increase the risk of generalised infection (possibly life-threatening) when given with **platinum compounds**. Public Health England advises avoid (refer to Green Book). [Severe] Theoretical

Polatuzumab vedotin → see monoclonal antibodies

Polymyxin b → see TABLE 2 p. 907 (nephrotoxicity), TABLE 20 p. 911 (neuromuscular blocking effects)

ROUTE-SPECIFIC INFORMATION Since systemic absorption can follow topical application, the possibility of interactions should be borne in mind.

Polystyrene sulfonate

SEPARATION OF ADMINISTRATION Manufacturers advise take other drugs at least 3 hours before or after calcium- or sodium-polystyrene sulfonate; a 6-hour separation should be considered in gastroparesis.

- **Antacids** increase the risk of metabolic alkalosis when given with **polystyrene sulfonate.** Severe Anecdotal

Pomalidomide → see TABLE 15 p. 910 (myelosuppression), TABLE 5 p. 907 (thromboembolism)
- **Combined hormonal contraceptives** are predicted to increase the risk of venous thromboembolism when given with **pomalidomide.** Avoid. Severe Theoretical
- **Hormone replacement therapy** is predicted to increase the risk of venous thromboembolism when given with **pomalidomide.** Severe Theoretical
- Quinolones **(ciprofloxacin)** are predicted to increase the exposure to **pomalidomide.** Adjust **pomalidomide** dose. Moderate Theoretical
- **SSRIs (fluvoxamine)** moderately increase the exposure to **pomalidomide.** Adjust **pomalidomide** dose. Moderate Study

Ponatinib
- Antiepileptics **(carbamazepine, fosphenytoin, phenobarbital, phenytoin, primidone)** are predicted to decrease the exposure to **ponatinib.** Avoid. Moderate Theoretical
- Antifungals, azoles **(itraconazole, ketoconazole, voriconazole)** are predicted to slightly increase the exposure to **ponatinib.** Monitor and adjust **ponatinib** dose. Moderate Study
- **Apalutamide** is predicted to decrease the exposure to **ponatinib.** Avoid. Moderate Theoretical
- **Cobicistat** is predicted to slightly increase the exposure to **ponatinib.** Monitor and adjust **ponatinib** dose. Moderate Study
- **Ponatinib** is predicted to increase the risk of bleeding events when given with **coumarins.** Severe Theoretical
- **Enzalutamide** is predicted to decrease the exposure to **ponatinib.** Avoid. Moderate Theoretical
- **Grapefruit juice** is predicted to increase the exposure to **ponatinib.** Moderate Theoretical
- **HIV-protease inhibitors** are predicted to slightly increase the exposure to **ponatinib.** Monitor and adjust **ponatinib** dose. Moderate Study
- **Idelalisib** is predicted to slightly increase the exposure to **ponatinib.** Monitor and adjust **ponatinib** dose. Moderate Study
- Macrolides **(clarithromycin)** are predicted to slightly increase the exposure to **ponatinib.** Monitor and adjust **ponatinib** dose. Moderate Study
- **Mitotane** is predicted to decrease the exposure to **ponatinib.** Avoid. Moderate Theoretical
- **Ponatinib** is predicted to increase the risk of bleeding events when given with **phenindione.** Severe Theoretical
- **Rifampicin** is predicted to decrease the exposure to **ponatinib.** Avoid. Moderate Theoretical
- **St John's Wort** is predicted to decrease the exposure to **ponatinib.** Avoid. Severe Theoretical

Posaconazole → see antifungals, azoles

Potassium aminobenzoate → see TABLE 16 p. 911 (increased serum potassium)
- **Potassium aminobenzoate** increases the concentration of **methotrexate.** Moderate Theoretical
- **Potassium aminobenzoate** is predicted to affect the efficacy of **sulfonamides.** Avoid. Severe Theoretical

Potassium canrenoate → see TABLE 16 p. 911 (increased serum potassium)

Potassium chloride → see TABLE 16 p. 911 (increased serum potassium)

Potassium citrate
- **Potassium citrate** is predicted to decrease the efficacy of **methenamine.** Avoid. Moderate Theoretical
- **Potassium citrate** increases the risk of side-effects when given with **sucralfate.** Avoid. Moderate Theoretical

Potassium-sparing diuretics → see TABLE 18 p. 911 (hyponatraemia), TABLE 16 p. 911 (increased serum potassium)

amiloride · triamterene

- **Triamterene** potentially increases the clearance of **lithium.** Moderate Study

Pramipexole → see dopamine receptor agonists

Prasugrel → see TABLE 4 p. 907 (antiplatelet effects)

Pravastatin → see statins

Praziquantel
- Antiepileptics **(carbamazepine, fosphenytoin, phenobarbital, phenytoin, primidone)** are predicted to markedly decrease the exposure to **praziquantel.** Avoid. Moderate Study
- Antifungals, azoles **(itraconazole, ketoconazole, voriconazole)** are predicted to moderately increase the exposure to **praziquantel.** Mild Study
- Antimalarials **(chloroquine)** moderately decrease the exposure to **praziquantel.** Use with caution and adjust dose. Moderate Study
- **Apalutamide** is predicted to markedly decrease the exposure to **praziquantel.** Avoid. Moderate Study
- **Cobicistat** is predicted to moderately increase the exposure to **praziquantel.** Mild Study
- Corticosteroids **(dexamethasone)** decrease the exposure to **praziquantel.** Moderate Study
- **Enzalutamide** is predicted to markedly decrease the exposure to **praziquantel.** Avoid. Moderate Study
- **Grapefruit juice** is predicted to increase the exposure to **praziquantel.** Moderate Study
- H_2 receptor antagonists **(cimetidine)** moderately increase the exposure to **praziquantel.** Moderate Study
- **HIV-protease inhibitors** are predicted to moderately increase the exposure to **praziquantel.** Mild Study
- **Idelalisib** is predicted to moderately increase the exposure to **praziquantel.** Mild Study
- Macrolides **(clarithromycin)** are predicted to moderately increase the exposure to **praziquantel.** Mild Study
- **Mitotane** is predicted to markedly decrease the exposure to **praziquantel.** Avoid. Moderate Study
- **Rifampicin** is predicted to markedly decrease the exposure to **praziquantel.** Avoid. Moderate Study

Prazosin → see alpha blockers

Prednisolone → see corticosteroids

Pregabalin → see antiepileptics

Prilocaine → see anaesthetics, local

Primaquine → see antimalarials

Primidone → see antiepileptics

Procarbazine → see TABLE 15 p. 910 (myelosuppression), TABLE 13 p. 910 (serotonin syndrome)

FOOD AND LIFESTYLE Procarbazine is a mild monoamine-oxidase inhibitor and might rarely interact with tyramine-rich foods (such as mature cheese, salami, pickled herring, *Bovril*®, *Oxo*®, *Marmite*® or any similar meat or yeast extract or fermented soya bean extract, and some beers, lagers or wines).

- **Alcohol (beverage)** potentially causes a disulfiram-like reaction when given with **procarbazine.** Moderate Anecdotal
- Antiepileptics **(carbamazepine, phenobarbital, phenytoin, primidone)** are predicted to increase the risk of hypersensitivity reactions when given with **procarbazine.** Severe Anecdotal
- Antiepileptics **(fosphenytoin)** are predicted to increase the risk of hypersensitivity when given with **procarbazine.** Severe Anecdotal
- **Live vaccines** are predicted to increase the risk of generalised infection (possibly life-threatening) when given with **procarbazine.** Public Health England advises avoid (refer to Green Book). Severe Theoretical

Prochlorperazine → see phenothiazines

Procyclidine → see TABLE 10 p. 909 (antimuscarinics)
- SSRIs **(paroxetine)** slightly increase the exposure to **procyclidine.** Monitor and adjust dose. Moderate Study

Proguanil → see antimalarials

Promazine → see phenothiazines

Promethazine → see antihistamines, sedating

Propafenone → see antiarrhythmics

Propantheline → see TABLE 10 p. 909 (antimuscarinics)

Propiverine → see TABLE 10 p. 909 (antimuscarinics)
- Antifungals, azoles **(itraconazole, ketoconazole, voriconazole)** given with carbimazole are predicted to increase the exposure to **propiverine.** Adjust starting dose. Moderate Theoretical
- **Carbimazole** given with a potent CYP3A4 inhibitor is predicted to increase the exposure to **propiverine.** Adjust starting dose. Moderate Theoretical
- **Cobicistat** given with carbimazole is predicted to increase the exposure to **propiverine.** Adjust starting dose. Moderate Theoretical

Propiverine (continued)
- HIV-protease inhibitors given with carbimazole are predicted to increase the exposure to **propiverine**. Adjust starting dose. Moderate Theoretical
- Idelalisib given with carbimazole is predicted to increase the exposure to **propiverine**. Adjust starting dose. Moderate Theoretical
- **Propiverine** is predicted to increase the exposure to lomitapide. Separate administration by 12 hours. Moderate Theoretical
- Macrolides **(clarithromycin)** given with carbimazole are predicted to increase the exposure to **propiverine**. Adjust starting dose. Moderate Theoretical

Propofol → see TABLE 8 p. 908 (hypotension), TABLE 11 p. 909 (CNS depressant effects)
- Antiepileptics **(valproate)** potentially increase the concentration of **propofol**. Adjust dose. Severe Theoretical

Propranolol → see beta blockers, non-selective

Propylthiouracil → see TABLE 15 p. 910 (myelosuppression)
- **Propylthiouracil** is predicted to decrease the effects of metyrapone. Avoid. Moderate Theoretical

Proton pump inhibitors

esomeprazole · lansoprazole · omeprazole · pantoprazole · rabeprazole

- Antifungals, azoles **(voriconazole)** increase the exposure to proton pump inhibitors **(esomeprazole, omeprazole)**. Adjust dose. Moderate Study
- **Proton pump inhibitors** decrease the absorption of antifungals, azoles **(itraconazole)**. Administer itraconazole capsules with an acidic beverage. Moderate Study
- **Proton pump inhibitors** decrease the absorption of antifungals, azoles **(ketoconazole)**. Administer ketoconazole with an acidic beverage. Moderate Study
- **Proton pump inhibitors** decrease the absorption of antifungals, azoles **(posaconazole)** (oral suspension). Avoid. Moderate Study
- **Apalutamide** markedly decreases the exposure to **omeprazole**. Avoid or monitor. Moderate Study
- **Apalutamide** is predicted to decrease the exposure to proton pump inhibitors **(lansoprazole, rabeprazole)**. Avoid or monitor. Mild Study
- **Proton pump inhibitors** are predicted to decrease the absorption of bosutinib. Moderate Study
- **Esomeprazole** is predicted to increase the exposure to cannabidiol. Moderate Theoretical
- **Proton pump inhibitors** are predicted to decrease the absorption of ceritinib. Moderate Theoretical
- **Esomeprazole** is predicted to increase the exposure to cilostazol. Moderate Theoretical
- **Omeprazole** is predicted to increase the exposure to **cilostazol**. Adjust **cilostazol** dose. Moderate Study
- Proton pump inhibitors **(esomeprazole, omeprazole)** potentially increase the exposure to clobazam. Adjust dose. Moderate Theoretical
- Proton pump inhibitors **(esomeprazole, omeprazole)** are predicted to decrease the efficacy of **clopidogrel**. Avoid. Moderate Study
- **Proton pump inhibitors** are predicted to decrease the exposure to **dacomitinib**. Avoid. Moderate Study
- **Proton pump inhibitors** are predicted to slightly to moderately decrease the exposure to dasatinib. Avoid. Severe Study
- **Proton pump inhibitors** are predicted to decrease the absorption of dipyridamole (immediate release tablets). Moderate Theoretical
- **Proton pump inhibitors** are predicted to slightly decrease the exposure to erlotinib. Avoid. Moderate Study
- **Proton pump inhibitors** are predicted to decrease the exposure to **gefitinib**. Severe Theoretical
- HIV-protease inhibitors **(tipranavir)** decrease the exposure to **proton pump inhibitors**. Avoid. Severe Study
- **Proton pump inhibitors** decrease the exposure to HIV-protease inhibitors **(atazanavir)**. Avoid or adjust dose. Severe Study
- **Proton pump inhibitors** increase the exposure to HIV-protease inhibitors **(saquinavir)**. Avoid. Severe Study
- **Proton pump inhibitors** are predicted to decrease the exposure to ledipasvir. Adjust dose, see ledipasvir with sofosbuvir p. 436. Moderate Theoretical
- **Proton pump inhibitors** decrease the clearance of **methotrexate** (high-dose). Use with caution or avoid. Severe Study
- **Proton pump inhibitors** are predicted to decrease the exposure to neratinib. Avoid. Severe Study
- **Proton pump inhibitors** are predicted to decrease the exposure to pazopanib. Avoid or administer concurrently without food. Moderate Study
- **Proton pump inhibitors** are predicted to decrease the exposure to rilpivirine. Avoid. Severe Study
- **Proton pump inhibitors** potentially decrease the exposure to sofosbuvir. Adjust dose, see ledipasvir with sofosbuvir, sofosbuvir with velpatasvir, and sofosbuvir with velpatasvir and voxilaprevir. Moderate Study
- **Esomeprazole** is predicted to slightly to moderately increase the exposure to SSRIs **(citalopram, escitalopram)**. Monitor and adjust dose. Severe Theoretical
- **Omeprazole** slightly to moderately increases the exposure to SSRIs **(citalopram, escitalopram)**. Monitor and adjust dose. Severe Study
- **Proton pump inhibitors** are predicted to decrease the concentration of velpatasvir. Adjust dose, see sofosbuvir with velpatasvir. Moderate Study
- **Proton pump inhibitors** are predicted to decrease the exposure to voxilaprevir. Adjust dose, see sofosbuvir with velpatasvir and voxilaprevir. Moderate Study

Proxymetacaine → see anaesthetics, local

Pseudoephedrine → see sympathomimetics, vasoconstrictor

Pyrazinamide
- Allopurinol is predicted to increase the risk of hyperuricaemia when given with **pyrazinamide**. Moderate Theoretical

Pyridostigmine → see TABLE 6 p. 908 (bradycardia)
- Aminoglycosides are predicted to decrease the effects of **pyridostigmine**. Moderate Theoretical

Pyrimethamine → see antimalarials

Quetiapine → see TABLE 8 p. 908 (hypotension), TABLE 11 p. 909 (CNS depressant effects)
- Antiarrhythmics **(dronedarone)** are predicted to increase the exposure to **quetiapine**. Avoid. Moderate Study
- Antiepileptics **(carbamazepine, fosphenytoin, phenobarbital, phenytoin, primidone)** are predicted to decrease the exposure to **quetiapine**. Moderate Study → Also see TABLE 11 p. 909
- Antiepileptics **(valproate)** potentially increase the risk of neutropenia when given with **quetiapine**. Moderate Study
- Antifungals, azoles **(fluconazole, isavuconazole, posaconazole)** are predicted to increase the exposure to **quetiapine**. Avoid. Moderate Study
- Antifungals, azoles **(itraconazole, ketoconazole, voriconazole)** are predicted to increase the exposure to **quetiapine**. Avoid. Severe Study
- **Apalutamide** is predicted to decrease the exposure to **quetiapine**. Moderate Study
- **Aprepitant** is predicted to increase the exposure to **quetiapine**. Avoid. Moderate Study
- **Bosentan** is predicted to decrease the exposure to **quetiapine**. Moderate Study
- Calcium channel blockers **(diltiazem, verapamil)** are predicted to increase the exposure to **quetiapine**. Avoid. Moderate Study → Also see TABLE 8 p. 908
- **Cobicistat** is predicted to increase the exposure to **quetiapine**. Avoid. Severe Study
- **Crizotinib** is predicted to increase the exposure to **quetiapine**. Avoid. Moderate Study
- **Quetiapine** is predicted to decrease the effects of dopamine receptor agonists. Avoid. Moderate Theoretical → Also see TABLE 8 p. 908
- **Efavirenz** is predicted to decrease the exposure to **quetiapine**. Moderate Study
- **Enzalutamide** is predicted to decrease the exposure to **quetiapine**. Moderate Study
- **Grapefruit juice** is predicted to increase the exposure to **quetiapine**. Avoid. Severe Theoretical
- **HIV-protease inhibitors** are predicted to increase the exposure to **quetiapine**. Avoid. Severe Study

- **Idelalisib** is predicted to increase the exposure to **quetiapine**. Avoid. [Severe] Study
- **Imatinib** is predicted to increase the exposure to **quetiapine**. Avoid. [Moderate] Study
- **Quetiapine** decreases the effects of **levodopa**. [Severe] Anecdotal → Also see TABLE 8 p. 908
- **Quetiapine** potentially increases the risk of neurotoxicity when given with **lithium**. [Severe] Anecdotal
- Macrolides **(clarithromycin)** are predicted to increase the exposure to **quetiapine**. Avoid. [Severe] Study
- Macrolides **(erythromycin)** are predicted to increase the exposure to **quetiapine**. Avoid. [Moderate] Study
- **Mitotane** is predicted to decrease the exposure to **quetiapine**. [Moderate] Study
- **Netupitant** is predicted to increase the exposure to **quetiapine**. Avoid. [Moderate] Study
- **Nevirapine** is predicted to decrease the exposure to **quetiapine**. [Moderate] Study
- **Nilotinib** is predicted to increase the exposure to **quetiapine**. Avoid. [Moderate] Study
- **Ribociclib** (high-dose) is predicted to increase the exposure to **quetiapine**. Avoid. [Moderate] Theoretical
- **Rifampicin** is predicted to decrease the exposure to **quetiapine**. [Moderate] Study
- **St John's Wort** is predicted to decrease the exposure to **quetiapine**. [Moderate] Study

Quinagolide → see dopamine receptor agonists

Quinapril → see ACE inhibitors

Quinine → see antimalarials

Quinolones → see TABLE 9 p. 909 (QT-interval prolongation)

ciprofloxacin · levofloxacin · moxifloxacin · ofloxacin

- Avoid concurrent administration of dairy products and mineral-fortified drinks with *oral* **ciprofloxacin** due to reduced exposure.
- Since systemic absorption can follow topical application of **ciprofloxacin, levofloxacin**, and **ofloxacin**, the possibility of interactions should be borne in mind.
- Interactions do not generally apply to topical use of **moxifloxacin** unless specified.

- **Ciprofloxacin** is predicted to increase the exposure to **agomelatine**. [Moderate] Study
- **Ciprofloxacin** is predicted to increase the exposure to **aminophylline**. Adjust dose. [Moderate] Theoretical
- **Ciprofloxacin** is predicted to increase the exposure to **anagrelide**. [Moderate] Theoretical
- **Antacids** decrease the absorption of **quinolones**. **Quinolones** should be taken 2 hours before or 4 hours after antacids. [Moderate] Study
- **Ciprofloxacin** slightly increases the exposure to antiarrhythmics **(lidocaine)**. [Mild] Study
- **Ciprofloxacin** affects the concentration of antiepileptics **(fosphenytoin, phenytoin)**. Monitor concentration and adjust dose. [Severe] Study
- Calcium salts **(calcium carbonate)** decrease the absorption of **ciprofloxacin**. Separate administration by 2 hours. [Moderate] Study
- **Ciprofloxacin** increases the concentration of **clozapine**. Monitor side effects and adjust dose. [Severe] Study
- **Quinolones** increase the anticoagulant effect of **coumarins**. [Severe] Anecdotal
- **Ciprofloxacin** is predicted to increase the exposure to dopamine receptor agonists **(ropinirole)**. Adjust dose. [Moderate] Study
- **Ciprofloxacin** is predicted to increase the exposure to **duloxetine**. Avoid. [Moderate] Theoretical
- **Ciprofloxacin** is predicted to increase the exposure to **eliglustat**. Avoid or adjust dose—consult product literature. [Severe] Theoretical
- **Enteral feeds** decrease the exposure to **ciprofloxacin**. [Moderate] Study
- **Ciprofloxacin** slightly increases the exposure to **erlotinib**. Monitor side effects and adjust dose. [Moderate] Study
- **Ciprofloxacin** is predicted to increase the exposure to **ibrutinib**. Adjust **ibrutinib** dose. [Severe] Theoretical
- **Iron (oral)** decreases the exposure to **quinolones**. Separate administration by at least 2 hours. [Moderate] Study
- **Lanthanum** moderately decreases the exposure to **quinolones**. **Quinolones** should be taken 2 hours before or 4 hours after **lanthanum**. [Moderate] Study
- **Leflunomide** is predicted to increase the exposure to **ciprofloxacin**. [Moderate] Theoretical
- **Ciprofloxacin** is predicted to increase the exposure to **loxapine**. Avoid. [Unknown] Theoretical
- **Ciprofloxacin** slightly increases the exposure to MAO-B inhibitors **(rasagiline)**. [Moderate] Study
- **Ciprofloxacin** is predicted to increase the exposure to **melatonin**. [Moderate] Theoretical
- **Ciprofloxacin** potentially increases the risk of toxicity when given with **methotrexate**. [Severe] Anecdotal
- **NSAIDs** potentially increase the risk of seizures when given with **quinolones**. [Severe] Theoretical
- **Ciprofloxacin** is predicted to increase the exposure to **olanzapine**. Adjust dose. [Moderate] Anecdotal
- **Ciprofloxacin** very slightly increases the exposure to **pentoxifylline**. [Moderate] Study
- **Ciprofloxacin** is predicted to increase the exposure to phenothiazines **(chlorpromazine)**. [Moderate] Theoretical
- **Ciprofloxacin** is predicted to increase the exposure to **pirfenidone**. Use with caution and adjust dose. [Moderate] Study
- **Ciprofloxacin** is predicted to increase the exposure to **pomalidomide**. Adjust **pomalidomide** dose. [Moderate] Theoretical
- **Ciprofloxacin** is predicted to increase the exposure to **riluzole**. [Moderate] Theoretical
- **Ciprofloxacin** is predicted to increase the exposure to **roflumilast**. [Moderate] Theoretical
- **Strontium** is predicted to decrease the absorption of **quinolones**. Avoid. [Moderate] Theoretical
- **Sucralfate** decreases the exposure to **quinolones**. Separate administration by 2 hours. [Moderate] Study
- **Teriflunomide** is predicted to increase the exposure to **ciprofloxacin**. [Moderate] Theoretical
- **Ciprofloxacin** is predicted to increase the exposure to **theophylline**. Monitor and adjust dose. [Moderate] Theoretical
- **Ciprofloxacin** increases the exposure to **tizanidine**. Avoid. [Moderate] Study
- **Ciprofloxacin** is predicted to increase the exposure to **tolvaptan**. Use with caution and adjust **tolvaptan** dose. [Moderate] Theoretical
- **Zinc** is predicted to decrease the exposure to **quinolones**. Separate administration by 2 hours. [Moderate] Study
- **Ciprofloxacin** is predicted to increase the exposure to **zolmitriptan**. Adjust **zolmitriptan** dose, p. 310. [Moderate] Theoretical

Rabeprazole → see proton pump inhibitors

Rabies immunoglobulin → see immunoglobulins

Rabies vaccine

- Antimalarials **(chloroquine)** decrease the efficacy of **rabies vaccine** (intradermal). Avoid. [Moderate] Study
- **Hydroxychloroquine** is predicted to decrease efficacy **rabies vaccine**. [Moderate] Theoretical

Raloxifene → see TABLE 5 p. 907 (thromboembolism)

- **Combined hormonal contraceptives** potentially oppose the effects of **raloxifene**. Avoid. [Severe] Theoretical
- **Hormone replacement therapy** potentially opposes the effects of **raloxifene**. Avoid. [Severe] Theoretical

Raltegravir

- **Antacids** slightly decrease the exposure to **raltegravir**. Avoid. [Moderate] Study
- Antiepileptics **(carbamazepine)** are predicted to affect the exposure to **raltegravir**. [Moderate] Theoretical
- Antiepileptics **(fosphenytoin, phenobarbital, phenytoin, primidone)** are predicted to affect the exposure to **raltegravir**. Use with caution or avoid. [Moderate] Theoretical
- Calcium salts **(calcium carbonate)** greatly decrease the exposure to **raltegravir** (high-dose). Avoid. [Severe] Study
- **Encorafenib** is predicted to increase the exposure to **raltegravir**. [Moderate] Theoretical
- HIV-protease inhibitors **(atazanavir)** increase the exposure to **raltegravir** (high-dose). Avoid. [Moderate] Study

Raltegravir (continued)

- HIV-protease inhibitors **(darunavir)** increase the risk of rash when given with **raltegravir**. Moderate Study
- HIV-protease inhibitors **(fosamprenavir)** boosted with ritonavir decrease the exposure to **raltegravir** and **raltegravir** decreases the exposure to HIV-protease inhibitors **(fosamprenavir)** boosted with ritonavir. Avoid. Severe Study
- HIV-protease inhibitors **(tipranavir)** boosted with ritonavir are predicted to decrease the exposure to **raltegravir** (high-dose). Avoid. Moderate Study
- **Rifampicin** slightly decreases the exposure to **raltegravir**. Avoid or adjust dose—consult product literature. Moderate Study
- **Sodium zirconium cyclosilicate** is predicted to decrease the exposure to **raltegravir**. Separate administration by at least 2 hours. Moderate Theoretical

Raltitrexed → see TABLE 15 p. 910 (myelosuppression)

- **Folates** are predicted to alter the effects of **raltitrexed**. Avoid. Moderate Study
- **Live vaccines** are predicted to increase the risk of generalised infection (possibly life-threatening) when given with **raltitrexed**. Public Health England advises avoid (refer to Green Book). Severe Theoretical

Ramipril → see ACE inhibitors

Ramucirumab → see monoclonal antibodies

Ranibizumab

- **Ranibizumab** is predicted to increase the risk of bleeding events when given with **argatroban**. Severe Theoretical
- **Ranibizumab** is predicted to increase the risk of bleeding events when given with **bivalirudin**. Moderate Theoretical
- **Ranibizumab** increases the risk of bleeding events when given with **coumarins**. Severe Theoretical
- **Ranibizumab** is predicted to increase the risk of bleeding events when given with **danaparoid**. Severe Theoretical
- **Ranibizumab** increases the risk of bleeding events when given with **heparin (unfractionated)**. Severe Theoretical
- **Ranibizumab** increases the risk of bleeding events when given with **low molecular-weight heparins**. Severe Theoretical
- **Ranibizumab** is predicted to increase the risk of bleeding events when given with **phenindione**. Severe Theoretical

Ranitidine → see H_2 receptor antagonists

Ranolazine → see TABLE 9 p. 909 (QT-interval prolongation)

- **Ranolazine** is predicted to increase the exposure to **afatinib**. Separate administration by 12 hours. Moderate Study
- **Ranolazine** is predicted to increase the exposure to **aliskiren**. Moderate Theoretical
- Antiarrhythmics **(dronedarone)** are predicted to increase the exposure to **ranolazine**. Severe Study → Also see TABLE 9 p. 909
- Antiepileptics **(carbamazepine, fosphenytoin, phenobarbital, phenytoin, primidone)** are predicted to decrease the exposure to **ranolazine**. Avoid. Severe Study
- Antifungals, azoles **(fluconazole, isavuconazole, posaconazole)** are predicted to increase the exposure to **ranolazine**. Severe Study → Also see TABLE 9 p. 909
- Antifungals, azoles **(itraconazole, ketoconazole, voriconazole)** are predicted to increase the exposure to **ranolazine**. Avoid. Severe Study → Also see TABLE 9 p. 909
- **Apalutamide** is predicted to decrease the exposure to **ranolazine**. Avoid. Severe Study → Also see TABLE 9 p. 909
- **Aprepitant** is predicted to increase the exposure to **ranolazine**. Severe Study
- **Ranolazine** is predicted to increase the exposure to beta blockers, non-selective **(nadolol)**. Moderate Study
- **Ranolazine** is predicted to increase the exposure to **bictegravir**. Use with caution or avoid. Moderate Theoretical
- Calcium channel blockers **(diltiazem, verapamil)** are predicted to increase the exposure to **ranolazine**. Severe Study
- **Ranolazine** is predicted to increase the exposure to **ceritinib**. Moderate Theoretical → Also see TABLE 9 p. 909
- **Ciclosporin** is predicted to increase the concentration of **ranolazine** and **ranolazine** is predicted to increase the concentration of **ciclosporin**. Moderate Theoretical
- **Cobicistat** is predicted to increase the exposure to **ranolazine**. Avoid. Severe Study
- **Ranolazine** is predicted to increase the exposure to **colchicine**. Avoid P-glycoprotein inhibitors or adjust **colchicine** dose. Severe Theoretical
- **Crizotinib** is predicted to increase the exposure to **ranolazine**. Severe Study → Also see TABLE 9 p. 909
- **Ranolazine** is predicted to increase the exposure to **dabigatran**. Severe Theoretical
- **Ranolazine** increases the concentration of **digoxin**. Moderate Study
- **Ranolazine** is predicted to increase the exposure to dopamine receptor agonists **(pramipexole)**. Adjust dose. Moderate Study
- **Ranolazine** is predicted to slightly increase the exposure to **edoxaban**. Severe Theoretical
- **Enzalutamide** is predicted to decrease the exposure to **ranolazine**. Avoid. Severe Study
- **Ranolazine** is predicted to increase the exposure to **erlotinib**. Moderate Theoretical
- **Ranolazine** is predicted to increase the exposure to **fidaxomicin**. Avoid. Moderate Study
- **Grapefruit juice** is predicted to increase the concentration of **ranolazine**. Avoid. Severe Theoretical
- **HIV-protease inhibitors** are predicted to increase the exposure to **ranolazine**. Avoid. Severe Study → Also see TABLE 9 p. 909
- **Idelalisib** is predicted to increase the exposure to **ranolazine**. Avoid. Severe Study
- **Imatinib** is predicted to increase the exposure to **ranolazine**. Severe Study
- **Ranolazine** is predicted to increase the exposure to **larotrectinib**. Mild Theoretical
- **Ranolazine** is predicted to increase the exposure to **lomitapide**. Separate administration by 12 hours. Moderate Theoretical
- Macrolides **(clarithromycin)** are predicted to increase the exposure to **ranolazine**. Avoid. Severe Study → Also see TABLE 9 p. 909
- Macrolides **(erythromycin)** are predicted to increase the exposure to **ranolazine**. Severe Study → Also see TABLE 9 p. 909
- **Mitotane** is predicted to decrease the exposure to **ranolazine**. Avoid. Severe Study
- **Ranolazine** is predicted to increase the exposure to **naldemedine**. Moderate Study
- **Netupitant** is predicted to increase the exposure to **ranolazine**. Severe Study
- **Nilotinib** is predicted to increase the exposure to **ranolazine**. Severe Study → Also see TABLE 9 p. 909
- **Ranolazine** is predicted to increase the exposure to **nintedanib**. Moderate Study
- **Ranolazine** is predicted to increase the exposure to **panobinostat**. Adjust dose. Moderate Theoretical → Also see TABLE 9 p. 909
- **Ranolazine** is predicted to increase the exposure to **pibrentasvir**. Moderate Theoretical
- **Rifampicin** is predicted to decrease the exposure to **ranolazine**. Avoid. Severe Study
- **St John's Wort** is predicted to decrease the exposure to **ranolazine**. Avoid. Severe Study
- **Ranolazine** is predicted to increase the exposure to statins **(atorvastatin)**. Moderate Theoretical
- **Ranolazine** slightly increases the exposure to statins **(simvastatin)**. Adjust **simvastatin** dose, p. 141. Moderate Study
- **Ranolazine** increases the concentration of **tacrolimus**. Adjust dose. Severe Anecdotal
- **Ranolazine** is predicted to slightly increase the exposure to **talazoparib**. Avoid or adjust **talazoparib** dose. Severe Study
- **Ranolazine** is predicted to increase the exposure to **ticagrelor**. Use with caution or avoid. Severe Study
- **Ranolazine** is predicted to increase the exposure to **topotecan**. Severe Study
- **Ranolazine** is predicted to increase the concentration of **trametinib**. Moderate Theoretical
- **Ranolazine** is predicted to increase the exposure to **venetoclax**. Avoid or monitor for toxicity. Severe Theoretical

Rasagiline → see MAO-B inhibitors

A1 Interactions | Appendix 1

Reboxetine
- Antiepileptics **(carbamazepine, fosphenytoin, phenobarbital, phenytoin, primidone)** are predicted to decrease the exposure to **reboxetine**. Moderate Anecdotal
- Antifungals, azoles **(itraconazole, ketoconazole, voriconazole)** are predicted to increase the exposure to **reboxetine**. Avoid. Moderate Study
- Antifungals, azoles **(miconazole)** are predicted to increase the concentration of **reboxetine**. Use with caution and adjust dose. Moderate Theoretical
- **Apalutamide** is predicted to decrease the exposure to **reboxetine**. Moderate Anecdotal
- **Cobicistat** is predicted to increase the exposure to **reboxetine**. Avoid. Moderate Study
- **Enzalutamide** is predicted to decrease the exposure to **reboxetine**. Moderate Anecdotal
- **HIV-protease inhibitors** are predicted to increase the exposure to **reboxetine**. Avoid. Moderate Study
- **Idelalisib** is predicted to increase the exposure to **reboxetine**. Avoid. Moderate Study
- **Reboxetine** is predicted to increase the risk of a hypertensive crisis when given with **linezolid**. Avoid. Severe Theoretical
- **Reboxetine** is predicted to increase the risk of hypokalaemia when given with **loop diuretics**. Moderate Theoretical
- Macrolides **(clarithromycin)** are predicted to increase the exposure to **reboxetine**. Avoid. Moderate Study
- **Reboxetine** is predicted to increase the risk of a hypertensive crisis when given with MAO-B inhibitors **(rasagiline, selegiline)**. Avoid. Severe Theoretical
- **Reboxetine** is predicted to increase the risk of a hypertensive crisis when given with **MAOIs, irreversible**. Avoid. Severe Theoretical
- **Mitotane** is predicted to decrease the exposure to **reboxetine**. Moderate Anecdotal
- **Reboxetine** is predicted to increase the risk of a hypertensive crisis when given with **moclobemide**. Avoid. Severe Theoretical
- **Rifampicin** is predicted to decrease the exposure to **reboxetine**. Moderate Anecdotal
- **Reboxetine** is predicted to increase the risk of hypokalaemia when given with **thiazide diuretics**. Moderate Anecdotal

Regorafenib → see **TABLE 15** p. 910 (myelosuppression), **TABLE 4** p. 907 (antiplatelet effects)
- Antiepileptics **(carbamazepine, fosphenytoin, phenobarbital, phenytoin, primidone)** are predicted to decrease the exposure to **regorafenib**. Avoid. Moderate Study
- Antifungals, azoles **(itraconazole, ketoconazole, voriconazole)** are predicted to increase the exposure to **regorafenib**. Avoid. Moderate Study
- **Apalutamide** is predicted to decrease the exposure to **regorafenib**. Avoid. Moderate Study
- **Cobicistat** is predicted to increase the exposure to **regorafenib**. Avoid. Moderate Study
- **Regorafenib** is predicted to increase the risk of bleeding events when given with **coumarins**. Severe Study
- **Enzalutamide** is predicted to decrease the exposure to **regorafenib**. Avoid. Moderate Study
- **Grapefruit juice** is predicted to increase the exposure to **regorafenib**. Avoid. Moderate Theoretical
- **HIV-protease inhibitors** are predicted to increase the exposure to **regorafenib**. Avoid. Moderate Study
- **Idelalisib** is predicted to increase the exposure to **regorafenib**. Avoid. Moderate Study → Also see **TABLE 15** p. 910
- Macrolides **(clarithromycin)** are predicted to increase the exposure to **regorafenib**. Avoid. Moderate Study
- **Regorafenib** is predicted to increase the exposure to **methotrexate**. Moderate Theoretical → Also see **TABLE 15** p. 910
- **Mitotane** is predicted to decrease the exposure to **regorafenib**. Avoid. Moderate Study → Also see **TABLE 15** p. 910
- **Regorafenib** is predicted to increase the exposure to NSAIDs **(mefenamic acid)**. Avoid. Moderate Theoretical → Also see **TABLE 4** p. 907
- **Regorafenib** is predicted to increase the risk of bleeding events when given with **phenindione**. Severe Theoretical
- **Rifampicin** is predicted to decrease the exposure to **regorafenib**. Avoid. Moderate Study
- **Regorafenib** is predicted to increase the exposure to statins **(atorvastatin, fluvastatin, rosuvastatin)**. Moderate Study
- **Regorafenib** is predicted to increase the exposure to **sulfasalazine**. Moderate Study → Also see **TABLE 15** p. 910
- **Regorafenib** is predicted to increase the exposure to **topotecan**. Moderate Study → Also see **TABLE 15** p. 910

Remifentanil → see opioids

Repaglinide → see **TABLE 14** p. 910 (antidiabetic drugs)
- Antiepileptics **(carbamazepine, fosphenytoin, phenobarbital, phenytoin, primidone)** are predicted to decrease the exposure to **repaglinide**. Monitor blood glucose and adjust dose. Moderate Study
- Antifungals, azoles **(itraconazole, ketoconazole, voriconazole)** are predicted to increase the exposure to **repaglinide**. Moderate Study
- **Apalutamide** is predicted to decrease the exposure to **repaglinide**. Monitor blood glucose and adjust dose. Moderate Study
- **Ciclosporin** moderately increases the exposure to **repaglinide**. Moderate Study
- **Clopidogrel** increases the exposure to **repaglinide**. Avoid. Severe Study
- **Cobicistat** is predicted to increase the exposure to **repaglinide**. Moderate Study
- **Enzalutamide** is predicted to decrease the exposure to **repaglinide**. Monitor blood glucose and adjust dose. Moderate Study
- Fibrates **(gemfibrozil)** increase the exposure to **repaglinide**. Avoid. Severe Study
- **HIV-protease inhibitors** are predicted to increase the exposure to **repaglinide**. Moderate Study
- **Idelalisib** is predicted to increase the exposure to **repaglinide**. Moderate Study
- Iron chelators **(deferasirox)** moderately increase the exposure to **repaglinide**. Avoid. Moderate Study
- **Leflunomide** is predicted to increase the exposure to **repaglinide**. Moderate Study
- **Letermovir** is predicted to increase the concentration of **repaglinide**. Avoid. Moderate Theoretical
- Macrolides **(clarithromycin)** are predicted to increase the exposure to **repaglinide**. Moderate Study
- **Mitotane** is predicted to decrease the exposure to **repaglinide**. Monitor blood glucose and adjust dose. Moderate Study
- **Opicapone** is predicted to increase the exposure to **repaglinide**. Avoid. Moderate Study
- **Pitolisant** is predicted to decrease the exposure to **repaglinide**. Mild Theoretical
- **Rifampicin** is predicted to decrease the exposure to **repaglinide**. Monitor blood glucose and adjust dose. Moderate Study
- **Teriflunomide** is predicted to increase the exposure to **repaglinide**. Moderate Study
- **Trimethoprim** slightly increases the exposure to **repaglinide**. Avoid or monitor blood glucose. Moderate Study
- **Venetoclax** is predicted to increase the exposure to **repaglinide**. Moderate Theoretical

Retigabine → see antiepileptics

Retinoids → see **TABLE 5** p. 907 (thromboembolism)

acitretin · adapalene · alitretinoin · bexarotene · isotretinoin · tazarotene · tretinoin

- Avoid concomitant use of keratolytics in patients taking **acitretin** and **isotretinoin**.
- Since systemic absorption can follow topical application of **isotretinoin** and **tretinoin**, the possibility of interactions should be borne in mind.

- **Alcohol (beverage)** potentially increases the concentration of **acitretin**. Avoid and for 2 months after stopping **acitretin**. Moderate Study
- Antiarrhythmics **(amiodarone)** are predicted to increase the exposure to **alitretinoin**. Adjust **alitretinoin** dose. Moderate Theoretical
- Antifungals, azoles **(fluconazole, itraconazole, ketoconazole, miconazole, voriconazole)** are predicted to increase the

Retinoids (continued)
exposure to **alitretinoin.** Adjust **alitretinoin** dose. [Moderate] Theoretical
- Antifungals, azoles **(fluconazole, ketoconazole, voriconazole)** are predicted to increase the risk of tretinoin toxicity when given with **tretinoin.** [Moderate] Study
- **Clopidogrel** is predicted to increase the exposure to **alitretinoin.** Adjust **alitretinoin** dose. [Moderate] Theoretical
- **Cobicistat** is predicted to increase the exposure to **alitretinoin.** Adjust **alitretinoin** dose. [Moderate] Theoretical
- Fibrates **(gemfibrozil)** are predicted to increase the exposure to **alitretinoin.** Adjust **alitretinoin** dose. [Moderate] Theoretical
- Fibrates **(gemfibrozil)** increase the concentration of **bexarotene.** Avoid. [Severe] Study
- **HIV-protease inhibitors** are predicted to increase the exposure to **alitretinoin.** Adjust **alitretinoin** dose. [Moderate] Theoretical
- **Idelalisib** is predicted to increase the exposure to **alitretinoin.** Adjust **alitretinoin** dose. [Moderate] Theoretical
- Macrolides **(clarithromycin)** are predicted to increase the exposure to **alitretinoin.** Adjust **alitretinoin** dose. [Moderate] Theoretical
- **Acitretin** is predicted to increase the concentration of **methotrexate.** Avoid. [Moderate] Anecdotal
- Retinoids **(acitretin, alitretinoin, isotretinoin, tretinoin)** increase the risk of benign intracranial hypertension when given with **tetracyclines.** Avoid. [Severe] Anecdotal
- Retinoids **(acitretin, alitretinoin, isotretinoin, tretinoin)** increase the risk of benign intracranial hypertension when given with **tigecycline.** Avoid. [Severe] Anecdotal
- **Bexarotene** is predicted to increase the risk of toxicity when given with **vitamin A.** Adjust dose. [Moderate] Theoretical
- Retinoids **(acitretin, alitretinoin, isotretinoin)** are predicted to increase the risk of vitamin A toxicity when given with **vitamin A.** Avoid. [Severe] Theoretical
- **Tretinoin** is predicted to increase the risk of vitamin A toxicity when given with **vitamin A.** Avoid. [Severe] Study

Ribavirin
- **Ribavirin** increases the risk of toxicity when given with **stavudine.** Avoid. [Severe] Study
- **Ribavirin** increases the risk of anaemia and/or leucopenia when given with **zidovudine.** Avoid. [Severe] Study

Ribociclib → see TABLE 9 p. 909 (QT-interval prolongation)

FOOD AND LIFESTYLE Avoid concomitant use of pomegranate or pomegranate juice as it is predicted to increase ribociclib exposure.

- **Ribociclib** (high-dose) is predicted to increase the exposure to alpha blockers **(alfuzosin).** Avoid. [Moderate] Theoretical
- Antiarrhythmics **(dronedarone)** are predicted to increase the exposure to **ribociclib.** [Moderate] Study → Also see TABLE 9 p. 909
- **Ribociclib** (high-dose) is predicted to increase the exposure to antiarrhythmics **(amiodarone).** Avoid. [Moderate] Theoretical → Also see TABLE 9 p. 909
- Antiepileptics **(carbamazepine, fosphenytoin, phenobarbital, phenytoin, primidone)** are predicted to markedly decrease the exposure to **ribociclib.** Avoid. [Severe] Study
- Antifungals, azoles **(fluconazole, isavuconazole, posaconazole)** are predicted to increase the exposure to **ribociclib.** [Moderate] Study → Also see TABLE 9 p. 909
- Antifungals, azoles **(itraconazole, ketoconazole, voriconazole)** are predicted to increase the exposure to **ribociclib.** Avoid or adjust **ribociclib** dose. [Moderate] Study → Also see TABLE 9 p. 909
- **Apalutamide** is predicted to markedly decrease the exposure to **ribociclib.** Avoid. [Severe] Study → Also see TABLE 9 p. 909
- **Aprepitant** is predicted to increase the exposure to **ribociclib.** [Moderate] Study
- **Bosentan** is predicted to decrease the exposure to **ribociclib.** [Moderate] Study
- Calcium channel blockers **(diltiazem, verapamil)** are predicted to increase the exposure to **ribociclib.** [Moderate] Study
- **Ribociclib** is predicted to increase the exposure to **ciclosporin.** Use with caution and adjust dose. [Moderate] Theoretical
- **Cobicistat** is predicted to increase the exposure to **ribociclib.** Avoid or adjust **ribociclib** dose. [Moderate] Study
- **Crizotinib** is predicted to increase the exposure to **ribociclib.** [Moderate] Study → Also see TABLE 9 p. 909
- **Ribociclib** is predicted to increase the exposure to **digoxin.** [Moderate] Theoretical
- **Efavirenz** is predicted to decrease the exposure to **ribociclib.** [Moderate] Study → Also see TABLE 9 p. 909
- **Enzalutamide** is predicted to markedly decrease the exposure to **ribociclib.** Avoid. [Severe] Study
- **Ribociclib** (high-dose) is predicted to increase the exposure to **ergotamine.** Avoid. [Moderate] Theoretical
- **Ribociclib** is predicted to increase the exposure to **everolimus.** Use with caution and adjust dose. [Moderate] Theoretical
- **Grapefruit juice** is predicted to increase the exposure to **ribociclib.** Avoid. [Moderate] Theoretical
- **HIV-protease inhibitors** are predicted to increase the exposure to **ribociclib.** Avoid or adjust **ribociclib** dose. [Moderate] Study → Also see TABLE 9 p. 909
- **Idelalisib** is predicted to increase the exposure to **ribociclib.** Avoid or adjust **ribociclib** dose. [Moderate] Study
- **Imatinib** is predicted to increase the exposure to **ribociclib.** [Moderate] Study
- Macrolides **(clarithromycin)** are predicted to increase the exposure to **ribociclib.** Avoid or adjust **ribociclib** dose. [Moderate] Study → Also see TABLE 9 p. 909
- Macrolides **(erythromycin)** are predicted to increase the exposure to **ribociclib.** [Moderate] Study → Also see TABLE 9 p. 909
- **Ribociclib** is predicted to increase the exposure to **metformin.** [Moderate] Theoretical
- **Ribociclib** moderately increases the exposure to **midazolam.** Avoid. [Moderate] Study
- **Mitotane** is predicted to markedly decrease the exposure to **ribociclib.** Avoid. [Severe] Study
- **Netupitant** is predicted to increase the exposure to **ribociclib.** [Moderate] Study
- **Nevirapine** is predicted to decrease the exposure to **ribociclib.** [Moderate] Study
- **Nilotinib** is predicted to increase the exposure to **ribociclib.** [Moderate] Study → Also see TABLE 9 p. 909
- **Ribociclib** is predicted to increase the exposure to opioids **(alfentanil, fentanyl).** Use with caution and adjust dose. [Moderate] Theoretical
- **Ribociclib** is predicted to increase the exposure to phosphodiesterase type-5 inhibitors **(sildenafil).** Avoid. [Moderate] Theoretical → Also see TABLE 9 p. 909
- **Ribociclib** (high-dose) is predicted to increase the exposure to **pimozide.** Avoid. [Moderate] Theoretical → Also see TABLE 9 p. 909
- **Ribociclib** (high-dose) is predicted to increase the exposure to **quetiapine.** Avoid. [Moderate] Theoretical
- **Rifampicin** is predicted to markedly decrease the exposure to **ribociclib.** Avoid. [Severe] Study
- **Ribociclib** is predicted to increase the exposure to **sirolimus.** Use with caution and adjust dose. [Moderate] Theoretical
- **St John's Wort** is predicted to decrease the exposure to **ribociclib.** Avoid. [Severe] Study
- **Ribociclib** is predicted to increase the exposure to statins **(pravastatin, rosuvastatin).** [Moderate] Theoretical
- **Ribociclib** (high-dose) is predicted to increase the exposure to statins **(simvastatin).** Avoid. [Moderate] Theoretical
- **Ribociclib** is predicted to increase the exposure to **tacrolimus.** Use with caution and adjust dose. [Moderate] Theoretical

Rifabutin

GENERAL INFORMATION Although some manufacturers class rifabutin as a potent inducer of CYP3A4, clinical data suggests it is potentially a weak inducer, and therefore the BNF does not extrapolate the interactions of potent CYP3A4 inducers to rifabutin. For those who wish to err on the side of caution, see the interactions of rifampicin but bear in mind other mechanisms might be involved.

- Antifungals, azoles **(fluconazole)** increase the risk of uveitis when given with **rifabutin.** Adjust dose. [Severe] Study
- Antifungals, azoles **(itraconazole, posaconazole)** increase the concentration of **rifabutin** and **rifabutin** decreases the concentration of antifungals, azoles **(itraconazole, posaconazole).** Avoid. [Severe] Study
- Antifungals, azoles **(ketoconazole)** are predicted to increase the concentration of **rifabutin** and **rifabutin** is predicted to

decrease the concentration of antifungals, azoles **(ketoconazole)**. Avoid. [Severe] Theoretical
- Antifungals, azoles **(miconazole)** are predicted to increase the concentration of **rifabutin**. Use with caution and adjust dose. [Moderate] Theoretical
- **Rifabutin** is predicted to decrease the exposure to antifungals, azoles **(isavuconazole)**. Avoid. [Severe] Theoretical
- **Rifabutin** decreases the concentration of antifungals, azoles **(voriconazole)** and antifungals, azoles **(voriconazole)** increase the concentration of **rifabutin**. Avoid or adjust **voriconazole** dose, p. 410. [Severe] Study
- **Rifabutin** slightly decreases the exposure to antimalarials **(atovaquone)**. Avoid. [Moderate] Study
- **Rifabutin** slightly decreases the exposure to **bictegravir**. Avoid. [Moderate] Study
- **Rifabutin** is predicted to decrease the exposure to **brigatinib**. Avoid. [Moderate] Theoretical
- **Rifabutin** decreases the concentration of **cobicistat** and **cobicistat** increases the exposure to **rifabutin**. Avoid or adjust dose. [Severe] Study
- **Rifabutin** is predicted to decrease the efficacy of **combined hormonal contraceptives**. For FSRH guidance, see Contraceptives, interactions p. 536. [Severe] Study
- **Rifabutin** decreases the exposure to **dapsone**. [Moderate] Study
- **Rifabutin** is predicted to decrease the efficacy of **desogestrel**. For FSRH guidance, see Contraceptives, interactions p. 536. [Severe] Theoretical
- **Rifabutin** moderately decreases the exposure to **doravirine**. Adjust doravirine or lamivudine with tenofovir disoproxil and doravirine dose. [Moderate] Study
- **Efavirenz** slightly decreases the exposure to **rifabutin**. Adjust dose. [Severe] Study
- **Rifabutin** is predicted to decrease the efficacy of **etonogestrel**. For FSRH guidance, see Contraceptives, interactions p. 536. [Severe] Theoretical
- **Rifabutin** decreases the exposure to **etravirine**. [Moderate] Study
- HIV-protease inhibitors **(atazanavir, darunavir, fosamprenavir, lopinavir, saquinavir, tipranavir)** boosted with ritonavir increase the exposure to **rifabutin**. Monitor and adjust dose. [Severe] Study
- HIV-protease inhibitors **(ritonavir)** markedly increase the exposure to **rifabutin**. Avoid or adjust dose. [Severe] Study
- **Rifabutin** is predicted to decrease the effects of **hormone replacement therapy**. [Moderate] Anecdotal
- **Rifabutin** is predicted to decrease the exposure to **ledipasvir**. Avoid. [Severe] Theoretical
- **Rifabutin** is predicted to decrease the concentration of **letermovir**. [Moderate] Theoretical
- **Rifabutin** is predicted to decrease the efficacy of **levonorgestrel**. For FSRH guidance, see Contraceptives, interactions p. 536. [Severe] Theoretical
- **Lumacaftor** is predicted to decrease the exposure to **rifabutin**. Adjust dose. [Moderate] Theoretical
- Macrolides **(azithromycin)** increase the risk of neutropenia when given with **rifabutin**. [Severe] Study
- Macrolides **(clarithromycin)** increase the risk of uveitis when given with **rifabutin**. Adjust dose. [Severe] Study
- Macrolides **(erythromycin)** are predicted to increase the risk of uveitis when given with **rifabutin**. Adjust dose. [Severe] Theoretical
- **Rifabutin** is predicted to decrease the efficacy of **norethisterone**. For FSRH guidance, see Contraceptives, interactions p. 536. [Severe] Anecdotal
- **Rifabutin** slightly decreases the exposure to **rilpivirine**. Adjust dose. [Severe] Study
- **Rifabutin** is predicted to decrease the exposure to **rolapitant**. Avoid. [Moderate] Theoretical
- **Rifabutin** is predicted to decrease the exposure to **tenofovir alafenamide**. Avoid. [Moderate] Theoretical
- **Rifabutin** is predicted to decrease the exposure to **tezacaftor**. Avoid. [Severe] Theoretical
- **Rifabutin** decreases the efficacy of **ulipristal**. For FSRH guidance, see Contraceptives, interactions p. 536. [Severe] Anecdotal
- **Rifabutin** is predicted to decrease the concentration of **voxilaprevir**. Avoid. [Severe] Theoretical

Rifampicin

- **Rifampicin** is predicted to markedly decrease the exposure to **abemaciclib**. Avoid. [Severe] Study
- **Rifampicin** is predicted to decrease the exposure to **abiraterone**. Avoid. [Severe] Study
- **Rifampicin** is predicted to decrease the exposure to **afatinib**. [Moderate] Study
- **Rifampicin** is predicted to decrease the exposure to **agomelatine**. [Moderate] Theoretical
- **Rifampicin** is predicted to decrease the exposure to aldosterone antagonists **(eplerenone)**. Avoid. [Moderate] Theoretical
- **Rifampicin** decreases the exposure to **aliskiren**. [Moderate] Study
- **Rifampicin** is predicted to decrease the exposure to **alprazolam**. Adjust dose. [Moderate] Theoretical
- **Rifampicin** transiently increases the exposure to **ambrisentan**. [Moderate] Study
- **Rifampicin** decreases the exposure to **aminophylline**. Adjust dose. [Moderate] Study
- **Rifampicin** is predicted to decrease the exposure to anaesthetics, local **(ropivacaine)**. [Moderate] Theoretical
- **Antacids** decrease the absorption of **rifampicin**. **Rifampicin** should be taken 1 hour before antacids. [Moderate] Study
- **Rifampicin** is predicted to decrease the exposure to antiarrhythmics **(disopyramide, dronedarone)**. Avoid. [Severe] Study
- **Rifampicin** is predicted to decrease the efficacy of antiarrhythmics **(propafenone)**. [Moderate] Study
- **Rifampicin** is predicted to decrease the exposure to anticholinesterases, centrally acting **(donepezil)**. [Mild] Study
- Antiepileptics **(phenobarbital, primidone)** are predicted to decrease the exposure to **rifampicin** and **rifampicin** is predicted to decrease the exposure to antiepileptics **(phenobarbital, primidone)**. Use with caution and adjust dose. [Moderate] Study
- **Rifampicin** slightly decreases the exposure to antiepileptics **(brivaracetam)**. Adjust dose. [Moderate] Study
- **Rifampicin** decreases the concentration of antiepileptics **(fosphenytoin, phenytoin)**. Use with caution and adjust dose. [Moderate] Study
- **Rifampicin** markedly increases the clearance of antiepileptics **(lamotrigine)**. Adjust **lamotrigine** dose, p. 216. [Moderate] Study
- **Rifampicin** is predicted to decrease the exposure to antiepileptics **(perampanel)**. Monitor and adjust dose. [Moderate] Study
- **Rifampicin** slightly decreases the exposure to antifungals, azoles **(fluconazole)**. Adjust dose. [Moderate] Study
- **Rifampicin** is predicted to decrease the exposure to antifungals, azoles **(isavuconazole)**. Avoid. [Severe] Study
- **Rifampicin** markedly decreases the exposure to antifungals, azoles **(itraconazole)**. Avoid and for 14 days after stopping **rifampicin**. [Moderate] Study
- **Rifampicin** markedly decreases the exposure to antifungals, azoles **(ketoconazole)** and antifungals, azoles **(ketoconazole)** potentially decrease the exposure to **rifampicin**. Avoid. [Moderate] Study
- **Rifampicin** is predicted to decrease the exposure to antifungals, azoles **(posaconazole)**. Avoid. [Moderate] Anecdotal
- **Rifampicin** very markedly decreases the exposure to antifungals, azoles **(voriconazole)**. Avoid. [Moderate] Study
- **Rifampicin** is predicted to decrease the exposure to antihistamines, non-sedating **(bilastine)**. [Moderate] Theoretical
- **Rifampicin** increases the clearance of antihistamines, non-sedating **(fexofenadine)**. [Moderate] Study
- **Rifampicin** is predicted to decrease the exposure to antimalarials **(artemether)** (with lumefantrine). Avoid. [Severe] Study
- **Rifampicin** moderately decreases the exposure to antimalarials **(atovaquone)** and antimalarials **(atovaquone)** slightly increase the exposure to **rifampicin**. Avoid. [Moderate] Study
- **Rifampicin** moderately decreases the exposure to antimalarials **(mefloquine)**. [Severe] Study
- **Rifampicin** is predicted to decrease the concentration of antimalarials **(piperaquine)**. Avoid. [Moderate] Theoretical

Rifampicin (continued)
- **Rifampicin** decreases the exposure to antimalarials **(quinine)**. Severe Study
- **Rifampicin** is predicted to moderately decrease the exposure to apixaban. Use with caution or avoid. Severe Study
- **Rifampicin** moderately decreases the exposure to **apremilast**. Avoid. Severe Study
- **Rifampicin** is predicted to markedly decrease the exposure to aprepitant. Avoid. Moderate Study
- **Rifampicin** is predicted to moderately decrease the exposure to aripiprazole. Adjust **aripiprazole** dose, p. 265. Moderate Study
- **Rifampicin** decreases the exposure to ataluren. Moderate Study
- **Rifampicin** is predicted to decrease the exposure to **axitinib**. Avoid or adjust dose. Moderate Study
- **Rifampicin** is predicted to decrease the exposure to bazedoxifene. Moderate Theoretical
- **Rifampicin** decreases the exposure to **bedaquiline**. Avoid. Severe Study
- **Rifampicin** moderately decreases the exposure to beta blockers, non-selective **(carvedilol)**. Moderate Study
- **Rifampicin** decreases the exposure to beta blockers, non-selective **(propranolol)**. Monitor and adjust dose. Moderate Study
- **Rifampicin** slightly decreases the exposure to beta blockers, selective **(bisoprolol, metoprolol)**. Mild Study
- **Rifampicin** moderately decreases the exposure to beta blockers, selective **(celiprolol)**. Moderate Study
- **Rifampicin** is predicted to decrease the exposure to **bictegravir**. Avoid. Moderate Study
- **Rifampicin** slightly decreases the exposure to **bortezomib**. Avoid. Severe Study
- **Rifampicin** affects the exposure to bosentan. Avoid. Severe Study
- **Rifampicin** is predicted to very markedly decrease the exposure to **bosutinib**. Avoid. Severe Study
- **Rifampicin** is predicted to decrease the exposure to **brigatinib**. Avoid. Severe Study
- **Rifampicin** is predicted to decrease the exposure to **bupropion**. Moderate Study
- **Rifampicin** is predicted to decrease the exposure to **buspirone**. Use with caution and adjust dose. Severe Study
- **Rifampicin** moderately decreases the exposure to **cabozantinib**. Avoid. Moderate Study
- **Rifampicin** is predicted to moderately increase the clearance of **caffeine citrate**. Monitor and adjust dose. Moderate Study
- **Rifampicin** is predicted to decrease the exposure to calcium channel blockers **(amlodipine, felodipine, lacidipine, lercanidipine, nicardipine, nimodipine)**. Monitor and adjust dose. Moderate Study
- **Rifampicin** greatly decreases the exposure to calcium channel blockers **(diltiazem, verapamil)**. Severe Study
- **Rifampicin** moderately decreases the exposure to calcium channel blockers **(nifedipine)**. Avoid. Severe Study
- **Rifampicin** moderately decreases the exposure to **canagliflozin**. Adjust **canagliflozin** dose. Moderate Study
- **Rifampicin** is predicted to decrease the exposure to cannabidiol. Adjust dose. Moderate Study
- **Rifampicin** is predicted to decrease the exposure to cariprazine. Avoid. Severe Theoretical
- **Rifampicin** decreases the concentration of **caspofungin**. Adjust **caspofungin** dose, p. 405. Moderate Study
- **Rifampicin** is predicted to decrease the exposure to **ceritinib**. Avoid. Severe Study
- **Rifampicin** decreases the concentration of **chloramphenicol**. Moderate Study
- **Rifampicin** is predicted to decrease the exposure to **chlordiazepoxide**. Moderate Theoretical
- **Rifampicin** decreases the concentration of **ciclosporin**. Severe Study
- **Rifampicin** is predicted to alter the effects of **cilostazol**. Moderate Theoretical
- **Rifampicin** is predicted to decrease the exposure to **cinacalcet**. Monitor and adjust dose. Moderate Study
- **Rifampicin** decreases the exposure to **clomethiazole**. Monitor and adjust dose. Moderate Study
- **Rifampicin** decreases the exposure to **clozapine**. Severe Anecdotal
- **Rifampicin** is predicted to decrease the exposure to **cobicistat**. Avoid. Severe Theoretical
- **Rifampicin** is predicted to decrease the exposure to **cobimetinib**. Avoid. Severe Theoretical
- **Rifampicin** is predicted to decrease the efficacy of **combined hormonal contraceptives**. For FSRH guidance, see Contraceptives, interactions p. 536. Severe Study
- **Rifampicin** is predicted to decrease the exposure to corticosteroids **(budesonide, deflazacort, dexamethasone, fludrocortisone, hydrocortisone, methylprednisolone, prednisolone, triamcinolone)**. Monitor and adjust dose. Moderate Study
- **Rifampicin** is predicted to decrease the exposure to corticosteroids **(fluticasone)**. Unknown Theoretical
- **Rifampicin** decreases the anticoagulant effect of **coumarins**. Severe Study
- **Rifampicin** is predicted to markedly decrease the exposure to crizotinib. Avoid. Severe Study
- **Rifampicin** is predicted to decrease the exposure to **dabigatran**. Avoid. Severe Study
- **Rifampicin** is predicted to decrease the exposure to **dabrafenib**. Avoid. Moderate Theoretical
- **Rifampicin** decreases the exposure to **dapsone**. Moderate Study
- **Rifampicin** is predicted to decrease the exposure to darifenacin. Moderate Theoretical
- **Rifampicin** is predicted to decrease the exposure to **dasabuvir**. Avoid. Severe Theoretical
- **Rifampicin** is predicted to markedly decrease the exposure to dasatinib. Avoid. Severe Study
- **Rifampicin** is predicted to slightly decrease the exposure to delamanid. Avoid. Moderate Study
- **Rifampicin** is predicted to decrease the efficacy of **desogestrel**. For FSRH guidance, see Contraceptives, interactions p. 536. Severe Theoretical
- **Rifampicin** moderately decreases the exposure to **diazepam**. Avoid. Moderate Study
- **Rifampicin** is predicted to markedly decrease the exposure to dienogest. Severe Study
- **Rifampicin** decreases the concentration of **digoxin**. Moderate Study
- **Rifampicin** decreases the exposure to **dolutegravir**. Adjust dose. Severe Study
- **Rifampicin** is predicted to decrease the exposure to **doravirine**. Avoid. Severe Study
- **Rifampicin** is predicted to decrease the exposure to **dronabinol**. Avoid or adjust dose. Mild Study
- **Rifampicin** is predicted to decrease the exposure to **duloxetine**. Moderate Theoretical
- **Rifampicin** is predicted to decrease the exposure to **edoxaban**. Moderate Study
- **Rifampicin** slightly decreases the exposure to **efavirenz**. Adjust dose. Severe Study
- **Rifampicin** is predicted to decrease the exposure to **elbasvir**. Avoid. Severe Study
- **Rifampicin** is predicted to decrease the exposure to **eliglustat**. Avoid. Severe Study
- **Rifampicin** is predicted to decrease the exposure to eltrombopag and eltrombopag is predicted to increase the concentration of **rifampicin**. Moderate Theoretical
- **Rifampicin** is predicted to decrease the concentration of elvitegravir. Avoid. Severe Theoretical
- **Rifampicin** is predicted to decrease the exposure to encorafenib. Severe Theoretical
- **Rifampicin** is predicted to decrease the effects of **ergotamine**. Moderate Theoretical
- **Rifampicin** is predicted to decrease the exposure to **erlotinib**. Avoid or adjust **erlotinib** dose. Severe Study
- **Rifampicin** is predicted to decrease the exposure to esketamine. Adjust dose. Moderate Theoretical
- **Rifampicin** is predicted to decrease the efficacy of **etonogestrel**. For FSRH guidance, see Contraceptives, interactions p. 536. Severe Theoretical

- **Rifampicin** is predicted to decrease the exposure to **etravirine**. Avoid. Severe Theoretical
- **Rifampicin** is predicted to decrease the concentration of **everolimus**. Avoid or adjust dose. Severe Study
- **Rifampicin** moderately decreases the exposure to **exemestane**. Moderate Study
- **Rifampicin** is predicted to decrease the exposure to **fesoterodine**. Avoid. Moderate Study
- **Rifampicin** is predicted to decrease the exposure to **fingolimod**. Moderate Study
- **Rifampicin** is predicted to decrease the exposure to **fosaprepitant**. Avoid. Moderate Theoretical
- **Rifampicin** is predicted to decrease the exposure to **gefitinib**. Avoid. Severe Study
- **Rifampicin** moderately decreases the exposure to **gilteritinib**. Avoid. Severe Study
- **Rifampicin** markedly affects the exposure to **glecaprevir**. Avoid. Severe Study
- **Rifampicin** is predicted to decrease the exposure to **grazoprevir**. Avoid. Severe Study
- **Rifampicin** is predicted to decrease the concentration of **guanfacine**. Adjust **guanfacine** dose, p. 247. Moderate Study
- **Rifampicin** decreases the concentration of **haloperidol**. Adjust dose. Moderate Study
- **Rifampicin** is predicted to moderately to markedly decrease the exposure to HIV-protease inhibitors **(atazanavir, darunavir, fosamprenavir, lopinavir, saquinavir)**. Avoid. Severe Study
- **Rifampicin** slightly decreases the exposure to HIV-protease inhibitors **(ritonavir)**. Severe Study
- **Rifampicin** is predicted to decrease the exposure to HIV-protease inhibitors **(tipranavir)**. Avoid. Severe Study
- **Rifampicin** is predicted to decrease the effects of **hormone replacement therapy**. Moderate Anecdotal
- **Rifampicin** is predicted to decrease the exposure to **ibrutinib**. Avoid or adjust **ibrutinib** dose. Severe Study
- **Rifampicin** is predicted to decrease the exposure to **idelalisib**. Avoid. Severe Study
- **Rifampicin** is predicted to decrease the exposure to **imatinib**. Avoid. Moderate Study
- **Rifampicin** is predicted to decrease the exposure to **irinotecan**. Avoid. Severe Study
- **Rifampicin** is predicted to decrease the exposure to iron chelators **(deferasirox)**. Monitor serum ferritin and adjust dose. Moderate Study
- **Rifampicin** is predicted to decrease the exposure to **ivabradine**. Adjust dose. Moderate Theoretical
- **Rifampicin** is predicted to moderately to markedly decrease the exposure to **ivacaftor**. Avoid. Severe Study
- **Rifampicin** is predicted to decrease the exposure to **ixazomib**. Avoid. Severe Study
- **Rifampicin** is predicted to decrease the exposure to **lapatinib**. Avoid. Severe Study
- **Rifampicin** is predicted to moderately decrease the exposure to **larotrectinib**. Avoid. Moderate Study
- **Rifampicin** is predicted to decrease the exposure to **ledipasvir**. Avoid. Severe Study
- **Leflunomide** is predicted to increase the exposure to **rifampicin**. Moderate Theoretical
- **Rifampicin** is predicted to affect the concentration of **letermovir**. Severe Theoretical
- **Rifampicin** is predicted to decrease the efficacy of **levonorgestrel**. For FSRH guidance, see Contraceptives, interactions p. 536. Severe Theoretical
- **Rifampicin** is predicted to decrease the exposure to **linagliptin**. Moderate Study
- **Rifampicin** slightly decreases the exposure to **linezolid**. Moderate Study
- **Rifampicin** is predicted to decrease the exposure to **lomitapide**. Monitor and adjust dose. Moderate Theoretical
- **Rifampicin** increases the clearance of **lorazepam**. Moderate Study
- **Rifampicin** is predicted to decrease the exposure to **lorlatinib**. Avoid. Severe Study
- **Rifampicin** is predicted to decrease the exposure to **lurasidone**. Avoid. Moderate Study
- **Rifampicin** is predicted to decrease the exposure to **macitentan**. Avoid. Severe Study
- **Rifampicin** decreases the concentration of macrolides **(clarithromycin)**. Severe Study
- **Rifampicin** is predicted to decrease the exposure to **maraviroc**. Adjust dose. Severe Study
- **Rifampicin** is predicted to decrease the exposure to **melatonin**. Moderate Theoretical
- **Rifampicin** is predicted to increase the clearance of **mexiletine**. Monitor and adjust dose. Moderate Study
- **Rifampicin** is predicted to decrease the exposure to **midazolam**. Monitor and adjust dose. Moderate Study
- **Rifampicin** is predicted to decrease the exposure to **midostaurin**. Avoid. Severe Study
- **Rifampicin** is predicted to decrease the exposure to **mirtazapine**. Adjust dose. Moderate Study
- **Rifampicin** is predicted to decrease the exposure to **modafinil**. Moderate Theoretical
- **Rifampicin** decreases the effects of monoclonal antibodies **(brentuximab vedotin)**. Severe Study
- **Rifampicin** is predicted to decrease the exposure to monoclonal antibodies **(polatuzumab vedotin)**. Moderate Theoretical
- **Rifampicin** is predicted to decrease the exposure to **montelukast**. Mild Study
- **Rifampicin** decreases the concentration of **mycophenolate**. Monitor and adjust dose. Severe Study
- **Rifampicin** is predicted to markedly decrease the exposure to **naldemedine**. Avoid. Severe Study
- **Rifampicin** is predicted to markedly decrease the exposure to **naloxegol**. Avoid. Moderate Study
- **Rifampicin** is predicted to slightly decrease the exposure to **nateglinide**. Mild Study
- **Rifampicin** is predicted to decrease the exposure to **neratinib**. Avoid. Severe Study
- **Rifampicin** is predicted to decrease the exposure to **netupitant**. Avoid. Severe Study
- **Rifampicin** decreases the concentration of **nevirapine**. Avoid. Severe Study
- **Rifampicin** is predicted to moderately decrease the exposure to **nilotinib**. Avoid. Severe Study
- **Rifampicin** is predicted to decrease the exposure to **nintedanib**. Moderate Study
- **Rifampicin** is predicted to decrease the exposure to **nitisinone**. Adjust dose. Moderate Theoretical
- **Rifampicin** increases the clearance of **nitrazepam**. Moderate Study
- **Rifampicin** is predicted to decrease the efficacy of **norethisterone**. For FSRH guidance, see Contraceptives, interactions p. 536. Severe Anecdotal
- **Rifampicin** moderately decreases the exposure to NSAIDs **(celecoxib, diclofenac, etoricoxib)**. Moderate Study
- **Rifampicin** is predicted to decrease the exposure to **olanzapine**. Monitor and adjust dose. Moderate Study
- **Rifampicin** is predicted to decrease the exposure to **olaparib**. Avoid. Moderate Theoretical
- **Rifampicin** is predicted to decrease the exposure to **ombitasvir**. Avoid. Severe Theoretical
- **Rifampicin** is predicted to decrease the exposure to **ondansetron**. Moderate Study
- **Rifampicin** is predicted to decrease the exposure to opioids **(alfentanil, fentanyl)**. Moderate Study
- **Rifampicin** is predicted to decrease the exposure to opioids **(buprenorphine)**. Monitor and adjust dose. Moderate Theoretical
- **Rifampicin** decreases the exposure to opioids **(codeine, morphine)**. Moderate Study
- **Rifampicin** decreases the exposure to opioids **(methadone)**. Monitor and adjust dose. Severe Study
- **Rifampicin** is predicted to decrease the exposure to opioids **(oxycodone)**. Monitor and adjust dose. Moderate Study
- **Rifampicin** is predicted to moderately decrease the exposure to **osimertinib**. Avoid. Moderate Study
- **Rifampicin** is predicted to moderately decrease the exposure to **ospemifene**. Moderate Study
- **Rifampicin** is predicted to decrease the exposure to **palbociclib**. Avoid. Severe Study

Rifampicin (continued)

- **Rifampicin** is predicted to decrease the exposure to **paliperidone**. Monitor and adjust dose. Severe Study
- **Rifampicin** is predicted to decrease the exposure to **panobinostat**. Avoid. Moderate Theoretical
- **Rifampicin** decreases the exposure to **paracetamol**. Moderate Study
- **Rifampicin** is predicted to decrease the exposure to **paritaprevir** (with ritonavir and ombitasvir). Avoid. Severe Study
- **Rifampicin** is predicted to decrease the exposure to **pazopanib**. Avoid. Severe Theoretical
- **Rifampicin** is predicted to decrease the exposure to phosphodiesterase type-5 inhibitors **(avanafil, tadalafil)**. Avoid. Severe Study
- **Rifampicin** is predicted to decrease the exposure to phosphodiesterase type-5 inhibitors **(sildenafil, vardenafil)**. Moderate Theoretical
- **Rifampicin** is predicted to moderately to markedly decrease the exposure to **pibrentasvir**. Avoid. Severe Study
- **Rifampicin** moderately decreases the exposure to **pioglitazone**. Monitor and adjust dose. Moderate Study
- **Rifampicin** is predicted to decrease the exposure to **pirfenidone**. Avoid. Moderate Theoretical
- **Rifampicin** is predicted to moderately decrease the exposure to **pitolisant**. Moderate Study
- **Rifampicin** is predicted to decrease the exposure to **ponatinib**. Avoid. Moderate Theoretical
- **Rifampicin** is predicted to markedly decrease the exposure to **praziquantel**. Avoid. Moderate Study
- **Rifampicin** is predicted to decrease the exposure to **quetiapine**. Moderate Study
- **Rifampicin** slightly decreases the exposure to **raltegravir**. Avoid or adjust dose—consult product literature. Moderate Study
- **Rifampicin** is predicted to decrease the exposure to **ranolazine**. Avoid. Severe Study
- **Rifampicin** is predicted to decrease the exposure to **reboxetine**. Moderate Anecdotal
- **Rifampicin** is predicted to decrease the exposure to **regorafenib**. Avoid. Moderate Study
- **Rifampicin** is predicted to decrease the exposure to **repaglinide**. Monitor blood glucose and adjust dose. Moderate Study
- **Rifampicin** is predicted to markedly decrease the exposure to **ribociclib**. Avoid. Severe Study
- **Rifampicin** markedly decreases the exposure to **rilpivirine**. Avoid. Severe Study
- **Rifampicin** is predicted to decrease the exposure to **risperidone**. Adjust dose. Moderate Study
- **Rifampicin** is predicted to moderately decrease the exposure to **rivaroxaban**. Avoid unless patient can be monitored for signs of thrombosis. Severe Study
- **Rifampicin** is predicted to decrease the exposure to **roflumilast**. Avoid. Moderate Study
- **Rifampicin** is predicted to markedly decrease the exposure to **rolapitant**. Avoid. Severe Study
- **Rifampicin** is predicted to decrease the exposure to **ruxolitinib**. Monitor and adjust dose. Moderate Study
- **Rifampicin** is predicted to moderately decrease the exposure to **saxagliptin**. Moderate Study
- **Rifampicin** moderately decreases the exposure to the active metabolite of **selexipag**. Adjust dose. Moderate Study
- **Rifampicin** is predicted to decrease the exposure to **siponimod**. Severe Study
- **Rifampicin** is predicted to decrease the concentration of **sirolimus**. Avoid. Severe Study
- **Rifampicin** is predicted to decrease the exposure to **sofosbuvir**. Avoid. Severe Study
- **Rifampicin** is predicted to decrease the exposure to **solifenacin**. Moderate Theoretical
- **Rifampicin** is predicted to decrease the exposure to **sorafenib**. Moderate Theoretical
- **Rifampicin** markedly decreases the exposure to statins **(atorvastatin)**. Manufacturer advises take both drugs at the same time. Moderate Study
- **Rifampicin** moderately decreases the exposure to statins **(fluvastatin)**. Monitor and adjust dose. Moderate Study
- **Rifampicin** very markedly decreases the exposure to statins **(simvastatin)**. Moderate Study
- **Rifampicin** is predicted to decrease the exposure to **sulfonylureas**. Moderate Study
- **Rifampicin** is predicted to decrease the exposure to **sunitinib**. Avoid or adjust **sunitinib** dose. Moderate Study
- **Rifampicin** decreases the concentration of **tacrolimus**. Monitor and adjust dose. Severe Study
- **Rifampicin** markedly decreases the exposure to **tamoxifen**. Unknown Study
- **Rifampicin** is predicted to decrease the exposure to taxanes **(cabazitaxel, paclitaxel)**. Avoid. Severe Study
- **Rifampicin** is predicted to decrease the exposure to taxanes **(docetaxel)**. Severe Theoretical
- **Rifampicin** is predicted to decrease the concentration of **temsirolimus**. Avoid. Severe Study
- **Rifampicin** is predicted to decrease the exposure to **tenofovir alafenamide**. Avoid. Moderate Theoretical
- **Rifampicin** decreases the exposure to **terbinafine**. Adjust dose. Moderate Study
- **Teriflunomide** is predicted to increase the exposure to **rifampicin**. Moderate Theoretical
- **Rifampicin** decreases the exposure to tetracyclines **(doxycycline)**. Monitor and adjust dose. Moderate Study
- **Rifampicin** is predicted to decrease the exposure to **tezacaftor**. Avoid. Severe Theoretical
- **Rifampicin** is predicted to decrease the exposure to **theophylline**. Adjust dose. Moderate Study
- **Rifampicin** is predicted to markedly decrease the exposure to **ticagrelor**. Avoid. Severe Study
- **Rifampicin** is predicted to decrease the exposure to **tivozanib**. Severe Study
- **Rifampicin** moderately decreases the exposure to **tizanidine**. Mild Study
- **Rifampicin** is predicted to decrease the exposure to **tofacitinib**. Avoid. Severe Study
- **Rifampicin** is predicted to decrease the exposure to **tolvaptan**. Use with caution or avoid depending on indication. Severe Study
- **Rifampicin** is predicted to decrease the exposure to **toremifene**. Adjust dose. Moderate Study
- **Rifampicin** is predicted to decrease the exposure to **trabectedin**. Avoid. Severe Theoretical
- **Rifampicin** decreases the exposure to **trimethoprim**. Moderate Study
- **Rifampicin** decreases the efficacy of **ulipristal**. For FSRH guidance, see Contraceptives, interactions p. 536. Severe Anecdotal
- **Rifampicin** is predicted to decrease the exposure to **upadacitinib**. Moderate Study
- **Rifampicin** is predicted to decrease the exposure to **vandetanib**. Avoid. Moderate Study
- **Rifampicin** is predicted to moderately decrease the exposure to **velpatasvir**. Avoid. Severe Study
- **Rifampicin** is predicted to decrease the exposure to **vemurafenib**. Avoid. Severe Theoretical
- **Rifampicin** is predicted to decrease the exposure to **venetoclax**. Avoid. Severe Study
- **Rifampicin** is predicted to decrease the exposure to vinca alkaloids **(vinblastine, vincristine, vindesine)**. Severe Theoretical
- **Rifampicin** is predicted to decrease the exposure to vinca alkaloids **(vinflunine)**. Avoid. Severe Theoretical
- **Rifampicin** is predicted to decrease the exposure to vinca alkaloids **(vinorelbine)**. Use with caution or avoid. Severe Theoretical
- **Rifampicin** is predicted to decrease the exposure to **vismodegib**. Avoid. Moderate Theoretical
- **Rifampicin** potentially increases the risk of nephrotoxicity when given with volatile halogenated anaesthetics **(methoxyflurane)**. Avoid. Severe Theoretical

- **Rifampicin** is predicted to decrease the exposure to vortioxetine. Monitor and adjust dose. [Moderate] Study
- **Rifampicin** is predicted to decrease the concentration of voxilaprevir. Avoid. [Severe] Study
- **Rifampicin** moderately decreases the exposure to **zolpidem.** [Moderate] Study
- **Rifampicin** is predicted to decrease the exposure to **zopiclone.** Adjust dose. [Moderate] Study

Rifaximin

- **Ciclosporin** very markedly increases the exposure to **rifaximin.** [Severe] Study

Rilpivirine

- **Antacids** are predicted to decrease the exposure to **rilpivirine. Rilpivirine** should be taken 4 hours before or 2 hours after antacids. [Severe] Theoretical
- Antiepileptics **(carbamazepine, fosphenytoin, phenobarbital, phenytoin, primidone)** markedly decrease the exposure to **rilpivirine.** Avoid. [Severe] Study
- Antiepileptics **(oxcarbazepine)** are predicted to decrease the concentration of **rilpivirine.** Avoid. [Severe] Theoretical
- **Apalutamide** markedly decreases the exposure to **rilpivirine.** Avoid. [Severe] Study
- **Bosentan** is predicted to decrease the exposure to **rilpivirine.** Avoid. [Severe] Theoretical
- Calcium salts **(calcium carbonate)** are predicted to slightly decrease the exposure to **rilpivirine. Calcium carbonate** should be taken 2 hours before or 4 hours after **rilpivirine.** [Severe] Theoretical
- Corticosteroids **(dexamethasone)** are predicted to decrease the concentration of **rilpivirine.** Avoid multiple-dose dexamethasone. [Severe] Theoretical
- **Efavirenz** is predicted to decrease the exposure to **rilpivirine.** Avoid. [Severe] Theoretical
- **Enzalutamide** markedly decreases the exposure to **rilpivirine.** Avoid. [Severe] Study
- **Etravirine** is predicted to decrease the exposure to **rilpivirine.** Avoid. [Severe] Theoretical
- **H_2 receptor antagonists** are predicted to decrease the exposure to **rilpivirine. H_2 receptor antagonists** should be taken 12 hours before or 4 hours after **rilpivirine.** [Severe] Study
- **Mitotane** markedly decreases the exposure to **rilpivirine.** Avoid. [Severe] Study
- **Nevirapine** is predicted to decrease the exposure to **rilpivirine.** Avoid. [Severe] Theoretical
- **Proton pump inhibitors** are predicted to decrease the exposure to **rilpivirine.** Avoid. [Severe] Study
- **Rifabutin** slightly decreases the exposure to **rilpivirine.** Adjust dose. [Severe] Study
- **Rifampicin** markedly decreases the exposure to **rilpivirine.** Avoid. [Severe] Study
- **Sodium zirconium cyclosilicate** is predicted to decrease the exposure to **rilpivirine.** Separate administration by at least 2 hours. [Moderate] Theoretical
- **St John's Wort** is predicted to decrease the exposure to **rilpivirine.** Avoid. [Severe] Theoretical

Riluzole

FOOD AND LIFESTYLE Charcoal-grilled foods are predicted to decrease the exposure to riluzole.

- **Mexiletine** is predicted to increase the exposure to **riluzole.** [Moderate] Theoretical
- Quinolones **(ciprofloxacin)** are predicted to increase the exposure to **riluzole.** [Moderate] Theoretical
- SSRIs **(fluvoxamine)** are predicted to increase the exposure to **riluzole.** [Moderate] Theoretical

Riociguat → see **TABLE 8** p. 908 (hypotension)

FOOD AND LIFESTYLE Dose adjustment might be necessary if smoking is started or stopped during treatment.

- **Antacids** slightly decrease the exposure to **riociguat. Riociguat** should be taken 1 hour before or 2 hours after antacids. [Mild] Study
- Antifungals, azoles **(itraconazole, posaconazole)** are predicted to increase the exposure to **riociguat.** Adjust **riociguat** dose and monitor blood pressure. [Moderate] Theoretical
- Antifungals, azoles **(ketoconazole)** moderately increase the exposure to **riociguat.** Adjust **riociguat** dose and monitor blood pressure. [Moderate] Study
- **Ciclosporin** is predicted to increase the exposure to **riociguat.** [Moderate] Theoretical
- HIV-protease inhibitors **(ritonavir)** are predicted to increase the exposure to **riociguat.** Adjust dose and monitor blood pressure. [Moderate] Theoretical
- **Riociguat** is predicted to increase the risk of hypotension when given with **phosphodiesterase type-5 inhibitors.** Avoid. [Severe] Theoretical → Also see **TABLE 8** p. 908

Risankizumab → see monoclonal antibodies

Risedronate → see bisphosphonates

Risperidone → see **TABLE 8** p. 908 (hypotension), **TABLE 9** p. 909 (QT-interval prolongation), **TABLE 11** p. 909 (CNS depressant effects)

- Antiepileptics **(carbamazepine, fosphenytoin, phenobarbital, phenytoin, primidone)** are predicted to decrease the exposure to **risperidone.** Adjust dose. [Moderate] Study → Also see **TABLE 11** p. 909
- Antifungals, azoles **(itraconazole, ketoconazole, voriconazole)** are predicted to increase the exposure to **risperidone.** Adjust dose. [Moderate] Study → Also see **TABLE 9** p. 909
- **Apalutamide** is predicted to decrease the exposure to **risperidone.** Adjust dose. [Moderate] Study → Also see **TABLE 9** p. 909
- **Bupropion** is predicted to increase the exposure to **risperidone.** Adjust dose. [Moderate] Study
- **Cinacalcet** is predicted to increase the exposure to **risperidone.** Adjust dose. [Moderate] Study
- **Cobicistat** is predicted to increase the exposure to **risperidone.** Adjust dose. [Moderate] Study
- **Risperidone** is predicted to decrease the effects of **dopamine receptor agonists.** Avoid. [Moderate] Theoretical → Also see **TABLE 8** p. 908 → Also see **TABLE 9** p. 909
- **Enzalutamide** is predicted to decrease the exposure to **risperidone.** Adjust dose. [Moderate] Study
- **HIV-protease inhibitors** are predicted to increase the exposure to **risperidone.** Adjust dose. [Moderate] Study → Also see **TABLE 9** p. 909
- **Idelalisib** is predicted to increase the exposure to **risperidone.** Adjust dose. [Moderate] Study
- **Risperidone** is predicted to decrease the effects of **levodopa.** Avoid or adjust dose. [Severe] Anecdotal → Also see **TABLE 8** p. 908
- **Risperidone** potentially increases the risk of neurotoxicity when given with **lithium.** [Severe] Anecdotal → Also see **TABLE 9** p. 909
- Macrolides **(clarithromycin)** are predicted to increase the exposure to **risperidone.** Adjust dose. [Moderate] Study → Also see **TABLE 9** p. 909
- **Risperidone** increases the risk of dyskinesias when given with **methylphenidate.** [Severe] Anecdotal
- **Mitotane** is predicted to decrease the exposure to **risperidone.** Adjust dose. [Moderate] Study
- **Rifampicin** is predicted to decrease the exposure to **risperidone.** Adjust dose. [Moderate] Study
- SSRIs **(fluoxetine, paroxetine)** are predicted to increase the exposure to **risperidone.** Adjust dose. [Moderate] Study
- **Terbinafine** is predicted to increase the exposure to **risperidone.** Adjust dose. [Moderate] Study

Ritonavir → see HIV-protease inhibitors

Rituximab → see monoclonal antibodies

Rivaroxaban → see **TABLE 3** p. 907 (anticoagulant effects)

- Antiarrhythmics **(dronedarone)** are predicted to increase the exposure to **rivaroxaban.** Avoid. [Moderate] Theoretical
- Antiepileptics **(carbamazepine, fosphenytoin, phenobarbital, phenytoin, primidone)** are predicted to moderately decrease the exposure to **rivaroxaban.** Avoid unless patient can be monitored for signs of thrombosis. [Severe] Study
- Antifungals, azoles **(itraconazole, ketoconazole)** are predicted to moderately increase the exposure to **rivaroxaban.** Avoid. [Severe] Study
- **Apalutamide** is predicted to moderately decrease the exposure to **rivaroxaban.** Avoid unless patient can be monitored for signs of thrombosis. [Severe] Study

Rivaroxaban (continued)
- Cobicistat is predicted to increase the exposure to **rivaroxaban**. Avoid. [Severe] Theoretical
- Enzalutamide is predicted to moderately decrease the exposure to **rivaroxaban**. Avoid unless patient can be monitored for signs of thrombosis. [Severe] Study
- HIV-protease inhibitors **(ritonavir)** moderately increase the exposure to **rivaroxaban**. Avoid. [Severe] Study
- Mitotane is predicted to moderately decrease the exposure to **rivaroxaban**. Avoid unless patient can be monitored for signs of thrombosis. [Severe] Study
- Rifampicin is predicted to moderately decrease the exposure to **rivaroxaban**. Avoid unless patient can be monitored for signs of thrombosis. [Severe] Study

Rivastigmine → see anticholinesterases, centrally acting

Rizatriptan → see TABLE 13 p. 910 (serotonin syndrome)
- Beta blockers, non-selective **(propranolol)** slightly to moderately increase the exposure to **rizatriptan**. Adjust **rizatriptan** dose and separate administration by at least 2 hours. [Moderate] Study
- **Rizatriptan** is predicted to increase the risk of vasoconstriction when given with **ergotamine**. **Ergotamine** should be taken at least 24 hours before or 6 hours after **rizatriptan**. [Severe] Theoretical
- MAOIs, irreversible are predicted to increase the exposure to **rizatriptan**. Avoid and for 14 days after stopping the MAOI. [Severe] Theoretical → Also see TABLE 13 p. 910
- Moclobemide moderately increases the exposure to **rizatriptan**. Avoid. [Moderate] Study → Also see TABLE 13 p. 910

Rocuronium → see neuromuscular blocking drugs, non-depolarising

Roflumilast
- Aminophylline is predicted to slightly increase the exposure to **roflumilast**. Avoid. [Moderate] Theoretical
- Antiepileptics **(carbamazepine, fosphenytoin, phenobarbital, phenytoin, primidone)** are predicted to decrease the exposure to **roflumilast**. Avoid. [Moderate] Study
- Apalutamide is predicted to decrease the exposure to **roflumilast**. Avoid. [Moderate] Study
- Combined hormonal contraceptives are predicted to increase the exposure to **roflumilast**. [Moderate] Theoretical
- Enzalutamide is predicted to decrease the exposure to **roflumilast**. Avoid. [Moderate] Study
- H_2 receptor antagonists **(cimetidine)** slightly increase the exposure to **roflumilast**. [Moderate] Study
- Mexiletine is predicted to increase the exposure to **roflumilast**. [Moderate] Theoretical
- Mitotane is predicted to decrease the exposure to **roflumilast**. Avoid. [Moderate] Study
- Quinolones **(ciprofloxacin)** are predicted to increase the exposure to **roflumilast**. [Moderate] Theoretical
- Rifampicin is predicted to decrease the exposure to **roflumilast**. Avoid. [Moderate] Study
- SSRIs **(fluvoxamine)** are predicted to increase the exposure to **roflumilast**. [Moderate] Study
- Theophylline is predicted to slightly increase the exposure to **roflumilast**. Avoid. [Moderate] Theoretical

Rolapitant
- **Rolapitant** is predicted to increase the exposure to alkylating agents **(bendamustine)**. Avoid or monitor. [Moderate] Study
- **Rolapitant** is predicted to increase the exposure to anthracyclines **(doxorubicin, mitoxantrone)**. Avoid or monitor. [Moderate] Study
- **Rolapitant** is predicted to increase the exposure to antiarrhythmics **(propafenone)**. [Severe] Study
- Antiepileptics **(carbamazepine, fosphenytoin, phenobarbital, phenytoin, primidone)** are predicted to markedly decrease the exposure to **rolapitant**. Avoid. [Severe] Study
- Apalutamide is predicted to markedly decrease the exposure to **rolapitant**. Avoid. [Severe] Study
- **Rolapitant** is predicted to moderately increase the exposure to beta blockers, selective **(metoprolol)**. [Severe] Study
- Bosentan is predicted to decrease the exposure to **rolapitant**. Avoid. [Severe] Study
- **Rolapitant** is predicted to increase the exposure to colchicine. [Moderate] Study
- **Rolapitant** is predicted to increase the exposure to **dabigatran**. [Moderate] Study
- **Rolapitant** slightly increases the exposure to **digoxin**. [Moderate] Study
- Efavirenz is predicted to decrease the exposure to **rolapitant**. Avoid. [Severe] Study
- Enzalutamide is predicted to markedly decrease the exposure to **rolapitant**. Avoid. [Severe] Study
- **Rolapitant** is predicted to increase the exposure to **irinotecan**. Avoid or monitor. [Moderate] Study
- **Rolapitant** is predicted to increase the exposure to methotrexate. Avoid or monitor. [Moderate] Study
- Mitotane is predicted to markedly decrease the exposure to **rolapitant**. Avoid. [Severe] Study
- Nevirapine is predicted to decrease the exposure to **rolapitant**. Avoid. [Severe] Study
- **Rolapitant** is predicted to increase the exposure to **pimozide**. [Severe] Study
- Rifabutin is predicted to decrease the exposure to **rolapitant**. Avoid. [Moderate] Theoretical
- Rifampicin is predicted to markedly decrease the exposure to **rolapitant**. Avoid. [Severe] Study
- St John's Wort is predicted to decrease the exposure to **rolapitant**. Avoid. [Severe] Study
- **Rolapitant** is predicted to increase the exposure to statins **(rosuvastatin)**. Monitor and adjust dose. [Severe] Study
- **Rolapitant** increases the exposure to **sulfasalazine**. [Severe] Study
- **Rolapitant** is predicted to increase the exposure to **tamoxifen**. [Severe] Study
- **Rolapitant** is predicted to increase the exposure to **topotecan**. Avoid or monitor. [Moderate] Study

Ropinirole → see dopamine receptor agonists

Ropivacaine → see anaesthetics, local

Rosuvastatin → see statins

Rotavirus vaccine → see live vaccines

Rotigotine → see dopamine receptor agonists

Rucaparib
- **Rucaparib** is predicted to increase the exposure to aminophylline. Monitor and adjust dose. [Moderate] Study
- **Rucaparib** is predicted to increase the exposure to antiepileptics **(phenytoin)**. Monitor and adjust dose. [Moderate] Study
- **Rucaparib** is predicted to increase the exposure to **ciclosporin**. Monitor and adjust dose. [Moderate] Study
- **Rucaparib** slightly increases the exposure to coumarins **(warfarin)**. Monitor and adjust dose. [Severe] Study
- **Rucaparib** is predicted to increase the exposure to **ergotamine**. Monitor and adjust dose. [Moderate] Study
- **Rucaparib** slightly increases the exposure to **midazolam**. Monitor and adjust dose. [Severe] Study
- **Rucaparib** is predicted to increase the exposure to opioids **(alfentanil, fentanyl)**. Monitor and adjust dose. [Moderate] Study
- **Rucaparib** is predicted to increase the exposure to **pimozide**. Monitor and adjust dose. [Moderate] Study
- **Rucaparib** is predicted to increase the exposure to **sirolimus**. Monitor and adjust dose. [Moderate] Study
- **Rucaparib** is predicted to increase the exposure to **tacrolimus**. Monitor and adjust dose. [Moderate] Study
- **Rucaparib** is predicted to increase the exposure to theophylline. Monitor and adjust dose. [Moderate] Study
- **Rucaparib** is predicted to increase the exposure to **tizanidine**. Monitor and adjust dose. [Moderate] Study

Rufinamide → see antiepileptics

Rupatadine → see antihistamines, non-sedating

Ruxolitinib → see TABLE 15 p. 910 (myelosuppression)
- Antiarrhythmics **(dronedarone)** are predicted to increase the exposure to **ruxolitinib**. [Moderate] Theoretical
- Antiepileptics **(carbamazepine, fosphenytoin, phenobarbital, phenytoin, primidone)** are predicted to decrease the exposure to **ruxolitinib**. Monitor and adjust dose. [Moderate] Study
- Antifungals, azoles **(fluconazole, isavuconazole, posaconazole)** are predicted to increase the exposure to **ruxolitinib**. [Moderate] Theoretical
- Antifungals, azoles **(itraconazole, ketoconazole, voriconazole)** are predicted to increase the exposure to **ruxolitinib**. Adjust dose and monitor side effects. [Moderate] Study

- Apalutamide is predicted to decrease the exposure to **ruxolitinib**. Monitor and adjust dose. Moderate Study
- Aprepitant is predicted to increase the exposure to **ruxolitinib**. Moderate Theoretical
- Bosentan is predicted to decrease the exposure to **ruxolitinib**. Monitor and adjust dose. Moderate Theoretical
- Calcium channel blockers **(diltiazem, verapamil)** are predicted to increase the exposure to **ruxolitinib**. Moderate Theoretical
- Cobicistat is predicted to increase the exposure to **ruxolitinib**. Adjust dose and monitor side effects. Moderate Study
- **Ruxolitinib** is predicted to increase the risk of bleeding events when given with **coumarins**. Severe Theoretical
- Crizotinib is predicted to increase the exposure to **ruxolitinib**. Moderate Theoretical → Also see TABLE 15 p. 910
- Efavirenz is predicted to decrease the exposure to **ruxolitinib**. Monitor and adjust dose. Moderate Theoretical
- Enzalutamide is predicted to decrease the exposure to **ruxolitinib**. Monitor and adjust dose. Moderate Study
- Grapefruit juice is predicted to increase the exposure to **ruxolitinib**. Severe Theoretical
- HIV-protease inhibitors are predicted to increase the exposure to **ruxolitinib**. Adjust dose and monitor side effects. Moderate Study
- Idelalisib is predicted to increase the exposure to **ruxolitinib**. Adjust dose and monitor side effects. Moderate Study → Also see TABLE 15 p. 910
- Imatinib is predicted to increase the exposure to **ruxolitinib**. Moderate Theoretical → Also see TABLE 15 p. 910
- Macrolides **(clarithromycin)** are predicted to increase the exposure to **ruxolitinib**. Adjust dose and monitor side effects. Moderate Study
- Macrolides **(erythromycin)** are predicted to increase the exposure to **ruxolitinib**. Moderate Theoretical
- Mitotane is predicted to decrease the exposure to **ruxolitinib**. Monitor and adjust dose. Moderate Study → Also see TABLE 15 p. 910
- Netupitant is predicted to increase the exposure to **ruxolitinib**. Moderate Theoretical
- Nevirapine is predicted to decrease the exposure to **ruxolitinib**. Monitor and adjust dose. Moderate Theoretical
- Nilotinib is predicted to increase the exposure to **ruxolitinib**. Moderate Theoretical → Also see TABLE 15 p. 910
- **Ruxolitinib** is predicted to increase the risk of bleeding events when given with **phenindione**. Severe Theoretical
- Rifampicin is predicted to decrease the exposure to **ruxolitinib**. Monitor and adjust dose. Moderate Study
- St John's Wort is predicted to decrease the exposure to **ruxolitinib**. Monitor and adjust dose. Moderate Theoretical

Sacubitril → see TABLE 8 p. 908 (hypotension)

- Sacubitril is predicted to increase the exposure to statins. Severe Study

Safinamide → see MAO-B inhibitors
Salbutamol → see $beta_2$ agonists
Salmeterol → see $beta_2$ agonists
Sapropterin → see TABLE 8 p. 908 (hypotension)

- Methotrexate is predicted to decrease the efficacy of **sapropterin**. Moderate Theoretical
- Phosphodiesterase type-5 inhibitors are predicted to increase the risk of hypotension when given with **sapropterin**. Moderate Theoretical → Also see TABLE 8 p. 908
- Trimethoprim is predicted to decrease the efficacy of **sapropterin**. Moderate Theoretical

Saquinavir → see HIV-protease inhibitors
Sarilumab → see monoclonal antibodies
Saxagliptin → see TABLE 14 p. 910 (antidiabetic drugs)

- Antiarrhythmics **(dronedarone)** are predicted to increase the exposure to **saxagliptin**. Mild Study
- Antiepileptics **(carbamazepine, fosphenytoin, phenobarbital, phenytoin, primidone)** are predicted to moderately decrease the exposure to **saxagliptin**. Moderate Study
- Antifungals, azoles **(fluconazole, isavuconazole, posaconazole)** are predicted to increase the exposure to **saxagliptin**. Mild Study
- Antifungals, azoles **(itraconazole, ketoconazole, voriconazole)** are predicted to increase the exposure to **saxagliptin**. Moderate Study
- Apalutamide is predicted to moderately decrease the exposure to **saxagliptin**. Moderate Study
- Aprepitant is predicted to increase the exposure to **saxagliptin**. Mild Study
- Calcium channel blockers **(diltiazem, verapamil)** are predicted to increase the exposure to **saxagliptin**. Mild Study
- Cobicistat is predicted to increase the exposure to **saxagliptin**. Moderate Study
- Crizotinib is predicted to increase the exposure to **saxagliptin**. Mild Study
- Enzalutamide is predicted to moderately decrease the exposure to **saxagliptin**. Moderate Study
- Grapefruit juice is predicted to increase the exposure to **saxagliptin**. Mild Theoretical
- HIV-protease inhibitors are predicted to increase the exposure to **saxagliptin**. Moderate Study
- Idelalisib is predicted to increase the exposure to **saxagliptin**. Moderate Study
- Imatinib is predicted to increase the exposure to **saxagliptin**. Mild Study
- Macrolides **(clarithromycin)** are predicted to increase the exposure to **saxagliptin**. Moderate Study
- Macrolides **(erythromycin)** are predicted to increase the exposure to **saxagliptin**. Mild Study
- Mitotane is predicted to moderately decrease the exposure to **saxagliptin**. Moderate Study
- Netupitant is predicted to increase the exposure to **saxagliptin**. Mild Study
- Nilotinib is predicted to increase the exposure to **saxagliptin**. Mild Study
- Rifampicin is predicted to moderately decrease the exposure to **saxagliptin**. Moderate Study

Secukinumab → see monoclonal antibodies
Selegiline → see MAO-B inhibitors
Selenium

ROUTE-SPECIFIC INFORMATION Interactions do not generally apply to topical use unless specified.

- Oral **selenium** is predicted to decrease the absorption of eltrombopag. **Eltrombopag** should be taken 2 hours before or 4 hours after **selenium**. Severe Theoretical

Selexipag

- Antiepileptics **(carbamazepine, fosphenytoin, phenytoin)** are predicted to decrease the exposure to the active metabolite of **selexipag**. Adjust dose. Moderate Study
- Antiepileptics **(valproate)** are predicted to increase the exposure to **selexipag**. Unknown Theoretical
- Antifungals, azoles **(fluconazole)** are predicted to increase the exposure to **selexipag**. Unknown Theoretical
- Clopidogrel is predicted to increase the exposure to **selexipag**. Adjust **selexipag** dose. Moderate Study
- Fibrates **(gemfibrozil)** increase the exposure to **selexipag**. Avoid. Severe Study
- Iron chelators **(deferasirox)** are predicted to increase the exposure to **selexipag**. Adjust **selexipag** dose. Moderate Study
- Leflunomide is predicted to increase the exposure to **selexipag**. Adjust **selexipag** dose. Moderate Study
- Rifampicin moderately decreases the exposure to the active metabolite of **selexipag**. Adjust dose. Moderate Study
- Teriflunomide is predicted to increase the exposure to **selexipag**. Adjust **selexipag** dose. Moderate Study

Semaglutide → see TABLE 14 p. 910 (antidiabetic drugs)
Sertraline → see SSRIs
Sevoflurane → see volatile halogenated anaesthetics
Sildenafil → see phosphodiesterase type-5 inhibitors
Siltuximab → see monoclonal antibodies
Silver sulfadiazine

PHARMACOLOGY Silver might inactivate enzymatic debriding agents—concurrent use might not be appropriate.

Simvastatin → see statins
Siponimod → see TABLE 6 p. 908 (bradycardia), TABLE 9 p. 909 (QT-interval prolongation)

Siponimod (continued)
- Antiarrhythmics **(amiodarone)** are predicted to increase the exposure to **siponimod.** Avoid depending on other drugs taken—consult product literature. Severe Study → Also see TABLE 6 p. 908
- Antiepileptics **(carbamazepine, fosphenytoin, phenobarbital, phenytoin, primidone)** are predicted to decrease the exposure to **siponimod.** Severe Study
- Antifungals, azoles **(itraconazole, ketoconazole, voriconazole)** are predicted to increase the exposure to **siponimod.** Avoid depending on other drugs taken—consult product literature. Severe Theoretical
- Antifungals, azoles **(miconazole)** are predicted to increase the exposure to **siponimod.** Avoid depending on other drugs taken—consult product literature. Severe Study
- **Apalutamide** is predicted to decrease the exposure to **siponimod.** Severe Study
- **Bosentan** is predicted to decrease the exposure to **siponimod.** Manufacturer advises caution depending on genotype—consult product literature. Severe Theoretical
- **Cobicistat** is predicted to increase the exposure to **siponimod.** Avoid depending on other drugs taken—consult product literature. Severe Theoretical
- **Efavirenz** is predicted to decrease the exposure to **siponimod.** Manufacturer advises caution depending on genotype—consult product literature. Severe Theoretical
- **Enzalutamide** is predicted to decrease the exposure to **siponimod.** Severe Study
- **HIV-protease inhibitors** are predicted to increase the exposure to **siponimod.** Avoid depending on other drugs taken—consult product literature. Severe Theoretical
- **Idelalisib** is predicted to increase the exposure to **siponimod.** Avoid depending on other drugs taken—consult product literature. Severe Theoretical
- **Live vaccines** are predicted to increase the risk of generalised infection (possibly life-threatening) when given with **siponimod.** Avoid and for 4 weeks after stopping **siponimod.** Severe Theoretical
- Macrolides **(clarithromycin)** are predicted to increase the exposure to **siponimod.** Avoid depending on other drugs taken—consult product literature. Severe Theoretical
- **Mitotane** is predicted to decrease the exposure to **siponimod.** Severe Study
- **Siponimod** potentially increases the risk of immunosuppression when given with monoclonal antibodies **(alemtuzumab).** Avoid. Severe Theoretical
- **Nevirapine** is predicted to decrease the exposure to **siponimod.** Manufacturer advises caution depending on genotype—consult product literature. Severe Theoretical
- **Rifampicin** is predicted to decrease the exposure to **siponimod.** Severe Study
- **St John's Wort** is predicted to decrease the exposure to **siponimod.** Manufacturer advises caution depending on genotype—consult product literature. Severe Theoretical

Sirolimus
- Antiarrhythmics **(amiodarone)** are predicted to increase the concentration of **sirolimus.** Severe Anecdotal
- Antiarrhythmics **(dronedarone)** increase the concentration of **sirolimus.** Monitor and adjust dose. Moderate Study
- Antiepileptics **(carbamazepine, fosphenytoin, phenobarbital, phenytoin, primidone)** are predicted to decrease the concentration of **sirolimus.** Avoid. Severe Study
- Antifungals, azoles **(fluconazole, isavuconazole, posaconazole)** increase the concentration of **sirolimus.** Monitor and adjust dose. Moderate Study
- Antifungals, azoles **(itraconazole, ketoconazole, voriconazole)** are predicted to increase the concentration of **sirolimus.** Avoid. Severe Study
- Antifungals, azoles **(miconazole)** are predicted to increase the concentration of **sirolimus.** Monitor and adjust dose. Moderate Study
- **Apalutamide** is predicted to decrease the concentration of **sirolimus.** Avoid. Severe Study
- **Aprepitant** increases the concentration of **sirolimus.** Monitor and adjust dose. Moderate Study
- **Bosentan** is predicted to decrease the concentration of **sirolimus** and **sirolimus** potentially increases the concentration of bosentan. Avoid. Severe Theoretical
- **Brigatinib** potentially decreases the concentration of **sirolimus.** Avoid. Moderate Theoretical
- Calcium channel blockers **(diltiazem, verapamil)** increase the concentration of **sirolimus.** Monitor and adjust dose. Moderate Study
- **Ceritinib** is predicted to increase the exposure to **sirolimus.** Avoid. Severe Theoretical
- **Sirolimus** is predicted to affect the efficacy of **chenodeoxycholic acid.** Monitor and adjust dose. Moderate Theoretical
- **Ciclosporin** moderately increases the exposure to **sirolimus.** Separate administration by 4 hours. Severe Study
- **Cobicistat** is predicted to increase the concentration of **sirolimus.** Avoid. Severe Study
- **Crizotinib** increases the concentration of **sirolimus.** Monitor and adjust dose. Moderate Study
- **Doravirine** is predicted to decrease the exposure to **sirolimus.** Monitor **sirolimus** concentration and adjust dose, p. 561. Moderate Theoretical
- **Efavirenz** is predicted to decrease the concentration of **sirolimus.** Monitor and adjust dose. Moderate Theoretical
- **Eliglustat** is predicted to increase the exposure to **sirolimus.** Adjust dose. Moderate Study
- **Enzalutamide** is predicted to decrease the concentration of **sirolimus.** Avoid. Severe Study
- **Grapefruit juice** increases the concentration of **sirolimus.** Avoid. Moderate Study
- **HIV-protease inhibitors** are predicted to increase the concentration of **sirolimus.** Avoid. Severe Study
- **Idelalisib** is predicted to increase the concentration of **sirolimus.** Avoid. Severe Study
- **Imatinib** increases the concentration of **sirolimus.** Monitor and adjust dose. Moderate Study
- **Lapatinib** is predicted to increase the exposure to **sirolimus.** Moderate Theoretical
- **Larotrectinib** is predicted to increase the exposure to **sirolimus.** Use with caution and adjust dose. Mild Theoretical
- **Letermovir** moderately increases the exposure to **sirolimus.** Monitor and adjust dose. Severe Study
- **Live vaccines** are predicted to increase the risk of generalised infection (possibly life-threatening) when given with **sirolimus.** Public Health England advises avoid (refer to Green Book). Severe Theoretical
- **Lorlatinib** is predicted to decrease the exposure to **sirolimus.** Avoid. Moderate Theoretical
- **Lumacaftor** is predicted to decrease the exposure to **sirolimus.** Avoid. Severe Theoretical
- Macrolides **(clarithromycin)** are predicted to increase the concentration of **sirolimus.** Avoid. Severe Study
- Macrolides **(erythromycin)** increase the concentration of **sirolimus.** Monitor and adjust dose. Moderate Study
- **Sirolimus** is predicted to decrease the efficacy of **mifamurtide.** Avoid. Severe Theoretical
- **Mirabegron** is predicted to increase the exposure to **sirolimus.** Mild Theoretical
- **Mitotane** is predicted to decrease the concentration of **sirolimus.** Avoid. Severe Study
- Monoclonal antibodies **(sarilumab)** potentially affect the exposure to **sirolimus.** Monitor and adjust dose. Moderate Theoretical
- **Neratinib** is predicted to increase the exposure to **sirolimus.** Moderate Study
- **Netupitant** increases the concentration of **sirolimus.** Monitor and adjust dose. Moderate Study
- **Nevirapine** is predicted to decrease the concentration of **sirolimus.** Monitor and adjust dose. Moderate Theoretical
- **Nilotinib** increases the concentration of **sirolimus.** Monitor and adjust dose. Moderate Study
- **Palbociclib** is predicted to increase the exposure to **sirolimus.** Adjust dose. Moderate Theoretical
- **Pibrentasvir** (with glecaprevir) is predicted to increase the exposure to **sirolimus.** Moderate Study

- Pitolisant is predicted to decrease the exposure to **sirolimus**. Avoid. [Severe] Theoretical
- Ribociclib is predicted to increase the exposure to **sirolimus**. Use with caution and adjust dose. [Moderate] Theoretical
- Rifampicin is predicted to decrease the concentration of **sirolimus**. Avoid. [Severe] Study
- Rucaparib is predicted to increase the exposure to **sirolimus**. Monitor and adjust dose. [Moderate] Study
- St John's Wort is predicted to decrease the concentration of **sirolimus**. Monitor and adjust dose. [Severe] Theoretical
- **Sirolimus** is predicted to decrease the concentration of tacrolimus and tacrolimus increases the exposure to **sirolimus**. [Severe] Study
- Velpatasvir is predicted to increase the exposure to **sirolimus**. [Severe] Theoretical
- Venetoclax is predicted to increase the exposure to **sirolimus**. Avoid or adjust dose. [Severe] Study

Sitagliptin → see TABLE 14 p. 910 (antidiabetic drugs)

Sodium aurothiomalate

- ACE inhibitors are predicted to increase the risk of hypersensitivity when given with **sodium aurothiomalate**. [Severe] Anecdotal
- **Sodium aurothiomalate** potentially increases the risk of side-effects when given with penicillamine (in those who have had previous adverse reactions to gold). Avoid. [Severe] Study

Sodium bicarbonate

ROUTE-SPECIFIC INFORMATION Interactions do not generally apply to topical use unless specified.

- Oral **sodium bicarbonate** decreases the absorption of antifungals, azoles (ketoconazole). [Moderate] Study
- **Sodium bicarbonate** decreases the concentration of lithium. [Severe] Anecdotal
- **Sodium bicarbonate** is predicted to decrease the efficacy of methenamine. Avoid. [Moderate] Theoretical

Sodium citrate

- **Sodium citrate** is predicted to decrease the efficacy of methenamine. Avoid. [Moderate] Theoretical
- **Sodium citrate** is predicted to increase the risk of side-effects when given with sucralfate. Avoid. [Moderate] Theoretical

Sodium feredetate → see iron (oral)

Sodium oxybate → see TABLE 8 p. 908 (hypotension), TABLE 11 p. 909 (CNS depressant effects)

- Antiepileptics (valproate) increase the exposure to **sodium oxybate**. Adjust **sodium oxybate** dose. [Moderate] Study

Sodium phenylbutyrate

- Antiepileptics (valproate) potentially decrease the effects of **sodium phenylbutyrate**. [Moderate] Anecdotal
- Corticosteroids potentially decrease the effects of **sodium phenylbutyrate**. [Moderate] Anecdotal
- Haloperidol potentially decreases the effects of **sodium phenylbutyrate**. [Moderate] Anecdotal

Sodium picosulfate → see TABLE 18 p. 911 (hyponatraemia)

Sodium stibogluconate

- **Sodium stibogluconate** increases the risk of cardiovascular side-effects when given with amphotericin. Separate administration by 14 days. [Severe] Study

Sodium zirconium cyclosilicate

- **Sodium zirconium cyclosilicate** is predicted to decrease the exposure to antifungals, azoles. Separate administration by at least 2 hours. [Moderate] Theoretical
- **Sodium zirconium cyclosilicate** is predicted to decrease the exposure to dasatinib. Separate administration by at least 2 hours. [Moderate] Theoretical
- **Sodium zirconium cyclosilicate** is predicted to decrease the exposure to erlotinib. Separate administration by at least 2 hours. [Moderate] Theoretical
- **Sodium zirconium cyclosilicate** is predicted to decrease the exposure to HIV-protease inhibitors. Separate administration by at least 2 hours. [Moderate] Theoretical
- **Sodium zirconium cyclosilicate** is predicted to decrease the exposure to ledipasvir. Separate administration by at least 2 hours. [Moderate] Theoretical
- **Sodium zirconium cyclosilicate** is predicted to decrease the exposure to nilotinib. Separate administration by at least 2 hours. [Moderate] Theoretical
- **Sodium zirconium cyclosilicate** is predicted to decrease the exposure to raltegravir. Separate administration by at least 2 hours. [Moderate] Theoretical
- **Sodium zirconium cyclosilicate** is predicted to decrease the exposure to rilpivirine. Separate administration by at least 2 hours. [Moderate] Theoretical

Sofosbuvir

- **Sofosbuvir** is predicted to increase the risk of severe bradycardia or heart block when given with antiarrhythmics (amiodarone). Refer to specialist literature. [Severe] Anecdotal
- Antiepileptics (carbamazepine) are predicted to decrease the exposure to **sofosbuvir**. Avoid. [Severe] Study
- Antiepileptics (fosphenytoin, oxcarbazepine, phenobarbital, phenytoin, primidone) are predicted to decrease the exposure to **sofosbuvir**. Avoid. [Severe] Theoretical
- H_2 receptor antagonists potentially decrease the exposure to **sofosbuvir**. Adjust dose, see ledipasvir with sofosbuvir sofosbuvir with velpatasvir, and sofosbuvir with velpatasvir and voxilaprevir. [Moderate] Study
- HIV-protease inhibitors (tipranavir) are predicted to decrease the exposure to **sofosbuvir**. Avoid. [Severe] Theoretical
- Modafinil is predicted to decrease the exposure to **sofosbuvir**. Avoid. [Severe] Theoretical
- Proton pump inhibitors potentially decrease the exposure to **sofosbuvir**. Adjust dose, see ledipasvir with sofosbuvir sofosbuvir with velpatasvir, and sofosbuvir with velpatasvir and voxilaprevir. [Moderate] Study
- Rifampicin is predicted to decrease the exposure to **sofosbuvir**. Avoid. [Severe] Study
- St John's Wort is predicted to decrease the exposure to **sofosbuvir**. Avoid. [Severe] Study

Solifenacin → see TABLE 10 p. 909 (antimuscarinics)

- Antiepileptics (carbamazepine, fosphenytoin, phenobarbital, phenytoin, primidone) are predicted to decrease the exposure to **solifenacin**. [Moderate] Theoretical
- Antifungals, azoles (itraconazole, ketoconazole, voriconazole) are predicted to increase the exposure to **solifenacin**. Adjust solifenacin or tamsulosin with solifenacin dose; avoid in hepatic and renal impairment. [Severe] Study
- Apalutamide is predicted to decrease the exposure to **solifenacin**. [Moderate] Theoretical
- Cobicistat is predicted to increase the exposure to **solifenacin**. Adjust solifenacin or tamsulosin with solifenacin dose; avoid in hepatic and renal impairment. [Severe] Study
- Enzalutamide is predicted to decrease the exposure to **solifenacin**. [Moderate] Theoretical
- HIV-protease inhibitors are predicted to increase the exposure to **solifenacin**. Adjust solifenacin or tamsulosin with solifenacin dose; avoid in hepatic and renal impairment. [Severe] Study
- Idelalisib is predicted to increase the exposure to **solifenacin**. Adjust solifenacin or tamsulosin with solifenacin dose; avoid in hepatic and renal impairment. [Severe] Study
- Macrolides (clarithromycin) are predicted to increase the exposure to **solifenacin**. Adjust solifenacin or tamsulosin with solifenacin dose; avoid in hepatic and renal impairment. [Severe] Study
- Mitotane is predicted to decrease the exposure to **solifenacin**. [Moderate] Theoretical
- Rifampicin is predicted to decrease the exposure to **solifenacin**. [Moderate] Theoretical

Somatropin

- Corticosteroids are predicted to decrease the effects of **somatropin**. [Moderate] Theoretical

Sorafenib → see TABLE 15 p. 910 (myelosuppression), TABLE 9 p. 909 (QT-interval prolongation)

- Antiepileptics (carbamazepine, fosphenytoin, phenobarbital, phenytoin, primidone) are predicted to decrease the exposure to **sorafenib**. [Moderate] Theoretical
- Apalutamide is predicted to decrease the exposure to **sorafenib**. [Moderate] Theoretical → Also see TABLE 9 p. 909
- **Sorafenib** increases the anticoagulant effect of coumarins. [Severe] Anecdotal
- Enzalutamide is predicted to decrease the exposure to **sorafenib**. [Moderate] Theoretical

Sorafenib (continued)
- **Mitotane** is predicted to decrease the exposure to **sorafenib**. [Moderate] Theoretical → Also see **TABLE 15** p. 910
- **Neomycin** moderately decreases the exposure to **sorafenib**. [Moderate] Study
- **Sorafenib** is predicted to increase the risk of bleeding events when given with phenindione. [Severe] Theoretical
- **Rifampicin** is predicted to decrease the exposure to **sorafenib**. [Moderate] Theoretical

Sotalol → see beta blockers, non-selective
Spironolactone → see aldosterone antagonists
SSRIs → see **TABLE 18** p. 911 (hyponatraemia), **TABLE 13** p. 910 (serotonin syndrome), **TABLE 9** p. 909 (QT-interval prolongation), **TABLE 4** p. 907 (antiplatelet effects)

citalopram · dapoxetine · escitalopram · fluoxetine · fluvoxamine · paroxetine · sertraline

- **Fluvoxamine** very markedly increases the exposure to agomelatine. Avoid. [Severe] Study
- **Fluvoxamine** moderately increases the exposure to alprazolam. Adjust dose. [Moderate] Study
- SSRIs **(fluoxetine, paroxetine)** are predicted to increase the exposure to amfetamines. [Severe] Theoretical → Also see **TABLE 13** p. 910
- **Fluvoxamine** moderately to markedly increases the exposure to aminophylline. Avoid. [Severe] Study
- **Fluvoxamine** decreases the clearance of anaesthetics, local **(ropivacaine)**. Avoid prolonged use. [Moderate] Study
- **Fluvoxamine** is predicted to increase the exposure to anagrelide. [Moderate] Theoretical → Also see **TABLE 4** p. 907
- Antiarrhythmics **(dronedarone)** are predicted to increase the exposure to **dapoxetine**. Adjust **dapoxetine** dose with moderate inhibitors of CYP3A4. [Moderate] Theoretical
- Antiarrhythmics **(dronedarone)** are predicted to increase the exposure to SSRIs **(citalopram, escitalopram, fluoxetine, fluvoxamine, paroxetine, sertraline)**. [Severe] Theoretical → Also see **TABLE 9** p. 909
- **Fluvoxamine** is predicted to increase the exposure to antiarrhythmics **(propafenone)**. Monitor and adjust dose. [Moderate] Study
- SSRIs **(fluoxetine, paroxetine)** are predicted to increase the exposure to anticholinesterases, centrally acting **(galantamine)**. Monitor and adjust dose. [Moderate] Study
- Antiepileptics **(fosphenytoin, phenytoin)** decrease the concentration of **paroxetine**. [Moderate] Study
- **Sertraline** potentially increases the risk of toxicity when given with antiepileptics **(fosphenytoin, phenytoin)**. Monitor concentration and adjust dose. [Severe] Anecdotal
- SSRIs **(fluoxetine, fluvoxamine)** are predicted to increase the concentration of antiepileptics **(fosphenytoin, phenytoin)**. Monitor and adjust dose. [Severe] Anecdotal
- Antifungals, azoles **(fluconazole, isavuconazole, posaconazole)** are predicted to increase the exposure to **dapoxetine**. Adjust **dapoxetine** dose with moderate inhibitors of CYP3A4. [Moderate] Theoretical
- Antifungals, azoles **(itraconazole, ketoconazole, voriconazole)** are predicted to moderately increase the exposure to **dapoxetine**. Avoid potent inhibitors of CYP3A4 or adjust **dapoxetine** dose. [Severe] Study
- Antifungals, azoles **(voriconazole)** are predicted to increase the exposure to **citalopram**. [Severe] Theoretical → Also see **TABLE 9** p. 909
- Antihistamines, sedating **(cyproheptadine)** potentially decrease the effects of **SSRIs**. [Moderate] Anecdotal
- **Apalutamide** is predicted to decrease the exposure to **citalopram**. Avoid or monitor. [Mild] Study → Also see **TABLE 9** p. 909
- **Aprepitant** is predicted to increase the exposure to **dapoxetine**. Adjust **dapoxetine** dose with moderate inhibitors of CYP3A4. [Moderate] Theoretical
- SSRIs **(fluoxetine, paroxetine)** are predicted to moderately increase the exposure to aripiprazole. Adjust **aripiprazole** dose, p. 265. [Moderate] Study
- **Fluvoxamine** increases the exposure to **asenapine**. [Moderate] Study
- **Paroxetine** moderately increases the exposure to **asenapine**. [Moderate] Study
- SSRIs **(fluoxetine, paroxetine)** are predicted to markedly increase the exposure to **atomoxetine**. Adjust dose. [Severe] Study
- **Fluvoxamine** moderately increases the concentration of beta blockers, non-selective **(propranolol)**. [Moderate] Study
- SSRIs **(fluoxetine, paroxetine)** are predicted to increase the exposure to beta blockers, selective **(metoprolol, nebivolol)**. [Moderate] Study
- **Bupropion** is predicted to increase the exposure to **dapoxetine**. [Moderate] Theoretical → Also see **TABLE 13** p. 910
- **Fluvoxamine** markedly decreases the clearance of **caffeine citrate**. Monitor and adjust dose. [Severe] Study
- Calcium channel blockers **(diltiazem, verapamil)** are predicted to increase the exposure to **dapoxetine**. Adjust **dapoxetine** dose with moderate inhibitors of CYP3A4. [Moderate] Theoretical
- SSRIs **(fluoxetine, fluvoxamine)** are predicted to increase the exposure to **cannabidiol**. [Moderate] Theoretical
- SSRIs **(fluoxetine, fluvoxamine)** are predicted to increase the exposure to **cilostazol**. Adjust **cilostazol** dose. [Moderate] Theoretical → Also see **TABLE 4** p. 907
- **Cinacalcet** is predicted to increase the exposure to **dapoxetine**. [Moderate] Theoretical
- **Fluvoxamine** is predicted to increase the exposure to cinacalcet. Adjust dose. [Moderate] Theoretical
- SSRIs **(fluoxetine, fluvoxamine)** potentially increase the exposure to **clobazam**. Adjust dose. [Moderate] Theoretical
- SSRIs **(fluoxetine, fluvoxamine)** are predicted to decrease the efficacy of **clopidogrel**. Avoid. [Severe] Theoretical → Also see **TABLE 4** p. 907
- **Fluvoxamine** increases the concentration of **clozapine**. Monitor side effects and adjust dose. [Severe] Study
- **Cobicistat** is predicted to moderately increase the exposure to **dapoxetine**. Avoid potent inhibitors of CYP3A4 or adjust **dapoxetine** dose. [Severe] Study
- **Crizotinib** is predicted to increase the exposure to **dapoxetine**. Adjust **dapoxetine** dose with moderate inhibitors of CYP3A4. [Moderate] Theoretical
- SSRIs **(fluoxetine, paroxetine)** are predicted to slightly increase the exposure to **darifenacin**. [Mild] Study
- **Fluvoxamine** moderately increases the exposure to **diazepam**. [Moderate] Study
- **Fluvoxamine** is predicted to increase the exposure to dopamine receptor agonists **(ropinirole)**. Adjust dose. [Moderate] Study
- **Fluvoxamine** markedly increases the exposure to **duloxetine**. Avoid. [Severe] Study → Also see **TABLE 18** p. 911 → Also see **TABLE 13** p. 910 → Also see **TABLE 4** p. 907
- SSRIs **(fluoxetine, paroxetine)** are predicted to increase the exposure to **eliglustat**. Avoid or adjust dose—consult product literature. [Severe] Study
- **Fluvoxamine** is predicted to increase the exposure to **eltrombopag**. [Moderate] Theoretical
- **Fluvoxamine** is predicted to increase the exposure to **erlotinib**. Monitor side effects and adjust dose. [Moderate] Theoretical
- **Fluvoxamine** increases the concentration of **frovatriptan**. [Severe] Study → Also see **TABLE 13** p. 910
- **Gilteritinib** is predicted to decrease the efficacy of SSRIs **(escitalopram, fluoxetine, sertraline)**. Avoid. [Moderate] Theoretical
- **Grapefruit juice** moderately increases the exposure to **sertraline**. Avoid. [Moderate] Study
- H_2 receptor antagonists **(cimetidine)** slightly increase the exposure to SSRIs **(citalopram, escitalopram)**. Adjust dose. [Moderate] Study
- H_2 receptor antagonists **(cimetidine)** slightly increase the exposure to SSRIs **(paroxetine, sertraline)**. [Moderate] Study
- **Fluoxetine** increases the concentration of **haloperidol**. Adjust dose. [Moderate] Anecdotal
- **Fluvoxamine** increases the concentration of **haloperidol**. Adjust dose. [Moderate] Study
- **HIV-protease inhibitors** are predicted to moderately increase the exposure to **dapoxetine**. Avoid potent inhibitors of CYP3A4 or adjust **dapoxetine** dose. [Severe] Study

A1

- Idelalisib is predicted to moderately increase the exposure to **dapoxetine**. Avoid potent inhibitors of CYP3A4 or adjust **dapoxetine** dose. Severe Study
- Imatinib is predicted to increase the exposure to **dapoxetine**. Adjust **dapoxetine** dose with moderate inhibitors of CYP3A4. Moderate Theoretical
- **Fluoxetine** is predicted to increase the exposure to **lomitapide**. Separate administration by 12 hours. Unknown Theoretical
- **Fluvoxamine** is predicted to increase the exposure to lomitapide. Separate administration by 12 hours. Moderate Theoretical
- **Fluvoxamine** is predicted to increase the exposure to **loxapine**. Avoid. Unknown Theoretical
- Macrolides **(clarithromycin)** are predicted to moderately increase the exposure to **dapoxetine**. Avoid potent inhibitors of CYP3A4 or adjust **dapoxetine** dose. Severe Study
- Macrolides **(erythromycin)** are predicted to increase the exposure to **dapoxetine**. Adjust **dapoxetine** dose with moderate inhibitors of CYP3A4. Moderate Theoretical
- **Fluvoxamine** very markedly increases the exposure to melatonin. Avoid. Severe Study
- SSRIs **(fluoxetine, fluvoxamine, paroxetine)** are predicted to increase the exposure to **mexiletine**. Moderate Study
- Netupitant is predicted to increase the exposure to **dapoxetine**. Adjust **dapoxetine** dose with moderate inhibitors of CYP3A4. Moderate Theoretical
- **SSRIs** potentially increase the risk of prolonged neuromuscular blockade when given with neuromuscular blocking drugs, non-depolarising **(mivacurium)**. Unknown Theoretical
- Nilotinib is predicted to increase the exposure to **dapoxetine**. Adjust **dapoxetine** dose with moderate inhibitors of CYP3A4. Moderate Theoretical
- **Fluvoxamine** moderately increases the exposure to **olanzapine**. Adjust dose. Severe Anecdotal
- SSRIs **(fluoxetine, paroxetine)** are predicted to decrease the efficacy of opioids **(codeine)**. Moderate Theoretical
- SSRIs **(fluoxetine, paroxetine)** are predicted to decrease the efficacy of opioids **(tramadol)**. Severe Study → Also see **TABLE 13** p. 910
- **Fluvoxamine** is predicted to increase the exposure to **pentoxifylline**. Moderate Theoretical
- **Fluvoxamine** is predicted to increase the exposure to phenothiazines **(chlorpromazine)**. Moderate Theoretical
- **Fluvoxamine** is predicted to moderately increase the exposure to pirfenidone. Avoid. Moderate Study
- SSRIs **(fluoxetine, paroxetine)** are predicted to moderately increase the exposure to **pitolisant**. Use with caution and adjust dose. Moderate Study
- **Fluvoxamine** moderately increases the exposure to pomalidomide. Adjust **pomalidomide** dose. Moderate Study
- **Paroxetine** slightly increases the exposure to **procyclidine**. Monitor and adjust dose. Moderate Study
- Proton pump inhibitors **(esomeprazole)** are predicted to slightly to moderately increase the exposure to SSRIs **(citalopram, escitalopram)**. Monitor and adjust dose. Severe Theoretical
- Proton pump inhibitors **(omeprazole)** slightly to moderately increase the exposure to SSRIs **(citalopram, escitalopram)**. Monitor and adjust dose. Severe Study
- **Fluvoxamine** is predicted to increase the exposure to **riluzole**. Moderate Theoretical
- SSRIs **(fluoxetine, paroxetine)** are predicted to increase the exposure to **risperidone**. Adjust dose. Moderate Study
- **Fluvoxamine** is predicted to increase the exposure to **roflumilast**. Moderate Study
- SSRIs **(fluoxetine, paroxetine)** are predicted to increase the exposure to SSRIs **(dapoxetine)**. Moderate Theoretical → Also see **TABLE 18** p. 911 → Also see **TABLE 13** p. 910 → Also see **TABLE 4** p. 907
- **SSRIs** potentially increase the risk of prolonged neuromuscular blockade when given with **suxamethonium**. Unknown Theoretical
- SSRIs **(fluoxetine, paroxetine)** are predicted to decrease the efficacy of **tamoxifen**. Avoid. Severe Study
- Terbinafine is predicted to increase the exposure to **fluoxetine**. Adjust dose. Moderate Theoretical
- Terbinafine moderately increases the exposure to **paroxetine**. Moderate Study
- Terbinafine is predicted to increase the exposure to SSRIs **(citalopram, dapoxetine, escitalopram, fluvoxamine, sertraline)**. Moderate Theoretical
- SSRIs **(fluoxetine, paroxetine)** are predicted to increase the exposure to the active metabolite of **tetrabenazine**. Moderate Study
- **Fluvoxamine** moderately to markedly increases the exposure to **theophylline**. Avoid. Severe Study
- **Fluvoxamine** very markedly increases the exposure to tizanidine. Avoid. Severe Study
- SSRIs **(fluoxetine, fluvoxamine)** given with a moderate CYP3A4 inhibitor are predicted to increase the exposure to **tofacitinib**. Adjust **tofacitinib** dose. Moderate Study
- SSRIs **(fluoxetine, paroxetine)** are predicted to increase the exposure to **tricyclic antidepressants**. Monitor for toxicity and adjust dose. Severe Study → Also see **TABLE 18** p. 911 → Also see **TABLE 13** p. 910
- **Fluvoxamine** increases the exposure to tricyclic antidepressants **(amitriptyline, imipramine)**. Adjust dose. Severe Study → Also see **TABLE 18** p. 911 → Also see **TABLE 13** p. 910
- **Fluvoxamine** markedly increases the exposure to tricyclic antidepressants **(clomipramine)**. Adjust dose. Severe Study → Also see **TABLE 18** p. 911 → Also see **TABLE 13** p. 910
- SSRIs **(fluoxetine, paroxetine)** are predicted to increase the exposure to **vortioxetine**. Monitor and adjust dose. Moderate Study → Also see **TABLE 13** p. 910 → Also see **TABLE 4** p. 907
- **Fluvoxamine** is predicted to increase the exposure to zolmitriptan. Adjust **zolmitriptan** dose, p. 310. Severe Theoretical → Also see **TABLE 13** p. 910

St John's Wort → see **TABLE 13** p. 910 (serotonin syndrome)

- **St John's Wort** is predicted to decrease the exposure to abemaciclib. Avoid. Severe Study
- **St John's Wort** is predicted to decrease the exposure to afatinib. Moderate Study
- **St John's Wort** is predicted to slightly decrease the exposure to aldosterone antagonists **(eplerenone)**. Avoid. Moderate Study
- **St John's Wort** decreases the exposure to **aliskiren**. Moderate Study
- **St John's Wort** moderately decreases the exposure to alprazolam. Moderate Study
- **St John's Wort** is predicted to decrease the concentration of **aminophylline**. Severe Theoretical
- **St John's Wort** is predicted to decrease the exposure to antiarrhythmics **(dronedarone)**. Avoid. Severe Theoretical
- **St John's Wort** is predicted to decrease the exposure to antiepileptics **(brivaracetam)**. Moderate Theoretical
- **St John's Wort** is predicted to decrease the concentration of antiepileptics **(carbamazepine)**. Monitor and adjust dose. Moderate Theoretical
- **St John's Wort** is predicted to decrease the concentration of antiepileptics **(fosphenytoin, phenobarbital, phenytoin, primidone)**. Avoid. Severe Theoretical
- **St John's Wort** is predicted to decrease the exposure to antiepileptics **(perampanel)**. Monitor and adjust dose. Moderate Theoretical
- **St John's Wort** is predicted to decrease the exposure to antiepileptics **(tiagabine)**. Avoid. Mild Theoretical
- **St John's Wort** is predicted to decrease the exposure to antifungals, azoles **(isavuconazole)**. Avoid. Severe Theoretical
- **St John's Wort** moderately decreases the exposure to antifungals, azoles **(voriconazole)**. Avoid. Moderate Study
- **St John's Wort** is predicted to decrease the concentration of antimalarials **(piperaquine)**. Avoid. Moderate Theoretical
- **St John's Wort** is predicted to decrease the exposure to apixaban. Use with caution or avoid. Moderate Theoretical
- **St John's Wort** is predicted to decrease the exposure to apremilast. Avoid. Severe Theoretical
- **St John's Wort** is predicted to decrease the exposure to aprepitant. Avoid. Moderate Theoretical
- **St John's Wort** is predicted to decrease the exposure to **axitinib**. Moderate Theoretical
- **St John's Wort** is predicted to decrease the exposure to bedaquiline. Avoid. Severe Study

St John's Wort (continued)

- **St John's Wort** is predicted to decrease the exposure to bictegravir. Avoid. [Moderate] Theoretical
- **St John's Wort** is predicted to decrease the exposure to bosentan. Avoid. [Moderate] Theoretical
- **St John's Wort** is predicted to decrease the exposure to bosutinib. Avoid. [Severe] Theoretical
- **St John's Wort** is predicted to decrease the exposure to brigatinib. Avoid. [Severe] Study
- **St John's Wort** is predicted to decrease the exposure to cabozantinib. [Moderate] Theoretical
- **St John's Wort** is predicted to decrease the exposure to calcium channel blockers **(amlodipine, felodipine, lacidipine, lercanidipine, nicardipine, nifedipine, nimodipine)**. Monitor and adjust dose. [Moderate] Theoretical
- **St John's Wort** is predicted to decrease the exposure to calcium channel blockers **(diltiazem, verapamil)**. [Moderate] Theoretical
- **St John's Wort** is predicted to decrease the exposure to cannabidiol. Adjust dose. [Mild] Study
- **St John's Wort** is predicted to decrease the exposure to cariprazine. Avoid. [Severe] Theoretical
- **St John's Wort** is predicted to decrease the exposure to ceritinib. Avoid. [Severe] Theoretical
- **St John's Wort** decreases the concentration of ciclosporin. Avoid. [Moderate] Study
- **St John's Wort** is predicted to alter the effects of cilostazol. [Moderate] Theoretical
- **St John's Wort** is predicted to decrease the exposure to cobicistat. Avoid. [Severe] Theoretical
- **St John's Wort** is predicted to decrease the exposure to cobimetinib. Avoid. [Severe] Theoretical
- **St John's Wort** decreases the efficacy of combined hormonal contraceptives. MHRA advises avoid. For FSRH guidance, see Contraceptives, interactions p. 536. [Severe] Anecdotal
- **St John's Wort** decreases the anticoagulant effect of coumarins. Avoid. [Severe] Anecdotal
- **St John's Wort** is predicted to decrease the exposure to crizotinib. Avoid. [Severe] Theoretical
- **St John's Wort** is predicted to decrease the exposure to dabigatran. Avoid. [Severe] Study
- **St John's Wort** is predicted to decrease the exposure to darifenacin. [Moderate] Theoretical
- **St John's Wort** is predicted to decrease the exposure to dasabuvir. Avoid. [Severe] Theoretical
- **St John's Wort** is predicted to decrease the exposure to dasatinib. [Severe] Study
- **St John's Wort** is predicted to decrease the efficacy of desogestrel. MHRA advises avoid. For FSRH guidance, see Contraceptives, interactions p. 536. [Severe] Theoretical
- **St John's Wort** decreases the concentration of digoxin. Avoid. [Severe] Anecdotal
- **St John's Wort** decreases the exposure to dolutegravir. Adjust dose. [Severe] Study
- **St John's Wort** is predicted to decrease the exposure to doravirine. Avoid. [Severe] Theoretical
- **St John's Wort** is predicted to decrease the exposure to dronabinol. Avoid or adjust dose. [Mild] Study
- **St John's Wort** is predicted to decrease the exposure to edoxaban. [Moderate] Study
- **St John's Wort** is predicted to decrease the concentration of efavirenz. Avoid. [Severe] Theoretical
- **St John's Wort** is predicted to moderately decrease the exposure to elbasvir. Avoid. [Severe] Study
- **St John's Wort** is predicted to increase the exposure to eliglustat. Avoid. [Severe] Study
- **St John's Wort** is predicted to decrease the concentration of elvitegravir. Avoid. [Severe] Theoretical
- **St John's Wort** is predicted to decrease the exposure to encorafenib. [Severe] Theoretical
- **St John's Wort** is predicted to decrease the effects of ergotamine. [Moderate] Theoretical
- **St John's Wort** is predicted to decrease the exposure to erlotinib. [Severe] Theoretical
- **St John's Wort** is predicted to decrease the efficacy of etonogestrel. MHRA advises avoid. For FSRH guidance, see Contraceptives, interactions p. 536. [Severe] Theoretical
- **St John's Wort** is predicted to decrease the exposure to etravirine. Avoid. [Severe] Study
- **St John's Wort** is predicted to decrease the concentration of everolimus. Avoid or adjust dose. [Severe] Study
- **St John's Wort** is predicted to decrease the exposure to exemestane. [Moderate] Theoretical
- **St John's Wort** is predicted to decrease the exposure to fesoterodine. Avoid. [Severe] Theoretical
- **St John's Wort** is predicted to decrease the exposure to fingolimod. Avoid. [Moderate] Theoretical
- **St John's Wort** is predicted to decrease the exposure to fosaprepitant. Avoid. [Moderate] Theoretical
- **St John's Wort** is predicted to decrease the exposure to gefitinib. Avoid. [Severe] Theoretical
- **St John's Wort** is predicted to decrease the exposure to gilteritinib. Avoid. [Severe] Study
- **St John's Wort** is predicted to decrease the exposure to glecaprevir. Avoid. [Severe] Study
- **St John's Wort** is predicted to markedly decrease the exposure to grazoprevir. Avoid. [Severe] Study
- **St John's Wort** is predicted to decrease the concentration of guanfacine. Adjust dose. [Moderate] Theoretical
- **St John's Wort** is predicted to decrease the exposure to **HIV-protease inhibitors**. Avoid. [Severe] Study
- **St John's Wort** is predicted to decrease the efficacy of **hormone replacement therapy**. [Moderate] Theoretical
- **St John's Wort** is predicted to decrease the exposure to ibrutinib. Avoid. [Severe] Theoretical
- **St John's Wort** is predicted to decrease the exposure to idelalisib. Avoid. [Moderate] Theoretical
- **St John's Wort** is predicted to decrease the exposure to imatinib. [Moderate] Study
- **St John's Wort** slightly decreases the exposure to **irinotecan**. Avoid. [Severe] Study
- **St John's Wort** decreases the exposure to **ivabradine**. Avoid. [Moderate] Study
- **St John's Wort** is predicted to decrease the exposure to ivacaftor. Avoid. [Severe] Study
- **St John's Wort** is predicted to decrease the exposure to ixazomib. Avoid. [Severe] Theoretical
- **St John's Wort** is predicted to decrease the exposure to lapatinib. Avoid. [Severe] Study
- **St John's Wort** is predicted to decrease the exposure to larotrectinib. Avoid. [Moderate] Study
- **St John's Wort** is predicted to decrease the exposure to ledipasvir. Avoid. [Severe] Study
- **St John's Wort** is predicted to decrease the concentration of letermovir. [Moderate] Theoretical
- **St John's Wort** is predicted to decrease the efficacy of levonorgestrel. MHRA advises avoid. For FSRH guidance, see Contraceptives, interactions p. 536. [Severe] Theoretical
- **St John's Wort** is predicted to decrease the exposure to lorlatinib. Avoid. [Severe] Theoretical
- **St John's Wort** is predicted to decrease the exposure to lurasidone. Monitor and adjust dose. [Moderate] Theoretical
- **St John's Wort** is predicted to decrease the exposure to macitentan. Avoid. [Severe] Theoretical
- **St John's Wort** is predicted to decrease the exposure to maraviroc. Avoid. [Severe] Theoretical
- **St John's Wort** moderately decreases the exposure to midazolam. Monitor and adjust dose. [Moderate] Study
- **St John's Wort** is predicted to decrease the exposure to midostaurin. Avoid. [Severe] Theoretical
- **St John's Wort** is predicted to decrease the exposure to naldemedine. Avoid. [Severe] Study
- **St John's Wort** is predicted to decrease the exposure to naloxegol. Avoid. [Moderate] Theoretical
- **St John's Wort** is predicted to decrease the exposure to neratinib. Avoid. [Severe] Theoretical
- **St John's Wort** is predicted to decrease the exposure to netupitant. [Moderate] Theoretical

- **St John's Wort** is predicted to decrease the concentration of nevirapine. Avoid. Severe Theoretical
- **St John's Wort** is predicted to decrease the exposure to nilotinib. Avoid. Severe Theoretical
- **St John's Wort** is predicted to decrease the exposure to nintedanib. Moderate Study
- **St John's Wort** is predicted to decrease the efficacy of norethisterone. MHRA advises avoid. For FSRH guidance, see Contraceptives, interactions p. 536. Severe Anecdotal
- **St John's Wort** is predicted to decrease the exposure to olaparib. Avoid. Moderate Theoretical
- **St John's Wort** is predicted to decrease the exposure to ombitasvir. Avoid. Severe Theoretical
- **St John's Wort** decreases the exposure to opioids **(methadone)**. Monitor and adjust dose. Severe Study → Also see TABLE 13 p. 910
- **St John's Wort** moderately decreases the exposure to opioids (oxycodone). Adjust dose. Moderate Study
- **St John's Wort** is predicted to decrease the exposure to osimertinib. Avoid. Moderate Theoretical
- **St John's Wort** is predicted to decrease the exposure to ospemifene. Moderate Study
- **St John's Wort** is predicted to decrease the exposure to palbociclib. Avoid. Severe Theoretical
- **St John's Wort** is predicted to decrease the exposure to paliperidone. Severe Theoretical
- **St John's Wort** is predicted to decrease the exposure to panobinostat. Avoid. Moderate Theoretical
- **St John's Wort** is predicted to decrease the exposure to paritaprevir (with ritonavir and ombitasvir). Avoid. Severe Study
- **St John's Wort** is predicted to decrease the exposure to phosphodiesterase type-5 inhibitors. Moderate Theoretical
- **St John's Wort** is predicted to decrease the exposure to pibrentasvir. Avoid. Severe Study
- **St John's Wort** slightly decreases the exposure to **pioglitazone**. Mild Study
- **St John's Wort** is predicted to decrease the exposure to pitolisant. Monitor and adjust dose. Moderate Theoretical
- **St John's Wort** is predicted to decrease the exposure to ponatinib. Avoid. Severe Theoretical
- **St John's Wort** is predicted to decrease the exposure to quetiapine. Moderate Study
- **St John's Wort** is predicted to decrease the exposure to ranolazine. Avoid. Severe Study
- **St John's Wort** is predicted to decrease the exposure to ribociclib. Avoid. Severe Study
- **St John's Wort** is predicted to decrease the exposure to rilpivirine. Avoid. Severe Theoretical
- **St John's Wort** is predicted to decrease the exposure to rolapitant. Avoid. Severe Study
- **St John's Wort** is predicted to decrease the exposure to ruxolitinib. Monitor and adjust dose. Moderate Theoretical
- **St John's Wort** is predicted to decrease the exposure to siponimod. Manufacturer advises caution depending on genotype—consult product literature. Severe Theoretical
- **St John's Wort** is predicted to decrease the concentration of sirolimus. Monitor and adjust dose. Severe Theoretical
- **St John's Wort** is predicted to decrease the exposure to sofosbuvir. Avoid. Severe Study
- **St John's Wort** slightly decreases the exposure to statins (atorvastatin). Mild Study
- **St John's Wort** moderately decreases the exposure to statins (simvastatin). Moderate Study
- **St John's Wort** decreases the concentration of **tacrolimus**. Avoid. Severe Study
- **St John's Wort** is predicted to decrease the exposure to taxanes (cabazitaxel). Avoid. Severe Study
- **St John's Wort** is predicted to decrease the concentration of temsirolimus. Avoid. Severe Theoretical
- **St John's Wort** is predicted to decrease the exposure to tenofovir alafenamide. Avoid. Moderate Theoretical
- **St John's Wort** is predicted to decrease the exposure to tezacaftor. Avoid. Severe Theoretical
- **St John's Wort** potentially decreases the exposure to theophylline. Severe Anecdotal
- **St John's Wort** is predicted to decrease the exposure to ticagrelor. Moderate Theoretical
- **St John's Wort** is predicted to decrease the exposure to tivozanib. Avoid. Severe Study
- **St John's Wort** is predicted to decrease the exposure to tofacitinib. Moderate Study
- **St John's Wort** is predicted to decrease the exposure to tolvaptan. Avoid. Moderate Theoretical
- **St John's Wort** is predicted to decrease the exposure to topotecan. Severe Theoretical
- **St John's Wort** decreases the efficacy of ulipristal. For FSRH guidance, see Contraceptives, interactions p. 536. Severe Anecdotal
- **St John's Wort** is predicted to decrease the exposure to velpatasvir. Avoid. Moderate Theoretical
- **St John's Wort** is predicted to decrease the exposure to venetoclax. Avoid. Severe Study
- **St John's Wort** is predicted to decrease the exposure to vismodegib. Avoid. Moderate Theoretical
- **St John's Wort** is predicted to decrease the concentration of voxilaprevir. Avoid. Severe Theoretical

Statins → see TABLE 1 p. 907 (hepatotoxicity)

atorvastatin · fluvastatin · pravastatin · rosuvastatin · simvastatin

- **Atorvastatin** slightly to moderately increases the exposure to aliskiren. Moderate Study
- Antacids moderately decrease the absorption of **rosuvastatin**. Separate administration by 2 hours. Moderate Study
- Antiarrhythmics **(amiodarone)** are predicted to increase the risk of rhabdomyolysis when given with **atorvastatin**. Monitor and adjust dose. Moderate Theoretical
- Antiarrhythmics **(amiodarone)** are predicted to increase the exposure to **fluvastatin**. Severe Theoretical
- Antiarrhythmics **(amiodarone)** increase the risk of rhabdomyolysis when given with **simvastatin**. Adjust **simvastatin** dose, p. 141. Severe Study
- Antiarrhythmics **(dronedarone)** slightly increase the exposure to **atorvastatin**. Monitor and adjust dose. Severe Study
- Antiarrhythmics **(dronedarone)** slightly increase the exposure to **rosuvastatin**. Adjust dose. Severe Study
- Antiarrhythmics **(dronedarone)** moderately increase the exposure to **simvastatin**. Monitor and adjust dose. Severe Study
- Antiepileptics **(carbamazepine)** moderately decrease the exposure to **simvastatin**. Monitor and adjust dose. Severe Study → Also see TABLE 1 p. 907
- Antiepileptics **(carbamazepine, eslicarbazepine)** are predicted to decrease the exposure to **atorvastatin**. Monitor and adjust dose. Moderate Theoretical → Also see TABLE 1 p. 907
- Antiepileptics **(eslicarbazepine)** moderately decrease the exposure to **simvastatin**. Monitor and adjust dose. Moderate Study
- Antiepileptics **(fosphenytoin, phenytoin)** potentially decrease the exposure to statins **(atorvastatin, simvastatin)**. Moderate Anecdotal
- Antifungals, azoles **(fluconazole)** potentially increase the risk of rhabdomyolysis when given with **atorvastatin**. Monitor and adjust dose. Severe Anecdotal → Also see TABLE 1 p. 907
- Antifungals, azoles **(fluconazole)** are predicted to increase the exposure to **simvastatin**. Monitor and adjust dose. Severe Anecdotal → Also see TABLE 1 p. 907
- Antifungals, azoles **(fluconazole, miconazole)** are predicted to increase the exposure to **fluvastatin**. Severe Theoretical → Also see TABLE 1 p. 907
- Antifungals, azoles **(isavuconazole)** slightly increase the exposure to **atorvastatin**. Moderate Study
- Antifungals, azoles **(isavuconazole)** are predicted to increase the exposure to **simvastatin**. Monitor and adjust dose. Severe Theoretical
- Antifungals, azoles **(itraconazole, ketoconazole, voriconazole)** are predicted to increase the exposure to **atorvastatin**. Avoid or adjust dose and monitor rhabdomyolysis. Severe Study → Also see TABLE 1 p. 907
- Antifungals, azoles **(itraconazole, ketoconazole, voriconazole)** are predicted to increase the exposure to **simvastatin**. Avoid. Severe Study → Also see TABLE 1 p. 907

Statins (continued)

- Antifungals, azoles **(miconazole)** potentially increase the exposure to **atorvastatin**. [Severe] Anecdotal
- Antifungals, azoles **(miconazole)** are predicted to increase the exposure to **simvastatin**. Avoid. [Severe] Theoretical
- Antifungals, azoles **(posaconazole)** are predicted to increase the exposure to **atorvastatin**. Avoid. [Severe] Anecdotal
- Antifungals, azoles **(posaconazole)** markedly to very markedly increase the exposure to **simvastatin**. Avoid. [Severe] Study
- Antifungals, azoles **(isavuconazole)** are predicted to increase the exposure to statins **(fluvastatin, rosuvastatin)**. [Moderate] Theoretical
- **Apalutamide** slightly decreases the exposure to **rosuvastatin**. [Mild] Study
- **Apalutamide** is predicted to decrease the exposure to **simvastatin**. Avoid or monitor. [Moderate] Study
- **Aprepitant** is predicted to increase the exposure to statins **(atorvastatin, simvastatin)**. Monitor and adjust dose. [Severe] Theoretical
- **Bosentan** slightly decreases the exposure to **atorvastatin**. [Mild] Study
- **Bosentan** moderately decreases the exposure to **simvastatin**. [Moderate] Study
- Calcium channel blockers **(amlodipine)** slightly increase the exposure to **simvastatin**. Adjust **simvastatin** dose, p. 141. [Mild] Study
- Calcium channel blockers **(diltiazem)** slightly to moderately increase the exposure to **atorvastatin**. Monitor and adjust dose. [Severe] Anecdotal
- Calcium channel blockers **(diltiazem, verapamil)** moderately increase the exposure to **simvastatin**. Monitor and adjust dose. [Severe] Study
- Calcium channel blockers **(verapamil)** are predicted to slightly to moderately increase the exposure to **atorvastatin**. Monitor and adjust dose. [Severe] Theoretical
- Cephalosporins **(ceftobiprole)** are predicted to increase the concentration of **statins**. [Moderate] Theoretical
- **Ciclosporin** very markedly increases the exposure to **atorvastatin**. Avoid or adjust **atorvastatin** dose, p. 139. [Severe] Study
- **Ciclosporin** moderately increases the exposure to **fluvastatin**. [Severe] Study
- **Ciclosporin** markedly to very markedly increases the exposure to **pravastatin**. Adjust dose. [Severe] Study
- **Ciclosporin** markedly increases the exposure to statins **(rosuvastatin, simvastatin)**. Avoid. [Severe] Study
- **Clopidogrel** increases the exposure to **rosuvastatin**. Adjust **rosuvastatin** dose, p. 140. [Moderate] Study
- **Cobicistat** is predicted to increase the exposure to **atorvastatin**. Avoid or adjust dose and monitor rhabdomyolysis. [Severe] Study
- **Cobicistat** is predicted to increase the exposure to **simvastatin**. Avoid. [Severe] Study
- **Colchicine** increases the risk of rhabdomyolysis when given with **statins**. [Severe] Anecdotal
- Statins **(fluvastatin, rosuvastatin)** increase the anticoagulant effect of **coumarins**. Monitor INR and adjust dose. [Severe] Study
- **Crizotinib** is predicted to increase the exposure to statins **(atorvastatin, simvastatin)**. Monitor and adjust dose. [Severe] Theoretical
- **Danazol** is predicted to increase the risk of rhabdomyolysis when given with **atorvastatin**. [Severe] Theoretical
- **Danazol** increases the risk of rhabdomyolysis when given with **simvastatin**. Avoid. [Severe] Anecdotal
- **Statins** are predicted to increase the risk of rhabdomyolysis when given with **daptomycin**. [Severe] Theoretical
- **Dasabuvir** increases the exposure to **rosuvastatin**. Adjust **rosuvastatin** dose, p. 140. [Moderate] Study
- **Dasatinib** is predicted to increase the exposure to **simvastatin**. [Moderate] Theoretical
- **Efavirenz** slightly decreases the exposure to **atorvastatin**. [Mild] Study
- **Efavirenz** moderately decreases the exposure to **simvastatin**. [Moderate] Study
- **Elbasvir** increases the exposure to **atorvastatin**. Adjust **atorvastatin** dose, p. 139. [Moderate] Study
- **Elbasvir** is predicted to increase the exposure to **fluvastatin**. Adjust **fluvastatin** dose, p. 139. [Unknown] Theoretical
- **Elbasvir** increases the exposure to **rosuvastatin**. Adjust **rosuvastatin** dose, p. 140. [Moderate] Study
- **Elbasvir** is predicted to increase the exposure to **simvastatin**. Adjust **simvastatin** dose, p. 141. [Unknown] Theoretical
- **Eltrombopag** is predicted to increase the exposure to **statins**. Monitor and adjust dose. [Moderate] Study
- **Enzalutamide** is predicted to decrease the exposure to **simvastatin**. [Severe] Study
- **Ezetimibe** potentially increases the risk of rhabdomyolysis when given with **statins**. [Severe] Anecdotal
- Fibrates **(bezafibrate, ciprofibrate)** increase the risk of rhabdomyolysis when given with **pravastatin**. Avoid. [Severe] Study
- Fibrates **(bezafibrate, ciprofibrate)** increase the risk of rhabdomyolysis when given with **rosuvastatin**. Adjust **rosuvastatin** dose, p. 140. [Severe] Study
- Fibrates **(bezafibrate, ciprofibrate)** increase the risk of rhabdomyolysis when given with **simvastatin**. Adjust **simvastatin** dose, p. 141. [Severe] Study
- Fibrates **(ciprofibrate)** increase the risk of rhabdomyolysis when given with **atorvastatin**. Avoid or adjust dose. [Severe] Study
- Fibrates **(ciprofibrate)** increase the risk of rhabdomyolysis when given with **fluvastatin**. [Severe] Study
- Fibrates **(fenofibrate)** are predicted to increase the risk of rhabdomyolysis when given with **fluvastatin**. Adjust **fenofibrate** dose, p. 138. [Severe] Theoretical
- Fibrates **(fenofibrate)** are predicted to increase the risk of rhabdomyolysis when given with **pravastatin**. Avoid. [Severe] Theoretical
- Fibrates **(fenofibrate)** increase the risk of rhabdomyolysis when given with **rosuvastatin**. Adjust **fenofibrate** and **rosuvastatin** doses, p. 138, p. 140. [Severe] Anecdotal
- Fibrates **(gemfibrozil)** increase the risk of rhabdomyolysis when given with **statins**. Avoid. [Severe] Anecdotal
- Fibrates **(bezafibrate)** increase the risk of rhabdomyolysis when given with statins **(atorvastatin, fluvastatin)**. [Severe] Study
- Fibrates **(fenofibrate)** increase the risk of rhabdomyolysis when given with statins **(atorvastatin, simvastatin)**. Adjust **fenofibrate** dose, p. 138. [Severe] Anecdotal
- **Fusidate** increases the risk of rhabdomyolysis when given with **statins**. Avoid. [Severe] Anecdotal
- **Glecaprevir** (with pibrentasvir) markedly increases the exposure to **atorvastatin**. Avoid. [Severe] Study
- **Glecaprevir** (with pibrentasvir) is predicted to increase the exposure to **fluvastatin**. [Moderate] Theoretical
- **Glecaprevir** (with pibrentasvir) increases the exposure to **pravastatin**. Use with caution and adjust **pravastatin** dose, p. 140. [Moderate] Study
- **Glecaprevir** (with pibrentasvir) increases the exposure to **rosuvastatin**. Use with caution and adjust **rosuvastatin** dose, p. 140. [Moderate] Study
- **Glecaprevir** (with pibrentasvir) increases the exposure to **simvastatin**. Avoid. [Moderate] Study
- **Grapefruit juice** increases the exposure to **atorvastatin**. [Mild] Study
- **Grapefruit juice** increases the exposure to **simvastatin**. Avoid. [Severe] Study
- **Grazoprevir** increases the exposure to **atorvastatin**. Adjust **atorvastatin** dose, p. 139. [Moderate] Study
- **Grazoprevir** is predicted to increase the exposure to **fluvastatin**. Adjust **fluvastatin** dose, p. 139. [Unknown] Theoretical
- **Grazoprevir** increases the exposure to **rosuvastatin**. Adjust **rosuvastatin** dose, p. 140. [Moderate] Study
- **Grazoprevir** is predicted to increase the exposure to **simvastatin**. Adjust **simvastatin** dose, p. 141. [Unknown] Theoretical
- **HIV-protease inhibitors** are predicted to increase the exposure to **atorvastatin**. Avoid or adjust dose and monitor rhabdomyolysis. [Severe] Study
- **HIV-protease inhibitors** slightly to moderately increase the exposure to **rosuvastatin**. Avoid or adjust dose. [Severe] Study

- **HIV-protease inhibitors** are predicted to increase the exposure to **simvastatin**. Avoid. Severe Study
- **Idelalisib** is predicted to increase the exposure to **atorvastatin**. Avoid or adjust dose and monitor rhabdomyolysis. Severe Study
- **Idelalisib** is predicted to increase the exposure to **simvastatin**. Avoid. Severe Study
- **Imatinib** is predicted to increase the exposure to **atorvastatin**. Monitor and adjust dose. Severe Theoretical
- **Imatinib** moderately increases the exposure to **simvastatin**. Monitor and adjust dose. Severe Study
- **Ledipasvir** is predicted to increase the exposure to **rosuvastatin**. Avoid. Severe Theoretical
- **Ledipasvir** is predicted to increase the exposure to statins **(atorvastatin, fluvastatin, pravastatin, simvastatin)**. Monitor and adjust dose. Moderate Theoretical
- **Leflunomide** is predicted to increase the exposure to **rosuvastatin**. Adjust dose. Moderate Study → Also see **TABLE 1** p. 907
- **Leflunomide** is predicted to increase the exposure to statins **(atorvastatin, fluvastatin, pravastatin, simvastatin)**. Moderate Study → Also see **TABLE 1** p. 907
- **Letermovir** moderately increases the exposure to **atorvastatin**. Avoid or adjust **atorvastatin** dose, p. 139. Severe Study
- **Letermovir** is predicted to increase the exposure to **fluvastatin**. Monitor and adjust dose. Moderate Theoretical
- **Letermovir** is predicted to increase the exposure to **pravastatin**. Avoid or adjust dose. Moderate Theoretical
- **Letermovir** is predicted to increase the exposure to statins **(rosuvastatin, simvastatin)**. Avoid. Severe Study
- **Lomitapide** increases the exposure to **atorvastatin**. Adjust **lomitapide** dose or separate administration by 12 hours. Mild Study → Also see **TABLE 1** p. 907
- **Lomitapide** increases the exposure to **simvastatin**. Monitor and adjust **simvastatin** dose, p. 141. Moderate Study → Also see **TABLE 1** p. 907
- Macrolides **(clarithromycin)** are predicted to increase the exposure to **atorvastatin**. Avoid or adjust dose and monitor rhabdomyolysis. Severe Study
- Macrolides **(clarithromycin)** moderately increase the exposure to **pravastatin**. Severe Study
- Macrolides **(clarithromycin)** are predicted to increase the exposure to **simvastatin**. Avoid. Severe Study
- Macrolides **(erythromycin)** slightly increase the exposure to **atorvastatin**. Monitor and adjust dose. Severe Anecdotal
- Macrolides **(erythromycin)** are predicted to increase the exposure to **pravastatin**. Severe Study
- Macrolides **(erythromycin)** markedly increase the exposure to **simvastatin**. Avoid. Severe Study
- **Mitotane** is predicted to decrease the exposure to **simvastatin**. Severe Study
- Monoclonal antibodies **(sarilumab)** are predicted to decrease the exposure to statins **(atorvastatin, simvastatin)**. Moderate Study
- Monoclonal antibodies **(tocilizumab)** are predicted to decrease the exposure to statins **(atorvastatin, simvastatin)**. Monitor and adjust dose. Moderate Study
- **Netupitant** is predicted to increase the exposure to statins **(atorvastatin, simvastatin)**. Monitor and adjust dose. Severe Theoretical
- **Nevirapine** slightly decreases the exposure to **atorvastatin**. Mild Study
- **Nevirapine** moderately decreases the exposure to **simvastatin**. Moderate Study
- **Nicotinic acid** is predicted to increase the risk of rhabdomyolysis when given with **statins**. Severe Theoretical
- **Nilotinib** is predicted to slightly increase the exposure to **atorvastatin**. Monitor and adjust dose. Severe Theoretical
- **Nilotinib** is predicted to increase the exposure to **simvastatin**. Monitor and adjust dose. Severe Theoretical
- **Osimertinib** slightly increases the exposure to **rosuvastatin**. Moderate Study
- **Paritaprevir** (in fixed-dose combination) is predicted to increase the risk of rhabdomyolysis when given with **atorvastatin**. Avoid. Severe Theoretical
- **Paritaprevir** (with ritonavir and ombitasvir) is predicted to increase the exposure to **fluvastatin**. Avoid. Moderate Theoretical
- **Paritaprevir** (with ritonavir and ombitasvir) increases the exposure to **pravastatin**. Adjust **pravastatin** dose, p. 140. Moderate Study
- **Paritaprevir** (with ritonavir and ombitasvir) slightly to moderately increases the exposure to **rosuvastatin**. Adjust **rosuvastatin** dose, p. 140. Moderate Study
- **Paritaprevir** (in fixed-dose combination) is predicted to increase the risk of rhabdomyolysis when given with **simvastatin**. Avoid. Severe Theoretical
- **Pazopanib** is predicted to affect the exposure to **atorvastatin**. Moderate Anecdotal
- **Pazopanib** is predicted to affect the exposure to statins **(pravastatin, rosuvastatin, simvastatin)**. Moderate Theoretical
- **Rosuvastatin** is predicted to increase the anticoagulant effect of **phenindione**. Monitor INR and adjust dose. Severe Theoretical
- **Pibrentasvir** (with glecaprevir) markedly increases the exposure to **atorvastatin**. Avoid. Severe Study
- **Pibrentasvir** (with glecaprevir) is predicted to increase the exposure to **fluvastatin**. Moderate Theoretical
- **Pibrentasvir** (with glecaprevir) increases the exposure to **pravastatin**. Use with caution and adjust **pravastatin** dose, p. 140. Moderate Study
- **Pibrentasvir** (with glecaprevir) increases the exposure to **rosuvastatin**. Use with caution and adjust **rosuvastatin** dose, p. 140. Moderate Study
- **Pibrentasvir** (with glecaprevir) increases the exposure to **simvastatin**. Avoid. Moderate Study
- **Ranolazine** is predicted to increase the exposure to **atorvastatin**. Moderate Theoretical
- **Ranolazine** slightly increases the exposure to **simvastatin**. Adjust **simvastatin** dose, p. 141. Moderate Study
- **Regorafenib** is predicted to increase the exposure to statins **(atorvastatin, fluvastatin, rosuvastatin)**. Moderate Study
- **Ribociclib** (high-dose) is predicted to increase the exposure to **simvastatin**. Avoid. Moderate Theoretical
- **Ribociclib** is predicted to increase the exposure to statins **(pravastatin, rosuvastatin)**. Moderate Theoretical
- **Rifampicin** markedly decreases the exposure to **atorvastatin**. Manufacturer advises take both drugs at the same time. Moderate Study
- **Rifampicin** moderately decreases the exposure to **fluvastatin**. Monitor and adjust dose. Moderate Study
- **Rifampicin** very markedly decreases the exposure to **simvastatin**. Moderate Study
- **Rolapitant** is predicted to increase the exposure to **rosuvastatin**. Monitor and adjust dose. Severe Study
- **Sacubitril** is predicted to increase the exposure to **statins**. Severe Study
- **St John's Wort** slightly decreases the exposure to **atorvastatin**. Mild Study
- **St John's Wort** moderately decreases the exposure to **simvastatin**. Moderate Study
- **Fluvastatin** slightly increases the exposure to sulfonylureas **(glibenclamide)**. Mild Study
- **Tedizolid** is predicted to increase the exposure to statins **(atorvastatin, fluvastatin, rosuvastatin)**. Avoid. Moderate Study
- **Teriflunomide** moderately increases the exposure to **rosuvastatin**. Adjust **rosuvastatin** dose, p. 140. Moderate Study → Also see **TABLE 1** p. 907
- **Teriflunomide** is predicted to increase the exposure to statins **(atorvastatin, fluvastatin, pravastatin, simvastatin)**. Moderate Study → Also see **TABLE 1** p. 907
- **Ticagrelor** slightly increases the exposure to **simvastatin**. Adjust **simvastatin** dose, p. 141. Moderate Study
- **Tivozanib** is predicted to decrease the exposure to **rosuvastatin**. Moderate Theoretical
- **Velpatasvir** increases the exposure to **rosuvastatin**. Adjust **rosuvastatin** dose and monitor side effects, p. 140. Severe Study
- **Velpatasvir** is predicted to increase the exposure to **simvastatin**. Monitor side effects and adjust dose. Severe Theoretical

Statins (continued)
- Venetoclax is predicted to increase the exposure to **atorvastatin.** Moderate Study
- Venetoclax is predicted to increase the exposure to statins **(fluvastatin, pravastatin, rosuvastatin, simvastatin).** Moderate Theoretical
- Voxilaprevir (with sofosbuvir and velpatasvir) is predicted to increase the exposure to **atorvastatin**. Adjust **atorvastatin** dose, p. 139. Moderate Theoretical
- Voxilaprevir (with sofosbuvir and velpatasvir) moderately increases the exposure to **pravastatin**. Monitor and adjust **pravastatin** dose, p. 140. Moderate Study
- Voxilaprevir (with sofosbuvir and velpatasvir) markedly increases the exposure to **rosuvastatin**. Avoid. Severe Study
- Voxilaprevir (with sofosbuvir and velpatasvir) is predicted to increase the exposure to statins **(fluvastatin, simvastatin).** Avoid. Moderate Theoretical

Stavudine → see TABLE 12 p. 910 (peripheral neuropathy)
- Hydroxycarbamide increases the risk of toxicity when given with **stavudine.** Avoid. Severe Study
- Isoniazid is predicted to increase the risk of peripheral neuropathy when given with **stavudine.** Severe Theoretical → Also see TABLE 12 p. 910
- Ribavirin increases the risk of toxicity when given with **stavudine.** Avoid. Severe Study
- Zidovudine is predicted to decrease the efficacy of **stavudine.** Avoid. Severe Theoretical

Stiripentol → see antiepileptics
Streptokinase → see TABLE 3 p. 907 (anticoagulant effects)
Streptomycin → see aminoglycosides
Streptozocin → see TABLE 1 p. 907 (hepatotoxicity), TABLE 2 p. 907 (nephrotoxicity)
- Live vaccines are predicted to increase the risk of generalised infection (possibly life-threatening) when given with **streptozocin.** Public Health England advises avoid (refer to Green Book). Severe Theoretical

Strontium → see TABLE 5 p. 907 (thromboembolism)
- Antacids decrease the absorption of **strontium**. Separate administration by 2 hours. Moderate Study
- Oral calcium salts decrease the exposure to **strontium.** Separate administration by 2 hours. Moderate Study
- **Strontium** is predicted to decrease the absorption of quinolones. Avoid. Moderate Theoretical
- **Strontium** is predicted to decrease the absorption of tetracyclines. Avoid. Moderate Theoretical

Sucralfate
- **Sucralfate** is predicted to decrease the exposure to bictegravir. Avoid. Moderate Theoretical
- **Sucralfate** potentially decreases the effects of coumarins (warfarin). Separate administration by 2 hours. Moderate Anecdotal
- **Sucralfate** decreases the absorption of digoxin. Separate administration by 2 hours. Severe Anecdotal
- **Sucralfate** decreases the absorption of dolutegravir. Moderate Study
- **Sucralfate** increases the risk of blocked enteral or nasogastric tubes when given with enteral feeds. Separate administration by 1 hour. Moderate Study
- Potassium citrate increases the risk of side-effects when given with **sucralfate.** Avoid. Moderate Theoretical
- **Sucralfate** decreases the exposure to quinolones. Separate administration by 2 hours. Moderate Study
- Sodium citrate is predicted to increase the risk of side-effects when given with **sucralfate**. Avoid. Moderate Theoretical
- **Sucralfate** decreases the absorption of sulpiride. Separate administration by 2 hours. Moderate Study
- **Sucralfate** potentially decreases the absorption of theophylline. Separate administration by at least 2 hours. Moderate Study
- **Sucralfate** decreases the absorption of thyroid hormones (levothyroxine). Separate administration by at least 4 hours. Moderate Study
- **Sucralfate** is predicted to decrease the absorption of tricyclic antidepressants. Moderate Study

Sugammadex
- **Sugammadex** is predicted to decrease the exposure to oral combined hormonal contraceptives. Refer to patient information leaflet for missed pill advice. Severe Theoretical
- **Sugammadex** is predicted to decrease the exposure to desogestrel. Refer to patient information leaflet for missed pill advice. Severe Theoretical
- **Sugammadex** is predicted to decrease the efficacy of etonogestrel. Use additional contraceptive precautions. Severe Theoretical
- **Sugammadex** is predicted to decrease the exposure to levonorgestrel. Use additional contraceptive precautions. Severe Theoretical
- **Sugammadex** is predicted to decrease the exposure to medroxyprogesterone. Use additional contraceptive precautions. Severe Theoretical
- **Sugammadex** is predicted to decrease the exposure to norethisterone. Use additional contraceptive precautions. Severe Theoretical

Sulfadiazine → see sulfonamides
Sulfadoxine → see sulfonamides
Sulfamethoxazole → see sulfonamides
Sulfasalazine → see TABLE 1 p. 907 (hepatotoxicity), TABLE 15 p. 910 (myelosuppression)
- Antifungals, azoles (isavuconazole) are predicted to increase the exposure to **sulfasalazine.** Moderate Theoretical
- **Sulfasalazine** decreases the concentration of digoxin. Moderate Study
- **Sulfasalazine** is predicted to decrease the absorption of folates. Moderate Study
- Leflunomide is predicted to increase the exposure to **sulfasalazine.** Moderate Study → Also see TABLE 1 p. 907 → Also see TABLE 15 p. 910
- Regorafenib is predicted to increase the exposure to **sulfasalazine.** Moderate Study → Also see TABLE 15 p. 910
- Rolapitant increases the exposure to **sulfasalazine.** Severe Study
- Tedizolid is predicted to increase the exposure to **sulfasalazine.** Avoid. Moderate Study
- Teriflunomide is predicted to increase the exposure to **sulfasalazine.** Moderate Study → Also see TABLE 1 p. 907
- Velpatasvir is predicted to increase the exposure to **sulfasalazine.** Moderate Theoretical
- Venetoclax is predicted to increase the exposure to **sulfasalazine.** Moderate Theoretical
- Voxilaprevir is predicted to increase the concentration of **sulfasalazine.** Avoid. Severe Theoretical

Sulfonamides → see TABLE 15 p. 910 (myelosuppression)

sulfadiazine · sulfadoxine · sulfamethoxazole

- **Sulfonamides** potentially increase the risk of methaemoglobinaemia when given with topical anaesthetics, local (prilocaine). Use with caution or avoid. Severe Anecdotal
- **Sulfadiazine** is predicted to increase the concentration of antiepileptics (fosphenytoin). Monitor and adjust dose. Moderate Study
- **Sulfadiazine** increases the concentration of antiepileptics (phenytoin). Monitor and adjust dose. Moderate Study
- Antimalarials (pyrimethamine) increase the risk of side-effects when given with **sulfonamides.** Severe Study → Also see TABLE 15 p. 910
- Chloroprocaine is predicted to decrease the effects of **sulfonamides.** Avoid. Severe Theoretical
- **Sulfadiazine** is predicted to increase the anticoagulant effect of coumarins. Severe Theoretical
- **Sulfamethoxazole** increases the anticoagulant effect of coumarins. Severe Study
- **Sulfonamides** are predicted to increase the risk of methaemoglobinaemia when given with dapsone. Severe Theoretical
- **Sulfonamides** are predicted to increase the exposure to methotrexate. Use with caution or avoid. Severe Theoretical → Also see TABLE 15 p. 910
- Potassium aminobenzoate is predicted to affect the efficacy of **sulfonamides.** Avoid. Severe Theoretical
- **Sulfonamides** are predicted to increase the exposure to sulfonylureas. Moderate Study

- **Sulfonamides** are predicted to increase the effects of **thiopental**. Moderate Theoretical

Sulfonylureas → see TABLE 14 p. 910 (antidiabetic drugs)

glibenclamide · gliclazide · glimepiride · glipizide · tolbutamide

- Antiarrhythmics **(amiodarone)** are predicted to increase the exposure to **sulfonylureas**. Use with caution and adjust dose. Moderate Study
- Antifungals, azoles **(fluconazole, miconazole)** are predicted to increase the exposure to **sulfonylureas**. Use with caution and adjust dose. Moderate Study
- Antifungals, azoles **(voriconazole)** are predicted to increase the concentration of **sulfonylureas**. Use with caution and adjust dose. Moderate Study
- **Bosentan** increases the risk of hepatotoxicity when given with **glibenclamide**. Avoid. Severe Study
- Cephalosporins **(ceftobiprole)** are predicted to increase the concentration of **glibenclamide**. Moderate Theoretical
- **Ceritinib** is predicted to increase the exposure to **glimepiride**. Adjust dose. Moderate Theoretical
- **Chloramphenicol** is predicted to increase the exposure to **sulfonylureas**. Severe Study
- **Fibrates** are predicted to increase the risk of hypoglycaemia when given with **sulfonylureas**. Moderate Theoretical
- **Leflunomide** is predicted to increase the exposure to **glibenclamide**. Moderate Study
- **Letermovir** is predicted to increase the concentration of **glibenclamide**. Moderate Theoretical
- Macrolides **(clarithromycin)** are predicted to slightly increase the exposure to **sulfonylureas**. Moderate Theoretical
- **Nitisinone** is predicted to increase the exposure to sulfonylureas **(glimepiride, tolbutamide)**. Moderate Study
- **Rifampicin** is predicted to decrease the exposure to **sulfonylureas**. Moderate Study
- Statins **(fluvastatin)** slightly increase the exposure to **glibenclamide**. Mild Study
- **Sulfonamides** are predicted to increase the exposure to **sulfonylureas**. Moderate Study
- **Teriflunomide** is predicted to increase the exposure to **glibenclamide**. Moderate Study
- **Venetoclax** is predicted to increase the exposure to **glibenclamide**. Moderate Theoretical

Sulindac → see NSAIDs

Sulpiride → see TABLE 8 p. 908 (hypotension), TABLE 9 p. 909 (QT-interval prolongation), TABLE 11 p. 909 (CNS depressant effects)

- **Antacids** decrease the absorption of **sulpiride**. Separate administration by 2 hours. Moderate Study
- **Sulpiride** is predicted to decrease the effects of **dopamine receptor agonists**. Avoid. Moderate Theoretical → Also see TABLE 8 p. 908 → Also see TABLE 9 p. 909
- **Sulpiride** is predicted to decrease the effects of **levodopa**. Avoid. Severe Theoretical → Also see TABLE 8 p. 908
- **Sulpiride** potentially increases the risk of neurotoxicity when given with **lithium**. Severe Anecdotal → Also see TABLE 9 p. 909
- **Sucralfate** decreases the absorption of **sulpiride**. Separate administration by 2 hours. Moderate Study

Sumatriptan → see TABLE 13 p. 910 (serotonin syndrome)

- **Sumatriptan** increases the risk of vasoconstriction when given with **ergotamine**. **Ergotamine** should be taken at least 24 hours before or 6 hours after **sumatriptan**. Severe Study
- **MAOIs, irreversible** are predicted to increase the exposure to **sumatriptan**. Avoid and for 14 days after stopping the MAOI. Severe Theoretical → Also see TABLE 13 p. 910
- **Moclobemide** moderately increases the exposure to **sumatriptan**. Avoid. Moderate Study → Also see TABLE 13 p. 910

Sunitinib → see TABLE 15 p. 910 (myelosuppression), TABLE 9 p. 909 (QT-interval prolongation)

- Antiarrhythmics **(dronedarone)** are predicted to increase the exposure to **sunitinib**. Moderate Theoretical → Also see TABLE 9 p. 909
- Antiepileptics **(carbamazepine, fosphenytoin, phenobarbital, phenytoin, primidone)** are predicted to decrease the exposure to **sunitinib**. Avoid or adjust **sunitinib** dose. Moderate Study
- Antifungals, azoles **(fluconazole, isavuconazole, posaconazole)** are predicted to increase the exposure to **sunitinib**. Moderate Theoretical → Also see TABLE 9 p. 909
- Antifungals, azoles **(itraconazole, ketoconazole, voriconazole)** are predicted to slightly increase the exposure to **sunitinib**. Avoid or adjust **sunitinib** dose. Moderate Study → Also see TABLE 9 p. 909
- **Apalutamide** is predicted to decrease the exposure to **sunitinib**. Avoid or adjust **sunitinib** dose. Moderate Study → Also see TABLE 9 p. 909
- **Aprepitant** is predicted to increase the exposure to **sunitinib**. Moderate Theoretical
- Calcium channel blockers **(diltiazem, verapamil)** are predicted to increase the exposure to **sunitinib**. Moderate Theoretical
- **Cobicistat** is predicted to slightly increase the exposure to **sunitinib**. Avoid or adjust **sunitinib** dose. Moderate Study
- **Sunitinib** is predicted to increase the risk of bleeding events when given with **coumarins**. Severe Theoretical
- **Crizotinib** is predicted to increase the exposure to **sunitinib**. Moderate Theoretical → Also see TABLE 15 p. 910 → Also see TABLE 9 p. 909
- **Elbasvir** is predicted to increase the concentration of **sunitinib**. Use with caution and adjust dose. Moderate Theoretical
- **Enzalutamide** is predicted to decrease the exposure to **sunitinib**. Avoid or adjust **sunitinib** dose. Moderate Study
- **Grapefruit juice** is predicted to increase the exposure to **sunitinib**. Avoid. Moderate Theoretical
- **Grazoprevir** is predicted to increase the concentration of **sunitinib**. Use with caution and adjust dose. Moderate Theoretical
- **HIV-protease inhibitors** are predicted to slightly increase the exposure to **sunitinib**. Avoid or adjust **sunitinib** dose. Moderate Study → Also see TABLE 9 p. 909
- **Idelalisib** is predicted to slightly increase the exposure to **sunitinib**. Avoid or adjust **sunitinib** dose. Moderate Study → Also see TABLE 15 p. 910
- **Imatinib** is predicted to increase the exposure to **sunitinib**. Moderate Theoretical → Also see TABLE 15 p. 910
- Macrolides **(clarithromycin)** are predicted to slightly increase the exposure to **sunitinib**. Avoid or adjust **sunitinib** dose. Moderate Study → Also see TABLE 9 p. 909
- Macrolides **(erythromycin)** are predicted to increase the exposure to **sunitinib**. Moderate Theoretical → Also see TABLE 9 p. 909
- **Mitotane** is predicted to decrease the exposure to **sunitinib**. Avoid or adjust **sunitinib** dose. Moderate Study → Also see TABLE 15 p. 910
- **Netupitant** is predicted to increase the exposure to **sunitinib**. Moderate Theoretical
- **Nilotinib** is predicted to increase the exposure to **sunitinib**. Moderate Theoretical → Also see TABLE 15 p. 910 → Also see TABLE 9 p. 909
- **Sunitinib** is predicted to increase the risk of bleeding events when given with **phenindione**. Severe Theoretical
- **Rifampicin** is predicted to decrease the exposure to **sunitinib**. Avoid or adjust **sunitinib** dose. Moderate Study

Suxamethonium → see TABLE 20 p. 911 (neuromuscular blocking effects)

- Alkylating agents **(cyclophosphamide)** increase the risk of prolonged neuromuscular blockade when given with **suxamethonium**. Moderate Study
- Antiarrhythmics **(lidocaine)** are predicted to increase the effects of **suxamethonium**. Moderate Study
- **Anticholinesterases, centrally acting** increase the effects of **suxamethonium**. Moderate Theoretical
- Antiepileptics **(carbamazepine)** increase the risk of prolonged neuromuscular blockade when given with **suxamethonium**. Moderate Study
- Antiepileptics **(fosphenytoin, phenytoin)** increase the effects of **suxamethonium**. Moderate Study
- **Clindamycin** increases the effects of **suxamethonium**. Severe Anecdotal
- **Corticosteroids** are predicted to decrease the effects of **suxamethonium**. Severe Anecdotal
- **Suxamethonium** is predicted to increase the risk of cardiovascular side-effects when given with **digoxin**. Severe Anecdotal

Suxamethonium (continued)
- **Irinotecan** is predicted to increase the risk of prolonged neuromuscular blockade when given with **suxamethonium.** [Moderate] Theoretical
- Intravenous **magnesium** is predicted to increase the effects of **suxamethonium.** [Moderate] Study
- **Metoclopramide** increases the effects of **suxamethonium.** [Moderate] Study
- Penicillins **(piperacillin)** increase the effects of **suxamethonium.** [Moderate] Study
- **SSRIs** potentially increase the risk of prolonged neuromuscular blockade when given with **suxamethonium.** [Unknown] Theoretical

Sympathomimetics, inotropic

dobutamine · dopamine

- **Sympathomimetics, inotropic** are predicted to decrease the effects of **apraclonidine**. Avoid. [Severe] Theoretical
- **Beta blockers, non-selective** increase the risk of hypertension and bradycardia when given with **dobutamine.** [Severe] Theoretical
- **Beta blockers, selective** increase the risk of hypertension and bradycardia when given with **dobutamine.** [Moderate] Theoretical
- **Entacapone** is predicted to increase the risk of cardiovascular side-effects when given with **sympathomimetics, inotropic.** [Moderate] Theoretical
- **Ergometrine** potentially increases the risk of peripheral vasoconstriction when given with **dopamine.** Avoid. [Severe] Anecdotal
- **Sympathomimetics, inotropic** are predicted to increase the risk of elevated blood pressure when given with **linezolid**. Avoid. [Severe] Theoretical
- **MAO-B inhibitors** are predicted to increase the risk of a hypertensive crisis when given with **sympathomimetics, inotropic**. Avoid. [Severe] Anecdotal
- **MAOIs, irreversible** are predicted to increase the risk of a hypertensive crisis when given with **sympathomimetics, inotropic**. Avoid and for 14 days after stopping the MAOI. [Severe] Theoretical
- **Opicapone** is predicted to increase the risk of cardiovascular side-effects when given with **sympathomimetics, inotropic.** [Severe] Theoretical
- **Tolcapone** is predicted to increase the risk of cardiovascular side-effects when given with **sympathomimetics, inotropic.** [Moderate] Theoretical

Sympathomimetics, vasoconstrictor

adrenaline/epinephrine · ephedrine · isometheptene · metaraminol · midodrine · noradrenaline/norepinephrine · phenylephrine · pseudoephedrine · xylometazoline

ROUTE-SPECIFIC INFORMATION Since systemic absorption can follow topical application, the possibility of interactions should be borne in mind.

- **Ephedrine** increases the risk of side-effects when given with **aminophylline**. Avoid in children. [Moderate] Study
- **Sympathomimetics, vasoconstrictor** are predicted to decrease the effects of **apraclonidine**. Avoid. [Severe] Theoretical
- **Atropine** increases the risk of severe hypertension when given with **phenylephrine.** [Severe] Study
- **Beta blockers, non-selective** are predicted to increase the risk of hypertension and bradycardia when given with sympathomimetics, vasoconstrictor **(adrenaline/epinephrine, noradrenaline/norepinephrine).** [Severe] Study
- **Beta blockers, selective** are predicted to increase the risk of hypertension and bradycardia when given with sympathomimetics, vasoconstrictor **(adrenaline/epinephrine, noradrenaline/norepinephrine).** [Severe] Study
- **Isometheptene** potentially increases the risk of side-effects when given with dopamine receptor agonists **(bromocriptine)**. Avoid. [Severe] Anecdotal
- **Entacapone** is predicted to increase the risk of cardiovascular side-effects when given with sympathomimetics, vasoconstrictor **(adrenaline/epinephrine, noradrenaline/norepinephrine).** [Moderate] Study
- **Ergometrine** is predicted to increase the risk of peripheral vasoconstriction when given with **noradrenaline/norepinephrine.** [Severe] Anecdotal
- **Pseudoephedrine** increases the risk of elevated blood pressure when given with **linezolid**. Avoid. [Severe] Study
- Sympathomimetics, vasoconstrictor **(adrenaline/epinephrine, ephedrine, isometheptene, noradrenaline/norepinephrine, phenylephrine)** are predicted to increase the risk of elevated blood pressure when given with **linezolid**. Avoid. [Severe] Theoretical
- **MAO-B inhibitors** are predicted to increase the risk of a hypertensive crisis when given with **sympathomimetics, vasoconstrictor**. Avoid. [Severe] Anecdotal
- **MAOIs, irreversible** are predicted to increase the risk of a hypertensive crisis when given with **sympathomimetics, vasoconstrictor**. Avoid and for 14 days after stopping the MAOI. [Severe] Study
- **Mianserin** decreases the effects of **ephedrine.** [Severe] Anecdotal
- **Moclobemide** is predicted to increase the risk of a hypertensive crisis when given with sympathomimetics, vasoconstrictor **(ephedrine, isometheptene, phenylephrine, pseudoephedrine).** Avoid. [Severe] Study
- **Opicapone** is predicted to increase the risk of cardiovascular side-effects when given with sympathomimetics, vasoconstrictor **(adrenaline/epinephrine, noradrenaline/norepinephrine).** [Severe] Theoretical
- **Ephedrine** increases the risk of side-effects when given with **theophylline**. Avoid in children. [Moderate] Study
- **Tolcapone** is predicted to increase the effects of sympathomimetics, vasoconstrictor **(adrenaline/epinephrine, noradrenaline/norepinephrine).** [Moderate] Theoretical
- **Tricyclic antidepressants** are predicted to decrease the effects of **ephedrine**. Avoid. [Severe] Study
- **Tricyclic antidepressants** increase the effects of sympathomimetics, vasoconstrictor **(adrenaline/epinephrine, noradrenaline/norepinephrine, phenylephrine)**. Avoid. [Severe] Study

Tacalcitol → see vitamin D substances

Tacrolimus → see TABLE 2 p. 907 (nephrotoxicity), TABLE 16 p. 911 (increased serum potassium)

- Pomelo and pomegranate juices might greatly increase the concentration of tacrolimus.
- Since systemic absorption can follow topical application, the possibility of interactions should be borne in mind.

- **Alcohol (beverage)** increases the risk of facial flushing and skin irritation when given with topical **tacrolimus.** [Moderate] Study
- Antiarrhythmics **(amiodarone)** are predicted to increase the concentration of **tacrolimus.** [Severe] Anecdotal
- Antiarrhythmics **(dronedarone)** are predicted to increase the concentration of **tacrolimus.** [Severe] Study
- Antiepileptics **(carbamazepine, fosphenytoin, phenobarbital, phenytoin, primidone)** decrease the concentration of **tacrolimus**. Monitor and adjust dose. [Severe] Study
- Antifungals, azoles **(fluconazole, isavuconazole, posaconazole)** are predicted to increase the concentration of **tacrolimus.** [Severe] Study
- Antifungals, azoles **(itraconazole, ketoconazole, voriconazole)** are predicted to increase the concentration of **tacrolimus**. Monitor and adjust dose. [Severe] Study
- Antifungals, azoles **(miconazole)** are predicted to increase the concentration of **tacrolimus**. Monitor and adjust dose. [Severe] Theoretical
- **Apalutamide** decreases the concentration of **tacrolimus.** Monitor and adjust dose. [Severe] Study
- **Aprepitant** is predicted to increase the concentration of **tacrolimus.** [Severe] Study
- **Bosentan** is predicted to decrease the concentration of **tacrolimus** and **tacrolimus** potentially increases the concentration of **bosentan**. Avoid. [Severe] Theoretical
- **Brigatinib** potentially decreases the concentration of **tacrolimus**. Avoid. [Moderate] Theoretical
- Calcium channel blockers **(diltiazem, verapamil)** are predicted to increase the concentration of **tacrolimus.** [Severe] Study

- Calcium channel blockers **(nicardipine)** potentially increase the concentration of **tacrolimus**. Monitor concentration and adjust dose. [Severe] Anecdotal
- **Ceritinib** is predicted to increase the exposure to **tacrolimus**. Avoid. [Severe] Theoretical
- **Chloramphenicol** increases the concentration of **tacrolimus**. [Severe] Study
- **Ciclosporin** increases the concentration of **tacrolimus**. Avoid. [Severe] Study → Also see TABLE 2 p. 907 → Also see TABLE 16 p. 911
- **Cobicistat** is predicted to increase the concentration of **tacrolimus**. Monitor and adjust dose. [Severe] Study
- **Crizotinib** is predicted to increase the concentration of **tacrolimus**. [Severe] Study
- **Tacrolimus** is predicted to increase the exposure to **dabigatran**. Avoid. [Severe] Theoretical
- **Danazol** potentially increases the concentration of **tacrolimus**. [Severe] Anecdotal
- **Doravirine** is predicted to decrease the exposure to **tacrolimus**. Monitor **tacrolimus** concentration and adjust dose, p. 562. [Moderate] Theoretical
- **Efavirenz** is predicted to decrease the concentration of **tacrolimus**. Monitor and adjust dose. [Moderate] Theoretical
- **Enzalutamide** decreases the concentration of **tacrolimus**. Monitor and adjust dose. [Severe] Study
- **Glecaprevir** (with pibrentasvir) slightly increases the exposure to **tacrolimus**. Monitor and adjust dose. [Mild] Study
- **Grapefruit juice** greatly increases the concentration of **tacrolimus**. Avoid. [Severe] Study
- **Grazoprevir** increases the exposure to **tacrolimus**. [Moderate] Study
- **HIV-protease inhibitors** are predicted to increase the concentration of **tacrolimus**. Monitor and adjust dose. [Severe] Study
- **Idelalisib** is predicted to increase the concentration of **tacrolimus**. Monitor and adjust dose. [Severe] Study
- **Imatinib** is predicted to increase the concentration of **tacrolimus**. [Severe] Study
- **Larotrectinib** is predicted to increase the exposure to **tacrolimus**. Use with caution and adjust dose. [Mild] Theoretical
- **Letermovir** moderately increases the exposure to **tacrolimus**. Monitor and adjust dose. [Severe] Study
- **Live vaccines** are predicted to increase the risk of generalised infection (possibly life-threatening) when given with **tacrolimus**. Public Health England advises avoid (refer to Green Book). [Severe] Theoretical
- **Tacrolimus** is predicted to increase the exposure to **lomitapide**. Separate administration by 12 hours. [Moderate] Theoretical
- **Lorlatinib** is predicted to decrease the exposure to **tacrolimus**. Avoid. [Moderate] Theoretical
- **Lumacaftor** is predicted to decrease the exposure to **tacrolimus**. Avoid. [Severe] Theoretical
- Macrolides **(clarithromycin)** are predicted to increase the concentration of **tacrolimus**. Monitor and adjust dose. [Severe] Study
- Macrolides **(erythromycin)** are predicted to increase the concentration of **tacrolimus**. [Severe] Study
- **Tacrolimus** is predicted to affect the efficacy of **mifamurtide**. Avoid. [Severe] Theoretical
- **Mitotane** decreases the concentration of **tacrolimus**. Monitor and adjust dose. [Severe] Study
- Monoclonal antibodies **(sarilumab)** potentially affect the exposure to **tacrolimus**. Monitor and adjust dose. [Moderate] Theoretical
- **Netupitant** is predicted to increase the concentration of **tacrolimus**. [Severe] Study
- **Nevirapine** is predicted to decrease the concentration of **tacrolimus**. Monitor and adjust dose. [Moderate] Theoretical
- **Nilotinib** is predicted to increase the concentration of **tacrolimus**. [Severe] Study
- **Palbociclib** is predicted to increase the exposure to **tacrolimus**. Adjust dose. [Moderate] Theoretical
- **Pibrentasvir** (with glecaprevir) slightly increases the exposure to **tacrolimus**. Monitor and adjust dose. [Mild] Study
- **Pitolisant** is predicted to decrease the exposure to **tacrolimus**. Avoid. [Severe] Theoretical
- **Ranolazine** increases the concentration of **tacrolimus**. Adjust dose. [Severe] Anecdotal
- **Ribociclib** is predicted to increase the exposure to **tacrolimus**. Use with caution and adjust dose. [Moderate] Theoretical
- **Rifampicin** decreases the concentration of **tacrolimus**. Monitor and adjust dose. [Severe] Study
- **Rucaparib** is predicted to increase the exposure to **tacrolimus**. Monitor and adjust dose. [Moderate] Study
- **Sirolimus** is predicted to decrease the concentration of **tacrolimus** and **tacrolimus** increases the exposure to **sirolimus**. [Severe] Study
- **St John's Wort** decreases the concentration of **tacrolimus**. Avoid. [Severe] Study
- **Tacrolimus** increases the exposure to **tofacitinib**. Avoid. [Severe] Study
- **Tacrolimus** potentially increases the risk of serotonin syndrome when given with **venlafaxine**. [Severe] Anecdotal

Tadalafil → see phosphodiesterase type-5 inhibitors

Talazoparib

- Antiarrhythmics **(amiodarone, dronedarone)** are predicted to slightly increase the exposure to **talazoparib**. Avoid or adjust **talazoparib** dose. [Severe] Study
- Antifungals, azoles **(itraconazole, ketoconazole)** are predicted to slightly increase the exposure to **talazoparib**. Avoid or adjust **talazoparib** dose. [Severe] Study
- Calcium channel blockers **(verapamil)** are predicted to slightly increase the exposure to **talazoparib**. Avoid or adjust **talazoparib** dose. [Severe] Study
- **Ciclosporin** is predicted to slightly increase the exposure to **talazoparib**. Avoid or adjust **talazoparib** dose. [Severe] Study
- **Eltrombopag** potentially increases the exposure to **talazoparib**. Avoid or monitor. [Moderate] Theoretical
- HIV-protease inhibitors **(lopinavir, ritonavir, saquinavir)** are predicted to slightly increase the exposure to **talazoparib**. Avoid or adjust **talazoparib** dose. [Severe] Study
- **Lapatinib** is predicted to slightly increase the exposure to **talazoparib**. Avoid or adjust **talazoparib** dose. [Severe] Study
- **Leflunomide** potentially increases the exposure to **talazoparib**. Avoid or monitor. [Moderate] Theoretical
- **Macrolides** are predicted to slightly increase the exposure to **talazoparib**. Avoid or adjust **talazoparib** dose. [Severe] Study
- **Ranolazine** is predicted to slightly increase the exposure to **talazoparib**. Avoid or adjust **talazoparib** dose. [Severe] Study
- **Teriflunomide** potentially increases the exposure to **talazoparib**. Avoid or monitor. [Moderate] Theoretical
- **Vemurafenib** is predicted to slightly increase the exposure to **talazoparib**. Avoid or adjust **talazoparib** dose. [Severe] Study

Tamoxifen → see TABLE 5 p. 907 (thromboembolism)

- **Bupropion** is predicted to decrease the efficacy of **tamoxifen**. Avoid. [Severe] Study
- **Cinacalcet** is predicted to decrease the efficacy of **tamoxifen**. Avoid. [Severe] Study
- **Tamoxifen** increases the anticoagulant effect of **coumarins**. [Severe] Study
- **Rifampicin** markedly decreases the exposure to **tamoxifen**. [Unknown] Study
- **Rolapitant** is predicted to increase the exposure to **tamoxifen**. [Severe] Study
- SSRIs **(fluoxetine, paroxetine)** are predicted to decrease the efficacy of **tamoxifen**. Avoid. [Severe] Study
- **Terbinafine** is predicted to decrease the efficacy of **tamoxifen**. Avoid. [Severe] Study

Tamsulosin → see alpha blockers

Tapentadol → see opioids

Taxanes → see TABLE 15 p. 910 (myelosuppression), TABLE 12 p. 910 (peripheral neuropathy)

cabazitaxel · docetaxel · paclitaxel

- Antiarrhythmics **(dronedarone)** are predicted to increase the exposure to **cabazitaxel**. [Moderate] Theoretical
- Antiarrhythmics **(dronedarone)** are predicted to increase the exposure to **paclitaxel**. [Severe] Theoretical
- Antiepileptics **(carbamazepine, fosphenytoin, phenobarbital, phenytoin, primidone)** are predicted to decrease the exposure to **docetaxel**. [Severe] Theoretical → Also see TABLE 12 p. 910

Taxanes (continued)

- Antiepileptics **(carbamazepine, fosphenytoin, phenobarbital, phenytoin, primidone)** are predicted to decrease the exposure to taxanes **(cabazitaxel, paclitaxel)**. Avoid. Severe Study → Also see **TABLE 12** p. 910
- Antifungals, azoles **(fluconazole, isavuconazole, posaconazole)** are predicted to increase the exposure to **cabazitaxel.** Moderate Theoretical
- Antifungals, azoles **(itraconazole, ketoconazole, voriconazole)** are predicted to increase the exposure to **cabazitaxel.** Avoid. Severe Study
- Antifungals, azoles **(itraconazole, ketoconazole, voriconazole)** are predicted to moderately increase the exposure to **docetaxel.** Avoid or adjust dose. Severe Study
- Antifungals, azoles **(itraconazole, ketoconazole, voriconazole)** are predicted to increase the exposure to **paclitaxel.** Severe Theoretical
- Antifungals, azoles **(miconazole)** are predicted to increase the concentration of **docetaxel**. Use with caution and adjust dose. Moderate Theoretical
- **Apalutamide** is predicted to decrease the exposure to **docetaxel.** Severe Theoretical
- **Apalutamide** is predicted to decrease the exposure to taxanes **(cabazitaxel, paclitaxel)**. Avoid. Severe Study
- **Aprepitant** is predicted to increase the exposure to **cabazitaxel.** Moderate Theoretical
- **Bosentan** is predicted to decrease the exposure to **cabazitaxel.** Avoid. Severe Study
- Calcium channel blockers **(diltiazem, verapamil)** are predicted to increase the exposure to **cabazitaxel.** Moderate Theoretical
- **Ceritinib** is predicted to increase the exposure to **paclitaxel.** Moderate Theoretical → Also see **TABLE 15** p. 910
- **Clopidogrel** is predicted to increase the concentration of **paclitaxel.** Severe Anecdotal
- **Cobicistat** is predicted to increase the exposure to **cabazitaxel.** Avoid. Severe Study
- **Cobicistat** is predicted to moderately increase the exposure to **docetaxel.** Avoid or adjust dose. Severe Study
- **Cobicistat** is predicted to increase the exposure to **paclitaxel.** Severe Theoretical
- **Crizotinib** is predicted to increase the exposure to **cabazitaxel.** Moderate Theoretical → Also see **TABLE 15** p. 910
- **Efavirenz** is predicted to decrease the exposure to **cabazitaxel.** Avoid. Severe Study
- **Eliglustat** is predicted to increase the exposure to **paclitaxel.** Adjust dose. Moderate Study
- **Enzalutamide** is predicted to decrease the exposure to **docetaxel.** Severe Theoretical
- **Enzalutamide** is predicted to decrease the exposure to taxanes **(cabazitaxel, paclitaxel)**. Avoid. Severe Study
- Fibrates **(gemfibrozil)** are predicted to increase the concentration of **paclitaxel.** Severe Anecdotal
- **HIV-protease inhibitors** are predicted to increase the exposure to **cabazitaxel.** Avoid. Severe Study
- **HIV-protease inhibitors** are predicted to moderately increase the exposure to **docetaxel**. Avoid or adjust dose. Severe Study
- **HIV-protease inhibitors** are predicted to increase the exposure to **paclitaxel.** Severe Theoretical
- **Idelalisib** is predicted to increase the exposure to **cabazitaxel.** Avoid. Severe Study → Also see **TABLE 15** p. 910
- **Idelalisib** is predicted to moderately increase the exposure to **docetaxel**. Avoid or adjust dose. Severe Study → Also see **TABLE 15** p. 910
- **Idelalisib** is predicted to increase the exposure to **paclitaxel.** Severe Theoretical → Also see **TABLE 15** p. 910
- **Imatinib** is predicted to increase the exposure to **cabazitaxel.** Moderate Theoretical → Also see **TABLE 15** p. 910
- Iron chelators **(deferasirox)** are predicted to increase the concentration of **paclitaxel.** Severe Anecdotal
- **Lapatinib** slightly increases the exposure to **paclitaxel.** Severe Study
- **Leflunomide** is predicted to increase the concentration of **paclitaxel.** Severe Anecdotal → Also see **TABLE 15** p. 910
- **Live vaccines** are predicted to increase the risk of generalised infection (possibly life-threatening) when given with taxanes **(docetaxel, paclitaxel)**. Public Health England advises avoid (refer to Green Book). Severe Theoretical
- Macrolides **(clarithromycin)** are predicted to increase the exposure to **cabazitaxel**. Avoid. Severe Study
- Macrolides **(clarithromycin)** are predicted to moderately increase the exposure to **docetaxel**. Avoid or adjust dose. Severe Study
- Macrolides **(clarithromycin)** are predicted to increase the exposure to **paclitaxel.** Severe Theoretical
- Macrolides **(erythromycin)** are predicted to increase the exposure to **cabazitaxel.** Moderate Theoretical
- **Mirabegron** is predicted to increase the exposure to **paclitaxel.** Mild Theoretical
- **Mitotane** is predicted to decrease the exposure to **docetaxel.** Severe Theoretical → Also see **TABLE 15** p. 910
- **Mitotane** is predicted to decrease the exposure to taxanes **(cabazitaxel, paclitaxel)**. Avoid. Severe Study → Also see **TABLE 15** p. 910
- **Netupitant** is predicted to increase the exposure to **cabazitaxel.** Moderate Theoretical
- **Netupitant** slightly increases the exposure to **docetaxel.** Moderate Study
- **Netupitant** is predicted to increase the exposure to **paclitaxel.** Moderate Study
- **Nevirapine** is predicted to decrease the exposure to **cabazitaxel.** Avoid. Severe Study
- **Nilotinib** is predicted to increase the exposure to **cabazitaxel.** Moderate Theoretical → Also see **TABLE 15** p. 910
- **Paritaprevir** (with ritonavir and ombitasvir) is predicted to increase the exposure to **paclitaxel.** Moderate Study
- **Pibrentasvir** (with glecaprevir) is predicted to increase the exposure to **paclitaxel.** Moderate Study
- **Pitolisant** is predicted to decrease the exposure to **docetaxel.** Avoid. Severe Theoretical
- **Pitolisant** is predicted to decrease the exposure to **paclitaxel.** Mild Theoretical
- **Rifampicin** is predicted to decrease the exposure to **docetaxel.** Severe Theoretical
- **Rifampicin** is predicted to decrease the exposure to taxanes **(cabazitaxel, paclitaxel)**. Avoid. Severe Study
- **St John's Wort** is predicted to decrease the exposure to **cabazitaxel.** Avoid. Severe Study
- **Teriflunomide** is predicted to increase the concentration of **paclitaxel.** Severe Anecdotal
- **Velpatasvir** is predicted to increase the exposure to **paclitaxel.** Severe Theoretical

Tazarotene → see retinoids

Tedizolid

- **Tedizolid** is predicted to increase the exposure to **imatinib.** Avoid. Moderate Theoretical
- **Tedizolid** is predicted to increase the exposure to **lapatinib.** Avoid. Moderate Theoretical
- **Tedizolid** is predicted to increase the exposure to **methotrexate.** Avoid. Moderate Theoretical
- **Tedizolid** is predicted to increase the exposure to statins **(atorvastatin, fluvastatin, rosuvastatin)**. Avoid. Moderate Study
- **Tedizolid** is predicted to increase the exposure to **sulfasalazine.** Avoid. Moderate Study
- **Tedizolid** is predicted to increase the exposure to **topotecan.** Avoid. Moderate Study

Tegafur

- **Tegafur** potentially increases the concentration of antiepileptics **(fosphenytoin, phenytoin)**. Monitor concentration and adjust dose. Severe Anecdotal
- **Tegafur** increases the anticoagulant effect of **coumarins.** Moderate Theoretical
- **Folates** are predicted to increase the risk of toxicity when given with **tegafur.** Severe Theoretical
- H_2 receptor antagonists **(cimetidine)** are predicted to increase the risk of toxicity when given with **tegafur.** Severe Theoretical
- **Live vaccines** are predicted to increase the risk of generalised infection (possibly life-threatening) when given with **tegafur.** Public Health England advises avoid (refer to Green Book). Severe Theoretical

- Methotrexate is predicted to increase the risk of toxicity when given with **tegafur**. [Severe] Theoretical

Teicoplanin

GENERAL INFORMATION If other nephrotoxic or neurotoxic drugs are given, monitor renal and auditory function on prolonged administration.

Telavancin → see TABLE 2 p. 907 (nephrotoxicity), TABLE 19 p. 911 (ototoxicity), TABLE 9 p. 909 (QT-interval prolongation)

Telbivudine

- Interferons **(interferon alfa)** are predicted to increase the risk of peripheral neuropathy when given with **telbivudine**. Avoid. [Severe] Theoretical
- Interferons **(peginterferon alfa)** increase the risk of peripheral neuropathy when given with **telbivudine**. Avoid. [Severe] Study

Telmisartan → see angiotensin-II receptor antagonists

Telotristat ethyl

- **Telotristat ethyl** is predicted to decrease the exposure to doravirine. Avoid or adjust doravirine or lamivudine with tenofovir disoproxil and doravirine dose. [Severe] Theoretical
- **Telotristat ethyl** decreases the exposure to **midazolam**. [Moderate] Study
- Octreotide (short-acting) decreases the exposure to **telotristat ethyl**. **Telotristat ethyl** should be taken at least 30 minutes before **octreotide**, p. 504. [Moderate] Study

Temazepam → see TABLE 11 p. 909 (CNS depressant effects)

Temocillin → see penicillins

Temozolomide → see alkylating agents

Temsirolimus → see TABLE 15 p. 910 (myelosuppression)

- ACE inhibitors are predicted to increase the risk of angioedema when given with **temsirolimus**. [Moderate] Theoretical
- Antiarrhythmics **(dronedarone)** are predicted to increase the concentration of **temsirolimus**. Use with caution or avoid. [Moderate] Theoretical
- Antiepileptics **(carbamazepine, fosphenytoin, phenobarbital, phenytoin, primidone)** are predicted to decrease the concentration of **temsirolimus**. Avoid. [Severe] Study
- Antifungals, azoles **(fluconazole, isavuconazole, posaconazole)** are predicted to increase the concentration of **temsirolimus**. Use with caution or avoid. [Moderate] Theoretical
- Antifungals, azoles **(itraconazole, ketoconazole, voriconazole)** are predicted to increase the concentration of **temsirolimus**. Avoid. [Severe] Theoretical
- Apalutamide is predicted to decrease the concentration of **temsirolimus**. Avoid. [Severe] Study
- Aprepitant is predicted to increase the concentration of **temsirolimus**. Use with caution or avoid. [Moderate] Theoretical
- Bosentan is predicted to decrease the concentration of **temsirolimus**. Avoid. [Severe] Theoretical
- Calcium channel blockers **(diltiazem, verapamil)** are predicted to increase the concentration of and the risk of angioedema when given with **temsirolimus**. Use with caution or avoid. [Moderate] Theoretical
- **Temsirolimus** is predicted to increase the risk of angioedema when given with calcium channel blockers **(amlodipine, felodipine, lacidipine, lercanidipine, nicardipine, nifedipine, nimodipine)**. [Moderate] Theoretical
- Cobicistat is predicted to increase the concentration of **temsirolimus**. Avoid. [Severe] Theoretical
- Crizotinib is predicted to increase the concentration of **temsirolimus**. Use with caution or avoid. [Moderate] Theoretical → Also see TABLE 15 p. 910
- Efavirenz is predicted to decrease the concentration of **temsirolimus**. Avoid. [Severe] Theoretical
- Enzalutamide is predicted to decrease the concentration of **temsirolimus**. Avoid. [Severe] Study
- Grapefruit juice is predicted to increase the concentration of **temsirolimus**. Use with caution or avoid. [Moderate] Theoretical
- HIV-protease inhibitors are predicted to increase the concentration of **temsirolimus**. Avoid. [Severe] Theoretical
- Idelalisib is predicted to increase the concentration of **temsirolimus**. Avoid. [Severe] Theoretical → Also see TABLE 15 p. 910
- Imatinib is predicted to increase the concentration of **temsirolimus**. Use with caution or avoid. [Moderate] Theoretical → Also see TABLE 15 p. 910
- Live vaccines are predicted to increase the risk of generalised infection (possibly life-threatening) when given with **temsirolimus**. Public Health England advises avoid (refer to Green Book). [Severe] Theoretical
- Lumacaftor is predicted to decrease the exposure to **temsirolimus**. Avoid. [Severe] Theoretical
- Macrolides **(clarithromycin)** are predicted to increase the concentration of **temsirolimus**. Avoid. [Severe] Theoretical
- Macrolides **(erythromycin)** are predicted to increase the concentration of **temsirolimus**. Use with caution or avoid. [Moderate] Theoretical
- Mitotane is predicted to decrease the concentration of **temsirolimus**. Avoid. [Severe] Study → Also see TABLE 15 p. 910
- Netupitant is predicted to increase the concentration of **temsirolimus**. Use with caution or avoid. [Moderate] Theoretical
- Nevirapine is predicted to decrease the concentration of **temsirolimus**. Avoid. [Severe] Theoretical
- Nilotinib is predicted to increase the concentration of **temsirolimus**. Use with caution or avoid. [Moderate] Theoretical → Also see TABLE 15 p. 910
- Pitolisant is predicted to decrease the exposure to **temsirolimus**. Avoid. [Severe] Theoretical
- Rifampicin is predicted to decrease the concentration of **temsirolimus**. Avoid. [Severe] Study
- St John's Wort is predicted to decrease the concentration of **temsirolimus**. Avoid. [Severe] Theoretical

Tenecteplase → see TABLE 3 p. 907 (anticoagulant effects)

Tenofovir alafenamide

- Antiepileptics **(carbamazepine, fosphenytoin, oxcarbazepine, phenobarbital, phenytoin, primidone)** are predicted to decrease the exposure to **tenofovir alafenamide**. Avoid. [Moderate] Theoretical
- Ciclosporin is predicted to increase the exposure to **tenofovir alafenamide**. [Moderate] Theoretical
- Eltrombopag is predicted to increase the exposure to **tenofovir alafenamide**. [Moderate] Theoretical
- HIV-protease inhibitors **(atazanavir, darunavir, lopinavir)** increase the exposure to **tenofovir alafenamide**. Avoid or adjust dose. [Moderate] Study
- HIV-protease inhibitors **(tipranavir)** are predicted to decrease the exposure to **tenofovir alafenamide**. Avoid. [Moderate] Theoretical
- Leflunomide is predicted to increase the exposure to **tenofovir alafenamide**. [Moderate] Theoretical
- Rifabutin is predicted to decrease the exposure to **tenofovir alafenamide**. Avoid. [Moderate] Theoretical
- Rifampicin is predicted to decrease the exposure to **tenofovir alafenamide**. Avoid. [Moderate] Theoretical
- St John's Wort is predicted to decrease the exposure to **tenofovir alafenamide**. Avoid. [Moderate] Theoretical
- Teriflunomide is predicted to increase the exposure to **tenofovir alafenamide**. [Moderate] Theoretical

Tenofovir disoproxil → see TABLE 2 p. 907 (nephrotoxicity)

- Ciclosporin is predicted to increase the exposure to **tenofovir disoproxil**. [Moderate] Theoretical → Also see TABLE 2 p. 907
- Eltrombopag is predicted to increase the exposure to **tenofovir disoproxil**. [Moderate] Theoretical
- HIV-protease inhibitors **(atazanavir, darunavir, lopinavir)** are predicted to increase the risk of renal impairment when given with **tenofovir disoproxil**. [Severe] Anecdotal
- Ledipasvir (with sofosbuvir) slightly increases the exposure to **tenofovir disoproxil**. [Moderate] Study
- Leflunomide is predicted to increase the exposure to **tenofovir disoproxil**. [Moderate] Theoretical
- Teriflunomide is predicted to increase the exposure to **tenofovir disoproxil**. [Moderate] Theoretical
- Velpatasvir is predicted to increase the exposure to **tenofovir disoproxil**. [Severe] Study
- Voxilaprevir (with sofosbuvir and velpatasvir) potentially increases the concentration of **tenofovir disoproxil**. [Severe] Study

Tenoxicam → see NSAIDs

Terazosin → see alpha blockers

Terbinafine

ROUTE-SPECIFIC INFORMATION Since systemic absorption can follow topical application, the possibility of interactions should be borne in mind.

- **Terbinafine** is predicted to increase the exposure to anticholinesterases, centrally acting **(galantamine)**. Monitor and adjust dose. Moderate Study
- **Terbinafine** is predicted to moderately increase the exposure to aripiprazole. Adjust **aripiprazole** dose, p. 265. Moderate Study
- **Terbinafine** is predicted to markedly increase the exposure to atomoxetine. Adjust dose. Severe Study
- **Terbinafine** is predicted to increase the exposure to beta blockers, selective **(metoprolol, nebivolol)**. Moderate Study
- **Terbinafine** is predicted to slightly increase the exposure to darifenacin. Mild Study
- **Terbinafine** is predicted to increase the exposure to **eliglustat**. Avoid or adjust dose—consult product literature. Severe Study
- **Terbinafine** is predicted to increase the exposure to **mexiletine**. Moderate Study
- **Terbinafine** is predicted to decrease the efficacy of opioids **(codeine)**. Moderate Theoretical
- **Terbinafine** is predicted to decrease the efficacy of opioids **(tramadol)**. Severe Study
- **Terbinafine** is predicted to moderately increase the exposure to pitolisant. Use with caution and adjust dose. Moderate Study
- Rifampicin decreases the exposure to **terbinafine**. Adjust dose. Moderate Study
- **Terbinafine** is predicted to increase the exposure to risperidone. Adjust dose. Moderate Study
- **Terbinafine** is predicted to increase the exposure to SSRIs **(citalopram, dapoxetine, escitalopram, fluvoxamine, sertraline)**. Moderate Theoretical
- **Terbinafine** is predicted to increase the exposure to SSRIs **(fluoxetine)**. Adjust dose. Moderate Theoretical
- **Terbinafine** moderately increases the exposure to SSRIs **(paroxetine)**. Moderate Study
- **Terbinafine** is predicted to decrease the efficacy of tamoxifen. Avoid. Severe Study
- **Terbinafine** is predicted to increase the exposure to the active metabolite of tetrabenazine. Moderate Study
- **Terbinafine** is predicted to increase the exposure to tricyclic antidepressants. Monitor for toxicity and adjust dose. Severe Study
- **Terbinafine** is predicted to increase the exposure to vortioxetine. Monitor and adjust dose. Moderate Study

Terbutaline → see beta$_2$ agonists

Teriflunomide → see **TABLE 1** p. 907 (hepatotoxicity)

- **Teriflunomide** is predicted to increase the exposure to adefovir. Moderate Study
- **Teriflunomide** is predicted to decrease the exposure to agomelatine. Moderate Theoretical
- **Teriflunomide** decreases the exposure to aminophylline. Adjust dose. Moderate Study
- **Teriflunomide** is predicted to decrease the exposure to anaesthetics, local **(ropivacaine)**. Moderate Theoretical
- **Teriflunomide** is predicted to increase the exposure to anthracyclines **(daunorubicin, doxorubicin, mitoxantrone)**. Moderate Theoretical
- **Teriflunomide** is predicted to increase the exposure to antihistamines, non-sedating **(fexofenadine)**. Moderate Study
- **Teriflunomide** potentially increases the exposure to baricitinib. Moderate Theoretical
- **Teriflunomide** is predicted to increase the exposure to bosentan. Moderate Study
- **Teriflunomide** is predicted to moderately increase the clearance of caffeine citrate. Monitor and adjust dose. Moderate Study
- **Teriflunomide** is predicted to increase the exposure to cephalosporins **(cefaclor)**. Moderate Study
- **Teriflunomide** is predicted to decrease the exposure to clozapine. Moderate Theoretical
- **Teriflunomide** affects the anticoagulant effect of coumarins. Severe Study
- **Teriflunomide** is predicted to decrease the exposure to duloxetine. Moderate Theoretical
- **Teriflunomide** is predicted to increase the exposure to ganciclovir. Moderate Study
- **Teriflunomide** is predicted to increase the exposure to H$_2$ receptor antagonists **(cimetidine, famotidine)**. Moderate Study
- **Teriflunomide** is predicted to increase the exposure to larotrectinib. Mild Study
- **Teriflunomide** is predicted to increase the concentration of letermovir. Moderate Study
- Live vaccines are predicted to increase the risk of generalised infection (possibly life-threatening) when given with **teriflunomide**. Public Health England advises avoid (refer to Green Book). Severe Theoretical
- **Teriflunomide** is predicted to increase the exposure to loop diuretics **(furosemide)**. Moderate Study
- **Teriflunomide** is predicted to decrease the exposure to melatonin. Moderate Theoretical
- **Teriflunomide** is predicted to increase the exposure to methotrexate. Moderate Study → Also see **TABLE 1** p. 907
- **Teriflunomide** is predicted to increase the clearance of mexiletine. Monitor and adjust dose. Moderate Study
- **Teriflunomide** is predicted to increase the exposure to montelukast. Moderate Theoretical
- **Teriflunomide** is predicted to increase the exposure to nateglinide. Moderate Theoretical
- **Teriflunomide** is predicted to increase the exposure to NSAIDs **(indometacin, ketoprofen)**. Moderate Theoretical
- **Teriflunomide** is predicted to decrease the exposure to olanzapine. Monitor and adjust dose. Moderate Study
- **Teriflunomide** is predicted to increase the exposure to oseltamivir. Moderate Study
- **Teriflunomide** is predicted to increase the exposure to penicillins **(benzylpenicillin)**. Moderate Study
- **Teriflunomide** is predicted to increase the exposure to pioglitazone. Moderate Study
- **Teriflunomide** is predicted to decrease the exposure to pirfenidone. Moderate Theoretical
- **Teriflunomide** is predicted to increase the exposure to quinolones **(ciprofloxacin)**. Moderate Theoretical
- **Teriflunomide** is predicted to increase the exposure to repaglinide. Moderate Study
- **Teriflunomide** is predicted to increase the exposure to rifampicin. Moderate Theoretical
- **Teriflunomide** is predicted to increase the exposure to selexipag. Adjust **selexipag** dose. Moderate Study
- **Teriflunomide** is predicted to increase the exposure to statins **(atorvastatin, fluvastatin, pravastatin, simvastatin)**. Moderate Study → Also see **TABLE 1** p. 907
- **Teriflunomide** moderately increases the exposure to statins **(rosuvastatin)**. Adjust **rosuvastatin** dose, p. 140. Moderate Study → Also see **TABLE 1** p. 907
- **Teriflunomide** is predicted to increase the exposure to sulfasalazine. Moderate Study → Also see **TABLE 1** p. 907
- **Teriflunomide** is predicted to increase the exposure to sulfonylureas **(glibenclamide)**. Moderate Study
- **Teriflunomide** potentially increases the exposure to talazoparib. Avoid or monitor. Moderate Theoretical
- **Teriflunomide** is predicted to increase the concentration of taxanes **(paclitaxel)**. Severe Anecdotal
- **Teriflunomide** is predicted to increase the exposure to tenofovir alafenamide. Moderate Theoretical
- **Teriflunomide** is predicted to increase the exposure to tenofovir disoproxil. Moderate Theoretical
- **Teriflunomide** is predicted to decrease the exposure to theophylline. Adjust dose. Moderate Study
- **Teriflunomide** moderately decreases the exposure to tizanidine. Mild Study
- **Teriflunomide** is predicted to increase the exposure to topotecan. Moderate Study
- **Teriflunomide** is predicted to increase the exposure to zidovudine. Moderate Theoretical

Tetanus immunoglobulin → see immunoglobulins

Tetrabenazine → see **TABLE 9** p. 909 (QT-interval prolongation), **TABLE 11** p. 909 (CNS depressant effects)

- Bupropion is predicted to increase the exposure to the active metabolite of **tetrabenazine**. Moderate Study

A1 Interactions | **Appendix 1**

- Cinacalcet is predicted to increase the exposure to the active metabolite of **tetrabenazine.** Moderate Study
- **Tetrabenazine** is predicted to decrease the effects of **levodopa.** Use with caution or avoid. Moderate Theoretical
- **Tetrabenazine** potentially increases the risk of CNS excitation and hypertension when given with **MAO-B inhibitors.** Severe Theoretical
- **Tetrabenazine** potentially increases the risk of CNS excitation and hypertension when given with **MAOIs, irreversible.** Avoid and for 14 days after stopping the MAOI. Severe Theoretical
- **Tetrabenazine** potentially increases the risk of CNS excitation and hypertension when given with **moclobemide.** Severe Theoretical
- SSRIs **(fluoxetine, paroxetine)** are predicted to increase the exposure to the active metabolite of **tetrabenazine.** Moderate Study
- Terbinafine is predicted to increase the exposure to the active metabolite of **tetrabenazine.** Moderate Study

Tetracaine → see anaesthetics, local

Tetracycline → see tetracyclines

Tetracyclines → see **TABLE 1** p. 907 (hepatotoxicity)

demeclocycline · doxycycline · lymecycline · minocycline · oxytetracycline · tetracycline

ROUTE-SPECIFIC INFORMATION Interactions do not generally apply to topical use of **oxytetracycline** unless specified.

- ACE inhibitors **(quinapril)** (tablet) decrease the absorption of oral **tetracycline.** Avoid. Moderate Study
- **Antacids** decrease the absorption of **tetracyclines.** Separate administration by 2 to 3 hours. Moderate Study
- Antiepileptics **(carbamazepine, fosphenytoin, phenobarbital, phenytoin, primidone)** decrease the exposure to **doxycycline.** Monitor and adjust dose. Moderate Study → Also see **TABLE 1** p. 907
- **Tetracycline** decreases the concentration of antimalarials **(atovaquone).** Moderate Study
- **Apalutamide** decreases the exposure to **doxycycline.** Monitor and adjust dose. Moderate Study
- **Bismuth** greatly decreases the efficacy of **tetracyclines.** Separate administration by 2 hours. Moderate Study
- Calcium salts **(calcium carbonate)** are predicted to decrease the absorption of **tetracyclines.** Separate administration by 2 to 3 hours. Moderate Theoretical
- **Tetracyclines** increase the risk of bleeding events when given with **coumarins.** Moderate Anecdotal
- **Dairy products** decrease the exposure to tetracyclines **(demeclocycline, oxytetracycline, tetracycline).** Avoid. Moderate Study
- **Enzalutamide** decreases the exposure to **doxycycline.** Monitor and adjust dose. Moderate Study
- **Iron (oral)** decreases the absorption of **tetracyclines. Tetracyclines** should be taken 2 to 3 hours after **iron (oral).** Moderate Study
- **Kaolin** is predicted to decrease the absorption of **tetracyclines.** Moderate Theoretical
- **Lanthanum** is predicted to decrease the absorption of **tetracyclines.** Separate administration by 2 hours. Moderate Theoretical
- **Tetracyclines** are predicted to increase the risk of lithium (lithium carbonate p. 250, lithium citrate p. 250) toxicity when given with **lithium.** Avoid or adjust dose. Severe Anecdotal
- **Mitotane** decreases the exposure to **doxycycline.** Monitor and adjust dose. Moderate Study
- Retinoids **(acitretin, alitretinoin, isotretinoin, tretinoin)** increase the risk of benign intracranial hypertension when given with **tetracyclines.** Avoid. Severe Anecdotal
- **Rifampicin** decreases the exposure to **doxycycline.** Monitor and adjust dose. Moderate Study
- **Strontium** is predicted to decrease the absorption of **tetracyclines.** Avoid. Moderate Theoretical
- **Oral zinc** is predicted to decrease the absorption of **tetracyclines.** Separate administration by 2 to 3 hours. Moderate Theoretical

Tezacaftor

FOOD AND LIFESTYLE Avoid bitter (Seville) oranges as they are predicted to increase the exposure to tezacaftor.

- Antiarrhythmics **(dronedarone)** are predicted to increase the exposure to **tezacaftor.** Adjust tezacaftor with ivacaftor p. 198 dose with moderate inhibitors of CYP3A4. Severe Study
- Antiepileptics **(carbamazepine, fosphenytoin, phenobarbital, phenytoin, primidone)** are predicted to decrease the exposure to **tezacaftor.** Avoid. Severe Theoretical
- Antifungals, azoles **(fluconazole, isavuconazole, posaconazole)** are predicted to increase the exposure to **tezacaftor.** Adjust tezacaftor with ivacaftor p. 198 dose with moderate inhibitors of CYP3A4. Severe Study
- Antifungals, azoles **(itraconazole, ketoconazole, voriconazole)** are predicted to increase the exposure to **tezacaftor.** Adjust tezacaftor with ivacaftor p. 198 dose with potent inhibitors of CYP3A4. Severe Study
- **Apalutamide** is predicted to decrease the exposure to **tezacaftor.** Avoid. Severe Theoretical
- **Aprepitant** is predicted to increase the exposure to **tezacaftor.** Adjust tezacaftor with ivacaftor p. 198 dose with moderate inhibitors of CYP3A4. Severe Study
- Calcium channel blockers **(diltiazem, verapamil)** are predicted to increase the exposure to **tezacaftor.** Adjust tezacaftor with ivacaftor p. 198 dose with moderate inhibitors of CYP3A4. Severe Study
- **Cobicistat** is predicted to increase the exposure to **tezacaftor.** Adjust tezacaftor with ivacaftor p. 198 dose with potent inhibitors of CYP3A4. Severe Study
- **Crizotinib** is predicted to increase the exposure to **tezacaftor.** Adjust tezacaftor with ivacaftor p. 198 dose with moderate inhibitors of CYP3A4. Severe Study
- **Enzalutamide** is predicted to decrease the exposure to **tezacaftor.** Avoid. Severe Theoretical
- **Grapefruit juice** is predicted to increase the exposure to **tezacaftor.** Avoid. Severe Study
- **HIV-protease inhibitors** are predicted to increase the exposure to **tezacaftor.** Adjust tezacaftor with ivacaftor p. 198 dose with potent inhibitors of CYP3A4. Severe Study
- **Idelalisib** is predicted to increase the exposure to **tezacaftor.** Adjust tezacaftor with ivacaftor p. 198 dose with potent inhibitors of CYP3A4. Severe Study
- **Imatinib** is predicted to increase the exposure to **tezacaftor.** Adjust tezacaftor with ivacaftor p. 198 dose with moderate inhibitors of CYP3A4. Severe Study
- Macrolides **(clarithromycin)** are predicted to increase the exposure to **tezacaftor.** Adjust tezacaftor with ivacaftor p. 198 dose with potent inhibitors of CYP3A4. Severe Study
- Macrolides **(erythromycin)** are predicted to increase the exposure to **tezacaftor.** Adjust tezacaftor with ivacaftor p. 198 dose with moderate inhibitors of CYP3A4. Severe Study
- **Mitotane** is predicted to decrease the exposure to **tezacaftor.** Avoid. Severe Theoretical
- **Netupitant** is predicted to increase the exposure to **tezacaftor.** Adjust tezacaftor with ivacaftor p. 198 dose with moderate inhibitors of CYP3A4. Severe Study
- **Nilotinib** is predicted to increase the exposure to **tezacaftor.** Adjust tezacaftor with ivacaftor p. 198 dose with moderate inhibitors of CYP3A4. Severe Study
- **Rifabutin** is predicted to decrease the exposure to **tezacaftor.** Avoid. Severe Theoretical
- **Rifampicin** is predicted to decrease the exposure to **tezacaftor.** Avoid. Severe Theoretical
- **St John's Wort** is predicted to decrease the exposure to **tezacaftor.** Avoid. Severe Theoretical

Thalidomide → see **TABLE 6** p. 908 (bradycardia), **TABLE 15** p. 910 (myelosuppression), **TABLE 12** p. 910 (peripheral neuropathy), **TABLE 5** p. 907 (thromboembolism), **TABLE 11** p. 909 (CNS depressant effects)

- **Combined hormonal contraceptives** are predicted to increase the risk of venous thromboembolism when given with **thalidomide.** Avoid. Severe Study
- **Hormone replacement therapy** is predicted to increase the risk of venous thromboembolism when given with **thalidomide.** Severe Theoretical

Theophylline → see TABLE 17 p. 911 (reduced serum potassium)

FOOD AND LIFESTYLE Smoking can increase theophylline clearance and increased doses of theophylline are therefore required; dose adjustments are likely to be necessary if smoking started or stopped during treatment.

- Aciclovir is predicted to increase the exposure to **theophylline**. Monitor and adjust dose. Severe Theoretical
- **Theophylline** decreases the efficacy of antiarrhythmics **(adenosine)**. Separate administration by 24 hours. Mild Study
- Antiepileptics **(carbamazepine)** potentially increase the clearance of **theophylline** and **theophylline** decreases the exposure to antiepileptics **(carbamazepine)**. Adjust dose. Moderate Anecdotal
- Antiepileptics **(fosphenytoin, phenytoin)** are predicted to decrease the exposure to **theophylline**. Adjust dose. Moderate Study
- Antiepileptics **(phenobarbital, primidone)** are predicted to increase the clearance of **theophylline**. Adjust dose. Moderate Theoretical
- Antiepileptics **(stiripentol)** are predicted to increase the exposure to **theophylline**. Avoid. Moderate Theoretical
- Beta blockers, non-selective are predicted to increase the risk of bronchospasm when given with **theophylline**. Avoid. Severe Theoretical
- Beta blockers, selective are predicted to increase the risk of bronchospasm when given with **theophylline**. Avoid. Severe Theoretical
- Caffeine citrate decreases the clearance of **theophylline**. Moderate Study
- Combined hormonal contraceptives are predicted to increase the exposure to **theophylline**. Monitor and adjust dose. Moderate Theoretical
- **Theophylline** increases the risk of agitation when given with **doxapram**. Moderate Study
- Enteral feeds decrease the exposure to **theophylline**. Moderate Study
- Esketamine is predicted to increase the risk of seizures when given with **theophylline**. Avoid. Severe Theoretical
- H_2 receptor antagonists **(cimetidine)** increase the concentration of **theophylline**. Adjust dose. Severe Study
- HIV-protease inhibitors **(ritonavir)** are predicted to decrease the exposure to **theophylline**. Adjust dose. Moderate Study
- Interferons slightly increase the exposure to **theophylline**. Adjust dose. Moderate Study
- Iron chelators **(deferasirox)** increase the exposure to **theophylline**. Avoid. Moderate Study
- Isoniazid is predicted to affect the clearance of **theophylline**. Severe Anecdotal
- Leflunomide is predicted to decrease the exposure to **theophylline**. Adjust dose. Moderate Study
- **Theophylline** is predicted to decrease the concentration of **lithium**. Monitor concentration and adjust dose. Moderate Anecdotal
- Macrolides **(azithromycin, clarithromycin)** are predicted to increase the exposure to **theophylline**. Adjust dose. Moderate Anecdotal
- Macrolides **(erythromycin)** decrease the clearance of **theophylline** and **theophylline** potentially decreases the clearance of macrolides **(erythromycin)**. Adjust dose. Severe Study
- Methotrexate decreases the clearance of **theophylline**. Moderate Study
- Mexiletine is predicted to increase the exposure to **theophylline**. Monitor and adjust dose. Moderate Theoretical
- Monoclonal antibodies **(blinatumomab)** are predicted to transiently increase the exposure to **theophylline**. Monitor and adjust dose. Moderate Theoretical
- Monoclonal antibodies **(sarilumab)** potentially affect the exposure to **theophylline**. Monitor and adjust dose. Moderate Theoretical
- Monoclonal antibodies **(tocilizumab)** are predicted to decrease the exposure to **theophylline**. Monitor and adjust dose. Moderate Theoretical
- Obeticholic acid is predicted to increase the exposure to **theophylline**. Severe Theoretical
- Pentoxifylline increases the concentration of **theophylline**. Monitor and adjust dose. Severe Study
- Quinolones **(ciprofloxacin)** are predicted to increase the exposure to **theophylline**. Monitor and adjust dose. Moderate Theoretical
- Rifampicin is predicted to decrease the exposure to **theophylline**. Adjust dose. Moderate Study
- **Theophylline** is predicted to slightly increase the exposure to **roflumilast**. Avoid. Moderate Theoretical
- Rucaparib is predicted to increase the exposure to **theophylline**. Monitor and adjust dose. Moderate Study
- SSRIs **(fluvoxamine)** moderately to markedly increase the exposure to **theophylline**. Avoid. Severe Study
- St John's Wort potentially decreases the exposure to **theophylline**. Severe Anecdotal
- Sucralfate potentially decreases the absorption of **theophylline**. Separate administration by at least 2 hours. Moderate Study
- Sympathomimetics, vasoconstrictor **(ephedrine)** increase the risk of side-effects when given with **theophylline**. Avoid in children. Moderate Study
- Teriflunomide is predicted to decrease the exposure to **theophylline**. Adjust dose. Moderate Study
- Valaciclovir is predicted to increase the exposure to **theophylline**. Severe Theoretical

Thiazide diuretics → see TABLE 18 p. 911 (hyponatraemia), TABLE 8 p. 908 (hypotension), TABLE 17 p. 911 (reduced serum potassium)

bendroflumethiazide · chlorothiazide · chlortalidone · hydrochlorothiazide · hydroflumethiazide · indapamide · metolazone · xipamide

- **Thiazide diuretics** are predicted to increase the risk of hypersensitivity reactions when given with **allopurinol**. Severe Theoretical
- Aspirin (high-dose) increases the risk of acute renal failure when given with **thiazide diuretics**. Severe Theoretical
- **Thiazide diuretics** increase the risk of hypercalcaemia when given with **calcium salts**. Severe Anecdotal
- **Thiazide diuretics** increase the concentration of **lithium**. Avoid or adjust dose and monitor concentration. Severe Study
- NSAIDs increase the risk of acute renal failure when given with **thiazide diuretics**. Severe Theoretical → Also see TABLE 18 p. 911
- Reboxetine is predicted to increase the risk of hypokalaemia when given with **thiazide diuretics**. Moderate Anecdotal
- **Thiazide diuretics** are predicted to increase the risk of hypercalcaemia when given with **toremifene**. Severe Theoretical
- **Thiazide diuretics** increase the risk of hypercalcaemia when given with **vitamin D substances**. Moderate Theoretical

Thiopental → see TABLE 8 p. 908 (hypotension), TABLE 11 p. 909 (CNS depressant effects)

- Sulfonamides are predicted to increase the effects of **thiopental**. Moderate Theoretical
- Tricyclic antidepressants increase the risk of cardiac arrhythmias and hypotension when given with **thiopental**. Moderate Study → Also see TABLE 8 p. 908 → Also see TABLE 11 p. 909

Thiotepa → see alkylating agents

Thyroid hormones

levothyroxine · liothyronine

- Antacids are predicted to decrease the absorption of **levothyroxine**. Separate administration by at least 4 hours. Moderate Anecdotal
- Antiarrhythmics **(amiodarone)** are predicted to increase the risk of thyroid dysfunction when given with **thyroid hormones**. Avoid. Moderate Study
- Antiepileptics **(carbamazepine, fosphenytoin, phenytoin)** are predicted to increase the risk of hypothyroidism when given with **thyroid hormones**. Moderate Study
- Antiepileptics **(phenobarbital, primidone)** are predicted to decrease the effects of **thyroid hormones**. Moderate Theoretical
- Apalutamide potentially decreases the exposure to **levothyroxine**. Mild Theoretical
- Oral calcium salts are predicted to decrease the absorption of **levothyroxine**. Separate administration by at least 4 hours. Moderate Anecdotal

- **Thyroid hormones** are predicted to affect the concentration of digoxin. Monitor and adjust dose. Moderate Theoretical
- HIV-protease inhibitors (ritonavir) decrease the concentration of **levothyroxine**. MHRA advises monitor TSH for at least one month after starting or stopping ritonavir. Moderate Anecdotal
- Oral hormone replacement therapy is predicted to decrease the effects of **thyroid hormones**. Moderate Theoretical
- Iron (oral) decreases the absorption of **levothyroxine**. Separate administration by at least 4 hours. Moderate Study
- Lanthanum decreases the absorption of **thyroid hormones**. Separate administration by 2 hours. Moderate Study
- Paritaprevir (with ritonavir and ombitasvir) is predicted to increase the exposure to **levothyroxine**. Monitor and adjust dose. Moderate Theoretical
- Sucralfate decreases the absorption of **levothyroxine**. Separate administration by at least 4 hours. Moderate Study

Tiagabine → see antiepileptics

Tiaprofenic acid → see NSAIDs

Tibolone → see TABLE 5 p. 907 (thromboembolism)

Ticagrelor → see TABLE 4 p. 907 (antiplatelet effects)

- Antiarrhythmics (amiodarone) are predicted to increase the exposure to **ticagrelor**. Use with caution or avoid. Severe Study
- Antiepileptics (carbamazepine, fosphenytoin, phenobarbital, phenytoin, primidone) are predicted to markedly decrease the exposure to **ticagrelor**. Avoid. Severe Study
- Antifungals, azoles (itraconazole, ketoconazole, voriconazole) are predicted to markedly increase the exposure to **ticagrelor**. Avoid. Severe Study
- Apalutamide is predicted to markedly decrease the exposure to **ticagrelor**. Avoid. Severe Study
- Bosentan is predicted to decrease the exposure to **ticagrelor**. Moderate Theoretical
- Ciclosporin is predicted to increase the exposure to **ticagrelor**. Use with caution or avoid. Severe Study
- Cobicistat is predicted to markedly increase the exposure to **ticagrelor**. Avoid. Severe Study
- **Ticagrelor** increases the concentration of digoxin. Moderate Study
- Efavirenz is predicted to decrease the exposure to **ticagrelor**. Moderate Theoretical
- Enzalutamide is predicted to markedly decrease the exposure to **ticagrelor**. Avoid. Severe Study
- **Ticagrelor** is predicted to increase the exposure to ergotamine. Avoid. Severe Theoretical
- Grapefruit juice moderately increases the exposure to **ticagrelor**. Moderate Study
- HIV-protease inhibitors are predicted to markedly increase the exposure to **ticagrelor**. Avoid. Severe Study
- Idelalisib is predicted to markedly increase the exposure to **ticagrelor**. Avoid. Severe Study
- **Ticagrelor** is predicted to increase the exposure to lomitapide. Separate administration by 12 hours. Moderate Theoretical
- Macrolides (azithromycin) are predicted to increase the exposure to **ticagrelor**. Use with caution or avoid. Severe Study
- Macrolides (clarithromycin) are predicted to markedly increase the exposure to **ticagrelor**. Avoid. Severe Study
- Mitotane is predicted to markedly decrease the exposure to **ticagrelor**. Avoid. Severe Study
- Nevirapine is predicted to decrease the exposure to **ticagrelor**. Moderate Theoretical
- Ranolazine is predicted to increase the exposure to **ticagrelor**. Use with caution or avoid. Severe Study
- Rifampicin is predicted to markedly decrease the exposure to **ticagrelor**. Avoid. Severe Study
- St John's Wort is predicted to decrease the exposure to **ticagrelor**. Moderate Theoretical
- **Ticagrelor** slightly increases the exposure to statins (simvastatin). Adjust **simvastatin** dose, p. 141. Moderate Study
- Vemurafenib is predicted to increase the exposure to **ticagrelor**. Use with caution or avoid. Severe Study

Ticarcillin → see penicillins

Tigecycline → see TABLE 1 p. 907 (hepatotoxicity)

- **Tigecycline** increases the risk of bleeding events when given with coumarins. Moderate Anecdotal
- Retinoids (acitretin, alitretinoin, isotretinoin, tretinoin) increase the risk of benign intracranial hypertension when given with **tigecycline**. Avoid. Severe Anecdotal

Tildrakizumab → see monoclonal antibodies

Timolol → see beta blockers, non-selective

Tinidazole

- Alcohol (beverage) potentially causes a disulfiram-like reaction when given with **tinidazole**. Avoid for 72 hours stopping treatment. Moderate Theoretical
- **Tinidazole** is predicted to increase the anticoagulant effect of coumarins. Monitor INR and adjust dose. Severe Theoretical

Tinzaparin → see low molecular-weight heparins

Tioguanine → see TABLE 15 p. 910 (myelosuppression)

- Live vaccines are predicted to increase the risk of generalised infection (possibly life-threatening) when given with **tioguanine**. Public Health England advises avoid (refer to Green Book). Severe Theoretical

Tiotropium → see TABLE 10 p. 909 (antimuscarinics)

Tipranavir → see HIV-protease inhibitors

Tirofiban → see TABLE 4 p. 907 (antiplatelet effects)

Tivozanib

- Antiepileptics (carbamazepine, fosphenytoin, phenobarbital, phenytoin, primidone) are predicted to decrease the exposure to **tivozanib**. Severe Study
- Apalutamide is predicted to decrease the exposure to **tivozanib**. Severe Study
- Enzalutamide is predicted to decrease the exposure to **tivozanib**. Severe Study
- Mitotane is predicted to decrease the exposure to **tivozanib**. Severe Study
- Rifampicin is predicted to decrease the exposure to **tivozanib**. Severe Study
- St John's Wort is predicted to decrease the exposure to **tivozanib**. Avoid. Severe Study
- **Tivozanib** is predicted to decrease the exposure to statins (rosuvastatin). Moderate Theoretical

Tizanidine → see TABLE 6 p. 908 (bradycardia), TABLE 8 p. 908 (hypotension), TABLE 9 p. 909 (QT-interval prolongation), TABLE 11 p. 909 (CNS depressant effects)

- Antiepileptics (fosphenytoin, phenytoin) moderately decrease the exposure to **tizanidine**. Mild Study
- Combined hormonal contraceptives increase the exposure to **tizanidine**. Avoid. Moderate Study
- HIV-protease inhibitors (ritonavir) moderately decrease the exposure to **tizanidine**. Mild Study
- Iron chelators (deferasirox) are predicted to increase the exposure to **tizanidine**. Avoid. Moderate Theoretical
- Leflunomide moderately decreases the exposure to **tizanidine**. Mild Study
- Mexiletine increases the exposure to **tizanidine**. Avoid. Moderate Study
- Obeticholic acid is predicted to increase the exposure to **tizanidine**. Severe Theoretical
- Quinolones (ciprofloxacin) increase the exposure to **tizanidine**. Avoid. Moderate Study
- Rifampicin moderately decreases the exposure to **tizanidine**. Mild Study
- Rucaparib is predicted to increase the exposure to **tizanidine**. Monitor and adjust dose. Moderate Study
- SSRIs (fluvoxamine) very markedly increase the exposure to **tizanidine**. Avoid. Severe Study
- Teriflunomide moderately decreases the exposure to **tizanidine**. Mild Study

Tobramycin → see aminoglycosides

Tocilizumab → see monoclonal antibodies

Tofacitinib

- Antiarrhythmics (dronedarone) given with a potent CYP2C19 inhibitor are predicted to increase the exposure to **tofacitinib**. Adjust **tofacitinib** dose. Moderate Study
- Antiepileptics (carbamazepine, fosphenytoin, phenobarbital, phenytoin, primidone) are predicted to decrease the exposure to **tofacitinib**. Avoid. Severe Study
- Antifungals, azoles (fluconazole) increase the exposure to **tofacitinib**. Adjust **tofacitinib** dose. Moderate Study

Tofacitinib (continued)
- Antifungals, azoles **(isavuconazole)** given with a potent CYP2C19 inhibitor are predicted to increase the exposure to **tofacitinib**. Adjust **tofacitinib** dose. Moderate Study
- Antifungals, azoles **(itraconazole, ketoconazole, voriconazole)** are predicted to increase the exposure to **tofacitinib**. Adjust **tofacitinib** dose. Moderate Study
- Antifungals, azoles **(posaconazole)** given with a potent CYP2C19 inhibitor are predicted to increase the exposure to **tofacitinib**. Adjust **tofacitinib** dose. Moderate Theoretical
- **Apalutamide** is predicted to decrease the exposure to **tofacitinib**. Avoid. Severe Study
- **Aprepitant** given with a potent CYP2C19 inhibitor is predicted to increase the exposure to **tofacitinib**. Adjust **tofacitinib** dose. Moderate Study
- **Bosentan** is predicted to decrease the exposure to **tofacitinib**. Moderate Study
- Calcium channel blockers **(diltiazem, verapamil)** given with a potent CYP2C19 inhibitor are predicted to increase the exposure to **tofacitinib**. Adjust **tofacitinib** dose. Moderate Study
- **Ciclosporin** increases the exposure to **tofacitinib**. Avoid. Severe Study
- **Cobicistat** is predicted to increase the exposure to **tofacitinib**. Adjust **tofacitinib** dose. Moderate Study
- **Crizotinib** given with a potent CYP2C19 inhibitor is predicted to increase the exposure to **tofacitinib**. Adjust **tofacitinib** dose. Moderate Study
- **Efavirenz** is predicted to decrease the exposure to **tofacitinib**. Moderate Study
- **Enzalutamide** is predicted to decrease the exposure to **tofacitinib**. Avoid. Severe Study
- **HIV-protease inhibitors** are predicted to increase the exposure to **tofacitinib**. Adjust **tofacitinib** dose. Moderate Study
- **Idelalisib** is predicted to increase the exposure to **tofacitinib**. Adjust **tofacitinib** dose. Moderate Study
- **Imatinib** given with a potent CYP2C19 inhibitor is predicted to increase the exposure to **tofacitinib**. Adjust **tofacitinib** dose. Moderate Study
- **Live vaccines** potentially increase the risk of generalised infection (possibly life-threatening) when given with **tofacitinib**. Avoid. Severe Theoretical
- Macrolides **(clarithromycin)** are predicted to increase the exposure to **tofacitinib**. Adjust **tofacitinib** dose. Moderate Study
- Macrolides **(erythromycin)** given with a potent CYP2C19 inhibitor are predicted to increase the exposure to **tofacitinib**. Adjust **tofacitinib** dose. Moderate Study
- **Mitotane** is predicted to decrease the exposure to **tofacitinib**. Avoid. Severe Study
- **Netupitant** given with a potent CYP2C19 inhibitor is predicted to increase the exposure to **tofacitinib**. Adjust **tofacitinib** dose. Moderate Study
- **Nevirapine** is predicted to decrease the exposure to **tofacitinib**. Moderate Study
- **Nilotinib** given with a potent CYP2C19 inhibitor is predicted to increase the exposure to **tofacitinib**. Adjust **tofacitinib** dose. Moderate Study
- **Rifampicin** is predicted to decrease the exposure to **tofacitinib**. Avoid. Severe Study
- SSRIs **(fluoxetine, fluvoxamine)** given with a moderate CYP3A4 inhibitor are predicted to increase the exposure to **tofacitinib**. Adjust **tofacitinib** dose. Moderate Study
- **St John's Wort** is predicted to decrease the exposure to **tofacitinib**. Moderate Study
- **Tacrolimus** increases the exposure to **tofacitinib**. Avoid. Severe Study

Tolbutamide → see sulfonylureas

Tolcapone
- **Tolcapone** increases the exposure to **levodopa**. Monitor and adjust dose. Moderate Study
- **Tolcapone** is predicted to increase the effects of **MAOIs, irreversible**. Avoid. Severe Theoretical
- **Tolcapone** is predicted to increase the risk of cardiovascular side-effects when given with **sympathomimetics, inotropic**. Moderate Theoretical
- **Tolcapone** is predicted to increase the effects of sympathomimetics, vasoconstrictor **(adrenaline/epinephrine, noradrenaline/norepinephrine)**. Moderate Theoretical

Tolfenamic acid → see NSAIDs

Tolterodine → see TABLE 9 p. 909 (QT-interval prolongation), TABLE 10 p. 909 (antimuscarinics)
- Antiarrhythmics **(dronedarone)** are predicted to increase the exposure to **tolterodine**. Mild Theoretical → Also see TABLE 9 p. 909
- Antifungals, azoles **(fluconazole, isavuconazole, posaconazole)** are predicted to increase the exposure to **tolterodine**. Mild Theoretical → Also see TABLE 9 p. 909
- Antifungals, azoles **(itraconazole, ketoconazole, voriconazole)** are predicted to increase the exposure to **tolterodine**. Avoid. Severe Study → Also see TABLE 9 p. 909
- **Aprepitant** is predicted to increase the exposure to **tolterodine**. Mild Theoretical
- Calcium channel blockers **(diltiazem, verapamil)** are predicted to increase the exposure to **tolterodine**. Mild Theoretical
- **Cobicistat** is predicted to increase the exposure to **tolterodine**. Avoid. Severe Study
- **Crizotinib** is predicted to increase the exposure to **tolterodine**. Mild Theoretical → Also see TABLE 9 p. 909
- **Dacomitinib** is predicted to markedly increase the exposure to **tolterodine**. Avoid. Severe Study
- **Eliglustat** is predicted to increase the exposure to **tolterodine**. Adjust dose. Moderate Theoretical
- **HIV-protease inhibitors** are predicted to increase the exposure to **tolterodine**. Avoid. Severe Study → Also see TABLE 9 p. 909
- **Idelalisib** is predicted to increase the exposure to **tolterodine**. Avoid. Severe Study
- **Imatinib** is predicted to increase the exposure to **tolterodine**. Mild Theoretical
- Macrolides **(clarithromycin)** are predicted to increase the exposure to **tolterodine**. Avoid. Severe Study → Also see TABLE 9 p. 909
- Macrolides **(erythromycin)** are predicted to increase the exposure to **tolterodine**. Mild Theoretical → Also see TABLE 9 p. 909
- **Netupitant** is predicted to increase the exposure to **tolterodine**. Mild Theoretical
- **Nilotinib** is predicted to increase the exposure to **tolterodine**. Mild Theoretical → Also see TABLE 9 p. 909

Tolvaptan → see TABLE 16 p. 911 (increased serum potassium)

GENERAL INFORMATION Avoid concurrent use of drugs that increase serum-sodium concentrations.

- Antiarrhythmics **(dronedarone)** are predicted to increase the exposure to **tolvaptan**. Manufacturer advises caution or adjust **tolvaptan** dose with moderate inhibitors of CYP3A4. Moderate Study
- Antiepileptics **(carbamazepine, fosphenytoin, phenobarbital, phenytoin, primidone)** are predicted to decrease the exposure to **tolvaptan**. Use with caution or avoid depending on indication. Severe Study
- Antifungals, azoles **(fluconazole, isavuconazole, posaconazole)** are predicted to increase the exposure to **tolvaptan**. Manufacturer advises caution or adjust **tolvaptan** dose with moderate inhibitors of CYP3A4. Moderate Study
- Antifungals, azoles **(itraconazole, ketoconazole, voriconazole)** are predicted to increase the exposure to **tolvaptan**. Manufacturer advises caution or adjust **tolvaptan** dose with potent inhibitors of CYP3A4. Severe Study
- **Apalutamide** is predicted to decrease the exposure to **tolvaptan**. Use with caution or avoid depending on indication. Severe Study
- **Aprepitant** is predicted to increase the exposure to **tolvaptan**. Manufacturer advises caution or adjust **tolvaptan** dose with moderate inhibitors of CYP3A4. Moderate Study
- Calcium channel blockers **(diltiazem, verapamil)** are predicted to increase the exposure to **tolvaptan**. Manufacturer advises caution or adjust **tolvaptan** dose with moderate inhibitors of CYP3A4. Moderate Study
- **Cobicistat** is predicted to increase the exposure to **tolvaptan**. Manufacturer advises caution or adjust **tolvaptan** dose with potent inhibitors of CYP3A4. Severe Study

- **Crizotinib** is predicted to increase the exposure to **tolvaptan**. Manufacturer advises caution or adjust **tolvaptan** dose with moderate inhibitors of CYP3A4. Moderate Study
- **Tolvaptan** increases the concentration of **digoxin**. Mild Study
- **Enzalutamide** is predicted to decrease the exposure to **tolvaptan**. Use with caution or avoid depending on indication. Severe Study
- **Grapefruit juice** increases the exposure to **tolvaptan**. Avoid. Moderate Study
- **HIV-protease inhibitors** are predicted to increase the exposure to **tolvaptan**. Manufacturer advises caution or adjust **tolvaptan** dose with potent inhibitors of CYP3A4. Severe Study
- **Idelalisib** is predicted to increase the exposure to **tolvaptan**. Manufacturer advises caution or adjust **tolvaptan** dose with potent inhibitors of CYP3A4. Severe Study
- **Imatinib** is predicted to increase the exposure to **tolvaptan**. Manufacturer advises caution or adjust **tolvaptan** dose with moderate inhibitors of CYP3A4. Moderate Study
- **Tolvaptan** is predicted to increase the exposure to **lomitapide**. Separate administration by 12 hours. Moderate Theoretical
- Macrolides **(clarithromycin)** are predicted to increase the exposure to **tolvaptan**. Manufacturer advises caution or adjust **tolvaptan** dose with potent inhibitors of CYP3A4. Severe Study
- Macrolides **(erythromycin)** are predicted to increase the exposure to **tolvaptan**. Manufacturer advises caution or adjust **tolvaptan** dose with moderate inhibitors of CYP3A4. Moderate Study
- **Mitotane** is predicted to decrease the exposure to **tolvaptan**. Use with caution or avoid depending on indication. Severe Study
- **Netupitant** is predicted to increase the exposure to **tolvaptan**. Manufacturer advises caution or adjust **tolvaptan** dose with moderate inhibitors of CYP3A4. Moderate Study
- **Nilotinib** is predicted to increase the exposure to **tolvaptan**. Manufacturer advises caution or adjust **tolvaptan** dose with moderate inhibitors of CYP3A4. Moderate Study
- Quinolones **(ciprofloxacin)** are predicted to increase the exposure to **tolvaptan**. Use with caution and adjust **tolvaptan** dose. Moderate Theoretical
- **Rifampicin** is predicted to decrease the exposure to **tolvaptan**. Use with caution or avoid depending on indication. Severe Study
- **St John's Wort** is predicted to decrease the exposure to **tolvaptan**. Avoid. Moderate Theoretical

Topiramate → see antiepileptics

Topotecan → see TABLE 15 p. 910 (myelosuppression)

- Antiarrhythmics **(amiodarone, dronedarone)** are predicted to increase the exposure to **topotecan**. Severe Study
- Antiepileptics **(fosphenytoin, phenytoin)** increase the clearance of **topotecan**. Moderate Study
- Antifungals, azoles **(isavuconazole)** are predicted to increase the exposure to **topotecan**. Moderate Theoretical
- Antifungals, azoles **(itraconazole, ketoconazole)** are predicted to increase the exposure to **topotecan**. Severe Study
- Calcium channel blockers **(verapamil)** are predicted to increase the exposure to **topotecan**. Severe Study
- **Ceritinib** is predicted to increase the exposure to **topotecan**. Moderate Theoretical → Also see TABLE 15 p. 910
- **Ciclosporin** is predicted to increase the exposure to **topotecan**. Severe Study
- **Eliglustat** is predicted to increase the exposure to **topotecan**. Adjust dose. Moderate Study
- HIV-protease inhibitors **(lopinavir, ritonavir, saquinavir)** are predicted to increase the exposure to **topotecan**. Severe Study
- **Lapatinib** is predicted to increase the exposure to **topotecan**. Severe Study
- **Leflunomide** is predicted to increase the exposure to **topotecan**. Moderate Study → Also see TABLE 15 p. 910
- **Live vaccines** are predicted to increase the risk of generalised infection (possibly life-threatening) when given with **topotecan**. Public Health England advises avoid (refer to Green Book). Severe Theoretical
- **Macrolides** are predicted to increase the exposure to **topotecan**. Severe Study
- **Mirabegron** is predicted to increase the exposure to **topotecan**. Mild Theoretical
- **Paritaprevir** (with ritonavir and ombitasvir) is predicted to increase the exposure to **topotecan**. Moderate Study
- **Pibrentasvir** (with glecaprevir) is predicted to increase the exposure to **topotecan**. Moderate Study
- **Pitolisant** is predicted to decrease the exposure to **topotecan**. Mild Theoretical
- **Ranolazine** is predicted to increase the exposure to **topotecan**. Severe Study
- **Regorafenib** is predicted to increase the exposure to **topotecan**. Moderate Study → Also see TABLE 15 p. 910
- **Rolapitant** is predicted to increase the exposure to **topotecan**. Avoid or monitor. Moderate Study
- **St John's Wort** is predicted to decrease the exposure to **topotecan**. Severe Theoretical
- **Tedizolid** is predicted to increase the exposure to **topotecan**. Avoid. Moderate Study
- **Teriflunomide** is predicted to increase the exposure to **topotecan**. Moderate Study
- **Velpatasvir** is predicted to increase the exposure to **topotecan**. Severe Theoretical
- **Vemurafenib** is predicted to increase the exposure to **topotecan**. Severe Study
- **Venetoclax** is predicted to increase the exposure to **topotecan**. Moderate Theoretical
- **Voxilaprevir** is predicted to increase the concentration of **topotecan**. Avoid. Severe Theoretical

Torasemide → see loop diuretics

Toremifene → see TABLE 5 p. 907 (thromboembolism), TABLE 9 p. 909 (QT-interval prolongation)

- Antiepileptics **(carbamazepine, fosphenytoin, phenobarbital, phenytoin, primidone)** are predicted to decrease the exposure to **toremifene**. Adjust dose. Moderate Study
- Antifungals, azoles **(itraconazole, ketoconazole, voriconazole)** are predicted to increase the exposure to **toremifene**. Moderate Theoretical → Also see TABLE 9 p. 909
- **Apalutamide** is predicted to decrease the exposure to **toremifene**. Adjust dose. Moderate Study → Also see TABLE 9 p. 909
- **Cobicistat** is predicted to increase the exposure to **toremifene**. Moderate Theoretical
- **Toremifene** is predicted to increase the anticoagulant effect of **coumarins**. Severe Theoretical
- **Enzalutamide** is predicted to decrease the exposure to **toremifene**. Adjust dose. Moderate Study
- **HIV-protease inhibitors** are predicted to increase the exposure to **toremifene**. Moderate Theoretical → Also see TABLE 9 p. 909
- **Idelalisib** is predicted to increase the exposure to **toremifene**. Moderate Theoretical
- Macrolides **(clarithromycin)** are predicted to increase the exposure to **toremifene**. Moderate Theoretical → Also see TABLE 9 p. 909
- **Mitotane** is predicted to decrease the exposure to **toremifene**. Adjust dose. Moderate Study
- **Rifampicin** is predicted to decrease the exposure to **toremifene**. Adjust dose. Moderate Study
- **Thiazide diuretics** are predicted to increase the risk of hypercalcaemia when given with **toremifene**. Severe Theoretical

Trabectedin → see TABLE 1 p. 907 (hepatotoxicity), TABLE 15 p. 910 (myelosuppression)

- Antiepileptics **(carbamazepine, fosphenytoin, phenobarbital, phenytoin, primidone)** are predicted to decrease the exposure to **trabectedin**. Avoid. Severe Theoretical → Also see TABLE 1 p. 907
- Antifungals, azoles **(itraconazole, ketoconazole, voriconazole)** are predicted to increase the exposure to **trabectedin**. Avoid or adjust dose. Severe Theoretical → Also see TABLE 1 p. 907
- **Apalutamide** is predicted to decrease the exposure to **trabectedin**. Avoid. Severe Theoretical
- **Cobicistat** is predicted to increase the exposure to **trabectedin**. Avoid or adjust dose. Severe Theoretical
- **Enzalutamide** is predicted to decrease the exposure to **trabectedin**. Avoid. Severe Theoretical
- **HIV-protease inhibitors** are predicted to increase the exposure to **trabectedin**. Avoid or adjust dose. Severe Theoretical

Trabectedin (continued)
- **Idelalisib** is predicted to increase the exposure to **trabectedin**. Avoid or adjust dose. [Severe] Theoretical → Also see **TABLE 15** p. 910
- **Live vaccines** are predicted to increase the risk of generalised infection (possibly life-threatening) when given with **trabectedin**. Public Health England advises avoid (refer to Green Book). [Severe] Theoretical
- Macrolides **(clarithromycin)** are predicted to increase the exposure to **trabectedin**. Avoid or adjust dose. [Severe] Theoretical
- **Mitotane** is predicted to decrease the exposure to **trabectedin**. Avoid. [Severe] Theoretical → Also see **TABLE 15** p. 910
- **Rifampicin** is predicted to decrease the exposure to **trabectedin**. Avoid. [Severe] Theoretical

Tramadol → see opioids

Trametinib
- Antiarrhythmics **(amiodarone, dronedarone)** are predicted to increase the concentration of **trametinib**. [Moderate] Theoretical
- Antifungals, azoles **(itraconazole, ketoconazole)** are predicted to increase the concentration of **trametinib**. [Moderate] Theoretical
- Calcium channel blockers **(verapamil)** are predicted to increase the concentration of **trametinib**. [Moderate] Theoretical
- **Ciclosporin** is predicted to increase the concentration of **trametinib**. [Moderate] Theoretical
- HIV-protease inhibitors **(lopinavir, ritonavir, saquinavir)** are predicted to increase the concentration of **trametinib**. [Moderate] Theoretical
- **Lapatinib** is predicted to increase the concentration of **trametinib**. [Moderate] Theoretical
- **Macrolides** are predicted to increase the concentration of **trametinib**. [Moderate] Theoretical
- **Ranolazine** is predicted to increase the concentration of **trametinib**. [Moderate] Theoretical
- **Vemurafenib** is predicted to increase the concentration of **trametinib**. [Moderate] Theoretical

Trandolapril → see ACE inhibitors

Tranexamic acid → see **TABLE 5** p. 907 (thromboembolism)

Tranylcypromine → see MAOIs, irreversible

Trastuzumab → see monoclonal antibodies

Trastuzumab emtansine → see monoclonal antibodies

Trazodone → see **TABLE 13** p. 910 (serotonin syndrome), **TABLE 11** p. 909 (CNS depressant effects)
- Antiarrhythmics **(dronedarone)** are predicted to increase the exposure to **trazodone**. [Moderate] Theoretical
- Antiepileptics **(carbamazepine)** decrease the concentration of **trazodone**. Adjust dose. [Moderate] Anecdotal
- Antifungals, azoles **(fluconazole, isavuconazole, posaconazole)** are predicted to increase the exposure to **trazodone**. [Moderate] Theoretical
- Antifungals, azoles **(itraconazole, ketoconazole, voriconazole)** are predicted to moderately increase the exposure to **trazodone**. Avoid or adjust dose. [Moderate] Study
- **Aprepitant** is predicted to increase the exposure to **trazodone**. [Moderate] Theoretical
- Calcium channel blockers **(diltiazem, verapamil)** are predicted to increase the exposure to **trazodone**. [Moderate] Theoretical
- **Cobicistat** is predicted to moderately increase the exposure to **trazodone**. Avoid or adjust dose. [Moderate] Study
- **Crizotinib** is predicted to increase the exposure to **trazodone**. [Moderate] Theoretical
- **HIV-protease inhibitors** are predicted to moderately increase the exposure to **trazodone**. Avoid or adjust dose. [Moderate] Study
- **Idelalisib** is predicted to moderately increase the exposure to **trazodone**. Avoid or adjust dose. [Moderate] Study
- **Imatinib** is predicted to increase the exposure to **trazodone**. [Moderate] Theoretical
- Macrolides **(clarithromycin)** are predicted to moderately increase the exposure to **trazodone**. Avoid or adjust dose. [Moderate] Study
- Macrolides **(erythromycin)** are predicted to increase the exposure to **trazodone**. [Moderate] Theoretical
- **Netupitant** is predicted to increase the exposure to **trazodone**. [Moderate] Theoretical
- **Nilotinib** is predicted to increase the exposure to **trazodone**. [Moderate] Theoretical

Tree pollen extract

GENERAL INFORMATION Desensitising vaccines should be avoided in patients taking beta-blockers (adrenaline might be ineffective in case of a hypersensitivity reaction) or ACE inhibitors (risk of severe anaphylactoid reactions).

Treosulfan → see alkylating agents

Tretinoin → see retinoids

Triamcinolone → see corticosteroids

Triamterene → see potassium-sparing diuretics

Tricyclic antidepressants → see **TABLE 18** p. 911 (hyponatraemia), **TABLE 8** p. 908 (hypotension), **TABLE 13** p. 910 (serotonin syndrome), **TABLE 9** p. 909 (QT-interval prolongation), **TABLE 11** p. 909 (CNS depressant effects), **TABLE 10** p. 909 (antimuscarinics)

amitriptyline · clomipramine · dosulepin · doxepin · imipramine · lofepramine · nortriptyline · trimipramine

ROUTE-SPECIFIC INFORMATION Since systemic absorption can follow topical application, the possibility of interactions of topical **doxepin** should be borne in mind.

- Antiarrhythmics **(dronedarone)** are predicted to increase the exposure to **tricyclic antidepressants**. Avoid. [Severe] Theoretical → Also see **TABLE 9** p. 909
- Antiarrhythmics **(propafenone)** are predicted to increase the concentration of **tricyclic antidepressants**. [Moderate] Theoretical → Also see **TABLE 10** p. 909
- Antiepileptics **(carbamazepine)** decrease the exposure to **tricyclic antidepressants**. Adjust dose. [Moderate] Study → Also see **TABLE 18** p. 911
- Antiepileptics **(phenobarbital, primidone)** are predicted to decrease the exposure to **tricyclic antidepressants**. [Moderate] Study → Also see **TABLE 11** p. 909
- Tricyclic antidepressants **(clomipramine, imipramine)** potentially increase the risk of overheating and dehydration when given with antiepileptics **(zonisamide)**. Avoid in children. [Severe] Theoretical
- **Bupropion** is predicted to increase the exposure to **tricyclic antidepressants**. Monitor for toxicity and adjust dose. [Severe] Study → Also see **TABLE 13** p. 910
- **Cinacalcet** is predicted to increase the exposure to **tricyclic antidepressants**. Monitor for toxicity and adjust dose. [Severe] Study
- **Tricyclic antidepressants** decrease the antihypertensive effects of clonidine. Monitor and adjust dose. [Moderate] Anecdotal → Also see **TABLE 8** p. 908 → Also see **TABLE 11** p. 909
- **Cobicistat** is predicted to slightly increase the exposure to **tricyclic antidepressants**. [Mild] Study
- **Dacomitinib** is predicted to markedly increase the exposure to tricyclic antidepressants **(imipramine, nortriptyline)**. Avoid. [Severe] Study
- **Darifenacin** is predicted to increase the exposure to **tricyclic antidepressants**. [Moderate] Theoretical → Also see **TABLE 10** p. 909
- **Eliglustat** is predicted to increase the exposure to **nortriptyline**. Adjust dose. [Moderate] Theoretical
- H_2 receptor antagonists **(cimetidine)** increase the exposure to **tricyclic antidepressants**. [Moderate] Study
- HIV-protease inhibitors **(ritonavir, tipranavir)** are predicted to increase the exposure to **tricyclic antidepressants**. [Moderate] Theoretical
- **Tricyclic antidepressants** potentially increase the risk of neurotoxicity when given with lithium. [Severe] Anecdotal → Also see **TABLE 13** p. 910 → Also see **TABLE 9** p. 909
- **Tricyclic antidepressants** are predicted to increase the risk of severe toxic reaction when given with **MAOIs, irreversible**. Avoid and for 14 days after stopping the MAOI. [Severe] Theoretical → Also see **TABLE 8** p. 908 → Also see **TABLE 13** p. 910
- **Amitriptyline** decreases the effects of metyrapone. Avoid. [Moderate] Theoretical
- **Tricyclic antidepressants** are predicted to increase the risk of severe toxic reaction when given with moclobemide. Avoid. [Severe] Theoretical → Also see **TABLE 13** p. 910

- **Tricyclic antidepressants** are predicted to decrease the effects of moxonidine. Avoid. Moderate Theoretical → Also see **TABLE 8** p. 908 → Also see **TABLE 11** p. 909
- **Tricyclic antidepressants** are predicted to decrease the efficacy of pitolisant. Mild Theoretical
- SSRIs **(fluoxetine, paroxetine)** are predicted to increase the exposure to **tricyclic antidepressants**. Monitor for toxicity and adjust dose. Severe Study → Also see **TABLE 18** p. 911 → Also see **TABLE 13** p. 910
- SSRIs **(fluvoxamine)** markedly increase the exposure to **clomipramine**. Adjust dose. Severe Study → Also see **TABLE 18** p. 911 → Also see **TABLE 13** p. 910
- SSRIs **(fluvoxamine)** increase the exposure to tricyclic antidepressants **(amitriptyline, imipramine)**. Adjust dose. Severe Study → Also see **TABLE 18** p. 911 → Also see **TABLE 13** p. 910
- **Sucralfate** is predicted to decrease the absorption of **tricyclic antidepressants**. Moderate Study
- **Tricyclic antidepressants** increase the effects of sympathomimetics, vasoconstrictor **(adrenaline/epinephrine, noradrenaline/norepinephrine, phenylephrine)**. Avoid. Severe Study
- **Tricyclic antidepressants** are predicted to decrease the effects of sympathomimetics, vasoconstrictor **(ephedrine)**. Avoid. Severe Study
- **Terbinafine** is predicted to increase the exposure to **tricyclic antidepressants**. Monitor for toxicity and adjust dose. Severe Study
- **Tricyclic antidepressants** increase the risk of cardiac arrhythmias and hypotension when given with **thiopental**. Moderate Study → Also see **TABLE 8** p. 908 → Also see **TABLE 11** p. 909

Trientine
- **Trientine** potentially decreases the absorption of **iron (oral)**. Moderate Theoretical
- **Trientine** potentially decreases the absorption of **zinc**. Moderate Theoretical

Trifluoperazine → see phenothiazines

Trihexyphenidyl → see **TABLE 10** p. 909 (antimuscarinics)

Trimethoprim → see **TABLE 18** p. 911 (hyponatraemia), **TABLE 15** p. 910 (myelosuppression), **TABLE 2** p. 907 (nephrotoxicity), **TABLE 16** p. 911 (increased serum potassium)
- **Trimethoprim** increases the concentration of antiepileptics **(fosphenytoin, phenytoin)**. Moderate Study
- Antimalarials **(pyrimethamine)** increase the risk of side-effects when given with **trimethoprim**. Severe Study → Also see **TABLE 15** p. 910
- **Trimethoprim** is predicted to increase the anticoagulant effect of **coumarins**. Severe Study
- **Dapsone** increases the exposure to **trimethoprim** and **trimethoprim** increases the exposure to **dapsone**. Severe Study
- **Trimethoprim** increases the concentration of **digoxin**. Moderate Study
- **Trimethoprim** is predicted to increase the exposure to dopamine receptor agonists **(pramipexole)**. Adjust dose. Moderate Study
- **Trimethoprim** slightly increases the exposure to **lamivudine**. Moderate Study
- **Trimethoprim** increases the risk of side-effects when given with **methotrexate**. Avoid. Severe Anecdotal → Also see **TABLE 15** p. 910 → Also see **TABLE 2** p. 907
- **Trimethoprim** slightly increases the exposure to **repaglinide**. Avoid or monitor blood glucose. Moderate Study
- **Rifampicin** decreases the exposure to **trimethoprim**. Moderate Study
- **Trimethoprim** is predicted to decrease the efficacy of **sapropterin**. Moderate Theoretical

Trimipramine → see tricyclic antidepressants

Tropicamide → see **TABLE 10** p. 909 (antimuscarinics)

Trospium → see **TABLE 10** p. 909 (antimuscarinics)

Tryptophan → see **TABLE 13** p. 910 (serotonin syndrome)
- **Tryptophan** greatly decreases the concentration of **levodopa**. Moderate Study
- **Tryptophan** increases the risk of side-effects when given with **MAOIs, irreversible**. Severe Anecdotal → Also see **TABLE 13** p. 910

Typhoid vaccine, oral → see live vaccines

Ulipristal
- Antiarrhythmics **(dronedarone)** are predicted to increase the exposure to **ulipristal**. Avoid if used for uterine fibroids. Moderate Study
- Antiepileptics **(carbamazepine, eslicarbazepine, fosphenytoin, oxcarbazepine, perampanel, phenobarbital, phenytoin, primidone, rufinamide, topiramate)** decrease the efficacy of **ulipristal**. For FSRH guidance, see Contraceptives, interactions p. 536. Severe Anecdotal
- Antifungals, azoles **(fluconazole, isavuconazole, posaconazole)** are predicted to increase the exposure to **ulipristal**. Avoid if used for uterine fibroids. Moderate Study
- Antifungals, azoles **(itraconazole, ketoconazole, voriconazole)** are predicted to increase the exposure to **ulipristal**. Avoid if used for uterine fibroids. Severe Study
- **Aprepitant** decreases the efficacy of **ulipristal**. For FSRH guidance, see Contraceptives, interactions p. 536. Severe Anecdotal
- **Bosentan** decreases the efficacy of **ulipristal**. For FSRH guidance, see Contraceptives, interactions p. 536. Severe Anecdotal
- Calcium channel blockers **(diltiazem, verapamil)** are predicted to increase the exposure to **ulipristal**. Avoid if used for uterine fibroids. Moderate Study
- **Cobicistat** is predicted to increase the exposure to **ulipristal**. Avoid if used for uterine fibroids. Severe Study
- **Ulipristal** is predicted to decrease the efficacy of **combined hormonal contraceptives**. Avoid. Severe Theoretical
- **Crizotinib** is predicted to increase the exposure to **ulipristal**. Avoid if used for uterine fibroids. Moderate Study
- **Ulipristal** is predicted to decrease the efficacy of **desogestrel**. Avoid. Severe Theoretical
- **Efavirenz** decreases the efficacy of **ulipristal**. For FSRH guidance, see Contraceptives, interactions p. 536. Severe Anecdotal
- **Enzalutamide** is predicted to markedly decrease the exposure to **ulipristal**. Avoid and for 4 weeks after stopping **ulipristal**. Severe Theoretical
- **Ulipristal** is predicted to decrease the efficacy of **etonogestrel**. Avoid. Severe Theoretical
- **Fosaprepitant** decreases the efficacy of **ulipristal**. For FSRH guidance, see Contraceptives, interactions p. 536. Severe Anecdotal
- **Grapefruit juice** is predicted to increase the exposure to **ulipristal**. Avoid if used for uterine fibroids. Moderate Theoretical
- **Griseofulvin** potentially decreases the efficacy of **ulipristal**. For FSRH guidance, see Contraceptives, interactions p. 536. Severe Anecdotal
- HIV-protease inhibitors **(atazanavir, darunavir, fosamprenavir, lopinavir, saquinavir, tipranavir)** are predicted to increase the exposure to **ulipristal**. Avoid if used for uterine fibroids. Severe Study
- HIV-protease inhibitors **(ritonavir)** decrease the efficacy of **ulipristal**. For FSRH guidance, see Contraceptives, interactions p. 536. Severe Anecdotal
- **Idelalisib** is predicted to increase the exposure to **ulipristal**. Avoid if used for uterine fibroids. Severe Study
- **Imatinib** is predicted to increase the exposure to **ulipristal**. Avoid if used for uterine fibroids. Moderate Study
- **Ulipristal** is predicted to decrease the efficacy of **levonorgestrel**. Avoid. Severe Theoretical
- **Lumacaftor** is predicted to decrease the efficacy of **ulipristal**. Use additional contraceptive precautions. Severe Theoretical
- Macrolides **(clarithromycin)** are predicted to increase the exposure to **ulipristal**. Avoid if used for uterine fibroids. Severe Study
- Macrolides **(erythromycin)** are predicted to increase the exposure to **ulipristal**. Avoid if used for uterine fibroids. Moderate Study
- **Modafinil** decreases the efficacy of **ulipristal**. For FSRH guidance, see Contraceptives, interactions p. 536. Severe Anecdotal
- **Netupitant** is predicted to increase the exposure to **ulipristal**. Avoid if used for uterine fibroids. Moderate Study

Ulipristal (continued)
- **Nevirapine** decreases the efficacy of **ulipristal**. For FSRH guidance, see Contraceptives, interactions p. 536. Severe Anecdotal
- **Nilotinib** is predicted to increase the exposure to **ulipristal**. Avoid if used for uterine fibroids. Moderate Study
- **Ulipristal** is predicted to decrease the efficacy of **norethisterone**. Avoid. Severe Theoretical
- **Rifabutin** decreases the efficacy of **ulipristal**. For FSRH guidance, see Contraceptives, interactions p. 536. Severe Anecdotal
- **Rifampicin** decreases the efficacy of **ulipristal**. For FSRH guidance, see Contraceptives, interactions p. 536. Severe Anecdotal
- **St John's Wort** decreases the efficacy of **ulipristal**. For FSRH guidance, see Contraceptives, interactions p. 536. Severe Anecdotal

Umeclidinium → see TABLE 10 p. 909 (antimuscarinics)

Upadacitinib
- Antiepileptics **(carbamazepine, fosphenytoin, phenobarbital, phenytoin, primidone)** are predicted to decrease the exposure to **upadacitinib**. Moderate Study
- Antifungals, azoles **(itraconazole, ketoconazole, voriconazole)** are predicted to increase the exposure to **upadacitinib**. Use with caution or avoid. Severe Study
- Antifungals, azoles **(posaconazole)** are predicted to increase the exposure to **upadacitinib**. Use with caution or avoid. Moderate Study
- **Apalutamide** is predicted to decrease the exposure to **upadacitinib**. Moderate Study
- **Cobicistat** is predicted to increase the exposure to **upadacitinib**. Use with caution or avoid. Severe Study
- **Enzalutamide** is predicted to decrease the exposure to **upadacitinib**. Moderate Study
- **HIV-protease inhibitors** are predicted to increase the exposure to **upadacitinib**. Use with caution or avoid. Severe Study
- **Idelalisib** is predicted to increase the exposure to **upadacitinib**. Use with caution or avoid. Severe Study
- **Live vaccines** are predicted to increase the risk of generalised infection (possibly life-threatening) when given with **upadacitinib**. Avoid. Severe Theoretical
- Macrolides **(clarithromycin)** are predicted to increase the exposure to **upadacitinib**. Use with caution or avoid. Severe Study
- **Mitotane** is predicted to decrease the exposure to **upadacitinib**. Moderate Study
- **Rifampicin** is predicted to decrease the exposure to **upadacitinib**. Moderate Study

Urokinase → see TABLE 3 p. 907 (anticoagulant effects)

Ursodeoxycholic acid
- **Antacids** are predicted to decrease the absorption of **ursodeoxycholic acid**. Separate administration by 2 hours. Moderate Theoretical
- **Ursodeoxycholic acid** affects the concentration of **ciclosporin**. Use with caution and adjust dose. Severe Anecdotal
- **Fibrates** are predicted to decrease the efficacy of **ursodeoxycholic acid**. Avoid. Severe Theoretical

Ustekinumab → see monoclonal antibodies

Vaborbactam
- **Vaborbactam** is predicted to increase the concentration of beta blockers, selective **(metoprolol)**. Unknown Theoretical
- **Vaborbactam** is predicted to increase the concentration of **venlafaxine**. Unknown Theoretical

Valaciclovir → see TABLE 2 p. 907 (nephrotoxicity)
- **Valaciclovir** is predicted to increase the exposure to **aminophylline**. Severe Anecdotal
- **Mycophenolate** is predicted to increase the risk of haematological toxicity when given with **valaciclovir**. Moderate Theoretical
- **Valaciclovir** is predicted to increase the exposure to **theophylline**. Severe Theoretical

Valganciclovir → see TABLE 15 p. 910 (myelosuppression), TABLE 2 p. 907 (nephrotoxicity)
- **Valganciclovir** is predicted to increase the risk of seizures when given with carbapenems **(imipenem)**. Avoid. Severe Anecdotal
- **Mycophenolate** is predicted to increase the risk of haematological toxicity when given with **valganciclovir**. Moderate Theoretical → Also see TABLE 15 p. 910

Valproate → see antiepileptics

Valsartan → see angiotensin-II receptor antagonists

Vancomycin → see TABLE 2 p. 907 (nephrotoxicity), TABLE 19 p. 911 (ototoxicity)

Vandetanib → see TABLE 9 p. 909 (QT-interval prolongation)
- Antiepileptics **(carbamazepine, fosphenytoin, phenobarbital, phenytoin, primidone)** are predicted to decrease the exposure to **vandetanib**. Avoid. Moderate Study
- **Apalutamide** is predicted to decrease the exposure to **vandetanib**. Avoid. Moderate Study → Also see TABLE 9 p. 909
- **Vandetanib** is predicted to increase the risk of bleeding events when given with **coumarins**. Severe Theoretical
- **Vandetanib** slightly increases the exposure to digoxin. Monitor ECG and adjust dose. Moderate Study
- **Vandetanib** is predicted to increase the exposure to dopamine receptor agonists **(pramipexole)**. Adjust dose. Moderate Study
- **Enzalutamide** is predicted to decrease the exposure to **vandetanib**. Avoid. Moderate Study
- **Vandetanib** increases the exposure to **metformin**. Monitor and adjust dose. Moderate Study
- **Mitotane** is predicted to decrease the exposure to **vandetanib**. Avoid. Moderate Study
- **Vandetanib** is predicted to increase the risk of bleeding events when given with **phenindione**. Severe Theoretical
- **Rifampicin** is predicted to decrease the exposure to **vandetanib**. Avoid. Moderate Study

Vardenafil → see phosphodiesterase type-5 inhibitors

Varicella-zoster immunoglobulin → see immunoglobulins

Varicella-zoster vaccine → see live vaccines

Vecuronium → see neuromuscular blocking drugs, non-depolarising

Vedolizumab → see monoclonal antibodies

Velpatasvir
- **Velpatasvir** is predicted to increase the exposure to **aliskiren**. Severe Theoretical
- **Antacids** are predicted to decrease the concentration of **velpatasvir**. Separate administration by 4 hours. Moderate Theoretical
- Antiarrhythmics **(amiodarone)** are predicted to increase the concentration of **velpatasvir**. Avoid or monitor. Moderate Theoretical
- Antiepileptics **(carbamazepine, fosphenytoin, phenobarbital, phenytoin, primidone)** are predicted to moderately decrease the exposure to **velpatasvir**. Avoid. Severe Study
- Antiepileptics **(oxcarbazepine)** are predicted to decrease the exposure to **velpatasvir**. Avoid. Severe Theoretical
- **Velpatasvir** is predicted to increase the exposure to antihistamines, non-sedating **(fexofenadine)**. Severe Theoretical
- **Apalutamide** is predicted to moderately decrease the exposure to **velpatasvir**. Avoid. Severe Study
- **Bosentan** is predicted to decrease the exposure to **velpatasvir**. Avoid. Moderate Theoretical
- Calcium salts **(calcium carbonate)** are predicted to decrease the concentration of **velpatasvir**. Separate administration by 4 hours. Moderate Anecdotal
- **Velpatasvir** is predicted to increase the exposure to **colchicine**. Severe Theoretical
- **Velpatasvir** increases the exposure to **dabigatran**. Avoid. Severe Study
- **Velpatasvir** is predicted to increase the exposure to **digoxin**. Severe Study
- **Velpatasvir** is predicted to increase the exposure to **edoxaban**. Severe Theoretical
- **Efavirenz** is predicted to decrease the exposure to **velpatasvir**. Avoid. Moderate Theoretical
- **Enzalutamide** is predicted to moderately decrease the exposure to **velpatasvir**. Avoid. Severe Study
- **Velpatasvir** is predicted to increase the exposure to **everolimus**. Severe Theoretical
- **H_2 receptor antagonists** are predicted to decrease the concentration of **velpatasvir**. Adjust dose, see sofosbuvir with velpatasvir. Moderate Study

- HIV-protease inhibitors **(tipranavir)** are predicted to increase the exposure to **velpatasvir**. Severe Theoretical
- **Velpatasvir** is predicted to increase the exposure to **loperamide**. Severe Theoretical
- **Mitotane** is predicted to moderately decrease the exposure to **velpatasvir**. Avoid. Severe Study
- **Modafinil** is predicted to decrease the exposure to **velpatasvir**. Avoid. Severe Theoretical
- **Nevirapine** is predicted to decrease the exposure to **velpatasvir**. Avoid. Moderate Theoretical
- **Proton pump inhibitors** are predicted to decrease the concentration of **velpatasvir**. Adjust dose, see sofosbuvir with velpatasvir. Moderate Study
- **Rifampicin** is predicted to moderately decrease the exposure to **velpatasvir**. Avoid. Severe Study
- **Velpatasvir** is predicted to increase the exposure to **sirolimus**. Severe Theoretical
- **St John's Wort** is predicted to decrease the exposure to **velpatasvir**. Avoid. Moderate Theoretical
- **Velpatasvir** increases the exposure to statins **(rosuvastatin)**. Adjust **rosuvastatin** dose and monitor side effects, p. 140. Severe Study
- **Velpatasvir** is predicted to increase the exposure to statins **(simvastatin)**. Monitor side effects and adjust dose. Severe Theoretical
- **Velpatasvir** is predicted to increase the exposure to **sulfasalazine**. Moderate Theoretical
- **Velpatasvir** is predicted to increase the exposure to taxanes **(paclitaxel)**. Severe Theoretical
- **Velpatasvir** is predicted to increase the exposure to **tenofovir disoproxil**. Severe Study
- **Velpatasvir** is predicted to increase the exposure to **topotecan**. Severe Theoretical

Vemurafenib → see **TABLE 9** p. 909 (QT-interval prolongation)

- **Vemurafenib** is predicted to increase the exposure to **afatinib**. Separate administration by 12 hours. Moderate Study
- **Vemurafenib** is predicted to increase the exposure to **aliskiren**. Use with caution and adjust dose. Moderate Theoretical
- Antiepileptics **(carbamazepine, fosphenytoin, phenobarbital, phenytoin, primidone)** are predicted to decrease the exposure to **vemurafenib**. Avoid. Severe Theoretical
- Antifungals, azoles **(itraconazole, ketoconazole, voriconazole)** are predicted to increase the exposure to **vemurafenib**. Severe Theoretical → Also see **TABLE 9** p. 909
- **Apalutamide** is predicted to decrease the exposure to **vemurafenib**. Avoid. Severe Theoretical → Also see **TABLE 9** p. 909
- **Vemurafenib** is predicted to increase the exposure to beta blockers, non-selective **(nadolol)**. Moderate Study
- **Vemurafenib** is predicted to increase the exposure to **bictegravir**. Use with caution or avoid. Moderate Theoretical
- **Cobicistat** is predicted to increase the exposure to **vemurafenib**. Severe Theoretical
- **Vemurafenib** is predicted to increase the exposure to **colchicine**. Avoid P-glycoprotein inhibitors or adjust **colchicine** dose. Severe Theoretical
- **Vemurafenib** increases the exposure to **dabigatran**. Use with caution and adjust dose. Severe Theoretical
- **Vemurafenib** is predicted to slightly increase the exposure to **edoxaban**. Severe Theoretical
- **Enzalutamide** is predicted to decrease the exposure to **vemurafenib**. Avoid. Severe Theoretical
- **Vemurafenib** is predicted to increase the exposure to **erlotinib**. Moderate Theoretical
- **Vemurafenib** is predicted to increase the exposure to **fidaxomicin**. Avoid. Moderate Study
- **HIV-protease inhibitors** are predicted to increase the exposure to **vemurafenib**. Severe Theoretical → Also see **TABLE 9** p. 909
- **Idelalisib** is predicted to increase the exposure to **vemurafenib**. Severe Theoretical
- **Vemurafenib** is predicted to increase the exposure to **larotrectinib**. Mild Theoretical
- Macrolides **(clarithromycin)** are predicted to increase the exposure to **vemurafenib**. Severe Theoretical → Also see **TABLE 9** p. 909
- **Mitotane** is predicted to decrease the exposure to **vemurafenib**. Avoid. Severe Theoretical
- **Vemurafenib** is predicted to increase the exposure to **naldemedine**. Moderate Study
- **Vemurafenib** is predicted to increase the exposure to **nintedanib**. Moderate Study
- **Vemurafenib** is predicted to increase the exposure to **panobinostat**. Adjust dose. Moderate Theoretical → Also see **TABLE 9** p. 909
- **Vemurafenib** is predicted to increase the exposure to **pibrentasvir**. Moderate Theoretical
- **Rifampicin** is predicted to decrease the exposure to **vemurafenib**. Avoid. Severe Theoretical
- **Vemurafenib** is predicted to slightly increase the exposure to **talazoparib**. Avoid or adjust **talazoparib** dose. Severe Study
- **Vemurafenib** is predicted to increase the exposure to **ticagrelor**. Use with caution or avoid. Severe Study
- **Vemurafenib** is predicted to increase the exposure to **topotecan**. Severe Study
- **Vemurafenib** is predicted to increase the concentration of **trametinib**. Moderate Theoretical
- **Vemurafenib** is predicted to increase the exposure to **venetoclax**. Avoid or monitor for toxicity. Severe Theoretical

Venetoclax

FOOD AND LIFESTYLE Avoid Seville (bitter orange) and star fruit as they might increase the exposure to venetoclax.

- Antiarrhythmics **(amiodarone)** are predicted to increase the exposure to **venetoclax**. Avoid or monitor for toxicity. Severe Theoretical
- Antiarrhythmics **(dronedarone)** are predicted to increase the exposure to **venetoclax**. Avoid or adjust dose—consult product literature. Severe Study
- Antiepileptics **(carbamazepine, fosphenytoin, phenobarbital, phenytoin, primidone)** are predicted to decrease the exposure to **venetoclax**. Avoid. Severe Study
- Antifungals, azoles **(fluconazole, isavuconazole, itraconazole, ketoconazole, posaconazole, voriconazole)** are predicted to increase the exposure to **venetoclax**. Avoid or adjust dose—consult product literature. Severe Study
- **Venetoclax** is predicted to increase the exposure to antihistamines, non-sedating **(fexofenadine)**. Moderate Theoretical
- **Apalutamide** is predicted to decrease the exposure to **venetoclax**. Avoid. Severe Study
- **Aprepitant** is predicted to increase the exposure to **venetoclax**. Avoid or adjust dose—consult product literature. Severe Study
- **Bosentan** is predicted to decrease the exposure to **venetoclax**. Avoid. Severe Study
- **Venetoclax** is predicted to increase the exposure to **bosentan**. Moderate Theoretical
- Calcium channel blockers **(diltiazem, verapamil)** are predicted to increase the exposure to **venetoclax**. Avoid or adjust dose—consult product literature. Severe Study
- **Ciclosporin** is predicted to increase the exposure to **venetoclax**. Avoid or monitor for toxicity. Severe Theoretical
- **Cobicistat** is predicted to increase the exposure to **venetoclax**. Avoid or adjust dose—consult product literature. Severe Study
- **Venetoclax** slightly increases the exposure to coumarins **(warfarin)**. Moderate Study
- **Crizotinib** is predicted to increase the exposure to **venetoclax**. Avoid or adjust dose—consult product literature. Severe Study
- **Venetoclax** is predicted to increase the exposure to **dabigatran**. Avoid or adjust dose. Severe Study
- **Venetoclax** increases the exposure to **digoxin**. Avoid or adjust dose. Severe Study
- **Efavirenz** is predicted to decrease the exposure to **venetoclax**. Avoid. Severe Study
- **Enzalutamide** is predicted to decrease the exposure to **venetoclax**. Avoid. Severe Study
- **Venetoclax** is predicted to increase the exposure to **everolimus**. Avoid or adjust dose. Severe Study
- **Grapefruit juice** is predicted to increase the exposure to **venetoclax**. Avoid. Severe Theoretical
- **HIV-protease inhibitors** are predicted to increase the exposure to **venetoclax**. Avoid or adjust dose—consult product literature. Severe Study

Venetoclax (continued)

- **Idelalisib** is predicted to increase the exposure to **venetoclax**. Avoid or adjust dose—consult product literature. Severe Study
- **Imatinib** is predicted to increase the exposure to **venetoclax**. Avoid or adjust dose—consult product literature. Severe Study
- **Lapatinib** is predicted to increase the exposure to **venetoclax**. Avoid or monitor for toxicity. Severe Theoretical
- **Venetoclax** potentially decreases the efficacy of **live vaccines**. Avoid. Severe Theoretical
- Macrolides **(clarithromycin, erythromycin)** are predicted to increase the exposure to **venetoclax**. Avoid or adjust dose—consult product literature. Severe Study
- **Mitotane** is predicted to decrease the exposure to **venetoclax**. Avoid. Severe Study
- **Netupitant** is predicted to increase the exposure to **venetoclax**. Avoid or adjust dose—consult product literature. Severe Study
- **Nevirapine** is predicted to decrease the exposure to **venetoclax**. Avoid. Severe Study
- **Nilotinib** is predicted to increase the exposure to **venetoclax**. Avoid or adjust dose—consult product literature. Severe Study
- **Ranolazine** is predicted to increase the exposure to **venetoclax**. Avoid or monitor for toxicity. Severe Theoretical
- **Venetoclax** is predicted to increase the exposure to **repaglinide**. Moderate Theoretical
- **Rifampicin** is predicted to decrease the exposure to **venetoclax**. Avoid. Severe Study
- **Venetoclax** is predicted to increase the exposure to **sirolimus**. Avoid or adjust dose. Severe Study
- **St John's Wort** is predicted to decrease the exposure to **venetoclax**. Avoid. Severe Study
- **Venetoclax** is predicted to increase the exposure to statins **(atorvastatin)**. Moderate Study
- **Venetoclax** is predicted to increase the exposure to statins **(fluvastatin, pravastatin, rosuvastatin, simvastatin)**. Moderate Theoretical
- **Venetoclax** is predicted to increase the exposure to **sulfasalazine**. Moderate Theoretical
- **Venetoclax** is predicted to increase the exposure to sulfonylureas **(glibenclamide)**. Moderate Theoretical
- **Venetoclax** is predicted to increase the exposure to **topotecan**. Moderate Theoretical
- **Vemurafenib** is predicted to increase the exposure to **venetoclax**. Avoid or monitor for toxicity. Severe Theoretical

Venlafaxine → see **TABLE 13** p. 910 (serotonin syndrome), **TABLE 9** p. 909 (QT-interval prolongation), **TABLE 11** p. 909 (CNS depressant effects), **TABLE 4** p. 907 (antiplatelet effects)

- Antifungals, azoles **(itraconazole, ketoconazole, voriconazole)** are predicted to increase the exposure to **venlafaxine**. Moderate Study → Also see **TABLE 9** p. 909
- **Cobicistat** is predicted to increase the exposure to **venlafaxine**. Moderate Study
- H_2 receptor antagonists **(cimetidine)** slightly increase the exposure to **venlafaxine**. Mild Study
- **Venlafaxine** slightly increases the exposure to **haloperidol**. Severe Study → Also see **TABLE 9** p. 909 → Also see **TABLE 11** p. 909
- **HIV-protease inhibitors** are predicted to increase the exposure to **venlafaxine**. Moderate Study → Also see **TABLE 9** p. 909
- **Idelalisib** is predicted to increase the exposure to **venlafaxine**. Moderate Study
- Macrolides **(clarithromycin)** are predicted to increase the exposure to **venlafaxine**. Moderate Study → Also see **TABLE 9** p. 909
- **Venlafaxine** is predicted to increase the exposure to **pitolisant**. Use with caution and adjust dose. Mild Theoretical
- **Tacrolimus** potentially increases the risk of serotonin syndrome when given with **venlafaxine**. Severe Anecdotal
- **Vaborbactam** is predicted to increase the concentration of **venlafaxine**. Unknown Theoretical

Verapamil → see calcium channel blockers

Vernakalant → see antiarrhythmics

Verteporfin

GENERAL INFORMATION Caution on concurrent use with other photosensitising drugs.

Vigabatrin → see antiepileptics

Vilanterol → see beta$_2$ agonists

Vildagliptin → see **TABLE 14** p. 910 (antidiabetic drugs)

Vinblastine → see vinca alkaloids

Vinca alkaloids → see **TABLE 1** p. 907 (hepatotoxicity), **TABLE 15** p. 910 (myelosuppression), **TABLE 19** p. 911 (ototoxicity), **TABLE 12** p. 910 (peripheral neuropathy), **TABLE 5** p. 907 (thromboembolism), **TABLE 9** p. 909 (QT-interval prolongation)

vinblastine · vincristine · vindesine · vinflunine · vinorelbine

- Antiarrhythmics **(dronedarone)** are predicted to increase the exposure to **vinca alkaloids**. Severe Theoretical → Also see **TABLE 9** p. 909
- Antiepileptics **(carbamazepine, fosphenytoin, phenobarbital, phenytoin, primidone)** are predicted to decrease the exposure to **vinflunine**. Avoid. Severe Theoretical → Also see **TABLE 12** p. 910
- Antiepileptics **(carbamazepine, fosphenytoin, phenobarbital, phenytoin, primidone)** are predicted to decrease the exposure to **vinorelbine**. Use with caution or avoid. Severe Theoretical → Also see **TABLE 12** p. 910
- Antiepileptics **(carbamazepine, fosphenytoin, phenobarbital, phenytoin, primidone)** are predicted to decrease the exposure to vinca alkaloids **(vinblastine, vincristine, vindesine)**. Severe Theoretical → Also see **TABLE 1** p. 907 → Also see **TABLE 12** p. 910
- Antifungals, azoles **(fluconazole, isavuconazole, itraconazole, ketoconazole, posaconazole, voriconazole)** are predicted to increase the exposure to **vinca alkaloids**. Severe Theoretical → Also see **TABLE 1** p. 907 → Also see **TABLE 9** p. 909
- Antifungals, azoles **(miconazole)** are predicted to increase the concentration of **vinca alkaloids**. Use with caution and adjust dose. Moderate Theoretical
- **Apalutamide** is predicted to decrease the exposure to vinca alkaloids **(vinblastine, vincristine, vindesine)**. Severe Theoretical
- **Apalutamide** is predicted to decrease the exposure to **vinflunine**. Avoid. Severe Theoretical → Also see **TABLE 9** p. 909
- **Apalutamide** is predicted to decrease the exposure to **vinorelbine**. Use with caution or avoid. Severe Theoretical
- **Aprepitant** is predicted to increase the exposure to **vinca alkaloids**. Severe Theoretical
- **Asparaginase** potentially increases the risk of neurotoxicity when given with **vincristine**. **Vincristine** should be taken 3 to 24 hours before **asparaginase**. Severe Anecdotal → Also see **TABLE 1** p. 907 → Also see **TABLE 15** p. 910
- Calcium channel blockers **(diltiazem, verapamil)** are predicted to increase the exposure to **vinca alkaloids**. Severe Theoretical
- **Cobicistat** is predicted to increase the exposure to **vinca alkaloids**. Severe Theoretical
- **Crisantaspase** potentially increases the risk of neurotoxicity when given with **vincristine**. **Vincristine** should be taken 3 to 24 hours before **crisantaspase**. Severe Anecdotal → Also see **TABLE 1** p. 907 → Also see **TABLE 15** p. 910
- **Crizotinib** is predicted to increase the exposure to **vinca alkaloids**. Severe Theoretical → Also see **TABLE 15** p. 910 → Also see **TABLE 9** p. 909
- **Enzalutamide** is predicted to decrease the exposure to vinca alkaloids **(vinblastine, vincristine, vindesine)**. Severe Theoretical
- **Enzalutamide** is predicted to decrease the exposure to **vinflunine**. Avoid. Severe Theoretical
- **Enzalutamide** is predicted to decrease the exposure to **vinorelbine**. Use with caution or avoid. Severe Theoretical
- **Fosaprepitant** is predicted to increase the exposure to **vinca alkaloids**. Severe Theoretical
- **HIV-protease inhibitors** are predicted to increase the exposure to **vinca alkaloids**. Severe Theoretical → Also see **TABLE 9** p. 909
- **Idelalisib** is predicted to increase the exposure to **vinca alkaloids**. Severe Theoretical → Also see **TABLE 15** p. 910
- **Imatinib** is predicted to increase the exposure to **vinca alkaloids**. Severe Theoretical → Also see **TABLE 15** p. 910
- **Live vaccines** are predicted to increase the risk of generalised infection (possibly life-threatening) when given with **vinca alkaloids**. Public Health England advises avoid (refer to Green Book). Severe Theoretical
- Macrolides **(clarithromycin, erythromycin)** are predicted to increase the exposure to **vinca alkaloids**. Severe Theoretical → Also see **TABLE 9** p. 909
- **Mitotane** is predicted to decrease the exposure to vinca alkaloids **(vinblastine, vincristine, vindesine)**. Severe Theoretical → Also see **TABLE 15** p. 910

- Mitotane is predicted to decrease the exposure to **vinflunine**. Avoid. Severe Theoretical → Also see TABLE 15 p. 910
- Mitotane is predicted to decrease the exposure to **vinorelbine**. Use with caution or avoid. Severe Theoretical → Also see TABLE 15 p. 910
- Netupitant is predicted to increase the exposure to **vinca alkaloids**. Severe Theoretical
- Nilotinib is predicted to increase the exposure to **vinca alkaloids**. Severe Theoretical → Also see TABLE 15 p. 910 → Also see TABLE 9 p. 909
- Pegaspargase potentially increases the risk of neurotoxicity when given with **vincristine**. **Vincristine** should be taken 3 to 24 hours before **pegaspargase**, p. 594, p. 597. Severe Anecdotal → Also see TABLE 1 p. 907 → Also see TABLE 15 p. 910
- Rifampicin is predicted to decrease the exposure to vinca alkaloids **(vinblastine, vincristine, vindesine)**. Severe Theoretical
- Rifampicin is predicted to decrease the exposure to **vinflunine**. Avoid. Severe Theoretical
- Rifampicin is predicted to decrease the exposure to **vinorelbine**. Use with caution or avoid. Severe Theoretical

Vincristine → see vinca alkaloids
Vindesine → see vinca alkaloids
Vinflunine → see vinca alkaloids
Vinorelbine → see vinca alkaloids
Vismodegib → see TABLE 15 p. 910 (myelosuppression)

- Antiepileptics **(carbamazepine, fosphenytoin, phenobarbital, phenytoin, primidone)** are predicted to decrease the exposure to **vismodegib**. Avoid. Moderate Theoretical
- Apalutamide is predicted to decrease the exposure to **vismodegib**. Avoid. Moderate Theoretical
- Enzalutamide is predicted to decrease the exposure to **vismodegib**. Avoid. Moderate Theoretical
- Mitotane is predicted to decrease the exposure to **vismodegib**. Avoid. Moderate Theoretical → Also see TABLE 15 p. 910
- Rifampicin is predicted to decrease the exposure to **vismodegib**. Avoid. Moderate Theoretical
- St John's Wort is predicted to decrease the exposure to **vismodegib**. Avoid. Moderate Theoretical

Vitamin A

- Retinoids **(acitretin, alitretinoin, isotretinoin)** are predicted to increase the risk of vitamin A toxicity when given with **vitamin A**. Avoid. Severe Theoretical
- Retinoids **(bexarotene)** are predicted to increase the risk of toxicity when given with **vitamin A**. Adjust dose. Moderate Theoretical
- Retinoids **(tretinoin)** are predicted to increase the risk of vitamin A toxicity when given with **vitamin A**. Avoid. Severe Study

Vitamin D substances

alfacalcidol · calcipotriol · calcitriol · colecalciferol · dihydrotachysterol · ergocalciferol · paricalcitol · tacalcitol

ROUTE-SPECIFIC INFORMATION Since systemic absorption can follow topical application, the possibility of interactions with topical **calcitriol** should be borne in mind.

- Antiepileptics **(carbamazepine)** are predicted to decrease the effects of **vitamin D substances**. Moderate Study
- Antiepileptics **(fosphenytoin, phenytoin)** decrease the effects of **vitamin D substances**. Moderate Study
- Antiepileptics **(phenobarbital, primidone)** are predicted to decrease the effects of **vitamin D substances**. Moderate Theoretical
- Antifungals, azoles **(clotrimazole, ketoconazole)** are predicted to decrease the exposure to **colecalciferol**. Moderate Theoretical
- Antifungals, azoles **(itraconazole, ketoconazole, voriconazole)** are predicted to increase the exposure to **paricalcitol**. Moderate Study
- Cobicistat is predicted to increase the exposure to **paricalcitol**. Moderate Study
- **Vitamin D substances** are predicted to increase the risk of toxicity when given with **digoxin**. Severe Theoretical
- HIV-protease inhibitors are predicted to increase the exposure to **paricalcitol**. Moderate Study
- Idelalisib is predicted to increase the exposure to **paricalcitol**. Moderate Study
- Macrolides **(clarithromycin)** are predicted to increase the exposure to **paricalcitol**. Moderate Study
- Thiazide diuretics increase the risk of hypercalcaemia when given with **vitamin D substances**. Moderate Theoretical

Vitamin E substances

alpha tocopherol · alpha tocopheryl acetate

- **Vitamin E substances** affect the exposure to **ciclosporin**. Moderate Study

Volanesorsen

- **Volanesorsen** potentially increases the risk of bleeding events when given with **drugs with anticoagulant effects** (see TABLE 3 p. 907). Avoid depending on platelet count—consult product literature. Severe Theoretical
- **Volanesorsen** potentially increases the risk of bleeding events when given with **drugs with antiplatelet effects** (see TABLE 4 p. 907). Avoid depending on platelet count—consult product literature. Severe Theoretical

Volatile halogenated anaesthetics → see TABLE 8 p. 908 (hypotension), TABLE 11 p. 909 (CNS depressant effects)

desflurane · isoflurane · methoxyflurane · sevoflurane

- Antiepileptics **(phenobarbital, primidone)** potentially increase the risk of nephrotoxicity when given with **methoxyflurane**. Avoid. Severe Theoretical → Also see TABLE 11 p. 909
- Isoniazid potentially increases the risk of nephrotoxicity when given with **methoxyflurane**. Avoid. Severe Theoretical
- Rifampicin potentially increases the risk of nephrotoxicity when given with **methoxyflurane**. Avoid. Severe Theoretical

Voriconazole → see antifungals, azoles
Vortioxetine → see TABLE 13 p. 910 (serotonin syndrome), TABLE 4 p. 907 (antiplatelet effects)

- Antiepileptics **(carbamazepine, fosphenytoin, phenobarbital, phenytoin, primidone)** are predicted to decrease the exposure to **vortioxetine**. Monitor and adjust dose. Moderate Study
- Apalutamide is predicted to decrease the exposure to **vortioxetine**. Monitor and adjust dose. Moderate Study
- Bupropion is predicted to increase the exposure to **vortioxetine**. Monitor and adjust dose. Moderate Study → Also see TABLE 13 p. 910
- Cinacalcet is predicted to increase the exposure to **vortioxetine**. Monitor and adjust dose. Moderate Study
- Enzalutamide is predicted to decrease the exposure to **vortioxetine**. Monitor and adjust dose. Moderate Study
- Mitotane is predicted to decrease the exposure to **vortioxetine**. Monitor and adjust dose. Moderate Study
- Rifampicin is predicted to decrease the exposure to **vortioxetine**. Monitor and adjust dose. Moderate Study
- SSRIs **(fluoxetine, paroxetine)** are predicted to increase the exposure to **vortioxetine**. Monitor and adjust dose. Moderate Study → Also see TABLE 13 p. 910 → Also see TABLE 4 p. 907
- Terbinafine is predicted to increase the exposure to **vortioxetine**. Monitor and adjust dose. Moderate Study

Voxilaprevir

- Antiepileptics **(carbamazepine, fosphenytoin, phenobarbital, phenytoin, primidone)** are predicted to decrease the concentration of **voxilaprevir**. Avoid. Severe Study
- Antiepileptics **(oxcarbazepine)** are predicted to decrease the concentration of **voxilaprevir**. Avoid. Severe Theoretical
- Apalutamide is predicted to decrease the concentration of **voxilaprevir**. Avoid. Severe Study
- Bosentan is predicted to decrease the concentration of **voxilaprevir**. Avoid. Severe Theoretical
- Ciclosporin increases the concentration of **voxilaprevir**. Avoid. Severe Study
- Combined hormonal contraceptives (containing ethinylestradiol) are predicted to increase the risk of increased ALT concentrations when given with **voxilaprevir** (with sofosbuvir and velpatasvir). Avoid. Severe Study
- **Voxilaprevir** (with sofosbuvir and velpatasvir) increases the concentration of dabigatran. Avoid. Severe Study
- **Voxilaprevir** (with sofosbuvir and velpatasvir) is predicted to increase the exposure to digoxin. Monitor and adjust dose. Severe Theoretical

Voxilaprevir (continued)
- **Voxilaprevir** (with sofosbuvir and velpatasvir) is predicted to increase the concentration of **edoxaban**. Avoid. Severe Theoretical
- Efavirenz is predicted to decrease the concentration of **voxilaprevir**. Avoid. Severe Theoretical
- Enzalutamide is predicted to decrease the concentration of **voxilaprevir**. Avoid. Severe Study
- HIV-protease inhibitors **(atazanavir)** boosted with ritonavir increase the concentration of **voxilaprevir**. Avoid. Severe Study
- HIV-protease inhibitors **(lopinavir)** boosted with ritonavir are predicted to increase the concentration of **voxilaprevir**. Avoid. Severe Theoretical
- HIV-protease inhibitors **(tipranavir)** boosted with ritonavir are predicted to increase the concentration of **voxilaprevir**. Severe Theoretical
- **Mitotane** is predicted to decrease the concentration of **voxilaprevir**. Avoid. Severe Study
- **Modafinil** is predicted to decrease the concentration of **voxilaprevir**. Avoid. Severe Theoretical
- **Nevirapine** is predicted to decrease the concentration of **voxilaprevir**. Avoid. Severe Theoretical
- **Proton pump inhibitors** are predicted to decrease the exposure to **voxilaprevir**. Adjust dose, see sofosbuvir with velpatasvir and voxilaprevir. Moderate Study
- **Rifabutin** is predicted to decrease the concentration of **voxilaprevir**. Avoid. Severe Theoretical
- **Rifampicin** is predicted to decrease the concentration of **voxilaprevir**. Avoid. Severe Study
- **St John's Wort** is predicted to decrease the concentration of **voxilaprevir**. Avoid. Severe Theoretical
- **Voxilaprevir** (with sofosbuvir and velpatasvir) is predicted to increase the exposure to statins **(atorvastatin)**. Adjust **atorvastatin** dose, p. 139. Moderate Theoretical
- **Voxilaprevir** (with sofosbuvir and velpatasvir) is predicted to increase the exposure to statins **(fluvastatin, simvastatin)**. Avoid. Moderate Theoretical
- **Voxilaprevir** (with sofosbuvir and velpatasvir) moderately increases the exposure to statins **(pravastatin)**. Monitor and adjust **pravastatin** dose. Moderate Study
- **Voxilaprevir** (with sofosbuvir and velpatasvir) markedly increases the exposure to statins **(rosuvastatin)**. Avoid. Severe Study
- **Voxilaprevir** is predicted to increase the concentration of **sulfasalazine**. Avoid. Severe Theoretical
- **Voxilaprevir** (with sofosbuvir and velpatasvir) potentially increases the concentration of **tenofovir disoproxil**. Severe Study
- **Voxilaprevir** is predicted to increase the concentration of **topotecan**. Avoid. Severe Theoretical

Warfarin → see coumarins

Wasp venom extract

GENERAL INFORMATION Desensitising vaccines should be avoided in patients taking beta-blockers (adrenaline might be ineffective in case of a hypersensitivity reaction) or ACE inhibitors (risk of severe anaphylactoid reactions).

Xipamide → see thiazide diuretics

Xylometazoline → see sympathomimetics, vasoconstrictor

Yellow fever vaccine, live → see live vaccines

Zidovudine → see TABLE 15 p. 910 (myelosuppression), TABLE 2 p. 907 (nephrotoxicity)
- Antiepileptics **(valproate)** slightly increase the exposure to **zidovudine**. Moderate Study
- Antifungals, azoles **(fluconazole)** slightly increase the exposure to **zidovudine**. Moderate Study
- Antimalarials **(pyrimethamine)** are predicted to increase the risk of side-effects when given with **zidovudine**. Severe Theoretical → Also see TABLE 15 p. 910
- **Zidovudine** increases the risk of haematological toxicity when given with **aspirin (high-dose)**. Severe Study
- **Zidovudine** increases the risk of haematological toxicity when given with **flucytosine**. Monitor and adjust dose. Severe Theoretical
- HIV-protease inhibitors **(tipranavir)** slightly decrease the exposure to **zidovudine**. Avoid. Moderate Study
- **Zidovudine** increases the risk of toxicity when given with **lamivudine**. Severe Anecdotal
- **Leflunomide** is predicted to increase the exposure to **zidovudine**. Moderate Theoretical → Also see TABLE 15 p. 910
- Macrolides **(clarithromycin)** decrease the absorption of **zidovudine**. Separate administration by at least 2 hours. Moderate Study
- **Nevirapine** is predicted to decrease the concentration of **zidovudine**. Refer to specialist literature. Severe Theoretical
- **Zidovudine** increases the risk of haematological toxicity when given with **NSAIDs**. Severe Study → Also see TABLE 2 p. 907
- **Ribavirin** increases the risk of anaemia and/or leucopenia when given with **zidovudine**. Avoid. Severe Study
- **Zidovudine** is predicted to decrease the efficacy of **stavudine**. Avoid. Severe Theoretical
- **Teriflunomide** is predicted to increase the exposure to **zidovudine**. Moderate Theoretical

Zinc

ROUTE-SPECIFIC INFORMATION Interactions do not generally apply to topical use unless specified.

- Oral **zinc** decreases the absorption of oral bisphosphonates **(alendronate)**. **Alendronate** should be taken at least 30 minutes before **zinc** . Moderate Study
- Oral **zinc** decreases the absorption of oral bisphosphonates **(clodronate)**. Avoid **zinc** for 2 hours before or 1 hour after **clodronate**. Moderate Study
- Oral **zinc** is predicted to decrease the absorption of oral bisphosphonates **(ibandronate)**. Avoid **zinc** for at least 6 hours before or 1 hour after **ibandronate**. Moderate Theoretical
- Oral **zinc** decreases the absorption of oral bisphosphonates **(risedronate)**. Separate administration by at least 2 hours. Moderate Study
- Oral **calcium salts** decrease the absorption of **zinc**. Moderate Study
- Oral **zinc** is predicted to decrease the absorption of **eltrombopag**. **Eltrombopag** should be taken 2 hours before or 4 hours after **zinc** . Severe Theoretical
- **Zinc** is predicted to decrease the efficacy of **iron (oral)** and **iron (oral)** is predicted to decrease the efficacy of **zinc**. Moderate Study
- Oral **zinc** is predicted to decrease the absorption of oral iron chelators **(deferiprone)**. Moderate Theoretical
- **Zinc** is predicted to decrease the absorption of **penicillamine**. Mild Theoretical
- **Zinc** is predicted to decrease the exposure to **quinolones**. Separate administration by 2 hours. Moderate Study
- Oral **zinc** is predicted to decrease the absorption of **tetracyclines**. Separate administration by 2 to 3 hours. Moderate Theoretical
- **Trientine** potentially decreases the absorption of **zinc**. Moderate Theoretical

Zoledronate → see bisphosphonates

Zolmitriptan → see TABLE 13 p. 910 (serotonin syndrome)
- **Combined hormonal contraceptives** are predicted to increase the exposure to **zolmitriptan**. Adjust **zolmitriptan** dose, p. 310. Moderate Theoretical
- **Zolmitriptan** is predicted to increase the risk of vasoconstriction when given with **ergotamine**. **Ergotamine** should be taken at least 24 hours before or 6 hours after **zolmitriptan**, p. 310. Severe Theoretical
- H_2 receptor antagonists **(cimetidine)** slightly increase the exposure to **zolmitriptan**. Adjust **zolmitriptan** dose, p. 310. Mild Study
- **MAOIs, irreversible** are predicted to increase the exposure to **zolmitriptan**. Severe Theoretical → Also see TABLE 13 p. 910
- **Mexiletine** is predicted to increase the exposure to **zolmitriptan**. Adjust **zolmitriptan** dose, p. 310. Moderate Theoretical
- **Moclobemide** slightly increases the exposure to **zolmitriptan**. Adjust **zolmitriptan** dose, p. 310. Moderate Study → Also see TABLE 13 p. 910
- Quinolones **(ciprofloxacin)** are predicted to increase the exposure to **zolmitriptan**. Adjust **zolmitriptan** dose, p. 310. Moderate Theoretical

A1 Interactions | Appendix 1

- SSRIs (fluvoxamine) are predicted to increase the exposure to **zolmitriptan**. Adjust **zolmitriptan** dose, p. 310. [Severe] Theoretical → Also see **TABLE 13** p. 910

Zolpidem → see **TABLE 11** p. 909 (CNS depressant effects)

- Antiepileptics **(carbamazepine)** moderately decrease the exposure to **zolpidem**. [Moderate] Study
- Rifampicin moderately decreases the exposure to **zolpidem**. [Moderate] Study

Zonisamide → see antiepileptics

Zopiclone → see **TABLE 11** p. 909 (CNS depressant effects)

- Antiarrhythmics **(dronedarone)** are predicted to increase the exposure to **zopiclone**. Adjust dose. [Moderate] Study
- Antiepileptics **(carbamazepine, fosphenytoin, phenobarbital, phenytoin, primidone)** are predicted to decrease the exposure to **zopiclone**. Adjust dose. [Moderate] Study → Also see **TABLE 11** p. 909
- Antifungals, azoles **(fluconazole, isavuconazole, posaconazole)** are predicted to increase the exposure to **zopiclone**. Adjust dose. [Moderate] Study
- Antifungals, azoles **(itraconazole, ketoconazole, voriconazole)** are predicted to increase the exposure to **zopiclone**. Adjust dose. [Moderate] Theoretical
- Apalutamide is predicted to decrease the exposure to **zopiclone**. Adjust dose. [Moderate] Study
- Aprepitant is predicted to increase the exposure to **zopiclone**. Adjust dose. [Moderate] Study
- Calcium channel blockers **(diltiazem, verapamil)** are predicted to increase the exposure to **zopiclone**. Adjust dose. [Moderate] Study
- Cobicistat is predicted to increase the exposure to **zopiclone**. Adjust dose. [Moderate] Theoretical
- Crizotinib is predicted to increase the exposure to **zopiclone**. Adjust dose. [Moderate] Study
- Enzalutamide is predicted to decrease the exposure to **zopiclone**. Adjust dose. [Moderate] Study
- HIV-protease inhibitors are predicted to increase the exposure to **zopiclone**. Adjust dose. [Moderate] Theoretical
- Idelalisib is predicted to increase the exposure to **zopiclone**. Adjust dose. [Moderate] Theoretical
- Imatinib is predicted to increase the exposure to **zopiclone**. Adjust dose. [Moderate] Study
- Macrolides **(clarithromycin)** are predicted to increase the exposure to **zopiclone**. Adjust dose. [Moderate] Theoretical
- Macrolides **(erythromycin)** are predicted to increase the exposure to **zopiclone**. Adjust dose. [Moderate] Study
- Mitotane is predicted to decrease the exposure to **zopiclone**. Adjust dose. [Moderate] Study
- Netupitant is predicted to increase the exposure to **zopiclone**. Adjust dose. [Moderate] Study
- Nilotinib is predicted to increase the exposure to **zopiclone**. Adjust dose. [Moderate] Study
- Rifampicin is predicted to decrease the exposure to **zopiclone**. Adjust dose. [Moderate] Study

Zuclopenthixol → see **TABLE 8** p. 908 (hypotension), **TABLE 9** p. 909 (QT-interval prolongation), **TABLE 11** p. 909 (CNS depressant effects)

- **Zuclopenthixol** is predicted to decrease the effects of dopamine receptor agonists. Avoid. [Moderate] Theoretical → Also see **TABLE 8** p. 908 → Also see **TABLE 9** p. 909
- **Zuclopenthixol** is predicted to decrease the effects of levodopa. Avoid or monitor worsening parkinsonian symptoms. [Severe] Theoretical → Also see **TABLE 8** p. 908
- **Zuclopenthixol** potentially increases the risk of neurotoxicity when given with lithium. [Severe] Anecdotal → Also see **TABLE 9** p. 909

Appendix 2
Borderline substances

CONTENTS

In certain conditions some foods (and toilet preparations) have characteristics of drugs and the Advisory Committee on Borderline Substances (ACBS) advises as to the circumstances in which such substances may be regarded as drugs. Prescriptions issued in accordance with the Committee's advice and endorsed 'ACBS' will normally not be investigated.

Information

General Practitioners are reminded that the ACBS recommends products on the basis that they may be regarded as drugs for the management of specified conditions. Doctors should satisfy themselves that the products can safely be prescribed, that patients are adequately monitored and that, where necessary, expert hospital supervision is available.

Foods which may be prescribed on FP10, GP10 (Scotland), or WP10 (Wales)

All the food products listed in this appendix have ACBS approval. Some products may not be approved in all three countries. The clinical condition for which the product has been approved is included with each entry.

Note Foods included in this appendix may contain cariogenic sugars and patients should be advised to take appropriate oral hygiene measures.

Enteral feeds and supplements

For most enteral feeds and nutritional supplements, the main source of **carbohydrate** is either maltodextrin or glucose syrup; other carbohydrate sources are listed in the relevant table, below. Feeds containing residual lactose (less than 1 g lactose/100 mL formula) are described as 'clinically lactose-free' or 'lactose-free' by some manufacturers. The presence of lactose (including residual lactose) in feeds is indicated in the relevant table, below. The primary sources of **protein** or **amino acids** are included with each product entry. The **fat** or **oil** content is derived from a variety of sources such as vegetables, soya bean, corn, palm nuts, and seeds; where the fat content is derived from animal or fish sources, this information is included in the relevant table, below. The presence of medium chain triglycerides (MCT) is also noted where the quantity exceeds 30% of the fat content.

Enteral feeds and nutritional supplements can contain varying amounts of **vitamins, minerals**, and **trace elements**—the manufacturer's product literature should be consulted for more detailed information. Feeds containing vitamin K may affect the INR in patients receiving warfarin. The suitability of food products for patients requiring a vegan, kosher, halal, or other compliant diet should be confirmed with individual manufacturers.

Note Feeds containing more than 6 g/100 mL protein or 2 g/100 mL fibre should be avoided in children unless recommended by an appropriate specialist or dietician.

Nutritional values

Nutritional values of products vary with flavour and pack size—consult product literature.

Paediatric ACBS indications: Disease-related malnutrition, intractable malabsorption, growth failure, pre-operative preparation of malnourished patients, dysphagia, short-bowel syndrome, bowel fistula.

Standard ACBS indications: Disease-related malnutrition, intractable malabsorption, pre-operative preparation of malnourished patients, dysphagia, proven inflammatory bowel disease, following total gastrectomy, short-bowel syndrome, bowel fistula.

Other conditions for which ACBS products can be prescribed

This is a list of clinical conditions for which the ACBS has approved toilet preparations.

Dermatitis, Eczema and Pruritus

Aveeno® Cream; *Aveeno*® Lotion; *E45*® Emollient Bath Oil; *E45*® Emollient Wash Cream

Disfiguring skin lesions (birthmarks, mutilating lesions, scars, vitiligo)

Covermark® classic foundation and finishing powder; *Dermacolor*® Camouflage cream and fixing powder; *Keromask*® finishing powder and masking cream; *Veil*® Cover cream and Finishing Powder. (Cleansing Creams, Cleansing Milks, and Cleansing Lotions are excluded).

Disinfectants (antiseptics)
May be prescribed on an FP10 only when ordered in such quantities and with such directions as are appropriate for the treatment of patients, but not if ordered for general hygenic purposes.
Dry mouth (xerostomia)
For patients suffering from dry mouth as a result of having (or having undergone) radiotherapy, or sicca syndrome.
AS Saliva Orthana®; *Biotène Oralbalance*®; *Glandosane*®; *Saliveze*®
Photodermatoses (skin protection in)
LA Roche-Posay Anthelios® XL SPF 50+ cream; *Sunsense*® Ultra (Ego) SPF 50+; *Uvistat*® Lipscreen SPF 50, *Uvistat*® Suncream SPF 30 and 50

Table 1 Enteral feeds (non-disease specific)

Less than 5 g protein/100 mL

Enteral feeds: 1 kcal/mL and less than 5 g protein/100 mL

Not suitable for use in child under 1 year unless otherwise stated; not recommended for child 1–6 years

Product	Formulation	Energy	Protein	Carbohydrate	Fat	Fibre	Special Characteristics	ACBS Indications	Presentation & Flavour
Fresubin® 1500 Complete (Fresenius Kabi Ltd)	Liquid (tube feed) per 100 mL	420 kJ (100 kcal)	3.8 g cows' milk soya	13 g (sugars 0.9 g)	3.4 g	1.5 g	Gluten-free Residual lactose Contains fish oil	Borderline substances standard ACBS indications p. 1098 except bowel fistula and pre-operative preparation of malnourished patients. Not suitable for child under 2 years	Fresubin 1500 Complete liquid: 1.5 litre = £15.00
Fresubin® Original (Fresenius Kabi Ltd)	Liquid (sip or tube feed) per 100 mL	420 kJ (100 kcal)	3.8 g cows' milk soya	13.8 g (sugars 3.5 g)	3.4 g	Nil	Gluten-free Residual lactose Contains fish gelatin Feed in flexible pack contains fish oil and fish gelatin	Borderline substances standard ACBS indications p. 1098	Fresubin Original drink: blackcurrant, chocolate, nut, peach, vanilla 200 ml = £2.43; Fresubin Original tube feed liquid: 500 ml = £4.70; 1000 ml = £9.33; 1500 ml = £13.99
Fresubin® Original Fibre (Fresenius Kabi Ltd)	Liquid (tube feed) per 100 mL	420 kJ (100 kcal)	3.8 g cows' milk soya	13 g (sugars 0.9 g)	3.4 g	1.5 g	Gluten-free Residual lactose Contains fish oil	Borderline substances standard ACBS indications p. 1098 except bowel fistula and pre-operative preparation of malnourished patients. Not suitable for child under 2 years	Fresubin Original Fibre liquid: 500 ml = £5.33; 1000 ml = £10.64
Jevity® (Abbott Laboratories Ltd)	Liquid (tube feed) per 100 mL	449 kJ (107 kcal)	4 g caseinates	14.1 g (sugars 470 mg)	3.47 g	1.76 g	Gluten-free Residual lactose	Borderline substances standard ACBS indications p. 1098 except bowel fistula. Not suitable for child under 2 years	Jevity liquid: 500 ml = £5.98; 1000 ml = £11.28; 1500 ml = £16.89
Nutrison® (Nutricia Ltd)	Liquid (tube feed) per 100 mL	420 kJ (100 kcal)	4 g cows' milk	12.3 g (sugars 1 g)	3.9 g	Nil	Gluten-free Residual lactose	Borderline substances standard ACBS indications p. 1098	Nutrison liquid: 500 ml = £5.55; 1000 ml = £9.75; 1500 ml = £14.63
Nutrison® Multi Fibre (Nutricia Ltd)	Liquid (tube feed) per 100 mL	420 kJ (100 kcal)	4 g cows' milk	12.3 g (sugars 1 g)	3.9 g	1.5 g	Gluten-free Residual lactose	Borderline substances standard ACBS indications p. 1098 except bowel fistula	Nutrison Multi Fibre liquid: 500 ml = £6.00; 1000 ml = £11.30; 1500 ml = £16.92
Osmolite® (Abbott Laboratories Ltd)	Liquid (tube feed) per 100 mL	424 kJ (100 kcal)	4 g caseinates soy isolate	13.6 g (sugars 630 mg)	3.4 g	Nil	Gluten-free Residual lactose	Borderline substances standard ACBS indications p. 1098	Osmolite liquid: 500 ml = £5.54; 1000 ml = £9.73; 1500 ml = £14.60

SOYA PROTEIN FORMULA

Not suitable for use in child under 1 year; not recommended for child 1–6 years

Product	Formulation	Energy	Protein	Carbohydrate	Fat	Fibre	Special Characteristics	ACBS Indications	Presentation & Flavour
Fresubin® Soya Fibre (Fresenius Kabi Ltd)	Liquid (tube feed) **per 100 mL**	420 kJ (100 kcal)	3.8 g soya protein	13.3 g (sugars 4.1 g)	3.6 g	2 g	Gluten-free Lactose-free Contains fish oil	Borderline substances standard ACBS indications p. 1098; also cows' milk protein intolerance, lactose intolerance	Fresubin Soya Fibre liquid: 500 ml = £5.51
Nutrison® Soya (Nutricia Ltd)	Liquid (tube feed) **per 100 mL**	420 kJ (100 kcal)	4 g soy isolate	12.3 g (sugars 1 g)	3.9 g	Nil	Gluten-free Residual lactose Milk protein-free	Borderline substances standard ACBS indications p. 1098; also cows' milk protein and lactose intolerance	Nutrison Soya liquid: 500 ml = £5.99; 1000 ml = £12.01
Nutrison® Soya Multi Fibre (Nutricia Ltd)	Liquid (tube feed) **per 100 mL**	420 kJ (100 kcal)	4 g soy isolate	12.3 g (sugars 700 mg)	3.9 g	1.5 g	Gluten-free Residual lactose Milk protein-free	Borderline substances standard ACBS indications p. 1098 except bowel fistula; also cows' milk protein and lactose intolerance	Nutrison Soya Multi Fibre liquid: 1.5 litre = £19.97

PEPTIDE-BASED FORMULA

Not suitable for use in child under 1 year; not recommended for child 1–6 years

Product	Formulation	Energy	Protein	Carbohydrate	Fat	Fibre	Special Characteristics	ACBS Indications	Presentation & Flavour
Nutrison Peptisorb® (Nutricia Ltd)	Liquid (tube feed) **per 100 mL**	425 kJ (100 kcal)	4 g whey protein hydrolysate	17.6 g (sugars 1.7 g)	1.7 g (MCT 47 %)	Nil	Gluten-free Residual lactose	Short bowel syndrome, intractable malabsorption, proven inflammatory bowel disease, bowel fistula	Nutrison Peptisorb liquid: 500 ml = £8.74; 1000 ml = £15.76
Peptamen® (Nestle Health Science)	Liquid (sip or tube feed) **per 100 mL**	420 kJ (100 kcal)	4 g whey peptides	12.7 g (sugars 480 mg)	3.7 g (MCT 70 %)	Nil	Gluten-free Residual lactose	Short bowel syndrome, intractable malabsorption, proven inflammatory bowel disease, bowel fistula	Peptamen liquid: vanilla 800 ml = £13.38; unflavoured 500 ml = £7.52; 1000 ml = £14.12
Survimed® OPD (Fresenius Kabi Ltd)	Liquid (tube feed) **per 100 mL**	420 kJ (100 kcal)	4.5 g whey protein hydrolysate	14.3 g (sugars 1.1 g)	2.8 g (MCT 51 %)	0.1 g	Gluten-free Residual lactose Contains fish oil	Borderline substances standard ACBS indications p. 1098; also growth failure	Survimed OPD: liquid 500 ml = £7.86; 800 ml = £13.56; 1000 ml = £15.72; HN liquid 500 ml = £7.57

Enteral feeds: Less than 1 kcal/mL and less than 5 g protein/100 mL

AMINO ACID FORMULA (ESSENTIAL AND NON-ESSENTIAL AMINO ACIDS)

Not suitable for use in child under 1 year; not recommended for child 1–6 years

Product	Formulation	Energy	Protein	Carbohydrate	Fat	Fibre	Special Characteristics	ACBS Indications	Presentation & Flavour
Elemental 028® Extra (Nutricia Ltd)	Liquid (sip feed) **per 100 mL**	360 kJ (86 kcal)	2.5 g (protein equivalent)	11 g (sugars 4.7 g)	3.5 g (MCT 35 %)	Nil		Short bowel syndrome, intractable malabsorption, proven inflammatory bowel disease, bowel fistula	Elemental 028 Extra liquid: grapefruit, orange & pineapple, summer fruits 250 ml = £4.11
	Standard dilution (20 %) of powder (sip or tube feed) **per 100 mL**	374 kJ (89 kcal)	2.5 g (protein equivalent)	11.8 g (sugars 1.8 g)	3.5 g (MCT 35 %)	Nil		Short bowel syndrome, intractable malabsorption, proven inflammatory bowel disease, bowel fistula.	Elemental 028 Extra powder: banana, orange, plain 100 gram = £7.99

Powder provides protein equivalent 12.5 g, carbohydrate 59 g, fat 17.45 g, energy 1871 kJ (443 kcal)/100 g. To flavour unflavoured products, see Modjul® Flavour System p. 1126.

Enteral feeds (non-disease specific): 5 g (or more) protein/100 mL

Enteral feeds: 1.5 kcal/mL and 5 g (or more) protein/100 mL

Not suitable for use in child under 1 year unless otherwise stated; not recommended for child 1–6 years unless otherwise stated

Product	Formulation	Energy	Protein	Carbohydrate	Fat	Fibre	Special Characteristics	ACBS Indications	Presentation & Flavour
Fresubin® 2250 Complete (Fresenius Kabi Ltd)	Liquid (tube feed) per 100 mL	630 kJ (150 kcal)	5.6 g cows' milk	18.8 g (sugars 1.5 g)	5.8 g	2 g	Gluten-free Residual lactose Contains fish oil and fish gelatin	Borderline substances standard ACBS indications p. 1098	Fresubin 2250 Complete liquid: 1.5 litre = £16.75
Fresubin® Energy (Fresenius Kabi Ltd)	Liquid (sip feed) per 100 mL	630 kJ (150 kcal)	5.6 g cows' milk	18.8 g (sugars)	5.8 g	Nil	Gluten-free Residual lactose Contains fish gelatin	Borderline substances standard ACBS indications p. 1098 Strawberry flavour may contain traces of wheat starch and egg.	Fresubin Energy liquid: banana, blackcurrant, cappuccino, chocolate, lemon, strawberry, tropical fruits, vanilla 200 ml = £1.40; unflavoured 200 ml = £1.40; 500 ml = £6.27; 1000 ml = £11.80; 1500 ml = £16.99
	Liquid (tube feed) per 100 mL	630 kJ (150 kcal)	5.6 g cows' milk	18.8 g (sugars 1.4 g)	5.8 g	Nil	Gluten-free Residual lactose Contains fish oil and fish gelatin	Borderline substances standard ACBS indications p. 1098	
Fresubin® Energy Fibre (Fresenius Kabi Ltd)	Liquid (sip feed) per 100 mL	630 kJ (150 kcal)	5.6 g cows' milk	18.8 g (sugars)	5.8 g	2 g	Gluten-free Residual lactose Contains fish gelatin	Borderline substances standard ACBS indications p. 1098	Fresubin Energy Fibre liquid: banana, caramel, cherry, chocolate, strawberry 200 ml = £2.23; unflavoured 500 ml = £6.97; 1000 ml = £13.14; 1500 ml = £15.68
	Liquid (tube feed) per 100 mL	630 kJ (150 kcal)	5.6 g cows' milk	18.8 g (sugars 1.5 g)	5.8 g	2 g	Gluten-free Residual lactose Contains fish oil and fish gelatin	Borderline substances standard ACBS indications p. 1098	Fresubin Energy Fibre liquid unflavoured: 500 ml = £6.97; 1000 ml = £13.14; 1500 ml = £15.68
Fresubin® HP Energy (Fresenius Kabi Ltd)	Liquid (tube feed) per 100 mL	630 kJ (150 kcal)	7.5 g cows' milk	17 g (sugars 1 g)	5.8 g (MCT 57 %)	Nil	Gluten-free Residual lactose Contains fish oil and fish gelatin	Borderline substances standard ACBS indications p. 1098; also CAPD and haemodialysis	Fresubin HP Energy liquid: 500 ml = £6.45; 1000 ml = £12.16
Jevity® 1.5 kcal (Abbott Laboratories Ltd)	Liquid (tube feed) per 100 mL	649 kJ (154 kcal)	6.38 g caseinates and soy isolate	20.1 g (sugars 1.47 g)	4.9 g	2.2 g	Gluten-free Residual lactose	Borderline substances standard ACBS indications p. 1098 Not suitable for child under 2 years; not recommended for child 2–10 years	Jevity 1.5kcal liquid: 500 ml = £7.16; 1000 ml = £13.50; 1500 ml = £20.83
Nutrison® Energy (Nutricia Ltd)	Liquid (tube feed) per 100 mL	630 kJ (150 kcal)	6 g cows' milk	18.5 g (sugars 1.5 g)	5.8 g	Nil	Gluten-free Residual lactose	Borderline substances standard ACBS indications p. 1098	Nutrison Energy liquid: 500 ml = £6.47; 1000 ml = £12.17; 1500 ml = £18.21
Nutrison® Energy Multi Fibre (Nutricia Ltd)	Liquid (tube feed) per 100 mL	630 kJ (150 kcal)	6 g cows' milk	18.5 g (sugars 1.5 g)	5.8 g	1.5 g	Gluten-free Residual lactose	Borderline substances standard ACBS indications p. 1098	Nutrison Energy Multi Fibre liquid: 500 ml = £7.18; 1000 ml = £13.51; 1500 ml = £20.86

Osmolite® 1.5 kcal (Abbott Laboratories Ltd)	Liquid (tube feed) per 100 mL	632 kJ (150 kcal)	6.25 g cows' milk soya protein isolate	20 g (sugars 4.9 g)	5 g	Nil	Gluten-free Residual lactose	Borderline substances standard ACBS indications p. 1098	Osmolite 1.5kcal tube feed liquid: 500 ml = £6.44; 1000 ml = £12.15; 1500 ml = £18.18;
Resource® Energy (Nestle Health Science)	Liquid (sip feed) per 100 mL	630 kJ (150 kcal)	5.6 g cows' milk	21 g (sugars 5.2 g)	5 g	less than 0.5 g	Gluten-free Residual lactose	Borderline substances standard ACBS indications p. 1098 Not suitable for use in child under 3 years	Resource Energy liquid: apricot, chocolate, coffee, strawberry and raspberry, vanilla 800 ml = £8.45

Enteral feeds: Less than 1.5 kcal/mL and 5 g (or more) protein/100 mL

Not suitable for use in child under 1 year unless otherwise stated; not recommended for child 1-6 years unless otherwise stated

Product	Formulation	Energy	Protein	Carbohydrate	Fat	Fibre	Special Characteristics	ACBS Indications	Presentation & Flavour
Fresubin® 1000 Complete (Fresenius Kabi Ltd)	Liquid (tube feed) per 100 mL	420 kJ (100 kcal)	5.5 g cows' milk	12.5 g (sugars 1.1 g)	3.1 g	2 g	Gluten-free Residual lactose Contains fish oil	Borderline substances standard ACBS indications p. 1098	Fresubin 1000 Complete liquid: 1 litre = £12.07
Fresubin® 1200 Complete (Fresenius Kabi Ltd)	Liquid (tube feed) per 100 mL	500 kJ (120 kcal)	6 g cows' milk	15 g (sugars 1.22 g)	4.1 g	2 g	Gluten-free Residual lactose Contains fish oil	Borderline substances standard ACBS indications p. 1098	Fresubin 1200 Complete liquid: 1 litre = £15.36
Fresubin® 1800 Complete (Fresenius Kabi Ltd)	Liquid (tube feed) per 100 mL	500 kJ (120 kcal)	6 g cows' milk	15 g (sugars 1.22 g)	4.1 g	2 g	Gluten-free Residual lactose Contains fish oil	Borderline substances standard ACBS indications p. 1098	Fresubin 1800 Complete liquid: 1.5 litre = £15.36
Jevity® Plus (Abbott Laboratories Ltd)	Liquid (tube feed) per 100 mL	514 kJ (122 kcal)	5.5 g caseinates soy isolates	15.1 g (sugars 0.89 g)	3.93 g	2.2 g	Gluten-free Residual lactose	Borderline substances standard ACBS indications p. 1098 Not suitable for child under 2 years; not recommended for child 2-10 years	Jevity Plus liquid: 500 ml = £7.17; 1000 ml = £13.07; 1500 ml = £19.54
Jevity® Plus HP (Abbott Laboratories Ltd)	Liquid (tube feed) per 100 mL	551 kJ (131 kcal)	8.13 g cows' milk soy isolates	14.2 g (sugars 0.95 g)	4.33 g	1.5 g	Gluten-free Residual lactose	Borderline substances standard ACBS indications p. 1098; also CAPD, haemodialysis Not suitable for child under 2 years; not recommended for child 2-10 years	Jevity Plus HP gluten free liquid: 500 ml = £7.03
Jevity® Promote (Abbott Laboratories Ltd)	Liquid (tube feed) per 100 mL	434 kJ (103 kcal)	5.55 g caseinates soy isolates	12 g (sugars 0.67 g)	3.32 g	1.7 g	Gluten-free Residual lactose	Borderline substances standard ACBS indications p. 1098 Not suitable for child under 2 years; not recommended for child 2-10 years	Jevity Promote liquid: 1 litre = £12.50
Nutrison® 800 Complete Multi Fibre (Nutricia Ltd)	Liquid (tube feed) per 100 mL	345 kJ (83 kcal)	5.5 g cows' milk pea protein soya protein	8.8 g (sugars 0.6 g)	2.5 g	1.5 g	Gluten-free Residual lactose Contains fish oil	Borderline substances standard ACBS indications p. 1098 except bowel fistula Not suitable for child under 6 years; not recommended for child 6-12 years	Nutrison 800 Complete Multi Fibre liquid: 1 litre = £11.81
Nutrison® 1000 Complete Multi Fibre (Nutricia Ltd)	Liquid (tube feed) per 100 mL	420 kJ (100 kcal)	5.5 g cows' milk	11.3 g (sugars 0.7 g)	3.7 g	2 g	Gluten-free Residual lactose	Disease related malnutrition in patients with low energy and/or low fluid requirements	Nutrison 1000 Complete Multi Fibre liquid: 1 litre = £12.54

Enteral feeds: Less than 1.5 kcal/mL and 5 g (or more) protein/100 mL (product list continued)

Not suitable for use in child under 1 year unless otherwise stated; not recommended for child 1–6 years unless otherwise stated

Product	Formulation	Energy	Protein	Carbohydrate	Fat	Fibre	Special Characteristics	ACBS Indications	Presentation & Flavour
Nutrison® 1200 Complete Multi Fibre (Nutricia Ltd)	Liquid (tube feed) per 100 mL	505 kJ (120 kcal)	5.5 g cows' milk	15 g (sugars 1.2 g)	4.3 g	2 g	Gluten-free Residual lactose	Borderline substances standard ACBS indications p. 1098 except bowel fistula	Nutrison 1200 Complete Multi Fibre liquid: 1000 ml = £13.26; 1500 ml = £19.91
Nutrison® MCT (Nutricia Ltd)	Liquid (tube feed) per 100 mL	420 kJ (100 kcal)	5 g cows' milk	12.6 g (sugars 1 g)	3.3 g (MCT 61%)	Nil	Gluten-free Residual lactose	Borderline substances standard ACBS indications p. 1098	Nutrison MCT liquid: 1000 ml = £11.29
Nutrison® Protein Plus (Nutricia Ltd)	Liquid (tube feed) per 100 mL	525 kJ (125 kcal)	6.3 g cows' milk	14.2 g (sugars 1.1 g)	4.9 g	Nil	Gluten-free Residual lactose	Borderline substances standard ACBS indications p. 1098	Nutrison Protein Plus liquid: 500 ml = £5.98; 1 litre = £11.59
Nutrison® Protein Plus Multi Fibre (Nutricia Ltd)	Liquid (tube feed) per 100 mL	535 kJ (128 kcal)	6.3 g cow's milk	14.1 g (sugars 1.0 g)	4.9 g	1.5 g	Gluten-free Residual lactose	For use as dietary management of disease related malnutrition.	Nutrison Protein Plus Multifibre liquid: 1 litre = £12.92; 500 ml = £6.66
Osmolite® Plus (Abbott Laboratories Ltd)	Liquid (tube feed) per 100 mL	508 kJ (121 kcal)	5.55 g caseinates	15.8 g (sugars 0.73 g)	3.93 g	Nil	Gluten-free Residual lactose	Borderline substances standard ACBS indications p. 1098 Not suitable for child under 10 years	Osmolite Plus liquid: 500 ml = £6.02; 1000 ml = £10.95; 1500 ml = £16.40
Peptamen® HN (Nestle Health Science)	Liquid (tube feed) per 100 mL	556 kJ (133 kcal)	6.6 g whey protein hydrolysates	15.6 g (sugars 1.4 g)	4.9 g (MCT 70%)	Nil	Gluten-free Residual lactose Hydrolysed with pork trypsin	Short bowel syndrome, intractable malabsorption, proven inflammatory bowel disease, bowel fistula Not suitable for child under 3 years	Peptamen HN liquid: 500 ml = £8.09; 1000 ml = £15.20
Perative® (Abbott Laboratories Ltd)	Liquid (sip or tube feed) per 100 mL	552 kJ (131 kcal)	6.7 g caseinate whey protein hydrolysates	17.7 g (sugars 0.66 g)	3.7 g (MCT 42%)	Nil	Gluten-free Residual lactose	Borderline substances standard ACBS indications p. 1098 Not suitable for child under 5 years	Perative liquid: 500 ml = £8.52; 1000 ml = £15.73

Enteral feeds: More than 1.5 kcal/mL and 5 g (or more) protein/100 mL

Not suitable for use in child under 1 year; not recommended for child 1–6 years

Product	Formulation	Energy	Protein	Carbohydrate	Fat	Fibre	Special Characteristics	ACBS Indications	Presentation & Flavour
Ensure® Twocal (Abbott Laboratories Ltd)	Liquid (sip or tube feed) per 100 mL	838 kJ (200 kcal)	8.4 g cows' milk	21 g (sugars 4.5 g)	8.9 g	1 g	Gluten-free Residual lactose	Borderline substances standard ACBS indications p. 1098; also haemodialysis and CAPD	Ensure TwoCal liquid: banana, neutral, strawberry, vanilla 200 ml = £2.22

Enteral feeds (non-disease specific): Child under 12 years

Enteral feeds, Child: Less than 1 kcal/mL and less than 4 g protein/100 mL

Product	Formulation	Energy	Protein	Carbohydrate	Fat	Fibre	Special Characteristics	ACBS Indications	Presentation & Flavour
Nutrini® Low Energy Multi Fibre (Nutricia Ltd)	Liquid (tube feed) per 100 mL	315 kJ (75 kcal)	2.1 g whey protein and caseinate	9.3 g (sugars 0.6 g)	3.3 g	0.8 g	Gluten-free Residual lactose Contains fish oil	Borderline substances paediatric ACBS indications p. 1098 except bowel fistula, in child 1–6 years, body-weight 8–20 kg	Nutrini Low Energy Multifibre liquid: 200 ml = £2.97; 500 ml = £7.57
Nutriprem® 1 (Cow & Gate Ltd)	Liquid (sip feed) per 100 mL	335 kJ (80 kcal)	2.5 g whey protein and casein	7.6 g (lactose 6.3 g)	4.4 g	0.8 g	Contains soya, fish oil and egg lipid	Low birth-weight formula	Nutriprem 1 liquid: 70 ml

Product	Formulation	Energy	Protein	Carbohydrate	Fat	Fibre	Special Characteristics	ACBS Indications	Presentation & Flavour
Nutriprem® 2 (Cow & Gate Ltd)	Liquid (sip feed) **per 100 mL**	310 kJ (75 kcal)	2 g whey protein and casein	7.4 g (lactose 5.8 g)	4 g	0.6 g	Contains soya, fish oil and egg lipid	Catch-up growth in pre-term infants (less than 35 weeks at birth) and small for gestational-age infants up to 6 months corrected age.	Nutriprem 2 liquid: 200 ml = £1.78
	Standard dilution (15.3%) of powder (sip feed) **per 100 mL**	315 kJ (75 kcal)	2 g whey protein and casein	7.4 g (lactose 5.9 g)	4 g (including MCT oil)	0.6 g			Nutriprem 2 powder: 800 gram = £10.64

Powder provides: protein 13 g, carbohydrate 48.3 g, fat 26.7 g, fibre 5.2 g, energy 2030 kJ (485 kcal)/100 g.

AMINO ACID FORMULA (ESSENTIAL AND NON-ESSENTIAL AMINO ACIDS)

Product	Formulation	Energy	Protein	Carbohydrate	Fat	Fibre	Special Characteristics	ACBS Indications	Presentation & Flavour
Emsogen® (Nutricia Ltd)	Standard dilution (20 %) of powder (sip or tube feed) **per 100 mL**	368 kJ (88 kcal)	2.5 g protein equivalent (essential and non-essential amino acids)	12 g (sugars 1.6 g)	3.3 g (MCT 83 %)	Nil	Lactose-free	Short-bowel syndrome, intractable malabsorption, proven inflammatory bowel disease, bowel fistula Not suitable for child under 1 year or as sole source of nutrition in child 1-5 years	Emsogen powder unflavoured: 100 gram = £8.22

Powder provides: protein equivalent 12.5 g, carbohydrate 60 g, fat 16.4 g, energy 1839 kJ (438 kcal)/100 g. Additional source of alpha linolenic acid needed if used as sole source of nutrition. To flavour unflavoured products, see Modjul® Flavour System p. 1126.

Enteral feeds, Child: 1 kcal/mL and less than 4 g protein/100 mL

Not suitable for use in child under 1 year unless otherwise stated

Product	Formulation	Energy	Protein	Carbohydrate	Fat	Fibre	Special Characteristics	ACBS Indications	Presentation & Flavour
Fortini® 1.0 Multi Fibre (Nutricia Ltd)	Liquid (sip feed) **per 100 mL**	420 kJ (100 kcal)	2.4 g cows' milk	11.8 g (sugars 4.7 g)	4.5 g	1.5 g	Gluten-free Residual lactose	Disease-related malnutrition and growth failure in child 1-6 years, body-weight 8-20 kg	Fortini 1.0 Multi Fibre liquid: banana, chocolate, strawberry, vanilla 200 ml = £2.85
Frebini® Original (Fresenius Kabi Ltd)	Liquid (tube feed) **per 100 mL**	420 kJ (100 kcal)	2.5 g cows' milk	12.5 g (sugars 0.7 g)	4.4 g	Nil	Gluten-free Residual lactose Contains fish oils and fish gelatin	Borderline substances standard ACBS indications p. 1098 and growth failure in child 1-10 years, body-weight 8-30 kg	Frebini Original liquid: 500 ml = £6.96
Frebini® Original Fibre (Fresenius Kabi Ltd)	Liquid (tube feed) **per 100 mL**	420 kJ (100 kcal)	2.5 g cows' milk	12.5 g (sugars 0.7 g)	4.4 g	0.75 g	Gluten-free Residual lactose Contains fish oils and fish gelatin	Borderline substances standard ACBS indications p. 1098 and growth failure in child 1-10 years, body-weight 8-30 kg	Frebini Original Fibre liquid: 500 ml = £7.74
Infatrini® (Nutricia Ltd)	Liquid (sip or tube feed) **per 100 mL**	415 kJ (100 kcal)	2.6 g cows' milk	10.3 g (lactose 5.2 g)	5.4 g	0.8 g	Gluten-free Contains fish oil	Failure to thrive, disease-related malnutrition and malabsorption, in child from birth up to body-weight 8 kg	Infatrini liquid: 125 ml = £1.60; 200 ml = £2.56; 500 ml = £6.97
Nutrini® (Nutricia Ltd)	Liquid (tube feed) **per 100 mL**	420 kJ (100 kcal)	2.8 g cows' milk	12.3 g (sugars 1 g)	4.4 g	Nil	Gluten-free Residual lactose	Borderline substances standard ACBS indications p. 1098 and growth failure in child 1-6 years, body-weight 8-20 kg	Nutrini liquid: 200 ml = £3.11; 500 ml = £7.71

Enteral feeds, Child: 1 kcal/mL and less than 4 g protein/100 mL (product list continued)

Not suitable for use in child under 1 year unless otherwise stated

Product	Formulation	Energy	Protein	Carbohydrate	Fat	Fibre	Special Characteristics	ACBS Indications	Presentation & Flavour
Nutrini® Multi Fibre (Nutricia Ltd)	Liquid (tube feed) **per 100 mL**	420 kJ (100 kcal)	2.8 g whey protein and caseinate	12.3 g (sugars 0.8 g)	4.4 g	0.8 g	Gluten-free Residual lactose Contains fish oil	Borderline substances standard ACBS indications p. 1098 and growth failure in child 1-6 years, body-weight 8-20 kg	Nutrini Multifibre liquid: 200 ml = £3.44; 500 ml = £8.56
Paediasure® (Abbott Laboratories Ltd)	Liquid (sip or tube feed) **per 100 mL**	422 kJ (100 kcal)	2.8 g cows' milk	11.2 g (sugars 3.92 g)	4.98 g	Nil	Gluten-free Residual lactose	Borderline substances paediatric ACBS indications p. 1098 in child 1-10 years, body-weight 8-30 kg	PaediaSure liquid: banana, chocolate, strawberry 200 ml = £2.78; vanilla 200 ml = £2.78; 500 ml = £7.71
Paediasure® Fibre (Abbott Laboratories Ltd)	Liquid (sip or tube feed) **per 100 mL**	424 kJ (101 kcal)	2.8 g caseinates and whey protein	10.9 g (sugars 3.84 g)	4.98 g	0.73 g	Gluten-free Residual lactose	Borderline substances paediatric ACBS indications p. 1098 in child 1-10 years, body-weight 8-30 kg	PaediaSure fibre liquid: banana, strawberry 200 ml = £2.93; vanilla 200 ml = £2.93; 500 ml = £8.55
Paediasure® Peptide (Abbott Laboratories Ltd)	Liquid (sip or tube feed) **per 100 mL**	420 kJ (100 kcal)	3 g whey protein and caseinate	13 g (sugars 2.98 g)	4g (MCT 50%)	Nil	Gluten-free Residual lactose	Borderline substances standard ACBS indications p. 1098 and growth failure in child 1-10 years, body-weight 8-30 kg	PaediaSure Peptide liquid: 200 ml = £4.33; 500 ml = £12.02
Similac® High Energy (Abbott Laboratories Ltd)	Liquid (sip or tube feed) **per 100 mL**	419 kJ (100 kcal)	2.6 g cows' milk and whey protein	10.1 g (sugars 5.6 g)	5.2 g	0.4 g	Gluten-free Contains lactose and soy oil	Increased energy requirements, faltering growth, and/or need for fluid restriction, in child body-weight up to 8 kg	Similac High Energy liquid: 60 ml = £0.74; 200 ml = £2.50
Tentrini® (Nutricia Ltd)	Liquid (tube feed) **per 100 mL**	420 kJ (100 kcal)	3.3 g whey protein and caseinate	12.3 g (sugars 0.8 g)	4.2 g	Nil	Gluten-free Residual lactose Contains fish oil	Borderline substances standard ACBS indications p. 1098 and growth failure in child 7-12 years, body-weight 21-45 kg	Tentrini liquid: 500 ml = £6.80
Tentrini® Multi Fibre (Nutricia Ltd)	Liquid (tube feed) **per 100 mL**	420 kJ (100 kcal)	3.3 g whey protein and caseinate	12.3 g (sugars 0.8 g)	4.2 g	1.1 g	Gluten-free Residual lactose Contains fish oil	Borderline substances standard ACBS indications p. 1098 except bowel fistula, and growth failure in child 7-12 years body-weight 21-45 kg	Tentrini Multifibre liquid: 500 ml = £7.48

HYDROLYSATE FORMULA

Not suitable for use in child under 1 year

Product	Formulation	Energy	Protein	Carbohydrate	Fat	Fibre	Special Characteristics	ACBS Indications	Presentation & Flavour
Nutrini® Peptisorb (Nutricia Ltd)	Liquid (tube feed) **per 100 mL**	420 kJ (100 kcal)	2.8 g whey protein hydrolysate	13.7 g (sugars 0.8 g)	3.9 g (MCT 46 %)	Nil	Gluten-free Residual lactose	Borderline substances standard ACBS indications p. 1098 and growth failure in child 1-6 years, body-weight 8-20 kg	Nutrini Peptisorb liquid: 500 ml = £12.05

Peptamen® Junior (Nestle Health Science)	Liquid (tube feed) **per 100 mL**	420 kJ (100 kcal)	3 g whey protein hydrolysate	13.2 g	4 g (MCT 60 %)	Nil	Gluten-free Residual lactose Hydrolysed with pork trypsin	Short bowel syndrome, intractable malabsorption, proven inflammatory bowel disease, bowel fistula, in child 1-10 years	Peptamen Junior liquid: 500 ml = £7.51
	Standard dilution (22%) of powder (sip or tube feed) **per 100 mL**	420 kJ (100 kcal)	3 g whey protein hydrolysate	13.8 g	3.85 g (MCT 60 %)	Nil	Gluten-free Residual lactose Hydrolysed with bacterial trypsin		Peptamen Junior powder: 400 gram = £19.71

Powder provides: protein 13.7 g, carbohydrate 62.9 g, fat 17.5 g, energy 1910 kJ (457 kcal)/100 g.

Enteral feeds, Child: More than 1 kcal/mL and less than 4 g protein/100 mL

Not suitable for use in child under 1 year unless otherwise stated

Product	Formulation	Energy	Protein	Carbohydrate	Fat	Fibre	Special Characteristics	ACBS Indications	Presentation & Flavour
Fortini® (Nutricia Ltd)	Liquid (sip feed) **per 100 mL**	630 kJ (150 kcal)	3.4 g cows' milk	18.8 g (sugars 7.4 g)	6.8 g	Nil	Gluten-free Residual lactose	Disease-related malnutrition and growth failure in child 1-6 years, body-weight 8-20 kg	Fortini liquid: strawberry, vanilla 200 ml = £3.69
Fortini® Multifibre (Nutricia Ltd)	Liquid (sip feed) **per 100 mL**	630 kJ (150 kcal)	3.4 g cows' milk	18.8 g (sugars 7.4 g)	6.8 g	1.5 g	Gluten-free Residual lactose	Disease-related malnutrition and growth failure in child 1-6 years, body-weight 8-20 kg	Fortini Multi Fibre liquid: banana, chocolate, strawberry, unflavoured, vanilla 200 ml = £3.87
Frebini® Energy (Fresenius Kabi Ltd)	Liquid (tube feed) **per 100 mL**	630 kJ (150 kcal)	3.75 g cows' milk	18.75 g (sugars 0.83 g)	6.7 g	Nil	Gluten-free Residual lactose Contains fish oil and fish gelatin	Borderline substances standard ACBS indications p. 1098 and failure in child 1-10 years, body-weight 8-30 kg	Frebini Energy Drink: banana, strawberry 200 ml = £3.29
Frebini® Energy Drink (Fresenius Kabi Ltd)	Liquid (sip feed) **per 100 mL**	630 kJ (150 kcal)	3.8 g cows' milk	18.7 g (sugars 4.5 g)	6.7 g	Nil	Gluten-free Residual lactose	Disease-related malnutrition and growth failure in child 1-10 years, body-weight 8-30 kg	Frebini Energy Drink: banana, strawberry 200 ml = £3.29
Frebini® Energy Fibre (Fresenius Kabi Ltd)	Liquid (tube feed) **per 100 mL**	630 kJ (150 kcal)	3.75 g cows' milk	18.75 g (sugars 0.83 g)	6.7 g	1.13 g	Gluten-free Residual lactose Contains fish oils and fish gelatin	Borderline substances standard ACBS indications p. 1098 and growth failure in child 1-10 years, body-weight 8-30 kg	Frebini Energy Fibre liquid unflavoured: 500 ml = £9.34
Frebini® Energy Fibre Drink (Fresenius Kabi Ltd)	Liquid (sip feed) **per 100 mL**	630 kJ (150 kcal)	3.8 g cows' milk	18.75 g (sugars 4.5 g)	6.7 g	1.1 g	Gluten-free Residual lactose	Disease-related malnutrition and growth failure in child 1-10 years, body-weight 8-30 kg	Frebini Energy Fibre liquid: chocolate, vanilla 200 ml = £3.36
Resource® Junior (Nestle Health Science)	Liquid (sip feed) **per 100 mL**	630 kJ (150 kcal)	3 g cows' milk	20.6 g (sugars 4.9 g)	6.2 g	Nil	Gluten-free Residual lactose	Borderline substances standard ACBS indications p. 1098 in child 1-10 years. Not suitable for use in child under 1 year	Resource Junior complete sip feed: chocolate, strawberry, vanilla 200 ml = £2.27

Enteral feeds, Child: 1.5 kcal/mL and more than 4 g protein/100 mL
Not suitable for use in child under 1 year

Product	Formulation	Energy	Protein	Carbohydrate	Fat	Fibre	Special Characteristics	ACBS Indications	Presentation & Flavour
Nutrini® Energy (Nutricia Ltd)	Liquid (tube feed) **per 100 mL**	630 kJ (150 kcal)	4.1 g caseinate whey protein	18.5 g (sugars 1.1 g)	6.7 g	Nil	Gluten-free Residual lactose Contains fish oil	Borderline substances standard ACBS indications p. 1098 and growth failure in child 1-6 years, body-weight 8-20 kg	Nutrini Energy liquid: 500 ml = £9.68; 200 ml = £3.78
Nutrini® Energy Multi Fibre (Nutricia Ltd)	Liquid (tube feed) **per 100 mL**	630 kJ (150 kcal)	4.1 g caseinate whey protein	18.5 g (sugars 1.1 g)	6.7 g	0.8 g	Gluten-free Residual lactose Contains fish oil	Borderline substances paediatric ACBS indications p. 1098 except bowel fistula; also total gastrectomy, in child 1-6 years, body-weight 8-20 kg	Nutrini Energy Multifibre liquid: 200 ml = £3.99; 500 ml = £10.00
Paediasure® Plus (Abbott Laboratories Ltd)	Liquid (sip or tube feed) **per 100 mL**	632 kJ (151 kcal)	4.2 g caseinates whey protein	16.7 g	7.47 g	Nil	Gluten-free Residual lactose	Borderline substances paediatric ACBS indications p. 1098 in child 1-10 years, body-weight 8-30 kg	PaediaSure Plus liquid: banana, strawberry, unflavoured, vanilla 200 ml = £3.59
Paediasure® Plus Fibre (Abbott Laboratories Ltd)	Liquid (sip or tube feed) **per 100 mL**	635 kJ (152 kcal)	4.2 g caseinates whey protein	16.4 g (sugars 5.3 g)	7.47 g	1.1 g	Gluten-free Residual lactose	Borderline substances paediatric ACBS indications p. 1098 in child 1-10 years, body-weight 8-30 kg. Not suitable for use in child under 1 year.	PaediaSure Plus fibre liquid: banana, strawberry 200 ml = £3.87; vanilla 200 ml = £3.87; 500 ml = £9.99
Peptamen® Junior Advance (Nestle Health Science)	Liquid (tube feed) **per 100 mL**	630 kJ (150 kcal)	4.5 g whey protein	18 g (sugars 2.1 g)	6.6 g (MCT 61%)	0.54 g	Gluten-free Residual lactose Hydrolysed with pork trypsin Contains fish oil	Intractable malabsorption, short-bowel syndrome, bowel fistula, and proven inflammatory bowel disease in child 1-10 years	Peptamen Junior Advance liquid: 500 ml = £8.57
Tentrini® Energy (Nutricia Ltd)	Liquid (tube feed) **per 100 mL**	630 kJ (150 kcal)	4.9 g whey protein and caseinate	18.5 g (sugars 1.1 g)	6.3 g	Nil	Gluten-free Residual lactose Contains fish oil	Borderline substances standard ACBS indications p. 1098 and growth failure, in child 7-12 years, body-weight 21-45 kg	Tentrini Energy liquid: 500 ml = £8.40
Tentrini® Energy Multi Fibre (Nutricia Ltd)	Liquid (tube feed) **per 100 mL**	630 kJ (150 kcal)	4.9 g whey protein and caseinate	18.5 g (sugars 1.1 g)	6.3 g	1.1 g	Gluten-free Residual lactose Contains fish oil	Borderline substances paediatric ACBS indications p. 1098 and proven inflammatory bowel disease, in child 7-12 years, body-weight 21-45 kg	Tentrini Energy Multifibre liquid: 500 ml = £9.25

Table 2 Nutritional supplements (non-disease specific)

Less than 5 g protein/100 mL

Nutritional supplements: 1 kcal/mL and less than 5 g protein/100 mL
Not suitable for use in child under 1 year; use with caution in child 1-5 years

Product	Formulation	Energy	Protein	Carbohydrate	Fat	Fibre	Special Characteristics	ACBS Indications	Presentation & Flavour
Ensure® (Abbott Laboratories Ltd)	Liquid (sip or tube feed) **per 100 mL**	423 kJ (100 kcal)	4 g caseinates soy isolate	13.6 g (sugars 3.93 g)	3.36 g	Nil	Gluten-free Residual lactose	Borderline substances standard ACBS indications p. 1098	Ensure liquid: chocolate, coffee, vanilla 250 ml = £2.45

Nutritional supplements: More than 1 kcal/mL and less than 5 g protein/100 mL

Not suitable for use in child under 1 year unless otherwise stated; use with caution in child 1-5 years unless otherwise stated

Product	Formulation	Energy	Protein	Carbohydrate	Fat	Fibre	Special Characteristics	ACBS Indications	Presentation & Flavour
Ensure® Plus Juce (Abbott Laboratories Ltd)	Liquid (sip feed) per 100 mL	638 kJ (150 kcal)	4.8 g whey protein isolate	32.7 g (sugars 9.4 g)	Nil	Nil	Gluten-free Residual lactose Non-milk taste	Borderline substances standard ACBS indications p. 1098	Ensure Plus Juce liquid: apple, fruit punch, lemon & lime, orange, peach, strawberry 220 ml = £1.97
Fortijuce® (Nutricia Ltd)	Liquid (sip feed) per 100 mL	640 kJ (150 kcal)	4.0 g cows' milk	33.5 g (sugars 13.1 g)	Nil	Nil	Gluten-free Residual lactose Non-milk taste	Borderline substances standard ACBS indications p. 1098 Not suitable for child under 3 years	Fortijuce Starter Pack liquid: assorted 800 ml = £8.08; Fortijuce liquid: apple, blackcurrant, forest fruits, lemon, orange, strawberry, tropical 200 ml = £2.02. Sugar content varies with flavour
Fresubin® Jucy Drink (Fresenius Kabi Ltd)	Liquid (sip feed) per 100 mL	630 kJ (150 kcal)	4 g whey protein	33.5 g (sugars 8 g)	Nil	Nil	Gluten-free Residual lactose	Borderline substances standard ACBS indications p. 1098; also CAPD, haemodialysis	Fresubin Jucy drink: apple, blackcurrant, cherry, orange, pineapple 800 ml = £8.04
Paediasure® Plus Juce (Abbott Laboratories Ltd)	Liquid (sip feed) per 100 mL	638 kJ (150 kcal)	4.2 g cows' milk	33.3 g (sugars 9.4 g)	Nil	Nil	Gluten-free Residual lactose Non-milk taste	Nutritional supplement in child 1-10 years, body-weight 8-30 kg with disease-related malnutrition and, or growth failure	PaediaSure Plus Juce liquid: apple, very berry 200 ml = £3.57

Nutritional supplements: 5 g (or more) protein/100 mL

Nutritional supplements: 1.5 kcal/mL and 5 g (or more) protein/100 mL

Not suitable for child under 3 years; use with caution in child under 11 years unless otherwise stated.

Product	Formulation	Energy	Protein	Carbohydrate	Fat	Fibre	Special Characteristics	ACBS Indications	Presentation & Flavour
Altraplen® Protein (Nualtra Ltd)	Liquid (sip feed) per 100 mL	632 kJ (150 kcal)	10 g cows' milk soya protein	15 g (sugars 4.6 g)	5.6 g	Nil	Gluten-free Residual lactose	Borderline substances standard ACBS indications p. 1098	Altraplen Protein Starter Pack liquid: 400 ml = £3.29; Altraplen Protein liquid: strawberry, vanilla 800 ml = £6.78
AYMES® ActaCal Creme (Aymes International Ltd)	Semi-solid per 100 g	632 kJ (150 kcal)	7.5 g caseinates, milk protein	19.0 g (sugars 8.1 g)	4.9 g	Nil	Contains residual lactose. Gluten-free.	Borderline substances standard ACBS indications p. 1098 except dysphagia.	Aymes Creme dessert: chocolate, vanilla 500 gram = £4.68
AYMES® Complete (Aymes International Ltd)	Liquid per 100 mL	630 kJ (150 kcal)	6 g milk protein	18 g (sugars 6.8 g)	6 g	Nil	Contains residual lactose. Gluten-free	Borderline substances standard ACBS indications p. 1098.	Aymes Complete Starter Pack liquid: 800 ml = £5.60; Aymes Complete liquid: banana, chocolate, strawberry, vanilla 800 ml = £4.20
Ensure® Plus Commence (Abbott Laboratories Ltd)	Starter pack (5–10 days supply), contains: Ensure® Plus Commence (liquid assorted), 1 pack (10 × 200 ml) = £11.10								
Ensure® Plus Fibre (Abbott Laboratories Ltd)	Liquid (sip or tube feed) per 100 mL	652 kJ (155 kcal)	6.25 g cows' milk soya protein isolate	20.2 g (sugars 5.5 g)	4.92 g	2.5 g	Gluten-free Residual lactose	Borderline substances standard ACBS indications p. 1098; also CAPD, haemodialysis.	Ensure Plus Fibre liquid: banana, chocolate, raspberry, strawberry 200 ml = £2.19

Nutritional supplements: 1.5 kcal/mL and 5 g (or more) protein/100 mL (product list continued)

Not suitable for child under 3 years; use with caution in child under 11 years unless otherwise stated.

Product	Formulation	Energy	Protein	Carbohydrate	Fat	Fibre	Special Characteristics	ACBS Indications	Presentation & Flavour
Ensure® Plus Milkshake style (Abbott Laboratories Ltd)	Liquid (sip or tube feed) per 100 mL	632 kJ (150 kcal)	6.25 g cows' milk soya protein isolate	20.2 g (sugars 6.89 g)	4.92 g	Nil	Gluten-free Residual lactose	Borderline substances standard ACBS indications p. 1098; also CAPD, haemodialysis	Ensure Plus milkshake style liquid: banana, chocolate, coffee, fruits of the forest, neutral, peach, raspberry, strawberry, vanilla 200 ml = £1.11
Ensure® Plus Yoghurt style (Abbott Laboratories Ltd)	Liquid (sip feed) per 100 mL	632 kJ (150 kcal)	6.25 g cows' milk	20.2 g (sugars 11.7 g)	4.92 g	Nil	Gluten-free Residual lactose	Borderline substances standard ACBS indications p. 1098; also CAPD, haemodialysis	Ensure Plus yoghurt style liquid: orchard peach, strawberry swirl 200 ml = £1.14
Fortisip® Bottle (Nutricia Ltd)	Liquid (sip feed) per 100 mL	630 kJ (150 kcal)	6 g cows' milk	18.4 g	5.8 g	Nil	Gluten-free Residual lactose	Borderline substances standard ACBS indications p. 1098 Not suitable for child under 3 years; use with caution in child 3–5 years.	Fortisip Bottle: banana, caramel, chocolate, neutral, orange, strawberry, tropical fruit, vanilla, 200 ml = £1.12. Sugar content varies with flavour
Fortisip® Range (Nutricia Ltd)	Starter pack contains 4×Fortisip® Bottle, 4×Fortijuce®, 2×Fortisip® Yoghurt Style, 1 pack (10×200 ml) = £20.20								
Fortisip® Yoghurt Style (Nutricia Ltd)	Liquid (sip feed) per 100 mL	630 kJ (150 kcal)	6 g cows' milk	18.7 g (sugars 10.8 g)	5.8 g	0.2 g	Gluten-free Contains lactose	Borderline substances standard ACBS indications p. 1098 Not suitable for child under 3 years	Fortisip Yogurt Style liquid: raspberry, vanilla & lemon 200 ml = £2.28
Fresubin® Protein Energy Drink (Fresenius Kabi Ltd)	Liquid (sip feed) per 100 mL	630 kJ (150 kcal)	10 g cows' milk	12.4 g (sugars 6.4 g)	6.7 g	Nil	Gluten-free Residual lactose Contains fish gelatin	Borderline substances standard ACBS indications p. 1098; also CAPD, haemodialysis.	Fresubin Protein Energy drink: cappuccino, chocolate, tropical fruits, vanilla, wild strawberry 200 ml = £2.15
Fresubin® Thickened (Fresenius Kabi Ltd)	Liquid (sip feed) per 100 mL	630 kJ (150 kcal)	10 g cows' milk	12 g (sugars 7.3 g)	6.7 g	0.83 g	Gluten-free Residual lactose	Dysphagia or disease-related malnutrition.	Fresubin Thickened Level 2: vanilla, wild strawberry 800 ml = £9.40; Fresubin Thickened Level 3: vanilla, wild strawberry 800 ml = £9.40
Fresubin® YOcrème (Fresenius Kabi Ltd)	Semi-solid per 100 g	630 kJ (150 kcal)	7.5 g whey protein	19.5 g (sugars 16.8 g)	4.7 g	Nil	Gluten-free Contains lactose	Dysphagia, or presence or risk of malnutrition Not suitable for child under 3 years	Fresubin YOcreme dessert: apricot-peach, biscuit, lemon, raspberry 500 gram = £8.68

Nutritional supplements: Less than 1.5 kcal/mL and 5 g (or more) protein/100 mL

Not suitable for infants below 1 year unless otherwise stated.

Product	Formulation	Energy	Protein	Carbohydrate	Fat	Fibre	Special Characteristics	ACBS Indications	Presentation & Flavour
Ensure® Plus Crème (Abbott Laboratories Ltd)	Semi-solid per 100 g	574 kJ (137 kcal)	5.68 g cow's milk soy protein isolates	18.4 g (sugars 12.4 g)	4.47 g	Nil	Gluten-free Residual lactose Contains soya	Borderline substances standard ACBS indications p. 1098; also CAPD, haemodialysis. Not suitable for child under 3 years; use with caution in child 3–5 years.	Ensure Plus Creme: banana, chocolate, neutral, vanilla 500 gram = £8.20

Product	Formulation	Energy	Protein	Carbohydrate	Fat	Fibre	Special Characteristics	ACBS Indications	Presentation & Flavour
Nutilis® Fruit Dessert Level 4 (Nutricia Ltd)	Semi-Solid per 100 g	560 kJ (133 kcal)	7 g whey isolate	16.7 g (sugars 11.3 g)	4 g	2.6 g	Gluten-free Residual lactose	Borderline substances standard ACBS indications p. 1098 except bowel fistula; also CAPD, haemodialysis. Not suitable for child under 3 years; use with caution in child 3–5 years.	Nutilis Fruit Dessert Level 4: apple, strawberry 450 gram = £7.56
Oral Impact® (Nestle Health Science)	Standard dilution of powder (74 g in 250 mL water) (sip feed) per 100 mL	425 kJ (101 kcal)	5.6 g cows' milk	13.4 g (sugars 7.4 g)	2.8 g	1 g	Residual lactose Contains fish oil	Pre-operative nutritional supplement for malnourished patients or patients at risk of malnourishment Not suitable for child under 3 years; use with caution in child 3–5 years.	Oral Impact oral powder 74g sachets tropical: 5 sachet = £18.20
Powder provides: protein 16.8 g, carbohydrate 40.2 g, fat 8.3 g, fibre 3 g, energy 1276 kJ (303 kcal)/74 g.									
Renapro Shot® (Stanningley Pharma Ltd)	Liquid (sip feed) per 100ml	583 kJ (137 kcal)	33 g	2.0 g (fructose 2.0 g)	0.1 g	Nil	Gluten-free	For the dietary management of dialysis patients with biochemically proven hypoproteinaemia on the recommendation of a specialist dietician.	Renapro Shot 60ml bottles wild berry: 30 bottle = £69.60

Nutritional supplements: More than 1.5 kcal/mL and 5 g (or more) protein/100 mL

Not suitable for use in child under 6 years unless otherwise stated; not recommended for child under 11 years unless otherwise stated

Product	Formulation	Energy	Protein	Carbohydrate	Fat	Fibre	Special Characteristics	ACBS Indications	Presentation & Flavour
Altraplen® Compact (Nualtra Ltd)	Liquid (sip feed) per 100 mL	1008 kJ (240 kcal)	9.6 g cows' milk soya protein	28.8 g (sugars 11.3 g)	9.6 g	Nil	Gluten-free Residual lactose	Borderline substances standard ACBS indications p. 1098	Altraplen Compact Starter Pack liquid: 500 ml = £5.96; Altraplen Compact liquid: banana, hazel chocolate, strawberry, vanilla 500 ml = £5.32
AYMES® 2.0KCAL (Aymes International Ltd)	Liquid per 100 ml	840 kJ (200 kcal)	8 g milk protein	24 g (sugars 10.0 g)	8 g	Nil	Contains residual lactose	Borderline substances standard ACBS indications p. 1098 except dysphagia.	Aymes 2.0kcal liquid: banana, strawberry, vanilla 800 ml = £6.40
AYMES® ActaGain 2.4 Complete Maxi (Aymes International Ltd)	Liquid per 100 ml serving	1008 kJ (240 kcal)	9.6 g milk protein	28.8 g (sugars 8.0 g)	9.6 g	Nil	Contains residual lactose. Gluten-free	Borderline substances standard ACBS indications p. 1098 except dysphagia.	Aymes ActaGain 2.4 Complete Maxi liquid: strawberry, vanilla 800 ml = £5.32
AYMES® ActaSolve Smoothie (Aymes International Ltd)	Powder per 100 g	1892 kJ (450 kcal)	16.2 g soya protein isolate	62.8 g (sugars 24.8 g)	14.6 g	0.7 g	Contains soya. Gluten-free	Borderline substances standard ACBS indications p. 1098 except dysphagia.	Aymes ActaSolve Smoothie Starter Pack powder: 4 sachet = £5.15; Aymes ActaSolve Smoothie powder 66g sachets: mango, peach, pineapple, strawberry & cranberry 7 sachet = £7.00
Powder 66 g reconstituted with 150ml water provides: protein 10.7 g, carbohydrate 41.5 g, fat 9.7 g, energy 1249 kJ (297 kcal)									
Complan® Shake (Nutricia Ltd)	Powder per 57 g	1065.9 kJ (253.7 kcal)	8.8 g cows' milk	35.6 g (sugars 18.8 g)	8.4 g	Trace g	Gluten-free Contains lactose	Borderline substances standard ACBS indications p. 1098	Complan Shake Starter Pack sachets: 5 sachet = £4.39; Complan Shake oral powder 57g sachets: banana, chocolate, milk, strawberry, vanilla 4 sachet = £2.80
Powder 57 g reconstituted with 200 mL whole milk provides: protein 15.5 g, carbohydrate 44.7 g, fat 15.5 g, energy 1595 kJ (380 kcal).									

Nutritional supplements: More than 1.5 kcal/mL and 5 g (or more) protein/100 mL (product list continued)

Not suitable for use in child under 6 years unless otherwise stated; not recommended for child under 11 years unless otherwise stated

Product	Formulation	Energy	Protein	Carbohydrate	Fat	Fibre	Special Characteristics	ACBS Indications	Presentation & Flavour
Foodlink® Complete (Nualtra Ltd)	Powder **per 100 g**	1869 kJ (444 kcal)	21 g cows' milk soya protein	56 g (sugars 43 g)	15 g	Nil	Contains lactose Gluten-free Contains soya	Borderline substances standard ACBS indications p. 1098 Not to be prescribed for any child under one year; use with caution for young children up to five years of age.	Foodlink Complete powder: banana, chocolate, natural, strawberry, vanilla 1596 gram = £13.72
Recommended serving = the contents of a 57-g sachet in 200 mL full cream milk provides: protein 19 g, carbohydrate 41 g, fat 16 g, energy 161 kJ (383kcal).									
Foodlink® Complete with Fibre (Nualtra Ltd)	Powder **per 100 g**	1779 kJ (423 kcal)	19 g cows' milk soya protein	52 g (sugars 40 g)	14 g	7.2 g	Contains lactose Gluten-free	Borderline substances standard ACBS indications p. 1098 Not to be prescribed for any child under one year; use with caution for young children up to five years of age.	Foodlink Complete powder with fibre Starter Pack: 5 sachet = £3.67 Foodlink Complete powder with fibre 63g sachets: banana, chocolate, natural, strawberry, vanilla 7 sachet = £4.97
Recommended serving = the contents of a 63-g sachet in 200 mL full cream milk provides: protein 19 g, carbohydrate 42 g, fat 16 g, fibre 4.5 g, energy 1667 kJ (397 kcal).									
Forticreme® Complete (Nutricia Ltd)	Semi-solid **per 100 g**	675 kJ (160 kcal)	9.5 g cows' milk	19.2 g (sugars 10.6 g)	5 g	0.1 g	Gluten-free Residual lactose	Borderline substances standard ACBS indications p. 1098; also CAPD, haemodialysis. Not suitable for child under 3 years; use with caution in child 3-5 years.	Forticreme Complete dessert: banana, chocolate, forest fruits, vanilla 500 gram = £8.04
Fortisip® 2kcal (Nutricia Ltd)	Liquid (sip feed) **per 100 mL**	845 kJ (201 kcal)	10.1 g milk proteins	21 g (sugars 15.6 g)	8.6 g	Nil	Contains residual lactose, soya. Gluten-free	Borderline substances standard ACBS indications p. 1098; also CAPD and haemodialysis.	Fortisip 2kcal liquid: chocolate-caramel, forest fruit, mocha, strawberry, vanilla 200 ml = £2.22
Fortisip® Compact (Nutricia Ltd)	Liquid (sip feed) **per 100 mL**	1010 kJ (240 kcal)	9.6 g milk proteins	29.7 g (sugars 15.0 g)	9.3 g	Nil	Contains residual lactose, soya. Gluten-free	Borderline substances standard ACBS indications p. 1098	Fortisip Compact Starter Pack liquid: 750 ml = £7.98; Fortisip Compact liquid: apricot, banana, chocolate, forest fruit, mocha, neutral, strawberry, vanilla 500 ml = £5.32
Fortisip® Compact Fibre (Nutricia Ltd)	Liquid (sip feed) **per 100 mL**	1000 kJ (240 kcal)	9.4 g cows' milk	25.2 g (sugars 13.9 g)	10.4 g	3.6 g	Gluten-free Residual lactose	Borderline substances standard ACBS indications p. 1098 Not suitable for child under 3 years; use with caution in child 3-5 years.	Fortisip Compact Fibre Starter Pack liquid: 500 ml = £8.60; Fortisip Compact Fibre liquid: mocha, strawberry, vanilla 500 ml = £8.60
Fortisip® Compact Protein (Nutricia Ltd)	Liquid (sip feed) **per 100 mL**	1010 kJ (240 kcal)	14.4 g cows' milk	24.4 g (sugars 13.3 g)	9.4 g	Nil	Gluten-free Residual lactose	Borderline substances standard ACBS indications p. 1098	Fortisip Compact Protein Starter Pack liquid: 750 ml = £12.00; 1000 ml = £16.00; Fortisip Compact Protein liquid: banana, berries, hot tropical ginger, mocha, neutral, peach & mango, vanilla 500 ml = £8.00
Fortisip® Extra (Nutricia Ltd)	Liquid (sip feed) **per 100 mL**	675 kJ (160 kcal)	10 g cows' milk	18.1 g (sugars 9 g)	5.3 g	Nil	Gluten-free Contains lactose	Borderline substances standard ACBS indications p. 1098 Not suitable for child under 3 years; use with caution in child 3-5 years.	Fortisip Extra liquid: strawberry, vanilla 200 ml = £2.37

Fresubin® 2 kcal Drink	Liquid (sip feed) **per 100 mL**	840 kJ (200 kcal)	10 g cows' milk	22.5 g (sugars 5.8 g)	7.8 g	Nil	Gluten-free Residual lactose	Borderline substances standard ACBS indications p. 1098; also CAPD, haemodialysis	Fresubin 2kcal drink: apricot-peach, cappuccino, fruits of the forest, neutral, toffee, vanilla 200 ml = £2.23
Fresubin® 2 kcal Fibre Drink (Fresenius Kabi Ltd)	Liquid (sip feed) **per 100 mL**	840 kJ (200 kcal)	10 g cows' milk	22.5 g (sugars 5.8 g)	7.8 g	1.6 g	Gluten-free Residual lactose	Borderline substances standard ACBS indications p. 1098; also CAPD, haemodialysis. Not suitable for use in child under 1 year; use with caution in child 1-5 years.	Fresubin 2kcal Fibre drink: apricot-peach, cappuccino, lemon, neutral 200 ml = £2.23
Fresubin® Powder Extra (Fresenius Kabi Ltd)	Powder **per 100 g**	1764 kJ (420 kcal)	17.5 g cows' milk whey protein	63 g (sugars 24.7 g)	10.9 g	Nil	Gluten-free Contains lactose	Borderline substances standard ACBS indications p. 1098 Not suitable for child under 1 year; use with caution in child 1-5 years.	Fresubin Powder Extra oral powder 62g sachets: chocolate, neutral, strawberry, vanilla 7 sachet = £4.90
62 g reconstituted with 200 ml whole milk provides: protein 17.7 g, carbohydrate 48.5 g, fat 14.8 g, energy 1658 kJ (397 kcal).									
Nutilis® Complete Crème Level 3 (Nutricia Ltd)	Semi-solid **per 100 g**	1030 kJ (245 kcal)	9.6 g cows' milk	29.1 g (sugars 11.8 g)	9.4 g	3.2 g	Gluten-free Residual lactose	Borderline substances standard ACBS indications p. 1098 Not suitable for child under 3 years; use with caution in child 3-6 years.	Nutilis Complete Creme Level 3 custard: chocolate, strawberry, vanilla 500 gram = £9.08
Nutilis® Complete Drink Level 3 (Nutricia Ltd)	Liquid (pre-thickened) **per 100 mL**	1010 kJ (240 kcal)	9.6 g cows' milk	29.1 g (sugars 5.4 g)	9.3 g	3.2 g	Residual lactose	Borderline substances standard ACBS indications p. 1098 Not suitable for child under 3 years; use with caution in child 3-5 years.	Nutilis Complete Drink Level 3 liquid: chocolate, lemon tea, mango & passionfruit, strawberry, vanilla 500 ml = £9.08
Nutricrem® (Nualtra Ltd)	Semi-solid **per 100 g**	756 kJ (180 kcal)	10 g cows' milk soya protein	18.8 g (sugars 9.7 g)	7.2 g	Nil	Gluten-free Residual lactose	Borderline substances standard ACBS indications p. 1098 Not suitable for child under 3 years; use with caution in child 3-6 years.	Nutricrem dessert: strawberry, vanilla 500 gram = £6.78
Renilon® 7.5 (Nutricia Ltd)	Liquid (sip feed) **per 100 mL**	840 kJ (200 kcal)	7.5 g cows' milk	20 g (sugars 4.8 g)	10 g	Nil	Gluten-free Residual lactose	Borderline substances standard ACBS indications p. 1098 Not suitable for child under 3 years; use with caution in child 3-5 years.	Renilon 7.5 liquid: apricot, caramel 500 ml = £9.72
Resource® 2.0 Fibre (Nestle Health Science)	Liquid (sip feed) **per 100 mL**	836 kJ (200 kcal)	9 g cows' milk	21.4 g (sugars 5.5 g)	8.7 g	2.5 g	Gluten-free Residual lactose	Borderline substances standard ACBS indications p. 1098 Not suitable for child under 6 years; caution in child 6-10 years.	Resource Fibre 2.0 liquid: apricot, coffee, neutral, strawberry, summer fruit, vanilla 200 ml = £2.08

Table 3 Specialised formulas

Specialised formulas: Infant and child

Specialised formulas: Infant and child: Amino acid-based formula

Not suitable for child under 1 year of age unless otherwise stated.

Product	Formulation	Energy	Protein	Carbohydrate	Fat	Fibre	Special Characteristics	ACBS Indications	Presentation & Flavour
Neocate® Junior (Nutricia Ltd)	Standard dilution (21.1 %) of powder **per 100ml serving**	420 kJ (100 kcal)	2.8 g protein equivalent (essential and non-essential amino acids)	12 g (sugars 1.1 g)	4.6 g	Nil	Milk protein-free	For the dietary management of proven whole protein allergy, short bowel syndrome, intractable malabsorption and other gastrointestinal disorders where an amino acid diet is recommended, for children from 1 year onwards.	Neocate Junior powder: strawberry, unflavoured, vanilla 400 gram = £30.62
Powder provides protein equivalent 13.3 g, carbohydrate 56 g, fat 22 g, energy 1992 kJ (475 kcal)/100 g.									
Neocate® LCP (Nutricia Ltd)	Standard dilution (13.8%) of powder **per 100 mL**	279 kJ (67 kcal)	1.8 g protein equivalent (essential and non-essential amino acids)	7.2 g (sugars 0.65 g)	3.4 g	Nil	Milk protein and lactose free	For the dietary management of cow's milk allergy, multiple food protein allergies and other conditions where an elemental diet is recommended.	Neocate LCP powder: 400 gram = £22.98
Powder provides: protein equivalent 13 g, carbohydrate 52.5 g, fat 24.5 g, energy 2020 kJ (483 kcal)/100 g.									
Neocate® Spoon (Nutricia Ltd)	Standard dilution of powder **per 97 g serving (37-g sachet diluted with 60 mL water)**	733 kJ (175 kcal)	3 g protein equivalent (essential and non-essential amino acids)	24.9 g (sugars 4.6 g)	7 g	Nil	Milk protein-free	For the dietary management of cow's milk allergy, multiple food protein allergy and other conditions requiring an amino acid-based food.	Neocate Spoon powder 37g sachets: 15 sachet = £43.95
Powder provides protein equivalent 8.2 g, carbohydrate 67.4 g, fat 18.8 g, energy 1981 kJ (472 kcal)/100 g.									
Neocate® Syneo (Nutricia Ltd)	Standard dilution (14.7%) of powder **per 100ml serving**	285 kJ (68.2 kcal)	1.9 g protein equivalent (essential and non-essential amino acids)	7.2 g (sugars 0.68 g)	3.4 g	0.66 g	Milk Protein Free	For the dietary management of cow's milk allergy, multiple food protein allergies and other conditions requiring an amino acid-based diet.	Neocate Syneo powder: 400 gram = £29.56
Powder provides protein equivalent 13 g, carbohydrate 49 g, fat 23 g, energy 1941 kJ (464 kcal)/100 g.									
Nutramigen® Puramino (Reckitt Benckiser Healthcare (UK) Ltd)	Standard dilution (13.6 %) of powder **per 100 mL**	290 kJ (68 kcal)	1.89 g essential and non-essential amino acids	7.2 g	3.6 g	Nil	Gluten-free Lactose-free	For use in the management of severe protein intolerance, multiple food intolerance and other gastro-intestinal disorders where an amino acid based diet is specifically indicated for infants and young children.	Nutramigen PurAmino powder: 400 gram = £23.00
Powder provides: protein 13.9 g, carbohydrate 53 g, fat 26 g, energy 2100 kJ (500 kcal)/100 g.									

SMA Alfamino® (Nestle Health Science)	Standard dilution (13.8 %) of powder **per 100 mL**	291 kJ (69 kcal)	1.8 g protein equivalent (essential and non-essential amino acids)	7.9 g (sugars 2.2 g)	3.4 g	Nil		Severe cows' milk allergy and or multiple food allergies	SMA Alfamino powder: 400 gram = £22.98
Powder provides protein equivalent 13.3 g, carbohydrate 57 g, fat 24.6 g, energy 2105 kJ (503 kcal)/100 g.									

Specialised formulas: Infant and child: Hydrolysate formula

Product	Formulation	Energy	Protein	Carbohydrate	Fat	Fibre	Special Characteristics	ACBS Indications	Presentation & Flavour
Aptamil Pepti-Junior® (Nutricia Early Life Nutrition Ltd)	Standard dilution (12.8 %) of powder **per 100 mL**	275 kJ (66 kcal)	1.8 g whey hydrolysed	6.8 g (sugars 1.1 g)	3.5 g	Nil	Residual lactose Contains fish oil	Disaccharide and/or whole protein intolerance, or where amino acids and peptides are indicated in conjunction with medium chain triglycerides.	Aptamil Pepti-Junior powder: 450 gram = £14.03
Powder provides: protein 14 g, carbohydrate 53.4 g, fat 27.3 g, energy 2155 kJ (515 kcal)/100 g.									
Aptamil Pepti® 1 (Nutricia Early Life Nutrition Ltd)	Standard dilution (13.64 %) of powder **per 100 mL**	276 kJ (66 kcal)	1.6 g whey hydrolysate	7.1 g (sugars 3.5 g)	3.4 g	0.5 g	Contains fish oil, lactose	Established cows' milk allergy with/without proven secondary lactose intolerance.	Aptamil Pepti 1 powder: 400 gram = £9.87; 800 gram = £19.73
Powder provides: protein 11.6 g, carbohydrate 51.8 g, fat 24.7 g, energy 2024 kJ (484 kcal)/100 g.									
Aptamil Pepti® 2 (Nutricia Early Life Nutrition Ltd)	Standard dilution (14.43 %) of powder **per 100 mL**	285 kJ (68 kcal)	1.6 g whey protein hydrolysate	7.8 g (sugars 3.6 g)	3.2 g	0.6 g	Contains fish oil, lactose	Established cows' milk allergy.	Aptamil Pepti 2 powder: 400 gram = £9.41; 800 gram = £18.82
Powder provides: protein 11.4 g, carbohydrate 54.3 g, fat 22.3 g, energy 1974 kJ (471 kcal)/100 g.									
Infatrini® Peptisorb (Nutricia Ltd)	Liquid (sip or tube feed) **per 100 mL**	420 kJ (100 kcal)	2.6 g whey protein hydrolysate	10.3 g (sugars 2.7 g)	5.4 g (MCT 50%)	Nil	Gluten-free Residual lactose Contains fish oil	Disease-related malnutrition, intractable malabsorption, proven inflammatory bowel disease, short bowel syndrome, bowel fistula, and intolerance to whole protein feeds in child from birth to 18 months or body-weight up to 9 kg	Infatrini Peptisorb liquid: 200 ml = £3.92
Nutramigen 1 with LGG® (Reckitt Benckiser Healthcare (UK) Ltd)	Standard dilution (13.5 %) of powder **per 100 mL**	280 kJ (68 kcal)	1.9 g casein hydrolysed	7.5 g	3.4 g	Nil	Residual lactose	For the dietary management of cow's milk allergy with / or without lactose intolerance.	Nutramigen 1 with LGG powder: 400 gram = £11.21
Powder provides: protein 14 g, carbohydrate 55 g, fat 25 g, energy 2100 kJ (500 kcal)/100 g.									
Nutramigen 2 with LGG® (Reckitt Benckiser Healthcare (UK) Ltd)	Standard dilution (14.2 %) of powder **per 100 mL**	280 kJ (68 kcal)	1.7 g casein hydrolysed	8.8 g	2.8 g	Nil	Gluten-free Residual lactose	For the dietary management of cow's milk allergy with / or without lactose intolerance.	Nutramigen 2 with LGG powder: 400 gram = £11.21
Powder provides: protein 12 g, carbohydrate 62 g, fat 20 g, energy 2000 kJ (480 kcal)/100 g.									

Specialised formulas: Infant and child: Hydrolysate formula (product list continued)

Product	Formulation	Energy	Protein	Carbohydrate	Fat	Fibre	Special Characteristics	ACBS Indications	Presentation & Flavour
Pregestimil® Lipil (Reckitt Benckiser Healthcare (UK) Ltd)	Standard dilution (13.5 %) of powder per 100 mL	280 kJ (68 kcal)	1.89 g casein hydrolysed	6.9 g	3.8 g (MCT 54 %)	Nil	Gluten-free Lactose-free	Disaccharide and/or whole protein intolerance, or where amino acids or peptides are indicated in conjunction with medium chain triglycerides.	Pregestimil LIPIL powder: 400 gram = £12.43
Powder provides: protein 14 g, carbohydrate 51 g, fat 28 g, energy 2100 kJ (500 kcal)/100 g.									
Similac® Alimentum (Abbott Laboratories Ltd)	Standard dilution (14%) of powder per 100 mL	283 kJ (67.6 kcal)	1.86 g casein hydrolysed	6.62 g (sugars 1.5 g)	3.75 g (MCT 33%)	Nil	Gluten-free Lactose-free Contains meat derivatives	Cows' milk protein allergy and other conditions where an extensively hydrolysed formula is indicated.	Alimentum powder: 400 gram = £9.69
Powder provides: protein 14.4 g, carbohydrate 51.4 g, fat 29.1 g, energy 2196 kJ (525 kcal)/100 g.									
SMA Althéra® (Nestle Health Science)	Standard dilution (13.2%) of powder per 100 mL	280 kJ (67 kcal)	1.7 g whey hydrolysed	7.3 g (sugars 4 g)	3.4 g	Nil	Contains lactose	Complete nutritional support from birth to 3 years or supplementary feeding from 6 months to 3 years, in cow's milk protein allergy or multiple food protein allergies	SMA Althera powder: 400 gram = £9.86
Powder provides: protein 12.5 g, carbohydrate 55.5 g, fat 26 g, energy 2119 kJ (506 kcal)/100 g.									

Specialised formulas: Infant and child: Residual lactose formula

Product	Formulation	Energy	Protein	Carbohydrate	Fat	Fibre	Special Characteristics	ACBS Indications	Presentation & Flavour
Enfamil® O-Lac (Reckitt Benckiser Healthcare (UK) Ltd)	Standard dilution (13%) of powder per 100 mL	280 kJ (68 kcal)	1.42 g cows' milk	7.2 g	3.7 g	Nil	Gluten-free Residual lactose	Proven lactose intolerance	Enfamil O-Lac powder: 400 gram = £5.08
Powder provides: protein 10.9 g, carbohydrate 55 g, fat 28 g, energy 2200 kJ (524 kcal)/100 g.									
Galactomin 17® (Nutricia Ltd)	Standard dilution (13.6%) of powder per 100 mL	295 kJ (70 kcal)	1.7 g protein equivalent (cows' milk)	7.5 g (sugars 1.4 g)	3.7 g	Nil	Residual lactose	Proven lactose intolerance in pre-school children, galactosaemia, and galactokinase deficiency.	Galactomin 17 powder: 400 gram = £18.79
Powder provides: protein equivalent 12.3 g, carbohydrate 55.3 g, fat 27.2 g, energy 2155 kJ (515 kcal)/100 g. To flavour unflavoured products, see Modjul® Flavour System p. 1126.									
SMA® LF (SMA Nutrition)	Standard dilution (13 %) of powder per 100 mL	281 kJ (67 kcal)	1.5 g casein, whey	7.2 g (sugars 2.6 g)	3.6 g	Nil	Residual lactose	Proven lactose intolerance	SMA LF powder: 400 gram = £5.32
Powder provides: protein 12 g, carbohydrate 55.6 g, fat 28 g, energy 2185 kJ (522 kcal)/100 g.									

Specialised formulas: Infant and child: MCT-enhanced formula

Suitable for infants from birth; Child under 12 years.

Product	Formulation	Energy	Protein	Carbohydrate	Fat	Fibre	Special Characteristics	ACBS Indications	Presentation & Flavour
Lipistart® (Vitaflo International Ltd)	Standard dilution (15%) of powder per 100 mL	282 kJ (68 kcal)	2.1 g protein equivalent (whey, soya)	8.3 g (sugars 0.7 g)	3.1 g (MCT 81%)	Nil	Residual lactose	Dietary management of fat malabsorption, long-chain fatty acid oxidation disorders, and other disorders requiring a high MCT, low LCT formula.	Lipistart powder: 400 gram = £21.90
Powder provides: protein equivalent 13.7 g, carbohydrate 55.3 g, fat 20.6 g, energy 1883 kJ (450 kcal)/100 g.									
Monogen® (Nutricia Ltd)	Standard dilution (17.5%) of powder per 100 mL	310 kJ (74 kcal)	2.2 g protein equivalent (whey)	12 g (sugars 1.2 g)	1.9 g (MCT 80 %)	Nil	Residual lactose Supplementation with essential fatty acids may be needed	Long-chain acyl-CoA dehydrogenase deficiency (LCAD), carnitine palmitoyl transferase deficiency (CPTD), primary and secondary lipoprotein lipase deficiency, chylothorax, and lymphangiectasia	Monogen powder: 400 gram = £22.71
Powder provides: protein equivalent 12.5 g, carbohydrate 68 g, fat 11 g, energy 1769 kJ (420 kcal)/100 g.									

Specialised formulas: Infant and child: Soya-based formula

Product	Formulation	Energy	Protein	Carbohydrate	Fat	Fibre	Special Characteristics	ACBS Indications	Presentation & Flavour
Wysoy® (SMA Nutrition)	Standard dilution (13.2%) of powder per 100 mL	280 kJ (67 kcal)	1.8 g soya protein isolate	6.9 g (sugars 2.5 g)	3.6 g	Nil	Lactose-free	Proven lactose and associated sucrose intolerance in pre-school children, galactokinase deficiency, galactosaemia, and proven whole cows' milk sensitivity.	SMA Wysoy powder: 800 gram = £10.45; 860 gram = £10.93
Powder provides: protein 14 g, carbohydrate 54 g, fat 27 g, energy 2155 kJ (515 kcal)/100 g.									

Specialised formulas: Infant and child: Low calcium formula

Product	Formulation	Energy	Protein	Carbohydrate	Fat	Fibre	Special Characteristics	ACBS Indications	Presentation & Flavour
Locasol® (Nutricia Ltd)	Standard dilution (13.1%) of powder per 100 mL	278 kJ (66 kcal)	1.9 g cows' milk	7 g (sugars 6.9 g)	3.4 g	Nil	Contains lactose Calcium less than 7 mg/100 mL No added vitamin D	Conditions of calcium intolerance requiring restriction of calcium and vitamin D intake	Locasol powder: 400 gram = £26.14
Powder provides: protein 14.6 g, carbohydrate 53.7 g, fat 26.1 g, energy 2125 kJ (508 kcal)/100 g.									

Specialised formulas: Infant and child: Fructose-based formula

Product	Formulation	Energy	Protein	Carbohydrate	Fat	Fibre	Special Characteristics	ACBS Indications	Presentation & Flavour
Galactomin 19® (Nutricia Ltd)	Standard dilution (12.9%) of powder per 100 mL	288 kJ (69 kcal)	1.9 g protein equivalent (cows' milk)	6.4 g (fructose 6.3 g)	4 g	Nil	Residual lactose, galactose and glucose	Conditions of glucose plus galactose intolerance	Galactomin 19 powder: 400 gram = £49.48
Powder provides: protein equivalent 14.6 g, carbohydrate 49.7 g, fat 30.8 g, energy 2233 kJ (534 kcal)/100 g.									

Specialised formulas: Infant and child: Pre-thickened infant feeds

Product	Formulation	Energy	Protein	Carbohydrate	Fat	Fibre	Special Characteristics	ACBS Indications	Presentation & Flavour
Enfamil® AR (Reckitt Benckiser Healthcare (UK) Ltd)	Standard dilution (13.5%) of powder per 100 mL	285 kJ (68 kcal)	1.7 g cows' milk	7.6 g (lactose 4.6 g)	3.5 g	Nil	Contains lactose, pregelatinised rice starch	Significant gastro-oesophageal reflux	Enfamil AR powder: 400 gram = £3.80
Powder provides: protein 12.5 g, carbohydrate 56 g, fat 26 g, energy 2093 kJ (500 kcal)/100 g.									

Specialised formulas for specific clinical conditions

Not suitable for child under 1 year unless otherwise stated; use with caution in child 1–4 years unless otherwise stated.

Product	Formulation	Energy	Protein	Carbohydrate	Fat	Fibre	Special Characteristics	ACBS Indications	Presentation & Flavour
Alicalm® (Nutricia Ltd)	Standard dilution (30%) of powder per 100 mL	567 kJ (135 kcal)	4.5 g caseinate whey	17.4 g (sugars 3.2 g)	5.3 g	Nil	Residual lactose	Crohn's disease Not suitable for child under 1 year; use as nutritional supplement only in children 1-6 years.	Alicalm oral powder: 400 gram = £24.04
Powder provides: protein 15 g, carbohydrate 58 g, fat 17.5 g, energy 1889 kJ (450 kcal)/100 g.									
Forticare® (Nutricia Ltd)	Liquid (sip feed) per 100 mL.	675 kJ (160 kcal)	9 g cows' milk	19.1 g (sugars 13.6 g)	5.3 g	2.1 g	Gluten-free Residual lactose Contains fish oil	Nutritional supplement in patients with lung cancer undergoing chemotherapy, or with pancreatic cancer Not suitable in child under 3 years	Forticare liquid: cappuccino, orange & lemon, peach & ginger 500 ml = £10.04
Heparon® Junior (Nutricia Ltd)	Standard dilution (18%) of powder per 100 mL	363 kJ (86 kcal)	2 g cows' milk	11.6 g (sugars 2.9 g)	3.6 g	Nil	Contains lactose Electrolytes/100 mL: Na^+ 0.56 mmol K^+ 1.9 mmol Ca^{2+} 2.3 mmol P^+ 1.6 mmol	Enteral feed or nutritional supplement for children with acute or chronic liver failure	Heparon Junior powder: 400 gram = £24.22
Powder provides: protein 11.1 g, carbohydrate 64.2 g, fat 19.9 g, energy 2016 kJ (480 kcal)/100 g.									
KetoCal® (Nutricia Ltd)	Standard dilution (20 %) of powder per 100 mL	602 kJ (146 kcal)	3.1 g cows' milk with additional amino acids	0.6 g (sugars 0.12 g)	14.6 g (LCT 100 %)	Nil	Electrolytes/100 mL: Na^+ 4.3 mmol K^+ 4.1 mmol Ca^{2+} 2.15 mmol P^+ 2.77 mmol	Enteral feed or nutritional supplement as part of ketogenic diet in management of epilepsy resistant to drug therapy, in children over 1 year, only on the advice of secondary care physician with experience of ketogenic diet.	KetoCal 4:1 powder: unflavoured, vanilla 300 gram = £34.10
Powder provides: protein 15.25 g, carbohydrate 3 g, fat 73 g, energy 3011 kJ (730 kcal)/100 g.									
KetoCal® 3:1 (Nutricia Ltd)	Standard dilution (9.5%) of powder per 100 mL	276 kJ (66 kcal)	1.5 g	0.68 g (sugars 0.57 g)	6.4 g	Nil	Electrolytes/100 mL: Na^+ 1.3 mmol K^+ 2.4 mmol Ca^{2+} 2 mmol P^+ 1.7 mmol	Enteral feed or nutritional supplement as part of ketogenic diet in management of drug resistant epilepsy or other conditions for which a ketogenic diet is indicated in children from birth to 6 years; as a nutritional supplement in children over 6 years.	KetoCal 3:1 powder: 300 gram = £33.01
Powder provides: protein 15.3 g, carbohydrate 7.2 g, fat 67.7 g, energy 2927 kJ (699 kcal)/100 g.									

KetoCal® 4:1 LQ (Nutricia Ltd)	Liquid (sip or tube feed) **per 100 mL**	620 kJ (150 kcal)	3.09 g casein and whey with additional amino acids	0.61 g (sugars 0.23 g)	14.8 g (LCT 100 %)	1.12 g	Residual lactose Electrolytes/100 mL: Na^+ 4.9 mmol K^+ 4.7 mmol Ca^{2+} 2.4 mmol P^+ 3.1 mmol	Enteral feed or nutritional supplement as part of ketogenic diet in management of drug resistant epilepsy or other conditions for which a ketogenic diet is indicated in children 1-10 years; as a nutritional supplement in children over 10 years.	KetoCal 4:1LQ liquid: unflavoured, vanilla 200 ml = £4.86
Kindergen® (Nutricia Ltd)	Standard dilution (20 %) of powder **per 100 mL**	421 kJ (101 kcal)	1.5 g whey protein	11.8 g (sugars 1.2 g)	5.3 g (LCT 93 %)	Nil	Electrolytes/100 mL: Na^+ 2 mmol K^+ 0.6 mmol Ca^{2+} 2.8 mmol P^+ 3 mmol Low Vitamin A	Enteral feed or nutritional supplement for children with chronic renal failure receiving peritoneal rapid overnight dialysis.	Kindergen powder: 400 gram = £32.51
Powder provides: protein 7.5 g, carbohydrate 59 g, fat 26.3 g, energy 2104 kJ (504 kcal)/100 g.									
Modulen IBD® (Nestle Health Science)	Standard dilution (20%) of powder (sip or tube feed) **per 100 mL**	420 kJ (100 kcal)	3.6 g casein	11 g (sugars 3.98 g)	4.7 g	Nil	Gluten-free Residual lactose	Crohn's disease active phase, and in remission if malnourished	Modulen IBD powder: 400 gram = £16.19
Powder provides: protein 18 g, carbohydrate 54 g, fat 23 g, energy 2070 kJ (500 kcal)/100 g.									
Nepro® (Abbott Laboratories Ltd)	Liquid (sip or tube feed) **per 100 mL**	838 kJ (200 kcal)	7 g cows' milk	20.6 g (sugars 3.26 g)	9.6 g	1.56 g	Gluten-free Residual lactose Electrolytes/100 mL: Na^+ 3.67 mmol K^+ 2.72 mmol Ca^{2+} 3.43 mmol P^+ 2.23 mmol	Enteral feed or nutritional supplement in patients with chronic renal failure who are on haemodialysis or CAPD, or with cirrhosis, or other conditions requiring a high energy, low fluid, low electrolyte diet. Not suitable for child under 1 year; use with caution in child 1-5 years.	Nepro HP liquid: strawberry 220 ml = £3.60; vanilla 220 ml = £3.60; 500 ml = £8.24
ProSure® (Abbott Laboratories Ltd)	Liquid (sip or tube feed) **per 100 mL**	536 kJ (127 kcal)	6.65 g	18.3 g (sugars 6.5 g)	2.56 g	2.07 g	Gluten-free Residual lactose Contains fish oil	For pancreatic cancer, oesophageal cancer and patients with lung cancer who are undergoing chemotherapy.	ProSure liquid: 220 ml = £3.69
Renamil® (Stanningley Pharma Ltd)	Powder (sip or tube feed when reconstituted) **per 100 g**	2003 kJ (477 kcal)	4.6 g cows' milk	70.8 g	19.3 g	Nil	Contains lactose Gluten-free Electrolytes/100 g: Na^+ 1.04 mmol K^+ 0.13 mmol Ca^{2+} 10.22 mmol P^+ 1.06 mmol Contains no vitamin A or vitamin D	Enteral feed or nutritional supplement for adults and children over 1 year with chronic renal failure.	Renapro powder 100g sachets: 10 sachet = £25.40

Specialised formulas for specific clinical conditions (product list continued)

Not suitable for child under 1 year unless otherwise stated; use with caution in child 1–4 years unless otherwise stated.

Product	Formulation	Energy	Protein	Carbohydrate	Fat	Fibre	Special Characteristics	ACBS Indications	Presentation & Flavour
Renapro® (Stanningley Pharma Ltd)	Powder **per 100 g**	1558 kJ (372 kcal)	90 g whey protein	3.4 g	1 g	Nil	Gluten-free Do not use in cow's milk allergy, or where absorption and digestive problems are present Electrolytes/100 g: Na^+ 15.65 mmol K^+ 4.60 mmol Ca^{2+} 4.74 mmol Mg^+ 0.82 mmol P^+ 3.55 mmol	Nutritional supplement for biochemically proven hypoproteinaemia and patients undergoing dialysis. Not suitable for child under 1 year.	Renapro powder 20g sachets: 30 sachet = £69.60
Powder provides: protein 18 g, energy 312 kJ (74 kcal)/20-g sachet.									
Renastart® (Vitaflo International Ltd)	Standard dilution (20%) of powder **per 100 mL**	414 kJ (99 kcal)	1.5 g cows' milk soya	12.5 g (sugars 1.3 g)	4.8 g	Nil	Contains lactose Electrolytes/100 mL: Na^+ 2.1 mmol K^+ 0.6 mmol Ca^{2+} 0.6 mmol P^+ 0.6 mmol	Dietary management of renal failure in child from birth to 10 years.	Renastart powder: 400 gram = £29.81
Powder provides: protein 7.5 g, carbohydrate 62.5 g, fat 23.8 g, energy 2071 kJ (494 kcal)/100 g.									
Supportan® (Fresenius Kabi Ltd)	Liquid (sip feed) **per 100 mL**	630 kJ (150 kcal)	10 g cows' milk	12.4 g (sugars 7.5 g)	6.7 g	1.5 g	Gluten-free Residual lactose Contains fish oil	Nutritional supplement in patients with pancreatic cancer or with lung cancer undergoing chemotherapy Not suitable for child under 1 year; use with caution in child 1–4 years	Supportan drink: cappuccino 800 ml = £11.60; tropical fruits 200 ml = £2.90; 800 ml = £11.60

Table 4 Feed supplements

High-energy supplements

High-energy supplements: carbohydrate

Flavoured carbohydrate supplements are not suitable for child under 1 year; liquid supplements should be diluted before use in child under 5 years.

Product	Formulation	Energy	Protein	Carbohydrate	Fat	Fibre	Special Characteristics	ACBS Indications	Presentation & Flavour
Maxijul® Super Soluble (Nutricia Ltd)	Powder **per 100 g**	1615 kJ (380 kcal)	Nil	95 g Glucose polymer (sugars 8.6 g)	Nil	Nil	Gluten-free Lactose-free	Disease-related malnutrition, malabsorption states, or other conditions requiring fortification with a high or readily available carbohydrate supplement.	Maxijul Super Soluble powder: 4x132g sachets = £7.25; 1x200 gram = £2.91; 1x25000 gram = £174.08
Polycal® (Nutricia Ltd)	Powder **per 100 g**	1630 kJ (384 kcal)	Nil	96 g Maltodextrin (sugars 6 g)	Nil	Nil	Gluten-free Lactose-free	Disease-related malnutrition, malabsorption states, or other conditions requiring fortification with a high or readily available carbohydrate supplement.	Polycal powder: 400 gram = £4.84

	Liquid **per 100 mL**	1050 kJ (247 kcal)	Nil	61.9 g Maltodextrin (sugars 12.2 g)	Nil	Nil		Disease-related malnutrition, malabsorption states, or other conditions requiring fortification with a high or readily available carbohydrate supplement.	Polycal liquid: neutral, orange 200 ml = £1.92
S.O.S.® (Vitaflo International Ltd)	Powder **per 100 g**	1590 kJ (380 kcal)	Nil	95 g (sugars 9 g)	Nil	Nil		For use as an emergency regimen in the dietary management of inborn errors of metabolism in adults and children from birth.	S.O.S10 oral powder 30x21g sachets = £8.26; S.O.S15 oral powder 30x31g sachets = £12.19; S.O.S20 oral powder 30x42g sachets = £16.53; S.O.S25 oral powder 30x52g sachets = £20.44
Contents of each sachet should be reconstituted with water to a total volume of 200 mL									
Vitajoule® (Vitaflo International Ltd)	Powder **per 100 g**	1590 kJ (380 kcal)	Nil	95 g Dried glucose syrup (sugars 9 g)	Nil	Nil	Gluten-free Lactose-free	Disease-related malnutrition, malabsorption states, or other conditions requiring fortification with a high or readily available carbohydrate supplement. Flavoured carbohydrate supplements are not suitable for child under 1 year; liquid supplements should be diluted before use in child under 5 years.	Vitajoule powder: 500 gram = £4.94

High-energy supplements: fat

Liquid supplements should be diluted before use in child under 5 years

Product	Formulation	Energy	Protein	Carbohydrate	Fat	Fibre	Special Characteristics	ACBS Indications	Presentation & Flavour
Calogen® (Nutricia Ltd)	Liquid (sip or tube feed) **per 100 mL**	1850 kJ (450 kcal)	Nil	0.1 g (sugar nil)	50.0 g	Nil	Banana and strawberry flavours not suitable for child under 3 years. Gluten-free. Lactose-free	Disease-related malnutrition, malabsorption states, or other conditions requiring fortification with a high fat supplement, with or without fluid and electrolyte restrictions.	Calogen emulsion: banana 500 ml = £12.11; neutral, strawberry 200 ml = £4.92; 500 ml = £12.11
Fresubin® 5 kcal Shot (Fresenius Kabi Ltd)	Liquid (emulsion) **per 100 mL**	2100 kJ (500 kcal)	Nil	4.0 g (sucrose)	53.8 g	0.4 g	Gluten-free Lactose-free	Disease-related malnutrition, malabsorption states, or other conditions requiring fortification with a high fat (or fat and carbohydrate) supplement. Liquid supplements should be diluted before use in child under 5 years. Not suitable for child under 3 years.	Fresubin 5kcal shot drink: lemon, neutral 480 ml = £11.96
Liquigen® (Nutricia Ltd)	Liquid (emulsion) **per 100 mL**	1850 kJ (450 kcal)	Nil	Nil	50 g (MCT 97 %) Fractionated coconut oil	Nil	Gluten-free Lactose-free	Steatorrhoea associated with cystic fibrosis of the pancreas, intestinal lymphangiectasia, intestinal surgery, chronic liver disease, liver cirrhosis, other proven malabsorption syndromes, ketogenic diet in epilepsy, and in type 1 lipoproteinaemia Not suitable for child under 1 year	Liquigen emulsion: 250 ml = £10.36

High-energy supplements: fat (product list continued)

Liquid supplements should be diluted before use in child under 5 years

Product	Formulation	Energy	Protein	Carbohydrate	Fat	Fibre	Special Characteristics	ACBS Indications	Presentation & Flavour
Medium-chain Triglyceride (MCT) Oil (Nutricia Ltd)	Liquid **per 100 mL**	3515 kJ (855 kcal)	Nil	Nil	MCT 100 %	Nil		Nutritional supplement for steatorrhoea associated with cystic fibrosis of the pancreas, intestinal lymphangiectasia, intestinal surgery, chronic liver disease and liver cirrhosis, other proven malabsorption syndromes, ketogenic diet in management of epilepsy, type 1 hyperlipoproteinaemia	MCT oil: 500 ml = £16.43

FAT AND CARBOHYDRATE

Product	Formulation	Energy	Protein	Carbohydrate	Fat	Fibre	Special Characteristics	ACBS Indications	Presentation & Flavour
Duocal® Super Soluble (Nutricia Ltd)	Powder **per 100 g**	2061 kJ (492 kcal)	Nil	72.7 g (sugars 6.5 g)	22.3 g (MCT 35 %)	Nil		Disease-related malnutrition, malabsorption states, or other conditions requiring fortification with a high fat (or fat and carbohydrate) supplement.	Duocal Super Soluble powder: 400 gram = £20.23
Energivit® (Nutricia Ltd)	Standard dilution (15%) of powder **per 100 mL**	309 kJ (74 kcal)	Nil	10 g (sugars 900 mg)	3.75 g	Nil	Lactose-free With vitamins, minerals, and trace elements	For children requiring additional energy, vitamins, minerals, and trace elements following a protein-restricted diet	Energivit powder: 400 gram = £24.60

Powder provides: carbohydrate 66.7 g, fat 25 g, energy 2059 kJ (492 kcal)/100 g.

High-energy supplements: protein

Product	Formulation	Energy	Protein	Carbohydrate	Fat	Fibre	Special Characteristics	ACBS Indications	Presentation & Flavour
ProSource® Jelly (Nutrinovo Ltd)	Semi-solid **per 100 mL**	315 kJ (75 kcal)	16.9 g collagen protein hydrolysate whey protein isolate	Less than 1 g	Nil	Less than 1 g	Gluten-free Lactose-free Contains porcine derivatives	Hypoproteinaemia Not recommended for child under 3 years	ProSource jelly: fruit punch, orange 118 ml = £1.99
Protifar® (Nutricia Ltd)	Powder **per 100 g**	1580 kJ (373 kcal)	88.5 g cows' milk	less than 1.5 g	1.6 g	Nil	Gluten-free Residual lactose Electrolytes/100 mL: Na^{+} 1.3 mmol K^{+} 1.28 mmol Ca^{2+} 33.75 mmol P^{+} 22.58 mmol	Nutritional supplement for use in biochemically proven hypoproteinaemia.	Protifar powder: 225 gram = £9.84

Powder provides: protein 2.2 g per 2.5 g.

PROTEIN AND CARBOHYDRATE
Not recommended for child under 3 years

Product	Formulation	Energy	Protein	Carbohydrate	Fat	Fibre	Special Characteristics	ACBS Indications	Presentation & Flavour
Dialamine® (Nutricia Ltd)	Standard dilution (20%) of powder **per 100 mL**	264 kJ (62 kcal)	4.3 g protein equivalent (essential and non-essential amino acids)	11.2 g (sugars 10.2 g)	Nil	Nil	Contains vitamin C	Hypoproteinaemia, chronic renal failure, wound fistula leakage with excessive protein loss, conditions requiring a controlled nitrogen intake, and haemodialysis. Not suitable for child under 6 months.	Dialamine powder: 400 gram = £82.20
Powder provides: protein equivalent 25 g, carbohydrate 65 g, vitamin C 125 mg, energy 1530 kJ (360 kcal)/100 g.									
ProSource® Liquid (Nutrinovo Ltd)	Liquid **per 30 mL**	420 kJ (100 kcal)	10 g collagen protein whey protein isolate	15 g (sugars 8 g)	Nil	Nil	Gluten-free Lactose-free May contain porcine derivatives	Biochemically proven hypoproteinaemia Not recommended for child under 3 years.	ProSource liquid 30ml sachets: citrus berry, lemon, neutral, orange creme 100 sachet = £107.32
ProSource® Plus (Nutrinovo Ltd)	Liquid **per 30 mL**	420 kJ (100 kcal)	15 g collagen protein whey protein isolate	11 g (sugars 10 g)	Nil	Nil	Gluten-free Residual lactose Contains porcine derivatives	Hypoproteinaemia	ProSource Plus liquid 30ml sachets: citrus berry, neutral, orange creme 50 sachet = £76.33; 100 sachet = £152.66

PROTEIN, FAT, AND CARBOHYDRATE
Not suitable for use in child under 3 years unless otherwise stated; not recommended for child 3-6 years unless otherwise stated

Product	Formulation	Energy	Protein	Carbohydrate	Fat	Fibre	Special Characteristics	ACBS Indications	Presentation & Flavour
Calogen® Extra (Nutricia Ltd)	Liquid (sip or tube feed) **per 100 mL**	1650 kJ (400 kcal)	5.0 g caseinates, whey protein hydrolysate	4.5 g (sugars 3.5 g)	40.3 g	Nil	Contains residual lactose. Gluten-free	Disease related malnutrition, malabsorption states or other conditions requiring fortification with a high fat supplement with or without fluid restriction.	Calogen Extra Shots emulsion: neutral, strawberry 240 ml = £5.88; Calogen Extra emulsion: neutral, strawberry 200 ml = £4.98
Calshake® (Fresenius Kabi Ltd)	Powder **per 87 g**	2504 kJ (598.5 kcal)	12 g cows' milk	70.2 g (sugars 22.4 g)	29.9 g	Nil	Contains lactose Gluten-free	Disease related malnutrition, malabsorption states or other conditions requiring fortification with a fat/carbohydrate supplement.	Calshake powder 87g sachets: banana, neutral, strawberry, vanilla 7 sachet = £18.41; Calshake powder 90g sachets chocolate: 7 sachet = £18.41
Powder: one sachet reconstituted with 240 mL whole milk provides approx. 600 kcal and 12 g protein.									
Enshake® (Abbott Laboratories Ltd)	Powder **per 100 g**	1893 kJ (450 kcal)	8.4 g cows' milk, soy protein isolate	69 g (sugars14.5 g)	15.6 g	Nil	Residual lactose Contains vitamins and minerals	Disease-related malnutrition, malabsorption states, or other conditions requiring fortification with a high fat or carbohydrate (with protein) supplement. Not suitable for child under 1 year; use with caution in child 1-6 years.	Enshake oral powder 96.5g sachets: banana, chocolate, strawberry, vanilla 6 sachet = £15.65
Powder: 96.5 g reconstituted with 240 mL whole milk provides approx. 2 kcal/mL and protein 16 g.									

PROTEIN, FAT, AND CARBOHYDRATE (PRODUCT LIST CONTINUED)

Not suitable for use in child under 3 years unless otherwise stated; not recommended for child 3-6 years unless otherwise stated

Product	Formulation	Energy	Protein	Carbohydrate	Fat	Fibre	Special Characteristics	ACBS Indications	Presentation & Flavour
MCT Procal® (Vitaflo International Ltd)	Powder **per 100 g**	2742 kJ (657 kcal)	12.5 g cows' milk	20.6 g (sugars 3.1 g)	63.1 g (MCT 99%)	Nil	Contains lactose	Dietary management of disorders of long-chain fatty acid oxidation, fat malabsorption, and other disorders requiring a low LCT, high MCT supplement. Not suitable for child under 1 year.	MCTprocal oral powder 16g sachets: 30 sachet = £26.85
Powder 16 g provides: protein 2 g, carbohydrate 3.3 g, fat 10.1 g, energy 439 kJ (105 kcal).									
Pro-Cal® (Vitaflo International Ltd)	Powder **per 100 g**	2764 kJ (667 kcal)	13.6 g cows' milk	28.2 g (sugars 16 g)	55.5 g	Nil	Contains lactose Gluten-free	Disease-related malnutrition, malabsorption states or other conditions requiring fortification with a fat / carbohydrate supplement (with protein). Suitable from one year of age.	Pro-Cal powder: 510 gram = £16.58; 1500 gram = £33.78; 12500 gram = £240.16
Powder 15 g provides: protein 2 g, carbohydrate 4.2 g, fat 8.3 g, energy 415 kJ (100 kcal).									
Pro-Cal® Shot (Vitaflo International Ltd)	Liquid **per 100 mL**	1385 kJ (334 kcal)	6.7 g cows' milk	13.4 g (sugars 13.3 g)	28.2 g	Nil	Contains lactose Gluten-free Contains soya	Disease-related malnutrition, malabsorption states, or other conditions requiring fortification with a high fat or carbohydrate (with protein) supplement. Not suitable for child under 3 years.	Pro-Cal Shot: banana, neutral, strawberry 720 ml = £15.71; starter pack 360 ml = £7.86
Scandishake® Mix (Nutricia Ltd)	Powder **per 100 g**	2099 kJ (500 kcal)	4.7 g cows' milk	65 g (sugars 14.3 g)	24.7 g	Nil	Gluten-free Contains lactose	Disease-related malnutrition, malabsorption states, or other conditions requiring fortification with a high fat or carbohydrate (with protein) supplement. Not suitable for child under 3 years.	Scandishake Mix oral powder 85g sachets: banana, caramel, chocolate, strawberry, unflavoured, vanilla 6 sachet = £15.96
Powder: 85 g reconstituted with 240 mL whole milk provides: protein 11.7 g, carbohydrate 66.8 g, fat 30.4 g, energy 2457 kJ (588 kcal).									
Vitasavoury® (Vitaflo International Ltd)	Powder **per 100 g**	2562 kJ (619 kcal)	12 g cows' milk	22.5 g (sugars 1.4 g Chicken/2.7 g Golden Vegetable)	52 g	6.4 g	Contains lactose Contains soya (chicken flavour) Contains gluten (wheat) (chicken flavour) Contains celery (golden vegetable flavour)	Disease-related malnutrition, malabsorption states, or other conditions requiring fortification with a high fat or carbohydrate (with protein) supplement. Not suitable for child under 3 years.	Vitasavoury powder 50g sachets: chicken, golden vegetable 10 sachet = £21.44

Fibre, vitamin, and mineral supplements

Vitamin and Mineral supplements

Not suitable for child under 4 years
Chewable tablets not suitable for child under 4 years. Liquid not suitable for child over 3 years. Softgels not suitable for child under 10 years.

Product	Formulation	Energy	Protein	Carbohydrate	Fat	Fibre	Special Characteristics	ACBS Indications	Presentation & Flavour
DEKAS® Essential (Alveolus Biomedical B.V.)	Capsule per 100 g	2642 kJ (631 kcal)	Nil	50 g	49 g	Nil	Contains fish gelatin	For the dietary management of patients with cystic fibrosis on the specific recommendation of a specialist in cystic fibrosis.	DEKAs Essential capsules: 60 capsule = £36.51
DEKAS® Plus (Alveolus Biomedical B.V.)	Solid per 100 g	1577 kJ (377 kcal)	2.5 g	88 g (sugars 70 g)	1.8 g	Nil		For the dietary management of patients with cystic fibrosis on the specific recommendation of a specialist in cystic fibrosis.	DEKAs Plus chewable tablets: 60 tablet = £42.58
	Liquid per 100 mL	400 kJ (100 kcal)	2 g	22 g	Nil	Nil		For the dietary management of patients with cystic fibrosis on the specific recommendation of a specialist in cystic fibrosis.	DEKAs Plus liquid: 60 ml = £33.24
	Solid per 100 g	2090 kJ (500 kcal)	25 g	22 g (sugars less than 100 mg)	43 g	Nil	Contains bovine gelatin Contains soy	For the dietary management of patients with cystic fibrosis on the specific recommendation of a specialist in cystic fibrosis.	DEKAs Plus softgels capsules: 60 capsule = £42.58
FruitiVits® (Vitaflo International Ltd)	Powder per 100 g	133 kJ (33 kcal)	Nil	8.3 g (sugars 400 mg)	0.1 g	3.3 g		Vitamin, mineral, and trace element supplement in children 3–10 years with restrictive therapeutic diets	FruitiVits oral powder 6g sachets: 30 sachet = £72.63
Paediatric Seravit® (Nutricia Ltd)	Powder per 100 g	1275 kJ (300 kcal)	Nil	75 g (sugars 6.75 g)	Nil	Nil	Pineapple flavour not suitable for child under 6 months	Vitamin, mineral, and trace element supplement in infants and children with restrictive therapeutic diets.	Seravit Paediatric powder: pineapple 200 gram = £21.35; unflavoured 200 gram = £20.03

To flavour unflavoured products, see Modjul® Flavour System p. 1126.

Feed additives

Special additives for conditions of intolerance

Colief®

▸ Transient Lactase Deficiency. For dosage and administration details, consult product literature.
LIQUID, lactase 50 000 units/g

Colief 50,000units/g infant drops (Crosscare Ltd)
7 ml (ACBS) · NHS indicative price = £8.40

Fructose

▸ (Laevulose) For proven glucose/galactose intolerance

Dietade dietary foods fruit sugar (Margetts)
250 gram · No NHS indicative price available

Glucose

▸ (Dextrose monohydrate) For use as an energy supplement in sucrose-isomaltase deficiency

Glucose powder for oral use BP 1980 (Ennogen Healthcare Ltd)
500 gram (ACBS) · No NHS indicative price available · Drug Tariff (Part VIIIA Category C) price = £1.75

Glucose powder for oral use BP 1980 (Thornton & Ross Ltd)
500 gram (ACBS) · NHS indicative price = £1.75 · Drug Tariff (Part VIIIA Category C) price = £1.75

Feed thickeners and pre-thickened drinks

Carobel, Instant®

▸ For thickening feeds in the treatment of vomiting.
POWDER, carob seed flour.

Instant Carobel powder (Cow & Gate Ltd)
135 gram (ACBS) · NHS indicative price = £2.98

Multi-thick®

▸ For thickening of liquids and foods in dysphagia. Not suitable for child under 3 years.
POWDER, modified maize starch, gluten and lactose-free.

Multi-thick powder (Abbott Laboratories Ltd)
250 gram (ACBS) · NHS indicative price = £4.83

Nutilis® Clear

▸ For thickening of liquids or foods in dysphagia. Not suitable for children under 3 years.
POWDER, dried glucose syrup, xanthan gum, guar gum, gluten- and lactose-free.

Nutilis Clear powder (Nutricia Ltd)
175 gram (ACBS) · NHS indicative price = £8.46

Nutilis® Powder

▸ For thickening of food and fluidin dysphagia. Not suitable for child under 3 years.
POWDER, carbohydrate 87.5 g, energy 1545 kJ (363 kcal)/100 g, contains modified starch. Gluten-free and lactose-free.

Nutilis powder (Nutricia Ltd)
300 gram (ACBS) · NHS indicative price = £5.66

Resource® Thickened Drink

▸ For dysphagia. Not suitable for children under 3 years.
LIQUID, carbohydrate: orange 21 g; apple 23 g, energy: orange 376 kJ (89 kcal); apple 396 kJ (93 kcal)/100 mL.

Resource Thickened Drink custard apple (Nestle Health Science)
114 ml (ACBS) · NHS indicative price = £0.78

Resource Thickened Drink custard orange (Nestle Health Science)
114 ml (ACBS) · NHS indicative price = £0.78

Resource Thickened Drink syrup orange (Nestle Health Science)
114 ml (ACBS) · NHS indicative price = £0.78

Resource® ThickenUp Clear

▸ For thickening of liquids or foods in dysphagia. Not suitable for children under 3 years.
POWDER, maltodextrin (corn, potato), xanthan gum, potassium chloride. Gluten-free. May contain milk (tin only).

Resource ThickenUp Clear powder (Nestle Health Science)
127 gram (ACBS) · NHS indicative price = £8.46

Resource® ThickenUp®

▸ For thickening of foods in dysphagia. Suitable for children above 3 years of age.
POWDER, modified maize starch. Gluten-free.

Resource ThickenUp powder (Nestle Health Science)
227 gram (ACBS) · NHS indicative price = £4.66

SLO Drinks®

▸ Nutritional supplement for patient hydration in the dietary management of dysphagia. Not suitable for children under 3 years.
POWDER, carbohydrate content varies with flavour and chosen consistency (3 consistencies available), see product literature.

SLO Drink Stage 1: IDDSI 2 Mildly Thick oral powder blackcurrant (SLO Drinks Ltd)
25 cup (ACBS) · NHS indicative price = £7.50

SLO Drink Stage 1: IDDSI 2 Mildly Thick oral powder orange (SLO Drinks Ltd)
25 cup (ACBS) · NHS indicative price = £7.50

SLO Drink Stage 2: IDDSI 3 Moderately Thick oral powder blackcurrant (SLO Drinks Ltd)
25 cup (ACBS) · NHS indicative price = £7.50

SLO Drink Stage 2: IDDSI 3 Moderately Thick oral powder orange (SLO Drinks Ltd)
25 cup (ACBS) · NHS indicative price = £7.50

Thick and Easy®

▸ For thickening of foods in dysphagia. Not suitable for children under 1 year except in cases of failure to thrive.
POWDERModified maize starch

Thick & Easy Original powder (Fresenius Kabi Ltd)
225 gram (ACBS) · NHS indicative price = £5.57 | 4540 gram (ACBS) · NHS indicative price = £96.75

Thicken Aid®

▸ For thickening of foods in dysphagia. Not suitable for children under 1 year.
POWDER, modified maize starch, maltodextrin, gluten- and lactose-free.

Thicken Aid powder (Aymes International Ltd)
225 gram (ACBS) · NHS indicative price = £3.71

Thicken Aid powder 9g sachets (Aymes International Ltd)
100 sachet (ACBS) · NHS indicative price = £22.40

Thixo-D®

▸ For thickening of foods in dysphagia. Not suitable for children under 1 year except in cases of failure to thrive.
POWDER, modified maize starch, gluten-free.

Thixo-D Original powder (Ecogreen Technologies Ltd)
375 gram (ACBS) · NHS indicative price = £8.10

Thixo-D Cal-Free powder (Ecogreen Technologies Ltd)
30 gram · NHS indicative price = £3.00

Flavouring preparations

FlavourPac®

▸ For use with Vitaflo's range of unflavoured protein substitutes for metabolic diseases; not suitable for child under 3 years.
POWDER

FlavourPac oral powder 4g sachets blackcurrant (Vitaflo International Ltd)
30 sachet (ACBS) · NHS indicative price = £15.58

FlavourPac oral powder 4g sachets orange (Vitaflo International Ltd)
30 sachet (ACBS) · NHS indicative price = £15.58

FlavourPac oral powder 4g sachets raspberry (Vitaflo International Ltd)
30 sachet (ACBS) · NHS indicative price = £15.58

FlavourPac oral powder 4g sachets tropical (Vitaflo International Ltd)
30 sachet (ACBS) · NHS indicative price = £15.58

Modjul® Flavour System

▸ For use with unflavoured amino acid and peptide-based Nutricia products used for the dietary management of various conditions including metabolic disorders and gastrointestinal disease.

POWDER

Nutricia Flavour Modjul powder blackcurrant (Nutricia Ltd)
100 gram (ACBS) · NHS indicative price = £13.62

Nutricia Flavour Modjul powder orange (Nutricia Ltd)
100 gram (ACBS) · NHS indicative price = £13.62

Nutricia Flavour Modjul powder pineapple (Nutricia Ltd)
100 gram (ACBS) · NHS indicative price = £13.62

Foods for special diets

Gluten-free foods

ACBS indications: established gluten-sensitive enteropathies including steatorrhoea due to gluten sensitivity, coeliac disease, and dermatitis herpetiformis.

Bread

LOAVES

Barkat® Loaf
GLUTEN-FREE

Barkat gluten free brown rice bread (Gluten Free Foods Ltd)
500 gram (ACBS) · NHS indicative price = £5.84

Barkat gluten free par baked white bread sliced (Gluten Free Foods Ltd)
300 gram (ACBS) · NHS indicative price = £4.21

Barkat gluten free home fresh country loaf (Gluten Free Foods Ltd)
250 gram · NHS indicative price = £4.43

Barkat gluten free multigrain rice bread (Gluten Free Foods Ltd)
500 gram (ACBS) · NHS indicative price = £5.84

Barkat gluten free wholemeal bread sliced (Gluten Free Foods Ltd)
500 gram (ACBS) · NHS indicative price = £4.05

Barkat gluten free white rice bread (Gluten Free Foods Ltd)
500 gram (ACBS) · NHS indicative price = £5.84

Genius Gluten Free® Loaf
GLUTEN-FREE

Genius gluten free brown sandwich bread sliced (Genius Foods Ltd)
535 gram (ACBS) · NHS indicative price = £3.80

Genius gluten free white sandwich bread sliced (Genius Foods Ltd)
535 gram (ACBS) · NHS indicative price = £3.80

Glutafin® Loaves
GLUTEN-FREE

Glutafin gluten free fibre loaf sliced (Dr Schar UK Ltd)
300 gram (ACBS) · NHS indicative price = £2.89

Glutafin gluten free white loaf sliced (Dr Schar UK Ltd)
300 gram (ACBS) · NHS indicative price = £2.89

Glutafin® Select Loaves
GLUTEN-FREE

Glutafin gluten free Select fibre loaf sliced (Dr Schar UK Ltd)
400 gram (ACBS) · NHS indicative price = £3.43

Glutafin gluten free Select fresh brown loaf sliced (Dr Schar UK Ltd)
400 gram (ACBS) · NHS indicative price = £3.43

Glutafin gluten free Select fresh white loaf sliced (Dr Schar UK Ltd)
400 gram (ACBS) · NHS indicative price = £3.43

Glutafin gluten free Select seeded loaf sliced (Dr Schar UK Ltd)
400 gram (ACBS) · NHS indicative price = £3.72

Glutafin gluten free Select white loaf sliced (Dr Schar UK Ltd)
400 gram (ACBS) · NHS indicative price = £3.43

Juvela® Loaf
GLUTEN-FREE

Juvela gluten free fresh fibre loaf sliced (Hero UK Ltd)
400 gram (ACBS) · NHS indicative price = £3.39

Juvela gluten free fresh white loaf sliced (Hero UK Ltd)
400 gram (ACBS) · NHS indicative price = £3.69

Juvela gluten free fibre loaf sliced (Hero UK Ltd)
400 gram (ACBS) · NHS indicative price = £3.54

Juvela gluten free part baked loaf (Hero UK Ltd)
400 gram (ACBS) · NHS indicative price = £3.95

Juvela gluten free part baked fibre loaf (Hero UK Ltd)
400 gram (ACBS) · NHS indicative price = £3.80

Juvela gluten free loaf unsliced (Hero UK Ltd)
400 gram (ACBS) · NHS indicative price = £3.54

Juvela gluten free fibre loaf unsliced (Hero UK Ltd)
400 gram (ACBS) · NHS indicative price = £3.54

Lifestyle® Loaf
GLUTEN-FREE

Lifestyle gluten free brown bread sliced (Ultrapharm Ltd)
400 gram (ACBS) · NHS indicative price = £2.82

Lifestyle gluten free high fibre bread sliced (Ultrapharm Ltd)
400 gram · NHS indicative price = £2.82

Lifestyle gluten free white bread sliced (Ultrapharm Ltd)
400 gram · NHS indicative price = £2.82

Warburtons® Loaf
GLUTEN-FREE

Warburtons gluten free brown bread sliced (Warburtons Ltd)
400 gram (ACBS) · NHS indicative price = £3.06

Warburtons gluten free white bread sliced (Warburtons Ltd)
400 gram (ACBS) · NHS indicative price = £3.06

BAGUETTES, BUNS AND ROLLS

Barkat® Baguettes and rolls
GLUTEN-FREE

Barkat gluten free par baked rolls (Gluten Free Foods Ltd)
200 gram (ACBS) · NHS indicative price = £4.05

Barkat gluten free par baked baguettes (Gluten Free Foods Ltd)
200 gram (ACBS) · NHS indicative price = £4.05

Glutafin® Baguettes and rolls
GLUTEN-FREE

Glutafin gluten free baguettes (Dr Schar UK Ltd)
350 gram (ACBS) · NHS indicative price = £3.51

Glutafin gluten free 4 white rolls (Dr Schar UK Ltd)
200 gram (ACBS) · NHS indicative price = £3.68

Glutafin gluten free part baked 4 fibre rolls (Dr Schar UK Ltd)
200 gram (ACBS) · NHS indicative price = £3.68

Glutafin® Select Rolls
GLUTEN-FREE

Glutafin gluten free part baked 4 white rolls (Dr Schar UK Ltd)
200 gram (ACBS) · NHS indicative price = £3.68

Glutafin gluten free part baked 2 long white rolls (Dr Schar UK Ltd)
150 gram (ACBS) · NHS indicative price = £2.81

Juvela® Rolls
GLUTEN-FREE

Juvela gluten free fresh fibre rolls (Hero UK Ltd)
425 gram (ACBS) · NHS indicative price = £4.42

Juvela gluten free fresh white rolls (Hero UK Ltd)
425 gram (ACBS) · NHS indicative price = £4.42

Juvela gluten free fibre bread rolls (Hero UK Ltd)
425 gram (ACBS) · NHS indicative price = £4.77

Juvela gluten free bread rolls (Hero UK Ltd)
425 gram (ACBS) · NHS indicative price = £4.77

Juvela gluten free part baked fibre bread rolls (Hero UK Ltd)
375 gram (ACBS) · NHS indicative price = £4.94

Juvela gluten free part baked white bread rolls (Hero UK Ltd)
375 gram (ACBS) · NHS indicative price = £4.94

Lifestyle® Rolls
GLUTEN-FREE

Lifestyle gluten free brown bread rolls (Ultrapharm Ltd)
400 gram (ACBS) · NHS indicative price = £2.82

Lifestyle gluten free high fibre bread rolls (Ultrapharm Ltd)
400 gram (ACBS) · NHS indicative price = £2.82

Lifestyle gluten free white bread rolls (Ultrapharm Ltd)
400 gram (ACBS) · NHS indicative price = £2.82

Proceli® Baguettes, buns and rolls
GLUTEN-FREE

Proceli gluten free part baked baguettes (Ambe Ltd)
250 gram (ACBS) · NHS indicative price = £3.24

Warburtons ® Baguettes and rolls
GLUTEN-FREE

Warburtons gluten free brown rolls (Warburtons Ltd)
220 gram (ACBS) • NHS indicative price = £2.55

Warburtons gluten free white rolls (Warburtons Ltd)
220 gram (ACBS) • NHS indicative price = £2.55

Cereals

Juvela ® Fibre flakes and oats
GLUTEN-FREE

Juvela gluten free fibre flakes (Hero UK Ltd)
300 gram • NHS indicative price = £2.78

Juvela gluten free flakes (Hero UK Ltd)
300 gram • NHS indicative price = £2.78

Juvela gluten free pure oats (Hero UK Ltd)
500 gram • NHS indicative price = £2.78

Nairns ® Porridge
GLUTEN-FREE

Nairn's gluten free oat porridge (Nairn's Oatcakes Ltd)
500 gram • NHS indicative price = £3.05

Cookies and biscuits

Barkat ® Biscuits
GLUTEN-FREE

Barkat gluten free digestive biscuits (Gluten Free Foods Ltd)
175 gram • NHS indicative price = £2.66

Ener-G ® Cookies
GLUTEN-FREE

Glutafin ® Cookies and biscuits
GLUTEN-FREE

Glutafin gluten free digestive biscuits (Dr Schar UK Ltd)
150 gram • NHS indicative price = £2.13

Glutafin gluten free shortbread biscuits (Dr Schar UK Ltd)
100 gram • NHS indicative price = £1.73

Juvela ® Biscuits
GLUTEN-FREE

Juvela gluten free digestive biscuits (Hero UK Ltd)
150 gram • NHS indicative price = £3.05

Juvela gluten free savoury biscuits (Hero UK Ltd)
150 gram • NHS indicative price = £3.82

Juvela gluten free sweet biscuits (Hero UK Ltd)
150 gram • NHS indicative price = £2.88

Juvela gluten free tea biscuits (Hero UK Ltd)
150 gram • NHS indicative price = £3.05

Crackers, crispbreads, and breadsticks

Barkat ® Crackers
GLUTEN-FREE

Barkat gluten free matzo crackers (Gluten Free Foods Ltd)
200 gram • NHS indicative price = £3.59

Glutafin ® Crackers
GLUTEN-FREE

Glutafin gluten free crackers (Dr Schar UK Ltd)
200 gram • NHS indicative price = £3.46

Glutafin gluten free mini crackers (Dr Schar UK Ltd)
175 gram • NHS indicative price = £2.96

Juvela ® Crispbread
GLUTEN-FREE

Juvela gluten free crispbread (Hero UK Ltd)
200 gram • NHS indicative price = £4.64

Flour mixes and xanthan gum

FLOUR MIXES

Barkat ® Flour mix
GLUTEN-FREE

Barkat gluten free high fibre bread mix (Gluten Free Foods Ltd)
500 gram (ACBS) • NHS indicative price = £9.13

Barkat gluten free all purpose flour mix (Gluten Free Foods Ltd)
500 gram (ACBS) • NHS indicative price = £4.74

Finax ® Flour mix
GLUTEN-FREE

Finax gluten free coarse flour mix (Drossa Ltd)
900 gram (ACBS) • NHS indicative price = £8.85

Finax gluten free fibre bread mix (Drossa Ltd)
1000 gram (ACBS) • NHS indicative price = £10.14

Finax gluten free flour mix (Drossa Ltd)
900 gram (ACBS) • NHS indicative price = £8.85

Glutafin Select ® Flour mix
GLUTEN-FREE

Glutafin gluten free Select bread mix (Dr Schar UK Ltd)
500 gram (ACBS) • NHS indicative price = £6.66

Glutafin gluten free Select fibre bread mix (Dr Schar UK Ltd)
500 gram (ACBS) • NHS indicative price = £6.66

Glutafin gluten free Select multipurpose fibre mix (Dr Schar UK Ltd)
500 gram (ACBS) • NHS indicative price = £6.66

Glutafin gluten free Select multipurpose white mix (Dr Schar UK Ltd)
500 gram (ACBS) • NHS indicative price = £6.66

Glutafin ® Flour mix
GLUTEN-FREE

Glutafin gluten free multipurpose white mix (Dr Schar UK Ltd)
500 gram (ACBS) • NHS indicative price = £6.66

Juvela ® Flour mix
GLUTEN-FREE

Juvela gluten free fibre mix (Hero UK Ltd)
500 gram (ACBS) • NHS indicative price = £7.35

Juvela gluten free harvest mix (Hero UK Ltd)
500 gram (ACBS) • NHS indicative price = £7.35

Juvela gluten free mix (Hero UK Ltd)
500 gram (ACBS) • NHS indicative price = £7.35

Mrs Crimbles ® Flour mixes
GLUTEN-FREE

Mrs Crimble's gluten free bread mix (Stiletto Foods (UK) Ltd)
275 gram • NHS indicative price = £1.09

Mrs Crimble's gluten free pastry mix (Stiletto Foods (UK) Ltd)
200 gram • NHS indicative price = £1.09

Orgran ® Flour mix
GLUTEN-FREE

Orgran gluten free self-raising flour (Naturally Good Food Ltd)
500 gram • NHS indicative price = £3.10

Orgran gluten free all purpose plain flour (Naturally Good Food Ltd)
500 gram • NHS indicative price = £3.10

Proceli ® Flour mix
GLUTEN-FREE

Proceli gluten free basic mix (Ambe Ltd)
1000 gram (ACBS) • NHS indicative price = £9.95

Tobia ® Flour mix
GLUTEN-FREE

Tobia Teff gluten free brown bread mix (Tobia Teff UK Ltd)
1000 gram (ACBS) • NHS indicative price = £3.85

Tobia Teff gluten free white bread mix (Tobia Teff UK Ltd)
1000 gram (ACBS) • NHS indicative price = £3.85

Tritamyl ® Flour mix
GLUTEN-FREE

Tritamyl gluten free brown bread mix (Gluten Free Foods Ltd)
1000 gram (ACBS) • NHS indicative price = £7.24

Tritamyl gluten free flour mix (Gluten Free Foods Ltd)
2000 gram (ACBS) • NHS indicative price = £14.54

Tritamyl gluten free white bread mix (Gluten Free Foods Ltd)
2000 gram (ACBS) • NHS indicative price = £14.54

XANTHAN GUM

Ener-G ® Xanthan gum
GLUTEN-FREE

Pure® Xanthan gum
GLUTEN-FREE

Innovative Solutions Pure xanthan gum (Innovative Solutions (UK) Ltd)
100 gram · NHS indicative price = £7.12

Pasta

Barkat® Pasta
GLUTEN-FREE

Barkat gluten free pasta animal shapes (Gluten Free Foods Ltd)
500 gram · NHS indicative price = £5.99

Barkat gluten free pasta macaroni (Gluten Free Foods Ltd)
500 gram · NHS indicative price = £5.99

Barkat gluten free pasta spaghetti (Gluten Free Foods Ltd)
500 gram · NHS indicative price = £5.99

Barkat gluten free pasta spirals (Gluten Free Foods Ltd)
500 gram · NHS indicative price = £5.99

Barkat gluten free pasta tagliatelle (Gluten Free Foods Ltd)
500 gram · NHS indicative price = £5.99

Barkat gluten free pasta buckwheat penne (Gluten Free Foods Ltd)
250 gram · NHS indicative price = £2.98

Barkat gluten free pasta buckwheat spirals (Gluten Free Foods Ltd)
250 gram · NHS indicative price = £2.98

BiAlimenta® Pasta
GLUTEN-FREE

BiAlimenta gluten free pasta acini di pepe (Drossa Ltd)
500 gram · NHS indicative price = £6.11 | 1000 gram · No NHS indicative price available

BiAlimenta gluten free pasta formati misti (Drossa Ltd)
3000 gram · NHS indicative price = £36.63

BiAlimenta gluten free pasta penne (Drossa Ltd)
500 gram · NHS indicative price = £6.11 | 1000 gram · No NHS indicative price available

BiAlimenta gluten free pasta sagnette (Drossa Ltd)
500 gram · NHS indicative price = £6.11

BiAlimenta gluten free pasta spirali (Drossa Ltd)
500 gram · NHS indicative price = £6.11

BiAlimenta gluten free pasta tubetti (Drossa Ltd)
500 gram · NHS indicative price = £6.03

BiAlimenta gluten free potato pasta gnocchi (Drossa Ltd)
500 gram · NHS indicative price = £5.71

BiAlimenta gluten free potato pasta perle di gnocchi (Drossa Ltd)
500 gram · NHS indicative price = £5.72

Glutafin® Pasta
GLUTEN-FREE

Glutafin gluten free pasta macaroni penne (Dr Schar UK Ltd)
500 gram · NHS indicative price = £6.73

Glutafin gluten free pasta spirals (Dr Schar UK Ltd)
500 gram · NHS indicative price = £6.73

Glutafin gluten free pasta long-cut spaghetti (Dr Schar UK Ltd)
500 gram · NHS indicative price = £6.73

Juvela® Pasta
GLUTEN-FREE

Juvela gluten free fibre penne (Hero UK Ltd)
500 gram · NHS indicative price = £6.61

Juvela gluten free pasta fusilli (Hero UK Ltd)
500 gram · NHS indicative price = £7.21

Juvela gluten free pasta lasagne (Hero UK Ltd)
250 gram · NHS indicative price = £3.68

Juvela gluten free pasta macaroni (Hero UK Ltd)
500 gram · NHS indicative price = £7.21

Juvela gluten free pasta spaghetti (Hero UK Ltd)
500 gram · NHS indicative price = £7.21

Juvela gluten free pasta tagliatelle (Hero UK Ltd)
250 gram · NHS indicative price = £3.47

Orgran® Pasta
GLUTEN-FREE

Orgran gluten free pasta rice & corn lasagne (Naturally Good Food Ltd)
200 gram · NHS indicative price = £3.13

Orgran gluten free pasta rice & corn macaroni (Naturally Good Food Ltd)
250 gram · NHS indicative price = £2.42

Orgran gluten free pasta buckwheat spirals (Naturally Good Food Ltd)
250 gram · NHS indicative price = £2.42

Orgran gluten free pasta brown rice spirals (Naturally Good Food Ltd)
250 gram · NHS indicative price = £2.42

Orgran gluten free pasta rice & corn spirals (Naturally Good Food Ltd)
250 gram · NHS indicative price = £2.42

Rizopia® Pasta
GLUTEN-FREE

Rizopia gluten free organic brown rice pasta fusilli (PGR Health Foods Ltd)
500 gram · NHS indicative price = £2.72

Rizopia gluten free organic brown rice pasta lasagne (PGR Health Foods Ltd)
375 gram · NHS indicative price = £2.72

Rizopia gluten free organic brown rice pasta penne (PGR Health Foods Ltd)
500 gram · NHS indicative price = £2.72

Rizopia gluten free organic brown rice pasta spaghetti (PGR Health Foods Ltd)
500 gram · NHS indicative price = £2.72

Pizza bases

Barkat®, Pizza crust
GLUTEN-FREE

Barkat gluten free brown rice pizza crust (Gluten Free Foods Ltd)
150 gram · NHS indicative price = £5.10

Barkat gluten free white rice pizza crust (Gluten Free Foods Ltd)
150 gram · NHS indicative price = £5.10

Glutafin® Pizza base
GLUTEN-FREE

Glutafin gluten free pizza base (Dr Schar UK Ltd)
300 gram · NHS indicative price = £6.56

Juvela® Pizza base
GLUTEN-FREE

Juvela gluten free pizza base (Hero UK Ltd)
360 gram · NHS indicative price = £8.78

Proceli® Pizza base
GLUTEN-FREE

Proceli gluten free pizza base (Ambe Ltd)
250 gram · NHS indicative price = £3.90

Gluten- and wheat-free foods

Ener-G® Bread loaves, rolls and pizza bases
GLUTEN-FREE, WHEAT-FREE

Glutafin® Flour mix, fibre and crispbread
GLUTEN-FREE, WHEAT-FREE

Glutafin gluten free crispbread (Dr Schar UK Ltd)
150 gram · NHS indicative price = £3.25

Glutafin gluten free bread mix (Dr Schar UK Ltd)
500 gram (ACBS) · NHS indicative price = £6.66

Glutafin gluten free fibre bread mix (Dr Schar UK Ltd)
500 gram (ACBS) · NHS indicative price = £6.66

Glutafin gluten free wheat free fibre mix (Dr Schar UK Ltd)
500 gram (ACBS) · NHS indicative price = £6.66

Low-protein foods

ACBS indications: inherited metabolic disorders, renal or liver failure, requiring a low-protein diet.

Bread

Juvela® Loaf and rolls
LOW PROTEIN
Juvela gluten free loaf sliced (Hero UK Ltd)
400 gram (ACBS) · NHS indicative price = £3.54
Juvela low protein bread rolls (Hero UK Ltd)
350 gram (ACBS) · NHS indicative price = £4.52
Juvela low protein loaf sliced (Hero UK Ltd)
400 gram (ACBS) · NHS indicative price = £3.64
Loprofin® Bread
LOW-PROTEIN
Loprofin low protein part baked bread rolls (Nutricia Ltd)
260 gram (ACBS) · NHS indicative price = £4.48
Loprofin low protein part baked loaf sliced (Nutricia Ltd)
400 gram (ACBS) · NHS indicative price = £4.26
PK Foods® Loaf
LOW PROTEIN
PK Foods low protein white bread sliced (Gluten Free Foods Ltd)
300 gram · NHS indicative price = £4.84

Cake, biscuits, and snacks

▶ Not recommended for any child under 1 year.
Loprofin® Wafers
LOW-PROTEIN
Loprofin low protein crackers (Nutricia Ltd)
150 gram (ACBS) · NHS indicative price = £3.91
Loprofin low protein herb crackers (Nutricia Ltd)
150 gram (ACBS) · NHS indicative price = £3.91
PK Foods® Biscuits
LOW-PROTEIN
PK Foods Aminex low protein rusks (Gluten Free Foods Ltd)
200 gram (ACBS) · NHS indicative price = £5.14
PK Foods low protein crispbread (Gluten Free Foods Ltd)
75 gram (ACBS) · NHS indicative price = £2.46
Promin® Cooked and flavoured pasta snax
LOW-PROTEIN
Promin low protein Snax salt & vinegar 25g sachets (Firstplay Dietary Foods Ltd)
3 sachet · No NHS indicative price available | 12 sachet (ACBS) · NHS indicative price = £11.25
Promin low protein Snax ready salted 25g sachets (Firstplay Dietary Foods Ltd)
3 sachet · No NHS indicative price available | 12 sachet (ACBS) · NHS indicative price = £11.25
Promin low protein Snax jalapeno 25g sachets (Firstplay Dietary Foods Ltd)
3 sachet · No NHS indicative price available | 12 sachet (ACBS) · NHS indicative price = £11.25
Promin low protein Snax cheese & onion 25g sachets (Firstplay Dietary Foods Ltd)
3 sachet · No NHS indicative price available | 12 sachet (ACBS) · NHS indicative price = £11.25
Taranis® Cake bars
LOW-PROTEIN
Taranis low protein apricot cake (Lactalis Nutrition Sante)
240 gram (ACBS) · NHS indicative price = £6.24
Taranis low protein lemon cake (Lactalis Nutrition Sante)
240 gram (ACBS) · NHS indicative price = £6.24
Taranis low protein pear cake (Lactalis Nutrition Sante)
240 gram (ACBS) · NHS indicative price = £6.24
Vita Bite®
▶ Not recommended for any child under 1 year.
LOW PROTEIN.
Bar, protein 30 mg (less than 2.5 mg phenylalanine), carbohydrate 15.35 g, fat 8.4 g, energy 572 kJ (137 kcal)/25 g.
VitaBite bar (Vitaflo International Ltd)
175 gram (ACBS) · NHS indicative price = £9.72
Vitaflo Choices® Mini crackers
LOW-PROTEIN
Vitaflo Choices mini crackers (Vitaflo International Ltd)
40 gram (ACBS) · NHS indicative price = £0.96

Cereals

Loprofin® Breakfast cereal
LOW-PROTEIN
Loprofin low protein breakfast cereal flakes (Flavour Not Specified)
375 gram (ACBS) · No NHS indicative price available
Loprofin low protein breakfast cereal flakes chocolate (Nutricia Ltd)
375 gram (ACBS) · NHS indicative price = £8.65
Loprofin low protein breakfast cereal flakes strawberry (Nutricia Ltd)
375 gram (ACBS) · NHS indicative price = £8.65
Loprofin low protein breakfast cereal loops (Nutricia Ltd)
375 gram (ACBS) · NHS indicative price = £8.97
Promin® Hot breakfast
LOW-PROTEIN
Promin low protein hot breakfast powder 56g sachets original (Firstplay Dietary Foods Ltd)
6 sachet (ACBS) · NHS indicative price = £8.55
Promin low protein hot breakfast powder 57g sachets apple & cinnamon (Firstplay Dietary Foods Ltd)
6 sachet (ACBS) · NHS indicative price = £8.55
Promin low protein hot breakfast powder 57g sachets banana (Firstplay Dietary Foods Ltd)
6 sachet (ACBS) · NHS indicative price = £8.55
Promin low protein hot breakfast powder 57g sachets chocolate (Firstplay Dietary Foods Ltd)
6 sachet (ACBS) · NHS indicative price = £8.55

Desserts

PK Foods® Jelly
LOW-PROTEIN
PK Foods low protein jelly mix dessert cherry (Gluten Free Foods Ltd)
320 gram (ACBS) · NHS indicative price = £8.19
PK Foods low protein jelly mix dessert orange (Gluten Free Foods Ltd)
320 gram (ACBS) · NHS indicative price = £8.19
Promin® Desserts
LOW-PROTEIN
Promin low protein dessert 36.5g sachets caramel (Firstplay Dietary Foods Ltd)
6 sachet (ACBS) · NHS indicative price = £6.72
Promin low protein dessert 36.5g sachets chocolate & banana (Firstplay Dietary Foods Ltd)
6 sachet (ACBS) · NHS indicative price = £6.72
Promin low protein dessert 36.5g sachets custard (Firstplay Dietary Foods Ltd)
6 sachet (ACBS) · NHS indicative price = £6.72
Promin low protein dessert 36.5g sachets strawberry & vanilla (Firstplay Dietary Foods Ltd)
6 sachet (ACBS) · NHS indicative price = £6.72

Flour mixes and egg substitutes

Fate® Flour mix
LOW PROTEIN
Fate low protein all purpose mix (Fate Special Foods)
500 gram (ACBS) · NHS indicative price = £6.97
Fate low protein chocolate cake mix (Fate Special Foods)
500 gram (ACBS) · NHS indicative price = £6.97
Fate low protein plain cake mix (Fate Special Foods)
500 gram (ACBS) · NHS indicative price = £6.97
Juvela® Mix
LOW-PROTEIN
Juvela low protein mix (Hero UK Ltd)
500 gram (ACBS) · NHS indicative price = £7.79

Loprofin ® Flour mixes and egg substitutes
LOW-PROTEIN

Loprofin low protein egg replacer (Nutricia Ltd)
500 gram (ACBS) · NHS indicative price = £16.81

Loprofin low protein egg white replacer (Nutricia Ltd)
100 gram (ACBS) · NHS indicative price = £10.81

Loprofin low protein cake mix chocolate (Nutricia Ltd)
500 gram (ACBS) · NHS indicative price = £9.68

Loprofin low protein mix (Nutricia Ltd)
500 gram (ACBS) · NHS indicative price = £9.01

PK Foods ® Flour mix and egg substitute
LOW-PROTEIN

PK Foods low protein egg replacer (Gluten Free Foods Ltd)
200 gram (ACBS) · NHS indicative price = £4.16

PK Foods low protein flour mix (Gluten Free Foods Ltd)
750 gram (ACBS) · NHS indicative price = £10.92

Pasta

Loprofin ® Pasta
LOW-PROTEIN

Loprofin low protein pasta animal shapes (Nutricia Ltd)
500 gram (ACBS) · NHS indicative price = £9.20

Loprofin low protein pasta lasagne (Nutricia Ltd)
250 gram (ACBS) · NHS indicative price = £4.65

Loprofin low protein pasta penne (Nutricia Ltd)
500 gram (ACBS) · NHS indicative price = £9.55

Loprofin low protein pasta tagliatelle (Nutricia Ltd)
250 gram (ACBS) · NHS indicative price = £4.60

Loprofin low protein pasta macaroni elbows (Nutricia Ltd)
250 gram (ACBS) · NHS indicative price = £4.60

Loprofin low protein pasta long cut spaghetti (Nutricia Ltd)
500 gram (ACBS) · NHS indicative price = £9.55

Promin ® Pasta
LOW-PROTEIN

Promin low protein pasta alphabets (Firstplay Dietary Foods Ltd)
500 gram (ACBS) · NHS indicative price = £7.39

Promin Plus low protein pasta macaroni (Firstplay Dietary Foods Ltd)
500 gram (ACBS) · NHS indicative price = £7.39

Promin Plus low protein pasta flat noodles (Firstplay Dietary Foods Ltd)
500 gram (ACBS) · NHS indicative price = £7.39

Promin low protein pasta shells (Firstplay Dietary Foods Ltd)
500 gram (ACBS) · NHS indicative price = £7.39

Promin low protein pasta short cut spaghetti (Firstplay Dietary Foods Ltd)
500 gram (ACBS) · NHS indicative price = £7.39

Promin low protein tricolour pasta spirals (Firstplay Dietary Foods Ltd)
500 gram (ACBS) · NHS indicative price = £7.39

Promin low protein pasta spirals (Firstplay Dietary Foods Ltd)
500 gram (ACBS) · NHS indicative price = £7.39

Promin low protein imitation rice (Firstplay Dietary Foods Ltd)
500 gram (ACBS) · NHS indicative price = £7.43

Promin low protein tricolour pasta alphabets (Firstplay Dietary Foods Ltd)
500 gram (ACBS) · NHS indicative price = £7.39

Promin low protein tricolour pasta shells (Firstplay Dietary Foods Ltd)
500 gram (ACBS) · NHS indicative price = £7.39

Promin low protein lasagne sheets (Firstplay Dietary Foods Ltd)
200 gram (ACBS) · NHS indicative price = £3.22

Pizza bases

Juvela ® Pizza base
LOW-PROTEIN

Juvela low protein pizza base (Hero UK Ltd)
360 gram (ACBS) · NHS indicative price = £8.61

Savoury meals and mixes

Promin ® Savoury meals and mixes
LOW-PROTEIN

Promin low protein cous cous (Firstplay Dietary Foods Ltd)
500 gram (ACBS) · NHS indicative price = £7.43

Promin low protein pasta elbows (Firstplay Dietary Foods Ltd)
500 gram · NHS indicative price = £7.39

Promin low protein pastameal (Firstplay Dietary Foods Ltd)
500 gram (ACBS) · NHS indicative price = £7.43

Promin low protein pasta macaroni (Firstplay Dietary Foods Ltd)
500 gram (ACBS) · NHS indicative price = £7.39

Promin Plus low protein pasta spirals (Firstplay Dietary Foods Ltd)
500 gram (ACBS) · NHS indicative price = £7.39

Promin low protein potato pot with croutons onion (Firstplay Dietary Foods Ltd)
200 gram (ACBS) · NHS indicative price = £17.45

Promin low protein potato pot with croutons cabbage & bacon (Firstplay Dietary Foods Ltd)
200 gram (ACBS) · NHS indicative price = £17.45

Promin low protein potato pot with croutons sausage (Firstplay Dietary Foods Ltd)
200 gram (ACBS) · NHS indicative price = £17.45

Promin low protein X-Pot all day scramble (Firstplay Dietary Foods Ltd)
240 gram (ACBS) · NHS indicative price = £22.20

Promin low protein X-Pot beef & tomato (Firstplay Dietary Foods Ltd)
240 gram (ACBS) · NHS indicative price = £22.20

Promin low protein X-Pot chip shop curry (Firstplay Dietary Foods Ltd)
240 gram (ACBS) · NHS indicative price = £22.20

Promin low protein X-Pot rogan style curry (Firstplay Dietary Foods Ltd)
240 gram (ACBS) · NHS indicative price = £22.20

Spreads

Taranis ® Spread
LOW-PROTEIN

Taranis low protein hazelnut spread (Lactalis Nutrition Sante)
230 gram (ACBS) · NHS indicative price = £8.15

Nutritional supplements for metabolic diseases

Glutaric aciduria (type 1)

GA1 Anamix ® Infant

▸ Nutritional supplement for the dietary management of proven glutaric aciduria (type 1) in children from birth to 3 years.

POWDER, protein equivalent (essential and non-essential amino acids except lysine, and low tryptophan) 13.1 g, carbohydrate 49.5 g, fat 23 g, fibre 5.3 g, energy 1915 kJ (457 kcal)/100 g, with vitamins, minerals, and trace elements; standard dilution (15%) provides protein equivalent 2 g, carbohydrate 7.4 g, fat 3.5 g, fibre 800 mg, energy 287 kJ (69 kcal)/100 mL.

GA1 Anamix Infant powder (Nutricia Ltd)
400 gram (ACBS) · NHS indicative price = £43.52

GA Gel ®

▸ Nutritional supplement for dietary management of type 1 glutaric aciduria in children 6 months–10 years.

GEL, protein equivalent (essential and non-essential amino acids except lysine, and low tryptophan) 10 g, carbohydrate 10.3 g, fat trace, energy 339 kJ (81 kcal)/24 g, with vitamins, minerals, and trace elements. To flavour unflavoured products, see FlavourPac p. 1126.

GA gel oral powder 24g sachets (Vitaflo International Ltd)
30 sachet (ACBS) · NHS indicative price = £240.23

XLYS, TRY Glutaridon ®

▸ Nutritional supplement for the dietary management of type 1 glutaric aciduria in children and adults; requires additional source of vitamins, minerals, and trace elements.

POWDER, protein equivalent (essential and non-essential amino acids except lysine and tryptophan) 79 g, carbohydrate 4 g, energy 1411 kJ (332 kcal)/100 g. To flavour unflavoured products, see Modjul Flavour System p. 1126.

XLYS TRY Glutaridon powder (Nutricia Ltd)
500 gram (ACBS) · NHS indicative price = £208.24

Glycogen storage disease

Corn flour and corn starch
- For glycogen storage disease

Glycosade®
- A nutritional supplement for use in the dietary management of glycogen storage disease and other metabolic conditions where a constant supply of glucose is essential. Not suitable for use in children under 2 years.

POWDER, protein 200 mg, carbohydrate (maize starch) 47.6 g, fat 100 mg, fibre less than 600 mg, energy 803 kJ (192 kcal)/60 g.

Glycosade oral powder 60g sachets unflavoured (Vitaflo International Ltd)
30 sachet (ACBS) · NHS indicative price = £126.25

Homocystinuria or hypermethioninaemia

HCU Anamix® Infant
- Nutritional supplement for the dietary management of proven vitamin B6 non-responsive homocystinuria or hypermethioninaemia in children from birth to 3 years.

POWDER, protein equivalent (essential and non-essential amino acids except methionine) 13.1 g, carbohydrate 49.5 g, fat 23 g, fibre 5.3 g, energy 1915 kJ (457 kcal)/100 g, with vitamins, minerals, and trace elements; standard dilution (15%) provides protein equivalent 2 g, carbohydrate 7.4 g, fat 3.5 g, fibre 800 mg, energy 287 kJ (69 kcal)/100 mL.

HCU Anamix Infant powder (Nutricia Ltd)
400 gram (ACBS) · NHS indicative price = £43.52

HCU cooler® 15
- A methionine-free protein substitute for use as a nutritional supplement in children over 3 years with homocystinuria.

LIQUID, protein (essential and non-essential amino acids except methionine) 15 g, carbohydrate 7 g, fat 500 mg, energy 393 kJ (92 kcal)/130 mL, with vitamins, minerals, and trace elements.

HCU orange cooler15 liquid (Vitaflo International Ltd)
130 ml (ACBS) · NHS indicative price = £12.68

HCU Express® 15
- A methionine-free protein substitute for use as a nutritional supplement in children over 8 years with homocystinuria.

POWDER, protein (essential and non-essential amino acids except methionine) 15 g, carbohydrate 3.8 g, fat 30 mg, energy 315 kJ (75.3 kcal)/25 g with vitamins, minerals, and trace elements. To flavour unflavoured products, see FlavourPac p. 1126.

HCU express15 oral powder 25g sachets (Vitaflo International Ltd)
30 sachet (ACBS) · NHS indicative price = £373.05

HCU Express® 20
- A methionine-free protein substitute for use as a nutritional supplement in children over 8 years with homocystinuria.

POWDER, protein (essential and non-essential amino acids except methionine) 20 g, carbohydrate 4.7 g, fat 70 mg, energy 416 kJ (99 kcal)/34 g with vitamins, minerals, and trace elements. To flavour unflavoured products, see FlavourPac p. 1126

HCU express20 oral powder 34g sachets (Vitaflo International Ltd)
30 sachet (ACBS) · NHS indicative price = £481.98

HCU gel®
- A methionine-free protein substitute for use as a nutritional supplement for the dietary management of children 1–10 years with homocystinuria.

POWDER, protein (essential and non-essential amino acids except methionine) 10 g, carbohydrate 10.3 g, fat 20 mg, energy 339 kJ (81 kcal)/24 g with vitamins, minerals, and trace elements. To flavour unflavoured products, see FlavourPac p. 1126.

HCU gel oral powder 24g sachets (Vitaflo International Ltd)
30 sachet (ACBS) · NHS indicative price = £240.17

HCU Lophlex® LQ 20
- Nutritional supplement for the dietary management of homocystinuria in children over 3 years.

LIQUID, protein equivalent (essential and non-essential amino acids except methionine) 20 g, carbohydrate 8.8 g, fat 440 mg, energy 509 kJ (120 kcal)/125 mL, with vitamins, minerals, and trace elements.

HCU Lophlex LQ 20 liquid (Nutricia Ltd)
125 ml (ACBS) · NHS indicative price = £17.94

HCU LV®
- Nutritional supplement for the dietary management of hypermethioninaemia or vitamin B6 non-responsive homocystinuria in children over 8 years.

POWDER, protein (essential and non-essential amino acids except methionine) 20 g, carbohydrate 2.5 g, fat 190 mg, energy 390 kJ (92 kcal)/27.8-g sachet, with vitamins, minerals, and trace elements. To flavour unflavoured products, see Modjul Flavour System p. 1126.

HCU-LV oral powder 27.8g sachets tropical (Nutricia Ltd)
30 sachet (ACBS) · NHS indicative price = £551.70

HCU-LV oral powder 27.8g sachets unflavoured (Nutricia Ltd)
30 sachet (ACBS) · NHS indicative price = £551.70

XMET Homidon®
- Nutritional supplement for the dietary management of hypermethioninaemia or homocystinuria in children and adults.

POWDER, protein equivalent (essential and non-essential amino acids, except methionine) 77 g, carbohydrate 4.5 g, fat nil, energy 1386 kJ (326 kcal)/100 g. To flavour unflavoured products, see Modjul Flavour System p. 1126.

XMET Homidon powder (Nutricia Ltd)
500 gram (ACBS) · NHS indicative price = £208.24

XMET Maxamum®
- Nutritional supplement for the dietary management of hypermethioninaemia or homocystinuria.

POWDER, protein equivalent (essential and non-essential amino acids except methionine) 39 g, carbohydrate 34 g, fat less than 500 mg, energy 1260 kJ (297 kcal)/100 g, with vitamins, minerals, and trace elements. To flavour unflavoured products, see Modjul Flavour System p. 1126.
Maxamum products are generally intended for use in children over 8 years.

HCU Maxamum powder (Nutricia Ltd)
500 gram (ACBS) · NHS indicative price = £176.20

Hyperlysinaemia

HYPER LYS Anamix® Infant
- Nutritional supplement for the dietary management of proven hyperlysinaemia in children from birth to 3 years.

POWDER, protein equivalent (essential and non-essential amino acids except lysine) 13.1 g, carbohydrate 49.5 g, fat 23 g, fibre 5.3 g, energy 1915 kJ (457 kcal)/100 g, with vitamins, minerals, and trace elements; standard dilution (15%) provides protein equivalent 2 g, carbohydrate 7.4 g, fat 3.5 g, fibre 800 mg, energy 287 kJ (69 kcal)/100 mL.

HYPER LYS Anamix Infant powder (Nutricia Ltd)
400 gram (ACBS) · NHS indicative price = £43.52

Isovaleric acidaemia

IVA Anamix® Infant
- Nutritional supplement for the dietary management of proven isovaleric acidaemia or other proven disorders of leucine metabolism in children from birth to 3 years.

POWDER, protein equivalent (essential and non-essential amino acids except leucine) 13.1 g, carbohydrate 49.5 g, fat 23 g, fibre

5.3 g, energy 1915 kJ (457 kcal)/100 g, with vitamins, minerals, and trace elements; standard dilution (15%) provides protein equivalent 2 g, carbohydrate 7.4 g, fat 3.5 g, fibre 800 mg, energy 287 kJ (69 kcal)/100 mL.

IVA Anamix Infant powder (Nutricia Ltd)
400 gram (ACBS) · NHS indicative price = £43.52

Maple syrup urine disease

MSUD Aid III ®

▸ Nutritional supplement for the dietary management of maple syrup urine disease and related conditions in children and adults where it is necessary to limit the intake of branched chain amino acids.
POWDER, protein equivalent (essential and non-essential amino acids except isoleucine, leucine, and valine) 77 g, carbohydrate 4.5 g, fat nil, energy 1386 kJ (326 kcal)/100 g. To flavour unflavoured products, see Modjul Flavour System p. 1126.

MSUD Aid 111 powder (Nutricia Ltd)
500 gram (ACBS) · NHS indicative price = £208.24

MSUD Anamix ® Infant

▸ Nutritional supplement for the dietary management of proven maple syrup urine disease in children from birth to 3 years.
POWDER, protein equivalent (essential and non-essential amino acids except isoleucine, leucine, and valine) 13.1 g, carbohydrate 49.5 g, fat 23 g, fibre 5.3 g, energy 1915 kJ (457 kcal)/100 g, with vitamins, minerals, and trace elements; standard dilution (15%) provides protein equivalent 2 g, carbohydrate 7.4 g, fat 3.5 g, fibre 800 mg, energy 287 kJ (69 kcal)/100 mL.

MSUD Anamix Infant powder (Nutricia Ltd)
400 gram (ACBS) · NHS indicative price = £43.52

MSUD Anamix ® Junior

▸ Nutritional supplement for the dietary management of maple syrup urine disease in children 1–10 years.
POWDER, protein equivalent (essential and non-essential amino acids except isoleucine, leucine, and valine) 10 g, carbohydrate 11.5 g, fat 4.5 g, energy 566 kJ (135 kcal)/36-g sachet, with vitamins, minerals, and trace elements. To flavour unflavoured products, see Modjul Flavour System p. 1126.

MSUD Anamix Junior oral powder 36g sachets (Nutricia Ltd)
30 sachet (ACBS) · NHS indicative price = £232.50

MSUD Anamix ® Junior LQ

▸ Nutritional supplement for the dietary management of maple syrup urine disease in children 1–10 years.
LIQUID, protein equivalent (essential and non-essential amino acids except isoleucine, leucine, and valine) 10 g, carbohydrate 8.8 g, fat 4.8 g, fibre 310 mg, energy 497 kJ (118 kcal)/125 mL, with vitamins, minerals, and trace elements. Lactose-free.

MSUD Anamix Junior LQ liquid (Nutricia Ltd)
125 ml (ACBS) · NHS indicative price = £10.09

MSUD cooler ® 15

▸ Nutritional supplement for the dietary management of maple syrup urine disease in children over 3 years and adults.
LIQUID, protein equivalent (essential and non-essential amino acids except leucine, isoleucine, and valine) 15 g, carbohydrate 7 g, fat 500 mg, energy 393 kJ (92 kcal)/130-mL pouch, with vitamins, minerals, and trace elements.

MSUD orange cooler15 liquid (Vitaflo International Ltd)
130 ml (ACBS) · NHS indicative price = £12.68

MSUD red cooler15 liquid (Vitaflo International Ltd)
130 ml (ACBS) · NHS indicative price = £12.68

MSUD express ® 15

▸ Nutritional supplement for the dietary management of maple syrup urine disease in children over 8 years and adults.
POWDER, protein equivalent (essential and non-essential amino acids except leucine, isoleucine, and valine) 15 g, carbohydrate 3.8 g, fat less than 100 mg, energy 315 kJ (75 kcal)/25 g, with vitamins, minerals, and trace elements. To flavour unflavoured products, see FlavourPac p. 1126.

MSUD express15 oral powder 25g sachets (Vitaflo International Ltd)
30 sachet (ACBS) · NHS indicative price = £373.05

MSUD express ® 20

▸ Nutritional supplement for the dietary management of maple syrup urine disease in children over 8 years and adults.
POWDER, protein equivalent (essential and non-essential amino acids except leucine, isoleucine, and valine) 20 g, carbohydrate 4.7 g, fat less than 100 mg, energy 416 kJ (99 kcal)/34 g, with vitamins, minerals, and trace elements. To flavour unflavoured products, see FlavourPac p. 1126.

MSUD express20 oral powder 34g sachets (Vitaflo International Ltd)
30 sachet (ACBS) · NHS indicative price = £481.98

MSUD Gel ®

▸ Nutritional supplement for the dietary management of maple syrup urine disease in children 1–10 years.
POWDER, protein equivalent (essential and non-essential amino acids except leucine, isoleucine, and valine) 10 g, carbohydrate 10.3 g, fat less than 100 mg, energy 339 kJ (81 kcal)/24 g, with vitamins, minerals, and trace elements. To flavour unflavoured products, see FlavourPac p. 1126.

MSUD gel 24g sachets (Vitaflo International Ltd)
30 sachet (ACBS) · NHS indicative price = £242.99

MSUD Lophlex ® LQ 20

▸ Nutritional supplement for the dietary management of maple syrup urine disease in children over 3 years.
LIQUID, protein equivalent (essential and non-essential amino acids except isoleucine, leucine, and valine) 20 g, carbohydrate 8.8 g, fat less than 500 mg, energy 509 kJ (120 kcal)/125 mL, with vitamins, minerals, and trace elements.

MSUD Lophlex LQ 20 liquid (Nutricia Ltd)
125 ml (ACBS) · NHS indicative price = £17.94

MSUD Maxamum ®

▸ Nutritional supplement for the dietary management of maple syrup urine disease.
POWDER, protein equivalent (essential and non-essential amino acids except isoleucine, leucine, and valine) 39 g, carbohydrate 34 g, fat less than 500 mg, energy 1260 kJ (297 kcal)/100 g, with vitamins, minerals, and trace elements. To flavour unflavoured products, see Modjul Flavour System p. 1126.
Maxamum products are generally intended for use in children over 8 years.

MSUD Maxamum powder orange (Nutricia Ltd)
500 gram (ACBS) · NHS indicative price = £176.20

MSUD Maxamum powder unflavoured (Nutricia Ltd)
500 gram (ACBS) · NHS indicative price = £176.20

Methylmalonic or propionic acidaemia

MMA/PA Anamix ® Infant

▸ Nutritional supplement for the dietary management of proven methylmalonic acidaemia or propionic acidaemia in children from birth to 3 years.
POWDER, protein equivalent (essential and non-essential amino acids except methionine, threonine, and valine, and low isoleucine) 13.1 g, carbohydrate 49.5 g, fat 23 g, fibre 5.3 g, energy 1915 kJ (457 kcal)/100 g, with vitamins, minerals, and trace elements; standard dilution (15%) provides protein equivalent 2 g, carbohydrate 7.4 g, fat 3.5 g, fibre 800 mg, energy 287 kJ (69 kcal)/100 mL.

MMA / PA Anamix Infant powder (Nutricia Ltd)
400 gram (ACBS) · NHS indicative price = £43.52

XMTVI Asadon ®

▸ Nutritional supplement for the dietary management of methylmalonic acidaemia or propionic acidaemia in children and adults.
POWDER, protein equivalent (essential and non-essential amino acids except methionine, threonine, and valine, and low isoleucine) 77 g, carbohydrate 4.5 g, fat nil, energy 1386 kJ (326 kcal)/100 g. To flavour unflavoured products, see Modjul Flavour System p. 1126.

XMTVI Asadon powder (Nutricia Ltd)
200 gram (ACBS) · NHS indicative price = £83.29

XMTVI Maxamum ®

▸ Nutritional supplement for the dietary management of methylmalonic acidaemia or propionic acidaemia.
POWDER, protein equivalent (essential and non-essential amino acids except methionine, threonine, and valine, and low isoleucine) 39 g, carbohydrate 34 g, fat less than 500 mg, energy 1260 kJ (297 kcal)/100 g, with vitamins, minerals, and trace elements. To flavour unflavoured products, see Modjul Flavour System p. 1126. Maxamum products are generally intended for use in children over 8 years.

MMA/PA Maxamum powder (Nutricia Ltd)
500 gram (ACBS) · NHS indicative price = £176.20

Other inborn errors of metabolism

Cystine500 ®

▸ Nutritional supplement for the dietary management of inborn errors of amino acid metabolism in adults and children from 3 years.
POWDER, cystine 500 mg, carbohydrate 3.3 g, fat nil, energy 64 kJ (15 kcal)/4 g

Cystine500 oral powder sachets (Vitaflo International Ltd)
30 sachet (ACBS) · NHS indicative price = £61.02

DocOmega ®

▸ Nutritional supplement for the dietary management of inborn errors of metabolism for adults and children from birth.
POWDER, protein (cows' milk, soya) 100 mg, carbohydrate 3.2 g, fat 500 mg (of which docosahexaenoic acid 200 mg), fibre nil, energy 74 kJ (18 kcal)/4 g, with minerals

DocOmega oral powder 4g sachets (Vitaflo International Ltd)
30 sachet (ACBS) · NHS indicative price = £44.16

EAA ® Supplement

▸ Nutritional supplement for the dietary management of disorders of protein metabolism including urea cycle disorders in children over 3 years.
POWDER, protein equivalent (essential amino acids) 5 g, carbohydrate 4 g, fat nil, energy 151 kJ (36 kcal)/12.5 g, with vitamins, minerals, and trace elements.

EAA Supplement oral powder 12.5g sachets (Vitaflo International Ltd)
50 sachet (ACBS) · NHS indicative price = £230.27

Isoleucine50 ®

▸ Nutritional supplement for use in the dietary management of inborn errors of amino acid metabolism in adults and children from birth.
POWDER, isoleucine 50 mg, carbohydrate 3.8 g, fat nil, energy 63 kJ (15 kcal)/4 g

Isoleucine50 oral powder 4g sachets (Vitaflo International Ltd)
30 sachet (ACBS) · NHS indicative price = £61.02

KeyOmega ®

▸ Nutritional supplement for the dietary management of inborn errors of metabolism.
POWDER, protein (cows' milk, soya) 170 mg, carbohydrate 2.8 g, fat 800 mg (of which arachidonic acid 200 mg, docosahexaenoic acid 100 mg), energy 80 kJ (19 kcal)/4 g.

KeyOmega oral powder 4g sachets (Vitaflo International Ltd)
30 sachet (ACBS) · NHS indicative price = £45.16

Leucine100 ®

▸ Nutritional supplement for the dietary management of inborn errors of amino acid metabolism in adults and children from birth.
POWDER, leucine 100 mg, carbohydrate 3.7 g, fat nil, energy 63 kJ (15 kcal)/4 g

Leucine100 oral powder sachets (Vitaflo International Ltd)
30 sachet (ACBS) · NHS indicative price = £61.02

Low protein drink

▸ Nutritional supplement for the dietary management of inborn errors of amino acid metabolism in adults and children over 1 year.
POWDER, protein (cows' milk) 4.5 g (phenylalanine 100 mg), carbohydrate 59.5 g, fat 29.9 g, fibre nil, energy 2194 kJ (528 kcal)/100 g, with vitamins, minerals, and trace elements. Contains lactose.
Termed *Milupa® lp-drink* by manufacturer.

Milupa LP drink (Nutricia Ltd)
400 gram (ACBS) · NHS indicative price = £10.00

Phenylalanine50 ®

▸ Nutritional supplement for use in the dietary management of inborn errors of metabolism in adults and children from birth.
POWDER, phenylalanine 50 mg, carbohydrate 3.8 g, fat nil, energy 63 kJ (15 kcal)/4 g

Phenylalanine50 oral powder sachets (Vitaflo International Ltd)
30 sachet (ACBS) · NHS indicative price = £59.25

ProZero ®

▸ A protein-free nutritional supplement for the dietary management of inborn errors of metabolism in children over 6 months and adults.
LIQUID, carbohydrate 8.1 g (of which sugars 3.5 g), fat 3.8 g, energy 278 kJ (66 kcal)/100 mL. Contains lactose.

ProZero liquid (Vitaflo International Ltd)
250 ml (ACBS) · NHS indicative price = £1.62 | 1000 ml (ACBS) · NHS indicative price = £6.50

Tyrosine1000 ®

▸ Nutritional supplement for the dietary management of inborn errors of amino acid metabolism in adults and children from birth.
POWDER, tyrosine 1 g, carbohydrate 2.9 g, fat nil, energy 63 kJ (15 kcal)/4-g sachet.

Tyrosine1000 oral powder 4g sachets (Vitaflo International Ltd)
30 sachet (ACBS) · NHS indicative price = £5.57

Valine50 ®

▸ Nutritional supplement for the dietary management of inborn errors of amino acid metabolism in adults and children from birth.
POWDER, valine 50 mg, carbohydrate 3.8 g, fat nil, energy 63 kJ (15 kcal)/4 g

Valine50 oral powder 4g sachets (Vitaflo International Ltd)
30 sachet (ACBS) · NHS indicative price = £61.02

Phenylketonuria

Easiphen ®

▸ Nutritional supplement for the dietary management of proven phenylketonuria in children over 8 years.
LIQUID, protein equivalent (containing essential and non-essential amino acids except phenylalanine) 6.7 g, carbohydrate 5.1 g, fat 2 g, energy 275 kJ (65 kcal)/100 mL with vitamins, minerals, and trace elements.

Easiphen liquid (Nutricia Ltd)
250 ml (ACBS) · NHS indicative price = £10.46

L-Tyrosine

▸ Nutritional supplement for the dietary management of phenylketonuria in pregnant women with low plasma tyrosine concentrations.
POWDER, L-tyrosine 20 g, carbohydrate 76.8 g, fat nil, energy 1612 kJ (379 kcal)/100 g.

L-Tyrosine powder (Nutricia Ltd)
100 gram (ACBS) · NHS indicative price = £24.52

Lophlex ®

▸ Nutritional supplement for the dietary management of proven phenylketonuria in children over 8 years and adults including pregnant women.
POWDER, protein equivalent (essential and non-essential amino acids except phenylalanine) 20 g, carbohydrate 2.5 g, fat 60 mg, fibre 220 mg, energy 385 kJ (91 kcal)/27.8-g sachet, with vitamins, minerals, and trace elements.

Lophlex powder 27.8g sachets berry (Nutricia Ltd)
30 sachet (ACBS) · NHS indicative price = £314.10

Lophlex powder 27.8g sachets orange (Nutricia Ltd)
30 sachet (ACBS) · NHS indicative price = £314.10

Lophlex powder 27.8g sachets unflavoured (Nutricia Ltd)
30 sachet (ACBS) · NHS indicative price = £314.10

Loprofin ® PKU Drink

▸ Nutritional supplement for the dietary management of phenylketonuria in children over 1 year and adults.
LIQUID, protein (cows' milk) 400 mg (phenylalanine 10 mg), lactose 9.4 g, fat 2 g, energy 165 kJ (40 kcal)/100 mL.

Loprofin PKU drink (Nutricia Ltd)
200 ml (ACBS) · NHS indicative price = £0.81

Loprofin ® Sno-Pro

▸ Nutritional supplement for the dietary management of phenylketonuria, chronic renal failure and other inborn errors of amino acid metabolism.
LIQUID, protein (cows' milk) 220 mg (phenylalanine 12.5 mg), carbohydrate 8 g, fat 3.8 g, energy 273 kJ (65 kcal)/100 mL. Contains lactose.

Loprofin SNO-PRO drink (Nutricia Ltd)
200 ml (ACBS) · NHS indicative price = £1.35

Phlexy-10 ® Exchange System

▸ Nutritional supplement for the dietary management of phenylketonuria.

CAPSULES, protein equivalent (essential and non-essential amino acids except phenylalanine) 416.5 mg/capsule.

Phlexy-10 600mg capsules (Nutricia Ltd)
200 capsule (ACBS) · NHS indicative price = £47.03

TABLETS, protein equivalent (essential and non-essential amino acids except phenylalanine) 833 mg tablet.

Phlexy-10 tablets (Nutricia Ltd)
75 tablet (ACBS) · NHS indicative price = £30.24

DRINK MIX, powder, protein equivalent (essential and non-essential amino acids except phenylalanine) 8.33 g, carbohydrate 8.8 g/20-g sachet.

Phlexy-10 drink mix 20g sachets apple & blackcurrant (Nutricia Ltd)
30 sachet (ACBS) · NHS indicative price = £139.28

Phlexy-10 drink mix 20g sachets citrus burst (Nutricia Ltd)
30 sachet (ACBS) · NHS indicative price = £139.28

Phlexy-10 drink mix 20g sachets tropical surprise (Nutricia Ltd)
30 sachet (ACBS) · NHS indicative price = £139.28

Phlexy-Vits ®

▸ For use as a vitamin and mineral component of restricted therapeutic diets in children over 11 years and adults with phenylketonuria and similar amino acid abnormalities.
POWDER, vitamins, minerals, and trace elements

Phlexy-Vits powder 7g sachets (Nutricia Ltd)
30 sachet (ACBS) · NHS indicative price = £77.23
TABLETS, vitamins, minerals, and trace elements

Phlexy-Vits tablets (Nutricia Ltd)
180 tablet (ACBS) · NHS indicative price = £88.51

PK Aid 4 ®

▸ Nutritional supplement for the dietary management of phenylketonuria in children and adults.
POWDER, protein equivalent (essential and non-essential amino acids except phenylalanine) 79 g, carbohydrate 4.5 g, fat nil, energy 1420 kJ (334 kcal)/100 g. To flavour unflavoured products, see Modjul Flavour System p. 1126

PK Aid 4 powder (Nutricia Ltd)
500 gram (ACBS) · NHS indicative price = £155.07

PKU Anamix ® First Spoon

▸ Nutritional supplement for the dietary management of proven phenylketonuria in children from 6 months to 5 years.
POWDER, protein equivalent (essential and non-essential amino acids except phenylalanine) 5 g, carbohydrate 4.8 g, fat 150 mg, fibre nil, energy 172 kJ (41 kcal)/12.5-g sachet, with vitamins, minerals, and trace elements

PKU Anamix First Spoon oral powder 12.5g sachets (Nutricia Ltd)
30 sachet (ACBS) · NHS indicative price = £96.30

PKU Anamix ® Infant

▸ Nutritional supplement for the dietary management of proven phenylketonuria in children from birth to 3 years.
POWDER, protein equivalent (essential and non-essential amino acids except phenylalanine) 13.1 g, carbohydrate 49.5 g, fat 23 g, fibre 5.3 g, energy 1915 kJ (457 kcal)/100 g, with vitamins, minerals, and trace elements; standard dilution (15%) provides protein equivalent 2 g, carbohydrate 7.4 g, fat 3.5 g, fibre 800 mg, energy 287 kJ (69 kcal)/100 mL

PKU Anamix Infant powder (Nutricia Ltd)
400 gram (ACBS) · NHS indicative price = £37.08

PKU Anamix ® Junior

▸ Nutritional supplement for the dietary management of phenylketonuria in children 1–10 years.
POWDER, protein equivalent (essential and non-essential amino acids except phenylalanine) 10 g, carbohydrate 11.5 g, fat 4.5 g, energy 566 kJ (135 kcal)/36-g sachet, with vitamins, minerals, and trace elements

PKU Anamix Junior powder 36g sachets chocolate (Nutricia Ltd)
30 sachet (ACBS) · NHS indicative price = £137.10

PKU Anamix Junior powder 36g sachets neutral (Nutricia Ltd)
30 sachet (ACBS) · NHS indicative price = £137.10

PKU Anamix Junior powder 36g sachets berry (Nutricia Ltd)
30 sachet (ACBS) · NHS indicative price = £137.10

PKU Anamix Junior powder 36g sachets orange (Nutricia Ltd)
30 sachet (ACBS) · NHS indicative price = £137.10

PKU Anamix ® Junior LQ

▸ Nutritional supplement for the dietary supplement of phenyketonuria in children 1–10 years.
LIQUID, protein equivalent (essential and non-essential amino acids except phenylalanine) 10 g, carbohydrate 8.8 g, fat 4.8 g, fibre 310 mg, energy 497 kJ (118 kcal)/125 mL, with vitamins, minerals, and trace elements. Lactose-free.

PKU Anamix Junior LQ liquid berry (Nutricia Ltd)
125 ml (ACBS) · NHS indicative price = £6.08

PKU Anamix Junior LQ liquid orange (Nutricia Ltd)
125 ml (ACBS) · NHS indicative price = £6.08

PKU cooler10 ®

▸ Nutritional supplement for the dietary management of phenylketonuria in children over 3 years.
LIQUID, protein equivalent (essential and non-essential amino acids except phenylalanine) 10 g, carbohydrate 4.7 g, energy 258 kJ (62 kcal)/87-mL pouch, with vitamins, minerals, and trace elements.

PKU orange cooler10 liquid (Vitaflo International Ltd)
87 ml (ACBS) · NHS indicative price = £5.16

PKU purple cooler10 liquid (Vitaflo International Ltd)
87 ml (ACBS) · NHS indicative price = £5.16

PKU red cooler10 liquid (Vitaflo International Ltd)
87 ml (ACBS) · NHS indicative price = £5.16

PKU white cooler10 liquid (Vitaflo International Ltd)
87 ml (ACBS) · NHS indicative price = £5.16

PKU yellow cooler10 liquid (Vitaflo International Ltd)
87 ml (ACBS) · NHS indicative price = £5.16

PKU cooler15 ®

▸ Nutritional supplement for the dietary management of phenylketonuria in children over 3 years.
LIQUID, protein equivalent (essential and non-essential amino acids except phenylalanine) 15 g, carbohydrate 7 g, energy 386 kJ (92 kcal)/130-mL pouch, with vitamins, minerals, and trace elements.

PKU orange cooler15 liquid (Vitaflo International Ltd)
130 ml (ACBS) · NHS indicative price = £7.68

PKU purple cooler15 liquid (Vitaflo International Ltd)
130 ml (ACBS) · NHS indicative price = £7.68

PKU red cooler15 liquid (Vitaflo International Ltd)
130 ml (ACBS) · NHS indicative price = £7.68

PKU white cooler15 liquid (Vitaflo International Ltd)
130 ml (ACBS) · NHS indicative price = £7.68

PKU yellow cooler15 liquid (Vitaflo International Ltd)
130 ml (ACBS) · NHS indicative price = £7.68

PKU cooler20®

▶ Nutritional supplement for the dietary management of phenylketonuria in children over 3 years.
LIQUID, protein equivalent (essential and non-essential amino acids except phenylalanine) 20 g, carbohydrate 9.4 g, energy 517 kJ (124 kcal)/174-mL pouch, with vitamins, minerals, and trace elements.

PKU orange cooler20 liquid (Vitaflo International Ltd)
174 ml (ACBS) · NHS indicative price = £10.32

PKU purple cooler20 liquid (Vitaflo International Ltd)
174 ml (ACBS) · NHS indicative price = £10.32

PKU red cooler20 liquid (Vitaflo International Ltd)
174 ml (ACBS) · NHS indicative price = £10.32

PKU white cooler20 liquid (Vitaflo International Ltd)
174 ml (ACBS) · NHS indicative price = £10.32

PKU yellow cooler20 liquid (Vitaflo International Ltd)
174 ml (ACBS) · NHS indicative price = £10.32

PKU express15®

▶ Nutritional supplement for the dietary management of phenylketonuria. Not recommended for children under 3 years.
POWDER, protein equivalent (essential and non-essential amino acids except phenylalanine) 15 g, carbohydrate 3.4 g, energy 310 kJ (74 kcal)/25 g, with vitamins, minerals, and trace elements. To flavour unflavoured products, see FlavourPac p. 1126.

PKU express15 powder 25g sachets lemon (Vitaflo International Ltd)
30 sachet (ACBS) · NHS indicative price = £226.17

PKU express15 powder 25g sachets orange (Vitaflo International Ltd)
30 sachet (ACBS) · NHS indicative price = £226.17

PKU express15 powder 25g sachets tropical (Vitaflo International Ltd)
30 sachet (ACBS) · NHS indicative price = £226.17

PKU express15 powder 25g sachets unflavoured (Vitaflo International Ltd)
30 sachet (ACBS) · NHS indicative price = £226.17

PKU express20®

▶ Nutritional supplement for the dietary management of phenylketonuria. Not recommended for children under 3 years.
POWDER, protein equivalent (essential and non-essential amino acids except phenylalanine) 20 g, carbohydrate 4.7 g, energy 422 kJ (101 kcal)/34 g, with vitamins, minerals, and trace elements. To flavour unflavoured products, see FlavourPac p. 1126.

PKU express20 powder 34g sachets lemon (Vitaflo International Ltd)
30 sachet (ACBS) · NHS indicative price = £292.20

PKU express20 powder 34g sachets orange (Vitaflo International Ltd)
30 sachet (ACBS) · NHS indicative price = £292.20

PKU express20 powder 34g sachets tropical (Vitaflo International Ltd)
30 sachet (ACBS) · NHS indicative price = £292.20

PKU express20 powder 34g sachets unflavoured (Vitaflo International Ltd)
30 sachet (ACBS) · NHS indicative price = £292.20

PKU gel®

▶ For use as part of the low-protein dietary management of phenylketonuria in children 6 months–10 years (unflavoured), 1–10 years (flavoured).
POWDER, protein equivalent (essential and non-essential amino acids except phenylalanine) 10 g, carbohydrate 10.3 g (unflavoured)/8.9 g (flavoured), fat less than 100 mg, energy 346 kJ (81 kcal) (unflavoured)/322 kJ (76 kcal) (flavoured)/24 g, with vitamins, minerals, and trace elements. PKU Orange contains soya. To flavour unflavoured products, see FlavourPac p. 1126.

PKU gel powder 24g sachets unflavoured (Vitaflo International Ltd)
30 sachet (ACBS) · NHS indicative price = £156.46

PKU gel powder 24g sachets orange (Vitaflo International Ltd)
30 sachet (ACBS) · NHS indicative price = £156.46

PKU gel powder 24g sachets raspberry (Vitaflo International Ltd)
30 sachet (ACBS) · NHS indicative price = £156.46

PKU Lophlex® **LQ 10**

▶ Nutritional supplement for the dietary management of phenylketonuria in children over 4 years and adults including pregnant women.
LIQUID, protein equivalent (essential and non-essential amino acids except phenylalanine) 10 g, carbohydrate 4.4 g, fibre 250 mg, energy 245 kJ (58 kcal)/62.5 mL, with vitamins, minerals, and trace elements.

PKU Lophlex LQ 10 liquid berry (Nutricia Ltd)
62.5 ml (ACBS) · NHS indicative price = £5.61

PKU Lophlex LQ 10 liquid juicy berries (Nutricia Ltd)
62.5 ml (ACBS) · NHS indicative price = £5.61

PKU Lophlex LQ 10 liquid juicy citrus (Nutricia Ltd)
62.5 ml (ACBS) · NHS indicative price = £5.61

PKU Lophlex LQ 10 liquid juicy orange (Nutricia Ltd)
62.5 ml (ACBS) · NHS indicative price = £5.61

PKU Lophlex LQ 10 liquid juicy tropical (Nutricia Ltd)
62.5 ml (ACBS) · NHS indicative price = £5.61

PKU Lophlex® **LQ 20**

▶ Nutritional supplement for the dietary management of phenylketonuria in children over 4 years and adults including pregnant women.
LIQUID, protein equivalent (essential and non-essential amino acids except phenylalanine) 20 g, carbohydrate 8.8 g, fibre 500 mg, energy 490 kJ (115 kcal)/125 mL, with vitamins, minerals, and trace elements.

PKU Lophlex LQ 20 liquid berry (Nutricia Ltd)
125 ml (ACBS) · NHS indicative price = £11.19

PKU Lophlex LQ 20 liquid juicy berries (Nutricia Ltd)
125 ml (ACBS) · NHS indicative price = £11.19

PKU Lophlex LQ 20 liquid juicy citrus (Nutricia Ltd)
125 ml (ACBS) · NHS indicative price = £11.19

PKU Lophlex LQ 20 liquid juicy orange (Nutricia Ltd)
125 ml (ACBS) · NHS indicative price = £11.19

PKU Lophlex LQ 20 liquid juicy tropical (Nutricia Ltd)
125 ml (ACBS) · NHS indicative price = £11.19

PKU Lophlex LQ 20 liquid orange (Nutricia Ltd)
125 ml (ACBS) · NHS indicative price = £11.19

PKU Lophlex® **Sensation 20**

▶ Nutritional supplement for the dietary management of phenylketonuria in children over 4 years and adults including pregnant women.
SEMI-SOLID, protein equivalent (containing essential and non-essential amino acids except phenylalanine) 20 g, carbohydrate 20.2 g, fibre 1 g, energy 706 kJ (166 kcal)/109 g, with vitamins, minerals, and trace elements.

PKU Lophlex Sensation 20 berries (Nutricia Ltd)
327 gram (ACBS) · NHS indicative price = £35.76

PKU squeezie®

▶ Nutritional supplement for the dietary management of phenylketonuria in children from 6 months to 10 years.
LIQUID, protein equivalent (essential and non-essential amino acids except phenylalanine) 10 g, carbohydrate 22.5 g, fat 500 mg, energy 575 kJ (135 kcal)/85 g, with vitamins, minerals, and trace elements.

PKU squeezie liquid 85g pouches (Vitaflo International Ltd)
30 pouch (ACBS) · NHS indicative price = £149.57

PKU Maxamum®

▶ Nutritional supplement for the dietary management of phenylketonuria in children over 8 years and adults.
POWDER, protein equivalent (essential and non-essential amino acids except phenylalanine) 39 g, carbohydrate 34 g, fat less than 500 mg, energy 1260 kJ (297 kcal)/100 g, with vitamins, minerals, and trace elements. To flavour unflavoured products, see Modjul Flavour System p. 1126.

PKU Maxamum oral powder 50g sachets orange (Nutricia Ltd)
30 sachet (ACBS) · NHS indicative price = £292.20

PKU Maxamum oral powder 50g sachets unflavoured (Nutricia Ltd)
30 sachet (ACBS) · NHS indicative price = £292.20

PKU Maxamum powder orange (Nutricia Ltd)
500 gram (ACBS) · NHS indicative price = £97.44

PKU Maxamum powder unflavoured (Nutricia Ltd)
500 gram (ACBS) · NHS indicative price = £97.44

Tyrosinaemia

Methionine-free TYR Anamix ® Infant

▸ Nutritional supplement for the dietary management of proven tyrosinaemia type 1 in children from birth to 3 years.
POWDER, protein equivalent (essential and non-essential amino acids except methionine, phenylalanine, and tyrosine) 13.1 g, carbohydrate 49.5 g, fat 23 g, fibre 5.3 g, energy 1915 kJ (457 kcal)/100 g, with vitamins, minerals, and trace elements; standard dilution (15%) provides protein equivalent 2 g, carbohydrate 7.4 g, fat 3.5 g, fibre 800 mg, energy 287 kJ (69 kcal)/100 mL.

TYR Anamix Infant methionine free powder (Nutricia Ltd)
400 gram (ACBS) · NHS indicative price = £43.52

TYR Anamix ® Infant

▸ Nutritional supplement for the dietary management of proven tyrosinaemia where plasma-methionine concentrations are normal in children from birth to 3 years.
POWDER, protein equivalent (essential and non-essential amino acids except phenylalanine and tyrosine) 13.1 g, carbohydrate 49.5 g, fat 23 g, fibre 5.3 g, energy 1915 kJ (457 kcal)/100 g, with vitamins, minerals, and trace elements; standard dilution (15%) provides protein equivalent 2 g, carbohydrate 7.4 g, fat 3.5 g, fibre 800 mg, energy 287 kJ (69 kcal)/100 mL.

TYR Anamix Infant methionine free powder (Nutricia Ltd)
400 gram (ACBS) · NHS indicative price = £43.52

TYR Anamix Infant powder (Nutricia Ltd)
400 gram (ACBS) · NHS indicative price = £43.52

TYR Anamix ® Junior

▸ Nutritional supplement for the dietary management of proven tyrosinaemia in children 1–10 years.
POWDER, protein equivalent (essential and non-essential amino acids except phenylalanine and tyrosine) 8.4 g, carbohydrate 11 g, fat 3.9 g, energy 475 kJ (113 kcal)/29-g sachet, with vitamins, minerals, and trace elements.

TYR Anamix Junior oral powder 29g sachets (Nutricia Ltd)
30 sachet (ACBS) · NHS indicative price = £206.40

TYR Anamix ® Junior LQ

▸ Nutritional supplement for the dietary management of tyrosinaemia type 1 (when nitisinone (NTBC) is used, see nitisinone p. 662), type II, and type III, in children over 1 year.
LIQUID, protein equivalent (essential and non-essential amino acids except phenylalanine and tyrosine) 10 g,carbohydrate 8.8 g, fat 4.8 g, fibre 310 mg, energy 500 kJ (119 kcal)/125 mL, with vitamins, minerals and trace elements.

TYR Anamix Junior LQ liquid (Nutricia Ltd)
125 ml (ACBS) · NHS indicative price = £10.09

TYR cooler ® 15

▸ Nutritional supplement for the dietary management of tyrosinaemia in children over 3 years and adults.
LIQUID, protein equivalent (essential and non-essential amino acids except tyrosine and phenylalanine) 15 g, carbohydrate 7 g, fat 500 mg, energy 393 kJ (92 kcal)/130 mL, with vitamins, minerals, and trace elements.

TYR orange cooler15 liquid (Vitaflo International Ltd)
130 ml (ACBS) · NHS indicative price = £12.68

TYR red cooler10 liquid (Vitaflo International Ltd)
87 ml (ACBS) · NHS indicative price = £7.89

TYR red cooler15 liquid (Vitaflo International Ltd)
130 ml (ACBS) · NHS indicative price = £12.68

TYR red cooler20 liquid (Vitaflo International Ltd)
174 ml (ACBS) · NHS indicative price = £16.48

TYR express15 ®

▸ Nutritional supplement for the dietary management of tyrosinaemia in children over 8 years and adults.
POWDER, protein equivalent (essential and non-essential amino acids except tyrosine and phenylalanine) 15 g, carbohydrate 3.4 g, fat less than 100 mg, energy 310 kJ (74 kcal)/25 g, with vitamins, minerals, and trace elements. To flavour unflavoured products, see FlavourPac p. 1126.

TYR express15 oral powder 25g sachets (Vitaflo International Ltd)
30 sachet (ACBS) · NHS indicative price = £373.05

TYR express20 ®

▸ Nutritional supplement for the dietary management of tyrosinaemia in children over 8 years.
POWDER, protein equivalent (essential and non-essential amino acids except tyrosine and phenylalanine) 20 g, carbohydrate 4.7 g, fat less than 100 mg, energy 416 kJ (99 kcal)/34 g, with vitamins, minerals, and trace elements. To flavour unflavoured products, see FlavourPac p. 1126.

TYR express20 oral powder 34g sachets (Vitaflo International Ltd)
30 sachet (ACBS) · NHS indicative price = £481.98

TYR Gel ®

▸ Nutritional supplement for the dietary management of tyrosinaemia in children 1–10 years.
GEL, protein equivalent (essential and non-essential amino acids except tyrosine and phenylalanine) 10 g, carbohydrate 10.3 g, fat less than 100 mg, energy 339 kJ (81 kcal)/24 g, with vitamins, minerals and trace elements. To flavour unflavoured products, see FlavourPac p. 1126.

TYR gel oral powder 24g sachets (Vitaflo International Ltd)
30 sachet (ACBS) · NHS indicative price = £240.17

TYR Lophlex ® LQ 20

▸ Nutritional supplement for the dietary management of tyrosinaemia in children over 4 years and adults, including pregnant women (in conjunction with standard folic acid supplementation).
LIQUID, protein equivalent (essential and non-essential amino acids except phenylalanine and tyrosine) 20 g, carbohydrate 8.8 g, fat less than 500 mg, fibre 500 mg, energy 509 kJ (120 kcal)/125 mL, with vitamins, minerals, and trace elements.

TYR Lophlex LQ 20 liquid (Nutricia Ltd)
125 ml (ACBS) · NHS indicative price = £17.94

XPHEN TYR Tyrosidon ®

▸ Nutritional supplement for the management of tyrosinaemia in children and adults where plasma-methionine concentrations are normal.
POWDER, protein equivalent (essential and non-essential amino acids except phenylalanine and tyrosine) 77 g, carbohydrate 4.5 g, fat nil, energy 1386 kJ (326 kcal)/100 g. To flavour unflavoured products, see Modjul Flavour System p. 1126.

XPHEN TYR Tyrosidon Free AA Mix powder (Nutricia Ltd)
500 gram (ACBS) · NHS indicative price = £208.24

XPTM Tyrosidon ®

▸ Nutritional supplement for the dietary management of tyrosinaemia type I in children and adults where plasma-methionine concentrations are above normal.
POWDER, protein equivalent (essential and non-essential amino acids except methionine, phenylalanine, and tyrosine) 77 g, carbohydrate 4.5 g, fat nil, energy 1386 kJ (326 kcal)/100 g. To flavour unflavoured products, see Modjul Flavour System p. 1126.

XPTM Tyrosidon powder (Nutricia Ltd)
500 gram · NHS indicative price = £91.31

Appendix 3
Cautionary and advisory labels for dispensed medicines

Guidance for cautionary and advisory labels

Medicinal forms within BNF publications include code numbers of the cautionary labels that pharmacists are recommended to add when dispensing. It is also expected that pharmacists will counsel patients and carers when necessary.

Counselling needs to be related to the age, experience, background, and understanding of the individual patient or carer. The pharmacist should ensure understanding of how to take or use the medicine and how to follow the correct dosage schedule. Any effects of the medicine on co-ordination, performance of skilled tasks (e.g. driving or work), any foods or medicines to be avoided, and what to do if a dose is missed should also be explained. Other matters, such as the possibility of staining of the clothes or skin, or discolouration of urine or stools by a medicine should also be mentioned.

For some medicines there is a special need for counselling, such as an unusual method or time of administration or a potential interaction with a common food or domestic remedy, and this should be mentioned where necessary.

Original packs

Most preparations are dispensed in unbroken original packs that include further advice for the patient in the form of patient information leaflets. The advice in patient information leaflets may be less appropriate when the medicine is for a child, particularly for unlicensed medicines or indications. Pharmacists should explain discrepancies to carers, if necessary. The patient information leaflet should only be withheld in exceptional circumstances because it contains other information that should be provided. Label 10 may be of value where appropriate. More general leaflets advising on the administration of preparations such as eye drops, eye ointments, inhalers, and suppositories are also available.

Scope of labels

In general no label recommendations have been made for injections on the assumption that they will be administered by a healthcare professional or a well-instructed patient. The labelling is not exhaustive and pharmacists are recommended to use their professional discretion in labelling new preparations and those for which no labels are shown.

Individual labelling advice is not given on the administration of the large variety of antacids. In the absence of instructions from the prescriber, and if on enquiry the patient has had no verbal instructions, the directions given under 'Dose' should be used on the label.

It is recognised that there may be occasions when pharmacists will use their knowledge and professional discretion and decide to omit one or more of the recommended labels for a particular patient. In this case counselling is of the utmost importance. There may also be an occasion when a prescriber does not wish additional cautionary labels to be used, in which case the prescription should be endorsed 'NCL' (no cautionary labels). The exact wording that is required instead should then be specified on the prescription.

Pharmacists label medicines with various wordings in addition to those directions specified on the prescription. Such labels include 'Shake the bottle', 'For external use only', and 'Store in a cool place', as well as 'Discard.... days after opening' and 'Do not use after....', which apply particularly to antibiotic mixtures, diluted liquid and topical preparations, and to eye-drops. Although not listed in the *BNF for Children* these labels should continue to be used when appropriate; indeed, 'For external use only' is a legal requirement on external liquid preparations, while 'Keep out of the reach of children' is a legal requirement on all dispensed medicines. Care should be taken not to obscure other relevant information with adhesive labelling.

It is the usual practice for patients to take standard tablets with water or other liquid and for this reason no separate label has been recommended.

The label wordings recommended by the *BNF for Children* apply to medicines dispensed against a prescription. Children and carers should be aware that a dispensed medicine should never be taken by, or shared with, anyone other than for whom the prescriber intended it. Therefore, the *BNF for Children* does not include warnings against the use of a dispensed medicine by persons other than for whom it was specifically prescribed.

The label or labels for each preparation are recommended after careful consideration of the information available. However, it is recognised that in some cases this information may be either incomplete or open to a different interpretation. The *BNF for Children* will therefore be grateful to receive any constructive comments on the labelling suggested for any preparation.

Recommended label wordings

For *BNF for Children* 2011–2012, a revised set of cautionary and advisory labels were introduced. All of the existing labels were user-tested, and the revised wording selected reflects terminology that is better understood by patients.

Wordings which can be given as separate warnings are labels 1–19, 29–30, and 32. Wordings which can be incorporated in an appropriate position in the directions for dosage or administration are labels 21–28. A label has been omitted for number 20; labels 31 and 33 no longer apply to any medicines in the *BNF for Children* and have therefore been deleted.

If separate labels are used it is recommended that the wordings be used without modification. If changes are made to suit computer requirements, care should be taken to retain the sense of the original.

Welsh labels

Comprehensive Welsh translations are available for each cautionary and advisory label.

Labels

1 Warning: This medicine may make you sleepy

Rhybudd: Gall y feddyginiaeth hon eich gwneud yn gysglyd

To be used on *preparations for children* containing antihistamines, or other preparations given to children where the warnings of label 2 on driving or alcohol would not be appropriate.

2 Warning: This medicine may make you sleepy. If this happens, do not drive or use tools or machines. Do not drink alcohol

Rhybudd: Gall y feddyginiaeth hon eich gwneud yn gysglyd. Peidiwch â gyrru, defnyddio offer llaw neu beiriannau os yw hyn yn digwydd. Peidiwch ag yfed alcohol

To be used on *preparations for adults that can cause drowsiness*, thereby affecting coordination and the ability to drive and operate hazardous machinery; label 1 is more appropriate for children. *It is an offence to drive while under the influence of drink or drugs.*

Some of these preparations only cause drowsiness in the first few days of treatment and some only cause drowsiness in higher doses.

In such cases the patient should be told that the advice applies until the effects have worn off. However many of these preparations can produce a slowing of reaction time and a loss of mental concentration that can have the same effects as drowsiness.

Avoidance of alcoholic drink is recommended because the effects of CNS depressants are enhanced by alcohol. Strict prohibition however could lead to some patients not taking the medicine. Pharmacists should therefore explain the risk and encourage compliance, particularly in patients who may think they already tolerate the effects of alcohol (see also label 3). Queries from patients with epilepsy regarding fitness to drive should be referred back to the patient's doctor.

Side-effects unrelated to drowsiness that may affect a patient's ability to drive or operate machinery safely include *blurred vision, dizziness, or nausea*. In general, no label has been recommended to cover these cases, but the patient should be suitably counselled.

3 Warning: This medicine may make you sleepy. If this happens, do not drive or use tools or machines

Rhybudd: Gall y feddyginiaeth hon eich gwneud yn gysglyd. Peidiwch â gyrru, defnyddio offer llaw neu beiriannau os yw hyn yn digwydd

To be used on *preparations containing monoamine-oxidase inhibitors*; the warning to avoid alcohol and dealcoholised (low alcohol) drink is covered by the patient information leaflet.

Also to be used as for label 2 but where alcohol is not an issue.

4 Warning: Do not drink alcohol

Rhybudd: Peidiwch ag yfed alcohol

To be used on *preparations where a reaction such as flushing may occur if alcohol is taken* (e.g. metronidazole). Alcohol may also enhance the hypoglycaemia produced by some oral antidiabetic drugs but routine application of a warning label is not considered necessary.

Patients should be advised not to drink alcohol for as long as they are receiving/using a course of medication, and in some cases for a period of time after the course is finished.

5 Do not take indigestion remedies 2 hours before or after you take this medicine

Peidiwch â chymryd meddyginiaethau camdreuliad 2 awr cyn neu ar ôl y feddyginiaeth hon

To be used with label 25 on *preparations coated to resist gastric acid* (e.g. enteric-coated tablets). This is to avoid the possibility of premature dissolution of the coating in the presence of an alkaline pH.

Label 5 also applies to drugs such as gabapentin *where the absorption is significantly affected by antacids*. Pharmacists will be aware (from a knowledge of physiology) that the usual time during which indigestion remedies should be avoided is at least 2 hours before and after the majority of medicines have been taken; when a manufacturer advises a different time period, this can be followed, and should be explained to the patient.

6 Do not take indigestion remedies, or medicines containing iron or zinc, 2 hours before or after you take this medicine

Peidiwch â chymryd meddyginiaethau camdreuliad neu feddyginiaethau sy'n cynnwys haearn neu sinc, 2 awr cyn neu ar ôl y feddyginiaeth hon

To be used on *preparations containing ofloxacin and some other quinolones, doxycycline, lymecycline, minocycline, and penicillamine*. These drugs chelate calcium, iron, and zinc and are less well absorbed when taken with calcium-containing antacids or preparations containing iron or zinc. Pharmacists will be aware (from a knowledge of physiology) that these incompatible preparations should be taken at least 2 hours apart for the majority of medicines; when a manufacturer advises a different time period, this can be followed, and should be explained to the patient.

7 Do not take milk, indigestion remedies, or medicines containing iron or zinc, 2 hours before or after you take this medicine

Peidiwch â chymryd llaeth, meddyginiaethau camdreuliad, neu feddyginiaeth sy'n cynnwys haearn neu sinc, 2 awr cyn neu ar ôl cymryd y feddyginiaeth hon

To be used on *preparations containing ciprofloxacin, norfloxacin, or tetracyclines that chelate calcium, iron, magnesium, and zinc,* and are thus less available for absorption. Pharmacists will be aware (from a knowledge of physiology) that these incompatible preparations should be taken at least 2 hours apart for the majority of medicines; when a manufacturer advises a different time period, this can be followed, and should be explained to the patient. Doxycycline, lymecycline, and minocycline are less liable to form chelates and therefore only require label 6 (see above).

8 Warning: Do not stop taking this medicine unless your doctor tells you to stop

Rhybudd: Peidiwch â stopio cymryd y feddyginiaeth hon, oni bai fod eich meddyg yn dweud wrthych am stopio

To be used on *preparations that contain a drug which is required to be taken over long periods without the patient necessarily perceiving any benefit* (e.g. antituberculous drugs).

Also to be used on *preparations that contain a drug whose withdrawal is likely to be a particular hazard* (e.g. clonidine for hypertension). Label 10 (see below) is more appropriate for corticosteroids.

9 Space the doses evenly throughout the day. Keep taking this medicine until the course is finished, unless you are told to stop

Gadewch yr un faint o amser rhwng pob dôs yn ystod y dydd. Parhewch i gymryd y feddyginiaeth nes bod y cyfan wedi'i orffen, oni bai eich bod yn cael cyngor i stopio

To be used on *preparations where a course of treatment should be completed* to reduce the incidence of relapse or failure of treatment.

The preparations are antimicrobial drugs given by mouth. Very occasionally, some may have severe side-effects (e.g. diarrhoea in patients receiving clindamycin) and in such cases the patient may need to be advised of reasons for stopping treatment quickly and returning to the doctor.

10 Warning: Read the additional information given with this medicine

Rhybudd: Darllenwch y wybodaeth ychwanegol gyda'r feddyginiaeth hon

To be used particularly on *preparations containing anticoagulants, lithium, and oral corticosteroids*. The appropriate treatment card should be given to the patient and any necessary explanations given.

This label may also be used on other preparations to remind the patient of the instructions that have been given.

11 Protect your skin from sunlight—even on a bright but cloudy day. Do not use sunbeds

Diogelwch eich croen rhag golau'r haul, hyd yn oed ar ddiwrnod braf ond cymylog. Peidiwch â defnyddio gwely haul

To be used on *preparations that may cause phototoxic or photoallergic reactions* if the patient is exposed to ultraviolet radiation. Exposure to high intensity ultraviolet radiation from sunray lamps and sunbeds is particularly likely to cause reactions.

12 Do not take anything containing aspirin while taking this medicine

Peidiwch â chymryd unrhyw beth sy'n cynnwys aspirin gyda'r feddyginiaeth hon

To be used on *preparations containing sulfinpyrazone* whose activity is reduced by aspirin.

Label 12 should not be used for anticoagulants since label 10 is more appropriate.

13 Dissolve or mix with water before taking

Gadewch i doddi mewn dŵr cyn ei gymryd

To be used on *preparations that are intended to be dissolved in water* (e.g. soluble tablets) or *mixed with water* (e.g. powders, granules) before use. In a few cases other liquids such as fruit juice or milk may be used.

14 This medicine may colour your urine. This is harmless
Gall y feddyginiaeth hon liwio eich dŵr. Nid yw hyn yn arwydd o ddrwg
To be used on *preparations that may cause the patient's urine to turn an unusual colour.* These include triamterene (blue under some lights), levodopa (dark reddish), and rifampicin (red).

15 Caution: flammable. Keep your body away from fire or flames after you have put on the medicine

Rhybudd: Fflamadwy. Ar ôl rhoi'r feddyginiaeth ymlaen, cadwch yn glir o dân neu fflamau
To be used on *preparations containing sufficient flammable solvent to render them flammable if exposed to a naked flame.*

16 Dissolve the tablet under your tongue—do not swallow. Store the tablets in this bottle with the cap tightly closed. Get a new supply 8 weeks after opening

Rhowch y dabled i doddi dan eich tafod - peidiwch â'i lyncu. Cadwch y tabledi yn y botel yma gyda'r caead wedi'i gau yn dynn. Gofynnwch am dabledi newydd 8 wythnos ar ôl ei hagor
To be used on *glyceryl trinitrate tablets* to remind the patient not to transfer the tablets to plastic or less suitable containers.

17 Do not take more than... in 24 hours
Peidiwch â chymryd mwy na... mewn 24 awr
To be used on *preparations for the treatment of acute migraine* except those containing ergotamine, for which label 18 is used. The dose form should be specified, e.g. tablets or capsules.

It may also be used on preparations for which no dose has been specified by the prescriber.

18 Do not take more than... in 24 hours. Also, do not take more than... in any one week

Peidiwch â chymryd mwy na... mewn 24 awr. Hefyd, peidiwch â chymryd mwy na... mewn wythnos
To be used on preparations containing ergotamine. The dose form should be specified, e.g. tablets or suppositories.

19 Warning: This medicine makes you sleepy. If you still feel sleepy the next day, do not drive or use tools or machines. Do not drink alcohol

Rhybudd: Bydd y feddyginiaeth hon yn eich gwneud yn gysglyd. Os ydych yn dal i deimlo'n gysglyd drannoeth, peidiwch â gyrru, defnyddio offer llaw neu beiriannau. Peidiwch ag yfed alcohol
To be used on *preparations containing hypnotics (or some other drugs with sedative effects) prescribed to be taken at night.* On the rare occasions when hypnotics are prescribed for daytime administration (e.g. nitrazepam in epilepsy), this label would clearly not be appropriate. Also to be used as an *alternative to the label 2 wording* (the choice being at the discretion of the pharmacist) *for anxiolytics prescribed to be taken at night.*

It is hoped that this wording will convey adequately the problem of residual morning sedation after taking 'sleeping tablets'.

21 Take with or just after food, or a meal

Cymerwch gyda neu ar ôl bwyd
To be used on *preparations that are liable to cause gastric irritation, or those that are better absorbed with food.*

Patients should be advised that a *small amount of food is sufficient.*

22 Take 30 to 60 minutes before food

Cymerwch 30 i 60 munud cyn bwyd
To be used on some preparations *whose absorption is thereby improved.*

Most oral antibacterials require label 23 instead (see below).

23 Take this medicine when your stomach is empty. This means an hour before food or 2 hours after food

Cymerwch y feddyginiaeth hon ar stumog wag. Mae hyn yn golygu awr cyn, neu 2 awr ar ôl bwyd
To be used on *oral antibacterials whose absorption may be reduced by the presence of food and acid in the stomach.*

24 Suck or chew this medicine

Bydd angen cnoi neu sugno'r feddyginiaeth hon
To be used on *preparations that should be sucked or chewed.*

The pharmacist should use discretion as to which of these words is appropriate.

25 Swallow this medicine whole. Do not chew or crush

Llyncwch yn gyfan. Peidiwch â chnoi neu falu'n fân
To be used on *preparations that are enteric-coated or designed for modified-release.*

Also to be used on *preparations that taste very unpleasant or may damage the mouth* if not swallowed whole.

Patients should be advised (where relevant) that some modified-release preparations can be broken in half, but that the halved tablet should still be swallowed whole, and not chewed or crushed.

26 Dissolve this medicine under your tongue

Gadewch i'r feddyginiaeth hon doddi o dan y tafod
To be used on *preparations designed for sublingual use.* Patients should be advised to hold under the tongue and avoid swallowing until dissolved. The buccal mucosa between the gum and cheek is occasionally specified by the prescriber.

27 Take with a full glass of water

Cymerwch gyda llond gwydr o ddŵr
To be used on *preparations that should be well diluted* (e.g. chloral hydrate), *where a high fluid intake is required* (e.g. sulfonamides), or *where water is required to aid the action* (e.g. methylcellulose). The patient should be advised that 'a full glass' means at least 150 mL. In most cases fruit juice, tea, or coffee may be used.

28 Spread thinly on the affected skin only

Taenwch yn denau ar y croen sydd wedi'i effeithio yn unig
To be used on *external preparations* that should be applied sparingly (e.g. corticosteroids, dithranol).

29 Do not take more than 2 at any one time. Do not take more than 8 in 24 hours

Peidiwch â chymryd mwy na 2 ar unrhyw un adeg. Peidiwch â chymryd mwy nag 8 mewn 24 awr
To be used on containers of dispensed *solid dose preparations containing paracetamol for adults when the instruction on the label indicates that the dose can be taken on an 'as required' basis.* The dose form should be specified, e.g. tablets or capsules.

This label has been introduced because of the serious consequences of overdosage with paracetamol.

30 Contains paracetamol. Do not take anything else containing paracetamol while taking this medicine. Talk to a doctor at once if you take too much of this medicine, even if you feel well

Yn cynnwys paracetamol. Peidiwch â chymryd unrhyw beth arall sy'n cynnwys paracetamol tra'n cymryd y feddyginiaeth hon. Siaradwch gyda'ch meddyg ar unwaith os ydych yn cymryd gormod, hyd yn oed os ydych yn teimlo'n iawn
To be used on all containers of dispensed *preparations containing paracetamol.*

32 Contains aspirin. Do not take anything else containing aspirin while taking this medicine

Yn cynnwys aspirin. Peidiwch â chymryd unrhyw beth arall sy'n cynnwys aspirin tra'n cymryd y feddyginiaeth hon
To be used on containers of dispensed *preparations containing aspirin when the name on the label does not include the word 'aspirin'.*

Dental Practitioners' Formulary

List of Dental Preparations

The following list has been approved by the appropriate Secretaries of State, and the preparations therein may be prescribed by dental practitioners on form FP10D (GP14 in Scotland, WP10D in Wales).
Licensed **sugar-free** versions, where available, are preferred.
Licensed **alcohol-free** mouthwashes, where available, are preferred.

Aciclovir Cream, BP
Aciclovir Oral Suspension, BP, 200 mg/5 mL
Aciclovir Tablets, BP, 200 mg
Aciclovir Tablets, BP, 800 mg
Amoxicillin Capsules, BP
Amoxicillin Oral Powder, DPF
Amoxicillin Oral Suspension, BP
Artificial Saliva Gel, DPF
Artificial Saliva Oral Spray, DPF
Artificial Saliva Pastilles, DPF
Artificial Saliva Protective Spray, DPF
Artificial Saliva Substitutes as listed below (to be prescribed only for indications approved by ACBS (patients suffering from dry mouth as a result of having or, having undergone, radiotherapy or sicca syndrome):
BioXtra® Gel Mouthspray
BioXtra® Moisturising Gel
Glandosane®
Saliveze®
Artificial Saliva Substitute Spray, DPF
Aspirin Tablets, Dispersible, BP
Azithromycin Capsules, 250 mg, DPF
Azithromycin Oral Suspension, 200 mg/5 mL, DPF
Azithromycin Tablets, 250 mg, DPF
Azithromycin Tablets, 500 mg, DPF
Beclometasone Pressurised Inhalation, BP, 50 micrograms/metered inhalation, CFC-free, as: *Clenil Modulite*®
Benzydamine Mouthwash, BP 0.15%
Benzydamine Oromucosal Spray, BP 0.15%
Betamethasone Soluble Tablets, 500 micrograms, DPF
Carbamazepine Tablets, BP
Cefalexin Capsules, BP
Cefalexin Oral Suspension, BP
Cefalexin Tablets, BP
Cefradine Capsules, BP
Cetirizine Oral Solution, BP, 5 mg/5 mL
Cetirizine Tablets, BP, 10 mg
Chlorhexidine Gluconate Gel, BP
Chlorhexidine Mouthwash, BP
Chlorhexidine Oral Spray, DPF
Chlorphenamine Oral Solution, BP
Chlorphenamine Tablets, BP
Choline Salicylate Dental Gel, BP
Clarithromycin Oral Suspension, 125 mg/5 mL, DPF
Clarithromycin Oral Suspension, 250 mg/5 mL, DPF
Clarithromycin Tablets, BP
Clindamycin Capsules, BP
Co-amoxiclav Tablets, BP, 250/125 (amoxicillin 250 mg as trihydrate, clavulanic acid 125 mg as potassium salt)
Co-amoxiclav Oral Suspension, BP, 125/31 (amoxicillin 125 mg as trihydrate, clavulanic acid 31.25 mg as potassium salt)/5 mL
Co-amoxiclav Oral Suspension, BP, 250/62 (amoxicillin 250 mg as trihydrate, clavulanic acid 62.5 mg as potassium salt)/5 mL
Diazepam Oral Solution, BP, 2 mg/5 mL
Diazepam Tablets, BP
Diclofenac Sodium Tablets, Gastro-resistant, BP
Dihydrocodeine Tablets, BP, 30 mg
Doxycycline Tablets, Dispersible, BP
Doxycycline Capsules, BP, 100 mg
Doxycycline Tablets, 20 mg, DPF
Ephedrine Nasal Drops, BP
Erythromycin Ethyl Succinate Oral Suspension, BP
Erythromycin Ethyl Succinate Tablets, BP
Erythromycin Stearate Tablets, BP
Erythromycin Tablets, Gastro-resistant, BP
Fluconazole Capsules, 50 mg, DPF
Fluconazole Oral Suspension, 50 mg/5 mL, DPF
Hydrocortisone Cream, BP, 1%
Hydrocortisone Oromucosal Tablets, BP
Hydrogen Peroxide Mouthwash, BP, 6%
Ibuprofen Oral Suspension, BP, sugar-free
Ibuprofen Tablets, BP
Lansoprazole Capsules, Gastro-resistant, BP
Lidocaine Ointment, BP, 5%
Lidocaine Spray 10%, DPF
Loratadine Syrup, 5 mg/5 mL, DPF
Loratadine Tablets, BP, 10 mg
Menthol and Eucalyptus Inhalation, BP 1980
Metronidazole Oral Suspension, BP
Metronidazole Tablets, BP
Miconazole Cream, BP
Miconazole Oromucosal Gel, BP
Miconazole and Hydrocortisone Cream, BP
Miconazole and Hydrocortisone Ointment, BP
Nystatin Oral Suspension, BP
Omeprazole Capsules, Gastro-resistant, BP
Oxytetracycline Tablets, BP
Paracetamol Oral Suspension, BP
Paracetamol Tablets, BP
Paracetamol Tablets, Soluble, BP
Phenoxymethylpenicillin Oral Solution, BP
Phenoxymethylpenicillin Tablets, BP
Promethazine Hydrochloride Tablets, BP
Promethazine Oral Solution, BP
Saliva Stimulating Tablets, DPF
Sodium Chloride Mouthwash, Compound, BP
Sodium Fluoride Mouthwash, BP
Sodium Fluoride Oral Drops, BP
Sodium Fluoride Tablets, BP
Sodium Fluoride Toothpaste 0.619%, DPF
Sodium Fluoride Toothpaste 1.1%, DPF
Sodium Fusidate Ointment, BP
Temazepam Oral Solution, BP
Temazepam Tablets, BP
Tetracycline Tablets, BP

Preparations in this list which are not included in the BP or BPC are described under Details of DPF preparations.
For details of preparations that can be prescribed, see individual entries under the relevant drug monographs throughout the BNF publications.

Details of DPF preparations

Preparations on the List of Dental Preparations which are specified as DPF are described as follows in the DPF.
Although brand names have sometimes been included for identification purposes preparations on the list should be prescribed by non-proprietary name.

Amoxicillin Oral Powder
amoxicillin (as trihydrate) 3 g sachet

Artificial Saliva Gel
consists of lactoperoxidase, lactoferrin, lysozyme, glucose oxidase, xylitol in a gel basis
Artificial Saliva Oral Spray
(proprietary product: *Xerotin*) consists of water, sorbitol, carmellose (carboxymethylcellulose), potassium chloride, sodium chloride, potassium phosphate, magnesium chloride, calcium chloride and other ingredients, pH neutral
Artificial Saliva Pastilles
(proprietary product: *Salivix*), consists of acacia, malic acid, and other ingredients
Artificial Saliva Protective Spray
(proprietary product: *Aequasyal*) consists of oxidised glycerol triesters, silicon dioxide, flavouring agents, aspartame
Artificial Saliva Substitute Spray
(proprietary product: *AS Saliva Orthana Spray*) consists of mucin, methylparaben, benzalkonium chloride, EDTA, xylitol, peppermint oil, spearmint oil, mineral salts
Azithromycin Capsules
azithromycin 250 mg
Azithromycin Oral Suspension 200 mg/5 mL
azithromycin 200 mg/5 mL when reconstituted with water
Azithromycin Tablets
azithromycin 250 mg and 500 mg
Betamethasone Soluble Tablets 500 micrograms
betamethasone (as sodium phosphate) 500 micrograms
Chlorhexidine Oral Spray
(proprietary product: *Corsodyl Oral Spray*), chlorhexidine gluconate 0.2%
Clarithromycin Oral Suspension 125 mg/5 mL
clarithromycin 125 mg/5 mL when reconstituted with water
Clarithromycin Oral Suspension 250 mg/5 mL
clarithromycin 250 mg/5 mL when reconstituted with water
Doxycycline Tablets 20 mg
(proprietary product: *Periostat*), doxycycline (as hyclate) 20 mg
Fluconazole Capsules 50 mg
fluconazole 50 mg
Fluconazole Oral Suspension 50 mg/5 mL
(proprietary product: *Diflucan*), fluconazole 50 mg/5 mL when reconstituted with water
Lidocaine Spray 10%
(proprietary product: *Xylocaine Spray*), lidocaine 10% supplying 10 mg lidocaine/spray
Loratadine Syrup 5 mg/5 mL
loratadine 5 mg/5 mL
Saliva Stimulating Tablets
(proprietary product: *SST*), citric acid, malic acid and other ingredients in a sorbitol base
Sodium Fluoride Toothpaste 0.619%
(proprietary product: *Duraphat '2800 ppm' Toothpaste*), sodium fluoride 0.619%
Sodium Fluoride Toothpaste 1.1%
(proprietary product: *Duraphat '5000 ppm' Toothpaste*), sodium fluoride 1.1%

Nurse Prescribers' Formulary (NPF)

Nurse Prescribers' Formulary for Community Practitioners

List of preparations approved by the Secretary of State which may be prescribed on form FP10P (form HS21(N) in Northern Ireland, form GP10(N) in Scotland, forms WP10CN and WP10PN in Wales) by Nurses for National Health Service patients.

Community practitioners who have completed the necessary training may only prescribe items appearing in the nurse prescribers' list set out below. Community Practitioner Nurse Prescribers are recommended to prescribe generically, except where this would not be clinically appropriate or where there is no approved generic name.

This list is for reference only; see the BNF for full prescribing information.

Medicinal Preparations

Preparations on this list which are not included in the BP or BPC are described under Details of NPF preparations.

Almond Oil Ear Drops, BP
Arachis Oil Enema, NPF
Aspirin Tablets, Dispersible, 300 mg, BP (max. 96 tablets; max. pack size 32 tablets)
Bisacodyl Suppositories, BP (includes 5-mg and 10-mg strengths)
Bisacodyl Tablets, BP
Catheter Maintenance Solution, Sodium Chloride, NPF
Catheter Maintenance Solution, 'Solution G', NPF
Catheter Maintenance Solution, 'Solution R', NPF
Chlorhexidine Gluconate Alcoholic Solutions containing at least 0.05%
Chlorhexidine Gluconate Aqueous Solutions containing at least 0.05%
Choline Salicylate Dental Gel, BP
Clotrimazole Cream 1%, BP
Co-danthramer Capsules, NPF
Co-danthramer Capsules, Strong, NPF
Co-danthramer Oral Suspension, NPF
Co-danthramer Oral Suspension, Strong, NPF
Co-danthrusate Capsules, BP
Co-danthrusate Oral Suspension, NPF
Crotamiton Cream, BP
Crotamiton Lotion, BP
Dimeticone barrier creams containing at least 10%
Dimeticone Lotion, NPF
Docusate Capsules, BP
Docusate Enema, NPF
Docusate Oral Solution, BP
Docusate Oral Solution, Paediatric, BP
Econazole Cream 1%, BP
Emollients as listed below:
- Aquadrate® 10% w/w Cream
- Arachis Oil, BP
- Balneum® Plus Cream
- Cetraben® Emollient Cream
- Dermamist®
- Diprobase® Cream
- Diprobase® Ointment
- Doublebase®
- Doublebase® Dayleve Gel
- E45® Cream
- E45® Itch Relief Cream
- Emulsifying Ointment, BP
- Eucerin® Intensive 10% w/w Urea Treatment Cream
- Eucerin® Intensive 10% w/w Urea Treatment Lotion
- Hydromol® Cream
- Hydromol® Intensive
- Hydrous Ointment, BP
- Lipobase®
- Liquid and White Soft Paraffin Ointment, NPF
- Neutrogena® Norwegian Formula Dermatological Cream
- Nutraplus® Cream
- Oilatum® Cream
- Oilatum® Junior Cream
- Paraffin, White Soft, BP
- Paraffin, Yellow Soft, BP
- Ultrabase®
- Unguentum M®

Emollient bath and shower preparations as listed below:
- Aqueous Cream, BP
- Balneum® (except pack sizes that are not to be prescribed under the NHS (see Part XVIIIA of the Drug Tariff, Part XI of the Northern Ireland Drug Tariff))
- Balneum Plus® Bath Oil (except pack sizes that are not to be prescribed under the NHS (see Part XVIIIA of the Drug Tariff, Part XI of the Northern Ireland Drug Tariff))
- Cetraben® Emollient Bath Additive
- Dermalo® Bath Emollient
- Doublebase® Emollient Bath Additive
- Doublebase® Emollient Shower Gel
- Doublebase® Emollient Wash Gel
- Hydromol® Bath and Shower Emollient
- Oilatum® Emollient
- Oilatum® Gel
- Oilatum® Junior Bath Additive
- Zerolatum® Emollient Medicinal Bath Oil

Folic Acid Tablets 400 micrograms, BP
Glycerol Suppositories, BP
Ibuprofen Oral Suspension, BP (except for indications and doses that are prescription-only)
Ibuprofen Tablets, BP (except for indications and doses that are prescription-only)
Ispaghula Husk Granules, BP
Ispaghula Husk Granules, Effervescent, BP
Ispaghula Husk Oral Powder, BP
Lactulose Solution, BP
Lidocaine Ointment, BP
Lidocaine and Chlorhexidine Gel, BP
Macrogol Oral Liquid, Compound, NPF
Macrogol Oral Powder, Compound, NPF
Macrogol Oral Powder, Compound, Half-strength, NPF
Magnesium Hydroxide Mixture, BP
Magnesium Sulfate Paste, BP
Malathion aqueous lotions containing at least 0.5%
Mebendazole Oral Suspension, NPF
Mebendazole Tablets, NPF
Methylcellulose Tablets, BP
Miconazole Cream 2%, BP
Miconazole Oromucosal Gel, BP
Mouthwash Solution-tablets, NPF
Nicotine Inhalation Cartridge for Oromucosal Use, NPF
Nicotine Lozenge, NPF
Nicotine Medicated Chewing Gum, NPF
Nicotine Nasal Spray, NPF
Nicotine Oral Spray, NPF
Nicotine Sublingual Tablets, NPF
Nicotine Transdermal Patches, NPF
Nystatin Oral Suspension, BP
Olive Oil Ear Drops, BP

Paracetamol Oral Suspension, BP (includes 120 mg/5 mL and 250 mg/5 mL strengths—both of which are available as sugar-free formulations)
Paracetamol Tablets, BP (max. 96 tablets; max. pack size 32 tablets)
Paracetamol Tablets, Soluble, BP (max. 96 tablets; max. pack size 32 tablets)
Permethrin Cream, NPF
Phosphates Enema, BP
Povidone–Iodine Solution, BP
Senna Oral Solution, NPF
Senna Tablets, BP
Senna and Ispaghula Granules, NPF
Sodium Chloride Solution, Sterile, BP
Sodium Citrate Compound Enema, NPF
Sodium Picosulfate Capsules, NPF
Sodium Picosulfate Elixir, NPF
Spermicidal contraceptives as listed below:
Gygel® Contraceptive Jelly
Sterculia Granules, NPF
Sterculia and Frangula Granules, NPF
Titanium Ointment, BP
Water for Injections, BP
Zinc and Castor Oil Ointment, BP
Zinc Oxide and Dimeticone Spray, NPF
Zinc Oxide Impregnated Medicated Bandage, NPF
Zinc Oxide Impregnated Medicated Stocking, NPF
Zinc Paste Bandage, BP 1993
Zinc Paste and Ichthammol Bandage, BP 1993

Appliances and Reagents (including Wound Management Products)

Community Practitioner Nurse Prescribers in England, Wales and Northern Ireland can prescribe any appliance or reagent in the relevant Drug Tariff. In the Scottish Drug Tariff, Appliances and Reagents which may **not** be prescribed by Nurses are annotated **Nx.**

Appliances (including Contraceptive Devices) as listed in Part IXA of the Drug Tariff (Part III of the Northern Ireland Drug Tariff, Part 3 (Appliances) and Part 2 (Dressings) of the Scottish Drug Tariff). (Where it is not appropriate for nurse prescribers in family planning clinics to prescribe contraceptive devices using form FP10(P) (forms WP10CN and WP10PN in Wales), they may prescribe using the same system as doctors in the clinic.)

Incontinence Appliances as listed in Part IXB of the Drug Tariff (Part III of the Northern Ireland Drug Tariff, Part 5 of the Scottish Drug Tariff).

Stoma Appliances and Associated Products as listed in Part IXC of the Drug Tariff (Part III of the Northern Ireland Drug Tariff, Part 6 of the Scottish Drug Tariff).

Chemical Reagents as listed in Part IXR of the Drug Tariff (Part II of the Northern Ireland Drug Tariff, Part 9 of the Scottish Drug Tariff).

The Drug Tariffs can be accessed online at:

National Health Service Drug Tariff for England and Wales: www.ppa.org.uk/ppa/edt_intro.htm

Health and Personal Social Services for Northern Ireland Drug Tariff: www.hscbusiness.hscni.net/services/2034.htm

Scottish Drug Tariff: www.isdscotland.org/Health-topics/Prescribing-and-Medicines/Scottish-Drug-Tariff/

Details of NPF preparations

Preparations on the Nurse Prescribers' Formulary which are not included in the BP or BPC are described as follows in the Nurse Prescribers' Formulary. Although brand names have sometimes been included for identification purposes, it is recommended that non-proprietary names should be used for prescribing medicinal preparations in the NPF except where a non-proprietary name is not available.

Arachis Oil Enema
arachis oil 100%

Catheter Maintenance Solution, Sodium Chloride
(proprietary products: *OptiFlo S; Uro-Tainer Sodium Chloride; Uriflex-S*), sodium chloride 0.9%

Catheter Maintenance Solution, 'Solution G'
(proprietary products: *OptiFlo G; Uro-Tainer Suby G; Uriflex G*), citric acid 3.23%, magnesium oxide 0.38%, sodium bicarbonate 0.7%, disodium edetate 0.01%

Catheter Maintenance Solution, 'Solution R'
(proprietary products: *OptiFlo R; Uro-Tainer Solutio R; Uriflex R*), citric acid 6%, gluconolactone 0.6%, magnesium carbonate 2.8%, disodium edetate 0.01%

Chlorhexidine gluconate alcoholic solutions
(proprietary products: *ChloraPrep; Hydrex Solution; Hydrex spray*), chlorhexidine gluconate in alcoholic solution

Chlorhexidine gluconate aqueous solutions
(proprietary product: *Unisept*), chlorhexidine gluconate in aqueous solution

Co-danthramer Capsules PoM
co-danthramer 25/200 (dantron 25 mg, poloxamer '188' 200 mg)

Co-danthramer Capsules, Strong PoM
co-danthramer 37.5/500 (dantron 37.5 mg, poloxamer '188' 500 mg)

Co-danthramer Oral Suspension PoM
co-danthramer 25/200 in 5 mL (dantron 25 mg, poloxamer '188' 200 mg/5 mL)

Co-danthramer Oral Suspension, Strong PoM
co-danthramer 75/1000 in 5 mL (dantron 75 mg, poloxamer '188' 1 g/5 mL)

Co-danthrusate Oral Suspension PoM
(proprietary product: *Normax*), co-danthrusate 50/60 (dantron 50 mg, docusate sodium 60 mg/5 mL)

Dimeticone barrier creams
(proprietary products *Conotrane Cream*, dimeticone '350' 22%; *Siopel Barrier Cream*, dimeticone '1000' 10%), dimeticone 10–22%

Dimeticone Lotion
(proprietary product: *Hedrin*), dimeticone 4%

Docusate Enema
(proprietary product: *Norgalax Micro-enema*), docusate sodium 120 mg in 10 g

Liquid and White Soft Paraffin Ointment
liquid paraffin 50%, white soft paraffin 50%

Macrogol Oral Liquid, Compound
(proprietary product: *Movicol Liquid*), macrogol '3350' (polyethylene glycol '3350') 13.125 g, sodium bicarbonate 178.5 mg, sodium chloride 350.7 mg, potassium chloride 46.6 mg/25 mL

Macrogol Oral Powder, Compound
(proprietary products: *Laxido Orange, Molaxole, Movicol*), macrogol '3350' (polyethylene glycol '3350') 13.125 g, sodium bicarbonate 178.5 mg, sodium chloride 350.7 mg, potassium chloride 46.6 mg/sachet; (amount of potassium chloride varies according to flavour of *Movicol®* as follows: plain-flavour (sugar-free) = 50.2 mg/sachet; lime and lemon flavour = 46.6 mg/sachet; chocolate flavour = 31.7 mg/sachet. 1 sachet when reconstituted with 125 mL water provides K^+ 5.4 mmol/litre)

Macrogol Oral Powder, Compound, Half-strength
(proprietary product: *Movicol-Half*), macrogol '3350' (polyethylene glycol '3350') 6.563 g, sodium bicarbonate 89.3 g, sodium chloride 175.4 mg, potassium chloride 23.3 mg/sachet

Malathion aqueous lotions
(proprietary products: *Derbac-M Liquid*), malathion 0.5% in an aqueous basis

Mebendazole Oral Suspension PoM
(proprietary product: *Vermox*), mebendazole 100 mg/5 mL

Mebendazole Tablets PoM
(proprietary products: *Ovex, Vermox*), mebendazole 100 mg (can be supplied for oral use in the treatment of enterobiasis in adults and children over 2 years provided its container or package is labelled to show a max. single dose of 100 mg and it is supplied in a container or package containing not more than 800 mg)

Mouthwash Solution-tablets
consist of tablets which may contain antimicrobial, colouring and flavouring agents in a suitable soluble effervescent basis to make a mouthwash

Nicotine Inhalation Cartridge for Oromucosal Use
(proprietary products: *NicAssist Inhalator, Nicorette Inhalator*), nicotine 15 mg (for use with inhalation mouthpiece; to be prescribed as either a starter pack (6 cartridges with inhalator device and holder) or refill pack (42 cartridges with inhalator device)

Nicotine Lozenge
nicotine (as bitartrate) 1 mg or 2 mg (proprietary product: *Nicorette Mint Lozenge, Nicotinell Mint Lozenge*), or nicotine (as resinate) 1.5 mg, 2 mg, or 4 mg (proprietary product: *NiQuitin Lozenges, NiQuitin Minis, NiQuitin Pre-quit*)

Nicotine Medicated Chewing Gum
(proprietary products: *NicAssist Gum, Nicorette Gum, Nicotinell Gum, NiQuitin Gum*), nicotine 2 mg or 4 mg

Nicotine Nasal Spray
(proprietary product: *NicAssist Nasal Spray, Nicorette Nasal Spray*), nicotine 500 micrograms/metered spray

Nicotine Oral Spray
(proprietary product: *Nicorette Quickmist*), nicotine 1 mg/metered spray

Nicotine Sublingual Tablets
(proprietary product: *NicAssist Microtab, Nicorette Microtab*), nicotine (as a cyclodextrin complex) 2 mg (to be prescribed as either a starter pack (2 × 15-tablet discs with dispenser) or refill pack (7 × 15-tablet discs))

Nicotine Transdermal Patches
releasing in each 16 hours, nicotine approx. 5 mg, 10 mg, or 15 mg (proprietary products: *Boots NicAssist Patch, Nicorette Patch*), or releasing in each 16 hours approx. 10 mg, 15 mg, or 25 mg (proprietary products: *NicAssist Translucent Patch, Nicorette Invisi Patch*), or releasing in each 24 hours nicotine approx. 7 mg, 14 mg, or 21 mg (proprietary products: *Nicopatch, Nicotinell TTS, NiQuitin, NiQuitin Clear*) (prescriber should specify the brand to be dispensed)

Permethrin Cream
(proprietary product: *Lyclear Dermal Cream*), permethrin 5%

Senna Oral Solution
(proprietary product: *Senokot Syrup*), sennosides 7.5 mg/5 mL

Senna and Ispaghula Granules
(proprietary product: *Manevac Granules*), senna fruit 12.4%, ispaghula 54.2%

Sodium Citrate Compound Enema
(proprietary products: *Micolette Micro-enema; Micralax Micro-enema; Relaxit Micro-enema*),sodium citrate 450 mg with glycerol, sorbitol and an anionic surfactant

Sodium Picosulfate Capsules
(proprietary products: *Dulcolax Perles*), sodium picosulfate 2.5 mg

Sodium Picosulfate Elixir
(proprietary product: *Dulcolax Liquid*), sodium picosulfate 5 mg/5 mL

Sterculia Granules
(proprietary product: *Normacol Granules*), sterculia 62%

Sterculia and Frangula Granules
(proprietary product: *Normacol Plus Granules*), sterculia 62%, frangula (standardised) 8%

Zinc Oxide and Dimeticone Spray
(proprietary product: *Sprilon*), dimeticone 1.04%, zinc oxide 12.5% in a pressurised aerosol unit

Zinc Oxide Impregnated Medicated Bandage
(proprietary product: *Steripaste*), sterile cotton bandage impregnated with paste containing zinc oxide 15%

Zinc Oxide Impregnated Medicated Stocking
(proprietary product: *Zipzoc*), sterile rayon stocking impregnated with ointment containing zinc oxide 20%

Non-medical prescribing

Overview

A range of non-medical healthcare professionals can prescribe medicines for patients as either Independent or Supplementary Prescribers.

Independent prescribers are practitioners responsible and accountable for the assessment of patients with previously undiagnosed or diagnosed conditions and for decisions about the clinical management required, including prescribing. They are recommended to prescribe generically, except where this would not be clinically appropriate or where there is no approved non-proprietary name.

Supplementary prescribing is a partnership between an independent prescriber (a doctor or a dentist) and a supplementary prescriber to implement an agreed Clinical Management Plan for an individual patient with that patient's agreement.

Independent and Supplementary Prescribers are identified by an annotation next to their name in the relevant professional register.

Information and guidance on non-medical prescribing is available on the Department of Health website at www.dh.gov.uk/health/2012/04/prescribing-change.

For information on the mixing of medicines by Independent and Supplementary Prescribers, see *Mixing of medicines prior to administration in clinical practice: medical and non-medical prescribing*, National Prescribing Centre, May 2010 (available at www.gov.uk/government/uploads/system/uploads/attachment_data/file/213885/dh_116360.pdf).

For information on the supply and administration of medicines to groups of patients using Patient Group Directions see Guidance on prescribing p. 1.

In order to protect patient safety, the initial prescribing and supply of medicines prescribed should normally remain separate functions performed by separate healthcare professionals.

Nurses

Nurse Independent Prescribers (formerly known as Extended Formulary Nurse Prescribers) are able to prescribe any medicine for any medical condition. Unlicensed medicines are excluded from the Nurse Prescribing Formulary in Scotland.

Nurse Independent Prescribers are able to prescribe, administer, and give directions for the administration of Schedule 2, 3, 4, and 5 Controlled Drugs. This extends to diamorphine hydrochloride p. 294, dipipanone, or cocaine for treating organic disease or injury, but not for treating addiction.

Nurse Independent Prescribers must work within their own level of professional competence and expertise.

The Nurse Prescribers' Formulary (NPF) p. 1143 for Community Practitioners provides information on prescribing.

Pharmacists

Pharmacist Independent Prescribers can prescribe any medicine for any medical condition. This includes unlicensed medicines, subject to accepted clinical good practice.

They are also able to prescribe, administer, and give directions for the administration of Schedule 2, 3, 4, and 5 Controlled Drugs. This extends to diamorphine hydrochloride p. 294, dipipanone, or cocaine for treating organic disease or injury, but not for treating addiction.

Pharmacist Independent Prescribers must work within their own level of professional competence and expertise.

Physiotherapists

Physiotherapist Independent Prescribers can prescribe any medicine for any medical condition. This includes "off-label" medicines subject to accepted clinical good practice. They are also allowed to prescribe the following Controlled Drugs: oral or injectable morphine p. 299, transdermal fentanyl p. 296 and oral diazepam p. 236, dihydrocodeine tartrate p. 295, lorazepam p. 238, oxycodone hydrochloride p. 302 or temazepam p. 879.

Physiotherapist Independent Prescribers must work within their own level of professional competence and expertise.

Therapeutic radiographers

Therapeutic Radiographer Independent Prescribers can prescribe any medicine for any medical condition. This includes "off-label" medicines subject to accepted clinical good practice. Therapeutic Radiographer Independent Prescribers must work within their own level of professional competence and expertise.

Optometrists

Optometrist Independent Prescribers can prescribe any licensed medicine for ocular conditions affecting the eye and the tissues surrounding the eye, except Controlled Drugs or medicines for parenteral administration. Optometrist Independent Prescribers must work within their own level of professional competence and expertise.

Podiatrists

Podiatrist Independent Prescribers can prescribe any medicine for any medical condition. This includes "off-label" medicines subject to accepted clinical good practice. They are also allowed to prescribe the following Controlled Drugs for oral administration: diazepam p. 236, dihydrocodeine tartrate p. 295, lorazepam p. 238 and temazepam p. 879.

Podiatrist Independent Prescribers must work within their own level of professional competence and expertise.

Further Information

For further details about the different types of prescribers, see *Medicines, Ethics and Practice*, London, Pharmaceutical Press (always consult latest edition).

Index of manufacturers

The following is an alphabetical list of manufacturers and other companies referenced in the BNF, with their medicines information or general contact details. For information on 'special-order' manufacturers and specialist importing companies see 'Special-order manufacturers'.

3M Health Care Ltd, Tel: 01509 611611

A. Menarini Farmaceutica Internazionale SRL, Tel: 0800 0858678, menarini@medinformation.co.uk

A S Pharma Ltd, Tel: 01264 332172, info@ccmed.co.uk

A1 Pharmaceuticals, Tel: 01708 528900, enquiries@a1plc.co.uk

Abbott Healthcare Products Ltd, Tel: 0800 1701177, ukabbottnutrition@abbott.com

AbbVie Ltd, Tel: 01628 561092, ukmedinfo@abbvie.com

Accord Healthcare Ltd, Tel: 01271 385257, medinfo@accord-healthcare.com

Actavis UK Ltd, Tel: 01271 385257, medinfo@accord-healthcare.com

Actelion Pharmaceuticals UK Ltd, Tel: 0208 9873333, medinfo_uk@its.jnj.com

Advanced Medical Solutions Ltd, Tel: 01606 863500

Advancis Medical, Tel: 01623 751500

Advanz Pharma, Tel: 08700 703033, medicalinformation@advanzpharma.com

AgaMatrix Europe Ltd, Tel: 0800 0931812, info@agamatrix.co.uk

Aguettant Ltd, Tel: 01275 463691, info@aguettant.co.uk

Alan Pharmaceuticals, Tel: 020 72842887, info@alanpharmaceuticals.com

Alcon Eye Care Ltd, Tel: 0345 2669363, gb.medicaldepartment@alcon.com

Alexion Pharma UK Ltd, Tel: 0800 6891592, MedicalInformation.UK@alexion.com

Alimera Sciences Ltd, Tel: 0800 0191253, medicalinformation@alimerasciences.com

Alissa Healthcare Research Ltd, Tel: 01489 564069, enquiries@alissahealthcare.com

ALK-Abello Ltd, Tel: 0118 9037940, info@uk.alk-abello.com

Allergan Ltd, Tel: 01628 494026, UK_MedInfo@Allergan.com

Allergy Therapeutics (UK) Ltd, Tel: 01903 844700, marketsupport@allergytherapeutics.com

Alliance Pharmaceuticals Ltd, Tel: 01249 466966, medinfo@alliancepharma.co.uk

Almirall Ltd, Tel: 0800 0087399, Almirall@EU.ProPharmaGroup.com

Almus Pharmaceuticals Ltd, Tel: 0800 9177983, med.info@almus.co.uk

Altacor Ltd, Tel: 01189 026766, info@altacor-pharma.com

Ambe Ltd, Tel: 01732 760900, info@ambemedical.com

Amgen Ltd, Tel: 01223 436441, gbinfoline@amgen.com

Amicus Therapeutics UK Ltd, Tel: 01753 888567

AMO UK Ltd, Tel: 01344 864042, crc@its.jnj.com

Amryt Pharma, Tel: 01604 549952, medinfo@amrytpharma.com

AOP Orphan Pharmaceuticals AG, Tel: 0121 2624119, anne.worrallo-hickman@aoporphan.com

Aristo Pharma Ltd, Tel: 01483 920754, medinfo@aristo-pharma.co.uk

Arjun Products Ltd, Tel: 0800 0157806, info@arjunproducts.co.uk

Ascot Laboratories Ltd, Tel: 01923 711971, specials@ascotpharma.com

Aspar Pharmaceuticals Ltd, Tel: 020 82059846, info@aspar.co.uk

Aspen Pharma Trading Ltd, Tel: 0800 0087392, aspenmedinfo@professionalinformation.co.uk

Aspire Pharma Ltd, Tel: 01730 231148, medinfo@aspirepharma.co.uk

Astellas Pharma Ltd, Tel: 0800 7835018, medinfo.gb@astellas.com

AstraZeneca UK Ltd, Tel: 0800 7830033, medical.informationuk@astrazeneca.com

Atlantic Pharma Ltd, Tel: 0845 5191609, enquiries@atlanticpharma.co.uk

Atnahs Pharma UK Ltd, Tel: 01279 406759, pvservices@diamondpharmaservices.com

Auden McKenzie (Pharma Division) Ltd, Tel: 01271 385257, Medinfo@accord-healthcare.com

Aurobindo Pharma Ltd, Tel: 0208 8458811, medinfo@aurobindo.com

AYMES International Ltd, Tel: 0845 6805496, info@aymes.com

B. Braun Medical Ltd, Tel: 0114 2259000, info.bbmuk@bbraun.com

B. Braun Melsungen AG, Tel: +49 5661 710, info@bbraun.com

Bard Ltd, Tel: 01293 527888, customer.services@crbard.com

Bausch & Lomb UK Ltd, Tel: 01748 828849, medicalinformationuk@bausch.com

Baxter Healthcare Ltd, Tel: 01635 206345, medinfo_uki@baxter.com

Bayer Plc, Tel: 0118 2063000, medical.information@bayer.co.uk

BBI Healthcare Ltd, Tel: 01656 868930, info@bbihealthcare.com

Beacon Pharmaceuticals Ltd, Tel: 01233 506574, medical@athlone-laboratories.com

Beiersdorf UK Ltd, Tel: 0121 329 8800

Bell, Sons & Co (Druggists) Ltd, Tel: 0151 4221200, Med-info@bells-healthcare.com

Besins Healthcare (UK) Ltd, Tel: 01748 828789, BHUK@professionalinformation.co.uk

BHR Pharmaceuticals Ltd, Tel: 02476 377210

BIAL Pharma UK Ltd, Tel: 01753 916010, medinfo.uk@bial.com

Bio Med Sciences, Tel: +1 610 5303193, info@silon.com

Bio Products Laboratory Ltd, Tel: 020 89572622, medinfo@bpl.co.uk

Bio-Diagnostics Ltd, Tel: 01684 592262, enquiries@bio-diagnostics.co.uk

Biogen Idec Ltd, Tel: 0800 0087401, MedInfoUKI@biogen.com

Biolitec Pharma Ltd, Tel: +49 3641 5195330, medinfo@biolitecpharma.com

BioMarin Europe Ltd, Tel: 0845 0177013, medinfoeu@bmrn.com

Bio-Tech Pharmacal Inc, Tel: +1 800 3451199, customerservice@bio-tech-pharm.com

Biotest (UK) Ltd, Tel: 0121 7448444, medicinesinformation.uk@biotest.com

Blumont Pharma Ltd, Tel: 01476 978568

BOC Medical, Tel: 0800 136603, healthcare.home-uk@boc.com

Boehringer Ingelheim Ltd, Tel: 01344 742579, medinfo@bra.boehringer-ingelheim.com

Boston Healthcare Ltd, Tel: 01908 363499, medinfo@bostonhealthcare.co.uk

Brancaster Pharma Ltd, Tel: 01737 243407, safety@brancasterpharma.com

Bray Group Ltd, Tel: 01367 240736, info@bray-healthcare.com

Bristol Laboratories Ltd, Tel: 01442 200922, info@bristol-labs.co.uk

Bristol-Myers Squibb Pharmaceuticals Ltd, Tel: 0800 7311736, medical.information@bms.com

Britannia Pharmaceuticals Ltd, Tel: 01483 920763, enquiries@medinformation.co.uk

Brown & Burk UK Ltd, Tel: 0208 5778200, bbukqa@bbukltd.com

BSN Medical Ltd, Tel: 01482 670100, orders.uk@bsnmedical.com

BTG International Ltd, Tel: +1 877 6269989, medical.services@btgplc.com

C D Medical Ltd, Tel: 01942 813933

Cambridge Healthcare Supplies Ltd, Tel: 01908 363434, medinfo@cambridge-healthcare.co.uk

Cambridge Sensors Ltd, Tel: 0800 0883920, info@microdotcs.com

CareFusion UK Ltd, Tel: 0800 0437546, carefusionGB@professionalinformation.co.uk

Carinopharm GmbH, Tel: 01748 828812, carinopharm@professionalinformation.co.uk

Casen Recordati S.L., Tel: +34 91 3517964, info@casenrecordati.com

CD Pharma Srl, Tel: +39 02 43980539, info@cdpharmagroup.one

Celgene Ltd, Tel: 08448 010045, medinfo.uk.ire@celgene.com

Chanelle Medical UK Ltd, Tel: 0870 1923283, chanelle@medinformation.co.uk

Charles S. Bullen Stomacare Ltd, Tel: 0800 888501

Chattem UK Ltd, consumer.affairs@chattem.com

Chemidex Pharma Ltd, Tel: 01784 477167, info@chemidex.co.uk

Cheplapharm Arzneimittel GmbH, Tel: 0800 1455034, cheplapharm@redlinepv.co.uk

Chiesi Ltd, Tel: 0161 4885555, medinfo.uk@chiesi.com

Chugai Pharma UK Ltd, Tel: 020 89875600, medinfo@chugai-pharm.co.uk

Church & Dwight UK Ltd, Tel: 0800 0281454, AESIP@sipdrugsafety.com

Cipla EU Ltd, Tel: 0203 6847710, Drugsafety@cipla.com

Clement Clarke International Ltd, Tel: 01279 414969, resp@clement-clarke.com

Clinigen Healthcare Ltd, Tel: 01748 828375, medicalinformation@clinigengroup.com

CliniMed Ltd, Tel: 0808 1596017, info@clinimed.co.uk

Clinisupplies Ltd, Tel: 020 88634168, info@clinisupplies.co.uk

Colgate-Palmolive (UK) Ltd, Tel: 00800 32132132

Colonis Pharma Ltd, Tel: 01892 739403, medinfo@colonis.co.uk

Coloplast Ltd, Tel: 0800 374654, hcp@coloplastcharter.co.uk

Combe International Ltd, care@combe.co.uk

Consilient Health Ltd, Tel: 020 37511888, drugsafety@consilienthealth.com

Contura Ltd, Tel: 0207 4217400, info@contura.com

ConvaTec Ltd, Tel: 0800 289738, wound.webcare@convatec.com

Correvio UK Ltd, Tel: +41 848 007870, medinfo@correvio.com

Covidien (UK) Commercial Ltd, Tel: 0203 0271757, email.csUK@covidien.com

Cow & Gate, Tel: 0800 9778880

Crawford Healthcare Ltd, Tel: 01565 654920, customercomments@acelity.com

Creo Pharma Ltd, Tel: 01371 823933, pv@creopharma.com

Crescent Pharma Ltd, Tel: 01256 772730, info@crescentpharma.com

CSL Behring UK Ltd, Tel: 01444 447405, medinfo@cslbehring.com

Cubic Pharmaceuticals Ltd, Tel: 01634 726628, orders@cubicpharmacy.co.uk

Curaprox (UK) Ltd, Tel: 01480 862084, contact@curaprox.co.uk

Daiichi Sankyo UK Ltd, Tel: 0800 0285122, medinfo@daiichi-sankyo.co.uk

Dendron Ltd, Tel: 01923 229251, info@dddltd.co.uk

Dentsply Ltd, Tel: 01932 838338, UKD-CustomerServices@dentsplysirona.com

Derma Sciences Europe Ltd, Tel: +1 800 8254325, cs@dermasciences.com

Derma UK Ltd, Tel: 0191 3759020, info@dermauk.co.uk

Dermacea Ltd, Tel: 01562 884898, info@skinniesuk.com

Dermal Laboratories Ltd, Tel: 01462 458866

Dermato Logical Ltd, Tel: 01730 231148, info@dermato-logical.co.uk

Dermatonics Ltd, Tel: 01480 462910

Desitin Pharma Ltd, Tel: 01908 488817, medinfo@desitin.co.uk

Dexcel-Pharma Ltd, Tel: 01748 828784, Dexcel@EU.ProPharmaGroup.com

DHP Healthcare Ltd, Tel: 01908 363437, dhphealthcare@redlinepv.co.uk

Discovery Pharmaceuticals, Tel: 01748 827266, medinfo@discoverypharma.co.uk

Dompé UK Ltd, Tel: +39 02 583831, info@dompe.com

Dr. Falk Pharma UK Ltd, Tel: 01628 536616, office@drfalkpharma.co.uk

Dr. Reddy's Laboratories (UK) Ltd, Tel: 01748 828873, DrReddys@professionalinformation.co.uk

Dr. Schär Ltd (UK), Tel: 0800 1615838, foodservice.it@drschaer.com

Dreamskin Health Ltd, Tel: 01707 260505

Drossa Ltd, Tel: 020 3393 0859

Dunelm Pharmaceuticals Ltd, Tel: 0800 0614116

Durbin Plc, Tel: 020 88696500, products@durbin.co.uk

E M Pharma, Tel: 01664 820347

E Sallis Ltd, Tel: 0115 9787841, info@sallis.co.uk

Easigrip Ltd, Tel: 01926 497108, info@easigrip.co.uk

Ecogen Europe Ltd, Tel: 0116 2897162, info@ecogen-europe.co.uk

Ecolab Healthcare Division, Tel: 0113 2322480, info.healthcare@ecolab.co.uk

Eisai Ltd, Tel: 0845 6761400, EUMedInfo@eisai.net

Eli Lilly and Company Ltd, Tel: 01256 315000, ukmedinfo@lilly.com

Endo Ventures Ltd, Tel: 0800 0698421, medinfoEU@endo.com

Ennogen Healthcare Ltd, Tel: 01322 629220, info@ennogen.com

Ennogen Pharma Ltd, Tel: 01322 629220, info@ennogen.com

Entra Health Systems, Tel: +1 619 6846232, info@entrahealth.com

Espère Healthcare Ltd, Tel: 01462 346100, info@esperehealth.co.uk

Essential Pharmaceuticals Ltd, Tel: 01784 477167, info@essentialpharmaceuticals.com

Essential-Healthcare Ltd, Tel: 01277 286199, info@essential-healthcare.co.uk

Ethicon Ltd, Tel: +1 877 3844266, customersupport@eesus.jnj.com

Ethypharm UK Ltd, Tel: 01277 266600, medinfo@martindalepharma.co.uk

Eumedica Pharmaceuticals, Tel: +32 64 448859, MIR@eumedica.com

Eurocept International bv, Tel: +31 35 5288377, info@eurocept.nl

EUSA Pharma Ltd, Tel: 0330 5001155, medicalinformation-uk@eusapharma.com

Evolan Pharma AB, Tel: +46 8 54496030, info@evolan.se

Farla Medical Ltd, Tel: 0345 1935193, sales@farla.co.uk

Farmigea S.p.A., Tel: 0208 8946601, info@farmigea.co.uk

Fate Special Foods, Tel: 01384 233230, admin@fatespecialfoods.com

Fenton Pharmaceuticals Ltd, Tel: 0207 4338595, mail@fent-pharm.co.uk

Ferndale Pharmaceuticals Ltd, Tel: 01937 541122, info@ferndalepharma.co.uk

Ferring Pharmaceuticals Ltd, Tel: 0800 1114125, medical.uk@ferring.com

Firstplay Dietary Foods Ltd, Tel: 0161 4804602, info@promin-metabolics.com

Flen Health UK Ltd, Tel: 0207 8725460, info@flenhealth.com

Flynn Pharma Ltd, Tel: 01438 727822, medinfo@flynnpharma.com

Fontus Health Ltd, Tel: 0121 6614615, Medinfo.uk@fontushealth.com

Ford Medical Associates Ltd, Tel: 01233 633224, enquiries@fordmedical.co.uk

Forest Laboratories UK Ltd, Tel: 01271 385257, Medinfo@accord-healthcare.com

Forum Health Products Ltd, Tel: 01737 857700

Fresenius Kabi Ltd, Tel: 01928 533533, communication@fresenius-kabi.com

Fyne Dynamics Ltd, Tel: 01279 423423

Galderma (UK) Ltd, Tel: 01923 208950, info.uk@galderma.com

Galen Ltd, Tel: 028 38334974, customer.services@galen-pharma.com

Galpharm International Ltd, Tel: 01226 704743, customerservice@galpharm.co.uk

Gebro Pharma GmbH, Tel: +43 5354 53000, pharma@gebro.com

Gedeon Richter (UK) Ltd, Tel: 0207 6048806, medinfo.uk@gedeonrichter.eu

Geistlich Sons Ltd, Tel: 0161 4902038, info@geistlich.co.uk

Genesis Pharmaceuticals Ltd, Tel: 020 72010400, info@genesis-pharma.com

Genius Foods Ltd, Tel: 0800 0192736

Genus Pharmaceuticals Ltd, Tel: 01484 848164, thorntonross@medinformation.co.uk

Genzyme Therapeutics Ltd, Tel: 0845 3727101, uk-medicalinformation@sanofi.com

Gilead Sciences International Ltd, Tel: 08000 113700, ukmedinfo@gilead.com

GlaxoSmithKline Consumer Healthcare, Tel: 0800 7838881, customer.relations@gsk.com

GlaxoSmithKline UK Ltd, Tel: 0800 221441, ukmedinfo@gsk.com

Glenmark Pharmaceuticals Europe Ltd, Tel: 0800 4580383, Medical_information@glenmarkpharma.com

Glenwood GmbH, Tel: +49 89 18935363, info@glenwood.de

GlucoRx Ltd, Tel: 01483 755133, info@glucorx.co.uk

Gluten Free Foods Ltd, Tel: 0208 9534444, info@glutenfree-foods.co.uk

G.R. Lane Health Products Ltd, Tel: info@laneshealth.com, 01452 524012

Grifols UK Ltd, Tel: 01223 395700, medinfo.uk@grifols.com

Grünenthal Ltd, Tel: 0870 3518960, medicalinformationuk@grunenthal.com

H&R Healthcare Ltd, Tel: 01482 631606, customerservices@hrhealthcare.co.uk

Haddenham Healthcare Ltd, Tel: 01844 208842, sales@hadhealth.com

Hameln Pharmaceuticals Ltd, Tel: 01452 621661, drugsafety@hameln.co.uk

HBS Healthcare Ltd, Tel: 01480 279481, mi@hbshealthcare.com

Health+Plus Ltd, Tel: 01323 872277, contact@healthplus.co.uk

Hennig Arzneimittel GmbH & Co. KG, info@hennig-am.de

Henry Schein Ltd, Tel: 0800 0304169, info@henryscheinmedical.co.uk

Heraeus, Tel: +49 06181/35-0

Hero UK Ltd, Tel: 0800 7831992, info@juvela.co.uk

HFA Healthcare Products Ltd, Tel: 0844 3358270, uk@movianto.com

Horizon Pharma Ireland Ltd, Tel: +31 20 5726516, medicalinformationEU@horizonpharma.com

Hospira UK Ltd, Tel: 01304 616161

HRA Pharma UK Ltd, Tel: 0800 9179548, med.info.uk@hra-pharma.com

Huntleigh Healthcare Ltd, Tel: 029 20485885

Huxley Europe Ltd, Tel: 0161 7730485

Ideal Medical Solutions Ltd, Tel: 020 87737844, info@ideal-ms.com

Incyte Biosciences UK Ltd, Tel: 00800 00027423, eumedinfo@incyte.com

Indivior UK Ltd, Tel: +1 800 27081901, PatientSafetyROW@indivior.com

INFAI UK Ltd, Tel: 01904 435228, info@infai.co.uk

infirst Healthcare Ltd, Tel: 0808 2810143, medinfo@infirst.co.uk

Innovative Solutions UK Ltd, Tel: 01706 746713, keeley@pureglutenfree.co.uk

Insight Medical Products Ltd, Tel: 01666 500055, info@insightmedical.net

Intercept Pharma UK & Ireland Ltd, Tel: 0330 1003694, medinfo@interceptpharma.com

Internis Pharmaceuticals Ltd, Tel: 01484 848164, thorntonross@medinformation.co.uk

Intrapharm Laboratories Ltd, Tel: 0800 1455031, medinfo@intrapharmlabs.com

Ipsen Ltd, Tel: 01753 627777, medical.information.uk@ipsen.com

J M Loveridge Ltd, Tel: 01264 367610

Janssen-Cilag Ltd, Tel: 0800 7318450, medinfo@janssen-cilag.co.uk

Jazz Pharmaceuticals UK, Tel: 0845 0305089, Medinfo-uk@jazzpharma.com

Jobskin Ltd, Tel: 0115 9734300, enquiries@jobskin.co.uk

Johnson & Johnson Ltd, Tel: 01344 864042, crc@its.jnj.com

JR Biomedical Ltd, Tel: 01745 535207, help@jrbiomedical.com

Juvela (Hero UK) Ltd, Tel: 0800 7831992, info@juvela.co.uk

KCI Medical Ltd, Tel: 0800 9808880, UKCUSTSERV@kci-medical.com

Kent Pharmaceuticals Ltd, Tel: 01233 506574, medical@athlone-laboratories.com

Kestrel Ophthalmics Ltd, Tel: 01202 696963, info@kestrelophthalmics.co.uk

King Pharmaceuticals Ltd, Tel: 01438 356924

kL Pharmaceuticals Ltd, Tel: 01294 215951, enquiries@klpharm.co.uk

Kora Healthcare, Tel: 0845 3038631, medinfo@korahealthcare.com

Kyowa Kirin Ltd, Tel: 01896 664000, medinfo@kyowakirin.com

L&R Medical UK Ltd, Tel: 01283 576800, customersolutions@uk.lrmed.com

Laboratoires CTRS, Tel: +33 1 41220970, ctrs@ctrs.fr

Lactalis Nutrition Santé, Tel: +33 2 9492000, info@lns-privatelabel.com

L.D. Collins & Co. Ltd, Tel: 02071 298660, medicalinfo@ldcollins.com

LEO Pharma, Tel: 01844 347333, medical-info.uk@leo-pharma.com

Leyden Delta B.V., Tel: +31 24 3726272, Medical.information@leydendelta.nl

LifeScan, Tel: +1 800 227 8862, customercare@LifeScan.co.uk

Lincoln Medical Ltd, Tel: 01722 742900, medicalinformation@lincolnmedical.co.uk

Lipomed GmbH, Tel: +41 61 7020200, lipomed@lipomed.com

Logixx Pharma Solutions Ltd, Tel: 01908 363454, mi@logixxpharma.com

Lohmann & Rauscher, Tel: +49 2634 990, info@de.LRmed.com

Lucane Pharma Ltd, Tel: +33 1 53868750, info@lucanepharma.com

Lundbeck Ltd, Tel: 01908 638972, ukmedicalinformation@lundbeck.com

Lupin Healthcare (UK) Ltd, Tel: 01748 828380, EU-PV@lupin.com

M & A Pharmachem Ltd, Tel: 01942 852085, safety@mapharmachem.co.uk

Mallinckrodt Specialty Pharmaceuticals Ireland Ltd, Tel: 00800 55444777, mallinckrodt@professionalinformation.co.uk

Manuka Medical Ltd, Tel: +1 615 6567852, supportUSA@manukamed.com

Manx Healthcare Ltd, Tel: 01926 482511, info@manxhealthcare.co.uk

Marlborough Pharmaceuticals Ltd, Tel: 01268 594777, info@atnahs.com

Martindale Pharmaceuticals Ltd, Tel: 01277 266600, medinfo@martindalepharma.co.uk

Mayors Healthcare Ltd, Tel: 020 82156200, info@mayorspharma.com

McNeil Products Ltd, Tel: 01344 864042, crc@its.jnj.com

Meadow Laboratories Ltd, enquiries@meadowlabs.co.uk

MeCoBo Ltd, Tel: 0844 8001705, enquiries@mecobo.com

Meda Pharmaceuticals Ltd, Tel: 01748 828810, meda@professionalinformation.co.uk

medac UK, Tel: 01786 458086, info@medacpharma.co.uk

Medical Developments UK Ltd, Tel: 01279 504055, info@medicaldev.co.uk

Medicareplus International Ltd, Tel: 020 88108811, info@medicareplus.co.uk

Medicom Healthcare Ltd, Tel: 01489 574119, info@medicomhealthcare.com

Medreich Plc, info@medreich.co.uk

Merck Serono Ltd, Tel: 020 88187373, medinfo.uk@merckgroup.com

Merck Sharp & Dohme Ltd, Tel: 01992 467272, medicalinformationuk@merck.com

Merus Labs Luxco S.a R.L., Tel: +352 2637 5878, medinfo@meruslabs.com

Merz Pharma UK Ltd, Tel: 0333 2004143, medical.information@merz.com

Millpledge Healthcare, Tel: 01777 708440, sales@millpledge.com

Milpharm Ltd, Tel: 0208 8458811, medinfo@aurobindo.com

Milupa Ltd, Tel: 0800 9961000

Mitsubishi Tanabe Pharma Europe Ltd, Tel: 0207 3829000, medinfo@mitsubishi-pharma.eu

Mölnlycke Health Care Ltd, Tel: 01908 355200

Morningside Healthcare Ltd, Tel: 0345 4592137, medicalenquiry@morningsidehealthcare.com

Movianto UK, Tel: 01234 248500, Customercare.UK@movianto.com

Mylan, Tel: 01707 853000, info.uk@mylan.co.uk

Nagor Ltd, Tel: 01236 780780, enquiries@nagor.com

Nairn's Oatcakes Ltd, Tel: 0131 6207000, info@nairns-oatcakes.com

Napp Pharmaceuticals Ltd, Tel: 01223 424444, medicalinformationuk@napp.co.uk

Naturally Good Food Ltd, Tel: 02476 541990, orders@naturallygoodfood.co.uk

Neoceuticals Ltd, Tel: 01748 828865, neoceuticals@professionalinformation.co.uk

Neomedic Ltd, Tel: 01923 836379, marketing@neomedic.co.uk

Neon Diagnostics Ltd, Tel: 01376 500720

Nestlé Health Science, Tel: 00800 68874846, nestlehealthcarenutrition@uk.nestle.com

Nipro Diagnostics (UK) Ltd, Tel: 0800 0858808, diagnostics-uk@nipro-group.com

Noden Pharma DAC, Tel: +1 844 3995701, Medinfo@nodenpharma.com

Nordic Pharma Ltd, Tel: 0800 1218924, nordic@professionalinformation.co.uk

Norgine Pharmaceuticals Ltd, Tel: 01895 826600, medinfo@norgine.com

Nova Laboratories Ltd, Tel: 08707 120655, xaluprine@aptivsolutions.com

Novartis Pharmaceuticals UK Ltd, Tel: 01276 698370, medinfo.uk@novartis.com

Novo Nordisk Ltd, Tel: 0845 6005055, CustomerCare@novonordisk.com

nSPIRE Health Ltd, Tel: 01992 526300, info@nspirehealth.com

Nualtra Ltd, Tel: 0118 4532853, support@nualtra.co.uk

Nutraconcepts Ltd, Tel: 0800 1123085, info@nutraconcepts.com

Nutri Advanced Ltd, Tel: 0800 0435777, advice@nutriadvanced.co.uk

Nutricia, Tel: 01225 751098, resourcecentre@nutricia.com

Nutrinovo Ltd, Tel: 01304 829068, info@nutrinovo.com

OakMed Ltd, Tel: 01604 586529, info@oakmed.co.uk

Octapharma Ltd, Tel: 0845 1300522, medinfo.uk@octapharma.com

Omega Pharma Ltd, Tel: 0203 5989603, UKLOcustomerservice@perrigo.com

Optima Consumer Health Ltd, Tel: 01274 526360, generalenquiries@optimah.com

Oralieve UK, Tel: 01582 439122, hello@oralieve.co.uk

Orexigen Therapeutics Ireland Ltd, Tel: 0800 0516402, mysimba@druginfo.com

Orion Pharma (UK) Ltd, Tel: 01635 520300, uk.medicalinformation@orionpharma.com

Orphan Europe (UK) Ltd, Tel: +1 888 5758344, medinfo@recordatirarediseases.com

Otsuka Novel Products GmbH, Tel: +49 89 206020500, medical@otsuka-onpg.com

Otsuka Pharmaceuticals UK Ltd, Tel: 0203 7475300, medical.information@otsuka-europe.com

Owen Mumford Ltd, Tel: 01993 812021, info@owenmumford.com

Pari Medical Ltd, Tel: +49 89 742846832, verena.prusinovsky@pari.com

Paul Hartmann Ltd, Tel: 01706 363200, info@uk.hartmann.info

PaxVax Ltd, Tel: 0800 0885449, medinfo.paxvax@apcerls.com

Peckforton Pharmaceuticals Ltd, Tel: 01908 363498, medinfo@peckforton.com

Pelican Healthcare Ltd, Tel: 0800 318282, contactus@pelicanhealthcare.co.uk

Pern Consumer Products Ltd, Tel: 0800 5999022, business_support@pern-consumer.co.uk

Pfizer Consumer Healthcare Ltd, Tel: 0333 5552526, carelineuk@pfizer.com

Pfizer Ltd, Tel: 01304 616161, Medical.Information@Pfizer.com

PGR Health Foods Ltd, Tel: 01992 581715, info@pgrhealthfoods.co.uk

Pharma Mar, S.A., Tel: +34 91 8466000, pharmamar@pharmamar.com

Pharma Nord (UK) Ltd, Tel: 01670 534900, info@pharmanord.co.uk

Pharmacosmos UK Ltd, Tel: 01844 269007, medinfo@pharmacosmos.co.uk

Pharmasure Ltd, Tel: 01923 233466, customercare@pharmasure.co.uk

Pharming Group N.V., Tel: 0161 6961478, medicalinformation@pharming.com

Phoenix Labs, Tel: +353 1 4688917, medicalinformation@phoenixlabs.ie

Pierre Fabre Ltd, Tel: 0800 0855292, medicalinformation@pierre-fabre.co.uk

Pinewood Healthcare, Tel: 01978 661261, drug.safety@wockhardt.co.uk

Pinnacle Biologics BV, Tel: +1 866 2482039, productinfo@concordialaboratories.com

Piramal Critical Care Ltd, Tel: 0800 7563979, medical.information@piramal.com

Pound International Ltd, Tel: 020 79353735, info@poundinternational.net

Proceli, Tel: 902 364334, info@proceli.com

Profile Pharma Ltd, Tel: 0800 0288942, info.profilepharma@zambongroup.com

Protex Healthcare (UK) Ltd, Tel: +32 475 548581, info@protexhealthcare.com

Proveca Ltd, Tel: 0333 2001866, medinfo@proveca.com

PTC Therapeutics Ltd, Tel: 0345 0754864, medinfo@ptcbio.com

Qdem Pharmaceuticals Ltd, Tel: 01223 426929, medicalinformationUKQdem@qdem.co.uk

Ranbaxy (UK) Ltd, Tel: 0208 8485052, medinfoeurope@sunpharma.com

Rayner Pharmaceuticals Ltd, Tel: 01279 406759, feedback@rayner.com

Reckitt Benckiser Healthcare (UK) Ltd, Tel: 0333 2005345

Recordati Pharmaceuticals Ltd, Tel: 01491 576336, medinfo@recordati.co.uk

Recordati Rare Diseases UK Ltd, Tel: 01491 414333, infoRRDUK@recordati.com

Reig Jofre UK Ltd, Tel: +34 93 4806710, medinfouk@reigjofre.com

Relonchem Ltd, Tel: 0151 556 1860, info@relonchem.com

Respironics (UK) Ltd, Tel: 0870 6077677

R.F. Medical Supplies Ltd, Tel: 01744 882206, enquiries@rfmedicalsupplies.co.uk

Richardson Healthcare Ltd, Tel: 0800 1701126, info@richardsonhealthcare.com

R.I.S. Products Ltd, Tel: 01438 840135, info@risproducts.co.uk

Rivopharm (UK) Ltd, Tel: 01279 406759, PVServices@diamondpharmaservices.com

Robinson Healthcare Ltd, Tel: 01909 735000, orders@robinsonhealthcare.com

Roche Products Ltd, Tel: 0800 3281629, medinfo.uk@roche.com

Rosemont Pharmaceuticals Ltd, Tel: 0113 2441400, rosemont.infodesk@perrigouk.com

RPH Pharmaceuticals AB, Tel: 0207 8621716, safety@elc-group.com

Sai-Meds Ltd, Talk2me@saimeds.com

Sandoz Ltd, Tel: 01276 698101, sandoz@professionalinformation.co.uk

Sanochemia Diagnostics UK Ltd, Tel: 0117 9290287, info@sanochemia.co.uk

Sanofi, Tel: 0845 3727101, uk-medicalinformation@sanofi.com

SanoMed Manufacturing bv, Tel: +32 50 393627, info@naturalsales.nl

Santen UK Ltd, Tel: 0345 0754863, medinfo@santen.co.uk

Santhera (UK) Ltd, Tel: 01423 850733, santhera@pi-arm.co.uk

Scope Ophthalmics Ltd, Tel: 0800 2700253, info@scopeophthalmics.com

Septodont Ltd, Tel: 01622 695520

Seqirus Vaccines Ltd, Tel: 01748 828816, Seqirus@eu.propharmagroup.com

SERB, Tel: 0033 173032000, medinfo.uk1@serb.eu

Servier Laboratories Ltd, Tel: 01753 666409, medical.information-uk@servier.com

Seven Seas Ltd, Tel: 08000 728777, info@sseas.com

Shermond, Tel: 01530 278111

Shield Therapeutics (UK) Ltd, Tel: 0207 1868500, info@shieldtx.com

Shire Pharmaceuticals Ltd, Tel: 08000 556614, medinfoemea@shire.com

Siemens Healthcare Diagnostics Ltd, Tel: 01276 696000, custcare-service.healthcare.gb@siemens.com

Sintetica Ltd, Tel: 01748 827269, SinteticaGB@EU.PropharmaGroup.com

Slõ Drinks Ltd, Tel: 0345 2222205, support@slodrinks.com

Smith & Nephew Healthcare Ltd, Tel: 0800 590173, customer.services.uki@smith-nephew.com

Sovereign Medical Ltd, Tel: 01268 823049, medinfo@amdipharm.com

SpePharm UK Ltd, Tel: +31 20 5670900

Spirit Healthcare Ltd, Tel: 0116 2865000, info@spirit-healthcare.co.uk

SSL International Plc, Tel: 0333 2005345

Stanningley Pharma Ltd, Tel: 01159 124253, medinfo@stanningleypharma.co.uk

STD Pharmaceutical Products Ltd, Tel: 01432 373555, enquiries@stdpharm.co.uk

Steroplast Healthcare Ltd, Tel: 0161 9023030, enquiries@steroplast.co.uk

Stiefel Laboratories (UK) Ltd, Tel: 0800 7838881, customercontactuk@gsk.com

Stiletto Foods (UK) Ltd, Tel: 0345 6021519, info@mrscrimbles.com

Stirling Anglian Pharmaceuticals Ltd, Tel: 0141 5856352, medinfo@stirlinganglianpharmaceuticals.com

Stragen UK Ltd, Tel: 0173 7735029, info@stragenuk.com

Strides Pharma (UK) Ltd, Tel: +91 80 67840000, sadiq.basha@stridesshasun.com

Su-Med International UK Ltd, Tel: 01457 890980

Sun Pharmaceutical Industries Europe B.V., Tel: +46 40 354854, info.se@sunpharma.com

Sunovion Pharmaceuticals Europe Ltd, Tel: 0207 8212840, Med.InfoEU@sunovion.com

SunVit-D3 Ltd, Tel: 0844 4822193, customerservice@sunvitd3.co.uk

Supra Enterprises Ltd, Tel: 0116 2222555, info@supra.org.uk

Sutherland Health Ltd, Tel: 01635 874488, info@sutherlandhealth.com

Swedish Orphan Biovitrum Ltd, Tel: 01748 828863, sobi@professionalinformation.co.uk

Synergy Biologics Ltd, Tel: 01922 705102, info@synergybiologics.co.uk

Synergy Pharmaceuticals, Tel: +1 212 2970020, info@synergypharma.com

Syner-Med (Pharmaceutical Products) Ltd, Tel: 0208 6556380, medicalinformation@syner-med.com

Systagenix Wound Management, Tel: 02030 278716, customercareuk@systagenix.com

Takeda UK Ltd, Tel: 01628 537900, DSO-UK@takeda.com

Talley Group Ltd, Tel: 01794 503500

Techdow Pharma England Ltd, Tel: 01271 334609, medinfouk@eu.techdow.com

Teofarma, servizioclienti@teofarma.it

Tesaro UK Ltd, Tel: 03303 328100, contact-ukinor@tesarobio.com

Teva UK Ltd, Tel: 0207 5407117, medinfo@tevauk.com

Thame Laboratories Ltd, Tel: 0208 5153700, medinfo@bnsthamelabs.co.uk

The Boots Company Plc, Tel: 01159 595165

Thea Pharmaceuticals Ltd, Tel: 0345 5211290, thea-pharma@medinformation.co.uk

Theramex HQ UK Ltd, Tel: 0333 0096795, medinfo.uk@theramex.com

Thomas Blake Cosmetic Creams Ltd, Tel: 01207 272311

Thornton & Ross Ltd, Tel: 01484 848164, thorntonross@medinformation.co.uk

Tillomed Laboratories Ltd, Tel: 01480 402400, medical.information@tillomed.co.uk

Tillotts Pharma Ltd, Tel: 01522 813500, ukmedinfo@tillotts.com

Tobia Teff UK Ltd, Tel: 0207 0181210, info@tobiateff.co.uk

TopRidge Pharma (Ireland) Ltd, Tel: 0800 443252, drugsafety@navamedic.com

Torbet Laboratories Ltd, Tel: 01953 607856, enquiries@torbetlaboratories.co.uk

Transdermal Ltd, Tel: 0148 3920749, transdermal.mi@primevigilance.com

TRB Chemidica (UK) Ltd, Tel: 0845 3307556, info@trbchemedica.co.uk

TriOn Pharma Ltd, Tel: 02392 255770, info@trionpharma.co.uk

Trudell Medical UK Ltd, Tel: 01256 338400, info@trudellmedical.co.uk

Typharm Ltd, Tel: 02037 694160, medinfo@typharm.com

UCB Pharma Ltd, Tel: 01753 777100, UCBCares.UK@ucb.com

Ultrapharm Ltd, Tel: 01495 765570, info@ultrapharm.eu

Unilever UK Home & Personal Care, Tel: 01372 945001

Univar Ltd, Tel: 0151 4226240

Unomedical Ltd, Tel: 0800 289738, wound.webcare@convatec.com

Urgo Ltd, Tel: 01509 502051, woundcare@uk.urgo.com

Valneva UK Ltd, Tel: 01506 446608, medinfo@valneva.com

Vega Nutritionals Ltd, Tel: 01639 825107, info@vegavitamins.co.uk

Veriton Pharma Ltd, Tel: 01932 690325, centralmedicalinformation@veritonpharma.com

Vertex Pharmaceuticals (UK) Ltd, Tel: 01923 437672, vertexmedicalinfo@vrtx.com

Vifor Pharma UK Ltd, Tel: 01276 853633, medicalinfo_UK@viforpharma.com

ViiV Healthcare UK Ltd, Tel: 020 83806200

Visufarma UK Ltd, Tel: 0113 4680661, UKMedicalinformation@VISUfarma.com

Vitaflo International Ltd, Tel: 0151 7099020, vitaflo@vitaflo.co.uk

Vitalograph Ltd, Tel: 01280 827110

Wallace, Cameron & Company Ltd, Tel: 01698 354600, sales@wallacecameron.com

Wallace Manufacturing Chemists Ltd, Tel: 01235 538700

Warburtons, Tel: 0800 243684, customercare@warburtons.co.uk

Warner Chilcott UK Ltd, Tel: 01271 385257, Medinfo@accord-healthcare.com

Waymade Healthcare Plc, Tel: 01268 535200, info@waymade.co.uk

Welland Medical Ltd, Tel: 01293 615455, info@wellandmedical.com

Wellfoods Ltd, Tel: 01226 382877, salesforce@fostersbakery.co.uk

Williams Medical Supplies Ltd, Tel: 01685 846666, medicalservices@wms.co.uk

Wockhardt UK Ltd, Tel: 01978 661261

Wyvern Medical Ltd, Tel: 01264 332172, info@wyvernmedical.co.uk

Zentiva, Tel: 0800 0902408, UKMedInfo@zentiva.com

Zeroderma Ltd, Tel: 01484 848164, thorntonross@medinformation.co.uk

Special-order manufacturers

Unlicensed medicines are available from 'special-order' manufacturers and specialist-importing companies; the MHRA maintains a register of these companies at tinyurl.com/cdslke.

Licensed **hospital manufacturing units** also manufacture 'special-order' products as unlicensed medicines, the principal NHS units are listed below. A database (*Pro-File*; www.pro-file.nhs.uk) provides information on medicines manufactured in the NHS; access is restricted to NHS pharmacy staff.

The Association of Pharmaceutical Specials Manufacturers may also be able to provide further information about commercial companies (www.apsm-uk.com).

The MHRA recommends that an unlicensed medicine should only be used when a patient has special requirements that cannot be met by use of a licensed medicine.

As well as being available direct from the hospital manufacturer(s) concerned, many NHS-manufactured Specials may be bought from the Oxford Pharmacy Store, owned and operated by Oxford Health NHS Foundation Trust.

England

London

Barts and the London NHS Trust

Mr J. A. Rickard, Head of Barts Health Pharmaceuticals
Barts Health NHS Trust
The Royal London Hospital
Pathology and Pharmacy Building
80 Newark St
Whitechapel
London
E1 2ES
(020) 3246 0394 (order/enquiry)
barts.pharmaceuticals@bartshealth.nhs.uk

Guy's and St. Thomas' NHS Foundation Trust

Mr P. Forsey, Associate Chief Pharmacist
Guy's and St. Thomas' NHS Foundation Trust
Guy's Hospital
Pharmacy Department
Great Maze Pond
London
SE1 9RT
(020) 7188 4992 (order)
(020) 7188 5003 (enquiry)
Fax: (020) 7188 5013
paul.forsey@gstt.nhs.uk

Moorfields Pharmaceuticals

Mr. T. Record, Technical Director
Moorfields Pharmaceuticals
25 Provost St
London
N1 7NH
(020) 7684 9090 (order/enquiry)
Fax: (020) 7502 2332

London North West Healthcare NHS Trust

Mr K. Wong
London North West Healthcare NHS Trust
Northwick Park Hospital
Watford Rd
Harrow
Middlesex
HA1 3UJ
(020) 8869 2295 (order)
(020) 8869 2204/2223 (enquiry)
kwong@nhs.net

Royal Free London NHS Foundation Trust

Mr J. Singh, Principal Pharmacist Technical Services
Royal Free Hospital Pharmacy Technical Services
Pond St
Hampstead
London
NW3 2QG
(020) 7830 2424 (order)
(020) 7830 2282 (enquiry)
Fax: (020) 7794 1875
rf.specials@nhs.net
jasdeep.singh1@nhs.net

St George's Healthcare NHS Trust

Mr V. Kumar, Assistant Chief Pharmacist
St George's Hospital
Technical Services
Blackshaw Rd
Tooting
London
SW17 0QT
(020) 8725 1770/1768
Fax: (020) 8725 3947
vinodh.kumar@stgeorges.nhs.uk

University College Hospital NHS Foundation Trust

Mr T. Murphy, Production Manager
University College Hospital
235 Euston Rd
London
NW1 2BU
(020) 7380 9723 (order)
(020) 7380 9472 (enquiry)
Fax: (020) 7380 9726
tony.murphy@uclh.nhs.uk

Midlands and Eastern

Barking, Havering and Redbridge University Trust

Mr N. Fisher, Senior Principal Pharmacist
Queen's Hospital
Pharmacy Department
Romford
Essex
RM7 0AG
(01708) 435 463 (order)
(01708) 435 042 (enquiry)
neil.fisher@bhrhospitals.nhs.uk

Burton Hospitals NHS Foundation Trust

Mr D. Raynor, Head of Pharmacy Manufacturing Unit
Queens Hospital
Burton Hospitals NHS Foundation Trust
Pharmacy Manufacturing Unit
Belvedere Rd
Burton-on-Trent
DE13 0RB
(01283) 511 511 ext: 5275 (order/enquiry)
Fax: (01283) 593 036
david.raynor@burtonft.nhs.uk

Colchester Hospital University NHS Foundation Trust

Mr S. Pullen, Pharmacy Production Manager
Colchester General Hospital
Main Pharmacy
Turner Rd
Colchester
Essex
C04 5JL
(01206) 742 007 (order)
(01206) 744 208 (enquiry)
Fax: (01206) 841 249
pharmacy.stores@colchesterhospital.nhs.uk (order)
psu.enquiries@colchesterhospital.nhs.uk (enquiry)

Ipswich Hospital NHS Trust

Dr J. Harwood, Production Manager
Ipswich Hospital NHS Trust
Pharmacy Manufacturing Unit
Heath Rd
Ipswich
IP4 5PD
(01473) 703 440 (order)
(01473) 703 603 (enquiry)
Fax: (01473) 703 609
john.harwood@ipswichhospital.nhs.uk

Nottingham University Hospitals NHS Trust

Mr J. Graham, Senior Pharmacist, Production
Nottingham University Hospitals NHS Trust
Pharmacy Production Units
Queens Medical Centre Campus
Nottingham
NG7 2UH
(0115) 924 9924 ext: 66521 (enquiry/order)
Fax: (0115) 970 9780
jeff.graham@nuh.nhs.uk

University Hospital of North Midlands NHS Trust

Ms K. Milner, Chief Technician
Royal Stoke University Hospital
University Hospital of North Midlands NHS Trust
Pharmacy Technical Services
Newcastle Road
Stoke-on-Trent
Staffordshire
ST4 6QG
(01782) 674 568 (order)
(01782) 674 568 (enquiry)
pharmacymanu@uhnm.nhs.uk
kate.milner@uhnm.nhs.uk

North East

The Newcastle upon Tyne Hospitals NHS Foundation Trust

Mr Y. Hunter-Blair, Production Manager
Royal Victoria Infirmary
Newcastle Specials
Pharmacy Production Unit
Queen Victoria Rd
Newcastle-upon-Tyne
NE1 4LP
(0191) 282 0395 (order)
(0191) 282 0389 (enquiry)
Fax: (0191) 282 0469
yan.hunter-blair@nuth.nhs.uk

North West

Preston Pharmaceuticals

Ms A. Bolch, Deputy Chief Pharmacist (PMU)
Preston Pharmaceuticals
Royal Preston Hospital
Fulwood
Preston
PR2 9HT
(01772) 523 617 (order)
(01772) 522 593 (enquiry)
Fax: (01772) 523 645
angela.bolch@lthtr.nhs.uk

Stockport Pharmaceuticals

Mr A. Singleton, Head of Production
Stepping Hill Hospital
Stockport NHS Foundation Trust
Stockport Pharmaceuticals
Stockport
SK2 7JE
(0161) 419 5666 (order)
(0161) 419 5657 (enquiry)
Fax: (0161) 419 5426
andrew.singleton@stockport.nhs.uk

South

Portsmouth Hospitals NHS Trust

Mr R. Lucas, Product Development Manager
Portsmouth Hospitals NHS Trust
Pharmacy Manufacturing Unit
Unit D2, Railway Triangle Industrial Estate
Walton Road
Farlington
Portsmouth
PO6 1TF
(02392) 389 078 (order)
(02392) 316 312 (enquiry)
Fax: (02392) 316 316
robert.lucas@porthosp.nhs.uk

South West

Torbay Pharmaceuticals

Mr Leon Rudd, Commercial Strategy Director
Torbay and South Devon Healthcare NHS Foundation Trust
Torbay Pharmaceuticals
Wilkins Drive
Paignton
TQ4 7FG
(01803) 664 707
Fax: (01803) 664 354
leon.rudd@nhs.net

Yorkshire

Calderdale and Huddersfield NHS Foundation Trust

Dr B. Grewal, Managing Director
Calderdale and Huddersfield NHS Foundation Trust
Huddersfield Pharmacy Specials
Gate 2 - Acre Mills, School St West
Huddersfield
HD3 3ET
(01484) 355 388 (order/enquiry)
info.hps@cht.nhs.uk

Northern Ireland

Victoria Pharmaceuticals

Mr S. Cameron, Production Manager - Pharmacy
Victoria Pharmaceuticals
Royal Hospitals
Plenum Building
Grosvenor Road
Belfast
BT12 6BA
(028) 9615 1000 (order/enquiry)
Fax: (028) 9063 5282 (order/enquiry)
samuel.cameron@belfasttrust.hscni.net

Scotland

NHS Greater Glasgow and Clyde

Ms K. Pollock, Acting Production Manager
Pharmacy Production Unit
University Place
Glasgow
G12 8TA
(0141) 451 5820 (order)
(0141) 451 5822 (enquiry)
Fax: (0141) 334 9137
pharmacyproductionunit@ggc.scot.nhs.uk

Tayside Pharmaceuticals

Mr S. Bath, Production Manager
Ninewells Hospital
Tayside Pharmaceuticals
Dundee
DD1 9SY
(01382) 632 052 (order)
(01382) 632 273 (enquiry)
Fax: (01382) 632 060
sbath@nhs.net

Wales

Cardiff and Vale University Health Board

Mr P. Spark, Principal Pharmacist (Production)
Cardiff and Vale University Health Board
20 Fieldway
Cardiff
CF14 4HY
(029) 2074 8120
Fax: (029) 2074 8130
paul.spark@wales.nhs.uk

Index

A

D

E

N

U

V

In Confidence

BNFC

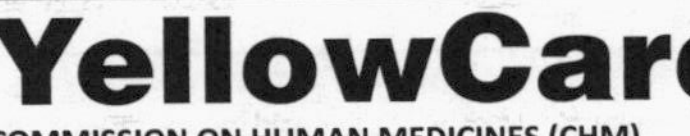

COMMISSION ON HUMAN MEDICINES (CHM)

It's easy to report online at:
www.mhra.gov.uk/yellowcard

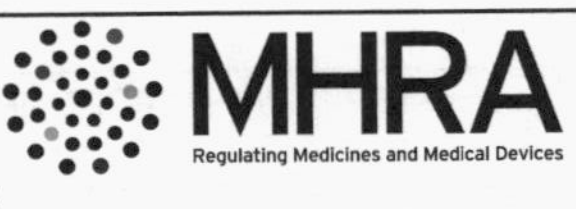

REPORT OF SUSPECTED ADVERSE DRUG REACTIONS

If you suspect an adverse reaction may be related to one or more drugs/vaccines/complementary remedies, please complete this Yellow Card. See 'Adverse reactions to drugs' section in BNFC or **www.mhra.gov.uk/yellowcard** for guidance. Do not be put off reporting because some details are not known.

PATIENT DETAILS

Patient Initials:________ Sex: M / F Is the patient pregnant? Y / N Ethnicity:________

Age (at time of reaction):________ Weight (kg):________ Identification number (e.g. Practice or Hospital Ref):________

SUSPECTED DRUG(S)/VACCINE(S)

Drug/Vaccine (Brand if known)	Batch	Route	Dosage	Date started	Date stopped	Prescribed for

SUSPECTED REACTION(S)

Please describe the reaction(s) and any treatment given. (Please attach additional pages if necessary):

Outcome

- ☐ Recovered
- ☐ Recovering
- ☐ Continuing
- ☐ Other

Date reaction(s) started:________ Date reaction(s) stopped: ________

Do you consider the reactions to be serious? Yes / No

If yes, please indicate why the reaction is considered to be serious (please tick all that apply):

- ☐ Patient died due to reaction
- ☐ Life threatening
- ☐ Congenital abnormality
- ☐ Involved or prolonged inpatient hospitalisation
- ☐ Involved persistent or significant disability or incapacity
- Medically significant; please give details: ________

If the reactions were not serious according to the categories above, how bad was the suspected reaction?

☐ Mild ☐ Unpleasant, but did not affect everyday activities ☐ Bad enough to affect everyday activities

It's easy to report online: **www.mhra.gov.uk/yellowcard**

OTHER DRUG(S) (including self-medication and complementary remedies)

Did the patient take any other medicines/vaccines/complementary remedies in the last 3 months prior to the reaction? Yes / No

If yes, please give the following information if known:

Drug/Vaccine (Brand if known)	Batch	Route	Dosage	Date started	Date stopped	Prescribed for

Additional relevant information e.g. medical history, test results, known allergies, rechallenge (if performed). For reactions relating to use of a medicine during pregnancy please state all other drugs taken during pregnancy, the last menstrual period, information on previous pregnancies, ultrasound scans, any delivery complications, birth defects or developmental concerns.

Please list any medicines obtained from the internet:

REPORTER DETAILS

Name and Professional Address: ________________

Postcode: ________ Tel No: ________

Email: ________

Speciality: ________

Signature: ________ Date: ________

CLINICIAN (if not the reporter)

Name and Professional Address: ________________

Postcode: ________ Tel No: ________

Email: ________

Speciality: ________

Date: ________

Information on adverse drug reactions received by the MHRA can be downloaded at **www.mhra.gov.uk/daps**

Stay up-to-date on the latest advice for the safe use of medicines with our monthly bulletin *Drug Safety Update* at: **www.mhra.gov.uk/drugsafetyupdate**

Please attach additional pages if necessary. Send to: FREEPOST YELLOW CARD (no other address details required)

BNFC

In Confidence

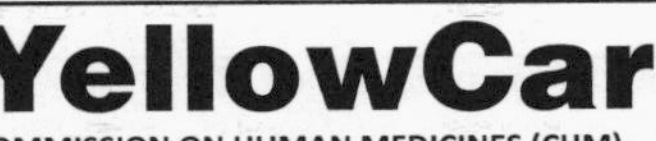

COMMISSION ON HUMAN MEDICINES (CHM)

It's easy to report online at:
www.mhra.gov.uk/yellowcard

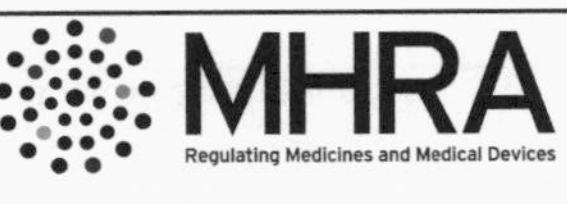

REPORT OF SUSPECTED ADVERSE DRUG REACTIONS

If you suspect an adverse reaction may be related to one or more drugs/vaccines/complementary remedies, please complete this Yellow Card. See `Adverse reactions to drugs' section in BNFC or **www.mhra.gov.uk/yellowcard** for guidance. Do not be put off reporting because some details are not known.

PATIENT DETAILS

Patient Initials:______________ Sex: M / F Is the patient pregnant? Y / N Ethnicity:____________________

Age (at time of reaction):__________ Weight (kg):__________ Identification number (e.g. Practice or Hospital Ref):____________________

SUSPECTED DRUG(S)/VACCINE(S)

Drug/Vaccine (Brand if known)	Batch	Route	Dosage	Date started	Date stopped	Prescribed for

SUSPECTED REACTION(S)

Please describe the reaction(s) and any treatment given. (Please attach additional pages if necessary):

Outcome

- ☐ Recovered
- ☐ Recovering
- ☐ Continuing
- ☐ Other

Date reaction(s) started:____________________ Date reaction(s) stopped: ____________________

Do you consider the reactions to be serious? Yes / No

If yes, please indicate why the reaction is considered to be serious (please tick all that apply):

- ☐ Patient died due to reaction
- ☐ Life threatening
- ☐ Congenital abnormality
- ☐ Involved or prolonged inpatient hospitalisation
- ☐ Involved persistent or significant disability or incapacity
- Medically significant; please give details: ____________________

If the reactions were not serious according to the categories above, how bad was the suspected reaction?

☐ Mild ☐ Unpleasant, but did not affect everyday activities ☐ Bad enough to affect everyday activities

It's easy to report online: www.mhra.gov.uk/yellowcard

OTHER DRUG(S) (including self-medication and complementary remedies)

Did the patient take any other medicines/vaccines/complementary remedies in the last 3 months prior to the reaction? Yes / No

If yes, please give the following information if known:

Drug/Vaccine (Brand if known)	Batch	Route	Dosage	Date started	Date stopped	Prescribed for

Additional relevant information e.g. medical history, test results, known allergies, rechallenge (if performed). For reactions relating to use of a medicine during pregnancy please state all other drugs taken during pregnancy, the last menstrual period, information on previous pregnancies, ultrasound scans, any delivery complications, birth defects or developmental concerns.

Please list any medicines obtained from the internet:

REPORTER DETAILS

Name and Professional Address:__________

Postcode:__________ Tel No:__________

Email:__________

Speciality:__________

Signature:__________ Date:__________

CLINICIAN (if not the reporter)

Name and Professional Address:__________

Postcode:__________ Tel No:__________

Email:__________

Speciality:__________

Date:__________

Information on adverse drug reactions received by the MHRA can be downloaded at **www.mhra.gov.uk/daps**

Stay up-to-date on the latest advice for the safe use of medicines with our monthly bulletin *Drug Safety Update* at: **www.mhra.gov.uk/drugsafetyupdate**

Please attach additional pages if necessary. Send to: FREEPOST YELLOW CARD (no other address details required)

In Confidence

BNFC

YellowCard

COMMISSION ON HUMAN MEDICINES (CHM)

It's easy to report online at:
www.mhra.gov.uk/yellowcard

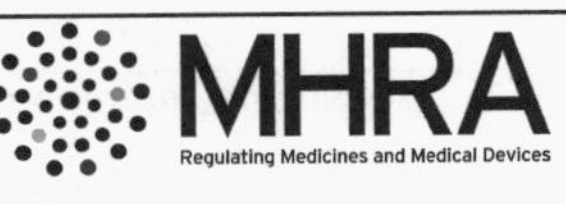

REPORT OF SUSPECTED ADVERSE DRUG REACTIONS

If you suspect an adverse reaction may be related to one or more drugs/vaccines/complementary remedies, please complete this Yellow Card. See `Adverse reactions to drugs' section in BNFC or **www.mhra.gov.uk/yellowcard** for guidance. Do not be put off reporting because some details are not known.

PATIENT DETAILS Patient Initials:________ Sex: M / F Is the patient pregnant? Y / N Ethnicity:________

Age (at time of reaction):________ Weight (kg):________ Identification number (e.g. Practice or Hospital Ref):________

SUSPECTED DRUG(S)/VACCINE(S)

Drug/Vaccine (Brand if known)	Batch	Route	Dosage	Date started	Date stopped	Prescribed for

SUSPECTED REACTION(S) Please describe the reaction(s) and any treatment given. (Please attach additional pages if necessary):

Outcome

- ☐ Recovered
- ☐ Recovering
- ☐ Continuing
- ☐ Other

Date reaction(s) started:________ Date reaction(s) stopped: ________

Do you consider the reactions to be serious? Yes / No

If yes, please indicate why the reaction is considered to be serious (please tick all that apply):

- ☐ Patient died due to reaction
- ☐ Life threatening
- ☐ Congenital abnormality
- ☐ Involved or prolonged inpatient hospitalisation
- ☐ Involved persistent or significant disability or incapacity
- Medically significant; please give details: ________

If the reactions were not serious according to the categories above, how bad was the suspected reaction?

☐ Mild ☐ Unpleasant, but did not affect everyday activities ☐ Bad enough to affect everyday activities

It's easy to report online: www.mhra.gov.uk/yellowcard

OTHER DRUG(S) (including self-medication and complementary remedies)

Did the patient take any other medicines/vaccines/complementary remedies in the last 3 months prior to the reaction? Yes / No
If yes, please give the following information if known:

Drug/Vaccine (Brand if known)	Batch	Route	Dosage	Date started	Date stopped	Prescribed for

Additional relevant information e.g. medical history, test results, known allergies, rechallenge (if performed). For reactions relating to use of a medicine during pregnancy please state all other drugs taken during pregnancy, the last menstrual period, information on previous pregnancies, ultrasound scans, any delivery complications, birth defects or developmental concerns.

Please list any medicines obtained from the internet:

REPORTER DETAILS

Name and Professional Address:____________________

Postcode:__________ Tel No:__________
Email:__________
Speciality:__________
Signature:__________ Date:__________

CLINICIAN (if not the reporter)

Name and Professional Address:____________________

Postcode:__________ Tel No:__________
Email:__________
Speciality:__________
Date:__________

Information on adverse drug reactions received by the MHRA can be downloaded at **www.mhra.gov.uk/daps**
Stay up-to-date on the latest advice for the safe use of medicines with our monthly bulletin *Drug Safety Update* at: **www.mhra.gov.uk/drugsafetyupdate**

Please attach additional pages if necessary. Send to: FREEPOST YELLOW CARD (no other address details required)

BNFC

In Confidence

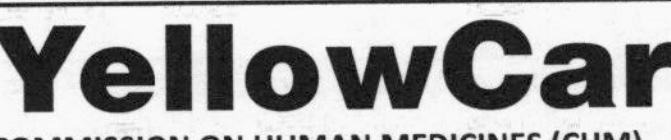

COMMISSION ON HUMAN MEDICINES (CHM)

It's easy to report online at:
www.mhra.gov.uk/yellowcard

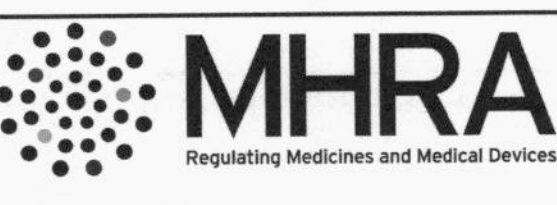

REPORT OF SUSPECTED ADVERSE DRUG REACTIONS

If you suspect an adverse reaction may be related to one or more drugs/vaccines/complementary remedies, please complete this Yellow Card. See `Adverse reactions to drugs' section in BNFC or **www.mhra.gov.uk/yellowcard** for guidance. Do not be put off reporting because some details are not known.

PATIENT DETAILS Patient Initials:________ Sex: M / F Is the patient pregnant? Y / N Ethnicity:________

Age (at time of reaction):________ Weight (kg):________ Identification number (e.g. Practice or Hospital Ref):________

SUSPECTED DRUG(S)/VACCINE(S)

Drug/Vaccine (Brand if known)	Batch	Route	Dosage	Date started	Date stopped	Prescribed for

SUSPECTED REACTION(S) Please describe the reaction(s) and any treatment given. (Please attach additional pages if necessary):

Outcome

- Recovered ☐
- Recovering ☐
- Continuing ☐
- Other ☐

Date reaction(s) started:________ Date reaction(s) stopped: ________

Do you consider the reactions to be serious? Yes / No

If yes, please indicate why the reaction is considered to be serious (please tick all that apply):

☐ Patient died due to reaction
☐ Involved or prolonged inpatient hospitalisation
☐ Life threatening
☐ Involved persistent or significant disability or incapacity
☐ Congenital abnormality
Medically significant; please give details: ________

If the reactions were not serious according to the categories above, how bad was the suspected reaction?

☐ Mild ☐ Unpleasant, but did not affect everyday activities ☐ Bad enough to affect everyday activities

It's easy to report online: www.mhra.gov.uk/yellowcard

OTHER DRUG(S) (including self-medication and complementary remedies)

Did the patient take any other medicines/vaccines/complementary remedies in the last 3 months prior to the reaction? Yes / No

If yes, please give the following information if known:

Drug/Vaccine (Brand if known)	Batch	Route	Dosage	Date started	Date stopped	Prescribed for

Additional relevant information e.g. medical history, test results, known allergies, rechallenge (if performed). For reactions relating to use of a medicine during pregnancy please state all other drugs taken during pregnancy, the last menstrual period, information on previous pregnancies, ultrasound scans, any delivery complications, birth defects or developmental concerns.

Please list any medicines obtained from the internet:

REPORTER DETAILS

Name and Professional Address:__________

Postcode:__________ Tel No:__________

Email:__________

Speciality:__________

Signature:__________ Date:__________

CLINICIAN (if not the reporter)

Name and Professional Address:__________

Postcode:__________ Tel No:__________

Email:__________

Speciality:__________

Date:__________

Information on adverse drug reactions received by the MHRA can be downloaded at **www.mhra.gov.uk/daps**

Stay up-to-date on the latest advice for the safe use of medicines with our monthly bulletin *Drug Safety Update* at: **www.mhra.gov.uk/drugsafetyupdate**

Please attach additional pages if necessary. Send to: FREEPOST YELLOW CARD (no other address details required)

Newborn Life Support

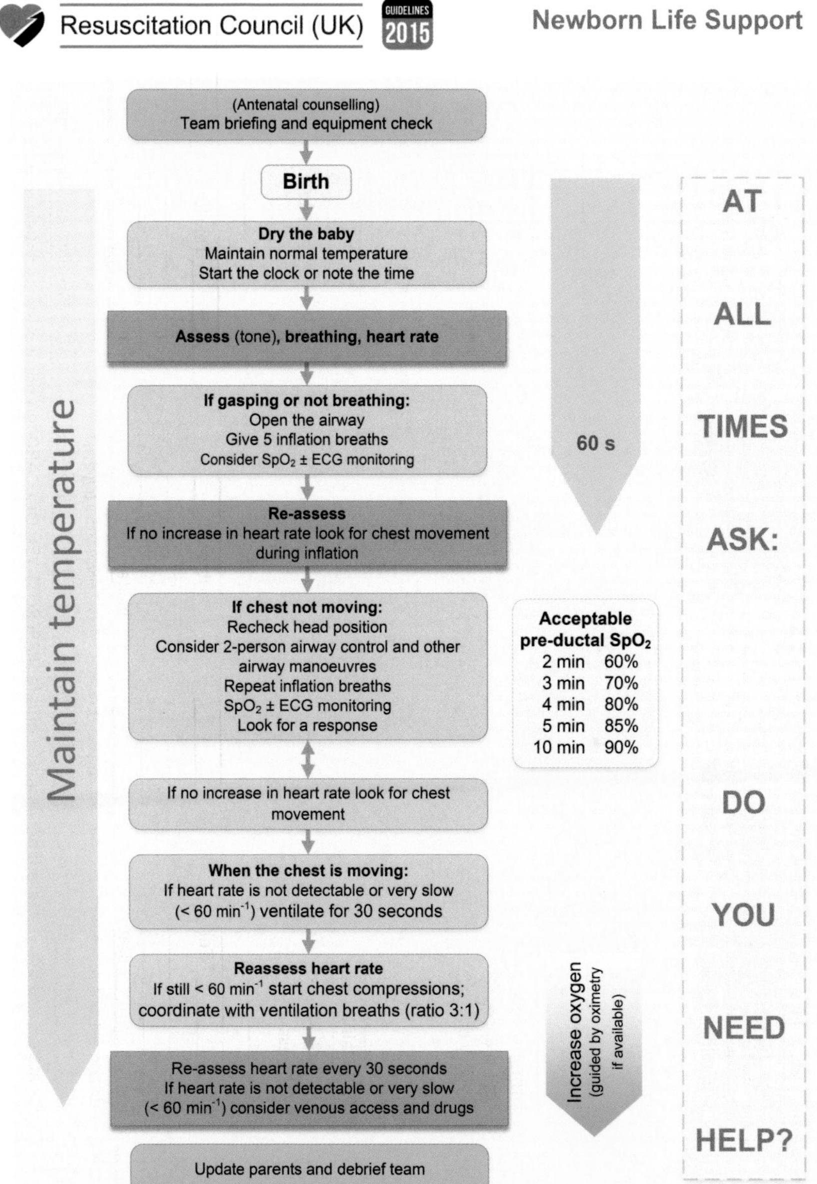

Reproduced with the kind permission of the Resuscitation Council (UK) from Resuscitation Guidelines, 2015

Paediatric Basic Life Support

(Healthcare professionals with a duty to respond)

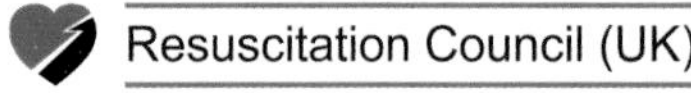

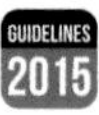

Paediatric Basic Life Support

(Healthcare professionals with a duty to respond)

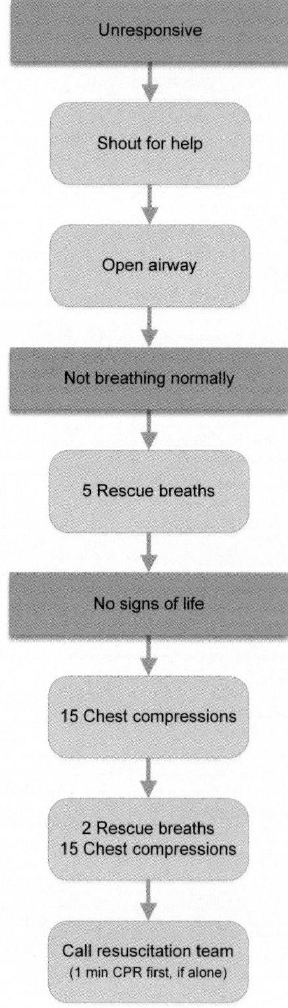

- OR **if history of immediate hypersensitivity reaction (including anaphylaxis, angioedema, urticaria, or rash immediately after administration) to penicillin or to cephalosporins**

  Chloramphenicol injection p. 385 (1 g)

  BY INTRAVENOUS INJECTION

  - Child 1 month–17 years: 12.5–25 mg/kg

  NOTE A single dose can be given before urgent transfer to hospital, so long as this does not delay the transfer.
  See also Central nervous system infections, antibacterial therapy p. 323.

Hypoglycaemia

- **DIABETIC HYPOGLYCAEMIA**

  Glucose or sucrose

  BY MOUTH

  - Child over 2 years: approx. 10–20 g (110–220 mL *Lucozade® Energy Original or* 100–200 mL *Coca-Cola®*—both non-diet versions *or* 2–4 teaspoonfuls of sugar *or* 3–6 sugar lumps) repeated after 10–15 minutes if necessary

- OR **if hypoglycaemia unresponsive *or* if oral route cannot be used**

  Glucagon injection p. 502 (1 mg/mL)

  BY SUBCUTANEOUS OR INTRAMUSCULAR INJECTION

  - Child body-weight up to 25 kg: 500 micrograms (0.5 mL)
  - Child body-weight 25 kg and over: 1 mg (1 mL)

- OR **if hypoglycaemia prolonged *or* unresponsive to glucagon after 10 minutes**

  Glucose intravenous infusion p. 638 (10%)

  BY INTRAVENOUS INJECTION INTO LARGE VEIN

  - Child 1 month–17 years: 5 mL/kg (glucose 500 mg/kg)

Seizures

- **CONVULSIVE (INCLUDING FEBRILE) SEIZURES LASTING LONGER THAN 5 MINUTES**

- EITHER **Diazepam rectal solution p. 236** (2 mg/mL, 4 mg/mL)

  BY RECTUM

  - Neonate: 1.25–2.5 mg, repeated once after 10–15 minutes if necessary
  - Child 1 month–1 year: 5 mg, repeated once after 10–15 minutes if necessary
  - Child 2–11 years: 5–10 mg, repeated once after 10–15 minutes if necessary
  - Child 12–17 years: 10–20 mg, repeated once after 10–15 minutes if necessary

- OR **Midazolam oromucosal solution p. 239**

  BY BUCCAL ADMINISTRATION, REPEATED ONCE AFTER 10 MINUTES IF NECESSARY

  - Neonate: 300 micrograms/kg [unlicensed]
  - Child 1–2 months: 300 micrograms/kg (max. 2.5 mg) [unlicensed]
  - Child 3 months–11 months: 2.5 mg
  - Child 1–4 years: 5 mg
  - Child 5–9 years: 7.5 mg
  - Child 10–17 years: 10 mg

Approximate Conversions and Units

Conversion of pounds to kilograms

lb	kg
1	0.45
2	0.91
3	1.36
4	1.81
5	2.27
6	2.72
7	3.18
8	3.63
9	4.08
10	4.54
11	4.99
12	5.44
13	5.90
14	6.35

Conversion of stones to kilograms

stones	kg
1	6.35
2	12.70
3	19.05
4	25.40
5	31.75
6	38.10
7	44.45
8	50.80
9	57.15
10	63.50
11	69.85
12	76.20
13	82.55
14	88.90
15	95.25

Conversion from millilitres to fluid ounces

mL	fl oz
50	1.8
100	3.5
150	5.3
200	7.0
500	17.6
1000	35.2

Length

1 metre (m) = 1000 millimetres (mm)
1 centimetre (cm) = 10 mm
1 inch (in) = 25.4 mm
1 foot (ft) = 12 inches
12 inches = 304.8 mm

Mass

1 kilogram (kg) = 1000 grams (g)
1 gram (g) = 1000 milligrams (mg)
1 milligram (mg) = 1000 micrograms
1 microgram = 1000 nanograms
1 nanogram = 1000 picograms

Volume

1 litre = 1000 millilitres (mL)
1 millilitre (1 mL) = 1000 microlitres
1 pint ≈ 568 mL

Other units

1 kilocalorie (kcal) = 4186.8 joules (J)
1000 kilocalories (kcal) = 4.1868 megajoules (MJ)
1 megajoule (MJ) = 238.8 kilocalories (kcal)
1 millimetre of mercury (mmHg) = 133.3 pascals (Pa)
1 kilopascal (kPa) = 7.5 mmHg (pressure)

Plasma-drug concentrations

Plasma-drug concentrations in BNF publications are expressed in mass units per litre (e.g. mg/litre). The approximate equivalent in terms of amount of substance units (e.g. micromol/litre) is given in brackets.

Prescribing for children: weight, height, and gender

The table below shows the **mean values** for weight, height and gender by age; these values have been derived from the UK-WHO growth charts 2009 and UK1990 standard centile charts, by extrapolating the 50th centile, and may be used to calculate doses in the absence of actual measurements. However, the child's actual weight and height might vary considerably from the values in the table and it is important to see the child to ensure that the value chosen is appropriate. In most cases the child's actual measurement should be obtained as soon as possible and the dose re-calculated.

Age	Weight (kg)	Height (cm)
Full-term neonate	3.5	51
1 month	4.3	55
2 months	5.4	58
3 months	6.1	61
4 months	6.7	63
6 months	7.6	67
1 year	9	75
3 years	14	96
5 years	18	109
7 years	23	122
10 years	32	138
12 years	39	149
14 year old boy	49	163
14 year old girl	50	159
Adult male	68	176
Adult female	58	164